Peyman's
Principles and Practice of
OPHTHALMOLOGY

Peyman's Principles and Practice of OPHTHALMOLOGY

SECOND EDITION

VOLUME 1

Editor-in-Chief

N Venkatesh Prajna DNB FRCOphth

Academic Director

Aravind Eye Care System

Madurai, Tamil Nadu, India

Foreword

Morton F Goldberg

JAYPEE

JAYPEE BROTHERS MEDICAL PUBLISHERS

The Health Sciences Publisher

New Delhi | London | Panama

Jaypee Brothers Medical Publishers (P) Ltd.

Headquarters
Jaypee Brothers Medical Publishers (P) Ltd.
4838/24, Ansari Road, Daryaganj
New Delhi 110 002, India
Phone: +91-11-43574357
Fax: +91-11-43574314
Email: jaypee@jaypeebrothers.com

Overseas Offices
JP Medical Ltd.
83, Victoria Street, London
SW1H 0HW (UK)
Phone: +44 20 3170 8910
Fax: +44 (0)20 3008 6180
E-mail: info@jpmedpub.com

Jaypee-Highlights Medical Publishers Inc.
City of Knowledge, Bld. 235, 2nd Floor, Clayton
Panama City, Panama
Phone: +1 507-301-0496
Fax: +1 507-301-0499
E-mail: cservice@jphmedical.com

Jaypee Brothers Medical Publishers (P) Ltd.
Bhotahity, Kathmandu, Nepal
Phone: +977-9741283608
E-mail: kathmandu@jaypeebrothers.com

Website: www.jaypeebrothers.com
Website: www.jaypeedigital.com

Inquiries for bulk sales may be solicited at: jaypee@jaypeebrothers.com

Peyman's Principles and Practice of Ophthalmology (Vols 1 and 2)

First Edition: 1987
Second Edition: **2019,** Reprint: 2023

ISBN: 978-93-5270-291-6

Printed in India

Dedicated to

The Founders of the Aravind Eye Care System
for creating one of the largest, efficient, compassionate and equitable eye care delivery system of global standards.

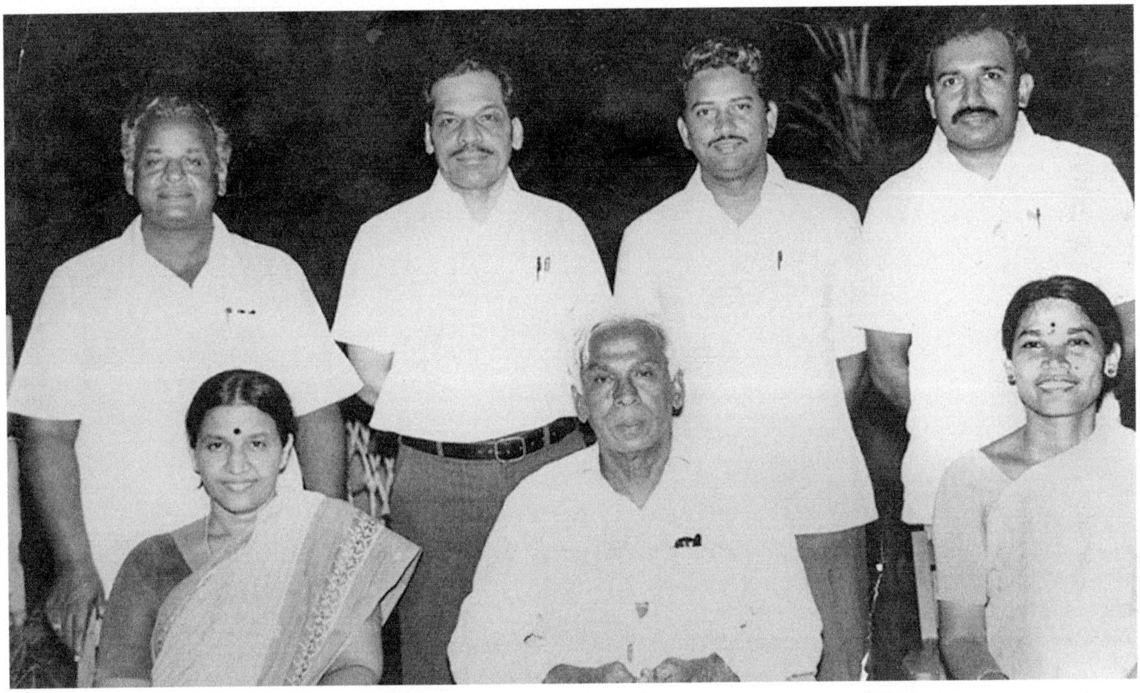

Standing from left to right
Mr G Srinivasan, Dr P Namperumalsamy, Dr M Srinivasan and Mr RD Thulasiraj

Sitting from left to right
Dr G Natchiar, Dr G Venkataswamy and Dr P Vijayalakshmi

Section Editors

Vision Rehabilitation

August Colenbrander MD PhD
Affiliate Senior Scientist
Smith-Kettlewell Eye Research Institute
San Francisco, USA

The Lens, Cataract and its Management

Uday Devgan MD FACS FRCS (Glasg)
Cataract and Refractive Surgeon
Devgan Eye Surgery, Los Angeles, California, USA
Partner, Speciality Surgical Center, Beverly Hills, California, USA
Chief of Ophthalmology, Olive View—UCLA Medical Center
Professor of Ophthalmology, Jules Stein Eye Institute
UCLA School of Medicine, Los Angeles, California, USA

Ocular Pathology

Deepak P Edward MD FACS FARVO
Professor (Ophthalmology and Pathology)
Department of Ophthalmology and Visual Sciences
University of Illinois Eye and Ear Infirmary
UIC College of Medicine
Chicago, Illinois, USA
King Khaled Eye Specialist Hospital
Riyadh, Kingdom of Saudi Arabia

Orbit and Oculoplasty

Shannon S Joseph MD
Assistant Professor
Department of Ophthalmology
Division of Oculoplastic Surgery
WK Kellogg Eye Center
University of Michigan
Ann Arbor, Michigan, USA

Optics and Rehabilitation

Joseph M Miller MD MPH
Professor of Ophthalmology
Optical Sciences and Public Health
University of Arizona College of Medicine
Tucson, Arizona, USA

Pediatric Ophthalmology and Strabismus

Michael O'Keeffe FRCS
Consultant Ophthalmic Surgeon
Mater Private Hospital and Beacon Hospital
Dublin, Ireland

Conjunctiva and Cornea

N Venkatesh Prajna DNB FRCOphth
Academic Director
Aravind Eye Care System
Madurai, Tamil Nadu, India

Glaucoma

Pradeep Ramulu MD PhD MHS
Professor of Ophthalmology (Glaucoma)
Wilmer Eye Institute
Johns Hopkins Hospital
Baltimore, Maryland, USA

Scleritis and Uveitis

SR Rathinam FAMS PhD
Professor of Ophthalmology and Head of Uveitis Service
Aravind Eye Hospital and Postgraduate Institute
of Ophthalmology
Madurai, Tamil Nadu, India

Retina and Vitreous

Srinivas R Sadda MD
President and Chief Scientific Officer
Doheny Eye Institute
Professor of Ophthalmology
University of California-Los Angeles
Los Angeles, California, USA

Neuro-ophthalmology

Prem S Subramanian MD PhD
Professor of Ophthalmology, Neurology and Neurosurgery
and Vice Chair for Academic Affairs
UC Health/Sue Anschutz-Rodgers Eye Center
Department of Ophthalmology
University of Colorado School of Medicine
Aurora, Colorado, USA

Contributors

Tushar Agarwal
Professor (Ophthalmology)
Dr Rajendra Prasad Centre for Ophthalmic Sciences
All India Institute of Medical Sciences (AIIMS)
New Delhi, India

Shweta Agarwal MD
Consultant
CJ Shah Cornea Services
Dr G Sitalakshmi Memorial Clinic for Ocular Surface Disorders
Sankara Nethralaya
Chennai, Tamil Nadu, India

Aniruddha Agarwal MS
Clinical Fellow in Vitreoretinal and Uveitis
Postgraduate Institute of Medical Education and Research (PGIMER)
Chandigarh, India

Kanika Aggarwal MS
Senior Research Associate
Postgraduate Institute of Medical Education and Research (PGIMER)
Chandigarh, India

Md Shahid Alam MS
Consultant Ophthalmologist
Orbit, Oculoplasty, Reconstructive and Aesthetic Services
Sankara Nethralaya
Kolkata, West Bengal, India

Mohammad Javed Ali FRCS PhD
Head
Govindram Seksaria Institute of Dacryology
LV Prasad Eye Institute (LVPEI)
Hyderabad, Telangana, India

A Yasin Alibhai MD
OCT Research Fellow
New England Eye Center
Tufts Medical Center
Boston, Massachusetts, USA

Hind Alkatan MD
Assistant Professor and Consultant
Director, Ophthalmology Training Programs
College of Medicine
Associate Director for External Accreditation Unit
Departments of Ophthalmology/ Pathology and Postgraduate Medical Education (PGME)
King Saud University-Medical City
Riyadh, Saudi Arabia

Eleftherios Anastasopoulos MD PhD
Consultant in Ophthalmology
2nd Department of Ophthalmology
Papageorgiou General Hospital
Aristotle University of Thessaloniki
Greece

Pamela Anketell PhD
Lead in Pediatric Orthoptics
Belfast Health and Social Care Trust (BHSCT)
Eye and Ear Clinic
Royal Victoria Hospital
Belfast, Ireland

Amreen Aslam MD
Senior Resident (Cornea)
Cataract and Refractive Surgery Services
Dr Rajendra Prasad Centre for Ophthalmic Sciences
All India Institute of Medical Sciences (AIIMS)
New Delhi, India

Ariana Austin MS
Study Coordinator
Francis I Proctor Foundation
University of California
San Francisco, California, USA

James T Banta MD
Bascom Palmer Eye Institute
Miami, Florida, USA

John Bartlett MD
Assistant Clinical Professor (Ophthalmology)
Jules Stein Eye Institute
UCLA School of Medicine
Los Angeles, California, USA

Rodanthi Christina Bartzoulianou MD
1st Department of Ophthalmology
AHEPA Hospital
Aristotle University of Thessaloniki
Greece

M Tariq Bhatti MD
Professor
Departments of Ophthalmology
Neurology and Neurosurgery
Duke Eye Center
Duke University Hospital
Durham, North Carolina, USA

Ferdinando Bottoni MD FEBO
Department of Biomedical and Clinical Science "Luigi Sacco"
Luigi Sacco Hospital, University of Milan
Milan, Italy

Marc A Bouffard MD
Instructor
Department of Neurology
Beth Israel Deaconess Medical Center
Boston, Massachusetts, USA

Richard Bowman MA MD FRCOphth
Consultant Ophthalmologist
Great Ormond Street Hospital
London, UK

Anthony Brune
Clinical Lecturer
Department of Ophthalmology and Visual Sciences
University of Michigan
Ann Arbor, Michigan, USA

Matthew J Burton PhD FRCOphth
Professor
International Eye Health
London School of Hygiene and Tropical Medicine
London, UK

Stathopoulos C MD
Ocular Oncology, Pathology and Genetics
Jules-Gonin Eye Hospital
Switzerland

Benjamin C Campbell MD
Resident (Physician Ophthalmology)
Jules Stein Eye Institute
UCLA School of Medicine
Los Angeles, California, USA

Jayne E Camuglia MBBS BSc FRANZCO
Visiting Medical Officer
Department of Ophthalmology
Children's Health Queensland
South Brisbane, Queensland, Australia

Dean Cestari MD
Associate Professor of Ophthalmology, Neuro-ophthalmology and Adult Strabismus
Harvard Medical School
Boston, Massachusetts, USA
Director, Adult Strabismus Service
Director, Ophthalmology Fellowship Education
Co-Director, Center for Thyroid Eye Disease and Orbital Surgery

Tiffany Chan OD
Associate
Drs Chan, Moon and Associates
Family Vision Care
Clinical Faculty
Frank Stein and Paul S May Center for Low Vision Rehabilitation
Department of Ophthalmology
California Pacific Medical Center
San Francisco, California, USA

Jessica R Chang MD
Assistant Professor of Ophthalmology
University of Southern California
Roski Eye Institute
Keck School of Medicine of USC
Los Angeles, California, USA

Ta Chen Peter Chang MD
Associate Professor of Clinical Ophthalmology and Pediatrics
Bascom Palmer Eye Institute
University of Miami
Miller School of Medicine
Miami, Florida, USA

Yanjun Chen MD PhD
Assistant Professor
Department of Ophthalmology and Visual Sciences
University of Wisconsin School of Medicine and Public Health
Madison, Wisconsin, USA

Emily Chew MD
Deputy Director
Division of Epidemiology and Clinical Research at NIH
Washington DC Metro Area Research
NIH

Catherine J Choi MD MS
Department of Ophthalmology
University of Miami, Miller School of Medicine
Miami, Florida, USA

Natalie N Chung MD
Research Scholar (Ophthalmology)
Shiley Eye Institute
University of California
San Diego, California, USA

August Colenbrander MD PhD
Affiliate Senior Scientist
Smith-Kettlewell Eye Research Institute
San Francisco, USA

Federico Corvi MD
Resident (Ophthalmology)
Eye Clinic
Department of Biomedical and Clinical Science "Luigi Sacco"
Luigi Sacco Hospital, University of Milan
Milan, Italy

Roberta Dalley MD
Associate Professor
Department of Radiology
University of Washington
Seattle, Washington, USA

Kunal K Dansingani MA FRCOphth
Associate Professor (Ophthalmology)
Department of Ophthalmology
University of Pittsburgh Medical Center
Pittsburgh, Pennsylvania, USA

Manoranjan Das DNB
Professor
Department of Cornea and Refractive Surgery
Aravind Eye Hospital
Madurai, Tamil Nadu, India

Shilpa Das MBBS MS
Cornea Consultant
Cornea and Cataract Services
Nethradhama Superspecialty Eye Hospital
Bengaluru, Karnataka, India
Fellow-Cornea/Anterior Segment
LV Prasad Eye Institute (LVPEI)
Hyderabad, Telangana, India

Janet L Davis MD
Leach Distinguished Professor of Ophthalmology
Bascom Palmer Eye Institute
University of Miami, Miller School of Medicine
Miami, Florida, USA

Hakan Demirci MD
Associate Professor
Richard N and Marilyn K Witham Professor
WK Kellogg Eye Center
University of Michigan
Ann Arbor, Michigan, USA

Uday Devgan MD FACS FRCS (Glasg)
Cataract and Refractive Surgeon
Devgan Eye Surgery, Los Angeles
California, USA
Partner, Speciality Surgical Center
Beverly Hills, California, USA
Chief of Ophthalmology
Olive View—UCLA Medical Center
Professor of Ophthalmology
Jules Stein Eye Institute
UCLA School of Medicine, Los Angeles
California, USA

K Dharmalingam MSc PhD
Director (Research)
Aravind Medical Research Foundation
Madurai, Tamil Nadu, India

Stephanie Ding BA
Orbital Oncology and Ophthalmic Plastic Surgery
Department of Plastic Surgery
The University of Texas
MD Anderson Cancer Center
Houston, Texas, USA

Raymond S Douglas MD PhD
Department of Surgery
Cedars-Sinai Medical Center
Los Angeles, California, USA

Todd Driver MD
PGY-4, UCLA Stein Eye Institute
University of California, San Francisco
San Francisco, California, USA

Vikram Durairaj MD
Oculoplastic Surgeon
TOC Eye and Face
Austin, Texas, USA

Deepak P Edward MD FACS FARVO
Professor
(Ophthalmology and Pathology)
Department of Ophthalmology and Visual Sciences
University of Illinois Eye and Ear Infirmary
UIC College of Medicine
Chicago, Illinois, USA
King Khaled Eye Specialist Hospital
Riyadh, Kingdom of Saudi Arabia

Dean Eliott MD
Stelios Evangelos Gragoudas Associate Professor
Department of Ophthalmology
Harvard Medical School
Associate Director
Retina Service
Massachusetts Eye and Ear
Boston, Massachusetts, USA

Zachary P Elkin MD MPH
Assistant Professor of Ophthalmology
New York University Langone Eye Center
New York, USA

Monica Ertel MD PhD
Resident
Department of Ophthalmology
Weil Cornell Medical College
New York, USA

Bita Esmaeli MD
Orbital Oncology and Ophthalmic Plastic Surgery
Department of Plastic Surgery
The University of Texas
MD Anderson Cancer Center
Houston, Texas, USA

Juliet Essilfie MD
Ophthalmology
Jules Stein Eye Institute
UCLA School of Medicine
Los Angeles, California, USA

Nina M Farivari MD
Ophthalmology Resident, PGY-4
Vanderbilt University Medical Center
Nashville, Tennessee, USA

Katrin Fasler MD
Honorary Fellow
Moorfields Eye Clinic
London, UK

Munier FL MD
Professor
Head of Ocular Oncology, Pathology and Genetics
Jules-Gonin Eye Hospital
Switzerland

Monika Fleckenstein MD
Consultant
Department of Ophthalmology
University of Bonn
Bonn, Germany

David Fleischman MD MS FACS
Assistant Professor
Department of Ophthalmology
University of North Carolina
Chapel Hill, North Carolina, USA

Donald C Fletcher MD
Envision Center for Low Vision Rehabilitation
Wichita, Kansas, USA

Allen Foster
MB ChB (Hons) FRCS FRCOphth FHEA
Professor of International Eye Health
International Centre of Eye Health
London School of Hygiene and Tropical Medicine
London, UK

Courtney Francis MD
Associate Professor
Department of Ophthalmology
University of Washington
Seattle, Washington, USA

Suzanne K Freitag MD
Director
Ophthalmic Plastic Surgery
Massachusetts Eye and Ear Infirmary
Harvard Medical School
Boston, Massachusetts, USA

K Bailey Freund MD
Clinical Professor
Department of Ophthalmology
The New York University School of Medicine
Vitreous Retina Macula Consultants
New York, USA

Scott J Fudemberg MD
Assistant Professor
Wills Eye Hospital
Philadelphia, Pennsylvania, USA

James G Fujimoto PhD
Elihu Thomson Professor of Electrical Engineering
Department of Electrical Engineering and Computer Science
Massachusetts Institute of Technology
Cambridge, Massachusetts, USA

Orly Gal-Or MD
Medical Retina Consultant
Department of Ophthalmology
Rabin Medical Center
Petah-Tikva, Israel

Elisha Garg MD
Resident (Ophthalmology)
Jules Stein Eye Institute
UCLA School of Medicine
Los Angeles, California, USA

Prashant Garg MS (Ophthalmology)
Consultant
Cornea and Anterior Segment Services
Tej Kohli Cornea Service, KAR Campus
LV Prasad Eye Institute (LVPEI)
Hyderabad, Telangana, India

Alain Gaudric MD
Emeritus Professor
Department of Ophthalmology
Lariboisière Hospital
University of Paris 7-Denis Diderot
Paris, France

Andrea Giani MD
Assistant Professor
Eye Clinic
Department of Biomedical and Clinical Science "Luigi Sacco"
Luigi Sacco Hospital, University of Milan
Milan, Italy

Dimitrios Giannoulis MD MSc
1st Department of Ophthalmology
AHEPA Hospital
Aristotle University of Thessaloniki
Greece

Kimberly K Gokoffski MD PhD
Assistant Professor
University of Southern California
Roski Eye Institute
Los Angeles, California, USA

Daniel Gold DO
Assistant Professor of Neurology
Division of Neuro-Visual and Vestibular Disorders
Ophthalmology, Neurosurgery, Otolaryngology—Head and Neck Surgery
Emergency Medicine
Director, Vestibular and Ocular Motor Oto-Neurology Fellowship
Director, Urgent Neurology
The Johns Hopkins Hospital
Baltimore, Maryland, USA

Glen A Gole
MBBS MD (NSW) FRANZCO FRACS FRCOphth
Professor/Director of Ophthalmology
Department of Ophthalmology
Lady Cilento Children's Hospital (LCCH)
South Brisbane, Queensland, Australia

John A Gonzales MD
Associate Professor
Francis I Proctor Foundation
University of California
San Francisco, California, USA

Rameshkumar Gunasekaran MSc
Microbiologist
Department of Ocular Microbiology
Aravind Eye Hospital
Madurai, Tamil Nadu, India

Noopur Gupta MS (Ophthalmology) PhD
Assistant Professor (Cornea, Cataract and Refractive Surgery Services)
Dr Rajendra Prasad Centre for Ophthalmic Sciences
All India Institute of Medical Sciences (AIIMS)
New Delhi, India

Vishali Gupta MS
Professor
Postgraduate Institute of Medical Education and Research (PGIMER)
Chandigarh, India

Samer Hamada
MD MSc DO (Hons) FRCSEd FRCOphth
Consultant Ophthalmic Surgeon (Adults and Children)
Corneoplastic Unit and Eye Bank
Queen Victoria Hospital NHS Trust
East Grinstead, Sussex, UK

D Rex Hamilton MD MS
Ophthalmology
Jules Stein Eye Institute
UCLA School of Medicine
Los Angeles, California, USA

B Hansen MD
Ophthalmology
UT Southwestern Medical Center
Dallas, Texas, USA

Manali Hazarika MBBS MS (Ophthalmology)
Fellow
Department of Cornea and Anterior Segment Services
Aravind Eye Hospital
Madurai, Tamil Nadu, India

Paul R Healey
BMedSc MBBS (Hons) MMed PhD FRANZCO
Clinical Associate Professor
Sydney Medical School
University of Sydney
Sydney, NSW, Australia

Martina C Herwig-Carl MD
Consultant
Department of Ophthalmology
University Clinic Bonn
Bonn, NRW, Germany

Jeremy JSL Hoffman FRCOphth
Clinical Research Fellow
London School of Hygiene and Tropical Medicine
London, UK

Frank G Holz MD
Chairman and Professor
Department of Ophthalmology
University of Bonn
Bonn, Germany

Jean Pierre Hubschman MD
Ophthalmology
Jules Stein Eye Institute
UCLA School of Medicine
Los Angeles, California, USA

Sarah Hull MBBS MA FRCOphth PhD
Specialist Registrar
Moorfields Eye Hospital NHS Foundation Trust
Honorary Research Associate
UCL Institute of Ophthalmology
London, UK

Alessandro Invernizzi MD
Assistant Professor
Eye Clinic
Department of Biomedical and Clinical Science "Luigi Sacco"
Luigi Sacco Hospital, University of Milan
Milan, Italy

Peter Charbel Issa MD DPhil
Oxford Eye Hospital and Nuffield Laboratory of Ophthalmology
Department of Clinical Neurosciences
University of Oxford
Oxford, UK

Sabita M Ittoop MD MS
Inova Fair Oaks Hospital
Herndon, Virginia, USA

Geetha Iyer MD FRCS
Senior Consultant
CJ Shah Cornea Services
Dr G Sitalakshmi Memorial Clinic for Ocular Surface Disorders
Sankara Nethralaya
Chennai, Tamil Nadu, India

Cunha-Vaz J MD PhD
Association for Innovation and Biomedical Research on Light and Image (AIBILI)
Faculty of Medicine
University of Coimbra (FMUC)
Coimbra, Portugal

Divya Janakiraman
MBBS MD (Ophthalmology)
Clinical Fellow
Department of Cornea and Anterior Segment Services
Aravind Eye Hospital
Madurai, Tamil Nadu, India

Pimkwan Jaru-ampornpan MD
Clinical Instructor
Department of Ophthalmology
Faculty of Medicine
Siriraj Hospital
Mahidol University
Bangkok, Thailand

Bennie H Jeng MD
Professor and Chair
Department of Ophthalmology and Visual Sciences
University of Maryland School of Medicine
Baltimore, Maryland, USA

Imran Jivraj MD
Neuro-ophthalmologist
Department of Ophthalmology
University of Alberta
Edmonton, Alberta, USA

Chris A Johnson PhD DSc
Professor
Department of Ophthalmology and Visual Sciences
University of Iowa Hospitals and Clinics
Iowa City, Iowa, USA

Michael Jordan MD MS
University of Minnesota
Department of Ophthalmology and Visual Sciences
Minneapolis, Minnesota, USA

Shannon S Joseph MD
Assistant Professor
Department of Ophthalmology
Division of Oculoplastic Surgery
WK Kellogg Eye Center
University of Michigan
Ann Arbor, Michigan, USA

Marques JP MD MSc FEBO
Association for Innovation and Biomedical Research on Light and Image (AIBILI)
Faculty of Medicine
University of Coimbra (FMUC)
Coimbra, Portugal

Albert S Jun MD PhD
Wilmer Eye Institute
Johns Hopkins Medical Institutions
Baltimore, Maryland, USA

Malik Y Kahook MD
Professor
Department of Ophthalmology
University of Colorado School of Medicine
Aurora, Colorado, USA

Paavan Kalra MS (Ophthalmology)
Consultant
Cornea and Anterior Segment Services
Tej Kohli Cornea Service, KAR Campus
LV Prasad Eye Institute (LVPEI)
Hyderabad, Telangana, India

Thomas J Kandl MD
Orbital Oncology and Ophthalmic Plastic Surgery
Department of Plastic Surgery
The University of Texas
MD Anderson Cancer Center
Houston, Texas, USA

L Jay Katz MD
Professor
Department of Ophthalmology
Wills Eye Hospital
Thomas Jefferson University
Philadelphia, Pennsylvania, USA

Srinivasan Kavitha MD PhD MS
Consultant
Glaucoma Services
Aravind Eye Hospital and Postgraduate Institute of Ophthalmology
Puducherry, India

Aki Kawasaki MD PhD
Professor
Hôpital Ophtalmique
University of Lausanne
Lausanne, Switzerland

Pearse A Keane MD
Consultant Ophthalmologist
Moorfields Eye Hospital
NIHR Clinician Scientist
University College London
Institute of Ophthalmology
London, UK

Jeremy Keenan MD MPH
Professor of Ophthalmology
Francis I Proctor Foundation and
Department of Ophthalmology
San Francisco, California, USA

Tiarnan Kennan MD PhD
Staff Clinician
Division of Epidemiology and Clinical Applications
National Eye Institute
National Institutes of Health
Bethesda, Maryland, USA

Christina Keskini MD MSc
Laboratory of Research and Clinical Applications in Ophthalmology (LaRCAO)
1st Department of Ophthalmology
AHEPA Hospital
Aristotle University of Thessaloniki
Greece

Peng Tee Khaw PhD FRCS FRCP FRCOphth FRCPath FRSB FCOptom Hon DSc FARVO FMedSci
Director
NIHR Biomedical Research Centre
Moorfields Eye Hospital and UCL Institute of Ophthalmology
Research and Development
Eyes and Vision Programme
UCL Partners Academic Health Science Centre
Emeritus NIHR Senior Investigator

Kay T Khine MD
Voluntary Assistant Professor
Bascom Palmer Eye Institute
University of Miami
Miami, Florida, USA

Don O Kikkawa MD FACS
Professor of Ophthalmology and Plastic Surgery
Chief, Division of Oculofacial Plastic Surgery and Vice Chairman
UC San Diego Department of Ophthalmology
Shiley Eye Institute
La Jolla, California, USA

Caitriona Kirwan FRCS
Consultant Ophthalmic Surgeon and Pediatric Ophthalmologist
Mater Private Hospital
Dublin, Ireland

Natasha Nayak Kolomeyer MD
Clinical Instructor
Wills Eye Hospital
Philadelphia, Pennsylvania, USA

Bobby S Korn MD PhD
Professor of Ophthalmology and Plastic Surgery
Department of Ophthalmology
UC San Diego School of Medicine
Shiley Eye Institute
La Jolla, California, USA

Agnieszka Kudasiewicz-Kardaszewska MD PhD
Ophthalmology Consultant and Surgeon
Zagorski Eye Surgery Centers
Nałęczów, Poland

Ferenc Kuhn MD PhD
President
International Society of Ocular Trauma
Associate Professor of Ophthalmology
University of Alabama, Birmingham, UK
Vice President for Clinical Research
Helen Keller Foundation for Research and Education
Consultant and Chief
Vitreoretinal Surgeon
Milos Eye Clinic
Belgrade, Serbia
Consultant and Vitreoretinal Surgeon
Zagorski Eye Surgery Center
Nałęczów, Poland

Ashish Kumar DNB
Consultant
Department of Cornea and Refractive Surgery
Aravind Eye Hospital
Madurai, Tamil Nadu, India

Nathan Kung MD
Neuro-ophthalmologist
Blue Sky Neurology
Denver, Colorado, USA

Pallak Kusumgar MS FAICO
Cornea, Refractive Surgeon
Narayana Nethralaya
Bengaluru, Karnataka, India

Jocelyn Lam MD
Department of Ophthalmology
University of Washington
Seattle, Washington, USA

Scott R Lambert MD
Professor of Ophthalmology and Pediatrics
Department of Ophthalmology
Stanford University School of Medicine
Chief of Pediatric Ophthalmology
Lucile Packard Children's Hospital
Palo Alto, California, USA

Suzanne W van Landingham MD
University of Wisconsin
Department of Ophthalmology and Vision Sciences
Madison, Wisconsin, USA

Michael S Lee MD
Department of Ophthalmology and Visual Neurosciences
University of Minnesota
Minneapolis, Minnesota, USA

Gary J Lelli MD
Vice Chair and Associate Professor of Ophthalmology
Director of Ophthalmic Plastic and Reconstructive Surgery
Department of Ophthalmology
Weil Cornell Medical College
New York, USA

S Fabian Lerner MD
Professor of Ophthalmology
University Favaloro
School of Medical Sciences
Buenos Aires, Argentina

Vaitheeswaran LG MBBS MD FICO
Cataract, Cornea and Refractive Surgeon
Narayana Nethralaya
Bengaluru, Karnataka, India

Edward P Lin MD MBA
Assistant Professor
Department of Imaging Sciences
University of Rochester Medical Center
Rochester, New York, USA

Shawn R Lin MD MS MBA
UCLA Jules Stein Eye Institute
UCLA School of Medicine
Los Angeles, California, USA

Katy C Liu MD PhD
Clinical Associate (Ophthalmology)
Duke Eye Center
Duke University Hospital
Durham, North Carolina, USA

James Liu MD
Resident in Ophthalmology
Department of Ophthalmology and Visual Sciences
Washington University
St Louis School of Medicine
St Louis, Missouri, USA

Karin U Loeffler MD
Consultant
Department of Ophthalmology
University Clinic Bonn
Bonn, NRW, Germany

Eibhlín Mc Loone MB BCh BAO FRCOphth
Consultant Pediatric Ophthalmologist
Belfast Health and Social Care Trust (BHSCT)
Eye and Ear Clinic
Royal Victoria Hospital
Belfast, Ireland

Mark J Lucarelli MD FACS
Dortzbach Professor of Ophthalmic Facial Plastic Surgery
Director, Oculoplastic, Facial Cosmetic and Orbital Surgery
University of Wisconsin-Madison
Madison, Wisconsin, USA

Rajeswari Mahadevan PhD
Head of Contact Lens Clinic
Assistant Professor
Elite School of Optometry
Sankara Nethralaya
Chennai, Tamil Nadu, India

Prafulla K Maharana MD DNB
Assistant Professor (Ophthalmology)
Dr Rajendra Prasad Centre for Ophthalmic Sciences
All India Institute of Medical Sciences (AIIMS)
New Delhi, India

Nicholas R Mahoney MD
Wilmer Eye Institute
Johns Hopkins University School of Medicine
Baltimore, Maryland, USA

Siddharth Malaiya MBBS MS
Comprehensive Clinical Fellow
LV Prasad Eye Institute (LVPEI)
KAR Campus
Hyderabad, Telangana, India

Sundas Maqsood MBBS
Consultant Ophthalmic Surgeon (Adults and Children)
Corneoplastic Unit and Eye Bank
Queen Victoria Hospital NHS Trust
East Grinstead, Sussex, UK

Ian Marsh
MD PhD MB ChB FRCS (Ed) FRCOphth
Consultant Ophthalmologist
Department of Ophthalmology
Aintree University Hospitals NHS Foundation Trust
Liverpool, UK

Louise A Mawn MD
Professor of Ophthalmology and Neurological Surgery
Vanderbilt Medical Centre
Nashville, Tennessee, USA

Tara A McCannel MD PhD
Ophthalmic Oncology Center
Stein Eye and Doheny Eye Institutes
Department of Ophthalmology
University of California
Los Angeles, California, USA

Collin M McClelland MD
Associate Professor
Department of Ophthalmology and Visual Neurosciences
University of Minnesota
Minneapolis, Minnesota, USA

John McSoley OD
Bascom Palmer Eye Institute
Miami, Florida, USA

Joseph M Miller MD MPH
Professor of Ophthalmology
Optical Sciences and Public Health
University of Arizona College of Medicine
Tucson, Arizona, USA

Kevin M Miller MD
Professor of Clinical Ophthalmology
Jules Stein Eye Institute
UCLA School of Medicine
Los Angeles, California, USA
Kolokotrones Chair in Ophthalmology
Chief, Cataract and Refractive Surgery Division
Director, Anterior Segment Diagnostic Laboratory

Anthony T Moore
MA FRCS FRCOphth FMedSci
Michael Vilensky Endowed Chair in Ophthalmology
The University of California, San Francisco (UCSF) School of Medicine
Koret Vision Center
San Francisco, California, USA

VV Mootha MD
Ophthalmology
UT Southwestern Medical Center
Dallas, Texas, USA

Eric M Moult BSc
Research Assistant
Department of Electrical Engineering and Computer Science
Massachusetts Institute of Technology
Cambridge, Massachusetts, USA

Bipasha Mukherjee MS DNB
Consultant Ophthalmologist
Orbit, Oculoplasty, Reconstructive and Aesthetic Services
Sankara Nethralaya
Medical Research Foundation
Chennai, Tamil Nadu, India

Harsha Nagaraja MBBS MS
Consultant Ophthalmolgist
Cornea and External Eye Diseases
Narayana Nethralaya
Bengaluru, Karnataka, India

Paolo Nucci PROF
Director
Department of Ophthalmology
San Giuseppe Hospital
University of Milan
Milan, Italy

Michael O'Keeffe FRCS
Consultant Ophthalmic Surgeon
Mater Private Hospital and Beacon Hospital
Dublin, Ireland

Patrick Oellers MD
Thomas J Madden Fellow in Vitreoretinal Surgery
Massachusetts Eye and Ear
Harvard Medical School
Boston, Massachusetts, USA

Hilal Eser Ozturk MD
Assistant Professor (Ophthalmology)
Faculty of Medicine
Ondokuz Mayis University
Samsun, Turkey

Srikanta Kumar Padhy MD
Resident (Ophthalmology)
Dr Rajendra Prasad Centre for Ophthalmic Sciences
All India Institute of Medical Sciences (AIIMS)
New Delhi, India

Prema Padmanabhan MD
Head
Department of Cornea Services and Refractive Surgery
Medical Research Foundation
Chennai, Tamil Nadu, India

Arun Kumar Panigrahi MS
Consultant
Department of Cornea and Refractive Surgery
Aravind Eye Hospital
Madurai, Tamil Nadu, India

Maria Papadopoulos MB BS FRACO
Consultant Ophthalmic Surgeon
Glaucoma Service
Moorfields Eye Hospital NHS Foundation Trust
London, UK

Vivek R Patel MD
Associate Professor
University of Southern California
Roski Eye Institute
Los Angeles, California, USA

Marco Pellegrini MD
Eye Clinic
Department of Biomedical and Clinical Science "Luigi Sacco"
Luigi Sacco Hospital, University of Milan
Milan, Italy

Mark E Pennesi MD PhD
Associate Professor (Ophthalmology)
Casey Eye Institute
Oregon Health and Science University
Portland, Oregon, USA

Monica S Perlmutter OTD OTR/L SCLV FAOTA
Associate Professor
Occupational Therapy and Ophthalmology
Lead OT (Low Vision in Home and Community Services)
Washington University Program in Occupational Therapy
St Louis, Missouri, USA

Chee Soon Phaik MBBS FRCS(G) MMed(Ophth) FRCS(Ed) FRCOphth
Head of Department and Senior Consultant
Cataract Subspecialty Service and Ocular Inflammation and Immunology Service
Singapore National Eye Centre
Singapore

Elise Philippakis MD
Consultant
Department of Ophthalmology
Lariboisière Hospital
University of Paris 7-Denis Diderot
Paris, France

Cameron Pole MD
Jules Stein Eye Institute
UCLA School of Medicine
Los Angeles, California, USA

Zia S Pradhan DNB FRCOphth
Consultant
Glaucoma Services
Narayana Nethralaya
Bengaluru, Karnataka, India

N Venkatesh Prajna DNB FRCOphth
Academic Director
Aravind Eye Care System
Madurai, Tamil Nadu, India

Lalitha Prajna MD (Microbiology)
Chief Microbiologist
Department of Ocular Microbiology
Aravind Eye Hospital and Postgraduate Institute of Ophthalmology
Madurai, Tamil Nadu, India

Narendra K Puttaiah DNB
Consultant
Glaucoma Services
Narayana Nethralaya
Bengaluru, Karnataka, India

Naveen Radhakrishnan MS FICO
Consultant
Department of Cornea and Refractive Surgery
Aravind Eye Care System
Madurai, Tamil Nadu, India

Pradeep Ramulu MD PhD MHS
Professor of Ophthalmology (Glaucoma)
Wilmer Eye Institute
Johns Hopkins Hospital
Baltimore, Maryland, USA

Harsha L Rao MD DNB PhD
Consultant
Glaucoma Services
Narayana Nethralaya
Bengaluru, Karnataka, India

SR Rathinam FAMS PhD
Professor of Ophthalmology and Head of Uveitis Service
Aravind Eye Hospital and Postgraduate Institute of Ophthalmology
Madurai, Tamil Nadu, India

Thulasiraj Ravilla MBA
Executive Director
Lions Aravind Institute of Community Ophthalmology (LAICO)
Madurai, Tamil Nadu, India

Sathya T Ravilla MS (Ophthalmology)
Consultant
Pediatric Ophthalmology and Strabismus Clinic
Aravind Eye Hospital
Madurai, Tamil Nadu, India

Hasika Ravula MS FICO
Cornea and Refractive Surgeon
Department of Cornea
Nayana Eye Care
Kakinada, Andhra Pradesh, India

Michael X Repka MD MBA
David L Guyton, MD, and Feduniak Family
Professor of Ophthalmology
Wilmer Eye Institute
Johns Hopkins University School of Medicine
Baltimore, Maryland, USA

Rajaraman Revathi MS
Professor
Department of Cornea and Refractive Surgery Services
Aravind Eye Hospital
Coimbatore, Tamil Nadu, India

Alan L Robin MD
Professor
Department of Ophthalmology and Visual Sciences
University of Michigan
Ann Arbor, Michigan, USA

V Romano MD
Consultant Ophthalmic Surgeon
Royal Liverpool University Hospital
Liverpool, UK

James T Rosenbaum MD
Professor of Ophthalmology, Medicine and Cell Biology
Edward E Rosenbaum Professor of Inflammation Research
Oregon Health and Science University
Portland, Oregon, USA

Jennifer Rose-Nussbaumer
MD (Medical Doctor)
Assistant Professor
Francis I Proctor Foundation
University of California
San Francisco, California, USA

Aravind Roy MS (Ophthalmology)
Consultant
Cornea and Anterior Segment Services
Tej Kohli Cornea Service, KVC Campus
LV Prasad Eye Institute (LVPEI)
Vijayawada, Andhra Pradesh, India

Srinivas R Sadda MD
President and Chief Scientific Officer
Doheny Eye Institute
Professor of Ophthalmology
University of California-Los Angeles
Los Angeles, California, USA

Oded Sagiv MD
Orbital Oncology and Ophthalmic Plastic Surgery
Department of Plastic Surgery
The University of Texas
MD Anderson Cancer Center
Houston, Texas, USA

Pranita Sahay MD
Senior Resident
Dr Rajendra Prasad Centre for Ophthalmic Sciences
All India Institute of Medical Sciences (AIIMS)
New Delhi, India

Sherveen S Salek BS MD
Vitreoretinal Fellow
Department of Ophthalmology
Emory University School of Medicine
Atlanta, Georgia, USA

Gunjan Saluja MD
Senior Resident
Dr Rajendra Prasad Centre for Ophthalmic Sciences
All India Institute of Medical Sciences (AIIMS)
New Delhi, India

Virender S Sangwan MS
Dr Paul Dubord Chair in Cornea
Tej Kohli Cornea Institute
Director, Center for Ocular Regeneration (CORE)
Director, Srujana-Center for Innovation
LV Prasad Eye Institute, KAR Campus
Hyderabad, Telangana, India

Steven S Saraf MD
Instructor
Bascom Palmer Eye Institute
University of Miami
Miller School of Medicine
Miami, Florida USA

VR Saravanan DNB
Consultant
Department of Retina and Vitreous
Aravind Eye Hospital and Postgraduate Institute of Ophthalmology
Coimbatore, Tamil Nadu, India

David Sarraf MD
Ophthalmology
Jules Stein Eye Institute
UCLA School of Medicine
Los Angeles, California, USA

Matteo Scaramuzzi MD
Resident
Department of Ophthalmology
San Giuseppe Hospital
University of Milan
Milan, Italy

Emily M Schehlein MD
Department of Ophthalmology and Visual Sciences
University of Michigan
Ann Arbor, Michigan, USA

Steffen Schmitz-Valckenberg MD
Consultant
Department of Ophthalmology
University of Bonn
Bonn, Germany

Hendrik PN Scholl MD MA
Director
Institute of Molecular and Clinical Ophthalmology Basel (IOB)
Professor and Chairman
Department of Ophthalmology
University of Basel, Switzerland
Adjunct Professor of Ophthalmology
Wilmer Eye Institute
Johns Hopkins University, USA

Etienne M Schönbach MD
Resident (Ophthalmology)
Department of Ophthalmology and Visual Sciences
Case Western Reserve University
Cleveland, Ohio, USA

Leonard K Seibold MD
Associate Professor
Department of Ophthalmology
University of Colorado School of Medicine
Aurora, Colorado, USA

Juan Carlos Serna-Ojeda MD MSc
Cornea, Refractive Surgery and Ocular Surface Specialist
Banco de Ojos de Aguascalientes
Aguascalientes, Mexico

Ayad Shafiq
FRCOphth MRCPPaeds DCH MA BM & BCh
Consultant Ophthalmologist
Royal Victoria Infirmary
Newcastle Upon Tyne, UK

Parag K Shah DNB
Consultant
Department of Retina and Vitreous
Aravind Eye Hospital and Postgraduate Institute of Ophthalmology
Coimbatore, Tamil Nadu, India

Namrata Sharma
Professor of Ophthalmology
Dr Rajendra Prasad Centre for Ophthalmic Sciences
All India Institute of Medical Sciences (AIIMS)
New Delhi, India

Sankalp Singh Sharma DO DNB
Medical Consultant (Ophthalmology)
Aravind Eye Hospital and Postgraduate Institute of Ophthalmology
Madurai, Tamil Nadu, India

Rohit Shetty FRCS PhD
Vice Chair and Translational Scientist
Narayana Nethralaya
Bengaluru, Karnataka, India

Eric Shieh MD
Physician
Jules Stein Eye Institute
UCLA School of Medicine
Los Angeles, California, USA

Aazim A Siddiqui MD
Resident Physician
Department of Ophthalmology and Visual Sciences
Montefiore Medical Center
Albert Einstein College of Medicine
New York, USA

Joseph M Simonett MD
Resident (Ophthalmology)
Casey Eye Institute
Oregon Health and Science University
Portland, Oregon, USA

Rashmi Singh MD (Ophthalmology)
Senior Resident (Cornea, Cataract and Refractive Surgery Services)
Dr Rajendra Prasad Centre for Ophthalmic Sciences
All India Institute of Medical Sciences (AIIMS)
New Delhi, India

Vidal Soberon
Retina and Oncology Fellow
Jules Stein Eye Institute
University of California-Los Angeles
Los Angeles, USA

Marie Somogyi MD
Oculoplastic Surgeon
TOC Eye and Face
Austin, Texas, USA

Bhaskar Srinivasan MD
Senior Consultant
CJ Shah Cornea Services
Dr G Sitalakshmi Memorial Clinic for Ocular Surface Disorders
Sankara Nethralaya
Chennai, Tamil Nadu, India

K Srinivasarao MS
Resident
Postgraduate Institute of Medical Education and Research (PGIMER)
Chandigarh, India

Giovanni Staurenghi MD FARVO FEBO
Chairman–Director
Eye Clinic
Department of Biomedical and Clinical Science "Luigi Sacco"
Luigi Sacco Hospital, University of Milan
Milan, Italy

Greg Van Stavern MD
Professor of Ophthalmology and Visual Sciences and Neurology
Department of Ophthalmology and Visual Sciences
Washington University in St Louis School of Medicine
St Louis, Missouri, USA

B Steger MD
Assistant Professor (Ophthalmology)
Department of Ophthalmology
Innsbruck, Austria

Prem S Subramanian MD PhD
Professor of Ophthalmology, Neurology and Neurosurgery and Vice Chair for Academic Affairs
UC Health/Sue Anschutz-Rodgers Eye Center
Department of Ophthalmology
University of Colorado School of Medicine
Aurora, Colorado, USA

Sandip Suresh MD
Jules Stein Eye Institute
UCLA School of Medicine
Los Angeles, California, USA

Colin S Tan
MBBS MMed (Ophth) FRCSEd (Ophth)
Associate Professor and Senior Consultant (Ophthalmology)
National Healthcare Group Eye Institute
Singapore

Erika Tanaka MD
Ophthalmology
Jules Stein Eye Institute
UCLA School of Medicine
Los Angeles, California, USA

Radhika Tandon
MD DNB FRCSEd FRCOphth
Professor of Ophthalmology
Faculty In-charge
Unit 6—Cornea and External Diseases Cataract and Refractive, Ocular Oncology and Low Vision Services
Co-Chairperson National Eye Bank
Dr Rajendra Prasad Centre for Ophthalmic Sciences
All India Institute of Medical Sciences (AIIMS)
New Delhi, India

David Taylor FRCOphth DSc (Med)
Professor Emeritus
The UCL Great Ormond Street Institute of Child Health
London, UK

Honeylen Maryl T Teo MD
Fellow (Ocular Oncology)
WK Kellogg Eye Center
University of Michigan
Ann Arbor, Michigan, USA

Sudip D Thakar MD
Orbital Oncology and Ophthalmic Plastic Surgery
Department of Plastic Surgery
The University of Texas
MD Anderson Cancer Center
Houston, Texas, USA

Fotis Topouzis MD MSc PhD
Professor of Ophthalmology
Chair 1st Department of Ophthalmology
AHEPA Hospital
Aristotle University of Thessaloniki
Greece

Roksolyana Tourkevich MD
Instructor of Neurology
Division of Neuro-Visual and Vestibular Disorders
Departments of Neurology, Otolaryngology—Head and Neck Surgery
The Johns Hopkins Hospital
Baltimore, Maryland, USA

David T Tse MD
Bascom Palmer Eye Institute
University of Miami,
Miller School of Medicine
Miami, Florida, USA

Ilknur Tugal-Tutkun MD
Professor (Ophthalmology)
Istanbul University
Istanbul Faculty of Medicine
Istanbul, Turkey

Mayjane Joan Tumulak Diplomate, Philippine Board of Ophthalmology
Consultant in Ocular Inflammation and Immunology
Maria Reyna-Xavier University Hospital
Cagayan de Oro City, Misamis Oriental
Philippines

Swati Upadhyaya MD PhD DNB
Consultant
Glaucoma Services
Aravind Eye Hospital and Postgraduate Institute of Ophthalmology
Puducherry, India

Prabhu V MS FICO
Consultant
Department of Cornea and Refractive Surgery Services
Aravind Eye Hospital
Coimbatore, Tamil Nadu, India

Saujanya Vadoothker MD
Clinical Fellow
Department of Ophthalmology and Visual Sciences
University of Maryland School of Medicine
Baltimore, Maryland, USA

Vikram Vaidee DNB FRCS (Glasg)
Consultant
Department of Cornea and Refractive Surgery Services
Aravind Eye Hospital
Coimbatore, Tamil Nadu, India

M Vanathi MD
Professor
Department of Ophthalmology
All India Institute of Medical Sciences (AIIMS)
New Delhi, India

Nithya Vijayakumar BS
Department of Ophthalmology and Visual Sciences
WK Kellogg Eye Center
University of Michigan
Ann Arbor, Michigan, USA

Perumalsamy Vijayalakshmi MS (Ophthalmology)
Professor of Ophthalmology
Pediatric Ophthalmology and Strabismus Clinic
Aravind Eye Hospital
Madurai, Tamil Nadu, India

Suneetha Viswanathaiah MBBS MD (Medical Microbiology)
Consultant Microbiologist
Department of Ocular Microbiology
Aravind Eye Hospital
Salem, Tamil Nadu, India

Ivan Vrcek MD
Oculoplastic Surgeon
Texas Eye Plastics
Dallas, Texas, USA

Nadia K Waheed MD MPH
Tufts Medical Center
Boston, Massachusetts, USA

Orli Weisser-Pike
Doctor of Occupational Therapy
OTD, OTR/L, CLVT, SCLV, CAPS
Department of Occupational Therapy
University of Tennessee Health Science Center
Memphis, Tennessee, USA

Zoë R Williams MD
Associate Professor
Departments of Ophthalmology, Neurology and Neurosurgery
Flaum Eye Institute
University of Rochester Medical Center
Rochester, New York, USA

CE Willoughby BSc MD FRCOphth
Professor
Department of Ophthalmology
Ulster University
Northern Ireland, UK

Kimberly M Winges MD
Assistant Professor (Neuro-ophthalmology)
Casey Eye Institute
Oregon Health and Science University and VA Portland Health Care System
Portland, Oregon, USA

Natalie Wolkow MD PhD
Ophthalmic Plastic Surgery Service
Massachusetts Eye and Ear Infirmary
Harvard Medical School
Boston, Massachusetts, USA

Maria A Woodward MD MS
Assistant Professor
Ophthalmology and Visual Sciences
WK Kellogg Eye Center,
University of Michigan
Ann Arbor, Michigan, USA

Fasika A Woreta MD MPH
Assistant Professor of Ophthalmology
Associate Residency Program Director
Director, Eye Trauma Center
Wilmer Ophthalmological Institute
Johns Hopkins University School of
Medicine, Baltimore, Maryland, USA

David Xu MD
Ophthalmology
Jules Stein Eye Institute
UCLA School of Medicine
Los Angeles, California, USA

Sung Jae Yang MD PhD
Associate Professor
Department of Ophthalmology
Gangneung Asan Hospital
University of Ulsan
College of Medicine
South Korea

Tamara Zompa MD
Glaucoma Service
Centro Oftalmológico Charles
Buenos Aires, Argentina

Foreword

Four decades have elapsed since the writing of the first edition, *Principles and Practice of Ophthalmology*. Quite a bit has happened since then! The time has clearly come for a reincarnation.

When Gholam A Peyman, Donald R Sanders and I compiled and edited the initial version of this multi-volume book in 1980, we utilized the considerable talents of our colleagues and students, all of whom were based in North America. Many of them were affiliated with the University of Illinois in Chicago (our academic home at the time). Now, the Editor-in-Chief is Dr N Venkatesh Prajna, the Chief, Department of Education, and the Director of Academics at the justifiably famous Aravind Eye System (*www.aravind.org*), headquartered in Madurai, Tamil Nadu, India. He has obtained 116 totally new chapters (almost 3 times as many as in the 1980 version).

These chapters have been written by experts from 10 countries, not just the USA. The results reflect the latest opinions from international authorities on diagnostic and therapeutic principles and techniques. Indeed, many of the subjects represent knowledge that did not even exist at all in 1980, such as the following: innovative techniques of cataract surgery; imaging modalities including OCT, for both retinal disease and glaucoma; pharmacotherapy for retinal and macular diseases; new forms of medical and surgical therapy for glaucoma; immunosuppression for uveitis; and many others.

Interestingly, reviews of the original book could equally well apply to this latest version. For example, Professor David Cogan of Harvard University and the National Eye Institute said the following in the New England Journal of Medicine: the book has "a high order of excellence for readers who want a modern and relatively complete thesaurus of ophthalmology…". In the Archives of Ophthalmology, reviewers concluded that "this is a comprehensive…textbook…for residents and practicing physicians…with well-written (chapters)…excellent photographs, drawings, and tables, (that) are well referenced…these volumes fill a need for a comprehensive review of general ophthalmology…and various subspecialty areas."

Our 1987's preface stated: "This book is intended to be a readable and comprehensive textbook for residents and practicing ophthalmologists. It is also meant to be a current, practical guide to a variety of diagnostic and therapeutic approaches to ophthalmic diseases". Dr Prajna and his highly experienced contributors have more than fulfilled our original attempt.

Congratulations!

Morton F Goldberg
MD FAOS FACS Dr Hon Causa (Univ Coimbra)
Director Emeritus
Wilmer Eye Institute
Johns Hopkins University School of Medicine (JHUSOM)
Advisory Board Member
Aravind Eye Foundation

Preface to the Second Edition

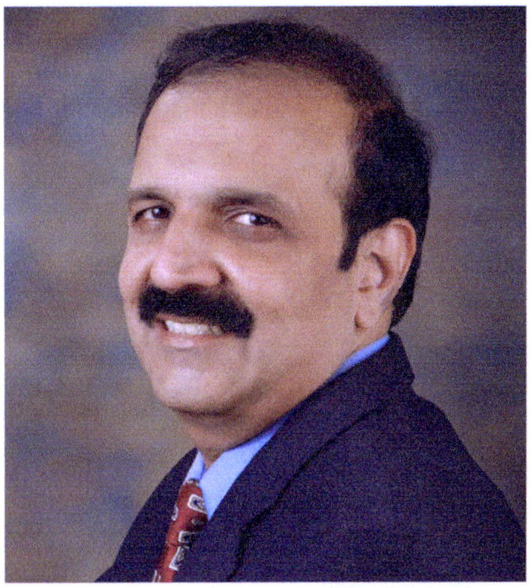

It is very rare to get an opportunity to become the Editor-in-Chief of the same book that one studied during the residency years I consider myself immensely fortunate to have got this chance to edit the book, which was my guiding force during my postgraduation career. The close personal and professional association of one of the previous editors, namely, Dr Morton F Goldberg , who has been a tremendous source of inspiration for all of us at Aravind Eye Care System, made this job an even more memorable one.

The previous edition of *Principles and Practice of Ophthalmology* was a comprehensive book for ophthalmologists in the 1980s. It was one of the most sought after books to get contemporary knowledge of the whole ophthalmology of those times and was presented with great lucidity. During these three decades ever since, ophthalmology has grown in leaps and bounds, and hence there was an urgent need to bring out a current edition of the book to reflect all these advances. The current edition has been designed to concentrate on the relevant practical details of all the advancements in the field and has been generously adorned with illustrations and photographs.

I am very thankful to all the esteemed Section Editors namely, Drs August Colenbrander (Vision Rehabilitation), Uday Devgan (Cataract), Deepak P Edward (Ocular Pathology), Shannon S Joseph (Orbit and Oculoplasty), Joseph M Miller (Optics and Refraction), Michael O'Keeffe (Pediatric Ophthalmology and Strabismus), Pradeep Ramulu (Glaucoma), Srinivas R Sadda (Retina and Vitreous), SR Rathinam (Scleritis and Uveitis) and Prem S Subramanian (Neuro-ophthalmology). All of them are well-respected doyens in their fields and the book has benefitted immensely due to their expertise. They have toiled hard to work with individual authors to produce excellent chapters.

It is always a challenge to mesh the basic concepts and the current advances straddling the entire specialty of ophthalmology in just two volumes. The expertise of heading a world class teaching program at Aravind Eye Hospitals for the past two decades, has helped me to understand the needs of the ophthalmology residents, and I do sincerely hope that this book would be a guiding force for them as well. The book would not have been possible without the blessings of my parents, Dr P Namperumalsamy and Dr G Natchiar; unwavering support of my wife, Dr Lalitha; and my children, Dr Meera Lakshmi and Aravind Krishna and I am very grateful for their love and affection. It is also a unique coincidence that my parents did their fellowships with Drs Gholam A Peyman and Morton F Goldberg in the 1970s in the University of Illinois, Chicago, USA. I am also extremely thankful for the management of the entire Aravind Eye Care System, which gave me all the support during this period.

N Venkatesh Prajna
Academic Director
Aravind Eye Care System
Madurai, Tamil Nadu, India

Preface to the First Edition

This book is intended to be a readable and comprehensive textbook for residents and practicing ophthalmologists. It is also meant to be a current, practical guide to a variety of diagnostic and therapeutic approaches to ophthalmic diseases.

Material is divided into large, well-defined subject areas: To maximize its practicality, the basic chapter style is standardized, containing, when applicable, (1) introduction, (2) basic anatomy and physiology, (3) techniques of examination, and (4) clinical entities with diagnostic procedures and medical and surgical therapies. Theoretical material is added only when it applies specifically to the clinical material under consideration.

Surgical techniques are presented in great detail and are extensively illustrated, so that the reader can easily visualize the recommended approaches. Most chapters are also liberally illustrated with clinical photographs and additional artists' drawings. Color plates are used for further clarity.

Contributors of chapters, while presenting their own approaches, do not neglect others' viewpoints. Alternatives are discussed in detail, or appropriate source material is referenced.

Completion of a project of the size required the cooperation of a great many people. We wish to thank all of the contributors for their time, effort, and patience, not only for composing their chapters initially, but also, in many cases, for revising them to conform to the standards and format of the book. Three talented medical Illustrators—Jean McConnell, Linda Warren, and Leonard Morgan, provided both valuable information and considerable beauty. Special thanks are due our Medical Editors—Maxine Gere and Jane Lantz, who did for the words of this book what our artists did for its illustrations. We appreciate the secretarial assistance of Diann Robinson, who helped bring order out of chaos. Finally, the painstaking efforts and, at times, almost daily cooperation of the WB Saunders Company are gratefully acknowledged.

Gholam A Peyman MD
Donald R Sanders MD
Morton F Goldberg MD

Acknowledgments

I have received tremendous support from all the section editors of this book and the entire Aravind Eye Care System (AECS) in bringing out this book. Without their help and insights, it would not have been possible to bring out a revised edition of this magnitude. I would also like to sincerely acknowledge and thank the disciplinary secretarial help rendered to me by Mrs S Kalyani, from the Department of Medical Education, Aravind Eye Care System, who patiently helped in coordinating with all the authors, section editors and the publishers. I am very grateful for the management of the Aravind Eye Care System for giving me unlimited time and support for making this exercise possible. I would also like to acknowledge the tremendous support of my immediate family for patiently supporting my professional career. My parents Dr P Namperumalsamy and Dr G Natchiar were excellent teachers in their own right and I have learnt a lot from them. My wife, Dr Lalitha and my children Dr Meera Lakshmi and Aravind Krishna have been a source of joy and pride in my professional journey. I do sincerely hope that the book becomes one of the widely used textbooks in ophthalmology globally.

Contents

VOLUME 1

Part 12: Orbit and Oculoplasty

Shannon S Joseph

Part 1 Basic Sciences and Ocular Pathology

■ *N Venkatesh Prajna, Deepak P Edward*

OUTLINE

Chapter 1 Anatomy and Embryology of the Eye

Kay T Khine, David Fleischman

ANATOMY OF THE ORBIT AND OCULAR ADNEXA

ORBITAL ANATOMY

The orbit is pear-shaped and it encloses the globe, extraocular muscles, nerves, fat, and blood vessels. The widest dimension of the orbit is approximately 1 cm posterior to the orbital rim (Table 1.1 and 1.2; and Fig. 1.1).

The orbital walls are perforated by important fissures and foramens (Table 1.3 and Fig. 1.2).

Innervation

The sensory innervation to the periorbital area is provided by the ophthalmic (CN V1) and maxillary (CN V2) divisions of the trigeminal nerve (CN V).

Ophthalmic Division (V1)

Branches can be remembered by mnemonic NFL—National Football League.

Nasociliary nerve enters the orbits through superior orbital fissure within the annulus of Zinn. There are five branches of the nasociliary nerve:

1. *Communicating branch to the ciliary ganglion*: Sensory fibers arise from the eye, exiting through the short ciliary nerves, and at the ciliary ganglion, splitting without synapse, as the sensory root or communicating branch to the nasociliary nerve. These sensory fibers serve the ciliary muscle, iris, and cornea.
2. *Long ciliary nerves*: There are two or three small branches arising from the nasociliary nerve while crossing the optic nerve. They travel alongside the short ciliary nerves and supply sensory information from the ciliary muscle, iris, and cornea.
3. *Posterior ethmoidal nerve*: Supplies ethmoidal and sphenoidal air sinuses.
4. *Infratrochlear nerve*: Terminal branch of the nasociliary nerve. Passes below the trochlea and innervates the skin of the medial aspect of the upper eyelid and the skin of the adjacent, superior aspect of the nose.
5. *Anterior ethmoidal nerve*:
   - Another terminal branch of the nasociliary nerve.
   - Passes through the anterior ethmoidal foramen.
   - Nerve enters the nasal cavity and supplies the nasal mucous membranes in this region.
   - The nerve continues to innervate the skin of the external nose down to the tip.
   - *Hutchinson's sign*: Due to coinnervation of the eye and the nasal skin, herpes zoster lesion on the nose is highly suspicious for ocular involvement.

Table 1.1: Adult orbital dimensions.

Volume	30 cc
Width	40 mm
Height	35 mm
Depth	45 mm
Distance from posterior globe to optic foramen	18 mm
Orbital portion of optic nerve	25–30 mm

Table 1.2: Orbital walls.

Wall	Bones	Additional information
Roof	Lesser wing of sphenoid, frontal	Contains lacrimal gland fossa
Lateral	Greater wing of sphenoid and zygomatic	Strongest orbital wall
Floor	Maxilla, palatine, and zygomatic	Shortest orbital wall
Medial	Lesser wing of sphenoid, maxilla, ethmoid, and lacrimal	Weakest orbital wall; ethmoidal contribution is called *lamina papyracea*; contains lacrimal sac fossa

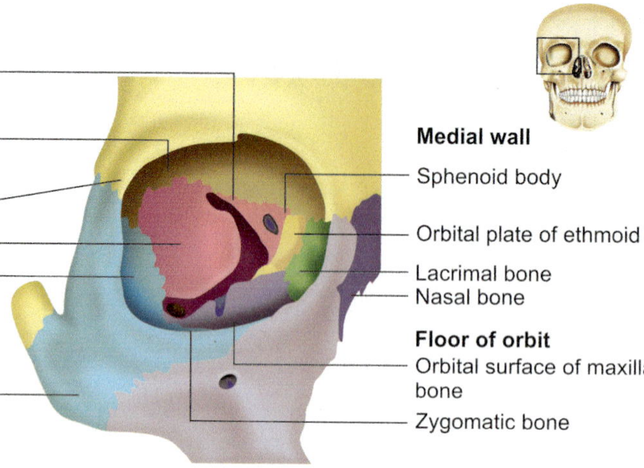

Fig. 1.1: Right orbit viewed along its axis.
Source: Reprinted with permission from Wolff.

Table 1.3: Apertures of orbit.

Name	Location	Transmits
Superior orbital fissure	Separates greater and lesser wings of the sphenoid	CN III, IV, V1, VI, sympathetic nerve fibers
Inferior orbital fissure	Lies between the lateral orbital wall and the orbital floor. Bordered by sphenoid, maxillary, and palatine bones	Infraorbital and zygomatic branches of CNV2, orbital nerve from pterygopalatine ganglion, inferior ophthalmic vein leading to pterygoid plexus and then to cavernous sinus
Optic canal (orbital foramen)	8–10 mm long, within the lesser wing of the sphenoid. Separated from superior orbital fissure by bony optic strut	Optic nerve, ophthalmic artery, and sympathetic nerves
Zygomaticofacial and zygomaticotemporal canals	Lateral orbital wall	Vessels and branches of the zygomatic nerve
Nasolacrimal canal	Extends from the lacrimal sac fossa to the inferior meatus	Nasolacrimal duct
Ethmoidal foramina	Medial orbital wall along the frontoethmoidal suture	Anterior and posterior ethmoid arteries (potential route for spread of infections and neoplasms from sinuses)
Foramen rotundum	Sphenoid bone	CN V2
Foramen ovale	Sphenoid bone, posterolateral to foramen rotundum	CN V3
Foramen lacerum	Triangular crevice between the sphenoid, apex of petrous temporal bone, basilar part of occipital bone	Artery of pterygoid canal (terminal branches of descending pharyngeal artery), nerve of pterygoid canal (greater petrosal nerve, deep petrosal nerve) and venous drainage

(CN: Cranial nerve)

- Frontal nerve enters the orbits above annulus of Zinn and divides into supraorbital nerve and supratrochlear nerve to innervate medial canthus, upper lid, and forehead.
- Lacrimal nerve enters orbits above annulus of Zinn to innervate upper eyelid and lacrimal gland.

Maxillary Division (V2)

It passes through the foramen rotundum and followed by inferior orbital fissure. It branches into the infraorbital nerve, zygomatic nerve, and superior alveolar nerve.

- *Ciliary ganglion*: 1-2 mm in diameter. Located between optic nerve and lateral rectus muscle, about 1.5-2.0 cm behind the globe. Three roots are:
  1. *Sensory roots*: Short ciliary nerves penetrate the sclera and supply the ciliary muscle, iris, and cornea.
  2. Parasympathetic innervation is responsible for accommodation, pupillary constriction, and lacrimal gland stimulation. Parasympathetic fibers arise from Edinger–Westphal nucleus and synapse in the ciliary ganglion via the oculomotor nerve (CN III). The postganglionic parasympathetics leave the

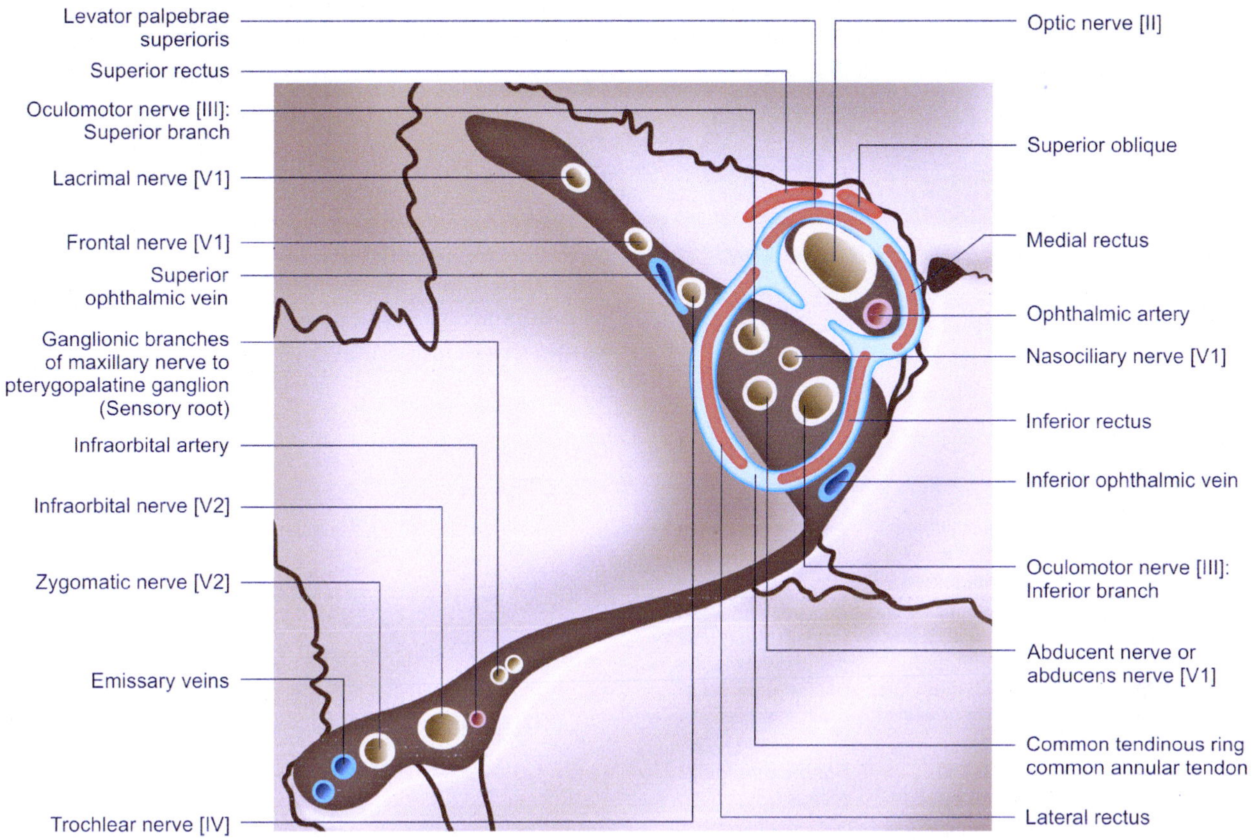

Fig. 1.2: Relationship of annulus of Zinn to structures passing through right superior orbital fissure and optic canal.

ciliary ganglion as short posterior ciliary nerves to supply ciliary body and iris sphincter.

3. Sympathetic innervation controls pupillary dilation, vasoconstriction, smooth muscle function of eyelids and orbit, and hidrosis. The sympathetic fibers arise from the superior cervical ganglion and enter the orbit via long ciliary nerves to the iris dilator and Muller's muscles. It does not synapse in the ciliary ganglion. Damage to any part of the system results in Horner syndrome.

Vasculature of the Orbit

The ophthalmic artery, which is the first branch of the internal carotid artery, is primarily responsible for blood supply to the orbit. Internal maxillary and facial arteries (branches of external carotid artery) also contribute minimally. The ophthalmic artery courses below the optic nerve through the optic canal to enter the orbit. The ophthalmic artery's major branches are—(1) central retinal artery, (2) posterior ciliary arteries (long posterior ciliary arteries supply to the anterior segment and about 20 short posterior ciliary arteries supply to the choroid).

The main venous drainage of the orbit is via the superior ophthalmic vein. It courses through the superior orbital fissure into the cavernous sinus.

Annulus of Zinn

The Annulus of Zinn is a fibrous ring formed by the common origin of the four rectus muscles. It also encircles the optic foramen and the central portion of the superior orbital fissure. Upper and lower divisions of CN III, CN VI, and the nasociliary branch of CN V1 transmit through the ring while the lacrimal and frontal branches of the CN V1, CN IV, and superior ophthalmic vein [mnemonic liver function tests ("LFTs")] travel outside the ring.

Sinuses (Fig. 1.3)

The orbital bones are pneumatized by the paranasal sinuses. The sinuses serve to decrease the weight of the skull and support the nasal passages by trapping irritants, warming, and humidifying the air.

The lateral wall of the nasal cavity has three bony projections called the superior, middle, and inferior turbinates. They overhang the corresponding meatuses. The nasolacrimal duct opens into the inferior meatus (Table 1.4).

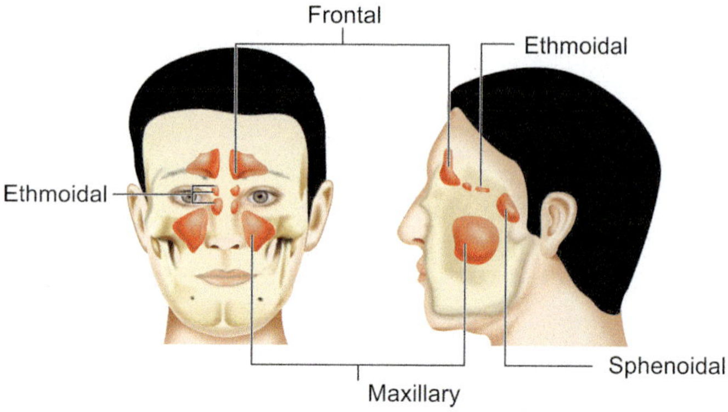

Fig. 1.3: Sinuses in relation to the orbits.

Table 1.4: Sinuses.

Sinus	Information	Drain to...
Frontal	Not visible radiologically until age 6, pneumatization is complete by early adulthood	Anterior portion of the middle meatus
Ethmoid	Lies between the medial orbital wall and the lateral wall of the nose. Presents at birth and expands as the child ages. First sinus to aerate. Often develops orbital cellulitis	Anterior and middle air cells drain into the middle meatus, posterior air cells drain into the superior meatus
Sphenoid	Rudimentary at birth and reaches full size after puberty. Optic canal is located superior and lateral to sphenoid sinus	Sphenoethmoidal recess
Maxillary	Largest sinus, the roofs form the orbital floor, which contains infraorbital nerve and artery	Middle meatus

Extraocular Muscles (Fig. 1.4)

An imaginary circle drawn through four rectus muscle insertions forms the spiral of Tillaux. All the rectus muscles are supplied by two anterior ciliary arteries except for lateral rectus, which is supplied by lacrimal artery. It is important to note that the value implies the tip of the tendinous insertion of the muscle. These values were averages of insertion sites from cadaveric eyes, and therefore these numbers are to serve as reference points and not exact landmarks in individual eyes (Table 1.5).

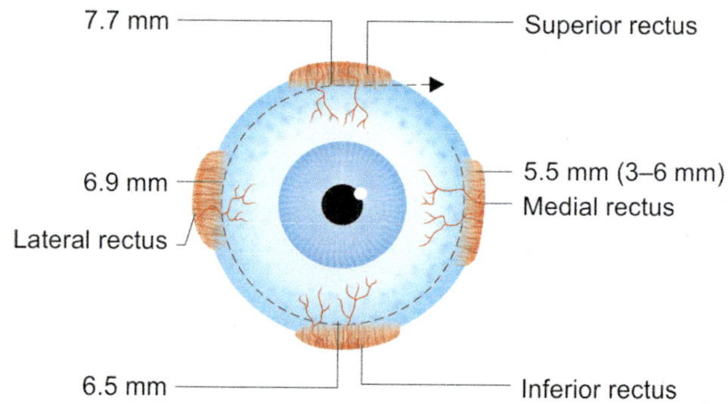

Fig. 1.4: Spiral of Tillaux. The insertions of rectus muscles in relation to limbus.

Table 1.5: Extraocular muscles.

Muscle	Origin	Insertion from limbus	Innervation	Muscle length (mm)	Tendon length (mm)	Primary position action	Note
Medial rectus	Annulus of Zinn	6.5 mm	Inferior division of CN III	40	4.5	Adduction	Most likely to get lost during strabismus surgery due to no fascial attachment
Inferior rectus	Annulus of Zinn	6.5 mm	Inferior division of CN III	40	7	• Depression • Extorsion • Adduction	
Lateral rectus	Annulus of Zinn	6.9 mm	CN VI	40	7	Abduction	
Superior rectus	Annulus of Zinn	7.7 mm	Superior division of CN III	40	6	• Elevation • Intorsion • Adduction	
Superior Oblique	Orbital apex (annulus of Zinn)	Superior temporal quadrant	CN IV	32	26	• Intorsion • Depression • Abduction	Has shortest muscle length but with longest tendon
Inferior oblique	Periosteum of maxillary bone, behind lacrimal fossa	Inferior temporal quadrant	Inferior division of CN III	37	1	• Extorsion • Elevation • Abduction	Shortest tendon
Levator palpebrae	Lesser wing of sphenoid	Tarsus	Superior division of CN 3	40	14–20 mm (aponeurotic portion)	Elevate the eyelid	Divides lacrimal gland into orbital and palpebral lobes

(CN: Cranial nerve)

EYELIDS

Palpebral fissure in adult is 27–30 mm long and 8–11 mm wide (Fig. 1.5).

Anterior and posterior lamellae are separated by the orbital septum:

- *Anterior*: Skin and orbicularis oculi
- *Posterior*: Palpebrae superioris muscle, Muller muscle, tarsus, and conjunctiva.

Eyelid Margin

The margin contains the punctum of the canaliculus medially. The superior punctum is located more medially compared to the lower punctum. The gray line (muscle of Riolan—the most superficial portion of the orbicularis oculi muscle) overlies the entire margin. Anterior to the gray line are the eyelashes and behind the lines are the openings of the tarsal (or meibomian) glands.

Orbicularis Oculi

Orbicularis oculi serves as the protractor of the eyelid. It is innervated by CN VII. The palpebral portion (pretarsal and preseptal) is responsible for involuntary and voluntary blinking. The orbital portion is responsible for voluntary lid closure.

Orbital Septum

Orbital septum is a sheet of connective tissue that provides a barrier between the orbit and eyelid, and is important in limiting the spread of infection. It originates from the periosteum of the superior and inferior orbital rims and inserts into levator aponeurosis and into lower eyelid retractors inferiorly. In Asians, the orbital septum fuses with levator aponeurosis between the eyelid margin and the superior border of the tarsus while in non-Asians, it inserts 2–5 mm above superior tarsal border into the levator aponeurosis.

Muller Muscle (Superior Tarsal Muscle)

The muscle is located posterior to levator aponeurosis. It is about 12–15 mm long and raises the eyelid 2 mm under sympathetic innervation. It originates from underneath levator at the level of Whitnall's ligament and inserts into upper border of tarsus. The 2 mm ptosis associated with Horner's syndrome is due to the denervation of Muller's muscle.

Tarsus

Tarsus is a dense-connective tissue plate in each eyelid that contains meibomian glands. The length is 29 mm long and 1 mm thick. The superior tarsal plate is 10 mm in height while the inferior tarsal plate is 4 mm in height.

Whitnall's Ligament (Superior Transverse Ligament)

This is a condensation of the levator muscle sheath. It functions to change direction of levator muscle and acts to prevent excessive lid elevation.

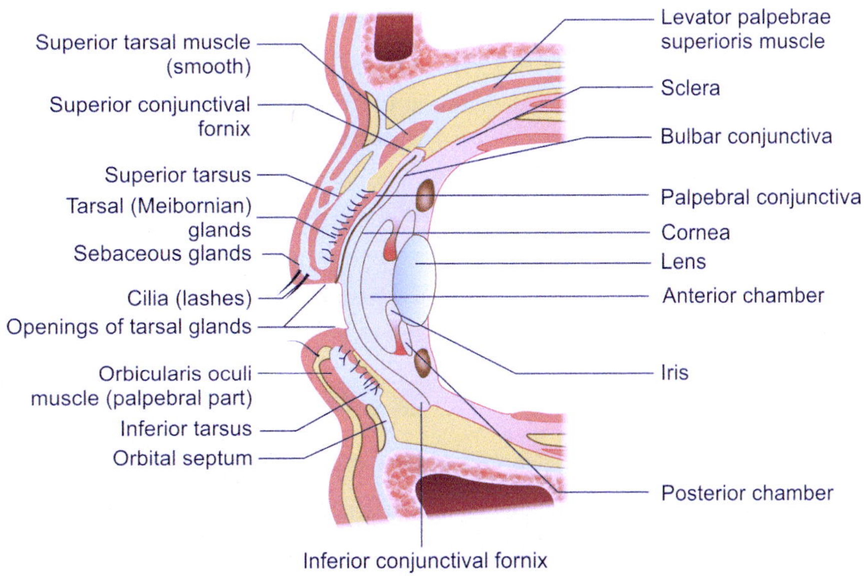

Fig. 1.5: Cross-section of upper and lower eyelids.

Lower Eyelid Retractors

Capsulopalpebral Fascia

It is analogous to levator aponeurosis. It originates from inferior rectus muscle sheath and inserts into inferior tarsus.

Lockwood's Suspensory Ligament

It is analogous to Whitnall's ligament. It originates from inferior rectus muscle and continues as capsulopalpebral fascia.

Inferior Tarsal Muscle

It is analogous to Muller's muscle and receives sympathetic innervation.

Innervation to Eyelid

- *Motor*: CN 3 (superior division), CN 7, and sympathetics
- *Sensory*: CN V1 (upper lid) and CN V2 (lower lid).

Lymphatic Drainage

It is classically believed that there are no lymphatic vessels or nodes within the orbit, although lymphatic capillaries have been well described in the meninges of the human optic nerve. Submandibular nodes drain medial one-third of upper lid and medial two-thirds of lower lid. Preauricular nodes drain lateral two-thirds of upper lid and lateral one-third of lower lid.

Glands of the Eye and Adnexa (Table 1.6)

Table 1.6: Glands of the eyelids.

Gland	Location	Secretion type	Content
Lacrimal (orbital and palpebral lobes separated by levator aponeurosis)	Superotemporal orbit	Exocrine	Aqueous
Accessory lacrimal: • Krause • Wolfring	• Fornix • Above tarsus	Exocrine	Aqueous
Meibomian	Tarsus	Holocrine	Lipid
Zeis	Lash follicles, eyelid, caruncle	Holocrine	Lipid
Moll	Eyelid	Apocrine	Sweat
Goblet cell	Conjunctiva, plica, caruncle	Holocrine	Mucus

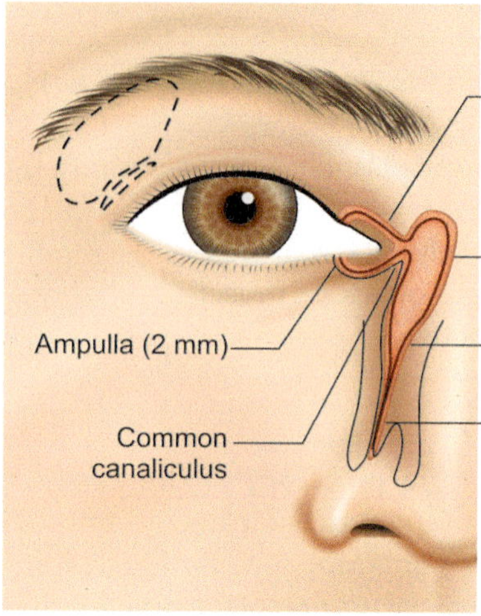

Fig. 1.6: The nasal lacrimal drainage system.

Lacrimal Excretory System (Fig. 1.6)

Puncta

Upper sits 6.0 mm from medial canthus, lower sits 6.5 mm from the medial canthus. These open into ampulla, which are 2 mm long and are oriented perpendicular to the eyelid margin.

Canaliculi

These are 10 mm long total (2 mm of ampulla and 8 mm horizontal portion), upper and lower canaliculi come together to form the common canaliculus in 90% of individual. Valve of Rosenmuller prevents reflux from lacrimal sac into canaliculi.

Nasolacrimal Sac

It is 10 mm long and occupies the lacrimal fossa between anterior and posterior crura of the medial canthal tendon.

Nasolacrimal Duct

It is 15 mm long and extends into inferior meatus, which is partially covered by valve of Hasner. It passes inferiorly, posteriorly, and laterally.

EYE

Topographic Features of the Globe (Fig. 1.7)

The globe is not a true sphere; the radius of curvature of the cornea is smaller than the radius of curvature of the

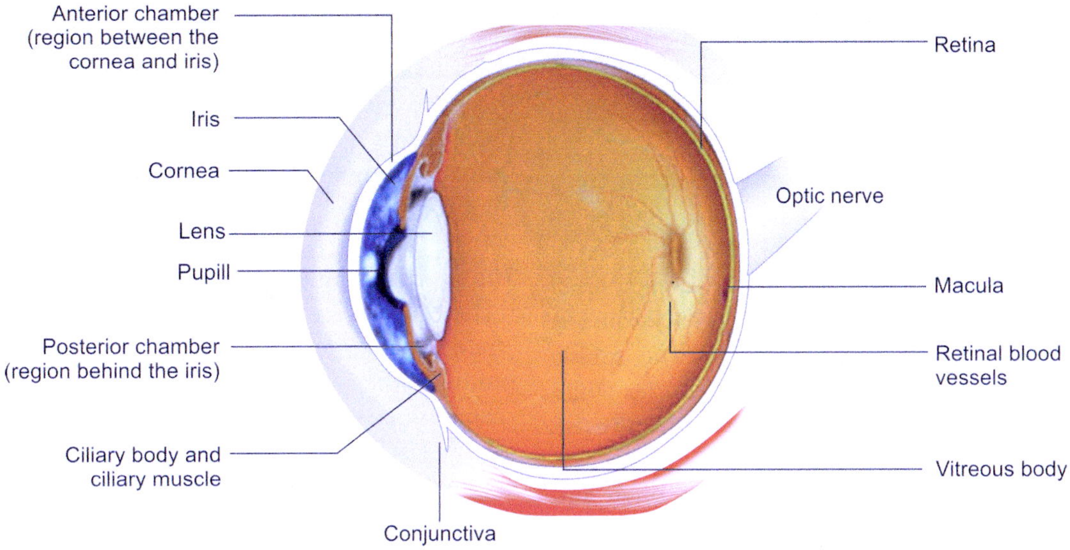

Fig. 1.7: Overview of the eye.

sclera. The anteroposterior diameter of the adult eye is approximately 23–25 mm. The average transverse diameter of the adult eye is 24 mm.

The eye contains three compartments: (1) the anterior chamber, (2) the posterior chamber, and (3) the vitreous cavity. The anterior chamber is 3 mm deep and has an average aqueous volume of 200 µL. It is the space between cornea and iris. The posterior chamber is filled with aqueous humor and has average volume of 60 µL. It is the space posterior to the iris and anterior to the vitreous. The vitreous cavity is the largest with volume of 5–6 mL, containing vitreous humor.

Cornea

The cornea becomes flatter in the periphery; flattening is more prominent nasally and superiorly than temporally and inferiorly (Table 1.7).

Table 1.7: Dimensions of cornea.

Power	Anterior surface = +49 D, posterior surface = −6 D, total = 43 D (75% of total power of eye)
Refractive index	1.36
Radius of curvature	7.8 mm anteriorly; 6.2–6.8 mm posteriorly
Thickness	Central = 550 µm, periphery = 1.0 mm
Diameter	At birth, horizontal diameter = 9.5–10.5 mm, reaches adult size by age 2. Vertical = 11.5 mm, horizontal = 12.5 mm

Layers of Cornea (Fig. 1.8)

- *Epithelium* is about 50 µm thick (5% of total corneal thickness) and is covered by nonkeratinized and stratified squamous epithelium. It has hydrophobic smooth surface and uses aerobic metabolism. Limbal stem cells regenerate with turn over time of 6–7 days. Cells are linked together by desmosomes tightly to form protective barrier and are anchored to basal lamina by hemidesmosomes.
- *Bowman layer* or membrane is 8–12 µm thick. It is not a true membrane and does not regenerate. It contains type I collagen.

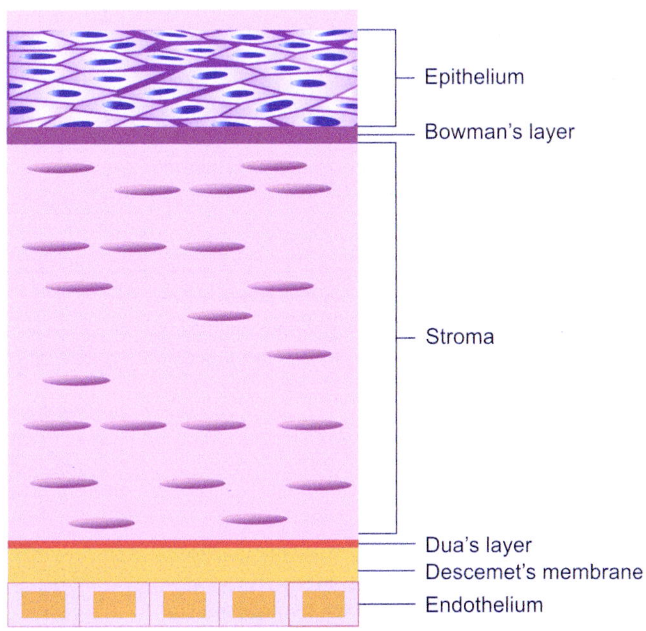

Fig. 1.8: Layers of cornea.

- *Stroma* is about 480 μm thick and constitutes 90% of total corneal thickness. It contains type I, III, V, and VI collagens. Collagen fibrils are carefully oriented to keep transparency of the cornea. Separation of the collagen fibrils by fluid results in stromal clouding.
- *Dua's layer* was reported in the literature in 2013 as a layer composed of type I collagen, measured to be 10 μm thick. The existence of this layer is controversial. It may have implication during corneal transplant. Small air bubbles can be injected into the corneal stroma in the "big-bubble technique". Occasionally, the bubble bursts. But, if the air bubble is injected under Dua's layer rather than above it, the layer can reduce the risk of tearing.
- *Descemet's membrane* is 3–4 μm thick at birth and increases to 10–12 μm at adulthood. It is a true basement membrane. Histologically, it is periodic acid–Schiff (PAS) positive. It contains type IV collagen like other basement membrane. It contains an anterior-banded layer, which develops in utero and a posterior nonbanded layer, which thickness increases with aging. It can regenerate as long as endothelium is intact.
- *Endothelium layer* is 4–6 μm thick and contains a single layer of hexagonal cells from neural crest. It functions to transport nutrients into cornea and to pump fluid out of cornea. At birth, there are approximately 3,800 endothelium cells/mm^2. Average corneal endothelium in adult is around 2,400 cells/mm^2. As loss of cells occurs with aging, there is no regeneration. Cells stretch to fill gaps.

Sclera

The scleral covers the posterior four-fifths of the surface of the globe with opening anteriorly for cornea and opening posteriorly for the optic nerve. The Tenon's capsule and bulbar conjunctiva cover the scleral anteriorly and fuse near the limbus. The scleral stroma contains bundles of collagen (mostly type I), fibroblasts, and ground substance. The sclera is thinnest (0.3 mm) behind the insertion of the rectus muscles and thickest (1.0 mm) near the optic nerve. The most common site of scleral rupture following blunt trauma is the superonasal quadrant near the limbus. The scleral is mostly avascular but contains superficial vessels of the episclera and intrascleral vascular plexus. Emissary channels penetrate the sclera to allow for the passage of the arteries, veins, and nerves. These perforations are also potential sites for extraocular extension in cases of malignant choroidal melanoma.

Innervation

The branches of ciliary nerve forms nerve loops called Axenfeld loops. These are appreciated as pigmented spots on slit-lamp examination.

Limbus

Limbus is the transition zone between the peripheral cornea and the sclera (Fig. 1.9). It is about 1–1.5 mm wide and is defined in multiple ways:

- *Anatomists*: Termination of Descemet's membrane and Bowman layer

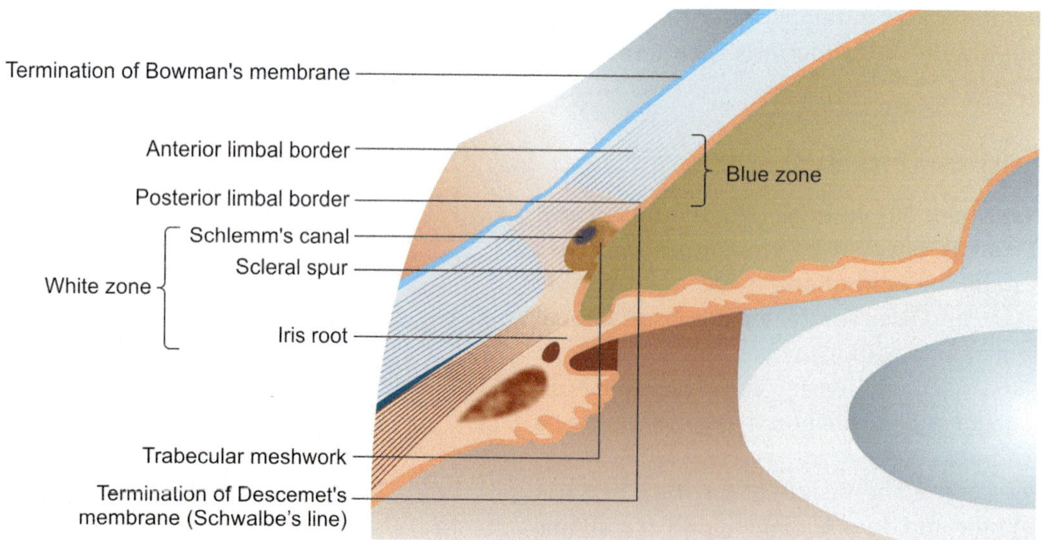

Fig. 1.9: Anterior chamber angle and its relationship to limbus.

- *Pathologists*: Anterior limbus is similar to anatomist's definition, posterior limbus is the line between iris root and Schlemm's canal.
- *Surgeons*: Surgical limbus is composed of: (1) anterior bluish-gray zone overlying the clear cornea, which extends from the Bowman layer to the Schwalbe line, and (2) a posterior white zone, which overlies the trabecular meshwork and extends from Schwalbe line to the scleral spur or iris root.

Conjunctiva

Conjunctiva is composed of stratified columnar epithelium with goblet cells. Palpebral conjunctiva covers the lid's inner surface and attached to tarsus and bulbar conjunctiva covers the scleral and fuses with Tenon's capsule at the limbus. Anterior ciliary arteries supply blood to the bulbar conjunctiva, while branches of the marginal arcades of the lids supply blood to the palpebral conjunctiva. The innervation is derived from CN V1. The conjunctiva also contains lymphatic vessels, plasma cells, macrophages, and mast cells.

Plica semilunaris is a narrow fold of medial bulbar conjunctiva and lateral to caruncle. It is a vestigial structure analogous to nictitating membrane or third eyelid of dogs and other animals. It contains goblet cells. Caruncle is at medial canthus and is located inferomedial to the plica semilunaris. It contains accessory dermal appendages and sebaceous glands. The surface is covered by nonkeratinized and stratified squamous epithelium.

Tenon Capsule

Tenon capsule forms a cavity, which the globe moves and is composed of collagen fibers and fibroblasts. It fuses posteriorly with the optic nerve sheath and anteriorly with a thin layer of tissue called intermuscular septum, which is located 3 mm posterior to the limbus.

Anterior Chamber

The anterior chamber angle lies between the junction of the cornea and the iris and consists of the following structures from anterior to posterior:

- Schwalbe's line (termination of Descemet's membrane)
- Schlemm's canal and trabecular meshwork
- Scleral spur (white band at which longitudinal fibers of ciliary muscle insert to sclera)
- Anterior border of the ciliary body
- Iris.

The chamber is approximately 3-mm deep centrally. It is deeper in aphakic, pseudophakic, and myopic eyes, while it is shallower in hyperopic eyes. An anterior chamber less than 2.5 mm is suspicious for angle closure. The volume of the anterior chamber is approximately 200 μL and is filled with aqueous humor from ciliary processes in the posterior chamber. The fluid passes through the pupil aperture and drains mainly through the conventional pathway via the trabecular meshwork. Then the outflow path continues to drain through Schlemm's canal, collector channels, aqueous veins, episcleral venous plexus, anterior ciliary, and superior ophthalmic veins, and finally to cavernous sinus. 15–50% of drainage outflow is via nontraditional pathway called uveoscleral drainage, although it may be higher in younger individuals. Aqueous goes to ciliary body and enters the suprachoroidal space and is drained by veins in the ciliary body, choroid, and sclera, or penetrates the sclera.

- *Trabecular meshwork*: Circular connective tissue lined by trabeculocytes. It can be divided into three layers. The pore size decreases toward Schlemm's canal.
  1. *Uveal meshwork*: Linked to ciliary muscle; pore size can be up to 70 μm.
  2. *Corneoscleral meshwork*: Connective tissue sheets inserted into scleral spur; pore size up to 30 μm.
  3. *Juxtacanalicular meshwork*: Connected to Schlemm's endothelium; site of the most aqueous outflow resistance.
- *Schlemm's canal*: Formed by monolayer of nonfenestrated endothelium and a thin connective tissue wall. Elevated episcleral venous pressure or pressure from a Goldmann three-mirror gonioscopy lens may cause blood to reflux, making Schlemm's canal visible as a faint red band.
- *Collector channels*: Approximately 25–30 collector channels arises from the Schlemm's canal and drain into the deep and episcleral venous plexus.

Uveal Tract

- Three parts are—(1) iris, (2) ciliary body, and (3) choroid
- Three sites of firm attachment to the sclera are at: (1) scleral spur, (2) vortex veins, and (3) optic nerve.

Iris

Iris is made of blood vessels and connective tissue. Iris stroma is composed of pigmented cells and nonpigmented cells. Melanocytes and pigment cells are responsible for its distinctive color. The amount of pigmentation in the anterior border layer and the deep stroma determine the differences in iris color. Blood vessels of the iris stroma follow a radial course. Myelinated and nonmyelinated nerve fibers serve as sensory, vasomotor, and muscular functions of the iris stroma. The posterior pigmented layer of iris is continuous with the nonpigmented epithelium of the ciliary body and with the neurosensory portion of the retina. It curves around the pupillary margin and extends for a short distance onto the anterior border layer of the iris stroma as the pigmented ruff. The dilator muscle lies parallel and anterior to the posterior pigmented layer. It has dual sympathetic (alpha-1 adrenergic) and parasympathetic innervation (cholinergic). The sphincter muscle is located near the pupillary margin in the deep stroma. Its primary innervation is via parasympathetic nerve fibers from CN III, which causes sphincter contraction.

Ciliary Body

The apex is directed toward ora serrata and the base gives rise to the iris. The ciliary body is 6–7 mm wide and consists of the pars plana and the pars plicata. The pars plana is an avascular, smooth, pigmented zone, and serves as the safest posterior surgical approach to the vitreous cavity through the pars plana or for intraocular injections. It is located 3–4 mm from the limbus in most eyes, but may be different in short or long eyes. The pars plicata is highly vascularized and contains ciliary processes.

The ciliary body is lined by the inner—nonpigmented epithelium and the outer—pigmented epithelium. The apices of the nonpigmented and pigmented layers are fused by tight junction to create the blood-aqueous barrier. The nonpigmented epithelium faces the posterior chamber while the pigmented epithelium faces the iris stroma. The major arterial supply to the ciliary body is from anterior and long posterior ciliary arteries, which ultimately drain into the vortex system.

- *Function*: (1) aqueous formation and (2) lens accommodation
- *Ciliary muscle*: (1) longitudinal, (2) radial, and (3) circular. Most of the ciliary muscle is the outer layer of longitudinal fibers, which attach to the scleral spur. The radial muscle is in the midportion while the circular fibers are located in the innermost portion. The contraction of the longitudinal muscle results in increase aqueous outflow by pulling the scleral spur and opening up the spaces of the meshwork. Radial and circular muscles are also involved in accommodation. Contraction of the longitudinal muscle pulls the lens forward and is shallowing the anterior chambers. Contraction of the circular fibers relaxes the zonules making the lens more spherical and increases its dioptric power while relaxation of the circular fibers tightens the zonules, trenching the lens and making it thinner, and decreasing its dioptric power.

Choroid (Fig. 1.10)

- Thickness—0.25 mm
- Three layers of vessels—(1) the choriocapillaris—the innermost layer, (2) middle layer of small-medium vessels (Sattler's layer), and (3) outer layer of large vessels (Haller's layer)

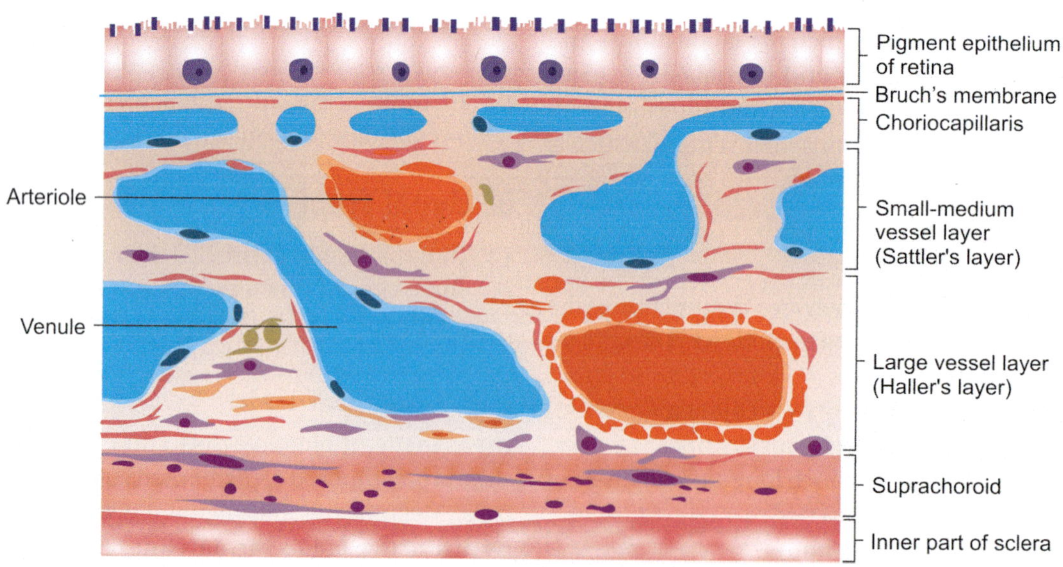

Fig. 1.10: Layers of choroid.

- *Perfusion*: Long and short posterior ciliary arteries and from perforating anterior ciliary arteries. Venous drainage is via vortex vein.
- Bruch's membrane is a PAS—positive basal lamina of retinal pigment epithelium (RPE) and choriocapillaris. It has five elements—(1) basal lamina of the RPE, (2) inner collagenous zone, (3) thicker and porous band of elastic fibers, (4) outer collagenous zone, and (5) basal lamina of the choriocapillaris.
- Choriocapillaris is a continuous layer of large capillaries lying below the RPE.

Lens (Fig. 1.11)

Lens has biconvex structure and is avascular. It lacks innervation and depends solely on the aqueous and vitreous for nourishment. The lens largely relies on anaerobic metabolism (Table 1.8).

Accommodation

At age of 8—accommodation power is 14.00 D, by age of 28 years—power decreases to 9 D, and it further decreases to 1.00 D by age of 64 years. Development of presbyopia is due to increased size of the lens, stiffness of the lens, and alterations in the zonular attachments with age.

Table 1.8: Dimensions of lens.

Refractive power	20.00 D in average adult eye
Adult equatorial diameter	9–10 mm, anteroposterior width –3 mm at birth and increases to 6 mm by age 80

Capsule Layer

Capsule layer composed of type IV collagen. Anterior lens capsule thickness increases throughout life whereas the posterior capsule remains stable with value of 2.8 µm. Average anterior capsule thickness is 15.5 µm.

Epithelium Layer

It lies below the anterior capsule and is absent under posterior capsule. In the periphery, there are rows of cuboidal pre-equatorial cells that form the germinative zone of the lens. There, cells divide, elongate, and differentiate into lens fibers; they lose their nuclei and most organelles.

Sutures

These are formed by the interdigitation of the anterior and posterior tips of the fibers. The Y suture is upright anteriorly and inverted posteriorly.

Zonules Hold Lens in Place

They originate from basal laminae of the nonpigmented epithelium of the pars plana and pars plicata of the ciliary body. In Marfan's syndrome, mutations in the fibrillin gene lead to weakening of the zonule and subluxation of the lens (Fig. 1.12).

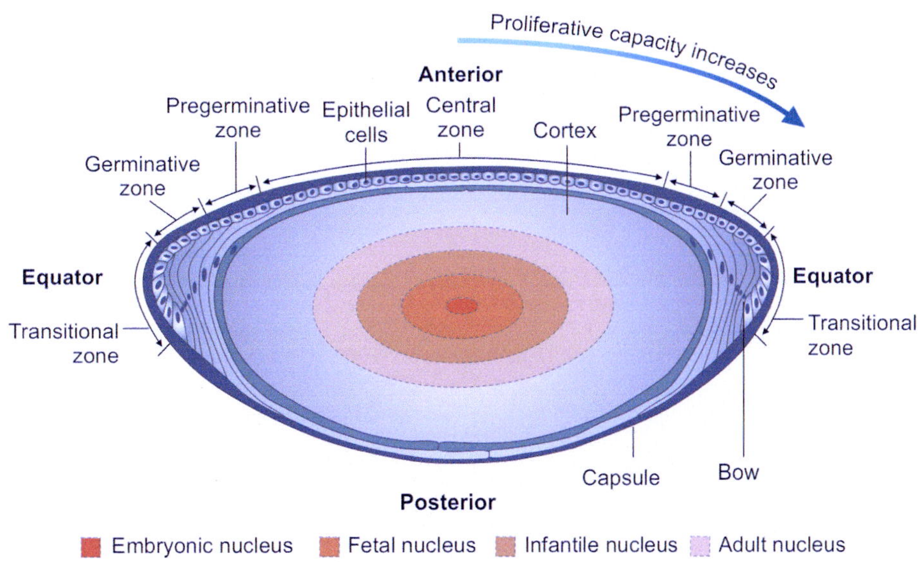

Fig. 1.11: Overview of the lens and its layer.

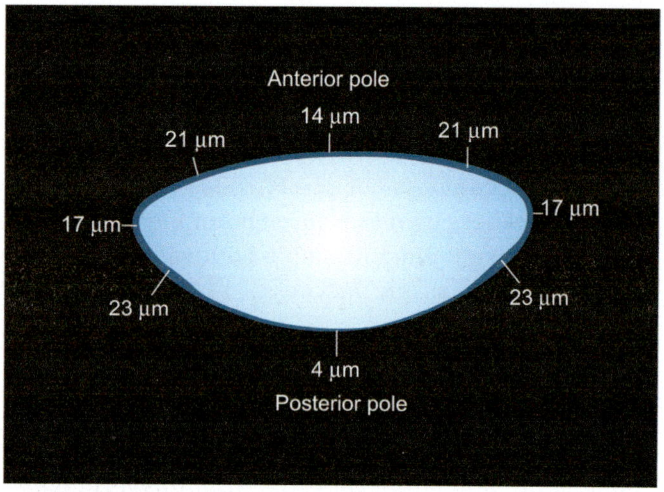

Fig. 1.12: Thickness of the lens capsule at different spot.

Retina

There are 10 layers of the neurosensory retina (from anterior to posterior retina) (Fig. 1.13).

1. Internal limiting membrane (ILM)
2. Nerve fiber layer (NFL)
3. Ganglion cell layer (GCL)
4. Inner plexiform layer (IPL)
5. Inner nuclear layer (INL)
6. Middle limiting membrane
7. Outer plexiform layer (OPL)
8. Outer nuclear layer (ONL)
9. External limiting membrane (ELM)
10. Rod and cone inner and outer segments (photoreceptor layer).

Retinal pigment epithelium is a monolayer of hexagonal cells that merges with the pigmented epithelium of the ciliary body, extending from the optic disk to the ora serrata. RPE serves functions in vitamin A metabolism, maintenance of the outer blood–retina barrier, phagocytosis of the photoreceptor outer segments, absorption of light, heat exchange, formation of the basal lamina of Bruch's membrane, production of the mucopolysaccharide matrix, and active transport of materials into and out of the neurosensory retina and RPE. Separation of the RPE from the neurosensory retina is a retinal detachment. RPE cells in the fovea are taller, thinner, contain more melanosomes, and have larger melanosomes. RPE cells in the periphery are shorter, broader, and less pigmented.

Photoreceptors

11-cis retinal is converted to all-trans retinol in photoreceptor layer outer segments and then is reverted back in RPE.

- *Rods*: 120 million (accounts for 95% of photoreceptors); maximally dense 20–40° around fovea; rods are 1,000 times more sensitive than cones in the dark. Rod disks are not attached to cell membrane. They provide vision in the dark.
- *Cones*: 6 million; maximally dense at fovea. There are three types of pigments (blue, green, and red). Cone disks are attached to cell membrane and undergo replacement. They provide color vision and high-quality acuity.

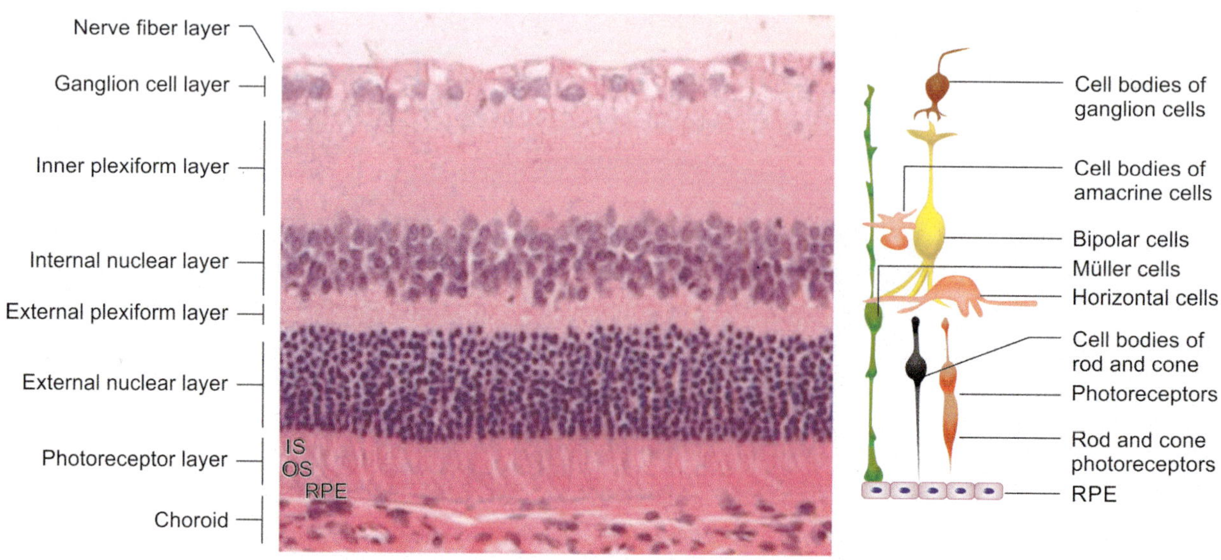

Fig. 1.13: Layers of retina.

Glial Elements

Muller cells are glial cells, which extend vertically from ELM to ILM. The nuclei are located in the INL. Muller cells, astrocytes, and microglia provide structural support and nutrition to the retina.

- *Vascular*: Inner two-thirds of retina is perfused by branches of the central retinal artery, while outer one-third of the retina is perfused by choroid. In 18–32% of eyes, cilioretinal artery from ciliary circulation also supplies the macula.
- ELM is not a true membrane, and formed by attachment sites of adjacent photoreceptors and Muller cells.
- ONL contains photoreceptor cell bodies and nuclei
- OPL contains horizontal and bipolar cells. In the macular region, OPL is thicker and contains more fibers and is known as Henle fiber layer.
- INL contains nuclei of bipolar, Muller, horizontal, and amacrine cells.
- IPL contains axons of the bipolar and amacrine cells and dendrites of the ganglion cells and their synapses.
- GCL consists of cell bodies of ganglion cells
- NFL is made up of axons of ganglion cells
- ILM is true membrane because it contains PAS-positive basement membrane. Formed by the footplates of the Muller cells.

Macula

Macula is histologically defined as an area of retina where there are more than 1 layer of ganglion nuclei. It is located 4 mm temporal and 0.8 mm inferior to optic nerve. The yellow color of central retina is due to presence of carotenoid pigments in the Henle fiber layers. Two major pigments are zeaxanthin and lutein with lutein being more concentrated in rod-dense areas and zeaxanthin being more concentrated in cone-dense areas.

- *Dimension*: 5–6 mm in diameter.
- *Histology*: Region with more than 1 layer of ganglion nuclei.
- *Fovea*: 1.5 mm in diameter within macula, concave central retinal depression. It consists of taller RPE cells and xanthophyll pigment, which block choroidal fluorescence during fluorescein angiography. Fovea is devoid of accessory neural elements.
- *Foveola*: Central area of fovea (350 μm in diameter). Only photoreceptor, Muller cells, and other glial cells are present in this area. Foveal avascular zone (FAZ) location is the same as fovea where it is devoid of capillaries. The diameter varies from 250 μm to 600 μm.

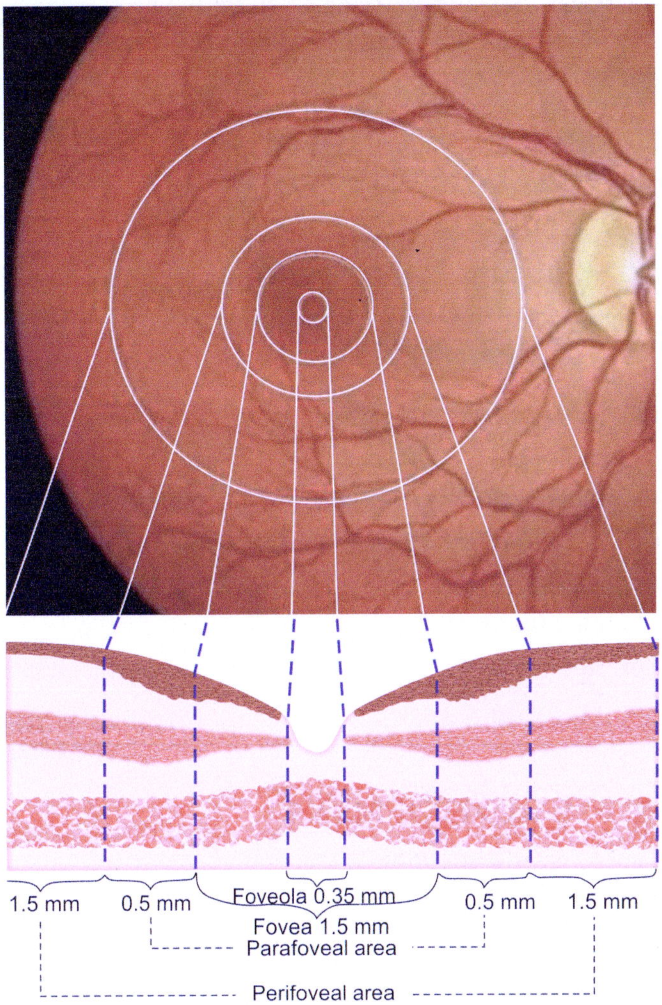

Fig. 1.14: Overview of macula.

The photoreceptor layer of foveola is only composed of cones.

- *Parafovea*: It is 0.5 mm wide around the fovea where GCL, INL, and OPL are thickest.
- *Perifoveal*: 1.5 mm wide on each side and adjacent to parafovea (Fig. 1.14).

Ora Serrata

It is a watershed zone between the anterior and posterior vascular systems and is located between the retina and the pars plana. The peripheral retina in the region is commonly attenuated.

Vitreous

The vitreous cavity is the four-fifths of the volume of the globe with volume around 4.0 mL. It provides a route for metabolites used by the lens, ciliary body, and retina.

- *Composition*: 99% water, and viscosity is due to presence of mucopolysaccharide hyaluronic acid. It contains type II collagen.
- *Degeneration*: The vitreous adheres strongly to the vitreous base in the periphery, which extends from 2.0 mm anterior to and 4.0 mm posterior to the ora serrata. It also has firm attachment to disk margin, perimacular region, along retinal vessels, and to the periphery of the posterior lens capsule. The vitreous liquefies with age and separates from the inner retina causing posterior vitreous detachment.

Optic Nerve

Optic nerve consists of 1.2 million nerve fibers. It is the same size as fovea with 1.5 mm in diameter and enlarges to 3.5 mm posterior to lamina cribrosa once myelination is acquired. The optic nerve insertion area appears as blind spot 15° temporal to fixation and slightly below horizontal meridian on the visual field. Three layers of meninges surrounding the optic nerve are outer layer of dura mater, middle layer of arachnoid, and inner layer of pia mater. Cerebrospinal fluid (CSF) flows between arachnoid and pia mater (Table 1.9).

Table 1.9: Blood supply to the optic nerve.

Location	Length (mm)	Blood supply
Intraocular	1	• NFL: Central retinal artery (CRA) • Prelaminar: Short posterior ciliary artery (SPCA), recurrent choroidal arteries • Laminar—SPCAs, branches of circle of Zinn–Haller • Retrolaminar—SPCAs and pia vessels
Intraorbital	25	• Distally/anteriorly—branches of CRA/pials and branches of ophthalmic artery • Proximally/posteriorly—pials and branches of ophthalmic artery
Intracanalicular	9	• Ophthalmic artery
Intracranial	10–15	• Ophthalmic artery and internal carotid artery

(NFL: Nerve fiber layer; SPCA: Short posterior ciliary arteries)

EMBRYOLOGY

EYE DEVELOPMENT

During the process of gastrulation, three germ layers form in human embryos:

1. Ectoderm (superficial layer)
2. Mesoderm (middle layer)
3. Endoderm (inner layer).

Following gastrulation, ectoderm is further divided into surface and neural ectoderm. Neural crest cells arise from neural ectoderm from the edge of the neural tube during neurulation. Neural crest cells are migratory stem cells that can form tissues with ectodermal and mesodermal characteristics. The globe and orbital tissues develop from ectoderm, mesoderm, and neural crest cells. Neural crest cells contribute the most to globe formation (Fig. 1.15; and Tables 1.10 and 1.11).

Development of Human Optic Cup (Fig. 1.16)

Summary: Neural plate → optic pits (day 23 of gestation) → optic vesicles (day 25) → optic cup → closing of embryonic fissure (day 33).

Optic pit has outpouching to form optic vesicles. Optic vesicle induces the lens placode at day 27, which is small surface ectoderm thickening on both sides of the developing head. The optic vesicle connects to the developing forebrain. When the optic vesicle touches the inner aspect of the surface ectoderm, the vesicle invaginates to form a bilayered optic cup. Inner layer becomes the

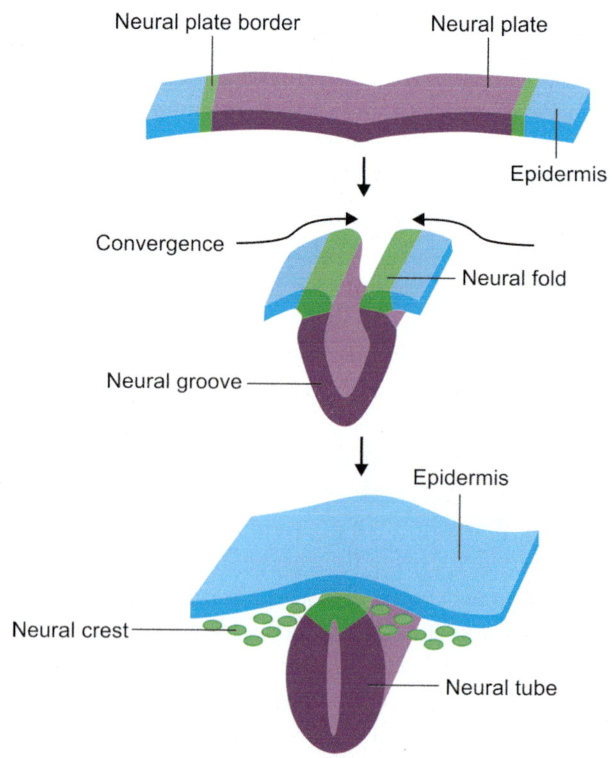

Fig. 1.15: Overview of neural crest migration.

Table 1.10: Derivatives of embryonic tissues.

	Ectoderm
Surface ectoderm	• Corneal epithelium layer • Conjunctival epithelium • Caruncle • Lacrimal drainage system • Lacrimal gland (also from neural crest) • Lens • Epithelium • Glands • Cilia of skin of eyelids
Neuroectoderm	*Retina*: • Sensory retina • Pigmented epithelium • Vitreous (also mesoderm) *Ciliary body*: • Inner nonpigmented layer • Outer pigmented layer • Optic nerve, axons, and glia *Iris*: • Sphincter • Dilator muscles
Neural creast	• Bones • Cartilage • Choroidal stroma • Ciliary ganglion • Ciliary body: – Stroma – Ciliary musculature • Connective tissue of orbit • *Corneal*: – Stroma – Endothelium • *Extraocular muscle*: – Sheaths – Tendons – Fat (also mesoderm) • Iris pigment epithelium • Melanocytes • Meningeal sheaths of optic nerve • Scleral (also mesoderm) • Trabecular meshwork • Vasculature, muscle and connective tissues sheaths of ocular and orbital vessels
	Mesoderm
	• Vascular endothelium • Vitreous (also neuroectoderm) • Temporal portion of scleral (also neural crest) • Extraocular muscles (also neural crest) • Remainder of eyelids (orbicularis oculi muscle, tarsus, orbital septum, etc.) • Schlemm's canal

inner neurosensory retinal layer; the outer layer becomes the RPE, which is continuous with the posterior pigment epithelium of the iris. The space between the two layers remains a potential space for subretinal fluid and retinal detachment.

Later on, the surface ectoderm begins to invaginate to form the lens. Meanwhile, mesoderm and neural crest cells fill up the space between the cup and the surface ectoderm to form much of the anterior segment of the eye. The fissure closes centrally, followed by anteriorly and posteriorly at day 33. Failure of embryonic fissure closure leads to coloboma. Most of the colobomas are found in inferonasal quadrant. Anterior colobomas are the most common followed by posterior colobomas and central colobomas.

Lids and Lacrimal Apparatus

The upper eyelid development begins around 4–5 weeks of gestation from surface ectoderm of the outer canthus, followed by development of lower lid. At 8 weeks, upper eyelid develops from fusion of medial and lateral frontonasal processes, while lower lid develops from fusion of maxillary processes and medial nasal processes. Around 10–12 weeks, eyelid fold fuses and orbicularis muscle migrates into the fold. At 20–24 weeks, separation of the eyelid begins nasally. This is also when secretion begins from sebaceous glands.

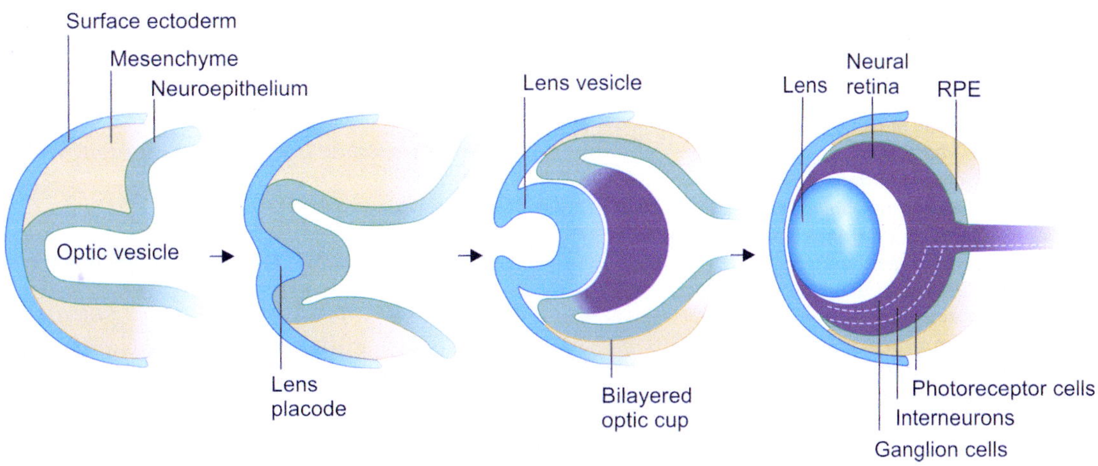

Fig. 1.16: Overview of formation of optic cup.
(RPE: Retinal pigment epithelium)

Table 1.11: Chronology of embryonic and fetal development of the eye.

Period after conception	Event
22nd day	Optic groove appears
23rd day	Optic pits form
25th day	Optic vesicle forms
27–28th day	Formation of lens placode
28th day	• Embryonic fissure forms • Pigment appears in RPE
33rd day	Closure of embryonic fissure
2nd month	• Hyaloid vessels develop • The beginning of lateral rectus and superior oblique muscles appears • Primary and secondary vitreous develop • Eyelid folds and nasolacrimal duct appear • Bone structures of the orbit begin to develop • Formation of primary lens fibers • Ciliary ganglion appears • Differentiation of RPE and proliferation of neural retinal cells • Corneal epithelial cells forms interconnections and neural crest cells of corneal endothelium migrate centrally • Choroid vessels develop • Migration of ganglion cells toward optic nerve • Formation of embryonic lens nucleus and tunica vasculosa lentis • Formation of sclera • Axons of ganglion cells migrate toward optic nerve • Laminal cribrosa forms • Bruch membrane appears • Three waves of neural crest migration: • *1st wave*: Formation of corneal endothelium and trabecular meshwork endothelium • *2nd wave*: Formation of iris stroma and pupillary membrane • *3rd wave*: Formation of corneal stroma and scleral
3rd month	• Precursors of rods and cones differentiate • Ciliary body develops • Sclera condenses and vortex vein pierce sclera • Eyelid folds fuse • Limbus appears
4th month	• Regression of hyaloid system and formation of retinal vasculature • Formation of tertiary vitreous • Formation of iris sphincter • Formation of Bowman's membrane and Descemet's membrane • Formation of longitudinal ciliary muscle and processes of ciliary body • Schlemm's canal appears • Glands and cilia develops • Formation of physiologic cup of optic disk
5th month	• Photoreceptors differentiate • Beginning of eyelid separation • Vascularization of iris stroma • Choroid vessels form layer
6th month	• Ganglion cells thicken in macula • Cones differentiate • Nasolacrimal system becomes patent • Formation of iris dilator muscle
7th month	• Rods differentiate • Formation of ora serrata • Formation of circular ciliary muscle fibers • Thinning of central fovea • Formation of lamina cribrosa • Choroid becomes pigmented • Migration of ganglion cells to form nerve fiber layer • Myelination of optic nerve • Orbicularis muscle differentiation
8th month	• Completion of anterior chamber angle formation • Hyaloid system disappears
9th month	• Retinal vessels reach the temporal periphery • Disappearance of pupillary membrane • Myelination of optic nerve to lamina cribrosa is complete
4 weeks after birth	Development of fovea

Lacrimal gland begins to develop around 6th–7th weeks of gestation. Neural crest cells differentiate into acini at the temporal region of the fornix. At 3 months, ducts of the gland form by vacuolation of the cord cells. However, lacrimal gland reflex tear production does not begin until 20 or more days after birth. As a result, newborn infants cry without tears secretion.

Development of nasolacrimal system begins at 6 weeks when surface ectoderm is buried in mesoderm between maxillary and lateral nasal processes. By 3rd month of gestation, the cord canalizes. 5% of infants can have obstruction of nasolacrimal duct system usually due to membrane covering the valve of Hasner. However, the obstruction usually opens spontaneously within 4–6 weeks of birth.

Anterior Segment Formation

Cornea develops from surface ectoderm (corneal epithelium) and neural crest cells (stroma and endothelium). First wave of neural crest grows between epithelium and lens, forming double layer of corneal endothelium. Second wave forms between epithelium and endothelium. At 4th month, Descemet's membrane develops. At 5th months, Bowman's membrane develops.

During 7th week, neural crest cells from peripheral cornea differentiate into angle. During 4th month, Schlemm's canal is formed from mesoderm. By 7th month, angle moves posteriorly. In 8th month, formation of angle is complete and trabecular meshwork appears before birth.

Pax-6 is an important regulatory protein involved in the development of the eye, encoded by the *PAX6* gene. Mutations in this gene can result in anterior segment dysgenesis syndromes such as aniridia and Peter's anomaly.

Lens

Lens placode is formed from surface ectoderm at day 27th, followed by inward invagination of the plate to form pits. By 6 weeks, basement membrane of the surface ectoderm forms the lens vesicle, which subsequently becomes lens capsule. Posterior epithelial cells elongate and migrate (primary lens fibers) and form embryonal nucleus which makes up the core of the lens. Later on, anterior cells migrate toward equator and form secondary lens fibers that encase the embryonal nucleus and form the Y sutures. Y sutures are the interdigitation of embryonal and fetal nuclei. It is upright anteriorly and inverted posteriorly. At 3 months, zonular fibers develop.

Sclera

Temporal portion of scleral derives from mesoderm, while the remaining portion is from neural crest cells. The blue hue in the neonate is from underlying uveal pigment due to scleral thinness. The scleral connects to cornea and to the optic cup.

Uvea

The uvea, consisting of the choroid, ciliary body, and iris, develops from a combination of neural ectoderm, mesoderm, and neural crest cells. Choroid vessel walls are from neural crest cells, while vascular endothelium is from mesoderm. RPE from neural crest cells contributes to the development of the choroidal stroma.

Iris is derived from neuroectoderm except for stroma, which is from neural crest cells. The five layers of iris are—(1) anterior border, (2) stroma, (3) muscular layer, (4) anterior pigmented epithelium, and (5) posterior pigmented epithelium. Iris pigment epithelia are from inner and outer layers of the optic cup and form part of the blood-aqueous barrier. By 7th week, stroma forms from neural crest cells and the tunica vasculosa lentis forms. In 6th month, sphincter and dilator muscles form from neuroectoderm. In 7th month, blood vessels enter iris, followed by disappearance of tunica vasculosa lentis in 9th month. Newborn iris is usually gray-blue because dendritic melanocytes from neural crest take weeks to months after birth to complete migration.

Ciliary body formation begins around 3rd month when a fold in the optic cup becomes the epithelial layers of the ciliary processes. The inner portion of the ciliary body is lined by an inner nonpigmented and outer pigmented layer. The inner nonpigmented layer faces the posterior chamber, while the outer pigmented layer faces the ciliary muscle. The orientation of these two layers is apex-to-apex, with the basement membranes directed outward and toward the posterior chamber, respectively between the pigmented and nonpigmented layers. The nonpigmented layer is derived from the inner nonpigmented layer of the optic cup. Around 4th month, zonules, longitudinal ciliary muscle, and the ciliary processes develop. The following month, formations of pars plana, ciliary body stroma, and ciliary muscle occur.

Retina and Posterior Segment

Retina is neuroectoderm. Foveal development is complete by 4-5 weeks after birth. Retina forms as two layers—(1) inner neurosensory layer and (2) outer RPEs. Retinal development begins in the center of the optic cup and extends out. RPEs are proliferating pseudostratified columnar epithelial cells and are the only pigmented tissue in the body that is not derived from neural crest cells.

Vitreous is formed from mesoderm and neuroectoderm. Primary vitreous is formed by the hyaloid vasculature and is surrounded by secondary vitreous, which is formed by retina. The secondary vitreous replaces primary vitreous. Failure to regress results in anomaly such as persistent hyperplastic primary vitreous (PHPV).

Optic Nerve

The optic nerve develops from the optic stalk, which connects the optic vesicle with the forebrain. The optic stalk forms from neuroectoderm cells and is surrounded by neural crest cells. In the 6th week, neuroectodermal cells begin to degenerate to provide space for axons from retinal ganglion cells. The surrounding neural crest cells form meninges while neuroectodermal cells form oligodendrocytes, which make myelin sheaths.

Mutations or abnormalities of the Pax-2 protein, essential for the development of the central nervous system, can result in optic nerve colobomas.

Extraocular Muscles

The extraocular muscles form from mesoderm following signals from the developing eye as well as from surrounding neural crest cells. By 2nd month, the beginning of lateral rectus and superior oblique muscles appear. Current literature suggests that the muscle and associated nerve develop jointly. As a result, a delay in the innervation of the muscle can lead to premature differentiation of the mesoderm into connective tissue and cause fibrosis. The delay or absence of innervation may cause inappropriate innervation by another cranial nerve (Marcus Gunn jaw-winking syndrome or Duane syndrome).

Blood Vessels (Hyaloid System)

Hyaloid artery enters embryonic fissure and forms vasa hyaloidea propria to supply blood to primary vitreous. Intravitreal portion regresses by 8.5 months of gestation, while intraneural portion becomes central retinal artery. Tunica vasculosa lentis supplies the lens. Vascularization of retinal begins at 4 months of gestation. Nasal ora serrata is completely vascularized by 36 weeks, while temporal periphery becomes vascularized by 40 weeks. Remnants of hyaloid vasculature system can form the following:

- *Bergmeister's papillae:* Located at optic nerve. It appears as a small tuft of fibrous tissue due to failure of fetal hyaloid artery to regress.
- *Mittendorf's dot:* Usually located inferonasally on the lens. Appears as a small opacity on the posterior capsule at which hyaloid artery is attached to posterior tunica vasculosa lentis.
- *Persistent pupillary membrane:* Appears as thin iris strands near pupils and the lens. It represents remnants of anterior tunica vasculosa lentis.

SUGGESTED READING

Orbital Anatomy and the Eyelids

1. Cassady JV. Developmental anatomy of nasolacrimal duct. AMA Arch Ophthalmol. 1952;47:141-58.
2. Demer JL. Mechanics of the orbita. Dev Ophthalmol. 2007;40:132-57.
3. Dutton JJ. Atlas of Clinical and Surgical Orbital Anatomy, 2nd edition. Philadelphia: Saunders; 2011.
4. Kakizaki H, Malhotra R, Madge SN, et al. Lower eyelid anatomy: an update. Ann Plast Surg. 2009;63:344.
5. Kakizaki H, Malhotra R, Selva D. Upper eyelid anatomy: an update. Ann Plast Surg. 2009;63:336.
6. Killer HE, Laeng HR, Groscurth P. Lymphatic capillaries in the meninges of the human optic nerve. J Neuroophthalmol. 1999;19:222-8.
7. Porter JD, Baker RS, Ragusa RJ, et al. Extraocular muscles: basic and clinical aspects of structure and function. Surv Ophthalmol. 1995;39:451-84.

Eye

1. Alio JL, Schimchak P, Negri HP, et al. Crystalline lens optical dysfunction through aging. Ophthalmology. 2005;112:2011.
2. Bourge JL, Robert AM, Robert L, et al. Zonular fibers, multimolecular composition as related to function (elasticity) and pathology. Pathol Biol (Paris). 2007;55:347-59.
3. Drexler W, Morgner U, Ghanta RK, et al. Ultrahigh resolution optical coherence tomography. Nature Med. 2001;7:502-7.
4. Dua HS, Said DG. Clinical evidence of the pre-Descemet's layer (Dua's layer) in corneal pathology. Eye (Lond). 2016;30:1144-5.
5. Jonas JB, Gusek GC, Naumann GO. Optic disc, cup and neuroretinal rim size, configuration and correlations in normal eyes. Invest Ophthalmol Vis Sci. 1988;29:1151-8.
6. Kaufman PL, Alm A, Levin LA, et al. Adler's physiology of the eye. New York: Saunders/Elsevier; 2011.
7. Krachmer JH, Mannis MJ, Holland EJ. Cornea, 3rd edition. St. Louis: Mosby; 2011.
8. Muller LJ, Pels L, Vrensen GF. Novel aspects of the ultrastructural organization of human corneal keratocytes. Invest Ophthalmol Vis Sci. 1995;36:2557-67.
9. Mustonen RK, McDonald MB, Srivannaboon S, et al. Normal human corneal cell populations evaluated by in vivo scanning slit confocal microscopy. Cornea. 1998;17:485-92.
10. Orth DH, Fine BS, Fagman W, et al. Clarification of foveomacular nomenclature and grid for quantitation of macular disorders. Trans Sect Ophthalmol Am Acad Ophthalmol Otolaryngol. 1977;83:OP506-14.
11. Pflugfelder SC. Tear dysfunction and the cornea: LXVIII Edward Jackson Memorial Lecture. Am J Ophthalmol. 2011;152:900-9.
12. Yannuzzi LA. The Retinal Atlas. Philadelphia: Saunders; 2010.
13. Yanoff M, Duker JS. Ophthalmology, 4th edition. Philadelphia: Saunders/Elsevier; 2014.

Embryology of the Eye

1. Jakobiec FA. Ocular Anatomy, Embryology, and Teratology. Philadelphia: Harper & Row; 1982.
2. O'Rahilly R, Muller F. Human Embryology and Teratology, 3rd edition. New York: Wiley-Liss; 2001.

Chapter 2 Physiology of the Eye

Manali Hazarika, N Venkatesh Prajna

PHYSIOLOGY OF TEAR FILM

An adequate quantity and an optimal quality of the tear film are important prerequisites for the health of the ocular surface.

Composition of the Tear Film

Traditionally, the tear film had been thought to consist of three discrete layers: an innermost mucin layer produced by the conjunctival goblet cells; an intermediate aqueous layer produced by the lacrimal glands, and an outermost lipid layer produced by the meibomian glands of the eyelids.[1]

However, over the last two decades, this concept has undergone a change with the advent of noninvasive investigative methods like the optical coherence tomography. The current concept of the tear–ocular surface structure is that of a metastable tear film consisting of four layers (Fig. 2.1). The innermost layer is a glycocalyx that extends from the superficial layer of the ocular surface epithelia. The second layer is a gradient of mucin, which, along with the third layer, i.e. the aqueous layer, forms a gel mixture. This mixture decreases from the ocular surface to the undersurface of the outermost lipid layer.[2] The fourth and the outermost layer is the tear film lipid layer (TFLL), which contributes to the stability of the tear film between blinks.[3] Figure 2.2 depicts the ocular structures that secrete the tear film.

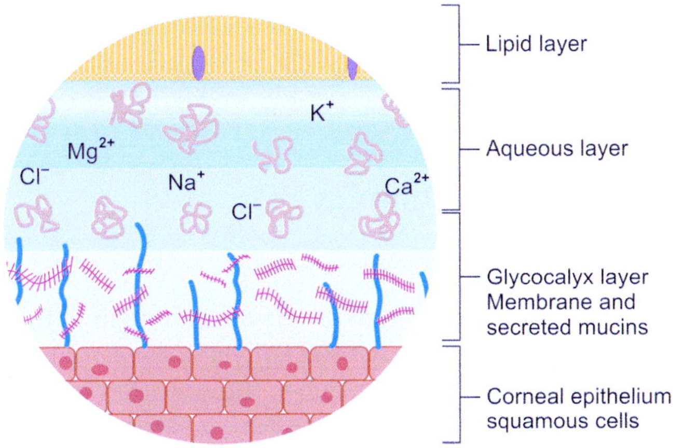

Fig. 2.1: Schematic diagram of the tear film.

Glycocalyx Layer

Mucins are a critical component of the glycocalyx and mucous layers. Three distinct types of mucins have been identified:

1. *Membrane-associated or transmembrane mucins*: MUCs 1, 4, and 16 (produced by the stratified squamous cells of the corneal and conjunctival epithelium).[4]
2. *Gel-forming mucins*: MUC5AC (produced by the conjunctival goblet cells).[4]
3. *Soluble mucins*: MUC7 (produced primarily from the lacrimal glands).[3,4]

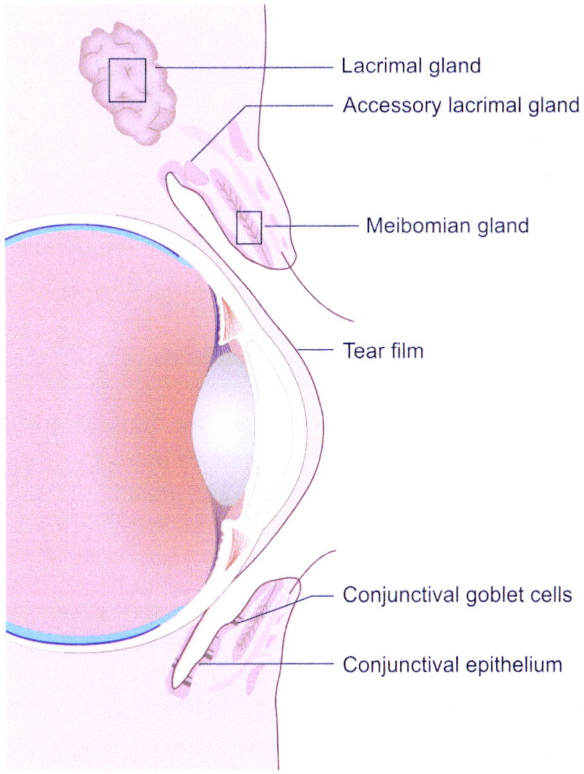

Fig. 2.2: Structures that secrete the tear film.

The membrane-associated or transmembrane mucins form the glycocalyx and are found on the apical portion of the microvilli that project from the plasma membrane of the superficial cell layer of the corneal epithelium.

Mucous Layer

The mucous layer is composed of the gel-forming mucin MUC5AC. It also contains ectodomains shed by membrane-associated mucins, soluble mucins, and other secretions of goblet and stratified squamous cells like proteins, electrolytes, and water.[5] The rate of mucin secretion by the conjunctival goblet cells is 2–3 μL/day.[6]

Aqueous Layer

The aqueous layer consists of electrolytes, water, protein, and a variety of other solutes.

The electrolyte composition of aqueous is similar to plasma except that it has a decreased $[Na^+]$ content and increased $[Cl^-]$ and $[K^+]$ content than the plasma.

Proteins in the aqueous layer include lysozyme, lactoferrin, secretory IgA, lipocalin, group II phospholipase A_2, and defensins. Also present in tears is lacritin, a protein unique to the lacrimal gland and surfactant proteins A–D.[7]

In addition, tears contain a wide array of cytokines and growth factors, including transforming growth factor (TGF)-β, epidermal growth factor (EGF)-β, fibroblast growth factor (FGF), interleukin-1α and 1β, tumor necrosis factor (TNF)-α, and interferon.

The main lacrimal gland is the major producer of the aqueous layer. It continuously secretes the fluid at the rate of approximately 1.2 μL/min. The conjunctiva, accessory lacrimal glands (glands of Krause and Wolfring), and to a small extent corneal epithelium also contribute to the aqueous layer.

Lipid Layer

The lipid layer is secreted by the Meibomian glands, that are modified sebaceous glands, and are located in the upper and lower eyelids in a single row. The bulk of the lipid layer is made by a mixture of nonpolar lipids (wax esters, cholesterol, and cholesterol esters) and polar lipids (mainly phospholipids).

Functions of the Tear Film

The functions of the tear film are elucidated in Box 2.1.[5,6]

Box 2.1: Functions of the tear film.

Functions of glycocalyx layer:
- Hydrates the ocular surface with help of the hydrophilic membrane-associated mucins
- Allows the mucin layer to evenly distribute over the ocular surface due to its nonadhesive property
- Provides a barrier against the penetrance of pathogens
- Influences epithelial activity through signaling pathways

Functions of mucous layer:
- Assists the tear film to respread after a blink
- Lowers the surface tension of the tear film by interacting with the lipid layer
- Helps in maintaining a healthy ocular surface via growth factors
- Traps exfoliated surface cells, foreign bodies, and pathogens by the loose mucin network covering the bulbar conjunctiva
- Lubricates the eyelids to reduce friction as they pass over the globe

Functions of aqueous layer:
- Provides an optically smooth surface for refraction
- Lubricates the ocular surface and thus prevents the underlying epithelia from desiccating
- Washes away debris and noxious substances through reflex secretion
- Protects the ocular surface from bacterial and viral infection
- Regulates wound healing of the ocular surface
- Regulates the pH by maintaining a constant electrolyte composition over the ocular surface epithelium
- Supplies oxygen to the avascular corneal epithelium
- Modulates the proliferation, migration, and differentiation of corneal and conjunctival epithelial cell function

Functions of lipid layer:
- Provides a hydrophobic barrier to prevent tear overflow onto the lids and sebum from the skin from entering into the tear film
- Reduces tear evaporation during eyelid opening
- Aids in lubrication of the eyelids during blinking
- Stabilizes the tear film and provides a smooth optical surface for the cornea at the air-lipid interface[1]

Properties of the Tear Film

The thickness of the tear film was originally estimated to be 8–9 μm, with the aqueous layer being the thickest layer (7 μm) and the lipid and mucous layers each relatively thin at 0.1 and 0.05 μm, respectively.[8]

However, current estimations of the thickness of the preocular tear film range between 3 μm and 11 μm. When the precorneal tear film was visualized with ultrahigh-resolution spectral domain optical coherence tomography, the average thickness was found to be 4.79 ± 0.88 μm.[9] Table 2.1 further elucidates the physical properties of the tear film.

Tear Film Dynamics

Tear Film Secretion

The lacrimal secretory system was once thought to have two components: *Basic secretors* and *reflex secretors*. Basic secretion was thought to be due to the accessory lacrimal glands of Krause and Wolfring; and reflex secretion, due to the main lacrimal gland. However, it is now established that

Table 2.1: Physical properties of tear film.

Volume of the tear film	*Unanesthetized eye*: 7.4 μL *Anesthetized eye*: 2.6 μL
Thickness	*Lipid layer*: 0.015–0.160 μm *Mucin layer*: 2.5–5 μm *Aqueous layer*: 4 μm
Secretory rate	*Unanesthetized eye*: • *Schirmer*: 3.8 μL/min • *Fluorophotometry*: 0.9 μL/min
	Anesthetized eye: • *Schirmer*: 1.8 μL/min • *Fluorophotometry*: 0.3 μL/min
Turnover rate	*Normal*: 12–16%/min *Stimulated*: 300%/min
Evaporation rate	1.4–39.3 x 10^7 g/cm^2/s
Osmolarity	296–308 mOsm/L
pH	6.5–7.6

the lacrimal glands (both main and accessory), the ocular surface (cornea, conjunctiva, and meibomian glands) and the interconnecting innervation respond to tear film secretion as a single component and are known as the lacrimal functional unit.[10]

Tearing occurs in response to stimulation of the afferent sensory nerves in cornea and conjunctiva by physical irritation due mechanical, thermal, or chemical means, psychogenic factors, and bright light via the optic nerve.[8] Afferent impulses pass through the ophthalmic branch of the trigeminal nerve to the trigeminal ganglion and on to the midbrain (pons) where they synapse and the signal is integrated with cortical and other neural inputs. The efferents, mainly parasympathetic and sympathetic, send fibers through the pterygopalatine ganglion and then to the main and accessory lacrimal glands.[10] The fibers interact with specific G-protein-linked receptors in the lacrimal glands, conjunctival goblet cells, and meibomian glands via neurotransmitters. These receptors then activate their respective signaling pathways. There are two main signaling pathways: a Ca^{2+}/protein kinase C-dependent pathway (Fig. 2.3) and a cyclic adenosine monophosphate (cAMP)-dependent pathway (Fig. 2.4).

1. *Ca^{2+}/Protein kinase C-dependent pathway*: This pathway is activated by acetylcholine everywhere except the main lacrimal gland, where it is activated by norepinephrine. Acetylcholine (released from para-

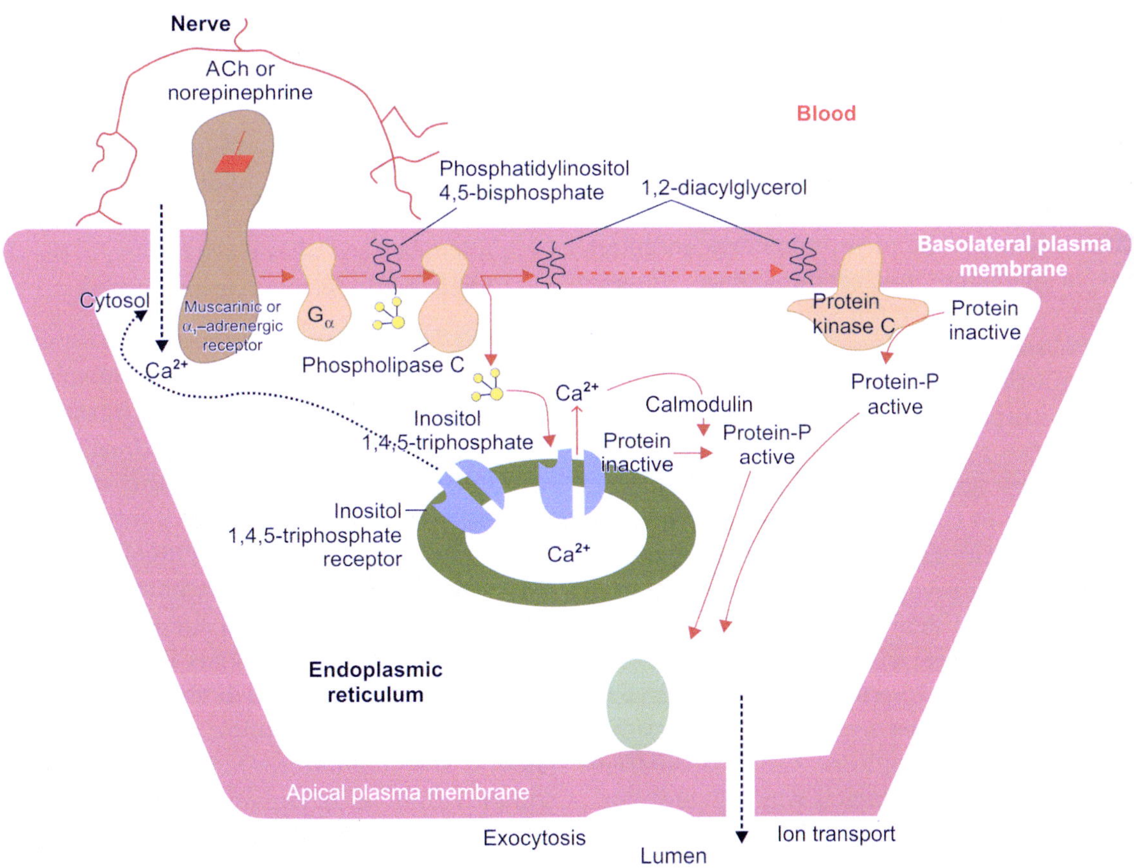

Fig. 2.3: Schematic diagram of Ca^{2+}/protein kinase C-dependent signal transduction pathway in the epithelial cell.

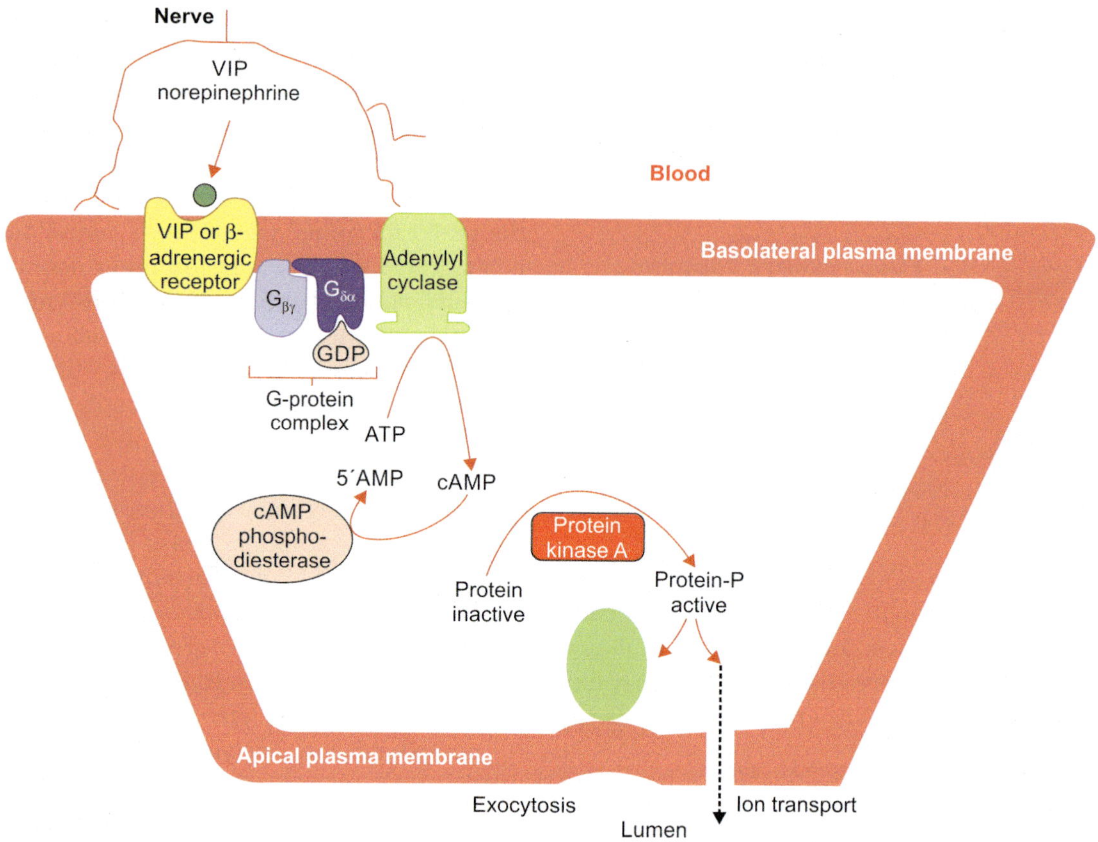

Fig. 2.4: Schematic diagram of 3′,5′-cyclic adenosine monophosphate (cAMP)-dependent signaling pathway in the epithelial cell.

sympathetic nerves) activates muscarinic receptors; while norepinephrine (released from sympathetic nerves) activates α_1-adrenergic receptors. The stimulation of muscarinic and α_1-adrenergic receptors activates a guanine nucleotide-binding protein (G protein), which leads to the activation of phospholipase C. Phospholipase C breaks down a membrane lipid—phosphatidylinositol 4,5,-bisphosphate into inositol 1,4,5-trisphosphate (IP3) and diacylglycerol. This leads to two sets of events. First, IP3 causes the depletion of Ca^{2+} from intracellular stores, thereby leading to influx of Ca^{2+} from extracellular stores to refill it. This leads to the secretion of protein and/or electrolyte and water. Secondly, diacylglycerol activates protein kinase C and this results in the secretion of protein and/or electrolyte and water.[6]

2. *Cyclic adenosine monophosphate-dependent pathway*: This pathway is activated by vasoactive intestinal peptide (VIP) and norepinephrine. VIP (released from parasympathetic nerves) interacts with VIP receptors and norepinephrine (released from sympathetic nerves) activates β-adrenergic receptors. This stimulation activates G proteins. This in turn stimulates adenylyl cyclase that produces cAMP from adenosine triphosphate (ATP). Activation of cAMP-dependent protein kinases takes place leading to the secretion of protein and/or electrolyte and water.[6]

Hormonal mechanism: In addition to neurologic pathways, peptide hormones, including α-melanocyte-stimulating hormone and adrenocorticotropic hormone, stimulate protein secretion from the main lacrimal gland.

These hormones activate the cAMP-dependent pathway described for VIP and β-adrenergic receptors. The steroid hormones, specifically the androgens, stimulate secretion of secretory immunoglobulin A (sIgA) from the main lacrimal gland and lipid secretion from the meibomian glands. Androgens diffuse into the nucleus and bind to receptors, which are members of the steroid or thyroid hormone or retinoic acid family of transcription factors. The monomeric-activated androgen-receptor complex then associates with the response elements in the regulating region of the target gene (e.g. for sIgA secretion, the target is the secretory component gene).

This association promotes dimerization of two androgen-receptor complexes, a process that then activates gene transcription and eventually protein synthesis.[6]

Alterations of any component of the lacrimal functional unit or of the hormonal or cytokine balance might result in dysfunctional tear film secretion.

Tear Film Stability

Once secreted, the tear film completely covers the preocular surface even though the underlying epithelial surface is hydrophobic. This is achieved as a result of the attractive forces between molecules on the surface of the tear film that act as an elastic membrane, constantly wanting to reduce its surface area and, therefore, its energy. This phenomenon is known as surface tension. Water forms beads on a hydrophobic surface because the rounded configuration reduces the interfacial area of contact between the water and the surface to be wet.

Such a surface could be wet by water or tears with the help of wetting (surface-active) agents. Mucin is a natural wetting agent. First, it is dissolved in the aqueous layer and interacts with the lipid layer to lower the surface tension of the tear film. Second, it is a large molecule with many sites where secondary bonds can be formed with a solid. These adsorption sites interact with sites located in the corneal epithelium. The adsorbed mucin thus creates a new surface. Not only does this new surface have a higher surface tension, and therefore is more readily wet by tears, but also, the hydrogen bonding capacity of the mucus layer is much higher than that of the epithelial surface and has a high affinity for the aqueous layer.

Tear Film Evaporation

The tear film interfaces with the external environment and thus is subject to evaporation. Environmental factors such as humidity, temperature, and air movement affect the rate of evaporation from the ocular surface.

Evaporation rates are related to the composition and distribution of the TFLL rather than being solely dependent on the thickness of the TFLL.[11] Higher evaporation rates could be a major contributor to tear film thinning and hence tear film instability and hyperosmolality.[12]

Tear Film Drainage

The excretory process begins at the lacrimal puncta, located at the nasal aspect of the eyelids, and proceeds through the upper and lower canaliculi, common canaliculus, lacrimal sac and on to the nasolacrimal duct, finally, emptying into the inferior meatus of the nose. The interaction of the eyelids, tarsal muscles, and preseptal muscles forms the lacrimal pump, which facilitates drainage of the lacrimal fluid. Normally, 90% of the lacrimal fluid is excreted by this system and 10% by evaporation between blinks.

With each blink, tears are moved nasally and toward the puncta.[8] The blink cycle is considered to be in four parts and is illustrated in Figure 2.5.[13]

1. The down stroke is the motion of the upper lid in the downward direction till where it stops. TFLL gets compressed during this event.
2. The point where it stops is called the turning point. The turning point is preceded by the downstroke and succeeded by the upstroke.
3. The upstroke is the upper lid motion in the upward direction along with the events that occur in the first 2 seconds following the lid motion. Here, tear film moves upward over the corneal surface by capillary action, but with a decaying velocity, and stabilizes after approximately 1 second.[14]
4. The interblink is the subsequent time until the next downstroke begins. During this event, the tear film first thins uniformly by evaporation. When it reaches a critical level, the lipid molecules migrate down to the mucin layer. This makes the mucin layer hydrophobic, thereby resulting in tear film break up.

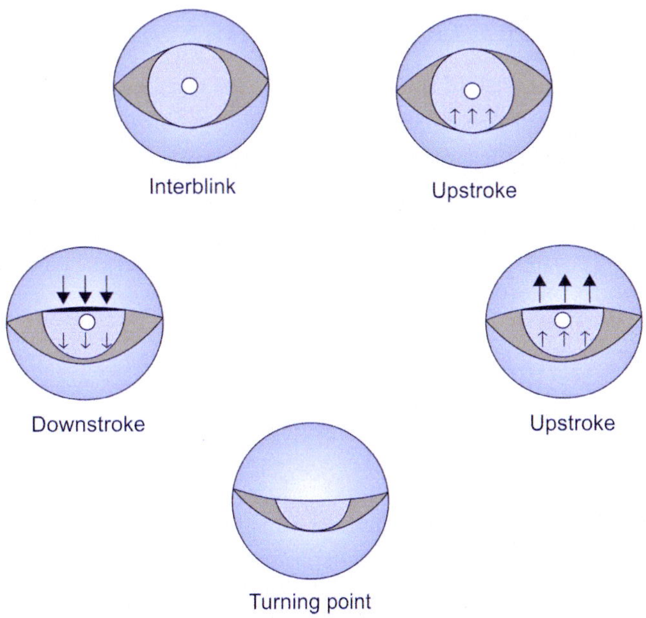

Fig. 2.5: Blink cycle.

A collection of all of these events forms a blink cycle.

The time of eyelid downstroke and upstroke in a spontaneous blink is approximately 100 ms and 250 ms, respectively.[14]

Average rate of the tear film compression and decompression is approximately 0.1 m/s and 0.04 m/s, respectively. After each blink, the tear film must respread at the surface of cornea. Factors such as osmolality, gravitational forces, and evaporation play a significant role during tear film spreading.

Tears are moved into the lacrimal puncta by negative pressure created within the lacrimal drainage system during a blink.[15] The majority of tears drain through the lower puncta via the action of gravity. However, if drainage is impaired in the lower puncta, sufficient compensatory drainage can be obtained through the upper puncta. In the presence of impaired drainage, reduced tear production has been observed.[16] This feedback mechanism between drainage and production of tears highlights the importance of tear elimination via drainage.

Tear Film Absorption

Tear film absorption occurs through the cornea, conjunctiva, and epithelium of the nasolacrimal duct. The bulk of the absorption occurs in the tissue of the nasolacrimal duct, while absorption via the cornea and conjunctiva plays only a minor role, possibly due to the tight junctions in these tissues.

PHYSIOLOGY OF CORNEA

More than 90% of the incident light is transmitted to the eye through the cornea. It contributes 43 diopters of the total refracting power, which is equivalent to two-thirds of the total dioptric power of the eye. Thus, the main function of the cornea is to act as a refracting medium, so that a clear retinal image is formed. Corneal transparency is an important pre-requisite for this optical function.

Corneal Transparency

The cornea possesses unique physiological properties that help in the efficient transmission of incident light. This is due to anatomical factors such as uniform and regular arrangement of the epithelium, the closely packed stromal lamellae of uniform size, transparency of cells that reside in the cornea, and a lack of blood and lymphatic vasculature. In addition, physiological factors that maintain corneal deturgescence are also important for corneal transparency.

The factors affecting corneal transparency are as follows:

- Anatomical factors
- Corneal vascularization
- Lymphangiogenesis
- Corneal hydration.

Anatomical Factors

Epithelium: The transparency of the normal epithelium is due to the homogeneity of the refractive index throughout this cellular layer. Normal epithelium is not observed by slit-lamp microscopy as it is, optically empty. Tight packing of epithelial cells ensures minimal light scattering. Tight junctions between superficial epithelial cells prevent penetration of tear fluid into the stroma. In conditions involving epithelial intercellular edema, the epithelial layer loses homogeneity and becomes visible by slit-lamp microscopy. This may cause symptoms of glare and halos around lights, because of light scattering. The effect of epithelial edema on vision depends upon ambient lighting conditions. In mesopic conditions, there may be a minimal effect upon visual acuity. However, in bright light, edematous epithelium causes light scattering and may have an appreciable effect upon vision. Surface irregularities such as those caused by keratoconus or epithelial edema will often be more damaging to vision than stromal edema or scarring.

Stroma: There are two theories that explain the role of the arrangement of stromal lamellae in corneal transparency. One, proposed by Maurice, states that corneal collagen fibrils of uniform diameter form a hexagonal lattice like structure, similar to a stack of diffraction gratings that eliminates light scattering by destructive interference. This is due to the fact that waves from all the collagen fibrils interfere with each other in a way that they cancel out in all directions except the forward direction. The adjacent fibrils have spacing less than the wavelength of visible light (4,000–7,000°A)[17] (Fig. 2.6). Loss of transparency will result if this regular arrangement is altered by stromal edema or mechanical stress as shown in Figure 2.7.

In 1968, after applying diffraction theory, Goldman and Benedek, introduced a second theory that the lattice arrangement is not a predominant requisite for stromal transparency. Rather, they postulated that the cornea is transparent because the fibrils are small in relationship to the light and do not interfere with light transmission unless the distance between collagen fibrils are larger than one-half a wavelength of light (2,000°A).

There is a difference in the arrangement of the collagen between the anterior and posterior stroma. While the collagen lamellae of the anterior stroma are short, narrow sheets with extensive interweaving between layers, the

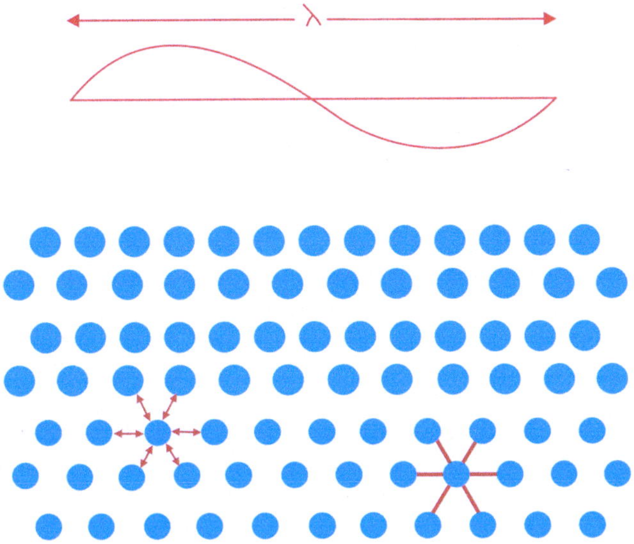

Fig. 2.6: Cross-sectional view of fibrils in lattice arrangement; size of wavelength of light is shown above for comparison. Forces of repulsion and rigid links between fibrils are shown.

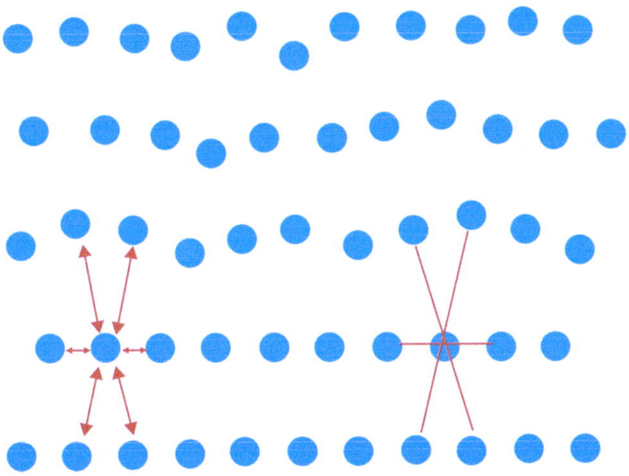

Fig. 2.7: Separation of rows of fibrils in swollen cornea. Their disarrangement is a result of weakening of forces of alignment disrupting lattice arrangement seen in Figure 2.6 with consequent loss of corneal transparency.

lamellae of the posterior stroma have long, wide, thick lamellae extending from limbus to limbus with minimal interlamellar connections. This makes light scattering greater, anteriorly; thereby resulting in a higher refractive index that decreases from 1.401 at the epithelium to 1.380 in the anterior stroma that further decreases to 1.373 in the posterior stroma.

The stroma also comprises of keratocytes that lie between the lamellae of these collagen bundles at a density of 23,000 cells/mm^3. The nucleus of the keratocyte mildly scatters some light, but the cell body does not. This is due to transparent intracellular cytoplasmic water-soluble corneal crystallins,[18] its thinness, and the even distribution of the keratocytes in a clock-wise circular arrangement. Thus light transmission is minimally affected.

The extracellular matrix (ECM) which lies between the collagen bundles and keratocytes is composed predominantly of water, proteoglycans, glycoproteins, and inorganic salts. By interacting with collagen fibrils, proteoglycans determine both the architecture of the corneal matrix and its water-retaining properties thereby having a bearing on light scattering.[19]

Endothelium: The corneal endothelium maintains corneal clarity through three functions. Firstly, it acts as a barrier to the aqueous humor; secondly it maintains normal corneal thickness by means of its deturgescence function through a metabolic pump and finally, because the endothelium is a single layer of homogeneous, closely packed cells, it possesses the property of transparency.

Corneal Vascularization

The cornea is largely avascular except for the peripheral capillary palisades at the limbus. When vessels are present, they are due to corneal pathology. It is the avascularity of the cornea that accounts, in part, for the immune privileged status it enjoys with respect to graft rejection. Its avascularity is also the reason for delayed wound healing after corneal lacerations and keratoplasty.

There is often a state of balance between pro- and antiangiogenic factors that keeps the cornea avascular. The process of angiogenesis involves the degradation of the ECM and the vascular basement membrane by matrix metalloproteinases (MMP) allowing vascular endothelial cells to invade and form vessels.

The following factors play a role in corneal neovascularization.

Inflammation: Proangiogenic factors are produced by macrophages under inflammatory conditions. Factors like macrophage migratory inhibitory factor promotes interactions between endothelial cells; increasing the angiogenic effects of leukocytes, while basic FGF (bFGF)[20] stimulates the proliferation and migration of endothelial cells into the cornea.[21]

The most significant role of macrophages in corneal neovascularization is their secretion of vascular endothelial growth factor (VEGF).[22] It is a potent proangiogenic factor. VEGF binds to its receptors expressed on the vascular endothelium. Upon VEGF binding, receptor transduction promotes endothelial cell proliferation and migration. VEGF further amplifies inflammatory corneal neovascularization by recruiting more macrophages.[23]

The Fas ligand is a transmembrane protein that is highly expressed on the corneal endothelial and epithelial layers. It causes apoptosis of the invading inflammatory cells and endothelial cells that are Fas positive[24] and thus provides a barrier against both inflammatory cells and new blood vessels.

Thrombospondin-1 (TSP-1) is a matrix protein expressed primarily in the endothelium that reduces angiogenesis in response to corneal injury. TSP-1 activates CD36, a transmembrane glycoprotein found on macrophages and endothelial cells. Activated CD36 on a macrophage reduces VEGF secretion, thus inhibiting endothelial cell proliferation, migration, and the recruitment of additional macrophages. In addition, activated CD36 on endothelial cells induces their apoptosis.[23]

The splicing of Fms-like tyrosine kinase (Flt) messenger RNA (mRNA) into a shorter fragment leads to the formation of soluble VEGF receptor-1 (sFlt-1). sFlt-1 inhibits angiogenic effects of VEGF by acting as a decoy receptor while also inactivating the membrane bound VEGF receptor, Flt.

Hypoxia: Clinically, continuous-wear hydrophilic contact lenses often induce corneal vascularization, presumably owing to hypoxia of the corneal epithelium that occurs under the contact lens. Under hypoxic conditions, proangiogenic factors are upregulated and antiangiogenic factors are downregulated. For example, pigment epithelium-derived factor effectively inhibits corneal neovascularization under normal conditions by hindering endothelial cell migration toward angiogenic inducers.[25] But under hypoxic conditions, pigment epithelium-derived factor is downregulated, thereby allowing neovascularization. Additionally, hypoxic conditions upregulate VEGF that stimulates angiogenesis.[20]

Lymphangiogenesis

Corneal lymphangiogenesis is induced along with corneal neovascularization and it correlates with the degree of corneal neovascularization, and thus affects transparency.[20]

Lymphangiogenesis is the creation of new lymphatics by lymphangioblasts or the sprouting of lymphatics from the pre-existing limbal lymphatics. In the cornea, lymphatics have been observed to arise either by extending from the limbal lymphatics or from within the cornea which then connect to the limbal lymphatic vessels.[26]

The following factors play a role in corneal lymphangiogenesis.

Homeobox gene prox1: The formation of lymphatics begins with the homeobox gene *prox1*.[20] Endothelial cells expressing this gene bud from veins and differentiate as lymphocyte endothelial cells which leads to the formation of the lymphatic system. *Prox1* also upregulates the gene encoding the tyrosine kinase receptor VEGFR-3 which regulates the growth and maintenance of lymphatic vessels.

Inflammation: Proinflammatory conditions recruit macrophages which further enhances lymphangiogenesis in two ways. First, macrophages release VEGF-C and VEGF-D which induces local sprouting of pre-existing lymphocyte endothelial cells. Second, CD11b positive macrophages transdifferentiate into lymphocyte endothelial cells which are integrated into sprouting lymphatic vessels.[20]

Fibroblast growth factor-2: It stimulates lymphangiogenesis more than angiogenesis by upregulating VEGF-C expression and promoting migration and proliferation of lymphocyte endothelial cells.

VEGF-A and neuropilin-2 also induce lymphangiogenic response.

Neostatin-7: This proteolytic fragment of collagen XVIII has antilymphangiogenic properties via reduction in bFGF-induced corneal lymphangiogenesis.

Endostatin: This is a proteolytic fragment of collagen XVII that also has the ability to diminish lymphangiogenesis.

Corneal Hydration

Corneal transparency is a resultant of maintaining the water content of the stroma at 78%.[27] An excised cornea placed in aqueous media will swell with the hydration increasing up to 98%. This is a significant finding, because even a 5% or more increase in corneal hydration from its normal physiologic level of 78%, leads to a significant amount of light scattering and loss of transparency.

The following factors affect corneal hydration:

Stromal swelling pressure: The tendency of the stroma to swell has been called the swelling pressure (SP). This is mainly due to the interfibrillary proteoglycans and other proteins that constitute the ground substance. The carbohydrate components of the proteoglycans consisting of negatively charged glycosaminoglycans (keratan sulfate, chondroitin sulfate, and dermatan sulfate) act like a sponge based upon electrostatic repulsion of anionic charges on its molecule. This is known as the Donnan effect.

The normal SP is +55 mm Hg because the corneal stroma has cohesive characteristics and tensile stiffness (elasticity) that resists expansion.[19] If the stroma is allowed to swell abnormally (edema), the SP drops rapidly; conversely, if the stroma is allowed to dry (because of tear film breakup), or if the stroma is compressed as occurs with increased IOP or mechanical applanation, the SP rises exponentially.

Fluid is drawn into the cornea by a negative pressure called the imbibition pressure (IP) of the corneal stroma. This occurs due to the negatively charged glycosaminoglycan side-chains that form a double-folded helix in aqueous solution (secondary structure) that attracts and binds Na^+ cations, resulting in an osmotic effect, leading to the diffusion and subsequent absorption of water.

Normally, the highly impermeable epithelium and the relatively lesser impermeable endothelium keep the diffusion of electrolytes and fluid flow in the stroma to such a low level that the endothelium's metabolic pumps can maintain stromal hydration in the normal range without significant effort.[19]

In the normal in vitro state, the IP equals the SP. However, in vivo, IP is modified by the intraocular pressure (IOP) according to the equation:

$$IP = IOP - SP$$

This is because, in vivo, a compressing effect of the IOP on the endothelium is seen in this relationship and thus it creates an IP of approximately –40 mm Hg (Fig. 2.8).

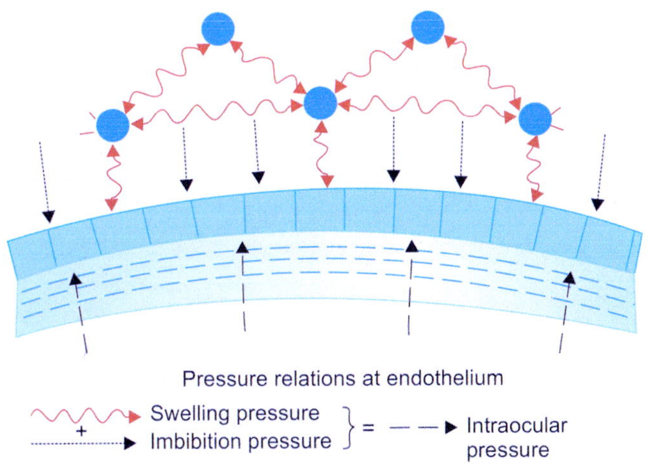

Fig. 2.8: Normal pressure relationships on endothelial surface. Tissue pressure is equal to swelling pressure. Fluid pressure is negative and equal to imbibition pressure. Swelling pressure plus imbibition pressure equals intraocular pressure.

Thus resistance is reduced when there is a loss of corneal barrier function, an IOP more than or equal to 55 mm Hg, or a combination of the two.[19] This increases corneal hydration causing corneal edema.

Function of the limiting layers: Both the epithelium and the endothelium act as semipermeable membranes that create a barrier to the diffusion of electrolytes and to the flow of water.

- Epithelial layer: The epithelium is 100 times less permeable than the endothelium. This is by virtue of a continuous band of apical zonula occludens tight junctions at the peripheral intercellular margins of the superficial squamous cells that form a high-resistance barrier to the external environment.[18] This prevents the movement of ions and thus fluid from the tears into the stroma.

  The epithelium also actively transports Cl^- from the stroma to tears. This transport is regulated by the beta-adrenergic receptor adenylate cyclase complex, with possible control by sympathetic nerve fibers.[28] The outward active Cl^- transport process competes with the inward active Na^+ transport process, leading to a net outward transport of solute and fluid that could account for a corneal thinning rate of 1.3 mm/hr.[29]
- Endothelial layer: The corneal endothelium maintains transparency by regulating corneal hydration and nutrition through a "leaky" barrier and metabolic pump function which was first described by Maurice.[19]
  - The "pump-leak" hypothesis suggests that an equilibrium is needed between the amount of passive fluid flow into the cornea and energy expended through pumping out excess fluid in order to maintain corneal transparency. The barrier function of the corneal endothelium is dependent upon two factors:
    1. *Number of endothelial cells*: Corneal endothelial permeability gradually increases as central endothelial cell density decreases below 2,000 cells/mm², but compensatory metabolic pump mechanisms keep the cornea at its normal dehydrated state until a central endothelial cell density of 500 cells/mm² is reached.
    2. *Intact macula occludens tight junctions*: These tight junctions between the endothelial cells result in a low electrical resistance (25 Ω·cm²) barrier to the aqueous humor flow.[19] This barrier prevents the bulk flow of fluid from the aqueous humor to the stroma, but it does still

allow moderate diffusion of small nutrients, water, and other metabolites to cross into the stroma through the 10 nm wide intercellular spaces. While this may seem counterproductive; however, most nutrients for all layers of the cornea come from the aqueous humor. Thus, leakiness of the endothelial cell monolayer is essential for corneal health.

Evaporation from the corneal surface: Evaporation of the tears (which happens at a rate of approximately 2.5 mL/cm^2/hr) makes the tear hypertonic resulting in an osmotic extraction, thereby thinning the cornea by 5%. This loss of fluid is readily replaced by aqueous and therefore matters little in corneal dehydration.

Intraocular pressure: With normal IOP there is no effect upon corneal thickness. However, when the IOP (>50–60 mm Hg) exceeds the SP, epithelial edema will occur. This can take place in two instances:

1. With a high IOP and normal stromal SP and thickness (for example, in acute glaucoma)
2. With normal IOP and low stromal SP (for example, in corneal edema secondary to endothelial dystrophy).

Corneal Wound Healing

Wound healing in the cornea differs from that in other tissues, primarily owing to its avascularity. In addition, the nature of the injury affects the course of wound healing. For instance, infectious ulcerations create special problems for wound repair not encountered in clean surgical wounds. Severe alkali burns often never heal. Other factors such as the nature of the suture material, location of the wound (central vs peripheral), and the presence of other corneal, ocular, or systemic disease may also affect corneal wound healing. Topical medications may have profound effects upon the reparative process. This is especially true of steroids, which are often used to modify the reparative process since scarring may more adversely affect vision than the original insult. Therefore, many factors are involved when considering corneal wound healing.

Wound healing in the cornea is brought about by epithelial, stromal, and endothelial cells by cell migration, growth factors, and ECM remodeling. However, there are significant differences in healing scenarios of these three types of corneal cells. The epithelium heals from itself, with continuous migration and differentiation of limbal stem cells, but it does not undergo transformation to different cell types. In contrast, stromal wounds heal with a sequence of transformation of stromal keratocytes to fibroblasts and myofibroblasts, and significant participation of resident and circulating immune system cells. Corneal endothelium, unlike other cell types, mostly heals by cell migration and spreading, and may undergo epithelial-mesenchymal transformation in this process, but cell proliferation plays a secondary role.[30]

Epithelial Wound Healing

Normally, the superficial squamous cells of the epithelium are continuously shed into the tear film. But this epithelium is continuously renewed every 7–10 days by the centripetal migration of the epithelial cells from the limbus at a rate of approximately 120 µm/week and the differentiation of basal proliferative cells into the superficial squamous cells as shown in Figure 2.9.[19]

Thoft and Friend suggested that an equilibrium exists between these three processes and called it the X, Y, Z hypothesis. According to this hypothesis, X, which is the basal corneal epithelial cell proliferation + Y which is the limbal cell proliferation = Z, which is the epithelial cell loss on the anterior surface from eyelid blinking.[31]

When this equilibrium is disrupted, corneal epithelial cell wound healing typically begins in two distinct phases: an initial latent phase and a closure phase. The initial phase includes cellular and subcellular reorganization to trigger migration of the epithelial cells at the wound edge. The closure phase includes several continuous processes starting with cell migration, which is independent of cell mitosis, followed by cell proliferation and differentiation and eventually, by stratification to restore the original multicellular epithelial layer.

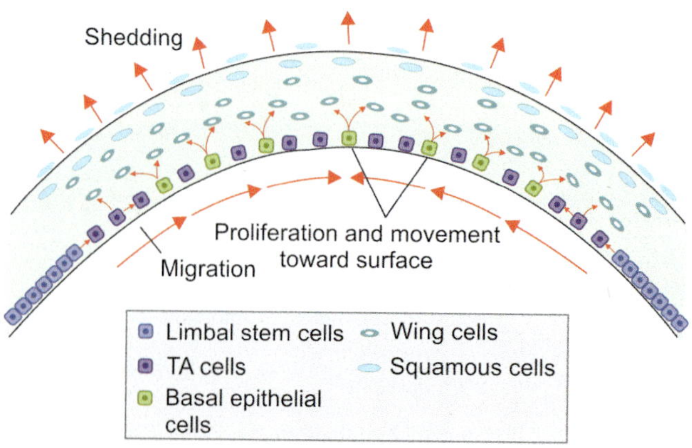

Fig. 2.9: XYZ hypothesis. The limbal stem cells give rise to transient amplifying (TA) cells that migrate centripetally to replenish the basal epithelial cells that undergo vertical proliferation.

Epithelial cells express several growth factors and cytokines that stimulate growth, proliferation, migration, differentiation, adhesion (cell to cell and cell to matrix), ECM deposition, and proteinase regulation of cells involved in wound healing. Factors activated during wound healing are EGF, platelet-derived (PDGF) and transforming (TGF) growth factors α and β, acidic (FGF-1) and basic (FGF-2) fibroblast growth factors, insulin-like (IGF-I), keratinocyte (KGF), hepatocyte (HGF) growth factors, thymosin-β4 (Tβ4), interleukins (IL)-1, -6, and -10, and tumor necrosis factor (TNF)-α.

The mechanisms by which corneal nerves maintain the ocular surface and promote healing are currently under active research. Corneal nerves secrete neuropeptides, such as substance P and calcitonin gene-related protein, and neurotransmitters, such as acetylcholine, vasoactive intestinal polypeptide, and neurotensin, which are believed to be important in corneal epithelial function and proliferation.[19]

Recently, there has been emerging evidence of the role of microRNAs (miRNAs) in epithelial wound healing. miRNAs are small noncoding RNAs that can specifically bind to complementary sequences of target mRNAs. They are natural and powerful gene expression regulators, and key mediators of delayed wound healing, especially in diabetic corneas. They are located in the limbal epithelial cells and help in migration and proliferation of corneal epithelial cells at the wound edge, by upregulating miR-205 that targets SH2-containing phosphoinositide-5-phosphatase (SHIP2), which in turn affects Akt signaling pathway and increases epithelial migration. In addition, the upregulated miR-205 can promote motility of epithelial cells through modification of F-actin organization.

Stromal Wound Healing

Normal stromal wound healing is important, as the stroma provides the major structural support for the cornea. The effect of corneal avascularity is most readily seen in this layer. Central avascular corneal wounds take much longer to heal than peripheral or limbal wounds. Cytokines and growth factors orchestrate cell behavior associated with the development of corneal neovascularization. VEGF and TGF-β thus contribute to injury-induced neovascularization, with ECM components supporting the growth of new vessels.[27] Thus vascularized corneas heal faster than nonvascularized corneas.

At the early stage of wound repair, damaged keratocytes undergo apoptosis.

The remaining viable keratocytes are activated from their quiescent state to proliferate into fibroblasts. This transformation is mediated by growth factors like FGF-2, PDGF-AB, and TGF-β. Other factors like IL-1 and IGF-1 mediate their mitogenic activity. Once transformed, these fibroblasts downregulate the expression of differentiated keratocyte proteins, such as corneal crystallins (transketolase and aldehyde dehydrogenase 1A1) and keratan sulfate proteoglycans, and start producing proteinases (mostly MMPs), needed to remodel the wounded ECM.

However, although these cells enter the cell cycle and acquire migratory properties necessary to repopulate and close the wound, they produce relatively little ECM and, as a result, form regions of hypercellularity between the recently migrated epithelium and the stroma.

The cytoplasm of these hypercellular cells start expressing α-smooth muscle actin (SMA) and desmin and upregulate the expression of vimentin. Thus they become highly motile and contractile myofibroblasts that remodel and contract the wound.[32]

Extracellular matrix remodeling during wound healing often accumulates aberrant proteins that include type III, VIII, XIV, and XVIII collagen, limbal isoforms of type IV collagen, embryonic fibronectin isoforms, TSP-1, tenascin-C, fibrillin-1, and hevin. As a result of slow turnover, these proteins may form scars that persist for years altogether.

The main signaling complex driving these processes in the stroma is TGF-β system. This system is tightly regulated, with profibrotic TGF-β1 and β2, and antifibrotic TGF-β3. The result of their interplay is unpredictable, as excessive healing may lead to stromal haze and/or ECM scar.

Endothelial Wound Healing

The corneal endothelial cells can be damaged both directly, e.g. by alkaline burns, surgical replacement, corneal transplantation or even cataract surgery, as well as indirectly. In the latter case, the healing of the wound primarily affecting epithelial and stromal cells can also provoke endothelial cell apoptosis.

But unlike many tissues, where wound repair entails cell proliferation as a major mechanism of reducing and remodeling the wound, the corneal endothelial cells have very limited capacity for mitosis. Thus the corneal endothelium closes the wound gap mainly by migration and increased cell spreading. During the process of wound healing, the endothelial cell transiently differentiates into fibroblastic morphology. This process is known as endothelial-mesenchymal transformation and encourages fibrotic changes in the endothelial layer. It is induced by FGF-2, IL-1β, and TGF-β. But endothelial-mesenchymal transformation may lead to fibrotic complications of healing such as the formation of retrocorneal fibrous membrane.

PHYSIOLOGY OF THE SCLERA

The sclera forms the outermost, fibrous tunic of the human eye and its principal function is to provide structural integrity to the globe and to protect the inner components of the eye from physical injury. The clear, transparent cornea covers the anterior one-sixth of the total surface area of the globe, while the white, opaque sclera covers the remaining five-sixths.

In comparison to the cornea, the sclera has the following differences:

- It has larger collagen fibril diameters and interfibrillar spaces.
- It is more opaque, interwoven, and rigid. The color of the sclera is opaquely white because it scatters all frequencies of visible light since the dimensions of the collagen fibrils are greater than a half-wavelength of visible light.[19]
- It has a regional zone of vascularity in the episclera.
- It does not have adjacent external or internal cellular barrier layers.

Functions of the Sclera

The sclera has the following functions:[19]

- Protects the delicate intraocular structures. The interwoven fibrils are rigid and they help maintain a stable shape.
- Facilitates aqueous outflow and resists the forces generated by IOP.
- Provides attachment sites for the extraocular muscles (EOMs) to rotate the eyeball.
- Provides a stable attachment for the ciliary muscle to accommodate the lens.
- Provides a conduit for vascular and neural pathways.
- Determines the absolute size of the eye and thus the refractive error of the eye. This is guided by a retino-RPE-scleral visual signaling pathway, which dynamically controls scleral extensibility under the stress of normal IOP and thus controls the innate biomechanical properties of the sclera.

Scleral Wound Healing

As is with the cornea, a scleral injury converts scleral fibrocytes to metabolically active fibroblasts. However, unlike the cornea, the presence of episcleral vasculature hastens wound healing here because episcleral fibrovascular granulation tissue migrates into and fills the superficial wound.[19]

Similarly, injuries involving the deeper portion of the sclera also heal predominantly through fibrovascular granulation tissue, which grows outward from the choroid, leading to fibrovascular scarring finally.

In later stages, the scar undergoes a gradual remodeling or reorganization.

PHYSIOLOGY OF AQUEOUS HUMOR

The aqueous humor is an optically clear fluid that fills the anterior and posterior chambers of the anterior segment.

Functions of Aqueous Humor

The aqueous humor has several important functions. These are described in Box 2.2.[33]

Properties of Aqueous Humor

Box 2.3 describes the physical properties of aqueous humor.[33]

Box 2.2: Functions of aqueous humor.

- Generates and maintains an intraocular pressure (IOP) of 15.5 ± 2.6 mm Hg that helps in the structural properties of the globe
- Provides nutrients to support the function of tissues of the anterior segment, such as the avascular lens, cornea, and trabecular meshwork
- Removes metabolic waste products (e.g. lactic acid and pyruvic acid) from tissues of the anterior segment
- Provides an optically clear medium for the transmission of light
- Has immunosuppressive effects as it contains multiple immunosuppressive factors like the soluble Fas ligand

Box 2.3: Properties of aqueous humor in normal human eye.

- *Aqueous formation rate*: ~2.5–3.0 μL/min
- *Volume of the aqueous humor*: ~250 μL (volume in the anterior chamber is 200 μL and posterior chamber is 50 μL)
- *Aqueous volume turnover rate*: 1.0–1.5%/min
- *Refractive index of aqueous*: 1.33332
- *Osmotic pressure*: 3–5 mOsm/L
- *pH of aqueous in the anterior chamber*: 7.2

Dynamics of Aqueous Humor

The dynamics of aqueous humor includes its mechanism of formation as well as outflow. The aqueous humor is produced from the substrate of the plasma by the nonpigmented ciliary epithelium, lining the ciliary processes. It then enters into the posterior chamber between the lens and the iris, flows through the pupil and then into the anterior chamber. The convectional currents present in the anterior chamber guide the flow of aqueous in a downward direction, on the side closer to the cornea where the temperature is cooler, and in an upward direction on the side near the lens where the temperature is warmer. Eventually the aqueous leaves the eye by passive bulk flow mainly via two pathways at the anterior chamber angle. The first pathway is called the "trabecular or conventional outflow route". In this pathway, aqueous exits through the trabecular meshwork, across the inner wall of Schlemm's canal into its lumen, and thence into collector channels, aqueous veins, and the episcleral venous circulation. The second pathway is called the "uveoscleral or unconventional outflow route". Here the aqueous passes across the root of the iris, into the uveal meshwork, and the anterior face of the ciliary muscle, through the connective tissue between the muscle bundles, into the suprachoroidal space, and thence out through the sclera. Figure 2.10 depicts the aqueous humor flow.[33]

Formation Mechanism

Aqueous humor formation results from active secretion, ultrafiltration, and simple diffusion. These three mechanisms contribute in varying degrees to the production of the aqueous humor.

1. *Active secretion*: This accounts for 80–90% of the total aqueous humor formation.

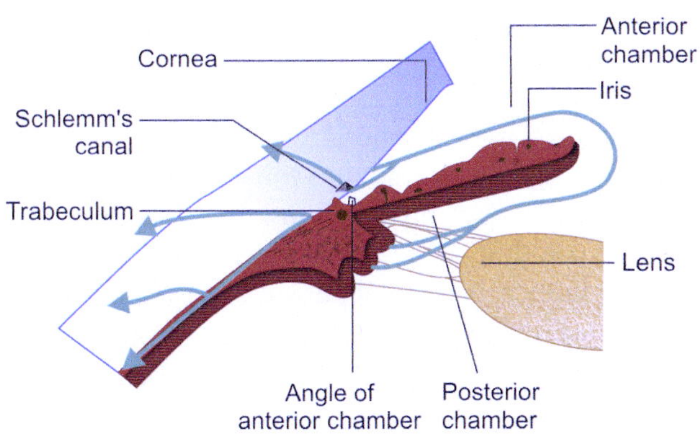

Fig. 2.10: Schematic representation of aqueous humor flow.

The basolateral membrane of the nonpigmented ciliary epithelium secretes aqueous by an energy-dependent process that actively transports sodium, chloride, and bicarbonate into the posterior chamber. Active secretion is independent of the IOP.[33]

2. *Ultrafiltration*: Ultrafiltration is a passive pressure-dependent movement along a pressure gradient. This component of aqueous formation decreases with increasing IOP.

   In the ciliary processes, the hydrostatic pressure difference between capillary pressure and IOP favors flow of water and water-soluble substances through the micropores in the cell membrane. At the same time, the oncotic gradient between the two pressures, however, resists this flow.[34]

3. *Diffusion*: In diffusion, certain ions, passively flow along an electrochemical gradient across a semipermeable membrane, from areas of high concentration toward areas of low concentration where the most negative potential is located.

Factors Regulating Aqueous Formation

Adrenergic mechanism: The vessels of the ciliary processes have a dense adrenergic innervation that regulates aqueous humor formation by influencing their permeability. However, adrenergic tone to the ciliary epithelium may be influenced by hormones rather than being just innervational. Two major hormones of the adrenal gland, epinephrine and cortisol, regulate aqueous formation.[35]

Adrenergic mechanisms regulate the rate of aqueous humor formation by receptor specificity.

- *Beta-adrenergic receptors*: Beta-adrenergic receptors (especially β2) are located in abundance in the ciliary epithelium. Stimulation of these receptors initiates a signal transduction cascade beginning with activation of a regulatory intramembranous G-protein. The G-protein activates the second messenger adenylyl cyclase, which is also localized to the ciliary body. This, in turn, leads to elevation of cAMP levels. cAMP activates protein kinase A by phosphorylation, which affects aqueous formation. Figure 2.11 elucidates this signal transduction pathway.

  The cAMP levels influence Na^+-K^+-ATPase activity that may regulate the extraction of Na^+ from stroma of nonpigmentary ciliary epithelium.[36]

  Beta-adrenergic antagonists may affect active transport by causing a decrease either in the efficiency of the Na^+-K^+ pump or in the number of pump sites.

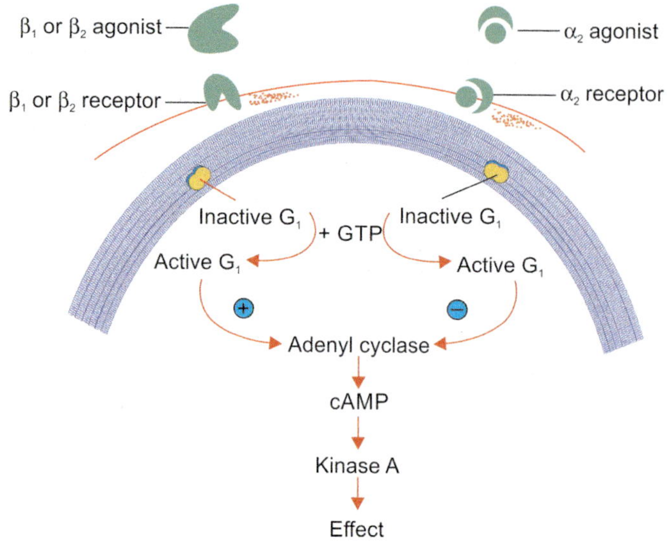

Fig. 2.11: Schematic diagram of signal transduction pathway following binding of β_1, β_2, and α_2 receptors.

- *Alpha-adrenergic receptors*: Majority of the receptors in the ciliary body are alpha2-adrenergic receptors. Like beta-receptors, they are also coupled through G proteins to adenylyl cyclase, but they inhibit the elevations of cAMP levels (Fig. 2.11). However, both alpha-adrenergic agonists and antagonists have been reported to lower IOP. They appear to act through suppression of aqueous inflow without an apparent effect on outflow facility. In addition, effects related to reductions in episcleral venous pressure and ciliary body vascular flow have also been reported with alpha adrenergic receptors.

Natriuretic peptide mechanism: A number of neuropeptides (e.g. VIP, neuropeptide Y, opioids, and substance P) present in the ciliary body have been identified to play a role in control of IOP, possibly mediated via nitric oxide. Nitric oxide donors have been shown to inhibit Na^+-K-ATPase activity in the nonpigmented ciliary epithelium.

Other factors: The passive mechanisms of aqueous formation like ultrafiltration and diffusion depend upon the level of blood pressure in the ciliary capillaries, the plasma osmotic pressure, and the level of the IOP.

Outflow Mechanism

The trabecular or conventional outflow pathway: Approximately 75–90% of the total aqueous is drained via this route. This pressure-driven outflow pathway regulates the bulk flow of aqueous humor out of the eye and limits flow back into the eye, by an energy-independent mechanism, thereby maintaining a constant IOP.

The trabecular meshwork is classically divided into three parts. The *uveal meshwork* is the innermost part of the trabecular meshwork that extends from the iris root and the ciliary body to the peripheral cornea. The *corneoscleral meshwork* consists of sheets of trabeculum that extend from the scleral spur to the lateral wall of the scleral sulcus. *The juxtacanalicular (endothelial) meshwork,* which is the part that offers outflow resistance, is adjacent to, and actually forms the inner wall of, the Schlemm's canal.

The contraction of the ciliary muscle causes expansion of the trabecular meshwork and opening of Schlemm's canal, which subsequently increases the flow of aqueous humor through the trabecular meshwork. Aqueous moves both across and between the endothelial cells lining the inner wall of the Schlemm canal.[33,35]

The uveoscleral or unconventional outflow pathway: This pathway is responsible for 10–25% of the total aqueous outflow. Aqueous flows from the anterior chamber into the ciliary muscle and then into the supraciliary and suprachoroidal spaces. The fluid is then drained by the venous circulation in the intact sclera. This pathway is pressure-independent and is affected by age, especially in young, normal eyes where the outflow is more. It is also increased by cycloplegia, adrenergic agents, prostaglandin analogs, and certain complications of surgery (e.g. cyclodialysis) and is decreased by miotics.[33]

Factors Regulating Aqueous Outflow

Cholinergic mechanisms:

- *Conventional (trabecular) outflow*: Topical, intracameral, or systemically administered cholinergic agonists (like pilocarpine) all decrease outflow resistance, while ganglionic blocking agents and cholinergic antagonists (such as atropine) increase resistance.

  Cholinergic nerve terminals induce contraction and relaxation of trabecular meshwork and scleral spur cells which might affect the area and configuration of the outflow pathways and thereby outflow resistance. These effects could be mediated by cAMP and/or increased intracellular calcium and phospholipase C activity.[33]
- *Unconventional (uveoscleral) outflow*: Cholinergic agonist agent like pilocarpine causes ciliary muscles to contract causing narrowing the space for perfusion, while cholinergic antagonist agent like atropine

induces muscle relaxation, thereby widening the space for perfusion causing increase in uveoscleral outflow.[33]

Adrenergic mechanisms:

- *Conventional (trabecular) outflow*: Topical and intracameral epinephrine increase outflow facility by stimulating adrenergic receptors that can alter intraocular, intrascleral, and extrascleral vascular tone, and also by directly affecting the outflow pathway. This action is mediated by β2-adrenergic receptors on the trabecular endothelial cells.[33]
- *Unconventional (uveoscleral) outflow*: The stimulation of β-adrenergic receptors relaxes the ciliary muscle. Thus epinephrine, not only increases trabecular outflow, but in addition, also increases uveoscleral outflow.

Alpha-2-adrenergic agonists such as brimonidine may enhance uveoscleral outflow.[33]

Corticosteroid mechanism: Glucocorticoid receptors are located in the cells of the outflow pathways. Corticosteroid regulation of IOP is proposed to occur via 11β-hydroxysteroid dehydrogenase (HSD)-1 expression which is localized in the nonpigmented ciliary epithelium. This enzyme catalyzes the conversion of cortisone to cortisol which, in turn, induces Na^+-K^+-ATPase, leading to sodium and water transport into the posterior chamber, resulting in aqueous production. However, over time, cortisol in the aqueous interacts with glucocorticoid receptors in the trabecular meshwork. In susceptible individuals known as steroid responders, this causes an alteration of hyaluronic acid, protein, and collagen synthesis and distribution in cells and tissues of the outflow systems, thereby causing an increase in outflow resistance.[33]

Prostaglandin mechanism: Prostaglandin F2α analog like latanoprost cause increase in aqueous outflow through the uveoscleral pathway by redirecting aqueous from the trabecular pathway. It also leads to the relaxation of the ciliary muscles, thereby causing widening of the intermuscular spaces. However, the major contribution to the outflow effect is due to remodeling of the ECM within the ciliary muscle, iris root, ciliary body, and sclera. This is achieved by an increase in matrix metalloproteinase -1, -2, and -3 and reduction in collagen types I, II, and IV.[33]

Glycosaminoglycan mechanism: Glycosaminoglycans cause a decrease in the outflow of aqueous through the trabecular meshwork by obstructing the pathway. This is more so with chondroitin sulfate. Hyaluronic acid, on the other hand, covers the surfaces of the outflow pathways, thereby discouraging adherence of molecules to ECM compounds within the meshwork. This prevents clogging of the outflow pathways. This is further reiterated by the fact that in patients with primary open angle glaucoma, there is depletion of hyaluronic acid and an accumulation of chondroitin sulfates in their trabecular meshwork.[33]

Other agents: Nitric oxide in the trabecular meshwork and ciliary muscle cause resistance to aqueous outflow either directly at the level of the trabecular meshwork, Schlemm's canal, and collecting channels, or indirectly through relaxation in the tone of the longitudinal ciliary muscle. Nitric oxide synthase released from nerve terminals could also cause relaxation of trabecular meshwork cells and allow an increase in outflow facility independent from the ciliary muscle.[35]

Age-related Changes of the Aqueous Humor

Intraocular Pressure

A study of aqueous humor dynamics in healthy subjects between two age groups, i.e. 20–30 years and more than 60 years of age, showed that in the healthy aging eye, there is a reduction in the production of aqueous humor and a reduction in its drainage through the uveoscleral outflow pathway, but there is no significant age-related IOP increase.[37]

Conversely, a study done in a Japanese population found that IOP decreases with age. But large demographic studies in the United States that included all eye conditions, found an increase in IOP with age.[38,39] All these differences were attributed to blood pressure, obesity, and other cardiac risk variables.[40]

- *Trabecular outflow*: In nonglaucomatous eyes, total outflow facility decreases by 30% with age.[40] There is slight but insignificant decrease in outflow facility from 0.25 mL/min/mm Hg in the 20–30 year age group to 0.19 mL/min/mm Hg, in those over 60 years.[33] This could, in part, be due to the increase in ocular rigidity with age.
- *Uveoscleral outflow*: This pathway accounts for 54% of total aqueous drainage in young healthy eyes from 20–30 years of age compared to 46% in older healthy eyes of above 60 years.[33]

Aqueous Humor Formation

Tonographic and fluorophotometric studies demonstrate an age-related decline in the rate of aqueous production which amounts to 15–35% over the 20–80 year age spectrum. The decline probably occurs throughout adult life and is estimated to be 0.003-0.015 mL/min/year or 2.4% per decade.[41] The reduction in aqueous humor formation with age counteracts the resistance to outflow with age so that the IOP normally does not substantially elevate, with age.

Episcleral Venous Pressure

Episcleral venous pressure does not appear to change with age.[41]

Ocular Rigidity

Ocular rigidity increases by about 25% in older compared to younger subjects.[41]

Iris Permeability

Iris permeability to intravenous fluorescein tends to increase by about 13% per decade between the ages of 20 years and 80 years.[41]

Aqueous Humor Turnover Rate

Although total aqueous flow decreases with age, there is a small but significant rise in the rate of anterior chamber refilling. This turnover rate of aqueous is estimated to be approximately 5% per decade which could be attributed to the decrease in anterior chamber depth and volume with age as a result of increased lenticular volume.

Trabecular Meshwork and Schlemm's Canal

A progressive decrease in trabecular meshwork cell counts occurs with age, at a rate of 0.58–0.85%/year. Also, there is an increase in pigmentation of trabecular meshwork cells, an increased incidence of cells detaching from trabeculae, and a progressively greater incidence of fusion between adjacent trabeculae. At 20 years of age the cell population in the trabecular meshwork is approximately 1,200,000 cells. This decreases to 500,000 cells by 80 years, indicating a loss of about 12,000 cells/year. This is because trabecular meshwork cells have a limited capacity for replication. With age, these cells become voracious phagocytes that remove increasing quantities of debris and eventually detach from the trabeculae, to be lost via the Schlemm's canal.

PHYSIOLOGY OF LENS

The crystalline lens is a key refractive element of the optical system and contributes approximately one-third (about 20 diopters) of the total optical power of the relaxed eye. The transparency, high refractive index property, and the capability to accommodate are responsible for the biconvex lens to help accomplish its function of focusing light rays onto the retina.

Lens Transparency

The transparency of the lens is an integral requirement for light to focus onto the retina. The lens transmits light with wavelengths ranging from 390 nm up to 1200 nm, efficiently.[42]

In order to be transparent, the lens needs to be efficient in minimizing both light scattering and absorption. The following factors aid in maintaining lens transparency.

Avascularity

The absence of blood vessels in the lens provides an unimpeded pathway for the light rays to reach the retina. It has to be remembered that the embryonic lens derives its nourishment from blood vessels namely, tunica vasculosa lentis. As lens development progresses, the vasculature disappears; the fibers produce the lens capsule, all of which leads to decreased light scattering.[43]

Cellular Content

The membrane-bound cellular organelles of the lens fibers are absent or relatively sparse in the central epithelium and are displaced to the equator, to avoid blocking of transmission of light.[44]

Lens crystallins make up about 90% of the water-soluble proteins, and are the main soluble components of lens fibers. It comprises of two major families: the βγ-crystallins and the α-crystallins. While the former are among the most stable proteins known, the latter exhibit a chaperone-like function. The high concentration of densely packed lens crystallins maintain a refractive index constant over distances approximating the wavelength of the light to be transmitted.[45] The other proteins found in the lens include actin, myosin, vimentin, α-actinin, and microtubules.[46]

These other proteins, along with metabolic activities of the lens are primarily organized to protect the crystallins from damage over time and to maintain homeostasis of the lens cells.[45]

Architecture of the Lens Fibers

In the lens cortex, transparency is enhanced by the high spatial order of the lens fiber architecture. A compact arrangement of the protein components coupled with the difference in the refractive indices of the nucleus and the cortical region, greatly aids in minimizing the scattering of light. Normally, membranes do not scatter light because their thickness is well below the dimensions of large spatial fluctuations that cause light scattering. As fiber membranes become closely apposed and tightly connected with lateral interdigitations, intercellular spacing is greatly decreased. This compensates for light-scattering caused by fluctuations of the refractive index between cell membranes and cytoplasm.[47,48]

Biochemical Factors

Membrane protein channels maintain osmotic and ionic balance across the lens. The metabolic activity in the lens is directed toward maintaining a reduced state, which shelters the lens crystallins and other cellular components from damage by the UV light and oxidative stress. In addition, due to the avascular nature of the lens, its energy requirements are largely met anaerobically by glycolysis and the pentose phosphate pathway.

Age-related Changes of the Crystallin Lens

Changes in Physical Behavior with Age

With aging and environmental insults such as ultraviolet (UV) light and other oxidative stresses, there is increase in light scattering, coloration, and stiffness of the lens.

Increasing light-scatter: After the age of 40 years, in the absence of cataract, there is a steady increase in the overall light scattering by the lens, which is greatest in the deep cortex, followed by nucleus and lastly in the superficial cortex.[44]

Decreasing elasticity: Accommodation is a function of the lens that allows a change in its shape so as to bring into focus, objects that are close to the eye. It is brought about by a change in the thickness and curvature of the lens, and is induced by ciliary muscle contraction. There is a steady increase in the stiffness of the lens with age, probably starting from birth[49] and eventually results in the condition of presbyopia, which occurs during middle age.

Helmholtz proposed a theory of accommodation in the 19th century, which is still accepted as standard. This theory proposed that ciliary muscle contraction causes a relaxation of the zonules that connect the ciliary body to the lens. This, in turn, causes the curvature of the lens to increase (Fig. 2.12).

Strenk[50] suggested another theory that the causal factor for age-related loss of accommodation amplitude is related to lens thickening. The lens grows mainly in the anterior direction which is accompanied by a displacement of the iris and ciliary muscle and results in muscle contraction being ineffective.

Thus, the factors determining the onset and progression of presbyopia are most likely to be both lenticular (e.g. increases in lens size, stiffness of the lens or lens capsule) and extralenticular (e.g. alterations in the ability of the ciliary muscles to shorten).

Up to the age of about 40 years, the lens nucleus is readily deformable and its stiffness is lower than that of the surrounding cortex; after this age, however, the situation is reversed. By the age of 50 years, ciliary muscle contraction is no longer able to change the shape of the lens.

Changes in the Lens Proteins with Age

Post-translational changes to the lens crystallins: From 10 years to 50 years of age, there is increased modification of crystallins and aggregation of high-molecular-weight and water-insoluble proteins.[51] Changes include thiolation, deamidation, glycation, carbamylation, cys-methylation, phosphorylation, acetylation and also proteolysis, leading to truncation and the release of crystallin fragments.[52]

The lens contains proteasomes, which preferentially degrade and remove oxidized proteins tagged with the protease cofactor ubiquitin.[53] Ubiquitin conjugation activity

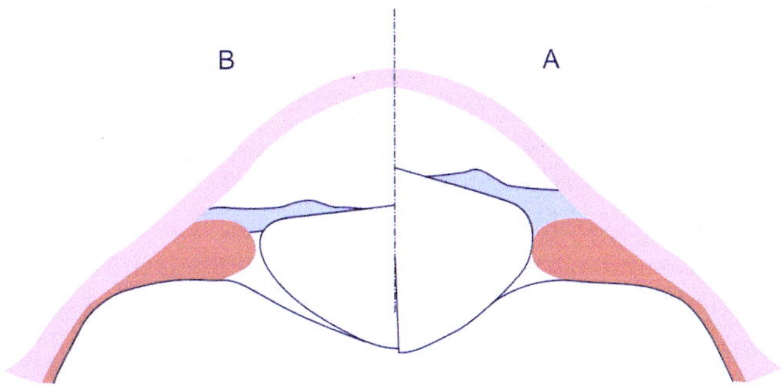

Fig. 2.12: Helmholtz drawing demonstrating his theory of accommodation. The image B shows relaxed accommodation. The image A shows the increase in lens thickness and decrease in equatorial diameter after ciliary muscle contraction.

fails in the ageing lens, thereby leading to the accumulation of oxidized crystallins.[54] This gives rise to aggregation and light-scattering.

Conformational changes: The oxidative insult on unfolded or modified crystallins results in cross-linking, insolubility, and the formation of high-molecular-weight aggregates. This leads to increased light-scatter and progressive hardening, particularly of the lens nucleus. In the nucleus, these changes gradually develop either into a grey-white nuclear opacity, or more often, to a yellow or brunescent nuclear opacity due to the accumulation of fluorescent chromophores.[44]

One major contributor to the accumulation of chromophores is advanced glycation end products (AGEs) that are the outcome of glycation or ascorbylation. Moreover, fluorescent chromophores are formed from tryptophan ("UV filter" compounds) such as GSH-3-OHKG, and 3-hydroxy kynurenine, which form cross-linked derivatives with the crystallins.[44]

Loss of chaperone function: The decline of α-crystallin chaperone activity with age leads to an increased aggregation β and γ crystallins, protein insolubility, light scattering, and loss of lens transparency. By middle age, there is absence of new protein synthesis, thereby leading to depletion of nuclear α-crystallin. The aggregates then contain mainly β- and γ-crystallins. Over time, the nucleus contains a larger proportion of both modified and cross-linked proteins than the cortex. These are precursors of cataract.[44]

Loss of antioxidant and free-radical scavenging capacity: The progressive loss of chaperone function with the process of ageing is accompanied by a corresponding fall in the free-radical scavenging capacity of the lens. The level of reduced glutathione decreases almost linearly with age[55] and the concentration of oxidized glutathione shows a corresponding increase. There is also a progressive fall of cysteine in the nucleus but not in the cortex. Decreases in the activity of these reducing enzymes make the lens vulnerable to oxidative damage, thereby exacerbating damage to crystallins.[56]

Enzymatic activity decreases especially in the central cells of the lens nucleus where the cells are older than those in the cortical nucleus and especially the anterior epithelial cells. This compromised intracellular homeostasis might be exacerbated by the decreased metabolic coupling of the active cortex and the inactive nucleus.[57]

Finally, as the lens ages, intracellular Na^+ and Ca^{2+} concentrations rise due to an increase in lens permeability or decrease in ion channel pumping efficiency.[58]

PHYSIOLOGY OF VITREOUS HUMOR

The vitreous humor is an optically transparent viscoelastic gel which fills the posterior segment of the eye, between the lens and the retina. Its volume is 4 mL which accounts for up to 80% of the volume of the eyeball.[59]

Functions of Vitreous Humor

The functions of the vitreous humor are as described here.

Support Function

The vitreous humor provides mechanical support to neighboring ocular tissues like the ciliary body, retina and lens, by occupying the largest space in the eyeball. Thus, it maintains appropriate ocular morphology and coordinates the growth of the eye.

It acts as an efficient shock absorber against external physical impact due to its viscoelastic properties. Thus it reduces mechanical deformation of the eyeball.[60,61]

Barrier Function

Being a gel, the vitreous has a considerable barrier function for bulk flow of substances between the anterior and posterior parts of the eye. Substances that are liberated from the anterior segment of the eye will not be able to reach high concentrations in the posterior part of the eye because of slow diffusion and limited movement in the gel. For example, topically administered substances are unable to reach the retina and the optic nerve head in significant concentrations. Entry of antibiotics from the bloodstream to the center of the vitreous is also impeded by the normal vitreous gel.[60]

Metabolic Buffer Function

The vitreous provides nutrients for the metabolic requirements of the ciliary body, lens, and especially the retina. Also, by virtue of its large size and central location within the eye, it allows the vascularized retina to be highly oxygenated while protecting tissues such as the lens and trabecular meshwork that are more sensitive to oxidative stress.[60]

Because of the tight blood–retina barrier, water-soluble substances located in the retina have easier access to the vitreous cavity than to the bloodstream when the transport across the barrier is limited.

Glucose and glycogen in the vitreous can supplement the metabolism of the retina, especially during anoxic conditions. The foot plates of the Müller cells also have close contact with the vitreous body. The vitreous body can thus act as a buffer in the physiological function of the Müller cells, for example in the potassium homeostasis of the retina.[62,63]

The mean concentration of ascorbate in the intact vitreous gel has been found to be remarkably high, i.e. approximately 2 mM. Blood levels are only 50–60 µM, thereby making it a 33- to 40-fold increase.[64] The high level of ascorbate in the vitreous is maintained by a sodium-dependent ascorbate transporter (SLC23A2) in the pigmented layer of the ciliary epithelium.[65]

This high ascorbate concentration has been thought to play a pivotal role in the regulation of intraocular oxygen concentration and distribution,[66] by consuming diffusing molecular oxygen before it reaches oxidative sensitive eye structures. Thus it acts as a reservoir of antioxidants in stress situations, protecting the retina from metabolic and light induced free radicals.

Optical Function

The vitreous body allows an unhindered passage of light to the retina. It guarantees this optical transparency by excluding possible interfering components by maintaining a low concentration of structural macromolecules and soluble proteins.[67] The transparency may also be maintained by the specific collagen or hyaluronic acid configuration, in analogy with the cornea. The scattering properties of the vitreous are increased when the vitreous swells.[68]

Age-related Changes in Vitreous Humor

With age, the vitreous body goes through considerable physiological changes like liquefaction and aggregation.[60] Incident light weakens collagen in vitreous through the production of free radicals and modifies the concentrations in glycosaminoglycans and chondroitin sulfate.

The process of vitreous liquefaction is known as synchysis. This process starts at around 4 years of age and progresses as an increase in the volume of vitreous liquid slowly into late age.[69,70] It is especially notable in the center of the vitreous where the collagen concentration is lowest.[71,72.]

The process of vitreous aggregation is known as syneresis. It results due to changes in the chemical or conformational state of hyaluronan and its interaction with collagen. These alterations lead to increased fibril concentration in the residual gel.[73]

PHYSIOLOGY OF RETINA

The retina is responsible for receiving photons of light that are translated into an electrical impulse and transmitted into the brain in order to finally result in the phenomenon of vision. For these events to take place, the major cellular components of the retina that are involved, are the retinal pigment epithelium (RPE), the photoreceptor (PR)cells, the interneurons, the ganglion cells, and the glial cells.

Physiology of Pigment Epithelial Cells

The RPE is a single layer of cuboidal epithelial cells that forms the outermost layer of the retina. It is located between the choriocapillaries and the light-sensitive PR outer segments. There are approximately 4–6 million RPE cells per eye. Although the RPE is not directly involved in vision, its role is essentially supportive. The loss of RPE results in secondary atrophy of adjacent PR and the choriocapillaris, while a healthy RPE is vital for their survival.

The RPE closely interacts with the multilayered Bruch's membrane on the basolateral side and forms the blood-retinal barrier. This is an important physiologic barrier to the free flow of molecules between the leaky choriocapillaris and the PR of the neuroretina. On the apical side, the RPE forms a functional unit with the PR. The ratio of PR cells to RPE cells is approximately 45:1.[74]

The RPE performs the following functions:

- Absorption of scattered light, i.e. role in photoprotection
- Transport of nutrients and ions to PR cells and removal of waste products from PRs, i.e. transport and barrier function
- Visual pigment regeneration, i.e. role in visual cycle
- Phagocytosis of PR outer segments
- Secretion of cytokines and growth factors
- Adhesion of the retina.

Role in Photoprotection

Light energy that is focused by the lens and concentrated onto the retina, is absorbed by melanin pigment in the RPE. This leads to an increase in the temperature of the RPE-choroid complex. The heat is transported away by the bloodstream in the choriocapillaris. But in the choriocapillaris, only small amounts of oxygen are extracted by the adjacent tissues although the choriocapillaris have a high blood perfusion. This leads to the formation of reactive oxygen species that in turn, lead to photo-oxidative damage.[75]

The RPE has three lines of defense against damage caused by scattered light:

1. *Absorption and filtering of light*: Melanin absorbs the scattered light, while pigments like carotenoids, lutein, and zeaxanthin selectively absorb blue light. Blue light is the most dangerous as it leads to the photooxidation of lipofuscin components to toxic substances.
2. *Antioxidants*: The RPE contains high amounts of enzymatic antioxidants, like superoxide dismutase and catalase as well as nonenzymatic antioxidants, like lutein and zeaxanthin, ascorbate, α-tocopherol, and β-carotene.
3. Ability to repair damaged DNA, lipids, and proteins.

Role in Transport

The tight intercellular junctional complexes of the outer blood retinal barrier formed by the RPE hinder the free passage of ions and larger molecules between the choriocapillaris and the RPE. At the same time, the RPE has active and facilitated transport mechanisms for ions and molecules that maintain the extracellular environment of the subretinal space, i.e. the RPE–PR interface.

Ion transport: RPE cells express ion channels on their apical and basolateral surfaces that mediate active transport of Na^+, K^+, Ca^{2+}, HCO_3^- and Cl^-. Na^+ is actively transported from the choriocapillaris toward the subretinal space, whereas K^+ is transported in the opposite direction. The apical membrane of the RPE is the major locus of this transport since the ouabain-sensitive Na^+, K^+-ATPase is present at the apical, but not the basal side. There is also an active bicarbonate-transport system that is associated with both the apical and basal sides of the cell.

Additionally, RPE cells maintain the volume and chemical composition of the subretinal space during the light and dark adaptation. For instance, in the dark, the concentration of K^+ in the subretinal space is approximately 5 mM. Under these conditions, there is a net transepithelial K^+ transport from the subretinal space to the choroid. Whereas with the transition to light, PRs hyperpolarize due to closure of Na^+ channels in the membrane of outer segments and K^+ efflux is diminished. The result is that K^+ concentration in the subretinal space decreases (2 mM) and the RPE apical membrane hyperpolarizes. But with the activation of K^+ channels and reversal of the Na^+-K^+-$2Cl^-$ cotransporter, movement of K^+ across the RPE changes direction so as to re-establish subretinal K^+ concentrations.

The ionic differences between the cytoplasm and the surrounding tissues results in a potential difference across the RPE cell. This transepithelial potential (~5–15 mV)[75] is the basis for the electrooculogram (EOG), which is the most common electrophysiologic test for evaluating the RPE.[76]

Transport of other molecules: The RPE eliminates waste produced by PRs such as lactic acid via a lactate–H^+ cotransporter, MCT1, in the apical membrane, and MCT3, in the basal membrane. Glucose is delivered from blood to PRs via its glucose transporters, GLUT1 and GLUT3. While, vitamin A is transported from the blood into the RPE.[77]

Fluid transport: The ion pumps help in the apposition of neural retina and RPE by keeping the subretinal space dehydrated. The RPE cell manages the subretinal volume by active water removal from the subretinal space via ion channels like the apical Na^+, K^+, $2Cl^-$ channel, basal Cl^- channels, and the H^+/lactate cotransporter. Recently, aquaporin 1, a membrane protein has also been identified to serve as a channel for water transport. RPE is estimated to transport water at a rate of 1.4 to 11 $\mu L\ cm^{-2}\ h^{-1}$.[78]

The transepithelial transport of ions, particularly Cl^-, in an apical to basal direction drives the movement of water through the water channels. This ionic movement is powered by the Na^+ gradient that is maintained by the Na^+-K^+-ATPase pump. Bicarbonate (HCO_3) transport can also provide an impetus for fluid elimination. In the dark, oxygen consumption by PR cells is considerably increased and the carbon dioxide (CO_2) and water that is produced proportionally, is transferred to the choriocapillaris by the RPE so as to prevent acidosis of the subretinal space. CO_2 can enter the RPE cell from the subretinal space both by diffusion across the RPE apical membrane and by carbonic anhydrase-mediated conversion to HCO_3 in the apical membrane followed by transmembrane transport via the electrogenic Na^+-HCO_3 cotransporter. The efflux of HCO_3 basolaterally is followed by fluid transport from the subretinal space to the choroid.[77]

The forces driving the fluid movement across the retina include IOP, osmotic or oncotic pressure, and the active solute-linked fluid transport by the RPE monolayer.

Role in Visual Cycle

Along with the PRs, the RPE plays a crucial role in the visual cycle (Fig. 2.13) by acquiring, storing, and mobilizing vitamin A.

Retinol (vitamin A) is an essential vitamin that humans cannot synthesize de novo. Therefore, it has to be supplied in the diet. It is stored in the liver and transported in the blood by a carrier protein called serum retinol-binding protein (RBP). The RPE cell absorbs retinol from the choroidal circulation across the basal surface and supplies the PRs via its apical surface.

In the RPE, retinol is converted to retinyl ester in the presence of the enzyme lecithin retinol acyltransferase (LRAT). Thus, all-*trans*-retinol is esterified to yield all-*trans*-retinyl esters (all-*trans*-RE), which are the substrates for RPE65 isomerase. RPE65 isomerase isomerizes the all-*trans*-RE to 11-*cis*-retinol, which is bound by cellular retinaldehyde-binding protein. This is reduced to 11-*cis*-retinal and transferred to the interphotoreceptor matrix (IPM) where it binds to interphotoreceptor binding protein (IRBP) and is translocated to the PRs.

In the PRs, 11-*cis*-retinal binds to the visual pigment (rhodopsin in rods and cone opsins in cones) to initiate the visual cycle. During phototransduction, absorption of light results in irreversible isomerization of 11-*cis*-retinal to all-*trans*-retinal. All-*trans*-retinal in the disk space is transported to the extradiscal space by an ATP-binding cassette protein (ABCR), known as ABCA4.

All-*trans* retinal leaves the disk membrane as N-retinylidene-phosphatidylethanolamine (N-retinylidene-PE) by the transport activity of ABCR4. Released from N-retinylidene-PE, all-*trans* retinal is reduced to all-*trans* retinol by RDH (all-*trans* retinol dehydrogenase), leaves the PR outer segments into subretinal space, is loaded onto the IRBP (IPM retinal binding protein) and transported to the RPE. In the cytosol of the RPE it binds to the CRBP (cellular retinol binding protein) and thus the cycle continues.[74,75,77,79,80] This pathway accounts for the reisomerization of retinal from rods. Cones might have an additional secondary pathway involving Müller cells.

Role in Phagocytosis

The PR outer segments are vulnerable to photo-oxidation due to constant exposure to light radiation, high levels of oxygen, and because they contain a very high proportion of polyunsaturated fatty acids mainly docosahexaenoic acid (DHA). Furthermore, photosensitizers like bisretinoid compounds that are the precursors of RPE lipofuscin, oxidatively damage protein and lipid. Also, as PRs do not contain the detoxifying enzyme glutathione reductase, they are under constant stress from free radical attack.[74,75,77,79,80]

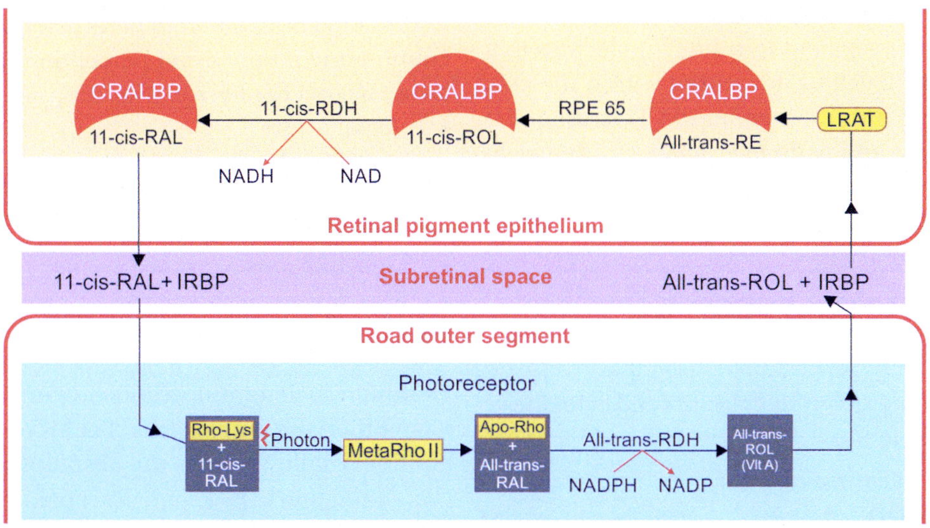

Fig. 2.13: Schematic diagram of the rod visual cycle.

(CRALBP: Cellular retinaldehyde-binding protein; IRBP: Interphotoreceptor retinoid binding protein; LRAT: Lecithin retinol acyltransferase; RDH: All trans retinol dehydrogenase; Rho: Rhodopsin; RAL: Retinal; ROL: Retinol; RE: Retinyl ester; Lys : Lysine; NAD: Nicotinamide adenine dinucleotide; NADP: Nicotinamide adenine dinucleotide phosphate; NADH: Reduced NAD; NADPH: Reduced NADP)

Thus, in order to maintain the excitability of the PR, the outer segments' oxidized membrane are shed and compensated by the addition of newly synthesized cellular components which maintains the cell at a constant overall length. The apical stacks of disks that are shed are ingested and degraded by RPE cells. This process of membrane turnover through phagocytosis is essential to the survival of both RPE and PR since from the ingested DHA, RPE synthesize neuroprotectin 1, a bioactive substance providing protection from oxidative insult.[76]

It has been calculated that each rod regenerates its outer segment within 7–12 days.[76] Each PR cell sheds approximately 100 outer segment disks per day. Because many PRs interdigitate with a single RPE cell, each RPE cell ingests or digests more than 4,000 disks daily.[79]

Phagocytosis may be triggered by the length of the outer segment, or the light-induced oxidized tips of outer segment. It then goes through the following stages: shedding, binding to RPE, internalization, migration to the basal cytoplasm, and digestion.[80]

The process of regeneration follows a circadian rhythm. In rods, shedding is most vigorous within 2 hours of light onset and in cones, shedding occurs most vigorously at the onset of darkness. The neurotransmitter dopamine acts within the PR-RPE complex to control disk shedding.[79] The shed outer segment disks are encapsulated within phagosomes, and transported basally. Then, a lysosome-phagosome interaction takes place in two steps. First, smaller lysosomes fuse with phagosomes. Subsequently, larger lysosomes interact with phagosomes via pore-like structures. Following fusion, lysosomal enzymes hydrolyze the sequestered outer segment into small molecules that diffuse out of the RPE cell or are reused within the cell. Of all the lysosomal enzymes, cathepsin D is the most important.[77] With age and pathologic changes, lipofuscin granules composed of rod outer segment residue are formed within the phagolysosomes.

Secretion of Cytokines and Growth Factors

The RPE secretes numerous growth factors and cytokines[77] that are summarized in Box 2.4 along with their functions.

Box 2.4: Growth factors produced by retinal pigment epithelium.

Neuronal growth factors:
- Pigment epithelial derived factor (PEDF)
- Nerve growth factor (NGF)
- Brain-derived neurotrophic factor (BDNF)
- Insulin-like growth factor (IGF-1)
- Neurotrophin-3 (NT-3)
- Neuroprotectin-1
- Interleukin-6

Cellular growth factors:
- Transforming growth factor-β (TGF-β)
- Granulocyte-macrophage colony-stimulating factor (GM-CSF)
- Monocyte chemotactic protein-1 (MCP-1)
- Hepatocyte growth factor (HGF)
- Erythropoietin (EPO)
- Platelet-activating factor (PAF)
- Fibroblast growth factor (FGF)
- Interleukin-6 and 8

Vascular growth factors:
- Vascular endothelial growth factor (VEGF)
- Endothelin-1
- Interleukin-6

Retinal Adhesion

During early development, the pigment epithelium and neurosensory retina are separated and although the subretinal space has no firm attachments, yet, the neural retina remains firmly adherent to the RPE throughout life.

This is mainly due to the fact that the RPE provides the pump function that keeps the subretinal space dehydrated, thereby maintaining the normal apposition of the neuroretina with the RPE. Other systems that keep the retina in place include passive hydrostatic forces, interdigitation of outer segments, and RPE microvilli, and the viscous binding properties of the IPM.[79]

Physiology of Neurosensory Retina

The neurosensory retina is responsible for integrating information from different parts of the visual pathway, and culminating it into visual perception. Its function can be tested by psychophysical tests such as:
- Visual acuity
- Visual field
- Contrast sensitivity
- Color vision
- Light and dark adaptation.

Visual Acuity

The ability to determine whether or not an object is present in an otherwise empty visual field is termed visibility. The limit of visibility reflects the absolute threshold of vision. Discrimination of two spatially separated targets is termed resolution. Measurement of the threshold of discrimination is essentially an assessment of the function of the foveola centralis and is termed visual acuity.

Thus, to determine visual acuity, the ability to resolve fine detail in a pattern, is tested by reducing the size of the test pattern until the smallest detail in the pattern can just be resolved. Visual acuity can be expressed numerically in terms of the reciprocal of the size of the smallest resolvable detail.

The distance between the two targets is specified by the angle subtended at the nodal point of the eye. The normal angular threshold of discrimination for resolution measures approximately 30–60 sec arc.

Visual acuity has many components that help to measure visual function. The following are definitions of terms used in the measurement of visual function.

- The *minimum legible threshold* refers to the point at which a patient's visual ability cannot further distinguish progressively smaller letters or forms from one another; Snellen visual acuity is the most common method of determining this threshold.[81]
- The *minimum visible threshold* is the minimum brightness of a target at which the patient can distinguish the target from the background.[81]
- The *minimum separable threshold* refers to the smallest visual angle formed by the eye and two separate objects at which a patient can discriminate them individually.[81]
- *Vernier acuity* is defined as the smallest detectable amount of misalignment of two line segments.[81]

In order to determine visual acuity, clinical tests measure the form sense or reading ability of the eye. Following are the tests for visual acuity:

- *Snellen's test types*: The distant central visual acuity is tested by Snellen's test types. The test letters (optotypes) are constructed such that each letter as a whole subtends an angle of 5 minutes of arc (arcmin) at the nodal point of the eye, whereas each stroke of the letter subtends 1 arcmin at the nodal point. Letters of different sizes are designated by the distance at which the letter subtends an angle of 5 arcmin (Fig. 2.14).[81]

  The Snellen chart is designed to measure visual acuity in angular terms.

  However, the accepted convention does not specify visual acuity in angular measure; instead, it uses a notation in which the numerator is the testing distance (in feet or meters) and the denominator is the distance at which a letter subtends the standard visual angle of 5 arcmin. Thus, on the 20/20 line (6/6 in meters), the letters subtend an angle of 5 arcmin when viewed at 20 ft (6 m).

  On the 20/40 (6/12) line, the letters subtend an angle of 10 arcmin when viewed at 20 ft, or 5 arcmin when viewed at 40 ft. The "40" in the 20/40 letter (or the "12" in the 6/12 letter) refers to the viewing distance at which this letter subtends the "normal" visual angle of 5 arcmin.

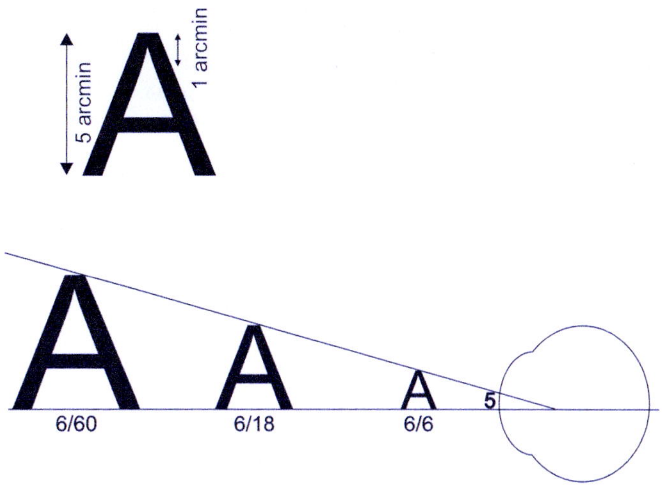

Fig. 2.14: Snellen letters are constructed such that they subtend an angle of 5 arcmin when located at the distance specified by the denominator. For example, if a Snellen A is 26 mm in height, it subtends 5 arcmin at 18 meters. Correspondingly, a 26-mm letter occupies the 20/60 (6/18) line of the Snellen chart at the standard testing distance of 20 ft (6 m).

- *Landolt's test types*: The test type uses broken circles instead of letters. Each broken ring subtends an angle of 5 arcmin at the nodal point and is constructed similar to letter of Snellen's test types. With Snellen's letters, the end point consists of letter recognition, but with Landolt's rings, it consists of the detection of the orientation of the break in the circle.[81] This method is useful in testing illiterates and children. But since the gap in the ring can be in only four positions, i.e. up, down, left, and right, the subject may makes guesses that may question the accuracy.

  Table 2.2 lists conversions of visual acuity measurements for the various methods in use—the Snellen fraction, decimal notation, visual angle minute of arc, and base-10 logarithm of the minimum angle of resolution (logMAR). LogMAR is useful for determining the mean of Snellen visual acuity in a series.
- *Early Treatment Diabetic Retinopathy Study (ETDRS) and Bailey-Lovie charts*: Although Snellen eye chart is used widely for testing of visual acuity, it suffers from certain shortcomings. The letters on different Snellen lines are not related to one another by size in any geometric or logarithmic sense.[81] Also, certain letters (such as C, D, O, and G) are inherently harder to recognize than others (such as A and J), partly because there are more letters of the alphabet with which they

Table 2.2: Visual acuity conversion chart.

Snellen fraction			
Feet (20/)	**Meters (6/)**	**Decimal notation**	**LogMAR (minimum angle of resolution)**
10	3.0	2.00	−0.30
15	4.5	1.33	−0.12
20	6.0	1.00	0.00
25	7.5	0.80	0.10
30	9.0	0.67	0.18
40	12.0	0.50	0.30
50	15.0	0.40	0.40
60	18.0	0.33	0.48
80	24.0	0.25	0.60
100	30.0	0.20	0.70
120	36	0.17	0.78
150	45.0	0.13	0.88
200	60.0	0.10	1.00

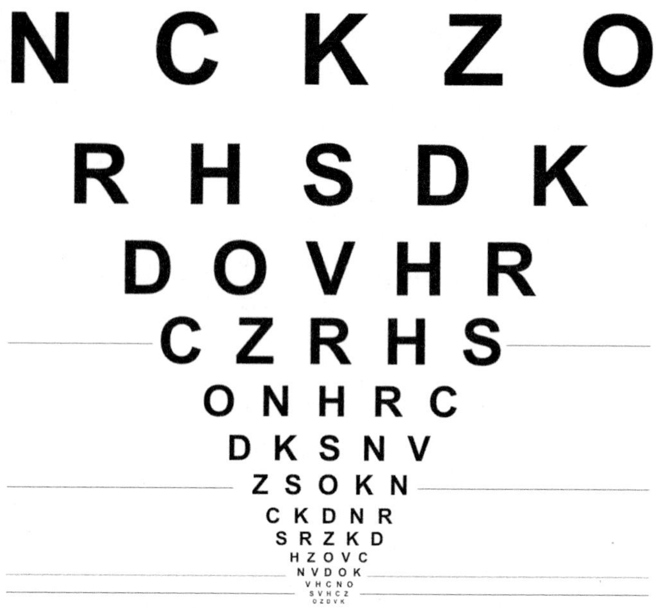

Fig. 2.15: Modified Early Treatment Diabetic Retinopathy Study (ETDRS) visual acuity chart. The chart is intended for use at 20 ft (6 m) but can also be used at 10 ft (3 m) or 5 ft (1.5 m) with appropriate scaling.

can be confused. For these reasons, alternative visual acuity charts like ETDRS (Fig. 2.15) or Bailey-Lovie charts have been developed and popularized in clinical trials. ETDRS chart uses the Sloan letter set (C, D, H, K, N, O, R, S, V, Z), while the Bailey-Lovie chart uses the British letter set (D, E, F, H, N, P, R, U, V, Z).

These charts have the same number of letters on each line; a constant ratio from one letter size to the next (i.e. each line is a fixed percentage smaller than the previous line); spacing between letters and lines are proportional to letter size, and nearly equal legibility to the optotypes. Each line is proportionally smaller than the preceding line. The constant ratio (logarithmic) size scaling is based on the psychophysical principle that just-noticeable differences and their variability scale logarithmically.

- *Testing in special situations*: Infants and other subjects who have limited capacity to respond to standard acuity charts require objective form of testing such as visual-evoked potentials (VEP), optokinetic nystagmus (OKN), and preferential looking (PL). For preschool children, various symbol and picture charts can be used to test vision.
- *Testing for near vision*: Near vision is tested by asking the patient to read a near vision chart which consists of a series of different sizes of optotypes arranged in increasing order and marked accordingly.
- *Jaeger's chart*: This chart was originally devised using ordinary printers' fonts of varying sizes, but was later modified to various sizes of modern fonts. In this chart, prints are marked from 1 to 7 and accordingly subject's acuity is labeled as J1 to J7 depending on the print read by the subject .
- *Roman test types*: To overcome the problem of font in Jaeger's charts, the Roman test type was developed that consisted of "Times Roman" type fonts with standard spacing. According to this chart, the near vision is recorded as N5, N6, N8, N10, N12, N18, N36, and N48.

Visual Field

The classic description of the visual field, given by Traquair (1875–1954), is "an island hill of vision in a sea of darkness".[83] The island of vision is usually described as a three-dimensional graphic representation of differential light sensitivity at different positions in space (Fig. 2.16A: Hill of vision). The shape of the normal visual field is oval. There is decreasing sensitivity with increasing eccentricity in the field, as the elevation corresponds to the sensitivity of the field, and the flat plane corresponds to location within the field. Visual acuity is sharpest at the very top of the hill (i.e. the fovea) and then declines progressively toward the periphery, the nasal slope being steeper than the temporal. From the point of fixation, the field extends 60° superiorly, 60° nasally, 70–75° inferiorly, and 100–110° temporally.

The blind spot is represented as a "bottomless pit" in the hill and is located temporally between 10° and 20, slightly below the horizontal.[83]

An isopter is a line connecting points of the same sensitivity, on a two-dimensional isopter plot encloses an area within which a stimulus of a given strength is visible.[83] An isopter plot of the right eye is shown in Figure 2.16B.

Testing of visual field: Perimetry is used to test the boundary of the hill of vision by systematically measuring the level of light sensitivity in the visual field.

Qualitative technique:

- *Confrontation test*: In severe retinal diseases, the vision may be extremely poor. In such instances visual fields may be obtained only by confrontation testing. Confrontation testing is performed with the examiner facing the patient, usually at about an arm's length. The peripheral vision of the patient is evaluated in relation to that of the examiner's. To test the patient's right eye, the examiner occludes the right eye and aligns the left eye so that both patient and examiner share a common visual axis. The examiner then moves the hand or test object from outside the field of vision toward the center of fixation. Relative preservation of peripheral vision can be established if the examiner places both hands or two test objects in different seeing quadrants of the patient and asking the patient to identify the clearer object. Central visual function is estimated by having the patient look toward the examiner's nose or, if vision is very poor, toward the direction of the examiner's voice. The patient describes which parts of the examiner's face are missing or most clearly seen.[84]
- *The Amsler grid test*: This test is useful for the evaluation of central 10° of vision in patients with macular degeneration or other progressive macular pathologies. There are seven variations of this chart, but in its original form, the subject fixates on the center dot of a white grid on a black background from a distance of 35.5 cm (14 inches) (Fig. 2.17). The patient describes the appearance of the grid pattern, especially in regard to missing areas (scotomata) and distortion (metamorphopsia). The sensitivity for detection of macular lesions can be increased with the use of red grids with or without the use of crossed polarizing lenses to decrease the light entering the patient's eye.[84]

Quantitative technique:

- *Kinetic perimetry using a Goldmann-type bowl perimeter*: Kinetic perimetry is a two-dimensional

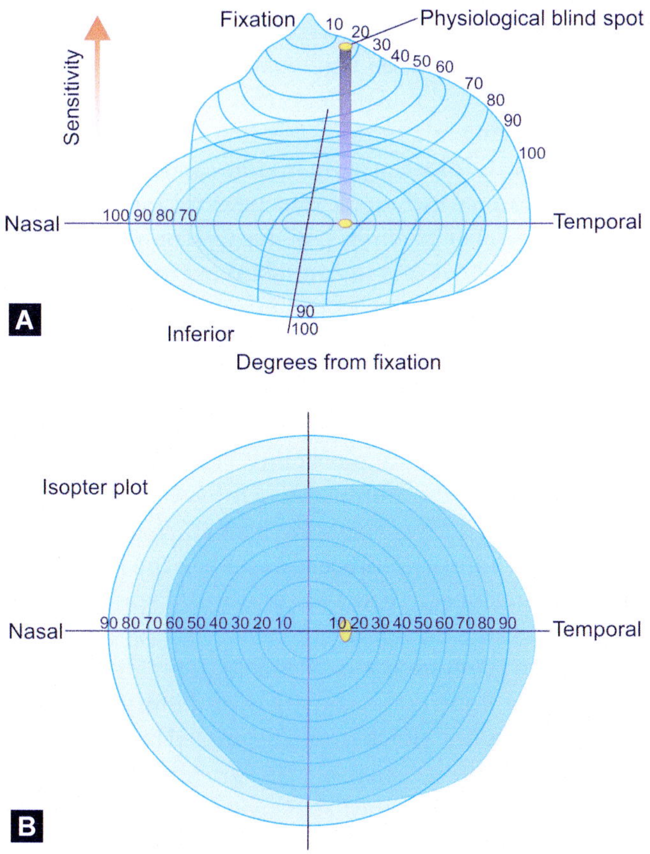

Figs. 2.16A and B: (A) Hill of vision; (B) Isopter plot.

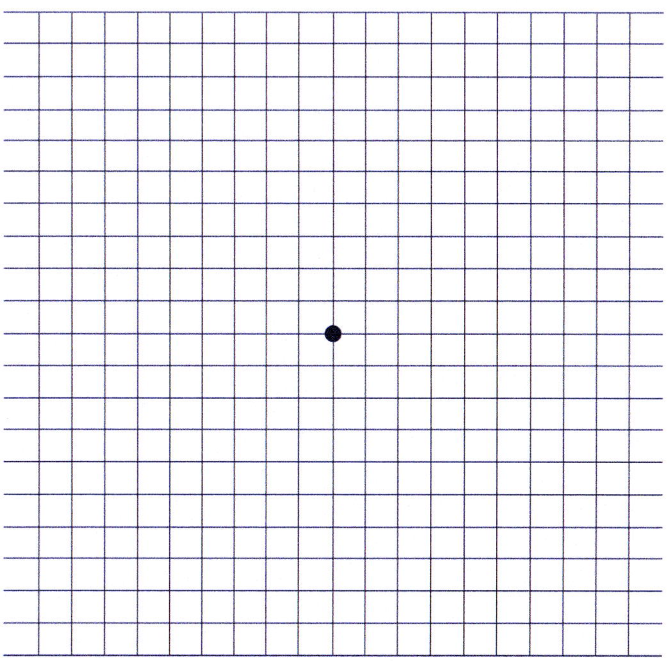

Fig. 2.17: The Amsler grid.

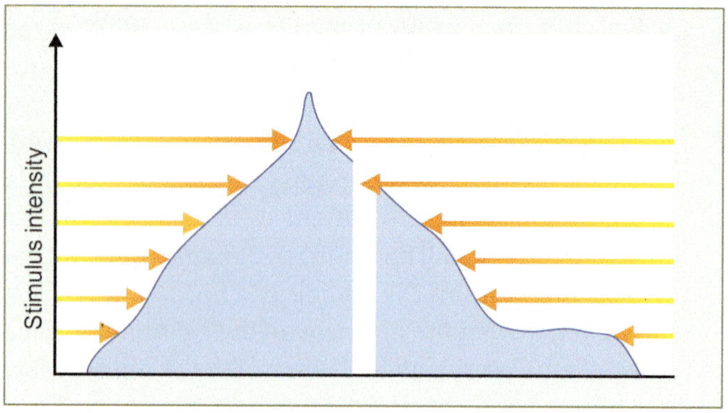

Fig. 2.18: Principle of kinetic perimetry.

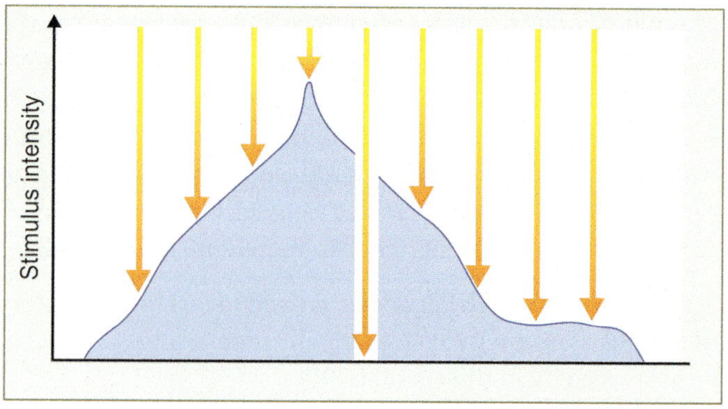

Fig. 2.19: Principle of static perimetry.

assessment of the visual field. A moving stimulus of known luminance or intensity from a non-seeing area to a seeing area is presented to the subject until it is perceived (Fig. 2.18). The stimulus is moved at a steady speed along various meridia (clock hours) and the point of perception is recorded on a chart. By joining these points along different meridians, an isopter is plotted for that stimulus intensity. Using stimuli of different intensities a contour map of the visual field with several different isopters can be plotted.[83]

- *Automated static perimetry using a bowl perimeter or video monitor*: A stimulus fixed at a certain location within the field is presented to the subject. The intensity of the stimulus is increased until it is seen by the subject (or decreased until it is no longer seen). In other words, the target intensity is increased (or decreased) until threshold is reached (Fig. 2.19). The most frequently used automated perimeter is the Humphrey Field Analyzer (HFA).[83]
- *Microperimetry*: It is a relatively new methodology for assessing visual fields that is especially helpful for evaluating and following macular disease. It is used to correlate anatomic pathology with function of the central visual field by combining fundus imaging, retinal sensitivity mapping, and fixation analysis while measuring computerized threshold perimetry at specific locations in the fundus.

There are two methods in microperimetry. In the first technique, a scanning laser ophthalmoscope is used to plot field defects within geographically defined regions of the retina. In the second technique, an infrared fundus camera that provides a 45° view and performs perimetry using a liquid crystal display with a special software. It also allows for eye tracking and color fundus image acquisition. Both the techniques have kinetic and static perimetric testing of the macula and permit simultaneous observation of the retina during perimetric testing. Similar to conventional perimetry, stimulus sizes range from Goldmann size I to V and the central 15–20° of visual field can be tested in both devices, although the second technique allows for a slightly larger field for testing.[84]

Contrast Sensitivity

The Snellen chart tests the visual acuity based on the ability to perceive sharp outlines of relatively small objects. It does not measure the ability to perceive subtleties of light and dark luminance between regions which are not separated by definite borders. Two patients can have the same acuity and yet have different middle- and low-frequency contrast sensitivities. The differences in middle- and low-frequency sensitivity can have dramatic effects on the patients' visual performances. For example, patients with only slight losses in acuity but with losses in contrast sensitivity over a wide range of spatial frequencies can experience difficulties in reading.[85]

Testing of contrast sensitivity function: Contrast sensitivity tests that have been developed primarily for clinical use include the functional acuity contrast test (FACT, replacement for the popular Vistech VCTS chart) and the CSV-1000, sine-wave grating tests in chart form, and various low-contrast optotype tests such as the Lea test, the Pelli–Robson letter chart, the Melbourne Edge Test, and the Mars Letter Contrast Sensitivity Test.[85]

In sine-wave grating tests, visual dysfunction can cause reductions in contrast sensitivity over a limited range of spatial frequencies, which would be missed by more global measures of contrast sensitivity like optotypes. On the other hand, in optotypes contrast sensitivities at specific spatial frequencies tend to be highly correlated with one another, and overall changes in contrast sensitivity are clinically more relevant than subtle changes in the contrast function that are subclinical.

- *Sine-wave grating test*: Contrast sensitivity is mostly related to spatial frequency, which refers to the width of the light-dark grating. To test the eye's ability to process spatial information, the observer is presented with a periodic pattern, usually a sine-wave grating of parallel light and dark bands, and is expected to adjust the contrast of the target until it can be just detected. When the observer is unable to resolve the grating frequency below a certain level, it is known as the threshold level, and the reciprocal of this contrast threshold gives the contrast sensitivity. Contrast sensitivity is then plotted as a function of the grating fineness, with the fineness of the grating expressed in terms of the number of bars in 1° of visual angle (cycles/degree). Because one cycle of a grating contains a dark and a light bar, a 30 cycles/degree grating has bars that subtend 1 minute of arc and corresponds in size to the strokes in the 20/20 letter. A high spatial frequency is implied by narrow bars, while a low spatial frequency is implied by wide bars. Individuals are normally most sensitive to contrast for objects that have a spatial frequency between 2 cycles and 5 cycles per degree, but this sensitivity can change in disease.[79]
- *Pelli-Robson contrast sensitivity chart*: This test uses letters or optotypes of varying dimness and size. It measures contrast sensitivity using a single, large letter size (20/60 optotype), with contrast varying across groups of letters (Fig. 2.20). The letters on the chart are organized as triplets, there being two groups of triplets on both sides.

Subjects read the letters, starting with the highest contrast, and continue until they are unable to read 2 or 3 letters in a single group. The subject is assigned a score based on the contrast of the last group in which 2 or 3 letters were correctly read.

The Pelli-Robson score is a logarithmic measure of the subject's contrast sensitivity. Thus, a score of 2.0 means that the subject was able to read at least 2 of the 3 letters with a contrast of 1% (contrast sensitivity = 100%, or $\log_{10} 2$); in other words, a score of 2.0 indicates normal contrast sensitivity of 100%. A Pelli-Robson contrast sensitivity score of less than 1.5 is consistent with visual impairment, and a score of less than 1.0 represents visual disability.

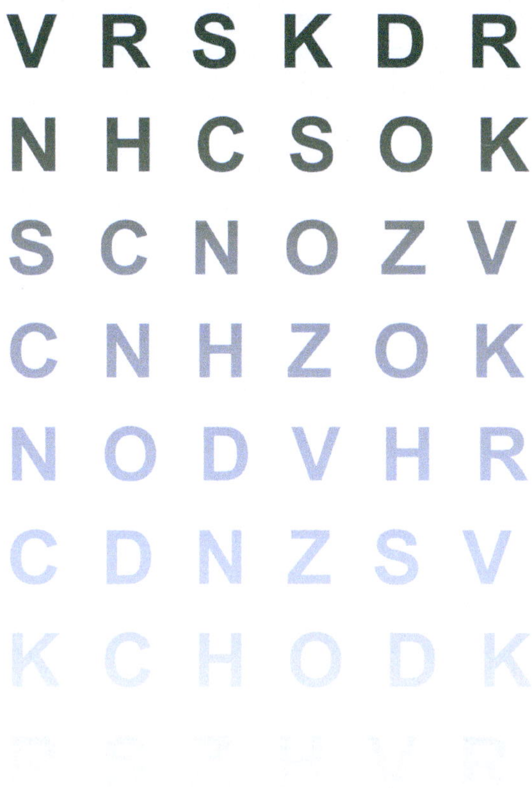

Fig. 2.20: Pelli-Robson contrast sensitivity chart.

Color Vision

Color can be described in terms of hue (determined by wavelength) and a degree of saturation (determined by the amount of white light mixed in). Two colored lights are complementary if their superimposition produces white. The perception of colors of objects depends on the spectral variations in light absorbed by the cone PRs, spectral composition of the light reflected from the object, and the state of light adaptation of the eye.

Theories of color vision:

- *Trichromatic theory*: The concept of trichromacy was first elaborated by Young in 1802. This was subsequently modified by Helmholtz. According to this theory, the human retina has three types of cone PRs that are responsible for trichromatic color vision: short-wavelength sensitive (S cone; blue), medium-wavelength (M cone; green), and long-wavelength sensitive (L cone; red) cones. Thus, a given color is an admixture of the three primary colors in different proportions. Loss of function of each individual cone class is associated with an inherited form of color vision deficiency: protan defects involve loss of L cone function, deutan defects with loss of M cone function, and tritan defects with loss of S cone function. Each type of color vision defect results from rearrangements, deletions, or mutations in the genes encoding the corresponding L, M, or S photopigment.

The gene for human rhodopsin is located on chromosome 3 and the gene for blue sensitive cone is located on chromosome 7. The genes for the red and green sensitive cones are arranged on the q arm of the X chromosome.[86]

- *Opponent color theory*: Hering suggested that some colors appear to be mutually exclusive; for instance, there is no color such as reddish green. This observation cannot be explained by the presence of three types of cone PRs. The neural circuitry for color vision extracts signals from just three cone types, but gives rise to six hues arranged in opponent pairs: blue-yellow, red-green, and black-white. Thus these "cone-opponent" cells increase their firing rate of receptor potential signals above baseline to activate one cone class and decrease their firing rate of receptor potential signals below baseline to activate a different cone class. For blue-yellow opponency, signals from S cones are combined antagonistically with an additive signal from M and L cones, abbreviated as S-(M+L); and for red-green opponency, signals from L cones are combined antagonistically with those from M cones (abbreviated as L-M). However, color vision testing in humans has established that the spectral signatures of hue perception actually involve contributions from all three cone types in the following manner: blue = (S+M)-L; yellow = L-(S+M); red = (S+L)-M; and green = M-(S+L).[86]

Long-to-middle wavelength sensitive cone type causes every midget ganglion cell in the retina, as well as the cells they project to in lateral geniculate nucleus (LGN), to respond to either spatially uniform red or green lights in addition to dark-light edges. Thus the red-green system outputs of the L and M cones constitute about 95% of the cone population, while the blue-yellow system is considered to be centered on the remaining 5% of cones, i.e. the S cones. Because an imbalance seems inherently implausible based on the similar perceptual acuities of both color systems, it has been proposed that the preponderance of L/M cones indicates that these cone types alone are used for luminance (dark-light) detection, suggesting that only a fraction of the spectrally opponent information from L/M cones actually contributes to color vision.

Also, at the level of the cortex, most of the chromatic signals become subtracted-out and disregarded, perhaps by a second round of lateral antagonism that is analogous to horizontal cell interactions at the level of the retina. This leads to the achromatic luminance circuitry or the black-white circuitry.

Neurophysiology of color vision:

- *Genesis of visual signals in cone photoreceptors*: The photochemical changes in the cone pigments produce visual signal in the form of cone receptor potential.
- *Processing and transmission of color vision signals in the retina*: The action potential generated in the PRs is transmitted by electronic conduction to the other cells of the retina across the synapses of PRs, bipolar cells, and horizontal cells and then across the synapses of bipolar cells, ganglion cells, and amacrine cells.
- *Ganglion cell color coding*: A single ganglion cell may be stimulated by a number of cones or by a few or even single cone. When all three types of cones (red, green, and blue) stimulate the same ganglion cell, the resultant signal is white. Some of the ganglion cells are excited by one color type of cone (e.g. red) and are inhibited by other (e.g. green) or vice versa. This system is called opponent color coding system.

  These ganglion cells also have a system of double opponent cells which have a receptive field with a center and concentric surrounding area. Here, in response to one color (e.g. red) in the center, the response may be "on" and "off" to it, in the surrounding area. At the same time, the response may be "off" to the color (e.g. green) in the center and "on" to it in the surrounding area.[86]
- *Processing of color signals in lateral geniculate body (LGB)*: Color information carried by the ganglion cell is relayed to the parvocellular portion of the LGB.

  Spectrally nonopponent cells which give the same type of response to any monochromatic light constitute about 30% of the LGB neurons.

  Spectrally opponent cells make up to 60% of LGB neurons. These cells are excited by some wavelengths and inhibited by others. These have been classified into four types:
  - Cells having red and green antagonism with +R/-G
  - Cells having red and green antagonism with +G/-R
  - Cells having blue and yellow antagonism with +B/-Y
  - Cells having blue and yellow antagonism with +Y/-B.
- *Analysis of color signals in the visual cortex:* Tests of color information from the parvocellular portion of the LGB are relayed up to the primary visual cortex (V1).

From V1, the signals are processed by the second visual area (V2); then by cells located in subcompartments ("globs") within the posterior inferior temporal (PIT) cortex, a brain region that encompasses area V4 and regions immediately anterior to V4. Color signals are then processed by regions deep within the inferior temporal (IT) cortex. Double-opponent neurons in the V1 generate local color contrast and are the building blocks for color constancy; glob cells elaborate the perception of hue; and IT integrates color perception in the context of behavior.[87]

Color deficiency: The term color blindness is unfortunate because it implies an inability to see colors. Most individuals with color deficiency can distinguish a great many colors but interpret them differently. If the ability to appreciate one or more primary colors is defective, the suffix used is *anomalous* and if absent, then the suffix used is *anopia.*

Classification of color deficiency:

- *Inherited*:
  - *Anomalous trichromacy*: It is the most common type of deficiency in which the affected individual has three cone pigments but one of them is abnormal.
    1. *Protanomaly*: Refers to defective red color appreciation
    2. *Deuteranomaly*: Refers to defective green color appreciation
    3. *Tritanomaly*: Refers to defective blue color appreciation.
  - *Dichromats*: They have only two cone pigments and thus cannot distinguish certain colors.
    - *Protanopia*: Refers to complete absence of red color appreciation
    - *Deuteranopia*: Refers to complete absence of green color appreciation
    - *Tritanopia*: Refers to complete absence of blue color appreciation.

    The most common forms are the red-green deficiencies, which are transmitted by X-linked inheritance. Impaired blue-yellow color vision defects are relatively rare. Tritan defects display incomplete penetrance, meaning there is variability in the degree to which color vision is impaired among individuals with the same underlying gene defect, even within a family.
  - *Monochromatism or achromatopsia*: This refers to individuals who have only a single cone pigment, or who lack cone pigments altogether (rod monochromatism). Rod monochromats can distinguish colored objects only in terms of brightness and have poor acuity (usually around 20/100 to 20/200) because they lack foveal cones. They are photophobic and even ordinary illumination dazzles them by saturating their rod system. The other features are irregular pendular nystagmus and a normal fundus.
- *Acquired*: Patients with an acquired deficiency may have test results that mimic an inherited deficiency. Particular confusion might occur with cone dystrophies (which can mimic monochromatism in the young) or congenital optic nerve disorders. However, since acquired diseases do not affect only red, green or blue sensitive cones, to the exclusion of others, the test results almost always show irregularities that are not seen in a congenital defect. Retinal diseases like central serous retinopathy, shallow retinal detachment, macular edema, etc. often manifest a relative blue-yellow deficiency while optic nerve disorders such as optic neuritis, Leber's optic atrophy, etc. show a relative red-green deficiency.

Testing of color vision: Color vision tests have been developed to detect changes in the cone complement.

- *Anomaloscope*: It is the most accurate instrument for classifying congenital red-green color defects, but it is not widely used.

  The anomaloscope exploits the observation that, within a narrow range, any two normal observers will accept each other's formula for matching a color. The subject views a split screen and is asked to mix varying proportions of red and green lights to match the appearance of a standard yellow light. Normal viewers and individuals with red-green color deficiency use characteristic proportions of red and green to match the yellow.
- *Pseudoisochromatic plates: Ishihara plates and Hardy-Rand-Rittler plates*: They depict colored numbers or figures that stand out from a background of colored dots (Fig. 2.21).

  The colors of the test figure and background are purposely pale and carefully chosen from hues that are difficult for a color-deficient person to distinguish. Thus individuals with defective color vision see either no pattern at all or an alternate pattern based on brightness rather than hue.

  Ishihara plates assess color discrimination along protan (red) and deutan (green) axes only; while Hardy-Rand-Rittler plates assess color discrimination along protan, deutan, and tritan (blue) axes.

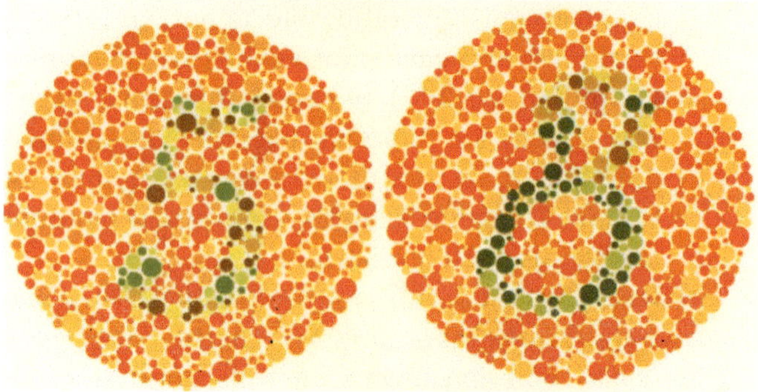

Fig. 2.21: Ishihara pseudoisochromatic plates.

However, these tests are sensitive only for screening color deficient people, and are not effective in classifying a deficiency.[88]

- *Panel tests*: *Farnsworth-Munsell 100 and Farnsworth Panel D-15 hue tests:* These tests are more accurate in classifying color deficiency because the subject's errors can be plotted to define an "axis" of color deficiency.
  The Farnsworth-Munsell (FM) 100-hue test consists of 85 colored tablets that are designed to approximate the minimum difference between hues that a normal observer can distinguish (1–4 nm). The spectrum is divided into four parts, with each part covering one-quarter of the color circle, during testing so that no confusion is possible between red and green or between blue and yellow. A normal observer arranges the tablets in sequence with few errors, but a color deficient subject has trouble with those parts of the spectrum complementary to the subject's deficiency. This occurs because the subtle differences between shades of blue and yellow are determined by the admixture of small amounts of red and green, which are poorly perceived by a red-green deficient subject.
  The 100 hue test is very sensitive to subtle deficiencies but suffers because the test is fatiguing and time-consuming.[88]
  The Farnsworth Panel D-15 test is more rapid and convenient for clinical use because it consists of only a single box of 15 colored tablets. The hues are more saturated and they cover the spectrum so that subjects are free to confuse the major colors for which they have deficient perception such as red and green. The subject is asked to arrange the colors in sequence, and the errors are plotted on a circular diagram to define the nature of the color deficiency. The D-15 test is not sensitive and may miss mildly affected individuals, but its speed and accuracy make it useful.
  Desaturated versions of the D-15 test, which recognize more subtle degrees of color deficiency, are also available. In addition, for patients with reduced visual acuity, enlarged versions (PV-16 tests) are also available.
  The D-15 test is useful in the evaluation of patients with retinal diseases because it enables discrimination between congenital and acquired defects. Individuals with major congenital color deficiencies typically make errors that show a very precise protan or deutan pattern on the D-15 scoring graph, whereas those with acquired optic nerve or retinal disease show an irregular pattern of errors.
  The D-15 test shows errors (blue-yellow confusion) very clearly; these results usually signify acquired disease.
- *The Sloan achromatopsia test* is designed to test for complete achromatopsia. The test consists of seven plates, each with a series of grey rectangles whose reflection increases gradually across the card. In the center of each rectangle appears a colored circle of fixed hue and reflectance. Subjects with complete achromatopsia can find an exact match of the colored circle with one of the rectangles on each card. Subjects who do not have complete achromatopsia can make only a brightness match of the colored circle to a rectangle.[88]
- *Computerized color vision tests*: These tests have been using a similar principle as the plate tests or discrimination ability tests like FM-100 hue test.
  As these tests are automated, they are easy to use. Also, these tests can avoid the issues with the illuminating light that exist for reflective materials because, in order to present the color accurately, the displays are calibrated for spectral distribution measurements and linearization.[88]

Light and Dark Adaptation

The eye possesses mechanisms for adjusting its sensitivity so that the eye can recognize objects both on a sunlit beach and on a cloudy night.

Mechanisms of adaptation:

- *Visual pigment mechanism*: The concentration of the visual pigments within the outer segments affects threshold visual sensitivity and this sensitivity increases as visual pigment regenerates in the dark (Fig. 2.22). This relationship is much more critical for rods than cones.

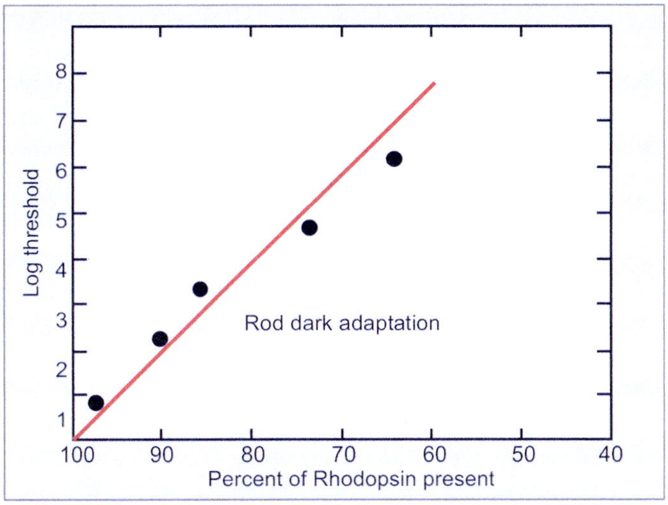

Fig. 2.22: Logarithmic relationship between visual sensitivity (measured as dark-adapted threshold) and concentration of rhodopsin.

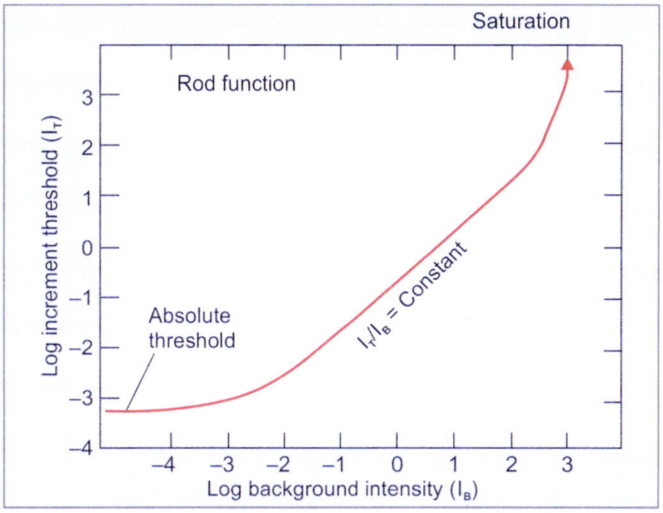

Fig. 2.23: Adjustment of rod increment threshold to different levels of background illumination in human eye. Under very dim conditions, increment and absolute thresholds are equal. At moderate intensities of background, increment sensitivity is a fixed percentage of background intensity. At very bright levels, rods "saturate" and fail to respond further. Cones (not shown) do not saturate but continue to adjust increment sensitivity to higher and higher backgrounds.

However, the relationship between visual sensitivity and pigment concentration accounts for only a portion of our range of sensitivity. For example, the bleaching or regeneration of visual pigment does not explain the adjustments of *increment sensitivity*, which are critical to the vision. The *increment threshold* is the additional light energy necessary just to perceive a difference in illumination—in dim light this energy is low, but in bright light, a large increment of energy is needed before we perceive any change. Adaptation provides a continual adjustment of retinal sensitivity so that the increment threshold remains a relatively constant percentage of the background level (Fig. 2.23).

- *Neural adaptation mechanism*: The adjustment of increment sensitivity and adaptation to bright lights are largely mediated by electrophysiologic changes in the retinal neurons and the synaptic connections. To some degree this is a general property of nerve cells, most of which show a burst of activity that soon fades to a lower level under a constant stimulus. The *adapted* neuron will not show another burst of activity unless the stimulus either increases or stops for a while to let the neuron recover. Another neurologic mechanism of adaptation is feedback inhibition, in which excitation of one cell stimulates other cells that make inhibitory connections to it. Thus, after a few milliseconds of activity, the excitation is turned off by the inhibitory feedback.

  A third mechanism of adaptation lies within the neuron itself, as much of the response to stimulation is nonlinear. For example, doubling the intensity of the stimulus may produce a response less than twice as large, and from a functional standpoint, this lessened response is an adaptation to the stimulus.

Light adaptation: The ability of the visual system to adjust its performance to the ambient level of illumination is known as light adaptation. This adjustment typically occurs very rapidly (within seconds), whether the light intensity is increasing or decreasing.

The bleaching of visual pigment in the light raises the threshold of both rods and cones, but not nearly enough to account for rapid decrease in visual sensitivity that occurs. The role of visual pigments in controlling sensitivity is mainly evident during dark adaptation, in which the slow regeneration of pigment becomes the rate limiting step. But when a light is turned on, the chemical changes are overshadowed by the more rapid neural adjustments, so that the light adaptation is primarily a neural phenomenon. Nonetheless, rod sensitivity (in contrast to that of cones) decreases dramatically as visual pigment is bleached, and loss of only 7% of rhodopsin brings cone function into play (as mesopic or mixed rod and cone vision).

The amplitude of receptor potential is not linearly related to light intensity, but follows an S-shaped function (Fig. 2.24), so it varies most critically near intensities of light that produce a half maximal response.

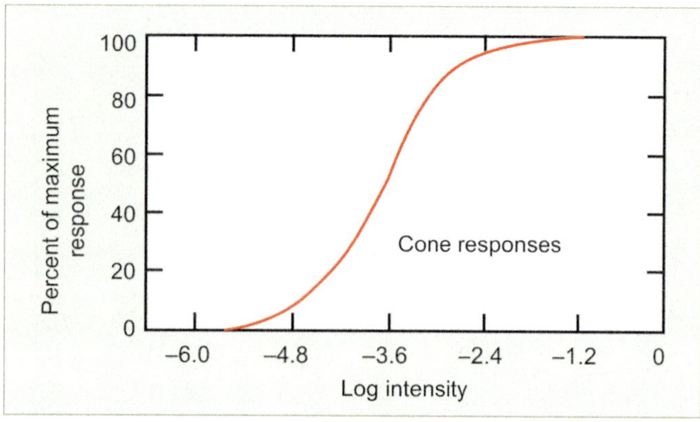

Fig. 2.24: Amplitude of receptor potential of cones to flashes of different intensity. Increasing or decreasing background light would shift this entire curve to right or left.

When a background light is turned on, the entire curve is shifted so that a higher range of intensities produces a most critical response. Thus, the receptor itself provides part of the adjustment of sensitivity and of increment threshold that occurs with the light adaptation. Additional adaptive effects are provided by the horizontal cells (which feedback upon the PRs with inhibitory signals) and probably by other retinal elements.

There are important differences between adaptation properties between rods and cones. Weber's law[89] states that sensitivity varies inversely with the intensity of the illumination. When intensity of illumination increases by, say, a factor of 10, the retinal sensitivity decreases by this same factor, and consequently the neural signal, which depends on the product of retinal illumination by retinal sensitivity, remains unchanged.

However, Weber's law fails when the background becomes so dim that it no longer affects sensitivity. At the other extreme, a bright background can overload the system by *saturation*.

Rods show light adaptation only over a limited range of light sensitivity. Once the light becomes moderately bright, the rod receptor potential *saturates* and fails to respond any further to bright light. Cones, on the other hand, continue to adapt; and to respond; to brighter and brighter light, and thereby completely avoid saturation. Furthermore, each of the three color systems (erythrolabe, chlorolabe, and cyanolabe) seem to be able to adapt independently of one another.

Light adaptation and neural adjustments of sensitivity, which take place rapidly and continuously as our gaze wanders between lighter and darker parts of the scenery, are just as critical to vision as the regeneration of visual pigment.

Consider how dark the inside of a tunnel looks (because we are light adapted) as we approach it on a sunny day, and how dazzled we find ourselves on coming into the sunlight from a cinema theatre. The rod monochromat lives with that disabling dazzle all the time, but the normal individual adjusts rapidly to these changing conditions.

Another important effect of light adaptation is not so obvious. Because the retina adjusts its increment sensitivity to whatever level of background illumination is present, it stops responding to an unchanging level of light. Images must change in intensity or move across the retina to register an impression on the brain, and for this reason, our eyes are never totally motionless. Very fine "microsaccades" take place continuously to move images on the retina. Then why do we not see our retinal blood vessels, which must cast a shadow on the PRs? Because, the retina and vessels always move together, the shadows are constant in location and are not perceived because of adaptation. We can see them by moving a small light close to the eye so that the shadows shift on the PRs.

Dark adaptation: The term "dark adaptation" is the recovery of sensitivity in darkness, following exposure of the eye to extremely bright and/or prolonged illumination that activates (and thereby bleaches) a substantial fraction of the visual pigment, rhodopsin or its cone equivalent. Dark adaptation occurs slowly and full recovery of the scotopic visual system after a very large bleach can take as much as an hour.

It involves a reversal of the mechanisms of light adaptation, but the reverse mechanisms are, in general, less efficient. The regeneration of visual pigment, for example, requires the expenditure of metabolic energy and an exchange of material with the pigment epithelium, whereas bleaching occurs spontaneously within the outer segment once light has been absorbed. Thus, pigment regeneration and photochemical dark adaptation are very slow phenomena in relation to the speed of light adaptation. Even the neural mechanisms of dark adaptation are slower than those of light adaptation, though they are rapid by comparison with pigment regeneration. Ongoing from a bright light to a dim environment, there is a rapid initial adjustment to the dim light that takes place in seconds and represents a reversal of the neural light adaptation of the PRs and other retinal cells. This rapid phase of dark adaptation may account for several log units of increase sensitivity if the initial conditions were very bright, but a point is soon reached at which further increases occurs slowly (over minutes) as the cone and rod visual pigments regenerate.

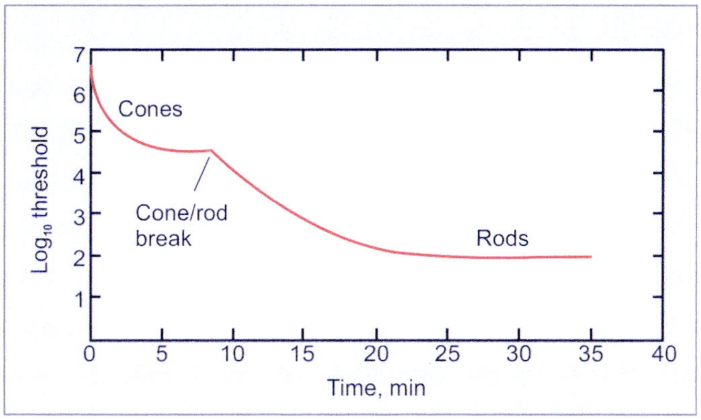

Fig. 2.25: Dark-adaptation testing yields a biphasic curve following preadaptation to bright light.

The relationship of threshold sensitivity to visual pigment concentration is logarithmic and is much more critical for rods than cone. Bleaching 50% of the appropriate pigment elevates the cone threshold by a factor of 30, but it elevates rod threshold by 100 million.

Dark adaptation is most commonly tested with the Goldmann-Weekers adaptometer. The patient is first light-adapted to a bright background light. This light is then extinguished, and the patient, now in the dark, is presented with a series of dim-light targets approximately 11° below fixation. The intensity of the test lights is controlled by neutral-density filters and the threshold at which the test light is first perceived is plotted against time. Under these conditions, the dark-adaptation curve,[89] illustrated in Figure 2.25, shows two plateaus: the first represents the cone threshold, which is usually reached in 5–10 minutes, and the second represents the rod threshold, which is reached after approximately 30 minutes.

The inflection of the dark adaptation curve where the rod limb begins is called the cone-rod break, or alpha point, and it usually occurs after 7–10 minutes of adaptation. The final rod phase of adaptation does not begin until 93% of rhodopsin has already been regenerated. If the test spot is focused on the foveola, where rods are absent, there is only a cone plateau. Dark adaptometry is useful clinically in the evaluation of retinal disorders, and is a necessity for patients complaining of night blindness. The test is subjective, but malingering and poor cooperation are easily recognized.

PHYSIOLOGY OF OCULAR MOVEMENTS

The main function of ocular movements is to precisely align the fovea of both eyes to the object in the visual field. It is important to understand certain terminologies which will help the reader to understand the physiology of ocular movements.

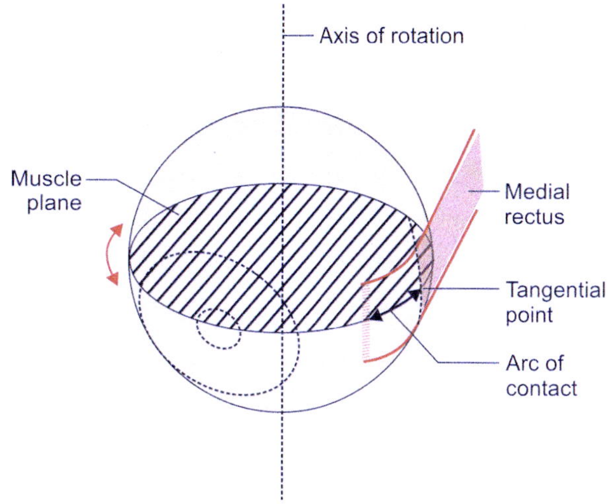

Fig. 2.26: Schematic diagram of muscle plane, rectus muscle, axis of rotation, tangential point, and arc of contact.

Terminologies

Tangential point: The point at which the center of the muscle or its tendon first touches the globe is the *tangential point.* This point indicates the direction of pull of that muscle. The position of this point changes when the muscle contracts or relaxes and the globe rotates (Fig. 2.26).

Arc of contact: It is the arc formed between the tangential point and the center of the insertion of the muscle on the sclera. The arc of contact changes in length as the muscle contracts. It is longest when the muscle is relaxed and shortest when the muscle is contracted.[90]

Muscle plane: It is an imaginary plane which passes through the centers of origin and insertion of the muscles and the center of rotation (Fig. 2.26).[90]

Axis of rotation: It is perpendicular to the muscle plane erected in the center of rotation, corresponds to each muscle plane. When the individual muscle makes an isolated contraction, the eye will rotate around this axis (Fig. 2.26).[90]

Muscle pulleys: The four recti muscles pass through condensations of connective tissue and smooth muscle just posterior to the equator. These condensations include fascial attachments, like anterior and posterior Tenon's capsule and conjunctiva. Although EOMs initiate the movement of the globe, these condensations act as pulleys and control the movements. For example, they stop the vertical movements of the medial and lateral recti muscles during upgaze and downgaze. Likewise, they stop the horizontal movements of the superior and inferior recti muscles in horizontal gazes.

The pull of the muscle on the globe occurs at the point of the insertion of the muscle. The pulling effect on the globe comes from the location of the pulley regardless of where the pull is initiated.

This new "post pulley" concept replaces the earlier held notion that the functional insertion of the EOM was at the point of tangency with the globe, which is anterior to the equator medially and just behind the equator laterally.[2] Thus pulleys act as check ligaments at extreme gazes (Figs. 2.27A and B). The individual muscles work as agonists or antagonists to initiate ocular movement.[90,91]

Agonist: It is the muscle responsible for moving the eye in a given direction. For example, for abduction in the right eye, the right lateral rectus muscle is the agonist.[90]

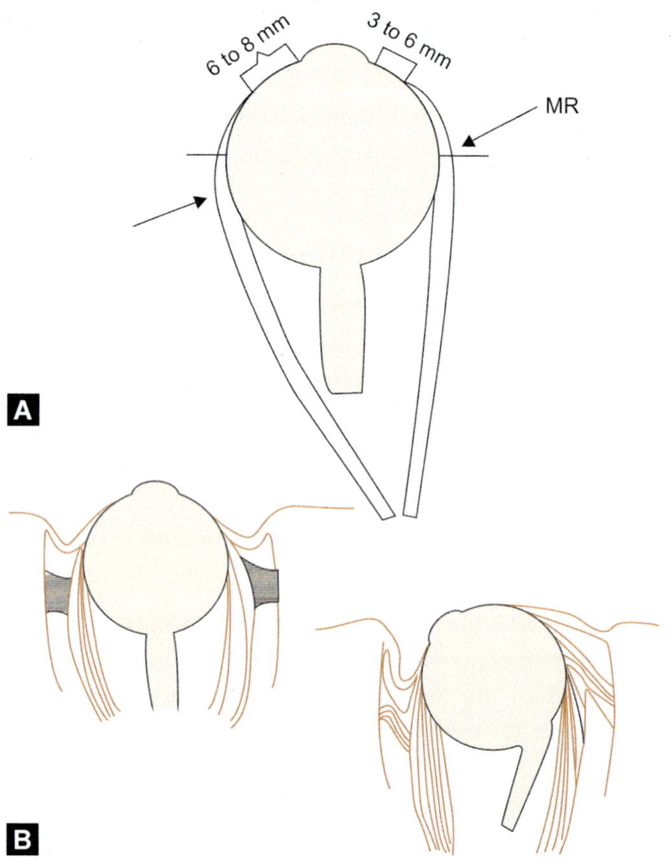

Figs. 2.27A and B: (A) The medial rectus (MR) inserts between 3 mm and 6 mm from the limbus; (B) Position of muscle pulley tissue.

Synergists: Pairs of muscles that move the eye in the same direction are known as *ipsilateral synergists*. For example, an ipsilateral synergist for the right superior rectus is right inferior oblique, both of which act together to move the eye directly up for elevation (Fig. 2.28).[90]

Ipsilateral antagonists: These are the muscles in the same eye with directly opposed main actions. For example, in the right eye these are lateral and medial recti.[90]

Contralateral synergists (also known as yoke muscles): These are pair of muscles (one from each eye) which contract simultaneously during conjugate binocular movements. For example, the contralateral synergist for the right superior rectus is left inferior oblique as both work as a pair to bring about binocular movement of up and to the right.[90]

Positions of Gaze

The positions of gaze determine the effect of extraocular movements, in their main field of action. There are nine positions of gaze that include one primary, four secondary and four tertiary positions.[90]

Primary position of gaze: This is the position of eyes with the individual looking straight ahead at a distant object with accommodation relaxed.

Secondary position of gaze: These are the positions of the eyes that lie along the horizontal or vertical meridian of the globe. The common secondary positions of gaze are elevation, depression, dextroversion, and levoversion.

Tertiary position of gaze: These are the positions assumed by the eyes assumed when combination of vertical and horizontal movements occur. These include dextroelevation, dextrodepression, levoelevation, levodepression, dextrocyclotorsion, and levocyclotorsion.

Cardinal position: Each of the six EOMs has different effects on the rotation based on the relationship between the visual axis of the eye and the orientation of the muscle plane to the visual axis.

In each cardinal position, the angle between the visual axis and the direction of pull of the muscle being tested is minimized. Thus, when the eyes are in one of the six cardinal positions, the ability of each of the six EOMs to move the eye can be isolated.

The six cardinal positions of gaze are: Dextroelevation, dextrodepression, levoelevation, levodepression, dextroversion, and levoversion (Fig. 2.28).

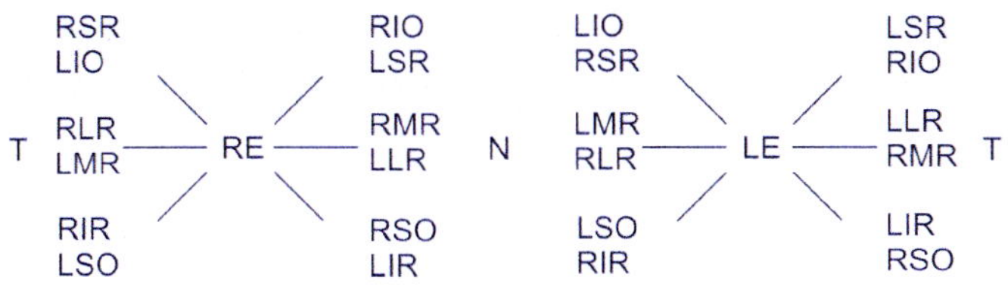

Fig. 2.28: Contralateral synergist muscles in the diagnostic positions of gaze.

Fick's Axis, Listing's, and Donder's Laws

When describing ocular rotations, three orthogonal axes known as *axes of Fick*[90] need to be considered. They enable the movement of the eye around a hypothetical center of rotation placed about 14 mm behind the apex of the cornea, at the intersection of the three axes. Thus, the six EOMs rotate the eye relative to the head about the three axes. The first axis is called the X-axis (also known as horizontal or transverse axis) and it crosses the eye horizontally. The second axis is called the Y-axis (also known as sagittal or anteroposterior axis) and it passes through the center of the pupil (through the "y" sutures of the lens). The third axis is called the Z-axis (also known as vertical axis) and it crosses the eye vertically. Vertical movements take place around the X-axis, torsion takes place around the Y-axis, and medial and lateral rotation takes place around the Z-axis.

However, there occurs a summation of the actions of all of the EOMs and all of the movements of the globe can be assumed to occur in a plane fixed in the orbit that passes through the center of rotation and the equator of the globe when the eye is in primary position. Thus the vertical and the horizontal axes are assumed to lie in this equatorial plane, called the *Listing's plane* (Fig. 2.29).[90]

Listing's law[90] states that virtually all positions of gaze can be achieved by rotations around axes that lie on Listing's plane.

Thus Listing's law reduces the rotational freedom of the eye from three planes (horizontal, vertical, and torsional) to only two planes (horizontal and vertical),[92] i.e. all eye movements from the primary position are true to the meridians and occur without "torsion" or cyclorotation with respect to the primary position.

Donder's law[90] states that there is a specific orientation of the retina and cornea for every position of gaze. This corneal orientation is specific for each position of gaze regardless of the path the eye took to achieve that position of gaze.[91]

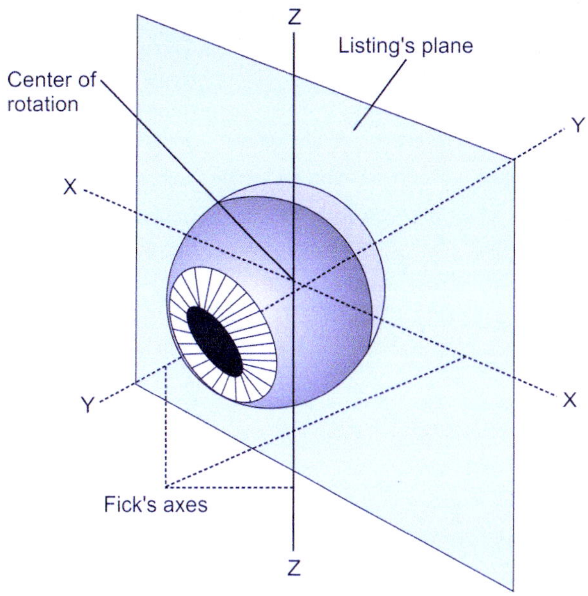

Fig. 2.29: Fick's axes and Listing's plane.

Thus this law implies that only one orientation of the retinal meridians is permissible with each position of the eyes. Thus, each gaze direction corresponds to a unique eye orientation regardless of previous movements and orientations.[93]

Types of Movements

Monocular Eye Movements[94]

Ductions: Ductions are the rotation of a single eye around the axes of Fick.

- *Abduction*: Movement of the eye outward
- *Adduction*: Movement of the eye inward
- *Supraduction (elevation or sursumduction)*: Movement of the eye upward
- *Infraduction (depression or deorsumduction)*: Movement of the eye downward
- *Intorsion (incycloduction)* is defined as a nasal rotation of the superior portion of the vertical corneal meridian
- *Extorsion (excycloduction)* is a temporal rotation of the superior portion of the vertical corneal meridian.

Actions of EOMs (Table 2.3)

- *Horizontal rectus muscles*: In primary position, the axis of rotation of the horizontal recti coincides with the z-axis of the Fick system. Hence, the contraction of one of the horizontal rectus muscles produces only one

Table 2.3: Actions of extraocular muscles.

Muscle	Main action	Secondary actions
Lateral rectus	Abduction	None
Medial rectus	Adduction	None
Superior rectus	Elevation on abduction	Intorsion on adduction
Inferior rectus	Depression on abduction	Extorsion on adduction
Superior oblique	Intorsion on abduction	Depression on adduction
Inferior oblique	Extorsion on abduction	Elevation on adduction

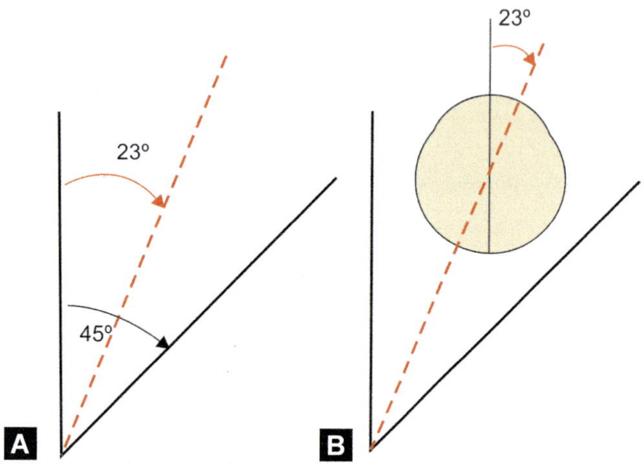

Figs. 2.30A and B: Schematic diagram showing lateral and medial orbital walls at an angle of 45° with each other; (B) Orbital axis forms an angle of 23° with visual axis.

unique primary action around the vertical axis, i.e. the lateral rectus abducts and the medial rectus adducts.[93,94]

- *Vertical rectus muscles*: The orbit forms a pyramid in which the lateral and medial walls are at 45° to each other, and the central axis is thus at 22.5° (approximated to 23°) (Fig. 2.30A). When the eye is looking straight ahead at a fixed point on the horizon with the head erect, i.e. in primary position of gaze, the visual axis forms an angle of 23° with the orbital axis (Fig. 2.30B).

  In primary position, the planes of the vertical rectus muscles do not include one of the axes of the Fick system. The planes of the *superior* and *inferior rectus muscles* form an acute angle of about 23° with the Y-axis (the median plane of the eye) (Fig. 2.31A).
- *Action of superior rectus muscle*: The primary action is elevation; secondary actions are adduction and intorsion.

  When the globe is abducted by 23°, the visual and orbital axes coincide. In this position of the globe, the superior rectus acts only as an elevator. Therefore, this is the optimal position of the globe for testing the function of the superior rectus muscle.

  When the globe is adducted by 67°, the angle between the visual and orbital axes would be 90°. In this position the superior rectus acts as an intortor.
- *Actions of inferior rectus muscle*: The primary action is depression; secondary actions are adduction and extorsion.

  When the globe is abducted by 23°, the inferior rectus acts purely as a depressor. This is the optimal position of the globe for testing the function of the inferior rectus muscle.

  If the globe is adducted by 67°, the inferior rectus acts only as an extortor.
- *Oblique muscles*: The muscle planes of the superior and inferior oblique go in a direction from the anteromedial aspect of the globe to the posterolateral aspect. Therefore, neither muscle plane coincides with the median plane of the globe, nor does the axis of rotation coincide with the X-axis. The muscle plane of the superior oblique and inferior oblique muscle forms an angle of approximately 51° with the median plane. Because of the large angles formed in primary position, the oblique muscles mainly produce cyclorotation (Fig. 2.31B).
- *Actions of superior oblique muscle*: The primary action is intorsion and secondary actions are depression and abduction.

  The angle between the median plane of the globe and the muscle plane increases with abduction of the eye. With 39° of abduction its action is one of pure intorsion.

  When the globe is adducted, the angle between the median plane of the eye and the muscle plane is reduced and the superior oblique muscle acts more and more as a depressor. With an adduction of 51°, the superior oblique would be a pure depressor.

  Thus, the maximum action of the superior oblique muscle as a depressor is in adduction; the maximum intorsion occurs in abduction.
- *Actions of inferior oblique muscle*: The primary action is extorsion; secondary actions are elevation and abduction.

With the globe adducted at 51°, the inferior oblique acts only as an elevator.

With the globe abducted at 39°, its action of extorsion is greatest.

Binocular Eye Movements (Fig. 2.32)[93]

Versions: Versions are conjugate eye movements in which both eyes move in the same direction. The functions of the versions are:

- To enlarge the field of view and
- To bring the object of attention onto the fovea.

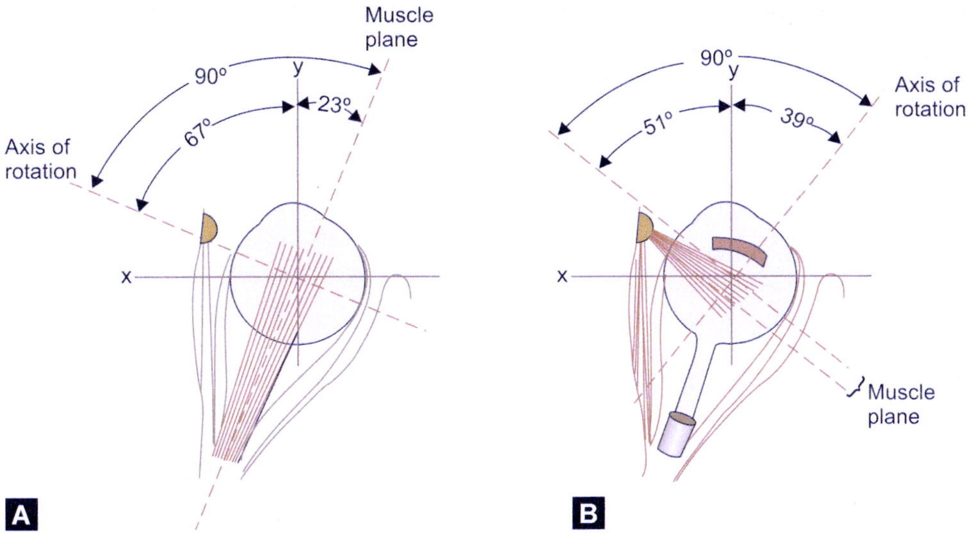

Figs. 2.31A and B: (A) Schematic diagram showing relation of muscle plane of superior and inferior recti with the visual axis in primary position; (B) Schematic diagram showing relation of muscle plane of superior and inferior obliques with the visual axis in primary position.

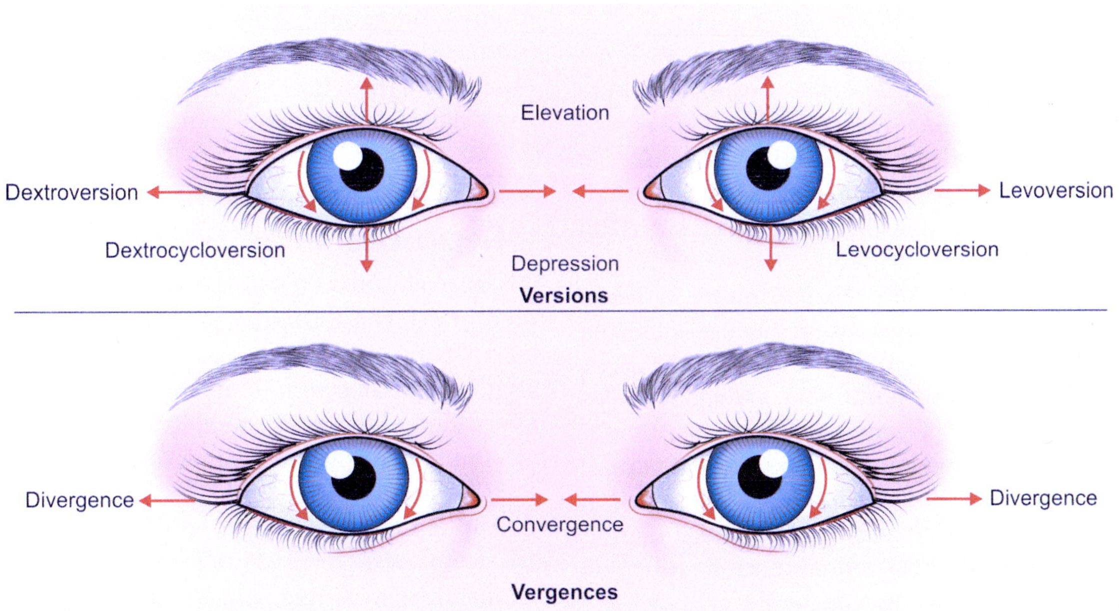

Fig. 2.32: Binocular movements.

Versions are described as:

- *Dextroversion*: Both eyes move to the right
- *Levoversion*: Both eyes move to the left
- *Dextroelevation*: Both eyes move up and to the right
- *Dextrodepression*: Both eyes move down and to the right
- *Levoelevation*: Both eyes move up and to the left
- *Levodepression*: Both eyes move down and to the left
- *Dextrocycloversion*: Both eyes rotate so that the superior portion of the vertical corneal meridian moves to the patient's right
- *Levocycloversion*: Both eyes rotate so that the superior portion of the vertical corneal meridian rotates to the patient's left.

Vergences: These are binocular eye movements that are dysconjugate wherein the eyes move in opposite directions. They align the eyes in such a way as to ensure and maintain binocular fixation and binocular vision.

Vergences are described as follows:

- *Convergence* is a movement wherein both eyes move nasally. Convergence has four components:

1. *Accommodative convergence* (AC): This is a part of the synkinetic near reflex. An increase in AC occurs for each diopter of accommodation (A), giving the accommodative convergence/accommodation (AC/A) ratio.
2. *Fusional convergence*: This is a movement to converge the eyes so that similar retinal images project on corresponding retinal areas of each eye. It is activated when a target in the midline is seen with bitemporal retinal image disparity.
3. *Proximal convergence*: This is an induced convergence movement caused by a psychological awareness of near; this movement is particularly apparent when a person looks through an instrument such as a binocular microscope.
4. *Tonic convergence*: This is an inherent innervational tone to the EOMs when a person is awake and alert to maintain eyes in straight gaze.

- *Divergence* is a movement wherein both the eyes move temporally. Divergence has two components:
  1. *Fusional divergence*: This is produced to align the eyes so that similar retinal images are projected onto corresponding retinal areas. Fusional divergence is a type of optomotor reflex and is accomplished without changing the refractive state of the eyes and is initiated when a target in the midline is seen with binasal retinal image disparity.
  2. *Nonfusional divergence*: An optomotor reflex to diverge the eyes when vision in one eye is blurred and fusion is disrupted on a long-term basis, as seen in cases of sensory exotropia or in spontaneous consecutive exotropia with amblyopia.
- *Vertical vergence*: An optomotor reflex to reduce vertical disparity as in vertical heterophorias. When fusion is disrupted, one eye rotates upward and the other downward, so that similar retinal images project on corresponding retinal areas.
- *Cyclovergence*: An optomotor reflex in which the vertical meridia of the two eyes move in opposite directions to each other. They are stimulated by cyclophoria, so that similar retinal images project on corresponding retinal areas. Cyclovergence includes two components: incyclovergence and excyclovergence.
  - *Incyclovergence* is a rotation of both eyes wherein the 12 o'clock corneal meridian rotates nasally
  - *Excyclovergence* is a rotation of both eyes wherein the 12 o'clock meridian of cornea rotates temporally.

Hering's Law of Equal Innervation

Hering's law of motor correspondence[93] states that when the eyes move into a conjugate gaze direction, equal and simultaneous innervation flows to the yoke muscle pair.

For example, during dextroversion, right lateral rectus and left medial rectus muscles receive equal and simultaneous innervation.

Hering's law is important for the understanding of paralytic or restrictive strabismus. Because the amount of innervation to both eyes is always determined by the fixating eye, the angle of deviation varies according to which eye is fixating.

When the unaffected eye is fixating, the amount of misalignment is called the *primary deviation*. When the paretic or restrictive eye is fixating, the amount of misalignment is called the *secondary deviation*.

The secondary deviation is larger than the primary deviation because of the increased innervation necessary to move the paretic or restrictive eye to the position of fixation. This extra innervation is transmitted to the yoke muscle(s) in the fellow eye, which causes excessive action of this muscle and a larger angle of deviation.

Sherrington's Law of Reciprocal Innervation

This law states that increased innervation and contraction force of a given EOM is accompanied by a reciprocal decrease in innervation and contraction force of its antagonist. For example, when the right eye abducts, innervation of the right lateral rectus muscle is increased but simultaneously, innervation of the right medial rectus is reduced.[93]

Application of Hering's and Sherrington's laws is also useful in the explanation of muscle palsy sequelae. For instance, in a right superior oblique muscle palsy, if the patient uses the right eye to fixate on an object that is located up and to the left, the innervation of the right inferior oblique muscle required to move the eye into this gaze position is reduced because the right inferior oblique does not have to overcome the normal antagonistic effect of the right superior oblique muscle (Sherrington's law). According to Hering's law, less innervation is also received by the yoke muscle of the right inferior oblique muscle, i.e. the left superior rectus muscle. This decreased innervation could lead to the incorrect impression that the left superior rectus muscle is paretic.

Supranuclear Eye Movement System

Supranuclear eye movement systems[94] are semireflex movements in response to optical, acoustic, or other stimuli. Each system is controlled by a different neural system but share a common pathway that finally supply the motor neurons of the EOMs. These systems are as follows:

- Saccadic system
- Smooth pursuit system
- Vestibular system [vestibulo-ocular reflex (VOR)]
- Optokinetic system (OKN)
- Vergence system.

Saccadic System

They are rapid movements that occur as the gaze shifts from one object to another, so as to place the image, quickly on the fovea. Velocity of these movements is 800–1,000°/sec.

Smooth Pursuit System

They are slow tracking movements that match the velocity of eye movement to the velocity of the target while following the moving target. They require a visual input of the object speed to be no greater than 30–40°/sec to match the velocity of tracking movements. Beyond this point, the eyes tend to fall behind and saccades have to be made to catch up.

Vestibulo-ocular Reflex

The VOR maintains a steady image on the retina during rotations of the head at great speed (for example, while spinning). VOR responses are driven by the semicircular canals (for angular movements) and the otoliths of the utricle and saccule (for linear acceleration). Neural activity (excitatory and inhibitory) from these structures passes along the vestibular nerves to the vestibular nuclei in the medulla of the brainstem; from there, the activity projects to the ocular motor neurons. Each of the semicircular canals innervates one pair of yoked EOMs, which move the two eyes in the same plane as the canal.

Optokinetic System

The optokinetic nystagmus (OKN) system maintains steady alignment of images on the retina by smooth pursuit during sustained rotation of the head. This system becomes operative after about 30 seconds, when the rotation-induced VOR attenuates. The OKN system provides a sustained output for eye position control that counters the effects of persistent rotations using a compensatory saccade to refixate. The vestibular and OKN systems act synergistically to align the eyes properly during head rotations.

Vergence System

They allow focusing of an object during dysconjugate eye movements, like convergence and divergence. These movements are driven primarily by a disparity in the relative location of images on the foveae. Vergence movements are very slow (about 20°/sec).

REFERENCES

1. Holly FJ, Lemp MA. Tear physiology and dry eyes. Surv Ophthalmol. 1977;22:69-87.
2. Lemp MA. Advances in understanding and managing dry eye disease. Am J Ophthalmol. 2008;146:350-6.
3. Gipson IK, Hori I, Argueso P. Character of ocular surface mucins and their alterations in dry eye disease. Ocular Surf. 2004;2:131-48.
4. Gipson IK, Argueso P. Role of mucins in the function of the corneal and conjunctival epithelia. Int Rev Cytol. 2003;231:1-49.
5. Dart DA. Formation and function of the tear film. In: Kaufman PL, Adler FH, Levin LA, et al. (Eds). Adler's Physiology of the Eye, illustrated edition. Edinburgh: Saunders-Elsevier; 2011. pp. 350-61.
6. Levin LM, Brar VS, Goldstein MH, et al. Tear film. In: American Academy of Ophthalmology. Fundamental and Principles of Ophthalmology. Basic and Clinical Science Course, 2015-2016. San Francisco; American Academy of Ophthalmology; 2015. pp. 258-69.
7. McKown RL, Wang N, Raab RW, et al. Lacritin and other new proteins of the lacrimal functional unit. Exp Eye Res. 2009;88:848-58.
8. Stahl U, Willcox M, Stapleton F. Osmolality and tear film dynamics. Clin Exp Optom. 2012;95:3-11.
9. Werkmeister RM, Alex A, Kaya S, et al. Measurement of tear film thickness using ultrahigh-resolution optical coherence tomography. Invest Ophthalmol Vis Sci. 2013;54:5578-83.
10. Stern ME, Gao J, Siemasko KF, et al. The role of the lacrimal functional unit in the pathophysiology of dry eye. Exp Eye Res. 2004;78:409-16.
11. Ring MH, Rabensteiner DF, Horwath-Winter J, et al. Non-invasive assessment of the human tear film dynamics. Ann Anat. 2015;202:61-70.
12. King-Smith PE, Nichols JJ, Nichols KK, et al. Contributions of evaporation and other mechanisms to tear film thinning and break-up. Optom Vis Sci. 2008;85:623-30.

13. Braun RJ, King-Smith PE, Begley CG, et al. Dynamics and function of the tear film in relation to the blink cycle. Prog Retin Eye Res. 2015;45:132-64.
14. Cwiklik L. Tear film lipid layer: A molecular level view. Biochim Biophys Acta. 2016;1858:2421-30.
15. Lemp MA, Weiler HH. How do tears exit? Invest Ophthalmol Vis Sci. 1983;24:619-22.
16. Francois J, Neetens A. Tear flow in man. Am J Ophthalmol 1973;76:351-8.
17. Maurice DM. The structure and transparency of the cornea. J Physiol (Lond). 1957;136:263-86.
18. Jester JV, Budge A, Fisher S, et al. Corneal keratocytes: phenotypic and species differences in abundant protein expression and in vitro light-scattering. Invest Ophthalmol Vis Sci. 2005;46:2369-78.
19. Dawson DG, Ubels JL, Edelhauser HF. Cornea and sclera. In: Kaufman PL, Adler FH, Levin LA, et al. (Eds). Adler's Physiology of the Eye, illustrated edition. Edinburgh: Saunders-Elsevier; 2011. pp. 71-122.
20. Qazi Y, Wong G, Monson B, et al. Corneal transparency: genesis, maintenance and dysfunction. Brain Res Bull. 2010;81:198-210.
21. Usui T, Yamagami S, Kishimoto S, et al. Role of macrophage migration inhibitory factor in corneal neovascularization. Invest Ophthalmol Vis Sci. 2007;48:3545-50.
22. Ambati BK, Anand A, Joussen AM, et al. Sustained inhibition of corneal neovascularization by genetic ablation of CCR5. Invest Ophthalmol Vis Sci. 2003;44:590-3.
23. Mwaikambo BR, Sennlaub F, Ong H, et al. Activation of CD36 inhibits and induces regression of inflammatory corneal neovascularization. Invest Ophthalmol Vis Sci. 2006;47:4356-64.
24. Stuart PM, Pan F, Plambeck S, et al. FasL-Fas interactions regulate neovascularization in the cornea. Invest Ophthalmol Vis Sci. 2003;44:93-8.
25. Dawson DW, Volpert OV, Gillis P, et al. Pigment epithelium-derived factor: a potent inhibitor of angiogenesis. Science. 1999;285:245-8.
26. Maruyama K, Ii M, Cursiefen C, et al. Inflammation-induced lymphangiogenesis in the cornea arises from CD11b-positive macrophages. J Clin Invest. 2005;115:2363-72.
27. Nishida T, Saika S. Cornea and sclera: Anatomy and Physiology. In: Krachmer JH, Mannis MJ, Holland EJ, Edward J (Eds). Cornea, Volume 1, 3rd edition. USA: Elsevier Mosby; 2010. pp. 13-9.
28. Klyce SD, Beuerman RW, Crosson CE. Alteration of corneal epithelial ion transport by sympathectomy. Invest Ophthalmol Vis Sci. 1985;26:434-42.
29. Klyce SD, Dohlman CH, Martinez CE. Corneal form and function: clinical perspective. In: Albert DM, Jakobiec FA (Eds). Principles and Practice of Ophthalmology, Volume 1, 3rd edition. Philadelphia: WB Saunders Company; 2000. pp. 441-5.
30. Ljubimov AV, Saghizadeh M. Progress in corneal wound healing. Prog Retin Eye Res. 2015;49:17-45.
31. Thoft RA, Friend J. The X, Y, Z hypothesis of corneal epithelial maintenance. Invest Ophthalmol Vis Sci. 198;24:1442-3.
32. Hassell JR, Birk DE. The molecular basis of corneal transparency. Exp Eye Res. 2010;91:326-35.
33. Gabelt BT, Kaufman P. Production and flow of aqueous humour. In: Kaufman PL, Adler FH, Levin LA, et al. (Eds). Adler's Physiology of the Eye, illustrated edition. Edinburgh: Saunders-Elsevier; 2011. pp. 274-99.
34. Cioffi GA, Durcan FJ, Girkin CA, et al. Intraocular pressure and aqueous humour dynamics. In: American Academy of Ophthalmology. Glaucoma. Basic and Clinical Science Course, 2015-2016. San Francisco: American Academy of Ophthalmology; 2015. pp. 25-31.
35. Roy Chowdhury U, Hann CR, Stamer WD, et al. Aqueous humor outflow: dynamics and disease. Invest Ophthalmol Vis Sci. 2015;56(5):2993-3003.
36. Freddo TF, Civan M, Gong H. Aqueous humour and the dynamics of its flow: Mechanisms and routes of aqueous humour drainage. In: Albert DM, Jakobiec FA (Eds). Principles and Practice of ophthalmology, Vol 2, 3rd edition. Philadelphia: WB Saunders Company; 2000. pp. 2439-53.
37. Toris CB, Yablonski ME, Wang YL, et al. Aqueous humor dynamics in the aging human eye. Am J Ophthalmol. 1999;127(4):407-12.
38. Hiller R, Sperduto RD, Krueger DE. Race, iris pigmentation, and intraocular pressure. Am J Epidemiol. 1982;115(5): 674-83.
39. Nomura H, Ando F, Niino N, et al. The relationship between age and intraocular pressure in a Japanese population: the influence of central corneal thickness. Curr Eye Res. 2002;24(2):81-5 .
40. Gaasterland D, Kupfer C, Milton R, et al. Studies of aqueous humour dynamics in man. Effect of age upon parameters of intraocular pressure in normal human eyes. Exp Eye Res. 1978;26(6):651-6.
41. Gabelt BT, Kaufman PL. Changes in aqueous humor dynamics with age and glaucoma. Prog Retin Eye Res. 2005;24(5):612-37.
42. Hejtmancik JF, Shiels A. Overview of the Lens. Prog Mol Biol Transl Sci. 2015;134:119-27.
43. Bassnett S, Shi Y, Vrensen GFJM. Biological glass: structural determinants of eye lens transparency. Philos Trans R Soc Lond B Biol Sci. 2011;366(1568):1250-64.
44. Michael R, Bron AJ. The ageing lens and cataract: a model of normal and pathological ageing. Philos Trans R Soc Lond B Biol Sci. 2011;366:1278-92.
45. Hejtmancik JF, Riazuddin SA, McGreal R, et al. Lens Biology and Biochemistry. Prog Mol Biol Transl Sci. 2015;134: 169-201.
46. Ireland M, Maisel H. A family of lens fiber cell specific proteins. Lens Eye Toxic Res. 1989;6:623-38.
47. Michael R, van Marle J, Vrensen GFJM, et al. Changes in the refractive index of lens fibre membranes during maturation--impact on lens transparency. Exp Eye Res. 2003;77:93-9.
48. Costello MJ, Johnsen S, Metlapally S, et al. Ultrastructural analysis of damage to nuclear fiber cell membranes in advanced age-related cataracts from India. Exp Eye Res. 2008;87:147-58.

49. Truscott RJ. Presbyopia. Emerging from a blur towards an understanding of the molecular basis for this most common eye condition. Exp Eye Res. 2009;88:241-7
50. Strenk SA, Strenk LM, Koretz JF. The mechanism of presbyopia. Prog Retin Eye Res. 2005;24:379-93.
51. Datiles MB, Ansari RR, Suh KI, et al. Clinical detection of precataractous lens protein changes using dynamic light scattering. Arch Ophthalmol. 2008;126:1687-93.
52. Sharma KK, Santhoshkumar P. Lens aging: effects of crystallins. Biochim Biophys Acta. 2009;1790:1095-108.
53. Jahngen JH, Lipman RD, Eisenhauer DA, et al. Aging and cellular maturation cause changes in ubiquitin-eye lens protein conjugates. Arch Biochem Biophys. 1990;276:32-7.
54. Shang F, Gong X, Taylor A. Activity of ubiquitin-dependent pathway in response to oxidative stress. Ubiquitin-activating enzyme is transiently up-regulated. J Biol Chem. 1997;272:23086-93.
55. Harding JJ. Free and protein-bound glutathione in normal and cataractous human lenses. Biochem J. 1970;117:957-60.
56. Wei M, Xing K-Y, Fan Y-C, et al. Loss of thiol repair systems in human cataractous lenses. Invest Ophthalmol Vis Sci. 2014;56:598-605.
57. Ganea E, Harding JJ. Glutathione-related enzymes and the eye. Curr Eye Res. 2006;31:1-11.
58. Duncan G, Hightower KR, Gandolfi SA, et al. Human lens membrane cation permeability increases with age. Invest Ophthalmol Vis Sci. 1989;30:1855-9.
59. Grus FH, Joachim SC, Pfeiffer N. Proteomics in ocular fluids. Proteomics Clin Appl. 2007;1:876-88.
60. Lund-Andersen H, Sander B. The vitreous. In: Kaufman PL, Alm A, Adler FH (Eds). Adler's Physiology of the Eye: Clinical Application, 10th edition. St Louis, Mo: Mosby; 2003. pp. 291-6.
61. Berman ER. Vitreous. In: Berman ER (Ed). Biochemistry of the Eye. New York: Springer Science & Business Media; 1991. pp. 291-307.
62. Brew H, Attwell D. Is the potassium channel distribution in glial cells optimal for spatial buffering of potassium? Biophys J. 1985;48:843-7.
63. Chauhan DS, Antcliff RJ, Rai PA, et al. Papillofoveal traction in macular hole formation: the role of optical coherence tomography. Arch Ophthalmol. 2000;118:32-8.
64. Duarte TL, Lunec J. Review: When is an antioxidant not an antioxidant? A review of novel actions and reactions of vitamin C. Free Radic Res. 2005;39:671-86.
65. Tsukaguchi H, Tokui T, Mackenzie B, et al. A family of mammalian Na^+-dependent L-ascorbic acid transporters. Nature. 1999;399:70-5.
66. Shui Y-B, Holekamp NM, Kramer BC, et al. The gel state of the vitreous and ascorbate-dependent oxygen consumption: relationship to the etiology of nuclear cataracts. Arch Ophthalmol. 2009;127:475-82.
67. Gao B-B, Chen X, Timothy N, et al. Characterization of the vitreous proteome in diabetes without diabetic retinopathy and diabetes with proliferative diabetic retinopathy. J Proteome Res. 2008;7:2516-25.
68. Bttelheim FA, Balazs EA. Light-scattering patterns of the vitreous humor. Biochim Biophys Acta. 1968;158:309-12.
69. Johnson MW. How should we release vitreomacular traction: surgically, pharmacologically, or pneumatically? Am J Ophthalmol. 2013;155:203-5.
70. Johnson MW. Posterior vitreous detachment: evolution and complications of its early stages. Am J Ophthalmol. 2010;149:371-82.
71. Swann DA. Chemistry and biology of the vitreous body. Int Rev Exp Pathol. 1980;22:1-64.
72. Swann DA, Constable IJ. Vitreous structure. I. Distribution of hyaluronate and protein. Invest Ophthalmol. 1972;11:159-63.
73. de Smet MD, Gad Elkareem AM, Zwinderman AH. The vitreous, the retinal interface in ocular health and disease. Ophthalmologica. 2013;230:165-78.
74. Levin LM, Brar VS, Goldstein MH, et al. Retinal Pigment epithelium. In: American Academy of Ophthalmology. Fundamentals and Principles of Ophthalmology. Basic and Clinical Science Course, 2015-2016. San Francisco: American Academy of Ophthalmology; 2015. pp. 324-9.
75. Strauss O, Helbig H. The function of the retinal pigment epithelium. In: Levin LA, Nilsson SFE, Hoeve JV, et al. (Eds). Adler's Physiology of the Eye, 11th edition. Edinburgh: Saunders-Elsevier; 2011.
76. Sparrow JR, Hicks D, Hamel CP. The retinal pigment epithelium in health and disease. Curr Mol Med. 2010;10:802-23.
77. Thumann G, Dou G, Wang Y, et al. Cell biology of the retinal pigment epithelium. In: Schachat AP, Wilkinson CP, Hinton DR, et al. (Eds). Ryan's Retina, 6th edition. Edinburgh: Elsevier Health Sciences; 2018. pp. 401-10.
78. Strauss O. The retinal pigment epithelium in visual function. Physiol Rev. 2005;85:845-81.
79. McCannel CA, Atebara NH, Kim SJ, et al. Retina and Vitreous American Academy of Ophthalmology. Basic and Clinical Science Course, 2015-2016. San Francisco: American Academy of Ophthalmology; 2015. pp. 69-75.
80. Gullapalli VK, Sugino IK, Zarbin MA. Muller cells and the retinal pigment epithelium. In: Albert DM, Jakobiec FA (Eds). Principles and Practice of Ophthalmology, Vol 2, 3rd edition. Philadelphia: WB Saunders Company; 2000. pp. 1633-48.
81. Azar DT, Azar NF, Brodie SE, et al. Optics of the human eye. In: American Academy of Ophthalmology. Fundamentals and Principles of Ophthalmology. Basic and Clinical Science Course, 2015-2016. San Francisco: American Academy of Ophthalmology; 2015. pp. 114-9.
82. Levi DM. Visual acuity. In: Kaufman PL, Adler FH, Levin LA, et al. (Eds). Adler's Physiology of the Eye, illustrated edition. Edinburgh: Saunders-Elsevier; 2011. pp. 627-45.
83. KanskiJJ, Bowling B. Glaucoma. In: Clinical Ophthalmology: a Systematic Approach, 7th edition. New Delhi: Elsevier; 2011. pp. 331-3.
84. Ramchandran RS, Feldon SE. Visual fields in retinal disease. In: Schachat AP, Wilkinson CP, Hinton DR, et al (Eds). Ryan's Retina, 6th edition. Edinburgh: Elsevier Health Sciences; 2018. pp. 308-12.

85. Rubin GS. Visual acuity and contrast sensitivity. In: Schachat AP, Wilkinson CP, Hinton DR, et al (Eds). Ryan's Retina, 6th edition. Edinburgh: Elsevier Health Sciences; 2018. pp. 300-5.
86. Neitz J, Mancuso K, Kuchenbecker JA, et al. Color vision. In: Kaufman PL, Adler FH, Levin LA, Alm A et al. Adler's Physiology of the Eye, illustrated edition. Edinburgh: Saunders-Elsevier; 2011. pp. 648-53.
87. Conway BR. Color vision, cones, and color-coding in the cortex. Neuroscientist. 2009;15:274-90.
88. Cao D. Color vision and night vision. In: Schachat AP, Wilkinson CP, Hinton DR, et al. (Eds). Ryan's Retina, 6th edition. Edinburgh: Elsevier Health Sciences; 2018. pp. 285-98.
89. Lamb TD. Light adaptation in photoreceptors. In: Kaufman PL, Adler FH, Levin LA, et al. (Eds). Adler's Physiology of the Eye, illustrated edition. Edinburgh: Saunders-Elsevier; 2011. pp. 429-36.
90. Von Noorden GK, Campos EC. Physiology of ocular movements. In: Von Noorden GK (Ed). Binocular vision and ocular motility: theory and management of strabismus, 6th edition. St Louis: Mosby; 2002. pp. 52-70.
91. Helveston EM. Surgical anatomy. In: Surgical Management of Strabismus: An Atlas of Strabismus Surgery, 4th edition. St Louis: Mosby; 1993. pp. 31-3.
92. Tweed D, Vilis T. Geometric relations of eye position and velocity vectors during saccades. Vision Res. 1990;30:111-27.
93. Quaia C, Optican LM. Three-dimensional rotations of the eye. In: Kaufman PL, Adler FH, Levin LA, Alm A (Eds). Adler's Physiology of the Eye, illustrated edition. Edinburgh: Saunders-Elsevier; 2011. pp. 208-15.
94. Lueder GT, Archer SM, Hered RW. Motor physiology. In: American Academy of Ophthalmology. Pediatric Ophthalmology and Strabismus. Basic and Clinical Science Course, 2015-2016. San Francisco: American Academy of Ophthalmology; 2015. pp. 59-73.

Chapter 3 Ocular Biochemistry

Divya Janakiraman, N Venkatesh Prajna

INTRODUCTION

A study of ocular biochemistry provides the ophthalmologist an opportunity to gain in-depth knowledge regarding the role of various ocular cellular structures in the maintenance of normal homeostasis. With recent technological advances, biochemical analytical methods have undergone a paradigm shift. There have been additional developments in the field of proteomics and lipidomics, which have enhanced our knowledge resulting in a better understanding of the biochemical mechanisms at the molecular level and their changes in disease conditions. This chapter discusses the biochemical characteristics of various structures of the eye and their role in the normal physiology of the eye.

TEAR FILM

Introduction

The tear film is an integral part of optical interface connecting the ocular surface with the external environment. The complexity of tear film structure, composition, and function has attracted researchers throughout the world. This section focuses on the normal biochemical composition of the tear film and their alterations in disease conditions.

Biochemical Composition of Tear Film

Traditionally, tear film has been classified into three layers, namely—the outer lipid layer, the middle aqueous layer, and the inner mucin layer.[1] Human tear film consists of 98.2% water and 1.8% dissolved solids (Table 3.1).[2]

Layers of Tear Film

Lipid Layer

Lipid layer, which forms the outermost layer of the tear film, consists of lipids primarily secreted by the meibomian glands. It consists of nonpolar lipids such as wax and cholesterol esters, which forms the major portion of this layer and polar lipids such as phospholipids, which interacts with the adjacent aqueous layer.[3] The lipid layer of tear film retards the evaporation of tears[4] and specifically the polar lipids help in distribution of tear film.[3]

Aqueous Layer

The components of aqueous layer are secreted mainly by main and accessory lacrimal glands. Water is the main component of aqueous layer of tear film. In addition, it also contains proteins, immunoglobulins (Igs), enzymes, electrolytes, growth factors, metabolites secreted by the lacrimal gland, corneal, and conjunctival epithelium (Box 3.1).

The tear film electrolytes, especially bicarbonate (HCO_3^-), regulate the movement of fluids between the cornea and the tear film and thus play an important role in the maintenance of osmolarity and pH of the tear film.

Albumin is the predominant protein found in the tear. The other proteins include globulins, prealbumin, Igs (with IgA being the predominant Ig), and various growth factors.

The major antimicrobial components in tears are lysozyme, lactoferrin, lipocalin, secretory IgA, and complement[18] (components Clq, C3, factor B, C4, C5, and C9), and they form the first line of defense of the ocular surface against pathogens. Phospholipase A2, serum

Table 3.1: Components of various layers of tear film.

Layers of tear film	Components
Lipid layer	Wax, cholesterol esters, phospholipids
Aqueous layer	Water, proteins, immunoglobulins, enzymes, electrolytes, growth factors, metabolites
Mucin layer	Gel-forming mucins (MUC5AC), membrane forming mucins, water, proteins, electrolytes, solutes

Box 3.1: Composition of aqueous layer of tear film.

- Water
- *Electrolytes (mmol/L)*:[5]
  - Sodium: 134–170
  - Potassium: 26–42
  - Magnesium: 0.3–0.6
  - Calcium: 0.5
  - Chloride: 120–135
  - Bicarbonate: 26
- *Proteins (mg/100 mL)*:[6]
  - Albumin: 394
  - Globulin: 275
- *Immunoglobulins*:[6]
  - IgG: 15 mg/100 mL
  - IgA: 17 mg/100 mL
  - IgM: 5 mg/100 mL
  - IgD: 1 mg/100 mL
  - IgE: 200 ng/100 mL
- Lactoferrin[7]
- Transferrin[7]
- Ceruloplasmin[7]
- Lacritin[8]
- Lipocalin[9]
- Defensins[9]
- Phospholipase A2[9]
- Interferons[10]
- Epithelial growth factor[11]
- Hepatocyte growth factor[12]
- Fibroblast growth factor[13]
- Tumor growth factor α,[14] β_1, β_2[15]
- Vascular endothelial growth factor[16]
- Tumor necrosis factor[16]
- Interleukin-1α, -1β[16]
- *Enzymes*:[7]
  - Lactate dehydrogenase
  - Lysozyme
  - Amylase
  - Peroxidase
  - Plasminogen activator
- *Metabolites*:
  - Glucose[7]
  - Lactate[7]
  - Urea[7]
  - Catecholamines[7]
  - Histamine[7]
  - Prostaglandins[7]
  - Ascorbate[17]
  - Amino acids[7]
- Mucins

leukocyte protease inhibitor, surfactant protein A and D, and defensins also support the antimicrobial activity in a minor capacity.[9]

Lacritin, a novel glycoprotein found in tears is thought to have many roles.[8] Encoded by *LACRT* gene;[8] it promotes tear secretion, corneal epithelial cell proliferation, and corneal wound healing. In addition, it is also found to express antimicrobial properties.

The tear film metabolites include glucose, lactate, urea, prostaglandins (PGs), ascorbate, and amino acids. Studies have demonstrated tear film glucose levels to be high in diabetics when compared to normal individuals. The mean tear glucose levels were found to be 6.34 ± 0.7 mg/dL and 2.9 ± 0.5 mg/dL in diabetics and nondiabetics, respectively.[19] It is being explored as an alternative tool for monitoring glucose levels in diabetics.

Tears also contain various cytokines and growth factors, which includes epidermal growth factor (EGF), transforming growth factor-alpha (TGF-α), TGF-β1, -β2, hepatocyte growth factor (HGF), fibroblast growth factor (FGF-2), vascular endothelial growth factor (VEGF), tumor necrosis factor (TNF), interleukin (IL)-1α, and IL-1β. They promote cell proliferation, cell migration, and wound healing.

Mucin Layer

Ocular mucins are produced predominantly by the conjunctival goblet cells, while a minor role is played by the conjunctival and corneal epithelial cells and the accessory lacrimal glands. This layer is composed of gel-forming mucin, the extracellular domain of membrane-forming mucin, proteins, solutes, electrolytes, and water.

The structural arrangements of the different chemical components in the mucin layer play an important role in the stability of the tear film. The protein backbone of the mucins consists of tandem repeats of amino acids, which are rich in serine and threonine. These amino acids serve as sites for O-glycosylation. Heavy glycosylation increases the molecular weight and also induces an overall negative charge, thus making them hydrophilic, which in turn helps the mucin layer to mix with the adjacent aqueous layer.

Ocular mucins can be classified into membrane forming and secretory mucins.

- *Membrane-forming mucins*: The most common membrane-forming mucins, which are expressed in the ocular surface are MUC-1, -4, -15, -16, and -20.[20] Soluble forms of MUC-1, -4, -16 have been detected in tears. These mucins have three domains, namely—cytoplasmic domain, transmembrane domain, and extracellular domain. Of these, the extracellular domain forms the glycocalyx, which is anchored to the microvilli on the cell membrane of corneal epithelial cells.[21]
- *Secretory mucins*: Secretory mucins are further classified into large gel-forming mucins and small soluble mucins. The various gel-forming mucins, which are known to be expressed on the ocular surface, are

MUC-2, -5AC, -5B, and -6 and -19.[20] Of these, MUC-2 and -5AC have been detected in tears as well. MUC-5AC forms the major backbone of tear film mucin layer and is secreted by goblet cells of the conjunctiva. The only soluble mucin expressed in the eye is MUC-7 and has been detected in lacrimal gland acinar cells and conjunctiva, but not expressed in tears.

Tear Film Biochemistry in Diseases

Ocular surface disorders can result from either an aqueous deficiency, mucin excess or deficiency, or lipid layer dysfunction. Inflammation is also thought to play a role as shown by the increased levels of various cytokines in dry eye conditions. The noninvasive nature of tear film collection has encouraged researchers to embark on studies to look for the presence of biomarkers. In fact, the biomarkers for ocular diseases like Graves ophthalmopathy, keratoconus, glaucoma, and Sjögren syndrome; and for systemic diseases like diabetic retinopathy, cancer, systemic sclerosis, Parkinson disease, and cystic fibrosis have been found to be expressed in the tears.[22] Continuous monitoring of tear glucose using glucose-sensing contact lenses is being experimented.

CORNEA

Introduction

Cornea covers the anterior one-sixth of the surface of eyeball and is a clear and transparent structure. Its primary function is to act as a powerful optical lens of fixed focus that transmits light in an orderly fashion for proper image formation. The tear film-corneal interface contributes to approximately two-thirds of the total refractive power of the eye. The cornea is richly supplied with nerves and is avascular. The avascular nature plays an important role in corneal transparency and confers the property of immunologic privilege to the cornea. The cornea also has a major role in the absorption of the topically applied drugs. This section deals with the biochemical characteristics of cornea, which aids in its transparency and physiologic function, the nutrition and metabolic pathways, and drug permeability through the cornea.

Biochemistry of Different Corneal Layers

The biochemical concentrations of water and electrolytes are dependent upon the state of corneal hydration. Generally speaking, the hydration of cornea in most species varies between 75% and 80%.

As seen in the Table 3.2, the concentration of potassium (K^+) is high in the epithelium, while the concentration of sodium (Na^+) is high in the stroma. In the stroma, the sum of the diffusible cations (sodium and potassium) is in excess of that of the diffusible anion [chloride (Cl^-)] (Table 3.2).

Table 3.2: Composition of the cornea.*

Component	Concentration	Species
Electrolytes		
Sodium:		
• Whole cornea	147 mEq/L	Ox, Pig
	155 mEq/L	Rabbit
• Epithelium	57 mEq/L	Rabbit
• Stroma	165 mEq/L	Rabbit
Potassium:		
• Whole cornea	35 mEq/L	Pig
	31.5 mEq/L	Rabbit
• Epithelium	109 mEq/L	Rabbit
• Stroma	21 mEq/L	Rabbit
Chloride:		
• Whole cornea	76 mEq/L	Calf
	94 mEq/L	Rabbit
• Epithelium	23 mEq/L	Rabbit
• Stroma	104 mEq/L	Rabbit
Bicarbonate:		
• Whole cornea	25–35 mEq/L	Not specified[23]
Calcium:		
• Whole cornea	2 mEq/L	Calf
	5–33 mEq/L	Rabbit
Magnesium:		
• Whole cornea	2 mEq/L	Pig
	1.5 mEq/L	Calf, Ox
Iron:		
• Whole cornea	2.6 µg/g	Ox
Copper:		
• Whole cornea	10–70 µg/g	Human
Zinc:		
• Whole cornea	9 µg/g	Human
Manganese:		
• Whole cornea	0.11 µg/g	Ox
Nonelectrolytes		
Glucose:		
• Whole cornea	16 µmol/g	Ox
	4.2 µmol/g	Rabbit
Glycogen:		
• Whole cornea	12–13 µmol/g	Ox
	8 µmol/g	Rabbit
Ascorbic acid:		
• Epithelium	6.5 µmol/g	Rabbit
• Stroma	1.4 µmol/g	Rabbit
Glutathione:		
• Epithelium	3.9 µmol/g	Ox
• Stroma	0.16 µmol/g	Ox

*Except as noted, all data from Maurice and Riley.[24]
Source: Peyman, 1st edition.

The cornea is chemically heterogeneous due to variations in cellularity among the different layers.

Epithelium

The 4–6-layered corneal epithelium is about 50 microns thick and is composed of three types of cells, namely—superficial cells, wing cells, and basal cells. The superficial layer is covered by a nonkeratinized stratified squamous epithelium. Water constitutes 70% of wet weight of corneal epithelium.

1. *Superficial cells*: The cells in this layer are arranged in 1–2 layers, flattened, and are approximately 40–60 microns in diameter. The external cell wall of the most superficial cells has numerous microvilli, which interact with the mucin layer of tear film. The microvilli are covered with membrane associated mucins (MUC-1, MUC-4, MUC-16), thus forming an effective barrier to fluid transport. Unique to this layer is the presence of zonula occludens, which are tight junctions that effectively contributes to the barrier function of the epithelium. In addition, these cells also have desmosomal and adherens junction attachment, which also enhances the barrier effect.
2. *Wing cells*: These cells constitute 2–3 layers beneath the superficial cells. They are rich in keratin and have numerous desmosomes, gap junctions, and adherens junction attachment.
3. *Basal cells*: The basal cells are attached with the fellow basal cells through desmosomes, gap junctions, and adherens junction attachments. These cells are unique in that they are the only component of the corneal epithelium, which exhibit mitotic activity. The basal cells are attached to the basement membrane via keratin filaments, hemidesmosomes, type-VII collagen fibrils, and laminin. They also express integrins, which are involved in the cellular adhesion with the extracellular matrix and also play a vital role in wound healing.

The cytoplasmic filaments expressed within corneal epithelial cells are actin, keratin, and microtubules. Keratin filaments are the major cytoplasmic filaments in human corneal epithelium. K12 keratin, present in the suprabasal layer of the epithelium, is considered cornea specific.[25,26] The other subtypes present in the corneal epithelium are K3, K5, and K14.[27,28] The gap junctional communication in human corneal epithelium is mediated by proteins called connexins. Connexins 43, 26, and 30 are expressed in the corneal epithelium.[29]

There exists a two-way process of electrolyte transport between the tears and the corneal epithelium. Na^+ is passively transported from the tears to the epithelium and Cl^- is transported from epithelium to tears. Na^+ from epithelium is transported to stroma through Na^+–K^+ adenosine triphosphatase (ATPase), which is coupled with Cl^- transport in the opposite direction.

Basement Membrane

The basement membrane, which is a periodic acid-Schiff (PAS) positive structure is formed by basal epithelial cells. Although type IV collagen is the major component of basement membrane, differences have been noted in the type IV collagen chains between the basement membrane of central cornea, limbus, and conjunctival epithelium. It plays an important role in cell adhesion.

Bowman's Layer

It is an acellular matrix situated beneath the epithelial basal lamina. It is composed of type I, type III, and type V collagen fibers embedded in proteoglycan and glycoprotein matrix.[30,31] The collagen fibrils in Bowman's layer are small, randomly dispersed, and densely packed when compared to stroma.

Stroma

Stroma is the thick collagenous layer situated between the Bowman's layer and Descemet's membrane. It constitutes 90% of corneal thickness and consists of predominantly water, which contributes to about 78–80% of its wet weight. The important components of the stroma are the collagen, keratocytes, and the proteoglycans.

Collagen: Type I collagen is the predominant collagen in the corneal stroma.[31] Type III, V, VI, XII, and XIV[32-35] are the other types which are also present. Like collagen from other sites, corneal collagen contains 33% glycine. It also has high proline and hydroxyproline content. The collagen molecules first arrange into fibrils and the fibrils assemble into collagen fibers, which then assemble to form around 300 lamellae. Each lamella runs across the cornea from limbus to limbus. Each fibril shows 64-nm periodicity typical of collagen.

Collagen synthesis begin on the ribosomes of the keratocytes with the translation of collagen messenger ribonucleic acid (mRNA) resulting in the formation of preprocollagen. After post-translational modifications in rough endoplasmic reticulum and Golgi apparatus, procollagen (composed of a helix of three alpha chains) is

Flowchart 3.1: Secretion of collagen.

Collagen gene in nucleus
↓
mRNA transcription
↓
mRNA translation in ribosomes
↓
Preprocollagen in rough endoplasmic reticulum
↓
Cleavage of signal peptide on N-terminal
↓
Hydroxylation of lysine and proline
↓
Glycosylation of hydroxylysine
↓
Disulfide bond formation
↓
C-terminal propeptide extension
↓
3 Pro alpha peptide chains assembly to procollagen triple helix with untrimmed ends
↓
Last post-translational modification in Golgi apparatus—addition of oligosaccharides
↓
Release into extracellular matrix
↓
Cleavage of terminal N and C propeptides
↓
Tropocollagen
↓
Formation of covalent cross-links
↓
Collagen fibrils

(mRNA: Messenger ribonucleic acid)

secreted into the extracellular medium. This procollagen undergoes modification to form insoluble tropocollagen, and finally, insoluble fibrillar collagen is formed by end-to-end bonding (Flowchart 3.1).

Each of these steps involves one or more enzymes, cofactors, and trace elements that, if blocked or deficient, can inhibit collagen synthesis. For instance, ascorbic acid is necessary for hydroxylation of proline. This collagen is vulnerable to proteolytic enzymes such as collagenase, which has important implications in corneal ulcerations.

The uniform diameter of stromal collagen fibrils (25-35 nm)[36] and uniform spacing (41.4 ± 0.5 nm)[37] along with parallel arrangement of the fibrils are one of the major factors responsible for corneal transparency.

Keratocytes: These modified fibroblasts are derived from the neural crest and are found in the stroma scattered between the collagen lamellae. In response to corneal stromal injury, they transform into myofibroblasts and contribute to extracellular matrix formation. In addition, they produce cytokines and metalloproteinases, which play a major role in wound repair.

Proteoglycans: They belong to a family of glycoproteins, which have a protein core covalently attached to glycosaminoglycans (GAGs). The GAG consists of long unbranched polysaccharide chains with repeating disaccharide units. They can absorb and retain large amounts of water and are responsible for the stromal swelling pressure. The predominant GAG in the human cornea is keratan sulfate (50%), while the other GAGs, which are found are dermatan sulfate and chondroitin sulfate.[38] Of these, dermatan sulfate is found more predominantly in the anterior stroma, while keratan sulfate is present more in the posterior stroma.[38,39] They are highly anionic and are present in the interfibrillary space. The proteoglycans core proteins present in the corneal stroma are decorin, keratocan, lumican, mimecan (osteoglycin), and biglycan.[40,41]

Descemet's Membrane

Descemet's membrane is made up of predominantly small diameter collagen fibers and a glycoprotein matrix. The absence of typical 64-nm-banded collagen fibrils and a higher concentration of glucose, galactose, and hydroxyproline and the presence of mannose differentiates the collagen present in the Descemet's membrane from the typical connective tissue collagen present elsewhere in the body. No uronic acid or sulfate is present, indicating the absence of GAG. This structure is extremely resistant to chemical and enzymatic actions and is clinically important as a strong supporting layer withstanding perforation associated with corneal ulceration.

Endothelium

The endothelium is metabolically active and contains all the enzymes necessary for glycolysis, hexose monophosphate (HMP) shunt, and Krebs cycle.

This structure has a metabolic pump, which is one of the factors responsible for maintaining the cornea in the dehydrated state. There is a constant counterbalancing between the stromal swelling pressure (denoted as "leak") and the pump effect of the corneal endothelium. Bonanno et al. have proposed the HCO_3^- and Cl^- secretion model for endothelial pump.[42,43] The endothelial pump is dependent on primary and secondary active transport mechanisms. The basolateral Na^+-K^+ ATPase creates a negative membrane potential inside the endothelial cell by Na^+ efflux and K^+ influx. This negative membrane potential drives the transendothelial net flux of HCO_3^- and Cl^- from basolateral and apical side. This movement of anions creates a net negative charge, which generates a small potential difference (0.5 mV, apical side negative). This potential difference results in Na^+ movement through the paracellular pathway and across the tight junction from the stromal to the endothelial side. The net flux of sodium bicarbonate ($NaHCO_3^-$) and/or sodium chloride (NaCl) drives the movement of water.

Na^+ enters the cell through various modes such as Na^+/H^+ exchanger, Na^+/HCO_3^- and $Na^+/K^+/2Cl^-$ cotransporters, and Na^+ permeable channels. K^+ leaves the cell via K^+ channels and through the nonselective cation channel.

Bicarbonate uptake on the basolateral membrane occurs through a Na^+/HCO_3^- cotransporter and indirectly through Na^+/H^+ exchanger, which loads the cell with HCO_3^- by increasing the rate of formation of HCO_3^- from CO_2 by carbonic anhydrase-II (CA-II) enzyme. This Na^+/H^+ exchanger helps in maintaining the intracellular pH by driving H^+ out of the cell. The transport of HCO_3^- across the apical membrane takes place through anion channels, which also include cystic fibrosis transmembrane conductance regulator (CFTR) channels and Ca^{2+} activated Cl^- channels (CaCC). The high intracellular HCO_3^- gets converted to CO_2 by the action of CA-II. This results in apical CO_2 diffusion where it is converted back to HCO_3^-, by carbonic anhydrase-IV (CA-IV) situated at the apical surface. This is an additional route for HCO_3^- flux. Endothelial Cl^- transport occurs through both transporters and channels, with Cl^- entering the cell from the stroma via a basal $Na^+/K^+/2Cl^-$ transporter and the HCO_3^-/Cl^- exchanger, and exiting into the aqueous humor via apical anion channels (including CFTR and CaCC channels) (Fig. 3.1).

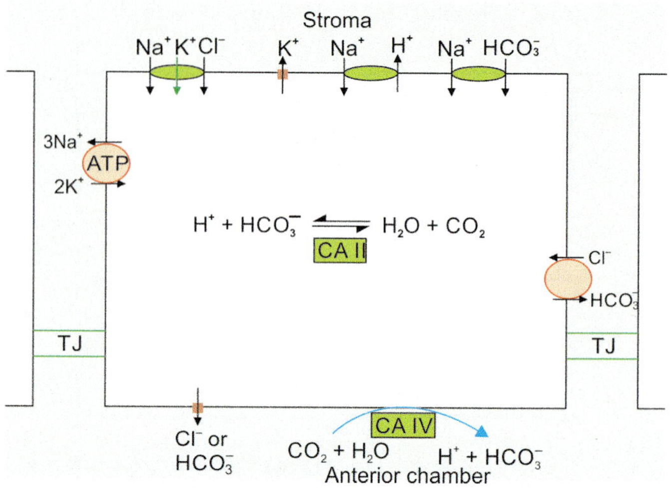

Fig. 3.1: Schematic representation of various mechanisms of ionic transport in the corneal endothelium

Sources of Nutrition to Cornea

Oxygen

The rate of oxygen consumption (QO_2) of the human cornea varies from 0.8 μL/h/mg to 1.0 μL/h/mg dry tissue. The consumption phenomena are maximum in the epithelium and minimum in the stroma, mainly attributable to the increased cellular content in the epithelial layer. When corrected for actual cell count, the rate of consumption is similar in each cell layer including the endothelium. The epithelium derives oxygen from the atmosphere across the tears as well as from the limbal capillaries, whereas the endothelium depends upon oxygen from the anterior chamber, which maintains a partial pressure of 50 mm Hg. This is not altered by covering the corneal surface with a contact lens.

The oxygen tension is highest at the anterior corneal surface (155 mm Hg), with an uptake of 5 μL/h/cm² in humans. Upon eyelid closure, the oxygen tension decreases to 55 mm Hg, similar to that found at the tarsal conjunctival surface, just enough to support the metabolism of the epithelium. A tight-fitting contact lens made of nonoxygen permeable plastic such as polymethyl methacrylate interferes with oxygen uptake of the epithelium and will cause intracellular edema, a decrease in epithelial glycogen, and an increase in lactic acid.

Glucose

Glucose is the primary source of energy in the cornea. Tear film contains only small amounts of glucose and, because of the slow turnover rate of the tear film, it cannot supply the needs of the epithelium. In addition, glucose is water soluble and penetrates the epithelium very poorly. The limbal vessels can supply, at most, 20% of the needs of the cornea and that too only the peripheral 1–2 mm. All evidence points to the aqueous humor as fulfilling the needs not only of the endothelium but of the stroma and epithelium as well. Thoft et al. have estimated that the minimal requirements of epithelial glucose consumption to be 50–60 μg/cm²/h.[44] Glycogen is formed only in the epithelium of the cornea, and represents 7% of the dry weight of the cornea. In the absence of an exogenous supply of glucose, glycogen is broken down to glucose and represents a reserve energy source especially after injury or trauma.

Metabolic Pathways in Cornea[45,24]

Epithelium

Glucose is metabolized by the corneal epithelium mainly by anaerobic glycolysis. However, HMP shunt is also active in the corneal epithelium.[46] Under aerobic conditions, the pyruvate from glycolysis can enter the Krebs cycle resulting in generation of 36 adenosine triphosphate (ATP) molecules. However, the activity of Krebs cycle in the epithelium is low due to the scanty number of mitochondria. Under hypoxic conditions like contact lens wear, pyruvate is converted to lactate, which results in lactate accumulation in the epithelium and stroma, which results in epithelial anoxia and epithelial edema. The HMP shunt does not generate ATP but has the following functions:

- Produces pentose sugars for nucleic acid synthesis and many nucleotides.
- Produces high-energy reducing agent nicotinamide adenine dinucleotide phosphate (NADPH) required for various metabolic reactions including fatty acid synthesis, reduced glutathione formation.

Stroma

The metabolic activity of stroma is slower due to its low-cell count, negligible turnover of collagen, and slow turnover of proteins. It has been proposed that the cellular activity of enzymes involved in glucose metabolism may be similar in epithelium and stroma except for the HMP shunt, which has a negligible part to play in the corneal stroma.

Endothelium

Endothelium mainly uses glycolysis and Krebs cycle for the metabolism of glucose. It has been proposed that glycolysis results in the conversion of 93% of glucose-6-phosphate to pyruvate in the endothelium. 30% of the pyruvate enters the Krebs cycle to produce ATP, whereas the remaining 70% becomes lactic acid by the anaerobic pathway with the help of lactate dehydrogenase.[47] Under hypoxic conditions like contact lens wear, there is an increase in the production of lactic acid resulting in its accumulation in stroma. This accumulation causes a drop in pH, which can result in alterations in endothelial cell function and morphology (Fig. 3.2).

Drug Permeability in Cornea

The cornea plays a major role in the control of the absorption of topically applied drugs. The permeability of the drug through cornea depends on various factors.

Precorneal Factors Affecting Corneal Absorption

Absorption of drugs through the cornea depends on tear film production, drainage, tear film turnover, and drug binding to proteins in tears. All these factors influence the drug retention time in the tear reservoir, which influence the amount of drug available for corneal absorption.

Drug-related Factors Related to Corneal Absorption

Lipid and water solubility of the drug: The permeability of the drug through the cornea depends primarily on its lipid or water solubility. As the lipid content of the corneal epithelium and endothelium is high, the fat-soluble drugs readily pass through these layers. Lipid-soluble molecules pass through the phospholipid portion of the cell membrane by dissolving in it and diffusing through it irrespective of molecular size and shape. The penetration of hydrophilic molecules through the epithelium is poor.

However, water-soluble drugs readily pass through the stroma. Therefore, a drug should exhibit both lipophilic and hydrophilic characteristics to penetrate all layers of cornea. Since the corneal epithelium is one of the major barriers for intraocular drug penetration, discontinuity in this barrier following trauma or ulcer can increase the rate of drug permeability through the cornea.

Molecular size and structure: Lipid-soluble molecules readily penetrate the epithelial cell membrane irrespective of their size and shape. Water-soluble molecules, on the other hand, are restricted to size 0.4 nm and filter through pores that may exist in or around the globular protein molecules in the cell membrane. The size of the pore restricts the flow of water-soluble molecules. To overcome

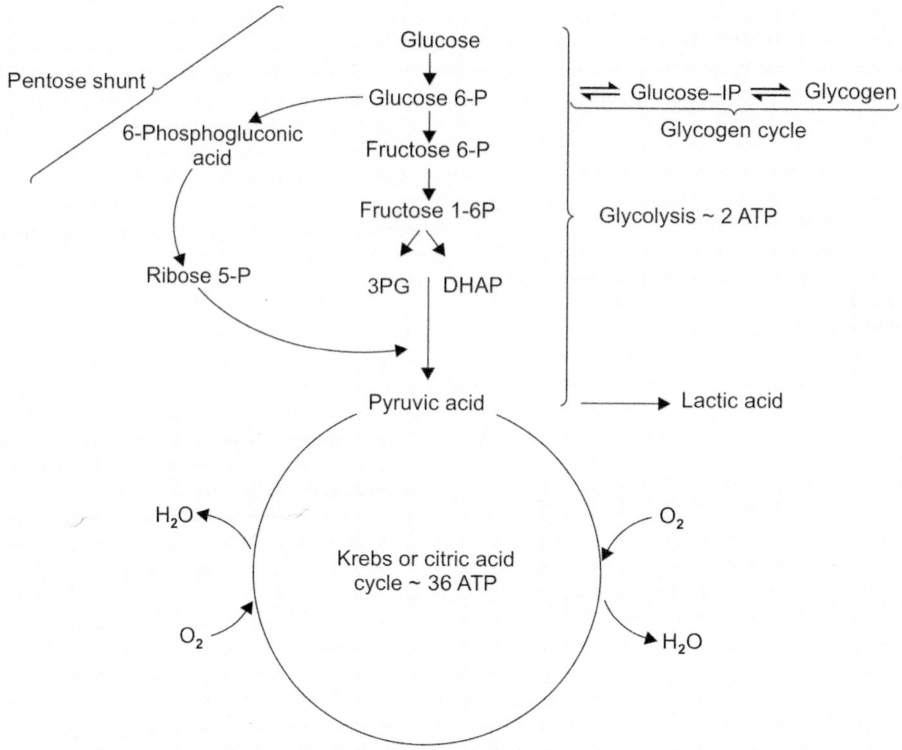

Fig. 3.2: Pathways for glucose metabolism in cornea.
Source: Peyman, 1st edition.

this limitation in molecular size, some ophthalmic drugs are prepared in high concentrations, so that by the laws of mass action a small percentage will still reach the anterior chamber and an effect will be obtained.

Ionic charge: Only nonionized drugs can penetrate the lipid cellular layers, whereas ionized drugs readily traverse the water-soluble stroma. Therefore, a drug should be able to exist in both an ionized and nonionized form to penetrate the cornea. Fluorescein, a negatively charged ion, will not penetrate the epithelium. This property is the basis of the fluorescein dye test. If the epithelium is intact, fluorescein will not stain the cornea; if the epithelium is damaged or absent, fluorescein will stain the stroma. As many ophthalmic medications such as tropicamide and atropine are weak bases, they prevail as both uncharged and charged forms at the alkaline pH of tears (7.4). The penetration of these drugs through the epithelium can be maximized by raising the water phase pH, thereby increasing the number of molecules in uncharged form.

Altering the permeability characteristics of the epithelium: Hypotonic solutions will increase the permeability of the epithelium. Surface-active agents that reduce the surface tension will increase epithelial permeability. Benzalkonium chloride, for example, acts to reduce surface tension, allowing carbachol, a compound of low-lipid solubility, to penetrate the epithelium.

Viscosity: The addition of highly viscous substances, such as methyl cellulose, increases the drug retention in the conjunctival cul-de-sac aiding drug permeability.

SCLERA

Introduction

Sclera is an opaque and dense connective tissue, which forms the posterior five-sixths of the outer fibrous tunic of the eyeball. Its primary function is to provide strong external structural framework to the eye, thus providing protection to the delicate intraocular structures and maintaining structural integrity of the globe. The differences in the functions and characteristics of cornea and sclera can be related to their biochemical composition.

Table 3.3: Comparison between collagen fibers of cornea and sclera.[50]

Corneal collagen	Scleral collagen
Collagen fibrils have diameter of around 25–35 nm[36]	Wider collagen fibrils (28–300 nm)
Uniform distance between the collagen fibers	Nonuniform spacing
Each collagen lamellae parallelly arranged to surface of cornea	Randomly directed, highly interweaving
Secreted by keratocytes	Secreted by stromal fibroblasts

Biochemical Composition

Water constitutes 68% of sclera.[48] Collagen contributes to 75% of dry weight of the sclera. The other constituents, which contribute to its dry weight, include proteoglycans (0.7–0.9%), elastin (2%), fibrocyte (2%), glycoproteins, and other salts.[49]

Collagen

Collagen is the major extracellular component of the scleral stroma. The predominant collagen in human sclera is type I.[48] Other types, which have been detected in human sclera are type III, IV, V, VI, and VIII[48,49] (Table 3.3).

Proteoglycans

The GAG, which is predominantly found in sclera, is dermatan sulfate. The other GAGs, which are found are chondroitin sulfate, hyaluronic acid, and heparan sulfate.[49] The core proteins, which are found in proteoglycans in sclera are decorin, biglycan, and aggrecan.[50]

AQUEOUS HUMOR, IRIS, AND CILIARY BODY

Introduction

Aqueous humor is a transparent clear fluid and forms an integral part of the optical system. It is secreted by the nonpigmented epithelium of the ciliary process from plasma by selective transport of solutes and water across the ciliary epithelium into the posterior chamber of the eye. The maintenance of intraocular pressure depends on the aqueous humor dynamics.

Biochemical Processes involved in Aqueous Humor Secretion

The formation of aqueous humor involves three physiological mechanisms—(1) diffusion, (2) ultrafiltration, and (3) active secretion.[51] All these mechanisms occur simultaneously. The first two mechanisms are passive and active secretion is an energy-dependent process, fuelled mainly by ATP. Even though active secretion accounts for 90% of production,[52,53] a seamless integration of all the three mechanisms, as described below, take place to contribute to the aqueous humor formation.

1. Exchange of solutes and water between the blood plasma, which flows through the fenestrated capillaries of ciliary processes and the ciliary stroma by ultrafiltration and diffusion results in the formation of stromal ultrafiltrate.
2. Selective transport of a number of solutes and ions across the ciliary epithelium to the posterior chamber mainly by active secretion.
3. This ionic transport creates an osmotic difference and results in flow of water by osmosis.

The apical adherence of pigmented and nonpigmented ciliary epithelium and the presence of tight junctions in the apex of nonpigmented ciliary epithelium deter the paracellular diffusion of ions and solutes. These tight junctions form the major component of blood–aqueous barrier.

Ionic Transport

Though there are numerous models, which have been proposed for ionic transport across ciliary epithelium,[54-56] it has been identified that the nonpigmented and pigmented ciliary epithelium acts as a syncytium and are involved in ionic and water transport.

The basic events, which are involved, are:

- Transport of ions and solutes from ciliary stroma into the pigment epithelial cells
- Movement of ions and solutes from pigment epithelial cells into the nonpigmented epithelial cells through the gap junctions
- Translocation of ions and solutes from nonpigmented cells to the posterior chamber by active or carrier-mediated transport systems.

It has been proposed that active transport of Na^+ is the main process in aqueous humor secretion, which has been supported by studies in which usage of Na^+–K^+ ATPase inhibitors caused reduction in intraocular pressure.[57-59] In recent years, it has been postulated that Cl^- transport across the ciliary epithelium from ciliary stroma to posterior chamber is equally important in aqueous humor secretion.[60-63] The major active transport systems involved in Na^+, Cl^- transport across the ciliary epithelium, which

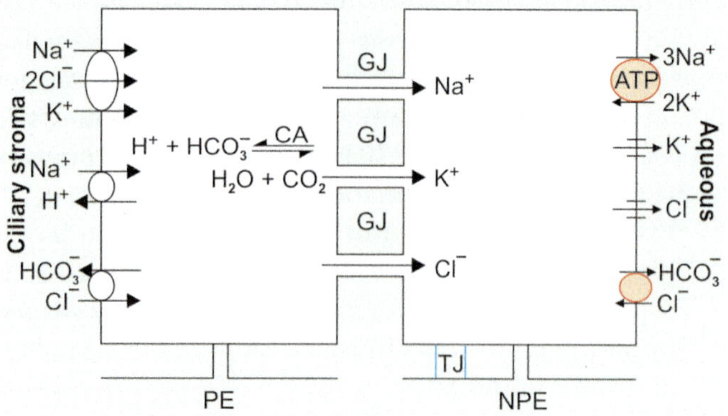

Fig. 3.3: Schematic representation of transporters and ion channels in pigmented epithelium (PE) and nonpigmented epithelium (NPE).
(TJ: Tight junctions; GJ: Gap junctions)

are involved in Na^+, Cl^- uptake from the ciliary stroma are the Na^+/H^+ antiport and Cl^-/HCO_3^- exchanger, and the $Na^+/K^+/2Cl^-$ cotransporter.[64-66] The energy for this Cl^- accumulation in ciliary epithelium is provided by Na^+–K^+ ATPase. The Cl^- channels are involved in transport from nonpigmented ciliary epithelium to the posterior chamber (Fig. 3.3).[62,63]

Role of Na+–K+ ATPase

Na^+–K^+ ATPase is an enzyme, which is found in the ciliary epithelium, predominantly in nonpigmented epithelial cells.[58] The enzyme activity is also detected to a lesser extent in the pigmented epithelial cells as well. This enzyme provides the energy for the transport of ions across the ciliary epithelium.

Role of Carbonic Anhydrase

Carbonic anhydrase (CA) is an enzyme, which is found in the cell membrane and cytoplasm of pigmented and nonpigmented epithelial cells. It catalyzes the reaction:

$$CO_2 + H_2O \rightleftarrows H_2CO_3 \rightleftarrows H^+ + HCO_3^-$$

Although the exact role of CA and mechanism of action of CA inhibitors is a subject of debate, it has been postulated that the enzyme plays an important role in intracellular buffering mechanism by providing H^+ and HCO_3^- and inhibition of the enzyme decreases Na^+ and HCO_3^- secretion into the aqueous.[67]

Transport of Water and Other Substances

Aquaporins 1 and 4 have been detected in the nonpigmented ciliary epithelium apical and basolateral membrane.[68] They are involved in water transport across nonpigmented ciliary epithelium for aqueous humor secretion. Transport systems for glucose,[69,70] amino acids,[71] and ascorbate[72] have also been reported in the nonpigmented ciliary epithelium.

Biochemical Composition of Aqueous Humor

Water is the main and major constituent of aqueous humor. It constitutes about 99.9% of aqueous humor under normal conditions. Aqueous humor is optically clear because of the relatively very low-protein content when compared to plasma and absence of red blood cells. It also contains various organic and inorganic ions, glucose, amino acids, and growth factors.

The ions are transported into the posterior chamber mainly by various active transport systems. A small amount is contributed by ultrafiltration and diffusion. The concentration of cations such as Na^+, K^+, magnesium (Mg^+) are almost nearly similar to the plasma concentration[73] (Table 3.4). Cl^- concentration is relatively high when compared to plasma.[74] Ascorbate concentration is 10–50 times more than plasma.[73] The concentration of lactate is high when compared to plasma probably due to anaerobic glycolysis. The level of calcium is 50% when compared to plasma.[73] The concentration of proteins in aqueous humor is 200 times less than the concentration of the same in plasma.[75,76] When compared to plasma, glucose concentration in the aqueous humor is mildly low.[77] Glutathione is also present in aqueous humor and it plays a role in protecting from oxidative damage.[78] Various growth factors like TGF-β,[79] FGF,[80] insulin like growth factor,[81] VEGF,[82] and enzymes of coagulation and fibrinolytic systems have also been identified in aqueous humor. In addition, oxygen[83] and carbon dioxide[73] is also present in aqueous humor. The corneal endothelium, lens, and the trabecular meshwork endothelial cells derive their oxygen supply from aqueous (Table 3.4).

Blood–Aqueous Barrier

Blood-aqueous barrier is more of a functional, rather than an anatomical concept. In the classical model, it was

Table 3.4: Biochemical composition of aqueous humor.

Component	Aqueous humor	Plasma
Na^+ (mM)	142	130–145
K^+ (mM)	4	3.5–5.
Ca^+ (mM)	1.2	2.–2.6
Mg^{2+} (mM)	1	0.7–1.1
Cl^- (mM)	131	92–125
HCO_3^- (mM)	20	24–30
Ascorbate (mM)	1.1	0.04–0.06
Lactate (mM)	4.5	0.5–0.8
Glucose (mM)	2.7–3.9	5.6–6.4

Source: Adapted from Riley MV. The Chemistry of Aqueous Humor. In: Anderson RE (Ed). Biochemistry of the Eye. San Francisco: American Academy of Ophthalmology; 1983.

proposed that blood-aqueous barrier is formed by the iris vascular endothelium and tight junctions connecting apical portions of nonpigmented ciliary epithelium.[84-86] It has also been suggested that tight junctions in the posterior iris epithelium is another key component of blood-aqueous barrier.[85,87] This barrier prevents the entry of high-molecular weight substances from entering the aqueous humor, which results in optical clarity of aqueous humor. Many factors can disrupt this barrier and result in various clinical implications. Factors affecting blood-aqueous barrier include ocular trauma, paracentesis, chemical irritants like acid, alkali, endogenous mediators like histamine, bradykinin, PGs, acetylcholine, and radiation exposure.[88,89] With the breakdown of blood-aqueous barrier, the level of proteins, inflammatory mediators, and fibrin in the aqueous rise rapidly. Chronic disruption of this barrier can result in cataract, posterior synechiae, and a neovascular response. Breakdown is accompanied by a transient rise in intraocular pressure followed by hypotony.

Iris and Ciliary Body

Iris and ciliary body are highly specialized tissues, which play important role in aqueous humor formation and dynamics, eicosanoid production, and drug metabolism.

Eicosanoids in the Iris and Ciliary Body

Eicosanoids include PGs, prostacyclins, thromboxane, and leukotrienes, which are arachidonic acid derivatives. PGs have important implications in maintenance of blood-aqueous barrier and aqueous humor dynamics. In the eye, they mediate several actions like pupillary miosis (PGE2), control of intraocular pressure (PGF2α), and inflammatory responses. Elevated levels of PGs are detected following anterior uveitis and high concentration can result in breakdown of blood-aqueous barrier and increase in intraocular pressure.

Inflammatory stimuli can release arachidonic acid from phospholipids in the plasma membrane by the action of phospholipase A2. The arachidonic acid, by the action of cyclooxygenase (COX) is converted to PGs. Cyclooxygenase exists in two forms—COX1 as the constitutive form, and COX2 as the inducible form. Classical nonsteroidal anti inflammatory drugs (NSAIDs) like aspirin and indomethacin block both forms of enzymes. Topical NSAIDs are useful in conditions such as postoperative inflammation, allergic conjunctivitis, pseudophakic cystoid macular edema, and also to prevent pupillary miosis during intraocular surgery. Trials are also currently underway regarding usage of topical NSAIDs in the management of diabetic macular edema.

The classical experiment of Camras et al.[90] in 1977 found that topically administered PGs (mainly PGF2α) produced an initial hypertensive followed by a prolong hypotensive phase. Since then, the evolution of PGs derivatives of PGF2α for the treatment of glaucoma has come a long way, and currently, they are one of the first lines of drugs in glaucoma management. They act by increasing aqueous outflow, mainly through the uveoscleral pathway.

Detoxification and Production of Antioxidants

Many enzymes, which are involved in the detoxification of endogenous and exogenous substances, have been identified in the ciliary body. The cytochrome P450 group of proteins plays a major role in the drug detoxification in the anterior segment. They convert the hydrophobic substances to hydroxylated hydrophilic substances, which can be easily metabolized. The ciliary body mediates secretion of ascorbic acid and reduced glutathione into the aqueous humor. It also has key antioxidant enzymes like catalase, superoxide dismutase, glutathione reductase, and glutathione peroxidase type I and type II enzymes. Thus the ciliary body delivers antioxidants and antioxidant enzymes to the aqueous humor.

LENS

Introduction

Lens is a transparent, biconvex, and avascular structure placed in the patellar fossa and plays an important role in the optical system of the eye by refracting light and focusing the incident light at the level of retinal photoreceptors. It is able to perform this function due to its high refractive index (1.42 centrally and 1.36 peripherally) and its biconvex structure. This high refractive index can be attributed to the relatively high concentration of proteins in the human lens. The lens is susceptible to oxidative damage by reactive oxygen species resulting in the development of cataract. The economic burden due to cataract and cataract surgery is huge; and as a consequence, there is an enormous interest among researchers to understand the molecular and biochemical processes involved in cataract formation. This section deals with the biochemical composition, metabolic pathways, transport mechanisms, antioxidants in the lens, and biochemical changes in cataract.

Biochemical Composition of Lens

The biochemical composition can vary with aging and different subtypes of cataract. The following section explains about the biochemical composition of a normal young crystalline lens.

Water

Water constitutes 65% of wet weight of the lens making it a relatively dehydrated structure. The low concentration of water, along with high protein content, is responsible for its optical clarity and refractive index.

Lipids[91-93]

The lipids form the major component of plasma membrane of lens fibers. The major lipids in the lens fiber plasma membrane include phospholipids (with dihydrosphingomyelin being the most abundant) and cholesterol. The amount of cholesterol in the human lens is higher than any other organ in the body.

Proteins

Proteins constitute 33% of wet weight of lens. In 1894, Morner classified lens proteins as water soluble and water insoluble.[94] Water-soluble proteins constitute up to 80–90% of lens proteins in young age. The crystallins are the major water-soluble proteins in the human lens. Water-insoluble proteins are further classified on the basis of urea solubility.

Crystallins: Crystallin lens proteins are one of the major determinant for transparency and optical properties of the lens. Vertebrate crystallins can be classified into α-crystallin, β-, and γ-crystallins. They are very stable proteins and are crucial to the lens where new protein synthesis is not possible.

- *α-crystallins*: It comprises about 40% of all lens proteins.[95] It consists of two subunits αA and αB with each subunit having a molecular mass of 20 kDa. The α-crystallins exist as heterodimers of αA and αB subunit in the ratio of 3:1, with a molecular weight of about 600–900 kDa. They belong to the family of heat shock proteins and act as a lens chaperone.[96] They help in keeping the lens proteins in their native state by preventing the unfolding and conformational changes, thereby minimizing denaturation of proteins.[95-97] With aging, due to post-translational changes to the lens crystallins, there is a formation of high-molecular weight water-insoluble aggregates of α-crystallin accompanied by a decrease in the chaperone activity resulting in increased susceptibility of lens proteins to oxidative damage due to protein denaturation and unfolding. All these factors contribute to protein aggregation, water insolubility resulting in light scattering and eventual loss of transparency.[98]
- *β-, γ-crystallins*: These compact and stable crystallins are believed to be products of same gene family. β-crystallins, which are the most abundant crystallins in the eye, have a molecular mass of around 23–32 kDa. γ-crystallin is monomeric with molecular mass of around 20 kDa. The exact biological function of these crystallins is not known.

Membrane proteins and cytoskeletal proteins: Membrane proteins are insoluble in water and urea. The major membrane protein found in lens is major intrinsic protein 26 (MIP), which belongs to the family of aquaporins (aquaporin 0). Earlier, MIP 26 was thought to be a gap junction protein. However, in recent times, it is considered to act as a water channel.[99,100] *LIM2* gene is a novel gene whose product MP19 is a novel integral membrane protein in lens fiber cells. MP19 has been proposed to play a role in junctional communication. Mutations in *LIM2* gene can lead to congenital cataracts.[101]

The cytoskeletal proteins, which provide the structural stability to the lens cells, are water insoluble and urea soluble. Actin, vimentin, tubulin, filensins, and phakinin are important members of this group.[102] Of these, the last two proteins are unique to the lens.

Electrolytes[103]

The lens has low-Na^+ levels and high-K^+ levels when compared to vitreous and aqueous humor. The lens Ca^{2+} level is also very low. However, this electrolyte balance is deranged in senile cataract and the Na^+ and Ca^{2+} levels are increased in this condition (Fig. 3.4).

Ascorbic Acid[104]

Ascorbic acid is present in the lens where it acts as an antioxidant. However, a product of it formed during free radical scavenging, called dehydroascorbic acid can cause oxidative damage. The dehydroascorbic acid is reduced to ascorbic acid by either glutathione-dependent enzymes or by reduced glutathione, which helps in maintaining low levels of dehydroascorbic acid.

Glutathione[104-106]

Glutathione is the major antioxidant in the lens. It is produced in the lens epithelium and superficial fiber cells where it exists in the reduced form (GSH). There is also evidence that some amount of glutathione is transported into lens from aqueous humor. GSH has sulfhydryl group, which can be readily oxidized, thereby protecting exposed thiols of lens protein from oxidation by reactive oxygen species. The oxidized form (GSSG) is reduced by NADPH-dependent glutathione reductase. However, the cells situated deep in the lens have minimal capacity for production or reduction of glutathione and they depend on diffusion from the superficial cells for reduced glutathione. The GSSG from the deeper cells diffuses back to the superficial cells for regeneration of GSH. This two-way diffusion decreases with age, making the proteins and lipids in the deeper fiber cells, and lens nuclei more susceptible to oxidative damage.

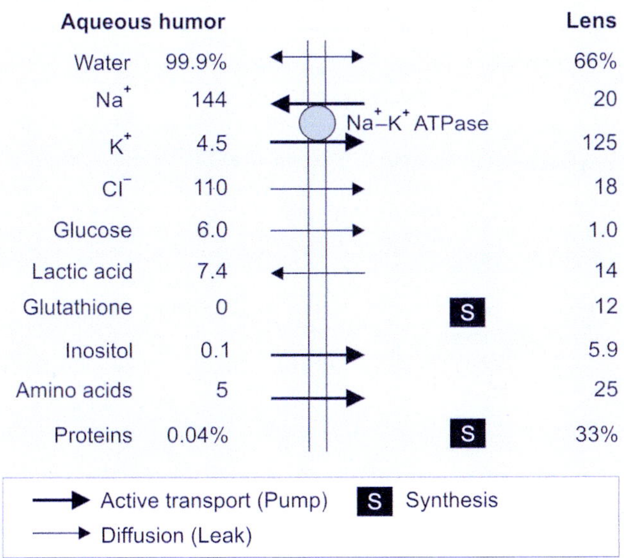

Fig. 3.4: Chemical composition of the rabbit lens. The values are similar to those in the human lens. All values are given in mmol/kg of lens water unless otherwise stated.
Source: Peyman, 1st edition.

Amino Acids

Lens epithelium also has various transporters for amino acid transport into the lens.

Inositol[107,108]

The concentration of inositol in the lens is high. Inositol is postulated to help in maintenance of osmotic balance and membrane integrity.

Metabolic Pathways in the Lens[109]

Lens being an avascular structure is mainly dependent on anaerobic glycolysis for energy production. The lens gets its glucose and oxygen primarily through diffusion from aqueous humor.

Glucose is metabolized in normal lens by these four pathways:

1. Anaerobic glycolysis
2. Krebs cycle (aerobic metabolism)
3. Hexose monophosphate shunt
4. Sorbitol pathway.

Anaerobic Glycolysis

Since the lens has low-oxygen tension and is mainly dependent on aqueous humor for oxygen, anaerobic glycolysis contributes to about 80% of glucose metabolism. Glucose is converted to glucose 6-phosphate by the enzyme hexokinase. The enzyme hexokinase is present at very low levels in the lens. It controls the production of glucose 6-phosphate for both glycolysis and HMP shunt and also regulates the rate of lactate formation. Hence, hexokinase appears to be the rate-limiting factor in lens glycolysis. The end product of anaerobic glycolysis is lactate, which can either be metabolized further by Krebs cycle or gets diffused into the aqueous humor. Two molecules of ATP are generated by one molecule of glucose by anaerobic glycolysis.

Krebs Cycle

Due to paucity of oxygen in the human lens, only around 3% of glucose is metabolized by Krebs cycle. This cycle is active mainly in the lens epithelium and equatorial cells. Metabolism of one molecule of glucose through Krebs cycle generates 36 ATP. Due to this efficient ATP generation, 20% of total ATP production in human lens is through the Krebs cycle.

Hexose Monophosphate Shunt

Hexose monophosphate shunt becomes active at times of oxidative stress to restore the NADPH levels, which is decreased due to oxidation by glutathione reductase.

Sorbitol Pathway

A small percentage of glucose (5%) is converted to sorbitol by the enzyme aldose reductase. Sorbitol is converted to fructose by the enzyme polyol dehydrogenase, which can enter the glycolytic pathway after conversion to fructose 6-phosphate by the enzyme fructokinase. The conversion of sorbitol to fructose is slow and hence during conditions of high-glucose levels, sorbitol accumulates causing osmotic stress, which can cause large movement of water into the lens resulting in lens hydration and opacification. The activation of this pathway also results in increase in NADP levels, which can stimulate HMP shunt (Fig. 3.5).

Transport Mechanisms in the Lens

The lens fibers function like a single cell or a syncytium and hence nutrition and support to the non-nucleated deep fiber cells is provided by the epithelial and surface nucleated fiber cells through gap junction communication between the cells. Gap junction channels are composed of proteins, which are member of connexins family. While connexin 43 is the predominant connexin in epithelial cells, connexin 46 and connexin 50 are involved in the intra-lens fiber communication.[110]

It has been proposed that the lens has an internal ionic current, which drives the circulation of water and ions inside the lens. According to this model, the current enters the lens at the anterior and posterior poles and flow outward at the lens equator. This current arises due to the differences in the distribution of ionic pumps inside the lens.[111]

Maintenance of electrolyte balance inside the lens is critical for its transparency. The predominant transport system in the lens is Na^+–K^+ ATPase, which is located mainly in the anterior lens epithelium and superficial cortical fibers. This system pumps K^+ into the lens and Na^+ out of the lens at the anterior surface, which in turn, generates a chemical gradient that stimulates diffusion of Na^+ into the lens and K^+ out of the lens mainly through the posterior surface. This process of active transport (pump) stimulating passive diffusion was termed by Kinsey and Reddy in 1965 as "pump leak theory".[112] Inhibition of Na^+–K^+ ATPase system can make

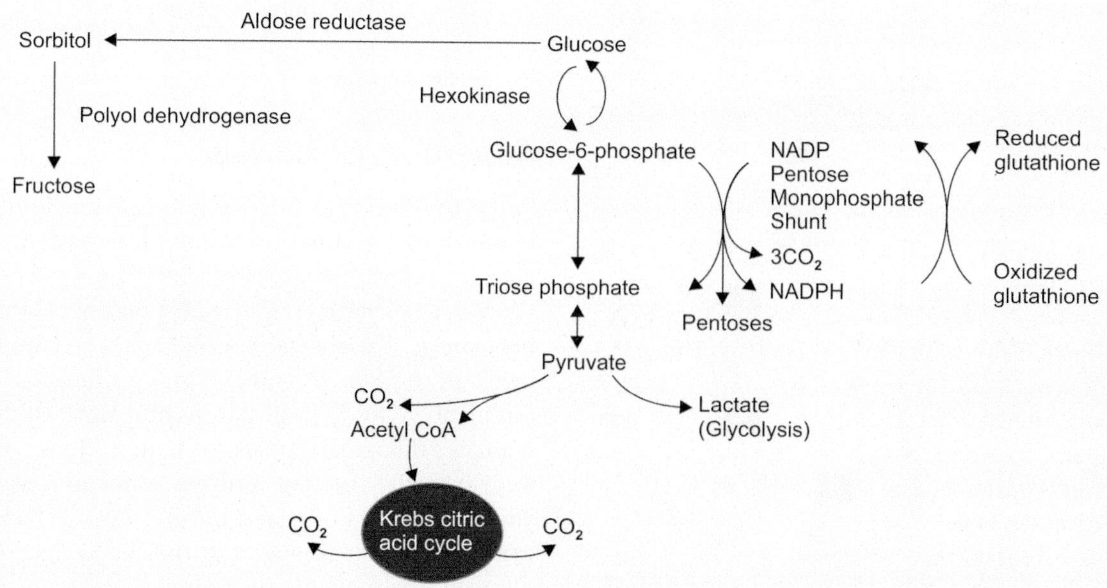

Fig. 3.5: Pathways for glucose metabolism in lens.
Source: Peyman, 1st edition.

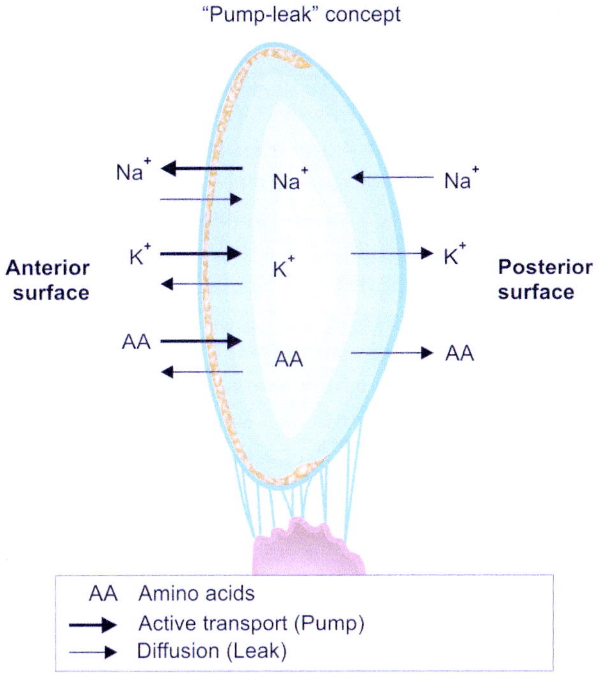

Fig. 3.6: The lens "pump leak" mechanism of active transport at anterior epithelial surface generates a diffusion gradient, resulting in leak of actively transported materials through the anterior and posterior surfaces.
Source: Peyman, 1st edition.

the cells to lose K^+ and gain Na^+. Water then enters the lens driven by the osmotic gradient, which causes swelling of cells resulting in loss of transparency (Fig. 3.6).

Antioxidants in the Lens[104-106,113]

The human cells are constantly exposed to oxidative stress from reactive oxygen species. The reactive oxygen species include superoxide anion (O_2^-), hydroxyl radical ($OH^\bullet$), hydrogen peroxide (H_2O_2), and singlet oxygen. They are produced in the mitochondria, peroxisomes, and cytoplasm through normal metabolic reactions, and/or by exposure to ionizing radiation, ultraviolet light, and anticancer drugs. Although free radicals and other reactive oxygen intermediates are essential for normal cellular metabolism, they can also result in lipid peroxidation and oxidation of critical proteins, which can lead to alteration of cell membrane permeability, and inhibition of membrane ionic pumps ultimately resulting in cellular dysfunction.

Even though lens has low-oxygen tension, it derives a part of its energy from oxidative phosphorylation making it vulnerable to oxidative damage. Although most of the ultraviolet light is absorbed by the cornea, some amount can reach the lens where it can react with chromophores and pigments to produce free radicals. The potential free radicals in the lens include oxidized glutathione (GSSG), dehydroascorbic acid, and hydrogen peroxide. These free radicals, by oxidation of critical proteins and lipids, can result in alteration of membrane permeability, crosslinking of proteins, increase in proportion of insoluble proteins, and ultimately it results in loss of transparency. Hence, it is critical that the lens proteins and lipids should be maintained in a reduced state.

The lens has numerous antioxidant systems to maintain the redox environment. This includes the enzymes superoxide dismutase, catalase, and glutathione peroxidase. The other antioxidants in the lens include ascorbic acid and vitamin E. The superoxide anion, which is produced as a result of oxidative damage, is converted to hydrogen peroxide (H_2O_2) by superoxide dismutase. The hydrogen peroxide in the presence of Fe^{++} or heavy metals can become hydroxyl radical, which is the most reactive free radical and can damage the cell membranes and deoxyribonucleic acid (DNA). The enzymes catalase and selenium-dependent glutathione peroxidase converts hydrogen peroxide to water, thus decreasing oxidative damage from these reactive oxygen species. In the process of conversion of H_2O_2 to water by glutathione peroxidase, glutathione is oxidized. Oxidized glutathione (GSSG) by the action of NADPH-dependent glutathione reductase is converted to its reduced form (GSH). In the normal young lens, the levels of GSH decrease from the cortex to nucleus.

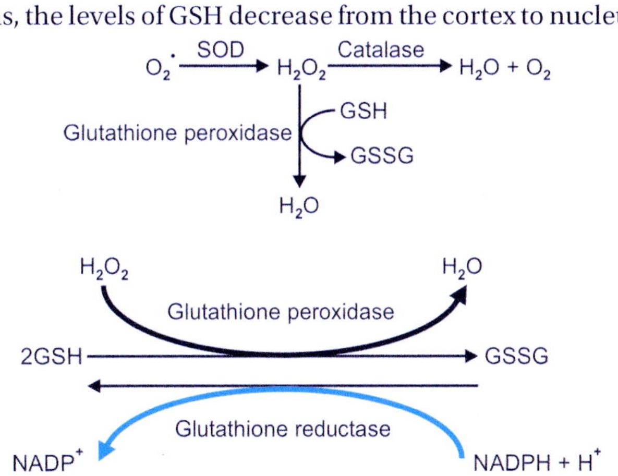

(SOD: Superoxide dismutase; GSH: Reduced glutathione; GSSG: Oxidized glutathione)

With increasing age, there is low activity of glutathione redox cycle. There is decrease in the level of glutathione reductase and reduced glutathione, rendering the lens susceptible to oxidative damage. Thiolation of proteins by GSSG, cysteine, and gamma glutamyl cysteine results in the formation of mixed disulfides. Further oxidation of these mixed disulfides results in protein-protein disulfides. These are found in the large water-insoluble protein aggregates, which cause light scattering and decrease in transparency.

The lens also has several mechanisms for repair of proteins after oxidative stress. It involves the GSH-dependent thioltransferase, NADPH-dependent thioredoxin and thioredoxin reductase system, and methionine sulfoxide reductases. These systems can partially restore the mixed disulfides and protein disulfides to their original form. Their activity also reduces with age.

Biochemical Changes Leading to Cataract Formation

As age progresses, there occurs various changes in the lens physically and biochemically. In many cases, aging changes may be accelerated and/or cellular metabolism may be deranged resulting in initiation of cataract formation. The cataractous changes can superimpose on the normal aging changes making it difficult to differentiate between these two processes.

Several studies have identified various risk factors for cataract development. These include heredity, exposure to ultraviolet radiation, ionizing radiation, diabetes, dietary factors, drugs like steroids and inborn error of metabolism.[114-116]

The etiology of age-related cataract is multifactorial and is not understood fully. The following changes are thought to aid in the process of cataract formation.

- Alterations in lens protein biochemistry[106] and lipid biochemistry[91]
- Decrease in reduced glutathione levels[105,106,113,117]
- Decreased activity of enzymes like catalase, superoxide dismutase, glutathione peroxidase, and glutathione reductase[113,118,119]
- Formation of advanced glycation end products[120]
- Decreased ATP production and alterations in water and ionic transport and electrolyte composition.[106]

Numerous evidence points to the oxidative damage as one of the primary biochemical mechanism responsible for cataract formation.[105,106,113,121,122] With aging, there occurs decrease in the activity of antioxidants in the lens resulting in increased susceptibility of lens proteins to oxidative damage. As a result of this oxidative stress, the following changes happen in proteins, namely—denaturation and unfolding, formation of high-molecular weight aggregates, and water insolubility resulting in loss of transparency. The protein thiol and protein disulfides, which are formed due to oxidation, are reported to be part of protein aggregates found in cataract.

In nuclear cataract, oxidative damage is postulated to be the key factor, which causes nucleus hardening, accumulation of pigments and light scattering resulting in loss of transparency.[122] In cortical cataract, increase in membrane permeability along with decreased activity of Na^+–K^+ ATPase results in increase in intralenticular Na^+ and Ca^{2+} levels, decrease in K^+ levels, hydration of lens fibers, and protein loss.[123]

As mentioned previously, under normal conditions sorbitol pathway is less active. With high-glucose levels, aldose reductase competes with hexokinase and more glucose is metabolized through this pathway. Accumulation of sorbitol occurs because it is neither metabolized nor transported out of the lens. This results in increase in osmolarity of lens causing water shift into the lens resulting in lens opacification.[124]

In addition to polyol pathway, increased level of free radicals,[125] decrease levels of antioxidants,[119] and formation of advanced glycation end products[126] are also postulated in the pathogenesis of diabetic cataract. In galactosemia, deficiency of galactokinase or galactose-1-phosphate uridyltransferase results in shunting of galactose through a pathway mediated by aldose reductase. This results in accumulation of galactitol inside the lens, which causes increased intralenticular osmolarity, influx of water into lens cells, eventually leading to opacification (Flowchart 3.2).[124]

Flowchart 3.2: Metabolic pathways for galactose metabolism in lens.

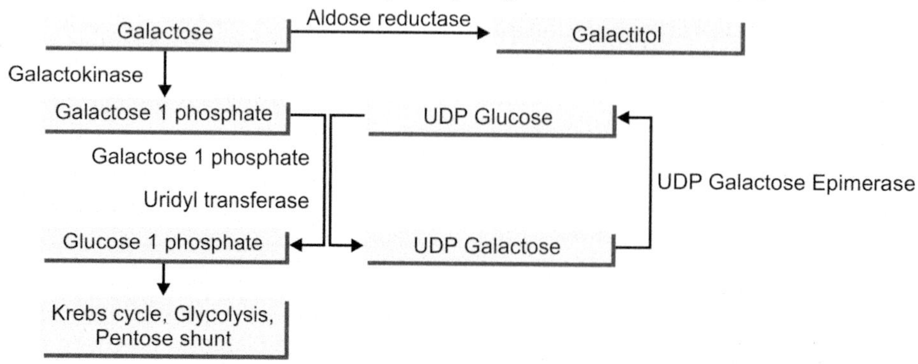

(UDP: Uridine diphosphate)
Source: Peyman, 1st edition.

In human lens, 3-hydroxykynurenine, a product of tryptophan metabolism is the major ultraviolet light-absorbing compound. Most of the ultraviolet light is absorbed by the cornea. The remaining UV rays, which enter the lens, are predominantly UVA. The 3-hydroxykynurenine can cause modification of crystallins resulting in structural and functional changes, which may play a role in cataractogenesis.[127]

VITREOUS

Introduction

Vitreous humor is a transparent, clear, and inert specialized connective tissue gel, which acts as a major supporting structure to the eyeball. The biochemical composition of the vitreous determines whether it exists as a gel or liquid. Biochemical changes in vitreous due to aging or disease conditions like myopia can manifest as clinically recognizable manifestations in retina and vitreous.

Biochemical Composition

The major structural components of vitreous are—water, collagen, and hyaluronic acid. Vitreous consists of approximately 98–99% water and 0.1% macromolecules such as collagen, proteoglycans, GAGs, and glycoproteins. The ions and low-molecular weight solutes constitute the remaining solid matter.

Collagen[128]

Vitreous collagen fibrils are heterotypic and predominantly consists of type II, type IX, and type V/XI. They are similar to cartilage collagen fibrils. The diameter of collagen fibrils in the vitreous is approximately 10–20 nm. Type II collagen is the major collagen type in the human vitreous and accounts for about 60–75% of the total collagen. Type IX collagen contributes to around 25% of vitreous collagen. It is found on the surface of heterotypic fibrils. Type IX collagen can occur as proteoglycan and nonproteoglycan form. The proteoglycan form carries a single chondroitin sulfate side chain. Type V/XI collagen is a minor fibril forming collagen (around 10%). This collagen along with type II collagen forms the core of heterotypic fibril.

Hyaluronic Acid[128]

Hyaluronic acid is the predominant GAG in the human vitreous. It consists of repeating disaccharide units composed of β1–4 glucuronic acid β1–3N-acetylglucosamine. It exists as a linear unbranched polymer, which can coil upon itself, forming a large sponge-like network amongst the collagen fibers. The negative charges in the hyaluronic acid contribute to its ability to adsorb water. The volume of nonhydrated hyaluronic acid is 0.66 cm^3/g, in contrast with the volume of the hydrated molecule, which is 2,000–3,000 cm^3/g. Thus the degree of hydration determines the size and extension of hyaluronic acid molecular network. A decline in surrounding ionic strength results in repulsion of anionic charges within the hyaluronic acid molecule resulting in expansion of vitreous gel, while an elevation of the ionic strength results in contraction of the molecule, thus resulting in vitreous gel contraction. The hyaluronic acid confers the property of viscoelasticity to the vitreous gel.

Chondroitin Sulfate Proteoglycans[128]

Two chondroitin sulfate proteoglycan forms exist in the vitreous—versican and type IX collagen. Versican is a proteoglycan with central domain, which carry chondroitin sulfate chains. Mutations that alter the splicing of the central chondroitin sulfate bearing domains of versican have been implicated in Wagner syndrome.

Noncollagenous Proteins

Soluble proteins:[129] The major soluble proteins of the vitreous include albumin, acid glycoprotein, and transferrin. Other proteins, which have been detected, are neutrophil elastase inhibitor, tissue plasminogen activator, retinol binding protein, alpha-1 antitrypsin, proapolipoprotein, beta-2 crystallin, and transthyretin. Albumin forms the majority of soluble protein in vitreous in many species. While the source of albumin is thought to be plasma, transferrin is presumed to be obtained from the ocular tissues surrounding the vitreous.

Fibrillin:[130,131] Glycoprotein fibrillin is an integral component of ciliary zonules and plays an important role in elasticity and stability of ocular connective tissue. Vitreous has fibrillin 1 and fibrillin 2, which assemble into beaded microfibrils. Mutations in fibrillin 1 result in Marfan's syndrome, which has various ophthalmic and systemic manifestations. Due to defective fibrillin, there is vitreous liquefaction and increased propensity for rhegmatogenous retinal detachment in these patients.

Fibulin:[132] Fibulin belongs to a family of extracellular matrix glycoproteins and helps in collagen fibers assembly.

Opticin:[132,133] Opticin is a novel glycoprotein, which has been associated with vitreous collagen fibrils. It belongs to a family of extracellular matrix proteins, which has leucine-rich repeats. It has been proposed to have important role in collagen fibrillar assembly and inhibition of aggregation of adjacent collagen fibrils into bundles. Decrease in activity of opticin protein may be related to vitreous liquefaction and age-related vitreous degeneration, which are characterized by collagen fibrillar aggregation. Opticin also has antiangiogenic properties and inhibits preretinal neovascularization.

VIT 1:[134] It is a novel protein, which helps in maintaining the structure of vitreous gel.

Matrix metalloproteinases (MMPs):[135] These are a group of zinc-dependent enzymes, which are involved in the degradation of basement membrane and extracellular matrix components along with other enzymes and hence play a key role in wound healing. It has been proposed that MMP can also increase VEGF bioavailability. Their activity is kept in check by the tissue inhibitors of matrix metalloproteinases (TIMP). These enzymes have both physiological and pathological roles in the vitreous. In vitreous, they play a major role in the initiation of angiogenesis and are upregulated in conditions causing neovascularization like proliferative diabetic retinopathy, retinopathy of prematurity, and other conditions causing retinal neovascularization. They are also upregulated in proliferative vitreoretinopathy. MMP-1, -2, -3, and -9 are expressed in vitreous. TIMP-1, -2, and -3 have also been detected in vitreous.

Biochemical Changes with Aging

With aging, there is progressive vitreous liquefaction and concurrent lowering in volume of vitreous gel. These changes result in the formation of pockets of liquid vitreous, called lacunae. There is exponential loss of type IX collagen, which is found on the surface of type II collagen fibril with age leading to exposure of sticky type II collagen resulting in intrafibrillar aggregation and condensation. There is increase in hyaluronic acid concentration in the liquid phase and decrease in levels in the gel phase. All these changes result in posterior vitreous detachment.

RETINA

Introduction

Human retina has specialized photoreceptors called rods and cones, which convert a photon of light into a neural signal by a cascade of biochemical events called phototransduction. Rods are responsible for scotopic vision (night vision) and cones are responsible for vision in bright light as well as color vision. This section explains about the visual pigments, visual cycle, and the biochemical events involved in phototransduction.

Vitamin A and Its Role in the Eye

The photosensitive pigments of the eye (rod and cone pigments) have 11-cis retinal, a compound derived from vitamin A, as its chromophore. Vitamin A obtained from dietary sources is stored in liver as retinol. Retinol is bound to plasma retinol binding protein (RBP), which is the carrier protein and it plays a significant role in retinol metabolism. It has been proposed that cellular uptake of retinol into retinal cells is mediated by a multidomain membrane protein encoded by *STRA* gene.[136] The retinol is esterified with fatty acids inside the Retinal Pigment Epithelium (RPE) and stored as retinyl esters (mainly palmitate esters). These esters serve as substrate for formation of 11-cis retinal, which acts as the chromophore in rod and cone pigments.

Visual Cycle

Visual cycle is the process by which the photosensitive pigments are recycled. It takes place simultaneously in the outer segment of the retinal photoreceptors, interphotoreceptor matrix, and RPE cells. While the classic visual cycle takes place both in rod and cone photoreceptors, additional mechanism called cone visual cycle happens exclusively in cones.[137]

Classic Visual Cycle[137-139]

As previously described, rhodopsin molecule consists of opsin and chromophore 11-cis retinal. When a photon strikes the rod photoreceptors, through a series of photochemical reactions, 11-cis retinal undergoes isomerization to all-transretinal. One of the intermediates during isomerization process, namely—metarhodopsin II triggers a series of biochemical reactions ultimately resulting in impulse transmission to the second order cells of the retina.

For visual perception and impulse transmission to continue, the 11-cis retinal should be continuously regenerated.

The all-transretinal gets released from opsin and reduced to *all-transretinol* by the action of retinol dehydrogenase, which is NADPH dependent. The all-transretinol is transported to RPE with interphotoreceptor retinol binding protein (IRBP). In the RPE, all-transretinol binds to cellular retinol binding protein (CRBP) type 1 and is esterified by the action of lecithin retinol acyltransferase (LRAT) and converted to *retinyl esters*. These retinyl esters become *11-cis retinol* by the action of an enzyme isomerohydrolase (RPE65). 11-cis retinol, thus formed, is bound to cellular retinaldehyde binding protein (CRALBP) and is oxidized to *11-cis retinal* by the action of a dehydrogenase enzyme. 11-cis retinal is transported back to the photoreceptor with the help of IRBP (Flowchart 3.3).

Role of ABCA4 in Visual Cycle and Lipofuscin Accumulation[140,141]

ABCA4, which is a member of subfamily of ATP-binding cassette transporters proteins, plays a major role in visual cycle. It processes all-transretinal and prevents accumulation of A2E (pyridinium bisretinoid), which is the major lipofuscin fluorophore. In the absence of ABCA4, A2E accumulates in lipofuscin. Lipofuscin, which accumulates in RPE with age, has been attributed to age-related decline in cellular function. Mutations in *ABCA4* gene can lead to Stargardt disease, which is the most common childhood inherited macular dystrophy.

ABCA4 may enhance the clearance of all-transretinal. It has been proposed that it may flip the Schiff-base N-retinylidene phosphatidylethanolamine to the cytoplasmic side where it can dissociate and form all-transretinal, thereby preventing the accumulation of phosphatidylethanolamine-bisretinoid (A2PE). The following events are involved in the formation of A2E as shown in the flowchart (Flowchart 3.4).

Flowchart 3.3: Schematic representation of classical visual cycle.

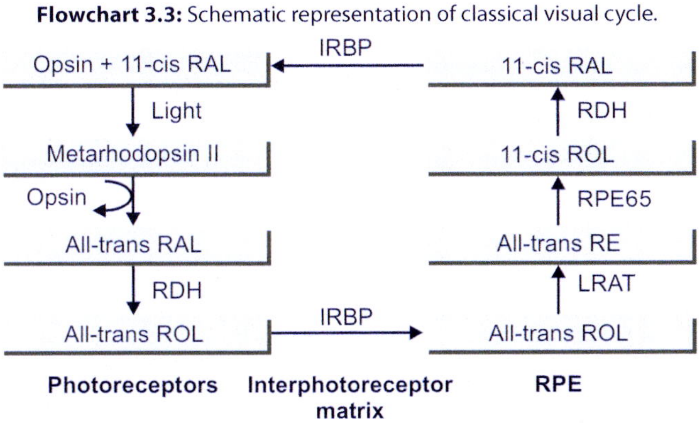

(RAL: Retinaldehyde; ROL: Retinol; RE: Retinyl esters; RDH: Retinol dehydrogenase; IRBP: Interphotoreceptor retinoid binding protein; LRAT: Lecithin retinol acyltransferase)

Flowchart 3.4: Events involved in the formation of pyridinium bisretinoid (A2E).

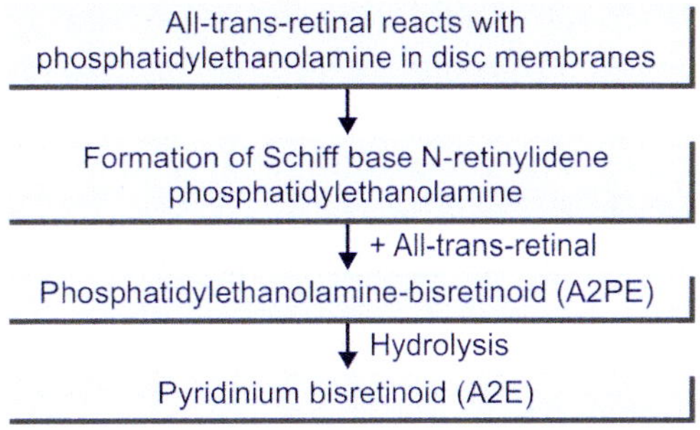

Cone Visual Cycle[137]

It has been postulated that there exists a separate mechanism in cones for recycling of chromophore, which is independent of RPE and involves the Muller cells in the retina.

Structure of Photoreceptors

The photoreceptors have outer segments (OS), inner segments (IS), and a cell body with nucleus and a synaptic terminal. All components, which are required for phototransduction, are found in the rod OS, while the metabolic requirements and the protein synthesis is taken care of by the rod IS. The rod OS have multiple lamellar disks, which are arranged along the OS long axis and a central connecting cilium, which has a characteristic 9-plus-0 configuration. The lamellar disks contain rhodopsin. The rod IS has an ellipsoid portion consisting of mitochondria and a myoid portion containing glycogen.

The cone OS is conical and the disks are continuous with the plasma membrane. The cone IS has ellipsoid and myoid portions like rods. It has been postulated that, as the cone disks are continuous with the plasma membrane, it increases the surface area and facilitates rapid phototransduction reaction in cones.[142]

Visual Pigments[139,143]

The photosensitizers in the human retina are the visual pigments namely rhodopsin (in rods) and cone pigments (in cones), which are found in the respective outer segment lamellar disks. The pigment consists of a protein called opsin attached to a chromophore 11-cis retinal.

Rhodopsin is an integral protein involved in rod phototransduction. It belongs to a family of G-protein-coupled receptors and consists of protein opsin and chromophore 11-cis retinal. It has seven transmembrane helical loops and contains ligand binding site for chromophore 11-cis retinal. The chromophore is attached to lysine residue 296 in rhodopsin's transmembrane domain through Schiff's base linkage. Rhodopsin has the ability to activate phototransduction cascade. However, this activity is inhibited by the chromophore 11-cis retinal, which is attached to it during dark, thus making the chromophore an inverse agonist. Rhodopsin is most sensitive to green portion of visible spectrum with maximum absorption at wavelengths close to 510 nm. When a photon of light strikes a rhodopsin molecule, the chromophore 11-cis retinal absorbs it and it undergoes photoisomerization to all-transretinal. The all-transretinal acts as a strong agonist for opsin resulting in a series of conformational changes in the opsin molecule ultimately resulting in formation of metarhodopsin II, which has been regarded as the activated form of rhodopsin molecule. This triggers a serious of biochemical responses resulting in hyperpolarization of rod photoreceptors, initiating a neural response.

There are three kinds of cone pigments in human, namely—S cones (which are short wavelength sensitive), M cones (for medium wavelength), and L cones for (long wavelength). Their absorption spectrum is different from rod absorption spectra and it gives rise to color vision. The chromophore 11-cis retinal is similar to rods and the difference in light absorption spectrum between rods and cones is due to the difference in the structure of protein opsin and also due to the difference in its interaction with the chromophore.

Events involved in Rod Phototransduction[144-146]

Phototransduction is the series of biochemical reactions by which absorption of a photon of light by the retinal photoreceptors results in a neural response. It consists of an activation phase and deactivation phase. The deactivation or termination response is essential for the subsequent light absorption by photoreceptors.

Many proteins are involved in phototransduction. Some of the transmembrane proteins, which are involved in rod phototransduction are rhodopsin, guanylate cyclase, and ABCR (ATP-binding cassette transporter) superfamily proteins. Peripherin and Rod outer segment protein-1 (Rom-1) are disk membrane components, which stabilize the structure of OS disks. Transducin and phosphodiesterase-6 (PDE6) are important peripheral membrane proteins involved in phototransduction.

When a photon of light is absorbed by rod photoreceptors, *11-cis retinal* found in the rod outer segment becomes *all-transretinal* by photoisomerization reactions. This triggers a serious of conformational changes in the opsin protein molecule. The intermediates, which are formed by these conformational changes in order, are bathorhodopsin, lumirhodopsin, metarhodopsin I, metarhodopsin II, and finally metarhodopsin III. *Metarhodopsin II* is considered as the activated form of rhodopsin and it results in various biochemical events finally leading to a neural response. Shortly after decay of metarhodopsin II, all-transretinal gets released from opsin. As explained above, the visual cycle converts the all-transretinal to 11-cis retinal and opsin combines with it to form rhodopsin (Flowchart 3.5).

Events Involved in Activation Phase When a Photon of Light Strikes the Rhodopsin Molecule[144-147]

Step 1: Formation of Activated Rhodopsin

As previously described, on absorption of a light photon by 11-cis retinal, photoisomerization and subsequent conformational changes in opsin molecule result in the formation of activated form metarhodopsin II (R^*).

Step 2: Activation of G Protein (Transducin)

The G protein, which is a peripheral membrane protein has 3 subunits α, β, and γ. In dark conditions, G protein remains in an inactive state and guanosine diphosphate (GDP) is attached to α subunit. On light stimulus, R* (the activated form) causes GDP to guanosine triphosphate (GTP) nucleotide exchange in α subunit. The G protein with GTP attached is the activated form. R* activates numerous transducin molecule till its deactivation.

Step 3: Phosphodiesterase Activation and Decrease in cGMP Levels

Phosphodiesterase-6 is a peripheral membrane protein with α, β, and 2γ subunits. When activated transducin is

Flowchart 3.5: Events involved when a photon of light strikes the rod photoreceptors.

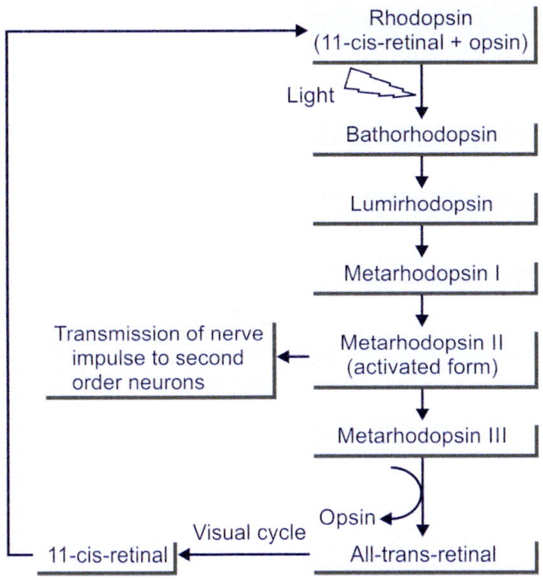

Flowchart 3.6: Events involved in rod phototransduction in the activation phase.

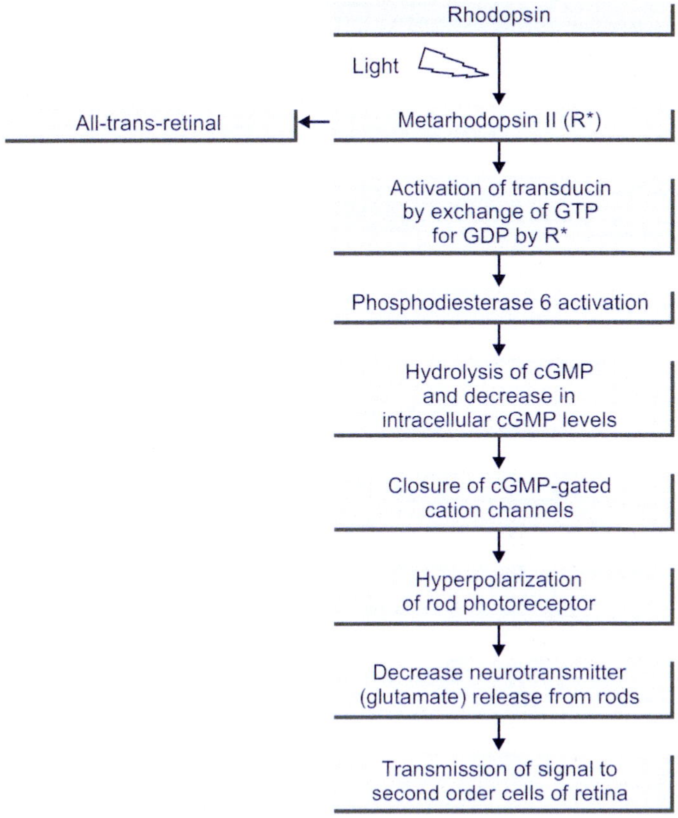

(cGMP: Cyclic guanosine monophosphate; GDP: Guanosine diphosphate; GTP: Guanosine triphosphate)

attached to PDE6, the catalytic activity of PDE6 increases many fold and it causes hydrolysis of cyclic guanosine monophosphate (cGMP) resulting in fall in concentration of cGMP.

Step 4: Closure of cGMP-gated Channels

Cyclic GMP-gated cation channel also known as CNG (cyclic nucleotide-gated channel) maintain the negative resting membrane potential of the rods. These channels allow passage of cations Na^+, K^+, and Ca^{2+}. In the dark, increased concentration of cGMP keeps these channels open. Ionic balance in rods is maintained by Na^+–K^+ ATPase in the inner segment, which causes Na^+ efflux and K^+ influx into cells and by Na^+/Ca^{2+}, K^+ (NCKX2) exchanger protein in the outer segment which pumps Ca^{2+} ions extracellularly. Phosphodiesterase activation results in decrease in cGMP concentration causing closure of cation channels, resulting in hyperpolarization. Hyperpolarization results in decreased glutamate release from rods, thus signaling light absorption to bipolar cells (Flowchart 3.6). The closure of cation channels along with continued action of NCKX2 protein results in decrease in intracellular Ca^{2+}, which triggers a feedback signal, which is essential for light adaptation.

Deactivation Phase of Rod Phototransduction[144-146]

The deactivation phase is essential to bring back the photoreceptors to its dark state. This phase consists of deactivation of activated rhodopsin, transducin, phosphodiesterase, and restoration of intracellular cGMP levels.

Deactivation of Activated Rhodopsin (R*)

For its deactivation, R* is phosphorylated by rhodopsin kinase-1. Recoverin is a protein belonging to calcium-binding protein family. In the dark state, when the calcium concentration is high, recoverin-Ca^{2+} binds to rhodopsin kinase and inhibits phosphorylation. As a result of decrease in intracellular Ca^{2+} levels following closure of cGMP-gated channels, recoverin affinity to rhodopsin kinase-1 decreases resulting in R* phosphorylation by rhodopsin kinase. Arrestins are a group of cytoplasmic proteins, which bind to G protein-coupled receptors and inhibit its activation and cellular signaling. Arrestins in the eye bind to phosphorylated rhodopsin and terminate its activation. The rhodopsin phosphorylation by rhodopsin kinase by itself cannot shut down the activity of R* completely and the binding of protein arrestin ends its activity fully.

Flowchart 3.7: Events involved in deactivation phase of rod phototransduction: (A) deactivation of activated rhodopsin (R*); (B) deactivation of transducin and phosphodiesterase-6 (PDE6); and (C) restoration of cyclic guanosine monophosphate (cGMP) levels.

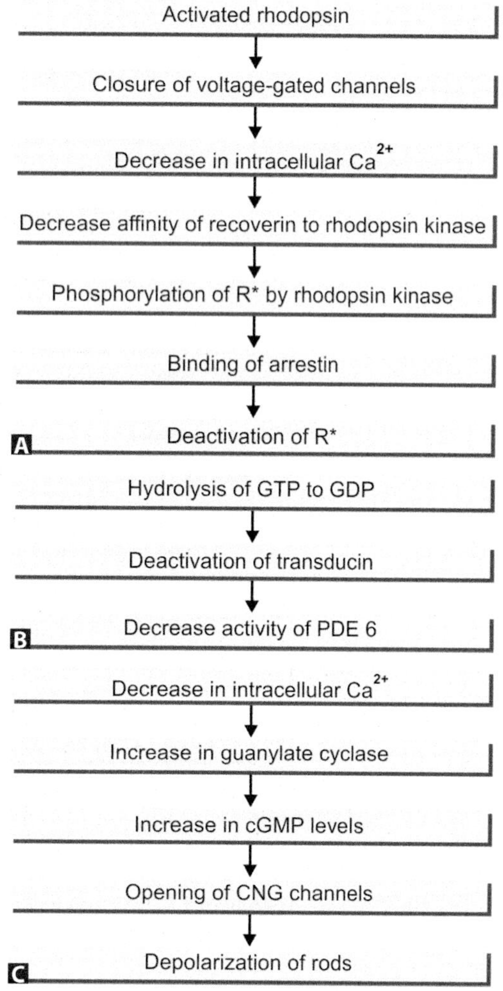

(GDP: Guanosine diphosphate; GTP: Guanosine triphosphate; CNG: Cyclic nucleotide-gated)

Deactivation of Transducin and Phosphodiesterase

Hydrolysis of GTP to GDP by GTPase-accelerating protein complex causes deactivation of transducin. This complex consists of RGS9-1 (G-protein signaling protein), Gβ5 subunit long form and R9AP (membrane anchor protein). Following hydrolysis of GTP, transducin affinity to PDE6 decreases, thus decreasing activation of PDE6.

Restoration of cGMP Levels

Decrease in intracellular calcium following closure of CNG channels activates guanylate cyclase. This activation is mediated by a group of proteins called GCAP (guanylate cyclase-binding proteins). When they are bound to Ca^{2+}, they bind to guanylate cyclase and decrease its activity. Hence, when the Ca^{2+} level decreases, it increases the guanylate cyclase activity. Activation of guanylate cyclase increases cGMP levels, which in turn open CNG channels and cause depolarization of rods (Flowchart 3.7).

Cone Phototransduction

The molecules and proteins involved in cone phototransduction are closely related to rod phototransduction proteins. Although the cones are less sensitive, they are fast and are capable of quick adaptation to the surrounding illumination. The paucity of data in cone phototransduction can be attributed to the less number of cones and decreased sensitivity of cones.

REFERENCES

1. Holly FJ, Lemp MA. Tear physiology and dry eyes. Surv Ophthalmol. 1977;22(2):69-87.
2. Kikkawa T. [Studies on the mechanism of tear secretion. I. On the salt and water secretion from the lacrimal gland and its secretion. (potential measured by external leading)]. Nippon Ganka Gakkai Zasshi. 1968;72(7):1005-9.
3. McCulley JP, Shine W. A compositional based model for the tear film lipid layer. Trans Am Ophthalmol Soc. 1997;95:79-88; discussion 88-93.
4. Iwata S, Lemp MA, Holly FJ, et al. Evaporation rate of water from the precorneal tear film and cornea in the rabbit. Invest Ophthalmol. 1969;8(6):613-9.
5. Tear Film. Fundamentals and principles of ophthalmology, American Academy of Ophthalmology basic and clinical science course. 2016-2017.
6. Allansmith M. Immunology of the Tears. Int Ophthalmol Clin. 1973;13(1):47-72.
7. Van Haeringen NJ. Clinical biochemistry of tears. Surv Ophthalmol. 1981;26(2):84-96.
8. Sanghi S, Kumar R, Lumsden A, et al. cDNA and genomic cloning of lacritin, a novel secretion enhancing factor from the human lacrimal gland. J Mol Biol. 2001;310(1):127-39.
9. McDermott AM. Antimicrobial compounds in tears. Exp Eye Res. 2013;117:53-61.
10. Massingale ML, Li X, Vallabhajosyula M, et al. Analysis of inflammatory cytokines in the tears of dry eye patients. Cornea. 2009;28(9):1023-7.
11. Ohashi Y, Motokura M, Kinoshita Y, et al. Presence of epidermal growth factor in human tears. Invest Ophthalmol Vis Sci. 1989;30(8):1879-82.
12. Li Q, Weng J, Mohan RR, et al. Hepatocyte growth factor and hepatocyte growth factor receptor in the lacrimal gland, tears, and cornea. Invest Ophthalmol Vis Sci. 1996;37(5):727-39.

13. Van Setten GB. Basic fibroblast growth factor in human tear fluid: detection of another growth factor. Graefes Arch Clin Exp Ophthalmol. 1996;234(4):275-7.
14. van Setten GB, Macauley S, Humphreys-Beher M, et al. Detection of transforming growth factor-alpha mRNA and protein in rat lacrimal glands and characterization of transforming growth factor-alpha in human tears. Invest Ophthalmol Vis Sci. 1996;37(1):166-73.
15. Gupta A, Monroy D, Ji Z, et al. Transforming growth factor beta-1 and beta-2 in human tear fluid. Curr Eye Res. 1996;15(6):605-14.
16. Carreño E, Enríquez-de-Salamanca A, Tesón M, et al. Cytokine and chemokine levels in tears from healthy subjects. Acta Ophthalmol. 2010;88(7):e250-8.
17. Paterson CA, O'Rourke MC. Vitamin C levels in human tears. Arch Ophthalmol. 1987;105(3):376-7.
18. Willcox MD, Morris CA, Thakur A, et al. Complement and complement regulatory proteins in human tears. Invest Ophthalmol Vis Sci. 1997;38(1):1-8.
19. Lane JD, Krumholz DM, Sack RA, et al. Tear glucose dynamics in diabetes mellitus. Curr Eye Res. 2006;31(11):895-901.
20. Hodges RR, Dartt DA. Tear film mucins: front line defenders of the ocular surface; comparison with airway and gastrointestinal tract mucins. Exp Eye Res. 2013;117:62-78.
21. Gipson IK. Distribution of mucins at the ocular surface. Exp Eye Res. 2004;78(3):379-88.
22. Hagan S, Martin E, Enríquez-de-Salamanca A. Tear fluid biomarkers in ocular and systemic disease: potential use for predictive, preventive and personalised medicine. EPMA J. 2016;7:15.
23. Cotlier E. The cornea. In: Moses RA (Ed). Adler's Physiology of the Eye: Clinical Application. StLouis: CV Mosby Company; 1975.
24. Maurice DM, Riley MV. The cornea. In: Graymore CN (Ed). Biochemistry of the Eye. New York: Academic Press Inc; 1970.
25. Kao WW, Liu CY, Converse RL, et al. Keratin 12-deficient mice have fragile corneal epithelia. Invest Ophthalmol Vis Sci. 1996;37(13):2572-84.
26. Sun TT, Tseng SC, Huang AJ, et al. Monoclonal antibody studies of mammalian epithelial keratins: a review. Ann N Y Acad Sci. 1985;455:307-29.
27. Chen B, Mi S, Wright B, et al. Investigation of K14/K5 as a stem cell marker in the limbal region of the bovine cornea. PLoS ONE. 2010;5(10):e13192.
28. Kurpakus MA, Stock EL, Jones JC. Expression of the 55-kD/64-kD corneal keratins in ocular surface epithelium. Invest Ophthalmol Vis Sci. 1990;31(3):448-56.
29. Hurman DL, Glazewski L, Gumpert A, et al. In vivo and in vitro expression of connexins in the human corneal epithelium. Invest Ophthalmol Vis Sci. 2005;46(6):1957-65.
30. Marshall GE, Konstas AG, Lee WR. Immunogold fine structural localization of extracellular matrix components in aged human cornea. I. Types I-IV collagen and laminin. Graefes Arch Clin Exp Ophthalmol. 1991;229(2):157-63.
31. Nakayasu K, Tanaka M, Konomi H, et al. Distribution of types I, II, III, IV and V collagen in normal and keratoconus corneas. Ophthalmic Res. 1986;18(1):1-10.
32. Newsome DA, Gross J, Hassell JR. Human corneal stroma contains three distinct collagens. Invest Ophthalmol Vis Sci. 1982;22(3):376-81.
33. Doane KJ, Yang G, Birk DE. Corneal cell-matrix interactions: type VI collagen promotes adhesion and spreading of corneal fibroblasts. Exp Cell Res. 1992;200(2):490-9.
34. Gordon MK, Foley JW, Lisenmayer TF, et al. Temporal expression of types XII and XIV collagen mRNA and protein during avian corneal development. Dev Dyn. 1996;206(1):49-58.
35. Michelacci YM. Collagens and proteoglycans of the corneal extracellular matrix. Braz J Med Biol Res. 2003;36(8): 1037-46.
36. Komai Y, Ushiki T. The three-dimensional organization of collagen fibrils in the human cornea and sclera. Invest Ophthalmol Vis Sci. 1991;32(8):2244-58.
37. Hamada R, Pouliquen Y, Giranud JP, et al. Quantitative analysis on the ultrastructure of human fetal cornea. In: Yamada E, Mishima S (Eds). The structure of the eye III. Tokyo: Japanese Journal of Ophthalmology; 1976. pp. 49-62.
38. Bron AJ. The architecture of the corneal stroma. Br J Ophthalmol. 2001;85(4):379-81.
39. Castoro JA, Bettelheim AA, Bettelheim FA. Water gradients across bovine cornea. Invest Ophthalmol Vis Sci. 1988;29(6):963-8.
40. Hassell JR, Birk DE. The molecular basis of corneal transparency. Exp Eye Res. 2010;91(3):326-35.
41. Zhang G, Chen S, Goldoni S, et al. Genetic evidence for the coordinated regulation of collagen fibrillogenesis in the cornea by decorin and biglycan. J Biol Chem. 2009;284(13):8888-97.
42. Bonanno JA. Molecular mechanisms underlying the corneal endothelial pump. Exp Eye Res. 2012;95(1):2-7.
43. Bonanno JA. Identity and regulation of ion transport mechanisms in the corneal endothelium. Prog Retin Eye Res. 2003;22(1):69-94.
44. Thoft RA, Friend J, Dohlman CH. Corneal glucose concentration. Arch Ophthalmol. 1971;85:467.
45. Kinoshita JH. Some aspects of the carbohydrate etabolism of the cornea. Invest Ophthalmol. 1962;1:178-86.
46. Kinoshita JH, Masurat T, Helfant M. Pathways of metabolism in corneal epithelium. Science. 1955;122(3158):72-3.
47. Riley MV. Transport of ions and metabolites across the corneal endothelium. In: McDevitt DS (Ed). Cell Biology of the Eye. New York: Academic Press; 1982. p. 53.
48. Watson PG, Young RD. Scleral structure, organisation and disease. A review. Exp Eye Res. 2004;78(3):609-23.
49. Foster CS, De la Maza MS. Structural considerations of the sclera. In: Foster CS, De la Maza MS (Ed). The Sclera. New York: Springer; 1994.
50. Rada JA, Achen VR, Penugonda S, et al. Proteoglycan composition in the human sclera during growth and aging. Invest Ophthalmol Vis Sci. 2000;41(7):1639-48.

51. Millar C, Kaufman PL. Aqueous humor: secretion and dynamics. In: Tasman W, Jaeger EA (Eds). Duane's foundations of clinical ophthalmology. Philadelphia: Lippincott-Raven; 1995.
52. Bill A. Blood circulation and fluid dynamics in the eye. Physiol Rev. 1975;55(3):383-417.
53. Mark HH. Aqueous humor dynamics in historical perspective. Surv Ophthalmol. 2010;55(1):89-100.
54. Jacob TJ, Civan MM. Role of ion channels in aqueous humor formation. Am J Physiol. 1996;271(3):C703-20.
55. Civan MM, Peterson-Yantorno K, Sánchez-Torres J, et al. Potential contribution of epithelial Na+ channel to net secretion of aqueous humor. J Exp Zool. 1997;279(5): 498-503.
56. Wiederholt M, Zadunaisky JA. Membrane potentials and intracellular chloride activity in the ciliary body of the shark. Pflügers Archiv. 1986;407(2):S112-5.
57. Becker B. Ouabain and aqueous humor dynamics in the rabbit eye. Invest Ophthalmol. 1963;2:325-31.
58. Becker B. Vanadate and aqueous humor dynamics. Proctor Lecture. Invest Ophthalmol Vis Sci. 1980;19(10):1156-65.
59. Maren TH. Ion secretion into the posterior aqueous humor of dogs and monkeys. Exp Eye Res. 1977;25:245-7.
60. Civan MM, Macknight AD. The ins and outs of aqueous humour secretion. Exp Eye Res. 2004;78(3):625-31.
61. Civan MM. The fall and rise of active chloride transport: implications for regulation of intraocular pressure. J Exp Zoolog Part A Comp Exp Biol. 2003;300(1):5-13.
62. Kong CW, Li KK, To CH. Chloride secretion by porcine ciliary epithelium: New insight into species similarities and differences in aqueous humor formation. Invest Ophthalmol Vis Sci. 2006;47(12):5428-36.
63. Do CW, Civan MM. Swelling-activated chloride channels in aqueous humour formation: on the one side and the other. Acta Physiol (Oxf). 2006;187(1-2):345-52.
64. Usukura J, Fain GL, Bok D. [3H]ouabain localization of Na+-K+ ATPase in the epithelium of rabbit ciliary body pars plicata. Invest Ophthalmol Vis Sci. 1988;29(4):606-14.
65. Edelman JL, Loo DD, Sachs G. Characterization of potassium and chloride channels in the basolateral membrane of bovine nonpigmented ciliary epithelial cells. Invest Ophthalmol Vis Sci. 1995;36(13):2706-16.
66. Helbig H, Korbmacher C, Kühner D, et al. Characterization of Cl--HCO3- exchange in cultured bovine pigmented ciliary epithelium. Exp Eye Res. 1988;47(4):515-23.
67. Maren TH. The rates of movement of Na+, Cl-, and HCO3- from plasma to posterior chamber: effect of acetazolamide and relation to the treatment of glaucoma. Invest Ophthalmol. 1976;15(5):356-64.
68. Schey KL, Wang Z, Wenke JL, et al. Aquaporins in the eye: expression, function, and roles in ocular disease. Biochim Biophys Acta. 2014;1840(5):1513-23.
69. Shin BC, Suzuki T, Tanaka S, et al. Connexin 43 and the glucose transporter, GLUT1, in the ciliary body of the rat. Histochem Cell Biol. 1996;106(2):209-14.
70. Tsukamoto H, Mishima HK, Kurokawa T, et al. Isoforms of glucose transporter in the iris-ciliary body. Jpn J Ophthalmol. 1995;39(3):242-7.
71. Hu RG, Lim JC, Kalloniatis M, et al. Cellular localization of glutamate and glutamine metabolism and transport pathways in the rat ciliary epithelium. Invest Ophthalmol Vis Sci. 2011;52(6):3345-53.
72. Chu TC, Candia OA. Active transport of ascorbate across the isolated rabbit ciliary epithelium. Invest Ophthalmol Vis Sci. 1988;29(4):594-9.
73. Aqueous humor, Iris,and ciliary body. In: Fundamentals and principles of ophthalmology, American Academy of Ophthalmology basic and clinical science course. 2016-2017.
74. Davson H. The aqueous humor and the intraocular pressure. In: Davson H, (Ed). Physiology of the Eye. New York: Pergamon Press; 1990. pp. 3.
75. Krause U, Raunio V. Proteins of the normal human aqueous humour. Ophthalmologica. 1969;159(1):178-85.
76. Goel M, Picciani RG, Lee RK, et al. Aqueous humor dynamics: a review. Open Ophthalmol J. 2010;4:52-9.
77. Duke-Elder S. The aqueous humor. In: Duke-Elder S (Ed). The physiology of the eye and of vision. System of ophthalmology, Volume 4. St Louis: CV Mosby; 1968. pp.104.
78. Riley MV, Meyer RF, Yates EM. Glutathione in the aqueous humor of human and other species. Invest Ophthalmol Vis Sci. 1980;19(1):94-6.
79. Jampel HD, Roche N, Stark WJ, et al. Transforming growth factor-beta in human aqueous humor. Curr Eye Res. 1990;9(10):963-9.
80. Tripathi RC, Borisuth NS, Tripathi BJ. Detection, quantification, and significance of basic fibroblast growth factor in the aqueous humor of man, cat, dog and pig. Exp Eye Res. 1992;54(3):447-54.
81. Koliakos GG, Schlötzer-Schrehardt U, Konstas AG, et al. Transforming and insulin-like growth factors in the aqueous humour of patients with exfoliation syndrome. Graefes Arch Clin Exp Ophthalmol. 2001; 239(7):482-7.
82. Tong JP, Chan WM, Liu DT, et al. Aqueous humor levels of vascular endothelial growth factor and pigment epithelium–derived factor in polypoidal choroidal vasculopathy and choroidal neovascularization. Am J Ophthalmol. 2006;141(3):456-62.
83. Sharifipour F, Idani E, Zamani M, et al. Oxygen Tension in the Aqueous Humor of Human Eyes under different Oxygenation Conditions. J Ophthalmic Vis Res. 2013;8(2):119-25.
84. Vegge T. An epithelial blood-aqueous barrier to horseradish peroxidase in the ciliary processes of the vervet monkey (Cercopithecus aethiops). Z Zellforsch Mikrosk Anat. 1971;114(3):309-20.
85. Cunha-Vaz J. The blood-ocular barriers. Surv Ophthalmol. 1979;23(5):279-96.
86. Smith RL, Raviola G. The structural basis of the blood-aqueous barrier in the chicken eye. Invest Ophthalmol Vis Sci. 1983;24(3):326-38.

87. Freddo TF. A contemporary concept of the blood-aqueous barrier. Prog Retin Eye Res. 2013;32:181-95.
88. Stamper RL. Aqueous humor: secretion and dynamics. In: Tasman W, Jaeger EA (Eds). Clinical ophthalmology, Volume 2. Philadelphia: Lippincott; 1979.
89. Eakins KE. Prostaglandin and non-prostaglandin mediated breakdown of the blood-aqueous barrier. Exp Eye Res. 1977;25 Suppl:483-98.
90. Camras CB, Bito LZ, Eakins KE. Reduction of intraocular pressure by prostaglandins applied topically to the eyes of conscious rabbits. Invest Ophthalmol Vis Sci. 1977;16(12):1125-34.
91. Borchman D, Yappert MC. Lipids and the ocular lens. J Lipid Res. 2010;51(9):2473-88.
92. Zigman S, Paxhia T, Marinetti G, et al. Lipids of human lens fiber cell membranes. Curr Eye Res. 1984;3(7):887-96.
93. Zelenka PS. Lens lipids. Curr Eye Res. 1984;3(11):1337-59.
94. Morner CT. Untersuchungen der Proteinsubstanzen in den lichtbrechended medien des Auges M. I. Hoppe-Seylers Z Physiol Chem. 1894;18:61.
95. Horwitz J, Bova MP, Ding LL, et al. Lens alpha-crystallin: function and structure. Eye (Lond). 1999;13 (Pt 3b):403-8.
96. Horwitz J. Alpha-crystallin can function as a molecular chaperone. Proc Natl Acad Sci U S A. 1992;89(21):10449-53.
97. Andley UP. Crystallins in the eye: function and pathology. Prog Retin Eye Res. 2007;26(1):78-98.
98. Sharma KK, Santhoshkumar P. Lens aging: effects of crystallins. Biochim Biophys Acta. 2009;1790(10):1095-108.
99. Mulders SM, Preston GM, Deen PM, et al. Water channel properties of major intrinsic protein of lens. J Biol Chem. 1995;270(15):9010-6.
100. Varadaraj K, Kushmerick C, Baldo GJ, et al. The role of MIP in lens fiber cell membrane transport. J Membr Biol. 1999;170(3):191-203.
101. Irum B, Khan SY, Ali M, et al. Mutation in LIM2 is Responsible for Autosomal Recessive Congenital Cataracts. PLoS ONE. 2016;11(11):e0162620.
102. Clark JI, Matsushima H, David LL, et al. Lens cytoskeleton and transparency: a model. Eye (Lond). 1999;13 (Pt 3b): 417-24.
103. Dilsiz N, Olcucu A, Atas M. Determination of calcium, sodium, potassium and magnesium concentrations in human senile cataractous lenses. Cell Biochem Funct. 2000;18(4):259-62.
104. Umapathy A, Donaldson P, Lim J. Antioxidant delivery pathways in the anterior eye. Biomed Res Int. 2013;2013:207250.
105. Giblin FJ. Glutathione: a vital lens antioxidant. J Ocul Pharmacol Ther. 2000;16(2):121-35.
106. Michael R, Bron AJ. The ageing lens and cataract: a model of normal and pathological ageing. Philos Trans R Soc Lond B Biol Sci. 2011;366(1568):1278-92.
107. Dickerson JE, Lou MF. Micro-quantitation of lens myo-inositol by anion exchange chromatography. Curr Eye Res. 1990;9(2):201-5.
108. Cammarata PR, Zhou C, Chen G, et al. A transgenic animal model of osmotic cataract. Part 1: over-expression of bovine Na+/myo-inositol cotransporter in lens fibers. Invest Ophthalmol Vis Sci. 1999;40(8):1727-37.
109. Kinoshita JH. Pathways of glucose metabolism in the lens. Invest Ophthalmol Vis Sci. 1965;4(4):619-28.
110. Beyer EC, Berthoud VM. Connexin hemichannels in the lens. Front Physiol. 2014;5:20.
111. Mathias RT, Kistler J, Donaldson P. The lens circulation. J Membr Biol. 2007;216(1):1-16.
112. Kinsey VE, Reddy DV. Studies on the crystalline lens. XI. the relative role of the epithelium and capsule in transport. Invest Ophthalmol. 1965;4:104-16.
113. Berthoud VM, Beyer EC. Oxidative stress, lens gap junctions, and cataracts. Antioxid Redox Signal. 2009;11(2):339-53.
114. West SK, Valmadrid CT. Epidemiology of risk factors for age-related cataract. Surv Ophthalmol. 1995;39(4):323-34.
115. Harding JJ. Recent studies of risk factors and protective factors for cataract. Curr Opin Ophthalmol. 1997;8(1):46-9.
116. Klein BE, Klein R, Lee KE. Diabetes, cardiovascular disease, selected cardiovascular disease risk factors, and the 5-year incidence of age-related cataract and progression of lens opacities: the Beaver Dam Eye Study. Am J Ophthalmol. 1998;126(6):782-90.
117. Harding JJ. Free and protein-bound glutathione in normal and cataractous human lenses. Biochem J. 1970;117(5): 957-60.
118. Fecondo JV, Augusteyn RC. Superoxide dismutase, catalase and glutathione peroxidase in the human cataractous lens. Exp Eye Res. 1983;36(1):15-23.
119. Özmen B, Özmen D, Erkin E, et al. Lens superoxide dismutase and catalase activities in diabetic cataract. Clin Biochem. 2002;35(1):69-72.
120. Nagaraj RH, Linetsky M, Stitt AW. The pathogenic role of Maillard reaction in the aging eye. Amino Acids. 2012;42(4):1205-20.
121. Spector A. Oxidative stress-induced cataract: mechanism of action. FASEB J. 1995;9(12):1173-82.
122. Truscott RJ. Age-related nuclear cataract—oxidation is the key. Exp Eye Res. 2005;80(5):709-25.
123. Duncan G, Bushell AR. Ion analyses of human cataractous lenses. Exp Eye Res. 1975;20(3):223-30.
124. Kinoshita JH. Mechanisms initiating cataract formation proctor lecture. Invest Ophthalmol Vis Sci. 1974;13(10): 713-24.
125. Mulhern ML, Madson CJ, Danford A, et al. The unfolded protein response in lens epithelial cells from galactosemic rat lenses. Invest Ophthalmol Vis Sci. 2006;47(9):3951-9.
126. Stitt AW. The Maillard reaction in eye diseases. Ann N Y Acad Sci. 2005;1043(1):582-97.
127. Aquilina JA, Carverja, Truscott RJ. Oxidation products of 3-hydroxykynurenine bind to lens proteins: relevance for nuclear cataract. Exp Eye Res. 1997;64(5):727-35.
128. Le Goff MM, Bishop PN. Adult vitreous structure and postnatal changes. Eye. 2008;22(10):1214.
129. Wu CW, Sauter JL, Johnson PK, et al. Identification and localization of major soluble vitreous proteins in human ocular tissue. Am J Ophthalmol. 2004;137(4):655-61.

130. Ashworth JL, Kielty CM, McLeod D. Fibrillin and the eye. Br J Ophthalmol. 2000;84(11):1312-7.
131. Ren ZX, Brewton RG, Mayne R. An analysis by rotary shadowing of the structure of the mammalian vitreous humor and zonular apparatus. J Struct Biol. 1991;106(1): 57-63.
132. Bishop PN. Vitreous proteins. In: Sebag J (Ed). Vitreous in health and disease. New York: Springer; 2014.
133. Reardon AJ, Le Goff M, Briggs MD, et al. Identification in vitreous and molecular cloning of opticin, a novel member of the family of leucine-rich repeat proteins of the extracellular matrix. J Biol Chem. 2000;275(3):2123-9.
134. Mayne R, Ren ZX, Liu J, et al. VIT-1: the second member of a new branch of the von Willebrand factor A domain superfamily. Biochem Soc Trans. 1999;27(6):832.
135. Plantner JM, Smine A, Quinn TA. Matrix metalloproteinases and metalloproteinase inhibitors in human interphotoreceptor matrix and vitreous. Curr Eye Res. 1998;17(2):132-40.
136. Kelly M, von Lintig J. STRA6: role in cellular retinol uptake and efflux. Hepatobiliary Surg Nutr. 2015;4(4):229-42.
137. Wang JS, Kefalov VJ. The cone-specific visual cycle. Prog Retin Eye Res. 2011;30(2):115-28.
138. Thumann G, Dou G, Wang Y, et al. Cell biology of the retinal pigment epithelium. In: Ryan SJ (Ed). Retina. London: Saunders/Elsevier; 2013.
139. Tang PH, Kono M, Koutalos Y, et al. New insights into retinoid metabolism and cycling within the retina. Prog Retin Eye Res. 2013;32:48-63.
140. Tsybovsky Y, Molday RS, Palczewski K. The ATP-binding cassette transporter ABCA4: structural and functional properties and role in retinal disease. Adv Exp Med Biol. 2010;703:105-25.
141. Liu J, Itagaki Y, Ben-Shabat S, et al. The biosynthesis of A2E, a fluorophore of aging retina, involves the formation of the precursor, A2-PE, in the photoreceptor outer segment membrane. J Biol Chem. 2000;275(38):29354-60.
142. Yau KW. Phototransduction mechanism in retinal rods and cones. The Friedenwald Lecture. Invest Ophthalmol Vis Sci. 1994;35(1):9-32.
143. Palczewski K. G protein-coupled receptor rhodopsin. Annu Rev Biochem. 2006;75:743-67.
144. Fu Y, Yau KW. Phototransduction in mouse rods and cones. Pflugers Arch. 2007;454(5):805-19.
145. Hargrave PA. Rhodopsin structure, function, and topography the Friedenwald lecture. Invest Ophthalmol Vis Sci. 2001;42(1):3-9.
146. Chen J, Sampath AP. Structure and function of rod and cone photoreceptors. In: Ryan SJ (Ed). Retina. London: Saunders/ Elsevier; 2013.
147. Lamb TD, Pugh EN. A quantitative account of the activation steps involved in phototransduction in amphibian photoreceptors. J Physiol. 1992;449(1):719-58.

Chapter 4 Ocular Pharmacotherapy

Sankalp Singh Sharma, N Venkatesh Prajna

INTRODUCTION

With the advancement of science, a large number of drugs have been made available for the use of the ophthalmologist. A judicious use of these drugs is essential for the ultimate benefit of the patient. The often quoted maxim, "*the difference between a drug and a poison, is the dose*" should always be kept in mind when one contemplates the use of these medications. An ideal therapeutic regimen should have the following characteristics:

- The selection of the drug should be appropriate.
- The concentration should be efficacious depending on the indication and the severity of the condition.
- The time duration of therapy should be optimized.
- When the drugs are not working to the optimal level, a principle of substitution rather than addition should be considered.
- Lastly, the side effects should be least possible.

A good knowledge of the pharmacologic agents that are available is therefore vital to an ophthalmologist to treat the patients, without exposing them to potential side effects of the drugs. This chapter aims to give the basic knowledge regarding the commonly available drugs in day-to-day use in an ophthalmologic clinic so that the practicing ophthalmologists can make the best decision for their patients.

ANESTHETIC AGENTS

For performing most of the ophthalmic procedures, it is necessary to have a good anesthesia. Anesthetic agents in ophthalmic practice can be used in the form of: (1) local injectable anesthesia (LIA), (2) topical anesthesia (TA), (3) intracameral anesthesia (IA), and (4) general anesthesia (GA).

Local Injectable Anesthesia

The LIA can be classified based on their duration of action (short, intermediate, long), or depending on their chemical structure (amides and esters) (Tables 4.1 and 4.2).

All LIAs are weak bases which have a hydrophilic secondary or tertiary amine attached to one side and a lipophilic aromatic residue which is attached to the other, and joined by an alkyl chain through an ester or amide bond.[1]

Table 4.1: Classification of local injectable anesthesia based on duration of action.

Short duration	Intermediate duration	Long duration
1. Procaine 2. Chloroprocaine	1. Lignocaine 2. Prilocaine	1. Tetracaine 2. Bupivacaine 3. Ropivacaine 4. Dibucaine

Source: Peyman GA, Sanders DR, Goldberg MF. Principles and Practice of Ophthalmology, 1st edition. Philadelphia: Saunders Ltd; 1980.

Table 4.2: Classification of local injectable anesthesia based on side chain.

Amides	Esters
1. Lignocaine 2. Bupivacaine 3. Mepivacaine 4. Prilocaine	1. Cocaine 2. Proparacaine 3. Tetracaine 4. Chloroprocaine

Source: Peyman GA, Sanders DR, Goldberg MF. Principles and Practice of Ophthalmology, 1st edition. Philadelphia: Saunders Ltd.; 1980.

Mechanism of Action of LIA

These agents block the conduction of impulses in the nerve by altering the entry of sodium ions during an action potential. The increase in concentration of the LIA is directly proportional to the decrease in height of action potential and inversely proportional to the rate of depolarization of the nerve fibers. The interplay of these activities prevents the generation of nerve impulses.

Amide anesthetics like lignocaine and bupivacaine are preferred in LIA due to their longer duration of action.

The various commonly used LIAs in ophthalmology are listed in Table 4.3.

Topical Anesthetics

Topical anesthetics in the form of eye drops are convenient to use in various procedures like applanation tonometry and also in cataract surgeries to provide a painless experience. They are used as eye drops and gels. The stinging sensation of the anesthetic agents is lessened when combined with methylcellulose as a gel form.

Table 4.3: Common local injectable anesthesia (LIA).

Drug	Maximum dose	Onset of action	Duration of action	Side effects	Remarks
Lignocaine	15 mL of a 2% given alone (300 mg) or 25 mL mixed with adrenaline (500 mg)	Fast	60 minutes when given alone; 90 minutes when mixed with adrenaline	Methemoglobinemia	
Mepivacaine	25 mL of 2% solution (400 mg)	Fast	90–120 minutes		Does not cause vasodilation like lignocaine so adrenaline not required
Bupivacaine	25 mL of 0.75% or 30 mL of 0.5% solution (175 mg)	Moderate (7–10 minutes)	300–720 minutes	Cardiotoxic Myotoxic	
Procaine	25 mL of 2% solution (500 mg)	Fast	30 minutes when given alone; 60 minutes when mixed with adrenaline.		Relatively nontoxic
Tetracaine	100 mg	Slow	90–120 minutes	Cardiac asystole Ventricular fibrillations	Protect solution from sunlight

Source: Peyman GA, Sanders DR, Goldberg MF. Principles and Practice of Ophthalmology, 1st edition. Philadelphia: Saunders Ltd.; 1980.

Table 4.4: Classification based on solubility of topical anesthetics.

Soluble	Insoluble
1. Cocaine 2. Lignocaine 3. Tetracaine 4. Benoxinate 5. Proparacaine	1. Benzocaine 2. Butyl aminobenzoate 3. Oxetacaine

Source: Peyman GA, Sanders DR, Goldberg MF. Principles and Practice of Ophthalmology, 1st edition. Philadelphia: Saunders Ltd.; 1980.

Topical anesthetics can be classified based on their solubility[2] as shown in Table 4.4.

Cocaine

Cocaine was the first anesthetic to be used in the year 1884 for a corneal surgery.[1] Solutions of 1% and 2% were used for corneal anesthesia. The duration of action is 30 minutes. It causes mydriasis of the pupil and also is very toxic to the corneal epithelium. It is rarely used now due to regulatory concerns.

Proparacaine

It is available as 0.5% solution. It is less irritating than other topical anesthetics when instilled onto the cornea and is also associated with lesser epithelial erosions of the cornea.[3] Hence it has become the drug of choice for performing contact investigations like applanation tonometry.

Tetracaine

It is used to obtain corneal analgesia in a concentration of 0.5% solution. The solution should be kept in bottles protected from light. It has a longer duration of action than proparacaine, but is more toxic to the corneal epithelium.[3]

Lignocaine

Lignocaine in a 4% solution can be used for TA. It causes corneal epithelial erosions and causes more stinging sensation on instillation onto the cornea. It is not preferred to use before corneal scraping as it inhibits the growth of microorganisms and can thus interfere with the results of culture testing.[4]

Intracameral Anesthetics

Lignocaine

Lignocaine as a 1% preservative-free solution is used intracamerally to enhance the analgesia during phacoemulsification surgeries. This allows for a pain-free phacoemulsification surgery without the need for peribulbar or retrobulbar injections. The potential complications associated with the other types of regional nerve blocks are thus avoided. Prior to the use of this mode of application, the cornea is initially anesthetized using topical anesthetic drops. A paracentesis is then made and the lignocaine injected into the anterior chamber as a solution. Newer techniques using a mixture of 1% lignocaine with 2.25% hydroxypropyl methylcellulose (HPMC); and 1% lignocaine with 1.5% sodium hyaluronate are also being used to provide anesthesia during phacoemulsification.

Another new method utilizing intracameral anesthetic that has been described, uses a mixture known as *"epi-Shugarcaine"*,[5] which comprises of a 0.025% epinephrine, 0.75% lignocaine and fortified Balanced Salt Solution plus (BSS plus). These new techniques help to provide analgesia as well as maintaining pupillary dilatation. The analgesia is sufficient to ensure that the patient has a pain-free cataract surgery.

General Anesthetics

The decision of using general anesthetics is dictated by the age of the patient, type of procedure, the duration of the procedure, the ability of the patient to cooperate during the procedure and also the comfort of the surgeon. In case gases like sulfur hexafluoride (SF_6) or perfluoropropane (C_3F_8) are going to be left inside the eye, nitrous oxide should be avoided to prevent postoperative rise in intraocular pressure (IOP). Adrenaline use should be avoided if Halothane has been used.

The effect of general anesthetics, both inhalational agents and intravenous agents, is to decrease the IOP. However, succinylcholine which is used as a muscle relaxant to enhance the anesthesia leads to an increase in the IOP and hence should best be avoided during open globe procedures.

The details of general anesthetics are beyond the scope of this book and the interested reader is advised to refer textbooks of Anesthesiology for the same.

ANTIBACTERIALS

With a large number of antibiotics available nowadays, it is important for the ophthalmologist to understand the benefits and side effects before initiating treatment. The sensitivity of the microorganism to the drug determines the efficacy, while the dosing frequency and the side effects dictates patient adherence to the treatment.

Unique to the eye is the blood-eye barrier (BEB) that resists penetration of most antibiotics. The BEB is the significant obstacle to the treatment of infections of the vitreous and aqueous cavities and the lens. The sclera and uveal tract are external to the BEB and hence the systemic antibiotics can be more efficacious in reaching these areas. The degree of disruption of the BEB by injury or infection can be estimated by the amount of flare in anterior chamber. When large protein molecules leak freely into the eye, so do the antibiotic molecules. The clinically significant problems arise when minimal damage has been done by the organism introduced via the trauma, surgery or metastatic entry. At this early stage, the microorganism is relatively sheltered from systemic and topical antibiotics, yet this is the most critical time for effective therapy. Strategies available to the ophthalmologist to achieve appropriate intraocular penetration of antibiotics include intraocular injection, subconjunctival injection, use of very high and frequent dosages of systemic or topical antibiotics, and selection of antibiotics based on their differential solubility characteristics.

The different classes of antibacterial that are available to the ophthalmologist are given in Table 4.5.

Table 4.5: Commonly available ophthalmic antibiotics.

Topical antibacterial	Topical drug strength	Mechanism of action	Susceptible organisms	Ocular side effects	Systemic side effects
Fluoroquinolones: 1. Ciprofloxacin 2. Ofloxacin 3. Levofloxacin 4. Gatifloxacin 5. Moxifloxacin 6. Besifloxacin	 0.3% solution 0.3% solution 0.5% solution 0.3% solution 0.5% solution 0.6% emulsion	Inhibit the enzymes DNA gyrase and topoisomerase IV, which take part in the DNA replication in bacterial cells	Broad-spectrum. All have good activity against Gram-negative rods; ciprofloxacin may have better activity against *Pseudomonas aeruginosa*; gatifloxacin and moxifloxacin have better activity against Gram-positive cocci	*Ocular:* Transient stinging sensation on instillation, tearing, redness Ciprofloxacin and Norfloxacin lead to corneal deposits on prolonged use	1. Gastrointestinal upset in the form of nausea, vomiting, diarrhea, metallic taste and anorexia. 2. Skin rash, pruritus, urticaria, photosensitivity 3. Tendinitis, arthropathy and rarely tendon rupture 4. Occasionally headache, dizziness and tremors
Tetracyclines: 1. Tetracycline 2. Oxytetracycline 3. Doxycycline 4. Minocycline 5. Tigecycline	1% ophthalmic solution and ointment	The drug combines with the 30S ribosomes of the bacteria. This prevents the binding of aminoacyl transferase RNA to the mRNA ribosome complex hence preventing the elongation of the peptide chains	Broad-spectrum, active against many Gram-positive and Gram-negative bacteria and *Chlamydia*. Not active against *P. aeruginosa* and Group B streptococci		*Systemic:* gastric symptoms like nausea, epigastric pain and vomiting. Diarrhea is more common with the older tetracyclines. Dose-related hepatotoxicity Contraindicated in children and pregnancy, as it is associated with suppression of bone growth

Contd...

Contd...

Topical antibacterial	Topical drug strength	Mechanism of action	Susceptible organisms	Ocular side effects	Systemic side effects
Aminoglycosides: 1. *Systemic aminoglycosides:* Streptomycin Gentamicin Tobramycin Amikacin Sisomicin 2. *Topical aminoglycosides (applied on skin):* Neomycin Kanamycin Framycetin	 0.3% solution 0.3% solution	They bind to 30S and 50S subunits and the interface between the two subunits Streptomycin binds to the 30S subunit only, stop the initiation of protein synthesis and also cause misreading of the codons by binding to the subunit interface	Aerobic Gram-negative bacteria; gentamicin and tobramycin have good activity against Staphylococci		1. All aminoglycosides are ototoxic and nephrotoxic 2. Can produce neuromuscular blockade and may result in respiratory paralysis
Macrolides: 1. Erythromycin 2. Azithromycin	Not available topically 1% solution and ointment	They act by inhibiting the synthesis of protein chains in bacteria. They bind to to the 50S ribosomal RNA of the bacteria thus blocking the aminoacyl translocation reaction and initiation complexes	Gram-positive cocci		1. Nausea, epigastric pain and diarrhea are common 2. Allergic reactions such as rashes, eosinophilia dermatitis and lymphadenopathy
Chloramphenicol	0.5% solution, 1% ointment	Inhibits bacterial protein synthesis by attaching to the 50S ribosome and prevents peptide bond formation between the newly formed amino acid	Broad-spectrum; active against Gram-negative and Gram-positive bacteria as well as *Chlamydia*		1. Bone marrow depression 2. Hypersensitivity reactions like rashes,fever and angioedema 3. *Gray baby syndrome:* encountered earlier when high-dose chloramphenicol was used in neonates as prophylaxis 4. Rare cases of aplastic anemia due to idiosyncratic reactions have been described after topical instillation
Glycopeptides: Vancomycin	25–50 mg/mL; not available commercially in topical form.	Inhibits the bacterial cell wall synthesis by binding to the terminal dipeptide D-Ala-D-Ala sequence of the peptidoglycan unit. This inhibits the Transglycolase enzyme, thus preventing the elongation of peptidoglycan chain and cross-linking	Gram-positive bacteria		1. Irritation and phlebitis at the site of injection 2. Dose-dependent sensorineural hearing loss and nephrotoxicity 3. If given rapidly, patient may suffer from chills, fever urticaria and flushing of the skin, the so-called "Red man syndrome"
Polymyxin B	10,000–25,000 units/mL	Drug molecules orient themselves between the phospholipid and protein layer of the Gram-negative bacterial cell wall and lead to the formation of pores	Gram-negative bacilli, good activity against *Pseudomonas*	Hypersensitivity	1. Nausea, vomiting and diarrhea 2. It is too toxic to be given parenterally
Bacitracin	10,000 units/mL (500 units/g)	Inhibits the cell wall formation by interfering with the functioning of the lipid carrier which transfers peptidoglycans to the cell wall	Gram-positive bacteria (group B beta-hemolytic *Streptococci* are resistant)	Hypersensitivity	Highly nephrotoxic if used systemically and hence available in topical formulations only

Source: Peyman GA, Sanders DR, Goldberg MF. Principles and Practice of Ophthalmology, 1st edition. Philadelphia: Saunders Ltd; 1980.

Table 4.6: Common antibiotic drugs and their doses.

Drug	Topical dose	Subconjunctival dose	Intravitreal dose (mg/0.1 mL)	Systemic dose
Norfloxacin	0.3% solution 0.3% ointment	—	0.1	*Oral:* 400 mg BID
Ciprofloxacin	0.3% solution 0.3% ointment	—	0.1	*Oral:* 500/750 mg BID Intravenous: 200–400 mg BID
Ofloxacin	0.3% solution 0.3% ointment	—	0.1	*Oral:* 200–400 mg BID
Levofloxacin	0.5% solution 1.5% ointment	—	—	*Oral:* 500 mg
Gatifloxacin	0.3% solution 0.3% ointment	—	—	Withdrawn due to toxicity
Moxifloxacin	0.5% solution 0.5% ointment	—	—	*Oral:* 400 mg OD
Besifloxacin	0.6% suspension	—	—	—
Gentamicin	0.3% solution	10–20 mg	0.02	5–6 mg/kg/day in 3 divided doses IV
Tobramycin	0.3% solution	10–20 mg	0.02	5–6 mg/kg/day IV or IM in 3 divided doses
Amikacin	0.5–1% solution	125 mg	0.04	15 mg/kg/day in 2 divided doses
Vancomycin	—	25 mg	1.0	1 g
Erythromycin	—	50–100 mg	—	250–500 mg TID to QID
Azithromycin	1% solution	—	—	*Oral:* 500 mg OD loading dose then 250 mg OD for 4 days
Chloramphenicol	0.5% solution 0.5% ointment	50–100 mg	2.0	50–100 mg/kg/day
Bacitracin		5,000–10,000 units		

Source: Peyman GA, Sanders DR, Goldberg MF. Principles and Practice of Ophthalmology, 1st edition. Philadelphia: Saunders Ltd; 1980.

The doses of the antibiotics in the different routes of administration are given in Table 4.6.

Principles of Therapy

- If a bacterial infection has been suspected clinically, empirical therapy can be started after taking the necessary swabs/samples for culture and sensitivity as required. A broad-spectrum antibiotic like a fluoroquinolone is usually preferred in these settings.[6] It is not advisable to combine a bacteriostatic drug with a bactericidal one as it brings down the efficacy of the latter.[7]
- Once the culture and sensitivity reports are available, the appropriate drugs can be used to eliminate the infection.
- On initiation frequent instillation, sometimes as often as one drop every half hourly in cases of severe infections, is advised as the induction dose. This is then reduced as per the severity of the lesion and the response as judged clinically by performing slit lamp biomicroscopic examination.
- In case the lesion shows response to a particular antibiotic, the therapy should continue till the signs of infection have resolved.
- If however the lesion does not seem to be resolving, other factors such as mixed infections, presence of foreign body, presence of a local focus of infections like blepharitis and dacryocystitis, and immune deficiencies should be ruled out.

Antibiotics in Common Ophthalmic Use

Fluoroquinolones

These are synthetic antibiotics and are fluorinated derivatives of nalidixic acid. They have a broad-spectrum of activity and excellent corneal penetration. The following are the important fluoroquinolones:

Ciprofloxacin: Among the quinolones, this is most effective against Gram-negative aerobic bacteria. Bacteria which are highly sensitive to ciprofloxacin include *Escherichia coli, Klebsiella pneumoniae, Enterobacter, Salmonella, Shigella, Neisseria species, Haemophilus influenzae, Campylobacter jejuni*. Moderately sensitive bacteria include *Pseudomonas aeruginosa, Staphylococcus aureus, Staphylococcus epidermidis, Branhamella catarrhalis, Legionella, Mycobacterium tuberculosis. Streptococcus pneumoniae, Streptococcus pyogenes, Mycoplasma, Chlamydia, Mycobacterium kansasii,* and *Mycobacterium avium* have low sensitivity.[8] Gram-positive bacteria usually require higher concentrations for inhibition.

Bacteroides fragilis and Clostridia are largely resistant.

It is used systemically in the treatment of urinary tract infections, bacterial gastroenteritis, typhoid fever, respiratory infections, tuberculosis, gonococcal and chlamydial urethritis and soft tissue infections. In ophthalmology, it is used as topical formulations to treat bacterial conjunctivitis and corneal ulcers resulting from susceptible bacteria. It is also used systemically as a prophylaxis against bacterial endophthalmitis.

Ofloxacin: It is more active against Gram-positive bacteria than ciprofloxacin but has lesser activity against Gram-negative organisms. It has good activity against Chlamydia and *M. tuberculosis*. However, it has lower efficacy than ciprofloxacin against *P. aeruginosa*.

It is used systemically for the treatment of respiratory tract infections, atypical pneumonias caused by *Chlamydia trachomatis* and *Mycoplasma*, and *Neisseria gonorrhoeae*. In ophthalmology, it is used topically to treat bacterial conjunctivitis and corneal ulcers due to susceptible organisms. It is used orally in a dose of 200–400 mg as empirical therapy against bacterial endophthalmitis.

Unlike ciprofloxacin, it does not lead to formation of deposits on the corneal epithelium due to its excellent solubility. It has a high oral bioavailability and its absorption is not influenced by the presence of food in the gastrointestinal tract. Its plasma half-life is around 5–7 hours. It is eliminated unchanged in the urine. The dose needs to be reduced in renal disorders.

Levofloxacin: It is an isomer of ofloxacin. It has a broader spectrum of action against *S. pneumoniae*, in addition to Gram-negative and Gram-positive bacteria. It is used systemically in the treatment of respiratory tract infections, urinary tract infections and soft tissue infections. In ophthalmology, it is used as topical drops for the treatment of bacterial conjunctivitis caused by susceptible bacteria.

It has nearly 95% bioavailability on oral regimens. Its longer plasma half-life of 7 hours allows once daily dosing in systemic therapy.

Gatifloxacin: It has excellent activity against *P. aeruginosa*, *Staphylococci* and other Gram-positive cocci. In ophthalmology, it is used as a topical formulation for treatment of corneal ulcers and bacterial conjunctivitis.[9] Since it has excellent penetration into the anterior chamber, it is also used in postoperative prophylaxis after ocular surgeries. It is not used systemically due to the adverse effects of QT prolongation, photosensitivity and hypoglycemic episodes in diabetic patients.[8]

Moxifloxacin: It has excellent activity against Gram-positive bacteria including *S. pneumoniae* and many penicillin-resistant bacteria and also some anaerobes. It is mainly used systemically to treat respiratory tract infections and ear, nose and throat (ENT) infections. It is also known to prolong QT interval and hence should be avoided in patients having arrhythmias and patients known to suffer from epilepsy. It is metabolized in the liver and should not be given to patients with liver disease. In ophthalmology, topical moxifloxacin is widely used for treating corneal ulcers caused by sensitive bacteria. It has very good penetration into the anterior chamber after topical instillation.[10] As it does not require preservative, it is increasingly being used intracamerally as prophylaxis after anterior segment surgical procedures. Its intravitreal use in patients with suspected bacterial endophthalmitis is under study. It has the added advantage that the formulation does not need a preservative for storage.

Besifloxacin: It is a new broad-spectrum fluoroquinolone which is formulated for ocular use only. It has good activity against Gram-negative and Gram-positive bacteria and also anaerobic bacteria.[11] Since it is being used only for ocular indications, the risk of the development of antibiotic resistance is less.

Cephalosporins

These are semisynthetic antibiotics, having a beta-lactam ring. They are chemically related to penicillins but bind to different bacterial proteins and thus their spectrum of action and potency is different. They are obtained from the fungus *Acremonium* (previously called *Cephalosporium*).

Cephalosporins are widely used systemically for respiratory tract infections, skin and soft tissue infections, pre- and postoperative prophylaxis for major surgeries and urinary tract infections caused by susceptible bacteria.

In ophthalmology, cefazolin is used as fortified eye drops, prepared by diluting the intravenous preparation. It is used in conjunction with aminoglycoside eye drops to treat corneal ulcers due to susceptible bacteria. Oral cefaclor has been used to treat early preseptal cellulitis. Intravenous cefuroxime with a beta-lactamase inhibitor has been used to treat severe preseptal cellulitis due to susceptible bacteria. Ceftazidime has been used in cases of bacterial endophthalmitis to cover the Gram-negative bacteria including *P. aeruginosa*. Parenteral ceftriaxone in combination with vancomycin is used to treat severe preseptal cellulitis. Ceftazidime or ceftriaxone in combination with nafcillin has been used to treat orbital cellulitis. For patients with gonococcal conjunctivitis, intramuscular ceftriaxone has been recommended. Intravenous or intramuscular ceftriaxone is also used for ophthalmia neonatorum caused by *Gonococcus*.

The different cephalosporins available and their spectrum are discussed in Table 4.7.

Glycopeptide Antibiotics

Vancomycin: It is a glycopeptide antibiotic produced from *Streptococcus orientalis*. Its spectrum of action is mainly against Gram-positive bacteria and has good activity against *S. aureus, Streptococcus viridans, Enterococcus* and *Clostridium difficile*. It is also active against cocci like *Neisseria, Clostridia* and *Diphtheroids*. It is used systemically for the treatment of pseudomembranous enterocolitis and for serious infections caused by methicillin-resistant *S. aureus* (MRSA). It is also used as empirical therapy for bacterial meningitis in combination with third-generation intravenous cephalosporins and in patients undergoing dialysis and chemotherapy for cancer. In ophthalmology, it is used intravitreally and as eye drops to treat patients with bacterial endophthalmitis[12] and corneal ulcers due to MRSA.[13]

Macrolides

They are a group of closely related compounds which have a macrocyclic lactone ring with attached deoxy sugars. Macrolides used in ophthalmology include:

Table 4.7: Classification of cephalosporins and their spectrum.

Generation	Parenterally administered	Orally administered	Spectrum of action
First generation	Cefazolin	Cefadroxil, cephalexin, cephalothin, cephradine, cephapirin	Active against Gram-positive cocci like *Staphylococci*, *Streptococci* and *Pneumococci* and some anaerobic cocci. Limited activity against *Escherichia coli*, *Klebsiella*, *Proteus*. Not active against MRSA
Second generation	Cefuroxime, cefoxitin	Cefaclor, cefuroxime axetil, cefprozil, loracarbef	Active against beta-lactamase producing *Haemophilus influenzae*, *Moraxella catarrhalis*, *Klebsiella pneumoniae* and penicillin-resistant *pneumoniae*
Third generation	Cefotaxime, ceftizoxime, ceftriaxone, ceftazidime, cefoperazone, moxalactam	Cefixime, cefpodoxime proxetil, cefdinir, ceftibuten, cefetamet pivoxil	Compared to the second-generation agents, these have better Gram-negative coverage and are able to cross the blood-brain barrier. They are active against *Citrobacter*, *Providencia*, beta-lactamase producing strains of *Haemophilus* and *Neisseria*. Only ceftazidime and cefoperazone are active against *Pseudomonas*. Ceftizoxime and moxalactam are active against *Bacteroides fragilis*. The oral agents are less active against *Pneumococci* and *Staphylococcus aureus*
Fourth generation	Cefepime, cefpirome		More resistant to beta-lactamases, have good activity against *Pseudomonas aeruginosa*, *Staphylococcus aureus*, *Streptococcus pneumoniae*, *Enterobacteriaceae*, *Haemophilus* and *Neisseria*. They have good penetration into the cerebrospinal fluid

Source: Peyman GA, Sanders DR, Goldberg MF. Principles and Practice of Ophthalmology, 1st edition. Philadelphia: Saunders Ltd; 1980.

Erythromycin: It is mainly active against Gram-positive bacteria and a few Gram-negative bacteria. *S. pneumoniae, S. pyogenes, N. gonorrhoeae, Corynebacterium diphtheriae, Listeria, B. catarrhalis* are sensitive.

It is systemically useful in abscesses caused by susceptible bacteria; community acquired upper respiratory tract infections, chlamydial infections and diphtheria. It can also be used as an alternative for prophylaxis in rheumatic fever and bacterial endocarditis. In ophthalmology, it is useful in cases of staphylococcal lid infections and as a prophylaxis for ophthalmia neonatorum.[14]

Azithromycin: Systemically, it has become the drug of choice for infections like *C. trachomatis, Legionnaires* pneumonia, donovanosis and chancroid. It is also indicated in cases of pharyngitis, tonsillitis, sinusitis due to *Streptococci* and *Staphylococci*; and also in toxoplasmosis. A single 1 g dose of oral azithromycin is recommended for chlamydial urethritis. The same can be used for chlamydial conjunctivitis in adults and a single dose of 20 mg/kg body weight can be used for children.[15] It is effective against Gram-positive organisms especially *Pneumococci, Streptococci, Staphylococci* and *Corynebacterium*. Azithromycin is more effective against *Chlamydia* and *H. influenzae* than the other macrolides.[16] It is not active against erythromycin-resistant bacteria and MRSA.

Spiramycin: It is the systemic drug of choice for toxoplasmosis in pregnancy. It has a similar spectrum of action like erythromycin and has been found to decrease the chances of development of lesions in the newborn after the transplacental spread of Toxoplasma gondii.[17,18]

Tetracyclines

These are a group of antibiotics which have a chemical structure comprising of four cyclic rings. They are all obtained from actinomycetes from the soil. They comprise of tetracycline, oxytetracycline, doxycycline, minocycline and demeclocycline.

They are systemically used as the first choice of drugs for treating chlamydial urethritis/cervicitis, lymphogranuloma venereum, atypical pneumonias due to *Mycoplasma pneumoniae*, brucellosis, plague, rickettsial infections, and cholera.

In ophthalmology, tetracycline is used as a topical prophylactic agent for ophthalmia neonatorum due to bacterial infections.[19] They are also known to inhibit staphylococcal lipases and hence are used in staphylococcal blepharitis.[20] Doxycycline is commonly used in ophthalmic practice. It is used in cases of chlamydial infections of the lids and conjunctiva, and in toxoplasmosis. It is also used orally in ocular rosacea and meibomian gland infections and after severe chemical injuries, for its anticollagenolytic effects.[21]

The term "Broad-spectrum" is used for this group of drugs as initially they had good activity against majority of Gram-positive and Gram-negative cocci and many Gram-negative bacilli. In addition, they have very good activity against *Chlamydia, Actinomyces, Spirochetes* and *Rickettsiae*. Some protozoa are also sensitive at high concentrations. Partial cross resistance between the different members of tetracycline family and chloramphenicol has been reported.

Aminoglycosides

They are compounds having a hexose ring to which various amino sugars are attached by glycosidic linkages. The hexose ring is either streptidine, in case of streptomycin, and 2-deoxystreptamine in other aminoglycosides.

Gentamicin: It is very active against Gram-negative organisms especially *E. coli, K. pneumoniae, H. influenzae, P. aeruginosa, Enterobacter* and *Proteus*. It is also active against Gram-positive bacteria like *S. aureus*, some *Streptococci* and *Listeria*. It has synergistic activity with beta-lactam antibiotics against *Pseudomonas, Enterobacter, Klebsiella, Proteus, Serratia* and Gram-negative bacilli. Bacteria that are resistant to gentamicin usually show cross resistance to tobramycin and sisomicin, but may still be sensitive to amikacin. Systemically, it is useful in respiratory tract infections due to Gram-negative bacilli, life-threatening infections due to *Pseudomonas, Proteus* or *Klebsiella* like meningitis, septicemia and also in the treatment of subacute bacterial endocarditis. It is recommended to combine the use of gentamicin with a cephalosporin as they act synergistically and also prevent the development of resistant strains.

In ophthalmology, it is used in topical formulations for the treatment of conjunctivitis and corneal ulcers caused by susceptible bacteria. The commercially available eye drops have to be fortified to use in corneal ulcers to be effective. It was used subconjunctivally earlier but this use was stopped following reports of macular infarction associated with its subconjunctival use.[22]

Tobramycin: Systemically, it has the same indications as gentamicin.

For ophthalmic use, it is available both as topical eye drops and ointment form. The eye drops are fortified for the use in corneal ulcers.

Tobramycin is more active against *Pseudomonas* and *Proteus* whereas gentamicin is more active against *Serratia*.

Amikacin: It is used systemically for the same indications as gentamicin. In addition, it is used for treatment of tuberculosis, especially for multidrug-resistant strains.

For Ophthalmic use, fortified topical eye drops can be prepared from the intravenous preparations for topical therapy in susceptible bacteria causing corneal ulcers. As it is found to be less toxic when injected into the vitreous cavity, it is one of the drugs of choice for intravitreal injection along with vancomycin in bacterial endophthalmitis. It is specifically useful for infections caused by *Nocardia*.

It has the widest spectrum of activity compared to other aminoglycosides. It is resistant to many aminoglycoside inactivating enzymes and so is found to be active against many bacteria that are resistant to gentamicin and tobramycin.[23] It is found to be more ototoxic than nephrotoxic and its serum concentrations should be monitored in long-term systemic therapy.

Penicillins[24,25]

They are beta-lactam antibiotics which contain a nucleus composed of fused thiazolidine ring attached to a beta-lactam ring which carries a secondary amino group.

The classification of the penicillins is given in Box 4.1.

Systemically, they are used for treatment of respiratory tract infections, skin and soft tissue infections, urinary tract infections, gonorrhea, meningitis, bacterial endocarditis and syphilis.

Box 4.1: Classification of penicillins.

1. *Penicillin G and its esters:*
   - Penicillin G
   - Procaine penicillin G
   - Benzathine penicillin G
2. *Acid-resistant penicillins:*
   - Penicillin V (phenoxymethyl penicillin)
   - Phenoxyethyl penicillin
3. *Penicillinase-resistant penicillins:*
   - Methicillin, cloxacillin, dicloxacillin
4. *Extended spectrum penicillins:*
   - *Aminopenicillins:* Ampicillin, amoxicillin, bacampicillin
   - *Carboxypenicillins:* Carbenicillin, ticarcillin
   - *Ureidopenicillins:* Piperacillin, mezlocillin

Source: Peyman GA, Sanders DR, Goldberg MF. Principles and Practice of Ophthalmology, 1st edition. Philadelphia: Saunders Ltd; 1980.

In ophthalmology, they are used orally for treatment of lid infections and preseptal cellulitis caused by susceptible bacteria.

Penicillin G has excellent action on infections caused by *Streptococci, Meningococci, Spirochaetes, Actinomyces*, sensitive *Pneumococci*, non-beta-lactamase producing *Staphylococci* and non-beta-lactamase producing Gram-negative anaerobic bacteria. It is given intravenously in a dose of 4–24 million units per day given in four divided doses.

Penicillin V can be given orally and is usually indicated for minor infections by susceptible organisms due to its poor bioavailability.

Benzathine penicillin and procaine penicillin are given intramuscularly and produce sustained duration of drug concentration in the plasma.

Extended spectrum penicillins are so called as they have greater activity against Gram-negative bacteria due to their ability to penetrate the cell membrane of these organisms.

These comprise of: (1) aminopenicillins, (2) beta-lactamase-resistant penicillins, (3) carboxypenicillins, and (4) ureidopenicillins.

The aminopenicillins comprising of ampicillin and amoxicillin, have similar spectrum of action but amoxicillin is absorbed better when given orally. Both are active against *Pneumococci* which are resistant to other penicillins and are commonly used for respiratory tract infections, urinary tract infections and otitis media. Ampicillin is active against *Shigella*.

Combined with beta-lactamase inhibitors like sulbactam, clavulanic acid and tazobactam, these amino-penicilllins can be used against infections caused by beta-lactamase producing *H. influenzae, S. aureus, S. epidermidis* and *S. pneumoniae*. These infections include preseptal cellulitis, orbital cellulitis and dacryocystitis.

Beta-lactamase-resistant penicillins such as nafcillin and methicillin are semisynthetic penicillins and are indicated for infections by beta-lactamase producing *Staphylococci*. They also have good activity against *Streptococci* and *Pneumococci*. Oxacillin and cloxacillin belong to the same group and are given orally for treatment of staphylococcal infections which are not life-threatening. They are reasonably well-absorbed from the gastrointestinal tract but the intake of food interferes with their absorption. For severe staphylococcal infections which may be life-threatening, oxacillin or nafcillin is given intravenously in a dose of 8–12 g/day in three divided doses. Methicillin use has been stopped due to its association with interstitial nephritis.

Carboxypenicillins, which includes carbenicillin and ticarcillin, have been termed as the antipseudomonas penicillins due to their action against *P. aeruginosa* as well as many *Enterobacter* and *Proteus species*. Carbenicillin has now become obsolete but all the other drugs in this group are still in use. They are usually used in combination with an aminoglycoside or fluoroquinolone in severe infections caused by *Pseudomonas*.

Ureidopenicillins comprise of mezlocillin and piperacillin, have been used as topical preparations in combination with aminoglycosides for treatment of corneal ulcer caused by *Pseudomonas*.

Chloramphenicol

It contains a nitrobenzene moiety, which is thought to be responsible for its antibacterial activity. It was earlier derived from *Streptomyces venezuelae* but is now prepared synthetically.

It can be considered for the treatment of severe rickettsial diseases like typhus and rocky mountain spotted fever but due to its severe adverse effects on the bone marrow, it is usually not used widely.[26,27]

For ophthalmic purposes, it is used for the treatment of conjunctivitis, corneal ulcer and lid infections caused by susceptible bacteria. Given systemically, it reaches high concentrations in the eye and may be indicated in cases of endophthalmitis by sensitive organisms.

It is a broad-spectrum antibiotic and has good coverage against many Gram-positive and Gram-negative cocci and bacilli, *Rickettsia, Chlamydia, Mycoplasma* and *Spirochetes. H. influenzae, Klebsiella, Neisseria meningitidis* and anaerobes are usually more sensitive to chloramphenicol than tetracyclines. It is inactive against *Pseudomonas*, mycobacteria and protozoal organisms.

Polymyxin B

It is obtained from *Bacillus polymyxa*. It is a basic peptide compound which has detergent-like activity on bacterial cell membrane. It is active predominantly against Gram-negative bacteria, except *Proteus, Serratia* and *Neisseria*. It is usually available as a mixture with bacitracin or neomycin in the form of ointment or eye drops for use in conjunctivitis caused by Gram-negative bacteria.

Bacitracin

It is a cyclic peptide compound. It was first obtained from the Tracy strain of *Bacillus subtilis*.

It is too toxic to use systemically.

Topical eye drops and ointment in combination with polymyxin B are used for superficial ocular infections. It is especially useful for staphylococcal blepharitis, as *Staphylococci* are seldom resistant to this drug.

It is active against Gram-positive bacteria, *Neisseria* and *Actinomyces*.

ANTIFUNGAL AGENTS

Fungal infections of the eye have become increasingly more common due to the rampant abuse of broad-spectrum antibiotics and steroids, without proper information. This alters the normal flora of the conjunctival sac and allows fungi to invade the ocular tissue. The increased prevalence of immune deficiency disorders has also lead to an increase in the susceptibility of host tissue to fungal infections.

Classification

There are three main classes of antifungals which are used in the ophthalmologic practice.

1. *Polyenes*: They have a large number of double bond in the chemical structure and hence are called "polyenes". Amphotericin B (AmB) and natamycin are the prototypes for this group of drugs. These preferentially bind to the ergosterol in the fungal plasma membrane.
2. *Azoles*: They are synthetic compounds and inhibit the fungal cytochrome P450 enzyme called lanosterol 14 alpha-demethylase. Azoles are classified based on the number of nitrogen atoms in the five-membered azole nucleus as:
   a. *Imidazoles*: Ketoconazole, miconazole and clotrimazole
   b. *Triazoles*: Itraconazole, fluconazole and voriconazole.
3. *Pyrimidines*: They are heterocyclic aromatic compounds with a six-membered nitrogen containing carbon ring structure. The prototype for this group is flucytosine. It is a water-soluble pyrimidine analog. Structurally, it is related to the chemotherapeutic agent 5-fluorouracil but it has no anticancer properties. It is converted to fluorouracil in susceptible fungi and blocks thymidine synthesis.

   The properties of antifungal drugs are given in Table 4.8.

Table 4.8: Properties of commonly used ocular antifungal agents.

Drug	Dose	Mechanism of action	Susceptible fungi	Systemic side effects	Local side effects
Polyenes:					
1. Amphotericin B	Topical: 0.1–0.2% solution in water for injection or 5% dextrose (0.5% solution too toxic) given every hour Intravitreal: 5 µg Intravenous: 0.5–1 mg/kg/day	Amphotericin B binds to the ergosterol, in the fungal cell membrane selectively. It then alters the permeability of the fungal cell membrane by forming micropores in it and leading to cell lysis	Highly effective for *Candida*; moderately effective against some filamentous fungi. Excellent for systemic use against *Candida*	Infusion-related: fever, chills, muscle spasms, vomiting, hypotension, renal damage	Hypersensitivity, corneal epithelial toxicity
2. Natamycin	5% suspension every hour	Similar mechanism of action like that of amphotericin B	Good effect against *Fusarium*, *Candida*, *Aspergillus*	Not used systemically	Hyperemia, corneal epithelial toxicity, precipitates on the epithelium
Imidazoles:		Azoles inhibit the fungal cytochrome P450 enzyme called lanosterol 14 alpha-demethylase. This impairs ergosterol synthesis, which is an important component of the fungal cell membrane. Thus resulting in defective cell membrane formation			
1. Ketoconazole	Topical: 1% suspension in arachis oil Oral: 200–400 mg/day		*Candida, Blastomyces, Coccidioides, Histoplasma*	Pruritus, gastrointestinal upset, abnormalities of liver enzymes, rarely cause hepatitis. Ketoconazole on long use causes gynecomastia	Corneal toxicity
2. Miconazole	Topical: 1% solution in arachis oil Subconjunctival: 5 mg Intravitreal: 10 µg		Active against many filamentous fungi and *Candida*		
Triazoles:		Similar to imidazoles			
1. Fluconazole	Topical: 1% solution in water Oral: 200 mg/day		*Candida, Aspergillus*		
2. Itraconazole	Oral: 200 mg/day		*Aspergillus, Candida species, Coccidioides, Paracoccidioides*	Hypokalemia, hyperlipidemia	
3. Voriconazole	Topical: 1% solution		*Aspergillus, Fusarium*	Rash, hepatic enzyme disorders, photopsia	
Pyrimidines:				Bone marrow and liver toxicity	
Flucytosine	Topical: 1.5% solution Oral: Begin at 50–100 mg/kg/day, increase to 200 mg/kg/day in divided doses		*Candida, Cryptococcus*		

Source: Peyman GA, Sanders DR, Goldberg MF. Principles and Practice of Ophthalmology, 1st edition. Philadelphia: Saunders Ltd; 1980.

Principles of Therapy

- Antifungal treatment should be started as soon as the results of the Gram stain and KOH mount become available.
- In case the test results are not very suggestive but the clinical findings are highly suggestive of a fungal infection, treatment should be started, especially if the patient is from areas where fungal infections are common.
- Topical therapy proves to be more effective than systemic therapy.
- Systemic therapy is considered as an adjunct in cases when there is an anterior chamber involvement or the ulcer threatens to perforate or there is limbal involvement, or there are multiple foci of the fungal infection in the body.
- Steroid therapy should be avoided if a fungal etiology for an ulcer is suspected.
- In case the ulcer is not responsive to medical therapy, the ophthalmologist should be ready to advise a therapeutic keratoplasty at the earliest.

Antifungal Agents Used in Ophthalmology

Polyenes

They are derived from *Streptomyces* species. They bind with the ergosterols in the cell wall of fungi which leads to the lysis of fungal cell. They also bind with the cholesterol (though with low intensity) which is found in human cell membrane and this interaction may lead to toxicity in humans.

They can be divided based on the number of the carbon atoms and the number of double bonds in their chemical structure into:

1. *Large molecule polyenes (e.g. AmB)*: They have concentration-dependent lytic activity on the fungal cell wall by forming pores in it. These pores allow the cellular contents to extrude causing the lysis of the fungi.
2. *Small molecule polyenes (e.g. natamycin)*: These drugs cause nonconcentration-dependent cell wall lysis by damaging the cell wall.

Amphotericin B:[28,29] It is obtained from Streptomyces nodosus. It has the broadest spectrum of action among the antifungal drugs and is active against a wide range of yeasts and filamentous fungi. It is active against yeasts like *Candida albicans* and *Cryptococcus neoformans*; molds like *Aspergillus fumigatus* and *Mucor* and also organisms causing endemic mycoses like *Blastomyces dermatitidis*, *Coccidioides immitis* and *Histoplasma capsulatum*. It is also known to be active on the protozoa and *Leishmania*. As it has a broad-spectrum of action, it is used systemically in nearly all life-threatening fungal infections.

Systemically, it is used in all serious fungal infections as an intravenous infusion and is also used for empirical therapy in febrile neutropenia not responding to intravenous higher antibacterials and in resistant cases of leishmaniasis. In ocular conditions, due to its higher toxicity, it is used for the initial few days as induction therapy and then substituted by an azole antifungal drug for long-term therapy.

A readymade topical form of AmB is not available for use as eye drops but the intravenous preparation can be diluted appropriately for topical as well as intravitreal route. Once reconstituted with water for injection, the solution has to be stored in the dark at 2–8°C. When the stock solution is further diluted with dextrose, the drug should be used promptly and the unused drug discarded. The topical preparation is used especially in all candidal corneal ulcers and may be supplemented with subconjunctival injections of the drug. In cases of fungal endophthalmitis, the drug is injected directly into the vitreous cavity to increase the drug concentration at the site of infection. In cases of orbital mycotic infections, the intravenous route is used.

Nystatin: It is obtained from *Streptomyces noursei*, it shares its structural properties and mechanism of action with AmB. Due to its high systemic toxicity, it is only used as topical preparations for superficial candidiasis. It is active against most *Candida*. It is currently available for use in oral thrush, vaginal candidiasis and intertriginous candidal infections. It is not absorbed from the skin, gastrointestinal tract and mucous membranes. For use in extraocular infections, it is available as a 100,000 units/g dermatologic ointment in some countries for candidal infection. It is too toxic for subconjunctival injection. Its intravitreal use is still in experimental stages.

Natamycin: It is a tetrene which is semisynthetically prepared. It is available as a 5% suspension. It has a broad-spectrum of activity and has good activity against *Fusarium* species.[30]

It is available only for topical use. It has better corneal penetration compared to AmB, but its penetration can be enhanced by scraping of the corneal epithelium.

Azoles

These are synthetic compounds and are classified into imidazoles and triazoles based on the number of nitrogen atoms in the five membered azole ring. These drugs reduce the synthesis of ergosterol in the fungal cells by inhibiting the fungal cytochrome P450 enzymes. They have higher affinity to the fungal cytochromes than the human counterpart and hence have a higher degree of specificity and better tolerability. The following are the various drugs available in this class:

Fluconazole: It has good water solubility and cerebrospinal fluid (CSF) penetration. Its bioavailability after oral administration is also high. It is available both for oral use and intravenous use.

It is the azole of choice for cryptococcal meningitis treatment; it is also effective in treatment of candidemia in patients with normal white blood cell count. It is commonly used to treat mucocutaneous candidiasis. It has no activity against *Aspergillus* or other filamentous fungi.

For topical use in ophthalmology, a 2 mg/mL eye drop can be formulated from the intravenous preparation and has been used to treat candidal corneal ulcers. A subconjunctival injection can also be given in cases of severe corneal ulcers caused by susceptible *Candida* species. Oral therapy also has been found to be effective.[31]

Itraconazole: It has a low water solubility and lower bioavailability. Its penetration into the CSF is also poor as compared to fluconazole. It has a broader spectrum of activity than ketoconazole and fluconazole.

It has good activity against *Candida* species, *Aspergillus, Coccidioides, Paracoccidioides*, and *Paecilomyces*. It is not very effective against *Fusarium* species.

It is preferred for systemic mycosis caused by susceptible fungi, except those associated with meningitis. It is also used in vaginal candidiasis and in onychomycosis.

For use in ophthalmology, it can be formulated into a 1–2% suspension from the intravenous preparation.[32] Corneal penetration as eye drops is very poor and it does not penetrate ocular tissues if given systemically.

Voriconazole: It is a newer triazole having a broad-spectrum of action. It has good activity against *Candida* species and dimorphic fungi; it has been used to treat invasive aspergillosis, disseminated infections due to fluconazole-resistant *Candida* and *Fusarium* infections. Severe infections are first treated by intravenous route and then oral voriconazole is used for maintenance therapy till the infection is eliminated.

Topical eye drops can be formulated from the intravenous preparation. The eye drops have been used to treat corneal ulcers due to susceptible *Candida* and dimorphic fungi.[33] It is also effective against *Aspergillus*, but may not work as efficiently against *Fusarium*.

Pyrimidines

5-flucytosine: It is a water-soluble pyrimidine analog. It has good penetration into all body compartments and in CSF. Its spectrum of action is limited to *C. neoformans* and few species of *Candida*. It is also used in chromoblastomycosis. To avoid development of resistance, it is always used in conjunction with AmB for cryptococcal meningitis or with itraconazole for chromoblastomycosis.

A 1% topical solution can be formulated for ophthalmic use.[34] It is used to treat superficial infections like blepharitis, conjunctivitis, canaliculitis and superficial ulcers of candidal origin.

ANTIVIRALS

The commonly used antiviral agents in ophthalmology are enumerated in Table 4.9.

Table 4.9: Common antiviral agents in ophthalmology.

Drug	Dose	Mechanism of action	Indications	Systemic side effects	Local side effects
Idoxuridine	*Topical:* 0.1% solution	Being a thymidine analog, it competes with thymidine and gets incorporated in the viral DNA. The new DNA formed is defective	*Herpes simplex* virus (HSV) keratitis, used for superficial dendritic ulcers	None reported	Conjunctival congestion and scarring, punctate epithelial keratopathy, follicular conjunctivitis, superficial vascularization, punctal occlusion, contact dermatitis, preauricular lymphadenopathy
Trifluridine	• *Topical:* 1% solution, given 9 times a day for 5 days and if improvement occurs, continued 5 times a day for 2–3 weeks • Needs to be stored between 2°C and 8°C	Similar to idoxuridine, it inhibits thymidine synthetase by incorporating into the viral DNA during replication and renders the new viruses formed noninfectious	HSV keratitis	None reported	Conjunctival congestion and scarring, punctate epithelial keratopathy, follicular conjunctivitis, superficial vascularization, punctal occlusion, contact dermatitis, preauricular lymphadenopathy
Vidarabine	*Topical:* 3% ointment, used 5 times a day for 1 week	It appears to interfere with early steps of viral replication and prevents the viral DNA chain elongation	HSV keratitis		Conjunctival congestion and scarring, punctate epithelial keratopathy, follicular conjunctivitis, superficial vascularization, punctal occlusion, contact dermatitis, preauricular lymphadenopathy
Acyclovir	*Topical:* 3% ointment *Oral:* 1. HSV keratitis: 200–400 mg 5 times per day for 7 days 2. Herpes zoster ophthalmicus: 800 mg 5 times a day for 10 days *Intravenous:* 10 mg/kg q8h for 7 days in immunocompromised	Activated acyclovir triphosphate binds to the DNA template by competing with the deoxy-GTP for the viral DNA polymerase and forming an irreversible complex, this leads to the early chain termination	1. HSV keratitis/ uveitis 2. Herpes zoster ophthalmicus 3. Prevention of recurrences • Has no effect on postherpetic neuralgia	Nausea, diarrhea, headache, reversible renal dysfunction, tremors, delirium and seizures also have been reported	Punctate epithelial erosions, follicular conjunctivitis, lid margin thickening
Valacyclovir	*Oral:* 1 g TID for 7–10 days Relieves postherpetic neuralgia	It is a prodrug of acyclovir and has similar mechanism of action against herpes viruses	HSV keratitis, uveitis, scleritis Herpes zoster ophthalmicus	Nausea, vomiting, rash, liver enzyme elevation, anemia, neutropenia	
Famciclovir	*Oral:* 1. HSV 250–500 mg BID for 7 days 2. Herpes zoster ophthalmicus: 500 mg TID for 7 days	Activated by phosphorylation by the thymidine kinase in the virus-infected cells. Once active it competitively inhibits the viral DNA polymerase thus stopping viral DNA synthesis	1. HSV keratitis, uveitis, scleritis 2. Herpes zoster ophthalmicus 3. Reduces the duration of postherpetc neuralgia	Nausea, vomiting, Headache	

Contd...

Contd...

Drug	Dose	Mechanism of action	Indications	Systemic side effects	Local side effects
Ganciclovir	*Intravenous:* *Induction:* 5 mg/kg q12h for 14 days *Maintenance:* 5 mg/kg/day, or 6 mg/kg 5 times a week *Oral:* 1 g TID can be used as maintenance therapy after induction	Activated by virus-specific thymidine kinase and the resultant phosphorylated products inhibit the viral DNA polymerase	1. *Intravenous:* Cytomegalovirus (CMV) retinitis 2. *Topical:* HSV keratitis	Myelosuppression (common cause of drug discontinuation), nausea, insomnia, peripheral neuropathy Once treatment is stopped, the CMV activity resumes	
Foscarnet	*Intravenous:* *Induction:* 60 mg/kg q8h, or 90 mg/kg q12h for 14 days *Maintenance:* 90–120 mg/kg/day	Affects the pyrophosphate binding site of the DNA	CMV retinitis	Renal impairment, serum calcium and phosphate disorders, anemia, penile ulcerations	
Cidofovir	*Intravenous:* 5 mg/kg every 7 days for 2 consecutive weeks *Maintenance:* 5 mg/kg every 14 days	It undergoes phosphorylation to its active biphosphate form which acts as an alternative substrate for the viral DNA polymerase and becomes incorporated into the viral DNA chain. It thus competitively inhibits viral DNA synthesis	CMV retinitis Also active against HSV, varicells-zoster virus, Epstein-Barr virus, Kaposi's sarcoma-associated herpesvirus (KSHV), adenovirus, poxvirus and human papillomavirus	Dose-related nephrotoxicity	Uveitis, ocular hypotony

Source: Peyman GA, Sanders DR, Goldberg MF. Principles and Practice of Ophthalmology, 1st edition. Philadelphia: Saunders Ltd; 1980

Properties of Commonly Used Antivirals in Ophthalmology

Idoxuridine

Chemically, it is 5-Iodo-2'-deoxyuridine. It acts as a thymidine analog and gets incorporated in the viral DNA.

Ophthalmic use: Its use was limited for topical treatment of superficial herpetic keratitis.[35] Due to its toxicity to the corneal epithelium it has largely been replaced by newer drugs and is no longer available for therapeutic use.

It is not used systemically.

Vidarabine

Chemically, it is 9-β-D-arabinofuranosyladenine. It was earlier known as adenine arabinoside. It is obtained from Streptomyces species and was initially synthesized as an antimetabolite drug. It is active against *herpes simplex viruses 1 and 2, herpes zoster virus* and *vaccinia virus.*[36] It is metabolized to hypoxanthine arabinoside, which is a lesser active by-product.

Ophthalmic use: It is relatively insoluble in water and available as an ointment form for topical use. It penetrates the cornea to enter the aqueous and has been rarely used to treat herpetic uveitis, though it is not the preferred agent for this. It is usually used five times a day for a week and titrated based on response. If there is no epithelialization after 2 weeks of treatment, its use should be abandoned. In case the lesion is epithelized, the treatment is continued at a lower frequency for an additional 1 week. The treatment should not be continued more than 3 weeks. It has rarely been used systemically for herpetic encephalitis.

Trifluridine

Chemically, it is 5-trifluoromethyl-2'-deoxyuridine. It is a fluorinated nucleoside analog of thymidine. It is a potent inhibitor of thymidylate synthetase and inhibits the synthesis of viral DNA. It has effect on all viruses belonging to the herpesvirus family including *herpes simplex viruses 1 and 2, cytomegalovirus (CMV)* and *vaccinia virus*. However, it is not very selective for the virus-infected cells and also damages the normal host cells. It is said to be twice as potent as idoxuridine and also is more soluble. It is also soluble in lipids and this biphasic solubility allows it to have better corneal penetration.

In ophthalmology, it is used to treat herpetic dendritic ulcers.[37] It is used initially for nine to ten times a day for the first 5 days and then five times a day for the next 2–3 weeks. It has a lesser corneal toxicity when compared to idoxuridine and has now become the preferred drug for topical therapy of dendritic ulcer in many developed countries. It is known to enter the aqueous humor but does not have proven efficacy in treating keratouveitis. The solution is supplied in a dose of 1% and needs to be stored between 2°C and 8°C.

It undergoes rapid metabolism when given systemically, with a half-life of 12–15 minutes and hence not used for systemic infections.

Acyclovir

Chemically, it is 9-2-hydroxyethoxymethyl guanine. It is a synthetic purine nucleoside analog. It is active against *herpetic viruses* only. *Herpesvirus type 1* is the most sensitive, followed by *herpesvirus type 2, varicella-zoster* and *Epstein-Barr virus*. It has no effect on *CMV*.
It is used systemically for:

- Treatment of genital herpes simplex in a dose of 400 mg orally for primary episodes. In case of recurrent disease, it is initially given intravenously in a dose of 5 mg/kg body weight, three times a day for 10 days and then as a maintenance therapy of 400 mg twice a day orally to keep the disease suppressed.
- In cases of herpes simplex encephalitis, 15–20 mg/kg intravenous infusion is given three times a day for 10–15 days.
- Herpes zoster treatment requires higher doses as the virus is affected by the drug to a lesser extent. Orally 800 mg tablets, five times a day for 7–10 days are useful if started early during the onset of the disease. In immunocompromised individuals, 10 mg/kg three times a day is given intravenously.
- Mucocutaneous herpes usually responds to treatment with skin cream formulation. In severe cases or spreading lesions, oral treatment for 10 days in a dose of 400 mg five times a day can be used.

It is used in ophthalmology for:

- *For herpes simplex virus keratitis*, it can be used as 3% ointment form administered five times a day.[38] Oral acyclovir in a dose of 400 mg has been used to prevent relapse of stromal keratitis.[39]
- *Herpes zoster ophthalmicus:* Oral acyclovir at a dose of 800 mg five times a day, usually for 7–10 days is used. It is suggested to start the treatment within 72 hours of the onset of the rash to prevent the severe ocular complications of zoster ophthalmicus like keratitis, scleritis, optic neuritis and acute retinal necrosis.[40]

Valacyclovir

Chemically, it is an L-valyl ester of acyclovir.
It is used systemically for:

- Treatment of herpes zoster, in a dose of 1 g three times a day for 7–14 days.
- Treatment of herpes simplex genitalis, initially in a dose of 1 g twice a day for 10 days in case of primary disease. In case of recurrence, an initial oral dose of 500 mg twice a day for 5 days is given followed by 500 mg/day dose to suppress the disease.
- For orolabial herpes, 2 g twice a day are given systemically followed by application of the skin cream on the lesions.
- It is helpful in preventing the infection from CMV after organ transplantation.

In ophthalmology, it has been used for:

- Herpetic keratitis as an ointment form and the oral formulation is used for the treatment of herpes zoster ophthalmicus.
- Used orally in a dose of 1 g TID for 7–14 days in herpes zoster ophthalmicus, it is reported to decrease the incidence of postherpetic neuralgia.[41]

Famciclovir

Chemically, it is the diacetyl ester prodrug of 6-deoxypenciclovir. It has activity against *herpes simplex* and *herpes zoster* viruses. It is being investigated for its action on *hepatitis B virus*.

Systemically, it is used for the treatment of genital herpes, both as the initial mode of treatment and also for preventing recurrence.[42] It is the US Food and Drug Administration (FDA)-approved for the treatment of zoster at doses of 500 mg thrice a day for 7 days. The treatment should preferably be initiated within 72 hours of the onset of the rash.

For ocular herpes infection, a dose of 250 mg thrice a day for 7–10 days is used. For recurrent episodes, 125–250 mg thrice a day for 7 days has been used.

Ganciclovir

Chemically, it is the synthetic purine nucleoside analog of guanine. Although it is active against nearly all viruses of herpesvirus family, its main clinical use has been against CMV.

It is used systemically for:

- Treatment of severe CMV infections like pneumonia or colitis.
- As a prophylaxis in transplant patients.

In ophthalmology, it is used for:

- *Intravenous use*: It is mainly used for the treatment of *CMV* retinitis in immunocompromised patients. As it is only virostatic, and does not eliminate the virus, the retinitis resumes once the therapy is stopped. Long-term maintenance therapy is thus needed in the immunocompromised patients till the immune system recovers. It is used at a dose of 5 mg/kg body weight, given twice a day for 1–3 weeks, followed by 5 mg/kg given once a day. The solution is reconstituted in sterile water for injection and once reconstituted can be stored between 15°C and 30°C for maximum of 12 hours. It should not be refrigerated.
- *Intravitreal*:[43] It is available as an intravitreal implant which contains 4.5 mg of the drug, which gets eluted for a period of about 8 months. It has the advantage of making high concentration of the drug available at the local site of infection, without the systemic toxicity and also does not require frequent injection repetitions. Once the implant has stopped eluting the drug, it can be replaced surgically with a new one.
- *Oral*: Orally it is available as valganciclovir, which is given in the dose of 900 mg twice a day. It is the L-valyl ester prodrug of ganciclovir. It has good oral absorption with a bioavailability of about 60%. It is recommended that the drug be taken along with food. It is used for the maintenance phase of the therapy in the treatment of CMV retinitis in immunocompromised patients and in those who have undergone solid organ transplantations.
- *Topical gel*: A 0.15% topical gel formulation has been used for the treatment of herpetic corneal ulcers.[44] In this form, it causes less irritation on application as compared to acyclovir ointment, even as the efficacy is comparable between both the agents.

As it is not virucidal, it does not remove the virus from the retina but only suppresses its activity. Once the therapy is stopped, the virus continues to proliferate. It is phosphorylated by healthy host cells also, especially rapidly dividing cells in the bone marrow thus increasing the toxicity to the bone marrow.

Topical therapy should not be continued if there is no significant improvement after 2–3 weeks of starting therapy.

Foscarnet

Chemically, it is phosphonomethanoic acid. It does not share structural similarities with the other available antiviral agents. It has in vitro activity against *herpes simplex virus, varicella-zoster virus, CMV, human herpesvirus-6, Kaposi's sarcoma-associated herpesvirus (KSHV)* and *human immunodeficiency virus type-1 (HIV-1)*. It can be used to treat acyclovir-resistant strains of herpesviruses and varicella-zoster virus.

It is used systemically for the treatment of CMV colitis, CMV esophagitis and for *herpesvirus* and *varicella-zoster viruses* that are resistant to acyclovir.

Intravenous: Foscarnet is used to treat immunocompromised patients with CMV retinitis. It is given at an induction dose of 60 mg/kg thrice a day or 90 mg/kg twice a day for 2 to 3 week period. This is followed by a maintenance dose of 90–120 mg/kg/day. It has been found to have synergistic action when given in combination with ganciclovir. However, the adverse reactions also increase when the drugs are given together.

Intravitreal: This route is used in patients who cannot be given intravenous foscarnet due to renal toxicity or cannot be given intravitreal ganciclovir due to allergy to its components.[45] The usual induction dose is 1,200 μg twice a week for 3 weeks which is followed by a one injection per weeks for maintenance.

Box 4.2 lists the common side effects which are encountered due to the use of topical antivirals.

Intravitreal preparations are preferred in cases of posterior segment virus infections as high concentrations can be achieved at the site of infection with no systemic side effects. The drawback of intravitreal injections is that the fellow eye is not protected against the infection and

Box 4.2: Common side effects of topical antiviral agent use.

- Contact dermatitis
- Punctal occlusion
- Ptosis
- Follicular conjunctivitis
- Perilimbal edema
- Conjunctival scarring
- Punctate epithelial erosions of cornea
- Stromal corneal ulceration
- Filamentary keratitis
- Toxic keratitis

Source: Peyman GA, Sanders DR, Goldberg MF. Principles and Practice of Ophthalmology, 1st edition. Philadelphia: Saunders Ltd; 1980.

the systemic infection remains unchecked. Intravitreal injections also raise the chances of iatrogenic retinal detachment and vitreous hemorrhage. The intravitreal dosages are indicated in Table 4.10.

ANTIPROTOZOALS

The eye can also be infected by protozoa which are commonly found in soil and dirty water. Immunocompromised patients are at increased risk. The commonly encountered protozoal infections in the eye are due to *Acanthamoeba, Microsporidium* and *T. gondii.*

Principles of Treatment of Ocular Protozoal Infections

The principles of treatment for these organisms are as follows:

Acanthamoeba

It is known to cause a very painful keratitis which is very difficult to treat. The keratitis commonly occurs in patients using contact lenses, who fail to take proper care of the lenses. In developing countries, it is commonly encountered in patients who are exposed to infested waters.

Principles of therapy: No single drug has been found to be effective in all the variants of *Acanthamoeba*. Multiple drugs are used simultaneously to increase the chances of affecting a cure. Usually combination therapies of topical drops along with systemic drugs are used. After the initiation of the therapy, patient is closely followed up to monitor the response of the ulcer to the therapy. In case the ulcer does not show signs of resolution or the cornea is at risk of perforation, a surgical intervention in the form of therapeutic keratoplasty may be needed.

Table 4.10: Intravitreal dosages of antiviral drugs.

Intravitreal antiviral drug	Dosage
Ganciclovir	200–400 μg in 0.1 mL
Foscarnet	1,200 μg in 0.05 mL
Cidofovir	20 μg in 0.1 mL

Source: Peyman GA, Sanders DR, Goldberg MF. Principles and Practice of Ophthalmology, 1st edition. Philadelphia: Saunders Ltd; 1980.

The various drugs which are available for the treatment are:

- Dibrompropamidine 0.15% ointment (Brolene ointment) in combination with neomycin-polymyxin B-gramicidin has been used topically. Topical paromomycin 10 mg/mL eye drops can also be used instead of neomycin.
- 0.1% propamidine isethionate (Brolene solution) with pentamidine isethionate 0.05–0.1% topically.
- Miconazole solution 10 mg/mL or clotrimazole 1% solution topically.
- Polyhexamethylene biguanide (PHMB) 0.02% topically is known to destroy the trophozoites as well as the cyst forms. It is usually given on an hourly basis initially and then is gradually tapered over months.
- Chlorhexidine digluconate (0.02%) topically is an effective drug which is used either as a monotherapy or as a combination therapy with PHMB.
- Ketoconazole 400 mg orally daily or itraconazole 200 mg daily.

Polyhexamethylene biguanide and chlorhexidine used topically have become the preferred agents for topical therapy.[46,47]

Microsporidial Infection

The infection in the eye can manifest in two forms:

1. *Superficial keratoconjunctivitis*: It is caused by *Encephalitozoon hellem*, and rarely *E. cuniculi* or *E. intestinalis* or *Trachipleistophora hominis.*
2. *Focal stromal keratitis*: It occurs after corneal trauma due to infection by *Vittaforma corneae* (earlier called Nosema), *Microsporifium africanum* or *Microsporidium ceylonensis.*

Principles of therapy: In cases of superficial lesions, local debridement of the lesions followed by topical fumagillin 70 μg/mL. In cases of stromal keratitis, topical fumagillin therapy is combined with systemic albendazole or itraconazole given orally.

In the experience of the authors, good clinical response is seen with the use of 0.3% fluconazole eye drops used four times a day in case of superficial lesions and conjunctivitis caused by microsporidia.[48]

In cases of nonresolving lesions, therapeutic keratoplasty may be needed.

Toxoplasma gondii

Toxoplasma gondii is an obligate intracellular parasite, with the domestic cat as its definitive host. It commonly leads to posterior uveitis, papillitis and sometimes a granulomatous anterior uveitis. The infection in most immunocompetent individuals is a self-limiting one and the goal of the therapy is to reduce ocular damage occurring due to the associated inflammation till the infection slowly gets contained. In immunocompromised individuals however the infection can be more devastating and also associated with systemic involvement, and may need a more active approach. The therapy should be monitored keeping in mind the severe inflammatory reaction that may follow the death of the protozoa and release of proinflammatory mediators.

Principles of therapy:[49] The usual approach is to start antimicrobials if any of the following factors are present:

- Significant decrease in visual acuity
- Lesions involving the posterior pole especially if threatening the optic disk or macula
- Presence of severe vitritis
- Presence of lesion greater than one disk diameter or multicentric lesions
- Persistent lesions which are active even after a month.

Lesions which are in the peripheral region with 6/6 vision are closely monitored.

Systemic steroids can be started after an antimicrobial therapy has been initiated at least 24–48 hours prior.

An initial regimen using sulfadiazine and pyrimethamine, followed by systemic prednisone has been found to be effective.

Another regimen using sulfonamide, clindamycin, pyrimethamine and prednisone has been suggested for advanced disease.

In pregnant patients, spiramycin is the preferred agent, if antimicrobial therapy is needed.

Folinic acid in a dose of 5–20 mg/day should be given whenever pyrimethamine is used in therapy and the blood cell count and platelet count should be monitored.

The various drugs that are used in the treatment of ocular toxoplasmosis are listed here:[50]

- *Sulfadiazine*: A loading dose of 2 g TDS orally, followed by a maintenance dose of 1 g TID to QID for up to 60 days. Children are given a dose of 100 mg/kg/day divided in four doses.
- *Pyrimethamine*: A loading dose of 100 mg orally is given, followed by a maintenance dose of 25 mg/day for up to 60 days. Children are given 4 mg/kg/day as a loading dose followed by 1 mg/kg/day as maintenance dose.
- Azithromycin 500–1,000 mg/day orally for up to 20 days has also been tried.
- Atovaquone 750 mg QID orally for up to 6 weeks has been tried. It is said to be more effective against the cysts.
- Clindamycin 300 mg QID orally for 4 weeks can be used along with sulfadiazine and pyrimethamine.
- Spiramycin 300–450 mg QID orally for up to 4 weeks has been used in pregnant patients. In children, it can be given in a dose of 100 mg/kg/day in four divided doses.

Prednisone in a dose of 1–2 mg/kg/day orally can be used to suppress the inflammation 24–48 hours after starting the antimicrobial therapy.

CORTICOSTEROIDS[51]

Corticosteroids play a vital role in the day-to-day ophthalmology practice. They are potent anti-inflammatory agents and can help to control ocular inflammation encountered postoperatively or due to any pathology.

Some of the common ocular indications for use of corticosteroids are enumerated in Box 4.3.

Mechanism of Action

Corticosteroids are used in ophthalmology mainly for their strong anti-inflammatory actions. The anti-inflammatory effects are due to the action of the drugs at multiple levels of the inflammatory reaction. They have effect over the cellular as well as the chemical component of inflammatory reactions.

The exact mechanism of action of steroids is still under evaluation, but the following reasons are known to contribute to their action:

- They stabilize the membranes of lysosomes, basophils and macrophages, and prevent them from degranulation.
- They decrease the production of chemotactic cytokines and prevent the aggregation of inflammatory cells at the site of lesion.

Box 4.3: Indications of corticosteroid use in ophthalmology.

1. *Lids:*
   - Contact dermatitis
   - Allergic blepharitis
   - Small chalazions/granulomas
   - Myasthenia gravis
2. *Conjunctiva:*
   - Allergic/vernal conjunctivitis
   - Phlyctenular conjunctivitis
   - Ocular cicatricial pemphigoid
   - Chemical injuries
   - After conjunctival surgeries like pterygium excision
3. *Cornea:*
   - Interstitial keratitis
   - Marginal keratitis
   - Mooren's ulcer
   - Disciform keratitis
   - Sclerokeratitis
   - Acne rosacea keratitis
   - Postcorneal surgeries
   - Acute graft rejection
   - Dry eyes
4. *Sclera:*
   - Scleritis and episcleritis
5. *Uveal involvement:*
   - Iritis, iridocyclitis
   - Postoperative uveitis
   - Posterior uveitis
   - Sympathetic ophthalmia
   - Endophthalmitis
6. *Others:*
   - Idiopathic inflammatory orbital disease
   - Thyroid eye disease
   - Post-glaucoma surgeries to regulate the fibrosis
   - Giant cell arteritis
   - Optic neuritis
   - Capillary hemangiomas
   - Juvenile xanthogranulomas

Source: Peyman GA, Sanders DR, Goldberg MF. Principles and Practice of Ophthalmology, 1st edition. Philadelphia: Saunders Ltd; 1980.

- They suppress the generation and release of inflammatory neutrophils from the bone marrow.
- Decrease the production of acute phase reactants from the macrophages and endothelial cells, prevent generation of cytokines, and inhibit proinflammatory complement system.
- They also decrease the production of collagenases and other tissue destructive enzymes.

Table 4.11 lists the common corticosteroids that are used in ophthalmology.

Principles of Therapy

- The principle of "start early, start strong" is usually applied to the use of corticosteroids in ophthalmology. The time duration between the disease onset and the start of therapy can make a huge difference especially in sight-threatening conditions like arteritic anterior ischemic optic neuropathy (AION). The therapy is started usually at high dose and then tapered gradually.
- In cases of infections, the starting of therapy needs careful assessment, weighing the risks versus the benefits of the therapy. It is a good practice to start the therapy under adequate antibiotic cover.
- The use of systemic steroids for more than 20 days mandates a gradual taper in the dose over the next few days. Sudden withdrawal risks precipitating an adrenergic crisis.
- Corticosteroids used in topical eye drops form, if not tapered, risk in the recurrence of the inflammation.
- They are absolutely contraindicated in cases of fungal infections and herpetic corneal ulcers.
- If long-term therapy is required, steroid-sparing agents can be employed, to prevent the development of ocular as well as systemic side effects of long-term corticosteroid use.

Routes of Corticosteroid Administration

Topical: The steroids are available in the aqueous, suspension and ointment forms. The dosing depends on the indication and the severity of the inflammation. The acetate form is preferred in severe inflammation. Preparations like medrysone and loteprednol, the so-called "soft steroids", do not penetrate the cornea and are useful only in superficial lesions. Other steroids like prednisolone have excellent corneal penetration and preferred for use in iridocyclitis. The disadvantage of the penetration into the anterior chamber is that these steroids are more likely to cause an increase in the IOP of the eye. The ointment forms are not very effective in drug delivery as the petroleum base hinders the release of the steroids hence reducing their availability.

Periocular injectable steroids: The sites of injection can be subconjunctival, anterior or posterior sub-Tenon's and rarely retrobulbar, depending on the indication for the steroid use. Usually triamcinolone acetonide, 4 mg depot preparation, is used for periocular injections.

Table 4.11: Common corticosteroids in use.

Drug	Indication	Dose	Side effects	Remarks
Dexamethasone	Anti-inflammatory (oral, IV, topical, subconjunctival)	*Oral and parenteral:* 0.75 mg is equivalent to 5 mg prednisone *Topical:* 0.05% ophthalmic ointment; 0.1% ophthalmic solution *Subconjunctival:* 4 mg (8 or 10 mg/mL solution may be used to decrease volume of injection) *Intravitreal:* Sustained release implants of 0.35 mg and 0.7 mg	*Oral and parenteral:* 1. Delays wound healing 2. Decreased bone density 3. Gastointestinal distress 4. Decreased wound strength 5. Increased risk of bacterial, fungal, yeast infections *Topical and subconjunctival:* 1. Corneal thinning 2. Increased incidence of infection 3. Intraocular pressure (IOP) increase in steroid responders 4. Decreased wound strength 5. Increased risk of bacterial, fungal, and yeast infections 6. Mydriasis (1–2 mm) 7. Ptosis (irreversible)	*Oral and parenteral:* 1. No mineralocorticoid activity 2. Cannot be used for alternate day therapy due to long duration of action *Topical and subconjunctival:* 1. Significant delay in corneal healing when used more than 6 times/day 5 2. If used 4 times/day for 6 weeks plasma cortisol levels can be decreased but the axis remains intact 3. When using steroids, infectious processes must be ruled out or the most likely anti-infective agent must be administered concurrently 4. Penetration of suspension into eye is greater than that of solution 5. Shake suspension 6. Can be used for prevention of adrenal crisis
Fluorometholone	Anti-inflammatory	*Topical:* 0.1% ophthalmic solution	See dexamethasone, topical and subconjunctival	1. Less IOP increase in steroid responders 2. Most potent of "non-IOP-raising" topical steroids
Loteprednol etabonate	Used in severe allergic conjunctivitis and vernal keratoconjunctivitis	0.5% solution available for topical instillation	Lesser propensity to cause raise in IOP, cataract formation, corneal epithelial toxicity	Most of the drug is metabolized in the anterior chamber and hence lesser concentration is present to have toxic effects on the anterior segment of eye
Hydrocortisone	Anti-inflammatory (IV, IM, topical), prevention of adrenal crisis in patients who are adrenally suppressed	*Parenteral:* To prevent adrenal crisis in patients with adrenal suppression, 100 mg IM 6-hour preoperatively. 100 mg IM 1-hour preoperatively. 100 mg IV drip during surgery, if needed. 100 mg 1-hour postoperatively either IV drip or IM	See prednisone	20 mg equals 5 mg prednisone
Medrysone	Anti-inflammatory (very anterior) for treatment of contact irritants, e.g. pollen, smoke, smog, epinephrine	*Topical:* 1% ophthalmic solution	See dexamethasone, topical and subconjunctival	1. No elevation of IOP 2. No reactivation of herpes 3. Not for intraocular inflammation—does not penetrate cornea adequately 4. Less effective than dexamethasone
Rimexolone	1. Postoperative inflammation 2. Allergic kerato-conjunctivitis 3. Anterior uveitis	1% solution	• Blurred vision • Lesser propensity to cause IOP rise • Conjunctival edema and hyperemia	

Contd...

Contd...

Drug	Indication	Dose	Side effects	Remarks
Methylpredniso-lone	Anti-inflammatory	Intravenous: 1 gram per day for 3 days, then tapered with oral methylprednisolone	1. Subconjunctival deposit usually lasts 2–4 weeks 2. See dexamethasone	1. Pain and tenderness for 6–12 hours after injection 2. Transient chemosis may appear 3. Prolonged increase in IOP in steroid responders may result from extended duration of action 4. Probably better choice than triamcinolone for first subconjunctival steroid injection in patients in whom steroid pressure response has not yet been ruled out (this product lasts for weeks while triamcinolone lasts for months)
Prednisolone	Anti-inflammatory	*Topical:* 0.125–1% ophthalmic solution or suspension. 0.25% ophthalmic ointment *Oral:* Dose same as for prednisone	*Topical:* See dexamethasone Oral: Minimal but more gastrointestinal distress than dexamethasone	1. Suspension is more potent than solution in eyes with intact corneal epithelium 2. Increased IOP in steroid responders can occur regardless of concentration of solution used[59] 3. Shake suspension
Prednisone	Anti-inflammatory (oral), immunosuppres-sion, prevention of graft rejection (e.g. corneal)	*Oral:* 20–100 mg/day can be given in divided dose for acute inflammation, returning to 1 dose a day when inflammation is under control. Optic neuritis (may speed resolution of active disease): 100 mg day 1, 80 mg day 2, 60 mg days 3–5, 30 mg days 6 and 7.	*Oral:* 1. Adrenal insufficiency after therapy 2. Edema 3. Hypokalemia (alkalosis) 4. Cushingoid symptoms 5. Increased likelihood of infections 6. Possibility of exacerbating pre-existing peptic ulcer 7. Myopathy 8. Osteoporosis 9. Behavioral changes 10. Increased IOP in steroid responders 11. Cataracts 12. Decreased long bone growth in children	1. Therapy on alternate days is generally ineffective for acute inflammatory conditions 2. Ineffective topically 3. Less frequent cataracts with alternate day therapy[61] 4. Granulocytosis with lymphopenia may be confused with infectious process
Difluprednate	Used in postoperative inflammation	0.5% emulsion for topical instillation	Increased IOP	• Requires QID dosage • Good ocular penetration
Triamcinolone	Anti-inflammatory (subconjunctival)	Subconjunctival: 20 mg (0.5 mL of 40 mg/mL)	1. Subconjunctival deposit may last several months 2. See dexamethasone	1. Use acetonide salt 2. Slow onset, very long duration (up to several months) 3. Prolonged increase in IOP in steroid responders may result from long duration of action (see methylprednisolone)

Source: Peyman GA, Sanders DR, Goldberg MF. Principles and Practice of Ophthalmology, 1st edition. Philadelphia: Saunders Ltd; 1980.

The advantage of periocular injections is that high concentrations of the drug can reach the sites of inflammation and also that the frequency of dosing is reduced. The disadvantage of the injections is that in case the patient has an IOP rise due to the steroid preparation, the steroid depot has to be removed by dissecting out the fat in the area of the injection. The other side effects are: periorbital fat atrophy, chances of orbital hemorrhage, globe perforation and atrophy of the periocular muscles. They are absolutely contraindicated in patients with scleritis; patients who are known "steroid responders" and those who are having active periocular or ocular infections.

Systemic steroids

Oral: This route is preferred in cases of severe inflammation and as maintenance therapy following initial intravenous loading dose of corticosteroids. Usually prednisolone in a dose of 1–2 mg/kg/day is used. The doses are tapered gradually if the therapy is continued for more than 20 days to prevent insufficiency due to adrenal suppression.

Parenteral: This route is preferred when high doses have to be administered especially in sight-threatening emergencies. These conditions comprise of the following:

- Temporal arteritis
- Sympathetic ophthalmia
- Vogt-Koyanagi-Harada syndrome
- Optic neuritis
- Post-traumatic optic nerve compression
- Has been tried for treatment of nonarteritic AION (NA-AION), though controversial.

Intravitreal: Used in cases of intermediate and posterior uveitis, bacterial endophthalmitis and in cases of macular edema. It provides high doses of the drug needed at the site of action without the systemic side effects. Dexamethasone and triamcinolone acetate are used for this route. Depot preparations of dexamethasone and fluorometholone are also available now for continuous supply of the drug for longer durations.

Chemical Formulation of Steroids

The steroid base which is used has a large effect on the efficacy of the topical drug. Majority of the topical steroids are available as acetate, alcohol or sodium phosphate preparations. The phosphate formulations are readily soluble in water and available as clear solutions. The acetate and alcohol formulations are not soluble in water freely and are available in suspension form. The acetate form penetrates cornea easily and these formulations are found to be more potent with a longer lasting therapeutic effect in comparison to the phosphate and alcohol formulations. The next in terms of potency are the alcohol formulations followed last by the phosphate formulations. For example, prednisolone acetate is found to be more potent with a longer action than prednisolone in phosphate formulation.

The common side effects of corticosteroid use are enumerated in Box 4.4.

Box 4.4: Complications of corticosteroid use in ophthalmology.

Topical therapy:
1. Raised intraocular pressure
2. Steroid-induced cataract formation
3. Blepharoptosis
4. Mydriasis (on long-term use)
5. Poor wound healing
6. Susceptibility to bacterial/fungal infections
7. Reactivation/increased intensity of viral keratitis

Periocular/intraocular injection:
1. Increased intraocular pressure
2. Chances of scleral thinning
3. Irreversible blepharoptosis

Systemic therapy:
Gastrointestinal complications:
1. Gastric ulceration
2. Pancreatitis
3. Visceral perforation

Cardiovascular system:
1. Hypertension

Metabolic:
1. Raised sugar levels in blood
2. Dyslipidemia

Endocrinal:
1. Cushingoid appearance
2. Growth retardation in children
3. Hypothalamic-pituitary axis suppression
4. Secondary amenorrhea

Musculoskeletal:
1. Aseptic necrosis of femoral head
2. Osteoporosis, increased susceptibility to fractures
3. Tendon ruptures

Renal:
1. Generalized puffiness due to fluid retention
2. Sodium retention, potassium loss

General:
1. Intracranial hypertension
2. Suppression of immune system leading to infections
3. Hirsutism
4. Subcutaneous tissue loss
5. Decreased wound healing

Source: Peyman GA, Sanders DR, Goldberg MF. Principles and Practice of Ophthalmology, 1st edition. Philadelphia: Saunders Ltd; 1980.

NONSTEROIDAL ANTI-INFLAMMATORY DRUGS

Nonsteroidal anti-inflammatory drugs (NSAIDs) are a vital addition to the armamentarium of the ophthalmologist against inflammatory diseases of the eye and adnexa. They not only help to alleviate the pain associated with the inflammatory diseases but also help in reducing the need for steroids as for some common eye problems. They have also proven to be beneficial in preventing cystoid macular edema (CME) associated with cataract surgery and prevent pupillary miosis during cataract surgery.

Mechanism of Action of NSAIDs[52]

The inflammatory reaction in the body is controlled by the generation of prostaglandins (PGs) by a cyclooxygenase (COX) enzyme-mediated pathway and leukotrienes (LKs) through a lipoxygenase-mediated pathway. The NSAIDs target the COX pathway and prevent the generation of PGs, which are vital for the inflammatory process. Unlike NSAIDs, corticosteroids target both the COX pathway and the lipoxygenase pathway and hence are more potent anti-inflammatory agents.

The various NSAIDs available are listed in Table 4.12.

Principles of Therapy

To prevent intraocular miosis during cataract surgery,[53] topical flurbiprofen or suprofen is started in QID dosage a day before the surgery. It has also been found to decrease the chances of development of postoperative CME[54] if the NSAID is continued for few days after the surgery.

To deal with postoperative pain, topical NSAIDs like ketorolac, nepafenac and bromfenac are used for a period of 20 days postoperatively.[55-57] These also help to decrease the need for topical corticosteroid eye drops and help in faster tapering of the corticosteroid eye drops if needed.

Table 4.12: Commonly used nonsteroidal anti-inflammatory drugs (NSAIDs) in ophthalmology.

Drug	Indication	Dose	Systemic side effects	Topical side effects
Diclofenac	*Topical:* 1. Preoperatively to maintain mydriasis during surgery 2. Postcataract surgery, corneal surgery inflammation 3. Postoperative cystoid macular edema (CME) *Systemic:* 1. Soft tissue inflammation 2. Post orbital surgeries to alleviate pain	*Topical:* 0.1% solution *Oral:* 50 mg BID to TID *IM:* 75 mg deep IM	1. Gastrointestinal upset 2. Gastric ulceration and bleeding 3. Increase risk of cardio-vascular incidents 4. Rarely, renal damage	1. Irritation and stinging 2. Keratolysis was documented (blamed on the preservative in the early generic forms)
Ketorolac	*Topical:* 1. Postocular surgeries and refractive surgeries 2. Allergic conjunctivitis 3. Episcleritis 4. Postoperative CME *Systemic:* • Alleviate postoperative pain	*Topical:* 0.4% solution (0.5% solution was earlier used) *Systemic:* 15–30 mg IM or IV TID, (maximum 90 mg a day)	1. Nausea 2. Drowsiness and dizziness 3. Gastric ulceration 4. Renal toxicity with chronic usage	1. Stinging and burning sensation on instillation
Flurbiprofen	*Topical:* 1. Maintain intraoperative mydriasis 2. Postcataract surgery and laser procedure pain alleviation 3. Prophylaxis against CME development *Systemic:* • Postoperative pain	*Topical:* 0.03% solution *Systemic:* orally 50–100 mg tablets BID to QID	1. Gastrointestinal upset 2. Gastric ulceration 3. Cogwheel rigidity, myoclonus, ataxia and tremors	1. Transient irritation on instillation
Nepafenac	*Topical:* 1. Alleviate postcataract surgery pain 2. Prophylaxis against CME development Not available systemically	*Topical:* 0.1% suspension, TID-QID	Not available systemically	1. Increased intraocular pressure 2. Opacification of the capsule 3. Corneal ulceration
Bromfenac	*Topical:* • Postcataract surgery pain alleviation Not available systemically	*Topical:* 0.09% solution, BID	Not available systemically	1. Stinging on instillation 2. Corneal ulceration
Indomethacin	*Topical:* 1. Postoperative CME treatment 2. Episcleritis *Systemic:* *Oral:* • Pain following orbital surgery • Pain in arthropathies	*Topical:* 0.5% solution *Systemic:* Oral: 25–50 mg BID to QID	• Abdominal pain, gastric ulceration, diarrhea • Pancreatitis • Headache, dizziness, depression • Rarely, thrombocytopenia, aplastic anemia, renal papillary necrosis	• Corneal ulceration • Stinging on instillation
Suprofen	*Topical:* • Prevent intraoperative mydriasis	Topical: 1% solution	Not available systemically	• Stinging on instillation

Source: Peyman GA, Sanders DR, Goldberg MF. Principles and Practice of Ophthalmology, 1st edition. Philadelphia: Saunders Ltd; 1980.

Topical NSAIDs are generally avoided in cases of corneal thinning or large corneal epithelial defects because of the risk of causing a corneal melt.

Systemic NSAIDs are useful to alleviate pain after orbital and ocular surgeries, acute orbital inflammations and lid infections.

ANTIALLERGIC DRUGS

Allergies or hypersensitivities, as they are called, are an exaggerated reaction of the immune system to foreign substances, usually proteins. These proteins are called allergens. The allergens enter the body tissue through various routes and once inside, are picked up by the leukocytes which lead to a immunoglobulin E (IgE) antibody-related immune reaction and mast cell degranulation.[58] The release of histamine and leukotrienes that follow is responsible for the range of signs and symptoms which vary from a mild itch to a devastating anaphylaxis.

In regular practice, ophthalmologists deal with seasonal allergic conjunctivitis (SAC) and perennial allergic conjunctivitis (PAC) which though troubling can easily be controlled with topical therapy,[59] and potentially vision-threatening forms of vernal keratoconjunctivitis (VKC) and atopic keratoconjunctivitis (AKC), which often run a chronic course.

Principles of Therapy[59]

In cases of SAC, drugs like olopatadine which have both antihistaminic effect as well as mast cell stabilizing action have become the agents of choice. The topical drug can be combined with an oral antihistaminic drug in cases where there is severe itching.

The topical antihistaminics can be combined with ketorolac eye drops in SAC and PAC treatment. Ketorolac greatly reduces the itching sensation associated with both these forms.

In severe forms of chronic conjunctivitis, VKC and AKC, topical steroids like loteprednol or rimexolone may be started along with antihistamines. The steroids can then be tapered gradually while the antihistamine drugs continued. Severe cicatrizing forms of allergic conjunctivitis may need potent steroids like prednisolone acetate topically or triamcinolone acetonide as subconjunctival injections.

In hay fever and contact dermatitis, topical antihistamines may not prove useful. The patient may require systemic therapy and avoidance of the allergen. In case the allergen cannot be totally avoided, desensitization therapy can be tried under the care of an immunologist.

Vasoconstrictors and decongestants are associated with "rebound congestion" if used for a long time. They should be used only for short-term relief in SAC.

The various antiallergic eye drops available are mentioned in Table 4.13.

Table 4.13: Antiallergy eye drops.

Drug	Indications	Dose	Systemic side effects	Local side effects	Mechanism of action
Azelastine	Seasonal allergic conjunctivitis	0.05% solution BID	Drowsiness and weight gain on systemic use	• Stinging sensation • Metallic taste	H1 blocker and also inhibits histamine release and leukotriene activity
Cromolyn sodium	Vernal keratoconjunctivitis	4% solution BID to TID	Poor absorption into circulation and hence no significant systemic effects	• Stinging on instillation • Hyperemia • Dryness • Puffiness around eyes	Mast cell stabilizer
Epinastine	Seasonal allergic conjunctivitis	0.05% solution BID	Flu-like syndrome	• Stinging on instillation	Mast cell stabilizer and antihistaminic
Ketorolac	Seasonal allergic conjunctivitis	0.5% solution TID to QID	Not absorbed significantly through topical route	• Burning sensation on instillation • Rarely, superficial keratitis	Inhibits the activity of cyclooxygenases, thus reducing prostaglandin production
Ketotifen	Seasonal allergic conjunctivitis	0.25% solution BID	• Headache • Flu-like syndrome	• Stinging on instillation • Dryness of eyes	Mast cell stabilizer and antihistaminic

Contd...

Contd...

Drug	Indications	Dose	Systemic side effects	Local side effects	Mechanism of action
Lodoxamide tromethamine	Vernal keratoconjunctivitis	0.1% solution BID	• Headache • Flu-like syndrome	• Hyperemia • Irritation • Dryness	Mast cell stabilizer
Naphazoline hydrochloride	Allergic conjunctivitis	0.025–0.1% solution QID	Caution in patients with cardiovascular diseases	• Pupillary dilatation • Epithelial erosions • Rebound congestion on prolonged use • May precipitate angle closure in susceptible individuals	Adrenergic decongestants
Nedocromil	Seasonal allergic conjunctivitis	2.0% solution BID	• Metallic taste • Headache	• Stinging sensation • Hyperemia	Mast cell stabilizer
Olopatadine	Seasonal allergic conjunctivitis	0.1% and 0.2% solution BID	• Flu-like syndrome • Metallic taste	• Stinging sensation/irritation on instillation • Dryness	Mast cell stabilizer and antihistaminic
Pemirolast	Seasonal allergic conjunctivitis	0.1% solution BID	Flu-like symptoms	• Stinging on instillation	Mast cell stabilizer

Source: Peyman GA, Sanders DR, Goldberg MF. Principles and Practice of Ophthalmology, 1st edition. Philadelphia: Saunders Ltd; 1980.

OCULAR LUBRICANTS

Ocular lubricants or *"artificial tears"* are indicated in conditions where there is a disruption of the tear film layer over the eye. This could be due to decrease in tear production from the glands, alteration in the ocular surface or due to abnormal tear drainage/evaporation due to lid abnormalities.

The properties of any ocular lubricant are determined by the following:[60-62]

- Demulcent agent
- Viscosity
- Preservative
- Osmolarity.

Demulcents

They are compounds that coat the irregularities of the ocular surface and thus make the surface smooth. These agents fill in the gaps like irregularities and thus help in the frictionless gliding action of the lids over the ocular surface. This prevents further damage to the abraded ocular surface. The various demulcents commonly used are: cellulose esters, dextran 70, polyvinyl alcohol, povidone and liquid polyols.

Viscosity

The viscosity of a lubricant determines the amount of time the agent is going to stay in the tear film. The more the viscosity, the longer it is going to help in lubrication of the ocular surface. On the other hand, drugs with higher viscosity also cause blurring of the vision due to formation of a layer in front of the cornea and also the more its tendency to leave behind crust-like deposits on the eyelashes. Viscosity is measured in centipoise units.

Osmolarity

It gives an indication about the crystalloid concentration of the tear film. Higher osmolarity of tear film indicates more evaporation of the aqueous layer. Increased osmolarity is also associated with more damage to the corneal epithelium. An ideal lubricating agent aims at maintaining a low tear osmolarity.

Preservatives

They are added to lubricant eye drops to prevent the growth of microorganisms. These agents also prove to have mild toxicity to the corneal epithelium and may damage the fragile epithelium of patients suffering from dry eyes or other tear film disorders.

The common preservatives used are:[63]

- Benzalkonium chloride (BAK)
- Chlorobutanol
- Ethylenediaminetetraacetic acid (EDTA)
- Sorbate
- Thimerosal
- Polyquaternium
- Stabilized oxychloro complex (SOC)
- Sodium perborate.

Out of these preservatives, only polyquaternium and SOC are found to be ideal for use in dry eye patients. All the rest have proven to produce ocular toxicity. SOC and sodium perborate, both get broken down when exposed to tear film. Sodium perborate gets broken down to hydrogen peroxide which proves to be toxic to the epithelium.

Polyquaternium has now become the preferred agent for use in lubricants for dry eye patients.

The commonly available ocular lubricants are mentioned in Table 4.14.

MYDRIATICS AND CYCLOPLEGICS

The iris contains a sphincter muscle which runs in a concentric fashion along the pupillary margin and dilator muscles that run radially away from the pupil. The interplay between these two muscles is responsible for the various pupillary reactions that occur in reaction to stimulus of any kind.

The sphincter muscle is controlled by the parasympathetic nervous system while the dilator responds to stimulation by the sympathetic portion of autonomic nervous system.

Sympathomimetic drugs that activate the adrenergic receptors of the dilator pupillae resulting in the dilation of the pupil, called mydriasis. Phenylephrine is a true mydriatic, with no cycloplegic effect.

Cycloplegics are agents that result in the relaxation of the ciliary muscle leading to paralysis of accommodation, by inhibiting the actions of acetylcholine which is released by the stimulation of the parasympathetic nervous system. All known cycloplegics also result in mydriasis as they result in the relaxation of the sphincter papillae muscles. The tone of the dilator pupillae muscle thus leads to the dilation of the pupil size passively.

Commonly Used Mydriatics in Ophthalmology Practice

Phenylephrine

It is a sympathomimetic agent, similar to epinephrine. It acts directly on the alpha receptors of the pupil mainly, with little effect on the beta receptors of the eye. It also acts on the Müller's muscle of the lids, leading to temporary widening of the palpebral fissure; and causes blanching of the conjunctival vessels, a property which can be used to differentiate conjunctival hyperemia from circumciliary

Table 4.14: Ocular lubricating agents.

Artificial tears	Indication	Dose	Side effects	Remarks
Cellulose esters (i.e. methylcellulose, hydroxy-propyl methylcellulose, hydroxyethyl cellulose) Methulose (0.25%), Visculose (0.5%, 1%)	Exposure keratopathy, keratoconjunctivitis sicca	Topical: 0.25–1% drops. Drop 4–6 times/day	Generally safe, the preservatives are the reason for corneal epithelial toxicity in cases of abuse. May form crusts on the lashes when used in 1% concentration	In general, cellulose esters are more effective as tear replacements than polyvinyl alcohol. Sticky eyelid debris is more pronounced, however, with the former Polyvinyl alcohol may suffice for patients with mild symptoms. The combination products probably produce a more natural tear film replacement than cellulose esters and are preferred in more severe cases Price differences may account for the popularity of the single agents
Polyvinyl alcohol	More efficacious in cases of mucin layer disorders	Same as above	Some people may complain of initial stinging on applying the drops	Same as above

Source: Peyman GA, Sanders DR, Goldberg MF. Principles and Practice of Ophthalmology, 1st edition. Philadelphia: Saunders Ltd; 1980.

congestion. It has to be stored protected from direct light and heat to prevent its oxidation.

Atropine[64]

It is a strong anticholinergic agent which was initially extracted from the plant *Atropa belladonna*. Its major uses in ophthalmology are for:

- Cycloplegic refraction in children.
- Treatment of uveitis by:
  - Inducing cycloplegia to relieve pain
  - Prevention of synechiae formation/breaking formed synechiae
  - Increasing the blood supply in the uveal tissue.
- Atropine penalization for treatment of mild refractive amblyopia.[65,66]
- To slow the progression of myopia.[67]

In children, usually the ointment form is preferred for use to decrease the systemic absorption through the nasolacrimal duct.

Homatropine

It is a semisynthetic anticholinergic agent. It is not as potent as atropine or cyclopentolate in causing cycloplegia. Thus, it is not the agent of choice for performing cycloplegic refraction. It is available as a salt of hydrobromide for ocular use.

Cyclopentolate

It is an anticholinergic agent which has cycloplegic effect comparable to that of atropine. It has become the agent of choice for cycloplegic refraction in children as it has a shorter duration of action as compared to atropine. It is also used as a substitute for atropine in treatment of uveitis if the patient is sensitive to atropine.

Scopolamine

It is derived from the shrub *Scopolia carniolica* and *Hyoscyamus niger*. It has cycloplegic effects comparable to atropine with a shorter duration of action. As it crosses the blood-brain barrier easily and is associated with idiosyncratic effects, it is not used commonly for cycloplegic refraction. It is usually used only in patients who are sensitive to atropine.

The commonly used mydriatics and cycloplegics in ophthalmology are mentioned in Table 4.15.

The duration of action of mydriatics and cycloplegics are mentioned in Table 4.16.

Table 4.15: Ocular mydriatics and cycloplegics.

Drug	Indication	Dose	Systemic side effects	Local side effects	Remarks
Phenyle-phrine	*Topical:* 1. Ocular fundus examination 2. Differentiate ciliary congestion from conjunctival hyperemia	5–10% solution	Increase in systemic blood pressure with possible reflex bradycardia, headache, trembling, cardiovascular collapse (with 10% solution)	Stinging, irritation, rebound miosis, release of iris pigments	• Mydriatric only, no cycloplegic effect • Usually used in combination with tropicamide • Use 2.5% solution in children less than 1 year of age • Contraindicated in patients taking mono-amine oxidase (MAO) inhibitors, methyldopa, tricyclic antidepres-sants, guanethidine and reserpine
Tropicamide	*Topical:* 1. Ocular fundus examination 2. Refraction in adolescents	0.5–1% solution	Systemic: Hypersensitvity has been described	Stinging, local hypersensitivity reactions, rise in intraocular pressure in patients with open angle closure glaucoma, can precipitate angle closure attack in predisposed individuals	• Dilatation not affected by iris pigmentation • One of the safer drugs for use in patients with cardiovascular disorders

Contd...

Contd...

Drug	Indication	Dose	Systemic side effects	Local side effects	Remarks
Homatropine hydrobromide	*Topical:* 1. Treatment of painful conditions like anterior uveitis	2–5% solution	Similar to atropine, though less frequent and less severe	Contact dermatitis, angle closure in predisposed individuals, increase in intraocular pressure in patients with open angle glaucoma	Due to its relatively weak cycloplegic effect, not recommended for refraction in children
Cyclopen-tolate	*Topical:* Agent of choice for cycloplegic refraction in school-aged children	0.5–2% solution (2% solution is not recommended)	Causes more central nervous system (CNS) toxicity than atropine and includes drowsiness, slurred speech, ataxia, disorientation and psychotic reactions Grand malseizures have been reported in children	Stinging on instillation of the drops Increased intraocular pressure in open angle glaucoma May lead to angle closure if anatomically narrow angles are present	• Frequent side effects are reported in children with 2% solution • Contraindicated in infants, preschool children and children with CNS diseases
Scopolamine	*Topical:* Used as an alternative to atropine in patients with atropine hypersensitivity *Transdermal patch:* Used in patients who suffer from motion sickness	0.25% solution	CNS toxicity is more severe as compared to other agents. Restlessness, confusion, hallucinations, incoherence, spastic muscle paralysis, vomiting, urinary incontinence	Local irritation occurs though less common than atropine Intraocular pressure may increase in patients with open angle glaucoma	• Causes lesser tachycardia than atropine • CNS toxicity more than atropine • Duration of action shorter than atropine • Due to idiosyncratic reactions on the CNS, not preferred for routine refraction or cycloplegic indications
Atropine sulfate	*Topical:* 1. Refraction in children 2. Cycloplegia in painful eye conditions like uveitis and keratitis 3. Prevent the formation of synechiae 4. Treatment of refractive amblyopia by penalization *Systemic:* 1. Preoperative medication 2. Antidote for cholinesterase poisoning 3. Cardiovascular collapse	*Topical dose:* Solution and ointment of 1% strength. 0.5% ointment is used in children *Parenteral:* Pre-operative dose: 0.02 mg/kg/day *Maximum dose:* 0.6 mg	Flushing, tachycardia, confusion, hyper-thermia, dryness of mucous membranes, constipation, urinary retention	Photophobia, decreased accommodation, contact dermatitis, may lead to angle closure in predisposed individuals	• Enters systemic circulation by absorption through the conjunctiva and nasal mucosal • Topical use also associated with severe side effects in children, especially those with NS disorders • Treatment of toxicity is initially symptomatic. In severe poisoning, physostigmine 2 mg IM is used as antidote

Source: Peyman GA, Sanders DR, Goldberg MF. Principles and Practice of Ophthalmology, 1st edition. Philadelphia: Saunders Ltd; 1980.

Table 4.16: Duration of action of mydriatics and cycloplegics.

Agent	Onset of mydriasis	Duration of mydriasis	Onset of cycloplegia	Duration of cycloplegia
Phenylephrine	15–30 minutes	3 hours	Not a cycloplegic	Not a cycloplegic
Tropicamide	20–25 minutes	4 hours	20–25 minutes	6 hours
Homatropine	10–30 minutes	6 hours to 4 days	30–90 minutes	10–48 hours
Cyclopentolate	15–30 minutes	24 hours	15–45 minutes	24 hours
Scopolamine	20–30 minutes	3–7 days	30–60 minutes	3–7 days
Atropine sulfate	30–40 minutes	7–12 days	3–4 hours	2 weeks

Source: Peyman GA, Sanders DR, Goldberg MF. Principles and Practice of Ophthalmology, 1st edition. Philadelphia: Saunders Ltd; 1980.

MIOTIC AGENTS

These are parasympathomimetic agents that bring about the constriction of the pupil by acting on the sphincter pupillae muscles and also lead to the contraction of the ciliary muscle resulting in induction of accommodation. The directly acting agents like pilocarpine act on the muscarinic receptors similar to acetylcholine.

The commonly used miotic agents in ophthalmology are mentioned in Table 4.17.

Two other agents have been developed, which bring about miosis through noncholinergic actions. These were developed to reverse the mydriasis caused by anticholinergic agents as it was found that using pilocarpine to reverse mydriasis leads to increased risk of angle closure attacks.

Dapiprazole and thymoxamine, the two agents have similar mechanism of action by blocking the alpha receptors on the iris. As they do not act on the sphincter pupillae, high IOPs do not seem to affect the action of these agents.

Dapiprazole[67] has been approved for the reversal of pupillary mydriasis. It is available as a 25 mg vial which is reconstituted in 5 mL of the provided diluents. Once reconstituted, it can be stored for 21 days. Its common side effects are irritation on instillation, congestion and chemosis of the conjunctiva and punctate erosions of the corneal epithelium.

DYES IN OPHTHALMOLOGY

The commonly used dyes in ophthalmology are mentioned in Table 4.18.

Ocular hypotensives and immunomodulators will be dealt in detail in the Sections of Glaucoma and Uvea, respectively.

Table 4.17: Miotic agents used in ophthalmology.

Drug	Indications	Dose	Systemic toxicity	Local side effects	Comments
Pilocarpine	1. Acute angle closure glaucoma (acts once the intraocular pressure is less than 30 mmHg) 2. Preoperative miosis for keratoplasty, anterior chamber lens implantation, iridectomy 3. Intraoperative miosis in cases of posterior capsular rupture 4. Diagnosis of Adie's pupil 5. Primary open angle glaucoma (rarely used for this indication solely now)	0.5–10% topical solution	Increased salivation, increased urination, hypotension, bradycardia	Cataract formation, brow ache, congestive iritis, retinal detachment, near accommodative spasm, iris cysts, blepharospasm	• Reverses mydriasis from phenylephrine but not atropine and cyclopentolate • Associated with shallowing of anterior chamber on chronic use • Causes increased lens diameter • To be used with caution in patients with asthma, coronary artery diseases and hyperthyroidism
Carbachol	1. Intraoperative miosis 2. Angle-closure glaucoma	*Topical:* 1.5% and 3% solution *Intracameral:* 0.01% solution, 0.5 mL in anterior chamber	Bradycardia, gastrointestinal distress, diarrhea, muscle weakness	Conjunctival hyperemia, nasal stuffiness, blurred vision, brow ache	To be used with caution in patients with asthma, coronary artery diseases and hyperthyroidism

Source: Peyman GA, Sanders DR, Goldberg MF. Principles and Practice of Ophthalmology, 1st edition. Philadelphia: Saunders Ltd.; 1980.

Table 4.18: Dyes in ophthalmology.

Dye	Indications	Dose	Adverse effects	Remarks
Fluorescein	*Intravenous:* Retinal angiography, iris angiography, vitreous fluorophotometry *Topical:* Diagnostics (e.g. corneal defects, tear duct patency), Seidel's test to rule out aqueous leak, for applanation tonometry, contact lens fitting	*Parenteral:* 10–25% ampoules. 500 mg rapid IV *Topical:* 2% ophthalmic drops, impregnated paper strips	*Parenteral:* 1. Nausea, vomiting, apprehension 2. Temporarily stains skin, urine 3. Anaphylactoid reaction (not a true anaphylaxis) may occur (rare)	1. Resuscitation equipment must be on hand 2. Solutions prepared just before use, must be checked for Pseudomonas growth 3. Absorbs light at 493 nm maximally and emits at 520 nm

Contd...

Contd...

Dye	Indications	Dose	Adverse effects	Remarks
Fluorexon, fluorescein complexon	*Topical:* Diagnostic as above (for patients wearing soft lenses)	*Topical:* 0.25% ophthalmic drops		1. Use when fluorescein is needed in patients who wear soft contact lenses 2. Fluorescent lesser than fluorescein—higher concentration as to be used 3. Has a molecular weight of about 710 Da, twice that of normal fluorescein 4. Solutions prepared just before use, must be checked for *Pseudomonas* growth
Rose bengal	Topical diagnostic agent used in diagnosis and grading of Dry eyes and staining neurotrophic ulcers. Stains devitalized tissue	*Topical:* 1% ophthalmic drops	Severe stinging, should be used after anesthetizing the eye with topical proparacaine solution	Has mild bactericidal and virucidal effect, may interfere with culture testing
Lissamine green	Stains devitalized tissue	*Topical:* Sterile strips having 15 mg stain	Mid irritation may occur, otherwise no frequently associated side effect has been noted	Has the same indications as Rose Bengal and may be preferred over it for diagnosis of dry eyes
Methylene blue	To stain the lacrimal sac before dacryocystorhinostomy To mark the margins of filtering blebs, gonioscopic laser sclerostomy		Causes much irritation and using a topical anesthetic before using the dye is suggested	Can stain mucus and devitalized cells as well as corneal nerves
Indocyanine green	To study the choroidal vasculature especially in cases of choroidal neovascular membrane (CNVM) Angiography-guided photocoagulation	25–50 mg in 1–2 mL water for injection	1. Relatively well tolerated, may cause occasional nausea and vomiting 2. Contains sodium iodide and should not be used in patients allergic to iodine and shellfish	1. Water-soluble tricarbocyanine dye 2. Peak absorption at 805 nm and emits radiation at 835 nm, at this range the absorption of light by the retinal pigment epithelium (RPE) and choroid is about 30% only 3. Completely bound by the plasma proteins so does not leak through the choriocapillaris
Trypan blue	Used to stain the anterior lens capsule during cataract surgeries	Available as 1 mL vial with a concentration of 0.06%	1. Fairly well tolerated but the effect on the endothelium is a concern 2. Washed out within seconds of injection into the anterior chamber to prevent endothelial damage and staining	Usually used in cataract surgeries where there is no clear fundal glow to assist in capsulorhexis/capsulotomy
Verteporfin	Photodynamic therapy for age-related macular degeneration (ARMD) especially classic CNVM involving the macula	15 mg freeze dried powder, reconstituted with sterile water and 5% dextrose. Total drug dose 6 mg/m^2 body surface area	*Ocular:* Photophobia, pain in the eye, transient blurring of vision and subretinal/vitreous hemorrhage can be attributed to the photodynamic therapy *Systemic effects due to injection* of verteporfin: Flu-like symptoms, nausea, headache, dizziness, inflammation and pain at the site of injection are common	1. Is a photosensitive porphyrin 2. Absorbs light of wavelength 680–695 nm well 3. Exposure to bright sunlight should be avoided for the next 48 hours after the injection

Source: Peyman GA, Sanders DR, Goldberg MF. Principles and Practice of Ophthalmology, 1st edition. Philadelphia: Saunders Ltd; 1980.

REFERENCES

1. McLeod G. Local anaesthetic agents. In: Davies NJ, Cashman JN (Eds). Lee's Synopsis of Anaesthesia, 13th edition. London: Elsevier Health Sciences; 2005. pp. 369-74.
2. Tripathi KD. Local anaesthetics. In: Tripathi K2D (Ed). Essentials of Medical Pharmacology, 7th edition. New Delhi, India: Jaypee Brothers Medical Publishers (P) Ltd; 2013. p. 360.
3. Than TP, Bartlett JD. Local anesthetics. In: Bartlett JD, Jaanus SD, Fiscella RG, Holdeman NR, Prokopich CL (Eds). Clinical Ocular Pharmacology, 5th edition. St. Louis: Butterworth-Heinemann Elsevier Inc.; 2008. p. 85.
4. Schmidt RM, Rosenkranz HS. Antimicrobial activity of local anesthetics: lidocaine and procaine. J Infect Dis. 1970; 121(6):597-607.
5. Myers WG, Shugar JK. Optimizing the intracameral dilation regimen for cataract surgery: prospective randomized comparison of 2 solutions. J Cataract Refract Surg. 2009;35(2):273-6.
6. Hyndiuk RA, Eiferman RA, Caldwell DR, et al. Comparison of ciprofloxacin ophthalmic solution 0.3% to fortified tobramycin-cefazolin in treating bacterial corneal ulcers. Ophthalmology. 1996;103(11):1854-63.
7. Lampiris HW, Maddix DS. Clinical use of antimicrobial agents. In: Katzung BG, Masters SB, Trevor AJ (Eds). Basic and Clinical Pharmacology, 10th edition. New York: McGraw-Hill; 2007. Chapter 51, p. 837.
8. Deck DH, Winston LG. Sulfonamides, trimethoprim, and quinolones. In: Katzung BG, Masters SB, Trevor AJ (Eds). Basic and Clinical Pharmacology, 10th edition. New York: McGraw-Hill; 2007. Chapter 46, pp. 766-7.
9. Prajna V, Vajpayee R, Trocme S, et al. Safety and efficacy of gatifloxacin 0.3% as compared with ciprofloxacin 0.3% for the treatment of acute bacterial corneal ulcers. Invest Ophthalmol Vis Sci. 2006;47(13):1916.
10. Kim DH, Stark WJ, O'Brien TP, et al. Aqueous penetration and biological activity of moxifloxacin 0.5% ophthalmic solution and gatifloxacin 0.3% solution in cataract surgery patients. Ophthalmology. 2005;112(11):1992-6.
11. Haas W, Pillar CM, Zurenko GE, et al. Besifloxacin, a novel fluoroquinolone, has broad-spectrum in vitro activity against aerobic and anaerobic bacteria. Antimicrob Agents Chemother. 2009;53(8):3552-60.
12. Pflugfelder SC, Hernández E, Fliesler SJ, et al. Intravitreal vancomycin: retinal toxicity, clearance, and interaction with gentamicin. Arch Ophthalmol. 1987;105(6):831-7.
13. Chang VS, Dhaliwal DK, Raju L, et al. Antibiotic resistance in the treatment of Staphylococcus aureus keratitis: a 20-year review. Cornea. 2015;34(6):698-703.
14. Hammerschlag MR, Chandler JW, Alexander ER, et al. Erythromycin ointment for ocular prophylaxis of neonatal chlamydial infection. JAMA. 1980;244(20):2291-3.
15. Chidambaram JD, Alemayehu W, Melese M, et al. Effect of a single mass antibiotic distribution on the prevalence of infectious trachoma. JAMA. 2006;295(10):1142-6.
16. Barry AL, Jones RN, Thornsberry C. In vitro activities of azithromycin (CP 62,993), clarithromycin (A-56268; TE-031), erythromycin, roxithromycin, and clindamycin. Antimicrob Agents Chemother. 1988;32(5):752-4.
17. Peyron F, Wallon M, Liou C, et al. Treatments for toxoplasmosis in pregnancy. Cochrane Database Syst Rev. 2000;(2):CD001684.
18. Hohlfeld P, Daffos F, Thulliez PA, et al. Fetal toxoplasmosis: outcome of pregnancy and infant follow-up after in utero treatment. J Pediatr. 1989;115(5):765-9.
19. David M, Rumelt S, Weintraub Z. Efficacy comparison between povidone iodine 2.5% and tetracycline 1% in prevention of ophthalmia neonatorum. Ophthalmology. 2011;118(7):1454-8.
20. Dougherty JM, McCulley JP, Silvany RE, et al. The role of tetracycline in chronic blepharitis. Inhibition of lipase production in staphylococci. Invest Ophthalmol Vis Sci. 1991;32(11):2970-5.
21. Perry HD, Hodes LW, Seedor JA, et al. Effect of doxycycline hyclate on corneal epithelial wound healing in the rabbit alkali-burn model. Preliminary observations. Cornea. 1993;12(5):379-82.
22. Campochiaro PA, Conway BP. Aminoglycoside toxicity—a survey of retinal specialists: implications for ocular use. Arch Ophthalmol. 1991;109(7):946-50.
23. Moellering RC, Wennersten C, Kunz LJ, Resistance to gentamicin, tobramycin and amikacin among clinical isolates of bacteria. Am J Med. 1977;62(6):873-81.
24. Deck DH, Winston LG. Beta-lactam and other cell wall- and membrane-active antibiotics. In: Katzung BG, Masters SB, Trevor AJ (Eds). Basic and Clinical Pharmacology, 10th edition. New York: McGraw-Hill; 2007. Chapter 43, pp. 726-33.
25. Yolton DP, Haesaert SP. Anti-infective drugs. In: Bartlett JD, Jaanus SD, Fiscella RG, Holdeman NR, Prokopich CL (Eds). Clinical Ocular Pharmacology, 5th edition. St. Louis: Butterworth-Heinemann Elsevier Inc.; 2008. pp. 179-82.
26. Fraunfelder FT, Bagby GC, Kelly DJ. Fatal aplastic anemia following topical administration of ophthalmic chloramphenicol. Am J Ophthalmol. 1982;93(3):356-60.
27. Kucers A. Chloramphenicol, erythromycin, vancomycin, tetracyclines. Lancet. 1982;320(8295):425-9.
28. Yolton DP, Haesaert SP. Anti-infective drugs. In: Bartlett JD, Jaanus SD, Fiscella RG, Holdeman NR, Prokopich CL (Eds). Clinical Ocular Pharmacology, 5th edition. St. Louis: Butterworth-Heinemann Elsevier Inc.; 2008. p. 208.
29. Sheppard D, Lampiris HW. Antifungal agents. In: Katzung BG, Masters SB, Trevor AJ (Eds). Basic and Clinical Pharmacology, 10th edition. New York: McGraw-Hill; 2007. Chapter 48, pp. 781-3.
30. Kalavathy CM, Parmar P, Kaliamurthy J, et al. Comparison of topical itraconazole 1% with topical natamycin 5% for the treatment of filamentous fungal keratitis. Cornea. 2005;24(4):449-52.
31. Wan WL, Kubak BM, Smith MD, et al. Treatment of ocular fungal infections with oral fluconazole. Am J Ophthalmol. 1995;119(4):477-81.
32. Agarwal PK, Roy P, Das A, et al. Efficacy of topical and systemic itraconazole as a broad-spectrum antifungal agent in mycotic corneal ulcer: a preliminary study. Indian J Ophthalmol. 2001;49(3):173.
33. Durand ML, Kim IK, D'Amico DJ, et al. Successful treatment of Fusarium endophthalmitis with voriconazole and Aspergillus endophthalmitis with voriconazole plus caspofungin. Am J Ophthalmol. 2005;140(3):552-4.

34. O'day DM, Head WS, Robinson RD, et al. Intraocular penetration of systemically administered antifungal agents. Curr Eye Res. 1985;4(2):131-4.
35. Kaufman HE, Martola EL, Dohlman C. Use of 5-Iodo-2'-deoxyuridine (IDU) in treatment of herpes simplex keratitis. Arch Ophthalmol. 1962;68(2):235-9.
36. Hyndiuk RA, Okumoto M, Damiano RA, et al. Treatment of vaccinial keratitis with vidarabine. Arch Ophthalmol. 1976;94(8):1363-4.
37. La Lau C, Oosterhuis JA, Versteeg J, et al. Acyclovir and trifluorothymidine in herpetic keratitis: a multicentre trial. Br J Ophthalmol. 1982;66(8):506.
38. McCulley JP, Binder PS, Kaufman HE, et al. A double-blind, multicenter clinical trial of acyclovir vs idoxuridine for treatment of epithelial herpes simplex keratitis. Ophthalmology. 1982;89(10):1195-200.
39. Barron BA, Gee L, Hauck WW, et al. Herpetic Eye Disease Study. A controlled trial of oral acyclovir for herpes simplex stromal keratitis. Ophthalmology. 1994;101(12):1871-82.
40. Hoang-Xuan T, Büchi ER, Herbort CP, et al. Oral acyclovir for herpes zoster ophthalmicus. Ophthalmology. 1992;99(7):1062-71.
41. Beutner KR, Friedman DJ, Forszpaniak C, et al. Valaciclovir compared with acyclovir for improved therapy for herpes zoster in immunocompetent adults. Antimicrob Agents Chemother. 1995;39(7):1546-53.
42. Tyring S, Barbarash RA, Nahlik JE, et al. Famciclovir for the treatment of acute herpes zoster: effects on acute disease and postherpetic neuralgia: a randomized, double-blind, placebo-controlled trial. Ann Intern Med. 1995;123(2):89-96.
43. Dhillon B, Kamal A, Leen C. Intravitreal sustained-release ganciclovir implantation to control cytomegalovirus retinitis in AIDS. Int J STD AIDS. 1998;9:227-30.
44. Colin J, Hoh HB, Easty DL, et al. Ganciclovir ophthalmic gel (Virgan; 0.15%) in the treatment of herpes simplex keratitis. Cornea. 1997;16(4):393-9.
45. Diaz-Llopis M, España E, Muñoz G, et al. High dose intravitreal foscarnet in the treatment of cytomegalovirus retinitis in AIDS. Br J Ophthalmol. 1994;78(2):120-4.
46. Duguid IG, Dart JK, Morlet N, et al. Outcome of Acanthamoeba keratitis treated with polyhexamethyl biguanide and propamidine. Ophthalmology. 1997;104(10):1587-92.
47. Kosrirukvongs P, Wanachiwanawin D, Visvesvara GS. Treatment of Acanthamoeba keratitis with chlorhexidine. Ophthalmology. 1999;106(4):798-802.
48. Agashe R, Radhakrishnan N, Pradhan S, et al. Clinical and demographic study of microsporidial keratoconjunctivitis in South India: a 3-year study (2013–2015). Br J Ophthalmol. 2017;101(10):1436-9.
49. Engstrom RE, Holland GN, Nussenblatt RB, et al. Current practices in the management of ocular toxoplasmosis. Am J Ophthalmol. 1991;111(5):601-10.
50. Rothova A, Meenken C, Buitenhuis HJ, et al. Therapy for ocular toxoplasmosis. Am J Ophthalmol. 1993;115(4):517-23.
51. Tripathi KD. Corticosteroids. In: Tripathi KD (Ed). Essentials of Medical Pharmacology, 7th edition. New Delhi, India: Jaypee Brothers Medical Publishers (P) Ltd.; 2013. pp. 282-95.
52. Borazan NH, Furst DE. Nonsteroidal anti-inflammatory drugs, disease-modifying antirheumatic drugs, nonopioid analgesics, and drugs used in gout. In: Katzung BG, Masters SB, Trevor AJ (Eds). Basic and Clinical Pharmacology, 10th edition. New York: McGraw-Hill; 2007. Chapter 36, pp. 574-83.
53. Rodríguez-García A, Hernández-Camarena JC, López-Jaime GR, et al. Effect of topical nonsteroidal anti-inflammatory drugs on pupillary size during uncomplicated cataract surgery. J Refract Surg. 2017;33(4):236-42.
54. Flach AJ, Jampol LM, Weinberg D, et al. Improvement in visual acuity in chronic aphakic and pseudophakic cystoid macular edema after treatment with topical 0.5% ketorolac tromethamine. Am J Ophthalmol. 1991;112(5):514-9.
55. Assouline M, Renard G, Arne JL, et al. A prospective randomized trial of topical soluble 0.1% indomethacin versus 0.1% diclofenac versus placebo for the control of pain following excimer laser photorefractive keratectomy. Ophthalmic Surg Lasers Imaging Retina. 1998;29(5):365-74.
56. Lane SS, Modi SS, Lehmann RP, et al. Nepafenac ophthalmic suspension 0.1% for the prevention and treatment of ocular inflammation associated with cataract surgery. J Cataract Refract Surg. 2007;33(1):53-8.
57. Lindstrom R. The pharmacologic and pathophysiologic rationale for using NSAIDs in ocular inflammatory disease and ocular surgery. Int Ophthalmol Clin. 2006;46(4):7-11.
58. Abelson MB, Schaefer K. Conjunctivitis of allergic origin: immunologic mechanisms and current approaches to therapy. Surv Ophthalmol. 1993;38:115-32.
59. Bielory L, Lien KW, Bigelsen S. Efficacy and tolerability of newer antihistamines in the treatment of allergic conjunctivitis. Drugs. 2005;65(2):215-28.
60. Bernal DL, Ubels JL. Artificial tear composition and promotion of recovery of the damaged corneal epithelium. Cornea. 1993;12(2):115-20.
61. Code of Federal Regulations: title 21, section. 349.12, 349.3, 349.6.
62. Meyer AE, Baier RE, Chen H, et al. Differential tissue-on-tissue lubrication by ophthalmic formulations. J Biomed Mater Res B Appl Biomater. 2007;82(1):74-88.
63. Pfister RR, Burstein N. The effects of ophthalmic drugs, vehicles, and preservatives on corneal epithelium: a scanning electron microscope study. Invest Ophthalmol Vis Sci. 1976;15(4):246-59.
64. Brown JH. Atropine, scopolamine and related antimuscarinic drugs. In: Goodman LS, Gilman AG (Eds). Goodman and Gilman's the Pharmacological Basis of Therapeutics. New York: McGraw-Hill; 1990.
65. Von Noorden GK, Milam JB. Penalization in the treatment of amblyopia. Am J Ophthalmol. 1979;88(3):511-8.
66. Chou AC, Shih YF, Ho TC, et al. The effectiveness of 0.5% atropine in controlling high myopia in children. J Ocul Pharmacol Ther. 1997;13(1):61-7.
67. Anicho UM, Cooper J, Feldman J, et al. The clinical efficacy of paremyd with and without dapiprazole in subjects with light and dark brown irides. Optom Vis Sci. 1999;76(2):94-101.

Chapter 5 Ocular Microbiology

Lalitha Prajna, Suneetha Viswanathaiah, Hasika Ravula, Rameshkumar Gunasekaran

INTRODUCTION

The knowledge of ocular microbiology is very important to understand the characteristics of the microorganisms causing ocular morbidity. Bacteria, viruses, fungi, and parasites may cause profound infections in susceptible humans and may cause significant loss of many years of productivity.

OCULAR BACTERIOLOGY

Bacterial infections of the eye are very prevalent and can vary from mild infections, such as conjunctivitis to sight-threatening endophthalmitis. Bacteria are part of the normal flora of the conjunctiva. Any break in host defense mechanisms allows them to invade the tissue and cause infection. This section describes the morphological characteristics, pathogenic mechanisms, and identification of common bacteria that cause ocular infections. Table 5.1 lists the bacteria that are commonly associated with ocular infections.

Gram-positive Cocci

Staphylococcus Species

The genus *Staphylococcus* comprises gram-positive cocci arranged in grape-like clusters (Fig. 5.1). More than 30 different species of *Staphylococci* have been identified;[1] among these, *Staphylococcus aureus* is recognized as the most clinically significant bacterium to cause eye infection. Based on the coagulase test, *Staphylococcus* species are classified into coagulase positive and coagulase-negative organisms (CoNS). *S. aureus* is coagulase-positive and produces a variety of toxins and other virulence factors. Resistance to antibiotics develops very quickly and resistance to fourth-generation quinolones is also very high. Moreover, methicillin-resistant *S. aureus* (MRSA) is one of the major concerns during management of any eye infection. *S. aureus* causes keratitis, conjunctivitis, blepharitis, lid abscess, and endophthalmitis. Among the CoNS, *S. epidermidis* is the most common organism causing ocular infection; it is the predominant cause of early postoperative endophthalmitis globally.

Streptococcus Species

The *Streptococcus* species are gram-positive cocci which appear in chains or pairs; occasionally, a *Streptococcus* species may present as a single organism (Fig. 5.2). Based on the hemolytic activity on 5% sheep blood agar, *Streptococcus* species are classified as:

- *α-hemolytic streptococci*, e.g. *Streptococcus pneumonia, viridans streptococci*
- *β-hemolytic streptococci*, e.g. *Streptococcus pyogenes*; and
- *Nonhemolytic streptococci* (*Enterococcus* group).

Most human hemolytic streptococcal pathogens belong to *β-hemolytic Lancefield group A streptococci*, which are extremely virulent; the principal human pathogen in this group is *S. pyogenes*. It causes a highly virulent acute postoperative endophthalmitis.

Lancefield group B *Streptococcus* is called *Streptococcus agalactiae*, which causes endophthalmitis occasionally, and can cause conjunctivitis in neonates. Lancefield group C and G streptococci are β-hemolytic and cause endophthalmitis in immunocompromised individuals.

Among the *α-hemolytic streptococci*, *Streptococcus pneumoniae* (commonly referred to as *pneumococcus*) is a very common cause of keratitis and endophthalmitis.

Nonpneumococcal α-hemolytic *streptococci*, formerly referred to as a single species, namely, *Streptococcus viridans*, are now collectively called "*viridans streptococci*"; they include *Streptococcus mitis* and *Streptococcus sanguinis*. These are usually associated with traumatic endophthalmitis.

Enterococcus species, such as *Enterococcus faecalis* and *Enterococcus faecium*, which are also known to cause endophthalmitis to a lesser extent, are now receiving major

Table 5.1: Common bacterial pathogens associated with ocular infections.

Ocular infections	Infectious agent				
	Gram-positive bacteria	Gram-negative bacteria	Actinomycetes and related organisms	Anaerobes	Others
Blepharitis	*Staphylococcus epidermidis, S. aureus*				
Canaliculitis		*Haemophilus influenza*	*Actinomyces israelii*		
Conjunctivitis—Neonates	*S. aureus, S. pneumoniae*	*H. influenza, Neisseria gonorrhoeae*			*Chlamydia trachomatis*
Conjunctivitis—Children	*S. pneumoniae, S. aureus, S. epidermidis, S. viridans*	*H. influenza, Moraxella catarrhalis, gram-negative intestinal bacteria*			
Conjunctivitis—Adults	*S. aureus, coagulase-negative Staphylococcus, S. pneumoniae, Corynebacterium ulcerans*	*H. influenza, N. gonorrhoeae*			
Corneal ulcer	*S. aureus, Coagulase negative staphylococci, S. pneumoniae, S. viridians, C. ulcerans, Bacillus cereus*	*Pseudomonas aeruginosa, N. gonorrhoeae, Branhamella catarrhalis, Escherichia coli, H. influenzae, Klebsiella pneumoniae, M. catarrhalis, Proteus mirabilis, Serratia marcescens, Acinetobacter* species	*Nocardia asteroides, Mycobacterium chelonae, Actinomyces israelii*	*Clostridium perfringens, Flavobacterium indologenes, Listeria monocytogenes*	
Dacryocystitis	*S. aureus, alpha and beta-haemolytic streptococci*				
Endophthalmitis—postoperative	*S. aureus, group B streptococci, S. pneumoniae, Corynebacterium* species	*H. influenzae , Klebsiella* species, *Serratia* species, *Proteus* species, *Morganella* species, *Vibrio vulnificus, Acinetobacter* species	*Actinomyces* species	*Clostridium* species, *Propionibacterium acnes, Listeria monocytogenes*	
Endophthalmitis—Traumatic	*B. cereus*	*P. aeruginosa*		*Clostridium* species	
Endogenous endophthalmitis	*B. cereus*	*N. meningitidis*			
Orbital cellulitis	*S. pneumoniae, S. aureus*	*H. influenzae, Eikenella corrodens*	*Atypical mycobacterium, M. tuberculosis*	*Peptostreptococcus, Veillonella, Fusobacterium, Eubacterium*	
Panophthamitis		*Pseudomonas* species		*C. septicum*	
Uveitis—Anterior			*M. tuberculosis*		*Treponema pallidum, Borrelia burgdorferi, Bartonella henselae, Tropheryma whipplei*
Uveitis—Posterior	*B. cereus*		*Actinobacillus* species	*L. monocytogenes, C. perfringens*	*Treponema pallidum, Borrelia burgdorferi, Tropheryma whipplei, Bartonella henselae*

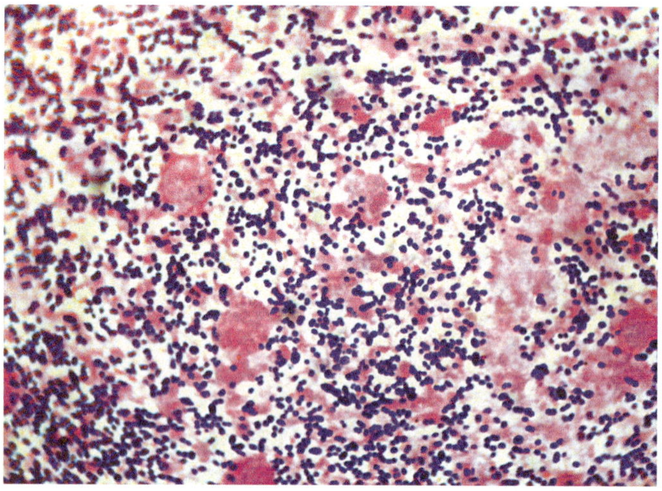

Fig. 5.1: Gram stain showing gram-positive cocci in clusters suggestive of *Staphylococcus aureus* (1000X magnification).

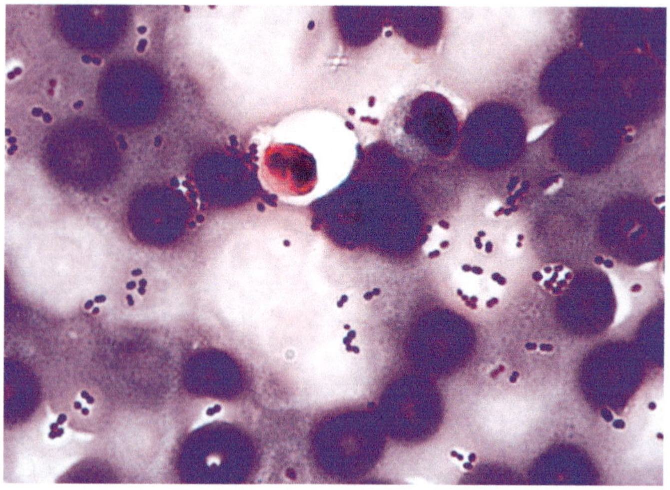

Fig. 5.2: Gram stain showing gram-positive cocci in pairs suggestive of *Streptococcus pneumoniae* (1000X magnification).

attention due to resistance to multiple antimicrobial drugs and their contributory role in nosocomial infections.

Gram-positive Bacilli

The gram-positive bacilli are ubiquitous in the environment. They are mainly grouped based on their spore-forming ability. A bacterial spore is a rigid structure that is formed either external to (exospores) or within (endospore) the bacterial cell; such spores are highly resistant to a hostile environment. Amongst the gram-positive bacilli, nondiphtheria *Corynebacterium* species. (which do not form spores) and nonanthrax *Bacillus* species. (which form spores) are considered as commensals when isolated from the external eye; these organisms must be reported only if heavy growth is present on the culture plate.[1]

Propionibacterium Species

These are anaerobic, non-spore forming gram-positive bacilli known to cause acne. These species are present as a part of the normal flora on the skin, conjunctiva, nasopharynx, oral cavity, and in the gastrointestinal and genitourinary tracts. Being anaerobic, they are difficult to isolate and grow on routinely-used culture media. Their colonies grow well on blood agar kept in an anaerobic or microaerophilic environment, with a minimum of 14 days incubation. Under the microscope, they appear as clumps and also show branched, filamentous structures. *Propionibacterium acnes* are most often implicated in ocular infections as causative agents of chronic postoperative endophthalmitis.[1]

Spore Bearers

Bacillus species are aerobic, gram-positive, spore-forming, and motile (*Bacillus anthracis* is nonmotile) bacilli that form large, gray-white colonies with irregular margins on blood agar. Most *Bacillus* species are nonpathogenic, except for *B. anthracis* and *Bacillus cereus*. *B. anthracis* causes anthrax in cattle, but is a rare cause of ocular infection; mainly, cutaneous anthrax leads to corneal scarring from a cicatricial ectropion, as well as preseptal cellulitis. *B. cereus* is associated with food poisoning due to its exotoxin; it can also cause traumatic endophthalmitis. *B. cereus* produces β-lactamases and is thus resistant to β-lactams, including third-generation cephalosporin.[1]

Clostridium species are anaerobic, gram-positive, spore-forming, motile (*Clostridium welchii* is nonmotile) bacilli found ubiquitously but especially in soil. *Clostridium* species are reported to cause exogenous and endogenous endophthalmitis, panophthalmitis, and rarely, keratitis. *Clostridium botulinum* toxin type A has been used to treat strabismus, eyelid retraction and spastic entropion. Microbiological surveillance of operation theaters is done to exclude presence of *Clostridium tetani* which, if present, could possibly infect operative wounds and cause tetanus in the affected individual.

Corynebacterium Species

Corynebacterium species (80 reported species) are aerobic, pleomorphic gram-positive bacilli that produce palisading or cuneiform patterns on smear (Fig. 5.3). Non-*Corynebacterium diphtheriae Corynebacterium* species are

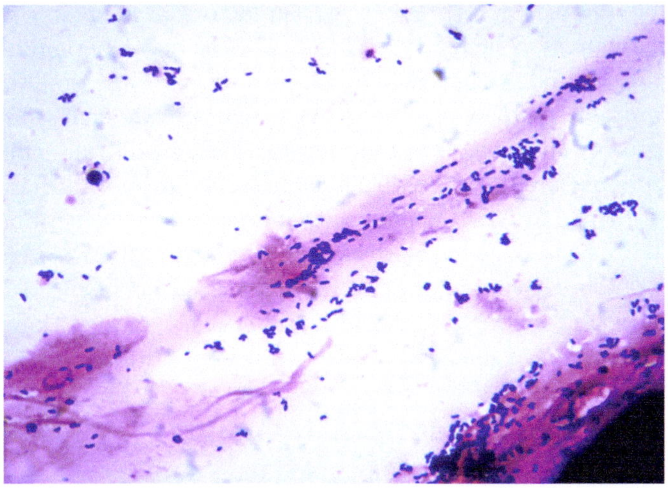

Fig. 5.3: Gram stain showing gram-positive bacilli suggestive of *Corynebacterium* species (1000X magnification).

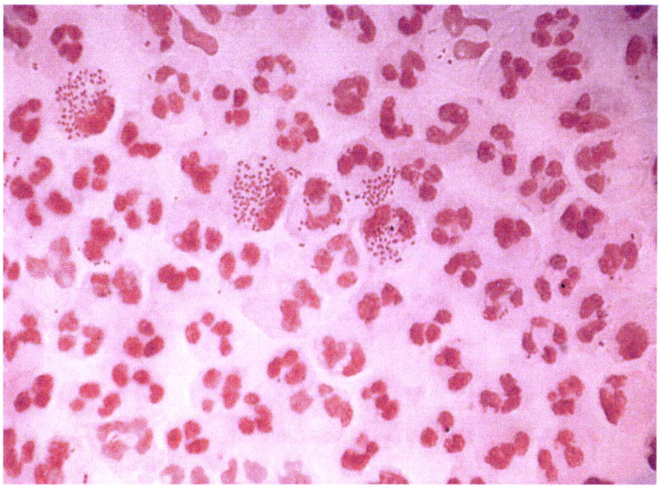

Fig. 5.4: Gram stain showing gram-negative cocci seen under 1000X magnification.

referred to as "*coryneforms*" or diphtheroids, and are part of the normal flora of the skin, mucous membrane and also ocular surface. *C. diphtheriae* is of clinical relevance since it produces an exotoxin that causes diphtheria; in the eye, it causes membranous conjunctivitis. *Corynebacterium xerosis* is associated with vitamin A-induced conjunctival Bitot spots. *Corynebacterium* species have been recently reported from keratitis and endophthalmitis.[1]

Listeria monocytogenes, a non-spore-forming aerobic gram-positive bacillus which causes listeriosis, is reported to cause endogenous endophthalmitis in immunocompromised hosts, typically with elevated intraocular pressure, pigment dispersion and dark hypopyon.

Gram-negative Cocci

Neisseria Species

Neisseria species are gram-negative, strictly aerobic, capsulated diplococci, present as part of the normal microflora in humans (Fig. 5.4); of these species, *Neisseria gonorrhoeae* and *Neisseria meningitidis* are clinically important. *N. meningitidis* is classified based on capsular polysaccharides; it mainly causes meningitis, but is also reported to cause conjunctivitis and rarely, endogenous endophthalmitis.[1] *N. gonorrhoeae* strains are pathogenic and cause gonococcal ophthalmia neonatorum; hitherto, no intraocular manifestation has been reported.

Gram-negative Bacilli

Enterobacteriaceae

Members of the family *Enterobacteriaceae* are aerobic and facultatively anaerobic gram-negative bacilli that are found in all natural habitats (Fig. 5.5). They are oxidase-negative, catalase-positive and easy to grow, producing acid, with or without gas, and reducing nitrates. *Enterobacteriaceae* of ocular importance include *Proteus* species, *Serratia marcescens, Morganella morganii, Citrobacter* species, *Escherichia coli* and *Klebsiella pneumoniae*. These organisms are known to cause keratitis, and endogenous and exogenous endophthalmitis. *Klebsiella* and *Serratia* species are the most common organisms within this group that cause endophthalmitis.[1]

Pseudomonas Species

Pseudomonas species are oxidase-positive, strictly aerobic, motile, gram-negative bacilli that are found in many habitats including soil and water. They thrive easily over a wide range of temperature. *Pseudomonas aeruginosa* is the most common human opportunistic pathogen. *P. aeruginosa* differs from other pseudomonads in being able to grow at 42°C, producing various pigments (pyocyanin, pyoverdin, and pyorubin) and emanating a distinctive fruity odor. It is resistant to chemical disinfectants and grows well in certain antiseptics (e.g. cetrimide and chloroxylenol).

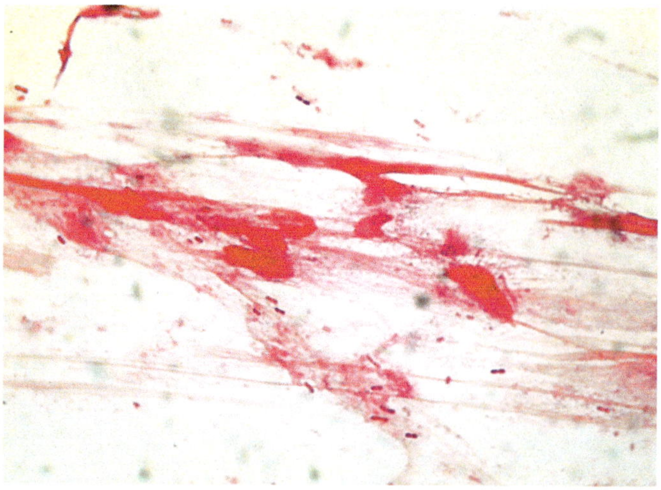

Fig. 5.5: Gram stain showing gram-negative bacilli seen under 1000X magnification.

P. aeruginosa exhibits multiple antibiotic resistance as well as immune evasion mechanisms to survive within a host.

Pseudomonas species are a major cause of nosocomial infections especially in immunocompromised patients; burn wound infections, cystic fibrosis patients, and patients on respirators or catheters. They thrive very well in solutions and, hence, have been implicated in extensive postoperative endophthalmitis outbreaks caused by use of contaminated irrigating fluids. They are also one of the major gram-negative organisms causing ocular infections, such as contact lens-associated keratitis, endogenous and exogenous endophthalmitis, and panophthalmitis.[1]

Acinetobacter Species

Acinetobacter species are gram-negative, nonmotile, oxidase-negative coccobacilli. While several *Acinetobacter* species can cause infection, the most frequently encountered is *Acinetobacter baumannii*, which causes skin and wound infections, pneumonia, and meningitis. Sporadic cases of ocular infection, especially exogenous endophthalmitis, have been reported.[1]

Vibrio organisms are obligate aerobic, curved (comma-shaped) gram-negative bacilli which are motile by a single polar flagellum. They may infect humans via infected water or fecal transmission. Ocular infection (including exogenous endophthalmitis) by *Vibrio vulnificus* following trauma involving contaminated seawater or shellfish has been reported.

Haemophilus organisms comprise a significant part of normal commensal flora of the upper respiratory tract. These gram-negative bacilli have an affinity to grow in blood since blood provides two key factors for their growth; namely, (1) X-factor (hemin) and (2) V-factor (nicotinamide dinucleotide). *Haemophilus* colonies, usually form satellites around staphylococcal colonies which provide factors for growth, appear as tiny gram-negative coccobacilli under the microscope. *Haemophilus influenzae*, the most important species, causes invasive upper respiratory infections with systemic sequelae. *H. influenzae* is a major cause of bleb-associated endophthalmitis, and may also cause infection following strabismus surgery and trauma. Other *Haemophilus* species may also cause endophthalmitis.

Anaerobic Gram-positive and Gram-negative Organisms

Anaerobic organisms are those which do not grow in the presence of oxygen. They require specialized oxygen-free environment to grow. Ocular infections by anaerobic organisms are very rare and constitute only 5–10% of all clinical infections. They are mostly difficult to culture. Some common anaerobic organisms recovered from eye infections are *P. acnes, Peptostreptococcus* species, *Clostridium* species, *Prevotella* species, and *Fusobacterium.*

Actinomycetes Species

Actinomycetes are anaerobic, gram-positive, non-spore-forming, and rod-shaped bacteria. They form filamentous branching structures, and are difficult to culture. In thioglycolate broth, they grow as "bread crumb"-like colonies below the fluid surface, where they can grow in a microaerophilic environment. Ocular infections by these species are infrequent, with only a few cases of postoperative endophthalmitis and canaliculitis reported so far.[2]

Nocardia Species

Nocardia is an aerobic actinomycete (gram-positive filamentous bacillus) that is found in soil, wet mud, decomposing plant material, dust, and air. They are endemic in dry and humid regions. Patients who acquire a systemic infection with *Nocardia*, such as pulmonary or disseminated infections, are mostly immunosuppressed. Endogenous *Nocardia* endophthalmitis also occurs in immunosuppressed individuals, whereas exogenous endophthalmitis occurs due to intraocular entry of organisms following trauma in individuals who may not be immunosuppressed.

There are currently more than 30 species of *Nocardia* of human clinical significance, with the majority of isolates being *N. nova complex, N. abscessus, N. transvalensis complex, N. farcinica, N. asteroides type VI (N. cyriacigeorgica),* and *N. brasiliensis.* These species cause a wide variety of diseases and have variable drug susceptibilities. Most systemic *Nocardia* infections are acquired through inhalation. Ocular infections can be either due to exogenous traumatic introduction of organisms or endogenous spread. In the eye, they commonly cause keratitis, postoperative, traumatic, and endogenous endophthalmitis.

Nocardia grows very well on most media. On 10% KOH wet mount preparation branching filamentous bacteria can be seen (Fig. 5.6A). On Gram stain, they are gram-positive, bacillary, branching bacteria whose hyphae often fragment to coccobacillary forms (Fig. 5.6B). On 1% acid fast stain, they are filamentous forms are partially acid fast with a branched beaded appearance (Fig. 5.6C). As they are slow growing pathogens, plates have to be kept for extended period of time and regularly examined. Colonies are typically dry and chalky which may later produce colored pigments (Fig. 5.6D). The antibacterials commonly tested in in vitro susceptibility tests include amikacin, gentamicin, vancomycin, cefazolin, ceftazidime, ciprofloxacin, ofloxacin, and sulfonamides or trimethoprim-sulfamethoxazole.[2] Amikacin is the drug of choice for treatment of *Nocardia* keratitis.

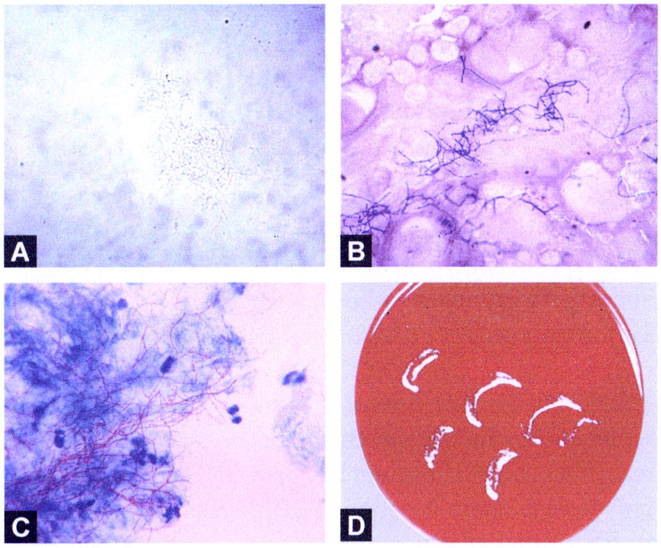

Figs. 5.6A to D: (A) 10% KOH wet mount preparation of branching filamentous bacteria suggestive of *Nocardia* species seen; (B) Gram stain showing gram-positive filamentous bacteria—*Nocardia* species under oil immersion; (C) 1% acid-fast stain (Kinyoun stain) showing the acid fast with a branched beaded appearance; and (D) A significant growth of *Nocardia* species growth was seen on blood agar plates.

Mycobacterium tuberculosis

Epidemiology and transmission: *Mycobacterium tuberculosis* belongs to the genus *Mycobacterium* in family *Mycobacteriaceae.* The same family includes *Mycobacterium leprae* and other *nontuberculous mycobacteria* (NTM). *M. tuberculosis* causes tuberculosis which remains a major global public health problem.

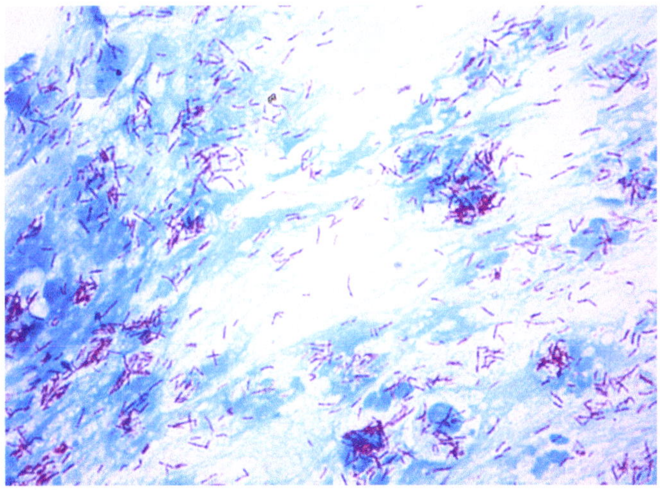

Fig. 5.7: 20% acid-fast stain (Ziehl-Neelsen acid-fast stain) showing *Mycobacterium tuberculosis* under 1,000X magnification.

Morphology and culture characteristics: *Mycobacterium tuberculosis* is straight or slightly curved, rod-shaped, 3 × 0.3 µm in size, occurring singly, in pairs or in small clumps; (Fig. 5.7) it is nonmotile and noncapsulated. *Mycobacteria* are neither gram-positive nor gram-negative. They are characterized by large amounts of fatty acids, such as mycolic acid, in their cell wall. After staining with strong carbol fuchsin, *M. tuberculosis* resists decolorization with acid-alcohol, and is therefore termed an "acid-alcohol-fast bacillus." *M. tuberculosis* is an obligate aerobe which grows slowly, the generation time in vitro being 14–15 hours. Colonies appear in about 2 weeks, but may sometimes even take up to 8 weeks. The organisms grow optimally in Lowenstein-Jensen (LJ) medium at 37°C; growth does not occur below 25°C or above 40°C. *M. tuberculosis* can be identified by various biochemical tests.[3]

Clinical significance: *Mycobacterium tuberculosis* causes primary and postprimary (secondary) tuberculosis. The postprimary type is due to reactivation of a latent infection or exogenous reinfection. The eye can be involved, even in the absence of any systemic tuberculous involvement.

Typical presentations of ocular tuberculosis include retinal vasculitis, serpiginous-like choroiditis, vitritis, retinal vasculitis, optic neuritis, choroidal tubercles, stromal keratitis, scleral nodules, and rarely, endophthalmitis.

Laboratory diagnosis of tuberculosis: Microscopic examination of acid-alcohol-fast stained smears of ocular samples is the most rapid and inexpensive way to diagnose tuberculosis. Growth of *M. tuberculosis* on LJ medium takes about 6–8 weeks. Several automated methods are available for the diagnosis of tuberculosis, such as liquid automated culture systems (Bactec 460, MB/BacT system and BACTEC MGIT 960) for isolation of *M. tuberculosis*, and modern molecular techniques such as nucleic acid amplification test (NAAT), deoxyribonucleic acid (DNA) hybridization, polymerase chain reaction (PCR), ligase chain reaction, strain displacement amplification and loop mediated isothermal amplification (LAMP), to detect *M. tuberculosis* nucleic acid in ocular samples.

Immunodiagnostic tests for tuberculosis, such as the tuberculin skin test (TST) or Mantoux skin test have been used for decades to detect latent disease. IFN-γ release *M. tuberculosis* assays (IGRAs) are based on gamma interferon production by T-cells sensitized to *M. tuberculosis*-specific antigens; such assays are not influenced by BCG and most NTMs. These tests include QuantiFERON-TB Gold In-Tube and The T-SPOT.TB test is an Enzyme-linked immunospot (ELISpot) assay-based test.[4]

Atypical Mycobacteria

Rapidly growing mycobacteria, also called *atypical* or NTM, are generally defined as mycobacterial species that grow within 7 days on laboratory media. They belong to the genus *Mycobacterium,* family *Mycobacteriaceae.* They have been classified into four groups by Runyon on the basis of pigment production and rate of growth (Table 5.2). There are more than 130 species of NTM, of which *M. chelonei, M. fortuitum,* and *M. abscessus* are the most common species associated with ocular infections. NTM can be identified and speciated by biochemical tests which are laborious. In recent times, molecular identification methods are more accurate and easier to perform.

Nontuberculous mycobacteria are opportunistic pathogens that produce diseases in a variety of clinical settings. They are ubiquitous in the environment and are most commonly found in tap water. In the eye, NTM can cause posterior uveitis. *M. fortuitum* and *M. chelonei* have been reported from ulcerative keratitis, particularly following refractive surgery. NTM can also cause suture-related infections and postoperative endophthalmitis.[2]

Chlamydiae

Morphology and life cycle: *Chlamydiae* are obligate intracellular bacterial parasites. The genus *Chlamydia* is composed of four species, namely, *C. trachomatis, C. psittaci, C. pneumoniae,* and *C. pecorum*. Transmission is human- to-human in the case of *C. trachomatis* and *C. pneumonia,* with no known animal reservoir. Transmission of *C. psittaci* in humans follows contact with infected birds. These species classically form intracytoplasmic inclusion bodies, which can be seen in Giemsa-stained smears. Inclusions of *C. trachomatis* contain glycogen and can be detected by staining with Lugol's iodine. These characteristic inclusion bodies are termed Halberstaedter-Prowazek or HP bodies. *Chlamydiae* were originally classified as viruses due to their small size (diameter 200–1,500 nm) and ability to replicate only in living cells. It has been taught that chlamydial cell walls do not contain peptidoglycan, and hence the β-lactam antibiotics are ineffective against chlamydial infections; however, previous study reported that when a new metabolic cell-wall labeling method was used, functional peptidoglycan was detected in *C. trachomatis*. Technological advances have led to the classification of *Chlamydia* as bacteria with the following characteristics namely, the presence of both DNA and

Table 5.2: Runyon classification of nontuberculous mycobacterium (NTM) based on pigment production and rate of growth.

Group	Group I Photochromogens	Group II Scotochromogens	Group III Nonphotochromogens	Group IV Rapid growers
Pigment	Form pigment after exposure to light	Pigment produced in dark	No pigment production	Colonies appear within seven days
Habitat	Water and animals	Water, soil, and fomites	Soil, Seawater, and animals	Water, soil, and animals
Diseases	Pulmonary, skin, systemic, lymph node infection	Cervical lymphadenitis in children	Pulmonary, gastrointestinal, renal, systemic, lymph node infections	Pulmonary, gastrointestinal, renal, systemic, lymph node infections
Example	*M. kansasii, M. simiae, and M. balnei*	*M. scrofulaceum and M. gordonae*	*M. intracellulare, M. avium and M. xenopi*	*M. fortuitum and M. cheloneii*

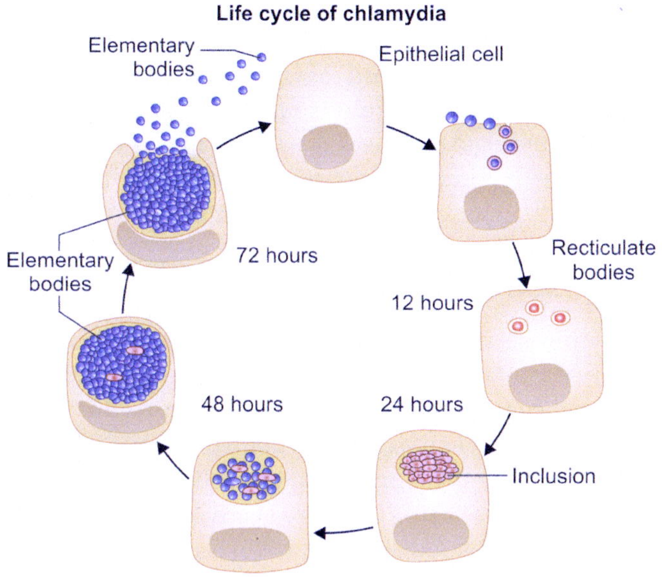

Fig. 5.8: Schematic diagram of the life cycle of *Chlamydia* species.
Source: California STD/HIV Prevention Training Center.

ribonucleic acid (RNA), replication by binary fission, presence of cell wall and inhibition of replication by several antimicrobial drugs. The life cycle comprises two stages: the infectious form is the elementary body (EB) and noninfectious form is the reticulate body (RB). The EB develops into an intracellular replicating RB within an infected eukaryotic host cell (Fig. 5.8). *C. trachomatis* can infect any columnar or transitional epithelial cell; it causes conjunctivitis in the eye and systemic presentations such as urethritis, cervicitis, and proctitis.[5]

Natural history and epidemiology: *Chlamydia trachomatis* is classified into two biovars: (1) TRIC (causing Trachoma and inclusion conjunctivitis) and (2) LGV (lymphogranuloma venereum). TRIC biovar is the only known cause of ocular chlamydial infections which includes 12 serovars; A, B, Ba, and C causing endemic blinding trachoma and serovars D through K causing less severe adult/neonatal inclusion conjunctivitis. Trachoma, an infectious disease that mainly occurs in communities with poor hygiene and inadequate sanitation, is the leading cause of preventable blindness worldwide; nearly 150 million individuals are affected, with the disease being prevalent in some regions of Africa, the Middle East and parts of Southeast Asia. Most of these infections are transmitted from eye to eye, while some may be transmitted through flies and other household fomites.

Laboratory diagnosis: *Chlamydia trachomatis* is detected by direct cytological examination of Giemsa-stained smears of

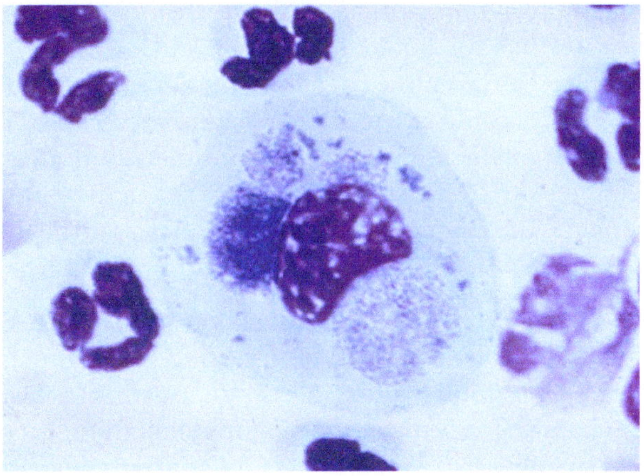

Fig. 5.9: Giemsa stain showing the *Chlamydia* inclusion bodies under 1,000X magnification.
Source: Vicky Chavalos, Proctor foundation; San Francisco: University of California.

conjunctival cell scrapings (Fig. 5.9). Additionally, staining of specimens isolated by cell culture techniques (McCoy cell culture and HeLa cells) for detection of inclusion bodies is also useful. Antigen detection is done by direct staining of specimens by fluorescent conjugated monoclonal antibody (DFA) and enzyme immunoassay. Serologic diagnosis to measure immunoglobulin G (IgG), IgA, IgM, or total classes of antibodies to individual or multiple Chlamydia serovars, is done by microimmunofluorescence. Molecular diagnostic tests using nucleic acid amplification results in better sensitivity of detection when compared to other non-culture methods.[6]

Spirochetes

Spirochetes are uniquely mobile, corkscrew (spiral)-shaped bacteria that represent a phylogenetically ancient bacterial group. They are also of great clinical importance. These organisms cannot be cultured easily in the clinical laboratory; hence, the diagnosis of spirochetal diseases mainly depends on serologic tests or microscopy using special techniques (e.g. silver stain, dark-field microscopy). *Treponema*, *Borrelia*, *Leptospira*, and *Spirillum* are the major human pathogens belonging to this group. They cause systemic illnesses such as syphilis, Lyme disease, relapsing fever, and leptospirosis that may also involve the eye during their infectious stages.

Treponema

Epidemiology and transmission: Treponema pallidum is a well-known human pathogen which causes syphilis. It has a worldwide distribution.

Morphology and culture characteristics: *Treponema pallidum* has an outer membrane and an inner thin peptidoglycan layer. The flagella for motility are embedded in the periplasmic space. The molecular mechanism of *T. pallidum* pathogenesis is very poorly understood. They are called "stealth organisms" since they escape the immune clearance. The main mode of infecting a host is through any break in the mucous membranes or skin.

Clinical significance: The disease manifests in 4 stages: (1) primary, (2) secondary, (3) tertiary, and (4) latent stage. In primary syphilis, after 3 weeks incubation, a lesion, the "chancre" appears at the site of inoculation; there is spread to other parts, especially the central nervous system (CNS). During this time, serologic tests may be negative, but treponemes can be detected in scrapings from the chancre, using either dark-field microscopy or immunostaining with fluorescent antibodies (DFA-TP). After 2–8 weeks, the chancre disappears, and secondary syphilis develops; this usually manifests with appearance of a rash on palms and soles. Painless moist plaques (condylomata lata) can develop in intertriginous areas and can be associated with fever, sore throat, arthralgia, and malaise. Once the CNS is involved, it is called acute neurosyphilis. Symptoms of secondary syphilis tend to resolve; however, relapses occur, usually with milder symptoms.

Some patients become asymptomatic with a positive serology, which leads to development of latent syphilis; the disease may relapse in later years. Tertiary syphilis, also called "late syphilis", is primarily manifested by cardiovascular or CNS symptoms. Ocular syphilis may occur either during secondary or tertiary syphilis. Congenital syphilis varies in severity based on the stage of maternal syphilis. In early maternal syphilis, the risk of transmission is very high; this risk decreases in the later stages of maternal syphilis. Characteristic stigmata of congenital syphilis include Hutchinson's teeth, abnormal facies, sensorineural deafness, and ocular disease, namely, interstitial keratitis, optic atrophy and chorioretinitis. Diagnosis of ocular syphilis is highly variable (Table 5.3). General serologic diagnosis is used for the screening. The patients with human immunodeficiency virus (HIV) have a higher risk of developing ocular syphilis.[7]

Leptospirosis

Leptospirosis is zoonotic, water-borne illness seen most commonly in tropical countries. It is caused by *Leptospira,* a gram-negative bacterium that belongs to the family *Spirochaetaceae*. Leptospires are thin, spiral-shaped, highly motile bacteria that can only be visualized by dark-field microscopy (Fig. 5.10). There are nearly 270 serovars, with antigenically-related serovars (which cross-agglutinate with each other) being grouped into 23 serogroups. There are seven pathogenic leptospiral species, of which *Leptospira interrogans* is the most common.

They are difficult to culture; being cultured only on semiliquid polysorbate albumin media. The leptospires are maintained in nature by chronic renal infection of carrier animals, such as rodents and cattle, and human infection usually occurs after exposure to contaminated water or damp soil. Clinical disease manifests either as a self-limited flu-like illness or as a severe illness characterized by renal and liver failure as well as hemorrhagic pneumonia (Weil's disease). Initially it presents as an acute febrile illness which may be followed by a symptomatic latent period and a late onset of ocular morbidity in the form of uveitis. Retinal vasculitis is seen in 5% of cases. The microscopic agglutination test (MAT) is used as a serologic diagnostic test and is considered as the "gold standard". Other serological tests include enzyme-linked immunosorbent assay (ELISA),

Table 5.3: Laboratory diagnosis of syphilis depending on the stage of the disease.

Stage of disease	Diagnostic methods	Test used for specimen type
Primary (10 days to 3 months after exposure)	Dark field (DF), direct fluorescent antibody test of *Treponema palladium* (DFA-TP), PCR	Lesion exudates, lymph node aspirate
Secondary (1–3 months later)	DF, DFA-TP, PCR, silver stain, immunohistochemistry test (IHC), DFAT-TP, venereal disease research laboratory (VDRL)	Lesion exudates, lymph node aspirate, tissue biopsy, blood/plasma/serum, cerebrospinal fluid (CSF)
Latent	Direct fluorescent antibody tissue test of *T. palladium* (DFAT-TP), Hemagglutination assay (HA), VDRL	CSF
Tertiary	Silver stain, IHC, DFAT-TP	Tissue biopsy, CSF
Fetal/congenital	DF, DFA-TP, PCR, silver stain, IHC, DFAT-TP, VDRL	Lesion exudates, tissue biopsy, blood/plasma/serum, CSF, amniotic fluid and placenta or cord

Source: Radolf JD, Pillay A, Cox DL. *Treponema* and *Brachyspira*, human host-associated spirochetes. In: Versalovic J, Carroll KC. Funke G, Jorgensen JH, Landry ML, Warnock DW (Eds). Manual of Clinical Microbiology, 10th edition. Washington, DC: ASM Press; 2011. pp. 941-63.

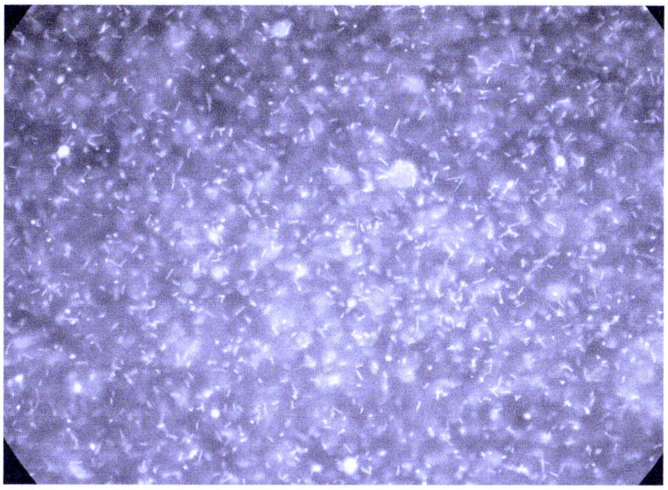

Fig. 5.10: Dark-field microscopic picture of *Leptospira* species seen under low power magnification.

macroscopic agglutination, indirect hemagglutination, "lepto dipstick", and immunofluorescence assay.[8]

Borrelia

Borrelia is a large, motile spirochete with wide-open and irregular coils. They are gram-negative organisms readily stained by ordinary methods. Of significance in ocular disease is *Borrelia burgdorferi*, the causative agent of Lyme disease. The disease is widespread in the United States, where it is the most commonly-reported vector-borne infection. *Ixodes dammini* and related species of tick are the vectors of Lyme disease. Infection occurs by regurgitation of gut contents of the tick while biting. Lyme disease commonly evolves in three stages. Stage 1 is characterized by localized erythema migrans. Ocular manifestations in this stage include mild follicular conjunctivitis and photophobia. Stage 2 is characterized by disseminated infection and Stage 3 by persistent infection. Ocular manifestations are severe in the latter two stages with reported presentations of Bell's palsy (one-fourth cases bilateral), idiopathic chronic uveitis, pars planitis, unexplained bilateral keratitis, optic nerve inflammation or papilledema. Diagnosis of Lyme disease is dependent on serological methods which includes an indirect immunofluorescence assay and ELISA.[9]

OCULAR VIROLOGY

Viruses are obligate intracellular pathogenic organisms. They are 18–400 nm in size with a nucleocapsid core which may be surrounded by a lipoprotein membrane, termed as the envelope. They are broadly classified into DNA (single or double stranded) and RNA viruses based on their nucleic acid composition. The double layered lipoprotein envelope is composed of host cell membrane and viral specific protein subunits. Initial immunologic immunity of the virus is attributed to the mixed host-virus composition of the envelope. Additionally, enveloped viruses, such as the HIV and herpes simplex virus (HSV), are intrinsically susceptible to damage by ultraviolet (UV) light, alcohol, detergents, and antiseptics. Nonenveloped viruses like adenovirus are comparatively resistant to such environmental insult and hence are more prone to spread via fomites or medical instruments. Viruses differ greatly in structure, genome organization and expression, and strategies of replication and transmission. They lack the independent means for energy metabolism, molecular biosynthesis or replication and hence exploit the host cell metabolic machinery.

Deoxyribonucleic Acid Viruses

Herpes Viruses

Morphology: The members of the family Herpesviridae share a common structure. They have linear double stranded DNA surrounded by icosahedral protein capsid, an amorphous appearing protein tegument and finally an envelope studded with viral glycoprotein (Fig. 5.11). Table 5.4 describes the different groups of DNA viruses that can cause ocular infections.

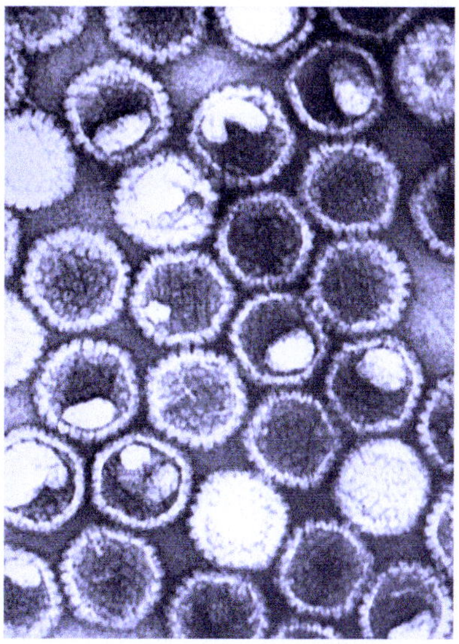

Fig. 5.11: Transmission electron microscopic (TEM) image revealed the presence of numerous herpes simplex virions, members of the herpesviridae virus family.

Source: Public Health Image Library.

Table 5.4: Deoxyribonucleic acid viruses classification and genome.

Viruses of ophthalmic importance	Family	Genera	Viral genome
Herpes simplex virus type 1 (HSV-1)	Herpesviridae	Alphaherpesvirinae HHV-1	Double-stranded deoxyribonucleic acid DNA with icosahedral capsid, with envelope
Herpes simplex virus type 2 (HSV-2)		Alphaherpesvirinae HHV-2	
Varicella-zoster virus		HHV-3	
Epstein-Barr virus		HHV-4 Gammaherpesvirinae	
Cytomegalovirus		HHV-5 Betaherpesvirinae	
Adenovirus	Adenoviridae	Mastadenovirus	Double-stranded DNA viruses, Non enveloped with icosahedral symmetry
Vaccinia	Poxviridae	Orthopoxvirus	Enveloped, double-stranded DNA viruses, with a distinctive large, brick or ovoid complex capsid structure
Molluscum contagiosum		Molluscipoxvirus	
Human papilloma virus	Papovaviridae	Papillomavirus	Double-stranded DNA genome and non enveloped capsid showing icosahedral symmetry

Epidemiology: Herpes simplex virus infections pose a major public health problem worldwide. The virus is ubiquitous. About one-third of world population suffers from recurrent infection.

Pathogenesis and transmission: The production of viral progeny invariably destroys the infected cell. All herpes viruses establish latency in their natural hosts, but the site of latency varies. For example, HSV types 1 and 2 and the varicella-zoster virus (VZV) establish latent infections in dorsal root ganglia, such as the trigeminal ganglion, whereas Epstein-Barr virus (EBV) latency occurs in B lymphocytes.[10]

Herpes Simplex Viruses

Herpes simplex virus type 1 (HSV-1) and type 2 (HSV-2) are antigenically related and may coinfect the same nerve ganglion. HSV is now more commonly acquired in adolescence than in childhood. It is spread by direct contact with infected lesions or their secretions but, most commonly, occurs as a result of exposure to viruses shed asymptomatically. It can also be vertically transmitted to neonates and can cause both cutaneous and systemic infections, including encephalitis.

Primary HSV-1 infection in humans occurs most commonly on skin and mucosal surfaces innervated by the trigeminal nerve. It usually manifests as a nonspecific upper respiratory tract infection. HSV traverses from infected mucocutaneous lesions via sensory nerve axons to establish a latent infection in the associated trigeminal ganglion. Latent infection of the trigeminal ganglion may often occur in the absence of recognized primary infection and reactivation of the virus may follow in any branch of the trigeminal nerve.[10]

Herpes simplex virus type 1 (HSV-1) and HSV-2 are one of the most common viruses causing ocular infections, ranging from keratitis to anterior and posterior uveitis, including acute retinal necrosis (ARN) and progressive outer retinal necrosis.

Varicella-Zoster Virus

Varicella-zoster virus infection can manifest as one of two clinical syndromes: chicken pox and shingles (herpes zoster). The former occurs more commonly in childhood, while the latter manifests in the sixth to seventh decade of life; in immune-compromised patients, it may manifest in younger age patients. The virus enters through inhalation, source being either a patient with chicken pox or a patient with herpes zoster. Chicken pox is highly contagious, characterized by vesicular rashes with centripetal distribution. Ocular manifestations include dermatoblepharitis, conjunctivitis, and keratitis.

Reactivation of VZV is associated with highly painful neuritis. The vesicles are usually confined to the area innervated by a single sensory ganglion. When the ophthalmic branch of the trigeminal nerve is affected, herpes zoster ophthalmicus (HZO) results. Generally, the rash appears within a few hours to days after the sensation of pain or tingling has begun; rarely, pain and tingling with ocular complications occur without a rash ever appearing (herpes zoster sine herpeticum). Uveitis (posterior) occurs in about 40% of patients with HZO, and generally starts 1–3 weeks after the onset of rash.

Epstein-Barr Virus

It is transmitted through saliva, blood, and bone marrow. EBV usually infects young adults, causing infectious mononucleosis, which is characterized by fever, sore throat, lymphadenopathy, and atypical lymphocytes in blood. It is also associated with several tumors, such as Burkitt's lymphoma, gastric, and nasopharyngeal carcinoma. Around 90% of the people are EBV-seropositive. In the eye it can cause conjunctivitis, episcleritis, keratitis, optic neuritis, ARN, and retinal vasculitis.

Cytomegalovirus

It is distributed worldwide, being present in blood, saliva, urine, semen, and breast milk of infected persons. Cytomegalovirus (CMV) is transmitted through blood transfusion, organ transplant, and sexual contact; in neonates, it spreads either by vertical transmission or via breast milk. Around 60–100% people worldwide show seropositivity. CMV causes a wide spectrum of disorders in older children and adults, ranging from asymptomatic subclinical or mild infections in healthy individuals to disseminated disease in immunocompromised patients. The hallmark of primary CMV infection is the appearance of atypical lymphocytes in peripheral blood. The virus persists indefinitely in host tissues and hence, may be activated to cause disease when immunity is compromised. The most frequent ocular manifestation of CMV infection is retinitis and is the most common cause of blindness in patients with advanced HIV disease. Rarely, the virus may cause ARN and optic neuritis.[11]

Adenoviruses

The Adenoviridae are double-stranded DNA, nonenveloped viruses with an icosahedral shape. Based on genetic sequencing, 49 serotypes of the family subdivide into six distinct subgroups (A–F) (Fig. 5.12). Ocular disease transmission is mainly through direct contact with infected material. It manifests commonly in three classical forms, pharyngoconjunctival fever, epidemic keratoconjunctivitis, and acute hemorrhagic conjunctivitis (AHC).

Adenoviruses are hardy, not susceptible to standard disinfection and easily transmissible in settings with a high population density. Different adenoviral syndromes are indistinguishable early in infection and may be unilateral or bilateral.

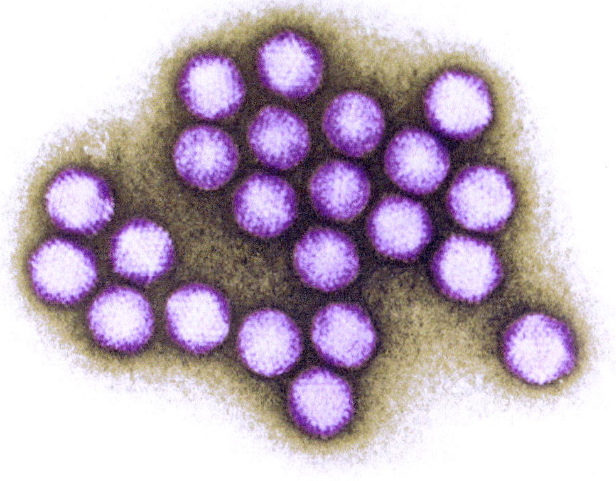

Fig. 5.12: Transmission electron microscopic (TEM) image of adenovirus. *Source*: Public Health Image Library.

Poxviruses

The Poxviridae constitutes a large family of enveloped, double-stranded DNA viruses, with a distinctive large, brick or ovoid complex capsid structure. The best-known poxviruses are molluscum contagiosum, vaccinia, and smallpox (variola) viruses.

Molluscum Contagiosum

Molluscum contagiosum virus is spread by direct contact with infected individuals. Infection produces one or more umbilicated nodules on the skin and eyelid margin and, less commonly, on the conjunctiva. Eyelid nodules release viral particles into the tear film.

A molluscum nodule is smooth with an umbilicated central core. It is smaller and associated with less inflammation than a keratoacanthoma. Punctate epithelial erosions and, in rare cases, a corneal pannus, may occur. Any chronic follicular conjunctivitis should prompt a careful search for lid margin molluscum lesions.

Vaccinia

Vaccinia virus is a large, complex, and enveloped virus belonging to the Poxvirus family. It was used as the small pox vaccine. Since the era of global eradication of small pox, there has been a marked reduction of vaccinia virus use and the vaccination program using this virus was halted.

More recently, concerns of bioterrorism have prompted the reinstitution of a vaccination program, especially for military personnel. Ocular complications from self-inoculation, including potentially severe periorbital pustules, conjunctivitis, and keratitis, can occur.

Papovaviruses

Viruses belonging to the family Papovaviridae contain double-stranded DNA genome and nonenveloped capsid showing icosahedral symmetry. Human papilloma virus (HPV) is the most important virus in this family. It has an affinity to infect squamous epithelial cells. Persistent HPV infection can result in malignant transformation of susceptible epithelial cells. HPV subtypes 6 and 11 are maintained in a latent state as circular episomes within basal epithelial cells with very limited viral gene transcription and low copy number. Early viral gene products stimulate cell growth and lead to a skin wart or a conjunctival papilloma. As HPV containing basal epithelial cells mature and differentiate into superficial epithelial cells, they become permissive for complete viral gene expression and produce infectious virus. Neoplastic transformation due to HPV 6 or 11 is very rare. In contrast, HPV 16 and 18 stereotypically integrate their viral genome into host chromosomal DNA, and this in turn is associated with malignant transformation and squamous cell carcinoma. Recently, developed immunization strategies specifically targeted against HPV oncogenes may result in a decreased incidence of these tumors in the future.

Verrucae and papillomas are caused by papilloma virus infection of the skin and conjunctival epithelium. Venereally-acquired conjunctival papillomas resemble those on the larynx and urogenital tract. Papilloma virus-associated conjunctival intraepithelial neoplasia and squamous cell carcinoma share many histological features with similar lesions in the uterine cervix. Another neoplasm, Kaposi sarcoma of the skin or conjunctiva, is associated with infection by human herpesvirus type 8.

Ribonucleic Acid Viruses

Eye infections due to RNA viruses (Table 5.5) present to the ophthalmologist less often than those due to DNA viruses. These viruses commonly cause follicular conjunctivitis associated with an upper respiratory infection. However, certain RNA virus infections may cause pathologic changes in virtually any ocular tissue. For example, influenza virus can induce inflammation in the cornea, lacrimal gland, iris, retina, optic nerve, and other cranial nerves. Certain arboviruses, such as West Nile virus (WNV), dengue, chikungunya, and Rift valley fever virus, are associated with uveitis and other ocular manifestations are emerging in recent times.

Paramyxoviruses

The paramyxoviruses comprise the viruses causing mumps, measles, and rubella. Due to effective immunization, there is a substantial decrease in the number of people suffering from infections due to these viruses.

Table 5.5: Ribonucleic acid viruses classification and genome.

Viruses of ophthalmic importance	Family	Genera	Viral genome
Measles	Paramyxoviridae	Morbillivirus	Single stranded RNA genome with helical nucleocapsid enveloped
Mumps	Paramyxoviridae	Rubulavirus	
Rubella	Togaviridae	Rubivirus	Positive sense single-stranded RNA, enveloped
Enterovirus	Picornaviridae		Single stranded RNA, with icosahedral symmetry, nonenveloped
West Nile virus	Flaviviridae	Flavivirus	Positive sense single stranded RNA, enveloped
Dengue virus			
Zika virus			
Rift valley fever virus	Bunyaviridae	Phlebovirus	Single-stranded RNA genome with envelope
Chikungunya virus	Togaviridae	Alpha virus	Positive sense single stranded RNA with envelope
HIV	Retroviridae	Lentivirus	RNA virus containing reverse transcriptase enzyme
Ebola virus	Filoviridae	Filovirus	Negative sense single stranded RNA with envelope
Rabies virus	Rhabdoviridae	Lyssavirus	Single stranded enveloped RNA

(RNA: Ribonucleic acid; HIV: Human immunodeficiency virus)

Measles: It is a highly contagious disease characterized by fever, cough, coryza, and conjunctivitis followed by appearance of generalized maculopapular rash. The virus is transmitted by direct contact with infected secretions through droplet inhalation. Chain of transmission is seen amongst household contacts, schoolchildren, and amongst the people in overcrowded areas. Infection is initiated when the measles virus proliferates and is deposited on epithelial cells of the respiratory tract, oropharynx, and conjunctiva. The most common ocular manifestation is mild epithelial keratitis; rarely, it causes optic neuritis, retinal vascular occlusion, and pigmentary retinopathy. Measles keratopathy, a major source of blindness in the developing world, typically presents as corneal ulceration in malnourished and vitamin A-deficient children.

Mumps: Mumps is an acute, self-limited, and systemic viral illness of children that primarily affects the parotid glands; it is also seen in adults who usually present with extra-salivary manifestations, the commonest being orchitis and pancreatitis. The virus spreads through saliva, nasal secretions, and close personal contact. Mumps occurs worldwide and is highly infectious to nonimmune individuals. Humans are the only known natural hosts. Ocular complications of mumps are rare, the commonest being dacryoadenitis, which is usually bilateral and begins with sudden pain in the orbits, chemosis of the bulbar conjunctiva, and enlarged tense painful lacrimal glands. In its milder form it causes conjunctivitis.

Rubella virus: The rubella virus causes the highly contagious disease, rubella or German measles. It is transmitted through droplet inhalation and vertical transmission. The disease is generally mild, with self-limiting fever, cervical lymphadenopathy, and a transient scarlatiniform rash in adults. Around 100,000 babies are born with congenital rubella infection. Fetal infection occurs transplacentally during the maternal viremic phase, which is more severe during first trimester. The teratogenic property of rubella was discovered by an Australian ophthalmologist, Gregg, who, in 1941, observed a sudden increase in congenital cataract in infants and related it to maternal rubella. Congenital rubella syndrome (CRS) is characterized by a triad of auditory, ocular (cataracts, microphthalmos, and pigmentary retinopathy), and cardiac defects. Pigmentary retinopathy secondary to rubella is seen in about 20–60% of children, with a pale fundus with scattered irregular spots of pigment.

Human Enteroviruses

These are a group of viruses (poliovirus, coxsackievirus, echovirus, and enterovirus) belonging to the family Picornaviridae; these encompass more than 100 serotypes, distributed worldwide. Most of the infections are subclinical, being transmitted by the faeco-oral route. Certain enteroviruses, such as enterovirus 70, can be transmitted by direct inoculation from the fingers to the eye. Enteroviruses causing ocular manifestations include enterovirus type 70 and coxsackievirus A24 variant. These viruses causes AHC, which is characterized by sudden onset of follicular conjunctivitis associated with multiple petechial hemorrhages of the bulbar and tarsal conjunctiva. The hemorrhages may become confluent. Edema of the eyelids, preauricular adenopathy, chemosis, and punctate epithelial keratitis may be associated with infection. AHC is highly contagious and occurs in large and rapidly spreading epidemics.

Human Immunodeficiency Virus

The HIV is a single-stranded RNA retrovirus that causes acquired immunodeficiency syndrome (AIDS). HIV is spread by sexual contact, blood and body fluids, or vertical transmission from mother to child. AIDS is a multisystem disease associated with progressive failure of the immune system that can cause opportunistic infections and viral-induced cancers.

Human immunodeficiency virus is a retrovirus. It consists of two types—HIV 1 and HIV 2. The common cause of HIV disease throughout the world is HIV 1 (groups M, N, O, and P); this is likely to have originated in chimpanzees. HIV 1 group M is responsible for the AIDS pandemic. HIV 2 (groups A to H) was first identified in 1986 in West African patients.

The replication of HIV virus binds to receptors on the surface of a CD4 cells with the function of gp120/gp41 glycoproteins present in the virus envelope. Cell tropism is mediated by two coreceptor molecules. Following fusion, the HIV genome is integrated into host cell genome by the action of the enzyme integrase establishing latent infection. Lytic infection is mediated intermittently by releasing progeny virions to infect other cells (Fig. 5.13).

The hallmark of HIV disease is profound immunodeficiency resulting from qualitative and quantitative depletion of T helper cells. Patients with CD4 cells below certain thresholds values are at high risk of developing opportunistic infections and neoplasms. HIV is unique

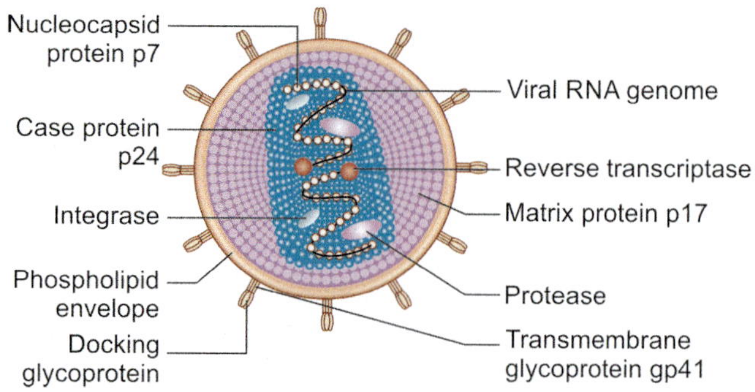

Fig. 5.13: Schematic representation of mature human immunodeficiency virus virion showing the location of viral proteins.
(RNA: Ribonucleic acid)

because once infection is established; it escapes complete immune-mediated clearance and thrives on immune activation; hence, virus always persists resulting in chronic infection and is never completely eliminated from the body.

Clinical features of human immunodeficiency virus infections: The course of a HIV infection has many stages:

1. *Seroconversion stage:* Acute HIV infection manifests within 3–6 weeks of infection with fever, lymphadenopathy, rash, and arthropathy. This stage may resolve spontaneously.
2. *Latent infection:* This is the symptomless latent period which may last for many years. The infection progresses in the course of time through various stages, such as CD4 lymphocytopenia, opportunistic infections, generalized lymphadenopathy, AIDS-related complex, and finally full-blown AIDS with immunodeficiency, infections, and malignancies.
3. Persistent generalized lymphadenopathy.
4. AIDS-related complex.
5. *AIDS:* End stage disease manifestations.

Ocular disease: Around 70% of AIDS patients have ocular manifestations during the natural course of the disease; both anterior and posterior segments of the eye may be affected. In patients with early-stage HIV disease (CD4 count >300 cells/μL), ocular syndromes associated with immunosuppression are uncommon. Anterior segment findings include tumors of the periocular tissues and a variety of external infections, such as Kaposi's sarcoma, HZO and HSV keratitis, molluscum contagiosum, and microsporidial keratoconjunctivitis. The common manifestations of posterior uveitis in AIDS patients are CMV retinitis, retinal microvasculopathy, choroiditis and progressive outer retinal necrosis, and rarely, HSV-related ARN.[12]

Arboviruses

Arboviruses are a taxonomically diverse group of viruses that are transmitted biologically to the vertebrate host by the bite of arthropod vectors (mosquitoes, ticks, sand flies, etc.). There are more than 500 viruses from diverse families, such as the Flaviviridae, Togaviridae, Bunyaviridae, Orthomyxoviridae, and Rhabdoviridae. Dengue, West Nile, and Japanese encephalitis are the most important viruses in the Flaviviridae family that are important causes of ocular diseases.

Dengue Virus

This is an arbovirus causing a mosquito-borne disease called dengue fever. The virus is transmitted by *Aedes aegypti*. Dengue fever and its complications are a major health burden in endemic areas. It has gained much importance in the current era due to growing urbanization and deforestation which favors the breeding of the vector.

There are four antigenically distinct serotypes (DEN-1, DEN-2, DEN-3, and DEN-4). Immunity to dengue virus is type-specific and as there are four serotypes, a person might be infected even four times. Dengue virus can cause spectrum of manifestations ranging from mild flu like symptoms to the dreaded dengue hemorrhagic fever and dengue shock syndrome. The mechanism behind this may be due to both humoral and cell-mediated immune response, of the virus, and host genetic determinants. Circulating IgM antibodies appear within 2–5 days of onset of illness and persist for 1–2 months.

Ocular signs and symptoms features: The first case of dengue fever-related posterior uveitis was described by Deutman and colleagues in 1979 among tourists who returned from dengue endemic countries. Since 2000, many cases have been reported, especially in the South East Asian countries. Dengue-related posterior uveitis is acute, bilateral in 75% of cases, and occurs in immunocompetent individuals.[12] Ocular symptoms frequently occur 1 week after the onset of dengue fever at the nadir of thrombocytopenia. Dengue-related posterior uveitis may presents as chorioretinitis or a hemorrhagic retinopathy.

West Nile Virus

West Nile virus is an emerging arbovirus, commonly found in all the continents except South America. It was first isolated from a woman in the West Nile district of Uganda in 1937 (Fig. 5.14). The virus is usually transmitted between birds

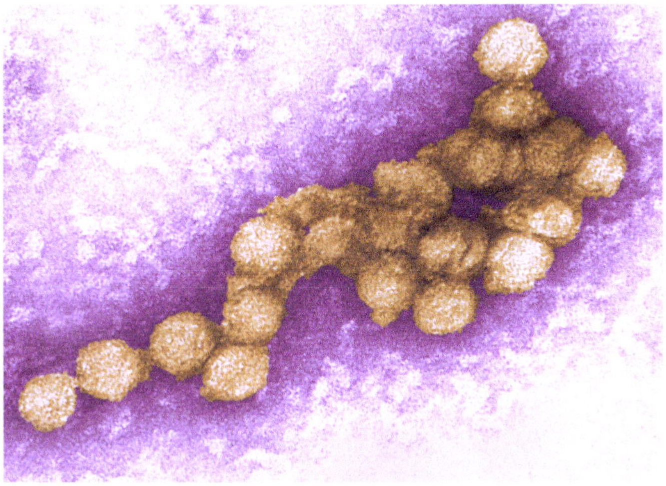

Fig. 5.14: West Nile virus (WNV)—this is a digitally-colorized transmission electron microscopic (TEM) image of the WNV.
Source: Public Health Image Library.

and mosquitoes in nature and humans acquire infection by the bite of such infected mosquitoes. In most of the cases it causes mild self-limiting febrile illness with headache and myalgia. In eye, it causes posterior uveitis which is associated with meningoencephalitis. Old age and diabetes can increase the occurrence of WNV chorioretinitis.

Chikungunya Virus

It is a mosquito-borne arbovirus prevalent in Africa and Asia, known to cause intermittent epidemics. *Aedes aegypti* are the usual vectors for the disease in urban areas, adults being most commonly affected. The abrupt onset of disease follows an incubation period of 2–10 days with saddleback fever, severe arthralgia, and constitutional symptoms. In eye, it can cause conjunctivitis, retinitis, and optic neuritis. It can cause posterior uveitis in immunocompetent individuals. Usually it resembles herpetic retinitis, but presence of associated symptoms such as fever, joint pain, and rash helps to differentiate the two conditions.[13]

Rift Valley Fever Virus

It is one of the causative agents of viral hemorrhagic fever and is confined to Sub Saharan Africa and Madagascar. It has caused major epidemics in Egypt during 1977-1979. The virus is maintained in nature in flood water. Transmission increases during heavy rainfall. Most of the infection manifests with fever and myalgia, while few presents with complications of hemorrhage. 10% individuals may have retinal vasculitis and some have permanent visual impairment.

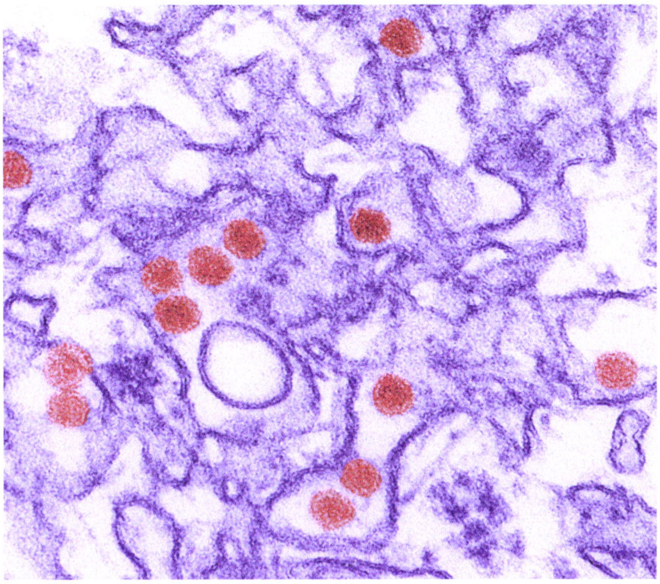

Fig. 5.15: Zika virus—this is a digitally-colorized transmission electron microscopic (TEM) image of Zika virus, which is a member of the family Flaviviridae.
Source: Public Health Image Library.

Zika Virus

The Zika virus is an emerging neurotropic pathogen that is transmitted among nonhuman primates and humans by *Aedes* mosquitoes. Outbreaks of the disease have been recorded in Africa, the America, Asia, and the Pacific. It is primarily transmitted to people through the bite of an infected *Aedes aegypti* mosquito in tropical regions; sexual transmission, congenital transmission, and through blood transfusion have been reported. Studies from Brazil in 2015 have reported the association of Zika virus infection with Guillain-Barré syndrome and microcephaly (Fig. 5.15).[14] In most cases, it causes subclinical illness. It can manifest like other arboviral infections with fever, conjunctivitis, arthralgias, and headache, which may confound the diagnosis. Ocular manifestations are seen in children with microcephaly. On examination there may be mild to gross macular pigment mottling, foveal reflex loss, well-demarcated circular areas of neuroretinal or chorioretinal atrophy with a predilection for the posterior pole and macula, posterior pole pigmentary clumping, and optic nerve hypoplasia with a double ring sign, pallor, and increased cup-to-disk ratio.[15] In addition, there may also be pigmentary and hemorrhagic retinopathy, extensive vascular tortuosity, vascular absence, early abnormal vascular termination, and torpedo maculopathy. It is still difficult to determine whether the ocular manifestations are due to Zika virus or caused by microcephaly.

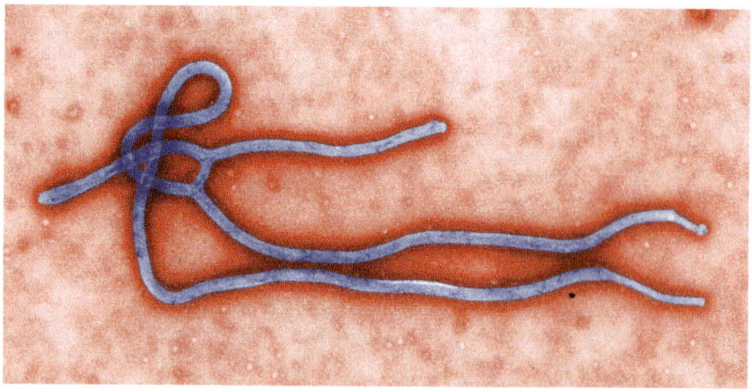

Fig. 5.16: Ebola virus—created by Centers for Disease Control and Prevention (CDC) microbiologist Cynthia Goldsmith, this transmission electron microscopic (TEM) image revealed some of the ultrastructural morphology displayed by an Ebola virus virion.
Source: Public Health Image Library.

Ebola Virus

Ebola virus, a zoonotic (from fruit bats) filovirus consisting of 5 species causes a deadly hemorrhagic disease called Ebola virus disease (EVD); it is characterized by profuse internal and external bleeding. Large outbreak of EVD happened in 2013 in West Africa with some spread to US and Europe (Fig. 5.16). The virus is transmitted through blood and body fluid contact. The pathogenic hallmark of filovirus infections is pronounced immune suppression and impaired vascular integrity. It manifests as biphasic disease. The first phase mimics influenza. The second phase involves vascular system, respiratory tract, and gastrointestinal tract. Patients usually succumb to disease 4–14 days after the infection. Patients who survive can manifest with sequelae such as hearing loss, arthralgia, and orchitis, parotitis and psychosis. During the convalescent phase, ocular involvement, such as anterior uveitis and vitritis can occur. Both blood and urine samples are negative for Ebola virus in this phase, whereas the virus persists in eye and semen for a long time. The immune privilege mechanism in the eye and testis explains the persistence of the virus in these organs.[16]

OCULAR PARASITOLOGY

Introduction

Parasitic infections of the eye can manifest either as ocular involvement alone, or as part of a generalized systemic infection. The prevalence of parasitic disease reflects the geographical distribution of the parasite, presence of vector for transmission, and life style of the affected human patient. Many parasites are endemic; hence, a history of travel is important in the diagnosis, as well as in knowledge of epidemiology and life cycle of parasites. Risks factors for acquiring the parasitic infections are closely related to epidemiological aspect of illness. Figure 5.17 provides a schematic diagram of classification of ocular parasites. Table 5.6 describes the miscellaneous parasites of ocular importance.-

Protozoan Parasitic Diseases

Acanthamoeba

Acanthamoeba, a free living protozoan parasite, is pervasive in the environment either as a trophozoite or a cyst. Of the several species of *Acanthamoeba*, the once implicated in keratitis are *A. culbertsoni*, *A. polyphaga*, and *A. castellanii*.

Distribution: This ubiquitous parasite is present in fresh water, soil, and air; it may contaminate contact lens solutions. It can enter the eye when a contaminated contact lens solution or water is applied to the eye; it can

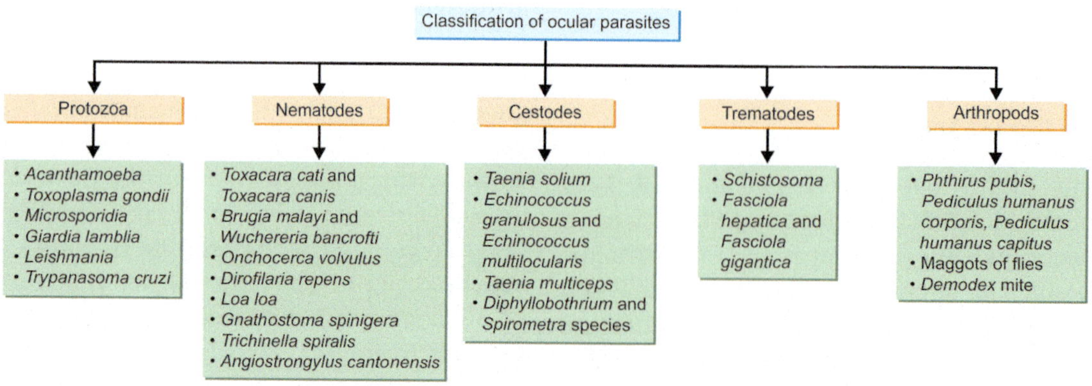

Fig. 5.17: A schematic diagram of classification of ocular parasites.

Table 5.6: Miscellaneous parasites of ocular importance.

Human disease	Causative agent	Mode of transmission	Geographical distribution	Ocular condition
Giardiasis	*Giardia lamblia*	Exists as Trophozoites and cyst Infective form—Cyst Route—Ingestion of contaminated food and water	South-East Asia, Europe, USA, and South Africa	Uveitis, salt, and pepper type of retinal degeneration, retinal arteritis, and retinal hemorrhages
Brugian filariasis	Lymphatic filariasis caused by *Brugia malayi*	Route—Bite by mosquitoes of the genera Mansonia, Anopheles, and Aedes	South-West India, China, Indonesia, Malaysia, Korea, Philippines, and Vietnam	Chemosis, lid edema, orbital cellulitis, anterior uveitis, or worm in anterior chamber, subconjunctival space and vitreous cavity
Bancroftian filariasis	*Wuchereria bancrofti*	The infection spreads from person to person by mosquitoes (*Culex*, *Anopheles*, *Mansonia*, and *Aedes*)	Asia, Africa, and Latin America.	The worm can localize in subconjunctival space, anterior chamber, iris, vitreous, retina, subretinal space, or choroid, resulting in uveitis and subretinal yellow lesions in the peripheral retina as well as pigment epithelial tracts
Dirofilariasis	*Dirofilaria repens*	By mosquito vectors (*Culex*, *Aedes*, *Anopheles*)	Endemic foci in Southern and Eastern Europe, Asia minor, Central Asia, Sri Lanka, and Italy	Eyelids are commonly involved, followed by orbit, sub-conjunctival tissue, anterior chamber, and vitreous. The worm usually remains encapsulated in a nodule in the conjunctiva or eyelid or it can migrate across the conjunctiva
Gnathostomiasis	Food-borne zoonotic parasitic infection *Gnathostoma spinigerum*	Man gets infected accidentally by ingestion of raw or undercooked meat of intermediate or paratenic hosts	South-East Asia (Thailand, China, Japan, and India), Central and South America, and Southern Africa	Rare, may affect the eyelids, conjunctiva, cornea, anterior chamber, uvea, and vitreous cavity. Associated with a unique unilateral form of ocular larva migrans, actively motile parasite can be seen more often in the anterior and less frequently in the posterior segment of the eye
Thelaziasis: Zoonotic parasitic disease	Agents—*Thelazia callipaeda* and *Thelazia californiensis*. Route—By drosophilid flies	Transmission occurs when a nonbiting flies feed on ocular secretions, tear, and conjunctiva of definitive host which harbors the first stage larvae	South Asian countries and Russia known as oriental eye worm. It is a disease of poor hygiene seen more in rural areas	Superficial pathologies such as conjunctivitis, keratitis, and corneal ulcers
Angiostrongyliasis	*Angiostrongylus cantonensis*, rat lungworm	Ingestion of raw infected mollusks, vegetables contaminated by mollusk slime or crabs, fresh water shrimps	South East Asia, Pacific Basin, and Caribbean islands and also has spread to countries in Central and South America and Southern United States	The worm can penetrate and gain access to the anterior chamber, vitreous, or sub retinal space, causing pigmentary retinal degeneration and optic atrophy
Echinococcosis	*Echinococcus granulosus* complex and *Echinococcus multilocularis*	Consumption of contaminated food and water with fecal matter containing eggs of *Echinococcus* parasites.	Asia, Africa, Latin America, Russia, Australia and the Mediterranean regions	Ocular manifestations occur approximately in 1% of the cases suffering from hydatid disease. Can cause proptosis due to the presence of intraorbital space-occupying lesion. This may further lead to exposure to keratitis and ulceration of the cornea.
Chagas disease	*Trypanosoma cruzi*, a protozoon flagellate	Man acquires infection by the bite of obligate hematophagous vector Triatomines belonging to the family Reduviidae	Chagas disease is also called as American Trypanosomiasis since its distribution is limited to temperate, sub tropical and tropical region in Western hemisphere	Trypomastigotes produce an erythematous nodule known as Chagoma in the skin. After few days, it infects the tissues such as heart, skeletal muscles, nervous system and adipose tissue. If the initial bite is near the orbit, the patient may experience significant painless palpebral and periorbital edema with associated constitutional symptoms; like fever, malaise, and anorexia (Romana sign).
Leishmania	Promastigotes in vector sand fly and amastigote in humans	Humans acquire infection by the bite of sand fly	Ocular Leishmaniasis has been reported from various countries such as India, Sudan, Italy, Norway, Turkey, and Iran.[8]	The ocular manifestations of VL are relatively uncommon and include chorioretinitis, central retinal vein thrombosis, iritis, papillitis, and keratitis and anterior uveitis.

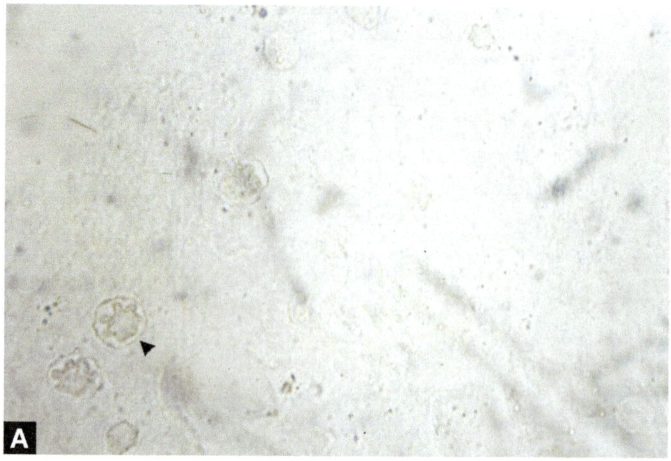

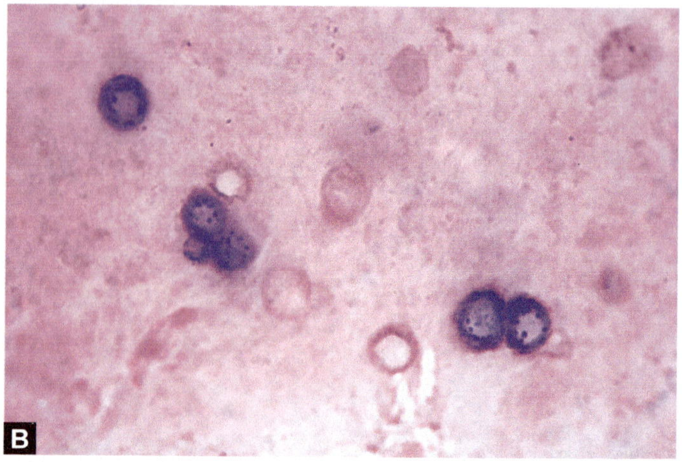

Figs. 5.18A and B: (A) 10% KOH wet mount showing the double walled (arrowhead), polygonal *Acanthamoeba* cyst under 400X magnification; and (B) Gram stain image showing *Acanthamoeba* in the form of double-walled cyst was seen under 1,000X magnification.

also enter following trauma, surgery or use of traditional eye medicines. The incidence of corneal ulcers with *Acanthamoeba* has been reported from around the world. In western literature, the major risk factor is contact lens wearing whereas in tropical countries it is mostly due to trauma to the eye.

Morphology and life cycle: *Acanthamoeba* exists in two forms; namely the trophozoite and cyst forms. The trophozoite, the active form of the parasite, can phagocytose bacteria and yeasts. Trophozoites measure approximately 8–40 μm in diameter with a single nucleus, dense nucleolus, and filamentous projections called acanthopodia (Figs. 5.18A and B).[17]

When the conditions are unfavorable to thrive, these trophozoites transform to cystic forms. Cystic forms allow survival of the parasite because these are resistant to many biocidal agents and can survive harsh environmental conditions such as desiccation and extreme temperatures.

Clinical features: In the eye, *Acanthamoeba* can cause keratitis, uveitis, and endophthalmitis.[18] Patients with *Acanthamoeba* keratitis present with severe ocular pain and photophobia. In the early stages, the disease is localized to the corneal epithelium and can present as dendritic epithelial lesions similar to those of herpetic keratitis. Later, as the disease progresses, there is a unilateral central or paracentral corneal infiltrate with a ring-shaped peripheral infiltrate.

Toxoplasma

Distribution: Toxoplasma gondii is the most common zoonotic protozoon to infect the eye. About one-third of the world's population is infected by *T. gondii.* The disease affects extremes of age in both immunocompetent and immunocompromised individuals.[19]

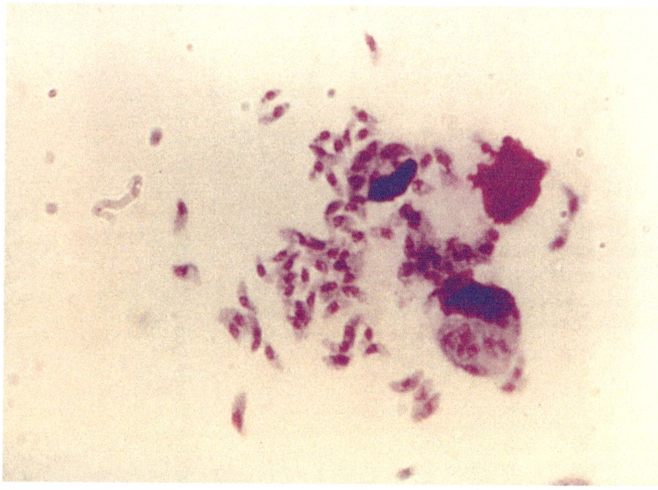

Fig. 5.19: Giemsa stain showing the crescent-shaped trophozoites of the parasitic protozoan organism, *Toxoplasma gondii* from murine ascitic fluid sample.
Source: Public Health Image Library.

Morphology and life cycle: It is an obligate intracellular parasite which exists as tachyzoites, bradyzoites, and oocyst (Fig. 5.19). Oocysts are produced sexually in feline enterocytes. Humans become infected when oocysts enter the body through ingestion of contaminated food and water, or by vertical transmission. The infective stage is the sporulated oocyst. Tachyzoites, the active intracellular forms which are capable of invading the host tissue, are produced from oocysts. They provoke a strong immune response and are responsible for clinical disease.

Under immune pressure, the tachyzoites, within 6–8 days, transform to slow-dividing bradyzoites, which are also called tissue cysts. The tissue cyst persists in a viable state in multiple tissues and establishes a lifelong chronic infection. When host immunity wanes, the bradyzoites are released from tissue cysts to form tachyzoites and recrudescent infection sets in.[20]

Clinical features: Ocular toxoplasmosis usually manifests in immunocompromised individuals and in neonates (who acquire infection transplacentally). Ocular manifestations of toxoplasmosis are the same in both congenital and acquired infections. Tachyzoites reach the eye via the retinal, rather than choroidal, circulation, and then migrate within the retina. The most common form of ocular toxoplasmosis is acute focal necrotizing retinochoroiditis.[21]

Helminthic Parasitic Diseases

Toxocariasis

Distribution: Toxocariasis is a zoonotic helminthic disease caused by *Toxocara canis* (dog ascarid) and *Toxocara cati* (cat ascarid). It has a worldwide distribution.

Morphology and life cycle: Adult worms are cylindrical and long, measuring about 75–120 mm. *Toxocara* larvae are approximately 400 × 20 µm. *Toxocara* eggs are found in the soil throughout tropical and temperate regions. Humans are accidental hosts and can acquire infection by ingesting soil or food that is contaminated with *Toxocara* eggs. Pets act as important sources of infection in children. After ingestion, the eggs mature to second-stage larvae in the small intestine. The larvae penetrate the intestinal wall and enter the lymphatic and portal circulation to reach liver and lungs. They may also disseminate to the heart and other organs, such as the brain, kidneys, muscle, and eyes, where they provoke an intense local eosinophilic granulomatous response; after reaching these organs, the parasite does not evolve further.[22]

Clinical features: Toxocariasis can present as either visceral larva migrans (VLM) or ocular toxocariasis. The manifestation depends on factors such as host immunological condition, inflammatory response, parasite load, and localization of second-stage larvae in human tissue. Most of the ocular damage results from the inflammatory response that occurs following the death of the larva, and is unilateral in 90% of cases.[21,23]

Onchocerciasis

Distribution: Onchocerciasis is caused by *Onchocerca volvulus*, a filarial nematode. It is transmitted from person-to-person by repeated bites of infected black flies (*Simulium* species). It is named "river blindness" because the black flies breed and propagate near fast-flowing rivers and streams, therein transmitting infection to individuals residing in nearby remote villages. The majority of cases occur in sub-Saharan Africa. Onchocerciasis is the second commonest infectious cause of blindness worldwide.[21,23]

Morphology and life cycle: The larvae migrate within the body for approximately 1 year before they settle in a subcutaneous nodule. Adult worms can survive in the nodules for around 15 years. Here, the male and female mate and periodically release millions of unsheathed microfilariae into the systemic circulation for years; these microfilariae (220–360 µm × 5–9 µm) have a life span of 2 years. They are occasionally found in peripheral blood, urine, and sputum, but are typically found in the skin and in the lymphatics of connective tissues, from where they invade the eyes. Onchocerciasis primarily affects the skin, eyes, and lymph nodes. In contrast to lymphatic filariasis, the damage is elicited by microfilariae, and not by adult worms. The ocular tissues are involved via migration of the microfilariae from neighboring tissues, through the bloodstream, or along the nerves. Most microfilariae die as immature worms and trigger an immune response, which damages the ocular tissue of localization (Fig. 5.20).

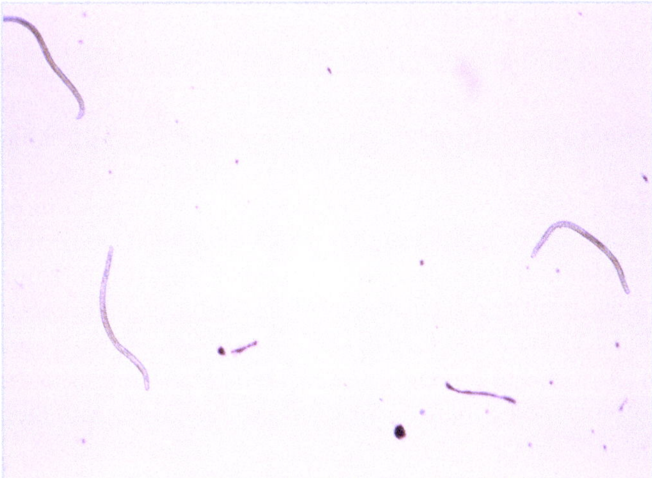

Fig. 5.20: This is a glycerin mount photomicrograph of the microfilarial pathogen *Onchocerca volvulus* in its larval form.
Source: Public Health Image Library.

The inflammatory response initiated against dying microfilariae causes gradual and progressive loss of vision due to sclerosing keratitis. Apart from causing keratitis, clinical features may also manifest as iridocyclitis, chorioretinitis, and optic atrophy. Autoimmune mechanisms have also been postulated to cause inflammation in the posterior part of eye.

Loiasis

Loiasis is caused by *Loa loa*, an African eye worm, endemic in the rain forests of west and central Africa. It is transmitted by the bite of tabanid flies of the genus *Chrysops.* Adult worms live in the subcutaneous tissues while microfilariae circulate in the blood with diurnal periodicity that peaks around midday. A hypersensitivity reaction to the excretory products of the parasite can occur in the form of episodic Calabar swellings during the movement of the parasite in the body. While the microfilaria enters the eye in onchocerciasis, it is the adult worm that enters the eye in loiasis. The parasite is most commonly found beneath the bulbar conjunctiva. The migrating worm in the periorbital area causes intense itching, swelling, and a sensation of a moving foreign body. A dead worm can incite inflammation, causing conjunctival congestion, chemosis, pruritus, keratitis, iritis, and, sometimes, blindness. Removal of worms alive from accessible location is the treatment of choice.[21,23]

Cestodes

Ocular Cysticercosis

Distribution: It is a helminthic infection caused by *Cysticercus cellulosae*, which is the larval form of *Taenia solium*. Human cysticercosis infection results from drinking contaminated water, eating uncooked vegetables infested with eggs of the worm, and autoinfection. Ingestion of poorly-cooked pork infested with *T. solium* larvae results in intestinal taeniasis, but not cysticercosis. It is a major public health problem, especially in the developing world, and is found worldwide in areas where pigs are raised and have access to human feces. It is most prevalent in Latin America, sub-Saharan Africa, China, India, and South East Asia.[21,23]

Morphology and life cycle: Humans are the only definitive hosts for *T. solium*, swine being the intermediate hosts. The adult worm resides in the upper part of the jejunum. The excreted eggs of *T. solium* can be consumed by swine or man. *Cysticercus cellulosae,* the larval stage of *T. solium,* develops from the eggs within the muscles of pigs. A mature cyst appears as an opalescent ellipsoidal body with a dense milky-white spot within the muscle fibers. Similarly, if man acts as an intermediate host and consumes eggs of *T. solium* in contaminated food or water, *Cysticercus cellulosae* is formed.

Clinical features: Cysticerci can lodge at various sites in the body, but are most commonly detected in the brain, cerebrospinal fluid (CSF), skeletal muscle, subcutaneous tissue, or eye. When cysticerci infect the eye, almost any part can be affected; in about 10% of cases, there is concomitant CNS involvement. The cyst can be traced in subconjunctival space, anterior and posterior orbit, and eyelid. It can also be present in sub retinal space and vitreous.

Trematodes

Schistosomiasis

Schistosomiasis, an infestation caused by the trematode genus *Schistosoma,* is prevalent in sub-Saharan Africa, China, and South Asia; the species involved include *S. mansoni, S. japonicum, S. mekongi, and S intercalatum.* Infective cercariae, armed with suckers to facilitate penetration of skin of definitive hosts, are released from fresh water snails (intermediate hosts). The risk of infection is high in people coming in contact with fresh water. After penetration, based on the species, the cercariae migrate to a specific target system via veins and lymphatics. They mature and directly lay eggs in the veins; these eggs disseminate and reach skin, brain, muscles, adrenal glands, genitalia, and rarely eye. Eggs released by female worms are passed out of the body in the urine or feces to complete the life cycle. Some eggs are trapped within tissue and induce a granulomatous reaction. Ocular involvement, which is rare, includes conjunctivitis, eyelids, orbital or sub retinal granuloma, keratouveitis, and vasculitis. Procerovum varium, a trematode of the family Heterophyidae, causes pediatric granulomatous anterior uveitis and is reported to be endemic in South India.[24]

Parasitic Infestations by Ectoparasites

Ophthalmomyiasis

Infestation of living or necrotic tissues or body cavities by larvae of flies (maggots) is called myiasis. All the flies are oviparous and eject their eggs, which hatch to larvae.

Ophthalmomyiasis, which can involve almost any ocular tissue, is categorized as external, internal, or orbital.[23] Orbital myiasis may be due to a number of fly species and is generally seen in debilitated patients who are unable to care for themselves. Diagnosis is established by the identification of the maggots. Flies are most commonly attracted to open wounds; some species can infest unbroken skin as well. Human myiasis usually follows a seasonal pattern, reflecting the insect life cycle. Ophthalmomyiasis externa accounts for the majority of cases of ophthalmomyiasis and can be subclassified into palpebral and conjunctival myiasis. It is generally caused by *Oestrus ovis* and *Dermatobia hominis*. Symptoms start abruptly with itching, pain, conjunctival hyperemia, lid edema, soreness, lacrimation, and a sensation of something moving on the ocular surface.

Rarely, they can gain intraocular access via a hematogenous route and optic nerve. The maggots can reach and wander in the subretinal space, creating gray-white criss-crossing tracks in the retinal pigment epithelium, and may perforate the retina to reach the vitreous, causing severe vitritis, and the anterior chamber, causing iridocyclitis.

Ocular Phthiriasis

Ocular phthiriasis is an ocular infestation by *Phthirus pubis*, a hematophagous ectoparasite of humans. *Phthirus pubis* is found predominantly in pubic hair and, less frequently, on axillary or facial hair, including the eyelashes (Fig. 5.21). The lice are mainly transmitted by sexual contact. *Phthirus pubis* is 2 mm long and has a broad crab-like body. Their thick and clawed legs allow them to navigate on smooth skin surfaces and to infest areas where the adjacent hairs are within their grasp.[21]

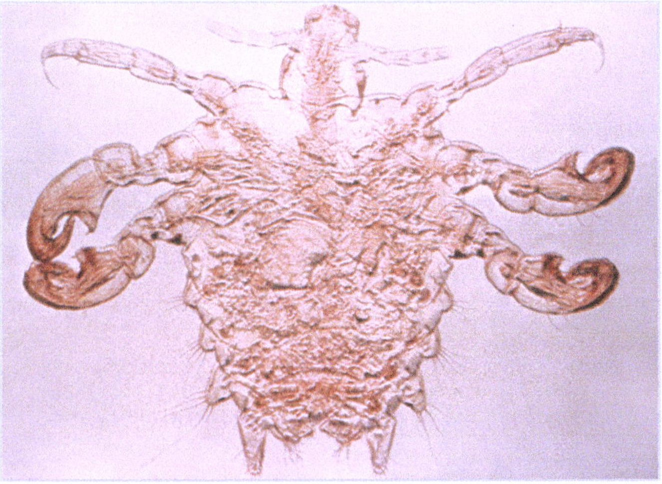

Fig. 5.21: Adult male of *Phthirus pubis*.
Source: Public Health Image Library.

Pediculosis palpebrarum is an eyelid infestation caused by *Pediculus humanus corporis* (body lice) or *Pediculus humanus capitis* (head lice). Pediculus species typically infest the hair, and infestation of the cilia and eyelid is rare. Phthiriasis palpebrarum frequently comes to an ophthalmologist's attention because it mimics lid eczema, blepharitis, nonresolving conjunctivitis, or rarely keratitis.[21] Intense pruritus caused by dermal hypersensitivity to louse saliva leads to scratching, inflammation, eczema, and superimposed bacterial infection. Slit lamp examination can show lice and nits anchored to the eyelashes, making the diagnosis easy.

Demodicosis

Demodex mite is an ectoparasite that belongs to the phylum Arthropoda and can infest the meibomian and sebaceous glands. Although they normally inhabit the hair and eyelash follicles in low numbers, an overproliferation may lead to lid margin infection, causing ocular surface irritation and symptoms of itching, foreign body, or stinging sensation. It may also exacerbate coexisting lid margin diseases, such as blepharitis. The adult *Demodex* mite is cigar-shaped, with several pairs of legs, and has a mouth with a biting apparatus. *Demodex* infestation is diagnosed using a light microscope by identification of the parasite at the root of the lashes.

OCULAR MYCOLOGY

Introduction

Fungi are eukaryotic organisms with a separate membrane-bound nucleus having multiple chromosomes containing both DNA and RNA. They possess certain distinct characteristics in that their rigid cell wall contains polysaccharides such as chitin, while their cell membrane contains ergosterol. Fungi grow in two basic forms as yeasts and molds.

Yeasts

Yeasts and yeast-like fungi are unicellular fungi which occur as spherical or ellipsoidal cells. They reproduce by budding. Yeasts (e.g. *Cryptococcus*) form buds but not pseudohyphae while yeast-like fungi (e.g. *Candida*) form buds which elongate to form pseudohyphae. Pseudohyphae are so-called since, unlike true hyphae, their cell walls have constrictions and are not parallel to each other.

Most episodes of ocular infection due to yeasts and yeast-like fungi are due to various *Candida* species, predominantly *Candida albicans.* They tend to occur in immunocompromised patients suffering from uncontrolled diabetes or from malignancies, or who are undergoing prolonged treatment with either topical or oral steroids. Patients with pre-existing ocular conditions, such as lid abnormalities or dry eye, are also at increased risk of becoming infected with *Candida. Cryptococcus* species, particularly *Cryptococcus neoformans*, are yeasts that can also cause ocular lesions.[25]

Molds (Filamentous Fungi)

Molds, also called filamentous fungi, are multicellular and composed of hyphae. These hyphae grow and branch to become an intertwined structure, the mycelium. They produce feathery, cottony, or powdery aerial growth. Reproduction may be by sexual or asexual (formation of external spores) mechanisms. The filamentous fungi form hyphae that are septate or nonseptate, and pigmented or nonpigmented. In septate hyphae, septa (cross-walls) are formed distal to the tip of the growing hypha during elongation. Fungi forming septate hyphae may be nonpigmented e.g. *Aspergillus* or *Fusarium* species, or pigmented, e.g. *Alternaria* or *Curvularia* species. In nonseptate hyphae, cross-walls are not formed.

While most fungi exist in either yeast or a mold form, there is a specific category, the dimorphic fungi, which exhibit both forms. These fungi occur in a yeast form in human tissue and in culture at 37°C and transform into a mold form in the soil and when grown in cultures at 22–25°C.[25]

Epidemiology and Transmission of Ocular Fungi

Ocular mycoses may manifest as serious debilitating infections leading to blindness. Any part of the eye may be infected; however the major ocular mycoses are mycotic keratitis and endophthalmitis. Common risk factors include trauma, ocular surgery, chronic eye disease, contact lens wear, and exposure to contaminated medical products. Diabetics and immunocompromised individuals are also prone to suffer from fungal infections.[26] Tables 5.7 and 5.8 describe the key characteristic features of hyaline filamentous fungi and pigmented fungi causing ocular infections, respectively.

Yeasts and Yeast-like Fungi Causing Ocular Mycoses

Candida

Candida species are ubiquitous in the environment and are present as resident flora of the gastrointestinal and genitourinary tracts, the oropharynx, and the skin (with *C. albicans* being the most common species at these sites). These species are true opportunistic pathogens that take advantage of the host's debilitated condition and gain access to the circulation and deep tissues. *C. albicans* and occasionally other species cause candidiasis, a major infection in immunocompromised hosts. *C. albicans* is the most common cause of endogenous endophthalmitis.

There are more than 80 species of *Candida*, but only a few are pathogenic in humans; these include *C. albicans,* C. *tropicalis,* C. *Parapsilosis,* C. *pseudotropicalis* (now called *C. keyfr*)*, and* C. *guilliermondii.*

Table 5.7: Key characteristic features of other hyaline filamentous fungi causing ocular infections

Etiologic agent	Microscopic morphology	Culture morphology
Scedosporium species (S. apiospermum, S. prolificans)	Conidiophores which are long and slender, single or branched, and sometimes aggregated into bundles (Graphium state). Conidia (6–12 µm by 3.5–6 µm) are yellow to pale brown, oval with a scar at base, and usually abundant for *S. apiospermum* and *S. prolificans* conidiophores are short with inflated base and tapering tip; oval conidia (3–7 µm by 2.5 µm) frequently occur in groups	Rapid growth at 25°C, texture is woolly to cottony, initially the colony color white becoming brownish on the surface, reverse pale with brownish black zones
Paecilomyces (P. lilacinus, P. variotii)	Septate hyphae, branched conidiophores, phialides thin and elongate at the tip, grouped in brush-like clusters at the end of the conidiophores, conidia oval to fusoid, in long chains, Chlamydospores sometimes present	Rapid growth. Texture woolly to powdery, color rusty, olive brown, lilac, pinkish, beige or white on surface, reverse pale
Acremonium species (A. kiliense, A. potronii)	Hyphae septate, hyaline; phialides solitary, long and narrow, typically with a septum at the base and a scarely visible collarate at the apex; conidia oblong to ovoid, unicellular or bicellular, often accumulating in heads at the apices of the phialides. Chlamydospores may be present	Slow growing, texture glabrous to lightly downy, sometimes powdery, color white, pale gray, or pale pink on the surface; reverse pale

Table 5.8: Dematiaceous fungi frequently implicated in ophthalmic infections.

Etiologic agent	Microscopic morphology			Culture morphology
	Hyphae	Conidiophores	Conidia	
Alternaria	Septate appear brown	Brown, septate simple or branched, scarcely if even geniculate	Large conidia (7–10 μm by 23–24 μm) appear brown, muriform, ovoid or obclavate, with an elongated, beak-like apical cell, often in chains and sometimes solitary	Rapid growth, texture downy to woolly, color pale gray to olive brown on surface, brown to black on reverse
Bipolaris	Septate appear brown	4.5–6 μm wide, brown, simple or branched, geniculate or sympodial, bending at the points	3–6 celled fusoid to cylindrical in shape, light to dark brown, sympodial geniculate growth pattern. The proconidium (30–35 μm by 11–13.5 μm) is distoseptate and scarcely protuberant, darkly pigmented hilum	Rapid growth, texture velvety to woolly, white to grayish brown and becomes olive green to black on surface, darkly pigmented and olive to black on reverse
Curvularia	Septate appear brown	Simple or branched and are bent at the points—sympodial geniculate growth	4–5 cells, Conidia (8–14 μm by 21–35 μm), straight, to pyriform, brown, multiseptate, and have dark basal protuberant hila	Rapid growth, colonies dark olive green to brown to black; surface pink-grey and woolly; the reverse is dark
Cladosporium	Septate appear brown	Simple or branched, with or without nodes or swellings	Ramoconidia (shield cells) give rise to branching chains of fragile, dark mostly 1–2 celled conidia with prominent attachment scares (hila)	Moderate growth, texture olivaceous to black, velvety to powdery
Exophiala	Septate appear brown	brown, cylindrical to flask shaped, with a narrow apex with or without collarettes; apical or borne on the side of hyphae	Single cell condia (2.5–5.9 μm by 1–3 μm), colorless to pale brown, and ellipsoidal; they may accumulate in clusters	Slow growing, initially yeast-like and black, becoming suede-like, olivaceous-grey with the development of aerial mycelium with age
Exserohilum	Septate appear pale brown	Brown, sympodial geniculate growth at the apex	Ellipsoidal to fusoid (30–128 μm by 9–23 μm): the basal cell of the conidium is round to conical, and the hilum protrudes markedly and is truncate; 7–9 pseudosepta present	Moderate rapid growth, texture velvety, dark olive to black on the surface and reverse
Lasiodiplodia theobromae	Septate appear brown		Conidia (20–30 μm by 10–15 μm) are initially colorless, ellipsoidal, nonseptate; later they are dark brown and septate, with longitudinal striations and truncate bases	Rapid growth, colonies greyish sepia to mouse grey to black, fluffy with abundant aerial mycelium, reverse fuscous black to black
Phialophora	Septate	Brown, cylindrical to flask shaped, with a very distinct flared, funnel-shaped, or cup-shaped collarette	Conidia (2.5–6 μm by 1–3 μm) are hyaline to pale brown, thick or thin walled, and oval to slightly kidney shaped; they may accumulate in slimy clusters	Slow growing, initially dome-shaped, later becoming flat, suede-like and olivaceous to black in color

The various species probably have a predilection for different clinical sites. Endogenous *Candida* endophthalmitis occurs as a direct result of usage of broad-spectrum antibiotics, indwelling central venous lines, parenteral nutrition, abdominal surgery, and cytotoxic chemotherapy. While any part of the eye may be affected by *Candida* species, the major ocular infections are *Candida* keratitis and endophthalmitis.[26]

Mycology of Candida:

Direct microscopy: The presence of small (3-4 μm) budding yeast cells and pseudohyphae is almost diagnostic for *Candida* species. The bud exhibits an off-axis position and a narrow base at the point of attachment; the yeast cell appears asymmetrical.

Cultural characteristics: *C. albicans* grows rapidly on Sabouraud dextrose agar, forming cream colored, raised, entire, and smooth and butyrous colonies that usually appear after 24-48 hours incubation at 35-37°C (Fig. 5.22A). On enriched media such as blood agar or chocolate agar, the colonies may develop small striations or outgrowths often referred to as "feet" which are indicative of the *C. albicans* species. The colonies have a distinctive yeast smell.

A smear made from colonies taken from Sabouraud dextrose agar, or blood agar reveal round to oval cells that are 4-8 μm in size. Yeast cells retain the crystal-violet stain of the routine Gram stain and therefore appear purple (Fig. 5.22B). The yeast cell divides by budding. On primary media (reduced nutritionally) the budding can create elongated

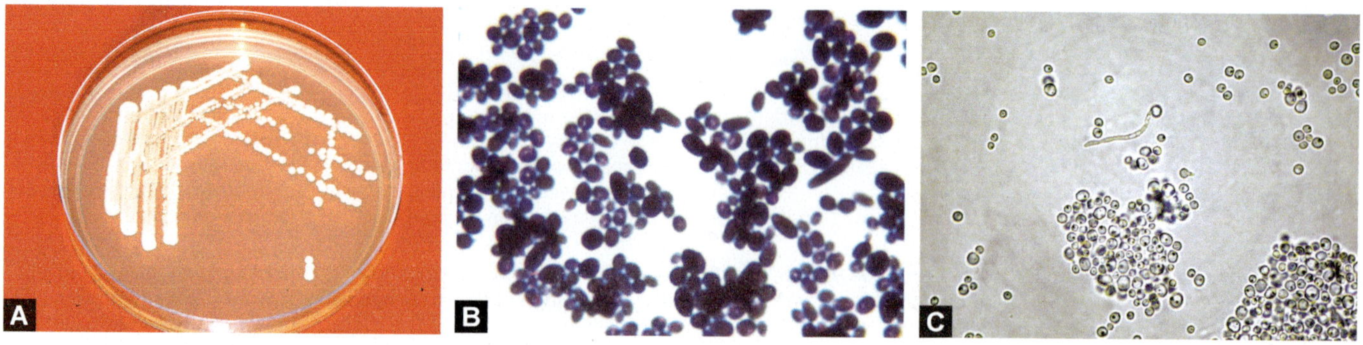

Figs. 5.22A to C: (A) *Candida albicans* growth on potato dextrose agar after 48 hours incubation at 35–37°C; (B) Gram-stained image showing the budding yeast like fungus seen under oil immersion; and (C) Germ tube formation of *C. albicans*.
Source: Prajna L, Kumar V, Prajna NV, et al. Aravind's Atlas of Fungal Corneal Ulcers: Clinical Features and Laboratory Identification Methods. New Delhi: Jaypee Brothers Medical Publishers (P) Ltd; 2008.

cells which when lined up along the dividing plane, mimic the appearance of a hypha; however, these inline individual cells are referred to as pseudohyphae. Some true hyphae may also be formed. *C. albicans* also forms blastoconidia adjacent to the "septa". These appear as smaller round "grape-like" clusters. *C. albicans* produces true germ tubes when incubated in serum for 2–3 hours at 37°C (Fig. 5.22C). Germ tubes appear as outgrowths from the side of the yeast cell. These are parallel-sided tubes which are formed at right angles to the parent cell and are at least twice as long as the parent cell before cross walls are formed. *Candida* species are susceptible to amphotericin B, voriconazole, and caspofungin.

Cryptococcus

C. neoformans and *Cryptococcus gattii* are etiologic agents of cryptococcosis. They belong to the phylum basidiomycota and can be readily distinguished from other pathogenic yeasts by the presence of a polysaccharide capsule, formation of melanin, and urease activity, which all function as virulence determinants. *C. neoformans* occurs worldwide in nature and is isolated readily from dry pigeon feces, as well as trees, soil, and other sites. The most common risk for cryptococcosis caused by *C. neoformans* is AIDS, whereas infections caused by *C. gattii* are more often reported in immunocompetent patients with undefined risk than in the immunocompromised.

Cryptococcus is transmitted to humans mainly by inhalation through the respiratory tract resulting in pulmonary lesions, but entry through the skin or gastrointestinal system by direct contact or ingestion respectively can occur.

Ocular manifestations: Most ocular cryptococcal infections are endogenous infections from a hematogenous source or by leptomeningeal spread down the optic nerve from an associated meningitis. *C. neoformans* can cause uveitis, retinitis, optic atrophy, and papilledema and neuro-ophthalmic manifestations such as cranial nerve palsies.[26]

Mycology of Cryptococcus:
Direct microscopy: Globose to ovoid budding yeast-like cells, that are typically 2–20 mm in diameter, are seen. The presence of teardrop-shaped, narrow-based budding of *C. neoformans var. neoformans* is a useful cytologic feature.

Cultural characteristics: In culture, *Cryptococcus* species produce smooth, whitish, or cream colored mucoid colonies within 2–3 days. The ability to grow at 37°C and hydrolyze urea differentiates C. *neoformans* from nonpathogenic *Cryptococcus* species. Culture smear shows globose to elongate gram-positive budding yeast-like cells or blastoconidia (5–10 mm in diameter). They are surrounded by a thick nonstaining capsule. The capsules stand out in India ink preparations. Pseudohyphae are absent or rudimentary.

Molds

Fusarium

Fusarium species are widely distributed in soil, subterranean and aerial plant parts, plant debris, and other organic matter. *Fusarium* species cause a broad spectrum of infections in humans such as keratitis and onychomycosis, as well as locally invasive and disseminated infections, particularly in immunocompromised patients. Trauma is the major predisposing factor for infection. The common *Fusarium* species include *F. solani, F. oxysporum, F. moniliforme, F. dimerum, and F. proliferatum*. In the eye, *Fusarium* species causes keratitis, scleritis, and intraocular infections. *Fusarium* keratitis may develop following the traumatic introduction of *Fusarium*-contaminated soil or plant material or due to poor hygiene practices of soft contact lens wearers. The incidence of fungal keratitis caused by *Fusarium* species is highly variable; these variable rates are probably related to climate characteristics, with tropical and subtropical areas exhibiting the highest rates.[25-28] Table 5.9 describes the microscopic and culture characteristic features of *Fusarium* species causing ocular infections (Figs. 5.23A to C). *Fusarium* species are considered resistant to amphotericin B and echinocandins. Voriconazole, isavuconazole, and posaconazole generally are more active than itraconazole against *Fusarium* species.

Aspergillus Species

Aspergillus species are hyaline filamentous fungi found ubiquitously in the environment, thriving on a variety of substrates such as corn, decaying vegetation, and soil. There are over 200 *Aspergillus* species described, of which at least 50 cause disease in humans. *Aspergillus* species may cause disseminated infections in immunocompromised patients, and may also cause a pulmonary or sinus fungus ball, allergic bronchopulmonary aspergillosis, external otomycosis, mycotic keratitis, onychomycosis, sinusitis, endocarditis, and CNS infections. These fungi are also common contaminants in hospital air.[29] The most common species in this group are *A. fumigatus, A. flavus, A. terreus,* and *A. niger*. Ocular infections include keratitis following occupational trauma or surgery, orbital lesions, dacryocystitis, scleritis, and endophthalmitis.[26] Table 5.10 describes the key characteristic feature of *Aspergillus* species causing ocular infections (Figs. 5.24A and B).

Scedosporium

Scedosporium is a common opportunistic pathogen found ubiquitously in the environment, including in soil, sewage, polluted water, and from the manure of farm animals. Two members of this genus, *Scedosporium apiospermum* and *Scedosporium prolificans*, are considered major human pathogens. Both *S. apiospermum* complex and *S. prolificans* are found distributed all over the world. Nosocomial outbreaks of *Scedosporium*

Table 5.9: Microscopic and culture characteristic features of *Fusarium* species causing ocular infection

Etiologic agent	Microscopic features				Macroscopic features
	Conidiogenous	Macroconidia	Microconidia	Chlamydospores	
F. solani	Long or short, cylindrical, simple or branched philalides	Curved, multicellular, with foot cell at the base	Unicellular or bicellular, hyaline, ovoid to ellipsoid	Present, hyaline, globose, single or pairs, smooth to rough walled	Rapid growth, mostly cream colored, occasionally blue-green, red or lavender, texture usually woolly
F. oxysporum	Short, single, monophilalides	Slightly sickle shaped, multicellular, thin walled, delicate	Non-septate, ellipsoidal to cylindrical, straight or often curved	Present, terminal or intercalary, hyaline, smooth or rough walled	Rapid growth, aerial mycelium white, becoming purple, with discrete orange sporodochia present in some strains, reverse hyaline to dark blue or dark purple

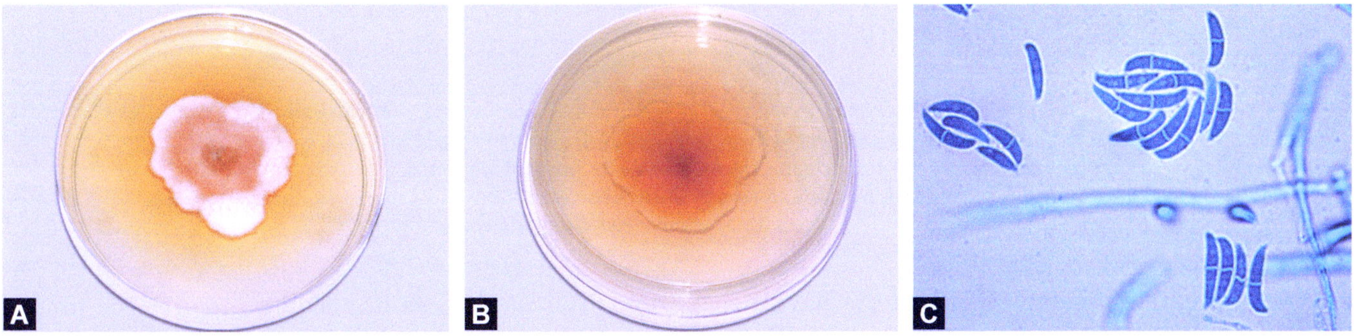

Figs. 5.23A to C: (A and B) *Fusarium* species growth on potato dextrose agar, 25°C, 5 days (A—surface; B—reverse); and (C) Macroconidium with foot cell of *Fusarium* species.

Source: Prajna L, Kumar V, Prajna NV, et al. Aravind's Atlas of Fungal Corneal Ulcers: Clinical Features and Laboratory Identification Methods. New Delhi: Jaypee Brothers Medical Publishers (P) Ltd; 2008.

Table 5.10: Key characteristic features of *Aspergillus species* causing ocular infections

Etiologic agent	Microscopic feature					Culture characteristic
	Conidial head	Phialides	Conidiophore stripes	Vesicle	Conidia	
***Aspergillus* species**						
Aspergillus flavus	Radiate	Uniseriate and biseriate	Rough walled, hyaline, yellow green	Spherical in shape, 24–45 µm in diameter	Sub-spherical, 3–5 µm in diameter, Sclerotia may be present	Yellow to dark yellowish green on surface and reverse goldish to red brown
Aspergillus fumigatus	Compactly columnar	Uniseriate	Short, smooth-walled, often green in the upper part	Subclavate, 20–30 µm wide	Sub-spherical, 2.5-3.0 µm in diameter, cleistothecia	Blue-green to gray on surface and reverse white to tan
Aspergillus terreus	Densely columnar	Biseriate	Smooth-walled hyaline, colorless	Sub-spherical, 10–20 µm in diameter	Smooth walled, spherical to broadly ellipsoidal, 1.5–2.5 µm hyaline	Cinnamon to brown on surface and reverse white to brown
Aspergillus niger	Radiate	Uniseriate and biseriate	Long smooth walled, brown to black	Spherical, 40–60 µm in diameter	Spherical to sub-spherical (3.5–5.0 µm in diameter), dark brown to black and rough walled	Black on surface and reverse white to yellow
Aspergillus nidulans	Short, columnar	Biseriate	Brownish in color	Hemispherical, 8–10 µm diameter	Spherical, rugulose, subhyaline, green in mass, Hulle cells present	Green, buff to yellow on surface and reverse purplish red to olive

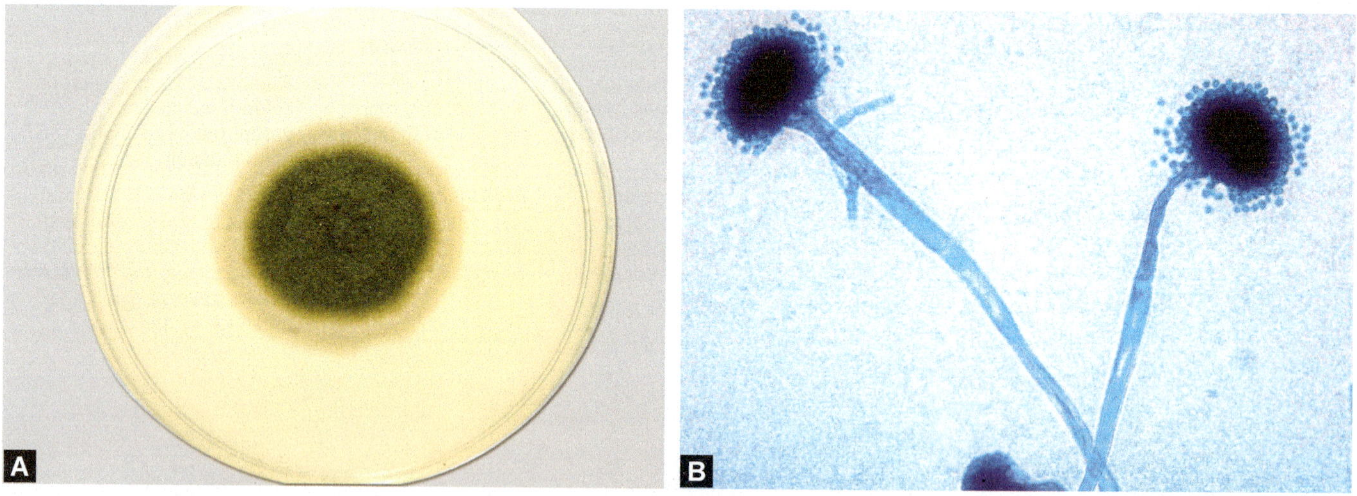

Figs. 5.24A and B: (A) *Aspergillus flavus* growth on potato dextrose agar, 25°C, 5 days; and (B) *A. flavus* conidial head supported by rough-walled conidiophores.
Source: Prajna L, Kumar V, Prajna NV, et al. Aravind's Atlas of Fungal Corneal Ulcers: Clinical Features and Laboratory Identification Methods. New Delhi: Jaypee Brothers Medical Publishers (P) Ltd; 2008.

infection in immunocompromised hosts have been linked to contaminated ambient air in hospitals. Human infection often results from inhalation of spores from the environment into the lungs or paranasal sinuses or through direct inoculation, as in a skin puncture. The fungus *S. prolificans* was first described as a human pathogen in 1984 and is reported as a cause of sclerokeratitis (Figs. 5.25A to C).[26] *Scedosporium* species are inherently resistant

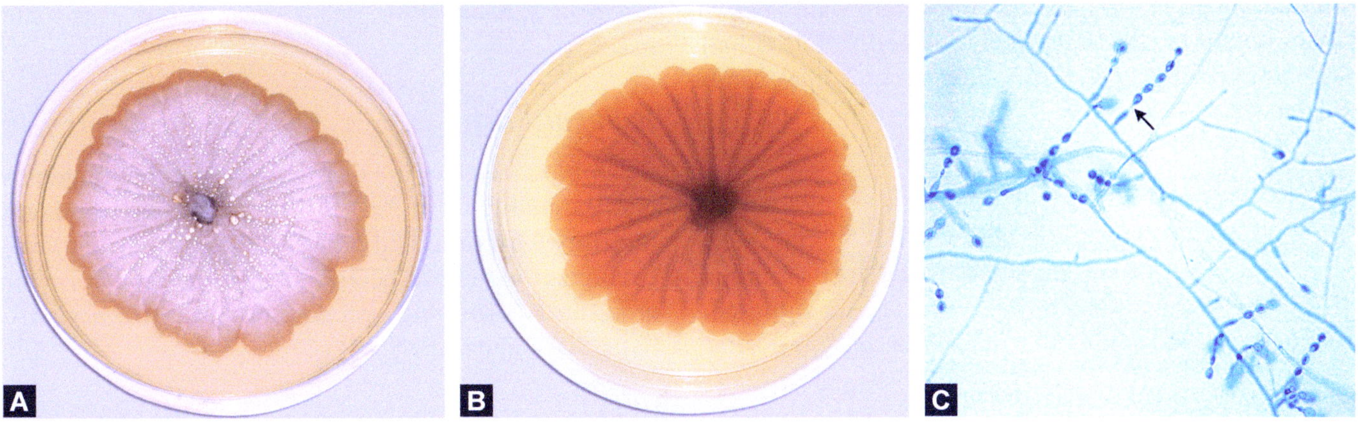

Figs. 5.25A to C: (A and B) *Scedosporium apiospermum* growth on potato dextrose agar, 25°C, 5 days (A—surface and B—reverse); and (C) *S. apiospermum* conidia at the tip of the more or elongate conidiophores (arrow).
Source: Prajna L, Kumar V, Prajna NV, et al. Aravind's Atlas of Fungal Corneal Ulcers: Clinical Features and Laboratory Identification Methods. New Delhi: Jaypee Brothers Medical Publishers (P) Ltd; 2008

to amphotericin B and, frequently, to azoles. The broad-spectrum azole voriconazole is the drug of choice for *S. apiospermum* infections.[25]

Paecilomyces

Paecilomyces species are saprophytic filamentous fungi found worldwide in soil and on decomposing plants. Occasionally airborne, this environmental mold occasionally contaminates biomaterials. *Paecilomyces* keratitis accounts for about 5% of keratomycosis in tropical and subtropical locales. While the cornea may rarely become infected by mycotic extension from the sclera or anterior chamber, *P. lilacinus* keratitis typically occurs by external invasion. It can also cause endophthalmitis. The common species in this group are *P. lilacinus and P. variotii.*[25,26]

Acremonium

Acremonium species are filamentous cosmopolitan fungi mostly isolated from plant debris, soil, and heating ventilation air conditioning systems in building materials. The common species in this group are *A. recifei, A. strictum, etc.* Infection generally occurs following abrogation of ocular defenses. Several cases of keratitis and occasional cases of endophthalmitis due to *Acremonium* species have been reported in the literature.[25,26]

Melanized Fungi (Fungi which contain Melanin)

Melanin is a ubiquitous compound found in many microbes, including fungi. Melanized fungi are those that have melanin or melanin-like pigment in the wall of their hyphae and/or spores and can cause a variety of infections in humans. The terms used to describe melanized fungi have evolved over several decades. "*Phaeo*" in Greek means "dark"; therefore, phaeohyphomycosis means infection caused by dark-walled fungi; "melanized" and "dematiaceous" are used synonymously as well, although it has been suggested that "dematiaceous" is not appropriate to describe such fungi. However, the term "dematiaceous fungi" is used very commonly in medical mycological literature and is likely to persist in nomenclature. Hence, in this chapter, the terms "dematiaceous", "dark", "phaeoid", and "melanized' are used interchangeably melanin in the cell wall is implicated as an important virulence factor. Over 150 species and 70 genera of these fungi are implicated in human and animal diseases. These group of infections though rare, are being reported increasingly, both in immunocompromised and immunocompetent settings.

The dematiaceous (brown-pigmented) fungi cause a wide range of diseases including phaeohyphomycosis, chromoblastomycosis, and eumycotic mycetoma. Among the more important human pathogens are *Alternaria* species, *Bipolaris* species, *Cladophialophora bantiana, Curvularia* species, *Exophiala* species, *Fonsecaea pedrosoi, Madurella* species, *Phialophora* species, *Scedosporium prolificans, Scytalidium dimidiatum,* and *Exophiala* (formerly *Wangiella*) *dermatitidis.* These organisms are widespread in the environment, being found in soil, wood, and decomposing plant debris. Cutaneous, subcutaneous, and corneal infections with dematiaceous fungi occur worldwide, but are more common in tropical and subtropical climates. Infection results from traumatic implantation. These fungi are important pathogens in immunocompromised patients, although individuals with apparently "normal" immune systems may also be affected.[30]

Bipolaris

Bipolaris is a large genus of dematiaceous hyphomycetes with more than 100 species, most of them being saprobes in soil and plants; some of these species infect humans and animals. The commonest species in this group are *B. spicifera, B. hawaiiensis, and B. australiensis* (Figs. 5.26A to C).[26,30]

Exserohilum

Exserohilum species are common environmental molds, often encountered in the soil, grass or rotting wood, and they thrive in warm and humid climates. They are rarely pathogenic for human beings. The common species in this group are *E. rostratum, E. longirostratum,* and *E. mcginnisii* (Figs. 5.27A and B).[26,30]

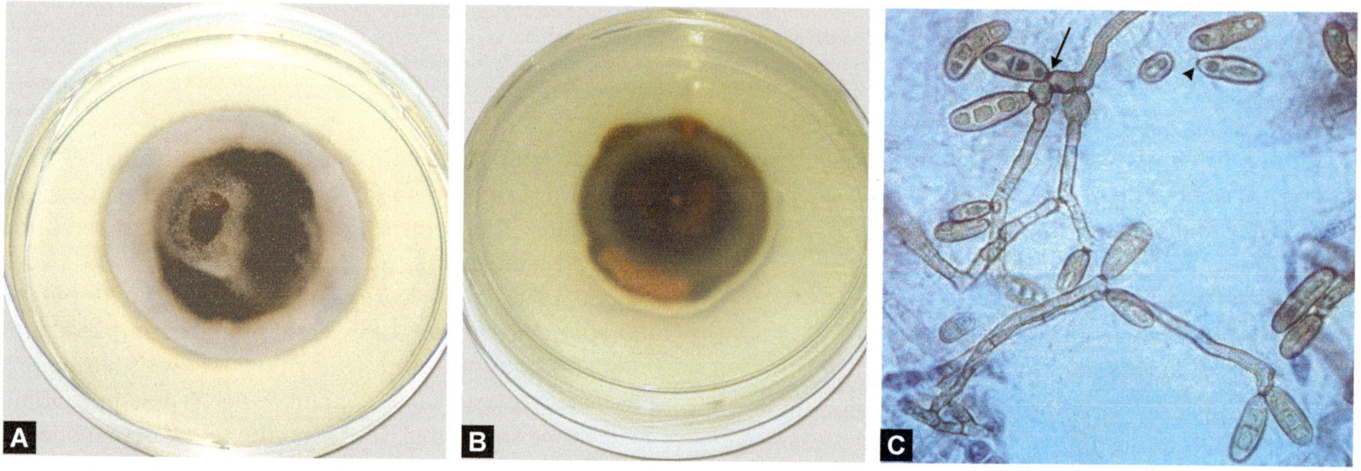

Figs. 5.26A to C: (A and B) *Bipolaris* species growth on potato dextrose agar, 25°C, 5 days (A—surface; B—reverse); and (C) *Bipolaris* species conidiophores geniculate with fusoid multiseptate conidia (arrow) scarcely protuberant hilum (arrowhead)
Source: Prajna L, Kumar V, Prajna NV, et al. Aravind's Atlas of Fungal Corneal Ulcers: Clinical Features and Laboratory Identification Methods. New Delhi: Jaypee Brothers Medical Publishers (P) Ltd; 2008.

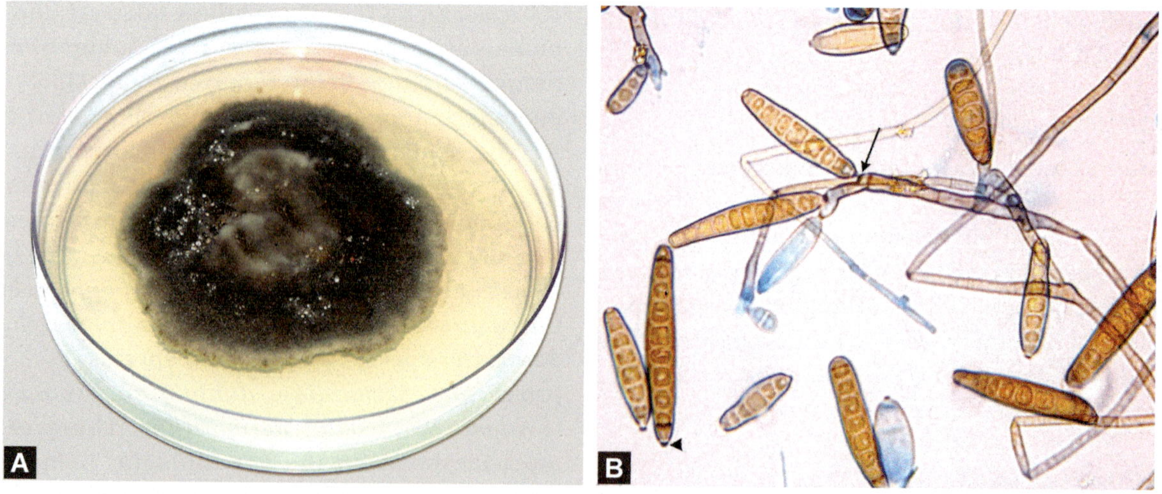

Figs. 5.27A and B: (A) *Exserohilum* species growth on potato dextrose agar, 25°C, 5 days; and (B) *Exserohilum* species geniculate conidiophores, poroconidium with protuberant hilum (arrow) and darker septa at the ends (arrowhead).
Source: Prajna L, Kumar V, Prajna NV, et al. Aravind's Atlas of Fungal Corneal Ulcers: Clinical Features and Laboratory Identification Methods. New Delhi: Jaypee Brothers Medical Publishers (P) Ltd; 2008.

Curvularia

Curvularia species are common in dead plant material and may cause a variety of human mycoses. The common species causing ocular infections in this group are *C. geniculata, C. lunata, C. senegalensis, and C. verruculosa. C. lunata* is the most common clinical species, and may produce large, upright stroma in culture that is visible with the naked eye. Infection of the cornea, reported in 1959, was the first human disease proved to be caused by *Curvularia* (Figs. 5.28A and B).[26,30]

Cladosporium

Members of the genus *Cladosporium* are dematiaceous hyphomycetes characterized by a unique coronate structure of the conidiogenous loci and conidial hila, consisting of a central convex dome surrounded by a raised periclinal rim (Figs. 5.29A to C). The genus belongs to the family Cladosporiaceae. The genus *Cladosporium* has recently has undergone molecular and morphologic scrutiny, with many organisms being reassigned to other genera. The genus is extremely ubiquitous, and although it is an agent of allergic disease in indoor settings, few species are documented to cause disease. The common species causing ocular infections in this group are *C. cladosporioides and C. oxysporum.*[26,30]

Alternaria

Alternaria is a genus of ascomycete fungi. *Alternaria* species are known as major plant pathogens. Cutaneous and subcutaneous phaeohyphomycosis in immunosuppressed individuals is the most common presentation. Ocular

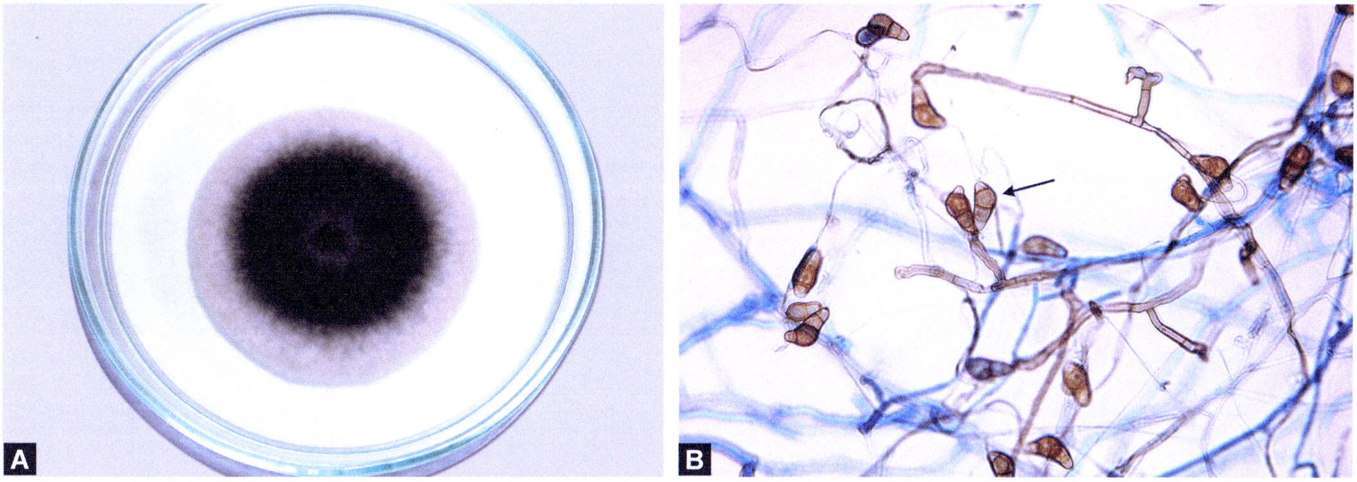

Figs. 5.28A and B: (A) *Curvularia* species growth on potato dextrose agar, 25°C, 5 days; and (B) *Curvularia* species growth curved poroconidia with larger and darker central cell (arrow).

Source: Prajna L, Kumar V, Prajna NV, et al. Aravind's Atlas of Fungal Corneal Ulcers: Clinical Features and Laboratory Identification Methods. New Delhi: Jaypee Brothers Medical Publishers (P) Ltd; 2008.

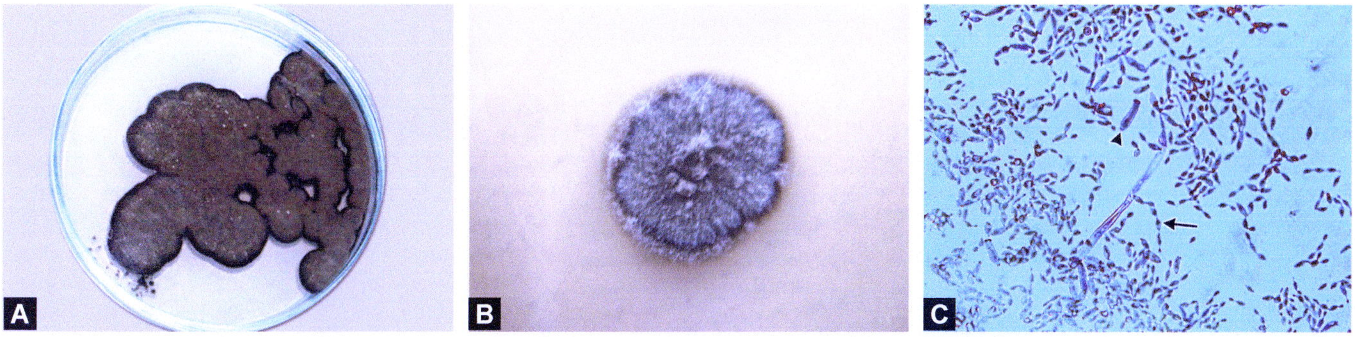

Figs. 5.29A to C: (A and B) *Cladosporium* species growth on potato dextrose agar, 25°C, 5 days; and (C) *Cladosporium* species shield-shaped conidia with scars (arrowhead) at points of attachment and (arrow) bicellular conidium.

Source: Prajna L, Kumar V, Prajna NV, et al. Aravind's Atlas of Fungal Corneal Ulcers: Clinical Features and Laboratory Identification Methods. New Delhi: Jaypee Brothers Medical Publishers (P) Ltd; 2008.

disease in individuals exposed to soil and garbage is the next most common presentation, while onychomycosis is rarely reported. *Alternaria* species, in particular *A. alternate and A. Infectoria,* are recognized as an infectious agent of subcutaneous phaeohyphomycosis and mycotic keratitis.[26,30]

Lasiodiplodia

Lasiodiplodia is a dematiaceous fungus belonging to the family Botryosphaeriaceae, subphylum Pezizomycotina of Ascomycota. It is a common plant pathogen causing rot in fruits and plants, mainly in tropical regions. Infections in human are extremely unusual and most frequently involve the eye, primarily the cornea. There are 21 species; *Lasiodiplodia theobromae* is the species implicated in human disease, affecting both immunocompetent and immunocompromised individuals. This organism was formerly known as *Botryodiplodia theobromae* (Figs. 5.30A and B).[26,30]

Mucor

Species of *Mucor* are widely distributed in the environment and frequently cause infections in plants and animals. In humans, these affect mostly immunocompromised individuals, causing infections of the skin, sinuses, and lungs. The genus *Mucor* contains about 50 recognized taxa. Recent studies have documented the increasing incidence of diabetic associated infection due to Mucormycosis. Risk factors for *Mucor* infections include solid-organ transplant recipients, renal failure, diabetes mellitus, and prior antifungal. Ocular manifestations of mucormycosis include rhino-orbito-cerebral mucormycosis and keratitis (Figs. 5.31A to C).[26,30]

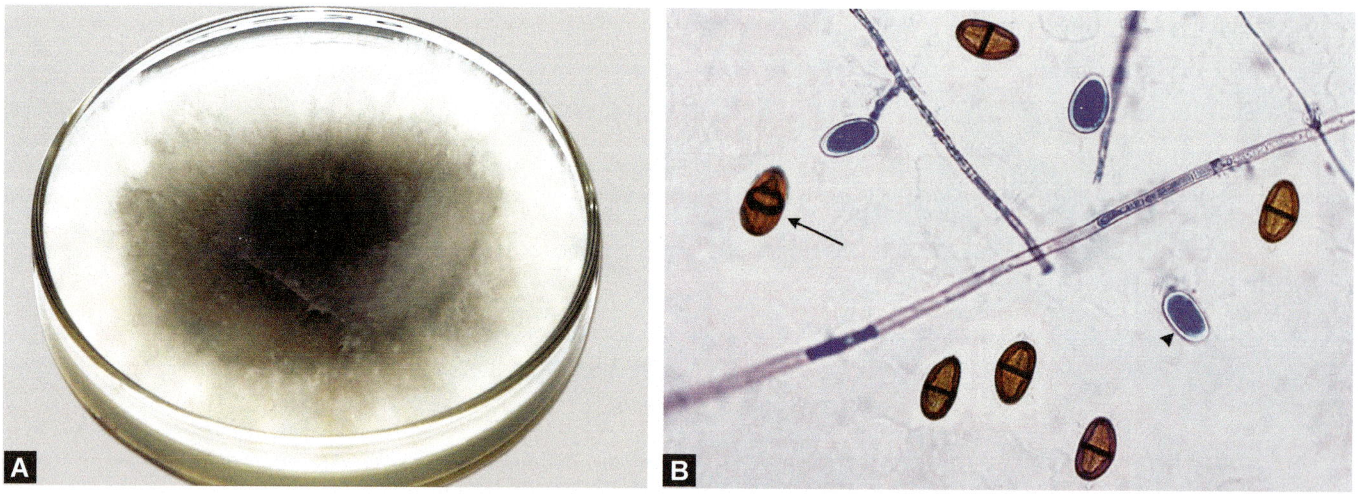

Figs. 5.30A and B: (A) *Lasiodiplodia theobromae* growth on potato dextrose agar, 25°C, 5 days; and (B) Two-celled, pigmented pycnidia and conidia of *L. theobromae.* (arrow head – Young conidia; arrow – Matured conidia)

Source: Prajna L, Kumar V, Prajna NV, et al. Aravind's Atlas of Fungal Corneal Ulcers: Clinical Features and Laboratory Identification Methods. New Delhi: Jaypee Brothers Medical Publishers (P) Ltd; 2008.

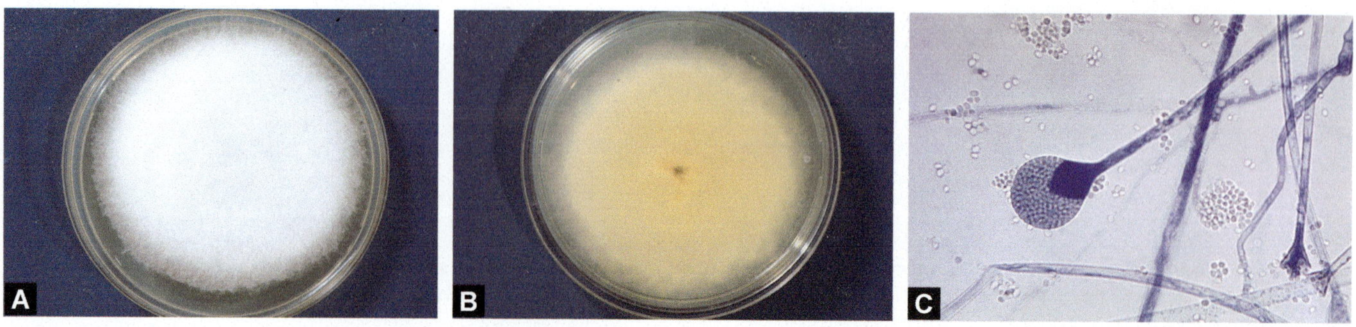

Figs. 5.31A to C: (A and B) *Mucor* species growth on potato dextrose agar, 25°C, 5 days (A—surface; B—reverse); and (C) Branching sporangiophores with a columella at the tip; the sporangia having dispersed their spores into the aqueous mounting medium.

Dimorphic Fungi

Dimorphic fungi are fungi that can exist as mold/hyphal/filamentous form or as yeast. An example is *Penicillium marneffei*, a human pathogen that grows as a mold at room temperature, and as yeast at human body temperature. Several species of dimorphic fungi are important pathogens of humans and the species that affect the eye are *Blastomyces dermatitidis, Coccidioides immitis, Histoplasma capsulatum* and *Paracoccidioides brasiliensis*. Table 5.11 describes the key characteristic feature of clinically relevant dimorphic fungi that affect the eye.

Microsporidia

Epidemiology and distribution: *Microsporidia* are diverse group of obligate intracellular parasites closely related to fungi that infect animals and cause disease in humans. Microsporidiosis in humans occurs worldwide, with prevalence rates between 0% and 50% depending on the region, method of diagnosis, and demographic characteristics of the population. Microsporidiosis has been consistently identified in patients with AIDS and additional risk factors that include poor sanitary conditions and exposure to animals.[31]

Microsporidiosis continues to be increasingly recognized in non-HIV-infected persons such as travellers, children, the elderly, and organ transplant recipients. The genotypes that infect humans have now been identified in animals, suggesting that microsporidiosis is a zoonotic disease. *Microsporidia* may spread through contact with water sources. The first case of ocular microsporidiosis was reported by Ashton and Wirashinha in 1973. Domestic animals, such as cats, may harbor the organism; hence, close contact with them may cause ocular infection.

Table 5.11: Key characteristic feature of clinically relevant dimorphic fungi.

Etiologic agent	Microscopic features (at 25–30°C)	Colony morphology (at 25–30°C)	Microscopic features (at 37°C)	Culture morphology (at 37°C)	Ocular manifestation
Blastomyces dermatitidis	Hyaline, ovoid to pyriform, one-celled, smooth-walled conidia (2–10 µm) of the *Chrysosporium* type, are borne on short lateral or terminal hyphal branches	Rapid growth, producing a fluffy white mycelium or slowly as glabrous, tan, nonsporulating colonies	Yeast cells are hyaline, smooth walled and thick walled, (8–15 µm) with the bud connected to the parent cell	Wrinkled and folded, glabrous and yeast-like	Lesion of the eyelids, cornea, conjunctiva, and orbit Intraocular lesions and endophthalmitis
Coccidioides immitis	Thin, and septate with spore producing hyphae, arthroconidia are hyaline, one celled, short, cylindrical to barrel-shaped, moderately thick and smooth walled and 2–8 µm by 3–5 µm	Moist, glabrous, and greyish to abundant, floccose, and white initially and become tan and even red			Anterior segment lesions—phlyctenular conjunctivitis, episcleritis, scleritis, and keratoconjunctivitis
Histoplasma capsulatum	Large, rounded, single-celled, 8–14 µm in diameter, tuberculate macroconidia formed on short, hyaline, undifferentiated conidiophores. Small, round to pyriform microconidia, 2–4 µm in diameter, borne on short branches or directly on the sides of the hyphae may also be present	Slow growing, white or buff-brown, suede-like to cottony with a pale yellow-brown reverse. Other colony types are glabrous or verrucose, and a red pigmented strain	Numerous small round to oval budding yeast-like cells, 3–4 × 2–3 µm in size	Smooth, moist, white, and yeast-like	Endogenous and exogenous endophthalmitis; choroiditis, retinitis and optic neuritis in patients with acquired immunodeficiency syndrome (AIDS) and anterior segment lesions are rare
Paracoccidioides brasiliensis	A variety of conidia including pyriform microconidia, chlamydospores and arthroconidia	Slow growing, colonies may be flat, wrinkled and folded, glabrous, suede-like or downy in texture, white to brownish with a tan or brown reverse	large, 20–60 µm, round, narrow base budding yeast cells, single and multiple budding occurs, the latter are thick-walled cells that form the classical "steering wheel" or "mickey mouse" structures	Colonies are white to tan, moist and glabrous and become wrinkled, folded and heaped	Lesions of eyelids, cornea and bulbar conjunctiva, anterior uveitis and granulomatous uveitis

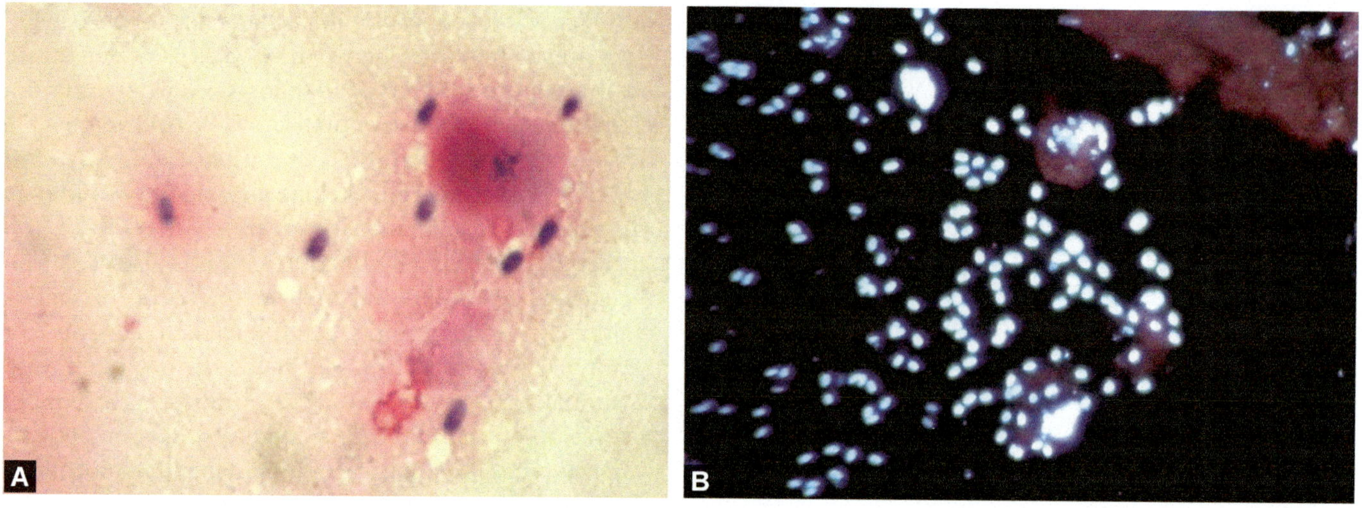

Figs. 5.32A and B: (A) Gram stain showing the intracellular gram-positive, oval, well-defined microsporidia spores with characteristic paracentral or polar dark staining; and (B) KOH/Calcofluor white stain of the corneal scraping showing oval fluorescing microsporidial spores (1,000X magnification).

Encephalitozoon and *Nosema* are the two genera that are important in ocular disease.

Morphology and life cycle: *Microsporidia* exist as single, highly organized spores that range in size from 1 mm to 40 mm. A normal unit membrane and two rigid extracellular walls bind the spore. Within the spore membrane is the sporoplasm, which is the infective material of microsporidia. The polaroplast is a large organization of membranes occupying the anterior part of the spore. The most obvious organelle associated with infection is the polar filament or the polar tube (diameter 0.1–0.2 mm). The polar filament is attached at the apex of the spore via an umbrella-shaped structure, called the anchoring disk, from which it extends to the posterior of the spore (Figs. 5.32A and B).

Ocular infection occurs either by direct inoculation of spores through contaminated water or soil, after trauma or by systemic dissemination seen in immunocompromised individuals. Ocular manifestations caused by *Microsporidia* are mainly superficial punctate keratoconjunctivitis, and corneal stromal keratitis. Keratoconjunctivitis mimicking adenoviral keratoconjunctivitis may occur especially in the rainy season.[31]

LABORATORY DIAGNOSTIC METHODS FOR OCULAR INFECTIONS

Collection and processing of clinical samples from the eye: Proper sample collection and transportation to the laboratory is the key to accurate identification. Specimens can be sent for microbiology, histopathology, or molecular diagnostic tests. Materials or scrapings for cultures should be collected as soon as possible after the onset of infection and from the actual site of the infection.[32,33] Table 5.12 describes the types of infections, specimens that are collected, specimen collection methods, and media used for culture of microorganism.

Ocular materials must be inoculated directly onto the appropriate media for optimum recovery of organisms (Figs. 5.33 and 5.34). It is ideal that the ophthalmologist collects the samples under magnification and directly inoculates onto the culture media. Vitreous and aqueous humor samples, which are collected in the operating room, must be transported to the laboratory as quickly as possible for inoculation into various media. Serum samples are rarely helpful in the diagnosis of eye infections. Some important points that must be remembered in sending samples are listed in Box 5.1.

Direct Microscopic Examination

Direct microscopy examination of ocular samples is a very rapid and inexpensive test that can provide preliminary results within a very short time so that treatment can be started. Some stains that are commonly performed are Gram stain, 10% potassium hydroxide (KOH), calcofluor, Giemsa, Ziehl-Neelsen (acid-fast), and some special stains. The sensitivity and specificity of Gram stain and 10% KOH with or without calcofluor white in the identification of bacterial and fungal filaments, respectively, are very good. This should be routinely done on specimens from

Table 5.12: Types of infections, types of specimens, specimen collection methods, and media used for culture of microorganism.

Infections	Specimens	Specimen collection device or procedure	Culture media	Expected organisms
Blepharitis	Discharge from lid margin	Sterile cotton swab	5% sheep blood agar, Thioglycollate broth, MacConkey agar, potato dextrose agar	*Staphylococcus* species, *Moraxella* species, *Phthirus pubis, Molluscum contagiosum, Herpes simplex virus*
Conjunctivitis	Conjunctival swab	Using sterile cotton swab gently swab across the lower tarsal conjunctiva	5% sheep blood agar, chocolate agar	*Staphylococcus aureus, Streptococcus* species, *Neisseria gonorrhoeae, Haemophilus influenzae, Moraxella* species, *Adenovirus, Herpes simplex virus, Chlamydia*
Canaliculitis	Expressed material	Compression of the canaliculus or incision into horizontal portion of canaliculus	5% sheep blood agar, chocolate agar, Thioglycollate broth, MacConkey agar	*Actinomycetes*
Dacryocystitis	Drainage from lacrimal sac	Pressure on the lacrimal sac is applied to drain or aspirate the specimen	5% sheep blood agar, chocolate agar, Thioglycollate broth, MacConkey agar	*Staphylococcus* species, *Streptococcus* species
Orbital cellulitis	Drainage from wound or abscess	Sterile syringe and a needle	5% sheep blood agar, chocolate agar, Thioglycollate broth, MacConkey agar	*Staphylococcus* species, *Streptococcus* species
Endophthalmitis	Anterior chamber fluid, vitreous aspirate, vitreous biopsy	Paracentesis (anterior chamber tap) with tuberculin syringe	5% sheep blood agar, chocolate agar, Thioglycollate broth, brain heart infusion broth, potato dextrose agar	*Staphylococcus epidermidis, Bacillus* species, very rarely GNB, *Fusarium* species, *Aspergillus* species
Keratitis	Corneal scraping	Sterile Kimura spatula, No. 15 surgical blade, bent needle	5% sheep blood agar, chocolate agar, potato dextrose agar	*Streptococcus pneumoniae, Pseudomonas aeruginosa, Fusarium* species, *Aspergillus flavus, Acanthamoeba, Microsporidia*

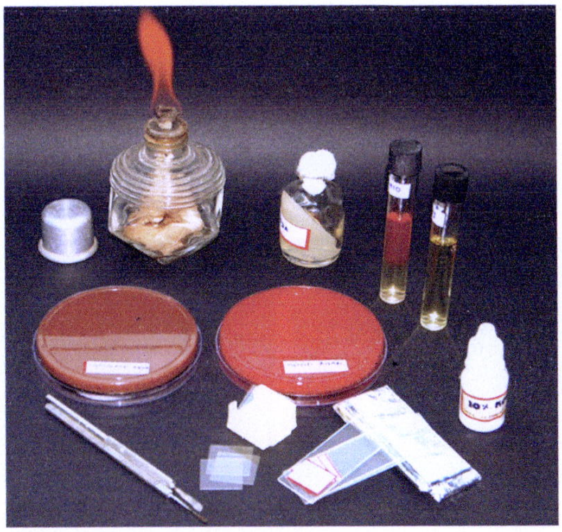

Fig. 5.33: Materials used for collecting specimens from corneal ulcers.

Source: Prajna L, Kumar V, Prajna NV, et al. Aravind's Atlas of Fungal Corneal Ulcers: Clinical Features and Laboratory Identification Methods. New Delhi: Jaypee Brothers Medical Publishers (P) Ltd; 2008.

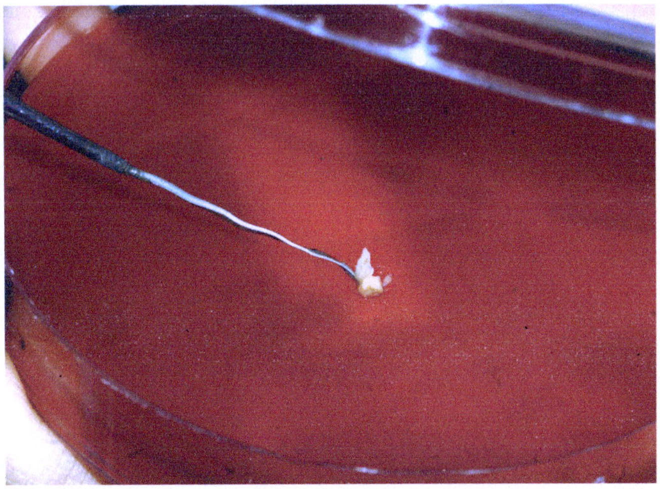

Fig. 5.34: Corneal scraped material inoculated on blood agar in multiple "C" streak form.

Source: Prajna L, Kumar V, Prajna NV, et al. Aravind's Atlas of Fungal Corneal Ulcers: Clinical Features and Laboratory Identification Methods. New Delhi: Jaypee Brothers Medical Publishers (P) Ltd; 2008.

Box 5.1: Important points that must be remembered in sending samples.

- For corneal ulcers, direct inoculation into the culture media is very important for optimum recovery of organisms
- Fastidious organisms like *Streptococcus pneumonia* may not withstand transportation
- As ocular sample volume is very limited, it may dry out during transportation
- A microbiology collection set comprising of clean slides and required medias can be stored in the ophthalmologist office for quick collection and inoculation
- Sample collection for detection of parasites and viruses require special procedures
- Samples such as corneal buttons/biopsies, eviscerated contents, or any other tissues can also be tested and correlated with the clinical diagnosis
- Samples for molecular diagnosis with polymerase chain reaction (PCR) should be transported in sterile phosphate buffered saline in an ice pack. In the laboratory if testing will be delayed samples must be stored at –20°C

conjunctivitis, keratitis, and endophthalmitis. Gram stain is the most commonly used stain that demonstrates the presence of bacteria, fungi, and parasites (Figs. 5.35A to H). Table 5.13 lists the different types of stains used in ocular microbiology.[34]

Culture Techniques

Processing for culture involves inoculation of the sample on appropriate culture media. Prior knowledge of expected organisms helps in determining the type of media to be included. Most samples are processed for isolation of bacteria and fungi. Fungi associated with eye infections are usually fast growing saprobes that can grow on media, such as blood and chocolate agar, traditionally meant for bacteria. Non-nutrient agar with *E. coli* overlay must be used for isolating *Acanthamoeba* (Figs. 5.36A to F).

All media are incubated at 37°C except Sabouraud dextrose agar, which requires 25–27°C [biochemical oxygen demand (BOD) incubator]. Media are examined for growth daily and are incubated for 1–2 weeks before discarding. Bacteria such as *Nocardia* species and *atypical* NTM, as well as *Acanthamoeba* species, grow slowly and require prolonged incubation.

Bacterial and fungal colonies are examined with the naked eye, whereas *Acanthamoeba* has to be observed under a microscope and the presence of trophozoites is looked for in the vicinity of the inoculation mark on the surface of the medium. *Acanthamoeba* forms no colonies.

For culture of ocular samples for viruses the sample must be transported to the laboratory in a viral transport medium, such as Hank's balanced salt solution. Samples for viral culture are processed using cell line like HeLa, Vero, HEp 2, MRC-5, etc. These cell lines have been used for isolation of HSV from corneal scrapings and other ocular samples.

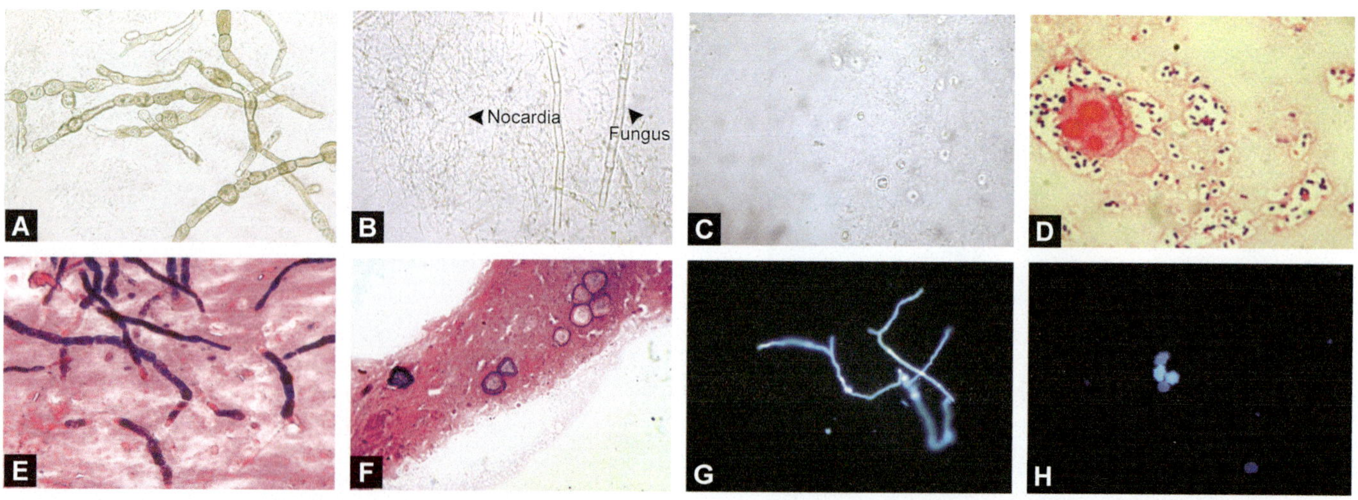

Figs. 5.35A to H: (A) Pigmented, septate fungal filaments in 10% KOH wet mount of corneal scrapings (400X magnification); (B) A 10% KOH wet mount showing hyaline septate fungal filaments and thin *Nocardia* filaments (400X magnification); (C) A 10% KOH wet mount showing double-walled cyst of *Acanthamoeba* species (400X magnification); (D) Gram stain showing capsulated gram-positive cocci in pairs suggestive of *Streptococcus pneumoniae* from corneal scraping (1,000X magnification); (E) Gram stain showing branching fungal filaments from corneal scraping (1,000X magnification); (F) Gram stain showing the double walled, polygonal *Acanthamoeba* cyst; (G) Blue white fluorescence of fungal hyphae of corneal scraping in KOH Calcofluor white staining (200X magnification); and (H) KOH Calcofluor white stain showing cyst of *Acanthamoeba* species under fluorescent microscope (200X magnification).

Table 5.13: Direct smear examination methods used for the diagnosis of ocular infections.

Type of specimens	Type of staining method performed	Type of organisms to be detected
Conjunctival swab/scraping	Gram stain, Giemsa stain, Calcofluor white stain	Bacteria, fungi, and parasites (microsporidia)
Aqueous/vitreous fluid	Gram stain, Giemsa stain, Calcofluor white stain	Bacteria and fungi
Corneal scraping	Gram stain, Giemsa stain, Calcofluor white stain, 1% acid-fast stain	Bacteria, fungi, parasites (*Acanthamoeba* and microsporidia), and *Nocardia* species

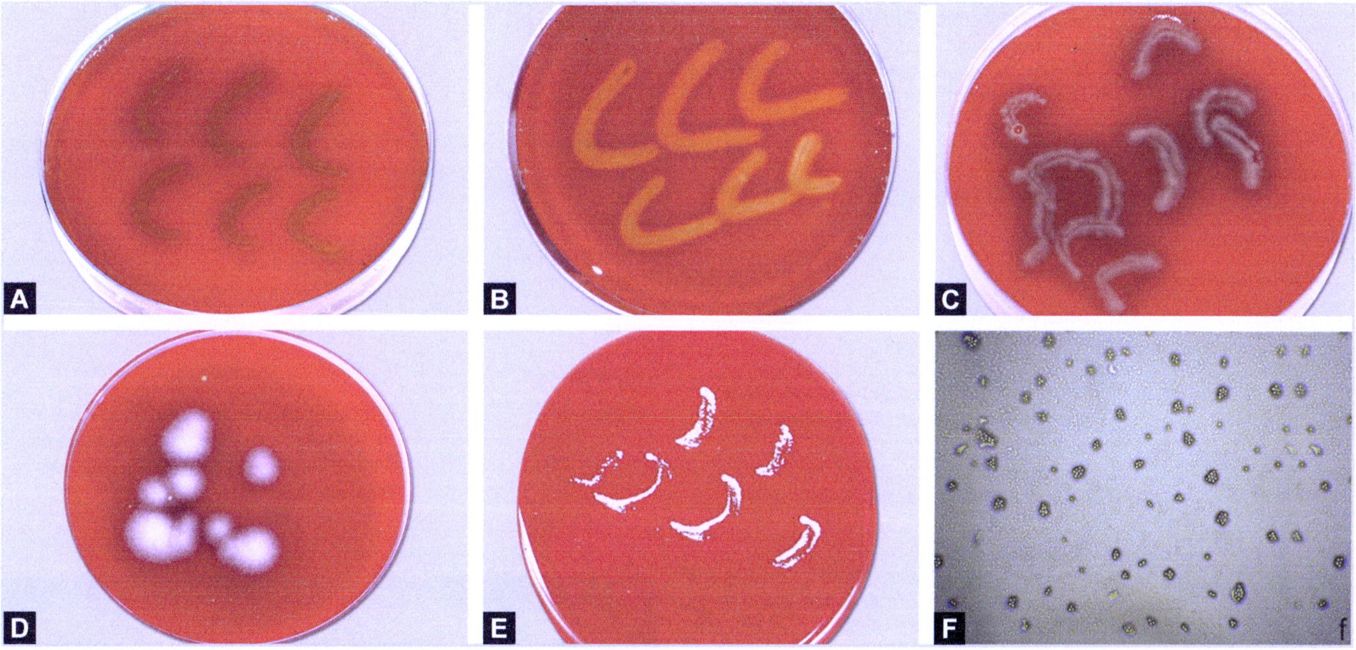

Figs. 5.36A to F: (A) A significant growth of alpha-hemolytic colony of *Streptococcus pneumoniae* growth on 5% sheep blood agar; (B) A significant growth of β-hemolytic colony of *Staphylococcus aureus* growth on 5% sheep blood agar; (C) A significant growth of *Pseudomonas aeruginosa* was seen in culture on blood agar of the corneal scraping; (D) A significant growth of *Fusarium* species was seen in culture on blood agar of the corneal scarping; (E) *Nocardia* species growth on multiple "C" streak of corneal scraping material; and (F) *Acanthamoeba* cyst (400X) growth on non-nutrient agar plates.

Laboratory criteria for identification:

The growth of bacteria or fungus in culture is considered significant if:

- The growth is confluent (more than 10 colonies) on the site of inoculation on solid media or
- The organism was seen in the smears, or
- The same organism was grown in more than one medium.

Antibiotic Susceptibility Testing

Antibiotic susceptibility testing is done according to the Clinical and Laboratory Standard Institute (CLSI) guidelines which are updated annually.[35] The antibiotics that are routinely tested for ocular infections are listed in Table 5.14. By doing susceptibility tests, the most effective antibiotics that can be used for an ocular infection can be determined. Susceptibility testing can be done by several methods such as broth microdilution, disk diffusion, and automated methods. Although, automated methods are more commonly used nowadays, disk diffusion testing is still preferred for its low cost, flexibility, and the ease for testing new antibiotics.

In the disk diffusion testing method, paper disks impregnated with the antibiotic are placed on the agar surface inoculated with a culture of the organism to be tested and the zone of inhibition around the disk is read (Fig. 5.37). All antibiotics that are available and used routinely for ocular infections must be tested. Some antimicrobials, such as chloramphenicol, polymyxin B, bacitracin, and neomycin are no longer tested routinely, but they remain important ocular therapeutic agents.

Minimum inhibitory concentration (MIC) provides a measure of the activity of an antimicrobial agent against

Table 5.14: List of antibacterial agents routinely used for susceptibility testing of ocular isolates.

Name of the antibacterial agents	Testing organisms
Aminoglycosides	
Amikacin	*Pseudomonas* species, other gram-negative bacteria, *Nocardia* species and atypical *mycobacterium*
Gentamicin Tobramycin	*Pseudomonas* species, other gram-negative bacteria, *Staphylococcus* species, *Nocardia* species, *Corynebacterium* species and atypical *Mycobacterium*
Carbapenem	
Imipenem	*Pseudomonas* species, other gram-negative bacteria
Cephalosporin	
1st generation:	
Cefazolin	*Staphylococcus* species, *Streptococcus* species, *Nocardia* species, *Corynebacterium* species, all gram-negative bacteria except *Pseudomonas* species and atypical *Mycobacterium*
2nd generation:	
Cefuroxime	All gram-positive bacteria
3rd generation:	
Cefotaxime	*Pseudomonas* species, other gram-negative bacteria, *Staphylococcus* species, *Nocardia* species, *Corynebacterium* species and atypical *mycobacteria*
Ceftazidime	*Pseudomonas* species, other gram-negative bacteria, *Nocardia* species and atypical *Mycobacterium*
Glycopeptides	
Vancomycin	*Staphylococcus* species, *Streptococcus* species, *Nocardia* species, and *Corynebacterium* species
Penicillin	
Ampicillin	*Haemophilus* species
Oxacillin	*Staphylococcus* species and *Streptococcus* species
Penicillin G	*Streptococcus* species
Penicillin combination	
Piperacillin/tazobactam	All gram-negative bacteria
Polypeptides	
Polymyxin B	All gram-negative bacteria
Quinolones/Fluoroquinolones	
2nd generation:	
Ciprofloxacin	All gram-positive, gram-negative bacteria and atypical *Mycobacterium*
Norfloxacin	All gram-negative bacteria (tested against urine isolates)
Ofloxacin	All gram-positive, gram-negative bacteria and atypical *mycobacterium*
3rd generation:	
Levofloxacin	All gram-positive and gram-negative bacteria
4th generation:	
Gatifloxacin Moxifloxacin	All gram-positive, gram-negative bacteria and atypical *mycobacterium*
Sulfonamides	
Trimethoprim-Sulfamethoxazole (Co-trimoxazole) (TMP-SMX)	*Nocardia* species
Tetracyclines	
Tetracycline	All gram-positive and gram-negative bacteria except *Pseudomonas* species, *Corynebacterium* species and atypical *Mycobacterium*

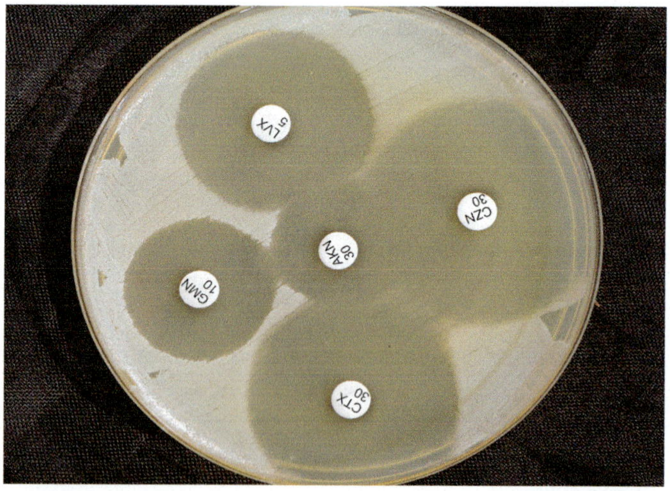

Fig. 5.37: Zone of inhibition obtained on Mueller-Hinton agar against commonly tested antibiotics.

an organism. It is defined as the lowest concentration that will inhibit the growth of a test organisms over a defined interval related to the organism's growth rate, most commonly 18–24 hours. The results can be obtained for a range of antibiotic concentrations. Interpretation of MIC data is confusing to many clinicians and laboratories must include interpretative data along with the report.

Susceptibility testing against antifungal drugs is performed for yeasts and filamentous fungi by broth or agar dilution methods, where MIC is determined, and by disk diffusion method. Drugs commonly tested include 5FC (flucytosine), ketoconazole, miconazole, fluconazole, itraconazole, and amphotericin B; more recently, voriconazole is also tested.

One important point to remember when performing antibiotic susceptibility testing on ocular isolates is that the disks only reflect the usually obtainable serum concentrations and not the higher levels obtainable within the tear film or cornea or intraocular milieu. Therefore, organisms reported as resistant may be susceptible in the ophthalmic setting. The organisms may still be killed by topical antibiotic due to the high drug levels achieved with frequent topical applications. Also, in infectious microbial keratitis, fortified antibiotic eye drops are used and sensitivity testing does not take into account the antibiotic levels obtainable. Hence, a clinical correlation is very important and should also be kept in mind in tandem with the laboratory reports for continuing or altering the existing therapeutic regimen.

Molecular Diagnostic Tests in Ocular Infections

Introduction: The confirmation of any ocular infection relies on microbiology identification of the causative organism. Although, cultures are still considered the gold standard, there are some limitation to the conventional culture techniques mainly, low sensitivity, time required to grow, and difficulty in culturing fastidious organisms like *Acanthamoeba* and viruses.

Molecular diagnostic tests can be used to overcome some of these limitations. The PCR is a molecular technique that is used for detection and analysis of specific DNA sequences. This technique has a very significant utility in the diagnosis of various ocular infectious like toxoplasmosis, various viruses, bacteria, or fungi involving both the anterior and posterior segment. With recent technical advances, as well as increased scope of application, PCR has become a useful tool in the clinic for diagnosis of ocular infectious disease. It has helped in changing the clinical treatment on the basis of PCR testing. It is now considered a gold standard especially for diagnosing ocular tuberculosis. This section describes the principle, various types of PCR that are available, application of PCR in infectious ocular diseases, and advantages and disadvantages.[36,37]

Polymerase chain reaction: Polymerase chain reaction is an in vitro enzymatic method of amplifying specific nucleic acid sequences of DNA or RNA. First described by Saiki et al. in 1985, the technique was perfected by Kary Mullis, who was awarded the Nobel Prize in 1993 in recognition of the impact of this technology on the scientific community. The concept of the PCR relies upon the repeated synthesis of the targeted DNA by DNA polymerase enzyme. In PCR reaction, two short DNA oligonucleotides complementary to the sequence in the organism of interest are used to amplify the intervening DNA using a thermostable DNA polymerase. The resulting DNA fragment may be analyzed by gel electrophoresis to document the presence of DNA from the suspected pathogen or sequenced to confirm its presence.[38] A basic PCR setup requires several components and reagents, and is described in Box 5.2.

Step in a polymerase chain reaction: The PCR cycle consist of three basic steps in one amplification cycles i.e. denaturation (melting), annealing, and polymerization (extension) (Fig. 5.38).

Denaturation—melting of desired deoxyribonucleic acid: In the first step, the target DNA containing sequence (between 100 bases and 5,000 bases) to be amplified is heat denatured (95°C for 15 seconds) to separate complementary strands. This process is called melting of desired DNA. After separation each strands acts as a template for subsequent DNA synthesis.

Primer annealing: The second step is the annealing (binding) of two oligonucleotide primers to the denatured DNA strands. Since, the nucleotide sequence of each oligonucleotide primer is complementary to 3' end of single stranded template, the primer anneals (hybridize) the each template. The reaction temperature is lowered to 50–65°C for 20–40 seconds. Consequently the primers form hydrogen bonds that anneals to the DNA on both sides of the DNA sequence.

Primer extension (polymerization): Finally, nucleoside triphosphate (dATP, dTTP, dGTP, and dCTP) and thermostable DNA polymerases are added to the reaction mixture. The enzyme DNA polymerase accelerates the polymerization process of primers and extends the primers

Box 5.2: Polymerase chain reaction components

- Template DNA
- Primers (Forward and reverse)
- dNTPs (dATP, dTTP, dCTP, and dGTP)
- Taq DNA polymerase enzyme
- $MgCl_2$
- PCR buffer, pH 8

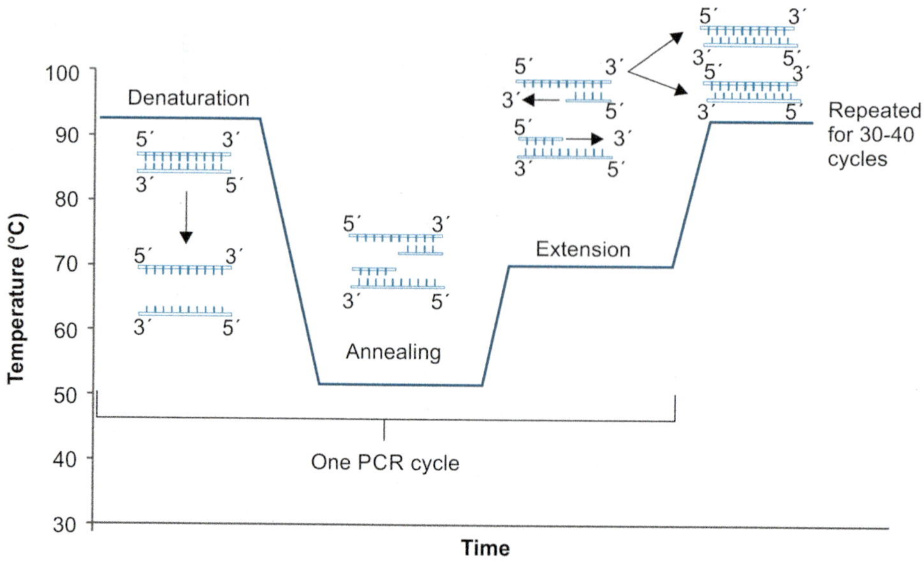

Fig. 5.38: Schematic diagram of polymerase chain reaction profile. (PCR: Polymerase chain reaction)

at 68°C resulting in synthesis of copies of the desired DNA sequences.

Types of polymerase chain reaction: Several modifications of PCR methods have been developed to enhance the utility of this method in diagnostic settings based on their applications. Some of the common types of PCR are uniplex PCR, multiplex PCR, nested PCR, and real-time PCR.

The *NAATs* generally are uniplex PCR, nested PCR, real-time reverse transcription PCR (RT-PCR), and RT loop-mediated isothermal gene amplification (RT-LAMP) assays. NAAT is usually followed by post amplification analysis such as DNA sequencing, pyrosequencing, melt curve analysis, and single strand conformation polymorphism to identify the organism at the species level.

Monoplex or uniplex assays amplify a single target region in the given DNA sample and help in rapid identification of the pathogen. Generally, the primers are designed to amplify the ribosomal DNA and internal transcribed spacer (ITS) regions or a specific gene target unique for the pathogen.

In a multiplex PCR, more than one target region is amplified in a single assay using different sets of primers. The different products could be identified based on their size in an electrophoretogram. These assays can detect multiple organisms simultaneously, but the interactions between the primers need to be validated, which may otherwise lead to nonspecific amplifications.

In a nested PCR reaction, the PCR product from the first reaction (uniplex PCR) is used as a template for a subsequent PCR reaction. Two sets of primers are used in a nested PCR reaction, where one set is nested within the other set of primers. The technique is more specific and sensitive, and particularly suited for ocular infections where we expect the DNA sample to be very small.

Real-time polymerase chain reaction: This technique of PCR is used to quantify the amount of genomes of a pathogen in a given sample. Low level of genomes of a pathogen in a given sample may indicate decreased presence of that particular pathogen. Thus this may help to differentiate between active infection and latent infections to quantify the mount of pathogens. PCR is performed in a thermocycler provided with real-time fluorescence detection unit in each well. In molecular biology it is also known as quantitative real-time PCR (Q-PCR/q PCR) or kinetic PCR.[37]

Applications of Polymerase Chain Reaction in the Diagnosis of Ocular Infections (Anterior and Posterior Segment Infections)

- *Polymerase chain reaction in the diagnosis of infectious keratitis and conjunctivitis*:
  - Polymerase chain reaction can be used in the diagnosis of infective keratitis and may help in differentiating bacterial and fungal organisms more rapidly than cultures. It is important to remember when testing for bacteria and fungi, normal flora

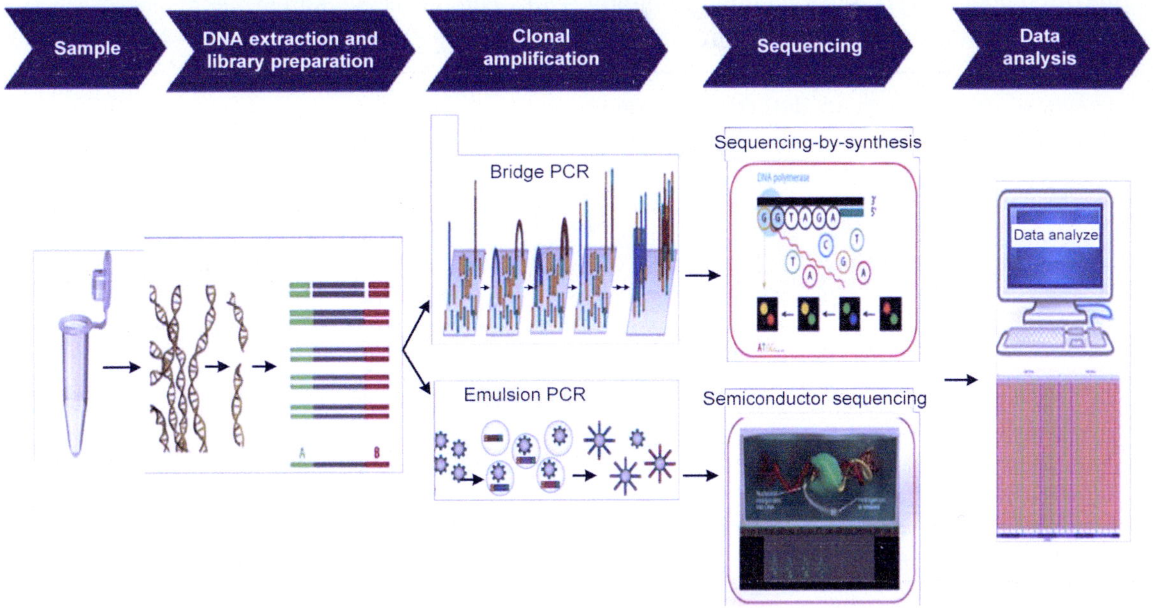

Fig. 5.39: Schematic workflow of next generation sequencing analysis.
(DNA: Deoxyribonucleic acid; PCR: Polymerase chain reaction)

will also be amplified and give false positive results. PCR for *Acanthamoeba* keratitis has demonstrated a much higher sensitivity than direct microscopy and culture in making the diagnosis of *Acanthamoeba* keratitis.

- Viral infections of the ocular surface, such as conjunctivitis and keratitis, are usually diagnosed clinically. But, in cases where a laboratory diagnosis is needed then PCR-based tests are very useful with high sensitivity and specificity. Multiplex PCR are available for the detection of adenovirus, HSV, and *C. trachomatis*.[36]

- *Polymerase chain reaction in the diagnosis of uveitis and endophthalmitis:* Polymerase chain reaction for posterior segment disease is often used to confirm the clinical diagnosis, such as, viral retinitis, ocular toxoplasmosis, tuberculosis, bacterial, and fungal endophthalmitis. Posterior segment uveitis of viral etiology was the initial condition where PCR was first used in ophthalmic disease. Since that time, the use of PCR for diagnosis has become a relatively routine test. A small sample of aqueous (as little as 10 μl) from the anterior chamber can be used to detect HSV, VZV, CMV, and *T. gondii* DNA. Additionally quantitative PCR may be useful in monitoring disease and treatment response.[36] The advantages and disadvantages of PCR as a diagnostic tool are listed in Table 5.15.

Table 5.15: Advantages and disadvantages of polymerase chain reaction

Advantages	Disadvantages
Very sensitive technique	High rate of false negatives
Highly specific	Requires skill
Rapid and accurate diagnosis	Expensive and not easily available
Defined, easy-to-follow protocols	Chance of laboratory contamination
Required small quantity of specimen	PCR can detect DNA of dead colonizing normal flora of the conjunctiva

- *Future direction: next generation sequencing (Fig. 5.39):* One drawback of current PCR techniques is the necessity of knowing the infecting organism. PCR cannot identify unexpected and unknown organisms in the way that culture can. Apart from PCR techniques, recent developments of techniques like next generation sequencing (NGS) or deep sequencing is a DNA sequencing technology which has revolutionized genomic research. Deep DNA sequencing for pathogen detection allows detection of all foreign DNA within a sample, and may allow discovery of novel pathogens.[39]

Such techniques will likely expand the range of molecular biology in the diagnosis of ocular inflammatory and infectious disease in the future. The main utility of NGS in clinical microbiology is to replace conventional characterization of pathogens by morphology, staining properties, and metabolic criteria with a genomic definition of pathogens. NGS technology has wide potential. In ophthalmology, NGS technology apart from infectious diseases has lots of applications in detection of novel mutations in various genetic and cancer-related diseases.

REFERENCES

1. Topley WWC. Topley and Wilson's Microbiology and Microbial Infections, 10th edition. London; New York: Wiley-Blackwell; 2007.
2. Moorthy RS, Valluri S, Rao NA. Nontuberculous mycobacterial ocular and adnexal infections. Surv Ophthalmol. 2012;57:202-35.
3. Goyal JL, Jain P, Arora R, et al. Ocular manifestations of tuberculosis. Indian J Tuberc. 2015;62:66-73.
4. Dunn JJ, Starke JR, Revell PA. Laboratory Diagnosis of Mycobacterium Tuberculosis Infection and Disease in Children. J Clin Microbiol. 2016;54:1434-41.
5. Hooppaw AJ, Fisher DJ. A Coming of Age Story: Chlamydia in the Post-Genetic Era. Infect Immun. 2015;84:612-21.
6. Domeika M, Savicheva A, Sokolovskiy E, et al. Guidelines for the laboratory diagnosis of Chlamydia trachomatis infections in East European countries. J Eur Acad Dermatol Venereol. 2009;23:1353-63.
7. Davis JL. Ocular syphilis. Curr Opin Ophthalmol. 2014;25:513-8.
8. Rathinam SR. Ocular leptospirosis. Curr Opin Ophthalmol. 2002;13:381-6.
9. Mikkilä HO, Seppälä IJ, Viljanen MK, et al. The expanding clinical spectrum of ocular lymeborreliosis. Ophthalmology. 2000;107:581-7.
10. Knipe DM, Howley PM. Fields Virology, 5th edition. Philadelphia: Lippincott Williams & Wilkins; 2006.
11. Rafailidis PI, Mourtzoukou EG, Varbobitis IC, et al. Severe cytomegalovirus infection in apparently immunocompetent patients: a systematic review. Virol J. 2008;5:47.
12. Lee JH, Agarwal A, Mahendradas P, et al. Viral posterioruveitis. Surv Ophthalmol. 2017;62:404-45.
13. Mahendradas P, Ranganna SK, Shetty R, et al. Ocular manifestations associated with chikungunya. Ophthalmology. 2008;115:287-91.
14. de Paula Freitas B, de Oliveira Dias JR, Prazeres J, et al. Ocular Findings in Infants With Microcephaly Associated with Presumed Zika Virus Congenital Infection in Salvador, Brazil. JAMA Ophthalmol. 2016.
15. Ventura CV, Maia M, Bravo-Filho V, et al. Zika virus in Brazil and macular atrophy in a child with microcephaly. Lancet. 2016;387:228.
16. Shantha JG, Yeh S, Nguyen QD. Ebola virus disease and the eye. Curr Opin Ophthalmol. 2016;27:538-44.
17. Lorenzo-Morales J, Martín-Navarro CM, López-Arencibia A, et al. Acanthamoeba keratitis: an emerging disease gathering importance worldwide? Trends Parasitol. 2013;29:181-7.
18. Illingworth CD, Cook SD. Acanthamoeba keratitis. Surv Ophthalmol. 1998;42:493-508.
19. Lim SJ, Lee SE, Kim SH, et al. Prevalence of Toxoplasma gondii and Toxocaracanis among patients with uveitis. Ocul Immunol Inflamm. 2014;22:360-6.
20. Dubey JP, Lindsay DS, Speer CA. Structures of Toxoplasma gondiitachyzoites, bradyzoites, and sporozoites and biology and development of tissue cysts. Clin Microbiol Rev. 1998;11:267-99.
21. Padhi TR, Das S, Sharma S, et al. Ocular parasitoses: A comprehensive review. Surv Ophthalmol. 2017;62:161-89.
22. Otranto D, Eberhard ML. Zoonotic helminths affecting the human eye. Parasit Vectors. 2011;4:41.
23. Nimir AR, Saliem A, Ibrahim IA. Ophthalmic parasitosis: a review article. Interdiscip Perspect Infect Dis. 2012; 2012:587402.
24. Rathinam SR, Usha KR, Rao NA. Presumed trematode-induced granulomatous anterior uveitis: a newly recognized cause of intraocular inflammation in children from south India. Am J Ophthalmol. 2002;133:773-9.
25. Versalovic J, Carroll KC, Funke G, et al. Manual of Clinical Microbiology, 10th edition. Washington, DC: ASM Press; 2011.
26. Thomas PA. Current perspectives on ophthalmic mycoses. Clin Microbiol Rev. 2003;16:730-97.
27. Diepeningen AD van, Al-Hatmi AMS, Brankovics B, et al. Taxonomy and Clinical Spectra of Fusarium Species: Where Do We Stand in 2014? Curr Clin Micro Rpt. 2014;1:10-8.
28. Larone DH. Medically Important Fungi: A Guide to Identification, 2nd edition. Washington, DC: American Society of Microbiology; 1986.
29. Richardson MD, Kokki M. Aspergillus. In: Annaissie EJ, McGinnis MR, Pfaller MA (Eds). Clinical Mycology. New York: Churchill Livingstone; 2003. p. 273.
30. Revankar SG, Sutton DA. Melanized fungi in human disease. Clin Microbiol Rev. 2010;23:884-928.
31. Sharma S, Das S, Joseph J, et al. Microsporidial keratitis: need for increased awareness. Surv Ophthalmol. 2011; 56:1-22.
32. Byrne KA, Burd E, Tabbara K, et al. Diagnostic microbiology and cytology of the eye. Boston: Butterworth-Heinemann; 1995.
33. Specter S. Laboratory diagnosis of ocular infections. Washington, DC: American Society for Microbiology; 1994.
34. Sharma S. Diagnosis of infectious diseases of the eye. Eye (Lond). 2012;26:177-84.
35. CLSI. Performance Standards for Antimicrobial Susceptibility Testing, 27th edition. CLSI supplement M100. Wayne, PA: Clinical and Laboratory Standards Institute; 2017.
36. Taravati P, Lam D, Van Gelder RN. Role of molecular diagnostics in ocular microbiology. Curr Ophthalmol Rep. 2013;1(4):10.
37. Yeung SN, Butler A, Mackenzie PJ. Applications of the polymerase chain reaction in clinical ophthalmology. Can J Ophthalmol. 2009;44:23-30.
38. Saiki RK, Gelfand DH, Stoffel S, et al. Primer-directedenzymatic amplification of DNA with a thermostable DNA polymerase. Science. 1988;239:487-91.
39. Behjati S, Tarpey PS. What is next generation sequencing? Arch Dis Child Educ Pract Ed. 2013;98:236-8.

Chapter 6 Immunology of the Eye

K Dharmalingam

The immune system of eukaryotes is a highly evolved multicellular and multifactor system of defense that recognizes foreign invaders and antigens. The immune system differentiates the self-antigens (from that of the host) and avoids development of immune response against them. This self versus non-self recognition is the hallmark of vertebrate immunity. Under normal conditions, the immune response elicited against foreign antigens returns to basal level once the antigen is cleared. Because of this, excess damage to the host tissue is prevented from an exuberant immune response. This dual requirement of defense against foreign antigens and at the same avoiding undue destruction of self-tissue makes this system one of the highly regulated processes in humans. This mutually exclusive and paradoxical immune equilibrium is well-studied in the immune regulation of the eye. The downmodulation of the immune functions in the eye is a unique property and is called as "immune privilege." Immune privilege is essential to keep the immune-mediated damage to the eye tissues to a minimum in order to keep the visual axis completely free of obstruction due to the damaged cells. At the same time, the defense functions of the immune system are not compromised in the eye. The eye being an organ that processes more than 70% of the information reaching the brain, the importance of immune privilege and prevention of self-destruction is of paramount importance. Surprisingly even with this limitation imposed by immune privilege, most infections of the eye are easily controlled by our immune system.

OVERVIEW OF VERTEBRATE IMMUNITY

Immune system in vertebrates is classically divided into two arms, namely innate immunity and adaptive immunity. Innate immunity, also called as natural immunity, exists in the host even before the encounter of foreign antigens or pathogens. This type of immunity includes immune barriers such as physical barriers, cellular defense systems mediated by phagocytes and dendritic cells, NK cells, complement system, immunoglobulins, and defense peptides.

Cells of the Innate Immune System

Cells of the immune system are derived from two precursor cells namely—common myeloid progenitor (CMP) cells and common lymphoid progenitor (CLP) cells. These precursor cells are produced in the bone marrow. While macrophages, granulocytes (neutrophils, basophils, and eosinophils), mast cells, and dendritic cells are derived from CMPs, antigen-specific lymphocytes (T-cells and B-cells) are derived from CLPs. There are cells such as natural killer (NK) cells, which also are derived from CLPs and these cells are involved in early stages of innate immune response and adaptive immune response.

There are two different types of macrophages namely—tissue macrophages and classical monocytes. Tissue macrophages that arise during embryonic development and localized to specific tissue are called by various names. Liver macrophages are called Kupffer cells and the macrophages residing in the neural tissue are called microglial cells. These cells are self-renewed in the tissue and their self-renewal is dependent on interleukin-34 (IL-34). The other class of macrophages is called classical monocytes and they are found in circulating blood. Upon entry into tissue from blood, they differentiate into macrophages. These are called monocyte-derived macrophages. Macrophages are the first cells recognizing the foreign pathogens and engulf them by phagocytosis. Phagocytosis results in pathogen killing and this process also leads to inflammation and induction of cytokines and chemokines, which recruit more monocytes and granulocytes, to the site of infection.

Granulocytes have dense granules that are filled with lytic enzymes and toxic proteins. These are released upon phagocytosis of the pathogens and these effectively kill the pathogens. While neutrophils predominantly kill invading bacteria and fungi, the eosinophils and basophils kill parasites. Neutrophils are short-lived and represent the major class of granulocytes. As in the case of macrophages, the process of phagocytosis and destruction of invading organisms leads to inflammation. Granulocytes are also called as polymorphonuclear phagocytes because of the shape of their nucleus.

Another group of cells that are involved in innate immune response are mast cells and these are localized predominantly in peripheral tissues including skin, mucosal lining of intestine, and other organs. These develop in the bone marrow and enter as immature cells and further differentiate in the tissues.

Dendritic cells are also phagocytic and they engulf organisms as well as particle suspended in fluid. This process of taking up extracellular fluid along with suspended particles is called macropinocytosis. Even though dendritic cells can kill organisms, their main function is activation of naïve T-cells and B-cells. In the absence of dendritic cells, adaptive immunity cannot develop.

Receptors Recognizing Foreign Antigens

Cells of the innate immune system recognize the pathogen-associated molecular patterns (PAMPs). PAMPs are conserved molecular structures of specific pattern found in the pathogens but not in the host and hence, the pathogen-specific nature of PAMPs allows recognition of the pathogen and avoids self-destruction. Host cells carry receptors that recognize PAMPs and these are called pattern recognition receptors (PRRs).

Table 6.1 shows the list of PAMPs and the PRRs. The signaling mediated through the PAMP and PRR interaction leads to the activation of several functions such as antiviral state, induction of acute inflammation, and stimulation of adaptive immunity.

Table 6.1: Pathogen-associated molecular patterns (PAMPs) and their pattern recognition receptors (PRRs).

Pathogen associated molecular patterns	Pattern recognition receptors
Toll-like receptors (TLRS)	
TLR1/TLR2	Triacyl lipopeptides
TLR6	Diacyl lipopeptides
TLR5	Flagellin
TLR4	Lipopolysaccharide/Mannan
C-type lectin receptors (CLRS)	
MR	Mannans, N-linked mannans, and mannoproteins
DC-SIGN	Galactomannans and mannans
Dectin-1	Beta 1, 3-glucans
Dectin-2	Alpha-mannans
MINCLE	Alpha-mannosyl residues

(MR: Mannose receptor; DC-SIGN: Dendritic cell-specific intercellular adhesion; MINCLE: Macrophage inducible Ca^{2+}-dependent lectin receptor)

Activation of Innate Immune Response

There are two different ways by which the innate cells such as neutrophils and macrophages, also called as professional phagocytes, are activated from their resting stage.

Direct Activation by Bacterial and Fungal Components

Cell wall components such as lipopolysaccharides (LPS) (also called as endotoxin) of bacterial and glucans of fungal cell wall are the predominant activators of innate immune cells. LPS binds to toll-like receptor 4 (TLR4) and TLR2 on the surface of the phagocytes and activate the signaling events. Fungal components predominantly initiate signaling through C-type lectin receptors (CLRs). Secreted components of the pathogens also contribute significantly to the initiation of innate response.

Indirect Activation of Innate Response

Nonimmune cells including corneal and conjunctival epithelia, retinal pigment epithelia, retinal Müller cells, and ciliary body epithelial cells can sense the pathogen and initiate synthesis and secretion of cytokines and other activators of immune system. For example, tear fluid bathing the corneal epithelium helps in the interaction and induction of gene expression leading to production of proteins which in turn initiate immune defense by phagocytes. Interestingly, corneal epithelial cells in vitro are sensitive to infection whereas the same cells in vivo are resistant to bacterial infection. Recent findings show the tear fluid covering the cornea help the corneal epithelium to deal with the infection by activating epithelial cell defense against bacteria. Infection of epithelial cells at conjunctival-limbal region of the cornea also creates a cytokine gradient and attracts the neutrophils from circulation.

Initiation of Innate Immune Response

Innate immune response is predominantly controlled by two phagocytes. Their recruitment and conversion into effector cell populations is described below.

Recruitment, Activation, and Maturation of Resting Neutrophils

Circulating neutrophils are resting cells and infection activates them in a series of well-orchestrated sequential events. Resting neutrophils roll slowly on the surface of the endothelium using the L-selectins binding to their cognate receptors on the endothelial cells. Upon infection, E- and P-selectins are induced and displayed on the surface of the endothelial cells. Neutrophils recognize these using their receptors and they slow down on the endothelial surface. This is followed by transmigration of the neutrophils across the vascular endothelial wall into the site of infection. The bacterial components and toxins as well as the host-derived components such as complement factor C3a, chemokines (IL-8) and several other factors are responsible for the transmigration and activation of neutrophils. Neutrophils are short-lived and once they enter the tissue, they stay in the infection site and ultimately die.

Recruitment, Activation, and Maturation of Circulating Monocytes

The resident macrophages recognize the pathogen and initiate the innate response to begin with. Further, the chemokines produced by these cells recruit the monocytes as well as neutrophils from blood circulation. These monocyte-derived macrophages amplify the innate immune response. Monocytes are the resting phagocytes and several factors activate them. Factors that activate the macrophages include—chemokines, cytokines, bacterial components (already discussed), complement proteins, and other foreign bodies. There are distinct stages of maturation of monocytes to macrophages. These stages are distinguishable based on their gene expression program. Resting, primed, stimulated, and activated macrophages are some of the common distinguishable classes of macrophages. Activated macrophages are effector cells. The migration of monocytes into the site of infection follows a similar pathway followed by neutrophils.

Activated macrophages also present antigen to antigen-specific effector T-cells. During this interaction, T-cells produce cytokines which in turn help the macrophages to kill the pathogens effectively. Unlike dendritic cells, macrophages can present antigens to antigen-specific T-cells and not to naïve T-cells. Partially activated macrophages also called as stimulated macrophages help in wound healing and angiogenesis by producing appropriate factors. Platelet-derived growth factors and metalloproteinases produced by macrophages are involved in wound healing and vascular endothelial growth factor produced by macrophages help in angiogenesis.

MOLECULES INVOLVED IN INNATE IMMUNITY

Apart from the cells described above, there are some specific set of molecules either alone or as a group participating in a pathway that also play significant role in innate immune response. These systems of molecules amplify the immune response to infection. The common ones are listed below:

1. Complement system
2. Coagulation system
3. Cytokines
4. Lipid mediators
5. Reactive nitrogen and reactive oxygen species
6. Vasoactive products (histamines and serotonins)
7. Neutrophil granules
8. Neutrophil extracellular traps (NETs)

Complement System

Complement system gets activated very early in immune response against pathogens. The classical pathway of complement cascade requires antigen-specific antibodies, whereas the alternate pathway and lectin pathway can be activated without the antibodies. Figure 6.1 shows the three pathways of complement system.

Activation of complement pathways leads to the formation of membrane attack complex on the surface of the foreign invaders and kills the cells. Apart from cell lysis, the components of the complement system have several other functions. Inflammation induced by the complement proteins contributes to the control and elimination of the pathogens. The role of other innate defense systems which could differ at different sites will be discussed under the section of immune response of the ocular surface.

ADAPTIVE IMMUNITY

Adaptive or acquired immunity is induced immunity, and is elicited during the sustained exposure of the host to foreign antigens or pathogens and takes about 5–7 days to develop fully. Those pathogens that survive the innate defense systems and continue to exist in the host ultimately induce the adaptive immunity. Adaptive immune response is elaborated only when dendritic cells present the foreign antigen to unstimulated or naïve T and B lymphocytes in specialized organs, namely spleen and lymph nodes. The development of adaptive immunity is shaped by the innate immune response. Among the organs involved in shaping

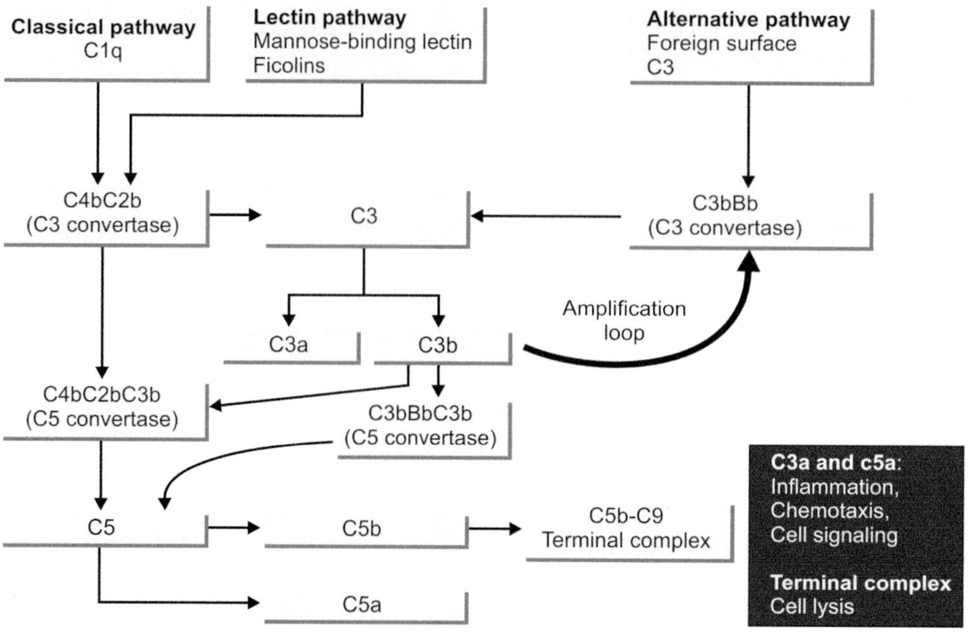

Fig. 6.1: Three pathways of complement system.

the adaptive immunity—bone marrow, spleen, lymph nodes, and specialized cells play a significant role. This response is much quicker against the secondary infection of the same pathogen and also is much more robust against reinfection. The importance of adaptive immunity for the subsequent infections is significant since this arm of immunity has immunological memory, which is the hallmark of vertebrate immune regulation. The response to vaccines is primarily through adaptive immunity. Lymphocytes constituting B-cells and T-cells are the central players in this arm of immunity. Adaptive immune system has the following important characteristics:

1. Production of B-cells and T-cells with appropriate receptors to recognize parts (epitopes) of foreign antigens.
2. Removal of B and T-cells recognizing self-antigens.
3. Ability to eliminate the pathogens once recognized as foreign.
4. Regulation of the immune response to avoid overt reaction in specialized organs such as eye. The phenomenon of tolerance is discussed detail in later.
5. Adaptive immune cells can be transferred from one individual to the other and the recipient will have the adaptive response against the antigen against which the B and T-cells were elaborated in the donor. This transferable immunity and other properties are specific for adaptive immunity and not innate immune response. Important components of the immune system are summarized in Table 6.2.

Table 6.2: Characteristics of innate versus adaptive immunity.

	Innate immunity	Adaptive immunity
Specificity	Not antigen-specific	Antigen-specific
Efficiency	Rapid	Primary responses slower
Memory	Absent	Present
Chief effectors	Neutrophils, macrophages, natural killer (NKT) T-cells	Lymphocytes

Phases of Adaptive Immune Response

Adaptive immune response is a multi-stage process. Since the development of antigen-specific T and B-cells occur in lymphoid organs, the invading pathogen and its components need to be transported to these specialized organs. In these organs, a complex interaction with several cell types and cytokines leads to the development of antigen-specific T-cells and B-cells. The stages of development of these cells take place through a series of well-defined phases.

Afferent Phase

The process of capturing, degradation, and processing occurs at the site of infection and is carried out by dendritic cells and macrophages. These antigen-loaded dendritic cells migrate via the afferent lymphatic vessels and enter the lymphoid organs (lymph nodes or spleen). Foreign antigens picked up by the dendritic cells are degraded and then displayed on major histocompatibility complex (MHC) class I and class II molecules. Protein molecules are cleaved into smaller peptides of 7–11 amino acids and then are displayed on MHC molecules.

There are two groups of MHC molecules that play a major role in the development of T-cell differentiation. MHC class I molecules are present in all nucleated cells and the foreign antigens synthesized within the host alone are displayed on the MHC class I molecules. If the displayed peptide is from the host, the T-cells recognizing these (CD8 T-cells) are removed early during development of T-cells by a process called negative selection. Proteins that are synthesized in tumor cells and the viral proteins are the foreign proteins processed in the dendritic cells and presented to CD8 T-cells.

Proteins from invading pathogens are phagocytosed and processed by the dendritic cells and presented along with MHC II complex molecules. As in the case described above, the processed peptides are presented along with the MHC II to CD4 T-cells. Only dendritic cells are proficient in presenting antigens to naïve T-cells. Even though the macrophages, which also can capture, process, and present antigens, they are not capable of activating naïve T-cells.

Processing Phase

In this phase, the Antigen Presenting Cell-T-cell interaction leads to the differentiation of T-cells and conversion of CD4 helper T-cells into different classes. Starting as Th0 cells, these cells become Th1, Th2 or Th17 cells. These are predominant classes and there are additional classes demonstrated. Some of the CD4-cells also become regulatory T-cells.

The process that leads to the maturation of Th0 into different classes is complex and factors such as the microenvironment and the type and quantity of antigens are important components which orchestrate this. These cells can be distinguished easily by the cytokines they secrete. Th1 cells secrete interferon gamma, tumor necrosis factor beta. Th2 cells secrete Il-4, IL-5, and IL-10. Th17 cells secrete Il-17, IL-21, and IL-22. It is important to remember that Th1 cells do not produce Th2 cytokines and vice versa. Further, Th1 cells can inhibit development of Th2 cells and vice versa. Therefore, the regulatory systems operating in these cells are tightly controlled.

B-cell Development

As described earlier, B-cells are also excellent APCs. In the lymphoid organs, the antigens entering through the afferent lymphatics will be captured and processed by the B-cells. The processed antigens are presented along with MHC class II molecules. If a CD4 T-cell carrying the receptor recognizes the MHC–peptide combination (antigen-specific T-cell) on the B-cells, the interacting B-cell is activated to differentiate to produce antibodies. The interaction between the T-cell and the B-cell leads to the production of necessary costimulatory events. The first costimulatory signal comes from the interaction of B7–CD28 interaction and the second stimulation comes from the cytokines. These activated B-cells will then produce antibodies. Further, these cells once activated can produce other classes of antibodies. This process is called isotype switch. The process of B-cell development results in clonal expansion of antigen-specific antibody producing plasma cells. Another class of B-cells called memory cells resides in the system and they respond to the secondary challenge with the same antigen. Vaccination efficacy depends on this production of memory cells. Surprisingly during the primary infection, 1 in 100,000 cells end up as antigen-specific cells and roughly 1 in 10,000 T-cells become antigen-specific T-cells. Those B-cells which fail to find the appropriate CD T-cell will not develop and are removed from the lymphoid organ. Similarly, the T-cells that fail to find appropriate dendritic cell with correct MHC–peptide complex will not be selected.

Unlike the primary response, which is slow, the second exposure to the same antigen elicits robust and specific defense during the secondary infection. The development of naïve cells takes place in the lymphoid organs and they are resident in these organs whereas the memory cells migrate to the tissues and engage the invading pathogens. This selective migration of cells from the lymphoid organs is called *homing*.

Effector Phase: Integrated View of Innate and Adaptive Immune Effector Functions

Early in infection, phagocytes are resting or inactive. Innate lymphoid cells, NK cells, and other innate lymphoid cells (ILCs) produce cytokines to activate tissue-resident macrophages, neutrophils, basophils, eosinophils, and mast cells. These lymphoid innate cells do not have the receptors carried by the T-cells and B-cells but their origin is from common lymphoid progenitor cells. When the antigen-specific T-cell and B-cell development is completed in lymph nodes and spleen, they enter the periphery upon infection. Once in the peripheral tissue, the CD4 Th1 cells produce IFN gamma and IL-12 when the macrophages present the antigen they phagocytosed. This interaction and the consequent production of IFN gamma and TNF alpha improves the killing of pathogens by activated macrophages. CD4 Th2 cells activate mast cells, basophils, and eosinophils to produce immunoglobulin E (IgE) and they are involved in killing parasites. CD4 Th17 cells are activators of neutrophils. CD8 T-cells are cytotoxic by themselves and they produce IL-12 and also kill the tumor cells and virus infected cells directly.

IMMEDIATE AND DELAYED TYPE HYPERSENSITIVITY REACTION

Normal immune response against invading pathogens is critical for the safety of the host. The immune response at times is elaborated against the antigens that are inherently harmless, such as pollens, food and drugs, and other environmental antigens. These are called immunologically mediated hypersensitivity reactions and are also called as allergic reactions. The hypersensitivity reactions are classified by Gell and Coombs into four types. Type I hypersensitivity reaction is mediated by IgE antibodies and type II and type III are mediated by IgG antibodies and the type IV hypersensitivity reaction is mediated by cellular effectors. Both lymphocytes and myeloid cells participate in type IV hypersensitivity reaction. Antibody-mediated hypersensitivity reactions are immediate hypersensitivity reactions and the cell-mediated reactions are called delayed-type hypersensitivity reactions (DTH).

Delayed-type Hypersensitivity Reactions

Delayed-type hypersensitivity reactions are mediated by antigen-specific CD4 T helper cells as well as CD8 cytotoxic T-cells. In the T helper cells, Th1 cells are the predominant type of cells involved in DTH. The mechanism of DTH is similar to the normal immune response to foreign antigens. For example, the DTH reaction is transferrable between experimental animals by purified T-cells. Chronic inflammation is also mediated by the cellular DTH. In DTH reaction, antigen-specific T-cells enter the site of antigen presence. On recognition of the antigen through the APCs, the T-cells secrete cytokines, which act on the vascular endothelium. Th1 cells produced during the previous exposure to the antigen are rare and since there is no inflammation, the recruitment of T-cells to the site is very slow. Hence, the delay in the appearance of immune reaction. Generally, it takes about 12–24 hours or even more for the appearance of DTH.

The cytokines released and acted on the vascular endothelium lead to the recruitment of additional macrophages to the site, and this will enhance the hypersensitivity reaction. A classic example is the Mantoux reaction where mycobacterial peptide–carbohydrate complex is injected into the skin and the result is observed after 72 hours. In this case, Th1 cells enter the site and recognize these antigens presented on APCs. This interaction induces the release of interferon gamma, TNF alpha, and lymphotoxin. These mediators act on vascular endothelium and increase the permeability of plasma and other cells to enter the site. This process leads to swelling and inflammation. This whole process takes about 72 hours. Contact hypersensitivity and gluten-sensitive enteropathy (Celiac disease) are also cell-mediated DTH reactions.

Inflammation and Immune Response

Inflammation is induced by several factors such as infection, tissue injury, stress, and other metabolic disturbances. The tissues and organs exposed to external environment such as gastrointestinal tract, pulmonary tissue, skin, cornea, limbus, and conjunctiva are prone to develop excessive inflammation. Under normal conditions, inflammation is well-regulated and self-limiting and hence many organs can withstand inflammatory damage. However, inflammation and the collateral damages due to inflammation have serious effect on the tissues of the eye including corneal stroma, vitreous, and retina (in particular macula). Paradoxically, inflammation is a necessary prerequisite for immune defense against infection. On the other hand, even minor inflammatory response can damage the eye and affect the visual axis if it is not controlled. In order to prevent the visual axis from inflammation, induced destruction specialized mechanisms operate to minimize and limit inflammatory damage.

IMMUNE RESPONSE IN THE OCULAR SURFACE

The ocular surface consists of cornea, limbus, bulbar and palpebral conjunctiva, glandular tissue, and the tear film. Conjunctiva and the limbus have well-organized immune systems including myeloid cells (dendritic cells, macrophages, and neutrophils), whereas the cornea is avascular and dendritic cells and macrophages are sparsely distributed. Absence of a full complement of dense population of immune cells is to avoid impeding the optical axis. However, the tear film and the multilayered corneal epithelium are armed with robust first-line of defense against pathogens and injury. Constitutive innate defense is adequate to control most infections. In addition, the epithelial cells can actively orchestrate the immune defense by recruiting other myeloid cells.

Tear Film and their Role in Immunity

Tear film is an organized structure external to the cornea and consists of an external lipid layer, middle aqueous layer, and inner glycocalyx. Tear film is about ten microns in thickness. Lipid layer is the product of meibomian glands and the components of the aqueous layer are predominantly produced by lacrimal glands. Epithelial cells of cornea and conjunctiva may also contribute to the proteins of the aqueous layer. The composition of the aqueous layer changes according to the external conditions including infections and disease. The innermost layer that covers the surface of the epithelium is made of mucins secreted by conjunctival goblet cells. There are at least 20 mucin-encoding genes. Mucins are highly glycosylated and more than 70% of the protein weight is due to the oligosaccharides. The membrane-spanning mucins that traverse the apical cells of the epithelium form the glycocalyx and these are produced by corneal and conjunctival epithelial cells. The secreted mucins in the tear are produced by goblet cells in the conjunctiva. Apart from forming the barrier to pathogen attachment and entry, pathogens bound to the glycocalyx will initiate signaling in the epithelial cells. Mucins also help in the clearance of the pathogens by trapping them in their network and expedite their passage through the nasolacrimal duct. There are several proteins of the tear film that are involved in innate immune response against infections. Many of these proteins are induced in response to infection and not found in the tear film of healthy individuals. Tear film composition and cellular content are different in closed eye (or night time) tear compared to open eye tear. More neutrophils are found in the night time tear. Rapid blinking movements also prevent permanent adherence of the pathogens to the corneal surface epithelium. Proteins and peptides either directly act against pathogens or activate immune effector cells to kill the invading organisms. Major antimicrobial proteins of the tear which have proven defense activities are lysozyme, lactoferrin, lipocalin, secretory immunoglobulins, lacritin, and complement proteins. Secretory phospholipase A2 (sPLA2) and surfactant protein (SA) also have antibacterial and antifungal properties. Major tear proteins and their functions are given in Table 6.3.

Table 6.3: Major tear proteins and their defense functions.

Tear protein	Function
Lysozyme	Antibacterial and antifungal
Lactoferrin	Ion chelator and bacteriostatic
Lipocalin	Binds siderophores and bacteriostatic
Secretory IgA	Pathogen clearance, prevents pathogen binding to cells
Complement	Antibacterial and antifungal. Complete pathway is found in mycotic patient tear but not in reflex tear
Lacritin	Promotes survival of stressed epithelial cells, basal tearing, and antimicrobial.

Antimicrobial Peptides in the Tear

Some of the peptides that have antimicrobial properties are produced constitutively and others are induced. Alpha-defensins and beta-defensins, psoriasin (S100A7), dermcidin, and histatin are constitutively produced and RNase 7, ST2 and cathelicidins are induced upon infection. Each of these antifungal peptides individually may be less effective in controlling the invading pathogen. However, all these together acting in concert are very effective in the elimination of the invading pathogen. Common pathogens infecting the ocular surface are shown in Table 6.4. Diversity of pathogens capable of infecting the eye implies the importance of the first-line of ocular surface immune efficacy, especially under the stringent condition of attenuated inflammatory response.

An array of antimicrobial protein defense systems such as NETs and complement pathway proteins are induced upon infection and released into the tear film. Therefore, the corneal surface is an effective barrier to infection for many pathogens.

The Epithelial Layer

Corneal epithelial cells are excellent physical barriers, and at the same time they are active immune defense system as well. Apart from the antimicrobial peptides and mucins synthesized by epithelial cells, they are also capable of phagocytosis and immunomodulation. Unlike the in vitro cultured corneal epithelial cells, live cornea in vivo is resistant to infection. Epithelial cells are capable of responding to the PRRs of pathogens through

Table 6.4: Pathogens causing corneal disease. Pathogens within each class of microorganism are listed in descending order of prevalence.

Bacteria
Gram-positive bacteria
Staphylococcus spp *(aureus, epidermidis)* *Streptococcus pneumoniae* *Streptococcus pyogenes* *Streptococcus viridians* *Corynebacterium diphtheriae* *Nocardia* spp *Propionibacterium acnes* *Bacillus* spp *Mycobacterium* spp *Micrococcus* spp
Gram-negative bacteria
Pseudomonas aeruginosa *Moraxella* spp *Klebsiella pneumoniae* *Enterobacter aerogenes* *Serratia* spp *(marcescens, liquefaciens)* *Acinetobacter* spp *Enterococcus* spp *Burkholderia cepacia* *Escherichia coli* *Stenotrophomonas maltophilia* *Neisseria gonorrhoeae* *Haemophilus* spp *Kingella kingae* *Pseudomonas* spp *(non-aeruginosa)* *Citrobacter* spp *Aeromonas* spp
Chlamydial
C. trachomatis, psittaci
Fungi
Fusarium spp *Aspergillus* spp *(flavus, fumigatus, niger, terreus and nidulans)* *Alternaria* spp *Curvularia* spp *Lasiodiplodia theobromae* *Paecilomyces* spp *Penicillium* spp *Scedosporium apiospermum* *Cephalophora irregularis* *Cladosporium cladosporioides* *Cylindrocarpon* spp *Exserohilum rostratum* *Bipolaris* spp *Candida* spp *Pythium insidiosum*
Virus
Herpes simplex virus type 1 Varicella zoster virus Human adenovirus (serotypes 8, 19 and 37) Enterovirus type 760 Coxsackievirus type 24 Echovirus type 13 Poliovirus type 3 Cytomegalovirus

Contd...

Contd...

Bacteria
Parasite
Acanthamoeba spp*(castellani, polyphaga, and culbertsoni)* *Microsporidia* spp *Hartmannella* spp *Vahlkampfia* spp *Dictyostelium polycephalum* *Phthiriasis palpebrarum* *Oestrus ovis*
Nematode
Loa loa *Onchocerca volvulus*

TLRs and danger-associated molecular patterns (DAMP) (activated by the infection of the host) through NOD-like receptors (NLRs) of the host. Conjunctival epithelial cells which differ from corneal epithelial cells particularly produce chemokines such as CCL20, CXCL9, CXCL10 and CXCL11in response to infection, which in turn recruit T helper cells. Epithelial cells respond to TLR and IL-1R mediated signaling by secreting beta-defensin-2, a potent antimicrobial peptide. The TLR-mediated activation of epithelial cells also leads to enhanced barrier function by way of preventing the penetration of bacteria and also inhibiting the traversal of the pathogen through the epithelial layers. In addition, epithelia might be a requisite for the recruitment of myeloid cells and recognition of pathogens by the myeloid cells.

Tear Fluid Corneal Epithelial Cell Interaction In Vivo

Contrary to the common belief unlike the epithelial cultured in vivo, epithelial cells from live corneal are resistant to infection by *Pseudomonas*. In animal models, mice infected with *A. flavus* spores are refractory to infection even after scrapping of epithelial cells. These studies show there is an active constitutive defense function elaborated by tear film and epithelial cells. Tear proteins interact with corneal epithelial cells and make them resistant to infection by increasing their barrier function leading to inhibition of penetration and traversal of the pathogens. Tear film induces stress response factors such as nuclear factor-kappa B (NF-κβ) and activating protein (AP-1). Tear fluid upregulates RNase7 and immunomodulator ST2. The cytokines and chemokines secreted by epithelial cells upon induction by tear film proteins are needed for the recruitment of myeloid cells.

Immune Modulation in the Eye

Dendritic cells (DCs) are the initiators of immune response against invading pathogens. In the lymphoid organs including draining lymph nodes, dendritic cells prime naïve T-cells which were not exposed previously to antigens, and activate them. These activated cells are the effector cells which upon antigen presentation by macrophages, B-cells or dendritic cells respond appropriately. The types of DCs present in the tissue are different and exist as multiple subtypes. $CD11^{+}$, $CD103^{+}$, and plasmacytoid DC are three tissue-specific subtypes in conjunctiva and to a lesser extent in corneal stroma. Inflammation either pathogen-induced or disease mediated can lead to DC migration and activation of T-cells. CD8, NK and $\gamma\ \delta$ T-cells are present in ocular surface including epithelia and are primed by DC. Another class of T-cells, called T regulatory cells (T reg) whose function is to establish immune non-responsiveness and immune tolerance are also found in the ocular surface. Blinking, sleep, infection, and environmental impact alter the physiology of the ocular surface. During sleep, neutrophil influx is demonstrated but these are physiologically different from activated neutrophils.

Cells of the Ocular Surface

Even though the cornea is devoid of highly dense multiple cell types, epithelial layer has macrophages and dendritic cells. These three cell types—epithelial, macrophages, and dendritic cells orchestrate the early immune response. Epithelial cells produce antimicrobial peptides and the chemokine gradient produced by the epithelial, macrophages, and DC recruit neutrophils from limbal vasculature. Majority of the studies using cultured epithelial cells give conflicting reports, as it is well-known that cultured cells and tissue epithelial cells in vivo behave differently, all these studies indicate a unified sequence of events which lead the epithelial cells to express TLR2, TLR3, TLR4, and TLR5. Therefore, they can sense the pathogen (particularly bacterial pathogens) as has been shown for *Pseudomonas* keratitis. Cell surface-associated mucins recognize bacterial pathogens and initiate signal transduction leading to NFkβ-mediated production of pro-inflammatory cytotoxins. Neutrophils are recruited to the site of infection through these chemokines and cytokines. In case of disruption, exposure of bacteria to macrophages amplifies this cascade further, ultimately resulting in neutrophil recruitment. Neutrophils and macrophages are the major sources of IL-1β, which is an important inflammatory cytokine. Early in infection, the recruited polymorphonuclear phagocytes are the primary source of IL-1β and the mature active form of IL-1β is processed by elastase. Caspase-1 activated by inflammasome can also process IL-1β to its mature form. However, caspase-1-mediated processing of active IL-Iβ occurs at late stages of infection.

MODULATION OF IMMUNE RESPONSE BY HOST NEUROPEPTIDES

Cornea has the densest innervation in human body. Neuropeptides form the major effectors of neural control of immunity in the ocular surface. Substance P (SP), calcitonin 4 gene-related protein (CGRP), vasoactive intestinal peptide (VIP), and neuropeptide Y are the major neuropeptides that regulate the immune response.

In the context of infection, particularly in pseudomonal keratitis, SP activates pro-inflammatory network. Macrophages, neutrophils, epithelial cells, and NK cells are activated to produce cytokines. IL-1, IL-6, IL-12, and TNF-λ levels are increased. Unlike SP, neuropeptide VIP downregulates the inflammatory response. VIP also increases wound healing in pseudomonal keratitis.

Modulation of Immune Response by the Pathogen

Pseudomonas effectively disrupt epithelial cell barrier and prevents phagocytosis by expressing type III secretion system (T3SS). T3SS infects exoenzymes of *Pseudomonas* directly into host cytoplasm through a needle-like structure to prevent neutrophil response against the pathogen.

In the epithelial cells, these exoenzymes sequester the pathogen in membrane blebs and the pathogen utilizes this niche for replication. Yet another common method to overcome host defense is biofilm formation.

IMMUNE TOLERANCE AT THE OCULAR SURFACE

Ocular immune tolerance is an active, antigen-specific local immune unresponsiveness to a given antigen that has systemic implication apart from local immune tolerance. Ocular immune tolerance is primarily mediated by dendritic cells, which sample antigens which are airborne or of microbial origin. Unknown factors condition these

DC into a tolerogenic profile and these imprinted DC migrate to the draining submandibular lymph node. The CCR7 expression in DC to follow the chemokine gradient is essential for their migrations. In the lymph node, the DC present antigen to the T-cells carrying the specific T-cell receptor and this leads to conversion of these T-cells to T-reg cells and this expansion follows in the lymph node. Some of these T-cells eventually reach the systemic circulation. After entering the ocular surface vasculature, they transit to the tissue and activate the DC if they present the same antigen. In this case, macrophages as well as DC can present antigen to these effector cells, since these are T-reg cells. The APC–T-cell interactions prevent local inflammatory response.

During infection, inflammatory response is generated by the activation of signaling by recognition of TLRs by the bacterial antigens or CLRs by the fungi. Both DC and epithelial cells respond by producing inflammatory cytokines. NK cells contribute in this by a burst of IFNγ which in turn can activate DC and epithelial cells in the production of pro-inflammatory signaling. These recruit Th1 or Th17 producing T-cells to the periphery from draining lymph nodes. These T-cells can prime antigen loading DC and macrophages elaborate pro-inflammatory response and pathogen clearance.

IMMUNE HOMEOSTASIS IN THE EYE

More than 70% of the information reaching the brain goes through the eye. Consequently, keeping the visual axis free of obstruction is of paramount importance for the host. Excessive immune response leading to cell death could be a major drawback in the eye since this will affect the functioning of the eye. The immunological property that circumvents this problem is called immune privilege. Immune privilege has been defined by Peter Medawar and colleagues in the 1940s and this is based on the survival of the allografts placed in the anterior chamber of the eye. Mismatched human cadaver cornea grafts are accepted 60–70% of the times indicating the immune tolerance in the anterior chamber. Apart from the anterior chamber, other parts of the eye including cornea, vitreous cavity, and subretinal space are also sites of immune privilege (Fig. 6.2). Based on the transplantation experiments, he concluded that the survival of the allograft is due to the sequestration of the foreign antigen from systemic lymphatic system. He also noted the absence of lymphatic system in the immune privileged sites. Further, antigens placed in the anterior chamber do not induce immune response. The concept of immune privilege however underwent considerable change.

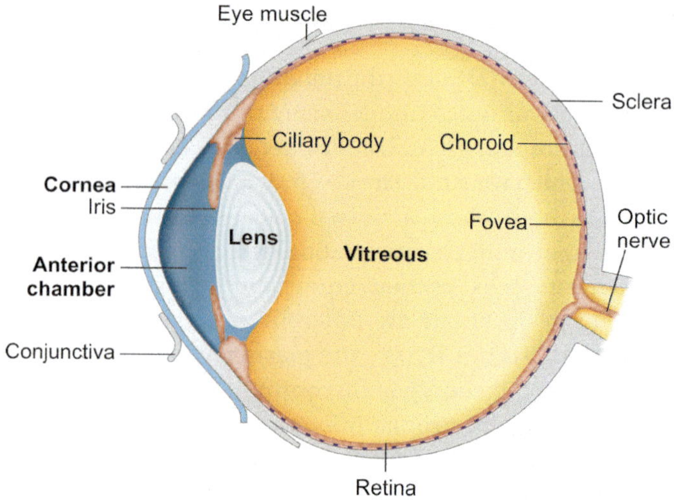

Fig. 6.2: Immune-privileged regions and tissues of the eye. Cornea, anterior chamber, iris and lens of the anterior segment and vitreous, retina and choroid of the posterior segment of the eye are the immune privileged sites of the eye.

Source: Modified from Reyes NL, Koren EGO, Saban DR. Nature Reviews Immunology. 2017;17(5):322-32.

Major components involved in immune privilege are given below:
1. Suppression of innate immune response.
2. Limitation of breach of blood–brain barrier by T-cells.
3. Activation of immune regulatory network to suppress immune response.
4. Prevention of lymphangiogenesis.
5. Activation of regulatory immune cells that lead to anterior chamber-associated immune deviation (ACAID).

Factors causing immune tolerance in the eye are listed in Table 6.5.

The process of ocular immune response to microbes and foreign antigens and the formation of tolerogenic response is summarized below:
1. Microbes and foreign antigens enter the epithelial layer and encounter APCs (dendritic cells).
2. Antigen-loaded dendritic cells migrate to the eye draining lymph node through the afferent lymphatic vessel.
3. Dendritic cells present antigen to naïve T-cells in the lymph node.
4. T-cells differentiate into tolerogenic T-reg cells.
5. T-reg cells enter into circulation through efferent lymphatic vessel.
6. T-reg cells migrate through ocular blood vessel to ocular surface.
7. T-reg cells inhibit maturation of APCs (DC and macrophages).
8. T-reg cells inhibit effective functioning of effector T-cells.

Table 6.5: Factors causing immune tolerance in the eye.

Factor	Effect	Eye
TCF-β	Suppresses activation of T-cells, NK cells, macrophages, induces tolerance-inducing APCs	Yes
VIP	Inhibits T-cell activation and proliferation, inhibits DTH	Yes
CGRP	Inhibits elaboration of pro-inflammatory factors by macrophages	Yes
α-MSH	Inhibits DTH and release of inflammatory factors of by macrophages, inhibits activation of neutrophils, induces CD4+, CD25-regulatory cells	Yes
SOM	Suppress interferon-γ production by activated T-cells, induces proliferation of α-MSH	Yes
MIF	Suppresses NK cell activity	Yes
sFasL	Suppresses neutrophil recruitment and activation	Yes
CRP	Inhibits complement cascade	Yes
IDO	Depletes tryptophan and starves T-cells	Yes

(VIP: Vasointestinal peptide; CGRP: Calcitonin gene-related peptide; αMSH: α-melanocyte stimulating hormone; SOM: Somatostatin; MIF: Macrophage migration inhibitory factor; sFasL: Soluble FasL; CRP: C-reactive protein; IDO: Indoleamine 2,3-dioxygenase)

Immune system in the eye is one of the best regulated processes, since the immune defense against infection and foreign bodies has to be balanced against immune system-mediated destruction. In addition to this, keeping the visual axis clear is a primary requisite that cannot be compromised by the unregulated immune defense. There are multiple immune regulatory mechanisms that are responsible for the maintenance of this intricate process.

IMMUNOLOGY OF SELECTED EYE DISEASES

Ocular Surface Allergies

Allergic sensitization of conjunctiva to common allergens such as pollens, house dust mite, and animal danders are mediated through Th1 T-cells. Mast cells under the influence of IgE release the granules which are the major causative factors in allergic conjunctivitis. In atopic individuals (those predisposed to IgE sensitized to environmental allergen), seasonal conjunctivitis can lead to perennial conjunctivitis.

Cicatrizing Diseases of the Conjunctiva

Ocular pemphigoid is a disorder in which autoantibodies are present against conjunctival epithelial beta-4 integrin. Characteristic feature of this disorder is progressive cicatrization of stroma. The Stevens-Johnson syndrome is much more acute form of the condition, where antibodies to basement membrane proteins have been detected.

Some types of keratitis, such as postherpetic disciform keratitis are also immunological. In this disease, antibodies to herpes simplex virus antigens have been implicated. Other disorders of cornea where corneal thinning and ulceration occur are presumably T-reg cell mediated.

Inflammatory condition of the sclera (scleritis) is an autoimmune or an immune disorder. However, the scleral antigen responsible for this scleritis has not been demonstrated. Involvement of CD4 T-cells and CD8 T-cells has been demonstrated, indicating the immune nature of the disease. Both autoimmune scleritis and necrotizing scleritis are shown to have immune cell infiltration.

Deficiency of tear production by lacrimal glands leads to Sjögren syndrome. T-cell infiltration and activation of T-cells have been demonstrated to play a role in Sjögren syndrome.

IMMUNE PRIVILEGE AND IMMUNE TOLERANCE IN THE CONTEXT OF EYE DISORDERS

This is a clear indication of the active immune tolerance involved in ACAID. The antigen tracking studies demonstrating the presence of green fluorescent-labeled protein within two hours after application of the protein on the cornea in the submandibular draining lymph node prove the active role of draining lymphatics in the cornea. Active involvement of immunosuppressive factors and T-reg cells indicate ACAID is indeed another form of immunosuppression. This suppression in the eye in reality makes it susceptible to parasites such as toxoplasma and fungi such as candida. Certain viruses such as cytomegalovirus and herpes simplex virus proliferate profusely in the retina.

INTRAOCULAR INFLAMMATION

Infectious agents such as bacteria, viruses, fungi, and protozoa can cause intraocular inflammation. Apart from this, noninfectious uveitis may affect anterior or posterior segment as well. Autoimmune disorder has been demonstrated in many cases and HLA association also shows the immune disorder in the uveitis. Clear demonstration of autoimmunity using humanized mice proves the autoimmune nature of this disease. The clinical response of this disease to cyclosporine and other immunosuppressors also points to the evidence of the autoimmune nature of this disease.

Recent studies clearly indicate many of the ocular disorders, which were thought to be genetic, developmental, metabolic, age-related or even cancer, indeed have the involvement of immune processes. For example, retinitis pigmentosa, diabetes, and age-related macular degeneration all have strong immunological processes in the induction and progression of the disease. As the understanding of the immunology of the eye improves, more therapeutic opportunities also will be available to effectively manage the eye diseases.

SUGGESTED READING

1. Forrester JV, Dick AD, McManamin PG, et al. The Eye. Basic Sciences in Practice, 4th edition. Elsevier; 2016.
2. Galletti JG, Guzman M, Giordano MN. Mucosal immune tolerance at ocular surface in health and disease. Immunology. 2017;150(4):397-407.
3. Intraocular Inflammation and Uveitis 2016-2017. American Academy of Ophthalmology.
4. Murphy K, Weaver C. Janeway's Immunobiology, 9th edition. Garland Science; 2017.
5. Reyes NJ, O'Koren EG, Saban DR. New insights into mononuclear phagocyte biology from the visual system. Nat Rev Immunol. 2017;17(5):322-32.

Chapter 7 Ocular Genetics

B Hansen, VV Mootha

INTRODUCTION

Our genes and proteins are encoded in our DNA collectively known as the genome; they determine our physical and mental traits that make us unique as individuals, but they also contain information which influences our lifelong ocular and systemic health. Genetic disorders are caused by mutations in our approximately 20,000 genes. Mutations in coding sequences or exons modify the resulting proteins. Mutations in the noncoding sequences of the genome may act via numerous molecular mechanisms. These mutations may occur spontaneously in an individual (*de novo*) or are inherited through the parental chromosomes (Figs. 7.1A to D). They may manifest in the heterozygous state (be present on one chromosome, either paternal or maternal) or in the homozygous state (affecting both alleles). A mutation that is manifest in the heterozygous state leads to an autosomal dominant (AD) disorder, whereas mutations that manifest in the homozygous state are referred to as autosomal recessive (AR). X-linked conditions differ from autosomal types in that women are unaffected or only mildly affected carriers and affected

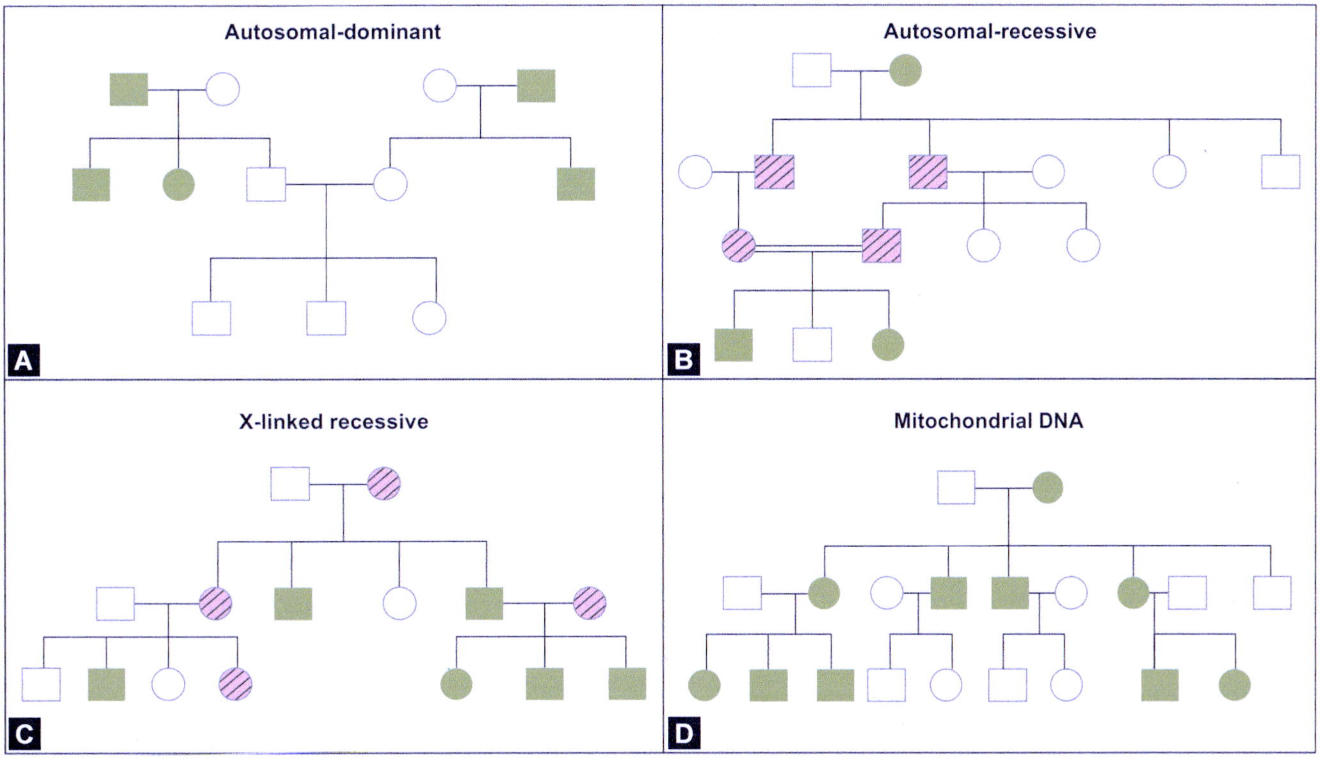

Figs. 7.1A to D: Example family pedigrees of Mendelian modes of inheritance. (A) Autosomal-dominant (AD) pedigree depicting affected parents with heterozygous mutations passing on trait to almost half of their offspring. Equal number of males and females offspring are affected; (B) In autosomal recessive (AR) pedigrees, subjects heterozygous for a mutation are unaffected. Parents of affected subjects are generally unaffected. Consanguinity increases the risk of affected children. Equal number of males and females are affected; (C) In X-linked recessive pedigrees, approximately half of male offspring are affected when mother is carrier of recessive allele on one of her sex chromosomes. All female offspring of affected father will be carriers of mutation. Female carriers may be unaffected or have mild/subclinical phenotype; (D) In pedigrees with maternal inheritance of mitochondrial DNA mutations, all children of affected mothers inherit the trait. (Square symbol = male subject; Circle symbol = female subject; Green symbol = affected subject; White symbol = unaffected subject; Shaded symbol = unaffected carrier of recessive allele (female carrier of recessive X-linked trait who may be unaffected or have mild/subclinical phenotype); Double line connecting male and female parents indicate consanguineous union in pedigree.)

persons are usually male. Other disorders may require the additive effect of mutations in several genes in order to become manifest or require an environmental component; they are then referred to as polygenic or multifactorial. Completion of the Human Genome Project and tools of modern genomics have accelerated ocular disease gene discovery. Some 6,000 human genetic diseases are known and nearly a third of these diseases are purely ocular or have ocular manifestations.[1]

DEFINITIONS[1]

A review of basic genetic terms is useful for an understanding of ocular genetics:

Allele: One or more different forms of a gene that are found at the same location on a chromosome.

Aneuploidy: The number of chromosomes are abnormal; examples include trisomy (3 homologous chromosomes) or monosomy (1 chromosome without a pair).

Anticipation: A disease in which the severity or onset of symptoms begins earlier in each successive generation. This is often observed in diseases with repeat expansion disorders.

Autosome: Any non-sex (X and Y) chromosomes, there are 22 pairs in the human body.

Carrier: A non-affected individual who has one mutated gene that they can pass on to progeny. Rarely, carriers may show partial expression of a disease.

Codominance: Expression of both heterozygous alleles (e.g. ABO blood groups).

Complex genetic disorder: A disease that does not follow Mendelian patterns of inheritance. The disease or trait is determined by genes at multiple loci, subject to environmental influence.

Compound heterozygote: A person who has two different mutations on each homologous chromosome.

Congenital: A disease present at birth, includes no information about the cause of the disease.

Expressivity: The phenomenon that people affected with the same disease can have different symptoms, age of onset, and even severity. An ocular disease that displays varying expressivity is neurofibromatosis type 1 (NF1). It often has different findings, present at different ages, and may develop over a span of many years.

Familial: Not necessarily genetic but a disease that occurs in more than one family member.

Genetic: A condition caused by a defect in genes which may be acquired or inherited.

Genetic heterogeneity: Mutations in different genes result in same phenotype.

Genotype: The genetic make-up of a particular locus.

Hereditary: A condition that results from a person's chromosomes that has potential to be passed on to future generations.

Heritability: Often evaluated through twin studies, a comparison of the impact genes have on the phenotypic expression of traits or diseases.

Infantile: A disease not present at birth but that develops soon thereafter.

Lyonization: The phenomenon that explains why some recessive X-linked traits are expressed in heterozygous females (only 1 X chromosome can be active at a time and so the other is turned off). This is seen in ophthalmology in choroideremia, X-linked RP, and color vision abnormalities.

Maternal inheritance: Suggestive of a mitochondrial DNA mutation; mother passes the trait or disease onto all children but no sons pass on the disease.

Mutation: An alteration in gene sequence or structure that results in disease.

Penetrance: Proportion of subjects with a particular genetic variant that exhibit associated phenotype.

Phenotype: Condition or trait resulting from a particular genotype which may be influenced by environment.

Sex-linked: A disease or gene carried on either the X or Y chromosome.

Variability: A genetic disease may affect different individuals to differing degrees (age of onset or severity may be variable).

X-linked: Genes expressed on X chromosome. Color vision defects, with absence of father-to-son transmission, were some of the early traits tied to a specific chromosome.

Y-linked: Gene expressed in males as they are found on Y chromosome.

CORNEA

Inheritance, clinical findings, pathology, and treatment of pertinent corneal disorders are summarized in Flowchart 7.1.

Flowchart 7.1: Corneal dystrophies excluding *TGFBI* gene: corneal layer involved gene, findings, typical symptoms, and treatments.

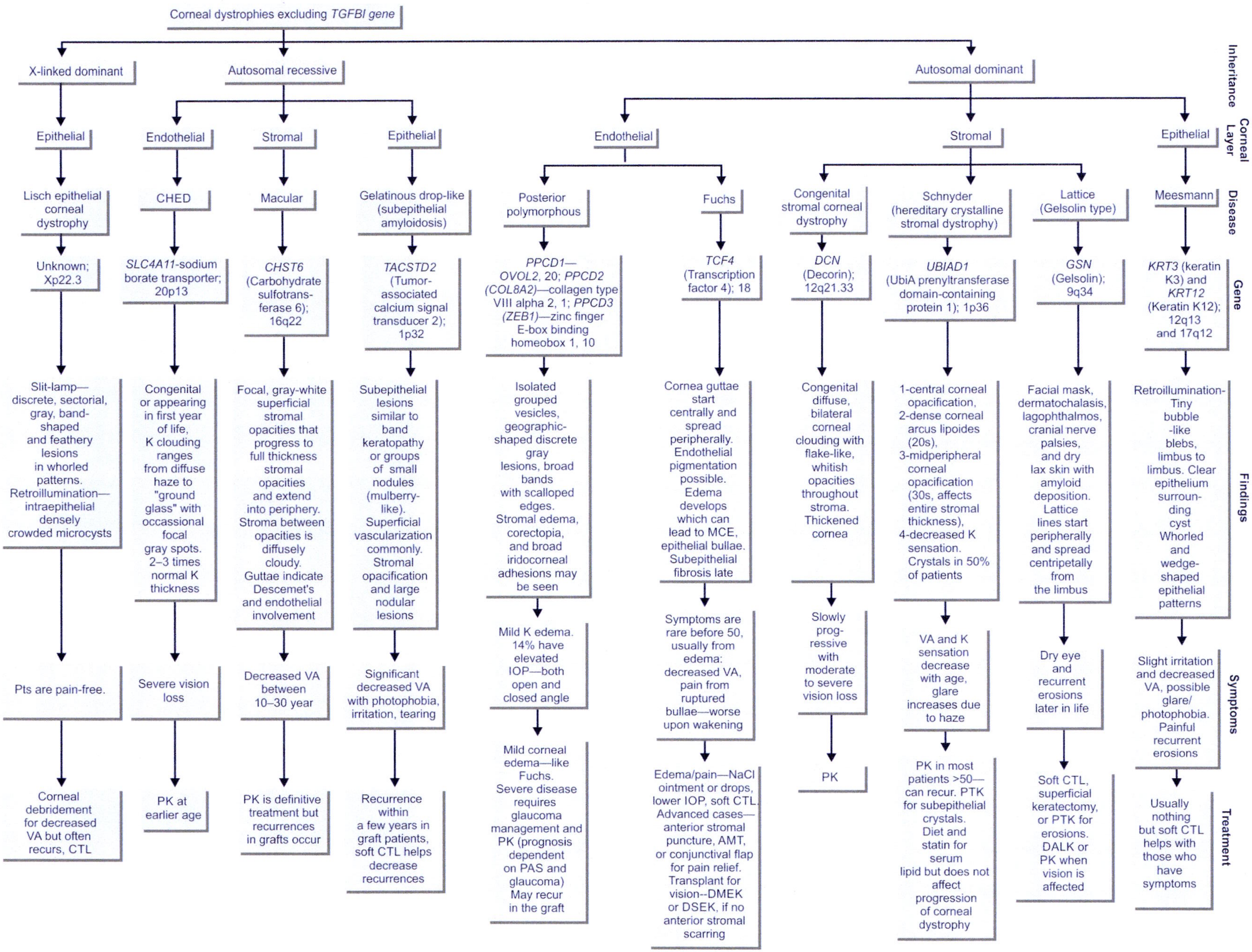

Epithelial and Subepithelial Dystrophies[2]

Meesmann

Inheritance: AD; chromosome: 12q13 and 17q12; gene: *KRT3* (keratin K3) and *KRT12* (keratin K12).[3]

Findings: Tiny bubble-like blebs (most numerous in interpalpebral fissure) are seen best with retroillumination. They extend from limbus to limbus. Epithelium surrounding the cysts is clear. Whorled and wedge-shaped epithelial patterns are observed throughout the superficial cornea. Sensation may be reduced. Slight irritation, decreased visual acuity, and possible glare/photophobia are frequent complaints but most notable are painful recurrent erosions (Figs. 7.2 and 7.3).[4]

Pathology: Epithelial microcysts (periodic acid Schiff-positive cellular debris). Epithelial cells contain accumulation of granular and filamentary material "peculiar substance".

Treatment: Usually observation but soft contact lens (CTL) helps with those who have symptoms.[2]

Lisch Epithelial

Inheritance: X-linked dominant; chromosome: Xp22.3; gene: Unknown.

Findings: Gray, discrete feathery lesions are seen in whorled pattern. Retroillumination shows densely crowded microcysts throughout epithelium. More crowded with no intervening clear space compared to Meesmann. Patients are pain-free.[5]

Pathology: Electron microscopy—diffuse cytoplasmic vacuolization. Immunohistochemistry—Ki67 scattered staining without increased mitotic activity. Confocal microscopy—solitary dark round and oval lesions.

Treatment: Corneal debridement for decreased visual acuity but often recurs, CTL may help.[6]

Gelatinous Drop-like (Subepithelial Amyloidosis)

Inheritance: AR; chromosome: 1p32; gene: *TACSTD2* (Tumor associated calcium signal transducer 2)

Findings: Subepithelial lesions similar to band keratopathy or with groups of small nodules (mulberry configuration)—visible on fluorescein staining. Significantly decreased visual acuity with photophobia, irritation, tearing, and progression of protruding subepithelial lesions is commonly observed. Superficial vascularization is observed. Stromal opacification and large nodular lesions are also seen.[7]

Pathology: Light microscopy—subepithelial and stromal amyloid deposits, disruption of epithelial tight junctions. Electron microscopy—amyloid deposition along basal epithelial layer.

Treatment: Recurrence within a few years in graft patients, soft CTL helps decrease recurrences.

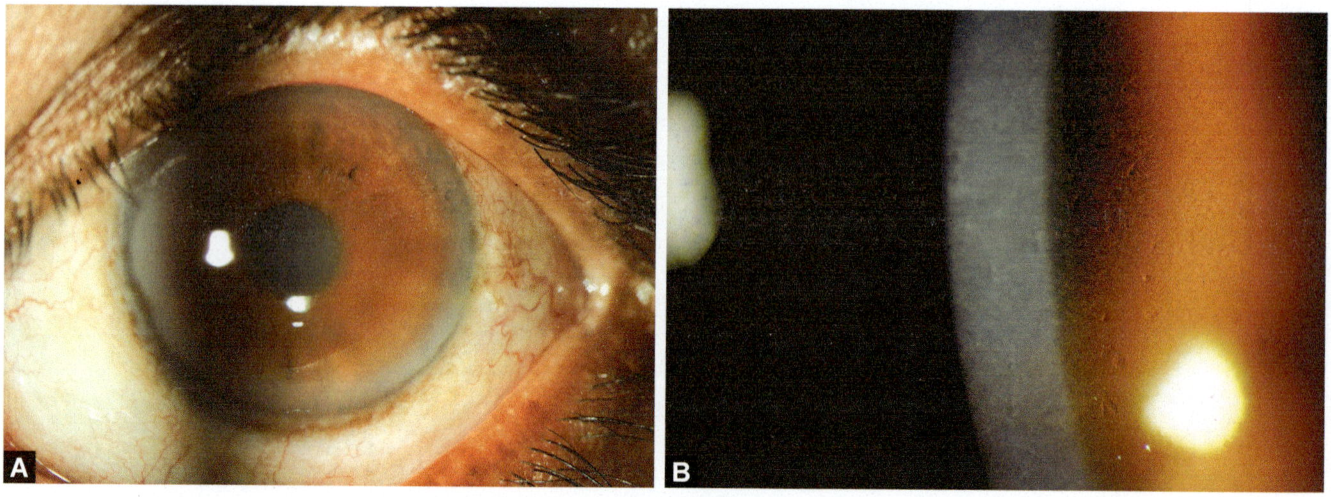

Figs. 7.2A and B: Slit-lamp photographs of Meesmann dystrophy.

Epithelial and Stromal *TGFBI* Dystrophies (Figs. 7.3A to E)

Reis-Bücklers

Inheritance: AD; chromosome: 5q31; gene: Transforming growth factor beta-induced (*TGFBI*) gene.[8]

Findings: Confluent, coarse, irregular geographic opacities with varying densities at Bowman's and superficial stroma—mostly central (may extend to limbus and deep stroma).

Patients have painful recurrent erosions in first or second decade of life (more severe and frequent then Thiel-Behnke). Decreased visual acuity from anterior scarring and anterior stromal edema causes symptoms (Fig. 7.4).[9,10]

Pathology: Light microscopy—Bowman layer is disrupted or absent. It may be replaced by sheet-like tissue layer with granular deposits, which stain with Masson trichrome red. Electron microscopy—rod-shaped bodies (versus curly fibers for Thiel-Behnke). Confocal—basal epithelial layer small granular highly reflective material without shadows.[9]

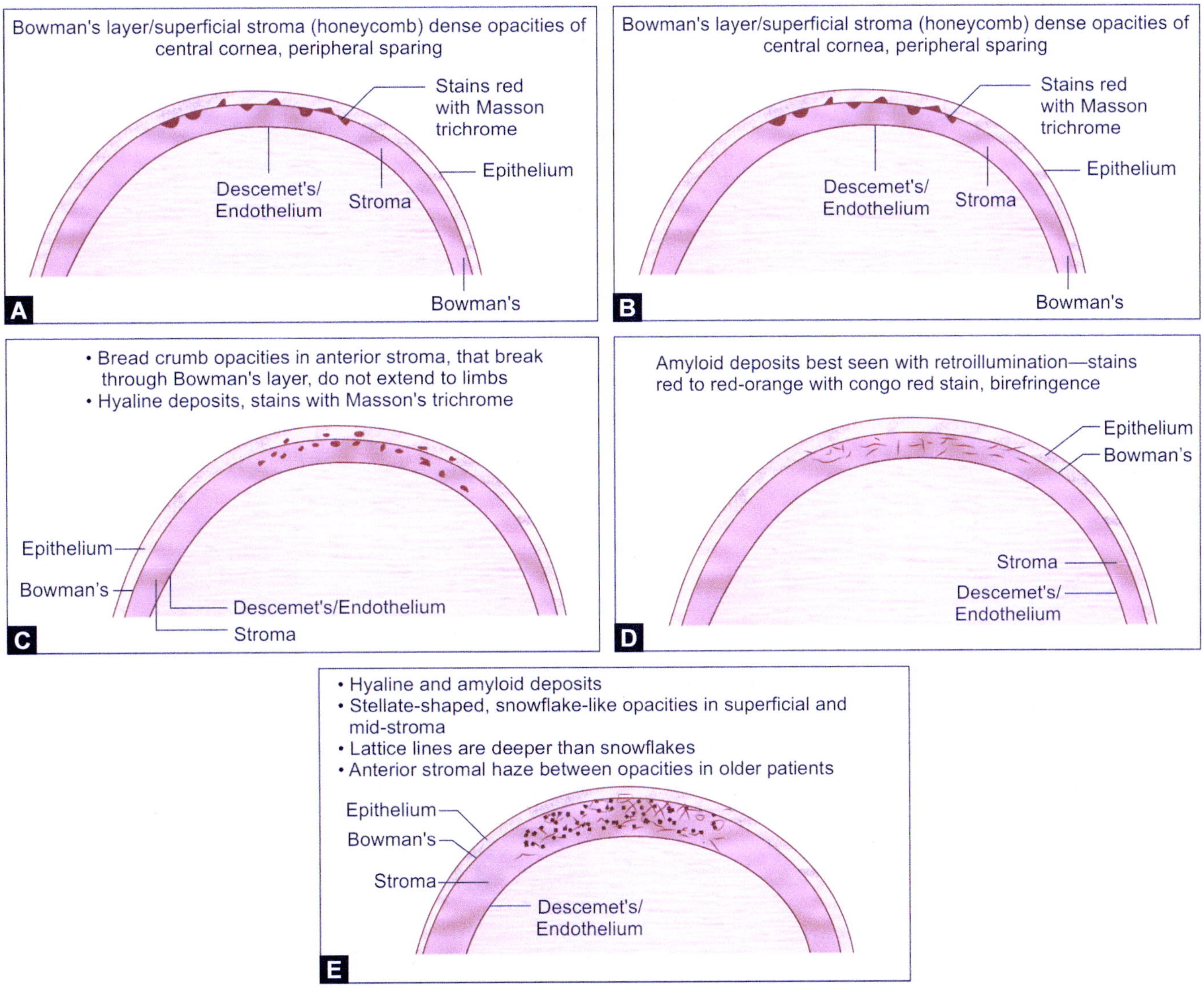

Figs. 7.3A to E: *TGFBI* Corneal Dystrophies: (A) Reis-Buckler depicting the Bowman layer and anterior stromal deposits in central cornea with peripheral sparing, this is more severe with more frequent corneal erosions than its related disease Thiel-Behnke; (B) Thiel-Behnke depicting Bowman layer deposits that stain with Masson Trichrome like A and curly fibers seen on electron microscopy (the differentiating diagnostic tool); (C) Granular Corneal Dystrophy with its central "bread crumb" opacities in the anterior stroma with some breaks in Bowman's layer allowing some of the opacities to creep into the deep epithelium; (D) Lattice Corneal Dystrophy characterized by the linear amyloid deposits, Congo red stains with birefringence, in the anterior and deep stromal layer seen best on retroillumination; (E) Avellino Corneal Dystrophy with deposits similar to Granular and Lattice with stromal haze in between opacities in older patients; however the granular deposits take on a more stellate appearance than those found in Granular dystrophy.

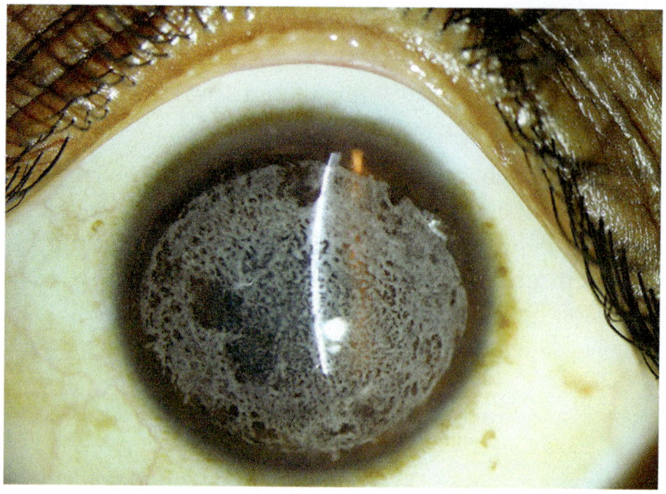

Fig. 7.4: Slit-lamp photograph of Reis-Bucklers dystrophy.

Treatment: Superficial keratectomy, deep anterior lamellar keratoplasty (DALK), phototherapeutic keratectomy (PTK) or rarely penetrating keratoplasty (PKP). Recurrence in graft is common.

Thiel-Behnke

Inheritance: AD; chromosome: 5q31; gene: *TGFBI.*

Findings: Symmetric subepithelial reticular (honeycomb) opacities that spare peripheral cornea. Recurrent corneal erosions are less frequent and severe than Reis-Bucklers. Patients develop worsening visual acuity from corneal opacification.

Pathology: Light microscopy—thickening of epithelium leads to ridges and furrows in underlying stroma; there may be focal absences of epithelial basement membrane. Bowman's layer is replaced by fibrocellular material with a characteristic *saw-toothed pattern.* Electron microscopy—curly fibers. Confocal—deposits in basal epithelial layer show reflectivity with dark shadows.[10]

Treatment: Similar to Reis-Bucklers.

Lattice

Inheritance: AD; chromosome: 5q31; gene: *TGFBI.*

Findings: Glass-like branching lines in stroma with broad spectrum from little involvement to severe. Refractile lines (seen best with retroillumination), start centrally and spread centrifugally and deeper. Central subepithelial ovoid white dots and diffuse anterior stromal haze appear early. Peripheral cornea remains clear. Recurrent erosions and decreased visual acuity affect patients (Figs. 7.5A to C)

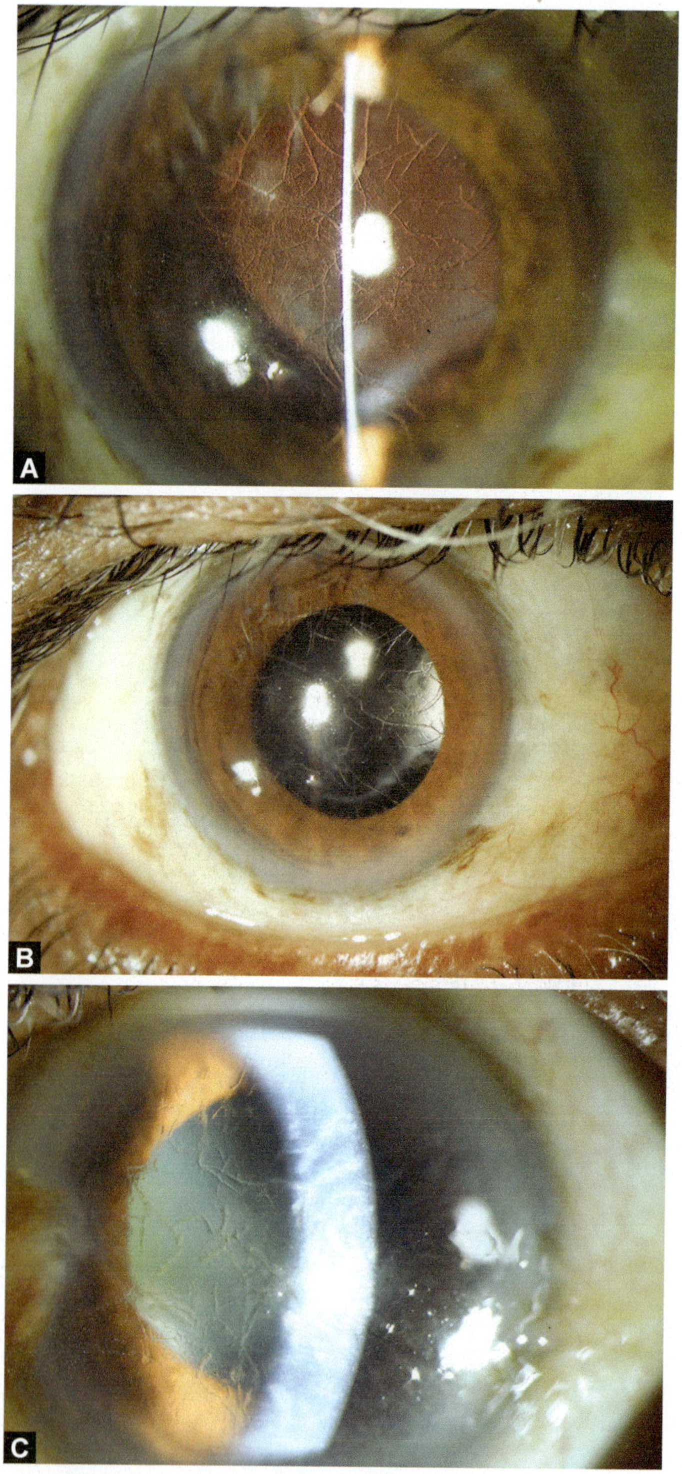

Figs. 7.5A to C: Slit-lamp photographs of lattice dystrophy.

Pathology: Light microscopy—amyloid deposits concentrated in anterior stroma (sometimes subepithelial area as well) lead to poor epithelial-stromal adhesion. Progressive focal thinning or absence of Bowman's layer, degeneration of basal epithelial cells, and epithelial atrophy occur because of amyloid deposition. Lesions stain red to red-orange with Congo. Crystal violet stain will metachromatically and birefringence staining pattern. Electron microscopy—extracellular masses of fibrils randomly aligned.

Treatment: Soft CTL, superficial keratectomy, or PTK for erosions. DALK or PKP is needed for severe cases. It recurs more than granular or macular.[11-13]

Granular

Inheritance: AD; chromosome: 5q31; gene: *TGFBI*.

Findings: Crumb-like lesions in superficial cornea with clear intervening stroma. Direct illumination—shows white opacities. Indirect illumination—demonstrate translucent dots with vacuoles and a *crushed breadcrumb* appearance. Crumbs do not extend to the limbus but through breaks in Bowman's. Patients maintain good visual acuity for a long time but report glare, photophobia, and recurrent erosions (Figs. 7.6A to C).

Pathology: Microscopically—hyaline that stains bright red with Masson. Electron microscopy—Shows a poorly defined matrix with bodies of election dense material shaped like a rod. Disease forms keratoepithelin derived from epithelium and keratocytes.

Stromal Dystrophies

Lattice-Gelsolin Type

Inheritance: AD; chromosome: 9q34; gene: Gelsolin *(GSN)*.

Findings: Amyloid deposition can cause dry lax skin, cranial nerve palsies, lagophthalmos, dermatochalasis, pendulous ears, facial mask. Lattice lines are less numerous and start peripherally. They spread centripetally from the

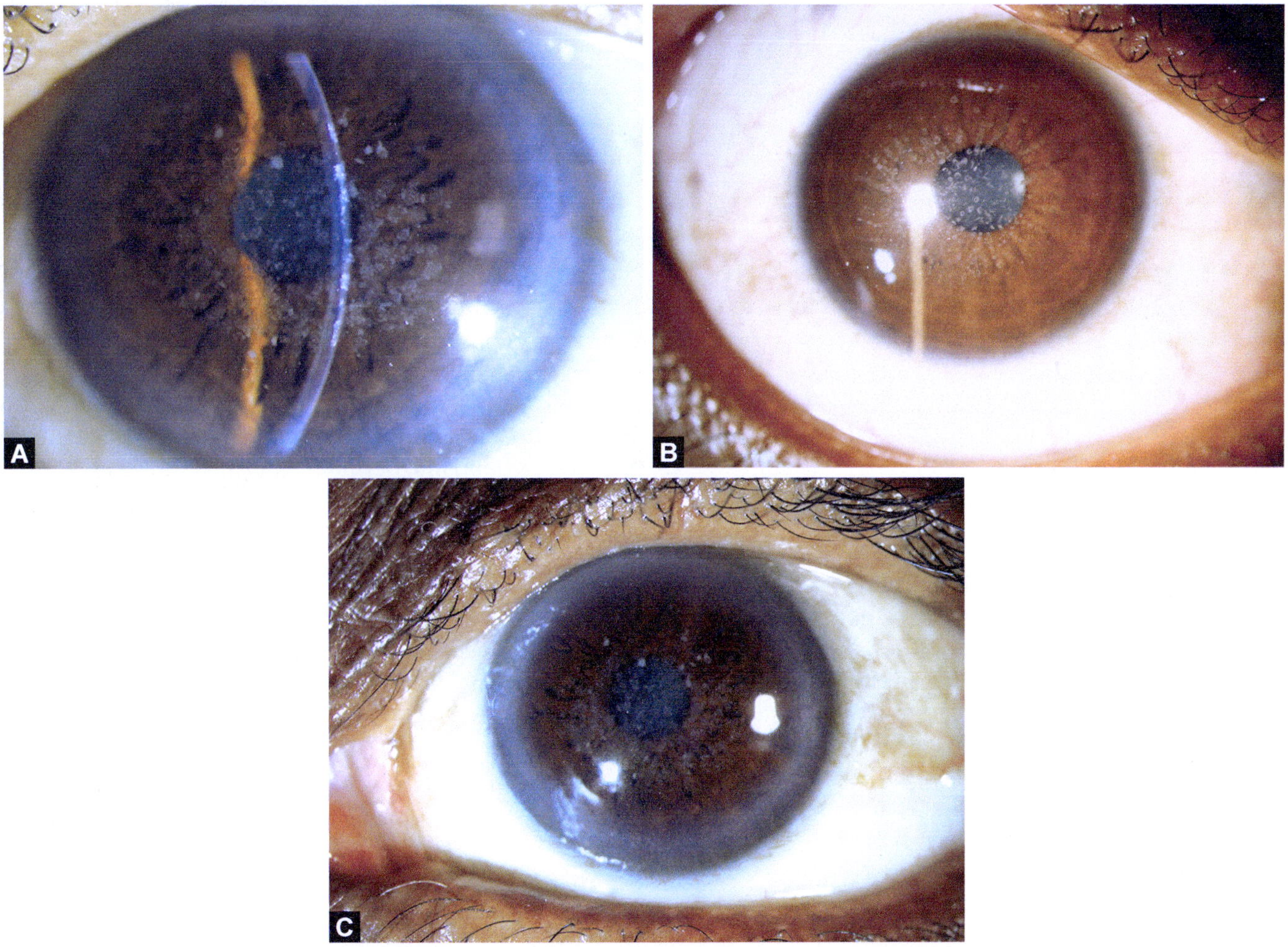

Figs. 7.6A to C: Slit-lamp photographs of granular dystrophy.

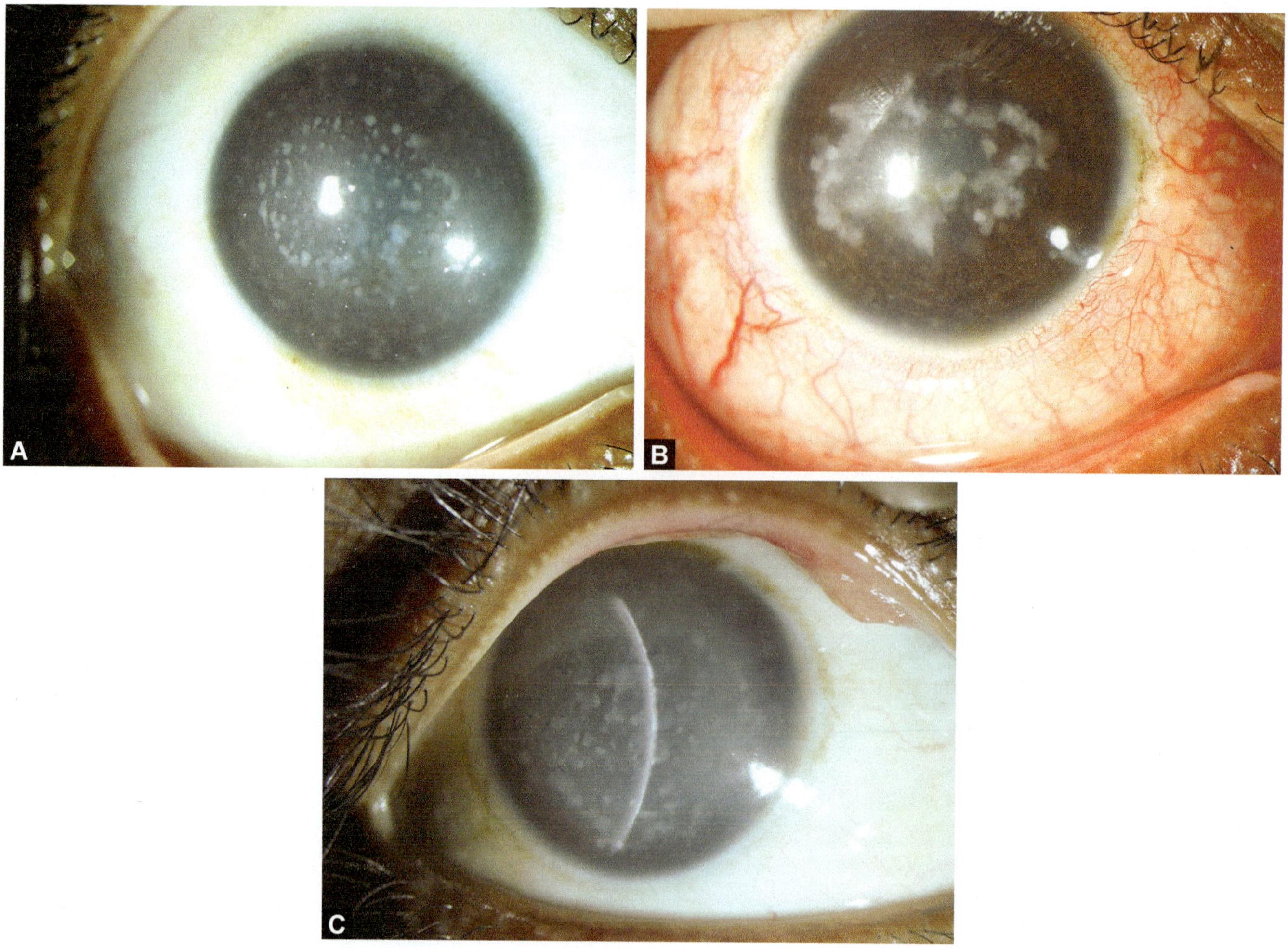

Figs. 7.7A to C: Slit-lamp photographs of macular dystrophy.

limbus. Central corneal sparing is often noted. Dry eye and recurrent erosions later in life affect patients.[14,15]

Pathology: Light microscopy—amyloid under Bowman's and within sclera appears as discontinuous band of lattice lines. Amyloid does not stain for amyloid A protein or amyloid P component. Altered gelsolin is seen in sclera, ciliary body, conjunctiva, and the optic nerve. Amyloid also present in arterial walls, glomeruli, and peripheral nerves.[16]

Treatment: Treat recurrent erosions as above. DALK or PKP performed when vision is affected. Recurrence after many years appears as fine subepithelial opacities.

Macular

Inheritance: AR; chromosome: 16q22; gene: Carbohydrate sulfotransferase 6 *(CHST6)*.

Findings: Involves entire stroma and periphery and sometimes the endothelium. Gray-white superficial stromal opacities extend into periphery and are visible via slit-lamp (Figs. 7.7A to C). Stroma between the opacities is cloudy. Guttae indicate Descemet's and endothelial involvement. Decreased visual acuity is noted between 10 years and 30 years of age. It is least common of the stromal dystrophies.[17]

Pathology: Glycosaminoglycans (GAGs) stain with colloidal iron and Alcian blue. Electron microscopy—keratocytes and endothelial cells stain positive for GAGs. Macular corneal dystrophy is disorder of keratan sulfate metabolism. In type 1, keratan sulfate is absent in serum and cornea. In type 2, keratan sulfate is present in serum and corneal stroma in decreased amounts. Type 1A has no keratan sulfate in serum but is present within stromal keratocytes.[17]

Treatment: PKP is definitive treatment but recurrences in grafts occur.

Schnyder

Inheritance: AD; chromosome: 1p36; gene: UbiA prenyltransferase domain-containing protein 1 *(UBIAD1)*.

Findings: Rare, slowly progressive—usually diagnosed in 10-20s (later with acrystalline form). Central subepithelial crystals occur in 50% (no epithelial involvement). Visual acuity and corneal sensation decrease with age, glare increase due to haze. Progression of the disease usually occurs: 1-Central opacification, 2-dense corneal arcus (20s), 3-mid-peripheral opacification affecting full stromal thickness (30s), 4-decreased sensation.

Pathology: A local disorder of corneal lipid metabolism. Phospholipids form opacities that stain with oil red O. Electron microscopy—cholesterol and phospholipid gather in epithelium, Bowman's, and throughout stroma.

Confocal: shows disruption of subepithelial nerve plexus and highly reflective intra and extracellular deposits.[18]

Treatment: PKP in most patients older than 50—can recur. PTK for subepithelial crystals but does not help panstromal haze. Diet and statin for serum lipid but does not affect progression of corneal dystrophy.

Congenital Stromal Corneal Dystrophy

Inheritance: AD; chromosome: 12q21.33; gene: Decorin (*DCN*).[19]

Findings: Children born with bilateral thickened cornea with flake-like lesions in the stroma. The cornea is cloudy and thickened. The vision loss is moderate to severe but nonprogessive.

Pathology: Separation of stromal lamellae. Electron microscopy—collagen fibrils are half of normal size. Normal epithelium, keratocytes and endothelium are observed.[20]

Treatment: PKP.

Endothelial Dystrophies

Fuchs Endothelial Corneal Dystrophy

Inheritance: AD; chromosome: 18q; gene: Transcription factor 4 *(TCF4)* triplet repeat expansions (CTG18.1) in majority of adult-onset cases; *SLC4A11, TCF8, LOXHD1*, and *AGBL1* in minority of adult-onset cases; *COL8A2* in rare, early-onset disease variant.[21,22]

Findings: Cornea guttae start centrally and spread peripherally. Endothelial pigmentation can be seen. Edema develops which can lead to stromal edema, which causes epithelial bullae. Subepithelial fibrosis occurs later. Symptoms are rare before 50 and are usually from edema. Corneal edema causes decreased visual acuity and pain (from ruptured bullae). Symptoms worse upon wakening (no evaporation while sleeping).

Pathology: Microscopically—large polymorphic endothelial cells. Descemet's membrane becomes thicker with focal excrescences (guttae) that result from collagen and extracellular matrix deposits. Reduced number of Na^+, K^+ -ATPase pumps and function.

Treatment: Reduce edema and pain—NaCl ointment or drops, soft CTL. Advanced cases require transplant for vision—Descemet membrane endothelial keratoplasty (DMEK) or Descemet stripping endothelial keratoplasty (DSEK), if no or minimal anterior stromal scarring; PKP with moderate or advanced stromal scarring.[21,23]

Posterior Polymorphous

Inheritance: AD; chromosome: 20, 1, 10; gene: PPCD1 *(OLOV2)* ; PPCD2 *(COL8A2)*—collagen type VIII alpha 2; PPCD3 *(ZEB1)*—zinc finger E-box binding homeobox 1.

Findings: Groups of vesicles, gray geographic-shaped opacities, bands with scalloped edges. Corectopia and broad iridocorneal adhesions may be seen. Elevated IOP secondary to both open and closed angle.

Pathology: Multilayered endothelial cells that act and appear like epithelial cells: microvilli, rapid and easy growth in culture, intercellular desmosomes, and proliferative tendencies. Descemets thickens taking on a laminated appearance with polymorphous changes (similar changes appear in ICE syndrome—sporadic and unilateral though). Specular microscopy—vesicles and bands, whereas ICE cells appear as dark areas with central area illuminated and light peripheral borders.[24]

Treatment: Mild corneal edema like Fuchs' dystrophy. More severe disease requires glaucoma management and DMEK/DSEK/PKP (prognosis dependent on PAS and glaucoma). May recur in the graft.

CHED

Inheritance: AR, chromosome: 2013; gene: *SLC4A11*—sodium borate transporter.

Findings: Diffuse corneal clouding seen at birth or in perinatal period resulting in profound vision loss and possible amblyopia.

Pathology: Marked thickening of Descemet's membrane and loss of endothelium. Stroma is markedly thickened.

Treatment: PKP/DSAEK.

LENS

Cataracts

Myotonic Dystrophy (DM)

Inheritance: AD; chromosome: 19; gene: DM1 *(DMPK)*—myotonic dystrophy protein kinase, a CTG triplet expansion—anticipation; DM2 *(ZNF9)*—CCTG quadruplet repeat, no anticipation.[25]

Findings: Affects eye (often first presenting symptoms), pulmonary, cardiac, endocrine, and central nervous systems—respiratory failure is the leading cause of death among those affected.[26] Cataract begins with iridescent colored opacities of the outer layer that later coalesce into spokes ("Christmas tree cataract"); cataract forms in 100% of these patients (Fig. 7.8). Ptosis, ophthalmoplegia (mostly adducting deficit) and extraocular myotonia (slowed and disconjugate saccades) are common. Patients also have miosis with slow pupil response. There is also an association with Fuchs' dystrophy.[25]

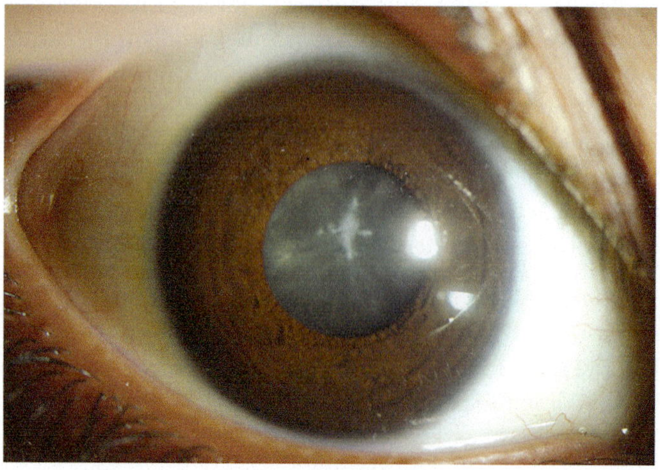

Fig. 7.8: Slit-lamp photograph of myotonic dystrophy.

Pathology: Increased level of gamma-glutamyl transpeptidase (GGT) is thought to be responsible for low levels of lenticular glutathione leading to cataract formation. Genetic testing is available with blood sample.[27]

Treatment: No known treatment for disease but surgeries to manage cataract and ptosis. Refer to specialist to manage systemic manifestations of the disease. Be aware that general anesthesia in particular can cause devastating complications and local anesthesia should be used judiciously.

Galactosemia

Inheritance: AR; chromosome: 9p13; 17q24; 1p36; gene: *Gal-1-PUT*: galactose-1-phosphate uridylyltransferase (most common and most severe); *galactokinase; UDP-*galactose-4-epimerase. All cause defect in enzyme to convert galactose to glucose.

Findings: If undiagnosed malnutrition, jaundice, hepatomegaly, and mental deficiency present in the first few weeks of life as will bilateral cataracts (accumulation of galactose and galactitol lead to influx of fluid into lens). The cataract is often described as an "oil droplet" appearance on retroillumination. Early cataract is reversed in some cases with treatment.[28]

Treatment: Elimination of all milk and milk products.

Wilson Disease

Inheritance: AR; chromosome: 13q14; gene: *ATP7B*—P type ATPase that transports copper into bile (Wilson Disease Protein).[29]

Findings: Deposits of copper is Descemet's membrane (Kayser-Fleischer ring used in diagnostic algorithms), sunflower cataract (rare and disappears with treatment). Ceruloplasmin is decreased in 85–90% of individuals but not the cause of symptoms. Patients have increased free copper and urinary copper.[30]

Treatment: Low-copper diet and life-long chelating agent (D-penicillamine is the drug of choice).

Dislocations

Marfan

Inheritance: AD; 15% no family history; chromosome: 15; gene: *FBN1*—fibrillin-1 a glycoprotein component of the extracellular matrix (particularly affect aorta, ligaments, and zonules).[31]

Findings: Systemic findings include: tall, arachnodactyly, chest wall deformities, aortic root dilation, and mitral valve prolapse. Ocular manifestations include: 50-80% with ectopia lentis (usually superior and temporal)—which can lead to amblyopia and pupillary block glaucoma; axial myopia and increased risk of retinal detachment.[32]

Treatment: Refer to cardiologist if not already. Glasses refraction of both phakic and aphakic portion to determine most helpful and a reading add are beneficial. Cataract surgery for those who do not benefit from glasses has many complications because of weak zonules and increased risk for retinal detachment. A higher rate of success has been achieved with lensectomy using vitrector although long-term analysis is still pending.[32]

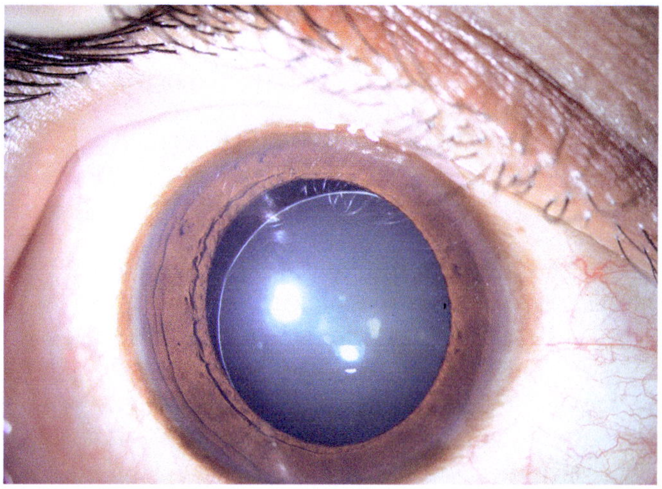

Fig. 7.9: Slit-lamp photograph of homocystinuria.

Homocystinuria

Inheritance: AR; gene: *CBS* (cystathionine-beta-synthase) is most common; *MTHFR* (methylenetetrahydrofolate reductase; *MTR* (methionine synthase); *MTRR* (methionine synthase reductase); and *MMADHC* (methylmalonic aciduria and homocystinuria, cblD) are less common.[33]

Findings: Absent brittle zonules (compared to stretched zonules of Marfan's) with a dislocated lens (down and nasally 50%, anteriorly 10%). Dislocated lens can cause pupillary block glaucoma. There is also an association with myopia, retinal detachment, and optic atrophy. Systemic involvement includes Marfanoid habitus, mental disability, seizures, flushed cheeks. There is an increased risk of life threatening thrombotic events (Figs. 7.9 and 7.10).[34]

Treatment: High dose vitamin B6 (works in 50% of patients). Those that do not respond to vitamin supplementation need a low methionine diet.

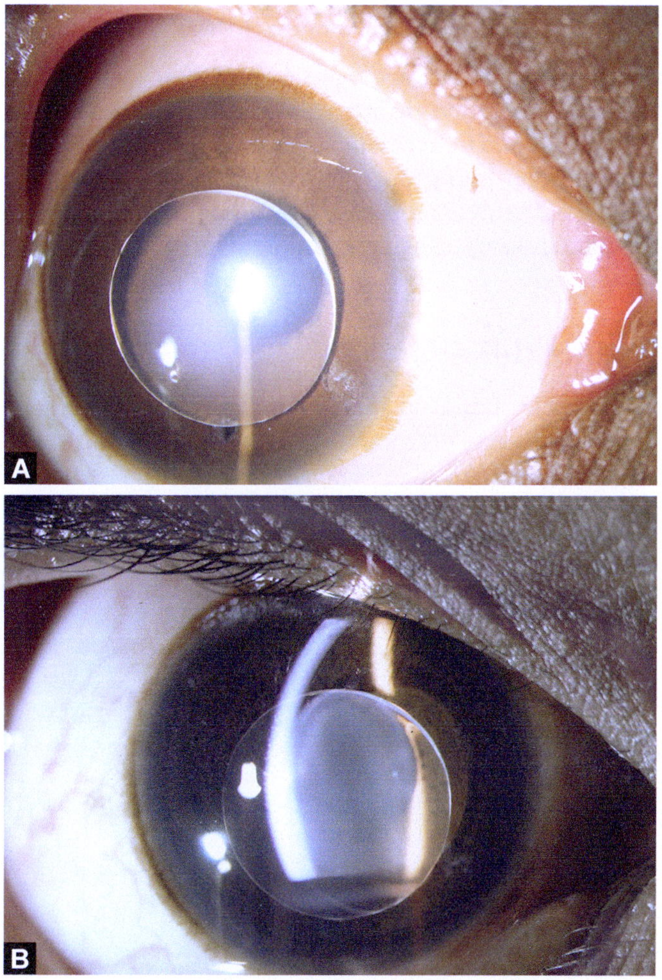

Figs. 7.10A and B: Slit-lamp photographs of a dislocated lens.

Ectopia Lentis et Pupillae

Inheritance: AR; chromosome: 7q31.32; gene: *AASS*—alpha-aminoadipic semialdehyde synthase.

Findings: Irregular pupil displaced from the normal position with the lens displaced in the opposite direction. The lens may bisect the pupil or be completely luxated from the pupillary axis. The disease is bilateral but asymmetric. Other ocular associations include abnormal iris transillumination, severe myopia, retinal detachment, enlarged corneal diameter, and cataract.[35]

GLAUCOMA

Primary Childhood-onset Glaucoma

Primary Congenital Glaucoma

Inheritance: AR; chromosome: 2p22.2; gene: *CYP1B1*—cytochrome P450 1B1.[36,37]

Findings: Classic triad of epiphora, photophobia, and blepharospam. Before age 3, increased IOP causes corneal stretch leading to: increased corneal diameter, buphthalmos (enlarged globe), *Haab striae* (breaks in Descemet's), and corneal edema/opacification (which leads to the photophobia). After age 3, increased IOP does not stretch the cornea but may cause scleral thinning and progressive myopia. Most cases are diagnosed in the first year (>75%), are bilateral (70%), has a worse prognosis the later it is diagnosed. There is newborn (25%) and infantile congenital glaucoma with the former having a much worse prognosis; almost half will progress to legal blindness.

Treatment: Angle surgery is necessary to treat the increased outflow resistance through the trabecular meshwork. Goniotomy and trabeculotomy *ab externo* are the preferred surgeries but trabeculotomy should be performed if the cornea is cloudy. Trabeculectomy and tubes are reserved for refractory cases where goniotomy or trabeculotomy have failed.

Axenfeld-Rieger

Inheritance: AD mostly, some sporadic; chromosome: 4q25 and 6p25.3; gene: *PITX2* and *FOXC1*—transcription factors regulating anterior chamber formation.[38,39]

Findings: Traditionally separated into Axenfeld anomaly, Rieger anomaly and Rieger syndrome. It is now viewed as a continuous spectrum ranging from: posterior embryotoxon with multiple peripheral adherent iris strands, that plus iris hypoplasia and corectopia, to all of that plus developmental defects of teeth, maxillary bone, pituitary gland, hypospadias, and redundant periumbilical skin (Figs. 7.11A and B).[28]

Peters Anomaly

Inheritance: Usually sporadic but AR and AD have been reported; chromosome: multiple; gene: *FOXC1*, *PITX2*, *PAX6*, or *CYP1B1* can all cause Peters' anomaly.[40]

Findings: Defect in possible corneal endothelium, (Descemet's and posterior stroma) that causes a central visual axis corneal opacity. Often there are adhesions between the cornea and iris. The lens can be normal or adherent to the posterior layers of the cornea with cataract. Corneolenticular adhesions lead to higher risk of angle abnormalities and microcornea and is associated with more systemic abnormalities (heart, GI, ear, palate, spine, and musculoskeletal). 50% of those affected have glaucoma—very difficult to treat glaucoma.[41]

Aniridia

Inheritance: AD (2/3), sporadic (1/3, 20% of which have WAGR); chromosome: 11p13; gene: *PAX6*—transcription factor involved in eye, spinal cord and pancreas development.

Findings: A bilateral congenital iris hypoplasia (only a rudimentary stump in most). It is associated with microcornea, cataracts, optic nerve hypoplasia, and foveal

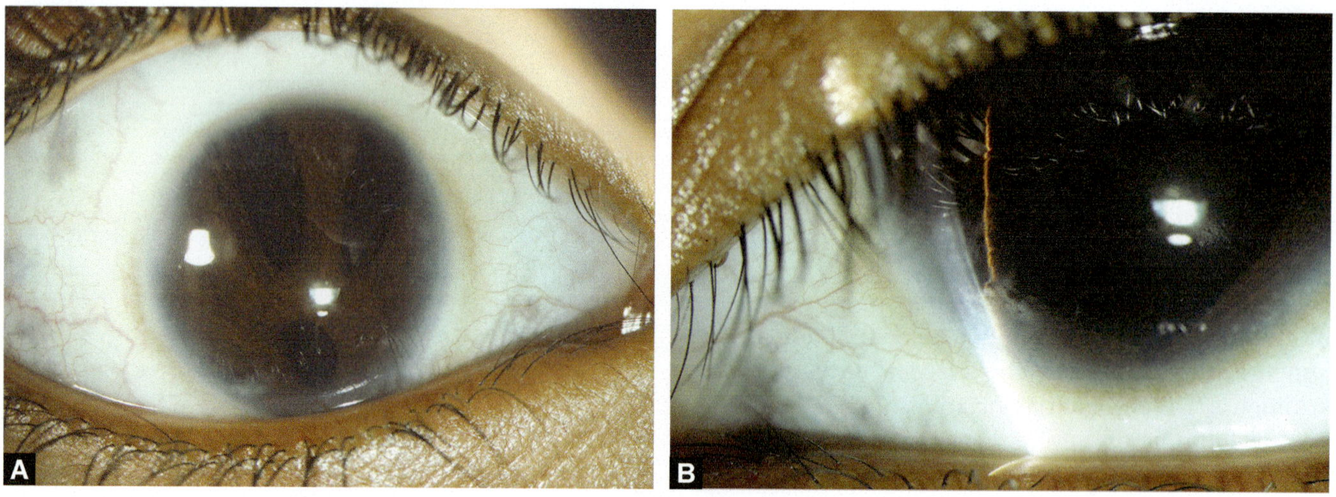

Figs. 7.11A and B: Slit-lamp photographs of Axenfeld-Rieger syndrome.

hypoplasia. The latter two findings lead to nystagmus (pendular) and reduced visual acuity. Almost 75% develop glaucoma from chronic angle closure. Patients have limbal stem cell deficiency that causes a pannus that moves centrally (some require limbal stem cell transplant). Besides WAGR in those with sporadic aniridia, Gillespie syndrome is an autosomal recessive variant with cerebellar ataxia and mental disability (occurs in 2% of patients with aniridia).[42]

Treatment: Angle surgery before it closes completely. Once angle is closed a trabeculectomy, tube, or cyclophotocoagulation will be required for long-term management.

NF1 (von Recklinghausen) (The Most Common Phakomatosis)

Inheritance: AD 50%, sporadic 50%; chromosome: 17q11.2; gene: *NF1*—neurofibromin a tumor suppressor protein.

Findings: Ectropion uveae in a neonate, Lisch nodules, optic nerve glioma, eyelid neurofibroma and glaucoma. Systemic findings include: cutaneous café-au-lait spots, axillary/inguinal freckling and cutaneous neurofibromas.[43]

Primary Open-Angle Glaucoma (POAG)

Inheritance: 5% AD, the rest unknown/sporadic; chromosome: 1q24.3, 1q24.1 and 3q25.31 gene: *MYOC*—myocilin protein found in ciliary body and trabecular meshwork but poorly understood; *OPTN*— optineurin protein involved in multiple pathways, notably maintenance of the golgi apparatus; *TMCO1; FNDC3B*.[44,45]

Findings and treatment discussion of POAG can be found in the glaucoma chapter. Genome-wide association studies for POAG have identified many genes including *ABCA1, AFAP1, GMDS, PMMZ, TGEBR3, FNDC3B, ARHGEF12, GAS7, FOXC1, ATXN2*, and *TXNRDZ*.[45a]

RETINA

Inheritance, clinical findings, pathology and treatment of pertinent retinal disorders are summarized (Flowcharts 7.2 and 7.3).[46]

Flowchart 7.2: Chart of macular dystrophies including inheritance, gene, and findings.

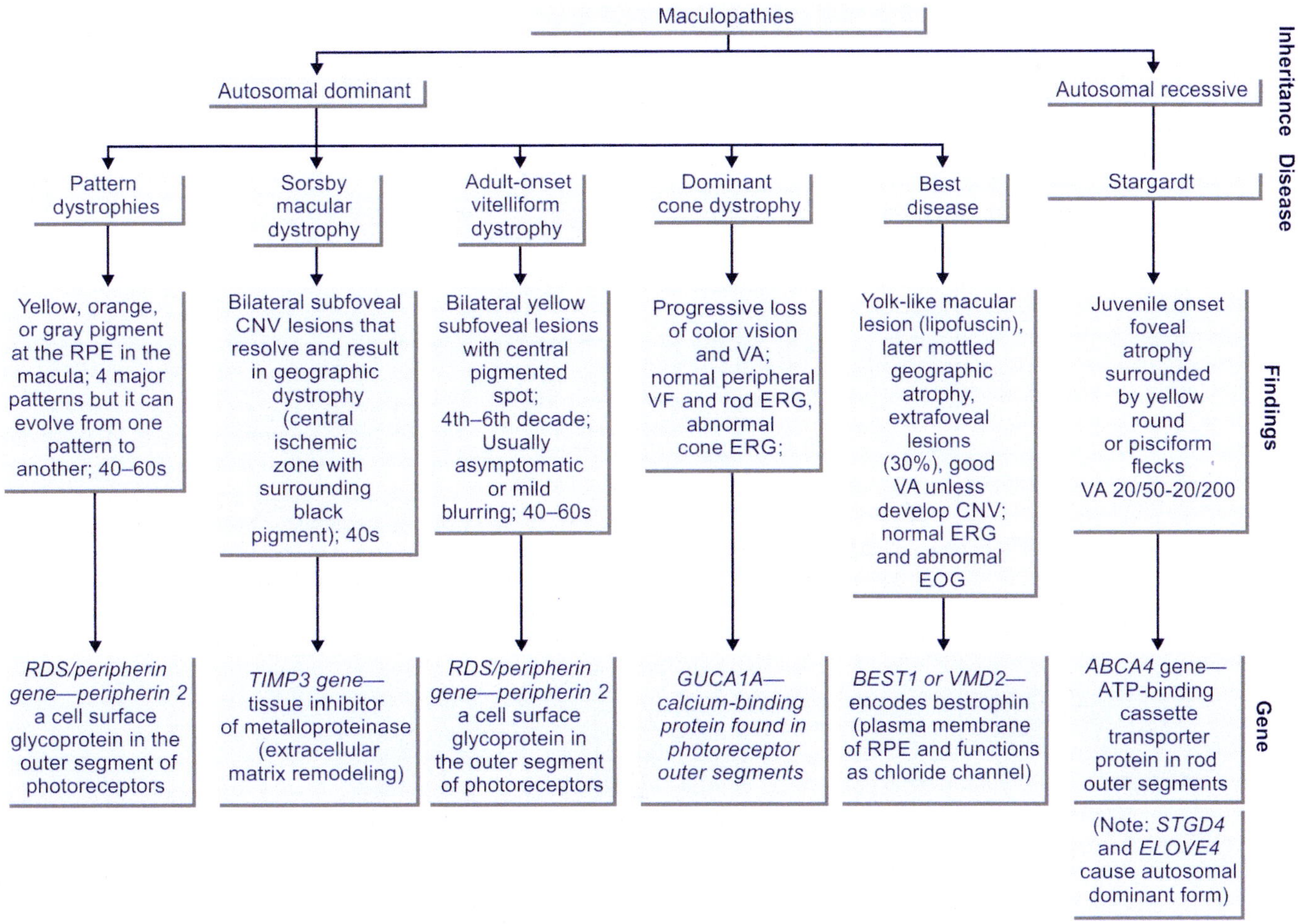

Flowchart 7.3: Chart of pigmentary retinopathies including inheritance, findings, and gene.

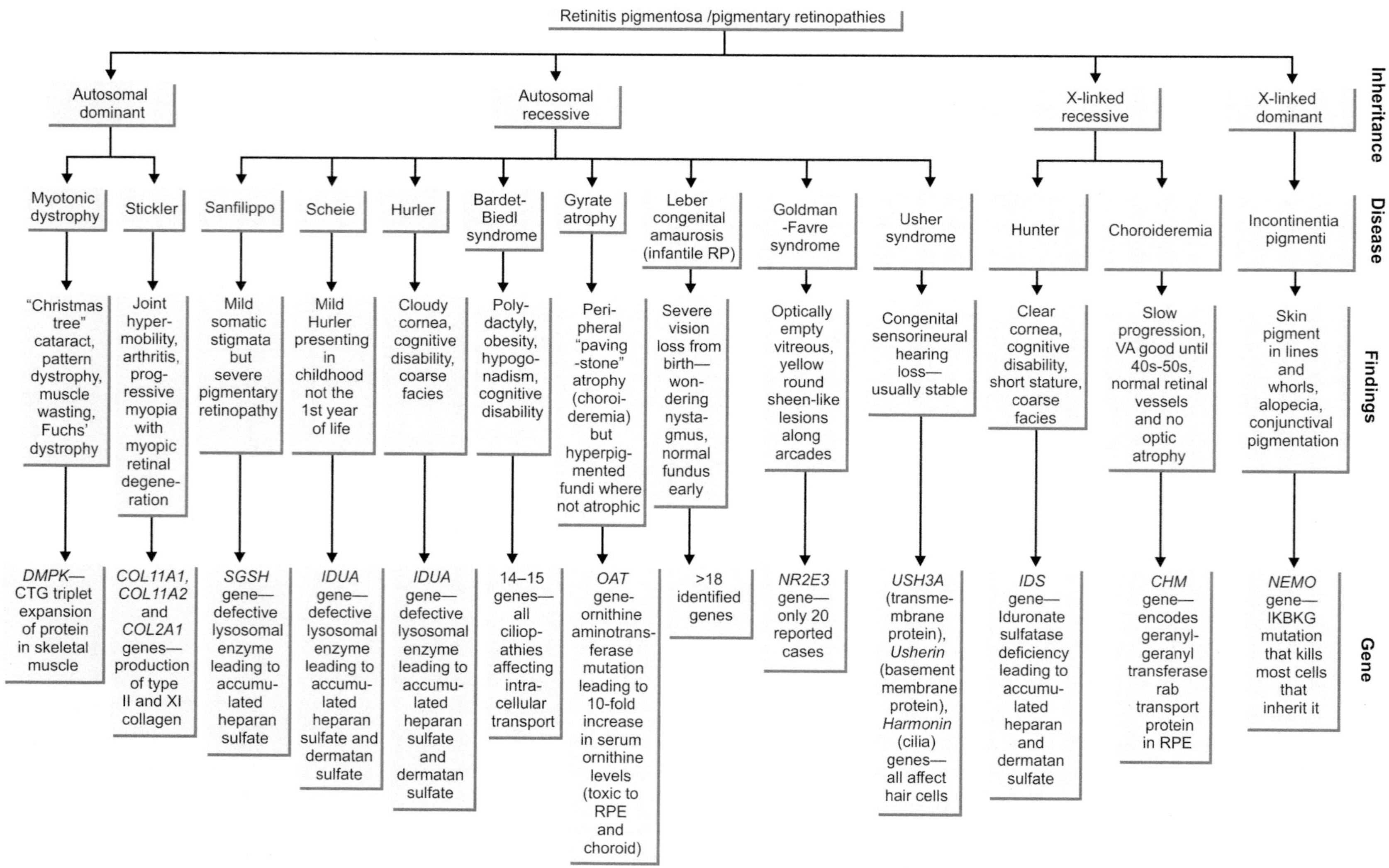

Retinoblastoma (RB) (The Most Common Intraocular Tumor of Childhood)

Inheritance: Germinal—40% (AD), Non-germinal--60% (Sporadic)—for parent with bilateral RB, offspring have 45% chance of having disease; for parent with unilateral RB, offspring have 7–15% probability of being affected; for unaffected parent the offspring have <1% chance of being affected; chromosome: 13q14.2; gene: *RB1*—tumor suppressor gene that keeps cells from replicating too fast.

Findings: 30–40% of cases are bilateral, similar among sexes, no predilection for race. Typically diagnosed in 1st year of life for bilateral and familial cases while sporadic unilateral cases are found between 1st year and 3rd year of life. Leukocoria is most common presenting sign, 25% of cases present with strabismus, and less commonly vitreous hemorrhage, inflammation, glaucoma, proptosis, or hyphema are the presenting signs. Trilateral RB is found in less than 0.5% in patients with unilateral RB and 5–15% in patients with bilateral RB.[46]

Diagnosis: Magnetic resonance imaging (MRI) and ultrasound is preferred to computed tomography (CT) because of increased risk of secondary malignancy due to radiation. Flexner-Wintersteiner rosettes are characteristic on histology. There is usually calcification which helps identify RB from other entities in the differential diagnosis.[47]

Treatment: If unlikely to salvage vision in patient with advanced unilateral RB, primary enucleation remains treatment of choice, which avoids systemic effects of chemotherapy (minimize manipulation of globe and take long amount of nerve to prevent seeding). Systemic chemotherapy followed by local therapy (cryotherapy, laser photocoagulation, thermotherapy, or plaque radiotherapy) for large RBs. Small RBs can be treated with laser photocoagulation. Intravitreal chemotherapy is consider for vitreous seeding in refractory cases. Long-term disease free survival is possible, if CNS is not involved.[47]

von Hippel-Lindau

Inheritance: Sporadic and hereditary forms—AD with incomplete penetrance and variable expression; chromosome: 3p25.3; Gene: *VHL*—von Hippel-Lindau protein which helps regulate hypoxia inducible factor 1-alpha, defect allows vascular endothelial growth factor (VEGF) and other growth factors to rise unchecked.[48]

Findings: Capillary hemangioblastoma in the retina and optic nerve that is bilateral in 50% of cases. Leakage of plasma from hemangioblastoma may lead to serous retinal detachment and accumulation in macula leading to decreased visual acuity. Neovascularization may develop following detachment.[49]

Systemic involvement: Central nervous system (CNS) tumors visceral lesions cysts of kidney, pancreas, liver, and ovary, renal cell carcinoma, meningiomas and pheochromocytomas.[50]

X-Linked Retinoschisis

Inheritance: X-linked recessive; chromosome: Xp22.13; gene: *RS1*—adhesion protein called retinoschisin found on all retinal neurons (especially Muller cells).[51]

Findings: Foveal schisis—cystoid spaces and fine striae in macula. FA shows no leakage in fovea. Visual acuity is good initially but decreases to 20/200. Peripheral retinoschisis occurs in 50% or more of males. Boys often present with vitreous hemorrhage from torn retinal vessels.[52]

Albinism: Oculocutaneous Versus Ocular

Inheritance: AR vs X-linked recessive; chromosome: 7q31.32; gene: *AASS*—alpha-aminoadipic semialdehyde synthase.

Findings:

1. Congenitally poor vision (20/100 or so) with nystagmus—fovea is hypoplastic.
2 Near normal vision (some call it albinoidism because it is milder). Photophobia, iris transillumination, and hypopigmented fundi are found in both.[53]

Congenital Stationary Night Blindness

Inheritance: X-linked (most common), gene: *NYX* and *CACNA1F*; AD, gene: *RHO*, *GNAT1*, or *PDE6B*; AR, gene: *GRM6* and *TRPM1*.

Findings: Life-long stable abnormal scotopic vision, visual acuity normally to 20/200, significant myopia, rhodopsin regeneration normal after bright light (not a loss of photoreceptors like RP but communication failure).[56]

Maculopathies (*see* Flowchart 7.2)

Stargardt Disease

Inheritance: AR majority, AD-a few; chromosome: 1p22.1; gene: *ABCA4* (rod outer segments), dominant genes *STGD4* (RDS/peripherin gene) and *ELOVL4*.[57]

Findings: Foveal atrophy surrounded by discrete, yellowish, round or pisciform flecks. Visual acuity ranges from 20/50-20/200.[58]

Best Disease

Inheritance: AD; chromosome: 11; gene: *Best1* or *VMD2*—encodes bestrophin.[59]

Findings: Lipofuscin accumulation leads to yolk like macular lesion which breaks down leading to the characteristic late mottled geographic atrophic appearance. Extrafoveal vitelliform lesions (up to 30% of patients) are observed. Affected individuals maintain good visual acuity in spite of the appearance on fundoscopy but may develop CNV leaving patient with 20/200 vision.[59,60]

Dominant Cone Dystrophy

Inheritance: AD; gene: *GUCA1A, GUCY2D, CRX*, and numerous others.

Findings: Abnormal or absent photopic electroretinogram (ERG) with normal rod-isolated ERG. Normal peripheral visual fields while having progressive loss of visual acuity and color discrimination help identify this disease.[61]

Sorsby Macular Dystrophy

Inheritance: AD; chromosome: 22; gene: *TIMP3* tissue inhibitor of metalloproteinase 3.[62,63]

Findings: Bilateral subfoveal choroidal neovascular lesions that resolve and become areas of geographic atrophy.[62] These areas have a central ischemic bone with surrounding black pigmentation.

Adult-onset Vitelliform Dystrophy

Inheritance: AD in some families; chromosome: 6p21.1; gene: *PRPH2*—Peripherin 2, cell surface glycoprotein in outer segment of photoreceptors.[64]

Findings: Bilateral round or oval subfoveal lesion that are yellow with a pigmented spot centrally.[65]

Pattern Dystrophies

Inheritance: AD; chromosome: 6p21.1; gene: *PRPH2*—Peripherin 2, cell surface glycoprotein in outer segment of photoreceptors.

Findings: Pigment in the macula, within RPE, has a yellow orange, or gray appearance. There are four major patterns but an individual can evolve from one pattern to another. Usually diagnosed from their 40s to 60s.

Pigmentary Retinopathies (*see* Flowchart 7.3)

Retinitis Pigmentosa (Figs. 7.12A and B)

Inheritance: AD 10–20%; AR 20%; 10% X-linked; 40% no family history; rarely X-linked dominant and mitochondrial have been reported; chromosome: multiple, one of the more common is 8q11.23; gene: *RP1*—oxygen-regulated protein 1 (one of hundreds identified).[66,67]

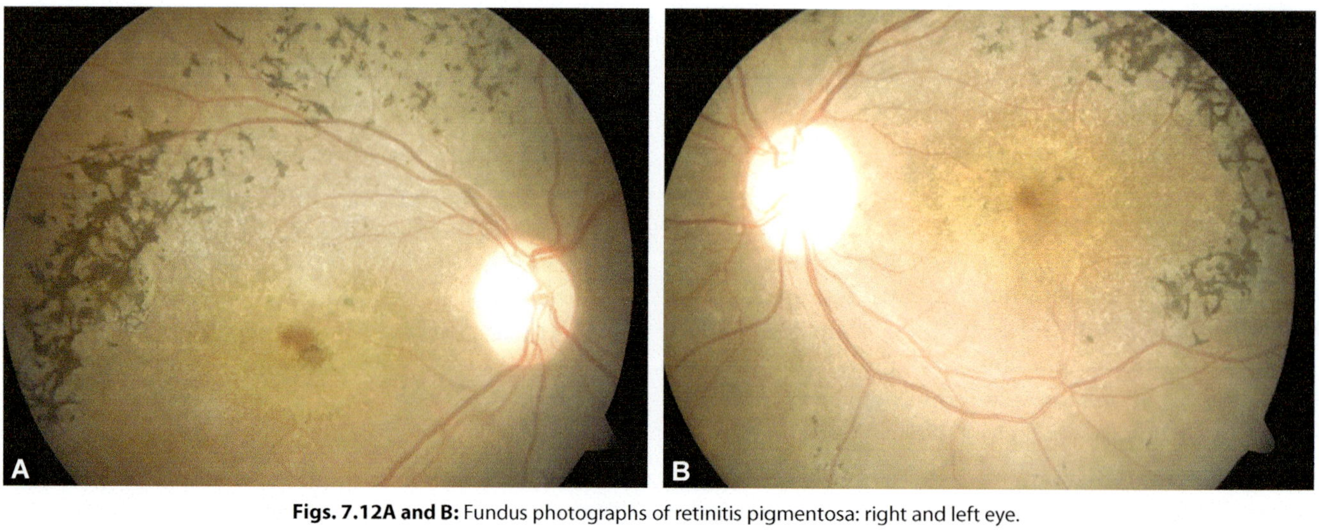

Figs. 7.12A and B: Fundus photographs of retinitis pigmentosa: right and left eye.

Findings: Diffusely involves photoreceptors and RPE function. Progressive visual field loss and abnormal ERG define disease. Divided into primary RP (confined to the eyes) and secondary RP (associated with single or multiple organ systems). Arteriolar narrowing, waxy pallor of the disc, +/-bone spicule-like pigment changes, atrophic peripheral retina and RPE, loss of foveal reflex are characteristic findings. CME occasionally occurs. Posterior subcapsular cataract commonly observed in older individuals.[68,69]

Enchanced S-cone Syndrome (Goldmann-Favre Syndrome)

Inheritance: AR; chromosome: 15q23; gene: *NR2E3*—ligand dependent transcription factor of a nuclear retinal receptor that activates rod development.[70]

Findings: Nyctalopia, blue light sensitivity, pigmentary retinal degeneration, optically empty vitreous, peripheral and midperipheral visual field loss. Round pigmented lesions are found along the arcades. Macular schisis is often present (no leak on FA).

Leber Congenital Amaurosis

Inheritance: AR mostly; chromosome: 12q21, 1q31.3, and 17p13; gene: > 14 *genes—CEP290, CRB1*, and *GUCY2D* most commonly.

Findings: Severe reduced VA (20/200 to NLP) from birth—wandering nystagmus, severely affected ERG cones and rods, normal fundus early on but black pigment clumps develop and, in some, bone spicules.

Choroideremia

Inheritance: X-linked recessive; chromosome: Xq21.2; gene: *CHM* encodes geranylgeranyltransferase Rab escort protein (in the RPE).

Findings: Chorioretinal dystrophy. Pigmentary changes in fundus, night blindness and progressive visual field loss but with atrophy of choroid and RPE. However, normal retinal vessels and absence of optic nerve atrophy set this a part from typical retinitis pigmentosa.[71]

Gyrate Atrophy

Inheritance: AR; chromosome: 10; gene: *OAT* gene—ornithine aminotransferase—10 fold increase in serum ornithine levels (toxic to RPE and choroid).

Findings: Hyperpigmented fundi in areas with no atrophy (distinguish it from choroideremia) with lobular loss of RPE and choroid (large geographic peripheral "paving stone" areas of atrophy). Nyctalopia during 1st decade with later visual field and visual acuity loss is typical.[72,73]

Usher Syndrome

Inheritance: AR; including numerous gene: *Clarin-1*—a transmembrane protein with role in hair cells and photoreceptors; *usherin*—basement membrane protein in many tissues including retina and inner ear; *USH1C*—cilia and microvilli gene.[74]

Findings: RP + congenital sensorineural hearing loss. The hearing loss is usually stable. Be aware of patients with nasal intonation or hearing aids as will likely not complain of hearing problems.[75]

Stickler

Inheritance: AD; chromosome: 12q13.11; gene: *COL2A1*—impairs collagen production.[75-77]

Findings: Progressive myopia with myopic retinal degeneration; empty vitreous, joint hypermobility, arthritis, and orofacial abnormalities; RD common.[76]

Bardet-Biedl Syndrome

Inheritance: AR or multigenic; chromosome: multiple; gene: 14 different genes, *BBS1* most common, all causing ciliopathy—affects microtubules-based intracellular transport.[78]

Findings: Ocular-peripheral retinal atrophy without bone spicules and pigment mottling in the macula.

Systemic findings: Polydactyly, obesity, hypogonadism, and cognitive improvement.[79]

Mucopolysaccharidoses

MPS I-H (Hurler syndrome), MPS I-S (Scheie syndrome), MPS II (Hunter syndrome), MPS III (Sanfilippo syndrome).

Inheritance: AR, except Hunter syndrome (type II) which is X-linked recessive; chromosome: 4p16.3; Xq28; Gene: *IDUA* (Hurler), *IDS* (Hunter)—Catabolic lysosomal enzymes that degrade glycosaminoglycans dermatan sulfate, keratan sulfate, and heparan sulfate.[80]

Findings: Heparan sulfate storage deficiency leads to retinal dystrophy. Hurler and Scheie are identified by coarse facies, cognitive disability, corneal clouding, retinal degeneration, and abnormal ERG. Hunter: pigmentary retinopathy but no corneal clouding, short stature, coarse facies, and cognitive disability. Sanfilippo: mild systemic changes but severe pigmentary retinopathy.[81-83]

Incontinentia Pigmenti

Inheritance: X-linked dominant; chromosome: Xq28; gene: *IKBKG*—makes a protein that regulates nuclear factor Kappa-B.[84]

Findings: Patchy mottling of retina, pigmented lines and whorls on skin, hair loss, dental anomalies, optic atrophy, cataract, nystagmus, conjunctival pigmentation.[85]

OPTIC NERVE

Leber Hereditary Optic Neuropathy

Inheritance: Maternal inheritance (Mitochondrial pattern); chromosome: mitochondrial DNA, most commonly 11778 position but also 3460 and 14484 (higher chance of late spontaneous recovery, up to 65%) positions; gene: *MT-ND1, MT-ND4, MT-ND4L*, or *MT-ND6* protein involved in mitochondrial function. It is occasionally a spontaneous mutation with no family history.[86,87]

Findings: 80–90% are boys or men usually 10–30 years old. Patients usually present with severe, acute, painless, sequential vision loss with triad of: hyperemia and elevation of optic disc (does not leak on FA), peripapillary telangiectasia, and tortuosity of medium-sized retinal arterioles. Fundus can also be entirely normal. The other eye usually becomes involved within weeks to months but occasionally years later.[86,88]

Diagnosis: Neuroimaging is advisable to rule out a treatable cause of disease.

Prognosis: No treatments are effective, corticosteroids do not work. Many think that alcohol and tobacco may play an inciting role, this theory remains controversial to some degree.

Autosomal Dominant Optic Atrophy

Inheritance: AD with variable penetrance and expression; chromosome: 7q31.32; gene: *OPA1*—protein involved in oxidative phosphorylation and maintenance of mitochondrial DNA.[89]

Findings: Chronic vision loss, 20/30–20/60 range, that is usual found during routine vision screening in 5–10 year olds. Majority maintain vision better than 20/200 but almost always have color deficiency (tritanopia-blue-yellow deficit, therefore they pass Ishihara color testing). Frequently, patients will have a central or cecocentral visual field deficit that does not respect the midline. Optic discs will show a focal, wedge-shaped optic atrophy that is frequently temporal but can be diffuse.[88]

Diagnosis: Based on negative imaging and clinical findings. Commercial genetic testing is available.

Prognosis: Generally stable to slowly progressive vision loss over decades. No current treatment.

EYE MOVEMENT

Chronic Progressive External Ophthalmoplegia

Inheritance: AD, AR, and mitochondrial patterns; chromosome: 15q26.1, 10q24.31, 8q22.3, mitochondrial DNA; gene: *POLG, TWNK, RRM2B*, and *MT-TL1*—all result in deletion/impairment of mitochondrial DNA.[90,91]

Findings: Presents in patients age 10–20 and displays slowly progressive restriction of extraocular muscles (ophthalmoplegia), ± ptosis, and trouble reading. Patients often present with ptosis and do not have diplopia because it is symmetric with slow onset. Initial presentation similar to myasthenia gravis (MG) but MG patients have variable signs and symptoms. Histology shows "ragged red fibers" and genetic testing is available to analyze mtDNA.[92]

Prognosis: Currently no treatment for the muscle weakness.

Kearns-Sayre

Inheritance: Sporadic, rarely mitochondrial pattern; chromosome: mitochondrial DNA; gene: large mitochondrial DNA deletion.[93]

Findings: Chronic progressive external ophthalmoplegia often with ptosis, pigmentary retinopathy ("salt and pepper" appearance of macula and midperiphery), and cardiac conduction problems. Sometimes it also includes deafness, cerebellar ataxia, and elevated CSF levels.

Prognosis: Essential to rule out conduction defects. No known treatment but symptoms can be managed with frontalis sling, prisms, defibrillator.

X-Linked Infantile Nystagmus (Congenital Motor Nystagmus)

Inheritance: X-linked recessive; chromosome: Xq26.2; gene: *FRMD7*—makes protein found in visual centers of the cortex and retina with an unknown role/function.[94,95]

Findings: Binocular conjugate nystagmus with no central nervous system abnormalities. Visual function remains near normal. There is no oscillopsia and the nystagmus disappears during sleep. The plane of nystagmus is usually horizontal even on up and downgaze (uniplanar). A null point is often present with an abnormal head position. The nystagmus improves with convergence which often leads to esotropia (nystagmus blockage syndrome—an esotropia that "eats up prism" and has an increased jerk nystagmus on lateral gaze). A paradoxical inversion of the OKN response is observed in 2/3 of patients—a patient with right jerk nystagmus that should have increased intensity of jerk when viewing a OKN drum rotating to the patient's left, instead has a damped right jerk nystagmus or even left jerk nystagmus (occurs only in congenital sensory nystagmus).[93-95]

Treatment: Prisms should always be attempted but an Anderson or Kestenbaum procedure to move the null point closer to primary position and eliminate the abnormal head position is utilized, if prisms fail.

ROLE FOR GENETIC TESTING

Genetic testing should be utilized when the results would affect clinical management or family planning. Currently those instances are limited but are developing and in the near future will become an important tool in an ophthalmologist's armamentarium.

Retinoblastoma (especially if the tumor represents a new genetic mutation), aniridia (often associated with Wilms tumor), *TGFBI* mutations (prior to keratorefractive surgery in high risk populations) are instances where genetic testing is commonly used today. There is also a role for genetic testing when a hereditary disease diagnosis is favored but not confirmed. A more accurate diagnosis will enable better counseling with patients and allow a more complete explanation of the disease. Genetic diseases bring a burden different from all others as guilt from parents are involved, treatment and prevention among family members, and family planning for future generations. Such life changing discussions require adequate time and expertise or a referral to a genetic counselor able to care for such patients. Avoid testing asymptomatic minors for untreatable disorders.

Treatment of genetic disorders consists of a few fundamental approaches. Dietary control is essential for many genetic diseases. Chelation of harmful metabolites slows down progression. Enzyme or gene product replacement can be beneficial. Vitamin and cofactor therapy can help augment a deficient enzyme. Drug therapy to reduce harmful by-products treats at another level of the disease process. Currently gene therapy is still in its embryonic origins with few clinical trials for a limited number of genes. There is a database of clinical trials that should be a reference to help ensure patients get the best and most innovative care, www.clinicaltrials.gov. However, the recent endorsement by the advisory committee of the Food and Drug Administration (FDA) in the United States of a gene therapy for *RPE65*-associated retinopathy[96,97] heralds a new era in the practice of medicine and ophthalmology (*see* Figs. 7.12A and B).

REFERENCES

1. Levine LM, Brar VS, Goldstein MH, et al. Basic and Clinical Science Course. Section 2. Part III. San Francisco: American Academy of Ophthalmology. 2014;131-208.
2. Weisenthal RW, Afshari NA, Bouchard CS, et al. Basic and Clinical Science Course. Section 8. Ch 10. San Francisco: American Academy of Ophthalmology. 2014;253-87.
3. Corden LD, Swensson O, Swensson B, et al. Molecular genetics of Meesmann's corneal dystrophy: ancestral and novel mutations in keratin 12 (K12) and complete sequence of the human KRT12 gene. Exp Eye Res. 2000;70(1):41-9.
4. Irvine AD, Corden LD, Swensson O, et al. Mutations in cornea-specific keratin K3 or K12 genes cause Meesmann's corneal dystrophy. Nat Genet. 1997;16(2):184-7.
5. Fischer MA, Toledo JA, Barraquer RI. Lisch corneal dystrophy. Cornea. 2005;24(4):494-5.
6. Lisch W, Büttner A, Oeffner F, et al. Lisch corneal dystrophy is genetically distinct from Meesmann corneal dystrophy and maps to xp22.3. Am J Ophthalmol. 2000;130(4):461-8.
7. Ide T, Nishida K, Maeda N, et al. A spectrum of clinical manifestations of gelatinous drop-like corneal dystrophy in Japan. Am J Ophthalmol. 2004;137(6):1081-4.
8. Kannabiran C, Klintworth GK. *TGFBI* gene mutations in corneal dystrophies. Hum Mutat. 2006; 27(7):615-25.

9. Yang J, Han X, Huang D, et al. Analysis of *TGFBI* gene mutations in Chinese patients with corneal dystrophies and review of the literature. Mol Vis. 2010;16:1186-93.
10. Kobayashi A, Sugiyama K. In vivo laser confocal microscopy findings for Bowman's layer dystrophies (Thiel-Behnke and Reis-Bucklers corneal dystrophies.) Ophthalmology. 2007;114(1):69-75.
11. Marcon AS, Cohen EJ, Rapuano CJ, et al. Recurrence of corneal stromal dystrophies after penetrating keratoplasty. Cornea. 2003;22(1):19-21.
12. Klintworth GK. Corneal dystrophies. Orphanet J Rare Dis. 2009;4:7.
13. Holland EJ, Daya SM, Stone EM, et al. Avellino corneal dystrophy. Clinical manifestations and natural history. Ophthalmology. 1992;99(10):1564-8.
14. Kim TI, Hong JP, Ha BJ, et al. Determination of treatment strategies for granular corneal dystrophy type 2 using Fourier-domain optical coherence tomography. Br J Opthalmol. 2010;94(3):341-5.
15. Levy E, Haltia M, Fernandez-Madrid I, et al. Mutation in gelsolin gene in Finnish hereditary amyloidosis. J Exp Med. 1990;172(6):1865-7.
16. Kwiatkowski DJ, Mehl R, Yin HL. Genomic organization and biosynthesis of secreted and cytoplasmic forms of gelsolin. J Cell Biol. 1988;106(2):375-84.
17. Jonasson F, Oshima, E, Thonar, et al. Macular corneal dystrophy in Iceland: a clinical, genealogic, and immunohistochemical study of 28 patients. Ophthalmology 1996;103:1111-7.
18. Weiss JS. Visual morbidity in thirty-four families with Schnyder crystalline corneal dystrophy (an American Ophthalmological Society thesis.) Trans Am Ophthalmol Soc. 2007;105:616-48.
19. Bredrup C, Knappskog PM, Majewski J, et al. Congenital stromal dystrophy of the cornea caused by a mutation in the decorin gene. Invest Ophthalmol Vis Sci. 2005;46(2):420-6.
20. Witschel H, Fine BS, Grützner P, et al. Congenital hereditary stromal dystrophy of the cornea. Arch Ophthalmol. 1978;96(6):1043-51.
21. Eghrari AO, Gottsch JD. Fuchs' corneal dystrophy. Expert Rev Ophthalmol. 2010;5(2):147-59.
22. Biswas S, Munier FL, Yardley J, et al. Missense mutations in COL8A2, the gene encoding the alpha2 chain of type VIII collagen, cause two forms of corneal endothelial dystrophy. Hum Mol Genet. 2001;10(21):2415-23.
23. Wright AF, Dhillon B. Major progress in Fuchs's corneal dystrophy. N Engl J Med. 2010(9);363(11):1072-5.
24. Weisenthal RW, Streeten BW. Posterior membrane dystrophies. In: Krachmer JH, Mannis MJ, Holland EJ (Eds) Cornea, 3rd edition. Philadelphia: Elsevier/Mosby; 2011. pp. 845-64.
25. Mootha VV, Hansen B, Rong Z, et al. Fuchs' endothelial corneal dystrophy and RNA foci in patients with myotonic dystrophy. Invest Ophthalmol Vis Sci. 2017;58:4579-85.
26. Machuca-Tzili L, Brook D, Hilton-Jones D. Clinical and molecular aspects of the myotonic dystrophies: a review. Muscle Nerve. 2005;32(1):1-18.
27. Ranum LP, Day JW. Myotonic dystrophy: RNA pathogenesis comes into focus. Am J Hum Genet. 2004;74(5):793-804.
28. Burke JP, O'Keefe M, Bowell R, et al. Ophthalmic findings in classical galactosemia: a screened population. J Pediatr Ophthalmol Strabismus. 1989;26(4):165-8.
29. Aggarwal A, Bhatt M. Update on Wilson disease. Int Rev Neurobiol. 2013;110:313-48.
30. Das SK, Ray K. Wilson's disease: an update. Nat Clin Pract Neurol. 2006;2(9):482-93.
31. Robinson PN, Arteaga-Solis E, Baldock C, et al. The molecular genetics of Marfan syndrome and related disorders. J Med Genet. 2006;43(10):769-87.
32. Pyeritz RE, Loeys B. The 8th international research symposium on the Marfan syndrome and related conditions. Am J Med Genet A. 2012;158A(1):42-9.
33. Sacharow SJ, Picker JD, Levy HL. (2017) Homocystinuria Caused by Cystathionine Beta-Synthase Deficiency. [online] Available from: *https://www.ncbi.nlm.nih.gov/books/NBK1524.* [Accessed November 2017]
34. Bobrow JC, Beardsley TL, Jick SL, et al. Basic and Clinical Science Course. Section 11. 2014:37-8.
35. Markovitz PJ, Chuang DT, Cox RP. Familial hyperlysinemias. Purification and characterization of the bifunctional aminoadipic semialdehyde synthase with lysine-ketoglutarate reductase and saccharopine dehydrogenase activities. J Biol Chem. 1984;259(19):11643-6.
36. Achary MS, Reddy AB, Chakrabarti S, et al. Disease-causing mutations in proteins: structural analysis of the CYP1B1 mutations causing primary congenital glaucoma in humans. Biophys J. 2006(15);91(12):4329-39.
37. Chavarria-Soley G, Sticht H, Aklillu E, et al. Mutations in CYP1B1 cause primary congenital glaucoma by reduction of either activity or abundance of the enzyme. Hum Mutat. 2008;29(9):1147-53.
38. Chang TC, Summers CG, Schimmenti LA, et al. Axenfeld-Rieger syndrome: new perspectives. Br J Ophthalmol. 2012;96(3):318-22.
39. D'haene B, Meire F, Claerhout I, et al. Expanding the spectrum of FOXC1 and PITX2 mutations and copy number changes in patients with anterior segment malformations. Invest Ophthalmol Vis Sci. 2011;52(1):324-33.
40. Vincent A, Billingsley G, Priston M, et al. Further support of the role of CYP1B1 in patients with Peters anomaly. Mol Vis. 2006;12:506-10.
41. Vincent A, Billingsley G, Priston M, et al. Phenotypic heterogeneity of CYP1B1: mutations in a patient with Peters' anomaly. J Med Genet. 2001;38(5):324-6.
42. Lee H, Khan R, O'Keefe M. Aniridia: current pathology and management. Acta Ophthalmol. 2008;86(7):708-15.
43. Korf BR. Clinical features and pathobiology of neurofibromatosis 1. J Child Neurol. 2002;17(8):573-7; discussion 602-4, 646-51.
44. Wiggs JL, Hauser MA, Abdrabou W, et al. The NEIGHBOR Consortium Primary Open-Angle glaucoma genome-wide association study: Rationale, study design, and clinical variables. J Glaucoma. 2013;22(7):517-25.

45. Hysi PG, Cheng CY, Springelkamp H, et al. Genome-wide analysis of multi-ancestry cohorts identifies new loci influencing intraocular pressure and susceptibility to glaucoma. Nat Genet. 2014;46(10):1126-30.
45a. Wiggs JL, Pasquale LR. Genetics of glaucoma. Hum Mol Genet. 2017;26(R1):R21-R27.
46. Schubert HD, Atebara NH, Kaiser RS, et al. Basic and Clinical Science Course. Section 12. 2014:221-70.
47. Lueder GT, Archer SM, Hered RW, et al. Basic and Clinical Science Course. Section 6. 2014:339-47.
48. Kaelin WG. Von Hippel-Lindau disease. Annu Rev Pathol. 2007;2:145-73.
49. Atebara NH. Retinal capillary hemangioma treated with verteporfin photodynamic therapy. Am J Ophthalmol. 2002;134(5):788-90.
50. Gass JD, Braunstein R. Sessile and exophytic capillary angiomas of the juxtapapillary retina and optic nerve head. Arch Ophthalmol. 1980;98(10):1790-7.
51. Molday LL, Hicks D, Sauer CG, et al. Expression of X-linked retinoschisis protein RS1 in photoreceptor and bipolar cells. Invest Ophthalmol Vis Sci. 2001;42(3):816-25.
52. Sieving PA, MacDonald IM, Trese MT. Congenital X-linked retinoschisis. In: Hartnett ME, Trese M, Capone A Jr, Keats BJB, Steidl SM (Eds). Pediatric Retina: Medical and Surgical Approaches. Philadelphia: Lippincott Williams & Wilkins; 2004. pp. 377-85.
53. Retina Albinism, Grønskov K, Ek J, et al. Oculocutaneous albinism. Orphanet J Rare Dis. 2007;2:43. Review.
54. Noble KG. Congenital stationary night blindness. In: Yanoff M, Duker JS (Eds). Ophthalmology, 2nd edition. St. Louis: Mosby; 2004. pp. 840-42.
55. Bech-Hansen NT, Naylor MJ, Maybaum TA, et al. Mutations in NYX, encoding the leucine-rich proteoglycan nyctalopin, cause X-linked complete congenital stationary night blindness. Nat Genet. 2000;26(3):319-23.
56. Boycott KM, Sauve Y, MacDonald IM. (2012) X-Linked Congenital Stationary Night Blindness. [online]. GeneReview. Available from: *https://www.ncbi.nlm.nih.gov/books/NBK1245.* [Accessed on November 2017].
57. Hamel CP. Cone rod dystrophies. Orphanet J Rare Dis. 2007;2:7-14.
58. Molday RS, Zhong M, Quazi F. The role of the photoreceptor ABC transporter ABCA4 in lipid transport and Stargardt macular degeneration. Biochim Biophys Acta. 2009;1791(7):573-83.
59. Boon CJ, Klevering BJ, Leroy BP, et al. The spectrum of ocular phenotypes caused by mutations in the BEST1 gene. Prog Retin Eye Res. 2009;28(3):187-205.
60. Fishman GA, Baca W, Alexander KR, et al. Visual acuity in patients with Best vitelliform macular dystrophy. Ophthalmology. 1993;100(11):1665-70.
61. Michaelides M, Hardcastle AJ, Hunt DM, et al. Progressive cone and cone-rod dystrophies: Phenotypes and underlying molecular genetic basis. Surv Ophthalmol. 2006;51(3):232-58.
62. Hamilton WK, Ewing CC, Ives EJ, et al. Sorsby's fundus dystrophy. Ophthalmology. 1989;96(12):1755-62.
63. Weber BH, Vogt G, Pruett RC, et al. Mutations in the tissue inhibitor of metalloproteinases-3 (TIMP3) in patients with Sorsby's fundus dystrophy. Nat Genet. 1994;8(4):352-6.
64. Felbor U, Schilling H, Weber BH. Adult vitelliform macular dystrophy is frequently associated with mutations in the peripherin/RDS gene. Hum Mutat. 1997;10(4):301-9.
65. Yang Z, Lin W, Moshfeghi DM, et al. A novel mutation in the RDS/Peripherin gene causes adult-onset foveomacular dystrophy. Am J Ophthalmol. 2003;135(2):213-8.
66. Daiger SP, Bowne SJ, Sullivan LS. Perspective on genes and mutations causing retinitis pigmentosa. Arch Ophthalmol. 2007;125(2):151-8.
67. Hamel C. Retinitis pigmentosa. Orphanet J Rare Dis. 2006;1:40.
68. Pelletier V, Jambou M, Delphin N, et al. Comprehensive survey of mutations in RP2 and RPGR in patients affected with distinct retinal dystrophies: genotype phenotype correlations and impact on genetic counseling. Hum Mutat. 2007;28(1):81-91.
69. Weleber RG, Gregory-Evans K. Retinitis pigmentosa and allied disorders. In: Ryan SJ, Hinton DR, Schachat AP, Wilkinson CP (Eds.) Retina, 4th edition. Philadelphia: Elsevier/Mosby;2006:395-498.
70. Milam AH, Rose L, Cideciyan AV, et al. The nuclear receptor NR2E3 plays a role in human retinal photoreceptor differentiation and degeneration. Proc Natl Acad Sci USA. 2002;99(1):473-8.
71. Roberts MF, Fishman GA, Roberts DK, et al. Retrospective, longitudinal, and cross sectional study of visual acuity impairment in choroideraemia. Br J Ophthalmol. 2002; 86(6):658-62.
72. Kaiser-Kupfer MI, Caruso RC, Valle D, et al. Use of an arginine-restricted diet to slow progression of visual loss in patients with gyrate atrophy. Arch Ophthalmol. 2004;122(7):982-4.
73. Santinelli R, Costagliola C, Tolone C, et al. Low-protein diet and progression of retinal degeneration in gyrate atrophy of the choroid and retina: a twenty-six-year follow-up. J Inherit Metab Dis. 2004;27(2):187-96.
74. Bonnet C, El-Amraoui A. Usher syndrome (sensorineural deafness and retinitis pigmentosa): pathogenesis, molecular diagnosis and therapeutic approaches. Curr Opin Neurol. 2012;25(1):42-9.
75. Saihan Z, Webster AR, Luxon L, et al. Update on Usher syndrome. Curr Opin Neurol. 2009;22(1):19-27.
76. Acke FR, Dhooge IJ, Malfait F, et al. Hearing impairment in Stickler syndrome: a systematic review. Orphanet J Rare Dis. 2012;7:84.
77. Faletra F, D'Adamo AP, Bruno I, et al. Autosomal recessive Stickler syndrome due to a loss of function mutation in the COL9A3 gene. Am J Med Genet A. 2014;164A(1):42-7.
78. Katsanis N, Ansley SJ, Badano JL, et al. Triallelic inheritance in Bardet-Biedl syndrome, a Mendelian recessive disorder. Science. 2001;293(5538):2256-9.

79. Zaghloul NA, Katsanis N. Mechanistic insights into Bardet-Biedl syndrome, a model ciliopathy. J Clin Invest. 2009;119(3):428-37.
80. Campos D, Monaga M. Mucopolysaccharidosis type I: current knowledge on its pathophysiological mechanisms. Metab Brain Dis. 2012;27(2):121-9.
81. Moore D, Connock MJ, Wraith E, et al. The prevalence of and survival in Mucopolysaccharidosis I: Hurler, Hurler-Scheie and Scheie syndromes in the UK. Orphanet J Rare Dis. 2008;3:24.
82. Wraith JE, Scarpa M, Beck M, et al. Mucopolysaccharidosis type II (Hunter syndrome): a clinical review and recommendations for treatment in the era of enzyme replacement therapy. Eur J Pediatr. 2008;167(3):267-77.
83. Clarke LA. The mucopolysaccharidoses: a success of molecular medicine. Expert Rev Mol Med. 2008;10:e1.
84. Ardelean D, Pope E. Incontinentia pigmenti in boys: a series and review of the literature. Pediatr Dermatol. 2006;23(6):523-7.
85. Goldberg MF. The skin is not the predominant problem in incontinentia pigmenti. Arch Dermatol. 2004;140(6):748-50.
86. Newman NJ, Biousse V, Newman SA, et al. Progression of visual field defects in Leber hereditary optic neuropathy: experience of the LHON treatment trial. Am J Ophthalmol. 2006;141(6):1061-7.
87. Spruijt L, Kolbach DN, de Coo RF, et al. Influence of mutation type on clinical expression of Leber hereditary optic neuropathy. Am J Ophthalmol. 2006;141(4):676-82.
88. Yu-Wai-Man P, Griffiths PG, Hudson G, et al. Inherited mitochondrial optic neuropathies. J Med Genet. 2009;46(3):145-58.
89. Cohn AC, Toomes C, Hewitt AW, et al. The natural history of OPA1-related autosomal dominant optic atrophy. Br J Ophthalmol. 2008;92(10):1333-6.
90. Goffart S, Cooper HM, Tyynismaa H, et al. Twinkle mutations associated with autosomal dominant progressive external ophthalmoplegia lead to impaired helicase function and in vivo mtDNA replication stalling. Hum Mol Genet. 2009;18(2):328-40.
91. Tyynismaa H, Ylikallio E, Patel M, et al. A heterozygous truncating mutation in RRM2B causes autosomal-dominant progressive external ophthalmoplegia with multiple mtDNA deletions. Am J Hum Genet. 2009;85(2):290-5.
92. DiMauro S, Hirano M. [2003]. Mitochondrial DNA Deletion Syndromes. Gene Review. Available from: *https://www.ncbi.nlm.nih.gov/books/NBK1203*. [Accessed November 2017].
93. Thomas S, Proudlock FA, Sarvananthan N, et al. Phenotypical characteristics of idiopathic infantile nystagmus with and without mutations in FRMD7. Brain. 2008;131(Pt 5):1259-67.
94. Self JE, Shawkat F, Malpas CT, et al. Allelic variation of the FRMD7 gene in congenital idiopathic nystagmus. Arch Ophthalmol. 2007;125(9):1255-63.
95. Foroozan R, Bhatti MT, Falardeau J, et al. Basic and Clinical Science Course. Section 5. 2014:229-30.
96. Stein L, Roy K, Lei L, et al. Clinical gene therapy for the treatment of RPE65-associated Leber congenital amaurosis. Expert Opin Biol Ther. 2011;11(3):429-39.
97. Weleber R, Pennesi M, Wilson D, et al. Results at 2 Years after Gene Therapy for RPE65-Deficient Leber Congenital Amaurosis and Severe Early-Childhood-onset Retinal Dystrophy. Ophthalmology. 2016;123(7):1606-20.

Chapter 8

Basic Principles of Ophthalmic Pathology and Molecular Ophthalmic Pathology

Deepak P Edward

INTRODUCTION

Tissue collection from biopsies and excision of periocular, orbital, and ocular specimens is often a routine process in the operating room. The purpose of this chapter is to provide practical guidelines and an understanding of how and why certain processes are followed when tissue is submitted to the laboratory for pathological examination. Following a standardized protocol maximizes the accuracy of diagnosis, and ultimately patient outcomes.

COMMUNICATION BETWEEN THE OPERATING SURGEON AND THE OPHTHALMIC PATHOLOGIST/ LABORATORY STAFF

Communication between the surgeon and ophthalmic pathology laboratories is critical, especially during the excision of small specimens, vitreous samples, intraocular and periocular tumors, and specimens where the clinical diagnosis and differential diagnosis is uncertain. In most instances, such communication takes place through accurate completion of the pathology requests that should state an accurate differential diagnosis and site of specimen. In cases where excised margins need to be carefully examined, the orientation of the specimen must be provided using a hand-drawn figure with appropriate markings or sutures to clearly define the lateral and deeper edges of excision. An example of such a diagram following a conjunctival biopsy for ocular surface neoplasia is shown (Fig. 8.1). In cases, where further history or information is to be provided to the ophthalmic pathologist or technician, verbal communication with the ophthalmic pathologist is essential. For example, intraocular lymphomas that affect the vitreous cavity might need a special cytology fixative that might not be routinely available in the laboratory or operating room, and to ensure availability of fixative prior communication is essential. Also for such specimens, DNA rearrangement studies might be needed, requiring collection of vitreous material in a specific manner.[1-3]

TYPES OF FIXATIVE USED IN OPHTHALMIC PATHOLOGY—PRACTICAL TIPS

The most common fixative used in ophthalmic pathology is 10% neutral buffered formalin that may be prepared or is available in the pre-prepared form commercially. It is essential that the formalin is adequately buffered to prevent tissue artifacts during processing and sectioning.

If multiple pieces of tissue are obtained from the same lesion, they can be submitted in the same specimen bottle. Tissue specimens must be submitted in separate containers using the same accession number with sub-accession numbers if (1) tissue specimens from the same lesion have different consistencies and the surgeon feels that this tissue might represent a different pathological process; (2) are from different areas of a widespread lesion; and (3) the surgeon would like to determine if a particular piece of tissue is involved in the disease process.

Tissue Processing for Electron Microscopy

Transmission electron microscopy is rarely used for tissue diagnosis today because of efficient immunohistochemistry, which can be performed on formalin-fixed paraffin-embedded tissue for diagnostic purposes. However, if transmission electron microscopy is needed, then small portions of tissue from the original specimen, i.e. fresh tissue

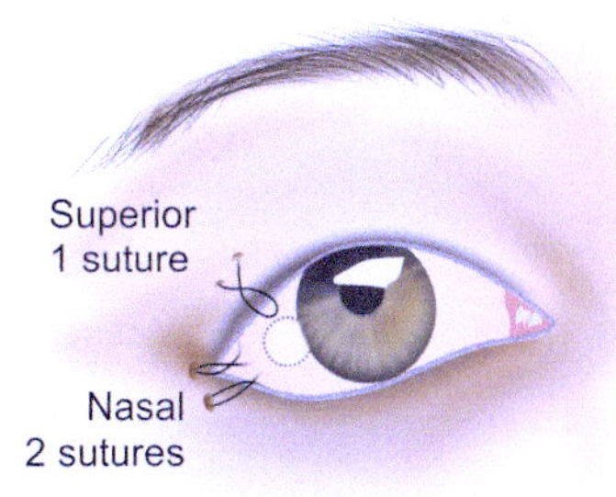

Fig. 8.1: Figure demonstrating an operating surgeons drawing of a conjunctival excision for ocular surface squamous neoplasia.

should be fixed in 2% glutaraldehyde fixative (or McDowell Trump fixative, which is also glutaraldehyde based). These fixatives provide better preservation of membranes and organelles for transmission electron microscopy.[4]

VOLUME OF FIXATIVE AND DURATION OF FIXATION[3,5,6]

- It is recommended that a 10:1 ratio of fixative volume to specimen volume is used to fix specimens. For example, if the volume of the eyeball is approximately 6 cc, 60 mL of formalin should be used to fix the eyeball.
- Small specimens, such as the cornea and small eyelid specimens, can be fixed for a few hours before processing. It is recommended that enucleated eyes are kept in fixative for at least 24 hours. Specimens with intraocular tumors, especially retinoblastoma should be fixed for at least 48 hours before grossing.[7] Larger orbital exenteration specimens may require 48 hours or more to obtain adequate fixation.
- Specimens that contain calcium; for example, bone specimens from the orbit, intraocular calcification, and phthisis bulbi—these tissues following fixation must undergo decalcification using chelating agents that might contain hydrochloric acid, formic acid, or ethylenediaminetetraacetic acid (EDTA). Following decalcification, the tissue is paraffin-embedded and sections are obtained. The degree of density of bone determines the type of chelating agent used to decalcify the tissue.[6]

Submission of Fresh Tissue in Ophthalmic Pathology

There are number of conditions in which fresh tissue might be needed for specific testing and ophthalmic pathology. These conditions and the rationale for obtaining fresh tissue is summarized in Table 8.1.

Specimens for Molecular Testing

- Molecular testing in ophthalmic pathology is performed on a limited basis. The most common test used for this purpose is immunohistochemistry, which identifies specific proteins expressed in certain tissues, especially neoplasms. Most immunohistochemical stains work on formalin-fixed paraffin-embedded tissue. However, antibody-antigen reactivity for antibodies (direct immunofluorescence) against the basement membrane in ocular cicatricial pemphigoid traditionally is done on fresh tissue;[8] although indirect immunoperoxidase has also been recommended in one study[9] (Fig. 8.2)
- Molecular testing on tissues might also be performed to identify infectious agents[10] or genetic mutations to

Table 8.1: The conditions and the rationale for submitting fresh tissue biopsies.

Condition/diagnosis	Tissue	Rationale	How to send specimen?	Tissue processing
Cystinosis	Conjunctiva	Crystals are water soluble	Send fresh in dry gauze	Frozen section
Ocular cicatricial pemphigoid	Conjunctiva	Immunohistochemistry for basement membrane antibodies best done and frozen sections	• Fresh tissue covered with wet gauze • Communicate with the pathologist as to which laboratory in the system performs this test	• Frozen sections • Immunofluorescence microscopy
Sebaceous cell carcinoma	Eyelid/ conjunctiva	To demonstrate lipid droplets and malignant cells; lipid dissolves during tissue processing	• Portion of the tissue sent as fresh tissue • Other portions sent as fixed tissue	Frozen sections performed on fresh tissue with oil red O staining to demonstrate lipid vacuoles
Identification of infectious agents by PCR	Any intraocular tissue/ocular fluid	PCR best performed on fresh tissue	• Fresh tissue or ocular fluid • Center molecular testing laboratory; suspect agents must be provided to the laboratory for accurate testing	Processing for PCR
Identification of tumor at excision margins	Any ocular, orbital or periorbital tissue	Rapid identification of tumors cells at the margin to plan treatment	Frozen sections arranged between the surgeon and ophthalmic pathologist; the location is usually in a room within the operating room or in an adjacent area	Frozen sections
Flow cytometry for lymphomas	Any ocular, orbital or periorbital tissue	Provides more quantitative assessment of cell types involved in neoplastic processes	Cells dissociated and fresh tissue and loaded onto a flow cytometry machine, labeled and quantified for analysis	Quantification of cell type by flow cytometry

(PCR: Polymerase chain reaction)

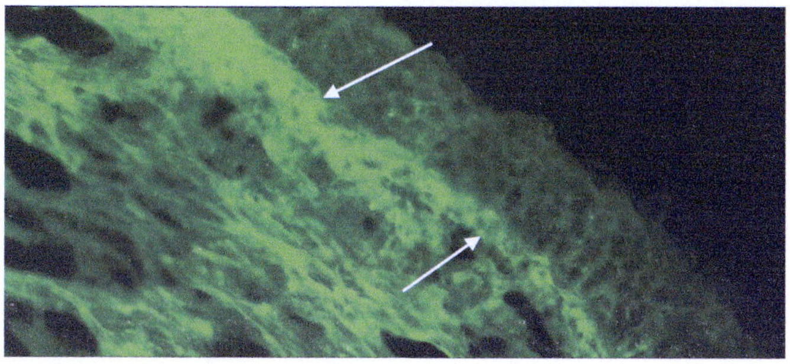

Fig. 8.2: Complement 3 immunofluorescence in a patient with ocular cicatricial pemphigoid. Note the bright immunofluorescence along the epithelial basement membrane (arrows).

determine prognosis such as in choroidal melanomas.[11] Molecualr testing for infectious diseases or genetic mutations are done in specialized testing laboratories. In this instance, additional communication with the ophthalmic pathologist is essential to determine specimen preparation and methods of submission prior to performing a biopsy on the tissue.

Container and Specimen Labeling

- To prevent medical errors, it is crucial that the container containing the specimen should be labeled accurately with the medical record number or other identifying data that match with the histopathology request form. Electronically generated bar-coded labels are often useful in preventing errors caused during the labeling process.
- Small tissue specimens, such as corneal biopsies, Descemet's membrane specimens and others, must be placed in large mouth containers, which allow easy retrieval of the specimen. Placing a specimen on a Weck-Cel sponge or cotton-tip should be avoided since the tissue might stick firmly to the sponge/cotton resulting in difficulty in specimen retrieval or tearing of the specimen, while retrieving it during the grossing process.

  Transparent membranous tissues such as lens capsule or Descemet's membrane can be placed in formalin followed by a drop of eosin put into the container. This enables easy visualization of the specimen.[12]

Specimen in the Laboratory: Technician's Responsibilities

In the laboratory, the ophthalmic laboratory technician plays a crucial role in the processing of the specimens. Ophthalmic pathology specimens are small, often need orientation, and sectioning at different levels. Therefore, a histology technician proficient in handling of ophthalmic specimens is the key to having an efficient laboratory that reports accurately on ophthalmic specimens. The role of the technician in the laboratory includes receiving samples, assisting in specimen grossing, tissue orientation during embedding, sectioning of the tissue, and performing routine histochemical and immunohistochemical stains. In addition, the technician must be proficient in cutting frozen sections, preparing cytology specimens, and have a working knowledge of electron microscopy and molecular pathology.

Specimen Grossing

- It is always useful to examine small specimens under a grossing/dissecting microscope to identify the lesion of interest. Grossing the specimen becomes easier when the lesion is identified in the excised tissue under magnification.
- Routine small specimens, such as the cornea, eyelid biopsy specimens, and conjunctival specimens, are grossed by bisecting the tissue through the lesion and having the technician embed these tissues on edge.
- In case of large specimens, where the lesion of interest might be embedded in a larger piece of excised tissue (for example recurrent infiltrating squamous cell carcinoma in the orbit in a exenteration specimen), the fixed tissue is often bread loafed, so that areas of interest in the tissue are represented when the bread-loafed sections is sectioned and stained.

Submission of Specimens from Neoplastic Tissue such as the Conjunctiva

- The excised conjunctiva must be spread on a piece of filter paper or cardboard in the operating room and air dried for 15–30 seconds. The flattened conjunctiva along with the filter paper or cardboard must then be placed in formalin and allowed to sink. In this way, the conjunctiva remains flattened and does not curl when dropped into the formalin container. A flattened conjunctiva specimen is essential to accurately determine, if there is involvement of the margins, both lateral and deep, by a neoplastic condition[6,13,14] (Fig. 8.3).
- Furthermore, if margin involvement by neoplastic cells is suspected, it is important that the margins be marked with sutures, and a clear drawing of the lesion with an adequate key explaining the marks applied to margins/orientation be provided to the ophthalmic pathologist. This will assist the ophthalmic pathologist in correctly sampling the tissues, so as to provide information on whether the margins were involved in the neoplastic process. (Fig. 8.1).

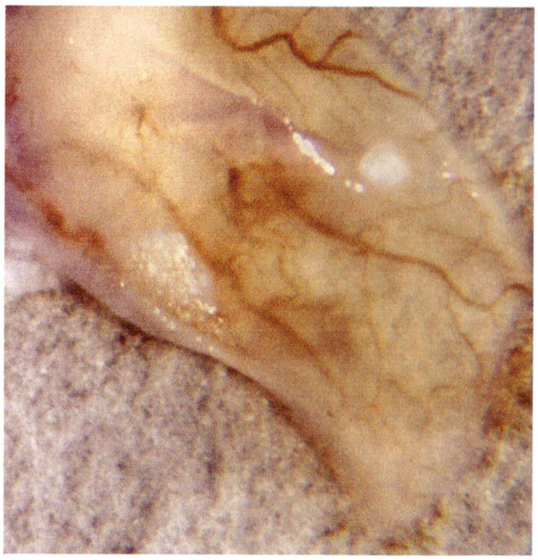

Fig. 8.3: Correct placement of conjunctiva on filter paper after excision. Note the manner in which the conjunctiva is flattened and air dried before fixation in formaldehyde.

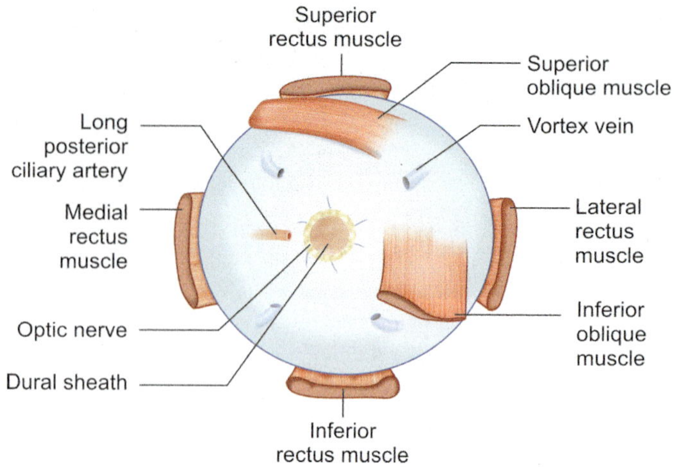

Fig. 8.4: Illustration depicting posterior surface of an enucleated globe. Note the positions of the superior oblique muscle tendon behind the superior rectus muscle and inferior oblique muscle attachment, which is close to the macular area.

ENUCLEATION

A detailed description of how to handle enucleated specimens is described in the referenced publications.[5,6,14] This portion of the chapter will highlight some of the important steps in handling of enucleation specimens:

- The orientation of the globe must first be identified by insertion of the extraocular muscles, specifically the superior oblique muscle tendon on the superior part of the globe behind the superior rectus and the inferior oblique muscle attachment that corresponds to the location of the macula posteriorly. By identifying the location of the cornea, optic nerve, and the oblique muscles, it is possible to distinguish between the right and left globe (Fig. 8.4).
- The dimensions of the globe and the length of the attached optic nerve must be measured.
- The external surface of the globe must be examined. For example, one should record, if the globe intact or distorted following injury. Any wounds, ruptures, extraocular spread of tumor must be identified and noted under the description.
- The globe is then transilluminated to determine tumor, blood, or other lesions that block light (Fig. 8.5). In a normal cadaver globe, the eyeball transilluminates uniformly with blockage of light seen only in the region of the ciliary body. Transillumination defects are circled using a surgical pen or pencil, since the globe is usually opened by transecting through the transillumination defect. The globe is best opened by a microtome blade or a sharp old-fashioned razor blade.
- Once the globe is opened, all the identifiable structures are described. If tumors are present, a detailed description of the tumor, including the extent, consistency, location, color, and gross invasion of surrounding structures is noted. Gross photography is suggested especially with neoplastic lesions in the globe.
- The two hemispheres of the transected globes (calottes) (Fig. 8.6) are further transected to create a pupillary optic nerve section (P-O section) (Fig. 8.6). The central

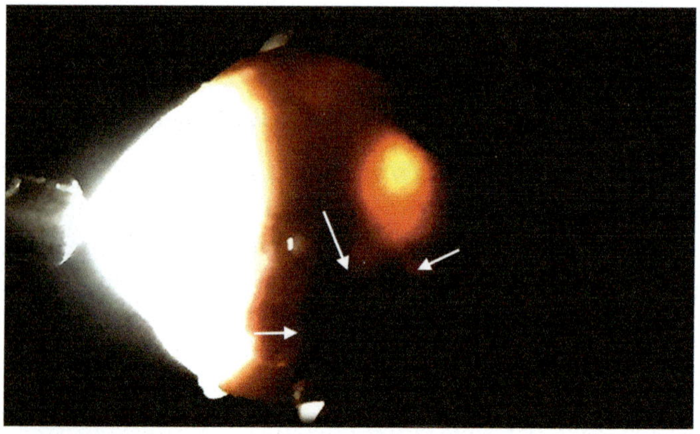

Fig. 8.5: Globe transillumination in an eye with retinoblastoma. Note areas of transillumination through the sclera and it is a blockage by tumor (arrows).

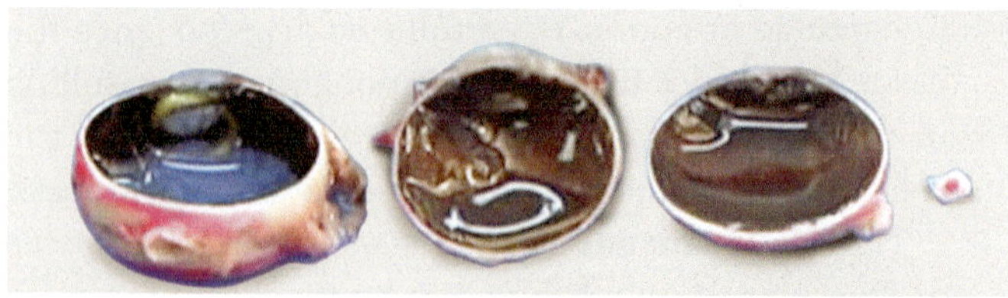

Fig. 8.6: The central pupillary optic nerve section (P-O section) the tissue to the left is the part of the traditionally submitted enucleated globe for processing. This section provides the opportunity for studying relationships between an eye lesion and other anterior and posterior structures of the globe.

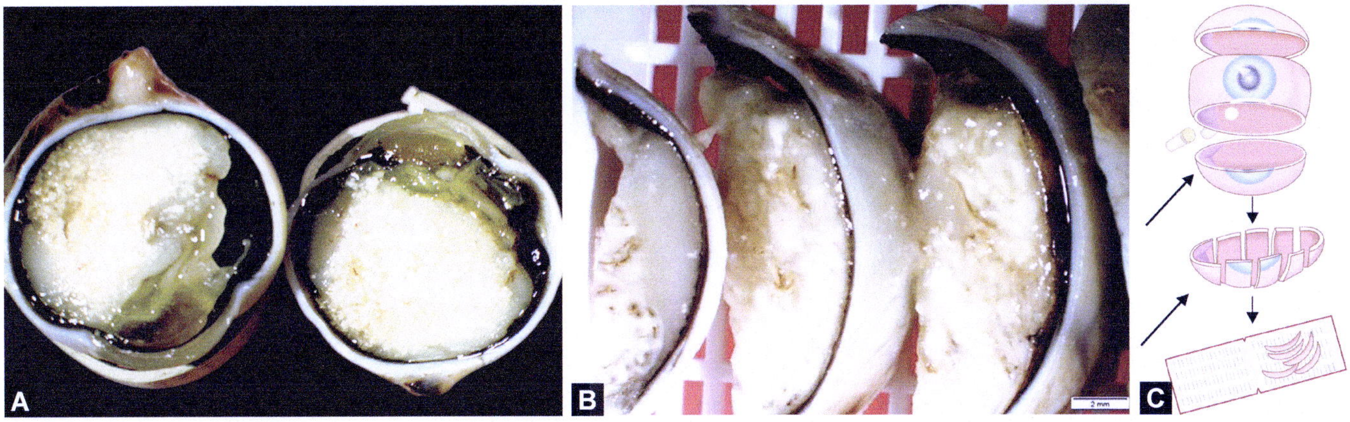

Figs. 8.7A to C: (A) Enucleation specimen with retinoblastoma. Following the transection of the globe, two calottes demonstrate eye filled with tumor; (B) Bread-loafed calottes from the two caps of an eye with retinoblastoma to detect choroid invasion; (C) Illustration depicting grossing of a globe with retinoblastoma. The two caps remaining after the central P-O section is obtained are bread loafed and submitted "en toto" to detect tumor invasion into the choroid.

piece of tissue (P-O sections) is what is submitted for processing. In case of retinoblastoma, the remaining portions of the calottes are also bread loafed (Figs. 8.7A to C) and submitted in entirety to look for choroidal invasion. Furthermore, in retinoblastoma, the distal end of the optic nerve is also sampled to examine the tissue for optic nerve infiltration by tumor at the resected edge.[15]

EXENTERATION SPECIMENS

Exenteration is a procedure performed when the entire globe along with the orbital contents with eyelids (total) or without the eyelids (partial) are excised. These procedures are usually done for infiltrating neoplasms such as squamous cell carcinoma, sebaceous cell carcinoma, or other malignant infiltrating orbital neoplasms. Specimens undergoing exenteration need at least 48-hour fixation in neutral buffered formalin. Grossing exenteration specimens includes sampling the edges of resection and submitting them for processing in separate cassettes. A central pupillary optic section of the eyeball is then made, so as to transect the globe and the surrounding tumor. The angle at which the globe is transected is dictated by the location of the bulk of extraocular tumor; the goal of this process is to transect the main tumor and to examine its relationship to the sclera and other surrounding ocular and extraocular structures (Fig. 8.8). These tissues are large and require special large glass slides on which sections can be placed for staining.

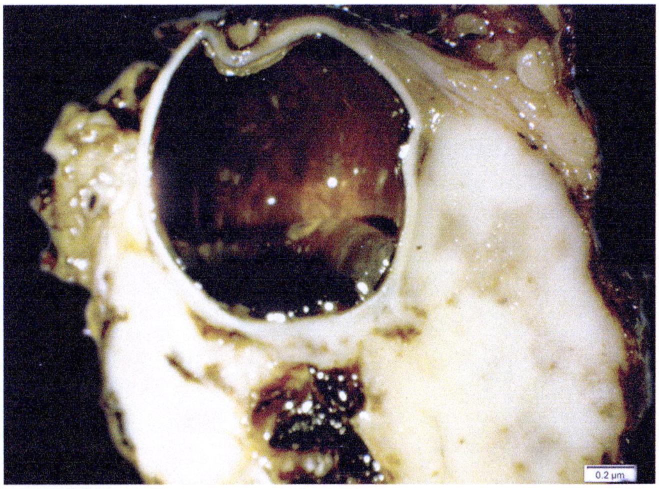

Fig. 8.8: Figure demonstrating grossing of an exenteration specimen in a case of invasive squamous cell carcinoma. Note the cross-section of the globe that is surrounded by tumor (T) invading the orbital tissues.

TISSUE PROCESSING, SECTIONING, AND STAINING

The principles of tissue processing are for the tissue to be dehydrated through a series of graded alcohols and then infiltrated by paraffin in the presence of an agent such as chloroform. Most tissue processing machines available today are automated. Slightly modified protocols are available for processing eyeballs, so as to prevent collapse or excess shrinkage of the globe during sectioning.[3]

Tissue sections are placed on glass slides for staining. The routine stain used is hematoxylin and eosin. Periodic acid–Schiff (PAS) stain is used when basement membrane identification is needed. In the eye, this would include the corneal epithelial basement membrane, Descemet's membrane, lens capsule, ciliary epithelial basement membranes, and Bruch's membrane. A summary of special stains used in ophthalmology, and the structures that they stain and the indications for what they are used as shown in Table 8.2.

Table 8.2: A summary of special stains used in ophthalmic pathology.

Name of stain	Structure stained	Application in ophthalmology	Figure
Periodic acid–Schiff (PAS)	Basement membranes	Ocular basement membranes	Fig. 8.9
Masson trichrome	Collagen	• Identify/delineate scars • Granular corneal dystrophy (negative stain)	Fig. 8.10
Congo red	Amyloid	Amyloid deposits in periocular and ocular structures *Specific examples:* • Lattice corneal dystrophy • Gelatinous drop-like corneal dystrophy	Fig. 8.11
Alcian blue (pH 2.5)/colloidal iron	Mucopolysaccharide	Stains abnormal keratan sulfate deposits in macular corneal dystrophy	Fig. 8.12
Prussian blue	Iron	• Iron lines in the cornea • Hemosiderosis	Fig. 8.13
von Kossa stain or Alizarin Red (not shown)	Calcium	• Band keratopathy • Intra- or extraocular calcification	Fig. 8.14
Verhoeff-van Gieson	Elastic tissue	• Elastoid degeneration in pterygium • Identifying disrupted internal elastic lamina in the artery in Giant cell arteritis	Figs. 8.15A and B
Gram stain	Bacteria	Identify bacteria in ocular tissues	Fig. 8.16
Gomori methenamine silver (GMS)	Fungus	Identify fungus in ocular tissues	Fig. 8.17
Ziehl–Neelsen stain/Fite stain	Acid-fast bacilli	Mycobacteria in ocular tissues	Fig. 8.18
Calcofluor white	Wall of *Acanthamoeba* cyst	*Acanthamoeba* keratitis	Fig. 8.19
Oil red O	Lipid in frozen sections	Sebaceous gland carcinoma to identify lipid	Fig. 8.20

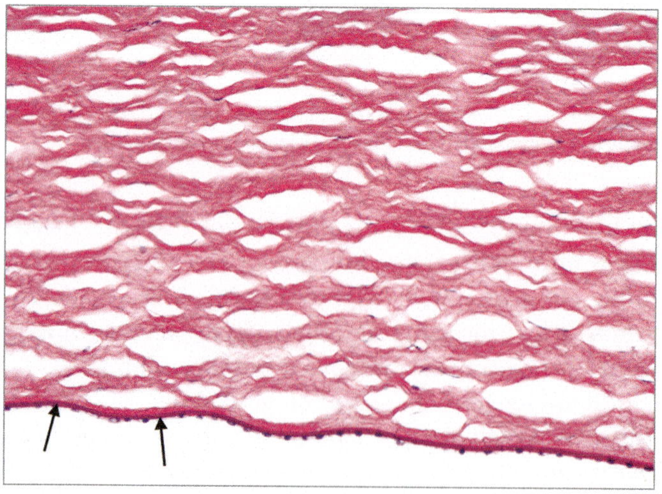

Fig. 8.9: Periodic acid–Schiff (PAS) stain used to stain basement membranes. Note positive purple color stain in Descemet's membrane (arrows).

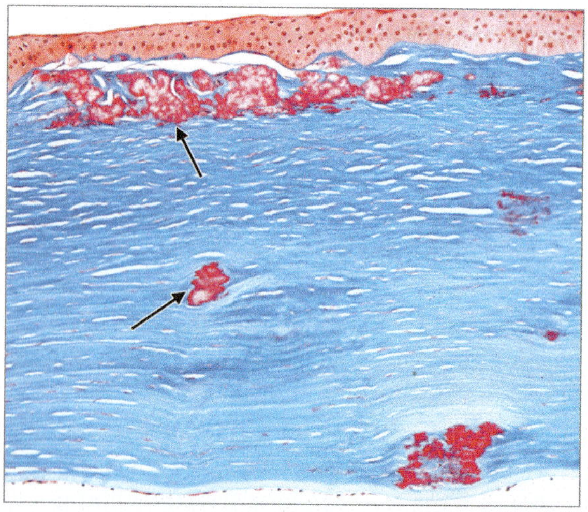

Fig. 8.10: Masson's trichrome stain used to stain collagen. Note the blue staining positive collagen in the corneal stroma in a case of granular corneal dystrophy. The hyaline deposits of granular dystrophy stain bright red (arrows).

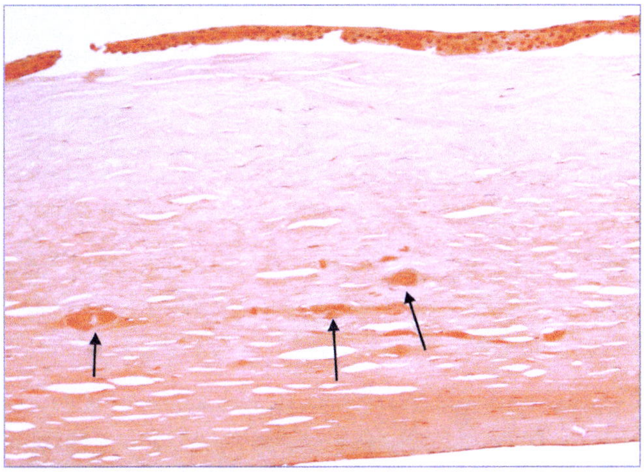

Fig. 8.11: Congo red stains amyloid. A case of lattice corneal dystrophy showing, Congo red positive deposits in the corneal stroma (arrows).

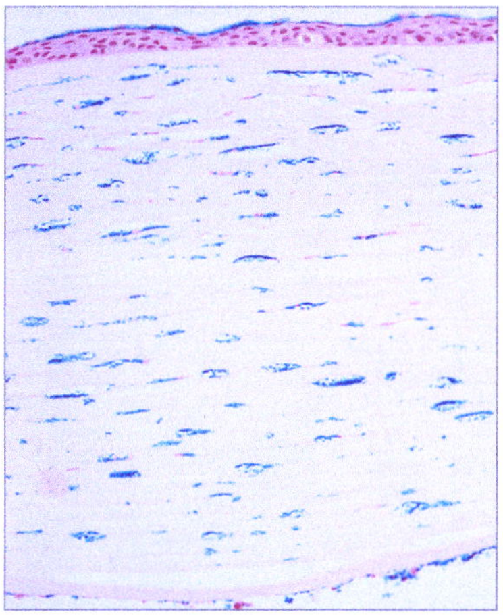

Fig. 8.12: Alcian blue stain used to stain mucopolysaccharides. A case of macular corneal dystrophy showing bluish deposits in the entire corneal stroma and the corneal endothelium.

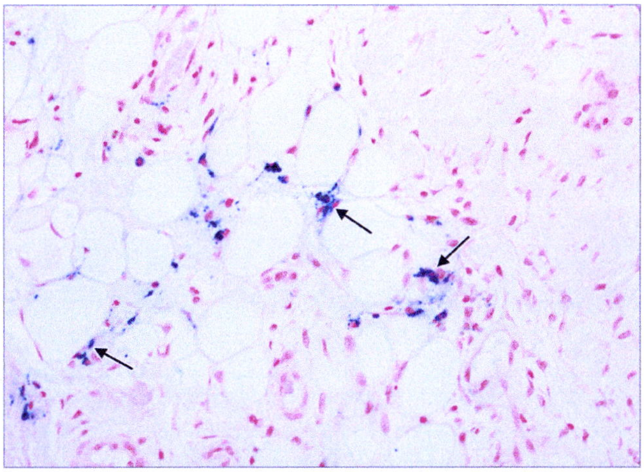

Fig. 8.13: Prussian blue stain used to stain iron. Note the blue staining hemosiderin deposits indicating old hemorrhage in orbital tissue (arrows).

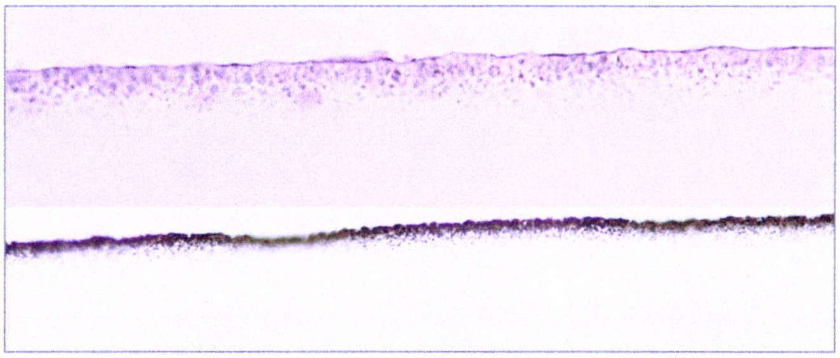

Fig. 8.14: *Upper panel*: Calcium deposition in lens capsule. Note the bluish stippled staining of the capsule with hematoxylin and eosin. *Lower panel*: von Kossa stain. The calcium deposits in the lens capsule are stained black confirming the presence of calcium.

Source: Dr Martina C Herwig-Carl.

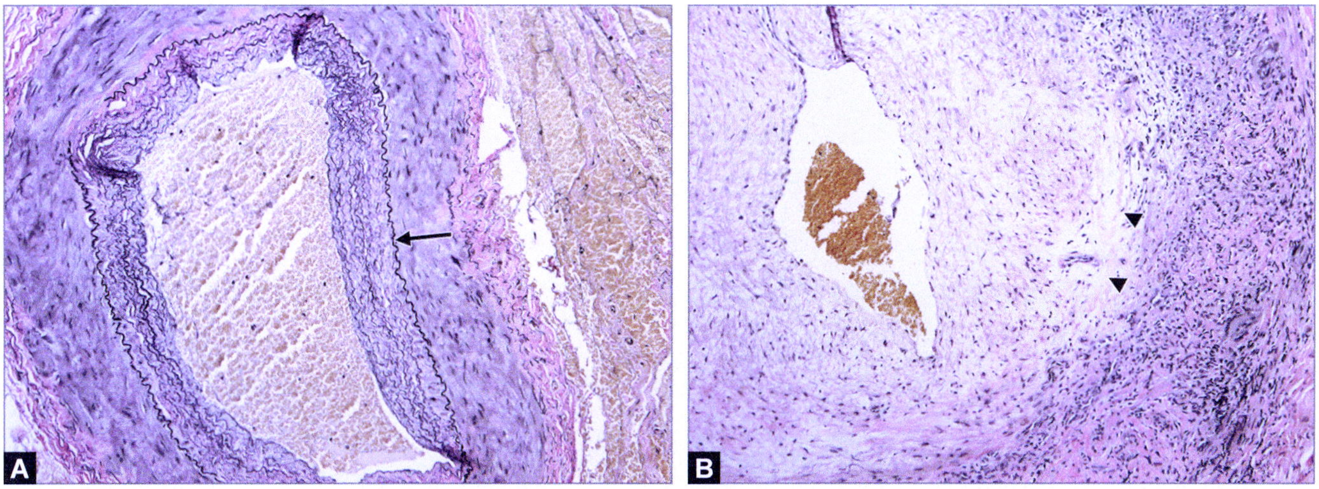

Figs. 8.15A and B: (A) Verhoeff-van Gieson stain for elastic tissue. Medium-size normal artery showing positive stain of the internal elastic lamina (arrow); (B) Temporal artery in giant cell arteritis. Note complete destruction and absence of internal elastic lamina (arrowheads).

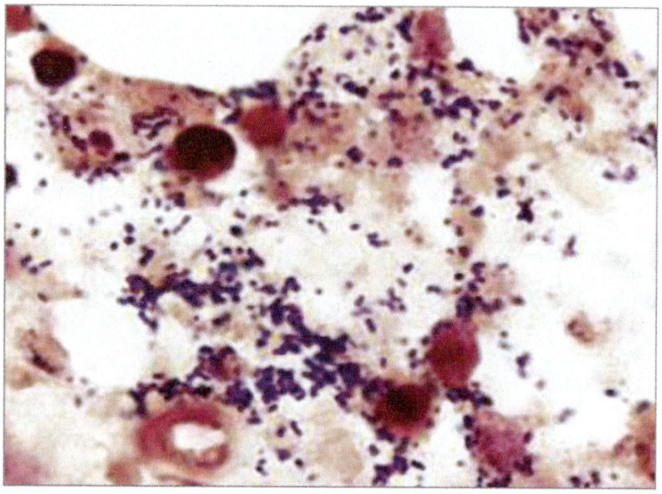

Fig. 8.16: Gram stain for bacteria. Not blue staining positive staphylococci.

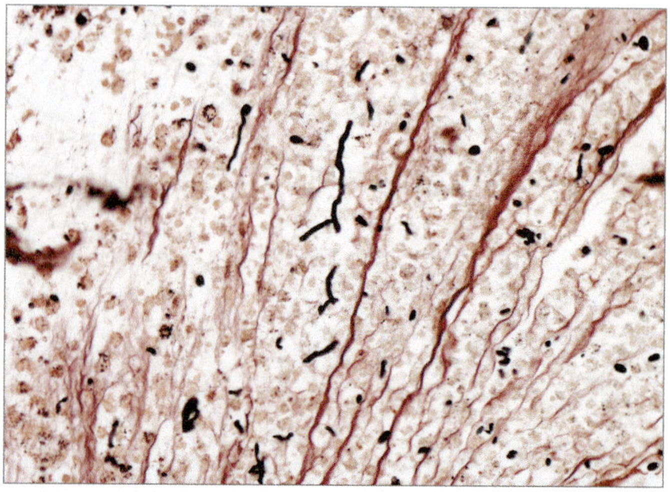

Fig. 8.17: Gomori methenamine silver stain for fungi. Note the black staining positive branching hyphae in the necrotic corneal stroma.

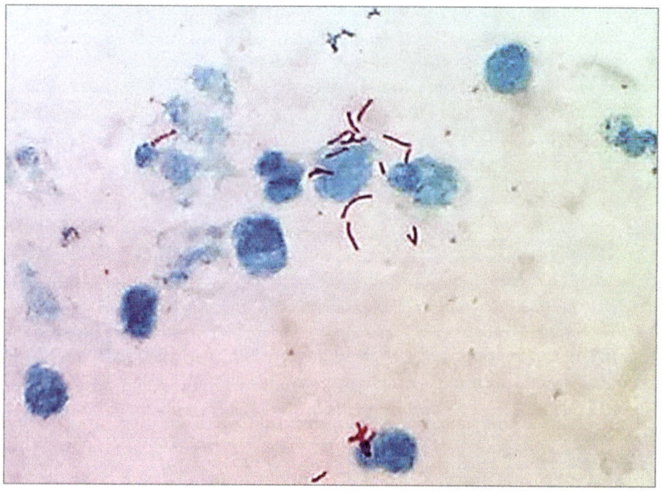

Fig. 8.18: Ziehl–Neelsen stain for mycobacteria. Note the pink staining slender mycobacteria in a tissue section.

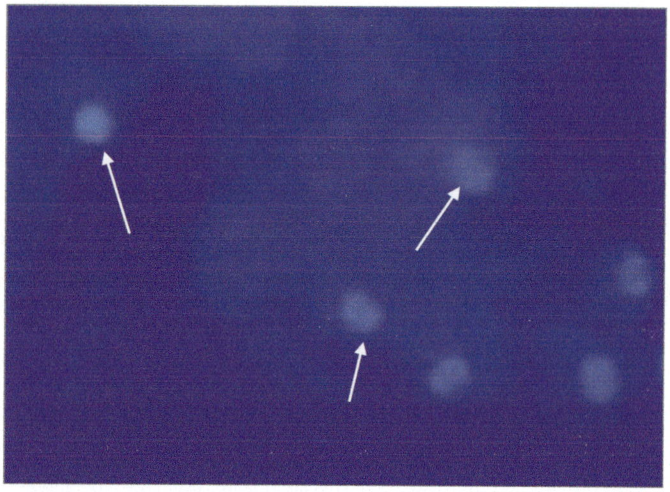

Fig. 8.19: Calcofluor stain for *Acanthamoeba*. Note the positive staining *Acanthamoeba* cyst wall under ultraviolet fluorescence (arrows).

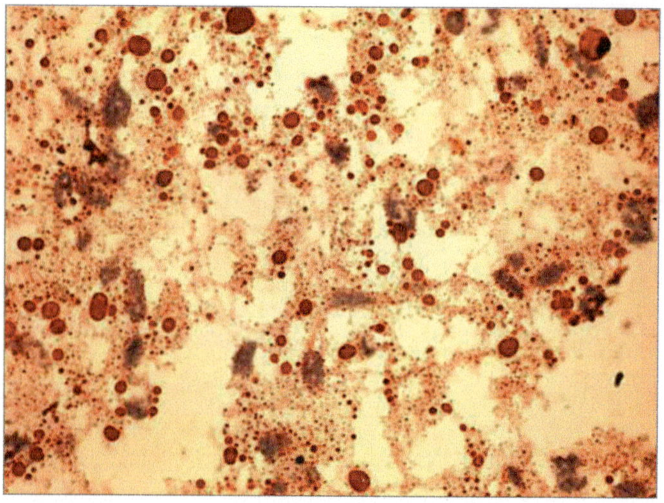

Fig. 8.20: Oil Red O stain for lipid. Frozen section demonstrating positive staining lipid droplets in sections from sebaceous gland carcinoma.

IMMUNOHISTOCHEMISTRY

Immunohistochemistry has become a vital tool in ophthalmic pathology, which assists in identification of cellular types and extracellular material, especially in neoplastic conditions. Immunohistochemistry involves the identification of a particular antigen/protein expressed in a cell or the extracellular matrix that is a signature for that particular cell or extracellular tissue. The antigen-antibody reaction is amplified and viewed by attaching a chromogen to the reaction and is visualized as a color. Common chromogenic use for immunohistochemistry includes diaminobenzidine (brown color) and 3-Amino-9-ethylcarbazole (AEC-pink/red).

Table 8.3 summarizes some of the common antibodies used to detect antigen/proteins in ophthalmic tissues and their clinical purpose.

Table 8.3: Some of the common antibodies used to detect antigen/proteins in ophthalmic tissues and their clinical purpose.

Antibody	Target cell/tissue	Purpose	Figure
Cytokeratin	Epithelial cells	Identify/delineate epithelial cells especially in squamous cell carcinoma or poorly differentiated tumors	Fig. 8.21
Myoglobin/myogenin/desmin	Muscle cells	For the diagnosis of rhabdomyosarcoma	Fig. 8.22
HMB-45/Melan A	Melanocytes/melanoma	For the diagnosis of ocular melanomas	Figs. 8.23A and B
S-100	Labels many cell types	*Identify*: • Spindle cells in schwannomas/melanomas/neurofibromas • Cells in juvenile xanthogranuloma • Cells in Rosai-Dorfman disease	Fig. 8.24
CD3	T-lymphocytes	• Determine type of inflammation • Lymphomas	Fig. 8.25
CD20	B-lymphocytes	• Determine type of inflammation • Lymphomas	Fig. 8.26
CD68	Macrophages/histiocytes	Identifying histiocytes in granulomatous inflammation	Fig. 8.27
Adipophilin	Sebaceous cells	Labeling malignant cells in sebaceous cell carcinoma	Fig. 8.28
Glial fibrillary acidic protein (GFAP)	Glial cells	Gliomas	Fig. 8.29

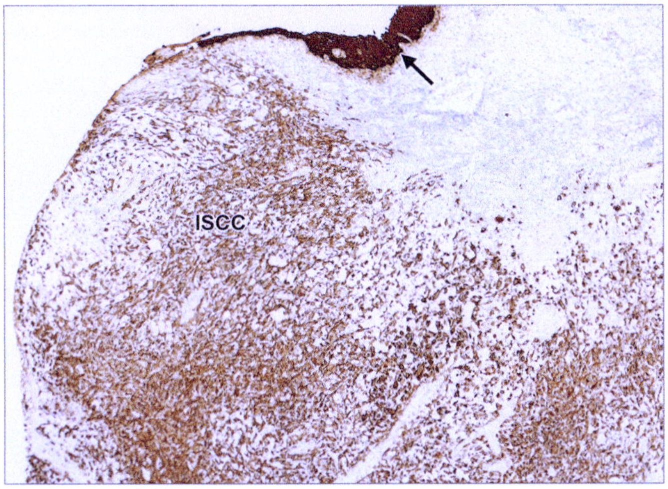

Fig. 8.21: Pancytokeratin immunostaining in a case of invasive conjunctiva squamous cell carcinoma (ISCC). Note the positive staining of the normal conjunctival epithelium (arrow) and the positive staining invasive spindle tumor cells in the conjunctival stroma (diaminobenzidine chromogen).

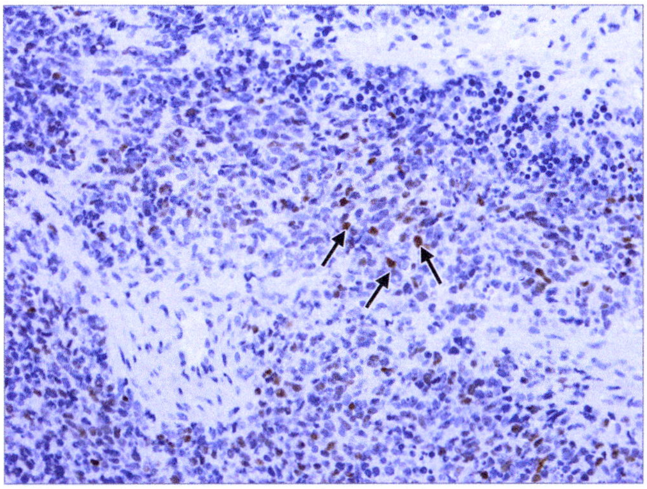

Fig. 8.22: Myogenin immunostaining in a case of rhabdomyosarcoma. Note scattered-positive staining (arrows) in the poorly differentiated cells (diaminobenzidine chromogen).

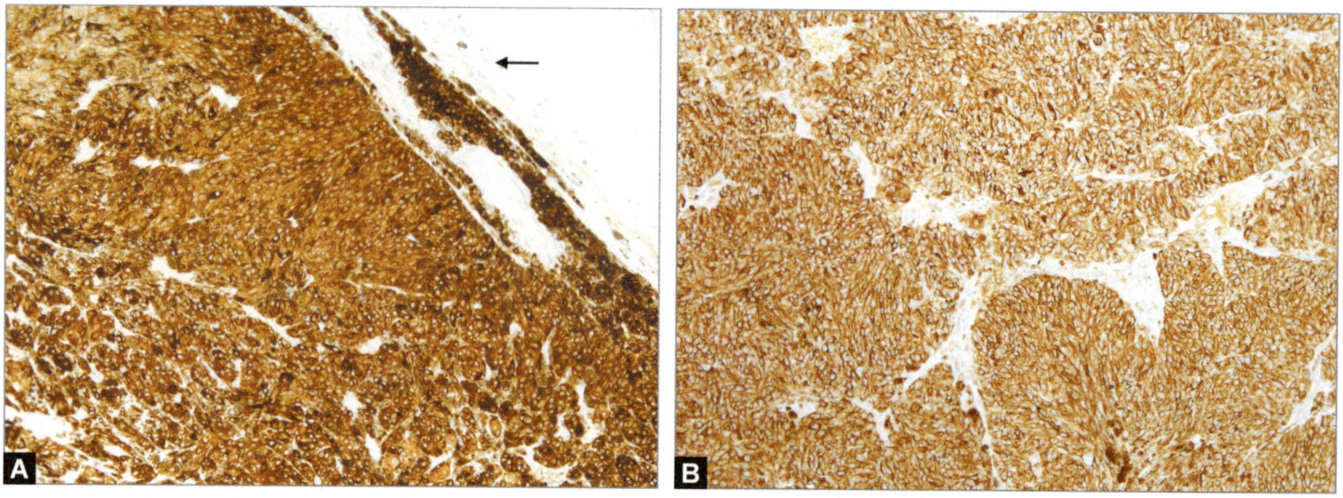

Figs. 8.23A and B: (A) Melan-A immunostaining for melanoma. Note the positive staining in the spindle melanoma cells that invade the overlying retina (arrow) (diaminobenzidine chromogen); (B) HMB-45 immunostaining for melanoma. Note the positive intracytoplasmic staining in the spindle-shaped tumor fascicles (diaminobenzidine chromogen).

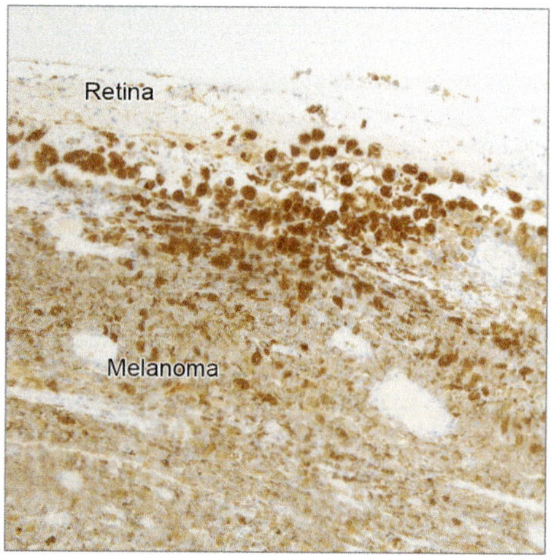

Fig. 8.24: S-100 immunostaining in an eye with choroidal melanoma. Note the positive staining tumor cells in the choroid and the subretinal space (diaminobenzidine chromogen).

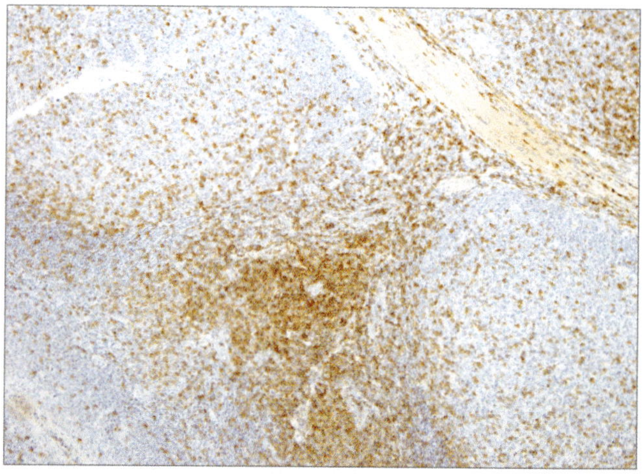

Fig. 8.25: CD3 immunostaining for T-lymphocytes. Note positive staining in scattered cells in idiopathic orbital inflammation (diaminobenzidine chromogen).

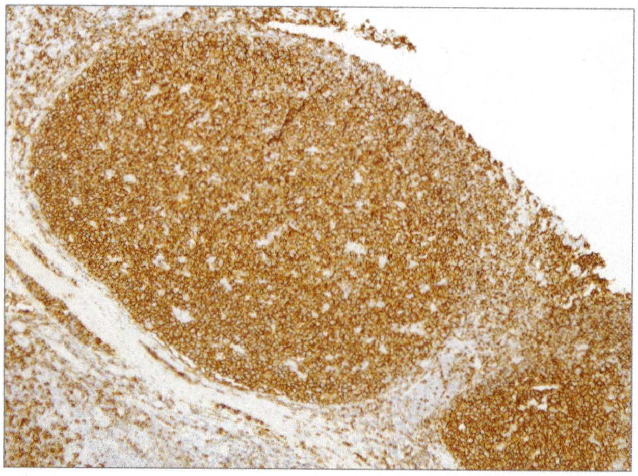

Fig. 8.26: CD20 immunostaining for B-lymphocytes. Note intense and diffuse positive staining in a conjunctiva lymphoma (diaminobenzidine chromogen).

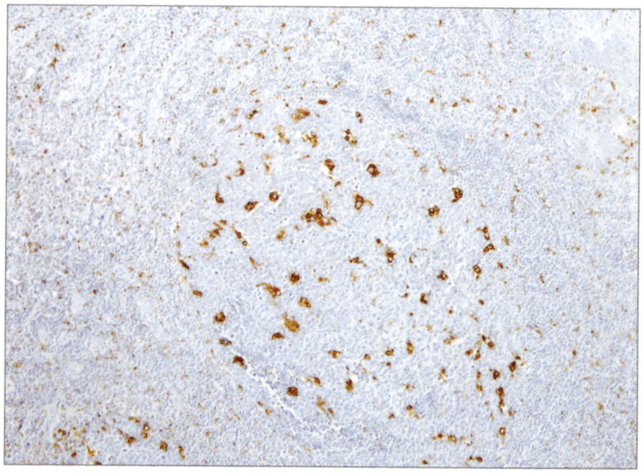

Fig. 8.27: CD68 immunostaining for macrophages/histiocytes. Note positive staining of the histiocytes in the germinal center of a follicle (diaminobenzidine chromogen).

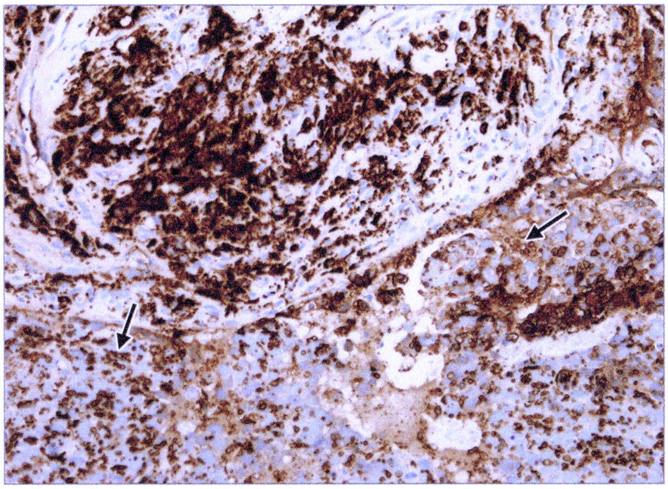

Fig. 8.28: Adipophilin immunostaining for lipid antigens. Note positive staining in the cytoplasm and lipid droplets (arrows) in a case of sebaceous gland carcinoma (diaminobenzidine chromogen).

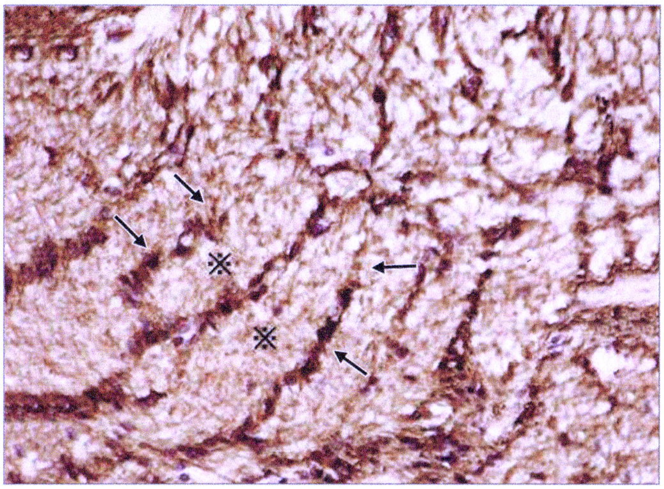

Fig. 8.29: Glial fibrillary acidic protein (GFAP) stain in the optic nerve. Note positive staining in glial cells in pial septae (arrows) and their processes (※) (diaminobenzidine chromogen).

REFERENCES

1. Araujo I, Coupland SE. Primary vitreoretinal lymphoma: a Review. Asia Pac J Ophthalmol (Phila). 2017;6:283-9.
2. Kase S, Namba K, Iwata D, et al. Diagnostic efficacy of cell block method for vitreoretinal lymphoma. Diagn Pathol. 2016;11:29.
3. Torczynski E. Preparation of ocular specimens for histopathologic examination. Ophthalmology. 1981;88:1367-71.
4. McDowell EM, Trump BF. Histologic fixatives suitable for diagnostic light and electron microscopy. Arch Pathol Lab Med. 1976;100:405-14.
5. Menocal NG, Ventura DB, Yanoff M. Routine processing of ophthalmic tissue for light microscopy. Am J Med Technol. 1977;43:156-60.
6. Azari AA, Syed NA, Albert DM. Examining and processing eye specimens. Methods Mol Biol. 2014;1180:377-96.
7. Albert D, Syed N, Cancer Committee CoAP. Protocol for the examination of specimens from patients with retinoblastoma: a basis for checklists. Arch Pathol Lab Med. 2001;125:1183-8.
8. Furey N, West C, Andrews T, et al. Immunofluorescent studies of ocular cicatricial pemphigoid. Am J Ophthalmol. 1975;80:825-31.
9. Demers PE, Robin H, Prost C, et al. Immunohistopathologic testing in patients suspected of ocular cicatricial pemphigoid. Curr Eye Res. 1998;17:823-7.
10. Bodaghi B, LeHoang P. Testing ocular fluids in uveitis. Ophthalmol Clin North Am. 2002;15:271-9.
11. Onken MD, Worley LA, Tuscan MD, et al. An accurate, clinically feasible multi-gene expression assay for predicting metastasis in uveal melanoma. J Mol Diagn. 2010;12:461-8.
12. Steven Houston SK, Morgan O, Olsakovsky LA, et al. A novel approach to processing descemet stripping automated endothelial keratoplasty specimens for histopathologic analysis. Cornea. 2010;29:1452-4.
13. Kiire CA, Srinivasan S, Karp CL. Ocular surface squamous neoplasia. Int Ophthalmol Clin. 2010;50:35-46.
14. Folberg R, Salomao D, Grossniklaus HE, et al. Recommendations for the reporting of tissues removed as part of the surgical treatment of common malignancies of the eye and its adnexa. The Association of Directors of Anatomic and Surgical Pathology. Hum Pathol. 2003;34:114-8.
15. Alkatan HM, ALBalawi H, Maktabi AM. The value of "en toto" globe submission in the assessment of high-risk retinoblastoma cases and staging. Int Ophthalmol. 2017. doi: 10.1007/s10792-016-0410-5. [Epub ahead of print].

Chapter 9 Ophthalmic Pathology

Martina C Herwig-Carl, Karin U Loeffler

CLINICOPATHOLOGICAL CORRELATION

How the pathologist can help with the clinical diagnosis and clinical management of the patient?

Ophthalmic pathologists not only provide a histologic diagnosis based on the submitted specimen, but correlate the histologic findings with the clinical picture and may also provide recommendations on treatment and follow-up. Basically, ophthalmic pathology represents an essential scaffold for understanding clinical appearances and tissue reactions in a disease process or a response to treatment. The study of enucleated eyes tells the "story" of the eye and provides a clear understanding of the underlying pathophysiologic changes of ocular tissues. It not only provides a clinical diagnosis but also clues on how local or systemic disease can be further investigated or treated.

Representative biopsies are helpful in selected cases not only to make a diagnosis but also to plan the further disease management or understand the prognosis. It is important that information is exchanged between the clinician and the pathologist especially in unusual cases. Surgeons may contact ophthalmic pathologists before surgery to discuss the clinical questions that are being asked through the biopsy. Such a conversation helps in planning the amount of tissue necessary for diagnosis, submission of fresh versus unfixed tissue, special stains on limited available material, and the timeframe for diagnosis.

This chapter focuses on some clinicopathologic correlations with special emphasis on clinical management.

REMNANTS OF FETAL DEVELOPMENT

The development of the eye is quite complex and will not be covered by this chapter. However, there are certain clinical findings in adults which are related to ocular development such as a delicate remnant of the pupillary membrane inserting at the iris collarette (Figs. 9.1A and B) or a posterior embryotoxon (prominent Schwalbe's line) which can occur as a physiologic variant or in association with syndromes, e.g. Axenfeld-Rieger syndrome (Figs. 9.2A and B).[1] Though pathologic material obtained during biopsies for such conditions are unusual,

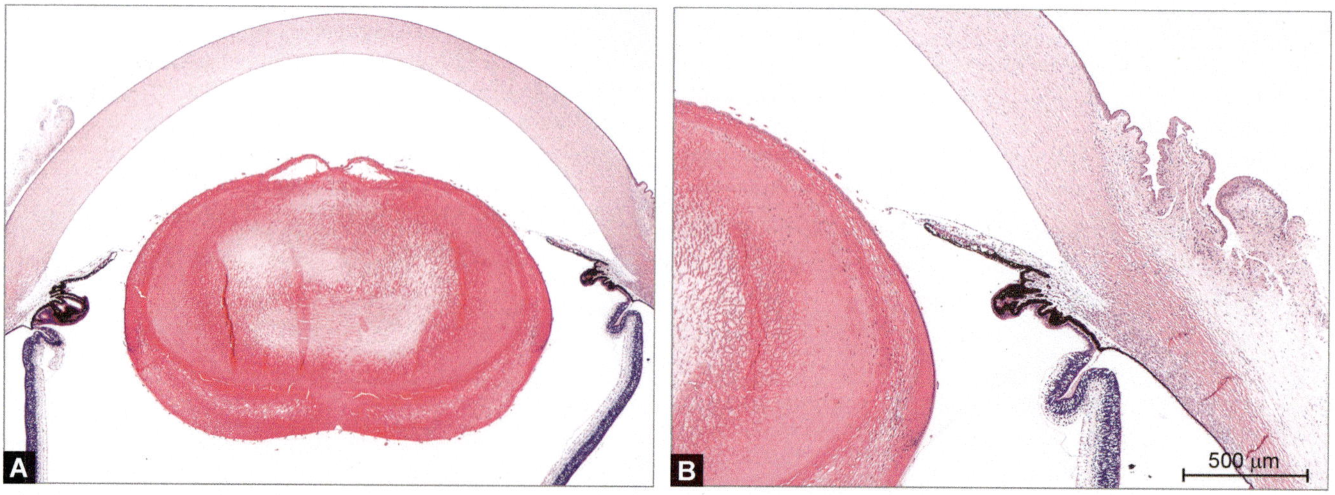

Figs. 9.1A and B: Tunica vasculosa lentis anterior. (A) Tunica vasculosa lentis anterior and posterior in a 24-week-old fetus; (B) Higher magnification of the fetal tunica vasculosa lentis anterior.

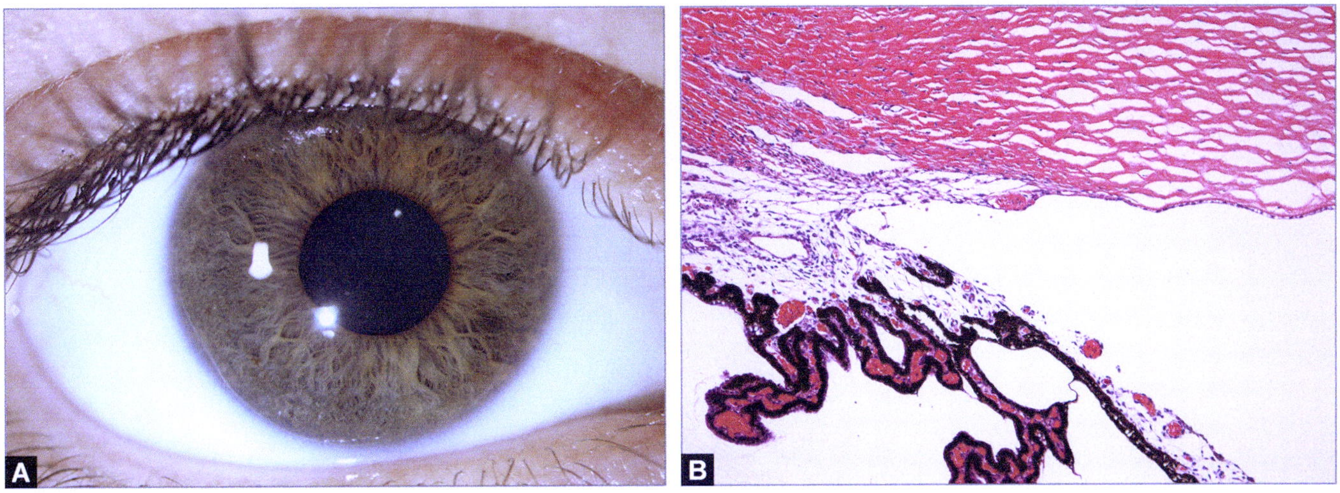

Figs. 9.2A and B: Posterior embryotoxon. (A) Delicate prominent Schwalbe's line (posterior embryotoxon) in a 22-year-old girl; (B) Histology shows a collagenous elevation embedded into the anterior trabecular meshwork, corresponding to posterior embryotoxon, in a 16-day-old newborn without additional ocular abnormalities.

it is important for the clinician to understand the pathophysiologic basis of these aberrations during development through clinicopathologic correlation.

Eyelid

Chronic blepharitis is a frequent condition which is characterized by Meibomian gland dysfunction and inflammation. Conjunctival concretions are often observed clinically which represent histologically inspissated secretions from goblet cells. Rarely, calcification is seen in these concretions. *Demodex* mites can be identified by ophthalmic pathologists in tissue specimens as a cofactor that may play a role in the inflammatory process in blepharitis.[2]

Several benign eyelid lesions are seen in ophthalmology clinics. The following paragraphs briefly highlight the important pathologic features of these entities.

While a hordeolum is histologically characterized by an acute inflammation with polymorphonuclear leukocytes, a chalazion on pathologic examination shows chronic lipogranulomatous inflammation with lipid vacuoles surrounded by epithelioid cells (macrophages), multinucleated giant cells and lymphocytes/plasma cells (Fig. 9.3). Several malignancies (e.g. sebaceous cell carcinoma, metastasis) can mimic a chalazion, thus justifying histological examination of all chalazia that are removed (Figs. 9.4A and B).[3,4]

Well-circumscribed papillomatous lesions of the eyelid skin can often be diagnosed as seborrheic keratosis (mostly in elderly) or basal cell papilloma showing histologically acanthosis and hyperkeratosis with occasional parakeratosis.

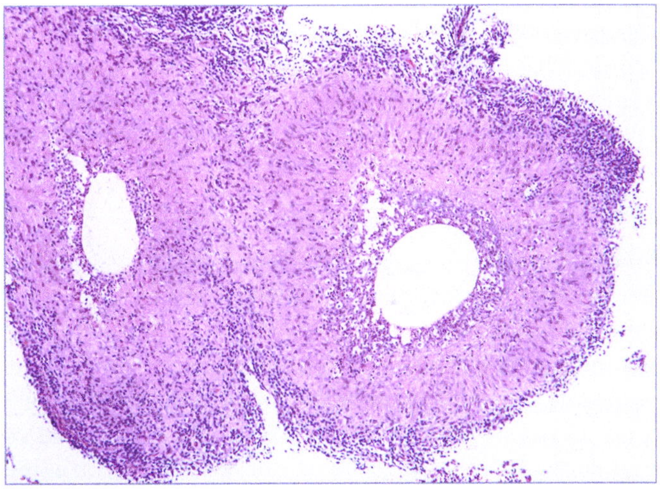

Fig. 9.3: Chalazion. Histologic picture of a chalazion showing a chronic granulomatous inflammation composed of epithelioid cells, multinucleated giant cells, plasma cells and leukocytes surrounding lipid vacuoles.

Molluscum contagiosum is a benign viral-induced lesion caused by a Pox virus. The lesion occurs as a pearly-white umbilicated lesion at the lid margin. Pathologically eosinophilic intracytoplasmic viral inclusion bodies are noted that can be shed onto the conjunctiva causing follicular conjunctivitis and corneal neovascularization. Disseminated molluscum contagiosum should raise the suspicion of immune deficiency.[5]

Cysts are frequently present in the eyelid, often close to the eyelid margin. They can arise from sweat gland ductal structures (eccrine or apocrine hidrocystomas), or represent an epithelial inclusion cyst. In contrast to simple cysts (epidermoid inclusion cysts) that are lined by stratified squamous epithelium, hidrocystomas show

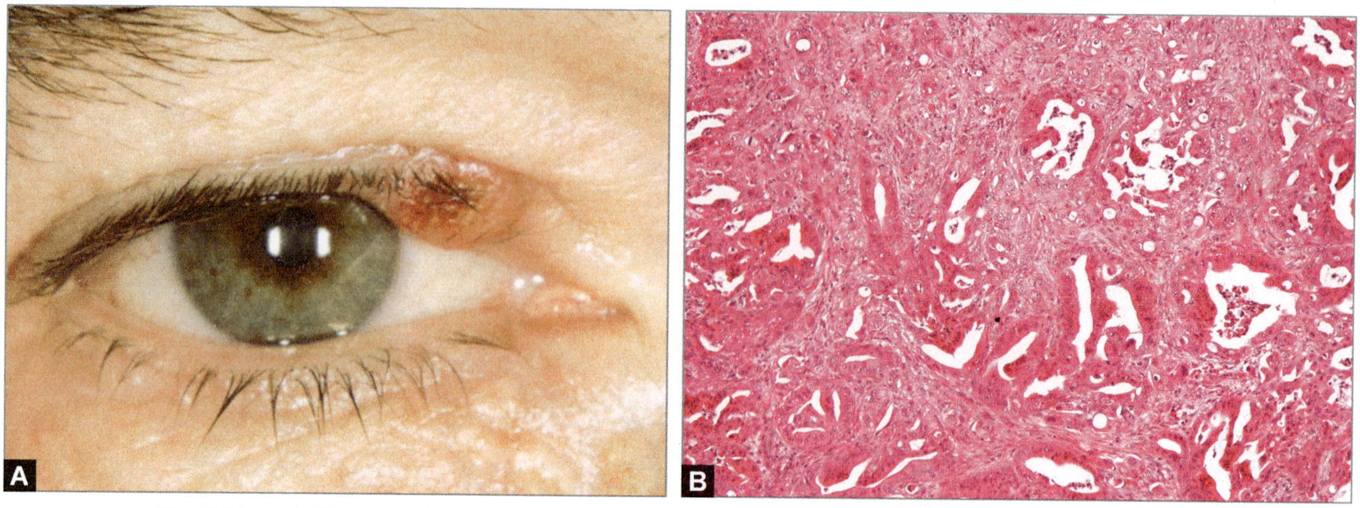

Figs. 9.4A and B: Metastasis of a pancreas carcinoma mimicking a chalazion. (A) Reddish nodule on the upper eyelid; (B) Histology shows an adenocarcinoma composed of polymorphous, atypical cells.

additional papillary projections into the lumen of the cyst. The objective of treatment of these cysts is to remove the entire epithelial lining during excision. Incision/puncture of cysts is not recommended as the cyst will recur shortly thereafter, once the epithelial lining has regenerated forming a new lumen. In rare cases, a basal cell carcinoma can clinically be mistaken for a cyst.[6]

Xanthelasmata are yellowish lesions on the upper and lower lid and represent accumulations of foam cells in the dermis. The cells can infiltrate deeper layers, such as the orbicularis muscle. Xanthelasmata which may be associated with disorders of the fat metabolism often recur and the patient should be advised to undergo a medical examination.[7]

A nevus of the eyelid margin can be pigmented or nonpigmented. Histologically, the nevus cells can be noted at the epidermal-dermal junction (a junctional component) and can be distinguished from an intradermal proportion. When both junctional and intradermal components are present, the nevus is known as a compound nevus. Most nevi are compound in nature. Junctional activity is typical in nevi of younger patients and should raise suspicion for melanoma in the elderly (junctional activity is illustrated in Figures 9.8A and B, Caruncle nevus).[8] There is usually no need for excision of nevi. However, if the lesion is to be excised a complete removal (e.g. wedge resection) should be attempted since the nevus cells frequently infiltrate deeper layers leading to recurrences with atypical clinical features similar to melanoma.

Conjunctiva

The conjunctival stroma normally contains lymphatics and mucosa-associated lymphoid tissue (MALT). Thus, infections (such as viral) and chronic irritating agents (e.g. glaucoma medications) can cause nonspecific reactions, such as follicles which are enlargement/expansion of normally occurring MALT in the conjunctiva. While unilateral chronic follicular conjunctivitis is suggestive of a chlamydia infection (agent: *Chlamydia trachomatis*, serotype: D-K), lymphoma should be excluded by a biopsy in therapy-resistant cases (Figs. 9.5A and B).[9] Conjunctival papillomas can be caused by human papillomavirus (HPV). In particular, HPV 16 and 18 are associated with squamous dysplasia and a higher recurrence rate.[10] A dysplastic dedifferentiation or sebaceous cell carcinoma should be excluded by histology in this usually benign lesion (Figs. 9.6A to C).

Pyogenic granulomas (vascularized granulation tissue) are reddish lesions of the conjunctiva that usually occur in conjunction with a chalazion or following enucleation, and can be the reason for spontaneous hemorrhage in such lesions after mild trauma. Pathologically these lesions represent granulation tissue that contains proliferating capillaries and infiltration of acute and chronic inflammatory cells. A deep excision including the base is mandatory to exclude associated lesions other than chalazion, in particular squamous (or sebaceous) cell carcinoma (Figs. 9.7A and B).

The benign conjunctival nevus typically harbors conjunctival inclusion cysts which are detectable clinically as well as histologically. This feature helps to distinguish nevi from primary acquired melanosis (PAM) or malignant melanoma. In nevi, junctional activity which is a sign of the growing capacity of a lesion is evaluated by ocular pathologists (Figs. 9.8A and B). While it usually occurs in

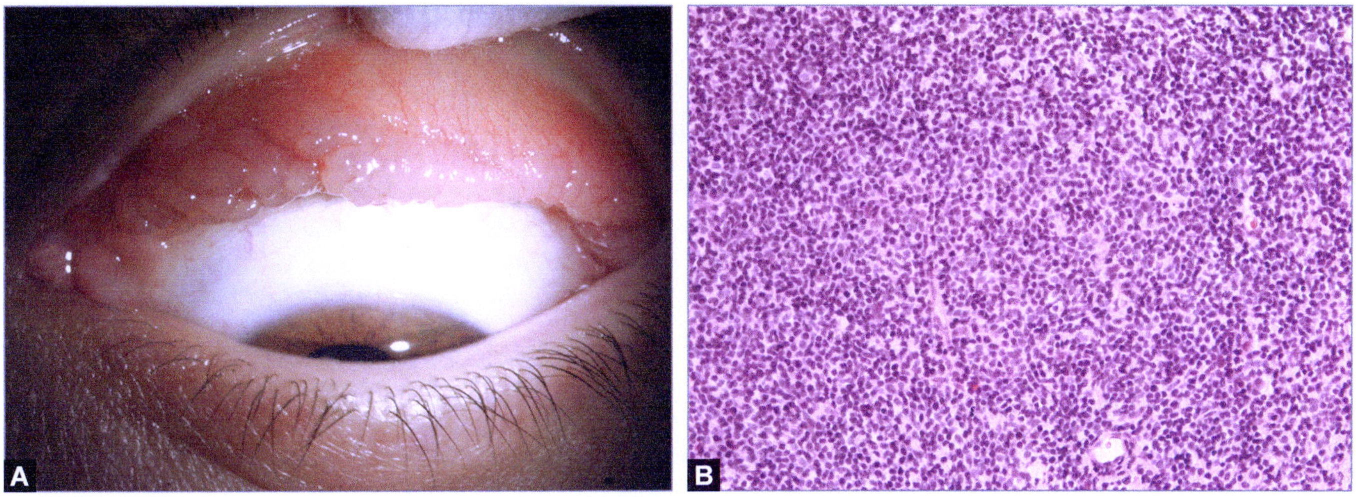

Figs. 9.5A and B: Mucosa-associated lymphatic tissue (MALT) lymphoma mimicking follicular conjunctivitis. (A) Follicular Chlamydia-negative conjunctivitis; (B) Histologically, a MALT lymphoma was diagnosed.

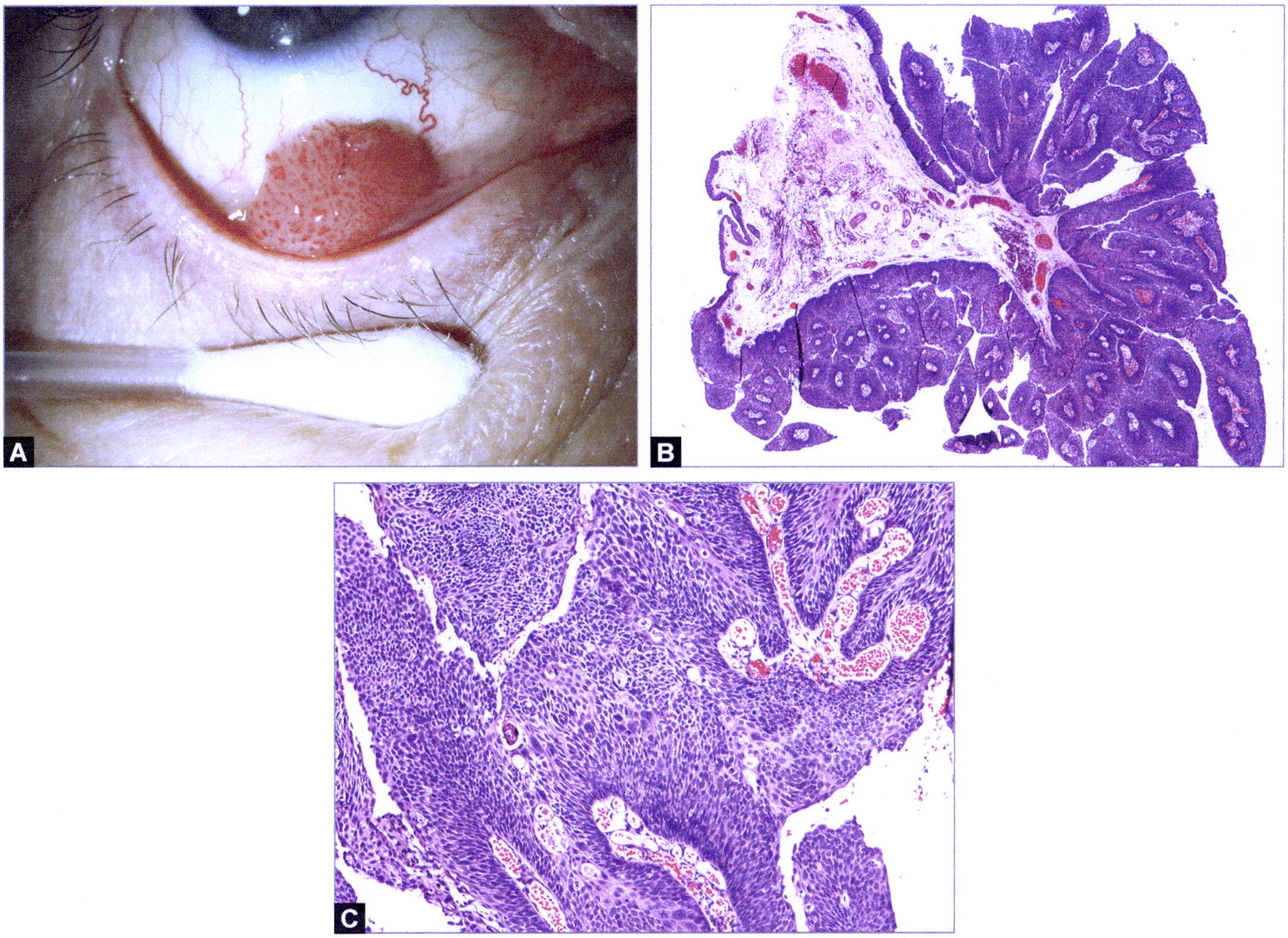

Figs. 9.6A to C: Conjunctival intraepithelial neoplasia (CIN) III in conjunctival human papillomavirus (HPV)-16 associated papilloma. (A) Conjunctival papillomatous lesion in the inferior fornix; (B) The histologic picture shows a fibrovascular core covered by dysplastic conjunctival epithelium; (C) Signs of severe dysplasia (polymorphous cells, atypia, no regular maturation) consistent with conjunctival intraepithelial neoplasia are present.

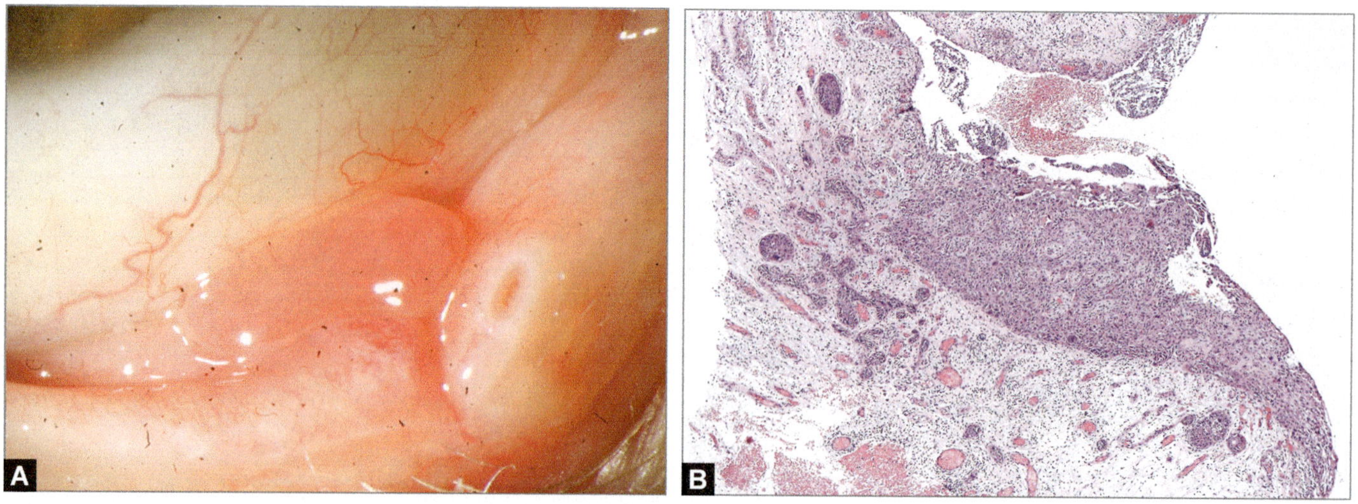

Figs. 9.7A and B: Pyogenic granuloma overlying a squamous cell carcinoma. (A) Pyogenic granuloma in the inferior fornix after wedge resection of squamous cell carcinoma; (B) Histopathologic analysis of the excised lesion shows a pyogenic granuloma with a squamous cell carcinoma on its base.

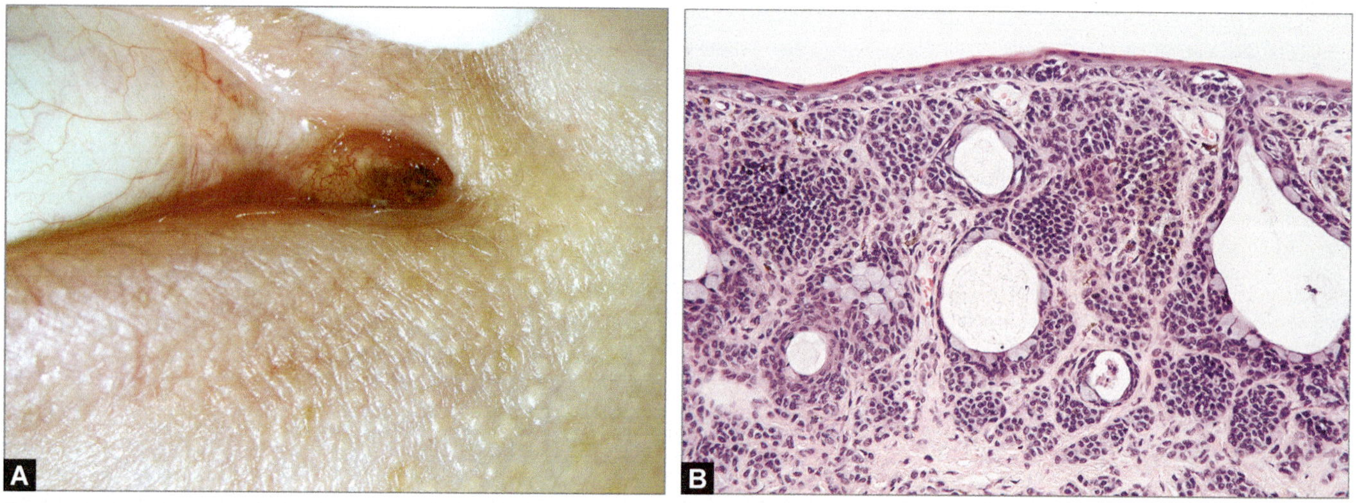

Figs. 9.8A and B: Conjunctival nevus. (A) Pigmented caruncle tumor with cysts; (B) Histology shows nevus cells and accompanying conjunctival inclusion cysts.

lesions in teenagers and young adults, it is a sign of potential malignancy in older patients. Primary acquired melanosis is characterized by melanocytic proliferation [rather than hypermelanosis (freckle or racial pigmentation) which represents increased transfer of melanin pigment to the basal epithelium from junctional melanocytes]. The presence of scattered melanocytes among the basal cells of the conjunctiva is considered normal. In PAM with atypia, nests of atypical melanocytes are observed in the conjunctival epithelium that often involve the entire thickness of the conjunctival epithelium. PAM with atypia is a pathologic diagnosis and may indicate a high risk (approximately 50%) of such lesions progressing to transformation into malignant melanoma. While intraepithelial lesions can be treated with an adjuvant therapy, such as topical mitomycin, a pathologic diagnosis through biopsy must be confirmed. Conjunctival malignant melanoma requires complete excision and if necessary followed by lymph node excision, if involved and possible radiation.[11]

The caruncle is also covered by conjunctival epithelium but contains additional adnexal structures, such as sebaceous glands and hair follicles. It is important to recognize this histologic difference since lesions that are often seen in the skin might at this site also be seen in the conjunctiva. Besides nevi and melanomas, there are some lesions which nearly exclusively (besides other nonocular locations) occur in the caruncle, such as oncocytoma or sebaceous gland hyperplasia/adenoma. Oncocytomas are reddish in color and histopathologically composed of eosinophilic, swollen cells which are packed with mitochondria and form gland like structures (Figs. 9.9A and B).[12]

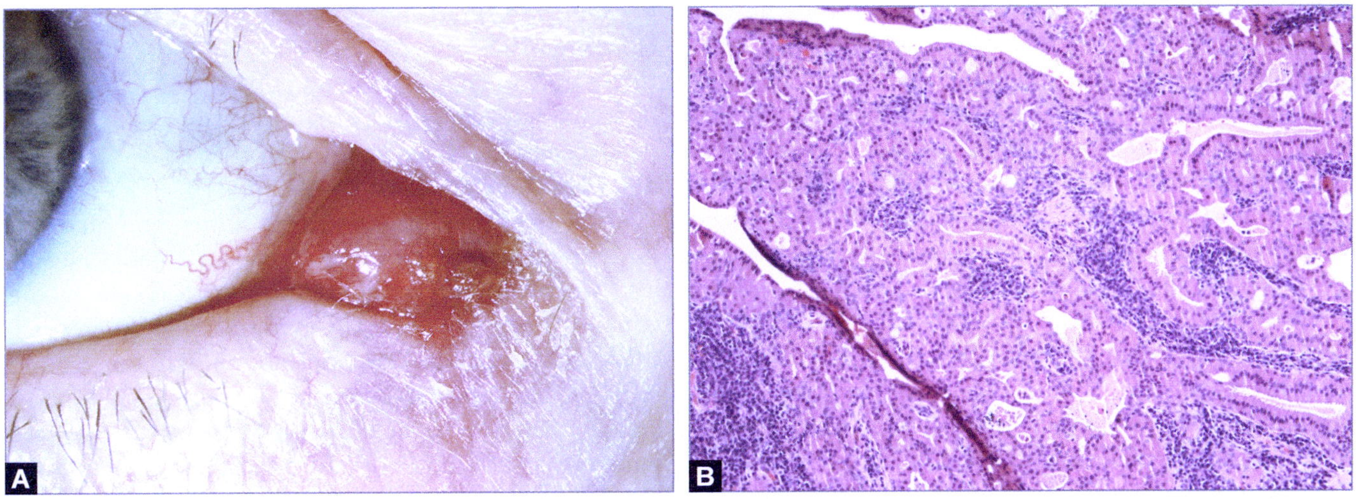

Figs. 9.9A and B: Oncocytoma. (A) Reddish lesion of the caruncle; (B) Oncocytic cells (eosinophilic epithelial cells) are present which show an adenoid pattern.

Cornea

Conjunctival (e.g. *Chlamydia*) and corneal infections can be detected by scrapings or corneal biopsies. Bacteria, fungi and *Acanthamoeba* can be identified by special stains, such as Gram stain, PAS stain, etc. (Table 9.1).[13] This is helpful in cases in which the microbiologists fail to detect an agent, when culture is difficult (e.g. in *Acanthamoeba*) or if an urgent result is needed. *Acanthamoeba* can be diagnosed by confocal microscopy by experienced investigators.[14] In penetrating grafts performed for *Acanthamoeba* keratitis, it is important that the clinician alerts the ophthalmic pathologist to the need to assess the margins of the excised corneal tissue for *Acanthamoeba* since recurrence or persistence of keratitis may occur with positive margins.

Fungi (e.g. *Fusarium* spp.) can penetrate Descemet's membrane and lens capsule in patients with fungal keratitis. In such cases, persistent inflammation despite long-term topical and systemic antifungal treatment highlights, these specialized membranes as a niche which may be an origin for recurrent or persistent inflammation (Fig. 9.10).[15] Presence of a long-standing fibrinous hypopyon, persistent posterior corneal stromal inflammation or a lens abscess should make the clinician suspicious of a fungal infection.

The corneal epithelium can also be examined histologically in cases where there is a suspicion of corneal intraepithelial neoplasia (CIN). These lesions are usually an extension of the neoplastic process from the adjacent conjunctiva.

The characteristic histologic finding in map-dot-fingerprint dystrophy is intraepithelial basement

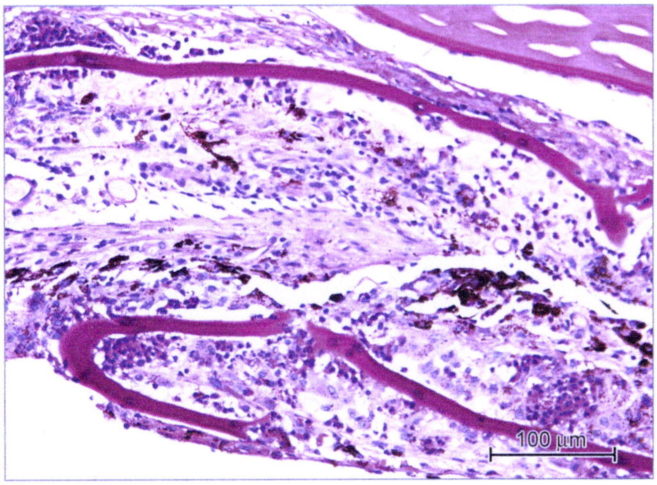

Fig. 9.10: *Fusarium* endophthalmitis. Histology shows *Fusarium* within the lens capsule despite aggressive topical, intracameral, and systemic treatment.

Table 9.1: List of selected infectious agents and how to detect them.

Agent	Special stain	Appearance
Bacteria	H&E/Giemsa, Gram stain	Blue (Gram-positive) Pink (Gram-negative)
Fungi	PAS, Grocott's methenamine silver (GMS) stain	PAS-positive, black with GMS stain
Acanthamoeba	H&E, PAS, calcofluor white (CW) stain and others[13]	Better visible on PAS stain than on H&E, fluorescence in CW stain
Mycobacterium tuberculosum	Ziehl-Neelsen stain/ Fite stain	Red/pink
Chlamydia	May-Grünwald + Giemsa stain	Cellular inclusions

(H&E: Hematoxylin-eosin; PAS: Periodic acid–Schiff reaction)

membrane thickening (Figs. 9.11A and B), while fibrotic tissue with partial destruction of Bowman's layer is seen in Salzmann's nodular degeneration.

Herpes keratitis is characterized by deep stromal vascularization and a stromal lymphocytic infiltrate. Chronic granulomatous inflammation with giant cells around Descemet's membrane may be noted on pathologic examination. Herpes simplex virus (HSV) infection can also be verified by immunostaining.[16]

Besides the characteristic deposits in the classical corneal dystrophies (in particular granular, lattice, and macular dystrophy) (Table 9.2), amyloid deposition can be found in chronic corneal scarring (Figs. 9.12A to C).[17] Knowledge regarding the molecular pathology of corneal dystrophies has significantly increased in the last few decades and is outside the scope of this chapter and a comprehensive review may be found in the literature.[17] In contrast to conjunctival and eyelid amyloid deposits in which systemic disease is more common, systemic involvement is extremely rare with corneal disease that is not a dystrophy but has to be excluded.[18]

New treatment options and resulting complications for corneal diseases can be evaluated pathologically and also in experimental settings. One example is keratoconus, which is histopathologically characterized by breaks in Bowman's layer, corneal stromal thinning and scarring and/or breaks in Descemet's membrane (corneal hydrops) in severe cases. After corneal crosslinking, loss of keratocytes and nerves in the anterior and midstroma is observed.[19,20] However, rare cases present a permanent loss of corneal

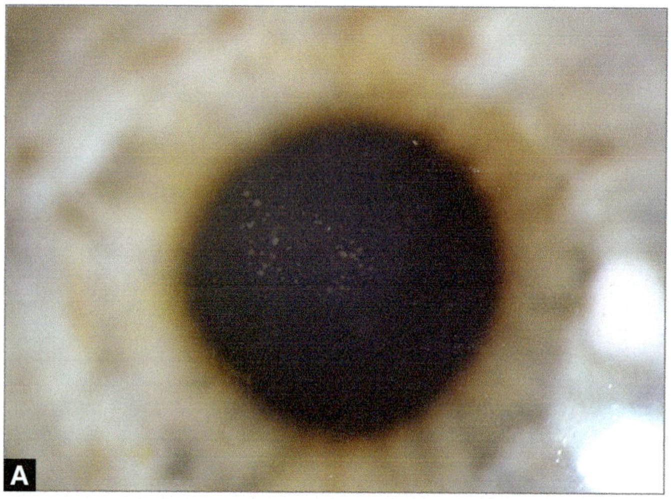

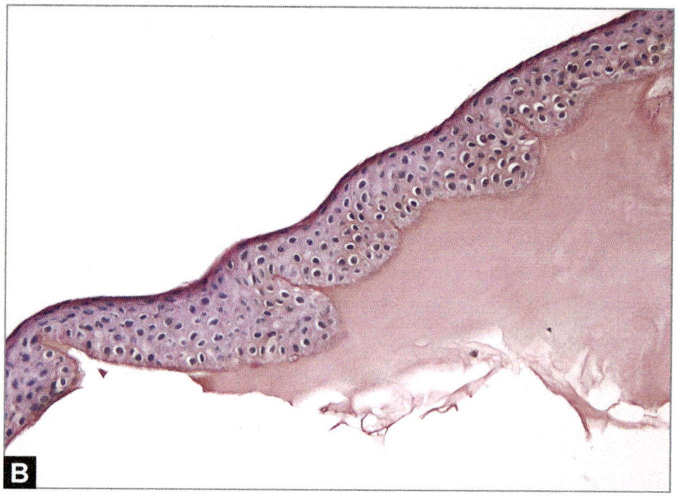

Figs. 9.11A and B: Map-dot-fingerprint dystrophy. (A) Clinical picture before corneal abrasion showing an irregular epithelium; (B) Histology shows basement membrane which is incorporated into the epithelium.

Table 9.2: Special stains of deposited material in selected corneal dystrophies.

Corneal disease	Localization	Deposited material	Special stain
Reis–Bücklers dystrophy	Anterior stroma	Granular extracellular eosinophilic deposits	Masson's trichrome stain (red deposits)
Thiel–Behnke dystrophy	Anterior stroma	Honeycomb pattern of degenerative changes	TEM (curly collagen fibrils)
Granular dystrophy	Throughout stroma with clear spaces between stroma	Granular extracellular eosinophilic deposits (protein keratoepithelin)	Masson's trichrome stain (red deposits)
Lattice dystrophy	Throughout stroma	Amyloid	Congo red stain (birefringence + dichroism under polarized light)
Macular dystrophy	Throughout stroma, endothelium	Amorphous intra- and extracellular deposits, abnormal keratan sulfate	Alcian blue, colloidal iron (stains for acid mucopolysaccharides)
Avellino dystrophy (combined granular-lattice dystrophy)	Throughout stroma	Granular dystrophy deposits and amyloid	Masson's trichrome stain and Congo red stain (birefringence + dichroism under polarized light)
Amyloid deposition in other conditions; gelatinous drop like dystrophy; scarring, etc.	Associated with other pathologic findings	Amyloid	Congo red stain (birefringence + dichroism under polarized light)

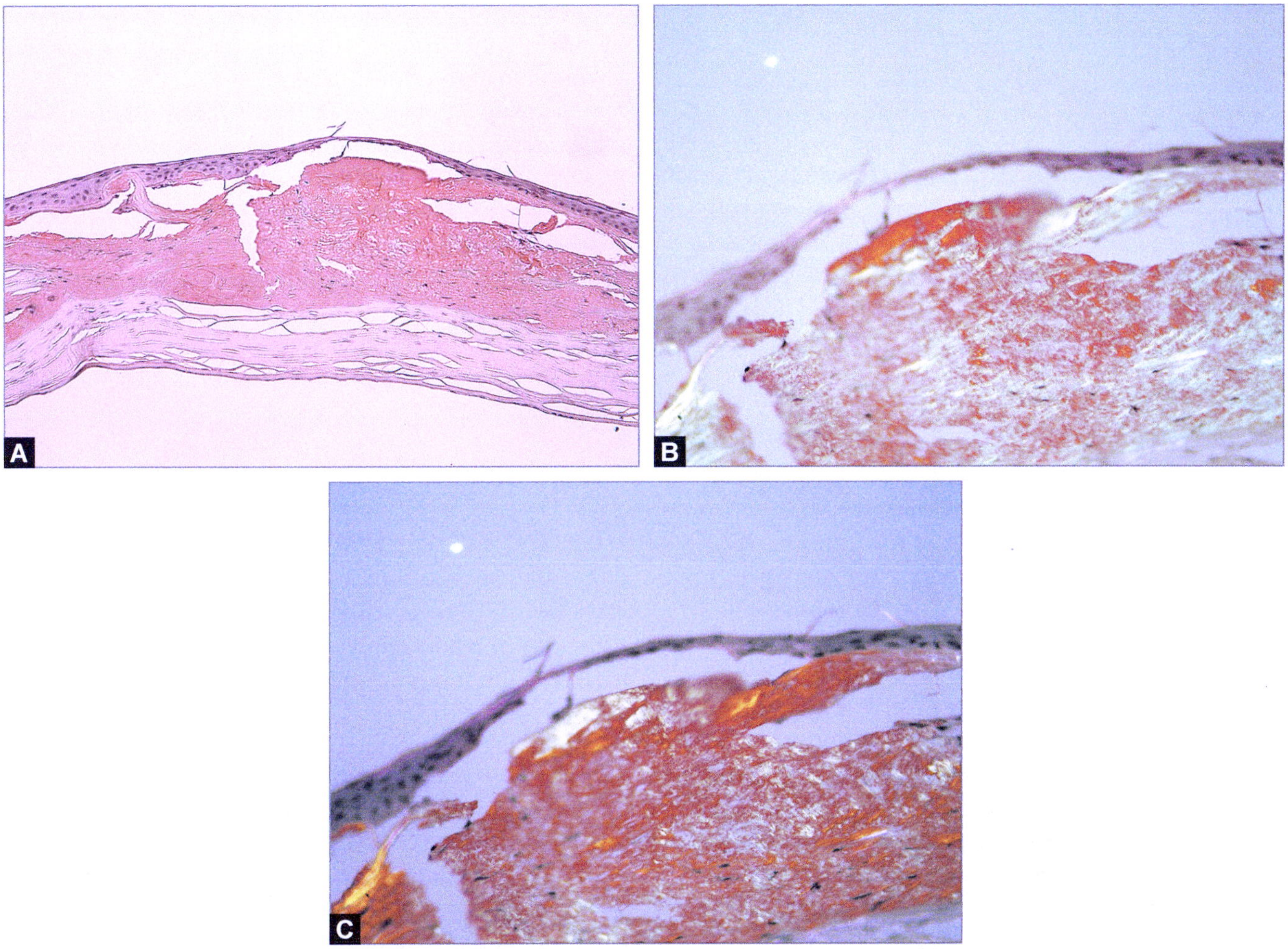

Figs. 9.12A to C: Corneal scar-associated amyloid deposition. (A) A Congo red stain shows a reddish-stained area in the anterior to mid-stroma; (B and C) Birefringence and dichroism are seen under polarized light.

keratocytes in this area, which may be a reason for a stromal scar after such treatment. Corneas that clear after "acute hydrops" illustrate that a new Descemet's membrane is secreted by corneal endothelial cells that enlarge to cover areas of focal Descemet's breaks.[20] Common corneal endothelial cell degenerations include Fuchs' corneal endothelial dystrophy and endothelial cell loss secondary to intraocular surgery such as cataract surgery. The clinical finding in these cases is corneal edema. Histologically, the two common causes of corneal endothelial cell loss can be distinguished by the presence of posterior excrescences of Descemet's membrane (guttae) in Fuchs' dystrophy. The number of endothelial cells is attenuated in both entities.

Glaucoma

In primary open angle glaucoma, the hallmark is glaucomatous optic nerve atrophy in which axonal atrophy without gliosis is seen in early stages and posterior/lateral bowing of the lamina cribrosa in later stages. Changes in the trabecular meshwork are only detectable by ultrastructural microscopy.[21] The secondary glaucomas show specific histopathologic findings: Pseudoexfoliation glaucoma exhibits material on the lens capsule and zonules (Fig. 9.13)[22] along with changes in the iris muscle and blood vessels. Neovascular glaucoma shows a neovascular membrane on the iris surface bridging the chamber angle (Fig. 9.14B) often associated with ectropion of the pupillary border secondary to dragging of the iris pigment epithelium by the fibrovascular membrane. Ghost cell glaucoma that occurs in patients with chronic vitreous hemorrhage or hyphema is characterized by rigid red blood cells that are partly devoid of hemoglobin with stiff cellular membranes that demonstrate Heinz bodies. These stiff cells fill the chamber angle, occlude the trabecular meshwork and cause elevated intraocular pressure. Tumor-related glaucoma[23]

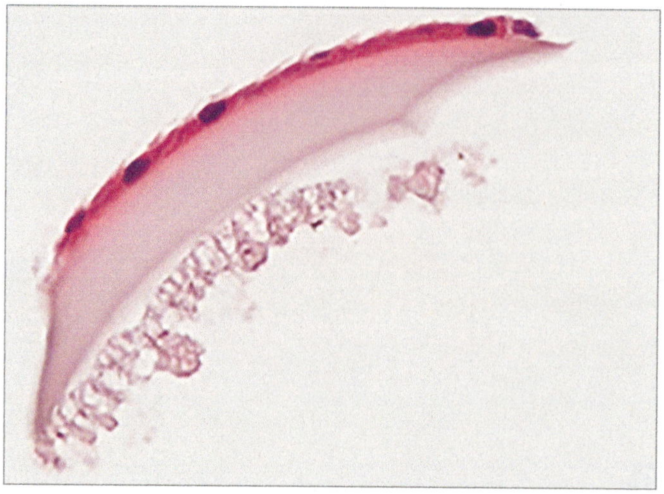

Fig. 9.13: Secondary glaucoma. Pseudoexfoliation material on the lens capsule.

may occur in a condition, such as melanomalytic glaucoma. It results from melanin containing macrophages from a necrotic melanoma congesting the trabecular meshwork. Tumor-related glaucoma may also occur from tumor invasion into the chamber angle in a tumor, such as a ciliary body melanoma. Other mechanisms of secondary angle closure may occur with epithelial downgrowth from surgical or traumatic wounds of the anterior segment resulting in a layer of epithelial cells covering the corneal endothelium, anterior chamber angle and iris surface.[24]

Lens

In adults, a cataract is characterized by Morgagnian globules, clefts in the lens cortex, and accumulations of crystals (e.g. calcium oxalate or other calcium salts). In anterior subcapsular cataract fibrous metaplasia of the anterior lens epithelium occurs from trauma or anterior segment inflammation. Capsulorhexis during cataract surgery can be challenging in presence of the fibrous tissue/metaplasia in anterior subcapsular cataract. An understanding of the pathologic process is important in the surgical planning in such cases. Posterior subcapsular cataract can occur from a variety of conditions and results from posterior migration of lens epithelial cells (the posterior capsule is normally devoid of lens epithelium) and may show bladder cell formation (Wedl cells).[25] This pathological change should be kept in mind during cortical cleanup in cataract surgery when the posterior capsule is polished to remove these epithelial cells and aberrant cortical material. Similarly, posterior capsule opacification results from migration of equatorial epithelial cells on to the posterior capsule. The cells attempt to form aberrant cortical material that appears as opalescent droplets (Elschnig's pearls) or epithelial sheets with fibrous metaplasia.

Histological changes in fetal eyes or children's eyes with cataract are more difficult to discern since artifacts which are similar to findings in adult cataracts often impair the diagnosis.[26] Cataracts may be associated with persistent hyperplastic primary vitreous (PHPV) with spontaneous rupture of the lens capsule. Rubella cataracts are typically nuclear type cataracts. The pathologic change that can be seen in this condition is persistence of lens nuclei (from the lens epithelium) in the lens nucleus and central cortical fibers.[25]

Retina

Diabetic Retinopathy (Figs. 9.14A to E)

Early diabetic retinopathy is characterized by vascular changes in the venous capillaries specifically degeneration of the pericytes lining the vessels resulting in loss of capillary tone and the formation of retinal microaneurysms. The arterial side of the retinal circulation is normally devoid of capillaries. These changes are followed by intraretinal and nerve fiber layer hemorrhages and exudates that predominantly occur in the outer plexiform layer.[27] Cotton wool spots (soft exudates) may also be present and represent microinfarctions of the nerve fiber layer. Histologically, cotton wool spots show localized axonal swelling with stasis of organelles in the axons (cytoid bodies). Diabetic macular edema results from transudation of protein and lipid into the extracellular areas in the retina that eventually leads to an irreversible change in macular architecture with atrophy in longstanding disease. Furthermore, with advancing disease and ischemia neovascular membranes develop that grow into the vitreous cavity. The neovascular membranes are an indicator of severe proliferative diabetic retinopathy and most often occur at the optic nerve, the iris surface/chamber angle but also in other areas of the retina. These neovascular membranes, having a fibrotic component, cause tractional retinal detachments, and angle closure in the anterior segment (resulting in neovascular glaucoma), both vision threatening and complications of the disease.

Age-related Macular Degeneration

The two types of macular degeneration [age-related macular degeneration (ARMD)] include *dry* ARMD (geographic atrophy) and *neovascular* ARMD. In dry

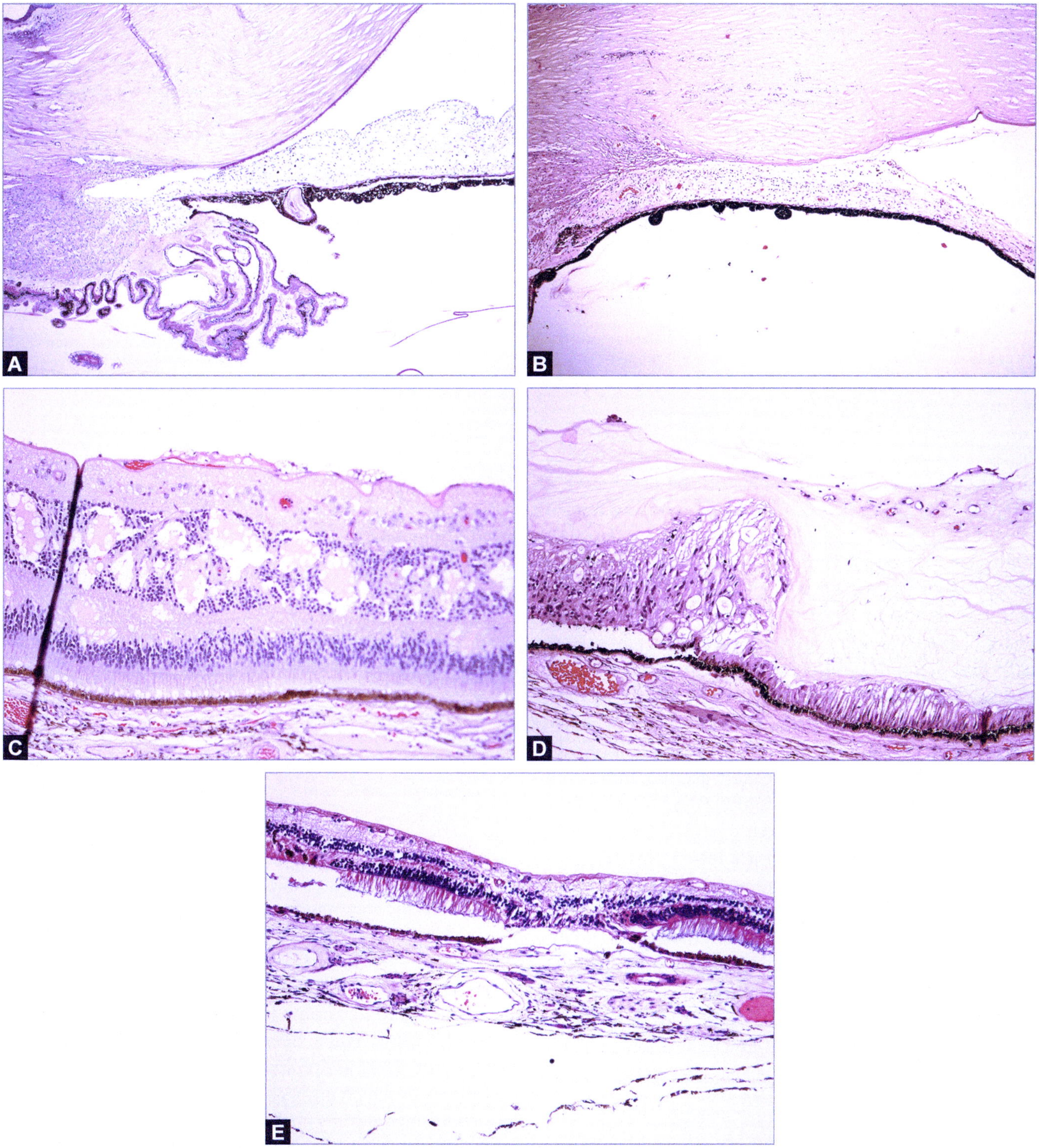

Figs. 9.14A to E: Diabetic changes. (A) Lacy iris vacuolization and thickening of the ciliary body's basement membrane; (B) Neovascular membrane on the iris surface bridging the chamber angle and thus leading to secondary glaucoma; (C) Neovascular epiretinal membrane and intraretinal edema; (D) Neovascularization into the anterior vitreous; (E) Laser lesion resulting in a scar at the outer retina, RPE and choriocapillaris.

Table 9.3: Overview of different types of drusen/deposits in age-related macular degeneration.

Drusen type	Clinical picture	Material	Histology	TEM
Hard drusen	Small, well-defined yellowish spots with sharp borders	Various components	Small homogeneous deposits of hyaline material beneath the RPE	Located between RPE basal lamina and inner collagenous layer of Bruch's membrane
Soft drusen	Larger than hard drusen, yellowish, with fluffy borders	Various components	Larger inhomogeneous deposits of hyaline material beneath the RPE	Located between RPE basal lamina and inner collagenous layer of Bruch's membrane
Basement membrane deposits	As yet to be determined	Similar to BM (e.g. laminin, fibronectin, collagen IV)	Palisade-like layer between RPE and Bruch's membrane	Located between RPE cell membrane and its basal lamina
Reticular pseudodrusen	Yellow, interlacing network occurring in the outer macula	As yet to be determined	As yet to be determined	As yet to be determined
Subretinal drusenoid deposits	As yet to be determined[29]	Similar to soft drusen	Between RPE and neural retina (determined in postmortem eyes)	Between RPE and neural retina (determined in postmortem eyes)

(BM: Basement membrane; RPE: Retinal pigment epithelium)

ARMD early stages are characterized by drusen which are located at the level of Bruch's membrane and beneath the retinal pigment epithelium. Hard and soft drusen as well as basal laminar deposits are typical for this disease (Table 9.3).[28,29] In the later stages of ARMD, the clinical picture is that of circumscribed geographic atrophy in the posterior pole. Pathologically this variant is characterized by retinal pigment epithelium (RPE) atrophy, extensive photoreceptor damage and loss of choriocapllaris. Neovascular or exudative ARMD is defined by neovascular choroidal membranes which may be subretinal (classic) and overlying the RPE or the neovascular membrane may be below the RPE (occult) (Fig. 9.15). These neovascular membranes have thin-walled blood vessels lined by endothelial cells that are leaky. This results in leakage of fluid into the retina and into the subretinal space which may be accompanied by hemorrhage.[30,31] These membranes are accompanied by damage of the RPE and the retinal architecture especially the photoreceptor layer. Retinal tubulations which have recently been described in ARMD are nonspecific and represent a misarrangement of the retinal layers in a longstanding disease. Such tubulations can be also observed in myopic neovascular membranes.[32]

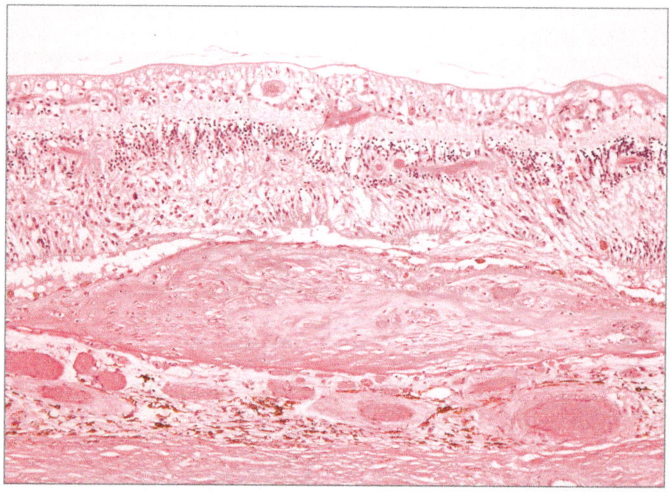

Fig. 9.15: Age-related macular degeneration. An occult neovascular membrane is seen. Basement membrane deposits are present beneath the residual RPE. The neurosensory retina shows loss of photoreceptors and gliotic degeneration of the outer retinal layers with beginning formation of degenerative pseudorosettes (retinal tubulations).

Uvea

The uvea (comprising iris, ciliary body and choroid) contains melanocytes, blood vessels and a stromal matrix. The ciliary body is lined by inner nonpigmented and outer pigmented epithelium, whereas the iris is posteriorly lined by two layers of pigmented epithelium. The melanocytes may give rise to uveal nevi which have to be distinguished from uveal melanoma. Nevi are typically composed of aggregates of spindle cells which are fusiform and have a bland nucleus (normal chromatin staining with absence of nucleoli). Folded nuclear chromatin may be present in some cells (Spindle A cells). Melanocytomas (magnocellular nevi) are subtypes of nevi and are typically heavily pigmented. The cells are large, polygonal, contain a lot of pigment, giant melanosomes, and have a bland nucleus. Bleaching of the sections is required to assess the cellular features.[33]

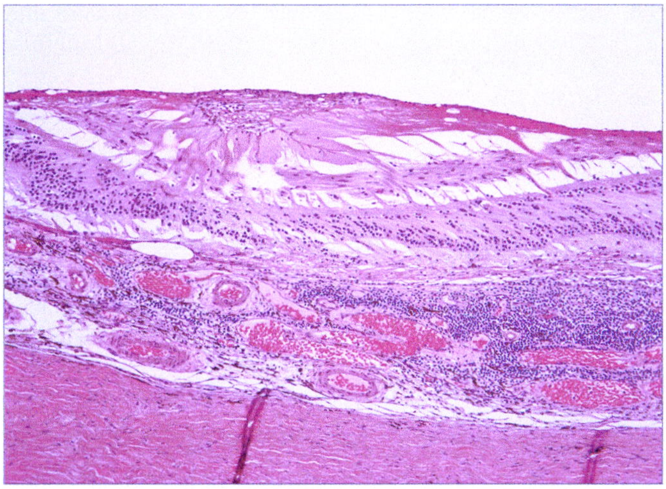

Fig. 9.16: Sympathetic ophthalmia. Chronic granulomatous inflammation of the choriocapillaris and neighboring choroid. The overlying retina and RPE are degenerated due to longstanding ocular disease.

Dalen-Fuchs nodules are pathognomonic for sympathetic ophthalmia, which is a diffuse granulomatous inflammation in the choroid (Fig. 9.16). They are situated between the retinal pigment epithelium and Bruch's membrane with overlying atrophic RPE.[34] Their detection in the affected eye with trauma can be vision-saving for the fellow eye, since treatment can be promptly instituted when the condition is identified. Clinically, Dalen-Fuchs nodules are yellowish dots at the posterior pole. The nodules can also be visualized by SD-OCT.[35]

Orbit

Clinicopathologic correlations of orbital lesions might be challenging but has improved with enhanced resolution of orbital imaging. Orbital neoplasms will be discussed elsewhere. Idiopathic inflammatory pseudotumor of the orbit (nonspecific orbital inflammation) is in the differential diagnosis of orbital lymphomas. Clinical findings include painful proptosis and a number of other symptoms depending on the type of tissue involved in the inflammatory process. Magnetic resonance imaging may show hypointense lesions on the T1- and T2-weighted images possibly suggesting the fibrotic changes, and the lesions show marked gadolinium enhancement suggesting vascularity. Fat suppression techniques can clearly detect an optic nerve sheath lesion and intraorbital inflammation.[36,37] Orbital pseudotumors can occur on their own or in association with IgG4-sclerosing disease.[38] A typical histologic finding is fibrosing orbital tissue interspersed with chronic inflammatory cells, in case of IgG4-sclerosing disease with a high IgG4/IgG ratio.

REFERENCES

1. Rennie CA, Chowdhury S, Khan J, et al. The prevalence and associated features of posterior embryotoxon in the general ophthalmic clinic. Eye (Lond). 2005;19:396-9.
2. Nicholls SG, Oakley CL, Tan A, et al. Demodex species in human ocular disease: new clinicopathological aspects. Int Ophthalmol. 2017;37:303-12.
3. Panda BB, Parija S, Pujahari S, et al. Sebaceous Gland Carcinoma of Eyelid—A Tarnished Masquerade. J Clin Diagn Res. 2016;10:ND3-5.
4. Ozdal PC, Codere F, Callejo S, et al. Accuracy of the clinical diagnosis of chalazion. Eye (Lond). 2004;18:135-8.
5. Leahey AB, Shane JJ, Listhaus A, et al. Molluscum contagiosum eyelid lesions as the initial manifestation of acquired immunodeficiency syndrome. Am J Ophthalmol. 1997;124:240-1.
6. Jakobiec FA, Zakka FR, Hatton MP. Eyelid basal cell carcinoma developing in an epidermoid cyst: a previously unreported event. Ophthal Plast Reconstr Surg. 2010;26: 491-4.
7. Dey A, Aggarwal R, Dwivedi S. Cardiovascular profile of xanthelasma palpebrarum. Biomed Res Int. 2013;2013: 932863.
8. Pfeiffer MJ. Eyelid nevi: differential diagnosis and surgical treatment. Klin Monbl Augenheilkd. 2013;230:36-42.
9. Duncan J, Chen Y, Fuchs D, et al. Follicular Lymphoma Presenting Solely as Chronic Follicular Conjunctivitis. Cornea. 2016;35:395-8.
10. Afrogheh AH, Jakobiec FA, Hammon R, et al. Evaluation for High-risk HPV in Squamous Cell Carcinomas and Precursor Lesions Arising in the Conjunctiva and Lacrimal Sac. Am J Surg Pathol. 2016;40:519-28.
11. Harooni H, Schoenfield LR, Singh AD. Current appraisal of conjunctival melanocytic tumors: classification and treatment. Future Oncol. 2011;7:435-46.
12. Say EA, Shields CL, Bianciotto C, et al. Oncocytic lesions (oncocytoma) of the ocular adnexa: report of 15 cases and review of literature. Ophthal Plast Reconstr Surg. 2012;28:14-21.
13. Grossniklaus HE, Waring GO 4th, Akor C, et al. Evaluation of hematoxylin and eosin and special stains for the detection of acanthamoeba keratitis in penetrating keratoplasties. Am J Ophthalmol. 2003;136:520-6.
14. Daas L, Viestenz A, Schnabel PA, et al. Confocal microscopy as an early relapse marker for acanthamoeba keratitis. Clin Anat. 2017.
15. Gao Y, Chen N, Dong XG, et al. Surgical management of fungal endophthalmitis resulting from fungal keratitis. Int J Ophthalmol. 2016;9:848-53.
16. Jansen AF, Rijneveld WJ, Remeijer L, et al. Five-year follow-up on the effect of oral acyclovir after penetrating keratoplasty for herpetic keratitis. Cornea. 2009;28:843-5.
17. Lin ZN, Chen J, Cui HP. Characteristics of corneal dystrophies: a review from clinical, histological and genetic perspectives. Int J Ophthalmol. 2016;9:904-13.
18. Suesskind D, Ziemssen F, Rohrbach JM. Conjunctival amyloidosis—clinical and histopathologic features. Graefes Arch Clin Exp Ophthalmol. 2015;253:1377-83.

19. Messmer EM, Meyer P, Herwig MC, et al. Morphological and immunohistochemical changes after corneal cross-linking. Cornea. 2013;32:111-7.
20. Muller PL, Loffler KU, Kohlhaas M, et al. Morphologic Corneal Changes after Crosslinking for Keratoconus. Klin Monbl Augenheilkd. 2017.
21. Tektas OY, Lutjen-Drecoll E. Structural changes of the trabecular meshwork in different kinds of glaucoma. Exp Eye Res. 2009;88:769-75.
22. Schlotzer-Schrehardt U, Naumann GO. Trabecular meshwork in pseudoexfoliation syndrome with and without open-angle glaucoma. A morphometric, ultrastructural study. Invest Ophthalmol Vis Sci. 1995;36:1750-64.
23. Stadigh A, Puska P, Vesti E, et al. Ring melanoma of the anterior chamber angle as a mimicker of pigmentary glaucoma. Surv Ophthalmol. 2017.
24. Smith MF, Doyle JW. Glaucoma secondary to epithelial and fibrous downgrowth. Semin Ophthalmol. 1994;9:248-53.
25. Yanoff M, Sassani JW. Ocular Pathology, 6th edition. New York: Elsevier Inc.; 2009.
26. Herwig MC, Müller AM, Klarmann-Schulz U, et al. Lens artifacts in human fetal eyes—the challenge of interpreting the histomorphology of human fetal lenses. Graefes Arch Clin Exp Ophthalmol. 2014;252:155-62.
27. Garner A. Histopathology of diabetic retinopathy in man. Eye (Lond). 1993;7(Pt 2):250-3.
28. Loeffler KU, Lee WR. Terminology of sub-RPE deposits: do we all speak the same language? Br J Ophthalmol. 1998;82:1104-5.
29. Curcio CA, Messinger JD, Sloan KR, et al. Subretinal drusenoid deposits in non-neovascular age-related macular degeneration: morphology, prevalence, topography, and biogenesis model. Retina. 2013;33:265-76.
30. Bird AC, Phillips RL, Hageman GS. Geographic atrophy: a histopathological assessment. JAMA Ophthalmol. 2014;132:338-45.
31. Spraul CW, Lang GE, Grossniklaus HE, et al. Histologic and morphometric analysis of the choroid, Bruch's membrane, and retinal pigment epithelium in postmortem eyes with age-related macular degeneration and histologic examination of surgically excised choroidal neovascular membranes. Surv Ophthalmol. 1999;44(Suppl 1): S10-32.
32. Litts KM, Ach T, Hammack KM, et al. Quantitative Analysis of Outer Retinal Tubulation in Age-Related Macular Degeneration From Spectral-Domain Optical Coherence Tomography and Histology. Invest Ophthalmol Vis Sci. 2016;57:2647-56.
33. Ahmad SS, Lad L, Ghani SA. A case of choroidal melanocytoma mimicking a choroidal melanoma. Saudi J Ophthalmol. 2015;29:242-5.
34. Chu XK, Chan CC. Sympathetic ophthalmia: to the twenty-first century and beyond. J Ophthalmic Inflamm Infect. 2013;3:49.
35. Muakkassa NW, Witkin AJ. Spectral-domain optical coherence tomography of sympathetic ophthalmia with Dalen-Fuchs nodules. Ophthalmic Surg Lasers Imaging Retina. 2014;45:610-2.
36. Valvassori GE, Sabnis SS, Mafee RF, et al. Imaging of orbital lymphoproliferative disorders. Radiol Clin North Am. 1999;37:135-50, x-xi.
37. Weber AL, Romo LV, Sabates NR. Pseudotumor of the orbit. Clinical, pathologic, and radiologic evaluation. Radiol Clin North Am. 1999;37:151-68, xi.
38. Sa HS, Lee JH, Woo KI, et al. IgG4-related disease in idiopathic sclerosing orbital inflammation. Br J Ophthalmol. 2015;99:1493-7.

Chapter 10 Practical Contributions of the Ophthalmic Pathologist to Ocular Oncology

Hind Alkatan, Deepak P Edward

INTRODUCTION

Ophthalmic pathology is an important subspecialty and a working knowledge of the subspecialty is important for all ophthalmologists but more so for those practicing ophthalmic oncology. In order for the ophthalmic pathologist to provide the highest level of accuracy and diagnosis, excellent communication between the oncologists and the pathologists is essential to provide quality clinical care.[1]

This chapter discusses the clinical and pathologic features of the following tumors:

- Orbital tumors
- External tumors
- Ocular surface
- Intraocular tumors.

10.1 ORBITAL TUMORS

Hind Alkatan

INTRODUCTION

The prevalence of orbital neoplasms varies in different geographical areas of the world depending on ethnicity, race, and study design reporting the incidence, but in general they are rare in an ophthalmic pathology practice. The literature suggests a prevalence of 3.5–4% in an oculoplastic practice.[2-4]

Orbital tumors can be classified based on the tissue of origin, site (lacrimal gland, eyelids), or clinical behavior.[5,6] Most researchers have classified orbital lesions into primary: arising from any anatomic structure in the orbit; or secondary where the tumor originates from surrounding tissue, or is metastatic via hematogenous or lymphatic spread.[5,6]

Primary orbital lesions are the most common ranging from 56% to 77.29%[5-7] of all orbital neoplasms. Secondary tumors range from 18.62% to 36%.[2,5-7] Finally, metastatic lesions are the least common accounting for 0.32% to 10% or oribital neoplasms.[5-8]

The frequency of malignant orbital lesions is reported to be as high as 86.17%.[5]

Demographically, orbital lesions are more common in adults with the majority of patients presenting in the 6th and 7th decades.[5,6] The median age for orbital tumors in the USA is 55 years.[7]

The frequency of orbital neoplasm differs depending on the age. The major presenting symptoms are proptosis, disturbance in extraocular muscle motility, diplopia, and lid dysfunction.[6]

The histopathopathological features of some of the common orbital tumors are discussed further below.

SECTION A: LACRIMAL GLAND LESIONS

The lacrimal gland is composed of glandular epithelium and its ducts, stroma, and lymphoid tissue. Neoplasms of this tissue are therefore classified into epithelial and nonepithelial tumors.

The epithelial lacrimal gland tumors account for about 10–16% of all orbital lesions and about half of the lacrimal gland lesions—with pleomorphic adenoma being the most common epithelial tumor.[8-10] In a 10-year survey from a tertiary referral center, the only epithelial tumors encountered were pleomorphic adenoma and adenoid cystic carcinoma, which are discussed in detail below.[11]

The most common benign epithelial lacrimal gland tumor is pleomorphic adenoma which accounts for approximately 20–50% of the epithelial lesions.[12,13] In South Asia, the prevalence of PA is much higher (75%) than in Caucasians.[14] The age range at diagnosis for patients with pleomorphic adenoma is wide (13–81 years) with long duration of symptoms.[12,15] The rate of recurrence following primary excision of pleopmorphic adenomas can reach up to 25%, and in one report, recurrences were significantly ($p < 0.03$) associated with positive tumor in the resection margins but not with preoperative incisional biopsy.[15] This further emphasizes the importance of histopathological examination of the primary excision. The pathologist should comment on the capsule that encases the neoplasm for infiltration with tumor cells, which may not be visible on preoperative imaging or during excision. The surgeon should look for comments on infiltration of the capsule, which would mandate careful patient follow-up.

Histopathologically, pleomorphic adenoma is a benign tumor surrounded by a pseudocapsule. The tumor consists of proliferating epithelial and mesenchymal components with variable proportions (Fig. 10.1.1). The epithelial component can show ductal structures and nonductal spindle, round, or stellate-shaped cells. Occasional squamous metaplasia is present in recurrent lesions. The stromal component can show myxoid, hyaline, cartilaginous, or even osseous differentiation.[12,15] When pleomorphic adenoma is suspected clinically, "en toto" surgical excision with intact capsule is the treatment of choice because of the risk of recurrence and malignant transformation. However, some reports claim that an incisional biopsy of pleomorphic adenoma can be performed provided that the biopsy tract is removed at the time of definitive surgery.[16,17] It is also recommended that pathology reports include a description of the presence or absence of high cellularity, atypia, and myoepithelial prominence when describing pleomorphic adenoma even though their relationship to possible malignant transformation of pleomorphic adenoma is not well established in comparison to the salivary gland pleomorphic adenomas.[18] Immunohistochemically, the epithelial cells in pleomorphic adenoma (and occasionally the myoepithelial cells) express cytokeratin while myoepithelial cells may express muscle-specific antigen and glial fibrillary acidic protein.[19] Recently, two nuclear markers, PLAG1 (pleomorphic adenoma gene 1) and MYB, that have been introduced into the immunohistochemical panel to accurately diagnose pleomorphic adenoma and adenoid cystic carcinoma. MYB belongs to a family of proteins that functions as transcriptional regulators. Translocation of t(6:9) (q22-23;p23-24) leads to fusion of the MYB oncogene to a transcription factor NF1B resulting in overexpression of the MYB protein in cases of ACC. *PLAG1* has been found to be strongly positive in pleomorphic adenoma while negative in all cases of adenoid cystic carcinoma.[13,20,21]

Malignant transformation in recurrent pleomorphic adenoma may show pathologic features of adenocarcinoma (more common), mucoepidermoid carcinoma, and carcinosarcomatous tumor (Fig. 10.1.2). Generally, the carcinomas are poorly differentiated with an infiltrative growth pattern and significant cytological atypia.[18] Regarding the terminology, carcinoma-ex-pleomorphic adenoma is defined as carcinoma arising in or from a pleomorphic adenoma, where histological examination

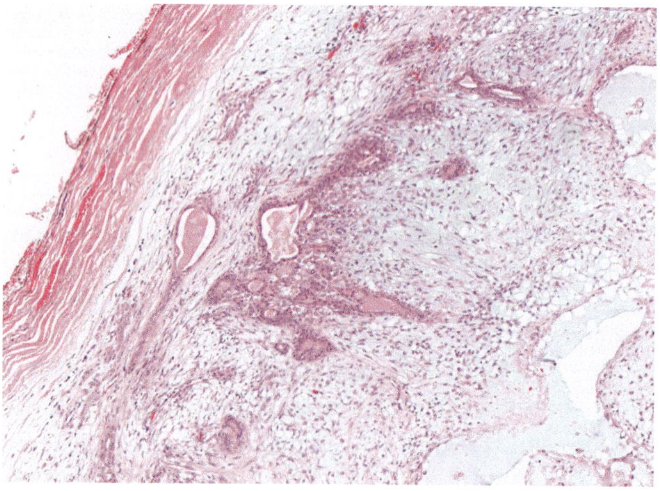

Fig. 10.1.1: Pleomorphic adenoma of the lacrimal gland showing fibrous pseudocapsule and mixed stromal and epithelial proliferation (Original magnification × 100; H and E).

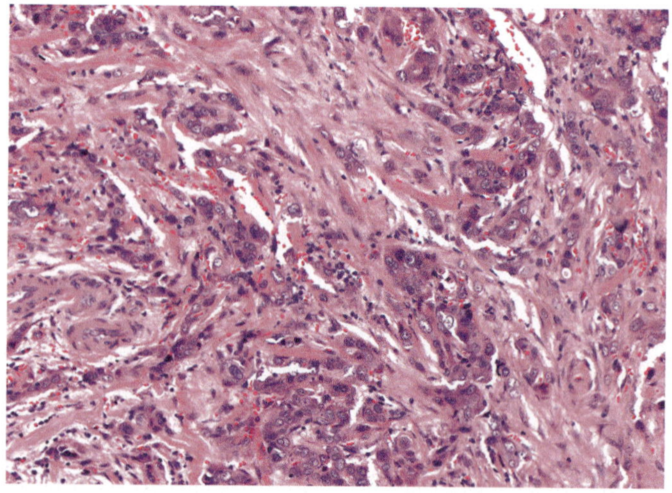

Fig. 10.1.2: Histopathology of a recurrent pleomorphic adenoma showing proliferation of atypical adenocarcinoma in the epithelial areas of the tumor (Original magnification × 200; H and E).

would show residual benign pleomorphic adenoma with transitional areas between the benign and malignant portions.[15] Also, immunohistochemical staining of other markers described in the salivary glands, such as androgen receptor, p53, and the HER-2⁄neu oncoprotein, has been be reported to be strongly and diffusely expressed in the malignant areas of carcinoma-ex-pleomorphic adenoma.[23]

Adneoid cystic carcinoma is the most common malignant epithelial tumor of the lacrimal gland. The tumor presents with short duration of symptoms (mean—7 months) and age ranging from 12 years to 75 years (mean; 44 years) in Saudi Arabia.[12] Pain is a cardinal symptom resulting from perineural invasion of the tumor.[12,13] Patients with adenoid cystic carcinoma are known to have a poor prognosis with reported 10-year overall survival (OS) and 10-year disease-specific survival (DSS) of 38.7 and 51.4% respectively in the USA.[23] Patients die from distant metastasis (mainly to the lung, brain, and bone) and intracranial spread.

Histopathologically, adenoid cystic carcinoma is typically nonencapsulated with infiltration of the surrounding orbital fat and muscle.[18] There are three known histological growth patterns: the cribriform or Swiss cheese, which is the most common, the solid and the tubular (Fig. 10.1.3). There is usually a mixture of more than one pattern within the same neoplasm.[21] The solid variant may show basaloid features and should be differentiated from basal cell carcinoma extending from nearby tissue.

Other lacrimal gland tumors are rare and include adenocarcinoma and mucoepidermoid carcinomas.

Adenocarcinoma is a rare lacrimal gland epithelial tumor. Histopathologically, the tumor shows variable glandular formation, necrosis, and mitotic rate.[18]

Mucoepidermoid carcinoma is another rare malignant epithelial tumor of the lacrimal gland accounting for less than 2% of lacrimal gland carcinomas.[24] The tumor histopathologically consists of squamous component, mucin-secreting cells in addition to intermediate cells (Fig. 10.1.4).

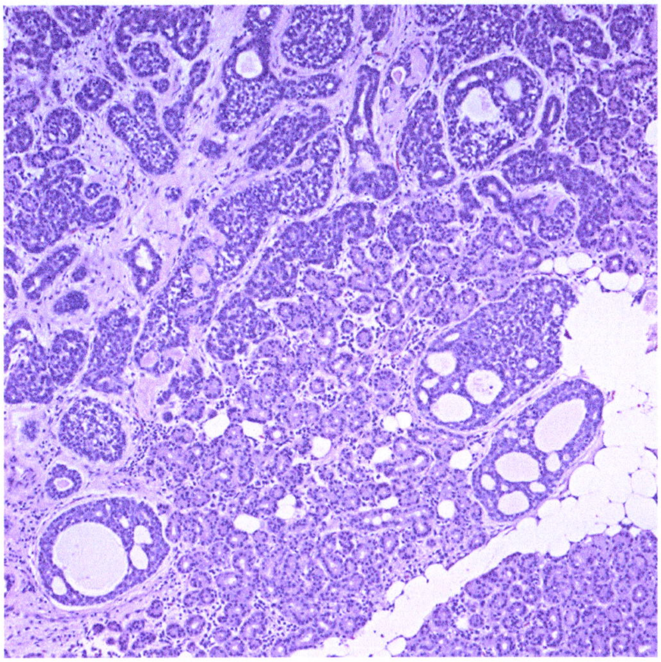

Fig. 10.1.3: Adenoid cystic carcinoma of the lacrimal gland with areas of typical Swiss-Cheese appearance (Original magnification × 100; H and E).

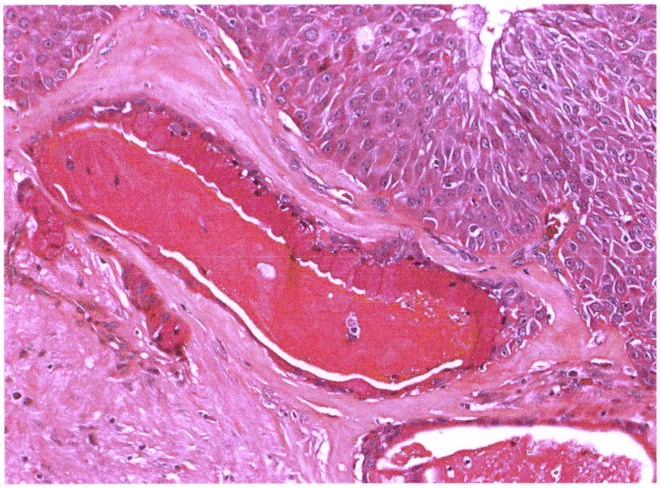

Fig. 10.1.4: Mucoepidermoid carcinoma of the lacrimal gland with mucous secreting cells (Original magnification × 200; H and E).

SECTION B: SOFT TISSUE ORBITAL TUMORS

Introduction

Various soft tissues in the orbit can be the source of orbital lesions seen in the clinic. These include muscle, vasculature, nerves, soft tissue, and lesions which could be from external/metastatic sources. In this chapter specific orbital tumors that are more common will be discussed.

An understanding of the pathology, biological behavior, and location may help the clinician to make a more accurate clinical assessment and also aid in determining the principles of management of these neoplasms.

The diagnosis of orbital tumors can be aided by imaging techniques such as computerized tomography (CT) and magnetic resonance imaging (MRI), but tissue diagnosis remains the mainstay for definitive diagnosis except when the tumor is in a location that is not easily accessible.[1,2]

Rhabdomyosarcoma

Rhabdomyosarcoma is a highly malignant mesenchymal tumor that accounts for 4–8% of all childhood malignancies.[3] Among pediatric orbital lesions, 25–35% of lesions are rhabdomyosarcomas.[4] The pathogenesis of orbital rhabdomyosarcoma (which is an extraskeletal variant) is unclear. It is believed to arise from pluripotent mesenchymal cells in the orbit and not the extraocular muscles.[4]

The most common clinical presentation is unilateral proptosis with rapid progression over few weeks.[5] A semi-urgent incisional biopsy is often needed to confirm the diagnosis. The histopathological examination of rhabdomyosarcoma incisional biopsies by an expert ophthalmic pathologist is critical not only for establishing the diagnosis, but also for decision making in management and to give information that might be helpful in determining prognosis. Orbital rhabdomyosarcoma is classified into several histological types—embryonal rhabdomyosarcoma with three subtypes—(1) conventional pattern (Fig. 10.1.5), (2) botryoid and spindle cell variant and an alveolar pattern.[6,7] Mixed cell populations are also known to occur. A pleomorphic type is seen in older patients.[4]

The embryonal rhabdomyosarcoma is the most common accounting for about two-thirds of tumors, and probably has the best prognosis while the alveolar type is less common, accounting for 20% of these tumors and carries a less favorable prognosis compared to the embryonal type. Immunohistochemistry (IHC) aids in confirming the diagnosis. Myogenin is more commonly expressed in the alveolar type, but generally IHC staining has no correlation with the different histopathologic types of rhabdomyosarcoma. Tumor cells also express desmin (Fig. 10.1.6), actin, and myogenic regulatory protein (MyoD1) in about 90% of cases.[8-10] From a genetic perspective, a relationship has been demonstrated between *DICER1* mutations and familial and, to a lesser extent, sporadic forms of embryonal rhabdomyosarcoma.[11] The survival rate is dependent on the disease extent with the orbital site having the best survival compared to other sites in the head and neck region.[12] The overall 5-year survival rate in the USA for rhabdomyosarcoma is around 90%, due to effective chemotherapy/radiation in treating these tumors. The embryonal type has a better survival rate than the alveolar type.[13] Recurrence or metastatic spread of rhabdomyosarcoma generally occurs within a period of 3 years after treatment. Metastatic sites include lungs, bone, skeletal muscles, skin (with most cases of skin metastasis originating from the alveolar subtype), in addition to regional lymph nodes.[4,14,15]

Orbital Soft Tissue Tumors

Fibrous Histiocytoma

Fibrous histiocytoma is the most common mesenchymal orbital tumor in adults.[16] Histopathologically, this tumor shows mixed proliferation of fibroblastic spindle-shaped cells and histiocytic cells with a variable intercellular collagenous background, fibrous matrix, or myxoid stroma (Fig. 10.1.7). It can be classified as benign, locally aggressive, or malignant (based on pleomorphism, atypia or mitosis). A malignant fibrohistiocytic tumor is also known as a pleomorphic undifferentiated sarcoma.[17]

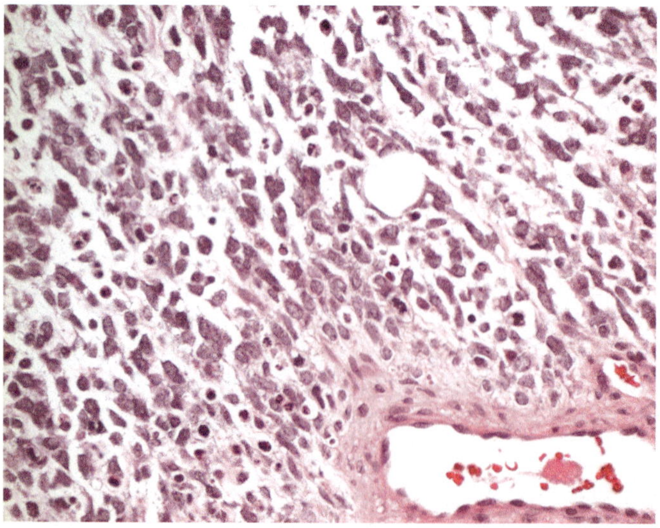

Fig. 10.1.5: Blue cell tumor representing embryonal rhabdomyosarcoma in a child (Original magnification × 400; H and E).

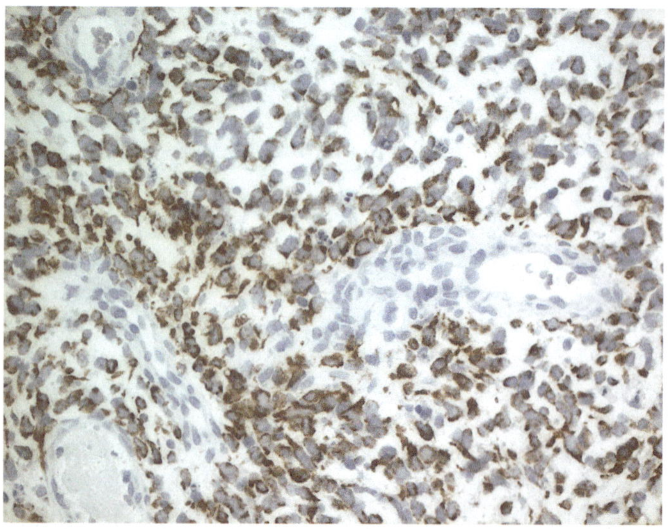

Fig. 10.1.6: Expression of muscle cell marker by the rhabdomyosarcoma tumor cells confirming the diagnosis [Original magnification × 400; Desmin; (brown DAB stain)].

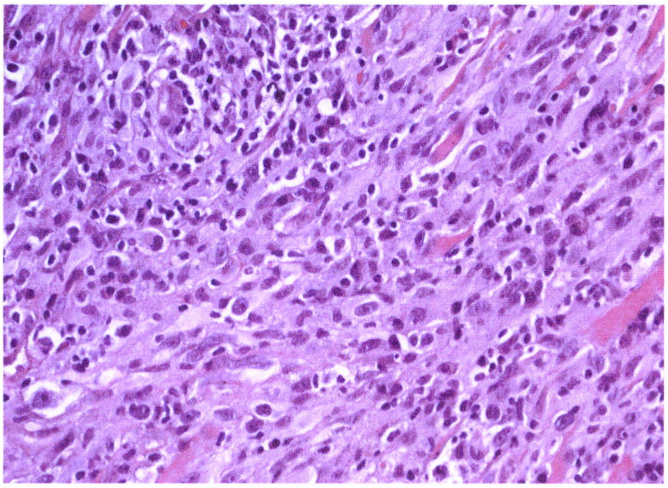

Fig. 10.1.7: Orbital malignant fibrous histiocytoma showing proliferation of cells with high degree of pleomorphism with a swirling arrangement in a fine collagen matrix (Original magnification × 200; H and E).

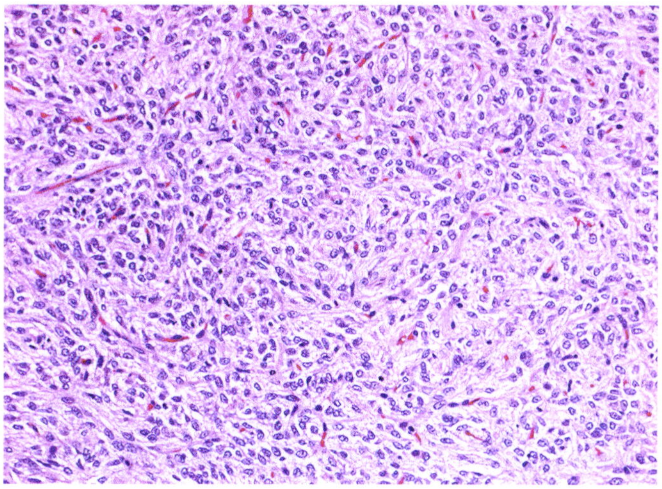

Fig. 10.1.8: Hypercellular area in solitary fibrous tumor of the orbit (Original magnification × 200; H and E).

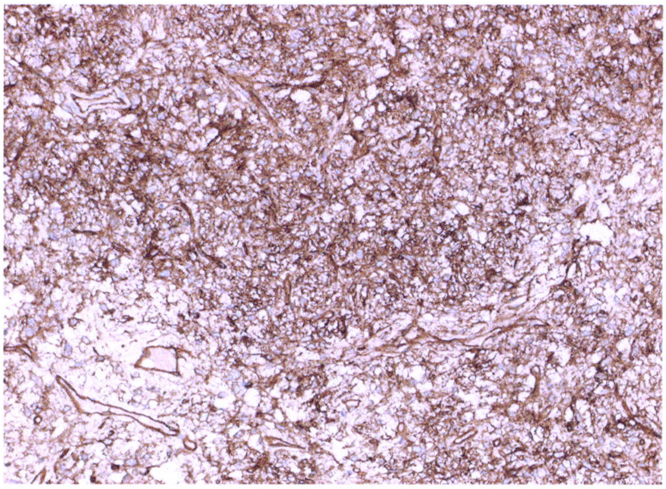

Fig. 10.1.9: Tumor cells in solitary fibrous tumor of the orbit showing cytoplasmic reactivity to CD34 (Original magnification × 200; CD34).

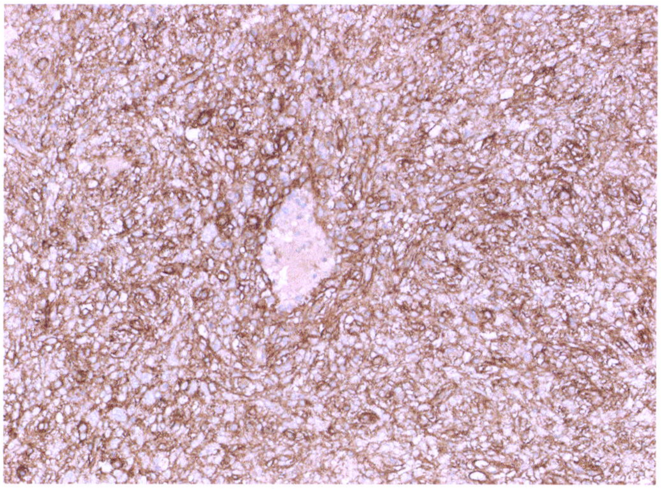

Fig. 10.1.10: Solitary fibrous tumor cells expressing CD99 (Original magnification × 200; CD99).

Solitary Fibrous Tumor

Solitary fibrous tumor (SFT) is a rare spindle cell tumor that is considered mesenchymal in origin and was originally described in the pleura and the peritoneum. It has been reported in 6% of head and neck lesions including the orbit.[18,19] The older terminology for this neoplasm was hemangiopericytoma. Histopathologically, the tumor consists of spindle cells with eosinophilic cytoplasm and indistinct cell borders separated by collagen fibers that are variable in thickness showing hypercellular and hypocellular areas (Fig. 10.1.8).[18,20-22] Immunohistochemical staining is helpful in confirming SFT tumors since they all express CD34 (Fig. 10.1.9), CD99 (Fig. 10.1.10), and STAT6 (nuclear reactivity).[23]

Neural Tumors

Schwannoma is a slowly progressing benign peripheral nerve sheath tumor originating from Schwann cells. Schwannomas are rare in the orbit, accounting for 1–6.5% of all orbital tumors.[24-26] They are usually solitary, have well-defined margins, and arise in relation to orbital sensory nerves, most frequently the supraorbital and supratrochlear nerves, but a lesion originating from the superior oblique muscle has been reported.[26,27]

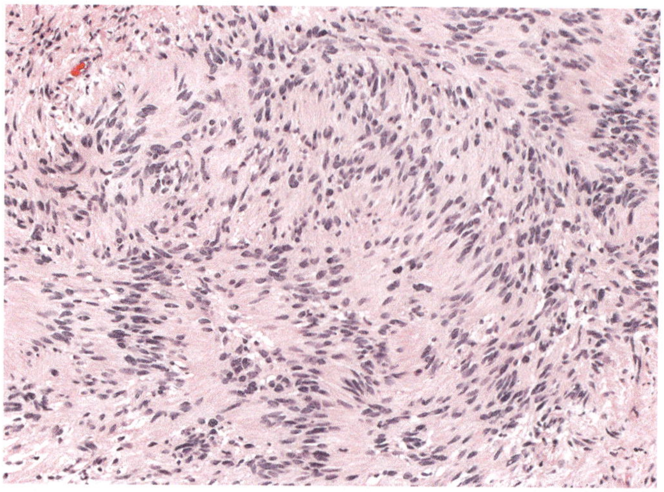

Fig. 10.1.11: Orbital schwannoma (Antoni Type A pattern) with proliferating spindle cells (Original magnification × 200; H and E).

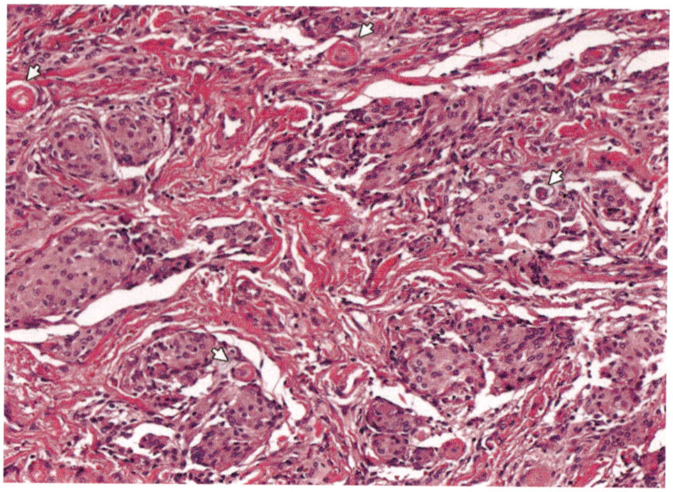

Fig. 10.1.12: Orbital meningioma with typical round structures representing psammoma bodies (arrowheads) (Original magnification × 200; H and E).

Clinically, orbital schwannoma can be asymptomatic (if small) or present with painless ocular proptosis.[25,26] Grossly, the tumor is encapsulated with a smooth outer surface, homogeneous grayish cut surface, often showing hemorrhage and/or cystic spaces. Histopathologically, these tumors show two patterns of cellular growth—Antoni A (consisting of closely packed spindle-shaped cells forming a pattern known as Verocay bodies, which are hyalinized acellular areas outlined by opposing rows of parallel nuclei), and Antoni B cells (characterized by distinct cytoplasmic margins and a myxoid matrix) (Fig. 10.1.11).[25,26] Immunohistochemical staining confirms the diagnosis by expression of calretinin and S100 protein in the tumor cells. Factor XIIIa, neurofilament, and CD56 can also aid in the diagnosis of these tumors.[28] CT scans may show variable hypodense to hyperdense appearance with diverse contrast enhancement owing to the mixed histological patterns.[25,29]

Meningioma

Other neurogenic orbital tumors include meningioma and optic nerve glioma. The meningioma may arise from intracranial cavity or the optic nerve sheath, where they might be associated with neurofibromatosis type-2 in children.[30] Optic nerve sheath meningiomas account for 1.7% of all orbital tumors and less than 2% are meningiomas.[31-33] Histopathologically, meningioma consists of proliferating meningothelial cells with a whorly configuration and possible presence of typical "psammoma bodies" that are formed of degenerating cells and may become calcified (Fig. 10.1.12). Optic nerve sheath meningioma morphologically shows four subgroups of growth patterns—(1) tubular, (2) globular, (3) fusiform, and (4) focal.[30] The growth patterns result in either thickening of the optic nerve sheaths without fusiform enlargement as seen in optic nerve gliomas. The compression of the nerve may cause disk edema, optic nerve atrophy, and appearance of optociliary shunts on the optic nerve head. Furthermore, optic nerve sheath meningioma can be infiltrative into the orbit and the peripapillary choroid. Calcification was seen in 31% of optic nerve sheath meningioma cases in a large series in Canada and was associated with slower rate of tumor growth.[34] The calcification in the meninges is responsible for the classic "tram track" appearance seen on computed axial tomography. It has been observed that using Ki-67 index as an additional marker along with WHO grading is valuable in predicting, meningioma behavior, especially in histologically borderline lesions.[33]

Optic Nerve Gliomas

Optic nerve glioma or pilocytic astrocytoma occurs mainly (75%) in children younger than 10 years and they are mostly isolated; however, when they are multifocal, they can be associated with neurofibromatosis type-1.[35] Expansion of the postlaminar optic nerve due to astrocytic proliferation and matrix results in fusiform/sausage-shaped enlargement of the orbital segment of the optic nerve. Axonal degeneration that accompanies tumor proliferation leads to optic nerve atrophy. Incisional biopsy is rarely needed for diagnosis, especially if vision is to be preserved.[36] Histopathologically, the tumor is composed of proliferating pilocytic astrocytes (Fig. 10.1.13). There has been a recent report of primary

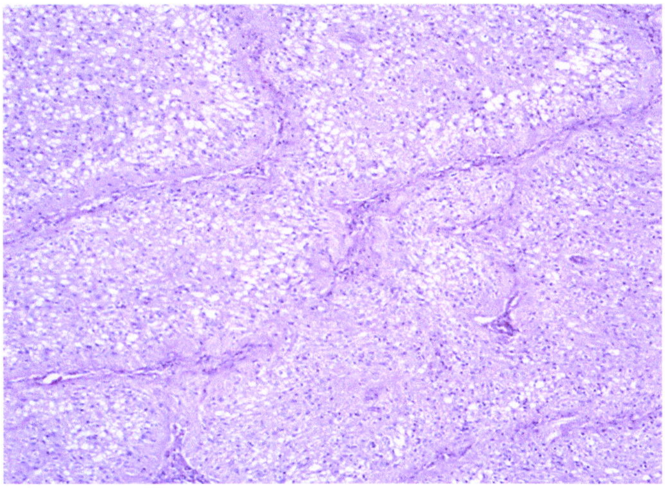

Fig. 10.1.13: A thickened optic nerve due to the proliferation of astrocytes (Original magnification × 200; H and E)
Source: Dr Charles Eberhart.

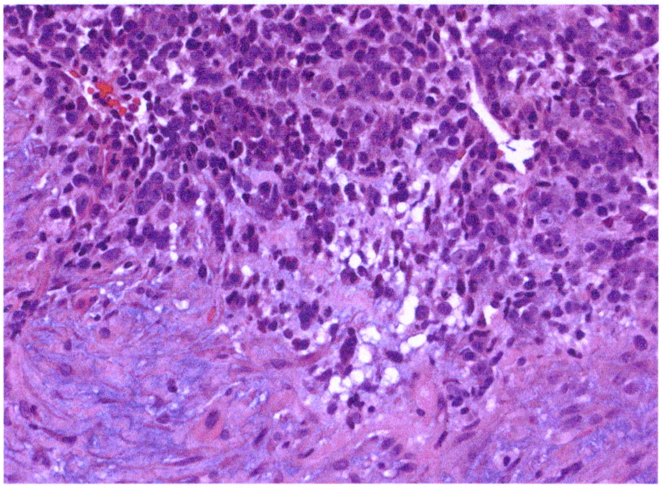

Fig. 10.1.14: Mesenchymal chondrosarcoma showing mesenchymal cells and adjacent immature cartilage (Original magnification × 400; H and E).

orbital pilocytic astrocytoma with typical histopathological features that was separate from the optic nerve and globe.[37] Mutations in the *NF1* gene as well as *BRAF* and *MAPK* mutations have been described in optic nerve glioma. Reports of the latter have opened up possible new therapies for treating this tumor.[38]

Vascular Tumors

Vascular tumors of the orbit are generally benign. These include cavernous hemangiomas, lymphangiomas, and capillary hemangiomas. These benign entities are not discussed in this Chapter. Reviews on the subject of vascular tumors are available in these comprehensive references.[39,40]

Rare Soft Tissue Tumors

Extraskeletal mesenchymal chondrosarcoma can occur in the orbit, which is the third most common site following the meninges and lower extremities. The tumor is more common in females and affects patients in their second and third decades of life.[41,42] The tumor shows mesenchymal cells that may be undifferentiated, small round or spindle-shaped or might show atypical islands of well-differentiated hyaline cartilage, endochondral ossification with bone formation, and coarse calcification (Fig. 10.1.14).[41,42] IHC staining is helpful in cases where typical pathologic features are absent with these tumors showing expression of S100 protein in the cartilaginous area and CD99 and vimentin in the cellular component.[43]

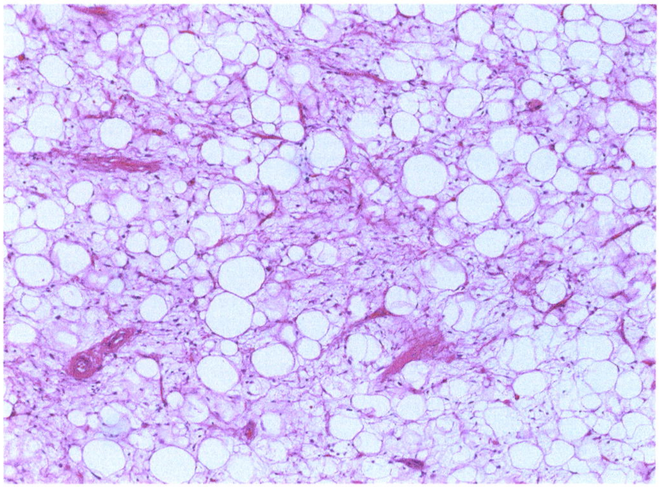

Fig. 10.1.15: A well-differentiated liposarcoma with fat cells of variable size (Original magnification × 100; H and E).

Liposarcoma is rare in the orbit and is believed to develop from mesenchymal cells rather than from a pre-existing lipoma. It is classified histopathologically into five subtypes—well-differentiated (Fig. 10.1.15), myxoid, round-cell, dedifferentiated, and pleomorphic. The myxoid type is the most common orbital liposarcoma subtype, and the presence of lipoblast is essential for making the diagnosis histopathologically.[44,45]

Alveolar soft part sarcoma is an uncommon malignant tumor of uncertain histogenesis that accounts for approximately 0.5–1% of all soft-tissue tumors. Histopathologically, the tumor shows epithelioid-looking cells separated by delicate fibrovascular septae with a

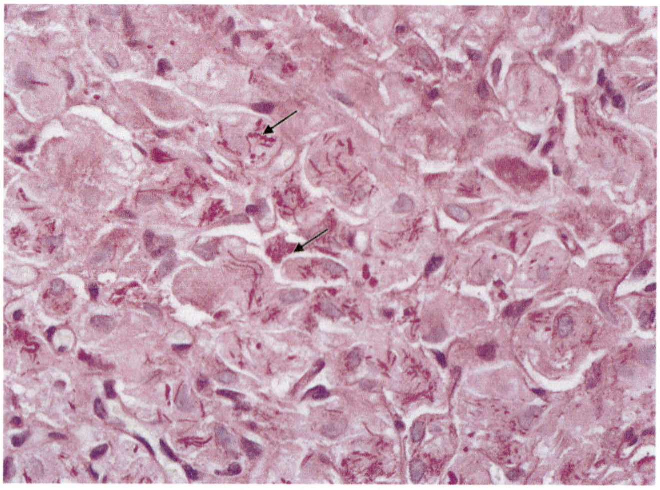

Fig. 10.1.16: Alveolar soft part sarcoma with intracellular periodic acid–Schiff (PAS)-positive, diastase-resistant crystalline structures (arrows). (Original magnification × 400; PAS).

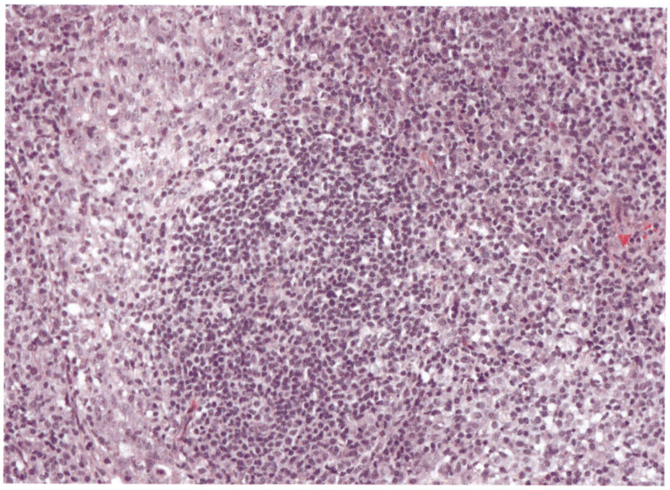

Fig. 10.1.17: Island of nasopharyngeal carcinoma with surrounding lymphocytic infiltrate (Original magnification × 200; H and E).

hemangiopericytoma-like pattern. Typically, intracellular periodic acid–Schiff (PAS)-positive, diastase-resistant crystalline structures are seen (Fig. 10.1.16). There are no specific IHC markers to confirm the diagnosis but electron microscopy shows diagnostic crystalline structures, lipid droplets, and paranuclear granules.[46-48]

Nasopharyngeal carcinoma is important in the differential diagnosis of secondary orbital neoplasms especially in Asians. It can reach the orbit by invading the inferior orbital fissure through the ethmoid or sphenoid sinus, as well as through the pterygopalatine fossa.[49-50] Three histopathological subtypes are identified: (1) keratinizing squamous cell carcinoma; (2) nonkeratinizing carcinoma (Figs. 10.1.17 and 10.1.18), which can be further divided into differentiated and undifferentiated (the most common); and basaloid squamous cell carcinoma. The undifferentiated NPC has a strong association with Epstein–Barr virus (EBV) in 100% of the cases.[50]

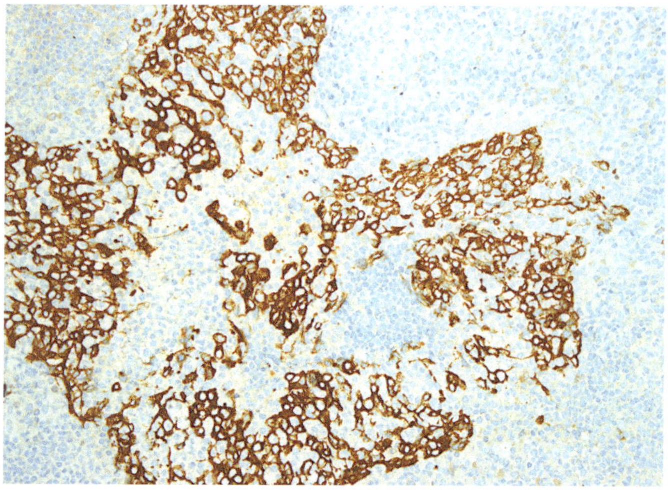

Fig. 10.1.18: The epithelial islands of the tumor in the same case of nasopharyngeal carcinoma are better identified with immunohistochemical stain (Original magnification × 200; cytokeratin).

Metastatic Tumors

Metastatic tumors to the orbit have different frequencies depending on the age, the most common being adenocarcinomas in adults and embryonal tumors/sarcomas (mainly neuroblastoma) in children. In children, neuroblastoma manifests as sudden-onset bilateral proptosis accompanied by periorbital ecchymosis.[51,52]

In adults, metastatic breast cancer is the most common in women (Figs. 10.1.19 and 10.1.20) often presenting with enophthalmos (retraction of the globe) and restriction of extraocular movements. The orbital biopsy in suspected metastatic carcinoma should be examined carefully using IHC staining for hormone receptors and Her-2 markers reactivity.[30] In men, the most common primary is in the the lungs. Other less common sites of primary tumors metastasizing to the orbit include—neuroendocrine tumor,[53] colorectal carcinoma,[54-56] and cutaneous melanoma.[57] Metastatic cutaneous melanoma to the orbit has been reported to involve the extraocular muscle in 35%, or intraconal soft tissue in 24% and presents as a painless circumscribed mass with overall survival of 25.1 months.[57] Orbital metastases of osteosarcoma is very rare.[58]

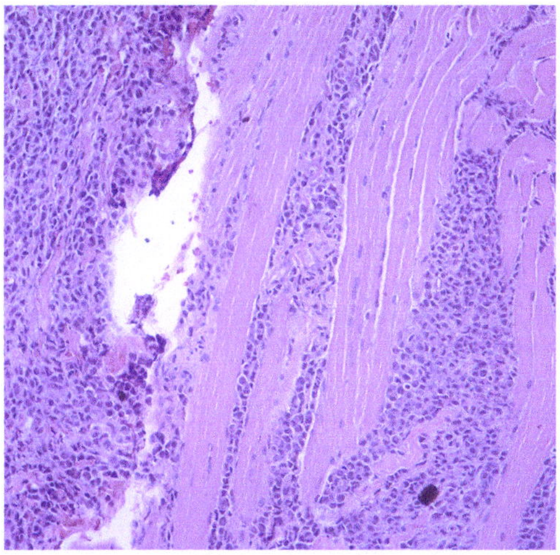

Fig. 10.1.19: Orbital metastatic breast carcinoma with Indian file configuration of the tumor cells. (Original magnification × 200; H and E).

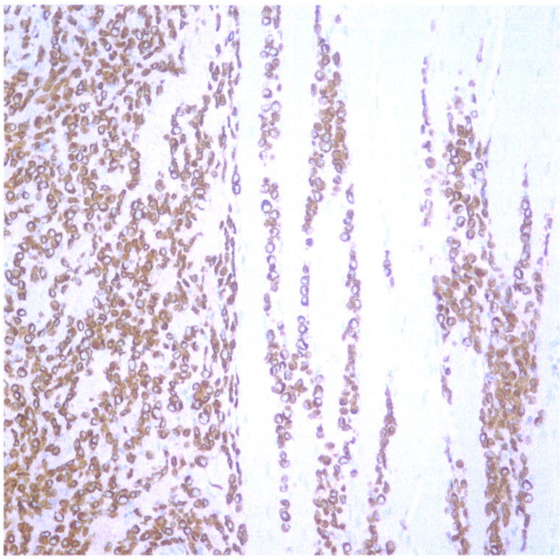

Fig. 10.1.20: The proliferating tumor cells in a case of orbital metastatic breast carcinoma showing expression of epithelial markers. (Original magnification × 200; cytokeratin 7).

REFERENCES

Section A

1. Saccani Jotti G, Bonadonna G. The pathologist and the clinical oncologist: a new effective partnership in assessing tumor prognosis. Eur J Cancer Clin Oncol. 1989;25(4): 585-98.
2. Khan AA, Sarwar S, Sadiq MA, et al. Analysis of orbital malignancies presenting in a tertiary care hospital in Pakistan. Pak J Med Sci. 2017;33(1):70-4.
3. Goldberg SH, Cantore WA. Tumors of the orbit. Curr Opin Ophthalmol. 1997;8(5):51-6.
4. Balabanov CH, Parashkevova B, Murgova S, et al. Tumors of the eye and adnexa. Bulgarian Review of Ophthalmology. 2005;49:12-20.
5. Khan AA, Sarwar S, Sadiq MA, et al. Analysis of 1246 cases of orbital lesions: a study of 17 years. Natural Science. 2015;7(6):324-37.
6. Parashkevova B, Balabanov C, Stateva D. Orbital tumors—clinical cases presentation. J IMAB Ann Proc Sci Paper. 2007;13(1):47-50.
7. Shinder R, Al-Zubidi N, Esmaeli B. Survey of orbital tumors at a comprehensive cancer center in the United States. Head Neck. 2011;33(5):610-4.
8. Bonavolontà G, Strianese D, Grassi P, et al. An analysis of 2,480 space-occupying lesions of the orbit from 1976 to 2011. Ophthal Plast Reconstr Surg. 2013;29(2):79-86.
9. Eldesouky MA, Elbakary MA, Sabik S, et al. Lacrimal fossa lesions: a review of 146 cases in Egypt. Clin Ophthalmol. 2014;8:1603-9.
10. Wang XN, Qian J, Yuan YF, et al. Space-occupying lesions of the lacrimal gland at one tertiary eye center in China: a retrospective clinical study of 95 patients. Int J Ophthalmol. 2012;5(2):208-11.
11. Teo L, Seah LL, Choo CT, et al. A survey of the histopathology of lacrimal gland lesions in a tertiary referral centre. Orbit. 2013;32(1):1-7.
12. Alkatan HM, Al-Harkan DH, Al-Mutlaq M, et al. Epithelial lacrimal gland tumors: a comprehensive clinicopathologic review of 26 lesions with radiologic correlation. Saudi J Ophthalmol. 2014;28(1):49-57.
13. Andreasen S, Esmaeli B, Holstein SL, et al. An update on tumors of the lacrimal gland. Asia Pac J Ophthalmol (Phila). 2017;6:159-72.
14. Chawla B, Kashyap S, Sen S, et al. Clinicopathologic review of epithelial tumors of the lacrimal gland. Ophthal Plast Reconstr Surg. 2013;29(6):440-5.
15. Von Holstein SL. Tumors of the lacrimal gland: epidemiological, clinical and genetic characteristics. Acta Ophthalmol. 2013;91(Thesis 6):1-28.
16. Lai T, Prabhakaran VC, Malhotra R, et al. Pleomorphic adenoma of the lacrimal gland: is there a role for biopsy? Eye (Lond). 2009;23(1):2-6.
17. Kaffenberger BH, Wakely PE, Mayerson JL.Local recurrence rate of fine-needle aspiration biopsy in primary high-grade sarcomas. J Surg Oncol. 2010;101:618-21.
18. Weis E, Rootman J, Joly TJ et al. Epithelial lacrimal gland tumors: pathologic classification and current understanding. Arch Ophthalmol. 2009;127(8):1016-28.
19. Grossniklaus HE, Specht CS, Allaire G, et al. Toxoplasma gondii retinochoroiditis and optic neuritis in acquired immune deficiency syndrome: report of a case. Ophthalmology. 1990;97(10):1342-6.
20. Rashid A, Jakobiec FA. Avoiding the major complication of ophthalmic pathology: misdiagnosis. A review of three common diagnostic challenges. Semin Ophthalmol. 2014;29(5-6):468-74.
21. Von Holstein SL, Coupland SE, Briscoe D, et al. Epithelial tumors of the lacrimal gland: a clinical, histopathological, surgical and oncological survey. Acta Ophthalmol. 2013;91:195-206.

22. McHugh JB, Visscher DW, Barnes EL. Update on selected salivary gland neoplasms. Arch Pathol Lab Med. 2009;133(11):1763-74.
23. Andreoli MT, Aakalu V, Setabutr P. Epidemiological trends in malignant lacrimal gland tumors. Otolaryngol Head Neck Surg. 2015;152(2):279-83.
24. Schwarcz RM, Coupland SE, Finger PT. Cancer of the orbit and adnexa. Am J Clin Oncol. 2013;36(2):197-205.

Section B

1. Heran MK, Rootman J, Sangha BS, et al. Dynamic arterial and Valsalva-augmented venous phase multidetector CT for orbital vascular lesions: a pictorial review. Ophthal Plast Reconstr Surg. 2014;30(2):180-5.
2. Gündüz K, Yanık Ö. Myths in the diagnosis and management of orbital tumors. Middle East Afr J Ophthalmol. 2015;22(4):415-20.
3. Wharam M, Beltangady M, Hays D. Localised rhabdomyosarcoma: an interim report of the Intergroup Rhabdomyosarcoma Study Committee. Ophthalmology. 1987;94:251-4.
4. Shields JA, Shields CL. Rhabdomyosarcoma: review for the ophthalmologist. Surv Ophthalmol. 2003;48:39-57.
5. Shields CL, Shields JA, Honavar SG, et al. Clinical spectrum of primary ophthalmic rhabdomyosarcoma. Ophthalmology. 2001;108(12):2284-92.
6. Newton WA Jr, Gehan EA, Webber BL. Classification of rhabdomyosarcoma and related sarcomas: pathologic aspects and proposals for a new classification—an Intergroup Rhabdomyosarcoma Study. Cancer. 1995;76:1073-85.
7. Rudzinski ER, Teot LA, Anderson JR, et al. Dense pattern of embryonal rhabdomyosarcoma, a lesion easily confused with alveolar rhabdomyosarcoma: a report from the Soft Tissue Sarcoma Committee of the Children's Oncology Group. 2013;140(1):82-90.
8. Dias P, Parham DM, David N, et al. Myogenic Regulatory Protein (MyoD1) expression in childhood solid tumors: diagnostic utility in rhabdomyosarcoma. Am J Path. 1990;137(6):1283-91.
9. Constine LS, Marcus RB Jr, Halperin EC. The future of therapy for childhood rhabdomyosarcoma: clues from molecular biology. Int J Radiat Oncol Biol Phys. 1995;32:1245-9.
10. Spahn B, Ducrey N, Nenadov-beck M. Orbital rhabdomyosarcoma: clinicopathologic correlation, management and follow-up in two newborns. A preliminary report. Orbit. 2001;20(2):149-56.
11. Doros L, Yang J, Dehner L, et al. DICER1 mutations in embryonal rhabdomyosarcomas from children with and without familial PPB-tumor predisposition syndrome. Pediatr Blood Cancer. 2012;59:558-60.
12. Crist WM, Garnsey L, Beltangady MS, et al. Prognosis in children with rhabdomyosarcoma: a report of the intergroup rhabdomyosarcoma studies I and II. Intergroup Rhabdomyosarcoma Committee. Clin Oncol. 1990;8:443-52.
13. Hassan WM, Alfaar AS, Bakry MS, et al. Orbital tumors in USA: difference in survival patterns. Cancer Epidemiol. 2014;38(5):515-22.
14. Amato MM, Esmaeli B, Shore JW. Orbital rhabdomyosarcoma metastatic to the contralateral orbit: a case report. Ophthalmology. 2002;109:753-6.
15. Elomrani F, Touri S, Ouziane I, et al. Orbital rhabdomyosarcoma with skin metastasis: a case report. BMC Res Notes. 2014;7:670.
16. Font RL, Hidayat AA. Fibrous histiocytoma of the orbit: a clinicopathologic study of 150 cases. Hum Pathol. 1982;13:199-209.
17. Lambade PN, Lambade D, Saha TK, et al. Malignant fibrous histiocytoma: an uncommon sarcoma with pathological fracture of mandible. J Maxillofac Oral Surg. 2015;14(Suppl 1):283-7.
18. Bauer JL, Miklos AZ, Thompson LDR. Parotid gland solitary fibrous tumor: a case report and clinicopathologic review of 22 cases from the literature. Head Neck Pathol. 2001;6: 21-31.
19. Gold JS, Antonescu CR, Hajdu C, et al. Clinicopathologic correlates of solitary fibrous tumors. Cancer. 2002;94(4): 1057-68.
20. Goldsmith JD, van de Rijn M, Syed N. Orbital hemangiopericytoma and solitary fibrous tumor: a morphologic continuum. Int J Surg Pathol. 2001;9(4): 295-302.
21. Seck SM, Agboton G, Gueye NN, et al. Epidemiological and clinical characteristics of primary ocular cancers in blacks: our experience with 111 cases. J Fr Ophtalmol. 2015;38(1):41-5.
22. Alkatan HM, Al Jarallah OJ, Fathaddin AA, et al. Solitary fibrous tumor of the lacrimal gland: a clinicopathological review of all reported cases in comparison to the salivary gland and a unique case report showing lacrimal gland entrapment mimicking pleomorphic adenoma. J Ponte. 2016;7(9):68.
23. Smith MH, Islam NM, Bhattacharyya I, et al. STAT6 reliably distinguishes solitary fibrous tumors from myofibromas. Head Neck Pathol. 2018;12(1):110-7.
24. Colapinto P, Sheth HG, Jain R, et al. Inferior oblique schwannoma: diagnosis and management. Orbit. 2007;26(4):287-9.
25. Pushker N, Khurana S, Kashyap S, et al. Orbital schwannoma: a clinicopathologic study. Int Ophthalmol. 2015;35:481-6.
26. Kim KS, Jung JW, Yoon KC, et al. Schwannoma of the orbit. Arch Craniofac Surg. 2015;16:67-72.
27. Li J, Lin J, Liu R, et al. Orbital schwannoma originating from the superior oblique muscle. J Craniofac Surg. 2015;26(2):559-60.
28. Miller RT. (2004). Immunohistochemistry in the Differential Diagnosis of Schwannoma and Neurofibroma. The focus—Immunohistochemistry. ProPath Oct 2004. [online] Available from: *http://www.ihcworld. com/_newsletter/2004/2004-10_NF_vs_schwannoma_v1.pdf.* [Accessed November, 2017].

29. Kantner BJ, Boldt B. Rare case of orbital schwannoma with intralesional haemorrhage and fluid-fluid levels. BMJ Case Rep. 2017.
30. Schwarz RM, Coupland SE, Finger PT. Cancer of the orbit and adnexa. Am J Clin Oncol. 2013;36(2):197-205.
31. Dutton JJ. Optic nerve sheath meningiomas. Surv Ophthalmol. 1992;37(03):167-83.
32. Castel A, Boschi A, Renard L, et al. Optic nerve sheath meningiomas: clinical features, functional prognosis and contro-versial treatment. Bull Soc Belge Ophtalmol. 2000;275:73-8.
33. Hunt PJ, DeMonte F, Tang RA, et al. Surgical resection of an optic nerve sheath meningioma: relevance of endoscopic endonasal approaches to the optic canal. J Neurol Surg Rep. 2017;78:e81-e85.
34. Saeed P, Rootman J, Nugent RA, et al. Optic nerve sheath meningiomas. Ophthalmology. 2003;110(10):2019-30.
35. Dutton JJ. Gliomas of the anterior visual pathway. Surv Ophthalmol. 1994;38:427-52.
36. Revere KE, Katowitz WR, Katowitz JA, et al. Childhood optic nerve glioma: vision loss due to biopsy. Ophthal Plast Reconstr Surg. 2017;33(3S Suppl 1):S107-9.
37. Mudhar HS, Nuruddin M, Roy S. Primary orbital cystic pilocytic astrocytoma. Ocul Oncol Pathol. 2016;2(4):280-4.
38. Rodriguez FJ, Ligon AH, Horkayne-Szakaly I, et al. BRAF duplications and MAPK pathway activation are frequent in gliomas of the optic nerveproper. J Neuropathol Exp Neurol. 2012;71:789-94.
39. Rootman J, Heran MKS, Graeb DA. Vascular malformations of the orbit: classification and the role of imaging in diagnosis and treatment strategies. Ophthal Plast Reconstr Surg. 2014;30(2):91-104.
40. Nassiri N, Rootman J, Rootman DB, et al. Orbital lymphaticovenous malformations: current and future treatments. Surv Ophthalmol. 2015;60(5):383-405.
41. Nakashima Y, Unni KK, Shives TC, et al. Mesenchymal chondrosarcoma of bone and soft tissue. A review of 111 cases. Cancer. 1986;57(12):2444-53.
42. Salvador AH, Beabout JW, DahlinDC. Mesenchymal chondrosarcoma observations on 30 new cases. Cancer. 1971;28:605-15.
43. Müller S, Söder S, Oliveira AM, et al. Type II collagen as specific marker for mesenchymal chondrosarcomas compared to other small cell sarcomas of the skeleton. Mod Pathol. 2005;18(8):1088-94.
44. Al-Qahtani AA, Al-Hussain H, Chaudhry I, et al. Primary orbital liposarcoma: histopathologic report of two cases. Middle East Afr J Ophthalmol. 2011;18(4):314-6.
45. Khurana S, Gupta AK, Sen S, et al. Primary liposarcoma of the orbit. Indian J Pathol Microbiol. 2014;57(4):617-9.
46. Alkatan H, Al-Shedoukhy AA, Chaudhry IA, et al. Orbital alveolar soft part sarcoma: Histopathologic report of two cases. Saudi J Ophthal. 2010;24:57-61.
47. Nava-Castañeda A, Tovilla-Canales JL, Zuazo F, et al. Alveolar so part sarcoma of the orbit. Nepal J Ophthalmol. 2017;9(17):70-3.
48. Mulay K, Ali MJ, Honavar SG, et al. Orbital alveolar soft-part sarcoma: clinico-pathological profiles, management and outcomes. J Can Res Therap. 2014;10(2):294-8.
49. Roh JL, Sung MW, Kim KH, et al. Nasopharyngeal carcinoma with skull base invasion: a necessity of staging subdivision. Am J Otolaryngol. 2004;25:26-32.
50. Kamio Y, Sakai N, Takahashi G, et al. Nasopharyngeal carcinoma presenting with rapidly progressive severe visual disturbance: a case report. J Med Case Rep. 2014;8:361.
51. Musarella MA, Chan HS, DeBoer G, et al. Ocular involvement in neuroblastoma: prognostic implications. Ophthalmology. 1984;91:936-40.
52. Shields JA, Shields CL, Scartozzi R. Survey of 1264 patients with orbital tumors and simulating lesions: the 2002 Montgomery Lecture, part 1. Ophthalmology. 2004;111: 997-1008.
53. Kamaleshwaran KK, Joseph J, Upadhya I, et al. Image findings of a rare case of neuroendocrine tumor metastatic to orbital extraocular muscle in gallium-68 DOTANOC positron emission tomography/computed tomography and therapy with lutetium-177 DOTATATE. Indian J Nucl Med. 2017;32(2):125-7.
54. Cherif E, Hassine LB, Azzabi S, et al. Orbital metastasis as the inaugural presentation of occult rectal cancer. BMJ Case Rep. 2014: bcr2013201428. Published online 2014 Jan 30. doi: 10.1136/bcr-2013-201428.
55. Chen S, Yii C, Chou J. Colon cancer with orbital metastasis. Clin Gastroenterol Hepatol. 2011;9(8):e76-e77.
56. Nabeel M, Farooqi R, Mohebtash M, et al. Rectal cancer in the eye: a case report of orbital metastasis. Cureus. 2017;9(8):e1589.
57. Greene DP, Shield DR, Shields CL, et al. Cutaneous melanoma metastatic to the orbit: review of 15 cases. Ophthal Plast Reconstr Surg. 2014;30:233-7.
58. Rajabi MT, Saeedi-Anari G, Ramezani F, et al. Metastatic tumors of the orbit and ocular adnexa. Curr Opin Ophthalmol. 2007;18:405-13.

SUGGESTED READING

1. Alkatan HM, Al-Falah MA, Elkhamary S, Al Shaikh O. “Prevalence of Orbital Vascular Lesions in Saudi Adults: A Tertiary Eye Hospital Experience.” Acta Bioethica June 2016; 22 (2): 1096-1105.
2. Belinsky I, Murchison AP, Evans JJ, et al. Spheno-Orbital Meningiomas: An Analysis Based on World Health Organization Classification and Ki-67 Proliferative Index. Ophthal Plast Reconstr Surg. 2017. doi: 10.1097/ IOP.0000000000000904. [Epub ahead of print].
3. Bhat V, Salins PC, Bhat V. Imaging Spectrum of Hemangioma and Vascular Malformations of the Head and Neck in Children and Adolescents. J Clin Imaging Sci. 2014; 4: 31. Published online 2014 Jun 24. doi: 10.4103/2156-7514.135179.
4. Das D, Deka P, Ramachandra V, et al. Profile of ocular and adnexal tumors at a tertiary institute of northeast India. Orbit. 2014;33(6):412-5.

5. Das JK, Tiwary BK, Paul SB, et al. Primary orbital rhabdomyosarcoma with skeletal muscle metastasis. Oman J Ophthalmol. 2010;3(2):91-3.
6. Domingo RE, Manganip LE, Castro RM. Tumors of the eye and ocular adnexa at the Philippine Eye Research Institute: a 10-year review. Clin Ophthalmol. 2015;9:1239-47.
7. Eivazi B, Werner JA. Extracranial vascular malformations (hemangiomas and vascular malformations) in children and adolescents - diagnosis, clinic, and therapy. GMS Curr Top Otorhinolaryngol Head Neck Surg. 2014; 13: Doc02. Published online 2014 Dec 1. doi: 10.3205/cto000105.
8. Kennedy A, Allan K, Rajak S. A primary squamous cell carcinoma of the orbit. CJO 2017. (In press).
9. Lee BB, Laredo J, Lee TS, Huh S, Neville R. Terminology and classification of congenital vascular malformations. Phlebology. 2007;22(6):249-252. doi: 10.1258/026835507782655236
10. Mendoza PR, Jakobiec FA, Krane JF. Immunohistochemical features of lacrimal gland epithelial tumors. Am J Ophthalmol. 2013;156(6):1147-58.e1.
11. Miyabe S, Okabe M, Nagatsuka H, et al. Prognostic significance of p27Kip1, Ki-67, and CRTC1-MAML2 fusion transcript in mucoepidermoid carcinoma: a molecular and clinicopathologic study of 101 cases. J Oral Maxillofac Surg. 2009;67:1432-41.
12. Woo KI, Yeom A, Esmaeli B. Management of Lacrimal Gland Carcinoma: Lessons From the Literature in the Past 40 Years. Ophthal Plast Reconstr Surg. 2016;32(1):1-10.

10.2 EXTERNAL TUMORS (EYELID)

Hind Alkatan

INTRODUCTION

The most common malignant eyelid tumors are sebaceous gland carcinoma in Asians and basal cell carcinoma (BCC) in Caucasians, while cutaneous squamous cell carcinoma and melanoma are relatively rare.

We will discuss the most common tumors in detail highlighting the impact of histopathology on patient care and proper management.

PERIOCULAR SEBACEOUS GLAND CARCINOMA

It accounts for 75% of all sebaceous gland carcinoma.[1,2] It can arise from the sebaceous glands of the eyelid skin, glands associated with the caruncle (in 12%), the glands of Zeiss, and the meibomian glands, which is the most common.[3] The frequency of sebaceous gland carcinoma is two to three times more in the upper eyelid than the lower eyelid, which is related to the greater number of meibomian glands in the upper eyelid.[4] The reported frequencies of sebaceous gland carcinoma vary in different populations, accounting for less than 1–5.5% of eyelid malignancies in Caucasians, while it has a higher frequency of 10.2–39% in Asians.[5-9]

Clinically, it can masquerade as a chalazion (in 42%), or chronic blepharoconjunctivitis (in 16%), or other tumors such as BCC.[3,10-12] Therefore, it is important to keep sebaceous gland carcinoma in the differential diagnosis of lesions in these locations (to avoid delay in the diagnosis and/or incomplete excision) and to perform histopathological examination on all lesions arising in these locations to rule out of sebaceous gland carcinoma.[3]

Complete surgical excision with frozen section control of the margins is recommended. In cases with extensive tumor, orbital exenteration, radiotherapy, and chemotherapy might be needed while wide surgical excision with 4 mm safe margin and radical neck dissection for lymph nodes is indicated for cases with regional metastases.[13]

Histopathologically, the tumor cells show distinct cell membranes, clear or vacuolated cytoplasm and vesicular nuclei with prominent nucleoli, arranged in sheets or lobules, and may show central comedo-necrosis in large tumor lobules (Fig. 10.2.1). Numerous mitotic figures and apoptotic cells are usually seen. Sebaceous gland carcinoma can be classified based on the degree by which neoplastic cells exhibit sebaceous differentiation into well, moderately, and poorly differentiated sebaceous gland carcinoma.[14] Oil red O or Sudan IV stains for intracytoplasmic lipid vacuoles staining can be performed on fresh or formalin-fixed tissues at the time of frozen sections, but this is less commonly used now because of emerging immunohistochemical (IHC) stains such as adipophilin, which stains residual lipid in the cytoplasmic granules of paraffin-embedded tissue (Fig. 10.2.2).[2]

Immunohistochemical staining is a challenge because of lack of specific markers, overlapping staining patterns, leading to conflicting conclusions.[15] Sebaceous gland carcinoma is known to be positive in most of the cases for CK5 and CK14 and negative for CK1, CK10, CK15, CK17, and CK20.[16] This, however, is not useful to differentiate between

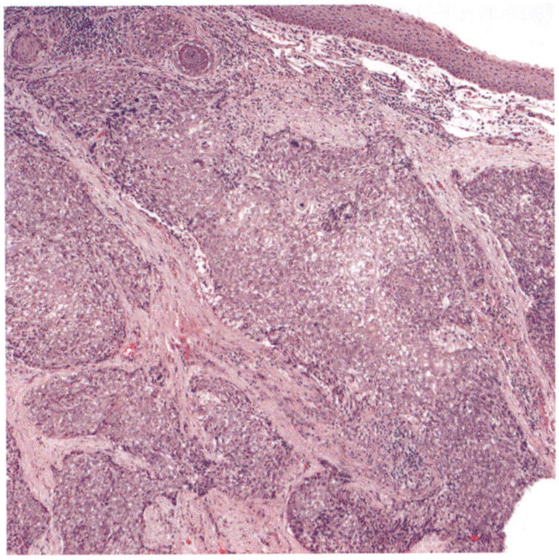

Fig. 10.2.1: Eyelid section showing malignant sebaceous gland proliferation (Original magnification × 100; H and E).

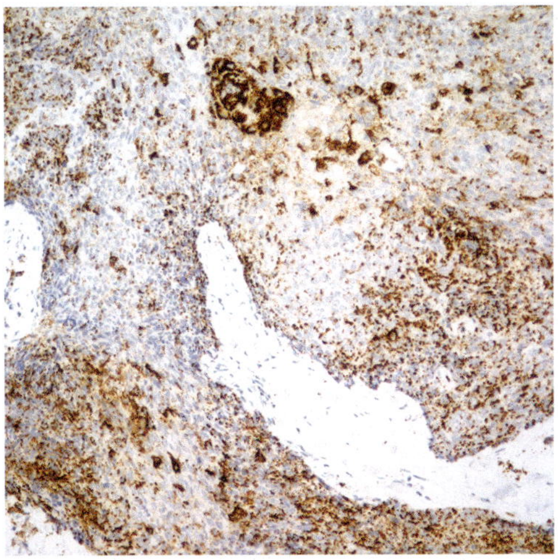

Fig. 10.2.2: A case of sebaceous gland carcinoma showing focal expression of adipophilin (Original magnification × 200; adipophilin).

sebaceous gland carcinoma and clear cell variants of BCC and squamous cell carcinoma leading to misdiagnosis, which can reach up to 77%.[17] Adipophilin is a highly sensitive marker of lipid droplets and is expressed in 45.5% up to 63% of the cases[3,15] It stains the well-differentiated tumor cells with strong vesicular pattern and is negative in basaloid cells. Therefore, it can differentiate between sebaceous gland carcinoma and BCC.[17] It is more challenging to differentiate between BCC with sebaceous differentiation and basaloid sebaceous gland carcinoma. In these cases, epithelial membrane antigen (EMA) [stem cells (SCs) are immune-reactive to EMA with restricted staining to the center of the nests, while BCC is negative] and Ber-EP4 (a monoclonal antibody used to detect EpCam, a transmembrane epithelial adhesion molecule, for which BCC is diffusely positive in contrast to sebaceous gland carcinoma and squamous cell carcinoma that are negative) are two helpful stains for diagnosis.[15,17,18] CK19 has been also reported to be useful in distinguishing these lesions, since BCC more often displaying strong positivity, whereas sebaceous lesions display only focal immunoreactivity.[17,19] The other more challenging scenario is differentiating between sebaceous gland carcinoma and epidermoid cell carcinoma, since both are stain positive with EMA and CK19.[17] Androgen hormones contribute to the activation of sebaceous glands, therefore immunostaining against the androgen receptor has been used especially in poorly differentiated sebaceous gland carcinoma that may not express EMA and other markers.[19] 35-beta-H11 is another useful marker, since it was found to be expressed in 81% of sebaceous gland carcinoma while negative in all cases of squamous cell carcinoma and basal cell epithelioma.[20] Perforin has been proposed as a new marker in the immunohistochemical staining panel for sebaceous gland carcinoma, as it was found to be strongly positive in 81% of sebaceous neoplasms including seven out of nine cases of sebaceous gland carcinoma. To distinguish benign from malignant sebaceous tumors, podoplanin (D2-40) is reported as a possible marker where basaloid cells in sebaceoma are immunopositive in contrast to sebaceous gland carcinoma (tend to be negative or focally positive).[21] Finally, Ki-67 is expressed in all eyelid malignant tumors; however, the highest Ki-67 labeling index was found in sebaceous gland carcinoma (mean 29.3%), followed by squamous cell carcinoma (mean 23.8%) and BCC (mean 4.2%).[15] Pagetoid/intraepithelial spread is a known feature in sebaceous gland carcinoma and occurs in approximately 39% of cases.[3] Pagetoid invasion is the spread of tumor cells into the conjunctival epithelium, often replacing the entire thickness of normal conjunctival epithelial cells. These cases, if biopsied, can be often misdiagnosed as squamous cell carcinoma in situ or Bowen's disease. Adipophilin is expressed within the infiltrative component and intraepithelial (pagetoid) component.[15,22] P53 is a tumor-suppressor gene. Immunohistochemical staining for nuclear p53 is increased in tumors with p53 mutations and it correlates with dysregulation of the signaling pathway. P53 staining was reported to be significantly associated with sebaceous gland carcinoma compared to benign sebaceous lesions in periocular tumors, and in another study its positivity was ranged from 22% to 68% in sebaceous gland carcinoma.[15,19] It is also reported to be less positive in squamous cell carcinoma and BCC (less than 20% of the cases).[17]

BASAL CELL CARCINOMA

Basal cell carcinoma accounts for 85–95% of all malignant eyelid epithelial tumors in non-Asian populations.[23,24] The most important risk factor for BCC is ultraviolet radiation, which explains the higher incidence in equatorial latitudes. The pathogenesis is related to the ultraviolet radiation damage of the DNA and its repair mechanism.

Clinical types of BCC include—nodular and noduloulcerative, pigmented, and infiltrative (morphea or sclerosing). The superficial spreading type of BCC is less common in the eyelid. BCC in the eyelid is usually painless and accompanied by loss of eyelashes and intraocular invasion is rare.[14]

For incisional biopsy preceding definitive surgery for BCC, it has been found that the accuracy was better for the diagnosis of aggressive subtypes of eyelid BCC using 2-mm punch biopsy in two sites rather than at one site.[25] Once the diagnosis of BCC is confirmed, it is essential to perform complete surgical excision with frozen section control of the margins. This is more important for recurrent BCC where frozen section-controlled excision is expected to lower the re-recurrence rate to approximately 5%.[26] For BCC in the periocular region, Mohs micrographic surgery is highly indicated where tissue blocks are 5–10 mm^2 and 2–4 mm thick are excised in a lamellar fashion until the surgical margins are free. Mohs micrographic surgery is considered by some as the treatment of choice for both primary and recurrent periocular BCC because of the increased recurrence rate.[27] However, the availability of this technique has been variable.[26] More extensive surgery using forehead skin flaps is used for treatment of large eyelid BCC.[28]

Histopathologically, previously reported data showed that inflammation in patients with BCC positively correlated with advanced age ($p < 0.01$), tumor diameter ($p < 0.05$), and the appearance of ulceration ($p < 0.001$).[29] The two main histopathological types of BCC are the solid type (corresponding to the clinical nodular type) and the morphea/sclerosing type (corresponding to the infiltrating type clinically) (Fig. 10.2.3).[30] The solid type is composed of epithelial lobules of cells with oval nuclei and scanty cytoplasm with prominent typical peripheral palisading of the nuclei and separation artifact because of the fixation and processing of the tumor. The larger solid nodules may show comedonecrosis (Fig. 10.2.4). The tumor proliferates in a desmoplastic stroma and may show several kinds of differentiation such as keratotic, cystic, pilar, or adenoid (Fig. 10.2.5). The sclerosing type shows elongated strands of basaloid cells embedded in a dense fibrous stroma. This type of BCC is aggressive, deeply infiltrative, and can be missed in frozen sections. The superficial type shows diffuse multicentric involvement of the epidermis with intervening areas that are free of tumor, which might also result in a false-negative frozen section margin. The differential diagnosis of BCC includes basosquamous carcinoma and adnexal tumors such as sebaceous carcinoma and trichoepithelioma.[14] In a histopathological study of 15 recurrent BCC lesions, the histopathological type did not change except in four cases where the recurrent tumor showed more invasive form. However, the values of Ki-67 index for primary BCC lesions ranged between 1% and 20%, and for relapsing lesions between 11% and 48%.[31] Prognostic factors include tumor location and size, histopathological type, and negative surgical margins of primary BCC

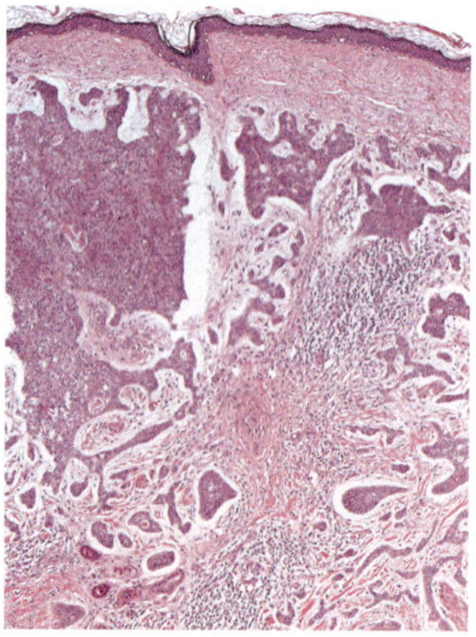

Fig. 10.2.3: Eyelid basal cell carcinoma showing combination of solid and sclerosing patterns of growth (Original magnification × 100; H and E).

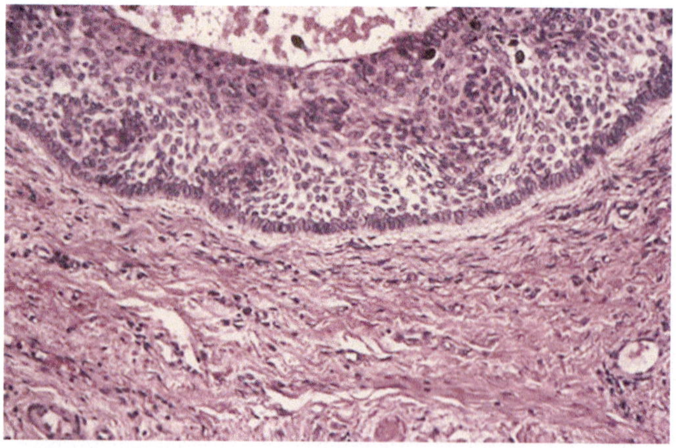

Fig. 10.2.4: Solid nodule of basal cell carcinoma showing peripheral palisading and central necrosis (Original magnification × 200; H and E).

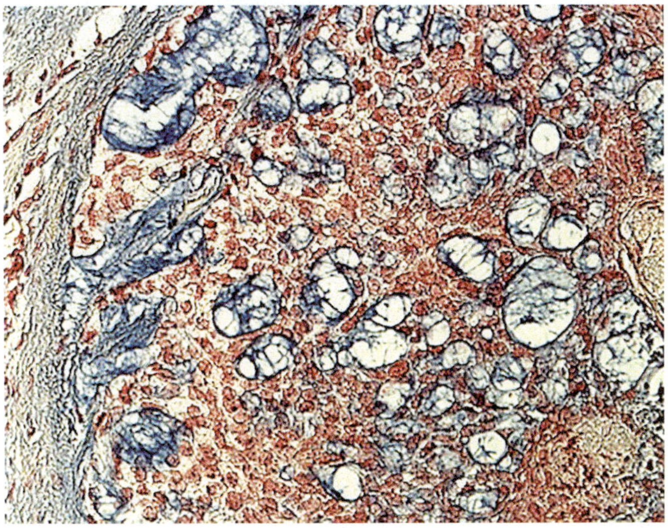

Fig. 10.2.5: Basal cell carcinoma with adenoid differentiation. Note alcian blue positive mucopolysaccharide in areas of glandular differentiation (Original magnification × 200; Alcian blue).

excision. Evaluation of proliferation index Ki-67 is essential for prognosis and choice of the appropriate treatment. It is particularly important in the histopathological evaluation particularly of recurrent BCC tumors.[31]

REFERENCES

1. Nelson BR, Hamlet KR, Gillard M, et al. Sebaceous carcinoma. J Am Acad Dermatol. 1995;33:1-15.
2. Shields JA, Demirci H, Marr BP, et al. Sebaceous carcinoma of the ocular region: a review. Surv Ophthalmol. 2005;50: 103-22.
3. Muqit MM, Foot B, Walters SJ, et al. Observational prospective cohort study of patients with newly-diagnosed ocular sebaceous carcinoma. Br J Ophthalmol. 2013;97:47-51.
4. Rao NA, Hidayat AA, McLean IW, et al. Sebaceous carcinomas of the ocular adnexa: a clinicopathologic study of 104 cases, with five-year follow-up data. Hum Pathol. 1982;13:113-22.
5. Cook BE Jr, Bartley GB. Epidemiologic characteristics and clinical course of patients with malignant eyelid tumors in an incidence cohort in Olmsted County. Minnesota Ophthalmol. 1999;106:746-50.
6. Kass LG, Hornblass A. Sebaceous carcinoma of the ocular adnexa. Surv Ophthalmol. 1989;33:477-90.
7. Lee SB, Saw SM, Au Eong KG, et al. Incidence of eyelid cancers in Singapore from 1968 to 1995. Br J Ophthalmol. 1999;83:595-7.
8. Kale SM, Patil SB, Khare N, et al. Clinicopathological analysis of eyelid malignancies—a review of 85 cases. Indian J Plast Surg. 2012;45:22-8.
9. Xu XL, Li B, Sun XL, et al. Eyelid neoplasmsin the Beijing Tongren eye centre between 1997 and 2006. Ophthalmic Surg Lasers Imaging. 2008;39:367-72.
10. Shet T, Kelkar G, Juvekar S, et al. Masquerade syndrome: sebaceous carcinoma presenting as an unknown primary with pagetoid spread to the nasal cavity. J Laryngol Otol. 2004;118(4):307-9.
11. Ozdal PC, Codère F, Callejo S, et al. Accuracy of the clinical diagnosis of chalazion. Eye (Lond). 2004;18(2):135-8.
12. Leibovitch I, Selva D, Huilgol S, et al. Intraepithelial sebaceous carcinoma of the eyelid misdiagnosed as Bowen's disease. J Cutan Pathol. 2006;33(4):303-8.
13. Zürchera M, Hintschichb CR, Garner A, et al. Sebaceous carcinoma of the eyelid: a clinicopathologic study. Br J Ophthalmol. 1998;82:1049-55.
14. Pe'er J. Pathology of eyelid tumors. Indian J Ophthalmol. 2016;64(3):177-90.
15. Mulay K, White VA, Shah SJ, et al. Sebaceous carcinoma: clinicopathologic features and diagnostic role of immunohistochemistry (including androgen receptor). Can J Ophthalmol. 2014;49:326-32.
16. Ansai S, Arase S, Kawana S, et al. Immunohistochemical findings of sebaceous carcinoma and sebaceoma: retrieval of cytokeratin expression by a panel of anti-cytokeratin monoclonal antibodies. J Dermatol. 2011;38:951-8.
17. Rashid A, Jakobiec FA. Avoiding the major complication of ophthalmic pathology: misdiagnosis. A review of three common diagnostic challenges. Semin Ophthalmol. 2014;29:46874.
18. Alhumaidi A. Practical immunohistochemistry of epithelial skin tumor. Indian J Dermatol Venereol Leprol. 2012;78(6):698-708.
19. Shalin SC, Sakharpe A, Lyle S, et al. p53 staining correlates with tumor type and location in sebaceous neoplasms. Am J Dermatopathol. 2012;34:129-35; quiz 136-8.
20. Murata T, Nakashima Y, Takeuchi M, et al. The diagnostic use of low molecular weight keratin expression in sebaceous carcinoma. Pathol Res Pract. 1993;189(8):888-93.
21. Yang HM, Cabral E, Dadras SS, et al. Immunohistochemical expression of D2-40 in benign and malignant sebaceous tumors and comparison to basal and squamous cell carcinomas. Am J Dermatopathol. 2008;30:549-54.
22. Muthusamy K, Halbert G, Roberts F. Immunohistochemical staining for adipophilin, perilipin and TIP47. J Clin Pathol. 2006;59:1166-70.
23. Font RL. Ophthalmic Pathology—An Atlas and Textbook, 3rd edition. Philadelphia: WB Saunders; 1996. pp. 2229-32.
24. Asproudis I, Sotiropoulos G, Gartzios C, et al. Eyelid Tumors at the University Eye Clinic of Ioannina, Greece: a 30-year retrospective study. Middle East Afr J Ophthalmol. 2015;22(2):230-2.
25. Rossato LA, Carneiro RC, Macedo EM, et al. Diagnosis of aggressive subtypes of eyelid basal cell carcinoma by 2-mm punch biopsy: prospective and comparative study. Rev Col Bras Cir. 2016;43(4):262-9.

26. şahan B, Çiftçi F, Özkan F, et al. The Importance of Frozen Section-Controlled Excision in Recurrent Basal Cell Carcinoma of the Eyelids. Turkish J Ophthalmol. 2016;46(6):277-81.
27. Sin CW, Barua A, Cook A. Recurrence rates of periocular basal cell carcinoma following Mohs micrographic surgery: a retrospective study. Int J Dermatol. 2016;55(9):1044-7.
28. Elshamma NA, Al Qabbani M, Alkatan HM, et al. "The use of forehead flaps in the management of large basal cell carcinomas of the medial canthus/medial Lower eyelid in Saudi patients". Saudi J Ophthalmol. 2013;27(3):223-6.
29. Tzoutzos K, Batistatou A, Kitsos G, Liasko R, et al. Retrospective clinicopathological study of 129 cancerous and 18 precancerous lesions of the eyelids in North-Western Greece. Int Ophthalmol. 2017;37:203-8.
30. Wu A, Sun MT, Huilgol SC, et al. Histological subtypes of periocular basal cell carcinoma. Clin Experiment Ophthalmol. 2014;42:603-7.
31. Iljin A, Zielin´ski T, Antoszewski B, et al. Clinicopathological analysis of recurrent basal cell carcinoma of the eyelid. Postepy Dermatol Alergol. 2016;33(1):42-6.

10.3 OCULAR SURFACE TUMORS

Hind Alkatan

INTRODUCTION

The conjunctiva is a mucous membrane that consists of nonkeratinized stratified squamous epithelium with goblet cells and an underlying stromal matrix (substantia propria). Melanocytes might be present at the epithelial/stromal conjunction.

The two most important malignant tumors discussed here are conjunctival squamous carcinoma and the conjunctival melanoma.

Conjunctival Squamous Cell Carcinoma

Conjunctival squamous cell carcinoma (SCC) is the most common nonmelanocytic malignant tumor of the conjunctiva. The incidence ranges from 0.02 to 3.5 per 100,000 per year.[1] This tumor is locally aggressive and can give rise to intraocular invasion in 2–15% of cases that result in enucleation, or even exenteration in a small proportion of cases, if associated with orbital invasion.[2,3] The tumor is typically seen in older individuals. If recurrent tumors are seen in a young individual, one should consider xeroderma pigmentosa as an underlying cause.

The spectrum of ocular surface squamous neoplasia includes conjunctival/corneal intraepithelial dysplasia, carcinoma in situ, and invasive SCC.[4]

Clinically, the appearance of conjunctival/corneal intraepithelial dysplasia and invasive SCC are almost identical. The tumor presents as a fleshy sessile, papillomatous, or plaque-like lesion in the interpalpebral conjunctiva adjacent to/or involving the limbus. The lesions have a gelatinous appearance or may have whitish surface (leukoplakia that likely represents hyperkeratosis or surface keratinization). Dilated conjunctival feeder blood vessels can be seen.[4]

The diagnosis of ocular surface squamous neoplasia by impression cytology is controversial and it depends on finding the typical cytological features that include pleomorphic cells with hyperchromatic nuclei, irregular nuclear outline, and prominent nucleoli.[5] Such features might be absent in the superficial layers of the affected conjunctiva. Interpretation of impression cytology should be made with caution since it is less sensitive in diagnosing SCC, and is of limited value in differentiating carcinoma-in-situ from infiltrating SCC. Therefore, it is strongly recommended that one performs an incisional biopsy in such cases or in hyperkeratotic lesions where impression cytology was negative.[6]

The histopathological examination (through an incisional or excisional biopsy) is the standard for ocular surface squamous neoplasia diagnosis and planning management. Mittal and colleagues have nicely demonstrated the technique of submitting with ocular surface squamous neoplasia samples for pathological examination. The excised lesion should be submitted on a filter paper aided by a diagram that describes the orientation of the specimen. The flattened conjunctiva with its mucosal surface facing up on the filter paper should be allowed to dry for approximately 2–3 minutes before being submitted in 10% buffered formalin. If margins of excision are submitted separately, proper labeling should indicate the location and orientation of the specimen as superior/inferior/medial, and/or lateral. Grossing the tumor specimen results in several samples, which should be submitted in separate cassettes.[4] Proper orientation and preventing curling of conjunctival tissue is critical for the pathologist to provide accurate interpretation on whether a tumor was excised with clear margins.

Histopathologically, the classification of dysplasia is based on the level of epithelial involvement and can be classifies into several grades—mild (abnormal transformation of epithelium in the lower one-third of the epithelium), moderate dysplasia (lower two-thirds). Loss of cellular polarity and/or maturation are important features of dysplasia. Carcinoma in situ indicates full thickness epithelial dysplasia with intact epithelial basement membrane (Fig. 10.3.1). Once the epithelial basement membrane is disrupted by tumor cells, the lesion is considered invasive. The invasion of tumor cells into the underlying stroma can be seen as invasion of malignant epithelial cells arranged in nodules, cords, or thin strands (Fig. 10.3.2).

Conjunctival SCC can show different degrees of differentiation depending on the amount of keratinization and preservation of the squamous morphology of the epithelial cells. Based on these features, conjunctival SCCs can be classified as well, moderately, and poorly differentiated tumors. Clear cells can be seen in SCC mimicking mucoepidermoid carcinoma or sebaceous carcinoma. Variants of SCC include mucoepidermoid carcinoma (Fig. 10.3.3) and spindle cell carcinoma (Fig. 10.3.4). Immunohistochemical stains such as cytokeratin (Fig. 10.3.5), adipophilin, p63, vimentin, and epithelial

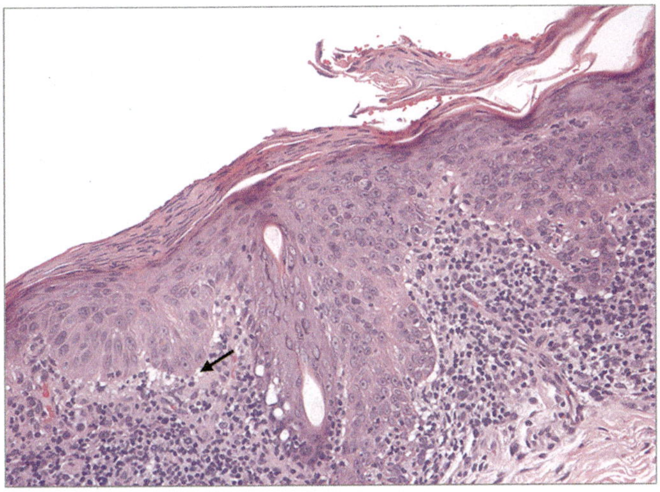

Fig. 10.3.1: Conjunctival squamous cell carcinoma in situ with an intact epithelial basement membrane (arrow). Note surface hyperkeratosis and inflammatory cell infiltrate in the underlying stroma (Original magnification × 200; H and E).

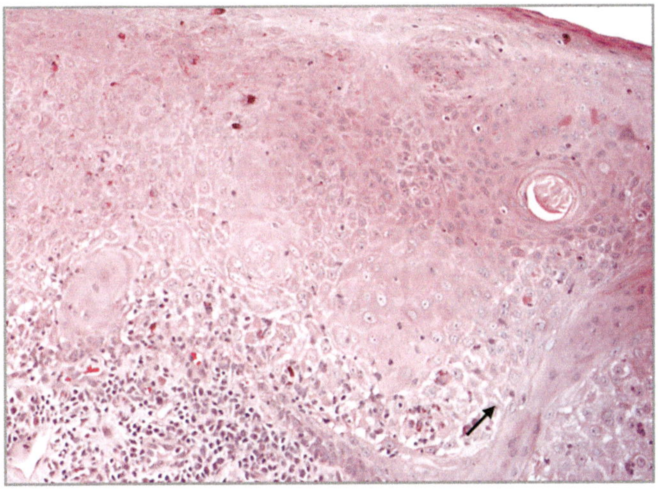

Fig. 10.3.2: Invasive squamous cell carcinoma arising from the limbus. Note invasion of malignant epithelial cells into the stroma (arrow) (Original magnification × 200; H and E).

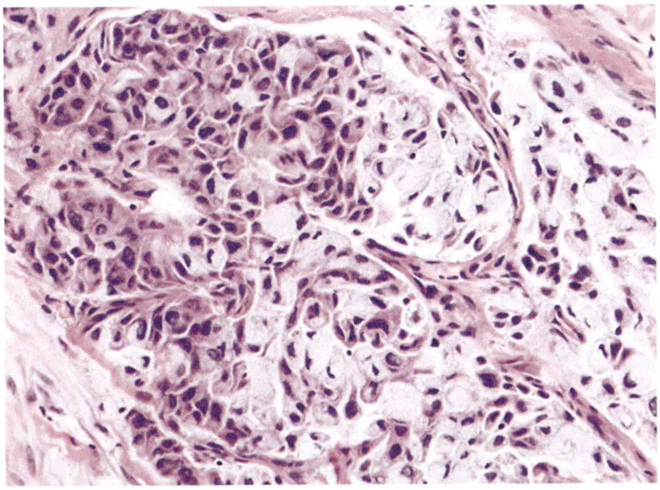

Fig. 10.3.3: Conjunctival mucoepidermoid carcinoma (Original magnification × 400; H and E).

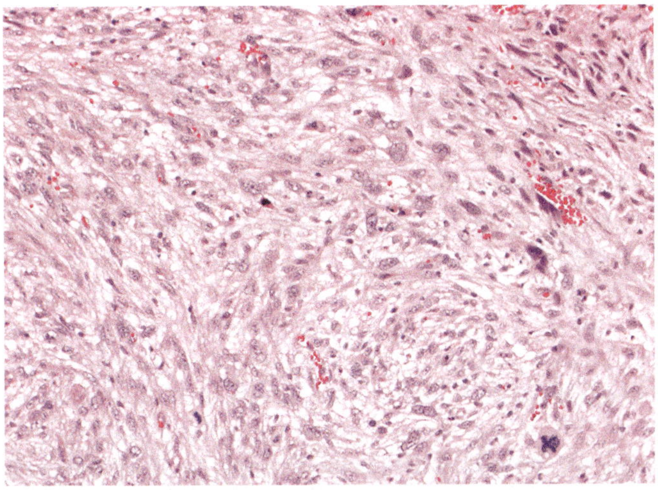

Fig. 10.3.4: Conjunctival spindle cell carcinoma with proliferating pleomorphic spindle-shaped cells (Original magnification × 200; H and E).

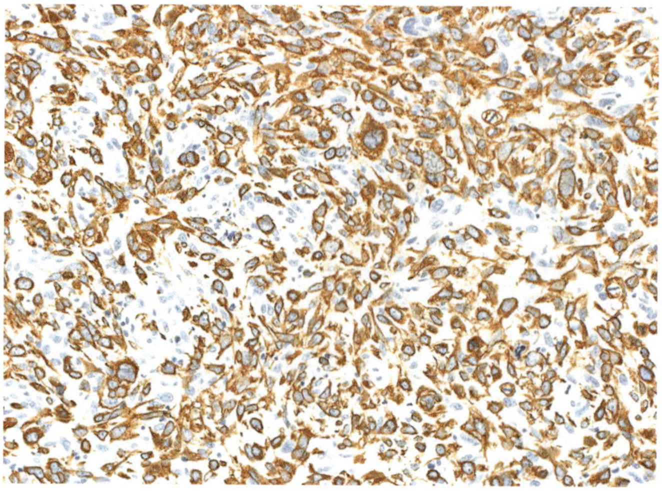

Fig. 10.3.5: Conjunctival spindle cell carcinoma showing squamous marker expression by the tumor cells (Original magnification × 200; cytokeratin).

membrane antigen (EMA) might be helpful for confirming the diagnosis, especially in poorly differentiated tumors.

Recurrence of ocular surface squamous neoplasia was previously common with significantly increased risk in the elderly, lesions with large diameter, high-Ki-67 proliferation index and positive surgical margins.[3] However, with modern effective therapeutic modalities, the overall prognosis is good, with local recurrence rate of 5% and regional lymph node metastasis of less than 2%.[4]

Regarding molecular genetic studies, variation on chromosome 8 with 8p11.22 amplification has been found in 75% of ocular surface squamous carcinomas. This region is known to contain genes that code for ADAM proteins, one of which is involved in oral SCC. Collagen type I alpha-1(*COL1A1*) which is known to be induced in oral SCC was also upregulated in ocular cases.[7,8]

Conjunctival Melanoma

Conjunctival melanoma is a uncommon conjunctival neoplasm with a higher incidence in Caucasians. Conjunctival melanomas can arise from a pre-existing nevus, primary acquired melanosis, or de novo. The histopathological classification and staging of conjunctival pigmented lesions including melanoma differ from that arising in the uveal tissue. A histological scoring for conjunctival melanocytic intraepithelial neoplasia has been advocated to replace the known grading of primary acquired melanosis (according to variable atypia). This suggested change aims at better therapeutic and prognostic correlation with histology.[9]

Clinically, conjunctival melanoma is suspected when there are alarming signs in relation to a pre-existing pigmented lesion. These signs include noticeable change in the size or color of a pre-existing nevus or primary acquired melanosis especially at the limbus, fornices or palpebral conjunctiva.[10]

Histopathologically, the lesions show proliferation of atypical melanocytes with abundant cytoplasm with granular pigment, prominent nucleoli, and atypical mitotic figures infiltrating the underlying substantia propria and the overlying epithelium (Figs. 10.3.6A and B). Lesions that arise from primary acquired melanosis can, in the early stages, be confined to the conjunctival epithelium (melanoma in situ), in which the tumor demonstrates radial spread similar to that seen in melanomas of the skin. Submission of biopsy specimen should follow guidelines described in the section on conjunctival SCCs. Additionally, as recommended by some ocular oncologists, care must be taken not to handle the main lesion with surgical instruments, so as to prevent inadvertent tumor cell seeding into the area of excision.

The pathologist should submit the entire surgical specimen for processing and note the presence of ulceration (absent epithelium), tumor thickness, predominant histological cell type (epithelioid or spindle), vertical growth phase, tumor infiltrating lymphocytes, microscopic satellitosis (discrete tumor nests that are separated from the main tumor mass), invasion (vascular or perineural), and most importantly the mitotic rate or KI-67 index.[11] Tumor location (bulbar vs nonbulbar) was not significantly correlated with regional lymph node metastasis or mortality in some reports with contradictory result in others. This inconsistency might be explained by the heterogeneity of the designations of the conjunctival melanoma anatomic sites.[11] Certain histological features correlate with worse disease-specific survival—tumor thickness more than 2 mm, mitotic figure count more than 1/mm^2, lymphovascular invasion, predominantly epithelioid histology in addition to histological evidence of ulceration, and microsatellitosis.[11] Using multivariate analysis, poor outcome was confirmed in patients with extrabulbar location of conjunctival melanoma.[10]

Immunohistochemistry stains that aid in the diagnosis of conjunctival melanoma include S-100 protein and the melanocytic markers HMB-45 and Melan-A (MART1) as well as the cell proliferative marker Ki-67. Immunohistochemistry labeling of HMB-45 and Ki-67 is increased in conjunctival melanomas compared to primary acquired melanosis or conjunctival nevi.[12]

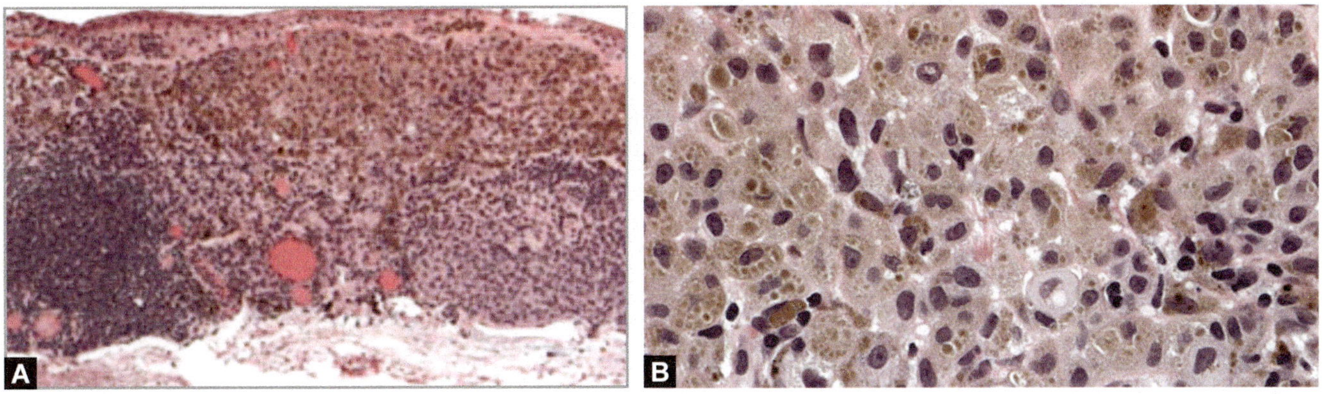

Figs. 10.3.6A and B: Conjunctival melanoma.

BRAF mutations are the predominant mutation described in conjunctival melanoma arising in the bulbar or caruncular location. *BRAF* mutation is also frequent in melanomas arising from a pre-existing nevus. Furthermore, conjunctival melanomas that harbor *BRAF* mutations might be associated with a higher chance of distant metastasis. The similarity between conjunctival melanoma and cutaneous melanoma in regards to the significance of *BRAF* mutations in relation to the clinical features has been also concluded.[10,13]

Beta-catenin expression in cutaneous melanoma has been found to be associated with more aggressive clinical disease. Recently, beta-catenin expression was investigated in conjunctival pigmented lesions, where it was found not to be preferentially expressed in benign conjunctival melanocytic lesions. This suggested that beta-catenin may play a different role in conjunctival atypia than what is known in cutaneous melanoma.[12]

Separate melanomas arising from the bulbar conjunctiva and eyelid skin have been reported in the same patient. These patients with multiple primary melanomas should be studied to determine whether possible low-penetrance susceptibility genes play a role in the pathogenesis of such lesions,[14] since identification of cellular pathways involved in conjunctival melanomas have identified new targets for possible intervention. The interaction of programmed cell death protein 1 (PD-1) and its ligand PD-L1 were recently investigated in conjunctival melanoma. PD-L1 expression was associated with distant metastases and a poorer conjunctival melanoma-related survival. Based on this finding, it was suggested that inhibitors of the PD-1/PD-L1 axis be evaluated as a potential therapy for conjunctival melanoma.[15]

Management of conjunctival melanoma has improved with the advances in cryotherapy, radiotherapy, and chemotherapy with less frequent need for exenteration. However, systemic screening is still needed in high-risk patients.[9] Incisional biopsy and excision without adjuvant therapy were found to be associated with poor outcome.[10] Tumor/node/metastasis (TNM) staging of conjunctival melanoma has been evolving and will assist in better correlations between therapeutic options and prognosis.[9,16] Recurrence rates of conjunctival melanomas can reach up to 50% especially in cases that have the following risk factors—multifocal and/or nonlimbal location, positive surgical margins, and absence of adjunctive therapy.[9,10] The use of BRAF/MEK inhibitors for metastatic or nonsurgical conjunctival melanoma has the potential to improve survival.[17]

REFERENCES

1. Yang J, Foster CS. Squamous cell carcinoma of the conjunctiva. Int Ophthalmol Clin. 1997;37(4):73-85.
2. Tunc M, Char DH, Crawford B, et al. Intraepithelial and invasive squamous cell carcinoma of the conjunctiva: analysis of 60 cases. Br J Ophthalmol. 1999;83(1):98-103.
3. McKelvie PA, Daniell M, McNab A, et al. Squamous cell carcinoma of the conjunctiva: a series of 26 cases. Br J Ophthalmol. 2002;86(2):168-73.
4. Mittal R, Rath S, Vemuganti GK. Ocular surface squamous neoplasia—Review of etiopathogenesis and an update on clinico-pathological diagnosis. Saudi J Ophthalmol. 2013;27:177-86.
5. Tole DM, McKelvie PA, Daniell M. Reliability of impression cytology for the diagnosis of ocular surface squamous neoplasia employing the Biopore membrane. Br J Ophthalmol. 2001;85(2):154-8.

6. Nolan GR, Hirst LW, Wright RG, et al. Application of impression cytology to the diagnosis of conjunctival neoplasms. Diag Cytopathol. 1994;11:246-9.
7. Asnaghi L, Alkatan H, Mahale A, et al. Identification of Multiple DNA Copy Number Alterations Including Frequent 8p11.22 Amplification in Conjunctival Squamous Cell Carcinoma. Invest Ophthalmol Vis Sci. 2014;55(12):8604-13.
8. Mahale A, Alkatan H, Alwadani S, et al. Altered Gene expression in conjunctival squamous cell carcinoma. Mod Pathol. 2016;29(5):452-60.
9. Kenawy N, Lake SL, Coupland SE, et al. Conjunctival melanoma and melanocytic intra-epithelial neoplasia. Eye (Lond). 2013;27(2):142-52.
10. Larsen AC, Dahmcke CM, Dahl C, et al. A Retrospective review of conjunctival melanoma presentation, treatment, and outcome and an investigation of features associated with BRAF Mutations. JAMA Ophthalmol. 2015;133(11):1295-303.
11. Esmaeli B, Roberts D, Merrick Ross M, et al. Histologic features of conjunctival melanoma predictive of metastasis and death (An American Ophthalmological Thesis). Trans Am Ophthalmol Soc. 2012;110:64-73.
12. Reddy HS, Keene CD, Chang SH, et al. Immunohistochemical profiling including beta-catenin in conjunctival melanocytic lesions. Exp Mol Pathol. 2017;102(2):198-202.
13. Larsen AC, Dahl C, Dahmcke CM, et al. BRAF mutations in conjunctival melanoma: investigation of incidence, clinicopathological features, prognosis and paired premalignant lesions. Acta Ophthalmol. 2016;94(5):463-70.
14. Jacinto FA, Fisher GH, Espana EM, et al. Separate primary melanomas of the bulbar conjunctiva and eyelid skin: clinical implications of multiple primary melanomas. Ocul Oncol Pathol. 2016;2(4):226-9.
15. Cao J, Brouwer NJ, Richards KE, et al. PD-L1/PD-1 expression and tumor-infiltrating lymphocytes in conjunctival melanoma. Oncotarget. 2017;8(33):54722-34.
16. Damato B, Coupland SE. Conjunctival melanoma and melanosis: a reappraisal of terminology, classification and staging. Clin Exp Ophthalmol. 2008;36(8):786-95.
17. Mor JM, Heindl LM. Systemic BRAF/MEK inhibitors as a potential treatment option in metastatic conjunctival melanoma. Ocul Oncol Pathol. 2017;3(2):133-141.

10.4 INTRAOCULAR TUMORS

Deepak P Edward

RETINOBLASTOMA

Retinoblastoma is the most common intraocular childhood tumor. It is estimated that 7,202–8,102 cases of new retinoblastoma cases are seen yearly on a global basis.[1,2] Retinoblastomas are more commonly seen in Southeast Asia, Africa, and South America compared to North America and Europe. In contrast, uveal melanomas are more common in the Western world. The mean age of presentation of retinoblastoma is 18 months.[2] Bilateral retinoblastoma is detected earlier, and unilateral retinoblastomas might be detected slightly later in life. A detailed description of genetics and the clinical features of retinoblastoma are outside the scope of this chapter. However, a brief description of the genetics and clinical pathological correlations will be included as part of the pathological description in the following paragraphs.

Retinoblastomas arise from a mutation in the *RB1* gene that is located on the long arm of chromosome 13(q1–4). The tumor gene is a recessive oncogene, which implies that retinoblastoma develops when both copies of the *RB1* gene are inactivated or deleted. In order for retinoblastoma to develop, two hits are required to inactivate the gene (Knudson's hypothesis).[3-5] Most retinoblastomas are sporadic in nature and mutations in these tumors are somatic. This translates to gene mutations being only detected in the tumor tissue/retinal cells, with other tissues of the body being spared. On the other hand, in germline mutations, which constitute about 25% of all new tumors, one copy of the gene is dysfunctional in all cells and the second "hit" is in the somatic retinal cell. These tumors are usually inherited in an autosomal dominant fashion. About 2% tumors which are negative for *RB1* mutations are initiated by amplification of the MYCN oncogene.[6] Hypermethylation of *RB1* promoter (which silences gene expression) may be seen in 10–12% of tumors that are sporadic, unilateral retinoblastomas.[7] Other cases negative for conventional *RB1* mutations may have low-level mosaic pathogenic variants.[8]

Retinoblastoma carriers are heterozygous for *RB1* mutations. Patients with germline mutations are at risk of developing secondary tumors such as osteosarcoma, melanomas, or other malignant neoplasms at a rate of approximately 1% a year.[9-12]

Pathology

Most eyes harboring retinoblastomas in recent years are not enucleated following the advent of effective chemotherapy and radiotherapy. The most common indications for enucleation include larger retinoblastomas, those that are resistant to adjuvant therapy and demonstrate recurrence, and tumors that have extended into the optic nerve or into the orbital tissues.

Tissue Handling

Following enucleation of an eye with retinoblastoma, many ocular oncologists will harvest fresh tissue from the tumor for genetic analysis. This is done by creating a trapdoor-like scleral incision using a 8-mm trephine or similar instrument in an area of transition between normal and tumor tissue (Fig. 10.4.1).[13] This procedure is preferably done in the operating room following which the globe is fixed in 10% neutral buffered formalin. Fixation for approximately 48 hours is recommended in such globes.

Retinoblastomas arise from the sensory retina, and their growth pattern often dictates the clinical appearance. Tumors that grow into the subretinal space will present with a retinal detachment (exophytic growth) (Fig. 10.4.2), and those that spread along the sensory retina or protrude as a mass into the vitreous (endophytic growth) appeared as a fluffy whitish mass in the vitreous cavity that seed the vitreous cavity (Fig. 10.4.3). In advanced cases, the tumor may fill the entire globe (Fig. 10.4.4). These presentations might result in an eye with a white pupil reflex or leukocoria. Tumors in younger children often affect the posterior pole and, because of sensory deprivation might present with

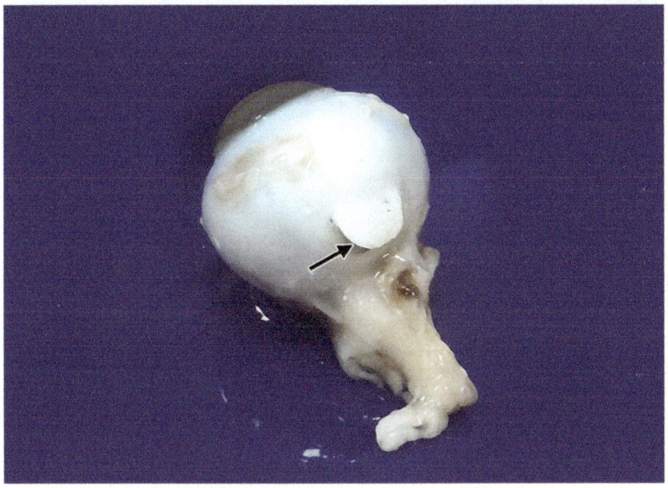

Fig. 10.4.1: Enucleated globe for retinoblastoma. Note scleral opening for harvesting fresh tissue for genetic studies (arrow).

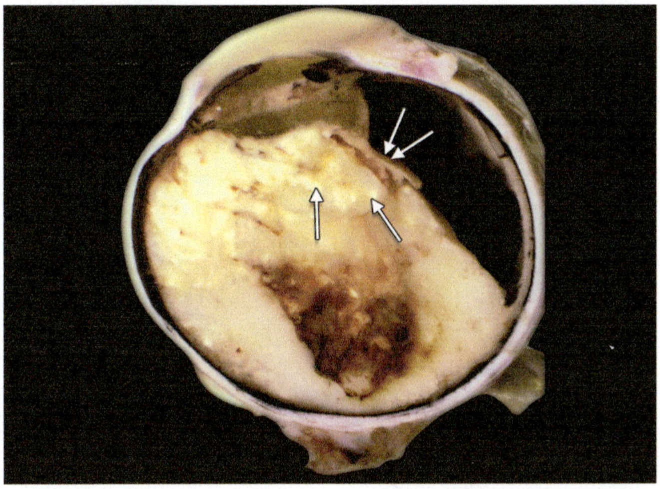

Fig. 10.4.2: Large whitish exophytic retinoblastoma mass with retinal detachment (double arrows). Areas of calcification are observed (arrows).

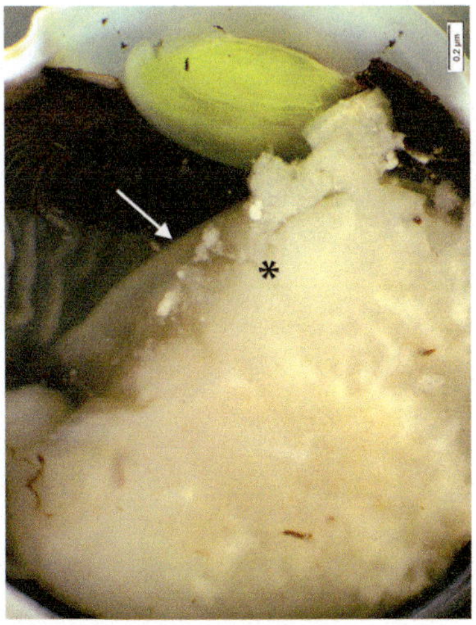

Fig. 10.4.3: Whitish fluffy endophytic retinoblastoma (*) with vitreous tumor seeds (arrow).

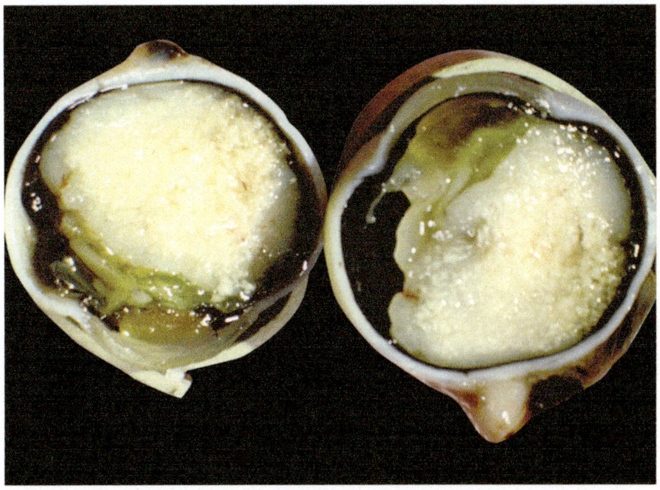

Fig. 10.4.4: Advanced retinoblastoma with tumor filling the entire vitreous cavity.

strabismus.[14,15] Rarely, tumors might undergo spontaneous massive necrosis and such eyes may present with phthisis bulbi.[16,17] Rare growth patterns of retinoblastoma, which are typically seen in older children or adults include diffuse infiltration of the retina without a definite mass with vitreous seeds[18-20] (Fig. 10.4.5), or very anteriorly located retinoblastoma there often presents with high-intraocular pressure, cells in the vitreous and anterior chamber and a tumor "pseudohypopyon"—a uveitis masquerade syndrome[21-24] (Fig. 10.4.6).

Tumors that demonstrate extraocular spread can present with proptosis.[22,25]

Microscopically, the tumor cells consist of small cells with hyperchromatic intensely basophilic nuclei with scant cytoplasm. Zones of ischemic necrosis that are eosinophilic often bridge zones of viable tumor (Fig. 10.4.7). Mitotic activity is variable. Calcification can be seen frequently on gross examination as whitish flecks (Fig. 10.4.4) and on microscopy as basophilic deposits among the tumor cells (Fig. 10.4.8).

The tumor cells might be undifferentiated or present with specific patterns of differentiation. Flexner-Wintersteiner rosettes that represents photoreceptor differentiation demonstrates a wreath of tumor cells lining a lumen that represents the subretinal space (Fig. 10.4.9). Flexner-Wintersteiner rosettes are typically seen in retinoblastomas, but may also be seen rarely in the teratoid variant of medulloepitheliomas.[26] Homer Wright rosettes

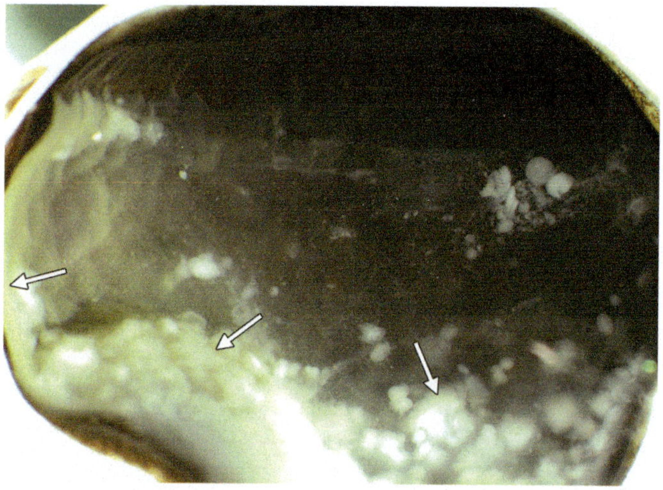

Fig. 10.4.5: Diffuse retinoblastoma affecting the posterior pole (long arrow) with extensive tumor vitreous seeding (small arrows).

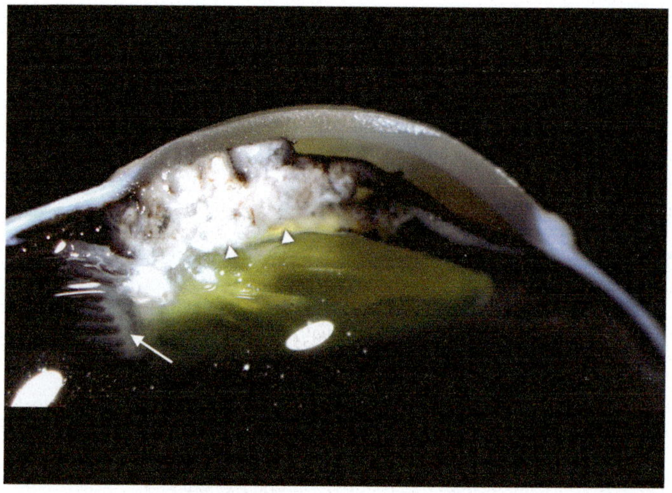

Fig. 10.4.6: Anterior retinoblastoma and an older child. The anterior chamber is filled with whitish tumor that demonstrates calcification, infiltrates the iris (arrowheads). Tumor cells are also seen covering the lens zonules (arrow).

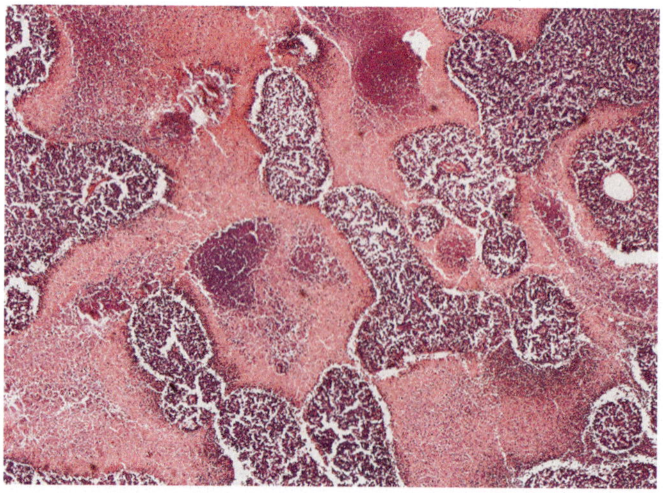

Fig. 10.4.7: Photomicrograph showing zones of small blue tumor cells with scant cytoplasm alternating with zones of necrosis.

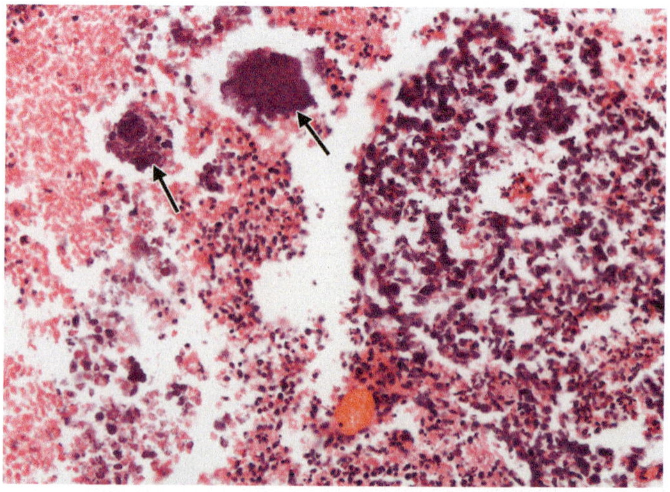

Fig. 10.4.8: Photomicrograph showing basophilic calcium deposits (arrows) around tumor cells and necrosis.

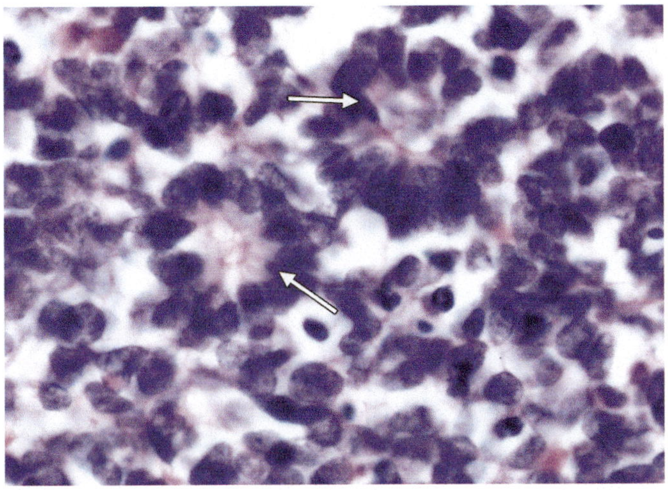

Fig. 10.4.9: Photomicrograph showing Flexner–Wintersteiner rosettes (arrows). Note the wreath of tumor cells lining a lumen. These represent photoreceptor differentiation.

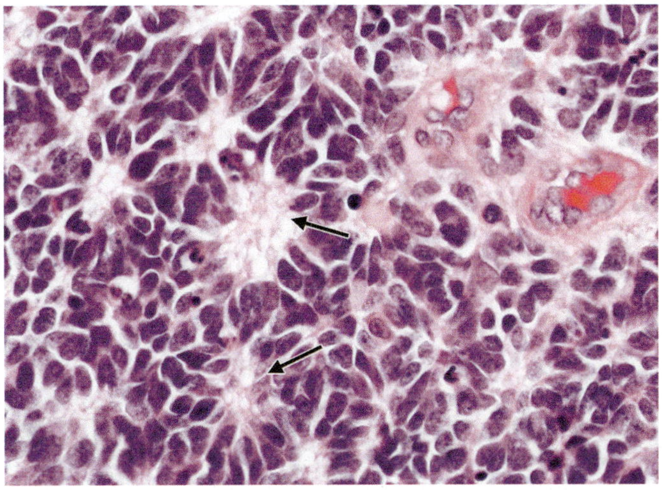

Fig. 10.4.10: Photomicrograph showing Homer Wright rosettes in retinoblastoma. Note the rosette consists of a ring of rumor cells surrounding a tangle of neural filamentous structures (arrows).

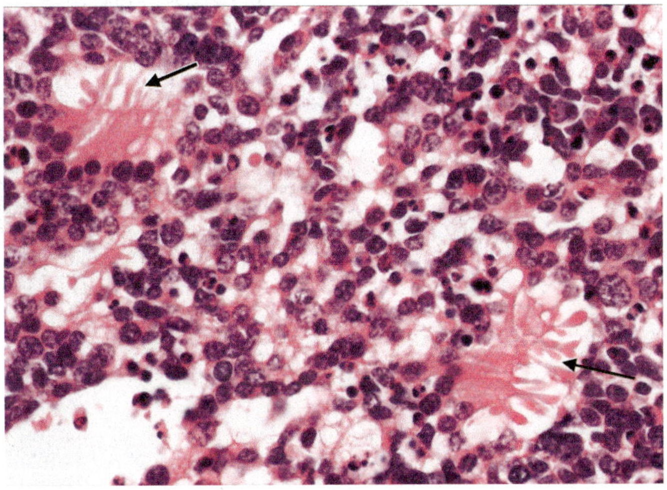

Fig. 10.4.11: Photomicrograph showing fleurettes (arrows). The eosinophilic bulbous/filamentous structures represent photoreceptor inner segments.

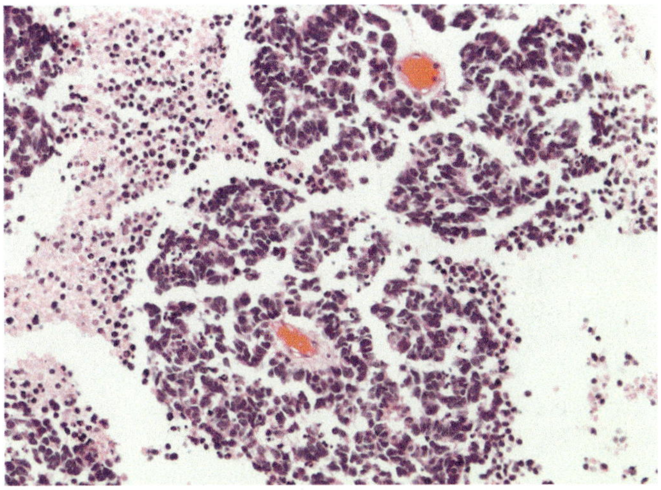

Fig. 10.4.12: Photomicrograph showing pseudorosettes. Layers of tumor cells arranged in a wreath-like fashion surround blood vessels.

represent more primitive neuroblastic differentiation of the tumor. This cell pattern is characterized by a ring of tumor cells without a distinct lumen surrounding a tangle of neural filamentous structures (Fig. 10.4.10). Flexner-Wintersteiner rosettes are more commonly seen in tumors that occur at a very young age, whereas tumors seen in older infants might harbor more poorly differentiated cells tumors that demonstrate cellular differentiation resembling photoreceptor cells are termed as fleurettes. Tumors mainly composed of fleurettes are called retinocytomas[27,28] (Fig. 10.4.11). Pseudorosettes are accumulation of layers of tumor cells around blood vessels (Fig. 10.4.12). In some tumors, basophilic material surrounds the tumor vasculature. The basophilic material represents DNA from the necrotic tumor cells (Fig. 10.4.13).

Pathological features of retinoblastoma that tend to increase the risk of metastatic disease are termed as "high-risk features" and often require chemotherapy or additional adjuvant therapy.[14,15,29-33] The following features are considered as high risk:

- Retinoblastoma has a predilection to spread via the optic nerve. Spread of tumor cells at the level of the lamina cribrosa increases the risk of the tumor cells (Fig. 10.4.14) coming in contact with the cerebrospinal

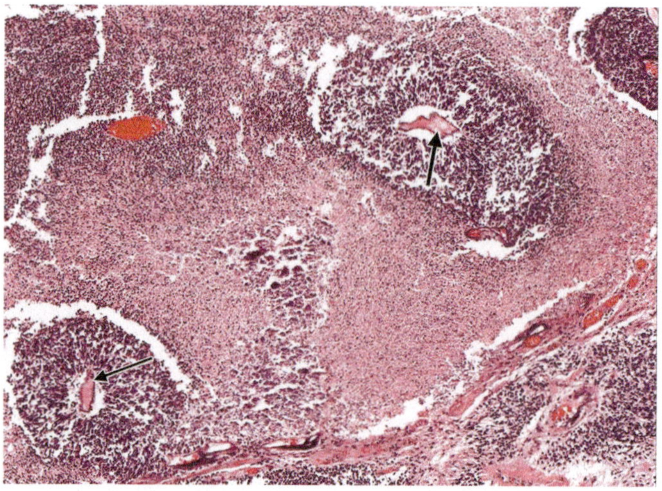

Fig. 10.4.13: Photomicrograph showing basophilic deposits in blood vessel wall (arrows) representing deoxyribonucleic acid (DNA) material from surrounding areas of tumor necrosis.

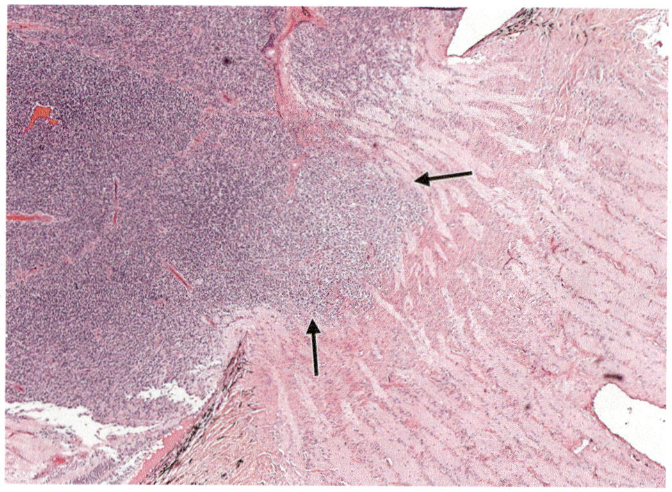

Fig. 10.4.14: Photomicrograph showing retinoblastoma tumor cells invading the lamina cribrosa (arrows).

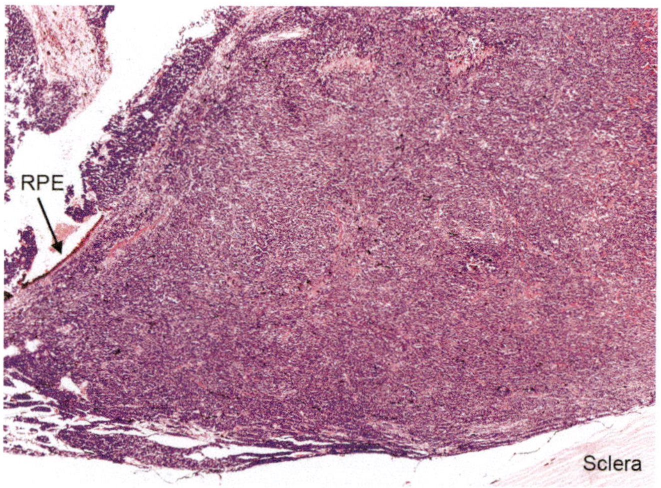

Fig. 10.4.15: Photomicrograph showing massive invasion of the choroid with retinoblastoma tumor cells.

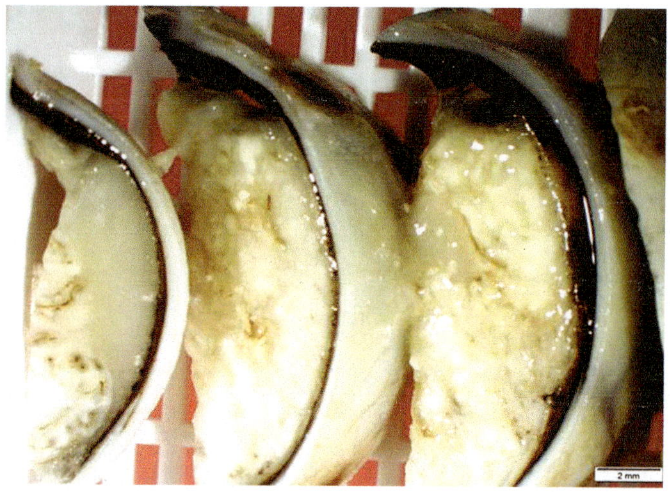

Fig. 10.4.16: Bread-loafing of calottes in retinoblastoma.

fluid, which circulates in the immediate vicinity of the lamina cribrosa. Spillage of tumor cells into the cerebrospinal fluid provides a direct channel for tumor metastasis into the brain. Furthermore, detection of tumor at the margin of optic nerve resection increases the chances of such a tumor spreading into the brain and surrounding structures and is considered a high-risk feature.

- The tumor cells may break through Bruch's membrane and infiltrate the vascular choroid. Massive infiltration of the choroid (greater than 3 mm in thickness) constitutes a high-risk feature (Fig. 10.4.15). In order to detect choroidal infiltration pathologically, the two caps of the enucleated globe that remain after a pupillary-optic section is obtained, is bread-loafed and submitted in its entirety for processing (Fig. 10.4.16).
- Tumor cells might access the scleral canals and spread into the orbit or subconjunctival space.
- Infiltration of tumor cells into the anterior chamber, trabecular meshwork and Schlemm's canal provide a conduit for tumor cells to enter the systemic circulation (Fig. 10.4.17).[15,34]

The American Joint Committee on Cancer (AJCC) has developed a tumor/node/metastasis (TNM) staging system

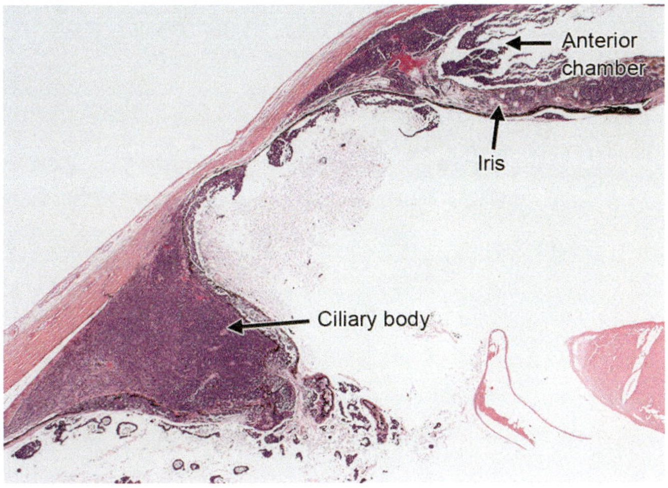

Fig. 10.4.17: Photomicrograph showing anterior retinoblastoma with invasion into the ciliary body, iris, and the anterior chamber angle.

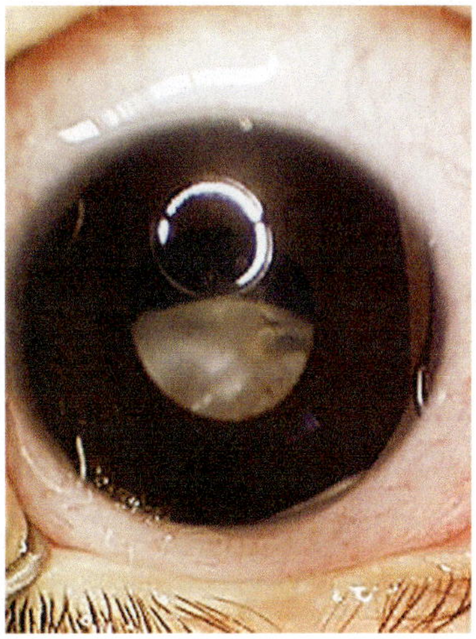

Fig. 10.4.18: Anterior segment photographs showing a retrolenticular whitish mass arising from the ciliary body consistent with a medulloepithelioma.

for retinoblastoma. Few studies have attempted to compare clinical staging group D and above with high-risk features as defined by the AJCC staging algorithm and determine its predictive value; the validation of staging is in evolution.[35,36]

MEDULLOEPITHELIOMA

Medulloepitheliomas are congenital tumors that arise mainly from the nonpigmented ciliary epithelium. They can rarely arise from the optic nerve or as a primary in the orbit. The term medulloepithelioma has been coined because the tumor is characterized by pseudostratified epithelium that resembles the medullary epithelium of the embryonic neural tube.[37-39]

Medulloepithelioma is typically seen in children older than children with retinoblastoma. The mean age in a large series was the 3.8 years. Rarely, the tumor might occur at an age older than 20 years. The tumor is typically unilateral and the eye is grossly normal but may show signs of persistent hyperplastic primary vitreous. Most medulloepitheliomas are sporadic. Rarely, the tumor may be associated with pleuropulmonary blastoma family tumor and dysplasia syndrome. This rare syndrome is associated with a germline mutation in the *DICER* gene.[40,41] Microribonucleic acid (miRNA) profiling has been reported in medulloepithelioma.[42]

The clinical presentation can be variable and depends on the size and how the tumor encroaches on intraocular tissues that cause visual impairment or causes distortion of intraocular structures.[38,43] The tumor is a slow-growing ciliary body mass that may present with leukokoria or lens displacement (Fig. 10.4.18) and can invade adjacent tissues. The tumor may have a cystic appearance (Figs. 10.4.19 and 10.4.20).

Pathology

Medulloepitheliomas typically show cords of primitive neuroepithelium or form tubular structures, which are seen adjacent to the ciliary body (Figs. 10.4.21 and 10.4.22). The cells typically have hyperchromatic nuclei with scant cytoplasm and might resemble neurosensory retina. The tumor cells are surrounded by mesenchymal matrix that is rich in hyaluronic acid.[38,44] Rosette-like structures might be seen in medulloepithelioma and include Flexner–Wintersteiner-type rosettes and Homer–Wright-type rosettes[45,46] (Fig. 10.4.23). The tubular structures in the tumor secrete at hyaluronic acid of rich matrix into the lumen that resembles vitreous. This material can be highlighted by staining the tumor with Alcian blue (Fig. 10.4.24).

Teratoid medulloepitheliomas are tumors that demonstrate heterotopic tissue. Hyaline type cartilage is the most common heterotopic element (Figs. 10.4.25 and 10.4.26). When this element is observed, calcification of the tumor might be seen on radiological studies. Other types of tissue include neuroglial tissue resembling brain, rhabdomyoblasts, or sarcomatous changes.[38,39,47]

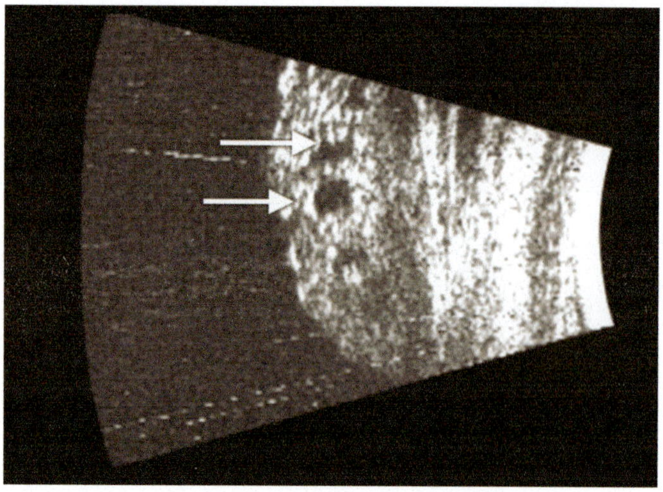

Fig. 10.4.19: B-scan ultrasound demonstrating ciliary body mass with cystic structure (arrows) consistent with a medulloepithelioma (arrows).

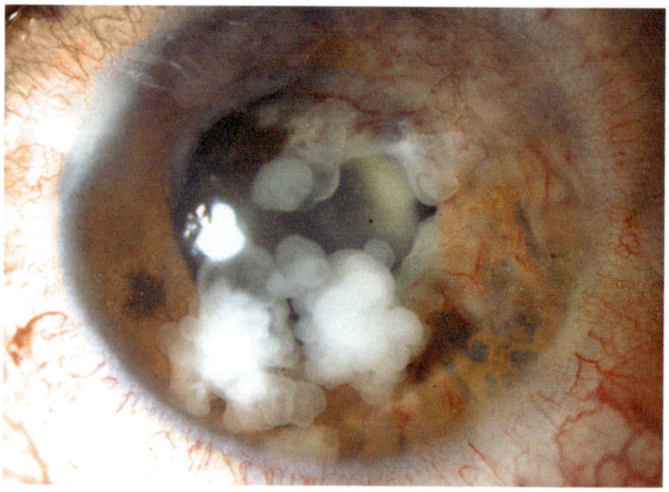

Fig. 10.4.20: Anterior segment photograph showing multiple whitish translucent cysts in the pupillary area in the anterior segment in a patient with medulloepithelioma.

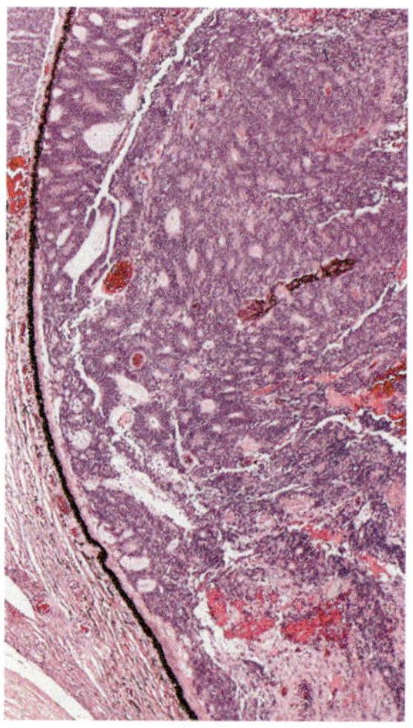

Fig. 10.4.21: Photomicrograph showing tumor arising from the ciliary body. The tumor consists of small neuroepithelial cells with hyperchromatic nuclei and scant cytoplasm. The tumor cells are arranged in cords and tubular structures.

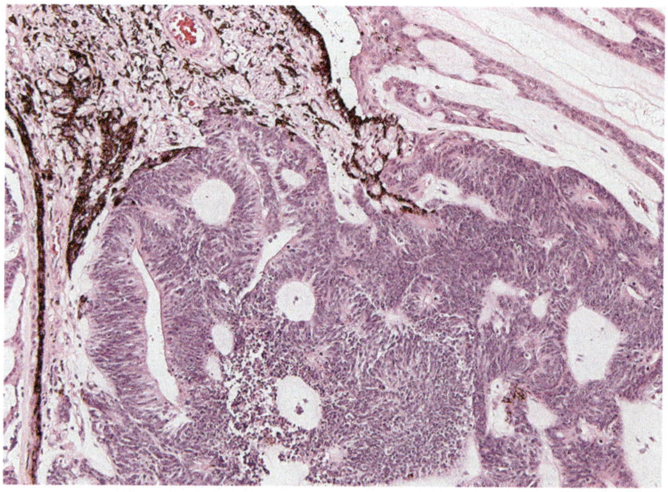

Fig. 10.4.22: Photomicrographs at higher magnification showing the tumor neuroepithelial cells arranged in a tubular fashion adjacent to the ciliary body.

The classification of medulloepitheliomas proposed by Zimmerman and colleagues is described in Table 10.4.1.[39]

There are no established criteria to designate a tumor as a malignant medulloepithelioma. Zimmerman et al. suggested that tumor cells that resemble retinoblastoma might be considered malignant.[39] Also, tumors that show an invasive behavior with extension into adjacent ocular structures or show extraocular extension (Fig. 10.4.27), sarcomatous change, and malignant features in the heteroplastic tissue (rhabdomyosarcoma or embryonal sarcoma-like change) may all be considered as features suggestive of malignancy. Immunohistochemistry is usually not helpful in the diagnosis but may be useful and delineating the teratoid elements in a tumor.

Table 10.4.1: The classification of medulloepitheliomas proposed by Zimmerman and colleagues.

Medulloepithelioma—nonteratoid	Medulloepithelioma—teratoid
Benign	Benign
Malignant	Malignant

Medulloepitheliomas that are small can be treated with iridocyclectomy, though recurrence rates are high.

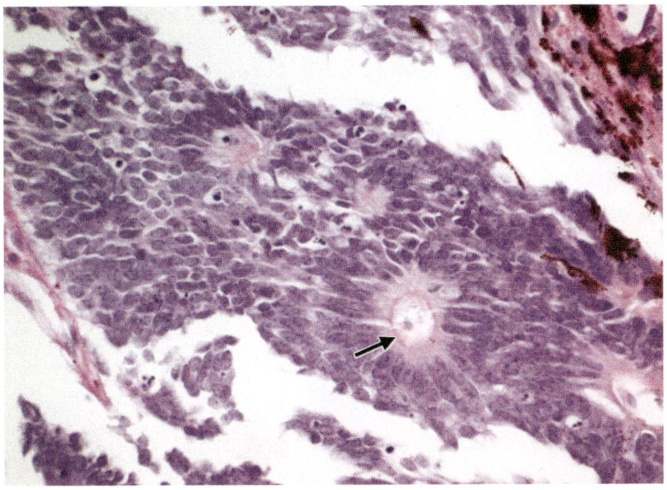

Fig. 10.4.23: Flexner–Wintersteiner rosette in a specimen of medulloepithelioma (arrow).

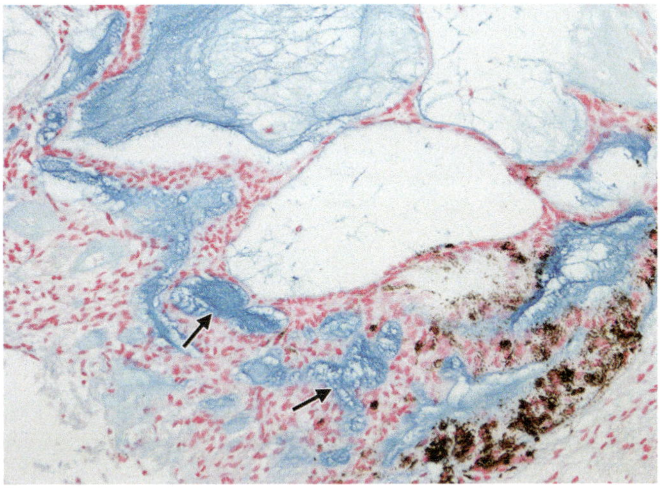

Fig. 10.4.24: Photomicrograph showing Alcian blue-positive material (arrows) (representing hyaluronic acid) in a lumen surrounded by tumor cells. The material represents vitreous-like material.

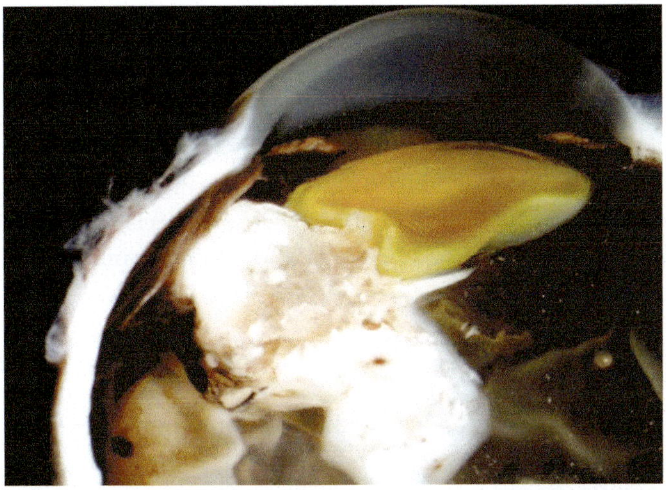

Fig. 10.4.25: Photographs from gross dissection of an enucleated with medulloepithelioma. Note the pedunculated mass arising from the ciliary body with calcification representing a teratoid medulloepithelioma.

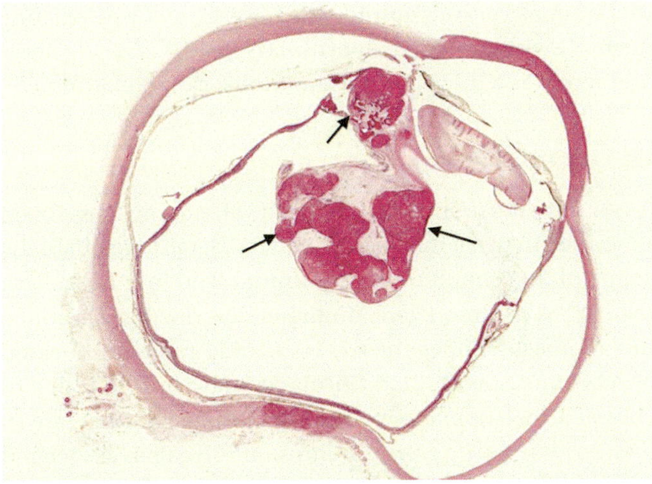

Fig. 10.4.26: Low-power microphotograph showing a cartilaginous tumor arising from the ciliary body consistent with a teratoid medulloepithelioma (arrows).

Enucleation otherwise is standard therapy for this tumor, once the diagnosis is made. Overall, the prognosis for this tumor is good based on the limited information on this rare tumor available in the literature. Local recurrence can occur in tumors that are resected. Tumor-related death is rare and is typically reported in patients that have malignant tumors with extraocular extension.[39,43,47]

UVEAL MELANOMA

Uveal melanoma is the most common adult intraocular neoplasm. Most tumors involve the choroid (90%) and the rest involve the ciliary body or the iris. The tumor is most often seen those of European descent in the 50–60-year-old age group. Melanomas account for 5% of all melanomas in the United States. Their age-adjusted risk is 5 per 1 million populations.[48,49]

The clinical appearance, risk factors have been discussed in great detail in the literature. This section will focus mainly on some of the more common clinical-pathological correlations genetics and other risk factors in choroidal melanomas.

Melanomas of the uvea have a distinct biological behavior that is different from cutaneous melanomas.

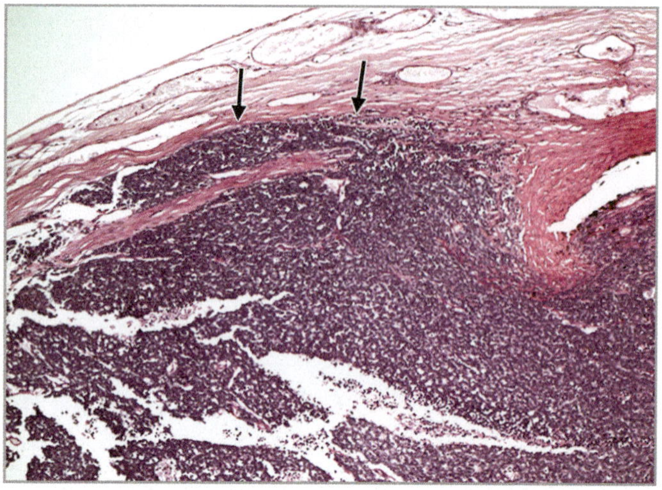

Fig. 10.4.27: Photomicrograph of a malignant nonteratoid medulloepithelioma showing invasion of the tumor into the sclera (arrows).

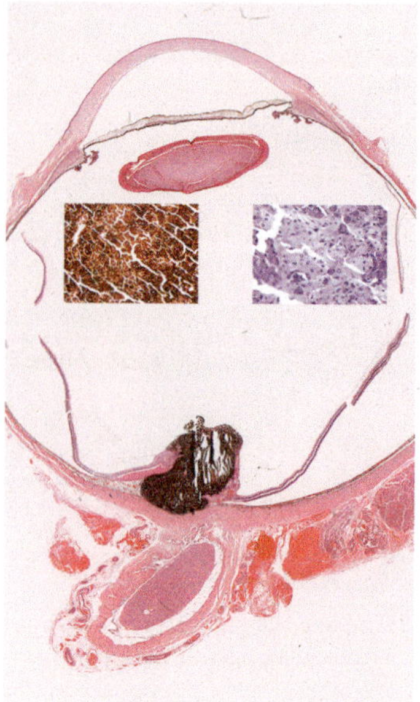

Fig. 10.4.28: Low-power microphotograph showing a densely melanotic mass arising from the optic nerve consistent with a melanocytoma (magnocellular nevus). *Inset left*: Large heavily pigmented nevus cells with bland nuclei. *Inset right*: Bleached section demonstrating the large cells with bland nuclei typical of a magnocellular nevus.

Melanomas of the choroid can arise from a pre-existing nevus[50] including a melanocytoma (Fig. 10.4.28),[51] de novo, and rarely as a metastatic lesion from a skin melanoma.[52]

Genetics

A number of genetic and epigenetic alterations have been described in uveal melanoma, and the details are out of the scope of this chapter but are summarized in an excellent review.[53] A common gene mutation described in choroidal melanomas includes the *GNAQ/GNA11* mutation located on chromosome 9p21.[48] Chromosomal abnormalities in choroidal melanomas that correlate with high mortality are 1p loss, 3p loss, and 8q gain. Chromosome 6B gain is associated with good prognosis.[53] Monosomy 3 is a chromosomal alteration commonly seen in uveal melanomas.[54,55]

Gene expression profiling studies were developed by Harbour and associates.[56,57] This test includes a 15-gene polymerase chain reaction (PCR)-based assay that discriminated choroidal melanomas into Class 1 and Class 2 tumors. Since the development of the assay, Class 1 tumors have been further subdivided in Class 1A and Class 1B. Reports suggest that Class 1A tumors have a 2% 5-year metastatic risk, while Class 1B tumors have a 21% 5-year metastatic risk. On the other hand, Class 2 tumors have a 72% 5-year metastatic risk.[58,59] This prognostic information has had helped in the clinical monitoring of patients with uveal melanomas. The test can be performed paraffin-embedded tissue, but is currently mainly done by fine-needle aspiration biopsy at the time when a radioactive plaque is placed for tumor therapy or immediately after enucleation for a choroidal melanoma. The test is now commercially available as DecisionDx-UM® (Castle Biosciences, Tucson, AZ) to provide patients with prognostic information about their tumor.

Pathology

Choroidal melanomas usually arise from melanocytes in the uveal tract. The tumor cells in this neoplasm can be spindle shaped or epithelioid cell in nature. The amount of melanin pigment in the cytoplasm of the melanoma cells is variable and in some tumors, the cells can be remarkably amelanotic. The Callender classification modified by McLean classifies these tumor cells into spindle cells, mixed cells, and epithelioid cell type[60] (Figs. 10.4.29A to C). The collaborative ocular melanoma study reported that in enucleated eyes with choroidal melanomas, spindle cell (9.0%), mixed cell (86.0%), and epithelioid cell (5.0%) types were observed. Tumor growth included lateral and vertical expansion of the tumor that resulted in increase in the size of the tumor base and tumor height. Vertical expansion includes rupture of Bruch's membrane resulting in a mushroom-shaped mass that protrudes into the subretinal space (Figs. 10.4.30 and 10.4.31). Tumor cells invade the scleral emissary canals and vortex veins, resulting in extraocular extension of the tumor

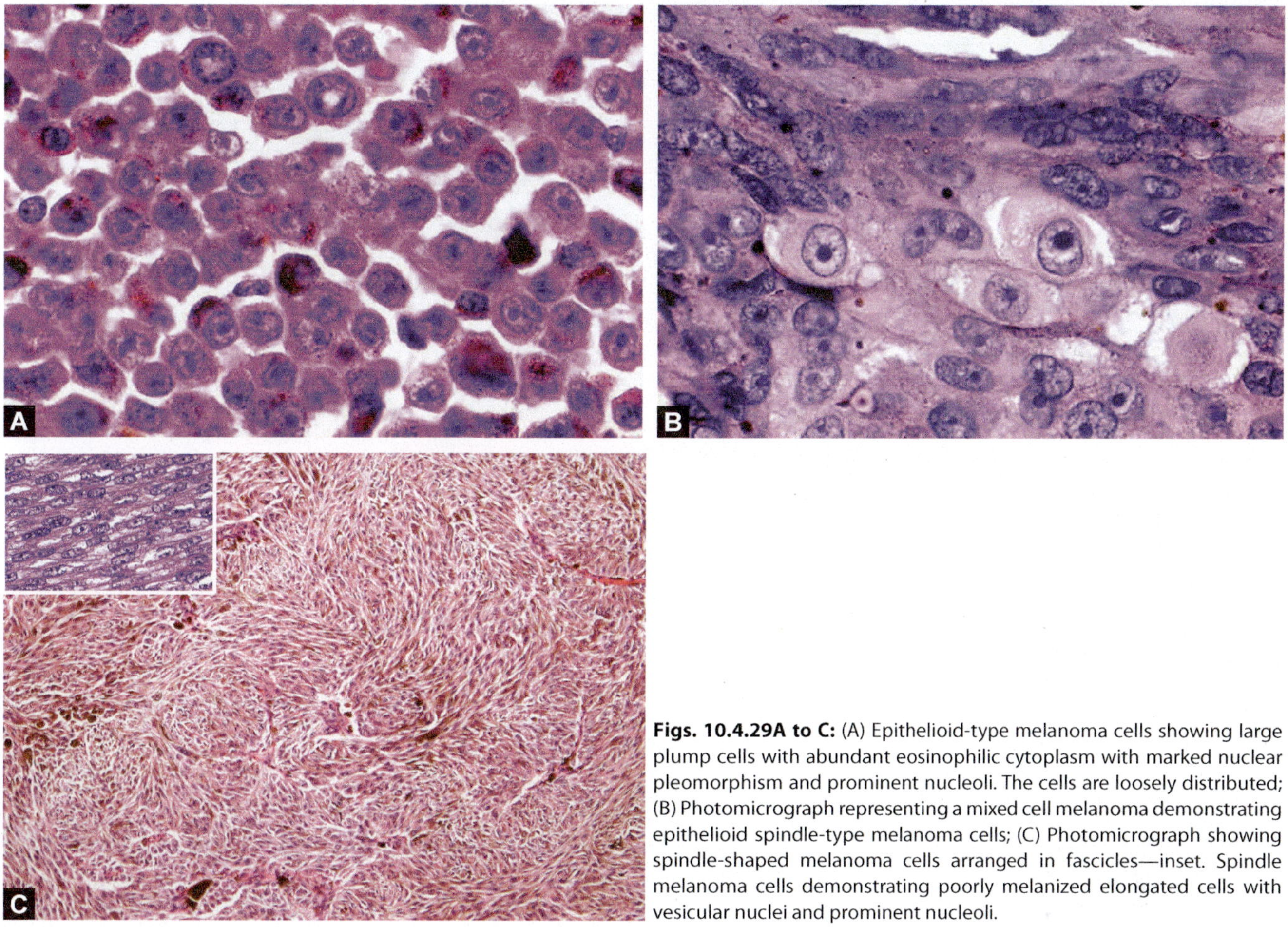

Figs. 10.4.29A to C: (A) Epithelioid-type melanoma cells showing large plump cells with abundant eosinophilic cytoplasm with marked nuclear pleomorphism and prominent nucleoli. The cells are loosely distributed; (B) Photomicrograph representing a mixed cell melanoma demonstrating epithelioid spindle-type melanoma cells; (C) Photomicrograph showing spindle-shaped melanoma cells arranged in fascicles—inset. Spindle melanoma cells demonstrating poorly melanized elongated cells with vesicular nuclei and prominent nucleoli.

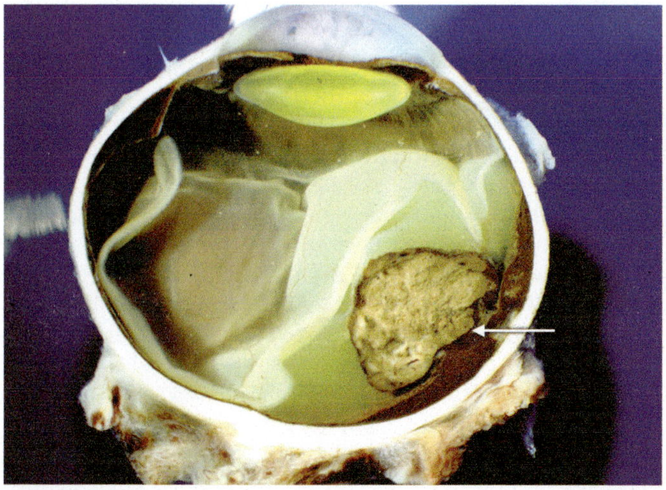

Fig. 10.4.30: Gross photograph showing a plaque-like pigmented melanoma in the choroid that has ruptured through Bruch's membrane (arrow) forming a mushroom-shaped mass in the subretinal space. The vessels in the subretinal tumor are slightly engorged. The surrounding retina shows an exudative retinal detachment.

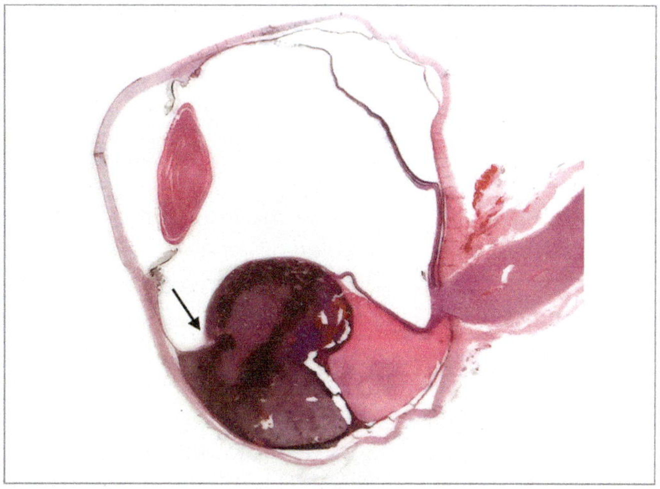

Fig. 10.4.31: Low-power photomicrograph showing densely pigmented choroidal melanoma rupturing through Bruch's membrane (arrow) into the subretinal space in a mushroom-shaped configuration.

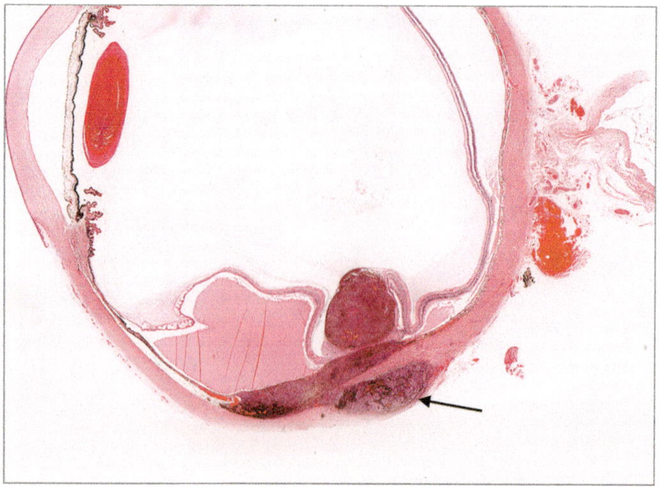

Fig. 10.4.32: Low-power photomicrograph showing choroidal melanoma with intrascleral infiltration through the emissary canals.

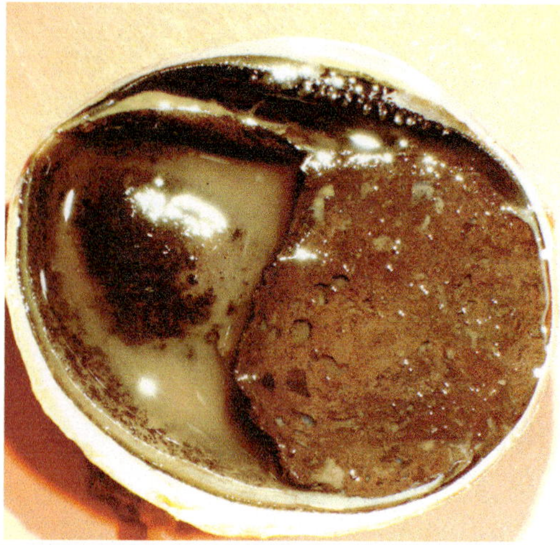

Fig. 10.4.33: Gross photograph showing a densely pigmented choroidal melanoma with a very large basal diameter that extends anteriorly to involve the ciliary body.

(Fig. 10.4.32). Local invasion of the retina and vitreous has also been noted. The Collaborative Ocular Melanoma Study pathology group reported Bruch's membrane rupture in 87.7%, retinal invasion in 49%, and vitreous invasion in 25% of the enucleated eyes.[61] The melanoma tumor cells demonstrate mitotic activity and in the older literature, a higher mitotic rate has been associated with higher mortality. A tourniquet-like effect of Bruch's membrane of the tumor that expands into the subretinal space leads to engorged vessels that might rupture and result in subretinal and vitreous hemorrhage. Large tumors may demonstrate necrosis. Extensive necrosis might result in a macrophagic response. These macrophages might enter the anterior chamber and block the trabecular pathways causing elevated intraocular pressure (melanomalytic glaucoma).[62]

Anteriorly located tumors and those with larger dimensions have a poor prognosis (Fig. 10.4.33). A number of histological prognostic factors have been described in the literature. Some of these include cell type (poor prognosis with epithelioid cell type), mitotic rate, specific vascular patterns, variation in nuclear size, and others. The usefulness of these the histological parameters in determining prognosis is variable.[15] Newer tests such as gene expression and nucleolar profiling, as described above have much greater specificity and sensitivity.

Apart from local extension of the tumor, the main organ that this tumor metastasizes in to the liver. With advances in treatment of uveal melanomas, local control rate exceeds 95%. However, the mortality rate from metastatic disease for medium and large-size tumors approaches 40–50%.[63,64]

REFERENCES

1. Kivela T. The epidemiological challenge of the most frequent eye cancer: retinoblastoma, an issue of birth and death. Br J Ophthalmol. 2009;93:1129-31.
2. Dimaras H, Kimani K, Dimba EA, et al. Retinoblastoma. Lancet. 2012;379(9824):1436-46.
3. Mallipatna A, Marino M, Singh AD. Genetics of Retinoblastoma. Asia Pac J Ophthalmol (Phila). 2016;5(4):260-4.
4. Soliman SE, Racher H, Zhang C, et al. Genetics and Molecular Diagnostics in Retinoblastoma—An Update. Asia Pac J Ophthalmol (Phila). 2017;6(2):197-207.
5. McEvoy JD, Dyer MA. Genetic and Epigenetic Discoveries in Human Retinoblastoma. Crit Rev Oncog. 2015;20(3-4):217-25.
6. Felsher DW. Role of MYCN in retinoblastoma. Lancet Oncol. 2013;14(4):270-1.
7. Zeschnigk M, Lohmann D, Horsthemke B. A PCR test for the detection of hypermethylated alleles at the retinoblastoma locus. J Med Genet. 1999;36(10):793-4.
8. Amitrano S, Marozza A, Somma S, et al. Next generation sequencing in sporadic retinoblastoma patients reveals somatic mosaicism. Eur J Hum Genet. 2015;23(11):1523-30.
9. Fidler MM, Reulen RC, Winter DL, et al. Risk of Subsequent Bone Cancers Among 69 460 Five-Year Survivors of Childhood and Adolescent Cancer in Europe. J Natl Cancer Inst. 2018;110(2). doi: 10.1093/jnci/djx165.
10. Sethi RV, Shih HA, Yeap BY, et al. Second nonocular tumors among survivors of retinoblastoma treated with contemporary photon and proton radiotherapy. Cancer. 2014;120(1):126-33.
11. Yamanaka R, Hayano A. Secondary Craniofacial Sarcomas Following Retinoblastoma: A Systematic Review. World Neurosurg. 2017;101:722-730 e724.

12. Temming P, Arendt M, Viehmann A, et al. Incidence of second cancers after radiotherapy and systemic chemotherapy in heritable retinoblastoma survivors: A report from the German reference center. Pediatr Blood Cancer. 2017;64(1):71-80.
13. Shields JA, Shields CL, De Potter P. Enucleation technique for children with retinoblastoma. J Pediatr Ophthalmol Strabismus. 1992;29(4):213-5.
14. Eagle RC Jr. High-risk features and tumor differentiation in retinoblastoma: a retrospective histopathologic study. Arch Pathol Lab Med. 2009;133(8):1203-9.
15. Eagle RC Jr. The pathology of ocular cancer. Eye (Lond). 2013;27(2):128-36.
16. Taha H, Amer HZ, El-Zomor H, et al. Phthisis bulbi: clinical and pathologic findings in retinoblastoma. Fetal Pediatr Pathol. 2015;34(3):176-84.
17. Kashyap S, Meel R, Pushker N, et al. Phthisis bulbi in retinoblastoma. Clin Exp Ophthalmol. 2011;39(2):105-110.
18. Schedler KJ, Traine PG, Lohmann DR, et al. Hereditary Diffuse Infiltrating Retinoblastoma. Ophthalmic Genet. 2016;37(1):95-7.
19. Khetan V, Al-Kharusi N, Ganesh A, et al. Diffuse infiltrating retinoblastoma with central nervous system metastasis. Arch Ophthalmol. 2011;129(3):375-7.
20. Shields CL, Ghassemi F, Tuncer S, et al. Clinical spectrum of diffuse infiltrating retinoblastoma in 34 consecutive eyes. Ophthalmology. 2008;115(12):2253-8.
21. Herwig MC, Hubbard GB, Wells JR, et al. [Diffuse anterior retinoblastoma]. Ophthalmologe. 2011;108(10):969-72.
22. Wilson MW, Qaddoumi I, Billups C, et al. A clinicopathological correlation of 67 eyes primarily enucleated for advanced intraocular retinoblastoma. Br J Ophthalmol. 2011;95(4):553-8.
23. Crosby MB, Hubbard GB, Gallie BL, et al. Anterior diffuse retinoblastoma: mutational analysis and immunofluorescence staining. Arch Pathol Lab Med. 2009;133(8):1215-8.
24. Shields CL, Lally SE, Manjandavida FP, et al. Diffuse Anterior Retinoblastoma with Globe Salvage and Visual Preservation in 3 Consecutive Cases. Ophthalmology. 2016;123(2):378-84.
25. Ray A, Gombos DS, Vats TS. Retinoblastoma: an overview. Indian J Pediatr. 2012;79(7):916-21.
26. Earl JB, Minckler DS, Lee TC, et al. Malignant teratoid medulloepithelioma with retinoblastic and rhabdomyoblastic differentiation. J AAPOS. 2013;17(3):328-31.
27. Tso MO. Clues to the cells of origin in retinoblastoma. Int Ophthalmol Clin. 1980;20(2):191-210.
28. Ts'o MO, Fine BS, Zimmerman LE. The nature of retinoblastoma. II. Photoreceptor differentiation: an electron microscopic study. Am J Ophthalmol. 1970;69(3):350-9.
29. Chantada GL, Gonzalez A, Fandino A, et al. Some clinical findings at presentation can predict high-risk pathology features in unilateral retinoblastoma. J Pediatr Hematol Oncol. 2009;31(5):325-9.
30. Chantada GL, Casco F, Fandino AC, et al. Outcome of patients with retinoblastoma and postlaminar optic nerve invasion. Ophthalmology. 2007;114(11):2083-9.
31. Kaliki S, Tahiliani P, Iram S, et al. Choroidal Infiltration by Retinoblastoma: Predictive Clinical Features and Outcome. J Pediatr Ophthalmol Strabismus. 2016;53(6):349-56.
32. Fabian ID, Stacey AW, Chowdhury T, et al. High-Risk Histopathology Features in Primary and Secondary Enucleated International Intraocular Retinoblastoma Classification Group D Eyes. Ophthalmology. 2017;124(6):851-8.
33. Kashyap S, Meel R, Pushker N, et al. Clinical predictors of high risk histopathology in retinoblastoma. Pediatr Blood Cancer. 2012;58(3):356-61.
34. Kaliki S, Shields CL, Rojanaporn D, et al. High-risk retinoblastoma based on international classification of retinoblastoma: analysis of 519 enucleated eyes. Ophthalmology. 2013;120(5):997-1003.
35. Alkatan HM, AL Balawi H, Maktabi AM. The value of "en toto" globe submission in the assessment of high-risk retinoblastoma cases and staging. Int Ophthalmol. 2017. doi: 10.1007/s10792-016-0410-5. [Epub ahead of print].
36. Yousef YA, Al-Hussaini M, Mehyar M, et al. Predictive Value of TNM Classification, International Classification, and Reese-Ellsworth Staging of Retinoblastoma for the Likelihood of High-Risk Pathologic Features. Retina. 2015;35(9):1883-9.
37. Becker LE, Hinton D. Primitive neuroectodermal tumors of the central nervous system. Hum Pathol. 1983;14(6):538-50.
38. Saunders T, Margo CE. Intraocular medulloepithelioma. Arch Pathol Lab Med. 2012;136(2):212-6.
39. Broughton WL, Zimmerman LE. A clinicopathologic study of 56 cases of intraocular medulloepitheliomas. Am J Ophthalmol. 1978;85(3):407-18.
40. Sahm F, Jakobiec FA, Meyer J, et al. Somatic mutations of DICER1 and KMT2D are frequent in intraocular medulloepitheliomas. Genes Chromosomes Cancer. 2016;55(5):418-27.
41. Kramer GD, Arepalli S, Shields CL, et al. Ciliary body medulloepithelioma association with pleuropulmonary blastoma in a familial tumor predisposition syndrome. J Pediatr Ophthalmol Strabismus. 2014;51:e48-50.
42. Edward DP, Alkatan H, Rafiq Q, et al. MicroRNA profiling in intraocular medulloepitheliomas. PLoS One. 2015;10(3):e0121706.
43. Shields JA, Eagle RC Jr., Ferguson K, et al. Tumors of the nonpigmented epithelium of the ciliary body: The Lorenz E. Zimmerman Tribute Lecture. Retina. 2015;35(5):957-65.
44. Zimmerman LE, Fine BS. Production of Hyaluronic Acid by Cysts and Tumors of the Ciliary Body. Arch Ophthalmol. 1964;72:365-79.
45. Korshunov A, Jakobiec FA, Eberhart CG, et al. Comparative integrated molecular analysis of intraocular medulloepitheliomas and central nervous system embryonal tumors with multilayered rosettes confirms that they are distinct nosologic entities. Neuropathology. 2015;35(6):538-44.
46. Jakobiec FA, Kool M, Stagner AM, et al. Intraocular Medulloepitheliomas and Embryonal Tumors With Multilayered Rosettes of the Brain: Comparative Roles of

LIN28A and C19MC. Am J Ophthalmol. 2015;159(6):1065-74 e1061.
47. Kaliki S, Shields CL, Eagle RC Jr., et al. Ciliary body medulloepithelioma: analysis of 41 cases. Ophthalmology. 2013;120(12):2552-9.
48. Chattopadhyay C, Kim DW, Gombos DS, et al. Uveal melanoma: From diagnosis to treatment and the science in between. Cancer. 2016;122(15):2299-312.
49. Kaliki S, Shields CL. Uveal melanoma: relatively rare but deadly cancer. Eye (Lond). 2017;31(2):241-57.
50. Chien JL, Sioufi K, Surakiatchanukul T, et al. Choroidal nevus: a review of prevalence, features, genetics, risks, and outcomes. Curr Opin Ophthalmol. 2017;28(3):228-37.
51. Shields JA, Shields CL, Eagle RC Jr. Melanocytoma (hyperpigmented magnocellular nevus) of the uveal tract: the 34th G. Victor Simpson lecture. Retina. 2007;27(6):730-9.
52. Grajewski RS, Schuler-Thurner B, Mauch C, et al. Ocular diseases in metastatic cutaneous melanoma: review of 108 consecutive patients in two German tertiary centers. Graefes Arch Clin Exp Ophthalmol. 2014;252(4):679-85.
53. Coupland SE, Lake SL, Zeschnigk M, et al. Molecular pathology of uveal melanoma. Eye (Lond). 2013;27(2):230-42.
54. Sandinha MT, Farquharson MA, Roberts F. Identification of monosomy 3 in choroidal melanoma by chromosome in situ hybridisation. Br J Ophthalmol. 2004;88(12):1527-32.
55. Mensink HW, Vaarwater J, Kilic E, et al. Chromosome 3 intratumor heterogeneity in uveal melanoma. Invest Ophthalmol Vis Sci. 2009;50(2):500-4.
56. Harbour JW, Chao DL. A molecular revolution in uveal melanoma: implications for patient care and targeted therapy. Ophthalmology. 2014;121(6):1281-8.
57. Harbour JW. Eye cancer: unique insights into oncogenesis: the Cogan Lecture. Invest Ophthalmol Vis Sci. 2006;47(5): 1736-45.
58. Field MG, Harbour JW. Recent developments in prognostic and predictive testing in uveal melanoma. Curr Opin Ophthalmol. 2014;25(3):234-9.
59. Walter SD, Chao DL, Feuer W, et al. Prognostic Implications of Tumor Diameter in Association With Gene Expression Profile for Uveal Melanoma. JAMA Ophthalmol. 2016;134(7):734-40.
60. McLean IW, Zimmerman LE, Evans RM. Reappraisal of Callender's spindle a type of malignant melanoma of choroid and ciliary body. Am J Ophthalmol. 1978;86(4):557-64.
61. Collaborative Ocular Melanoma Study. Histopathologic characteristics of uveal melanomas in eyes enucleated from the Collaborative Ocular Melanoma Study. COMS report no. 6. Am J Ophthalmol. 1998;125(6):745-66.
62. el Baba F, Hagler WS, De la Cruz A, et al. Choroidal melanoma with pigment dispersion in vitreous and melanomalytic glaucoma. Ophthalmology. 1988;95(3):370-7.
63. Kivela T, Kujala E. Prognostication in eye cancer: the latest tumor, node, metastasis classification and beyond. Eye (Lond). 2013;27(2):243-52.
64. Hawkins BS, Collaborative Ocular Melanoma Study Group. The Collaborative Ocular Melanoma Study (COMS) randomized trial of pre-enucleation radiation of large choroidal melanoma: IV. Ten-year mortality findings and prognostic factors. COMS report number 24. Am J Ophthalmol. 2004;138(6):936-51.

Part 2 Clinical Examination

N Venkatesh Prajna

OUTLINE

Chapter 11

Clinical Examination of the Anterior Segment

Geetha Iyer, Shweta Agarwal, Bhaskar Srinivasan

INTRODUCTION

Examination of the anterior segment includes a diffuse general examination of the eye, slit-lamp evaluation, intraocular pressure measurement using applanation tonometry and assessment of the angle with gonioscopy. A detailed evaluation of the anterior segment provides the required information to diagnose anterior segment disorders and can provide clues toward posterior segment abnormalities. In addition, it also provides subtle clues toward variations from normal anatomy that warrant further investigative modalities, e.g. shallow anterior chamber. Though, the anterior segment evaluation includes multiple tests. This chapter focuses on the primary uses of the slit lamp in the anterior segment examination.

GENERAL EXAMINATION OF THE EYE

Although multiple newer sophisticated instruments are available to examine the eye, general examination of the eye using a simple torch light can provide significant information, especially in small children who might not cooperate otherwise.

Lid abnormalities such as entropion, ectropion, lid notch, lid swellings, nodules and edema, the presence of ptosis and lagophthalmos can be better appreciated on torch light evaluation.

Bulbar conjunctiva can be evaluated for the type of congestion—diffuse or localized and site of congestion, associated discharge or foreign bodies if present. Upper and lower fornix can also be assessed for similar conditions by everting the upper lid or retracting the lower lid.

A torch placed temporally and directed across the anterior surface of the globe, might reveal any decrease in corneal luster as seen in corneal edema or superficial punctate keratitis or even a corneal infiltrate.

An external examination can highlight not only surface abnormalities but it can also give a brief idea about corneal opacities, depth of the anterior chamber and the lens status.

External examination helps document presence of squint, increased or reduced blink rate, the presence of features suggestive of blepharospasm or hemifacial spasm and any obvious external mass lesions.

A handheld light source capped with a cobalt blue filter demonstrates the presence of fluorescein staining when a corneal epithelial defect exists.

SLIT-LAMP BIOMICROSCOPY

Biomicroscopy is defined as microscopic examination of living tissue in the body. For the eye, it implies methodical examination of the ocular structures using the slit lamp to evaluate the eye in health and disease. An indispensible instrument for the ophthalmologist, and a valuable tool for detailed dynamic evaluation of the anterior segment, it is the most frequently used instrument for ocular examination. The slit beam provides an optical section of the ocular structures being evaluated.

The eye is evaluated by moving the machine both anteroposteriorly and horizontally using different permutations of angles, intensity and filters of illumination.

COMPONENTS OF THE SLIT LAMP

The two basic components of a slit lamp include an illuminating and observation system. In addition the other systems included are the mechanical and electrical components. The slit lamp and its different parts have been enumerated in Figures 11.1A and B.

The illuminating system can be adjusted to vary the width, height and angle of incidence of the light beam. The aim of the illuminating system is to produce a uniformly bright, accurately focused slit of light whose dimensions can be adjusted. This is usually obtained by using the Vogt-Koeller projection system.

The illuminating system consists of a light source (most of the recent slit lamps use halogen or LED bulbs, the shorter

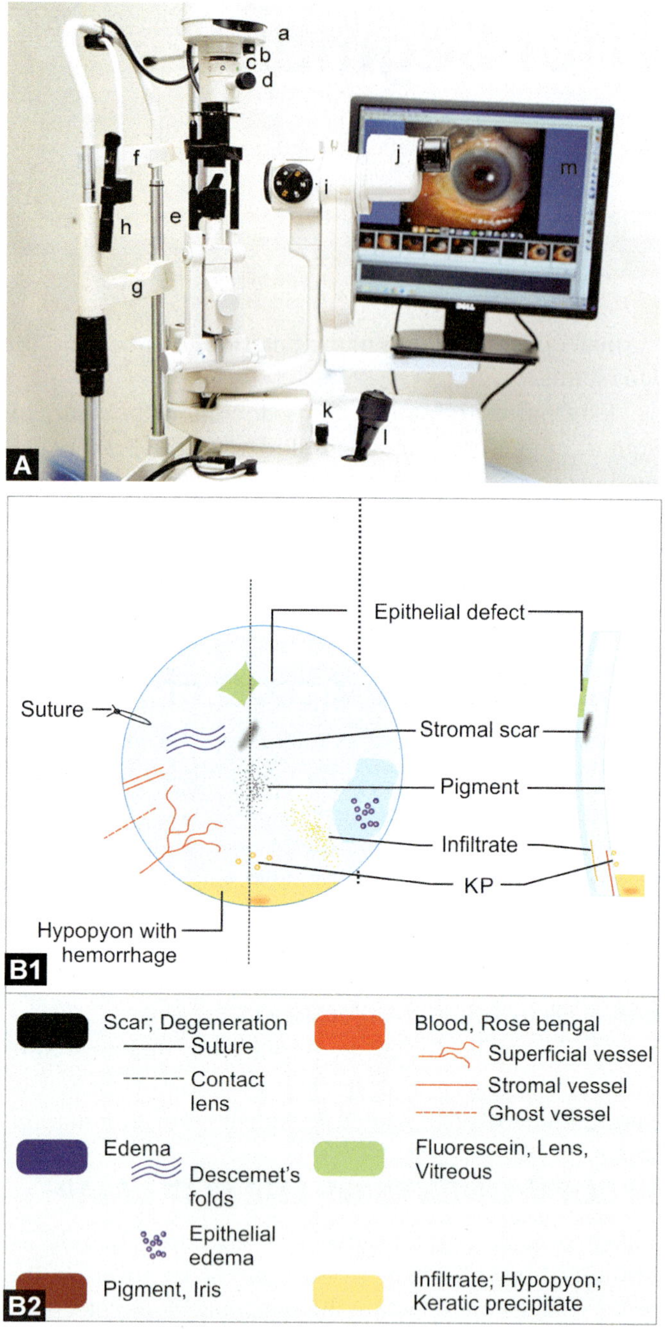

Figs. 11.1A and B: (A) Parts of a slit lamp: a—aperture/slit length display window, b—aperture/slit window selector knob, c—filters, d—filter selector knob, e—mirror, f—forehead rest, g—chin rest, h—fixation target, i—magnification index mark, j—eyepiece, k—brightness adjustment knob, l—control lever, m—computer screen; (B1) Waring scheme for drawing general pathologic corneal conditions. Example sketch displaying typical corneal pathologic changes. The dotted line indicates the optical section that is displayed in the slit view (KP = keratic precipitate). (For demonstration purposes, temporal and nasal changes from the slit-lamp are shown); (B2) Six-color code for drawing.

wavelength of LED spectrum allows better visualization and brighter illumination) and condensing lenses.

The features of illumination that can be altered based on the need and types of examination include:

- The intensity
- The width (narrow, broad)
- The angle (with respect to the biomicroscope)
- The orientation (vertical, horizontal or inclined)

These alterations are achieved with the help of the various knobs for adjusting the parameters as required on the body of the slit lamp.

The observation system is designed with the aim to providing an optimum stereopsis, maintaining an adequate field of view and depth of field. This is achieved by means of binocular eyepiece with telescopic lens systems. The eyepiece can be aligned to correspond to the examiner's interpupillary distance and adjustments allow the refractive error of the examiner to be adjusted for on the eyepiece to view without spectacles. The illuminator and the biomicroscope are mounted on a common axis in a co-pivotal arrangement in order to achieve a parfocal and isocentric relationship between the two systems. The illumination system can be located above or below the microscope based on the manufacturer.

The mechanical system includes the patient positioning frame (forehead strap and chin rest), the joystick and the lever to adjust the height of the slit lamp. The joystick allows anteroposterior and horizontal movements of the viewing system. The slit lamp can be locked in position with the help of a lock key.

The electrical system includes the main power pack and the rheostat.

SLIT-LAMP EXAMINATION TECHNIQUES

Berliner described six basic methods of illumination, which are reviewed below.

Diffuse Illumination

Using a wide beam that is slightly out of focus, the general topography and extent of gross alterations in the cornea can be determined by diffuse illumination. This technique provides information similar to that obtained with hand light and is best used in combination with other forms (Fig. 11.2).

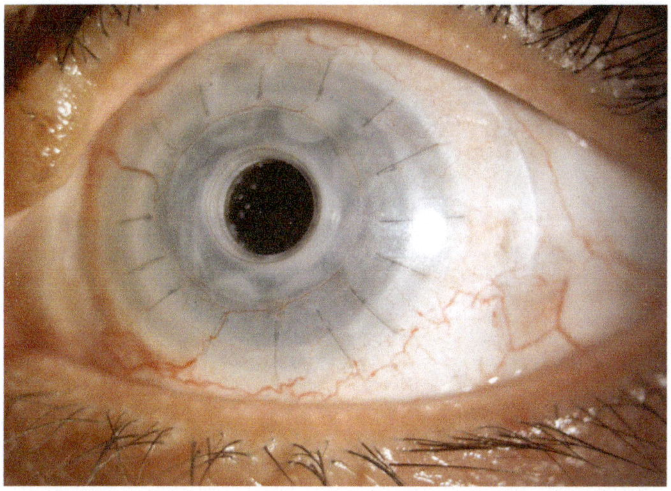

Fig. 11.2: Slit-lamp photograph of an eye with a Boston type 1 keratoprosthesis in diffuse illumination.

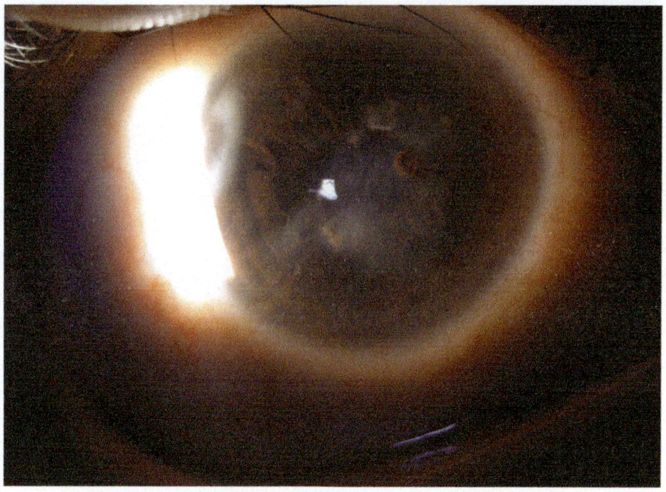

Fig. 11.3: Sclerotic scatter illumination highlighting the stromal corneal opacities.

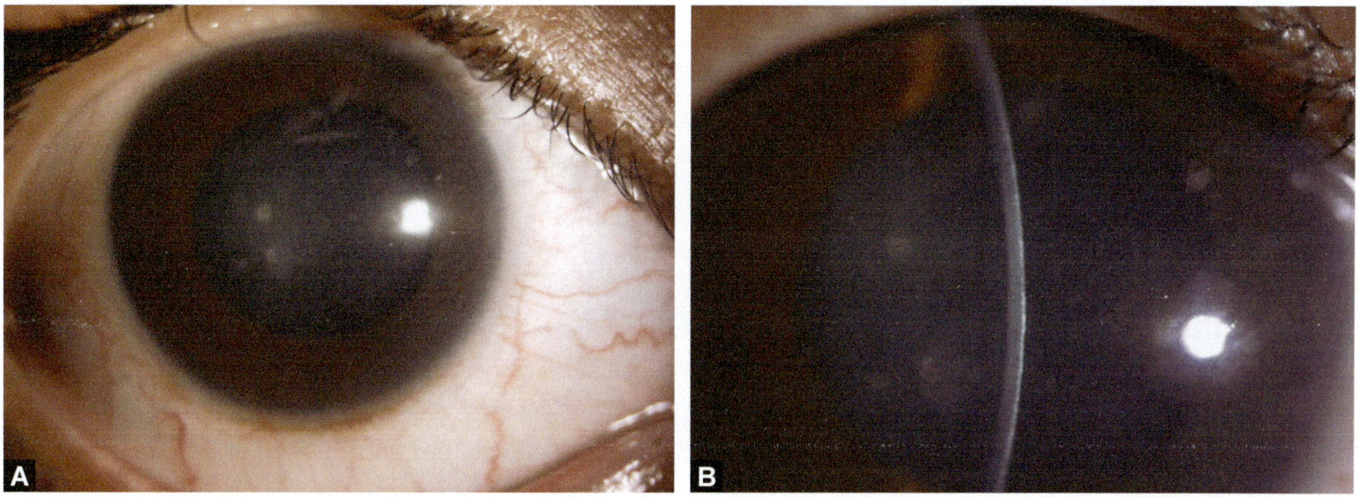

Figs. 11.4A and B: Diffuse illumination in corneal dystrophy (A) revealing the superficial depth of the opacities in direct focal illumination (B).

Sclerotic Scatter

This is an indirect form of illumination where a narrow beam is directed at the temporal limbus while the microscope is focused centrally on the cornea. Under these circumstances, light is transmitted within the cornea by total internal reflection (similar to the transmission of light in a fiber-optic bundle) and exits at the opposite limbus. In a normal clear cornea, no light is seen. However, if any structure obstructs light, it will become illuminated by altering the path of the internally reflected light beam. Thus, even subtle stromal and epithelial opacities or irregularities can be observed (Fig. 11.3). Sclerotic scatter is especially useful in evaluating minimal changes in corneal epithelium such as edema induced by contact lens wear. This is the only technique of evaluation wherein the illuminating and the viewing systems are decoupled.

Direct Focal

It is the most frequently used form of corneal illumination, focuses the slit beam and microscope at coincident points. This technique provides the observer with a direct view of the structure of interest. The angle of incidence of light beam can be altered by swinging the instrument arm, which carries the light source, thus decreasing reflections and giving clues that allow localization of the depth of lesions (Figs. 11.4A and B). The changes seen by altering the angle of incidence of the light allow accurate determination of the depth of lesions in the cornea.

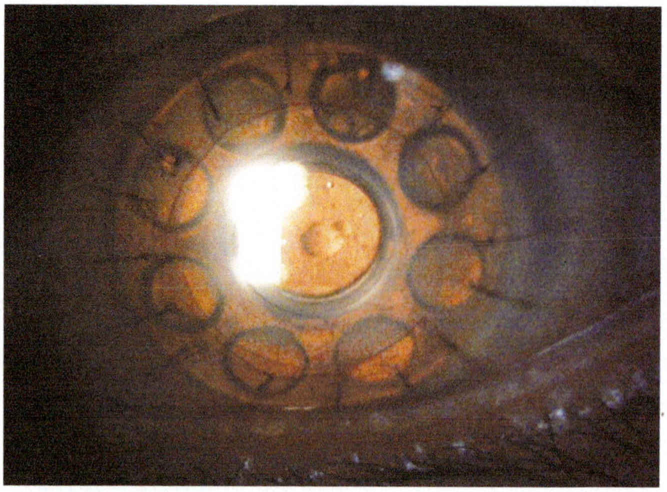

Fig. 11.5: Retroillumination in an eye with a Boston type 1 keratoprosthesis helps delineate presence and location of retroprosthetic membrane.

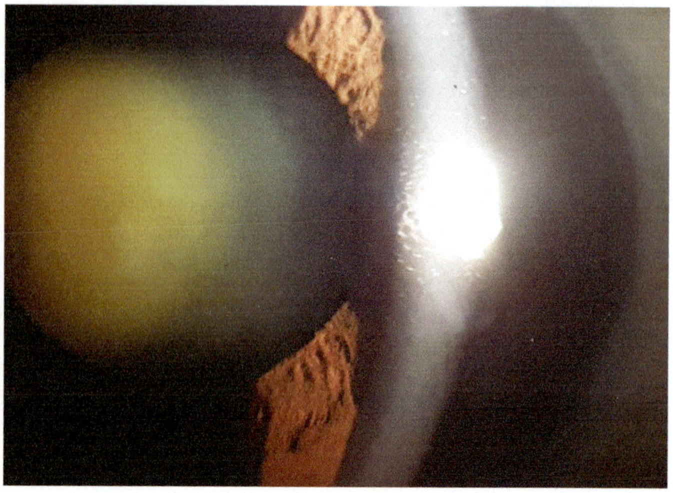

Fig. 11.6: Specular reflection imaging highlighting the guttate changes.

Indirect Illumination

Indirect illumination similar to sclerotic scatter depends on transmission of light in illuminated nontransparent tissue. A small beam of light directed at a corneal opacity will highlight such changes in the adjacent tissues as the presence of vessels, which will stand out in the scattered light.

Retroillumination

Retroillumination uses light reflected from intraocular structures, especially the iris and fundus, to illuminate the cornea. The beam is directed so that the microscope is focused on the corneal area of interest and the light beam is focused behind the cornea. This provides excellent illumination of fine epithelial alterations, small stromal opacities and endothelial alterations including guttata and keratic precipitates. One can look directly along the reflected beam of light (direct retroillumination), thus perceiving a greater contrast of dense or pigmented opacities (Fig. 11.5), or the microscope can be aligned to view the area of interest in reflected light against the black background of the pupil (indirect retroillumination). This is for viewing changes that scatter but do not totally obstruct light, such as epithelial edema.

Specular Reflection

It relies on the reflective properties of anterior and posterior corneal surfaces. By observing the cornea adjacent to the illuminating beam and altering the angle of the beam, a point will be reached at which the reflection of the posterior corneal surface will allow visualization of the endothelial cell mosaic pattern and endothelial changes, as well as folds in Descemet's membrane (Fig. 11.6).

Filters (Fig. 11.7)

Slit lamps may have some/all of the following filters. Each filter is indicated by a symbol specific to it. The different types of filters, their symbols and uses have been elaborated in Table 11.1.

Range of Magnification

The range of magnification can be divided into:

- *Low*: 6–10 X
- *Medium*: 16–25 X
- *High*: 40 X

The magnification of the viewing system can be changed by changing the objective or the eye-piece, based on the slit-lamp manufacturer. As the magnification increases, the depth of focus and the field of view decreases.

PREPARATION OF THE PATIENT FOR SLIT-LAMP EXAMINATION

There are no specific preexamination instructions for evaluating an adult patient. Based on the height of the patient, the position of the slit lamp as well as the chin rest is adjusted to the patient's position comfortably. The patient is instructed to look in a particular direction based on the part of the eye being examined. Everting the lid is not done as a part of routine examination. The patient is informed of the same and its associated minimal discomfort prior

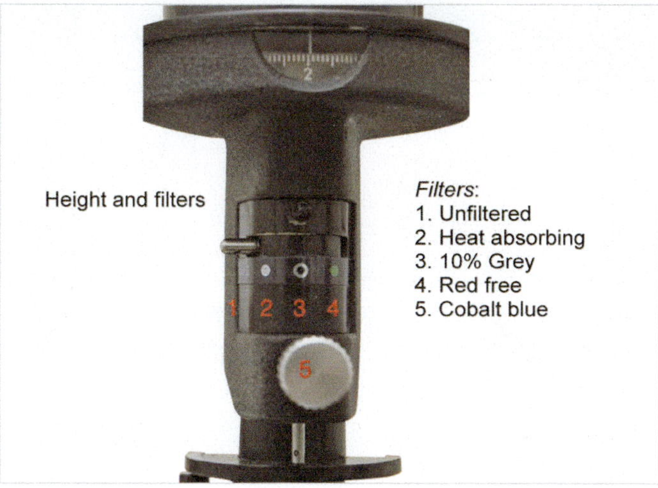
Height and filters
Filters:
1. Unfiltered
2. Heat absorbing
3. 10% Grey
4. Red free
5. Cobalt blue

Fig. 11.7: Different types of filters and knob to measure height of lesion.

to lid eversion, if required. Topical anesthetic drops for measuring the intraocular pressure using the applanation tonometer and various stains for assessing the ocular surface are instilled after informing the patient of the same. The fixation target helps the patient fix the gaze in a particular direction. For evaluating a pediatric patient on the slit lamp, it is important to build a rapport with the child and demonstrate the noninvasiveness of the technique to make the child comfortable and co-operate. The child is usually asked to kneel down on the chair in order to be able to place the chin on the chin rest.

SEQUENCE AND TIPS FOR SLIT-LAMP EXAMINATION

Prior to initiation of the examination, at the start of the day, it is important to check that the refractive error in the observation system is set at zero or in accordance with the examiner's refractive error.

For ease of documentation and in order to follow a fixed routine in all eyes, the slit-lamp evaluation is begun with examination of the eyelids, lid margin, puncta, the bulbar conjunctiva, and fornices are evaluated by asking the patient to look down and up, followed by the cornea (including the limbus), the anterior chamber, iris and the lens. The examination is first performed under low magnification with diffuse illumination. It is important to ensure that the light used for examination is not overly bright. This is followed by a slit evaluation of the cornea and the anterior chamber depth. Higher magnification is used to evaluate the corneal endothelium using a slit beam sweeped horizontally. Areas of abnormality identified on low magnification are further examined under higher magnification as well as using filters and illumination as deemed appropriate.

Table 11.1: different types of filters, their symbols and uses.

Filter	Symbol	Use
Neutral density 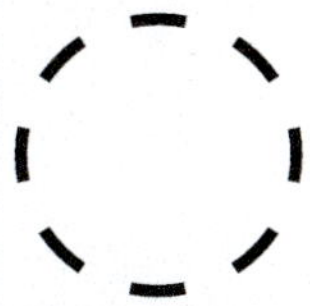	Circle with hashed line	Reduces illumination for photosensitive patients
Cobalt blue 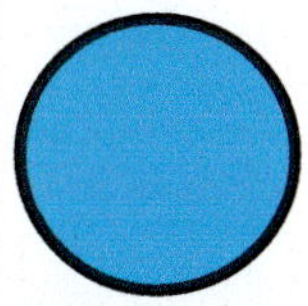	Blue-filled circle/ rotating knob	Fluorescein staining
Red free 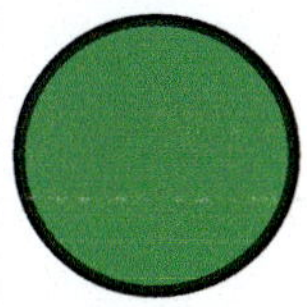	Green-filled circle	Differentiates vascular/ pigmented lesions. Enhances blood vessels/hemorrhages
Grey 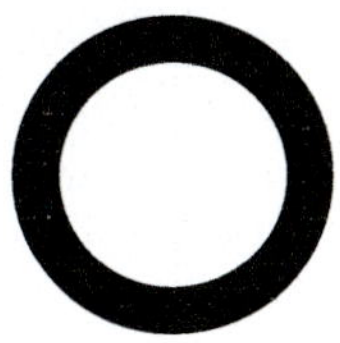	Circle with thick line	Photosensitive patients
Yellow 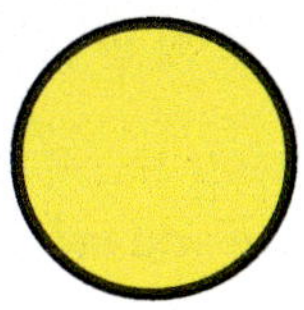	Yellow-filled circle on the observation system	Improves contrast while using fluorescein and cobalt blue filter
Diffuser	Flip-up filter placed on the illumination system	General observation of eye and adnexa, slit-lamp photography

Assessing the presence and extent of conjunctivochalasis is enhanced by moving the corresponding lid over the globe in order to appreciate the excess fold of conjunctiva.

Asking the patient to look in extremes of gaze in low magnification with diffuse illumination helps identify early conjunctival cicatricial changes and/or symblepharon bands (Fig. 11.8). This maneuver also completes evaluation of the sclera, at times inadvertently highlighting areas of scleral thinning or staphylomas hidden beneath the lids as well as pigmented conjunctival lesions.

Eversion of the lid helps to identify the presence of lid margin keratinization, papillae, scarring and foreign bodies (Figs. 11.9A and B).

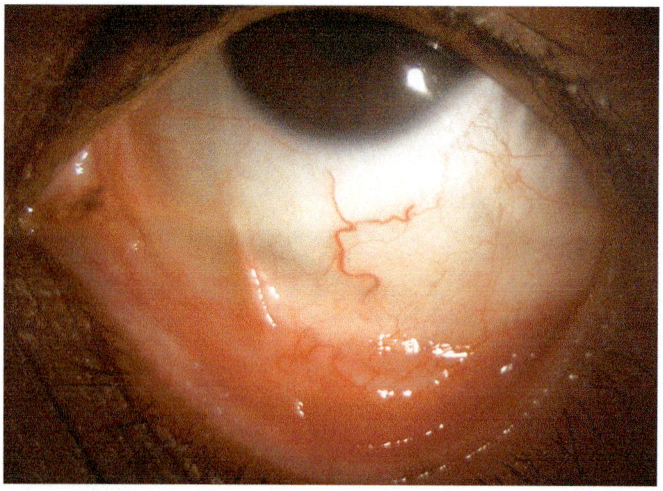

Fig. 11.8: Symblepharon bands being better appreciated on upgaze.

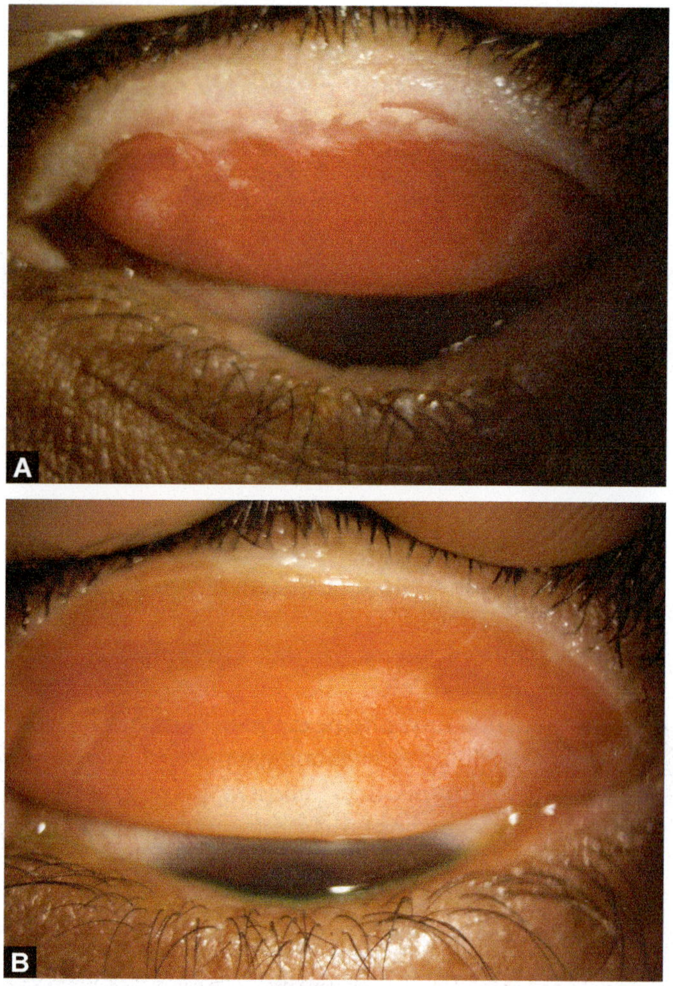

Figs. 11.9A and B: (A) Eversion of eyelid helps grade lid margin keratinization; (B) Assessment of the mucosal graft following mucous membrane grafting for lid margin keratinization with lid eversion.

Cobalt blue filter enhances the appearance of the Fleischer's ring in keratoconus and is used to view and grade fluorescein staining of the ocular surface (Fig. 11.10).

Red free filter enhances the ischemic areas and helps highlight the areas stained by Rose Bengal.

Intermittent pressure on the globe during examination helps appreciate the presence of Vogt's striae in keratoconus that reappears on releasing the pressure.

Applying pressure to blanch the vessels also helps in differentiating episcleritis from scleritis based on the direction of refilling of the vessels.

A high intensity, high magnification short wide beam in a dark room helps grade anterior chamber flare and cells.

The dimensions of the area of interest can be measured using the slit beam up to a maximum of 8 mm or 14 mm based on the slit-lamp type.

Prior to any contact evaluation, such as the applanation tonometry or gonioscopy, the head of the tonometer and the lens must be cleaned using 2% Bacillocid. The tonometer should be set to 1 in order to avoid causing corneal abrasions.

SLIT-LAMP DOCUMENTATION

The practice of slit-lamp documentation improves biomicroscopic skill, provides an easily reviewed record of the disease's course helps monitor observations and creates a standardized method of notation. It also, in addition, forms an integral part of teaching tool. It is important to indicate corneal pathologic conditions in the patient record by color-coded frontal and slit sketches. Though slit-lamp

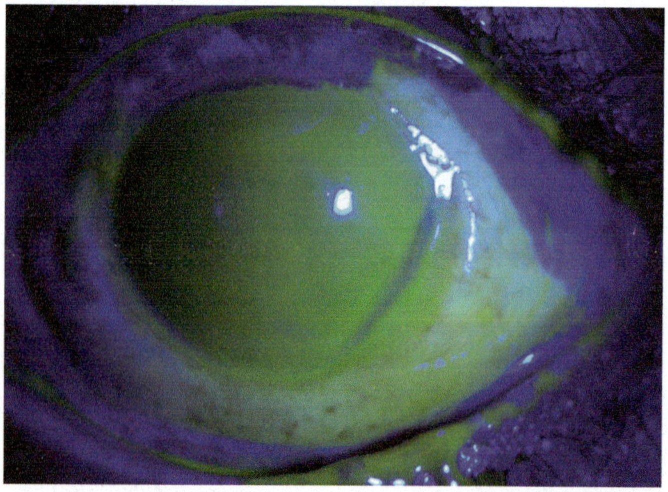

Fig. 11.10: Fluorescein staining of the ocular surface in acute chemical injury.

photography forms an important asset in documenting various findings, it is extremely important to include a detailed color-coded slit-lamp drawing. An approximately 30 mm diameter circle denoting the cornea with a central small brown round pupil and an outline of the upper and lower eyelid is used as a standard template to record slit-lamp findings using the color codes.

- Opacities such as scars and degenerations are drawn in black.
- Epithelial edema is represented by fine blue circles, stromal edema as blue shading and folds in Descemet's membrane as wavy blue lines.
- Hypopyon and corneal infiltrates are shown in yellow.
- Blood vessels are added in red. Superficial vessels are wavy lines that begin outside the limbus and deep vessels are straight lines that begin at the limbus.
- Pigmented lesions such as iron lines and Krukenberg spindles are shown in brown.
- Green is the color used to indicate epithelial defects and lenticular opacities.

ADDITIONAL USES OF THE SLIT LAMP

In addition slit lamp can also be used to assess anterior chamber angle using gonioscopy and measure intraocular pressure by applanation tonometry, and the posterior segment using handheld lenses.

Slit-lamp photography is an important value-addition to the slit lamp biomicroscope that helps capture images and store the same for documentation and future reference (Figs. 11.11A to D). These include in-built and externally attached camera options along with various storage software programs.

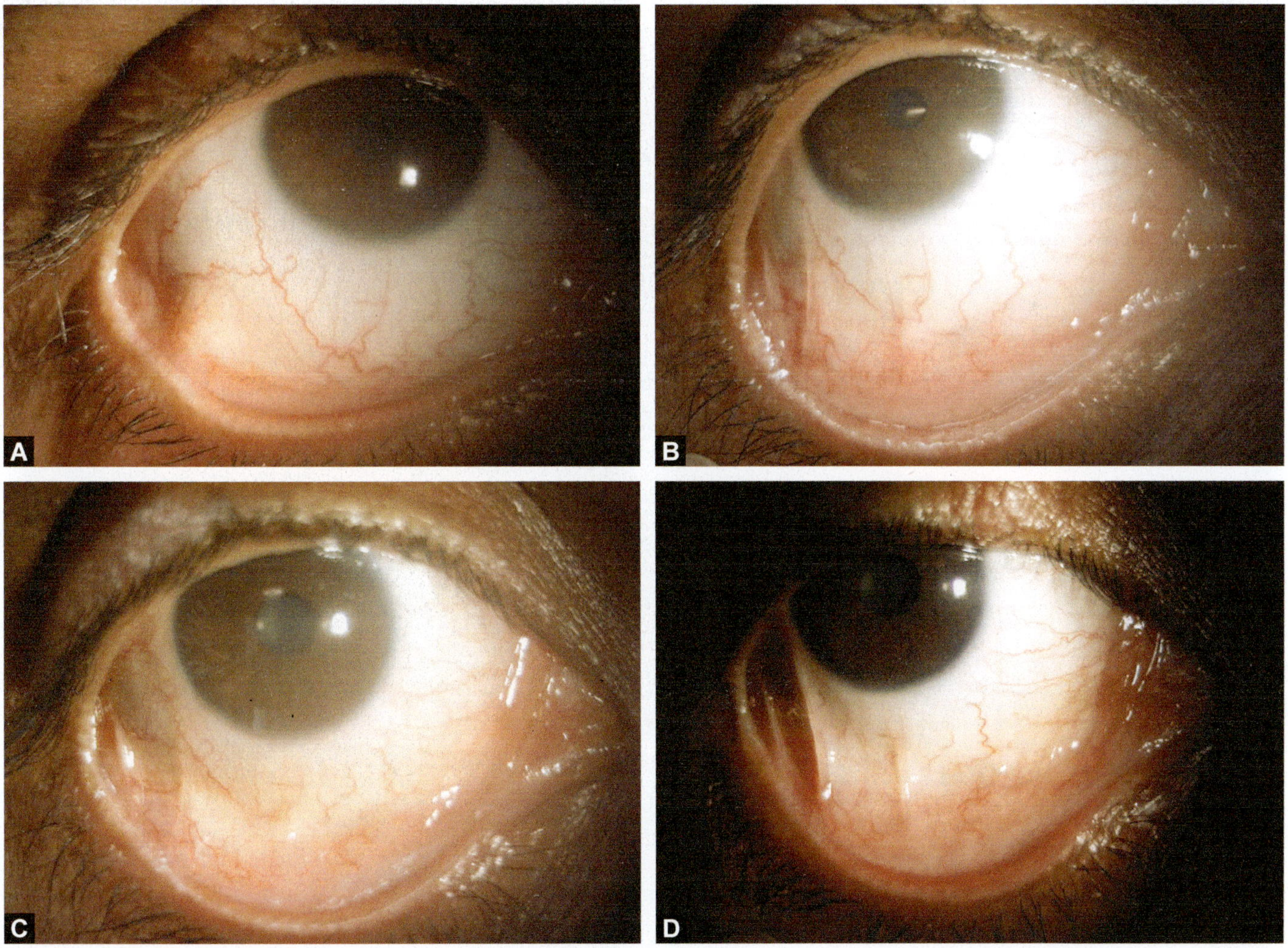

Figs. 11.11A to D: Importance of slit-lamp photography in serial documentation revealing progression of cicatricial changes in ocular cicatricial pemphigoid.

OUTPATIENT ANTERIOR SEGMENT SLIT-LAMP PROCEDURES

Apart from its utility for anterior segment examination, the slit lamp provides a platform for performing several outpatient diagnostic and therapeutic procedures. These include:

- *Manual epilation*: Therapeutic/diagnostic (for *Demodex*)
- Punctal plugs/Occlusion
- Pseudomembrane peeling in conjunctivitis
- Foreign body removal
- Suture removal
- Bandage contact lens removal (following refractive procedures/others)
- *Corneal debridement or scraping*: Diagnostic/therapeutic
- Cyanoacrylate glue application
- Anterior chamber tap—Diagnostic
- Air bubble release post-Descemet's stripping endothelial keratoplasty (DSEK)
- Other minor procedures as deemed appropriate.

CONCLUSION

Anterior segment examination forms the first and most important aspect of ophthalmic evaluation with slit-lamp biomicroscope being an essential tool to diagnose and document abnormalities. A meticulous and sequential examination forms the basis for a thorough investigative approach to several anterior and posterior segment disorders and in certain instances can provide the first sign of an underlying systemic condition.

SUGGESTED READING

1. Berliner ML. Development of biomicroscopy. In: Berliner ML (Ed). Biomicroscopy of the eye. Slit lamp biomicroscopy of living eye. New York: Paul B Holber; 1943.
2. Duke-Elder S, Abrams D. Ophthalmic optics and refraction, Vol V. In: Duke-Elder S (Ed): System of ophthalmology. St Louis: CV Mosby Co.; 1970. p. 30.
3. Henson DB. (1983). Optometric Instrumentation. Chapter 6. Oxford, Boston: Butterworth-Heinemann. [online] Available from: *http://www.worldcat.org/title/optometric-instrumentation/oclc/756480063*. [Accessed Nov, 2017]
4. Mondal B. Slit-Lamp Biomicroscopy in Primary Eye Care. New Delhi: Jaypee Brothers Medical Publishers (P) Ltd, 2013.
5. Sinhota R, Tandon R. Examination of the anterior segment. In: Sinhota R, Tandon R (Eds). Parson's Diseases of the eye. Gurugram, India: Reed Elsevier India Pvt Ltd; 2015.
6. Waring GO, Laibson PR. A systematic method of drawing corneal pathologic conditions.. Arch Ophthalmol. 1977;95 (9):1540-2.

Chapter 12 Clinical Examination of the Posterior Segment

Parag K Shah, VR Saravanan

INTRODUCTION

The posterior segment of the eye comprises of structures situated beyond the posterior capsule of lens and ciliary body and includes the vitreous (anterior and posterior), optic disk and retina (from posterior pole till the ora serrata). A part of this segment comprising of the optic disk and macular region is called as the posterior pole. Three basic techniques, which are useful in examining the posterior segment, are direct ophthalmoscopy, indirect ophthalmoscopy and slit-lamp biomicroscopy. In many instances, a thorough and systematic examination of the posterior segment may lead to the diagnosis of a hitherto undiagnosed systemic disease and hence, it is advisable to perform this examination in each and every patient.

ANATOMICAL LANDMARKS OF NORMAL FUNDUS

A practical understanding of the structures is imperative for a clinician to use these techniques in an optimal fashion. The important components of this segment are discussed here.

Vitreous Humor

It is a clear gel which fills the cavity from the posterior capsule of the lens till the optic disk. Clinically, it can be divided into the anterior vitreous face which is situated just behind the lens and posterior vitreous face which lies just in front of the optic disk. While the anterior face can be visualized with a slit-lamp, the posterior vitreous examination requires the use of additional condensing lenses (78 or 90 D) alongside the slit-lamp. The strongest attachment of the vitreous to the retina is at the vitreous base which is 2 mm anterior to ora serrata and 3–4 mm posterior to it. In addition, the vitreous is also firmly attached to optic disk, fovea, blood vessels, and areas of retinal degenerations. The tight adherence of the vitreous to the underlying retina may be a predisposing factor in several of the acquired retinal diseases such as rhegmatogenous retinal detachment, proliferative diabetic retinopathy, etc.

Posterior Pole

It is defined as the area comprising the optic disk and the macula.

Optic disk: It is pink in color, vertically oval with a size of approximate 1.75 mm vertically and 1.5 mm horizontally. It has a central depression called the physiological cup. Location and size of any retinal lesion can be well described in terms of the optic disk diameter (DD). Due to the complete absence of rods and cones, the optic disk is insensitive to light and corresponds to the blind spot seen in visual fields.[1] In pathological conditions such as papilledema, the nasal margin of the optic disk gets blurred first since the nerve fiber layer is thickest nasally.

Macula: It is an approximately 5.5 mm area just temporal to the disk and is enclosed by the arcade vessels (Fig. 12.1A). It has a yellowish hue due to presence of xanthophyll and hence also called as macula lutea. As compared to the rest of the macula, the nerve fiber layer is the thickest in the papillomacular bundle on optical coherence tomography (OCT) (Fig. 12.1B) and this gives a clue for the reader in determining which eye it is. The central region of the macula is a slightly hyperpigmented area called the fovea which is approximately 1.5 mm in size. OCT evaluation performed in this region depicts the beginning of the typical slope or the foveal dip. This slope is the result of the peripheral displacement of the inner retinal layers (ganglion cell, inner plexiform and inner nuclear layers) leaving only the photoreceptors (cones) in the center. The outer plexiform layer is called the Henle's layer and is arranged obliquely. This oblique arrangement of the Henle's layer is the reason for flower-petal appearance in cystoid macular edema and star configuration of macular hard exudates in conditions such as neuroretinitis and diabetic macular edema. While

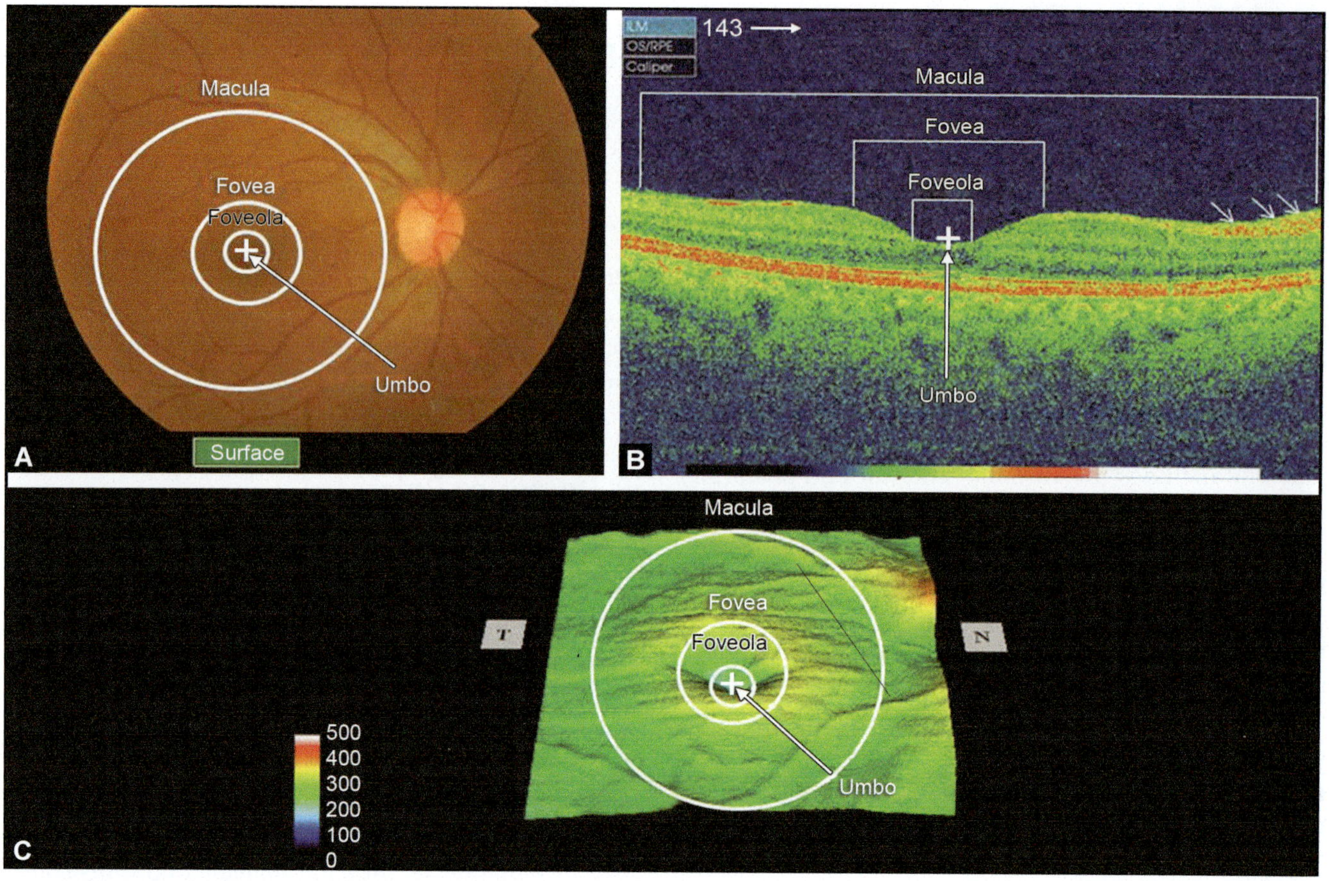

Figs. 12.1A to C: (A) Normal fundus of the right eyes showing the posterior pole consisting of disk, macula and blood vessels. Outermost white circle is the macula which is approximately of 5.5 mm in size. Middle circle is the fovea which is around 1.5 mm and innermost circle is the foveola around 400–500 μm which contains the foveal avascular zone. The central dot seen clinically as foveal reflex is called the umbo depicted as a white cross; (B and C) Two- and three-dimensional OCT scans of the same eye showing the macula, fovea, foveola and umbo (white cross). Small white arrows depict the thick nerve fiber layer in papillomacular bundle.

rods are completely absent in this area, the cones are present in the highest concentration. The center of the fovea is called the foveola which is approximately 400–500 μ in size. This area is avascular and shows up as the foveal avascular zone (FAZ) on fundus fluorescein angiography. The center of the foveola is the thinnest part of the retina (Fig. 12.1C) and is seen as a white dot on ophthalmoscopy known as the foveal reflex (umbo). Clinically, it is situated at the level of inferior disk margin, 2 DD temporally and about 1 mm below horizontal meridian. The foveal pit is present at the bottom of the slope. The normal foveal thickness is around 200 μ on OCT (ranging from 150 μm to 250 μm).

Arteries and veins: The central retinal artery and vein emerge from the optic nerve head, nasal to the physiological cup. It divides into superior and inferior branches, which subdivide into temporal and nasal branches near the optic disk margin. These, then divide dichotomously and supply the entire retina till the ora serrata. Clinically, the arteries are brighter red in color and narrower compared to the veins (A:V ratio being 2:3). The arteries are also less tortuous than veins and may have a white streak running through the center due to reflection of light. Normally, no visible pulsations are seen clinically. While arterial pulsations always indicate a pathology, venous pulsations over the optic disk may be seen in 20% of the normal individuals. These pulsations happen because of the collapse of the venular walls, which happens in systole due to the slight, but sudden, increase in intraocular pressure, as the veins pass through the narrow mesh of the lamina cribrosa.[2] This phenomenon is useful clinically, since the presence of venous pulsation rules out papilledema. Venous pulsations can be increased or made manifest by applying gentle pressure over the globe. This can be easily done with the help of the finger while examining the disk with 90 or 78 D lens on slit lamp. Arterial pulsations are always pathological.

Peripheral Retina

Clinically, it is subdivided into three zones.

- *Near periphery:* 1.5 mm area outside the macula[3,4].
- *Equatorial retina:* This region is present just anterior to the ampulla of the vortex veins which are seen as finger-like projections (Fig. 12.2). It is approximately 4 DD from ora serrata.
- *Peripheral retina:* This region extends from equator to the ora serrata. The posterior border of vitreous base is attached here and hence, most retinal tears occur in this region.
- *Ora serrata:* It is the region between the retina and pars plana, where the vitreous base is attached the strongest. It has a serrated border with retinal projections in between the oral bay called dentate processes which are more prominent nasally (Fig. 12.3). Sometimes, two adjoining dentate processes might join at the tip and this is called an enclosed oral bay which appears like a pseudohole. The base of a pseudohole is brownish in color (similar to ora) in contrast to the red color seen in the base of a true hole.
- *Pars plana:* It is the flat part of the ciliary body, anterior to the ora serrata. It is approximately 3 mm wide nasally and 4 mm temporally. It cannot be seen clinically by an ophthalmoscopic evaluation and its visualization requires the use of specialized instruments like the ultrasound biomicroscope (UBM). This is the surgical space through which intravitreal injections are given and sclerotomies are made for vitrectomy. In adults, the injections and the sclerotomy entries are made 3 mm from limbus in aphakic/pseudophakic eyes and 3.5–4 mm in phakic eyes.

EXAMINATION TECHNIQUES

Direct Ophthalmoscopy

Instrument: It is a handheld device, composed of a handle and head with a viewing aperture. It was invented by von Helmholtz in 1850. A light source is situated at the aperture along with various refractive lenses ranging from +35 D to –40 D. The light source has moved from older conventional light bulbs to xenon halogen bulbs to the latest LED light sources which are brighter and better. The latest rechargeable lithium batteries are also long lasting. Various additional in-built tools which are very useful include, red free and cobalt blue filters, fixation target, normal spot, small spot, D spot, and slit illumination. It is an ergonomically designed instrument where in all these lenses and filters can be easily rotated with the help of a dialer (Fig. 12.4). The direct ophthalmoscope provides an erect virtual image of the retina and gives approximately 15X magnification with a limited field of view of about 5°. Hence it is best suited to examine the area of the posterior pole. As stereopsis is only obtained with binocular vision, the height or depth of a lesion cannot be commented using a direct ophthalmoscope. However using the inbuilt refractive lenses, one can predict the height or depth of a lesion. The bottom of the optic cup is relatively myopic

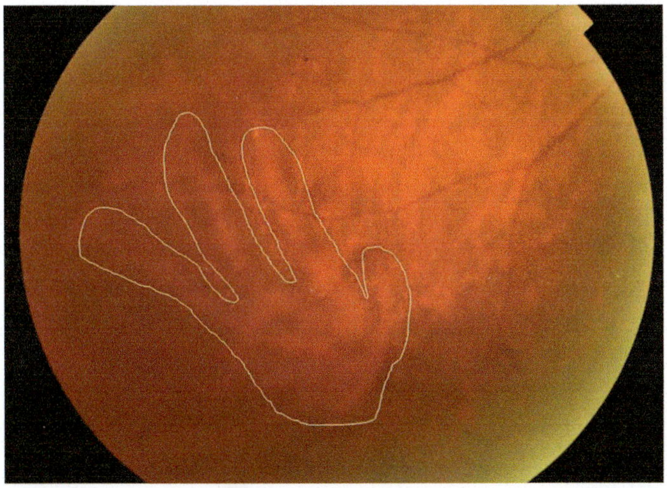

Fig. 12.2: Fundus picture showing the ampulla of the vortex vein which is seen having finger-like projections (white outline).

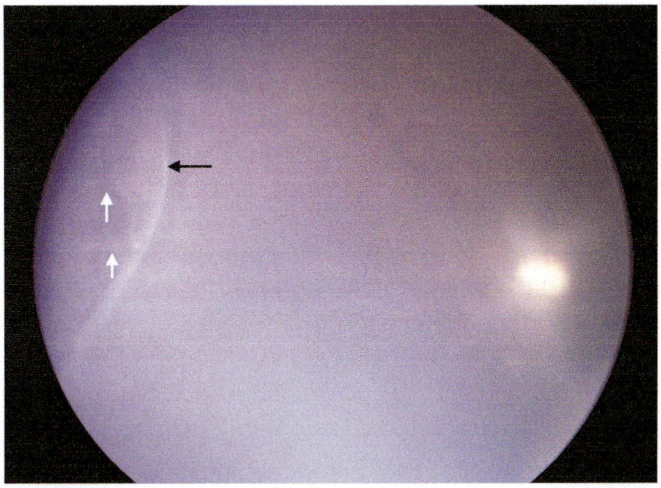

Fig. 12.3: Fundus picture of the extreme nasal periphery showing the dentate processes (white arrows) at the ora serrata. The dome-shaped projection (black arrow) is the scleral indentation effect.

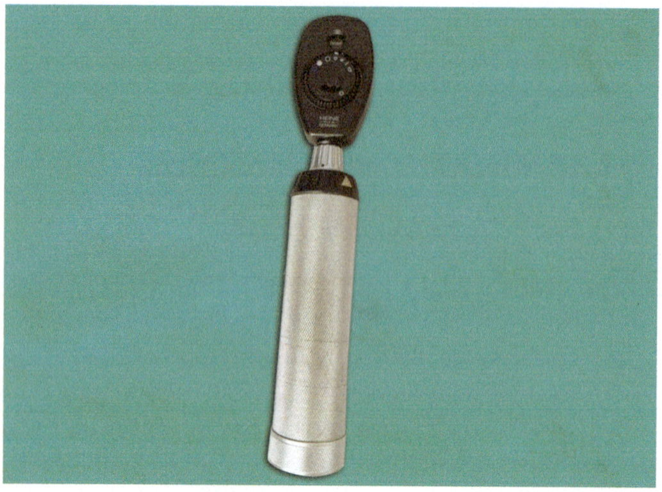

Fig. 12.4: Direct ophthalmoscope.

to the edge. Hence, more concave lenses are required to focus the vessels at the bottom of the cup. A depth of 1 mm corresponds to -3 D lens. Similarly, for an elevated lesion more convex lenses are required to focus. Thus, +3 D lens corresponds to an elevation of 1 mm.[5]

Technique: Examination should be done in a dark or dimly lit room. The patient is asked to look at a distant fixation object. The first step would be to perform a distant direct ophthalmoscopy. From a distance of two feet, the examiner, through the aperture of the ophthalmoscope examines the red glow emanating from the dilated pupil of the patient. The presence of gross opacities in the optical media can be identified by this technique. If the opacities move in the same direction of the eye movement then these opacities are present in front of the anterior lens capsule (e.g. corneal opacity). If the opacities move in the opposite direction of eye movement then these are situated behind the anterior lens capsule (e.g. posterior subcapsular cataract, vitreous opacities).

After completing the distant direct ophthalmoscopy, the examiner moves closer to the eye to be examined. The right eye of the examiner is used for examining the right eye of the patient and the left eye of the examiner is used for examining the left eye of the patient. While the examiner wears his/her refractive glasses on, it is better to ask the patient to remove their glasses as unwanted reflexes will come from their glasses and maximum view of the fundus can be obtained when the examiner is closest to the eye. Inbuilt refractive lenses within the ophthalmoscope can be used to adjust for the patient's refractive error. The patient is asked to continue fixing at the distance and the examiner should also avoid accommodation by keeping both the eyes open while going near to the patient's eye. By moving a little temporal to the patient, the optic disk is focused. The examiner then moves nasally to see the fovea. The nerve fiber layer is seen as thin striations fanning off the optic disk and is better visualized with red free filter. Near peripheral retina can be seen with a little bending by the examiner but equatorial retina and far periphery cannot be examined by direct ophthalmoscopy.

Indirect Ophthalmoscopy

The indirect ophthalmoscope offers the advantage of stereoscopic wide viewing of the central and the peripheral retina. It is called "indirect" because the fundus is viewed indirectly by holding a lens in front of the eye. Christian Ruete devised the first indirect ophthalmoscope using a concave mirror for focusing to enable a wider view of the posterior segment in 1852. Using Gullstrand's principle, Charles Schepens improvised and combined the illumination and bioscope into a single unit which can be worn on the head. This enabled the examiner to get a wide indirect reversed view of the fundus. This improvisation has stood the test of time and no big change in the design has happened since its invention in 1945.

Instrument: The device consists of a head unit which consists of a set of binocular lenses with an illumination or light source positioned above and in between the binoculars forming a triangle. Like the direct ophthalmoscope, now most indirect ophthalmoscopes also come with either xenon halogen or LED light source. Technology has moved the conventional plugin wired indirect to wired indirect with pocket transformers to totally wireless indirect with rechargeable lithium batteries. Teaching mirror attachment is also available in some models (Fig. 12.5). This unit is held in position with headbands with tightening screws to hold them in place. Lighter spectacle mounted indirect ophthalmoscope is also currently available. The binoculars and a set of plane mirrors help to effectively alter the interpupillary distance (IPD) from approximately 55 mm (varies according to the examiners IPD) to 15 mm thereby enabling simultaneous stereoscopic view of the fundus through the pupil (Fig. 12.6). Without this adjustment, simultaneous binocular viewing through the pupil would be impossible due to the small size of the pupil and wide separation of the eyes. The illumination is positioned slightly above the midpoint of the eyes according to Gullstrand's principle, to prevent reflection from the various refracting surfaces.

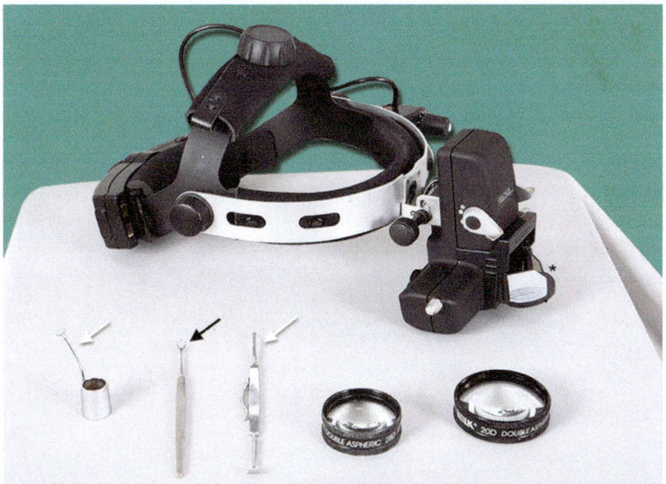

Fig. 12.5: Indirect ophthalmoscope with thimble and Schocket scleral depressors (white arrows), wire vectis (black arrow) used for ROP screening and 20 and 28 D lenses. Teaching mirror is also attached (asterisk).

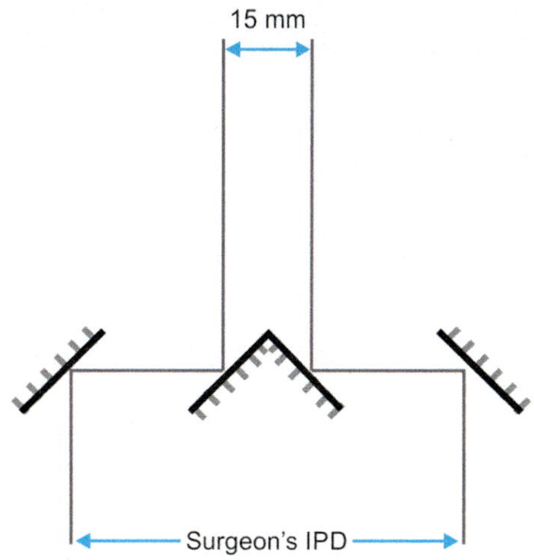

Fig. 12.6: Schematic diagram showing the plane mirror arrangements in an indirect ophthalmoscope.
(IPD: Interpupillary distance)

The second part of the device is the condensing lens which is held in the examiner's hand, a few inches from the patient's eye. The light rays emanating from the patient's eyes are divergent due to the refraction occurring at the cornea. The condensing lens captures this light and helps to focus them by converging and producing an indirect but real inverted and laterally reversed image between the lens and the examiner. The usual power of the condensing lens is +20 D. But the condensing lens is available in various powers ranging from +14 D to +30 D, +28 D being popular for the pediatric use. The viewing distance, field of view and magnification depend upon the power of the condensing lens used. A 20 D lens gives a 45° field of view and a magnification of 3X. As the power of the lens increases, field of view increases but magnification decreases. Hence for 14 D, 28 D and 30 D lenses, field of view is 40°, 47°, 50° and magnification is 4X, 2.27X, 2X respectively.[6] However, with the increase in power of the lens, the stereopsis decreases. Thus, stereopsis is best for +14 D lens and worst for 28 D lens.

The field of illumination is usually available in three levels, small, medium and large (Fig. 12.7A). Large field examinations have an obvious advantage of viewing a wider area of retina but they also produce the maximum amount of unwanted reflection. On the other hand, the smallest field enables to view clearly through media opacities such as cataract, asteroid hyalosis and small pupil. Newer indirect ophthalmoscopes also have continuous variation of field of illumination allowing the examiner, the choice of his/her field. There are two color filters available: the red-free (green) filter (which enables high contrast imaging of blood, blood vessels etc.) and a cobalt blue filter (which may be used to do fluorescein angioscopy of the peripheral retina, though the contrast of the image seen is poor owing the level of illumination and the absence of barrier filter). A diffuser is also available to spread and decrease the level of illumination and is useful for patients who have extreme photophobia (Fig. 12.7B).

Technique: The head unit is worn in such a way that the horizontal band is positioned just above the brow (Fig. 12.8A). The horizontal and vertical tightening screws are adjusted to obtain a snug and a comfortable fit. The knob that connects the binoculars to the headband is loosened and the binoculars are adjusted so that they are at the pupillary level. It is also tilted a little toward the surgeon's face rather than maintain a perpendicular orientation to the line of vision (Fig. 12.8B). The interpupillary distance of the examiner is adjusted to the desired measurement by focusing at an object at an arm's length. The illumination is adjusted so that it is a little above the center of the observation field to minimize reflections. The desired field of illumination is then set and the desired filter is also chosen if required. The level of illumination can also be adjusted using the rheostat (Fig. 12.9).

The pupil should ideally be dilated to the maximum to get a clear view of the peripheral retina. The examination can be done with the patient in either the sitting or lying position. While the sitting position is enough for a cursory screening, the examination of the peripheral retina is achieved well when the patient is examined in a lying position. The bed of the patient should ideally be at the hip level of the examiner to enable comfortable examination.

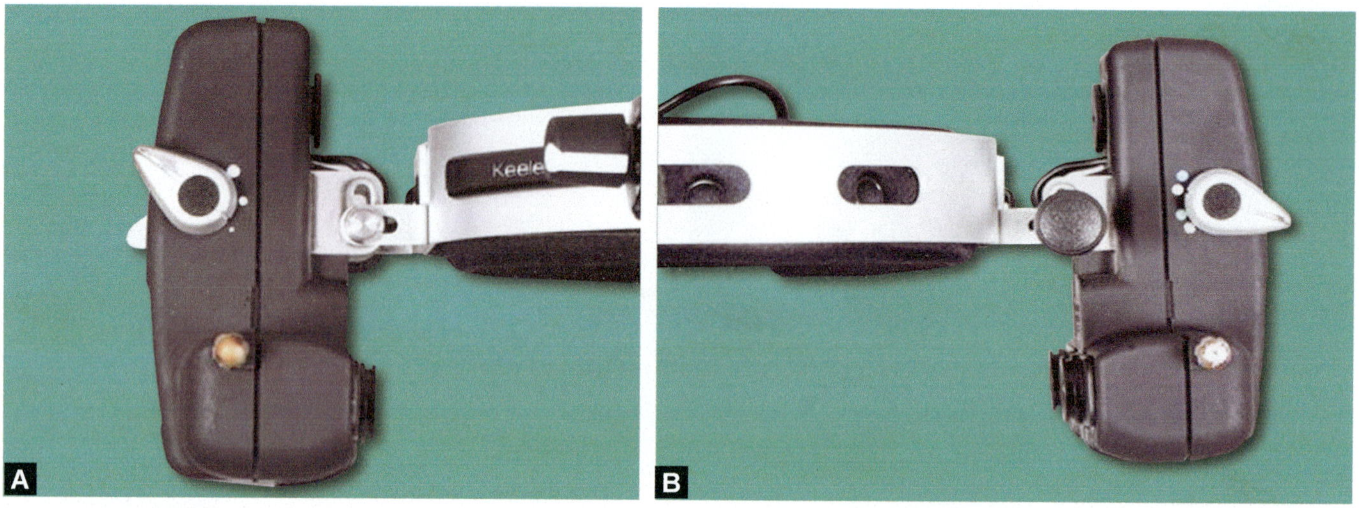

Figs. 12.7A and B: (A) The field of illumination of the three levels—small, medium and large can be adjusted by turning the knob as shown; (B) Knob used to change the filters from blue to green and to diffuse illumination.

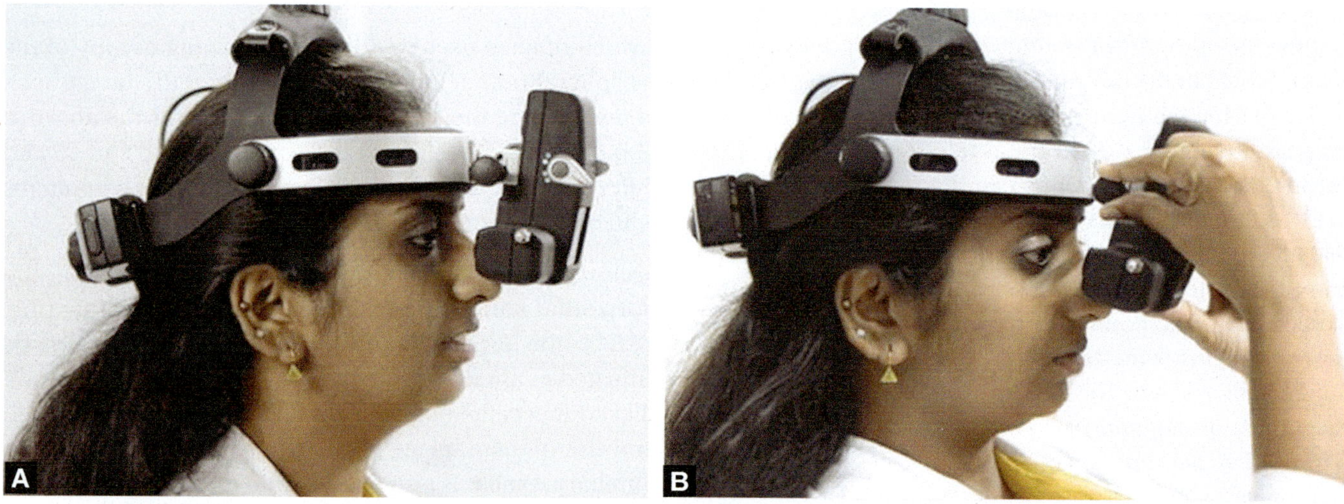

Figs.12.8A and B: (A) Photograph showing placement of head unit which is worn with the band positioned just above the brow; (B) Adjustment of the overhead binoculars to the pupillary level.

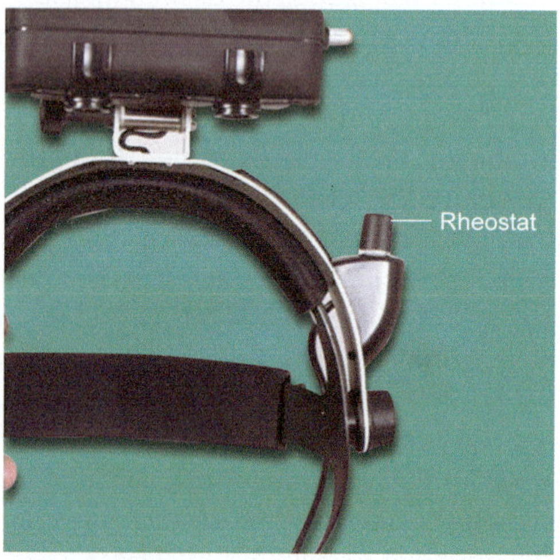

Fig. 12.9: Photograph showing rheostat to adjust the illumination.

When performing indirect ophthalmoscopy, alteration in the movements should be at the hip level of the examiner rather than at the neck. This helps to maintain the head-neck-torso axis to enable dynamic viewing of various quadrants of the retina without losing view of the eye. Even small movements at the neck level will make the examiner to lose the field of interest. The condensing lens is held between the thumb and index finger, while the ring finger or the middle finger rests on some part of the patient's face to provide a balance (Fig. 12.10A). This helps to hold the lens in position without wobbling and also pivot the lens, so that it always faces the examiner as he leans sideways to examine various quadrants of the retina. Holding the lens in midair causes excessive movement with consequent loss of visibility, whenever the lens moves. Resting the palm

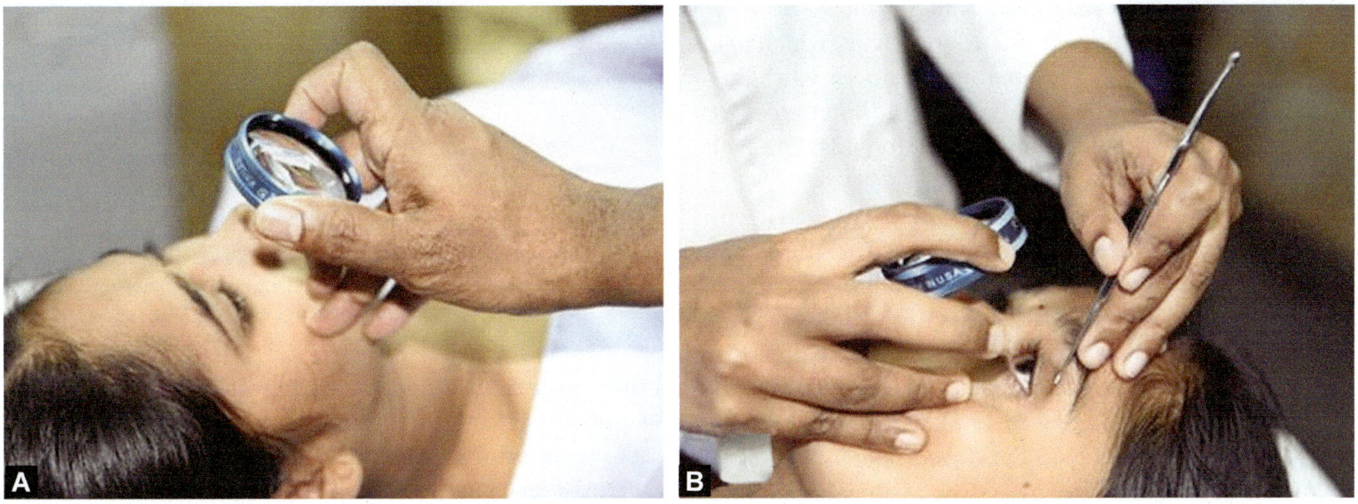

Figs. 12.10A and B: (A) Correct way of holding the indirect lens; (B) Use of scleral depressor.

on the patient's face will hamper adequate movement to achieve the proper focal length. The indirect lenses are plano-convex and the plano surface should always face the patient. To identify this easily, the rim of the plano surface is white in color. The image is distorted if the lens held vice versa.

When examining an indirect image, it is easy for beginners to get confused as to which quadrant of the retina is being examined. It is important to remember that the quadrant which is being aimed is the quadrant being examined. For example, if the examiner is standing at the patient's leg end and aiming at his head end, he is seeing the superior quadrant. But the lesions seen in that particular quadrant appear upside down due to inversion happening at the condensing lens.

There is no particular sequence on how to go about examining the various quadrants of the retina. One can start from the posterior pole and move on to the periphery or vice versa. It is advisable for the examiners to develop their own sequence and also to practice it consistently on each patient to avoid missing any particular part of the retina. For uncooperative patients, it is best to tell them to outstretch their hand with their fist closed and the thumb outstretched. Moving the thumb in the desired direction will help the examiner to navigate the patient's eye in the clock hour being examined (Fig. 12.11). When examining the retinal periphery, examination should be done in a way to overlap two adjacent quadrants to prevent missing out lesions in between the two quadrants.

While examining the peripheral retina, it should be remembered that stereoscopic three-dimensional view may not be possible. When the eye is rotated eccentrically, the pupil is no longer round. It appears as an oval shape to the examiner. So, if the examiner maintains the face on position (as during posterior pole examination), the illumination falls outside the pupil presenting a dark fundus. The examiner should tilt his neck in opposite direction in order to direct the light into the oval pupil to enable uniocular but clear view of the periphery. It should also be noted that owing to the oval shape of the pupil, half the field appears dark during examination of the peripheral retina.

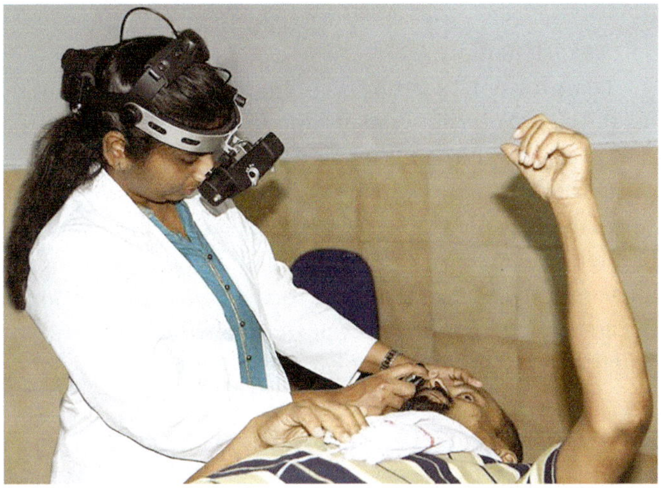

Fig. 12.11: Navigating patients eye using his outstretched hand and thumb in the clock hour to be examined.

Scleral depression: Scleral depression is an integral part of indirect ophthalmoscopy.[7] It serves two functions, namely:

1. It pushes peripheral parts of retina and pars plana into the field of examination.

2. It enables the examination of the retina in profile. It helps to see the retina from various angles, which helps the examiner to assess whether a lesion is elevated or excavated. This is more pertinent in the context that stereoscopic examination may not be possible while viewing the extreme periphery.

It also helps to enhance viewing areas of vitreous traction. Scleral depressors commonly used are the thimble depressor and schocket depressor (for adults) (*see* Fig. 12.5) and Flynn depressor (wire vectis) for retinopathy of prematurity screening in neonates. To examine an area of the periphery, the patient is asked to look at the opposite quadrant first. The depressor is placed preferably over the lid at the lid crease and depressed tangentially to the globe (*see* Fig. 12.10B). Depressing in a vertical orientation is avoided as this is more painful to the patient. Also, the orbital margins act like a fulcrum and push the tip of the depressor anteriorly when the depressor is handled in a vertical orientation.

Learning how to perform a proper depression is an art by itself. The process does not produce a color change in all the retinal areas. Whitening appears only in areas of white with pressure. Normally a small raised mound is visible at the site of depression. If this mound is not seen, it indicates that the depressor is not in the right quadrant. It may be in the adjacent quadrant or it may be too anterior or posterior to the area being examined. The position can then be corrected and the examination can be proceeded with.

Indirect Slit-lamp Biomicroscopy

Instrument: A slit-lamp is required along with a handheld condensing lens. The condensing lenses are either noncontact or contact. Noncontact lenses usually used are +78 D or +90 D. Indirect slit-lamp biomicroscopy uses the same principle of indirect ophthalmoscopy, where a real inverted and laterally reversed image is formed between the examiner and lens. The magnification is 7.5X and field of view is 40° (when 90 D lens is used) while it is 10X and 30° (when a 78 D lens is used). Magnification can be further increased by shifting from 10X to the 16X slit-lamp magnification. Thus, higher the power of lens, smaller the image size but larger the field of view. The 90 D lens is more popular than 78 D. It is mainly used to see the posterior pole. A unique advantage over the direct ophthalmoscope is the ability of obtaining a good stereopsis and the height and depth of lesions can be very well judged.

The Contact lens most commonly used is the Goldmann three mirror lens. It contains a central lens (–64 D) for posterior pole examination and three mirrors at different angles (59°, 67° and 73°) to view the mid periphery, periphery and the anterior chamber angle, respectively (Fig. 12.12). Other contact lenses available are the panfundoscopic lens, which is used mainly for laser photocoagulation.

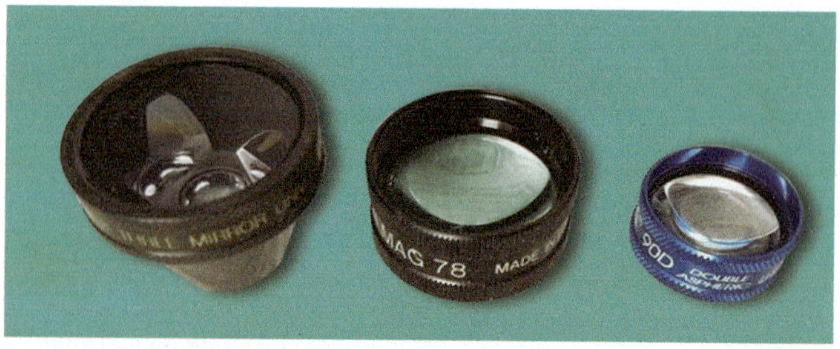

Fig. 12.12: Goldmann 3 mirror contact lens (left), 78 D noncontact lens (center) and 90 D noncontact lens (right).

Technique:

Noncontact method: Like direct and indirect ophthalmoscopy, fundus examination by slit-lamp microscopy should be carried out in a dimly lit room. While dilatation is ideal for a complete evaluation, this technique can be performed through a reactive pupil as well. The patient should be sitting comfortably with the chin resting on the chin rest. The forehead should touch the headband and if the patient is not cooperative then light pressure can be applied by the assistant behind the patient's head to keep it in place. The height of the chin rest should be adjusted so that the eyebrows come at the level of the marker. Examiner should be seated at a comfortable height and patient's right eye is examined by examiner holding the lens in left hand and vice versa. The lens rim is held between the thumb and the index finger with the elbow resting on the slit-lamp table. Most lenses are biconvex and hence any side can be used to examine the fundus. In case, they are plano-convex then again the white rim which signifies the plano surface, should face the patient. The patient should be told to look straight and fix at the examiner's ear. Some slit lamps have a fixation light which can be used. The illumination should be kept at the minimum and the vertical slit-lamp beam narrow. The beam is kept at an angle of 10–15° to get the maximum stereopsis. Wide beam hampers the image quality and stereopsis. Green filter can be used for better visualization of nerve fiber layer. A mild anterior defocusing from the optic disk using a narrow beam brings the posterior hyaloid to a focus. The movement of the vitreous can be appreciated by asking the patients to move their eyes. The inflammatory cells in the posterior hyaloid (such as in cases of optic neuritis) can be visualized by using higher magnification and reducing the height of the narrow beam.

Table 12.1: Comparison between direct ophthalmoscopy, indirect ophthalmoscopy, and indirect slit-lamp biomicroscopy.

Parameters	Direct ophthalmoscopy	Indirect ophthalmoscopy (using 20 D lens)	Indirect slit-lamp biomicroscopy (using 90 D lens)
Image	Virtual, erect	Real, inverted	Real, inverted
Magnification	15X	3X	7.5X
Field of view	5°	45°	40°
Stereopsis	Absent	Present	Present
Portability	Portable	Portable	Not portable
Uses	Examination of disk and fovea	Examination of posterior pole and periphery	Examination of posterior pole

Table 12.2: Tips and tricks of direct, indirect and slit-lamp biomicroscopy.

Tips and Tricks		
Direct ophthalmoscope	**Indirect ophthalmoscope**	**Slit-lamp biomicroscope**
• A highly magnified image of lid, lid margins, cornea, anterior chamber, iris and anterior and posterior capsule of lens can be examined using the +10 or +20 D lenses and going close to the patient's eye • Thus, anterior segment also can be viewed with direct ophthalmoscope in a setting where slit lamp is not available • Corneal epithelial defects can be seen by using the cobalt blue filter after using the fluorescein strip • Equatorial retina can be seen by fully dilating the pupil and by asking the patient to gaze in the quadrant to be examined with the examiner bending in opposite direction • Simultaneous red reflex test (Bruckner Test) in infants from three months age at a distance of 2–3 feet, can be used to identify various diseases such as retinoblastoma, Coat's disease, congenital cataracts, strabismus, refractive errors, etc.	• Condensing lens can be used to examine the anterior segment by going close to the eye keeping the lens in position and using it as a magnifying glass • Often ora serrata can be seen without scleral indentation and fully dilated eyes using 28 D lens • Elevated macular lesions such as CSCR are more appreciated using the red-free filter. This filter also helps in seeing the blood vessels especially to see the subtle peripheral avascular zone in Familial Exudative Vitro Retinopathy • Distant indirect ophthalmoscopy is a method of seeing the red eye reflex while focusing the indirect ophthalmoscopy light on the dilated eye without the condensing lens. It is very helpful in pediatric retinal diseases such as retinoblastoma, Coat's disease, etc.	• To appreciate the thickness or depth of a lesion at the macula more clearly, the slit beam can be kept horizontal at 180° (instead of vertical at 90°) but moving the rotating knob above the eyepiece by 90°. Then a horizontal tilt is made by releasing the clip which lies below in the center of the light width changing knob. Using red free filter will further enhance the macular elevations in CSCR • Retina till equator can be seen with eyes fully dilated and asking the patient to look in the direction of examining quadrant

Contact method: Being a contact lens, cornea of the patient is anesthetized using topical anesthetic drops and a coupling gel (methyl cellulose gel) needs to be used. As it is more cumbersome for both, the examiner and the patient, it is less popular than noncontact method for routine fundus examination in an outpatient setting and is mainly used for peripheral laser photocoagulation.

Comparison between direct ophthalmoscopy, indirect ophthalmoscopy and indirect slit-lamp biomicroscopy is shown in Table 12.1. Few tips and tricks of all these three techniques of examination are given in Table 12.2.

FUNDUS RECORDING AND COLOR CODING

Documentation

The findings noted in the examination should be documented on an Amsler-Dubois chart to aid in surgery or for further reference. Charting is particularly essential when a surgical procedure is planned. All the significant features like peripheral retinal degeneration should be integrated along with the extent of the retinal detachment

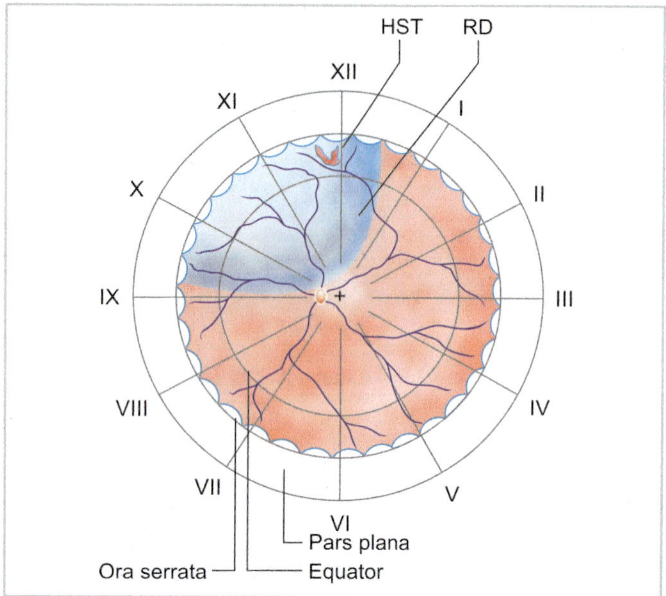

Fig. 12.13: Retinal chart showing fresh rhegmatogenous retinal detachment (RD) with superior horse shoe tear (HST). *Note:* The inner circle on a retinal chart denotes equator, middle circle is the ora serrata, where drawing of retinal vessels should end and the outermost zone is the pars plana, which should be left empty.

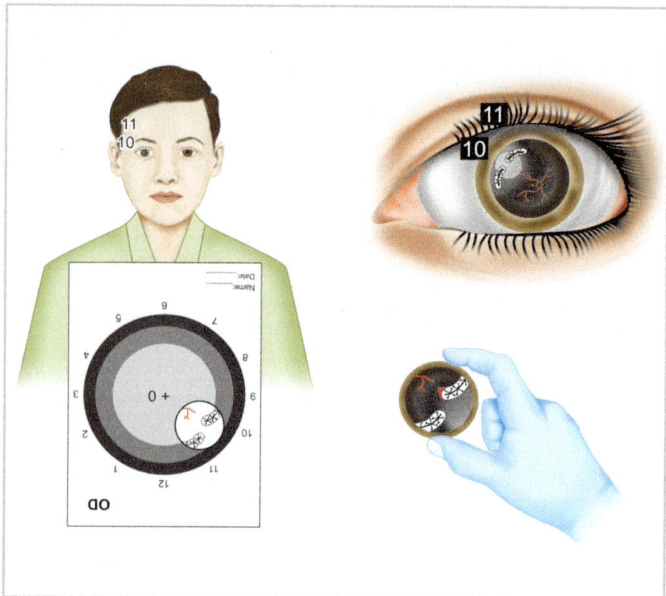

Fig. 12.14: Schematic diagram showing charting of right eye. The lesions seen in 10 and 11'O clock hours should be drawn in the same clock hour and not on the opposite 4 and 5'O clock hours.

to a get a comprehensive overview of the various factors at play (Fig. 12.13).

The chart is placed inversely oriented in relation to the patient. This is done, so that the lesions seen can be directly drawn onto the chart, without putting a mental effort to reinvert and draw. When viewing peripheral lesions, these should be drawn diametrically opposite to the quadrant being examined because any lesion viewed closer to the examiner is in the far periphery. A common mistake done by the beginners is that they tend to draw the lesions in the opposite clock hour, e.g. 12 O'clock lesions are drawn at 6 O'clock and vice versa. The lesions should be drawn on the clock hour being examined, 12 O'clock periphery lesions will remain at 12 O'clock and one should not draw lesions at 6 O'clock periphery in the chart. On an inverted chart, the lesions are drawn diametrically opposite to the quadrant being examined (which is the actual clock hour being examined) (Fig. 12.14).

The examiner then moves around the patient to view the entire 360° periphery noting down findings. The various retinal lesions are depicted in Figure 12.15. Recently direct and indirect ophthalmoscopy, virtual reality simulators have been developed that can give a highly realistic training experience (Figs. 12.16A and B). It can even gauge the pressure applied by the examiner and even gives hints and tips on where the examiner is going wrong. It can also be connected to a web based online teaching and monitoring module.[8] For practice of indirect ophthalmoscopy, special plastic eyes with replaceable thin retinal films (Fig.12.17A and B) have been developed.[9,10]

CONCLUSION

Examination of the posterior segment is an integral part of a holistic ocular examination. To get the best results the patient has to be fully dilated. Direct ophthalmoscopy is mainly used to examine the disk and fovea because of its restricted field of view. However, it is the most portable and handy instrument to use after a torchlight examination of the anterior segment. Fundus examination using indirect slit-lamp biomicroscopy is ideally used after finishing the slit-lamp examination of the anterior segment. It is mainly used to examine the disk and macula and a big advantage over direct ophthalmoscopy is that it has stereopsis. Indirect ophthalmoscopy is best suited to examine the periphery and gives a "bird's-eye view" of the entire fundus. It concludes the total eye examination.

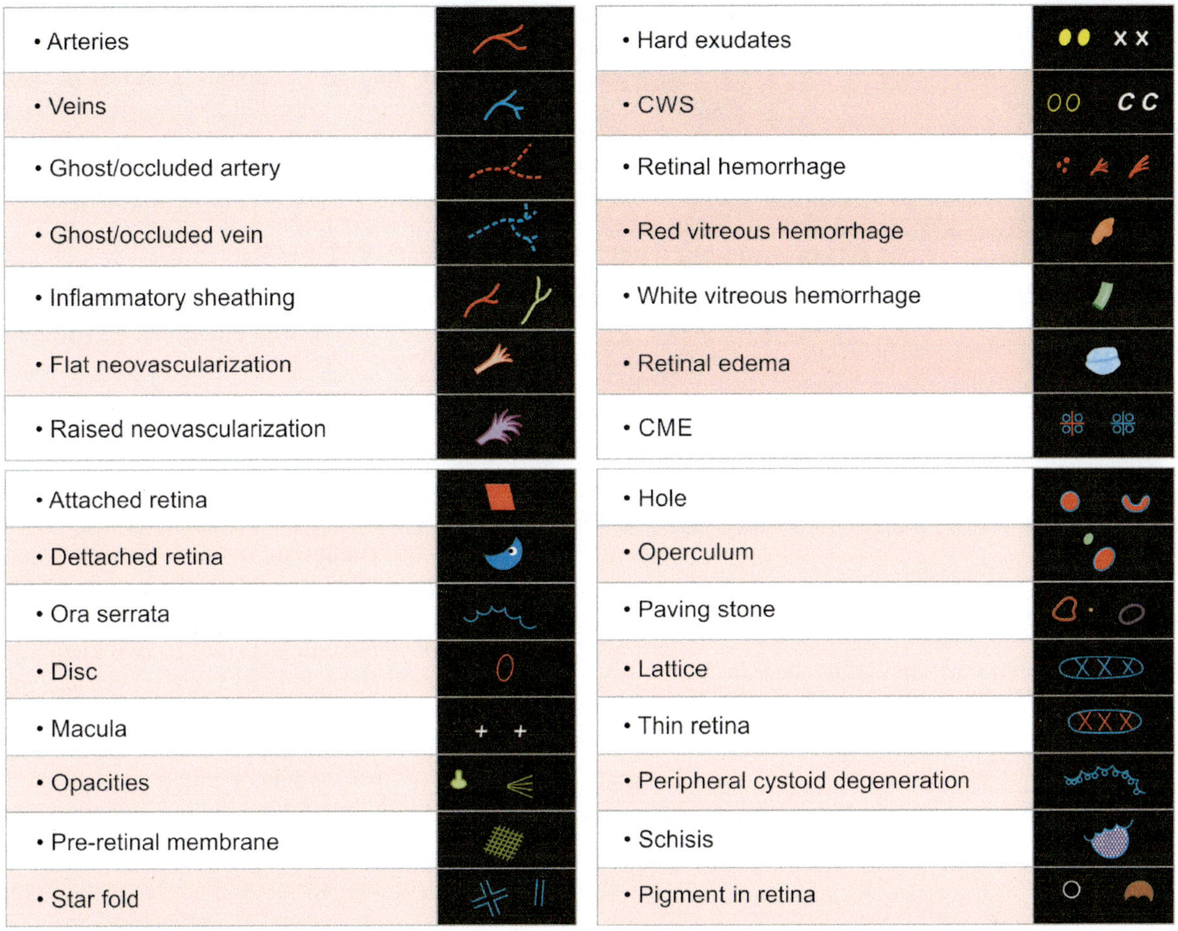

Fig. 12.15: Diagrammatic representation of various retinal lesions while documenting the fundus drawing.
(CWS: Cotton-wool spots; CME: Cystoid macular edema)

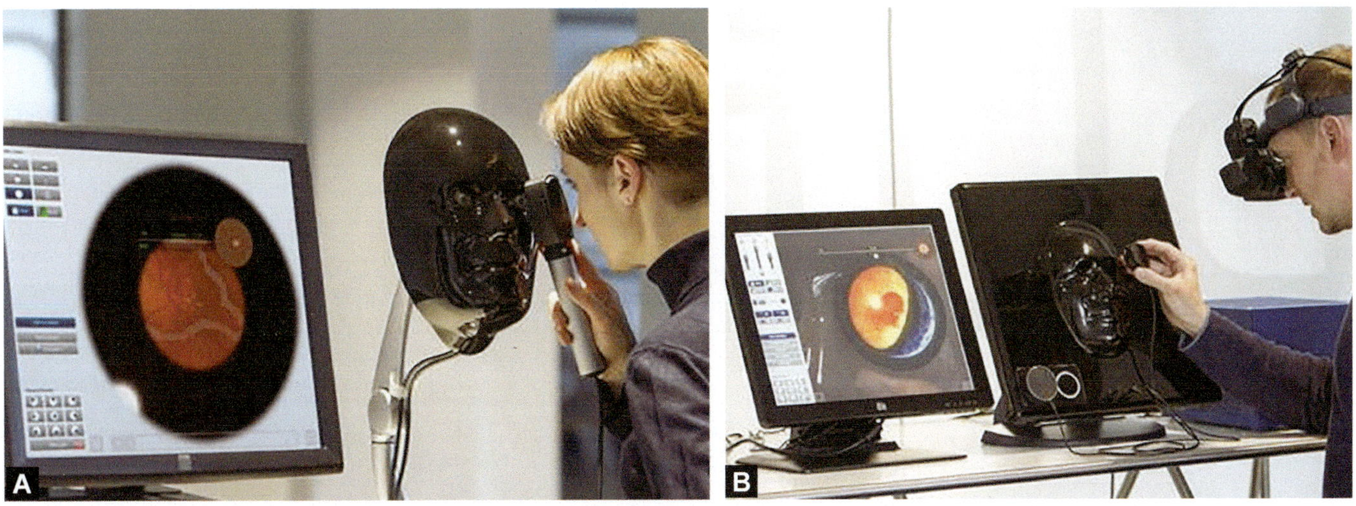

Figs. 12.16A and B: Direct and indirect ophthalmoscopy virtual reality simulators (by VRmagic Holding AG, Mannheim, Germany).

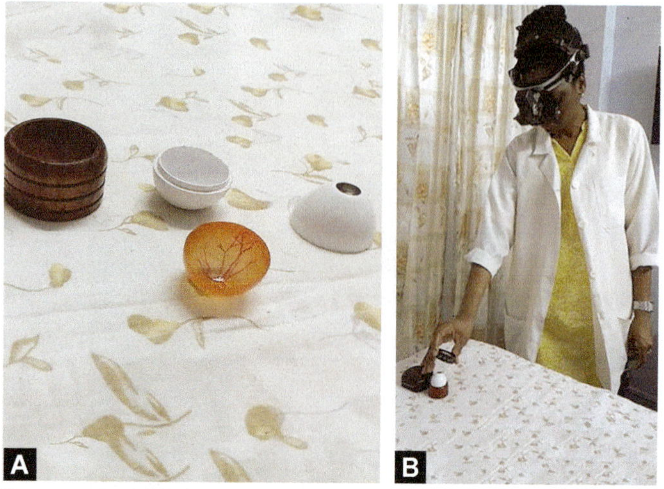

Fig. 12.17A and B: Special plastic model eye (Retieye, Aurolab, Madurai, India) with replaceable thin retinal films for practice of indirect ophthalmoscopy and laser.

REFERENCES

1. Wilson FM. Posterior segment examination. In: Blomquist PH (Ed). Practical Ophthalmology: A Manual for Beginning Residents, 7th edition. San Francisco: American Academy of Ophthalmology; 2015. pp. 229-74.
2. Snell RS, Lemp MA. The Eyeball. Clinical Anatomy of The Eye, 2nd edition. Hoboken, New jersey, United States: Wiley-Blackwell; 1998. pp. 132-214.
3. Snell RS, Lemp MA. The fundus oculi. Clinical Anatomy of the Eye, 2nd edition. Malden: Blackwell Science; 2013.
4. Sihota R, Tondon R. Parsons' Diseases of the Eye, 18th edition. London. Churchill Livingstone, 1990. pp. 103-5.
5. American Academy of Ophthalmology. Basic anatomy. In: Retina and Vitreous, Basic and Clinical Science Course 2016–2017. San Francisco: American Academy of Ophthalmology; 2016. pp. 8.
6. Khurana AK, Khurana I. Retina, visual pathway and physiology of vision. Anatomy and Physiology of Eye, 2nd edition. New Delhi: CBS Publishers & Distributors; 2008. pp. 139-270.
7. Miller SJ. Examination of the fundus. Parsons' Diseases of the Eye, 18th edition. London: Churchill-Livingstone; 1990. pp. 87-101.
8. Goldbaum MH, Joondeph H, Huamonte FU, et al. Retinal examination and surgery. In: Peyman GA, Sanders DR, Goldberg MF (Eds). Principles and Practice of Ophthalmology. New Delhi: Jaypee Brothers Medical Publishers (P) Ltd.; 1987. pp 988-1097.
9. Review of Ophthalmology. (2012). Two 21st Century Ways to Practice Surgery (Kent C). [online] Available from *https://www.reviewofophthalmology.com/article/two-21st-century-ways-to-practice-surgery*. [Accessed November, 2017]
10. Aurolab. (2016). Retieye. [online] Available from *http://www.aurolab.com/retieye_rp.asp*. [Accessed November, 2017]

Part 3 Optics and Refraction

Joseph M Miller

OUTLINE

Chapter 13 Optics of Clinical Refraction

Joseph M Miller

INTRODUCTION

First, light came from the sun, moon, stars and flames; later, light came from electricity; now, light comes from lasers and light-emitting diodes. At all times, the study of light has fascinated mankind. We study ophthalmology because we choose to work to preserve sight, the sense of light. We study optics because it gives us the tools to manipulate light, and shape it for our patients. With optics, we can refine the sight of our patients - through spectacles, contact lenses, intraocular lenses, and through the use of light as a surgical tool, perform laser surgery. This chapter will teach some of the principles of optics as they apply to refraction, and to explain the process of correcting refractive error through eyeglasses, contact lenses, intraocular lenses, and corneal refractive surgery.

LIGHT WAVES

A wave is a phenomenon that transfers energy from one place to another. Light waves transfer energy in a three-dimensional electromagnetic wave, but it is more familiar to start with a discussion of mechanical waves. In a pool of water, the wave generated by a dripping spigot expands radially and transfers the energy of the falling drop of water into the expanding circle of predominantly up and down motion of the surface of the water. Any little object floating atop the water largely moves up and down as a wave passes (the wave largely moves the water up and down, not radially, and so the object bobs). The water is the medium through which the energy of the wave travels, but the energy of the wave moves particles of water up and down, transferring the energy in the direction perpendicular to the up and down motion of the individual water particles. Each drop from the spigot creates a new impulse that sends out a radiating, expanding circular wave. The interval from one drop to the next defines the frequency at which a wave will pass a point on the surface of the water (Fig. 13.1).

Light waves are three-dimensional, and composed of an oscillating electromagnetic field (think radio waves). Unlike mechanical waves, electromagnetic radiation is created by vibrating electrically charged particles (electrons or protons). Electromagnetic waves can pass through a vacuum (and do so most readily at the speed of light) and can also pass through physical matter via a somewhat time-consuming process. When electromagnetic radiation encounters an atom, the atom absorbs the energy, causing the atom to vibrate at the frequency of wave that struck it. The vibration creates another electromagnetic wave. The energy of the wave is radiated and absorbed by the next atom down the line. This is why light travels more slowly when it passes through something other than a vacuum: the energy is absorbed by an atom, the atom vibrates a bit, and gives off radiation at the same frequency at which it was excited. This slows the light down. The more stuff, the greater the optical density, and the slower the rate of transmission (Fig. 13.2).

Frequency versus Wavelength

When the energy is absorbed and reradiated, the frequency of the electromagnetic wave (the number of oscillations of the electromagnetic field per second) does not change. However, depending upon the material, how far radiation can travel per unit time does change with the material that it is passing through—the greater the optical density of the material, the more atoms the wave interacts with, and the less distance the wave can travel per unit time.

The difference between frequency and wavelength is important to keep in mind when thinking about light in ophthalmic optics, for the frequency of the light is what determines what color the light appears to be. The easiest way to keep this straight is to remember that the color of the light does not change as it passes through vacuum, air or water; the frequency does not change, but as the light passes through different materials, it does so at different

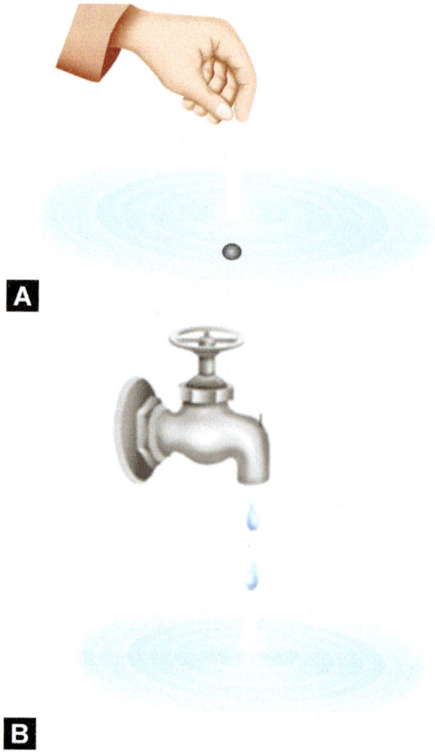

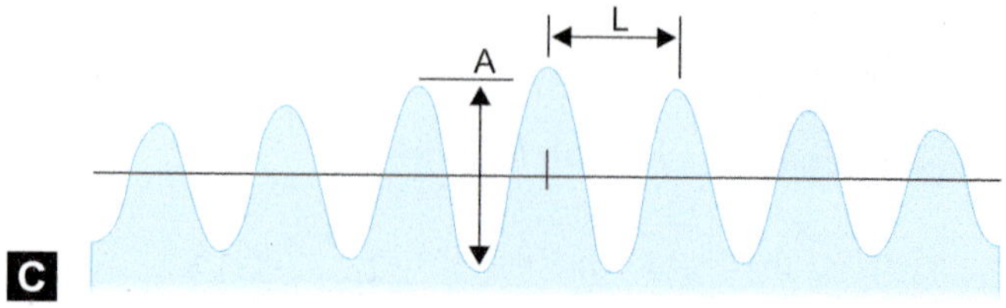

Figs. 13.1A to C: (A) When a pebble is dropped into a pool of water, the energy transferred by the falling pebble to the water sets up a series of waves that radiate from the center of impact. Even though only a single pebble was dropped, a series of waves are created and radiate outward. The distance between the crest of each wave is the same, but the height of each crest decreases with the distance from the point of impact. The waves produced by a single dropped pebble will eventually fade away. (B) A leaky faucet will drip water at a rate that periodically imparts energy to the pool of water underneath. If the drip rate is properly timed, the waves will continually be produced as long as the drops continue. (C) The waves are seen in cross section. The greatest amplitude is at the center of the concentrically radiating waves. While the wavelength (L, the distance between the crests of the waves) is a constant, the amplitude (A, the height between adjacent crest and trough) declines with the distance from the center. The same amount of energy is present in each concentric wave, but as the circumference of each wave increases, the amplitude of the wave at that radial distance decreases, keeping the total energy constant.

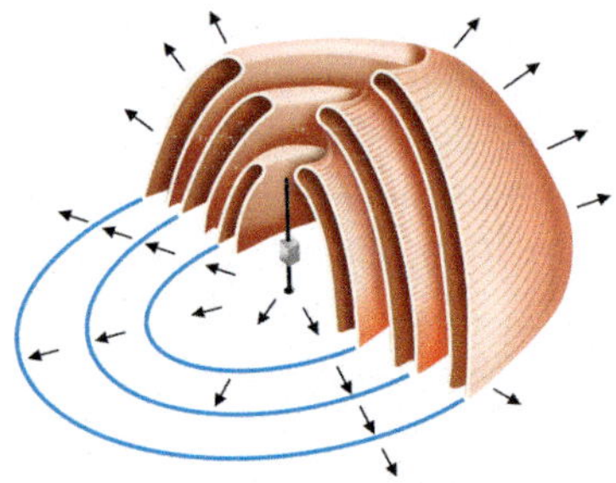

Fig. 13.2: Electromagnetic radiation in 3 dimensions. Electromagnetic radiation (e.g. radiowaves, or light) is created by a charged particle oscillating back and forth along the line of a radiator, or antenna. The electromagnetic field that is created by this oscillating particle is radiated in a three dimensional shell of waves. Half of the three-dimensional shell is shown. The radiation of light from a point source results in a spherical set of electromagnetic waves whose wavelength does not change, but whose amplitude decreases with distance.

rates of travel. Red light has a lower frequency than green light, which has a lower frequency than blue light.

The wavelength of light (in a vacuum) is related to the frequency, so red light with its low frequency vibration has a longer wavelength than blue light with its higher frequency of vibration and shorter wavelength. Not surprisingly, it takes more energy to make an atom vibrate fast than slow, so there is inherently more energy in higher frequency, shorter wavelength blue light than lower frequency, longer wavelength red light.

Expanding Wavefronts

There are some analogies of water waves that are useful to continue for a while longer. First, consider the amplitude of a wave on the surface of water, expanding from a point where a drip from a leaky faucet occurs. This thought experiment only holds up if you can imagine the drip occurring in the middle of a vast ocean, free of wind that would cause the water to ripple for any reason other than the steady drip... drip... drip of the faucet hanging in the sky. There is no shore anywhere to capture a wave that is generated—it just keeps going forever. This ocean is too big to fit on any planet, for even if the planet were covered completely with water, eventually a wave would travel to the other side of the planet and meet itself. No, this is a flat ocean that just keeps going forever, dead calm and flat other than the ripples that are generated by the steady drip... drip... drip.

Each drip creates a single wave, the leading edge of the wave being the wavefront. The rate of the drip (drips per second) defines the frequency of the wavefront. The height of the spigot determines how far the drop falls before it hits the water, and thus the energy that creates each wave.

Now, what happens right after the drip? The energy from the single falling drop turns into the energy that is in the entire wave. At first, the wave is in a very small portion of the vast ocean, right next to where the drop landed on the water. There is a lot of energy in a wave that has a very small circumference. All that energy causes the wave to be a big wave; big in terms of amplitude (very high to the top, a long distance to the bottom of the wave). As the wave expands outward, the energy of the wave is distributed over a larger and larger distance. As the distance increases, the circumference of the wavefront increases, but the total energy remains constant, so the amplitude of the wave falls as the wavefront expands.

The next step requires a little imagination, asking that you visualize what happens as the distance of the wavefront to the origin of wave increases to infinity. As the distance increases, the amplitude decreases but never goes away, it is always there, just very very small. As the distance increases, the curvature of the wavefront becomes less and less, to the point that when the distance is infinite, the curvature is zero, and the wavefront has changed from being curved to being flat. In two dimensions, the wavefront would describe a line. In three dimensions, the wavefront would describe a plane—a plane wave, arising from a point source at an infinite distance

Unlike drips into infinite oceans on infinite planets with no shores and no wind, light travels through an infinite universe filled with empty space and interesting things like eyeballs. Light can travel through a vacuum—filled with nothing. The vibrating charged atom that creates electromagnetic radiation light creates an expanding, spherical wavefront. A slice through this spherical wavefront (think taking a CT scan of a sphere) produces the two-dimensional set of concentric circles akin to our water drops. The vibration of the charged particle is akin to the periodic drips of water. However, this two-dimensional picture is misleading because it confuses how light travels—as radiation—with how waves in water travel—on the surface, in two dimensions. The recognition that light does not require a medium to travel through in 1887, was one of the great advances of physics, and was the stepping off point for the physics of Einstein (Fig. 13.3).

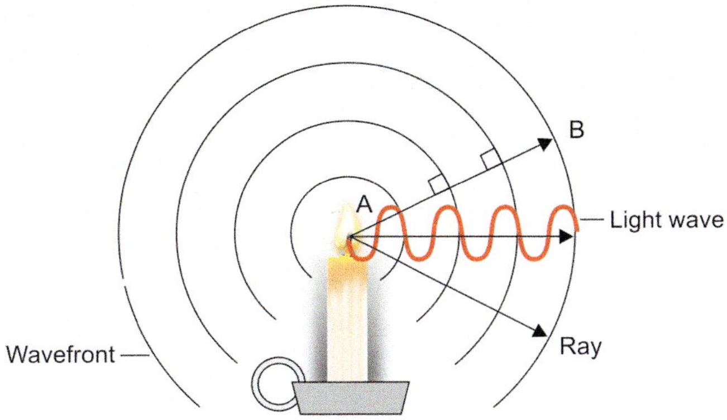

Fig. 13.3: A more familiar point source of light giving off a spherical wavefront is a candle. At each point on the wavefront, a line can be drawn perpendicular to the local wavefront, as shown in B. Each of the perpendicular lines are directed backward to the point of origin. A "Ray" of light is simply a line that is drawn from the point source through a series of wavefronts, intersecting each wavefront perpendicularly.

Wavefront Curvature, Light Rays, and Coherence

An expanding wavefront can be thought of in its entirety (like we have done so far, in thinking about how the entire wavefront expands outward toward infinity), or can be thought of a portion at a time. Any portion of the wavefront remains inexorably connected to all the other portions, as the entire wavefront is linked by the energy that is contained within it. Other than the simplest case of an expanding sphere extending infinitely outward, it becomes more relevant to think of portions of the wavefront, the direction of travel of these portions, and the amount of energy that is present in that portion. This permits us to think of another way of describing how light travels and interacts with matter, through the concept of light rays.

Just as we had to think of wavefront becoming infinitely distant from the point source to see how we can create a plane wave, we now have to think of infinitely small portions of the wavefront to describe the concept of a light ray. A light ray represents the direction of travel of an infinitely small portion of a wavefront of light. If every wavefront that comes from our vibrating charged particle is exactly the same, then at some point in space, every wavefront that passes through that point is moving in the same direction. The direction of travel is perpendicular to this infinitely small portion of the wavefront.

This definition is a little deceptive because in the real world, not every wavefront is the same. There may be variation in the frequency of the vibrating charged particle, and the contents of space that the wavefronts pass through may change over time, causing the distance from one wavefront to the next to vary. Such changes would cause variation within and between wavefronts.

Spatial coherence is the term used to describe similarity of portions of a single wavefront across space (all portions of a single wavefront were created at the same time).

Temporal coherence is the term used to describe how similar a corresponding portion of one wavefront is to the next across time. Coherence is an important concept because it is related to the ability of waves to interact with each other, either adding together to become a larger amplitude wave, or to cancel each other out. These concepts become important in describing such phenomenon as laser light, interference patterns, and antireflection coatings, but this is as far as we go in this chapter with respect to coherence and interference.

REFRACTION AND HUYGENS' PRINCIPLE (FIG. 13.4)

The ability of light waves to interact with each other constructively and destructively is explained by Huygens' principle that explains how the waves propagate in time. At any instant in time, every point on a wavefront serves as a point source for a new spherical wavefront that propagates for an instant in time. The wavefront at any given instant is defined by the envelope of wavefronts created from all points on the wave created the prior instant in time. This principle can be used to explain such phenomenon as why shadows are not absolutely black and white, and how light bends around corners to light up a room. Right now, it is important to explain how light rays change direction when the light passes from one material to another, across an interface that separates material of one optical density from another. This is the process of refraction, and explains how lenses and prisms work, and is something called Snell's Law.

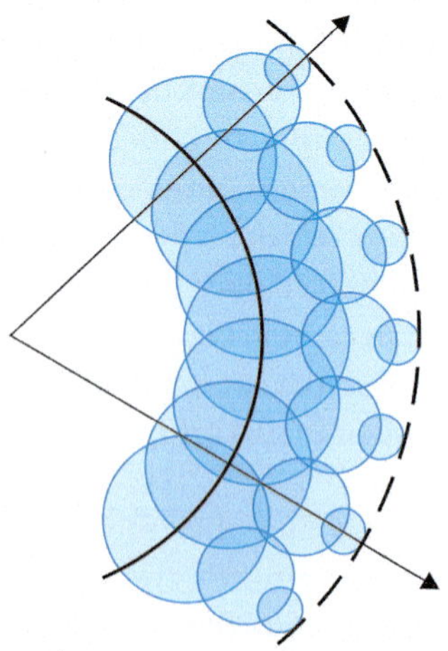

Fig. 13.4: Huygens' wavefront theory explains the propagation of waves as events separated by instants of time. At each instant, every leading point on a wave becomes a source for a new spherical wave to be generated during the next instant. The large circles give rise to the smaller circles to the smallest circles. At each instant, the simultaneously generated waves will have a leading edge that is furthest from the origin which describes the portions of the wave that originated at the same point in time. Two "rays" of light are show, leading backward to the point where wave first started.

Refraction Across an Interface (Fig. 13.5)

Consider what happens when light crosses an interface, boundary, or separating one material from another, for example, air and glass. The optical density of air is almost the same as the optical density of a vacuum: there are relatively few atoms in air, so there is very little delay in the light wave propagating through air. If we were to compare the speed of light in a vacuum, to the speed of light in air, they would be almost the same. In fact, if we took the ratio of the speed of light in a vacuum (in the numerator) and the speed of light in air (in the denominator) of a fraction, we would obtain 1.0003—the two numbers are almost exactly (to 3 decimal places) the same. Because the numerator and the denominator of this fraction have the same units (speed, or meters per second), this ratio of speeds has no units, but it does carry the information of much relative slowing occurs when light passes through air as compared to a vacuum. This number (1.0003 for air) is called the index of refraction for air.

Similarly, there is an index of refraction for glass. Compared to air, there are a lot of atoms in glass for the light to interact with, which considerably slows the light down as it passes through the glass. When we take the

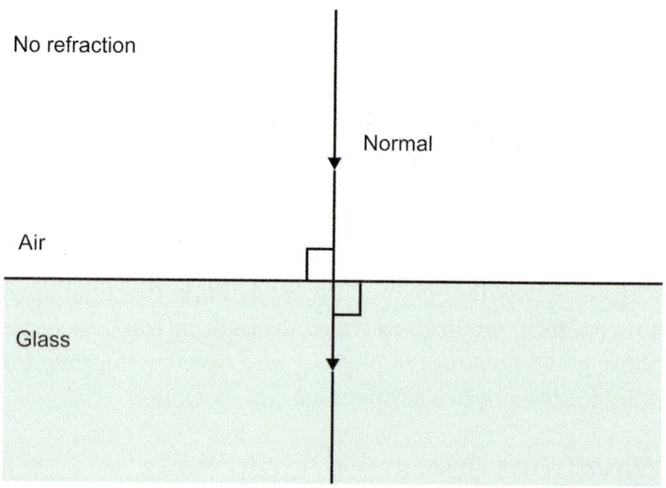

Fig. 13.5: Shows a light ray passing from one material to another. If the light ray (and hence the associated wavefront) directly approaches this interface between two materials (normal to the surface, rather that at an angle) the light ray does not change direction, nor does the wavefront change its direction.

ratio of how fast light travels through a vacuum to typical kinds of glass, the ratio is 1.5. Another way of saying this is that light travels about two-third the speed of light in a vacuum when it passes through typical glass. When light goes from air into glass, it slows down by a third, and the wavelength decreases proportionally. When light passes from glass to air, it speeds up, and the wavelength increases proportionally.

Huygens' principle tells us that at each instant, the wavefront generates new wavelets from every point on it, and those wavelets propagate at the speed appropriate for the material that the wave is passing through. Now imagine what happens when a plane wave of light directly strikes the transition from air to glass, passing from the air to the glass. Directly means that every portion of a given wavefront strikes every portion of the interface, or transition, from air to glass, at the same instant. Think head on or perpendicularly or normal to the surface; they all mean the same thing—all portions at the same time. When the entire wavefront strikes the interface, the wavelength of light to the next wave (behind in air) will be essentially the wavelength of light in a vacuum. However, an instant later, every point on the wavefront gives off a new wave, and the new wave is traveling through glass instead of air, so at the next instant, the wave has only traveled two-third as far (assuming the index of refraction of glass is 1.5). Drawing it a different way, using light rays, we would say that the light ray does not change direction when it passes from a material of one index of refraction into another as long as the ray is perpendicular to the interface (Fig. 13.6).

When the light strikes the interface other than perpendicularly, one portion the wavefront will enter the interface before another, and there will be a boundary that is at the interface that separates these two portions of the wavefront. Applying Huygens' principle in this instance results in something very interesting—the overall direction of the wavefront (and corresponding rays) are different on the two sides of the interface. At the interface, the wavefront changes direction. Snell's law tells how, but Huygens' principle tells why.

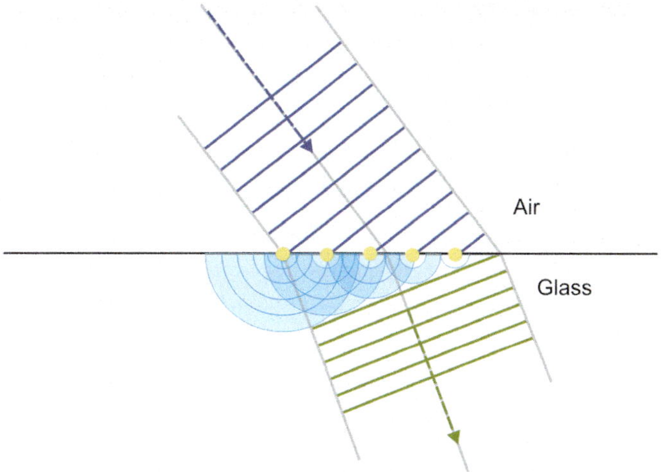

Fig. 13.6: Refraction of light as explained by Huygen's Principle notes that the wave's speed of transmission differs between materials. When a wavefront approaches an interface at an angle, the same wavefront is in materials of different speeds of propagation. At each instant, the wavefront in the faster medium of transmission can travel further than its corresponding portion in the material having the slower speed of transmission. The leading portions of each instant's propagation are knit together to define the direction of the wavefront for each material the wave is passing through. The wavefront, generated each instant by propagation at each point, changes direction at the interface.

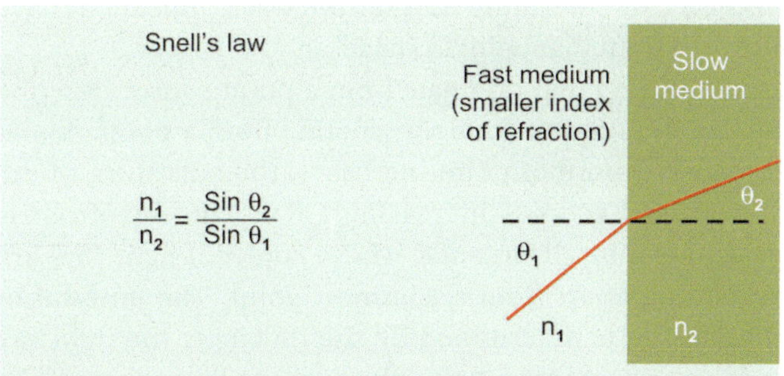

Fig. 13.7: Snell's law quantifies the relation between change in the velocity of wavefront propagation in the materials on either side of the refractive interface, and the change in direction of associated light rays. The index of refraction is the ratio of speed of transmission of light in a vacuum to the speed of the material of interest. Angles θ_1 and θ_2 describe the angle of incidence and angle of refraction. Given any three of these four quantities, the fourth can be determined.

Snell's Law (Fig. 13.7)

Snell's law says that the ratio of refractive indices is equal to the ratio of the sines of the two angles. While it is useful in designing lenses, we use it very little if at all in ophthalmic optics, other than to learn a basic principle from its application: when light travels from a material with lower index of refraction (e.g. air), into a material with a higher index of refraction (e.g. glass), the light ray is bent toward the normal (perpendicular) of the interface. When light travels the other way, from a material with a higher index of refraction (e.g. glass) into a material with a lower index of refraction (e.g. air), it is bent away from the normal with one catch, if the originating angle is too steep, beyond a critical angle for the two materials, the light ray does not escape from the higher index material, but instead is internally reflected. This is the basis of total internal reflection that is used in prisms to bend light every efficiently, and is also the principle by which glass fibers can be used to create fiber optics.

Vergence and Light Rays

A light ray is a very a useful construct, it represents the direction of travel of corresponding portions of wavefronts emanating from a source. For a spherical wavefront coming from a point source, following one light ray backwards will describe a line that will pass through the origin of the wave—a point source of light. That tells us something (the direction to the source) but far less than the information that we get from following two light rays backwards. Earlier we said that light rays represent the direction of travel of an infinitely small portion of a wavefront. If we take any two light rays coming from a point source and extend them infinitely far, they will intersect at some point. That point of intersection is the location of the point source. And once we know the distance that the wavefront has traveled from this point, we know how curved the wavefront is. This means that for any two portions of a wavefront, we can look at the direction of travel of those two portions (our light rays), and we can determine how far the wave appears to have traveled from that point in space.

Light rays that originate from a point source describe an expanding wavefront, originating from a point. As the distance from that point increases, the curvature of the wavefront becomes increasingly flat. The wavefront is said to exhibit divergence, where adjacent light rays are spreading apart from a common point. The amount of divergence is determined by the distance, the light ray is from the common point of origin of all portions of the wavefront.

So far, we have only considered light waves that are expanding from a point source, easy to visualize from the water drop analogy. Soon, we will see that the story is more interesting with light, because we can use lenses to change an expanding wavefront into a contracting wavefront, by passing the light through a lens. For now, rather than thinking about how that might occur, think about the consequences of having light rays pointing forward to a common point rather than emanating from a common point found by tracing the rays backwards.

Light rays, that when extended forward in the direction of travel of the wave come together to a common point, are said to exhibit convergence. Convergent light rays describe a wavefront that is contracting toward a single point as the wavefront moves forward through time and space. Again, it is the distance to which rays from the same wavefront come together that describes the curvature of the wavefront as it converges toward the single point.

The curvature of the wavefront and the spreading apart or coming together of light rays are described by the same entity—the distance for that wavefront to where it is coming from (for divergent rays) or heading toward (for converging rays). Vergence is described by the curvature of the wavefront either expanding (with divergent rays), shrinking (with convergent rays), or flat (with parallel rays).

Diopters

The units of vergence are Diopters (D), or the reciprocal, in meters, of the distance to the common point of two light rays from the same wavefront. If you trace a single wavefront from its origin, the curvature at the origin is infinite, the distance to the origin is infinitely small, and the Dioptric value of the vergence is infinite. As the wavefront expands and the distance increases, the vergence continually decreases. The magnitude of the vergence (in Diopters) is continually changing as the light moves from the source.

SPHERICAL LENSES AND THEIR IMAGES

Lenses

A lens is a piece of glass or other transparent material, which by virtue of its curved shape, changes the vergence of the light passing through. A discussion of lenses usually starts with spherical lenses, not because they produce an ideal image (they do not read about spherical aberration), but because by virtue of their shape (a section of a sphere), they interact with a spherical wavefront in a very convenient manner mathematically. Spherical lenses, by virtue of their spherical shape, can either add convergence to passing light (when the lens is a convex, or fat in the middle, lens) or divergence to passing light (when the lens is concave, or skinny in the middle) (Fig. 13.8).

It is actually very easy to calculate the dioptric power of a spherical refracting surface. Only three things are required to be known: the index of refraction for the material that the lens is in, the index of refraction of the material that the lens is made of, and the radius of curvature of the sphere, in meters, that describes the spherical interface. Almost always (the exception being something like a bubble in water) the lens is made of a material with

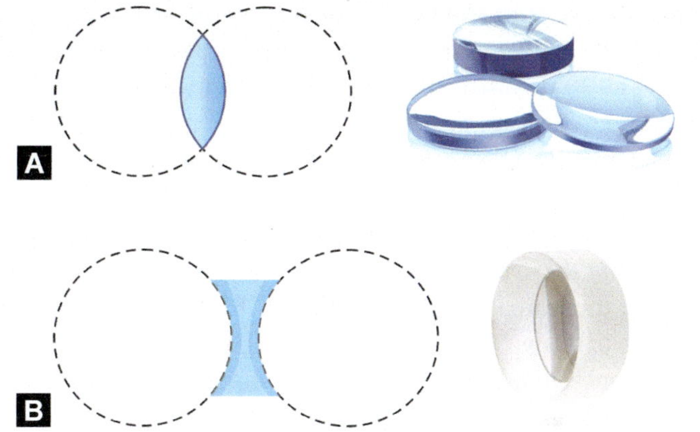

Figs. 13.8A and B: Spherical lenses can be conceptually thought of as the three dimensional intersection of two spheres. A "Plus" lens can be thought of as the volume of intersection between two spheres (A). A minus lens (B) can be thought of as the volume defined by the space between two spheres, where the lens is missing the material defined by the shape of the spheres. A plus sphere lens is called a convex lens, as the lens is thicker in the middle. A minus sphere lens is thinnest in the middle, and is called a concave lens.

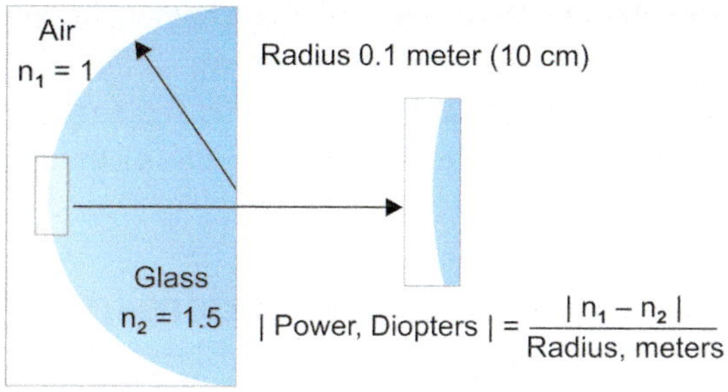

Fig. 13.9: Determining the optical power of an spherical interface. The first step is to establish the index of refraction of the two materials either side of the spherical interface, and the radius of curvature of the interface itself. In this example, a glass sphere of 10 cm diameter is resting in air. The index of refraction of air is 1.00, and glass (in this example) 1.50. The glass sphere has a radius of 10 cm. The first step is to determine if the optical interface describes a positive or negative lens. Look at the shape of the material having the higher index of refraction by enclosing the interface in an imaginary rectangle (13.9, right). Glass, having the higher index of refraction, describes a positive lens (thicker in the middle). Next, determine the absolute power of the interface, determined by taking the absolute difference of the indices of refraction, and dividing by the interface radius in meters.

a higher index of refraction than the material it is in. An example might be a lens made of glass (index of refraction 1.5) sitting in air (index of refraction 1) and sliced off a spherical piece of glass, having a diameter of say, 0.1 meter (10 cm). The lens would look something like this as shown in Figure 13.9.

The absolute value of the lens power is simply the difference in index of refraction of the two materials divided by the radius of the spherically curved interface, in meters. In the example given, the power of such a lens would be 5 D. To know if it is a plus or minus lens, simply look at the shape of the material having the higher index of refraction: if it is thicker in the middle, the lens is a plus lens; if it is thinner in the middle, the lens is a minus lens—but either way, the power is determined by the curvature and the two indices of refraction (Fig. 13.9).

Often, lenses are constructed with curvature both on the front and back, rather than one side being flat. When this occurs, the total lens power is the sum of the powers of the front and back surfaces (Fig. 13.10).

Now that we know how to make a plus lens of 5 D power, let us play with it. Let us see how we can use a lens to form an image of a point source of light. To do that, we will need to see how lenses change the vergence of light.

Objects and Images

We have been talking about point sources of light and describing the wavefront that emanates from the source.

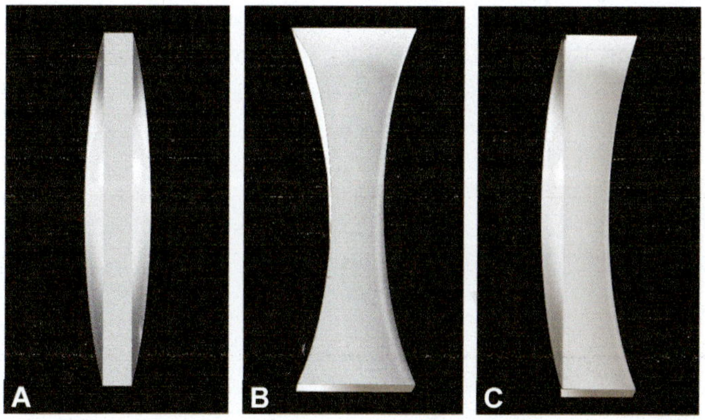

Figs. 13.10A to C: Biconvex (A), Biconcave (B), and Mensicus (C) lenses. In a biconvex lens (A), both surfaces add optical power, with the total power being the sum of the two powers. In a biconcave lens (B), both surfaces subtract optical power, again with the total power being the sum. A meniscus lens (C) has both concave and convex surfaces, and depending on which surface has the greater power, the net power can be either positive or negative. Spectacle lenses are often fabricated as meniscus lenses, as they minimize distortions as the eye moves in different positions of gaze.

The object is that thing which gives off light. The light from an object is manipulated by a lens to form an image of the object. There is a convention that light flows from left to right. Rays of light that leave an object are called object rays. Rays of light that leave a lens are called image rays. The optical axis passes through the center of curvature of the lens infinitely far in each direction, and the object and image are placed on this axis. Distances are measured with respect to the lens, so the object distance is the distance from the object to the lens, and the image distance is the distance of the lens to the image. As we will later see, it is possible for these distances to be negative, meaning that the object can be to the right of the lens, or the image to the left of the lens.

Real and Virtual Object and Images

When object rays, the rays of light entering a lens, are diverging, the rays point back to an object that is to the left of the lens. When the object rays are on the same side of the lens as the object, the object is said to be real. If the light entering the lens (the object rays) are converging when they enter the lens, then the object rays are pointing to a location on the opposite side of the lens, to the right of the lens. If the object is on the opposite side of the lens from the object rays, then the object is said to be virtual (Fig. 13.11).

The same goes for images: If the image is found to the right of the lens, on the same side of the lens as the image rays, it is said to be a real image. This happens when converging rays of light exit the lens. If diverging rays of light are exiting the lens, they would trace back to a point on the opposite side of the lens system. When the image is to the left of the lens, on the opposite side of the lens as the image rays, it is said to be a virtual image (Fig. 13.12).

It is not clear why the terms real and virtual were chosen long ago, for it makes the virtual image sound somewhat mystical. There is no mysticism at work, the term virtual is meant to imply that the object has the virtue of being located someplace other than where the light is coming from. For there to have been converging light rays entering a lens, there needed to be some sort of optical system not shown or drawn that created the converging rays of light, for we know that point sources radiate outward in a spherical manner, giving off divergent light. Some optical system—perhaps a lens, perhaps a mirror—changed the vergence of the light entering the lens was positive.

The Vergence Formula

A plus lens of 5 D power will add 5 D of vergence to any light that is passing through it. Another way of saying this is that the vergence of the light entering the lens (call it U), added to the power of the lens (call it D), equals the vergence of the light exiting the lens (call it V). In formula form,

$$U + D = V$$

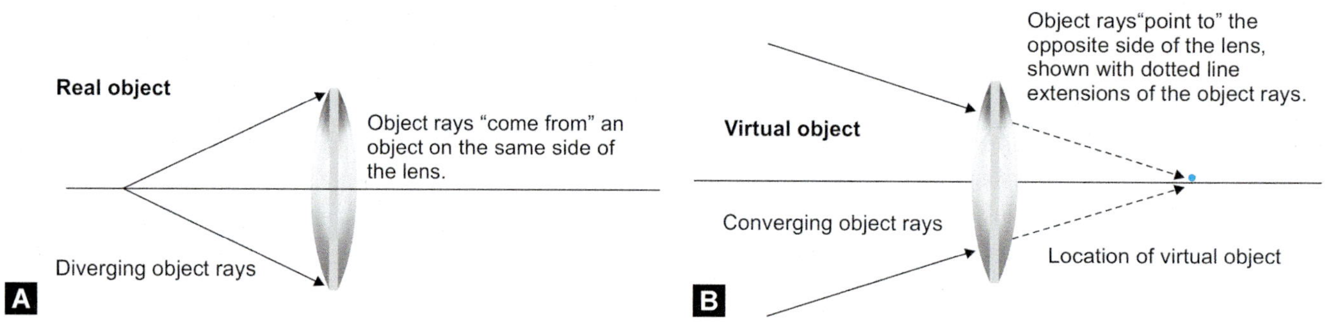

Figs. 13.11A and B: (A) Object rays are light rays that enter an optical system, in this case a plus lens. When the object rays are on the same side of the lens as the object emitting the light, the object is said to be a real object; (B) A virtual object is located on the opposite side of the lens system from the entering object rays. The location of the virtual object is found by dotted line extensions of the incoming rays through the lens system to the point where they converge towards.

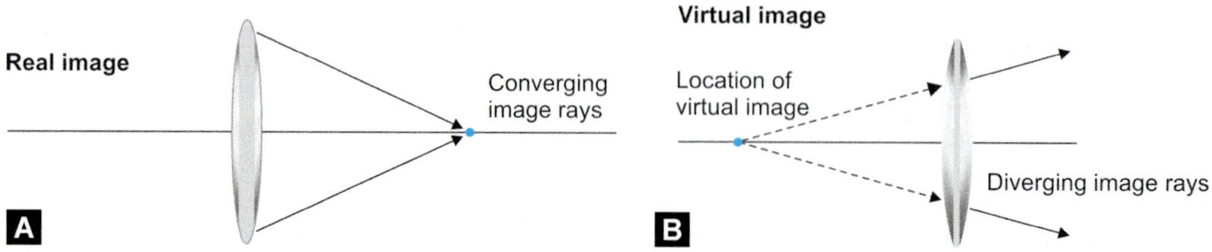

Figs. 13.12A and B: (A) A real image is located on the same side of the optical system as the image rays. It is shown by solid lines representing image rays exiting a lens system and converging to a point, the point being the real image; (B) Image rays "come from" the opposite side of the lens, shown with dotted line extensions of the image rays. The diverging image rays, exiting the lens, are traced backwards with dotted lines to show the point where they intersect. This intersection on the incoming side of the lens system is the location of the virtual image. A virtual image is located on the opposite side of the lens system as the image rays.

This simple formula, called the vergence formula, allows us to determine where an image will form when light from an object (the thing that gives off light) passes through a lens (which changes the vergence by a constant amount, that being the power of the lens). Remember that light leaving an object has its vergence that is constantly changing; the vergence (either convergence or divergence) is measured in Diopters, and is the reciprocal of the distance in meters from the object to the point in space where the value of the vergence is to be determined.

Image Formation with Plus Lenses (Fig. 13.13)

In Figure 13.13, a point source of light is located a half meter (50 cm) to the left of a +5 D lens. The image is found to be 33 cm to the right of the lens by the vergence formula. At 50 cm, the vergence of light entering the lens is –2 D, being minus because the light rays are diverging and being –2 D, because this is the reciprocal of half meter.

The lens power is 5 D, and the lens adds 5 D of vergence to the light that enters it. This results in the light that exits having vergence of +3 D. As the sign is positive, the light rays are converging to a point to the right of the lens. As the vergence, when the light leaves the lens is +3, the rays come to converge at a point one-third meter (33 cm) to the right of the lens.

In the above example, the vergence formula was used to solve for the location of an image, given the location of an object, and the power of the lens. The location of the object with respect to the lens was used to determine U, the vergence of the light from the object as it entered the lens. The power of the lens, D, was provided. Given two of the three unknowns (U and D), V, the vergence of the light exiting the lens was used to determine the location of the image. Without knowing two of the three components of the vergence formula, the third cannot be solved for. If U is unknown, then U = V – D. If D is unknown, then D = V – U.

Collimated Light

The vergence formula is a very powerful tool. It allows the location of an image to be determined for any plus or minus lens quite easily. The only trick is to remember that vergence is constantly changing, as the wavefront either converges or diverges towards a point. The only time the vergence stays constant is when the light is neither converging nor diverging. This is the case when the wavefront is flat, originating from optical infinity, and the rays of light are parallel to each other. Such light, with zero vergence, is said to be collimated. Let us see how to make collimated light with a point source and a +5 D lens, so we do not have to go all the way to infinity to do an experiment.

Primary and Secondary Focal Points

Here we have placed the object, a point source, 20 cm (1/5 m) from a +5 D lens. The vergence of the light entering from 20 cm to the left of the lens has –5 D vergence. The power of the lens is +5 D, so the divergence of the light entering is exactly countered by the convergence added by the lens. The light that exits has 0 D power, or is collimated, and the light forms an image at infinity (Fig. 13.14).

There is a term for the reciprocal of the power of a lens, and that is the focal length of the lens. This length, or

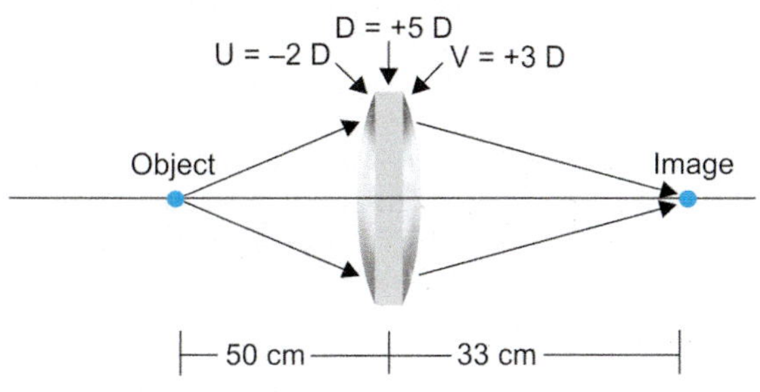

Fig. 13.13: Image formation with a plus lens and a real object. In this example, a real object is located a half meter (50 cm) to the left of a +5 D lens. The object is a real object as it is on the same side of the lens system as the incoming image rays. At a distance of 50 cm, the image rays have diverged over a distance of ½ meter, and so have –2 D vergence when entering the +5 D lens. By the vergence formula of U + D = V, the vergence of the light leaving the lens is +3 D. A real image will form 1/3 m to the right of the lens, as shown.

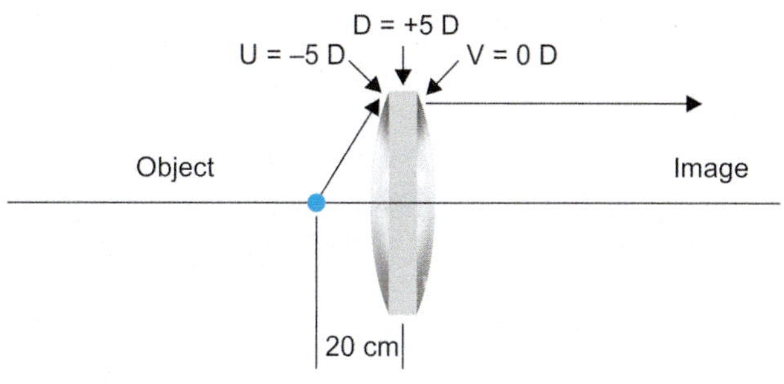

Fig. 13.14: As a real object approaches a lens an interesting phenomenon occurs when the real object is placed at the anterior focal point of the object. Here a real object is located 20 cm from a +5 D lens. The focal length of the lens is the inverse of the dioptric power, or in this case the inverse of 5 D, or 20 cm. When the vergence formula is used to determine the vergence of light exiting the lens in this example –5 D is entering, and the lens power is +5 D, so the vergence of light exiting is 0 D. Such light is said to be collimated, and the image that is formed is located at infinity.

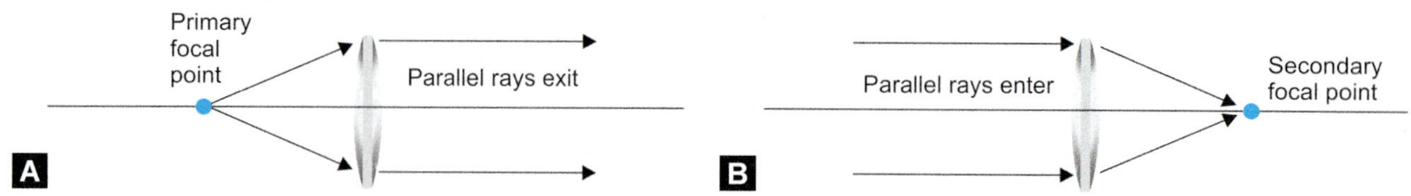

Figs. 13.15A and B: (A) The primary focal point is the location on the optical axis where an object will cause parallel rays of light to exit the lens system. It can be a real object, to the left of the lens, or it can be a virtual object, with the primary focal point being located to the right of the lens; (B) The secondary focal point is the location on the optical axis where an image is formed from the parallel rays of light entering the lens.

distance from the lens, can be used to describe two special locations for a given lens: the primary and secondary focal points.

The primary focal point of a lens is where an object would be placed to have parallel rays of light exit the lens, forming an image at infinity (Fig. 13.15A).

The secondary focal point of a lens is where an image is formed when parallel rays of light, coming from an object at infinity, enters a lens (Fig. 13.15B).

Usually, we think of the two focal points being the same distance from the center of the lens, and that is true for simple lens problems. However, the primary and secondary focal points can be very asymmetrically located with respect to the lens when a lens is comprised of multiple optical elements, or there are two different materials (say air and water) on either side of the lens. An example of the latter might be the human eye: the cornea forms an optical surface, air is on one side of the lens, and aqueous is on the other. More refraction will occur at the air-tear interface of the cornea than at the posterior corneal surface, where the difference in the cornea's index of refraction and the aqueous is quite small.

Minus Lenses (Fig. 13.16)

Minus lenses add negative vergence (divergence) to light, hence the name. They also make things look small and far away, unlike plus lenses that magnify and make things look bigger. The power of a minus lens is measured in Diopters and, not surprisingly, is always a negative number. In our plus lens, we determined the shape of a +5 D spherical lens. To make a -5 D lens, the shape is reversed but the radius of curvature remains the same. The lens becomes thinner in the middle instead of thicker.

In Figure 13.17, the minus lens is located 100 cm (1 m) from the object. The object rays have vergence of -1 D when they enter the -5 lens. The power of the lens (-5 D) is added to the vergence of the incoming light (-1 D) so the light exiting the lens has vergence of -6 D. The image rays exiting the lens are diverging (see the dotted line extensions of the image rays) and trace back to virtual image 16 cm (1/6 m) to the left of the lens.

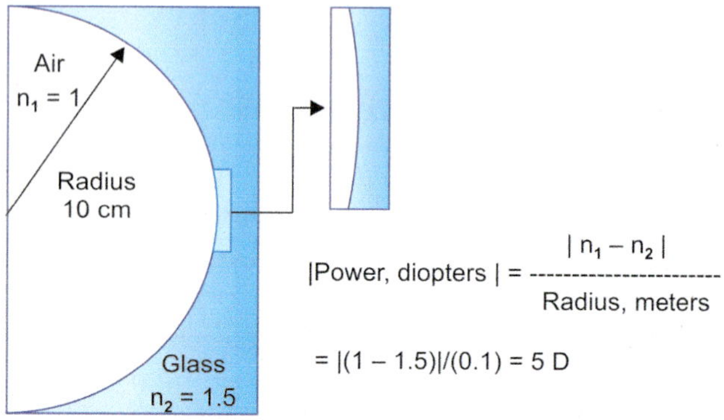

Fig. 13.16: A minus lens has a concave shape removed from the material having the higher index of refraction. The concave shape in the higher index material determines that the net power will be negative. The absolute value of the power is determined by the absolute value of the difference of refractive indices, divided by the radius of curvature in meters. In this example where the concave surface is described by a sphere of 10 cm radius, and with air (n = 1.00) and glass (n = 1.50), the absolute value of the power is 5 Diopters. The negative power is assigned by knowing the shape described by the higher index material, in this case negative.

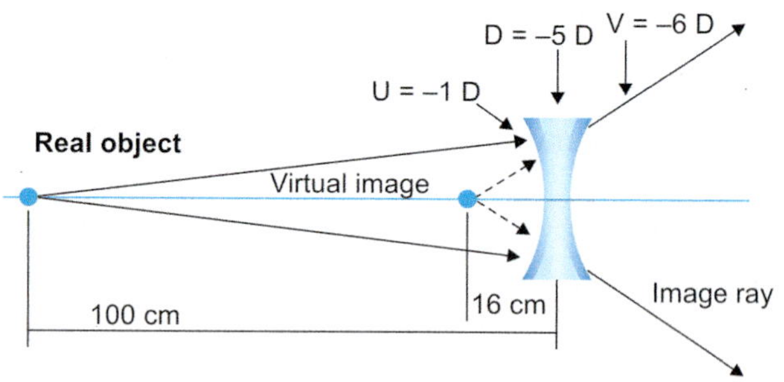

Fig. 13.17: A real object that is outside the focal length of a minus lens results in a virtual image located inside the focal length of the lens. In this example, a real object is located 100 cm from a –5 D lens. The vergence formula U + D = V is used to determine V from U (the vergence of the light entering the lens, in this case 1/1 or –1 D. The lens power is shown as –5 D. The vergence V is then (–1) + (–5) = –6 D. The light exiting the lens has 6 D of divergence, or power of –6D. The virtual image is located 1/6 m to the left of the lens, at 16 cm.

Just as with plus lenses, the vergence formula works with minus lenses. Given U + D = V, if you know two of the values, you can solve for the third. It is always important to remember that the vergence of light is always changing for other than collimated light, and that the vergence is the reciprocal of the distance to the point where light rays are converging toward, or diverging from.

Magnification and Minification

If you have looked through a plus lens, it is apparent that it makes things appear larger (a plus lens is a magnifying glass). If you have looked at a myopic individuals face through their spectacles, you have seen how the lenses make their eyes look smaller. Bigger and smaller are relative terms, but magnification and minification have mathematical meaning, and we use the terms in optics.

Thus far, we have only explored where images of point sources are formed. To discuss magnification, we must think about extended objects, something that is bigger than a point. No matter how much you magnify a point, it remains a point—it never gets any bigger. But two points, separated in space and joined by a line, represent an object that has measureable size. In optics, we represent such an extended object as an arrow that extends perpendicular to the optical axis.

If you got this far, the idea of things being infinitely far away but still giving off light that reaches us has not scared you off. We are about to make a similar kind of thought experiment to understand how paraxial optics allow us to define a central ray that makes determination of magnification and minification quite simple.

Now, think back to what happens when a light ray strikes an optical interface perpendicular to the interface. It passes through without changing direction. The optical axis defines this position, and why an object that is placed on the optical axis will form its image on the optical axis. If we imagine our lenses to be infinitely thin, and further imagine that a point source is infinitely close to, but not on, the optical axis, then something interesting happens. A light ray that passes through the optical axis at the location of the lens from that off axis (but very close, so close that it is called paraxial) passes through without being refracted.

Using this approximation, it is possible to envision an object plane that is perpendicular to the optical axis, located the object distance from lens, and an image plane, also perpendicular to the optical axis, located the image distance away from the lens. Any object that is located on the object plane will be imaged on the image plane. Consider a point on the object plane that defines the tip of

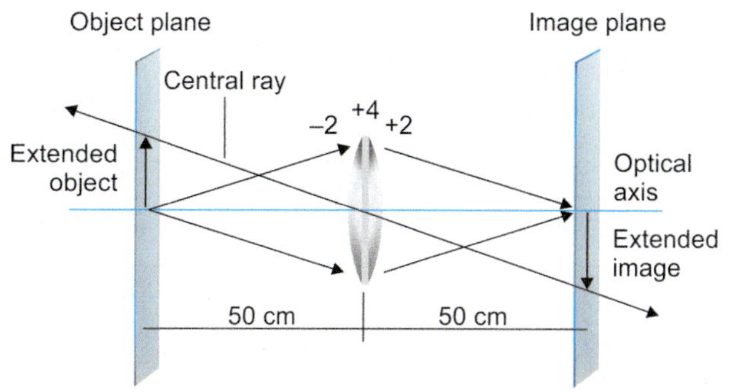

Fig. 13.18: Using the central ray to determine the image location and orientation for an extended object and a plus lens. Extended objects are objects that extend beyond a single point on the optical axis. They are indicated by an arrow, with the arrow having an arrowhead indicating direction. Any ray that passes through the optical center of a lens passes through without refraction. A ray exiting the tip of the extended object, and passes through the optical center, will have to intersect the image at the tip of the image area, and is known as the central ray. The position along the optical axis of the image is determined by the vergence formula. The central ray then is used to determine the orientation and size of the resultant image, with the size given by the ratio of image distance to object distance.

an extended object. This point gives off light in all directions, and one of those rays will find its way to the optical center of the lens where it intersects the optical axis. This ray, called the central ray, passes undeviated through the lens. The location on the image plane where the central ray strikes the image plane corresponds to the location of the tip of the extended object (Fig. 13.18).

Using the ratio of the object distance to the image distance, we can see magnification by using similar triangles. The ratio of the distances of the image planes is the same as the ratio of the heights of the extended object. It is conventional to assign an object height of one to the object. That way, the ratio of image to object distances gives the relative magnification (if greater than one) or minification (if less than one).

Additionally, the central ray provides a way to know if the image that is produced is upright, oriented in the same direction as the object, or inverted, oriented in the opposite direction as the object (Fig. 13.19).

When a minus lens is used to image a real object, as in Figure 13.20, a virtual image is formed. In this example, a -4 D lens is used to form an image of an extended object located 1 m from the lens. Using the vergence formula, the vergence of light leaving the lens is -5 D. The virtual image that is formed is 20 cm to the left of the lens. The ratio of the distances is 100 cm to 20 cm. The image, while upright, is one-fifth as large as the object. The image is minified, and it is one-fifth as large as the object.

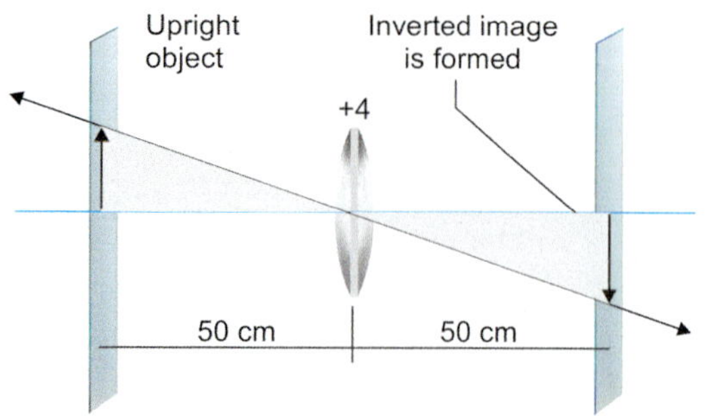

Fig. 13.19: Using the central ray to determine the magnification of an extended object and a plus lens. In this example, the vergence of the light entering the lens is −2 D, and the light exiting the lens is +2 D. The object is located as far from the lens as the image (50 cm). Because the object and image distance is the same the resultant image is as large as the object (the similar triangles are equal). The central ray, passing from the tip of the object through the optical center of the lens, intersects the tip of the inverted real image.

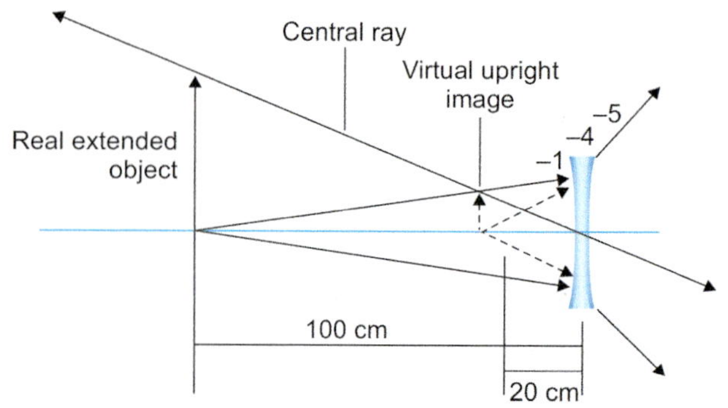

Fig. 13.20: Using the central ray to determine the image location and orientation for a minus lens. By using the vergence formula U + D = V, the location of the image is found to be on the optical axis 20 cm to the left of the lens. The central ray determines the image to be upright, in the same orientation as the real object. By similar triangles, the image is one fifth the size of the object. If the object has size of 1 unit, the image would have size of 0.20. The magnification would be said to be 0.20.

CYLINDER LENSES AND THEIR IMAGES

So far, we have considered spherical wavefronts and spherical lenses, and how a lens can change the curvature of a wavefront as it passes through the interfaces of the lens. However, not all lenses are perfectly spherical, so any spherical wavefront that passes through a nonspherical lens will emerge to some extent deviated from the spherical shape that went in.

Since we are learning optics to understand refraction and how to correct refractive error so patients can see better, it is time to start talking about optical surfaces other than slices off of perfect spheres that form a perfect image of a point source of light. Human eyes are mostly made of water, and they are basically inflated water balloons that hold a somewhat spherical shape and bring light to focus on the retina. When you think of all it does, it is a remarkable bag of water.

So, imagine filling a balloon with water, and then resting it in a tub of water. Since it is filled with water, and resting in water, the only thing that might cause it to sink or float would be the density of the balloon itself. If the balloon were less dense than water, it might tend to float; if the material of the balloon was denser than water, it might tend to sink, but at least for a little while, it would probably bob around submerged in the pool of water and assume a spherical shape. Now, imagine taking the balloon filled with water out of the tub and resting it on a table. It would likely flatten out a little on the bottom, and it would become wider than it is tall, with a steeper curve vertically than horizontally. And, if the balloon were made of a transparent material, when you looked through the balloon, the balloon would act as a lens—but not a spherical lens. Because it was steeper in one direction than another, there would be more dioptric power along the steeper, vertical orientation than along the flatter, horizontal orientation. Because eyeballs are basically a bag of water, and they are not floating in water, it is not surprising that some of them sag one way or another, depending on what is pushing on them and supporting them.

Astigmatic Lens Shape (Fig. 13.21)

A slice off a hard-boiled egg, or a slice off a donut: which would you prefer to think about? Either shape resembles the deviation from a spherical shape that is frequently seen in the corneas of humans, where the cornea is steeper along one orientation than another. A cornea that exhibits such a shape will not produce a point image on the retina. The patient will have a type of refractive error known as astigmatism, and their eyeglasses will need to have a similar shape to undo the inherent astigmatism present (most commonly) in the cornea. The correcting lens will need to be steeper in the same orientation that the cornea is flatter, and flatter where the cornea is steeper, to allow the combination of cornea and correcting lens to add up to a spherical shape that will bring a point of light to a point focus on the retina.

As you can imagine, it could be difficult to grind a lens into such a complicated shape, but there is another way to

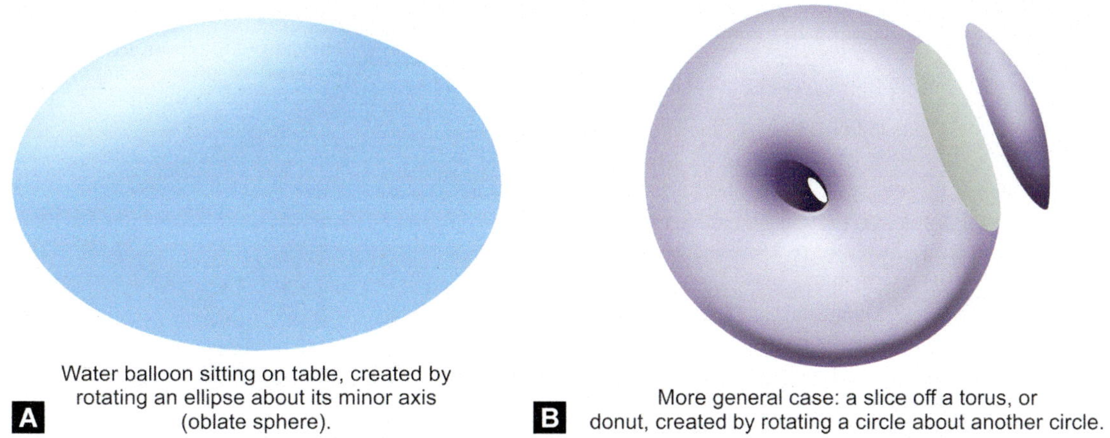

Figs. 13.21A and B: Shapes that describe an astigmatic lens surface. (A) A water balloon setting on a table, creates a shape describing that of an ellipse that rotates around its minor axis (an oblate sphere); (B) The more general case of a slice off of a torus, or donut, created by rotating a circle about another circle.

produce the same net curvature as a toric lens, and that is to combine a spherical lens with a cylinder lens.

Cylinder Lenses

A cylinder lens is created by taking a slice off a rod (for a plus cylinder) or a slice off a piece of glass that has a rod removed from it (for a minus cylinder). Such a lens has curvature along directions that are perpendicular to the axis that runs through the middle of the cylinder from which the lens was sliced, and no curvature in directions that run parallel to the cylinder axis (Fig. 13.22).

Spherical lenses derive their ability to change the vergence of light rays because of their curvature, and the difference in index of refraction between the index of the lens index, and index of the material that surrounds the lens. The same principle applies to cylinder lenses, with several complications.

First, there is no clearly defined optical center of a cylindrical lens. There is a line that defines a plane that is perpendicular to the flat (plano) side of the lens, that passes through the apex of the curved side of the lens, and any rays that pass along that line will pass through without deviation. Second, for the orientation that is perpendicular to the axis of rotation, there is a circle that has a radius that is used to determine the lens power in the orientation perpendicular to the axis.

Finally, for every other orientation that is neither parallel to nor perpendicular to the axis, the power is greater than 0 D, and less than the maximum power that is found perpendicular to the axis. There is sinusoidal power variation between 0 and the maximum power, given by the

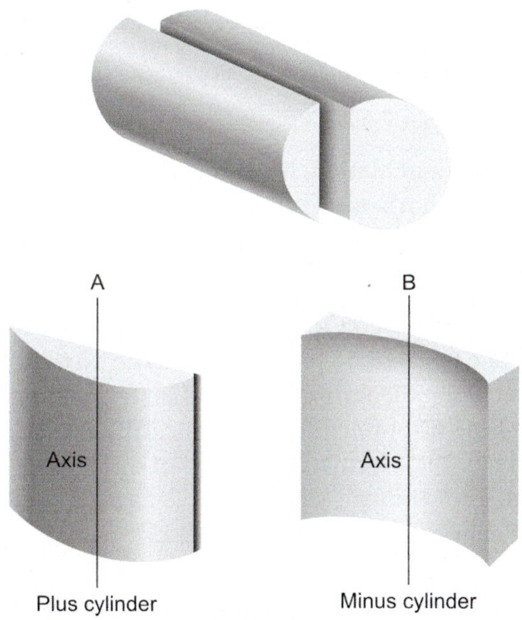

Fig. 13.22: Creating a cylindrical lens of either plus or minus power starts with creating a cylinder and then taking a slice off of a rod. A minus cylinder is slightly more difficult to create—take a cube of material, drill a hole through it (the removed material now describes a cylinder), and then carving out one portion of the cylinder.

radius of the circle that forms the cylinder, and difference between the indices of refraction.

Cylinder lenses are more complex to describe, as they have both a curvature (along one axis) and an orientation that describes the axis. For the moment, we will simply limit the orientation to vertical and horizontal for choices of axis rotation, but when we start describing actual eyes, we will find that any orientation is possible, and conventions to

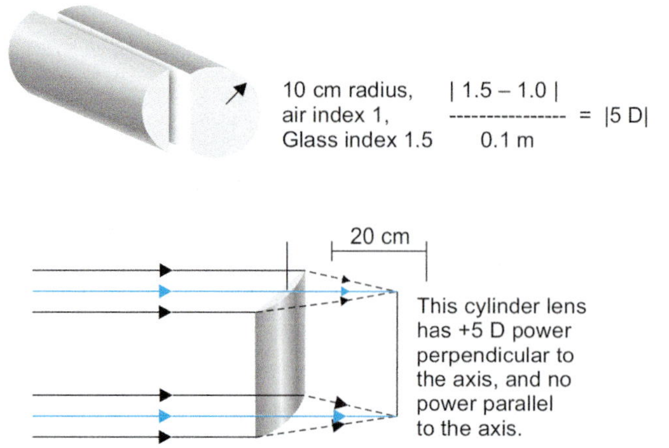

Fig. 13.23: The power of a cylinder lens is determined in the same manner as that of a spherical lens. First, determine the shape of the material having the higher index of refraction (in this case, a plus cylinder is carved out of glass, having index of refraction of 1.50). Take the absolute value of the the difference in indices of refraction divided by the radius of curvature in meters to determine the absolute power of the cylindrical lens in one orientation. Use the shape to determine the sign of the lens (plus or minus).

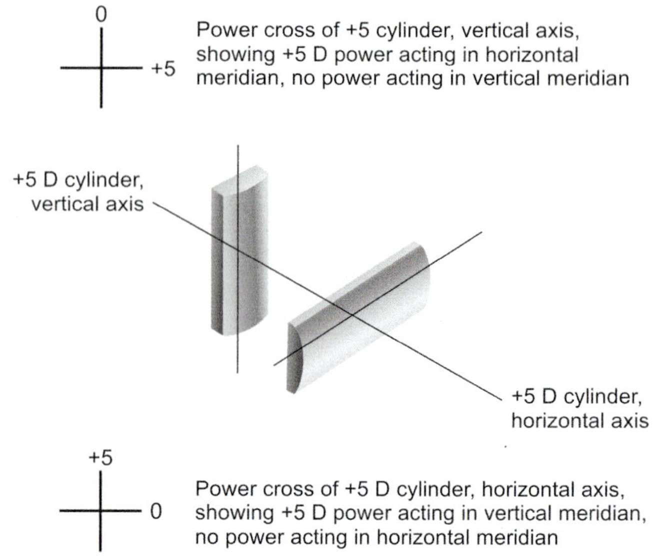

Fig. 13.24: Describing pairs of perpendicular lenses using power crosses. In this example, a +5 D cylinder lens is placed perpendicular to, and adjacent to, another cylinder lens of identical power. The power crosses showing horizontal and vertical power are shown.

describe the orientation. Now, however, let us stick with vertical and horizontal, with vertical being associated with 90°, and horizontal being associated with 180° (Fig. 13.23).

Combining cylinder lenses: Figure 13.24 shows two cylinder lenses. The first lens, to the left has a vertical axis. It has +5 D power along the horizontal meridian (perpendicular to the axis) and no power along the vertical meridian (parallel to the axis). The shorthand notation for this lens is +5.00 X 090, and would be read plus 5 D cylinder axis 90°, where the X is the abbreviation for axis. (Fig. 13.25)

Power Cross Diagrams

There is a diagrammatic way of describing the lens power and orientation that is much easier to draw than pictures of cylinders, and that is the power cross diagram that is shown above the drawing of the cylinder. In the power cross, two lines are drawn 90° apart at the approximate orientation of the greatest and least power associated with the lens. The vertical line indicates the power in the vertical direction, or meridian, and the horizontal line indicates the power along the horizontal meridian.

Similarly, the second cylinder lens to the right, having +5 D cylinder power with horizontal axis, would be written as +5 D X 180, and read as plus 5 D cylinder axis 180°. Its power cross is also shown, this time with the +5 noted to be along the vertical meridian, and now power along the horizontal, which is also the orientation of the axis (Fig. 13.25).

When two cylinder lenses are stacked atop each other and their axis are either parallel to each other or perpendicular to each other, the powers along each of the axes of the power crosses can be added to determine the resultant power. If the two cylinders are equal in power and perpendicular to each other, they combine to form a spherical lens, and regardless of the orientation, the power is constant. This only holds when the axes are perpendicular to each other. In the example shown, there is a new symbol introduced between the two cylinders. A pair of parentheses on their side, this symbol is read combined with, as in plus 5 D cylinder axis 090 combined with plus 5 D cylinder axis 180 gives +5 D sphere (Fig. 13.25).

SPHEROCYLINDRICAL LENSES

A spherocylindrical lens is created when two cylinders of unequal power are combined perpendicular to each other, as is seen in Figures 13.26. A +5 cylinder axis 90 is combined with a +8 cylinder axis 180. The resultant power cross shows +8 D in the vertical meridian and + 5 D in the horizontal meridian. One way to make this combination would be to use a +5 D sphere combined with a +3 D cylinder axis 180, and is shown. But that is not the only way to make this combination of two cylinder lenses. Instead of using

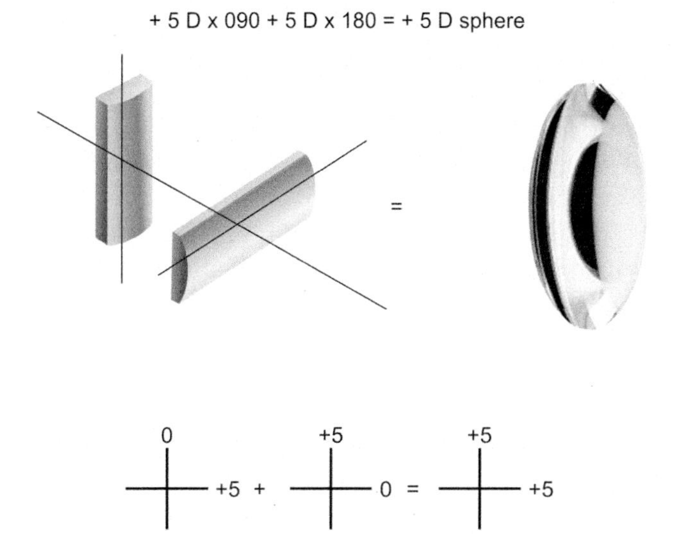

Fig. 13.25: Combining identically powered cylinder lenses at right angles to each other creates a spherical lens, as shown by adding the associated power crosses.

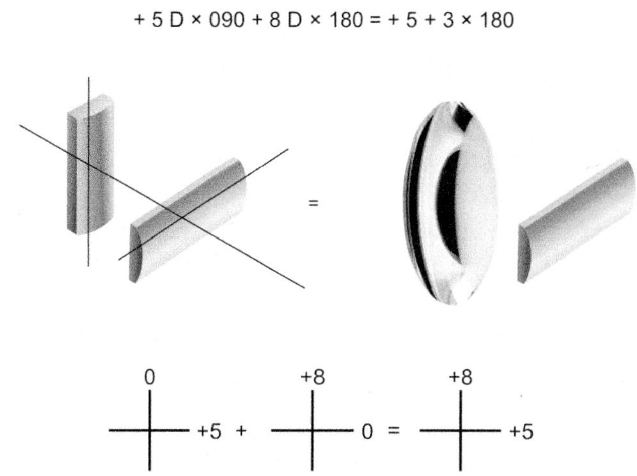

Fig. 13.26: Adding differently powered cylinder lenses perpendicular to each other creates a spherocylinder lens. In this instance, the +5 D and +8 D cylinders result in a +5 D sphere with additional +3 D cylinder.

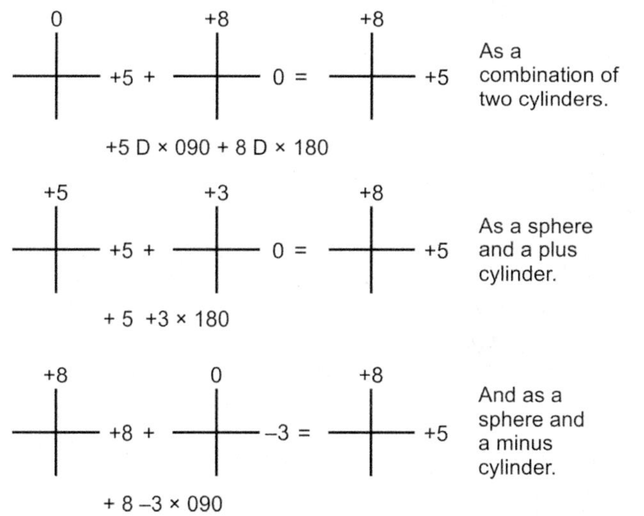

Fig. 13.27: Plus and minus sphereocylindrical lens notation. Figure 13.26 showed how two cylinders could be combined and described as crossed cylinders (top) or as a sphere with associated plus cylinder (middle). In the bottom, a third way is demonstrated showing how a minus cylinder can be combined with a sphere to create the same resultant power. Thus, there are three ways that a sphereocylindrical lens can be described: as a combination of two cylinders (top), as a sphere and a plus cylinder (middle), and as a sphere and a minus cylinder (bottom).

a plus cylinder lens atop a sphere to add power in one of the meridia, we can use a minus cylinder lens to take away power in one of the meridians of a sphere.

Transposition of Cylinders

In general, there are three ways to describe a spherocylindrical lens: as a combination of two cylinders (as we have seen), as a combination of a sphere and a plus cylinder (as we have seen), and as a combination of a sphere and a minus cylinder as is shown. All three combinations are equally valid, all work equally well, and all are acceptable ways of describing the lens combination. Some people prefer to write prescriptions in plus cylinder notation, and others prefer to write their prescriptions in minus cylinder notation. The plus cylinder notation for the example here is given in the middle, while the minus cylinder is given in the bottom of Figure 13.27.

Once you see how power crosses are created and describe the power of a spherocylindrical lens, you can understand why the rules given to change from one axis notation to the other work. Take a look at Figure 13.27 and see how the rules of transposition describe the conversion of the plus cylinder power cross to the minus cylinder power cross, and vice versa (Fig. 13.28).

Image Formation with a Cylinder Lens

A cylinder lens has power along one orientation, and no power along the other. To understand how a cylinder lens forms an image, it seems easiest to consider what happens to three rays that strike perpendicular to the back surface of a plano-convex cylinder lens, as shown in Figure 13.29.

In Figure 13.29A, three light rays are labeled rays 1, 2, and 3. Rays 1 and 2 both pass through the apex of the curved cylinder surface, through the axis of the cylinder, and perpendicular to the plano surface, and emerge undeviated. Ray 3 also enters perpendicular to the posterior

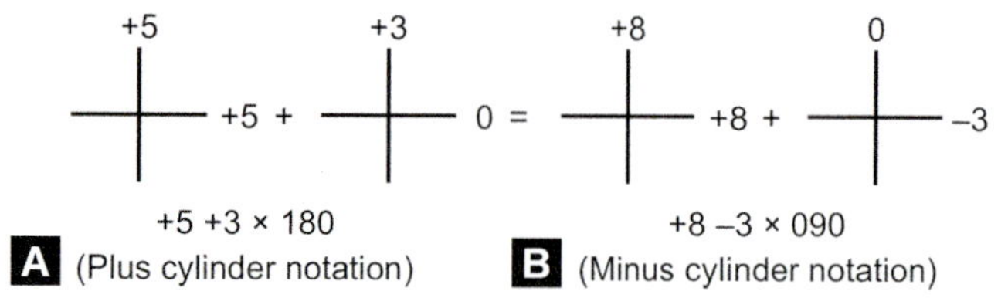

Figs. 13.28A and B: Power crosses showing two equivalent combinations of the same sphereocylindrical lens. In (A) a +5 D sphere is combined with a +3 D cylinder lens having axis 180° (remember, the power of a spherocylinder is perpendicular to the axis). In (B), a +8 D sphere is combined with a –3 D cylinder having axis 90°. In either case, the effective power is +8 D in the vertical meridian, and +5 D in the horizontal meridian. This combination of cylinders is +8 D axis 180 combined with +5 D axis 090.

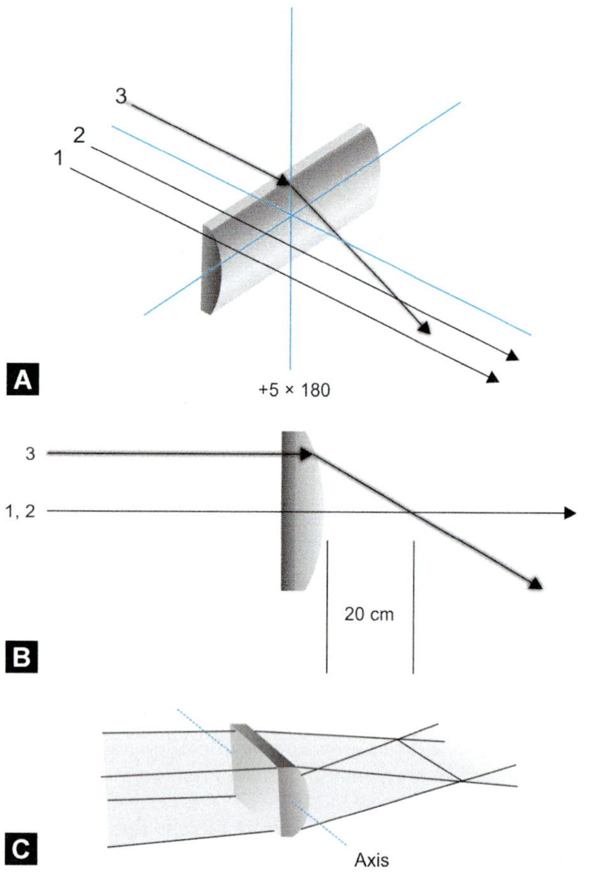

Figs. 13.29A to C: A focal line is formed by a cylinder lens. The focal line is parallel to the axis of the cylinder. In (A), rays 1 and 2 enter the cylinder and pass through the optical axis without refraction, as the rays enter the back surface of the cylinder perpendicular to its surface and exit the curved anterior face perpendicular to its surface. However, ray 3 (A) approaches the back surface perpendicular to it, but exits the lens at an interface angle that is not perpendicular, and is thus refracted. As the optical power of this cylinder lens is +5 D (B), ray 3 intersects the optical axis at a point 20 cm to the right of the lens. In (C), multiple parallel rays to ray 3 enter and similarly come to focus at the same distance from the lens, forming a focal line.

plano surface but enters above ray 2 and above the axis. When ray 3 exits the lens curvature (in this case, for our continuing example of 10 cm radius, air, and glass), there is 5 D of refracting power at the curved glass where ray 3 exits, and it refracts to intersect ray 2 at a distance of 20 cm from the cylinder lens.

Figure 13.29B, shows the three rays from the side of the lens. Rays 1 and 2 are superimposed in this view, but ray 3 is shown above, entering the lens, and refracting when the ray exits the lens.

In Figure 13.29C, a plethora of parallel rays of light (coming from infinity) strike the posterior surface of the cylinder lens perpendicular to the surface (as rays 1, 2 and 3 did). All of these rays head in the direction of a line that runs parallel to the axis of the cylinder.

The image that is formed by a cylinder lens is a line, not a point. For a spherical lens, the secondary focal point is the location of the image when collimated light enters the lens. Cylinder lenses do not have focal points, they have focal lines. The focal line is imaged at a distance corresponding to the power of the steepest orientation of the cylinder lens. The steepest curvature is perpendicular to the axis of rotation; this is why the focal line is parallel to the axis of the cylinder lens.

Image Formation with a Spherocylinder Lens

Seeing that a cylinder lens forms a focal line, it is not surprising that two cylinder lenses form two focal lines that are located at their respective focal distances. What is interesting is what happens to the places where the light rays are out of focus, at locations other than the distance to either of the focal lines (Fig. 13.30).

In Figure.13.31, two cylinder lenses (+5 D axis 90, and +3 D axis 180) are combined. We now know that this combination can also be written as a +3 D sphere lens, combined with a +2 D cylinder axis 90 (written as +3.00 +2,00 × 90), or as a +5 D sphere lens, combined with a –2 D cylinder axis 180 (written as +5.00 –2.00 × 180). All three combinations have the same effect of forming two focal lines, one vertical at 20 cm (the +5 D focal line), and one horizontal at 33 cm (the +3 D focal line).

The average of 3 D and 5 D is 4 D, and this represents the average power (in Diopters) of the spherocylinder lens. This average power produces an out of focus concentration of light between the two focal lines. The average power of the two cylinders is called the spherical equivalent power,

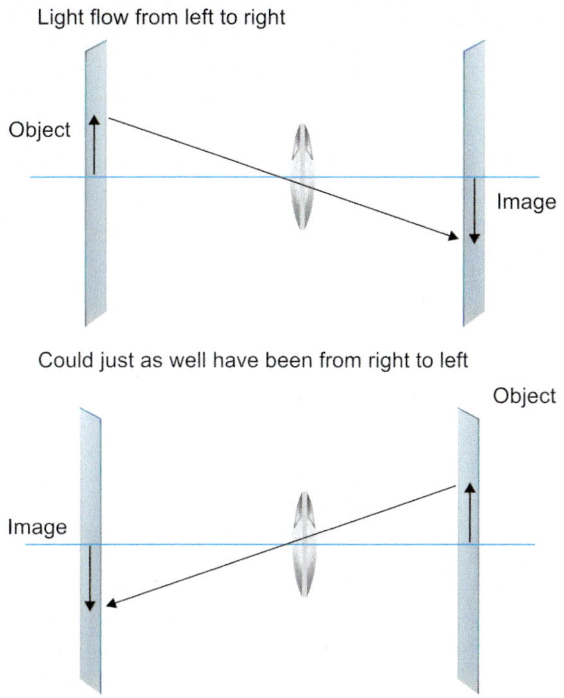

Fig. 13.30: Conjugate planes are frequently encountered in ophthalmology. The power of a lens does not depend upon the direction of light flow, and its effect on vergence is unchanged. Whether light flows from left to right, or right to left, the effect of the lens on the vergence of light is unchanged. For a given object and image, the distances and magnifications are interchangeable. The object can become image, and image become object, with no change in magnification or location.

and represents the location is space where a point source of light would have been imaged using a spherical lens of the same power. It is the best we can do to create an image with an uncorrected spherocylinder lens.

If the rays of light that enter the combination of the two lenses pass through a circular hole, the bounding rays that enclose the wavefront that is passing through the lens form a circle in cross section. The light rays that leave the spherocylinder lens start out as a circle (on the surface of the lens) but then start to become elliptical, leading to the formation of the anterior focal line, the focal line closest to the lens. As the rays continue past the anterior focal line, they again form a circular cross section (because the bounding rays are circular) at the reciprocal distance of the spherical equivalent of the lens power. This circular cross section of rays is called the Circle of Least Confusion. The bounding rays become elliptical leading to the formation of the second focal line, furthest from the lens, called the posterior focal line. The bounding image rays are collectively known as the Sturm's conoid and the interval between the two focal lines, containing the circle of least confusion, is known as the Sturm's Interval.

Why Astigmatic Lenses are Useful?

Optical system designers rarely create astigmatic lenses intentionally. Most optical systems are designed using spherical lenses, or other aspheric lenses that are rotationally symmetmric and bring point sources of light to a point focus.

As we will see, the primary purpose of astigmatic lenses is to correct the errors induced in an optical system by other astigmatic lenses. This finally leads us to the good part of this chapter, which is how we use lenses, both spherical and cylindrical, to correct refractive errors in our patients, allowing them to see clearly (Fig. 13.32).

TYPES OF REFRACTIVE ERROR

We now have enough knowledge of how lenses work to understand how an image is formed, and how sphere and cylinder lenses can be used to generate images. We know how to solve for the location of an image, given the location of an object and the power and location of the lens. Let us use these tools first to understand how light comes to focus inside the eye to see what should happen. We will then see what does, rather than should, happen in instances when people have refractive error and would benefit from spectacles. Finally, we will see how lenses can be used to put things right for those who would benefit from eyeglasses.

The Eye as an Optical System

As far as optical systems go, the eye is quite complex. It comes with its own built-in lens cleaner (the eyelids and tear film). There is a computer that automatically controls the aperture (pupil) and exposure time (retinal adaptation). There is an autofocus system that comes with a pretty good warranty (40 years or so). For the most part, it is maintenance free, but there are enough problems that we in eye care can find work.

The lenses of most optical systems are constructed of materials with a single, uniform index of refraction, and with shapes that are either very easy to manufacture (spherical lenses, for example) or at least specify in mathematics, so the surfaces can be readily manufactured. This is not the case with the eye, because the materials that are used to make the optical elements are not uniform, and the shapes that define these elements grow and then change over time.

We have so far considered a lens as being made of a material that has a different index of refraction than the

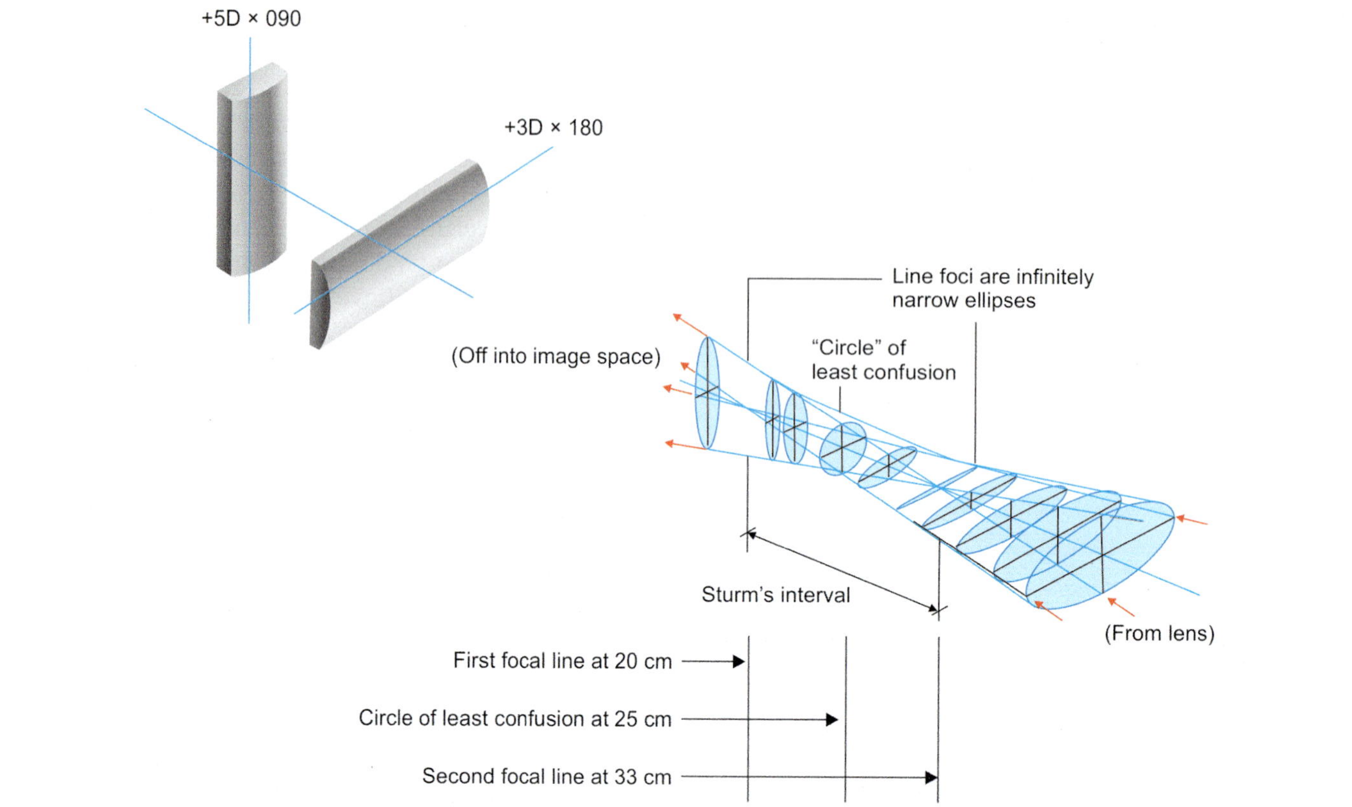

Fig. 13.31: Image formation with spherocylinder lenses. When two cylinder lenses are placed perpendicular to each other, the focal line for each lens forms as described in Figure 13.29. The transition from one focal line to the other is described by the transition from a line, to an ellipse, then to a circle (if the aperture is circular), and then again to an ellipse and line. The circle is located at the average dioptric value of the two cylinder lenses and is known as the circle of least confustion. The interval between the two focal lines that includes the circle of least confustion is called the Interval of Sturm.

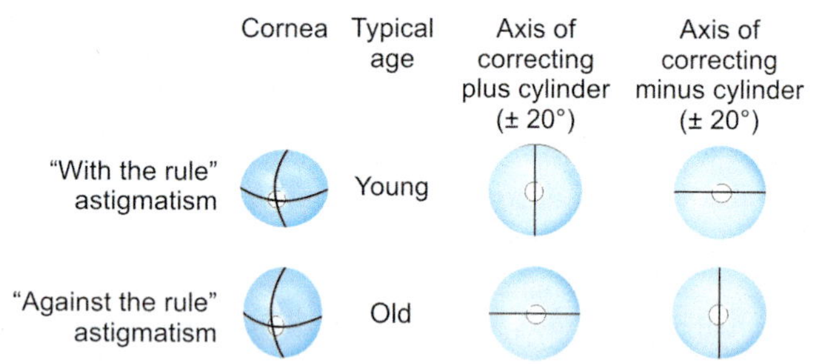

Fig. 13.32: Human eyes typically have a small amount of astigmatism at birth, become spherical with time, and then become astigmatic again with increasing age. Typically, young people have eyes that are steep vertically, and adults have eyes that are steep horizontally. Because correcting cylinders may be plus or minus in power, there can be confusion in differentiating these two states. For this reason, the term "with the rule" applies to the astigmatism arising from a vertically steep cornea, and "against the rule" is the term applied to a cornea that is horizontally steep.

material that surrounds it, and having a well-defined boundary of some shape that we can analyze using Snell's law to see how light would change direction when it crosses the interface. When we are dealing with materials such as air (refractive index of 1) and glass (refractive index about 1.5), it is very easy to say where the air stops and the glass starts.

The Optical Surfaces of the Eye

Finding similar, well-defined boundaries is not so easy with the eye. The only really clear boundary is between air (refractive index of 1) and the tears that coat the cornea (refractive index about 1.33). Inside the cornea, there are multiple layers of structure, all with slight variation in their contents. The aqueous is pretty much uniform in its refractive index, only slightly higher than water. The crystalline lens has a well-defined interface that separates it from the aqueous and the vitreous, but once past childhood, the lens is very complex in its interior distribution of materials of various refractive indices (the nucleus develops, and each layer of the cortex is a little different than the next). The vitreous, like the aqueous, is uniform for the most part (except for those troublesome

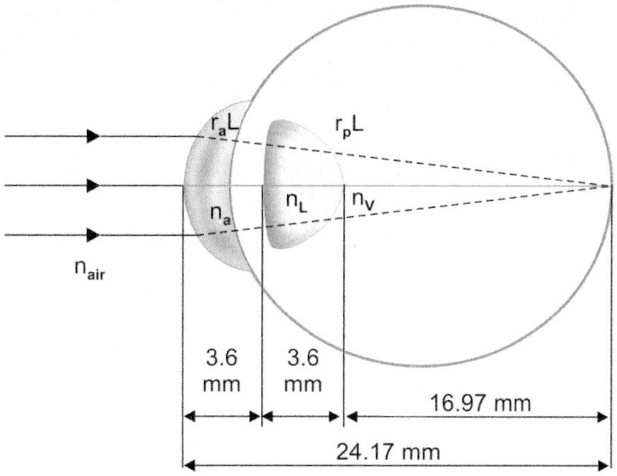

Fig. 13.33: Gullstrand's model eye. This description of the human eye assumes the eye is made of four different materials, each with a different index of refraction. The cornea has an anterior and posterior curvature, there is an anterior chamber filled with aqueous, and a lens that has a different anterior and posterior curvature. Behind the lens is the vitreous cavity leading to the retina. The curvatures and indices of refraction are shown.

floaters), and the retina has a lot of structure (cellular in nature) on top of the actual sensors (the rods and cones) that the light has to pass through before being detected.

Gullstrand's model eye (Fig. 13.33): If we try to make a model that incorporates knowledge of all this anatomy, the model will become very complex very quickly. Allvar Gullstrand (1852–1930) was awarded a Nobel Prize in 1911 for his work to characterize the typical human eye. His eye model simplified the complex anatomy into three refracting surfaces (cornea, front of the lens, and back of the lens) and uniform refractive indices for the aqueous, lens, and vitreous as shown. This model can be further simplified, if all the eye contents are considered to be water.

The reduced schematic eye (Fig. 13.34): The reduced schematic eye (model eye) is about as simple as an eye model can get, and is sufficient for understanding normal types of refractive error and spectacle correction. The eye is completely made of water (refractive index 13.33) and has optical power of 60 D. The focal length of a 60 D lens is 1/60 = 16.66 mm. (The 60 D power for the eye combines approximately 40 D of corneal power and 20 D of lens power into a single refracting surface).

We previously learned that the radius of curvature associated with 60 D power, and indices of refraction of 1 (air) and 4/3 (water) would be 60 = (4/3 -1) /(radius in meters), or 5.55 mm (check my mathematical), and this corresponds to the corneal radius of curvature in the reduced eye.

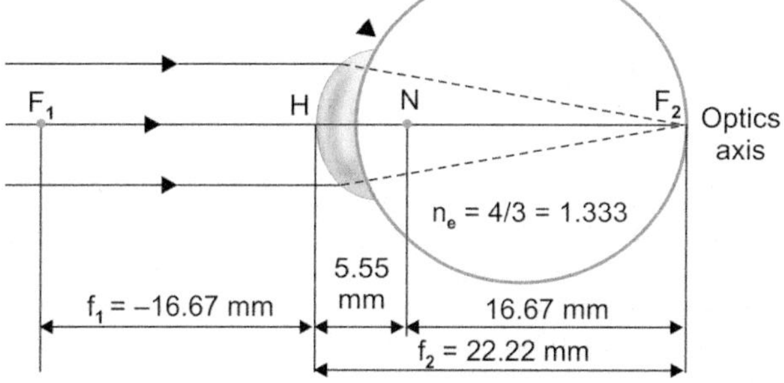

Fig. 13.34: The reduced schematic eye is a simplification of Gullstrand's eye. All refraction occurs at a single optical interface (the anterior cornea). The entire eye is made of water (index of refraction 1.33). The curvature of the cornea has +60 D power. With this simplified model eye, and by remembering that the nodal point of the eye is located 16.67 mm from the retina, it is possible to determine image sizes on the retina by drawing the central ray through the nodal point.

Up until now, we have considered lenses to have air on either side of the lens. This is the first we are considering where an image will form when there is a different refractive index on one side of the lens than the other. The model eye has a single refracting surface, with air on one side and water on the other. This asymmetry causes the nodal point of the eye to be displaced to a point 5.55 mm inside the eye; this is the position through which the central ray would pass, and from which the secondary focal point of the eye (where the retina is located) is measured.

Long and short eyes: This eye model is useful to us because it serves as a starting point for what constitutes normal vision, free of refractive error, and what happens when an individual eye diverges from normal.

An eye that is free of refractive error is said to exhibit emmetropia. In this instance, the optical power of the eye is balanced with the optical length of the eye, and light from infinity falls into focus on the retina.

If the eye is too long, then the 60 D of optical power provides too much optical power for the excessive axial length, and the light from infinity focuses in the vitreous. This condition is called axial myopia. Relatively normal optical power and relatively long axial length is the most commonly found type of myopia. In this circumstance, the secondary focal point of the eye is in the vitreous cavity.

If the eye is too short, the 60 D of optical power provides too little power to bring the light into focus on a retina that is too close to the cornea. This condition is called axial hyperopia, and is associated with nanophthalmos. Here the secondary focal point of the eye is behind the retina (Fig. 13.35).

Steep and flat corneas and lenses: Conversely, sometimes the eye has a relatively normal axial length, but the optical power of the eye is excessive. Causes might include an excessively steeply curved crystalline lens, as is found in lentiglobus. Regardless of the cause, the secondary focal point is again in the vitreous.

An eye that has a normal axial length but insufficient optical power might arise from a patient having a relatively flat cornea, or weak lens, the extreme example of which is aphakia, where the crystalline lens has been removed and not replaced with an intraocular lens (Fig. 13.36). The secondary focal point of the eye is behind the retina.

Astigmatic refractive errors: All these refractive errors can be associated with astigmatism, where the refracting power of the eye is not symmetric, and one orientation has more power than another. Astigmatic lenses produce focal lines rather than a point focus, and the secondary focal lines can either be located in the vitreous (myopic) or behind the retina (hyperopic). Sometimes both lines are myopic or hyperopic, sometimes only one, sometimes the two lines straddle the vitreous. These five conditions are named as shown in Figure 13.37.

Patterns of astigmatism: Astigmatism usually arises from unequal steepness of the cornea, and can change over one's

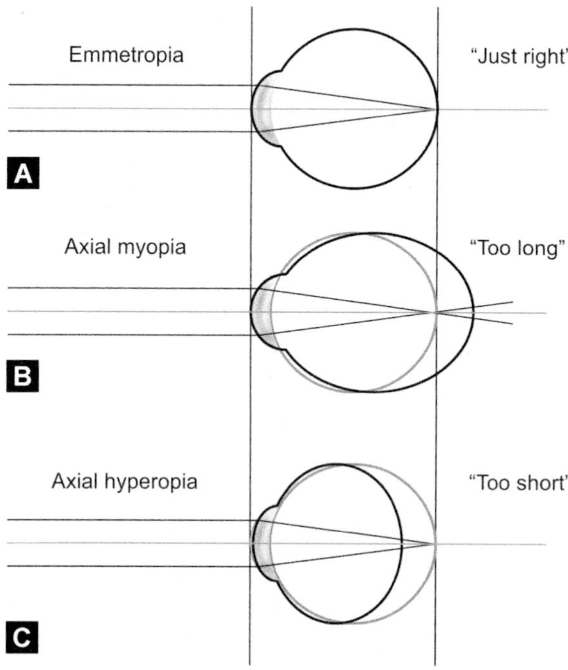

Figs. 13.35A to C: Axial refractive errors, where the eye is too long or too short. The emmetropic eye (A) is an eye that has sufficient optical power to bring light from infinity into focus on the retina. In the eye that is "too long" (B) the axial length is excessive for the optical power, and the eye is said to exhibit axial myopia. For the eye that is "too short" (C), the eye is too short for the optical power, and is said to exhibit axial hyperopia.

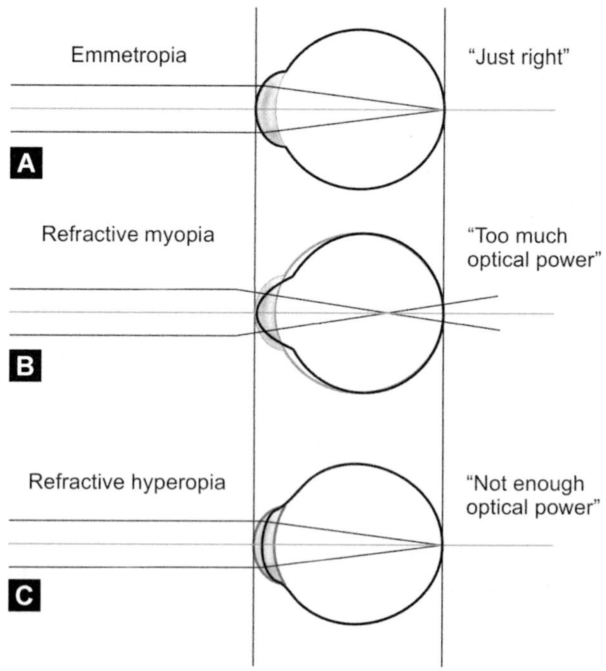

Figs. 13.36A to C: Refractive power errors, where the optical power is either excessive or insufficient. In emmetropia (A), the eye is balanced between the optical power and the axial length; light from infinity comes to focus on the retina. In refractive myopia (B), the eye has too much optical power for the normal axial length, and the light comes to focus in the vitreous. In refractive hyperopia (C), there is insufficient optical power for the normal axial length, and the light from infinity has not yet converged to focus when it strikes the retina.

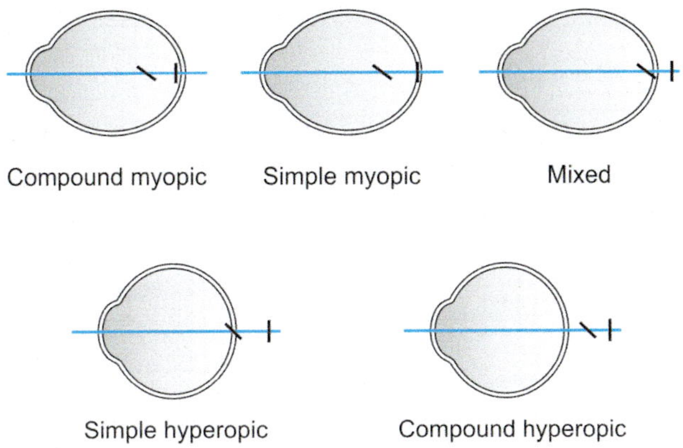

Fig. 13.37: In the presence of astigmatism, the naming of refractive errors becomes more complex. When both focal lines are in the vitreous (top left), the eye has compound myopic astigmatism. When one focal line is on the retina, and the other in the vitreous, the eye has simple myopic astigmatism (upper, middle). When the two focal lines straddle the retina, the astigmatism is mixed (top, right). When one focal line is on the retina, and the other behind the retina, the astigmatism is simple hyperopic astigmatism (bottom left). Finally, when both focal lines are behind the retina, the astigmatism is compound hyperopic astigmatism.

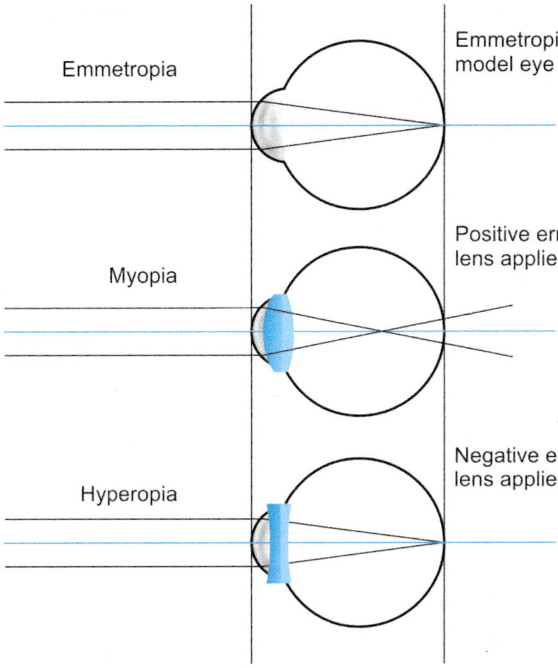

Fig. 13.38: Simple refractive errors can be modeled by thinking of the reduced schematic eye (top) being change to myopic (middle) or hyperopic (bottom) by the insertion of an error lens. This error lens can be thought of as a plus lens inserted into the eye (for myopia) or a minus lens inserted into the eye (for hyperopia). In practice, these changes are typically modelled by changing the optical power of the cornea in the reduced schematic eye but leaving the nodal point and axial length unaffected.

lifetime. Typically, when people are young, their corneas are steep vertically. As they go through adolescence, the corneas transition to spherical, and then as they age, the corneas sag and become steeper horizontally than vertically. This is only a generalization that applies to average values of astigmatism across the population and does not mean that each person goes through this transition, as many people with higher levels of astigmatism exhibit the same general shape throughout their lives. There is a convention that instead of saying corneas that are steep vertically, corneas that are steep vertically are said to exhibit with the rule astigmatism, and corneas that are steep horizontally are said to exhibit against the rule astigmatism (*see* Fig. 13.32).

A Simplified Model of Refractive Error (Fig. 13.38)

Why do we need to know all these terms to describe the types of refractive error? At this point, if your goal is to simply learn how the optics of spectacles work to correct refractive error, this information is not needed. However, an understanding of the origins of refractive error is essential when you are anticipating corrections to the eye, such as for refractive surgery, where the cornea is manipulated, or cataract surgery, where the intraocular lens power is determined as part of surgical planning. For right now, we can get back to the business of learning how glasses work by going back to the schematic eye and making it deviate from normal by placing an error lens on top of the model eye. We can add or subtract optical power by placing a lens on the cornea of the model eye. For example, we can make an emmetropic individual experience myopia by placing a plus power contact lens on their eye. The plus power contact lens is the error lens—it takes a normal eye and induces a refractive error. The correcting lens for this normal individual who was made to by myopic by placing a positively powered contact lens on their cornea would be a minus lens in their spectacles.

This is a very powerful tool, for it allows us to think of the difference between the underlying error of refraction, and then, how to correct that error. It also allows us to clear up some common errors that occur when discussing deviations from emmetropia. For example, it is not correct to say that an individual with 5 D of myopia, and who wears a correction of -5 D has a refractive error of minus 5 D. That individual has a refractive correction of minus 5 D, as their underlying refractive error is plus 5 D. It is much easier to simply say they have 5 D of myopia, which is clear, correct, and unambiguous.

Spectacle Correction of Refractive Error

We have considered the characteristics of refractive error as a defect of manufacturing, and while it helps us to understand that why people need to wear glasses, it does not help us to understand that how it affects their lives. To get to the impact that refractive error has on vision, we need to turn the light around and try and see things from the perspective of the patient. This is also a chance to introduce a new optical concept, that of conjugate planes.

Conjugate Points and Planes: Conventional lenses pass light in either direction. As a consequence, the image plane and the object plane can be interchanged as long as the respect positions are not changed. In Figure 13.30, on top, a plus lens is used to image an object, and the object distance is greater than the image distance. If we were to turn the light around, and place the object to the right (as in the bottom part of the illustration) the distances to the respective planes are unchanged. These planes are conjugal, the positions are fixed but either can serve for placing an object or image.

The far point of the eye: Knowing that we can reverse the direction of light flow, we can now consider what the visual experience of individuals with refractive error is like. Instead of thinking about refractive error in terms of where the secondary focal point of the eye is located with respect to the retina, think about where in space the patient's retina is conjugate with. This location in space is called the far point, and represents where an object would be placed and be seen by the patient without glasses (Fig. 13.39).

For the emmetropic individual, the far point is at infinity. Their eyes are such that light rays coming from infinity are focused on the retina.

The myopic individual has a far point that is said to be in from infinity, or located in space in front of the patient. For the myope, this is where they can see clearly when they are not wearing their glasses.

The hyperopic individual has a problem: nothing is in focus for them at any distance. The minus error lens causes rays of light exiting the eye (when we turned the light around, and passed it through the minus error lens, the light rays diverged). If we trace the rays back, we see that the far point is a virtual far point, located behind the eye, and found by following the dotted line extensions of the light rays leaving the eye.

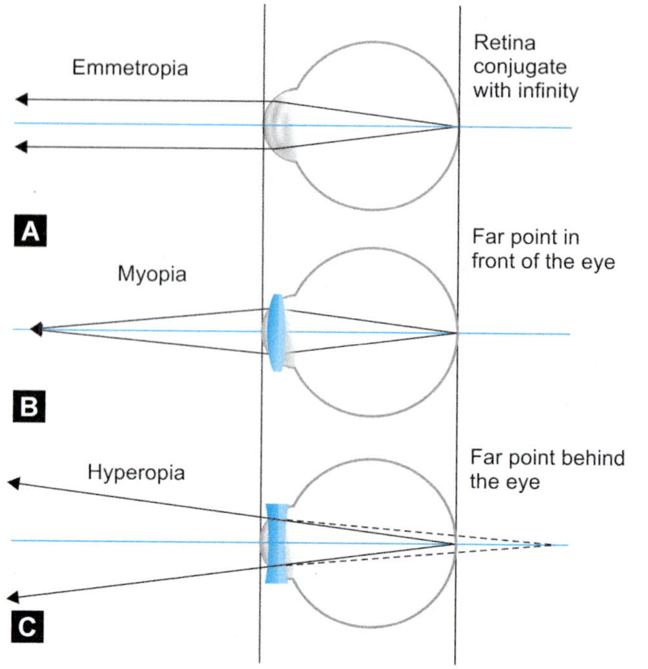

Figs. 13.39A to C: The far point as applied to the reduced schematic eye. For the emmetropic eye (A) the retina is conjugate with infinity: light emitted from the retina would come to focus at infinity. For the myopic eye (B), light from the retina would converge in response to the plus power error lens, and come to focus in front of the eye. For the hyperopic eye (C), light from the retina would never come to focus, because the minus error lens would cause diverging light rays to exit the eye. Tracing these rays backwards to behind the eye reveals the hyperopic far point to be behind the eye.

ACCOMMODATION

People with hyperopia are often not aware that they are hyperopic early in life, because accommodation provides a mechanism to increase the plus power of the eye via contraction of the ciliary muscle. By increasing the plus power of the eye, they are able to overcome the inherent imbalance that induced the hyperopia (either too short an eye for the optical power, or insufficient optical power when accommodation is relaxed). By increasing the internal plus power of the eye and adding that additional plus power to the negative error lens in the hyperopic eye model, the error lens is converted to a plano lens, and parallel rays of light emerge from the eye. For accommodation to overcome the negative hyperopic error lens, the hyperopic individual must be able to chronically accommodate sufficiently well to see at infinity, and intermittently accommodate an additional three or so Diopters for near vision.

An uncorrected hyperopic individual that accommodates does so at the risk of inducing accommodative esotropia, where the accommodation also stimulates convergence of the eyes, leading to an imbalance between where the eyes are focused, and where the eyes converge to in space.

Determining the Location of the Far Point

There are many ways to determine the far point of the eye, all of which fall under the general name of refraction. Yes, we have already used the term refraction to describe the change in the direction of light when it passes from one optical media to another by passing through an optical interface. The term is also used to determine a lens prescription to allow an individual to see clearly when they need spectacles.

The retinoscope is the far point finder, in that the flash of retinoscopic neutralization occurs when the peephole of the retinoscope is located at a position in space that corresponds with the patient's far point. With the additional use of handheld lenses, the patient's far point can be optically manipulated until it is moved to a convenient location, typically about arm's length from a patient.

For a myopic individual, the simplest way of locating the patient's far point is to tell them to move far enough away from an object that it is not seen clearly, and then to slowly move toward the object till it first comes into focus. Measure that distance in meters, and you have the distance to the far point for that eye.

Once the patient's far point has been identified, it is time to prescribe a pair of glasses.

Correcting Refractive Error Using the Far Point Method

As it turns out, there are only two steps to prescribing a distance correction:

1. Determine the location of the far point.
2. Choose a lens that places its secondary focal point at the patient's far point.

That is it—two steps. Of course, included in those two steps is a lot of background information. Let us work through those steps to see how these two rules can be used to select a prescription for spectacles.

Let us start with a myope.

MYOPIC SPECTACLE CORRECTION

Using a near card and a tape measure, we learned that until the near card was brought to 50 cm from a subject, they could not read the smallest letters. Our measurement provides the location of the far point, 50 cm from the cornea. We wish to prescribe a pair of eyeglasses and must take into account the vertex distance of the spectacles, or the distance between the correcting spectacle lens and the cornea. Allowing for 10 mm (1 cm) for the vertex distance, a correcting lens would need to be (1/0.49) D, or 2.04 D. Lenses are commonly prescribed to the nearest 0.25 D, so a prescription for -2.00 spectacles would be provided to the patient (Fig. 13.40).

Here, accounting for the 1 cm vertex distance had a minimal effect (0.04 D). That is not always the case.

Vertex Distance Conversion

There are any number of lenses, plus or minus, that can be used to satisfy the requirement to choose a lens that places its secondary focal point at the patient's far point. In this example, we are changing the vertex distance (actually, eliminating it) by moving the correction from the spectacle

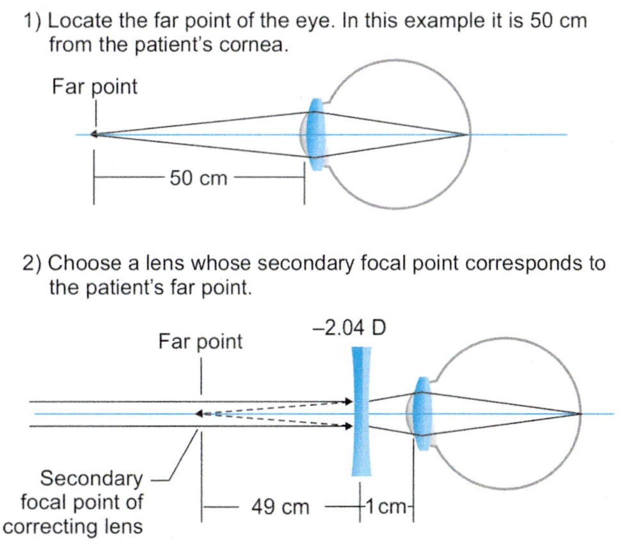

Fig. 13.40: Correction of myopic using the far point concept. To correct myopia, it is necessary to first find the far point of the eye by refraction, then place a lens whose secondary focal point coincides with the patient's far point. By doing so, the converging error for light exiting the eye heading to the far point is compensated by the minus power that brings light from infinity into matching divergence.

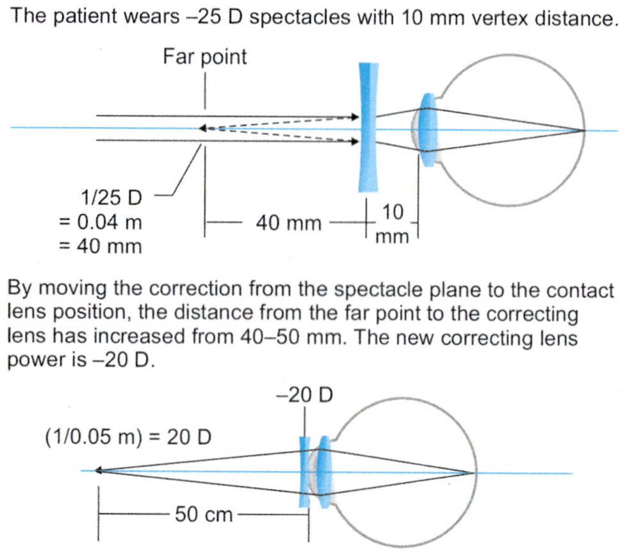

Fig. 13.41: Minus spectacle vergence distance correction. When a myopic patient's correction is moved from the spectacle plane to the contact lens position, the correcting lens is moved further from the far point. The greater the distance, the less power is required for the correcting lens. For this reason, minus spectacle lenses require less optical power for contact lens correction.

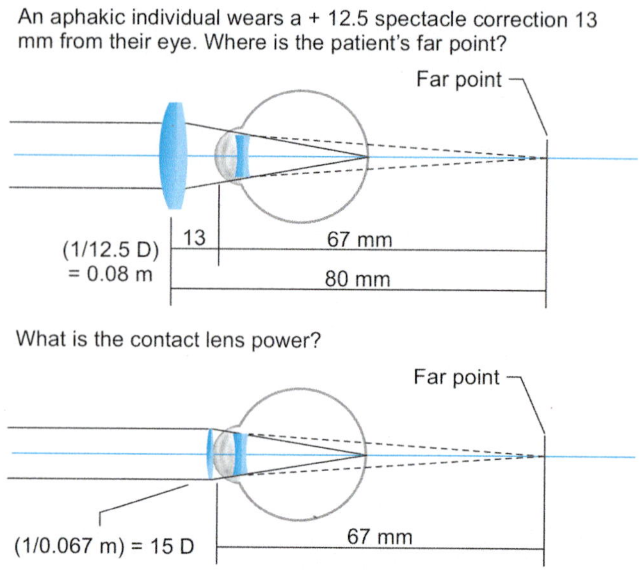

Fig. 13.42: Plus spectacle lens vertex distance correction. When a hyperopic patient's correction is moved from the spectacle plane to the contact lens position, the correcting lens is moved closer to the far point. The shorter distance is associated with a higher powered plus correcting lens. For this reason, plus spectacle lenses increase in power when moved from the spectacle plane to the contact lens position.

plane to the contact lens position. For this high myope, there is an additional ten of distance from the contact lens to the far point, as compared to the spectacle distance. This increased distance of the correction to the far point results in the required correcting power to decrease (Fig. 13.41).

In general, for a myope, moving the correction further from the patient decreases the distance of the correction to the far point, and increases the required correcting power. Moving a correction toward the patient increases the distance of the correction to the far point, and decreases the required correcting power.

The above generalization is true for myopes. As you have probably already figured out, it is the opposite for hyperopes. Let us see why.

Hyperopic Corrections

The hyperopic patient has a far point that is located behind the eye. If a patient comes in wearing spectacles, which is the correct prescription for that patient, the patient's far point is identified by the lens power and the vertex distance (Fig. 13.42).

A change in lens position will result in the new lens either being closer to, or further from, the patient's far point. For the hyperope, with a far point behind the eye, the contact lens is closer to the far point than the spectacle lens. Because the distance to the far point is less, the dioptric power of the contact lens is greater. In this example, for an aphakic individual, there is a 2.5 D difference between the contact lens (greater power) and spectacle (lesser power).

Astigmatic Correction

Patients with astigmatism have two far lines, rather than a single far point. There is a distance from each of these far lines to the patient's cornea, and the reciprocal of the distance of the far line to the cornea, in meters, is the associated cylinder power. Remember that the axis of astigmatism is parallel to the focal line that is created with a cylinder lens when attributing a line to an orientation of cylinder.

A final nuance is that not all cylinder powers are simply vertical or horizontal as we have largely used so far. Astigmatism axes are oriented the same for both the right and left eye, with the axes starting at zero to your right (or the patient's left) as you face the patient.

CONCLUSION

Prescribing spectacles really is as simple as finding the patient's far point, and then picking a lens whose secondary focal point coincides with the patient's far point. Understanding these concepts will allow you to visualize in your mind what is happening during activities such as retinoscopy and subjective refraction.

ACKNOWLEDGMENTS

The author is grateful to Paul Boeder, PhD and David Guyton, MD for refining the teaching of clinical optics through vergence concepts.

Part 4 Vision Rehabilitation

August Colenbrander

OUTLINE

Chapter 14 Why Vision Rehabilitation?

August Colenbrander, Donald C Fletcher

INTRODUCTION

Vision rehabilitation refers to the multidisciplinary effort of assisting those with various degrees of vision loss in coping with the *consequences* of that loss. To describe vision rehabilitation, the nature of vision itself must be understood.

Vision is the major source of information about our environment. The eyes alone contribute as much information to the brain as all other organs combined. It is not surprising, therefore, that many people fear loss of vision almost as much as loss of life.

Most people will state that "we see with our eyes". On closer examination, this is not true. An isolated eyeball cannot produce any vision; our brain, however, can produce exquisite visual imagery in our dreams, without any input from the eyes.

Vision rehabilitation cuts across all traditional subspecialties of ophthalmology, since it deals with the *consequences*, rather than with the *causes* of vision loss. This section will have three chapters. This first chapter will provide an overview. The second chapter will discuss the assessment and devices, needed to improve—*how the eyes function.* The third chapter will discuss ways to improve—*how the person functions.*

FOUR ASPECTS OF VISION LOSS

Vision is a complex phenomenon. A convenient framework for discussing the various impacts of vision loss is to consider four aspects of visual functioning (Fig. 14.1).[1]

First, we must consider how various external causes may result in *structural changes* to the eyes and the visual pathways. For this aspect, the focus is on the tissue; an ocular pathologist is needed to describe the pathological condition.

However, structural changes alone do not determine how well the eyes actually function. Clinicians need to measure *organ function*, such as visual acuity, visual field and contrast sensitivity.

Yet, even knowing how the eyes function, does not tell us how the person functions. In other words, the *abilities* of the person to perform tasks, such as reading, mobility, face recognition and activities of daily living, must be considered. Occupational therapists and other rehabilitation professionals work with patients to teach them how residual vision can be used most effectively. Occupational therapists also assess the person in a societal context.[2] For example, do the visual changes have an impact on the person's *participation* in society, on the ability to perform necessary tasks and on general satisfaction with one's quality of life? It is clear that to cover all aspects of vision rehabilitation a team approach is necessary, and that the patient must be part of that team.

Any single activity of daily living may exhibit several of the above aspects. When reading, the aspect of minimum print size falls under organ function (retinal resolution). Reading speed (words/minute) and reading endurance (hours/day) define abilities of the person; reading endurance may be poor, even if reading acuity is adequate. Reading enjoyment, finally, falls under the aspect of quality of life.

It is helpful to draw a line between the organ side of Figure 14.1 on the left, and the person side on the right.

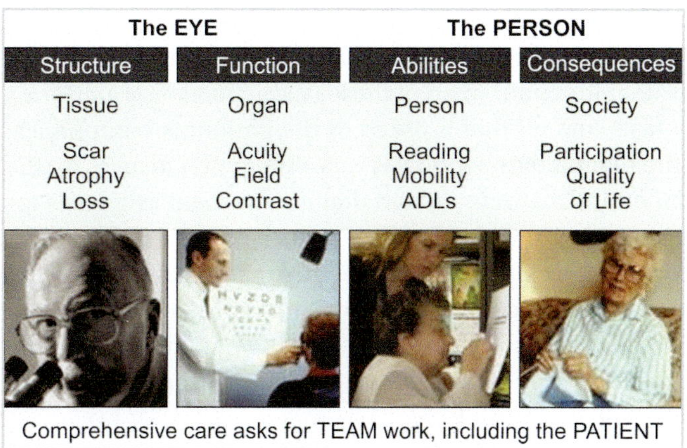

Fig. 14.1: Aspects of visual functioning.

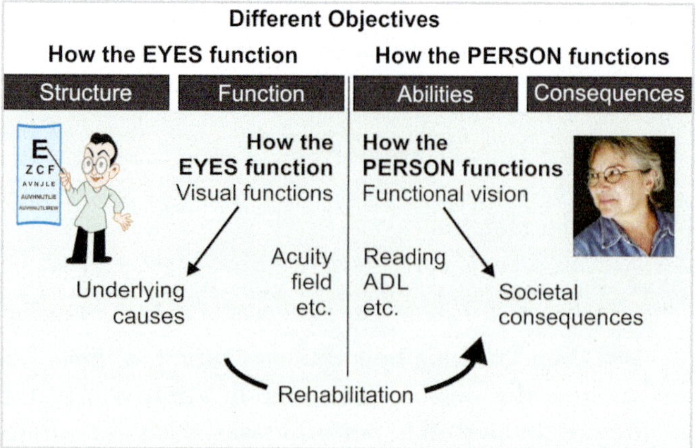

Fig. 14.2: The role of rehabilitation.

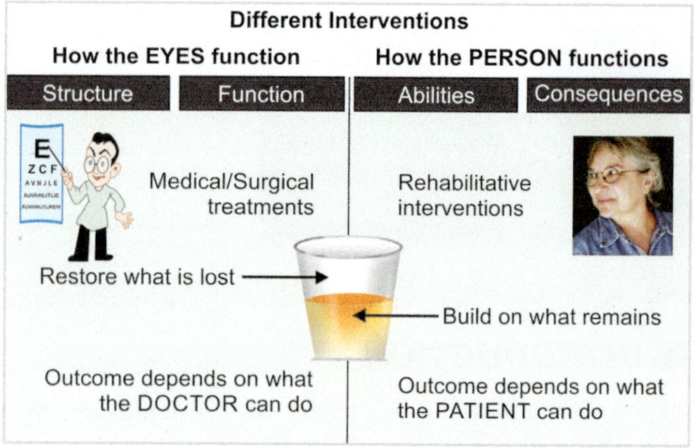

Fig. 14.3: Different interventions.

On the left side of the diagram, we discuss *visual functions*, such as visual acuity and visual field. Eye doctors are interested in these aspects, which describe *how the Eyes function*, since their task is to find the underlying *causes* of eye disease. On the right side, we speak of *functional vision*, which describes *how the person functions* in vision-related activities, such as reading, mobility and activities of daily living. Here, the goal is to address the societal *consequences* of eye disease, since the ultimate goal of all interventions is to improve the patient's quality of life. It is the function of vision rehabilitation to make sure that "eye" doctors become "people" doctors by extending their interest to the right side of the diagram as well (Fig. 14.2).

This is not just a theoretical distinction. It affects the interventions that are needed. On one side, we follow the *medical model*; on the other side, we follow the *rehabilitation model*. The medical model seeks to restore what is lost by focusing on the part of the glass that is half-empty. The most common example is the correction of refractive error, to restore lost focus. The oldest example may be the removal of cataracts to restore lost transparency. The latest examples are retinal implants that bypass lost retinal function. In all of these cases, the doctor performs a task, and all that is asked of the patient is compliance. The rehabilitation model is very different. It focuses on the functions that remain and that can be used as a basis for new skills. Here, the patient must perform the task, and the doctor's role shifts. Words, like treatment and prescription, must be replaced with support and guidance (Fig. 14.3). We can give the patient crutches; the patient must do the walking. We can give the patient a magnifier, the patient must do the reading.

Moving from the medical model to the rehabilitation model requires a *role reversal*. When either the doctor or the patient does not accept this shift in responsibilities, rehabilitation will not be optimal. An important part of rehabilitation counseling is to shift the focus from the part of the glass that is half-empty, to the part that is still half-full.

COMPREHENSIVE VISION REHABILITATION

Considering all of these aspects, comprehensive vision rehabilitation involves much more than the patient's performance on a letter chart and requires teamwork between different professionals who specialize in different aspects of vision loss. Since all vision loss starts with some medical condition, ophthalmologists are well positioned to coordinate team activities. Every physician needs to be aware of what other team members can contribute and should know where to locate vision rehabilitation resources and how to make appropriate referrals.

Individuals, who suffer a visual impairment that cannot be eliminated with refractive correction, yet are not blind, are said to have *low vision*. They may benefit from a broad variety of services, as indicated in Figure 14.4. Their needs differ from the needs of the blind and are more diverse. All those who are totally blind are equally blind; the residual visual functions of those with low vision can vary greatly.

Vision enhancement, which is the traditional focus of low vision care, is primarily oriented at improving the optical stage of visual processing, through visual aids, including a wide range of magnification devices. Additionally,

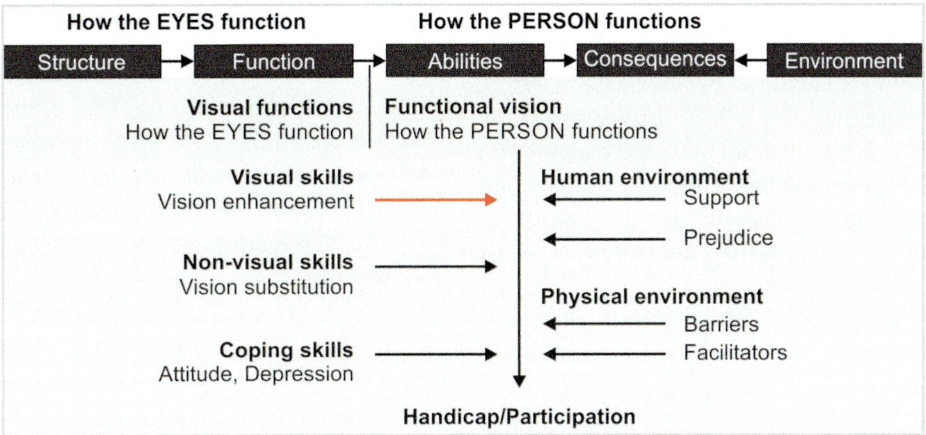

Fig. 14.4: Factors in comprehensive vision rehabilitation.

enhancement of contrast, illumination and filters need to be explored.

Vision substitution expands the options for rehabilitation by optimizing the use of other senses. This can range from using simple tactile markings to sense the position of a stove dial, to devices such as talking books, a long cane for travel and Braille for reading. Vision enhancement and vision substitution are not mutually exclusive. A patient may use a magnifier to read price tags, and may prefer talking books for recreational reading. A patient with retinitis pigmentosa, which causes reduced night vision, may have normal mobility in the day time, and need a cane at night. Digital audio books may have Braille labels.

Vision assistance is a special form of vision substitution that involves using the vision of others. Family members, care givers and office personnel should be familiar with *sighted guide* techniques to effectively assist visually impaired patients with minimal embarrassment. *Guide dogs* are also a possibility. Using a guide dog requires training of the patient as well as of the dog, so that they can work as a team. Dog users must also demonstrate mastery of independent travel skills.

Coping skills: How different patients will accept visual aids may differ greatly. It is important to recognize that vision loss often causes a reactive depression. On the one hand, a depressed patient will be less receptive to rehabilitative suggestions. On the other hand, demonstration of rehabilitative success can be a powerful tool to lift a reactive depression and to motivate the patient for further success. It has been shown that the teaching of problem solving skills may improve the effectiveness of vision rehabilitation.[3]

Many professionals may be involved in vision rehabilitation. Technicians may prescribe magnifiers; rehabilitation workers may teach daily living skills and psychologists may address depression. Acceptance of the work of these professionals will be improved if the trusted primary physician is credited for making the referrals.

Beyond the factors that directly involve the patient, the environment must also be considered.

The *human environment* is important. As patients go through the stages of adaptation, a supportive home environment is essential. As patients are counseled, it is important to include spouses, adult children or significant others, to make sure that they understand the condition, know what can be expected, and how to support the patient. Answering family and caregiver questions directly by including them in the consultation is often better than leaving this to the patient, who initially may not have absorbed everything that was said. An over-protective environment, which deprives patients of opportunities to do things for themselves, can be as detrimental as an over-demanding one that puts too much emphasis on the patient's shortcomings. The same holds for the work or school environment or for social groups.

Initially, patients often feel isolated and believe that they are the only ones experiencing these problems. *Peer support groups* can be helpful; in these groups, patients can experience how others are dealing with similar problems.

Finally, the *Physical environment* needs to be considered. An uncluttered environment, where things have a defined, fixed place is helpful because it reduces the need for searching. Good general illumination and task lighting often help, because at higher illumination levels retinal cells that are damaged but not dead can still contribute to vision. Good contrast is important: do not serve milk in a white Styrofoam cup; mark the edges of steps and stairs. Triangles and circles on men's and woman's bathrooms are designed to be visible for those with very low vision; Braille labels in elevators are useful for people who are totally blind.

The American Academy of Ophthalmology has developed a Preferred Practice Pattern for Vision Rehabilitation[4] and recently produced a video,[5] stating that vision rehabilitation is now the standard of care, and that all patients with vision problems should receive such care. These services may either be provided in the office, or by an appropriate agency. The LOVIT II study,[6] a study of vision rehabilitation with randomized controls, found that for simple cases (down to 20/60) simple refraction and magnifying aids may be sufficient, but that for more severe cases (20/80 and less) formal vision rehabilitation services are advantageous.

HOW BLIND IS BLIND?

The most common visual function test is the letter chart, developed by Snellen in 1862. That test determines how large a letter, or other symbol, must be to be recognized by the patient. That size is then compared to the size recognized by a standard observer.

The test is simple; unfortunately, the terminology used to describe various ranges of vision loss is confusing. The Figures 14.5A to D show progressively degraded pictures with examples of the labels used to describe different degrees of visual impairment. The visual acuity level represented by each picture can be determined from the number of lines is that is readable on the low vision letter chart.

The first picture shows the visual acuity level that is labeled as "low vision" by the World Health Organization (WHO). Although the bottom lines of the letter chart cannot be read, the appearance of the room is near normal. The next picture shows what the Social Security Administration in the US considers "Statutory Blindness" for its programs.

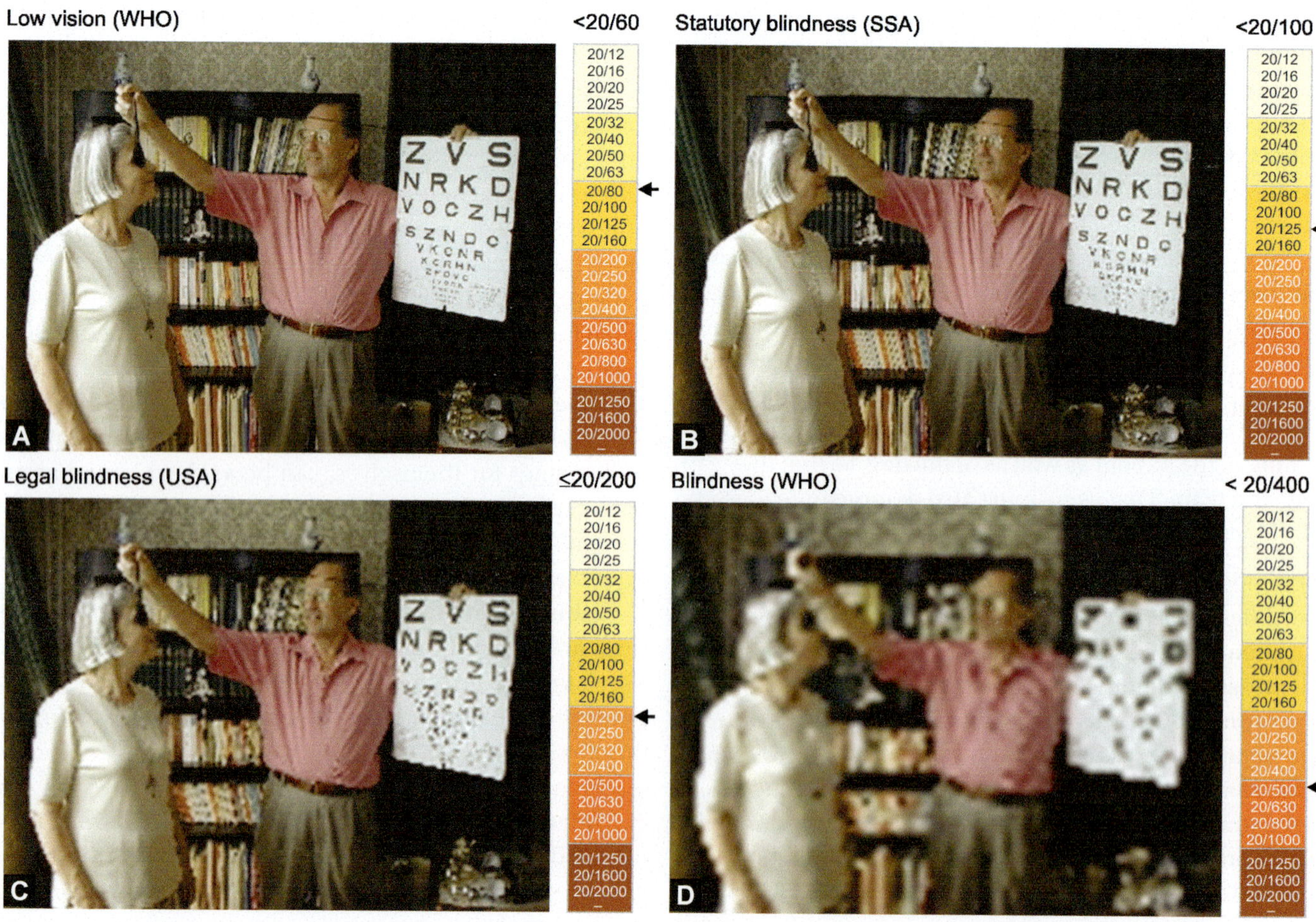

Figs. 14.5A to D: Labels for levels of vision loss. (A) Low vision; (B) Statutory blindness (SSA); (C) Legal blindness; (D) Blindness.

It is clear that this is far from actual blindness. Other US programs use a different definition, called "Legal Blindness", and the WHO does not consider a person "Blind" until they have reached the status of the last picture. At that level, reading even the special letter chart is not possible, but one can still navigate the room. Even this level of visual impairment does not constitute actual blindness.

The widespread use of the word blindness is unfortunate, since it emphasizes what has been lost, rather than the abilities that remain. Also, the term cannot be used with modifiers; one is either blind or sighted; one cannot be "a little bit blind". This negative emphasis and the associated black-and-white thinking have hampered the acceptance of vision rehabilitation. Terms such as vision loss or visual impairment are preferred, since they can be used with modifiers from mild and moderate to severe and profound and finally to total vision loss. Although "legal blindness" (USA) and "severe vision loss" (ICD-9-CM) have the same definition, there is a big difference between telling a patient *"You are legally blind"* and telling them *"You have a severe visual impairment".* The first statement might be followed by *"I am sorry, there is nothing more we can do for your eyes";* the second statement leads to the question *"What can we do to help you cope with this problem?"*

STAGES OF VISUAL PROCESSING

The visual process goes through three distinct stages. Each stage comes with its own specific problems.

- First is the *optical stage,* where the refractive media of the eye deliver an image to the retina. Familiar problems in this area include refractive errors and cataracts.
- Second is the *receptor stage,* where the optical image is translated into neural impulses. Age-related macular degeneration (AMD) is a significant problem of the receptor stage; it is becoming increasingly common as the population ages.
- Third are various stages of *neural processing,* initially in the inner retina, then in the visual cortex, and finally in higher cortical centers, where the visual input gives rise to visual perception and to visually-guided behaviors, actions and interactions.

The most common visual problems vary for different ages. Today, brain damage related vision problems [cerebral visual impairment (CVI)] are the most prevalent cause of visual impairment in *infants* and *young children.* Since vision is so important for normal development, vision loss in infants constitutes a developmental emergency and should be detected and addressed as early as possible. When a child does not smile back at the mother, the mother may be inclined to leave the baby in its crib, instead of holding it to provide extra tactile stimulation to compensate for missing visual stimulation.

At *school age* and later, visual health is critical because reading becomes important for academic development. For *adults,* vision is important for maintaining independence in activities of daily living (ADL) and for the development of vocational skills. For *seniors,* vision loss may exacerbate other age-related dysfunctions. Studies of the elderly have shown correlations between visual impairment and depression, falls and reduced longevity. In all of these instances early detection and early intervention are essential; intervention should not be delayed until a stage of advanced vision loss. General ophthalmologists and primary care physicians play a crucial role in this respect.

VISION REHABILITATION TECHNIQUES AND DEVICES

Having considered the general outlines of vision rehabilitation, some details of rehabilitative interventions can be mentioned briefly. They will be discussed in more detail in the next two chapters. Every ophthalmologist should know what types of vision rehabilitation techniques are available.

Optical Problems

The most commonly encountered visual problems are those involving the optical system of the eye.

Refractive errors are the easiest visual problems to deal with. Refractive errors can be corrected with glasses or contact lenses, and for those who hate glasses, by refractive surgery. Even if there are also other causes of vision loss, determining the best refractive correction is an important first step.

Uncorrected refractive error is a major cause of visual impairment worldwide.[7] In developed countries, the question may be why people do not avail themselves of the solutions that are available. In developing countries, availability of and accessibility to eye care and to the correction of refractive errors often do not exist. Providing these, is a matter of public infrastructure, not of individual health care.

Opacities disrupt visual image formation. Cataracts are the most familiar opacity; they can be removed by surgery. Other opacities of a temporary or permanent nature may occur in the cornea, in the anterior chamber or in the vitreous cavity. Trachoma and the resulting corneal scarring, is a condition that does not exist in the developed world anymore, but it still is a significant cause of vision loss worldwide.

Letter chart acuity is a good way to measure the severity of optical problems. It should be understood, however, that letter chart acuity assesses only the function of the retina where the letter read is projected. Even for a patient with 20/200 acuity, this area is less than 1 degree. For optical problems, this does not matter, since foveal defocus predicts equal defocus in other areas of the retina. But for retinal problems, visual acuity alone does not provide a comprehensive assessment.

Magnification is the primary way to compensate for reduced acuity. One way to provide magnification is to bring print closer to the eye. Young people may do this without aids; for the elderly, this requires reading glasses with extra power. Additionally, large print may be helpful. Larger print on medicine labels, as required in several states, can reduce medication errors by the elderly, who often take several medications. Hand-held magnifiers are another option; today, many have built-in LED illumination to provide more light. Video magnifiers with a table mounted large screen are ideal for prolonged reading; they can also enhance contrast and brightness, while some devices can even read the text out loud. Tablets and smartphone apps can provide similar advantages in a portable form and are increasingly popular as visual aids.

Retinal Problems

While primitive forms of cataract surgery have existed for centuries, the study of retinal disorders has only been possible since the invention of the ophthalmoscope in 1851. The ability to effectively treat some retinal disorders is even more recent. Important retinal disorders include the following.

Age-related macular degeneration is the most frequent diagnosis encountered in any low vision rehabilitation service in the developed world. Since the condition is age-related, its frequency will continue to increase as the population ages. This has caused profound changes in the nature of low vision care. Until the mid-20th century most low vision care was provided by special education teachers, serving young students in schools for the blind. Today the majority of low vision patients are seniors. This has contributed to a significant influx of occupational therapists (OTs) into the field, with skills in addressing multiple geriatric impairments. Yet, the needs of seniors to be served still outstrip the available services.

Since macular degeneration affects central vision and the ability to read, most patients will ultimately seek rehabilitation help. However, if only one eye is affected, age-related macular degeneration may go unnoticed.[8] The patient may only complain when the second eye starts to deteriorate; at that point, the damage in the first eye may be beyond help. Therefore, it is useful to ask patients to develop the habit of alternately covering one eye to see whether there is any difference in vision between the eyes. If there is, this asks for further exploration.

Glaucoma is another age-related condition. Glaucoma often goes undetected, because it causes loss of peripheral vision, which is not obvious to the patient. Therefore, glaucoma must be sought out, primarily by measuring the intraocular pressure.

Letter charts are not an effective screening tool for glaucoma, since visual acuity is only affected in end-stage glaucoma. More effect can be expected from screening tests for contrast sensitivity and for visual field defects. The MeyeSight visual fitness test provides the tools to do this in a smartphone app.[9]

Diabetic retinopathy is not limited to seniors. As the incidence of diabetes is rising worldwide, so is the incidence of diabetic retinopathy. Even if treated, it may affect central vision (visual acuity) and cause scattered blind spots throughout the periphery (visual field).

There are many other hereditary and nonhereditary retinal conditions that may cause vision loss, but they occur in smaller numbers. They all require the help of vision rehabilitation professionals to help patients cope effectively.

Scotomata: Whatever the cause, retinal conditions will generally cause localized blind spots (scotomata). Therefore, when retinal damage is suspected, visual acuity alone is no longer a sufficient descriptor of visual impairment, since the retinal area where the chart letter is projected does not predict anything about other retinal areas. In addition to letter chart acuity, the condition of the central visual field and the presence of blind spots (scotomata) must be considered.

The Figures 14.6A and B show a retinal image, where a long word is projected across a ring scotoma that leaves only a small central island of vision. This patient will be able to recognize the central letter, but will not be able to read the word. Clinicians must be careful when providing such patients with magnification, since too much magnification will mean that fewer letters fit into the central area. This example makes it clear that when retinal involvement is suspected, a reading test will be more informative than a letter chart test, since reading requires a larger retinal area.[10]

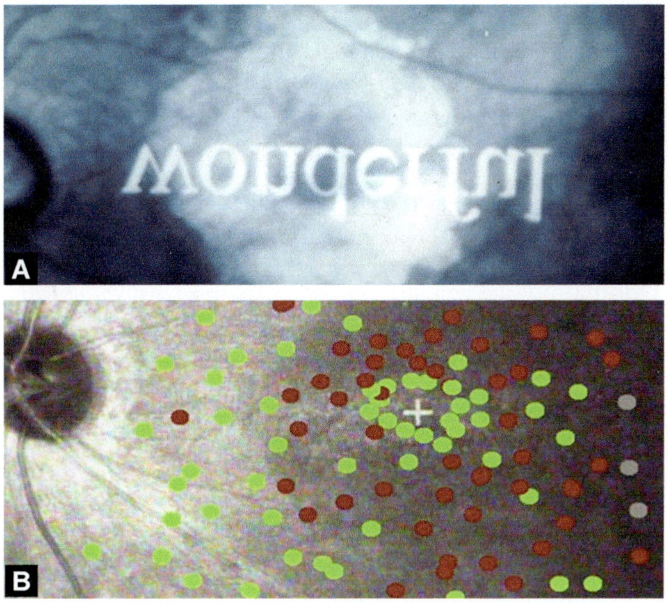

Figs. 14.6A and B: Ring scotoma. (A) Recognizing letters, but not words; (B) Micro-perimetry. Green = points seen; red = points missed.

Neural Processing Problems

As stated earlier, the most important stages of the visual process take place after the retinal receptors have translated the optical image into neural impulses.

The first transformations take place in the *inner retina*. Here, the input from 100 M receptors in each retina is compressed for transmission through 1 M nerve fibers in each optic nerve. The optic nerve fibers do not simply transmit a pixel-by-pixel image, as does a digital camera. Different retinal ganglion cells probably transmit different aspects of the image, such as edges (contrast enhancement), movement, color, brightness, etc. These separate "movies" are transmitted in parallel. Only at a later stage of neural processing, are these different aspects of the image combined again to trigger a single visual perception.

At the first synaptic station in the *lateral geniculate nucleus (LGN)* only 10–20% of the incoming connections come from the optic nerves, the other 80–90% come from other cortical centers and probably contribute to filtering based on attention and other factors.

Thus, the visual signal is heavily pre-processed when it arrives in the *visual cortex*, where it is further analyzed for shapes and contours.

In *higher cortical centers* the processing of the various parallel streams continues. Finally, the ascending visual information is matched with concepts stored in long-term memory. Only once the information is thus matched, can we recognize objects, and create a *mental model* of the environment (Fig. 14.7). That mental model is no longer limited to the retinal input, it is multisensory and contains all the information we ever collected about the object. With that accumulated information, we can now make decisions that lead to visually-guided action.

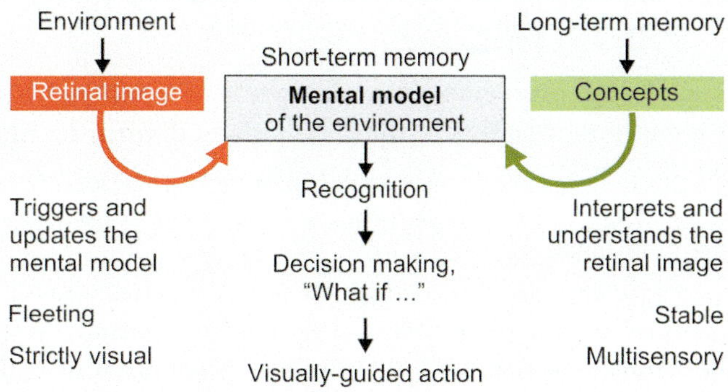

Fig. 14.7: The mental model.

In other words, the content of the mental model comes from concepts stored in memory. The retinal image serves to trigger those concepts and to keep the Mental Model consistent with the actual environment. While the retinal image is fleeting, the mental model of the environment provides a stable basis for our actions. When we move, and look around, we do not experience the retinal image moving across our retina, rather, we experience ourselves moving through a stable environment. Our detailed knowledge of these processes is still relatively new. It has been greatly helped by new modalities for neural and retinal imaging.

Today, neural processing problems are increasingly recognized in all age groups. In young children, CVI is now recognized as the most frequent cause of visual perceptual problems.[11] CVI effects are often not limited to the visual system. Schools for the blind have increasingly developed into schools for the multiply-handicapped.

In contact sports, the results of repeated subclinical injuries are now recognized. Traumatic brain injuries may cause problems that may be hard to define. Oculomotor system problems are common, while visual interpretation and decision making may also be impaired. Traffic accidents may cause similar damage. In the elderly, strokes may cause more localized problems and agnosias for specific tasks.

In all of these cases, the term *visual impairment* may be used when visual acuity and/or visual field are impaired. The term *visual dysfunction* may be more appropriate when the visual input to the brain is normal, but the processing of this information is not.

PATIENT-CENTERED FUNCTIONAL PRIORITIES

Since vision problems affect all aspects of a patient's life, it is no longer sufficient for clinicians to determine that *"nothing more can be done"* about the *causes* of vision loss, since *"much more can be done"* about the *consequences* of vision impairment.

To determine the range of services that may be appropriate for an individual with vision impairment, the American Academy of Ophthalmology recommends consideration of the following five functional priority areas:[8]

1. *Reading:* For many patients this is their foremost concern.
2. *Activities of daily living:* Even though reading may be the most prominent complaint, most people spend the larger part of their day performing a variety of vision dependent activities, other than reading, for self-care and home management.
3. *Safety:* Are people at risk for falls? How do they cross the street? Do they drive?
4. *Community participation:* Can the individual still participate in community events, including religious gatherings?
5. *Physical, cognitive and psychosocial well-being:* Since many patients with vision loss are elderly, this is an important aspect that should not be overlooked. If cognitive problems exist, it may affect the recommendations to be made.

Based on these considerations, patient-centered priorities can be set and specific rehabilitation goals formulated that reflect the patient's needs and desires.

CONCLUSION

Most of the chapters of this textbook deal with the *causes* of vision loss. Vision rehabilitation extends the perspective to its *consequences*. This extends the area of interest beyond the eye to the visual system, to the person as a whole and to the person's environment (*see* Fig. 14.4). The next chapter offers a discussion of factors relating to the eye, and by extension to the visual system. The last chapter discusses the interaction with the environment.

ADDITIONAL RESOURCES

The AFB Senior Site (*www.AFB.org/seniorsitehome.asp*) contains many resources for seniors. The MDsupport website (*www.MDsupport.org*) specializes in support and documentation for AMD patients and care givers. The Lighthouse Guild in New York (*www.lighthouseguild.org*) offers extensive resources for all forms of vision loss. These websites contain links to many more websites with additional information and often can provide information about local resources.

The Low Vision section of the American Academy of Ophthalmology website (*https://www.aao.org/low-vision-and-vision-rehab*) contains additional recommendations for ophthalmologists and links to its Vision Rehabilitation Preferred Practice Pattern and to handouts for patients.

REFERENCES

1. Colenbrander A. Measuring vision and vision loss. In: Duane's Clinical Ophthalmology. Philadelphia: Lippincott Williams & Wilkins; 2010.
2. Schoessow KA. Shifting from compensation to participation: a model for occupational therapy in low vision. Br J Occupat Ther. 2010;73(4):160-9.
3. Dreer LE, Fletcher DC, Swanson M, et al. Social problem-solving abilities and psychological adjustment of persons in low vision rehabilitation. Rehab Psychol. 2005;50(3): 232-8.
4. American Academy of Ophthalmology. (2013). Vision Rehabilitation PPP 2013. [online] Available from: *https://www.aao.org/preferred-practice-pattern/vision-rehabilitation*. [Accessed November, 2017].
5. American Academy of Ophthalmology. [2012]. Initiative in Vision Rehabilitation. [online] Available from: *https://www.aao.org/low-vision-and-vision-rehab*. [Accessed November, 2017].
6. Stelmack JA, Tang XC, Wei Y, et al. Outcomes of the Veterans Affairs Low Vision Intervention Trial II (LOVIT II): a randomized clinical trial. JAMA Ophthalmol. 2017;135(2): 96-104.
7. Naido KS, Leasher J, Bourne RR, et al. Global vision impairment and blindness due to uncorrected refractive error. Optom Vis Sci. 2016;93(3):227-34.
8. Neely DC, Bray KJ1, Huisingh CE, et al. Prevalence of undiagnosed age-related macular degeneration in primary eye care. JAMA Ophthalmol. 2017;135(6):570-5.
9. Colenbrander A, Fletcher C. The MeyeSight test, a comprehensive visual fitness test. ARVO. 2017.
10. Fletcher DC, Schuchard RA, Watson G. Relative locations of macular scotomas near the PRL: effect on low vision reading. J Rehabil Res Dev. 1999;36:356-64.
11. Huo R, Hoyt CS, Good WV, et al. Chronic cortical visual impairment in children: Etiology, prognosis, and associated neurological deficits. Br J Ophthalmol. 1999;83:670-5.

Chapter 15

Supporting How the Eyes Function

August Colenbrander, Tiffany Chan

INTRODUCTION

Any assessment of *"how the eyes function"* should address at least these basic functions:

- *Detail vision*: Usually characterized by letter chart visual acuity.
- *Contrast vision*: Often characterized by threshold performance, although supra-threshold performance is more relevant to most activities.
- *Surround vision*: The central field is relevant to reading and manipulation; the peripheral field is relevant to mobility.

Assessment of "how the person functions" will be discussed in the Chapter 16.

SUPPORTING DETAIL VISION

Detail vision is commonly measured as visual acuity. Unfortunately, this measure is so common that the visual acuity scale is often confused with the concept of vision. Detail vision is a concept, like length or weight. Concepts can be measured on various scales, like centimeters, inches or pounds; visual acuity, as defined by Snellen, is one of the scales used for detail vision.

To define visual acuity, Snellen compares the performance of an individual to that of a standard observer who can recognize letters subtending 5 min of arc (Figs. 15.1A and B).

When testing a patient, we determine the smallest letter size the subject can recognize and compare it to the size recognized by the standard observer. The resulting ratio is called the *MA*gnification *R*equirement (MAR).[a] This value is used for the prescription of magnification aids. Higher values imply poorer vision.

For clinical use, we prefer a scale where higher values indicate better vision.

We achieve this by using the reciprocal of MAR; we call it *visual acuity*: VA = 1/MAR.

The reverse formula is known as Kestenbaum's rule for magnification: MAR = 1/VA.

The visual acuity value can be expressed in different ways. In the United States, the numerator is commonly standardized to 20. In Britain and commonwealth countries 6 is used. In Europe, decimal notation is common.[b]

Thus: 1/2 = 20/40 = 6/12 = 0.5, 1/5 = 20/100 = 6/30 = 0.2, and 1/10 = 20/200 = 6/60 = 0.1.

MAR and VA are two scales to express *how the eye functions.*

To estimate *how the person functions*, it is common to use a logarithmic scale (Weber-Fechner's law). The logMAR scale [logMAR = log(MAR)] is mathematically simple, but can be clinically confusing, because larger values indicate poorer vision, and because of its decimal values. Simply using a log (VA) scale has similar problems. The *Visual Acuity Score* [VAS = 100 + 50 × log (VA)] provides a more intuitive estimate of visual ability. This scale has no decimals and is anchored at standard vision (20/20, 6/6, 1.0) = 100, often expressed as 100%. On a chart in Early Treatment Diabetic Retinopathy Study (ETDRS) format (logarithmic progression, 5 symbols on every line) it is a simple letter count score, since it increases by

---

a. When discussing the optical stage of vision, MAR is often interpreted as "minimum angle of resolution", and is based on the stroke width of optotypes. MAR as "MAgnification Requirement" applies to any need for magnification, and is based on the overall symbol size.

b. The use of different numerators harks back to Snellen's use of the fractional notation on printed charts with a fixed symbol size. In the original Snellen notation, the numerator indicated the actual viewing distance, often 20 ft or 6 m. Today, using monitors or projectors, the symbol size can be adjusted for any test distance, and. "Snellen equivalents" are used, in which the numerator is standardized, regardless of the test distance, whether for far or for near vision.

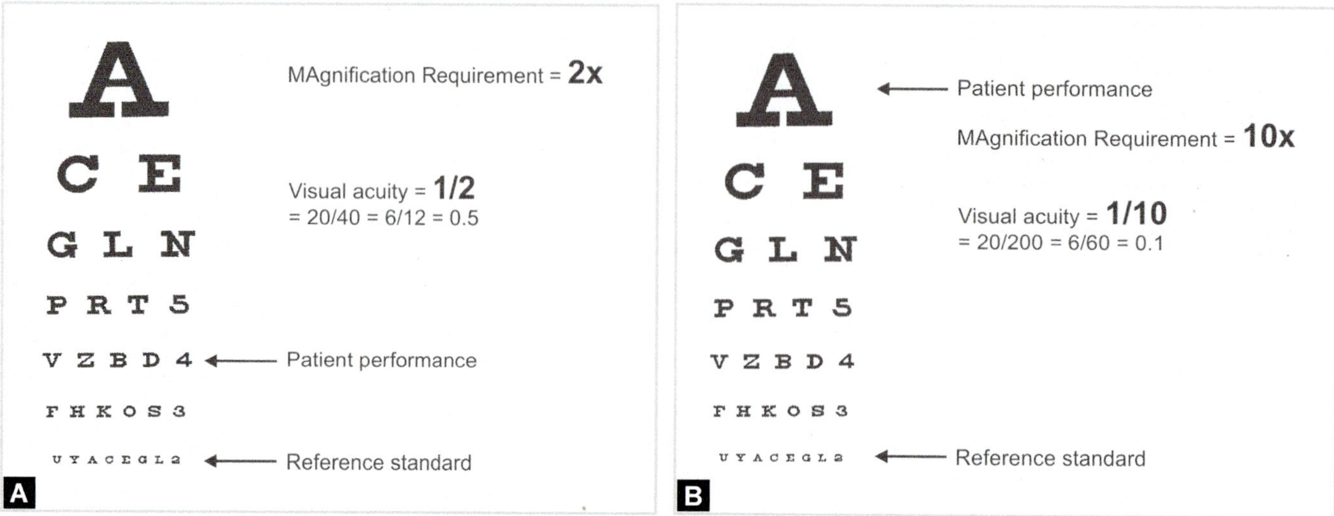

Figs. 15.1A and B: Defining visual acuity. Snellen defined visual acuity as the reciprocal of the magnification required for character recognition, relative to the performance of a standard observer.

1 point for every letter read correctly. The VAS value as an estimate of visual ability is used in the AMA *Guides to the Evaluation of Permanent Impairment.*[1] logMAR and VAS are two scales that provide an estimate of *how the person functions*.

Visual Acuity Measurement

For normally sighted patients, visual acuity is usually measured at a distance; for patients with low vision, this may not be feasible. For low vision, a distance of 1 meter is preferred, since this provides the simplest Snellen fraction (1/...); the distance can easily be verified with a cord attached to the chart (Fig. 15.2).

The 1-meter distance extends the range of measurement by seven lines, and makes vague statements such as "count fingers" and "hand movements" obsolete. The psychological effect of being able to read several lines at 1 meter for patients who previously "could not read the big E", should also not be underestimated.

Refraction

Verifying and if possible improving the refractive correction is the first thing that should be done for any patients with low vision. It is easier at 1 meter, since the patient can recognize more letters. A trial frame is recommended, since it gives the patient more freedom to search for the best retinal area; it also allows larger steps to be used. For most patients with low vision, the 0.25 phoropter steps are too small to be recognized.

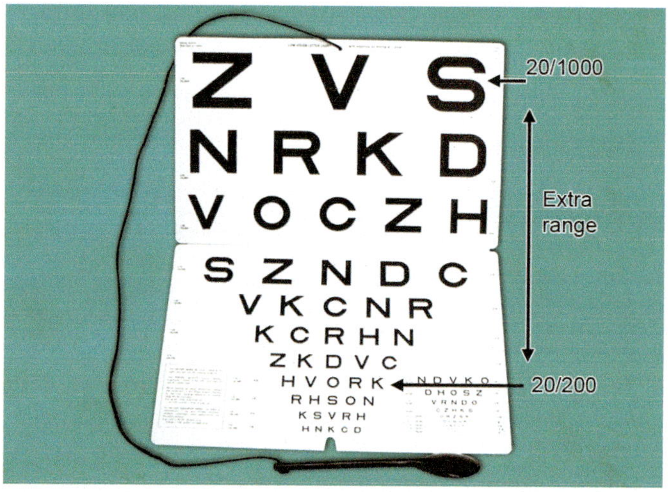

Fig. 15.2: Extended range of a 1-m chart. The chart extends the range by 7 lines (*see* also Chapter 14, Fig. 14.5).

Modified Snellen Fraction

For distance vision, Snellen's formula is:

VA = viewing distance (in meters)/letter size (in M-units)

One M-unit is the size of a letter, which subtends 5 minutes of arc at 1 meter (1.454 mm). Snellen defined a standard observer as someone able to recognize letters of that angular extent.

When calculating the magnification requirement, we can write:

MAR = letter size (in M-units)/viewing distance (in meters)

For near vision, this can further be changed to:

MAR = letter size (in M-units) X viewing distance (in diopters), or: MAR = M × D.

When a 1-meter letter chart is used, the numerator of the standard Snellen fraction is 1 (1/...) and the denominator is the letter size in M-units (1/M). For the modified Snellen formula, the viewing distance is measured in diopters (1/distance in meters), which is easily done with a ruler as included with most phoropters. The use of diopters has the advantage that it relates directly to the required reading add, and that multiplication is easier than division.

Reading

Having determined the refractive error, reading should be addressed next, since it is the most common complaint of most patients with low vision. Reading continuous text is a more relevant test of near vision than the use of a reduced letter chart, since the retinal area involved in reading is larger than that required for character recognition.

Starting with the patient's own reading glasses and the best reading distance for those glasses, determine whether MAR = M × D yields the same value as on the letter chart.

Next, increase the reading add and repeat the comparison. As the dioptric power (D) increases, the smallest size read (M) will decrease accordingly. As the focal point of the lens gets closer, the patient is required to hold the reading material closer. An increase of the M × D value may indicate that the patient is reluctant to bring the print close enough. In children and nonpresbyopic adults the available accommodation must also be taken into account.

The endpoint of this sequence will be the spectacle correction that allows the patient to read 1 M print (average newsprint). This is the starting point for other magnification options.

Magnification Options

Magnification can be provided in different ways.

Bringing Print Closer

For children, who have large amounts of accommodation, bringing print closer is a natural solution. Because of this, they may be able to resolve print much smaller than expected based on their distance visual acuity. However, since this requires a strong accommodative effort, they may experience visual fatigue. This is an important topic to discuss with the child, the parents, and the teacher, because adults may be inclined to interpret the behavior of a child that initially reads small print, but later claims not to be able to read it, as laziness. The print size at reading threshold (smallest print that can be resolved) and the print size for sustained reading could be very different. Visual aids may be useful to improve the resolution of small print, and to reduce visual fatigue. A reading add that replaces half of the accommodative effort may be a good starting point (Figs. 15.3 and 15.4).

Large Print

In many cases of mild vision impairment, the use of large print material is an easy and effective strategy. Many libraries carry a selection of large print books. For moderate

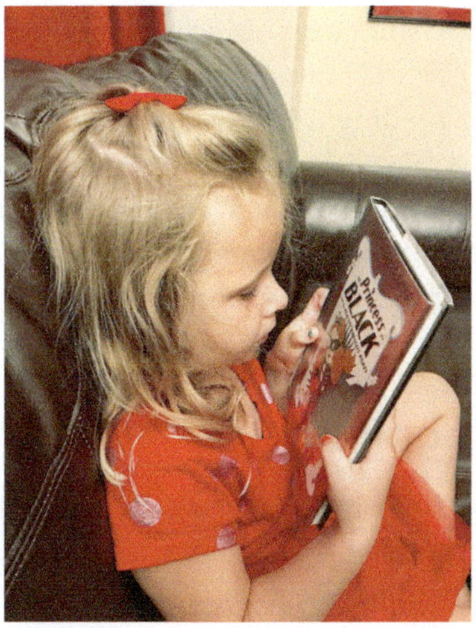

Fig. 15.3: Child, using accommodation.

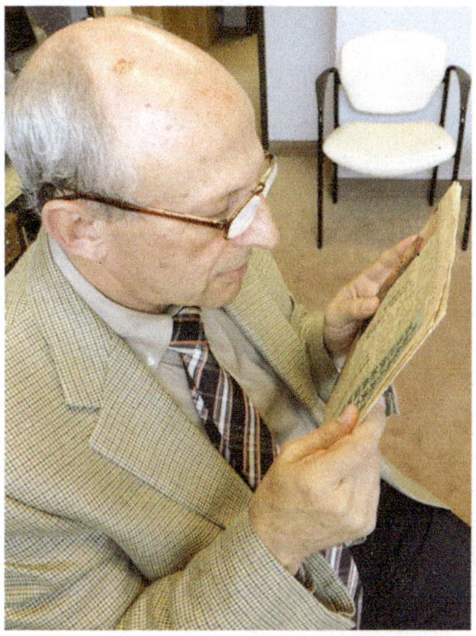

Fig. 15.4: Adult, using reading glasses.

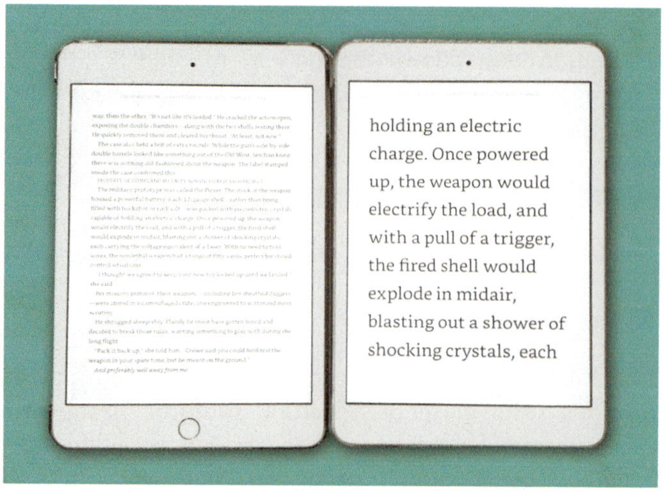

Fig. 15.5: Tablets provide an easy way to produce large print.

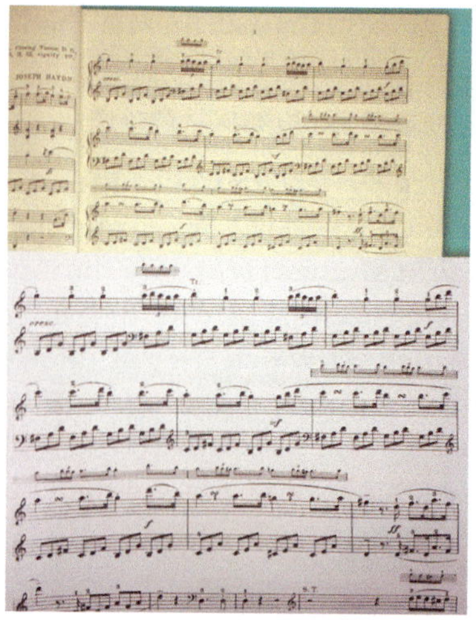

Fig. 15.6: Music can be enlarged on a standard copier.

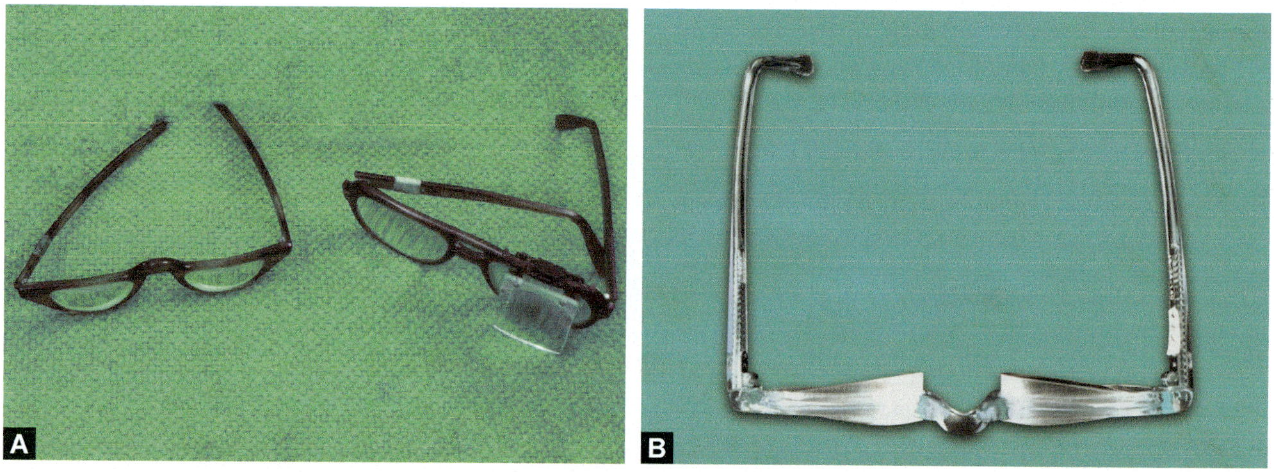

Figs. 15.7A and B: Medium power glasses. Pros: Familiar, maintain binocularity, can look over the top for orientation. Cons: Only for moderate power, needs prism to maintain fusion.

magnification demands, this may be sufficient. Reading tablets can also be used to provide large print (Fig. 15.5).

For musicians who have trouble reading music and cannot bend over to get closer, it can be helpful to use a photocopier to enlarge an 8.5 × 11 sheet to 11 × 17 (Fig. 15.6).

Spectacle Correction

As children get older, a larger proportion of their accommodative demand needs to be replaced. Patients may believe that the glasses magnify the image; the truth is that the glasses allow the object to be brought close, and that the closeness provides the magnified retinal image. It should be stressed that a short reading distance is the inevitable result of stronger reading glasses.

Binocular vision can be advantageous, since better areas in one eye may compensate for worse areas in the other eye. For reading adds up to 4 diopters (25 cm, 10″) this is still possible without further aids. In the range from 5 D to 10 D (down to 10 cm, 4″) the help of prisms is indicated. Closer than 10 diopters, the convergence demand becomes too much and vision with optical magnifiers must be monocular (Figs. 15.7 and 15.8).

Optical Magnifiers

The distance of the lens to the paper is dictated by the dioptric power of the lens. Therefore, when the patient resists a very short reading distance, a longer reading distance can only be achieved by moving both the lens and the

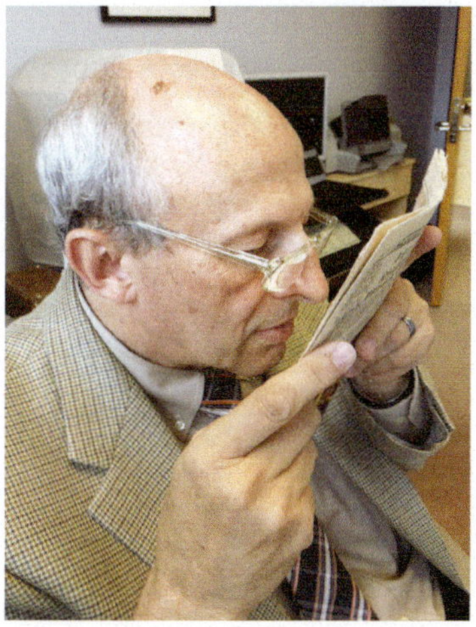

Fig. 15.8: High power reading glasses. Pros: More magnification, hands free, wider field than magnifiers. Cons: Very-short reading distance, monocular, requires adjustable light (other eye plano for orientation vision).

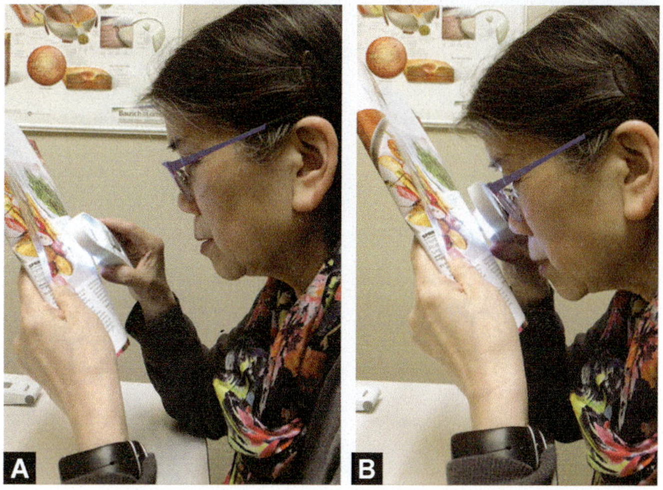

Figs. 15.9A and B: Hand-held magnifiers. Pros: Simple to use for spot reading, portable. Cons: Requires hand stability.

object away from the eye. At this point, the lens is called a magnifier.

As the lens is moved away, its field of coverage is reduced. Its effective power also becomes less, so the power of the magnifier lens must be somewhat higher than that of the spectacle lens. Whether a magnifier or a spectacle correction is more advantageous, will depend on the patient's preference and on the task to be performed. To achieve the widest possible field of view, all magnifiers need to be brought close to the eye (Figs. 15.9A and B).

The advent of LED lighting has made it possible to include brighter light in both hand and stand magnifiers (Fig. 15.10).

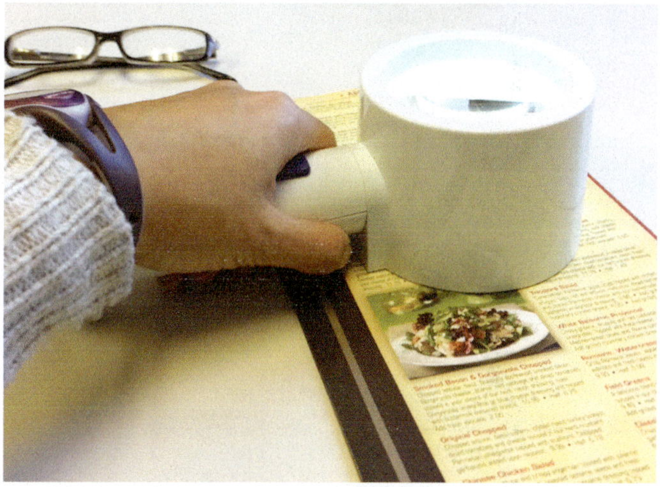

Fig. 15.10: Stand magnifier. Pros: More stable, often with illumination. Cons: Larger, must be moved when reading requires reading correction.

Electronic Magnifiers

Optical magnifiers create a virtual, optical image of the object; electronic magnifiers replace the original object with an enlarged actual image on a screen. This has eliminated the need for an uncomfortably short reading distance, and enables binocular viewing. Originally, electronic magnification was only available in table-mounted systems with a large screen (Fig. 15.11). Today, many portable versions are available with smaller screens. These devices cost more than optical magnifiers, but by increasing the electronic magnification, they allow a more comfortable viewing distance, enhanced contrast, adjustable magnification and binocular vision (Fig. 15.12).

For any magnification setting, a larger screen can display more words and will require less movement of the text or the magnifier. Thus, for prolonged reading tasks, desk-based models are preferred; for spot reading, portable models may be advantageous.

Telescopes

The magnifiers mentioned above address near vision. Magnifying distant objects requires a more complex system of lenses, called a telescope.

Magnification of the peripheral field disrupts the relation between the image seen and the actual object. This means that telescopes, whether hand-held or spectacle-mounted, are best used when the user is stationary, such as when watching TV at home or a movie or a play in a theater. For mobility purposes, telescopes can only be used intermittently, from a stationary position (Fig. 15.13).

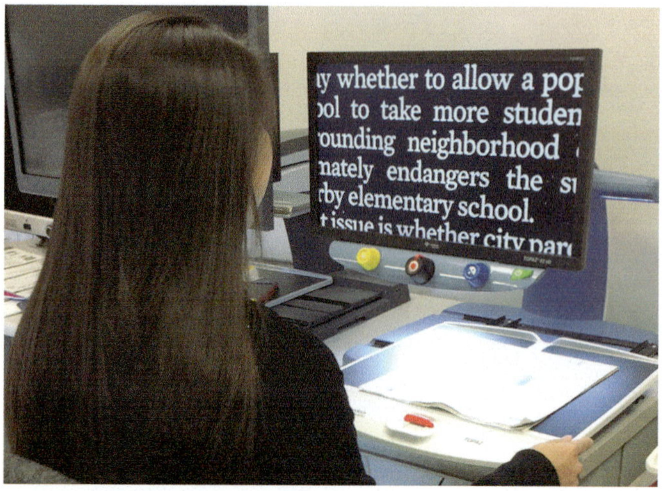

Fig. 15.11: Desk-based electronic magnifier. Pros: Larger field, higher magnification, preferable for sustained reading, text on moveable platform, newer models with text-to-speech. Cons: Takes up more space, not portable.

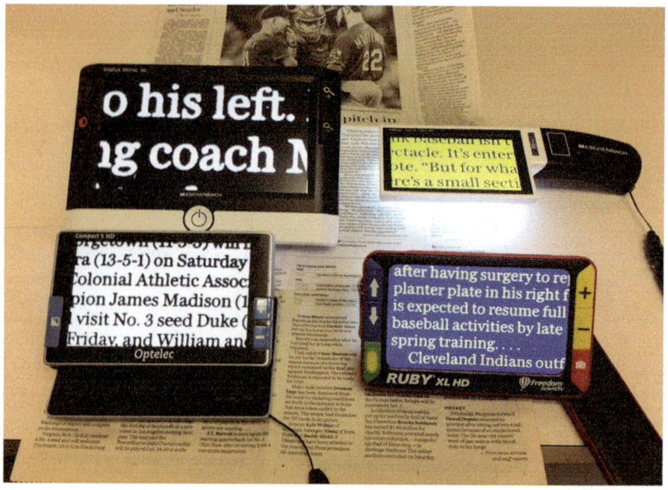

Fig. 15.12: Handheld electronic magnifiers. Pros: Portable, easy to use for spot reading, contrast enhancement. Cons: Small screen, more portable, larger screen, less portable.

Telescopes for continuous use

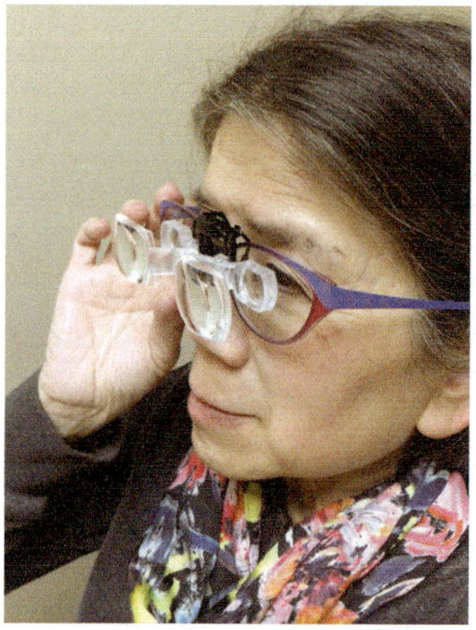

Fig. 15.13: Low power full-field telescopes for TV or theater. Pros: Light weight. Cons: Limited magnification.

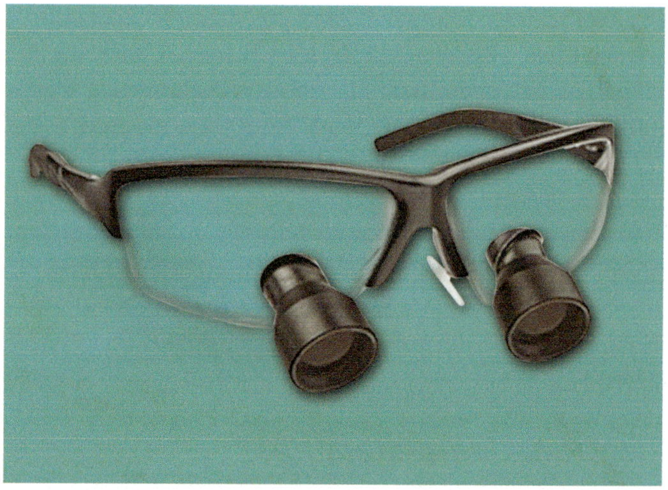

Fig. 15.14: Higher power, surgical loupes. Pros: Often with built-in illumination. Cons: Fixed focus, because of fixed convergence.

A pedestrian must stop to read a street sign with a telescope, then walk the next block using unmagnified vision. The same is true for bioptic telescopes,[c] which in some states can be legal for driving. The driver may briefly use the telescope to read a road sign, but must navigate using unrestricted, unmagnified vision through the carrier lens. The availability of GPS systems provides an alternative to visual recognition of road signs.

Spectacle-mounted telescopes may be placed centrally for continuous viewing, such as for TV or for surgical loupes (Figs. 15.13 and 15.14). For intermittent use, they should be placed outside the line of view (often called bioptic placement, Fig. 15.16), so that a head movement is required for their use.

An intermediate solution is the use of clip-on or flip-up telescopes. They may be cheaper, but are also

c. Bioptic telescopes are telescopes mounted like a bifocal lens, so that vision can be switched easily between the telescope and the unmagnified carrier lens.

Telescopes for intermittent use

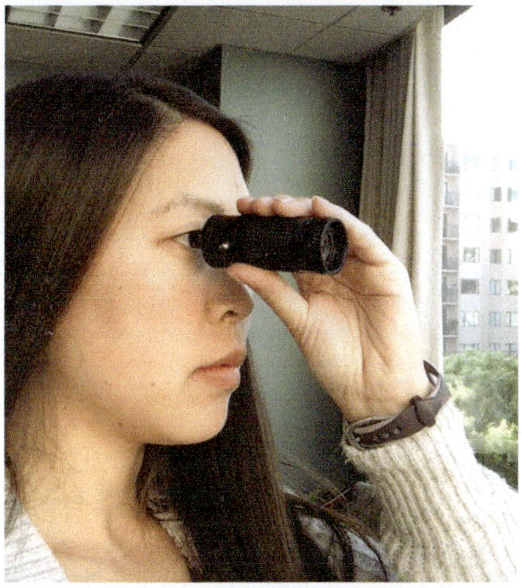

Fig. 15.15: Hand-held telescope. Pros: Best for intermittent use, many are focusable. Cons: Requires steady hands, must be carried separately.

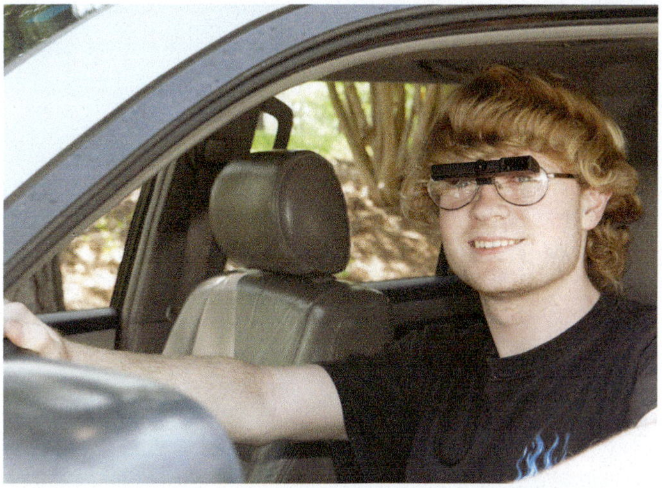

Fig. 15.16: Bioptic telescope. Pros: Hands-free, immediately available when needed. Cons: Conspicuous, often no or limited focusing.

less stable. Users should remember that a telescope does not only magnify the image, if also magnifies its movements. The stronger the telescope, the greater the need for stability. Most telescopes also reduce the amount of light entering the pupil, which may be a problem for patients with contrast deficits. Large diameter front lenses (night telescopes) can limit this, but they make the telescope heavier and more difficult to stabilize.

SUPPORTING CONTRAST VISION

Traditional letter charts,[d, 2-5] have very high contrast, since this makes them less sensitive to changes in illumination. Most activities of daily living, however, involve objects with lesser contrast. Assessing the ability to see at reduced contrast levels, therefore, is important for the evaluation of patients with low vision.

The traditional contrast tests (Pelli-Robson, Mars) measure the contrast threshold. Threshold measurements are easily defined and easily repeated. But for most activities of daily living, supra-threshold contrast is more relevant.

The use of separate tests to determine visual acuity and contrast sensitivity, may leave the impression that these two measurements are independent. They are not. The contrast sensitivity curve depicts their interaction: better contrast results in better visual acuity.

As shown in Figure 15.17, the Snellen chart measures one endpoint of the curve (threshold detail, with highest contrast); the Pelli-Robson and Mars cards measure the other endpoint (threshold contrast for large letters). Neither one covers the central area of the curve, where supra-threshold contrast and supra-threshold detail interact in activities of daily living (Fig. 15.18).

The *mixed contrast cards*[6] were developed to overcome this problem (Fig. 15.19). They present high contrast (HC) and low contrast (LC) print side by side. This ensures that the two tests are always presented at the same distance and with the same illumination, and makes it easy to assess the HC-LC difference, i.e. the trade-off between contrast and detail seen. This difference provides an estimate of the slope of the CS curve. An HC-LC difference of one or two lines is within normal limits; in AMD patients, differences of four or five lines are not uncommon; occasionally differences of up to 10 lines have been noted. This format also provides patients with a better insight into their contrast problem, and a better understanding of the benefits of providing more contrast in their environment.

---

d. The term "letter chart" is used as a generic term for visual acuity charts with single symbols, be it letters, numbers, pictures or symbols. Traditional charts (often called Snellen charts) have a rectangular shape with few large letters and many smaller ones. The ETDRS format, which is the current gold standard, was developed for the Early Treatment of Diabetic Retinopathy Study;[2] it has a triangular format with five symbols on every line (Bailey-Lovie layout, 1976[3]) and a strict logarithmic progression,[4] often implemented with nonserif Sloan letters[5]).

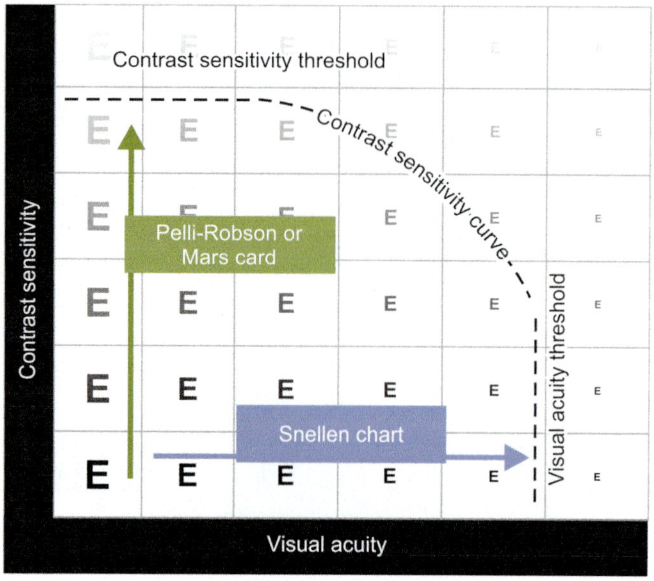

Fig. 15.17: Threshold measurements.

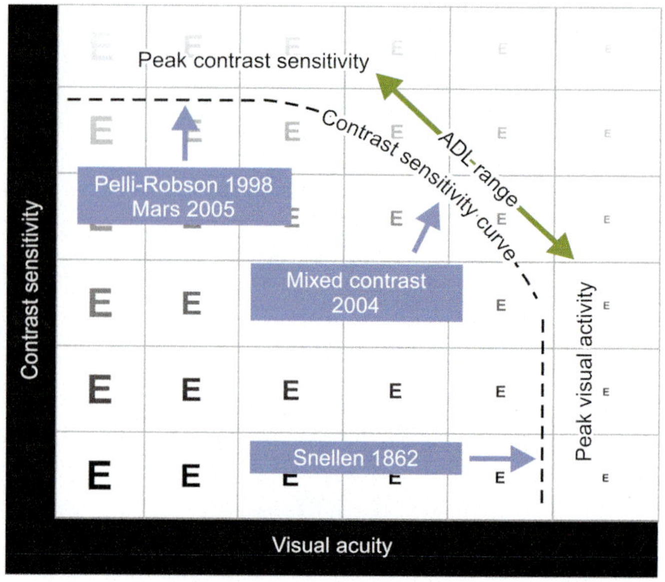

Fig. 15.18: Supra-threshold measurements.

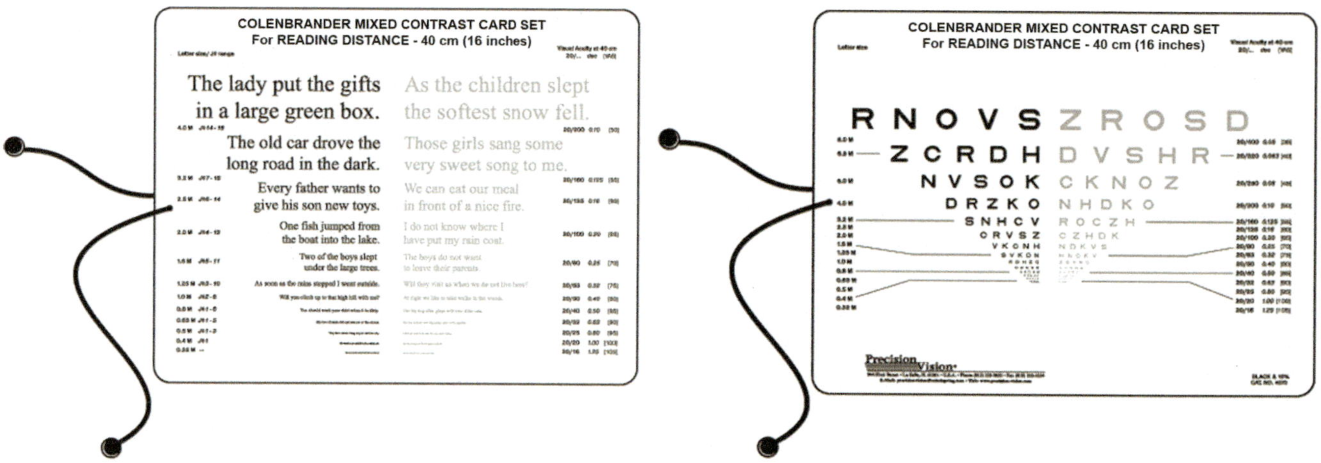
COLENBRANDER MIXED CONTRAST CARD SET
For READING DISTANCE - 40 cm (16 inches)
The lady put the gifts in a large green box.
As the children slept the softest snow fell.
The old car drove the long road in the dark.
Those girls sang some very sweet song to me.
Every father wants to give his son new toys.
We can eat our meal in front of a nice fire.
One fish jumped from the boat into the lake.
I do not know where I have put my rain coat.
Two of the boys slept under the large trees.
The boys do not want to leave their parents.
COLENBRANDER MIXED CONTRAST CARD SET
For READING DISTANCE - 40 cm (16 inches)
R N O V S Z R O S D
Z C R D H D V S H R
N V S O K C K N O Z
D R Z K O N H D K O
S N H C V R O C Z H

Fig. 15.19: Mixed contrast reading cards.

The HC-LC difference is largely independent of the visual acuity. There are patients with a good HC acuity and a large HC-LC difference; others have poor acuity and a small HC-LC difference. One hypothesis states that visual acuity reflects the density of the receptor mosaic, while the HC-LC difference reflects the sensitivity of the individual units.

Remediation of Contrast Problems

Changing the contrast sensitivity of the eye is not possible. But changes to the environment are possible.

The high contrast letter charts used in the office are not representative of the average contrast in the average home. Where possible, contrast in the environment should be increased. This is true in the work environment (Figs. 15.20A and B), as well as in the home. Do not serve white rice on a white plate on a white table cloth.

An advantage of electronic magnifiers is that they not only provide magnification, but can also enhance contrast. For some conditions, reverse contrast can also be beneficial. This is sometimes the case for glaucoma (Fig. 15.21). Yellow filters (blue-blockers) do not raise the threshold sensitivity, but tend to enhance the subjective perception of supra-threshold contrast.

Although increased illumination does not increase the *contrast* of objects, it does increase the *contrast sensitivity* of the eye. Print with poor contrast that cannot be read

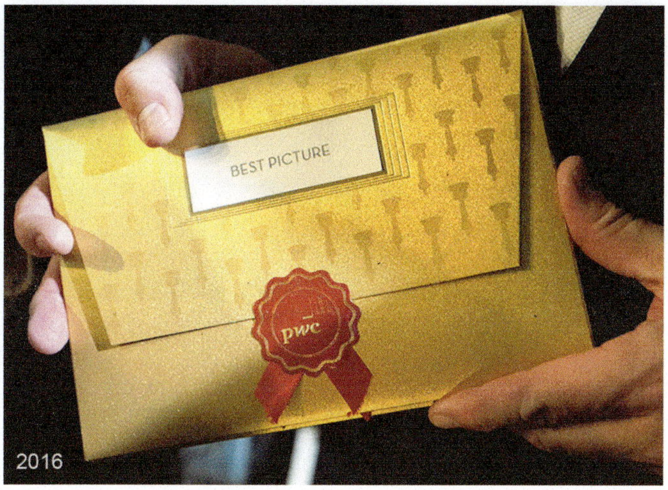

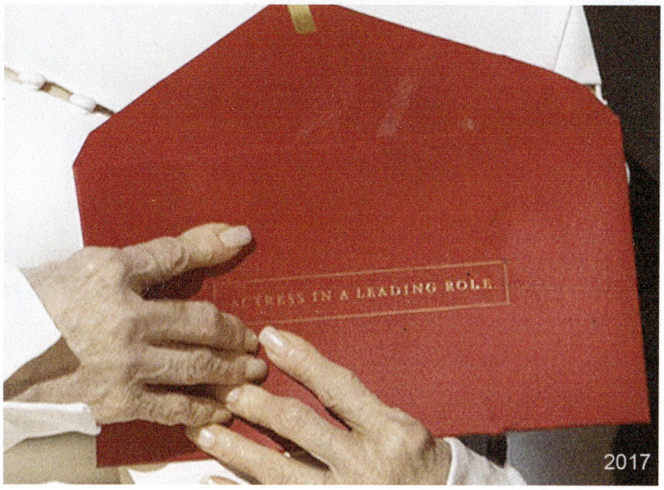

Figs. 15.20A and B: Low contrast on envelopes. Low contrast on envelopes contributed to naming the wrong winner at the 2017 Oscars.

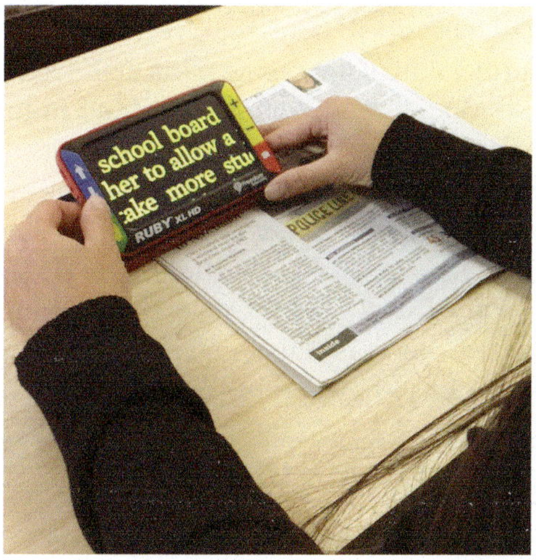

Fig. 15.21: Contrast enhancement. Video-magnifiers allow contrast enhancement on handheld and desk models.

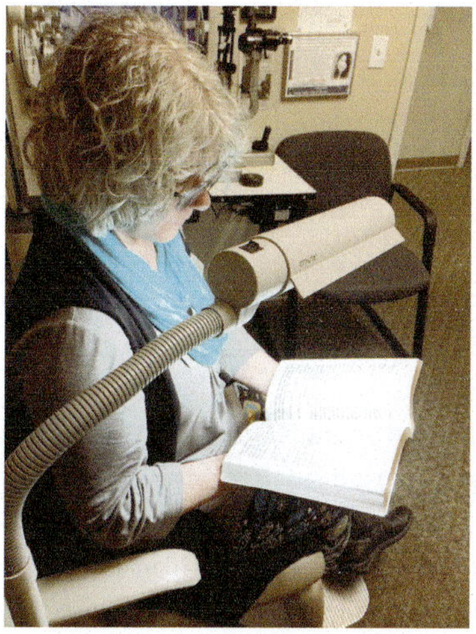

Fig. 15.22: Adjustable task lighting.

indoors, may be readable when taken to the window or outdoors. Receptors that are damaged, but not dead, may not respond at low light levels, but can contribute when the illumination is increased.

Illumination devices, therefore, are among the best devices for those with contrast problems. The advent of LED lights has made it possible to include brighter lights in hand-held magnifiers and to offer desk lamps that can be brought close to the object, without causing excessive heat (Figs. 15.22 and 15.23).

SUPPORTING SURROUND VISION

As stated earlier, letter chart acuity assesses only the retinal area where the letter is projected. Even for a 20/200 letter,

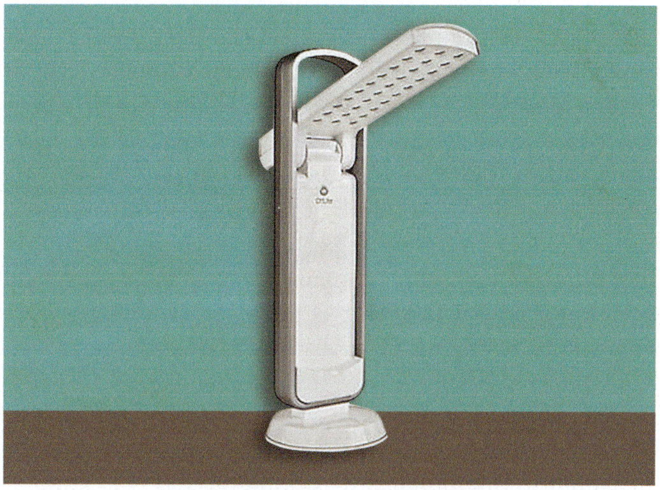

Fig. 15.23: Portable LED light.

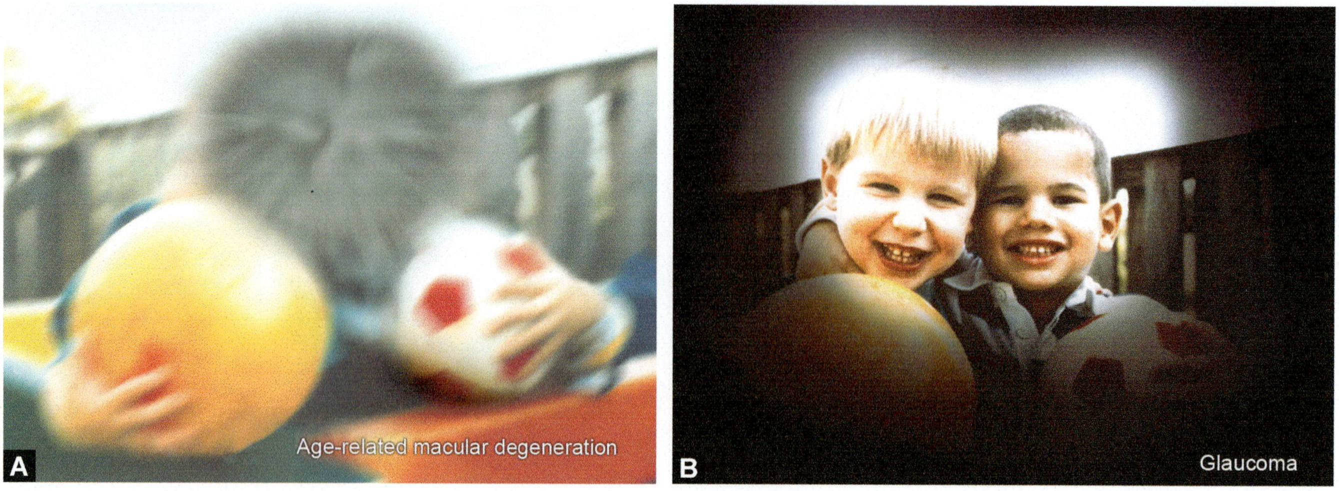

Figs. 15.24A and B: Misleading images. These commonly used images do not reflect what the patients' experience. They refer to the retinal image, not to the Mental Model, on which perception is based.

this is an area of less than 1-degree diameter. Everything beyond this area, from the immediate para-foveal area to the far periphery, is captured under the general term of surround vision. How surround vision is described, depends on one's point of view.

When considering *how the person functions,* we saw that interactions with the environment are based on the *mental model* of that environment (*see* Chapter 14, Fig. 14.7). The Mental Model is based on the accumulation and integration of many snapshots over time. It has no boundaries and no gaps. The Mental Model includes the area behind our back. That area may be less detailed, because our last look in that direction was a while ago; however, it is not experienced as an empty black hole or as a nonexistent space.

Therefore, the popular images (Figs. 15.24A and B) that describe field restrictions as black blotches, do not represent what people experience, because they represent the retinal image, rather than the Mental Model.

The Mental Model is stationary in space. We can direct our attention to various objects in that space, and make head and eye movements to foveate those objects for closer inspection. The ability to make goal directed eye movements is an essential part of normal visual ability. Those movements can be made, even if the target falls outside the visual field. It has been shown that persons with a very restricted field of view, frequently make eye movements to points outside their limited field.

The spatial awareness, based on the mental model, is entirely different from the clinical *visual field* that is measured to document disease progression. The clinical visual field describes *How the eye functions;* it is the outward projection of the seeing parts of the retina. Unlike the Mental Model, the visual field is fixed to the eye; its measurement cannot tolerate eye movements. If the eye moves during the test, the test is invalid. The visual field has no memory component. It ends at the limit of the functioning retina and has gaps where there are scotomata. The common clinical field tests have been optimized to follow diseases, such as glaucoma, not to explain how the person functions (*see* Chapter 14, Fig. 14.2).

Use of Surround Vision

Surround vision can serve different purposes.

One purpose, of spatial awareness, is to *explore the environment.* This happens continuously, as people, consciously or subconsciously, direct their attention and fixation to various points that are defined in their Mental Model. Since the Mental Model is not limited by the extent of the visual field, peripheral field loss will not impair this ability. When the remaining field is narrow, patients will need more scanning movements, but they will not be aware of their visual field loss, just as we are not consciously aware of the 180° blind spot behind our head.

Another purpose for which surround vision is used is for *guidance of the motor system.* This may involve eye movements, as in reading, or limb and body movements, as when walking or when grasping an object. This aspect of the system is also used almost continuously.

Reading would be impossible if we did not make regular eye movements from word to word. Yet, the control of these eye movements happens entirely outside our conscious awareness. When this system fails, for instance because of scotoma interference, the failure itself will not be recognized, but its consequences, such as a reduced reading speed, can be noticed.

When grasping an object, our hand automatically adjusts to its shape and position, and our fingers open just wide enough, but not too wide, to grasp it. This also happens outside our conscious awareness. When walking in a crowded environment, we avoid collisions with objects or people without consciously determining the location of each obstacle. This subconscious processing of peripheral visual input is similar to the autonomous regulation of breathing, heart rate, and other body functions, which happens continuously and reliably without the need for conscious involvement. Because they happen involuntary, we are rarely aware of these functions.

Finally, surround vision may *trigger central vision*. This happens occasionally; yet, it often is the only function mentioned when the role of peripheral vision is discussed. When a peripheral stimulus meets certain "saliency" criteria, it will trigger a fixational saccade to bring the object to the central field, where it can be examined more closely. If this system fails, because the stimulus falls in a scotomatous area, it may result in tripping over a pothole or bumping into an obstacle.

Conscious versus Subconscious Visual Processing

Unfortunately, the distinction between conscious and subconscious visual processing is rarely made. When reading, attention is mostly given to the correct recognition of words and to the understanding of the story, because these aspects feed directly into conscious awareness. Little attention is given to the eye movement control that makes reading possible.

The above examples make it clear why people with visual field defects are usually not aware of their deficits. This applies to peripheral losses (as in RP, glaucoma), as well as to scotomata in the central field (as in AMD). Therefore, the first step in dealing with visual field deficits must be to make people aware of their existence. This awareness requires training and practice; it cannot be provided by devices. As in other aspects of life, only when one is if aware of a problem, and understands its effects, can one make conscious efforts to compensate.

While devices are extremely important when dealing with deficits of detail vision, they have a far more limited role when dealing with visual field deficits.

When exploring the environment from a stationary position, various prism arrangements can help by making the shift in visual direction larger than the shift of the eye position. However, control of eye or body movements requires a consistent relationship between visual and tactile space. When fixation is consistently shifted from the fovea to an eccentric preferred retinal locus (PRL), the brain can adapt. When prisms are worn 24/7, the brain can adapt also. However, the adaptation to intermittent use of devices that remap the retinal image is more problematic.

Use of a telescope when scanning from a stationary position is possible because in that situation, localization is based on the location of objects relative to other objects. However, using the same telescope while walking is problematic, since foot and body movements now require absolute agreement between visual and tactile localization. It is well known that even the slight prismatic effect of bifocals can confuse some people when walking up or down stairs.

Central Field Defects

Central field defects will primarily affect tasks like reading, writing, drawing and manipulation.

When a scotoma includes the former fovea, there will be a loss of visual acuity. However, AMD does not always start in the fovea. When testing AMD patients, the fellow eyes, which still had normal visual acuity, were sometimes found to have islands of reduced contrast sensitivity surrounding the fovea.[7] Such spots are not detected by a letter chart or by a letter-based contrast sensitivity test, but may interfere with reading fluency. Since the advent of anti-vascular endothelial growth factor (VEGF) therapy, it is more common to find foveal and perifoveal areas that are defective, but are not totally lost. Such patients need magnification and extra light, but maintain central fixation, which makes rehabilitation easier than for those who need eccentric fixation.

A simple test to determine the position and extent of such scotomata, is to have the patient fixate a door knob or similar object, while moving a laser pointer around. When scotomata are found, it is useful to let the patient move the laser pointer. Their proprioceptive experience of their scotoma is much more convincing than any verbal description.

Patients with a small central functional area may show a characteristic speed pattern when reading the letter chart from the top down. On the largest letters, they may have difficulty, or read slowly, since they need scanning movements for letters that are larger than their functional area. As the letters get smaller, they will speed up, until they slow down again at their visual acuity limit.

Thus, when judging their performance, the reading *speed* is more informative than the reading *threshold*. Consider that the definition of 20/20 threshold acuity is the ability to recognize 1 M letters at 1 meter. But to read comfortably, we hold average newsprint (1 M) at 40 cm, which is 2.5X above threshold. Comfortable magnification should not be based on threshold acuity, but on the *critical print size*, that is the print size at which a comfortable reading speed can be maintained with the least amount of magnification.[8] Determining the critical print size requires a reading card with standardized paragraphs (MN-read, Colenbrander, Radner). It is well known that those with contrast deficits will need more magnification than estimated based on their letter chart acuity alone.

The configuration of the scotomata will also affect the reading speed. Sometimes, it is particularly difficult to track along the line. In those cases, underlining may be as important as magnification. Sometimes, patients may not start at the beginning of the line, or may not read to the end. In those cases, placing a finger or contrasting strip at the margin may help them to determine whether their eyes have moved far enough.

Peripheral Field Defects

Peripheral field defects will mostly affect mobility.

The visual demands of mobility are very different from those in reading. For reading and other central vision tasks, conscious recognition is of primary importance, and localization is based on the relative position of one object next to the other. For the rehabilitation of reading and related tasks, we have seen that devices play an important role.

For mobility, however, devices cannot substitute for a lack of awareness. Localization for mobility uses an absolute frame work. This need for absolute localization means that relocating the image to a different retinal area (magnification, eccentric viewing) will cause problems. If the visual estimate of a step does not exactly match the demand on the motor system, we stumble. The fact that patients will rarely be spontaneously aware of these effects as vision problems, was discussed earlier. Education and training for mobility will be discussed in the next chapter.

The use of prisms just outside the line of view can help in intermittently scanning peripheral areas. Prisms may be helpful as a training aid, but ultimately, the same effect can be obtained with natural eye movements. The essential element for those with peripheral deficits is the awareness of the need to use conscious eye movements to replace the natural subconscious, autonomous scanning.

CONCLUSION

Different visual deficits ask for different remedies. Visual acuity deficits are well-known; they require magnification, which can be provided by a variety of devices. Equally important, but often overlooked, are contrast deficits. They must be addressed through increased illumination, and increased contrast in the environment. Visual field deficits, in the central field for reading, or in the periphery for mobility, require education about their nature and teaching of better search strategies.

REFERENCES

1. Colenbrander A. The visual system. In: Rondinelli RD, Genovese E (Eds). Guides to the Evaluation of Permanent Impairment, 6th edition. Chicago: AMA Press; 2007.
2. Ferris FL, Kassov A, Bresnick GH, et al. New visual acuity charts for clinical research. Am J Ophthalmol. 1982;94: 91-6.
3. Bailey IL, Lovie JE. New design principles for visual acuity letter charts. Am J Optom Physiol Opt. 1976;53:740-5.
4. Green J. On a new series of test-letters for determining the acuteness of vision, Transact. Amer. Opth Soc. 1868:68-71.
5. Sloan LL. New test charts for the measurement of visual acuity at far and near distances. Am J Ophth. 1959;48: 807-13.
6. Precision Vision. Mixed Contrast cards. [online] Available from: *http://www.precision-vision.com/product-category/contrast-eye-charts/mixed-and-threshold-contrast-charts/*. [Accessed November, 2017].
7. Hahn GA, Messias A, MacKeben M, et al. Parafoveal letter recognition at reduced contrast in normal aging and in patients with risk factors for AMD. Graefes Arch Clin Exp Ophthalmol. 2009;247(1):43-51.
8. Whittaker SG, Lovie-Kitchin J. Visual requirements for reading. Optom Vis Sci. 1993;70:54-65.

Chapter 16 Supporting How the Person Functions

Orli Weisser-Pike, Monica S Perlmutter

INTRODUCTION

The previous chapter addressed *how the eyes function* and emphasized reading. Even the most ardent readers, however, spend more hours on other activities than they spend on reading. This chapter addresses *how the person functions.* It will discuss:

- The vision rehabilitation team
- Supporting the use of remaining vision
- Supporting activities of daily living
- Supporting a livable environment
- Supporting safe mobility
- Supporting psychosocial adjustment

VISION REHABILITATION TEAM

As previously mentioned, rehabilitation is a team effort. Knowing how and where to locate the players on the team, as well as understanding their roles and scopes of practice is essential. In many instances, low vision services require a referral by a physician, because reimbursement depends on a low vision diagnosis in addition to the ocular diagnoses. Rehabilitation specialists will rely on specific information from you *(How the eyes function)*, just as you will rely on them to manage the rehabilitation of your patients *(How the person functions)*.

Vision Rehabilitation Service Providers

Vision rehabilitation service providers can be found in the private, education, and healthcare systems. The following list may help you understand the alphabet soup.

Teachers of the visually impaired (TVI) are special education teachers in primary, secondary, and tertiary school systems who work with students with visual impairments to meet their unique educational needs. They frequently teach braille.

Certified vision rehabilitation therapists (CVRTs) often work in government and community agencies. Anne Sullivan, who taught Helen Keller, is their role model as a "home teacher" (Fig. 16.1). There are approximately 600 CVRTs in the US.

Certified low vision therapists (CLVTs) help patients use remaining vision more efficiently, through use of optical and electronic devices, and nonvisual strategies. They typically work in community agencies, veterans affairs (VA) locations, or under the auspices of optometry. There are approximately 300 CLVTs in the US.

Certified orientation and mobility specialist (COMS) provide systematic training in safe and independent mobility using a long white cane, as well as optical and electronic devices. Many of the 30,000 COMS in the US work in VA systems, school systems, and community organizations.

Certified assistive technology instructional specialists (CATISs) have emerged as a new professional certification in vision rehabilitation to address the unique knowledge and skills required to evaluate and recommend assistive technologies for the blind and visually impaired.

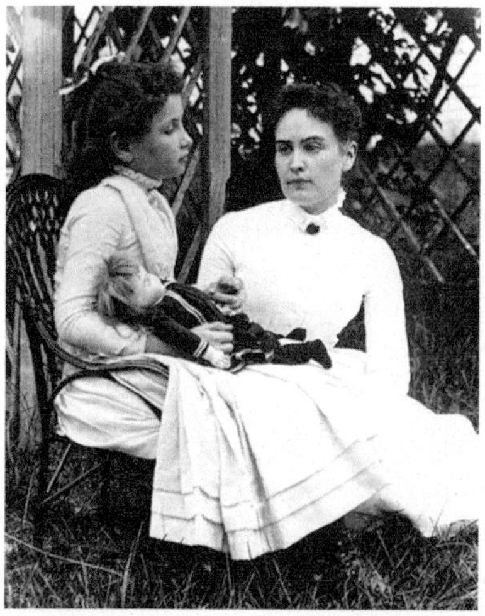

Fig. 16.1: Anne Sullivan with Helen Keller (1888).

The above professions evolved from the education system, where they worked mostly with students. Since these professionals are excluded from healthcare reimbursement, most of them work within various agencies collectively known as "the blindness system".

Occupational therapists (OTs) form a profession with a vast scope and a century of history. The OT profession evolved within the healthcare system, often working with adults and seniors. OTs are subject to state licensing, and mostly work in healthcare settings. As early as the late 1940s, occupational therapy practitioners were working with people disabled by vision loss. However, it was not until the early 1990s that the professions of occupational therapy and ophthalmology became bonded via a ruling from the Centers for Medicaid and Medicare Services which recognized that any sensory impairment (in this case, low vision) warranted medically necessary rehabilitation services. Since the end of the 1990s, low vision has been the third leading cause of disability amongst older Americans. With over 200,000 licensed OT practitioners in the US, occupational therapy is well positioned to cater to the needs of the aging population. Many OT practitioners receive specialized training in low vision and are well equipped to work with seniors, which represents the largest segment of the low vision population. In 2006, the American Occupational Therapy Association launched a Specialty Certification in Low Vision.

Not every patient with low vision will need all low vision rehabilitation service providers, and some services overlap with each other. In any event, you should strive to have a network of low vision rehabilitation service providers to help your patients, since no two patients have the same needs even if they have the same low vision diagnoses.

Order for Occupational Therapy

Date: *May 22, 2017*
Patient Name: *John Doe*
Ocular Condition: *Exudative Macular Degeneration*
ICD-10 Diagnosis: *H54.2*
Services Requested:
Occupational therapy evaluation and treatment

Physician: *Janet Deer, MD*

Fig. 16.2: Example of a referral to occupational therapy.

Referring for Low Vision Rehabilitation

The process of vision rehabilitation starts when your patients experience limitations in their daily activities because of their vision. The American Academy of Ophthalmology (AAO) recommends that the need for rehabilitation be considered for anyone with visual acuity of less than 20/40, but also for other conditions, such as field restrictions and contrast sensitivity loss. The AAO has stated that this now is a "standard of care". Patients may not voluntarily report their daily living concerns during an eye examination; thus, it is very important that ophthalmologists and other eye care specialists ask about these specifically.

Occupational therapy services can be provided following orders from an ophthalmologist or optometrist, similar to a prescription for medications (Fig. 16.2). The order specifies the patient's name, ocular condition and ICD-10 low vision diagnosis, service requested, frequency, and duration of occupational therapy services. OT services are reimbursable through Medicare and most private health insurance policies. After the initial evaluation of your patient, the occupational therapist will develop a plan of care requiring your approval in the form of a signature. As the referring physician, you can expect to receive an initial plan of care and monthly updates from the occupational therapist.

Unlike occupational therapy other vision rehabilitation services (low vision therapy, vision rehabilitation therapy, orientation and mobility, and assistive technology instruction) do not require orders or your signature on a plan of care. However, open communication is always encouraged with all service providers, and these service providers may have protocols requiring information from you about your patients. Rehabilitation is a team effort and communication amongst all team players is key to successful outcomes.

INTERVENTIONS IN VISION REHABILITATION

Vision rehabilitation is a comprehensive effort, which may require the knowledge, skills, and talents of a range of service providers. The following section is intended to provide an overview of common interventions in vision rehabilitation. Broadly, these include interventions to maximize use of remaining vision, support performance of activities of daily living, make environments more livable, facilitate safe mobility, and promote psychosocial adjustment to low vision. Henceforth, the term "vision rehabilitation service provider" is used to denote one or more of the professionals on the rehabilitation team.

Initial and Ongoing Patient Education

At the start and throughout the intervention process, the patient needs information about his or her eye condition and its possible prognosis. Facilitating health literacy is ongoing and includes education about the patient's condition, awareness of visual deficits, reinforcement of compensatory techniques, and dispelling common myths about use of vision (e.g. "if I use my vision for detailed tasks I will lose more vision").

Supporting the Use of Remaining Vision

Patients can learn to make better use of their remaining vision, it is not enough to prescribe an optical, electronic, or other device to a patient. Assuring that the device meets the patient's needs, habits, and abilities is vital for successful rehabilitation. Factors that need to be considered include the patient's cognitive and physical abilities, roles, routines, physical environment, social support, and culture.

Spectacle Design

Bifocal, trifocal, and progressive lenses combine various lens powers in one frame. This leaves the patient with smaller areas of the lens in which there is clarity for a specific distance. Patients with low vision may have difficulty locating the best position in the lens while simultaneously locating the best retinal position. Bifocal, trifocal, and progressive lenses have also been also found to impact a person's ability to estimate obstacles such as curbs and steps. They can impact the patient's posture resulting in exaggerated neck flexion and a downward gaze, presumably in an attempt to view obstacles in the inferior visual field via the upper segment of the lens (Figs. 16.3 and 16.4). This change in posture can negatively impact balance by shifting the center of gravity forward when stepping down from a higher surface to a lower one, increasing the risk of falls.

While many older people might wear bifocals, trifocals, or progressive lenses for convenience, the low vision rehabilitation provider may recommend single-vision spectacles for tasks at specific distances, particularly for near and intermediate activities. Wearing only single-vision distance glasses, or removing bifocals, trifocals, or progressives when walking, may help to reduce falls in older, active people.

Glare Control

Recommendations for glare control may include glare filters (Fig. 16.5). The choice of filter is subjective and may vary depending on the amount of illumination in the environment. Filters may be used to limit the amount of light entering the eyes, to provide contrast enhancement, to ease the transition between light and dark environments, and for eye protection. Strategies for timing of use of glare filters may also be provided. For example, a person with severe photophobia may be advised to clip light-colored filters over reading spectacles while performing reading tasks indoors, and to switch to darker polarized sunglasses before stepping outside on a sunny day. Persons with delayed dark adaptation may start their adaptation by

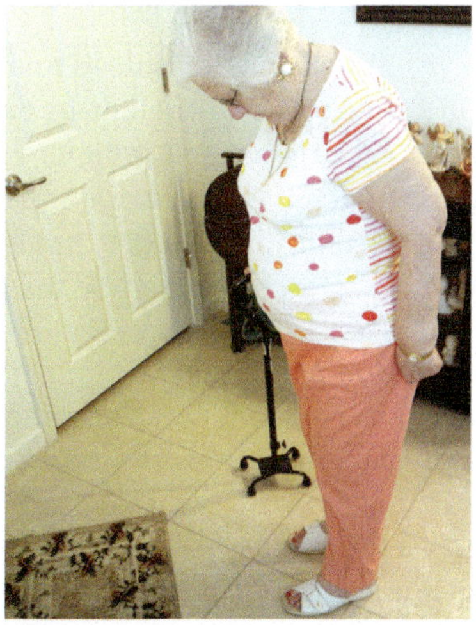

Fig. 16.3: Viewing the edge of the carpet with bifocals.

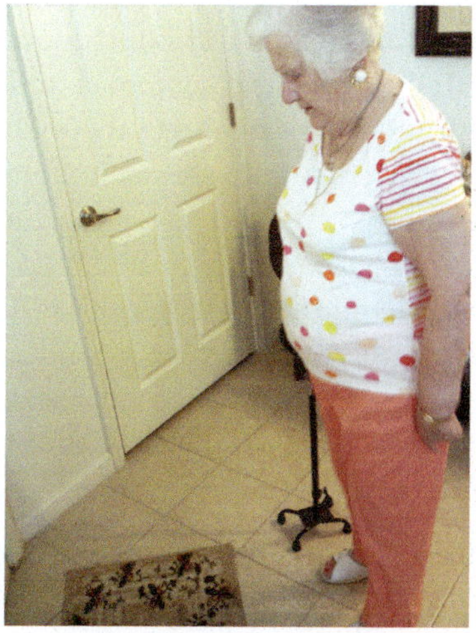

Fig. 16.4: Viewing the edge of the carpet without bifocals.

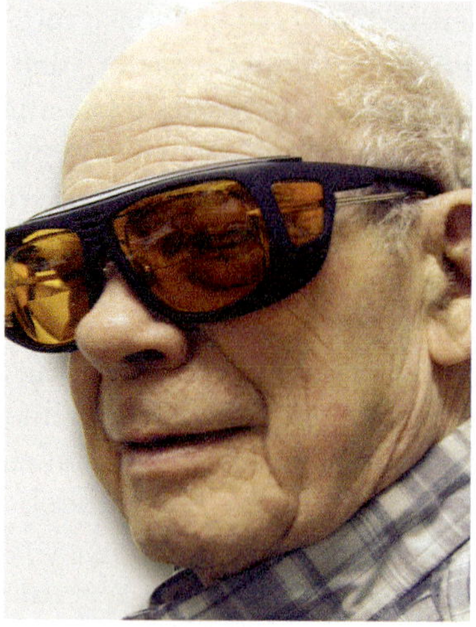

Fig. 16.5: Filters worn over glasses.

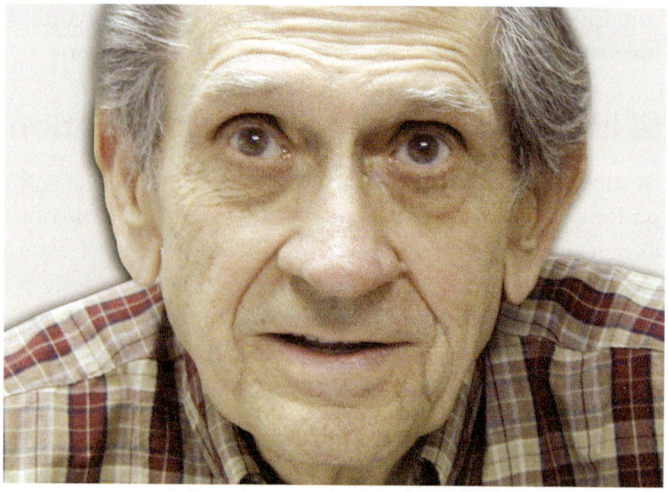

Fig. 16.6: A man viewing eccentrically.
Note: He stated, he was looking straight ahead into the camera. Notice how his gaze is directed upward.

putting on a dark filter before they enter a dark place, such as a theater; once inside, they may take it off. In addition to glare filters, hats, visors, and environmental modifications may be recommended to reduce glare.

Visual Skills Training

Visual skills training refer primarily to three techniques: (1) eccentric viewing, (2) steady eye strategy (SES), and (3) scanning. Learning these skills requires acceptance, awareness, conscious effort, and adaptation to new ways of looking at visual targets and the environment. The vision rehabilitation service provider uses a systematic approach when training these visual skills.

Eccentric viewing: Eccentric viewing refers to nonfoveal fixation that can be used for distance and near tasks, such as facial recognition and reading. This technique is beneficial for people with dense central scotomas. Individuals with a dense central scotoma may direct their gaze so that the visual target of interest falls on an undamaged retinal location, commonly referred to as a preferred retinal location for fixation, or simply preferred retinal locus (PRL) (Fig. 16.6). Some people naturally adopt a PRL while others require training to discover and use it. Studies have shown mixed results for the efficacy of eccentric viewing training, due in part to the lack of a standard protocol for the type, dosage, and frequency of training.

Steady eye strategy: Steady eye strategy is a reading technique that is frequently used in combination with eccentric fixation. The reader keeps his or her eyes in a fixed position of gaze while physically moving the reading material in front of the eyes to scroll it past the PRL. Some patients respond better than others. The success of this method may depend on the configuration of paracentral scotomas.

Scanning: Scanning is a visual skill used by individuals with visual field defects to improve awareness of the person's surroundings, systematically search the environment and determine location of items in the context of a functional activity. Instruction in scanning strategies is particularly relevant for individuals with hemianopia and constricted visual fields.

Training in Manual Skills for Using Optical Devices

In addition to visual skills, patients need to master certain motor skills in order to be proficient in handling their devices. Problems can arise when the better-seeing eye and the dominant hand are on contralateral sides. The patient will naturally use the dominant hand to hold the device up to the dominant eye, which may not be the better-seeing eye (Figs. 16.7 and 16.8). The vision rehabilitation service provider can help the patient learn to line the device up with the better eye during functional activities.

Moreover, the patient must learn where to position the optical device so that the visual target will appear sharpest, i.e. at the focal distance. As the power of the lens increases, the focal distance decreases. If the device is held too far from the target, it will appear upside down. Other manual skills

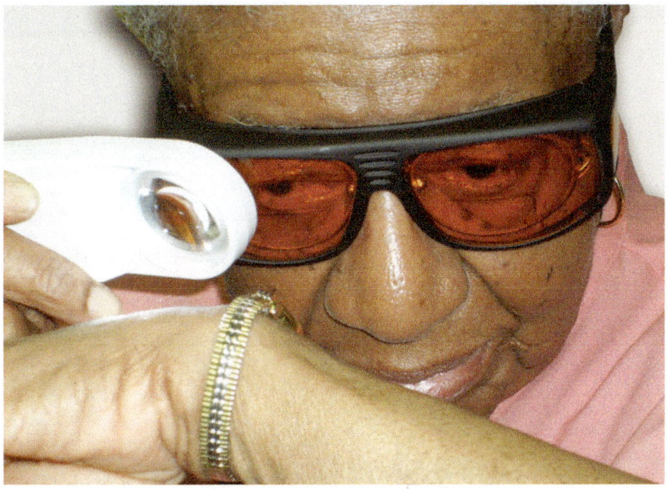

Fig. 16.7: Poor alignment of eye, device, and target.

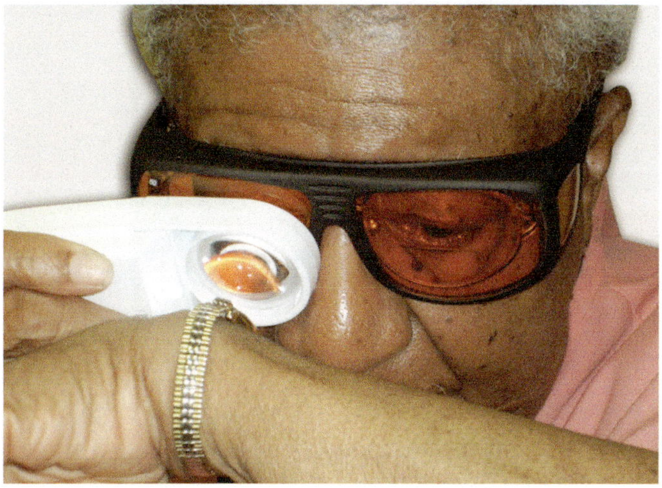

Fig. 16.8: Correct alignment of eye, device, and target.

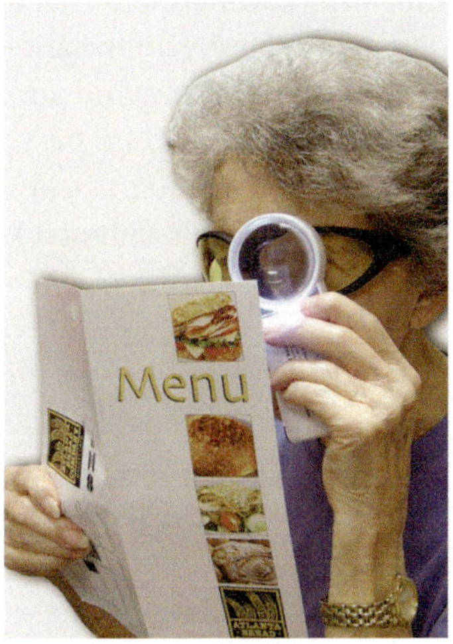

Fig. 16.9: For any lens system it is imperative to know where the visual target will appear sharpest, i.e. the focal distance.

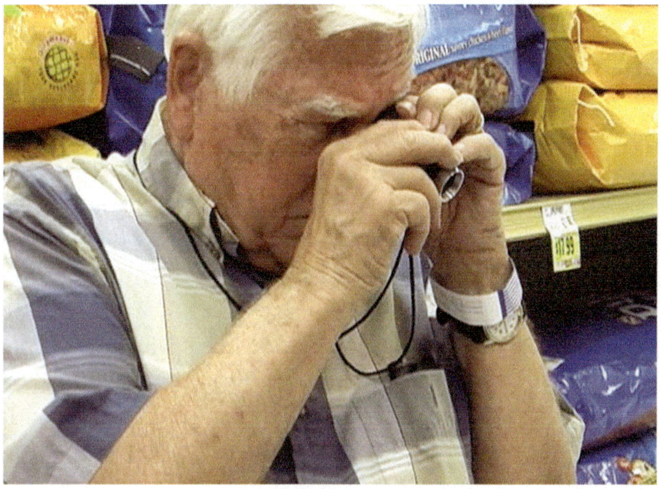

Fig. 16.10: Learning to focus a telescope for reading prices on the bottom shelf of the grocery store.

include moving the magnifier smoothly while maintaining the appropriate focal distance, as when reading. These manual skills of alignment, focus, and motion apply to use of hand held, stand, and telescopic magnification devices (Figs. 16.9 and 16.10).

Supporting Performance of Daily Living

Reading and Writing for Daily Communication

Reading is a complex task and requires a wide variety of strategies and interventions, depending on the type of visual impairment, the patient's habits, routines, and other factors. In addition, different forms of reading require different strategies. For example, continuous reading for pleasure (i.e. a book) presents greater demands than spot reading a grocery bill or price tag.

Patients with central scotomas may experience a variety of difficulties when reading. Central scotomas can distort text or "cut off" letters so the patient may misread a word, such as "how" instead of "show" or replace letters, such as "lake" instead of "take".

Writing is equally necessary for performance of common daily tasks, including those associated with recording and remembering information, paying bills, and completing correspondence. In addition to the visual

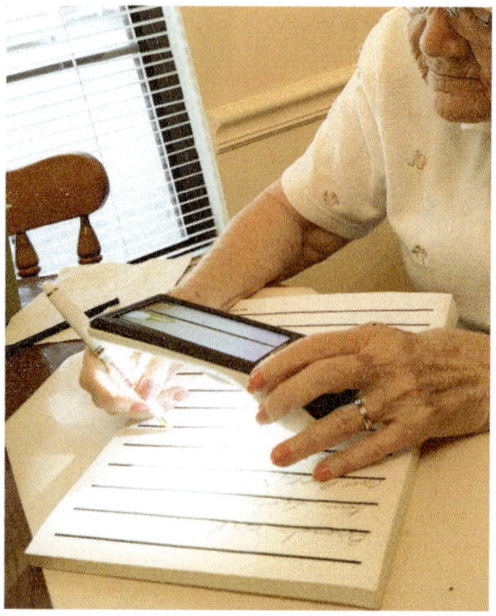

Fig. 16.11: Writing with a portable electronic magnifier.

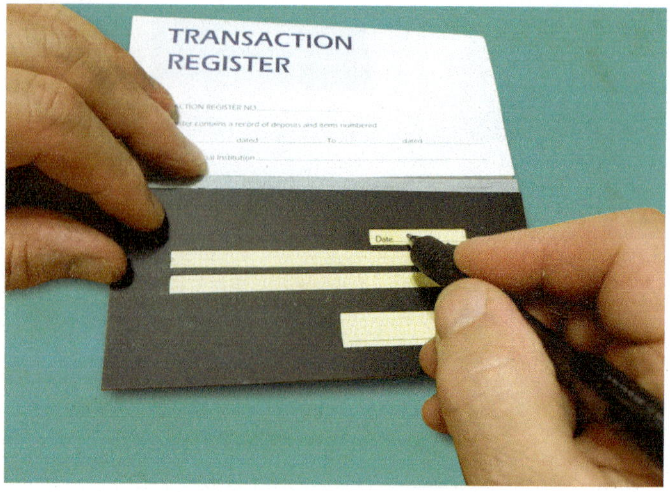

Fig. 16.12: Using a check writing template.

and cognitive demands of reading, writing includes motor demands such as eye-hand coordination of the pen tip as it is moved by the hand, proximal stability and distal control of the upper extremity, etc. When writing, the patient with central scotomas may have trouble viewing the tip of the writing instrument to visually guide motor actions.

Whether reading or writing, the patient may have difficulty staying on the same line of text, keeping place, or transitioning to the next row. In addition to training in visual and manual skills, and the selection of the appropriate optical or electronic devices (Fig. 16.11), the deliberate setup of ergonomic workstations for reading has been found to improve reading rates in older adults with macular degeneration. Practical considerations for reading and writing include use of task lighting, illuminated optical devices, bookmarks and other placekeeping strategies (such as using a finger or line guide), bold lined paper, thicker pens, writing templates (Fig. 16.12), and enlarged records (e.g. check ledger or blood pressure log).

Alternative, nonvisual reading and writing strategies may be useful for patients regardless of the level of visual impairment. Alternatives for reading include audio books, podcasts, and newspapers; text-to-speech software programs and applications; and braille. Alternatives for writing might include voice-recording systems for labeling or voice-activation features on a smartphone.

Computing, Smartphones, and Tablet Technologies

Computers, smartphones, and tablets can help patients retain independence in many aspects of daily living. Most operating systems are modifiable to meet the needs and abilities of the patient. Display of information on the screen, text and icon size, pointer options, and audio descriptions are some of the features that can be personalized to the user. Traditional computer keyboards can also be altered using contrasting stick-on labels for each key (Fig. 16.13), or the entire keyboard can be switched to a high contrast console.

These devices help patients stay connected to family and friends, but can also present challenges to older adults who, in addition to low vision, may have physical challenges, can be more skeptical of new technologies, and may require frequent repetition and practice to adopt these technologies. In the United States, older adults are more likely to use smartphones and tablets (Fig. 16.14) if they are college educated, have relatively high incomes and are in their sixties.

Phone Use

Efficient and accurate phone use is important for safety reasons and socialization. Vision loss may limit the individual's ability to read a personal phone book, dial the phone correctly, and contact emergency services. Large print, customized phone list, a large dial phone (Fig. 16.15), a phone with talk back features, use of voice activation on cell phones, and high contrast or tactile markings can promote independent phone use.

Self-care

Vision rehabilitation service providers can address concerns related to self-care tasks such as eating, dressing,

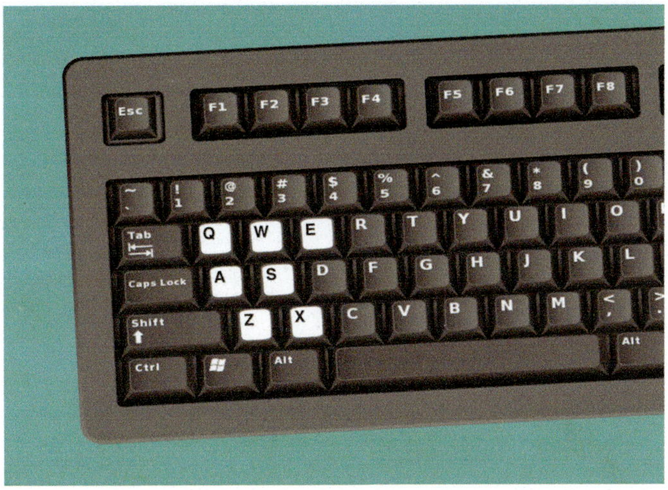

Fig. 16.13: Stickers with enlarged letters for computer keys.

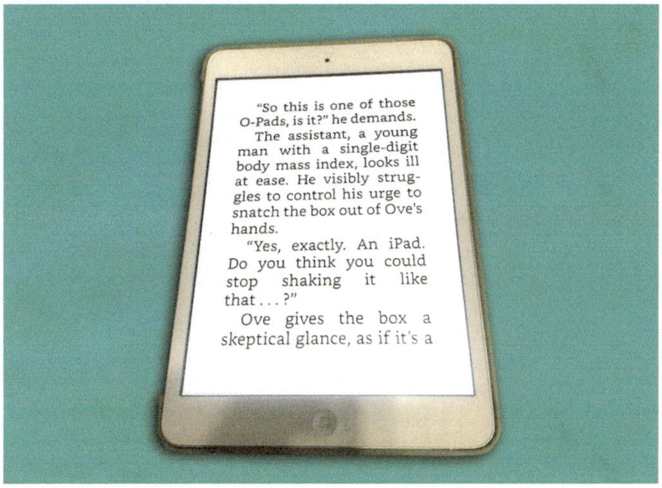

Fig. 16.14: Electronic reader (*see* also Chapter 15, Fig. 15.5)

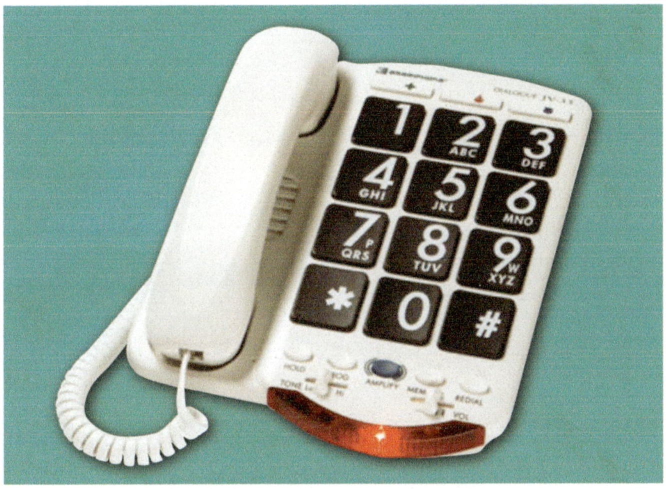

Fig. 16.15: Phone with enlarged numbers.

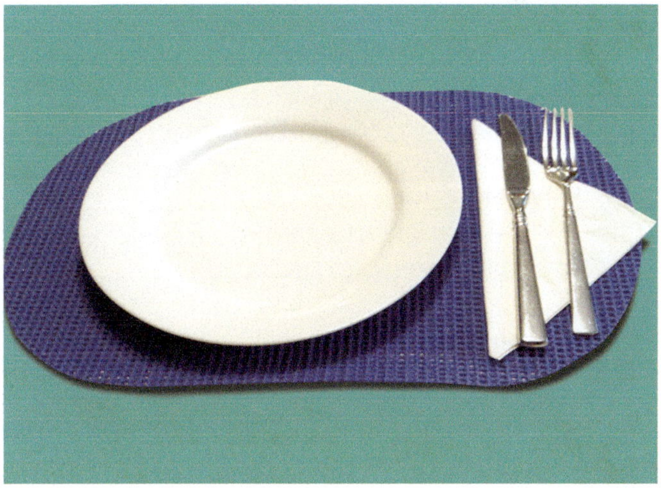

Fig. 16.16: Use of contrasting place mat increases visibility of plate.

and grooming. Difficulty locating food on a plate can be remedied through use of contrast strategies (Figs. 16.16 and 16.17), additional task lighting, and serving food in separate bowls. Adapted pouring and cutting methods are also useful.

Grooming tasks, such as shaving, makeup and toothpaste application (Fig. 16.18), and toiletry identification can be accomplished through use of lighted magnified makeup mirrors, marking and organization systems, and use of tactile input. Locating and matching clothing are common challenges that can be addressed by use of organization, lighting, and clothing marking strategies. Adapted needle threaders can assist with mending tasks (Fig. 16.19).

Health Management

The majority of adults with vision impairments have at least one additional chronic health condition, such as arthritis, hypertension, diabetes, and depression that impacts daily activity performance.[1] Thus, low vision rehabilitation providers address a variety of skills needed to foster health and wellness. Medication management strategies include use of medication bottle marking and organization strategies (Fig. 16.20), setting up a medication station, creating large print medication and dosage lists, optical device use, and task lighting. A study regarding physical activity levels found that only 25% of participants with age-related macular

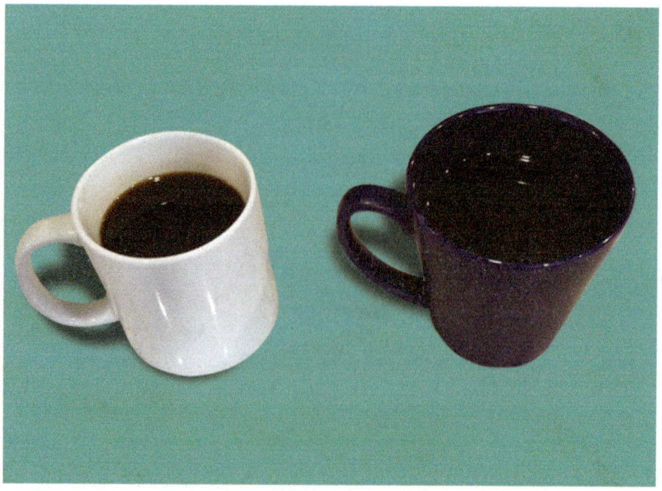

Fig. 16.17: Coffee in white cup is more visible.

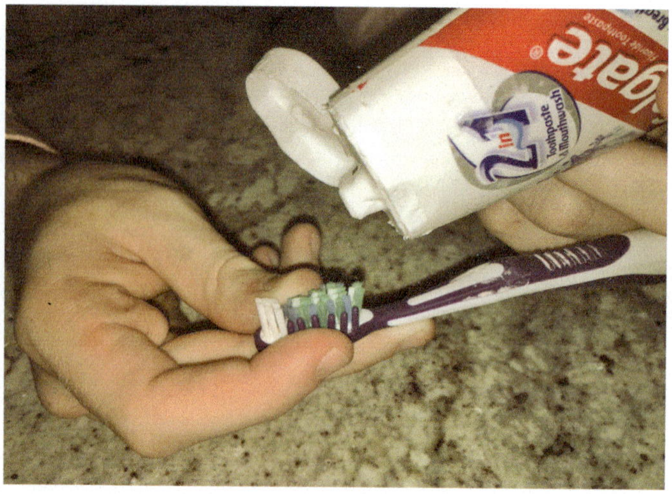

Fig. 16.18: Holding toothbrush at bristle end allows for tactile input while applying toothpaste.

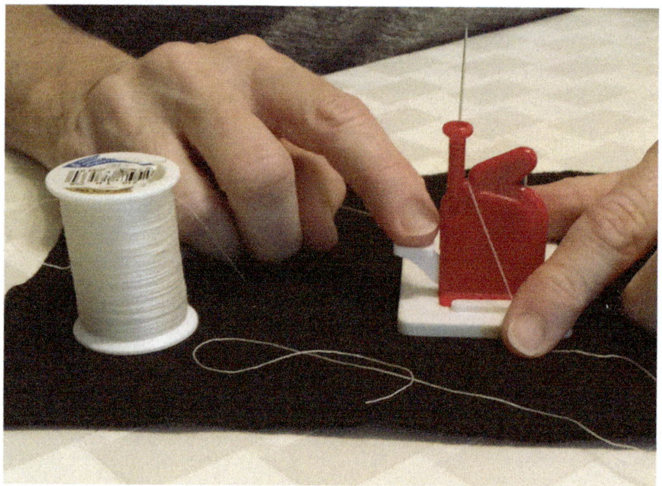

Fig. 16.19: Needle threader.

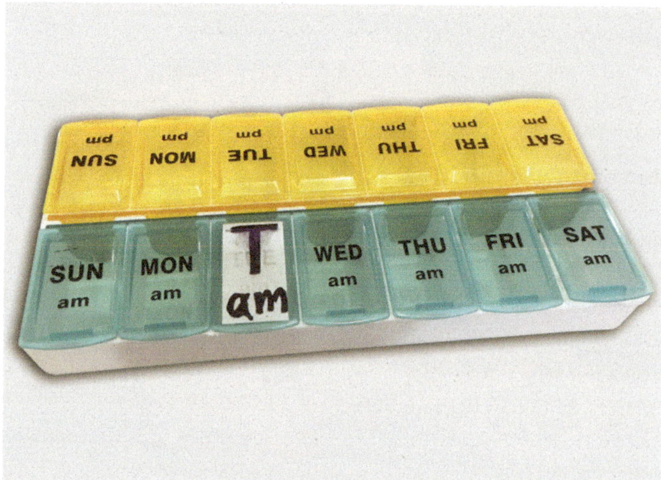

Fig. 16.20: Medication organizer with bold colors and enlarged print.

degeneration engaged in regular exercise.[2] Physical activity is strongly linked to better mental and physical health and can be promoted by instruction in safe, accessible methods such as chair exercise and yoga routines, walking with a partner, and incorporation of rigorous leisure activities such as gardening and dancing. Nutrition management is of great importance, particularly for individuals with diabetes. The American Diabetes Association's standards of care focuses on blood glucose and blood pressure control, both of which can be influenced by diet. Reinforcement of increasing intake of fruits and vegetables, implementing spot reading techniques for reading food labels and enabling individuals to prepare healthy meals safely and independently through use of adaptive strategies described in the following section allows individuals to manage their diabetes and other chronic conditions.

Meal Preparation

Safe and independent meal preparation is routinely addressed in low vision rehabilitation. Common limitations include difficulty seeing appliance controls, measuring ingredients, chopping and slicing, reading food labels and recipes, locating food items in the pantry and refrigerator, and determining when food is fully cooked or spoiled. High contrast and tactile markings can be added to kitchen appliances to increase visibility of controls. Measuring spoons and cups with high contrast markings can increase accuracy when measuring ingredients. High contrast

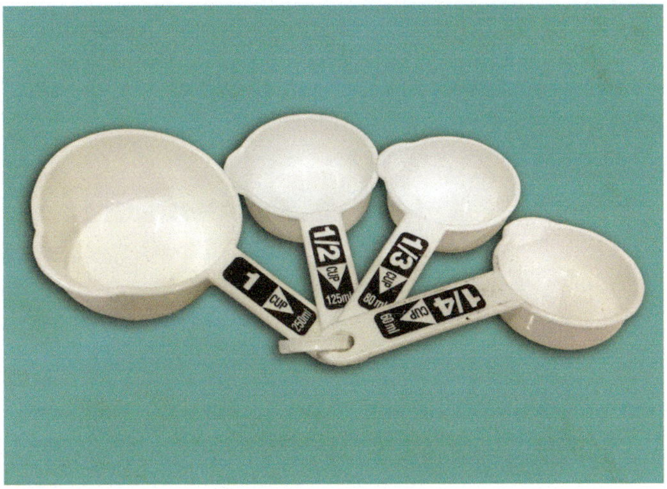

Fig. 16.21: High contrast, large print measuring cups.

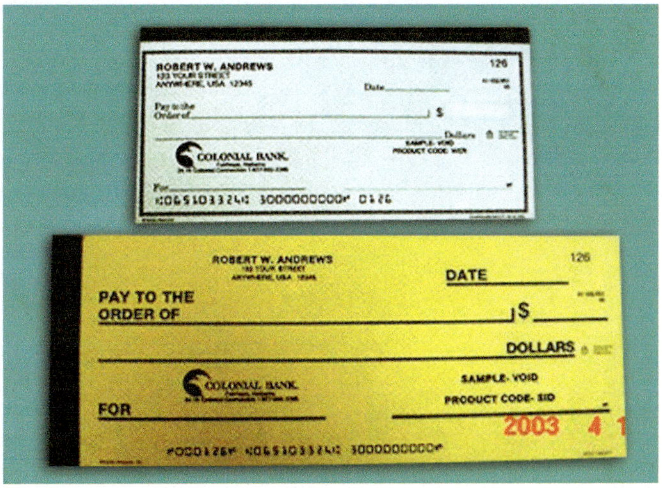

Fig. 16.22: Enlarged personal check.

cutting boards and a knife guard can help with safety when slicing foods. Recipe and food label reading can be promoted through use of task lighting, marking strategies, and optical device use. Use of timers, tactile sensation, added lighting, and large print expiration date markings increase food safety.

Money Management

Individuals with vision loss can continue to perform money management tasks, such as counting coins and currency, reading bills, writing checks and money orders, using computers for online banking, and organizing records through use of reading and writing strategies, enlarged checks and ledgers (Figs. 16.22 and 16.23), computer software and accessibility settings, and money organizers.

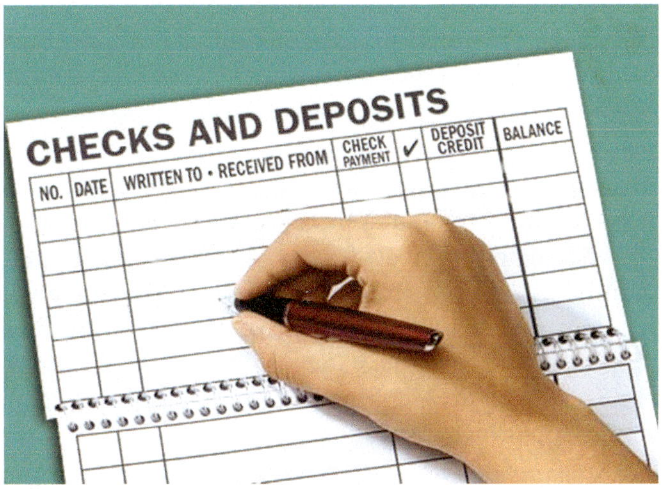

Fig. 16.23: Enlarged check ledger.

Work and Leisure Pursuits

People who have low vision can perform most jobs provided they have the tools, modifications, and accommodations necessary to safely execute their work duties. Typical workplace accommodations include glare reduction and adjusted lighting, computers with screen magnifying or screen-reading software, larger monitors, braille displays, talking calculators, and many of the strategies and environmental modifications mentioned in this chapter.

Continued engagement in leisure and physical activities promotes a greater sense of social self and well-being and is commonly addressed during low vision rehabilitation. Reading for pleasure can be augmented through use of optical devices, large print books, audiobooks, and task lighting (Fig. 16.24). Large print playing cards, adaptive board games, and crossword puzzles can be recommended. Gardening can be accomplished through use of colorful borders and gardening tools with contrasting handles, and selecting plants with scents and tactile qualities. Active leisure pursuits that are tailored for individuals with vision loss include tandem biking, beep ball, running with a guide or tether, and many more. If an individual must give up an activity, finding a satisfying replacement activity has been shown to decrease depressive symptoms.

Supporting a Livable Environment

Lighting

Home lighting should be addressed routinely because (1) the aging eye causes reduced amounts of light to reach

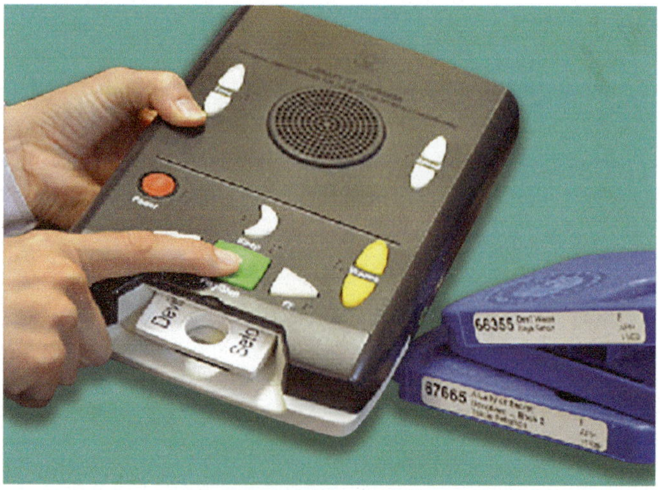

Fig. 16.24: Use of audio book player.

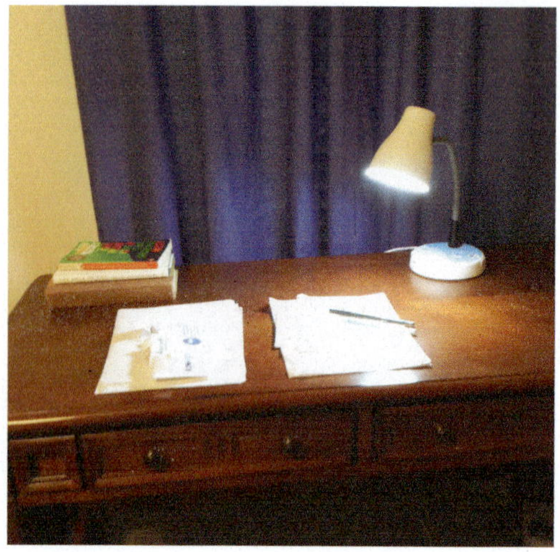

Fig. 16.25: Task lamp could be moved to left corner of desk surface for right handed person.

the retina,[3] (2) persons with ocular disease require high levels of illumination,[4] (3) some ocular diseases cause light sensitivity, and (4) home lighting is usually well below recommended levels.[5-7] Lighting levels can be measured using a light meter at the location that near tasks are performed and in key areas such as stairwell landings. A device (LuxIQ™) that can be used to determine lighting preferences in terms of illumination and color temperature. Lighting principles such as ensuring even lighting, positioning task lighting directly over and in close proximity to reading material, and situating the light source opposite the dominant hand for writing tasks serve as a guide to implementing lighting interventions that are tailored to the individual (Fig. 16.25). In addition, outdoor motion detector lighting, night lights, and below cabinet light-emitting diode (LED) lighting can enhance safety during mobility.

Labeling

Labeling of appliances, electronics, and other items can be accomplished through visual and/or tactile strategies. This includes using contrasting colors to mark control buttons, while tactile strategies make use of adhesive materials with unique textures, such as Velcro®, electrician's tape or textured paint (Figs. 16.26 to 16.28).

Supporting Safe Mobility

Safe mobility in the home and community can be impacted by central and peripheral vision loss, decreased contrast sensitivity, inappropriate glasses, and balance issues.[8] Conducting a falls history and questioning patients about frequency of falls and bumping into obstacles, difficulty with steps, and fear of falling will assist in identifying the impact of vision loss on mobility. Visual skills and scanning techniques, mentioned earlier in this chapter, can foster the patient's use of their retained vision and compensate for visual field loss. Training in the use of a white mobility cane can provide the patient with additional independence, particularly in unfamiliar environments. The cane serves to alert others, as well as to explore the environment. Telescopes are used to help read road signs and traffic signals once they have been spotted with unmagnified vision. Patients are advised to use telescopes while stationary because distorted perception of the location of objects is dangerous while moving.

Prisms may be requested for the purpose of "field expansion". Prisms do not reduce visual field loss, but may be used to create greater awareness of the missing visual field. Similar to telescopes, the patient cannot continuously view through the prisms when walking due to mismatch of actual and perceived location of objects because an object may appear off to the side, when in fact it is in front of the person, causing him or her to trip.

Fall Prevention

Falls are the leading cause of injury-related deaths in those over the age of 65; nearly one-third of people over 65 years of age fall each year.[9] Falls often result in decreases in activity, loss of mobility, pain, and death. Factors associated with falls can be categorized as internal (personal) and external

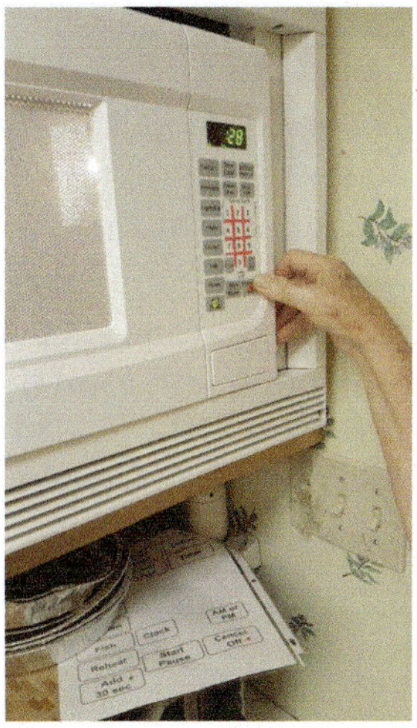

Fig. 16.26: High contrast and tactile markings on a microwave panel.

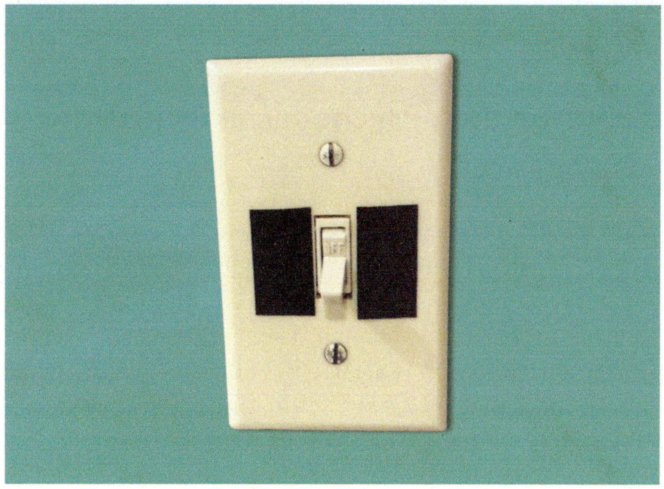

Fig. 16.27: High contrast marking on light switch.

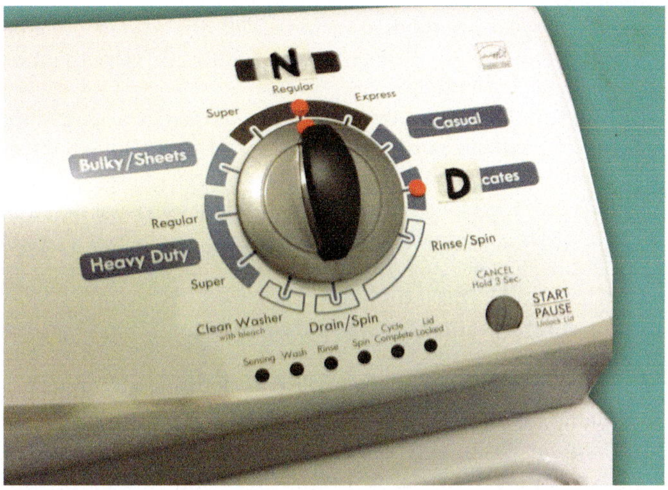

Fig. 16.28: High contrast and tactile markings on washer controls.

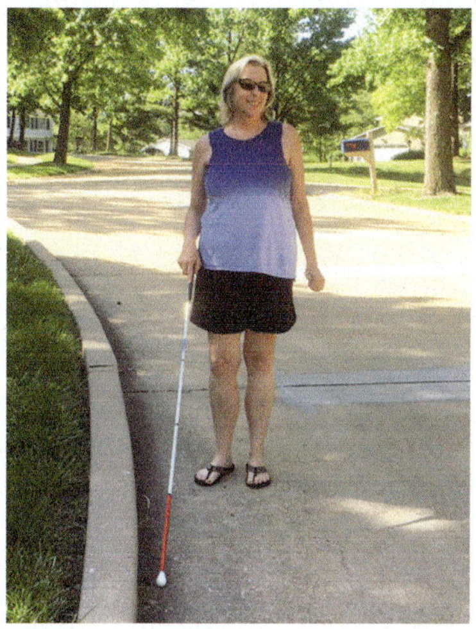

Fig. 16.29: Woman using a long white cane, for visibility (walking in the street), and for not straying away from the curb.

(environmental). Internal factors include age, medical conditions, frailty, visual impairment, balance, cognitive status, dizziness, incontinence, and depression. External factors include environmental hazards, poor footwear, and medications. Successful fall prevention programs address multiple factors including building strength, endurance and balance, improving lighting, reducing hazards, and consideration of vision.

Cane Travel

Certified orientation and mobility specialists (COMS) are specifically trained to provide systematic instruction to people with low vision and blindness in use of a long cane for safe travel. Cane skills are essential to the patient's safety and protection and include rhythmic movement of the cane, hand position, sensitivity to cane drop-off, safe negotiation of obstacles and stairs, and overriding visual misinformation (Fig. 16.29).

Guide Dogs

Like the long white cane, guide dogs are intended to help people with low vision and blindness travel safely. Guide dogs need more continued care than a cane, but have the additional benefit to the handler of companionship, improved self-esteem, and improved confidence. The dog and the owner form a team, so both need training. The handler should have prior skills in orientation and mobility, because the dog is reliant on its handler for instructions.

Matching a dog to a person with low vision or blindness is a crucial step toward this end.

Supporting Psychosocial Adjustment

Depression

Individuals with visual impairments are at increased risk of developing depression; research has found depression rates range between 25% and 40%.[10] Thus, it is important to quickly identify those at risk through use of screens such as the Geriatric Depression Scale (GDS)[11] and the Patient Health Questionnaire-9 (PHQ-9)[12] so that appropriate referrals and intervention decisions can be made. To complement medical care, low vision rehabilitation providers can assist by enabling valued activity performance, providing instruction in relaxation techniques, teaching coping strategies and exercise routines, and making referrals to support groups.

Dealing with Stress and Anxiety from Visual Hallucinations

Charles Bonnet syndrome (CBS) is the name given to phantom visual images or visual hallucinations, which can occur following vision loss due to conditions such as macular degeneration, cataract, glaucoma, or diabetic retinopathy. CBS is akin to phantom limb sensations that people can experience after a limb amputation. Estimates of the prevalence of CBS vary widely from 1% to 40% depending on the populations studied; however, it is also widely recognized as an under-reported condition since many people with low vision fear they will be ridiculed, labeled as "crazy", or lose their independence. While the patient may be aware that the images or hallucinations are not real, we need to recognize that people with low vision often experience a great deal of anxiety and stress if they are not reassured that these types of visual hallucinations can be expected to occur. Aside from educating people with low vision about the potential for them to experience visual hallucinations, there are no evidence-based tests or treatments for CBS.

SUMMARY

This chapter described the various professionals that can be members of a vision rehabilitation team along with the basic interventions used to make the most of the patient's remaining vision, environment, and engagement in life. There are, of course, many more strategies and resources which are continually evolving. It is imperative for the patient to have the support of such a team; other team members can also alleviate much of the anxiety and burden of care from the physician. Find out who the service providers are in your community and network with them. They will be eager to share in the care of your patients and become part of the support network you offer as part of your clinical care.

REFERENCES

1. Crews JE, Jones GC, Kim JH. Double jeopardy: the effects of comorbid conditions among older people with vision loss. J Vis Impair Blind. 2006;100:824-48.
2. Knudtson MD, Klein R, Klein BE. Physical activity and the 15-year cumulative incidence of age-related macular degeneration: the Beaver Dam Eye Study. Br J Ophthalmol. 2006;90(12):1461-3.
3. Watson GR. Low vision in the geriatric population: rehabilitation and management. J Am Geriatr Soc. 2001;49(3):317-30.
4. Haymes SA, Lee J. Effects of task lighting on visual function in age-related macular degeneration. Ophthalmic Physiol Opt. 2006;26(2):169-79.
5. Charness N, Dijkstra K. Age, luminance, and print legibility in homes, offices, and public places. Hum Factors. 1999;41(2):173-93.
6. Cullinan TR, Gould ES, Silver JH, et al. Visual disability and home lighting. Lancet. 1979;1(8117):642-4.
7. Lindner H, Rinnert T, Behrens-Baumann W. Illumination conditions of visually impaired people under private domestic circumstances-clinical study on 91 patients. Klin Monbl Augenheilkd. 2001;218(12):774-81.
8. Lord SR. Visual risk factors for falls in older people. Age Ageing. 2006;35(Suppl 2):ii42-5.
9. Blake AJ, Morgan K, Bendal MJ, et al. Falls by elderly people at home: prevalence and associated factors. Age Ageing. 1988;17(6):365-72.
10. Popescu M, Boisjoly H, Schmaltz H, et al. Explaining the relationship between three eye diseases and depressive symptoms in older adults. Invest Ophthalmol Vis Sci. 2012;53(4):2308-13.
11. Yesavage JA, Brink TL, Rose TL, et al. Development and validation of a geriatric depression screening scale: a preliminary report. J Psychiatr Res. 1983;17(1):37-49.
12. Kroencke K, Spitzer R, Williams J. The PHQ-9: validity of a brief depression severity measure. J Gen Intern Med. 2001;16(9):606-13.

Part 5 Conjunctiva and Cornea

■ *N Venkatesh Prajna*

OUTLINE

Chapter 17

Corneal Examination and Investigations

Ashish Kumar, Manoranjan Das, Arun Kumar Panigrahi

MEASUREMENT OF CORNEAL SHAPE

Introduction

More than three centuries have passed since the discovery that cornea is responsible for two-thirds of the refractive power of the eye but the quest for developing a single device which can describe and measure the shape of the cornea accurately is still continuing. In 1619, Father Christopher Scheiner determined the corneal curvature by comparing the apparent size of the window panes viewed by reflections from the cornea with the relative size of the images seen in glass marbles of various size.[1] Jesse Ramsden in 1796 built the first device to measure the corneal curvature.[2] The telescope was then used to magnify the images reflected off the cornea and a doubling device was incorporated to decrease the effects of the unintentional eye movements. The device did not gain significant scientific recognition until 1854 when Helmholtz further fine-tuned the instrument to measure corneal curvature more precisely.[3] Later Javal and schiotz in 1881 further modified to make this a more practical instrument to aid in clinical practice for the measurement of corneal curvature.[4] Since then the basic design of the keratometer has been the same. In 1932, Bausch and Lomb introduced certain modifications (Fig. 17.1) which made it more user-friendly and has almost been the gold standard for measuring corneal curvature for decades until the advent of newer topography machines. With all the limitations, keratometry still has considerable use in ophthalmology.

Various topography machines use the similar basic principle of measuring the patterns reflected by the corneal surface. With the advancement of the corneal laser surgery, it became essential to measure corneal surface over a wider area. This requirement ushered in the manufacture of keratoscope, which was then modified to a photokeratoscope and finally to a videokeratoscope. The term "*topography*" was introduced to represent the computerized corneal surface reconstruction of the photokeratoscopic images. In recent times, the ability to measure the posterior corneal surface along with the anterior corneal curvature has led to the introduction of a new terminology *"tomography"* which is more reflective of the three-dimensional characterization of the cornea.

Keratometry

Keratometry is the measurement of the radii of the curvature of the central cornea. It is based on the assumption that the anterior surface of the cornea acts as a perfect spherical convex mirror and the size of the image varies with the curvature of the cornea. The optics of the keratometer is explained with the help of a ray diagram (Fig. 17.2) and the magnification equation (M) as mentioned below:

$$M = \frac{\text{Image size}}{\text{Object size}} = \frac{\text{Image distance}}{\text{Object distance}}$$

$$M = \frac{i}{o} = \frac{v}{u}$$

where i is the height of the image, o is the height of the mire (target), v is the distance of the image from the mirror and u is the distance of the mire (target) from the mirror.

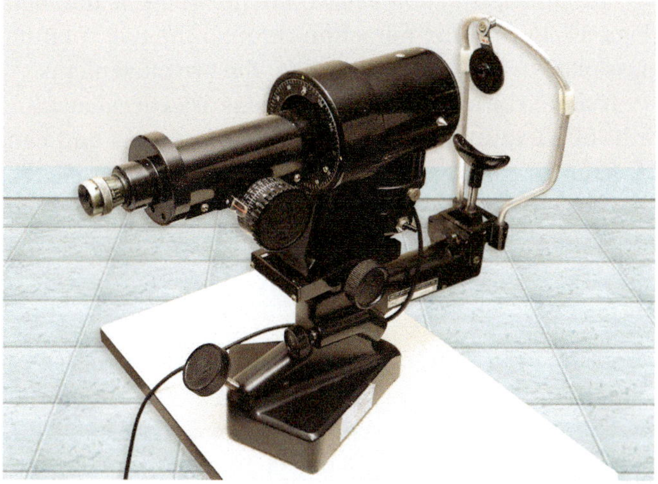

Fig. 17.1: Bausch and Lomb Keratometer.

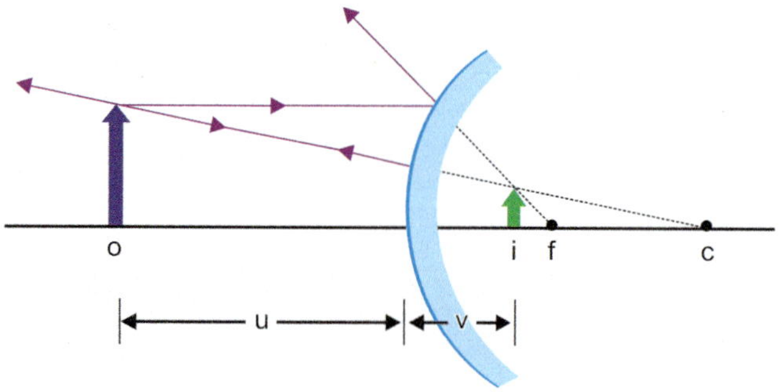

Fig. 17.2: Ray diagram to understand the optics of the keratometer. ("i" is the height of the image, "o" is the height of the mire (target), "v" is the distance of the image from the mirror and "u" is the distance of the mire (target) from the mirror, "f" is the focal length of the mirror and "c" is the center of curvature of the mirror).

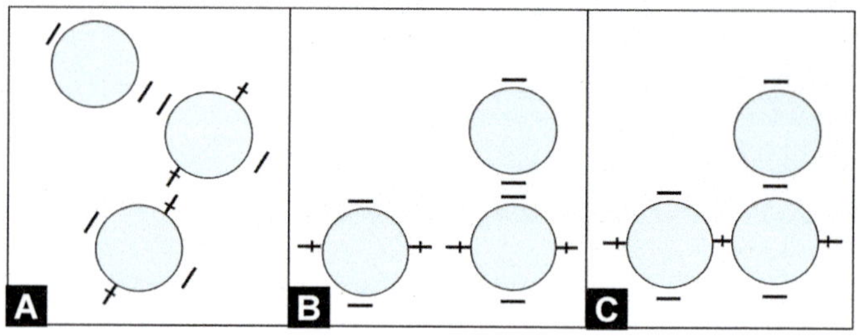

Figs. 17.3A to C: Alignment of the mires on a Bausch and Lomb keratometer using the principle of doubling. (A) The view when the mires are of the principal meridians; (B) The view when the mires are on the principal meridians; (C) The view when the plus and minus signs are overlapping to measure the "horizontal" and "vertical" radii of curvature/equivalent power.

An illuminated mire ring target is placed in front of the cornea. This distance (u) of the target is kept constant for any instrument by using short focus telescope in order to view the reflected image. The working distance (u) is large as compared to the radii of curvature of the cornea and so the image can be assumed to be located at the focal point. The focal length (f) of the convex mirror is half the radius of the curvature (r) of the mirror. So,

$$v = f, \quad f = \frac{r}{2}$$

Then,

$$\frac{i}{o} = \frac{r}{2u} \quad \text{or} \quad r = \frac{2ui}{o}$$

In theory, it is reasonable to assume that for a known target size, measuring the size of the image will give the radii of curvature of the cornea, while keeping the target distance constant. However, in actual clinical practice, measuring image size is a challenge due to the constant movement of the living eyes. To overcome this, the current keratometers use the *principle of doubling* where the image is doubled (Figs. 17.3A to C) by refraction through the two rotating glass plates which compensates for the eye movements.

It should be noted that the formulas used in calculating radii of curvature are approximation formulas and can sometimes results in minor errors which are not significant.

Corneal power can be derived from the radius of curvature shown as below.

$$P = \frac{(n' - n)}{r}$$

where P is the power of the cornea, n′ is the index of refraction of cornea and n is the index of refraction of air. Cornea has two refracting surfaces anterior and the posterior. In order to calculate the power of the cornea, the radii of curvature of the two surfaces should be known. However, it is not possible to measure the posterior corneal surface by keratometers. The corneal index of refraction is usually taken as 1.376 but to compensate for the posterior corneal curvature, a value of 1.3375 is generally used. Thus, the equation becomes:

$$P = \frac{(1.3375 - 1.000)}{r} = \frac{0.3375}{r}$$

Keratometry is useful in the fitting of contact lenses and in the measurement of the power of the intraocular lenses implanted during cataract surgery. However, keratometry has the following limitations.

1. It assumes the cornea to be an ideal spherocylindrical structure with a single radius of curvature in each meridian. However, the cornea is aspherical and flattens from center to periphery.
2. It only measures the area surrounding the four points on the cornea which are 3 mm apart. It does not take into the account the area peripheral or central to it. In steeper corneas, it measures a zone less than 3 mm, but assumes it to be 3 mm. On the other hand, in flatter corneas, it measures a zone greater than 3 mm, but still gives values assuming that it is measuring a 3 mm zone. It gives no information of the area inside or outside of the 3 mm ring and therefore the reliability of the keratometer in asymmetrical corneas like keratoconus and post refractive surgeries is questionable.

In spite of these limitations, keratometer is still widely used because of its low cost, ease of use and minimal maintenance.

Corneal Topography

In the last three decades, refractive surgical practice has undergone tremendous changes in terms of the procedure, predictability and the outcome. Much of this happened because of the advancement in the corneal topography. However still the yardsticks for evaluating the outcome of the refractive surgical procedure is the uncorrected and best corrected visual acuity. Corneal topography has become the standard of care for preoperative screening of a refractive surgical candidate and also for qualitative analysis of the postoperative patient to find out the causes of unexplained reduced vision after an uneventful surgery. With the advent of cross linking procedure for strengthening of the ectatic cornea, topography has become an essential tool in the armamentarium of management of these cases.

Currently there are mainly three corneal imaging techniques to assess corneal topography, i.e. Placido-disk based keratoscopy, Slit-scanning tomography and Scheimpflug imaging.

Placido-disk Based Keratoscopy

In 1847, Henry Goode described the first keratoscope, where the reflection of a square object from the cornea was observed from the side of the target.[5] Antonio Placido da Costa from Portugal in 1880 used a more complete target which covered a wider area of cornea, consisting of circular mires with alternating black and white concentric rings with a central hole to observe the reflections from the cornea (Fig. 17.4).[6] The goal was to decipher the information about the curvature of the cornea from the examination of the pattern of the reflected rings. A non-uniform reflection usually denotes astigmatism, keratoconus or a corneal scar. The reflective mires appear closer together on steeper areas of the cornea and farther apart in flatter areas (Figs. 17.5A and B). These examinations cannot identify subtle changes in the cornea and only gross curvature changes can be identified. Further advances led to the video capturing of these reflections and quantitative analysis of the corneal shape and power distribution were depicted as "maps". With the help of the computer software, these maps are represented in different color patterns to give an instant information about the corneal surface.[7] This became the basis for modern day corneal topography. Placido-disk keratoscopy in combination with other technologies like slit-scanning or Scheimpflug imaging is the standard of care for screening refractive surgical candidates and detection of keratoconus.

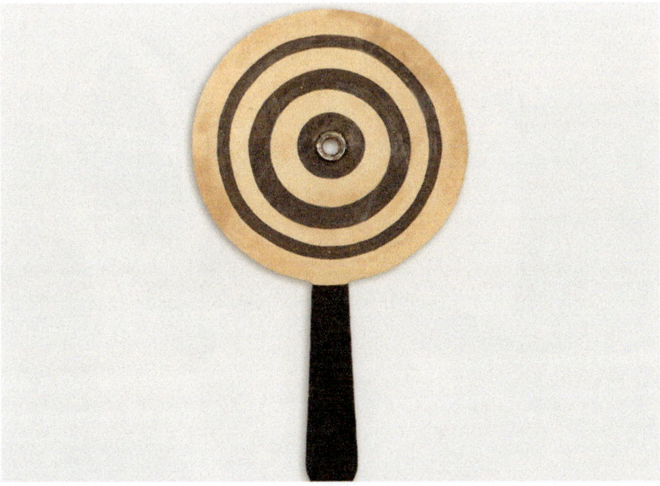

Fig. 17.4: Placido-disk. Circular mires with alternating black and white concentric rings with a central hole to observe the reflections from the cornea.

Slit-scanning Based Tomography

The slit-scanning system provides information about the anterior and posterior corneal surface elevations, corneal thickness as well as the anterior lens surface and iris. It uses the theorem of slit scan triangulation for the calculation of the corneal power. The same principle is applied in standard or normal photography where the plane of the camera lens is located in parallel with the image as explained in the Figure 17.6A. The device projects 40 vertical slits of light on the vertical meridian of the cornea, 20 from right and 20 from left covering the entire cornea at a fixed angle of 45° to the instrument axis. The digital video camera captures the slits and its anterior and posterior edges are analyzed. Each slit has 250 data points which makes a total of 9,600 analyzable data points. The presence of a tracking system attempts to minimize the influence of the involuntary eye movements during the acquisition time. The data for the areas in between the slits are extrapolated.

A significant advancement was the incorporation of a Placido-disk imaging into slit-scanning technology to directly measure the anterior corneal curvature and corneal power. The Orbscan II (TECHNOLAS perfect vision GmbH, Bausch + Lomb company, Salt Lake City, Utah, USA) (Fig. 17.7A) is the only device commercially available that utilizes this technology.[8] The common image obtained is a display containing four maps (often referred to as the quad map) that provides information about the curvature, anterior and posterior corneal elevation and pachymetry of the entire corneal surface (Figs. 17.8A and B).[9] The most recent upgrade is the Orbscan IIz which integrates with a Hartmann-Shack aberrometer (Fig. 17.7B) in the Zyoptix workstation for evaluating patients of refractive surgery.

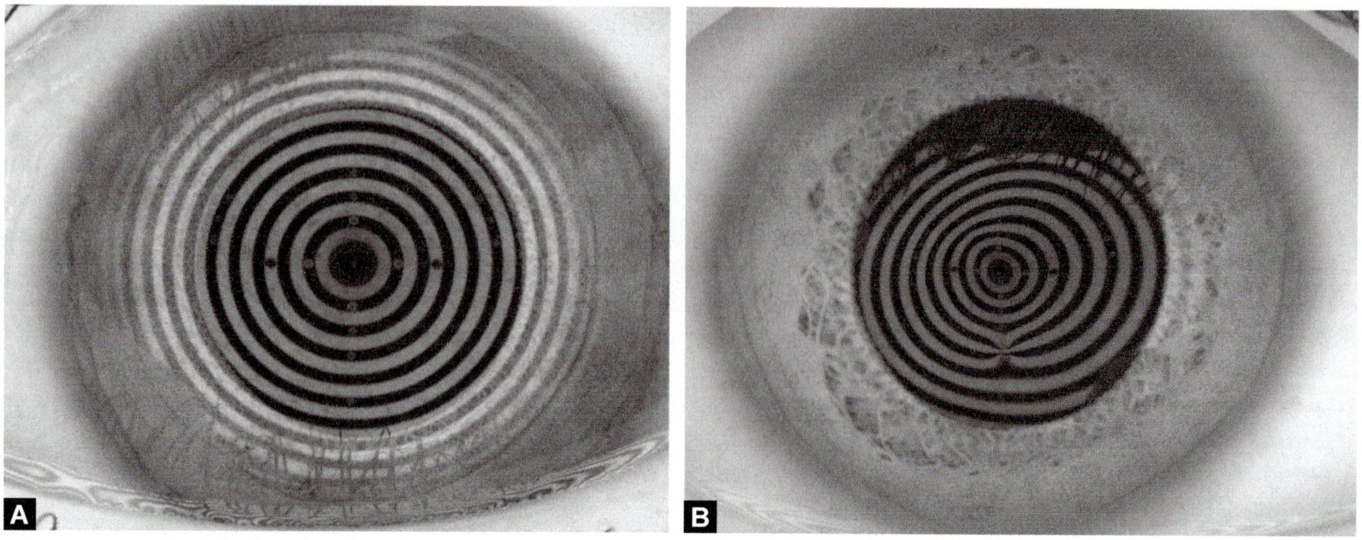

Figs. 17.5A and B: Placido-disk image of the cornea. (A) The concentric mires are of equal width and equidistant from each other; (B) The mires are of unequal width and appear closer superiorly and inferiorly.

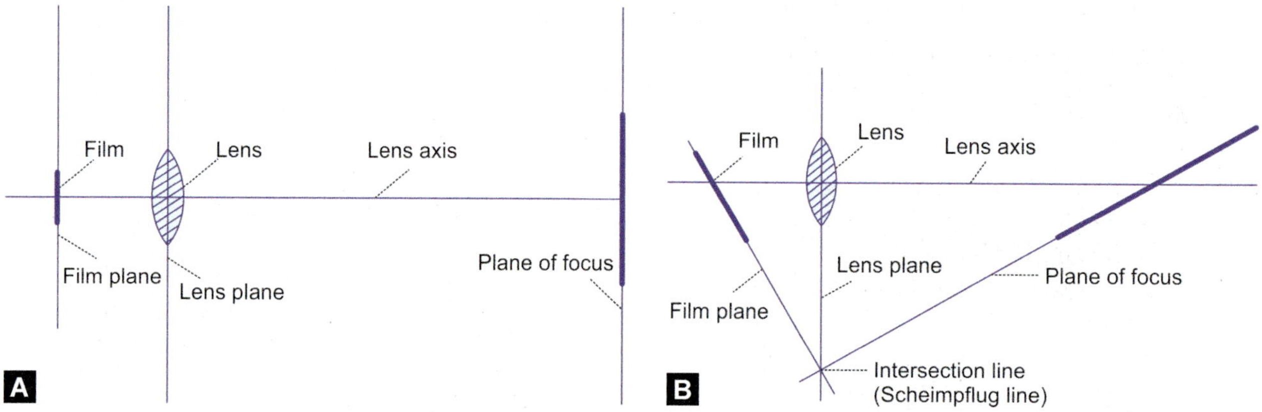

Figs. 17.6A and B: Principle of Photography. (A) Slit-scanning. Plane of camera lens is in parallel with the image; (B) Scheimpflug imaging. Plane of the camera lens is placed sideways to the image.

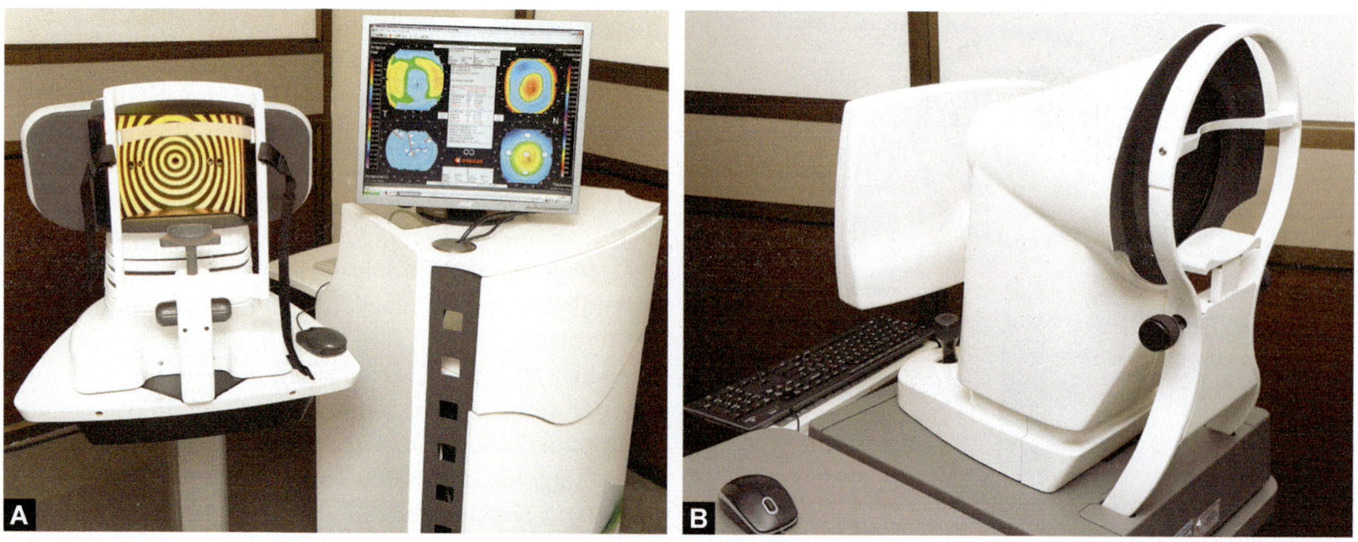

Figs. 17.7A and B: Orbscan II along with Hartmann-Shack aberrometer. (A) Orbscan II from TECHNOLAS perfect vision; (B) iDESIGN Advanced WaveScan Studio System using Hartmann-Shack sensor.

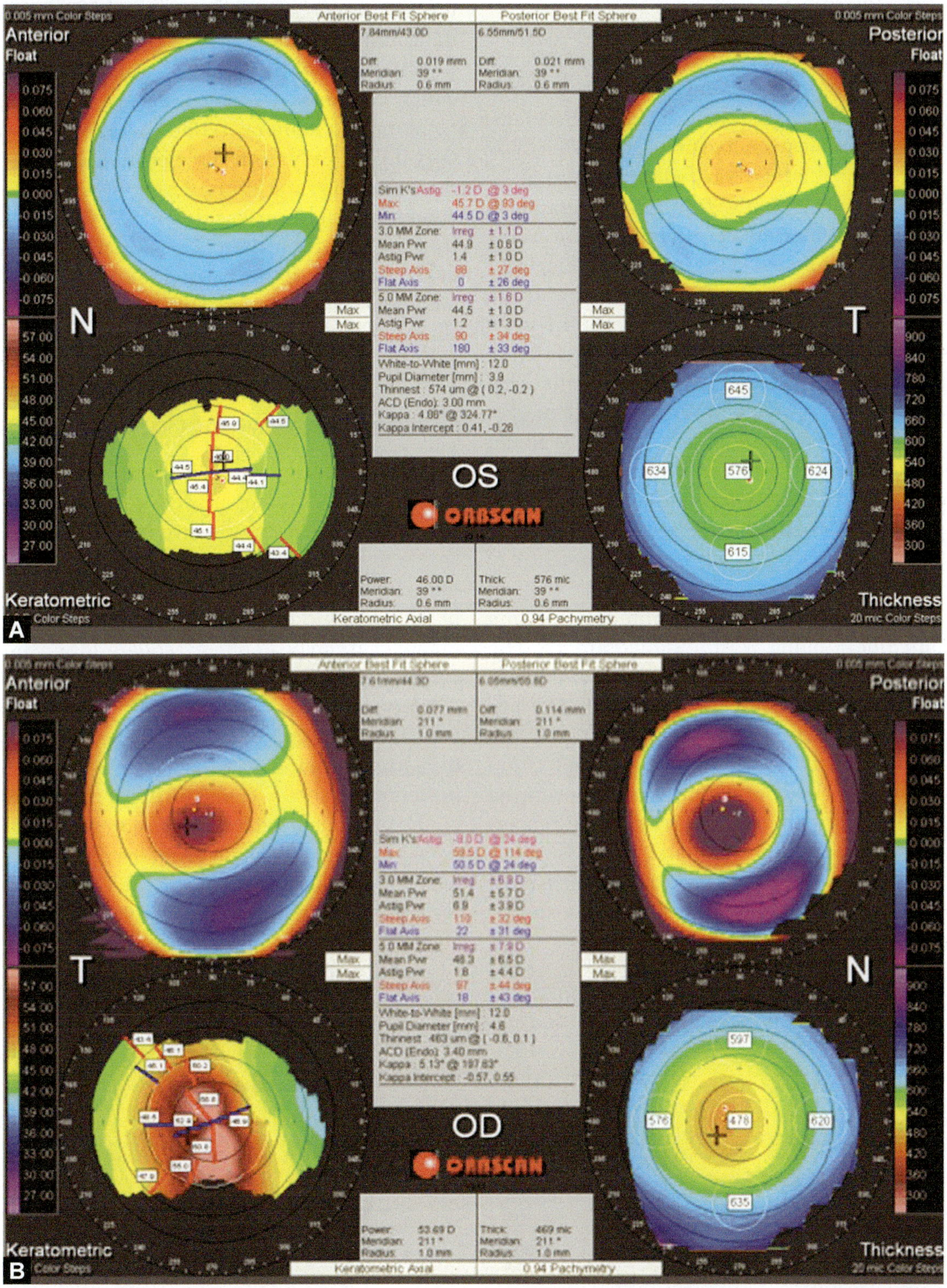

Figs. 17.8A and B: Orbscan printout showing quad map. (A) Normal cornea; (B) Keratoconic cornea. (Top left) anterior elevation, (Top right) posterior elevation, (Bottom left) Curvature/Keratometric map, (Bottom right) optical pachymetry. A few of the important differences to note are: (1) Posterior BFS: normal, 51.5D; Keratoconus (KCN), 55.8D; (2) Maximum posterior elevation: normal, 21 µm; keratoconus (KCN), 114 µm; (3) Irregularity index at 3 mm: normal, 1.1D; KCN, 6.9D; (4) Irregularity index at 5 mm: normal, 1.6D; KCN, 7.9 D; (5) Thinnest optical pachymetry: normal, 574 µm; KCN, 463 µm; (6) Skewing of the superior and inferior radial axis of astigmatism: normal, absent; KCN, significant skewing.

Scheimpflug Imaging

Scheimpflug imaging attains a wide depth of focus, providing information from the anterior corneal surface through to the posterior capsule of the crystalline lens. Theodor Scheimpflug, an Australian naval force officer, was a cartographer in the Austrian Navy who first introduced the Scheimpflug principle in the field of photography at the beginning of the 20th century.[10] Here the plane of the camera lens is placed sideways to the image. The imaginary extensions of the planes of the film, the lens and the focal plane are not parallel (Fig. 17.6B),[11] resulting in an increase in the region of focus as well as an increase in the sharpness of the image.[12-14] There are various commercial systems based on this principle available in the market like Pentacam (Oculus Optikgeräte GmbH, Wetzlar, Germany), Galilei (Ziemer, Port, Switzerland) and Sirius (CSO, Florence, Italy). These imaging modalities involve the acquisition of slices of the cornea by a rotating camera with each slice passing diametrically through the centre of the cornea (Fig. 17.9).

Oculus Pentacam (Fig. 17.10) combines a rotating scheimpflug camera along with a static camera. The rotating camera scans the cornea from 0° to 180° along with a monochromatic slit light source around the optical axis to acquire slit images. The static camera is placed in the center to record the contour of the pupil and act as fixation point. This keeps a check on the eye movements during the imaging process. Pentacam can take upto 50 slit images (up to 100,000 data points) in less than 2 seconds. These photographs are then reconstructed into three dimensional images (Fig. 17.11) to provide anterior and posterior corneal topographies along with several parameters which are generated by computer softwares.

The Galilei Dual Scheimpflug analyzer combines a Placido-disk and a dual rotating Scheimpflug system for obtaining anterior and posterior corneal topography data, the complete corneal pachymetry, and the lens densitometry. The Sirius is another bimodal device which combines a large cone placido-disk with a single Scheimpflug camera. While the Pentacam derives the curvature purely from the elevation data, the other two devices (Galilei and Sirius) derive the anterior curvature by combining data from Placido and Scheimpflug imaging. The readings from these devices are not strictly interchangeable as the technology for calculation of various data differs amongst different devices. The Scheimpflug scores over the slit-scanning devices due to better edge identification and reproducibility of data.[15-18]

Interpretation of Corneal Topography

Commonly the clinicians elucidate the elevation data not in its raw form but in comparison to some reference shape. The machine identifies the dimension of the selected reference shape that can best fit the examined cornea depending upon its individual characteristics. This is called the best fit reference surface (Fig. 17.12A) which is usually of 8 mm diameter. It can be a sphere, asphere, toric aspheroid or an ellipsoid with multiple options available and customizable in every device. The maps typically display how the actual elevation data compares or deviates from the this best fit reference shape. It is displayed for both anterior and posterior elevations. To make it easier to interpret, the maps on the printout are color coded representing the elevation data. Any points higher or lower in comparison to the best fit reference shape are represented by hot (red) or cool (blue) colors, respectively. The type of reference shape,

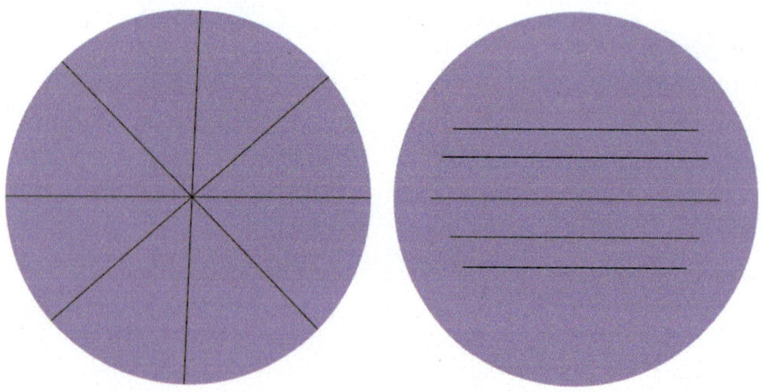

Fig. 17.9: Diagram of the Pentacam (left) and Orbscan (right) showing the radial imaging of the Pentacam and the parallel imaging of the Orbscan.

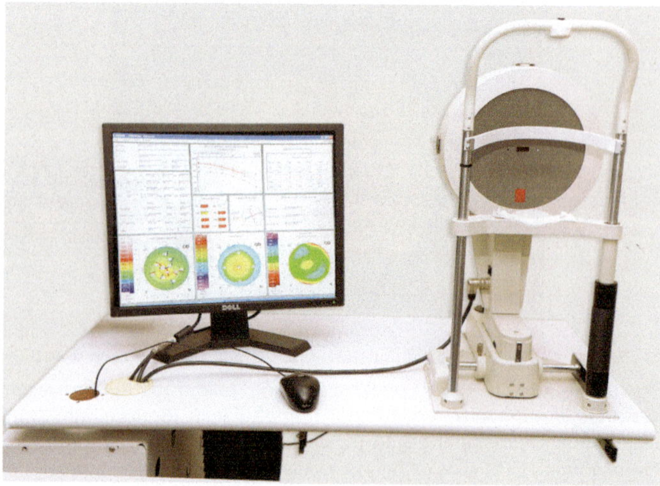

Fig. 17.10: Oculus Pentacam machine.

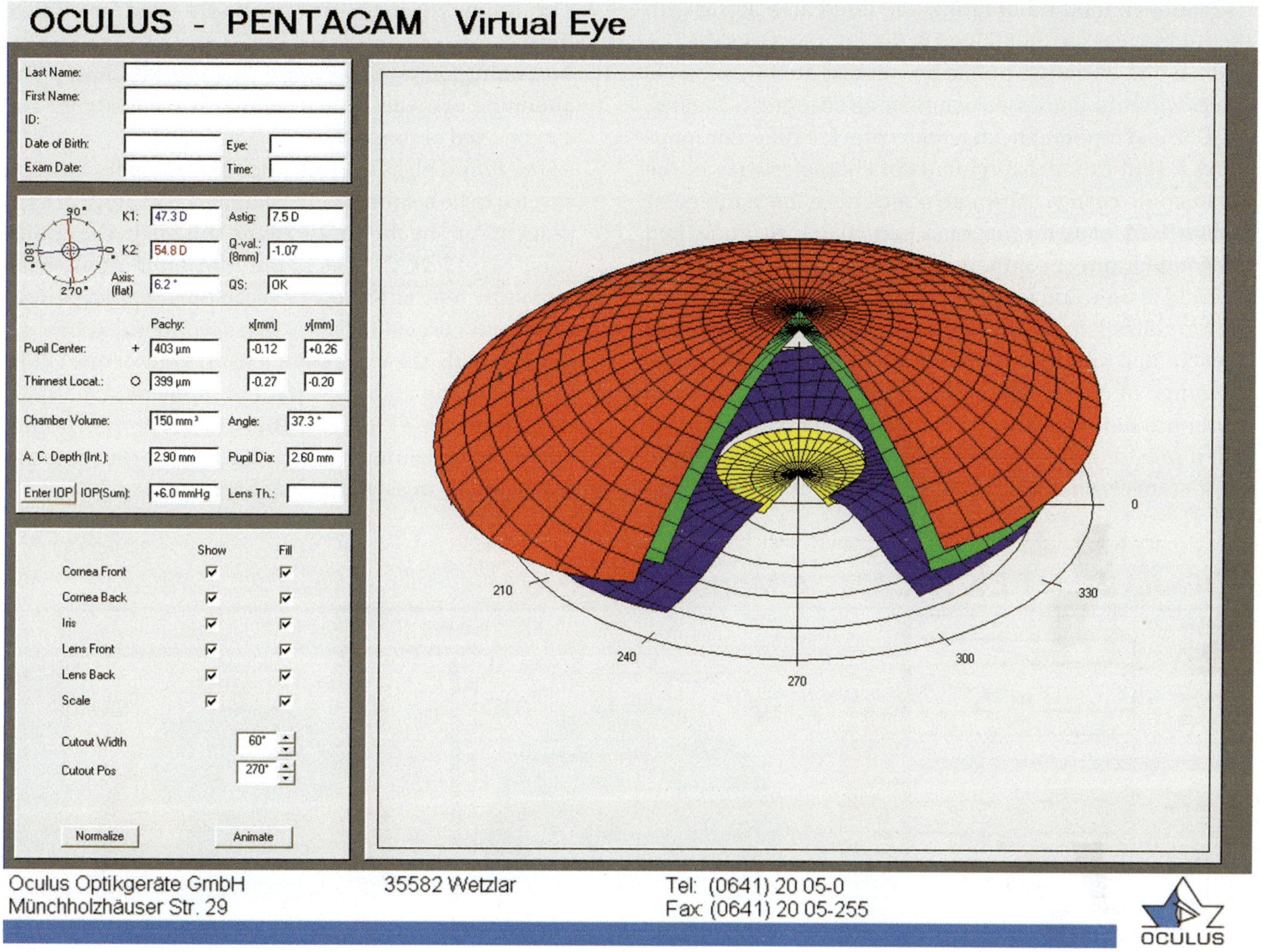

Fig. 17.11: Three-dimensional reconstruction of the anterior corneal surface (red), posterior corneal surface (green), iris (blue) and the lens (yellow).

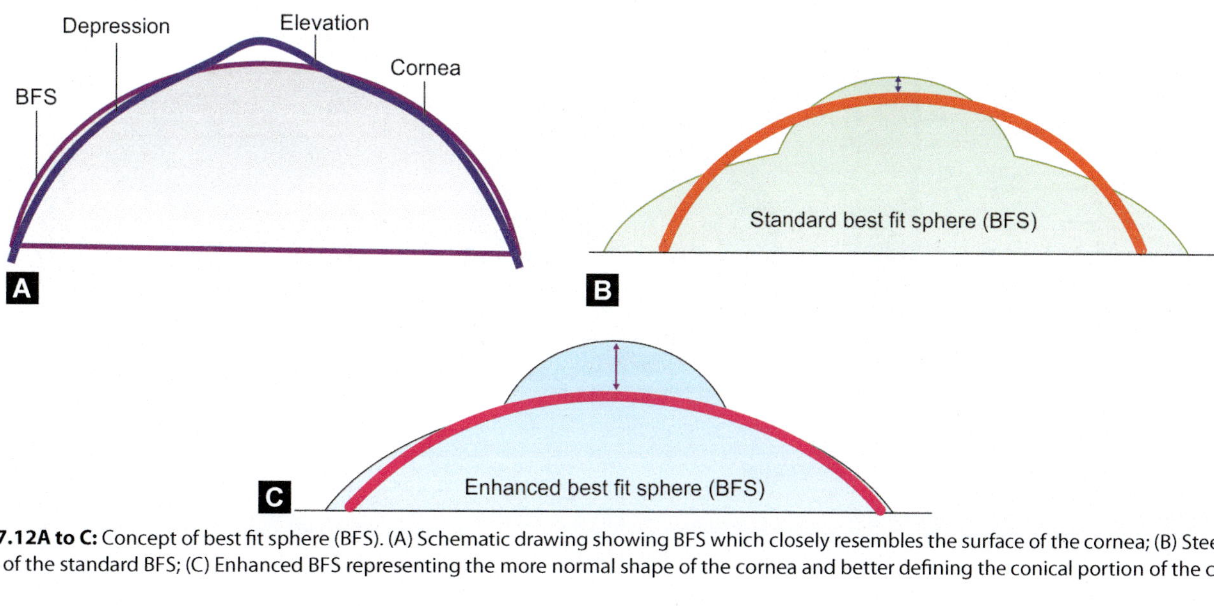

Figs. 17.12A to C: Concept of best fit sphere (BFS). (A) Schematic drawing showing BFS which closely resembles the surface of the cornea; (B) Steepening effect of the standard BFS; (C) Enhanced BFS representing the more normal shape of the cornea and better defining the conical portion of the cornea.

its diameter, method of fitting, the fitted area along with the color scales are mentioned in the printout (Figs. 17.13A and B). The elevation points are represented by plus (+) values while the depressed points are given minus (-) values.

Corneal topography machines provide different maps to represent the measurements of characteristics of the keratoconic cornea. Absolute scales have the same color coding fixed for all the maps in a particular instrument and are good for direct comparison of the different maps over a period of time and for population based studies. Relative or normalized steps have different color scales assigned to each map and the computer automatically distributes the range of colors depending upon the maximum and minimum diopters. The advantage of the relative scale is that it provides more topographic details as the steps are comparatively smaller.

The following maps are routinely used in clinical practice:

1. *Curvature/Keratometric map:* They provide information about the corneal surface curvature at each point and can be axial or tangential.
   Axial map (Figs. 17.13A and B) considers corneal surface to be a sphere and calculates curvature of each point assuming the center of the sphere on the optical axis (Fig. 17.14A). This is the most commonly used curvature map and shows typical topographic patterns of several corneal diseases like asymmetrical bow-tie pattern with skewed radial axis in keratoconus (Fig. 17.15A) or the crab-claw pattern in Pellucid marginal degeneration (Fig. 17.15B). However peripheral curvature measurement, and local or smaller changes can be easily missed in axial curvature map.

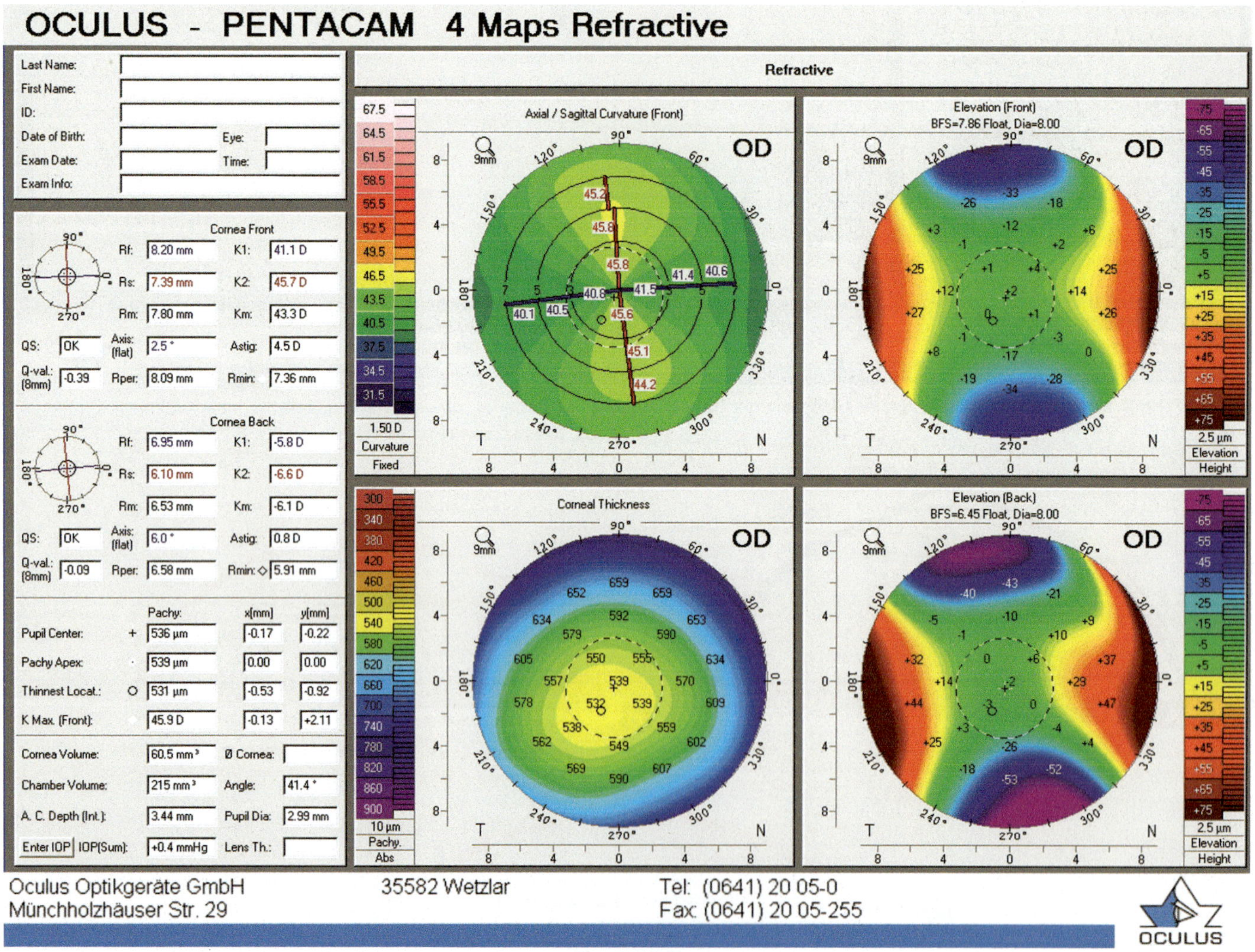

Fig. 17.13A

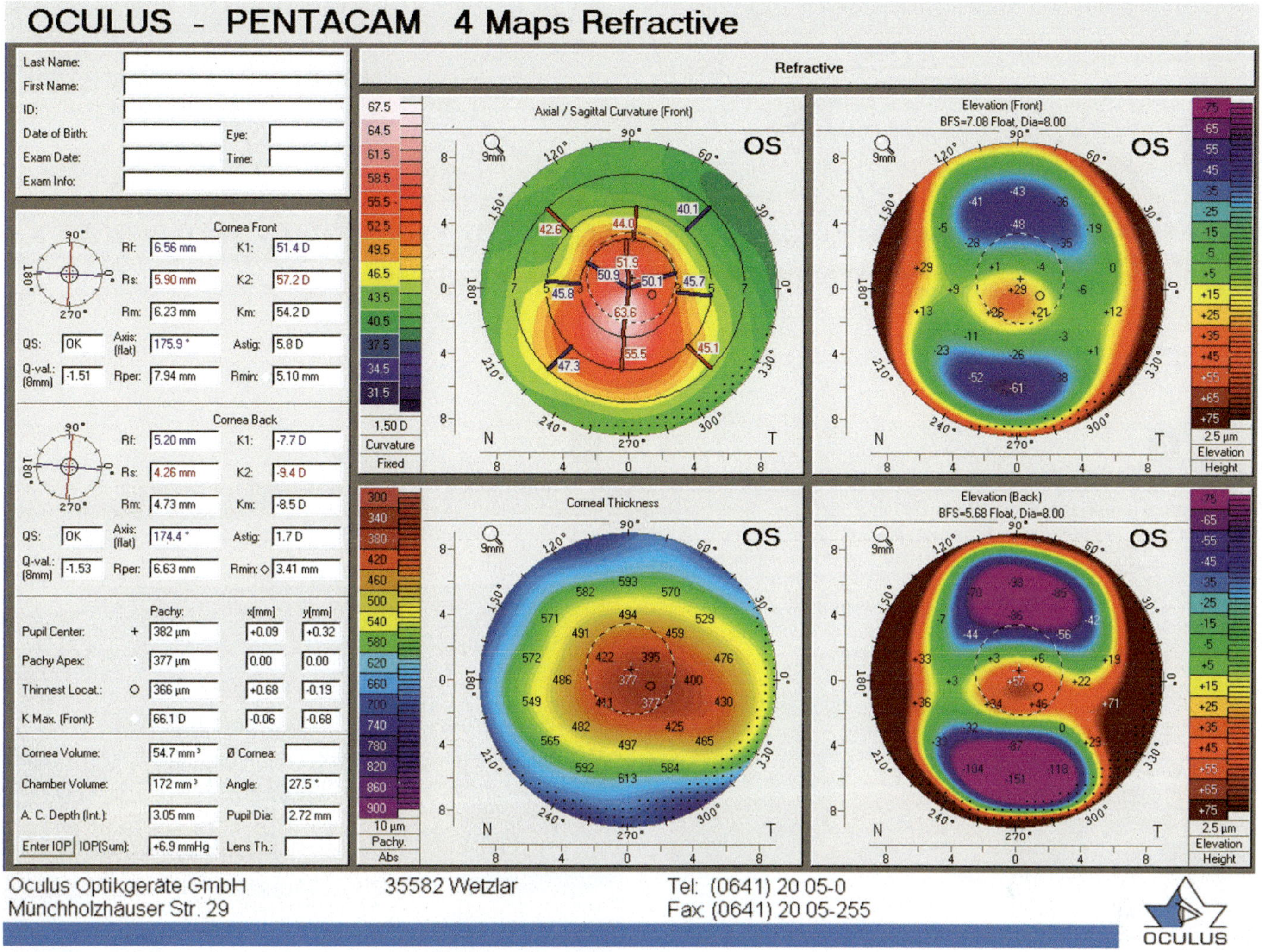

Fig. 17.13B

Figs. 17.13A and B: Pentacam topography refractive quad map. (A) Normal. Ks are less than 47.2 D, front elevation BFS max 4 mm zone (cut-off >12) and back elevation BFS max 4 mm zone (cut-off >22) are within normal range with thinnest point (TP) > 500 µm; (B) Keratoconus. Ks are more than 47.2 D, front and back elevation BFS max 4 mm zone are above the cut-off value with TP <500 µm. More importantly elevated points on the front and the back elevation maps corresponds to the highest power on axial curvature map and the thinnest point on the pachymetry map, i.e. the presence of four-point touch. (BFS: Best fit sphere)

Tangential map: It does not assume the spherical morphology of the corneal surface. Instead, it measures the curvature at a certain point on the corneal surface in a meridional direction relative to the other points on that particular ring (Fig. 17.14B). It can detect even localized changes in the corneal morphology and hence subjected to more variation. This implies that the same disease may not have same topographic pattern in tangential map.

2. *Elevation map:* These maps do not show the raw elevation data obtained by the corneal topography but the data in relation to the best fit corneal shape. It provides data separately for both anterior and posterior corneal surfaces (Figs. 17.8 and 17.13). Data from the posterior corneal surface is very useful for the early detection of keratoconus. A posterior best fit sphere (BFS) of greater than 54 D (*see* Fig. 17.8B) should arise suspicion even if the anterior BFS is within the normal range (41 to 46D).[19] The maximum posterior elevation (MPE) is the absolute magnitude in micrometers (µm) of the posterior corneal surface above the BFS. MPE more than 40 µm has been described as a diagnostic index for keratoconus (*see* Fig. 17.8B).[20,21]
3. *Thickness map (Figs. 17.8 and 17.13):* This map provides the thickness distribution of the cornea and is obtained from the reconstruction of the anterior and posterior

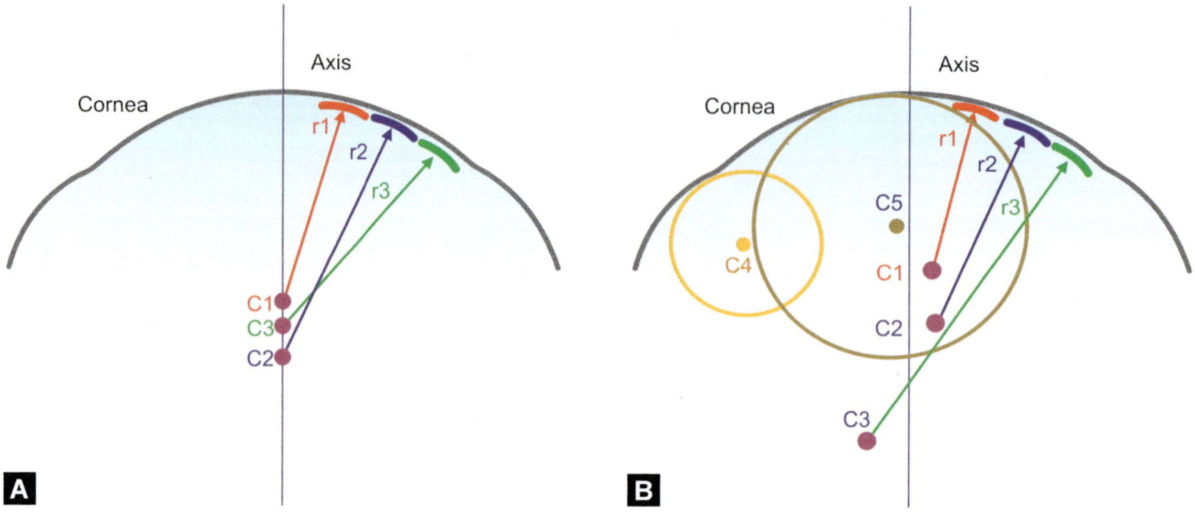

Figs. 17.14A and B: Geometric reconstruction of the corneal curvature map. (A) Axial map where the cornea is assumed as a sphere and the center of the curvature is fixed at the optical axis; (B) Tangential map where the cornea is not considered as a sphere and the corneal curvature is reconstructed by means of local curvature radii whose centers are not located on the optical axis.

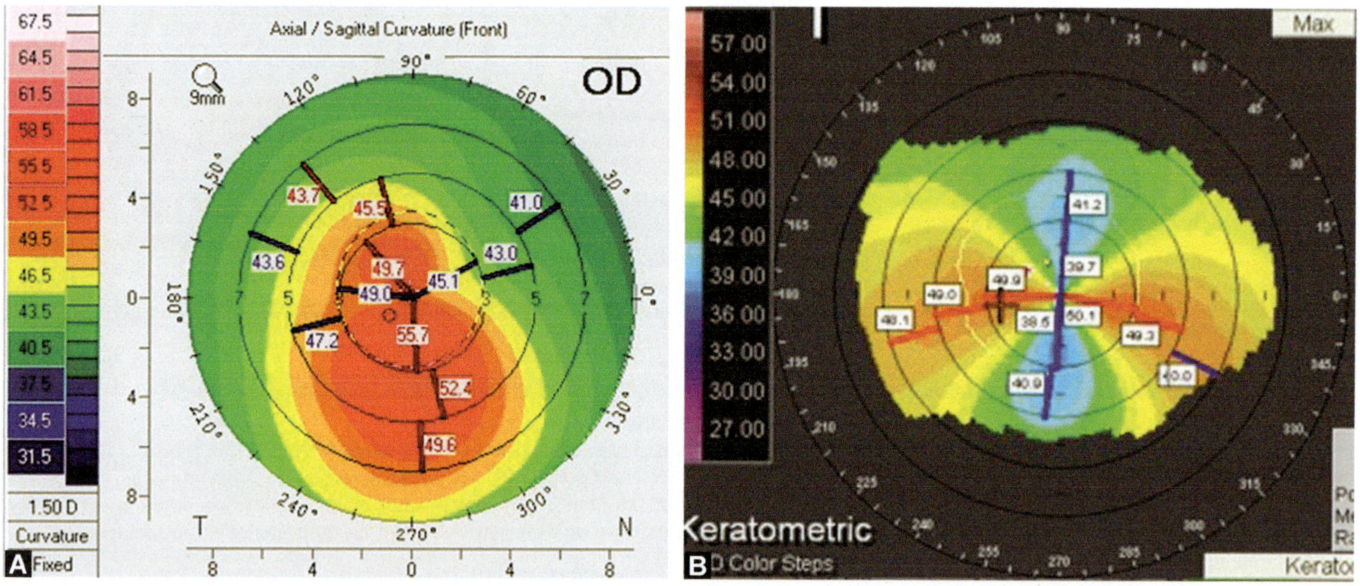

Figs. 17.15A and B: (A) Pentacam axial curvature map showing asymmetrical bow-tie pattern with skewed radial axis in keratoconus; (B) Orbscan axial curvature map showing the crab-claw pattern in Pellucid marginal degeneration.

corneal surfaces. It also provides information about the location of thinnest point (TP) and its position in comparison to the center of the cornea. If the area of thinning correlates with the area of steepening, then it assumes even greater significance in detecting ectatic corneal disorders. Serial measurements can be used to estimate the progression of keratoconus. Thickness less than 500 µm in the presence of other topographical asymmetry is commonly used as one of the diagnostic criteria for subclinical keratoconus.[22] Additional criteria like minimal thickness less than 460 µm or decentration of this point by more than 500 µm from the center or difference between the apical thickness and the minimal thickness more than 27 µm has been correlated with high probability of corneal ectasia (Fig. 17.16).[23] Also difference of more than 100 µm between the apex and the thickness at 7 mm ring is considered an additional point for suspecting ectasia. Several studies have shown Orbscan provides central corneal thickness (CCT) values higher than the

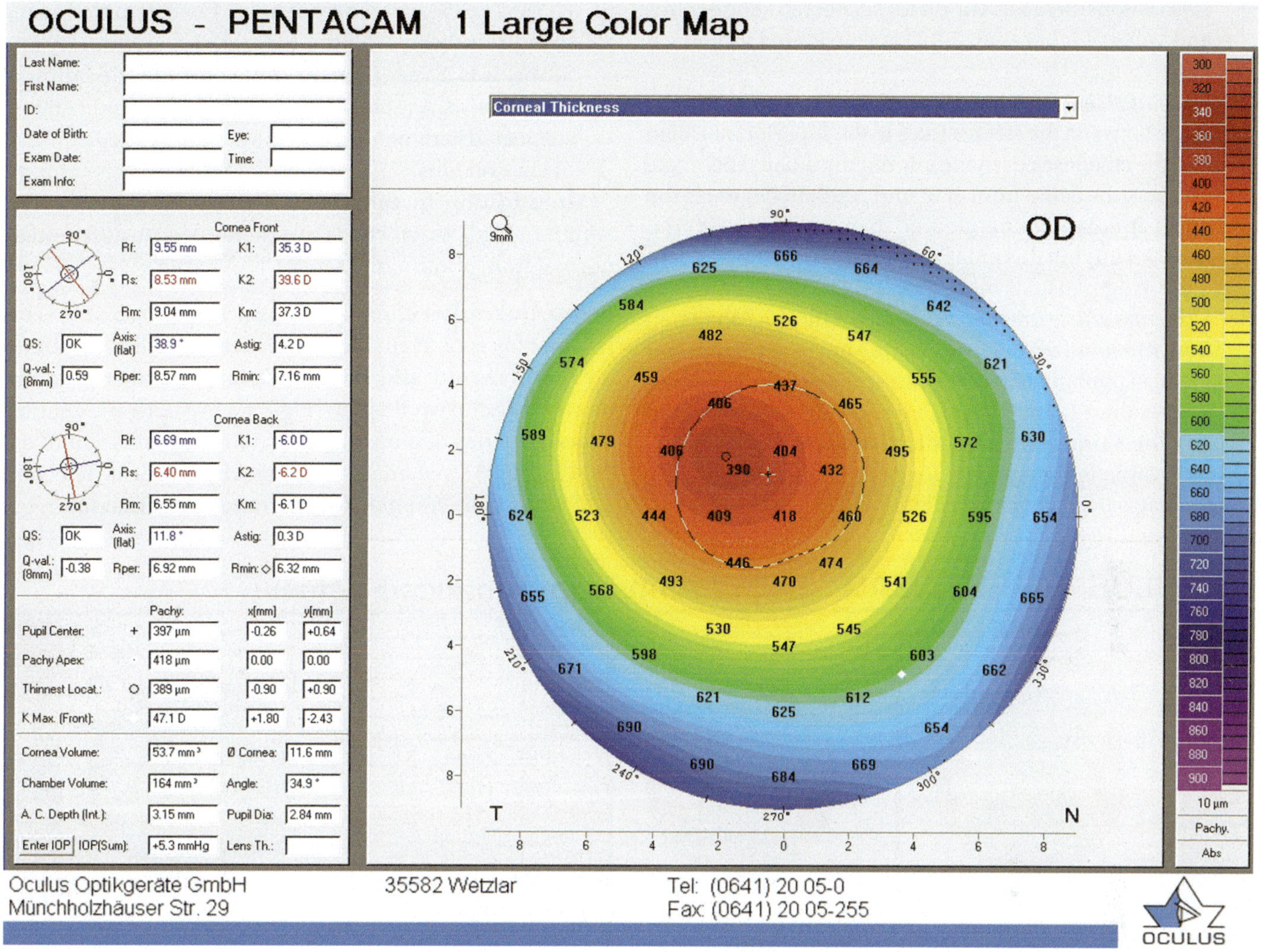

Fig. 17.16: Corneal thickness Pentacam map of post-LASIK ectasia. Minimal thickness is 389 μm, difference between the thickness at apex and the thinnest point is 29 μm and the thinnest point is decentered by 900 μm both horizontally and vertically.

ultrasound (USG) pachymeter[17,24-29] whereas Pentacam provides lower values compared to USG.[30,31] This difference becomes even more prominent in advanced keratoconus.[30] Orbscan manufacturers have provided a linear acoustic factor of 0.92 to compensate for overestimation of central pachymetry.

Statistical Indices

The following are the commonly used indices in corneal topography.

1. *Simulated keratometry (SimK):* This denotes the dioptric power derived from the corneal topography of the flattest and steepest meridians at four cardinal points 3–4 mm apart, akin to the keratometry mires on the cornea. It is represented by K1 and K2 and the difference between the two will denote the corneal astigmatism. A clinical study showed SimK mean values of 43.53 ± 1.02 D for normal corneas, and established a cut-off value for keratoconus group as twice the value of the standard deviation of the control group.[32,33]
2. *Central keratometry (Central K):* It is the average value of corneal power for the rings with diameters of 2, 3 and 4 mm. Values below 47.2 D are considered normal and values between 47.2 D and 48.7 D are considered probable keratoconus. Values above 48.7 D are clinical keratoconus.[32,34]
3. *Inferior-superior asymmetry (I-S asymmetry):* It denotes the power difference between the inferior meridian and the superior meridian, at a 3-mm zone from the centre at 30° interval. Values between 1.4 D and

1.8 D is considered as cut-off for suspected keratoconus and values higher than 1.8 D is considered as clinical keratoconus.[34,35]

4. *Skew of steepest radial axis (SRAX):* It represents the angle between the steepest axis in the superior meridian and the steepest axis in the inferior meridian. This angle is then subtracted from 180° and result in degree is the SRAX index. A value greater than 20° is considered keratoconus but this index is only considered significant if the astigmatism is more than 1.5 D.[36]
5. *Orbscan surface irregularity:* It is a coefficient calculated from the standard deviations of the mean curvature and mean astigmatism in the 3 mm and 5 mm zone. Values greater than 1.5 in 3 mm zone and values greater than 2 in the 5 mm zone are indicative of high irregularity. This value is not specific for keratoconus but merely indicates irregularity (*see* Fig. 17.8B).[36]
6. *KISA %:* KISA is an acronym and is calculated using the four indices—Central K, SimK, I-S asymmetry and SRAX. It is a very effective index for identification of keratoconus. A value between 60 and 100 is indicative of suspected keratoconus and more than 100 is diagnostic of keratoconus.[37]

In addition to the above, Pentacam provides few additional indices which are commonly used to differentiate normal from abnormal corneas.

Belin/Ambrósio-enhanced ectasia display (BAD): This is a display tool available in Pentacam, which combines elevation based and pachymetric corneal evaluation in an all-inclusive display (Figs. 17.17A and B). Clinical experience has demonstrated that the combination of the data in the BAD enhances the sensitivity of ectasia detection and is a useful screening tool for refractive surgeons.[38,39]

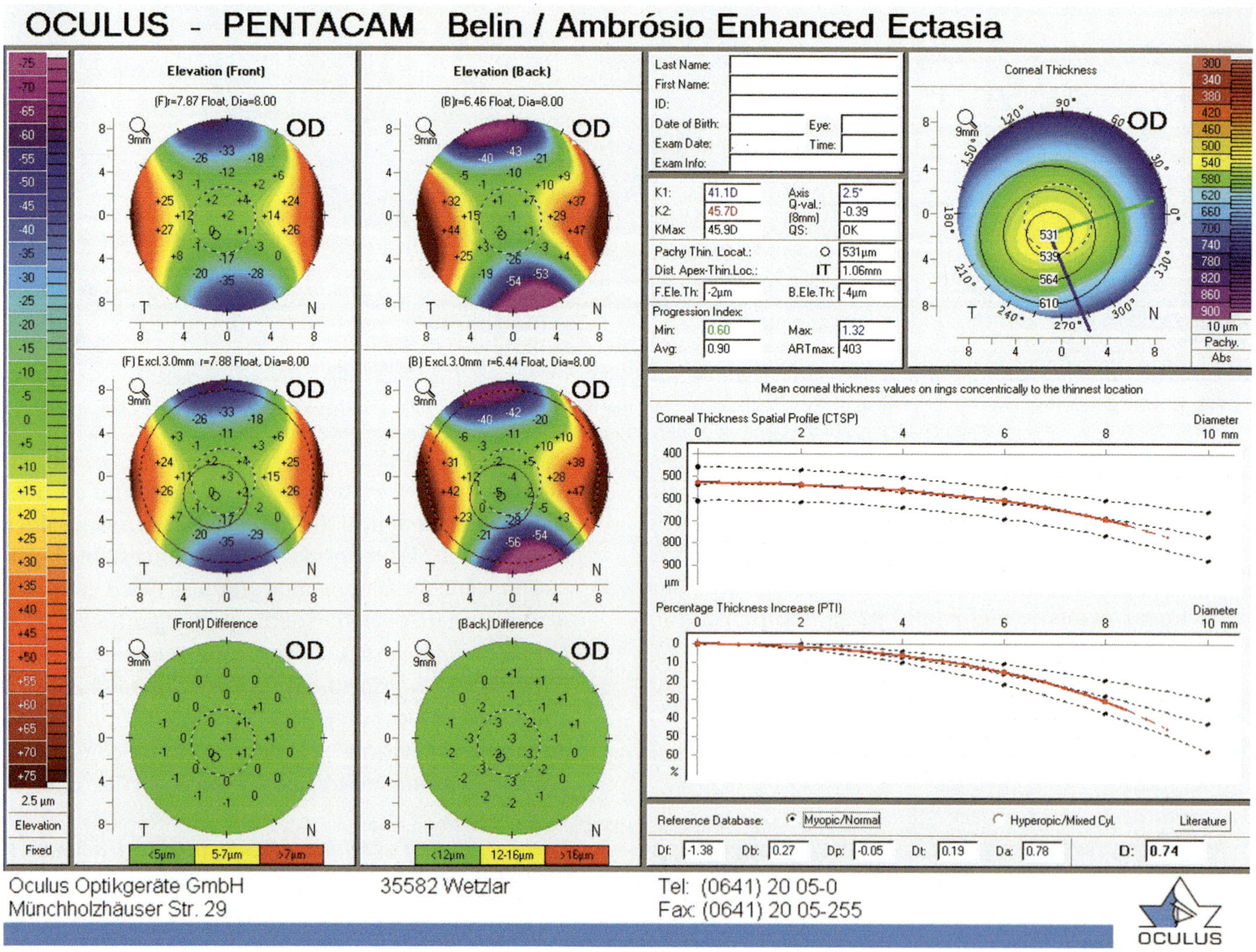

Fig. 17.17A

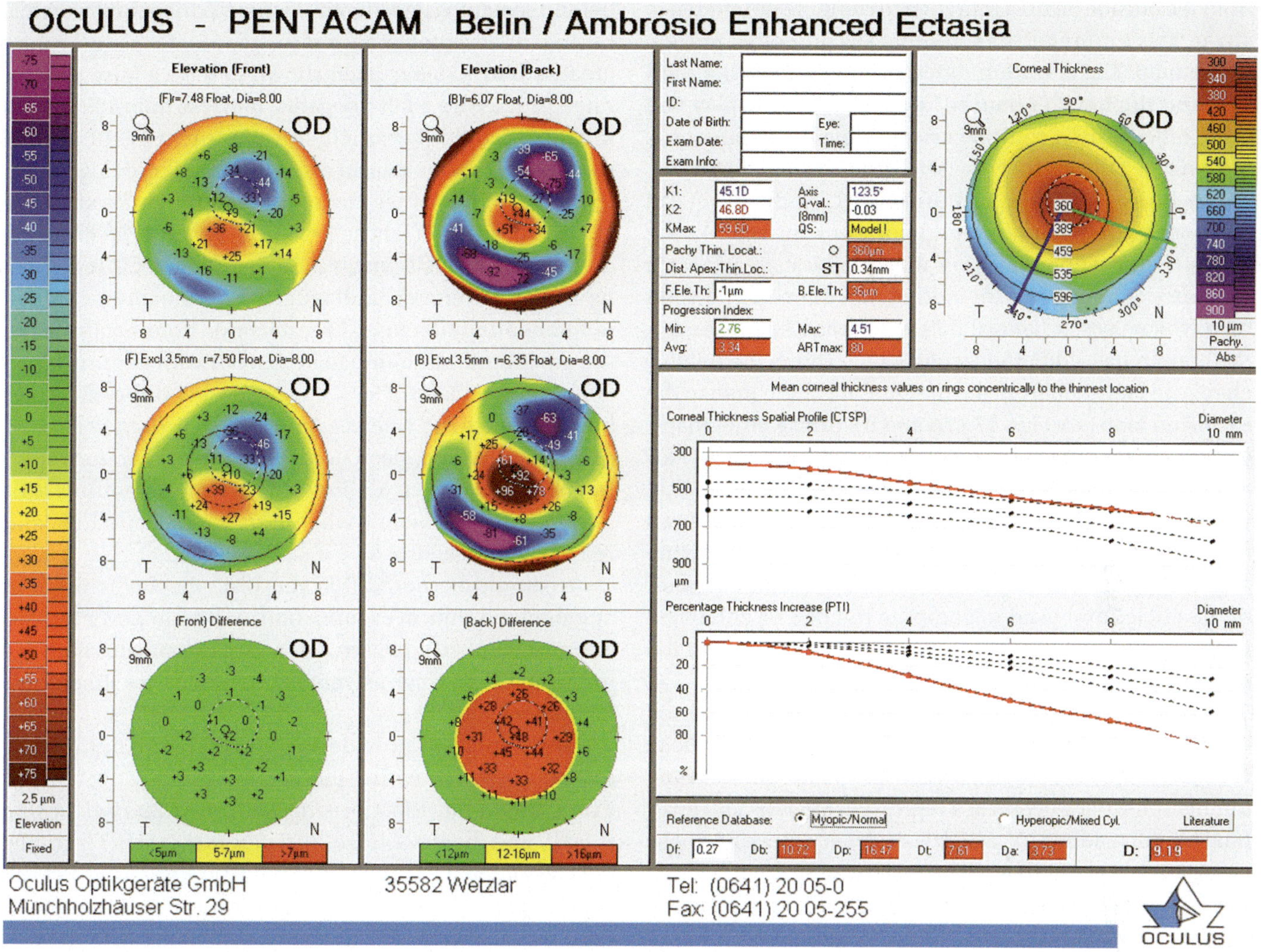

Fig. 17.17B

Figs. 17.17A and B: Belin/Ambrósio-enhanced ectasia display (BAD) in Pentacam. (A) In normal corneas elevation difference between a standard BFS and the new "enhanced" BFS elevation display is minimal; (B) In ectasia, this difference becomes significant as shown by the presence of red color in the difference map of the posterior elevation.

In BAD, elevation and pachymetry maps are placed side by side complementing each other in providing quick and effective screening of patients for suspected ectatic disease. Elevation maps are always viewed in reference to some standard shapes and hence raw elevation data as such lacks enough surface variability to differentiate between normal and abnormal corneas. Elevation maps when displayed after subtracting the reference shape from the raw elevation data highlights the deviation or differences between the normal and the abnormal corneas. The reference shapes commonly employed are best fit sphere (BFS) or best fit toric ellipsoid (BFTE). BFS as a reference shape gives the most useful qualitative map for the majority of the clinical situations and refractive surgery screening. Toric ellipsoid shape more closely resembles a cone and therefore will actually mask the cone.

While the BFS is quantitatively useful, in the cases of keratoconus or ectasia, the conical or apical protrusion of the cornea will have steepening effect on the BFS (*see* Fig. 17.12B). This will actually minimize the difference between the cone and the BFS. What we really expect from the reference shape is to represent the more normal shape of the individual's cornea. This would have the effect of better defining or exaggerating the ectatic regions of the cornea as in the case of enhanced BFS (*see* Fig. 17.12C).

To do this, Pentacam has been equipped with a new enhanced BFS. It basically excludes the 4 mm zone centered on the thinnest portion of the cornea and utilizes only data from the outside of this 4 mm zone to compute the reference shape. This 4 mm zone is represented by the dotted red line in the map. The elevation difference between a standard BFS and the new "enhanced" BFS elevation display will be significant for a conical cornea, while the difference is minimal in a normal cornea (*see* Figs. 17.17A and B).

In BAD, elevation is represented by three sets of maps for both the anterior and posterior surface. On the top is the baseline elevation map which uses BFS as a reference shape, while the mid region has the exclusion map which uses enhanced BFS as reference shape and in the bottom has a difference map which shows the relative change in elevation from the baseline elevation map to the exclusion map (*see* Figs. 17.17A and B). Unlike other maps, difference map uses only 3 colors (green, yellow, red) for representation of elevation data. Green represents normal eyes whereas yellow represents suspicious eyes and red represents keratoconic eyes. On the top of the baseline and exclusion map, radius of curvature (r) and diameter of the circle (dia) used to compute the BFS or enhanced BFS is mentioned. Float represents the positioning of the reference surface relative to the corneal surface.

Multiple tomographic parameters when combined together have shown increased sensitivity and specificity compared with any single parameter.[40-42] BAD III uses nine tomographic parameters in a regression analysis and gives final overall reading "D" which is designed to identify those preoperative maps that differ significantly from normal (*see* Figs. 17.17A and B).[43] The nine parameters used in the regression analysis are:

1. *Df*: This represents the change in anterior (front) elevation between two different reference surfaces.
2. *Db*: Change in posterior (back) elevation between two different reference surfaces.
3. Anterior elevation at the thinnest point.
4. Posterior elevation at the thinnest point.
5. *Dp*: Represents the rate of change in corneal thickness from the thinnest point to the periphery (progression index).
6. *Dt*: Corneal thickness at the thinnest point.
7. *Dy*: Vertical displacement of the thinnest point.
8. K_{max}: Maximal simulated keratometry.
9. ART_{max}: Corneal thickness at the thinnest point divided by the maximal progression index.

Each parameter is reported as a standard deviation based on comparison with a large published normative database.[43] D value is primarily used for refractive screening where identifying abnormal map is critical.[43] The goal behind screening is to identify as many patients at risk, while having an acceptable false positive rate. Final "D" values greater than 1.88 has been shown to have a false positive rate of 2.5% with a false negative rate less than 1%[26] which means it would potentially misidentify 2.5% of normal candidates as abnormal in exchange for identifying greater than 99% of the cones correctly.[44] Muftuoglu et al. found that the best cutoff for the D was 2.1, with 100% sensitivity and 100% specificity suggesting that the new D index can be a sole parameter in diagnosing keratoconus.[45] When differentiating subclinical keratoconus from healthy eyes, the best cutoff was found to be 1.3, but with a sensitivity of 60% and specificity of 90%, suggesting good specificity but limited sensitivity[45] whereas Ambrósio et al. suggested a cut-off point of 1.45 for detection of subclinical keratoconus.[46] In the Pentacam as defined by the manufacturer, this parameter turns yellow when D value exceeds 1.65, and red when it exceeds 2.6.

It should be noted that the BAD display is there to augment the clinical examination and it can never replace a clinician's own judgment. BAD display evaluates each eye individually, and high asymmetry between eyes should also raise suspicion.[47,48]

The Pentacam provides a detailed corneal thickness distribution map with 3 μm accuracy and repeatability. From this data, the *Corneal Thickness Spatial Profile (CTSP)* and the *Percentage Thickness Increase (PTI)* graphs are calculated. On the Belin/Ambrósio Enhanced Ectasia Display page, the pachymetry portion is displayed on the right which includes pachymetry map along with the two graphs (CTSP and PTI) and the various indices (*see* Figs. 17.17A and B). It displays the corneal thickness at the apex and thinnest point (TP) and their location and distance of the TP from the apex (*see* Figs. 17.17A and B). The direction of the TP is displayed as temporal (T), nasal (N), superior (S) and inferior (I) or intermediate [e.g. inferotemporal (IT)]. In 87.6% of the normal eyes the distance between the apex and thinnest point is less than 10 μm.[49] There is also a significant correlation between the distance difference and the pachymetry difference between these points.[38,50] The distance between the thinnest point (TP) and the apex (CCT) is significantly higher in keratoconus (0.98 ± 0.38 mm) than normals (0.74 ± 0.35 mm) ($p < 0.0001$).[49] TP is a statistically better index to diagnose keratoconus than CCT ($p < 0.0001$).[49]

The CTSP displays the average thickness of the cornea along the 22 concentric circles with a center at the thinnest point with increasing diameters of 0.4 mm.

In addition to the average values, the standard deviations of the pachymetry along each circle are also calculated. The second graph showing PTI is calculated using a simple formula: (CT@x – TP)/TP, where CT represents corneal thickness at a particular point *x* and *x* represents the diameter of the imaginary circle centered on the TP with increasing diameters as provided by the CTSP. The Pentacam reports CTSP and PTI of the examined cornea as red color in graphs along with the data of the mean and two standard deviations of a normal population as broken dark lines (Fig. 17.18).

Keratoconus has much higher rate of increase in thickness toward the periphery and therefore has a faster and more abrupt increase of the CTSP and PTI than normal corneas (Fig. 17.18).[51] The CTSP and PTI graphs were designed to provide at a glance identification of very early forms of ectasia, thereby further helping in screening candidates for refractive surgery.

The arithmetic average of thickness on the 1 mm, 2 mm, 3 mm, 4 mm and 5 mm diameter rings is represented as the average *pachymetric progression index (PPI ave)*. The pachymetric progression indexes (PPI) are calculated for all hemi-meridian 360 degrees, starting from the thinnest point. The meridians with maximal (PPI Max) and minimal (PPI Min) pachymetric increase are noted along with their axes. PPI ave has a statistical significance when comparing normal patients (0.87 ± 0.21 mm) to those with keratoconus (2.42 ± 1.74 mm) (p <0.0001).[49] The cutoff values for PPI Ave, PPI Max, PPI Min are 1.06 mm, 1.44 mm, 0.79 mm respectively for differentiating normal from keratoconic

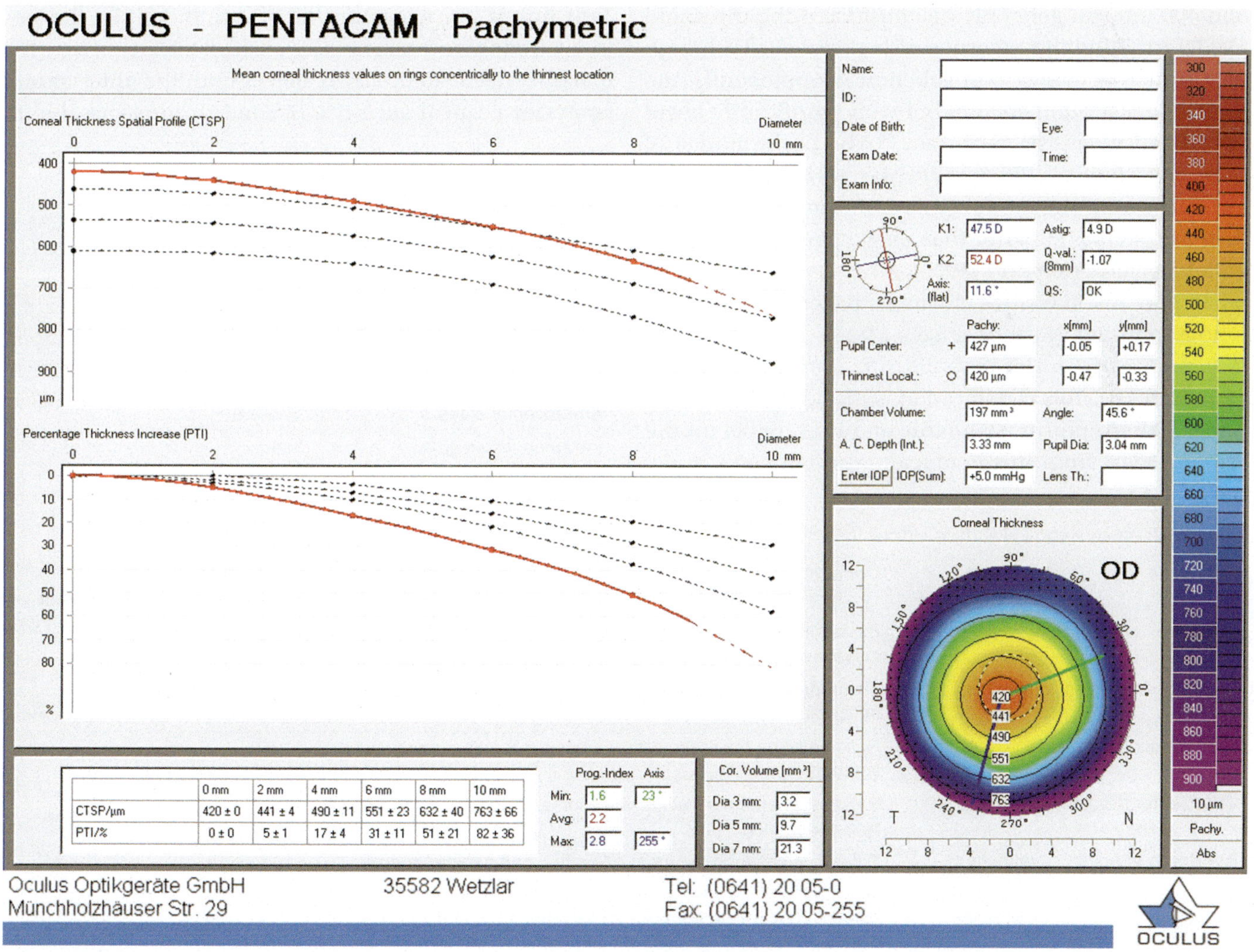

Fig. 17.18: Pentacam pachymetry map showing corneal thickness spatial profile (CTSP), percentage thickness increase (PTI), pachymetric progression index (PPI). CTSP and PTI of the patient are represented by broken red line in the graph which in case of keratoconus is outside the normal limit.

eyes.[49] Normal corneas typically have an average progression index lower than 1.2 and a CTSP and PTI lines within the 95% CI limits. The pachymetric index will be higher if the cornea gets thicker in a more accentuated pattern from the thinnest point out to the periphery as in the case of keratoconus where the PTI and CTSP graphs also falls down (*see* Fig. 17.18).

Ambrósio's relational thickness (ART) refers to the relational thickness of the TP with PPI Ave (ART Ave) and with PPI Max (ART Max) (*see* Figs. 17.17A and B). ART Ave and ART Max are among the best parameters for detecting ectasia with cutoffs of 424 μm and 339 μm, respectively.[49] ART Avg had 4.5% false negatives and 4.5% false positives, and ART Max had 0 false negatives and 4.4% false positives. ART Max offers greater diagnostic ability than ART Ave.[45,49,52-55] Although there is a variability between studies about the cut-off values, a value between 300 μm and 400 μm can generally be considered the threshold for determining the presence of keratoconus with high precision.[56] In contrast, in subclinical keratoconus, the threshold is around 400 μm but with significantly lower associated diagnostic accuracy.[56] The performance of these novel indices (PPI Avg, PPI Max, ART Ave, ART Max) for differentiating keratoconus from normal eyes was demonstrated as superior than single point pachymetric parameters like CCT and TP.[49]

Pentacam classifies corneas based on anterior topography into various stages (Table 17.1) called as *topographical keratoconus classification* (TKC) (Figs. 17.19A and B). This classification is the adaptation of the Amsler-Muckenhirn[57] standards and is available on the screen. Apart from this Pentacam also indicates if any corneal surgery has been done before or the maps are grossly abnormal. In some cases, intermediate stages (e.g. 1–2) are displayed when there is an overlap of minimum radius of curvature (R_{min}).

Pentacam software offers seven anterior corneal surface indices (Table 17.2 and Fig. 17.19) which are calculated according to an undisclosed formula that are yet to be validated in large series. This software compares the measured values with the means and standard deviations of a normal population, and provides color-coded flags. Measured values are highlighted as yellow color when it exceeds standard deviation by a factor of 2.5 and as red when it exceeds the standard deviation by a factor of 3.

Advantages and Disadvantages of Pentacam and Orbscan

Two things are necessary for the tomography devices to accurately reconstruct the corneal surface. First, the machine needs to precisely detect both the anterior and posterior corneal surfaces. Second, it must be able to

Table 17.1: Topographical Keratoconus Classification (TKC).

Topographical Keratoconus Classification	Minimum radius of curvature (R_{min}) in mm
Normal	> 7.8
Keratoconus suspect	7.8–6.7
Keratoconus stage 1	7.5– 6.5
Keratoconus stage 2	6.9–5.3
Keratoconus stage 3	6.6–4.8
Keratoconus stage 4	< 5

Table 17.2: Anterior corneal surface indices in Pentacam.

Index	Definition	Abnormal values from manufacturer's user manual
ISV (Index of surface variance)	Deviation of individual corneal sagittal radii from the mean curvature	>37
IVA (Index of vertical asymmetry)	The degree of symmetry of the corneal radii with respect to the horizontal meridian	>0.28 (mm)
KI (Keratoconus Index)	Ratio between the mean radius values in the upper and lower segment	>1.07
CKI (Center Keratoconus Index)	Ratio between mean radius values in a peripheral ring divided by a central ring	>1.03
IHA (Index of height asymmetry)	Difference between the mean elevation of the superior and inferior cornea	>19 (μm)
IHD (Index of height decentration)	The value of the decentration of elevation data in the vertical direction	>0.014 (μm)
R_{min} (minimum radius of curvature)	Smallest radius of sagittal corneal curvature	<6.71 (mm)

register each optical slice against the others. Pentacam accurately measures both the anterior and posterior corneal surfaces pre- and post-operatively.[58] Its ability to perform this measurement does not appear to be affected by previous surgery, haze, or superficial scarring. The Orbscan fails to correctly identify the postoperative posterior corneal surface and routinely locates the surface too anteriorly. As a result, its pachymetry reading is too thin, and its topography suggests ectasia in post-Lasik eyes which might give a false belief that change like this is a commonplace after Lasik.[15,17,18,59]

The rotating imaging technique of the Pentacam has inherent advantages as each optical cross section shares a common point (center of rotation), which makes image registration easier and more reliable. Serial slices used by the Orbscan does not share a common data point and hence image reconstruction is difficult and less reliable (*see* Fig. 17.9).

The addition of the placido-disk imaging to augment the Orbscan's elevation system was necessary because of the difficulty of achieving proper image registration. Normally, if the elevation data were accurate, there would be no need for a supplementary placido image, because curvature is simply the second derivative of elevation. Unfortunately, the placido image in the Orbscan does not identify or measure the posterior corneal surface.

Ultimately, it is the accuracy of the raw elevation data that will determine not only the diagnostic ability but also potential clinical therapeutic applications. Changes on the posterior corneal surface are critical and are often the first indicators for future ectatic disease, even when the anterior curvature is completely normal.

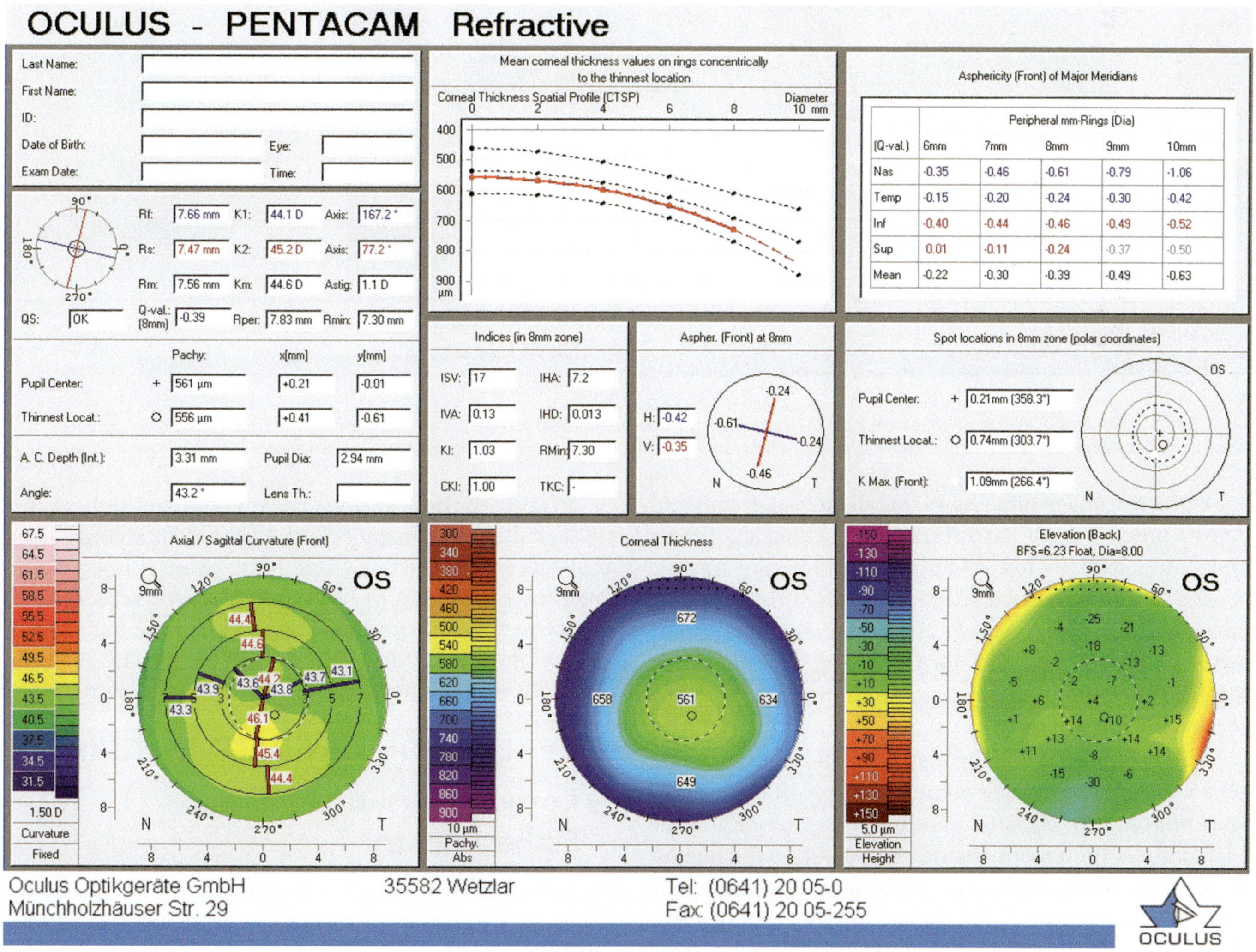

Fig. 17.19A

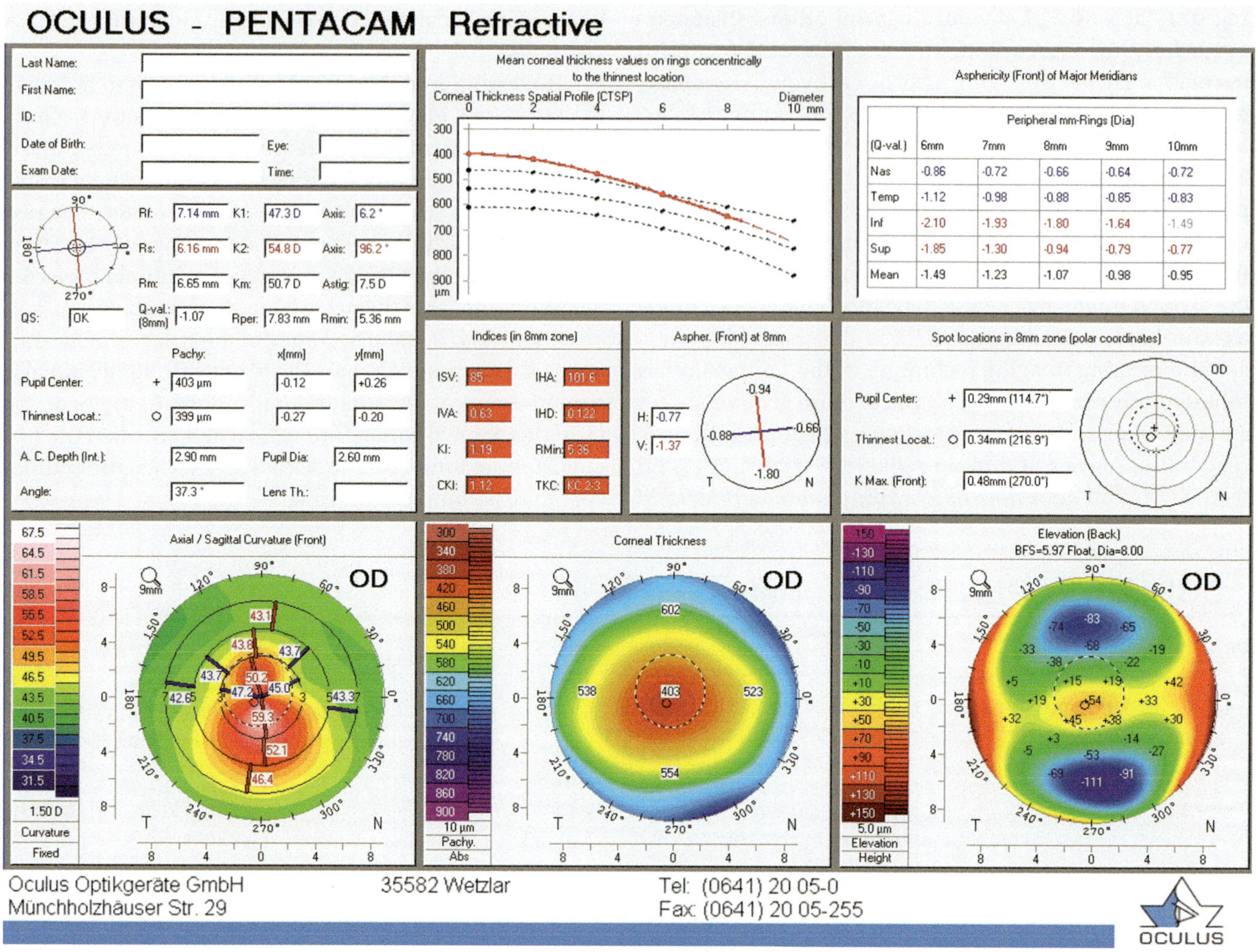

(Q-val.)	6mm	7mm	8mm	9mm	10mm
Nas	-0.86	-0.72	-0.66	-0.64	-0.72
Temp	-1.12	-0.98	-0.88	-0.85	-0.83
Inf	-2.10	-1.93	-1.80	-1.64	-1.49
Sup	-1.85	-1.30	-0.94	-0.79	-0.77
Mean	-1.49	-1.23	-1.07	-0.98	-0.95

Fig. 17.19B

Figs. 17.19A and B: Pentacam refractive map. (A) Normal. All the anterior corneal surface indices are within normal limits and topographical keratoconus classification (TKC) is not indicating ectasia; (B) Keratoconus. Anterior corneal indices and TKC are marked red as in the case of keratoconus.

Pentacam on the other hand over diagnose keratoconus many a times because of the built-in screening algorithms and could lead to the rejection of otherwise normal candidate for refractive surgery. Corneal thickness as measured in preoperative eyes by pentacam is commonly less as compared to USG pachymetry and Orbscan which can lead to conflicting information on minimal residual corneal thickness.

The readings from all the maps should be correlated to get a comprehensive idea about the shape of the cornea. Most importantly, elevated points on the anterior and the posterior elevation maps should correspond to the highest power on axial curvature map and the thinnest point on the pachymetry map to be considered significant. If all the above match, it is called as the *"four point touch"* and is a hallmark of a suspected corneal ectasia (*see* Figs. 17.8B and 17.13B).

In spite of these various parameters and indices it is still a challenge to diagnose very early ectatic changes such as subtle forme fruste keratoconus. There is not a single machine which can be fully relied on for screening of refractive surgical candidate. Every machine has its own limitations and the clinicians should be fully aware to the extent these machines can be relied upon.

EVALUATION OF CORNEAL SURFACE

Corneal Sensation Testing/ Esthesiometry

Esthesiometry is a measurement of corneal sensation which is a function of the ophthalmic branch of fifth cranial nerve. Corneal epithelium depends upon normal corneal sensation for maintenance of its healthy surface.

In conditions like viral keratitis, post refractive surgery, tumors like acoustic neuroma, Hansen's disease, chronic nonsteroidal anti-inflammatory drug (NSAID) usage, drug abuse (cocaine) corneal sensation may get affected. Reduced corneal sensations typically presents with an interpalpebral punctate corneal erosions which eventually progresses to epithelial defects if left untreated and causes neurotrophic ulcer. In a clinical practice the most important usage of corneal sensation testing is in making the diagnosis of herpes simplex keratitis.

Qualitative or Quantitative assessment of corneal sensation can be done by various methods:

Qualitative Measurement

The easiest and the widely used method of testing corneal sensation employ a cotton tipped swab. A wisp from the cotton tip is used to compare the sensation in each eye. Topical anesthetic drops should not be used before the testing. Proper care should be taken to bring the wisp of cotton from the sides to avoid frightening the patient. Response is noted by comparing the blink reflex and the patient's response between the two eyes. Sometimes it is helpful to ask the patient about the differences in the sensation felt. Ideally the testing should be done in all the four quadrants and recorded as normal, reduced or absent. It may be required to do the testing multiple times to arrive at a conclusion.

Quantitative Measurement

There are various ways to measure the corneal sensation quantitatively.

Cochet-Bonnet esthesiometer is a device with a 6 cm long adjustable nylon monofilament (Fig. 17.20). The tip of the nylon is brought on corneal surface perpendicularly and the response noted for each quadrant and recorded. Persons with normal corneal sensation will sense touch at 6 cm length. The length can be progressively reduced in steps of 0.5 cm till the sense of touch is felt. The length of the nylon filament directly correlates with the pressure (11–200 mg/mm^2).

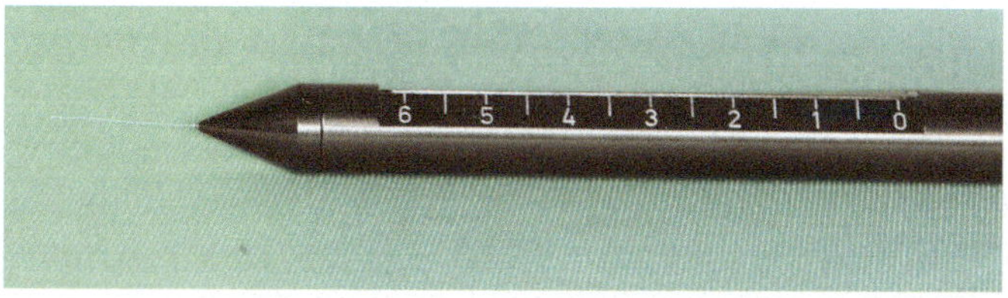

Fig. 17.20: Cochet-Bonnet esthesiometer.

Other methods find their usage mostly in research applications. A jet of warm saline solution is used to warm the cornea in a saline bath at ocular temperature. A 4.5°C increase in temperature elicited a response in a normal cornea.[60] Chemical stimulation of cornea with pungent substance like capsaicin is employed to quantify the corneal sensation.[61] In another technique, carbon dioxide laser is used to thermally stimulate the cornea and sensations are measured.[62] This is a highly controllable technique. A non-contact air puff technique has also been described to measure sensations.[63]

Clinical Application (Table 17.3)

Corneal sensation is greatest in the central cornea[64] except in the elderly in whom the peripheral cornea is most sensitive. Sensitivity reduces rapidly as the distance from the limbus increases. Temporal limbus is more sensitive than the inferior limbus. Sensation also decreases with aging process.[65]

Decreased corneal sensations in viral keratitis like herpes simplex and herpes zoster help in the diagnosis of these diseases. Long-term contact lens wearers have reduced corneal sensations with a drop of 150% in 6 months duration on usage of extended wear lenses.[66] Corneal sensation progressively improves with time following penetrating keratoplasty but central cornea will never regain back the normal sensitivity.[67] Refractive surgeries also affect cornea sensations. Patients who have undergone Lasik have significantly better corneal sensations than patients who have undergone photorefractive keratectomy (PRK).[65] Nasal hinge preserved corneal sensations better than superior hinge.[68]

Vital Dyes

Vital dyes are an important tool in corneal examination for the diagnosis and evaluation of various ocular surface disorders. Each dye has an unique chemical composition and, exhibits distinct characteristics which allows the preferential usage of the dye in specific conditions. They are called vital dyes as they stain cells and tissue in their living state.

There are three main vital dyes which are commonly used currently.

Fluorescein is a yellowish red dye that shows as a bright yellow-green hue in cobalt blue light (Fig. 17.21A).

Table 17.3: Causes of reduced corneal sensations.

Congenital	Ocular	Systemic	Central nervous system	Drugs
Riley–Day syndrome	Herpes simplex and herpes zoster keratitis	Diabetes	Neoplasia	Topical anesthetics abuse
Mobius syndrome	Thermochemical injury	Leprosy	Trauma	β-blockers (Timolol, betaxolol)
Familial corneal hypoesthesia	Corneal dystrophies (lattice and granular)	Vitamin A deficiency	Aneurysm	NSAIDs (Diclofenac Sodium)
Goldenhar–Gorlin syndrome	Contact lens wear	Aging	Stroke	Sulfacetamide
	Surgical trauma (PKP, lasik, large limbal incisions, Bowman's cautery)		Post neurosurgical procedures for acoustic neuroma, trigeminal ganglion	Cocaine abuse
	Ocular surface disorders			

(NSAIDs: Nonsteroidal anti-inflammatory drugs)

Fluorescein is hydrophilic and stains the tear film. It does not stain cells or mucus but if the intercellular junctions between epithelial cells are disrupted, the tear film and dye will pass into the intercellular spaces and stains the disruption. If an epithelial defect is present, the dye will readily pass into the hydrophilic stroma and eventually into the aqueous humor. The primary purpose of fluorescein staining is to detect epithelial defects, corneal erosions, abrasions and corneal ulcers. It is very useful in monitoring the rate of healing corneal epithelial lesions. Fluorescein staining should be differentiated from pooling. Pooling occurs in a depressed or irregular area of the cornea even if the epithelium is intact. The easiest way to differentiate between the two is by using a cotton wisp to absorb the fluorescein tear film in the area of concern. If the epithelium is intact, the pool of fluorescein will be removed and no staining will be left behind. Since it stains the pre-corneal tear film, it is used in different tests for evaluation of dry eyes like tear film height (TFH), tear film break up time (TBUT). It is also used for evaluating contact lens fitting and identifying subtle leaks in microcorneal perforations.

Contrary to historical belief, a study showed that fluorescein also stains healthy epithelium but it can only be detected by florescence microscopy.[69] Its staining is enhanced with cell degeneration or death which increases the cell permeability of the fluorescein. It lacks intrinsic cellular toxicity and is not blocked by tear components like mucin, albumin or tear substitutes like carboxycellulose.[69]

The dye can be applied by touching a fluorescein impregnated filter paper strip to the tear meniscus or by instilling a drop of 1 or 2% fluorescein solution into the conjunctival cul-de-sac. Excess fluorescein may be irrigated out or washed away in the tears. After a few moments, the cornea can be examined in cobalt blue light; epithelial defects or abrasions will be noted as areas of bright green stain.

Rose Bengal, a fluorescein derivative, is believed to stain dead and damaged cells, without penetrating into epithelial defects or intercellular spaces. It is used to detect and evaluate Keratoconjunctivitis sicca (KCS), squamous neoplasia, herpetic corneal epithelial dendrites (Fig. 17.21B), and various forms of superficial punctate keratitis. The dye is available as a 0.5 or 1% solution or impregnated filter paper strip and it can be applied after instilling a drop of topical anesthetic as rose Bengal stain can be quite irritating to the patient. Patients with dry eyes are more uncomfortable with rose Bengal instillations.

Rose Bengal in serial dilutions has also been shown to stain healthy epithelial cells but agents such as mucin, albumin or carboxycellulose can block this dose dependent staining.[69,70] Thus, it has a tendency to stain wherever there is a poor protection of the surface epithelium by precorneal tear film. In conditions like epithelial dysplasia, metaplasia or viral dendritic ulcer where the epithelium's ability to interact with the mucous layer of the tear film is disturbed, rose Bengal staining appears. There have also been questions raised on rose Bengal being a vital dye as it exerts a direct toxic effect on human corneal epithelial cells in a dose dependent manner.[71]

Fluorescein and rose Bengal may be used concurrently to give complementary information, as in the case of a geographic herpetic lesion, where fluorescein will stain the base of the ulcer while rose bengal stains the damaged surrounding cells that are infected with virus.

Lissamine green (Fig.17.21C) has similar staining profile as rose Bengal with an added advantage of being less irritating to the ocular surface.[72] Lissamine green stains only the membrane damaged cells and does not stain

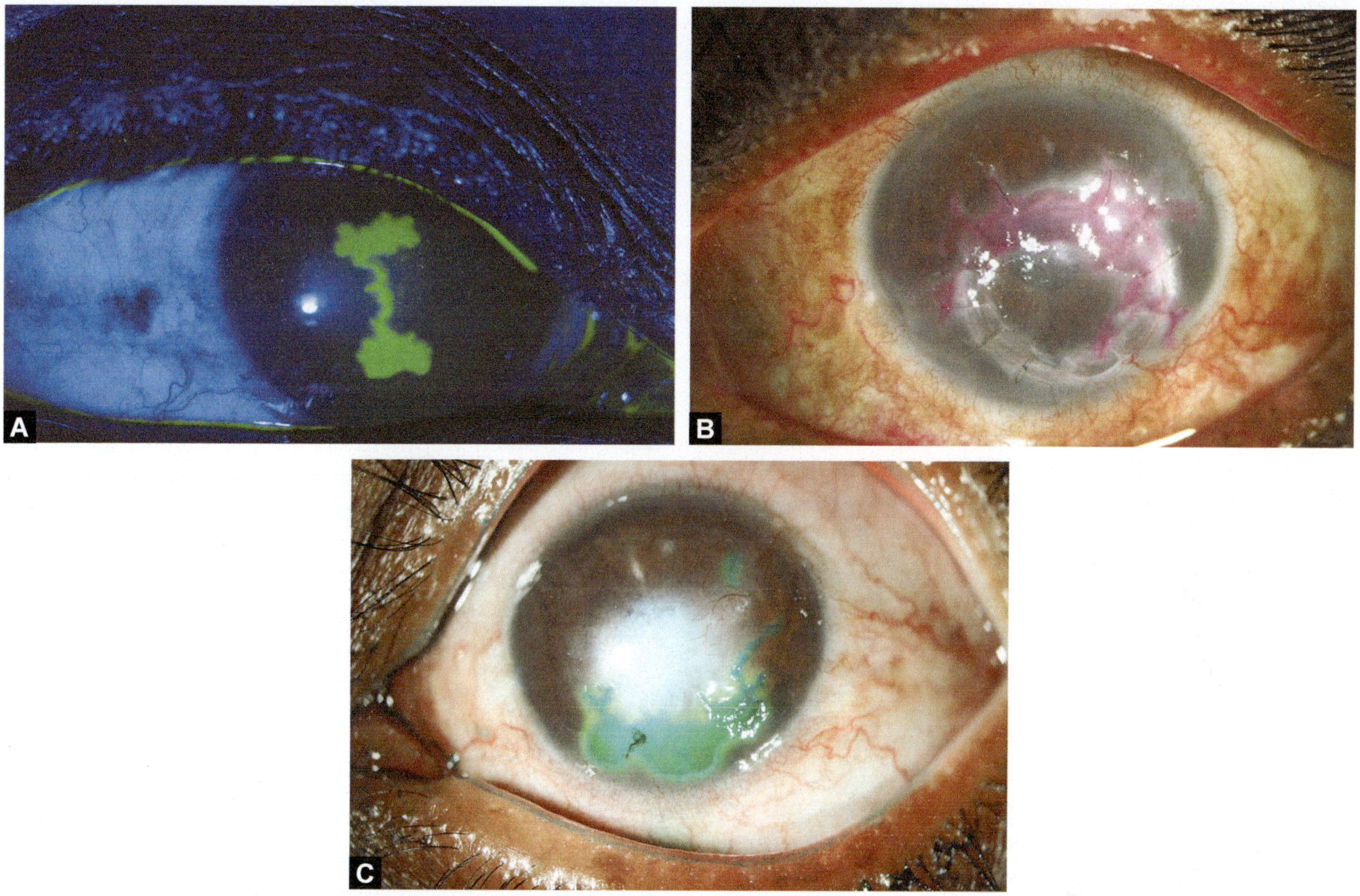

Figs. 17.21A to C: Vital stains. (A) Fluorescein staining pattern of herpes simplex viral (HSV) keratitis under a cobalt blue filter light; (B) Rose Bengal staining pattern of recurrent HSV keratitis in a post PKP eye under low illumination with no filter; (C) Lissamine green staining pattern of recurrent HSV keratitis under high illumination with no filter.

healthy corneal epithelium. Overall, lissamine stain can be considered a better dye compared to the rose Bengal as it is more tolerable and less toxic to the eyes.

MEASUREMENT OF CORNEAL THICKNESS

Pachymetry or measurement of corneal thickness can be of value in normal people as well as patients with certain corneal diseases. It may be used to evaluate the degree of corneal edema in various states of corneal decompensation, as in early Fuchs' corneal dystrophy or the thinness of the cornea, as in keratoconus. Refractive surgeons use central corneal thickness for planning the procedure, as adequate thickness is one of the most important factors in avoiding postoperative ectasia. Its role in influencing the accurate estimation of intraocular pressure (IOP) cannot be undermined. Serial measurements can be used as a surrogate measure of the corneal endothelial function and hence it is very useful in following up patients with corneal transplants to determine endothelial function and its recovery and to become alerted to graft decompensation.

There are two types of pachymetric techniques:

1. *Spot measurements:* In this technique only a small area of the cornea is measured to determine the corneal thickness. It includes traditional optical pachymetry, USG pachymetry, optical low-coherence reflectometry, specular and confocal microscopy.
2. *Wide area mapping:* It refers to the mapping of corneal thickness over a wide area. The techniques are slit-scanning optical pachymetry, Scheimpflug imaging, optical coherence tomography, and very high frequency USG imaging.

Ultrasound pachymetry: It is the most commonly used method and also considered as gold standard for measurement of corneal thickness. It depends upon the reflections of the ultrasonic signals from the anterior and posterior surfaces of the cornea. It is calculated by the time difference between reflected signals of the ultrasonic waves from the transducer of the probe to the front and back surfaces of the cornea.

Corneal thickness can be calculated by the following formulae:

$$\text{Corneal thickness} = \frac{\text{Transit time} \times \text{Ultrasonic velocity in cornea}}{2}$$

The propagation velocity through the cornea is taken as 1640 m/sec. The ultrasonic pachymeter consists of three components viz. the probe, the transducer and the tip. The probe consists of the piezoelectric crystal which vibrates at a frequency of 10–20 MHz. The transducer sends and receives the ultrasonic signals from the probe to the cornea. The tip is around 2 mm to improve the accuracy of the corneal thickness measurement and it should be kept perpendicular to the cornea surface without indentation of the cornea. It is widely used because of its simplicity, portability, less time consuming and intraoperative usability. USG pachymetry reproducibility depends upon the precise probe placement in the center of the cornea at each examination (Fig. 17.22).

Very high frequency (VHF) digital ultrasound biomicroscopy: This technology uses a broadband of 50 MHz VHF USG transducer (bandwidth approximately 10–60 MHz) that is swept by a reverse arc by a high precision mechanism to acquire B-scans that follow the surface contour of anterior and posterior structures of interest. The only device based on VHF technology is the Artemis (Arc Scan Inc., Morrison, CO, USA), which has shown high repeatability that validates the use of the system for in-vivo layered pachymetry. It has shown the best repeatability for central corneal thickness measurements. With the newer studies showing the importance of epithelial thickness in the screening of keratoconus, this technology seems to have a bright future.

Manual optical pachymetry: The most convenient instrument for measuring corneal thickness used to be the Haag-Streit depth measuring device (Haag-Streit AG, Koeniz, Switzerland). This instrument has two planoglass plates (the upper one is movable) that can be used to split the image of the corneal parallelepiped. The instrument is attached to the slit lamp and the slit beam is projected perpendicularly to the cornea through the narrow diaphragm of the instrument. The observer, looking through a split-image eyepiece that replaces the regular eyepiece of the slit lamp, moves the scale of the instrument until the focused upper half of the corneal image is positioned so that its posterior surface is in direct contact with the anterior surface of the lower image (Fig. 17.23). The corneal thickness can then be read directly from the scale on the instrument. However, it lacked accuracy with a wide unacceptable range of error, upto ± 2% which was a major disadvantage. This method is no more used these days.

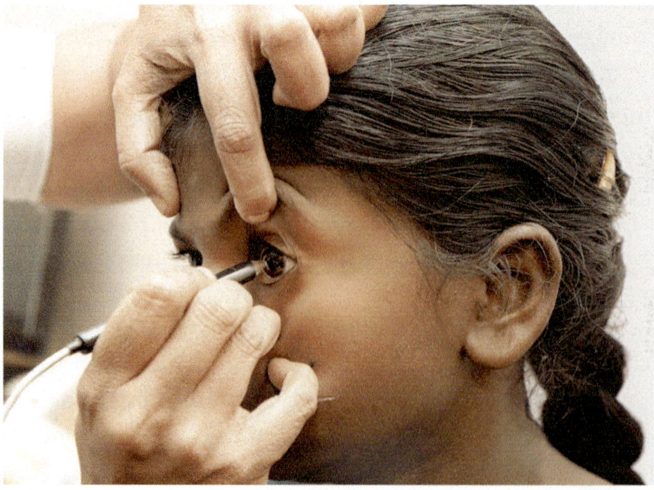

Fig. 17.22: Ultrasound pachymetry. Figure showing the placement of USG probe on the cornea.

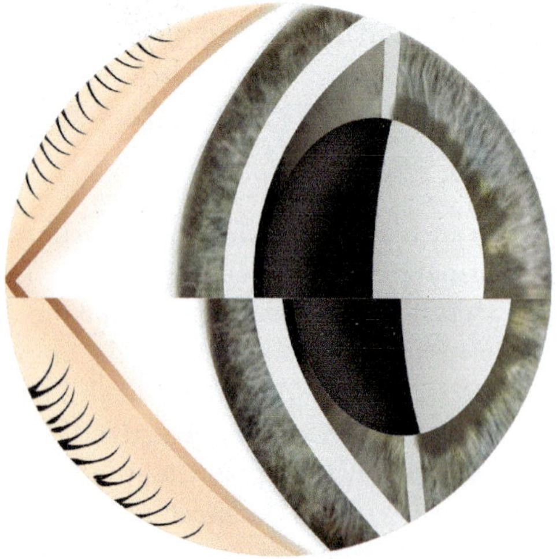

Fig. 17.23: Manual optical pachymetry. Figure showing the end point where the posterior surface of the upper half of the cornea is in direct contact with the anterior surface of the lower half of the cornea.

Anterior segment optical coherence tomography (ASOCT): Optical coherence tomography was first introduced in 1991 for imaging the posterior segment of eye. 3 years later, its use expanded and the first report of anterior segment imaging with OCT appeared. Since then ASOCT has been refined continuously and today it is one of the most essential tool for assessing the anterior segment structures. ASOCT is based on the principle of low coherence interferometry, which compares the time-delay of infrared light reflected from the anterior segment structures with the reference reflections. The interference pattern forms a cross-section image of the anterior segment with a high resolution of 2–20 µm. Multiple scans at a series of different locations are obtained to form a composite two-dimensional image.

There are currently two types of OCTs:

1. *Time domain ASOCT,* where varying the position of the reference mirror produces cross-sectional images.
2. *Fourier domain or spectral domain ASOCT,* where the Fourier transformation of the spectral interferogram produces the cross-sectional images. The spectral domain ASOCT has a faster acquisition time and higher resolution compared to time domain ASOCT. The advantage of time domain ASOCT is that all of anterior segment structures can be captured in a single image whereas spectral domain ASOCT captures only a small part of anterior segment structure in a single image.

ASOCT is most frequently used for pre- and post-operative assessment of the patients undergoing corneal surgeries (Figs. 17.24A to I).

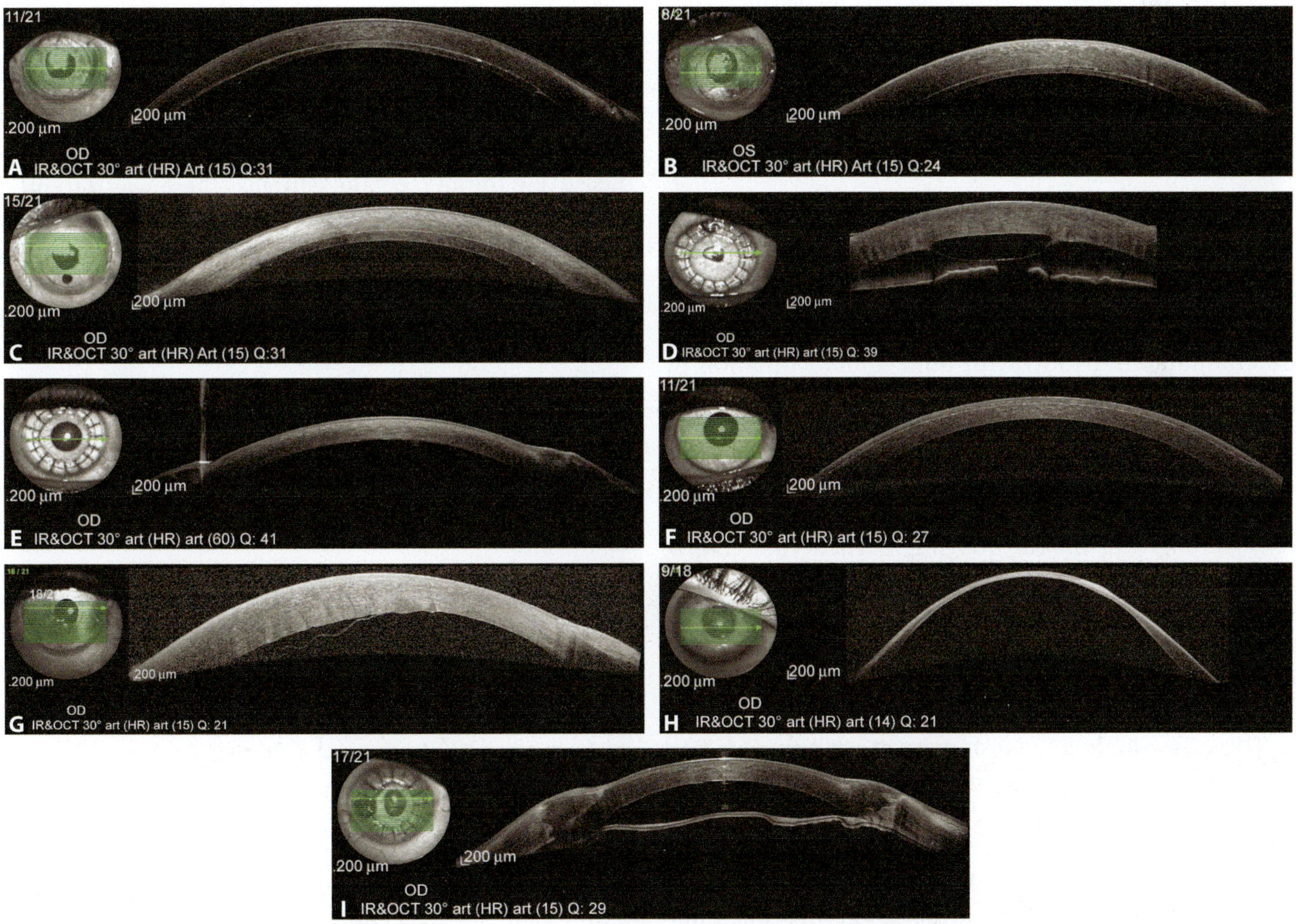

Figs. 17.24A to I: ASOCT images. (A) DSAEK lenticule well apposed to host stroma; (B) Interface gape between the host stroma and the DSAEK lenticule; (C) Uneven DSAEK lenticule; (D) Detached Descemet's membrane (DM) in DALK on postoperative day 1; (E) Spontaneously attached DM on postoperative Day 3; (F) Uniformly thick LASIK flap; (G) DM detachment postcataract surgery; (H) Thin cornea in keratoconus; (I) Remnant host DM following penetrating keratoplasty in congenital hereditary endothelial dystrophy.

I. In DSAEK, uniformity of the thickness of donor lenticule, any interface gape can be assessed and correlated with the postoperative outcome.
II. In DALK, OCT can be of great help in locating the site of perforation and assessment of double anterior chamber postoperatively thereby guiding in the management of these cases.
III. It can also be employed to measure the residual stromal bed and flap thickness following lasik before taking the patient for enhancement procedures to avoid post lasik ectasia.
IV. It is an excellent tool for localizing the site of Descemet's membrane detachment following cataract surgeries.
V. It can be used to measure the depth of demarcation line to find out the treatment effects of cross-linking.
VI. Extent of corneal ulcer and scar can be measured precisely and accordingly surgical intervention can be planned.
VII. Apart from corneal thickness, OCT also provides anterior chamber depth, anterior chamber angle, iris imaging, lens thickness and density. It serves a very important function in the management of phakic intraocular lenses. The vault distance can be measured by OCT.

OCT being a non-contact method with an acquisition time of less than 1 second allows easier patient fixation and fewer repeat scans due to blinking. OCT measurements are comparable to USG with mild underestimation of corneal thickness. The range of deviation from USG is similar to Pentacam. As with other optical devices, OCT measurements are not directly interchangeable with USG due to wide limits of agreements between the instruments.

Slit-scanning/Scheimpflug imaging: Corneal topography machines provide corneal thickness distribution by reconstruction of the anterior and the posterior corneal surfaces. Both slit-scanning and scheimpflug imaging measures central corneal thickness as well as minimum thickness of the cornea.

Orbscan which is the prototype of slit-scanning has been compared to USG for corneal thickness estimation in many studies[17,26,73-77] with variable and limited agreement.[78] Orbscan has been found to overestimate corneal thickness (approximately 8% higher) compared with USG. As a result, an acoustic factor of 0.92 was introduced in Orbscan by the manufacturer to compensate for this overestimation.[78]

It has been observed that in eyes with keratoconus, Orbscan II (with correction factor) underestimate CCT compared to USG.[79,80] This may have clinical implication. For example, some eyes may get rejected for collagen cross-linking which would have otherwise qualified for the treatment.

Studies comparing pachymetry data obtained by Orbscan and Pentacam (prototype for Scheimpflug imaging) have showed varied results. Some studies suggest that Orbscan II (with correction factor) underestimates CCT readings than those obtained by Pentacam systems.[81-83] whereas there are others which shows either no difference or slightly higher CCT readings.[84,85]

Interestingly in myopic eyes, pachymetry was comparable between Orbscan II (with correction factor) and Pentacam before surgery, whereas after PRK, Orbscan values were lesser as compared to Pentacam in the early and late postoperative period.[86]

There were more variations between Orbscan and Pentacam CCT measurements of keratoconic corneas as compared to non-keratoconic healthy corneas.[87] In Keratoconus, Orbscan pachymetry data more closely correlated with Pentacam when the acoustic factor was not applied.[87] Since the acoustic factor of 0.92 was derived using normal corneas, this factor may not be accurate when measuring thinner, ectatic corneas. There was a trend of underestimation of CCT in keratoconic eyes by Orbscan II (without acoustic factor applied) compared with Pentacam when measuring thinner corneas (below approximately 470 mm), whereas these values were overestimated by Orbscan II when measuring the thicker corneas.[87]

The accuracy of the Orbscan II-derived CCT thickness measurements remains a controversial subject.[15,78] Measurements of CCT obtained with the Pentacam have shown higher repeatability and interexaminer correlation compared with ultrasound pachymetry for eyes with keratoconus.[87]

Confocal microscopy: Confocal microscopy is a useful tool for studying corneal microscopy in-vivo with clinical applications in the diagnosis of acanthamoeba and fungal keratitis. Since it scans through the entire cornea from epithelium to endothelial surfaces, it is able to measure corneal thickness too. It is believed that the confocal microscopy measures the true thickness of the cornea since it directly visualizes the two limits of the corneal surface rather than relying on an unseen optical or ultrasonic energy. Comparative studies have shown varying results of CCT estimation by confocal microscopy. In a study by McLaren et al., CCT was found to be 34 µm less compared to USG pachymetry and 24 µm less compared to Orbscan.[74] It was suggested, the lack in precision of confocal microscopy could be due to the corneal motion in anteroposterior direction. Confocal microscopy was also found to have overestimated CCT in comparison to USG, Scheimpflug[88] and non-contact specular microscopy[89] in different studies. Although the difference was small in normal corneas.[88] Confocal microscopy is rarely used for estimation of CCT as there are very conflicting results about its accuracy. It is less preferred also since it is an expensive instrument, takes longer time for acquisition and requires a contact with a lens or adaptor ring.

Specular microscopy: Specular microscopy is used for analyzing corneal endothelium but can also measure corneal thickness by differential focusing on epithelial and endothelial surfaces. It operates on the similar principle of optical devices like Orbscan, Pentacam and OCT. It has the advantage of being non-contact and ability to measure both central and peripheral corneal thickness. Noncontact Specular microscopes underestimate the CCT by 10–33 µm, compared to USG in normal corneas[27,30,90-92] whereas in post lasik and keratoconus eyes this difference was 11 and 18 µm respectively.[30,93,94] In contrast the contact specular microscopes measures substantially thicker central pachymetry, ranging from 60 µm to 80 µm higher than USG.[27,92] Similar to other optical devices, specular microscopy provides close approximation of corneal thickness when compared to USG.

USG pachymetry has often been used as the standard to which newer modalities have been compared. However, there are significant limitations in using ultrasound as a reference, including different operating modes of various ultrasounds, probe design and sensitivity, effects of the contact procedure (topical anesthetic and corneal indentation), nonperpendicular probe position, and variability in the exact location of corneal measurement.[78] It also exhibits relatively higher interobserver variability.[24] Consequently, attempts to calibrate other devices with ultrasound pachymetry must be viewed with caution.

It has already been observed that pachymetry measurements obtained by different devices cannot be used interchangeably.[16,78,82,83,95,96] Since the true value is unknown, it is difficult to conclude which device obtains the most accurate pachymetry and therefore it is not possible to recommend one device absolutely over the others at the present time.

SPECULAR MICROSCOPY

Specular microscopy is a non-invasive technique to determine the density and the morphology of the corneal endothelial cells. The present day clinical specular microscopes are all derived from laboratory microscope designed by Maurice[97] to provide a high magnification view of specular reflected light from the corneal endothelium.

Optical Principles

The specular reflex occurs at the interface of two media with different refractive indices with the light from the source having an angle of incidence equal to the angle of reflection to the observer. The corneal endothelial cells can be imaged because the refractive index of these cells is greater than the aqueous humor, thus reflecting part of the projected light.[98]

A restriction in the area of the light reflex is caused by the proximity of the two concentric surfaces, i.e. epithelium and the endothelium. The epithelial surface is highly reflective because of the large refractive index difference between air and the tear/epithelium. The viewable specular area is a compromise between the beam width and the corneal thickness. As the slit beam of light passes through the corneal stroma, the light will be scattered from the collagen lamellae and keratocytes and will reduce the contrast of the endothelial cell image. The light scatter is compounded by increasing the width of the beam of light.

Types

All the presently available instruments use computer interface for image capture and endothelial cell morphology analysis. The instruments can be divided into contact or noncontact types. The contact instrument has an objective microscope lens that applanates the corneal surface, requiring a topical anesthetic. During corneal applanation, the corneal curvature is flattened and the specular reflex area is enlarged. The noncontact instruments use automatic image focusing technology. The specular reflex area obtained through non-contact imaging techniques is smaller than the contact specular microscopes because of the curved corneal reflecting surface.

Quantitative Analysis

Quantitative specular microscopy is the objective description of the attributes of the selected group of endothelial cells from the specular photomicrograph. The endothelial cell morphology analysis includes the following: mean cell area ± SD (µm²/cell), endothelial cell density (ECD) (measured as cells/mm²), coefficient of variation (CV) (standard deviation of cell areas/mean cell area), and pleomorphism (percentage of hexagonal cells).

In most individual ECD decreases throughout life.[99]Armitage et al.,[100] showed the cell loss to be bimodal, with 0–20 years showing a more rapid cell loss per year than subjects more than 20 years old. Published studies show that young children usually have 4,000 cells/mm^2,[101,102] while the cell count in middle-aged adult scan range from 2,700 cells/mm^2 to 2,900 cells/mm^2 and adults older than 75 years can have a range of ECD between 2,400 cells/mm^2 and 2,600 cells/mm^2.[101-104] CV represents the variation in endothelial cell areas as compared to the mean cell area. In a normal young adult, CV ranges from 0.22 to 0.31 and it increases in conditions when the endothelial cells are in stress and adopts different sizes to compensate for the endothelial damage.[104]

The ECD can be performed by following methods:

1. *Comparison method:* Here the patient's endothelial cell size pattern is compared to a known standard of hexagonal patterns for various cell densities.
2. *Frame method (fixed or variable):* In fixed frame method the number of cells lying in a given area is counted (Fig.17.25A). Not all the cells present at the boundary will be fully inside the frame and so to avoid overestimation, the total number of cells present at the boundary is either divided by two or only the cells lying at the two adjacent boundaries are counted. In variable frame method, the boundary of a largest possible group of nonadjoining cells is traced and the number of cells present in that area is counted (Fig. 17.25B). The variable frame analysis is more accurate than fixed frame since the cells lying completely within the given area are only counted.
3. *Automated method:* Most of the modern specular microscopes are capable of automatically analyzing cells and also enables users to remove and redraw lines if required (Fig. 17.25C).
4. *Corner method:* The corner of each cell is marked and then these points are connected to outline the cell borders leading to the determination of cell area (Fig. 17.25D).
5. *Centre method:* It is the most frequently employed technique in the specular microscope. It is also easier to approximate the center of the cells than determining the intersecting cell borders. The centre of each cell and its adjoining cell in a specular microphotograph image is accurately marked (Fig. 17.25E.). The average radius to the center of adjacent cells is determined to calculate the area of the cell. Newer specular microscopes have recently developed a new analysis, the *center flex method* which capitalizes on the advantage of both variable frame and center methods (Fig. 17.25F).

Comparison of the corner method and the center method have been reported in the literature to be equivalent.[105-107] Regardless of the technique, accuracy is dependent on the quality of the endothelial cell image to identify individual cells.

The noncontact specular microscope can capture 120–170 cells on a cornea with a cell density of 2,500 cells/mm^2. For a cornea with a cell density of 2,500 cells/mm^2, a single capture of 120 cells/per field is only 0.04% of a population of 325,000 cells per cornea which may not be representative of the entire endothelium. Hence it is equally important to do the qualitative assessment of the endothelial morphology.

Qualitative Analysis

It is a subjective evaluation of the health of the endothelial cells based on the visual assessment with focus on variability of endothelial structures. It is relatively fast clinical assessment of the endothelial status which helps in establishing a diagnosis.

Corneal guttae are excrescences of Descemet's membrane. They appear as dark structures varying in size often becoming larger than the adjacent endothelial cells (Fig. 17.26). Sometimes a bright spot can be seen within these dark structures. In Fuchs' endothelial corneal dystrophy, these dark spots are surrounded by abnormal endothelial cells. Guttae can also be seen normally in far periphery of the young individuals, called as Hassal-Henle warts with adjacent normal endothelial cells.

Other dark structures seen intracellularly are endothelial cilia which are small with sharp borders whereas vacuoles or blebs are relatively larger and less distinct.

Intracellular bright structures can be seen sometimes in the stressed cells. These bright structures are as large as the size of the cell, believed to represent cell nucleus. When these are spanning several endothelial cells and appear as structures with sharp borders, they are considered to be pigment deposits.

Besides the dark and bright spots, the cell borders and cell shape has to be given utmost importance when reading a specular microphotograph. The central endothelial

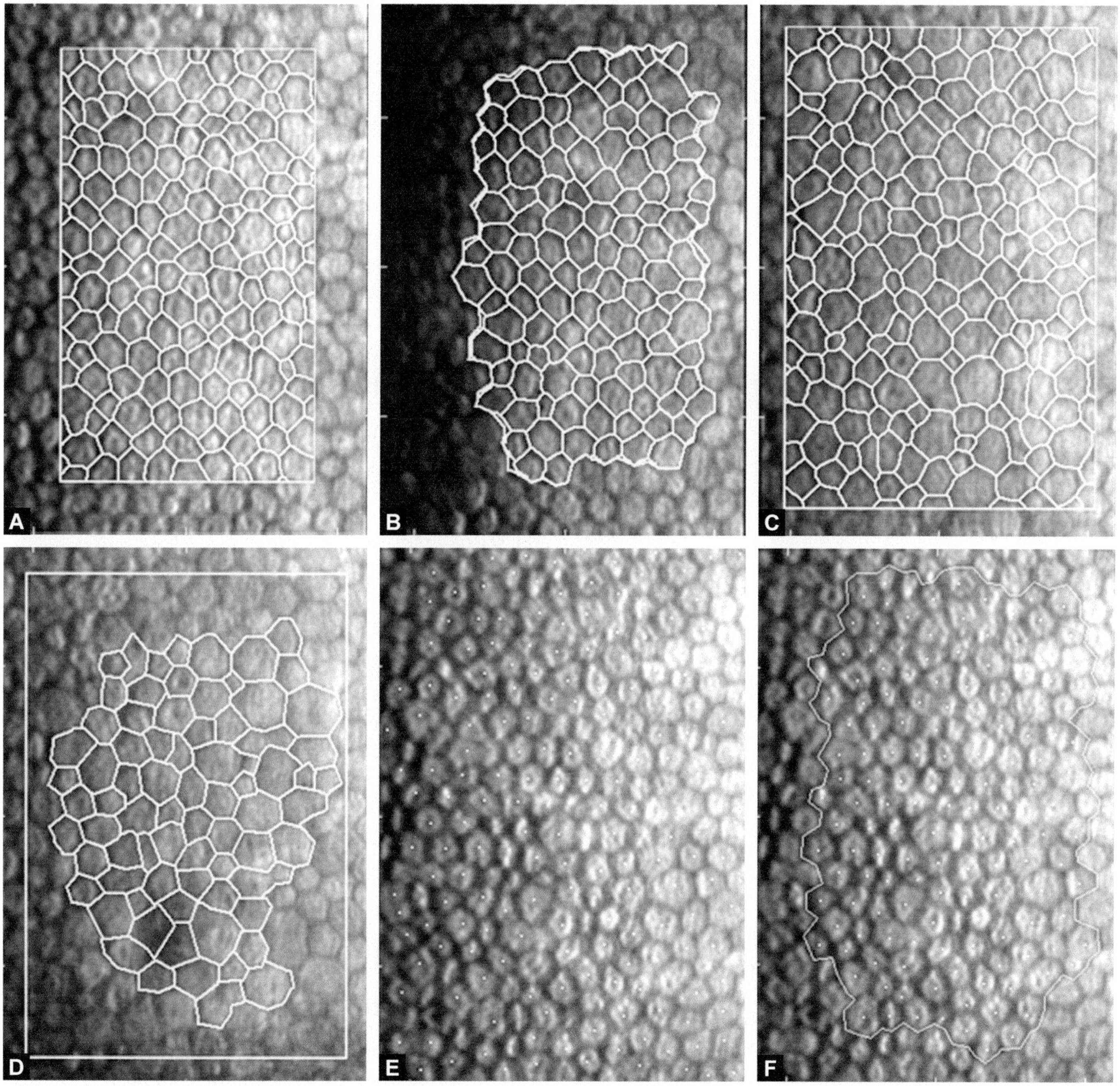

Figs. 17.25A to F: Various methods of analyzing endothelial cells. (A) *Fixed frame analysis*. Cells within the rectangular box and touching the two adjacent borders are counted; (B) *Variable frame analysis*. All the cells within the outlined border are counted; (C) *Automated method*. Instrument analyzes cells automatically; (D) *Corner method*. Corners of each cell are marked individually and all corner points are then connected and cell area determined; (E) *Center method*. Center of the adjacent cells are marked; (F) *Center flex method*. The center of the cells is marked within an outlined area.

cells of young people with normal eyes are hexagonal and approximately the same size with roughly equal side lengths. Any variations like pleomorphism (variation in cell shape) and polymegathism (variation in cell area) (Fig. 17.27) represents aging, reparative changes following injury or specific pathology.

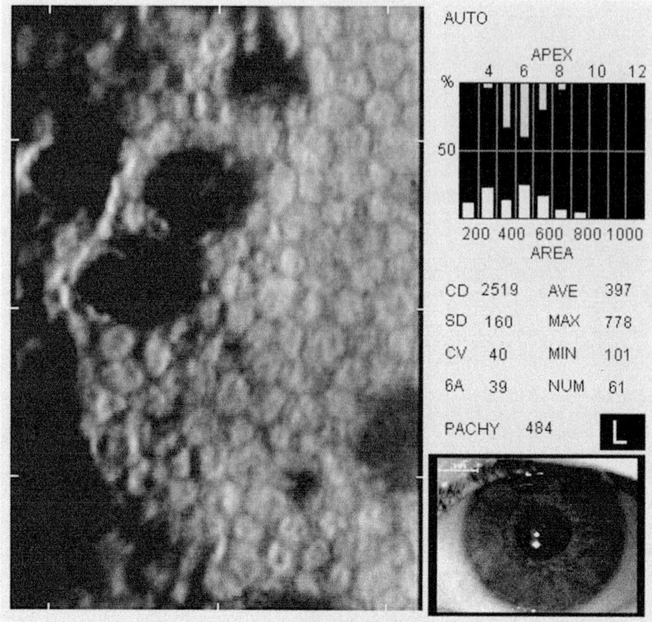

Fig. 17.26: Cornea guttae seen as dark hollow structures varying in size often becoming larger than the adjacent endothelial cells.

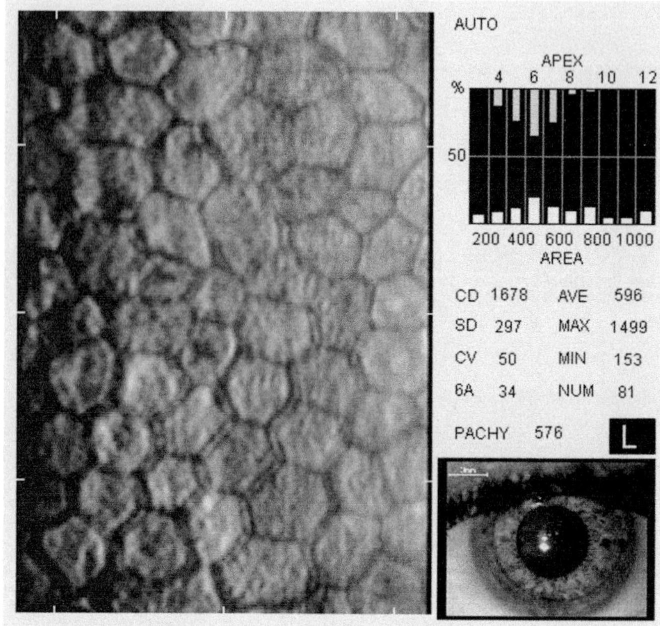

Fig. 17.27: Polymegathism is a variation in endothelial cell area denoted by increase in coefficient of variation (CV).

Clinical Application

Specular microscopy is an essential tool for evaluating donor corneas, monitoring corneal decompensation in endothelial corneal dystrophies, post-keratoplasty corneas and also for identifying subtle and macroscopic changes prior to intraocular surgery. Apart from the slit-lamp evaluation of the donor cornea, specular microscopy is routinely performed to measure the ECD and to note the morphology of the endothelial cells because it influences long-term corneal graft survival. A minimum ECD of 2,000 cells/mm^2 has been established as the lower limit for adequate PKP graft survival,[108] but a safe minimum ECD value for endothelial keratoplasty (EK) has not been validated in the literature but most of the EK surgeons prefer minimum donor ECD of at least 2,300 cells/mm^2 for EK although there are no good scientific data why the minimum was established at this level.

Specular microscopy plays an important role when planning an intraocular surgery. A clear cornea with a normal pachymetry is no guarantee of a normal endothelial morphology and cell density. In conditions where the endothelium is compromised extra precautions during the surgery like use of dispersive viscoelastics, and minimal ultrasonic energy during phacoemulsifications are considered. The ECD at which corneal edema occurs is quite variable ranging from 300 to 700 cells per mm^2. Assuming a cell loss in the range of 0–30% after any intraocular surgery, a patient should have at least 1,000–1,200 cells per mm^2 to safely undergo the procedure without an increased risk of postoperative corneal edema. An ECD of less than 750 cells/mm^2 is an indication to consider endothelial keratopalsty along with phacoemulsification. A patient with a cornea of CV greater than 0.40 or the presence of less than 50% hexagonal cells should be informed about increased risk of developing postoperative corneal edema and subsequent corneal decompensation.

CONFOCAL MICROSCOPY

Introduction

Confocal Microscopy enables noninvasive in-vivo imaging of the full thickness of the living cornea. It is a unique technique in which the tissue is imaged parallel to its surface as opposed to the majority of the devices where the images are oriented generally perpendicular to the surface of the tissues. Conventional light microscopes are limited by reflections and light scattered from structures outside of the focal plane, which degrade the image. The confocal microscope, first described by Goldmann in 1940[109] and later published as a patent by Minsky in 1957,[110] overcomes this problem of defocused light by using the *confocal principle.*

Optical Principle

In its simplest form, a point-source of light, created by a pinhole aperture, is focused by an objective lens on the tissue. The light reflected by the tissue is collected by a parallel objective lens and focused onto a separate pinhole aperture. Light that passes this second aperture is collected by a detector. Both the illuminating point source and the observation aperture of the detector are conjugate with the same point in the tissue, and are said to be *confocal* (Fig. 17.28).[110] With this optical system, illumination is brightest at the point of interest and decreases rapidly in front of and behind this point (focal plane). Light that originates at this point will be detected efficiently, because the image of this point is focused on the detection aperture. However, only a small amount of light that originates a small distance in front of or behind this focal point is detected, because it is imaged behind or in front of the detection aperture. This confocal design provides two important features for imaging the cornea: reduced depth of field (improving axial resolution) and improved lateral resolution as compared to conventional microscopes. This principle is called principle of Lukosz[111] which is based on the fact the resolution increases at the expense of field of view. Clinical confocal microscopes typically have a depth of field of 10–26 μm, depending on the design of the microscope, and lateral resolution of 1–2 μm.[74,112]

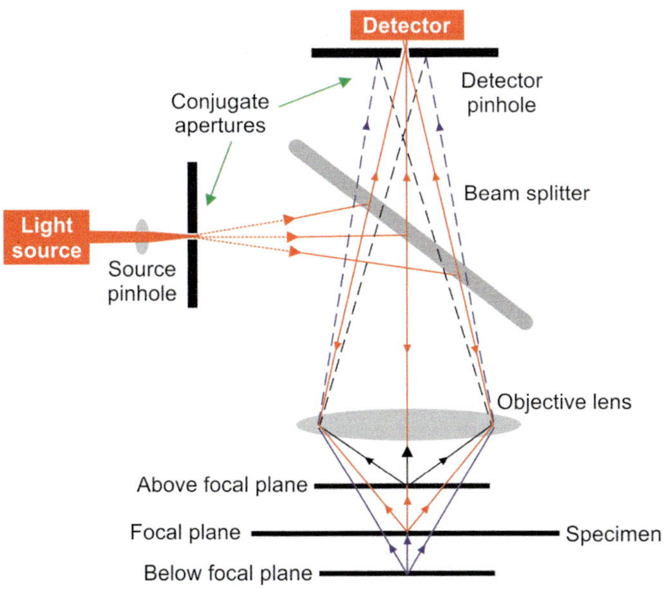

Fig. 17.28: Principles of confocal microscopy—both the light source pinhole and the detector pinhole are conjugate with the same point in the tissue, and are said to be confocal. Any point in front or behind the focal plane will be defocused and not detected.

Types

The three most common confocal microscopes are:
1. Tandem scanning confocal microscope (TSCM)
2. Slit scanning confocal microscope (SSCM)
3. Laser scanning confocal microscope (LSCM).

Tandem scanning confocal microscope: TSCM utilizes a rotating Nipkow disk that contains multiple pinhole apertures arranged in an Archimedean spiral (Fig. 17.29). The focal plane is illuminated through an array of apertures on one-side of the disk and imaged through a conjugate set of apertures on the opposite side. When this disk is rotated, the entire tissue plane can be scanned.[113,114] Because of the small pinhole diameters (typically 30 μm) and high numeric aperture of the objective lens, it has a narrow depth of field (approximately 11 microns) and produces images with a very thin optical section.[74] The focal plane can also be advanced at various speeds, enabling a scan through the full-thickness of the cornea in as quickly as 7 seconds.[74] The small pinhole diameters of the TSCM significantly limit light transmission (range, 0.5–1%),[115] which produces images with relatively poor contrast compared to those of confocal microscopes with larger apertures. Limited field brightness and contrast makes visualization of small structures (<5 μm diameter) difficult. Also, all though the illumination is inefficient, it appears very bright to the patient and may be discomforting and is not commercially available anymore.

Slit scanning confocal microscope: It uses vertical-slit apertures for illumination and observation of the field. A rapidly oscillating two-sided mirror is used to scan the image of the slit over the plane of the cornea to produce optical sectioning in real time. The wide slit aperture allows increased light throughput, which improves field brightness and contrast when compared to the TSCM. This is accomplished in part at the expense of an axial resolution. Increased light throughput also means that illumination need not be as bright as that of the Tandem Scanning microscope, and therefore improves patient comfort. The Confoscan 4 is a SSCM commercially available from Nidek Technologies, Greensboro, North Carolina, USA.

Laser scanning confocal microscope: The HRT III with Rostock Corneal Module (Heidelberg Engineering; GmbH, Heidelberg, Germany) is a laser scanning confocal microscope. It projects a 670-nm laser beam in a raster pattern over the area of interests with the help of two horizontally and vertically oriented scanning mirrors. The reflected light is descanned using the same two mirrors and

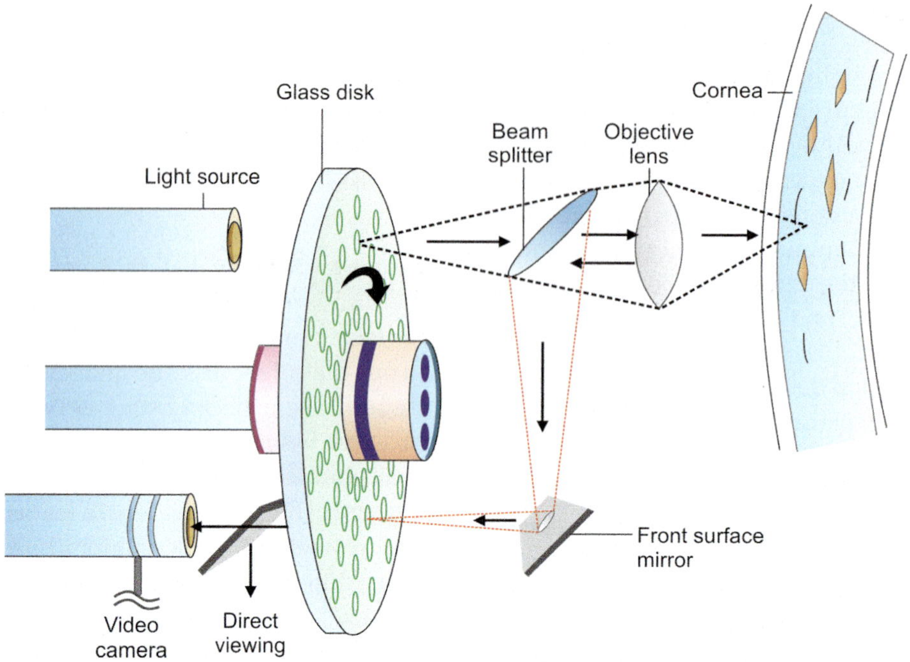

Fig. 17.29: Tandem scanning confocal microscope (TSCM). Light from a broadband source pass through the pinhole aperture on one side of the Nipkow disk and the beam splitter and is focused on the specimen by the objective lens. The reflected signal again passes through the beam splitter and the front surface of the mirror to the conjugate pinholes on the opposite side of the Nipkow disk, which prevents light from outside the optical volume from reaching the camera.

directed to the photodetectors using a beam splitter. It has an excellent lateral and axial resolution of 1 μm and 4 μm respectively.

Application

It is necessary to recognize the normal appearance of different layers of cornea in order to differentiate it from the pathologic condition. Most of the anatomical layers of cornea can be made out easily including epithelial cells, basal nerve plexus, stromal layers with keratocytes, Descemet's membrane, and endothelial cells (Fig. 17.30).

The most important use of confocal microscopy in clinical scenario is the detection and identification of the causative organism in corneal infections. In vivo confocal microscopy has shown high sensitivity, specificity for detecting fungal filaments (Fig. 17.31A) and Acanthamoeba cysts (Fig. 17.31B) in moderate-to-large corneal ulcers.[116] It is particularly useful for detecting organisms in deep ulcers in which culture and light microscopy results were negative. Apart from this, it is also possible to identify other organisms like Nocardia (Fig. 17.31C) and Microsporidia.

Confocal microscopy can also be used to monitor the cellular changes in different layers of the cornea following laser refractive surgeries and penetrating keratoplasty.[117] Besides this confocal microscopy is a useful tool for the diagnosis of various corneal dystrophies. Conjunctival and limbal structures may be monitored for cysts, inflammation and proliferation of different cell types.

CORNEAL BIOMECHANICS

Introduction

The study of the mechanical properties of cornea and its response to stress is corneal biomechanics. Cornea contributes to approximately two-thirds of the optical power of the eye and hence even the slightest changes in the corneal shape will substantially affect the visual function. The strength of the cornea also allows it to withstand the IOP and still maintain its shape. Corneal ectatic conditions and keratorefractive procedures can cause significant changes in the optical system by virtue of mechanical and structural modifications in the cornea. A study of the biomechanics of the cornea is useful to predict the consequences of laser refractive procedures and interventions such as collagen cross linking. It will also improve our capability to diagnose ectatic conditions at an earlier stage and correct estimation of IOP in these conditions.

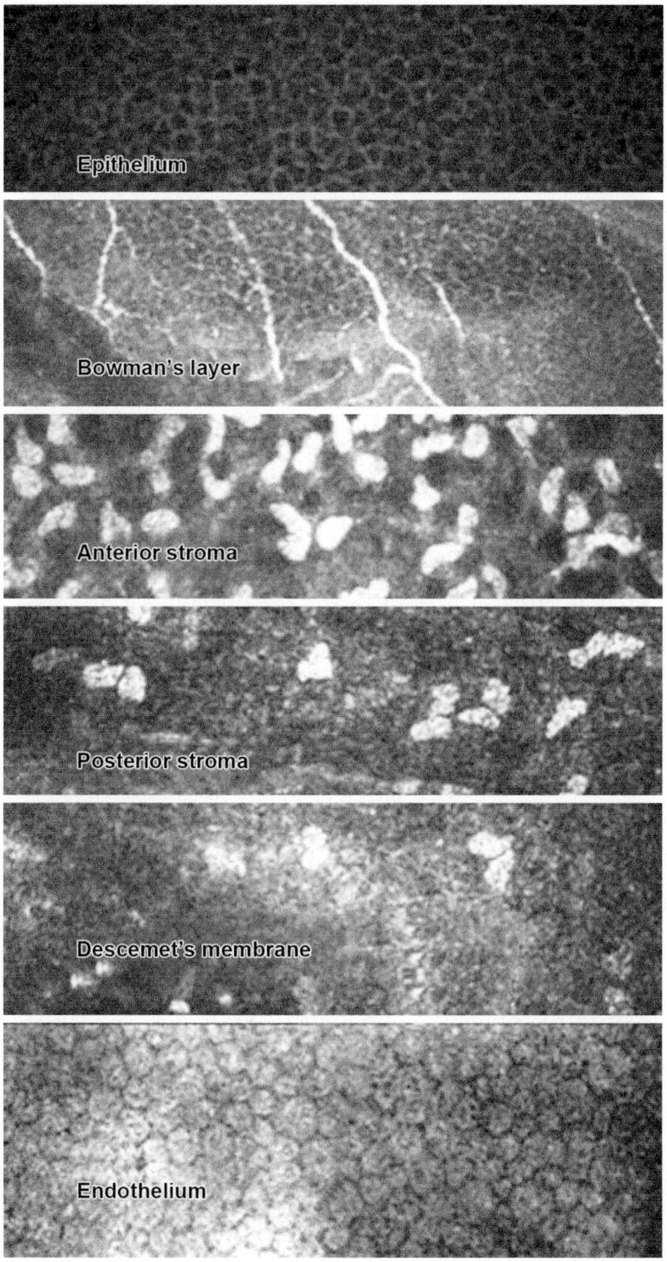

Fig. 17.30: The HRT III laser scanning confocal microscopy image showing different layers of the cornea.

General Concepts of Biomechanics

Assessing biomechanical properties of the living tissue is complex and requires some basic knowledge of the physics. The commonly used terminologies in the field of biomechanics are:

1. *Stress:* Stress is defined as the amount of force applied to a unit area of tissue.
2. *Strain:* Strain is defined as the amount of deformation of the tissue in the direction of the applied stress.
3. *Loading:* Application of force or stress to a material.
4. *Unloading:* Removal of force or stress from a material.
5. *Strength:* The maximum stress a tissue can sustain before breaking.
6. *Elastic properties:* Elastic material is a material in which, a change in stress results in an instantaneous change in strain. Elastic limit is the maximum limit beyond which permanent deformation of the material occur leading to material breakage. Below the elastic limit, the stress-strain relationship of an elastic material is linear. When the load is removed, the object immediately regains its original shape in a completely reversible displacement direction along the stress-strain plot (Fig. 17.32A).
7. *Elastic modulus or Young's modulus:* It is the ratio of stress and strain. The slope of the stress strain graph represents Young's modulus. The greater the slope is, higher the modulus and stiffer the material, i.e. more stress is required to deform the material.
8. *Viscous properties:* Viscous materials undergo a continuing deformation for as long as the load is maintained and unlike the elastic material do not regain their shape once the stress is discontinued.
9. *Viscoelasticity:* Viscoelastic materials have an immediate elastic response to a change in load followed by an ongoing viscous response. Most biological tissues are viscoelastic by nature. The stress-strain relationship of biological tissues is non-linear. These tissues absorb energy during loading and dissipate energy in the form of heat during unloading, resulting in a different stress-strain curve/relationship for loading and unloading (Fig. 17.32B).
10. *Hysteresis:* The energy absorbed and dissipated as heat by a biological tissue during the loading and unloading is known as hysteresis.
11. *Fatigue:* The failure or breakage of a tissue due to constant accumulation of micro damage over time caused by the energy absorbed and dissipated in hysteresis.
12. *Creep:* Progressive deformation of soft tissue due to constant loading over an extended period of time.

Cornea is a viscoelastic tissue with high tension and is difficult to stretch. The major contributing reasons for this stiffness are the highly resilient collagen fibrils and the crosslinking between these fibrils. The elasticity of cornea is dependent on the collagen fibrils, which allows the cornea to come back to its original shape after deformation. The viscosity of the corneal tissue is due to the proteoglycan matrix which absorbs the energy produced during stress and

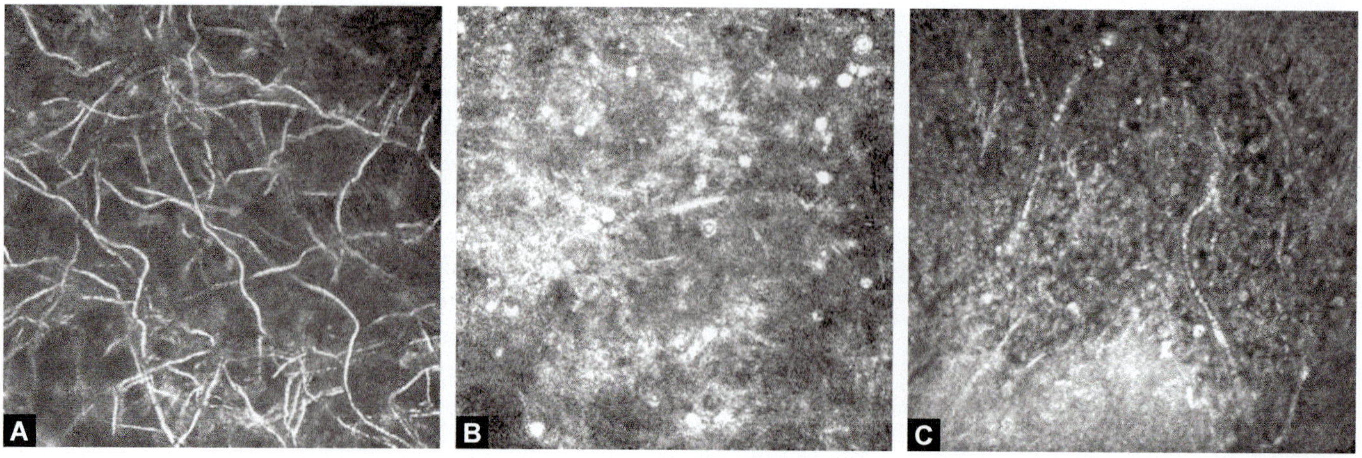

Figs. 17.31A to C: The HRT III laser scanning confocal microscopy images. (A) Fungal keratitis. Hyper-reflective branching filaments; (B) Acanthamoeba keratitis. Hyper-reflective double-walled cysts; (C) Nocardia keratitis. Hyper-reflective filamentous beaded structures.

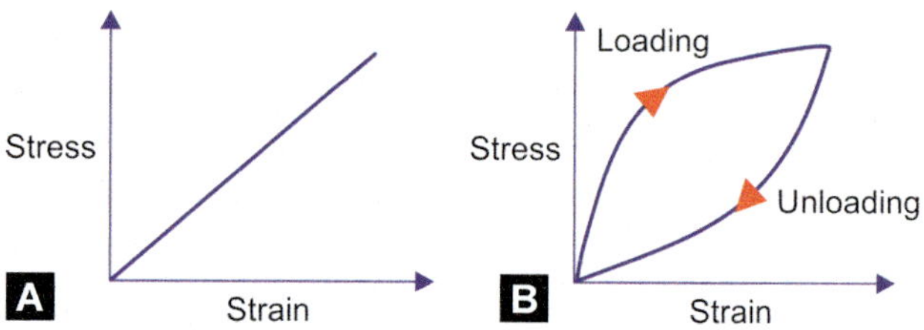

Figs. 17.32A and B: Stress/strain plot for an elastic and viscoelastic material. (A) Elastic material will return to its normal configuration once the external stress has been removed, reversing through the same pathway; (B) Viscoelastic material will also return to its original configuration but through a different pathway. The area between the two curves represents the energy dissipated and is termed hysteresis.

dissipates it. Elasticity and viscosity occur as a continuing process to stress and thus complicates the biomechanical assessment of cornea. However, cornea can undergo fatigue and creep and can lead to chronic biomechanical failure as in the case of corneal ectasia.

Applied Anatomy of Cornea with Reference to Corneal Biomechanics

The outermost layer of the eye is formed by cornea and sclera. It is these two layers which provides structural integrity to the globe and also protects the inner components from physical insults. The cornea is composed of five layers and each of these layers has a different structural and functional characteristic. All these five layers together are responsible for the optical properties, barrier and biomechanical function of the cornea.

The stratified squamous epithelium is thicker inferiorly and thinner superiorly. The tear film and corneal epithelium do not play a direct role in corneal biomechanics. Bowman's membrane is composed of highly interwoven type I collagen fibrils. Stroma forms 90% thickness of cornea and is predominantly responsible for the biomechanical properties of the cornea. Approximately 80% of stroma is made of water and the rest is comprised of collagen, proteoglycans and keratocytes. Collagen forms 10–15% of corneal stroma and is arranged as parallel lamellae across the stroma. These lamellae are thinner, smaller and highly interwoven in the anterior one-third of stroma. Posterior two-thirds of stroma have larger, wider and minimally interwoven lamellae. Hence the anterior stroma is much stiffer and stronger than posterior stroma.

Type I Collagen is the most common collagen seen in stroma proper. Type I collagen are extremely resilient, moderately stiff, slightly extensible and have high elasticity, i.e. they return to the original shape after stretching. Type VI collagen are interspersed between and connect type 1 collagen fibrils. The stromal thickness and the arrangement of lamellae vary from center to periphery. The central stroma proper consists of approximately 300 corneal lamellae, gradually increasing to approximately 500 lamellae in the peripheral cornea.[118] Consequently the central and the paracentral cornea is relatively weaker compared to the peripheral cornea. This rigid scaffold is intermixed with the softer, amorphous, hydrophilic interfibrillar matrix of bridging proteoglycans. At the limbus, corneal lamella interweaves with the scleral lamellae and takes a circular course thought to be responsible for the thickness of this region.[119] Descemet's membrane and the monolayered endothelium do not play a direct role in corneal biomechanics. The flap based refractive surgeries aim a cut in the stronger anterior stroma (90–120 μm) thereby inducing lesser changes in corneal biomechanics. Thicker flap involving the posterior stroma weakens the cornea and have a higher risk of post-lasik ectasia. Surgical procedures such as photorefractive keratectomy do not alter the corneal biomechanics since there is no flap created.

As a result of this complex organization, cornea is aspheric, anisotropic (displays different physical properties when stress is applied in different directions) and its thickness varies from center (thinner) to periphery (thicker).[120] These factors responsible for biomechanical properties are not constant and shows variations with age, hydration and various corneal conditions. Understanding of these concepts and their application to the cornea and eye as a whole explains why it is so difficult to define corneal biomechanics as a single number or scale.

Clinical Measurements of Biomechanics

Over the last three decades there has been continued effort in characterizing the biomechanical properties of the cornea but most of these assessments were confined to in-vitro studies[121,122] and to virtual mathematical corneal finite element models.[123-125] Two devices which are currently available for characterizing biomechanical properties of the cornea in-vivo used in clinical practice are ocular response analyzer (ORA) (Reichert, Buffalo, New York, USA) based on bidirectional applanation tonometry and Corvis ST (Oculus Optikgeräte GmbH, Wetzlar, Germany) based on corneal deformation measurement using Scheimpflug imaging.

There are few other techniques which can measure biomechanical properties but are still being tested includes radial shearing speckle pattern interferometry,[126,127] brillouin optical microscopy,[128] ocular coherence tomography (OCT),[129] and other forms of dynamic corneal imaging.[130,131] Their applicability to clinical practice is still undergoing a lot of evolution.

Bidirectional Applanation Tonometry

The first commercially available device capable of measuring biomechanical properties in a clinical setting is Ocular Response Analyzer (Fig. 17.33).[132] Initially considered as a device to measure IOP, it has developed into an instrument which can measure the innate corneal biomechanical properties in-vivo.

Principle: ORA analyzes the corneal response during the bidirectional applanation process induced by a high-speed air puff. Cornea being a viscoelastic tissue, absorbs energy during loading and dissipates it in the form of heat during unloading, resulting in a different stress-strain curve for loading and unloading and this difference or the energy dissipated represents corneal hysteresis (*see* Fig. 17.32B).

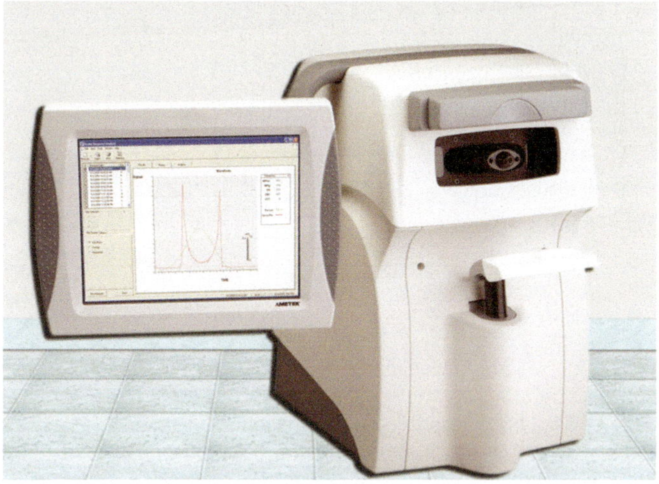

Fig. 17.33: Ocular response analyzer (ORA).

Mechanism: A high-speed pressurized air jet is applied, forcing the cornea to deform. As the air pressure causes cornea to move inwards, the cornea assumes a flattening or the first applanation (P1) state. Cornea indents further to a concave configuration until the air pressure decreases. Shortly within a microsecond, air pressure decreases and cornea again assumes a flattening or the second applanation state (P2) while becoming less concave and returning to the original convex state. The system monitors the complete process and records two pressure values during which the cornea started to applanate in either direction (P1 and P2). These two pressure values are not the same owing to the viscoelastic properties of the cornea.[132] The maximum air pressure applied with this instrument is not constant and is dependent on P1, a value determined by both the true IOP and the structural resistance of each individual eye.[132] Figure 17.34 illustrates the typical response waveform.

Parameters: The first version of the ORA provided only two biomechanical parameters namely corneal hysteresis (CH) and corneal resistance factor (CRF).

1. *Corneal hysteresis (CH)* is defined as the difference between the two pressures P1 and P2 recorded during the measurement. It represents the energy loss due to viscous damping in the cornea and extracorneal structures. This difference would be equal to 0 in an

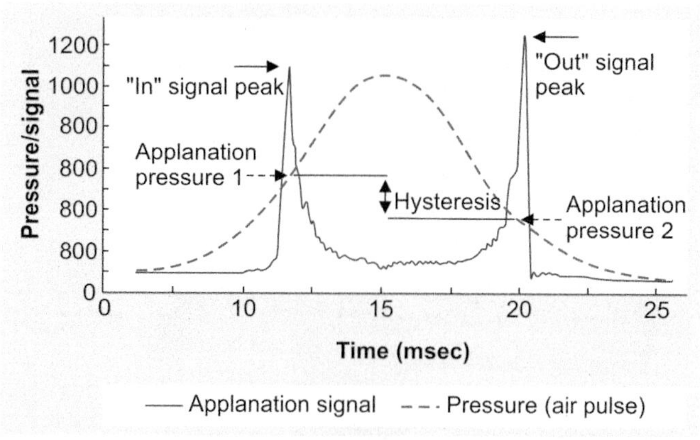

Fig. 17.34: Typical response waveform from ocular response analyzer (ORA). The solid line represents the applanation signal and the dashed line the pressure changes. The device delivers to the eye an air pulse, which causes the cornea to move inward achieving a specific applanation state or flattening (Pressure 1). Milliseconds after the first applanation, the pressure decreases and the cornea passes through a second applanated state (Pressure 2) while returning from concavity to its normal convex curvature. Both the applanation events are recognized by the peak of the corneal reflex signal which corresponds to two independent pressure valves on the air puff pressure profile. Corneal hysteresis represents the difference between these two pressures.

isotropic material and is always positive in a viscoelastic tissue. A higher CH indicates a greater capacity for absorption and dissipation of kinetic energy in the tissue.

2. *Corneal resistance factor (CRF)* is calculated using a linear equation and is related to the elastic properties of the cornea.[132] The CRF is derived from the formula (P1-kP2), where k is a constant. The constant k has a value determined from an empirical analysis of the relationship between both P1 and P2 and central corneal thickness.[133]

The ORA also reports 2 IOP values: The Goldmann-correlated IOP derived from the mean of P1 and P2 and the cornea-compensated IOP. The latter measurement is helpful in assessing IOP with some degree of compensation for atypical corneas.

Interpretation: In the normal healthy eye, the corneal hysteresis ranges between 9.3 ± 1.4 and 11.4 ± 1.5 mm Hg and CRF between 9.2 ± 1.4 and 11.9 ± 1.5 mm Hg.[134] Therefore, there is a significant variability in CH and CRF among normal healthy individuals that can be influenced by the variability of IOP in the same population. In spite of this variability, CH and CRF have been suggested to be potentially useful for discriminating healthy eyes from those suffering a pathological condition, such as corneal ectasia or glaucoma. Many authors have reported significantly lower CH in glaucomatous eyes compared to healthy eyes.[135-139] Similarly in cornea ectasia, many studies have reported significantly lower CH and CRF values compared to normal eyes[140-146] suggesting that viscous damping capacity and overall corneal resistance are reduced in these diseases.[132]

Limitations: CH and CRF have been demonstrated to be poor parameters for differentiating mild keratoconus from normal corneas.[145-146] In cross linked corneas, CH and CRF are expected to increase but several studies have demonstrated these parameters are not changed.[147] In an effort to address this issue, investigators and the manufacturers have come up with other characteristics provided by the ORA beyond CH and CRF. Because of the variability in air puff pressure in ORA, comparison cannot be made between eyes and across time and intervention.[148,149]

CorVis ST (Fig.17.35)

The combination of corneal topography, bidirectional applanation tonometry and high-speed photography has been suggested as a potentially useful concept for an integral analysis of the cornea, including corneal biomechanics. This combined technology has been called dynamic corneal topography. Corneal imaging can be obtained by means of a Scheimpflug camera or using spectral optical coherence tomography. Currently, the only device commercially available based on this concept is the CorVis ST from Oculus.

Principle: Similar to ORA.

Mechanism: A high speed pressurized air jet is applied to the cornea and is forced to deform. The corneal deformation is similar to that occurring in ORA. A high speed Scheimpflug camera (4,330 frames per second) records the bidirectional applanation movements of the cornea when subjected to air jet, which is then displayed in ultra-slow movement on the display panel. Specifically, the air jet of the tonometer forces the cornea through several distinct phases that are recorded on the Scheimpflug images (Fig. 17.36).

Parameters: The timing and corresponding pressure of the air puff at the first and second applanations and at the highest concavity (HC) are recorded (Fig. 17.36). Intraocular pressure is calculated based on the timing of the first applanation event. This initial IOP measurement is dependant of corneal resistance. Contrary to the ORA, in Corvis ST the air puff pressure remains constant. The deformation amplitude (DA) is represented by the maximum displacement of the apex in the highest concavity

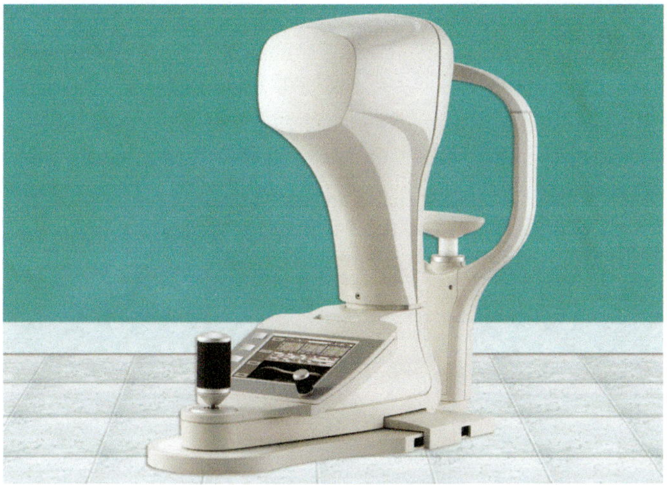

Fig. 17.35: Corvis® ST tonometer.

(HC) moment image (Fig. 17.36). The radius of curvature at HC is recorded. Applanation lengths (AL) and corneal velocities (CVel) are recorded during ingoing and outgoing phases (Figs. 17.36 and 17.37). Corneal thickness is also calculated through the horizontal Scheimpflug image. The lowest value is displayed. The above-mentioned parameters were computed in the first-generation software of the instrument. Several new parameters based on deformation cornea response (DCR) were introduced in the new software of the Corvis ST. Deformation amplitude ratio (DA Ratio 2 mm) is calculated as the ratio between the deformation of the apex and the average deformation amplitude 2 mm from the apex. The peak distance describes the distance between the two highest points of the cornea's temporal-nasal cross-section at the highest concavity moment

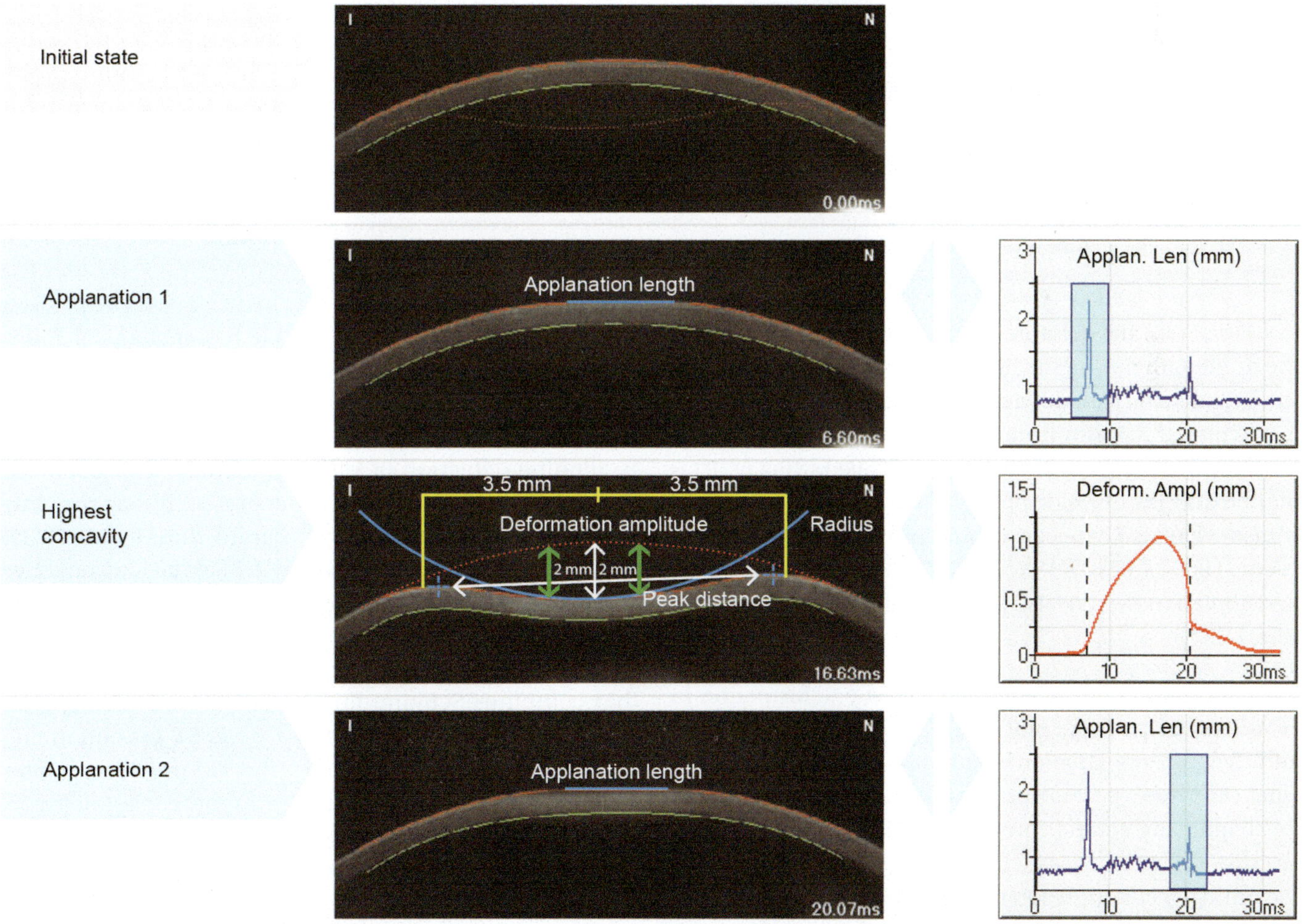

Fig. 17.36: Sequence of Scheimpflug images during Corvis ST measurement with different parameters mentioned along with their graphical representation.

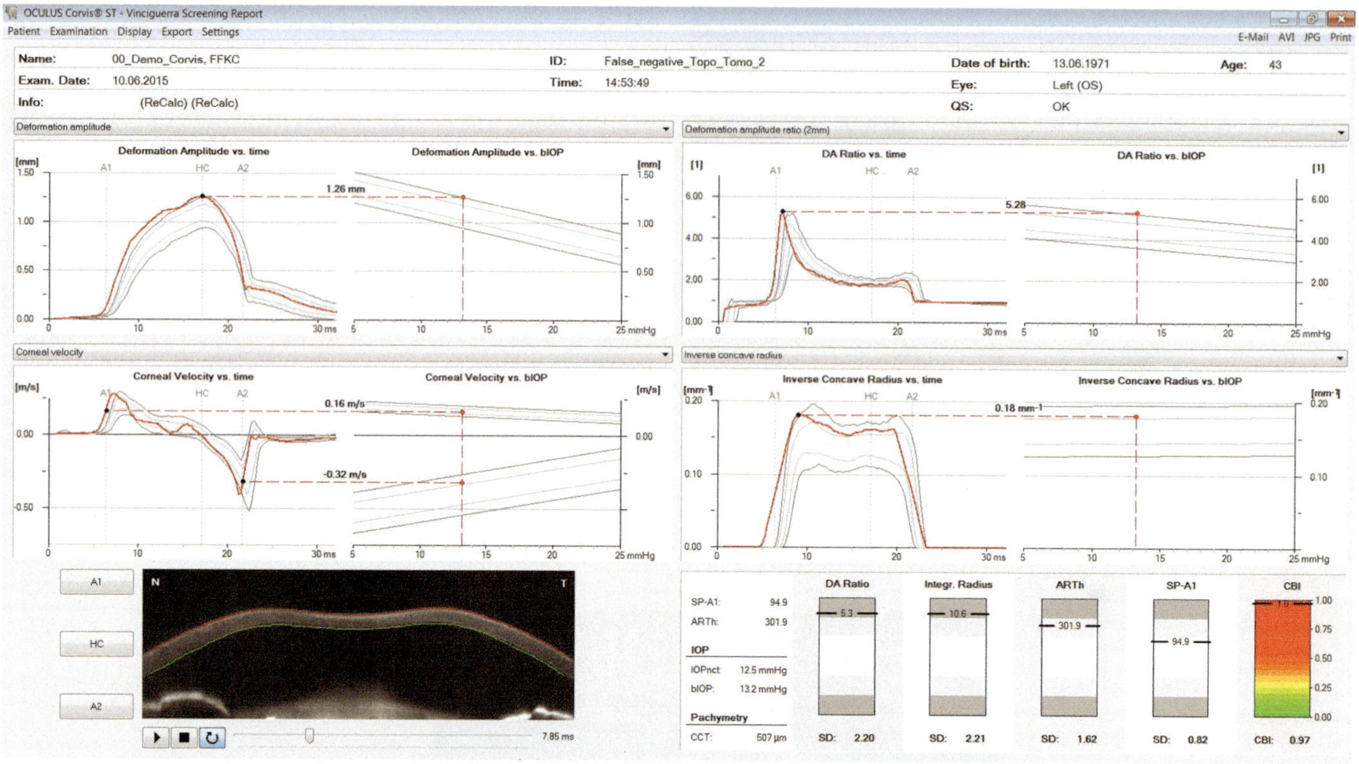

Fig. 17.37: Vinciguerra display for a forme fruste keratoconus showing the curves for different parameters such as deformation amplitude, corneal velocity, deformation amplitude ration 2 mm (DA ratio 2 mm) and inverse concave radius as against the time and biomechanic intraocular pressure (bIOP). The red line shows the patient's measurement and the faint black line shows the range of normative values (± 2SD). In addition, it also displays Corvis Biomechanical index (CBI) along with novel stiffness parameter like SP-A1 (stiffness parameter at first applanation).

(*see* Fig. 17.36) The delta arc-length describes the change of the arc-length during the highest concavity moment from the initial state, in a defined 7 mm zone. This parameter is calculated 3.5 mm from the apex to both sides in the horizontal direction. The inverse concave radius (1/R) is plotted over the duration of the air pulse and the integrated sum is calculated between the first and second applanation events (Fig. 17.37).[148,150] Novel stiffness parameters at the first applanation were also provided in the newer software (Fig. 17.37).

Interpretation: It has been found that the deformation in ectatic cornea is more pronounced along with higher DA and CVel. The applanation lengths in the ectatic cornea are smaller.[150] These parameters have been found to be useful for diagnosing ectatic corneas as well as for assessment of cross linked corneas. Greater negative magnitude in the radius of curvature after corneal collagen crosslinking or a flatter curvature at maximum deformation was observed.[150] The first set of parameters derived from the Corvis ST measurement had relatively low accuracy for keratoconus.[151-154] Later on Corvis Biomechanical Index (CBI) was developed using linear regression analysis which combined parameters from the deformation corneal response (DCR) and the horizontal thickness profile facilitating detection of keratoconus with high accuracy (Fig. 17.37).[155] With a cutoff value of 0.5 CBI has correctly classified 98.8% of the cases (keratoconus) with 98.4% specificity and 100% sensitivity.[155] CBI alone may not have such high sensitivity and specificity to separate healthy eyes from subclinical keratoconus. To overcome this tomographic/biomechanical index (TBI) was introduced that combines Scheimpflug-based corneal tomography and biomechanics analysis by Corvis ST for enhancing ectasia detection (Fig. 17.38).[156] The TBI provided greater accuracy for detecting ectasia than any other parameters.[156] The TBI was sensitive for detecting subclinical ectasia in eyes with normal topography where the fellow eye is clinically ectatic. A cut-off value of 0.35 correctly classified all ectasia cases from forme fruste to frank keratoconus.[156] It has been hypothesized that TBI may reflect the inherent susceptibility of the cornea to ectasia progression.

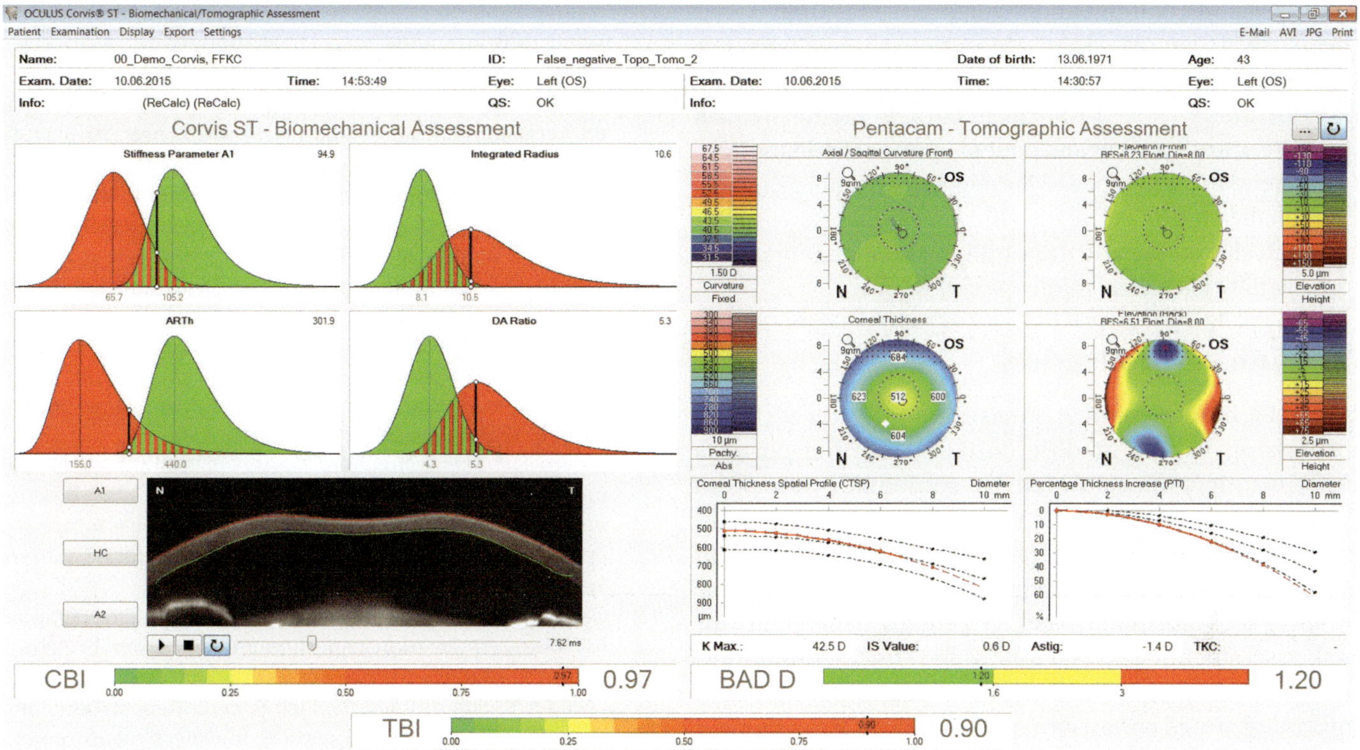

Fig. 17.38: Ambrósio, Roberts and Vinciguerra (ARV) Biomechanics and Tomographic Assessments which combines Scheimpflug based corneal tomographic and biomechanical analysis from Pentacam HR and Corvis ST exams respectively and gives a Tomographic/Biomechanical index (TBI) which has a very high accuracy for detecting early corneal ectatic diseases. In this example, the Pentacam seems to be normal whereas CBI and TBI values suggest ectasia.

Limitations: There are certain limitations to both ORA and Corvis ST as both are not designed to assess the spatial differences in the cornea properties across the width and depth of cornea and also extracorneal structures may have an influence in the corneal biomechanical measurements.[157]

Inspite of these limitations, both these devices have greatly helped in better understanding of the cornea biomechanical behavior. Corneal tomography when combined with corneal biomechanics has shown better refractive surgery screening potential.[158,159]

Brillouin Optical Microscopy

Brillouin optical microscopy is a technology that measure in-vivo corneal biomechanical properties through the analysis of light scatter.[128] The interaction of photons of the incident light with the acoustic phonons in the corneal tissue results in light scattering. A phonon is a unit of vibration of the lattice structure that makes up a material. Photons gain or lose energy from interaction with phonons, and this change corresponds with a shift in frequency in the Brillouin spectrum of the scattered light. Brillouin imaging have demonstrated to show differences between healthy and keratoconic corneas. It showed the mechanical loss was only concentrated in the area of corneal protrusion and outside this area the brillouin shift was comparable with the normal cornea.[160] Brillouin optical microscopy also showed increased stiffness following cross linking treatment and the differences between various protocols of cross linking.[161] Current limitations include a long acquisition time and the high cost of the equipment.

Finite Element Model

Finite element (FE) consists of a model which simulates the material or a design under study to be stressed and then later analyzed for specific results. For analysis, FE modeling uses a complex system of points called nodes that form a grid or mesh. The cornea and surrounding structures can be represented as a mesh of smaller geometric elements with specified material properties and interconnected at element nodes. The predictive value of any model depends on the validity of input and assumptions. FE analysis has been used to simulate surgical results in various refractive procedures as well as the biomechanical alterations in keratoconus.[135,162-165] Advances in corneal biomechanical property measurement and patient-specific modeling have the potential to enhance early keratoconus diagnosis, enable personalized, procedure-specific ectasia risk assessment through simulation and drive optimized treatment design for a variety of corneal refractive conditions.

Clinical Application

Corneal biomechanical measurements have shown promising results in differentiating normal corneas from ectatic corneas, which are sometimes missed on the regular topography. Its most important application would be in the field of refractive surgeries where it will help in improving the visual outcomes by providing better nomogram adjustments, and also enhance the ability for risk assessment of ectasia following refractive surgeries. It will help in decision making as to which laser refractive procedure would be best for a specific patient. Measurement of biomechanical changes after cross linking has reinforced the usefulness of these nonablative procedures and also made it possible to choose amongst the different cross-linking protocols. It also plays a major role inaccurate IOP measurement (which was till now dependant on the simple adjustment factor of central corneal thickness), by considering the innate biomechanical property of stiffness of the cornea.

REFERENCES

1. Scheiner C. O Oculus, hoc est: fundamentum opticum. Austria: Innsbruck; 1619.
2. Mandell R. Jesse: Inventor of the ophthalmometer. Am J Optom Arch Am Acad Optom. 1960;37:633-8.
3. Helmontz H von. Handbook per physiologicshen optik. Hamburg, Germany: Leopold Voss; 1909.
4. Javal L, Schiötz H. Un opthalmomètre pratique. Annales d'Oculistique, Paris. 1881;86:5-21.
5. Rio-Cristobal A, Martin R. Corneal assessment technologies: current status. Surv Ophthalmol. 2014;59:599-614.
6. Nover A. 100 years of ophthalmology. Fortschr Med. 1982;100(47-48):2222-7.
7. Maguire LJ, Singer DE, Klyce SD. Graphic Presentation of Computer-Analyzed Keratoscope Photographs. Arch Ophthalmol. 1987;105(2):223-30.
8. Oliveira CM, Ribeiro C, Franco S. Corneal imaging with slit-scanning and Scheimpflug imaging techniques. Clin Exp Optom. 2011;94:33-42.
9. Swartz T, Marten L, Wang M. Measuring the cornea: the latest developments in corneal topography. Curr Opin Ophthalmol. 2007;18:325-33.
10. Gomes JA, Tan D, Rapuano CJ, et al. Global consensus on keratoconus and ectatic diseases. Cornea. 2015;34(4):359-69.
11. Merklinger HM. Focusing the view camera: a scientific way to focus the view camera and estimate depth of field. Canada: Paperback; 1993.
12. Piñero DP. Technologies for anatomical and geometric characterization of the corneal structure and anterior segment: a review. Semin Ophthalmol. 2015;30(3):161-70.
13. Dubbelman M, Sicam VA, Van der Heijde GL. The shape of the anterior and posterior surface of the aging human cornea. Vision Res. 2006;46(6-7):993-1001.
14. Piñero DP, Saenz González C, Alió JL. Intraobserver and interobserver repeatability of curvature and aberrometric measurements of the posterior corneal surface in normal eyes using Scheimpflug photography. J Cataract Refract Surg. 2009;35(1):113-20.
15. Cairns G, McGhee CN. Orbscan computerized topography: Attributes, applications, and limitations. J Cataract Refract Surg. 2005;31:205-20.
16. Lackner B, Schmidinger G, Pieh S, et al. Repeatability and reproducibility of central corneal thickness measurement with Pentacam, Orbscan and ultrasound. Optom Vis Sci. 2005;82:892-9.
17. Charkrabarti HS, Craig JP, Brahma A, et al. Comparison of corneal thickness measurements using ultrasound and Orbscan slit-scanning topography in normal and post-LASIK eyes. J Cataract Refract Surg. 2001;27:1823-8.
18. Cairns G, Ormonde SE, Gray T, et al. Assessing the accuracy of Orbscan II post-LASIK: Apparent keratectasia is paradoxically associated with anterior chamber depth reduction in successful procedures. Clin Experiment Ophthalmol. 2005;33:147-52.
19. Arntz A, Dura JA, Pijoa JI. Subclinical keratoconus diagnosis by elevation topography. Arch Soc Esp Oftalmol. 2003;78:659-64.
20. Tanabe T, Oshika T, Tomodokoro A, et al. Standardized color-coded scales for anterior and posterior elevation maps of scanning slit corneal topography. Ophthalmology. 2002;109:1298-302.
21. Rao SN, Raviv T, Majmudar PA, et al. Role of Orbscan II in screening keratoconus suspects before refractive corneal surgery. Ophthalmology. 2002;109:1642-6.
22. Piñero DP, Alio JL, Aleso A, et al. Corneal volume, pachymetry, and correlation of anterior and posterior corneal shape in subclinical and different stages of clinical keratoconus. J Cataract Refract Surg. 2010;36:814-25.
23. Prakash G, Agarwal A, Mazhari AI, et al. A new, pachymetry-based approach for diagnostic cutoffs for normal, suspect and keratoconic cornea. Eye. 2012;26:650-7.
24. Marsich MW, Bullimore MA. The repeatability of corneal thickness measures. Cornea. 2000;19:792-5.

25. Gonzalez-Meijome JM, Cervino A, Yebra-Pimentel E, et al. Central and peripheral corneal thickness measurement with Orbscan II and topographical ultrasound pachymetry. J Cataract Refract Surg. 2003;29:125-32.
26. Giraldez Fernandez MJ, Diaz RA, Cervino A, et al. A comparison of two pachymetric systems: slit-scanning and ultrasonic. CLAO J. 2002;28:221-3.
27. Modis L Jr, Langenbucher A, Seitz B. Scanning-slit and specular microscopic pachymetry in comparison with ultrasonic determination of corneal thickness. Cornea. 2001;20(7):711-4.
28. Yaylali V, Kaufman SC, Thompson HW. Corneal thickness measurements with the Orbscan Topography System and ultrasonic pachymetry. J Cataract Refract Surg. 1997;23: 1345-50.
29. Basmak H, Sahin A, Yildirim N. The reliability of central corneal thickness measurements by ultrasound and by Orbscan system in school children. Curr Eye Res. 2006;31:569-75.
30. Uçakhan OO, Ozkan M, Kanpolat A. Corneal thickness measurements in normal and keratoconic eyes: Pentacam comprehensive eye scanner versus noncontact specular microscopy and ultrasound pachymetry. J Cataract Refract Surg. 2006;32(6):970-7.
31. de Sanctis U, Missolungi A, Mutani B, et al. Reproducibility and repeatability of central corneal thickness measurement in keratoconus using the rotating Scheimpflug camera and ultrasound pachymetry. Am J Ophthalmol. 2007;144:712-8.
32. Montalbán R. Caracterización y validación diagnóstica de la correlación de la geometría de las dos superficies de la córnea humana. Alicante: Universidad de Alicante; 2013.
33. Smolek MK, Klyce SD. Current keratoconus detection methods compared with a neural network approach. Invest Ophthalmol Vis Sci. 1997;38(11):2290-9.
34. Maeda N, Klyce SD, Smolek MK, et al. Automated keratoconus screening with corneal topography analysis. Invest Ophthalmol Vis Sci. 1994;35(6):2749-57.
35. Rabinowitz YS, McDonnell PJ. Computer-assisted corneal topography in keratoconus. Refract Corneal Surg. 1989;5(6):400-8.
36. Albertazzi R. Queratocono: pautas para su diagnóstico y tratamiento. Buenos Aires: Ediciones Científicas Argentinas; 2010.
37. Rabinowitz YS, Rasheed K. KISA% index: a quantitative videokeratography algorithm embodying minimal topographic criteria for diagnosing keratoconus. J Cataract Refract Surg. 1999;25(10):1327-35.
38. Ambrósio R Jr, Belin MW. Imaging of the cornea: topography vs tomography. J Refract Surg. 2010;26:847-9.
39. Belin MW, Ambrosio R. Corneal ectasia risk score system—"statistical validity and clinical relevance" J Refract Surg. 2010;26(4):238-40.
40. Maeda N, Klyce S, Smolek M. Comparison of methods for detecting keratoconus using videokeratography. Arch Ophthalmol. 1995;113:870-4.
41. Lopos B, Ramos IC, Correia FF, et al. Correlation of topometric and tomographic indices with visual acuity in patients with keratoconus. Int J Keratoco Ectatic Corneal Dis. 2012;1:167-72.
42. Correia FF, Ramos I, Lopes B, et al. Topometric and tomographic indices for the diagnosis of keratoconus. Int J Keratoco Ectatic Corneal Dis. 2012;1:92-9.
43. Gilani F, Cortese M, Ambrosio RR Jr, et al. Comprehensive anterior segment normal values generated by rotating Scheimpflug tomography. J Cat Refract Surg. 2013;39: 1707-12.
44. Villavicencio OF, Gilani F, Henriquez MA, et al. Independent population validation of the Belin/Ambrosio enhanced ectasia display: Implications for keratoconus studies and screening. Int J Keratoco Ectatic Corneal Dis. 2014;3:1-8.
45. Muftuoglu O, Ayar O, Hurmeric V, et al. Comparison of multimetric D index with keratometric, pachymetric, and posterior elevation parameters in diagnosing subclinical keratoconus in fellow eyes of asymmetric keratoconus patients. J Cataract Refract Surg. 2015;41:557-65.
46. Ambrósio Jr R, Faria-Correia F, Ramos I, et al. Enhanced screening for ectasia susceptibility among refractive candidates: the role of corneal tomography and biomechanics. Curr Ophthalmol Rep. 2013;1:28-38.
47. Saad A, Gatinel D. Bilateral corneal ectasia after laser in situ keratomileusis in patient with isolated difference in central corneal thickness between eyes. J Cataract Refract Surg. 2010;36:1033-5.
48. Khachikian SS, Belin MW, Ciolino JB. Intrasubject pachymetric asymmetry analysis. J Refract Surg. 2008;24: 606-9.
49. Ambrósio Jr R, Caiado AL, Guerra FP, et al. Novel Pachymetric Parameters based on corneal tomography for diagnosing keratoconus. J Refract Surg. 2011;27(10):753-8.
50. Jonsson M, Behndig A. Pachymetric evaluation prior to laser in situ keratomileusis. J Cataract Refract Surg. 2005;31: 701-6.
51. Ambrósio R Jr, Alonso RS, Luz A, et al. Corneal-thickness spatial profile and corneal-volume distribution: tomographic indices to detect keratoconus. J Cataract Refract Surg. 2006;32(11):1851-9.
52. Muftuoglu O, Ayar O, Ozulken K, et al. Posterior corneal elevation and back difference corneal elevation in diagnosing forme fruste keratoconus in the fellow eyes of unilateral keratoconus patients. J Cataract Refract Surg. 2013;39:1348-57.
53. Kovacs I, Mihaltz K, Kranitz K, et al. Accuracy of machine learning classifiers using bilateral data from a Scheimpflug camera for identifying eyes with preclinical signs of keratoconus. J Cataract Refract Surg. 2016;42:275-83.
54. Lim HB, Tan GS, Lim L, Htoon HM. Comparison of keratometric and pachymetric parameters with Scheimpflug imaging in normal and keratoconic Asian eyes. Clin Ophthalmol. 2014;8:2215-20.

55. Ruiseñor Vázquez PR, Galletti JD, Minguez N, et al. Pentacam Scheimpflug tomography findings in topographically normal patients and subclinical keratoconus cases. Am J Ophthalmol. 2014;158:32-40.
56. Martinez-Abad A, Pinero DP. New perspectives on the detection and progression of keratoconus. J Cataract Refract Surg. 2017;43(9):1213-27.
57. Muckenhirn D. Die Anpassung von asphérischen Kontaktlinsen bei Keratoconus unter Berücksichtigung der geometrisch-optischen Verhät-nissen der Hornhaut. Neues Optik J. 1984;5:67-94.
58. Ciolino J, Belin MW. Changes to the posterior cornea after LASIK and PRK. J Cataract Refract Surg. 2006;32:1426-31.
59. Giessler S, Duncker GI. Orbscan pachymetry after LASIK is not reliable [letter]. J Refract Surg. 2001;17:385-7.
60. Beuerman RW, Maurice DM, Tanelian DL. Thermal stimulation of the cornea. In: Anderson D, Mathews B (Ed). Pain in the trigeminal region. New York: North-Holland Biomedical; 1977.
61. Dupuy B, Thompson H, Beurman RW. Capsaicin: a psychophysical tool to explore corneal sensitivity. Invest Ophthalmol Vis Sci. 1988;29(Suppl):454.
62. Brennan NA, Maurice DM. Corneal esthesiometry with a carbon dioxide laser. Invest Ophthalmol Vis Sci. 1989;30(Suppl):148.
63. Zaidman G, Gould H, Weinstein C, et al. Corneal sensitivity mapping studies in postsurgical patients. Invest Ophthalmol Vis Sci. 1989;30(Suppl):338.
64. Thorgaard GL, Holland EJ, Krachmer JH. Corneal edema induced by cold in trigeminal nerve palsy. Am J Ophthalmol. 1987;103:641-6.
65. Lawrenson JG, Ruskell GL. Investigation of limbal touch sensitivity using a Cochet-Bonnet aesthesiometer. Br J Ophthalmol. 1993;77:339-43.
66. Brennan NA, Bruce AS. Esthesiometry as an indicator of corneal health. Optom Vis Sci. 1991;68:699-702.
67. Rao GN, John T, Ishida N, et al. Recovery of corneal sensitivity in grafts following penetrating keratoplasty. Ophthalmology. 1985;92:1408-11.
68. Donnenfeld ED, Solomon K, Perry HD, et al. The effect of hinge position on corneal sensation and dry eye after LASIK. Ophthalmology. 2003;110:1023-30.
69. Feenstra RPG, Tseng SCG. Comparison of fluorescein and rose Bengal staining. Ophthalmology. 1992;99:605-17.
70. Feenstra RPG, Tseng SCG. What's actually stained by rose Bengal? Arch Ophthalmol. 1992;110:984-93.
71. Kim J, Foulks GN. Evaluation of the effect of lissamine green and rose Bengal on human corneal epithelial cells. Cornea. 1999;18:328-32.
72. Khurana AK, Chaudhary R, Ahluwalia BK, et al. Tear film profile in dry eye. Acta Ophthalmol. 1991;69:79-86.
73. Fakhry MA, Artola A, Belda JI, et al. Comparison of corneal pachymetry using ultrasound and Orbscan II. J Cataract Refract Surg. 2002;28(2):248-52.
74. McLaren JW, Nau CB, Erie JC, et al. Corneal thickness measured by confocal microscopy, ultrasound, and scanning slit methods. Am J Ophthalmol. 2004;137(6): 1011-20.
75. Rainer G, Findl O, Petternel V, et al. Central corneal thickness measurements with partial coherence interferometry, ultrasound, and the Orbscan system. Ophthalmology. 2004;111(5):875-9.
76. Radford SW, Lim R, Salmon JF. Comparison of Orbscan and ultrasound pachymetry in the measurement of central corneal thickness. Eye. 2004;18(4):434-6.
77. Amano S, Honda N, Amano Y, et al. Comparison of central corneal thickness measurements by rotating Scheimpflug camera, ultrasonic pachymetry, and scanning-slit corneal topography. Ophthalmology. 2006;113(6):937-41.
78. Doughty MJ, Jonuscheit S. The Orbscan acoustic (correction) factor for central corneal thickness measures of normal human corneas. Eye Cont Lens. 2010;36(2):106-15.
79. Dutta D, Rao HL, Addepalli UK, et al. Corneal thickness in keratoconus: comparing optical, ultrasound, and optical coherence tomography pachymetry. Ophthalmology. 2013;120(3):457-63.
80. Gherghel D, Hosking SL, Mantry S, et al. Corneal pachymetry in normal and keratoconic eyes: Orbscan II versus ultrasound. J Cataract Refract Surg. 2004;30(6): 1272-7.
81. Crawford AZ, Patel DV, McGhee CN. Comparison and repeatability of keratometric and corneal power measurements obtained by Orbscan II, Pentacam, and Galilei corneal tomography systems. Am J Ophthalmol. 2013;156(1):53-60.
82. Faramarzi A, Karimian F, Jafarinasab MR, et al. Central corneal thickness measurements after myopic photorefractive keratectomy using Scheimpflug imaging, scanning-slit topography, and ultrasonic pachymetry. J Cataract Refract Surg. 2010;36(9):1543-9.
83. Rosa N, Lanza M, Borrelli M, et al. Comparison of central corneal thickness measured with Orbscan and Pentacam. J Refract Surg. 2007;23(9):895-9.
84. Sedaghat MR, Daneshvar R, Kargozar A, et al. Comparison of central corneal thickness measurement using ultrasonic pachymetry, rotating Scheimpflug camera, and scanning-slit topography. Am J Ophthalmol. 2010;150(6):780-9.
85. Buehl W, Stojanac D, Sacu S, et al. Comparison of three methods of measuring corneal thickness and anterior chamber depth. Am J Ophthalmol. 2006;141(1):7-12.
86. Kim SW, Byun YJ, Kim EK, Kim TI. Central corneal thickness measurements in unoperated eyes and eyes after PRK for myopia using Pentacam, Orbscan II, and ultrasonic pachymetry. J Refract Surg. 2007;23(9):888-94.
87. Meyer JJ, Gokul A, Vellara HR, et al. Repeatability and Agreement of Orbscan II, Pentacam HR, and Galilei Tomography Systems in Corneas With Keratoconus. Am J Ophthalmol. 2017;175:122-8.

88. Meenakshi Sundaram S, Sufi AR, Prajna NV, et al. Comparison of In Vivo Confocal Microscopy, Ultrasonic Pachymetry, and Scheimpflug Topography for Measuring Central Corneal Thickness. JAMA Ophthalmol. 2016;134(9):1057-9.
89. Salvetat ML, Zeppieri M, Miani F, et al. Comparison between laser scanning in vivo confocal microscopy and noncontact specular microscopy in assessing corneal endothelial cell density and central corneal thickness. Cornea. 2011;30(7):754-9.
90. Suzuki S, Oshikia T, Oki K, et al. Corneal thickness measurements: scanning-slit corneal topography and noncontact specular microscopy versus ultrasonic pachymetry. J Cataract Refract Surg. 2003;29(7):1313-8.
91. Bovelle R, Kaufman SC, Thompson HW, et al. Corneal thickness measurements with Topcon SP-2000P specular microscope and an ultrasound pachymeter. Arch Ophthalmol. 1999;117(7):868-70.
92. Módis L, Langenbucher A, Seitz B. Corneal thickness measurements with contact and noncontact specular microscopic and ultrasound pachymetry. Am J Ophthalmol. 2001;132(4):517-21.
93. Kawana K, Tokunaga T, Miyata K, et al. Comparison of corneal thickness measurements using Orbscan II, non-contact specular microscopy, and ultrasonic pachymetry in eye after laser in situ keratomileusis. Br J Ophthalmol. 2004;88(4):466-8.
94. Kawana K, Miyata K, Tokunaga T, et al. Central corneal thickness measurements using Orbscan II scanning slit topography, noncontact specular microscopy, and ultrasonic pachymetry in eyes with keratoconus. Cornea. 2005;24(8):967-71.
95. Huang J, Pesudovs K, Wen D, et al. Comparison of anterior segment measurements with rotating Scheimpflug photography and partial coherence reflectometry. J Cataract Refract Surg. 2011;37(2):341-8.
96. Hashemi H, Roshani M, Mehravaran S, et al. Effect of corneal thickness on the agreement between ultrasound and Orbscan II pachymetry. J Cataract Refract Surg. 2007;33(10):1694-700.
97. Maurice DM. Cellular membrane activity in the corneal endothelium of the intact eye. Experientia. 1968;24:1094-5.
98. Laing RA, Sandstrom MM, Leibowitz HM. Clinical specular microscopy. I. Optical principles. Arch Ophthalmol. 1979;97:1714-9.
99. Abib FC, Barreto Jr J. Behavior of corneal endothelial density over a lifetime. J Cataract Refract Surg. 2001;27:1574-8.
100. Armitage WJ, Dick AD, Bourne WM. Predicting endothelial cell loss and long-term corneal graph survival. Invest Ophthalmol Vis Sci. 2003;44:3326-31.
101. Laing RA, Sandstrom M, Leibowitz HM. In vivo photomicrography of the corneal endothelium. Arch Ophthalmol. 1975;93:143-5.
102. McCarey BE. Noncontact specular microscopy: a macrophotography technique and some endothelial cell findings. Ophthalmology. 1979;86:1848-60.
103. Hoffer KJ. Corneal decomposition after corneal endothelium cell count. Am J Ophthalmol. 1979;87:252-3.
104. Yee RW, Matsuda M, Schultz RO, et al. Changes in the normal corneal endothelial cellular pattern as a function of age. Curr Eye Res. 1985;4:671-8.
105. Bursell SE, Hultgren BH, Laing RA. Evaluation of the corneal endothelial mosaic using an analysis of nearest neighbor distances. Exp Eye Res. 1981;32:31-8.
106. Ohno K, Nelson LR, McLaren JW, et al. Comparison of recording systems and analysis methods in specular microscopy. Cornea. 1999;18:416-23.
107. Benetz BAM, Diaconu E, Bowlin SJ, et al. Comparison of corneal endothelial image analysis by Konan SP8000 noncontact and bio-optics Bambi systems. Cornea. 1999;18:67-72.
108. Borderie VM, Scheer S, Touzeau O, et al. Donor organ cultured corneal tissue selection before penetrating keratoplasty. Br J Ophthalmol. 1998;82:382-8.
109. Goldmann H. Spaltlampenphotographie und-photometrie. Ophthalmologica. 1940;98:257-70.
110. Minsky M. Memoir on inventing the confocal scanning microscope. Scanning. 1988;10:128-38.
111. Lukosz W. Optical systems with resolving powers exceeding the classical limit. J Opt Soc Am. 1966;57:1190.
112. McLaren JW, Nau CB, Patel SV, et al. Measuring corneal thickness with the Confoscan 4 and z-ring adapter. Eye Cont Lens. 2007;33:185-90.
113. Semwogerere D, Weeks ER. Confocal microscopy. In: Wnek GE, Bowlin GL (Eds). Encyclopedia of biomaterials and biomedical engineering. London: Taylor & Francis; 2005. pp. 1-10
114. Petran MH, Hadravsky M, Egger MD, et al. Tandem scanning reflected light microscope. J Optics Soc Am. 1968;58:661-4.
115. Cavanagh HD, Jester JV, Essepian J, et al. Confocal microscopy of the living eye. CLAO J. 1990;16:65-73.
116. Chidambaram JD, Prajna NV, Larke NL, et al. Prospective study of the diagnostic accuracy of the in vivo laser scanning confocal microscope for severe microbial keratitis. Ophthalmology. 2016;123:2285-93.
117. Patel SV, Erie JC, McLaren JW, et al. Confocal microscopy changes in epithelial and stromal thickness up to 7 years after LASIK and PRK for myopia. J Refract Surg. 2007;23: 385-92.
118. L Komai Y, Ushiki T. The three-dimensional organization of collagen fibrils in the human cornea and sclera. Invest Ophthalmol Vis Sci. 1991;32:2244-58.
119. Newton RH, Meek KM. The integration of the corneal and limbal fibrils in the human eye. Biophys J. 1998;75:2508-12.
120. De Stefano VS, Dupps WJ Jr. Biomechanical Diagnostics of the Cornea. Int Ophthalmol Clin. 2017;57(3):75-86.

121. Andreassen TT, Simonsen AH, Oxlund H. Biomechanical properties of keratoconus and normal corneas. Exp Eye Res. 1980;31(4):435-41.
122. Elsheikh A, Geraghty B, Rama P, et al. Characterization of age-related variation in corneal biomechanical properties. J R Soc Interface. 2010;7(51):1475-85.
123. Liu J, Roberts CJ. Influence of corneal biomechanical properties on intraocular pressure measurement: quantitative analysis. J Cataract Refract Surg. 2005;31(1):146-55.
124. Dupps WJ Jr. Biomechanical modeling of corneal ectasia. J Refract Surg. 2005;21(2):186-90.
125. Carvalho LA, Prado M, Cunha RH, et al. Keratoconus prediction using a finite element model of the cornea with local biomechanical properties. Arq Bras Oftalmol. 2009;72(2):139-45.
126. Knox Cartwright NE, Tyrer JR, Marshall J. Age-related differences in the elasticity of the human cornea. Invest Ophthalmol Vis Sci. 2011;52(7):4324-9.
127. Jaycock PD, Lobo L, Ibrahim J, et al. Interferometric technique to measure biomechanical changes in the cornea induced by refractive surgery. J Cataract Refract Surg. 2005;31(1):175-84.
128. Scarcelli G, Pineda R, Yun SH. Brillouin optical microscopy for corneal biomechanics. Invest Ophthalmol Vis Sci. 2012;53(1):185-90.
129. Dorronsoro C, Pascual D, Perez-Merino P, et al. Dynamic OCT measurement of corneal deformation by an air puff in normal and cross-linked corneas. Biomed Opt Express. 2012;3(3):473-87.
130. Grabner G, Eilmsteiner R, Steindl C, et al. Dynamic corneal imaging. J Cataract Refract Surg. 2005;31(1):163-74.
131. Bonatti JA, Bechara SJ, Carricondo PC, et al. Proposal for a new approach to corneal biomechanics: dynamic corneal topography. Arq Bras Oftalmol. 2009;72(2):264-7.
132. Luce DA. Determining in vivo biomechanical properties of the cornea with an ocular response analyzer. J Cataract Refract Surg. 2005;31(1):156-62.
133. Kotecha A. What biomechanical properties of the cornea are relevant for the clinician? Surv Ophthalmol 2007;52:S109-S114.
134. Piñero DP, Alcón N. In vivo characterization of corneal biomechanics. J Cataract Refract Surg. 2014;40:870-87.
135. Gatzioufas Z, Labiris G, Stachs O, et al. Biomechanical profile of the cornea in primary congenital glaucoma. Acta Ophthalmol. 2013;91:e29-e34.
136. Grise-Dulac A, Saad A, Abitbol O, et al. Assessment of corneal biomechanical properties in normal tension glaucoma and comparison with open-angle glaucoma, ocular hypertension, and normal eyes. J Glaucoma. 2012;21:486-9.
137. De Moraes CV, Hill V, Tello C, et al. Lower corneal hysteresis is associated with more rapid glaucomatous visual field progression. J Glaucoma. 2012;21:209-13.
138. Abitbol O, Bouden J, Doan S, et al. Corneal hysteresis measured with the Ocular Response Analyzer in normal and glaucomatous eyes. Acta Ophthalmol. 2010;88:116-9.
139. Sullivan-Mee M, Billingsley SC, Patel AD, et al. Ocular Response Analyzer in subjects with and without glaucoma. Optom Vis Sci. 2008;85:463-70.
140. Ortiz D, Piñero D, Shabayek MH, et al. Corneal biomechanical properties in normal, post-laser in situ keratomileusis, and keratoconic eyes. J Cataract Refract Surg. 2007;33:1371-5.
141. Galletti JG, Pförtner T, Bonthoux FF. Improved keratoconus detection by ocular response analyzer testing after consideration of corneal thickness as a confounding factor. J Refract Surg. 2012;28:202-8.
142. Touboul D, Benard A, Mahmoud AM, et al. Early biomechanical keratoconus pattern measured with an ocular response analyzer: curve analysis. J Cataract Refract Surg 2011;37:2144-22150.
143. Alió JL, Piñero DP, Alesón A, et al. Keratoconus-integrated characterization considering anterior corneal aberrations, internal astigmatism, and corneal biomechanics. J Cataract Refract Surg. 2011;37:552-68.
144. Fontes BM, Ambrósio R Jr, Velarde GC, et al. Corneal biomechanical evaluation in healthy thin corneas compared with matched keratoconus cases. Arq Bras Oftalmol. 2011;74:13-6.
145. Fontes BM, Ambrósio R Jr, Jardim D, et al. Corneal biomechanical metrics and anterior segment parameters in mild keratoconus. Ophthalmology. 2010;117:673-9.
146. Shah S, Laiquzzaman M, Bhojwani R, et al. Assessment of the biomechanical properties of the cornea with the ocular response analyzer in normal and keratoconic eyes. Invest Ophthalmol Vis Sci. 2007;48:3026-31.
147. Goldich Y, Marcovich AL, Barkana Y, et al. Clinical and corneal biomechanical changes after collagen cross-linking with riboflavin and UV irradiation in patients with progressive keratoconus: results after 2 years of follow-up. Cornea. 2012;31:609-14.
148. Roberts CJ. Concepts and misconceptions in corneal biomechanics. J Cataract Refract Surg. 2014;40:862-9.
149. Roberts CJ. Importance of accurately assessing biomechanics of the cornea. Curr Opin Ophthalmol. 2016;27:285-91.
150. Ambrósio R Jr, Ramos I, Luz A, et al. Dynamic ultra-high speed Scheimpflug imaging for assessing corneal biomechanical properties. Rev Bras Oftalmol. 2013;72:99-102.
151. Ali NQ, Patel DV, McGhee CN. Biomechanical responses of healthy and keratoconic corneas measured using a noncontact Scheimpflug based tonometer. Invest Ophthalmol Vis Sci. 2014;55:3651-9.
152. Bak-Nielsen S, Pedersen IB, Ivarsen A, et al. Dynamic Scheimpflug based assessment of keratoconus and the effects of corneal cross-linking. J Refract Surg. 2014;30:408-14.

153. Steinberg J, Katz T, Lucke K, et al. Screening for keratoconus with new dynamic biomechanical in vivo Scheimpflug analyses. Cornea. 2015;34:1404-12.
154. Ambrósio R Jr, Lopes B, Faria-Correia F, et al. Ectasia detection by the assessment of corneal biomechanics. Cornea. 2016;35:e18-e20.
155. Vinciguerra R, Ambrósio R Jr, Elsheikh A, et al. Detection of keratoconus with a new biomechanical index. J Refract Surg. 2016;32:803-10.
156. Ambrósio R Jr, Lopes B, Faria-Correia F, et al. Integration of Scheimpflug based corneal tomography and biomechanical assessments for enhancing ectasia detection. J Refract Surg. 2017;33(7):434-43.
157. Kling S, Marcos S. Contributing factors to corneal deformation in air puff measurements. Invest Ophthalmol Vis Sci. 2013;54:5078-85.
158. Luz A, Lopes B, Hallahan KM, et al. Discriminant value of custom ocular response analyzer waveform derivatives in forme fruste keratoconus. Am J Ophthalmol. 2016;164:14-21.
159. Vinciguerra R, Elsheikh A, Roberts CJ, et al. Influence of pachymetry and intraocular pressure on dynamic corneal response parameters in healthy patients. J Refract Surg. 2016;32:550-61.
160. Scarcelli G, Besner S, Pineda R, Yun SH. Biomechanical characterization of keratoconus corneas ex vivo with Brillouin microscopy. Invest Ophthalmol Vis Sci. 2014;55(7):4490-5.
161. Scarcelli G, Kling S, Quijano E, et al. Brillouin microscopy of collagen crosslinking: noncontact depth-dependent analysis of corneal elastic modulus. Invest Ophthalmol Vis Sci. 2013;54(2):1418-25.
162. Sinha Roy A, Dupps WJ, Roberts CJ. Comparison of biomechanical effects of small incision lenticule extraction and laser in situ keratomileusis: finite-element analysis. J Cataract Refract Surg. 2014;40:971-80.
163. Sinha Roy A, Dupps WJ. Effects of altered corneal stiffness on native and postoperative LASIK corneal biomechanical behavior: a whole-eye finite element analysis. J Refract Surg. 2009;25:875-87.
164. Seven I, Sinha Roy A, Dupps WJ. Patterned corneal collagen crosslinking for astigmatism: computational modeling study. J Cataract Refract Surg. 2014;40:943-53.
165. Seven I, Vahdati A, De Stefano VS, et al. Comparison of patient-specific computational modeling predictions and clinical outcomes of LASIK for myopia. Invest Ophthalmol Vis Sci. 2016;57:6287-97.

Chapter 18 Infectious Conjunctivitis

Jeremy JSL Hoffman, Matthew J Burton

INTRODUCTION

The conjunctivae are thin, predominantly squamous cell epithelial surfaces, that cover the anterior part of the sclera ("bulbar" conjunctiva), beginning at the corneal limbus and reflecting back on itself (forming the conjunctival fornices), to cover the inner surface of the eyelids ("palpebral" or "tarsal" conjunctiva). Infection, which is considered in this chapter, and non-infectious inflammation (*see* Chapter 19), of the conjunctiva is known as *conjunctivitis.* Conjunctivitis is characterized by conjunctival vascular vasodilation causing hyperemia, edema (chemosis) and frequently discharge.[1] Infectious causes of conjunctivitis include bacteria (including *Chlamydia trachomatis* and mycobacteria), viruses and fungi.

Infectious conjunctivitis is a common problem, affecting all ages: it is estimated to affect 6 million Americans annually.[2,3] Conjunctivitis accounts for approximately 1% of all primary care attendances in the UK and USA.[4,5] The overall incidence in England is approximately 13/1,000/year, with the rate highest in children under one-year-old (80 cases per 1,000-patient years).[6,7] There is also a considerable economic cost to the problem: data from 2005 suggest an annual cost of between $377 to $857 million per year for treating bacterial conjunctivitis in the United States alone.[8]

As infectious conjunctivitis is a common usually self-limiting presentation, particularly to non-ophthalmologists, it is important to be able to recognize it and exclude other, more serious pathology. It is also important to differentiate between the infectious and non-infectious causes of conjunctivitis, as well as between the various infectious agents as the management of these can be different. This chapter aims to present relevant background information on the condition in a pragmatic, clinically-orientated fashion to enable the reader to formulate an accurate differential diagnosis and management plan.

ETIOLOGY

Infectious conjunctivitis can be broadly divided by the responsible organism: bacterial, viral or rarely fungal (Table 18.1). These different infectious agents may have distinct clinical features, but it is often difficult to accurately distinguish the underlying organism on signs and symptoms alone. Investigations can therefore prove useful in the context of diagnostic uncertainty given equivocal clinical signs and symptoms. Each subtype of infectious conjunctivitis is described in detail later.

BACTERIAL CONJUNCTIVITIS

Conjunctival Microbiota

The conjunctiva is not a sterile site; it is populated by a diverse collection of bacterial organisms. Commensal bacteria typically include *Staphylococcus epidermidis, Staphylococcus aureus* and *Corynebacterium spp.* Less frequently isolated are *Propionibacterium acnes, Moraxella catarrhalis, Haemophilus influenzae* and *Streptococcus spp.*[9] This work was based on culture techniques; more recent microbiota studies using 16S rRNA sequencing identified the genera *Pseudomonas, Bradyrhizobium, Propionibacterium, Acinetobacter,* and *Corynebacterium* as the most frequently present organisms on the ocular surface.[10] On average there are 221 species of microorganisms present.[11] The proportion of different organisms varies with age and location, with gram negative species becoming more common with increasing age.[12] These organisms usually live in symbiosis with their host, only causing disease if the host defenses fail, or if there is an over proliferation of certain organisms.[13] There is also growing evidence that the normal conjunctival microbiota can help prevent ocular infections by preventing colonization by pathogenic species.[10] For example, a reduction in the homeostatic conjunctival microbiota has been associated with the emergence of a pathological microbiome dominated by *Pseudomonas aeruginosa,* leading to microbial keratitis.[14]

Epidemiology

An intact epithelium is usually able to prevent bacterial penetration; disorders that disrupt this such as dry eye

Table 18.1: Main causes of infectious conjunctivitis, microorganism, clinical presentation, investigations and management.

Category	Microorganism	Epidemiology	Symptoms	Signs	Investigations	Management	Photograph
Bacterial	• *Staphylococcus epidermidis* • *Staphylococcus aureus* • *Corynebacterium spp.* • *Propionibacterium acnes* • *Moraxella catarrhalis* • *Haemophilus influenza* • *Streptococcus spp.*	• 135 cases per 10,000 population in the USA • About 18–57% of all acute conjunctivitis • More common in young and elderly (bimodal distribution)	Mucopurulent discharge	• Conjunctival hyperemia • Papillae • Follicles • Mucopurulent discharge	• None routine • Conjunctival swabs for microscopy, culture and sensitivities (MCS), if not resolving or atypical/ sexually transmitted infection suspected	Topical antibiotics (particularly if contact lens wearer, ocular surface disease), e.g. chloramphenicol QDS 1/52	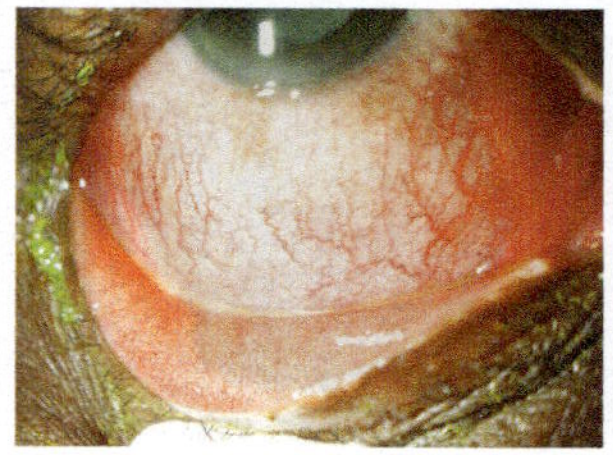
Chlamydial	• *C. trachomatis* • Serovars **A-C** – Trachoma • Serovars **D-K** – adult inclusion conjunctivitis	About 1.8–5.6% of all acute conjunctivitis	Variable	• Conjunctival hyperemia • Follicles	Swabs for PCR	PO azithromycin 1g stat G Azithromycin BD 3/7	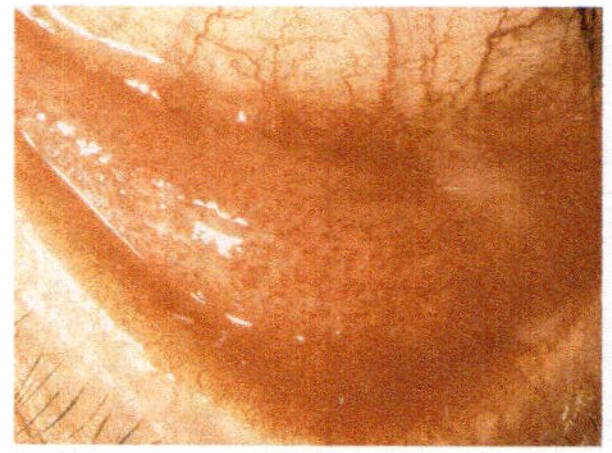
Viral	• Adenovirus (65%) • Herpes Simplex virus (HSV) • Molluscum contagiosum • *Numerous others: see* Box 18.1	• Up to 80.3% of all acute conjunctivitis • Young and middle aged	• Serous discharge • Foreign body sensation • Reduced vision and discomfort, if keratitis	• Conjunctival hyperemia • Tarsal conjunctival follicles • Tender pre-auricular lymphadenopathy • Conjunctival membranes or pseudomem-branes	• None, routine swabs for PCR and/or viral culture • Rapid diagnostic test	Symptomatic relief (cold compresses, artificial tears)	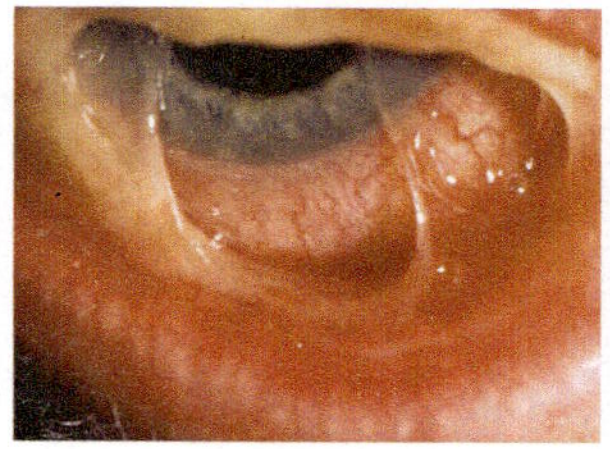
Fungal	*Candida* species *Paracoccidioides brasiliensis, Coccidioides immitis, Blastomyces Dermatitidis, Malassezia spp.* and *Rhinosporidium seeberi*	Very rare	• Often chronic symptoms (> 4 weeks), red eye, mucopurulent discharge, irritation, conjunctival masses	• Conjunctival hyperemia • Papillae • Follicles • Mucopurulent discharge • Necrotizing granulomata	• Histology of conjunctival granulomata • Smears for fungal hyphae • Swabs for culture • Swabs for PCR	Topical antifungals, e.g. 5% Natamycin or 2% fluconazole	

disease, contact-lens use, trauma and immunosuppression can increase the risk of developing bacterial conjunctivitis. Furthermore, pathogenic bacteria such as *Neisseria gonorrhoea, Neisseria meningitides, Corynebacterium diphtheriae, Listeria* and *Shigella* can cross intact conjunctival, and indeed corneal, epithelium. Organisms can be transmitted person-to-person through contaminated fingers, fomites or oculogenital contact.[4,13]

The incidence of bacterial conjunctivitis is estimated at approximately 135 per 10,000/year.[8] The most frequently isolated organisms causing bacterial conjunctivitis in adults are staphylococcal species (Table 18.1). The etiology is different in children, with *H. influenzae, Streptococcus pneumoniae* and *Moraxella catarahhalis* being implicated most frequently.[12]

Clinical Patterns

Bacterial conjunctivitis can be divided into different subtypes dependent on the amount and type of discharge (mucopurulent and purulent), the speed of onset of symptoms (hyperacute, less than 2 days until peak of discharge; acute, approximately 2–3 days until peak of discharge; and chronic, when the symptoms are present for 4 weeks or more) and by the presence of specific signs (papillary, follicular and membranous). The differential diagnoses for these various clinical signs are given in Table 18.2.

Acute mucopurulent bacterial conjunctivitis is the most common subtype, caused by the organisms listed in Table 18.1. Presentation is with a rapid of onset conjunctival injection, mucopurulent discharge and chemosis (Fig. 18.1), following an initial incubation period of between 1 and 7 days.[4] Often one eye is infected initially, with the fellow eye becoming infected through cross-inoculation after 2–3 days. The eyelids and lashes may be stuck together on waking, there is usually no history of previous conjunctivitis or itching.[15] Other signs on examination include subconjunctival hemorrhages and papillae visible on eyelid eversion. The condition is usually self-limiting after 7–10 days,[13] although treatment with topical antibiotics may speed resolution.[16] The condition remains infectious for approximately 2–7 days.[4]

In children, conjunctivitis caused by *H. influenzae* may present with petechial conjunctival hemorrhages and perilimbal corneal infiltrates, and can occasionally

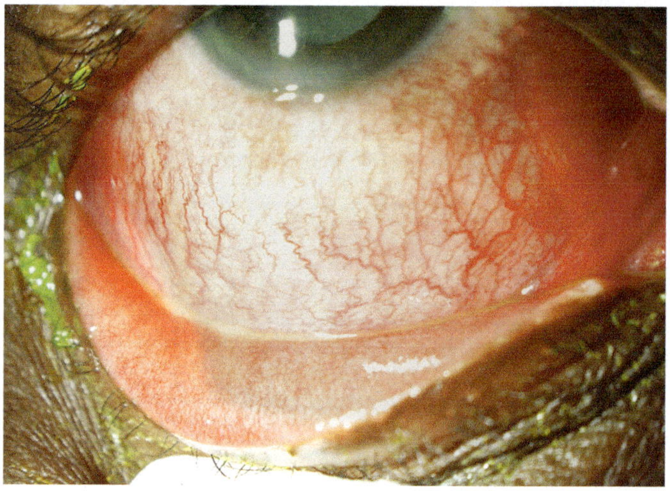

Fig. 18.1: Acute mucopurulent bacterial conjunctivitis.
Source: Scott Hau.

Table 18.2: Differential diagnosis for main clinical patterns of acute conjunctivitis.

Papillary	Follicular	Membranous
Acute	*Acute*	*Acute*
• *N. gonorrhoeae* • *N. meningitidis* • *S. aureus* • *H. influenzae* • Streptococci	• Adenovirus • Inclusion conjunctivitis • Herpes viruses (HSV, VZV) • Paramyxoviruses • Poxviruses • Picornaviruses • Orthomyxoviruses • Togaviruses	• Adenovirus • HSV • Beta-hemolytic streptococci • *S. aureus* • *C. diphtheria* • Chemical injury • Stevens–Johnson syndrome • Vernal conjunctivitis
Chronic	*Chronic*	*Chronic*
• Giant papillary conjunctivitis • Malignancy (masquerade syndrome) • Blepharoconjunctivitis • Toxic papillary keratoconjunctivitis • Atopic keratoconjunctivitis • Mucous membrane pemphigoid	• *Chlamydia trachomatis* (Trachoma, inclusion conjunctivitis) • Molluscum contagiosum • *Moraxella* • Parinaud's oculoglandular syndrome • Lyme disease • Toxic (drug-induced) conjunctivitis • Folliculosis	Ligneous conjunctivitis

be associated with otitis media (conjunctivitis-otitis syndrome).[17] The virulent *H. influenzae* type B (HiB) is a rare cause, largely due to the introduction of the HiB vaccine. However, it can rapidly spread to cause orbital cellulitis, sepsis and meningitis. *H. influenzae* type III conjunctivitis is also very rare; it has been reported to lead to fulminant purpuric sepsis in children in South America.[18]

Hyperacute purulent bacterial conjunctivitis presents rapidly with severe, copious discharge, eyelid edema, preauricular lymphadenopathy, reduced vision and pain on palpation, in addition to the symptoms and signs seen in acute conjunctivitis (Fig. 18.2). A membrane or pseudomembrane may be present. The organism most frequently responsible is *N. gonorrhoeae,* which can penetrate intact corneal epithelium leading to bacterial keratitis and perforation.[19,20] This form of infection is usually sexually transmitted, although not universally so,[21,22] and when there is copious discharge one should have a high index of suspicion for gonococcal infection, prompting the clinician to take conjunctival swabs for microscopy and culture. Treatment in adults is with a single dose of ceftriaxone 1 g intramuscular (IM), plus a single oral dose of azithromycin 1 g.[23,24] In true penicillin allergy, treatment with combination of oral gemifloxacin 320 mg plus oral azithromycin 2 g is suggested.[24] Ocular lavage should also be performed.

Rarely *N. meningitides* can cause hyperacute conjunctivitis (Fig. 18.3), either as an endogenous or exogenous infection.[25] This condition needs to be treated promptly with both systemic and topical antibiotics, as meningitis or meningosepticemia can ensue. There is limited evidence regarding the appropriate dose and regime for antibiotic treatment and systemic therapy should be commenced following discussion with a microbiologist. Previously reported antibiotic options for *N. meningitides* conjunctivitis include intravenous ceftriaxone 1 g once daily for 3 days intravenous (IV) or by deep IM injection, followed by phenoxymethyl penicillin 500 mg four times a day orally for 10 days, combined with ofloxacin eye drops.[26,27] However, it should be noted that the standard empirical treatment for suspected meningitis is higher at 2 g once a day of ceftriaxone for 10 days or longer.[28]

Membranous Conjunctivitis

Several infectious agents can cause a membranous or pseudomembranous conjunctivitis (Fig. 18.4). These membranes consist of fibrin, inflammatory cells and exudate. When the membrane penetrates into the epithelium, then it is considered a true membrane, causing bleeding when it is removed, whilst a pseudomembranes do not bleed when peeled. Bacterial infectious causes include *Corynebacterium diphtheria* and beta-hemolytic *streptococci*. Viral causes are adenoviral infection (particularly types 8 and 19) and primary herpes simplex infection. These are discussed in detail here. *Candida* infection has also been reported to cause a membranous conjunctivitis.[29]

Chronic Conjunctivitis

Chronic conjunctivitis is defined as conjunctivitis that lasts longer than 4 weeks. Symptoms include bilateral foreign

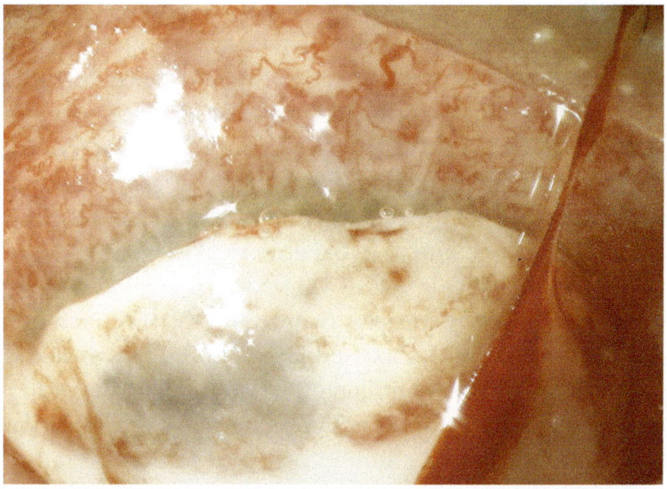

Fig. 18.2: Gonococcal conjunctivitis showing a mucous plaque.
Source: Steve Tuft.

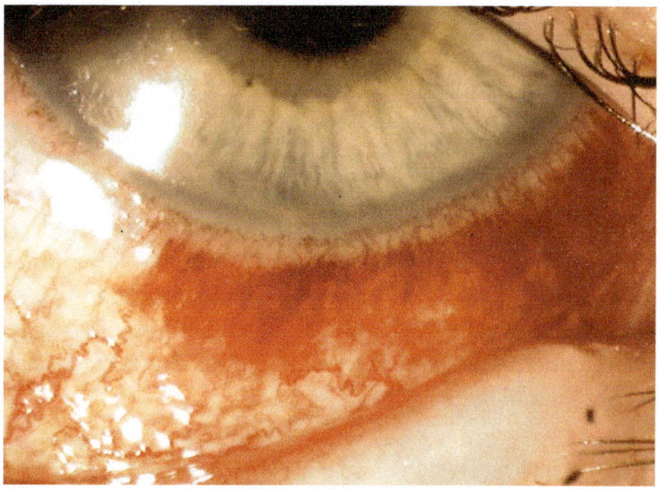

Fig. 18.3: *Meningococcus* conjunctivitis.
Source: Steve Tuft.

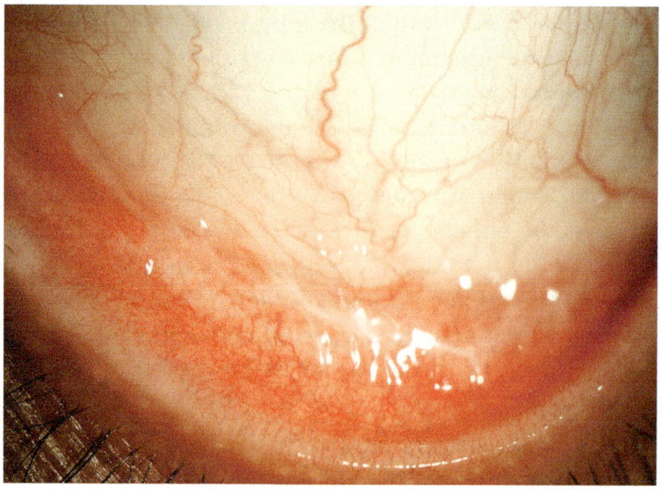

Fig. 18.4: Membranous conjunctivitis caused by adenovirus.
Source: Steve Tuft.

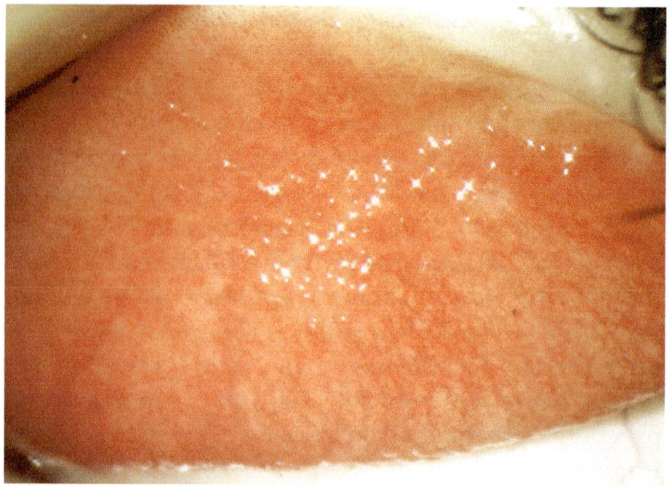

Fig. 18.5: Chronic blepharoconjunctivitis.
Source: Steve Tuft.

body sensation and crusting of eyelashes that are often stuck together in the morning with minimal discharge. It is often associated with blepharitis, presenting with thickened eyelids, eyelid margin erythema and blocked Meibomian glands. Other signs include mild conjunctival hyperemia in association with small follicles or papillae (Fig. 18.5).

The most common causative organism is *S. aureus*. Punctate epithelial erosions may form due to the production of exotoxins, whilst a type III hypersensitivity reaction against *Staphylococcal* antigens leading to immune complex deposition can cause marginal keratitis or phlyctenulosis. Chronic angular blepharoconjunctivitis is caused by *Moraxella lacunata* and presents with ulceration and crusting of the canthi. Other responsible organisms include enteric gram-negative bacteria such as *Proteus spp., Klebsiella pneumoniae* and *Escherichia coli.*

Treatment is with lid hygiene measures including hot compresses and eyelid massage in combination with empirical topical antibiotics such as chloramphenicol ointment applied four times a day for 1 week. If there is no resolution with this regimen, eyelid and conjunctival swabs for microscopy, culture and sensitivities should be taken after waiting 48 hours from stopping the original antibiotics. Treatment should then be targeted depending on these results. One should also consider the patency of the lacrimal system, as the lacrimal canaliculus and sac can act as a potential reservoir for reinfection. This is discussed in more detail later.

Investigations

Investigations for uncomplicated bacterial conjunctivitis are not usually required and empirical therapy can be commenced as discussed later. However, certain scenarios mandate laboratory investigations. Such situations include ophthalmia neonatorum (ON), hyperacute mucopurulent conjunctivitis (due to the risk of gonococcal infection), patients with symptom onset following a new sexual contact or with concurrent urogenital symptoms, and patients who have failed to respond to initial empirical therapy.

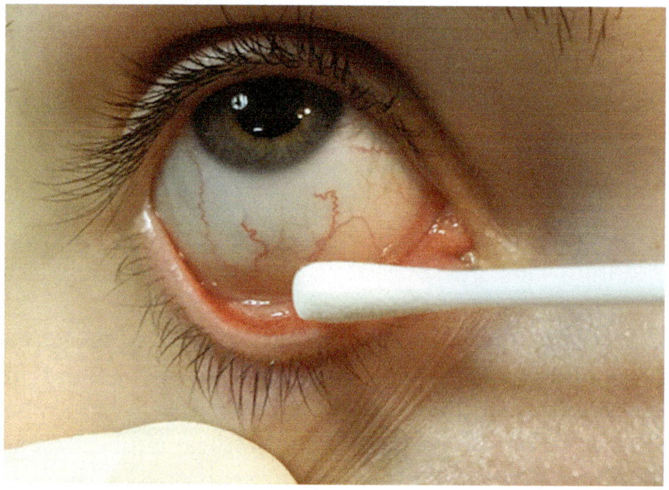

Fig. 18.6: Conjunctival swabs of the inferior fornix.

Initial investigations include conjunctival swabs for microscopy, culture and sensitivities and PCR for chlamydia and certain viruses (discussed later). Conjunctival swabs should be taken without bacteriostatic topical anesthetic and ideally before antibiotics have started. It is important to take good quality conjunctival swabs: these need to sweep relatively deeply into the inferior conjunctival fornix, which can be uncomfortable for the patient (Fig. 18.6). Care must be taken to avoid the eyelids and lashes, which can

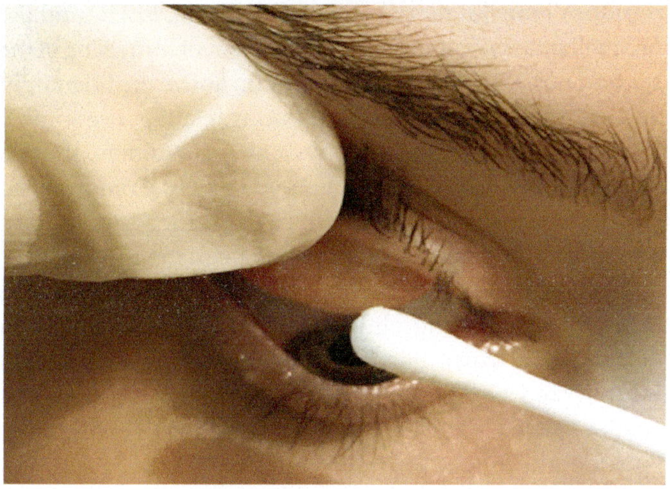

Fig. 18.7: Conjunctival swabs for chlamydia of the superior tarsal conjunctiva.

contaminate the culture with skin flora. Chlamydial swabs should also be considered, although the technique for this involves everting the upper lids and running the chlamydia-specific swab several times across the tarsal conjunctiva (Fig. 18.7).[22] Depending on the swabs used and local policy, these can either be inserted directly into transport medium or inoculated onto blood, chocolate and mannitol salt agar. For suspected *Gonococcus*, Thayer-Martin medium should be used.

Treatment

Bacterial conjunctivitis is often a self-limiting disease with good prognosis, and permanent visual loss is rare. Indeed, it is estimated that 60% of cases of bacterial conjunctivitis resolve spontaneously within 1–2 weeks of onset.[4] Topical antibiotic is the conventional treatment, although there has been some debate as to their role given the disease is often self-limiting. However, given that approximately 40% of cases do not resolve without treatment within 1–2 weeks,[4] topical antibiotic treatment is recommended in cases of clinically suspected or culture-proven bacterial conjunctivitis. Furthermore, a 2012 Cochrane review meta-analysis looking at a combined number of 3,673 patients treated for bacterial conjunctivitis in 11 randomized clinical trials, found there was a benefit in using topical antibiotics between days 2 and 5 of the disease in improving clinical (RR 1.36, 95% confidence interval (CI) 1.15–1.61) and microbiological remission (RR 1.55, 95% CI 1.37–1.76).[16] For days 6–10, topical antibiotics still conferred a modest benefit in terms of both clinical (RR 1.21, 95% CI 1.10–1.33) and microbiological (RR 1.37, 95% CI 1.24–1.52) cure rates.[16] This study also found that approximately 41% of cases resolved by days 6–10 with placebo alone. The study also concluded that treatment was unlikely to be associated with any significant adverse outcomes. It is reasonable to conclude that topical antibiotic treatment speeds resolution. It also decreases transmission and speeds return to school.[30,31]

Although it may be reasonable to defer treatment in some cases due to the available evidence suggesting no sight-threatening complications without treatment,[13] patients with purulent and mucopurulent conjunctivitis, those with discomfort, immunosuppressed individuals and contact lens-wearers should be treated empirically.[4,13] Additional factors to consider in the management of bacterial conjunctivitis in contact lens wearers include ensuring abstention from wearing lenses for at least 2 weeks following resolution of symptoms, as well as the use of new lenses when returning to lens wear, to reduce the risk of developing bacterial keratitis.[4] Patients in whom gonococcal or chlamydial conjunctivitis is suspected should be investigated and treated appropriately, as outlined earlier. Patients who have not responded to initial first-line therapy should be re-evaluated with laboratory studies including microscopy, culture and sensitivities as well as investigations for chlamydial infection, with antibiotic treatment directed by sensitivities.

All broad-spectrum topical antibiotics appear to adequately treat bacterial conjunctivitis, with no significant difference in cure rates between individual agents.[13] Choice of drug depends on local availability, resistance patterns, patient allergies and cost. Chloramphenicol is widely used as a first-line agent globally, but fears of a potential risk of aplastic anemia has restricted its use within some countries including the USA.[32,33] This rare side-effect is controversial and has been questioned recently.[34] If a causative relationship does exist, the risk is about 1 in 1,000,000.[34] Due to its low cost, good patient tolerability and broad-spectrum action, it is reasonable to use topical chloramphenicol as a first-line agent. Quinolone antibiotics, although effective, should ideally be held in reserve for treating bacterial keratitis to reduce the risk of quinolone-resistance. Topical steroids should be avoided as they can worsen the condition and lengthen the course.[13]

Special Cases of Bacterial Conjunctivitis

Trachoma

Trachoma is the most common infectious cause of blindness worldwide. It is caused by repeated re-infection of the conjunctiva by the ocular serovars of *Chlamydia trachomatis* (serovars A, B, Ba and C). It is an obligate intracellular bacterium with a biphasic developmental cycle: the transmissible elementary body phase (extracellular, hardy, metabolically inactive, and small) and the replicating reticulate body phase (intraepithelial cell, metabolically active, larger).

First episodes of infection occur early in life and result in a chronic, repeated follicular-papillary conjunctivitis, referred to as active trachoma. The upper tarsal conjunctiva is particularly affected, with the bulbar conjunctiva showing only minimal or no inflammation. The formal World Health Organization (WHO) definition of follicular trachoma (TF) requires the identification of 5+ follicles of at least 0.5 mm in diameter in the upper tarsal conjunctiva (Figs. 18.8A and B). The acquired immune response to ocular *C. trachomatis* are relatively weak and short lived, therefore within an endemic community repeated infections are the norm. With each episode of inflammation, particularly those with a severe papillary phenotype, the conjunctival stroma is damaged and resolution is typically associated with progressive scarring (TS) (Fig. 18.8C), which can in turn result in trachomatous trichiasis (TT) due to upper lid entropion (Fig. 18.8D). Trichiasis can also be due to metaplastic or misdirected lashes. Sight-threatening corneal opacification (CO) develops either as a result of the traumatic effect of the trichiasis, generalized ocular surface disease or secondary corneal infections (Fig. 18.8E).

Globally, there are about 2 million people with visual impairment and 0.45 million blind from trachoma.[35] Approximately, 3.2 million people have trichiasis requiring surgical or other interventions. Approximately, 190 million live in districts which require active disease control interventions at the population level. Trachoma is endemic in around 50 countries. The African continent carries about 90% of the global burden. Ethiopia is particularly affected, with 39% of the burden.

There is a worldwide effort to eliminate trachoma as a public health problem. This is coordinated through the WHO-led Alliance for the Global Elimination of Trachoma by 2020 (GET2020), a grouping of endemic communities, major donors, industry, international NGOs and academic groups. The control of Trachoma is primarily being achieved through the implementation of the *SAFE* Strategy: **S**urgery for trichiasis, **A**ntibiotics to treat infection and **F**acial Hygiene and **E**nvironmental Improvements to suppress its transmission.

Several alternative procedures have been used to correct TT.[36] Of these the two WHO-endorsed options are the posterior lamellar tarsal rotation (or Trabut, PLTR) and the bilamellar tarsal rotation (BLTR). Both involve incising of the scarred posterior lamellar about 3 mm above the lid margin and everting sutures for fixation during healing. The surgery is usually performed by non-physician practitioners. The two procedures were recently compared in a large randomized controlled trial which found the PLTR procedure to have about half the trichiasis recurrence rate of the BLTR.[37]

At the population level, there is a mismatch between individuals showing clinical signs of active trachoma and those in which current *C. trachomatis* infection can be detected by PCR.[38] This is because in children, the signs of disease develop several days into an infection episode and linger for many weeks after the resolution of infection. Moreover, infected adults do not develop prolonged episodes of clinical inflammation. Treatment targeted to only those with active disease signs will leave infected individuals untreated. Therefore, infection control measures need to be provided to the entire community.

Where the prevalence of TF in 1–9 year olds is above 5%, A, F and E control measures are indicated. The macrolide antibiotic azithromycin is given as a single annual oral dose through mass drug administration (MDA) to all community members above 6 months of age. This treatment is given for three to five annual rounds. MDA is discontinued after the community TF prevalence drops below 5%. Emphasis is placed on improving the facial cleanliness of children, to remove potentially infected ocular discharge, to reduce onward transmission. Improvement to water supply and sanitation is also considered to help suppress transmission.

Adult Inclusion Conjunctivitis

Adult inclusion conjunctivitis is caused by *C. trachomatis* serovars D-K. It is thought to account for between 1.8% and 5.6% of acute conjunctivitis.[13,39-41] The suspected diagnosis is usually confirmed by a PCR for *C. trachomatis.* It is most common in sexually active young adults, being acquired through genital to ocular transmission. It presents as a uni- or bilateral follicular conjunctivitis with a purulent or mucopurulent discharge and is often present for weeks or months (Fig. 18.9). Concurrent genital infection is common (54% in men and 74% in women).[42] Treatment with a single dose of oral azithromycin 1 g is effective.[43,44] The patient must be referred to a genitourinary specialist for investigations for other sexually transmitted infections as well as contact tracing.

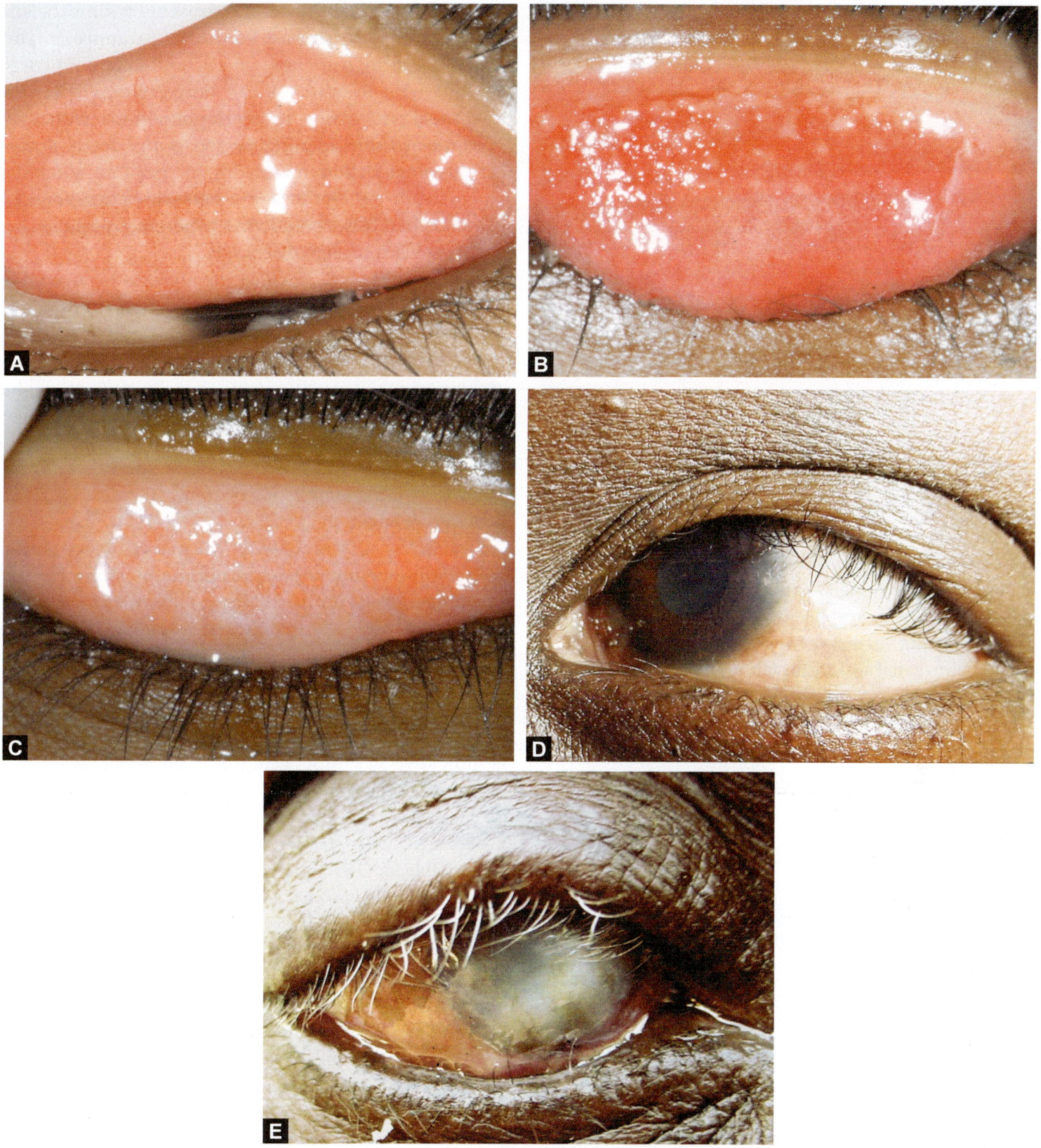

Figs. 18.8A to E: (A) Follicular trachoma (TF); (B) Inflammatory trachoma (TI); (C) Trachomatous scarring (TS); (D) Trachomatous trichiasis (TT); (E) Corneal opacity (CO).

Source: Matthew J Burton.

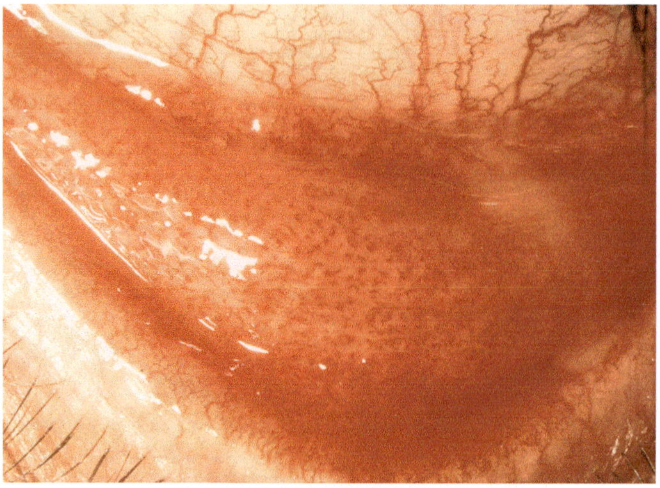

Fig. 18.9: Adult inclusion conjunctivitis.
Source: Steve Tuft.

Ophthalmia Neonatorum

Neonatal conjunctivitis or ON is defined as any conjunctivitis occurring within the first month after birth. It is an ophthalmic emergency. Viral and bacterial infections, in particular *N. meningitides* and *C. trachomatis,* as well as chemical agents are responsible. The infectious causes are acquired during vaginal delivery following exposure to an infected birth canal and are therefore not acquired following cesarean section. *C. trachomatis* is the leading cause of ON, accounting for up to 55% of cases.[45] The timeframe of onset can be helpful in establishing the causative agent (Table 18.3), although microbiological investigations are crucial.

Chemical conjunctivitis presents in the first few hours after delivery following the application of topical drops intended to prevent the more serious life- or vision-threatening causes of ON. It is most commonly seen following application of silver nitrate 1% (Crede's prophylaxis), when it can be seen in up to 90% of treated infants.[46] Signs include mild conjunctival injection and watering, resolving in 1–2 days.

Table 18.3: Timeframe for the most common causes of neonatal conjunctivitis. Note that the vesicular rash for herpes simplex virus (HSV) usually only appears between 6 and 14 days following birth.

Interval since birth	Potential cause
Hours	Chemical conjunctivitis
1–7 days	Gonococcal
5–7 days	Gonococcal or Chlamydial
7–14 days	Chlamydial
> 14 days	Non-sexually transmitted bacterial infection

Gonococcal conjunctivitis presents within the first 1–7 days after birth and accounts for approximately 1% of ON in high-income countries.[45] Like gonococcal conjunctivitis in adults, it can progress rapidly leading to corneal perforation and endophthalmitis, with a risk of septic arthritis, meningitis, sepsis and death, if there is systemic infection, mandating the need for admission and systemic antibiotics. It presents with a rapid onset of bilateral chemosis, conjunctival hyperemia, eyelid edema and a profuse purulent discharge.

ON caused by *C. trachomatis* presents between days 5 and 14 after birth. The signs are variable, ranging from mild conjunctival hyperemia with limited mucoid discharge to severe conjunctival injection and chemosis, eyelid edema and occasionally pseudomembranes. In contrast to adult chlamydial conjunctivitis, there are no follicular changes in infants due to the immaturity of the immune system. Unlike in adults, there is a risk of pneumonitis or otitis media and therefore systemic treatment is indicated as with gonococcal infection.

As ON is an emergency, all neonates presenting with conjunctivitis need appropriate investigation and treatment. Swabs for microscopy, culture and sensitivity must be sent urgently, together with conjunctival smears. PCR samples for *Gonococcus* and *C. trachomatis* should also be sent, as these allow for more rapid diagnosis compared to culture. With microscopy, the presence of Gram negative diplococci present on gram staining is indicative of gonococcal infection, whereas Giemsa staining is useful for demonstrating *Chlamydial* inclusions on cell culture monolayers.

Non-sexually transmitted bacteria may also be responsible for ON. Organisms include both Gram positive (*Staphylococcus aureus, Streptococcus pneumoniae,* and *Streptococcus viridans)* and Gram negative (*H. influenzae, E. coli, Enterobacter spp., Klebsiella spp.,* and *Proteus spp.*) bacteria. This usually presents later than either chlamydial or gonococcal ON.

Viral neonatal conjunctivitis is usually caused by either adenovirus or herpes simplex virus (HSV). The adult forms of viral conjunctivitis are discussed later. Adenoviral infection in neonates can lead to petechial hemorrhages or large subconjunctival hemorrhage and is associated with preauricular lymphadenopathy in 50% of cases.[47,48] As HSV conjunctivitis is often treated empirically as either gonococcal or chlamydial ON due to the overlap of signs and symptoms, it can be diagnosed late. The vesicular herpetic lesions commonly appear on days 6–14. These neonates are at risk of encephalitis and require pediatric inpatient care, lumbar puncture and treatment with systemic antivirals. A possible regime is acyclovir 60 mg/kg in divided doses three times per day for 2 weeks combined with topical acyclovir ointment.

Treatment of ON caused by both chlamydial and gonococcal infection requires admission and pediatric review due to the potential for systemic infection. Treatment is with oral erythromycin (50 mg/kg/day divided into four equal doses for 14 days) for chlamydial infection and IV or IM ceftriaxone as a once only injection (25–50 mg/kg, maximum 125 mg) for gonococcal infection, in addition to regular ocular lavage.

Prophylaxis against chlamydial and gonococcal ON is possible with either topical silver nitrate 1%, erythromycin 1% or tetracycline 1%.[48] Silver nitrate is the most likely agent to cause a chemical conjunctivitis and so its routine use is no longer recommended. Alternative agents that may be beneficial include fusidic acid and povidone-iodine 2.5%, although further research is needed to evaluate their efficacy.[48]

Canaliculitis

This is an uncommon condition that is usually caused by *Actinomyces israelii*. It presents with recurrent unilateral conjunctivitis, worse nasally, together with unilateral epiphora, canalicular inflammation, punctal "pouting", concretions in the canaliculi or expression of exudate (Fig. 18.10). *Actinomyces* infection characteristically causes bright yellow "sulfur granule" concretions. The nasolacrimal system is patent. Treatment for canaliculitis is surgical with an extended 1-snip punctoplasty. The canaliculus is opened fully and the concretions are removed with a curette. These should be sent for microscopy, culture and sensitivities. The canaliculus can then be irrigated with either benzylpenicillin or iodine 1%, ensuring that this drains through the nose and is not swallowed. Patients can then be discharged on topical antibiotics.

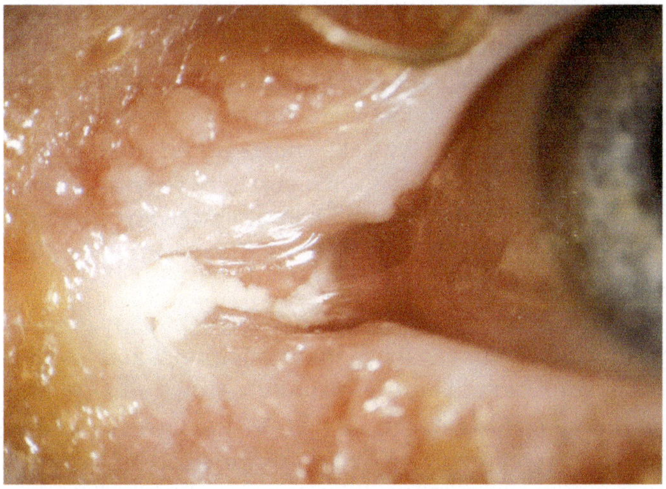

Fig.18.10: Canaliculitis caused by *Actinomyces israelii*.
Source: Steve Tuft.

Mycobacterial Conjunctivitis

Conjunctivitis caused by *Mycobacterium tuberculosis* is rare. However, at the end of the 19th century, tuberculous mycobacterial conjunctivitis was considerably more common than it is now. Eyre reviewed 206 cases between 1882 and 1912, and in his original description, classified it into ulcerative, nodular, hypertrophic granulomatous and pedunculated forms.[49] However, in the last few decades there have been only a handful of case reports of conjunctival tuberculosis.[50] It is usually unilateral, presenting as a chronic conjunctivitis with occasional discharge and most frequently a conjunctival mass, usually within the palpebral conjunctiva of the upper eyelid and associated with preauricular lymphadenopathy. Infection is thought to arise following contact between the contaminated sputum droplets and the conjunctiva, either from another individual or the patients' own respiratory secretions. It is important to consider the diagnosis in cases of recurrent chalazia.[51] With the rise of HIV/AIDS the incidence of *M. tuberculosis* infection has probably increased, although there is considerable geographic variation.[52] Cases of tuberculous conjunctivitis may therefore increase, although this still remains one of the rarer presentations of ocular tuberculosis accounting for 11.8% of cases in a recent case series from Malaysia.[53]

Diagnosis is histological and microbiological. Histology shows typical clusters of tubercles, epitheloid cells, giant cells, lymphocytes and plasma cells, with or without caseation. If acid-fast bacilli are seen then this is diagnostic of mycobacterial conjunctivitis. Confirmation of *Mycobacterium tuberculosis* infection can be made by culture and PCR.

Treatment is with systemic anti-tuberculous treatment under the care of an infectious diseases or respiratory physician. This is usually quadruple therapy for 2 months followed by two agents for 4 months.

Non-tuberculous mycobacterial (NTM) conjunctivitis is exceptionally rare, with only three cases reported in the literature.[54-56] Two of these cases did not have any risk factors for NTM infection whilst the third had AIDS and bacillary angiomatosis of the palpebral conjunctiva.

All these cases presented with a conjunctival mass that demonstrated-caseating granulomas with acid-fast bacilli present on histology.

VIRAL CONJUNCTIVITIS

Many different viral pathogens can cause conjunctivitis (*see* Table 18.2 and Box 18.1). Adenovirus is responsible for between 65% and 90% of cases.[30] Diagnostic accuracy is reported as less than 50% compared to laboratory investigations, with many cases being wrongly treated as bacterial conjunctivitis.[30] In general, viral conjunctivitis presents with bilateral conjunctival injection with a watery, clear discharge. There may be associated systemic features of viral infection including fever, rhinitis and malaise. It is estimated that viruses cause up to 80% of acute follicular conjunctivitis.[13] There is usually tender preauricular lymphadenopathy. Additionally, there are certain clinical signs and patterns of presentation that are associated with distinct clinical syndromes, although there is considerable overlap.

Adenovirus

The adenoviruses (Ad) comprise 51 distinct types of structurally similar but antigenically different double-stranded DNA viruses.[57] They are highly stable viruses that are found throughout the world causing respiratory tract, genitourinary, gastrointestinal and ocular infections. Adenoviral infection is usually self-limiting but can lead to fatal multiple-organ failure in the immunocompromised.

Natural immunity to adenovirus varies geographically: there is a low level of seropositivity in European populations to Ad type 8, whilst in Africa and Asia there is positive serology to the same virus in 25–85% of the population.[58] This observation helps explain the different patterns of disease in these two populations. In Europe and North America, it often occurs in epidemic form whilst in Asia and Africa, it is endemic. Whilst the overall incidence is estimated to be relatively low (0.03–1.10%), it can increase to as high as 35% in localized populations where there is close contact between individuals such as in prisons, boarding schools and nursing homes.[13,30,58]

Box 18.1: Causes of viral conjunctivitis.

- Adenovirus
  - EKC (Ad Types 8 and 19 predominantly)
  - PCF (Ad Types 3, 4 and 7 predominantly)
- Herpes simplex virus (HSV-1 and HSV-2)
- Varicella zoster virus
- Molluscum contagiosum
- Paramyxoviruses, e.g. measles, mumps
- Enteroviruses, e.g. EV70, Coxsackie A and B
- Flaviviruses, e.g. dengue virus, yellow fever, Zika viruses
  Filoviruses, e.g. Ebola, Marburg

Adenoviral infection, in common with most other causes of viral conjunctivitis, is highly contagious: the risk of interfamilial infection rates have been estimated at between 10% and 50%.[4,59] It is transmitted through contaminated hands, towels, swimming pools and medical devices as well as probably through contaminated nasal air droplets. It is very important to appreciate the highly contagious nature of adenovirus. Anything that the patient touches (or touches the patient) can act as a potential source. Good hand-hygiene technique between patients, cleaning ophthalmic equipment thoroughly with disinfectant wipes after patient contact, keeping suspected infectious cases in a separate waiting room and treating them in a separate examination room can help minimize the chance of spreading the virus.

There are four recognized clinical phenotypes for adenoviral conjunctivitis: epidemic keratoconjunctivitis (EKC), pharyngoconjunctival fever (PCF), acute nonspecific follicular conjunctivitis and chronic keratoconjunctivitis.

Epidemic Keratoconjunctivitis

It is the most serious of the adenoviral infections. It is associated with types 8 and 19, although associations with other types have been reported (types 2–4, 7–11, 14, 16 and 29).[60,61] These other types may have similar clinical phenotypes to EKC caused by 8 and 19, but rarely result in epidemic transmission.

As discussed earlier, transmission occurs amongst individuals in close contact with one another. However, it has also been reported that Ad type 19 transmission is associated with sexual contact; the incidence of genital infection in adults has been reported to correspond to the incidence of ocular infection by the same virus within the same population.[62] It typically effects young adults during autumn and winter and is unilateral in two-thirds of cases with no systemic features. This is in contrast with PCF which is usually bilateral and associated with systemic symptoms of sore throat and fever.

After an incubation period of 8 days, patients develop significant conjunctival hyperemia, epiphora and foreign-body sensation. There is usually tender preauricular lymphadenopathy (seen in over 50% of cases) together with tarsal conjunctival follicles—the presence of these two signs together is highly suggestive of viral conjunctivitis.[30] Other symptoms and signs that may be present include mild photophobia, chemosis, petechial subconjunctival hemorrhages and either pseudomembranes or true membranes that may bleed when removed (Fig. 18.11). Rarely symblephara may form and tarsal scarring can occur (Fig. 18.12). If the fellow eye becomes involved, this usually occurs 4–5 days into the disease and the signs are generally less severe than the first eye due to partial host immunity.[58]

Adenoviral keratitis, which is divided into four stages, occurs in approximately 80% of patients (Box 18.2 and Fig. 18.13).[58,60,63,64] Stage 1 occurs on or around day 8 with symptoms of worsening discomfort, photophobia and tearing. This is due to a diffuse superficial epithelial punctate keratitis caused directly by the live virus. Stage 2, characterized by larger, fluorescein-staining white punctate epithelial lesions follows soon after Stage 1. About 24–48 hours later, these areas develop into combined epithelial and subepithelial lesions (Stage 3). By Stage 4, the conjunctivitis is usually resolving and the patient is left with non-staining subepithelial macular lesions (Fig. 18.13). Stages 2–4 are thought to develop due to a delayed-type hypersensitivity reaction to the epithelial viral antigens.

The conjunctivitis has usually resolved by 2–3 weeks, whilst Stage 4 keratitis reaches its peak between weeks 3 and 4, at which point the visual acuity in these patients may be reduced by two lines. These subepithelial lesions may persist for months and rarely years, but usually resolve entirely without scarring, with visual acuity returning to baseline.

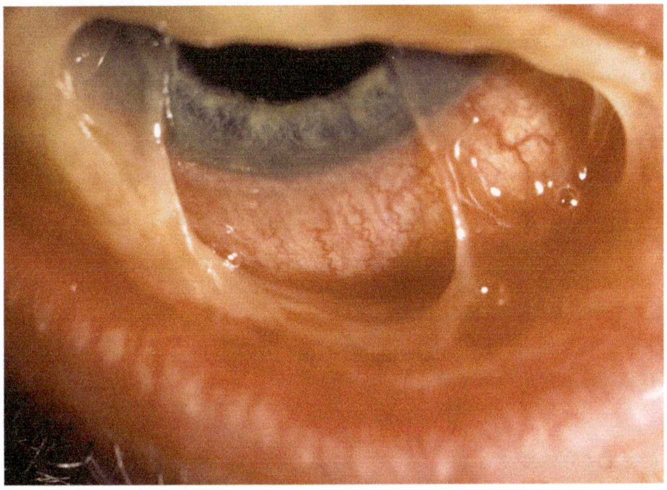

Fig. 18.11: Acute adenoviral conjunctivitis.
Source: Steve Tuft.

Pharyngoconjunctival Fever

It is associated with adenovirus types 3, 4 and 7.[57,58] It is highly contagious and spreads rapidly amongst individuals living or working in close proximity with one another such as schools, families, prisons and military personnel. Unlike EKC, systemic symptoms predominate with pharyngitis, tender preauricular lymphadenopathy, fever and an acute follicular conjunctivitis.

The incubation period is approximately 8 days following exposure (range 5–12 days), when patients develop a high fever with associated myalgia, malaise and occasionally gastrointestinal upset.[57,58] An acute follicular conjunctivitis

Box 18.2: Stages of adenoviral keratitis.

- *Stage 1:* Diffuse, fine, superficial epithelial punctate keratitis
- *Stage 2:* Staining focal punctate white epithelial lesions
- *Stage 3:* Combined epithelial and subepithelial areas
- *Stage 4:* Non-staining subepithelial macular lesions

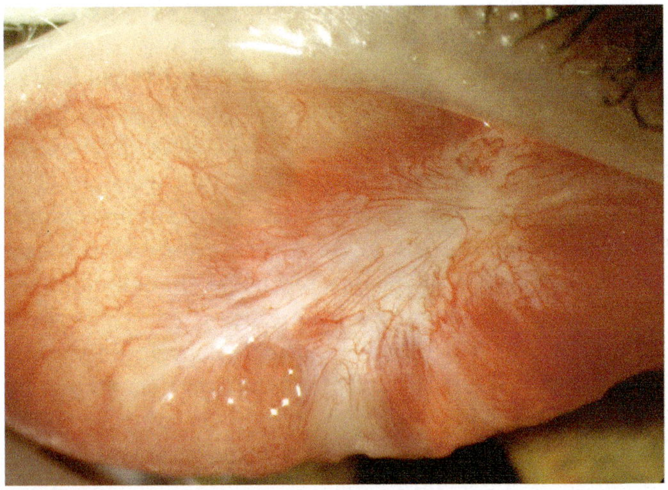

Fig. 18.12: Superior tarsal scarring following adenoviral infection.
Source: Matthew J Burton.

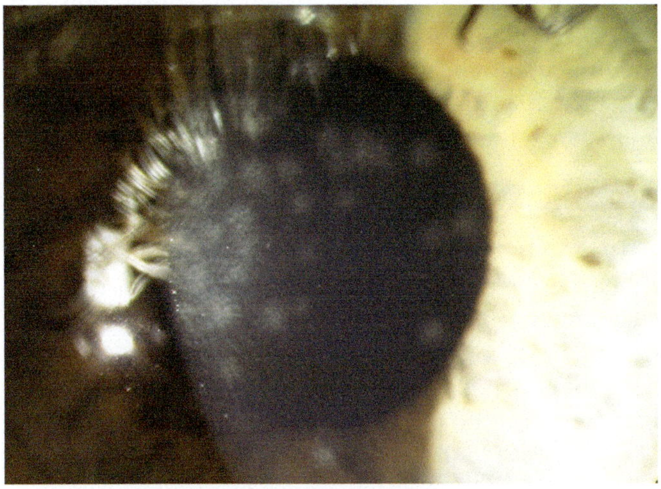

Fig. 18.13: Adenoviral keratoconjunctivitis.
Source: Matthew J Burton.

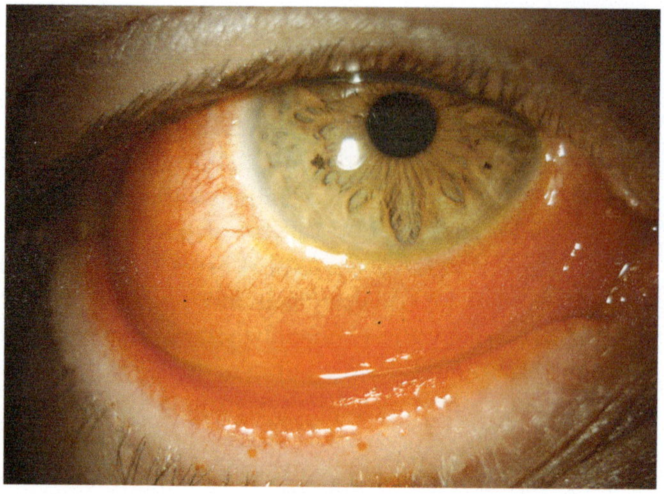

Fig. 18.14: Adenovirus pharyngoconjunctival fever.
Source: Scott Hau.

develops a few days into the symptomatic illness, with initial symptoms of irritation, burning and lacrimation. The conjunctivitis is usually worse in the lower fornix and can lead to a tender, swollen lower eyelid, occasionally with ecchymosis that can mimic orbital trauma. Both eyes are usually involved, although there may be a delay of 1–3 days before the fellow eye becomes symptomatic (Fig. 18.14).

Keratitis is less common than with EKC but if present, follows the same progressive stages as outlined earlier.

Acute Nonspecific Follicular Conjunctivitis

This form of viral conjunctivitis is caused by numerous types of adenovirus including those that cause EKC and PCF but is a mild, self-limiting condition commonly seen in children and young adults, which resolves within 7–10 days of symptom onset. As the symptoms are mild, it rarely requires ophthalmological input. However, one should consider chlamydial or HSV infection as a cause for acute follicular conjunctivitis.

Chronic Keratoconjunctivitis

Chronic keratoconjunctivitis caused by adenovirus is rare but has been reported.[65-67] Clinically, it presents as a relapsing and remitting prolonged course of intermittent conjunctival hyperemia, lacrimation and photophobia. There will be a history of previous viral conjunctivitis within the last 6–9 months. It can be a challenge to diagnose as unlike the other types of adenoviral conjunctivitis, papillae rather than follicles predominate. Diagnosis can be confirmed through laboratory investigations as discussed here.

Investigations

As with bacterial conjunctivitis, routine investigations are not always required for viral conjunctivitis as the diagnosis can be made clinically, particularly if there are conjunctival follicles and tender preauricular lymphadenopathy in the absence of significant discharge. When performing investigations for viral conjunctivitis, tests for bacterial and chlamydial infection should also be sent, and the testing for viruses should test for a range of different pathogens including adenovirus and HSV.

Real-time PCR has become the laboratory test of choice for viral conjunctivitis as it is rapid with high sensitivity and specificity. In addition, it can test for chlamydial infection. The sensitivity for adenovirus, HSV-1, VZV and *Chlamydia trachomatis* is 85%, 91%, 100% and 95% respectively, with specificity of 98%, 100%, 100% and 100% respectively.[68]

More recently, rapid antigen testing is available for adenovirus, with 89% reported sensitivity and 94% specificity.[69] This point-of-care testing can be very useful in a primary care setting and prevent the incorrect diagnosis of bacterial conjunctivitis and unnecessary antibiotic use. It is also a useful test in confirming adenoviral infection in healthcare workers.

Other investigations include viral culture and serology for virus-specific IgM. Serial testing showing an increase in virus-specific antibody titer over time can also be diagnostic.[58]

Treatment

There is no specific-licensed treatment for adenoviral conjunctivitis. Current advice is targeted at symptom relief with artificial tears and cold compresses to the eyes.[13] There is no role for antibiotics as they do not protect against secondary infection; unscrupulous use can lead to bacterial resistance and diagnostic confusion as the drops themselves can lead to local toxicity and allergy.[30,59] Beyond these recommendations, treatment is controversial.

Following promising *in vitro* and animal studies, clinical trials investigating the efficacy of the topical antiviral cidofovir were largely disappointing.[70] Although cidofovir was shown to reduce the frequency of severe corneal opacities, clinical use, and hence further development, was limited by local toxicity and concerns over the emergence of resistance.[71,72]

Ganciclovir has been shown to be effective against certain adenoviral strains *in vitro*.[70,71,73] Topical ganciclovir 0.15% gel is known to be effective for herpes simplex keratitis and is licensed and available for this in Europe and the USA.[74] A small randomized, double-blinded clinical trial of 18 patients in Saudi Arabia compared ganciclovir 0.15% gel with artificial tears and found the mean time of virus-shedding was 7.7 days in the ganciclovir group compared to 18.5 days in the control group ($p = <0.05$).[75] However, further work and larger studies are required in different geographic locations, where the adenoviral types may differ to explore the potential role of topical ganciclovir further.

There have been some promising results with the use of povidone-iodine (PVP-I) drops in the treatment of adenoviral conjunctivitis.[70] PVP-I is an established agent in preventing infection both before and after ocular surgery, as well as in preventing neonatal conjunctivitis.[76] *In vitro* PVP-I kills bacteria, viruses, protozoa and fungi. Studies investigating PVP-I in combination with topical steroids (0.1% dexamethasone) have shown a reduction in symptoms and viral titer in both humans and rabbit models.[77,78] One such protocol of using PVI-P includes anesthetizing the eye with topical anesthetics followed by a pretreatment topical nonsteroidal anti-inflammatory drug (NSAID) and then by 5 drops of 5% povidone-iodine. This is left to work for 1 minute before being irrigated with normal saline.[79]

Other than antivirals, there is also controversy surrounding the use of topical steroids to treat adenoviral infection. Although topical steroids can speed the resolution of the signs and relieve symptoms, it is associated with increased viral shedding and duration of active viral infection beyond the typical 12 days, meaning the patient is infectious for longer.[80,81] This can have public health implications as the viral reservoir is increased. If there is keratitis, topical steroids can rapidly reduce or eliminate the subepithelial opacities with a corresponding improvement in visual acuity. However, on cessation of the topical steroids, the opacities usually recur and it is only with time that they will fade.[63] The established side-effects of topical steroids of raised intraocular pressure and cataract formation should also be remembered. It is reasonable to treat patients with significant pseudomembranes or membranes with topical steroids to reduce the chance of symblephara formation. In addition, patients with significantly reduced vision due to keratitis, especially where it is limiting their daily activities, may benefit from treatment provided they are counseled regarding the side-effects and the potential rebound keratitis on cessation of treatment.

Other Viral Causes

As described in Box 18.1 and Table 18.2, there are several different viruses that can cause infectious keratitis. Herpes simplex virus and molluscum contagiosum (MC) are considered here in detail as there are specific therapies for these.

Herpes Simplex Virus

It is a double-stranded DNA virus that exists as two types (HSV-1 and HSV-2). HSV accounts for 1.3–4.8% of acute conjunctivitis.[13,41,82] It is typically a unilateral follicular conjunctivitis with a thin and watery discharge (Fig. 18.15). There may or may not be preauricular lymphadenopathy. Vesicular lesions may be present on the eyelid margin and occasionally, a conjunctival dendritic ulcer that stains with fluorescein may be present. Treatment is with either topical acyclovir or ganciclovir ointment 5 × day for 7–10 days, oral acyclovir 400 mg 5 × day for 7–10 days or oral valacyclovir 500 mg TDS for 7–10 days.[83] Resolution occurs between 7 days and 10 days.

Molluscum Contagiosum

It is a large DNA poxvirus that is ubiquitous but more common in children and the immunosuppressed. Infection causes growth of small, pearly-white skin lesions with an umbilicated center. If present within a few millimeters from the eyelid margin molluscum contagiosum (MC) can cause a chronic follicular conjunctivitis. The conjunctivitis resolves following excision of the MC lesions.

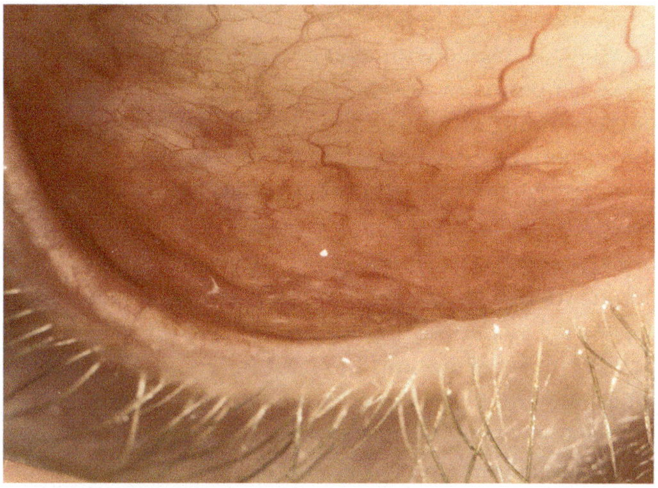

Fig. 18.15: Follicular conjunctivitis caused by primary herpes simplex virus (HSV) infection.

FUNGAL CONJUNCTIVITIS

Fungal organisms are infrequently present in the normal conjunctival microbiota, present in between 6% and 25% of normal individuals.[84-86] Under normal conditions, fungi do not remain or proliferate within the conjunctival sac.[87] *Candida* species are the most common organisms to cause conjunctivitis. Other organisms include *Paracoccidioides brasiliensis, Coccidioimmitis, Blastomyces dermatitidis, Malassezia spp.* and *Rhinosporidium seeberi*. Risk factors associated with fungal conjunctivitis include shared cosmetics, long-term use of broad-spectrum antibiotics and/or steroids, trauma involving vegetation and immunosuppression.[29]

Presentation is similar to that seen in chronic conjunctivitis. A necrotizing granulomatous conjunctivitis can be seen with *Malassezia spp.* infection, whilst black conjunctival secretions are seen with *Aspergillus niger* infection. *Rhinosporidium seeberi* infection can present with a fleshy, red, friable mass.[29] These should be investigated with conjunctival biopsy. Other investigations that may be helpful are conjunctival smears demonstrating fungal hyphae, culture and PCR.

Treatment is with topical antifungals such as natamycin 5%, amphotericin B 0.15%, fluconazole 2% or ketoconazole 2%. Deeper and necrotizing lesions may require systemic antifungals in combination with topical treatment.

DIAGNOSTIC STRATEGY

A focused, accurate history can be helpful in differentiating the cause of conjunctivitis. A history of mucopurulent discharge is often in keeping with bacterial conjunctivitis, whilst a watery discharge is typical of viral infection; itching is often associated with allergic conjunctivitis. However, these symptoms are not specific, with a large meta-analysis demonstrating no association between the symptoms and the underlying cause.[15] However, a prospective study found that a combination of no prior history of conjunctivitis, both eyelids being stuck together in the morning and no history of itching was associated with culture-positive bacterial conjunctivitis.[15] Systemic features that may be helpful in suggesting an underlying viral etiology include a history of recent coryzal symptoms or sore throat, particularly true for adenoviral PCF. Patient demographics can also assist in diagnosis: bacterial conjunctivitis often has a bimodal distribution, being more common in young children and the elderly; whilst viral conjunctivitis is more common in young to middle aged adults. Chlamydial or gonococcal infection should be considered in sexually active patients.

With this prior knowledge, we suggest a diagnostic and therapeutic algorithm in Flowchart 18.1. It is important to consider alternative causes of conjunctival hyperemia, particularly if there are atypical features such as severe pain, photophobia or loss of vision.

CONCLUSION

Infectious conjunctivitis is a very common problem with significant economic costs associated with it; conjunctivitis accounts for 1% of all patient visits to a General Practitioner and the estimated cost in the USA alone for bacterial conjunctivitis is between $377 and $857 million per annum.[5,8]

Nonherpetic viral conjunctivitis is the most common cause of infectious conjunctivitis (estimated up to 80.3% of cases), followed closely by bacterial conjunctivitis (estimated at up 57% of all cases).[13,30] Adenovirus is the most commonly implicated viral agent.[30] By following a diagnostic approach that considers the patients' age, signs and symptoms and any other risk factors, one should attempt to differentiate bacterial from viral conjunctivitis, as well as ruling out any alternative serious ocular condition (Flowchart 18.1). However, it should be remembered that relying on signs and symptoms alone is not always reliable, and investigations should be considered, if there is any uncertainty, and particularly if a sexually-transmitted infection is a possibility.

As there is no specific treatment for viral conjunctivitis other than symptomatic measures and bacterial conjunctivitis resolves spontaneously in over 60% of cases,[4] treatment of infectious conjunctivitis in a setting where viral conjunctivitis is the most likely cause, initial treatment should consist of cold compresses and artificial tears. Investigations including cultures should be taken when there is no response to therapy, cases of hyperacute conjunctivitis and suspected chlamydial infection. Topical antibiotics should only be used when the patient is a contact lens wearer, mucopurulent discharge and a painful eye, patients with known ocular surface disease and cases of suspected gonococcal and chlamydial infection when additional systemic antibiotics and a referral to a sexual health clinic are required.

Flowchart 18.1: Algorithm showing diagnostic strategy for conjunctivitis.

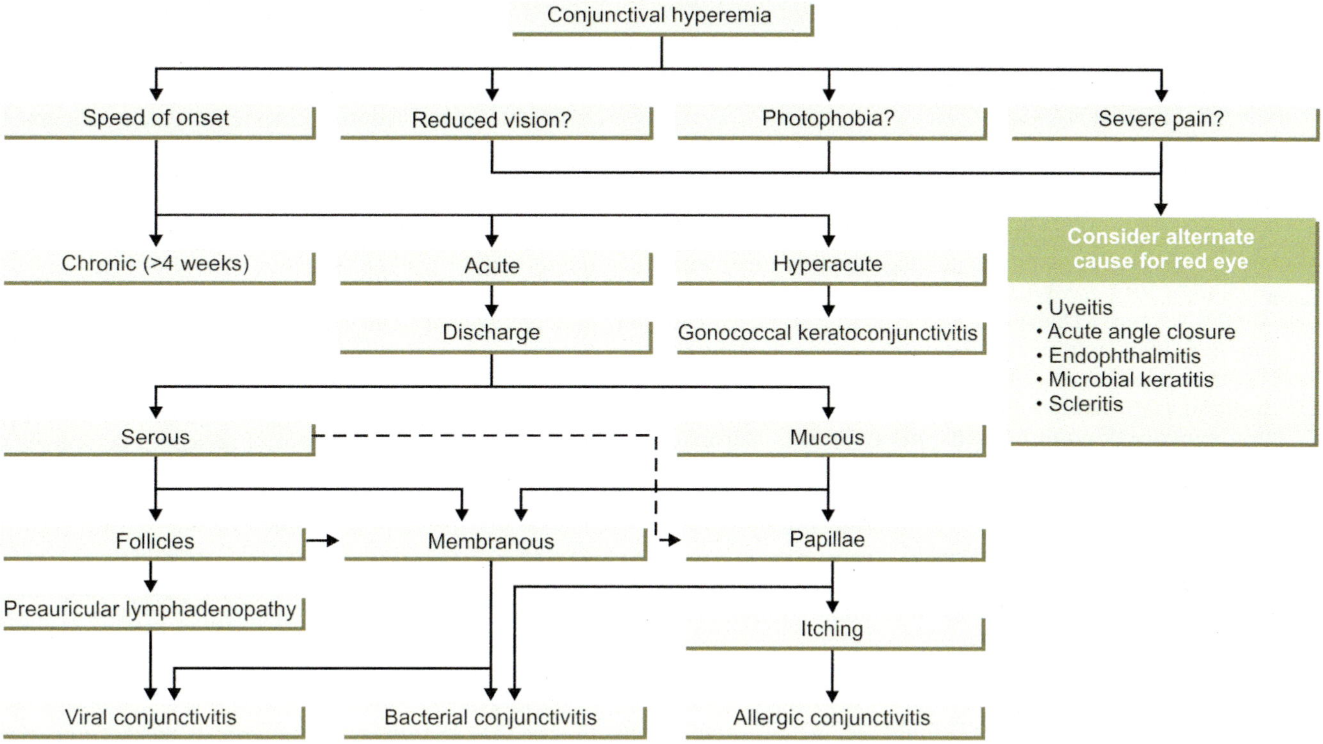

REFERENCES

1. Leibowitz HM. The red eye. N Engl J Med. 2000;343(5): 345-51.
2. Udeh BL, Schneider JE, Ohsfeldt RL. Cost effectiveness of a point-of-care test for adenoviral conjunctivitis. Am J Med Sci. 2008;336(3):254-64.
3. American Academy of Ophthalmology. Preferred practice pattern: conjunctivitis, 2nd edition. San Francisco: American Academy of Ophthalmology; 2003.
4. Høvding G. Acute bacterial conjunctivitis. Acta Ophthalmol. 2008;86(1):5-17.
5. Shields T, Sloane PD. A comparison of eye problems in primary care and ophthalmology practices. Fam Med. 1991;23(7):544-6.
6. Rietveld RP, Bindels PJE, Schellevis FG, et al. Do general practitioners adhere to the guideline on infectious conjunctivitis? Results of the Second Dutch National Survey of General Practice. BMC Fam Pract. 2007;8(1):54.
7. Manners T. Managing eye conditions in general practice. BMJ. 1997;315(7111):816-7.
8. Smith AF, Waycaster C. Estimate of the direct and indirect annual cost of bacterial conjunctivitis in the United States. BMC Ophthalmol. 2009;9(1):13.
9. Epling J, Smucny J. Bacterial conjunctivitis. Clin Evid. 2005;(14):756-61.
10. Lu LJ, Liu J. Human Microbiota and Ophthalmic Disease. Yale J Biol Med. 2016;89(3):325-30.
11. Dong Q, Brulc JM, Iovieno A, et al. Diversity of bacteria at healthy human conjunctiva. Invest Ophthalmol Vis Sci. 2011;52(8):5408-13.
12. Singer TR, Isenberg SJ, Apt L. Conjunctival anaerobic and aerobic bacterial flora in paediatric versus adult subjects. Br J Ophthalmol. 1988;72(6):448-51.
13. Azari AA, Barney NP. Conjunctivitis. JAMA. 2013;310(16):1721-9.
14. Tuzhikov A, Dong Q, Panchin A, et al. Keratitis-induced changes to the homeostatic microbiome at the human cornea. Invest Ophthalmol Vis Sci. 2013;54(15):1-5.
15. Rietveld RP, van Weert HCPM, Bindels PJE, et al. Diagnostic impact of signs and symptoms in acute infectious conjunctivitis: systematic literature search. BMJ. 2003;327(7418):789-9.
16. Sheikh A, Hurwitz B, van Schayck CP, et al. Antibiotics versus placebo for acute bacterial conjunctivitis. Cochrane Database Syst Rev. 2012;(9):CD001211.
17. Bodor FF, Marchant CD, Shurin PA, et al. Bacterial etiology of conjunctivitis-otitis media syndrome. Pediatrics. 1985;76(1):26-8.
18. Centers for Disease Control (CDC). Brazilian purpuric fever: Haemophilus aegyptius bacteremia complicating purulent conjunctivitis. Morb Mortal Wkly Rep. 1986;35(35):553-4.
19. Tarabishy AB, Jeng BH. Bacterial conjunctivitis: a review for internists. Cleve Clin J Med. 2008;75(7):507-12.
20. Day AC, Ramkissoon YD, George S, et al. Don't forget *Gonococcus*! Eye. 2006;20(12):1400-2.

21. Hoffman JJS, Ali B. Gonococcus—the culprit of refractory, severe conjunctivitis in an elderly patient. Cont Lens Anterior Eye. 2015;38(6):468-70.
22. Hoffman J, Ali B, Hoffman A, et al. Gonococcal conjunctivitis: the importance of good-quality conjunctival swabs. Br J Gen Pract. 2015;65(639):552-3.
23. Haimovici R, Roussel TJ. Treatment of gonococcal conjunctivitis with single-dose intramuscular ceftriaxone. AJOPHT. 1989;107(5):511-4.
24. Workowski KA, Bolan GA. Centers for Disease Control and Prevention. Sexually transmitted diseases treatment guidelines, 2015. MMWR. 2015;64:1-137.
25. Barquet N, Gasser I, Domingo P, et al. Primary meningococcal conjunctivitis: report of 21 patients and review. Rev Infect Dis. 1990;12(5):838-47.
26. Andreoli CM, Wiley HE, Durand ML, et al. Primary meningococcal conjunctivitis in an adult. Cornea. 2004;23(7):738-9.
27. Dryden AWS, Rana M, Pandey P. Primary meningococcal conjunctivitis: an unusual case of transmission by saliva. Digit J Ophthalmol. 2016;22(1):25-7.
28. Joint Formulary Committee. BNF 73 (British National Formulary) March 2017. London: BNF Publications; 2017. pp. 1.
29. Mishra D, Ranjan P, Mohan N, et al. Fungal conjunctivitis: How to Suspect and Diagnose. DOS Times. 2014;19:57-8.
30. O'Brien TP, Jeng BH, McDonald M, et al. Acute conjunctivitis: truth and misconceptions. Curr Med Res Opin. 2009;25(8):1953-61.
31. Ohnsman CM. Exclusion of students with conjunctivitis from school: policies of state departments of health. J Pediatr Ophthalmol Strabismus. 2007;44(2):101-5.
32. Fraunfelder FT, Bagby GC, Kelly DJ. Fatal aplastic anemia following topical administration of ophthalmic chloramphenicol. AJOPHT. 1982;93(3):356-60.
33. Flach AJ. Fatal aplastic anemia following topical administration of ophthalmic chloramphenicol. AJOPHT. 1982;94(3):420-2.
34. Fraunfelder FW, Fraunfelder FT. Restricting topical ocular chloramphenicol eye drop use in the United States. Did we overreact? Am J Ophthalmol. 2013;156(3):420-2.
35. World Health Organization. Weekly epidemiological record. Weekly epidemiological record. Geneva: WHO; 2017. pp. 357-68.
36. Burton M, Habtamu E, Ho D, et al. Interventions for trachoma trichiasis. Cochrane Database Syst Rev. 2015;40(11):CD004008.
37. Habtamu E, Wondie T, Aweke S, et al. Posterior lamellar versus bilamellar tarsal rotation surgery for trachomatous trichiasis in Ethiopia: a randomised controlled trial. Lancet Glob Health. 2016;4(3):e175-84.
38. Ramadhani AM, Derrick T, Macleod D, et al. The Relationship between active trachoma and ocular Chlamydia trachomatis infection before and after mass antibiotic treatment. PLoS Negl Trop Dis. 2016;10(10):e0005080.
39. Harding SP, Mallinson H, Smith JL, et al. Adult follicular conjunctivitis and neonatal ophthalmia in a Liverpool eye hospital, 1980-1984. Eye. 1987;1(Pt 4):512-21.
40. Rönnerstam R, Persson K, Hansson H, et al. Prevalence of chlamydial eye infection in patients attending an eye clinic, a VD clinic, and in healthy persons. Br J Ophthalmol. 1985;69(5):385-8.
41. Uchio E, Takeuchi S, Itoh N, et al. Clinical and epidemiological features of acute follicular conjunctivitis with special reference to that caused by herpes simplex virus type 1. Br J Ophthalmol. 2000;84(9):968-72.
42. Postema EJ, Remeijer L, van der Meijden WI. Epidemiology of genital chlamydial infections in patients with chlamydial conjunctivitis; a retrospective study. Genitourin Med. 1996;72(3):203-5.
43. Salopek-Rabatić J. Chlamydial conjunctivitis in contact lens wearers: successful treatment with single dose azithromycin. CLAO J. 2001;27(4):209-11.
44. Katusic D, Petricek I, Mandic Z, et al. Azithromycin vs doxycycline in the treatment of inclusion conjunctivitis. AJOPHT. 2003;135(4):447-51.
45. Hammerschlag MR, Rapoza P. Neonatal Conjunctivitis. In: Ocular Infection and Immunity. St Louis: Mosby; 1996. pp. 831-42.
46. Nishida H, Risemberg HM. Silver nitrate ophthalmic solution and chemical conjunctivities. Pediatrics. 1975;56(3):368-73.
47. Thanathanee O, O'Brien TP. Conjunctivitis: systematic approach to diagnosis and therapy. Curr Infect Dis Rep. 2011;13(2):141-8.
48. Zuppa AA, D'Andrea V, Catenazzi P, et al. Ophthalmia neonatorum: what kind of prophylaxis? J Matern Fetal Neonatal Med. 2011;24(6):769-73.
49. Eyre JW. Tuberculosis of the conjunctiva: its aetiology, pathology and diagnosis. Lancet. 1912;1:1319-28.
50. Jennings A, Bilous M, Asimakis P, et al. Mycobacterium tuberculosis presenting as chronic red eye. Cornea. 2006;25(9):1118-20.
51. Salas D, Murthy S, Champ C, et al. Primary tuberculosis of the conjunctiva. Eye. 2001;15(Pt 5):674-6.
52. World Health Organization. Global tuberculosis report 2017. Geneva: World Health Organization; 2017. pp. 262.
53. Shahidatul-Adha M, Zunaina E, Liza-Sharmini AT, et al. Ocular tuberculosis in Hospital Universiti Sains Malaysia—a case series. AnnMed Surg. 2017;24:25-30.
54. Merani R, Orekondy S, Gottlieb T, et al. Postoperative Mycobacterium abscessus nodular conjunctivitis. Clin Experiment Ophthalmol. 2008;36(4):371-3.
55. Edmonson BC, Morris WR, Osborn FD. Bacillary angiomatosis with cytomegaloviral and mycobacterial infections of the palpebral conjunctiva in a patient with AIDS. Ophthal Plast Reconstr Surg. 2004;20(2):168-70.
56. Jeng CJ, Hsiao CH, Hu FR, et al. Nontuberculous mycobacterial conjunctival granuloma detected by nested polymerase chain reaction. J Formos Med Assoc. 2014;113(10):760-1.
57. Baum S. Adenovirus. In: Mandell, Douglas, and Bennett's principles and practice of infectious diseases. Philadelphia: Churchill Livingstone; 2010.
58. Pavan-Langston D. Viral Disease of the Cornea and External Eye. In: Albert & Jakobiec's Principles and Practice of Ophthalmology. Philadelphia: Saunders; 2008.

59. Kaufman HE. Adenovirus advances: new diagnostic and therapeutic options. Curr OpinOphthalmol 2011;22(4): 290-3.
60. Murrah WF. Epidemic keratoconjunctivitis. Ann Ophthalmol. 1988;20(1):36-8.
61. O'Day DM, Guyer B, Hierholzer JC. Clinical and laboratory evaluation of epidemic keratoconjunctivitis due to adenovirus types 8 and 19. AJOPHT. 1976;81(2):207-15.
62. Harnett GB, Newnham WA. Isolation of adenovirus type 19 from the male and female genital tracts. Br J Vener Dis. 1981;57(1):55-7.
63. Laibson PR, Dhiri S, Oconer J, et al. Corneal infiltrates in epidemic keratoconjunctivitis. Response to double-blind corticosteroid therapy. Arch Ophthalmol. 1970;84(1): 36-40.
64. Dawson CR, Hanna L, Wood TR, et al. Adenovirus type 8 keratoconjunctivitis in the United States. 3. Epidemiologic, clinical, and microbiologic features. AJOPHT. 1970;69(3): 473-80.
65. Boniuk M, Phillips CA, Friedman JB. Chronic adenovirus type 2 keratitis in man. N Engl J Med. 1965;273(17):924-5.
66. Darougar S, Quinlan MP, Gibson JA, et al. Epidemic keratoconjunctivitis and chronic papillary conjunctivitis in London due to adenovirus type 19. Br J Ophthalmol. 1977;61(2):76-85.
67. Pettit TH, Holland GN. Chronic keratoconjunctivitis associated with ocular adenovirus infection. AJOPHT. 1979;88(4):748-51.
68. Kowalski RP, Thompson PP, Kinchington PR, et al. Evaluation of the SmartCycler II system for real-time detection of viruses and Chlamydia from ocular specimens. Arch Ophthalmol. 2006;124(8):1135-9.
69. Sambursky R, Tauber S, Schirra F, et al. The RPS adeno-detector for diagnosing adenoviral conjunctivitis. Ophthalmology. 2006;113(10):1758-64.
70. Pihos AM. Epidemic keratoconjunctivitis: areview of current concepts in management. J Optomet. 2013;6(2):69-74.
71. Kinchington PR, Romanowski EG, Jerold Gordon Y. Prospects for adenovirus antivirals. J Antimicrob Chemother. 2005;55(4):424-9.
72. Hillenkamp J, Reinhard T, Ross RS, et al. The effects of cidofovir 1% with and without cyclosporin a 1% as a topical treatment of acute adenoviral keratoconjunctivitis: a controlled clinical pilot study. Ophthalmology. 2002;109(5):845-50.
73. Huang J, Kadonosono K, Uchio E. Antiadenoviral effects of ganciclovir in types inducing keratoconjunctivitis by quantitative polymerase chain reaction methods. Clin Ophthalmol. 2014;8:315-20.
74. Tabbara KF, El-Sheikh HF, Aabed B. Extended wear contact lens related bacterial keratitis. Br J Ophthalmol. 2000;84(3):327-8.
75. Tabbara KF, Jarade EF. Ganciclovir effects in adenoviral keratoconjunctivitis. IOVS.2001:S579.
76. Isenberg SJ, Apt L, Campeas D. Ocular applications of povidone-iodine. Dermatology (Basel). 2002;204 (Suppl 1): 92-5.
77. Pelletier JS, Stewart K, Trattler W, et al. A combination povidone-iodine 0.4%/dexamethasone 0.1% ophthalmic suspension in the treatment of adenoviral conjunctivitis. Adv Ther. 2009;26(8):776-83.
78. Clement C, Capriotti JA, Kumar M, et al. Clinical and antiviral efficacy of an ophthalmic formulation of dexamethasone povidone-iodine in a rabbit model of adenoviral keratoconjunctivitis. Invest Ophthalmol Vis Sci. 2011;52(1):339-44.
79. Melton R, Thomas R. Stop EKC with a "silver bullet." Rev Optomet. 2008;145:80-1.
80. Romanowski EG, Roba LA, Wiley L, et al. The effects of corticosteroids of adenoviral replication. Arch Ophthalmol. 1996;114(5):581-5.
81. Romanowski EG, Yates KA, Gordon YJ. Topical corticosteroids of limited potency promote adenovirus replication in the Ad5/NZW rabbit ocular model. Cornea. 2002;21(3):289-91.
82. Woodland RM, Darougar S, Thaker U, et al. Causes of conjunctivitis and keratoconjunctivitis in Karachi, Pakistan. Trans R Soc Trop Med Hyg. 1992;86(3):317-20.
83. American Academy of Ophthalmology.Preferred Practice Pattern Guidelines: conjunctivitis-limited revision. San Francisco:American Academy of Ophthalmology; 2011.
84. Klotz SA, Penn CC, Negvesky GJ, et al. Fungal and parasitic infections of the eye. Clin Microbiol Rev. 2000;13(4):662-85.
85. Ando N, Takatori K. Fungal flora of the conjunctival sac. AJOPHT. 1982;94(1):67-74.
86. Segal E, Romano A, Eylan E, et al. Fungal flora of the normal conjunctival sac. Mycoses. 1977;20(1):9-14.
87. Fontes BM, Muccioli C, Príncipe AH, et al. Effect of chronic systemic use of trimethoprim-sulfamethoxazole in the conjunctival bacterial flora of patients with HIV infection. AJOPHT. 2004;138(4):678-9.

Chapter 19

Conjunctival Inflammatory Disorders

Aravind Roy, Paavan Kalra, Prashant Garg

INTRODUCTION

The conjunctiva along with the tear film forms an important immune barrier of the ocular surface. It consists of a thin epithelium lined mucous membrane with a substantia propria comprising of lymphoid and vascular connective tissue. While the conjunctiva is commonly affected in several acute infections, the present discussion deals with chronic disorders of the conjunctiva that may be caused due to external allergens, chemicals, immune-mediated mechanisms or as a toxic reaction to drugs/foreign bodies. The conjunctival chronic inflammatory conditions can typically be classified as per etiology, morphology or by their underlying pathology (Box 19.1).

It is important to appreciate the nature of the disease, its underlying immune mechanisms and the related pathology in the affected tissues. Several subtle symptoms and signs of the chronic nature of this disease aid the clinician to give appropriate diagnosis. These could be longstanding conjunctival injection, acute or chronic exacerbation followed by remission, nonspecific irritation, itching, discharge and watering. In the sections later, we provide an overview of the disease entities encompassing chronic inflammatory conjunctival disorders.

ALLERGIC CONJUNCTIVITIS

Allergic conjunctivitis is a immunoglobulin E (IgE) mediated type I hypersensitivity reaction to allergens which may be typically air borne, such as pollen, animal dander, dust, etc. When the allergen comes in contact with the tear film containing IgE antibodies, it triggers degranulation of the conjunctival mast cells. It leads to inflammatory cascade and release of histamines, leukotrienes and other inflammatory mediators that lead to vasodilation, conjunctival edema and recruitment of inflammatory cells. Repeated insults sensitize the immune mechanisms and lead to an earlier response. Typically, allergic conjunctivitis may consist of two types:

1. Seasonal allergic conjunctivitis (SAC) is the commonest form. It typically manifests in spring to summer on exposure to pollen.

Box 19.1: Classification of conjunctival inflammatory disorders.

Etiological Classification

Noninfectious

- *Mechanical/Irritative/Toxic*:
  - Superior limbic keratoconjunctivitis
  - Contact lens related
  - Foreign body related
  - Medication induced
  - Radiation induced
  - Pediculosis palpebrarum
  - Ophthalmia nodosum
  - Giant-Fornix syndrome
  - Floppy-eyelid syndrome
  - Factitious (self inflicted)
- *Immune-mediated*:
  - SJS/TEN
  - OCP/MMP
  - Graft vs host disease
  - Allergic
  - Seasonal
  - Vernal
  - Atopic
  - Giant papillary conjunctivitis
  - Phlycten
- *Neoplastic*:
  - Sebaceous carcinoma
  - OSSN
  - Lymphoma
  - Others-melanoma, angioma, angiosarcoma, fibrosarcoma
- Dry eye
- Idiopathic

Infectious

- Viral
- Bacterial
- Chlamydial
- Microsporidial
- Fungal
- Parasitic

Classification Based on Clinical Features

Onset

- Acute
- Subacute
- Chronic
- *Exudate*:
  - Serous
  - Mucoid
  - Purulent
  - Mucopurulent
- *Morphology*:
  - Follicular
  - Papillary
  - Giant papillary
  - Pseudomembranous/membranous
  - Cicatrizing

2. Perennial allergic conjunctivitis (PAC) is less common. It is chronic with periodic exacerbations especially in winter with exposure to dust and fungal spores.[1]

Patients with allergic conjunctivitis may also suffer from additional atopic conditions such as allergic rhinitis, asthma, eczema and atopic dermatitis. Typically attacks are short-lived and they consist of episodic attacks of ocular itching with runny nose, puffiness and redness of eyes. On examination there is conjunctival edema, hyperemia and mucoid discharge. Diagnosis is chiefly clinical and ocular impression cytology may yield eosinophils in the tear film. An immune challenge test may help detect sensitivity to any particular antigen.

Treatment

- Avoiding exposure to the inciting antigen through environmental modification, such as avoiding dusty places, cleaning of rugs, mattresses and linen.
- Cold compresses can be applied over the eye for symptomatic relief.
- Lubricant eye drops help to dilute the tear film and wash away inciting antigens and inflammatory mediators.
- Topical mast cell stabilizers, such as Cromolyn sodium and iodoxamide tromethamine help to prevent mast cell degranulation and may be used prior to the attacks, typically in seasonal allergic conjunctivitis. Topical cyclosporin, combined mast cell stabilizers and antihistamines, such as olopatadine, azelastine and ketotifen are also typically used to control and prevent attacks.
- Topical corticosteroids though rarely indicated are useful in acute attacks but need to be used under supervision and judiciously.[1,2] Hyposensitization injections have also been tried where the inciting allergen has been identified.

VERNAL KERATOCONJUNCTIVITIS

Vernal keratoconjunctivitis (VKC) is a recurring bilateral inflammatory disease of the cornea and conjunctiva. There is a predominant seasonal influence commonly in spring. However, a perennial variant with periodic exacerbations has also been reported. The disease predominantly affects male children typically until the completion of teenage. In the rare instances of the disease affecting females, it may persist beyond teenage. There is a positive personal and/family history of atopy.[3]

The immunopathogenesis is a type I and type IV hypersensitivity. The conjunctival biopsy specimens show inflammatory cells including eosinophils, plasma cells, lymphocytes and monocytes. The disease consists of palpebral, limbal and mixed palbepral and limbal forms with or without keratopathy.

Clinical Features

Vernal keratoconjunctivitis has a bilateral asymmetric presentation. The patient typically, a young boy presents with complaints of severe ocular itching, watering, redness and discharge. The hallmark sign of VKC is a papillary reaction on the upper tarsal plate. This may vary from small papillae to giant or cobblestone papillae.[4] The limbal variety consists of thickened gelatinous nodules of epithelial hyperplasia with chalky white excrescences, Horner-Trantas dots, with increased limbal pigmentation. The keratopathy typically starts as superficial punctate spots on the cornea that may coalesce to form macroerosions. Eye rubbing and the outpouring of inflammatory mediators aggravate this condition causing shield ulcers. Based on the stages of disease progression, Cameron[5] proposed a classification based on the degree of severity of shield ulcer as follows (Table 19.1):

1. Grade I ulcer having a transparent base.
2. Grade II being an ulcer with a translucent base or with white/yellowish deposits.
3. Grade III ulcers have an elevated plaque which is above the level of the adjacent normal epithelium (Figs. 19.1A to D).

Chronic VKC may cause limbal stem cell deficiency leading to corneal vascularization, pannus formation, poor ocular surface and persistent epithelial defects. VKC may be differentiated from PAC and SAC by the presence of giant/cobblestone papillae, limbal nodules and limbal stem cell deficiency. In contrast, atopic keratoconjunctivitis (AKC) is a more severe form of allergic eye disease and is seen in older children and young adults. This condition is also associated with a family/personal history of atopy.[6]

Table 19.1: Grades of shield ulcers.

Grade	Description
Grade I	Transparent base
Grade II	Translucent base or with whitish/ yellowish deposits
Grade III	Elevated plaque above normal epithelium

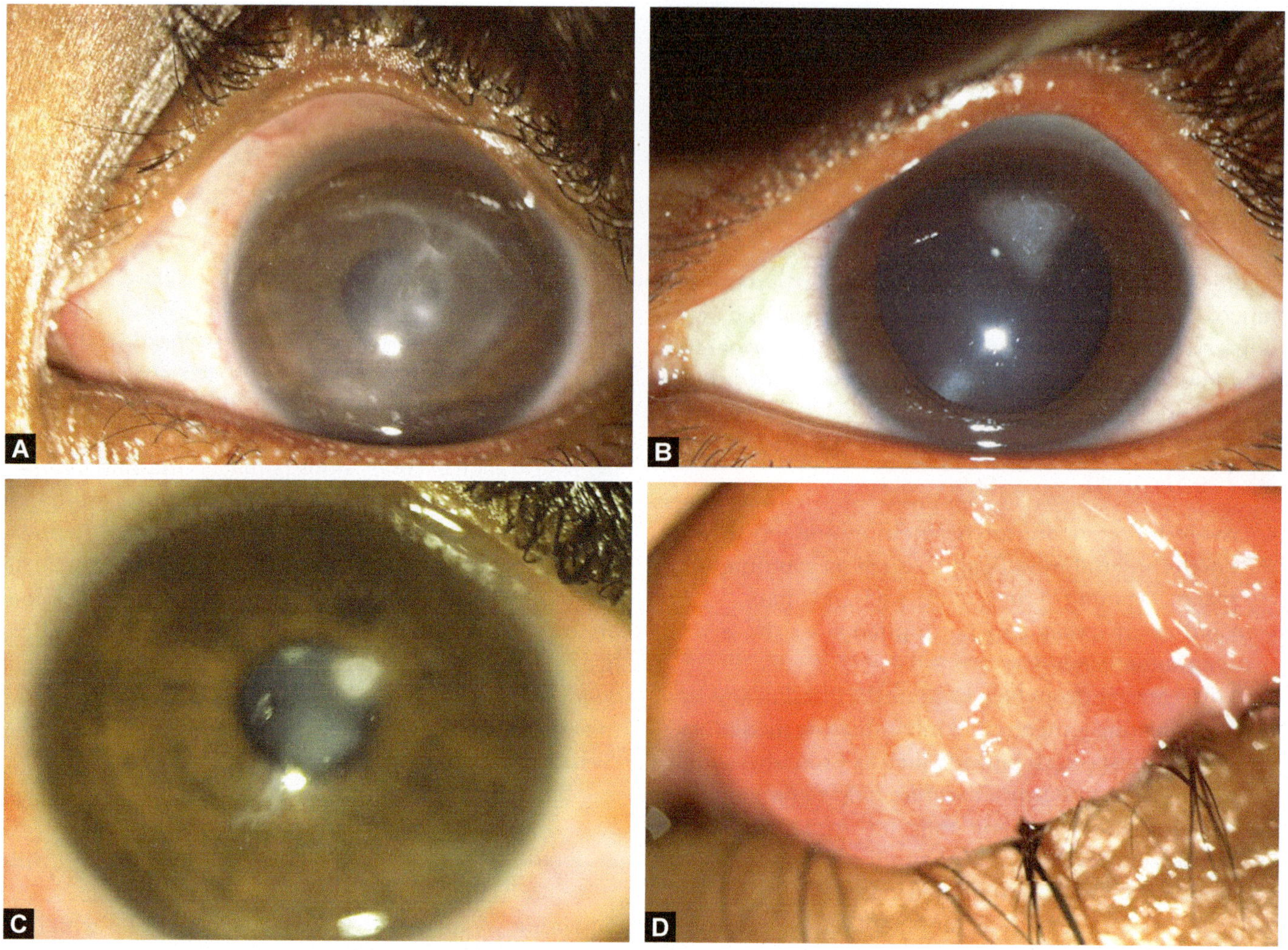

Figs. 19.1A to D: (A) Shield ulcer with a transparent base; (B) Translucent base with whitish deposits; (C) Elevated plaque; (D) Cobble-stone papillae on the upper tarsal conjunctiva in a patient of vernal keratoconjunctivitis.

Management

The disease runs a chronic course with periodic exacerbations and remission requiring regular follow-up:

- Topical antihistamines, such as levocabastine and emedastine remain the main stay of treatment for mild cases.[7]
- Mast cell stabilizers, such as cromolyn sodium, nedocromil sodium and lodoxamide prevent degranulation of the mast cells. They are used for prophylactic treatment and require a loading dose. Ketotifen and olopatadine have a dual action of antihistaminic effect and prevention of mast cell degranulation.
- Topical corticosteroids, such as prednisolone, dexamethasone, fluorometholone and loteprednol have been used in more severe cases. These agents need to be used under close supervision owing to the chance of secondary glaucoma, cataract and secondary infections.[8] Supratarsal injections of periocular steroids such as triamcinolone acetonide and dexamethasone sodium phosphate are very effective in the acute stage of the disease. It is important to identify patients who are steroid responders prior to injection. Shield ulcers especially those with opaque base respond well to corticosteroids and mechanical debridement.
- Cyclosporin, a T-cell and mast cell inhibitor has been used with varied success in VKC.[9] Tacrolimus is another potent immunomodulator that is effective in the management of VKC.[10] However, there is a chance of opportunistic infections and herpes simplex keratitis.

- Oral medications, such as Montelukast, a leukotriene antagonist and cyclosporin have been used for severe cases.[11]

The role of oral antihistamines and corticosteroids for the management of VKC is limited by systemic side effects. Cases not responding to medical treatment and those with persistent epithelial defects can be benefited by amniotic membrane graft.[6] It is important however, to rule out secondary infections in shield ulcers and treat as per the causative microbiological agent. Resultant corneal scar may need phototherapeutic keratectomy or superficial keratectomy. Severe cases of VKC with extensive limbal stem cell deficiency may need specialized contact lens and Boston keratoprosthesis.[12]

SUPERIOR LIMBIC KERATOCONJUNCTIVITIS

Superior limbic keratoconjunctivitis (SLKC) is an inflammatory conjunctival disorder with periods of exacerbations and remission. It is characterized by inflammation of the superior tarsal and bulbar conjunctiva, punctate staining of the adjacent cornea and superior limbus, corneal filaments and proliferating superior limbic epithelial cells.[13]

Etiopathogenesis

The etiology is multifactorial with several theories being proposed, such as mechanical, immune-mediated, infectious and environmental. Of these, the mechanical theory has the greatest acceptance. A thick taut lid with a prominent globe induces greater friction and tissue roll between the palpebral conjunctiva and the superior bulbar conjunctiva causing chronic mechanical rubbing resulting in thrusting of the tissue onto the superior cornea.[14]

Clinical Features

Typically, the disease presents in middle age during the 3rd to 5th decade of life with a female preponderance. It is bilateral but may have unilateral and asymmetric presentation. Patients may present with irritation, grittiness and redness of eyes. There may be associated burning sensations, dryness, foreign body sensations and mucoid discharge. Typically, the superior palberal conjunctiva is hyperemic with papillary reaction. There is proliferation of limbal cells. The superior cornea may have filaments and punctate staining that stain positive with Rose Bengal. Schirmer's test is decreased with abnormal corneal sensations. The disease runs a chronic course with exacerbations and remission (Figs. 19.2A and B). The diagnosis is clinical, however, impression cytology of the bulbar conjunctiva may show varying degrees of squamous metaplasia with irregular epithelial cells and scrapings from the superior tarsal conjunctiva may show keratinized and hyalinized epithelial cells with polymorphonuclear cells and lymphocytes. The in vivo confocal scanning laser microscopy is a useful adjunct to diagnosis and shows altered nuclear-cytoplasmic ratio and inflammatory cells in the superior bulbar conjunctiva.[15]

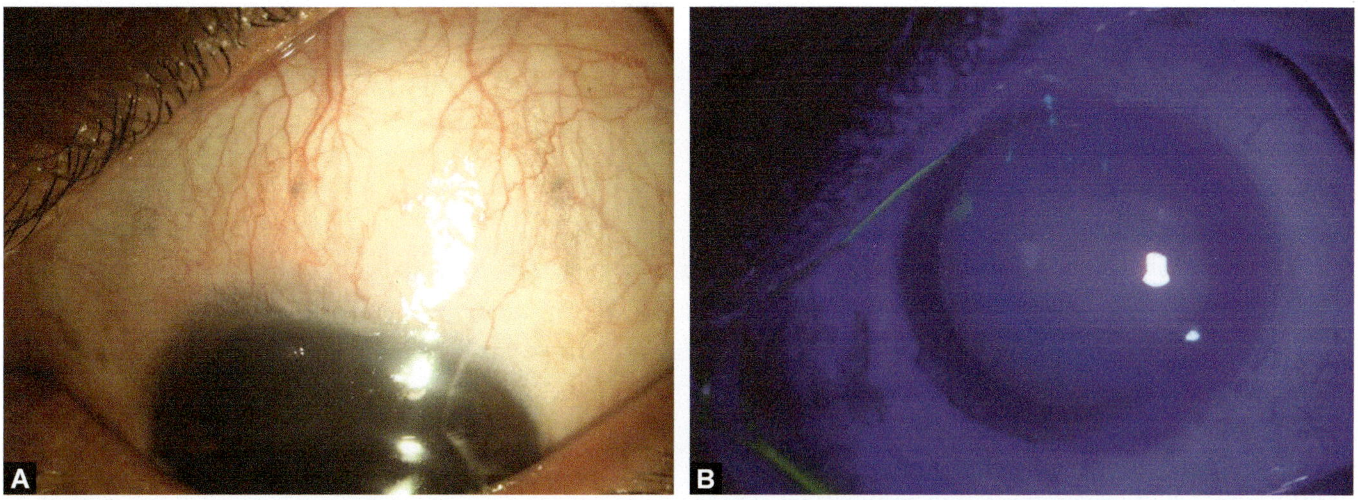

Figs. 19.2A and B: (A) Superior bulbar conjunctiva shows a thickening. (B) The adjacent cornea shows filaments with punctate staining.

Source: Dr C Jagadesh Reddy, Tej Kohli Cornea Institute, LV Prasad Eye Institute, KAR Campus, Hyderabad, Telangana, India.

Management

- The tarsal inflammation and mechanical trauma causes squamous metaplasia and proliferation of goblet cells. This may be managed by conservative treatment with topical lubricants, Vitamin A eye drops, and 5–10% acetylcysteine. Acetylcysteine breaks covalent bonds with dissolution of mucin, due to which it is used as a mucolytic and mucokinetic agent.
- Definitive treatment consists of local application of 0.5–1.0% freshly prepared silver nitrate to the superior palpebral conjunctiva. It is applied for 1minute with cotton tipped applicator or cellulose sponge. This results in relief of symptoms and the effect is sustained for 4–6 weeks but may be repeated in a week, if the symptoms relapse.
- Conjunctival resection with dissection of a broad flap of the superior bulbar conjunctiva has also been described. The underlying conjunctival defect is left unsutured and postoperative antibiotics are used. Patients have rapid improvement of symptoms, if the preoperative Schirmer's test was normal.[16]
- Supra tarsal triamcinolone and tacrolimus have also been used to control the local inflammation and induce remission.[17,18]
- Various other treatment modalities have also been discussed, such as application of diathermy to the superior bulbar conjunctiva to induce stromal shrinkage without affecting the sclera.

TOXIC CONJUNCTIVITIS

Toxic conjunctivitis is an inflammatory reaction of the conjunctiva to topical medications and preservatives. Antiglaucoma medications, preservatives containing lubricants, antivirals and some antibiotics usually when used chronically, cause this condition.[19,20] Toxicity is often related to concentration, duration and frequency of drugs. The pathophysiology includes direct toxicity of the ocular surface epithelium to the preservatives or directly to the pharmacologic agents as well as by immunologic mechanisms.

Clinical Features

Symptoms include watering, tearing, redness and grittiness of eyes. On examination there may be lid edema, thickening of lid margins and excoriations. The conjunctiva shows injection/congestion, chemosis, papillary reaction, mucoid discharge and erosions. Dua and coworkers describe an ocular "up-down" sign where there is an increased congestion of the inferior conjunctiva. A marked difference in the conjunctival redness may be noted on asking the patient to look up and down while noting the ocular surface congestion.[19] The cornea may show corneal punctate opacities, corneal erosions and pseudodendrites, which may be confused with herpetic viral keratitis. The treatment of this condition lies in recognizing this entity in the background of a chronic topical medication usage. Conservative management includes frequent instillation of preservative-free lubricants and advising a drug holiday by stopping the inciting medications.

GIANT PAPILLARY CONJUNCTIVITIS

Giant papillary conjunctivitis (GPC) is caused by chronic ocular allergy with formation of papillae in the tarsal conjunctiva. Papillae are classified as macropapillae, if they are 0.3–1.0 mm and giant papillae, if they are more than 1.0 mm.[21] GPC typically occurs due to contact lens wear, ocular prosthesis, filtering blebs, sutures, scleral buckles, tissue adhesives and foreign bodies (Fig. 19.3). Patients can present with excessive mucoid discharge, redness, discomfort and grittiness of eyes. Contact lens wearers experience increasing contact lens intolerance, excessive movement of contact lenses, blurring vision and contact lens coating with mucoid discharge. The degree of coating is influenced by the severity of the condition and type of contact lenses. The pathophysiology of this condition

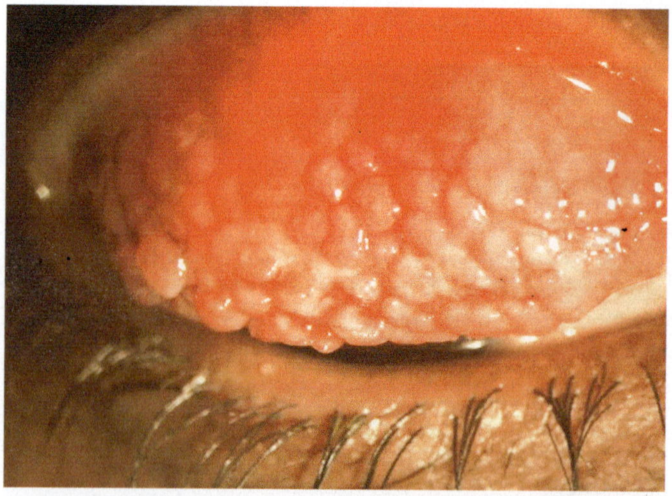

Fig. 19.3: Contact lens wearer with giant papillae on the superior tarsal conjunctiva.
Source: Dr Muralidhar Ramappa, Tej Kohli Cornea Institute, LV Prasad Eye Institute, KAR Campus, Hyderabad, Telangana, India.

is probably immune-mediated with increased tarsal inflammation and a mechanical component. The levels of inflammatory mediators, such as cytokines, chemokines, complement factors and neutrophil chemotactic factors (NCF) are elevated. The treatment of GPC consists of eliminating the inciting agent. Stopping contact lens usage for 2–4 weeks allows for inflammatory reaction to subside. Topical medications, such as loteprednol etabonate, mast cell stabilizers and lubricants help to control the initial discomfort.[22] Topical steroids are not found to be effective and may be avoided due to the potential side effects of glaucoma, cataract and secondary infections. Preventive strategies include improving the cleaning of contact lenses, shifting to daily wear contact lenses, decreasing the wearing time, and the use of alternative materials or designs.

PHLYCTENULAR KERATOCONJUNCTIVITIS

Phlyctenular keratoconjunctivitis (PKC) is a nonspecific unilateral allergic reaction to an antigen that is characterized by formation of a circumscribed nodular lesion at the limbus, cornea or adjacent conjunctiva (Fig. 19.4). PKC often manifests in the first two decades of life with a slightly female preponderance. There is often an association with hypersensitivity to tuberculoprotein with or without tubercular disease. In addition the other etiological agents include hypersensitivity to nematode antigens following worm infestation, staphylococcal antigens with attendant lid margin disease like blepharitis, fungi, viruses and parasites. There may be associated nutritional and vitamin deficiencies. The condition presents as a limbal nodule with a blister like appearance, which may be single or having multiple foci and involves the adjacent cornea and conjunctiva. It may ulcerate with necrosis and sloughing of the epithelium. The disease has a short self-limiting course and responds well to topical steroids. A short course of low potency steroids, such as 1% fluorometholone may be administered under close supervision. 2% cyclosporin A has also been found to be effective. Though the condition is self-limited it is important to identify and treat local and systemic causative factors.[23-25]

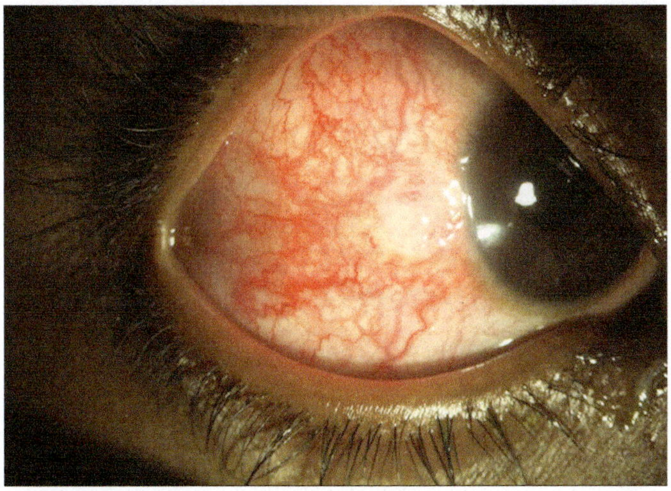

Fig. 19.4: Phlycten presents as a circumscribed nodular lesion at the limbus and adjacent conjunctiva.

SARCOIDOSIS

Sarcoidosis is a granulomatous inflammatory disease of unknown etiology that commonly involves the lungs, skin and eyes. Tissue biopsies showing noncaseating granulomas are the histopathologic hallmark of the disease. The etiology is poorly understood as exposure to microbial antigens, such as mycobacterium, occupational and environmental toxins and a genetic predisposition may have a causative role. Ocular involvement is noted in 25–50% of systemic sarcoidosis with formation of conjunctival granuloma, lacrimal gland involvement and uveitis.[26] Conjunctival involvement is common with the initial presentation being multiple discrete tiny palpebral, bulbar or perilimbal conjunctival deposits. Follicular conjunctivitis with irritation, redness and chronic cicatricial conjunctivitis with scarring and symblepharon has been reported. Large conjunctival granulomas may present as tumors.[27] Definitive diagnosis is made through conjunctival biopsy demonstrating the presence of noncaseating granuloma, giant cells with Schaumann bodies, asteroid bodies or both. The goals of treatment are control of inflammation and preservation of vision. Often corticosteroids are the main stay of treatment. They need to be administered through several routes, such as topical, periocular, regional implants and systemic modes. Other immunomodulators, such as methotrexate, azathioprine, mycophenolate mofetil, cyclosporin A and cyclophosphamide may be used in case of corticosteroid nonresponse or intolerance. Topical corticosteroids are used only for the anterior segment inflammation. In addition, there are reports of efficacy of topical cyclosporin for conjunctival lesions.[28]

OPHTHALMIA NODOSA

Ophthalmia nodosa is an inflammatory reaction to insect body parts, such as caterpillar setae, tarantula spider hairs etc. It presents as an inflamed conjunctival nodule. There is a typical history of exposure to an insect with sudden onset of redness, pain, grittiness, and foreign body sensations (Fig. 19.5). The setae can migrate into the anterior chamber, lens, vitreous and retina. The toxins within the spines cause an intense inflammatory reaction. Multiple hairs may get buried into the conjunctiva forming a follicular nodule with a part of the hair projecting out of the nodule, which in turn may rub into the cornea causing corneal abrasions and scars. In India, the clinical features are characterized by a seasonal incidence from September to January and the setae being sharp, smooth and without barbs.[29]

Cadera et al.[30] proposed an useful clinical classification:

- *Type 1:* An acute reaction with chemosis
- *Type 2:* Chronic mechanical keratoconjunctivitis with corneal abrasions
- *Type 3:* Conjunctival granulomas
- *Type 4:* Iritis with penetration of setae into the anterior segment
- *Type 5:* Vitreoretinal involvement with vitritis, cystoid macular edema and endophthalmitis.

The treatment is also based on this classification with type 1 and 2 needing immediate identification and prompt removal of setae. Type 3 with a subconjunctival or corneal penetration requires removal and symptomatic treatment with topical steroids. Type 4 iritis is treated with topical steroids and removal of any anterior chamber setae and iris nodules with iridectomy. Type 5 reactions need periocular and/or oral steroids and vitrectomy and removal of setae may be needed, if there is no response to conservative management.

LIGNEOUS CONJUNCTIVITIS

Ligneous conjunctivitis (LC) is rare bilateral chronic recurrent fibrinous reaction of the conjunctiva. It is characterized by formation of thick membranous reactions with a woody consistency over conjunctiva and other mucosal surfaces. It is commonly associated with type I plasminogen deficiency.

Clinical Features

The disease may affect children though it has also been reported to occur from birth to the 6th to 8th decade of life, with a slight female preponderance and an autosomal recessive pattern of inheritance.[31] The ocular involvement typically consists of congestion, watering, redness and formation of membranes on the palpebral conjunctiva that gradually gets replaced by yellow white or reddish thick wood like firm sessile or pedunculated masses on the conjunctival mucosa. Though referred in ophthalmic literature as a pseudomembrane, in pathologic terms it is a true membrane. With chronic inflammation, the initial friable fibrovascular membrane transforms into a fibrous vascular membrane with a mucoid discharge. It involves the palpebral conjunctiva of the upper lids more frequently than the lower lids; bulbar conjunctiva and cornea may get involved but less frequently from the adjacent conjunctival lesions (Fig. 19.6).

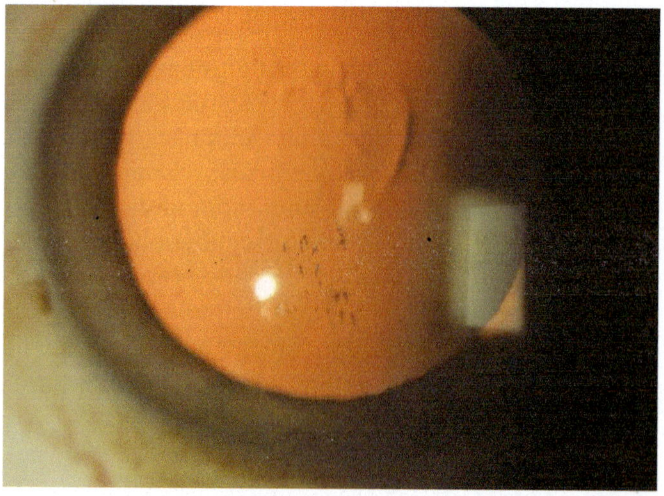

Fig. 19.5: Insect hairs on the cornea highlighted on retroillumination.
Source: Dr Mukesh Taneja, Tej Kohli Cornea Institute, LV Prasad Eye Institute, KAR Campus, Hyderabad, Telangana, India.

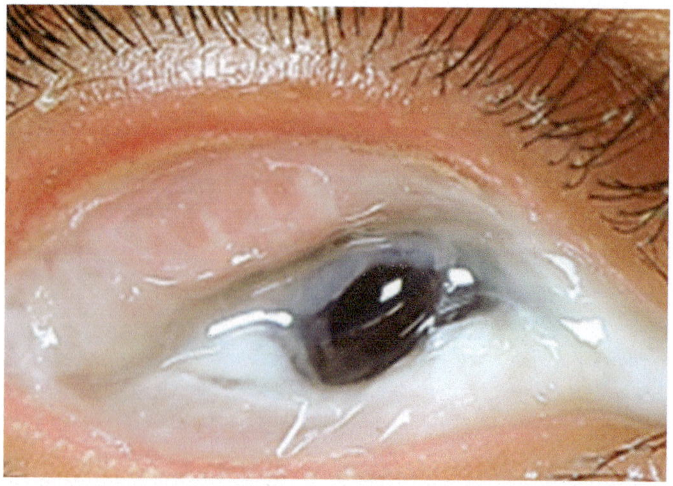

Fig. 19.6: Ligneous conjunctivitis with thick protruding sessile masses on the conjunctival mucosa.
Source: Dr Muralidhar Ramappa, Tej Kohli Cornea Institute, LV Prasad Eye Institute, KAR Campus, Hyderabad, Telangana, India.

Etiopathogenesis

In normal life, plasmin plays an important role in tissue healing and it regulates the migration, division and differentiation of keratinocytes. In ligneous conjunctivitis, there is limited ability to clear the fibrin in response to an environmental insult. This leads to formation of abundant granulation tissue and deposition of fibrin in the extracellular matrix. This is the reason for repeated recurrences inspite of excision of these masses and seemingly complete resolution on systemic plasminogen application. The histopathology of the excised tissues shows alternate areas of thick and thinned-out ulcerated epithelium, deposits of hyaline eosinophilic material, mucopolysaccharides with granulation tissue and inflammatory cells, such as lymphocytes, granulocytes and plasma cells. There may be extensive ulcerations with overlying exudates and irregular cord, cyst and gland-like extensions of the epithelium into the substantia propria.[32]

Treatment

The treatment is usually prolonged and marred by frequent recurrences. Several pharmacologic approaches have been attempted, including the use of cromolyn sodium, heparin, alpha-chymotrypsin, topical corticosteroids, cyclosporin and plasminogen.[33-36] Local excision of the lesions always leads to relapse of the condition; recurrent cases require excision of lesions and intensive medications for much longer duration.[37,38]

MASQUERADE SYNDROME

Masquerade syndromes are neoplastic lesions that mimic chronic inflammation. Theodore first used the term "masquerade syndrome" to describe a case of conjunctival neoplasia presenting as chronic conjunctivitis.[39] Masquerades of conjunctival inflammatory disorders include sebaceous gland carcinoma, ocular surface squamous neoplasia (OSSN), lymphoma, melanoma, angiomas, angiosarcoma and fibrosarcoma including Kaposi's sarcoma. Sebaceous gland carcinoma most commonly arises from the tarsal meibomian glands but can also arise from glands of Zeiss at eyelid margin and from the caruncle. The presenting features vary with the lesion appearing as chalazion, a small yellowish nodule, or as a blepharoconjunctivitis or as a keratoconjunctivitis. Sebaceous gland carcinoma with pagetoid (intraepithelial) spread presenting as blepharoconjunctivitis or keratoconjunctivitis can mimic chronic conjunctival inflammation. The lesion can be differentiated from chronic inflammation by a high index of suspicion combined with a comprehensive clinical examination which shows any or all of the following features—thick and deformed eyelid, loss of eyelashes, chronic disease and an unilateral involvement. The treatment is surgical comprising of excision with wide margins and confirmation with frozen section or Moh's microsurgery. Conjunctival map biopsy from palpebral, forniceal and bulbar conjunctiva and caruncle with a diagram and an identifier of the site of the biopsy are recommended in these cases. This helps in identifying the presence and extent of the pagetoid spread of the tumor. The management options for limited pagetoid spread of sebaceous gland carcinoma are cryotherapy and topical mitomycin C. Extensive pagetoid spread with involvement of contiguous structures may warrant orbital exenteration.[40] Conjunctival ocular squamous neoplasia has been reported to present as a blepharoconjunctivitis.[41] The lesions typically start at the limbus and present as a leukoplakic, gelatinous or a papilliform nodule. It may extend into the cornea as multiple finger-like or fimbriated extensions. The lesions stain with Rose Bengal that demarcates the extent of the tumor. The lesions need to be excised with a wide margin and application of cryotherapy to the base and margins in a double freeze- thaw method. Topical interferon alpha 2b, 5-flurouracil and mitomycin C may be used as a primary treatment or as an adjuvant to surgical excision.[42,43] Conjunctival lymphoma may present as chronic conjunctivitis with diffuse conjunctival involvement. The characteristic salmon pink nodular appearance of conjunctival lymphoma may not be always present. It can lead to chronic conjunctival inflammation and cicatrizing conjunctivitis.[44] Tissue biopsy is of diagnostic value. The lesion resolves with radiation therapy or systemic chemotherapy.[45]

STEVENS-JOHNSON SYNDROME

Stevens-Johnson syndrome (SJS) and toxic epidermal necrolysis (TEN) describe a spectrum of systemic diseases which involves acute immunological injury to skin and mucous membranes, usually in response to drugs most frequently due to sulfonamides and antiseizure medications. The annual incidences of SJS/TEN range from 1.2 to 12.35 new cases per million per year.[46] Though generally considered to be a part of the disease spectrum, TEN is thought to be a severe variant of SJS.

Etiopathogenesis

Various drugs have been implicated to cause SJS[47] (Box 19.2) although the reaction may also be triggered less commonly by systemic viral or Mycoplasma infection. Association with human leukocyte antigens HLAB12 and HLA-Bw44 has been noted[48] and a genetic predisposition probably contributes to the etiology of SJS/TEN.

Pathogenesis of acute phase involves activation of T-cell mediated type 4 hypersensitivity which leads to death of epithelial cells in skin (known as keratinocytes) and mucous membranes and hence, development of blisters and erosions at these sites.[49]

Box 19.2: Few important drugs implicated for Stevens-Johnson syndrome.

- *Anticonvulsants*:
  - Phenytoin
  - Phenobarbital
  - Carbamazapine
- *NSAIDs*:
  - Salicylates
  - Ibuprofen
  - Pyrazoline derivatives
- *Antimicrobials*:
  - Beta-lactam antibiotics
  - Macrolides
  - Tetracyclines
  - Quinolones
  - Griseofulvin
  - Nystatin
  - Chloroquine
  - Quinine
  - Nevirapine, Abacavir
- *Sulfa derivatives*:
  - Trimethoprim
  - Sulfasalazine
  - Sulfadiazine
- *Metals*:
  - Arsenic
  - Lithium
  - Mercury
  - Gold
- *Miscellaneous*:
  - Acetazolamide
  - Allopurinol
  - Cimetidine
  - Lamotrigine
  - Indapamide
  - Enalapril, Captopril
  - Calcium-channel blockers
  - Diuretics
  - Vaccinating agents

(NSAIDs: Nonsteroidal anti-inflammatory drugs)

Clinical Presentation

Acute

In the acute phase, the patient presents with an initial prodrome of malaise, fever and an upper respiratory tract infection followed by inflammation and ulceration of the ocular, oral and genital mucosa. Mucositis is associated with a painful generalized erythematous vesiculobullous rash. The bullae rupture leading to epidermal sloughing. There may be accompanying dysfunction of major body systems with mortality reaching up to 35%.[48] Intensive management is important as the acute manifestations of this condition may be life threatening. About 60 to 100% of adult patients may have ocular involvement during acute phase.[50] The ocular involvement ranges from self-limiting conjunctival hyperemia to near total denudation of the ocular surface epithelium. Apposing raw surfaces between palpebral and bulbar conjunctiva lead to early symblepharon and forniceal foreshortening. Pseudomembranes or frank membranes form because of intense inflammation. The corneal surface may have extensive ulceration leading to corneal melt and perforation.[51]

Chronic

Recovery from acute phase generally leads to resolution of skin lesions while some patients may continue to experience reduced quality of life because of systemic sequels like dryness of mouth and strictures of esophagus, urethra, vagina and anus.[52] However, chronic ocular complications, which may affect around one-third to half of the patients[50] are considered to be the most debilitating residual effects of SJS/TEN.

Conjunctival scarring leads to destruction of lubricating glands of surface (including goblet cells and meibomian glands), symblephera formation, eyelid malpositions and trichiasis (Figs. 19.7A to D). A persistent and prolonged ocular surface inflammation is the hallmark of SJS. Tear film abnormality, dry eyes, limbal stem cell deficiency (LSCD), mechanical trauma from lashes and lid margin keratinization contribute to corneal ulceration, perforation, vascularization and conjunctivalization. The end-stage disease is marked by the total keratinization of ocular surface.[50]

Management

Acute Phase

The acute treatment is usually performed in an ICU setting. It includes a meticulous examination including lid eversion

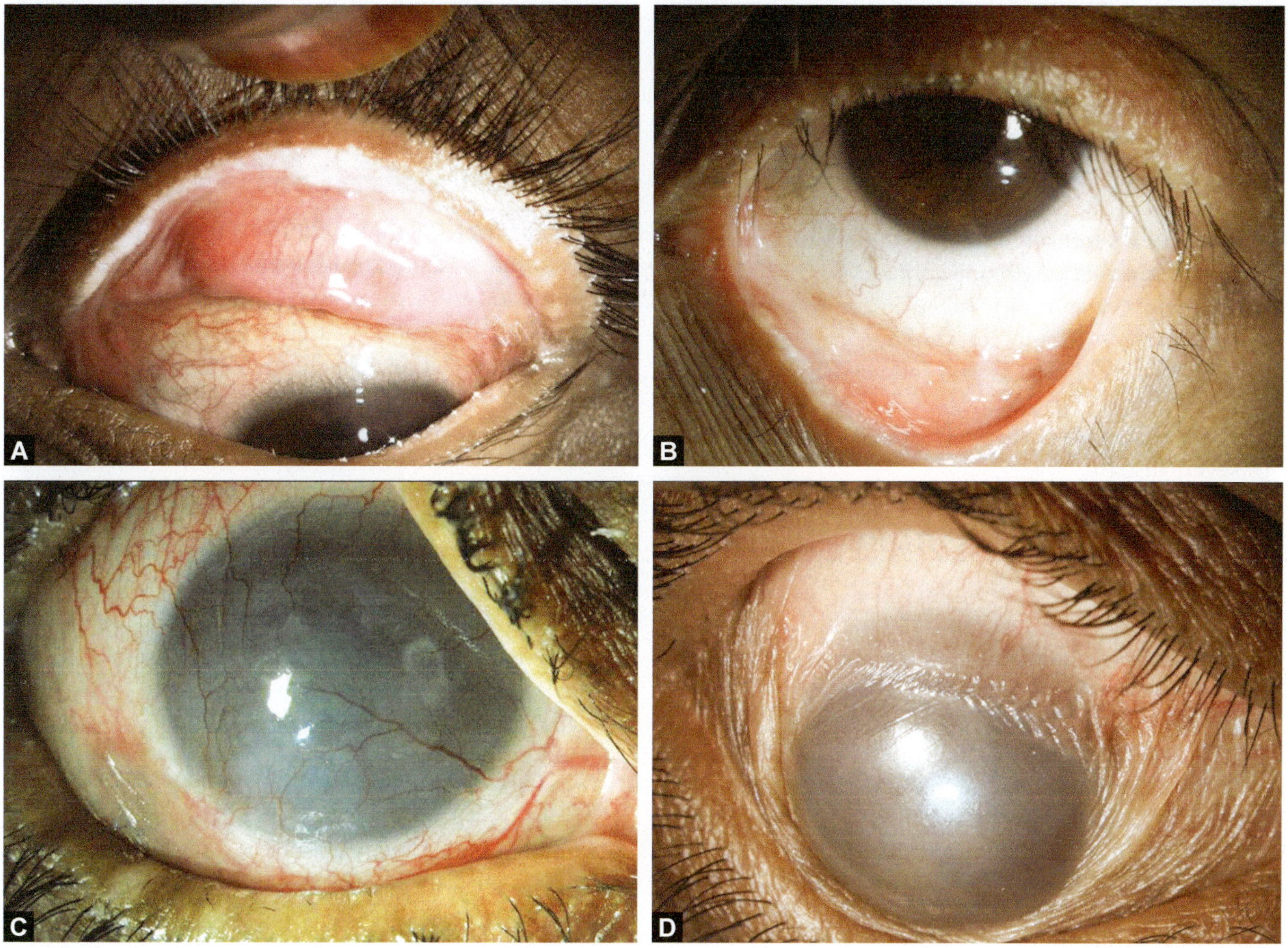

Figs. 19.7A to D: (A) Chronic debilitating sequelae of SJS with: Lid margin keratinization; (B) Extensive symblephara of the ocular surface in end stage disease; (C) SJS with Limbal stem cell deficiency; (D) End-stage disease with dermalization of ocular surface.
Source: Dr Sayan Basu, Tej Kohli Cornea Institute, LV Prasad Eye Institute, KAR Campus, Hyderabad, Telangana, India.

to look for membranes and fluorescein staining to assess defects on cornea, bulbar and palpebral conjunctiva and especially eyelid margin.

- Topical steroids, prophylactic antibiotics and intensive lubrication (with preservative-free artificial tears) are administered along with steroid ointment over lid margins.
- Supportive measures include saline rinses to remove debris, peeling of membranes, release of conjunctival adhesions and placement of bandage soft contact lens.[51]
- Lagophthalmos and exposure keratopathy needs to be assessed and prevented by tarsorrhaphy and frequent instillation of lubricants.
- *Amniotic membrane transplant (AMT)*: There is a considerable body of evidence indicating benefits of amniotic membrane transplantation during the acute phase of Stevens-Johnson syndrome. Indications of amniotic membrane transplantation includes presence of lid margin involvement, pseudomembrane and tarsal or forniceal conjunctival defects.[50]
- Adjuvant systemic treatment includes (systemic steroids, intravenous immunoglobulin (IVIG), plasmapheresis and immunomodulators) though, not conclusively shown to benefit ocular manifestations of SJS/TEN.[52]

Chronic Phase

The management of chronic phase of SJS/TEN chiefly includes restoring the ocular surface, eyelid and conjunctival anatomy and improving the tear film function.

- Control of dry eye manifestations includes frequent nonpreserved artificial tears, autologous serum, punctate occlusion and tarsorrhaphy.
- Exacerbations of inflammation need treatment with topical steroids.
- To prevent progressive worsening, lid margin keratinization, entropion, and trichiasis may have to be treated surgically, which includes conjunctival or buccal mucous membrane grafting.
- To restore vision, advanced cases require limbal stem cell transplantation (autologous, living-related or cadaveric limbal grafts) followed by penetrating keratoplasty.
- Keratoprosthesis is reserved for patients who have more severe disease.

OCULAR CICATRICIAL PEMPHIGOID

Ocular cicatricial pemphigoid (OCP) is a condition characterized by bilateral chronic conjunctivitis which leads to progressive ocular surface scarring and eventually, blinding keratopathy. It is a subset of mucous membrane pemphigoid (MMP), a term which includes heterogeneous, autoimmune, chronic inflammatory, subepithelial blistering diseases, which predominantly affects mucous membranes (ocular, oral, nasopharyngeal, laryngeal, genital, and perianal) and sometimes skin. These are characterized by linear deposition of IgG, IgA, or C3 along the epithelial basement membrane zone.[53] OCP has a female preponderance with most patients presenting in the 6th to 7th decade of life though it can also manifest in relatively younger age groups.

Pathogenesis

Mucus membrane pemphigoid is an autoimmune disease. In MMP, epithelial basement membrane proteins-BP180, laminin 332, BP230, $\alpha6\beta4$ integrin, laminin 311, type VII collagen, laminin $\gamma1$ have been identified as possible targets for the immune attack and it has been found that presence of *HLA-DQB*0301* gene is likely to predispose to the autoimmunity.[54,55] Beta-4 subunit of the alpha-6 beta-4 integrin of hemidesmosomes in the conjunctiva has been more particularly associated with OCP.[56] Type 2 hypersensitivity reactions due to autoantibodies and interaction of autoreactive T and B-cells lead to destruction of the basement membrane and blistering. The associated cellular inflammatory infiltrate manifests as chronic conjunctivitis. Fibroblast activation leads to subepithelial fibrosis, forniceal foreshortening, symblepharon, ankyloblepharon and entropion.

Clinical Presentation

Ocular cicatricial pemphigoid has a bilateral asymmetric presentation. It is often classified as four stages.

- *Stage 1:* Presenting symptoms of OCP could be nonspecific, such as irritation, burning, tearing, mucoid discharge and red eyes. High level of clinical suspicion in cases of unexplained chronic, recurrent conjunctivitis is warranted to diagnose this disease early, especially when the symptoms are accompanied by evidence of subepithelial fibrosis that appears as fine gray-white striae.
- *Stage 2:* Progressive inflammation leads to conjunctival scarring and inferior forniceal foreshortening.
- *Stage 3:* In later stages, the symblepharon begin in the lower lid (Stage 3) and eventually whole of ocular surface may get involved.
- *Stage 4:* End-stage disease presents with profound dry eyes, surface keratinization, motility restriction due to extensive symblephara and blindness due to corneal scarring and vascularization. Loss of goblet cells, tear film instability, entropion, trichiasis, limbal stem cell deficiency and persistent corneal epithelial defects overlap the various stages and contribute to disease etiopathogenesis (Figs. 19.8A to E).

Diagnosis

Early diagnosis is of paramount importance to prevent blinding complications of the disease. Demonstration of homogeneous linear deposition of immunoreactants (IgG, IgA, IgM,, C3) along the basement membrane zone on direct immunofluorescence (DIF) on a sample from perilesional biopsy (including both inflamed and noninflamed tissue) from conjunctiva or other mucosal lesions is diagnostic of OCP.[54] If the DIF is negative, circulating autoantibodies against basement membrane zone (BMZ) antigens may be of diagnostic value.[57] In the absence of positive immunopathology tests, this condition may also be diagnosed clinically in patients with progressive conjunctival scarring after ruling out other causes of cicatrizing conjunctivitis (Box 19.3).[54]

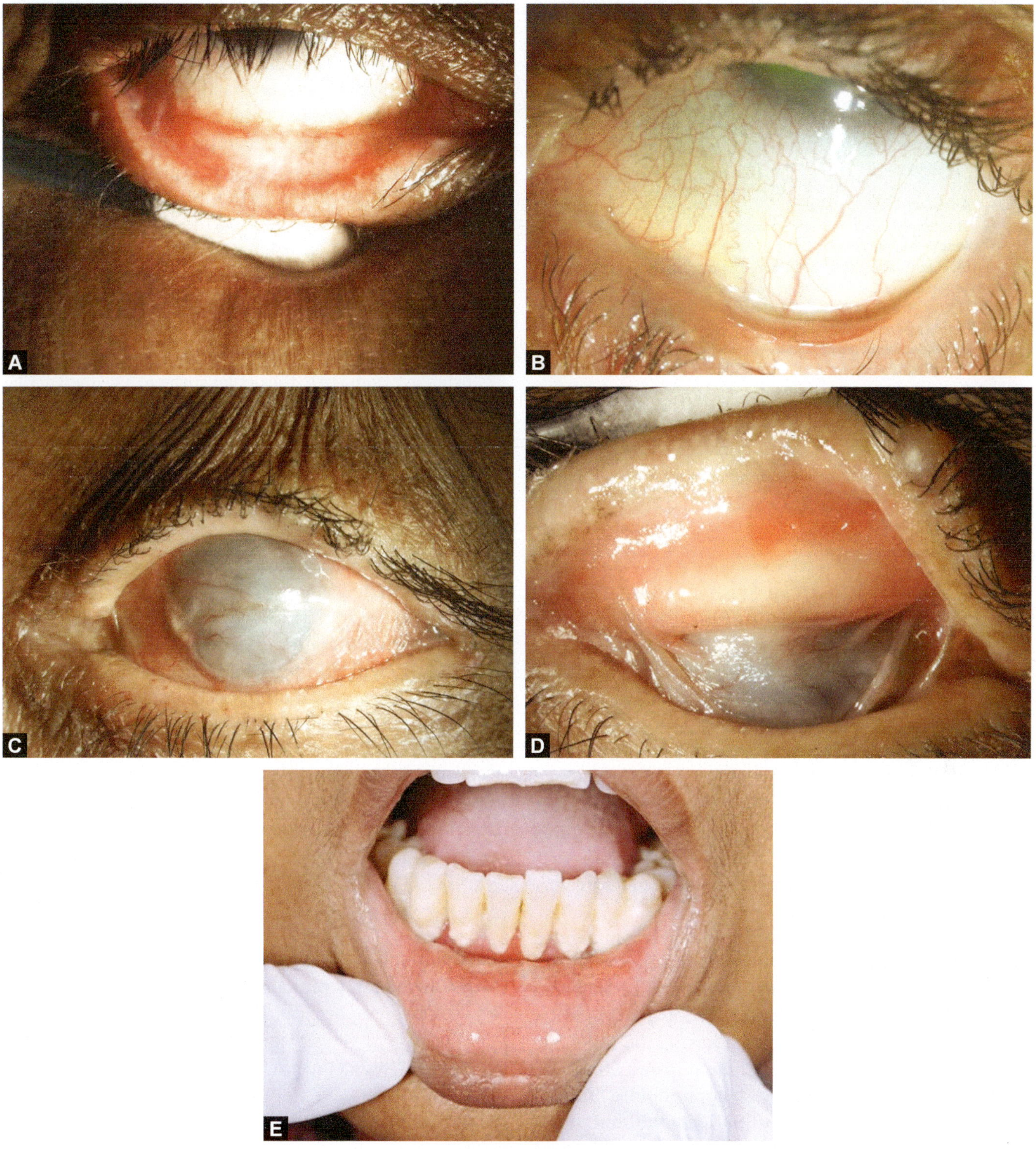

Figs. 19.8A to E: (A) Ocular cicatricial pemphigoid; (B) Subepithelial fibrosis; (C) Forniceal foreshortening; (D) End-stage disease with surface keratinization, extensive symblephara; (E) Buccal mucosal involvement with submucosal fibrosis.

Source: Dr Sayan Basu and Dr Virender S Sangwan, Tej Kohli Cornea Institute, LV Prasad Eye Institute, KAR Campus, Hyderabad, Telangana, India.

Box 19.3: Differential diagnosis of cicatrizing conjunctivitis.[52]

- *Blinding scarring diseases*:
  - Mucous membrane pemphigoid
  - SJS/TEN
  - Drug-induced progressive scarring
- *Ocular surface neoplasia*:
  - OSSN
  - Sebaceous cell carcinoma
- *Ocular disease with no systemic invovement*:
  - Adenoviral conjunctivitis
  - Trachoma
  - Atopic conjunctivitis
  - Conjunctival trauma (chemical, thermal, radiation, surgical)
- *Systemic diseases (other than MMP and SJS)*:
  - Ocular Rosacea
  - Bullous pemphigoid
  - Paraneoplastic pemphigoid
  - Pemphigus vulgaris
  - Paraneoplastic pemphigus
  - Lichen planus
  - Dermatitis herpetiformis
  - SLE
  - Sarcoidosis
  - Graft versus host disease

Management

- Management consists of control of inflammation and fibrosis. Management of local ocular surface issues contributing to inflammation like blepharitis, keratinization, trichiasis, entropion, lagophthalmos, dry eyes, corneal punctate epitheliopathy and persistent epithelial defects goes hand-in-hand with the control of ongoing systemic and immune mediated inflammation.[58]
- Topical corticosteroid instillation offers only symptomatic relief and is ineffective in controlling progression.[54] Systemic corticosteroids are used in OCP as a temporary measure until other immunomodulatory drugs can take effect.
- Immunosuppressive therapy is generally recommended for more severe grades of disease usually beyond stage 1.[57] Immunosuppressive agents are selected depending on disease activity with a step-ladder approach, starting with agents having the least side effects, progressing to more potent drugs with more severe adverse effects.[57] Mycophenolate mofetil is the preferred therapy in patients without sight-threatening complications.[57] Methotrexate is a second alternative. Cyclophosphamide is used for patients with treatment failure or that subset of patients with severe inflammation.[57] Administration of intravenous immunoglobulin and/or biologic agents (rituximab, antitumor necrosis factor alpha) may be considered in cases of inadequate response. Once complete control of inflammation has been achieved, immunosuppression is continued for at least 12 months.[54] Cases with end-stage ocular surface with a quiescent conjunctiva do not require immunosuppressive therapy unless conjunctival incisional surgery is planned.[54]
- On resolution of the ocular surface inflammation and control of disease progression, ocular surface reconstruction (forniceal reconstruction, pannus resection, limbal stem cell transplantation) with subsequent keratoplasty (lamellar/penetrating) may be attempted for restoring vision in patients with corneal blindness.[58] Advanced surface disease with extensive damage to the ocular surface may need ocular keratoprosthesis.

CONCLUSION

Inflammatory conjunctival disorders are chronic ocular conditions, which are characterized by a long-standing affliction. They have characteristic underlying disease mechanisms. These entities may present with a chronic course with exacerbations and remission. They may be typically unilateral than bilateral. It is important to detect early signs and symptoms and have a high index of suspicion to rule out ominous underlying conditions, such as neoplasia, collagen vascular diseases, atopy, etc. Conjunctival scraping and biopsy may help in diagnosis of granulomas, foreign bodies, neoplasia, etc. An understanding of the underlying disease pathology and directing specific treatment is crucial to achieve disease remission.

ACKNOWLEDGMENT

The authors would like to acknowledge Dr Swathi Kaliki (MD) Consultant, Ophthalmic Plastic Surgery, Orbit and Ocular Oncology Service, KAR Campus, LV Prasad Eye Institute, Hyderabad, Telangana, India, for her assistance in preparing the section on Masquerade syndromes.

REFERENCES

1. La Rosa M, Lionetti E, Reibaldi M, et al. Allergic Conjunctivitis: a comprehensive review of the literature. Ital J Pediatr. 2013;39:18.
2. Mishra GP, Tamboli V, Jwala J, et al. Recent patents and emerging therapeutics in the treatment of allergic

conjunctivitis. Recent Pat Inflamm Allergy Drug Discov. 2011;5(1):26-36.
3. De Smedt S, Wildner G, Kestelyn P. Vernal keratoconjunctivitis: an update. Br J Ophthalmol. 2013;97(1):9-14.
4. Bonini S, Sacchetti M, Mantelli F, et al. Clinical grading of vernal keratoconjunctivitis. Curr Opin Allergy Clin Immunol. 2007;7(5):436-41.
5. Cameron JA. Shield ulcers and plaques of the cornea in vernal keratoconjunctivitis. Ophthalmology. 1995;102(6):985-93.
6. Tuft SJ, Kemeny DM, Dart JK, et al. Clinical features of atopic keratoconjunctivitis. Ophthalmology. 1991;98(2):150-8.
7. Ono SJ, Abelson MB. Allergic conjunctivitis: update on pathophysiology and prospects for future treatment. J Allergy Clin Immunol. 2005;115(1):118-22.
8. Tabbara KF. Ocular complications of vernal keratoconjunctivitis. Can J Ophthalmol. 1999;34(2):88-92.
9. Kilic A, Gurler B. Topical 2% cyclosporine A in preservative-free artificial tears for the treatment of vernal keratoconjunctivitis. Can J Ophthalmol. 2006;41(6):693-8.
10. Ohashi Y, Ebihara N, Fujishima H, et al. A randomized, placebo-controlled clinical trial of tacrolimus ophthalmic suspension 0.1% in severe allergic conjunctivitis. J Ocul Pharmacol Ther. 2010;26(2):165-74.
11. Lambiase A, Bonini S, Rasi G, et al. Montelukast, a leukotriene receptor antagonist, in vernal keratoconjunctivitis associated with asthma. Arch Ophthalmol. 2003;121(5):615-20.
12. Basu S, Taneja M, Sangwan VS. Boston type 1 keratoprosthesis for severe blinding vernal keratoconjunctivitis and Mooren's ulcer. Int Ophthalmol. 2011;31(3):219-22.
13. Nelson JD. Superior limbic keratoconjunctivitis (SLK). Eye (Lond). 1989;3(Pt 2):180-9.
14. Cher I. Superior limbic keratoconjunctivitis: multifactorial mechanical pathogenesis. Clin Exp Ophthalmol. 2000;28(3):181-4.
15. Kojima T, Matsumoto Y, Ibrahim OM, et al. In vivo evaluation of superior limbic keratoconjunctivitis using laser scanning confocal microscopy and conjunctival impression cytology. Invest Ophthalmol Vis Sci. 2010;51(8):3986-92.
16. Passons GA, Wood TO. Conjunctival resection for superior limbic keratoconjunctivitis. Ophthalmology. 1984;91(8): 966-8.
17. Shen YC, Wang CY, Tsai HY, et al. Supratarsal triamcinolone injection in the treatment of superior limbic keratoconjunctivitis. Cornea. 2007;26(4):423-6.
18. Kymionis GD, Klados NE, Kontadakis GA, et al. Treatment of superior limbic keratoconjunctivitis with topical tacrolimus 0.03% ointment. Cornea. 2013;32(11):1499-501.
19. Dua HS, Otri AM, Said DG, et al. The "up-down" sign of acute ocular surface drug toxicity. Br J Ophthalmol. 2012;96(11):1439-40.
20. Hong J, Bielory L. Allergy to ophthalmic preservatives. Curr Opin Allergy Clin Immunol. 2009;9(5):447-53.
21. Korb DR, Allansmith MR, Greiner JV, et al. Prevalence of conjunctival changes in wearers of hard contact lenses. Am J Ophthalmol. 1980;90(3):336-41.
22. Asbell P, Howes J. A double-masked, placebo-controlled evaluation of the efficacy and safety of loteprednol etabonate in the treatment of giant papillary conjunctivitis. CLAO J. 1997;23(1):31-6.
23. Rohatgi J, Dhaliwal U. Phlyctenular eye disease: a reappraisal. Jpn J Opthalmology. 2000;44(2):146-50.
24. Gautam P, Shrestha GS, Sharma AK. Phlyctenular keratoconjunctivitis among children in the tertiary eye hospital of Kathmandu, Nepal. Oman J Ophthalmol. 2015;8(3):147-50.
25. Sorsby A. The etiology of phlyctenular ophthalmia. Br J Ophthalmol. 1942;26(5):189-215.
26. Kefella H, Luther D, Hainline C. Ophthalmic and neuro-ophthalmic manifestations of sarcoidosis. Curr Opin Ophthalmol. 2017:28(6):587-94.
27. Pasadhika S, Rosenbaum JT. Ocular Sarcoidosis. Clin Chest Med. 2015;36(4):669-83.
28. Han SB, Yang HK, Hyon JY, et al. Conjunctival sarcoidosis presenting as limbal conjunctival hypertrophy: a case report. J Med Case Rep. 2014;8:63.
29. Sethi PK, Dwivedi N. Ophthalmia nodosa. Indian J Ophthalmol. 1982;30(1):11-4.
30. Cadera W, Pachtman MA, Fountain JA, et al. Ocular lesions caused by caterpillar hairs (ophthalmia nodosa). Can J Ophthalmol. 1984;19(1):40-4.
31. Schuster V, Seregard S. Ligneous conjunctivitis. Surv Ophthalmol. 2003;48(4):369-88.
32. Hidayat AA, Riddle PJ. Ligneous conjunctivitis. A clinicopathologic study of 17 cases. Opthalmology. 1987;94(8):949-59.
33. Cooper TJ, Kazdan JJ, Cutz E. Lingeous conjunctivitis with tracheal obstruction. A case report, with light and electron microscopy findings. Can J Ophthalmol. 1979;14(1):57-62.
34. Holland EJ, Olsen TW, Ketcham JM, et al. Topical cyclosporin A in the treatment of anterior segment inflammatory disease. Cornea. 1993;12(5):413-9.
35. De Cock R, Ficker LA, Dart JG, et al. Topical heparin in the treatment of ligneous conjunctivitis. Ophthalmology. 1995;102(11):1654-9.
36. Mingers AM, Heimburger N, Zeitler P, et al. Homozygous type I plasminogen deficiency. Semin Thromb Hemost. 1997;23(3):259-69.
37. Barabino S, Rolando M. Amniotic membrane transplantation in a case of ligneous conjunctivitis. Am J Ophthalmol. 2004;137(4):752-3.
38. Krachmer JH, Mannis MJ, Holland EJ. Cornea. St. Louis/ London: Elsevier Mosby; 2011.
39. Theodore FH. Conjunctival carcinoma masquerading as chronic conjunctivitis. Eye Ear Nose Throat Mon. 1967;46(11):1419-20.
40. EyeRounds. (2006). Sebaceous Cell Carcinoma: A Masquerade Syndrome (Johnson S, Syed N, Nerad J). [online] Available from: *http://webeye.ophth.uiowa.edu/cases/eyeforum/62-Sebaceous-Cell-Carcinoma-A-Masquerade-Syndrome.htm.* [Accessed November, 2017].

41. Akpek EK, Polcharoen W, Chan R, et al. Ocular surface neoplasia masquerading as chronic blepharoconjunctivitis. Cornea. 1999;18(3):282-8.
42. Kim JW, Abramson DH. Topical treatment options for conjunctival neoplasms. Clin Ophthalmol. 2008;2(3):503-15.
43. Nanji AA, Moon CS, Galor A, et al. Surgical versus medical treatment of ocular surface squamous neoplasia: a comparison of recurrences and complications. Ophthalmology. 2014;121(5):994-1000.
44. Akpek EK, Polcharoen W, Ferry JA, et al. Conjunctival lymphoma masquerading as chronic conjunctivitis. Ophthalmology. 1999;106(4):757-60.
45. Duncan J, Chen Y, Fuchs D, et al .Follicular Lymphoma Presenting Solely as Chronic Follicular Conjunctivitis. Cornea. 2016;35(3):395-8.
46. White ML, Chodosh J, Jang J, et al. Incidence of Stevens-Johnson Syndrome and Chemical Burns to the Eye. Cornea. 2015;34(12):1527-33.
47. Mockenhaupt M, Viboud C, Dunant A, et al. Stevens-Johnson syndrome and toxic epidermal necrolysis: assessment of medication risks with emphasis on recently marketed drugs. The EuroSCAR study. J Invest Dermatol. 2008;128(1):35-44.
48. Jain R, Sharma N, Basu S, et al. Stevens-Johnson syndrome: the role of an ophthalmologist. Surv Ophthalmol. 2016;61(4):369-99.
49. Kinoshita Y, Saeki H. A Review of the Pathogenesis of Toxic Epidermal Necrolysis. J Nippon Med Sch. 2016;83(6):216-22.
50. Saeed HN, Chodosh J. Ocular manifestations of Stevens-Johnson syndrome and their management. Curr Opin Ophthalmol. 2016;27(6):522-9.
51. Kohanim S, Palioura S, Saeed HN, et al. Acute and chronic ophthalmic involvement in Stevens-Johnson syndrome/toxic epidermal necrolysis-a comprehensive review and guide to therapy. II. Ophthalmic Disease. Ocul Surf. 2016;14(2):168-88.
52. Kohanim S, Palioura S, Saeed HN, et al. Stevens-Johnson syndrome/toxic epidermal necrolysis—a comprehensive review and guide to therapy. I. Systemic Disease. Ocul Surf. 2016;14(1):2-19.
53. Chan LS, Ahmed AR, Anhalt GJ, et al. The first international consensus on mucous membrane pemphigoid: definition, diagnostic criteria, pathogenic factors, medical treatment, and prognostic indicators. Arch Dermatol. 2002;138(3):370-9.
54. Dart JK. The 2016 Bowman Lecture Conjunctival curses: scarring conjunctivitis 30 years on. Eye (Lond). 2017;31(2):301-32.
55. Setterfield J, Theron J, Vaughan RW, et al. Mucous membrane pemphigoid: HLA-DQB1*0301 is associated with all clinical sites of involvement and may be linked to antibasement membrane IgG production. Br J Dermatol. 2001;145(3):406-14.
56. Srikumaran D, Akpek EK. Mucous membrane pemphigoid: recent advances. Curr Opin Ophthalmol. 2012;23(6):523-7.
57. Sobolewska B, Deuter C, Zierhut M. Current medical treatment of ocular mucous membrane pemphigoid. Ocul Surf. 2013;11(4):259-66.
58. Saw VP, Dart JK. Ocular mucous membrane pemphigoid: diagnosis and management strategies. Ocul Surf. 2008;6(3):128-42.

Chapter 20 Pterygium

Amreen Aslam, Srikanta Kumar Padhy, Murugesan Vanathi

INTRODUCTION

Pterygium is derived from a Greek word *"pteryx"* which means *wing*. Pterygium is a benign triangular fibrovascular proliferation presenting as elevated, superficial wing-shaped lesion extending from the perilimbal bulbar conjunctiva onto the corneal surface.

A pterygium (Fig. 20.1) is commonly seen to extend from the nasal side of the bulbar conjunctiva, the reason being the increased actinic exposure of the nasal bulbar conjunctiva secondary to ultraviolet (UV) light reflection from nose. The light incident on temporal limbus gets focused intracamerally onto the nasal limbus. Pterygium is seen all over the world but its prevalence rates are higher in tropics than temperate latitudes with equatorial countries having the highest prevalence rates, commonly referred as "pterygium belt".[1] The pterygium belt described by Cameron[1] extends between the latitudes 37° north and south of the equator, occurring in the hot and dry regions. People at high risk for occurrence of pterygium include outdoor workers and those working in the setting of highly reflective surfaces like Eskimos.[2] The prevalence of pterygium in India ranges from 9.5%[3] to 13%[4] and is more common in rural parts of the country. The prevalence of pterygium in the world ranges from 2.8% to 33%.[5]

PSEUDOPTERYGIUM

Pseudopterygium (Fig. 20.2) refers to a fold of conjunctiva attached to cornea following injury to the cornea as in ocular trauma or thermochemical injury or peripheral corneal ulceration. It can occur in any age, any site unlike the 3 o'clock and 9 o'clock position in pterygium and is generally stationary. The "probe test" is used to differentiate it from true pterygium, i.e. a probe can be passed beneath a pseudopterygium.

STAGING SYSTEMS IN PTERYGIUM

Tan et al.[6] have elaborated a morphological grading system for pterygium as shown in Table 20.1.

Chao et al.[7] described another grading system (Figs. 20.6 and 20.7) based on the extent of the pterygium (Table 20.2).

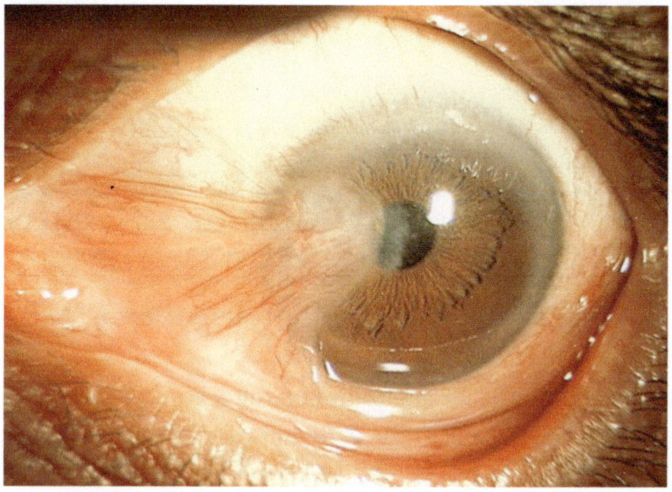

Fig. 20.1: Clinical photograph of nasal pterygium of left eye.

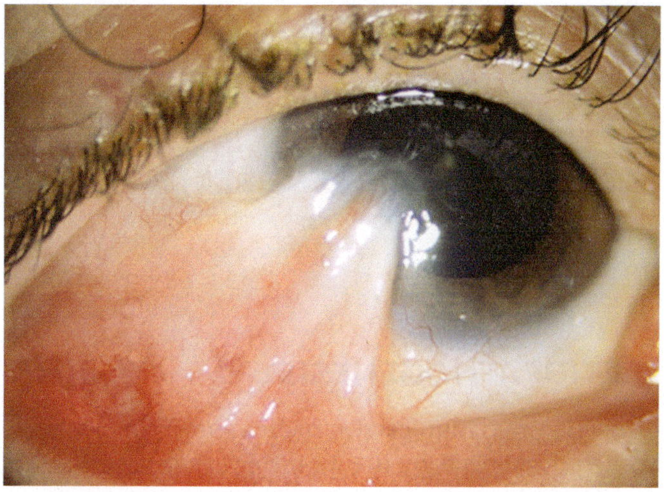

Fig. 20.2: Clinical photograph of pseudopterygium of right eye.

Table 20.1: Morphological grading system for pterygium.

T1	*Atrophic and transparent form* with episcleral vessels that are clearly visible (Fig. 20.3)
T2	*Intermediate* with episcleral vessels that are partially visible (Fig. 20.4)
T3	*Fleshy and opaque* form with episcleral vessels that are obscured totally (Fig. 20.5)

Table 20.2: Grading system for pterygium based on the extent of the pterygium.

Grade 1	Pterygium just crossing the limbus
Grade 2	Pterygium crossing the midway between limbus and pupillary margin
Grade 3	Pterygium crossing the pupillary margin

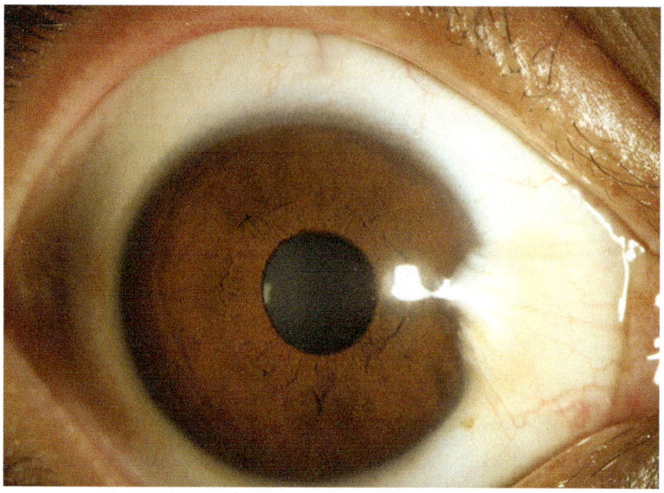

Fig. 20.3: Clinical photograph depicting atrophic type of pterygium of right eye.

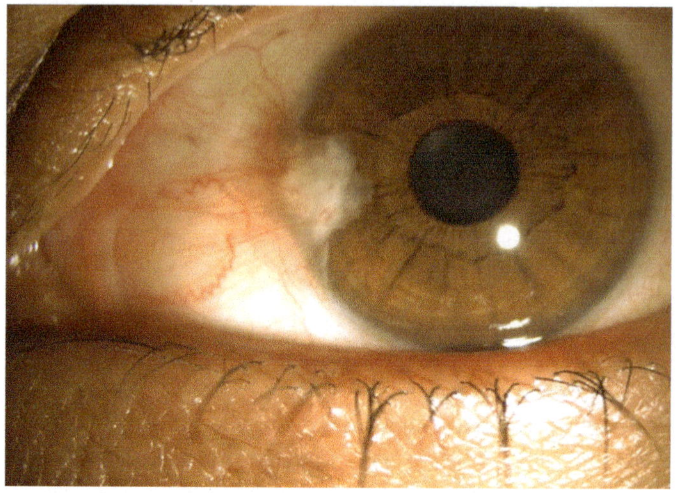

Fig. 20.4: Clinical photograph depicting an intermediate type of pterygium in the left eye.

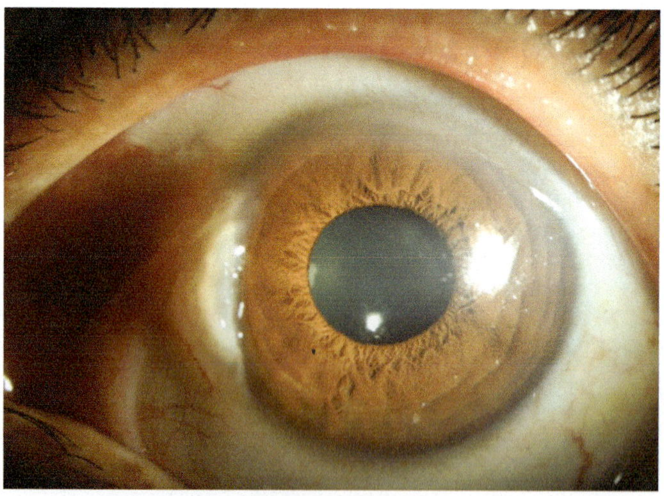

Fig. 20.5: Clinical photograph depicting a fleshy pterygium of left eye.

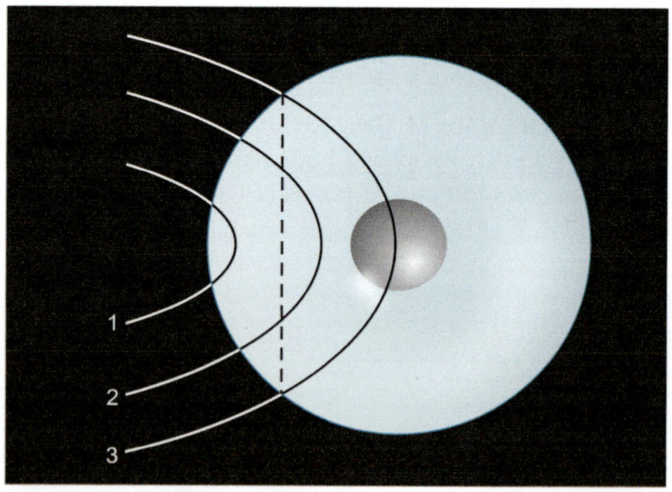

Fig. 20.6: Diagrammatic representation of Chao et al. staging system for pterygium according to the extent of the pterygium. (1—just crossing the limbus; 2—crossing the midway between limbus and pupillary margin; 3—crossing the pupillary margin)

ETIOPATHOGENESIS

Ultraviolet radiation carries higher energy than visible light, and its effects on tissues include deoxyribonucleic acid (DNA) damage, gene mutations, immunosuppression, oxidative stress and inflammatory responses. Pterygium is believed to be an environmental disease, UV radiation playing a major role in its pathogenesis due to the above mentioned reasons. Studies suggest that certain signaling pathways get activated by UV light resulting in induction of mediators that promote growth of the pterygium.[8]

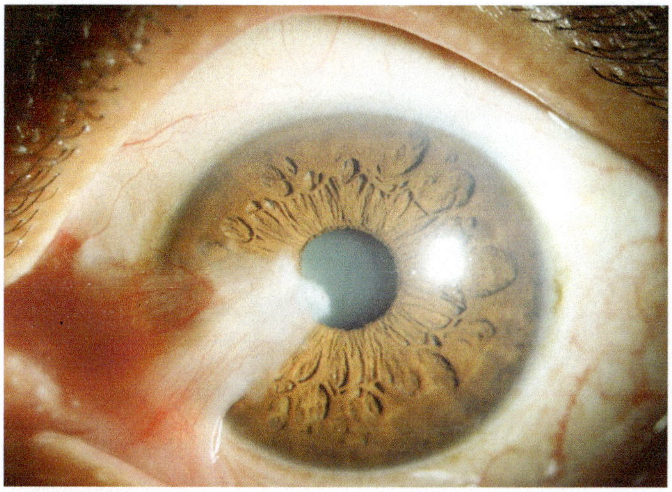

Fig. 20.7: Clinical photograph of nasal pterygium in the left eye crossing nasal pupillary margin.

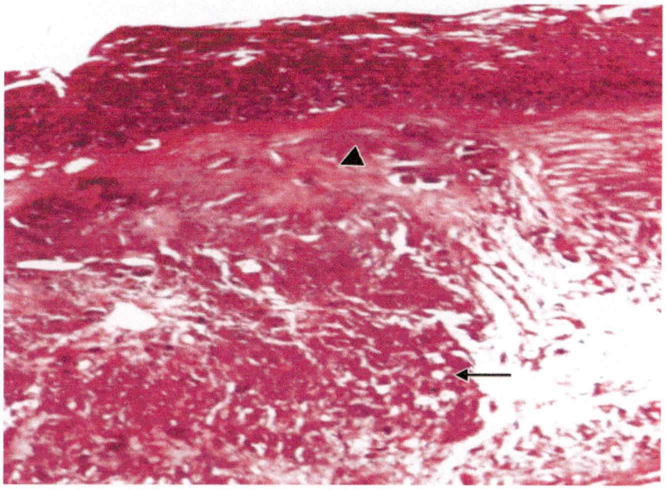

Fig. 20.8: Histopathological photograph (200x)—arrowhead depicting hyaline degeneration and arrow mark depicting elastoid degeneration.
Source: Dr Seema Sen, Professor of Pathology, Ocular Pathology, AIIMS, New Delhi, India.

Studies have also found that focal limbal stem cell deficiency can cause pterygium.[9] Such pterygia have more of underlying fibrotic tissue.

Genetic studies suggest that some molecular alterations including loss of heterozygosity, point mutations of proto-oncogenes, microsatellite instability and alterations in tumor suppressor genes are involved in the pathogenesis of pterygium.[10] It is also found that pterygia may result from disruption of the normal process of apoptosis occurring in the conjunctiva. The apoptotic cells in pterygium express significant levels of p53 and Bax, as well as the apoptosis inhibiting protein bcl-2 unlike the normal conjunctiva.[11]

Few others have noted an association of human papilloma virus (HPV) DNA with pterygium.[12] The detection of potentially oncogenic viruses, like herpes simplex virus (HSV) and HPV, supports the concept that pterygium can be considered a neoplastic condition. In such cases, there occurs greater postoperative recurrence and there is history of previous episode of conjunctivitis.[13]

The overexpression of angiogenic factors and the concurrent decreased expression of angiogenesis inhibitor probably supply one pathway for the pathogenic mechanism of pterygium. The overexpression of vascular endothelial growth factor (VEGF) in pterygium and the presence of abundant CD31-positive microvessels are seen in pterygium. Expression of VEGF in endothelial as well as in stromal cells of pterygium induces significant angiogenic activity, expressed by high microvessel density (MVD) values. On the other hand, thrombospondin-1 (TSP-1), an inhibitor of angiogenesis is absent in pterygium tissues.[14] Local bevacizumab may be effective in treatment of pterygium. Currently, data in the use of subconjunctival bevacizumab in the treatment of pterygia are not conclusive.

PATHOLOGY

Pterygium is characterized by elastotic degeneration of collagen (actinic elastosis) and fibrovascular proliferation. Histopathology specimen reveals loose fibrous connective tissue with fibrovascular ingrowth and destruction of Bowman's layer (Fig. 20.8). Matrix metalloproteinases (MMPs) and tissue inhibitors of MMPs (TIMPs) at the advancing pterygium edge may be responsible for the inflammation, tissue remodeling, destruction of Bowman's layer and pterygium invasion into the cornea.[15] A unique feature of the pterygium epithelial cell is its positive immunohistochemical staining for different types of MMPs that is absent in normal conjunctival, limbal or corneal cells.[16] The degenerated collagen produces hyalinization that results in eosinophilic granular material and concretions. The abnormal elastic fibers stain as elastin but do not degrade with elastase and hence the name elastotic degeneration.[17] Recurrent pterygium does not show elastotic degeneration.

SIGNS AND SYMPTOMS

Pterygium commonly located in the nasal interpalpebral region is comprised of a *"body"* which is a fleshy part connected to bulbar conjunctiva, a *"neck"* lying on limbus, a *"head"* which is highly vascular and proceeds anteriorly onto the cornea and a *"cap"* which is a fibrous nonvascular structure at the leading edge.

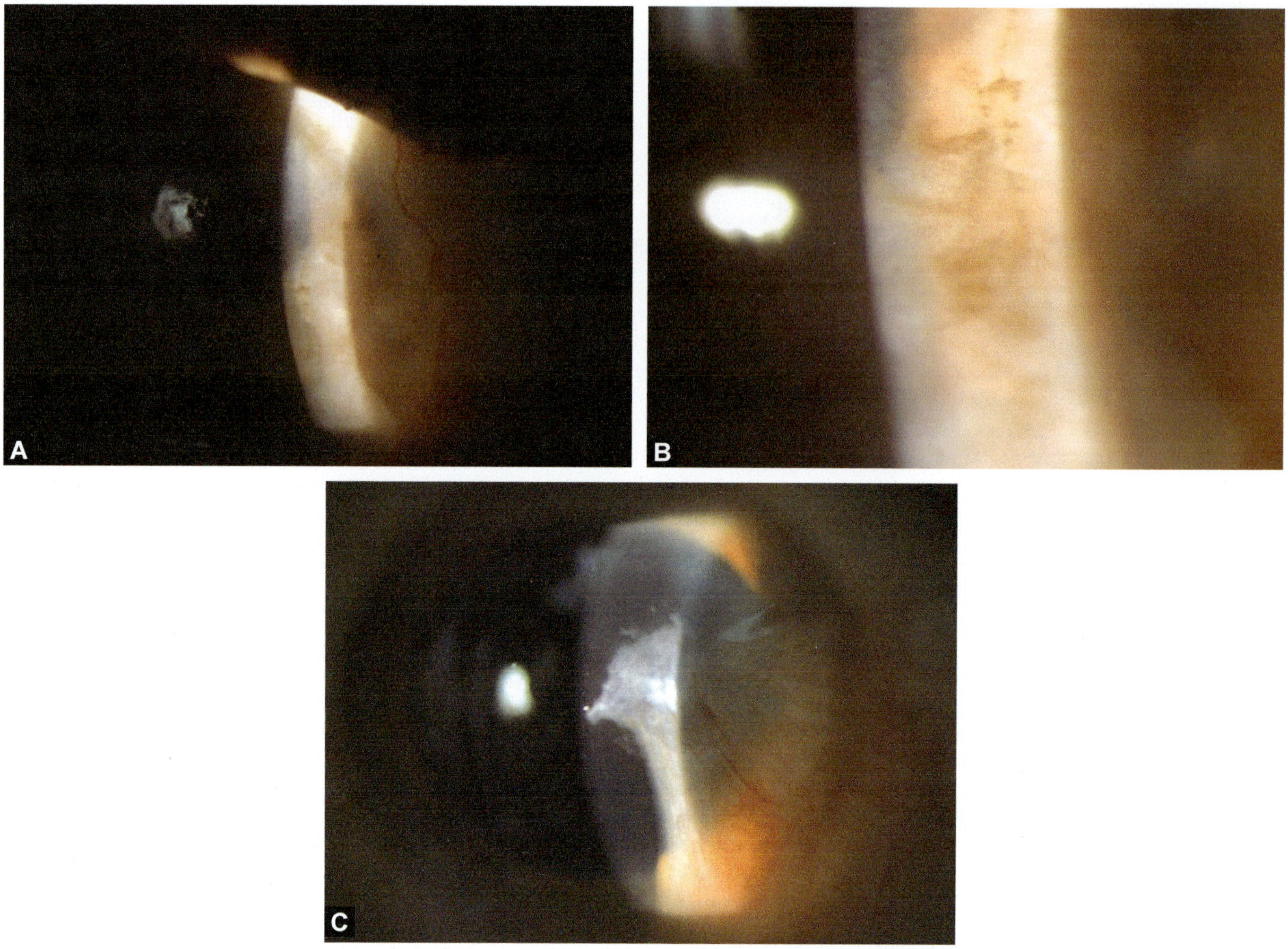

Figs. 20.9A to C: (A) Clinical photograph showing the pigmentation just ahead of the pterygium known as Stocker's line; (B) Magnified view of the same; (C) Clinical photograph showing Fuchs' patches at the head of the pterygium.

Stocker's line (Figs. 20.9A and B) is a brownish line of iron deposits found central to the leading edge where tear film is abnormal.[18] Its presence indicates chronicity and a stable position. Stocker's line generally rarely seen in atrophic pterygium. Fuchs' patches[19] are minute gray (Fig. 20.9C) blemishes that disperse near the pterygium head.

Inflammation and cystic degenerative changes (Fig. 20.10) can be seen in pterygium. Sometimes pterygium can present as fibrovascular growth both in nasal and temporal interpalpebral quadrant called as double-headed pterygium (Fig. 20.11). Symptoms include blurring of vision, irritation, lacrimation and foreign body sensation due to tear film disturbances. Visual acuity disturbances can occur due to the induced astigmatism, tear film disruption and in larger pterygium, due to the direct involvement of the central cornea with resultant scarring.

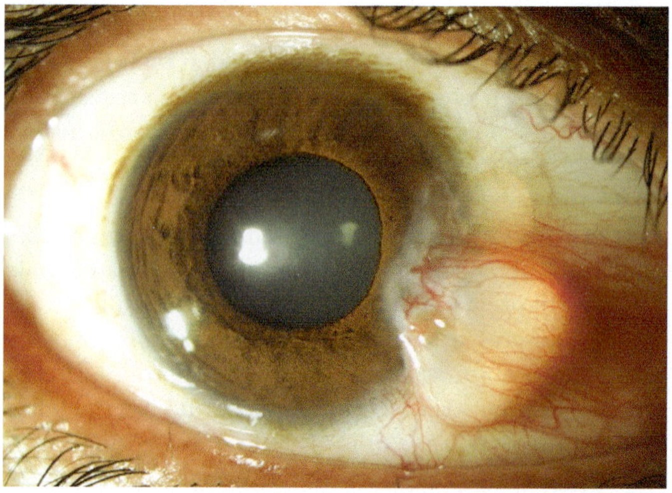

Fig. 20.10: Clinical photograph showing cystic degeneration in pterygium in the right eye.

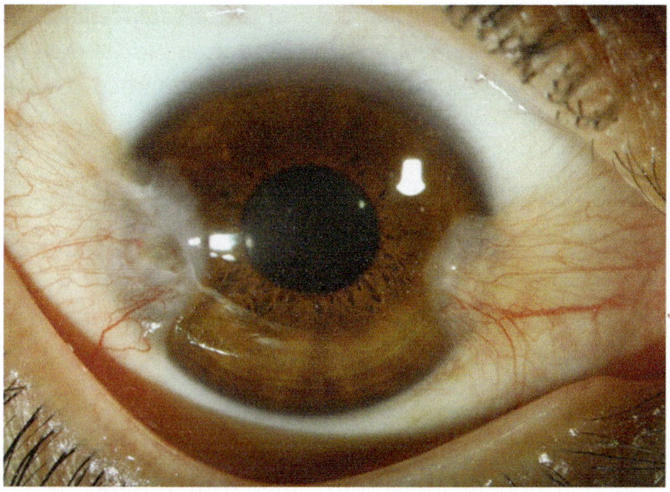

Fig. 20.11: Double-headed pterygium of right eye.

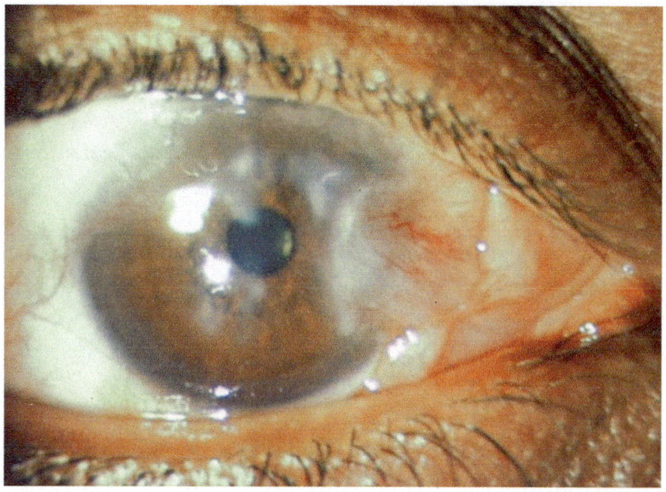

Fig. 20.12: Clinical photograph of a recurrent nasal pterygium in the right eye. Also seen altered limbal anatomy due to mild limbal stem cell deficiency (LSCD) in superotemporal region from where conjunctival graft had been harvested.

RECURRENT PTERYGIUM

Recurrent pterygium (Fig. 20.12) is characterized by increased underlying fibrotic changes with ocular movement restriction in cases where the medial rectus muscle has been damaged by recurrent surgery. The mechanism involved in recurrence is the reactivation of the inflammatory process present in the primary form. Compromised conjunctival epithelial integrity over the entire excised area of the pterygial tissue induces vigorous fibrovascular proliferation. Surgical trauma acts as an inflammatory response enhancer. The limbal stem cells remain activated and fibroblastic tissue is also active, there occurs an increase of proliferative cytokines and growth factors (VEGF), which induce the fibrovascular proliferation and increase in the synthesis of metalloproteinases that destroy the Bowman's membrane and stromal collagen, facilitating progress of pterygium. Regrowth of the remnant pterygial tissue is another reason for recurrence. The tissue can originate from the body of the pterygium or the remnant tissue at the limbal area. In cases of recurrence attributable to remnant pterygial tissue, the tissue usually adheres tightly to the surface and it cannot be easily removed. In cases in where conjunctival grafting or amniotic membrane grafts performed tissue retraction may be observed. The activity of a recurrent pterygium can be noted by UV fluorescence photography.

The described grading system[20] in recurrent pterygium takes into account the amount of conjunctival inflammation and is given in Table 20.3.

Table 20.3: Grading system in recurrent pterygium.

Grade 1	Normal
Grade 2	Fine episcleral vessels present but no fibrous tissue
Grade 3	Fibrovascular tissue reaching the limbus
Grade 4	Fibrovascular tissue invading the cornea

PTERYGIUM AND ASTIGMATISM

Corneal astigmatism is a result of cumulative effect of naturally occurring astigmatism and that due to pterygium itself. The contractile components in the pterygium produce tractional force that produces mechanical distortion and flattening of cornea. It is also said that the pooling of tear film at the apex of pterygium also contributes to the flattening effect. The common types of astigmatism induced by pterygium include with-the-rule astigmatism mainly followed by against the rule and oblique astigmatism. Length of extension of the pterygium into the cornea, total area and the width of the pterygium form important parameters in pterygium assessment. The size of pterygium is important in determining the amount of astigmatism induced by it, when it extends greater than 2.2 mm, greater than 5 mm wide, greater than 6.25 mm^2 area, it induces greater than 2 diopters astigmatism.[21] Most studies confirm an association between increasing size of pterygium and increasing degrees of corneal astigmatism.

Few studies recommend early surgical intervention when the pterygium size is 1 mm from limbus or greater than 16% of the corneal radius.[22] Posterior corneal surface has been shown to compensate 12.9–31% of front corneal astigmatism.[23] The size of pterygium has also been shown to significantly influence higher order aberrations of the eye especially total coma and total trefoil as compared to normal eyes.[24] The anterior corneal surface induces both lower and higher order aberrations while the posterior surface induces much of higher order aberrations.

PREVENTION

Wearing protective sunglasses with side shield or wide-brimmed hats can help to decrease the effects of UV radiation in outdoor environments. Eye protection gear is recommended in surfers and other water-sport athletes to enable blocking of almost 100% of the UV rays reflected from the water, as is often used by snow-sport athletes.

MANAGEMENT

Medical Management

Decrease in visual acuity requires refractive correction of the induced astigmatism with glasses. Early pterygium may be managed with refractive correction and topical lubricants. Associated inflammation may require topical anti-inflammatory agents. Topical corticosteroids such as loteprednol etabonate 0.5% have also gained importance in management of pterygium.[25] UV filters in glasses have also been recommended to be of help in early stages of pterygium.

Surgical Management

Indications for surgical intervention include:

- Proximity to the visual axis resulting in diminution of vision
- Encroachment of the visual axis
- Significant amount of astigmatism (>2 D)[21,26]
- Restriction of ocular movements
- Atypical appearance such as dysplasia
- Symptomatic growth
- Cosmetic concerns.

Preoperative Preparation

The surgery is best planned when the patient can avoid sunlight for at least 3 weeks postoperatively or for 6 weeks in cases with more inflammation or for recurrent cases. Preoperatively, all ocular surface inflammation should be controlled, including allergy, blepharitis, conjunctivitis and dry eye.

Intraoperative Considerations

The choice of anesthesia depends on the type of surgery. Peribulbar anesthesia is appropriate if extensive surgery, lengthy operative time, muscle manipulation, or when adjunctive lid procedures are anticipated. In cases of simple excision with grafting topical or light anterior subconjunctival anesthesia or even topical anesthesia should be sufficient in cooperative patients. Subconjunctival anesthetic injection is quite useful while harvesting graft from superior quadrant achieved by anterior subconjunctival lidocaine with 1:100,000 epinephrine, injected with a 30-gauge needle directly beneath the lesion, which helps to provide anesthesia and achieve excellent hemostasis.

In addition, topical dilating drops have been suggested to be useful in pterygium excision; the sympathomimetic promotes conjunctival vasoconstriction and hemostasis, while the parasympatholytic provides relief from ciliary spasm pain postoperatively. It is important to use atraumatic technique throughout, respecting the conjunctival tissues. Specially designed conjunctival forceps (Bausch and Lomb), with a Maumenee handle and Pierse tips (Fig. 20.13), are ideally suited for manipulation of the delicate conjunctiva, thereby reducing the risk of conjunctival tears or button holes. While harvesting the conjunctival graft, angled and straight Vannas scissors are useful.

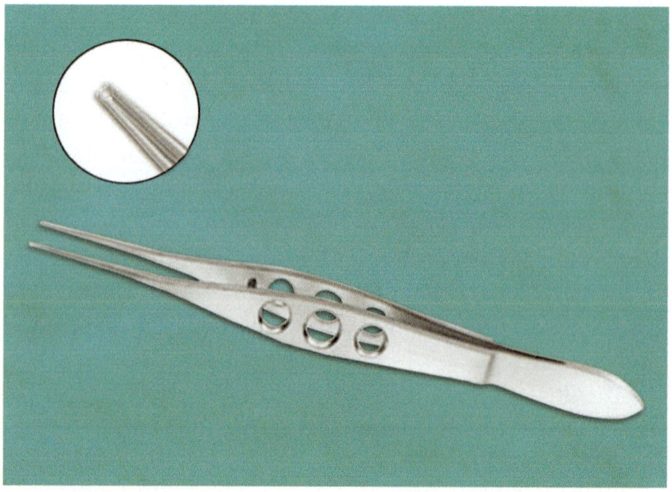

Fig. 20.13: Specially designed non-traumatizing forceps with Pierse tips.

The primary aim of treatment is to do a meticulous surgery, close the scleral defect with conjunctiva or biological equivalent tissue so as to prevent its recurrence. The decision to use biological replacements such as amniotic membrane, mucous membrane or bioengineered tissue (ex vivo cultivated conjunctival or mucosal epithelium) will depend on the size of the defect that needs to be covered and availability of autologous tissue for surgery.

Surgical Techniques

Currently there are a wide variety of surgical techniques described for surgical management of pterygium.

Excision of Pterygium

There are two techniques described for excision of the pterygium: (1) avulsion technique and (2) superficial keratectomy. Avulsion technique involves initial dissection of the body of pterygium from underlying sclera and then avulsing the head by grasping it with forceps and applying counter traction to assist shearing it off from cornea. Superficial keratectomy involves dissection starting from the head of the pterygium to achieve better smoothness of the cornea.

Several methods have been described based on the closure technique after excision of the pterygium.

Bare Sclera Closure

Following excision the resultant underlying defect may be left exposed leaving the defect to heal from surrounding conjunctiva with or without postoperative adjunctive therapy. Recurrence rates described are high as 30–80%.[27] This method is no longer in vogue for pterygium surgical management.

Simple Conjunctival Closure

Following excision of the pterygium the resultant defect is closed using the adjacent conjunctival tissue in primary closure. Recurrence rates range from 29.2% to 89%.[27]

Sliding Conjunctival Graft

Following excision the defect can be closed by employing a pedicle graft or sliding conjunctival flaps from superior or inferior conjunctiva. Recurrence rates described up to 6.9%[28] with minimal complications such as flap retraction and cyst formation.

Following pterygium excision the defect can also be closed by transposition of the pterygium head.

Conjunctival-Limbal Autografts (Limbal-Conjunctival Autograft Transplantation)

The first real advance in pterygium management was the description of the technique of conjunctival-limbal autograft transplantation after pterygium excision, by Kenyon in 1985.[29] In this technique, free conjunctival-limbal autograft from the superotemporal limbus is used to close the defect. The graft is preferably taken from the superior temporal bulbar conjunctiva, because of the technical difficulty in harvesting a graft from the inferior bulbar conjunctiva. The inferior limbus and inferior bulbar conjunctiva are more exposed to the deleterious effects of UV radiation, compared to the superior limbus and superior temporal bulbar conjunctiva which are shielded by the upper lid. Reported recurrence rates range from 2% to 40%.[27,30] This technique requires longer surgical time and greater ocular surface disruption. This is the most widely performed technique.

Free Conjunctival Autograft

In some situations, where there has been previous surgery or limbal damage due to any disease, surgical manipulations when removing a limbal graft may promote further damage to stem cells. In this situation, Tan et al. have suggested that the use of free conjunctival grafts (Fig. 20.14) may have equivalent outcomes.[31] This technique is also advantageous when surgery is performed in a patient with a subsequent risk of glaucoma and the need to preserve the superior bulbar conjunctiva. Reported recurrence rate is 2.6–39%[27,29,32-34] by this method.

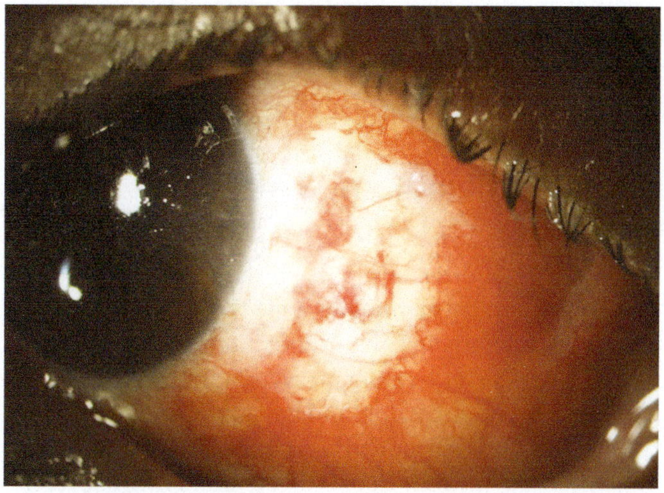

Fig. 20.14: Clinical photograph of pterygium excision with conjunctival autograft on postoperative day 1.

Pterygium Extended Removal Followed by Extended Conjunctival Transplant (P.E.R.F.E.C.T. for Pterygium)

Dr Hirst from Australia reported a recurrence rate of 0.5% with a technique named P.E.R.F.E.C.T.[35] In this approach, an extensive conjunctival autografting of about 15 mm by 12 mm which is substantially larger than usual and involves extensive removal of Tenon's layer. The advantages of this approach are less recurrence and a better cosmetic outcome as graft edge and the surgical scars are hidden in the fornices and caruncle. The main limitation is that this is time consuming, technically challenging procedure and patients experience a moderate amount of pain for 24 hours.

Conjunctival Rotational Autografts

This was first described by Tan et al.[36] and this method requires the removal of conjunctiva in the region of the body of the pterygium. This tissue is stored in saline and the rest of the surgery is completed. Then, the tissue is replaced and sutured in place in the bare scleral bed, with the limbal aspect of the graft facing the fornix and vice versa. This is a useful technique for cases in which it is not possible or desirable to use the superior conjunctiva as a donor source, such as with excision of extensive pterygium, which leaves insufficient conjunctival tissue for the autograft, double pterygium, previous glaucoma surgery.

Cultivated Conjunctival Graft

Another method of closing the surgical defect involves the use of an ex vivo expanded conjunctival epithelial sheet on an amniotic membrane substrate. Recurrence of 23%[37] noted by this method.

Amniotic Membrane Graft

The amniotic membrane, the placenta's inner lining, is composed of three layers: (1) a single epithelial layer; (2) a thick basement membrane; and (3) an avascular stroma. Several characteristics of amniotic membrane appear to make it suitable for treating pterygium, including its anti-inflammatory, antiscarring, and antiangiogenic properties. Once harvested, amniotic membrane can be used fresh or preserved (either freeze-dried or cryopreserved). Unfortunately, fresh amniotic membrane is usually not used in developed countries, due to the need to exclude infections, such as human immunodeficiency virus (HIV) and hepatitis. Clinical trials of amniotic membrane grafts for the treatment of pterygium reported recurrence rate between 2.6% and 10.7%[38] for primary pterygia and as high as 37.5%[27,39] for recurrent pterygia compared to closure with the use of conjunctival autograft (CAG) 2.6–39%. The use of amniotic membrane in combination with conjunctival autografting techniques has also been suggested in recurrent pterygium where the amniotic membrane in the subconjunctival space acts as a natural inhibitor of fibrosis, decreases vascularization and inflammation and promotes epithelialization.[40,41]

In cases in which the pterygium is wider and has multiple heads, enough tissue might not be available for harvesting CAGs. In such scenarios, amniotic membrane transplantation can be used to close the bare sclera area after the pterygium excision (Figs. 20.15A and B). Amniotic membrane grafts facilitate epithelialization, have anti-inflammatory action due to inhibition of fibroblast chemokine expression, antiangiogenic action due to VEGF inhibition.

Lamellar Corneal/Scleral Transplant

Following pterygium excision in cases with pterygium encroaching onto the pupillary region, the bare lamellar cornea grafting helps to achieve tectonic integrity of the underlying involved corneal surface. This has mostly been used to treat eyes with recurrent pterygium to restore corneal thickness in thinned, scarred corneas or associated corneal opacity in the visual axis (keyhole lamellar keratoplasty).[42] Limitations in this surgery include complex surgical approach, greater surgical time, need for donor cornea, risk of rejection and risk of transmission of infectious disease. Reported recurrence rates range from 6% to 30%.[43]

Other approaches include use of buccal mucous membrane grafts to close bare sclera,[44] full thickness keratoplasty or sclerokeratoplasty[45] in cases with extensive corneal involvement, yttrium-aluminum-garnet laser treatment,[46] Barraquer polishing technique.[47]

Fibrin Glue versus Sutures

The conjunctival graft can be fixated onto the bare sclera using absorbable vicryl sutures or human fibrin glue. Use of adjuvants like fibrin glue to fixate the graft is very

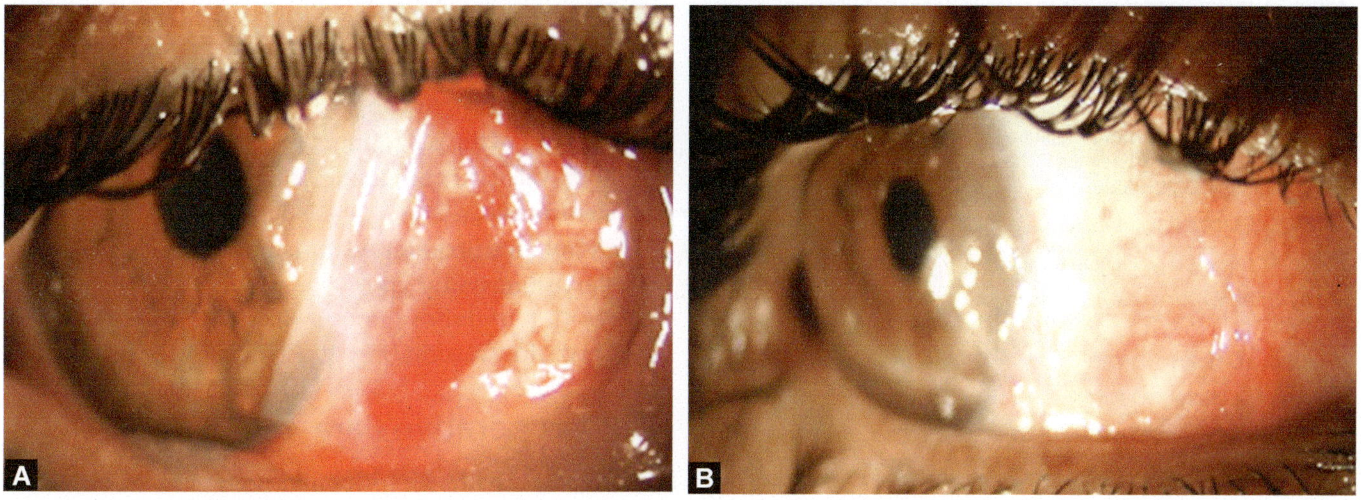

Figs. 20.15A and B: Clinical photograph after pterygium excision surgery with amniotic membrane grafting. (A) Immediate postoperative period; (B) Late postoperative period.
Source: Dr Uma Sridhar, ICARE Hospital, Noida, Uttar Pradesh, India.

useful in decreasing postoperative pain, surgical time and recurrence rate which is 5.3%[48] versus 13.5% with suture.[49-52] These heal with minimal inflammation. Fibrinogen part of fibrin glue is applied on graft and thrombin part on bare sclera. The major concerns include the cost and since fibrin adhesives are prepared from pooled donor sources, there is a small but finite risk of infection, such as hepatitis and HIV, but there are no such reported infections, as well as of anaphylactic reaction. The infection risk is reduced by testing donors for viral markers, at the time of donation and 6 months later, as well as by sterilization of the products by gamma irradiation and treatment with detergents or solvents. Recombinant biotechnology could provide an ideal source of fibrinogen and thrombin, thus completely bypassing the viral contamination issues.

Another technique of split-conjunctival grafting described in multiple headed pterygium, wherein the graft is split the largest or the nasal pterygium gets the limbal stem cells while the smaller one gets conjunctival graft without limbal stem cells.[40]

Autologous Serum

Patient's own blood is used as a bioadhesive in pterygium surgery (sutureless and glueless pterygium excision with conjunctival grafting)[53] and the recurrence rate was found to be similar to fibrin glue.[49,54] It is more cost-effective with no risk of transmission of infections. The drawback of this technique is that the complications like graft displacement, loss of the graft and graft retraction, which have been noted to be more common in patients with grafting with autologous blood than with the fibrin glue or suture fixation.

Adjuvant Treatment

Adjuvants like mitomycin C, 5-fluorouracil, daunorubicin and cyclosporin A have been noted to reduce the recurrence rates after pterygium excision when used in conjunction with CAG.[55,56]

In *beta irradiation* of the bare sclera, high-speed electrons induce radiation causing obliterative endarteritis of vessels. Dosage recommended is 15 Gy in single or divided doses.[57]

Mitomycin C is a potent alkylating agent that interferes with DNA replication, particularly in cells that are growing actively. It also interferes with ribonucleic acid (RNA) and protein synthesis. The use of topical mitomycin C as an adjunct to pterygium surgery to inhibit the growth of fibroblasts was first described in 1963 and actively investigated in the late 1980s. Two approaches have been developed for applying mitomycin C: (1) postoperative use of topical eye drops and (2) intraoperative use of mitomycin C-soaked sponges (0.4 mg/mL or 0.2 mg/mL four times daily for 1–2 weeks postoperatively and 0.2 mg/mL for 3 minutes intraoperatively).[55,56,58]

5-fluorouracil is a fluorinated pyrimidine, also inhibits the proliferation of fibroblasts, but through different mechanisms involving the inhibition of thymidylate synthetase and other enzymes related to nucleic acid biosynthesis.[59,60]

Table 20.4: Reported recurrence rates in various studies.

Study	Agent/tissue used	Recurrence rate (%)
Alp et al. 2002[27]	MMC Intraop	3.33–42.7
	Postop	0–54.5
	Beta radiation	0.5–33
	Excimer PTK	4.5–91
	AMG	3.8–37.5
	CAG	2.6–39
	LCAT	0–14.6
	Simple excision	29.2–89
Kenyon et al. 1985[29]	CAG	5.3
Pulte et al. 1998[67]	LCAT	2.9
Mutlu et al. 1999[68]	LCAT	14.6
Tekin et al. 2001[38]	AMT	10.7

(MMC: Mitomycin C; PTK: Excimer laser phototherapeutic keratectomy; AMG: Amniotic membrane graft; CAG: Conjunctival autograft; LCAT: Limbal-conjunctival autograft transplantation; AMT: Amniotic membrane transplantation)

Thiotepa is given in 1:2,000 concentration 3 hourly for 6 weeks postsurgery.[61,62]

Others including cyclosporin A and daunorubicin are also aimed at reducing the recurrence rates.

These adjuvant therapies are associated with complications such as poor epithelial healing, superficial punctate epitheliopathy, scleral melt, microbial infection, glaucoma, endophthalmitis, corectopia, iritis, sudden onset mature cataract, scleral calcification and incapacitating photophobia and pain.[63-65]

Subconjunctival bevacizumab may also be used as an adjuvant in pterygium surgery to prevent recurrence.[66]

The amount of subconjunctival tissue removed, type of suture used and the postoperative treatment influence the recurrence rates (Table 20.4).

Basic Steps of the Surgical Procedure

The basic steps in pterygium excision surgery (Figs. 20.16A to N) include the following:

1. Excision of the pterygium head from the cornea
2. Removal of subconjunctival fibrous degenerative tissue
3. Hemostasis
4. Donor area preparation and marking
5. Harvesting donor graft
6. Fixation of donor graft on the host bed with human fibrin glue/sutures (Fig. 20.17) or autologous blood.

Postoperative Care

A therapeutic bandage soft contact lens may be considered at the end to enhance patient conform and accelerate re-epithelialization.

As pterygia are both actinic and inflammatory in nature, progressive or recurrent degeneration can be avoided with aggressive UV protection and anti-inflammatory therapy.

- First, a subconjunctival triamcinolone acetonide injection can be given immediately postoperatively in the operating room.
- Second, the patient must be warned to never expose the eyes to sunlight without UV sunglasses protection.
- Third, aggressive postoperative application of topical steroids constitutes the mainstay to reduce recurrence rates by inflammation control and helps avoid scarring and neovascularization. Topical steroids should continue until all the signs of hypervascularity have vanished. The initial therapy with topical loteprednol suspension or gel up to QID and ointment at bedtime

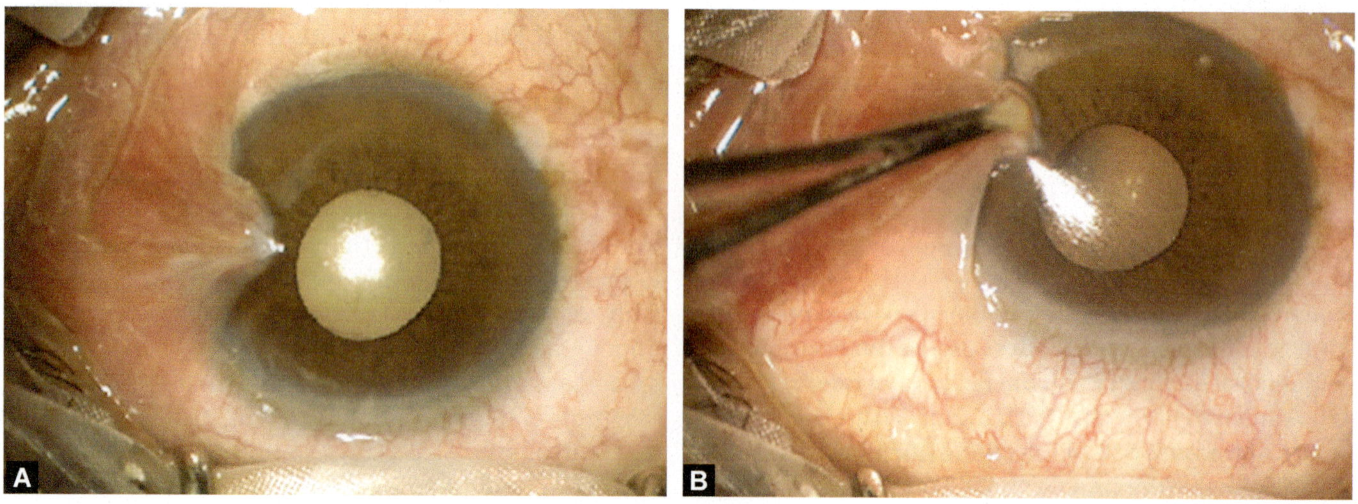

Figs. 20.16A and B

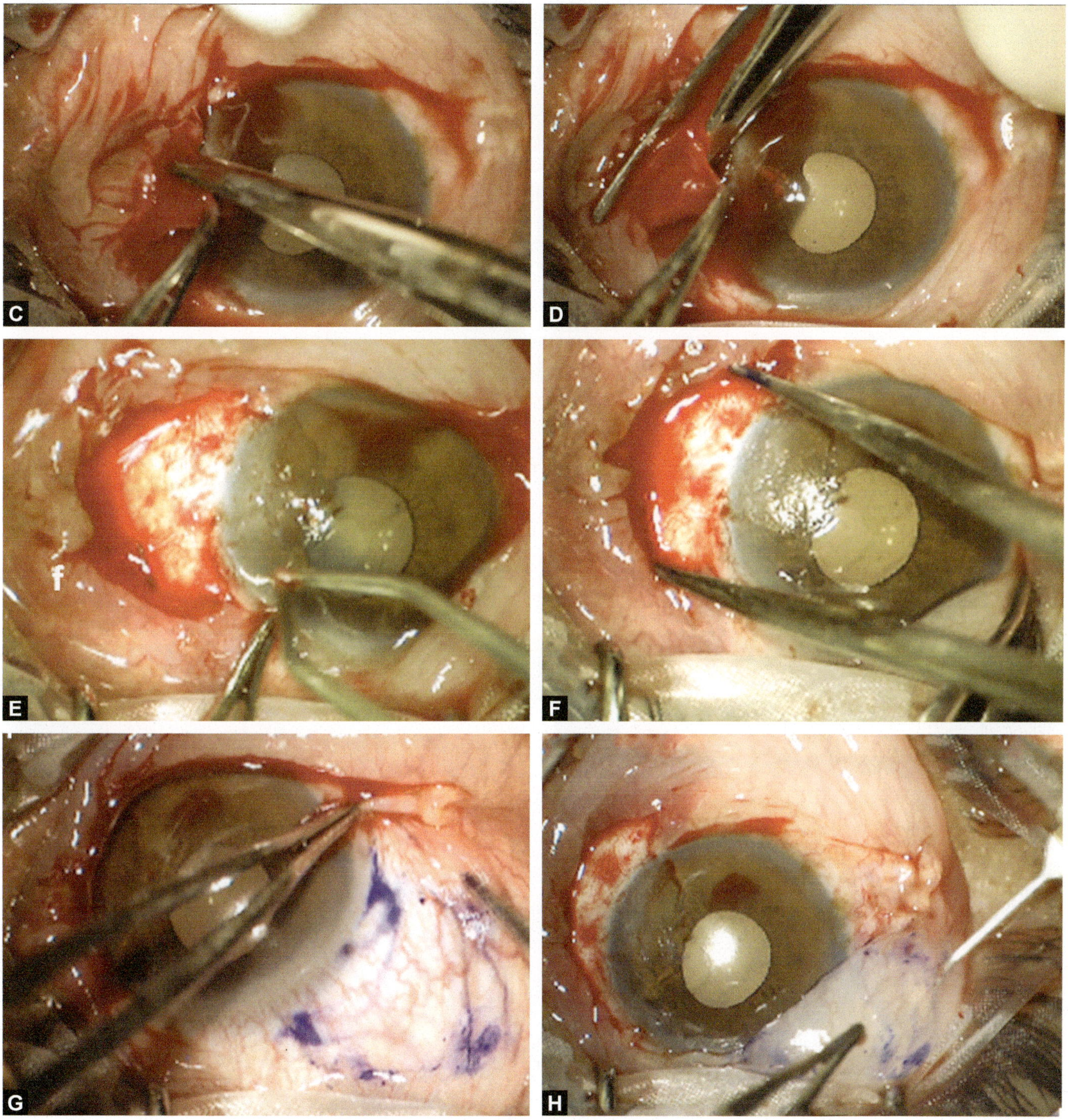

Figs. 20.16C to H

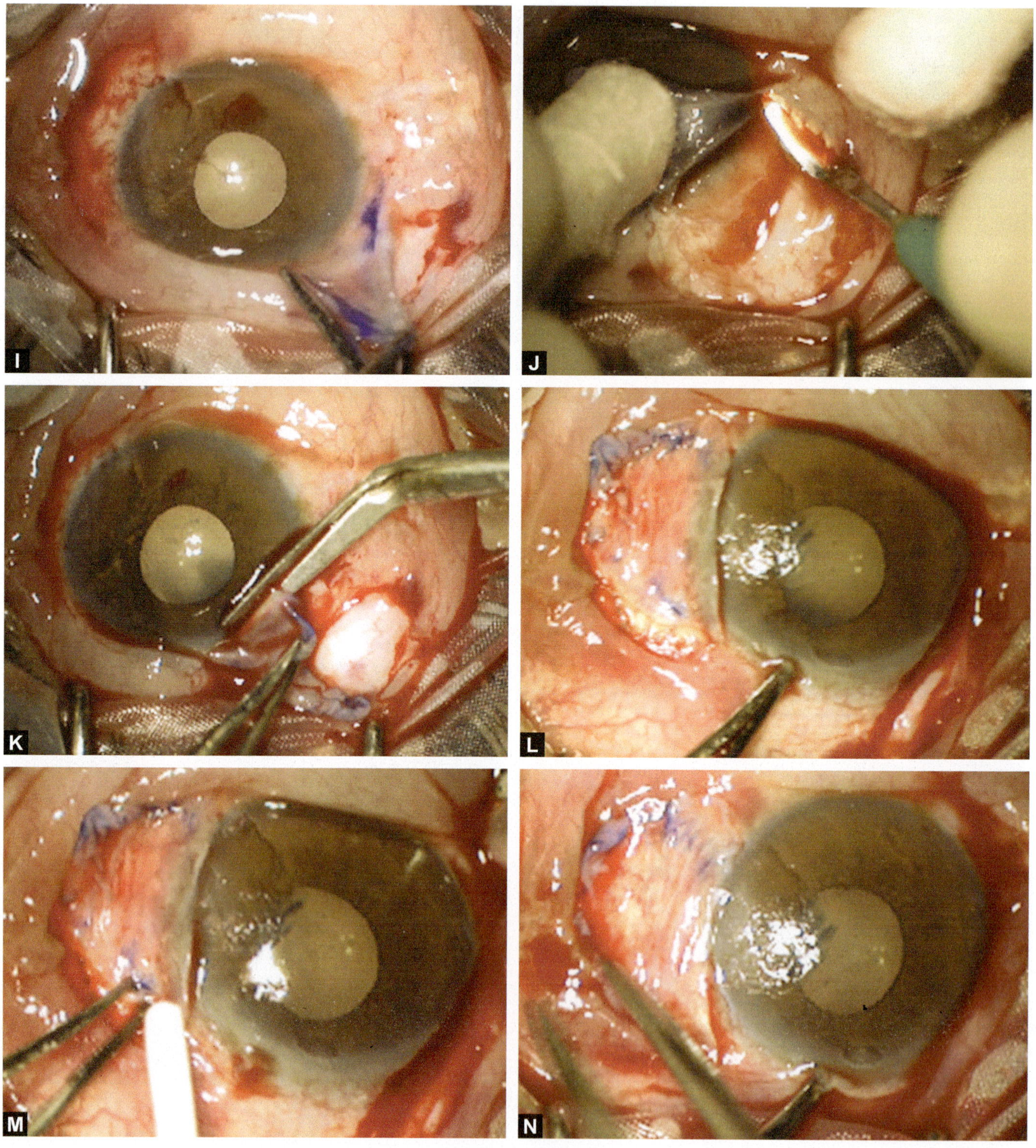

Figs. 20.16I to N

Figs. 20.16A to N: Surgical steps in pterygium excision with conjunctival-limbal autograft (surgeon's view). (A) Fleshy nasal pterygium encroaching into nasal paracentral cornea of the right eye; (B) Pterygium head being avulsed from the corneal surface; (C and D) Subconjunctival fibrous tissue being dissected out from the body of the pterygium and excised; (E) Sclera bed being cauterized to achieve adequate hemostasis; (F) Measurement of the size of the bare sclera host bed after excision of pterygium head; (G) Marking of the superotemporal donor conjunctival site; (H) Autologous donor conjunctival tissue being separated from underlying Tenon's capsule by subconjunctival lidocaine with adrenaline injection; (I) Donor conjunctival excision commenced with Vannas scissors; (J) Gentle dissection of the limbal conjunctival epithelium with crescent knife; (K) Conjunctival-limbal autograft (CLAG) being harvested with Vannas scissors; (L) CLAG tissue placed into position on the host scleral bed; (M) Injection of human fibrin glue under the CLAG graft; (N) CLAG gently stroked into position and apposed well with the surrounding conjunctival tissue to facilitate optimal adhesion.

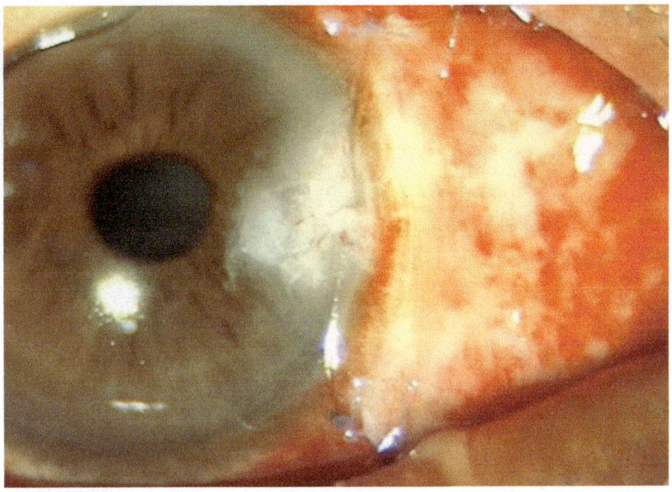

Fig. 20.17: Postoperative clinical photograph of conjunctival-limbal autograft (CLAG) fixated with sutures. Scarring of the nasal cornea is visible.

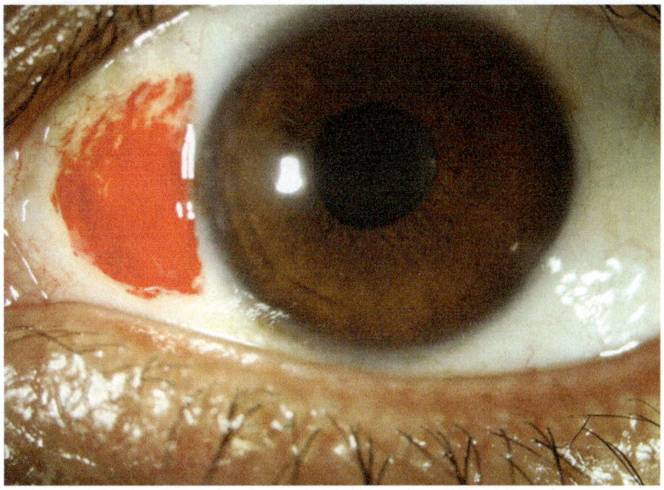

Fig. 20.18: Clinical photograph showing graft hemorrhage.

is prescribed until the eye is completely "quiet", all hemorrhage has resolved, full comfort is restored, and all vasculature has returned to normal caliber. This may require up to 3 months in routine cases or much longer in complicated or high recurrence risk cases. Once the desired level of anti-inflammatory control has been achieved, the daytime treatment can be discontinued and the preservative-free ointment sustained at night (for up to 1 year postoperatively). This ensures compliance and avoids the appearance of limbal vascular tufts that lead to recurrence.

Additional environmental, nutritional, and topical preservative-free tear replacement therapeutic measures to support dry eye therapy are also extremely important.

Complications of Pterygium Surgery

Intraoperative Complications

Intraoperative complications during pterygium surgery include the following:

- Excessive bleeding
- Inverted graft
- Button holing of the graft
- Damage to extraocular muscles by excessive dissection
- Loss of graft tissue
- Globe perforation.

Immediate Complications

Complications in the immediate postoperative period include the following:

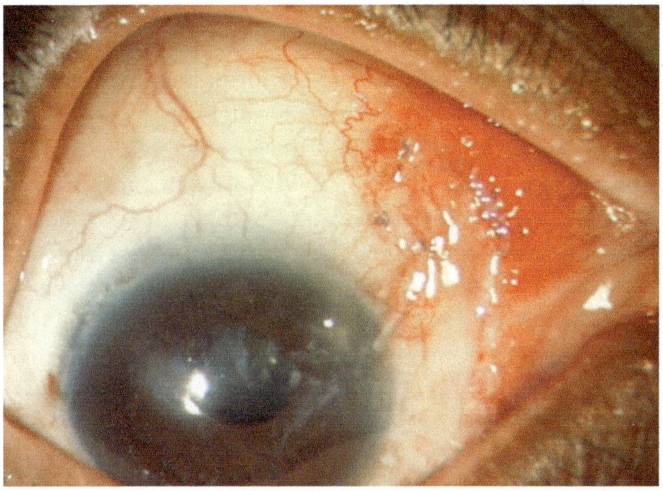

Fig. 20.19: Clinical photograph showing postoperative inflammation in conjunctival autograft.

- Conjunctival chemosis and hemorrhage
- Edema of the conjunctival graft
- Hematoma below the graft (Fig. 20.18)
- Localized epithelial defect
- Loose sutures (in cases where suture fixation of the graft is done)
- Conjunctival wound dehiscence
- Infection of the graft
- Postoperative inflammation (Fig. 20.19).

While some complications may resolve without intervention, such as a localized epithelial defect or conjunctival chemosis, others require specific management.

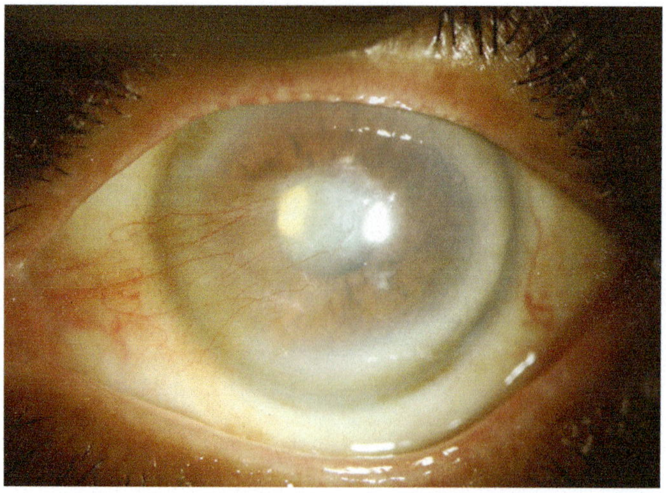

Fig. 20.20: Clinical photograph of recurrent pterygium.

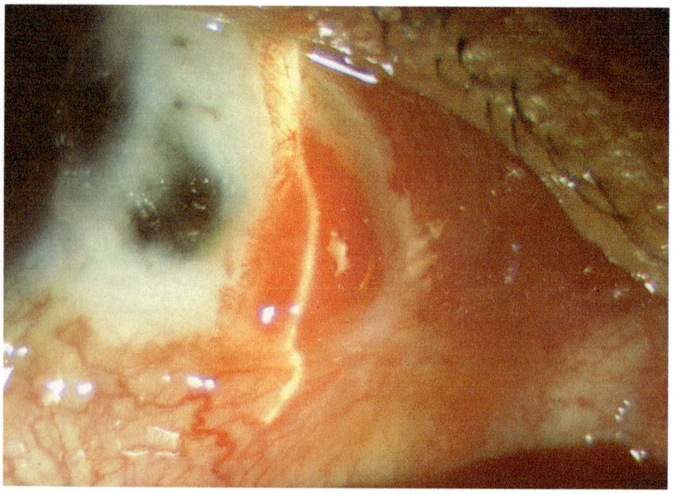

Fig. 20.21: Clinical photograph of post-pterygium excision scleral melt with pyogenic granuloma formation.

Late Complications

The major late complication following pterygium surgery is recurrence (Fig. 20.20). Recurrence rates vary by procedure (Table 20.4), with bare sclera excision having the highest rate, followed by excision with amniotic membrane grafting, and by conjunctival autografting. The risk factors for recurrence include male sex and a history of high sun exposure. Nontranslucent pterygia have been associated with an increased risk of recurrence.

Other late complications include those related to adjunct therapy (such as mitomycin C), suture-related inflammation (Fig. 20.18), Tenon's capsule cyst, diplopia and strabismus, episcleral pyogenic granuloma, limbal stem cell deficiency, dellen, scleral complications (Fig. 20.21), corneal perforation, graft retraction, lens changes (due to prolonged steroids and mitomycin use), and graft necrosis, as well as more unexpected complications, such as ptosis, entropion and symblepharon.

STRATEGIES FOR DECREASING PTERYGIUM RECURRENCE

Few strategies have been elaborated by Sheppard et al. with the objective to decrease the incidence of recurrence.[69] These include the following:

- Topical steroid prior to and following pterygium surgery can help to decrease inflammation and fibrosis.
- Oral doxycycline, especially in patients with ocular rosacea may be useful. Continuous oral doxycycline can be a useful adjunct due to its beneficial nonantimicrobial effects, including anti-inflammatory, anti-collagenase, meibomian lipid viscosity reduction, vascular stabilization, and anti-MMP-9 activities.
- Use of topical azithromycin may be considered particularly in patients intolerant to oral doxycycline. Many chronic patients benefit from 1 week per month of topical azithromycin HS, year round.
- Subconjunctival injection of antifibrotic agents such as dexamethasone or triamcinolone along with 5-fluorouracil and lidocaine may be given. Intraoperative subconjunctival steroid injections provide excellent control of postoperative inflammation in addition to topical therapy, thereby enabling significant reduction in the intensity of the postoperative steroid regimen. An excellent postoperative "cocktail" regimen for problematic patients includes 0.1 cc of 5-fluorouracil and 0.3 cc of dexamethasone, with 0.1 cc of lidocaine drawn into the syringe last, so the anesthetic reaches the eye first on the way into the subconjunctival space. This 0.5 cc injection can be given with a bevel-down, 30-gauge needle, tangential to the globe, and adjacent and posterior to the lurking recurrence site.
- Subconjunctival injection of an anti-VEGF agent, bevacizumab and topical bevacizumab drops, 1% solution can readily be prepared by a qualified compounding pharmacy and applied BID to QID over a period of several weeks to several months. This often enables a significant therapeutic antineovascular effect

in the cornea and conjunctiva—superficial vessels remain more susceptible to all therapeutic efforts, while deeper interstitial vessels prove more recalcitrant.

- Locally applied argon laser photocoagulation, enhanced by topical photosensitizer, such as sodium fluorescein can be used to obliterate specific conjunctival feeder vessels or intrastromal corneal vessels. The argon laser is typically set to repeat mode (as with a panretinal photocoagulation), 0.1 second duration, 100 μm spot size, and anywhere between 200 mW and 900 mW. The procedure is comfortable with topical anesthesia, and retinal safety can be enhanced with preoperative pilocarpine miosis. Interestingly, topical sodium fluorescein, routinely used on the ocular surface for clinical diagnostic purposes, is also activated at the 514 nm argon green wavelength incorporated into generations of therapeutic ophthalmic lasers; thus, the simple application of topical fluorescein acts as a photoactivator, significantly enhancing the local effects of the laser, particularly in foci where inflammation may potentiate fluorescein absorption through damaged ocular surface cells and compromised vascular endothelial junctions.

REFERENCES

1. Johnson GJ. Pterygium. In: Johnson GJ, Weale RA, Minassian DC, West SK (Eds). The Epidemiology of Eye Disease, 2nd edition. Arnold: London, UK; 2003. pp. 218-21.
2. Moran DJ, Hollows FC. Pterygium and ultraviolet radiation: a positive correlation. Br J Ophthalmol. 1984;68(5):343-6.
3. Asokan R, Venkatasubbu RS, Velumuri L, et al. Prevalence and associated factors for pterygium and pinguecula in a South Indian population. Ophthalmic Physiol Opt. 2012;32:39-44.
4. Nangia V, Jonas JB, Nair D, et al. Prevalence and associated factors for pterygium in rural Agrarian Central India. The Central India Eye and Medical Study. PLoS One. 2013;8(12):e82439.
5. McCarty CA, Fu CL, Taylor HR. Epidemiology of pterygium in Victoria, Australia. Br J Ophthalmol. 2000;84:289-92.
6. Tan DT, Chee SP, Dear KB, et al. Effect of pterygium morphology on pterygium recurrence in a controlled trial comparing conjunctival autografting with bare sclera excision. Arch Ophthalmol. 1997;115(10):1235-40.
7. Yang SF, Lin CY, Yang PY, et al. Increased expression of gelatinase (MMP-2 and MMP-9) in pterygia and pterygium fibroblasts with disease progression and activation of protein kinase C. Invest Ophthalmol Vis Sci. 2009;50:4588-96.
8. Moran DJ, Hollows FC. Pterygium and ultraviolet radiation: a positive correlation. Br J Ophthalmol. 1984;68:343-6.
9. Tseng SC. Concept and application of limbal stem cells. Eye (Lond). 1989;3:141-57.
10. Spandidos DA, Sourvinos G, Kiaris H, et al. Microsatellite instability and loss of heterozygosity in human pterygia. Br J Ophthalmol. 1997;81:493-6.
11. Tan DT, Tang WY, Liu YP, et al. Apoptosis and apoptosis-related gene expression in normal conjunctiva and pterygium. Br J Ophthalmol. 2000;84:212-6.
12. Gallagher MJ, Giannoudis A, Herrington CS, et al. Human papilloma virus in pterygium. Br J Ophthalmol. 2001;85:782-4.
13. Detorakis ET, Sourvinos G, Spandidos DA. Detection of herpes simplex virus and human papilloma virus in ophthalmic pterygium. Cornea. 2001;20(2):164-7.
14. Aspiotis M, Tsanou E, Gorezis S, et al. Angiogenesis in pterygium: study of microvessel density, vascular endothelial growth factor, and thrombospondin-1. Eye (Lond). 2007;21:1095-101.
15. Di Girolamo N, Chui J, Coroneo MT, et al. Pathogenesis of pterygia: role of cytokines, growth factors, and matrix metalloproteinases. Prog Retin Eye Res. 2004;23:195-228.
16. An MX, Wu KL, Lin SC. Detection and comparison of matrix metalloproteinase in primary and recurrent pterygium fibroblasts. Int J Ophthalmol. 2011;4(4):353-6.
17. Lemercier G, Cornand G, Burckhart MF. Pinguecula and pterygium: histologic and electron microscopic study (author's transl). Virchows Arch A Pathol Anat Histol. 1978;379:321-33.
18. Stocker FW, Prindle RE. A new type of pigment line in the cornea. Am J Ophthalmol. 1944;27(4):341-5.
19. Fuchs E. Ueber das pterygium (Concerning the pterygium): German. Graefes Arch Ophthalmol. 1892;38:1-89.
20. Anduze AL, Merritt JC. Pterygium: clinical classification and management in Virgin Islands. Ann Ophthalmol. 1985;17(1):92-5.
21. Mohammad-Salih PA, Sharif AF. Analysis of pterygium size and induced corneal astigmatism. Cornea. 2008;27(4):434-8.
22. Avisar R, Loya N, Yassur Y, et al. Pterygium induced corneal astigmatism. Isr Med Assoc J. 2000;2(1):14-5.
23. Prisant O, Hoang-Xuan T, Proano C, et al. Vector summation of anterior and posterior corneal topographical astigmatism. JCRS. 2002;28(9):1636-43.
24. Gumus K, Erkilic K, Topaktas D, et al. Effect of pterygia on refractive indices, corneal topography and ocular aberrations. Cornea. 2011;30(1):24-9.
25. Nguyen HT, Samudre SS, Lattanzio FA, et al. Loteprednol etabonate (Lotemax, 0.5%) reduces inflammatory response associated with pterygium progression. Invest Ophthalmol Vis Sci. 2008;49:6027.
26. Hsu MY, Lee HN, Liang CY, et al. Pterygium is related to a decrease in corneal endothelial cell density. Cornea. 2014;33:712-5.

27. Alp BN, Yanyali A, Ay GM, et al. Conjunctival rotation autograft for primary pterygium. Ophthalmologica. 2002;216:333-6.
28. Müller S, Stahn J, Schmitz K, et al. Recurrence rates after pterygium excision with sliding conjunctival flap versus free conjunctival autograft. Ophthalmologe. 2007;104(6):480-3.
29. Kenyon KR, Wagoner MD, Hettinger ME. Conjunctival autograft transplantation for advanced and recurrent pterygium. Ophthalmology. 1985;92:1461-70.
30. Rao SK, Lekha T, Mukesh BN, et al. Conjunctival-limbal autografts for primary and recurrent pterygia: technique and results. Indian J Ophthalmol. 1998;46:203-9.
31. Ang LP, Chua JL, Tan DT. Current concepts and techniques in pterygium treatment. Curr Opin Ophthalmol. 2007;18:308-13.
32. Dadeya S, Malik KP, Gulliani BP. Pterygium surgery: conjunctival rotation autograft versus conjunctival autograft. Ophthalmic Surg Lasers. 2002;33:269-74.
33. Riordan-Eva P, Kielhorn I, Ficker LA, et al. Conjunctival autografting in the surgical management of pterygium. Eye. 1993;7:634-8.
34. Allan BD, Short P, Crawford GJ, et al. Pterygium excision with conjunctival autografting: an effective and safe technique. Br J Ophthalmol. 1993;77:698-701.
35. Hirst LW. Prospective study of primary pterygium surgery using pterygium extended removal followed by extended conjunctival transplantation. Ophthalmology. 2008;115: 1663-72.
36. Jap A, Chan C, Lim L, et al. Conjunctival rotation autograft for pterygium: an alternative to conjunctival autografting. Ophthalmology. 1999;106(1):67-71.
37. Ang LP, Tan DT, Cajucom-Uy H, et al. Autologous cultivated conjunctival transplantation for pterygium surgery. Am J Ophthalmol. 2005;139:611-9.
38. Tekin NF, Kaynak S, Saatci AO, et al. Preserved human amniotic membrane transplantation in the treatment of primary pterygium. Ophthalmic Surg Lasers Imaging Retina. 2001;32(6):464-9.
39. Solomon A, Pires RT, Tseng SC. Amniotic membrane transplantation after extensive removal of primary and recurrent pterygia. Ophthalmology. 2001;108:449-60.
40. Xi XH, Jiang DY, Tang LS. Transplantation of amniotic membrane and amniotic membrane combined with limbal autograft for patients with complicated pterygium. Hunan Yi Ke Da Xue Xue Bao. 2003;28:149-51.
41. Shimazaki J, Shinozaki N, Tsubota K. Transplantation of amniotic membrane and limbal autograft for patients with recurrent pterygium associated with symblepharon. Br J Ophthalmol. 1998;82:235-40.
42. Dake CL, Crone RA, Keizer RJ. Treatment of (recurrent) pterygium oculi by lamellar keratoplasy. Documenta Ophthalmologica. 1980;48:223-30.
43. Simona F, Tabatabay CA, Leuenberger PM. Lamellar corneal graft in the treatment of pterygium. A 10-year retrospective study of the recurrence and changes of astigmatism. J Fr Ophtalmol. 1988;11(11):759-63.
44. Forbes J, Collin R, Dart J. Split thickness buccal mucous membrane grafts and β irradiation in the treatment of recurrent pterygium. Br J Ophthalmol. 1998;82:1420-3.
45. Süveges I. Sclerokeratoplasty in recurrent pterygium. Ger J Ophthalmol. 1992;1(2):114-6.
46. Nakammura K, Bissen-Meyajima H, Shimmura S, et al. Clinical application of Er:YAG laser for the treatment of pterygium. Ophthalmic Surg Lasers Imaging Retina. 2000;31:8-9.
47. Singh G, Rana RK. Evaluation of a new polishing technique in surgery of primary pterygium. Indian J Ophthalmol. 1982;30:281-4.
48. Koranyi G, Seregard S, Kopp ED. Cut and paste: a no suture, small incision approach to pterygium surgery. Br J Ophthalmol. 2004;88:911-4.
49. Hall RC, Logan AJ, Wells AP. Comparison of fibrin glue with sutures for pterygium excision surgery with conjunctival autografts. Clin Exp Ophthalmol. 2009;37(6):584-9.
50. Farid M, Pirnazar JR. Pterygium recurrence after excision with conjunctival autograft: a comparison of fibrin tissue adhesive to absorbable sutures. Cornea. 2009;28:43-5.
51. Karalezli A, Kucukerdonmez C, Akova YA, et al. Fibrin glue versus sutures for conjunctival autografting in pterygium surgery: a prospective comparative study. Br J Ophthalmol. 2008;92:1206-10.
52. Pan HW, Zhong JX, Jing CX. Comparison of fibrin glue versus suture for conjunctival autografting in pterygium surgery: a meta-analysis. Ophthalmology. 2011;118:1049-54.
53. Kurian A, Reghunadhan I, Nair KG. Autologous blood versus fibrin glue for conjunctival autograft adherence in sutureless pterygium surgery: a randomised controlled trial. Br J Ophthalmol. 2015;99(4):464-70.
54. Singh PK, Singh S, Vyas C, et al. Conjunctival autografting without fibrin glue or sutures for pterygium surgery. Cornea. 2013;32:104-7.
55. Chen PP, Ariyasu RG, Kaza V, et al. A randomized trial comparing mitomycin C and conjunctival autograft after excision of primary pterygium. Am J Ophthalmol. 1995; 120:151-60.
56. Singh G, Wilson MR, Foster CS. Long-term follow-up study of mitomycin eye drops as adjunctive treatment of pterygia and its comparison with conjunctival autograft transplantation. Cornea. 1990;9:331-4.
57. Paryani SB, Scott WP, Wells JW Jr, et al. Management of pterygium with surgery and radiation therapy. The North Florida Pterygium Study Group. Int J Radiat Oncol Biol Phys. 1994;28(1):101-3.
58. Young AL, Leung GY, Wong AK, et al. A randomised trial comparing 0.02% mitomycin C and limbal conjunctival autograft after excision of primary pterygium. Br J Ophthalmol. 2004;88:995-7.

59. Pikkel J, Porges Y, Ophir A. Halting pterygium recurrence by postoperative 5-fluorouracil. Cornea. 2001;20(2):168-71.
60. Prabhasawat P, Tesavibul N, Leelapatranura K, et al. Efficacy of subconjunctival 5-fluorouracil and triamcinolone injection in impending recurrent pterygium. Ophthalmology. 2006;113(7):1102-9.
61. Liddy BS, Morgan JF. Triethylene thiophosphoramide (thiotepa) and pterygium. Am J Ophthalmol. 1966;61(5 Pt 1):888-90.
62. Tassy A, Ribe D. Thiotepa eye drops for prevention of pterygium recurrence: 18 years of use. J Fr Ophtalmol. 1999;22(2):215-9.
63. Yamanouchi U. Scleral changes induced by instillation of mitomycin C. Acta Med Nagasaki. 1983;28:99-110.
64. Rubinfeld RS, Pfister RR, Stein RM, et al. Serious complications of topical mitomycin-C after pterygium surgery. Ophthalmology. 1992;99:1647-54.
65. Ibanez M, Eugarrios MF, Calderon DI. Topical cyclosporin A and mitomycin C injection as adjunctive therapy for prevention of primary pterygium recurrence. Ophthalmic Surg Lasers Imaging. 2009;40:239-44.
66. Ozgurhan EB, Agca A, Kara N, et al. Topical application of bevacizumab as an adjunct to recurrent pterygium surgery. Cornea. 2013;32:835-8.
67. Pulte P, Heiligenhaus A, Koch J, et al. Long-term results of autologous conjunctiva-limbus transplantation in pterygium. Klinische Monatsblatter fur Augenheilkunde. 1998;213(1):9-14.
68. Mutlu FM, Sobaci G, Tatar T, et al. A comparative study of recurrent pterygium surgery: limbal conjunctival autograft transplantation versus mitomycin C with conjunctival flap. Ophthalmology. 1999;106(4):817-21.
69. Sheppard JD, Mansur A, Comstock TL, et al. An update on the surgical management of pterygium and the role of loteprednol etabonate ointment. Clin Ophthalmol. 2014;8:1105-18.

Chapter 21 Ocular Surface Disorders

Virender S Sangwan, Siddharth Malaiya, Shilpa Das,
Juan Carlos Serna-Ojeda

INTRODUCTION

Ocular surface constitutes the anterior most part of the eyeball that is exposed to the environment. It consists of conjunctival mucosa that lines the bulbar and palpebral surfaces, the corneoscleral limbus, the corneal epithelium and the tear film.[1-4] These components work physiologically along with eyelids and lacrimal functional unit (LFU) to maintain a healthy ocular surface and form an "ocular surface system".[5-7] Ocular surface protects the eye from mechanical, toxic, infectious, and immunologic insults and ensures smooth movement of the globe against palpebral mucosa for visual tracking.[2,8] Figure 21.1 depicts a healthy ocular surface.

FUNCTIONAL ANATOMY

Lids

The eyelids form the first line of defense against trauma and desiccation. Eyelashes trap dust particles and prevent debris from entering the eye. Lids cover the ocular surface in its most part and when the eyes are maintained in closed position as in sleep they help in conjunctival and corneal epithelial healing. Normal blinking action also helps in tear film redistribution.[2,9]

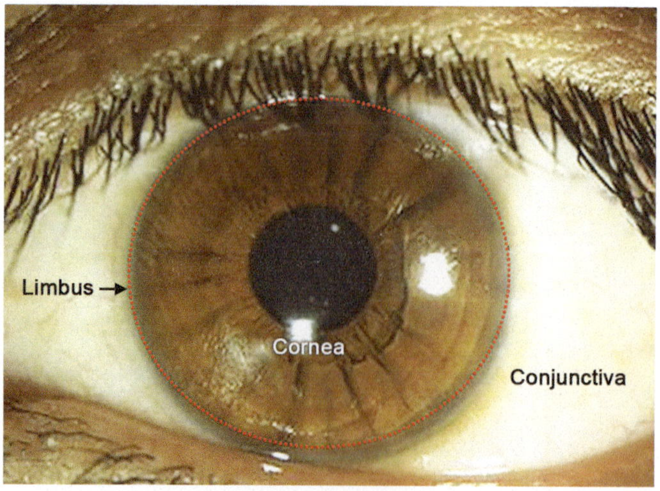

Fig. 21.1: Normal eye with healthy eyelids, tear film, conjunctiva, cornea, and limbus.

The outer surface of the eyelid can get involved pathologically as a part of systemic dermatological diseases. These include epithelial diseases (e.g. contact dermatitis), basement membrane diseases (e.g. pemphigus), connective tissue disorders [e.g. scleroderma, systemic lupus erythematosus (SLE)], and follicular diseases (e.g. folliculitis). Clinical sequelae to this result in scarring, retraction and trichiasis leading to exposure keratopathy and mechanical trauma to the surface. The meibomian glands, which are located within the tarsal plate, produce oily secretions that form the lipid layer of tear film. Lipid layer preserves the other layers by preventing evaporation and acts as surfactant to spread tear film all over the surface.[10] Meibomitis, i.e. inflammation of these glands, is a common condition encountered and is often difficult to treat permanently. These glands are also targets for chronic inflammatory diseases such as acne rosacea and ocular cicatricial pemphigoid (OCP).[2]

Conjunctiva

Conjunctiva is the mucosal membrane that extends from mucocutaneous junction of lid margins, reaches to the fornices and resurfaces the bulbar region back to end at the corneoscleral limbus. The conjunctival folds are especially pronounced in the fornices and facilitate the movement of globe against the lids and socket.[11] Ocular surface stem cells are spread all over the bulbar conjunctiva, limbus and fornices. Their cryptic location in fornices explains conjunctival regeneration in some cases even after sustaining severe injuries to the surface.[12] Conjunctival mucosa harbors accessory lacrimal glands and ducts of main lacrimal gland, which pass through it to open on its surface. They contribute to aqueous component of tear film and may get involved in various conjunctival diseases and lead to dry eye disorders (DEDs).[2] Goblet cells constitute 5–10% of conjunctival epithelial cells and contribute to mucin layer of tear film which firmly binds to ocular surface and provides base for aqueous layer to rest upon it. The tear film, conjunctiva-associated lymphoid tissue (CALT) and the rich conjunctival vascular supply contribute to surface immunity.[9]

Cornea

Cornea is an avascular tissue consisting of epithelium, Bowman's layer, stroma, Descemet's layer, Dua's layer and endothelium.[13] Its optical properties have a significant contribution in maintaining vision. Corneal has approximately 5–7 cells thick stratified squamous epithelium, which is devoid of keratinization unlike skin for maintenance of optical clarity. But, this also makes the surface more prone for dehydration and trauma. Functional corneal innervation provides trophic support to epithelium, mediates blinking process as well as reflex tear secretion from the main lacrimal gland.

Limbus

Limbus is the junction between sclera and cornea where conjunctival epithelium abruptly ends and corneal epithelium begins; both of which are significantly different in their phenotypes (Fig. 21.2).[2] Conjunctival mucosa manifests radial folds at limbus referred as "limbal palisades of Vogt". These palisades of Vogt and interpalisade rete ridges are nests for limbal stem cells (LSCs).[14,15]

Limbal stem cells are specifically involved in maintaining corneal clarity by renewal and regeneration of corneal epithelium in organized manner along with prevention of conjunctival overgrowth.[16,17] They are unique from other cells being undifferentiated and are capable of indefinite multiplication to form highly differentiated progeny.[14,15] Various characteristics of LSCs are given in Box 21.1.[14,17]

In 1983, Schofield proposed "niche hypothesis" for LSCs which states that these cells require optimal microenvironment for their survival and maintenance.[18] Compact limbal anatomy along with support of limbal vascular plexus for provision of nutrition and growth factor and other local cytokines constitutes limbal niche.[17,19] In 1971, Davanger and Evensen showed centripetal migration of limbal cells in regeneration of corneal epithelium.[20] In 1983, Thoft and Friend proposed XYZ hypothesis; where X represents basal proliferation, Y represents centripetal migration of stem cells toward center of cornea, and Z represents loss of superficial cells from surface (Fig. 21.3).[21]

Box 21.1: Characteristic features of limbal stem cells.

- Lack of differentiation
- High proliferative reserve
- Pluripotency
- Slow cell cycle
- Long lifespan
- Asymmetric division
- Require optimal microenvironment for survival

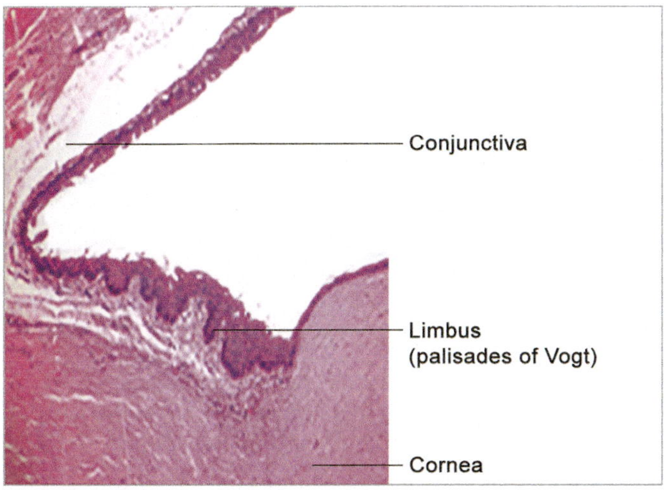

Fig. 21.2: Histological architecture of corneoscleral limbus showing limbal transition zone with undulated limbal epithelium between corneal and conjunctival layer epithelium.

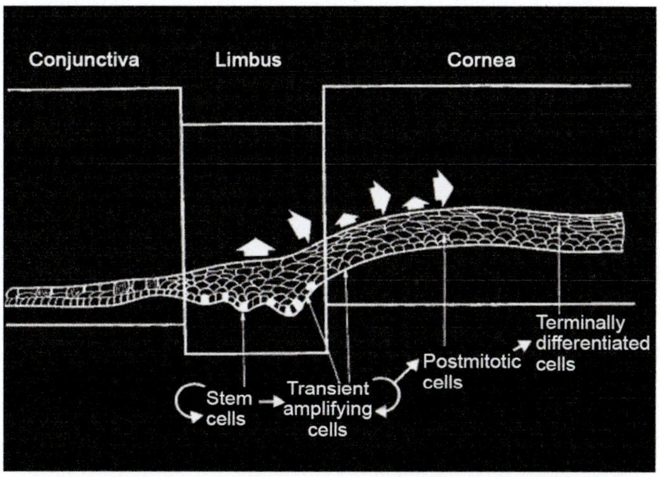

Fig. 21.3: Limbal stem cells differentiate through various stages into corneal epithelial cells.

The integrity of each of the components of the ocular surface is essential to maintain a balanced ocular surface ecosystem.

HALLMARK CLINICAL FEATURES OF OCULAR SURFACE DISEASES

Ocular surface disorders can have an array of presentations:

- The complex of overlapping symptoms of tear film disorder and goblet cell deficiency commonly referred as "dysfunctional tear syndrome" include ocular discomfort, burning, stinging, foreign body sensation, photophobia and blurred vision. This disorder may present with variable surface inflammation along with lusterless surface, increased blink rate and decreased tear meniscal height. In presence of impaired corneal sensations, the blink rate may also be decreased. Chronic cases undergo squamous metaplasia with goblet cell loss inviting more inflammation (Flowchart 21.1). The ocular surface response and sequelae to acute and chronic inflammation has been depicted in Flowchart 21.2.
- Conjunctival infections and allergic eye diseases present with discharge, conjunctival injection, papillae, and follicles. Chronic cases may also involve cornea such as shield ulcer in vernal keratoconjunctivitis.
- Limbal stem cell deficiency (LSCD) from various causes can lead to two classes of problems. First one results from improper healing which includes recurrent epithelial erosions and persistent epithelial defects (PEDs). Second class of problems occurs due to breach in LSC barrier, resulting in superficial vascularization and conjunctivalization of cornea, where conjunctival epithelium starts growing over cornea[14,22] (Flowchart 21.3 and Figs. 21.4A to D). Both classes of patients have variable irregular corneal surface.

The primary symptoms of these patients include decreased vision, photophobia and ocular discomfort.[22,23] Patients with partial LSCD would have milder symptoms with localized conjunctivalization, which may not involve visual axis. On the other hand, total LSCD has 360° of vascularization and conjunctivalization that usually involves visual axis, which leads to further deterioration in vision and increase photophobia. Pain, photophobia, and blepharospasm are marked, if epithelial healing problems are predominant presentations.[22,23]

Flowchart 21.1: Continued ocular surface damage after initial insult due to chronic inflammation resulting in a vicious cycle.

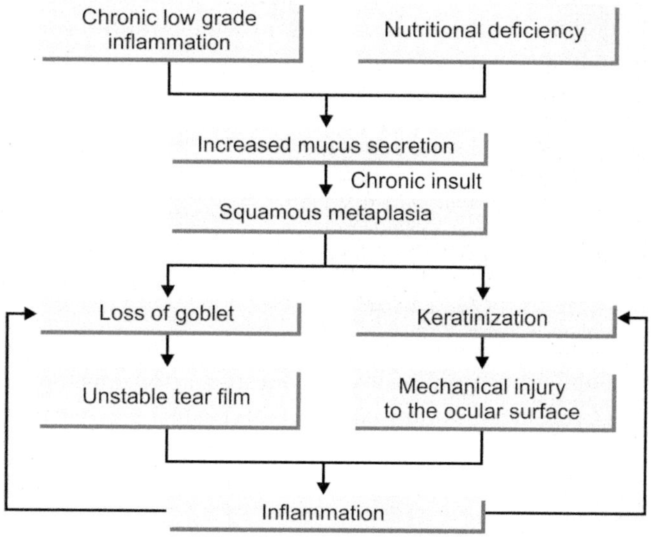

Flowchart 21.2: Anatomical changes and long-term sequel to ocular surface damage caused by acute and chronic insults.

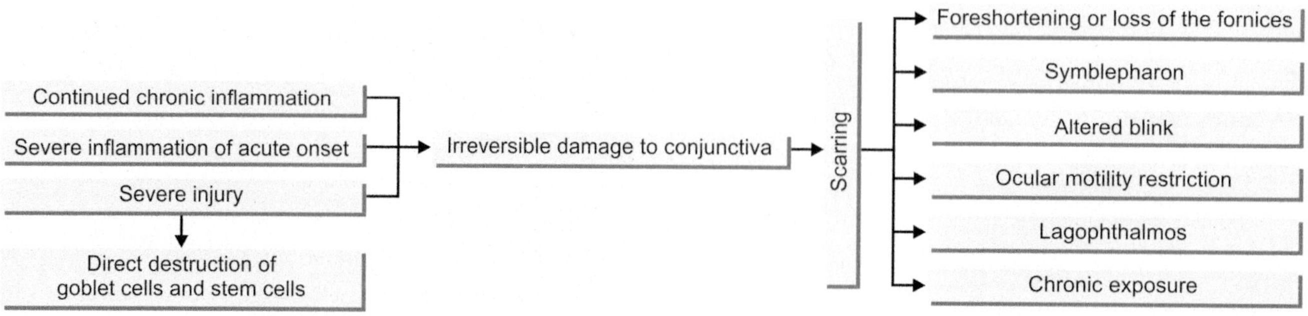

Flowchart 21.3: Characteristic clinical features of limbal stem cell deficiency.

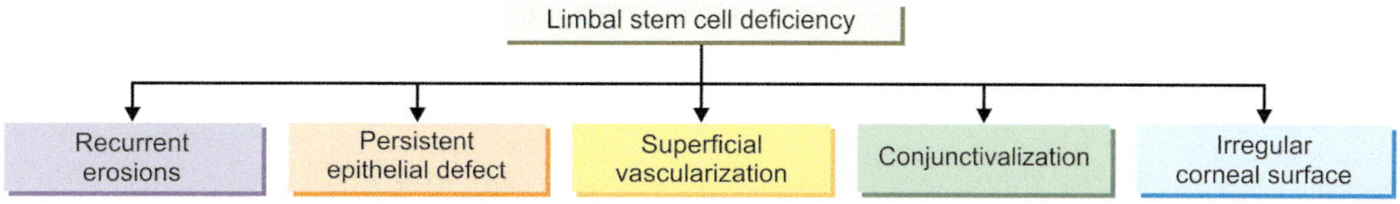

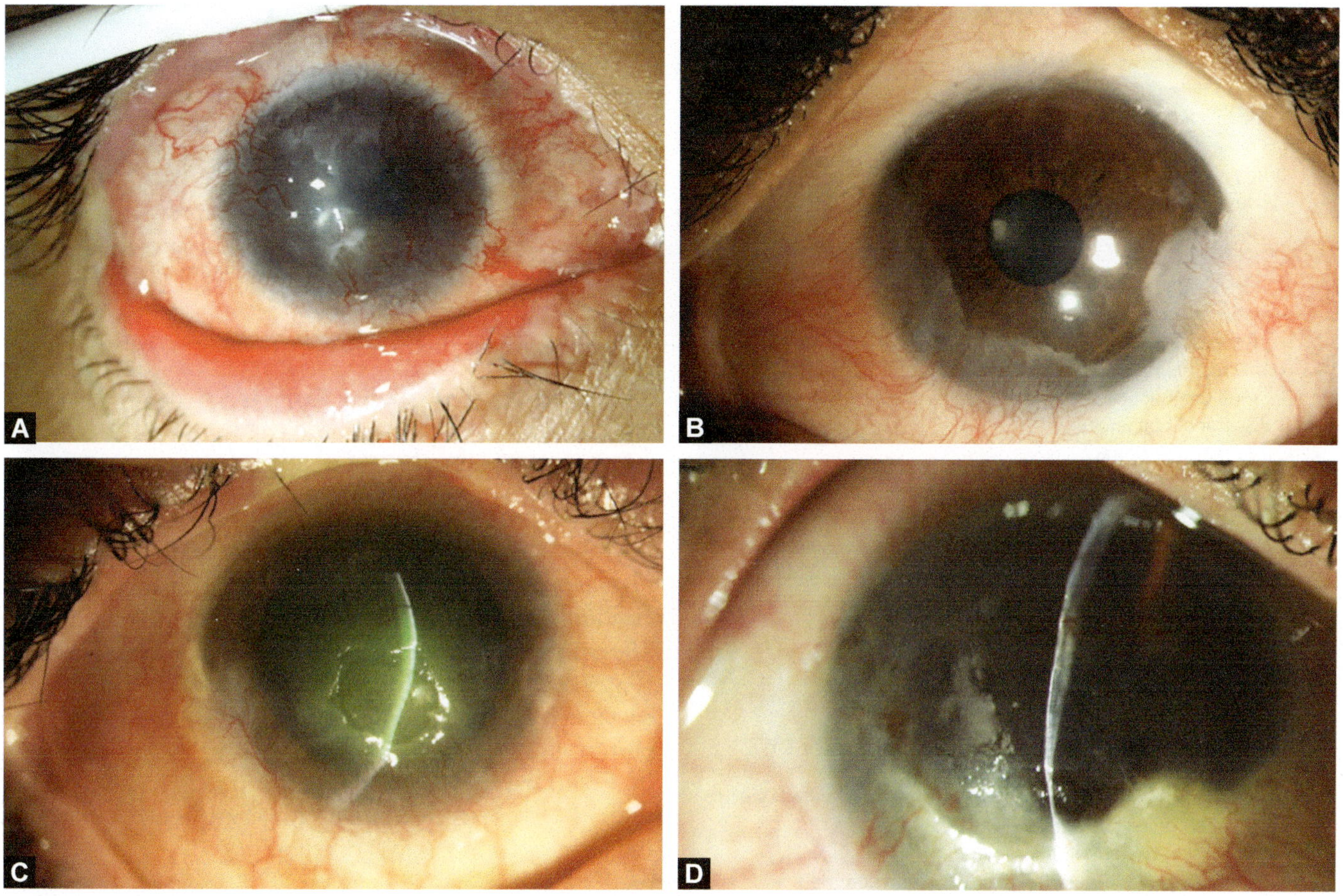

Figs. 21.4A to D: Different presentations of limbal stem cell deficiency (LSCD). (A) Total LSCD involving visual axis with predominant neovascularization; (B) Partial LSCD with sectoral conjunctivalization; (C) Persistent epithelial defect; (D) Peripheral corneal vascularization and lipid keratopathy, perforation with iris prolapse.

OCULAR SURFACE FAILURE

On the basis of epithelial phenotype assessed by impression cytology, ocular surface failure has been divided into two categories:

1. *Type I failure*: It is characterized by squamous metaplasia where, nonkeratinized corneal epithelium is replaced by keratinized one. It is usually accompanied with conjunctival squamous metaplasia.
2. *Type II failure*: It is characterized by LSCD in which normal corneal epithelium gets replaced by conjunctival epithelium.

There are a wide spectrum of surface disorders and on the basis of anatomic level of involvement and primary pathophysiology (Boxes 21.2 and 21.3).[11,24-26]

Individual description of each of these conditions is beyond the scope of this chapter. Three important ocular surface disorders are discussed below:

1. Stevens-Johnson syndrome (SJS)
2. Ocular cicatricial pemphigoid
3. Ocular surface chemical burns.

Box 21.2: Ocular surface failure type I/goblet cell insufficiency.

- *Malnutrition*:
  - Vitamin A deficiency
- *Oculocutaneous disease:*
  - Cicatricial pemphigoid
  - Bullous pemphigoid
  - Linear IgA disease
  - Dermatitis herpetiformis (Duhring)
  - Epidermolysis bullosa acquisita
  - Stevens-Johnson syndrome/toxic epidermal necrolysis
  - Toxic epidermal necrolysis (Lyell syndrome)
  - Porphyria cutanea tarda
  - Atopic keratoconjunctivitis
  - Acne rosacea
- Drugs (pseudopemphigoid)
- *Miscellaneous conjunctival inflammations:*
  - Sjögren's syndrome
  - Systemic sclerosis (scleroderma)
  - Graft-versus-host disease
  - Inflammatory bowel disease
  - Reiter's syndrome
- *Infectious membranous conjunctivitis:*
  - Viral conjunctivitis
  - Bacterial conjunctivitis
- Ocular surface burns

Box 21.3: Ocular surface failure type II/limbal stem cell deficiency (LSCD).

- *Primary LSCD:*
  - Aniridia
  - Sclerocornea
  - Multiple endocrine deficiency (MEN)
  - *Ectodermal dysplasia*:
    - Ectrodactyly-ectodermal dysplasia-clefting (EEC) syndrome
    - Senter's syndrome or keratitis-ichthyosis-deafness (KID) syndrome
  - Erythrokeratoderma
  - Lacrimo-auriculo-dento-digital (LADD) syndrome
  - Dominantly inherited keratitis
  - Dyskeratosis congenita
  - Epidermolysis bullosa
  - Turner's syndrome
  - Peter's anomaly
  - Xeroderma pigmentosum
- *Secondary LSCD:*
  - *Systemic conditions:*
    - Vitamin A deficiency
    - Stevens-Johnson syndrome (SJS)/toxic epidermal necrolysis (TEN)
    - Mucous membrane pemphigoid
    - Sjögren's syndrome
    - Graft-versus-host disease (GVHD)
    - Rosacea
    - Systemic chemotherapy (e.g. anticancer drug S-1 for treatment of gastric cancer)
  - Ocular conditions

Contd...

Contd...

- *Trauma:*
  - *Chemical:* acid, alkali, others
  - Thermal burns
  - Radiation
- *Ocular diseases:*
  - Postinfectious keratitis
  - Neurotropic keratitis
  - Keratoconjunctivitis sicca
  - Vernal keratoconjunctivitis
  - Ocular surface tumors
  - Pterygium and pseudopterygium
  - Contact lens use
  - Aphakic and pseudophakic bullous keratopathy
- *Iatrogenic:*
  - Multiple ocular surgeries
  - Pterygium excision
  - Cyclocryotherapy
  - Antimetabolites—topical mitomycin C, 5-fluorouracil
  - Toxicity from topical medications [benzalkonium chloride (BAC)]
- Idiopathic

Stevens-Johnson Syndrome

Spectrum of Disease

Stevens-Johnson syndrome, the more severe toxic epidermal necrolysis (TEN), and their intermediate (SJS/TEN overlap) characterize a severe immunologic dermatobullous condition. It is an acute, self-limiting vesicobullous disorder affecting the skin and at least two mucous membranes (Fig. 21.5).[5,6] Severe necrosis of external and internal body surfaces results in fatal systemic complications with lifelong comorbidities. When the disease involves less than 10% body surface area (BSA), it is referred as SJS, when greater than 30%, it is referred as TEN and between 10% and 30% the term given is SJS-TEN overlap.[27]

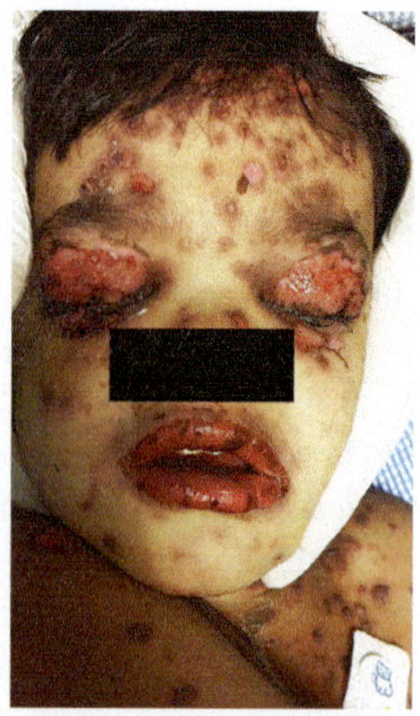

Fig. 21.5: A case of acute Stevens-Johnson syndrome (SJS), with extensive involvement of skin and mucous membranes showing multiple papules and target-like lesions with total necrosis of eyelid skin.

The SJS/TEN is quite rare, affecting 0.4–7 cases/million population/year. SJS affects more commonly children and adolescents, whereas TEN affects all age groups from infants to elderly. The mortality rate is high and ranges from 1–5% in SJS to 25–40% in TEN.[27]

Predisposing Factors

Idiosyncratic reaction to systemic drugs (sulfonamide most common) has been implicated.[27]

Pathophysiology

The SJS/TEN is considered essentially a type IV delayed hypersensitivity mediated by CD8+ cytotoxic T cells and natural killer cells which cause wide spread keratinocyte apoptosis and epidermal necrosis.[27] Numerous human leukocyte antigens (HLAs) have shown associations with different drugs in predisposing SJS/TEN; the intensity of which varies across different ethnic groups. HLA-B*1502 is strongly associated with carbamazepine-induced SJS/TEN in Asian population.[28]

Clinical Course

Ocular involvement is unrelated to systemic illness and ranges from self-limited conjunctival hyperemia to total sloughing of the ocular surface epithelium, inclusive of tarsal conjunctiva and lid margins. Severe conjunctival lesions result in pseudomembranous/membranous conjunctivitis coursing to cicatricial conjunctivitis in chronic phase (Table 21.1 and Figs. 21.6A to D).[29,30]

Table 21.1: Ocular complications of Stevens-Johnson syndrome (SJS)/toxic epidermal necrolysis (TEN).

Acute	Chronic
• Self-limited conjunctival hyperemia	• Symblepharon formation
• Near total/total ocular surface epithelial sloughing	• Ankyloblepharon formation
• Lid margin de-epithelialization	• Ectropion
• Pseudomembrane/membrane formation	• Entropion
• Early symblepharon formation	• Punctal occlusion
• Fornix foreshortening	• Lid margin keratinization
• Corneal ulceration/perforation	• Meibomian gland atrophy
	• Distichiasis
	• Trichiasis
	• Severe dry eye disease (DED)
	• Limbal stem cell deficiency (LSCD)
	• Persistent epithelial defect (PED)
	• Stromal scarring
	• Corneal perforation

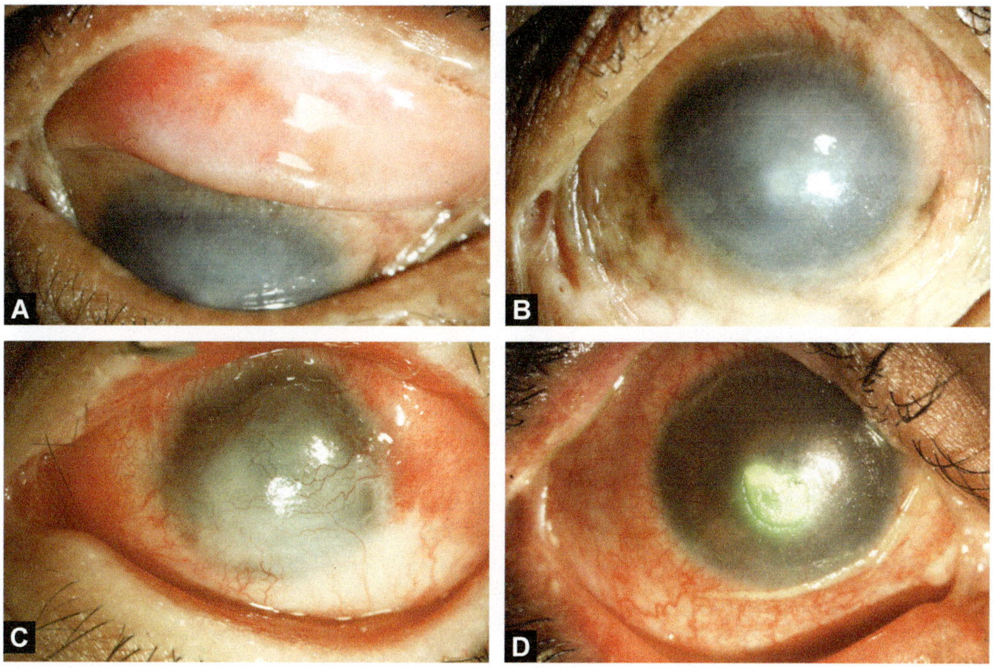

Figs. 21.6A to D: Ocular features of Stevens-Johnson syndrome (SJS)/toxic epidermal necrolysis (TEN) in chronic stage. (A) Keratinization of the superior lid margin; (B) Total limbal stem cell deficiency and keratinization of the ocular surface; (C) Total limbal stem cell deficiency and superficial vascularization of the cornea; (D) Persistent epithelial defect with a plaque of medication deposition.

Management of Acute Stevens-Johnson Syndrome

As SJS/TEN is a medical emergency, the supportive treatment is started in burn intensive care unit (ICU). High-dose pulse steroids, human intravenous (IV) immunoglobulin and immunomodulation drugs form the mainstay of systemic treatment in acute stage.[27,30]

Ocular examination is done to assess the extent of sloughing using fluorescein stain after rinsing away the debris (Figs. 21.7A to C). Topical steroids, broad-spectrum antibiotics and preservative-free lubricants are started. They help in reducing inflammation, preventing infection and improving ocular surface respectively. Bandage contact lens (BCL) and custom made amniotic membrane with tubing/symblepharon ring is extremely useful. It should be applied to cover complete ocular surface along with lid margins to achieve best outcomes. Flowchart 21.4 shows an algorithm for management of acute SJS.

Ocular involvement can be managed on the basis of Gregory's grading system (Table 21.2).[31]

Flowchart 21.4: Algorithm for ocular management of acute Stevens-Johnson syndrome (SJS)/toxic epidermal necrolysis (TEN).

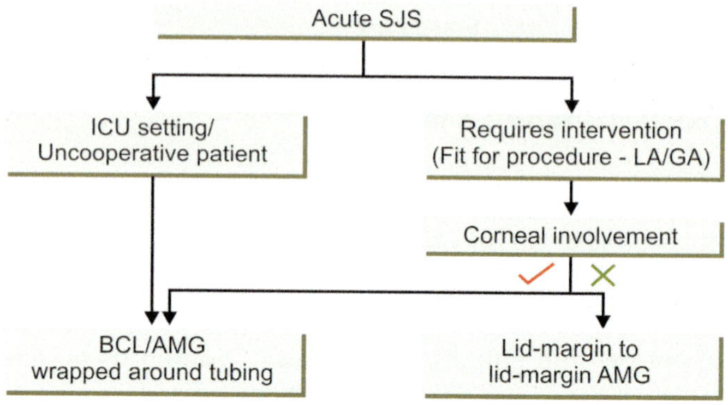

(BCL: Bandage contact lens; AMG: Amniotic membrane graft; LA: Local anesthesia; GA: General anesthesia)
Source: Dr Sahil Goel.

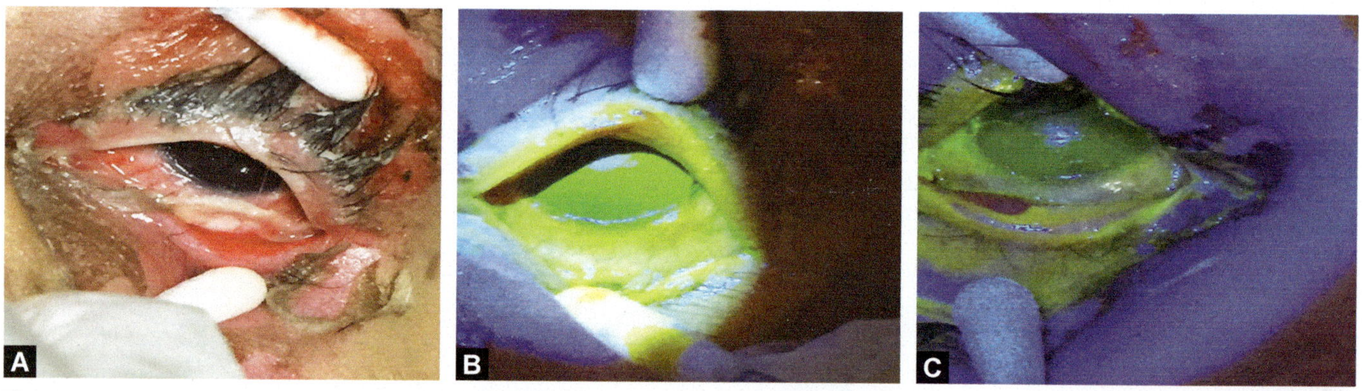

Figs. 21.7A to C: Ocular examination of SJS/TEN in acute stage. (A) Charred eyelid skin with erythematous margins, matted eyelashes and membranous conjunctivitis; (B) Variable involvement of lid margin and ocular surface seen on fluorescein staining; (C) Examining the palpebral conjunctival after lid eversion.

Table 21.2: Ophthalmologic grading criteria and treatment recommendations for acute Stevens-Johnson syndrome.

Staining location and treatment recommendations	Severity of eye involvement			
	Mild	**Moderate**	**Severe***	**Extremely severe†**
Lid margin	No stain	Stain <1/3 of lid margin length	Stain >1/3 of lid margin length on at least 1 lid	Stain >1/3 of lid margin length on more than 1 lid
Cornea	No stain	No stain	Any epithelial defect more than punctate staining	Any epithelial defect more than punctate staining
Conjunctiva (bulbar and palpebral)	Hyperemia, without stain	(+)Stain, <1 cm in greatest diameter	(+)Stain >1 cm	Multiple areas of stain >1 cm
Treatment recommendations	Medical	Medical and close observation	Medical and urgent amniotic membrane transplantation (AMT)	Medical and urgent AMT (may require repeat AMT)

*A case was considered severe if there was severe involvement of the lid margin, cornea, or conjunctiva. It was not required that all three areas have severe involvement simultaneously.
†Extremely severe cases had multiple areas of extensive fluorescein staining simultaneously.
Source: Gregory DG. New grading system and treatment guidelines for the acute ocular manifestations of Stevens-Johnson syndrome. Ophthalmology. 2016;123(8):1653-8.

Management of Chronic Stevens-Johnson Syndrome Sequelae

Systemic immunomodulators are preferred over systemic steroids to combat persistent ocular inflammation. Topical steroids are best avoided in long run though other preservative-free formulations can be continued. Different chronic sequelae are to be managed individually as shown in Table 21.3.[30]

Scleral contact lens: Application of prosthetic replacement of the ocular surface ecosystem (PROSE) scleral lenses in these patients reduces the pain, enhances vision and improves the surface over a period of time. It vaults over the cornea and protects the surface from blink-related microtrauma and provides it with a fluid-filled reservoir, which generates hydrated ocular environment and promotes healing.[30,32]

Mucous membrane graft (MMG): Lid margin keratinization repeatedly traumatizes the corneal surface. The MMG addresses to replace the keratinized surface with healthy mucous membrane harvested from oral mucosa. It can also be used to repair symblepharon and cicatricial entropion. The surgical steps are explained in Figures 21.8 to 21.10.[30,33,34]

Keratoprosthesis (K-Pro): K-Pro or artificial cornea as it is popularly known helps to restore vision in end-stage

Table 21.3: Management of chronic Stevens-Johnson syndrome (SJS) sequelae.

Complications	Management
Trichiasis	Hyfrecation, cryotherapy, eyelash bulb extirpation, mucous membrane grafting (MMG) if associated with entropion
Lagophthalmos	Release of cicatrix, tarsorrhaphy
Entropion/Ectropion	Lateral canthoplasty/tarsal strip, anterior lamellar repositioning, posterior lamellar tightening, transconjunctival advancement
Persistent epithelial defect	Lubrication, punctal occlusion, bandage contact lens, tarsorrhaphy, autologous serum tears, amniotic membrane transplantation (AMT), scleral lens, cultivated oral mucosal epithelial transplantation (COMET)
Dry eye	Preservation-free artificial tears, punctal cautery, minor salivary gland transplant
Posterior lid margin keratinization	All-trans-retinoic acid ointment, scleral lens, MMG
Symblephara	Lysis/fornix reconstruction with amnion/MMG
End-stage corneal blindness	MMG, COMET, keratoprosthesis

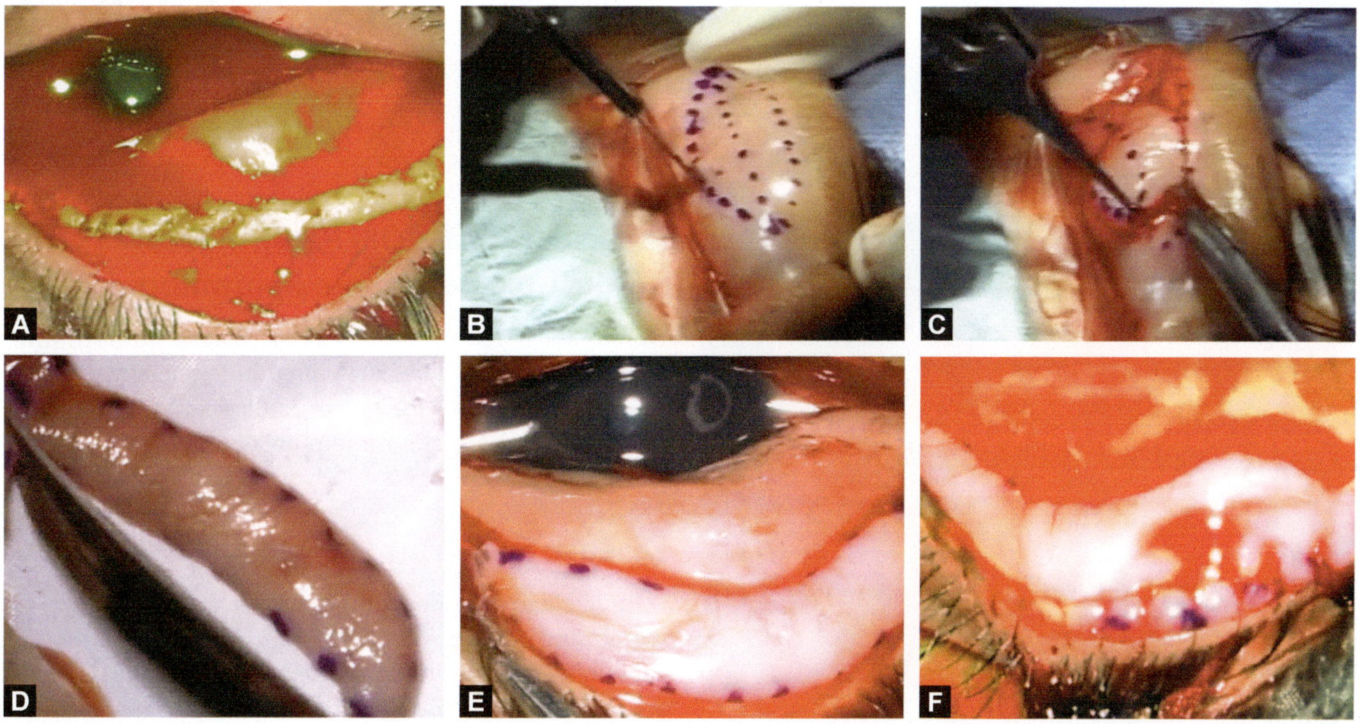

Figs. 21.8A to F: Surgical steps of mucous membrane grafting: Patient's lid margin is excised (Top left). The labial mucosa of the patient is marked, excised and trimmed sequentially (Bottom left). The harvested mucous membrane graft is sutured to the lid (Bottom right).

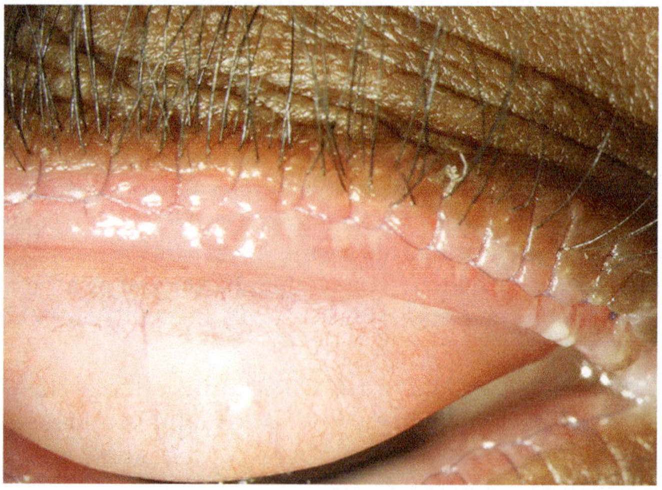

Fig. 21.9: Patient with chronic Stevens-Johnson syndrome, 1-month post lid margin mucous membrane grafting; graft well taken with sutures intact.

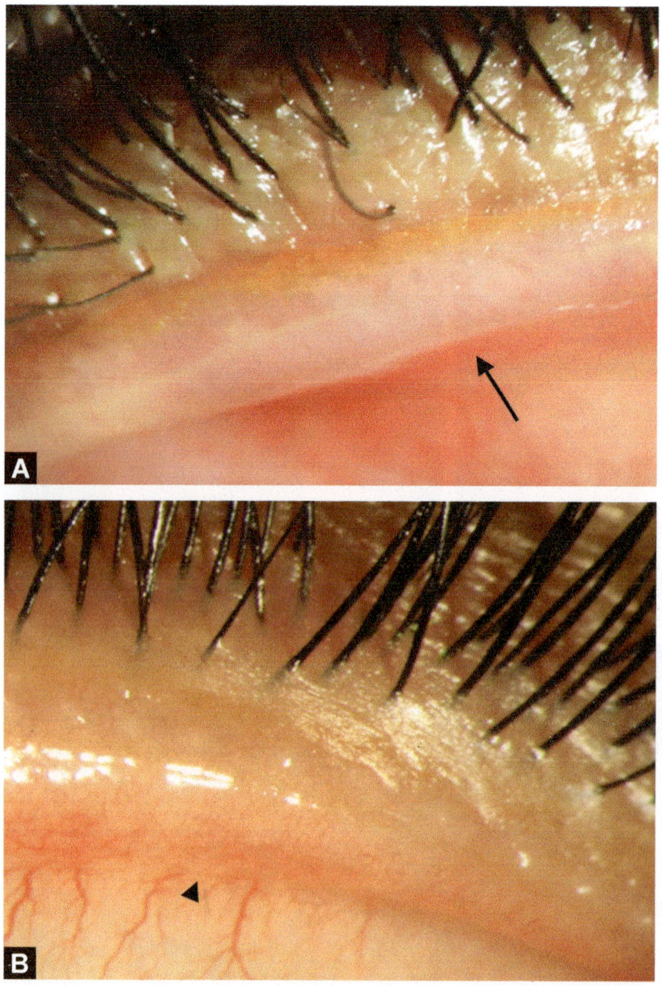

Figs. 21.10A and B: Mucous membrane graft (arrow) in a patient with Stevens-Johnson syndrome nearly resembling normal lid margin (arrowhead) anatomy.

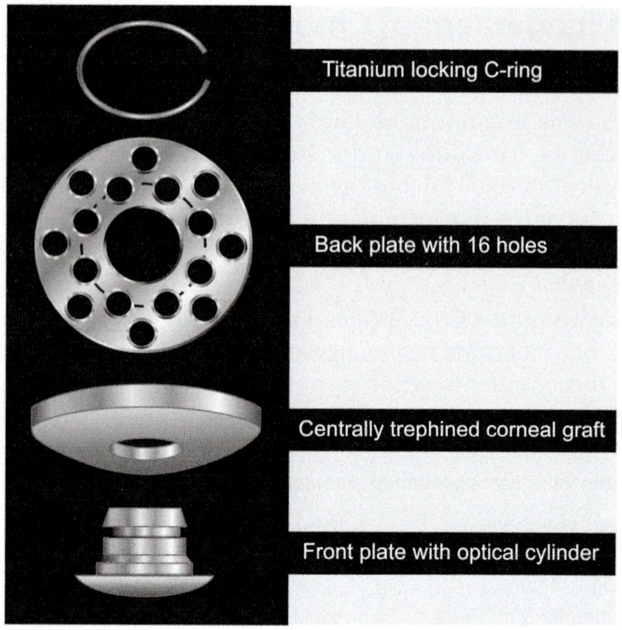

Fig. 21.11: Boston K-Pro assembly: Front plate with optical cylinder is placed facing down. The centrally 3 mm trephined cornea is placed over it; endothelium side up. The back plate is placed over corneal graft so that it gets sandwiched between front back plates. The titanium locking C-ring is attached over back plate to hold all the three structures together. The holes in back plate ensure adequate nutrition from the aqueous humor to overlying corneal graft when sutured onto the host eye.

diseases where keratoplasty procedures often fail due to a severely damaged ocular surface. Boston type I K-Pro (for wet surface), modified Boston type I K-Pro, Boston type II K-Pro (for total dry surface) and Osteo-odonto K-Pro have all been reported with good outcomes by various authors all over the world. Figures 21.11 to 21.13 explain the assembly as well as surgical steps.[30,35,36]

Ocular Cicatricial Pemphigoid/ Mucous Membrane Pemphigoid

Ocular cicatricial pemphigoid is a rare autoimmune disease of the eye. It has male preponderance (M:F = 1:2). The average age of incidence is 65 years though most patients have been reported to present late in the course of disease.[37]

Disease Spectrum

Ocular cicatricial pemphigoid is a variant of mucous membrane pemphigoid (MMP—a systemic autoimmune subepithelial blistering condition) where in ocular features are predominantly present. There may also be involvement of other mucous membranes of the body.[37]

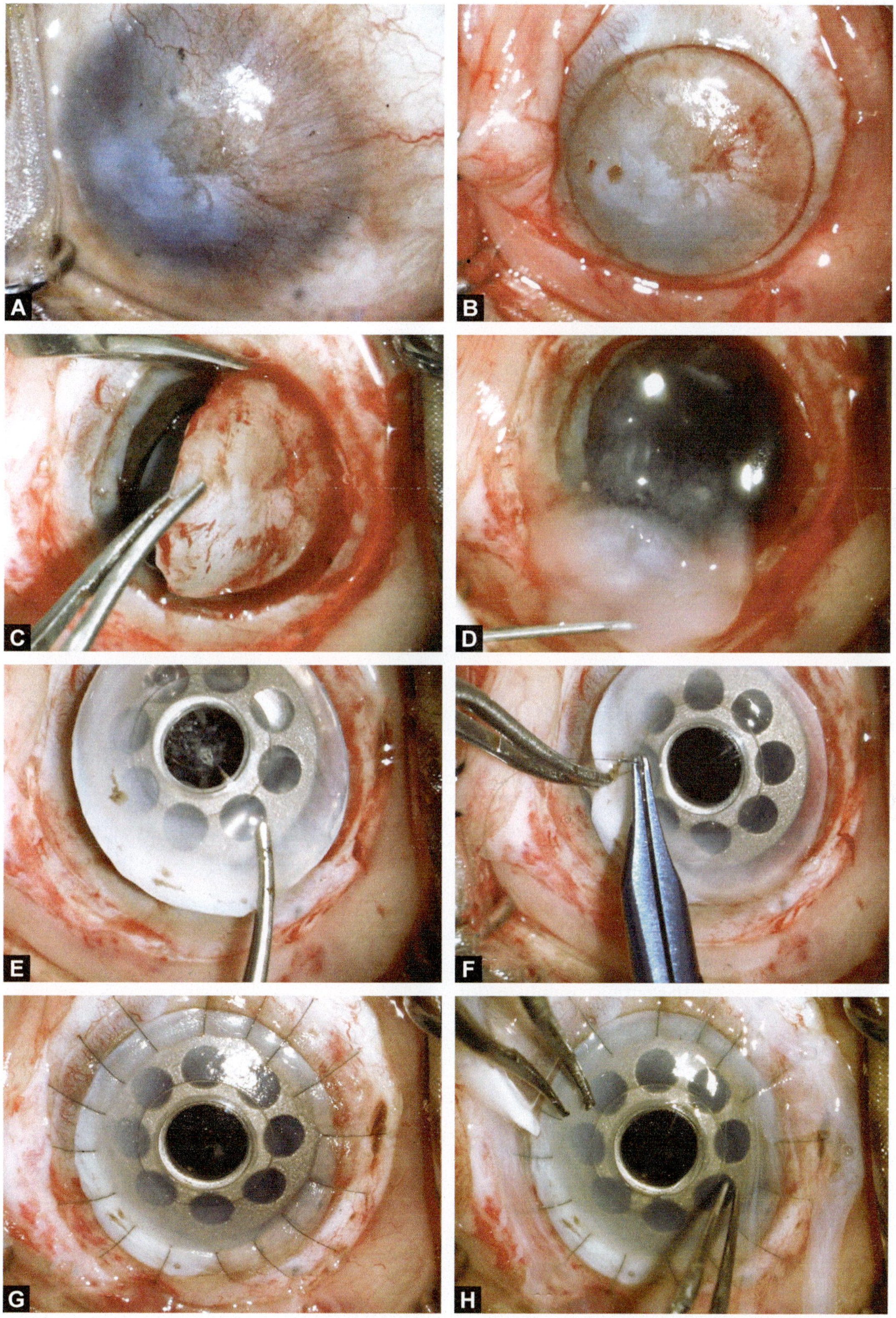

Figs. 21.12A to H: Clinical photographs showing the steps of surgical implantation of K-Pro. (A) Preoperative picture showing nearly 180° of limbal stem cell deficiency with central corneal scarring; (B) An 8 mm central trephination of host cornea is done; (C) Host cornea is excised using corneal scissors; (D) Open sky cataract extraction is done; (E) Placement of assembled K-Pro; (F) Placement of cardinal sutures; (G) Placement of 16 (10-0 nylon) sutures; (H) Application of amniotic membrane to aid early epithelialization of ocular surface.

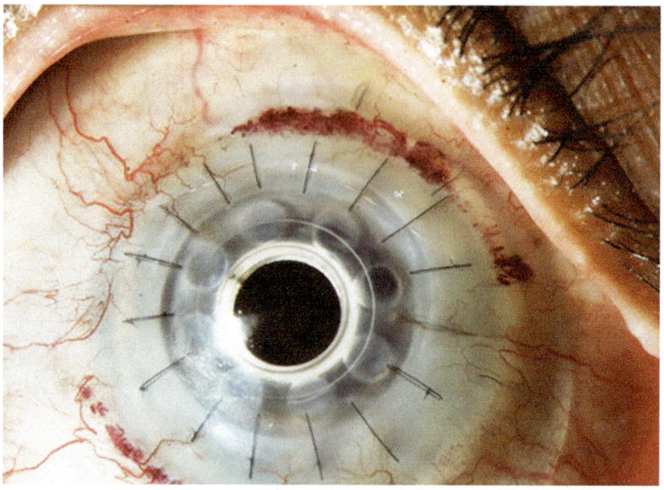

Fig. 21.13: Auro K-Pro in place in the eye of a patient with total limbal stem cell deficiency (LSCD).

Table 21.4: Foster's classification of ocular cicatricial pemphigoid (OCP) staging.

Stages	Ocular condition
I	Chronic conjunctivitis with subepithelial fibrosis
II	Forniceal shortening
III	Symblepharon appearance
IV	Ankyloblepharon, frozen globe

Table 21.5: Mondino and Brown classification of ocular cicatricial pemphigoid (OCP) staging.

Stages	Conjunctival forniceal shortening
I	≤25%
II	25–50%
III	~75%
IV	End-stage diseases: obliterated fornices

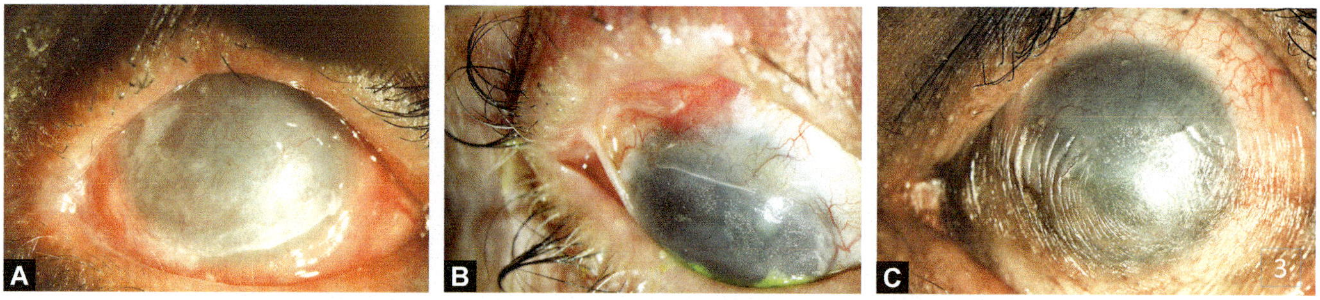

Figs. 21.14A to C: Patients with ocular cicatricial pemphigoid. (A) Total limbal stem cell deficiency and keratinization of the ocular surface; (B) Extensive symblepharon; (C) End-stage disease showing dermalization of the ocular surface.

Pathogenesis

The OCP/MMP is a type II immune reaction characterized by immunoreactants' deposition on epithelial basement membrane (EBM) inducing subepidermal split with subsequent blister formation. Specific β-4 integrin subunit antibodies are revealed in cases with exclusive involvement of ocular mucosa.[37]

Clinical Features

The initial findings in OCP are unilateral, chronic, recurrent, papillary conjunctivitis that progresses to involve both eyes. The condition is characterized by subepithelial fibrosis that relentlessly progresses to cicatricial conjunctivitis. The disease progresses gradually as described by Foster in his classification (Table 21.4).[38] The progression can also be assessed by Mondino and Brown's classification (Table 21.5).[39]

Inferior fornix is usually affected earlier than the superior one. Various ocular manifestations include entropion, lagophthalmos, symblepharon, surface and lid margin keratinization, trichiasis, distichiasis, severe dryness, corneal erosion, ulceration, vascularization, and perforation. In end-stage disease, with continued cicatrization there occurs total globe obliteration (Figs. 21.14A to C).[37,39]

Systemic Involvement

Skin involvement is seen in 4–15% of cases involving inguinal region, face, scalp, and extremities. Oral mucosa is commonly involved and most patients present with desquamative gingivitis. Epiglottic erosions cause dysphonia and hoarse voice. Esophageal strictures cause dysphagia and aspiration. Genital mucosae may also get affected.[37]

Diagnosis

As most cases are missed in early course of disease, high clinical suspicion is required to prevent late irreversible sequelae. Conjunctival biopsy reveals linear deposition of immunoglobulin G (IgG), IgA, IgM and/or C_3 complement on EBM (Fig. 21.15). Biopsy is taken, from an area involving both inflamed and noninflamed or scarred conjunctiva. The results should be correlated clinically. Negative result does not rule out the disease and may require another biopsy in suspicious cases.[37,40]

Medical Management

Local: Dry eyes and blepharoconjunctivitis are treated with preservative-free lubricants and warm compresses with antibiotics respectively. Topical calcineurin inhibitors have been used, but hardly halt the progression of the disease. Subconjunctival steroids may also offer only short-term symptomatic relief. Gas permeable limbal-fit corneal or scleral lenses improve vision and have shown to halt the progression of sterile corneal ulcer in such cases.[37,41,42]

Systemic: Systemic immunosuppressants are quite effective in controlling OCP severity and progression. They are started and are continued in cross consultation with dermatologist to monitor systemic disease and physician to monitor the serious adverse effects of these drugs. As adverse effects are a major concern, a step-ladder approach is practiced with series of available drugs. Systemic therapy is usually initiated in Stage II OCP as ocular involvement is considered as a "high risk" for MMP (Flowchart 21.5).[40]

Oral prednisone is useful in controlling ocular scarring. Dapsone and methotrexate are generally the first-line treatment in initial phase, but with lower side effects and better continuation rates, mycophenolate mofetil is preferred.[41] For resistant cases, pulsed IV cyclophosphamide (CPM) is highly efficacious, especially when combined with oral steroids, which controls inflammation.[37,41] Another promising combination for late stages, recognized in recent years is rituximab with intravenous immunoglobulin (IVIg) infusion.[37,40]

Surgical management: Surgical management mainly entails the correction of eyelid abnormalities and fornix reconstruction. Amniotic membrane grafting (AMG) and MMG remain most conducive. AMG is also effective in healing PEDs. Minor salivary gland transplantation (MIST) has been attempted with symptomatic relief in case of severe dryness, though salivary tears has been claimed to lack similar nutritional and visual properties. Penetrating keratoplasty (PK) and lamellar keratoplasty often fail in these cases and should be attempted cautiously. Ultimately K-Pro remains the last resort for visual rehabilitation, but is still associated with higher complication rates.[43]

Differential Diagnosis

Pemphigus vulgaris (PV): Ocular PV is an important differential diagnosis of OCP. It usually presents with catarrhal conjunctivitis and early cicatrization but does not progress to conjunctival scarring and symblepharon. Blisters in PV are flaccid and have erythematous base unlike MMP, which have tense bullae. The condition can be further differentiated on tissue biopsy, which shows intraepidermal split with diagnostic acantholytic cells. Ocular PV responds well to systemic steroids. Resistant cases may require adjuvant immunosuppressants.[44,45]

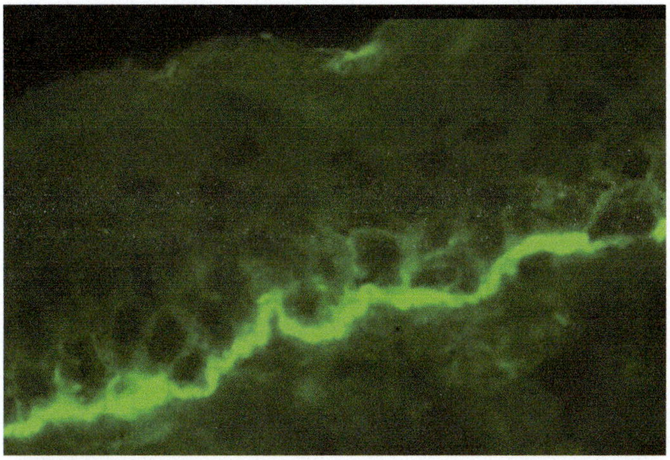

Fig. 21.15: Immunofluorescence staining of conjunctival biopsy specimen showing immunoglobulin G (IgG) positive basement membrane proteins in a case of ocular cicatricial pemphigoid.

Flowchart 21.5: A stepwise approach to the treatment of ocular cicatricial pemphigoid.

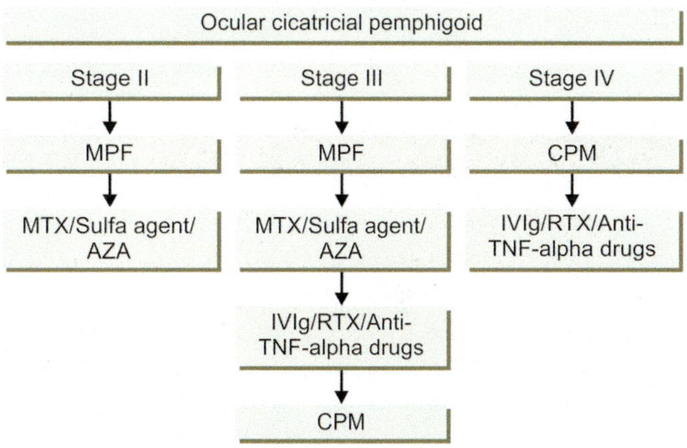

(MPF: Mycophenolate mofetil; MTX: Methotrexate; AZA: Azathioprine; RTX: Rituximab; IVIg: Intravenous immunoglobulin; CPM: Cyclophosphamide)

Dermatitis herpetiformis (DH): Ocular involvement in DH occurs in about 50% of cases and follows similar course to OCP. Because of this, all patients of DH should have ophthalmological examination to reveal subclinical disease. It is difficult to differentiate it from OCP by ocular features. Patients usually have prodrome of pruritus before emergence of cutaneous lesions. The lesions comprise of annular bullae resembling "string of pearls". Direct immunofluorescence and serology are diagnostic. Most cases respond well to dapsone. Refractory cases respond to IVIg.[45]

Pseudopemphigoid/drug-induced pemphigoid: Certain systemic and topical drugs result in vesicobullous condition resembling MMP/OCP. It is referred as pseudopemphigoid. Culpable drugs include:

- *Topical*: Timolol, brimonidine epinephrine, pilocarpine, iodide, and echothiophate.
- *Systemic*: Practolol, phenytoin, amiodarone, and vancomycin.

For topical medication, the features would restrict to same eye. Removal of causative agent and short course of steroids brings remission.[37,45]

Ocular Surface Chemical Burns

Chemical injuries constitute one of the major causes of ocular surface disease. Severity of injury depends on various factors including nature of chemical (acid or alkali), concentration of solution, amount of chemical exposed, duration of exposure, surface area of contact and associated thermal reaction. Usually, alkali injuries are more grievous than acids ones. The amount of damage and prognosis significantly depends on initial management of case after initial injury.[46,47]

They amount for 7.7–18% of all ocular traumas. In developing countries, the reported incidence of chemical injury ranges between 1.25% and 4.4%. They are more common in young males between 16 years and 45 years of age.[48,49] The chemicals are an integral part of commonly used detergents, cement material, paints, automobiles, bleach, dyes, etc. (Figs. 21.16A and B and Table 21.6).

Effect of Chemicals in the Eye

Chemical injuries in eyes can cause wide range of destruction involving ocular surface, stroma, Descemet's membrane, endothelium, trabecular meshwork, ciliary body, iris and lens.[47] Alkalis cause much more damage to eye against acid, because of their lipophilic nature and higher penetration (Flowchart 21.6 and Figs. 21.17A and B). In specific instances, certain acids may also have increased penetrability (Table 21.6).[46,47,50]

Following acute episode, the damage to ocular structures continues as a result of retained chemical, persistent inflammation and loss of epithelium.[47]

Smaller epithelial abrasions usually heal by migration of surrounding epithelial cells. Larger abrasions heal by centripetal migration of LSCs and take longer to heal. Limbal ischemia further delays epithelialization with inadequate oxygen and nutrient supply to proliferating stem cells. If there is LSC loss causing LSCD the process is further delayed and remaining stem cells and conjunctival tissue covers the cornea. Even, conjunctival epithelium covering the cornea carries better prognosis than denuded

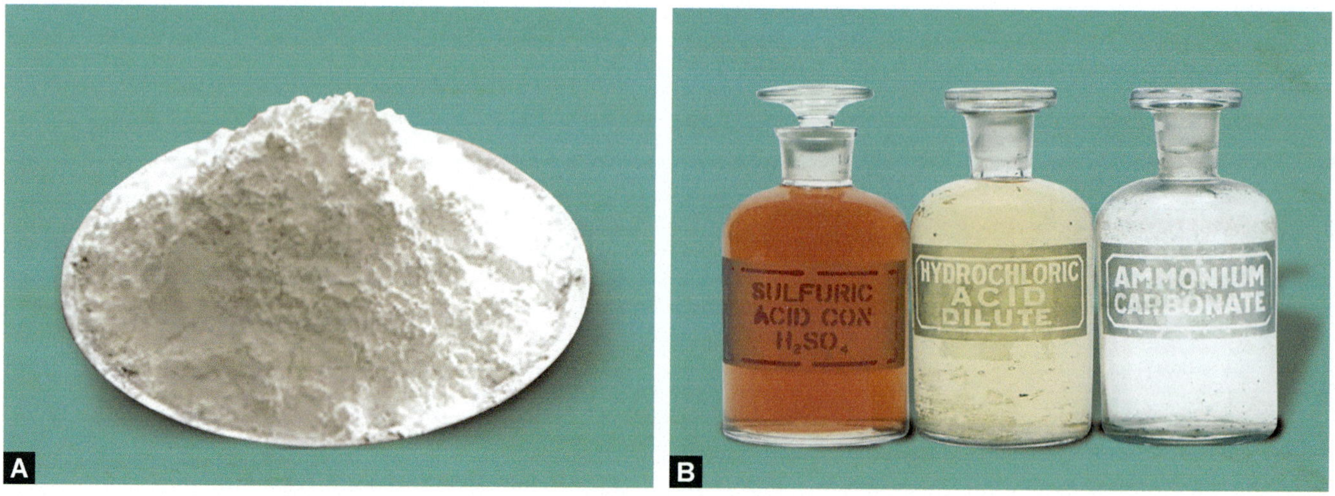

Figs. 21.16A and B: Common chemicals responsible for ocular surface burns. (A) Lime powder; (B) Strong acids and bases.

Table 21.6: Common causes of chemical injury.

Compound	Class	Common source/uses	Anterior chamber penetration
Ammonia	Alkali	Fertilizers, refrigerants, cleaning agents	Very high
Sodium hydroxide (Lye)	Alkali	Drain cleaners	Very high
Potassium hydroxide	Alkali	Caustic potash	Very high
Magnesium hydroxide	Alkali	Sparklers	Low
Calcium hydroxide (Lime)	Alkali	Plaster, cement, mortar	Very low
Sulfuric acid	Acid	Car batteries, industrial cleaners	Low
Sulfurous acid	Acid	Bleach, preservatives, refrigerants	High
Hydrofluoric acid	Acid	Glass polishing and frosting, etching, silicone production, rust removal	High
Hydrochloric acid	Acid	Fertilizers, bleach, process regulators, cleaning and furnishing products	Very low
Acetic acid	Acid	Vinegar and in its essence	Low
Chromic acid	Acid	Used for chrome plating	Very low

Flowchart 21.6: Mechanism of acid and alkali injury.

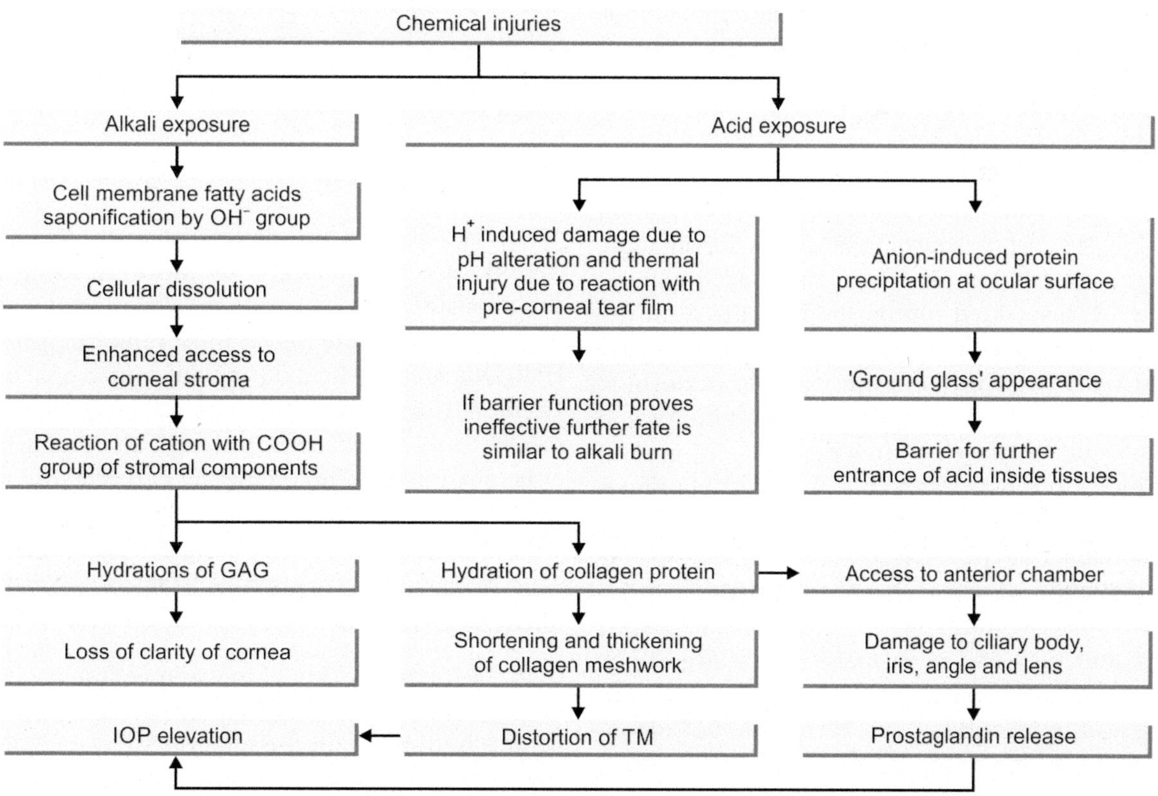

(GAG: Glycosaminoglycan; TM: Trabecular meshwork; IOP: Intraocular pressure)

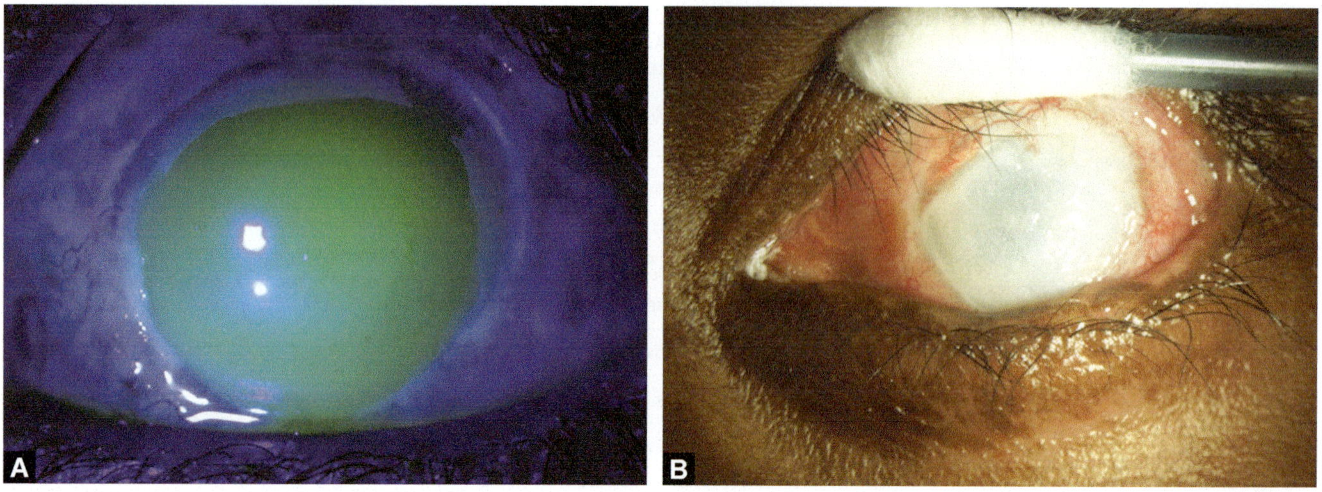

Figs. 21.17A and B: Chemical injuries. (A) Acid injury leading to total corneal epithelial defect; (B) Alkali injury resulting in a lusterless corneal surface, epithelial sloughing and whitening of cornea due to alkali penetration and edema.

surface. In acute phase, LSCD can be anticipated to certain extent looking at limbal ischemia, though both are not synonymous.[47,50]

Epithelialization is also hampered by continued inflammation, EBM damage and loss of fibronectin (EBM adhesion protein). Additional damage to ciliary body epithelium depletes the citrate levels in aqueous humor and affects the collagen synthesis further.[46,47]

Clinical Features

Chemical injury is an ocular emergency, where patient presents with severe pain, burning sensation, lacrimation, blepharospasm, and loss of vision. Upon examination, there may be associated foreign body apart from the chemical itself. Although, presentation varies from case to case, usually they present with variable periorbital edema, erythema, charred skin, with loss of eyebrows, and eyelashes. Ocular surface features include conjunctival congestion, chemosis, variable limbal ischemia, conjunctival and corneal epithelial defects, corneal haze, corneal edema, sterile corneal ulceration, and occasionally corneal perforation.[47,51]

In late phase, features of dry eye and LSCD start appearing and may end in formation of a large thick pannus. Periorbital skin burn and widespread conjunctival burn may lead to lagophthalmos, ectropion, entropion, trichiasis and symblepharon formation.[47,51] Figures 21.18 to 21.20 show different clinical presentations after ocular burn.

Evaluation and Grading

In 1965, Roper-Hall prognostic classification for chemical injuries based on limbal ischemia and corneal opacification was deployed (Table 21.7).[52] In 2001, Dua improved it and stated a classification emphasizing the importance of conjunctival loss (bulbar and forniceal) along with limbal involvement in deciding the prognosis of these cases (Table 21.8).[50,53]

Clinical Course

McCulley divided the course of postchemical injury period into four phases[46,54] as shown in Table 21.9. The prognosis of cases is good when managed well during the immediate acute phase. Most minor injuries (Roper-Hall, Dua grade I) heal during the course of acute phase. Grade II (Roper-Hall, Dua) injuries take some time to recover and epithelialization along with clearing of corneal opacification is complete by the end of early reparative phase. In higher grades, little or no epithelialization occurs and progressive corneal thinning and melting is seen.[46,47]

Management

Goals of treatment: Initial management aims at removal of retained chemical from the eye, neutralize the ocular surface and maintain the integrity of eyeball. Following successful irrigation, all steps must be taken to lessen inflammation, prevent infection, stop ulceration, promote epithelial wound healing, and control intraocular

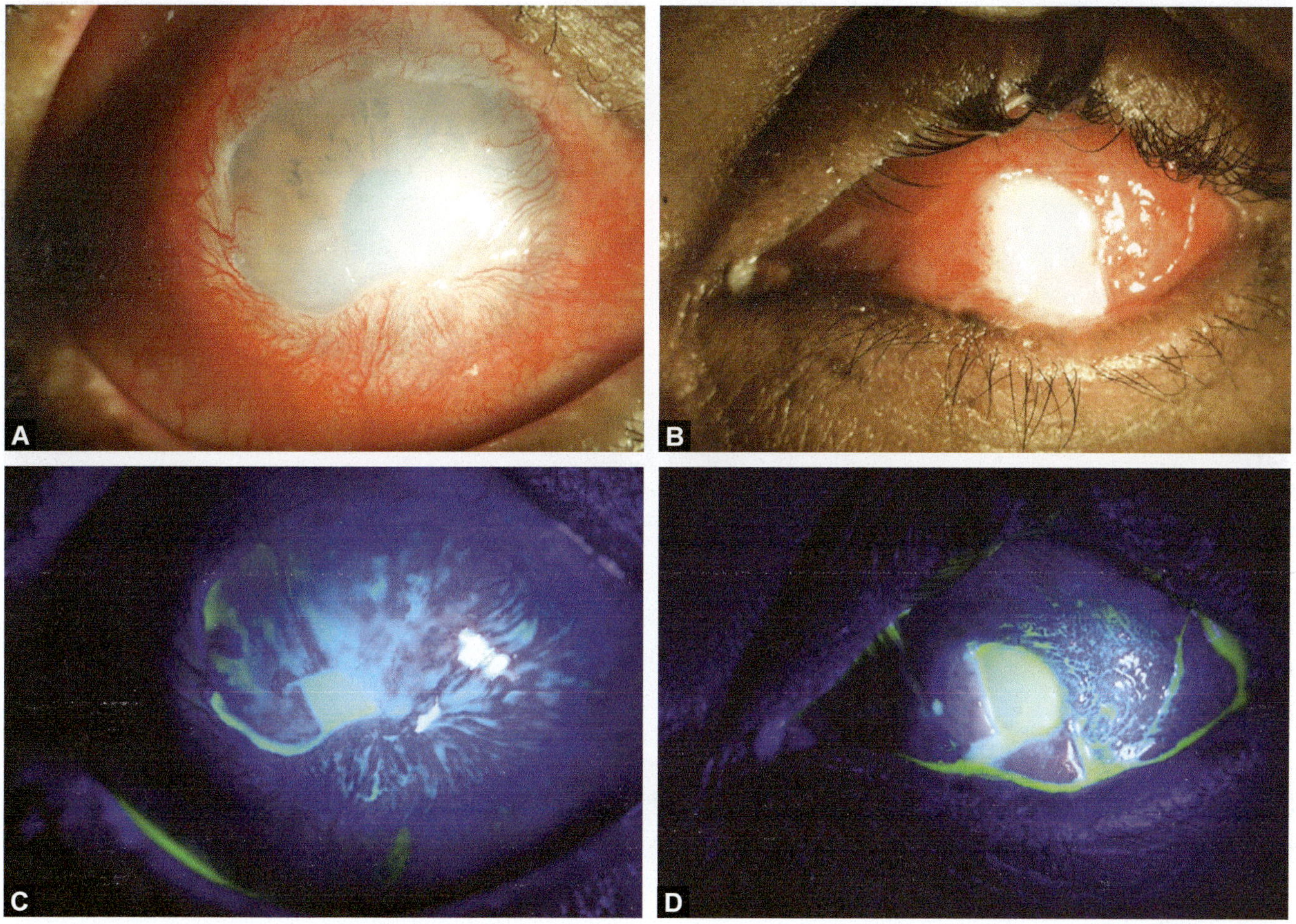

Figs. 21.18A to D: Ocular surface burn following fall of caustic soda on face. (A and C) *Right eye*: Pannus with mild corneal haze; fluorescein staining shows paracentral epithelial defect; (B and D) *Left eye*: Large pannus covering two-thirds of corneal surface with corneal whitening and central epithelial defect.

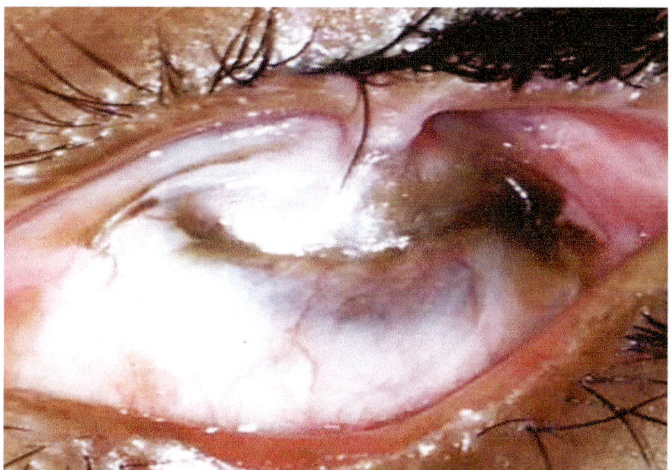

Fig. 21.19: Cicatrizing changes following ocular surface chemical injury: symblepharon formation with conjunctivalization of ocular surface.

pressure.[46,51] Long-term goals of therapy aim at promoting corneal re-epithelialization (by corneal or conjunctival epithelium), preventing symblepharon formation and managing persistent inflammation, dry eyes, LSCD, corneal scarring, glaucoma and treatment of symblepharon and associated lid problems.[51]

Acute phase management: Ocular surface is thoroughly irrigated with double eversion of lids exposing the fornices. Irrigation should be done with at least 1 L of irrigant for at least 15 minutes.[46] Normal saline can be used for irrigation, but BSS plus has been shown to be most effective. Amphoteric solutions can also be used.[46,51] After irrigation, a thorough clinical examination is done. Broad-spectrum antibiotics are started in presence of epithelial defect. For early re-epithelialization, frequent lubricants in form of drops and gels are started.[47,51] Other

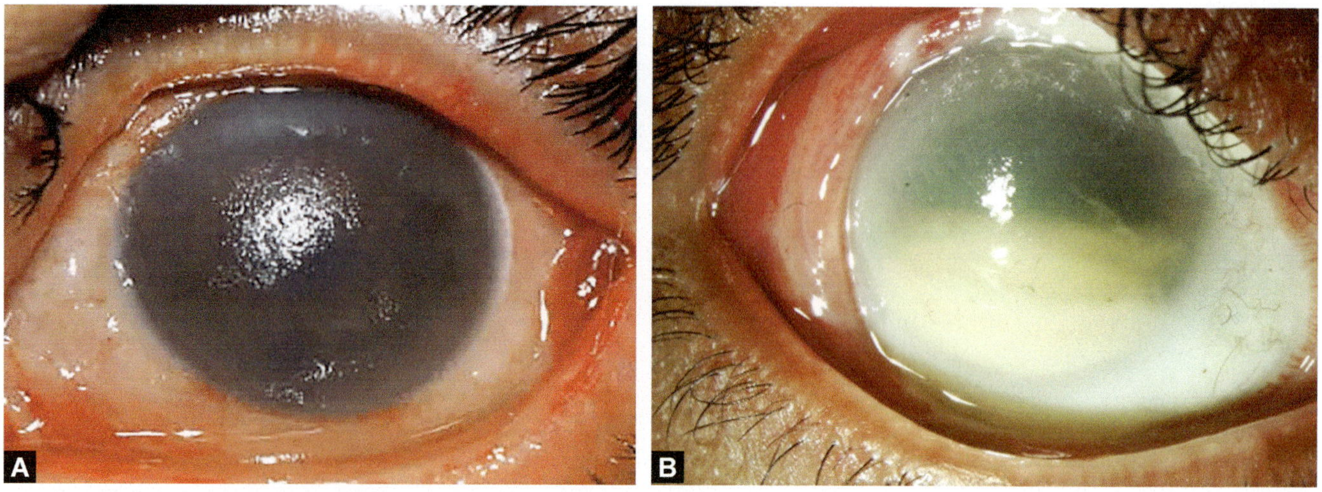

Figs. 21.20A and B: Chemical injury. (A) About 90% limbal ischemia with corneal edema, but retained conjunctiva; (B) Total limbal ischemia associated with hypopyon and more than 75% conjunctival loss suggestive of a poor prognosis.

Table 21.7: Classification of severity of ocular surface burns by Roper-Hall.

Grade	Prognosis	Cornea	Conjunctiva/limbus
I	Good	Corneal epithelial damage	No limbal ischemia
II	Good	Corneal haze, iris details visible	<1/3 limbal ischemia
III	Guarded	Total epithelial loss, stromal haze, iris details obscured	1/3–1⁄2 limbal ischemia
IV	Poor	Cornea opaque, iris and pupil obscured	>1⁄2 limbal ischemia

Table 21.8: Dua's classification of ocular surface burns.

Grade	Prognosis	Clinical findings	Conjunctival involvement	Analog scale*
I	Very good	0 clock hours of limbal involvement	0%	0/0%
II	Good	<3 clock hours of limbal involvement	<30%	0.1–3/1–29.9%
III	Good	>3–6 clock hours of limbal involvement	>30–50%	3.1–6/31–50%
IV	Good to guarded	>6–9 clock hours of limbal involvement	>50–75%	6.1–9/51–75%
V	Guarded to poor	>9–<12 clock hours of limbal involvement	>75–<100%	9.1–11.9/75.1–99.9%
VI	Very poor	Total limbus (12 clock hours) involved	Total conjunctiva (100%) involved	12/100%

*The analog scale records accurately the limbal involvement in clock hours of affected limbus/percentage of conjunctival involvement. While calculating percentage of conjunctival involvement, only involvement of bulbar conjunctiva, up to and including the conjunctival fornices is considered.

Table 21.9: Clinical phases after ocular burn by McCulley.

Phases	Duration
Immediate	Within few hours
Acute phase	0–7 days
Early reparative phase	7–21 days
Late reparative phase	>21 days

useful interventions to promote epithelialization are mentioned in Table 21.10.[46,51,55-62] Potent corticosteroids like *prednisolone acetate 1%* are started on hourly basis for at least 10 days, this helps in reducing inflammation and expedites healing.[46,47] After this period, if epithelialization is complete, steroids can be continued further. In presence of incomplete epithelialization and stromal thinning, they have to be tapered as they interfere with collagen

Table 21.10: Intervention in different situations in chemical injuries.

Condition		Intervention
Corneal epithelial defect	Small	Bandage contact lens (BCL)
	Large	Amniotic membrane grafting (AMG)
Corneal and conjunctival epithelial defect		Prosthetic replacement of the ocular surface ecosystem (PROSE) lens Amniotic membrane patch graft
Epithelial defect with dead necrotic tissue		Surgical debridement along with AMG/tarsorrhaphy/contact lens placement
Epithelial defect with significant limbal stem cell loss and limbal ischemia		Preferred AMG and/or tenoplasty along with conjunctival advancement/tarsorrhaphy
Significant limbal stem cell loss along with severe conjunctival loss	In acute phase	High-risk attempt of limbal stem cell transplantation (LSCT) procedures along with conjunctival transplantation/tenoplasty under immunosuppression cover
Anticipated symblepharon		Regular swipe of fornices with glass rod Symblepharon-amniotic membrane ring complex placement Sutured amniotic membrane
Progressive corneal thinning		Multilayer amniotic membrane Tissue adhesive + BCL
Small corneal perforation Impending perforation	Small	Tissue adhesive + BCL/AMG
Severe corneal thinning Large descemetocele Large corneal perforation Impending perforation		Tectonic keratoplasty
Limbal stem cell deficiency (LSCD)	Unilateral	Conjunctival limbal autograft (CLAU or CLAG), simple limbal epithelial transplantation (SLET)
	Bilateral	SLET-allograft/cultivated limbal epithelial transplantation (CLET)-allograft/keratolimbal allograft (KLAL)/combined conjunctival and keratolimbal allograft (C-KLAL)
Successful LSCT with stromal scarring		Lamellar keratoplasty (LK)/deep anterior lamellar keratoplasty (DALK)/penetrating keratoplasty (PK)
Multiple failed LSCT/keratoplasty	Satisfactory counseling	Boston K-PRO/LVPEI K-PRO (only in one eye)
Symblepharon		Symblepharon release + AMG + CLAG
Obliterated fornix Conjunctival scarring Cicatricial entropion	Unilateral	Reconstruction with bulbar conjunctival transplantation and AMG
	Bilateral	Reconstruction with tarsoconjunctival advancement and AMG Reconstruction with mucous membrane grafting (MMG) and AMG
Medically uncontrolled glaucoma		Ahmed glaucoma valve/trabeculectomy (less preferred)

synthesis. Topical ascorbate, citrate and oral vitamin C, and tetracycline have all shown to have positive effect on collagen synthesis.[46,47,51,63]

Amniotic membrane grafting should be done at the earliest to expedite recovery for large epithelial defects. It is extensively used in chemical burns in acute as well as chronic phase owing to its properties. It helps in epithelialization of corneal and conjunctival surface, enhances healing, reduces inflammation and prevents infection.[55,57,64,65] Tarsorrhaphy is an adjunct procedure to AMG which aids in healing. Tenoplasty becomes essential in cases with severe limbal ischemia (Dua's grade V, VI).[46]

Chronic phase management: In chronic phase, corneal tissue heals with scarring and conjunctivalization, especially in higher grades (Roper-Hall IV, Dua IV and V).[50] Various complications in chronic phase and management are shown in Table 21.10. But, before attempting any kind of limbal stem cell transplantation (LSCT) procedure, eyelid problems are to be addressed. After successful oculoplastic procedures, LSCT is attempted to restore deficiency. This can be combined with penetrating or lamellar keratoplasty but results are significantly better when keratoplasty follows successful LSCT.[50,66] Keratoprosthesis is reserved for patients with repeated failed keratoplasty and unsuccessful LSCT procedures.[58-60]

MANAGEMENT OF LIMBAL STEM CELL DEFICIENCY IN OCULAR SURFACE DISORDER

The management of LSCD is based on preservation and proliferation of remaining LSCs. When not feasible, transplanting stem cells from donor's tissue in form of autograft or allograft is necessary. LSCT is deemed to fail in active stages of disease and therefore should be attempted only after acute phase subsides. Various methods of ocular surface reconstruction include:[15,67,68]

- *Amniotic membrane grafting*: It provides nutrition, reduces inflammation, supports LSCs and enhances epithelial growth. It is used in acute stage of disease, in partial LSCD and as scaffold in LSCT procedures.[69,70]
- *Sequential sectorial conjunctival epitheliectomy (SSCE)*: It involves repeated debridement of conjunctiva over the corneal surface in cases of partial LSCD where area of recurrence reduces with subsequent debridement to disappear completely.[71,72]
- *Ipsilateral limbal stem cell translocation*: Limbal conjunctiva is harbored from healthy limbal area of same eye and transplanted with the help of sutures and fibrin glue onto the deficient area. The method is not often used because of pre-existing LSCD in the diseased eye.[73]
- *Conjunctival limbal autograft (CLAU)*: Limbal biopsy of 4 mm is taken from limbus extending up to 5–8 mm posteriorly onto the conjunctiva from the normal eye of patient. This is transplanted in the area of LSCD by sutures and fibrin glue. It poses some risk of LSCD to donor.[67]
- *Cultivated limbal epithelial stem cell transplantation (CLET)—autograft*: A small limbal biopsy (2 × 2 mm^2) is taken from healthy or relatively healthy eye of the patient and divided into multiple pieces. The LSCs are cultured in vitro in a stem cell laboratory on a de-epithelialized amniotic membrane by explant culture or suspension culture methods and allowed to proliferate. After the cells have grown, transplantation is done by attaching the amniotic membrane containing cultivated LSCs using fibrin glue onto the surface of the affected eye (Fig. 21.21).[65]
- *Cultivated limbal epithelial stem cell transplantation—living-related allograft*: Technique is similar to CLET—autograft, but the stem cells are harvested from the eye of a closely related family member or HLA-matched donor. There is an increased risk of rejection and mandates use of postoperative immunosuppression.[74,75]
- *Simple limbal epithelial transplantation (SLET)*: The CLAU and CLET are largely getting replaced by SLET because it gives better outcomes, there is lesser risk for donor eye LSCD, is easily repeatable and does not require a laboratory setup. The method employs harboring of limbal biopsy of 2 × 2 mm^2 from normal eye of patient and transplanting it directly into the diseased eye by dividing it in ten to fifteen pieces and spreading them over preplaced amniotic membrane [human amniotic membrane (hAM)] in concentric fashion avoiding the visual axis. Here, hAM acts as in vivo culture media for LSC proliferation (Figs. 21.22A to H).[56,68,76]

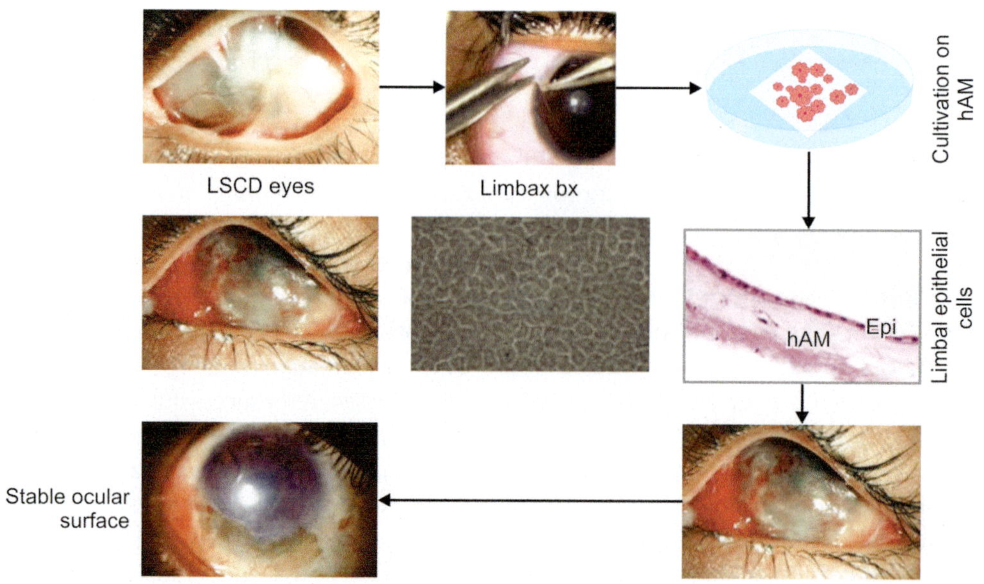

Fig. 21.21: Steps of cultivated limbal epithelial transplantation in a case of limbal stem cell deficiency (LSCD): After cultivation of limbal epithelial stem cells on human amniotic membrane (hAM), the membrane is transplanted onto the diseased eye resulting in a stable ocular surface.

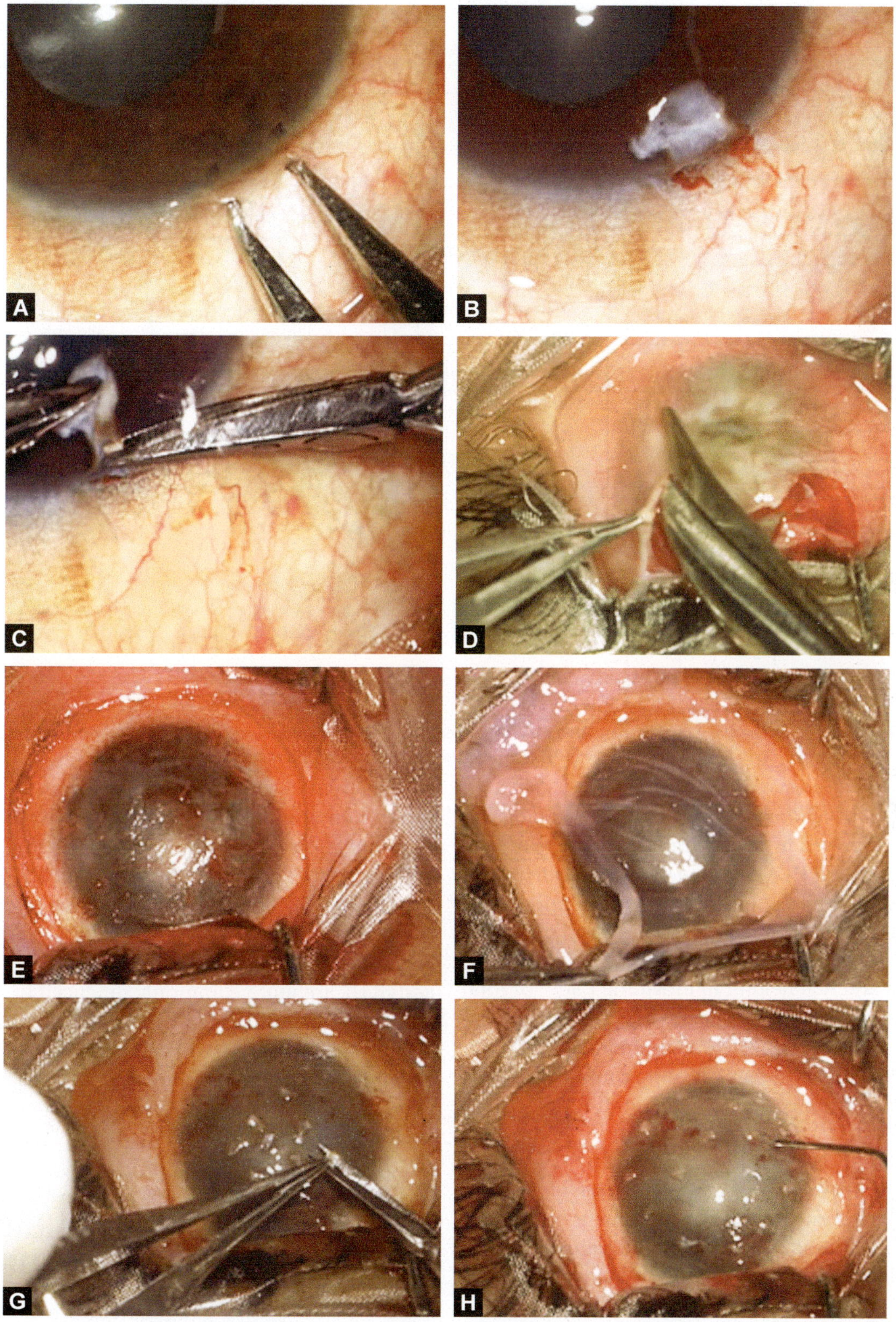

Figs. 21.22A to H: Clinical photographs showing the surgical technique of simple limbal epithelial transplantation. (A) A 2 × 2 mm^2 area is marked across the superior limbus of the donor eye; (B) A subconjunctival dissection is carried out 1 mm into clear cornea; (C) The limbal tissue is excised; (D and E) A peritomy is performed and the fibrovascular pannus is excised from the recipient ocular surface; (F) A human amniotic membrane graft is placed on the bare ocular surface and secured to it with fibrin glue; (G and H) The donor limbal tissue is cut into 10 to 15 small pieces and secured to the amniotic membrane overlying the cornea with fibrin glue.

Flowchart 21.7: Algorithm depicting approach and line of management in cases of limbal stem cell deficiency (LSCD).

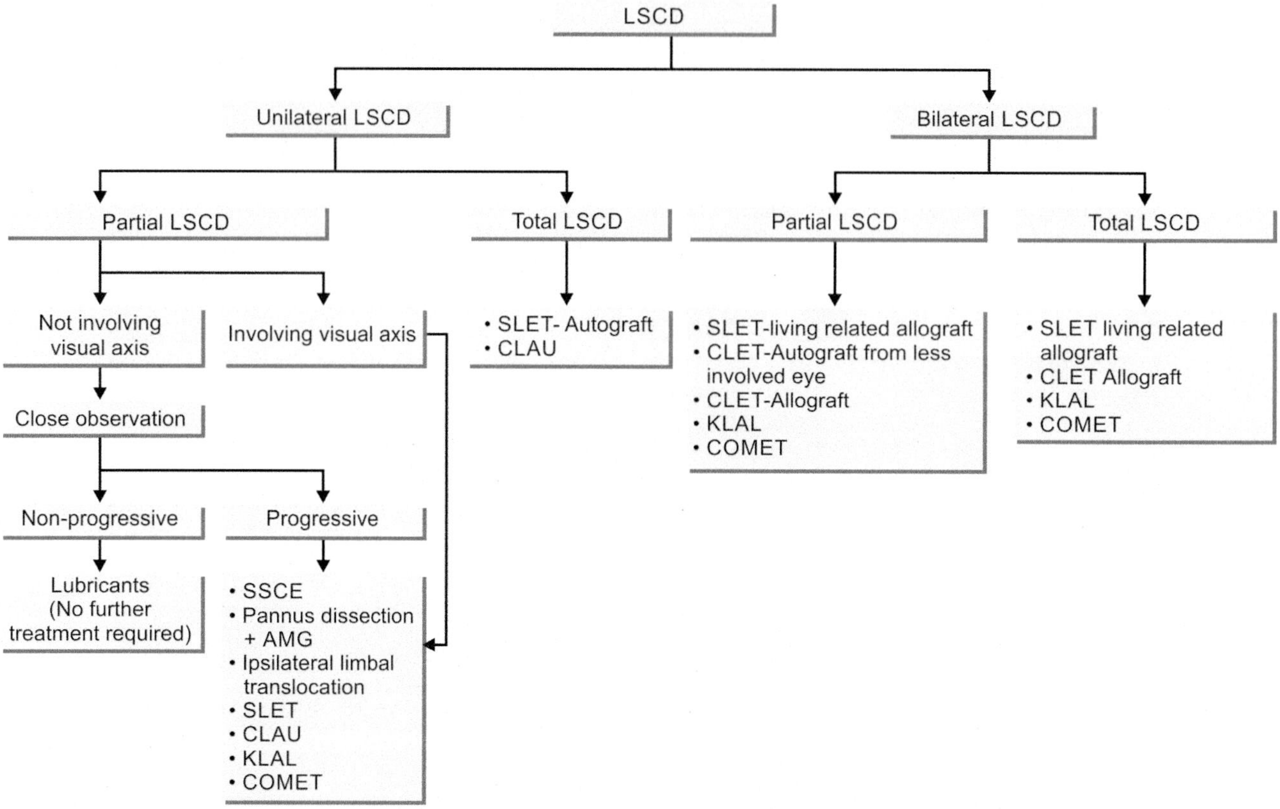

(SLET: Simple limbal epithelial transplantation; CLAU: Conjunctival limbal autograft; SSCE: Sequential sectoral conjunctival epitheliectomy; AMG: Amniotic membrane graft; KLAL: Keratolimbal allograft; COMET: Cultivated oral mucosal epithelial transplantation)

- *Simple limbal epithelial transplantation—allograft*: SLET is performed by taking graft from closely related family member or HLA-matched donor. It is indicated in bilateral LSCD and would require immunosuppression postoperatively.[68,77]
- *Keratolimbal allograft (KLAL)*: The donor tissue is cadaveric and it is helpful in providing LSCs for total LSCD cases especially in bilateral cases.[78,79]
- *Coculture KLAL-C*: It involves transplantation of living-related allograft comprising healthy conjunctival cells and LSCs in form of keratolimbal graft to effectively manage both LSCD and conjunctival damage simultaneously.[80,81]
- *Cultivated oral mucosal epithelial transplantation (COMET)*: Oral mucosal stem cells from the patient are harvested, cultured in laboratory and transplanted in the affected eye.[68,82]

Recent Research

Embryonic stem cells, induced pluripotent stem cells and dedifferentiated mesenchymal stem cells are other experimental modalities, which hold promise for LSCT in coming times. Recently, it is reported that partial LSCD has been successfully treated medically with topical interferon-α (IFN-α)-2b and all-trans-retinoic acid 0.01% in combination without recurrence.[83,84]

Of all the above-mentioned procedures, AMG, CLET and SLET are more commonly practiced with good long-term outcomes. The algorithm of LSCD management is shown in Flowchart 21.7. Postoperative follow-up entails examination of graft, conjunctival and corneal epithelial defects, evidence of rejection episodes in cases of allograft, evidence of donor LSCD, amount of inflammation and presence of other ocular surface problems.

MANAGEMENT OF CATARACT IN OCULAR SURFACE DISORDER

Formation of cataract in ocular surface disorders occurs early as a result of ongoing inflammation and/or prolonged use of topical steroids. In these cases, cataract surgery is difficult to perform in due to poor visibility and increased risk of postoperative complication or surface disorder aggravation. Cataract surgery should be attempted only after taking care of other surface problems including dry eyes and lid abnormalities. The disease should be well controlled with immunosuppressants and eye should be quiet.[85] Performing cataract surgery in the setting of active disease can worsen prognosis.

Peribulbar blocks are preferred for most cases anticipating a prolonged surgery due to compromised media clarity. In eyes with well-preserved corneal clarity, the preferred technique is phacoemulsification through a corneal incision, as this causes the least disruption to ocular surface. When central corneal scarring is too advanced, extracapsular extraction can be performed through a corneal or limbal incision. In cases with extensive peripheral corneal thinning, a limbal or scleral wound can be used. Trypan blue is an indispensable tool to enhance visibility during surgery when white cataract is combined with corneal opacity.[86] Dye staining allows capsulorhexis to be performed easily. Endoilluminator can be used in anterior chamber to enhance visualization of rhexis margins during phacoemulsification and intraocular lens (IOL) insertion.[87]

Postoperatively topical steroids should be administered for 6 weeks along with regular maintenance therapy of immunosuppressants. However, in this period, immunosuppressants both topical and systemic have to be tailored in accordance to disease status. PROSE/scleral lenses help in providing better vision by taking care of the irregular astigmatism that often exists.[88,89]

CONCLUSION

The array of clinical features of ocular surface diseases is vast; history and careful examination can help clinch the diagnosis of different conditions. Ocular surface reconstruction surgeries and immunosuppressive therapy are the main tools to manage such conditions. Timely identification and management is of utmost importance to salvage vision in such patients.

REFERENCES

1. Cher I. Ocular surface concepts: development and citation. Ocul Surf. 2014;12(1):10-3.
2. Tsubota K, Tseng SC, Nordlund ML. Anatomy and physiology of the ocular surface. In: Holland EJ, Mannis MJ (Eds). Ocular Surface Disease: Medical and Surgical Management. New York: Springer-Verlag; 2002. pp. 3-15.
3. Friend J, Thoft RA. Functional competence of regenerating ocular surface epithelium. Invest Ophthalmol Vis Sci. 1978;17(2):134-9.
4. The ocular surface. Basic science aspects. Clinical aspects. Int Ophthalmol Clin. 1979;19(2):1-283.
5. Cher I. Fluids of the ocular surface: concepts, functions and physics. Clin Exp Ophthalmol. 2012;40(6):634-43.
6. Gipson IK. The ocular surface: the challenge to enable and protect vision: the Friedenwald lecture. Invest Ophthalmol Vis Sci. 2007;48(10):4390;4391-8.
7. Stern ME, Gao J, Siemasko KF, et al. The role of the lacrimal functional unit in the pathophysiology of dry eye. Exp Eye Res. 2004;78(3):409-16.
8. Leong YY, Tong L. Barrier function in the ocular surface: from conventional paradigms to new opportunities. Ocul Surf. 2015;13(2):103-9.
9. Schwartz GS, Gomes LV, Holland EJ. Classification and staging of ocular surface disease. In: Mannis MJ, Holland EJ (Eds). Cornea, 4th edition. China: Elsevier; 2016.
10. Tiffany JM. The role of meibomian secretion in the tears. Trans Ophthalmol Soc UK. 1985;104(Pt 4):396-401.
11. Biber J. Classification of ocular surface disease. In: Holland EJ, Mannis MJ, Lee WB (Eds). Ocular Surface Disease: Cornea, Conjunctiva and Tear Film, 1st edition. China: Elsevier; 2013. pp. 35-43.
12. Wei ZG, Cotsarelis G, Sun TT, et al. Label-retaining cells are preferentially located in fornical epithelium: implications on conjunctival epithelial homeostasis. Invest Ophthalmol Vis Sci. 1995;36(1):236-46.
13. Dua HS, Said DG. Clinical evidence of the pre-Descemet's layer (Dua's layer) in corneal pathology. Eye (Lond). 2016;30(8):1144-5.
14. Dua HS, Azuara-Blanco A. Limbal stem cells of the corneal epithelium. Surv Ophthalmol. 2000;44(5):415-25.
15. Sangwan VS, Jain R, Basu S, et al. Transforming ocular surface stem cell research into successful clinical practice. Indian J Ophthalmol. 2014;62(1):29-40.
16. Tseng SC. Concept and application of limbal stem cells. Eye (Lond). 1989;3(Pt 2):141-57.
17. Singh V, Shukla S, Ramachandran C, et al. Science and art of cell-based ocular surface regeneration. Int Rev Cell Mol Biol. 2015;319:45-106.
18. Schofield R. The stem cell system. Biomed Pharmacother. 1983;37(8):375-80.
19. Dua HS, Shanmuganathan VA, Powell-Richards AO, et al. Limbal epithelial crypts: a novel anatomical structure and a putative limbal stem cell niche. Br J Ophthalmol. 2005;89(5):529-32.
20. Davanger M, Evensen A. Role of the pericorneal papillary structure in renewal of corneal epithelium. Nature. 1971;229(5286):560-1.
21. Thoft RA, Friend J. The X, Y, Z hypothesis of corneal epithelial maintenance. Invest Ophthalmol Vis Sci. 1983;24(10):1442-3.
22. Sangwan VS, Tseng SC. New perspectives in ocular surface disorders. An integrated approach for diagnosis and management. Indian J Ophthalmol. 2001;49(3):153-68.

23. Sejpal K, Bakhtiari P, Deng SX. Presentation, diagnosis and management of limbal stem cell deficiency. Middle East Afr J Ophthalmol. 2013;20(1):5-10.
24. Kruse F. Classification of ocular surface disease. In: Holland EJ, Mannis MJ (Eds). Ocular Surface Disease: Medical and Surgical Management. New York: Springer-Verlag; 2002. pp. 16-36.
25. The definition and classification of dry eye disease: report of the Definition and Classification Subcommittee of the International Dry Eye WorkShop. Ocul Surf. 2007;5(2):75-92.
26. Coursey TG, de Paiva CS. Managing Sjogren's syndrome and non-Sjogren syndrome dry eye with anti-inflammatory therapy. Clin Ophthalmol. 2014;8:1447-58.
27. Kohanim S, Palioura S, Saeed HN, et al. Stevens-Johnson syndrome/toxic epidermal necrolysis: a comprehensive review and guide to therapy. I. Systemic Disease. Ocul Surf. 2016;14(1):2-19.
28. Ueta M. Genetic predisposition to Stevens-Johnson syndrome with severe ocular surface complications. Cornea. 2015;34 Suppl 11:S158-65.
29. Pushker N, Tandon R, Vajpayee RB. Stevens-Johnson syndrome in India: risk factors, ocular manifestations and management. Ophthalmologica. 2000;214(4):285-8.
30. Kohanim S, Palioura S, Saeed HN, et al. Acute and chronic ophthalmic involvement in Stevens-Johnson syndrome/ toxic epidermal necrolysis: a comprehensive review and guide to therapy. II. Ophthalmic disease. Ocul Surf. 2016;14(2):168-88.
31. Gregory DG. New grading system and treatment guidelines for the acute ocular manifestations of Stevens-Johnson syndrome. Ophthalmology. 2016;123(8):1653-8.
32. Papakostas TD, Le HG, Chodosh J, et al. Prosthetic replacement of the ocular surface ecosystem as treatment for ocular surface disease in patients with a history of Stevens-Johnson syndrome/toxic epidermal necrolysis. Ophthalmology. 2015;122(2):248-53.
33. Saeed HN, Chodosh J. Ocular manifestations of Stevens-Johnson syndrome and their management. Curr Opin Ophthalmol. 2016;27(6):522-9.
34. Kheirkhah A, Ghaffari R, Kaghazkanani R, et al. A combined approach of amniotic membrane and oral mucosa transplantation for fornix reconstruction in severe symblepharon. Cornea. 2013;32(2):155-60.
35. Basu S, Sureka S, Shukla R, et al. Boston type 1 based keratoprosthesis (Auro Kpro) and its modification (LVP Kpro) in chronic Stevens-Johnson syndrome. BMJ Case Rep. 2014.
36. Tan A, Tan DT, Tan XW, et al. Osteo-odonto keratoprosthesis: systematic review of surgical outcomes and complication rates. Ocul Surf. 2012;10(1):15-25.
37. Kirzhner M, Jakobiec FA. Ocular cicatricial pemphigoid: a review of clinical features, immunopathology, differential diagnosis, and current management. Semin Ophthalmol. 2011;26(4-5):270-7.
38. Foster CS. Cicatricial pemphigoid. Trans Am Ophthalmol Soc. 1986;84:527-663.
39. Mondino BJ, Brown SI. Ocular cicatricial pemphigoid. Ophthalmology. 1981;88(2):95-100.
40. Sobolewska B, Deuter C, Zierhut M. Current medical treatment of ocular mucous membrane pemphigoid. Ocul Surf. 2013;11(4):259-66.
41. Queisi MM, Zein M, Lamba N, et al. Update on ocular cicatricial pemphigoid and emerging treatments. Surv Ophthalmol. 2016;61(3):314-7.
42. Schornack MM, Baratz KH. Ocular cicatricial pemphigoid: the role of scleral lenses in disease management. Cornea. 2009;28(10):1170-2.
43. Saw VP, Dart JK. Ocular mucous membrane pemphigoid: diagnosis and management strategies. Ocul Surf. 2008;6(3):128-42.
44. Hodak E, Kremer I, David M, et al. Conjunctival involvement in pemphigus vulgaris: a clinical, histopathological and immunofluorescence study. Br J Dermatol. 1990;123(5):615-20.
45. Elchahal S, Kavosh ER, Chu DS. Ocular manifestations of blistering diseases. Immunol Allergy Clin North Am. 2008;28(1):119-36, vii.
46. Rao NK, Goldstein MH. Acid and alkali burns. In: Yanoff M, Duker J (Eds). Ophthalmology. New Delhi, India: Elsevier Health Sciences; 2013. pp. 296-8.
47. Wagoner MD. Chemical injuries of the eye: current concepts in pathophysiology and therapy. Surv Ophthalmol. 1997;41(4):275-313.
48. Vajpayee RB, Shekhar H, Sharma N, et al. Demographic and clinical profile of ocular chemical injuries in the pediatric age group. Ophthalmology. 2014;121(1):377-80.
49. Kuckelkorn R, Schrage N, Keller G, et al. Emergency treatment of chemical and thermal eye burns. Acta Ophthalmol Scand. 2002;80(1):4-10.
50. Dua HS, King AJ, Joseph A. A new classification of ocular surface burns. Br J Ophthalmol. 2001;85(11):1379-83.
51. Eslani M, Baradaran-Rafii A, Movahedan A, et al. The ocular surface chemical burns. J Ophthalmol. 2014;(2014):196827.
52. Roper-Hall MJ. Thermal and chemical burns. Trans Ophthalmol Soc UK. 1965;85:631-53.
53. Gupta N, Kalaivani M, Tandon R. Comparison of prognostic value of Roper-Hall and Dua classification systems in acute ocular burns. Br J Ophthalmol. 2011;95(2):194-8.
54. McCulley J. Chemical injuries. In: Smolin G, Thoft RA (Eds). The Cornea: Scientific Foundations and Clinical Practice, 2nd edition. Boston: Little, Brown and Co.; 1987.
55. Clare G, Suleman H, Bunce C, et al. Amniotic membrane transplantation for acute ocular burns. Cochrane Database Syst Rev. 2012;(9):CD009379.
56. Sangwan VS, Basu S, MacNeil S, et al. Simple limbal epithelial transplantation (SLET): a novel surgical technique for the treatment of unilateral limbal stem cell deficiency. Br J Ophthalmol. 2012;96(7):931-4.
57. Dua HS, Gomes JA, King AJ, et al. The amniotic membrane in ophthalmology. Surv Ophthalmol. 2004;49(1):51-77.
58. Aldave AJ, Sangwan VS, Basu S, et al. International results with the Boston type I keratoprosthesis. Ophthalmology. 2012;119(8):1530-8.

59. Phillips DL, Hager JL, Goins KM, et al. Boston type 1 keratoprosthesis for chemical and thermal injury. Cornea. 2014;33(9):905-9.
60. Ranjan A, Senthil S, Sangwan V. Successful acute and late management of a chemical burn with primary implantation of Boston type 1 keratoprosthesis. BMJ Case Rep. 2015;2015. pii: bcr2014209247.
61. Iyer G, Srinivasan B, Rishi E, et al. Large lamellar corneoscleral grafts: tectonic role in initial management of severe ocular chemical injuries. Eur J Ophthalmol. 2016;26(1):12-7.
62. Kuckelkorn R, Redbrake C, Kottek A, et al. Tenon-plasty and early keratoplasty in severe chemical eye burns. Ophthalmologe. 1995;92(4):439-44.
63. Smith VA, Cook SD. Doxycycline: a role in ocular surface repair. Br J Ophthalmol. 2004;88(5):619-25.
64. Shimmura S, Shimazaki J, Ohashi Y, et al. Anti-inflammatory effects of amniotic membrane transplantation in ocular surface disorders. Cornea. 2001;20(4):408-13.
65. Sangwan VS, Basu S, Vemuganti GK, et al. Clinical outcomes of xeno-free autologous cultivated limbal epithelial transplantation: a 10-year study. Br J Ophthalmol. 2011;95(11):1525-9.
66. Basu S, Mohamed A, Chaurasia S, et al. Clinical outcomes of penetrating keratoplasty after autologous cultivated limbal epithelial transplantation for ocular surface burns. Am J Ophthalmol. 2011;152(6):917-24.e1.
67. Kenyon KR, Tseng SC. Limbal autograft transplantation for ocular surface disorders. Ophthalmology. 1989;96(5):709-22; discussion 722-3.
68. Ramachandran C, Basu S, Sangwan VS, et al. Concise review: the coming of age of stem cell treatment for corneal surface damage. Stem Cells Transl Med. 2014;3(10):1160-8.
69. Sangwan VS, Matalia HP, Vemuganti GK, et al. Amniotic membrane transplantation for reconstruction of corneal epithelial surface in cases of partial limbal stem cell deficiency. Indian J Ophthalmol. 2004;52(4):281-5.
70. Tseng SC, Prabhasawat P, Barton K, et al. Amniotic membrane transplantation with or without limbal allografts for corneal surface reconstruction in patients with limbal stem cell deficiency. Arch Ophthalmol. 1998;116(4):431-41.
71. Mataix B, Alcántara A, Caro M, et al. Variations in the technique for autologous limbal transplantation. Arch Soc Esp Oftalmol. 2016;91(10):501-4.
72. Dua HS. The conjunctiva in corneal epithelial wound healing. Br J Ophthalmol. 1998;82(12):1407-11.
73. Nishiwaki-Dantas MC, Dantas PE, Reggi JR. Ipsilateral limbal translocation for treatment of partial limbal deficiency secondary to ocular alkali burn. Br J Ophthalmol. 2001;85(9):1031-3.
74. Shortt AJ, Secker GA, Rajan MS, et al. Ex vivo expansion and transplantation of limbal epithelial stem cells. Ophthalmology. 2008;115(11):1989-97.
75. Basu S, Fernandez MM, Das S, et al. Clinical outcomes of xeno-free allogeneic cultivated limbal epithelial transplantation for bilateral limbal stem cell deficiency. Br J Ophthalmol. 2012;96(12):1504-9.
76. Basu S, Sureka SP, Shanbhag SS, et al. Simple limbal epithelial transplantation: long-term clinical outcomes in 125 cases of unilateral chronic ocular surface burns. Ophthalmology. 2016;123(5):1000-10.
77. Bhalekar S, Basu S, Sangwan VS. Successful management of immunological rejection following allogeneic simple limbal epithelial transplantation (SLET) for bilateral ocular burns. BMJ Case Rep. 2013;2013. pii: bcr2013009051.
78. Cheung AY, Holland EJ. Keratolimbal allograft. Curr Opin Ophthalmol. 2017;28(4):377-81.
79. Parihar JK, Parihar AS, Jain VK, et al. Allogenic cultivated limbal stem cell transplantation versus cadaveric keratolimbal allograft in ocular surface disorder: 1-year outcome. Int Ophthalmol. 2017;37(6):1323-31.
80. Subramaniam SV, Sejpal K, Fatima A, et al. Coculture of autologous limbal and conjunctival epithelial cells to treat severe ocular surface disorders: long-term survival analysis. Indian J Ophthalmol. 2013;61(5):202-7.
81. Tan DT, Ang LP, Beuerman RW. Reconstruction of the ocular surface by transplantation of a serum-free derived cultivated conjunctival epithelial equivalent. Transplantation. 2004;77(11):1729-34.
82. Inatomi T, Nakamura T, Koizumi N, et al. Midterm results on ocular surface reconstruction using cultivated autologous oral mucosal epithelial transplantation. Am J Ophthalmol. 2006;141(2):267-75.
83. Tan JC, Tat LT, Coroneo MT. Treatment of partial limbal stem cell deficiency with topical interferon alpha-2b and retinoic acid. Br J Ophthalmol. 2016;100(7):944-8.
84. Samarawickrama C, Chew S, Watson S. Retinoic acid and the ocular surface. Surv Ophthalmol. 2015;60(3):183-95.
85. Sangwan VS, Surender P, Burman S. Cataract surgery in patients with Mooren's ulcer. J Cataract Refract Surg. 2005;31(2):359-62.
86. Bhartiya P, Sharma N, Ray M, et al. Trypan blue assisted phacoemulsification in corneal opacities. Br J Ophthalmol. 2002;86:857-9.
87. Sharma N, Aron N, Venugopal R, et al. New surgical approach in cases of cataract with ocular Stevens-Johnson syndrome. J Cataract Refract Surg. 2016;42(11):1549-55.
88. Das S, Mohamed A, Sangwan VS. Clinical course and outcomes in patients with Mooren ulcer who had cataract surgery. J Cataract Refract Surg. 2017;43(8):1044-9.
89. Narang P, Mohamed A, Mittal V, et al. Cataract surgery in chronic Stevens-Johnson syndrome: aspects and outcomes. Br J Ophthalmol. 2016;100(11):1542-6.

Chapter 22 Dry Eye

Rashmi Singh, Noopur Gupta, M Vanathi, Radhika Tandon

INTRODUCTION

Dry eye is a common ocular problem seen in all age groups with a greater propensity in the elderly population. Known to have a complex etiopathogenesis with several etiological differential diagnoses, a thorough understanding of anatomy and physiology of the ocular surface, lids and adnexa is essential for properly understanding the disease. Patients may present with a variety of symptoms and signs with often nonspecific complaints such as general discomfort, feeling of tiredness in eyes, burning, foreign body sensation, itching, even watering in some cases, and dryness in others.

EPIDEMIOLOGY

It can be seen in both the genders but has been seen to be more common in women[1] and they tend to experience dry eye symptoms at an earlier age (nearing menopause) as compared to men.[2] 1 out of 7 people are seen to experience symptoms of dry eye between the age group of 65 to 84 years.[3] The prevalence of dry eye, as noted by Moss et al, is 14.4% in the age group of 48 to 91 years. He also reported the prevalence to get doubled after the age of 59 years.[4]

DEFINITION

To define dry eye is as complex as its pathogenesis. Various study groups have tried to define dry eye; the most commonly used definitions being described here:

The NEI (National Eye Institute)[5] definition of dry eye is:

"Dry eye is a disorder of the tear film due to tear deficiency or excessive tear evaporation, which causes damage to the interpalpebral ocular surface and is associated with symptoms of discomfort."

The newer Tear Film and Ocular Surface Society (TFOS) Dry Eye Workshop (DEWS II)[6] definition of dry eye is:

"Dry eye is a multifactorial disease of the ocular surface characterized by a loss of homeostasis of the tear film, and accompanied by ocular symptoms, in which tear film instability, and hyperosmolarity, ocular surface inflammation and damage and neurosensory abnormalities play etiological roles."

Before we go into the details of the pathophysiology and management of dry eye, there is a need to know about the normal structures involved in maintaining the ocular surface stability.

Lacrimal System

The normal lacrimal system consists of the main lacrimal gland and accessory glands of Wolfring and Krause. The basal secretion is controlled by the glands of Wolfring and Krause while the lacrimal gland contributes to reflex secretion. The secretions reach the superior fornix via multiple excretory ducts from the lacrimal gland. There are few (1–2) excretory ducts that open into the inferior fornix also. The eyelids play an important role in spreading the tear film over the ocular surface. The tear secretions are excreted into the lacrimal sac via the upper and lower punctum and canaliculi and then finally into the nasolacrimal duct as explained in Figure 22.1.

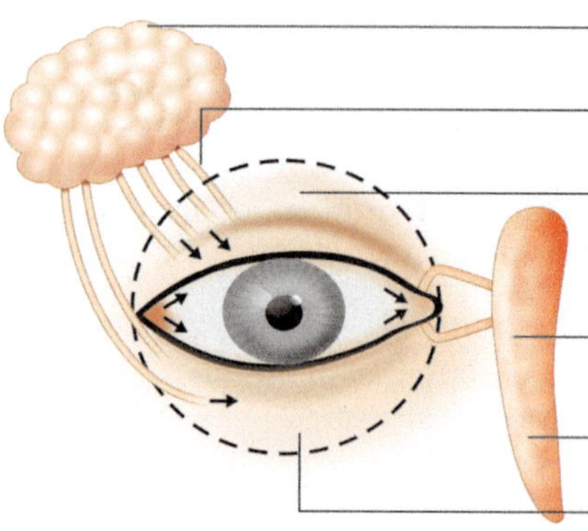

Fig. 22.1: Normal lacrimal apparatus.

Tear Film

The precorneal tear film is composed of three layers as explained in Figure 22.2. The outermost lipid layer, middle aqueous layer and innermost mucinous layer. There is no clear line of distinction between the three layers. While the mucin component is most concentrated close to the corneal epithelial cells, the aqueous layer also contains some amount of mucin interspersed within it. The outermost lipid layer is secreted by the meibomian glands, glands of Zeis and Moll, aqueous layer by lacrimal gland along with accessory lacrimal glands and the mucinous layer by the goblet cells. The tear film protects the ocular surface as well as provides nutrition, dilutes toxins or inflammatory mediators, and washes away debris.

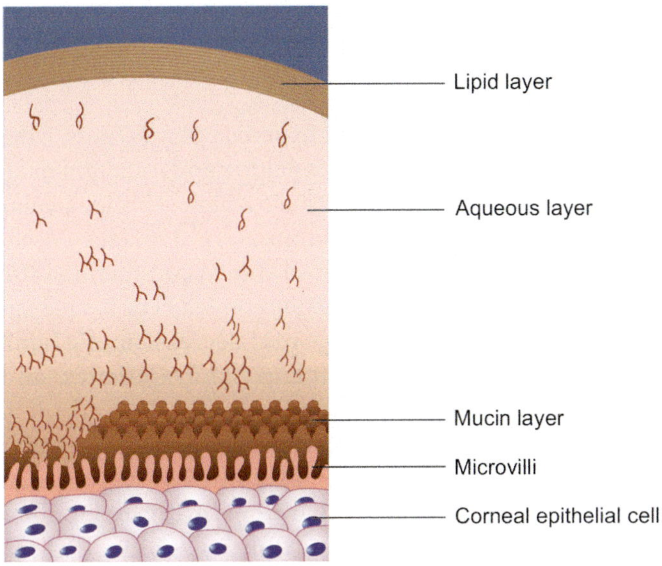

Fig. 22.2: The layers of tear film.

CLASSIFICATION OF DRY EYE

Dry eye can broadly be classified into two types: (1) the tear deficient type, and (2) the evaporative type (Fig. 22.3). The evaporative dry eye basically means an increase in the amount of evaporation from the ocular surface. It can further be affected by intrinsic ocular or extrinsic environmental factors. Sicca syndrome is a condition of reduced tear production which could be attributed to a variety of causes; most common cause being the normal aging process. Congenital absence of lacrimal gland, lacrimal gland obstruction can also lead to absence of tear production and secondary corneal and conjunctival changes. Another congenital condition familial dysautonomia or Riley-Day syndrome has also been seen to be associated with a severe sicca syndrome.

There are various secondary causes which lead to tear deficiency like chemical burns, Stevens-Johnson syndrome, ocular cicatricial pemphigoid, trachoma, irradiation, surgical removal of lacrimal gland or scarring of lacrimal ducts. It is also associated with the use of certain systemic drugs and systemic associations such as collagen vascular diseases, e.g. rheumatoid arthritis, systemic lupus erythematosus, systemic sclerosis, etc.

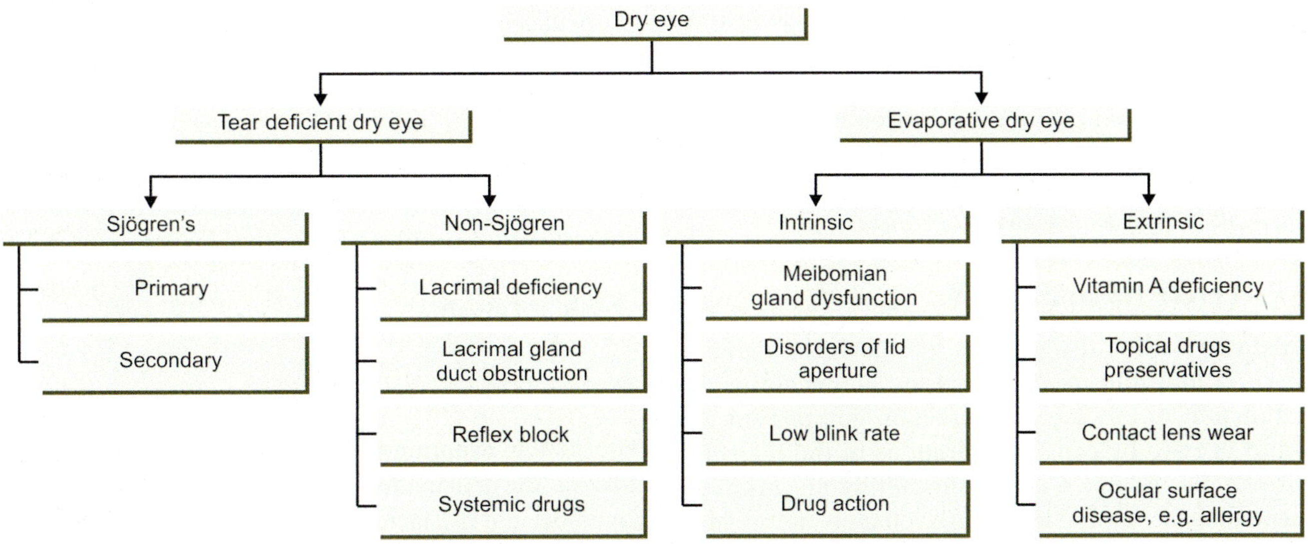

Fig. 22.3: Dry eye classification from the 2007 International Dry Eye WorkShop (DEWS) report.

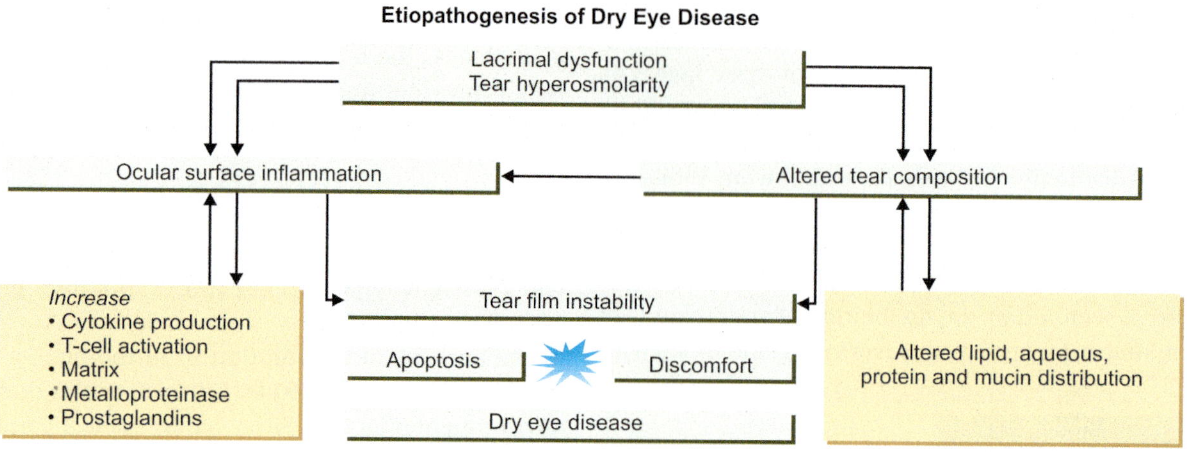

Fig. 22.4: Pathogenesis of dry eye.

Sjögren's syndrome is a triad of keratoconjunctivitis sicca, xerostomia and rheumatoid arthritis or any other collagen vascular disease. Salivary gland enlargement may or may not be seen. Histological features in the glands include atrophy of the acinar parenchyma and diffuse lymphoid infiltration.

There are various systemic medications which can increase the predisposition of dry eye. They include diuretics, beta-blockers, oral contraceptive pills, antihistaminics and antidepressants. Hormonal changes also play an important role thus, making postmenopausal women at high risk for developing dry eye.[7,8]

Lid disorders such as entropion, ectropion, lagophthalmos, trichiasis, distichiasis may lead to poor ocular surface and dry eye. Meibomian gland dysfunction leads to increase in inflammatory mediators and thus, precipitation of dry eye disease. The use of long-term topical medications especially their preservatives lead to ocular surface toxicity and dry eye. Frequent use of contact lens also poses a high risk for the development of dry eye. Another important cause for the development of dry eye, is history of previous ocular surgeries such as corneal transplantation and refractive procedures.

PATHOPHYSIOLOGY

As defined earlier, dry eye is a multifactorial disorder involving multiple mechanisms for its development. Dysfunction of any lacrimal function component can lead to dry eye by causing alterations in the tear film. Tear osmolarity and tear film instability are mutually potentiating factors and lead to precipitation of dry eye.[9]

1. *Tear hyperosmolarity:* Increase in osmolarity of tear film can occur either due to low aqueous component or high tear film evaporation. Tear hyperosmolarity leads to the release of inflammatory mediators and initiation of an inflammatory cascade. It causes damage to the ocular surface as increased inflammation damages goblet cells and leads to decreased mucin production. The presence of chronic inflammation leads to decreased corneal sensations which cause decrease in the blink rate which can lead to increased evaporation and contribute to tear film instability.[9]
2. *Tear film instability:* It can occur secondary to tear film hyperosmolarity as explained above or can be the initiating event like in cases of meibomian gland dysfunction. Tear film instability causes increased evaporation, which further increases tear hyperosmolarity.[9] Thus, the key factor in the causation and precipitation of dry eye is inflammation in the ocular surface.[10]

The pathophysiology of dry eye has been explained in Figure 22.4.

SIGNS AND SYMPTOMS

The patients present with very nonspecificocular symptoms like watering, mucoid discharge, burning sensation, foreign body sensation, stinging sensation, blurred vision (Figs. 22.5 to 22.7 and Box 22.1).

Examination

The ocular examination should start from the ocular adnexa. The ocular adnexa needs to be examined properly for associated risk factors like blepharitis, meibomitis, etc. as management of dry eye would first include managing the adnexal problems.

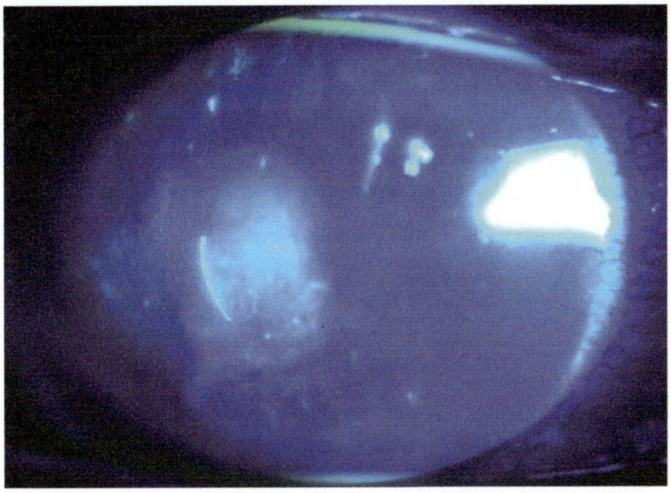

Fig. 22.5: Fluorescein staining showing filaments in a case of dry eye with filamentary keratopathy.

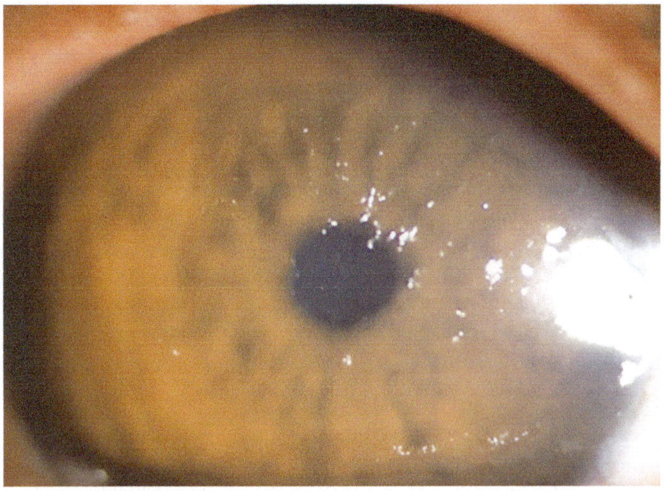

Fig. 22.6: Ocular surface showing lack of lustre and poor epithelium.

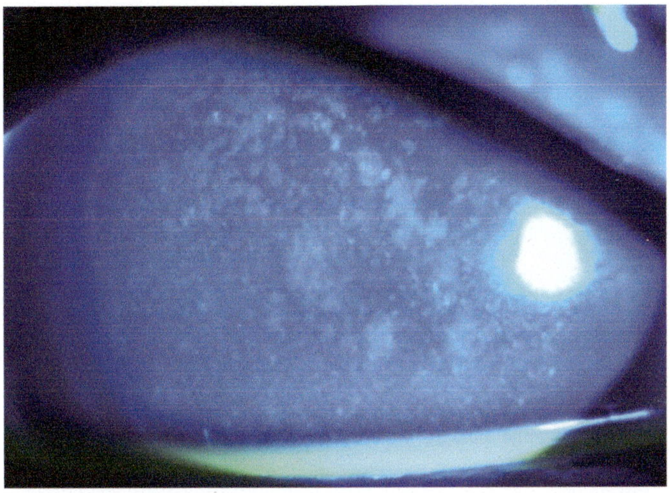

Fig. 22.7: Fluorescein staining showing superficial punctate epitheliopathy.

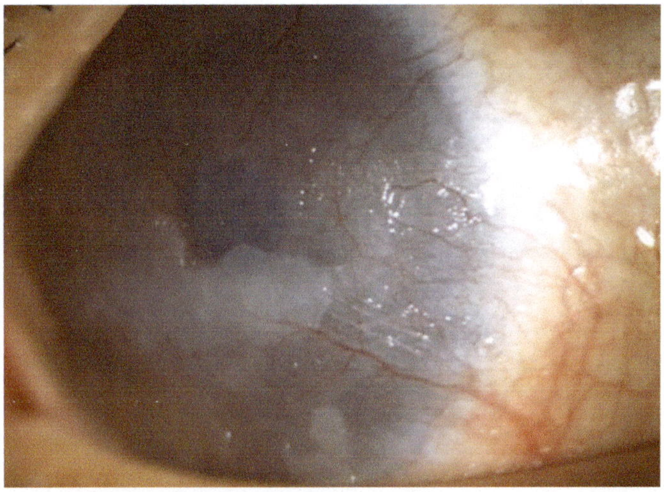

Fig. 22.8: A case of severe dry eye with corneal opacification, keratinization and vascularization.

Ocular surface shows very mild changes. A reduced tear film meniscus height on slit-lamp examination gives a hint towards the abnormal ocular surface.[11] It is further corroborated by the presence of mucus and debris in the tear film. Conjunctiva and cornea would appear lusterless along with the presence of exposure keratitis in the interpalpebral area. The exposure keratopathy initially starts in the inferior cornea in mild cases and becomes diffuse in severe cases of dry eye. Corneal filaments are also seen in severe cases of dry eye (Figs. 22.8 to 22.10).

DIAGNOSIS

There are various tests to evaluate tear secretion, tear film stability and tear clearance along with qualitative analysis of the tear film and ocular surface.

Tear Secretion Tests

Schirmer's Test

It was first introduced by Schirmer in 1903.[12] It was further modified by various investigators and De Roeth brought

Box 22.1: To diagnose and investigate a patient suspected to have dry eye disease.*

To start the process of confirming the diagnosis and plan further investigations for managing dry eye disease (DED) effectively, we have to assess the severity, risk factors and rule out secondary causes of dry eye. The following information needs to be elicited for further evaluation of the patient:

- Presence of eye discomfort and its severity
- Duration of symptoms and any event which might have aggravated the condition
- If these symptoms are associated with a diminution/blurring of vision and effect of blinking on vision
- If these symptoms are predominantly present in one eye or are similar in both eyes
- History of any itching, crusting or swelling in the eyes or the presence of any discharge
- Association of the ocular symptoms with any complaints of dryness of mouth or presence of swollen glands
- Any history of wearing contact lenses (If yes, duration and type to be noted)
- History of any associated systemic health condition/smoking or long-term systemic medications

Depending on the response to these questions, a comprehensive examination with detailed evaluation of lids, adnexa and anterior segment is undertaken. Thereafter, certain diagnostic tests for dry eye disease are performed. Dry eye symptom assessment questionnaires like DEQ-5 and OSDI are administered for the purpose of screening suspected patients. DEQ-5 score of more than 6 or OSDI score of more than 13 raises the likelihood of having dry eye disease. These symptom scores are corroborated by dry eye tests like noninvasive/invasive tear break up time < 10 seconds, tear osmolarity ≥ 308 mOsm/L in either eye or interocular osmolarity difference > 8 mOsm/L, ocular surface staining (> 5 corneal spots, > 9 conjunctival spots or lid margin staining). Results of these tests helps to subclassify dry eye into evaporative, aqueous deficient or mixed evaporative-aqueous deficient spectrum. Evaporative dry eye is further classified as mild, moderate and severe depending on the severity of meibomian gland dysfunction. Aqueous deficient dry eye can further be classified on the basis of tear meniscus height (TMH) as mild (0.2 mm), moderate (0.1 mm) and severe (0.00 mm).

*Adapted from Craig JP, Nelson JD, Azar DT, et al. TFOS DEWS II Report Executive Summary. Ocul Surf. 2017;15(4):802-12.

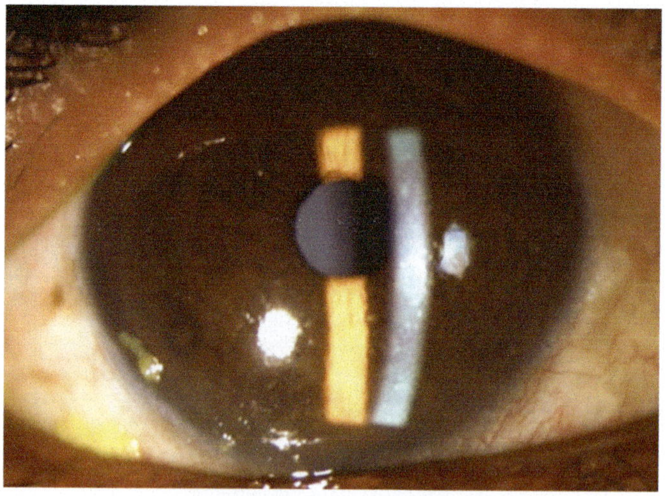

Fig. 22.9: Ocular surface showing mucus debris in the tear film and superficial epitheliopathy.

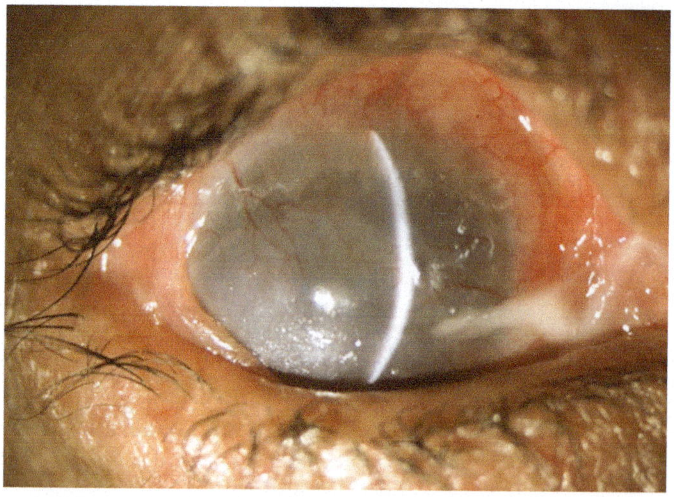

Fig. 22.10: A case of Stevens-Johnson syndrome showing severe dry eye with conjunctival inflammation, corneal opacification with superficial vascularization and mucus debris in tear film.

the Whatman standard No. 41 filter paper in 1953. The standardized Schirmer strips were given by Halberg and Berens.[13,14]

It is the most commonly used test for the assessment of tear secretion. It is performed by placing Schirmer strip over the lower lid margin at the junction of lateral one-third and medial two-thirds as explained in Figure 22.11. It is measured at the end of five minutes by observing the "mm" of strip wetted. It has been classified as Schirmer 1, Schirmer 2 and Schirmer 3.

- *Schirmer 1:* It detects the basal as well as reflex tear secretion. A value less than 5 mm at five minutes is considered abnormal.[15]
- *Schirmer 2:* It is done after anesthetizing the cornea with topical anesthesia medication like proparacaine. It measures only the basal secretion.[16,17] Some authors also describe it as a tactile reflex secretion as measurement is done after nasal stimulation with a cotton applicator. A value less than 10 mm at five minutes is considered abnormal.[15]

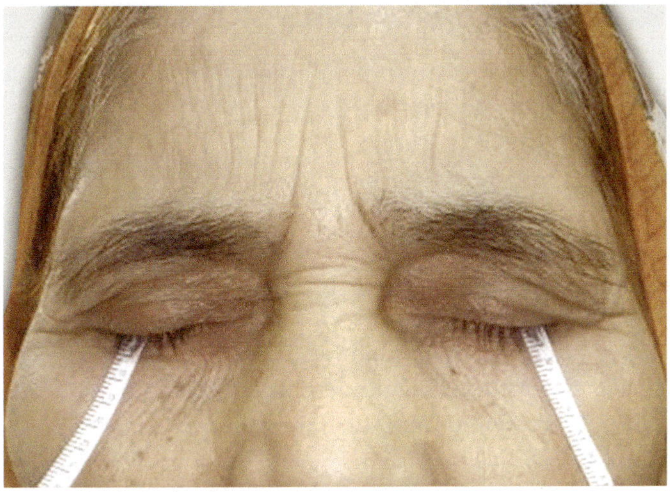

Fig. 22.11: Patient being evaluated for Schirmer's test.

- *Schirmer 3:* It is also called as photic reflex secretion as test is observed after asking the person to look at sun.

The average Schirmer test values in normal population as measured by various investigators has a range from 8.1 mm to 33.1 mm without anesthesia and from 3.5 mm to 11.9 mm with anesthesia.[18-20]

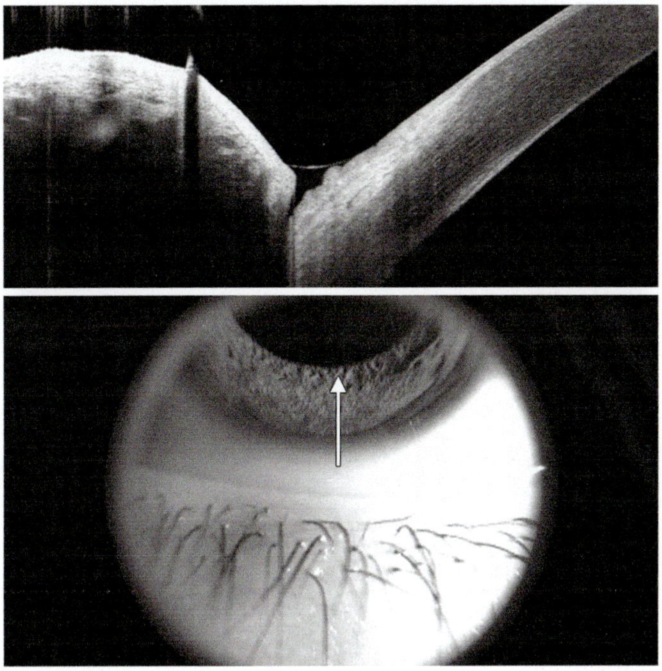

Fig. 22.12: Spectral domain anterior segment optical coherence tomography (SD-ASOCT) showing tear meniscus height (TMH). It can be used to measure the baseline TMH and objectively assess the improvement after initiation of dry eye treatment.

Phenol Red Thread Test

There is an increased incidence of conjunctival and lid irritation with placement of Schirmer strips. Therefore, Kurihashi et al.[21] introduced the concept of placing a fine thread instead of Schirmer strip. He used a white thread 0.25 mm in diameter and 70 mm length which was stained with fluorescein at one end. It is inserted into the conjunctival sac in temporal portion. As the thread gets wetted by tears, it is stained yellow because of the fluorescein dye. Further modification in this test was the introduction of cotton thread impregnated with phenol red dye and test was called "phenol red thread test". It was introduced by Hamano et al.[22] The thread changes color from yellow to red upon wetting by tears. The normal values described are 9–18 mm; but the thread acts as a rate limiting factor because it keeps absorbing tears even after removal from eye.

Tear Volume Assessment

Tear Meniscus Height

The height of the tear meniscus at the lower lid margin can provide us a clue about the tear film volume. A detailed look at the tear film and the presence of mucus/debris in the tear film points towards some component of meibomian gland dysfunction. There are recent advances in imaging techniques with the introduction of spectral domain anterior segment optical coherence tomography (SD-ASOCT) (Fig. 22.12) which can help in quantitatively measuring tear meniscus height. It can be used to objectively assess the baseline level of ocular surface and also the response to treatment.

Tear Film Stability

It can be assessed by tear break up time (TBUT). TBUT can be invasive or noninvasive. Invasive TBUT was first described by Norn. It is placed by putting fluorescein in the lower conjunctival sac and then asking the patient to blink. The time is recorded between the complete blink and the appearance of first random dry spot in the precorneal tear film. It should be repeated atleast three times and the appearance of random dry spot is to be taken into account as the appearance of a dry spot at the same position in every test could be because of a localized pathology. Noninvasive TBUT can be assessed by various modalities like xeroscope, Keeler tearscope, placido-based computerized videokeratoscopy.

For both the invasive and noninvasive TBUT, a value less than five sec is definite dry eye, 5–10 sec is marginal dry eye and more than 10 sec is normal.

There is another parameter called ocular protection index (OPI). It is equal to TBUT/IBI. IBI is interblink interval. OPI less than 1 is considered abnormal.

Tear Clearance Tests

In this test, fluorescein is instilled in the lower fornix and serial Schirmer's tests are done at one minute interval. The presence of dye at the end of 10 minutes is considered abnormal.

OCULAR SURFACE HEALTH

Dye staining: Corneal and conjunctival staining can give a clue towards the health status of the ocular surface. The various dyes used are sodium fluorescein 1%, rose Bengal 1%, lissamine green (LG). There are various grading systems that have been used to describe the staining patterns, i.e. van Bijsterveld staging, oxford grading, NEI grading.

Fluorescein staining: Fluorescein staining has long been used to detect epithelial defect but it has become an important staining dye for dry eye evaluation and management.[23,24] Fluorescein is a water soluble dye and does not penetrate the lipid layer of epithelium. It stains the corneal and conjunctival surface at the areas of disrupted cell junctions.[25] There are various types of fluorescein staining patterns seen in dry eye disease as explained in Figures 22.5 and 22.7. It ranges from mild superficial punctate erosions to involving the whole corneal surface. The staining is seen not just in cornea but also conjunctiva and some investigators report that corneal damage and staining is preceded by conjunctival damage.[26]

Rose Bengal staining: Rose Bengal does not stain the healthy epithelial cells but the dead and desquamated cells. It was based on this that the whole concept of rose bengal staining came into being.[27] Rose bengal staining to detect ocular surface damage has gained importance since 1960s after introduction by Norn. It is mainly helpful for the conjunctival damage.[28,29] There are other theories which state that rose bengal stains in the areas of ocular surface lacking the mucin component in patients of dry eye.[30]

Lissamine green: LG is a synthetic organic acid dye. It stains the ocular surface similar to rose bengal and they can be used interchangeably. But the one advantage that has been seen with LG dye is the less stinging and pain associated with it.[31-33]

STAINING SYSTEMS

The three most commonly employed methods to grade ocular surface staining are the,

1. Van Bijsterveld system
2. NEI/Industry workshop guidelines
3. Oxford scheme.

Van Bijsterveld System

The ocular surface is divided into three parts: cornea, nasal and temporal bulbar conjunctiva. The staining patterns are scored from 0 to 3 as explained in Figure 22.13. Zero indicating no staining and 3 indicating confluent staining. The final score is calculated out of nine.[33]

The NEI/Industry Workshop Guidelines

Designed to give a more detailed grading of the staining pattern of cornea and conjunctiva,[5] it divides the cornea into five areas (central, nasal temporal, superior, and inferior). Both nasal and temporal conjunctiva are divided into three areas each as shown in Figures 22.14A and B. Each area is scored on a scale of 0–3 where 0 is no staining and three is confluent staining. So, cornea is scored out of a total score of 15 and conjunctiva out of 18.

The Oxford Scheme

Intended to quantify the epithelial damage mainly, this consists of a series of pictures labeled from A to E and is used to classify dry eye as absent, mild, moderate, severe by comparing with the pictures available in the chart.[34]

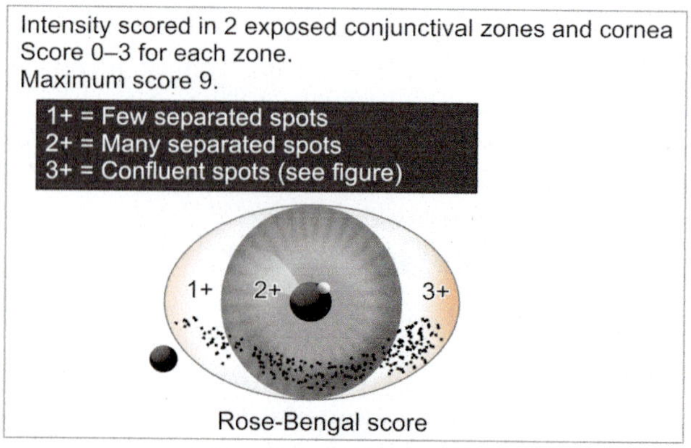

Fig. 22.13: van Bijsterveld staging.
Source: van Bijsterveld OP. Diagnostic tests in the Sicca syndrome. Arch Ophthalmol. 1969;82:10-4.

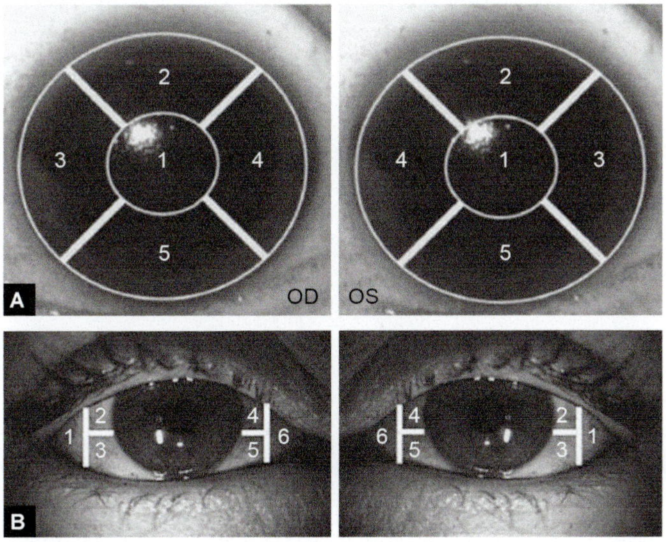

Figs. 22.14A and B: National Eye Institute (NEI)/industry workshop grading.

Panel	Grade	Criteria
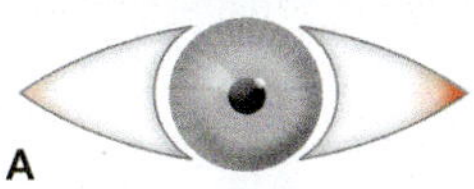 A	0	Equal to or less than panel A
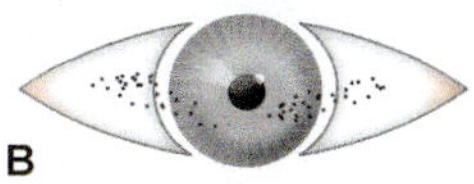 B	I	Equal to or less than panel B, greater than A
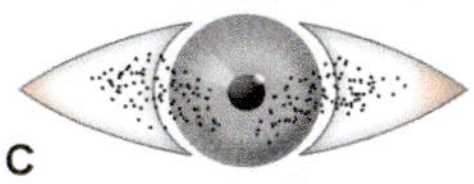 C	II	Equal to or less than panel C, greater than B
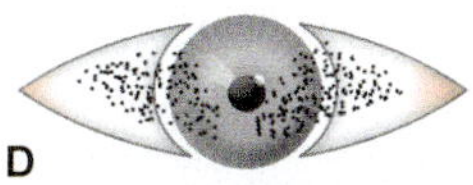 D	III	Equal to or less than panel D, greater than C
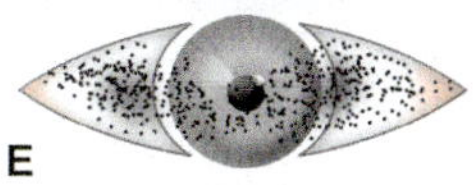 E	IV	Equal to or less than panel E, greater than D
>E	V	Greater than panel E

Fig. 22.15: Oxford grading [International Dry Eye WorkShop (DEWS 2007)—ocular surface].

In this chart, staining is depicted by the number of dots in the picture and the number of dots increase logarithmically from mild to severe as shown in Figure 22.15.

QUALITATIVE ASSAYS (LABORATORY TESTS)

Tear Osmolarity

There is a definite role of tear hyperosmolarity in the pathogenesis of dry eye as described in all definitions of dry eye. A disturbance in the equilibrium of tear secretion, evaporation and clearance leads to increased osmolarity and leads to inflammation and further symptoms of dry eye.[35] It has been identified by Pflugfelder et al. that there is a positive correlation between the severity of dry eye symptoms, staining patterns and conjunctival sqaumous metaplasia with the tear osmolarity.[36]

There are various ways of measuring tear osmolarity. The gold standard is the freezing point depression (FPD)[36,37] which requires very minute quantity, i.e. 0.1 mL.[38] The other two methods described are by measuring the vapor pressure[39,40] and electrical conductivity or impedance.[41]

The TearLab system (Tearlab Inc., San Diego, CA, USA) (Fig. 22.16) is an example of measurement by electrical impedance.[42] This method has the advantage of requiring a very small tear volume for testing, i.e. 0.05 mL and results being available in 30 seconds.

Tear Protein Assays

Proteolytic enzymes like matrix metalloproteinases (MMPs) are expressed in low quantity in normal eyes but their production is increased by the ocular surface in conditions of stress like in dry eye with increased inflammation.[43,44] The presence of high quantity of proteolytic enzymes leads to damage to the corneal epithelial barrier. The other conditions associated with increased quantity of MMP-9 are conjunctivochalasis,[45] meibomian gland dysfunction and Sjögren syndrome.[46]

MANAGEMENT

The management of dry eye is mainly symptomatic. It consists of making environmental changes, improving eyelid hygiene and tear supplementation (Box 22.2).

Environmental modifications include avoiding exacerbating factors, avoiding dry dusty areas, improving blinking, and taking breaks between work.

If there is associated meibomian gland dysfunction or blepharitis then, first efforts should be made towards improving lid hygiene. Patients should be explained about the importance of warm compresses and lid massage. Besides topical antibiotics and tear supplements, oral antibiotics should be started whenever needed.

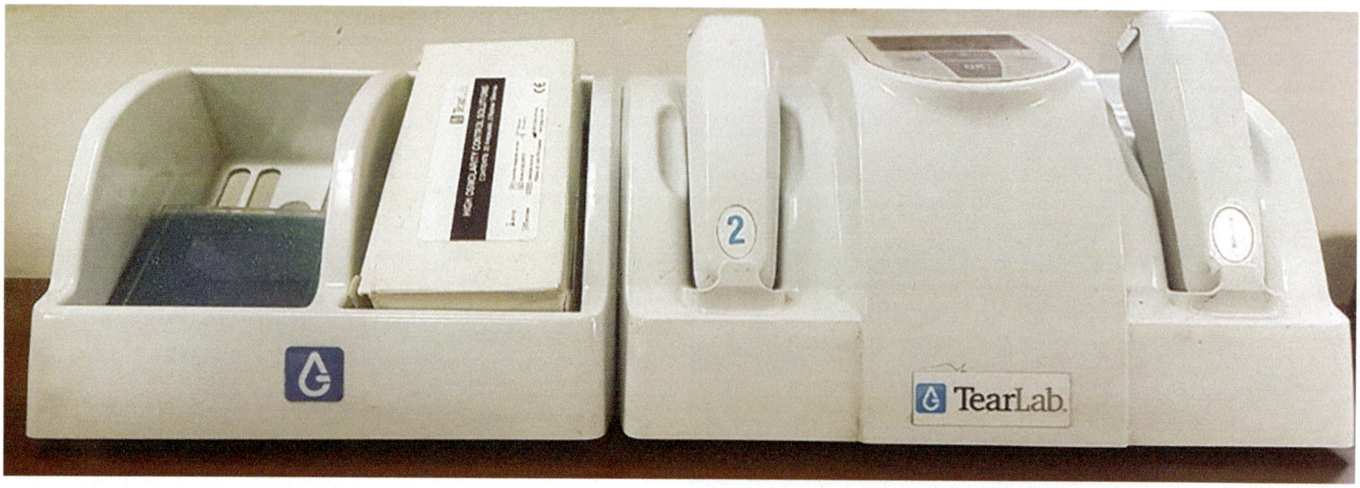

Fig. 22.16: Tear Lab osmolarity system. It is based on the principle of electrical impedance and provides a quick and simple method to measure osmolarity of human tears. It thus aids in the diagnosis of dry eye disease in conjunction with other methods of clinical evaluation. An elevated reading of more than 300 mOsm/liter indicate loss of homeostasis of the tear film.

Box 22.2: To decide management of a patient with dry eye.*

When a patient with suspected DED presents to the outpatient department/clinic, we ask the patient for the presence of any symptoms. The patient is then examined for signs of ocular surface disease.

1. If the patient is asymptomatic with no signs of ocular surface disease, he is confirmed to be normal and no treatment is required.
2. If the patient has signs in the absence of any symptoms, he is more likely to suffer from DED in presence of precipitating factors such as ocular surgery, air-conditioned environment or excessive use of digital screens. In such cases, preventive management and environmental modification is recommended.
3. If an asymptomatic person is found to have neurotrophic condition, i.e. decreased corneal sensations, it warrants timely and effective dry eye management.
4. If the patient is symptomatic in the absence of any ocular signs, it could mean a pre-clinical state which requires observation, and preventive therapy or the patient may be suffering from neuropathic pain (nonocular surface disease), for which the patient needs to be referred for pain management.
5. If the patient is symptomatic and has ocular signs, then the patient is suspected to have DED and is further evaluated for severity, duration, and precipitating local and systemic conditions as detailed in Box 22.1. Other differential diagnoses for ocular surface disease are ruled out before making a diagnosis of dry eye disease. Once the diagnosis of dry eye disease is confirmed, it is further classified as aqueous deficient or evaporative or mixed and is managed accordingly.

*Adapted from Craig JP, Nelson JD, Azar DT, et al. TFOS DEWS II Report Executive Summary. Ocul Surf. 2017;15(4):802-812.

Tear Supplementation

The most basic management starts with tear supplementation and maintaining the retention of tears. The ideal lubricant can be described as containing potassium and bicarbonate as the main electrolyte component with a neutral to alkaline pH. It should be preservative-free. Patients often complain of blurring of vision after using these topical medications therefore, besides being adequate pharmacologically, these should have the ability to spread easily over cornea and aid in good visual performance.

Another option in cases of moderate to severe dry eye, is autologous serum. It is preservative-free and contains essential components like epithelial growth factor, neurotrophic growth factor like nerve growth factor, substance P.

Various surgical procedures have been described for improving tear retention. Punctal occlusion is done in moderate to severe dry eye which is not getting improved by artificial tears. It consists of absorbable inserts and nonabsorbable inserts.

Tarsorrhaphy is done in severe or refractory dry eyes. It reduces the surface area of exposure and thus, helps decrease evaporation.

Anti-inflammatory Agents

The mainstay of anti-inflammatory therapy are topical nonsteroidal anti-inflammatory drugs (NSAIDs) and steroids. Steroids have been evaluated for their role in Sjögren's syndrome inspite of being associated with severe side effects like cataract, glaucoma and increased risk of infections.[47,48] Steroids are also described as mainly a pulse therapy during exacerbations. There is a speculation that the NSAIDs and steroids can themselves lead to dry eye by reducing corneal sensations.[49,50]

There is a naturally occurring peptide called thymosin β4 which is found in high concentrations in blood plasma, and ocular surface fluid. It has been known to have both woundhealing and anti-inflammatory properties[48,51] and has been seen to improve epithelial cell migration and healing of ocular surface.

Tetracyclines have antibacterial, antiprotease, antilipase, anti-inflammatory, and immunomodulatory actions. Their main role is in cases of meibomian gland dysfunction.

Essential fatty acids like Omega-3 fatty acids have an essential role in the synthesis of meibum which further forms the lipid layer of tear film. They improve the symptoms of dry eye by clearing and thinning the meibomian gland secretions.

There is a new topical substance called proteoglycan 4 (PRG4). It is a natural glycoprotein and also known as lubricin. It plays an important role as a boundary lubricant in several sites.[52,53]

Secretagogues

When the tear supplementation therapy does not work, there comes the role of secretagogues which stimulate tear production. It includes pilocarpine, cevilimine, eledosin, diquafosol and rebapimide. They can increase both the aqueous and mucin secretion.

Three percent diquafosol tetrasodium is a P2Y2 purinergic receptor agonist which works by activating P2Y2 receptors of the ocular surface. It stimulates the tear secretion and has been proved on imaging like ASOCT and meniscometry.[54] Diquafosol also stimulates the secretion of a mucin-like substance, i.e. sialic acid. It was seen in healthy individuals. Therefore, clinical trials have demonstrated a promising improvement of the ocular surface in patients with severe and refractory dry eyes.[55,56]

Topical Immunomodulators

Cyclosporine is a calcineurin inhibitor which reduces pro-inflammatory cytokines like interleukin-6 (IL-6), inflammatory and apoptotic markers and increases the release of anti-inflammatory cytokines.[57]

It is the first topical immunomodulator to be used as an ophthalmic emulsion as approved by the United States Food and Drug Administration (FDA) in 2002. The various conditions in which its topical administration has been seen to help are blepharitis, dry eye, keratoconjunctivitis, post-LASIK dry eye, graft versus host disease (GVHD), Steven-Johnson syndrome (SJS), and TEN.[56-59]

Newer Modalities

Topical Vitamin A

Lacrimal gland provides vitamin A/retinol for the ocular surface. Retinol has been seen to reverse the conjunctival squamous metaplasia and even keratinization in severe dry eyes.[60] Therefore, topical administration of vitamin A is a promising treatment option for very severe and advanced cases.

Janus Kinase Inhibitors

A new drug named Tofacitinib (CP-690,550) has been seen to show an optimal improvement in dry eye symptomatology. It is still under phase 1/2 trial.[61]

Antilymphangiogenic Agents

There have been experiments on the role of antivascular endothelial growth factor (antiVEGF) agents injected intraperitoneally in murine models. They have shown to improve the dry eye disease. It is based on the fact that low-grade inflammation found in dry eyes leads to the induction of lymphangiogenesis without accompanying hemangiogenesis and antiVEGF agents can be used to improve the inflammation and thus, dry eye symptoms.[62]

Lacritin and Tear Proteome

Lacritin which is a tear protein has been found to be deficient in dry eye and its replacement through topical medications can be used to improve dry eye.[63]

REFERENCES

1. McCarty CA, Bansal AK, Livingston PM, et al. The epidemiology of dry eye in Melbourne, Australia. Ophthalmology. 1998;105(6):1114-9.
2. Yazdani C, McLaughlin T, Smeeding JE, et al. Prevalence of treated dry eye disease in a managed care population. Clin Ther. 2001;23(10):1672-82.
3. Schein OD, Muñoz B, Tielsch JM, et al. Prevalence of dry eye among the elderly. Am J Ophthalmol. 1997;124(6):723-8.
4. Moss SE, Klein R, Klein BE. Prevalence of and risk factors for dry eye syndrome. Arch Ophthalmol. 2000;118(9):1264-8.

5. Lemp MA. Report of the national eye institute/industry workshop on clinical trials in dry eyes. CLAO J. 1995;21(4):221-32.
6. Gomes JAP, Azar DT, Baudouin C, et al. TFOS DEWS II iatrogenic report. Ocul Surf. 2017;15(3):511-38.
7. Ohashi Y, Ishida R, Kojima T, et al. Abnormal protein profiles in tears with dry eye syndrome. Am J Ophthalmol. 2003;136(2):291-9.
8. Solomon A, Dursun D, Liu Z, et al. Pro- and anti-inflammatory forms of interleukin-1 in the tear fluid and conjunctiva of patients with dry-eye disease. Invest Ophthalmol Vis Sci. 2001;42(10):2283-92.
9. The definition and classification of dry eye disease: report of the Definition and Classification Subcommittee of the International Dry Eye WorkShop. Ocul Surf. 2007;5(2): 75-92.
10. Behrens A, Doyle JJ, Stern L, et al. Dysfunctional tear syndrome: a Delphi approach to treatment recommendations. Cornea. 2006;25(8):900-7.
11. Nebbioso M, Del Regno P, Gharbiya M, et al. Analysis of the pathogenic factors and management of dry eye in ocular surface disorders. Int J Mol Sci. 2017;18:1764.
12. Schirmer O. Studien zur physiologie und pathologie der tranen-absonderung und tranenabfuhr. Graefes Arch Clin Exp Ophthalmol. 1903;56:197-91.
13. De Roetth A. Lacrimation in normal eyes. Arch Ophthalmol. 1953;49(2):185-9.
14. Halberg GP, Berens C. Standardized Schirmer tear test kit. Am J Ophthalmol. 1961;51:840-2.
15. Bron, AJ, Smith, JA, Calonge M. Methodologies to diagnose and monitor dry eye disease: report of the Diagnostic Methodology Subcommittee of the International Dry Eye WorkShop. Ocul Surf. 2007;5(2):108-23.
16. Clinch TE, Benedetto DA, Felberg NT, et al. Schirmer's test: a closer look. Arch Ophthalmol. 1983;101(9):1383-6.
17. Tsubota K, Yamada M. The importance of the Schirmer Test with nasal stimulation. Am J Ophthalmol. 1991;111(1): 106-8.
18. Wright JC, Meger GE. A review of the Schirmer test for tear production. Arch Ophthalmol. 1962;67:564-5.
19. Lamberts DW, Foster CS, Perry HD. Schirmer test after topical anesthesia and the tear meniscus height in normal eyes. Arch Ophthalmol. 1979;97(6):1082-5.
20. Lee JH, Kee CW. The significance of tear film break-up time in the diagnosis of dry eye syndrome. Korean J Ophthalmol. 1988;2(2):69-71.
21. Kurihashi K, Yanagihara N, Honda Y. A modified Schirmer test: the fine-thread method for measuring lacrimation. J Pediatr Ophthalmol. 1977;14(6):390-7.
22. Hamano H, Hori M, Hamano T, et al. A new method for measuring tears. CLAO J. 1983;9(3):281-9.
23. Behrens A, Doyle JJ, Chuck RS, et al. Dysfunctional tear syndrome: a Delphi approach to treatment recommendations. Cornea. 2006;25(8):900-7.
24. Turner AW, Layton CJ, Bron AJ. Survey of eye practitioners' attitudes towards diagnostic tests and therapies for dry eye disease. Clin Exp Ophthalmol. 2005;33(4):351-5.
25. Feenstra RP, Tseng SC. Comparison of fluorescein and rose bengal staining. Ophthalmology. 1992;99(4):605-17.
26. Yokoi N, Kinoshita S. Importance of conjunctival epithelial evaluation in the diagnostic differentiation of dry eye from drug-induced epithelial keratopathy. Adv Exp Med Biol. 1998;438:827-30.
27. Passmore JW, King JH Jr. Vital staining of conjunctiva and cornea: review of literature and critical study of certain dyes. AMA Arch Ophthalmol. 1954;53(4):568-74.
28. Norn MS. Vital staining of cornea and conjunctiva. Acta Ophthalmol (Copenh). 1962;40:389-401.
29. Norn MS. Dead, degenerate, and living cells in conjunctival fluid and mucous thread. Acta Ophthalmol (Copenh). 1969;47(5-6):1102-15.
30. Argüeso P, Tisdale A, Spurr-Michaud S, et al. Mucin characteristics of human corneal-limbal epithelial cells that exclude the rose Bengal anionic dye. Invest Ophthalmol Vis Sci. 2006;47(1):113-9.
31. Norn MS. Lissamine green: vital staining of cornea and conjunctiva. Acta Ophthalmol (Copenh). 1973;51(4):483-91.
32. Manning FJ, Wehrly SR, Foulks GN. Patient tolerance and ocular surface staining characteristics of lissamine green versus rose bengal. Ophthalmology. 1995;102(12):1953-7.
33. McCulley JP, Shine WE, Aronowicz J, et al. Presumed hyposecretory/hyperevaporative KCS: tear characteristics. Trans Am Ophthalmol Soc. 2003;101:141-52.
34. Bron AJ, Evans VE, Smith JA. Grading of corneal and conjunctival staining in the context of other dry eye tests. Cornea. 2003;22(7):640-50.
35. Farris RL. Tear osmolarity—a new gold standard? Adv Exp Med Biol. 1994;350:495-503.
36. Pflugfelder SC, Jones D, Ji Z, et al. Altered cytokine balance in the tear fluid and conjunctiva of patients with Sjogren's syndrome keratoconjunctivitis sicca. Curr Eye Res. 1999;19(3):201-11.
37. Farris RL, Gilbard JP, Stuchell RN, et al. Diagnostic tests in keratoconjunctivitis sicca. CLAO J. 1983;9(1):23-8.
38. Gilbard JP. Tear film osmolarity and keratoconjunctivitis sicca. Eye Contact Lens. 1985;11:243-50.
39. Gilbard JP, Farris RL, Santamaria J. Osmolarity of tear microvolumes in keratoconjunctivitis sicca. Arch Ophthalmol. 1978;96(4):677-81.
40. Miller WL, Doughty MJ, Narayanan S, et al. A comparison of tear volume (by tear meniscus height and phenol red thread test) and tear fluid osmolality measures in non-lens wearers and in contact lens wearers. Eye Contact Lens. 2004;30(3):132-7.
41. Pensyl CD, Benjamin WJ. Vapor pressure osmometry, minimum sample microvolumes. Acta Ophthalmol Scand. 1999;77(1):27-30.
42. Ogasawara K, Tsuru T, Mitsubayashi K, et al. Electrical conductivity of tear fluid in healthy persons and keratoconjunctivitis sicca patients measured by a flexible conductimetric sensor. Graefes Arch Clin Exp Ophthalmol. 1996;234(9):542-6.

43. Versura P, Profazio V, Campos E. Performance of tear osmolarity compared to previous diagnostic tests for dry eye diseases. Curr Eye Res. 2010;35(7):553-64.
44. Pflugfelder SC, Farley W, Luo L, et al. Matrix metalloproteinase-9 knockout confers resistance to corneal epithelial barrier disruption in experimental dry eye. Am J Pathol. 2005;166(1):61-71.
45. Smith V, Rishmawi H, Hussein H, et al. Tear film MMP accumulation and corneal disease. Br J Ophthalmol. 2001;85(2):147-53.
46. Acera A, Sua´rez T, Rodrı´guez-Agirretxe I, et al. Changes in tear protein profile in patients with conjunctivochalasis. Cornea. 2011;30(1):42-9.
47. Solomon A, Dursun D, Liu Z, et al. Pro- and anti-inflammatory forms of interleukin-1 in the tear fluid and conjunctiva of patients with dry eye disease. Invest Ophthalmol Vis Sci. 2001;42(10):2283-92.
48. Nebbioso M, Fameli V, Gharbiya M, et al. Investigational drugs for the treatment of dry eye disease. Expert Opin Investig Drugs. 2016;25(12):1437-46.
49. Liu X, Wang S, Kao AA, et al. The effect of topical pranoprofen 0.1% on the clinical evaluation and conjunctival HLA-DR expression in dry eyes. Cornea. 2012;31(11):1235-9.
50. Fujishima H, Fuseya M, Murat D, et al. Efficacy of bromfenac sodium ophthalmic solution for treatment of dry eye disease. Asia Pac J Ophtalmol (Phila). 2015;4(1):9-13.
51. Nassar A, Tabbara KF, Aljurf M. Ocular manifestations of graft versus disease. Saudi J Opthalmol. 2013;27(3):215-22.
52. Schmidt TA, Sullivan DA, Knop E, et al. Transcription, translation, and function of lubricin, a boundary lubricant, at the ocular surface. JAMA Ophthalmol. 2013;131(6):766-76.
53. Samsom ML, Morrison S, Masala N, et al. Characterization of full-length recombinant human Proteoglycan 4 as an ocular surface boundary lubricant. Exp Eye Res. 2014;127:14-9.
54. Bremond-Gignac D, Gicquel JJ, Chiambaretta F. Pharmacokinetic evaluation of diquafosol tetrasodium for the treatment of Sjögren's syndrome. Expert Opin Drug Metab Toxicol. 2014;10(6):905-13.
55. Stevenson W, Chauhan SK, Dana R. Dry eye disease: an immune-mediated ocular surface disorder. Arch Ophthalmol. 2012;130(1):90-100.
56. Wan KH, Chen LJ, Young AL. Efficacy and safety of topical 0.05% cyclosporine eye drops in the treatment of dry eye syndrome: a systematic review and meta-analysis. Ocul Surf. 2015;13(3):213-25.
57. Semba CP, Torkildsen GL, Lonsdale JD, et al. A phase 2 randomized, double-masked, placebo-controlled study of a novel integrin antagonist (sar 1118) for the treatment of dry eye. Am J Ophthalmol. 2012;153(6):1050-60.
58. Zhou XQ, Wei RL. Topical cyclosporine a in the treatment of dry eye: a systematic review and meta-analysis. Cornea. 2014;33(7):760-7.
59. Agarwal P, Rupenthal ID. Modern approaches to the ocular delivery of cyclosporine A. Drug Discov Today. 2016;21(6):977-88.
60. Murphy PT, Sivakumaran M, Fahy G, et al. Successful use of topical retinoic acid in severe dry eye due to chronic graft versus-host disease. Bone Marrow Transplant. 1996;18(3):641-2.
61. Liew SH, Nichols KK, Klamerus KJ, et al. Tofacitinib (CP-690,550), a Janus kinase inhibitor for dry eye disease: results from a phase 1/2. Ophthalmology. 2012;119(7):1328-35.
62. Goyal S, Chauhan SK, Dana R. Blockade of prolymphangiogenic vascular endothelial growth factor C in dry eye disease. Arch Ophthalmol. 2012;130(1):84-9.
63. Karnati R, Laurie DE, Laurie GW. Lacritin and the tear proteome as natural replacement therapy for dry eye. Exp Eye Res. 2013;117:39-52.

Chapter 23 Infectious Keratitis

Naveen Radhakrishnan, N Venkatesh Prajna

INTRODUCTION

Infectious keratitis is an important public health problem across the world, and more so in the developing countries. The common organisms implicated in this suppurative condition include bacteria, fungi and protozoa. The initial step in this condition is the development of a corneal ulcer, defined as an epithelial defect with an associated stromal infiltrate and stromal necrosis.

23.1 BACTERIAL KERATITIS

INTRODUCTION

Though fungi are replacing bacteria as a most common causative organism of infective keratitis in developing countries, bacteria remain the most common cause in developed nations.[1] Bacterial keratitis usually occurs following a predisposing factor which causes a breech in the host local defense mechanisms.

EPIDEMIOLOGY

The common pathogenic bacteria causing infectious keratitis are given in Table 23.1.1. *Pseudomonas* and staphylococci are the most common organisms causing bacterial keratitis in the developed countries whereas in developing countries, *Streptococcus pneumoniae* and *Pseudomonas* are the most common organisms.[2,3] Contact lens use is the most common predisposing factor for bacterial keratitis in the developed countries.[4] Trauma is the most common risk factor in developing countries.

PATHOGENESIS

The steps involved in pathogenesis of bacterial keratitis are illustrated in Flowchart 23.1.1. The pathogenesis depends on the interplay between the host defense mechanisms, intrinsic and extrinsic risk factors and the bacterial virulence.

Host Defense Factors and Predisposing Conditions

There are three lines of defense, working seamlessly and synchronously, in the ocular surface which provides protection against infection.

The *bony orbit, lids and lashes* form the first line of defense for the cornea. Blinking is an important protective phenomena, which helps in prevention of exposure to noxious stimuli. Disorders impacting the first line of defense,

Table 23.1.1: Pathogenic bacteria causing infective keratitis.

Gram-positive cocci	*Staphylococcus aureus* *Staphylococcus epidermidis* *Streptococcus pneumoniae* *Streptococcus viridans*
Gram-positive bacilli	*Corynebacterium diphtheriae* *Nocardia asteroides* Nontuberculous mycobacteria *Propionibacterium* spp
Gram-negative cocci	*Neisseria gonorrhoeae* *Neisseria meningitidis*
Gram-negative bacilli	*Pseudomonas aeruginosa* *Klebsiella* spp *Serratia marcescens* *Bartonella henselae* *Proteus mirabilis* *Escherichia coli*
Gram-negative coccobacilli	*Haemophilus* spp *Moraxella* spp

Flowchart 23.1.1: Pathogenesis of bacterial corneal ulcer.

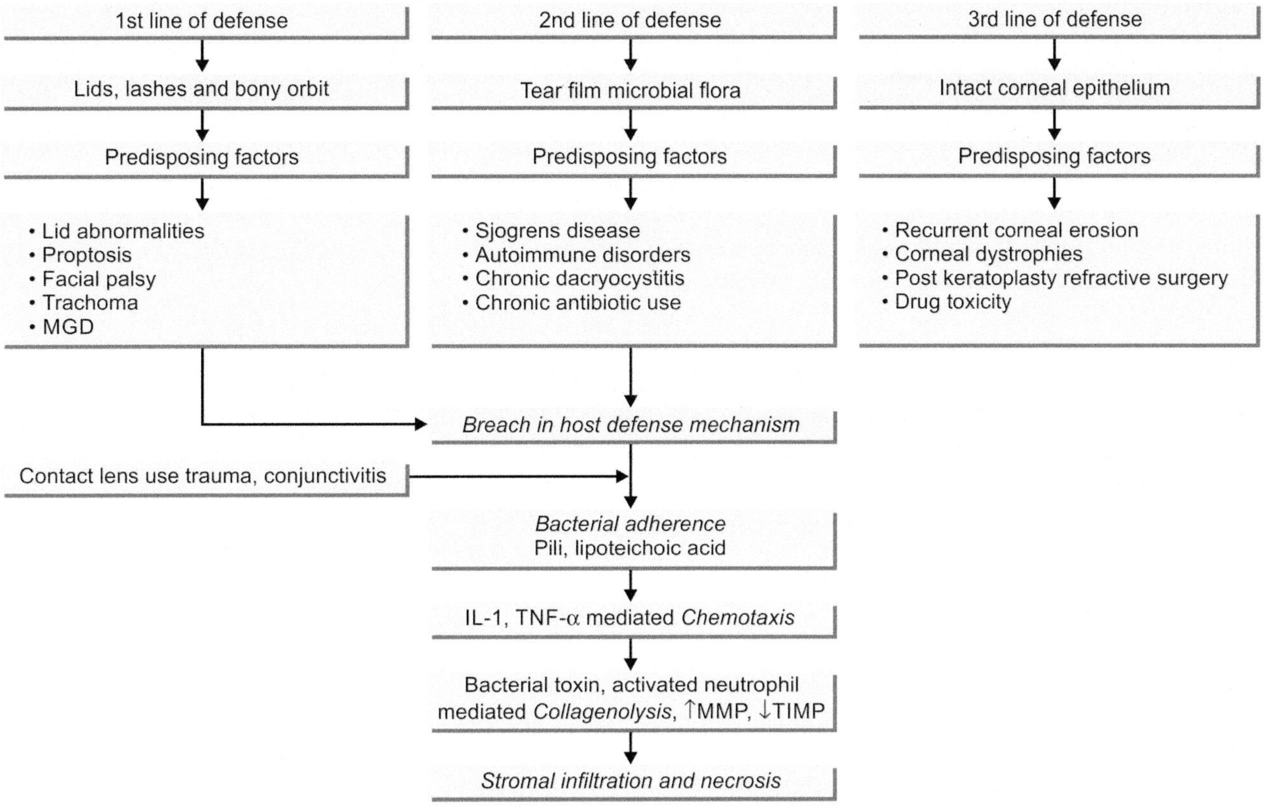

such as lagophthalmos, ectropion, trichiasis, trachoma and severe proptosis can predispose the cornea to infection.[5]

Tear film and its components along with the conjunctival mucosal-associated lymphoid tissue (MALT) constitute the second line of defense. Excess secretion of tear film in response to an offending stimuli and subsequent blinking clears the infective pathogen from the ocular surface. Tear film also contains various immunomodulatory proteins like secretory immunoglobulin A (IgA), complement factors, lysozymes, ceruloplasmin, orosomucoid acid, lactoferrin and betalysin, which inhibits the growth of pathogenic bacteria and also keeps the normal microbial flora intact.[6] The free-floating and sessile bacteria in the tear film over the ocular surface prevent the colonization of pathogenic bacteria by producing bacteriocins.[7] Conditions which cause compromise to tear function such as primary and secondary Sjögren's syndrome and conjunctival scarring can predispose to bacterial keratitis. Chronic topical antibiotic use (by altering the normal microbial flora) and chronic topical steroid use (by causing a focal immunosuppressed state) are important factors which might predispose to bacterial keratitis. Obstruction to the flow of tears and the subsequent accumulation of the microbes in the lacrimal sac in chronic dacryocystitis carries a high risk of bacterial keratitis.

An intact *corneal epithelium* forms the third line of defense with its tight junctions (through zonula occludens) and phagocytic activity. Most bacteria require a pre-existing epithelial defect for penetration into the corneal stroma. However, *Neisseria gonorrhoeae, Listeria monocytogenes, Corynebacterium diphtheriae* and *Haemophilus aegyptius* are known to cross an intact epithelium and set up an infection. Conditions resulting in compromised epithelium such as epithelial bullae, postherpetic corneal anesthesia, spheroidal degenerations, postkeratoplasty, recurrent corneal erosions, epithelial and Bowman's membrane dystrophies are some of the conditions that can predispose to bacterial keratitis.

External Risk Factors

Contact lens use is the most common predisposing factor for bacterial keratitis in the developed countries.[8] Infection can occur with all types of contact lens with an increased risk for extended wear lenses and therapeutic bandage contact lenses. Corneal hypoxia, repetitive microtrauma to the epithelium, collection of debris and the close proximity of bacterial biofilms are the pathogenic mechanisms for contact lens-induced keratitis. *Pseudomonas aeruginosa* is the most common organism associated with contact lens-induced keratitis.[4] With the help of pili, the bacteria adhere to the contact lens case, the contact lens and the cleaning solutions, and an unhealthy epithelium. The organism is capable of forming a biofilm which subsequently prevents the penetration of the antimicrobial agents in these settings.

Trauma, either with metal foreign bodies, contaminated soil and vegetable matter is the most common predisposing factor in developing countries.[9] Contaminated soil is associated with *Nocardia* keratitis and broomstick injury with *Bacillus* infection. Refractive surgeries are known to predispose to infections with nontuberculous mycobacteria with an indolent course.[10]

Bacterial Virulence

Once the host defense factors are breeched, the bacteria adhere to the margins of the epithelial defect and the stroma with the help of bacterial adhesins like lipoteichoic acid of *Staphylococcus* and pili of *Pseudomonas.* Some of the bacteria can evade the host complement system activation with the capsular lipopolysaccharides. The bacterial cell wall components and the toxins (exotoxin and endotoxin) secreted, trigger a potent host immune response. Activation of the local immune system and secretion of cytokines like interleukins (IL-1, IL-6, IL-8) and tumor necrosis factor-alpha (TNF-α) cause chemotaxis of leukocytes (neutrophils in the early stage and macrophages in the late stages), from the dilated limbal blood vessels.[11] Activated neutrophils cause collagenolysis by two pathways namely: (1) the matrix metalloproteinase-8 (MMP-8) degradation pathway and (2) plasminogen-mediated pathway. In addition, the tissue inhibitors of MMPs (TIMP-1 and TIMP-2) are also downregulated and thereby exacerbating the degradation of the collagen and leading to liquefactive necrosis.[12]

CLINICAL FEATURES

The symptoms and signs vary with the virulence of the bacteria and the existing predisposing factors.[13] Patients present with symptoms of sudden onset severe eye pain, redness, tearing, mucoid or purulent discharge, photophobia and defective vision. A history of trauma or contact lens use may be associated. Prior treatment with steroids and antimicrobials can alter the clinical appearance of the lesion and may reduce the microbial yield in smears and culture. Lid edema, severe blepharospasm, conjunctival injection with or without chemosis and discharge are the accompanying signs. An epithelial defect is invariably present in the early stages of the disease.

The initial stage is also known as the *stage of progressive infiltration* (Fig. 23.1.1) with an epithelial defect and rapidly increasing cellular infiltrate and edema. This stage progresses to a *stage of active ulceration* (Fig. 23.1.2) with the progression of the epithelial defect, stromal necrosis and dense corneal suppuration with fuzzy margins surrounded by corneal edema. Hypopyon is usually present and it is flat

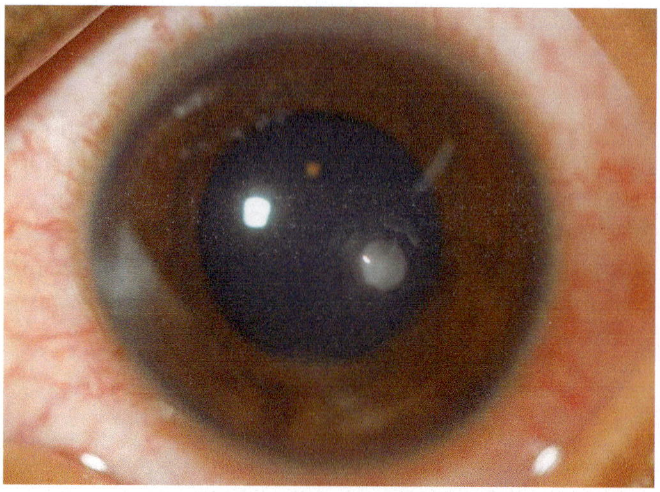

Fig. 23.1.1: Early bacterial keratitis. A 2 × 1 mm early dirty white infiltrate with rounded margins and wet surface.

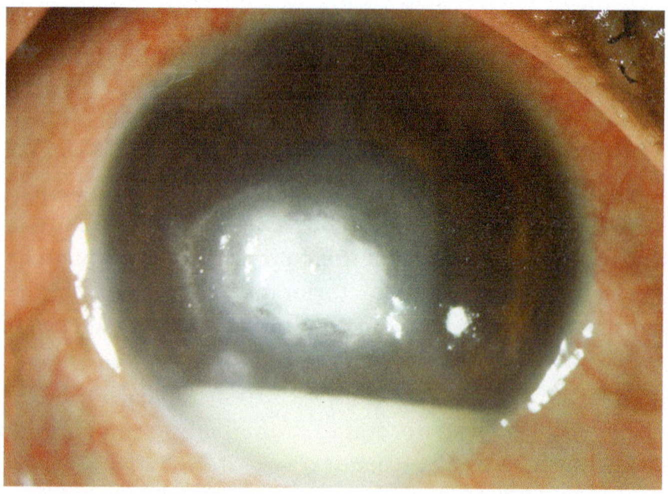

Fig. 23.1.2: Active bacterial keratitis with hypopyon. Central stromal necrosis with active edges and a flat dirty white hypopyon.

and mobile. The anterior chamber reaction is usually severe with dense fibrinary reaction. With appropriate therapy, the severity of the symptoms comes down; the ulcer margins get more defined with resolution of surrounding corneal edema in the *stage of regression and healing* (Fig. 23.1.3). This stage is characterized by re-epithelialization and graying of the ulcer suggestive of scarring which starts from the margins and the superficial anterior stroma and progresses to the entire infiltrate.

If the ulcer is not treated at appropriate time, further liquefactive necrosis leads to corneal thinning, descemetocele and corneal perforation. A small perforation may be self-sealed with plugging by the iris tissue. Pseudocornea formation with the exudates may be seen over a perforation. Extension of the infiltrate to sclera to form scleral abscess can occur in certain bacterial infection such as caused by *Nocardia*. The differential diagnosis for patients with symptoms of corneal ulcer is given in Table 23.1.2. Clinical features of bacterial keratitis, fungal keratitis and *Acanthamoeba* keratitis are compared in Table 23.1.3. Clinical features of specific bacteria are given in the Table 23.1.4 and in Figures 23.1.4 to 23.1.7.

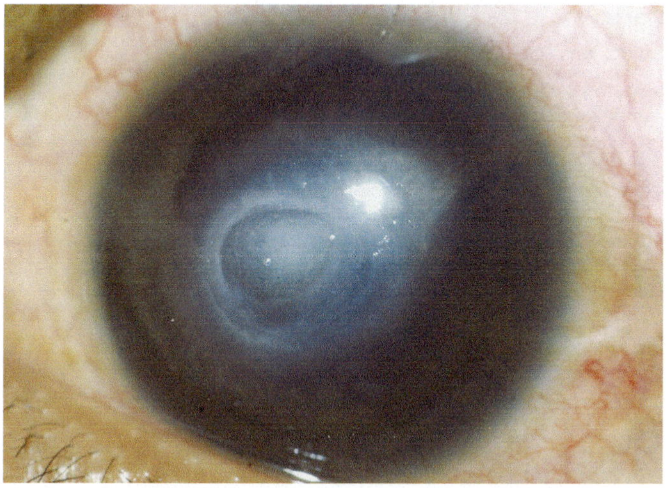

Fig. 23.1.3: Resolving bacterial keratitis. Well-defined epithelial defect smaller than the infiltrate. Gray infiltrate with scarred margins.

DIAGNOSIS

Microbial investigations ensure an appropriate therapy and enhance the knowledge of regional microbial profile and antibiotic sensitivity pattern.[14] The specimen from the corneal infection is obtained using a heat sterilized Kimura's spatula/Bard-Parker knife/26-gauge needle/Hockey stick knife after the application of topical anesthetics. Proparacaine is preferred as the topical anesthetic agent, since it does not interfere with the identification of the bacteria because of its lower antimicrobial activity. The scrapings are taken from the active edges and the base of the ulcer. Plating of the superficial slough alone may not

Table 23.1.2: Differential diagnosis of keratitis.

Infectious keratitis	Noninfectious keratitis
Bacterial keratitis	Shield ulcer of vernal keratoconjunctivitis
Fungal keratitis	Interstitial keratitis
Acanthamoeba keratitis	Peripheral ulcerative keratitis
Onchocerciasis	Keratomalacia
Viral keratitis	Fascicular ulcer
• Herpes simplex keratitis	Phlyctenular keratitis
• Herpes zoster keratitis	Marginal keratitis
• Epstein-Barr keratitis	Keratitis medicamentosa
Microsporidial keratitis	Factitious keratitis
	Chemical injury

Table 23.1.3: Comparison of clinical features of keratitis caused by bacteria, fungi, and *Acanthamoeba*.

	Bacterial keratitis	Fungal keratitis	*Acanthamoeba* keratitis
Predisposing factors	Contact lens use Decompensated cornea Immunocompromised status Trauma with metal foreign bodies	Trauma with vegetable matter Contaminated soil exposure	Contaminated fresh water bodies Contact lens use
Symptoms	Severe from early stage with watering, severe pain and photophobia	Relatively less severe pain in the initial stages	Pain disproportionate to signs due to perineuritis
Accompanying signs	Lid edema, mucopurulent to mucoid discharge, chemosis, conjunctival injection, photophobia	Minimal lid edema, tearing, conjunctival injection, photophobia	Lid edema, chemosis, conjunctival injection, tearing and photophobia
Keratitis	Dirty white dense suppuration with rounded margins, stromal abscess and surrounding corneal edema	Dry ulcer with feathery margins, plaque lesions, satellite lesions, endoexudate Pigmentation can be present	Epithelial irregularity, grayish white diffuse infiltrate in ring pattern, perineuritis, immune ring. Indolent course
Hypopyon	Thin, grayish white, flat, mobile	Thick immobile, dome-shaped	Minimal

Table 23.1.4: Clinical features of specific bacteria.

Bacteria	Clinical features
Gram-positive bacteria	
Staphylococcus aureus	Most common bacteria of ocular flora. Most common Gram-positive bacterial keratitis in developed countries. Commonly associated in compensated corneas like bullous keratopathy, dry eye, vernal keratoconjunctivitis, postherpetic keratitis, postkeratoplasty Rapid dense suppuration. Antibiotic resistance should be expected in nonresolving cases
Staphylococcus epidermidis	Slow indolent course. Common in compensated corneas
Streptococcus pneumoniae	Most common bacteria causing keratitis in developing countries. Associated with chronic dacryocystitis, filtering bleb infections and trauma. Rapidly progressive infiltrate with one advancing margin and one healing margin. Perforation is common
Nocardia asteroides	Associated with exposure to contaminated soil. Severe pain. Multiple tiny pinhead-shaped infiltrate arranged in classic wreath pattern. Protracted course of healing
Nontuberculous mycobacteria	Associated with postrefractive surgery, postcorneal tear repair. Slow indolent course with well-defined grayish white infiltrates. These infiltrates can develop radial projections leading to cracked windshield appearance
Gram-negative bacteria	
Pseudomonas aeruginosa	Most common Gram-negative bacteria causing keratitis in the world. Rapidly progressive dense infiltrate with severe necrosis and perforation. Surrounding corneal edema with ground-glass appearance. Greenish yellow discharge
Serratia marcescens	Pink hypopyon. Associated with contact lens use
Neisseria gonorrhoeae	Associated with hyperpurulent conjunctivitis. Severe chemosis, rapidly progressive infiltrate. Perforation is common. Systemic ceftriaxone is indicated
Others	
Infectious crystalline keratopathy	Mostly seen with α-hemolytic streptococci. Deep infiltrate with multiple needle-like extensions resembling snowflake especially in a postkeratoplasty patient. Bacterial colonies grow in the interlamellar spaces of the stroma to produce this pattern. Other causative organisms are *Pneumococcus, Staphylococcus epidermidis, Peptostreptococcus, Haemophilus, Pseudomonas*. Treatment is with fortified cephalosporin.

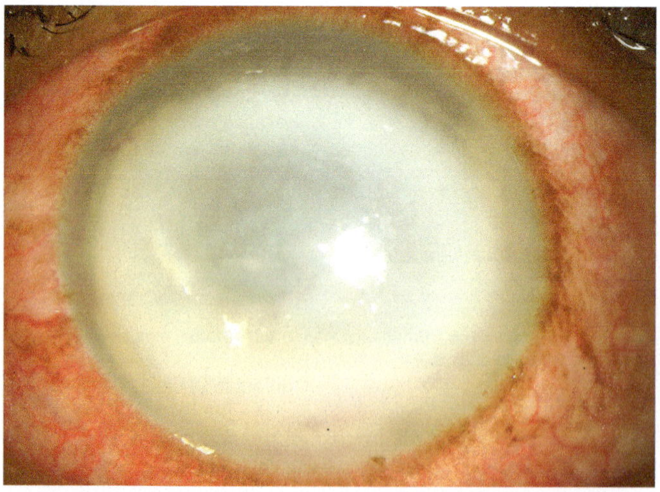

Fig. 23.1.4: *Bacillus cereus* keratitis. Subtotal corneal ulcer with dense infiltration and thick hypopyon.

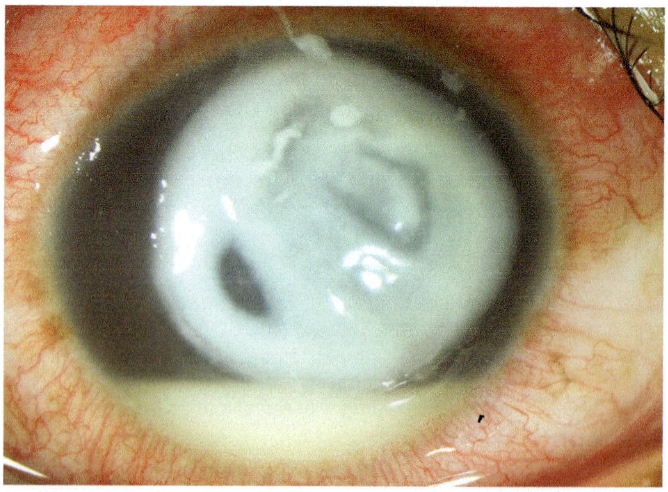

Fig. 23.1.5: *Pseudomonas* keratitis. Dense ring infiltrate with severe necrosis and surrounding corneal edema with discharge.

yield good microbial results. In the scenario of corneal thinning, scraping should be as gentle as possible, so as to avoid perforation. The first half of the specimen is smeared on one to two thin glass slides for direct smear examination and the second half is inoculated into the culture media in alternating "C" strokes. The specimen should be examined for the microbiological investigations within 30 minutes for better microbial yield. Gram stain and potassium hydroxide (KOH) wet mount are the routinely performed smear examinations. Other smears include Giemsa,

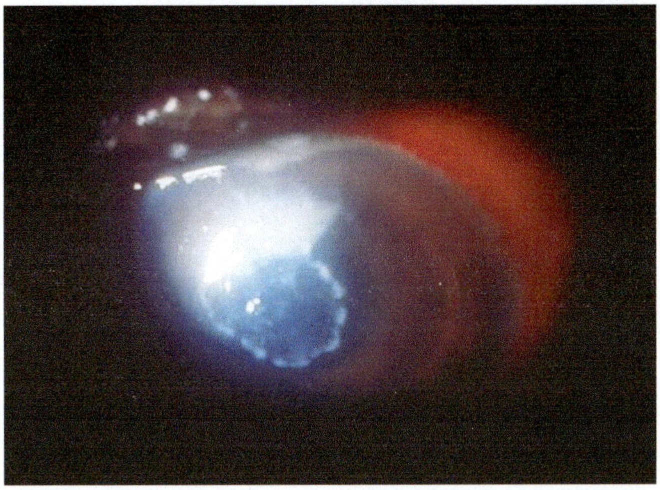

Fig. 23.1.6: *Nocardia* keratitis. Multiple tiny pinhead-shaped infiltrate arranged in classic wreath pattern.

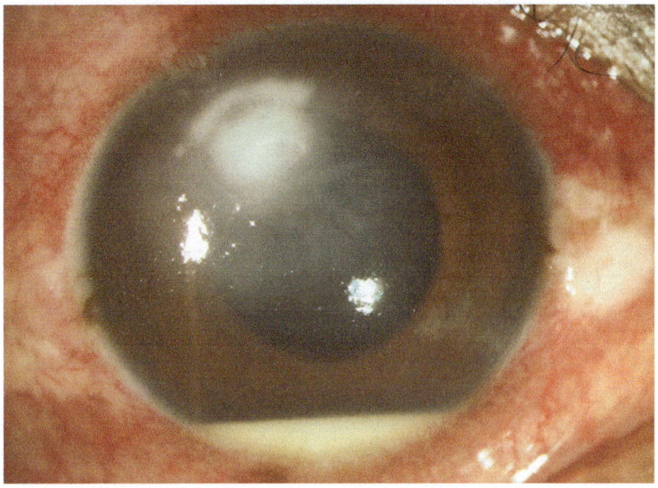

Fig. 23.1.7: Atypical mycobacteria keratitis. Paracentral grayish white infiltrate with surrounding satellite lesions.

Ziehl-Neelsen, modified Ziehl-Neelsen and acridine orange. Blood agar and chocolate agar are the most commonly used culture media for bacteria. Sabouraud dextrose agar is used for isolation of fungi. Special media like Thioglycolate broth for anaerobic bacteria, Löwenstein-Jensen medium for *Mycobacterium* and Thayer-Martin medium for *Neisseria*, are used for isolating organisms that are difficult to grow on routine media. In deeper corneal infiltrates, a corneal biopsy with 2–3 mm trephine may be needed for specimen collection. Alternatively, a sterile silk suture can be passed through the deep infiltrate and can be plated onto culture. Reculture is indicated if the initial culture is negative and the ulcer is progressing with empirical therapy. Cessation of the antibiotic 12–24 hours before reculture increases the microbial yield. The role of polymerase chain reaction in bacterial keratitis may help to exclude fungus but at the same time, its role is limited as many bacteria are normal conjunctival flora. The current resolution of in vivo confocal microscopy cannot identify bacteria except *Nocardia.*[15] Examination of the nasolacrimal duct passage by applying pressure over the lacrimal sac area and/or syringing is recommended in all the cases of corneal ulcers. Corneal sensation should also be checked carefully. Intraocular pressure measurement by digital tonometry may be useful to suspect secondary glaucoma. Systemic immunosuppression, if suspected, must be ruled out with appropriate blood investigations. Adequate control of blood glucose in diabetic patients is necessary for resolution of corneal ulcer.

TREATMENT (FLOWCHART 23.1.2)

Adequate and appropriate topical antibiotic application is the cornerstone of the treatment regimen in patients with bacterial keratitis. With frequent application through topical route, higher tissue concentrations of the drug are obtained. While clinical appearance may aid in the diagnosis, treatment should be based on microbiological examinations. The recommended smear-guided therapy for various bacteria is given in Table 23.1.5. If there is a delay in microbiological report or if the initial smear is negative, an empirical therapy with broad-spectrum fourth-generation fluoroquinolones (0.3% gatifloxacin or 0.5% moxifloxacin eye drops) or a combination of fortified cephalosporin with fortified aminoglycoside may be initiated.[13] The frequency of medication varies with the severity of the disease. A loading dose is usually preferred with application of topical antibiotics every minute for the first 5 minutes, followed by every 5 minutes for the first hour and then hourly during the waking hours and 2 hourly at night. If two antibiotics are used, then a minimum interval of 5–10 minutes between applications is needed between both the drops as immediate application might wash away the other antibiotic from the conjunctival cul-de-sac. Cycloplegics like topical homatropine or atropine is used to relieve the ciliary spasm and to break any synechiae formation. Systemic analgesic to reduce the severity of pain is a major adjuvant in treatment.

The patient is reviewed periodically depending on the severity to reassess the severity and to modify the

Flowchart 23.1.2: Treatment algorithm of bacterial corneal ulcer.

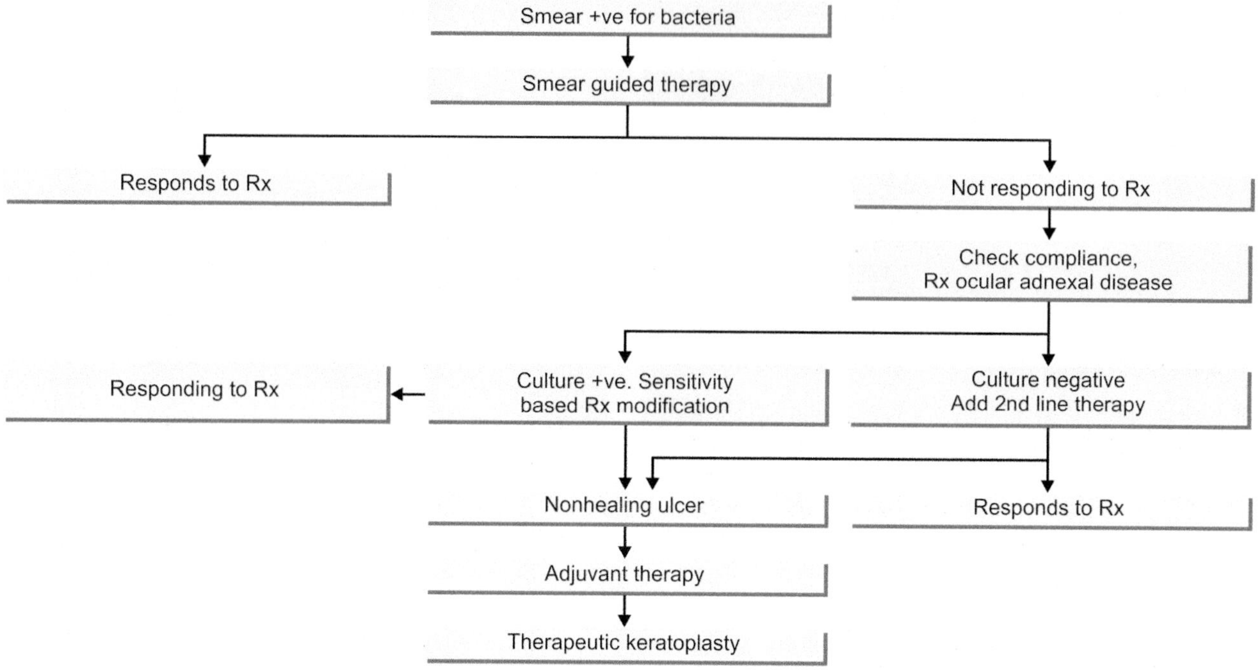

Table 23.1.5: Smear-guided therapy.

Organism	First line of therapy	Second line of therapy
Gram-positive cocci	Fortified cephalosporins 5% or 50 mg/mL cefazolin 0.5% chloramphenicol	0.5% moxifloxacin or 0.3% gatifloxacin 5% or 50 mg/mL vancomycin
Gram-positive bacilli	0.5% moxifloxacin or 0.3% gatifloxacin	1.4% or 14 mg/mL tobramycin/gentamicin
Nocardia asteroides	2–4% amikacin	Trimethoprim/sulfamethoxazole (16:80 mg/mL) 5% ampicillin
Nontuberculous mycobacteria	2–4% amikacin 0.5% moxifloxacin or 0.3% gatifloxacin	Clarithromycin
Gram-negative cocci	5% or 50 mg/mL ceftazidime or ceftriaxone	0.5% moxifloxacin or 0.3% gatifloxacin
Gram-negative bacilli	1.4% or 14 mg/mL tobramycin/gentamicin 0.5% moxifloxacin or 0.3% gatifloxacin	5% or 50 mg/mL ceftazidime
No organism	0.5% moxifloxacin or 0.3% gatifloxacin	5% or 50 mg/mL cefazolin with 1.4% or 14 mg/mL tobramycin/gentamicin

therapy based on culture reports. If the ulcer progresses with smear-guided therapy, then compliance of the patient should be checked with the quantity of leftover medication in the prescribed bottle. A careful re-examination to rule out the persistence of predisposing factors should be done. Progression despite smear-guided therapy also may indicate resistant bacterial strains and the second line of therapy should be initiated (Table 23.1.5). If the ulcer progresses in a patient with negative smear and culture report, then reculture is performed after stopping the antibiotic for 12–24 hours and the therapy is modified. In patients with persistence of symptoms, drug toxicity should be ruled out especially with fortified antibiotics.

With appropriate therapy, if the organism is susceptible, patients respond to treatment with reduction in the severity of symptoms. The margins of the ulcer become more blunted and demarcated and the edges begin to get scarred. The frequency of antibiotic drops is reduced gradually with the appearance of signs of resolution and stopped with complete resolution. Use of steroids in corneal ulcer is controversial. In a large randomized control trial, the steroids in corneal ulcer trial (SCUT) studying the efficacy of adjunctive topical steroid to topical antibiotics, there was no significant difference in the 3-month best-corrected visual acuity compared to a placebo.[16] Steroids, if indicated should be started in smear proven bacterial corneal ulcers after 48 hours of antibiotic use. In ulcers unresponsive to maximal medical therapy, progressive thinning can occur which further worsens to descemetocele and perforation. If the perforation is small and peripheral, iris plugs the wound. In general, there is a tendency for the ulcer to heal after such small perforations as there is associated fresh flow of aqueous with new antibodies. Adjuvant therapy with cyanoacrylate glue and bandage contact lens may be required in smaller perforations. Multilayered amniotic membrane graft can also be used in smaller perforation and nonhealing ulcers. In cases of persistent epithelial defect, a therapeutic contact lens or temporary tarsorrhaphy might help. Collagen cross-linking with ultraviolet A (UVA) and riboflavin has been tried with variable results in ulcers refractive to conventional therapy. Antibacterial activity of UVA and strengthening of collagen by cross-linking are the suggested mechanisms of action of corneal cross-linking (CXL) in bacterial keratitis. At present CXL is used as an adjuvant to conventional therapy in refractory cases caused by multidrug-resistant strains.[17] If the ulcer is persistent or the perforation is large, a therapeutic keratoplasty is performed for maintaining the structural integrity and reduction of the microbial load. The indications and steps of therapeutic keratoplasty are described in Table 23.1.6. Although the outcomes of keratoplasty in an acutely inflamed eye are poor with high chances of graft rejection and failure, the outcomes of therapeutic keratoplasty in bacterial keratitis are better compared to therapeutic keratoplasty for fungal keratitis.[18]

Table 23.1.6: Therapeutic keratoplasty.

Indications
- Perforated corneal ulcer
- Impending perforation
- Nonhealing corneal ulcer in spite of appropriate and adequate therapy
- Ulcer threatening to involve limbus

Preoperative work-up
- Informed consent with explanation of the purpose of the procedure is for preserving the structural integrity or reducing the load of infection
- Intravenous mannitol or oral acetazolamide to reduce intraoperative positive pressure
- Anesthesia—local anesthesia or general anesthesia. In local anesthesia, facial block is given first to prevent excess squeezing of the lids during peribulbar anesthesia. In complicated cases, general anesthesia is preferred

Procedure
- The size of the ulcer is measured. The excised corneal tissue should have at least 1 mm clear margin throughout. Peritomy should be done in large ulcers extending to the limbus
- Full-thickness donor button of size 0.5–1 mm larger than the host cornea is taken with the help of a handheld punch or guillotine punch
- Partial trephination of the host cornea is done with a trephine
- Careful and controlled entry into anterior chamber with a stab incision is made
- Host cornea is excised manually with corneal scissors
- Exudates over the iris, angle and the lens are removed carefully
- Retain the lens as much as possible. In case of obvious capsular rupture, lens removal may be done
- One to two peripheral iridectomies can be performed
- The donor cornea is sutured with the host rim with 10-0 or 9-0 nylon interrupted sutures. First four cardinal sutures at 12, 6, 3 and 9 o'clock position are placed respectively. The donor button is sutured with 16–24 interrupted sutured depending on the size of the graft

Postoperative management
- *Immediate postoperative period:*
  - Continue appropriate antimicrobials at least for the first 2 months
  - Topical or oral antiglaucoma drugs in cases of postoperative glaucoma
  - Frequent follow-up in the early postoperative period for early detection of complications is needed
  - Steroids can be used in the early postoperative period, if keratoplasty is done for bacterial ulcers. For keratoplasty done for fungal corneal ulcers, steroids can be withheld for the first postoperative month
- *Late postoperative period:*
  - Loose sutures to be selectively removed to prevent vascularization and reinfection
  - Sutures with obvious infiltration can be removed selectively
  - In failed grafts with at least 6 months of infection-free period, repeat optical keratoplasty can be performed for visual rehabilitation

REFERENCES

1. Lin CC, Lalitha P, Srinivasan M, et al. Seasonal trends of microbial keratitis in South India. Cornea. 2012;31(10):1123-7.
2. Lalitha P, Prajna NV, Manoharan G, et al. Trends in bacterial and fungal keratitis in South India, 2002–2012. Br J Ophthalmol. 2015;99:192-4.
3. Lichtinger A, Yeung SN, Kim P, et al. Shifting trends in bacterial keratitis in Toronto: an 11-year review. Ophthalmology. 2012;119(9):1785-90.
4. Cheung N, Nagra P, Hammersmith K. Emerging trends in contact lens-related infections. Curr Opin Ophthalmol. 2016;27(4):327-32.
5. Schaefer F, Bruttin O, Zografos L, et al. Bacterial keratitis: a prospective clinical and microbiological study. Br J Ophthalmol. 2001;85:842-7.
6. McDermott AM. Antimicrobial compounds in tears. Exp Eye Res. 2013;117:53-61.
7. McClellan KA. Mucosal defense of the outer eye. Surv Ophthalmol. 1997;42(3):233-46.
8. Bourcier T, Thomas F, Borderie V, et al. Bacterial keratitis: predisposing factors, clinical and microbiological review of 300 cases. Br J Ophthalmol. 2003;87:834-8.
9. Gopinathan U, Sharma S, Garg P, et al. Review of epidemiological features, microbiological diagnosis and treatment outcome of microbial keratitis: experience of over a decade. Indian J Ophthalmol. 2009;57(4):273-9.
10. Haq Z, Farooq AV, Huang AJ. Infections after refractive surgery. Curr Opin Ophthalmol. 2016;27(4):367-72.
11. Karthikeyan RS, Priya JL, Leal SM Jr, et al. Host response and bacterial virulence factor expression in *Pseudomonas aeruginosa* and *Streptococcus pneumoniae* corneal ulcers. PLoS One. 2013;8(6):e64867.
12. Xue ML, Wakefield D, Willcox MD, et al. Regulation of MMPs and TIMPs by IL-1b during corneal ulceration and infection. Invest Ophthalmol Vis Sci. 2003;44:2020-5.
13. American Academy of Ophthalmology. (2005). Bacterial keratitis, Preferred Practice Pattern. [online] Available from: *www.aao.org/ppp*. [Accessed November, 2017].
14. Garg P, Rao GN. Corneal ulcer: diagnosis and management. Community Eye Health. 1999;12(30):21-3.
15. Labbé A, Khammari C, Dupas B. Contribution of in vivo confocal microscopy to the diagnosis and management of infectious keratitis. Ocul Surf. 2009;7(1):41-52.
16. Srinivasan M, Mascarenhas J, Rajaraman R, et al. Corticosteroids for bacterial keratitis: the Steroids for Corneal Ulcers Trial (SCUT). Arch Ophthalmol. 2012;130(2):143-50.
17. Said DG, Elalfy MS, Gatzioufas Z, et al. Collagen cross-linking with photoactivated riboflavin (PACK-CXL) for the treatment of advanced infectious keratitis with corneal melting. Ophthalmology. 2014;121(7):1377-82.
18. Sharma N, Sachdev R, Jhanji V. Therapeutic keratoplasty for microbial keratitis. Curr Opin Ophthalmol. 2010;21:293-300.

23.2 FUNGAL KERATITIS

INTRODUCTION

Fungal keratitis is the most common cause of corneal ulcer in the developing countries.[1] Contrary to the historic concept of this problem affecting debilitated individuals, the bulk of the fungal corneal ulcers affecting this population happens in immunocompetent individuals engaged in agrarian activities. While the filamentous fungi (*Fusarium* and *Aspergillus*) are the most common etiological agents for causing fungal keratitis in tropical regions, yeasts like *Candida* play an important role in temperate climates.[2] The filamentous fungi gain access to the human cornea after a corneal abrasion or trauma, most commonly involving some kind of vegetable matter. The yeasts usually cause keratitis in immunocompromised individuals. Their pathogenicity is related to a decrease in the systemic or local defense mechanisms either by a direct effect on the immune system (topical steroids) or by an alteration in the normal epithelial barriers (i.e. persistent epithelial defects, bandage contact lenses, neurotrophic keratitis, topical anesthetics, etc.) with predisposing systemic and/or eye disease. The dimorphic fungi are a rare cause of keratitis.

The clinical outcomes of fungal keratitis are worse than bacterial keratitis due to delayed diagnosis, inappropriate use of antibiotics and/or steroids, virulence of the organism as well as a limited choice of antifungal drugs.[3] In spite of adequate treatment, a quarter of the patients with fungal keratitis fail medical treatment and will require surgical intervention like keratoplasty.[3]

CLASSIFICATION

Fungi are eukaryotic and heterotrophic organisms. Although numerous fungi have been implicated, the pathogenic fungi, which cause significant keratitis, can be divided into filamentous, yeast and dimorphic forms.

Filamentous Fungi

Also known as molds, they occur as long filaments, called hyphae, which grow by apical extension and produce feathery aerial colonies above the culture media. They can be further divided into septate and nonseptate organisms. The septate filamentary fungi are the most common cause of keratomycosis. They are divided into nonpigmented hyaline fungi (which include *Fusarium* spp, *Aspergillus* spp, and *Acremonium* spp) and pigmented dematiaceous fungi (*Curvularia* spp, *Lasiodiplodia* spp) varieties. The nonseptate filamentary fungi (*Mucor, Absidia* and *Rhizopus* spp) are important cause of orbital disease and endogenous endophthalmitis, but do not commonly produce corneal disease.

Yeasts

Yeasts are unicellular organisms and form creamy, pasty colonies, which may be mistaken for staphylococcal colonies. They divide by asexual budding, forming pseudohyphae and do not form mycelium in culture. The most common fungi in this category are the *Candida* spp and *Cryptococcus* spp, which are part of the normal flora of skin, respiratory tract and conjunctiva and act as opportunistic pathogens.

Dimorphic Fungi

They possess two distinct morphologic forms: (1) the yeast phase which occurs in tissues and (2) a mycelial phase which occurs in media and natural surfaces. These fungi, which include *Blastomyces, Coccidioides, Histoplasma* and *Sporothrix,* exhibit properties of molds at 25°C and of yeasts when grown at 37°C.

PATHOGENESIS

Stage of Fungal Entry and Adhesion

Fungal conidial spores gain access to the cornea through a breach in the corneal epithelium, often following a trivial shearing trauma with a vegetative foreign body like paddy husk, onion skin flakes or groundnut skin. Invasiveness of the fungi is directly related to the fungal load and immune response. After entry, the conidia shed the outer protective protein coat and expose the cell wall proteins namely β-glucans. The cell wall proteins bind with the mannose glycoproteins expressed on the corneal epithelial cells and this causes the fungus to adhere to the epithelial cells. The conidia elongate to produce hyphae which branch out and interconnect with surrounding hyphae to form large mycelia.

Activation of the Innate and Adaptive Immunity

The pattern recognition receptors (PRRs) on the corneal epithelium [Dectin 1 and 2, Toll-like receptor 2 (TLR2), TLR4 and nucleotide-binding oligomerization domain-like receptor, NOD2] identify the conserved microbial structures present in the fungus, called pathogen-associated molecular patterns (PAMPs) and activate the innate immunity.[4,5] Activation of the innate immunity leads to increased secretion of proinflammatory cytokines like IL-8, IL-1β, IL-17 and interferon-γ which are involved in neutrophil recruitment from the limbal vasculature and activation of adaptive immune response. Neutrophils form the major immune response in fungal keratitis followed by macrophages and lymphocytes.[6]

Sequelae of Immune Response

Neutrophil activation leads to secretion of proteases like matrix metalloproteinases (MMP-8, MMP-9), serine protease (Cathepsin) and cysteine protease which causes collagenolysis and disruption of extracellular matrix glycoproteins. The corneal collagen is degraded by the MMP activity, which in turn is regulated by tissue inhibitors of metalloproteinases (TIMPs). Increased activity of MMP-8 and MMP-9 associated with the infiltration of polymorphonuclear neutrophils (PMNs) and an insufficient increase in TIMP-1 and TIMP-2 may be actively involved in the excessive collagenolysis and stromal necrosis.[7] Neutrophils also wrap the fungal hyphae and produce reactive oxygen species (ROSs) at close proximity to the hyphae, through the nicotinamide adenine dinucleotide phosphate (NADPH) oxidase (NOX) system. These ROSs can interact with the cell membrane and the cytoplasmic components leading to fungal cell death. Thioredoxin and superoxide dismutase in the fungal hyphae are involved in metabolizing these ROSs to oxygen and water and hence resist the oxidative stress. Prolonged multiplication of the hyphae increases the fungal load and leads to increased immune response and further stromal necrosis. Certain fungi also produce toxins which help in its invasiveness. Aflatoxin in animal models can produce corneal haziness with edema, separation of corneal lamellae and neutrophil infiltration.[7]

CLINICAL FEATURES

When compared with bacterial keratitis, the symptoms in this condition (congestion, chemosis, pain, discharge) are correspondingly less as to what one traditionally expects out of an ulcer of a significant size. In the early stages of the fungal keratitis, there may even be no congestion. This is because the size of the fungi is much larger than the bacteria and hence the inflammatory cells are not able to phagocytose them rapidly and trigger off a complement cascade. The earliest finding may be a small nonspecific stromal infiltrate with a surrounding unhealthy epithelium, in which case it is indistinguishable from a bacterial infection. The lesion may mimic the dendrite of herpes simplex. These pseudodendritic lesions are shorter, stockier and are associated with surrounding stromal infiltration, edema and Descemet's membrane folds (Figs. 23.2.1A and B). Commonly, the patient presents with a central or a paracentral ulcer with feathery stromal margins (Fig. 23.2.2). The feathery margins are the characteristic hallmark of fungal keratitis.

With time, the ulcer starts to become larger and elevated above the level of the corneal surface (Fig. 23.2.3). The surface looks dirty white and dry and has a rough texture. In rare instances, the lesion may be entirely in the posterior aspect of the stroma without an accompanying epithelial defect. An endothelial plaque lesion is usually seen in the late stages (Fig. 23.2.4).

Foci of infiltration can be seen several millimeters away from the main area of involvement. These are called satellite lesions (Fig. 23.2.5). Like in many other keratitis, a ring infiltrate may surround the primary lesion, most likely

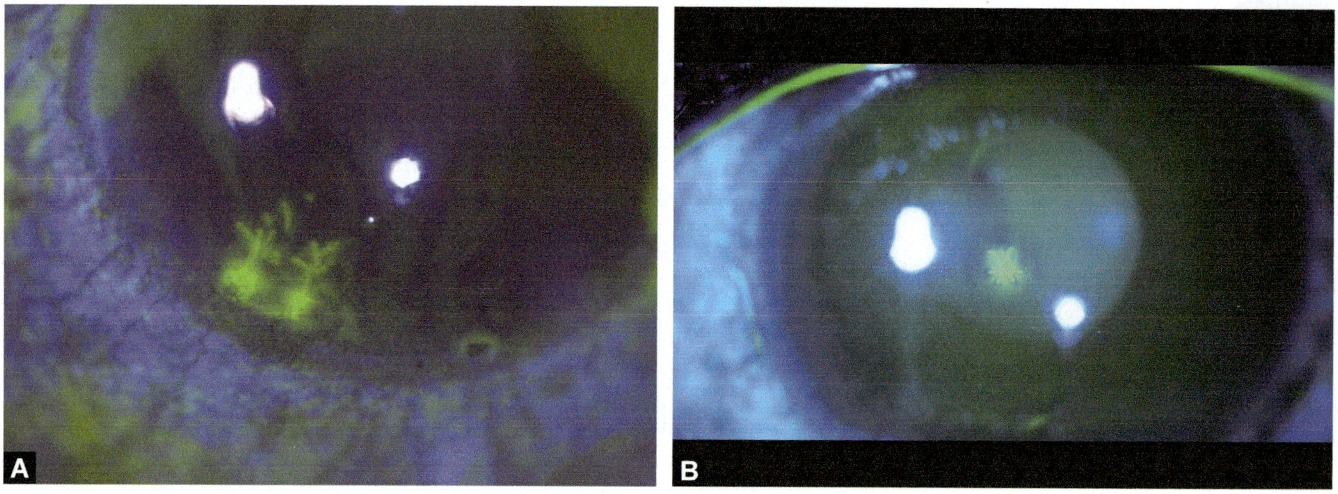

Figs. 23.2.1A and B: Fungal pseudodendrite versus viral dendrite. (A) Pseudodendrite of fungal keratitis; (B) Herpes simplex dendrite.

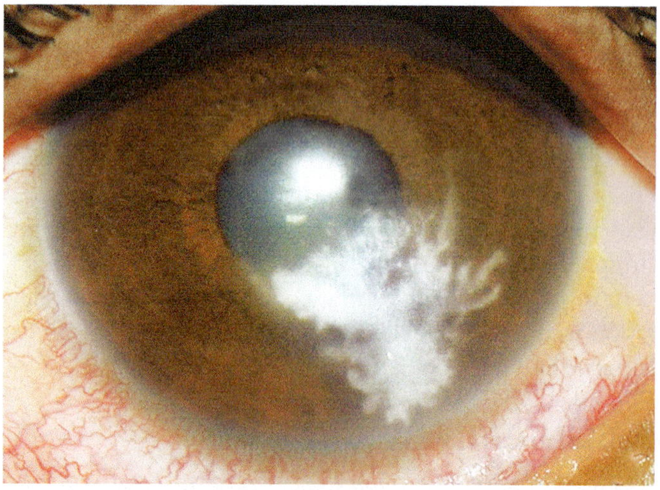

Fig. 23.2.2: Feathery margin. Active feathery margin ulcers. Characteristic of fungal keratitis.

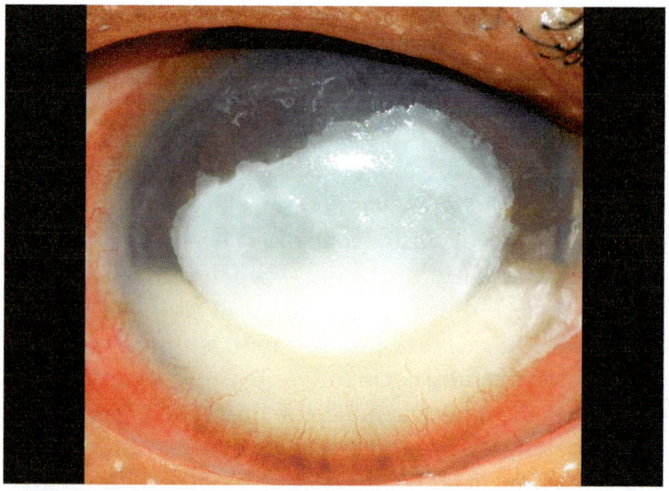

Fig. 23.2.3: Elevated plaque lesion. Thick leathery dirty white plaque lesion.

representing an antibody response to fungal antigen (Fig. 23.2.6). In certain instances, the entire lesion can start in the periphery and progress to form a ring infiltration and a ring abscess. The central cornea may be relatively spared. Hypopyon can be present in varying proportions and the amount is not directly proportional to the size of the ulcer (Fig. 23.2.7). The hypopyon is thick, immobile and has a dome-shaped configuration due the presence of fungal hyphae in it.

In the ulcers caused by the dematiaceous fungi, there may be macroscopic pigment deposition over the surface (Figs. 23.2.8A to C). The color may vary from a thick blackish brown pigmentary lesion to a less mottled greenish gray pigment dispersed over a whitish base. The denser lesion can be mistaken for a uveal prolapse (Figs. 23.2.9A and B). The lesion caused by dematiaceous fungi is more elevated than those caused by nonpigmentary filamentous fungi and has a characteristic mushroom head appearance. These lesions can be usually dissected from the surface using a Bard-Parker knife and has a tough, leathery attachment to the ulcer surface.

As the lesions progress, the pain starts to get intense and the ulcer starts to involve almost the whole of the cornea and starts to lose its characteristic pattern and becomes indistinguishable from advanced bacterial ulcer. A significant majority of the deeper stromal ulcers perforate over time.

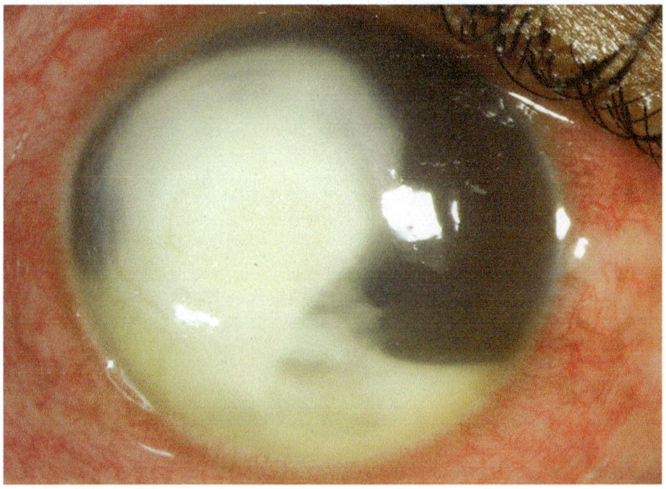

Fig. 23.2.4: Endothelial plaque. Dense posterior infiltrate with endothelial plaque and hypopyon.

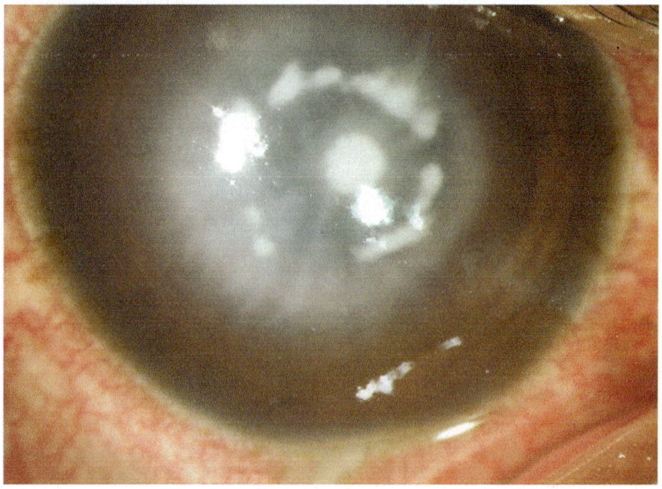

Fig. 23.2.5: Satellite lesions. Multiple pinpoint yellowish white lesions surrounding the central infiltrate.

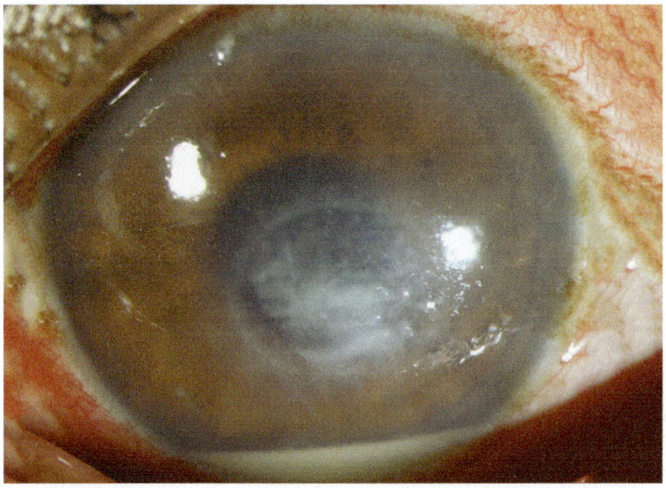

Fig. 23.2.6: Wessely's immune ring. Grayish white immune ring surrounding the infiltrate representing antigen-antibody reaction.

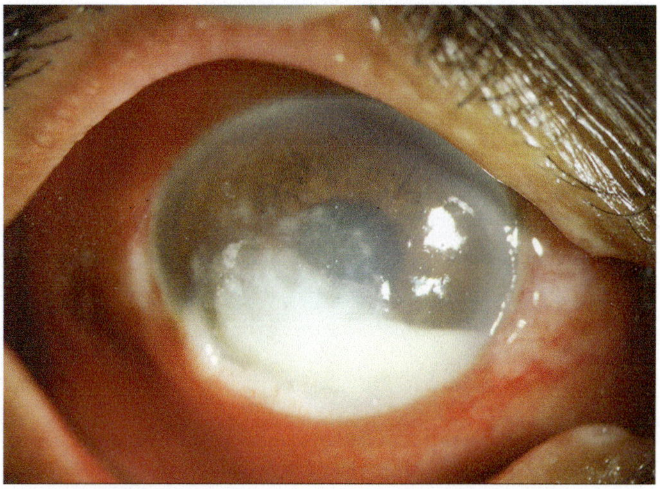

Fig. 23.2.7: Dome-shaped hypopyon. Thick yellowish white dome-shaped hypopyon.

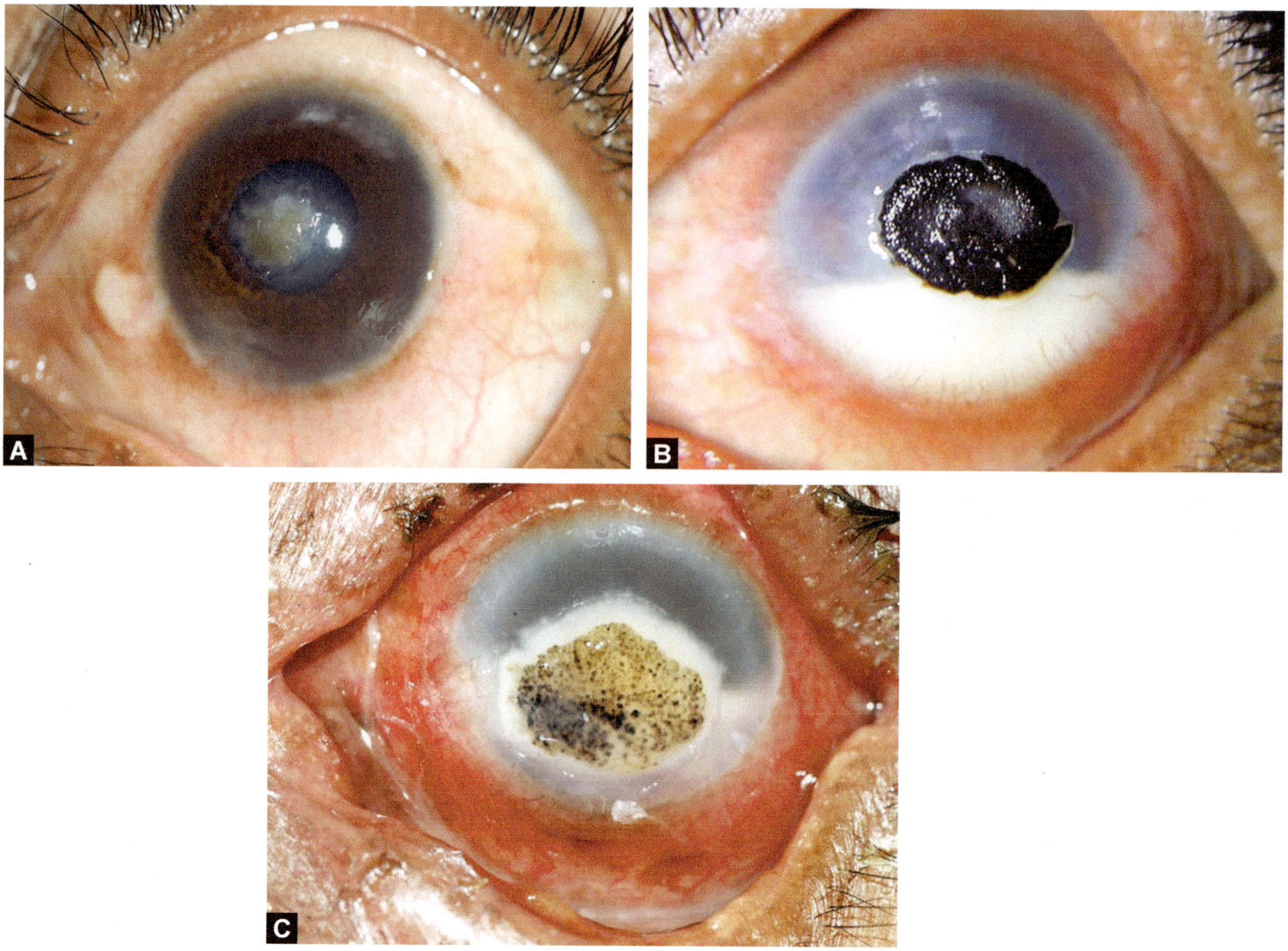

Figs. 23.2.8A to C: Dematiaceous fungal ulcer. Fungal corneal ulcer with various hues of pigmentation.

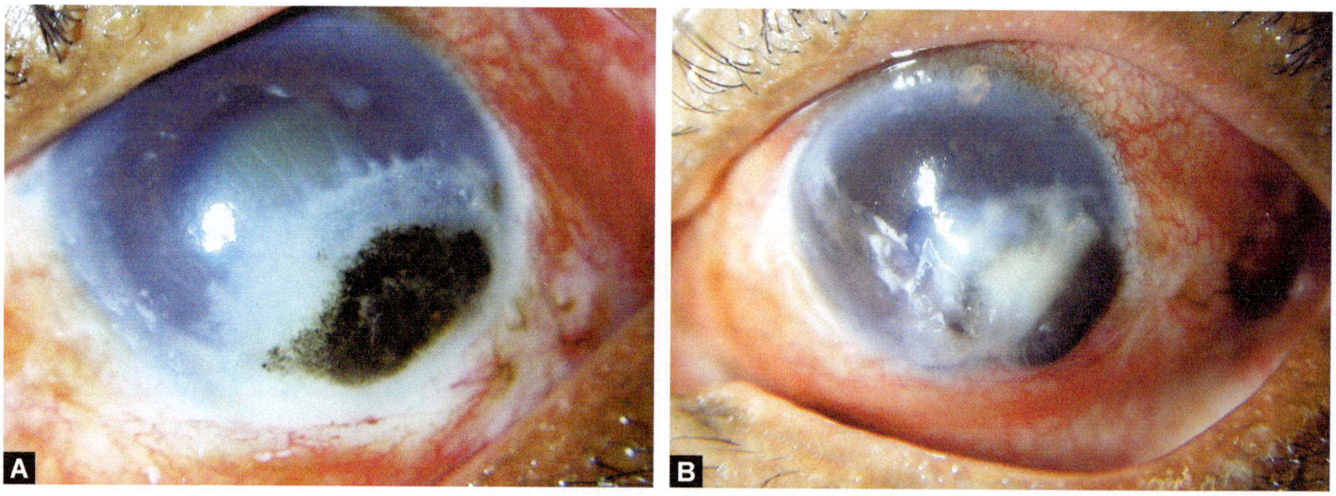

Figs. 23.2.9A and B: Dematiaceous keratitis versus iris prolapse. (A) Dematiaceous keratitis; (B) Iris prolapse.

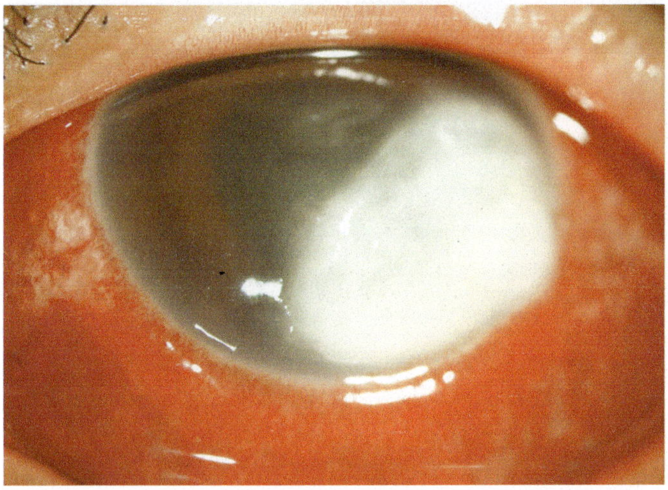

Fig. 23.2.10: *Candida* keratitis. Dense dirty white infiltrate with stromal necrosis.

In contrast to the fungal keratitis caused by filamentous fungi, stromal keratitis caused by *Candida* may be more localized and have a collar button configuration, often with a small ulceration and an expanding infiltrate (Fig. 23.2.10). They are usually superimposed on a chronic debilitative ocular condition. The lesions tend to be oval, plaque like and elevated. They are well outlined and surrounded by stromal edema and more closely resemble bacterial keratitis. If untreated, the keratitis evolves to produce dense suppuration and necrosis of the deep stroma.

INVESTIGATIONS

It should be emphasized that the differentiation between the advanced keratitis caused by bacteria and fungi can be very difficult to distinguish by clinical features alone (Figs. 23.2.11A to D). Despite these descriptive findings, studies to assess the clinical manifestations of bacterial versus fungal keratitis have demonstrated that it was not possible to differentiate between bacterial and fungal keratitis in all cases and microbiological investigations are essential to confirm the diagnosis.[8] This is even more crucial in the regions of the world, where fungi and bacteria cause keratitis, almost in equal proportions. Standard microbiological techniques such as smear examination and culture are more than enough in a majority of instances while sophisticated techniques like polymerase chain reaction (PCR) may be useful in some cases.

Specimen collection for microbiological evaluation: Scrapings are made from the base and the edges of the ulcer under topical anesthesia using a Bard-Parker knife/Kimura's spatula/26-gauge needle/Hockey stick knife. The lesions caused by fungi often feel gritty and have a leathery attachment to the base of the ulcer (Fig. 23.2.12). Calcium alginate swabs have been reported to increase the recovery rate of the organisms. In deeper lesions, a corneal biopsy using 2–3 mm trephine may be required for obtaining adequate specimen. Alternatively, a sterile silk suture can be passed through the deeper lesion and cultured.

Direct smear examination: The first half of the specimen is transferred to the glass slides for direct smear examination. Direct microscopic evaluation is the most valuable and rapid diagnostic tool for the detection of fungal elements in corneal scrapings.[9] The initial smears can be examined using a freshly prepared 10% KOH wet mount preparation and a Gram stain. The KOH preparation is a simple, reliable and reproducible screening method for identifying filamentary fungi (Fig. 23.2.13). KOH has been used as a 10–20% suspension, either as plain or with ink or with lactophenol cotton blue. Proteinaceous components such as host cells are partially digested by the alkali, leaving intact the polysaccharide-containing fungal cell walls. The sensitivity of KOH wet mount varies from 76% to 91% and is considered to be a simple and cost-effective procedure for diagnosis of fungal keratitis. The Gram stain does not stain the cell wall or septa of hyphal fragments but is absorbed by the protoplasm (Fig. 23.2.14). Yeasts typically stain dark blue and can be distinguished from bacteria, foreign material, precipitate and other artifacts.

Other stains which are useful include Giemsa stain, Gomori methenamine silver stain, acridine orange and calcofluor white. Hyphal fragments and yeasts appear dark blue or purple in Giemsa stain. Though the use of calcofluor white, acridine orange and fluorescein-conjugated lectins yield rapid results, special infrastructural requirements like fluorescent microscopes make them inapplicable in most situations (Fig. 23.2.15). Calcofluor white is a fabric whitener used in the textile industry and has an affinity for cellulose and chitin, which are common compounds of hyphal fragments and yeasts. The optical activity of acridine orange is due to the binding of the dye to the nuclear proteins of fungi to form a green fluorescing complex.

Fungal culture: Sabouraud dextrose agar (SDA), potato dextrose agar and Brain Heart infusion broth are the most commonly used primary isolation medium for fungi. Cycloheximide should never be incorporated in SDA, because it inhibits the saprophytic fungi predominantly responsible for keratitis. The media are kept at room

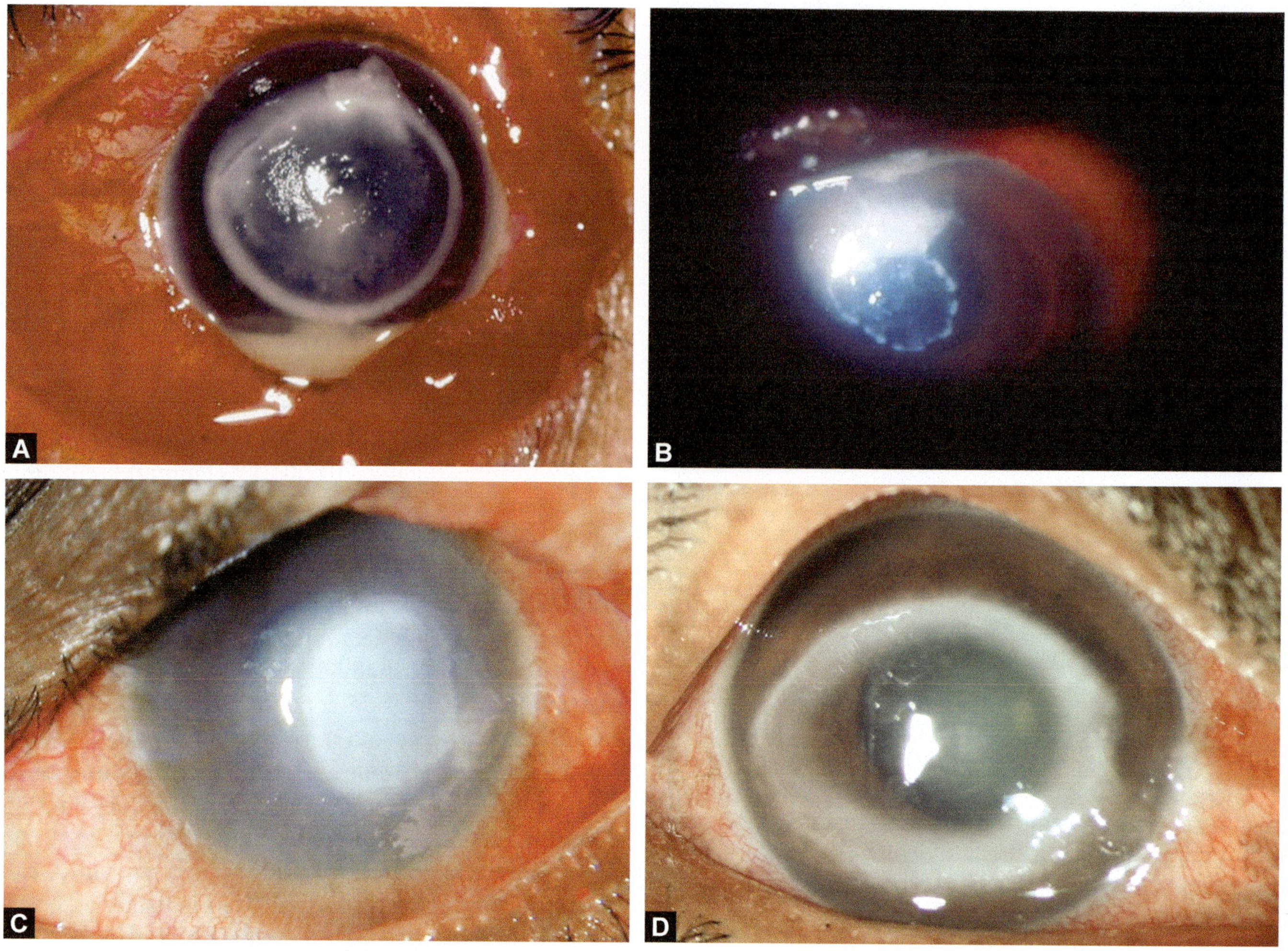

Figs. 23.2.11A to D: Differential diagnosis of ring infiltrate. (A) Fungal keratitis; (B) *Nocardia* keratitis; (C) Bacterial keratitis; (D) *Acanthamoeba* keratitis.

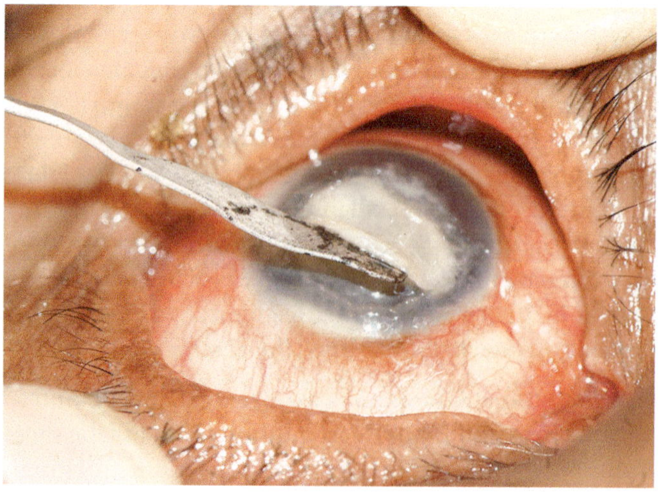

Fig. 23.2.12: Specimen collection with Kimura's spatula.

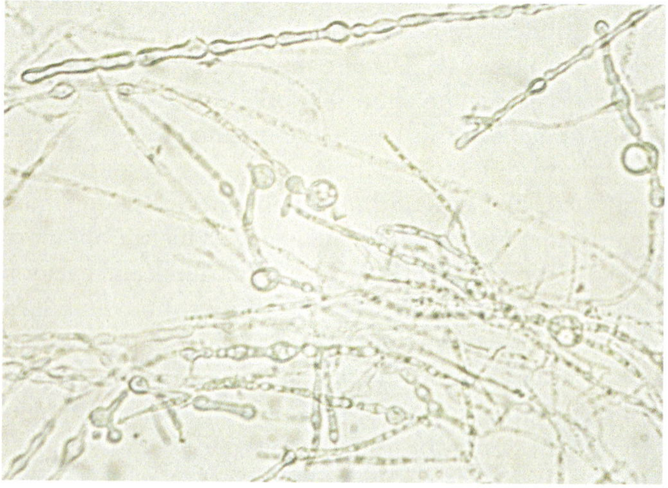

Fig. 23.2.13: Fungal filaments in potassium hydroxide (KOH) wet mount. Refractile septate branching fungal hyphae with spores.

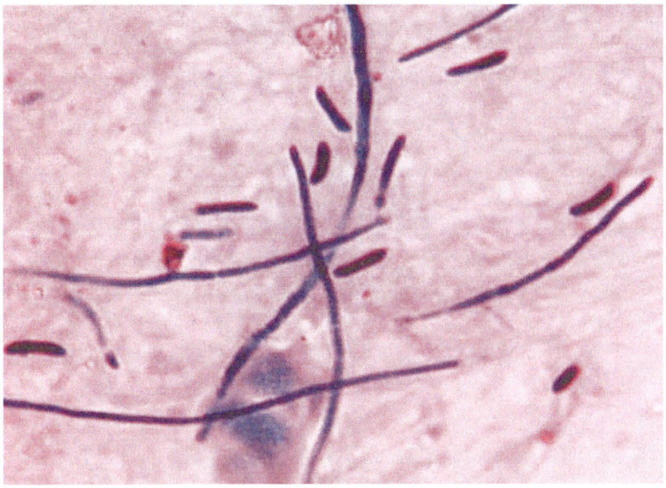

Fig. 23.2.14: Fungal filaments in Gram stain. Gram-positive fungal filaments.

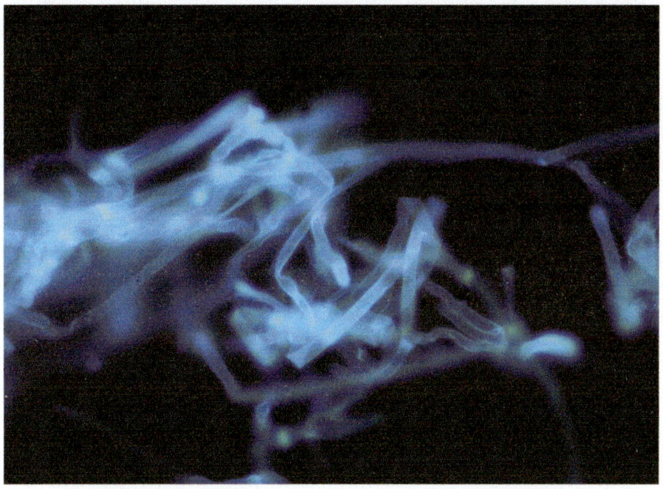

Fig. 23.2.15: Fungal filaments in calcofluor white. Blue-white fluorescence of fungal hyphae in calcofluor white.

temperature (25°C) for the isolation of fungi. Since bacterial pathogens are always a consideration in the differential diagnosis of suppurative keratitis, additional material is inoculated in a row of C-streaks on fresh sheep blood agar or chocolate agar. Most fungi show mycelial growth on blood agar within 24–72 hours. Yeasts grow on these media at 30°C and are visible in 18–24 hours. Colonies of *Fusarium* organisms are usually white in the early stages of development, but often acquire a buff coloration. As the colonies mature, a variety of color pigments ranging from yellow to red to purple are produced and are best seen on the undersurface of the colony. This is known as reverse pigmentation. The classification is based on microscopic features of conidia that form on specialized hyphae called conidiophores. *Fusarium* produces boat-shaped conidia. Colonies of *Aspergillus fumigatus* are white at first, but as spores are produced, they become velvet green owing to the pigmentation of the conidia. *Aspergillus niger* colonies are also white during the initial growth phase but turn completely black on sporulation (Figs. 23.2.16A to D). The typical colony of *Candida* organisms on SDA has a dirty white color. It is opaque with a smooth, flat, round contour and a pasty soft consistency. When grown on blood agar 35°C, they are slow growing and nonhemolytic. *Candida* colonies have a distinctive fruity, yeasty odor. Identification of *Candida albicans* is usually based on the formation of germ tubes in vitro and further speciation is based on sugar fermentation. Classification of noncandidial yeasts is based on biochemical testing.

Polymerase chain reaction: Panfungal PCR is rapid and highly sensitive for diagnosing fungi in smear- and culture-negative keratitis (Fig. 23.2.17). However, amplification of nonpathogenic organisms can give rise to high false-positive results. Other limiting factors are the availability and the cost-effectiveness of PCR in areas with predominant fungal keratitis.[10]

In vivo confocal microscopy (IVCM): IVCM has been used to identify fungal hyphae in corneal stroma (Fig. 23.2.18). Fungal hyphae are seen as high-contrast filaments with 4–6 μm thickness and 60–400 μm length. The depth of the corneal stromal infiltration with fungal hyphae and the response to treatment can be monitored. A comparative cohort study did not find any significant difference in the branching angles of the fungal hyphae of *Fusarium* and *Aspergillus*.[11]

TREATMENT

Medical Management

The development of new ocular antifungal agents has been hindered by the small market that fungal keratitis represents when compared with the systemic fungal infections. With the exception of natamycin, most of the antifungals used were developed for use in systemic mycoses. Before the advent of the first effective antifungal agents in the mid-1950s, the medical treatment of fungal keratitis included methods such as sulfacetamide iontophoresis and thimerosal. Frequently, cauterization and cryotherapy were used adjunctively. The advent of the current antifungals has made a good impact on the management of the surface corneal infections. Even today, however, they share certain common drawbacks. All the available antifungal agents are

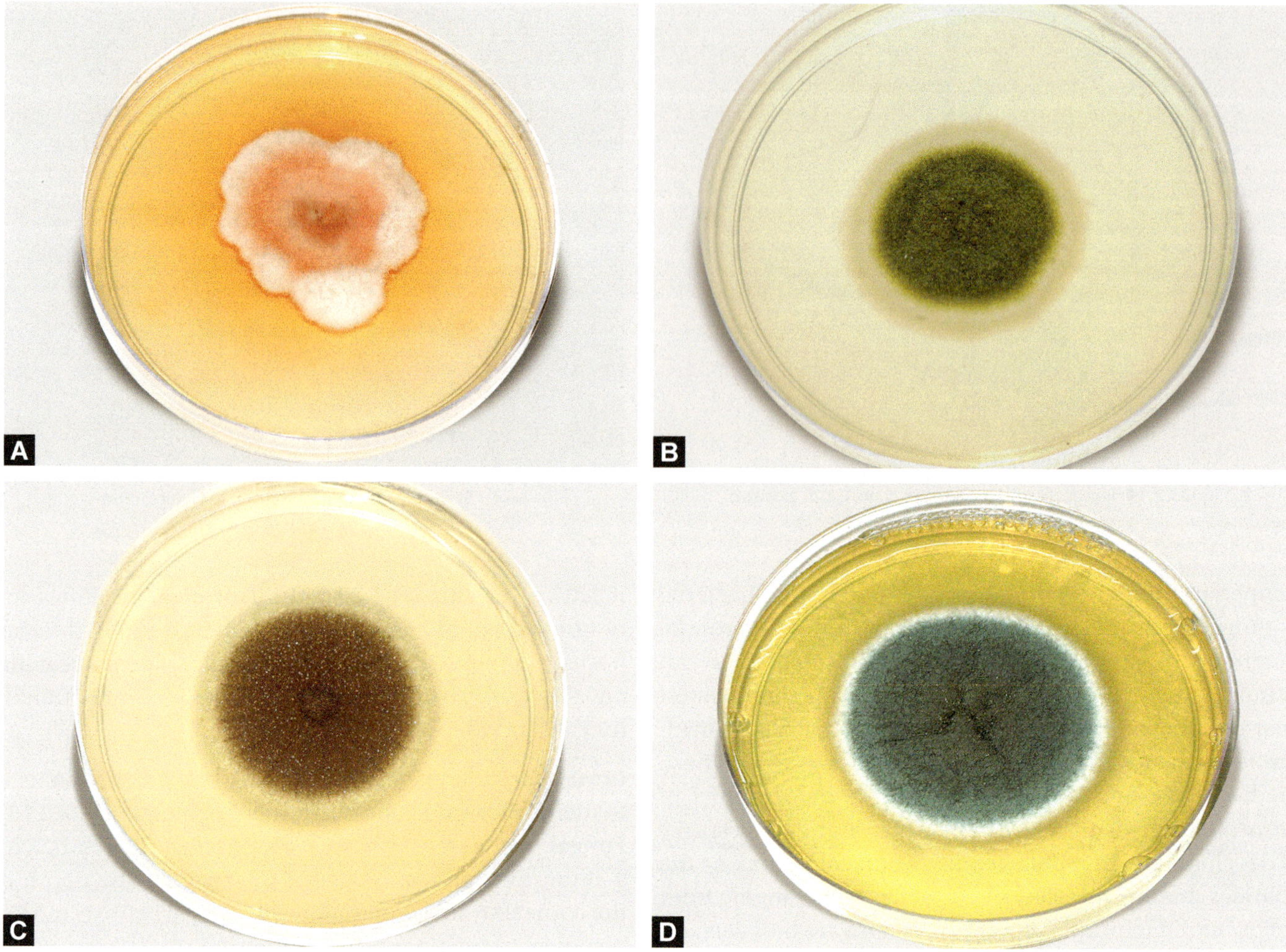

Figs. 23.2.16A to D: Fungal colonies in potato dextrose agar. (A) *Fusarium solani*—woolly to cottony, flat, spreading colonies. From the front, the color of the colony may be white, cream, tan, salmon, cinnamon, yellow, red, violet, pink, or purple. From the reverse, it may be colorless, tan, red, dark purple or brown; (B) *Aspergillus flavus*—colonies are granular, flat, often with radial grooves, yellow at first but quickly becoming bright to dark yellow-green with age; (C) *Aspergillus niger*—colonies consist of a compact white or yellow basal felt covered by a dense layer of dark brown to black conidial heads; (D) *Aspergillus fumigatus*—colonies show typical blue-green surface pigmentation with a suede-like surface consisting of a dense felt of conidiophores.

fungistatic and not fungicidal in tissue concentrations. The treatment schedules are often prolonged, often leading to poor compliance with medical therapy.

Most of the antifungal drugs exhibit their effect through their actions on the fungal cell membrane. In addition to its barrier function, the fungal cell membrane controls the movement of electrolytes and thereby controls the internal homeostasis of the cell. Ergosterol is the predominant sterol unique to the fungal cell membrane, while mammalian cell membranes are composed of cholesterol. Most antifungals capitalize on this important difference in plasma membrane constituents to damage the fungal cells, while minimizing damage to the host cells. There are three major classes of antifungal drugs available namely (1) polyenes, (2) imidazoles, and (3) fluorinated pyrimidines (Table 23.2.1).

Principles of Therapy (Flowchart 23.2.1)

The initiation of treatment can be performed as soon as the results of the KOH mount and the Gram stain are obtained. These tests can readily be performed at the office of the physician itself. If the smears and the culture results are negative, but the clinical features are strongly in favor of fungal keratitis, initiation of topical antifungal therapy especially in countries where there is a high prevalence is indicated (Table 23.2.1). For suspected filamentous fungal keratitis, natamycin 5% suspension should be administered hourly for the initial 24–48 hours and at 2-hour intervals. The dosage can then be gradually reduced depending upon the response. In severe or high-risk ulcers, 2% econazole or 1% voriconazole can be added to natamycin. The mycotic

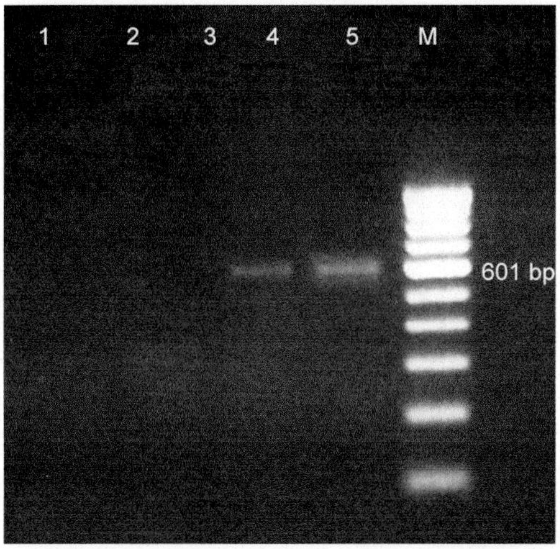

Fig. 23.2.17: Polymerase chain reaction. Lane 4 shows sample spiked with positive *Candida* DNA. Lane 5 positive control of *Candida* DNA showed specific band in 601 bp product.

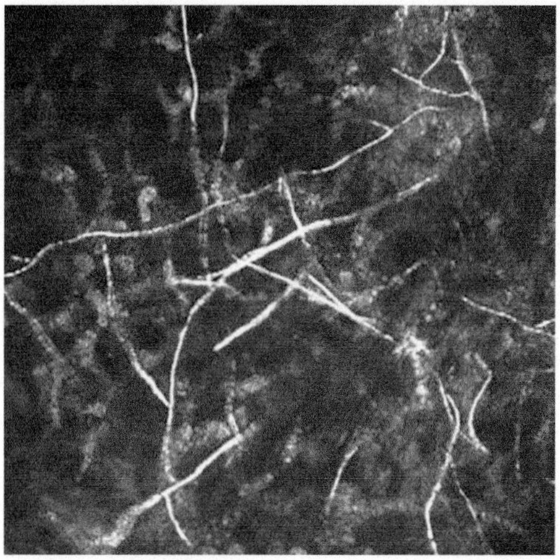

Fig. 23.2.18: Fungal filaments in *in vivo* confocal microscopy. High contrast branching fungal filaments in corneal stroma.

Table 23.2.1: Antifungal medications.

Drug category	Antifungal agents	Mechanism of action
Larger polyenes	Amphotericin (0.15%) Nystatin (50,000 units/mL)	Formation of pores in fungal cell membrane
Smaller polyenes	Natamycin (5%)	Alteration of cell permeability
Imidazoles	Ketoconazole (2%) Miconazole (1%) Econazole (2%) Clotrimazole (1%)	Inhibition of 14-alpha lanosterol demethylase
Triazoles	Itraconazole (1%) Fluconazole (0.3%) Voriconazole (1%) Posaconazole (10%)	Inhibition of 14-alpha lanosterol demethylase
Antimetabolites	Flucytosine (1%)	Inhibition of fungal RNA and DNA synthesis
Echinocandins	Caspofungin (0.5%) Anidulafungin Micafungin (0.1%)	Inhibition of 1,3-beta-glucan synthase

ulcer treatment trial I (MUTT I) compared the safety and efficacy of natamycin and voriconazole in the treatment of filamentary fungal keratitis. This trial concluded that natamycin was consistently superior than voriconazole and this difference was even more significant in ulcers caused by *Fusarium*. The study also recommended that voriconazole should not be used as monotherapy in filamentous fungal keratitis.[12] For yeast keratitis, amphotericin B 0.1–0.25% drops should be administered at 15-minute intervals for the first 24–48 hours and thereafter reduced during the next 4–6 days. In a randomized control study (MUTT II) from India, addition of systemic voriconazole to topical therapy did not add any benefit in the clinical outcomes of deep stromal severe filamentous keratitis.[13] Systemic antifungals are reserved for keratitis associated with scleritis and endophthalmitis. The most frequently used oral antifungals are ketoconazole 200–600 mg, voriconazole 200–400 mg, fluconazole 200–400 mg and itraconazole 200 mg. The course duration is for 14–21 days and liver function should be monitored. Intrastromal and intracameral antifungal medications are used in the treatment of recalcitrant keratitis.[14,15] Preservative-free voriconazole 50 µg in 0.1 mL or amphotericin 5–10 µg in 0.1 mL is used. The efficacy of intrastromal antifungals in nonhealing fungal keratitis is variable. Supplementary therapy includes a cycloplegic—mydriatic agent, such as atropine 1% twice a day. A topical beta-blocker or oral carbonic anhydrase inhibitor should be used to control secondary ocular hypertension. Corticosteroids do not have any role in the treatment regimen of fungal keratitis and is not recommended in any stage of the disease. Photoactivated chromophore for infectious keratitis cross-linking (PACK CXL) with riboflavin and UVA is not effective as adjuvant therapy in recalcitrant deep stromal fugal keratitis and is not recommended.[16] Its efficacy in early fungal keratitis is variable.

The treatment for fungal keratitis is usually prolonged. Improvement may not be visible for several days. Lack of progression of the stromal infiltrate is the first sign that the antifungal is effective. This is followed by a rounding of the feathery margins, blunting of the perimeters and reduction in cellular infiltrate and edema in surrounding stroma.

Flowchart 23.2.1: Treatment algorithm for fungal keratitis.

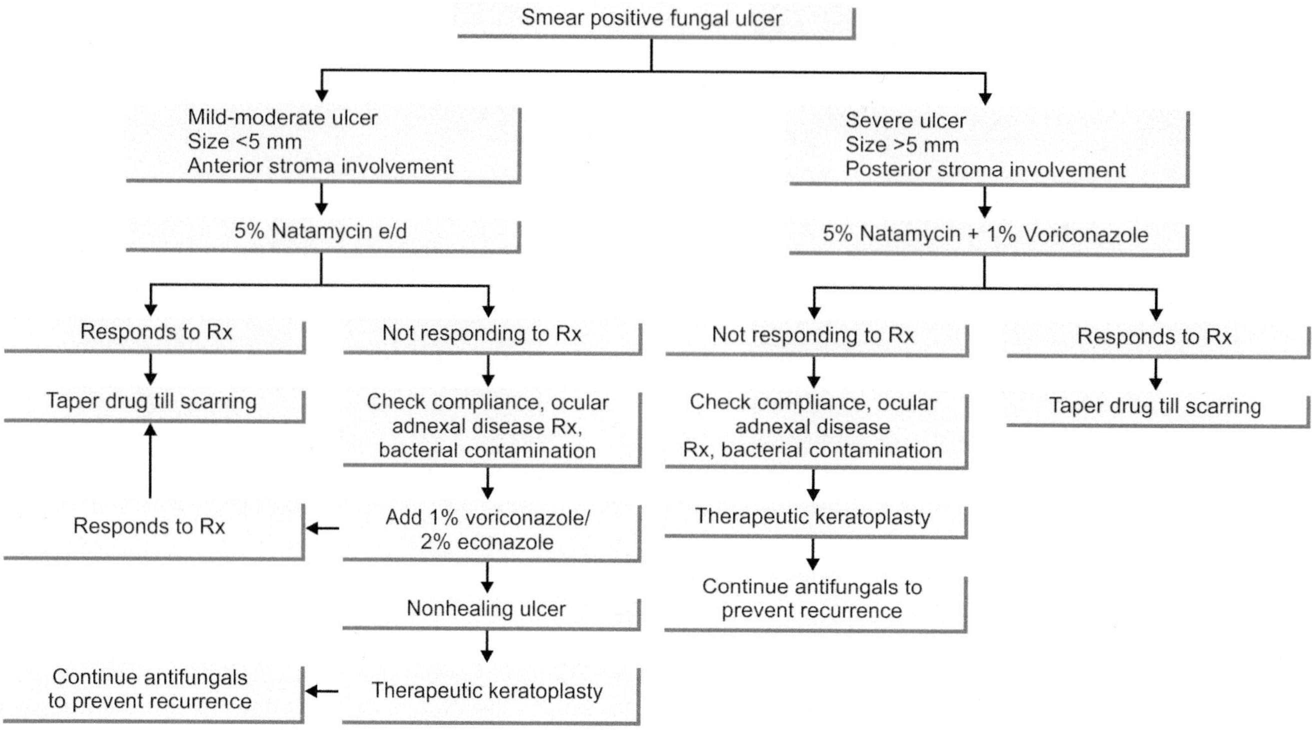

Prolonged conjunctival injection, protracted epithelial ulceration, punctate corneal epithelial erosion and diffuse stromal haze imply drug toxicity. The appearance of a transient hypopyon in the face of an improving corneal picture has been attributed to hypersensitivity or a toxic reaction. Bacterial contamination of the antifungal medication should be suspected in patients with sudden onset lid edema, chemosis, increase in corneal edema and hypopyon. Culture of the antifungal medication will help in clenching the diagnosis.

The poor prognostic factors identified are larger infiltrate size at presentation, larger epithelial defect, *Aspergillus* keratitis, presence of hypopyon and smear positivity in spite of prior antifungal treatment.[17] The MUTT II study defined a high-risk case with high chances of perforation/therapeutic penetrating keratoplasty (TPK) as an ulcer with geometric mean infiltrate size more than 6.63 mm, involving the posterior one-third of cornea and hypopyon.[18]

Therapeutic Keratoplasty

The goals of the therapeutic keratoplasty are to primarily eliminate the infection and restore the integrity of the globe. Local anesthesia may suffice in a majority of the cases. In these cases, O'Brien's facial nerve block is given first prior to the ciliary block to prevent squeezing of the eyelid and resultant inadvertent perforation. In cases of frank or impending perforation, general anesthesia may be preferred. If the area of suppuration is large and asymmetric, decentration of the trephination or a free hand dissection to encompass the infected areas should be done. The size of the trephination should preferably leave 1–1.5 mm clear zone of uninvolved cornea to reduce the possibility of residual organisms peripheral to the trephination. The graft is then secured with 9-0 or 10-0 nylon interrupted sutures. The advantage of these interrupted sutures is that they can be removed selectively if future infiltrations develop. The recurrence of the infection in the graft usually starts from the periphery. Postoperatively, topical natamycin 5% or econazole 2% is continued for a period of 1–2 months. The cure rate of TPK for fungal keratitis varies from 60% to 90% with a recurrence rate of 6–15%.[19]

PYTHIUM INSIDIOSUM KERATITIS

Pythium insidiosum is an oomycete resembling the morphology of fungal hyphae, commonly found in stagnant water bodies and occasionally in soil.[20] They are usually associated with cutaneous ulcers in equines and intestinal infection in dogs. They have been identified in 3-5% of unidentified fungal isolates in keratitis.[21] The oomycete filaments are broad, branching, nonparallel and thin walled with ribbon-like folds which lack ergosterol. They reproduce by biflagellate spores. There are no known risk factors associated with this disease. The clinical features of *Pythium* keratitis resembles to a large extent to that of fungal keratitis. The characteristic clinical features include multiple dot-like infiltrates surrounding the main infiltrate resembling satellite lesions (Fig. 23.2.19). They also present with hyphate edges and reticulate or mesh patterns with tentacle-like projections resembling the mycelium in higher magnification.[21] Rapid worsening of keratitis with antifungal therapy should raise the suspicion of *Pythium* keratitis. The oomycete filaments can be seen in KOH wet mount and calcofluor white. Potassium iodide-sulfuric acid (KI-H_2SO_4) stain helps in distinguishing between *Pythium* and fungal filaments as *Pythium* takes up blue stain and fungal filaments do not.[22] They grow in Sabouraud dextrose agar, blood agar and chocolate agar as flat, feathery, colorless or light brown colonies and are identified by production of biflagellate spores in liquid media. PCR has also been used for rapid diagnosis. Due to the lack of ergosterol, they respond poorly to commonly used antifungal drugs. In vitro and animal studies have shown susceptibility of *Pythium* to antibacterial antibiotics like tigecycline, linezolid, tetracycline and azithromycin.[23-25] Recurrence of infection is frequently seen after therapeutic keratoplasty. Lack of clinical suspicion, late diagnosis and poor response to medical and surgical therapy in *Pythium* keratitis often lead to poor structural and functional outcomes.

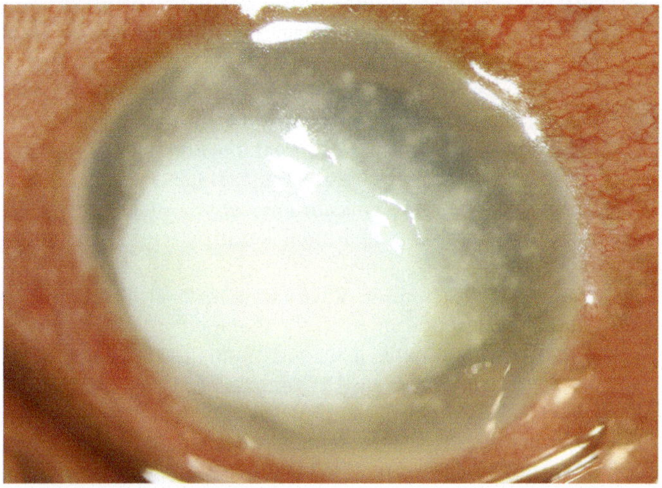

Fig. 23.2.19: *Pythium* keratitis. Multiple dot-like infiltrates surrounding the main lesion characteristic of *Pythium* keratitis.

REFERENCES

1. Whitcher JP, Srinivasan M. Corneal ulceration in the developing world—a silent epidemic. Br J Ophthalmol. 1997;81(8):622-3.
2. Srinivasan M. Fungal keratitis. Curr Opin Ophthalmol. 2004;15:321-7.
3. Prajna NV, Srinivasan M, Lalitha P, et al. Differences in clinical outcomes in keratitis due to fungus and bacteria. JAMA Ophthalmol. 2013;131(8):1088-9.
4. Leal SM, Pearlman E. The role of cytokines and pathogen recognition molecules in fungal keratitis—insights from human disease and animal models. Cytokine. 2012;58(1):107-11.
5. Sivaganesakarthikeyan R, Leal SM, Prajna NV, et al. Expression of innate and adaptive immune mediators in human corneal tissue infected with *Aspergillus* or Fusarium. J Infect Dis. 2011;204:942-50.
6. Rohini G, Murugeswari P, Prajna NV, et al. Matrix metalloproteinases (MMP-8, MMP-9) and the tissue inhibitors of metalloproteinases (TIMP-1 and TIMP-2) in patients with fungal keratitis. Cornea. 2007;26:207-11.
7. Leema G, Kaliamurthy J, Geraldine P, et al. Keratitis due to *Aspergillus flavus*: clinical profile, molecular identification of fungal strains and detection of aflatoxin production. Mol Vis. 2010;16:843-54.
8. Dalmon C, Porco TC, Lietman TM, et al. The clinical differentiation of bacterial and fungal keratitis: a photographic survey. Invest Ophthalmol Vis Sci. 2012;53:1787-91.
9. Sharma S, Kunimoto DY, Gopinathan U, et al. Evaluation of corneal scraping smear examination methods in the diagnosis of bacterial and fungal keratitis. A survey of 8 years of laboratory experience. Cornea. 2002;21(7): 643-7.
10. Kim E, Chidambaram JD, Srinivasan M, et al. Prospective comparison of microbial culture and polymerase chain reaction in the diagnosis of corneal ulcer. Am J Ophthalmol. 2008;148:714-23.
11. Chidambaram JD, Prajna NV, Larke N, et al. In vivo confocal microscopy appearance of Fusarium and Aspergillus species in fungal keratitis. Br J Ophthalmol. 2017;101(8):1119-23.
12. Prajna NV, Krishnan T, Mascarenhas J, et al. The mycotic ulcer treatment trial: a randomized trial comparing natamycin vs voriconazole. JAMA Ophthalmol. 2013;131(4):422-9.
13. Prajna NV, Krishnan T, Rajaraman R, et al. Effect of oral voriconazole on fungal keratitis in the mycotic ulcer treatment trial II (MUTT II): a randomized clinical trial. JAMA Ophthalmol. 2016;134(12):1365-72.
14. Prakash G, Sharma N, Goel M, et al. Evaluation of intrastromal injection of voriconazole as a therapeutic adjunctive for the management of deep recalcitrant fungal keratitis. Am J Ophthalmol. 2008;146:56-9.

15. Sharma N, Agarwal P, Sinha R, et al. Evaluation of intrastromal voriconazole injection in recalcitrant deep fungal keratitis: case series. Br J Ophthalmol. 2011;95(12):1735-7.
16. Uddaraju M, Mascarenhas J, Das MR, et al. Corneal cross-linking as an adjuvant therapy in the management of recalcitrant deep stromal fungal keratitis: a randomized trial. Am J Ophthalmol. 2015;160:131-4.e5.
17. Lalitha P, Prajna NV, Kabra A, et al. Risk factors for treatment outcome in fungal keratitis. Ophthalmology. 2006;113(4):526-30.
18. Prajna NV, Krishnan T, Rajaraman R, et al. Predictors of corneal perforation or need for therapeutic keratoplasty in severe fungal keratitis: a secondary analysis of the mycotic ulcer treatment trial II. JAMA Ophthalmol. 2017;135(9):987-91.
19. Sharma N, Sachdev R, Jhanji V. Therapeutic keratoplasty for microbial keratitis. Curr Opin Ophthalmol. 2010;21:293-300.
20. Gaastra W, Lipman LJA, Arthur WA, et al. Pythium insidiosum: an overview. Vet Microbiol. 2010;146:1-16.
21. Sharma S, Balne PK, Motukupally SR, et al. Pythium insidiosum keratitis: clinical profile and role of DNA sequencing and zoospore formation in diagnosis. Cornea. 2015;34:438-42.
22. Mittal R, Jena SK, Desai A, et al. Pythium insidiosum keratitis: histopathology and rapid novel diagnostic staining technique. Cornea. 2017;36(9):1124-32.
23. Jesus FP, Ferreiro L, Loreto ES, et al. In vitro synergism observed with azithromycin, clarithromycin, minocycline, or tigecycline in association with antifungal agents against Pythium insidiosum. Antimicrob Agents Chemother. 2014;58:5621-5.
24. Jesus FP, Loreto ES, Ferreiro L, et al. In vitro and in vivo antimicrobial activities of minocycline in combination with azithromycin, clarithromycin, or tigecycline against Pythium insidiosum. Antimicrob Agents Chemother. 2016;60:87-91.
25. Loreto ES, Tondolo JS, Pilotto MB, et al. New insights into the in vitro susceptibility of Pythium insidiosum. Antimicrob Agents Chemother. 2014;58:7534-7.

23.3 ACANTHAMOEBA KERATITIS

INTRODUCTION

Acanthamoeba is a free-living pathogenic protozoan commonly found in soil, and water resources like ponds, lakes, tap water and swimming pools. It is capable of causing infectious keratitis in immunocompetent patients and chronic granulomatous meningitis in immunocompromised patients. *Acanthamoeba* keratitis (AK) was first described in early 1970s and the incidence has been on the rise since then. Though contact lens wear is the most common risk factor associated with AK, it accounts for less than 5% of contact lens-induced keratitis.[1] Eight species of *Acanthamoeba* are associated with keratitis of which *Acanthamoeba castellani* and *Acanthamoeba polyphagia* are the most common species causing infectious keratitis.[2]

FORMS OF ACANTHAMOEBA

Acanthamoeba exists in two forms: (1) a motile trophozoite form and (2) a double-walled cyst form. Trophozoite is the metabolically active form, 25–40 µm in size with a single nucleus and a prominent nucleolus. The cytoplasm contains many cytoplasmic contractile vacuoles. Many finger-like projections called acanthopodia on its surface helps in motility. Trophozoite feeds on bacteria and other protozoa and it reproduces by mitosis.[3] They are also intracellular carriers for many obligate bacteria like *Legionella, Chlamydia, Pseudomonas, Mycobacterium,* etc. These endosymbionts are believed to increase the pathogenicity of *Acanthamoeba*.[3] When exposed to unfavorable conditions like lack of nutrition, extremes of temperature, pH alteration and exposure to amoebicidal drugs, the trophozoite encysts to form double-walled cysts of 15–25 µm. The double walls of the cyst are joined in places to give a polygonal appearance.[3] The cysts are resistant to antibiotics, chlorination, low temperature, etc. They can remain dormant in the corneal stroma and may reactivate to cause the disease.

RISK FACTORS

Contact lens wear is the most common risk factor for infectious keratitis. Poor contact lens hygiene, extended use of contact lens, biofilm over contact lens, use of tap water for contact lens cleaning, swimming with contact lens on, can predispose to AK.[4,5] Exposure to brackish water source like washing the eye with field water/pond water following a trauma is common in agrarian population and may predispose to AK. AK has also been reported following refractive surgery procedures like radial keratotomy and LASIK.[6]

PATHOGENESIS

A break in the epithelium like that caused by contact lens-induced microabrasion or trauma is a prerequisite for corneal infection. The primary step is the adhesion of *Acanthamoeba* to corneal epithelium with the help of glycoproteins like mannose-binding proteins and acanthopodia. On adhesion, *Acanthamoeba* causes desquamation of epithelial cells and penetrates the Bowman's membrane. They also secrete numerous substances like serine proteases, cysteine proteases, metalloproteases, elastase and phospholipase A, which cause collagenolysis and stromal degradation and thereby help in further penetration of the *Acanthamoeba* into the corneal stroma.[2,7] The trophozoites show chemotactic response toward neuronal cells and are seen to cluster around the corneal nerves leading to perineuritis.[8] With amoebicidal treatment, the trophozoites can form cysts and remain dormant in the stroma and cause reactivation at a later date.

CLINICAL FEATURES

It is traditionally felt that the patient often presents with severe pain out of proportion to clinical signs. Other symptoms are redness, photophobia, tearing, discharge and defective vision. Since the clinical features in the early stages may be indistinguishable from a viral or a fungal keratitis, delay in the commencement of appropriate therapy is common. *Acanthamoeba* should be suspected in all nonhealing or atypical presumed viral or fungal keratitis.

Early disease presents with epithelial disease with signs of punctate epithelitis, epithelial haze, pseudodendrite and microcysts. Radial infiltrates around one or two corneal nerves can be seen and these perineuritis lesions are considered pathognomonic of AK, though it can be seen even in *Pseudomonas* keratitis and fungal keratitis[3] (Fig. 23.3.1). AK can progress to anterior and posterior patchy grayish white infiltrates (Figs. 23.3.2 and 23.3.3). With time, these infiltrates coalesce to form arcuate and ring infiltrates (Fig. 23.3.4). Satellite lesions and immune rings may also be seen (Fig. 23.3.5). If untreated, deep stromal abscess, corneal melt and perforation may occur (Figs. 23.3.6 to 23.3.8). A sterile transient anterior uveitis with hypopyon can be present. Deep stromal disease and ring infiltrate at presentation carries poor prognosis. Noncorneal lesions include limbitis, episcleritis, anterior and posterior scleritis and choroiditis. The disease follows a prolonged course and can also lead to secondary glaucoma and cataract.

DIAGNOSIS

In vivo confocal microscopy (IVCM) can identify trophozoites and cysts in the corneal stroma. IVCM has the advantage of being noninvasive offers rapid diagnosis in contrast to culture. The depth, density and distribution of cysts can be quantified. The sensitivity and specificity of IVCM is more than 90% in microbiologically proven cases. Cysts can be seen as round/ovoid dense highly refractile bodies of 10–25 μm or as round/ovoid bodies with bright center and dark surrounding cyst wall or as bright cyst wall with dark center or coffee-bean shaped

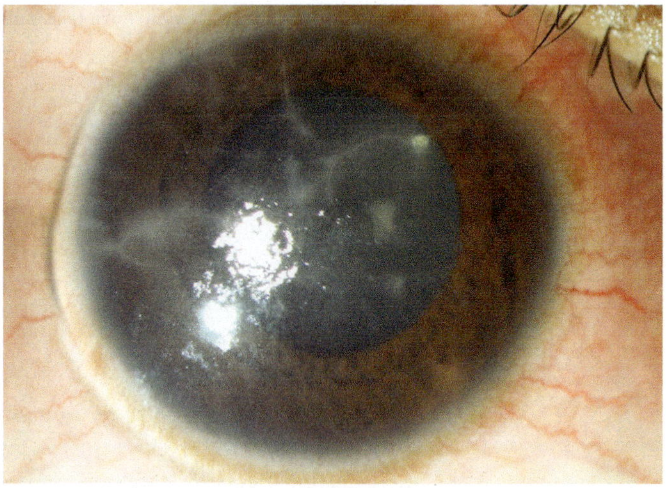

Fig. 23.3.1: Early epithelial keratitis with radial keratoneuritis. Diffuse epithelial irregularity with grayish white anterior stromal radial infiltrates along the corneal nerves.

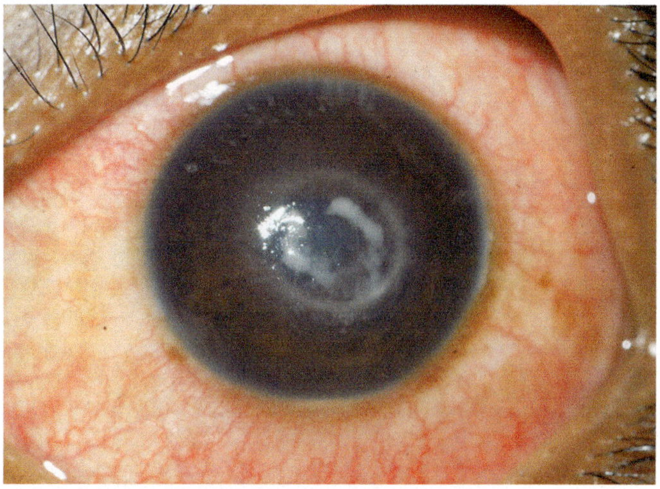

Fig. 23.3.2: Patchy anterior stromal infiltrate with early ring infiltrate.

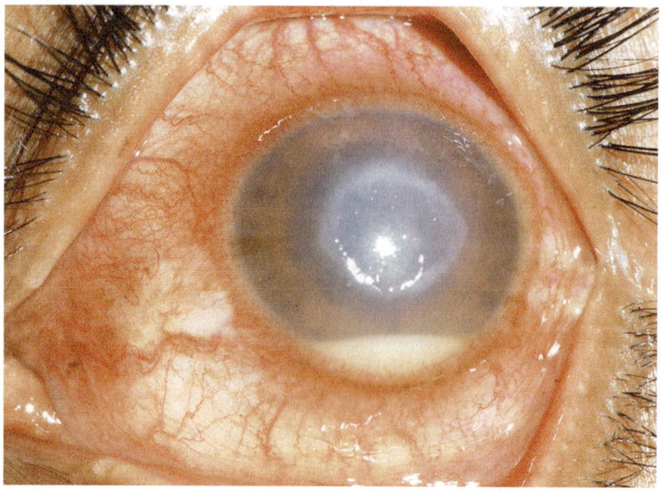

Fig. 23.3.3: Anterior stromal infiltrate. Central grayish white diffuse anterior stromal infiltrate with epithelial defect.

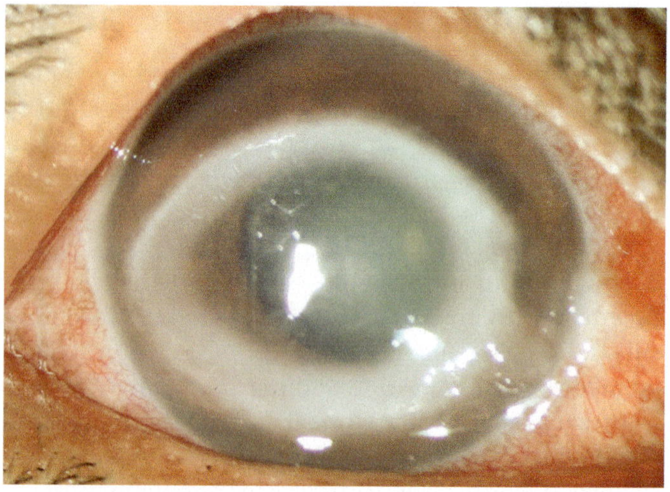

Fig. 23.3.4: Classic ring infiltrate of *Acanthamoeba* keratitis.

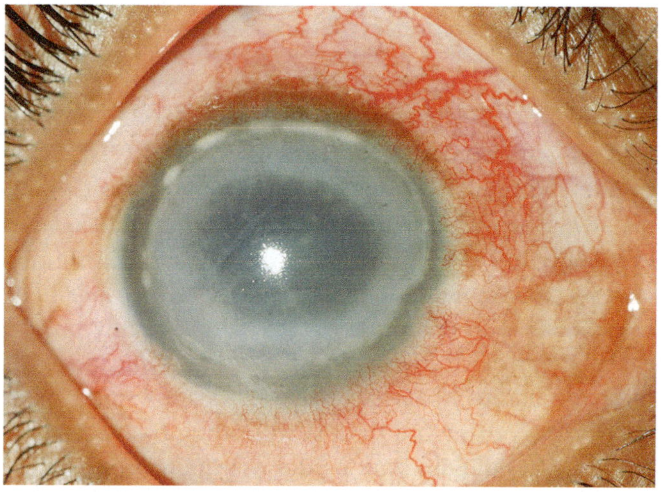

Fig. 23.3.5: Ring infiltrate with surrounding satellite lesions. Multiple grayish white satellite lesions seen surrounding the ring infiltrate.

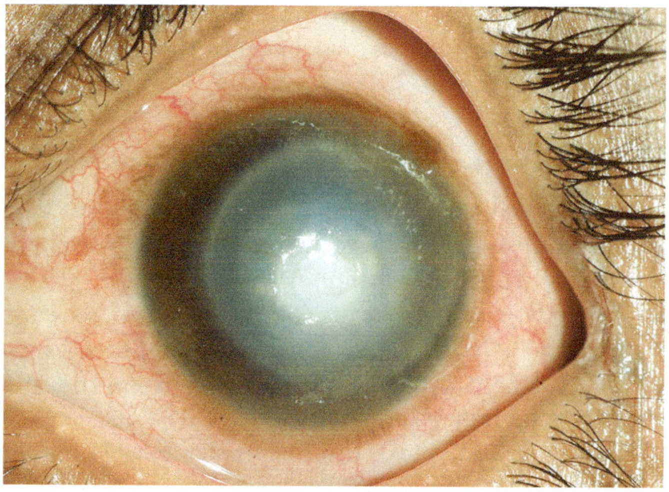

Fig. 23.3.6: Diffuse stromal infiltrate. Diffuse grayish white stromal infiltrate with dense anterior stromal infiltrate and peripheral ring lesion.

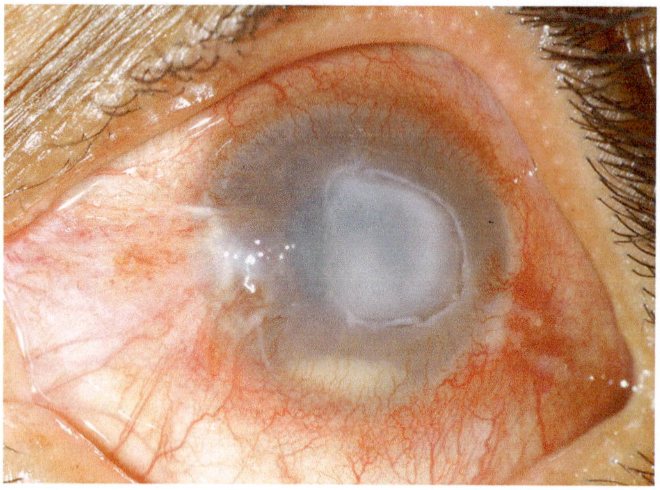

Fig. 23.3.7: Nonhealing *Acanthamoeba* keratitis. Chronic epithelial defect with heaped up edges, dense stromal infiltrate and 360° stromal vascularization.

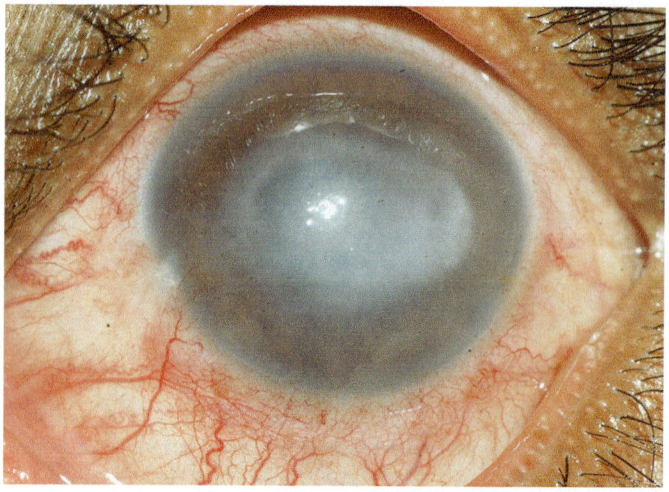

Fig. 23.3.8: Resolving *Acanthamoeba* keratitis. Resolving stromal infiltrate with rounded graying margins and healed epithelium.

structures.[8] Polymerase chain reaction can also be used for identification amoebic DNA in corneal tissue.[9]

As mentioned earlier, AK is often misdiagnosed and treated as viral or fungal keratitis. Culture of corneal scrapings is considered gold standard.[10] The corneal scrapings are obtained using a Kimura's spatula/Bard-Parker knife/26-gauge needle after anesthetizing the cornea with 0.5% proparacaine. One half of the specimen is smeared onto a glass slide and is subjected to direct microscopic examination. Gram stain, KOH wet mount, lactophenol cotton blue, Giemsa, calcofluor white, acridine orange and immunoperoxidase stains can be used for identification of trophozoites or cysts in corneal scrapings. The other half of the specimen is inoculated in the center of nonnutrient agar enriched with bacteria like *Escherichia coli* or *Enterobacter aerogenes*. *Acanthamoeba* feeds on the bacteria and migrate leaving behind trails. The non-nutrient nature of the agar prevents overgrowth of bacteria. The agar plates can be seen under light microscope for trophozoite.

Acanthamoeba can take 1–2 weeks to grow in the agar. The sensitivity of culture is reported to vary from 30% to 60%. In deeper lesions, corneal biopsy with a 2–3 mm trephine or a suture passed through the infiltrate can be used for culture. Also culture of contact lens and lens solution can be used to isolate the organism.

TREATMENT

The treatment of AK is a prolonged one and often takes months. Topical amoebicidal drugs with activity over both cysts and trophozoites are the treatment of choice. Biguanides are the most effective cysticidal amoebicides.[11] They are cationic disinfectants which disrupt the cell membrane and damage the cell components. Polyhexamethylene biguanide (PHMB, 0.02–0.06%) and chlorhexidine (0.02–0.2%) are the commonly used biguanides.[12] They have high cysticidal activity and are also less epitheliotoxic. They are used in combination with diamidine or neomycin. Propamidine isethionate 0.1% and hexamidine 0.1% are commonly used diaminidines. They alter cell membrane structure and cause denaturation of cytoplasmic proteins. Both biguanides and diaminidines are started as hourly drops and slowly tapered after clinical resolution. The medications should be continued for 3–4 months postscarring to prevent reactivation of the disease from dormant cysts. Neomycin has excellent amoebicidal activity on trophozoites and does not have cysticidal activity. It should not be used as monotherapy to avoid emergence of resistant strains. Use of corticosteroids in AK is controversial.

Epithelial debridement helps in drug penetration and complete removal of *Acanthamoeba* in epithelitis stage of the disease. Therapeutic keratoplasty is reserved for impending perforation, perforated corneal ulcer and nonhealing keratitis.[13] Deep anterior lamellar keratoplasty has been reported to be effective in recalcitrant AK, not involving the deeper stromal layers. The role of collagen cross-linking has not been fully elucidated in the treatment of AK.[14,15]

REFERENCES

1. Cheung N, Nagra P, Hammersmith K. Emerging trends in contact lens-related infections. Curr Opin Ophthalmol. 2016;27(4):327-32.
2. Clarke DW, Niederkorn JY. The pathophysiology of *Acanthamoeba* keratitis. Trends Parasitol. 2006;22: 175-80.
3. Illingworth CD, Cook SD. *Acanthamoeba* keratitis. Surv Ophthalmol. 1998;42:493-508.
4. Joslin CE, Tu EY, Shoff ME, et al. The association of contact lens solution and *Acanthamoeba* keratitis. Am J Ophthalmol. 2007;144:169-80.
5. Radford CF, Minassian DC, Dart JK. *Acanthamoeba* keratitis in England and Wales: incidence, outcome and risk factors. Br J Ophthalmol. 2002;86:536-42.
6. Balasubramanya R, Garg P, Sharma S, et al. *Acanthamoeba* keratitis after LASIK. J Refract Surg. 2006;22:616-7.
7. Niederkorn JY, Alizadeh H, Leher H, et al. The pathogenesis of *Acanthamoeba* keratitis. Microbes Infect. 1999;1(6): 437-43.
8. Huang P, Tepelus T, Vickers LA, et al. Quantitative analysis of depth, distribution, and density of cysts in *Acanthamoeba* keratitis using confocal microscopy. Cornea. 2017;36(8): 927-32.
9. Thompson PP, Kowalski RP, Shanks RM, et al. Validation of real-time PCR for laboratory diagnosis of *Acanthamoeba* keratitis. J Clin Microbiol. 2008;46:3232-6.
10. MaycocK JR, Rakesh J. Update on *Acanthamoeba* keratitis: diagnosis, treatment, and outcomes. Cornea. 2016;35(5): 713-20.
11. Dart JK, Saw VP, Kilvington S. *Acanthamoeba* keratitis: diagnosis and treatment update 2009. Am J Ophthalmol. 2009;148(4:)487-99.e2.
12. Lim N, Goh D, Bunce C, et al. Comparison of polyhexamethylene biguanide and chlorhexidine as monotherapy agents in the treatment of *Acanthamoeba* keratitis. Am J Ophthalmol. 2008;145(1):130-5.
13. Robaei D, Carnt N, Minassian DC, et al. Therapeutic and optical keratoplasty in the management of *Acanthamoeba* keratitis: risk factors, outcomes, and summary of the literature. Ophthalmology. 2015;122:17-24.
14. Demirci G, Ozdamar A. A case of medication-resistant *Acanthamoeba* keratitis treated by corneal crosslinking in Turkey. Case Rep Ophthalmol Med. 2013;608253.
15. Khan YA, Kashiwabuchi RT, Martins SA, et al. Riboflavin and ultraviolet light a therapy as an adjuvant treatment for medically refractive *Acanthamoeba* keratitis: report of 3 cases. Ophthalmology. 2011;118(2):324-31.

Chapter 24 Viral Keratitis

Namrata Sharma, Prafulla K Maharana, Pranita Sahay,
Gunjan Saluja, Tushar Agarwal

INTRODUCTION

Viral keratitis is a frequent cause of corneal blindness globally. In fact, it is the most common cause of keratitis in the developed world.[1] Both DNA and RNA viruses are implicated in the causation of this condition. There are now eight recognized human herpes viruses: herpes simplex virus type 1 (HSV-1), HSV-2, varicella-zoster virus (VZV), cytomegalovirus (CMV), Epstein-Barr virus (EBV), human herpes virus 6 (HHV-6), human herpes virus 7 (HHV-7) and human herpes virus 8 (HHV-8). Of these, HSV-1 is the most common agent and is responsible for 78–98% of cases.[2] In clinical practice, herpes simplex keratitis is often the most common type of viral keratitis seen.[1]

HERPES SIMPLEX VIRUS KERATITIS

Epidemiology

Herpes Simplex virus (HSV) is endemic throughout the world and humans are the only reservoir. Studies examining the presence of HSV-1 DNA in trigeminal ganglion have found that 90% of world's population is infected with asymptomatic HSV infection by age of 60 years.[1-3] The incidence of all episodes of herpes simplex keratitis reported was 20.7 cases/100,000 population. While the prevalence of ocular HSV disease in community is around 149/100,000 population, the incidence is reported to be 84/100,000/year.[1-4] HSV keratitis is predominantly unilateral. However, bilateral HSV keratitis is commonly seen in immunocompromised individuals with incidence of bilateral keratitis being about 11.9%.[5]

Etiopathogenesis

HSV is a double-stranded DNA virus with an icosahedral capsid. The virus can be subdivided into two types: HSV-1 and HSV-2 based on their clinical, biological and serological characteristics. HSV-1 is associated mainly with oral infections and blisters in mouth, face and upper body. HSV-2 causes genital herpes, which is a sexually transmitted disease and is primarily an infection of young adults. Thus, HSV-1 affects upper part of the body above the waist while HSV-2 affects the lower part of the body. Ocular herpes is caused chiefly by HSV-1. Infrequently, HSV-2 may be associated with neonatal herpetic keratitis, in the setting of the neonates acquiring the infection as they pass through the birth canal of mother infected with HSV-2 genital infection.[1,6]

Immunocompromised states such as malignancy, HIV infections and prolonged steroid usage serve as a setting for a greater risk of developing the disease and in some instances, may be life threatening as well.[1,2]

HSV genome has the ability to code for 50–75 different proteins. The possibility of the different unique combinations of gene results in each strain producing a dendritic ulcer with characteristic length pattern and depth. The viral envelope is highly immunogenic and can induce hypersensitivity reactions.[1]

Mode of Transmission

The virus can be transmitted from person to person by direct contact with infected lesions, by salivary and tear droplets, fomites from children and adults with active disease. It can also be transmitted from asymptomatic virus shedding carriers.[1,2] Primary infection occurs usually early in life and can be asymptomatic or symptomatic. Corneal epithelium is one of the major sites of primary infection.[5] HSV enters oral mucosa, eye and skin through small cuts and abrasions to reach the epithelial cells which represent the primary targets of HSV. The infection may also spread to the eye from the other sites most often from the mouth.[1,2] A common cause is the iatrogenic transmission of infection through contaminated Schiotz and applanation tonometer.[1]

Pathogenesis

After gaining entry into host, the virus first replicates at a peripheral site like eyes, skin or oral mucosa. It then spreads to the axonal terminals of sensory neurons and gains entry into the neuronal bodies in the sensory and autonomic ganglia through retrograde intra-axonal transport. The virus then becomes latent in the trigeminal ganglion.[1-3] During latency, the viral gene is completely repressed but the viral genome remains transcriptionally active. This activity results in the synthesis of latency associated transcripts (LAT), which has been implicated in establishment of latency and reactivation of virus. The virus does not generally replicate and damage neurons. Intermittent shedding of trigeminal ganglion-based virus can be detected in tears and saliva of adult humans without apparent clinical disease.[6] Immune control of viral infection and replication occurs at the level of skin or mucosa during primary or recurrent infection. The immune control of latency and reactivation happens within the dorsal root ganglion.[2,7]

The virus can get reactivated in any of the following settings: exposure to ultraviolet radiations, fever, stress, menstruation, hormonal changes, ocular trauma, LASIK, YAG-laser iridotomy and capsulotomy, argon laser trabeculoplasty, photorefractive keratectomy and cataract surgery.

Once reactivated, the virus gets transported anterogradely to a peripheral site and starts replicating. Disease severity and extension of lesions as well as latency and recurrence depends on viral genes encoded by specific strains and host immune system, both innate and adaptive.[1,2]

Clinical Manifestations

Herpes simplex viral keratitis can have a varied presentation and can involve all the corneal layers. A patient with HSV keratitis can present as either a primary case or a recurrent case of herpes simplex keratitis. Most ocular diseases are thought to represent recurrent HSV disease following the establishment of viral latency in the host, rather than a primary ocular infection as explained in Table 24.1, which summarizes the various clinical manifestations of HSV infection.

PRIMARY OCULAR HERPES

Primary ocular herpes presents as an acute infection of the nonimmune host, often missed and rarely affects the cornea. The most common presentation is blepharoconjunctivitis that often heals without scarring. Systemic symptoms such as fever, malaise may be more apparent than ocular complaints. Only 6% of the affected individuals develop ocular and perioral features.[7]

Table 24.1: Clinical manifestations of ocular herpes.

Anterior segment manifestations	Posterior segment manifestations
• Blepharitis • Conjunctivitis • Keratitis • Iridocyclitis • Trabeculitis	Chorioretinitis

The follicular conjunctivitis is often confused with adenoviral conjunctivitis, but unilateral and nonepidemic follicular conjunctivitis provides a clue towards herpetic conjunctivitis. Patients present with complains of redness, watering, discharge, itching, irritation, and lid swelling. In addition, there may be pain, photophobia, lid vesicles and blurring of vision but these symptoms are less frequent.

Slit-lamp examination shows presence of vesicles and ulcers on the lids, papillary responses and follicles in the conjunctiva. Corneal findings include presence of fine and coarse epithelial punctate keratitis and subepithelial punctate keratitis. Primary ocular herpes is usually mild and its course lasts for 10 days but life threatening ocular herpes may occur in immunocompromised individuals and newborns.

Facial area supplied by maxillary division of trigeminal nerve is the most common site of HSV infection and this results in latency of virus in trigeminal ganglion.

RECURRENT OCULAR HERPES

Recurrence rate of ocular herpes has been reported to be around 20% after 2 years, 40% after 5 years and 63% after 20 years of primary episode.[1-4]A large number of factors as stated previously can cause reactivation of viral infection. The HEDS study reported an 18% recurrence rate for epithelial keratitis and for stromal keratitis within 18 months in 346 patients with history of ocular HSV within the previous year.[8]

Recurrent viral keratitis can present as blepharitis, conjunctivitis, epithelial keratitis, stromal keratitis, uveitis, trabeculitis and chorioretinitis. Generally, recurrence follows the same pattern as that of the previous episode-, e.g. patients with epithelial keratitis usually have recurrence of epithelial keratitis and that of stromal keratitis will have recurrence of stromal keratitis. Recurrences are generally caused by same strain of virus.[1,2] Clinical types of recurrent ocular herpes include a variety of manifestations as shown in Table 24.2.[1]

Table 24.2: Clinical spectrum of herpetic keratitis.

Broad category	Subtypes
Infectious epithelial keratitis	Dendritic Geographic Marginal
Stromal keratitis	Immune stromal keratitis Necrotizing stromal keratitis
Endotheliitis	Disciform Diffuse Linear
Keratouveitis	Any form of keratitis with iritis or iridotrabeculitis
Neurotrophic keratitis	

INFECTIOUS EPITHELIAL KERATITIS

Infectious epithelial keratitis is caused by the replication of live virus. In recurrent infections, it can manifest along with stromal keratitis or endothelitis.[1,2] Patients at presentation can have watering, pain, photophobia, foreign body sensation and diminution of vision. The different manifestations are:

Punctate keratitis: This consists of opaque plaques of swollen epithelial cells due to active viral replication. Fluorescein staining shows the presence of fine or coarse superficial punctate lesions. Careful examination of these lesions demonstrates minute, raised, clear vesicles similar to the vesicular eruptions seen in the skin or mucous membranes elsewhere in the body.[1]

Dendritic keratitis: Active replication of the virus and the enlargement of plaques of swollen epithelial cells forms dendrites. The linear nature of the dendrite is the result of the corneal epithelium sliding in to cover the epithelial defect created by the proliferating virus at the edge of the ulcer.

Fluorescein staining shows irregular, zig-zag linear branching ulcer with knobbed ends (Figs. 24.1 and 24.2). By its property of being taken up into dead and degenerated cells, rose bengal dye can be used to stain the epithelial defect to the exact extent and demonstrates the ocular surface damage. However, rose Bengal dye can cause severe pain and hence, lissamine green dye can be used as an alternative. Corneal sensations are usually reduced.[1,2]

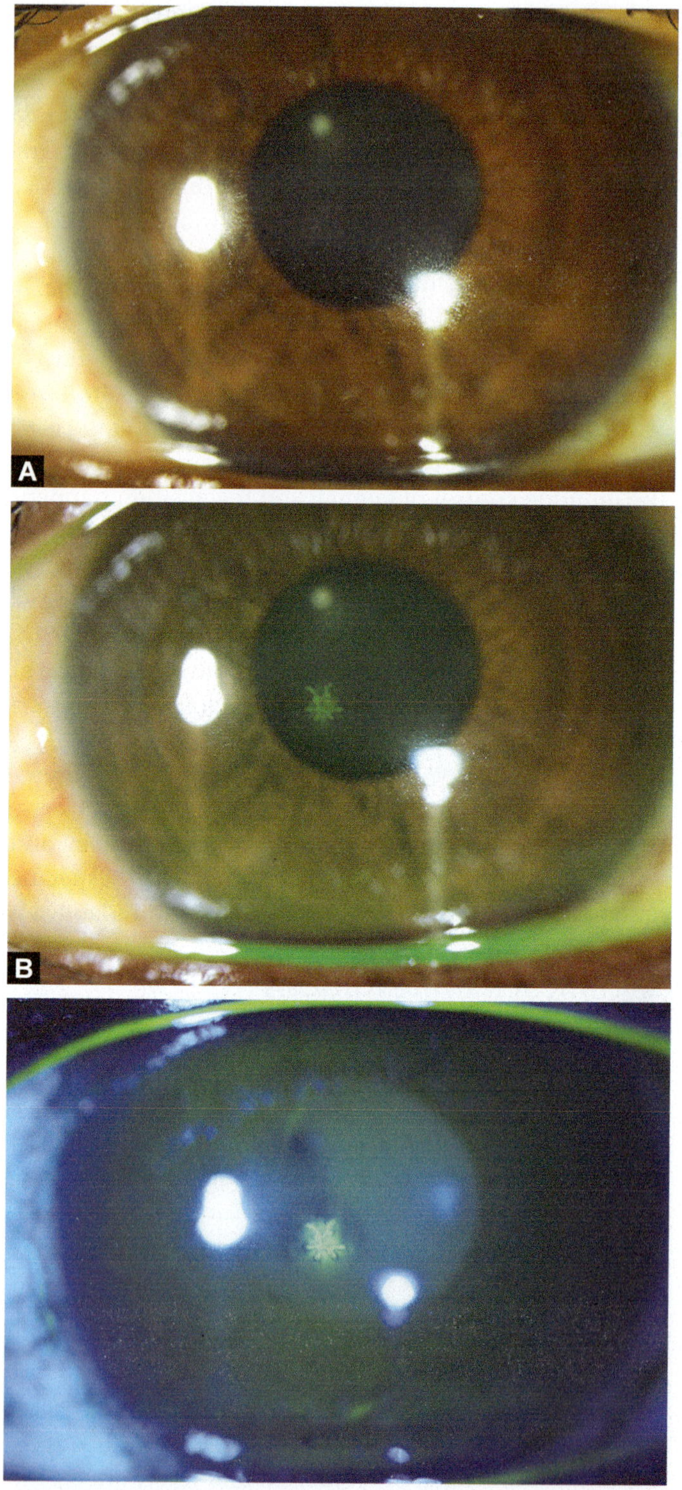

Figs. 24.1A to C: Dendritic ulcer—(A) without fluorescein stain; (B) with fluorescein stain; (C) with fluorescein stain using cobalt blue filter.

Geographical ulcer: A linear dendritic ulcer can further progress until there is a broad area of epithelial ulceration with irregular angulated borders like those of a map hence, given the term "geographic" or "amoeboid" ulcer (Figs. 24.3A and B). Not infrequently, a typical dendritic ulcer extends from the side of a geographic ulcer and has a much longer clinical course. A dendritic ulcer can progress to geographic ulcers if steroids are used to treat the dendrite.

Like a dendritic ulcer, it is a true ulcer as it extends through the basement membrane and it has swollen epithelial cells at its borders containing live virus. The scalloped or geographic borders of the HSV geographic ulcer differentiates it from healing abrasions and neurotrophic keratopathy that tends to have smooth borders.[2]

A dendritic or geographic ulcer may heal without any residual evidence of prior infection or more commonly leads to stromal scarring appearing as faint, gray-white, subepithelial opacities. These opacities are known as the "ghost figures" or "footprints" of HSV (Fig. 24.4) and an important sign for making the clinical diagnosis in future episodes especially in patients with recurrent unilateral keratoconjunctivitis.[1]

Marginal keratitis: HSV marginal keratitis is an uncommon manifestation of viral reactivation. It classically presents as a dendritic ulcer peripherally near limbus with associated vascularization and subepithelial infiltrates (Fig. 24.5).[1] The ulcer progresses centrally in a dendritic shape, typically followed by a leash of blood vessels and subepithelial infiltration. It is important to differentiate it from staphylococcal marginal keratitis (Table 24.3).[1]

Neurotrophic epithelial keratitis: Neurotrophic ulcers result from damage to the sensory nerves supplying the cornea. Corneal sensory nerve damage induces marked changes in the levels of neuromediators that lead to an impairment of epithelial cell vitality, which results in the development of recurrent or persistent epithelial defects. The ulcer typically

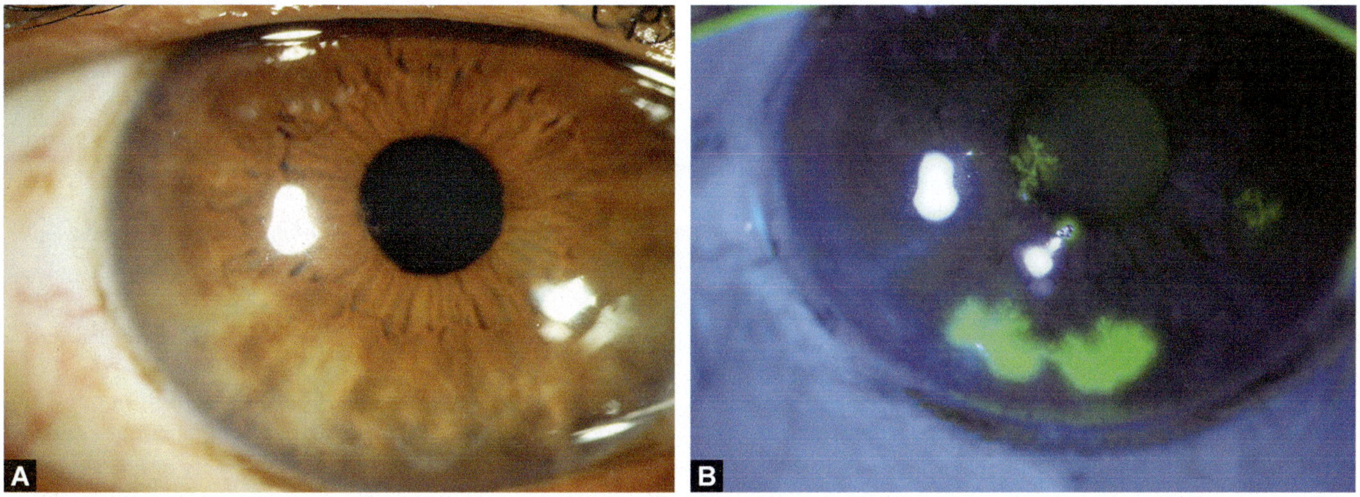

Figs. 24.2A and B: Dendritic ulcer—(A) without fluorescein stain; (B) with fluorescein stain.

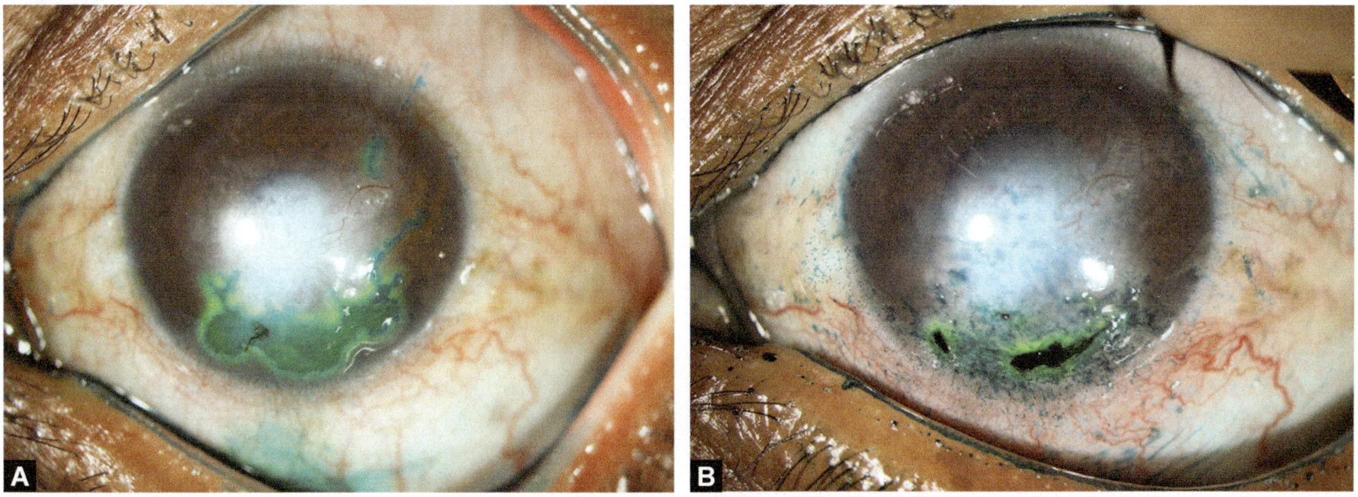

Figs. 24.3A and B: Geographic ulcer— (A) with fluorescein stain; (B) with fluorescein and lissamine green stain using cobalt blue filter.

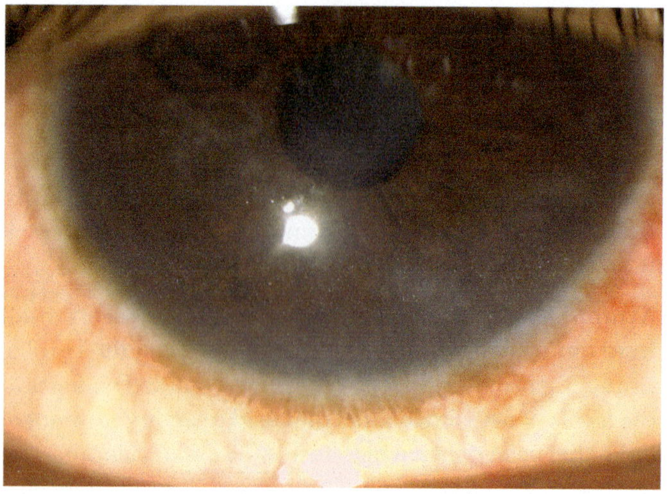

Fig. 24.4: Herpetic footprints.

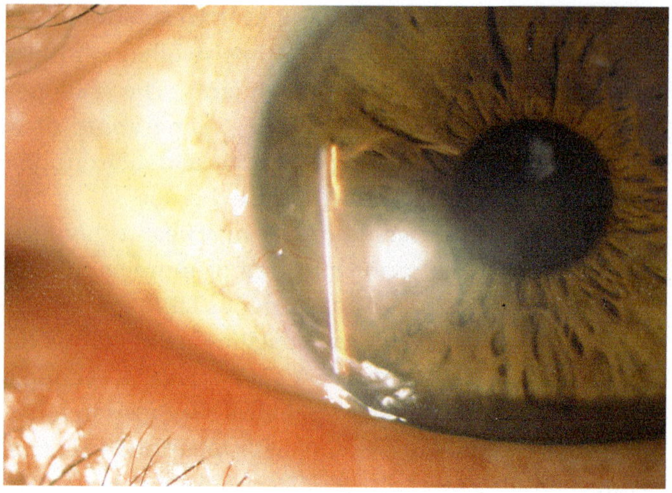

Fig. 24.5: Marginal keratitis.

Table 24.3: Difference between herpes simplex marginal keratitis and staphylococcal marginal keratitis.

Characteristics	Staphylococcal marginal keratitis	HSV marginal keratitis
Cause	Immunologic response to staphylococcal antigen	Active virus
Associated blepharitis	Associated	None
Location	2, 4, 8, 10 o'clock meridians (point of contact of lid)	Any meridian
Epithelial defect	Usually absent	Present often dendritic
Infiltration	Infiltrate develops first followed by ulceration in late stages	Begins as an ulcer in which later infiltrate develops
Neovascularization	Absent	Usually present
Progression	Circumferentially	Centrally

(HSV: Herpes simplex virus)

starts as an irregularity of the corneal surface and a lack of the normal corneal lusture that progress to punctate epithelial erosions, persistent epithelial defect and eventually stromal ulceration. The ulcer is usually oval with smooth borders (in contrast to irregular shape with scalloped borders of geographic ulcer). The ulcer bed typically develops a gray-white opacification with a thickened border formed by heaped-up epithelium (Fig. 24.6).[1] It usually follows a long indolent course and is exacerbated by the use of topical epitheliotoxic drugs like antivirals. Complications include stromal scarring, neovascularization, necrosis, perforation, and secondary bacterial infection.[1]

STROMAL KERATITIS

Herpes simplex stromal keratitis is responsible for 20–48% of cases of recurrent viral keratitis, although may rarely also occur in primary herpetic infections (around 2%).[1,10] Secondary stromal keratitis is the involvement of stroma secondarily to epithelial keratitis, neurotrophic keratopathy or endotheliitis. Stromal keratitis can manifest in two forms, either as necrotizing stromal keratitis, which occurs due to direct invasion of virus or as immune stromal keratitis, which is caused due to the hypersensitivity reaction within stroma.[1,2]

Necrotizing stromal keratitis: Necrotizing stromal keratitis is a severe and rare form of viral keratitis and results due to direct invasion of virus thus, causing involvement of all the layers of cornea. Combination of replicating virus and intense host inflammatory reaction can result in destructive intrastromal inflammation that often mimics bacterial keratitis. Clinical signs include necrosis, ulceration and severe stromal infiltration associated with overlying epithelial defect. The ulcer often responds poorly to standard therapy and can progress to thinning and perforation within a short period.[1]

*Immune stromal keratitis:*Immune stromal keratitis is a common chronic recurrent manifestation of ocular HSV, and results from type III hypersensitivity reaction. It occurs in around 20% of patients with ocular HSV.[1,2] The retained viral antigen within the stroma triggers an antigen-antibody complement cascade, which further

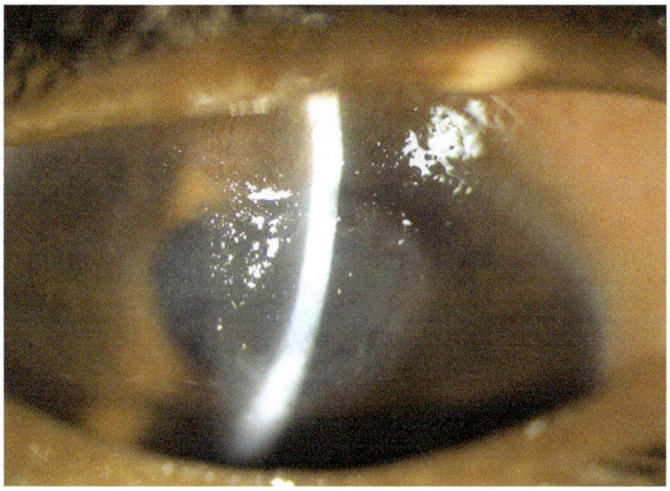

Fig. 24.6: Neurotrophic ulcers.

causes intrastromal inflammation. Overlying epithelium is usually intact. Immune stromal keratitis can present few days to years after an episode of infectious epithelial keratitis. However, in certain instances, there may not be a well-defined history of an epithelial keratitis. In such cases, meticulous history or the presence of ghost scars/herpetic footprints can help to clinch the diagnosis.[1]

The stromal keratitis is characterized by presence of stromal infiltrate, stromal haze, corneal edema and neovascularization (Fig. 24.7A). Stromal infiltration is the most common finding in immune stromal keratitis (Fig. 24.7B). These infiltrates are usually punctate that represent the antigen-antibody complexes. The stromal haze is due to inflammatory cellular infiltrates. The corneal edema is due to the associated inflammation rather than any endothelial malfunction.[1,2]

The HSV immune stromal keratitis can present with certain unique clinical features. Visual disturbances are very common in this condition. A specific form of immune stromal keratitis is the presence of immune ring of Wesley, which is due to the precipitation of the antigen-antibody complex in a circular manner. The ring can be complete or incomplete and can be present in mid- stroma of either the central or paracentral cornea. Another characteristic finding is presence of stromal neovascularization, which can be sectoral or can involve all the quadrants. After treatment, the neovascularization can resolve and leave behind empty vascular channels known as ghost vessels within stroma.[1] While the ghost vessels do not cause deterioration of the visual acuity themselves, the accompanying stromal scarring and thinning may do so. A prolonged inflammation accompanied by a persistent permanent neovascularization of the cornea puts any future corneal graft into high-risk category of rejection.[1] Lipid keratopathy can be associated with the accompanying stromal neovascularization that further increases the scarring and loss of visual acuity.

The clinical course of immune stromal keratitis is chronic, recurrent inflammation that responds to topical steroid therapy. Sometimes a constant low-grade inflammation may persist for years with intermittent flare-ups. Patients often need a prolonged topical corticosteroids regimen since uncontrolled or inadequately controlled inflammation can lead to stromal scarring, neovascularization, lipid keratopathy and severe loss of vision.[1]

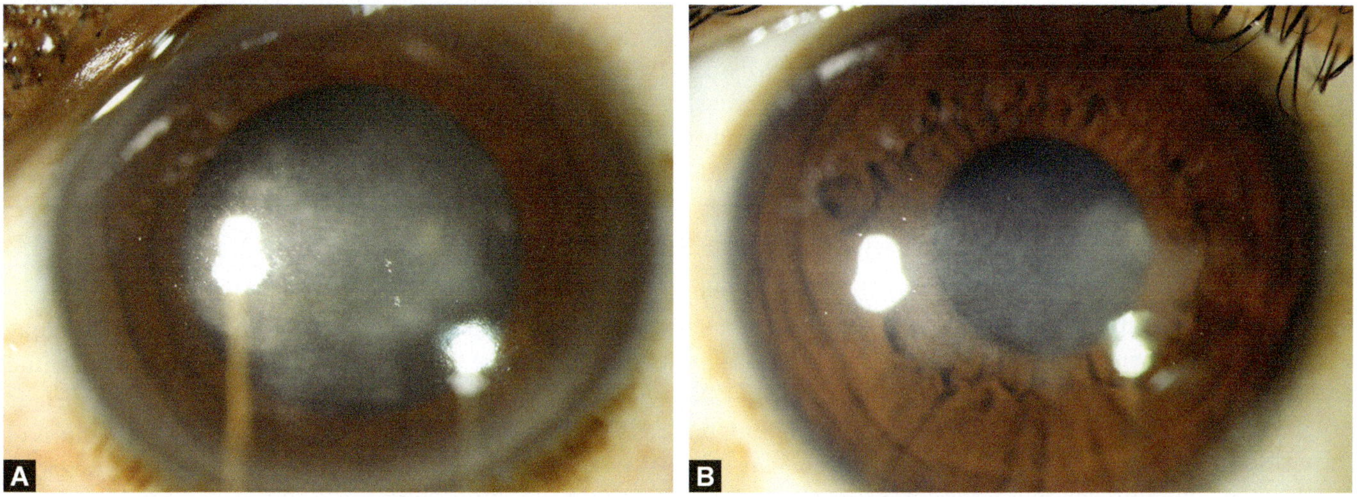

Figs. 24.7A and B: Stromal keratitis—(A) before; (B) after steroid therapy.

HERPETIC ENDOTHELIITIS

Herpetic endotheliitis is a result of delayed type of hypersensitivity reaction mediated by T- lymphocytes. It is characterized by presence of following findings: keratic precipitates (KP), overlying stromal and epithelial edema and iritis. Endotheliitis can be categorized as: disciform keratitis, diffuse endotheliitis and linear endotheliitis based on the distribution of KP and configuration of overlying stromal and epithelial edema.[1,2]

Disciform keratitis: In this condition, KPs are distributed in a disk-shaped pattern in the central or paracentral cornea. There is secondary edema of stroma and epithelium.[1] Corneal epithelium reveals microcystic edema, which corresponds to severe stromal edema. In late presentations, the stromal edema may mask the underlying KP, which may become evident after the edema has resolved. A mild to moderate iritis usually accompanies the disciform keratitis. It is important to remember that intraocular pressure (IOP) may be elevated, often severe in most cases. The rise in IOP is due to either inflammatory cells blocking aqueous outflow or primary trabeculitis. Patients present with complains of photophobia and ocular discomfort. There can be mild to severe reduction of vision depending on the location and severity of stromal and epithelial edema.[1]

Most cases are self-limiting and can resolve by their own, but severe cases can lead to permanent edema, scarring and neovascularization when left untreated. Similar to immune stromal keratitis, endotheliitis may occur months to years following an episode of infectious epithelial keratitis. At times there may not be any documented history and careful examination, looking for footprints of HSV or ghost scars is often helpful in making the proper diagnosis.[1]

Diffuse endotheliitis: This is a rare condition where KP are scattered all over the endothelium with overlying stromal edema and epithelial microcytic edema. Patient usually presents with complaints of pain, photophobia, redness and decreased vision. The clinical course of diffuse endotheliitis is similar to that of disciform endotheliitis.

Linear endotheliitis: Linear endotheliitis is also known by names of keratitis linearis migrans, progressive herpetic corneal endotheliitis and idiopathic corneal endotheliopathy.[1] It is characterized by a line of KP progressing from limbus to center, and is accompanied by peripheral stromal and epithelial edema between KP and limbus. This line can be sectoral, circumferential or rarely serpiginous in appearance. Similar to the differential edema and Khodadoust line seen in acute corneal graft rejection, there is often a well-demarcated line between the edematous and nonedematous cornea and the KP are present at the leading edge of the edema.[1] Presentation is similar to disciform keratitis, however, unlike the previous two types of endotheliitis, linear endotheliitis is quite difficult to treat.

DIAGNOSIS

The diagnosis of HSV keratitis is done mainly based on clinical examination but microbiological demonstration of the virus in culture and by staining will help to make a definite diagnosis.

Cytologic examination: Cytologic examination is done by staining specimens obtained by corneal scraping, with Wright or Giemsa stain. The characteristic finding is the presence of Cowdry type A intranuclear acidophilic inclusion bodies. In addition, multinucleated giant cells may also be seen. These staining techniques are rapid but not sensitive and hence, negative results do not exclude HSV infection.[1]

Electron microscopy: Corneal scrapings can be examined by electron microscopy for the presence of HSV particles in the nuclei of epithelial cells.[1]

Viral culture: The virus is relatively easy to isolate from corneal scrapings by the inoculation of the rabbit cornea, the brains of suckling mice, the chorioallantoic membrane of embryonated hen's eggs or a variety of tissue culture cells. Virus can be recovered readily from previously untreated dendritic ulcers.[1,2]

The lesion is swabbed and placed in viral transport media or into viral monolayer tubes and sent to laboratory where carrier medium is inoculated into cultures. A typical cytopathic effect is noticed in 5–10 days and the virus recovery rate is higher if the specimen is taken within 2–3 days of appearance of lesion. [11]

Polymerase chain reaction (PCR): PCR is a highly sensitive tool to demonstrate herpes viral DNA. It is less responsive in patients with atypical lesions. In stromal keratitis, PCR may be negative since the condition is due to the host immune response rather than direct viral infections. Dyes such as rose bengal and lissamine green inhibit the detection of HSV DNA by PCR assay and thus, may give false negative results.[12]

Viral load can be determined by obtaining the samples either by corneal scraping or from the tear film.[13]

Enzyme-linked immunosorbent assay (ELISA): ELISA and immunological tests like immunofiltration test, latex agglutination assays can be used to demonstrate antiviral antibodies and viral antigen. Immunologic tests for the detection of ocular HSV are commercially available and can detect HSV antigen in cell culture and direct specimens within 5 hours. Along with PCR, ELISA has also been used to detect virus in tear collections. However, the sensitivity of these tests is not that high, sensitivity of ELISA was found to be around 49.2% and specificity 82.6%.[14]

TREATMENT

Treatment of HSV ocular infections should be aimed at preserving the vision and reducing patient morbidity and as herpes simplex infections are recurrent in nature, prevention of recurrences is extremely important in long-term management.

MANAGEMENT OF EPITHELIAL KERATITIS

The infectious epithelial keratitis results from direct invasion of virus and responds well to the topical antiviral drugs. An adjuvant, often useful therapy is debriding the epithelium, which reduces the viral load.[1,15] This is performed by removal of the loose corneal epithelium with a dry, cotton-tipped applicator. The debrided epithelium can be sent for viral culture.[1]

Chemical debridement with such solutions as carbolic acid, iodine, alcohol and ether have been used in the past but all these chemical agents especially iodine, can damage the corneal stroma and may delay epithelial healing. Epithelial debridement is contraindicated in the coexistence of herpetic conjunctivitis and keratitis as conjunctiva provides a reservoir of virus, which can reinfect the exposed edge of the corneal epithelium.[1,2] It is also not advisable to debride when a neurotrophic component is suspected.

Topical antiviral drugs administered include 3% acyclovir ointment 5 times/day or 1% trifluridine solution 2 hourly when awake or ganciclovir gel 0.15% every 3 hours while awake.[1] Topical antivirals are usually continued for 10–14 days. After 5–7 days, ganciclovir is usually tapered to 3 times a day for the duration of the treatment period and trifluridine is usually tapered to 5 times a day for the rest of the treatment period.[1]

Epithelial lesions usually heal by 2 weeks as it takes 14 days for virus loaded basal epithelial cells to reach the surface and to shed off. Any epithelial keratitis persisting beyond 2 weeks with standard antiviral medication raises suspicion of epithelial toxicity or antiviral resistance rarely. Topical use of antiviral drugs in ocular herpes may cause a direct toxic effect on the corneal epithelium; "toxic" follicular conjunctivitis with conjunctival scarring and contact dermatitis of the lids.[1]

In addition to antivirals, a prophylactic antibiotic and lubricating eye drops can be added to the treatment regimen. Mild iridocyclitis may be associated with some cases and cycloplegics are added in such cases (2% Homatropine hydrobromide or 1% Cyclopentolate hydrochloride).[1]

MANAGEMENT OF NEUROTROPHIC KERATITIS

A long-standing nonhealing corneal ulcer characterizes neurotrophic keratitis. The goals of treatment of neurotrophic keratitis are to avoid potentially toxic medications, prevent progression of corneal damage and to promote epithelial healing. The therapy should be prompt and depends on clinical stage of the disease.[16]

The presence of punctate keratopathy, which represents *stage 1* requires the discontinuation of all topical antiviral medications and administration of topical preservative-free artificial tears.[1,2]

In *stage 2* of neurotrophic keratitis, an epithelial defect develops and management requires withdrawal of all topical epitheliotoxic drugs and preservative-free artificial tears can improve corneal surface. The patients should be carefully monitored because the progression of the disease is often without symptoms.[1,2]

In case of no improvement, corneal or scleral therapeutic contact lens can be used but their use may increase the risk of secondary infections.[17-19] If the ulcer is nonresponsive then, tarsorrhaphy or amniotic membrane transplantation can be done.[1,19]

In *stage 3* of neurotrophic keratitis, ulcer progresses quickly. Prophylactic topical antibiotic and preservative-free artificial tears are the initial treatment of choice. If stromal melting is present topical collagenase inhibitors such as N-acetylcysteine, tetracycline, or medroxyprogesterone may be administered. Tarsorrhaphy and conjunctival flap are effective surgical procedures in promoting corneal healing in cases of poor response. Small perforations can be treated with the application of cyanoacrylate glue followed by a soft bandage contact lens. Larger defects require either a patch graft (lamellar or full thickness) or a penetrating keratoplasty. The success rates of these corneal transplants are low because of poor wound healing and the persistent risk of epithelial defects owing to corneal anesthesia.[1,17-19]

MANAGEMENT OF STROMAL KERATITIS AND ENDOTHELIITIS

Immune Stromal Keratitis

Immune stromal keratitis is the result of hypersensitivity reaction and hence topical steroids are the treatment of choice. Often stromal keratitis may be associated with epithelial keratitis, in such cases, administration of topical steroids should be avoided and therapy should be directed towards managing epithelial lesions by topical antivirals as described earlier. Once the epithelial lesion heals, topical corticosteroids can be started.[20] Mild cases of stromal keratitis may resolve without the need of steroids. Although few clinicians do not find addition of prophylactic antivirals for immune stromal keratitis useful, we strongly suggest the use of antivirals since steroids can increase the risk of viral penetration into the cornea and individual keratocytes.[1]. It is usually recommended that topical antivirals should be administered along with corticosteroids with equal frequency (drop for drop) till the corticosteroids are tapered to once a day dose. However, topical antivirals are associated with significant toxicity and hence, we recommend oral acyclovir for few weeks in standard dose followed by prophylactic dose in cases where long-term antiviral cover is required.[1]

Dose of topical steroids: 0.1% dexamethasone or 1% prednisolone eye drops 4–6 times for severe disease and 0.12% prednisolone eye drops daily QID for less severe cases. Steroids are then tapered after 1-week-depending upon the clinical response. It is important to remember that steroids should never be tapered or stopped abruptly else rebound inflammation could occur.[1,2]

The major issue with immune stromal keratitis is recurrence of stromal keratitis or a chronic immunologic disease. These cases may need long-term steroid therapy, which predisposes them to steroid- induced complications such as glaucoma and cataract. However, it is important to remember that the control of inflammation outweighs the risk of such complications and steroids should never be withheld due to the unwanted fear of these complications.[1]

Topical cyclosporine 0.05% has also been found to treat effectively herpes simplex nonnecrotizing stromal keratitis which is unresponsive to topical prednisolone.[21]

Necrotizing stromal keratitis: In mild cases of necrotizing stromal keratitis, topical corticosteroids are administered. In all cases, administration of topical corticosteroids is to be accompanied with topical antiviral drugs like 1% trifluridine or 3% acyclovir ointment. Topical corticosteroids have to be tapered gradually over months usually 10 weeks to avoid reactivation of virus and rebound inflammation. Mydriatic-cycloplegic drugs like 2% homatropine and 1% cyclopentolate are added to reduce ciliary spasm.[2]

Role of oral antivirals: The different oral antivirals currently available are summarized in Table 24.4.[1,2] Oral antivirals are indicated in:

- Severe diffuse endotheliitis
- Herpetic iridocyclitis/trabeculitis
- Immunocompromised patients
- Prophylaxis in recurrent epithelial keratitis
- Prophylaxis for post-PK patients with history of HSV keratitis

Herpetic Eye Disease Study (HEDS), done in USA was a multi-armed set of five randomized placebo-controlled trials designed to determine best treatments and prophylaxis of HSV keratitis and one epidemiologic study to investigate for risk factors of HSV.[8,9,20] The conclusion of study has been summarized in Tables 24.5 and 24.6.[8,9,20]

Table 24.4: Oral antiviral drugs.

Drug	Mechanism of action	Treatment dose	Prophylactic dose
Acyclovir	Activated by viral thymidine kinase to inhibit DNA polymerase	400 mg 5 times/day	400 mg BD usually for 1 year
Famciclovir	Is a prodrug that is converted by first-pass metabolism to the antiviral drug penciclovir which further inhibits DNA polymerase of susceptible viruses	500 mg BD	250 mg BD
Valaciclovir	Activated by viral thymidine kinase to inhibit DNA polymerase	1,000 mg TDS	500 mg OD

Table 24.5: Summary of herpetic eye disease study-I.

Group	Comparison	Results
HSV stromal keratitis (On topical trifluridine but not on steroids)	*Group 1:* Topical 1% prednisolone acetate Group 2: Placebo	Faster resolution with steroids Final visual acuity same
HSV stromal keratitis (On topical trifluridine and prednisolone 1%)	*Group 1:* Oral acyclovir 400 mg 5 TID for 10 weeks *Group 2:* Placebo	No benefit of oral acyclovir
HSV iridocyclitis (On topical trifluridine and prednisolone 1%)	*Group 1:* Oral acyclovir 400 mg 5 TID for 10 weeks *Group 2:* Placebo	Decrease in treatment failure rate with oral acyclovir

Table 24.6: Summary of herpetic eye disease study-II.

Group	Comparison	Results
HSV epithelial keratitis trial (On topical trifluridine)	*Group 1:* Oral acyclovir 400 mg 5 TID *Group 2:* Placebo	No added advantage
HSV acyclovir prevention trial (Past history of keratitis with 1 year)	*Group 1:* Oral acyclovir 400 mg BD for 1 year *Group 2:* Oral placebo	41% decrease in recurrence 50% decrease in more severe keratitis
HSV risk factors study	Risk factors evaluated	*Risk factors:* History of epithelial keratitis

Surgical management: Surgical treatment in herpes keratitis is done only when the inflammation is subsided and eye is silent. Keratoplasty in herpetic disease is indicated in cases of corneal perforation to maintain corneal integrity and to restore vision in cases of healed keratitis. Keratoplasty done in cases of herpetic eye disease usually have a high failure rate and the recurrence of herpetic infection (Fig. 24.8) has been reported in 12–19% cases.[9] It is extremely important to differentiate post- keratoplasty graft rejection from viral reactivation. In cases of graft rejection, the inflammation is confined only to the donor cornea while in viral reactivation both host and donor cornea are involved. The KPs are typically seen on donor endothelium without affecting the host part in acute graft rejection while both host and graft are involved in case of viral reactivation. Also, epithelial rejection line and khodadoust endothelial rejection line are typically seen in cases of graft rejection. The raised epithelial rejection line can sometimes be misdiagnosed as viral dendritic keratitis. In addition, a typical khodadoust line may not be evident in all cases of endothelial graft rejection and can lead to misdiagnosis of viral keratouveitis. Therefore, a clear-cut distinction between graft rejection and viral reactivation is not always easy.

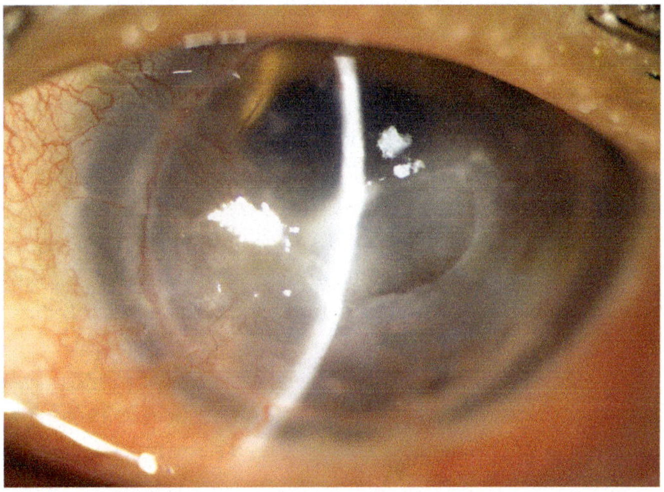

Fig. 24.8: Recurrence of viral keratitis in corneal graft.

HERPES ZOSTER OPHTHALMICUS

Varicella-zoster virus 9 (VZV-9), also known as herpes virus III, differs clinically and antigenically from herpes simplex. It causes varicella (chicken pox) and herpes zoster (shingles).[22]

Epidemiology

Annual incidence of herpes zoster is 1.5/1,000 to 3/1,000 cases and has no gender, race or seasonal variations.[1,22]

Etiopathogenesis

Chickenpox represents the primary infection after exposure of a nonimmune person to VZV. The virus then becomes latent in the cells of dorsal root ganglion. Reactivation results in characteristic dermatological eruptions, often resembling a dermatome. An eruption of herpes zoster in young adults should arouse the suspicion of immunosuppression.[22]

The virus commonly involves ophthalmic division of trigeminal nerve. Reactivation is preceded by a prodrome of malaise, fever and headache. Hutchinson's sign is the occurrence of vesicles at the side and tip of nose that indicates involvement of nasociliary branch of ophthalmic division of trigeminal nerve and is pathognomonic of herpes zoster ophthalmicus.[22] Nasociliary nerve involvement in herpes zoster ophthalmicus is associated with increased risk of ocular complications.

Clinical Features

Clinical manifestations are variable and include punctuate epithelial keratitis, pseudodendritic keratitis, anterior stromal infiltrates or nummular keratitis, keratouveitis and endotheliitis. Patient can also present with serpiginous ulceration, sclerokeratitis, corneal mucous plaques, disciform keratitis, neurotrophic keratopathy, exposure keratopathy and interstitial keratitis. Keratouveitis is usually accompanied and severity varies according to the immune status of patient.

Pseudodendrites are broader, more plaque-like and without central ulceration. Varicella-zoster Virus is present in these lesions.[22] Difference between true and pseudodendrites has been summarized in Table 24.7.

Other ocular features include conjunctival hyperemia, petechial hemorrhages, papillary or follicular reaction, pseudomembrane formation, episcleritis and scleritis. Patchy scleral atrophy can occur as a long-term complication of scleritis. Painful posterior scleritis because of infiltrative perivasculitis and perineuritis can also occur. Posterior segment complications include acute retinal vasculitis, acute retinal necrosis, progressive outer retinal necrosis and acute optic neuritis. Transient palsy of third, fourth and sixth cranial nerve is also seen as a result of vasculitis within the orbital apex or due to brain stem dysfunction. Postherpetic neuralgia (PHN) is a common long-term complication of VZ seen in 35% of cases not receiving antiviral therapy and in 15% of cases treated with antiviral drugs.[23]

Management

Management of herpes zoster ophthalmicus requires treatment to be started within 72 hours of onset of rash with high doses of oral acyclovir 800 mg 5 times/day or valacyclovir 1 g thrice a day or famciclovir 500 mg thrice a day for 7–10 days.[1,22] Oral valacyclovir and famciclovir have better oral bioavailability and compliance to medication considering the less frequent dosing. The only concern is that it is more expensive than acyclovir. This treatment protocol reduces the risk of ocular involvement from 50% to 30 % but there is no difference in the rate of PHN. Elderly patients and immunocompromised individuals affected with herpes zoster benefit the most, as they are at high risk for complications.Topical antivirals may be useful for the skin lesion, but are not very useful for the corneal condition. Topical steroids such as 1% prednisolone acetate are useful in nummular keratitis, sclerokeratitis and disciform keratitis.

In an ongoing multicenter randomized clinical trial, the Zoster Eye Disease Study (ZEDS), the role of prophylactic oral valacyclovir 1 g daily for 1 year in immunocompetent patients with an episode of dendritiform epithelial keratitis, stromal keratitis, endothelial keratitis and/or iritis due to Herpes Zoster Ophthalmicus (HZO) is being assessed. The pilot data of the proposed study concluded that cases of HZO treated with antivirals using acyclovir 400 mg orally twice daily or valacyclovir 500 mg daily lead to reduced recurrences in cases of HZO by 35%.[24,25]

Table 24.7: Difference between dendrites and pseudodendrites.

Feature	Dendrite	Pseudodendrite
Causative agent	Herpes simplex virus	Herpes zoster virus Others: Neurotrophic epitheliopathy, Acanthamoeba, healing epithelial defect, and recurrent erosion syndrome
Epithelium	Fine lacy linear epithelial defect with barred stroma, surrounded by edematous epithelial cells	Elevated painted on or "stuck on appearance" appearance
Staining pattern	Base stains with fluorescein and border epithelial cells stain with rose bengal	Shows minimal fluorescein staining
Location	More in central cornea	More in peripheral cornea
Depth	More deep	More superficial
Terminal bulbs	Frequently present	Absent

Zostavax, a live attenuated VZV vaccine has been approved by US-FDA in 2006 for prevention of herpes zoster in individuals 60 years of age and older. In a randomized controlled trial, Zostavax was found to reduce the incidence of herpes zoster by 51.3%and that of PHN by 66.5%. The most common adverse effect to this vaccine was injection site inflammation, seen more commonly in young patients. There have been few case reports of postvaccination stromal keratitis and endotheliitis and have been attributed to the immune reponse to vaccine.[26] PHN is a neuropathic pain due to damage to the sensory neurons by HZV. Patients present with either continuous or paroxysmal episodes of symptoms like allodynia and itching. Poor response to treatment has been noted in various studies. Drugs used for treatment of PHN include: tricyclic antidepressants (nortryptiline and amitriptyline), anticonvulsants (gabapentin and pregabalin), opioids (morphine), topical agents (lidocaine patch or gel, and capsaicin) and intrathecal steroids. Also, vaccine against herpes zoster (Zostavax) may reduce the incidence of PHN.[27]

ADENOVIRAL KERATITIS

Etiology

Adenoviral keratitis is commonly associated with fever and upper respiratory infection. The Keratitis is seen associated with pharyngoconjunctival fever (PCF) caused by type 3, 4, 7 adenoviruses and more commonly with epidemic keratoconjunctival fever.[28] It is highly contagious and transmits from person to person by direct contact, fomites, ophthalmic solutions and hands of health care workers.[28]

Clinical Manifestations

Stage I: Stage I is characterized by punctate epithelial erosions (7–10 days). Initially these lesions are small epithelial vesicle -like elevations, about 25–30 microns in size and are not visible in slit- lamp. After 2–5 days, these lesions coalesce and become clearly visible. This stage is self-limiting in 2 weeks and antivirals are not useful.

Stage II: Stage II is characterized by focal white subepithelial opacities (Fig. 24.9), which represent an immune response to the virus.

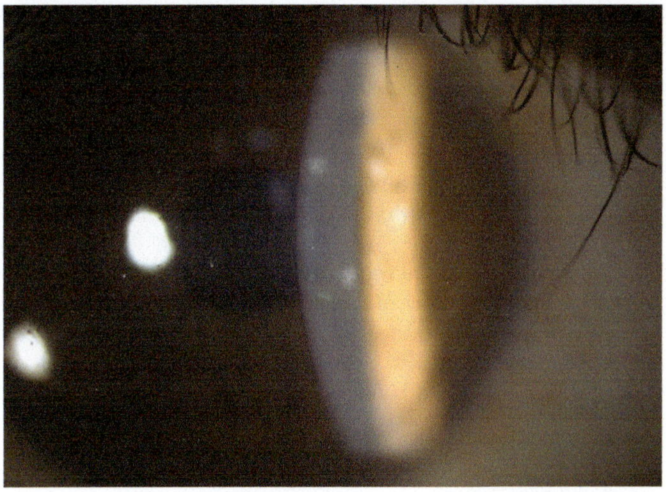

Fig. 24.9: Subepithelial infiltrates in adenoviral keratitis.

Stage III: Stage III is characterized by anterior stromal infiltrates, which fade over months or years. These lesions are typically associated with preauricular lymphadenopathy and needs supportive and symptomatic treatment. Steroids suppress inflammation but lesions can recur on tapering steroids.

Stage IV: Stage IV is characterized by nummular opacities and can be present months to weeks after initial episode.[28]

REFERENCES

1. Holland EJ, Brilakis HS, Schwartz GS. Herpes simplex keratitis. In: Krachmer JH, Mannis MJ, Holland EJ (Eds). Cornea, 2nd edition. St. Louis: Mosby; 2004. pp. 1043-74.
2. Pepose JS, Keadle TL, Morrison LA. Ocular herpes simplex: changing epidemiology, emerging disease patterns, and the potential of vaccine prevention and therapy. Am J Ophthalmol. 2006;141(3):547-57.
3. Cohrs R, Randall J, Smith J, et al. Analysis of individual human trigeminal ganglia for latent herpes simplex virus type 1 and varicella-zoster virus nucleic acid using real-time PCR. J Virol. 2000;74(24):11464-71.
4. Liesegang TJ. Herpes simplex virus epidemiology and ocular importance. Cornea. 2001;20(1):1-13.
5. Liesegang TJ. Epidemiology of ocular herpes simplex virus. Arch Ophthalmol. 1989;107(8):1160-5.
6. Jeffries DJ. Intra-uterine and neonatal herpes simplex virus infection. Scand J Infect Dis Suppl. 1991;80:21-6.
7. Kaufman, HE, Rayfield, MA. Viral conjunctivitis and keratitis. In: Kaufman HE, Barron BA, McDonald MB, Waltman SR (Eds.). Cornea. New York: Churchill Livingstone; 1988.
8. Barron BA. Herpetic Eye Disease Study. A controlled trial of oral acyclovir for herpes simplex stromal keratitis. Ophthalmology. 1994;101(12):1871-82.
9. The Herpetic Eye Disease Study Group. Oral acyclovir for herpes simplex virus eye disease. Effect on prevention of epithelial and stromal keratitis. Arch Ophthalmol. 2000;118(8):1030-6.

10. Wilhelmus KR. Diagnosis and management of herpes simplex stromal keratitis. Cornea. 1987;6(4):286-91.
11. Hanna L, Jawetz E, Coleman VR. Studies on herpes simplex VIII. The significance of isolating herpes simplex virus from the eye. Am J Ophthalmol. 1957;43(4):126-31.
12. Seitzman GD, Cevallos V, Margolis TP. Rose bengal and lissamine green inhibit detection of herpes simplex virus by PCR. Am J Ophthalmol. 2006;141(4):756-8.
13. Satpathy G, Mishra AK, Tandon R, et al. Evaluation of tear samples for herpes simplex virus 1 (HSV) detection in suspected cases of viral keratitis using PCR assay and conventional laboratory diagnostic tools. Br J Ophthalmol. 2011;95(3):415-8.
14. Shoji J, Sakimoto T, Inada N, et al. A diagnostic method for herpes simplex keratitis by simultaneous measurement of viral DNA and virus-specific secretory IgA in tears: an evaluation. Jpn J Opthalmol. 2016;60(4):294-301.
15. Wilhelmus KR. The treatment of herpes simplex virus epithelial keratitis. Trans Am Ophthalmol Soc. 2000;98:505-32.
16. Lambiase A, Rama P, Aloe L, et al. Management of neurotrophic keratopathy. Curr Opin Ophthalmol. 1999;10(4):270-6.
17. Gould HL. Treatment of neurotrophic keratitis with scleral contact lenses. Eye Ear Nose Throat Mon. 1967;46(11):1406-14.
18. Kent HD, Cohen EJ, Laibson PR, et al. Microbial keratitis and corneal ulceration associated with therapeutic soft contact lenses. CLAO J. 1990;16(1):49-52.
19. Pfister RR. Clinical measures to promote corneal epithelial healing. Acta Ophthalmol Suppl. 1992;202:73-83.
20. Wilhelmus KR, Gee L, Hauck WW, et al. Herpetic Eye Disease Study. A controlled trial of topical corticosteroids for herpes simplex stromal keratitis. Ophthalmology. 1994;101(12):1883-95.
21. Rao SN. Treatment of herpes simplex virus stromal keratitis unresponsive to topical prednisolone 1% with topical cyclosporine 0.05%. Am J Ophthalmol. 2006;141(4):771-2.
22. Kaufman HE. Treatment of viral diseases of the cornea and external eye. Prog Retin Eye Res. 2000;19(1):69-85.
23. Liesegang TJ. Herpes zoster ophthalmicus natural history, risk factors, clinical presentation, and morbidity. Ophthalmology. 2008;115(2 Suppl):S3-12.
24. ClinicalTrials. Zoster Eye Disease Study. [online] Available from: *https://clinicaltrials.gov/ct2/show/NCT03134196.* [Accessed November, 2017].
25. Miserocchi E, Fogliato G, Bianchi I, et al. Clinical features of ocular herpetic infection in an Italian referral center. Cornea. 2014;33(6):565-70.
26. Cohen EJ. Management and prevention of herpes zoster ocular disease. Cornea. 2015;34(Suppl 10):S3-8.
27. Johnson RW. Herpes zoster and postherpetic neuralgia. Expert Rev Vaccines. 2010;9(3Suppl):21-6.
28. Kaufman HE. Adenovirus advances: new diagnostic and therapeutic options. Curr Opin Ophthalmol. 2011;22(4):290-3.

Chapter 25 Immunological Disorders of Cornea

Jeremy Keenan

INTRODUCTION

The cornea is an immune privileged, avascular tissue, and thus has natural protection from immune-mediated diseases. Nonetheless, innate and adaptive immune responses of the ocular surface can lead to a host of diseases, either as a normal inflammatory response to infection or other stimuli, or as a dysregulation of the normal immune response as seen in systemic or localized autoimmune diseases. Immune-mediated corneal processes often start in the peripheral cornea which has more Langerhans cells and immunoglobulin M (IgM) than the central cornea and closer access to the limbal blood vessels. Several different immune mechanisms can cause ocular surface disease (Table 25.1). The major entities causing immune-mediated corneal disease are summarized below.

Table 25.1: Classification of hypersensitivity reactions.

Type	Pathophysiology	Examples
I	Allergic	Hay fever and allergic conjunctivitis
II	Cell mediated	Mucous membrane pemphigoid
III	Immune complex	Vasculitis, peripheral ulcerative keratitis, and scleritis
IV	Delayed type	Staphylococcal marginal keratitis and phlyctenulosis

PERIPHERAL ULCERATIVE KERATITIS

Peripheral ulcerative keratitis (PUK) is characterized by peripheral corneal stromal infiltration and thinning with an overlying epithelial defect. The chief symptoms of PUK are eye discomfort which can range from mild irritation to severe pain and photophobia, and decreased vision, usually from irregular astigmatism. Conjunctivitis or episcleritis is often present, and usually precedes the corneal findings. PUK often arises adjacent to a site of scleritis, especially in the case of necrotizing scleritis. Corneal stromal infiltrates, an overlying epithelial defect, and stromal thinning are present in a crescent-shaped pattern at the limbus (Figs. 25.1A and B). If untreated the inflammatory process will progress circumferentially and centrally, and can result in perforation. PUK is bilateral in about half of the cases.

The pathophysiology of PUK is not entirely clear, but it is thought that conjunctival vessels provide inflammatory mediators access to the peripheral cornea. Immune complexes are deposited in the peripheral cornea and activate the classical pathway of the complement system,

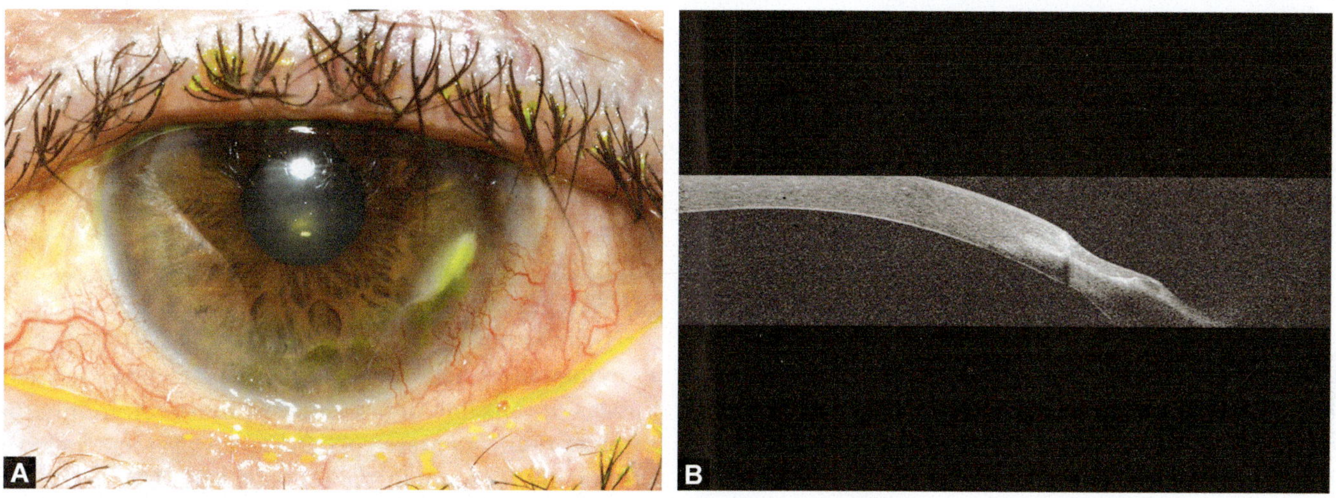

Figs. 25.1A and B: Idiopathic peripheral ulcerative keratitis.
Source: Nisha Acharya, MD.

Table 25.2: Disorders that can present with findings of peripheral ulcerative keratitis.

Category	Conditions
Aqueous deficiency	Keratoconjunctivitis sicca, mucous membrane pemphigoid, graft versus host disease, and Stevens-Johnson syndrome
Blepharitis-related	Rosacea and staphylococcal marginal keratitis
Burn	Chemical, thermal, and radiation
Exposure	Lagophthalmos, ectropion, and incomplete blink
Immune-mediated	Rheumatoid arthritis, granulomatosis with polyangiitis, polyarteritis nodosa, microscopic polyangiitis, eosinophilic granulomatosis with polyangiitis, relapsing polychondritis, systemic sclerosis, psoriatic arthritis, Sjögren's syndrome, sarcoidosis, systemic lupus erythematosus, inflammatory bowel disease, and Mooren's ulcer
Infectious, exogenous	Bacterial, fungal, viral, and amoebic
Infectious and endogenous	Gonorrhea, syphilis, tuberculosis, and zoster
Nutritional	Xerophthalmia
Postsurgical	Cataract surgery, laser refractive surgery, and glaucoma surgery
Other	Terrien's marginal degeneration and sarcoidosis

thereby recruiting proinflammatory cytokines and an immune cell infiltrate. Stromal keratocytes produce matrix metalloproteinases which in turn lead to stromal degradation and thinning.

The findings of PUK prompt consideration of a broad differential diagnosis (Table 25.2). Many causes can be ruled out with a thorough history. The review of systems should be targeted to detect possible systemic infection, collagen vascular disease, or vasculitis (Table 25.3). Exogenous bacterial and fungal pathogens can cause peripheral ulcers, and should be ruled out by sending corneal scrapings for smear and culture. Systemic infections such as syphilis and tuberculosis have been reported to cause peripheral corneal ulcers, and should be ruled out with serologic tests. Systemic immune-medicated conditions should be assessed with serologic testing.

Rheumatoid arthritis (RA) is the most common systemic disease causing PUK. RA usually affects the hands, wrists, knees, and feet, and unlike osteoarthritis, spares the distal interphalangeal joints. As with other inflammatory arthritides, the arthralgias are normally worse in the morning. The most common ocular complications of RA are keratoconjunctivitis sicca (KCS), scleritis, and PUK. Serologic tests include rheumatic factor (RF) and the more specific anti-cyclic citrullinated peptide (CCP). Ocular disease almost always occurs in people with known RA, although scleritis has been reported to occur as the initial clinical finding, so serologic tests should be performed. RA is treated with a variety of immunomodulatory agents, most commonly antimetabolites and tumor necrosis factor-α (TNF-α) inhibitors.

Table 25.3: Review of systems and testing in patients with peripheral ulcerative keratitis.

Disease	Review of systems	Screening tests
Syphilis	Known history, signs, or symptoms of syphilis or sexually transmitted infection	Treponemal antibody test
Tuberculosis	Known history, signs, or symptoms of pulmonary or extrapulmonary tuberculosis	IFN-γ release assay and tuberculin skin test
Rheumatoid arthritis	Arthralgias, inflammatory nodules especially in proximal interphalangeal or metacarpophalangeal joints or wrist	RF and anti-CCP
Polyangiitis with granulomatosis	Fever, weight loss, arthralgia, rhinosinusitis, cough, dyspnea, and urinary abnormalities	ANCA (usually anti-PR3)
Microscopic polyangiitis	Fever, weight loss, arthralgia, rhinosinusitis, cough, dyspnea, and urinary abnormalities	ANCA (usually anti-MPO)
Eosinophilic granulomatosis with polyangiitis	Atopy, allergic rhinitis, and asthma	ANCA
Relapsing polychondritis	Pain in cartilage of ears and nose, hearing loss, dyspnea, and arthritis	None
Systemic lupus erythematosus	Fatigue, rashes, skin photosensitivity, alopecia, and arthritis	ANA
Systemic inflammation		ESR and CRP

(ANA: Antinuclear antibody; ANCA: Anti-neutrophil cytoplasmic antibody; Anti-CCP: Anti-cyclic citrullinated peptide; CRP: C-reactive protein; ESR: Erythrocyte sedimentation rate; IFN-γ: Interferon-gamma; MPO: Myeloperoxidase; PR3: Proteinase-3; RF: Rheumatoid factor)

Granulomatosis with polyangiitis (GPA) is a granulomatous necrotizing vasculitis affecting the small vessels of multiple organ systems, most commonly the respiratory and renal systems. Ocular involvement includes orbitopathy, conjunctivitis, scleritis, and PUK (Fig. 25.2).

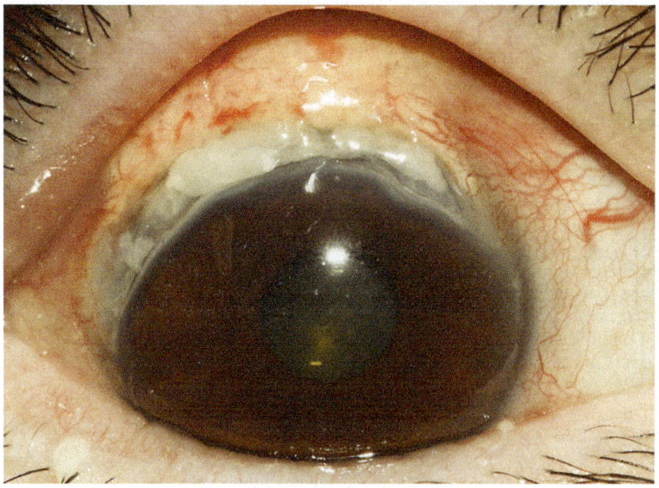

Fig. 25.2: Peripheral ulcerative keratitis due to granulomatosis with polyangiitis.
Source: Thuy Doan, MD.

GPA is the second most common disease causing PUK. The key diagnostic test for GPA is the anti-neutrophil cytoplasmic antibody (ANCA) test which usually reveals a cytoplasmic staining pattern on the indirect immunofluorescence assay (c-ANCA) and anti-proteinase-3 antibodies on the enzyme-linked immunosorbent assay (ELISA). PGA is fatal if not treated. First-line therapies include the anti-CD20 monoclonal antibody rituximab and the alkylating agent cyclophosphamide.

Mooren's ulcer is a PUK with no associated systemic immune disorder.[1] The key features that differentiate Mooren's ulcer from idiopathic PUK are severe pain and lack of scleritis; in addition, Mooren's ulcer may be more likely to involve the limbus than PUK, and the stromal melting classically leaves the uninvolved central cornea with a steep, overhanging edge. Despite the absence of an underlying immune condition, Mooren's ulcer often requires systemic therapy with cyclophosphamide, rituximab, or another immunosuppressive agent to gain control of inflammation.

Management of PUK begins with appropriate diagnostic tests. Infection should be ruled out through corneal scrapings and superinfection prevented with broad spectrum topical antibiotics. Prompt administration of oral or intravenous high-dose corticosteroids is important to quickly control inflammation and prevent progression and perforation. Institution or escalation of systemic immunosuppression is usually required with an antimetabolite, calcineurin inhibitor, alkylating agent, or biologic agent, with the therapy targeted to the underlying inflammatory condition. Immunosuppression is not only necessary for controlling ocular inflammation, but has also been shown to reduce mortality in conditions like RA and GPA. Topical corticosteroids are not effective at controlling the inflammation, and may even increase the risk of perforation by inhibiting collage production. In vitro studies have shown that doxycycline inhibits matrix metalloproteinase activity and that ascorbic acid enhances collagen synthesis, so oral doxycycline and topical ascorbate are often used in an attempt to prevent corneal thinning, although little clinical evidence exists demonstrating their efficacy. Conjunctival resection may be performed in an attempt to remove the inflammatory mediators present in the limbal conjunctiva, and has been especially advocated for Mooren's ulcer. Corneal perforations less than 2 mm should be managed with cyanoacrylate glue and a bandage contact lens. Larger perforations can be managed with amniotic membrane and fibrin glue or lamellar or full-thickness keratoplasty. Corneal grafts should be avoided until the inflammation is under control since transplanted tissue will rapidly melt in the absence of systemic immunosuppression.

KERATOCONJUNCTIVITIS SICCA

Dry eye syndromes can generally be classified into conditions of aqueous deficiency or excessive tear evaporation.[2] KCS is an aqueous deficiency dry eye syndrome that commonly accompanies systemic immune-mediated diseases such as RA, Sjögren's syndrome (SS), and systemic lupus erythematosus (SLE). Subclinical ocular surface inflammation is a key feature of KCS, although eyes rarely appear overtly inflamed. Like other dry eye syndromes, ocular symptoms in KCS are described in various ways including grittiness, burning, itchiness, soreness, and visual disturbance, though the key symptom descriptors for screening purposes are dryness and irritation.

Several examination techniques are helpful when evaluating dry eye disease. The eyelids are examined for evidence of lagophthalmos, blepharitis, and meibomitis. The tear film meniscus of the lower eyelid is measured with the slit lamp biomicroscope set to a thin beam; values of 1 mm or greater are considered normal. The tear film breakup time is measured by instilling fluorescein dye and counting the seconds until the appearance of a dark disruption of the tear film under the cobalt blue light; values of more than and equal to 10 seconds indicate a stable tear film. Approximately 1.5–3 minutes following instillation of

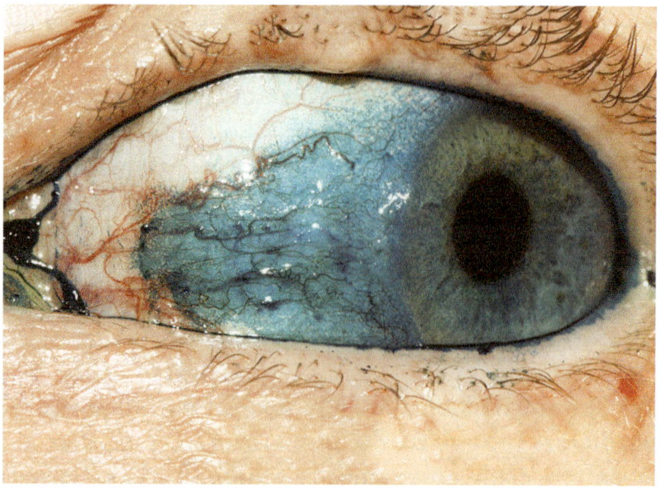

Fig. 25.3: Interpalpebral conjunctival lissamine green staining in keratoconjunctivitis sicca due to Sjögren's syndrome.
Source: John Gonzales, MD.

fluorescein, the cornea is examined for punctate epithelial erosions. The cornea should also be examined for filaments which are strands of epithelial cells and mucous that adhere to areas of irregular epithelium. Lissamine green dye is then instilled and the conjunctival staining pattern evaluated after 1–4 minutes; the key finding is staining in the interpalpebral area (Fig. 25.3). Several different systems have been designed to grade corneal and conjunctival staining; one of the most recent is the ocular staining score (OSS) (Table 25.4).[3] The Schirmer I test is performed by placing a piece of filter paper in the unanesthetized lower fornix for 5 minutes and counting the extent to which the paper wets; values of more than and equal to 10 mm are considered normal. The Schirmer I test measures basal tear secretion and reflex tearing. The same test performed in an anesthetized eye measures only baseline tearing with values of more than and equal to 5 mm considered normal. The phenol red thread test is analogous to the Schirmer's test but conducted for only 15 seconds; values of more than and equal to 10 mm are considered normal. In addition to these traditional tests, high tear osmolarity as assessed by an in-office device can be used as a test for dry eye disease. Although there is an overlap, aqueous tear deficiency is generally characterized by low tear meniscus, interpalpebral corneal and conjunctival staining, and low Schirmer's testing, whereas evaporative dry eye is characterized by the presence of blepharitis and short tear film breakup time.

Sjögren's syndrome is a chronic progressive autoimmune condition that causes dysfunction of the exocrine glands of mucosal membranes, primarily the lacrimal and salivary glands. Primary SS occurs in an otherwise healthy person; secondary SS in someone with a coexisting autoimmune disease such as RA or SLE. Approximately half of SS cases are secondary. Women are considerably more affected with SS with a female:male ratio of 9:1. Among women, the incidence of primary SS increases with age, peaking around age 60. Diagnosis of SS is based on ocular tests (OSS and Schirmer's tests), oral tests (minor salivary gland and salivary flow rate), and laboratory tests [anti-SS-A/Rho, anti-SS-B/La, antinuclear antibodies (ANAs), and RF]. The most recent consensus diagnostic classification for SS is shown in Table 25.5.[4] Although the management of KCS is similar in patients with and without SS, the diagnosis is important because of the possibility of multi-organ involvement as well as an increased risk of lymphoma.

The most common underlying immune-mediated conditions associated with secondary SS are RA and SLE. Conversely, KCS is the most common ocular complication for both RA and SLE. The key features of RA were summarized above. SLE is a multi-organ inflammatory disease that can affect many different parts of the eye. KCS is the most common ocular manifestation followed by retinopathy. While an ANA test is often sent to screen for SLE, this test has relatively high false positive rate and thus the clinician should consider the pretest probability of SLE before ordering this test.

Table 25.4: Ocular staining score (OSS).[3]

Points[a]	Cornea[b]	Conjunctiva[c]
0	0 dots	0 dots
1	1–5 dots	10–32 dots
2	6–30 dots	33–100 dots
3	>30 dots	>100 dots

[a]The nasal and temporal conjunctiva are graded separately, and an extra point is given for each of the following types of corneal staining: Patches of confluent staining, staining in pupillary area, or ≥1 filaments. Thus, OSS values can range from 0 to 12 points for each eye.
[b]Corneal staining is graded 1.5–3 minutes after instillation of fluorescein dye.
[c]Conjunctival staining is graded 1–4 minutes after instillation of lissamine green dye.

Table 25.5: Diagnosis of Sjögren's syndrome (SS).[4]

Weight	Test
3	Focal lymphocytic sialadenitis
3	anti-SS-A/Rho
1	Ocular staining score ≥5 in at least 1 eye
1	Schirmer's test ≥5 mm at 5 minutes in at least 1 eye
1	Unstimulated whole saliva flow rate ≤0.1 mL/min

Note: A summed weighted score of ≥4 points fulfills the diagnosis of SS.

Keratoconjunctivitis sicca is primarily managed with punctal occlusion, lubrication, and pharmacotherapy. Punctal occlusion of the lower and upper punctae can be performed either with temporary silicon punctal plugs or punctal cautery. A variety of artificial tear supplements are available in varying viscosities and with varying chemical vehicles. In general, artificial tears are instilled as needed for symptomatic relief; patients using artificial tears more than 4 times per day should use nonpreserved formulations, if possible. Several topical medications are available to address the subclinical ocular surface inflammation of KCS. Topical corticosteroids often provide symptomatic benefit, but their use must be closely monitored due to potential adverse effects. Topical cyclosporine is used in an attempt to decrease cell-mediated inflammatory responses; randomized trials of 0.05% cyclosporine have shown this medication to improve several dry eye syndrome parameters. Topical lifitegrast is also thought to play a role in cell-mediated immunity and has been shown to improve dry eye symptoms and corneal staining in randomized trials. Oral pilocarpine stimulates salivary and lacrimal gland secretion, though the high doses required for lacrimal secretion normally produce side effects such as sweating and palpitations and thus preclude its use specifically for eye disease.

INTERSTITIAL KERATITIS

Interstitial keratitis (IK) is characterized by corneal stromal white blood cell infiltration without primary epithelial involvement.[5] Several different infectious conditions ultimately result in IK (Table 25.6), either through an inflammatory response during active corneal infection or through an immune-mediated process after the active infection has been cleared. Symptoms during acute episodes of inflammation include photophobia, pain, tearing, and reduced vision. On slit lamp examination, a unilateral or bilateral corneal stromal white blood cell infiltrate is present. The infiltrate can be either focal or diffuse, and located at any level of the stroma. An epithelial defect does not precede the stromal infiltrate, although the epithelium can be involved as a result of adjacent stromal inflammation. Stromal vascularization is a common feature with vessels directed from the limbus towards the area of infiltration. Associated signs of inflammation such as conjunctival injection, fine keratic precipitates, and anterior chamber inflammation may be present. Resolution results in vascularized stromal scarring with variable corneal thinning, and occasionally in so-called 'ghost vessels'.

Table 25.6: Causes of interstitial keratitis.

Bacteria	Viruses	Parasitic	Noninfectious
Syphilis	Herpes simplex	Leishmaniasis	Cogan's syndrome
Tuberculosis	Herpes zoster	Onchocerciasis	Sarcoidosis
Chlamydia	Epstein-Barr	Trypanosomiasis	
Relapsing fever	Mumps	Acanthamoeba	
Brucellosis	Measles	Microsporidia	
Lyme disease			
Leprosy			

Historically, congenital syphilis was the most common cause of IK. Congenital syphilis is acquired transplacentally, but inflammation only becomes apparent at 5–20 years of age. The disease represents a host immune reaction to an unclear antigenic stimulus; treponemes are not found in the cornea or aqueous. Classically, the most prominent symptom is photophobia, and examination reveals a bilateral IK starting at the superior limbus with stromal involvement so deep that the accompanying blood vessels appear to be at the level of Descemet's membrane. Stromal vascularization and edema can cause the appearance of a so-called 'salmon patch'. Untreated congenital syphilis will resolve spontaneously within several months, leaving variable corneal scarring and ghost vessels. Corneal thinning can occur as can scrolls of Descemet's membrane. Acquired syphilis can also cause a delayed IK which is usually unilateral and milder in presentation. Diagnosis of syphilis is established with serologic tests. Treponemal antibody tests are highly specific and remain positive for life. The less specific rapid plasma reagin (RPR) and venereal disease research laboratory (VDRL) tests are used to determine recent or active disease. Evaluation of the cerebrospinal fluid is recommended in congenital syphilis or when neurosyphilis is suspected. Congenital syphilis should be distinguished from Cogan's syndrome which consists of bilateral IK and vestibuloauditory symptoms (Fig. 25.4). Syphilis is treated with a single intramuscular dose of penicillin for primary, secondary, or early latent syphilis and a 10-day course of intravenous penicillin for congenital, tertiary, and neurosyphilis. However, penicillin will not improve the immune-mediated corneal disease. Topical corticosteroids and cycloplegics reduce pain, speed resolution, and result in better visual outcomes.

Currently, the most common cause of IK is herpetic disease (Fig. 25.5). IK caused by herpes simplex virus (HSV)

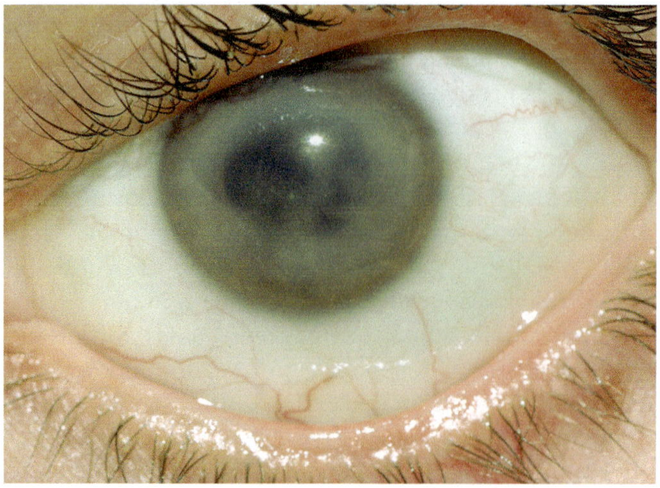

Fig. 25.4: Interstitial keratitis due to Cogan's syndrome.

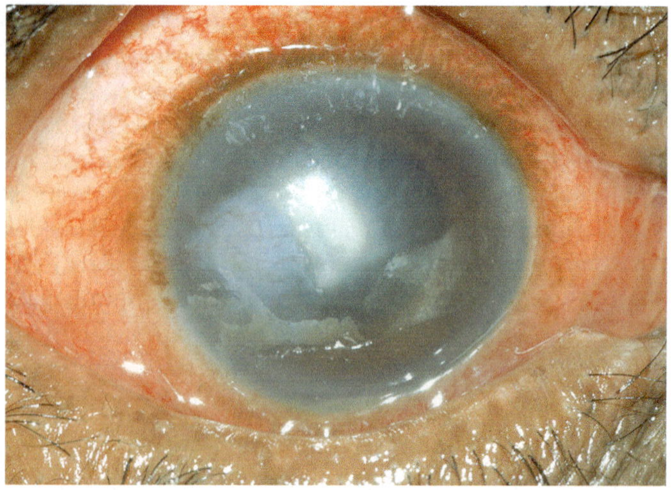

Fig. 25.5: Interstitial keratitis due to herpes simplex virus infection.

is usually unilateral with a focal vascularized infiltrate. Corneal sensation is often diminished near the infiltrate, but may be normal elsewhere. Other signs of anterior segment herpetic infection may be present including sectoral iris atrophy and hypertensive anterior uveitis. Herpetic IK is primarily an immune reaction to viral particles in the corneal stroma. Viral culture and polymerase chain reaction (PCR) tests are low yield unless the epithelium is also involved. Corneal inflammation is normally responsive to low-dose topical corticosteroid therapy, but an oral antiviral such as acyclovir must be used concurrently to suppress viral replication. Varicella-zoster virus (VZV) can cause a clinical picture similar to HSV keratitis although classically results in diminished corneal sensation diffusely throughout the cornea. The diagnosis is usually obvious based on a prior V1 dermatomal rash, though the virus can uncommonly cause corneal disease in the absence of skin involvement. Management principles for all forms of IK include corneal scrapings for appropriate culture, smear, and PCR testing followed by the treatment of any infections and subsequent topical corticosteroids. Low-dose anti-inflammatory therapy must often be continued for months, years, or even indefinitely.

OCULAR ROSACEA

Rosacea is a common progressive disease of the skin and pilosebaceous units that most often affects fair-skinned middle-aged individuals.[6] While the pathogenesis is not entirely clear, rosacea is thought to result from dysregulation of innate immune responses. The current classification scheme divides rosacea into four subtypes: (1) Erythematotelangiectactic, (2) Papulopustular, (3) Phymatous, and (4) Ocular. Rosacea primarily affects the central face in a so-called axial distribution (forehead, nose, cheeks, and chin). Inflammatory signs often flare after certain triggers including sun exposure, spicy food, alcohol, and temperature extremes. An association between rosacea and Demodex mites has been documented, although the causality and significance of this finding is unclear.

Ocular rosacea can occur with/without concomitant facial rosacea. Many ophthalmic manifestations are possible including hordeola and chalazia, blepharoconjunctivitis, cicatrizing conjunctivitis, episcleritis, and keratitis. Symptoms depend on the extent of involvement; patients with blepharoconjunctivitis usually complain of dryness and irritation, and those with keratitis complain additionally of photophobia and tearing. Disease is usually bilateral but can be asymmetric. Blepharitis is a key diagnostic feature of ocular rosacea, and usually consists of telangiectasias of the eyelid margins and dilated meibomian glands with excessive secretions resulting in a foamy, debris-laden tear film and abnormal tear film breakup time. Chronic papillary conjunctivitis and cicatricial conjunctival changes are common. The corneal manifestations present initially as an epitheliopathy, and then progress to marginal infiltrates and stromal vascularization, classically in a spade-shaped pattern on the inferior cornea (Fig. 25.6). Epithelial defects can occur over the infiltrates during flares. The inflammatory process will progress centrally if untreated, and results in vascularized corneal stromal scarring.

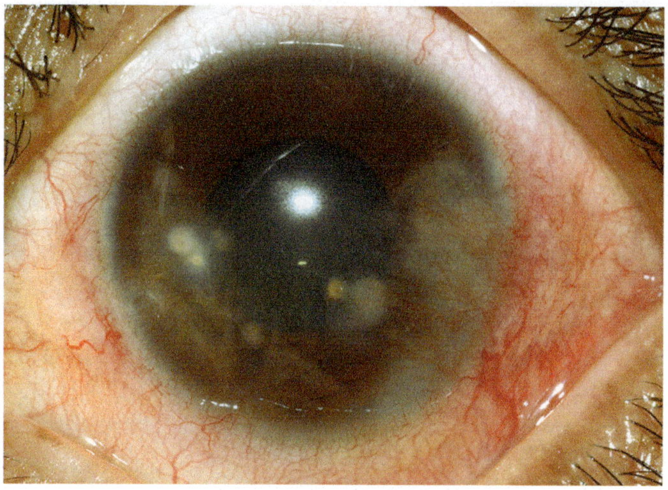

Fig. 25.6: Rosacea keratitis.
Source: Gerami Seitzman, MD.

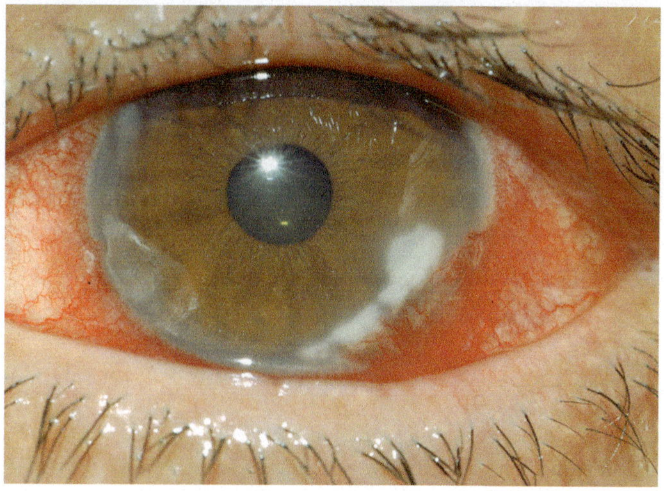

Fig. 25.7: Staphylococcal marginal keratitis.

Management of ocular rosacea depends on the severity and location of the findings. Facial rosacea can be treated with topical therapies such as metronidazole, azelaic acid, and ivermectin. Long-term oral tetracyclines especially doxycycline are effective for facial and ocular rosacea. Blepharitis and meibomitis can initially be managed with hot compresses and lid hygiene, and artificial tears can be prescribed in an attempt to stabilize the tear film. Ultimately anti-inflammatory therapy with a topical corticosteroid or cyclosporine may be required to provide symptomatic relief in cases of blepharoconjunctivitis. Keratitis also requires topical corticosteroids which hasten resolution of infiltrates and prevent progression and scarring. Secondary corneal infections must be ruled out and treated with appropriate antimicrobial therapy before starting topical corticosteroids.

STAPHYLOCOCCAL MARGINAL KERATITIS

Marginal or catarrhal ulcers are curvilinear infiltrates located at the peripheral cornea in the anterior stroma, with an intervening clear zone between the white blood cell infiltration and the limbus (Fig. 25.7).[7] An adjacent conjunctivitis is usually present. The chief symptoms are eye pain, foreign body sensation, and photophobia. The infiltrates are sterile, and thought to be a delayed-type hypersensitivity reaction caused by bacterial toxins from concomitant blepharitis. This theory has been supported by the isolation of *Staphylococcus aureus* from some eyes with catarrhal ulcers, and by their frequent occurrence at the 10, 2, 4, and 8 o'clock positions where the eyelids make contact with the cornea. If not treated promptly, the overlying corneal epithelium breaks down. The infiltrate normally heals spontaneously within a month, occasionally leaving mild superficial corneal vascularization. However, marginal infiltrates frequently recur. Staphylococcal marginal keratitis is managed with a topical broad-spectrum antibiotic to clear the eyelid margins from any colonizing bacterial organisms coupled with a topical corticosteroid. In recurrent cases, an oral tetracycline can be considered in an attempt to control the underlying blepharitis and prevent marginal ulcers from developing.

PHLYCTENULOSIS

A phlyctenule is a nodular inflammatory response of the peripheral cornea and/or conjunctiva usually in children.[8] Like staphylococcal marginal keratitis, phlyctenulosis is thought to be a delayed-type sensitivity reaction to a previously sensitized antigen. Several infectious organisms have been suggested to have an association with phlyctenulosis, especially *Mycobacterium tuberculosis* and *S. aureus*. Symptoms include foreign body sensation, tearing, and photophobia and are usually worse when the cornea is involved. An active phlyctenule usually appears as a raised anterior stromal infiltrate of the peripheral cornea with adjacent conjunctival hyperemia. An epithelial defect develops atop the infiltrate, and the lesion heals over a period of approximately 2 weeks leaving anterior stromal scarring and vascularization. Disease is frequently recurrent, and subsequent phlyctenules often occur

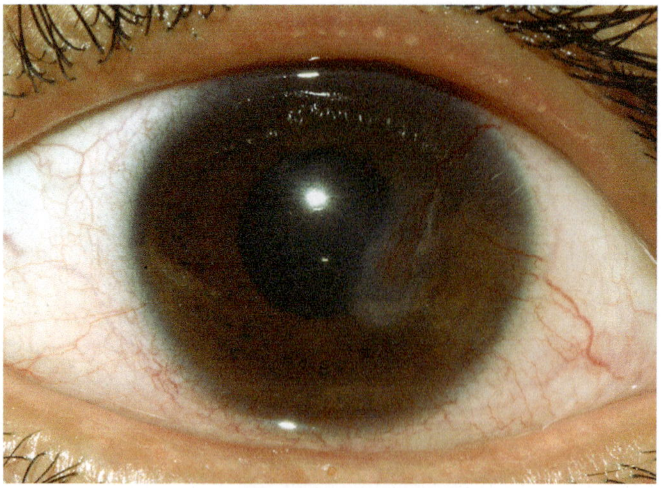

Fig. 25.8: Phlyctenulosis.
Source: John Gonzales, MD.

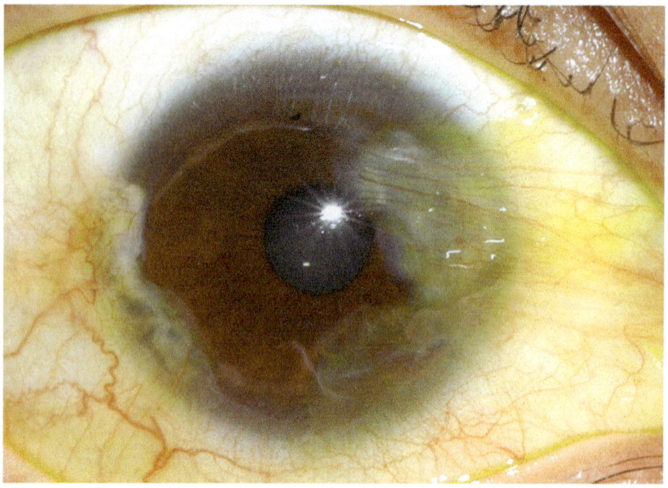

Fig. 25.9: Pseudopterygium in Fuchs' superficial marginal keratitis.

adjacent to sites of prior inflammation resulting in several fascicular opacities connected by a leash of blood vessels (Fig. 25.8). Phlyctenules confined to the conjunctiva also occur, but do not result in conjunctival scarring. Treatment of phlyctenules is generally similar to staphylococcal marginal keratitis: a broad-spectrum antibiotic to clear bacterial organisms colonizing the eyelid margins or conjunctiva plus a topical corticosteroid. Chronic oral tetracycline can be used to prevent flares.

FUCHS' SUPERFICIAL MARGINAL KERATITIS

Fuchs' superficial marginal keratitis is an uncommon inflammatory corneal disease consisting of relapsing episodes of peripheral corneal ulceration that results in a hazy thin peripheral cornea with irregular margins.[9] Disease is usually bilateral but may be asymmetric. The condition is often accompanied by a pseudopterygium which is an inflammatory overgrowth of conjunctiva onto the cornea that does not have the classic wing shape of a pterygium nor the usual 3 or 9 o'clock position of a pterygium (Fig. 25.9). Recurrent inflammatory episodes can lead to a marked peripheral corneal thinning and perforation. In addition, the pseudopterygium may mask the extent of thinning, so care should be taken during any surgical procedure to prevent inadvertent perforation. Flares of inflammation are treated with topical corticosteroids.

STEVENS-JOHNSON SYNDROME

Stevens-Johnson syndrome (SJS) is a rare autoimmune blistering disease of the skin and mucous membranes.[10] SJS most often occurs as an idiosyncratic reaction to a systemic medication, although infections and other chemical insults may also precipitate the disease. Sulfa antibiotics are the most common offending agent. After an initial prodrome, ulcers of the ocular, oral, and genital mucosa develop followed by a painful generalized rash. Epidermal detachment of more than 30%, 10–30%, and less than 10% is classified as toxic epidermal necrolysis (TEN), SJS/TEN overlap, and SJS, respectively. TEN is associated with increased mortality. In terms of eye findings, the acute stage is characterized by a bilateral conjunctivitis, often with membranes that can develop into symblephara if not removed. Conjunctival and corneal epithelial loss can occur, as can secondary infections. Chronic ocular SJS is characterized by a cicatricial conjunctivitis with symblephara, entropion, and trichiasis. KCS results from reductions in aqueous, mucin, and lipid due to scarring of the conjunctival goblet cells, lacrimal gland orifices, and meibomian glands, respectively.

Management of acute SJS/TEN includes systemic antibiotics and supportive care, and usually occurs in a burn intensive care unit (ICU). Systemic corticosteroids and intravenous immunoglobulin are advocated by some but remain controversial. Ocular management in the acute phase usually consists of lubrication, topical antibiotics, and removal of membranes. Some advocate topical corticosteroids, but the benefits remain unclear. Early application of an amniotic membrane graft may be the most important intervention for acute SJS. Although the optimal timing is not clear, the procedure should likely be done early during the disease course—at the bedside in the ICU if needed. The goal of the procedure is to cover the entire ocular surface from the superior eyelid margin to inferior eyelid margin. Chronic KCS and meibomian gland disease are managed with eyelid hygiene, preservative-free lubrication, and topical steroids. Keratinization of the ocular surface is common, and usually responds to topical formulations of all-trans retinoic acid. Scleral lenses are an indispensable treatment for the severe KCS that develops in chronic SJS and greatly improve patients' ocular symptoms and quality of life.

THYGESON'S SUPERFICIAL PUNCTATE KERATITIS

Thygeson's superficial punctate keratitis is a disease of unclear etiology characterized by multiple groups of evanescent corneal intraepithelial opacities.[11] The primary symptoms are irritation, foreign body sensation, photophobia, and blurry vision. Each group of opacities consists of smaller discrete white opacities, more dense in the center of the opacity and often staining with fluorescein (Fig. 25.10). Anterior stromal scarring occasionally develops under areas of opacities. The disease is usually bilateral. Treatment consists primarily of topical anti-inflammatories usually corticosteroids. Topical formulations of cyclosporine and tacrolimus can also be effective, and if so, these are preferred to avoid the complications of chronic corticosteroid use. Disease is usually chronic and many patients require long-term topical anti-inflammatory therapy.

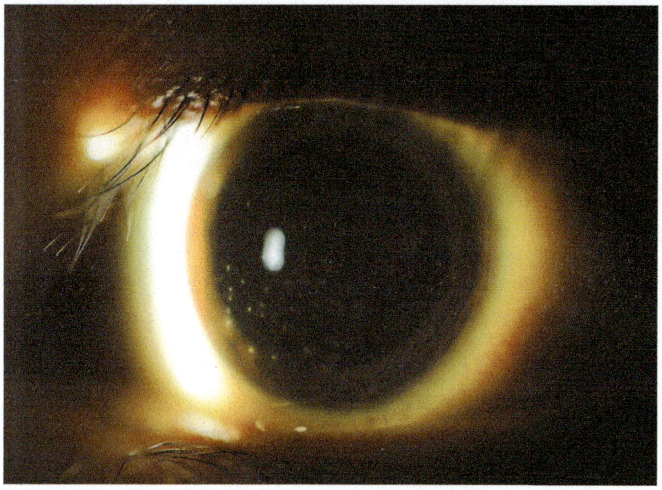

Fig. 25.10: Thygeson's superficial marginal keratitis.

SUPERIOR LIMBIC KERATOCONJUNCTIVITIS

Superior limbic keratoconjunctivitis (SLK) is characterized by bilateral inflammation of the superior bulbar and tarsal conjunctiva with accompanying epitheliopathy of the superior conjunctiva and cornea.[12] Symptoms are primarily irritation and foreign body sensation, and unlike many other forms of ocular irritation, patients are often able to identify the superior ocular surface as the site of irritation. The condition occasionally causes blepharospasm. The key findings are lissamine green or rose bengal staining of the superior bulbar conjunctiva and fluorescein staining of the superior cornea. The surrounding conjunctiva is inflamed, and redundant bulbar conjunctiva can be folded over the superior cornea. Filaments are often present on the superior cornea. The underlying etiology is unclear. An immune-mediated cause is supported by an association with thyroid disease, but laboratory studies have failed to find a significant inflammatory infiltrate, immunoglobulin deposition, or circulating antibodies. While the classic treatment is silver nitrate solution applied to the superior bulbar conjunctiva, many clinicians opt for topical corticosteroid therapy or supratarsal corticosteroid injection as an initial treatment, and proceed to conjunctival resection if anti-inflammatory therapy is not successful.

IMMUNE CORNEAL RING

A Wessely ring is sterile ring-shaped infiltrate in the corneal stroma. The ring of white blood cells is thought to be the result of antigen-antibody immune complex formation with resultant activation of the classical complement pathway and inflammation. The inciting antigen is not always clear, but rings have been reported in association with *Pseudomonas aeruginosa* and herpes simplex corneal ulcers. Antibodies are thought to diffuse into cornea from the conjunctival blood vessels. Ring infiltrates normally resolve spontaneously, but a topical corticosteroid may speed healing if not contraindicated by a coexisting corneal infection.

REFERENCES

1. Srinivasan M, Zegans ME, Zelefsky JR, et al. Clinical characteristics of Mooren's ulcer in South India. Br J Ophthalmol. 2007;91(5):570-5.
2. Craig JP, Nichols KK, Akpek EK, et al. TFOS DEWS II Definition and Classification Report. Ocul Surf. 2017;15(3): 276-83.
3. Whitcher JP, Shiboski CH, Shiboski SC, et al. A simplified quantitative method for assessing keratoconjunctivitis sicca from the Sjogren's Syndrome International Registry. Am J Ophthalmol. 2010;149(3):405-15.
4. Shiboski CH, Shiboski SC, Seror R, et al. 2016 American College of Rheumatology/European League Against Rheumatism Classification Criteria for Primary Sjogren's Syndrome: A Consensus and Data-Driven Methodology Involving Three International Patient Cohorts. Arthritis Rheumatol. 2017;69(1):35-45.
5. Knox CM, Holsclaw DS. Interstitial keratitis. Int Ophthalmol Clin. 1998;38(4):183-95.
6. Alvarenga LS, Mannis MJ. Ocular rosacea. Ocul Surf. 2005; 3(1):41-58.
7. Smolin G, Okumoto M. Staphylococcal blepharitis. Arch Ophthalmol. 1977;95(5):812-6.
8. Culbertson WW, Huang AJ, Mandelbaum SH, et al. Effective treatment of phlyctenular keratoconjunctivitis with oral tetracycline. Ophthalmology. 1993;100(9):1358-66.
9. Bierly JR, Dunn JP, Dawson CR, et al. Fuchs' superficial marginal keratitis. Am J Ophthalmol. 1992;113(5):541-5.
10. Jain R, Sharma N, Basu S, et al. Stevens-Johnson syndrome: The role of an ophthalmologist. Surv Ophthalmol. 2016;61(4):369-99.
11. Thygeson P. Superficial punctate keratitis. J Am Med Assoc. 1950;144(18):1544-9.
12. Nelson JD. Superior limbic keratoconjunctivitis (SLK). Eye (Lond). 1989;3(Pt 2):180-9.

Chapter 26 Corneal Ectatic Disorders

Rohit Shetty, Vaitheeswaran LG, Pallak Kusumgar, Harsha Nagaraja

INTRODUCTION

Corneal ectatic disorders are a group of disease entities which lead to progressive corneal thinning associated with areas of corneal steepening and high astigmatism and poor quality of vision. Though they can be managed in the initial stages with spectacles and contact lenses (CLs), further in the course of the disease they are known to cause contact lens intolerance, corneal scarring and risk of acute corneal hydrops or perforation and blindness if not managed appropriately.[1]

Keratoconus is the most common among the ectatic disorders, which will be discussed in detail. Pellucid marginal degeneration (PMD), Terrien's degeneration, keratoglobus and post-LASIK ectasia will also be highlighted with reference to their clinical features, topographic appearance and broad overview of their management.

The management of keratoconus and other ectasias has undergone a sea change from a time when the only option after contact lens intolerance was a full thickness keratoplasty. Topography and other imaging modalities have revolutionized the understanding of the disease process and criteria for early diagnosis have emerged. Currently, newer contact lens options have prolonged the time before invasive treatment options as they can fit much better in irregular corneas than the traditional rigid gas permeable (RGP) lenses.[2]

Crosslinking has emerged as a boon for these patients in stabilizing the disease process and preventing progression as well as flattening the steep cornea and enhancing contact lens fit.[3] The newer inventions in crosslinking in the form of accelerated and transepithelial options and availability of hypoosmolar riboflavin have expanded the range of patients who could benefit from crosslinking. Laser ablative modality in the form of topography-guided photorefractive keratectomy (PRK) and intracorneal ring segments (ICRS) have also in addition been able to provide visual rehabilitation and improved quality of vision for the stabilized ectatic corneas.[4,5]

Keratoplasty has also advanced with options of anterior lamellar surgeries in the form of deep anterior lamellar keratoplasty (DALK). These have improved visual outcomes with lesser risk of long-term graft rejection for patients with advanced ectasias, not amenable to other treatment modalities.

Readers are encouraged to use the appropriate references quoted for further reading in the areas of their interest as it is beyond the scope of any single source to give adequate information about everything.

EPIDEMIOLOGY

Keratoconus usually begins around puberty and has a variable course until stabilization around third to fourth decades. It affects both the genders and there is no final observation as to whether there are significant differences between males and females affected.[1,6] The prevalence of the disease is highly variable and is dependent on the diagnostic criteria used, the geography and population studied. It varies between 0.00003% and 2.3%.[7] It is greater among the Asians compared to the Caucasians.[8] It is mostly bilateral with asymmetry between the two eyes and there are a few reports of unilateral involvement as well. With the use of better imaging and screening criteria, the apparently normal eye of unilateral cases may also be detected to have early features of the disease.[9]

ETIOLOGY AND PATHOGENESIS

The debate regarding the pathogenesis of keratoconus is 'on' since several decades. Genetic predisposition, immunologic or structural or enzymatic alterations, inflammation, role of hormones and external factors as atopy, eye rubbing and contact lens use have all been described, but *what initiates and what follows* leading to the morphological changes are all hypothetical and remains unsettled. But all of these provide valuable insights into understanding the disease process from different perspectives and we will be describing the role each of these factors plays with special relevance to their application in managing keratoconus. These different mechanisms listed are all interlinked and are not water tight compartments, for example, a genetic defect in an enzyme, superoxide dismutase (SOD) as a possible cause for keratoconus could be described under genetic role or due to an imbalance of redox system, as two pathogenetic pathways for ectasia.

Role of Genetics

Though many of the cases of keratoconus that we see in our practice are sporadic, the association of the disease with multiple genetic syndromes—both ocular and systemic (covered separately) and the higher prevalence in families with one affected individual (up to 11%) and high concordance among monozygotic twins prove that there is a strong genetic component to the pathogenesis of the disease.[10]

Recently, with the availability of genome-wide linkage study (GWLS), genome-wide association study (GWAS) and next generation sequencing (NGS), numerous genes with strong predisposition to keratoconus have been identified, though the exact role played by them is not known in many cases.[11]

Lysyl oxidase (LOX) is a copper dependent enzyme responsible for initiating crosslinks between collagen and in turn the biomechanical strength of the cornea.[12] Polymorphism in the LOX gene has been identified, responsible for a linkage signal at 5q32-q33 chromosomal region.[13] This can lead to collagen framework weakness and ectasia. It is also functionally supported by the presence of lower amounts of LOX in the epithelium of the cones of keratoconus patients.[14]

Visual system homeobox 1 (VSX1) gene is responsible for the process of cell differentiation and maturation in the ocular regions.[15] A novel missense variation (p. Leu268His) in the coding region of VSX1 has been reported in Indian patients with keratoconus with a possible role in pathogenesis.[16]

The transforming growth factor beta-1 (TGF-β1) family of genes involved in the pathogenesis of corneal dystrophies has been found to be associated with keratoconus.[17,18] Collagen genes responsible for the development of the basic framework of the cornea: COL5A1, COL4A3, CoL4A4 have also been associated with keratoconus.[19] COL5A1 is found to have maximum association with keratoconus or central corneal thickness variation among patients. But this association is highly variable and not found to be consistent among those with this mutation.[20]

Loss of the structural component collagen or decrease in the number of its lamellae in cornea can predispose to distensibility of cornea by sliding of the lamellae.

Micro-RNA 184 mutations have been found to be associated with keratoconus and anterior polar cataracts, endothelial dystrophy, iris hypoplasia, congenital cataract and stromal thinning (EDICT) syndrome in different populations.[21,22]

Inflammatory/Immunologic Etiology

Though keratoconus has for long been considered noninflammatory, the role of inflammation is gradually being realized. The fact that it is associated with systemic autoimmune conditions such as Crohn's disease, ulcerative colitis, systemic lupus erythematosus (SLE), amyloidosis, autoimmune hepatitis as reported,[23], has raised thoughts about its etiology being contributed by inflammation or immunologic alteration.

Interleukin-1 (IL-1) is a proinflammatory cytokine and polymorphisms in *IL-1A* and *IL-1B* gene has been found to be associated with keratoconus.[24] Upregulation of these cytokines can contribute to stromal degradation and thinning of the cornea.[25]

Matrix metalloproteinase-9 (*MMP9*) group of enzymes which contribute to tissue remodeling in higher levels can cause stromal disintegration and weakening. MMP9 levels in a study were found to be an independent factor associated with the degree of keratoconus.[26]

Eye rubbing, contact lens use and mechanical stimulation of cornea have been found to over express IL-6, VCAM1, ICAM1, TNF-α all of which are proinflammatory.[27]

With the above evidences, role of inflammation is building up in the pathogenesis of keratoconus and recent evidence indicate the possible role of raised systemic immunoglobulin E (IgE) even in cases with no apparent ocular allergy to be associated with keratoconus.[28]

Role of Eye Rubbing

The role of eye rubbing as a stand-alone factor is being emphasized recently. When the biomechanical resistance capacity of the cornea is exceeded by repeated biomechanical stress (friction), irreversible weakening can occur. Rubbing or mechanical stress can induce the release of proinflammatory cytokines (*IL-1, IL-8*) and recruitment of cells that release further molecules that eventually may tilt the balance towards proteolysis of collagen.

Situations that simulate this apart from eye rubbing are contact lens use (RGP) and sleeping with face buried in a pillow onto one side which apart from mechanical stress can also expose the eye to local allergens, if any.

Role of Oxidative Stress

Corneal tissue like every other tissue goes through oxidative stress due to environment and innate factors like inflammation and routine cell turnover.

Antioxidants like glutathione, peroxidase, catalase and superoxide dismutase help in scavenging the free radicals and avoid tissue damage. Levels of some of these antioxidants (SOD) have been found to have decreased activity in a cohort of keratoconus patients.[29]

Role of aldehyde dehydrogenase (*ALDH3*) has been studied by measuring the level of the oxidative by-product malondialdehyde (MDA) that accumulates in the absence of ALDH3 and was found to be higher in the keratoconus eyes studied.[30]

This explains how corneal damage can occur in response to environmental ultraviolet (UV) rays by the process of accumulation of oxidative end products and mitochondrial DNA damage.[31]

Role of Hormones

Corneal tissue is known to express alpha and beta receptors for estrogen and receptors for progesterone and androgen.[32] Though some studies have shown no effect of hormonal interplay on the progression of keratoconus,[33] some have shown significant differences in corneal biomechanics and progression associated with pregnancy.[34] Even we see pregnancy and conditions like polycystic ovarian disease (PCOD) affecting keratoconus progression.

These hormones are steroidal and have been found to be present in tears and aqueous humor in half of the concentration to that of the plasma.[35] Their receptors are intranuclear and act by modifying gene expression. The probable mechanism through which estrogen acts is by induction of MMPs which in turn activates collagenases leading to degradation and weakening of the collagen framework.[36]

Progesterone inhibits the agents that activate collagenases, thereby causing the reverse of what estrogen does. Thus, they may contribute to the possible biomechanical stabilization towards the end of pregnancy.[37]

Thyroxin hormone is also postulated to play a role in the progression of keratoconus as they were found to be higher in the tears of keratoconus patients.[38]

Nature-Nurture Model

After having seen an exhausting list of causes ranging from genetic weakness of collagen to mechanical etiology and inflammation, it is time to understand that it is basically a combination of them with one of them (genetic) providing the first hit and an added second factor (rubbing or inflammation) delivering the second hit. We can call this the nature-nurture model where the genetic predisposition is nature and what we do to the eye as the nurture arms of the model (Fig. 26.1).

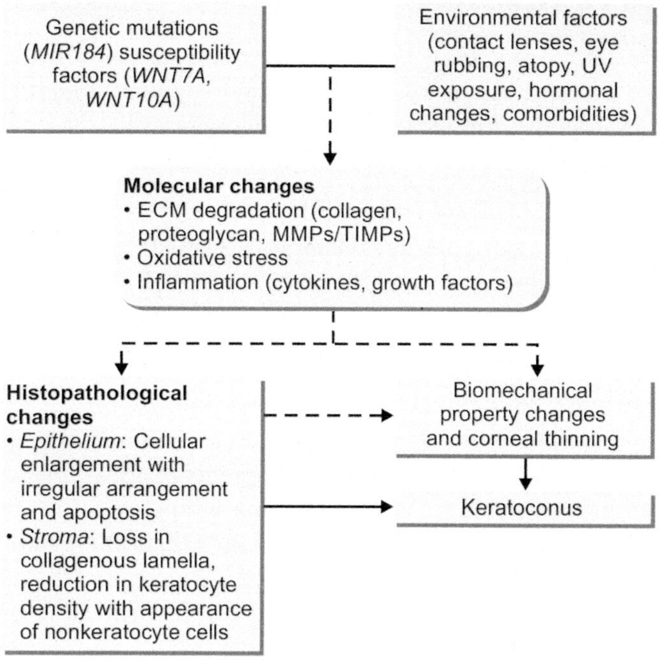

Fig. 26.1: Depicts a basic representation of a mixed etiology similar to the nature-nurture concept.[101]
(ECM: Extracellular matrix; MMPs: Matrix metalloproteinases; TIMPs: Tissue inhibitors of metalloproteinases; UV: Ultraviolet)
Source: Khaled ML, Helwa I, Drewry M, et al. Molecular and Histopathological Changes Associated with Keratoconus. Biomed Res Int. 2017;2017: 7803029.

Role of Tear Proteomics

With rapid developments in molecular biology techniques, it has been off late possible to quantify the level of various cytokines and enzymes from tears. IL levels, MMP9 levels in tears can be estimated quantitatively or qualitatively using tear strip tests.[39] The exact role and future of these is not known, but it holds possibilities in deciding the appropriate treatment targeted against the most dominant cytokine or molecule in the tear sample of a patient and helps in preventing the targeted progression of keratoconus.

Associated Ocular and Systemic Conditions

Common ocular conditions associated are vernal keratoconjunctivitis, PMD, Terrien, Fuchs' corneal dystrophy, iridocorneal endothelial syndrome, retinitis pigmentosa, aniridia, congenital cataract, Leber's congenital amaurosis.

Common systemic associations include Downs, Alagille syndrome, Marfan syndrome, Angelman syndrome, Ehlers-Danlos syndrome, osteogenesis imperfecta, and neurofibromatosis.[40]

DIAGNOSIS

Keratoconus can be diagnosed based on clinical suspicion and confirmed with various diagnostic tools like keratometry, topography and tomography.

CLINICAL FEATURES

Keratoconus is typically a bilateral disease with asymmetric presentation.

Symptoms

Patients typically present in teens and twenties with complaints of blurring of vision, and/or frequent change of glasses. Some present with complains of ghost images and unsatisfactory visual correction with glasses or soft CLs. They might have associated with ocular allergy and eye rubbing.

Patients may also present later in life and may be asymptomatic.

Signs

Early in the course of the disease visual acuity can be normal. Contrast sensitivity might decrease before drop in visual acuity. Retinoscopy shows irregular myopic astigmatism with a *Scissors reflex*.

In advanced keratoconus the corneal protrusion causes angulation of lower eyelid on down gaze, a nonspecific sign referred as *Munson's sign* (Fig. 26.2).

Rizzuti sign or conical reflection is sharply focused beam of light on nasal limbus produced by lateral illumination.

Slit lamp examination in earlier stages may be normal. Only in moderate-to-severe cases the signs become evident. *Corneal thinning and protrusion* can be seen in the area of cone. The cone is most commonly eccentric located inferonasally, while central cone and superior keratoconus are also seen.

Fleischer's ring (iron deposition line) is a partial or complete ring seen at the base of the cone (Fig. 26.3). It provides a landmark for peripheral edge of the cone and as the disease progresses it becomes denser and narrower. In early cases, subtle ring can be seen using cobalt filter illumination.

Fine vertical lines called *Vogt's striae* occur in posterior stroma and Descemet's membrane parallel to the axis of the cone and disappear with gentle pressure on globe (Fig. 26.4).

Charleux oil droplet reflex can be seen on retroillumination or with distant direct ophthalmoscope. Other accompanying signs include *prominent corneal*

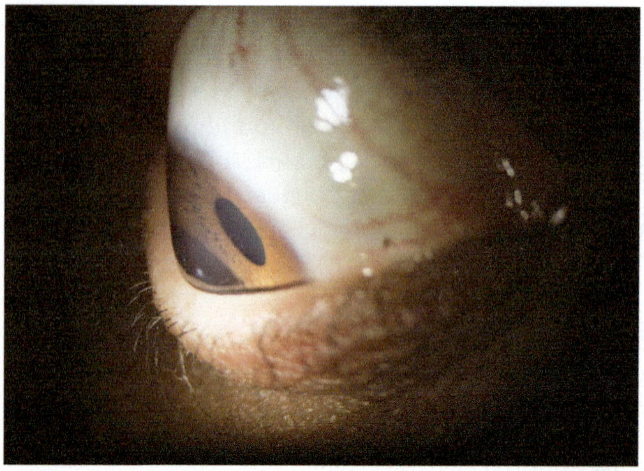

Fig. 26.2: Corneal protrusion causing angulation of the lower eyelid on down gaze known as Munson's sign.

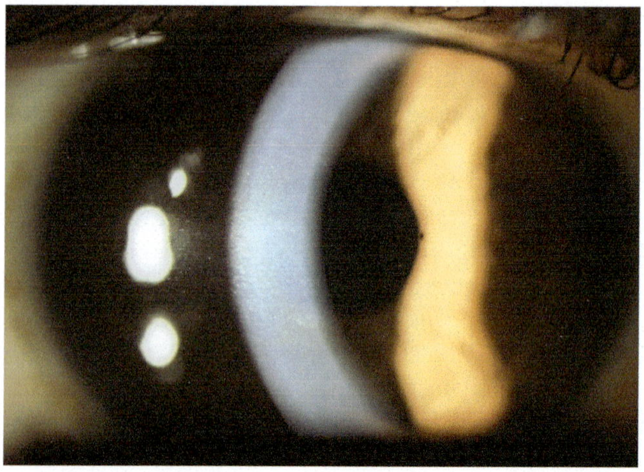

Fig. 26.3: The Fleischer ring—results from hemosiderin pigment deposited in the basal epithelium; a landmark indicating the location of the base of the cone.

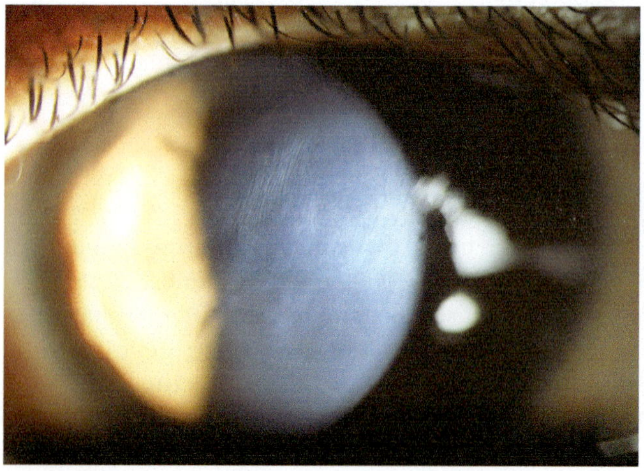

Fig. 26.4: Vogt's striae commonly found in and around apex. They are fine vertical lines in posterior stroma and Descemet's membrane, parallel to axis of the cone and disappears with pressure on globe.

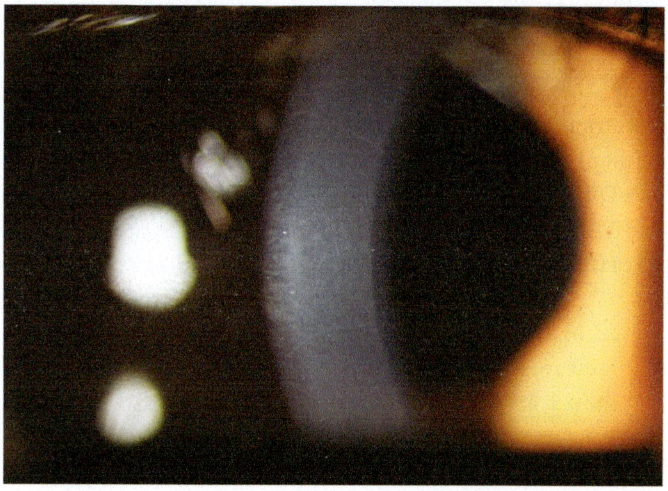

Fig. 26.5: Prominent corneal nerves superiorly and striae.

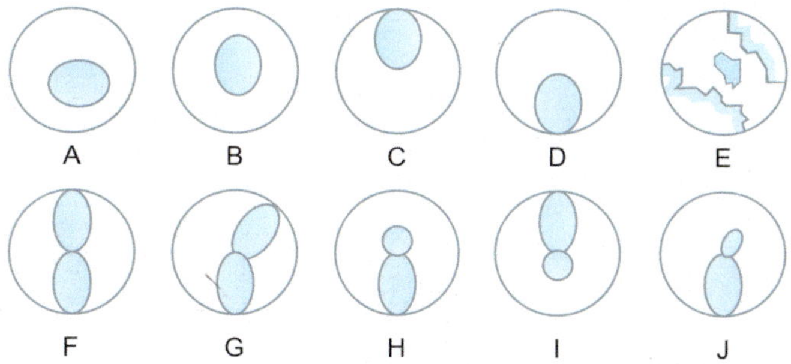

Fig. 26.6: Illustration of the curvature map showing different patterns of astigmatism: A, round; B, oval; C, superior steepening; D, inferior steepening; E, irregular; F, symmetric bow tie; G, symmetric bow tie with skewed radial axes; H, asymmetric bow tie with inferior steepening (AB/IS); I, asymmetric bow tie with superior steepening; J, asymmetric bow tie with skewed radial axes (AB/SRAX).

nerves (Fig. 26.5), subepithelial fibrillary lines, increased intensity of corneal endothelial reflex and apical scarring.

In cases of advanced ectasia patients might present with a sudden diminution of vision, pain and redness, called *hydrops*. This is due to a break in Descemet's membrane causing imbibition of aqueous into the stroma. Slit lamp examination will reveal diffuse stromal edema and Descemet's break may be seen. The edema may persist for weeks to months and eventually leads to stromal scarring.

INVESTIGATIONS

The clinical diagnosis of keratoconus is easy when it presents with classical signs and symptoms. The challenge is in diagnosing the disease at an early stage when prognosis is much better.

A variety of imaging modalities are available to detect subtle changes in cornea. It ranges from keratometry to placido-based devices like photokeratoscopy, computer-assisted videokeratography (CAVK) to slit scanning, scheimpflug and optical coherence based corneal tomography.[41]

Corneal Topography

The most common topographers used in clinical practices are placido based though elevation based topography is gaining popularity. Various patterns of corneal astigmatism like round, oval, symmetric and asymmetric bow tie are described on its axial map (Fig. 26.6).

Major drawback of placido system is its inability to pick up early changes occurring on the posterior corneal surface.

Table 26.1: Index-based systems for keratoconus detection. A higher value than the point of cut value suggests the presence of keratoconus.

Author	Index	Point of cut-off	Description
Rabinowitz/ McDonnell	K value I-S value	47.2 1.4	Diagnosis is performed based on the central keratometry and the inferior–superior asymmetry in keratometric power
Maeda/ Klyce	KPI KCI%	0.23 0%	KPI is derived from eight quantitative VKG indices. KCI% is derived from KPI and other four indexes
Smolek/ Klyce	KSI	0.25	Keratoconus detection and the level of severity is assessed using an artificial intelligent system
Rabinowitz/ Rasheed	KISA%	100%	Diagnosis is derived from K value, I-S value, AST and SRAX
Mc Mahon et al.	KSS	0.5	Diagnosis is performed based on slit-lamp findings, corneal topography, corneal power and higher order first corneal surface wavefront root mean square error.

(I-S: Inferior-superior; KPI: Keratoconus prediction index; KCI: Keratoconus index; KSI: Keratoconus severity index; KSS: Keratoconus severity score; SRAX: Skewed radial axes; KISA: Keratoconus percentage index; AST: Keratometric astigmatism; VKG: Videokeratography)

Several indices like Rabinowitz/McDonnell, Rabinowitz/Rasheed's KISA%, Maeda/Klyce, etc. are described to define diagnostic criteria for keratoconus (Table 26.1).

Rabinowitz[41] suggested four quantitative VKG indices as an aid for screening patients of keratoconus. These include:

1. Central corneal power value greater than 47.2 D
2. Inferior-superior dioptric asymmetry (I-S value) over 1.2 D
3. Sim-K astigmatism greater than 1.5 D
4. Skewed radial axes (SRAX) greater than 21° (Fig. 26.7).

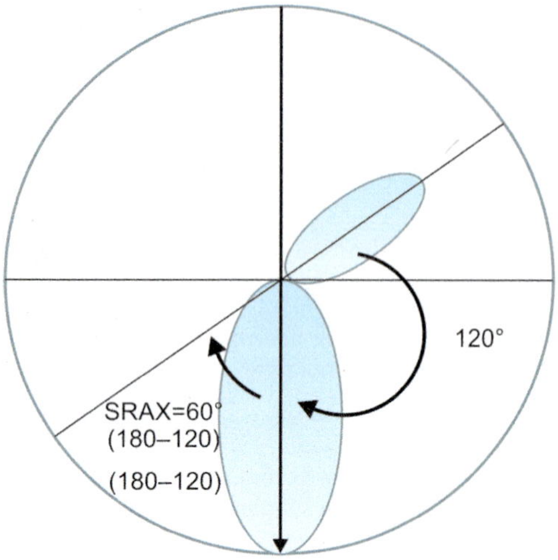

Fig. 26.7: *Calculation of SRAX:* SRAX is calculated from 180° angle between two steep axes above and below the horizontal meridian (smaller of the two angles). In this example, two steep axis form 120° angle, hence SRAX = 180–120 = 60.[41]

The Massachusetts Eye and Ear Infirmary (MEEI) keratoconus detection criteria use both topographic and clinical criteria which include:

- Difference in keratometry with the fellow eye: Less than 1.9, score 0 and greater than equal to 1.9, score 1
- Highest keratometry of the examined eye: Less than 47.2, score 0; 47.3–48.7, score 1 and greater than equal to 48.7, score 2
- Difference in inferior and superior keratometry: Less than 1.4, score 0; 1.4–1.9, score 1; greater than equal to 1.9, score 2
- Greater than equal to 2, findings on clinical examination: Atopy, Down's syndrome, family history of keratoconus or clinical signs of keratoconus (Fleischer, Vogt, Munson, nerves and scarring): No, score 0 and yes, score 2.
- Signs of corneal hydrops: Present, score 2 and no, score 0.

By this, a score of 0 is considered normal, 1–3 suspect, 4–5 early keratoconus and 5–9 advanced keratoconus[42,43] (Fig. 26.8).

MEEI KC Classification

Name____________________________

Patient ID #_________________________

			Score	Score			
KOD-KOS	≤ 1.9	0			0	≤ 1.9	KOS-KOD
	> 1.9	1			1	> 1.9	
KOD	< 47.2	0			0	< 47.2	KOS
	47.2-48.7	1			1	47.2-48.7	
	>48.7	2			2	>48.7	
ISOD	<1.4	0			0	<1.4	ISOS
	1.4-1.9	1			1	1.4-1.9	
	> 1.9	2			2	> 1.9	
≥ 2 Findings on hx (atopy, down), FH and exam (Fleisher, Vogt, Munson, nerves, scarring)	No	0			0	No	≥ 2 Findings on hx (atopy, down), FH and exam (Fleisher, Vogt, Munson, nerves, scarring)
	Yes	2			2	Yes	
Corneal hydrops (by exam or hx) OD	No	0			0	No	Corneal hydrops (by exam or hx) OS
	Yes	2			2	Yes	
		Total score	OD	OS	Total score		

SCORE	DIAGNOSIS
(Zero)	Normal
(1–3)	Suspect
(4–5)	Early KC
(6–9)	Advanced KC

Diagnosis:______________________OD **Diagnosis:**______________________OS

Fig. 26.8: The Massachusetts Eye and Ear Infirmary (MEEI) keratoconus detection criteria.
(hx: History; OD: Right eye; OS: Left eye; KC: Keratoconus)

Corneal Tomography

Tomography also provides information of posterior corneal surface, pachymetry, anterior and posterior elevation maps which help in detecting subtle changes. Orbscan is based on scanning slit and placido technology (Table 26.2).

Scheimpflug imaging is based on a rotating camera which is one of the most prevalent modalities for screening, diagnosis and staging keratoconus. Pentacam, Galilei and Sirius use this principle.

Corneal Optical Coherence Tomography

It is a noncontact imaging modality giving high resolution cross-sectional analysis of the corneal thickness. In cases where topography is not confirmatory, optical coherence tomography (OCT), pachymetry maps can detect the focal thinning characteristic of keratoconus.

Corneal Biomechanics

It is hypothesized that biomechanical changes occur before the topographical changes. Therefore, it could be useful for the detection of early/subclinical cases.

Currently, Corvis, ocular response analyzer (ORA) and Brillouin microscopy can measure the biomechanics.

The data from Corvis and Pentacam are combined to give two new indices—Corvis Biomechanical Index (CBI) and Tomographic Biomechanical Index (TBI) which can help in detecting early or subclinical cases.[44]

Confocal Microscopy

In vivo confocal microscopy (IVCM), a noninvasive modality allows imaging of the cornea at a microstructural level. Studies with IVCM have clearly demonstrated the involvement of corneal nerves in keratoconus. Alterations in corneal nerve morphology (decreased nerve fiber density and length in keratoconus eyes compared to controls) can be used as a marker for early diagnosis, monitoring of progression and prognostication of keratoconus[45] (Fig. 26.9).

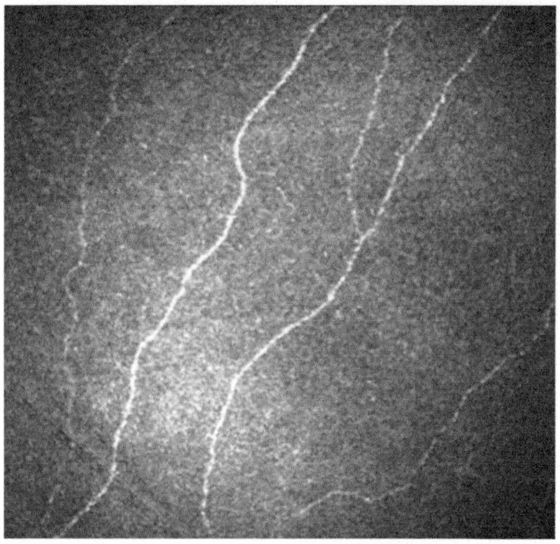

Fig. 26.9: In vivo confocal microscopic image of sub-basal nerve fiber plexus in patient of keratoconus with reduced nerve branching and nerve fiber density.

CLASSIFICATION

Keratconus can be classified based on morphology, evolution, ocular signs and topographic indices.

- *Amsler-Krumeich*: It is one of the oldest and commonly used systems (Table 26.3).
- *ABCD*: This is simple to use and dependent on tomography and is integrated in Pentacam[46] (Table 26.4).

Table 26.2: Red Flags on Orbscan (Roush criterion).

Stage	Findings
1	A thinnest point of <470 μm on pachymetry
2	A difference of >100 μm from the thinnest point to the values of the 7 mm optic zone implies a steep gradient of thinning from midperiphery to the thinnest point
3	The thinnest point on the cornea should correspond with the highest point of elevation of the posterior corneal surface. On posterior elevations map, a posterior high point >50 μm above best-fit sphere (BFS). BFS power is greater than 55 D on the posterior profile
4	Relative difference >100 μm between the highest and lowest point on the posterior elevation map. Keratometric mean power map >46 D. Bow-tie pattern or lazy C on the axial power map is suspect when the astigmatism shifts >20° from a straight line
5	A change within the central 3 mm optic zone of the cornea of more than 3 D from superior to inferior can be correlated to the presence of vertical coma (Most common aberration seen in keratoconus)
6	Composite integrated information which includes highest point on the posterior elevation coincides with the highest point on the anterior elevation, the thinnest point on pachymetry, and the point of steepest curvature on the power map

Table 26.3: Amsler-Krumeich Classification for grading of keratoconus.

Stage	Finding
1	• Eccentric steepening • Myopia, induced astigmatism, or both <5.00 D • Mean central K readings <48 D
2	• Myopia, induced astigmatism, or both from 5.00 D to 8.00 D • Mean central K readings <53.00 D • Absence of scarring • Corneal thickness >400 micron
3	• Myopia, induced astigmatism, or both from 8.00 D to 10.00 D • Mean central K readings >53.00 D • Absence of scarring • Corneal thickness 300–400 micron
4	• Refraction not measurable • Mean central K readings >55.00 D • Central corneal scarring • Corneal thickness <200 micron

Table 26.4: ABCD grading system for classifying keratoconus.

ABCD criteria	ARC (3 mm zone)	PRC (3 mm zone)	Thinnest pachy	BDVA	Scarring
Stage 0	>7.25 mm (<46.5 D)	>5.90 mm (<57.25 D)	>490	>20/20	
Stage 1	>7.05 mm (<48.0 D)	>5.70 mm (<59.25 D)	>450	>20/20	+++
Stage 2	>6.35 mm (<53.0 D)	>5.15 mm (<65.5 D)	>400	<20/40	+++
Stage 3	>6.15 mm (<55.0 D)	>4.95 mm (<68.5 D)	>300	<30/100	+++
Stage 4	<6.15 mm (>55.0 D)	<4.95 mm (>68.5 D)	<300	<20/400	+++

(ARC: Anterior radii of curvature; PRC: Posterior radii of curvature; BDVA: Best-corrected distance visual acuity)

TREATMENT

Treatment is focused on halting or stabilization of the disease and towards visual rehabilitation.

A five-point management algorithm has been described to simplify the management of keratoconus[47] (Fig. 26.10)

Modalities of Visual Rehabilitation

- *Spectacles*: Spectacles are usually the first choice, useful in early cases only. As the disease progresses irregular astigmatism results only in subnormal correction with spectacles.[40]

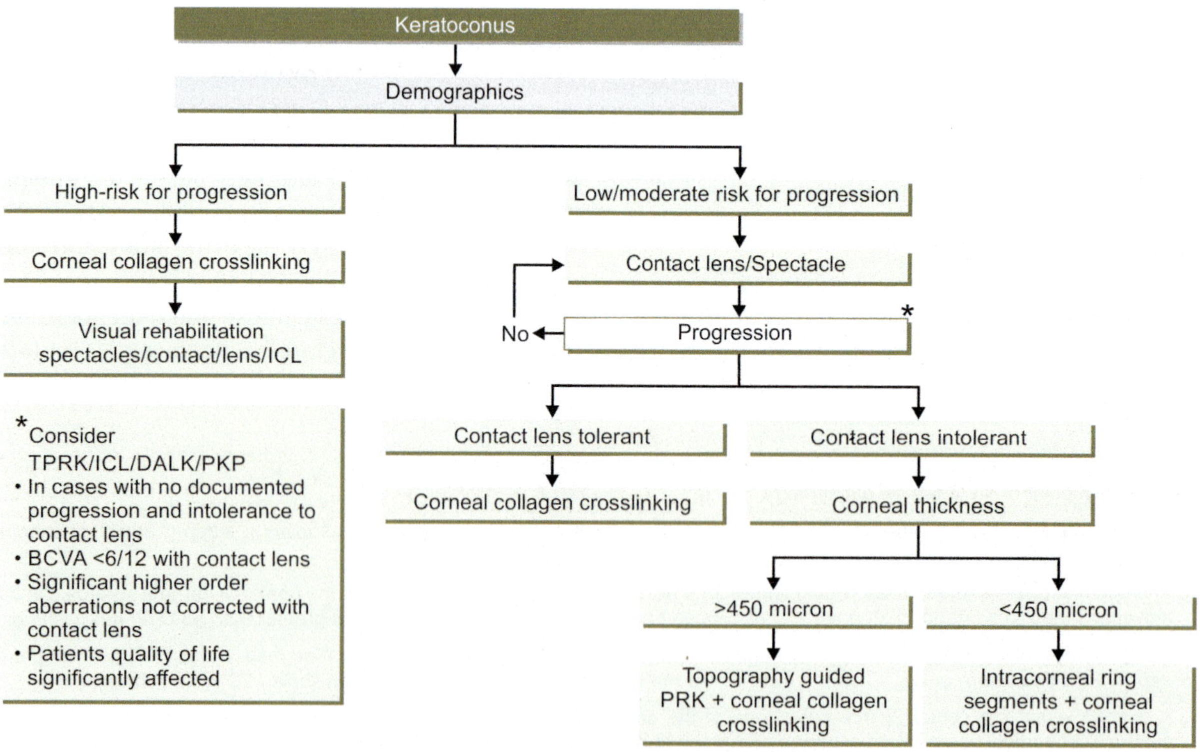

Fig. 26.10: Management protocol based on risk progression.[47]
(TPRK: Topography photoreactive keratectomy; ICL: Implantable collamer lens; DALK: Deep anterior lamellar keratoplasty; PKP: Penetrating keratoplasty; PRK: Photoreactive keratectomy; BCVA: Best-corrected visual acuity)

- *Contact lenses*: Adolf Fick first described the use of CLs in keratoconus.[48] In a long-term study CL proved to be a satisfactory modality and delayed the need for surgical intervention in almost 99% of cases.[49] Various CL options, such as soft and soft toric lenses, RGP, scleral and hybrid lenses (rigid center and soft skirt) are available. The main goal of CL fitting is to improve visual acuity without compromising the health of the cornea.[50]
    - *Soft spherical/soft toric CL*: They can be selected for early keratoconus cases, but as the disease progresses these might no longer be comfortable. They can also be used when there is discomfort/intolerance to RGP and as part of piggy back lenses.[50]
    - *Rigid gas permeable lens*: Amongst all, RGP is the most common one used.[51] The three different fitting strategies for RGP CL are:
        1. *Apical clearance*: Apex clear, lens support and bearing directed off apex onto paracentral cornea.
        2. *Apical touch*: Primary lens support at the apex of cornea. It provides good visual acuity but increases chances of scarring at apex.[52]
        3. *Three-point touch*: Most popular technique. Lens is supported at several points with light touch at apex and heavier on paracentral cornea.

        There are various materials and designs available for fitting these lenses such as traditional or customized lenses that are made locally.
    - *Rose K lenses*: They are multicurve lenses with a small optical zone which snugly fits the cone, for the so called 'feather touch' to the cornea. It closely mimics the cone like shape of cornea, thus is more comfortable and gives better visual acuity (Figs. 26.11A and B).

Further advances in technology have resulted in the following designs:

Rose K2—front surface aberration control and providing better vision

Rose K2 irregular cornea (IC)—for large areas of corneal distortion

Rose K2 post graft (PG)—post keratoplasty

Rose K2 XL (semi-scleral lenses)—for those who cannot tolerate smaller RGP, pellucid marginal degeneration and keratoglobus.

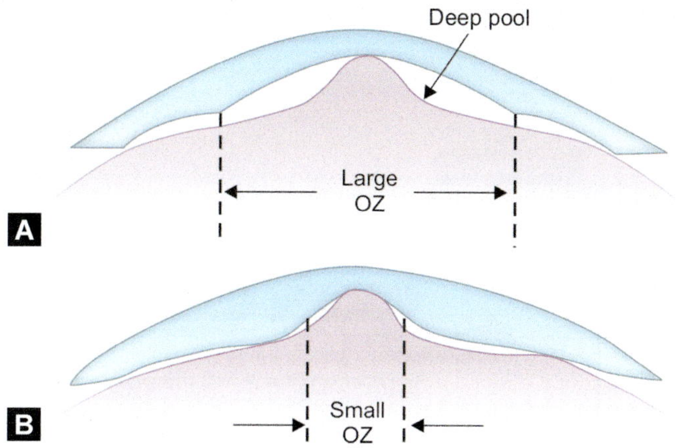

Figs. 26.11A and B: (A) A standard lens that will yield unwanted pooling at the base of the cone and peripheral bearing that can seal off and cause corneal problems; (B) Demonstrating the benefits of a smaller optical zone to fit the cone contour. The design results in little tear pooling at the base of the cone and show an event distribution of tears under the lens.

Recently reverse geometry CL design has been used with relative success in keratoconus.[53]

- *Piggyback lenses*: Piggyback contact lenses (PBCLs) include two lenses on one eye; the RGP lens piggybacks on a soft CL. PBCL is indicated in patients with RGP discomfort or intolerance, unstable RGP on the eye, popping out of lens, 3 and 9 o'clock staining with RGP fit and presence of scar.[50]
- *Scleral lenses*: They rest on the sclera not touching the cornea and limbus, leaving a clear area between the CLs and the cornea. This increases patients comfort level
- *Hybrid contact lenses*: These have a rigid lens in the center and a soft skirt in the periphery. The overall diameter is 14.5 mm. They are fitted with no or minimal apical touch in the central cornea.

Surgical Intervention

When patients cannot be managed by CL alone and/or progression is seen, surgical intervention is needed. The Global Consensus on Keratoconus and Ectatic Diseases concluded that surgery should be considered when patients are not fully satisfied with nonsurgical treatments or are intolerant to CL.[54]

Currently different modalities available are[55,56] (Fig. 26.12):

- Corneal collagen crosslinking (CXL)
- Intracorneal ring segment (Figs. 26.13A and B)
- Corneal transplants
- Bowman's layer (BL) transplantation

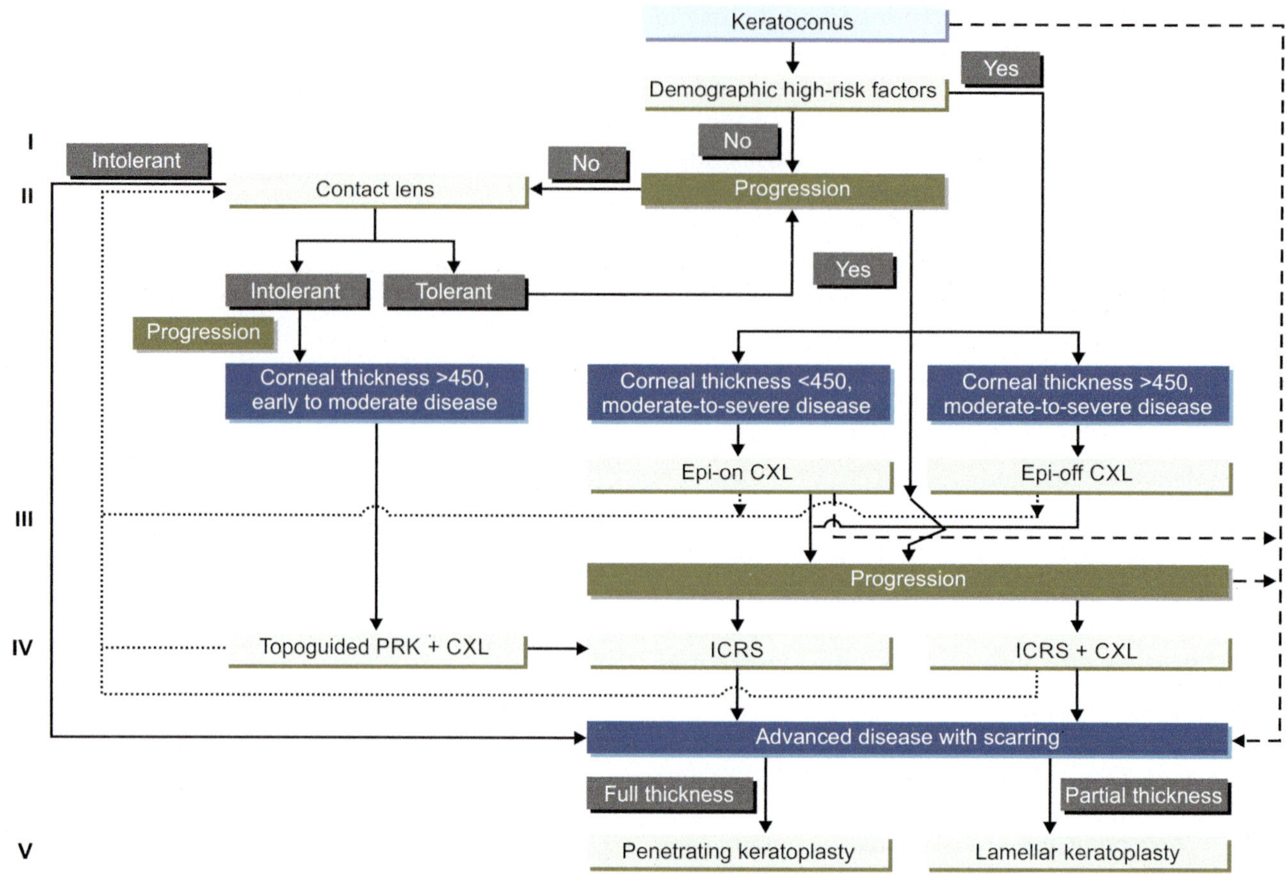

Fig. 26.12: The 5-point algorithm for management of keratoconus.[47]

(CXL: Corneal collagen crosslinking; PRK: Photoreactive keratectomy; ICRS: Intracorneal ring segments)

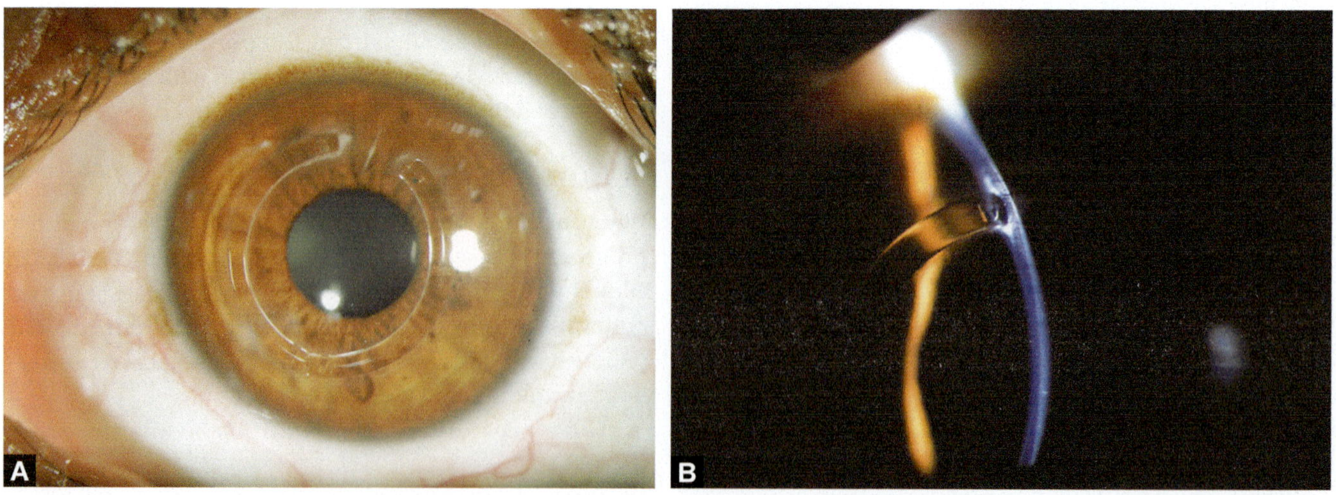

Figs. 26.13A and B: (A) Intracorneal ring segment (ICRS) placement in keratoconus; (B) *Slit view showing placement*: It is placed at around 60% stromal depth in keratoconus and causes central corneal regularization.

- Excimer laser ablation—for visual rehabilitation and regularization of corneal surface
- Toric and phakic intraocular lenses (IOLs).

Corneal Collagen Crosslinking

It is a treatment modality for eyes with documented clinical progression or with perceived risk of progression.[54] The procedure got United State Food and Drug Administration (USFDA) approval recently. Several studies have shown halting of progression and also flattening of keratometry.[57-62]

Principle: Riboflavin plays the role of a photosensitizer in the photopolymerization process and when combined with UVA (370 nm) irradiation increases the formation of intrafibrillar and interfibrillar carbonyl-based collagen covalent bonds through a molecular process that has still not been completely elucidated.

Procedure: Corneal collagen crosslinking was first performed at the Dresden Technical University in 1998 and its use in keratoconus was first reported by Wollensak and associates[57] in 2003. The standard Dresden protocol includes removal of the central 8–10 mm of the epithelium and application of a riboflavin solution (0.1% riboflavin-5-phosphate and 20% dextran T-500) to the corneal surface 30 minutes before irradiation and at 5-minutes intervals during the course of a 30-minutes exposure to 370 nm UVA with an irradiance of 3 mW/cm^2. There have been various modifications to the conventional CXL like increasing the intensity of ultraviolet-A (UVA) irradiation and shortening the exposure time (accelerated CXL) without altering the total energy delivered. Studies have concluded that accelerated crosslinking (9 and 18 mW/cm^2) has shown promising results similar to the conventional crosslinking (3 mW/cm^2 for 30 minutes).[3]

Corneal thickness of at least 400 micron is considered safe for the procedure.[63] Pachymetry should be obtained after epithelial removal and prior to the application of riboflavin and UVA light exposure in order to prevent UV toxicity to the endothelium.

The use of hypoosmolar riboflavin is indicated in patients with borderline corneal thickness to swell the tissue.

Transepithelial/epi-on CXL: Another modification has been to perform CXL through an intact epithelium. This technique causes less discomfort to the patient and reduces postoperative discomfort associated with epithelial removal.[64]

Iontophoresis-assisted transepithelial CXL: It is one of the epi-on approaches which increases the imbibition of riboflavin into the corneal stroma with a noninvasive delivery system via a small electric current.

Customized crosslinking[65,66]: keratoconus is proposed to be a focal disease and new studies suggest customized/selective crosslinking of the cone area (area of maximum weakness receiving maximum dosing and differential energy spread across rest of the cornea) to be safe, effective with better refractive outcomes. Though CXL is a safe and effective procedure, it sometimes has problems with epithelial healing, keratitis, postoperative corneal haze and scarring.

Intracorneal Ring Segment

Intracorneal rings are polymethylmethacrylate (PMMA) segments that were initially approved by the USFDA and the Communauté Europée ne for management of myopia and astigmatism.[67-70] It is now used in keratoconus.[4,71] It may delay progression[72], improve CL tolerance (by regularizing corneal surface) and also delay need for transplantation.[56]

Most of the studies suggest that the best indications for INTACS are in patients with mild-moderate keratoconus with a clear optical zone and CL intolerance. The upper limit of the steepest K reading should not exceed 58 D, with preferably no visual axis scarring and minimum pachymetry of 450 micron at the 7 mm zone or over the area in which the INTACS are to be placed.[73]

Three varieties are available: 1) Ferrara intracorneal ring; 2) Bisantis segments; and 3) Intrastromal rings most commonly used known as INTACS. Channels for ICRS can be made either manually or with femtosecond laser. Combining crosslinking with INTACS can augment the flattening effects of INTACS.[74]

Keratoplasty

Penetrating keratoplasty: Penetrating keratoplasty(PKP) has been the mainstay of treatment for keratoconus since many decades. Several studies have showed good outcomes of post-PKP for keratoconus. Same size of donor tissue and recipient can result in lesser myopia and astigmatism.[75,76]. Postoperative visual recovery is slow and is influenced by astigmatism and anisometropia. PKP is now reserved for patients with advanced keratoconus with significant scarring involving visual axis.

Lamellar keratoplasty: DALK aims to remove all or near total corneal stroma preserving only the host Descemet's membrane. The advantages are: Extraocular procedure, preservation of the host endothelium minimizing the risk of corneal rejection, better wound stability and faster postoperative recovery when done using femto assistance.

Bowman Layer Transplantation

Bowman layer transplantation was devised specifically for use in steep corneas. Van Dijk et al. published the results of BL transplantation in eyes with max K values greater than 70 D, where in 90% of eyes, disease progression was successfully arrested.[77-79]

Excimer Laser Ablation

Several groups have evaluated the role of phototherapeutic keratectomy,[80] photoastigmatic refractive keratectomy,[81] PRK,[82] topography-guided surface ablation[83] and circular keratotomy[84] in cases of keratoconus with variable results.

Combined Treatment

Various combinations have been used in management of keratoconus. Combination of topography-guided PRK with crosslinking has been studied with promising results in visual rehabilitation.[85-87] In addition to combining crosslinking with INTACS as described earlier, toric and phakic IOLs have been used to correct remnant myopia and astigmatism after INTACS.[5,88-90]

OTHER COMMON ECTATIC DISORDERS

Pellucid marginal degeneration and keratoglobus have been described with subtle points of differentiation from keratoconus. Terrien, posterior keratoconus and post-LASIK ectasia (PLE) are mentioned in brief.

Pellucid Marginal Degeneration

Pellucid marginal degeneration usually presents between 2nd and 5th decades and involves both males and females.[91] Genetic predisposition and association with keratoconus in the same patient or family has been reported for PMD.[92]

The word 'pellucid' means 'clear'. It mostly lacks scarring or vascularization or lipid deposition or Vogt's striae, unlike keratoconus or Terrien except when complicated by hydrops.

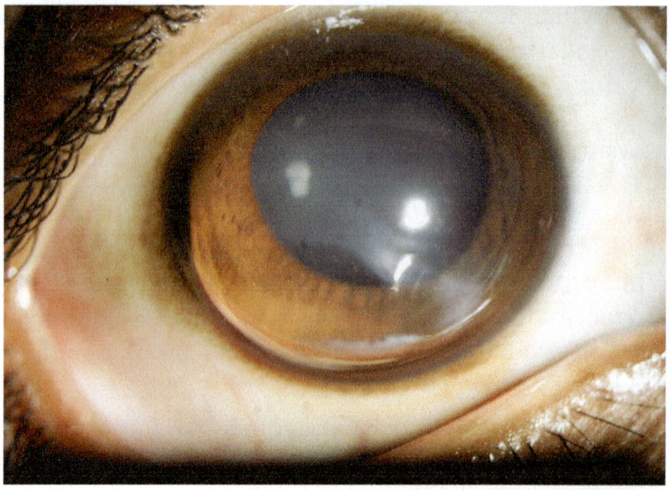

Fig. 26.14: Pellucid marginal degeneration in a 30-year old female showing typical inferior crescentic thinning with superior area of ectasia.

It is usually a bilateral peripheral inferior 4–8 o'clock hour ectasia measuring 1–2 mm width (Fig. 26.14). Atypical forms can have extension beyond 4 or 8 o'clock hours, even superiorly.[91,93]

In PMD, the area of steepening is above the area of thinning, resembling a *beer-belly* causing irregular against the rule astigmatism and a *crab claw* type pattern on topography,[94] which is nonspecific of PMD (Table 26.5).

Pellucid marginal degeneration usually does not develop hydrops or scars in comparison to keratoconus. Sometimes, it has to be differentiated from an inferior Terrien or a Mooren ulcer. While Mooren presents with pain and epithelial defect with circumferential involvement, Terrien usually involves males and area of thinning and steepening coincide with each other and shows vascularization and lipid deposition.

Management of PMD in the initial stages includes large diameter CL (scleral lenses),[95] hybrid and PROSE lenses. CXL has been tried for controlling progression and ICRS can also be done. But the results are not predictable. In advanced cases, large penetrating or lamellar eccentric grafts will be required. Crescentic grafts have also been done in PMD cases (Fig. 26.15). The long-term graft survival may not be very encouraging owing to its proximity to limbus.

Keratoglobus

Keratoglobus usually presents bilaterally within the first decade as a diffuse generalized corneal thinning and a globular protrusion, more marked in the periphery

Table 26.5: Differentiating keratoconus, pellucid marginal degeneration and keratoglobus.

	Keratoconus	Pellucid marginal degeneration	Keratoglobus
Onset/Presentation	Around the time of puberty, sometimes in the first decade also	Around 20–40 years of age	At birth/first decade
Gender	Males and females	Males and females	Males and females
Laterality	Bilateral, some unilateral reports also available	Bilateral	Bilateral
Vogt's striae/Fleischer ring/scarring	Common	Usually clear cornea except when complicated by hydrops	Can have striae and scarring rarely
Area of thinning and ectasia and relationship	Thinnest pachy usually coincides with steepest keratometry and is central or inferior	Usually inferior region of band-shaped thinning and area of ectasia is superior to the area of thinning	Uniform diffuse thinning and ectasia with thinning more pronounced in periphery

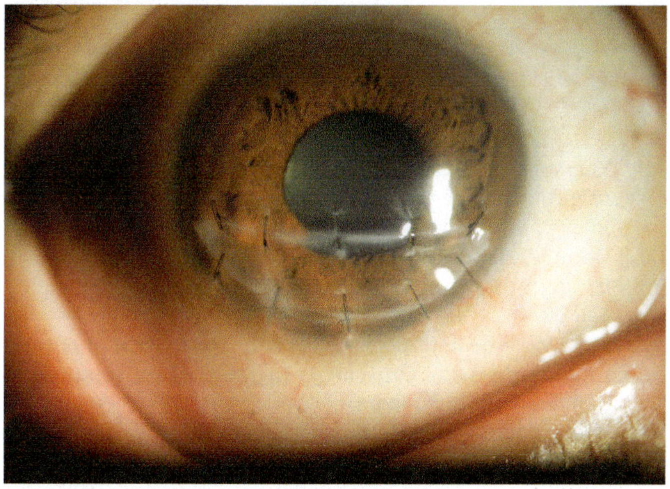

Fig. 26.15: Crescentic patch graft for PMD—done for extremely thin cornea in the inferior periphery.

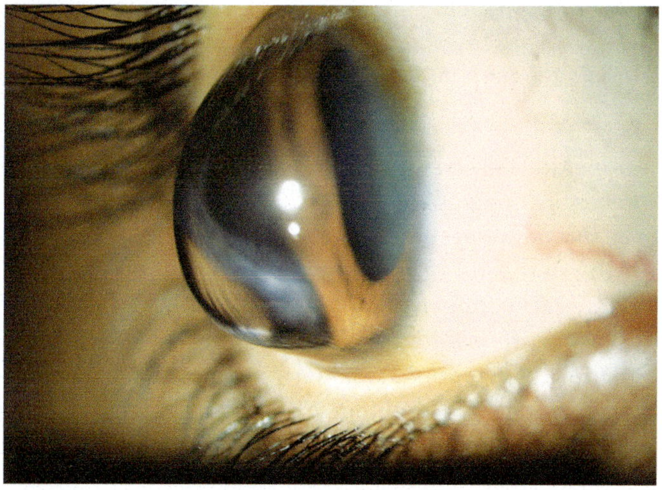

Fig. 26.16: Keratoglobus—showing diffuse thinning and steepening of the cornea in a young patient.

(Fig. 26.16). They are more prone to rupture with minor mechanical trauma.[96]

Cornea may be of normal or slightly larger diameter and can be differentiated from congenital glaucoma with the absence of Haab's striae or corneal edema. Topography shows a large area of diffuse (localized in keratoconus) steepening and thinning.

Some of the ocular factors associated are chronic blepharitis and eye rubbing[97] and orbital inflammatory pseudotumor. Systemic disorders with weak collagen and hyperextensible joints have been reportedly associated.[98,99]

Treatment is dependent on large CLs in the early phase and large and eccentric grafts later which increases the chance of rejection. Hence, surgical intervention is usually delayed until possible.

Terrien Marginal Degeneration

This is a usually a bilateral ectasia predominantly in males and commonly involving superior cornea with a clear gap from the limbus. The band of thinning and steepening can coincide and it has features of superficial vascularization crossing the area of thinning and lipid deposits central to the thinning area (Figs. 26.17A and B).

Posterior Keratoconus

It is a usually unilateral localized or generalized steepening of only the posterior cornea without any anterior involvement or other signs of keratoconus and neither does it progress to keratoconus.[1]

It rarely causes low vision due to astigmatism or scarring if the involved area is central. Even in such cases, correction of the same with CLs or keratoplasty may not be effective as most of them may be amblyopic at the time they reach us.

Post-keratorefractive Surgery Ectasia

With the advancements in refractive surgeries and greater number of patients ready to undergo these procedures, it

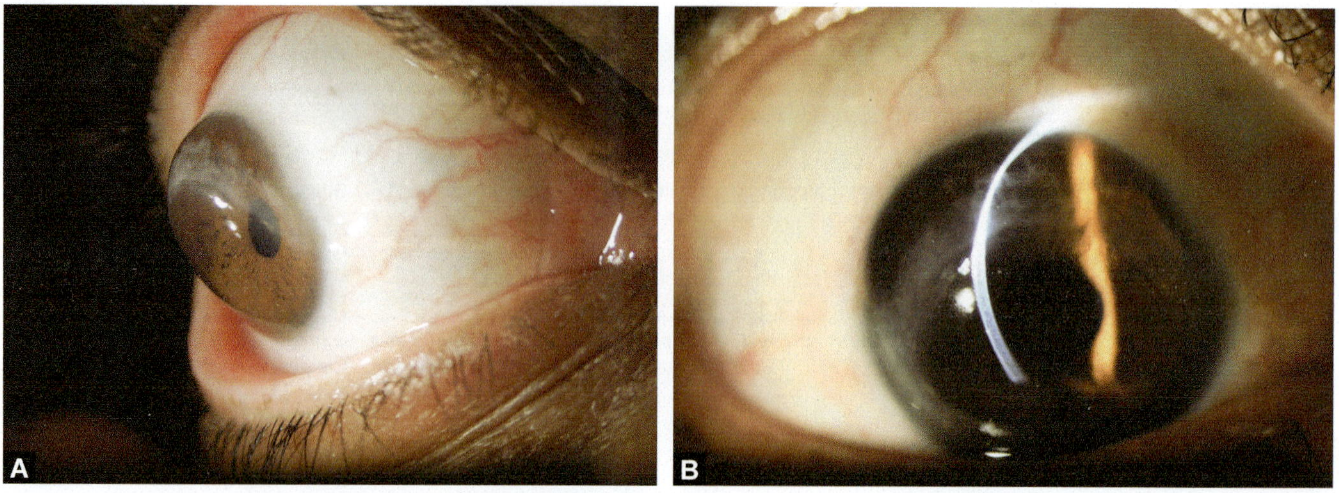

Figs. 26.17A and B: (A) Terrien degeneration in a young male who wanted refractive surgery for myopic astigmatism—showing lipid deposition and superior ectasia; (B) Slit view shows superior corneal thinning sparing the limbus.

is imperative to screen patients at risk meticulously. Many indices on topography, tomography and biomechanics are available nowadays in effective screening (described earlier) for the detection of forme fruste keratoconus patients. In general, younger patients, high myopia, those with abnormal preoperative topography or reduced thickness and those with reduced residual stromal bed thickness are predisposed to this condition.[100] The management is similar to that of keratoconus with options of CL, crosslinking, INTACS and keratoplasty if everything fails.

REFERENCES

1. Krachmer JH, Feder RS, Belin MW. Keratoconus and related noninflammatory corneal thinning disorders. Surv Ophthalmol. 1984;28(4):293-322.
2. Betts AM, Mitchell GL, Zadnik K. Visual performance and comfort with the Rose K lens for keratoconus. Optom Vis Sci. 2002;79(8):493-501.
3. Shetty R, Pahuja NK, Nuijts RM, et al. Current Protocols of Corneal Collagen Cross-Linking: Visual, Refractive, and Tomographic Outcomes. Am J Ophthalmol. 2015;160(2):243-9.
4. Colin J, Cochener B, Savary G, et al. INTACS inserts for treating keratoconus: one-year results. Ophthalmol. 2001;108(8):1409-14.
5. Colin J, Velou S. Implantation of Intacs and a refractive intraocular lens to correct keratoconus. J Cataract Refract Surg. 2003;29(4):832-4.
6. Jonas JB, Nangia V, Matin A, et al. Prevalence and associations of keratoconus in rural Maharashtra in central India: the central India eye and medical study. Am J Ophthalmol. 2009;148(5):760-5.
7. Gorskova EN, Sevost'ianov EN. Epidemiology of keratoconus in the Urals. Vestn Oftalmol. 1998;114(4):38-40.
8. Pearson AR, Soneji B, Sarvananthan N, et al. Does ethnic origin influence the incidence or severity of keratoconus? Eye (Lond). 2000;14 (Pt 4):625-8.
9. Chopra I, Jain AK. Between eye asymmetry in keratoconus in an Indian population. Clin Exp Optom. 2005;88(3):146-52.
10. Kaya V, Utine CA, Altunsoy M, et al. Evaluation of corneal topography with Orbscan II in first-degree relatives of patients with keratoconus. Cornea. 2008;27(5):531-4.
11. Jeyabalan N, Shetty R, Ghosh A, et al. Genetic and genomic perspective to understand the molecular pathogenesis of keratoconus. Indian J Ophthalmol. 2013;61(8):384-8.
12. Bykhovskaya Y, Li X, Epifantseva I, et al. Variation in the lysyl oxidase (LOX) gene is associated with keratoconus in family-based and case-control studies. Invest Ophthalmol Vis Sci. 2012;53(7):4152-7.
13. Bisceglia L, De Bonis P, Pizzicoli C, et al. Linkage analysis in keratoconus: replication of locus 5q21.2 and identification of other suggestive Loci. Invest Ophthalmol Vis Sci. 2009;50(3):1081-6.
14. Shetty R, Sathyanarayanamoorthy A, Ramachandra RA, et al. Attenuation of lysyl oxidase and collagen gene expression in keratoconus patient corneal epithelium corresponds to disease severity. Mol Vis. 2015;21:12-25.
15. Heon E, Greenberg A, Kopp KK, et al. VSX1: a gene for posterior polymorphous dystrophy and keratoconus. Hum Mol Genet. 2002;11(9):1029-36.
16. Shetty R, Nuijts RM, Nanaiah SG, et al. Two novel missense substitutions in the *VSX1* gene: clinical and genetic analysis of families with Keratoconus from India. BMC Med Genet. 2015;16:33.
17. Guan T, Liu C, Ma Z, et al. The point mutation and polymorphism in keratoconus candidate gene *TGFBI* in Chinese population. Gene. 2012;503(1):137-9.
18. Engler C, Chakravarti S, Doyle J, et al. Transforming growth factor-beta signaling pathway activation in Keratoconus. Am J Ophthalmol. 2011;151(5):752-9e2.

19. Stabuc-Silih M, Ravnik-Glavac M, Glavac D, et al. Polymorphisms in *COL4A3* and *COL4A4* genes associated with keratoconus. Mol Vis. 2009;15:2848-60.
20. Li X, Bykhovskaya Y, Canedo AL, et al. Genetic association of *COL5A1* variants in keratoconus patients suggests a complex connection between corneal thinning and keratoconus. Invest Ophthalmol Vis Sci. 2013;54(4):2696-704.
21. Hughes AE, Bradley DT, Campbell M, et al. Mutation altering the miR-184 seed region causes familial keratoconus with cataract. Am J Hum Genet. 2011;89(5):628-33.
22. Iliff BW, Riazuddin SA, Gottsch JD. A single-base substitution in the seed region of miR-184 causes EDICT syndrome. Invest Ophthalmol Vis Sci. 2012;53(1):348-53.
23. Nemet AY, Vinker S, Bahar I, et al. The association of keratoconus with immune disorders. Cornea. 2010;29(11):1261-4.
24. Mikami T, Meguro A, Teshigawara T, et al. Interleukin 1 beta promoter polymorphism is associated with keratoconus in a Japanese population. Mol Vis. 2013;19:845-51.
25. Olofsson EM, Marklund SL, Pedrosa-Domellof F, et al. Interleukin-1alpha downregulates extracellular-superoxide dismutase in human corneal keratoconus stromal cells. Mol Vis. 2007;13:1285-90.
26. Lema I, Duran JA. Inflammatory molecules in the tears of patients with keratoconus. Ophthalmology. 2005;112(4): 654-9.
27. Lema I, Duran JA, Ruiz C, et al. Inflammatory response to contact lenses in patients with keratoconus compared with myopic subjects. Cornea. 2008;27(7):758-63.
28. Shetty R, Sureka S, Kusumgar P, et al. Allergen-specific exposure associated with high immunoglobulin E and eye rubbing predisposes to progression of keratoconus. Indian J Ophthalmol. 2017;65(5):399-402.
29. Behndig A, Karlsson K, Johansson BO, et al. Superoxide dismutase isoenzymes in the normal and diseased human cornea. Invest Ophthalmol Vis Sci. 2001;42(10):2293-6.
30. Chwa M, Atilano SR, Reddy V, et al. Increased stress-induced generation of reactive oxygen species and apoptosis in human keratoconus fibroblasts. Invest Ophthalmol Vis Sci. 2006;47(5):1902-10.
31. Atilano SR, Coskun P, Chwa M, et al. Accumulation of mitochondrial DNA damage in keratoconus corneas. Invest Ophthalmol Vis Sci. 2005;46(4):1256-63.
32. Gupta PD, Johar K, Sr. Nagpal K, et al. Sex hormone receptors in the human eye. Surv Ophthalmol. 2005;50(3):274-84.
33. Fink BA, Sinnott LT, Wagner H, et al. The influence of gender and hormone status on the severity and progression of keratoconus. Cornea. 2010;29(1):65-72.
34. Gliceria J, Freitas Valbon B, Teixeira Santos R, et al. Pregnancy-induced progression of keratoconus in a 37-year-old Patient. Intern J Keratoconus Ectatic Corneal Dis. 2013;2:84-8.
35. Tachibana M, Kasukabe T, Kobayashi Y, et al. Expression of estrogen receptor alpha and beta in the mouse cornea. Invest Ophthalmol Vis Sci. 2000;41(3):668-70.
36. Spoerl E, Zubaty V, Raiskup-Wolf F, et al. Oestrogen-induced changes in biomechanics in the cornea as a possible reason for keratectasia. Br J Ophthalm. 2007;91(11):1547-50.
37. Koob T, Jeffrey J, Eisen A, et al. Hormonal interactions in mammalian collagenase regulation Comparative studies in human skin and rat uterus. Biochimica et Biophysica Acta (BBA)—General Subjects. 1980;629(1):13-23.
38. Kahán IL, Varsányi-Nagy M, Tóth M, et al. The possible role of tear fluid thyroxine in keratoconus development. Exp Eye Res. 1990;50(4):339-43.
39. Shetty R, Ghosh A, Lim RR, et al. Elevated expression of matrix metalloproteinase-9 and inflammatory cytokines in keratoconus patients is inhibited by cyclosporine A. Invest Ophthalmol Vis Sci. 2015;56(2):738-50.
40. Rabinowitz YS. Keratoconus. Surv Ophthalmol. 1998;42(4):297-319.
41. Matalia H, Swarup R. Imaging modalities in keratoconus. Indian J Ophthalmol. 2013;61(8):394-400.
42. Melki SA, Azar DT. LASIK complications: etiology, management, and prevention. Surv Ophthalmol. 2001;46(2):95-116.
43. Prakash G, Agarwal A, Mazhari AI, et al. A new, pachymetry-based approach for diagnostic cutoffs for normal, suspect and keratoconic cornea. Eye (Lond). 2012;26(5):650-7.
44. Ambrosio R, Jr Lopes BT, Faria-Correia F, et al. Integration of Scheimpflug-Based Corneal Tomography and Biomechanical Assessments for Enhancing Ectasia Detection. J Refract Surg. 2017;33(7):434-43.
45. Pahuja NK, Shetty R, Nuijts RM, et al. An In Vivo Confocal Microscopic Study of Corneal Nerve Morphology in Unilateral Keratoconus. Biomed Res Int. 2016;2016:5067853.
46. Belin MW, Duncan JK. Keratoconus: The ABCD Grading System. Klin Monbl Augenheilkd. 2016;233(6):701-7.
47. Shetty R, Kaweri L, Pahuja N, et al. Current review and a simplified "five-point management algorithm" for keratoconus. Indian J Ophthalmol. 2015;63(1):46-53.
48. Fick AE. A contact-lens. 1888 (translation). Arch Ophthalmol. 1988;106(10):1373-7.
49. Bilgin LK, Yilmaz S, Araz B, et al. 30 years of contact lens prescribing for keratoconic patients in Turkey. Cont Lens Anterior Eye. 2009;32(1):16-21.
50. Rathi VM, Mandathara PS, Dumpati S. Contact lens in keratoconus. Indian J Ophthalmol. 2013;61(8):410-5.
51. Lim N, Vogt U. Characteristics and functional outcomes of 130 patients with keratoconus attending a specialist contact lens clinic. Eye (Lond). 2002;16(1):54-9.
52. McMonnies CW. Keratoconus fittings: apical clearance or apical support? Eye Contact Lens. 2004;30(3):147-55.
53. Hu CY, Tung HC. Managing keratoconus with reverse-geometry and dual-geometry contact lenses: a case report. Eye Cont Lens. 2008;34(1):71-5.
54. Gomes JA, Tan D, Rapuano CJ, et al. Global consensus on keratoconus and ectatic diseases. Cornea. 2015;34(4): 359-69.

55. Parker JS, van Dijk K, Melles GR. Treatment options for advanced keratoconus: a review. Surv Ophthalmol. 2015; 60(5):459-80.
56. Jhanji V, Sharma N, Vajpayee RB. Management of keratoconus: current scenario. Br J Ophthalmol. 2011;95(8):1044-50.
57. Wollensak G, Sporl E, Seiler T. Treatment of keratoconus by collagen cross linking. Ophthalm. 2003;100(1):44-9.
58. Caporossi A, Baiocchi S, Mazzotta C, et al. Parasurgical therapy for keratoconus by riboflavin-ultraviolet type A rays induced cross-linking of corneal collagen: preliminary refractive results in an Italian study. J Cataract Refract Surg. 2006;32(5):837-45.
59. Wittig-Silva C, Whiting M, Lamoureux E, et al. A randomized controlled trial of corneal collagen cross-linking in progressive keratoconus: preliminary results. J Refract Surg. 2008;24(7):S720-5.
60. Hoyer A, Raiskup-Wolf F, Sporl E, et al. [Collagen cross-linking with riboflavin and UVA light in keratoconus. Results from Dresden]. Ophthalm. 2009;106(2):133-40.
61. Raiskup-Wolf F, Hoyer A, Spoerl E, et al. Collagen crosslinking with riboflavin and ultraviolet-A light in keratoconus: long-term results. J Cataract Refract Surg. 2008;34(5):796-801.
62. Jankov MR 2nd, Hafezi F, Beko M, et al. [Corneal Cross-linking for the treatment of keratoconus: preliminary results]. Arq Bras Oftalmol. 2008;71(6):813-8.
63. Kymionis GD, Portaliou DM, Diakonis VF, et al. Corneal collagen cross-linking with riboflavin and ultraviolet-A irradiation in patients with thin corneas. Am J Ophthalmol. 2012;153(1):24-8.
64. Sorkin N, Varssano D. Corneal collagen crosslinking: a systematic review. Ophthalmologica. 2014;232(1):10-27.
65. Seiler TG, Fischinger I, Koller T, et al. Customized Corneal Cross-linking: One-Year Results. Am J Ophthalmol. 2016;166:14-21.
66. Wernli J, Schumacher S, Spoerl E, et al. The efficacy of corneal cross-linking shows a sudden decrease with very high intensity UV light and short treatment time. Invest Ophthalmol Vis Sci. 2013;54(2):1176-80.
67. Fleming JF, Wan WL, Schanzlin DJ. The theory of corneal curvature change with the Intrastromal Corneal Ring. CLAOJ. 1989;15(2):146-50.
68. Nose W, Neves RA, Burris TE, et al. Intrastromal corneal ring: 12-month sighted myopic eyes. J Refract Surg. 1996;12(1):20-8.
69. Schanzlin DJ, Asbell PA, Burris TE, et al. The intrastromal corneal ring segments. Phase II results for the correction of myopia. Ophthalm. 1997;104(7):1067-78.
70. Asbell PA, Ucakhan OO, Durrie DS, et al. Adjustability of refractive effect for corneal ring segments. J Refract Surg. 1999;15(6):627-31.
71. Colin J, Cochener B, Savary G, et al. Correcting keratoconus with intracorneal rings. J Cataract Refract Surg. 2000;26(8):1117-22.
72. IbrahimTA, Elmor O. Intracorneal Rings (INTACS SK) Might be Beneficial in Keratoconus; A Prospective Nonrandomized Study. Med Hypothesis Discov Innov Ophthalmol. 2013;2(2):35-40.
73. Rabinowitz YS. INTACS for keratoconus and ectasia after LASIK. Int Ophthalmol Clin. 2013;53(1):27-39.
74. Chan CC, Sharma M, Wachler BS. Effect of inferior-segment Intacs with and without C3-R on keratoconus. J Cataract Refract Surg. 2007;33(1):75-80.
75. Bourne WM, Davison JA, O'Fallon WM. The effects of oversize donor buttons on postoperative intraocular pressure and corneal curvature in aphakic penetrating keratoplasty. Ophthalm. 1982;89(3):242-6.
76. Duran JA, Malvar A, Diez E. Corneal dioptric power after penetrating keratoplasty. Br J Ophthalmol. 1989;73(8): 657-60.
77. Abou Shousha M, Perez VL, Fraga Santini Canto AP, et al. The use of Bowman's layer vertical topographic thickness map in the diagnosis of keratoconus. Ophthalm. 2014;121(5):988-93.
78. van Dijk K, Liarakos VS, Parker J, et al. Bowman layer transplantation to reduce and stabilize progressive, advanced keratoconus. Ophthalm. 2015;122(5):909-17.
79. van Dijk K, Parker J, Tong CM, et al. Midstromal isolated Bowman layer graft for reduction of advanced keratoconus: a technique to postpone penetrating or deep anterior lamellar keratoplasty. JAMA Ophthalm. 2014;132(4): 495-501.
80. Elsahn AF, Rapuano CJ, Antunes VA, et al. Excimer laser phototherapeutic keratectomy for keratoconus nodules. Cornea. 2009;28(2):144-7.
81. Alpins N, Stamatelatos G. Customized photoastigmatic refractive keratectomy using combined topographic and refractive data for myopia and astigmatism in eyes with forme fruste and mild keratoconus. J Cataract Refract Surg. 2007;33(4):591-602.
82. Appiotti A, Gualdi M. Treatment of keratoconus with laser in situ keratomileusis, photorefractive keratectomy, and radial keratotomy. J Refract Surg. 1999;15(2 Suppl):S240-2.
83. Koller T, Iseli HP, Donitzky C, et al. Topography-guided surface ablation for forme fruste keratoconus. Ophthalm. 2006;113(12):2198-202.
84. Krumeich JH, Kezirian GM. Circular keratotomy to reduce astigmatism and improve vision in stage I and II keratoconus. J Refract Surg. 2009;25(4):357-65.
85. Kymionis GD, Kontadakis GA, Kounis GA, et al. Simultaneous topography-guided PRK followed by corneal collagen cross-linking for keratoconus. J Refract Surg. 2009;25(9):S807-11.
86. Kanellopoulos AJ. Comparison of sequential vs same-day simultaneous collagen cross-linking and topography-guided PRK for treatment of keratoconus. J Refract Surg. 2009;25(9):S812-8.
87. Kanellopoulos AJ, Binder PS. Collagen cross-linking (CCL) with sequential topography-guided PRK: a temporizing

alternative for keratoconus to penetrating keratoplasty. Cornea. 2007;26(7):891-5.
88. Kamburoglu G, Ertan A, Bahadir M. Implantation of Artisan toric phakic intraocular lens following Intacs in a patient with keratoconus. J Cataract Refract Surg. 2007;33(3):528-30.
89. El-Raggal TM, Abdel Fattah AA. Sequential Intacs and Verisyse phakic intraocular lens for refractive improvement in keratoconic eyes. J Cataract Refract Surg. 2007;33(6):966-70.
90. Coskunseven E, Onder M, Kymionis GD, et al. Combined Intacs and posterior chamber toric implantable Collamer lens implantation for keratoconic patients with extreme myopia. Am J Ophthalmol. 2007;144(3):387-9.
91. Rao SK, Fogla R, Padmanabhan P, et al. Corneal topography in atypical pellucid marginal degeneration. Cornea. 1999;18(3):265-72.
92. Santo RM, Bechara SJ, Kara-Jose N. Corneal topography in asymptomatic family members of a patient with pellucid marginal degeneration. Am J Ophthalmol. 1999;127(2):205-7.
93. Bower KS, Dhaliwal DK, Barnhorst DA, et al. Pellucid marginal degeneration with superior corneal thinning. Cornea. 1997;16(4):483-5.
94. Maguire LJ, Klyce SD, McDonald MB, Kaufman HE. Corneal topography of pellucid marginal degeneration. Ophthalm. 1987;94(5):519-24.
95. Pullum KW, Buckley RJ. A study of 530 patients referred for rigid gas permeable scleral contact lens assessment. Cornea. 1997;16(6):612-22.
96. Gupta VP, Jain RK, Angra SK. Acute hydrops in keratoglobus with vernal keratoconjunctivitis. Indian J Ophthalmol. 1985;33(2):121-3.
97. Cameron JA. Keratoglobus. Cornea. 1993;12(2):124-30.
98. Biglan AW, Brown SI, Johnson BL. Keratoglobus and blue sclera. Am J Ophthalmol. 1977;83(2):225-33.
99. Hyams SW, Kar H, Neumann E. Blue sclerae and keratoglobus. Ocular signs of a systemic connective tissue disorder. Br J Ophthalmol. 1969;53(1):53-8.
100. Randleman JB, Russell B, Ward MA, et al. Risk factors and prognosis for corneal ectasia after LASIK. Ophthalm. 2003;110(2):267-75.
101. Khaled ML, Helwa I, Drewry M, et al. Molecular and Histopathological Changes Associated with Keratoconus. BioMed Research International. 2017;2017:1-16.

Chapter 27 Corneal Degenerations

Saujanya Vadoothker, Bennie H Jeng

INTRODUCTION

Corneal degenerations can include both involutional or age-related changes to the cornea as well as changes to the cornea due to external factors such as depositions, trauma or environmental factors. Most importantly, corneal degenerations are different from corneal dystrophies as they can occur both bilaterally or unilaterally, occur at different age ranges, and may be related to aging or external factors. In contrast, corneal dystrophies tend to be bilateral, have a hereditary pattern and occur at a younger age. Age-related changes to the cornea can result in decreased corneal transparency, increased refractive index, increased against-the-rule astigmatism due to flattening of the vertical meridian and peripheral corneal thinning.[1]

Involutional or age-related corneal degenerations are described first in this chapter, followed by peripheral corneal degenerations, central corneal degenerations and degenerations due to external climatic factors.

INVOLUTIONAL OR AGE-RELATED CORNEAL DEGENERATIONS

Arcus Senilis

Arcus senilis (Fig. 27.1) is a peripheral corneal degeneration that occurs more in men and in aging population.[2] Studies have shown that 80% of patients over the age of 40 years and 100% of patients over the age of 80 years have this condition.[1,3] Arcus senilis has also been noted more often in African-American patients.[1] This condition can be found in the peripheral corneal stroma at the level of Bowman's layer and Descemet membrane and has also been noted in the perilimbal region of the sclera on histopathologic analysis.[2] Generally, it first appears in the inferior cornea and then in the superior cornea. With time, the inferior arc and superior arc form a peripheral corneal annulus.[3] The annulus itself is separated from the limbus by a clear interval called the clear zone of Vogt where limbal vessels enter the cornea and the borders of the arcus are distinct peripherally but diffuse interiorly.[1,3]

Associated with abnormal serum lipids and atherosclerosis, arcus senilis forms through the infiltration of the cornea by lipids from the limbal vasculature.[2,3] Atherosclerosis causes increased permeability in the limbal vasculature, allowing lipids to escape the bloodstream and deposit in the cornea.[3] This process occurs as low-density lipoprotein molecules modified by oxidation and glycation cause damage to the vascular endothelium and smooth muscle in the same manner that atherosclerosis affects all blood vessels in the body. The deposition of lipid exceeds the clearance of the lipids by the corneal vasculature resulting in increased corneal deposition.[3] Apart from atherosclerosis, limbal vessels also become increasingly permeable with age and large molecules such as IgM, fibrinogen and low density lipoproteins continue to deposit in the cornea resulting in the gray-white/yellow annulus.[1,2] The deposition first occurs anterior to Descemet membrane and then in Bowman's layer and with time, the anterior and posterior depositions fuse.[1]

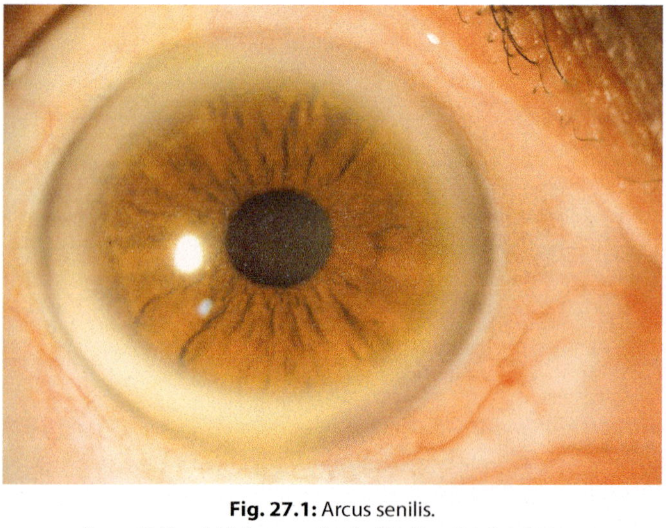

Fig. 27.1: Arcus senilis.
Source: Dr Revathi Rajaraman, Aravind Eye Hospital, Coimbatore.

Arcus senilis can also rarely develop in children in conjunction with familial hyperlipidemia and in blue sclera and megalocornea. This latter deposition is also referred to as juvenile arcus or anterior embryotoxon.[1] Another deposition resembling arcus senilis but depositing only in the anterior stroma is pseudogerontoxon. Pseudogerontoxon is a localized lipid deposition from prolonged hyperemia and changes in limbal vasculature due to inflammation at the limbus. It occurs in vernal and atopic keratoconjunctivitis, and its appearance resembles a segment of arcus senilis.[4]

On slit-lamp examination, the arcus senilis annulus appears as a gray-white or yellow opacity separated from the limbus by a clear zone. The deposited particles are cholesteryl ester-rich lipid particles 40–200 nm in size, low-density lipoproteins, phospholipids and triglycerides.[2] If arcus senilis develops in patients under the age of 50, it is a very likely sign of hyperlipidemia and the patient should be appropriately referred and managed with primary care physicians.[5]

As noted previously, arcus senilis is highly associated with not only atherosclerosis but also cardiovascular disease, coronary heart disease, hypertension, hyperlipidemia, diabetes mellitus, individuals with high body mass index, cigarette smoking, myocardial infarction and stroke. It has recently been shown to be associated with the above conditions even in low risk individuals of South-Asian descent who are young, nonsmoking, and nondiabetic with low risk Framingham scores.[3] The presence of arcus senilis is also important due to its ability to predict cardiovascular disease and coronary heart disease in the Framingham Study Cohort.[5]

Corneal Pigmentation

Corneal pigmentation can occur due to the deposition of melanin, iron, copper, silver or gold. Melanin deposits onto the inferior endothelium of the cornea in patients with Krukenberg spindle and is sometimes associated with pigmentary glaucoma.[6] In alkaptonuria, an autosomal recessive deficiency of homogentisic acid oxidase, elevated serum and tissue homogentisic acid causes a black-colored discoloration called ochronosis in the palpebral fissure in the peripheral cornea at the basal epithelium and Bowman's layer.[7] Iron lines occur due to changes in the tear film: the pooling of tears in areas of topographic abnormalities causes iron deposition.[8] For example, Hudson-Stahli line is a brown discoloration of the inferior cornea that occurs bilaterally in elderly individuals. Ferry line is a golden-brown line that appears anterior to a filtering bleb.[9] Fleischer rings appear at the base of a cone in keratoconus (Fig. 27.2) and Stocker line occurs at the leading edge of a pterygium.[6,9] More recently with the advent of refractive surgery, iron lines have also been found after laser in-situ keratomileusis, radial keratectomy, corneal inlay placement and many other refractive procedures.[10] In Wilson disease (hepatolenticular degeneration), low levels of ceruloplasmin, a copper transporting protein, leads to excess deposition of copper in the liver, brain, kidneys and eyes. Called the Kayser-Fleischer ring, the copper deposits in Descemet membrane and creates a 1–3 mm peripheral green-brown band after the age of 10 years.[7] Copper also deposits in the Descemet membrane as chalcosis after trauma with an intraocular foreign body.[11] Ocular chrysiasis is the deposition of gold in the cornea usually in the stroma or endothelium after gold therapy for rheumatoid arthritis.[7] Thus, corneal pigmentation can occur for a variety of causes.

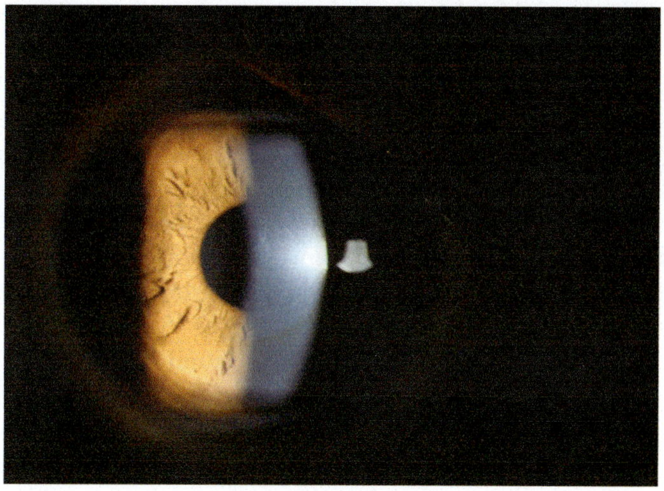

Fig. 27.2: Fleischer ring.
Source: Dr N Venkatesh Prajna, Aravind Eye Hospital, Madurai.

Crocodile Shagreen

Crocodile shagreen can be classified based on location as either anterior or posterior. Anterior crocodile shagreen appears as central, polygonal, gray-white opacities that are usually found bilaterally. These opacities form a mosaic pattern in the anterior stroma due to the arrangement of collagen lamella that attach obliquely to Bowman's layer. This arrangement then changes the tension on Bowman's layer causing the appearance of ridges that indent the epithelium and create the mosaic pattern. Calcium has been found to deposit on the apex of these ridges and the change in tension on Bowman's layer can cause ruptures in Bowman's layer that then allows for fibrous tissues to collect between the epithelium and Bowman's layer.[1]

The gray-white opacities that are characteristic of anterior crocodile shagreen may cause some decrease in vision. Furthermore, anterior crocodile shagreen can be classified as juvenile or traumatic in nature. Juvenile anterior crocodile shagreen can occur in megalocornea, peripheral band keratopathy and iris malformations, while traumatic anterior crocodile shagreen occurs from the loosening and folding of Bowman's layer after trauma.[1]

Posterior crocodile shagreen is found in the central cornea and posterior stroma in many elderly individuals.[12] Histologically, symmetric gray-white polygonal opacities with indistinct edges and intervening clear zones are found, and epithelium and endothelium are usually spared.[13,14] Vacuoles composed of electron dense fibrillogranular material arranged in a sawtooth pattern can be seen in the stroma and Bowman's layer. These vacuoles have been found to be most dense just anterior to Descemet membrane. Clinically, posterior crocodile shagreen appears very similar to central cloudy cornea of François. There is no associated visual loss.[12]

Peripheral Corneal Guttae

Peripheral corneal guttae, also known as Hassell-Henle bodies, are generally found in the corneas of elderly individuals. They are localized drop-like excrescences of hyaline material projecting into the anterior chamber and originating from Descemet membrane. They appear as dark round holes in the corneal periphery and have no relation to endothelial dysfunction in the corneal periphery.[7] Peripheral guttae are a very common aging change in the cornea and form as a result of hyaline overproduction by endothelial cells. They are identical histologically to central corneal guttata.[1]

White Limbal Girdle of Vogt

The white limbal girdle of Vogt is found in approximately 55% of patients between the ages of 40 and 60 years.[1,15] It occurs as a bilateral symmetric snow-white opacity in the peripheral cornea mostly in the interpalpebral area in the medial and temporal limbus although it can also occur as a ring or in a donut shape.[1,7,15] Generally, the opacities are in the superficial and inferior cornea and they manifest as minute discrete granules. The white limbal girdle of Vogt tends to be 0.5–1.0 mm in diameter. Peripherally this degeneration has a sharp demarcation however, the interior border is more diffuse.[15] Histopathologically, this opacity is a result of elastotic degeneration at Bowman's layer and the anterior stroma.[7] Subepithelial hyperelastosis associated with the destruction of Bowman's layer, calcium deposition and hypertrophy of the overlying epithelium have been noted in previous studies.[1]

Clinically, this degeneration occurs in two forms. Type I tends to have a chalky-white band with a perilimbal clear zone. Multiple holes can be seen in the band and it can also look like early band keratopathy.[1,7] Type II presents as a chalky-white band with no clear zone.[7]

PERIPHERAL CORNEAL DEGENERATIONS

Band Keratopathy

Band keratopathy results from the deposition of calcium salts in the subepithelial layers of the anterior portion of Bowman's layer and in the anterior corneal stroma that is associated with chronic eye disease (uveitis, glaucoma, keratitis, ocular hypotony/phthisis, trauma), systemic conditions with increased serum calcium and phosphates, corneal chemical burns, intraocular silicone oil and the injection of tissue plasminogen activator for intraocular inflammation[1,16,17] (Fig. 27.3). The band occurs horizontally due to the alkaline pH in the interpalpebral area that favors calcium precipitation, and it tends to be separated from the limbus by a clear zone and also has many holes from where the corneal nerves penetrate the cornea.[1] The disease has variable progression but tends to occur faster in dry eyes.[17] Calcium precipitates in the anterior stroma and Bowman's layer, and Bowman's layer can become fragmented or irregular.[17]

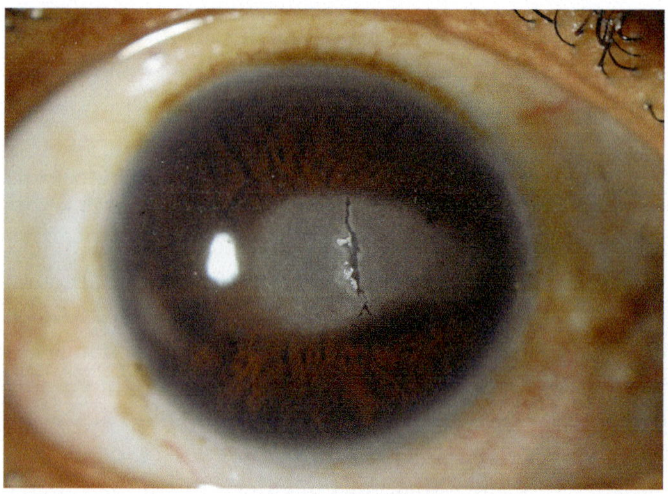

Fig. 27.3: Band keratopathy.

Clinically, band keratopathy can be seen as gray-white opacities in a "Swiss cheese" like pattern in the superficial cornea mostly interpalpebrally.[18] The opacities consist of calcium hydroxyapatite, noncrystalline phosphates and carbonate salts of calcium.[16] Patients can have recurrent erosions, photophobia and ocular irritation due to the disruption of the ocular surface.[18] Treatment consists of mechanical debridement of the corneal epithelium coupled with the chemical chelation of calcium with ethylenediaminetetraacetic acid (EDTA). This procedure can sometimes be painful, so creating an epithelial flap with alcohol can decrease the pain and hasten visual recovery.[17,18] Phototherapeutic keratectomy (PTK) is another option for treatment, however cost and refractive shifts are a concern. For children with band keratopathy, the main goal in treatment is to clear the visual axis and prevent amblyopia. Keeping uveitis (the primary cause of band keratopathy in children) under control in these children prevents worsening of the band keratopathy.[1,19]

Dellen

Dellen occur at areas of limbal elevation and are caused by localized evaporation and corneal dehydration due to a break in the oily tear film that protects against evaporation (Fig. 27.4). The speed of the evaporation tends to be greater than the lateral flow of water in the corneal stroma causing localized dehydration to occur. Stroma in general is resistant to fluid flow and this dehydration then leads to stromal thinning without actual tissue loss. Dellen usually occurs temporally as an ellipse concentric to the limbus and with clearly defined edges.[20]

Dellen often occurs after trabeculectomies, corneal surgery, excision of limbal malignancies, excision of pterygia, localized cocaine administration, chemosis, post-cataract surgery, post-strabismus surgery, subconjunctival hemorrhage and in the setting of Graves disease.[20,21] However, in an elderly population, dellen can occur spontaneously possibly due to a compromised limbal blood supply or thinning of the epithelium. With these conditions and any other procedures that can disrupt the tear film, dellen can occur appearing as small, saucer-like excavations at the margin of the cornea near an area of limbal or conjunctival elevation.[20,21] Dellen have well-defined borders where the central edge is steep and the limbal wall slopes gradually.[7] Patients are usually asymptomatic but can sometimes experience a foreign body sensation.[21] On examination, patients may have minimal to moderate hyperemia of the conjunctiva with no corneal infiltrate or anterior chamber reaction. Dellen can occur within 1–2 weeks after surgery as the precorneal tear film is disrupted.[7,20] The overlying epithelium is usually intact resulting in pooling of fluorescein, but sometimes a break in the epithelium can occur resulting in fluorescein staining.[20] Dellen were originally reported as being transient lesions lasting for 24–48 hours.[20,22]

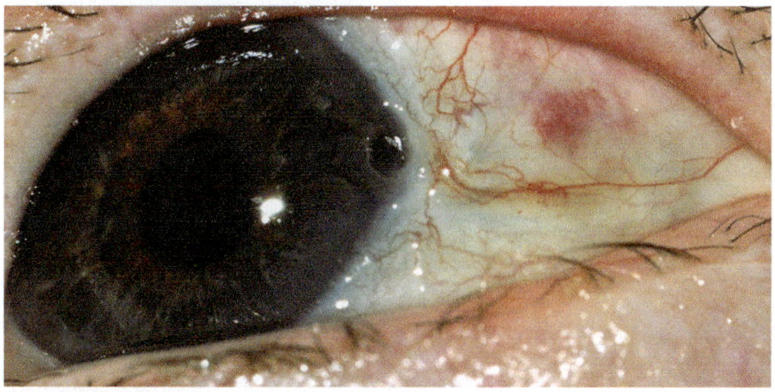

Fig. 27.4: Delle.
Source: Proctor Foundation, University of California, San Francisco.

Treatment of dellen is conservative. Increasing corneal lubrication with sodium hyaluronate drops, decreasing the elevation of the limbus, rehydration through patching of the eye, bandage contact lenses and topical steroids can be used to improve the corneal surface.[20-22] Diabetes and superficial punctate keratitis (possibly from topical glaucoma medications containing benzalkonium chloride) can worsen the clinical picture and impede rapid healing.[22]

Mooren's Ulcer

Mooren's ulcer is an idiopathic progressive inflammatory thinning of the peripheral cornea that manifests as a chronic serpiginous ulceration of the peripheral cornea (Fig. 27.5). Two types of Mooren's ulcer have been differentiated in previous studies. One type occurs in adults and responds well to therapy. A second type that occurs classically in young African males is aggressive and poorly responsive to therapy. Mooren's ulcer initially occurs as gray infiltrates in the peripheral perilimbal cornea in the interpalpebral zone. With time, epithelial breakdown occurs along with degeneration of the anterior stroma. The disease tends to progress circumferentially and centrally and is likely immune-mediated. Patients tend to experience severe pain, photophobia and tearing. The conjunctiva, episclera and sclera are generally inflamed. After the degeneration of the anterior lamella, blood vessels grow to cover the remaining stroma and Descemet membrane. This thin tissue can then perforate with minor trauma.[7]

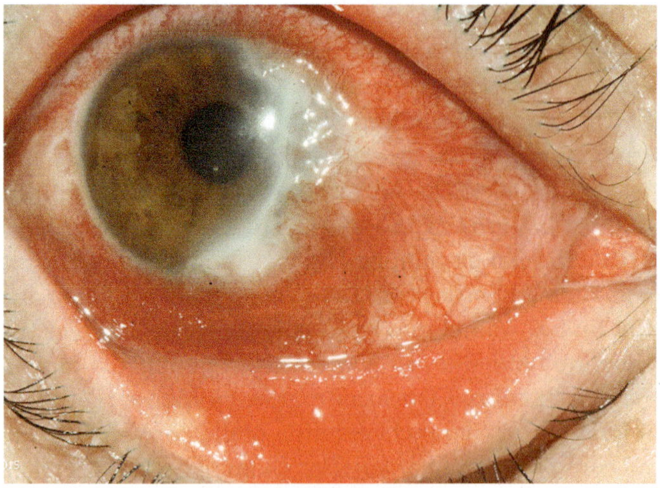

Fig. 27.5: Mooren's ulcer.
Source: Proctor Foundation, University of California, San Francisco.

Management centers on stopping the inflammatory process. Topical corticosteroids and systemic immunomodulators are the mainstay in therapy aiding in decreasing inflammation. Excision of the perilimbal conjunctiva or cryotherapy of the perilimbal conjunctiva aids in removing immunoglobulins. Lamellar keratoplasty and conjunctival flaps can also be used to provide tectonic support to thinned areas of the cornea.[7]

Peripheral Subepithelial Hypertrophic Degeneration

Peripheral subepithelial hypertrophic degeneration is generally bilateral, progresses slowly and can appear similar to Salzmann's nodular degeneration.[23] It appears as a superficial vascularization with grayish peripheral subepithelial fibrosis which can result in significant induced astigmatism and hyperopic shift.[24,25] Peripheral subepithelial hypertrophic degeneration occurs more in females.[25] Fibrosis can be seen on histology but no inflammation is present, and no cause has been isolated for this degeneration.[23,24] Patients can present with pain, irritation, blurred vision and monocular diplopia.[24] Astigmatism and hyperopic shift can be found on examination due to peripheral corneal elevation.[24] Treatment is initially conservative and involves lubrication, punctal occlusion, oral doxycycline and topical steroids however, superficial keratectomy (as with Salzmann's nodules) with or without mitomycin C has shown to be helpful in refractory cases and also to decrease induced astigmatism and hyperopic shift.[24,25]

Salzmann's Nodular Degeneration

Salzmann's nodular degeneration (Figs. 27.6A and B) is an uncommon, noninflammatory, slowly progressive disease that mostly occurs in the 50–60 years old age range, but has been reported to occur at any age from 4 years to 70 years. It tends to be more common in females, in Caucasians, and in those patients who had previously experienced corneal inflammation. Androgen deficiency causing meibomian gland dysfunction, evaporative dry eye and reduced tear production have been proposed in literature to further explain the female preponderance of the disease.[26,27] Currently, most cases of Salzmann's nodular degeneration are idiopathic although some studies have linked this condition to cataract surgery, anterior basement

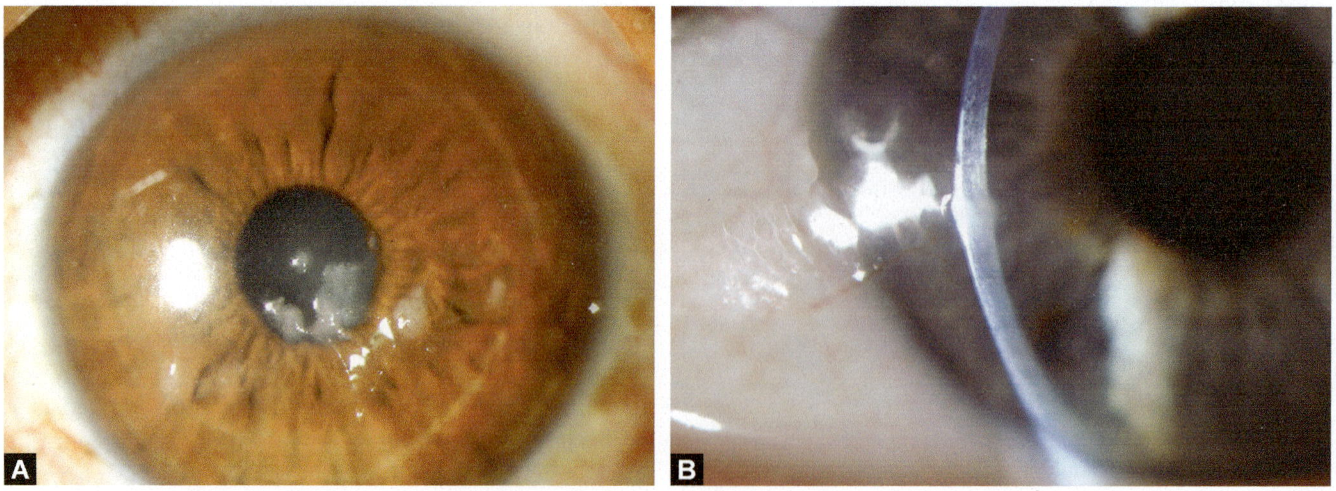

Figs. 27.6A and B: (A) Salzmann's nodules; (B) Slit-beam demonstrating elevation of the Salzmann's nodule.
Source: (A) Dr N Venkatesh Prajna, Aravind Eye Hospital, Madurai; (B) Proctor Foundation, University of California, San Francisco.

membrane disease, pterygia, long-term (monthly) contact lens wear, ocular trauma, measles, scarlet fever, previous surgery, trachoma, interstitial keratitis, vernal keratoconjunctivitis, meibomian gland dysfunction, and phlyctenular keratoconjunctivitis.[26,28,29]

Salzmann's nodules occur in the superior or inferior cornea if they are associated with inflammation (sometimes associated with pterygia) in the interpalpebral zone if in myopic contact lens wearers and at the apex of the cone in keratoconus patients.[26] The nodules are associated with destruction of Bowman's layer, thinning or denuded epithelium, duplication of the epithelial basement membrane, and disorganization of collagen of superficial anterior stroma.[27] Bowman's layer is generally replaced by periodic acid Schiff staining eosinophilic material that mimics basement membrane, and hyaline plaques can form between epithelium and Bowman's layer leading to a degenerative pannus. External irritation then causes the overgrowth of fibroblasts and a nodule then forms.[26] *In vivo* confocal microscopy shows an irregular network of activated keratocytes, irregularly arranged collagen fibers, hyaline deposits and irregularly shaped and elongated epithelial cells.[27]

The disease tends to be bilateral in most cases and the nodules appear as blue-gray opacities that vary in number from 1 to 8 and in size (usually 1–2 mm).[1,26] They can be round, conical or prismatic, and recurrences are rare. Patients are mostly asymptomatic but they can develop a foreign body sensation if the nodules are peripheral, and they can have decreased visual acuity if the nodules are mid-peripheral in the cornea.[26] Patients can also present with recurrent erosions, photophobia, blepharospasm and abnormal tearing.[29] Irregular astigmatism and hyperopic shift can occur along with disruption of the tear film. The nodules generally have negative fluorescein staining, are avascular and can have a pigmented iron line at the base of the nodule in the basal epithelial layer or Bowman's layer.[26] The nodules can fuse together if nearby, and the underlying cornea may be scarred, vascularized, edematous, or normal. Patients can also present with recurrent erosions, photophobia, blepharospasm, and abnormal tearing.[29]

Treatment of Salzmann's nodules can start with lubrication and management with preservative-free artificial tears, eyelid hygiene, cyclosporine 0.05%, autologous serum, collagen and silicone punctal plugs, topical steroids and oral doxycycline.[27] However, treatment may need to be escalated to superficial keratectomy or PTK with alcohol-assisted epithelial delamination, mitomycin C or amniotic membrane. Rarely, patients may need a keratoplasty.[26] Superficial keratectomy is completed by removing the epithelium and then peeling off the nodule. If the underlying cornea is not smooth, diamond burr polishing or PTK can decrease the irregularity of the underlying cornea.[26] PTK can improve visual acuity however, patients may experience a hyperopic shift after treatment.[30] In general, most patients with Salzmann's nodular degeneration respond to medical management alone.[27]

Terrien's Marginal Degeneration

Also called gutter dystrophy, peripheral furrow keratitis and senile marginal atrophy, Terrien's marginal degeneration can be found at any age but is often seen in the 20–40 years old age range.[7,31,32] Terrien's marginal degeneration first appears as a peripheral thinning in the superior cornea and with time spreads circumferentially. Generally, this results in thinning superiorly and a furrow inferior to the primary area of thinning. If corneal thinning progresses, perforation can occur in 15% of patients with Terrien.[32]

Histologically, one can see the loss of Bowman's layer and the anterior stromal lamella as the stroma undergoes fibrillar degeneration and the collagen fibers undergo lipid infiltration. This area of degeneration is then partially replaced with loosely vascularized connective tissue.[7,32]

Clinically, patients do not tend to experience regular, recurring attacks of acute pain and inflammation however, inflammatory Terrien's degeneration (associated with conjunctival hyperemia, lacrimation and photophobia) has been reported previously.[32] Terrien's marginal degeneration is a bilateral disease, but it does tend to progress asymmetrically in both eyes.[31,32] It first begins as fine yellow white punctate stromal opacities in the periphery that are associated with mild superficial corneal vascularization. Then very slowly, a progressive thinning occurs in the same area and a gutter is formed (Fig. 27.7). The overlying epithelium remains intact during this process.[7] No protrusion or iron line is seen in this disease. Occasionally, corneal hydrops has been reported to occur due to tears in Descemet membrane as aqueous humor seeps into the stroma.[31] Corneal topography can show flattening over the areas of thinned cornea and steepening of the cornea 90° away from the lesion. This tends to create against-the-rule or oblique astigmatism. In certain circumstances if corneal thinning is circumferential, corneal topography can remain spherical.[33]

The goal of treatment in Terrien's marginal degeneration is to improve visual acuity and provide tectonic support to the cornea. Contact lenses can improve visual acuity.[7] In

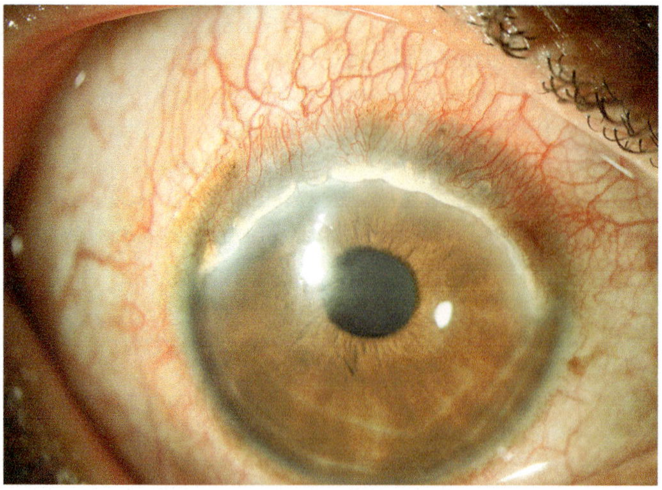

Fig. 27.7: Terrien's marginal degeneration.
Source: Dr N Venkatesh Prajna, Aravind Eye Hospital, Madurai.

the setting of hydrops, corneal edema can be treated with topical hypertonic saline, steroids, prophylactic antibiotic drops and antiglaucoma medications. Persistent edema however, can lead to infection, neovascularization and perforation. Surgical treatment involves the injection of air or isoexpansile gas, placement of compressive sutures or performing a penetrating keratoplasty. Oftentimes if the cornea is thin and perforation is imminent, prophylactic surgical treatment is recommended. Surgical maneuvers in these circumstances would include conjunctival flaps to cover the area of thinning, suturing the walls of the furrow, lamellar or penetrating keratoplasty, crescentic lamellar keratoplasty and compressive C-shaped lamellar keratoplasty.[31] The latter procedure while difficult technically, can decrease astigmatism and provide increased tectonic support to the cornea.[34]

CENTRAL CORNEAL DEGENERATIONS

Iridocorneal Endothelial Syndrome

Iridocorneal endothelial syndrome (ICE) is subdivided into three entities: essential iris atrophy, Chandler syndrome and iris nevus or Cogan Reese syndrome. In this condition, abnormal endothelial cells undergo epithelial transformation and grow over the endothelium, angle and iris. Patients can develop corneal edema and a secondary glaucoma due to peripheral anterior synechia.[35] Examination can reveal changes in the endothelium appearing with a "hammered silver" look, ectropion uvea, thickened iris stroma with increased pigmentation, iris atrophy and peripheral anterior synechiae.[35,36] ICE syndrome is usually unilateral although bilateral cases have been reported. Treatment involves corneal transplantation for corneal edema and intraocular pressure control with trabeculectomy or other types of glaucoma surgery.[35]

Lipid Keratopathy

Lipid keratopathy is secondary deposition of lipid in old corneal scars, especially vascularized scars, from diseases such as herpes simplex virus and varicella zoster virus infections or trachoma. Dense plaques of lipid containing keratin, neutral fats and glycoproteins are deposited in the corneal scar.[37] Corneal vascularization can occur after corneal insults. Initially it can facilitate healing however, as lipids begin leaking from the vessels into the cornea, corneal transparency can decrease.[37] If the visual axis is obscured, then treatment of neovascularization with argon laser, corneal and conjunctival injections of bevacizumab and photodynamic therapy with verteporfin have been shown to decrease feeder vessels and decrease lipid deposition.[37,38]

Polymorphic Amyloid Degeneration

Polymorphic amyloid degeneration is a localized amyloid degeneration that occurs primarily in the posterior corneal stroma. On examination, the cornea presents with filamentous and punctate-gray opacities however, these opacities do not decrease vision. The opacities generally occur bilaterally and may have a crystalline appearance on retroillumination. The degeneration is not hereditary and is not associated with systemic disease unlike lattice dystrophy.[39]

Vortex Degeneration

Vortex degeneration or corneal verticillata, occurs as a whorl-like pattern from the centripetal migration of epithelial cells from the limbus. These epithelial cells undergo deposition of intralysosomal lipid-filled inclusion bodies in the basal epithelium. Classically, patients with Fabry disease have the gray or golden-brown deposits of vortex degeneration due to an accumulation of trihexosylceramide. Many medications can also cause a similar corneal deposition and pattern including the chloroquine family of drugs (chloroquine, hydroxychloroquine, amodiaquine), suramin (an antitrypanosomal agent and reverse transcriptase inhibitor), tamoxifen (an estrogen antagonist), perhexiline maleate (an antianginal drug), atovaquone (an antiparasitic), phenothiazine, clofazimine, tilorone hydrochloride (antineoplastic), naproxen, indomethacin, ibuprofen, netarsudil and monobenzone. Of all medications, amiodarone is the most common cause of vortex degeneration. Corneal changes can be found in 60–100% of patients taking 600–1400 mg of amiodarone anywhere from 6 days to 4 months after initiation of therapy. The medications that cause vortex degeneration are cationic and amphiphilic, thus enabling them to penetrate lysosomes and then bind to lysosomal metabolites. Because these molecules then cannot be expelled from the lysosome, they form inclusion bodies. Visual acuity is not affected and once the medications are stopped, vortex keratopathy then recedes.[40]

CORNEAL DEGENERATIONS DUE TO EXTERNAL CLIMATIC FACTORS

Climatic Proteoglycan Stromal Keratopathy

Climatic proteoglycan stromal keratopathy results from climatic damage to the cornea. It occurs primarily in the interpalpebral fissure in the corneal stroma as a horizontally oval and diffuse opacification of that area. The central cornea can flatten due to the hydration from excess stromal proteoglycans, and the anterior stroma is more involved than the posterior stroma. Histological examination can show excess intracellular and extracellular stromal proteoglycans. Of note, this degeneration occurs primarily in older males in the Middle East likely due to environmental factors including the heat, sun, sand and solar radiation. It has been hypothesized that eye protection from the elements and urbanization away from the desert may protect from worsening of the degeneration. In cases where the central cornea is heavily opacified, penetrating keratoplasty has been shown to be helpful in regaining useful vision.[41]

Spheroidal Degeneration

Spheroidal degeneration also known as Bietti's corneal degeneration, Labrador keratopathy, climatic droplet keratopathy, droplet degeneration of the cornea, fisherman keratopathy, Eskimo corneal degeneration and elastotic degeneration of the cornea is more common in areas with increased ultraviolet light exposure or in tropical areas and in hot climates.[42,43] Welders have also been found to have increased prevalence of the condition.[44] Although the etiology is unknown, sunlight is involved in the pathology of the degeneration.[43] Spheroidal degeneration is usually bilateral unless it occurs unilaterally due to other conditions.[42]

In this condition, the cornea is usually hazy and opalescent, and small gold and yellow spherules can be found in the cornea and conjunctiva.[43,45] In the cornea, these spherules are of varying size (usually less than 8 microns) and are mostly found in the anterior stroma and Bowman's layer (Fig. 27.8). They do not extend into the epithelium.[42] On clinical examination, patients with spheroidal degeneration have homogenous, translucent, yellow-gold, spherical and oval lesions in the superficial cornea that first appear at the limbus at 3 and 9 o'clock in the interpalpebral zone. They are separated from the limbus by a clear zone initially, but this clear zone is lost as the degeneration progresses. Rarely the lesions can breach Bowman's layer and cause recurrent erosions.[42] As the condition progresses, patients may develop worsening corneal hypoesthesia, inferior iris depigmentation and atrophy.[46]

Four forms of spheroidal degeneration have been noted: primary corneal, secondary corneal, conjunctival and familial.[42] Spheroidal degeneration can also be graded. *Grade 1* displays many translucent droplets that are best seen on retroillumination and in the palpebral fissure with a clear zone at the limbus. In *Grade 2*, a hazy opacification develops across the cornea over the pupil decreasing visual acuity to approximately 20/100. In *Grade 3*, large yellow

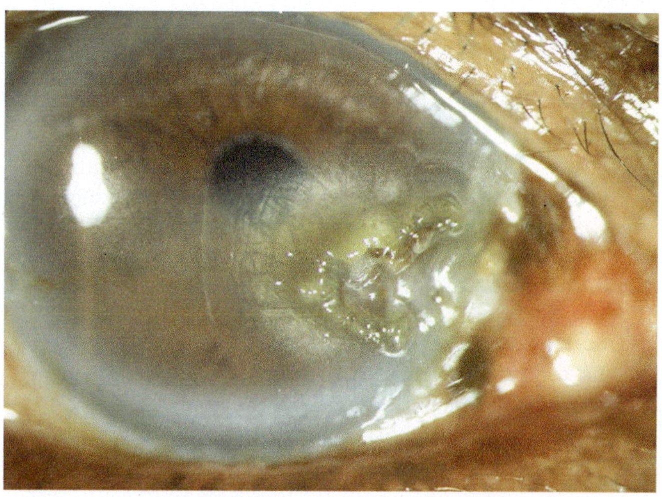

Fig. 27.8: Climatic droplet keratopathy.
Source: Dr N Venkatesh Prajna, Aravind Eye Hospital, Madurai.

opalescent nodules elevate the epithelium and decrease visual acuity to 20/200. These large nodules are up to 1 mm in diameter and disease progression leads to worsening corneal sensation.[1,45] In the advanced stages of spheroidal degeneration, subepithelial and stromal hyperreflective plaques develop, activating keratocytes and causing peripheral corneal vascularization.[45] It has been speculated in previous studies that the spherules form from plasma proteins, immunoglobulins and albumin that arrive in the cornea from the limbal circulation.[42]

Management hinges on visual acuity and irregular astigmatism as well as the presence of recurrent erosions. In advanced stages of the disease, PTK or mechanical debridement coupled with PTK is an option. Very severe disease may require penetrating or lamellar keratoplasty to improve vision.[42]

CONCLUSION

As presented here, corneal degenerations come varied in location, laterality and severity across the cornea. As noted above, most are related to older age or external factors, and visual prognosis can vary in individual eyes. Hereditary factors are not involved in the pathogenesis of corneal degenerations.

REFERENCES

1. Friedlaender MH, Smolin G. Corneal degenerations. Ann Ophthalmol. 1979;11(10):1485-95.
2. Ayhan Z, Ozturk T, Kaya M, et al. Corneal biomechanical properties in patients with arcus senilis. Cornea. 2014;35(7): 980-2.
3. Ang M, Wong W, Park J, et al. Corneal arcus is a sign of cardiovascular disease, even in low-risk persons. Am J Ophthalmol. 2011;152(5):844-71.
4. Jeng BH, Whitcher JP, Margolis TP. Pseudogerontoxon. Clinical and Exp Ophthalmol. 2004;32(4):433-4.
5. Fernandez AB, Keyes MJ, Pencina M, et al. Relation of corneal arcus to cardiovascular disease (from the Framingham Heart Study data set). Am J Cardiol. 2009;103(1):64-6.
6. Kriszt Á, Losonczy G, Berta A, et al. Presence of Fleischer ring and prominent corneal nerves in keratoconus relatives and normal controls. Int J Ophthalmol. 2015;8(5):922-7.
7. Friedlaender MH, Smolin G. Peripheral corneal disorders. Surv Ophthalmol. 1986;31(1):01-36.
8. Barraquer-Somersault E, Chan CC, Green R. Corneal epithelial iron deposition. Ophthalmology. 1983;90:729-34.
9. Rose GE, Lavin MJ. The Hudson-Stahli line. An epidemiological study. Eye (Lond). 1987;1(Pt 4):466-70.
10. Yeung L, Chen Y, Lin K, et al. Central corneal iron deposition after myopic laser assisted in situ keratomileusis. Cornea. 2006;25(3):291-5.
11. Rosenthal AR, Marmor MF, Leuenberger P, et al. Chalcosis: a study of natural history. Ophthalmology. 1979;86(11):1956-72.
12. Belliveau MJ, Brownstein S, Agapitos P, et al. Ultrastructural features of posterior crocodile shagreen of the cornea. Surv Ophthalmol. 2009;54(5):569-75.
13. Woodward M, Randleman JB, Larson PM. In vivo confocal microscopy of polymorphic amyloid degeneration and posterior crocodile shagreen. Cornea. 2007;26(1):98-101.
14. Goodside V. Posterior crocodile shagreen: a corneal dystrophy. Am J Ophthalmol. 1958;46(5 Part 1):748-50.
15. Nevins RC, Elliott JH. White ring of the cornea. Arch Ophthalmol. 1969;82(4):457-60.
16. Moisseiev E, Gal A, Addadi L, et al. Acute calcific band keratopathy: case report and literature review. J Cataract Refract Surg.2013;39(2):292-4.
17. de Ortueta D, Schreyger F, Baatz H. Band keratopathy:a modified treatment. Eur J Ophthalmol. 2006;16(4):618-20.
18. Najjar DM, Cohen EJ, Rapuano CJ, et al. EDTA chelation for calcific band keratopathy: results and long-term follow-up. Am J Ophthalmol. 2004;137(6):1056-64.
19. Nascimento H, Yasuta MK, Marquezan MC, et al. Uveitic band keratopathy:child and adult. J Ophthalmic Inflamm Infect. 2015;5(1):35.
20. Baum JL, Mishima S, Boruchoff SA. On the nature of Dellen. Arch Ophthalmol. 1968;79(6):657-62.
21. Kymionis GD, Plaka A, Kontadakis GA, et al. Treatment of corneal dellen with a large diameter soft contact lens. Cont Lens Anterior Eye. 2011;34(6):290-2.
22. Ono T, Yuki K, Ozeki N, et al. Ocular surface complications after trabeculectomy:incidence, risk factors, time course and prognosis. Ophthalmologica. 2013;230(2):93-9.
23. Rommel F, Grisanti S, Ranjbar M. Peripheral hypertrophic subepithelial corneal degeneration. JAMA Ophthalmol. 2017;135(6):509-676.
24. Järventausta PJ, Holopainen JM, Zalentein WN, et al. Peripheral hypertrophic subepithelial corneal degeneration:characterization, treatment and association with human leucocyte antigen genes. Acta Ophthalmol. 2014;92(1):71-6.
25. Jeng BH, Millstein ME. Reduction of hyperopia and astigmatism after superficial keratectomy of peripheral hypertrophic subepithelial corneal degeneration. Eye Contact Lens. 2006;32(3):153-6.
26. Maharana PK, Sharma N, Das S, et al. Salzmann's nodular degeneration. Ocul Surf. 2016;14(1):20-30.
27. Farjo AA, Halperin GI, Syed N, et al. Salzmann's nodular corneal degeneration clinical characteristics and surgical outcomes. Cornea. 2006;25(1):11-5.
28. Hamada S, Darrad K, McDonnell PJ. Salzmann's nodular corneal degeneration (SNCD): clinical findings, risk factors, prognosis and the role of previous contact lens wear. Cont Lens Anterior Eye. 2011;34(4):173-8.

29. Das S, Link B, Seitz B. Salzmann's nodular degeneration of the cornea: a review and case series. Cornea. 2005;24(7):772-7.
30. Das S, Langenbucher A, Pogorelov P, et al. Long-term outcome of excimer laser phototherapeutic keratectomy for treatment of Salzmann's nodular degeneration. J Cataract Refract Surg. 2005;31(7):1386-91.
31. Maharana PK, Dubey A, Jhanji V, et al. Management of advanced corneal ectasias. Br J Ophthalmol. 2016;100(1): 34-40.
32. Austin P, Brown SI. Inflammatory Terrien's marginal corneal disease. Am J Ophthalmol. 1981;92(2):189-92.
33. Wilson SE, Lin DT, Klyce SD, et al. Terrien's marginal degeneration: corneal topography. Refract Corneal Surg. 1990;6(1):15-20.
34. Cheng CL, Theng JT, Tan DT. Compressive C-shaped lamellar keratoplasty: a surgical alternative for the management of severe astigmatism from peripheral corneal degeneration. Ophthalmology. 2005;112(3):425-30.
35. Liu YK, Wang IJ, Hu FR, et al. Clinical and specular microscopic manifestations of iridocorneal endothelial syndrome. Jpn J Ophthalmol. 2001;45(3):281-7.
36. Laganowski HC, Sherrard ES, Muir MG, et al. Distinguishing features of the iridocorneal endothelial syndrome and posterior polymorphous dystrophy: value of endothelial specular microscopy. Br J Ophthalmol. 1991;75(4):212-6.
37. Oh JY, Kim MK, Wee WR. Subconjunctival and intracorneal bevacizumab injection for corneal neovascularization in lipid keratopathy. Cornea. 2009;28(9):1070-3.
38. You IC, Im SK, Lee SH, et al. Photodynamic therapy with verteporfin combined with subconjunctival injection of bevacizumab for corneal neovascularization. Cornea. 2011; 30(1):30-3.
39. Mannis MJ, Krachmer JH, Rodrigues MM, et al. Polymorphic amyloid degeneration of the cornea. A clinical and histopathologic study. Arch Ophthalmol. 1981;99(7):1217-23.
40. Hollander DA, Aldave AJ. Drug-induced corneal complications. Curr Opin Ophthalmol. 2004;15(6):541-8.
41. Waring GO, Malaty A, Grossniklaus H, et al. Climatic proteoglycan stromal keratopathy, a new corneal degeneration. Am J Ophthalmol. 1995;120(3):330-41.
42. Magovern M, Wright JD Jr, Mohammed A. Spheroidal degeneration of the cornea: a clinicopathologic case report. Cornea. 2004;23(1):84-8.
43. Garner A, Fraunfelder FT, Barras TC, et al. Spheroidal degeneration of cornea and conjunctiva. Br J Ophthalmol. 1976;60(6):473-8.
44. Norn M, Franck C. Long-term changes in the outer part of the eye in welders. Acta Ophthalmologica. 1991;69(3): 382-6.
45. Serra HM, Holopainen JM, Beuerman R, et al. Climatic droplet keratopathy: an old disease in new clothes. Acta Ophthalmol. 2015;93(6):496-504.
46. Urretts-Zavalia JA, Maccio JP, Knoll EG, et al. Surface alterations, corneal hypoesthesia, and iris atrophy in patients with climatic droplet keratopathy. Cornea. 2007;26(7):800-4.

Chapter 28 Corneal Dystrophies

V Romano, B Steger, CE Willoughby

INTRODUCTION

Corneal dystrophies are traditionally described as a group of inherited disorders that are slowly progressive, usually bilateral and symmetrical, noninflammatory in nature and not related to an environmental or a systemic cause.[1,2] The term dystrophy comes from the Greek, *dys* meaning *wrong* and *trophe* meaning *nourishment*; defective nourishment. In fact corneal dystrophies represent genetic disorders and this is reflected in The International Committee for Classification of Corneal Dystrophies (IC3D) which was introduced[1] and revised[2] to reflect the clinical phenotype, pathology and genetics of these corneal disorders.

Many historically reported corneal dystropies are in fact degenerations, and were described before the use of slit lamps or respresent systemic or complex (genes and environment) diseases. Corneal dystrophies were initially characterized on the basis of the anatomical involvement of the cornea and then histopathology. Advances in genetic analysis has revolutionized the classification of corneal dystrophies.[3,4] Genetic studies have detected both genotypic and phenotypic heterogeneity in corneal dystrophies. Genotypic heterogeneity is used to describe a single clinical entity, for example Meesmann corneal dystrophy, which results from mutations in more than one gene: *keratin 3 (KRT3)* and *keratin 12 (KRT12)*.[5] Phenotypic heterogeneity results, if mutations in a single gene, for example *TGFβI*, result in specific and distinct clinical entities or phenotypes: Reis-Bucklers corneal dystrophy (RBCD), Thiel-Behnke corneal dystrophy (TBCD), granular corneal dystrophies type 1 and 2 respectively (GCD1 and GCD2) and lattice corneal dystrophy (LCD).[4,6,7]

The IC3D has developed a classification system for corneal dystrophies based on levels of evidence from the clinical findings, histopathology and genetics.[1,2] The IC3D classification consists of categories 1 to 4 with decreasing levels of evidence. In this chapter, we will only cover corneal dystrophies in category 1 (a well-defined corneal dystrophy with a known gene in which pathogenic mutations have been identified) and category 2 (a well-defined corneal dystrophy mapped to one or more specific chromosomal loci but in which the causative or genes have not been identified yet).[2] Category 3 represents a well-defined corneal dystrophy but with no supporting genetic mapping, whereas category 4 is applied to corneal dystrophies lacking enough evidence to be classified as a distinct clinical entity.

EPITHELIAL AND SUBEPITHELIAL DYSTROPHIES

Epithelial Basement Membrane Dystrophy

Epithelial basement membrane dystrophy (EBMD, MIM#121820), also known as Cogan or map-dot-fingerprint dystrophy, is a predominantly degenerative or post-traumatic corneal disorder.[2] It is considered as corneal dystrophy as some isolated familial autosomal dominant cases reported in literature result from mutations in the *transforming growth factor β-induced gene (TGFβI)* on chromosome 5q31.[8] These mutations were only present in a small subset of patients; the rest of the EBMD cohort did not have any mutation in the *TGFβI* region. It is probable this mutation is only responsible for a subset of EBMD, but could be associated with as much as 10% of cases. In the familial cases recorded, the age of onset was younger (4 to 8 years of age) and shows a progressive nature as the frequency of erosions gradually increases with age.[9]

Epithelial basement membrane dystrophy is sometimes misdiagnosed due to its very varied appearance.[2] It is a bilateral disease, with an onset in the second decade; however, many patients remain asymptomatic throughout life and the disease is not usually progressive. It is known that 10% of patients will have recurrent idiopathic erosions and loss of vision due to surface irregularity. The erosions may be mild and transient, lasting minutes or occasionally characterized by severe pain; the pain is often present on awakening. Slit-lamp examination may reveal lesions, such as dot-like opacities, subepithelial map-like patterns, epithelial fingerprint lines, and blebs, either in isolation or in combination (Fig. 28.1). The clinical features may change frequently, which makes it difficult to identify a phenotypic pattern. Treatment is directed either at alleviating blurred vision or managing recurrent corneal erosion. Lubricating ointments are beneficial and more severe erosions can benefit from debridement of loosened epithelium.[10] Phototherapeutic keratectomy (PTK) ablates abnormal basement membrane.

This dystrophy produces a thickening of the basement membrane with deposition of fibrillary protein between the basement membrane and Bowman's Layer.[11,12] Recurrent corneal lesions are produced when the basal epithelial cells lose their hemidesmosomes. In light microscopy, maps show up as sheets of intraepithelial, multilamellar, basal laminar material.[11,12] Fingerprint lines are seen as rib-like intraepithelial extensions of basal laminar material, while dots correlate to intraepithelial pseudocysts containing cytoplasmic debris.[11,12]

Epithelial Recurrent Erosion Dystrophy

Epithelial recurrent erosion dystrophy (ERED) can show an autosomal dominant inheritance and a mutation in the *collagen type XVII alpha 1 (COL17A1)* gene located on chromosome 10q23-q24 was identified in a large family from Sweden.[13] Subsequent, genetic testing in further families identifed the same mutation in the *COL17A1* gene.[14] ERED presents with recurrent ocular pain episodes secondary to corneal epithelial erosions. Frequent, painful, recurrent corneal erosions begin in childhood. Although these episodes cease in the second decade, the resulting accumulation of corneal scarring impairs vision in some patients. The corneal features include small, fine gray anterior stromal flecks, with more unique larger gray-white opacities at the level of the Bowman's layer and the immediately subjacent anterior stroma, with increased prominence of the corneal nerves.[14] The use of soft contact lenses is advocated during painful episodes and PTK has a place in the management of ERED. Lamellar or penetrating keratoplasties may be required in cases with significant visual loss in adulthood.

Meesmann Corneal Dystrophy

Meesmann corneal dystrophy (MECD, MIM#122100), formerly known as juvenile hereditary epithelial dystrophy, is an autosomal dominant corneal dystrophy resulting from a mutations in the *keratin 3 (KRT3)* gene located on chromosome 12q13, or more rarely in the *keratin 12 (KRT12)* gene on chromosome 17q12.[5] *Keratin 3 & 12* are only expressed in the corneal epithelium[5] playing a critical role in the structural integrity and mechanical strength of the corneal epithelium.[5,15] MECD is characterized by multiple, small intraepithelial vesicles with clear surrounding epithelium which extend to the limbus (Fig. 28.2). On indirect illumination, the solitary transparent cysts are readily apparent. Cysts can coalesce to form gray serpiginous lines in the epithelium. Histopathology shows an irregularly thickened corneal epithelium with numerous intraepithelial cysts of uniform size.[16] These intraepithelial

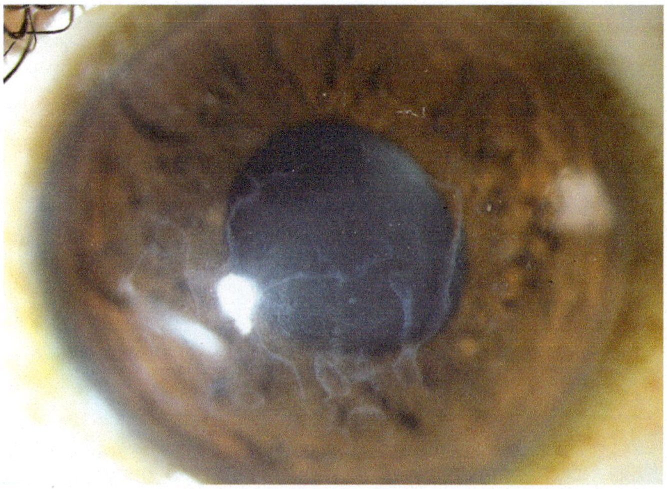

Fig. 28.1: Subepithelial map-like patterns and fingerprint lines characteristic of epithelial basement membrane dystrophy.
Source: Dr N Venkatesh Prajna, Aravind Eye Hospital, Madurai, Tamil Nadu, India.

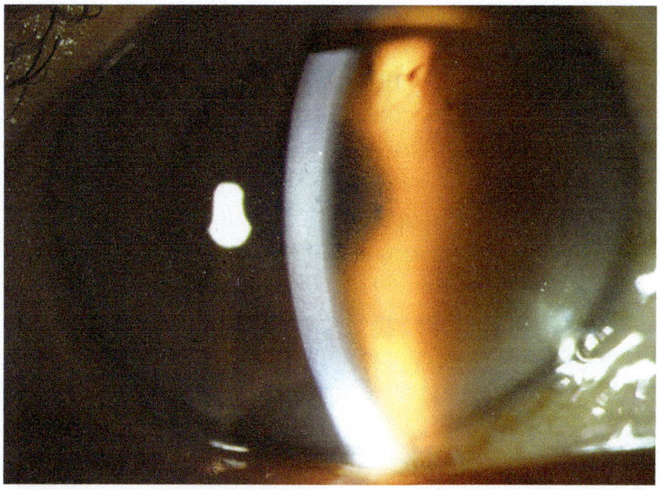

Fig. 28.2: Meesmann corneal dystrophy characterized by multiple, small intraepithelial vesicles with clear surrounding epithelium which extend to the limbus.
Source: Dr N Venkatesh Prajna, Aravind Eye Hospital, Madurai, Tamil Nadu, India.

cysts are filled with PAS-positive cellular debris and the corneal epithelial cells also contain PAS-positive and diastase-sensitive glycogen.[16] The corneal epithelial basement membrane may be thickened and multilaminar, projecting into the basal epithelium. Confocal microscopy can typically show multiple hyporeflective areas in the basal corneal epithelium and hyperreflective material thought to represent fibrillogranular material.[17] Patients may remain asymptomatic throughout life but MECD typically presents in early childhood.[18] Common symptoms are contact lens intolerance, pain and lacrimation, if erosions are present, intermittent blurred vision, photophobia. Notably, visual impairment is usually mild.[18,19] Treatment includes lubricants, cycloplegia and therapeutic contact lenses.[20] In severe cases, management with epithelial debridement, phototherapeutic keratectomy and lamellar keratoplasty has been advocated.[20] New gene silencing and editing techniques are being developed in cellular and mouse models of MECD and may represent a future gene-based therapy for this condition.[21-23]

Lisch Epithelial Corneal Dystrophy

Lisch epithelial corneal dystrophy (LECD, MIM#300778), also called band-shaped whorled microcystic corneal dystrophy,[24] is a X-linked corneal dystrophy mapped to chromosome Xp22.3;[25] no specific gene or mutation has been identified to date. Bilateral gray intraepithelial opacifications occur in the corneal epithelium in a banded, whorled pattern. Indirect illumination demonstrates multiple densely crowded clear cysts.[24] The onset occurs in the second decade of life. Patients become symptomatic with vision loss but no pain when opacities significantly involve the pupillary axis. Epithelial debridement offers a temporary improvement in vision but the opacities recur within months. Soft contact lenses have been reported to reduce the epithelial opacities over several months of wear[26] and photorefractive keratectomy has been reported to decrease epithelial opacities.[27] Histologically, the corneal epithelial basal cells are cuboidal and in the suprabasal and parabasal layers, vacuolated cells progress to the epithelial surface, where they adopt elongated flat squamous shapes.[24,27] These vacuoles contain glycogen and are PAS-positive, diastase-sensitive, and Sudan black negative.[24]

Gelatinous Drop-like Corneal Dystrophy

Gelatinous drop-like corneal dystrophy (GDLD, MIM# 204870), formerly known as subepithelial amyloidosis, is an autosomal recessive dystrophy caused by a mutations in the *tumor-associated calcium signal transducer 2 (TACSTD2)* gene located on chromosome 1p32.[28] Some families with GDLD cannot be linked to 1p31 and so GDLD shows locus heterogeneity.[29] *TACSTD2* acts as a cell surface receptor and mutations in *TACSTD2* significantly increase corneal epithelial permeability and alter cell junctions.[30] Histologically, there is disruption of epithelial tight junctions in the superficial epithelium and amyloid evident in the basal epithelium.[31] About twenty mutations in *TACSTD2* have been reported, with the majority resulting in a truncated protein product, eliminating the C-terminal transmembrane domain. Q118X is a recurring mutation, which was found to be present in 82% cases in Japan.[30] GDLD is highly prevalent in Japan and has its clinical onset within the first decade of life.[30] Flat subepithelial nodular deposits, which increase in number to form gray, raised gelatinous masses (mulberry), with surrounding dense subepithelial opacities (Fig. 28.3); this causes severe visual impairment.[30] Lamellar or penetrating keratoplasty may be required for visual rehabilitation. However, almost all patients will experience a recurrence of the disease within a few years[32] (Fig. 28.3).

Epithelial-stromal *TGFβI* Dystrophies

The epithelial-stromal *TGFβI* dystrophies are a group of autosomal dominant corneal dystrophies which result from mutations in the *transforming growth factor β-induced gene (TGFβI)* on chromosome 5q31.[3,4] TGFβI is an extracellular matrix protein which is predicted to bind fibronectin,

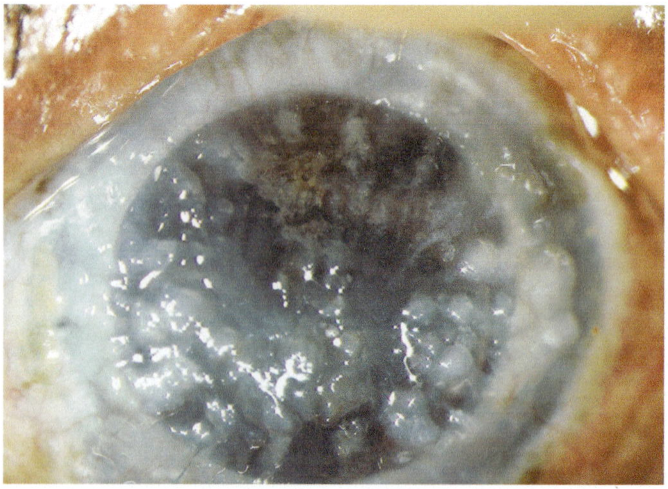

Fig. 28.3: Recurrence of gelatinous drop-like corneal dystrophy following penetrating keratoplasty showing nodular, gray, raised gelatinous deposits. *Source*: Dr N Venkatesh Prajna, Aravind Eye Hospital, Madurai, Tamil Nadu, India.

collagen and integrins.[33,34] The exact role of *TGFβI* in the pathogenesis of the 5q31-linked corneal dystrophies is still unclear.[33,35] Mutations in *TGFβI* result in specific and distinct phenotypes: Reis-Bucklers corneal dystrophy (RBCD), Thiel-Behnke corneal dystrophy (TBCD), granular corneal dystrophy type 1 and 2 respectively (GCD1 and GCD2) and lattice corneal dystrophy (LCD).[4,6,7] Previously, the *TGFβI* associated dystrophies were classified on the basis of the anatomical level of the cornea affected into Bowman's layer and stromal dystrophies.[1] The *TGFβI* associated dystrophies affect multiple layers wihtin the cornea and are now considered as a group: the epithelial-stromal *TGFβI* dystrophies.[2] In the *TGFβI* associated corneal dystrophies, aberrant accumulation of the *TGFβI* protein (*TGFβIp*) or its proteolytic fragments leads to cornea-specific insoluble protein deposits.[33] There is a strong correlation between *TGFβI* mutations and their associated phenotype: genotype-phenotype correlation.[6,7,34] Specifically, the clinical appearance and course, histopathology and location of the corneal deposits is related to the specific amino acid alterations in the *TGFβI* protein.[34]

Reis-Bücklers Corneal Dystrophy

In 1917, Reis reported an autosomal dominant corneal condition associated with corneal erosions and superficial corneal scarring occurring in the first two decades of life.[2] In 1949, Bucklers described similar features in this original family, previously studied by Reis.[2] Reis-Bücklers corneal dystrophy (RBCD; MIM608470) is usually associated with the p.Arg124Leu (R124L) mutation in the *TGFβI* gene.[6,7,34,36] RBCD commonly presents in childhood with the painful recurrent corneal erosions. The frequency and severity of erosions reduce with age but there is a progressive decline in vision due to progressive corneal opacification. Early clinical signs include the development of gray-white, irregular geographical or polygonal opacities in the Bowman's layer and superficial stroma (Fig. 28.4A). Over time, these lesions extend to the limbus and into the deeper stroma. Histologically, the Bowman's layer is replaced by multistratified granular material with projections into the epithelium and in the anterior stroma which stains red with Masson trichome stain.[34,37] Clinically, it is difficult to distinguish between RBCD and TBCD. Electron microscopy (EM) is required to confirm the diagnosis histopathologically. In RBCD there are electron dense rod or trapezoid shaped bodies in the Bowman's layer extending into the basal epithelium and anterior stroma.[37] The histopathological findings resemble granular corneal dystrophy, type 1 (GCD1).[37,38] Hyperreflective and homogeneous deposits at the level of the Bowman's layer and anterior stroma can be detected by anterior segment ocular coherence tomography (AS-OCT).[39] In vivo confocal microscopy (IVCM) may demonstrate that the Bowman's layer is replaced by a highly reflective amorphous material with scattered diffuse round refractile deposits in the epithelium and corneal stroma.[39] The reflectivity of this amorphous material is much higher in RBCD than in TBCD.[40]

Thiel-Behnke Corneal Dystrophy

In 1967, Thiel and Behnke described a corneal dystrophy of the Bowman's layer with honeycomb-shaped opacities.[41] Thiel-Behnke corneal dystrophy (TBCD; MIM#602082) usually results from a p.Arg555Gln (R555Q) mutation in *TGFβI*.[6] TBCD has a similar but usually less aggressive course than RBCD; presentation in childhood with painful recurrent corneal erosions and a progressive decline in vision. Early clinical signs include solitary flecks or irregular opacities in the Bowman's layer and subsequent appearance of irregular subepithelial opacities in a reticular or honeycomb pattern. Over time, these lesions extend to the limbus and into the deeper stroma. Histologically, the epithelial basement membrane may be focally absent with alternate areas of thinning and thickening corresponding and compensating for undulations in the underlying stroma.[42] The Bowman's layer is replaced by a saw-toothed undulating fibrocellular material;[42] the deposits do not stain with Masson trichrome. This saw-tooth pattern is detectable using AS-OCT as a hyperreflective undulating material;[43] this is a significant finding to differentiate TBCD from RBCD clinically. With IVCM the Bowman's layer is replaced by a highly reflective amorphous material which is less reflective in TBCD than RBCD.[40] In TBCD there are pathognomic culry collagen fibres (diameter 9–15 nm) with EM which also distinguish TBCD from RBCD.[42,44]

Lattice Corneal Dystrophy, Type 1

Lattice Corneal Dystrophy type 1 (LCD1; MIM#122200), the classic form of the dystrophy, is characterized by a network of branching refractile lines and/or subepithelial opacities of amyloid in the anterior and midstroma.[2,34] LCD1 usually results from a p.Arg124Cys (R124C) mutation in the first FAS1 domain of *TGFβI*.[6] Onset is in the first and second decade with recurrent corneal erosions and the development of progressive visual impairment.

Early clinical signs do not show the classic lattice lines but central superficial fleck-like deposits. Subsequently, subtle and sparse lattice lines develop in the superficial corneal stroma which are more obvious with slit-lamp retroillumination. The lattice lines develop centrally in the superficial stroma and evolve centrifugally spreading into the deeper stroma and outward from the central cornea (Figs. 28.4B and C). The degree of corneal involvement and number of lattice lines maybe asymmetrical and unilateral cases have been reported.[45] The peripheral stroma, Descemet's membrane and endothelium are spared. IVCM shows linear branches of variable reflectivity with poorly demarcated margins.[46] The interlattice line cornea develops a diffuse subepithelial haze which often causes visual impairment in the third and fourth decade requiring corneal transplantation.

Variations from the classic LCD1, clinical phenotype have been reported as LCD subtypes: type IIIA, I/IIIA, IV, and atypical polymorphic amyloidosis.[2] These lattice corneal dystrophies subtypes were proposed on the basis of genotypic and phenotypic variability[34] and the recent IC3D classification groups these subtypes as *variant* LCD.[2] These LCD variants result from heterozygous *TGFβI* mutations clustered in the fourth FAS1 domain and tend to have a later disease onset, show variations in lattice line morphology and distribution, variable severity on corneal erosions and are found in restricted geographical populations when compared to classic LCD1.[2,34] Lattice corneal dystrophy type 2 (LCD2) is not a true corneal dystrophy but represents a systemic amyloidosis with corneal involvement are hence is a familial amyloidosis (Finnish type or Meretoja's syndrome) which results from mutations in the *gelsolin (GSN) gene.*[47]

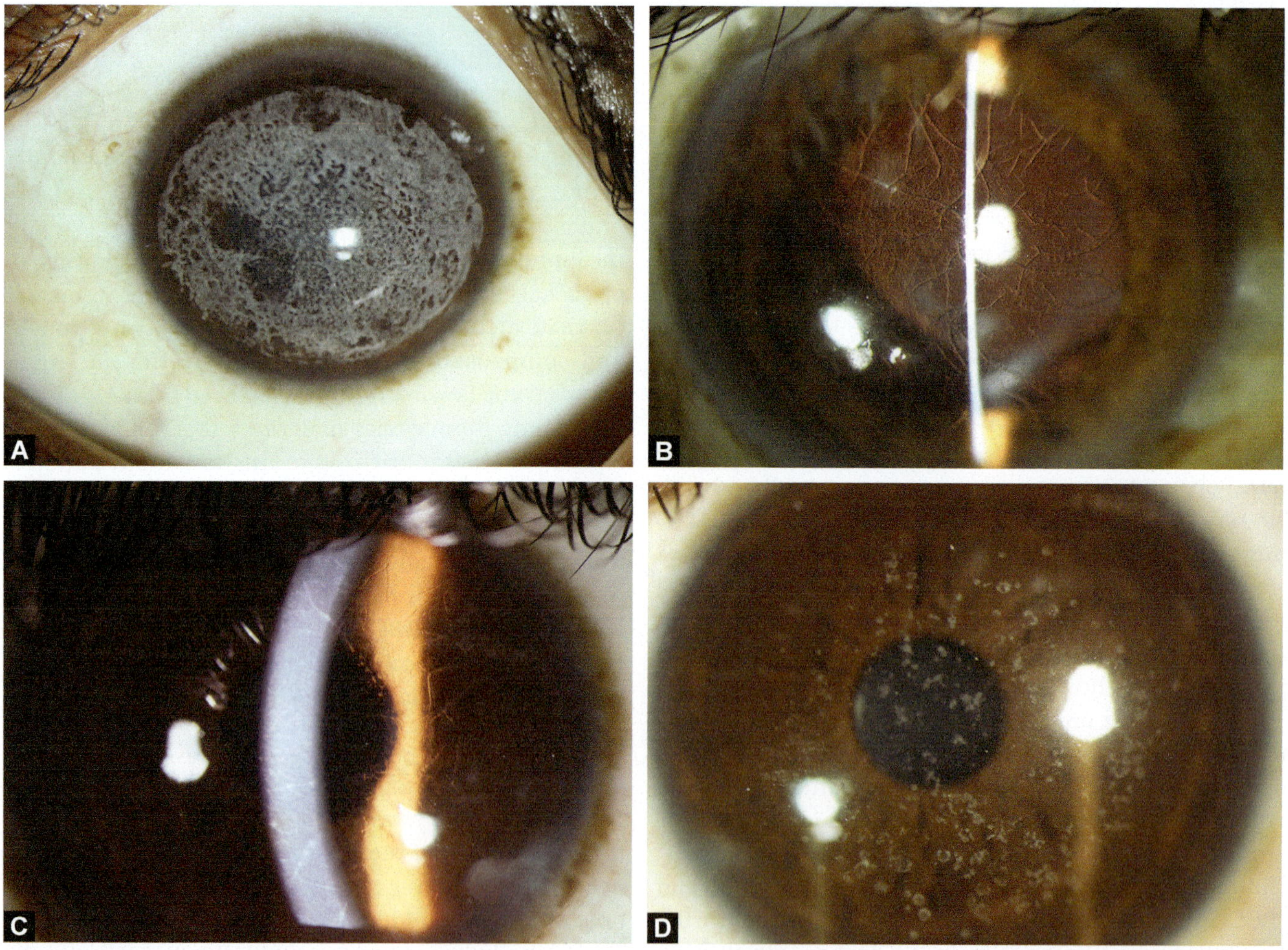

Figs. 28.4A to D: (A) Reis-Bücklers corneal dystrophy showing gray-white, irregular geographical or polygonal opacities in the Bowman's layer and superficial stroma; (B and C) Lattice corneal dystrophy type 1 (LCD1) with lattice lines centrifugally spreading into the deeper stroma and outward from the central cornea; (D) Granular corneal dystrophy type 1 (GCD1) characterized by small white, discrete, sharply demarcated opacities in the central anterior stroma which vary in shape (crumb-, drop- and ring- shaped) sparing the periphery of the cornea.

Source: Dr N Venkatesh Prajna, Aravind Eye Hospital, Madurai, Tamil Nadu, India.

Histolgically, there is disruption of the corneal epithelium and Bowman's layer with eosinophilic material between the epithelial basement membrane and Bowman's layer. The amyloid deposits in the cornea of LCD1 stain with Congo red and show apple green birefringence with polarized light.[48] The deposits also show metachromasia with crystal violet. EM shows characteristics of amyloid protein, electron dense fibrils of 8-10 nm diameter.[48]

Granular Corneal Dystrophy Type 1

Granular Corneal Dystrophy type 1 (GCD1; MIM#121900), is characterized by bilateral, multiple, discrete granular white opacities in the anterior stroma, sparing the periphery of the cornea which develop during the first or second decade of life.[2,34,49] GCD1 usually results from a heterozygous p.Arg555Trp (R555W) mutation in *TGFβI*.[6] Patients with homozygous mutations have been reported and this results in a severe phenotype characterized by a placoid type of corneal opacity with early recurrence after surgery.[50] The onset of GCD1 is usually in the first and patients develop recurrent corneal erosions.[2,49] The patients develop small white, sharply demarcated opacities in the central anterior stroma which vary in shape (crumb-, drop- and ring-shaped) and increase in size and number over time; the opacities do not extend to the limbus (Fig. 28.4D). On retroillumination, the granular opacities are composed of small, translucent dots resembling bread-crumbs. Initially, the stroma between opacities remains clear and vision is not usually affected, but mild photophobia and glare may occur. As the disease progresses visual acuity is affected, as the lesions coalesce and the cornea develops a ground-glass appearance, and corneal transplantation can be required in the third and fourth decade. Histopathologically, GCD1 is characterized by eosinophilic, rod-shaped hyaline deposits in the corneal stroma which stain bright red with Masson trichrome. EM shows stromal deposits are made up of rod-shaped or trapezoidal bodies which are similar to those seen in RBCD.[2,49,51]

Granular Corneal Dystrophy Type 2

Granular Corneal Dystrophy type 2 (GCD2; MIM#607541) is a distinct corneal dystrophy which was previously named Avellino corneal dystrophy.[2] This corneal dystrophy illustrates the impact of genetic analysis in the classification of corneal dystrophies and the ambiguity that can be perpetuated when really soley of clinical examination and/or histopathological investigation. This dystrophy was initially considered as mild subtype of granular corneal dystrophy type 1. Subsequent, histopathological investigation detected the presence of both amyloid and hyaline deposits suggestive of a combined granular-lattice dystrophy.[52] The term Avellino corneal dystrophy was introduced in 1992 to describe this dystrophy as it was characterized in patients originating from the Avellino area of Italy.[53] Genetically, Avellino corneal dystrophy results from a p.Arg124His (R124H) in *TGFβI*[6,7] and under the IC3D classification is termed granular dystrophy type 2 (GCD2) given the global occurrence of this dystrophy.[2] Most patients have heterozygous mutations in *TGFβI* but homozygous mutations have been reported which result in a severe phenotype often requiring earlier surgical intervention to restore vision.[54]

GCD2 shows clinical and histological features of both granular and lattice dystrophy.[2] Patients with the typical *TGFβI*, heterozygous mutations develop clinical features in the second decade which are slowly progressive resulting in recurrent erosions and subsequent visual impairment.[2,55] Clinically, the early lesions present as superficial stromal faint white opacities with spoke-like excrescences. More deposits accumulate with age and can appear stellate with spiky icicle or spider shaped mid-stromal deposits. When the superficial granular deposits result in recurrent ersoions the original deposits can alter in morphology forming ring-shaped opacities.[55] Patients with GCD2 typically have fewer granular deposits than patients with GCD1.[55] Histologically, granular deposits in the anterior stroma stain with Masson trichrome, and the latticelike lesions in the deep stroma stain with Congo red.

Treatment of Epithelial-Stromal *TGFβI* Dystrophies

The aim of treatment is to maintain visual function while minimising surgical intervention and a stage-related therapy for corneal dystrophies has been proposed based on the depth of corneal opacities. Excimer laser photorefractive keratectomy (PTK).[56,57] or femtosecond laser-assisted keratectomy (FLK).[58] for superficial lesions affecting the corneal epithelium, Bowman's layer, superficial and deep anterior lamellar keratoplasty (SALK and DALK)[59] for deeper stromal opacities sparing the corneal endothelium and penetrating keratoplasty (PK) for complete corneal involvement. Following PTK and corneal surgery the corneal deposits can recur in the *TGFβI* associated dystrophies and recurrence rates depend on the specifc phenotypes, genotypes and corneal procedures.[49] Whether PTK can exacerbate the clinical condition and lead to higher PK rates is debated in the literature.[55] As *TGFβI* associated corneal dystrophies are progressive conditions which can recur following surgical intervention pharmacological treatments (e.g. lithium and rapamycin) have been evaluated to reduce progression by decreasing the production of mutant *TGFβI* protein.[49,60,61] Gene therapy approaches using RNA interference (RNAi) have been assessed in *TGFβI* associated corneal dytrophies.[49,62] Decreased amyloid aggregation in vitro was achieved using a siRNA against the mutant allele Arg124Cys in LCD1.[62] The continued development of site-specific genome editing technologies using clustered regularly interspaced short palindromic repeat/Cas9 (CRISPR/Cas9) may offer other potential gene based therapies for corneal dystrophies.[23]

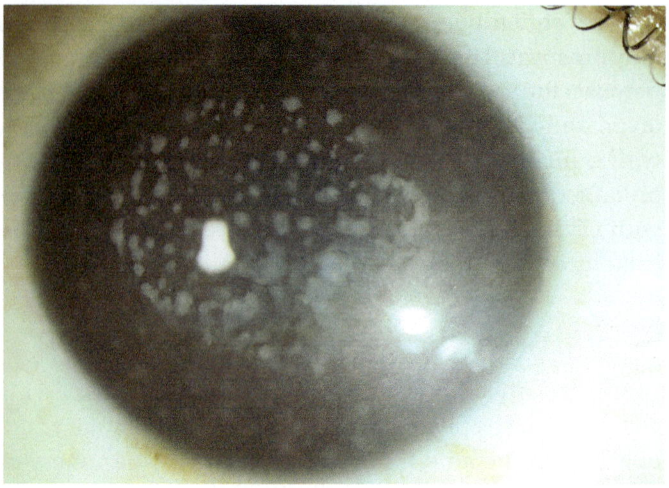

Fig. 28.5: Macular corneal dystrophy (MCD; MIM#217800) with superficial, gray-white fleck-like opacities and progressive corneal haze involving the limbus.
Source: Dr N Venkatesh Prajna, Aravind Eye Hospital, Madurai, Tamil Nadu, India.

STROMAL DYSTROPHIES

Macular Corneal Dystrophy

Macular corneal dystrophy (MCD; MIM#217800) is an autosomal recessive stromal corneal dystrophy which results from mutations in the *carbohydrate sulfotransferase 6 (CHST6)* gene which is located on chromosome 16q22.[63] *CHST6* encodes an enzyme designated corneal N-acetylglucosamine-6-sulphotransferase (C-GlcNAc6ST)[64] which transfers sulfate to position 6 of GlcNAc residues required for the biosynthesis of the proteoglycan keratan sulfate (KS) in the cornea.[63] MCD is common in India[65], Saudi Arabia[66] and Iceland[67] but is found throughout the world. Onset is in childhood with the occurrence of central, superficial, gray-white fleck-like opacities which progress to involve the limbus (Fig. 28.5) and the entire corneal stroma down to Descemet's membrane which help to differentiate MCD from GCD. The fleck-like lesions also differentiate MCD from systemic mucopolysaccharidoses (MPS; e.g. Hurler, Hurler-Scheie and Maroteaux-Lamy MPS types) which also normally have earlier diffuse corneal opacification.[68] The corneal stroma also shows a progressive diffuse haze (Fig. 28.5) and the cornea is markedly thinner than normal.[69,70] In the later stages, Descemet's membrane and endothelium[71] becomes involved with a grayish appearance and guttata; endothelial decompensation is rare. Severe visual impairment occurs in the second and third decades and visual rehabilitation requires corneal transplantation: PK or DALK outcomes have been reported.[72-75] DALK surgery shows higher recurrence rates[73] and if the endothelium is involved or likely to be involved with disease progression this may not offer the most successful long-term outcomes.[74,75]

Histologically, gylcosaminoglycans (GAG) which stain with Alcian blue accumulate as intra- and extra-cellular deposits in the stroma with involvement of Descemet's membrane and the corneal endothelium; this is a unique feature in the stromal dystrophies. With electron microscopy, the keratocytes and endothelial cells contain intracytoplasmatic vesicles and there are abnomarlities in the extracellular matrix.[71] Although clinically indistinguishable MCD is divided into three variants or immune phenotypes: types I, IA, and II.[76] This classification is based on the reaction of the patient's serum and corneal tissue to an antibody which binds to sulfated residues of antigenic keratan sulfate (AgKS).[76] In MCD type I, antigenic KS (AgKS) is undetectable in both the serum and cornea and results from missense mutations, insertions, and nonsense mutations in CHST6.[65,67,77] In MCD type II, AgKS is present in normal or subnormal levels in serum and cornea and results from deletions and/or rearrangements in the upstream region as well as missense mutations in CHST6.[65,67,77] In MCD type IA, AgKS is absent in the serum and in most of the cornea but can be detected in the keratocytes.[66]

Schnyder Corneal Dystrophy

Schnyder corneal dystrophy (SCCD; MIM#121800) is an autosomal dominant stromal corneal dystrophy which results from mutations in the *UbiA prenyltransferase domain containing 1* (*UBIAD1*) gene which is located on chromosome 1p36.[78] SCD is characterized by bilateral corneal clouding, oval or ring opacities, arcus lipoides and/or crystalline deposits of cholesterol in the stroma which can be unilateral.[78,79] As only 50% of patients have corneal crystals,[79] the more common name of Schnyder crystalline corneal dystrophy was replaced in the IC3D classification: Schnyder corneal dystrophy (SCD).[2] The absence of corneal crystals can make diagnosis more challenging. If corneal crystals are present then there are a number of genetic, metabolic and drug deposits which should be considered as potential alternative diagnoses.[80] Both affected and unaffected family members with SCD can show a systemic hyperlipoproteinaemia.[80] SCD usually presents in the second and third decade and the corneal changes show an age-related phenotype. Younger patients have oval or ring-like central opacities and/or corneal crystals (Fig. 28.6), arcus lipoides develops in the second and third decade and in midlife the cornea shows a generalized haze which increasing glare and loss of visual function requiring subsequent penetrating keratoplasty.[79] Tissue available following keratoplasty for histological analysis must be handled to allow an assessment of corneal lipids: fresh tissue can be stained with Oil Red O and Sudan black for light microscopy. Histologically, there are intra- and extracellular deposits of phospholipid and cholesterol in the corneal stroma. Confocal microscopy can detect brightly refractile deposits in the anterior and middle corneal stroma.[81]

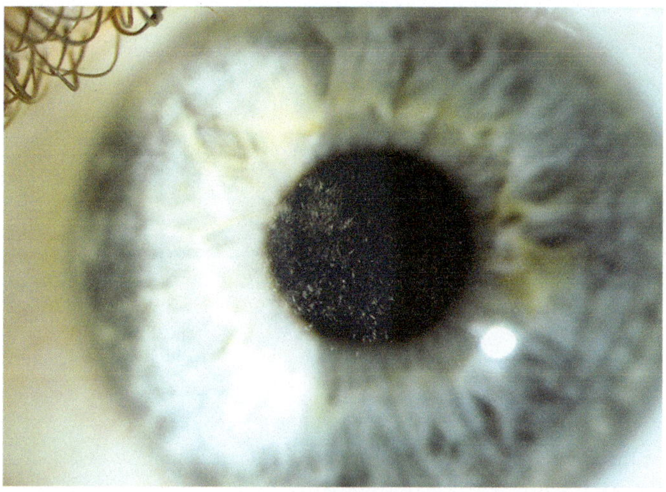

Fig. 28.6: Schnyder corneal dystrophy with crystalline deposits of cholesterol in the stroma.
Source: Dr B Steger, Department of Ophthalmology, Medical University of Innsbruck, Innsbruck, Austria.

Fleck Corneal Dystrophy

Fleck corneal dystrophy (FCD; MIM#121850) is an autosomal dominant condition which is also known as François-Neetens speckled corneal dystrophy.[82] Mutations have been reported in *PIP5K3* which is now called *PIKFYVE* (*phosphoinositide kinase FYVE finger- containing* gene).[83,84] FCD is a rare corneal dystrophy which can be present in the first decade and is asymptomatic and normally detected as a coincidental finding during a routine examination. It is characterized by nonprogressive, dis crete, small, translucent, gray-white flecks throughout the corneal stroma.[82,83,85] The corneal stroma between the flecks is typically clear and the corneal epithelium, Bowman's layer, Descemet's membrane and endothelium are normal. Retroillumination slit-lamp examination or confocal microscopy may aid diagnosis. Confocal microscopy shows bright reflective deposits in the keratocytes.[86] Histologically, the flecks are attributed to abnormal keratocytes swollen with complex lipids and glycosaminoglycans (GAGs).[87]

Congenital Stromal Corneal Dystrophy

Congenital stromal corneal dystrophy (CSCD; MIM# 610048) results from mutations in *decorin (DCN)*[88] and shows autosomal dominant inheritance.[88,89] Decorin is a small leucine-rich proteoglycan (SLRP) which has important roles in the extra-cellular matrix.[90] All reported mutations in decorin are predicted to cause a 33-amino-acid-deletion in the C-terminus of the decorin protein which impacts on collagen organization in the stroma with a resultant loss of transparency.[90] CSCD is a congenital dystrophy which results in diffuse, bilateral corneal clouding with an increase in corneal thickness.[88,89]

Posterior Amorphous Corneal Dystrophy

Posterior amorphous corneal dystrophy (PACD; MIM# 612868) is a rare, autosomal dominant disorder and clinically manifests with diffuse gray-white sheet-like opacities usually in the posterior lamella of the corneal stroma, decreased corneal thickness and flattening of the corneal curvature (<41 dioptres with consequent hyperopia).[91,92] The phenotype is variable and can include associated anomalies of the anterior segment: peripheral sclerocornea and abnormalities of the iris (pupillary remnants, correctopia, iridocorneal adhesions, iris atrophy and fine iris processes.[91-93] PACD was mapped to chromosome 12q21.33 and a hemizygous deletion in the PACD linkage interval containing 4 genes encoding keratocan, lumican, decorin and epiphycan.[92] These genes are small leucine-rich proteoglycans (SLRPs) and are involved in collagen fibrillogenesis and extracellular matrix assembly.[94]

ENDOTHELIAL DYSTROPHIES

Endothelial corneal dystrophies result from primary endothelial dysfunction and include Fuchs endothelial corneal dystrophy (FECD), posterior polymorphous corneal dystrophy (PPCD) and congenital hereditary endothelial dystrophy (CHED). These endothelial dystrophies are thought to result from defects in the terminal differentiation of neural crest.[95] As such, corneal endothelial dystrophies have many features in common including corneal decompensation, abnormal corneal endothelial cell morphology and the secretion of an abnormal collagenous layer in the posterior zone of Descemet's membrane.[96-98]

Fuchs' Endothelial Corneal Dystrophy

Fuchs' endothelial corneal dystrophy (FECD) is a genetically heterogenous, common, late-onset disorder of corneal endothelium. FECD is a leading cause of corneal transplantation and affects 4% of persons in the United States who are over the age of 40 years.[99,100] Early onset forms of FECD have been associated with mutations in *COL8A2* (FECD1; MIM#136800), *SLC4A11* (FECD4; MIM#613268), *ZEB1* (FECD6; MIM#613270) and *AGBL1* (FECD8; MIM#615523).[98,101] Other loci for late-onset FECD have been identified[101] and a genome-wide association study identified genetic variation near TGF4 on chromosome 18 which confer susceptibility to FECD.[102]

Fuchs endothelial corneal dystrophy passes through a series of clinical stages.[99] In stage 1 there is a gradual increase of central guttata with peripheral spread and confluence, giving rise to a beaten metal appearance. At this early stage, corneal guttae alone may result some aberration as light scattering. In stage 2 endothelial decompensation occurs, resulting in central stromal edema and epithelial edema develop when stromal thickness has increased by 30%. In stage 2 the patient usually complains of intermittent reduced vision from epithelial/stromal edema. Visual acuity worse in the morning because of increased stromal/ epithelial edema after overnight eyelid closure. Inducing hypertonicity of the tear film with sodium chloride 5% drops during the day and ointment night time to dehydrate early epithelial edema may help visual symptoms. In stage 3 (Fig. 28.7) bullae develop from the persistent epithelial edema which can result in pain, photophobia and epiphora due to epithelial erosions resulting from ruptured epithelial bullae. Bandage contact lenses may relieve discomfort but should be used with caution, due to the risk of microbial keratitis. Subsequently, a degenerative pannus is laid down on the Bowman's layer and the stroma gradually becomes opacified which results in progressive visual impairment. Specular microscopy and confocal microscopy are both able to image the changing in size (polymegethism), shape (pleomorphism or decreased hexagonality) and number of the corneal endothelial cells and the guttae.[103] Topographic corneal pachymetry can be used to follow these patients and corneal thickness is a surrogate marker of endothelial function. Histologically, Descemet's membrane becomes thickened (2–3 times size) and irregular; the size and shape of the corneal endothelial cells are altered as they are pushed between the developing guttae.[104]

Fuchs endothelial corneal dystrophy is a common indication for corneal transplantation to improve vision and comfort.[100] Endothelial keratoplasty (EK) is the treatment of choice as visual recovery is more rapid, surgically induced astigmatism (regular and irregular) is less and rates of transplant rejection are lower with EK compared to penetrating keratopasty.[100,105] EK procedures have evolved over the years and can be performed using different techniques.[105] Currently, the most common techniques are Descemet's stripping automated endothelial keratoplasty (DSAEK) and Descemet's membrane endothelial

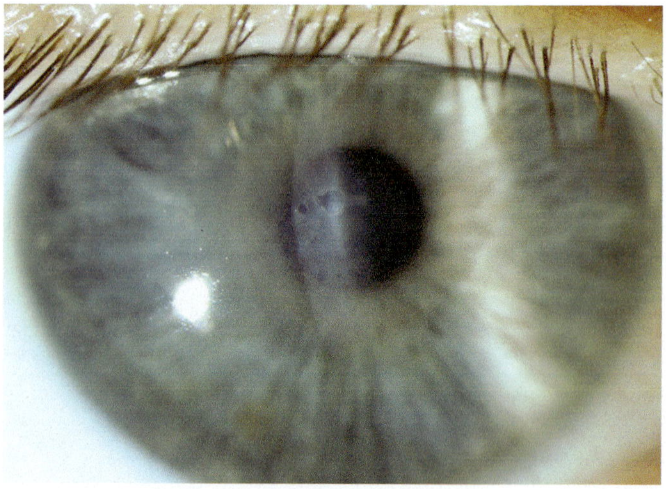

Fig. 28.7: Fuchs' endothelial corneal dystrophy with guttata giving rise to a *beaten-metal* appearance, stromal/epithelial edema with epithelial bullae.
Source: Dr B Steger, Department of Ophthalmology, Medical University of Innsbruck, Innsbruck, Austria.

keratoplasty (DMEK). Penetratring keratoplasty still has a place in cases with long-standing corneal edema and subsequent subepithelial fibrosis.

Posterior Polymorphous Corneal Dystrophy

Posterior polymorphous dystrophy (PPCD) is an autosomal dominant dystrophy with variable age of onset. It usually presents in adulthood, but can be severe and be present at birth.[106,107] The vast majority of patients are asymptomatic and stable, but some patients have a severe form of the disease complaining visual impairment secondary to corneal edema.[106,107] At slit-lamp opacities of Descemet's membrane and endothelium with peculiar morphologic features are detected. (Fig. 28.8). These opacities are often asymmetric and form distinct patterns: geographic gray opacities; vesicular lesions, either local or diffuse, often surrounded by gray circular opacity; parallel gray-white endothelial bands with white flaky material along the bands (railroad tracks), which may extend across the entire cornea. If severe corneal edema may develop necessitating corneal transplantation; PPCD can also recur after transplantation.[107,108] Peripheral iridocorneal adhesions occur in about 25% of cases and iris abnormalities can be present. There is an increased risk of glaucoma in PPCD as abnormal endothelial proliferate and obstruct the anterior chamber angle.[109]

Specular microscopy and confocal microscopy can image the peculiar morphological features of PPCD:

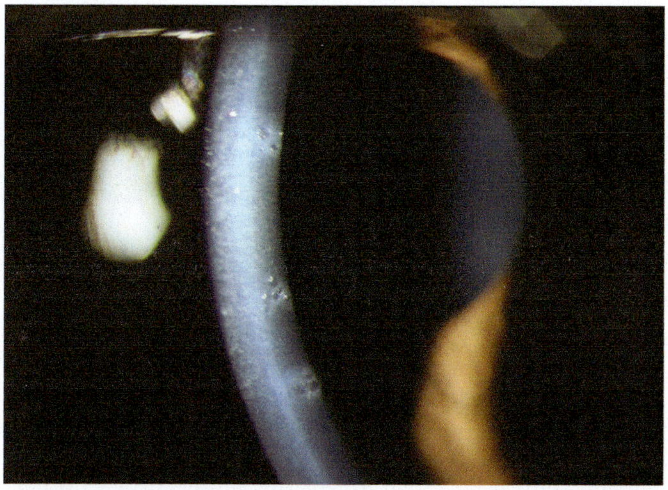

Fig. 28.8: Posterior polymorphous dystrophy with geographic gray opacities and vesicular lesions of Descemet's membrane and endothelium.
Source: Dr N Venkatesh Prajna, Aravind Eye Hospital, Madurai, Tamil Nadu, India.

vesicular lesions (rounded dark areas with some cell detail apparent in the middle giving a doughnut-like appearance), railroad track (band-like dark area with irregular edges enclosing some smaller lighter epithelial-like cells), including changes in the size (polymegethism), shape (pleomorphism or decreased hexagonality) and number of the corneal endothelial cells.[110] Pathologically, there is epithelialization of the endothelium.[111] With multilayering (2–5 cell layers) of endothelial cells with the presence of microvilli and desmosomes instead of tight junctions.[109,112] This layer stains positive for cytokeratins indicating the corneal endothelium has a epithelial phenotype. Transmission electron microscopy shows that the anterior banded portion of Descemet's membrane may be markedly abnormal, demonstrating alterations in thickness, a multilaminar appearance and occasional guttae.

Mutations in three genes result in PPCD: Noncoding mutations in the promoter of *OVOL2* (*ovo-like zinc finger 2*) result in PPCD1 (MIM#122000),[113] heterozygous mutation in the *COL8A2* gene result in PPCD2 (MIM#609140)[114] and heterozygous mutation in the *ZEB1 (zinc finger E-box binding homeobox 1)* gene result in PPCD3 (MIM# 609141).[115] Mutations in *ZEB1* causing PPCD are associated with extraocular features including hydroceles and abdominal and inguinal hernias.[115-117]

Congenital Hereditary Endothelial Dystrophy

Congenital hereditary endothelial dystrophy is an autosomal recessive severe dystrophy.[97] The IC3D classification in 2008 divided CHED into two types: autosomal dominant (CHED1) and autosomal recessive (CHED2).[1] CHED1 has been shown to be allelic with PPCD1 and both result from noncoding mutations in the promoter of *OVOL2* and as such CHED1 forms part of the PPCD spectrum and is not a separate entity,[113] as allelic conditions and show that CHED1 represents the extreme of what can be considered a disease spectrum. AD CHED (CHED1), does not form part of the current IC3D classification and has been eliminated.[2] AR CHED, which was previously called CHED2, is now the sole type of this endothelial disorder and is simply termed CHED.[2] CHED (MIM#217700) results from mutations homozygous or compound heterozygous mutation in the solute carrier family 4 (*sodium borate cotransporter*), *member 11 (SLC4A11)* gene.[118] CHED with sensorineural deafness also results from *SLC4A11* mutations and is termed Harboyan Syndrome.[119]

CHED presents with a ground glass, bluish-white opaque cornea due to diffuse corneal edema (Fig. 28.9).[97] The anterior segmented intraocular pressure is normal. The clinicial course in CHED is usually stationary or shows little progression.[97] Corneal pachymetry and microscopy reveal thickening of the cornea two or three times the normal corneal thickness and endothelial cell count reduced about 10-fold compared with age-matched controls.[120,121] Histologically, there is diffuse epithelial and stromal edema, defects in the Bowman's layer, a degenerated corneal endothelium with multinucleated sparse and atrophic endothelial cells and a thickened laminated Descemet's membrane.[121] DSAEK can be used successfully in the treatment of CHED in children as an alternative to PK.[122,123] DSAEK allows for a more rapid visual rehabilitation of patients and fewer postoperative complications.[123] Outcomes are limited by amblyopia and high risk of graft failure in this population.[124]

X-linked endothelial corneal dystrophy: X-linked endothelial corneal dystrophy (XECD) results in congenital corneal clouding and moon crater-like endothelial changes showing X-linked inheritance and mapped to Xq25.[125] Male patients present with congenital corneal clouding ranging from diffuse haze to ground-glass, milky appearance with moon crater-like endothelial changes and and nystagmus.[125] A subepithelial band keratopathy secondary to endothelial changes can develop. Female patients are asymptomatic with nonprogressive lesions. Histologically, there are atypical endothelial cells or cell loss and irregular thickening of Descemet's membrane with small excavations and pits. There is also irregular thinning of the corneal epithelium and Bowman's layer with irregularly arranged collagen lamellae in the anterior stroma.[125]

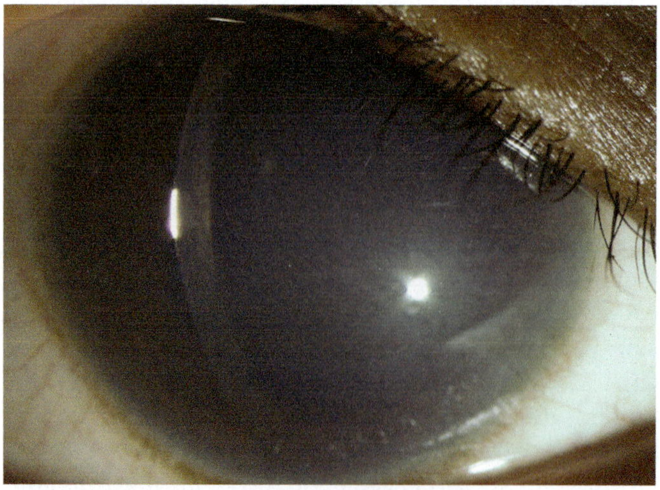

Fig. 28.9: Congenital hereditary endothelial dystrophy producing a ground glass, bluish-white opaque cornea due to diffuse corneal edema.
Source: Dr N Venkatesh Prajna, Aravind Eye Hospital, Madurai, Tamil Nadu, India.

CONCLUSION

Understanding the clinical, pathological and genetic basis of corneal dystrophies can be challenging. The ICD3 classification is a significant aid to the clinician in interpreting, understanding and managing these conditions.[1,2] Objective assessment is required to understand the classification of corneal dystrophies and the level of evidence required to definitively support the term.[2] With advances in genetic sequencing the molecular genetics of corneal dystrophies is rapidly evolving. There is also the emergence of new gene-based therapies.[21,62] and gene editing techniques,[23] which might prevent visual impairment or restore visual function in inherited corneal disease.

REFERENCES

1. Weiss JS, Moller HU, Lisch W, et al. The IC3D classification of the corneal dystrophies. Cornea. 2008;27(Suppl 2):S-83.
2. Weiss JS, Møller HU, Aldave AJ, et al. IC3D Classification of Corneal Dystrophies—Edition 2. Cornea. 2015;34(2): 117-59.
3. Stone EM, Mathers WD, Rosenwasser GO, et al. Three autosomal dominant corneal dystrophies map to chromosome 5q. Nat Genet. 1994;6(1):47-51.
4. Munier FL, Korvatska E, Djemaï A, et al. Kerato-epithelin mutations in four 5q31-linked corneal dystrophies. Nat Genet. 1997;15(3):247-51.
5. Irvine AD, Corden LD, Swensson O, et al. Mutations in cornea-specific keratin K3 or K12 genes cause Meesmann's corneal dystrophy. Nat Genet. 1997;16(2):184-7.
6. Munier FL, Frueh BE, Othenin-Girard P, et al. BIGH3 mutation spectrum in corneal dystrophies. Invest Ophthalmol Vis Sci. 2002;43(4):949-54.
7. Korvatska E, Munier FLL, Djemai A, et al. Mutation hot spots in 5q31-linked corneal dystrophies. Am J Hum Genet. 1998;62(2):320-4.
8. Boutboul S, Black GCM, Moore JE, et al. A subset of patients with epithelial basement membrane corneal dystrophy have mutations in *TGFβI/BIGH3*. Hum Mutat. 2006;27(6):553-7.
9. Laibson PR, Krachmer JH. Familial occurrence of dot (microcystic), map, fingerprint dystrophy of the cornea. Invest Ophthalmol. 1975;14(5):397-9.
10. Vo RC, Chen JL, Sanchez PJ, et al. Long-Term Outcomes of Epithelial Debridement and Diamond Burr Polishing for Corneal Epithelial Irregularity and Recurrent Corneal Erosion. Cornea. 2015;34(10):1259-65.
11. Rodrigues MM, Fine BS, Laibson PR, et al. Disorders of the corneal epithelium. A clinicopathologic study of dot,

geographic, and fingerprint patterns. Arch Ophthalmol. 1974;92(6):475-82.
12. Ehlers N, Møller HU. Pathology and pathomechanisms of epithelial microcystic and basement membrane abnormalities of the cornea. Acta Ophthalmol. 1988;66(3):318-26.
13. Jonsson F, Byström B, Davidson AE, et al. Mutations in Collagen, Type XVII, Alpha 1 (*COL17A1*) Cause Epithelial Recurrent Erosion Dystrophy (ERED). Hum Mutat. 2015; 36(4):463-73.
14. Oliver VF, van Bysterveldt KA, Cadzow M, et al. A *COL17A1* Splice-Altering Mutation Is Prevalent in Inherited Recurrent Corneal Erosions. Ophthalmology. 2016;123(4):709-22.
15. Allen EHA, Courtney DG, Atkinson SD, et al. Keratin 12 missense mutation induces the unfolded protein response and apoptosis in Meesmann epithelial corneal dystrophy. Hum Mol Genet. 2016;25(6):1176-91.
16. Javadi MA, Rezaei-Kanavi M, Javadi A, et al. Meesmann corneal dystrophy; a clinico-pathologic, ultrastructural and confocal scan report. J Ophthalmic Vis Res. 2010;5(2): 122-26.
17. Patel DV, Grupcheva CN, McGhee CNJ. Imaging the microstructural abnormalities of meesmann corneal dystrophy by in vivo confocal microscopy. Cornea. 2005;24(6):669-73.
18. Ehlers N, Hjortdal J, Nielsen K, et al. Phenotypic variability in Meesmann's dystrophy: clinical review of the literature and presentation of a family genetically identical to the original family. Acta Ophthalmol. 2008;86(1):40-4.
19. Szaflik JP, Oldak M, Maksym RB, et al. Genetics of Meesmann corneal dystrophy: a novel mutation in the keratin 3 gene in an asymptomatic family suggests genotype-phenotype correlation. Mol Vis. 2008;14:1713-8.
20. Jalbert I, Stapleton F. Management of Symptomatic Meesmann Dystrophy. Optom Vis Sci. 2009;86(10):E1202-6.
21. Allen EHA, Atkinson SD, Liao H, et al. Allele-Specific siRNA Silencing for the Common Keratin 12 Founder Mutation in Meesmann Epithelial Corneal Dystrophy. Investig Opthalmology Vis Sci. 2013;54(1):494-502.
22. Courtney DG, Atkinson SD, Allen EH, et al. siRNA Silencing of the Mutant Keratin 12 Allele in Corneal Limbal Epithelial Cells Grown From Patients With Meesmann's Epithelial Corneal Dystrophy. Investig Opthalmology Vis Sci. 2014;55(5):3352-60.
23. Courtney DG, Moore JE, Atkinson SD, et al. CRISPR/Cas9 DNA cleavage at SNP-derived PAM enables both in vitro and in vivo KRT12 mutation-specific targeting. Gene Ther. 2016;23(1):108-12.
24. Lisch W, Steuhl KP, Lisch C, et al. A new, band-shaped and whorled microcystic dystrophy of the corneal epithelium. Am J Ophthalmol. 1992;114(1):35-44.
25. Lisch W, Büttner A, Oeffner F, et al. Lisch corneal dystrophy is genetically distinct from Meesmann corneal dystrophy and maps to xp22.3. Am J Ophthalmol. 2000;130(4):461-8.
26. Lisch W, Wasielica-Poslednik J, Lisch C, et al. Contact Lens-Induced Regression of Lisch Epithelial Corneal Dystrophy. Cornea. 2010;29(3):342-5.
27. Wessel MM, Sarkar JS, Jakobiec FA, et al. Treatment of Lisch Corneal Dystrophy With Photorefractive Keratectomy and Mitomycin C. Cornea. 2011;30(4):481-5.
28. Nakamura Y, Tsujikawa M, Kurahashi H, et al. Identification of the gene responsible for gelatinous drop-like corneal dystrophy. Nat Genet. 1999;21(4):420-3.
29. Ren Z, Lin PY, Klintworth GK, et al. Allelic and locus heterogeneity in autosomal recessive gelatinous drop-like corneal dystrophy. Hum Genet. 2002;110(6):568-77.
30. Tsujikawa M. Gelatinous Drop-like corneal dystrophy. Cornea. 2012;31:S37-40.
31. Kinoshita S, Nishida K, Dota A, et al. Epithelial barrier function and ultrastructure of gelatinous drop-like corneal dystrophy. Cornea. 2000;19(4):551-5.
32. Kawasaki S, Kinoshita S. Clinical and basic aspects of gelatinous drop-like corneal dystrophy. Dev Ophthalmol. 2011;48:97-115.
33. Kim JE, Park RW, Choi JY, et al. Molecular properties of wild-type and mutant betaIG-H3 proteins. Invest Ophthalmol Vis Sci. 2002;43(3):656-61.
34. Lakshminarayanan R, Chaurasia SS, Anandalakshmi V, et al. Clinical and Genetic Aspects of the *TGFβI*-associated Corneal Dystrophies. Ocul Surf. 2014;12(4):234-51.
35. Lakshminarayanan R, Chaurasia SS, Murugan E, et al. Biochemical Properties and Aggregation Propensity of Transforming Growth Factor-Induced Protein (*TGFβIp*) and the Amyloid Forming Mutants. Ocul Surf. 2015;13(1): 9-25.
36. Yang J, Han X, Huang D, et al. Analysis of *TGFβI* gene mutations in Chinese patients with corneal dystrophies and review of the literature. Mol Vis. 2010;16:1186-93.
37. Qiu WY, Zheng LB, Pan F, et al. New histopathologic and ultrastructural findings in Reis-Bücklers corneal dystrophy caused by the Arg124Leu mutation of *TGFβI* gene. BMC Ophthalmol. 2016;16(1):158.
38. Lin ZN, Chen J, Cui HP. Characteristics of corneal dystrophies: a review from clinical, histological and genetic perspectives. Int J Ophthalmol. 2016;9(6):904-13.
39. Liang Q, Pan Z, Sun X, et al. Reis-Bücklers corneal dystrophy: a reappraisal using in vivo and ex vivo imaging techniques. Ophthalmic Res. 2014;51(4):187-95.
40. Kobayashi A, Sugiyama K. In Vivo Laser Confocal Microscopy Findings for Bowman's Layer Dystrophies (Thiel-Behnke and Reis-Bücklers Corneal Dystrophies). Ophthalmology. 2007;114(1):69-75.
41. Thiel HJ, Behnke H. A hitherto unknown subepithelial hereditary corneal dystrophy. Klin Monbl Augenheilkd. 1967;150(6):862-74.
42. Küchle M, Green WR, Völcker HE, et al. Reevaluation of corneal dystrophies of Bowman's layer and the anterior stroma (Reis-Bücklers and Thiel-Behnke types): a light and electron microscopic study of eight corneas and a review of the literature. Cornea. 1995;14(4):333-54.
43. Vajzovic LM, Karp CL, Haft P, et al. Ultra High-Resolution Anterior Segment Optical Coherence Tomography in the Evaluation of Anterior Corneal Dystrophies and Degenerations. Ophthalmology. 2011;118(7):1291-6.

44. Lohse E, Stock EL, Jones JC, et al. Reis-Bücklers' corneal dystrophy. Immunofluorescent and electron microscopic studies. Cornea. 1989;8(3):200-9.
45. Aldave AJ, Rayner SA, Kim BT, et al. Unilateral lattice corneal dystrophy associated with the novel His572del mutation in the TGFβI gene. Mol Vis. 2006;12:142-6.
46. Chiou AG, Beuerman RW, Kaufman SC, et al. Confocal microscopy in lattice corneal dystrophy. Graefes Arch Clin Exp Ophthalmol. 1999;237(8):697-701.
47. Maury CPJ, Kere J, Tolvanen R,et al. Finnish hereditary amyloidosis is caused by a single nucleotide substitution in the gelsolin gene. FEBS Lett. 1990;276(1-2):75-7.
48. Dighiero P, Niel F, Ellies P, et al. Histologic phenotype-genotype correlation of corneal dystrophies associated with eight distinct mutations in the *TGFβI* gene. Ophthalmology. 2001;108(4):818-23.
49. Han KE, Choi S, Kim T, et al. Pathogenesis and treatments of *TGFβI* corneal dystrophies. Prog Retin Eye Res. 2016;50: 67-88.
50. Okada M, Yamamoto S, Watanabe H, et al. Granular corneal dystrophy with homozygous mutations in the kerato-epithelin gene. Am J Ophthalmol. 1998;126(2):169-76.
51. Akiya S, Brown SI. Granular dystrophy of the cornea. Characteristic electron microscopic lesion. Arch Ophthalmol. 1970;84(2):179-92.
52. Folberg R, Alfonso E, Croxatto JO, et al. Clinically Atypical Granular Corneal Dystrophy with Pathologic Features of Lattice-like Amyloid Deposits. Ophthalmology. 1988;95(1):46-51.
53. Holland EJ, Daya SM, Stone EM, et al. Avellino Corneal Dystrophy. Ophthalmology. 1992;99(10):1564-8.
54. Mashima Y, Konishi M, Nakamura Y, et al. Severe form of juvenile corneal stromal dystrophy with homozygous R124H mutation in the keratoepithelin gene in five Japanese patients. Br J Ophthalmol. 1998;82(11):1280-4.
55. Han KE, Kim TL, Chung WS, et al. Clinical findings and treatments of granular corneal dystrophy type 2 (avellino corneal dystrophy): a review of the literature. Eye Contact Lens. 2010;36(5):296-9.
56. Woreta FA, Davis GW, Bower KS. LASIK and surface ablation in corneal dystrophies. Surv Ophthalmol. 2015;60(2): 115-22.
57. Lee ES, Kim EK. Surgical do's and don'ts of corneal dystrophies. Curr Opin Ophthalmol. 2003;14(4):186-91.
58. Steger B, Romano V, Biddolph S, et al. Femtosecond Laser-Assisted Lamellar Keratectomy for Corneal Opacities Secondary to Anterior Corneal Dystrophies. Cornea. 2016;35(1):6-13.
59. Kymionis GD, Mikropoulos DG, Portaliou DM, et al. New Perspectives on Lamellar Keratoplasty. Adv Ther. 2014;31(5):494-511.
60. Choi SI, Kim BY, Dadakhujaev S, et al. Inhibition of TGFβIp expression by lithium: implications for TGFβI-linked corneal dystrophy therapy. Invest Ophthalmol Vis Sci. 2011;52(6):3293-300.
61. Choi SI, Kim BY, Dadakhujaev S, et al. Impaired autophagy and delayed autophagic clearance of transforming growth factor β-induced protein (*TGFβI*) in granular corneal dystrophy type 2. Autophagy. 2012;8(12):1782-97.
62. Courtney DG, Atkinson SD, Moore JE, et al. Development of allele-specific gene-silencing siRNAs for *TGFβI* Arg124Cys in lattice corneal dystrophy type I. Invest Ophthalmol Vis Sci. 2014;55(2):977-85.
63. Akama TO, Nishida K, Nakayama J, et al. Macular corneal dystrophy type I and type II are caused by distinct mutations in a new sulphotransferase gene. Nat Genet. 2000;26(2): 237-41.
64. Musselmann K, Hassell JR. Focus on Molecules: *CHST6* (carbohydrate sulfotransferase 6; corneal N-acetylglucosamine-6-sulfotransferase). Exp Eye Res. 2006;83(4):707-8.
65. Sultana A, Sridhar MS, Jagannathan A, et al. Novel mutations of the carbohydrate sulfotransferase-6 (*CHST6*) gene causing macular corneal dystrophy in India. Mol Vis. 2003;9:730-4.
66. Klintworth GK, Oshima E, al-Rajhi A, et al. Macular corneal dystrophy in Saudi Arabia: a study of 56 cases and recognition of a new immunophenotype. Am J Ophthalmol. 1997;124(1):9-18.
67. Liu N-P, Smith CF, Bowling BL, et al. Macular corneal dystrophy types I and II are caused by distinct mutations in the *CHST6* gene in Iceland. Mol Vis. 2006;12:1148-52.
68. Fahnehjelm KT, Ashworth JL, Pitz S, et al. Clinical guidelines for diagnosing and managing ocular manifestations in children with mucopolysaccharidosis. Acta Ophthalmol. 2012;90(7):595-602.
69. Koçluk Y, Yalnız-Akkaya Z, Burcu A, et al. Topography Analysis of Stromal Corneal Dystrophies. Pak J Med Sci. 2014;31(1):116-20.
70. Nowinska AK, Teper SJ, Janiszewska DA, et al. Comparative Study of Anterior Eye Segment Measurements with Spectral Swept-Source and Time-Domain Optical Coherence Tomography in Eyes with Corneal Dystrophies. Biomed Res Int. 2015;2015:1-10.
71. Micali A, Pisani A, Puzzolo D, et al. Macular Corneal Dystrophy. Ophthalmology. 2014;121(6):1164-73.
72. Al-Swailem SA, Al-Rajhi AA, Wagoner MD. Penetrating keratoplasty for macular corneal dystrophy. Ophthalmology. 2005;112(2):220-4.
73. Cheng J, Qi X, Zhao J, et al. Comparison of Penetrating Keratoplasty and Deep Lamellar Keratoplasty for Macular Corneal Dystrophy and Risk Factors of Recurrence. Ophthalmology. 2013;120(1):34-9.
74. Sogutlu Sarı E, Kubaloglu A, Unal M, et al. Deep Anterior Lamellar Keratoplasty versus Penetrating Keratoplasty for Macular Corneal Dystrophy: A Randomized Trial. Am J Ophthalmol. 2013;156(2):267-74.
75. Kawashima M, Kawakita T, Den S, et al. Comparison of Deep Lamellar Keratoplasty and Penetrating Keratoplasty for Lattice and Macular Corneal Dystrophies. Am J Ophthalmol. 2006;142(2):304-9.
76. Jonasson F, Oshima E, Thonar EJ, et al. Macular corneal dystrophy in Iceland. A clinical, genealogic, and immunohistochemical study of 28 patients. Ophthalmology. 1996;103(7):1111-7.

77. Klintworth GK, Smith CF, Bowling BL. *CHST6* mutations in North American subjects with macular corneal dystrophy: a comprehensive molecular genetic review. Mol Vis. 2006;12:159-76.
78. Orr A, Dubé MP, Marcadier J, et al. Mutations in the *UBIAD1* gene, encoding a potential prenyltransferase, are causal for Schnyder crystalline corneal dystrophy. PLoS One. 2007;2(8):e685.
79. Weiss JS. Schnyder corneal dystrophy. Curr Opin Ophthalmol. 2009;20(4):292-8.
80. Weiss JS, Khemichian AJ. Differential Diagnosis of Schnyder Corneal Dystrophy. Dev Ophthalmol. 2011:67-96.
81. Ciancaglini M, Carpineto P, Doronzo E, et al. Morphological evaluation of Schnyder's central crystalline dystrophy by confocal microscopy before and after phototherapeutic keratectomy. J Cataract Refract Surg. 2001;27(11):1892-5.
82. Francois J, Neetens A. New hereditary-familial dystrophy of the corneal parenchyma (spotted hereditary dystrophy). Bull Soc Belge Ophtalmol. 1957;114:641-6.
83. Li S, Tiab L, Jiao X, et al. Mutations in PIP5K3 Are Associated with François-Neetens Mouchetée Fleck Corneal Dystrophy. Am J Hum Genet. 2005;77(1):54-63.
84. Kotoulas A, Kokotas H, Kopsidas K, et al. A novel PIKFYVE mutation in fleck corneal dystrophy. Mol Vis. 2011;17:2776-81.
85. Patten JT, Hyndiuk RA, Donaldson DD, et al. Fleck (Mouchetée) dystrophy of the cornea. Ann Ophthalmol. 1976;8(1):25-32.
86. Frueh BE, Böhnke M. In vivo confocal microscopy of fleck dystrophy. Cornea. 1999;18(6):658-60.
87. Nicholson DH, Green WR, Cross HE, et al. A clinical and histopathological study of François-Neetens speckled corneal dystrophy. Am J Ophthalmol. 1977;83(4):554-60.
88. Bredrup C, Knappskog PM, Majewski J, et al. Congenital Stromal Dystrophy of the Cornea Caused by a Mutation in the Decorin Gene. Investig Opthalmology Vis Sci. 2005;46(2):420.
89. Rødahl E, Knappskog PM, Bredrup C, et al. Congenital Stromal Corneal Dystrophy; 1993.
90. Kamma-Lorger CS, Pinali C, Martínez JC, et al. Role of Decorin Core Protein in Collagen Organisation in Congenital Stromal Corneal Dystrophy (CSCD). PLoS One. 2016;11(2):e0147948.
91. Carpel EF, Sigelman RJ, Doughman DJ. Posterior amorphous corneal dystrophy. Am J Ophthalmol. 1977;83(5):629-32.
92. Kim MJ, Frausto RF, Rosenwasser GOD, et al. Posterior Amorphous Corneal Dystrophy Is Associated with a Deletion of Small Leucine-rich Proteoglycans on Chromosome 12. Janecke AR, (Ed) PLoS One. 2014;9(4):e95037.
93. Dunn SP, Krachmer JH, Ching SS. New findings in posterior amorphous corneal dystrophy. Arch Ophthalmol. 1984;102(2):236-9.
94. Massoudi D, Malecaze F, Galiacy SD. Collagens and proteoglycans of the cornea: importance in transparency and visual disorders. Cell Tissue Res. 2016;363(2):337-49.
95. Bahn CF, Falls HF, Varley GA, et al. Classification of corneal endothelial disorders based on neural crest origin. Ophthalmology. 1984;91(6):558-63.
96. Zhang J, Patel DV. The pathophysiology of Fuchs' endothelial dystrophy – A review of molecular and cellular insights. Exp Eye Res. 2015;130:97-105.
97. Aldave AJ, Han J, Frausto RF. Genetics of the corneal endothelial dystrophies: an evidence-based review. Clin Genet. 2013;84(2):109-19.
98. Eghrari AO, Riazuddin SA, Gottsch JD. Fuchs Corneal Dystrophy. Prog Mol Biol and Transl Sci. 2015:79-97.
99. Elhalis H, Azizi B, Jurkunas U V. Fuchs endothelial corneal dystrophy. Ocul Surf. 2010;8(4):173-84.
100. Jun A, Vedana G, Villarreal G Jr. Fuchs endothelial corneal dystrophy: current perspectives. Clin Ophthalmol. 2016:321.
101. Schmedt T, Silva MM, Ziaei A, et al. Molecular bases of corneal endothelial dystrophies. Exp Eye Res. 2012;95(1):24-34.
102. Brown WL, Branham K, Chen W, et al. E2-2 Protein and Fuchs's Corneal Dystrophy. 2010,363(11):1016-24.
103. Huang J, Maram J, Tepelus TC, et al. Comparison of Noncontact Specular and Confocal Microscopy for Evaluation of Corneal Endothelium. Eye Contact Lens. 2017:1.
104. Adamis AP, Filatov V, Tripathi BJ, et al. Fuchs' endothelial dystrophy of the cornea. Surv Ophthalmol. 38(2):149-68.
105. Bruinsma M, Tong CM, Melles GR. What does the future hold for the treatment of Fuchs endothelial dystrophy; will "keratoplasty" still be a valid procedure? Eye (Lond). 2013;27(10):1115-22.
106. Ahn YJ, Choi S I, Yum HR, et al. Clinical Features in Children with Posterior Polymorphous Corneal Dystrophy. Optom Vis Sci. 2017;94(4):476-81.
107. Chaurasia S, Mittal R, Bichappa G, et al. Clinical characterization of posterior polymorphous corneal dystrophy in patients of Indian ethnicity. Int Ophthalmol. 2017;37(4):945-52.
108. Boruchoff SA, Weiner MJ, Albert DM. Recurrence of posterior polymorphous corneal dystrophy after penetrating keratoplasty. Am J Ophthalmol. 1990;109(3):323-8.
109. Rodrigues MM, Phelps CD, Krachmer JH, et al. Glaucoma due to endothelialization of the anterior chamber angle. A comparison of posterior polymorphous dystrophy of the cornea and Chandler's syndrome. Arch Ophthalmol. 1980;98(4):688-96.
110. Vincent AL, Niederer RL, Richards A, et al. Phenotypic characterisation and ZEB1 mutational analysis in posterior polymorphous corneal dystrophy in a New Zealand population. Mol Vis. 2009;15:2544-53.
111. Ross JR, Foulks GN, Sanfilippo FP, et al. Immunohistochemical analysis of the pathogenesis of posterior polymorphous dystrophy. Arch Ophthalmol. 1995;113(3):340-5.
112. Krachmer JH. Posterior polymorphous corneal dystrophy: a disease characterized by epithelial-like endothelial cells which influence management and prognosis. Trans Am Ophthalmol Soc. 1985;83:413-75.
113. Davidson AE, Liskova P, Evans CJ, et al. Autosomal-Dominant Corneal Endothelial Dystrophies *CHED1* and *PPCD1* Are Allelic Disorders Caused by Non-coding Mutations in the Promoter of *OVOL2*. Am J Hum Genet. 2016;98(1):75-89.

114. Biswas S, Munier FL, Yardley J, et al. Missense mutations in *COL8A2*, the gene encoding the α 2 chain of type VIII collagen, cause two forms of corneal endothelial dystrophy. Hum Mol Genet. 2001;10(21):2415-23.
115. Krafchak CM, Pawar H, Moroi SE, et al. Mutations in *TCF8* cause posterior polymorphous corneal dystrophy and ectopic expression of *COL4A3* by corneal endothelial cells. Am J Hum Genet. 2005;77(5):694-708.
116. Aldave AJ, Yellore VS, Yu F, et al. Posterior polymorphous corneal dystrophy is associated with *TCF8* gene mutations and abdominal hernia. Am J Med Genet A. 2007;143A(21):2549-56.
117. Nguyen DQ, Hosseini M, Billingsley G, et al. Clinical phenotype of posterior polymorphous corneal dystrophy in a family with a novel *ZEB1* mutation. Acta Ophthalmol. 2010;88(6):695-9.
118. Vithana EN, Morgan P, Sundaresan P, et al. Mutations in sodium-borate cotransporter SLC4A11 cause recessive congenital hereditary endothelial dystrophy (*CHED2*). Nat Genet. 2006;38(7):755-7.
119. Desir J, Moya G, Reish O, et al. Borate transporter SLC4A11 mutations cause both Harboyan syndrome and non-syndromic corneal endothelial dystrophy. J Med Genet. 2007;44(5):322-6.
120. Kirkness CM. The corneal endothelial dystrophies. Ann Acad Med Singapore. 1989;18(2):158-64.
121. Ehlers N, Módis L, Møller-Pedersen T. A morphological and functional study of Congenital Hereditary Endothelial Dystrophy. Acta Ophthalmol Scand. 1998;76(3):314-8.
122. Pineda R 2nd, Jain V, Shome D, et al. Descemet's stripping endothelial keratoplasty: is it an option for congenital hereditary endothelial dystrophy? Int Ophthalmol. 2010;30(3):307-10.
123. Ashar JN, Madhavi Latha K, Vaddavalli PK. Descemet's stripping endothelial keratoplasty (DSEK) for children with congenital hereditary endothelial dystrophy: surgical challenges and 1-year outcomes. Graefe's Arch Clin Exp Ophthalmol. 2012;250(9):1341-5.
124. AlArrayedh H, Collum L, Murphy CC. Outcomes of penetrating keratoplasty in congenital hereditary endothelial dystrophy. Br J Ophthalmol. 2017.
125. Schmid E, Lisch W, Philipp W, et al. A New, X-linked Endothelial Corneal Dystrophy. Am J Ophthalmol. 2006; 141(3):478-87.

Chapter 29 Eye Banking

Maria A Woodward, Nithya Vijayakumar

INTRODUCTION

Eye banks are organizations that recover, store, process, and distribute donations from deceased donors to transplant recipients. The most common indication is use of corneal tissue for corneal transplantation. This process allows recipient patients to have sight-restoring surgeries. Globally, there are more than 742 eye banks in 74 countries, and recent estimates indicated that 184,000 corneal transplants occur each year.[1] Eye banks have altered the way that corneal surgeries are performed. Since eye banks are dedicated, regulated institutions, eye banks can set standards for optimal recovery procedures, promote awareness of eye donation, and work closely with hospitals and donor families through the consent and recovery process. Eye banks can store corneal tissue, increasing available tissue supply. Eye banking allows corneal transplantation to become a scheduled procedure, no longer limited as much by tissue scarcity or its emergent nature. Figure 29.1 illustrates the standard steps taken by eye banks when handling ocular tissue. In recent years, improved technology has allowed eye banks to process corneal tissue for partial transplantation, further aiding corneal surgeons and recipient patients.

EYE BANK HISTORY

In 1905, Austrian physician Dr Eduard Zirm performed the first successful corneal transplant. The operation involved removing both corneas from a living boy who had suffered untreatable ocular trauma. The corneas were transplanted to the eyes of a 45-year-old farmer. Although the right eye graft developed complications, the left eye graft was successful.[2-4] The technique for corneal transplants (whole and partial) became more sophisticated with time and improving technology. However, tissue could not be stored, and each corneal surgery was emergent. Corneal tissue needed to be used as soon as it became available, much like organ transplants today.

Dr R Townley Paton created the first eye bank in the United States in 1944. The eye bank was called the Eye Bank for Sight Restoration.[4] Since then, the Lions Club has also played a large role in advocating for and founding eye banks. The Lions Club is an International Service Organization, challenged by Helen Keller in 1925 to "be the knights of the blind in the crusade against darkness".[5] They have established numerous eye banks internationally, and engage with preventing blindness more broadly.[5] At the time, eye banks focused on increasing the donor pool by raising awareness and working with hospitals. In the coming decades, various means of preserving corneal tissue postmortem were developed, including M-K medium and cryopreservation.[6,7] As these methods were tested and put to use, eye banks were able to store corneal tissue, and increase the pool of eligible tissue for surgery. In the decades since the formation of eye banks, regional and national associations have been created by

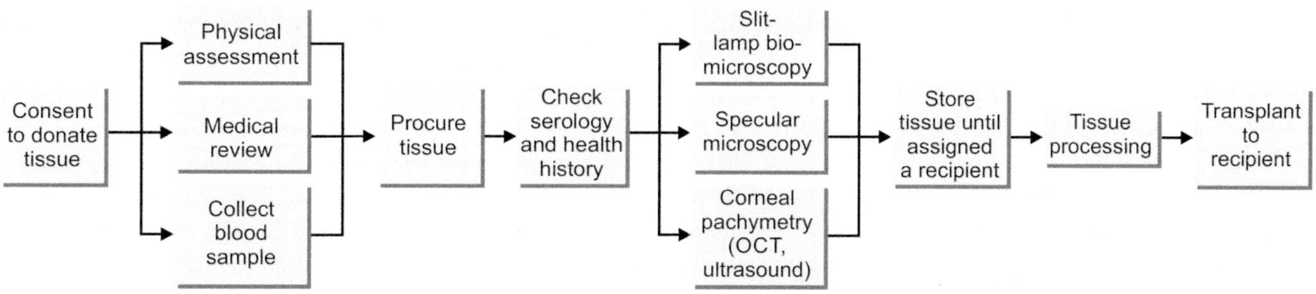

Fig. 29.1: The steps in which ocular tissue is handled by the eye bank, from consent and procurement to transplant. (OCT: Optical coherence tomography)

ophthalmologists and eye bank specialists, to ensure the safety and quality of corneal tissue.

EYE BANK STRUCTURE AND FUNCTION

Eye banks and their affiliated associations evolved from the ground up beginning in the 1940s. As the number of eye banks increased, the American Academy of Ophthalmology (AAO) felt a need to standardize practice across eye banks, leading to creation of the EBAA in 1961.[4,8] Eye banks across the world have done similarly, leading to the creation of several large regional associations, including the EBAA, European Eye Bank Association, Association of Eye Banks of Asia, Eye Bank Association of Australia and New Zealand, Pan American Association of Eye Banks, and the Eye Bank Association of India. Each of these associations works independently within their region, providing regulatory recommendations, guidelines and practice standards, and advocating for eye banks and eye donations. Many of these associations work with national or regional governments to create laws and regulations about tissue eligibility, handling, and procedures for safety and quality.[9-11]

Individual eye banks most often serve their own regions, but some do share and collaborate with other eye banks. Eye banks' main purposes are to recover and screen qualifying tissues, process procured corneal tissue, store donor ocular tissue, send qualified ocular tissue to surgeons, and advocate for tissue and eye donation. Many eye banks are either part of a hospital, or collaborate closely with hospitals. All are staffed with medical physician directors. In addition to managing donor corneal tissue for transplantation, eye banks may be involved in processing tissue not eligible for surgery and using this tissue for research or educational purposes at the discretion of eye bank leadership.[12]

The roles of staff in each eye banks varies from region to region based on local regulatory bodies, but share some basic commonalities. As per the EBAA, each eye bank has a director who oversees the day-to-day operations and determines the responsibilities and scope of the eye bank. The director handles administrative tasks and ensures compliance of the eye bank with the rules and regulations prescribed by its governing body or board of directors. The director is able to delegate some of these responsibilities to appropriate staff. Each eye bank also has a medical director, who is an ophthalmologist with training and cornea expertise. The medical director is tasked with overseeing and managing the medical procedures and policies performed by an eye bank, quality assurance, guiding training for technical staff in relevant procedures, and supervising these procedures periodically to ensure best practices.[12,13]

The medical director may assign and train a staff trainer, who can then train other technicians in the eye bank to perform medical procedures such as in situ corneoscleral excision from the whole eye, manual dissection, or posterior lamellar processing.[12]

In the United States, the eye bank must also have at least one Certified Eye Bank Technician (CEBT) in a supervisory and training role for other technicians and staff. The director may appoint other technical and supportive staff to ensure that eye bank operations can be conducted proficiently.[12]

EQUIPMENT REQUIRED FOR AN EYE BANK

Eye banks need a basic set of equipment to appropriately recover, process, and store donor corneal tissue, as well as to work with biological materials. A well-defined laboratory space is needed, with a stable electrical source, sufficient grounded outlets for laboratory equipment, a sink with drain and running water, adequate counter space for eye bank procedures, and clean walls, floor and sink.[12,14] The EBAA requires documentation of regular laboratory cleaning schedules to be kept for 3 years in the laboratory.[12]

In order to preserve tissue, the eye bank also needs a temperature controlled-space. For cold storage, an eye bank will need a refrigerator that can keep materials within the range of 2–8°C. If tissue is preserved using organ media storage, the eye bank will need to regulate temperatures at 30–37°C. In either case, an external temperature recorder should be calibrated against the appropriate region-specific calibration, such as the the National Institute of Standards and Technology standard thermometer in the United States. The daily variation in temperature should be recorded. If the temperature deviates outside of the prescribed range, an alarm system ought to be in place to alert appropriate staff.[11,12,14-17]

An eye bank also needs the appropriate equipment to maintain a sterile environment around the tissues. This includes a laminar airflow cabinet or alternate processing environment, an autoclave to sterilize equipment, and the appropriate instrumentation for sterile removal of whole eyes or corneas. There should be appropriate procedures and protocols to maintain personnel safety and prevent infection of tissue. Eye banks also need means to appropriately dispose of any remains or biological waste in a dignified manner, in line with local regulations.[12,14]

To ensure that these requirements are met, eye banks keep a procedures and policy manual within the building for reference. Further, records should be maintained of the appropriate inspection, cleaning, and maintenance of laboratory equipment.[12,14]

DONOR ELIGIBILITY

Determining donor eligibility is a multipart process: to ensure high quality, safe donor tissue and to ensure a complete record of donor and referral information. Donor eligibility can be performed partially through telephone screening and then completed with on-site screening. First, the eye bank agent must assume proper authorization from a legally authorized person (e.g. deceased, legal next of kin). In the United States, deceased persons may have registered their intent to donate organs prior to death. In this circumstance, documentation of the registered donation is needed, but further consent (from next of kin) is not. If not on record, the agency is required to obtain proper documentation from next of kin under the Uniform Anatomical Gift Act, a law enacted in all states. In the US, state laws vary in terms of specifics. In each country, laws surrounding consent vary where many have a presumed consent (opt-out) system so that donation occurs automatically after death, and others have opt-in systems for consent. Practicing ophthalmologists should review requirements for eye donor tissue applicable to their region.[12,18]

In addition to obtaining authorization, the eye bank agents perform the donor screening before proceeding, summarized in Table 29.1. The screening evaluation consists of many parts:

- The eye bank agent should perform a medical assessment of donor demographic characteristics, donor health history and medical records, donor health behaviors, and donor circumstances of death.
- The eye bank agent also performs a thorough physical assessment consisting of a head-to-toe body inspection to evaluate for risk factors (described in Quality Assurance). A physical assessment is to evaluate donor health and look for risk factors related to disease transmission to the recipient. Examples of risk factors include needle tracks from intravenous drug use, homemade tattoos, and external signs of transmissible diseases.

Table 29.1: Screening of the donor.*

Method	Examples
Medical assessment	
Diagnoses	Medical chart review reveals a condition not listed on problem list
Risk factors	Diagnosed with dementia of unknown etiology
Clinical evidence	*Indication of sepsis:* Temperature >100.4°F; HR >90 beats/min; RR >20 breaths/min; or WBC >12,000 cells/mm^3 (if have 2 of 4 signs)
Physical assessment	Evidence of nonmedical percutaneous drug use (e.g. needle tracks)

(HR: Heart rate; RR: Respiratory rate; WBC: White blood cells)
*Tissues determined to be ineligible—"any potential donor who exhibits one or more of the following conditions or behaviors."
Source: Eye Bank Association of America (EBAA). Medical Standards. Washington, DC: EBAA; 2015.

- The eye bank agent also reviews all medical documentation surrounding the cause of death from the medical examiner, coroner, or pathologist.[12,14,18]

QUALITY ASSURANCE

Quality assurance is the cornerstone of eye bank practices. Protecting the recipient and thereby honoring the deceased's gift of donation is paramount. Donor risk of transmission and tissue quality are the main factors evaluated. Based on the 2015 EBAA annual report, there are several main indications, related to the donor's health, that recovered tissues were not released for transplantation. Of tissues and donor screened in any capacity, only 66% were deemed suitable for transplantation.[19] In 2015, of the tissues not released for use, 29.5% of tissues not released for transplant were because of positive donor serology for communicable diseases; 23.1% of tissues not released because of medical record or autopsy findings; and 8.2% were not released because of the medical/social interview. The remaining tissues were not released because of concerns of tissue quality.[19]

Donor risk of disease transmission can be from infectious or noninfectious etiologies. Table 29.2 summarizes the current EBAA and US Federal Drug Administration standards for contraindications to transplantation. The most critical factor is the dynamic, active involvement of the eye bank and medical communities to keep standards current. In 2016, the outbreak of Zika virus prompted immediate action by the EBAA and other organizations and resulted in policy changes.[12] This is one of many examples of involved, where people focused on quality and patient safety. It should be noted, that some of the diseases listed

Table 29.2: Contraindications to transplant.*

Disease category	Disease
Infectious etiologies	
Viral disease	Rubella (congenital)
	Reye syndrome within 3 months
	Viral encephalitis (e.g. subacute sclerosing panencephalitis, progressive multifocal leukoencephalopathy, etc.)
	Viral meningitis
	Rabies
	Ebola virus disease
	Human immunodeficiency virus** (by anti-HIV-1, anti-HIV-2 or combination test)
	Hepatitis B [by Hepatitis B surface antigen (HBsAg)]**
	Hepatitis C (by anti-HCV)**
	West Nile virus
	Vaccinia
	Zika virus
Bacterial disease	Bacterial meningitis
	Bacterial endocarditis
	Syphilis (*Treponema pallidum*)**
Fungal disease	Fungal endocarditis
Prion disease	Human transmissible spongiform encephalopathy (TSE) including Creutzfeldt-Jakob disease (CJD)
Noninfectious etiologies	
Systemic	
	Leukemia
	Lymphomas
	Malignant melanoma
	Parkinson disease
	Amyotrophic lateral sclerosis
	Multiple sclerosis
	Alzheimer disease
	Down's syndrome
Ocular	
	Retinoblastoma
	Malignant anterior segment tumors
	Adenocarcinoma in the eye of primary or metastatic origin
	Active ocular or intraocular inflammation
	Congenital or acquired disorders (e.g. keratoconus)
Other	
	Sepsis
	Death of unknown causes

*EBAA and Food and Drug Administration (FDA) standards, combined.
**Diseases where donor blood testing required.
Source: Eye Bank Association of America (EBAA). Medical Standards. Washington, DC: EBAA; 2015.

in Table 29.2 are difficult to identify on screening. In some, there is no blood test or formalized screening criteria. Eye banks should employ best practices to attempt to screen for all contraindicated diseases.

Tissue quality standards exist to ensure the recipient will benefit from the tissue. Clearly, these standards vary by the indication. Tissue used for a corneal transplantation will have certain requirements. Tissues for a scleral patch graft or therapeutic keratoplasty will have different requirements. Overall, eye banks evaluate the tissue to make sure that there are no indicators of disease affecting the ultimate tissue purpose. In the case of corneal transplantation, the eye bank can determine its standards for endothelial cell density, limits of age of the donor, and limits on death-to-preservation and procurement times. Eye banks can also determine separate standards for tissue quality of specialized corneal transplantation tissues [e.g. Descemet's membrane endothelial keratoplasty (DMEK)]. The "proper" tissue standards are contended amongst corneal specialists, and numerous published studies investigate how tissue characteristics are related to recipient outcomes.[20-24] As a result, some surgeons are more restrictive with tissue requests than their eye bank standards. Ophthalmologists who are medical directors and affiliated eye banks are aware that meeting the requests of surgeons with tight tissue standards may affect the donor pool.[25,26]

TISSUE RETRIEVAL

Tissue retrieval should be conducted by a trained and certified person from the eye bank. They should have thorough understanding of proper retrieval protocols. Prior to tissue retrieval, if the donor is deemed eligible for tissue recovery, the on-site staff should be notified of optimal methods to maintain the eye prior to recovery. The on-site staff should moisten and close the eyes completely. If possible, eyelids should be lightly taped closed. The eye bank agent should assess, upon arrival, if the donor and eyes have been preserved in such a way to ensure tissue quality for the recipient. If so, they can proceed with the medical and physical assessment of the donor. If there are no donor eligibility or tissue quality concerns, the eye bank agent can proceed with the steps for tissue retrieval, shown in Box 29.1.[18]

The eye bank agent should collect a blood sample from the donor to screen for diseases that could affect the recipient (described in Quality Assurance). The blood sample should be obtained under sterile conditions using standard precautions. The EBAA lists the tests, shown in Box 29.2, to be included in the donor blood sample.[12]

Box 29.1: Tissue retrieval steps.

- Collection of blood sample
- Enucleation versus in situ corneal excision
- Transport to an eye bank

Box 29.2: Diseases screened by blood work from the donor, United States—Eye Bank Association of America.*

- HIV [anti-HIV-1, anti-HIV-2 (or combination test)]
- Hepatitis B [Hepatitis B surface antigen (HBsAg)]
- Hepatitis C (anti-HCV)
- Syphilis

**Also see Table 29.2*

Eye banks most commonly procure ocular tissue by enucleation or by in-situ corneal excision. Eye bank agents use sterile techniques and standard precautions in both procedures. The goal is to minimize ocular tissue damage. For in-situ corneal excision, the more specific goal is to minimize endothelial cell loss, minimize contamination risk, and provide adequate scleral rim for postprocessing requirements (e.g. for Descemet's stripping automated endothelial keratoplasty (DSAEK) or DMEK processing). Some eye banks perform cultures at the time of tissue recovery (Fig. 29.2).

After procurement, all ocular tissues and donor information should be safely and securely transported to the eye bank for evaluation and processing. Tissues and records should be labeled so all documentation to the donor is connected. Time stamps should be used throughout the process, so the eye bank and ophthalmic surgeon know the length of time between donor death and tissue preservation. These factors are related to tissue health, especially the risk of infection. The eye bank should have standard forms to collect information and to retain records. The eye bank should have protocols for tissue acceptance at the eye bank and registration of the donor tissue with the eye bank. The ophthalmic surgeon should have access to these complete records, as appropriate, upon request.[12,18]

LABORATORY PROCESSING

Once procured and brought to the eye bank, ocular tissue is evaluated to determine its suitability for transplant or graft (Table 29.3). Even before procurement, gross inspection of the tissue with a penlight is performed to look for any visible corneal scarring, corneal infiltrates, or other evidence of ocular disease. Since the tissue is recovered mainly for use in corneal transplantation, the cornea is then inspected more closely at the eye bank with slit-lamp biomicroscopy and specular microscopy.[27,28]

Table 29.3: Evaluation methods for tissue viability.

Evaluation methods	Tissue features
Gross inspection	Corneal scarring, infiltrates
Slit-lamp biomicroscopy	Corneal scars, significant arcus, edema, folds, striae, epithelial defects, guttata changes, foreign bodies, and infiltrates
Specular microscopy	Corneal endothelial morphology
Corneal pachymetry	Corneal thickness

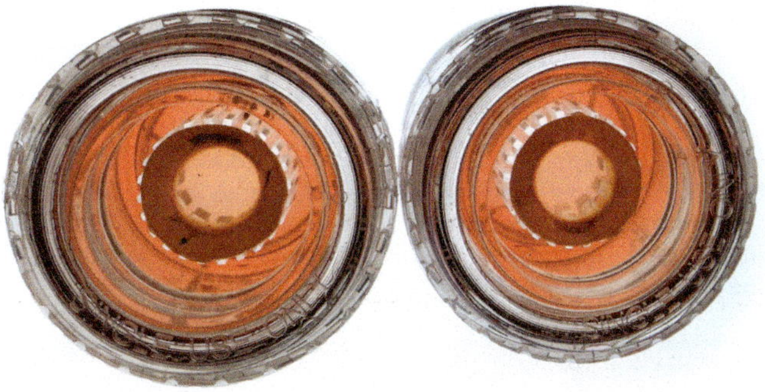

Fig. 29.2: Recovered tissues have been stored in tissue culture media, and will be kept in cold storage at the eye bank.

For the slit-lamp biomicroscope evaluation, the technician first examines with a diffuse light and low magnification, to obtain an overall view of the cornea. Next, a focal high power examination is conducted with a narrow slit beam. The eye bank technician looks for factors affecting corneal viability, including corneal scars, edema, significant corneal arcus, folds, striae, epithelial defects, guttata changes, foreign bodies, or infiltrates (Fig. 29.3).[29]

In addition to slit-lamp biomicroscopy, the technician performs imaging with specular microscopy to assess the health of the corneal endothelium. The specular microscope shines light in through the cornea and reflects on the corneal endothelium. The corneal endothelial cells are supposed to be hexagonal and evenly spaced when healthy (Fig. 29.4). Corneal endothelial cells degenerate over time, and are unable to regenerate. Corneas from older donors tend to have a lower endothelial cell count and more irregular spacing than corneas from younger donors. The endothelial cell density is often required to be greater than 2000 cells/mm^2 in order to proceed with penetrating or endothelial keratoplasty (i.e. DSAEK or DMEK). However, other ophthalmic surgeries do not need high cell counts to be successful, such as anterior lamellar keratoplasty or

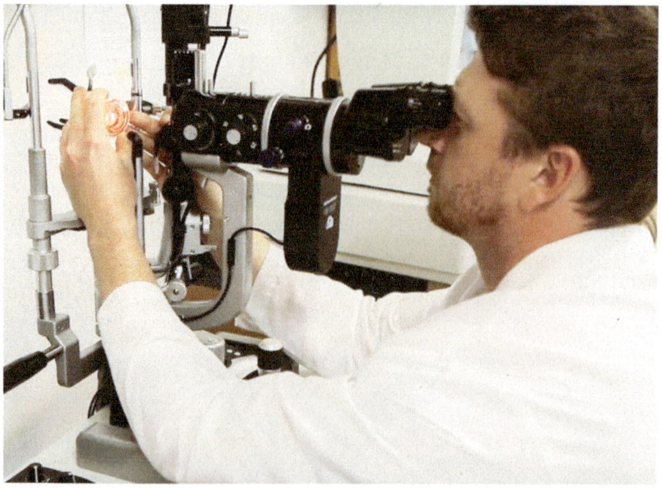

Fig. 29.3: Slit-lamp biomicroscopy evaluation of a donor cornea, to evaluate tissue for characteristics such as corneal scars, significant arcus, edema, folds, striae, epithelial defects, guttata changes, foreign bodies, and infiltrates (*see* Table 29.3).

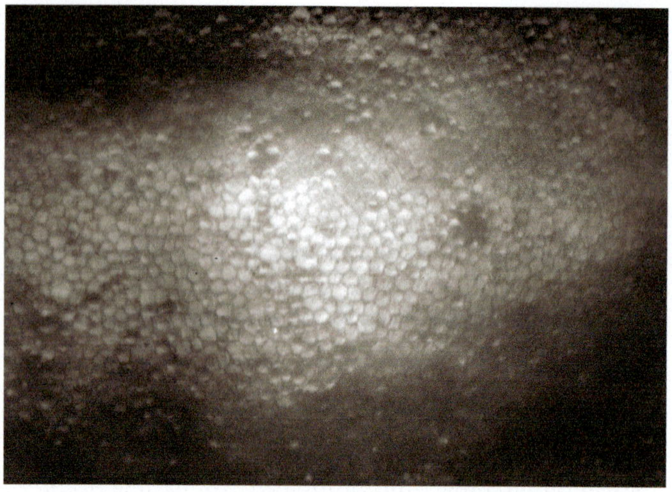

Fig. 29.4: Specular microscopy image of the corneal endothelium. This image shows healthy, evenly spaced hexagonal cells.

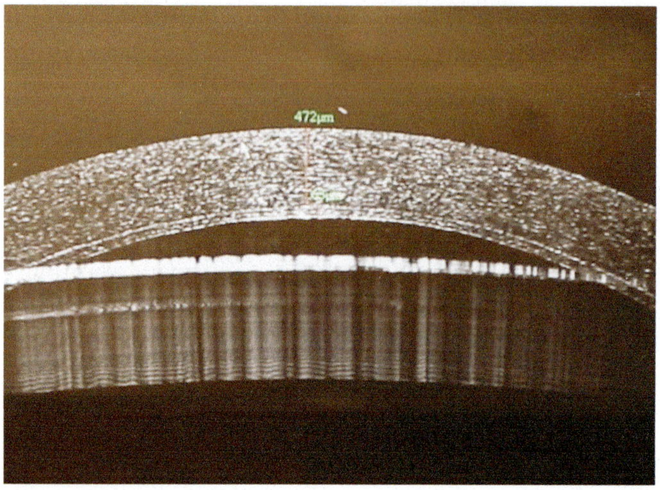

Fig. 29.5: Optical coherence tomography (OCT) image used in corneal pachymetry can visualize the thickness of the cornea. This thickness is measured using digital calipers within the OCT software.

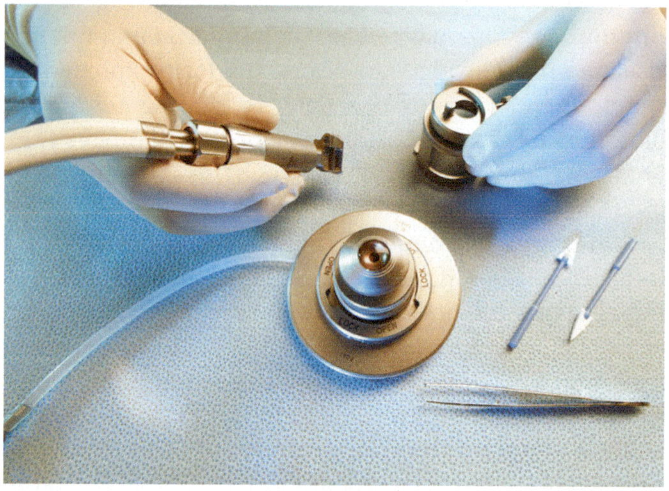

Fig. 29.6: Descemet's stripping automated endothelial keratoplasty (DSAEK) equipment used to process corneal tissue prior to surgical graft placement.

therapeutic keratoplasties in emergencies.[18,30] Specular microscopy also shows endothelial cell morphology—features such as guttae, polymegathism, pleomorphism, striae, folds, or areas of low density that should be factored for quality when determining tissue viability and quality.[18]

Corneal thickness is important for endothelial keratoplasty tissue processing, especially in DSAEK. Eye banks use various imaging techniques to measure corneal pachymetry including ocular coherence tomography (OCT), ultrasound, and topography.[27] Figure 29.5 shows an OCT image used to measure corneal thickness.

After viability assessment, suitable tissue is preserved in media and stored accordingly. If tissue is designated to be used for endothelial keratoplasty (either DSAEK or DMEK), it may need to be processed by the eye bank prior to use (Fig. 29.6). For DSAEK, the corneal tissue is sectioned by a microkeratome so a thin tissue of corneal stroma, Descemet's membrane, and endothelium remain to be used in surgery. For DMEK, the tissue is processed and only Descemet's membrane and the endothelium remain to be used in surgery.[31-39] All corneal tissues, processed and unprocessed, are transferred from the eye bank to the operating room for surgery on a recipient.[27] Both the eye bank and the surgeon can perform these processing procedures, with equivalent outcomes. However, eye banks tend to do more tissue processing, which allows for preoperative measurement of endothelial cell count and graft thickness, increases operating room efficiency and reduces tissue wastage.[24]

Cornea Preservation and Storage

A few different methods of corneal preservation have been developed, such as moist chamber, cryopreservation, cold storage, and organ culture. Currently, cold storage and organ culture are most commonly used to store ocular tissue, although all methods have their benefits and limitations.

Moist chamber preservation is the simplest means of storage, in which ocular tissue is stored in a moist environment at cold temperatures. The tissue lasts 1–2 days, and little else is needed to preserve the viability of tissue. This method, while effective, has largely been replaced by more current techniques.[40]

Cryopreservation is another technique used less commonly today, in which corneal tissue is frozen in the presence of a cryoprotectant. This preservation method sought to reduce tissue shortages, since frozen tissue can be stored for 12 years with 58% graft survival. However, cryopreservation also requires the tissue to be returned to organ culture after thawing to confirm viability, and its complexity has rendered it less convenient than cold storage preservation or organ culture preservation.[40]

The two most commonly used preservation methods today are cold storage and organ media preservation. Cold storage is more common, and used throughout the world, while organ media preservation is more common in Western Europe.[41] Both methods have been proven equally effective. In cold storage, the corneoscleral button is often examined and excised, and then stored in a specific tissue culture medium at 2–6ºC (Fig. 29.7).[41] The tissue culture media are commercially available, and include antibiotics, deturgescent agents to prevent corneal swelling, and other additives to improve storage capacity. M-K medium, the original for tissue storage, preserved tissue for 7–10 days. Today, commercially available media such as Optisol, Dexsol, K-sol, Lexosol, and 4-C media can preserve tissue for longer durations (up to 14–16 days). To limit tissue degeneration however, corneal tissue is stored for much less time than manufacturer claims; with Optisol, tissue is kept for 7–10 days. In storage, tissue retains its shape and size, and can be used immediately for transplant. However, as its stored for longer periods, degenerative changes in the endothelium and endothelial cell loss can

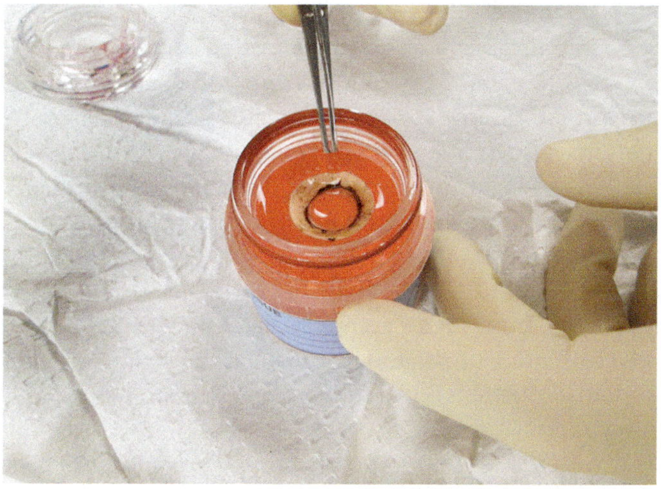

Fig. 29.7: The corneoscleral tissue is placed in tissue culture media for cold storage.

increase the risk for primary graft rejection. To ensure the best quality possible of tissue for transplant, all efforts are made to recover and store the tissue as quickly as possible postmortem, usually within 12 hours.[40,41]

Organ media preservation is equally as effective as cold storage, and used more frequently in Western Europe. This method relies on storing corneal tissue in traditional organ media, a tissue culture medium supplemented with antibiotics, antimycotics, and fetal or newborn calf serum.[41] The antimicrobials tend to be more effective, and viability of the corneal tissue is evident in this media. Tissue can last up to 4 weeks in this culture, although the endothelium must be inspected after storage to ensure its quality for transplant. Corneal tissue also tends to swell when stored in organ media, because the dehydrating macromolecules usually used to prevent swelling in vitro are taken up by the corneal cells. Tissue needs to be deswollen before transplant by placing it in a media with dextran (4–8%), which can take 1–7 days depending on the protocol of the eye banks. The main advantage to organ media preservation is the extended time available to recover and store tissue postmortem. The organ media culture allows for wound healing, so tissue can be recovered and stored even 24–48 hours after death.[41]

REGULATORY LAWS AND STANDARDS FOR AN EYE BANK

Eye bank regulations and standards around the world come from both their regional eye bank associations and the local government. Regional eye bank associations publish their medical standards and guidelines, and often consult with governmental organizations in the lawmaking process to ensure appropriate and accurate regulations for procurement, storage and use of ocular tissue. In countries such as the US or Australia, eye banking falls under the legal jurisdiction of the organization tasked with regulating medications and tissue handling. In Australia, this is the Therapeutic Goods Association; in the US, the Food and Drug Administration (FDA). The European Union has published a comprehensive directive (2004/23/EC) regulating organ and tissue donations.[15] Similarly, the Indian Parliament released the Transplantation of Human Organs and Tissue Rules, 2014.[42] Each of these regulations is directed at maintaining the ethical procurement, safe handling, and use of tissue.

Safety standards for the eye banks are often prescribed to ensure a sterile environment that protects laboratory personnel. These laws, such as the "current good tissue practice for manufacturers of human cellular and tissue-based products" in the US, have details about equipment, facilities, environmental control and supplies necessary in an eye bank.[8]

Regulatory laws also serve to prevent disease transmission from donor to recipient. Many laws focus on eligibility criteria of donors, to screen out tissues from individuals with transmissible blood-borne infections. All incoming tissue to an eye bank must be screened for communicable diseases such as hepatitis and HIV. Further, eye banks may be required to register with the government and pass an inquiry or inspection to ensure they meet all requirements before they can become operational.[12,13,42]

Current Supply and Distribution

Globally, different regions have their own eye banks and manage the supply and demand of tissue. Typically, good collaborations exist between eye banks to ensure that all eligible donor tissue is transplanted. Regional eye banks may collaborate with other neighboring regions, or even those across the globe to transport corneal tissue (Figs. 29.8A and B). About 89% of corneal transplants are performed with domestically sourced corneal tissue, and 37 countries use only nationally procured tissue. The remaining countries import tissue from other eye banks to meet local demand. Still, about 53% of the world's population does not have access to corneal tissue for transplant, and the majority of the remaining population still has to wait for tissue availability. Currently, the United States, Italy and Sri Lanka have more than sufficient supply of corneal tissue, and are able to export to other countries. Brazil, Canada, most of Europe and Australia are self-sufficient, while the rest of the world remains in need. Globally, about 12.7 million people were in need of corneal transplant in 2016.[1]

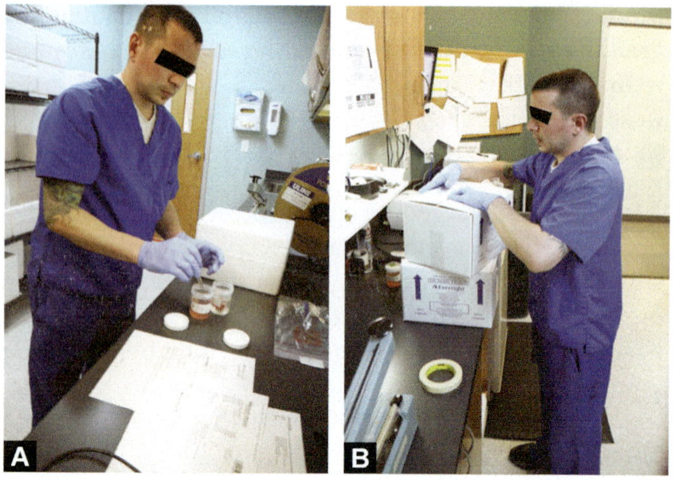

Figs. 29.8A and B: Tissue is prepared, placed in cold storage media, and stored in dry ice. It is packaged and ready to be shipped to another eye bank facility.

Strategies to Find Donors

Given the need for corneal tissue, particularly in the developing world, eye banks strive to encourage more individuals to enroll as eye donors and optimize procurement of eligible patients. Eye banks often coordinate with grief counselors to discuss the gift of donation for deceased patients' families. Since the request for tissue donation is made around the time of death, counselors need to time their request appropriately. Decoupling the death notification from the donation request has been shown to increase consent, by asking about tissue donation either before or after the death notice, but not at the same time. Other factors that increase the consent rate include the ability of the person who is discussing donation with the family and the quality of hospital care as perceived by the family.[43] A key barrier to donation is education and awareness. Patients with higher academic education level and education about eye banking are more likely to consent to organ donation.[44] Many eye banks hold awareness events to educate the public and encourage donation.[44]

The hospital corneal retrieval program is a means of encouraging donation. An eye donation counselor speaks with and educates eligible next of kin about eye donation.

Traditionally, eye donations occur when either the donor had already decided to donate his or her organs prior to death or the next of kin decides to do so and informs hospital staff. Hospital corneal retrieval programs take a more proactive approach than traditional methods, and have had a large impact on increasing donors in a hospital setting.[45]

Internationally, several laws have also been passed that both raise awareness of donation and facilitate the conversations with families. Countries with opt-in tissue and organ donation tend to have lower donation rates than countries with default donation and an opt-out policy. Several other laws have made the process easier. The Anatomical Donation Law in the United States allows an individual to state their wish to donate organs and tissue at the time of their death. The donor's wishes are to be followed and the medical and social interview with next of kin may not be needed for authorization. In some areas, this information is put on the driver's license, for easy identification of the donor's wishes. In another regulation, hospitals must ask all eligible patients or their next of kin about donation. All hospitals are required to at least contact organ procurement organizations for donations at the time of a person's death. The Medical Examiner or Justice of Peace Act, passed in the United States, also allows a medical examiner to excise corneal tissue in certain cases, such as autopsy, given that there is no objection from next of kin.[6]

Given the global shortage of corneal tissue, scientists are now looking to tissue engineering to create synthetic and naturally-derived corneal tissue for transplant. These strategies seek to recreate the layers of the cornea, or replace only certain cell types that can be grown in vitro.[46] These developing methods may be the next forefront to address the current need for corneal transplants.

ACKNOWLEDGMENTS

We would like to acknowledge Eversight eye bank and especially Michael Titus and Stephanie Sorenson of Eversight for help with editing, figures, and photographs of eye banking.

REFERENCES

1. Gain P, Jullienne R, He Z, et al. Global Survey of Corneal Transplantation and Eye Banking. JAMA Ophthalmol. 2016;134(2):167-73.
2. Robert Calendra. Why, how the eye bank has evolved. Ophthalmol Manag. 2016;20(22):25-6.
3. Eye Bank Assosciation of America. (2017). History of Corneal Transplantation, Eye Banking, and the EBAA. [Online] Available from: *http://restoresight.org/wp-content/uploads/2017/02/History-of-Eye-Banking-and-EBAA.pdf* [Accessed November, 2017].
4. Lambert NG, Chamberlain WD. The structure and evolution of eye banking: a review on eye banks' historical, present, and future contribution to corneal transplantation. J Bioreposit Sci App Med. 2017;5:23-40.
5. Lions Medical Eye Bank and Research Center of Eastern Virginia. (2012). How the Lions Helped. [Online] Available from: *http://www.lionseyebank.org/lions.htm* [Accessed November, 2017].
6. Albert D, Farge EJ. History of ophthalmology Eye Banking: 1944 to the Present. Surv Ophthalm. 1989;33(4):260-3.
7. Chu W. The past twenty-five years in eye banking. Cornea. 2000;19(5):754-65.
8. Eversight. Regulation of Eye Banking. Eversight Orientat Man. 2016:6-9.
9. Jones GLA, Dekaris I, Hjortdal J, et al. European Eye Bank Association: Past, Present, and Future. Int J Eye Bank. 2012; 1(1):1-6.
10. Pollock GA. The Eye Bank Association of Australia and New Zealand: Origins, History, Activity, and Future. Int J Eye Bank. 2013;1(2):1-6.
11. Jones GLA, Ponzin D, Pels E, et al. European Eye Bank Association. Dev Ophthalmol. 2009;43:15-21.
12. Eye Bank Association of America. Medical Standards. Washington DC; 2017.
13. Eye Bank Association of Australia and New Zealand. Medical and Quality Standards for Eye Donation and Eye Tissue Banking. 2009;(April).
14. Government of India. Standards of Eye Banking in India. New Delhi; 2009.
15. European Union. Directive 2004/23/EC of the European Parliament and of the Council of 31 March 2004 on setting standards of quality and safety for the donation, procurement, testing, processing, preservation, storage and distribution of human tissues and cells. Off J Eur Union. 2004:48-58.
16. European Union. Commission Directive 2006/17/EC. Off J Eur Union. 2006:40-52.
17. European Union. Commission Directive 2006/86/EC. Off J Eur Union. 2006:32-50.
18. Eye Bank Association of America. Procedures manual. Washington DC; 2017.
19. Eye Bank Association of America. 2015 Eye Banking Statistical Report. Washington DC. 2016;(202).
20. Terry MA, Straiko MD, Goshe JM, et al. Descemet's stripping automated endothelial keratoplasty: the tenuous relationship between donor thickness and postoperative vision. Ophthalm. 2012;119(10):1988-96.
21. Price MO, Price FW. Descemet's Stripping with Endothelial Keratoplasty. Ophthalm. 2006;113(11):1936-42.
22. Terry MA, Shamie N, Chen ES, et al. Precut Tissue for Descemet's Stripping Automated Endothelial Keratoplasty. Ophthalm. 2009;116(2):248-56.

23. Neff KD, Biber JM, Holland EJ. Comparison of Central Corneal Graft Thickness to Visual Acuity Outcomes in Endothelial Keratoplasty. Cornea. 2011;30(4):388-91.
24. Woodward MA, Titus MS, Shtein RM. Effect of microkeratome pass on tissue processing for Descemet stripping automated endothelial keratoplasty. Cornea. 2014;33(5):507-9.
25. Boynton GE, Woodward MA. Eye-bank preparation of endothelial tissue. Current Opinion in Ophthalmology. 2014:319-24.
26. Woodward MA, Ross KW, Requard JJ, et al. Impact of Surgeon Acceptance Parameters on Cost and Availability of Corneal Donor Tissue for Transplantation. Cornea. 2013;32(6):737-40.
27. Liaboe C, Vislisel JM, Schmidt GA, et al. (2015). Corneal Transplantation: From Donor to Recipient [Online] Available from: *http://webeye.ophth.uiowa.edu/eyeforum/tutorials/Cornea-transplant-donor-to-recipient/index.htm* [Accessed November, 2017].
28. Bonnel AJ, Cymbor M. (2012). Under the Specular Microscope. [Online] Available from: *https://www.reviewofoptometry.com/article/under-the-specular-microscope* [Accessed November, 2017].
29. Eversight. F1.211 Policy Statement Slit Lamp Evaluation of Corneas. 2015:1-4.
30. Eversight. F1.311 Specular Microscopy Procedure. 2012: 1-2.
31. Tourtas T, Laaser K, Bachmann BO, et al. Descemet membrane endothelial keratoplasty versus descemet stripping automated endothelial keratoplasty. Am J Ophthalmol. 2012;153(6):1082-90.e2.
32. Melles GRJ, Ong TS, Ververs B, et al. Descemet membrane endothelial keratoplasty (DMEK). Cornea. 2006;25(8):987-90.
33. Price MO, Giebel AW, Fairchild KM, et al. Descemet's membrane endothelial keratoplasty. Ophthalm. 2009;116(12): 2361-8.
34. Guerra FP, Anshu A, Price MO, et al. Descemet's membrane endothelial keratoplasty: prospective study of 1-year visual outcomes, graft survival, and endothelial cell loss. Ophthalm. 2011;118(12):2368-73.
35. Kruse FE, Laaser K, Cursiefen C, et al. A stepwise approach to donor preparation and insertion increases safety and outcome of descemet membrane endothelial keratoplasty. Cornea. 2011;30(5):580-7.
36. Schlötzer-Schrehardt U, Bachmann BO, Tourtas T, et al. Reproducibility of Graft Preparations in Descemet's Membrane Endothelial Keratoplasty. Ophthalmol. 2013;120(9):1769-77.
37. Anwar M, Teichmann KD. Big-bubble technique to bare descemet's membrane in anterior lamellar keratoplasty. J Cataract Refract Surg. 2002;28(3):398-403.
38. Yoeruek E, Bayyoud T, Hofmann J, et al. Comparison of Pneumatic Dissection and Forceps Dissection in Descemet Membrane Endothelial Keratoplasty. Cornea. 2012;31(8):920-5.
39. Muraine M, Gueudry J, He Z, et al. Novel Technique for the Preparation of Corneal Grafts for Descemet Membrane Endothelial Keratoplasty. Am J Ophthalmol. 2013;156(5): 851-9.
40. Ehlers N, Hjortdal J, Nielsen K. Corneal Grafting and Banking. Dev Ophthalmol. 2009;43:1-14.
41. Pels E, Beele H, Claerhout I. Eye bank issues: II. Preservation techniques: warm versus cold storage. Int Ophthalmol. 2008;28:155-63.
42. National Organ and Tissue Transplant Organization (NOTTO). (2014). Transplantation of Human Organs and Tissues Rules, 2014. [Online] Available from: *http://notto.nic.in/act-end-rules-of-thoa.htm* [Accessed November, 2017].
43. Simpkin AL, Robertson LC, Barber VS, et al. Modifiable factors influencing relatives' decision to offer organ donation: systematic review. BMJ. 2009:1-8.
44. Panwar R, Pal S, Dash NR, et al. Why are we Poor Organ Donors: A Survey Focusing on Attitudes of the Lay Public from Northern India. J Clin Exp Hepatol. 2016;6(2): 81-6.
45. Sharma N, Agrawal N, Maharana PK, et al. Comparison of hospital cornea retrieval and voluntary eye donation program in eye banking. Eye and Contact Lens. 2016;0(0): 1-5.
46. Ghezzi CE, Rnjak-Kovacina J, Kaplan DL. Corneal tissue engineering: recent advances and future perspectives. Tissue Eng Part B Rev. 2015;21(3):278-7.

Chapter 30 Corneal Transplantation

Jennifer Rose-Nussbaumer, Ariana Austin

INTRODUCTION

Corneal transplantation is one of the most commonly performed transplant surgeries in the world. In the United States, over 27,000 keratoplasties were performed in 2015, and a large international survey recently found that in 116 countries representing 89% of the world's population, approximately 185,000 keratoplasties were performed annually.[1,2] Corneal opacities are the fourth leading cause of blindness and it has been estimated that 12.7 million people globally are in need of a corneal transplant.[2,3] Originally pioneered over 100 years ago, corneal transplantation has evolved to include a variety of different surgeries and techniques. With the tools and techniques at our disposal today, opacification of the cornea no longer guarantees lifelong blindness as it once did.

HISTORY OF CORNEAL TRANSPLANTATION

Written references to corneal transplantation can be found as far back as 2000 BC in Egypt.[4] While the concept of cornea or eye transplants has appeared in many cultures since, it was usually in myths and legends requiring magic. It was not until 1760 that Charles Darwin's grandfather Erasmus Darwin first proposed removal of the opaque cornea.[5,6] Transplantation with a glass keratoprosthesis was suggested by Guillaume Pellier in 1789, although this procedure was never successfully performed.[6] Franz Reisinger conceived of using clear corneal tissue from a living donor in 1818, experimenting on chickens and rabbits and coining the term "keratoplasty".[6-8] In 1837, the first successful cornea transplant in an animal was performed by Samuel Bigger on a pet gazelle, and by 1886 Arthur von Hippel performed the first successful animal-to-human keratoplasty using a rabbit cornea.[9] Finally in 1905, Czech physician Eduard Zirm performed the first successful penetrating keratoplasty using corneas from a living 11-year-old donor.[4,10]

Since Zirm performed that first human-to-human transplant, there have been significant advances in corneal transplantation surgery. Anton Elschnig began performing lamellar keratoplasties in 1914 and although lamellar keratoplasty soon became the preferred technique, by midcentury it was abandoned in favor of penetrating keratoplasty due to complications such as scarring and interface haze.[6,11] Since then newer techniques, such as deep lamellar endothelial keratoplasty, Descemet's stripping endothelial keratoplasty and Descemet's membrane endothelial keratoplasty (EK) have been developed to improve vision, reduce recovery time and improve complication rates. These new techniques along with a growing global network of transplant surgeons and eye banks are responsible for our increasing ability to address the burden of reversible corneal blindness around the world. Flowchart 30.1 describes the decision-making algorithm of corneal transplantation.

PENETRATING KERATOPLASTY

Indications

Developed in the 1960s, penetrating keratoplasty (PKP) was long the standard of care for those requiring transplantation. Once the mainstay of corneal transplantation, PKP has declined in popularity in favor of partial thickness transplants due to long postoperative recovery, incidence of rejection, wound dehiscence and suture complications.[12-14] In developed countries, PKP used to be the treatment of choice for all corneal pathology requiring transplantation with the most common indications being Fuchs' dystrophy, Pseudophakic bullous keratopathy, Keratoconus (KCN) or regraft.[12,15] In developing countries, a large portion of penetrating keratoplasties continue to be performed for infection (ulceration and trachoma) or trauma.[16,17] Although largely replaced by lamellar keratoplasty in developed countries, PKP is still indicated for patients with concurrent endothelial and stromal

Flowchart 30.1: Corneal transplantation decision-making.

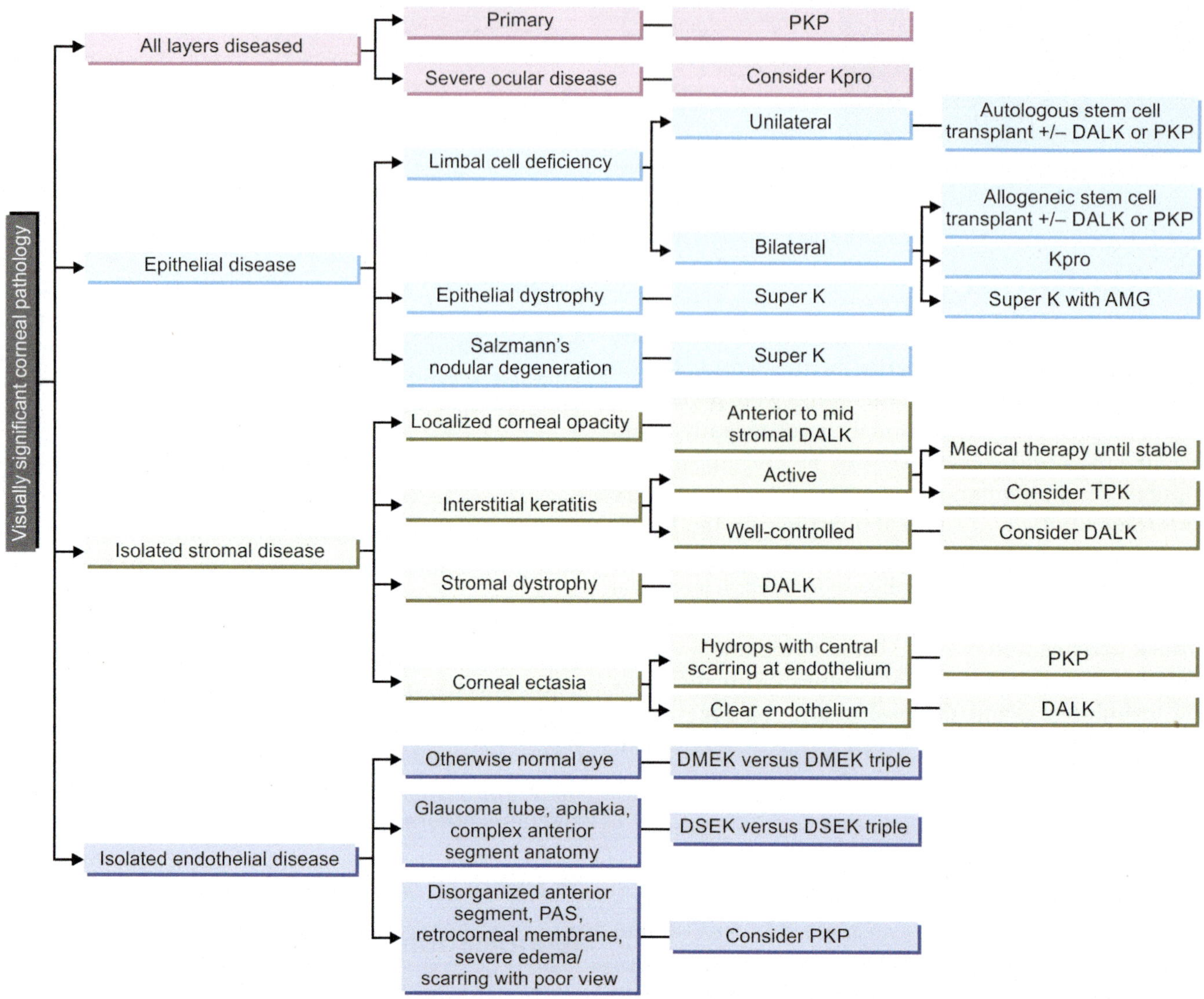

(AMG: Amniotic membrane graft; DALK: Deep anterior lamellar keratoplasty; DMEK: Descemet's membrane endothelial keratoplasty; DSEK: Descemet's stripping endothelial keratoplasty; Kpro: Keratoprosthesis; PAS: Peripheral anterior synechiae; PKP: Penetrating keratoplasty; Super K: Superficial keratectomy; TPK: Therapeutic penetrating keratoplasty)

disease, severe corneal opacity or for regrafting in cases where there is endothelial failure and high astigmatism in the original graft.

Techniques

A lid speculum must be used to open the lids with careful positioning so as to avoid placing any pressure on the globe. A scleral fixation ring is essential for young patients, patients with KCN and aphakic or effectively aphakic (such as scleral sutured intraocular lens) patients to reduce collapse of the eye once it is open. Both of these maneuvers are to reduce the risk of expulsion of intraoocular contents and collapse of the eye during the open-sky portion of the surgery. A hand-held trephine can be used to mark the cornea centering over the pupil in most cases. If the patient has ectasia, slightly decentering the cornea to encompass the ectasia is advised. On average the recipient cornea is trephined to approximately 8 mm. If the patient has a white-to-white measurement greater than 12.5 mm, an 8.25–8.50 mm trephine can be used. If the patient has a white-to-white measurement of less than 11.5 mm then a 7.5 mm or 7.75 mm trephine is preferred. Once the surgeon has determined the size of the recipient bed, the donor tissue must be prepared before proceeding by cutting from the endothelial side to avoid endothelial trauma. Usually the donor corneal button is oversized by approximately 0.25–0.50 mm. Some surgeons will not oversize a graft for KCN to reduce the steep corneal curvature and resultant myopia.

Once the donor tissue has been prepared, a small paracentesis incision is made and viscoelastic is infused into the anterior chamber. This allows sufficient intraocular pressure to ensure a perpendicular trephined edge and protects the iris and lens from damage. Once a partial thickness trephination has been achieved, a supersharp blade can be used to enter the anterior chamber in a controlled manner. Right and left cutting scissors should be used to complete the excision of the host tissue. The anterior chamber and corneal rim are then covered in viscoelastic and the donor button is transferred to the surgical field. Four interrupted 10-0 nylon cardinal sutures are placed. Suturing is then finished with an additional 12 radial interrupted sutures or alternatively a continuous suture technique can be employed. Suture depth should be approximately 90% of the corneal stroma to avoid full thickness penetration and possible endophthalmitis with later suture removal. It is imperative to bury all of the knots. A preferred technique is to bury them in the anterior stroma on the donor side with suture tails pointed away from the epithelium to aid in easy suture removal and reduce the number of broken sutures. Interrupted suturing technique is preferred in cases where there may be inflammation or neovascularization of the graft-host junction since these can be removed more easily than a running suture. Selective suture removal can begin around 4 months when there is adequate healing of the graft-host junction; however, wound dehiscence may occur if the sutures are all removed before 9–12 months.

Management of Intraoperative Complications

The complications of PKP have been outlined in Table 30.1. The incidence of explusive choroidal hemorrhage during PKP is approximately 1%.[18] The management involves rapid closure of the corneal wound and usually requires stronger suture, such as 7-0 or 8-0 nylon or even 7-0 silk. If the hemorrhage occurs during the open-sky period of the procedure, the wound should be occluded with either a finger or a Cobo temporary keratoprosthesis. In either case, a sclerotomy through the conjunctiva and sclera should be performed to drain blood clots and restore normal anatomy. Once the hemorrhage has been controlled, attention should be turned to the anterior segment where a lensectomy and vitrectomy can be performed as needed.

Table 30.1: Indications and complications of corneal transplantation.

Surgery	Indications	Intraoperative complications	Postoperative complications
PKP	Full thickness pathology, severe anterior segment disorganization (severe peripheral anterior synechiae, retrocorneal membrane)	Scleral perforation with fixation sutures, expulsive choroidal hemorrhage	Wound leaks, persistent epithelial defects, infection, inflammation, glaucoma, graft rejection, retinal detachment, endophthalmitis, wound dehiscence
TPK	Active keratitis not responding to medical therapy, perforation	Spread of infection intraocularly, expulsive choroidal hemorrhage, loss of lens or iris	Inflammation, increased IOP, glaucoma, endophthalmitis, recurrent infection, graft failure or rejection, retinal detachment
DALK	Isolated stromal disease	Rupture or perforation of Descemet's membrane	Pseudoanterior chamber, pupillary block, interface deposits and neovascularization
DSEK	Isolated endothelial disease	Complications with donor tissue preparation, retained Descemet's membrane, pupillary block	Donor dislocation, primary graft failure, graft rejection, pupillary block, endothelial cell loss, refractive change, interface deposits and epithelial ingrowth
DMEK	Isolated endothelial disease	Donor endothelial cell trauma	Donor dislocation, primary graft failure, graft rejection, pupillary block, endothelial cell loss, refractive change, interface deposits and epithelial ingrowth
Keratoprosthesis	Multiple failed grafts, severe ocular surface disease, aniridia or other limbal stem cell deficiency	Complications with donor assembly, scleral perforation with fixation sutures, expulsive choroidal hemorrhage	Retroprosthetic membrane, glaucoma, retinal detachment, endophthalmitis, loss of soft contact lens, sterile viritis, corneal melting

(PKP: Penetrating keratoplasty; TPK: Therapeutic penetrating keratoplasty; DALK: Deep anterior lamellar keratoplasty; DSEK: Descemet's stripping endothelial keratoplasty; DMEK: Descemet's membrane endothelial keratoplasty)

Postoperative Care

The early postoperative period is focused on decreasing inflammation and avoiding infection. Inflammation can be controlled with topical steroids drops, initially prednisolone 1% or equivalent is used every 2 hours while awake, then decreasing to 4 times daily for approximately 4 months before tapering further. Topical antibiotic drops, such as polymyxin B sulfate–trimethoprim can be used 4 times daily for approximately 1 month. Patients are typically seen or a follow up is done at postoperative day 1, week 1, month 1, and then every 6–8 weeks for the 1st year.

After approximately 4 months, selective suture removal can begin. Tight sutures that are causing astigmatism can be identified on topography. Pooling of fluorescein over a suture can be used to confirm that a suture is tight. It is most often beneficial to remove 2 sutures at time that are 180° from each other. Once the topography shows less than 3 diopters of astigmatism, a refraction can be performed. If the patient has satisfactory visual acuity with glasses, selective suture removal can cease and the manifest prescription can be prescribed. If there is significant astigmatism or anisometropia following lysis of all suture, rigid gas permeable contact lens fitting may be necessary for visual rehabilitation.

Graft Rejection

The cornea is an immune-privileged site in the body due to a lack of corneal blood vessels and lymphatics. Therefore, in the majority of corneal transplants, rejection can be avoided with low topical steroid drops. Postoperatively, patient education regarding the signs and symptoms of rejection as well as the importance of early treatment can improve outcomes. Acute corneal transplant rejection is characterized by pain, limbal injection, focal or diffuse corneal edema, keratic precipitates and anterior chamber flare and cells. Some patient may have a classic "Khodadoust line" which is a line of white blood cells moving across the endothelium (Figs. 30.1A and B). Treatment usually involves an hourly topical steroid drop, such as prednisolone 1% or a sub-Tenons steroid injection if it is felt that the patient will have difficulty with compliance.

The Collaborative Corneal Transplantation Studies (CCTS) have defined 'high-risk' transplant as a cornea with two or more quadrants of deep stromal vascularization. The risk of rejection appears to be doubled in grafts with 4 quadrants of vascularization. Prior graft failure, large diameter or eccentric grafts, age less than 40, previous surgery and presence of extensive peripheral anterior synechiae are also significant risk factors.

Strategies for optimizing outcomes in high-risk keratoplasty include treating preexistent ocular surface disease and inflammation as well as any infections, such as herpetic keratitis. Particular attention should also be given to recognition of aqueous deficiency or lid abnormalities, such as entropion, ectropion and trichiasis which can lead to poor wound healing. Early suture removal in areas of corneal vascularization can also decrease the probability

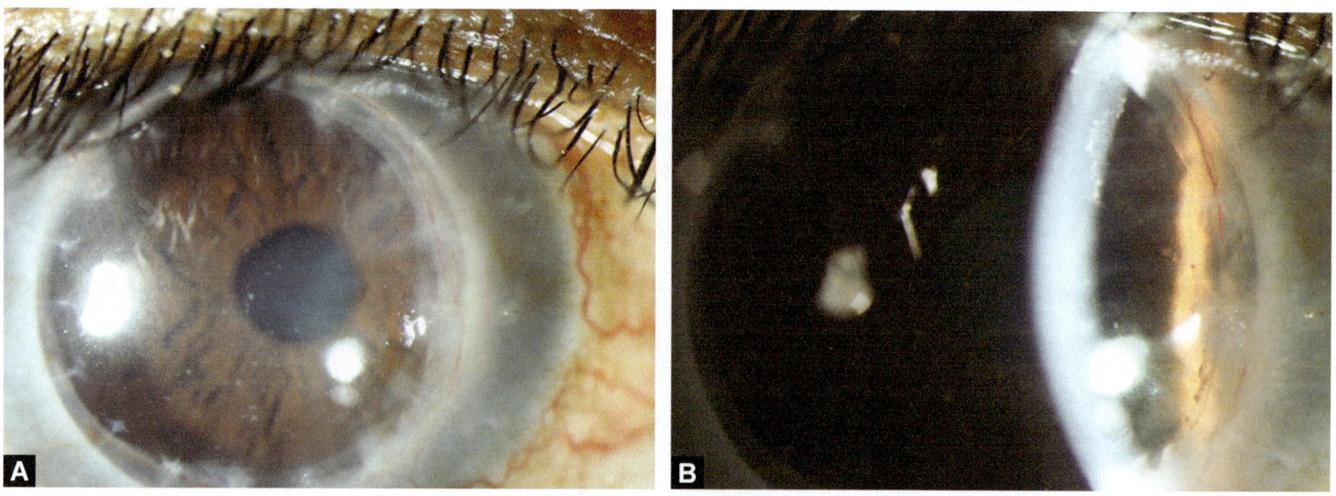

Figs. 30.1A and B: (A) Patient with acute graft rejection characterized by diffuse keratic precipitates on the graft and a Khodadoust line; (B) Close-up of Khodadoust line.

Source: N Venkatesh Prajna, Aravind Eye Hospitals, Madurai, Tamil Nadu, India.

of subsequent graft rejection. The role of systemic immunosuppression in the treatment of corneal allograft rejection is unknown.

Graft Failure

Graft failure is characterized by dysfunction of endothelial cells and subsequent irreversible corneal edema. Primary graft failure occurs in the early postoperative period and can be due to issues with the donor tissue or surgical trauma. Secondary graft failure occurs in a graft which was initially clear but becomes irreversibly cloudy. The risk of secondary graft failure can be related to a number of factors, including the indications for corneal transplant, donor characteristics such as age, episodes of rejection, or need for subsequent surgeries.[19] In the Corneal Donor Study, the largest prospective corneal transplant study to-date, the cumulative probability of graft failure in the low-risk condition Fuchs dystrophy was 20% compared to 37% for patients with pseudophakic bullous keratopathy.[19] Preexistent glaucoma requiring intraocular pressure lowering medications or with prior glaucoma surgery was also a significant risk factor for graft failure in this study with approximately 4 times the hazard of graft failure than those without glaucoma. Other large series have shown that indication for surgery is an important determinant of graft survival.[20-23] Table 30.2 outlines high and low-risk indications for corneal transplant.

The treatment for graft failure is repeat corneal transplant. Repeat EK is usually indicated for failed posterior lamellar transplant unless the anterior segment anatomy has become significantly distorted with extensive peripheral anterior synechiae. In the case of a failed penetrating keratoplasty, EK may be an option if the view is adequate and there is not a large amount of corneal astigmatism. It is advisable to avoid stripping Descemet's membrane (DM) in these cases since stripping could destabilize the graft-host junction. Undersizing the EK by 0.25–0.50 mm compared with the PKP will improve graft adherence. There may be an increased risk of graft dislocation in these cases therefore, placement of a retention suture can be beneficial. In the case of multiple failed grafts, a keratoprosthesis can be considered.

Table 30.2: Indication for surgery and prognosis.

Prognosis	Condition
Very favorable prognosis	• Keratoconus (graft <8 mm) • Fuchs' dystrophy • Localized corneal opacity (less than one half of cornea with clear, deep layers and without vascularization)
Favorable prognosis	• Keratoconus (graft of 8 mm or more) • Hereditary granular, macular, and lattice dystrophies • Aphakic bullous keratopathy • Lipid degeneration (without large vessels)
Less favorable prognosis	• Herpes zoster and simplex keratitis • Corneal opacity from infectious keratitis • Trachoma • Chemical burns (variable prognosis depending on area, density, and vascularization)
Unfavorable prognosis	• Active infectious keratitis • Multiple graft failures • Congenital hereditary dystrophy/opacity • Leprosy • Severe chemical burns • Pemphigoid • Stevens-Johnson syndrome • Severe graft-versus-host disease

Femtosecond Laser-assisted Penetrating Keratoplasty

Astigmatism is a significant concern when performing a PKP. Recently, the femtosecond laser has been proposed as a tool to reduce astigmatism during transplantation. It is theorized that by cutting the host and donor corneas with the laser into zigzag, top-hat, or mushroom shapes, graft-host congruence is enhanced, reducing suture tension and therefore, reducing astigmatism and improving vision.[24]

Therapeutic Penetrating Keratoplasty

Therapeutic penetrating keratoplasty (TPK) is performed "au chaud" for acute infectious keratitis in cases not responding to medical therapy, to avoid scleral extension or for tectonic support. Perforation and/or the need for TPK is more common in fungal than bacterial or herpetic keratitis. Baseline features such as presence of hypopyon and large, deep infiltrates are predictors of perforation and TPK. Culture positivity after starting therapy is also an early indicator of lack of response to therapy and is a risk factor for eventuating to TPK.[25]

These grafts are known to have a high risk of graft rejection and failure and the optimal timing of TPK to prevent these complications is unknown.[26] More recently, deep anterior lamellar keratoplasty (DALK) has been proposed as an alternative to traditional penetrating keratoplasty because it preserves the host endothelium and likely reduces the risk of intraocular spread of infection.[27]

ANTERIOR LAMELLAR KERATOPLASTY

Indications and Outcomes

In stromal diseases, such as KCN, other stromal dystrophies, such as granular, or postinfectious stromal scars, anterior lamellar keratoplasty is preferred. DALK removes diseased stromal layers while leaving healthy DM intact. Numerous case reports have suggested that potential advantages of this technique include fewer intraoperative risks, such as expulsive hemorrhage, decreased risk of wound dehiscence with ocular trauma, decreased rates of rejection and endothelial cell loss as well as early suture removal and earlier visual recovery.[28]

Several small clinical trials have randomized patients with stromal diseases to DALK versus PKP and have found relatively comparable visual acuity outcomes with reduced endothelial cell loss and rejection rates among the DALK patients.[29-31] From these data, a recent Cochrane review concluded that there was no evidence of a difference in visual acuity or graft survival between PKP and DALK, although they did find some moderate evidence of decreased immune rejection in DALK (Figs. 30.2 and 30.3).[32] Similarly, the American Academy of Ophthalmology has concluded that there is no advantage to DALK over PKP for best corrected visual acuity (BCVA) or refractive error, but may be an advantage in reduced endothelial cell loss and graft rejection.[33] In contrast the Australian Corneal Transplant Registry recently published the results of its cohort study, which showed that PKP grafts had improved survival over DALK in patients with KCN.[34]

Techniques

The techniques for performing DALK which have been described include the manual layer technique, and the big-bubble technique. Manual layer by layer stromal dissection generally results in residual posterior stroma which has been associated with interface scarring and decreased visual acuity compared with PKP. Anwar's big-bubble technique has increased in popularity as it significantly increases the rate of complete baring of DM and results in visual acuity outcomes more similar to PKP.

Figures 30.3A to H demonstrate the steps of DALK. Briefly after partial thickness trephination, a dissector is used to dissect through the layers of stroma to just anterior to DM advancing 2–4 mm to a pericentral location of the cornea. An air cannula is then placed in the track created by the dissector and advanced to just beyond the location of the dissector and air is injected forcefully separating DM from the overlying stroma. Once the big bubble has been created, a stab incision is used to release the air and allow for the anterior stromal layers to be removed in quadrants with blunt tipped scissors. Finally, the new cornea which is oversized by 0.25 mm is sutured into place (Fig. 30.4). Melles has described a DM barring technique which has similar outcomes but may have reduced contrast sensitivity compared with Anwar's technique.[35]

Management of Complications

If a big bubble is not achieved on the first try, further attempts can be performed in different locations of the cornea. Manual dissection of the most anterior layers of

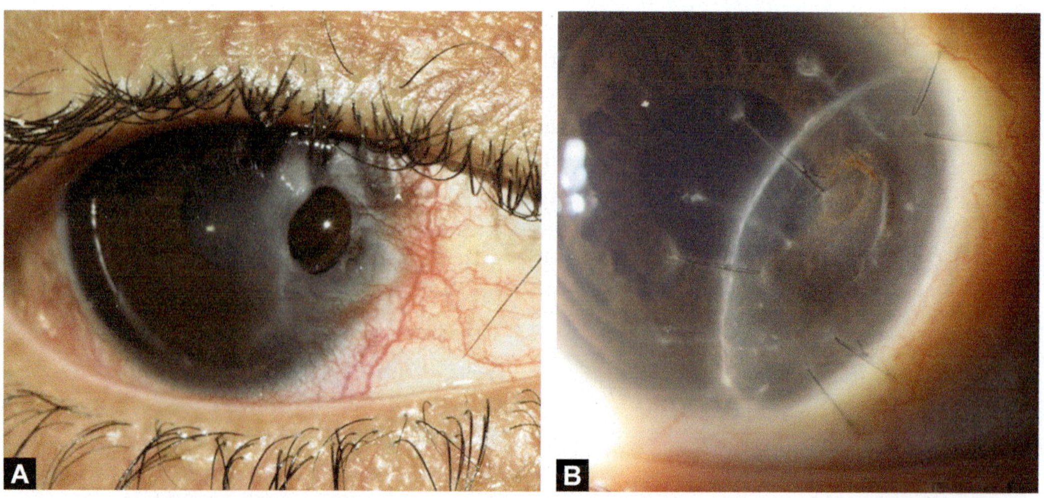

Figs. 30.2A and B: (A) Patient with interstitial keratitis presenting with decreased vision and corneal perforation; (B) 4 months postlamellar graft, visual acuity is 20/25.

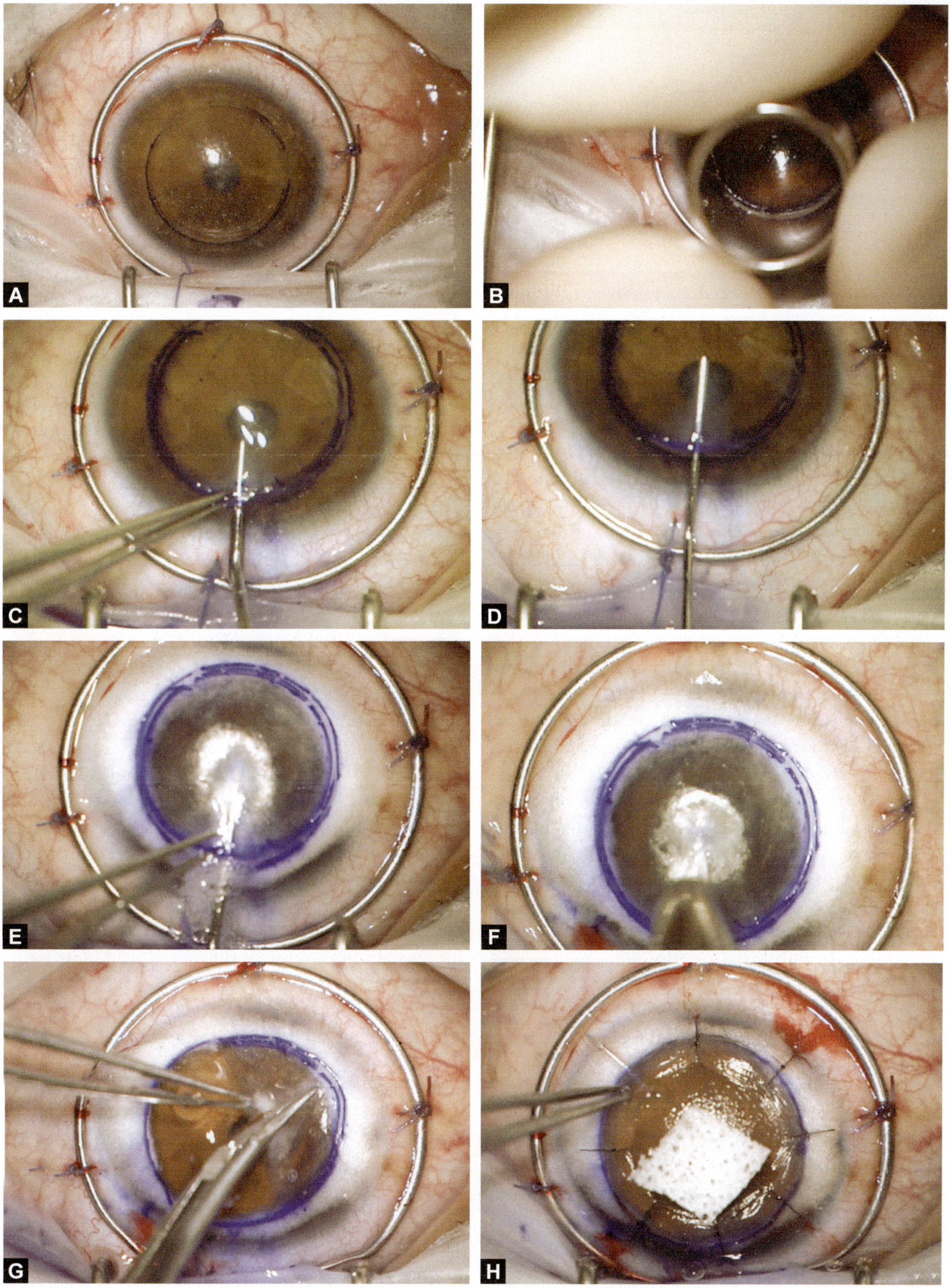

Figs. 30.3A to H: Surgical steps of DALK. (A) Encompass the ectasia; (B) Partial thickness trephination; (C) Fogla dissector; (D) Fogla 27 gauge air injector; (E) Use of air injector to create the big bubble; (F) Brave slash; (G) Removal of stroma in quadrants; (H) Donor secured with interrupted sutures.

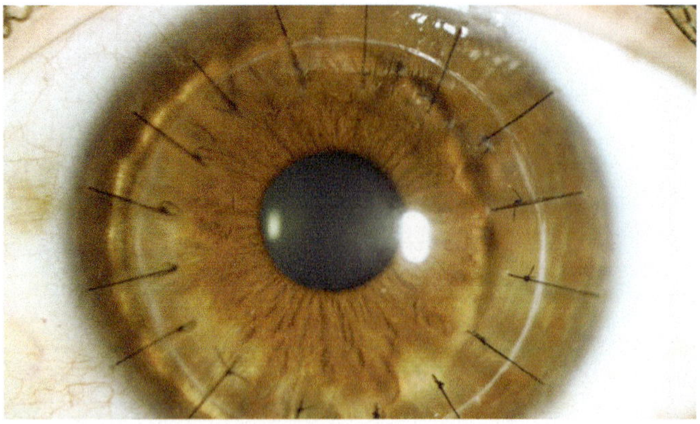

Fig. 30.4: Two-months postoperative after DALK with uncorrected visual acuity of 20/25 (same patient as Fig. 30.3).

the cornea may aid in visualization and increase the rate of successful big bubble in subsequent attempts.

Microperforation can occur at any stage in DALK. It is important not to use viscoelastic in the anterior chamber as it will likely exit the perforation and cause it to expand in size. An air bubble injected into the anterior chamber can serve the dual function of tamponading the perforation and aiding in locating the perforation so that further manipulation of the tissue in the area of perforation can be minimized. Dissection of stroma in the area of perforation should be left until the rest of DM has been fully barred. A small amount of residual stroma can be left over the perforation if it is outside of the central cornea where it might affect the visual outcome. In cases of microperforation, an approximately 80% air bubble should be left in the anterior chamber and the patient should be dilated with atropine to avoid pupillary block. The patient should be positioned supine postoperatively to prevent fluid from collecting between the new donor cornea and the patients DM, so-called "double anterior chamber." If a double anterior chamber is apparent postoperatively, injecting an air bubble into the anterior chamber behind DM and positioning the patient will resolve the problem mostly.

ENDOTHELIAL KERATOPLASTY

Posterior lamellar keratoplasty, which replaces only diseased endothelium and DM, has led to faster recovery times, fewer complications and better visual acuity outcomes compared to traditional PKP.[36] Studies have shown that cataract surgery combined with EK is safe and results in similar outcomes.[37,38] Currently in developed countries, Descemet's stripping automated endothelial keratoplasty (DSAEK) is the most common type of posterior lamellar keratoplasty, because of its relative ease and good outcomes.[39] In this surgery, the diseased endothelium and Descemet's membrane is replaced with donor tissue comprising of a little bit of stroma, DM and endothelium. The donor tissue is usually around 150 µm. Ultrathin-DSAEK (UT-DSAEK) involves similar surgical techniques to DSAEK but donor grafts are prepared to be less than 100 µm thick. UT-DSAEK has been shown in a recent well-designed randomized controlled trial to have superior visual acuity results compared with traditional DSAEK.[40] In this study, the average graft thickness for UT-DSAEK was 101 µm compared with an average of 209 µm for traditional DSAEK. At 12 months, the average visual acuity was 20/26 among UT-DSAEK and 20/31 for DSAEK ($P = 0.03$).

A newer technique, Descemet's membrane endothelial keratoplasty (DMEK), where only DM and the endothelium is transplanted, has the potential to further improve visual acuity outcomes, produce fewer higher-order corneal aberrations and decrease rejection rates.[41-45] A few large series in the literature report excellent outcomes with DMEK surgery. One such study by Melles' group published results of a large cohort of 500 DMEK procedures performed by 2 surgeons and reported that 41% of study participants had visual acuity of 20/20 or better by 6 months, while 75% achieved a visual acuity of 20/25 or better.[46] In this series only 2.2% of patients required repeat grafting.

These visual acuity results of DMEK, however, may not be generalizable. According to the Eye Bank Association of America, DMEK still accounted for less than 15% of endothelial keratoplasties in the United States in 2015, while DSAEK accounted for about 50% of all corneal transplants.[47,48] This suggests that the majority of endothelial keratoplasty surgeons in the United States have not yet adopted DMEK or are early on the DMEK learning curve. The surgeon-learning curve, which may be anywhere from 20–75 cases, is steep.[42] Donor preparation, increased intraoperative times and problems with donor attachment in DMEK are challenges.[49,50] A second Melles series reported outcomes of 431 DMEK's performed by 18 experienced Melles-trained corneal surgeons in 11 countries during the surgeon-learning curve.[51] In this study, only 43.8% of participants achieved 20/25 or better visual acuity by 6 months and only 18.8% achieved 20/20 visual acuity or better. It is important to note that almost 50% of study participants were excluded from visual acuity analysis in this series because they had a second surgery or had graft failure which means that these data are likely generous regarding visual acuity outcomes in DMEK. The re-bubble rate was also much higher at 20%.

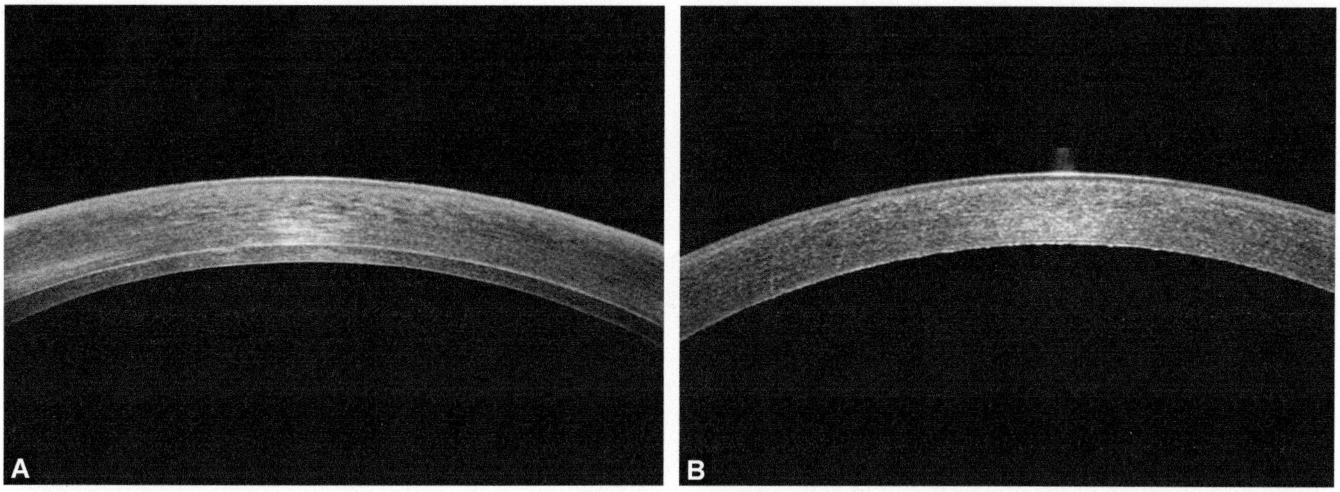

Figs. 30.5A and B: (A) Anterior segment optical coherence tomography—Descemet's stripping endothelial keratoplasty (DSEK), note the graft is of approximately 100 µm thickness; (B) Descemet's membrane endothelial keratoplasty (DMEK)—note near anatomic replacement of tissue.

Figures 30.5A and B compare anterior segment optical coherence tomography for DSAEK and DMEK. Given the added tissue thickness of the donor lenticule in DSAEK, there is a hyperopic shift of approximately 1.0 Diopter postoperatively. If a patient is undergoing cataract surgery but may require DSAEK in the future, it is advisable to target their refractive outcome to approximately -1.00 to avoid subsequent hyperopia. This is also true if combination cataract surgery and DSAEK are performed simultaneously. Although DMEK may also result in a mild hyperopic shift in some patients, it appears to be lessened compared with DSAEK.

Postoperative endothelial cell counts have been shown to correlate with risk of subsequent graft failure in PKP.[19] The rate and pattern of endothelial cell loss after endothelial keratoplasty is different than that of PKP with a larger initial drop but slower rate of subsequent cell loss. This may be due to differences in endothelial trauma during surgery with more central damage in DSAEK resulting in an initial decrease in endothelial cells.[52] More peripheral trauma during PKP results in better central endothelial counts at first but peripheral migration of residual endothelial cells may cause the continued decline in central endothelial counts seen over time.[53] Other possible factors include decreased rejection in endothelial keratoplasty. Rates of endothelial cell loss in DMEK appear to be around 39% at 5 years which may be improved compared with DSAEK and are much better than those reported in PKP.[19,54-56] These data must be interpreted with caution as a 5-year follow-up was available for only 4.2% of the initial cohort in the DMEK series and there was no mention of the number of graft failures during that time. This highlights the need for a more rigorous study of these techniques.

DMEK may provide better visual acuity outcomes in carefully selected patients, however it may also carry more risk of donor tissue damage, repeat surgery and higher cost to society. A randomized clinical trial comparing outcomes of DMEK and UT-DSAEK, Descemet Endothelial Thickness Comparison Trial (DETECT) found DMEK patients to have almost 2 lines improved visual acuity over UT-DSAEK 6 months postoperatively when correcting for baseline visual acuity.[57] This study is ongoing and will be following patients for 24 months postoperatively (*https://clinicaltrials.gov/show/NCT02373137*).

DSEK Techniques

Donor preparation includes mounting the donor corneal tissue on an artificial anterior chamber device. In DSEK, the surgeon creates the donor lenticule by performing a manual lamellar dissection while in DSAEK this dissection is created using a microkeratome to provide smooth interface at a prespecified depth with a single pass. The resultant donor lenticule is approximately 100–150 µm depending on surgeon preference. Standardization of surgical techniques likely reduces intraoperative and postoperative complications in endothelial keratoplasty.[57] Terry et al. have described a standardized approach to DSEK where Descemet's membrane is stripped from the receipt bed, peripheral stromal fibrils are roughened with a Terry Scrapper (Bausch & Lomb Surgical) to aid with donor attachment and the donor tissue is folded in a 60–40 taco configuration and inserted into the anterior chamber using forceps. The graft is opened using fluid and an air bubble is inserted into the anterior chamber. Interface fluid is swept away by compressing the cornea externally with a Cindy Sweeper (Bausch & Lomb Surgical).

Improving DSEK insertion techniques to reduce operative times, increased rates of donor attachment and reduced endothelial cell loss has been a significant research focus over the last 2 decades. In forceps insertion, variations in surgical technique may greatly influence endothelial cell loss. For example, larger incision sizes and clear corneal rather than scleral tunnels may result in less tissue compression.[59] Additionally, single-point fixation forceps result in less endothelial cell trauma than forceps which apply compression throughout the graft.[59]

Other techniques such as insertion of the donor lenticule with the Sheets Glide avoids the trauma associated with folding and grasping of the allograft and may be superior to forceps insertion.[60] However, a number of graft insertion devices have been developed which likely further reduce endothelial cell damage. Most have been shown to have less endothelial cell loss compared with forceps insertion.[60-63] EndoGlide has been shown to have less endothelial cell loss than Sheets glide.[64] The EndoSerter has been shown in one small trial to have equivalent cell loss and donor detachment rates compared to the EndoGlide.[65]

DMEK Techniques

Prepeeled corneal tissue prepared by eye banks has significantly improved upon the safety and ease of DMEK.[66] Vision Blue (DORC- Zuidland, Netherlands) can be used to identify the edge of Descemet membrane.

The central Descemet disk can be separated from stroma under Optisol GS using the SCUBA technique[42] by gently lifting the graft from Descemet side with a single tine of a McPherson tier and then grasping in 1 peripheral point to complete the peel. The scrolled central disc is stained with Vision blue for 5 minutes and then rinsed with balanced salt solution.

In preparing the recipient, inferior iridotomies can be made by passing a 30 g needle through the inferior peripheral iris in 3 separate locations. Other than the peripheral iridotomies, recipient preparation and stripping of Descemet's membrane is performed as described previously for DSEK however, scraping of recipient donor is unnecessary and may result in decreasing the chance of graft unscrolling and adherence in the stromal fibrils.

There have been a number of insertion techniques which have been described. Most commonly insertion is performed either with a truncated AMO intraocular lens injector (Abbott Medical Optics, Santa Ana, CA) attached with polypropylene tubing to a 3.0 cc syringe that was preloaded with balanced salt solution (BSS) or with a modified Jones Tube in a similar fashion.[58] The Geuder glass cannula (Geuder AG, Heidelberg, Germany) is a newer injection device that is gaining popularity. The incision is closed with 10.0 nylon suture and the chamber is shallowed to allow fluid waves generated by gentle peripheral corneal taps to orient and unfurl the graft under the host. A full air-fill is performed to a pressure of approximately 30–40 mm Hg for 10 minutes and then the air bubble is reduced to 80% volume and the anterior chamber returned to physiologic pressure.

Eyes with Complex Anatomy

Eyes with glaucoma tubes or complex anatomy such as peripheral anterior synechiae, aphakia or anterior chamber lenses are likely more appropriately managed with DSEK. In particular the pullthrough technique in which a preplaced 10-0 prolene suture pulls the graft into the eye and secures it. It can be used when there is a risk of the graft dislocating into the posterior chamber as in eyes with scleral-sutured intraocular lenses or aphakia. Figures 30.6A to F outline the steps of the pull through technique.

Management of Complications

Primary graft failure occurs approximately 1–3% of the time in DSAEK/UT-DSAEK and has been reported in 1- 20% of DMEKs.[40,58,67,68] The re-bubble rate for DSAEK is approximately 1–10% and DMEK is 2.2–20%.[40,58,68] Using standardized surgical techniques, switching to SF6 gas for the air bubble and positioning for 1 or more days postoperatively have all been advocated as techniques to minimize surgical complications and re-bubbling in endothelial keratoplasty (Figs. 30.7 and 30.8).[69]

PEDIATRIC PENETRATING KERATOPLASTY

Indications

Approximately 88 children are born annually in the United States with congenital corneal opacity.[70] Nischal et al. have proposed a novel classification of congenital corneal opacification.[71] Under this classification, conditions with well-defined genetics such as the endothelial dystrophies, sclerocornea, corneal dermoids and CYP1B1 cytopathy would be considered primary corneal diseases.

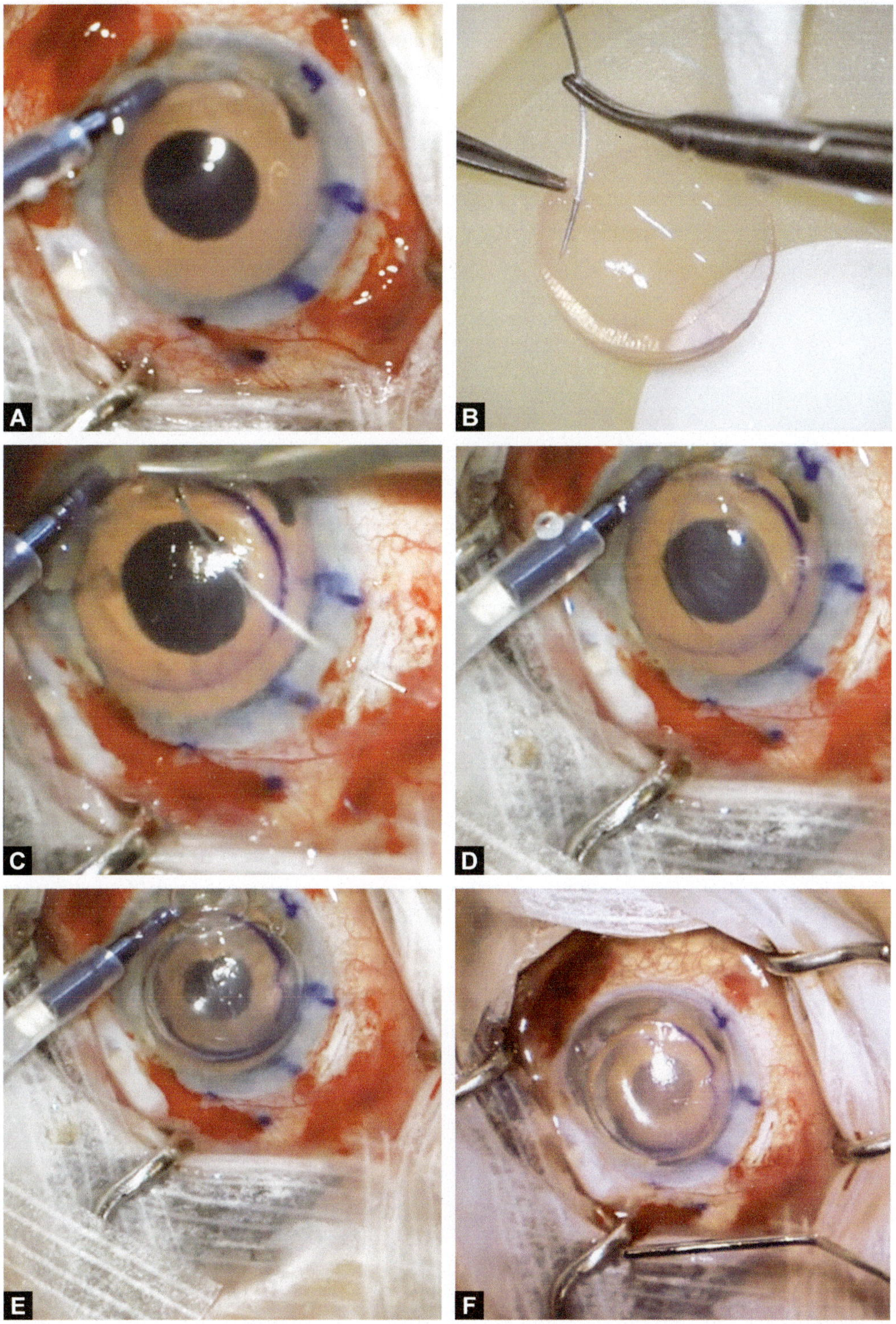

Figs. 30.6A to F: Surgical steps of EK pull through technique. (A) Patient with history of traumatic aniridia and corneal edema status-post iris reconstruction with a scleral sutured aniridia lens. Patient is set up for DSEK by creating a scleral tunnel, two paracenteses, and placing an anterior chamber maintainer; (B) Viscoelastic is placed on the donor endothelium and it is folded in a taco configuration. An anchoring stitch with double armed 10-0 prolene on a CIF-4 needle is passed through the stroma; (C) Both CIF-4 needles are passed through the scleral tunnel through the anterior chamber and out of the nasal cornea approximately 1 mm apart, keeping in mind the orientation of the tissue as this will form the retention suture; (D) The graft is pulled into the anterior chamber using the two ends of the prolene sutures; (E) An air bubble is injected into the anterior chamber to unfold the graft; (F) The two ends of the prolene suture are tied to form the retention suture.

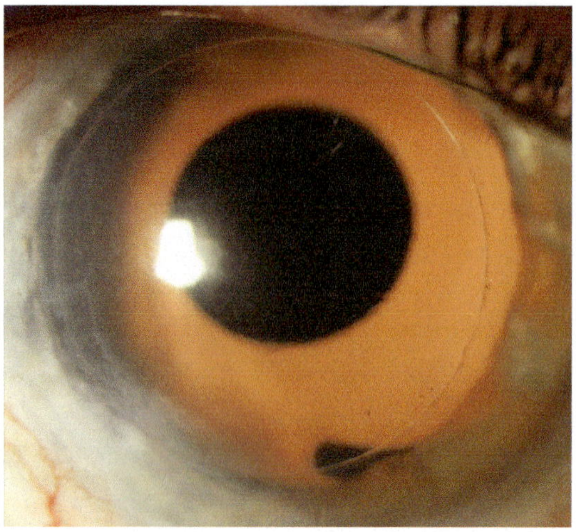

Fig. 30.7: Complex DSAEK in patient with history of traumatic aphakia and aniridia as well as glaucoma status post-trabeculectomy. He underwent placement of the Ophtec lens followed by DSAEK utilizing the pull through technique. 2 years postoperatively uncorrected visual acuity is 20/30 and BSCVA is 20/25 (Same patient as Fig. 30.6).

In secondary developmental corneal diseases, the genotype does not fully explain the phenotype and this includes conditions such as Peter's syndrome, congenital glaucoma with corneal edema, Axenfeld-Rieger syndrome and aniridia.[71] Other acquired conditions which may result in the need for pediatric corneal transplants include trauma, metabolic disorders, infection (Herpes, bacterial or fungal), neurotrophic keratitis and Stevens-Johnson syndrome.[72]

The majority of congenital opacity in the United States are due to Peters anomaly and associated with mutations in PAX6, PITX2 or FOXCI. Peters syndrome type 1 manifests with iridocorneal adhesions while type 2 has cataract or lenticular adhesions to the cornea. Peters plus syndrome has systemic manifestations such as cleft lip or palate, short stature, developmental delay or abnormalities of the ear, heart, brain or genitourinary system.

The etiology of Peter's syndrome relates to a primary mesodermal dysgenesis with incomplete mesenchymal cell migration and focal absence of DM and endothelium. If the opacity is central in location, optical iridectomy is the best option. Creating an eccentric opening in the iris allows the patient to see around the central scar while preserving their native cornea (Figs. 30.9A to C).

Perioperative Considerations

When optical iridectomy is not an option, PKP may be performed. Figures 30.10A to C demonstrate a patient with total corneal opacity from Peters syndrome who underwent PKP. This procedure presents with a number of challenges.[72,73] Preoperatively, one must consider the amount of amblyopia, concurrent ocular conditions such as glaucoma and place goals of care in the context of the patient's systemic condition. Intraoperatively, the surgery is technically demanding due to microphthalmia, low scleral rigidity and positive posterior pressure which can result in iris and lens extrusion, suprachoroidal hemorrhage and retinal detachment. Postoperatively, aggressive management of inflammation, suture removal, secondary glaucoma and increased risk of infections are all challenging and require repeated examination under anesthesia.

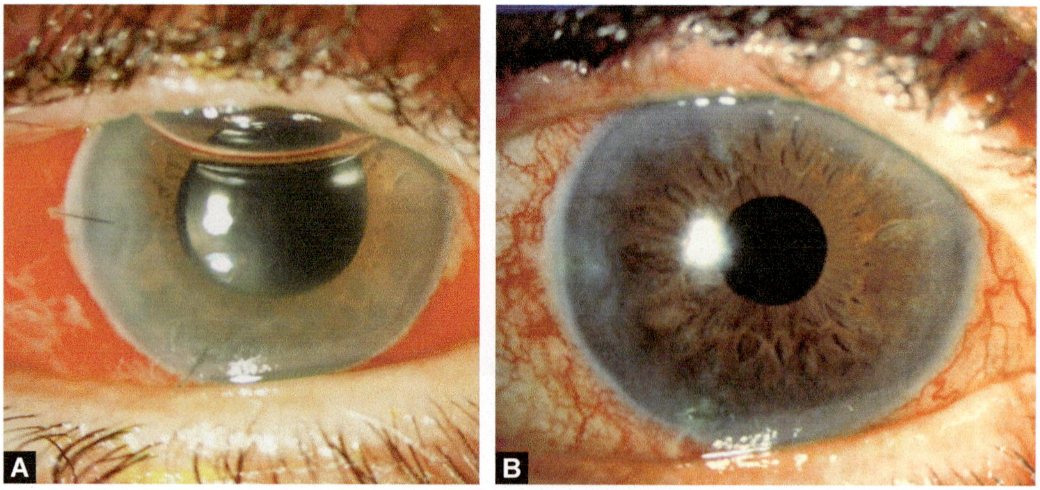

Figs. 30.8A and B: (A) 1 day post-DMEK triple with uncorrected visual acuity of 20/40; (B) 1 week post-DMEK triple with uncorrected visual acuity of 20/20.

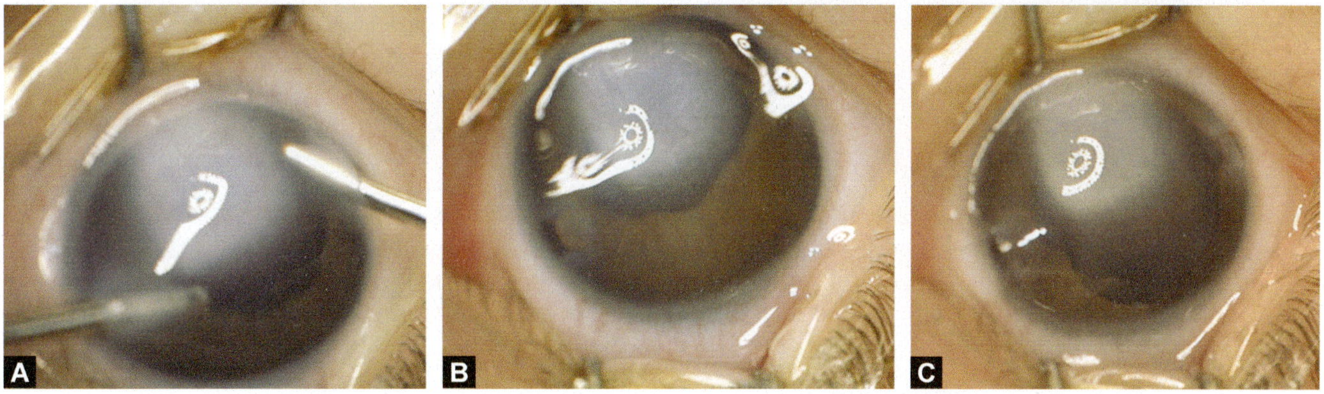

Figs. 30.9A to C: Surgical steps of a pediatric iridectomy. (A) Patient cannot see because of corneal opacity overlapping pupil; (B) Anterior vitrector is used to remove iris tissue; (C) Peripheral iridectomy allowing patient to see through clear cornea.
Source: Alejandra De Alba, UCSF Ophthalmology, USA.

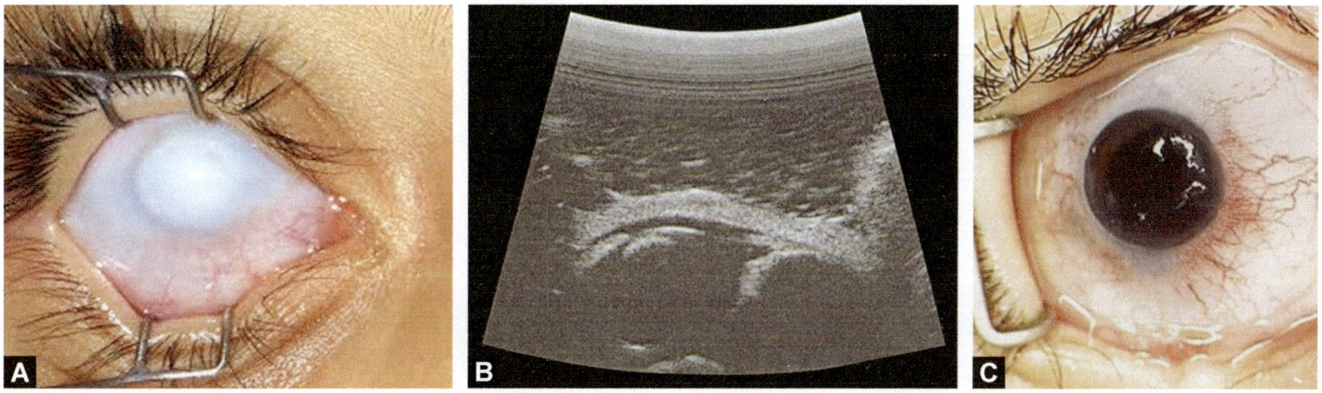

Figs. 30.10A to C: (A) A 2-year-old girl with cloudy corneas since birth. C section birth at 36-week gestational age. She had no family history of ocular disease and no known systemic abnormalities. UBM of the right eye reveals an absent anterior chamber, lenticular and iridocorneal touch and a cataractous lens; (B) UBM of the left eye revealed a shallow anterior chamber with iridocorneal touch, no lenticular-corneal touch and normal lens. The patient underwent penetrating keratoplasty with over-lay technique. She subsequently required Ahmed's tube placement and cataract extraction; (C) One year later, her vision had improved from LP to HM allowing her improved ambulation, her IOP was well controlled and corneal graft was clear and she wore aphakic spectacles.

Novel Techniques

A Mcneill-Goldmann scleral fixation ring or a Flerigaring can prevent scleral collapse and provide globe fixation to the drape. The donor diameter should be between 5.5 mm and 7 mm with donor tissue oversized by 0.5 -1.0 mm due to increased corneal and scleral elasticity which can cause cheese-wiring and compromise wound closure. Interrupted or running sutures can be appropriate during pediatric corneal transplants as they are typically removed quite early in the postoperative period. In babies under 6 months of age, all sutures should be removed within 4–6 weeks postoperatively. The overlay technique has been developed to minimize the risk of expulsion of intraocular contents as is so common with children. Figures 30.11A to H show a small child with Peters anomaly who underwent corneal transplantation with the overlay technique and outlines surgical steps.

Prognosis

Prognosis is poor and graft survival in the literature is reported at between 50% and 85% depending on indications for surgery and age at time of keratoplasty.[72,74,75] Common complications include loose sutures, corneal infections, graft failure, glaucoma and amblyopia.

Keratoprosthesis

The concept of Keratoprosthesis is over 200 years old and was first introduced by Pellier de Quengsy who described a

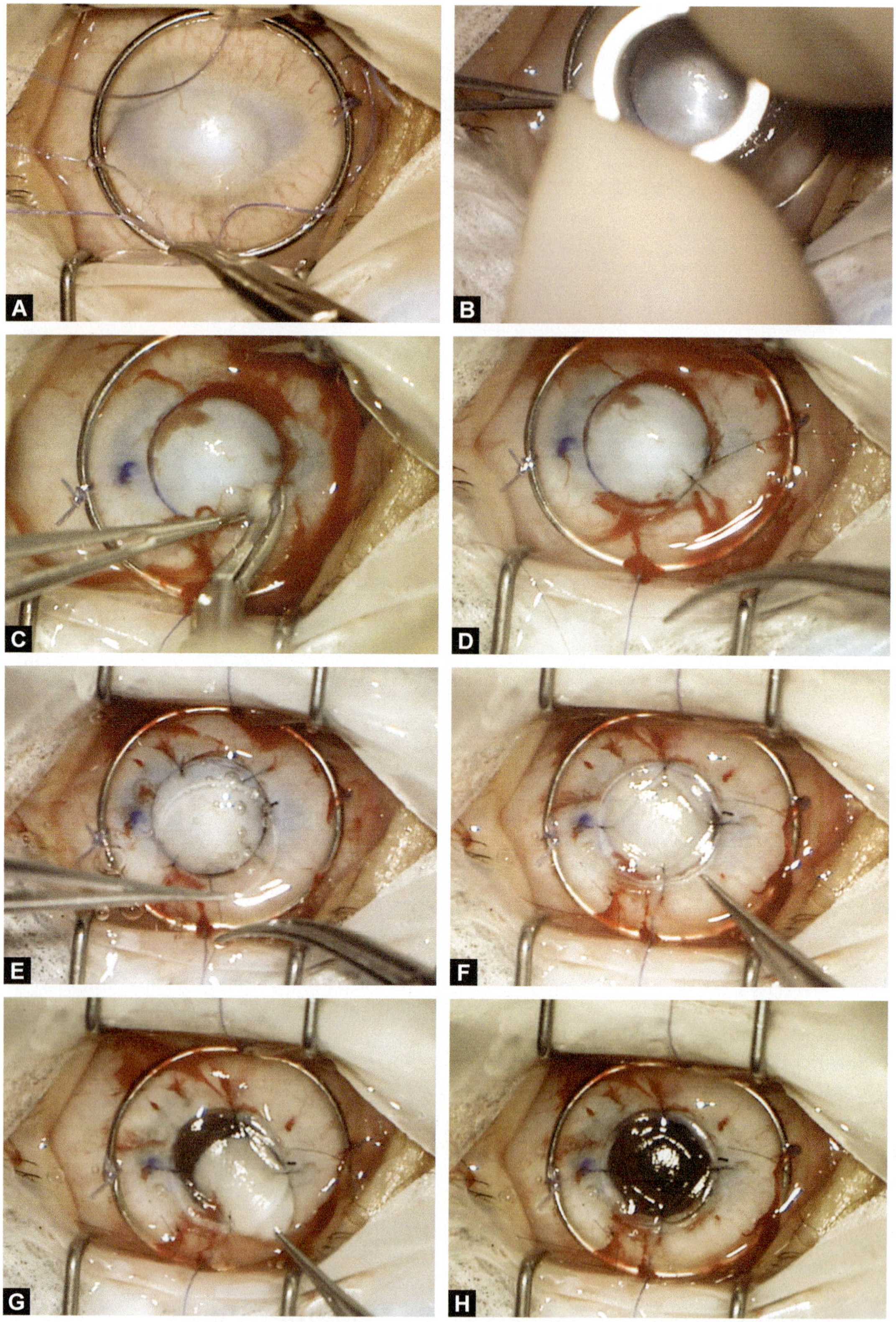

Figs. 30.11A to H: Surgical steps of pediatric keratoplasty with overlay technique on the patient from Figure 30.10. (A) Place Flieringa ring; (B) Partial thickness trephination; (C) Excise one quadrant at a time; (D) Place anchoring sutures in four quadrants; (E) Cover cornea with viscoelastic and overlay new cornea; (F) Place four cardinal sutures; (G) Remove the old cornea from underneath the new one; (H) This technique has preserved the patient's native lens and iris tissue.

quartz implant in 1789 that is strikingly similar to modern keratoprosthesis design.[76] The first to report implantation of a device was Nussbaum in 1853.[77] However, it was not until the discovery of inert plastic and antibiotics that retention rates were improved enough to make keratoprosthesis a viable alternative to cadaveric transplantation.

Current Keratoprosthesis Designs

In the 1960s, Claes Dohlman introduced the Boston Keratoprosthesis with its collar button design; now the Boston Type 1 Keratoprosthesis is the most popular type of keratoprosthesis implanted with over 4500 procedures performed worldwide (Fig. 30.12). Type 2 Keratoprosthesis Alternative Keratoprostheses include the Osteo-odonto Keratoprosthesis and AlphaCor.

Indications for Surgery and Preoperative Selection

Keratoprosthesis (Kpro) is indicated for patients with history of severe limbal stem cell deficiency from inherited conditions such as aniridia or from chemical injury and a history of multiple failed corneal grafts.[78,79] Patients with history of severe autoimmune disease such as Stevens-Johnson and ocular cicatricial pemphigoid are known to have inferior retention rates compared with other indications.[80] There is currently controversy surrounding the safety and efficacy of Kpro in children with proponents advocating that this could reduce amblyopia and graft failure that complicate pediatric corneal transplantation and opponents suggesting that complications of Kpro can result in devastating results such as complete loss of vision and/or the eye.[81]

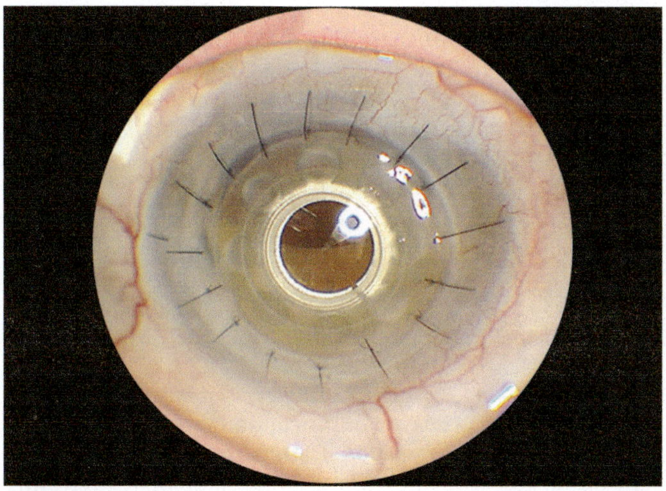

Fig. 30.12: Boston keratoprosthesis type 1 in a patient with history of multiple failed corneal transplants and visual acuity of bare hand motions. She underwent combined Boston Kpro and Ahmed tube shunt. Postoperative best corrected visual acuity remains 20/30 three years later with excellent glaucoma control on Cosopt.
(Kpro: Keratoprosthesis)

Preoperative patient selection is extremely important in these cases to reduce the occurence of postoperative complications. Excellent tear production, normal lid apposition, and consideration of comorbid ocular conditions such as glaucoma and autoimmune disease are essential to long-term retention of the prosthesis and optimal visual acuity results.[82]

Complications Unique to Boston Keratoprosthesis

The most common complication is retroprosthetic membrane (RPM) formation which can usually be managed with YAG-laser when addressed early on. Posterior offset and using no more than 3.0 mJ with a can-opener style approach reduces the likelihood of injury to the prosthesis.[83] When the RPM is dense it may require surgical membranectomy or even replacement of the prosthesis altogether.

Infection is another major concern due to a lack of biointegration. The lack of formation of a complete epithelial barrier allows for the introduction of bacteria or fungi resulting in keratitis or endophthalmitis. Prevention has been focused on reducing load of organisms on the surface of the eye by using prophylactic antibiotics and betadine rinses. Overall risk of endophthalmitis dramatically decreases with prophylactic topical antibiotics possibly as low as 0.35% per patient year. In one retrospective chart review, the topical vancomycin group had an endophthalmitis rate of 0.35% compared with 4.13% per patient year (P = 0.001).

Sterile corneal melt can occur and if not caught and managed aggressively early on can result in extrusion of the implant. Extended wear bandage contact lenses have reduced the occurrence of sterile melt.[84] Additionally, corneal crosslinking donor corneas may reduce this complication.[85]

Glaucoma is now the most common cause of visual loss among Boston Kpro patients.[86] Intraocular pressure monitoring is challenging. Concomitant glaucoma surgery is advised for all patients with preexisting glaucoma. Close optic nerve monitoring and collaboration with glaucoma colleagues familiar with kpro is essential to manage these patients.

Outcomes of Boston Keratoprosthesis

The largest multicenter cohort study-to-date followed 300 eyes from 19 surgeons at 18 medical centers.[87] Their main outcome measure was Kpro retention. With an average follow up of 17 months, the overall retention rate was 94% at 1 year and 89% at 2 years. Retroprosthetic membrane formation occurred 30% of the time and infectious keratitis occurred in 3% with 78% (7/9) of the infections being fungal in nature. Endophthalmitis occurred in 2 patients (0.6%). Risk factors for Kpro retention failure included autoimmune disease, greater than 3-prior graft failures and severe ocular surface disease requiring tarsorrhaphy. This cohort also reported improved visual acuity results with a mean final visual acuity of logMAR 0.64 (Snellen 20/150).[88] In other series, international eye centers have found similar retention rates to US centers.[89]

Keratoprosthesis appears to be a viable option in carefully selected patients in the appropriate settings with access to skilled glaucoma and retina colleagues who can manage potential complications. These patients require lifelong eye drops, contact lenses and monitoring for infectious keratitis, sterile melt, endophthalmitis and glaucoma. There is certainly room for improvement in the future and prostheses with improved biocompatibility would likely reduce the infectious complications.

CONCLUSION

Given the recent evolution of the field of corneal transplant, the cornea surgeon is now well-equipped to address visually significant corneal pathology. Selectively transplanting only the diseased layer of the cornea is leading to improved patient outcomes.

REFERENCES

1. America Eye Bank Association. 2015 Eye Banking Statistical Report. Washington: AEBA; 2016.
2. Gain P, Jullienne R, He Z, et al. Global Survey of Corneal Transplantation and Eye Banking. JAMA Ophthalmol. 2016;134(2):167-73.
3. Pascolini D, Mariotti SP. Global estimates of visual impairment: 2010. Br J Ophthalmol. 2012;96(5):614-8.
4. Moffatt SL, Cartwright VA, Stumpf TH. Centennial review of corneal transplantation. Clin Exp Ophthalmol. 2005;33(6):642-57.
5. Coster DJ. Doyne Lecture. Influences on the development of corneal transplantation. Eye. 1994;8(Pt 1):1-11.
6. Mannis MM, Albert, D. Corneal transplantation: a history in profiles. Belgium: JP Wayenborgh; 1999.
7. Mannis MJ, Krachmer JH. Keratoplasty: a historical perspective. Surv Ophthalmol. 1981;25(5):333-8.
8. Forstot SL, Kaufman HE. Corneal transplantation. Ann Rev Med. 1977;28:21-35.
9. Crawford AZ, Patel DV, McGhee C. A brief history of corneal transplantation: From ancient to modern. Oman J Ophthalmol. 2013;6(Suppl 1):S12-7.
10. Tan DT, Dart JK, Holland EJ, et al. Corneal transplantation. Lancet. 2012;379(9827):1749-61.
11. Terry MA. Endothelial keratoplasty: history, current state, and future directions. Cornea. 2006;25(8):873-8.
12. Maeno A, Naor J, Lee HM, et al. Three decades of corneal transplantation: indications and patient characteristics. Cornea. 2000;19(1):7-11.
13. Mamalis N, Anderson CW, Kreisler KR, et al. Changing trends in the indications for penetrating keratoplasty. Arch Ophthalmol. 1992;110(10):1409-11.
14. Pineros O, Cohen EJ, Rapuano CJ, et al. Long-term results after penetrating keratoplasty for Fuchs' endothelial dystrophy. Arch Ophthalmol. 1996;114(1):15-8.
15. Quigley C, McElnea E, Fahy G. Trends in corneal transplant surgery in Ireland: indications and outcomes of corneal transplant surgery and intraocular lens opacification following Descemet's stripping automated endothelial keratoplasty. Ir J Med Sci; 2017.
16. Ayalew M, Tilahun Y, Holsclaw D, et al. Penetrating Keratoplasty at a Tertiary Referral Center in Ethiopia: Indications and Outcomes. Cornea. 2017;36(6):665-8.
17. Chaudhry TA, Sadiq SN, Sirang Z, et al. A 10-year review of indications for penetrating keratoplasty in a tertiary care setting in Karachi, Pakistan. Pak Med Assoc. 2016;66(10 Suppl 3):S84-6.
18. Bandivadekar P, Gupta S, Sharma N. Intraoperative Suprachoroidal Hemorrhage After Penetrating Keratoplasty: Case Series and Review of Literature. Eye Contact Lens. 2016;42(3):206-10.
19. Writing Committee for the Cornea Donor Study Research Group. Sugar A, Gal RL. Factors associated with corneal graft survival in the cornea donor study. JAMA Ophthalmol. 2015;133(3):246-54.
20. Tilahun Y, Shimelash D. The outcome of corneal transplantation versus indications in a tertiary eye care center in Ethiopia. Ethiop J Med J. 2010;48(1):35-9.
21. Dandona L, Naduvilath TJ, Janarthanan M, et al. Survival analysis and visual outcome in a large series of corneal transplants in India. Br J Ophthalmol. 1997;81(9):726-31.
22. Wagoner MD, Gonnah el S, Al-Towerki AE. King Khaled Eye Specialist Hospital Cornea Transplant Study Group. Outcome of primary adult penetrating keratoplasty in a Saudi Arabian population. Cornea. 2009;28(8):882-90.
23. Tabin GC, Gurung R, Paudyal G, et al. Penetrating keratoplasty in Nepal. Cornea. 2004;23(6):589-96.
24. Chamberlain WD, Rush SW, Mathers WD, et al. Comparison of femtosecond laser-assisted keratoplasty versus conventional penetrating keratoplasty. Ophthalmology. 2011;118(3):486-91.

25. Ray KJ, Lalitha P, Prajna NV, et al. The Utility of Repeat Culture in Fungal Corneal Ulcer Management: A Secondary Analysis of the MUTT-I Randomized Clinical Trial. Am J Opthalmol. 2017;178:157-627.
26. Tan DT, Janardhanan P, Zhou H, et al. Penetrating keratoplasty in Asian eyes: the Singapore Corneal Transplant Study. Ophthalmology. 2008;115(6):975-82.e1.
27. Sarnicola E, Sarnicola C, Sabatino F, et al. Early Deep Anterior Lamellar Keratoplasty (DALK) for Acanthamoeba Keratitis Poorly Responsive to Medical Treatment. Cornea. 2016;35(1):1-5.
28. van Dooren BT, Mulder PG, Nieuwendaal CP, et al. Endothelial cell density after deep anterior lamellar keratoplasty (Melles technique). Am J Ophthalmol. 2004;137(3):397-400.
29. Cheng YY, Visser N, Schouten JS, et al. Endothelial cell loss and visual outcome of deep anterior lamellar keratoplasty versus penetrating keratoplasty: a randomized multicenter clinical trial. Ophthalmology. 2011;118(2):302-9.
30. Javadi MA, Feizi S, Yazdani S, et al. Deep anterior lamellar keratoplasty versus penetrating keratoplasty for keratoconus: a clinical trial. Cornea. 2010;29(4):365-71.
31. Sogutlu Sari E, Kubaloglu A, Unal M, et al. Deep anterior lamellar keratoplasty versus penetrating keratoplasty for macular corneal dystrophy: a randomized trial. Am J Ophthalmol. 2013;156(2):267-74.e1.
32. Keane M, Coster D, Ziaei M, et al. Deep anterior lamellar keratoplasty versus penetrating keratoplasty for treating keratoconus. Cochr Database Sys. 2014;22(7):CD009700.
33. Reinhart WJ, Musch DC, Jacobs DS, et al. Deep anterior lamellar keratoplasty as an alternative to penetrating keratoplasty a report by the am academy of ophthalmology. Ophthalmology. 2011;118(1):209-18.
34. Coster DJ, Lowe MT, Keane MC, et al. Australian Corneal Graft Registry Contributors. A comparison of lamellar and penetrating keratoplasty outcomes: a registry study. Ophthalmology. 2014;121(5):979-87.
35. Baradaran-Rafii A, Eslani M, Sadoughi MM, et al. Anwar versus Melles deep anterior lamellar keratoplasty for keratoconus: a prospective randomized clinical trial. Ophthalmology. 2013;120(2):252-9.
36. Price FW Jr, Price MO. Evolution of endothelial keratoplasty. Cornea. 2013;32(Suppl 1):S28-32.
37. Terry MA, Shamie N, Chen ES, et al. Endothelial keratoplasty for Fuchs' dystrophy with cataract: complications and clinical results with the new triple procedure. Ophthalmology. 2009;116(4):631-9.
38. Chaurasia S, Price FW Jr, Gunderson L, et al. Descemet's membrane endothelial keratoplasty: clinical results of single versus triple procedures (combined with cataract surgery). Ophthalmology. 2014;121(2):454-8.
39. Chen ES, Terry MA, Shamie N, et al. Descemet-Stripping Automated Endothelial Keratoplasty: Six-month Results in a Prospective Study of 100 eyes. Cornea. 2008;27(5): 514-20.
40. Dickman MM, Kruit PJ, Remeijer L, et al. A Randomized Multicenter Clinical Trial of Ultrathin Descemet Stripping Automated Endothelial Keratoplasty (DSAEK) versus DSAEK. Ophthalmology. 2016;123(11):2276-84.
41. Ham L, Dapena I, van Luijk C, et al. Descemet membrane endothelial keratoplasty (DMEK) for Fuchs endothelial dystrophy: review of the first 50 consecutive cases. Eye. 2009;23(10):1990-8.
42. Price MO, Giebel AW, Fairchild KM, et al. Descemet's membrane endothelial keratoplasty: prospective multicenter study of visual and refractive outcomes and endothelial survival. Ophthalmology. 2009;116(12):2361-8.
43. Guerra FP, Anshu A, Price MO, et al. Endothelial keratoplasty: fellow eyes comparison of Descemet stripping automated endothelial keratoplasty and Descemet membrane endothelial keratoplasty. Cornea. 2011;30(12):1382-6.
44. Anshu A, Price MO, Price FW Jr. Risk of corneal transplant rejection significantly reduced with Descemet's membrane endothelial keratoplasty. Ophthalmology. 2012;119(3): 536-40.
45. Dapena I, Ham L, Netukova M, et al. Incidence of early allograft rejection after Descemet membrane endothelial keratoplasty. Cornea. 2011;30(12):1341-5.
46. Rodriguez-Calvo-de-Mora M, Quilendrino R, Ham L, et al. Clinical outcome of 500 consecutive cases undergoing Descemet's membrane endothelial keratoplasty. Ophthalmology. 2015;122(3):464-70.
47. Park CY, Lee JK, Gore PK, et al. Keratoplasty in the United States : A 10-Year Review from 2005 through 2014. Ophthalmology. 2015;122(12):2432-42.
48. America Eye Bank Association. 2014 Eye Banking Statistical Report. Washington: AEBA; 2015.
49. Dirisamer M, van Dijk K, Dapena I, et al. Prevention and management of graft detachment in Descemet membrane endothelial keratoplasty. Arch Ophthalmol. 2012;130(3): 280-91.
50. Kruse FE, Laaser K, Cursiefen C, et al. A stepwise approach to donor preparation and insertion increases safety and outcome of Descemet membrane endothelial keratoplasty. Cornea. 2011;30(5):580-7.
51. Monnereau C, Quilendrino R, Dapena I, et al. Multicenter study of Descemet membrane endothelial keratoplasty: first case series of 18 surgeons. JAMA ophthalmol. 2014;132(10):1192-8.
52. Terry MA, Saad HA, Shamie N, et al. Endothelial keratoplasty: the influence of insertion techniques and incision size on donor endothelial survival. Cornea. 2009;28(1):24-31.
53. Alqudah AA, Terry MA, Straiko MD, et al. Immediate endothelial cell loss after penetrating keratoplasty. Cornea. 2013;32(12):1587-90.
54. Feng MT, Price MO, Miller JM, et al. Air reinjection and endothelial cell density in Descemet membrane endothelial keratoplasty: five-year follow-up. JCRS. 2014;40(7):1116-21.
55. Price MO, Fairchild KM, Price DA, et al. Descemet's stripping endothelial keratoplasty five-year graft survival and endothelial cell loss. Ophthalmology. 2011;118(4):725-9.
56. Ang M, Mehta JS, Lim F, et al. Endothelial cell loss and graft survival after Descemet's stripping automated endothelial

keratoplasty and penetrating keratoplasty. Ophthalmology. 2012;119(11):2239-44.
57. Chamberlain W, Lin CC, Austin A, Schubach N, Clover J, McLeod SD, Porco TC, Lietman TM, Rose-Nussbaumer J. Descemet Endothelial Thickness Comparison Trial: A Randomized Trial Comparing Ultrathin Descemet Stripping Automated Endothelial Keratoplasty to Descemet Membrane Endothelial Keratoplasty. Ophthalmology. 2018 (in press); doi: 10.1016/j.ophtha.2018.05.019.
58. Hamzaoglu EC, Straiko MD, Mayko ZM, et al. The First 100 Eyes of Standardized Descemet Stripping Automated Endothelial Keratoplasty versus Standardized Descemet Membrane Endothelial Keratoplasty. Ophthalmology. 2015;122(11):2193-9.
59. Price MO, Price FW Jr. Endothelial cell loss after Descemet stripping with endothelial keratoplasty influencing factors and 2-year trend. Ophthalmology. 2008;115(5):857-65.
60. Khor WB, Kim T. Descemet-stripping automated endothelial keratoplasty with a donor tissue injector. JCRS. 2014;40(11):1768-72.
61. Busin M, Bhatt PR, Scorcia V. A modified technique for Descemet membrane stripping automated endothelial keratoplasty to minimize endothelial cell loss. Arch Ophthalmol. 2008;126(8):1133-7.
62. Khor WB, Mehta JS, Tan DT. Descemet stripping automated endothelial keratoplasty with a graft insertion device: surgical technique and early clinical results. Am J Ophthalmol. 2011;151(2):223-32.e2.
63. Bahar I, Kaiserman I, Sansanayudh W, et al. Busin Guide vs Forceps for the Insertion of the Donor Lenticule in Descemet Stripping Automated Endothelial Keratoplasty. Am J Ophthalmol. 2009;147(2):220-6.e1.
64. Ang M, Saroj L, Htoon HM, et al. Comparison of a donor insertion device to sheets glide in Descemet stripping endothelial keratoplasty: 3-year outcomes. Am J Ophthalmol. 2014;157(6):1163-9.e3.
65. Elbaz U, Yeung SN, Lichtinger A, et al. EndoGlide versus EndoSerter for the insertion of donor graft in Descemet stripping automated endothelial keratoplasty. Am J Opthalmol. 2014;158(2):257-62.e1.
66. Jardine GJ, Holiman JD, Stoeger CG, et al. Imaging and quantification of endothelial cell loss in eye bank prepared DMEK grafts using trainable segmentation software. Curr Eye Res. 2014;39(9):894-901.
67. Busin M, Madi S, Santorum P, et al. Ultrathin Descemet's stripping automated endothelial keratoplasty with the microkeratome double-pass technique: two-year outcomes. Ophthalmology. 2013;120(6):1186-94.
68. Guerra FP, Anshu A, Price MO, et al. Descemet's membrane endothelial keratoplasty: prospective study of 1-year visual outcomes, graft survival, and endothelial cell loss. Ophthalmology. 2011;118(12):2368-73.
69. Terry MA, Straiko MD, Veldman PB, et al. Standardized DMEK Technique: Reducing Complications Using Prestripped Tissue, Novel Glass Injector, and Sulfur Hexafluoride (SF6) Gas. Cornea. 2015;34(8):845-52.
70. Kurilec JM, Zaidman GW. Incidence of Peters anomaly and congenital corneal opacities interfering with vision in the United States. Cornea. 2014;33(8):848-50.
71. Nischal KK. Genetics of Congenital Corneal Opacification-Impact on Diagnosis and Treatment. Cornea. 2015;34(Suppl 10):S24-34.
72. Huang C, O'Hara M, Mannis MJ. Primary pediatric keratoplasty: indications and outcomes. Cornea. 2009;28(9):1003-8.
73. Vanathi M, Panda A, Vengayil S, et al. Pediatric keratoplasty. Surv Ophthalmol. 2009;54(2):245-71.
74. Rao KV, Fernandes M, Gangopadhyay N, et al. Outcome of penetrating keratoplasty for Peters anomaly. Cornea. 2008;27(7):749-53.
75. Lowe MT, Keane MC, Coster DJ, et al. The outcome of corneal transplantation in infants, children, and adolescents. Ophthalmology. 2011;118(3):492-7.
76. Lund OE. Plastics in keratoplasty (Cornea artificialis). The past and the present. Munch Med Wochenschr. 1972; 114(23):1115-25.
77. Nussbaum JN. Cornea artificialis, ein Substitut fur die transplantatio cornea. Deutsch Klin. 1853;5:367-72.
78. Aldave AJ, Kamal KM, Vo RC, et al. The Boston type I keratoprosthesis: improving outcomes and expanding indications. Ophthalmology. 2009;116(4):640-51.
79. Aravena C, Bozkurt TK, Yu F, et al. Long-Term Outcomes of the Boston Type I Keratoprosthesis in the Management of Corneal Limbal Stem Cell Deficiency. Cornea. 2016;35(9):1156-64.
80. Alexander JK, Basak SK, Padilla MD, et al. International Outcomes of the Boston Type I Keratoprosthesis in Stevens-Johnson Syndrome. Cornea. 2015;34(11):1387-94.
81. Aquavella JV, Gearinger MD, Akpek EK, et al. Pediatric keratoprosthesis. Ophthalmology. 2007;114(5):989-94.
82. Rootman DB, Kim MJ, Aldave AJ, et al. Ocular surface, fornix, and eyelid rehabilitation in Boston type I keratoprosthesis patients with mucous membrane disease. Ophthal Plast Reconstr Surg. 2015;31(1):43-9.
83. Chak G, Aquavella JV. A safe Nd:YAG retroprosthetic membrane removal technique for keratoprosthesis. Cornea. 2010;29(10):1169-72.
84. Kammerdiener LL, Speiser JL, Aquavella JV, et al. Protective effect of soft contact lenses after Boston keratoprosthesis. Br J Ophthalmol. 2016;100(4):549-52.
85. Robert MC, Arafat SN, Ciolino JB. Collagen cross-linking of the Boston keratoprosthesis donor carrier to prevent corneal melting in high-risk patients. Eye Contact Lens. 2014;40(6):376-81.
86. Crnej A, Paschalis EI, Salvador-Culla B, et al. Glaucoma progression and role of glaucoma surgery in patients with Boston keratoprosthesis. Cornea. 2014;33(4):349-54.
87. Ciolino JB, Belin MW, Todani A, et al. Boston Keratoprosthesis Type 1 Study Group. Retention of the Boston keratoprosthesis type 1: multicenter study results. Ophthalmology. 2013;120(6):1195-200.
88. Rudnisky CJ, Belin MW, Guo R, et al. Boston Type 1 Keratoprosthesis Study Group. Visual Acuity Outcomes of the Boston Keratoprosthesis Type 1: Multicenter Study Results. Am J Ophthalmol. 2016;162:89-98.e1.
89. Aldave AJ, Sangwan VS, Basu S, et al. International results with the Boston type I keratoprosthesis. Ophthalmology. 2012;119(8):1530-8.

Chapter 31 Contact Lenses

Rajeswari Mahadevan, Prema Padmanabhan

INTRODUCTION

It is estimated that 140 million people wear contact lenses worldwide and this number is believed to be growing at 5–15% annually.[1] The constant development of newer materials and designs, along with novel lens care systems, has enhanced the patient comfort and safety, thus broadening the scope of it being used for newer options. While rigid gas permeable (RGP) lenses have withstood the test of time, silicone hydrogel materials have now become the most popular lenses, especially since they facilitate continuous wear. Astigmatism and presbyopia corrections using contact lenses are no longer as challenging as they were a couple of decades ago. The utility has expanded beyond cosmesis, and now includes addressing anisometropia and thereby facilitating binocularity, restoration of quality vision to an eye with an irregular cornea, improvement of the ocular surface health and proving useful as an effective drug delivery system. While contact lenses are also used as a part of certain diagnostic and treatment procedures, this chapter will focus on the optical and therapeutic applications alone.

INDICATIONS FOR CONTACT LENS WEAR

- *Optical*:
  - *Refractive errors*: Myopia, hyperopia, astigmatism, presbyopia
  - Irregular cornea
  - Postkeratoplasty
- *Therapeutic*:
  - Recurrent corneal erosions
  - Filamentary keratitis
  - Epithelial defect
  - Bullous keratopathy
  - Microperforations in cornea
  - Prevention of symblepharon (chemical injuries)
  - Trichiasis
  - Exposure keratitis
- *Diagnosis and Treatment*:
  - Gonioscopy
  - Fundus examination
  - Electroretinogram
  - *Laser treatments*: Iridotomy, capsulotomy, retinal photocoagulation
  - Drug delivery system
- *Cosmetic*:
  - Corneal scars
  - Phthisis bulbi.

EFFECT OF CONTACT LENS ON THE CORNEA AND OCULAR SURFACE

The contact lens alters the environment surrounding the normal cornea which may impact the corneal physiology. The extent of this effect would depend on the size of the contact lens, the material it is made of and the method of fitting. In 2012, the Tear Film and Ocular Surface Society (TFOS) sponsored a workshop on Contact Lens Discomfort (CLD), in which critical areas of contact lens wear were studied and discussed, the conclusions of which were published in 2013.[2] The following section draws from that report.

Effect of Contact Lens Wear on Biophysical Properties of Tear Film

Unstable Tear Film

This occurs due to a higher percentage of incomplete blinks observed in contact lens wearers,[3] which can induce changes in the ocular surface epithelium. This in turn aggravates the unstable tear film, creating a vicious cycle.

Thinning of the Lipid and Aqueous Layer

Contact lenses with higher water content are more vulnerable to drying after prolonged wear, resulting in thinning of tear film.[4] Disruption of the lipid layer predisposes to lipid deposits on the contact lens, which impair optical quality and render the contact lens surface hydrophobic. Depletion of the post-lens tear film also causes lens adherence and could be detrimental to epithelial integrity of the ocular surface.

Increased Tear Evaporation

An increase in tear evaporation is typically associated with a loss of integrity of the tear lipid layer.[5]

Osmolarity

After an initial transient decrease in osmolarity due to reflex tearing, the osmolarity of the tears increases due to the excessive evaporation and disrupted tear film stability.[6]

Reduction in pH

This has been attributed to the lens preventing loss of carbon dioxide and to lactic acid accumulation.[7]

Effect of Contact Lens Wear on Tear Composition

Lipids

An increase in the ratio of nonpolar to polar lipids has been reported in the tears of contact lens wearers.[8] The low level of polar lipids could contribute to the dryness and discomfort with contact lenses. Intolerance to contact lens wear has been found to be associated with increased levels of secretory phospholipases.[9]

Protein

Tear film proteomics has revealed varied results. While it is known that the tear film contains numerous inflammatory cytokines, mediators and enzymes, the effect of contact lenses on each of them is still not clear.

Mucin

Several studies have reported a decrease in MUC5AC in contact lens wearers,[10] suggesting damage to the glycocalyx.

Effect of Contact Lenses on Corneal Physiology

Corneal Metabolism

The cornea normally gets its oxygen from tears and aqueous; while its glucose requirement is met by the aqueous. All forms of contact lenses inhibit the supply of atmospheric oxygen. The oxygen permeability is a physical property of the contact lens material and refers to the rate of oxygen flow under specified conditions through unit area of contact lens material when subjected to unit pressure differences. It is denoted as the Dk value.[11] The oxygen transmissibility, denoted as Dk/t, defines the ability of the contact lens to allow oxygen to move from its anterior to posterior surface.

In practical terms, the oxygen transmissibility (Dk/t) of a lens to meet the physiological requirements of the cornea is: 24×10^{-9} Fatt units for daily wear contact lenses and 87×10^{-9} Fatt units for extended wear contact lenses (Box 31.1).[12]

Box 31.1: Oxygen supply to cornea with contact lens.

- Tear movement and exchange during blinking (Tear pump). More effective with rigid lenses
- Oxygen diffusion through the contact lens. More important for soft lenses

Corneal Tissue Fragility

The corneal hypoxia associated with prolonged contact lens wear could cause:

- *Reduced epithelial adhesion*[13] due to decrease in the number of hemidesmosomes
- *Reduced corneal sensitivity*
- *Refractive error*: A slight myopic shift could result from corneal edema. This phenomenon is more common with thick low water content hydrogel lenses. The rate of increase in myopia was reported to be significantly more with reusable and daily disposable hydrogel lenses than with silicone hydrogel lenses.[14]

Hypoxia-related Effects on the Cornea

Clinically observable hypoxia-related responses that typically occur with low Dk/t contact lenses include the following:

- *Corneal swelling*: This is an acute response that invariably occurs after overnight wear of contact lenses. It is more likely to occur with thick lens designs as with high refractive errors, presbyopic corrections and toric designs.[15] It manifests as vertical striae at the posterior stromal level.
- *Epithelial microcysts* usually develop with chronic hypoxia, more commonly with extended wear lenses.
- *Epithelial thinning* also more commonly seen with extended wear lenses.

- *Limbal hyperemia* is a clinical indicator of hypoxic stress and is a precursor to corneal vascularization. The oxygen transmissibility required to prevent limbal hyperemia is 125×10^{-9} Fatt units.
- *Corneal vascularization* is a response to chronic hypoxia. The prominent risk factors include thicker lenses (higher prescriptions), all day wear and hydrogel lenses. The introduction of silicone-hydrogel material with high Dk/t has reduced the incidence of corneal vascularization.[16]
- *Endothelial polymegathism:* The build-up of carbon dioxide and lactic acid causes the decrease in pH of the cornea which, in turn, can cause endothelial changes. These changes could be transient, without significantly altering corneal hydration.

BROAD GUIDELINES FOR CONTACT LENS FITTING

Prerequisites

Patient selection and pre-fitting evaluation are important prerequisites for successful contact lens practice. This begins with understanding the needs of the patients as well as their motivation to use the contact lenses and their willingness to adhere to the advice of the care provider.

Preliminary Examination and Prefitting Assessment

A detailed history of the patient's general health, occupation and lifestyle should include documentation of allergies, endocrine disorders and smoking. The use of systemic medications should specifically be asked for; estrogens, antihistaminics, psychotropic drugs and beta-blockers are often associated with dry eyes that may lead to contact lens intolerance and corneal staining. Certain systemic drugs such as tetracycline, rifampicin, nitrofurantoin can cause discoloration of contact lenses. The unaided and best spectacle corrected visual acuity after retinoscopic refraction should be recorded. A comprehensive ocular examination starts with a focus on lid margin and ocular surface disease. An assessment of the preocular tear film is very crucial since this is an important determinant for compliance. Conditions such as hordeolum, trichiasis, blepharitis and meibomian gland dysfunction should be treated before contact lens fitting is undertaken.

Ocular measurements relevant to contact lens fitting include vertical palpebral fissure height, tear meniscus height, pupil size horizontal visible iris diameter (HVID) and keratometry. Special investigations like corneal topography, specular microscopy and aberrometry are performed, if indicated.

Advantages and Disadvantages of Different Types of Lens

Contact lens indications vary with purpose of lens wear and the type of lens; Table 31.1 lists the advantages and disadvantages of different types of lens.

Terminologies Used for Different Lens Wear Modalities and Lens Replacement Schedules

Classification of Lenses Based on Wearing Schedule

- *Daily wear*: Can be worn during waking hours.
- *Extended wear*: Can be worn for 6 nights and 7 days without removing.
- *Continuous wear*: Can be worn for 29 nights and 30 days without removing.

Table 31.1: Advantages and disadvantages of different types of lens.

Lens type	Advantages	Disadvantages
Soft contact lens	• Short adaptation time • Increased comfort • Good stability in eye • Widely available • Good for active lifestyle	• Vision may not be as sharp as with RGP lenses • Chances of increased complications, if instructions are not followed • Cost
Rigid gas-permeable (RGP) Corneal lens	• Superior quality of vision • Durability and ease of care • Good tear exchange and oxygen supply	• Needs adaptation time and gives initial discomfort • Debris and foreign body trapping • Lens can dislodge or decenter
Scleral lens	• These are very stable and comfortable on the eye • No foreign body trapping • No distortion to the cornea • Helps in rendering the cornea moist in ocular surface disorders • Very useful in sports and activities involving high movements	• Needs training and requires prolonged professional time of the practitioner • Involves high cost

Classification of Lenses Based on Replacement Schedule

Daily disposable:
- Discarded after a single day or wear.
- Cannot be stored or preserved.
- May need rewetting with lubricants.

Monthly disposable or frequent replacement:
- Discarded monthly or quarterly.
- Need storage and preservation.

Conventional replacement:
- Discarded after 6 months or a year.
- Needs storage and preservation.

Soft-lens Fitting Steps

- The material, modality and the replacement period for the contact lens is decided according to the patient's need and refractive error. There are variety of lens material combinations—low or high water content with ionic and non-ionic options that are available. Generally, the replacement frequency of the lens is chosen depending on the estimated hours of use per day, lifestyle and environment exposed to, ocular hygiene and health, and availability of the power range. Contact lens spectrum publishes an annual guide every year that summarizes the available lenses with their respective power ranges and details of lens care solutions as well (*http://www.clspectrum.com/class*).
- Selection of base curve of the lens or off-the-shelf lens with manufacturer's guidelines. The general rule of thumb is 0.6–0.8 mm flatter than flat K reading.
- Select total diameter at least 2 mm more than the horizontal visible iris diameter (HVID).
- Selection of spherical power of the lens should be made after considering vertex distance. In case of toric soft lenses, select cylindrical axis nearest or similar to spectacle axis.

Table 31.2 describes the characteristics of the soft lens observed during optimal, flat and steep fitting on a normal cornea. The fitting steps and assessment hold good for all types of soft lens designs. Some manufacturers may provide a guideline and final optimal fitting characteristics based on their lens design and material.

Corneal Gas-permeable Lenses

Selection of Trial Lens (Tables 31.3 and 31.4)

- Selection of trial lens parameters can be done with keratometry or topography measurements as baseline reference. Table 31.3 illustrates the recommended selection of first trial lens base curve for gas-permeable lenses.[17]
- The selection of diameter is based on horizontal visible iris diameter. Ideally, the corneal gas-permeable lens should fit at least 2 mm smaller than the cornea.

Table 31.2: Characteristics of soft lens fit in normal cornea.

Parameter	Ideal fit	Tight fit	Loose fit
Comfort	Comfortable	Comfortable on insertion and uncomfortable after few hours of wear	Uncomfortable
Centration and coverage	Centers well extending at least 1 mm beyond the limbus (Fig. 31.1A)	Centers well and coverage might be excessive also	Poor centration and poor coverage during different gazes and at different quadrants (Fig. 31.1B)
Movement	0.3–0.5 mm movement on blink and different gazes	Movement less than 0.3 mm, or no movement	Excessive movement beyond 1 mm and decenters at different gazes (Fig. 31.1B)
Push-up movement (Fig. 31.1C)	Good movement and recentration on push-up test	Very less movement on push-up tests and recentration is slow	More movement on push-up tests and recentration is jerky or quick.
Edge	Well-aligned edge landing on the sclera	Well-aligned edge but shows conjunctival indentation (Fig. 31.1D)	Poorly aligned edge with fluting or lift in different few quadrants (Fig. 31.1E)
Vision	Stable vision with blink	Vision clears with blink	Vision blurs with blink or variable
Rotation – Additional steps for soft toric or bifocal design	Rotation of the lens is stable and markings in the lens repositions quickly with blink and in different gazes	Rotation of the lens is stable and markings in the lens show very slow recentration or decentration with blink and in different gazes	Rotation of the lens is unstable and markings in the lens show very jerky and decentration with blink and in different gazes

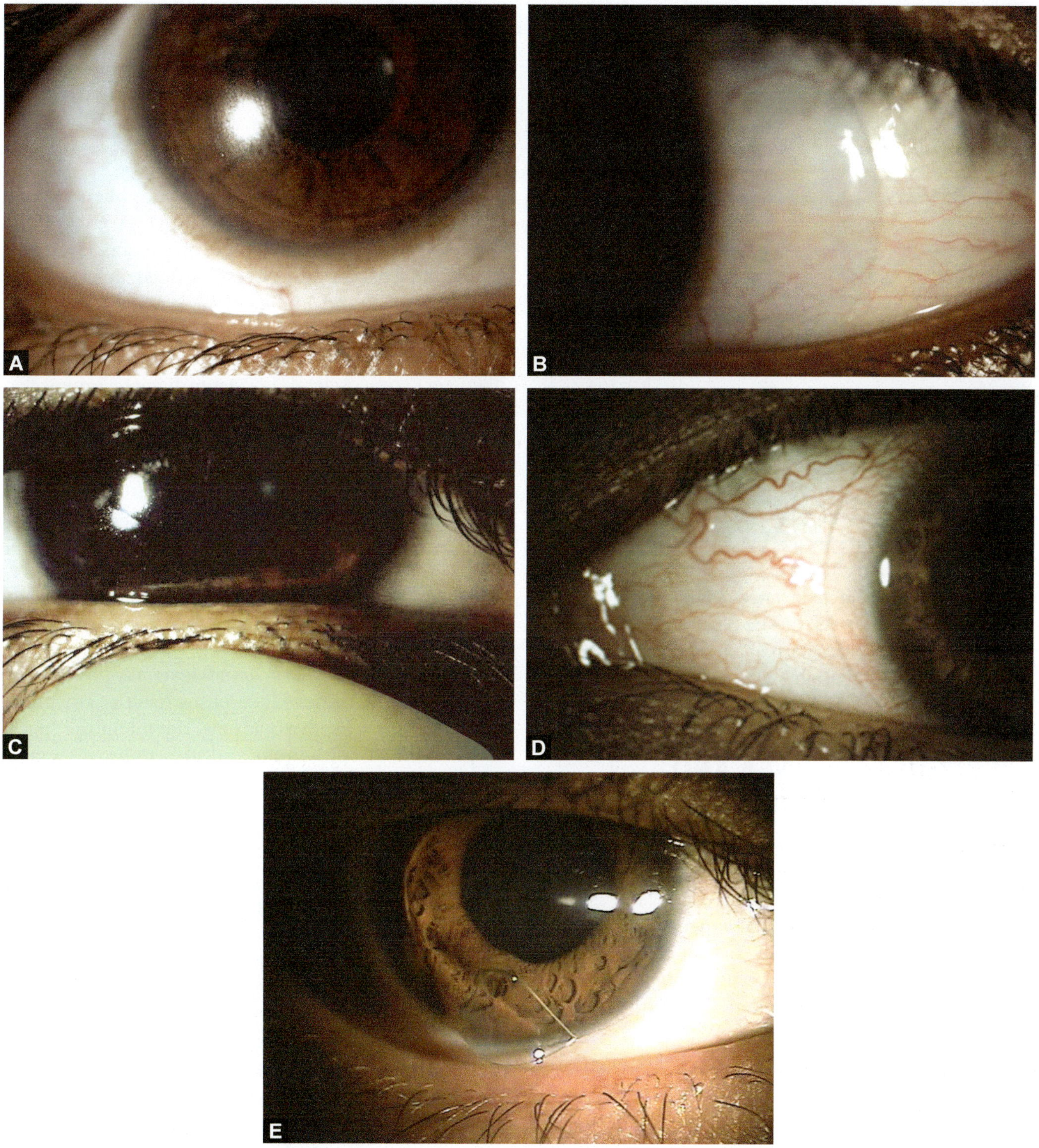

Figs. 31.1A to E: (A) Centered soft lens; (B) Decentered soft lens; (C) Soft lens push-up test; (D) Excessive tightness of soft lens; (E) Soft lens fluting—flat fit.

Table 31.3: Bennett's recommendation for selection of first trial lens base curve.[17]

Corneal cylinder (D)	Base curve
0–0.50	0.50–0.75 D flatter than K
0.75–1.25	0.25–0.50 D flatter than K
1.5	On K
1.75–2.00	0.25 D steeper than K
2.25–2.75	0.50 D steeper than K
3.00–3.50	0.75 D steeper than K

Table 31.4: Bennett's recommendation for selection of first trial lens diameter.[17]

Diameter (mm)	Pupil size (mm)	Corneal curvature (D)	Palpebral fissure size (mm)
8.8–9.0	≤6	≥45	≤9.0
9.2–9.4	6–8	42	9.0–10.5
9.6–9.8	≥8	≤42	≥10.5

Table 31.4 illustrates the recommended selection of first trial lens diameter for gas-permeable lenses.[17]

- Power of the lens must be calculated based on vertex conversion and respective over-refraction with a trial lens. Fluorescein pattern assessment is the handy tool for fitting gas permeable lenses. The fitting patterns in optimal, flat and steep fits are illustrated in Table 31.5 and the fluorescein pattern obtained in corneal ectasia are illustrated in the Table 31.6.[18]

CONTACT LENS FITTING IN IRREGULAR CORNEA AND POST-REFRACTIVE SURGERY

Contemporary contact lens designs, newer materials and advanced imaging technologies have expanded the options and enhanced the success of contact lenses in the functional visual rehabilitation of patients with irregular corneas, including all forms of corneal ectasia. From a contact-lens-fitting perspective, central (nipple) cones are easier to manage than oval (sagging) cones or globus cones.

Contact Lens Modalities

Soft Lenses

Although soft lenses are comfortable and well tolerated, their visual performance is compromised by the higher order aberrations and asymmetry in eyes with irregular corneas. Advances in technology have allowed the manufacture of newer quadrant-specific designs. Custom-made aberration-controlled soft contact lens designs have been developed and have undergone preliminary investigations.[19,20]

Rigid Gas-permeable Lenses

Rigid gas-permeable lenses (RGP) have been the most time-tested contact lens modality for visual correction in corneal ectasias. Based on fluorescein patterns, three major fitting philosophies have been described: apical bearing, apical clearance and 3-point touch.

RGP lenses could be specially designed with multicurve or aspheric contours. It could be corneal (7-12 mm diameter), corneoscleral (12-15 mm diameter), miniscleral (15-18 mm diameter) or scleral (>18 mm diameter). In recent years, there is a growing trend to fit large diameter contact lenses for corneal ectasias.

Corneoscleral lenses have a larger optic zone and are more stable than corneal lenses. The lens-bearing is shared between cornea and sclera and allows a moderate amount of tear exchange.

Piggyback Lenses

A piggyback contact lens system is generally possible with both corneal and corneoscleral lenses. A soft lens (hydrogel) forms the base beneath a rigid lens. This minimizes trauma to the corneal epithelium and also improves patient comfort.

SCLERAL LENSES

Advances in polymer science, the computer-aided design and manufacture (CAD/CAM) and clinical appreciation of the therapeutic value of large diameter contact lenses have resulted in renewed utilization of scleral lenses.[21]

Technically, any lens that extends beyond the limbus could be considered a scleral lens. To avoid confusion in terminology, the Scleral Lens Education Society proposed that scleral lenses be defined as RGP lenses that are supported entirely by the conjunctival tissue overlying the sclera, and vault the cornea and limbus. Further distinctions within the category of scleral lenses define minisclerals as lenses up to 6 mm larger than the horizontal visible iris diameter (HVID) (Fig. 31.3A) and full sclerals as lenses more than 6 mm larger than HVID (Figs. 31.2A and B).[22]

Table 31.5: Grading of fluorescein fit.[18]

	–2	–1	0	+1	+2
Central fit	Excessively steep	Slightly steep	Alignment	Slightly flat	Excessively flat
Peripheral fit	Thin edge-steep	Slightly thin edge	Adequate edge	Edge lift	Edge lift excessively
Width	Extremely wide (0.4 mm)	Slightly wide (0.3–0.4 mm)	Optimal (0.2–0.30 mm)	Slightly narrow (0.1–0.2 mm)	Extremely narrow (<0.1 mm)
Height	Excessive	More than optimal	Optimal	Less than optimal	Insufficient
Mid-peripheral fit	Hard well-defined contact	Poorly defined contact	No contact	Pooling	Excessive pooling
	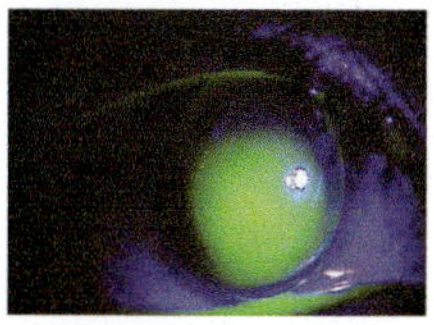	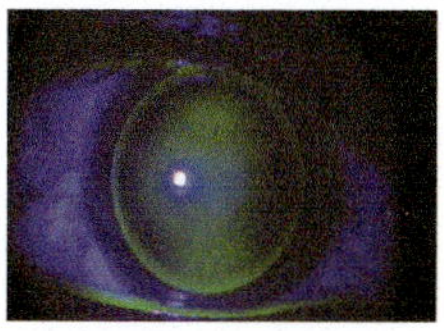	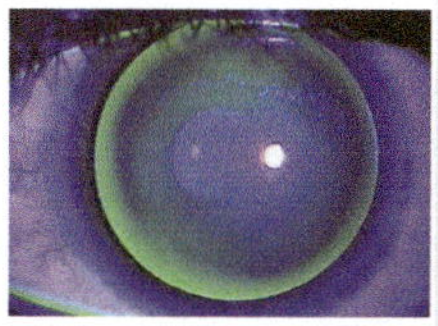	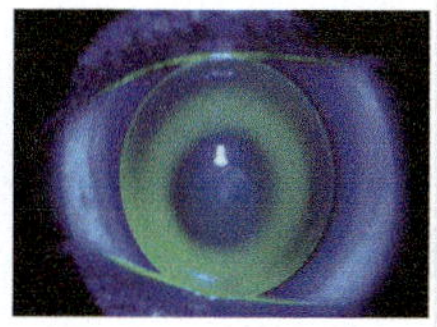	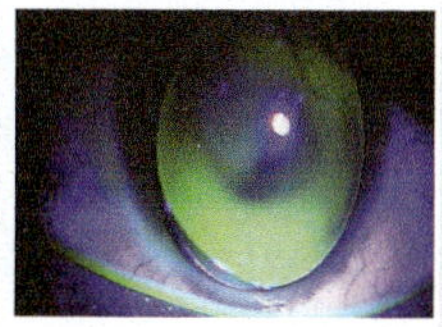

Source: Adapted from Reference 18.

Table 31.6: Fluorescein pattern of different fitting philosophies in corneal ectasia.

Fitting pattern	Support	Advantages	Disadvantages
Apical bearing 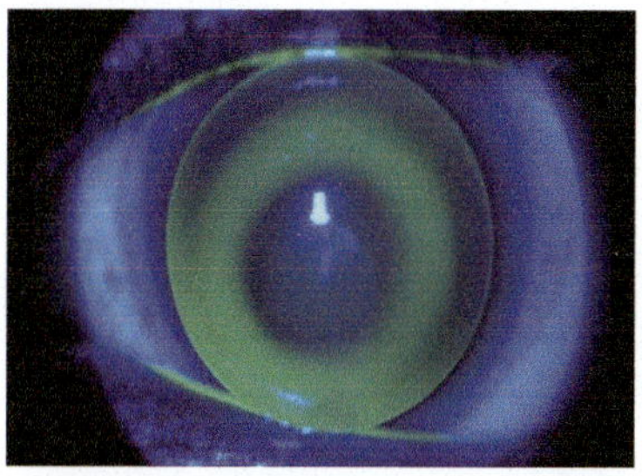	Directly on corneal apex	Visual improvement immediately after insertion	• Whorl epitheliopathy • Axial corneal scarring • May worsen pathology
Apical clearance 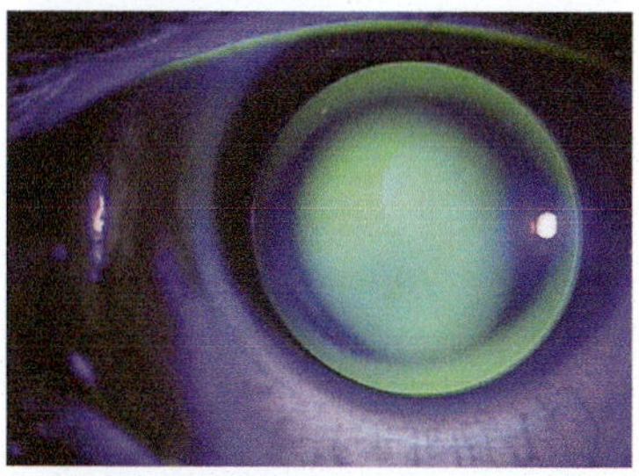	Apical vault support on paracentral cornea	No trauma to apical corneal epithelium	• Transient corneal moulding. • Peripheral corneal epithelial disruption
3-point touch 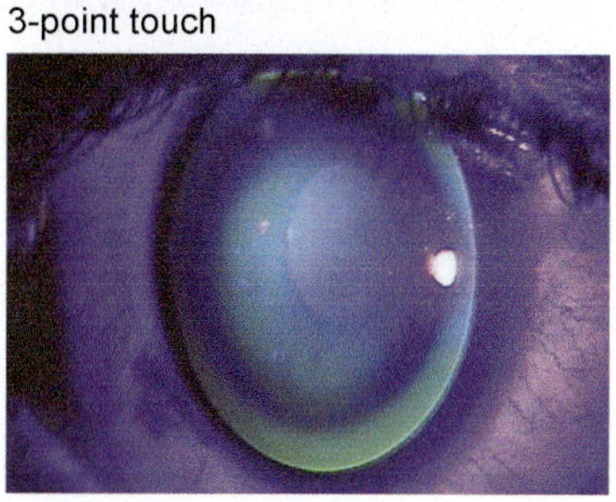	Feather touch on apex support on peripheral cornea	Optimal corneal touch stable	Nil

Major Indications for Scleral Lens Therapy

Ocular Surface Disease

- Stevens-Johnson syndrome
- Exposure keratopathy
- Neurotrophic keratopathy
- Cicatricial conjunctivitis
- Persistent epithelial defects
- Chronic graft versus host disease
- Sjogren's syndrome.

Visual Rehabilitation

- Primary corneal ectasias
- Post-keratoplasty
- Postrefractive surgery
- Corneal scarring
- Refractive instability.

Scleral lenses of different manufacturers vary in design but share the same basic lens geometry: a central optic zone, a transition zone and a landing (or haptic) zone. There is also an emerging consensus that all scleral lenses should have certain characteristics of fit, such as satisfactory tear exchange, absence of corneal touch, limbal vessel compression, edge lift and conjunctival impingement.[21]

The anterior segment optical coherence tomography (AS-OCT) allows precise measurement of anterior segment parameters, visualization of contact lens to cornea relationships, including the vault. It has become a useful tool to design as well as to assess the fitting of scleral lenses.[23,24]

Scleral lenses significantly reduce corneal higher order aberrations (HOA) when compared with spectacles or hydrogel contact lenses.[25,26]

The PROSE (Prosthetic Replacement of the ocular system ecosystem) uses scleral lenses which are customized during design and fabrication to address not only the patient's visual needs but also the physiological requirements of the eye. The CAD/CAM system used in the fabrication of devices is directly accessed by clinicians and uses mathematical spline functions to create junctionless contours.[21]

The physiological impact of scleral lenses and the fluid reservoir on the anterior segment has not been adequately reported. There is, however, growing evidence that scleral lenses using high DK material could be considered as a viable therapeutic option in several clinical conditions. The image sets in (Figs. 31.2 and 31.3) illustrate the fitting and vault in miniscleral and scleral lenses.

COMPLICATIONS WITH CONTACT LENS WEAR

Corneal Hypoxia-related Complications

- Corneal swelling
- Epithelial microcysts and vacuoles
- Corneal tissue fragility
- Limbal hyperemia
- Corneal haze
- Corneal striae
- Endothelial bleb.

Microbial Keratitis (MK)

The normal ocular surface has an arsenal of defense mechanisms that effectively protect the cornea from microbial invasion.

Tear Film

Apart from the mechanical effect of washing and wiping, the normal blinking ensures the tears also contain mucin, IgA, lysozyme, lactoferrin and surfactant protein D which have an antimicrobial effect.[27]

Corneal Epithelium

The tight junctions between cells prevent microbial penetration. Normal sloughing and exfoliation of epithelial cells is also believed to remove infected cells. The normal epithelium produces defensins that have an antimicrobial action[28] and also releases cytokines that orchestrate immune responses.

Basal Lamina

The intact basal lamina composed of extracellular matrix proteins acts as yet another barrier to prevent stromal entry of microbes.

Microbial keratitis is a sight-threatening complication of contact lens wear. While the contact lens itself provides a surface for microbial growth, it also renders the cornea more vulnerable to microbial infection by microdisruptions to the corneal epithelium and by altering ocular surface homeostasis. In addition, contaminated lens cases or lens care solutions could also endanger the eye of a contact lens user.

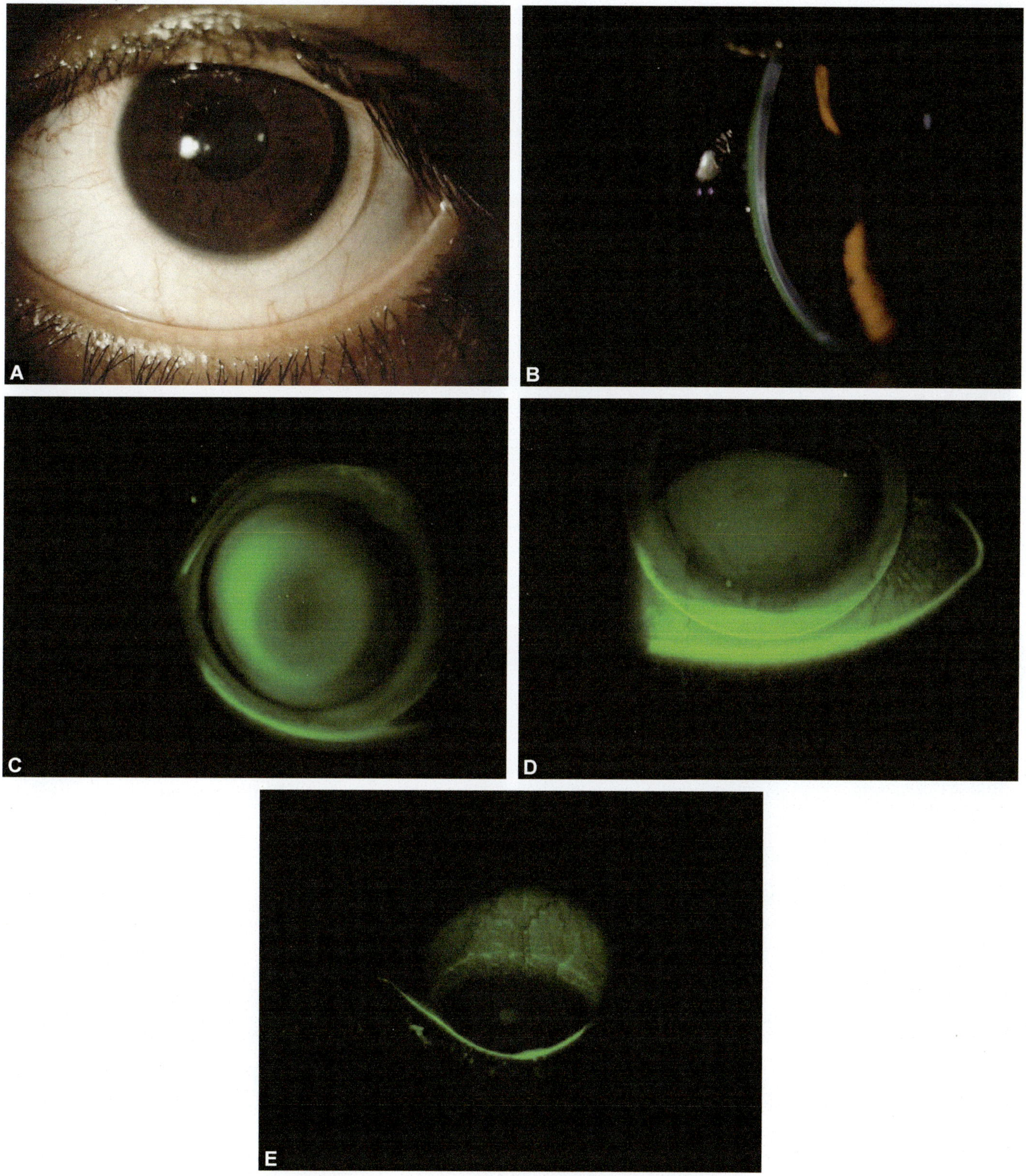

Figs. 31.2A to E: Miniscleral lenses. (A) Centered miniscleral lens; (B) Miniscleral vault 50–150 µm; (C) Fluorescein pattern with a well-centered miniscleral lens; (D) Edge lift with a miniscleral lens; (E) Impingement staining after miniscleral removal.

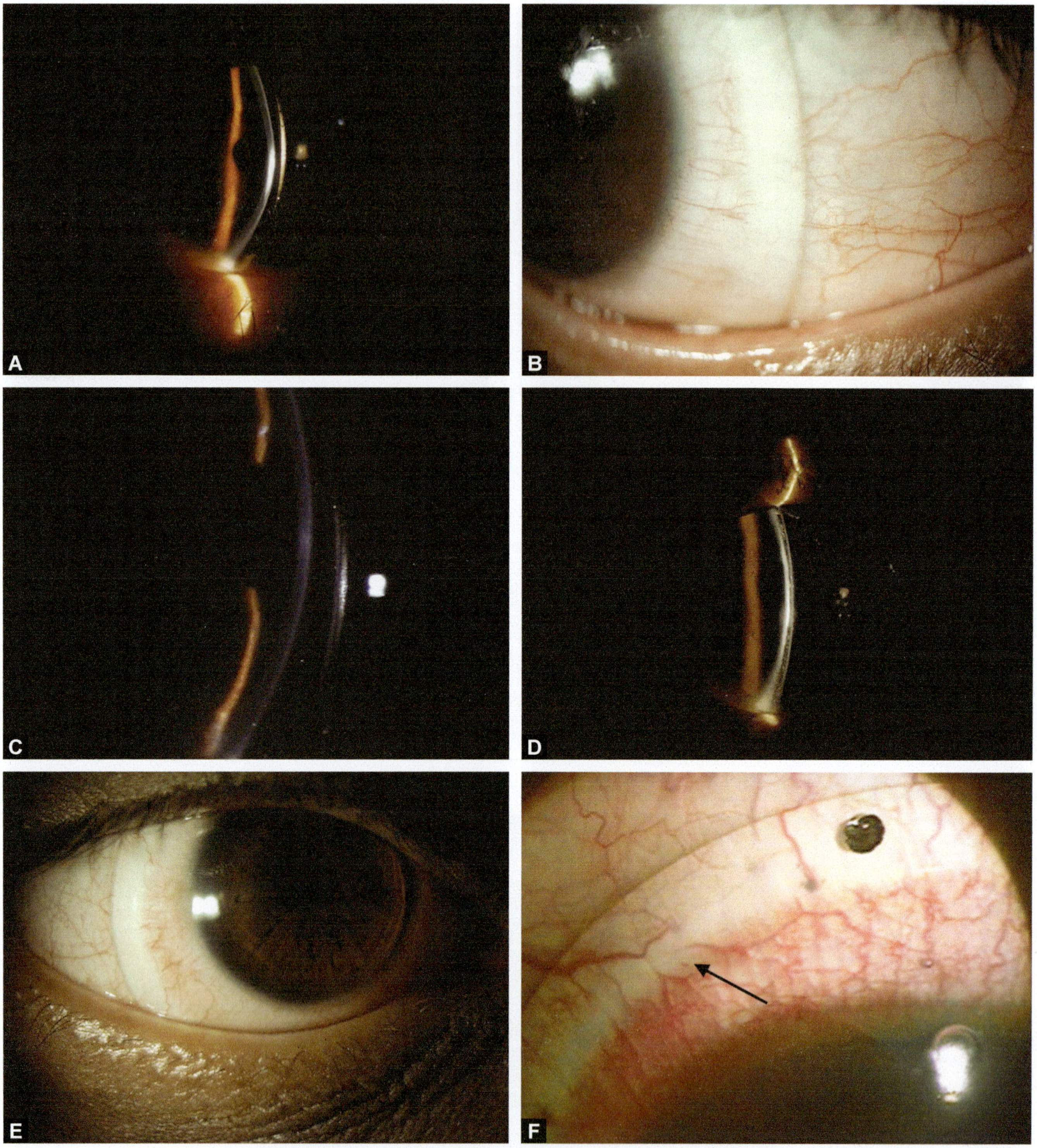

Figs. 31.3A to F

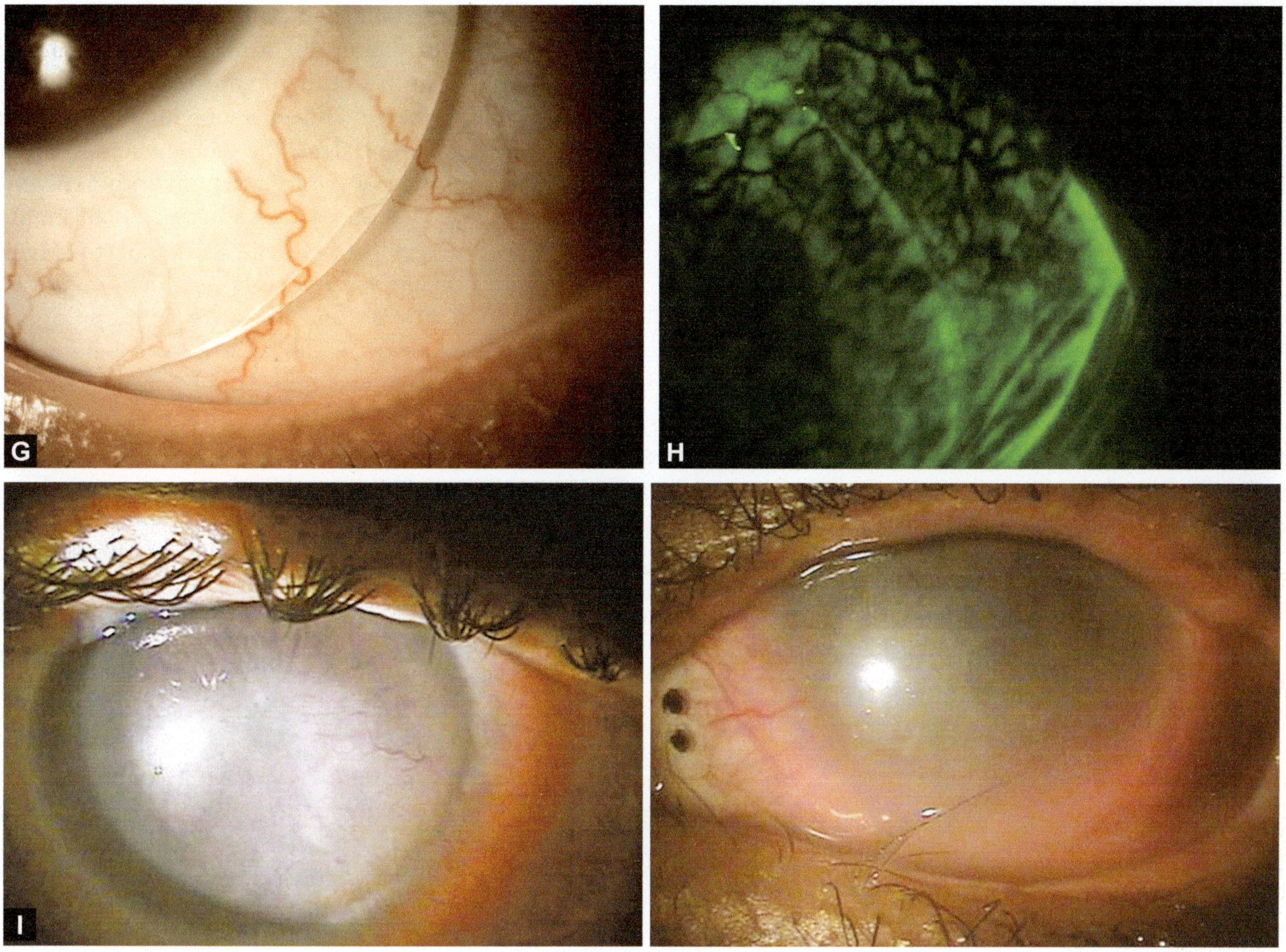

Figs. 31.3G to I

Figs. 31.3A to I: Full scleral lens. (A) Adequate vault of full scleral lens 200–300 μm; (B) Blanching in lateral gaze with full scleral lens; (C) Generous vault with full scleral lens; (D) Minimal inadequate vault in full scleral lens; (E) Blanching at the edges—impingement with full scleral lens; (F) Mid haptic compression with full scleral lens; (G) Edge lift with full scleral lens; (H) Impingement staining after scleral lens removal; (I) Scleral lens in dry eyes—ocular surface disorders.

Risk Factors for MK

- Overnight wear of contact lens.
- Extended wear contact lens.
- Poor patient compliance with lens care.
- Low DK lens.
- Contamination of lenses, lens cases and lens care solutions.
- Contact lens-related dry eye.

PATHOGENESIS

All forms of contact lens, regardless of material or modality of wear, do affect the tear film, ocular surface including the corneal epithelium and also alter corneal physiology—all of which could potentially trigger a chain of events that leaves the cornea susceptible to infection.[29]

Pseudomonas Keratitis

The most common bacterial pathogen in contact lens-related MK is *Pseudomonas aeruginosa*.[30] In the corneal epithelium, *P. aeruginosa* binds to the plasma membrane and also invades internally through fluid structures in the cell membrane known as lipid rafts.[31] Lipid rafts are cholesterol and glycosphingolipid-enriched microdomains which function as signaling platforms to mediate a host of cellular signaling functions including microbial internalization.[32]

The presence of a contact lens, the reduced availability of oxygen, the stagnation of the post-lens tear film contribute to bacterial binding.[33] The inhibition of apoptotic desquamation and slowed epithelial renewal associated with contact lens wear further compromise the corneal defenses.

The multipurpose solution (MPS) which is chemically preserved, also induces toxic staining which is associated with a three-fold greater risk of corneal infiltration events.[34]

A combination of all the above factors facilitates the localization of *P. aeruginosa* beneath the epithelium. Cytotoxins and factors secreted by epithelial cells in response to the damage then lead to eventual destruction of the basal lamina and microbial invasion into the corneal stroma.

Acanthamoeba Keratitis

Acanthamoeba keratitis is yet another vision threatening infection caused by a free-living pathogenic protozoa. Contact lens wear has been incriminated as the main risk factor; accounting for 80% of ocular *Acanthamoeba* infections.[35] Poorly fitting contact lenses leading to microtrauma to the corneal epithelium predispose patients to infection, the source of the organisms typically being contaminated water. Patients present with a broad range of clinical symptoms and signs. The overwhelming majority of patients complain of pain that is not commensurate with clinical signs. As with all cases of microbial keratitis, prompt diagnosis and treatment is the key to salvage the eye and prevent serious complications. Treatment involves immediate cessation of lens wear, the appropriate use of propamidine isetionate 0.1%, polyhexamethylene biguanide 0.02%, neomycin, mydriatics, topical steroids and oral analgesics. Persistence of the cyst form of the protozoa explains the recalcitrant course and the frequent recurrence that characterizes the infection. Resumption of contact lens wear can be considered only after a follow-up and complete eradication of infection, counseling the patient about avoiding risk factors and ensuring proper lens fitting and compliance.

The other contact lens complications are described in Table 31.7.[36]

Table 31.7: Contact lens complications.

Condition	Signs and symptoms	Pathology	Etiology	Treatment
Meibomian gland dysfunction (MGD) 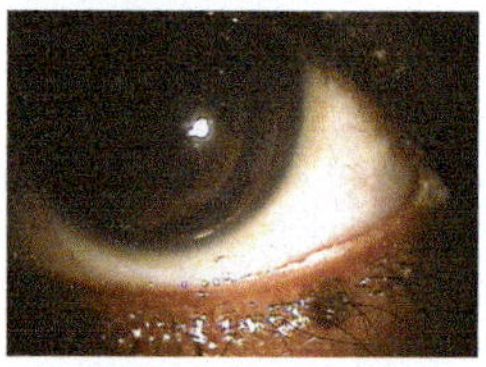	• Poor wetting of lens • Frothing of tear film • No secretion if blocked • Dry eye • Lens intolerance • Creamy yellowish discharge on expression	Hyperkeratinization of Meibomian ducts resulting in obstruction of ducts, loss of secretory meibocytes and altered meibum.	Toxic effect of chemicals, physical presence of contact lens	• Warm compresses • Heating devices • Lidscrubs/hygiene • Mechanical expression • Antibiotics • Tears/lipid supplements • Essential fatty acids • Surfactant lens cleaning
Conjunctival staining 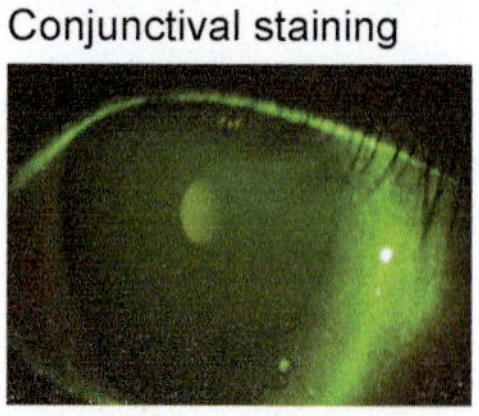	• Furrow staining • Diffuse stain • *Lens edge* stain may be associated with tight lens syndrome or lens edge design	Trauma to superficial epithelial cells	• Physical trauma of lens edge • Deposits on back of lens • Trauma induced by excessive movement of loose fitting lens	• Reassess lens fit • Improve care regimen to alleviate deposit formation
Conjunctival redness 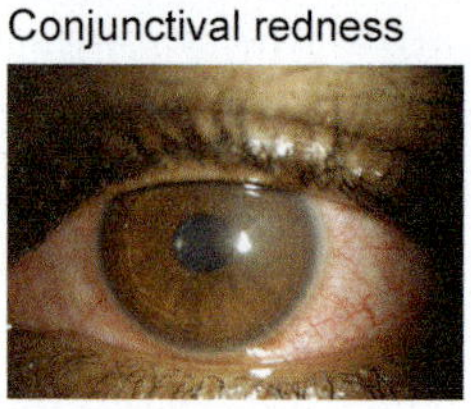	• Conjunctival redness may be associated with itchiness, congestion, mild irritation • Tight lens fit	Blocked blood vessels in case of tight lens	• Hypoxia and hypercapnia • Mechanical irritation • Infection • Inflammation • Acute red eye • Solution toxicity	• Depending on etiology remove cause • Decongestants • If > grade 2, discontinue lens wear

Contd...

Contd...

Condition	Signs and symptoms	Pathology	Etiology	Treatment
Papillary conjunctivitis 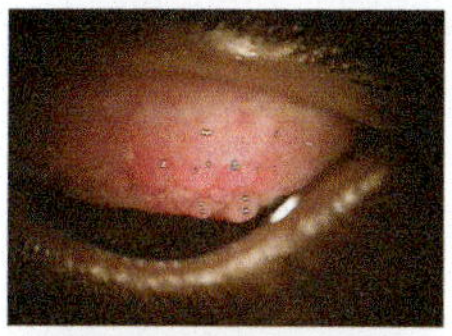 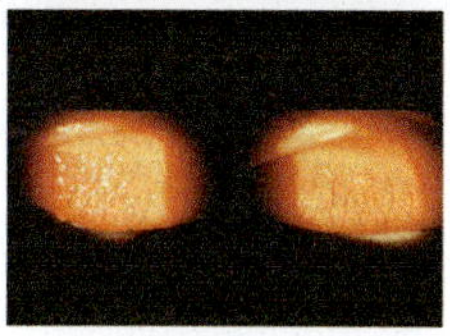	• Papillae on tarsal conjunctiva • Cobblestone appearance or otherwise called as giant papillae. • Excess lens movement • Mucus discharge • Lens awareness • Mild itching • Slight blur • Lens discomfort • Intense itching • Blur • Reduced wearing time	• Altered goblet cells • Inflammatory cells • Mast cells • Eosinophils • Basophils	• Lens deposits • Anterior lens surface • Mechanical irritation due to lens design or fit • Immunological reaction • Hypoxia under lid • Solution toxicity	• Discontinue lens wear until inflammation subsides • Reduce wearing time • Improve solutions • Ocular lubricant • Mast cell stabilizers • Nonsteroidal anti-inflammatory agents • Change to a lens material that deposits differently or lesser with more frequent lens replacement • Improve ocular hygiene
Limbal redness 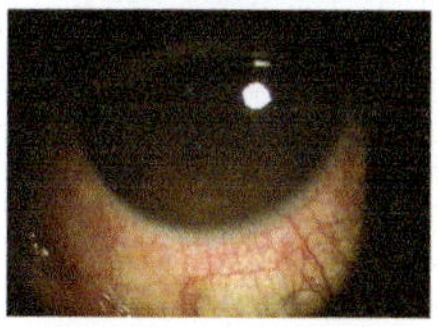	• Depends on lens type • Usually absent with silicone hydrogel lenses • May be associated with pain • Poor lens tolerance in case of hypoxia	Recurrent limbal vessels	• Hypoxia/overwear • Mechanical irritation • Immunological reaction • Infection • Inflammation • Acute red eye • Solution toxicity	• Remove cause (see etiology) • Change of lens material and DK may help.
3- and 9-O'clock corneal staining 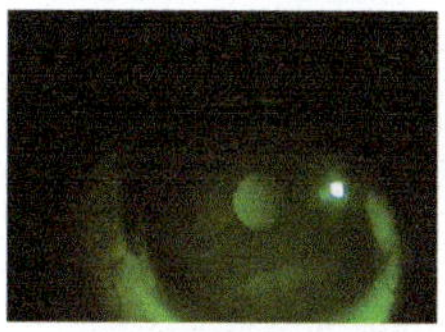	• Punctate or diffuse staining at the 3- and 9-O'clock limbal locations. • Only seen in rigid lens wearers. • Slight discomfort Or dryness	Epithelial disruption at limbus	• Rubbing of poor-fitting rigid lens • Ocular surface adjacent to lens edge not properly wetted • Incomplete blinking	• Alter lens design • Reduce thickness of lens edge • Smaller lens diameter • Blinking instructions
Superior epithelial arcuate lesion (SEAL) 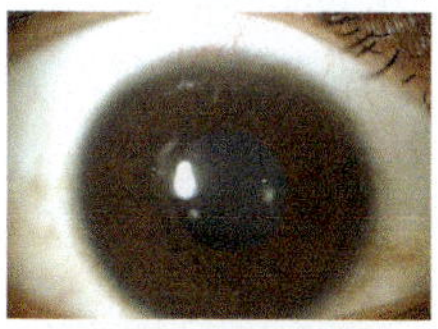	• Superior arcuate stain parallel to limbus also known as epithelial splitting commonly asymptomatic • Lens intolerance	Full thickness splitting of epithelium	• Mechanical chaffing of superior cornea • Inward pressure of upper lid • Rigid lens modulus • Mid-peripheral lens design	• Alter lens design or type • Alter lens type (lower modulus material) • Better surface characteristics
Solution-induced corneal staining (SICS) 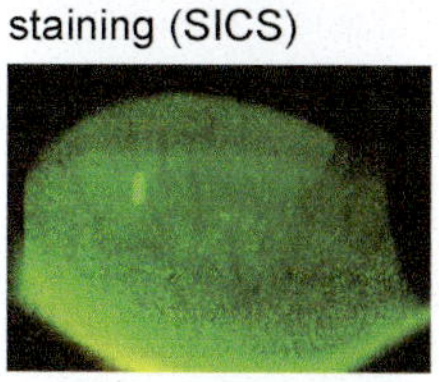	• Diffused corneal punctate staining • Usually bilateral • Asymptomatic if mild • Severe stinging or burning if severe	• Toxic reaction of epithelium • Epithelial cell damage	• Condition is rare with modern preservatives • Wrong use of solution • Exposure to hydrogen peroxide	• Discontinue lens wear until staining clears • Avoid noxious causative agent • Ocular lubricants • Prophylactic antibiotics, if severe epithelial disruption
Corneal infiltrative event (CIE) 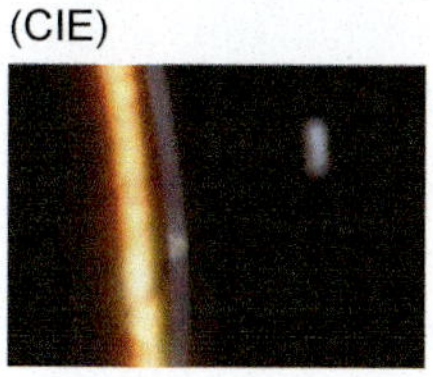	• Any condition whereby there are infiltrates in the cornea • Ranges from minute, barely detectable infiltrate to full-blown corneal ulcer	Infiltrates in the epithelium and/or stroma	• Toxic or allergic inflammatory reaction • Risk factors are contaminated lenses • Solution inefficacy • Patient non-compliance • Poor hygiene	• Discontinue lens wear immediately • If discomfort persists after lens removal, scrape to test for offending microorganisms

Contd...

Contd...

Condition	Signs and Symptoms	Pathology	Etiology	Treatment
	• Symptoms may range from being asymptomatic to excruciating pain • Watch for microbial keratitis in all contact lens wearers		• Hypoxia • Swimming with overnight lens use • Overnight ortho-K • Mechanical trauma • Smoking • Diabetes • Warm climates • Male gender • Socioeconomic class	• Assume bacterial until proven otherwise • Prescribe fluoroquinolones • Cold compresses • Analgesics • Continue appropriate treatment when microbiological result is known • Avoid risk factors, if lens wear is to be resumed
Corneal warpage	• Can manifest as change in corneal: curvature Symmetry Regularity • Corneal indentation • May be associated with corneal binding • Spectacle blur haze	• More likely with rigid lenses • Decentered or poorly fit lens flattens cornea • Distortion may be symmetrical • Corneal indentation • Pressure from lens edge	• Physical molding or change of shape due to rigid lenses • Pressure from eyelids • Associated pathology, e.g. Keratoconus	• Reassess lens fit, cleaning procedures and replacement frequency • Alleviate rigid bearing • Alleviate hypoxia • Corneal indentation

Table 31.8: Indications for bandage contact lens (BCL) in different ocular conditions and their benefits.

Pathology	Objective	Recommended lens material	Duration of bandage contact lens wear
Recurrent erosion	Pain relief, healing of epithelium	High or mid-water content soft lenses	*Mild cases*: few days *Recurrences*: 2–3 months
Filamentary keratitis	Pain relief	High or mid-water content soft lens	Few days to 2 weeks depending on healing and recurrence
Superficial punctate keratitis	Pain relief	High or mid-water content soft lens	1 month daily wear
Corneal perforation	Splint/seal leak	High water content	<1 month, may need a large diameter lens and slightly tighter fit
Bullous keratopathy	Pain relief	Mid-water content, high DK lenses preferably silicone hydrogel with frequent replacement lenses for regular use	Monthly or bimonthly follow-up to watch for corneal vascularization or problems due to lens deposits
Chemical burns: Acid or alkali	Pain relief and promotion of stable epithelialization, maintenance of the forniceal space to prevent symblepharon	High water content soft lens with scleral coverage or scleral lenses allowing added benefit of vision improvement	Variable (weeks/months) or continuous use of scleral lens for therapeutic purposes and vision improvement
Stevens-Johnson syndrome	Pain relief and mechanical protection	• Thick, medium water content soft lens • Large diameter lens to prevent symblepharon, or small diameter lens, if symblepharon already present	Indefinite

THERAPEUTIC (BANDAGE) CONTACT LENS

Silicone hydrogel or high water content hydrogel lenses are sometimes used therapeutically for pain relief, epithelial healing or structural support. The choice of the lens depends on the indication, clarity and regularity of the cornea, the health of the ocular surface, the likely duration of intended use and the estimated level of patient compliance and hygiene. Frequent replacement disposable lenses are generally preferred over conventional medium water content lenses. If previous K readings are available, the flat K is converted to millimeters and 0.8 mm added to get the nearest base curve for the lens to be fitted. The fit should be evaluated after 15 minutes, after 1 hour and again on the next day. The list of different ocular conditions indicated for bandage lens wear, the choice of lens and the duration for bandage lens wear, are tabulated in Table 31.8.

CONCLUSION

The contact lens field is constantly evolving—newer materials, newer designs and newer lens care products creating an industry that has geared itself to cater to a widening circle of potential beneficiaries, with an assurance of quality, comfort and safety. The prescription and fitting of contact lenses has become a specialized area of health care and requires skill and trained expertise.

REFERENCES

1. Cavanagh HD, Robertson DM, Petroll WM, et al. Forty Years in Search of the Perfect Contact Lens. Cornea. 2010;29(10):1075-85.
2. Nichols JJ, Willcox MD, Brno AJ, et al. The TFOS International Workshop on Contact Lens Discomfort: Executive Summary Executive Summary. Invest Ophthalmol Vis Sci. 54(11),(2013):TFOS7-13.
3. Van Der Worp E, De Brabander J, Hendrikse F. Eye blink Frequency and Type in Relation to 3- and 9-O'Clock Staining and Gas-permeable Contact Lens Variables. Optom Vis Sci. 2008;85(9):E857-66.
4. Maruyama K, Yokoi N, Taka Mata A, et al. Effect of Environmental Conditions on Tear Dynamics in Soft Contact Lens Wearers. Invest Ophthalmol Vis Sci. 2004; 45:2563-8.
5. Craig JP, Tomlinson A. Importance of the lipid layer in human tear film stability and evaporation. Optom Vis Sci. 1997;74(1):8-13.
6. Nichols JJ, Sinnott LT. Tear Film, Contact Lens, and Patient-related Factors Associated with Contact Lens-related Dry Eye. Invest Ophthalmol Vis Sci. 2006;47:1319-28.
7. Chen FS, Maurice DM. The pH in the precorneal tear film and under a contact lens measured with a fluorescent probe. Exp Eye Res. 1990;50:251-9.
8. Maïssa C, Guillon M, Girard-Claudon K, et al. Tear lipid composition of hydrogel contact lens wearers. Adv Exp Med Biol. 2002;506:935-8.
9. Glasson MJ, Stapleton F, Keay L, et al. Differences in clinical parameters and tear film of tolerant and intolerant contact wearers. Curr Eye Res. 2002;25:227-35.
10. Berry M, Pult H, Purslow C, et al. Mucins and Ocular Signs in Symptomatic and Asymptomatic Contact Lens Wear. Optom Vis Sci. 2008;85:E930-8.
11. Fatt I, St Helen R. Oxygen tension under an oxygen-permeable contact lens. Am J Optom Arch Am Acad Optom. 1971;48:545-55.
12. Holden BA, Mertz GW. Critical oxygen levels to avoid corneal oedema for daily and extended wear contact lenses. Invest Ophthalmol Vis Sci. 1984;25:1161-7.
13. Madigan MC, Holden BA. Reduced epithelial adhesion after extended contact lens wear correlates with reduced hemidesmosome density in cataract cornea. Invest Ophthalmol Vis Sci. 1992;33:314-23.
14. Kinoshita BT, Chalmers RL, Mitchell GL, et al. Rate of change and predictive factors for increasing minus contact lens powers in young myopes. Clin Exp Optom. 2015; 98:323-9.
15. Lira M, Pereira C, Real Oliveira ME, et al. Importance of contact lens power and thickness in oxygen transmissibility. Cont Lens Anterior Eye. 2015;38(2):120-6.
16. Bergenske P, Long B, Dillehay S, et al. Long-term clinical results: 3 years of up to 30-night continuous wear of lotrafilcon A silicone hydrogel and daily wear of low-Dk/t hydrogel lenses. Eye Contact Lens. 2007;33(2):74-80.
17. Bennett ES, Sorbara L. Lens design, fitting and evaluation. In: Clinical manual of contact lenses, 2nd edition. Philadelphia: Lippincott Williams & Wilkins; 2000. pp. 75-124.
18. Guillon. M. Basic contact lens fitting. In: Rub M, Guillon M (Eds). Contact lens practice. London: Chapman and Hall Medical; 1994. pp. 587-622.
19. Marsack JD, Parker KE, Applegate RA. Performance of wavefront-guided soft lenses in three keratoconus subjects. Optom Vis Sci. 2008;85:E1172-8.
20. Marsack JD, Parker KE, Niu Y, et al. On-eye performance of custom wavefront-guided soft contact lenses in a habitual soft lens-wearing keratoconic patient. J Refract Surg. 2007;23(9):960-4.
21. Parminder A, Jacobs DS. Advances in scleral lenses for refractive surgery complications. Curr Opin Ophthalmol. 2015;26(4):243-8.
22. Schornack MM. Scleral lenses: a literature review. Eye Contact Lens. 2015;41(1):3-11.
23. Van der Worp, E. A guide to scleral lens fitting. Oregon: Pacific University; 2015.
24. Luo ZK, Jacobs DS. Current and potential applications of anterior segment optical coherence tomography in contact lens fitting. Semin Ophthalmol. 2012;27:138-42.
25. Gumus K, Gire A, Pflugfelder SC. The Impact of the Boston Ocular Surface Prosthesis on Wavefront Higher-order Aberrations. Am J Ophthalmol. 2011;151:682-90.
26. Sabesan R, Johns L, Tomashevskaya O, et al. Wavefront-guided scleral lens prosthetic device for keratoconus. Optom Vis Sci. 2013;90:314-23.
27. McNamara NA, Andika R, Kwong M, et al. Interaction of *Pseudomonas aeruginosa* with human tear fluid components. Curr Eye Res. 2005;30:517-25.
28. McNamara NA, Van R, Tuchin OS, et al. Ocular Surface epithelia express mRNA for human beta defensin-2. Exp Eye Res. 1999;69:483-90.
29. Fleiszig SM. The Glenn A. Fry Award Lecture 2005. The pathogenesis of contact lens-related keratitis. Optom Vis Sci. 2006;83(12):e866-73.
30. Sharma S, Gopalakrishnan S, Aasuri MK, et al. Trends in contact lens-associated microbial keratitis in Southern Indian. Ophthalmology. 2003;110:138-43.
31. Yamamoto N, Yamamoto N, Jester JV, et al. Prolonged Hypoxia Induces Lipid Raft Formation and Increases *Pseudomonas* Internalization in vivo after Contact Lens Wear and Lid Closure. Eye Contact Lens. 2006;32(3):114-20.
32. Duncan MJ, Shin JS, Abraham SN. Microbial entry through caveolae: variations on a theme. Cell Microbiol. 2002;4(12):783-91.
33. Robertson DM, Cavanagh HD. The Clinical and Cellular Basis of Contact Lens-related Corneal Infections: A Review. Clin Ophthalmol. 2008;2(4):907-17.
34. Carnt N, Jalbert I, Stretton S, et al. Solution toxicity in soft contact lens daily wear is associated with corneal inflammation. Optom Vis Sci. 2007;84(4):309-15.
35. Hargrave SL, McCulley JP, Husseini Z, et al. Results of a trial of combined propamidine isethionate and neomycin therapy for *Acanthamoeba* keratitis. Ophthalmology. 1999;106(5):952-7.
36. Efron N. Contact Lens Complications (e-Book). Philadelphia: Elsevier Health Sciences; 2012.

Chapter 32 Refractive Surgeries

Revathi Rajaraman, Vikram Vaidee, Prabhu V

INTRODUCTION

Refractive surgeries are surgical procedures done to correct preexisting refractive errors of an eye. As the cornea and crystalline lens are the two most important refracting structures of the eye, these surgeries can either be cornea-based or lens-based procedures.

CORNEA-BASED PROCEDURES

A change in the corneal curvature achieves a significant refractive change as the cornea is responsible for 70% of the optical power of the eye. The basic principle of corneal refractive surgeries is to flatten the center in myopes and the mid periphery in hypermetropes to achieve the desired refractive correction. This corneal reshaping is achieved by:

- Mechanical incisional procedures
- Laser ablative procedures
- Additive procedures

Mechanical Incisional Procedures

Radial keratotomy and astigmatic keratotomy are the two corneal incisional refractive procedures. The deep corneal incision flattens the perpendicular meridian with a proportional steepening of the corresponding opposite meridian.

Radial Keratotomy

This incisional procedure was first proposed by Svyatoslav Fyodorov in 1974, to correct low myopia.

Principle: Deep radial incisions at regular intervals made at the midperiphery of the cornea in all quadrants produces a peripheral corneal bulge with an associated central flattening.

Procedure: About 4–8 incisions up to 90% depth of the cornea, leaving a central clear untouched optic zone of 3–4 mm are made. More incisions may compromise corneal biomechanical strength. Incisions are made either centripetally from the edge of the optic zone or centrifugally from the periphery or bidirectional to have uniform depth.

Advantages: This is a low cost procedure since no expensive equipment is needed. It is easy to learn for the surgeons since it is a familiar incisional technique.

Disadvantages:

- Low precision with high unpredictability
- Diurnal refractive fluctuation due to tissue swelling
- Accidental corneal perforation
- Glare and irregular astigmatism

Astigmatic Keratotomy

This incisional surgery is useful for treating corneal astigmatism. While radial keratotomy has fallen out of favour due to the advent of more predictable procedures, astigmatic keratotomy is still fairly used.

Principle: One or two deep arcuate incisions are made across a steep meridian in order to obtain a flattening of that meridian. This also causes a reciprocal steepening of the corresponding flat meridian, 90° away, by a phenomenon known as coupling effect.

Procedure: The steep meridian is marked with reference to 90° or 180° on the corneal periphery. Care is taken to leave the central 7 mm of the optic zone untouched. One or two arcuate incisions up to 80–90% depth, with 45–90° of arc length on both sides of the steep meridian are made with guarded diamond or steel blades. These incisions can be made even more precisely using femtosecond laser. The coupling effect can be enhanced by resecting a wedge of tissue and applying compression sutures in the opposite flat meridian (Figs. 32.1A and B). The amplitude of the refractive correction achieved depends on number, depth and arc length of the incisions. The effect will be more in younger patients.

Indications: This procedure is useful in correcting regular astigmatism. In post-keratoplasty scenario, astigmatic keratotomy, if indicated, should be planned after removing all sutures and confirming refractive stability.

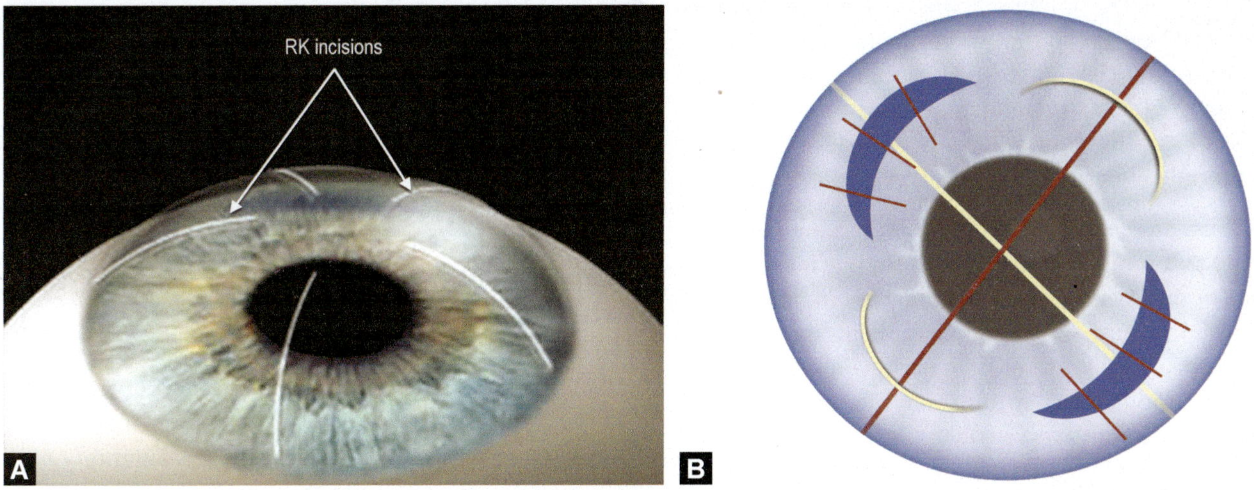

Figs. 32.1A and B: (A) Radial keratotomy (RK) to flatten the corneal center in myopia (Line drawing); (B) Arcuate keratotomy across the steep axis with wedge resection and compression sutures across the reciprocal flat axis-coupling effect to treat astigmatism (Line drawing).

***Advantages*:** Low cost procedure with rapid visual rehabilitation.

***Disadvantages*:**
- Poor predictability
- Regression of the effect

A variant of this technique is used as limbal relaxing incisions along with cataract surgery to address the preexisting astigmatism.

Laser Vision Correction

The evolution of laser refractive surgery: The modern and precise corneal refractive surgeries started with Barraquer keratomileusis. This procedure was further refined with the adjuvant use of the excimer laser[1] (Table 32.1).

Table 32.1: Evolution of laser refractive procedures.

Jose Barraquer (1950–60)	Keratomileusis by Cryo lathe
Luis Ruiz (1983–86)	Automated lamellar keratoplasty (ALK) by automated microkeratome
Trokel (1983)	Photoablation by excimer laser
Munnerlyn (1985)	Formula for accurate calculation of tissue removal to achieve a specific refractive change
Buratto & Pallikaris (1988)	In situ ablation of stromal bed after creating a lamellar free cap/hinged flap
Seiler and McDonald (1999)	First wavefront-customized ablation
2001 FDA approval	Introduction of femtosecond lasers

Principles of Laser Vision Correction

Laser energy is used to reshape the cornea, by precise tissue removal without compromising quality of vision and structural integrity of the cornea.

Laser biophysics: Laser energy is used in corneal refractive surgeries in three different modalities:

1. *Photoablation*: This is achieved by using the laser energy to break the carbon-carbon molecular bond in the corneal stroma and removing a precise amount of tissue. The laser used is a 193 nm excimer laser.
2. *Photodisruption*: This is achieved by using the laser energy to cause intrastromal optical breakdown and vaporization, which helps in flap creation by means of tissue removal. The laser used is the 1,053 nm infrared femtolaser.
3. *Photothermal*: This is achieved by using the laser energy to cause collagen shrinkage and localized flattening as in conductive keratoplasty (CK). The laser used is the 2.13 μm holmium: YAG laser.

Excimer—A Precise Surgical Tool

As mentioned previously, excimer laser works on the principle of photoablation.

Laser production: Excimer is a terminology derived from the words excited dimer. The lasing medium consists of argon and fluorine gas which are inherently stable molecules. On stimulation by electrical energy, unstable excited dimers are formed. When these dimers dissociate, laser in the far ultraviolet range is emitted. This nonmutagenic, high-energy photon breaks the molecular bonds of the corneal tissues, resulting in ablation with submicron level precision without thermal effect.

Laser delivery system: The laser beam emerging from the laser cavity is homogenized and delivered by a computer controlled optical system on to the target as either a pulsed broad beam, scanning slit beam or as a flying spot.

A broad beam will deliver high energy in a short time but is less homogenized, which may compromise the smoothness of the ablated surface. Scanning slit beam gives smoother surface after ablation. Both broad beam and scanning slit beam needs relatively complex delivery systems with masks and diaphragms to get a desired ablation pattern.

The commonly used delivery mode is a flying spot with energy in the range of 100–300 mJ/cm^2, pulse rate of 100–1,000 Hz and a spot size of 1–2 mm. The laser spot will be randomly projected in programmed pattern to chisel the tissue. The flying spot system will give a much smoother surface but needs eye tracking system as it takes longer time to ablate.

The eye tracking system uses infrared light reflection to identify the pupil and keeps the laser delivery centered to the pupil, even if the eye moves during ablation. However, this adjustment can be achieved only within a narrow range of eye movement.

Ablation calculation: The corneal biomechanical stability is affected by the amount of tissue ablated, which in turn depends on the area and the depth of ablation. Munnerlyn equation is used to calculate the depth of tissue need to be ablated to achieve a specific refractive change.[1]

$$\text{Ablation depth} = \frac{\text{Optic zone}^2 \times \text{Dioptric Correction required}}{3}$$

According to this formula, each spherical equivalent diopter of myopic correction performed at a 6 mm optical zone will ablate 12 μm of tissue.

The size of optic zone should be larger than the mesopic pupil diameter to avoid night vision problems like glare and distortions. A larger optic zone and a larger dioptric correction will result in deeper ablation with more tissue removal.

Corneal Biomechanics

Corneal biomechanical stability depends on compact and interwoven anterior stromal lamellae. It has been reported that when anterior 60% of the corneal stroma was cut as a flap, the residual posterior lamellae will bulge forward under intraocular pressure (IOP).

In laser-assisted in situ keratomileusis (LASIK) the anterior lamellae are cut from their peripheral anchorage as a flap. The laser ablation further removes some amount of stromal tissue, leaving the residual posterior stroma to be responsible for biomechanical strength of the cornea. It is recommended at least 50% of the stroma to be left untouched to preserve the biomechanical stability of the cornea. Hence, the amount of tissue which can be removed and the resultant dioptric error corrected, depend on the preoperative corneal thickness.

Effects of Wound Healing on Refractive Outcome

The healing response of the cornea varies as per the plane at which the laser is applied. The laser can either be applied on the surface of the cornea (surface ablations) or underneath a corneal flap (LASIK). Ideally there should be minimal healing response of the corneal tissues to maintain the effect of refractive correction.

Surface ablations: Initial re-epithelialization occurs within the first 2–3 days. After the initial keratocyte apoptosis, the stromal wound healing begins in 24 hours and continues up to 3 weeks, when activated keratocytes form new collagen and proteoglycan matrix. No significant changes have been found in the corneal endothelium or the Descemet's membrane. Myofibroblastic transformation of regenerating keratocytes and hyperplasia of the regenerating epithelium can lead on to regression and reticular haze formation.[2]

LASIK: Wound healing changes are maximal at the flap edge and minimal at the stromal bed, hence haze formation is very rare. The stromal interface remains as a potential space, and hence the flap can be relifted with ease even years after the procedure. Regression of the refractive results can occur due to epithelial hyperplasia and stromal remodeling. The subbasal corneal nerve plexus are cut during flap creation as well as laser ablation and takes more time to regenerate than in surface procedures.

Corneal Reshaping—Conventional versus Customized

Before we discuss about the conventional and customized form of ablations, it is essential to understand the concept of aberrations.

Aberrations: A homogenous light ray that enters the eye undergoes distortions by its complex optical components. These distortions are called aberrations. Chromatic and achromatic aberrations like spherical aberrations are present even in emmetropic eyes. The aberrations are described in several orders, using mathematical models like Zernike's polynomial. Spherocylindrical refractive errors like myopia, hyperopia and astigmatism constitute the second or lower order aberrations. Higher order aberrations beyond third order like spherical aberrations, coma and trefoil are considered important for optical quality of the image. Aberrations of an eye are measured by analyzing the distortions in an emerging wavefront from that eye using aberrometer and are expressed in root mean square value (RMS) and point spread function. Higher order aberrations more than 0.3 RMS are considered significant. The aberrations are dynamic for an eye and change with age, position of the head, position of the eye, corneal shape, pupil size and lens status. Corneal reshaping itself induces some higher order aberrations.

Types of laser ablations: The ablations can be classified conventional and customized based on the order of aberrations they correct.

- *Conventional laser ablation*: Laser ablation is done to correct the basic spherocylindrical refractive error. It does not address either preexisting or induced higher order aberrations.
- *Custom ablations*: Laser ablation based on wavefront pattern to correct higher order aberrations or corneal topography to correct corneal irregularities are custom ablations.[3] Wavefront based ablations can be of three types. They are:
  1. *Wavefront optimized custom ablations*: The conventional laser ablations change the corneal curvature and its shape from prolate to oblate profile. This change in the corneal shape itself will induce higher order aberrations. Wavefront optimized ablation pattern tries to minimize the shape change by delivering more laser pulses to the peripheral zone. Preexisting higher order aberrations are not addressed by this method.
  2. *Wavefront-guided custom ablations*: The treatment pattern is planned as per preoperative refraction and aberrometry to correct both pre-existing lower as well as higher order aberrations. This method is useful when the pre-existing higher order aberrations are significant. Since aberrations are dynamic, position change between capturing and correction may compromise the effect. Accurate registration of the planned treatment pattern on the cornea is important. This is usually achieved by iris registration, which will use reference points of the iris from a precaptured photo to compensate cyclotorsion of the globe and pupillary shift during the treatment. Moreover flap creation itself can induce aberration, which can affect the treatment plan.
  3. *Topo-guided custom ablation*: Ablations are based on topographical abnormalities as in decentered ablations, stable subclinical ectasias and postkeratoplasty astigmatism.

Preoperative Evaluation for Refractive Procedure

Since laser vision correction (LVC) is a precision surgery, proper patient selection is important to ensure a favourable outcome and to avoid complications. The following factors are the basic needs for a suitable candidate:

- Age above 18 years to ensure the eye does not change further in shape and form.
- Should have stable refraction for at least a year.

Since refractive surgery is a purely elective procedure, it is important to discuss the realistic goals like predictability, stability of the outcome and safety of the procedure. The risks and benefits should be discussed in complete detail so that the candidate does not have unrealistic expectations. The purpose of preoperative workup is to determine:

- Patient suitability for refractive procedures
- Selection and planning of the appropriate surgery.

Preoperative evaluation for a refractive procedure includes a detailed history (Table 32.2) and detailed clinical examination (Table 32.3) to assess the suitability and the need of patient.[4-7] LVC should be avoided in patients with some ocular and systemic conditions (Table 32.4).

Table 32.2: Preoperative history.

Ocular history	General history
• Years of spectacle usage • Frequency of spectacle change • Contact lens history (years of usage, type of lens, intolerance or any infections, and whether stopped using contact lens for adequate time prior to evaluation) • Medical or surgical management of other ocular problems such as viral keratitis, strabismus, glaucoma and retinal pathology.	• Age • Profession • Sports activities (contact sports and martial arts) • Any systemic disease and its treatment—diabetes, hypertension, autoimmune diseases and collagen vascular disorders.

Table 32.3: Clinical evaluation for laser vision correction (LVC).

Visual Acuity	• Uncorrected and best corrected • Suboptimal—rule out amblyopia, keratoconus, retinal pathologies
Refraction	• Precise refraction to plan correction • Cycloplegic refraction in accomodative spasm
Orthoptic examination	• Rule out phoria and tropia • Postoperative diplopia and need for squint correction
Diffuse light examination of the face	• Prominent bony orbital rim, narrow or tight palpebral fissures, prominent nasal bridge—difficulty in flap making, hence surface procedure is preferred
Slit-lamp biomicroscopy	• Conjunctival scarring, pingecula—difficulty in achieving vacuum • Cornea—Dystrophies, scaring, vascularization and ectatic disorders • Lens—rule out congenital or developmental cataract • Applanation tonometry and glaucoma evaluation • Tear film assessment—Baseline Schirmer's test and tear breakup test
Fundus examination	• Retinal degenerations like lattice and holes need to be treated first and LASIK should be considered only after adequate scarring. • History of previous retinal detachment (RD), post-RD surgery–to consider surface ablations
Computerized video keratometry (CVK)	• To exclude corneal ectatic disorders—A composite analysis of all three maps has to be done. Some topographers are incorporated with nomograms/softwares, which will give indices to aid in the diagnosis of potential ectatic disorders • To identify contact lens induced warping and advise the patient to stop contact lens for a considerable period and then to repeat the evaluation to ensure better outcomes • To asses corneal thickness to ensure adequate residual stromal thickness (RST) in LASIK • Corneal curvature steeper or flatter than the normal range can lead on to flap complications in LASIK. Axial keratometry map will help in planning the surgery to avoid these complications • Axis and amplitude of the refractive astigmatism can be confirmed from topography
Pupillometry	• Mesopic pupil size—measured by pupillometer by topography • Ablation zone diameter 2.4 mm larger than the pupil size • Large preoperative pupils—higher risk of postoperative glare and halos
Aberrometry	• Analyze wavefront pattern and higher order aberrations • Significant preoperative aberrations need wavefront-guided customized ablation
Pachymetry	• Below 480 microns is a contraindication • Calculate RST—should be more than 50% of corneal thickness

Table 32.4: Contraindications for laser vision correction (LVC).

Ocular	Systemic
• Keratoconus and other corneal ectatic disorders • Recurrent and recalcitrant viral or other immune diseases • Thin cornea or high refractive errors where minimum required RST cannot be maintained • Corneal dystrophies and scars • Glaucoma • Progressive vitreoretinal pathologies • Immune-mediated dry eye and ocular surface disorders (SJS, OCP) • Pediatric age group or unstable refraction	• *Absolute contraindications*: – Pregnancy – Lactating mothers – Collagen vascular diseases • *Relative contraindications*: – Hormonal therapy – Uncontrolled diabetes mellitus

(RST: Residual stromal thickness; SJS: Stevens-Johnson syndrome; OCP: Ocular cicatricial pemphigoid disease)

Procedures

The laser ablative procedures can be classified based on the anatomical plane at which they are done as surface ablative procedures and lamellar ablative procedures.

Surface ablations: According to the method of epithelial removal, the surface ablations are sub-classified as photorefractive keratectomy, laser-assisted subepithelial keratomileusis (LASEK) and Epi-LASIK.

Photorefractive Keratectomy/ Advanced Surface Ablation

Photorefractive keratectomy (PRK) consists of the application of excimer laser energy to the anterior corneal stroma after epithelial removal. The Bowman's membrane is also violated by the laser ablation.

***Indications*:**

- Myopia up to -6.0 D, astigmatism up to 3.0 D and hyperopia up to 4.0 D—higher corrections are associated with a greater risk of corneal haze formation and regression of the correction effect
- In thinner corneas to save tissue and to avoid compromised corneal biomechanical strength
- In steep or flat corneas to avoid flap related complications
- Deep set eyes
- LASIK complications in fellow eye
- In patients with a predisposition to trauma such as those engaged in contact sports or in armed forces
- Epithelial basement membrane disease—PRK can be therapeutic to reduce recurrent corneal erosions
- Dry eye syndrome—since corneal nerve damage is less in PRK further exacerbation of dry eye is minimal
- Enhancements following LASIK

Procedure: The first step is the removal of the epithelium by mechanical scrapping. About 20% alcohol application over the epithelial surface may aid in its removal. Epithelium can be ablated by the laser itself in phototherapeutic mode. The laser beam is centered for the entrance pupil and activated to ablate the anterior corneal stroma. The Bowman layer is destroyed in the process of PRK with no known deleterious consequences. A residual stromal thickness of 350 µm or more after PRK is necessary to prevent future corneal ectasia.

Once the ablation is completed, the surface is irrigated gently. Mitomycin 0.02% is applied over the ablated surface for 2 minutes and then thoroughly irrigated out. This step is useful for reducing the stromal haze formation, especially in higher corrections. A bandage contact lens is applied (Fig. 32.2).

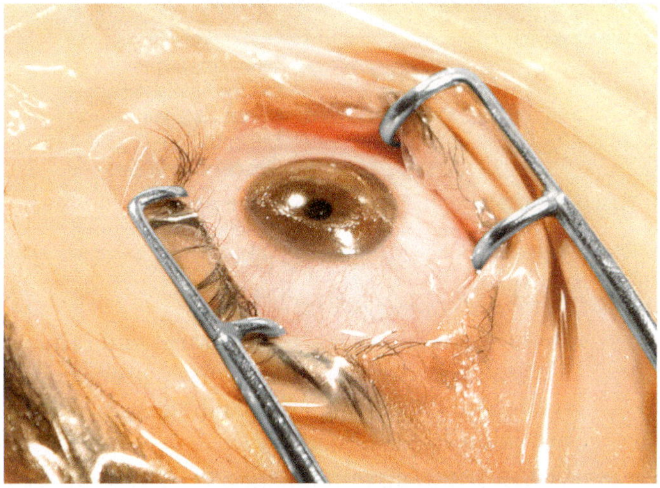

Fig. 32.2: PRK—Laser ablation done on the corneal surface after the epithelium is scrapped off.

***Postoperative care*:**

- Therapeutic bandage contact lens and a topical antibiotic drop are applied till the epithelial healing is completed
- Analgesic and antianxiety oral medications can be used during the first 24 hours postoperatively, to minimize pain and discomfort
- Topical steroids are started after epithelium heals and continued in tapering doses up to 1–3 months
- To enhance epithelial healing and to minimize stromal haze formation, nonpreserved tear supplements, oral vitamin C and avoiding sunlight exposure are recommended

***Advantages*:**

- Simple procedure
- Less invasive—no flap related complications
- Suitable for steep and thin corneas
- Less biomechanical compromise

***Disadvantages*:**

- Significant discomfort felt in the immediate postoperative period due to epithelial removal
- Abnormal wound healing response can result in haze formation and regression of the refractive correction
- Cannot be done for higher refractive errors

***Complications*:**

Complications of the surface procedures can be laser ablation related or tissue response related (Table 32.5).

Table 32.5: Complications of surface ablations.

Laser related	• Under corrections • Overcorrections • Induced astigmatism • Central islands • Decentration • Optical aberrations
Tissue response	• Regression • Reticular stromal haze

- *Laser-related complications*:
  - Under corrections, overcorrections, and induced astigmatism are due to improper preoperative refraction, data entry, laser calibration and tissue hydration
  - *Central islands* represent areas of unablated tissue in the central cornea. This phenomenon is common with broad beam lasers, where the plume from tissue destruction settles back on the corneal surface and reduces the effect of further ablation. This problem is rare in flying spot lasers
  - *Decentration* of the ablation zone may occur following decentered flap or inadequate centration on the entrance pupil at the time of laser application. The resulting irregular astigmatism, glare or ghosting of the images can be incapacitating. A topo-guided or wavefront guided retreatment may reduce the symptoms
  - *Night vision distortions* include glare, ghost images and haloes which are felt more in dim light conditions. Risk factors include smaller ablation zone than mesopic pupil diameter, and high refractive correction
- *Tissue response-related complications*:
  - *Persistent epithelial defects* are usually associated with dry eyes, underlying connective tissue disorders and diabetes mellitus. These underlying pathologies need to be addressed before the surgery.
    Management—postoperatively epithelial healing has to be supported with nonpreserved lubricants. As there is an increased risk of infectious keratitis, corneal haze and refractive irregularity, these patients need to be monitored closely.
  - *Regression* is the partial or total loss of the refractive correction achieved. The gradual refractive drift towards the original error will be noted 3–6 months later.[8-10] Hyperopic corrections, higher myopic corrections, delayed epithelial healing with stromal haze formation and patients with keloidal tendency are considered as risk factors for developing regression.

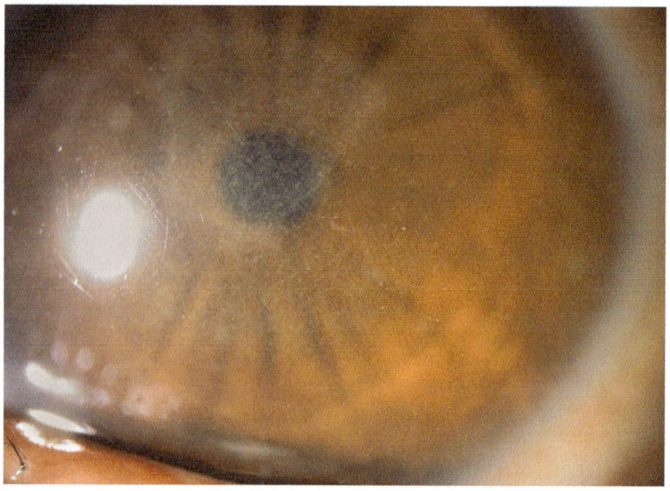

Fig. 32.3: Post-PRK reticular haze.
Source: Dr Jagadeesh Kumar Reddy.

Pathologically, the epithelial hyperplasia or stromal thickening fills up the ablated area and reduces the treatment effect. Early ectasia which is usually associated with corneal thinning has to be differentiated from regression due to tissue thickening, since both conditions present with reappearance of the refractive error. Progression of an unstable preoperative refractive error also mimics regression.

Management—refractive and topographical changes have to be documented periodically. Ectasia has to be ruled out. After the refractive error stabilized, retreatment can be attempted if there is adequate corneal thickness.

  - *Reticular stromal haze* is the most important complication of surface procedures. It is an abnormal wound healing response which is associated with higher ablations and delayed epithelial healing. It is often transient and does not affect visual acuity. Clinically, this is recognized by slit lamp biomicroscopic examination as a lace like anterior stromal opacity[11,12] (Fig. 32.3)

    Management of persistent moderate-to-severe haze includes topical steroids and liberal lubrication. If the haze is persistent and severe enough to cause visual problems laser ablation can be attempted.

    Prevention of haze—intraoperative application of mitomycin 0.02% for 30–120 seconds is recommended when more than 80 microns of tissue needs to be ablated. Postoperatively liberal lubrication, steroids, oral vitamin C and prevention of UV exposure are recommended.

Laser-assisted Subepithelial Keratomileusis

Laser-assisted subepithelial keratomileusis is a modified surface procedure in which the epithelium is loosened by using 15–25% alcohol as a sheet and is reflected back to expose the anterior stroma for laser ablation.

Epi-LASIK

A motorized epithelial separator mechanically separates the corneal epithelium at the layer of Bowman's membrane from the stroma, without the use of alcohol or chemicals. In both procedures the reflected epithelial flap is nonviable and will be replaced by regenerating epithelium. Since the denuded surface is covered with the reflected epithelial flap after the laser ablation the recovery time is expected to be reduced with less postoperative discomfort. There is less risk of infection and incidence of corneal haze.

Advanced surface ablation with better understanding of wound healing can achieve good results. It is a preferred procedure in patients with suspicious corneal biomechanics or where flap creation is expected to be difficult.

Lamellar ablative procedures: These include excimer and femtolaser-based procedures such as LASIK and SMILE.

Laser-assisted in situ Keratomileusis

Principle: Excimer laser ablation of the corneal stroma is done beneath a hinged corneal flap that is created with a mechanical microkeratome or a femtosecond laser. Since tissue healing response is minimal in LASIK, higher correction up to 12 D of myopia, 6 D of hyperopia, and 6 D of astigmatism are considered possible.

Procedure: LASIK involves a surgical step of flap creation in addition to laser ablation. Meticulous planning is imperative to achieve high quality results and to avoid serious complications.

Flap creation: An ideal flap should be hinged for stability, of optimal thickness with uniform parallel surfaces exposing a regular stromal bed. Currently flaps are made by automated microkeratomes or by femtosecond laser.

- *Flap creation by automated microkeratome*: In this procedure, the flap is created by mechanical means by using motorized equipment called microkeratome.
  - *Components of automated microkeratome (Fig. 32.4)*:
    - The suction ring holds the globe by creating vacuum at the limbus and applanates the cornea during flap cut by increasing IOP (Fig. 32.4)
    - The head holds the oscillating blade with a gauge which determines the thickness of the flap. The stainless steel blades are for single use. The flap thickness usually ranges from 100 microns to 140 microns (Fig. 32.5)
    - The motor moves the blade as well as the head across the cornea to create the flap. The movement is stopped at a predetermined stage to leave behind a hinge. The hinge can be located superiorly which makes the flap more stable or nasally which will minimize corneal nerve damage[13] (Fig. 32.6)

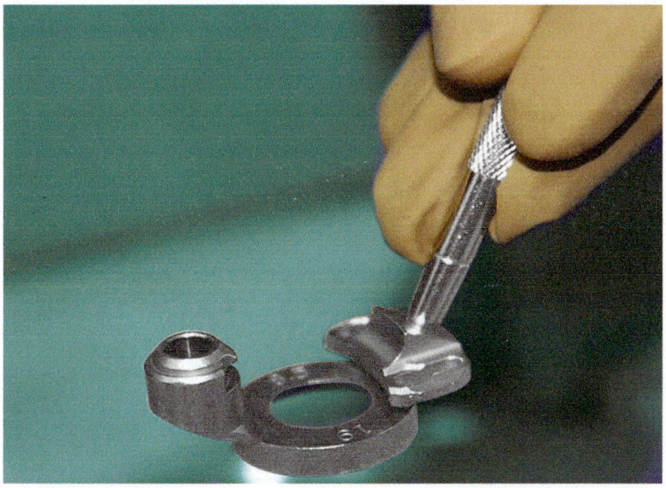

Fig. 32.4: Microkeratome suction ring determines the flap diameter.

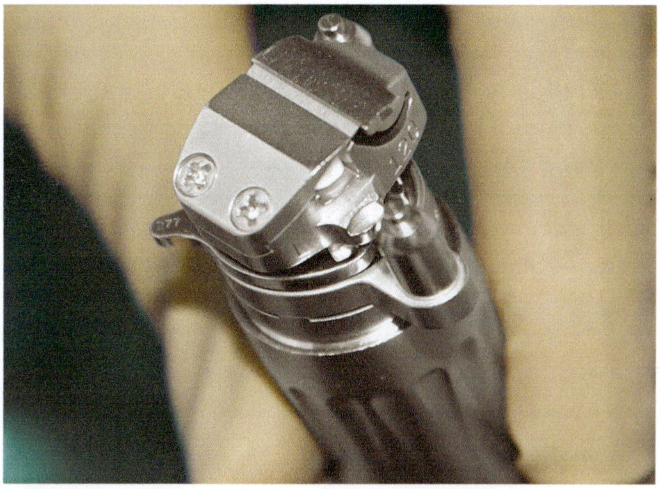

Fig. 32.5: Microkeratome head holds the blade and determines flap thickness.

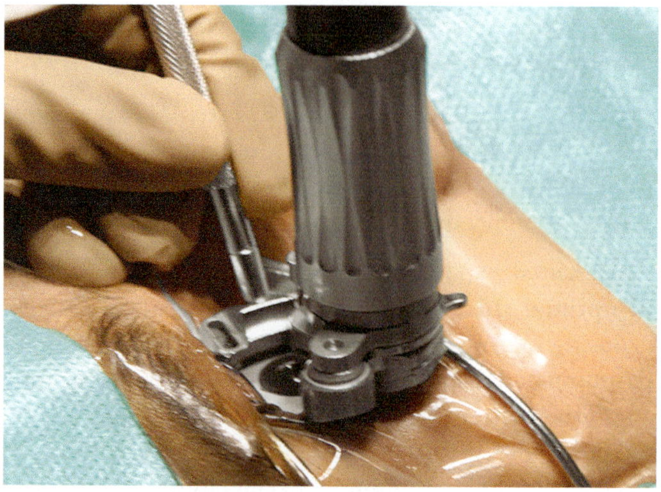

Fig. 32.6: Suction is activated to hold the globe and the microkeratome motor moves the head with oscillating blade forward and backward to create the flap.

- *Limitations of the microkeratome*:
    - Microkeratome can cut flaps thinner or thicker than the intended thickness. A thicker flap can compromise the preplanned residual stromal thickness after laser ablation
    - They can create flaps only within a narrow range of thickness and diameter
    - Mechanical failure of any of the microkeratome parts can lead on to higher incidence of flap related complications
    - High suction and raised IOP may rarely cause vascular occlusion and retinal detachment

• *Flap creation by femtosecond laser*:[14] In this procedure, a femtosecond laser is used to create the flap, instead of a mechanical device by a process of photodisruption. The cornea is held by a relatively lesser suction. Femtosecond laser pulses are focused at a desired depth in the stroma to create cavitation and bubble formation. Multiple cavities are formed in expanding spiral or raster pattern in the same plane. This lamellar cut is externalized by a side cut all around except at the hinge position. The flap is lifted by breaking the trabecular tissue formed by the cavitation with a spatula (Figs. 32.7A to C).

- *Advantages*:
    - Suction is much less compared to mechanical device thus problems associated with high IOP are rare

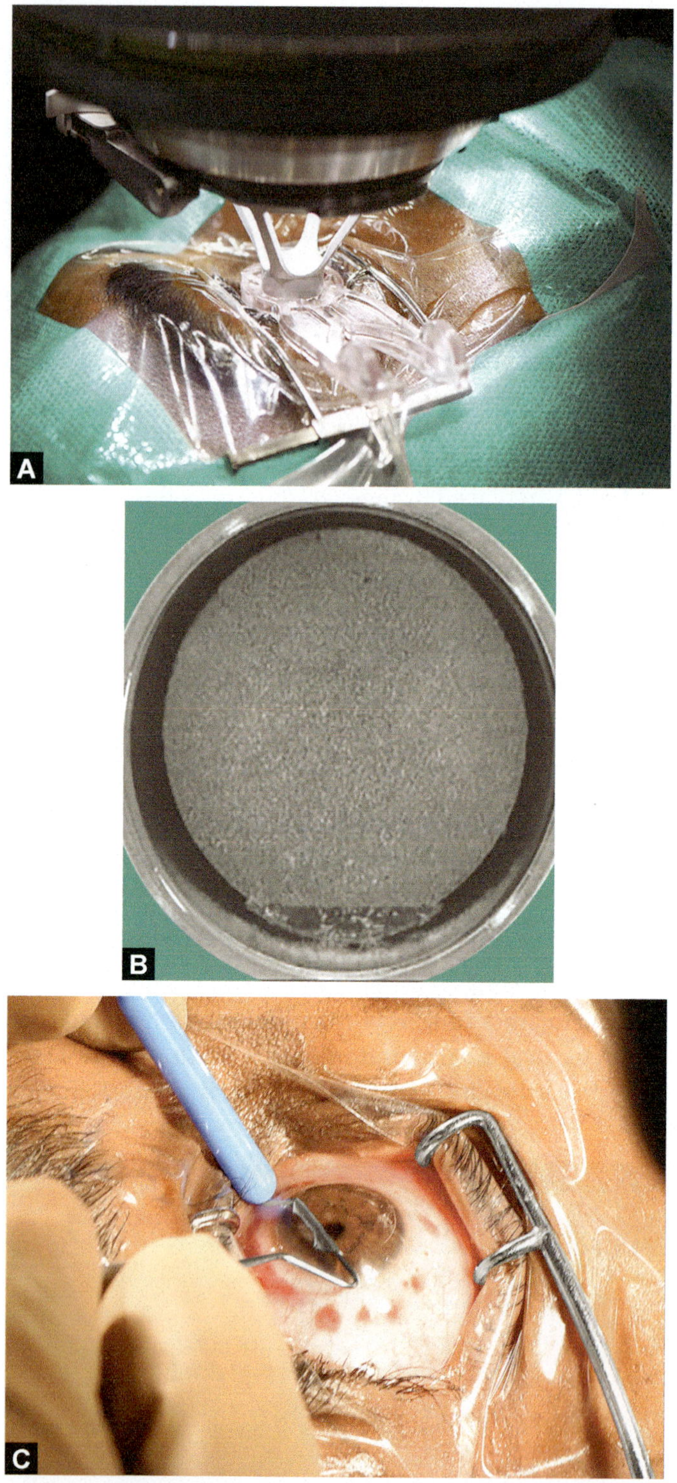

Figs. 32.7A to C: Femtolaser flap making. (A) A cone to applanates the cornea is docked in to suction ring; (B) Intrastromal cavities formed in a raster pattern with a side cut to create a flap. Air pocket at the hinge end to reduce opaque bubble formation; (C) The flap is lifted by breaking the cavities.

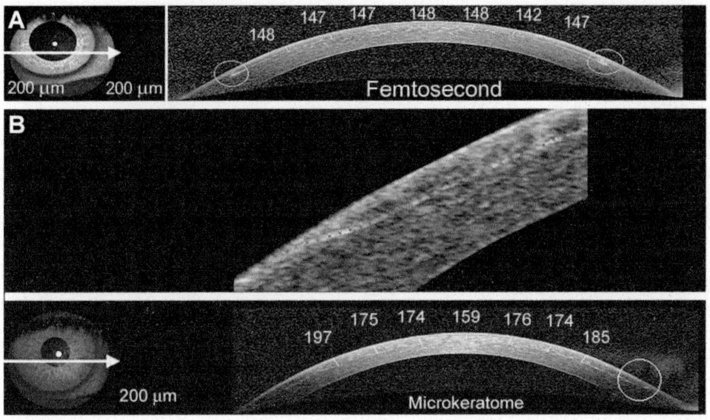

Figs. 32.8A and B: (A) Anterior segment optical coherence tomography (ASOCT) showing a femtoflap with uniform thickness and straight side cut; (B) Meniscus flap cut by microkeratome with sloping margin and thick periphery.
Source: Dr N Venkatesh Prajna.

- Wide range of flap thickness starting from 90 microns can be planned as laser beam can be focused at any depth
- The predictability of the flap thickness is more reliable than mechanical microkeratome
- Flaps are of uniform thickness with planar margins which allows better reposition compared to a meniscus flap created by microkeratome (Figs. 32.8A and B)
- Less chance for mechanical failures and contamination by the microkeratome parts. Hence, low incidence of flap related complications and infections are expected

- *Disadvantages*:
  - The excimer laser ablation cannot be processed as long as the opaque bubbles formed by cavitation remain in the optical zone. These bubbles are collected in an air pocket at the hinge end of the flap to prevent opaque bubble formation
  - Tissue beneath a corneal opacity will not be cut by femtosecond laser. Any superficial corneal opacity within the proposed flap area is a contraindication for femtolaser flap

Laser ablation procedure: Laser energy and homogeneity of the beam has to be checked at prescribed intervals before the procedure. Patient head has to be positioned with chin and forehead in the same plane. Once the flap is created either by microkeratome or femtolaser, a reference mark is made across the flap edge, which will help in replacing the flap with proper orientation after laser ablation. The flap is checked for any abnormalities before being lifted up. The lifted flap is folded on its stromal side and left to lie on the globe. The laser beam is activated after it is centered to the pupil. Once the ablation is completed, the interface is irrigated gently and the flap is floated in to the position. Excess fluid is milked out by cellulose sponge and the flap is allowed to dry for firm adhesion by natural endothelial pump mechanism (Figs. 32.9A to C).

- *Postoperative care*:
  - The flap adherence is checked again after about 30 minutes
  - Any kind of pressure over the lids should be avoided, including patching
  - The patient is advised to wear a pair of protective goggles for a week
  - Broad-spectrum antibiotic and steroid drops are applied for a week

The epithelium at the cut edge usually heals within few hours and the patient will be comfortable and begins to see relatively clear the same day. Lubricating drop is continued for several weeks. Topography is repeated to assess the centration and regularity of the treatment after a month and repeated periodically to rule out regression and ectasia. Refractive stability is usually achieved by 1 month.

- *Complications*: Laser related complications after lamellar procedures are similar to that of surface ablative procedures. The complications related to flap creation, flap adherence and the interface between the flap and the underlying stroma are unique to lamellar refractive surgeries (Table 32.6).

Flap-related complications:

Intraoperative complications: Intraoperative difficulty in obtaining adequate suction due to anatomical constraints like deep set eyes, narrow palpebral fissure with prominent bony orbital margins may warrant a conversion to surface procedure.

The following flap abnormalities can occur during flap cutting:

- Incomplete flap
- Irregular cut surface and thickness
- Decentered and inadequate stromal exposure
- Button hole of the flap leaving behind an island of uncut tissue on the bed
- Free cap—a flap cut all around without a hinge

Inadequate or loss of suction can result in small, irregular or incomplete flap. Conjunctival irregularities, mechanical failure of the vacuum system, faulty microkeratome head

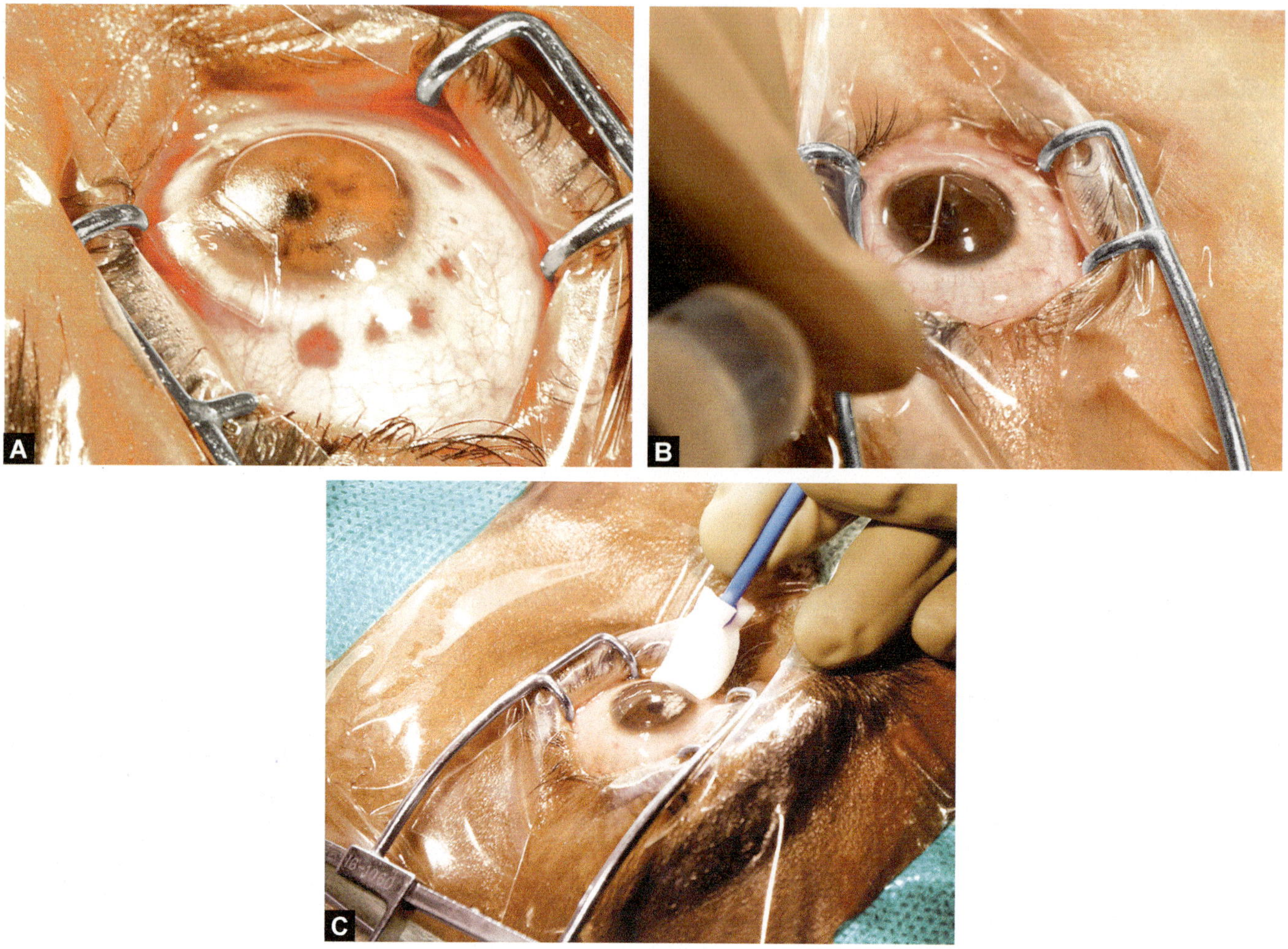

Figs. 32.9A to C: (A) Flap is lifted and folded on its stromal side on the globe during laser ablation; (B) Flap is repositioned and the interface is irrigated; (C) Excess interface fluid is milked out and the flap is allowed to adhere.

Table 32.6: Complications of LASIK.

Intraoperative	Flap related
Early postoperative	• Striae • Dislocation • DLK • PISK • Central toxic keratopathy • Infection
Late postoperative	• Epithelial ingrowth • Ectasia • Ocular surface problems • Posterior segment complications

(DLK: Diffuse lamellar keratitis; PISK: Pressure-induced stromal keratopathy)

or blade movement and reused blunt blades could lead to inadequate suction.[15,16]

Buckling of a cornea with steep curvature within a large ring may result in button holing of the flap. A flat corneal curvature can result in a free cap.

Management: Once the flap abnormality is recognized, the flap should not be disturbed and the procedure is ideally aborted without proceeding to laser ablation. A recut can be made at a different depth after a period of 3 months. A surface procedure is a safer alternative after the flap is healed and the refractive stability is confirmed.

If a free cap is large enough and exposes adequate stroma, laser ablation can be continued. The flap should be replaced and properly aligned. A bandage contact lens or sutures are used to keep it in place.

Early postoperative complications:

Flap folds: Fine microstriae are wrinkles in Bowman's membrane seen in the immediate postoperative period. Flap hydration and change in the corneal curvature are thought to be the causes for microstriae. They usually will not interfere with visual outcome.

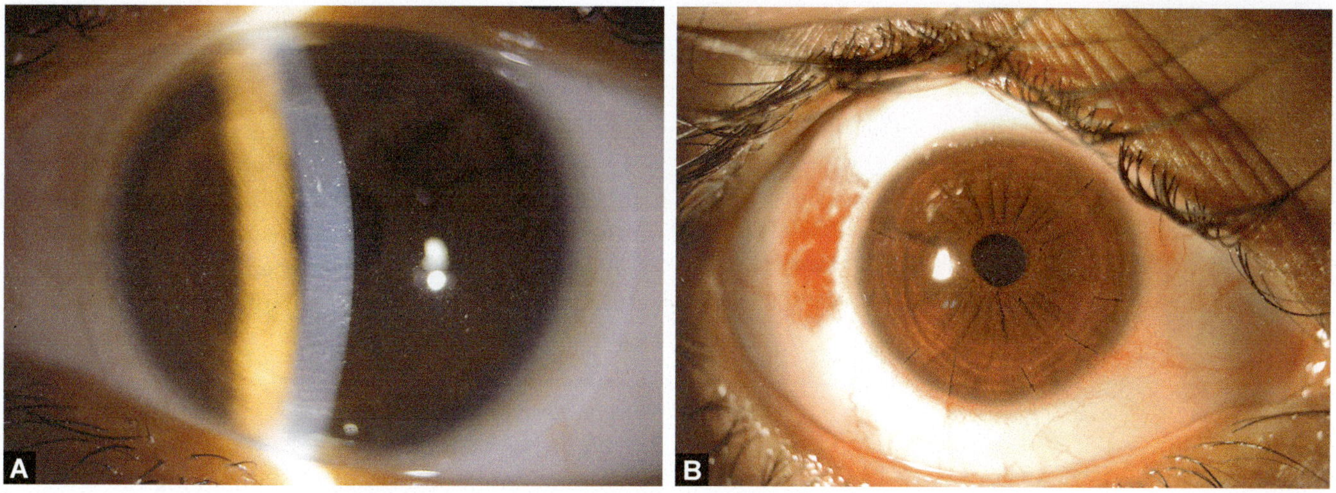

Figs. 32.10A and B: (A) Flap macrofolds need intervention; (B) Folds cleared after suturing.
Source for Fig. A: Dr Jagadeesh Kumar Reddy .

Macrofolds involve full thickness of the flap and interfere with visual outcome. They occur due to flap displacement either in the early postoperative period or later due to traumatic dislocation. Pooling of fluorescein in the gutters of the folds will differentiate them from microstriae.

Management:

- Flap has to be relifted and stretched by hydration
- Removal of epithelium will help to smooth out the folds
- Long standing folds need suturing
- The sutures can be removed after 3 weeks and the astigmatism usually disappears with suture removal (Figs. 32.10A and B)

Flap dislocation: Flap can get dislocated from the stromal bed due to poor adhesion or due to shear force like rubbing in the early postoperative period. LASIK flap can get dislocated even years after healing, by trauma (Fig. 32.11). Early repositioning will reduce further complications like epithelial in growth, flap folds, infection and interface inflammation.

Diffuse lamellar keratitis (DLK): It is also known as Sands of Sahara syndrome is a nonspecific inflammatory reaction and is usually due to the neutrophil collection in the interface.[17,18]

Early onset DLK—occurs in clusters within weeks after the procedure and is thought to be caused by toxins from the sterilizer, detergents used to clean the keratome parts and meibomian secretions.[19]

Late onset DLK—this is triggered by trauma, conjunctivitis or orbital infections.[20-22]

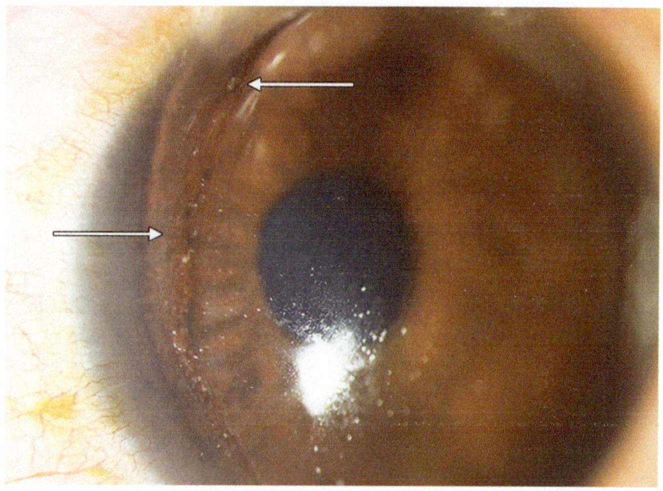

Fig. 32.11: Traumatic flap dislocation can occur even years after the procedure
Source: Dr N Venkatesh Prajna.

Mild cellular collection in the periphery of the interface may be noticed in the immediate postoperative period. It usually clears with regular postoperative steroid therapy. In DLK this inflammation and cellular deposition progresses to involve the center (Fig. 32.12). Collagenase secreted by the inflammatory cells can result in flap melt and scaring. The progressive stage needs more aggressive treatment. The management varies according to the severity which is graded as per the clinical picture (Table 32.7).

Pressure-induced stromal keratopathy (PISK): This phenomenon occurs as fluid collection in the interface due to raised intraocular pressure and presents with a

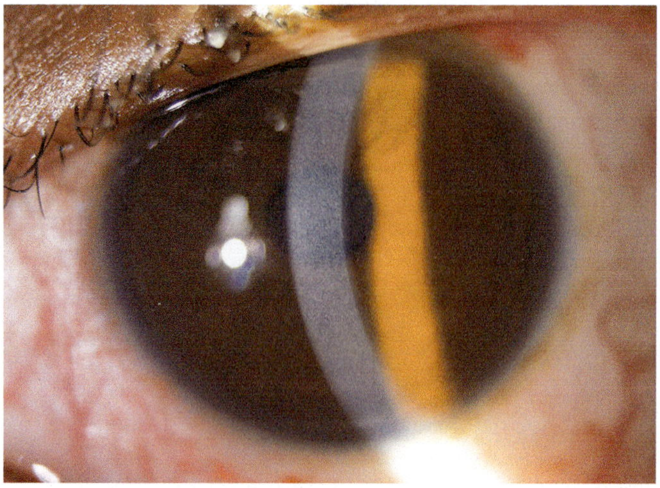

Fig. 32.12: Grade 2 DLK—with diffuse cellular deposition in the interface.

Table 32.7: Clinical grading and management of diffuse lamellar keratitis (DLK).

Grading	Management
• *Grade 1*: Diffuse cellular deposition in the periphery of the interphase • *Grade 2*: Cellular deposition which is diffuse and involves the visual axis • *Grade 3*: Clumps of aggregated cells with surrounding clear area. The collagenase released from the inflammatory cells can cause stromal and flap melts that result in permanent scar • *Grade 4*: Rare. Flap melt and scaring will give a mud-crack appearance. Hyperopic shift is seen	• *Grade 1 and 2*: – Medical management with hourly steroid application – Close monitoring to recognize progression to stage 3 which usually occurs at around 48–72 hours • *Grade 3*: – Surgical intervention to lift the flap and irrigate the interphase – A microbiological work-up also be done to rule out infection • *Grade 4*: The fragile flap should not be interfered at this stage

diffuse stromal and interface opacity. Careful slit lamp observation reveals a fluid cleft in the interface, which can be confirmed by anterior segment optical coherence tomography (OCT). Often this condition is misdiagnosed as DLK which presents early and with a normal IOP. PISK presents after a few weeks post corticosteroids treatment.[23]

Management: The management is entirely different from that of DLK. Cessation of corticosteroid drops with use of topical antiglaucoma medications will reverse the condition.

Central toxic keratopathy:

This is an acute central corneal opacification due to noninflammatory enzymatic degradation in the immediate postoperative period. This condition is usually not amenable to treatment and can result in flap wrinkling with hyperopic shift.[24,25]

Infection: The postrefractive surgery infection is a rare but devastating complication. Incidence varies from 0.02% to 1.5%. In PRK, the infection is on the surface whereas post-LASIK, it usually starts at the interface. Intraoperative contamination can occur during epithelial removal in PRK and flap making in LASIK. Late infections can occur after traumatic inoculation.

Risk factors for post-LASIK infection:

- Poor lid hygiene
- Dry eyes
- Intraoperative excessive manipulations
- Delayed epithelial healing
- Postoperative trauma

Causative pathogens: Early onset within first 2 weeks suggests virulent bacterial infections caused by organisms like *Staphylococcus*, *Streptococcus* and *Pseudomonas* species.

Late onset from 2 weeks to 3 months usually is due to atypical mycobacteria, nocardia, fungi or *Acanthamoeba*.

The incidence of atypical mycobacterial infections have come down with the use of fourth generation fluoroquinolones. However, methicillin resistant staphylococcal infections have increased especially in healthcare workers. Recurrence of herpetic keratitis can occur if preoperative dormant infection is missed out.

Clinical picture:

The patient presents with a history of sudden drop in vision with signs of anterior segment inflammation and a focal necrotic infiltration involving the stromal bed. This condition has to be differentiated from DLK, where the cellular deposition is confined to interface, with minimal or no anterior chamber reactions (Figs. 32.13A and B).

Management:

Empirical antimicrobial treatment should be avoided. The microbiological workup is done immediately by lifting the flap and scraping the material for laboratory tests. Interface irrigation with vancomycin in early onset infections and amikacin in late infections are recommended. Steroids have to be avoided.[26,27] Appropriate antimicrobial therapy as per the culture and sensitivity report should be started. Flap amputation may be needed to reduce the infection load and to improve drug penetration. In severe, progressive infections, a lamellar or full thickness therapeutic keratoplasty can be considered.

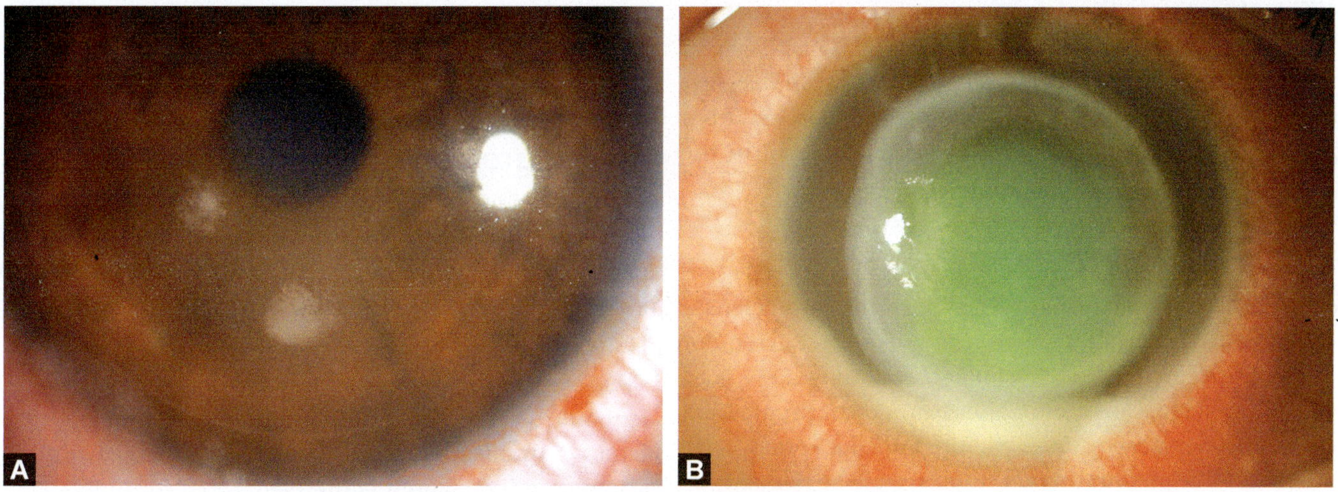

Figs. 32.13A and B: (A) Post-LASIK infection—interface infiltrate; (B) Post-PRK infection.
Source: Dr Jagadeesh Kumar Reddy.

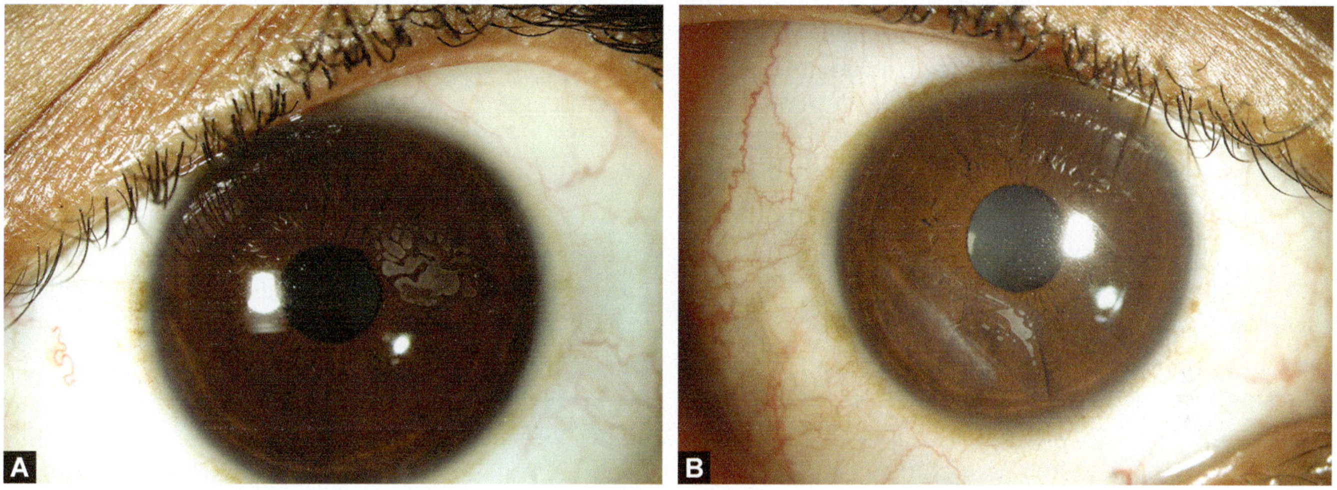

Figs. 32.14A and B: (A) Epithelial ingrowth at the periphery; (B) Epithelial ingrowth after trauma to the flap.
Source: Dr N Venkatesh Prajna.

Late postoperative complications:

Epithelial in-growth in the interface: Epithelial cell seedling in the interface can occur during flap making, through poorly adherent flap edge or by trauma. Often they present as grayish opaque Island of tissue, usually at the periphery unless they are associated with a central buttonhole (Figs. 32.14A and B). Predisposing conditions include:

- Flap dislocation
- Perioperative epithelial defects
- Buttonhole of the flap
- Trauma or relifting of the flap later

A lesion progressing towards the visual axis, can compromise vision. The collagenase secreted by the epithelial cells can cause flap melt.

Management: Conservative management is advised if epithelial ingrowth remains stationary. A progressive lesion involving visual axis needs to be scrapped off after lifting the flap. Aggressive and recurrent growth warrants use of intraoperative mitomycin and the flap margin should be sealed tightly with sutures or fibrin glue.

Post-LASIK ectasia: Iatrogenic ectasia is a rare but serious complication of LASIK.

Predisposing factors:

- Preexisting subclinical ectasia
- Inadequate residual stroma probably due to thin cornea, thicker flaps or excessive ablation.[28,29]

Clinical features: The time of onset of ectasia varies from immediate postoperative period to years after LASIK. Patient presents with gradual deterioration of vision with irregular astigmatism. This condition should be differentiated from regression. Serial topography is needed to confirm the diagnosis.

Management of post-LASIK ectasia:

- Early stages should be observed for progression
- Visual acuity can be improved with rigid contact lenses
- Intrastromal ring segments may stabilize irregular astigmatism and help in contact lens fitting
- Collagen crosslinking to stabilize the ectatic progression
- In advanced cases, deep anterior lamellar keratoplasty (DALK) or penetrating keratoplasty will be needed

LASIK induced changes in ocular surface: Refractive surgical procedures damage the corneal sensory nerve endings, which is more in superior hinged flaps. The resulting hypesthesia and interference in sensory feedback of lacrimal secretion can lead on to inadequate and unstable tear film and poor ocular surface repair. A poor ocular surface can affect the quality of vision and increases chances for regression.[30,31]

Management: Any tear film abnormalities should be treated before surgery. Postoperatively, nonpreserved lubricants may be needed for 3–6 months.

Posterior segment complications: Several posterior segment complications like retinal detachment, choroidal infarct and optic neuropathy have been reported.[32] Suction induces increase in IOP in the presence of vitreous syneresis, peripheral retinal degenerative changes is thought to be the cause for such posterior segment complications. Routine thorough preoperative examination of the retinal periphery is mandatory and any significant pathology has to be treated with prophylactic cryo- or laser-photocoagulation.

Lamellar Femtosecond Laser-based Procedures

Refractive corneal lenticule extraction/femtosecond lenticule extraction: Femtosecond laser is used to cut the flap as well as to effect the refractive correction. Corneal curvature is altered by cutting a lenticule of tissue using femtosecond laser beneath a flap.[33]

Small incision lenticule extraction: Small incision lenticule extraction (SMILE) is a procedure involves using femtosecond laser to create a corneal lenticule within the stromal pocket, which is then extracted through a small incision. It is reported to achieve effects similar to LASIK without a corneal lamellar flap being fashioned. But treating low refractive powers and high cylindrical corrections can be challenging[33,34] (Figs. 32.15A and B).

Indications: Myopia up to –11 D and astigmatism up to –5 D can be corrected. Since no flap is made in SMILE, it is a preferable procedure in patients with dry eyes, and those with high-risk of contact trauma.

Advantages: The incision is small and heals faster. Since it is a flapless procedure, there is no risk of flap related problems, less disruption to the sub-basal nerve plexus and less violation of corneal biomechanics.

Disadvantages: Incomplete lenticule dissection and removal can result in poor visual outcome. This is common in low corrections, where the lenticule will be too thin to handle.[35] Wavefront guided corrections are not possible. Femtosecond laser based lamellar procedure is showing better safety profile as a flapless procedure but are suitable for limited indications at present.

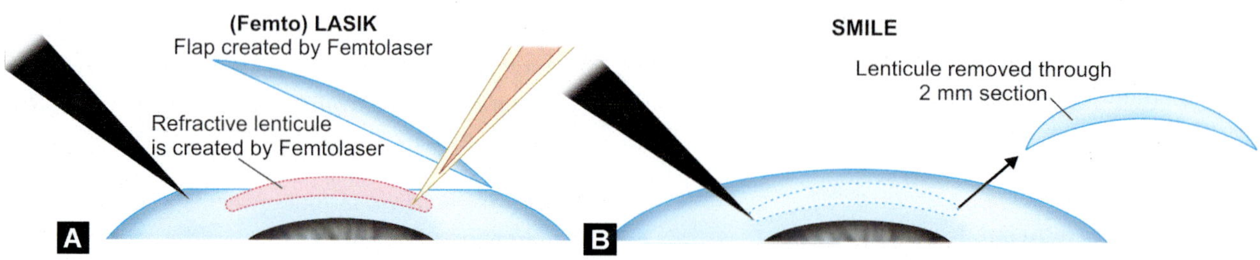

Figs. 32.15A and B: (A) Femto-based LASIK—Femtolaser flap is created and lifted up. A refractive lenticule is created by femtolaser in the stromal bed and removed. Flap is repositioned as in LASIK; (B) SMILE—Intrastromal refractive lenticule is created by femtolaser and removed through a 3 mm incision by dissection within the stromal pocket.

LENS-BASED REFRACTIVE SURGERIES

Replacing a cataractous crystalline lens with an artificial intraocular lens (IOL) is a well-known lens based refractive procedure. This concept evolved further to replacement of clear lens or IOL insertion in a phakic eye to correct high refractive errors.

Refractive Lens Exchange

This is an intraocular refractive surgery in which the natural clear lens is replaced with artificial IOL to correct refractive errors. In high myopia, removing the clear lens and rendering the eye aphakic itself will correct the refractive error. A clear lens extraction can be combined with monofocal, multifocal, toric and accommodative IOL to address myopia, hyperopia, astigmatism and also presbyopia.[36] This procedure can be combined with corneal refractive procedures (bioptics).

The procedure is similar to cataract removal and IOL insertion. High hyperopic correction may need insertion of two IOLs as piggyback system, if the calculated power is not available commercially. One lens will be placed within the bag and the second one will be sulcus fixated.

Refractive lens exchange is more suitable for older patients with high refractive errors who are presbyopic or likely to develop cataract soon.

***Advantages*:**
- The procedure is familiar for the surgeons and does not need expensive equipment
- Higher refractive errors can be corrected
- Since corneal contour is preserved, there is no night vision distortions or reduced contrast sensitivity

***Disadvantages*:**
- Chances for retinal detachment are more in myopic eyes when the natural crystalline lens is removed. It is advisable to insert even a zero power IOL within the capsular bag instead of leaving the eye aphakic
- Crowded anterior segment may lead on to angle closure and corneal endothelial compromise in hyperopic eyes with piggyback IOLs

Phakic Intraocular Lens

Phakic intraocular lens (PIOL) is a special lens that is implanted surgically into a phakic eye to correct higher refractive errors. This procedure is considered for patients who are not suitable for laser procedures due to high refractive errors or thin corneas.[37]

Table 32.8: Indications and contraindications for phakic IOL.

Indications for phakic IOL	Contraindications for phakic IOL
• Correction of myopia –3 D to –18 D • Hyperopia +0.5 D to +10.0 D • Astigmatism 1.0–4.0 D cyl • 21 years of age • AC depth 3.0 mm or greater • Stable refractive history with <0.5 D change for 12 months	• Progressive refractive error • Corneal endothelial count <2500 cells/mm³/pathology • Glaucoma • Narrow AC angle • Cataract or capsular opacification • AC Depth <2.8 mm • Iritis/synechiae/pigment dispersion/pseudoexfoliation • Individuals prone for injury by occupation or hobbies

(IOL: Intraocular Lens)

Since the PIOL is to be kept in addition to a natural lens, it should be of different dimensions from regular IOLs. Requirements of an ideal PIOL are:
- Thin enough not to cause anterior segment crowding
- Should be placed as far as away from corneal endothelium, iris and lens
- Should not damage angle structures

Indications and Contraindications

Phakic intraocular lens is more suitable for roomy myopic anterior segment than hyperopic eyes. They are not suitable for patients with certain intraocular diseases or those who do not have optimal anterior segment dimensions. Specific indications and contraindications are given in Table 32.8.

Types of PIOLs as per their placement:
- Anterior chamber angle supported
- Iris fixated—rigid polymethylmethacrylate (PMMA) lens
- Posterior chamber sulcus fixated—implantable collamer lens (ICL).

Posterior chamber ICL is the most commonly used PIOL because of better safety profile since it is away from sensitive corneal endothelium, iris and angle structures. The sulcus fixation is more close to nodal point. The posterior surface of the ICL is vaulted to avoid touching the crystalline lens (Figs. 32.16A to C)

Preoperative Evaluation

In addition to the routine investigations for other intraocular surgeries and refractive procedures, the following measurements are important in PIOL implantation.

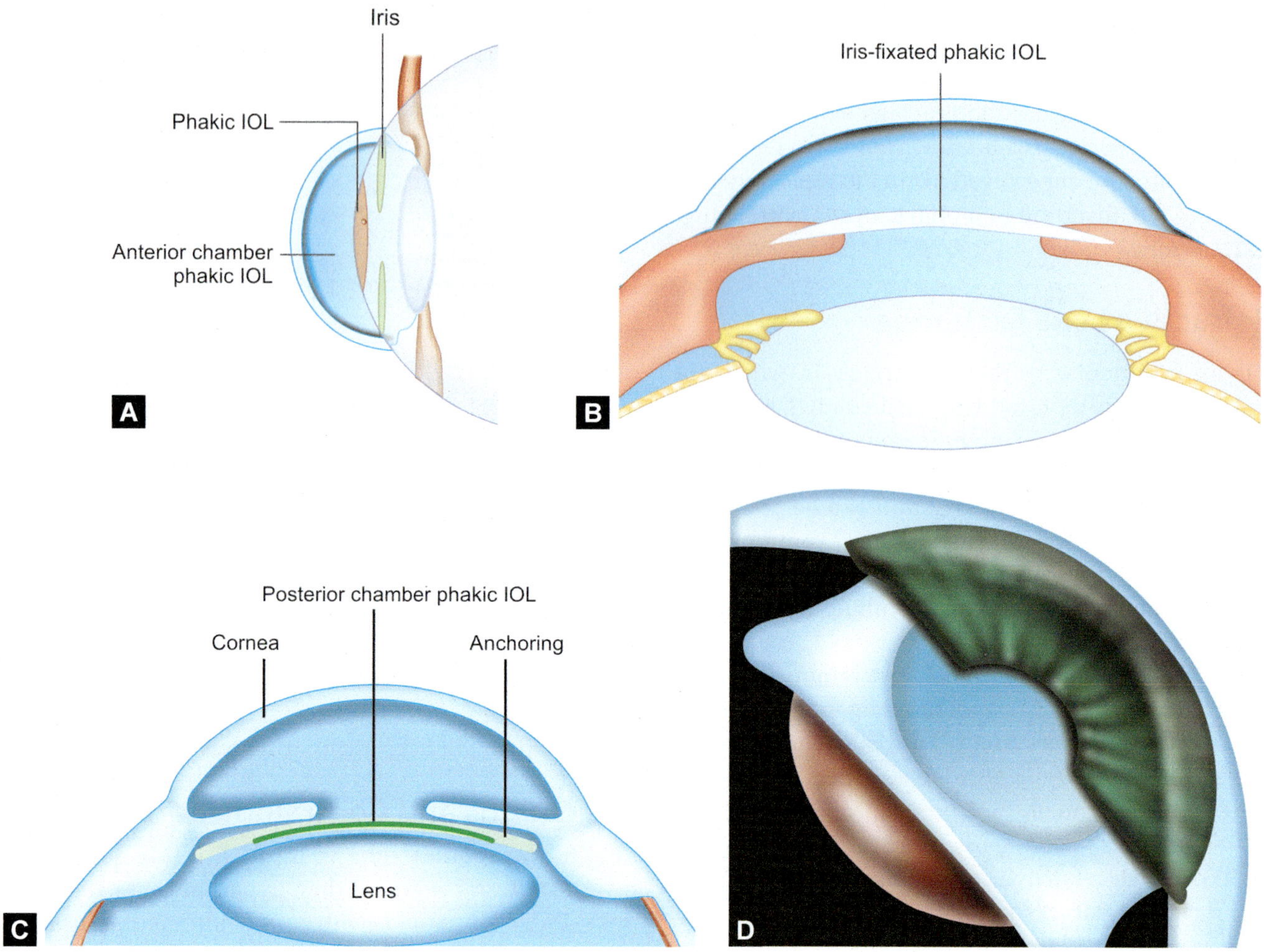

Figs. 32.16A to C: (A) Anterior chamber angle-fixated phakic IOL; (B) Iris-fixated phakic IOL; (C and D) Posterior chamber sulcus fixated PIOL (ICL). (IOL: Intraocular lens)

Corneal endothelial cell density and morphology should be analyzed by specular or confocal imaging. Gradual endothelial loss is documented with all 3 types of PIOL.

Adequate anterior chamber depth should be more than 3.2 mm to implant any type of PIOL. Anterior chamber depth is measured by anterior segment optical coherence tomography (ASOCT), scanning slit scan (Orbscan) or Scheimpflug imaging (Pentacam).

Measurement of sulcus diameter is crucial for the accurate IOL sizing in posterior chamber PIOL implantation. Sulcus diameter is usually measured by measuring white to white limbal diameter. This measurement is done by digital caliper or by topography by scanning slit beam. Direct sulcus measurement is also done by using ASOCT.

Procedure

A peripheral iridectomy is done either before or intraoperatively to avoid pupillary block. Both angle supported lens and posterior chamber PIOL are flexible and can be inserted through small, clear corneal sections whereas iris fixated PMMA lenses need a larger section.

Iris supported PIOL is fixed by a process called enclavation, using a second instrument passed through the limbal stab incisions.

Posterior chamber PIOL is injected in to anterior chamber under dispersive viscoelastic cover with its convexity facing posteriorly. The plate haptics are tucked beneath the iris without touching the optic center.

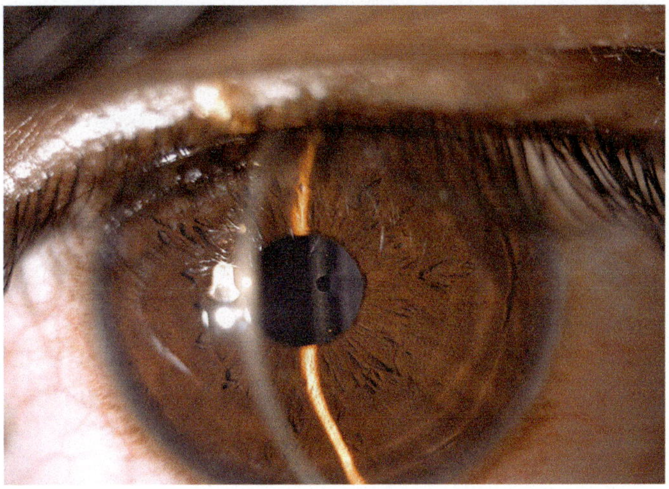

Fig. 32.17: ICL in the posterior chamber with a vault in front of anterior lens surface.

Table 32.9: Complications of implantable collamer lens (ICL).

Intra- and early postoperative	Late postoperative
• Damaged ICL • Reversal of the vault • Postoperative complications • Toric ICL rotation away from the desired axis • ICL decentration • Initial spike in IOP can be managed with pupillary dilatation and antiglaucoma medications. • *ICL vault*: If it is too low, chances for lenticular damage are more. If the vault is high, chances for angle-closure glaucoma should be kept in mind.	• Anterior subcapsular cataract • Pupil ovalization • Glare and halos • Glaucoma • Retinal detachment

(IOP: Intraocular pressure)

Viscoelastic material should be irrigated out thoroughly to reduce IOP spike postoperatively. Present day ICL with a central hole (center flow) does not need peripheral iridectomy (Fig. 32.17).

Complications

Specific complications occur with different types of PIOLs:

- *Angle supported PIOL*: Chronic angle structure damage, pupil ovalization and endothelial cell loss are the complications associated with this type of phakic lens
- *Iris fixated PIOL*: Iritis, IOL dislocation with endothelial decompensation are reported with iris supported PIOL
- *Posterior chamber ICL*: Transient increase in IOP in the immediate postoperative period due to entrapped viscoelastic and potential lens touch and late cataract formation are the common complications with ICL (Table 32.9)

Accurate sizing is very important in both anterior chamber PIOL and posterior chamber ICL. In posterior chamber PIOL, appropriate size determines its clearance from the anterior lens surface, called vault of the ICL. This vault is seen as a dark space in slit beam examination and is measured as in Van Herick's method in comparison to corneal thickness in a thin slit beam. Ideally, this vault should be of 0.5–1.5 corneal thickness (Fig. 32.17).

Phakic IOL implantation is suitable for patients with higher refractive errors with proper patient selection, proper preoperative planning and immediate recognition of complications.

Corneal Additive Procedure

The INTACS (intrastromal corneal ring segments or intracorneal rings) are made of biocompatible material, which are placed in deep corneal stromal tunnels made at midperiphery to correct low myopia up to 4 D. The placement of the rings involves the creation of a tunnel in the cornea with the use of a femtosecond laser. The increase in the stromal thickness at midperiphery will flatten the corneal center. However, this procedure is used in keratoconus management more often than in myopic correction. Single or double rings are placed to centralize the cone and to reduce the corneal irregularity, which helps in better contact lens fitting in keratoconus patients.

REFRACTIVE SURGERIES FOR PRESBYOPIA

Surgical correction of presbyopia can be achieved mainly by two approaches, namely nonaccommodative or accommodative methods. Treatment remains a challenge as the mechanism of accommodation is complex and it progressively increases with age (Table 32.10).

Nonaccommodative Procedures

Monovision

Principle: In monovision, one eye is made myopic to improve near vision. The dominant eye is corrected for distance and the nondominant eye for near vision, so that

Table 32.10: Procedures to correct presbyopia.

Nonaccommodative	• Monovision correction • Corneal inlays • Conductive keratoplasty • Multifocal LASIK • IntraCor • Multifocal intraocular lens
Accommodative	• Accomodative IOL • Flexible anterior ciliary sclerotomy (ACS) • Scleral expansion bands

(IOL: Intraocular lens)

patient does not need spectacles. Depending on the initial status of refraction, under correction or overcorrection of the refractive power is used to achieve a myopic shift of 0.5–1.5 D for good intermediate vision or 1.5–2.5 D for good near vision in the nondominant eye, as per the lifestyle requirement of the patient. Monovision can be obtained using contact lenses, intracorneal inlays, monofocal IOLs or monovision laser procedures.[38]

Indications: Presbyopes with simple myopia are good candidates than patients with astigmatism or hyperopia. Myopic patients have some amount of functional near vision in their presbyopic age group as well, and hence retaining it by means of monovision will be more acceptable than for hyperopic and astigmatic patients. A trial with monovision contact lens is advisable to develop cortical adaptation. Patients are given 1–2 D contact lens in nondominant eye for 3 weeks to assess their ability to adapt. This trial will also determine any compromise in vision which may affect routine work or hobbies.

Disadvantages: Binocular visual acuity may be reduced in monovision, more so during low illumination. This will affect the quality of night vision. Stereopsis is also reduced and the effect is more enhanced in those with poor adaptability. Monocular defocus will also reduce the contrast sensitivity especially in higher spatial frequencies. Monovision may affect those who require fine vision in routine work. Since presbyopia is progressive, the effect will be short lived in phakic patients.

Intracorneal Inlays

Corneal inlays are devices made of biocompatible material, with apertures for nutrient flow that are inserted in an intrastromal pocket made by femtosecond laser.[39] This procedure can be used as an adjunctive to LASIK and the inlays can be placed before replacing the flap.

Mechanism of action: Kamra inlay implants are 5–10 microns thick, diameter of 3–4 mm and a central aperture of 1.5–2 mm. An intracorneal pocket is made with a femtosecond laser into which the inlay is implanted at a depth of 170–200 μm. The inlay increases the depth of focus. The pupil size during distant vision is well beyond the opaque ring allowing peripheral rays to enter the eye. As pupil constricts in near activities, the diameter will be smaller than that of the inlay. This allows only paraxial rays to enter the eye, increasing depth of focus and improving near vision.

Raindrop inlay changes the radius of curvature of the anterior cornea to achieve presbyopic correction. These hydrogel lenses are implanted under a standard LASIK flap within the pupillary aperture.

Advantages: Inlays, which use biocompatible materials, are only minimally invasive. It can be combined with LASIK for simultaneous correction of refractive error and presbyopia. This is a reversible procedure without the need of tissue removal.

Disadvantages: These are currently used as a monovision implant. Patients may have night vision problems like halos and diplopia. High permeability of the material can also lead to variations in the thickness and refractive power of the implant.

Conductive Keratoplasty

Central corneal curvature is increased by causing conductive radiofrequency waves are used to cause relative increase in central corneal curvature. The procedure involves using radiofrequencies of 350 kHz to the cornea through probe that is 90 μ in diameter and 450 μ long. The tissue temperature in the cornea increases, leading to nonablative collagen shrinkage. The spots are made in a ring pattern at the midperiphery of the cornea, all around to produce localized tissue contraction that steepens the central cornea and increasing its refractive power.[40] It was initially used for hyperopic corrections, but later expanded to include treatment of presbyopia in emmetropes and hyperopes. However, long-term follow-up studies showed regression of the effect (Fig. 32.18).

Lasers

Both excimer and femtosecond lasers are used to create multifocal corneas. Excimer laser can be used to create a multifocal cornea, by fashioning a small steep zone within the ablated area, to improve near vision without compromising distant vision.

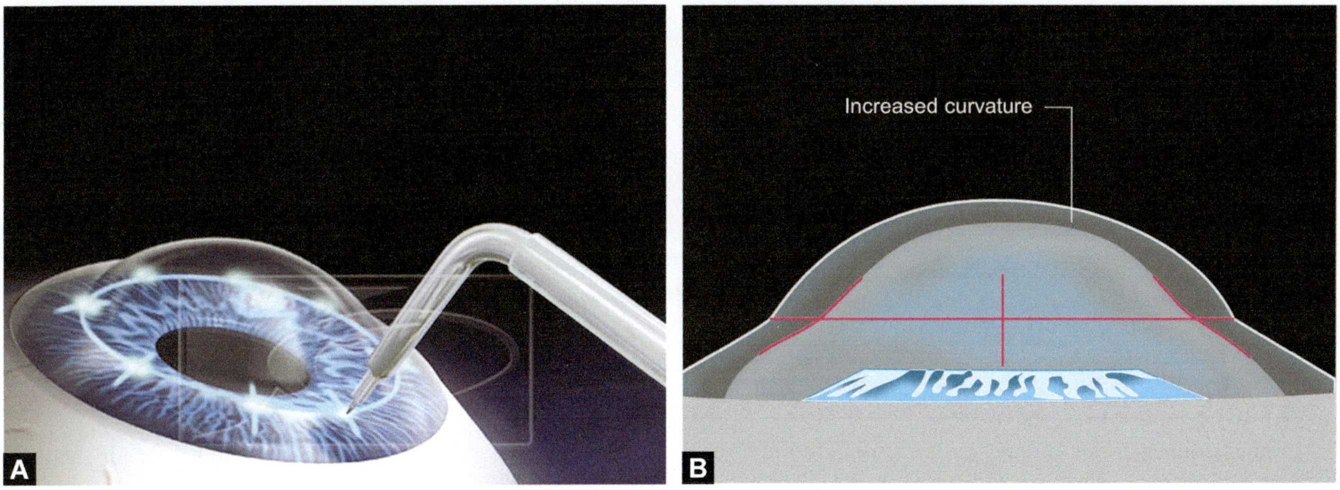

Fig. 32.18: Conductive keratoplasty—collagen shrinking by radiofrequency waves at corneal midperiphery results in central steepening.

The femtosecond laser makes 5 concentric rings within the stroma, from center to periphery.[41] IOP pushes the innermost part of the cornea slightly forward, to create a central steepening and the multifocal, hyperprolate, corneal shape enhances the depth of focus, improving near vision, while good distance vision is maintained. Quick intrastromal delivery avoids pain and inflammation. Biomechanical stability of the cornea is not compromised as the anterior fibers remains untouched.

Disadvantages: Quality of vision may be affected by induced hyperprolate aberration pattern. A proper centration and alignment is imperative. The rings may induce a diffractive pattern producing haloes. Long-term variation in corneal biomechanics will cause regression and the effect may be lost.

Binocular Nonaccommodative Presbyopic Correction

Multifocal Intraocular Lenses

Multifocal IOLs can be refractive and diffractive. The refractive lenses use different zones of power to correct near and distance vision. They are pupil dependent for their effect. The different regions are used to create differential focus of light rays to produce near as well as distance vision focus. Central region will have distance and paracentral region will have additions for near focus. More peripheral regions will have distance power. Thus, focus will depend on the pupil size.

The diffractive lenses have series of concentric rings with gradually tapered step heights.[42] They are not pupil dependent and give smooth transition of near, intermediate and distance focus. Light is split by the diffractive rings producing 2 distinct loci of focus for distance and for near. *Patient selection*: Patients with irregular astigmatism, media opacities other than cataract and macular pathologies are not suitable for multifocal IOL.

Disadvantages: Patient should be counseled preoperatively that these lenses cannot provide a seamless clear focus for all distances. They require a period of neuroadaptation to adjust to the multiple foci. The IOL should be placed within the capsular bag with a well-centered anterior capsulorhexis. Capsular phimosis or posterior capsular opacification can affect the vision significantly. Nd: YAG capsulotomy or an IOL exchange may be needed in highly symptomatic patients.[43] Compromised contrast sensitivity and night vision problems such as halos are common. Refractive IOL may have variation in focus with ambient light as it is pupil depended. Distance vision may be affected in bright surrounding as the near focus becomes dominant and vice versa in mesopic conditions.

Accommodative Methods of Presbyopia Correction

Accommodative Intraocular Lenses

Accommodative intraocular lenses (IOLs) work on the focus-shift principle.[44] Accommodative IOLs are made of flexible silicone or acrylate, and have flexible "hinge" at the haptic-optic junction which lets forward movement of the optic with haptic compression. The IOL optic shifts forward with ciliary muscle contraction and vitreous pressure. This shifts the focal plane, resulting in true pseudophakic accommodation. In normal eyes, an IOL displacement of 0.60 mm would cause 1 D of accommodation in the spectacle plane.

Types of accommodative IOLs:

- Single plate haptic
- Flexible optic-haptic hinge
- Double optics connected by struts
- Deformable IOL
- Injectable IOL
- Light adjustable IOL—silicon matrix in which photosensitive molecules are embedded. Postoperative customization of the IOL power can be done by using ultraviolet light

Disadvantages: Postoperative lens position shifts, IOL gets fixed in one position and fails to move forward with accommodation. Capsular opacification and fibrosis are issues that may compromise the outcomes.

Anterior Ciliary Sclerotomy and Scleral Expansion Bands

These scleral procedures are based on Schachar theory of accommodation which proposes that reduction in the distance between the lens and ciliary body is the reason for loss of accommodation with age.[45] Anterior sclerotomy and scleral expansion bands are aimed to expand the sclera over ciliary body area to increase the distance from the lens and to increase zonular tension to correct presbyopia. However, potentially dangerous complications like scleral weakening and anterior ciliary ischemia limit the usefulness of these procedures.

Refractive procedures for presbyopia are still evolving. Progressive nature of the presbyopia in phakic eyes is a challenge to give long-lasting results.

REFERENCES

1. Krueger RR, Rabinowitz YS, Binder PS. The 25th Anniversary of Excimer Lasers in Refractive Surgery: Historical Review. J Ref Surg. 2010;26:749-60.
2. Mohan RR, Hutcheon AE, Choi R, et al. Apoptosis, necrosis, proliferation, and myofibroblast generation in the stroma following LASIK and PRK. Exp Eye Res. 2003;76:71-87
3. Myrowitz EH, Chuck RS. A comparison of wavefront-optimized and wavefront-guided ablations. Curr Opin Ophthalmol. 2009;20:247-50.
4. Burratto L, Brint S. From Keratomileusis to LASIK, In: Lucio Buratto, Stephen Brint (Eds). Custom LASIK. New Jersey: Slack Incorporated; 2003. p. 8.
5. Shrivastava A, Madu A, Schultz J. Refractive surgery and the glaucoma patient. Curr Opin Ophthalmol. 2011;22:215-21.
6. Godts D, Tassignon MJ, Gobin L. Binocular vision impairment after refractive surgery. J Cataract Refract Surg. 2004;30:101-9.
7. Kushner BJ, Kowal L. Diplopia after refractive surgery: occurrence and prevention. Arch Ophthalmol. 2003;121: 315-21.
8. Albietz JM, Lenton LM, McLennan SG. Chronic dry eye and regression after laser in situ keartomileusis for myopia. J Cataract Refract Surg. 2004;30:675-84.
9. Reinstein DZ, Ameline B, Uech M, et al. VHF digital ultrasound three-dimensional scanning in the diagnosis of myopic regression after corneal refractive surgery. J Refract Surg. 2005;21:480-4.
10. Gauthier CA, Holden BA, Epstein D, et al. Role of epithelial hyperplasia in regression following photorefractive keratectomy. Br J Ophthalmol. 1996;80:545-8.
11. Wilson SE. Analysis of the keratocyte apoptosis, keratocyte proliferation, and myofibroblast transformation responses after photorefractive keratectomy and laser in situ keratomileusis. Trans Am Ophthalmol Soc. 2002;100:411-33.
12. Shah RA, Wilson SE. Use of mitomycin-C for phototherapeutic keratectomy and photorefractive keratectomy surgery. Curr Opin Ophthalmol. 2010;21:269-73.
13. Donnenfeld ED, Solomon K, Perry HD, et al. The effect of hinge position on corneal sensation and dry eye after LASIK. Ophthalmol. 2003;110:1023-9.
14. Vaddavalli PK, Yoo SH. Femtosecond laser in-situ keratomileusis flap configurations. Curr Opin Ophthalmol. 2011;22:245-50.
15. Schallhorn SC, Amesbury EC, Tanzer DJ. Avoidance, Recognition, and Management of LASIK Complications. Am J Ophthalmol. 2006;141:733-9.
16. Lee JK, Nkyekyer EW, Chuck RS. Microkeratome complications. Curr Opin Ophthalmol. 2009;20:260-3.
17. Smith RJ, Maloney RK. Diffuse lamellar keratitis. A new syndrome in lamellar refractive surgery. Ophthalmol. 1998;105:1721-6.
18. Gritz CD. LASIK interface keratitis: epidemiology, diagnosis and care. Curr Opin Ophthalmol. 2011;22:251-5.
19. Holland SP, Mathias RG. Diffuse lamellar keratitis related to endotoxins released from sterilizer reservoir biofilms. Opthalmol. 2000;107:1227-34.
20. Gris O, Guell JL, Wolley-Dod C, et al. Diffuse lamellar keratitis and corneal edema associated with viral keratoconjunctivitis 2 years after laser in situ keratomileusis. J Cataract Refract Surg. 2004;30:1366-70.
21. Symes RJ, Catt CJ, Males JJ. Diffuse lamellar keratitis associated with gonococcal keratoconjunctivitis 3 years

after laser in situ keratomileusis. J Cataract Refract Surg. 2007;33:323-5.
22. Kuo CL, Lin HF, Fang PC, et al. Late onset lamellar keratitis and epithelial ingrowth following orbital cellulitis. J Refract Surg. 2006;22:202-4.
23. Nordlund ML, Grimm S, Lane S, et al. Pressure-induced interface keratitis: a late complication following LASIK. Cornea. 2004;23:225-34.
24. Moshirfar M, Hazin R, Khalifa YM. Central toxic keratopathy. Curr Opin Ophthalmol. 2010;21:274-9.
25. Sonmez B, Maloney RK. Central toxic keratopathy: description of a syndrome in laser refractive surgery. Am J Ophthalmol. 2007;143:420-7.
26. Solomon R, Donnenfeld ED, Azar DT, et al. Infectious keratitis after laser in situ keratomileusis: results of an ASCRS survey. J Cataract Refract Surg. 2003;29:2001-6.
27. Donnenfeld ED, Kim T, Holland EJ, et al. ASCRS White Paper-Management of infectious keratitis following laser in situ keratomileusis. J Cataract Refract Surg. 2005;31:2008-11.
28. Binder PS. Ectasia after laser in situ keratomileusis. J Cataract Refract Surg. 2003;29:2419-29.
29. Miyata K, Tokunaga T, Nakahara M, et al. Residual bed thickness and corneal forward shift after laser in situ keratomileusis. J Cataract Refract Surg. 2004;30:1067-72.
30. Toda I. LASIK and the ocular surface. Cornea. 2008;27 (Suppl 1):S70-6.
31. Ambrosio R. LASIK-associated Dry Eye and Neurotrophic Epitheliopathy: Pathophysiology and Strategies for Prevention and Treatment. J Refract Surg. 2008;24:396-407.
32. Arevalo JF. Retinal complications after laser-assisted in situ keratomileusis (LASIK). Curr Opin Ophthalmol. 2004;15:184-91.
33. Blum M, Täubig K, Gruhn C, et al. Five-year results of Small Incision Lenticule Extraction (ReLEx SMILE). Br J Ophthalmol. 2016;100:1192-5.
34. Ang M, Mehta JS, Chan C, et al. Refractive lenticule extraction: Transition and comparison of 3 surgical techniques. Cataract Refract Surg. 2014;40:1415-24.
35. Dong Z, Zhou X. Irregular astigmatism after femtosecond laser refractive lenticule extraction. J Cataract Refract Surg. 2013;39:952-4.
36. Alio JL, Grzybowski A, Aswad AE, et al. Refractive lens exchange. Surv Ophthalmol. 2014;59:579-98.
37. Barsum A, Allan BD. Excimer laser refractive surgery versus phakic intraocular lenses for the correction of moderate to high myopia. Cochrane Database Sys Rev. 2012;1:CD007679.
38. Reilly CD, Barry Lee W, Alvarenga L, et al. Surgical Monovision and Monovision Reversal in LASIK. Cornea. 2006;25:136-8.
39. Torricelli AM, Junior JB, Santhiago MR, et al. Surgical management of presbyopia. Clin Ophthalmol. 2012:6: 1459-66.
40. McDonald MB, Durrie D, Asbell P, et al. Treatment of Presbyopia With Conductive Keratoplasty® Six-Month Results of the 1-Year United States FDA Clinical Trial. Cornea. 2004;23:661-8.
41. Ruiz LA, Cepeda LM, Fuentes VC. Intrastromal correction of presbyopia using a femtosecond laser system. J Refract Surg. 2009;25(10):847-54.
42. Cionni RJ, Chang DF, Donnenfeld ED, et al. Clinical outcomes and functional visual performance: comparison of the ReSTOR apodised diffractive intraocular lens to a monofocal control. Br J Ophthalmol. 2009;93(9):1215-9.
43. Woodward MA, Randleman JB, Stulting RD. Dissatisfaction after multifocal intraocular lens implantation. J Cataract Refract Surg. 2009;35(6):992-7.
44. Menapace R, Findl O, Kriechbaum K, et al. Accommodating intraocular lenses: a critical review of present and future concepts. Graefes Arch Clin Exp Ophthalmol. 2007;245(4):473-89.
45. Hamilton DR, Davidorf JM, Maloney RK. Anterior ciliary sclerotomy for treatment of presbyopia: a prospective controlled study. Ophthalmol. 2002;109(11):1970-6; discussion 1976-7.

Part 6

The Lens, Cataract and its Management

■ *Uday Devgan*

OUTLINE

Chapter 33

Femtosecond Laser in Cataract Surgery

Shawn R Lin, D Rex Hamilton

INTRODUCTION

Cataract removal is the most commonly performed surgery in the world, with over 3 million procedures completed annually in the United States.[1] Over the past three decades, the annual incidence of cataract surgery has risen rapidly from about 3,000 per million to over 10,000 per million. An aging population, an improved surgical safety profile, and a higher expectation for visual function all contribute to this dramatic increase.[2]

Numerous innovations have supported the development of modern cataract surgery. The first documented cataract operation dates back to the fifth century BC. A technique called "couching" involved pressing on the eye with enough force to break the zonules and cause lens dislocation into the vitreous cavity. These patients, though aphakic, were able to regain approximately 20/200 to count fingers vision.[3]

The first surgical removal of a lens occurred more than 2,000 years later, in 1748. This operation required a 180° circumferential scleral incision. As intraocular sutures did not exist at the time, a patient's head needed to be immobilized with sandbags for days to allow for scleral wound healing. A non-trivial incidence of pulmonary embolism was a known complication.[2]

Two hundred years later, in 1967, Dr Charles Kelman developed phacoemulsification. The inspiration for phacoemulsification came from ultrasonic instruments found in the dental office. Early models were crude, and phacoemulsification was not initially a widely accepted technology. Only with the development of foldable intraocular lenses did phacoemulsification become the standard of care.

In the mid-1980s, the development of foldable intraocular lenses allowed surgeons to insert lenses through a dramatically smaller incision. The combination of these two technologies, phacoemulsification and foldable intraocular lenses, marks the beginning of the modern cataract surgery era.

The last 30 years have witnessed a remarkable complement of new technologies addressing all aspects of cataract surgery. Advanced phacoemulsification technologies have improved surgical safety by reducing cumulative ultrasound energy, improving anterior chamber stability and reducing endothelial cell loss.[4-6] Significant advances in intraocular lens technology, including aspheric, toric, multifocal, and extended depth of focus lenses have improved the quality of vision.[7-10] Next generation lens power calculation formulas, together with intraoperative aberrometry, digital marking systems[11] and light adjustable lenses, have improved the precision of our refractive outcomes.[12,13] Finally, femtosecond laser technology is defining its role in this rapidly evolving era of refractive cataract surgery.

The first femtosecond laser, the LenSx (Alcon Laboratories, Ft. Worth, TX), was approved by the FDA in 2009 for capsulotomies and corneal incisions. A series of 50 femtosecond cataract surgeries was completed shortly thereafter.[14] The technology has the stated benefit of allowing for decreased phacoemulsification energy, increasing clear corneal and astigmatic incision precision and creating a perfectly round capsulorhexis.

In this chapter, we will explore the technology of femtosecond laser, examine studies comparing femtosecond laser-assisted cataract surgery (FLACS) to traditional cataract surgery, detail best practices, and discuss how FLACS may impact the future of cataract surgery.

TECHNOLOGY

There are three primary steps associated with FLACS, regardless of the system being utilized: docking, imaging, and laser application.

Docking

All FLACS systems on the market utilize an apparatus to stabilize the eye during the imaging and laser application process, which typically takes a few minutes. Some systems use a suction ring that is applied to the eye first, followed by docking of the laser to the suction ring. Other systems utilize a single laser interface that includes the suction device used to stabilize the eye. Devices that use a separate suction ring may be more familiar to refractive surgeons who have experience with femtosecond laser systems used to create LASIK flaps, as it has the advantage of stabilizing the eye prior to corneal applanation and imaging. These type of devices typically require wider exposure, and can be challenging to use in patients with narrow palpebral fissures. Systems that do not utilize a separate suction ring present less of a challenge in small orbits, but require a learning curve for centration as the eye is free to move during the applanation process. Because of the wide operating field required to place peripheral clear corneal incisions, the suction application with all of the systems occurs outside the limbus and can be associated with a variable amount of subconjunctival hemorrhage.

Imaging

Current FLACS systems utilize either three dimensional (3D) optical coherence tomography (OCT) or super-luminescent Scheimpflug technology to image the anterior segment. This requires that the cornea be clear without significant edema, folds, or scarring. Depending on the system, 2D or 3D representations of the anterior segment structures allow the surgeon to establish laser boundaries, cut depths and locations, as well as lens fragmentation patterns. This real-time imaging allows for implementation of an accurate, customized treatment plan.

Laser Application

Femtosecond lasers have been utilized for LASIK flap creation since the FDA approval of the IntraLase laser in 2001.[15] Although the first femtosecond laser systems fired at 10 kHz, modern femtosecond systems are more than an order of magnitude faster. In addition to being adapted for cataract surgery, the femtosecond laser is also used today for keratoplasty incisions, intrastromal pockets, intrastromal channels, and small incision lenticule extraction (SMILE) keratorefractive surgery.

Femtosecond lasers utilize pulses of near-infrared (1053 nm) light energy of ultrashort duration to photodisrupt tissue at a focused target location. In photodisruption, high-density energy absorption at the point of focus leads to the formation of a rapidly expanding cavitation bubble. This bubble separates tissue, and can be targeted accurately within the anterior segment with an error of less than 3 μm. This near-infrared energy is not absorbed by clear tissues at low energy densities, and is known to dissipate quickly outside of the target site.[15] FLACS systems fire at very fast rates, placing multiple cavitation bubbles adjacent to one another in specific orientations to create tissue planes of dissection for capsulotomy, lens fragmentation, clear corneal incisions, and astigmatic keratotomies (Figs. 33.1A to D).

OUTCOMES DATA

The literature on FLACS support its use in cataract surgery, with advantages in several steps.

Capsulotomy Precision

Most studies of capsulorhexis precision favor femtosecond laser over manual creation. This is an important metric for lens stability, as a decentered or aberrant capsulorhexis can induce lens tilt and introduce higher order aberrations. Numerous studies have demonstrated a statistically significant reduction in horizontal and vertical tilt with femtosecond laser capsulotomy versus traditional continuous curvilinear capsulorhexis.[16-18] In addition, circularity of the capsulorhexis is significantly better in

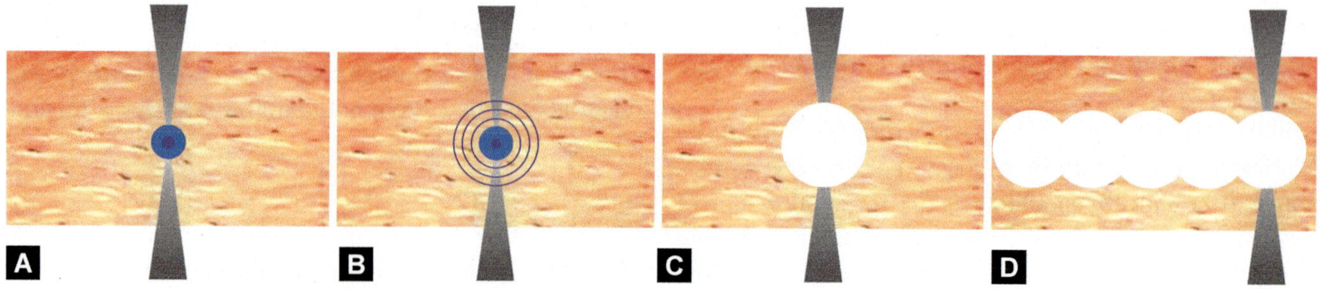

Figs. 33.1A to D: Expanding cavitation bubble cleaving tissue. (A) Plasma development; (B) Expansion of a shock wave; (C) Development of a cavitation bubble; (D) Formation of cavitation bubbles cleaves the tissue.

the femtosecond laser group.[19] Eyes with a femtosecond laser created capsulorhexis exhibit less intraocular lens decentration than manually created capsulorhexis at 1 year.[20] However, using the femtosecond laser to create the capsulotomy does not appear to decrease the rate of anterior capsular tear in a 2017 meta-analysis.[21]

Phacoemulsification Time

Several studies have compared total phacoemulsification time between traditional cataract surgery and FLACS. These studies demonstrate a lower effective phacoemulsification time in the FLACS group.[22-24]

Central Corneal Thickness/Anterior Chamber Inflammation

Measurements of corneal edema by central corneal thickness and anterior chamber inflammation show a significantly decreased central corneal thickness after FLACS compared to traditional cataract surgery during the initial postoperative period.[25] In addition, postoperative inflammation is decreased, with a decrease in postoperative flare in the FLACS group versus the traditional cataract surgery group.[26]

Endothelial Cell Loss

Studies have demonstrated a decreased rate of endothelial cell loss after FLACS in both early and advanced cataract groups.[25,27]

Visual Acuity

Studies aimed at comparing visual acuity between FLACS and traditional cataract surgery have delivered mixed results. While some report superior visual acuity during the postoperative period and out to 1 year,[17,28,29] others report no difference.[23,30-32]

BEST PRACTICES

All femtosecond lasers are stand-alone units at this time, and require patients to undergo a separate procedure prior to undergoing cataract removal under an operative microscope.

The following are the best practice considerations compiled from currently published literature and user focus groups. Although there are several different FLACS systems on the market, these comments are generalizable to all systems. We discuss these best practices in their standard order of completion, organized into workflow, docking, imaging, and laser application. In addition, we discuss how cataract removal differs following femtosecond laser treatment.

Workflow

Femtosecond Laser Positioning

Some FLACS systems, such as the Ziemer Z8, allow for patients to be positioned on the operative table, and incorporate an articulating arm to allow the laser to swing into the operative field to dock onto a patient's eye.

Other FLACS systems require the patient to be treated first at the femtosecond laser machine, then moved to the operating microscope for the remainder of the surgery. For these systems, there are two surgical center setups commonly used.

In the single room setup, the laser is placed in the operating room, and the patient is moved from the laser to the operative microscope. The benefit of this system is decreased total case time, as patients need not be moved between rooms. However, this setup does not allow multiple surgeons to utilize the laser for cataract surgery in multiple operating rooms. If the laser is in the operating room, other surgeons cannot utilize the laser until the entire cataract surgery is completed (Fig. 33.2).

In the multiroom setup, the femtosecond laser is kept outside the operating room, allowing multiple surgeons to access the laser sequentially. Following application of the laser, the patient is then brought to the operating room where the remainder of the cataract surgery is completed.

Case Duration

As with any technology, incorporation of FLACS into an operating room workflow will initially result in increased case duration. However, this increased case duration decreases rapidly over time, with most routine cases adding about 5 minutes to total case duration.

Staff Training

With current implementations of FLACS, a technician is commonly tasked with operating certain laser controls during docking. These staff need to be trained to perform this task accuracy and efficiently.

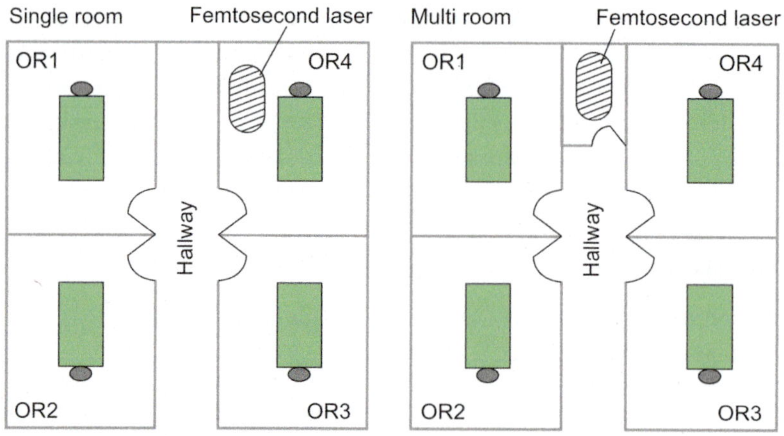

Fig. 33.2: In this single room setup example, only one operating room has access to the femtosecond laser. The laser cannot be used during room turnover or cataract surgery. In the multiple room setup, all 4 operating rooms can access the femtosecond laser, allowing for increased efficiency.

Programming the Femtosecond Laser

The treatment plan is entered into the system prior to laser docking, and there are multiple opportunities for transcription error while measurements are being transferred from preoperative calculations to the femtosecond laser. We like to employ a femtosecond laser "timeout" with designated operating room staff prior to docking to ensure the correct entry of patient and treatment information. Some laser systems have digital marking systems that are used in conjunction with the laser that allow for automatic uploading of patient data directly to the laser system's computer, eliminating possible transcriptional errors (e.g. Verion by Alcon and Streamline III by Lensar).

Docking

Anesthesia and Patient Fixation

Patients undergoing FLACS must be able to fixate during the docking portion of the case in order to achieve good corneal centration. Although all FLACS platforms allow the surgeon to adjust the size and position of incisions, capsulorhexis and lens fragmentation patterns, a decentered dock makes these tasks more challenging. In addition, the risk of suction loss increases during the planning and treatment steps, particularly if conjunctiva and/or eyelashes have been applanated (Fig. 33.3).

In our operating rooms, we direct anesthesiology to utilize fentanyl instead of Versed whenever possible in order to minimize patient sedation.

Lid Speculum

All FLACS systems must dock with the eye in order to maintain stability of the working space. A well-designed lid speculum is crucial, as it must allow sufficient exposure for the docking apparatus to engage the eye without putting unbalanced pressure on the globe. Oftentimes, an optimal lid speculum is matched to a particular laser, helping to facilitate the docking process while maximizing patient comfort.

Docking the Laser

With systems that utilize a suction ring prior to applanation, it is crucial to precisely center the suction ring. Surgeons who have utilized femtosecond lasers for LASIK flap creation (e.g. Intralase) are very familiar with this process. Once the suction ring is centered, the docking maneuver can be carried out easily. It is important to ensure that the laser head is in a neutral (x, y) position over the eye before commencing docking maneuvers. For gross alignment, this means moving the patient's bed to the correct spot so that the laser can have maximum range of motion after the bed is locked. After this step, the patient is instructed to fixate on the target light while the laser is docked onto the eye. Patients should be talked through this process, as the sight of a large docking head moving toward the eye can be unsettling.

The position of the suction tubing is important to monitor. Occasionally, the patient can experience pain from suction tubing pressure on the lateral corner of

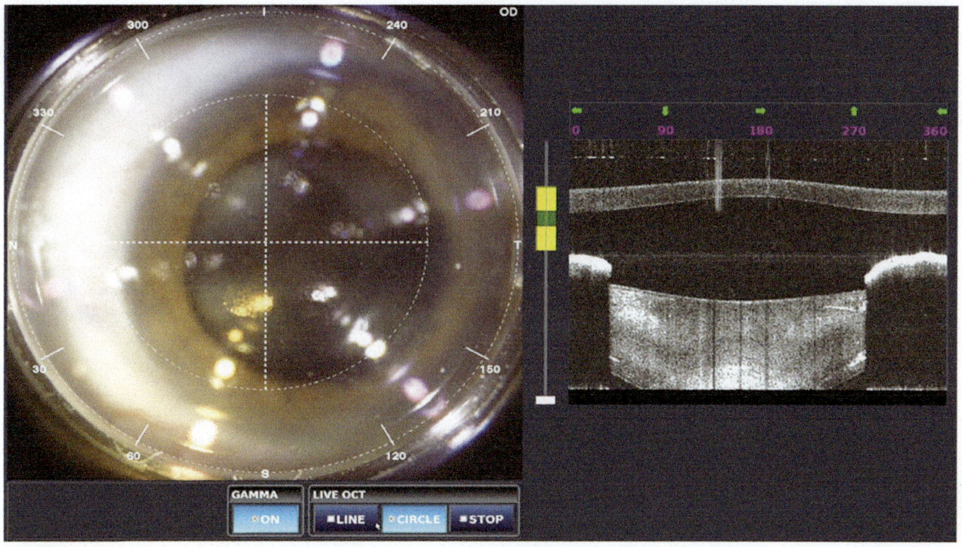

Fig. 33.3: Poor patient fixation prior to dock. The patient is encouraged to look at the fixation lights and is able to correct his/her misalignment. The operative images presented in this chapter are sequential, and illustrate progression of a single femtosecond laser-assisted cataract surgery (FLACS) case.

the globe. This can be ameliorated by adjusting the docking pressure, or repeating docking after minor head adjustment. Typically, the head should be tilted slightly inward to move the nose away from the docking cone apparatus. Care should be taken to ensure that no part of the eyelid or conjunctiva is caught in the suction apparatus. In addition to causing the patient discomfort, applying suction to the eyelid or conjunctiva typically results in unstable fixation of the eye. It is also very important to ensure there are no air bubbles trapped between the interface and the corneal surface. Gas bubbles may attenuate the laser energy, resulting in inconsistent cutting. This is most concerning during capsulorhexis creation as it can lead to an incomplete cut. If not noticed, an incomplete capsulorhexis can lead to radialization during removal. If gas bubbles are observed, gentle head movements can tease the bubbles out of the interface. If bubbles still remain, docking can be repeated.

Imaging

Anterior segment imaging is acquired immediately after a successful dock. The imaging should be clear and all anterior segment structures should be identifiable. The software can often automatically position cuts and set safety boundaries. However, it is always the role of the surgeon to thoroughly and efficiently check and fine-tune these boundaries. For example, the pupil may sometimes be poorly dilated and the surgeon will need to decide whether or not to forgo the capsulorhexis and/or fragmentation portion of the laser procedure. It is usually advisable to avoid both capsulorhexis and fragmentation if the pupil is insufficiently dilated. Fragmentation of the lens in a closed capsule can increase intracapsular pressure and make visualization for performing a manual capsulorhexis challenging. Once all settings are confirmed, the treatment plan is finalized, and the laser application can begin (Fig. 33.4).

Laser Application

Capsulorhexis

The first cut by most femtosecond laser systems is the capsulorhexis, as this allows for venting of intracapsular gas created during the subsequent lens fragmentation step. After fragmentation, the corneal incisions are created (Fig. 33.5).

It is important to ensure that the patient's eye is level and fixated. If the eye is tilted, laser energy may not completely penetrate the anterior capsule in certain spots, leading to an incomplete capsulorhexis and risk of radicalization.

Lens Fragmentation

The lens fragmentation can follow many predefined patterns, including quadrants, sextants, central cylindrical or any other conceivable pattern. In addition, the nucleus can also be "softened" using a "grid" or "waffle" pattern.

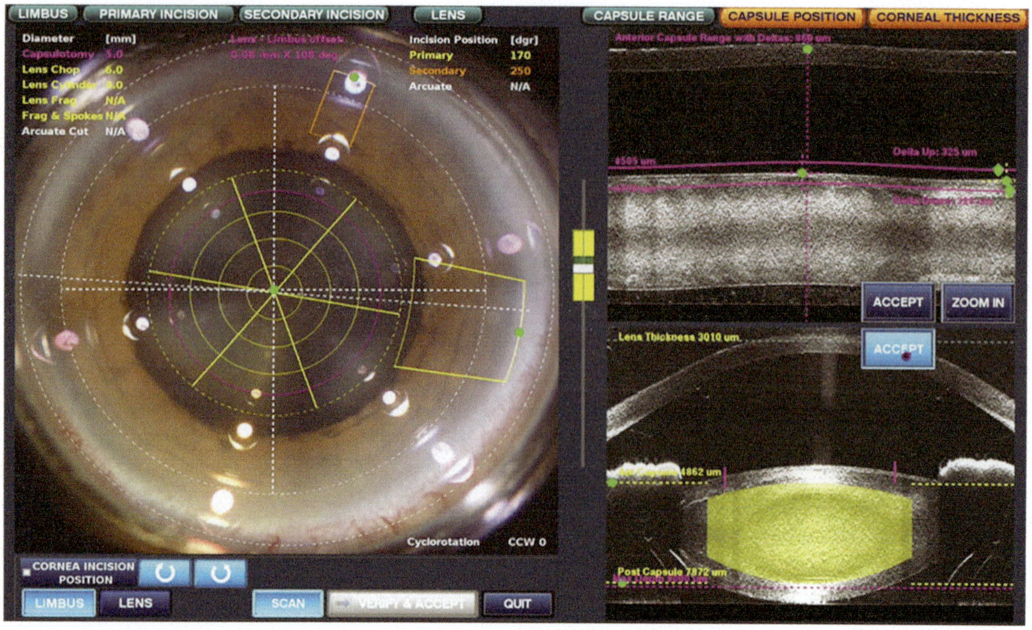

Fig. 33.4: A good dock, note that the eye is well-centered, and all anterior segment structures are horizontally level.

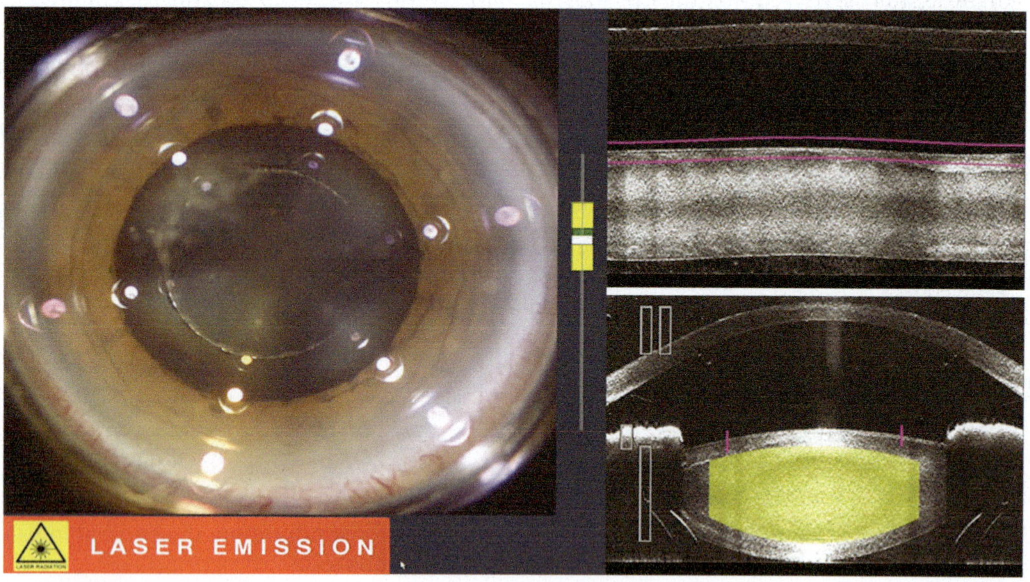

Fig. 33.5: The capsulorhexis is almost completely cut. The top right inset shows that the eye is relatively level, leading to a well cut and clean capsulorhexis.

The size of the cubes created by the laser in the grid pattern can be adjusted based on the density of the cataract being treated (Figs. 33.6 and 33.7).

Corneal Incisions/Arcuates

It is important to ensure the cornea is as well centered during the docking process as possible. Once suction is established, it becomes more challenging to identify centration of the arcuate incisions (Fig. 33.8). If the arcuates are not symmetrically positioned, one will be too posterior and the other too anterior, possibly leading to asymmetric astigmatism treatment. Additionally, a posterior arcuate may be difficult to open as the laser does not cut efficiently in opaque tissue such as peripheral pannus or limbus. If placed too anterior, the arcuate may induce more astigmatic effect than intended. Arcuates are generally set at 80% depth, and the femtosecond laser is able to cut at this depth precisely based on corneal thickness measurements taken during the imaging stage.

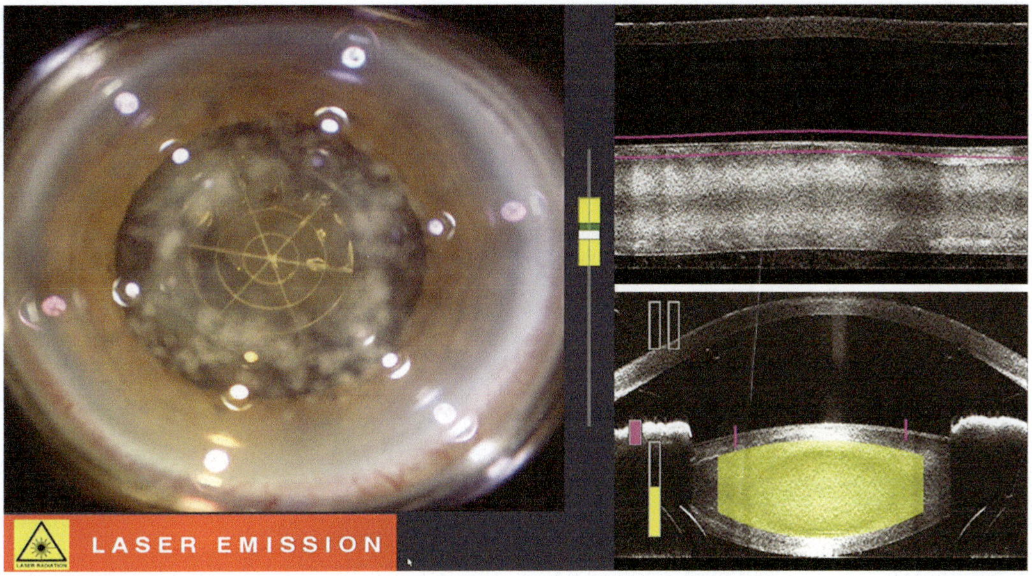

Fig. 33.6: Lens fragmentation: Here a 3-concentric cylinder, 6-radial spoke pattern facilitates easy chop and nucleus removal.

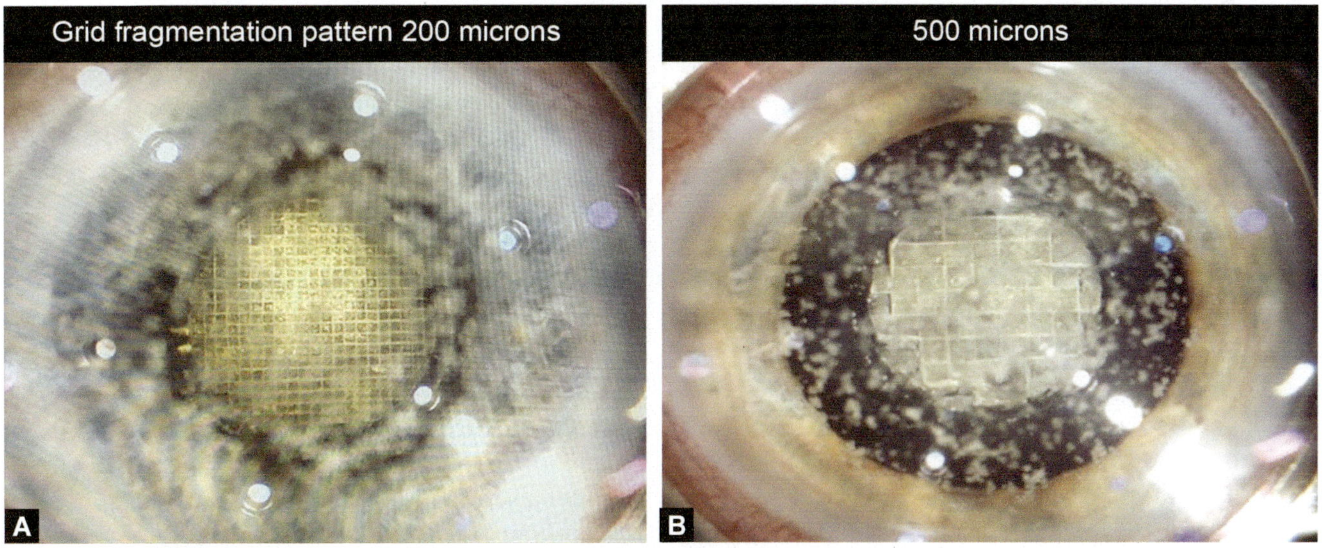

Figs. 33.7A and B: Grid fragmentation patterns.

CATARACT SURGERY FOLLOWING FEMTOSECOND LASER

While the principles of cataract surgery do not change, some nuances are introduced by use of the femtosecond laser.

Pupillary Miosis

The pupil often begins to constrict after femtosecond treatment, leading to need for reapplication of topical drops or intracameral epinephrine.[33] Due to this predictable miosis, it is prudent to ensure very good dilation prior to femtosecond laser treatment, and to have intracameral epinephrine available at the start of every case.

Opening of Incisions

As the femtosecond laser cuts with cavitation bubbles, it does not always create a smooth surface that separates easily. Thus, a flat spatula is utilized to open up the main incision and paracentesis. Occasionally, an incision placed too far posteriorly may not open, as the cut to the surface has occurred in opaque tissue (e.g. pannus or limbus). In this situation, a standard blade is used to cut through

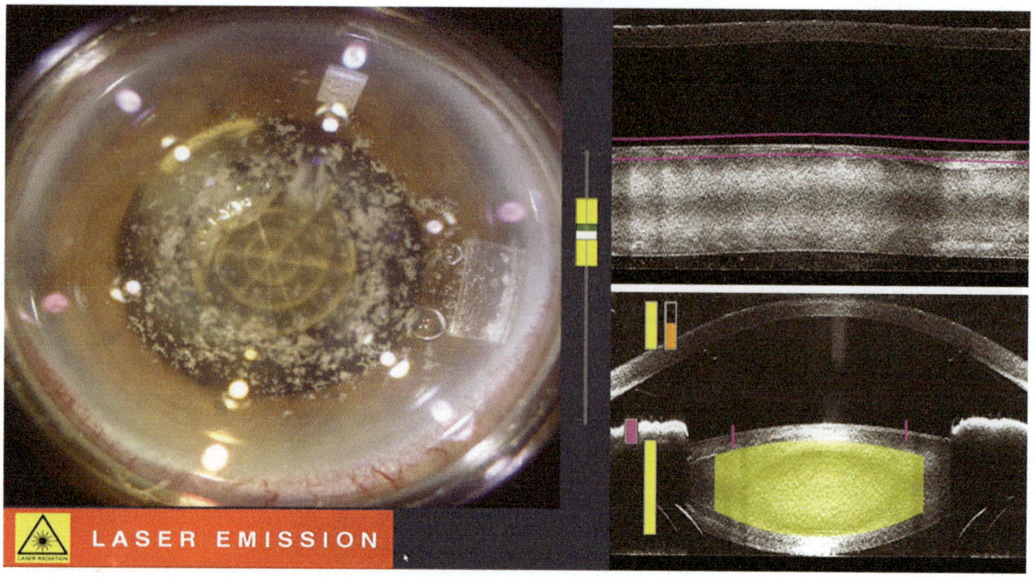

Fig. 33.8: A main incision is cut temporally, and a paracentesis is cut inferiorly for this left-handed surgeon.

the pannus and enter into the incision, after which point the incision can usually be opened using a flat spatula. Conversely, if the incision is positioned too anteriorly, a standard keratome blade can be used to enter the eye either posterior to the untouched FLACS incision or at an alternative location.

Removal of Capsulorhexis

It is prudent to carefully examine the edges of the femtosecond laser-cut capsulorhexis prior to removal of the capsule to ensure a free-floating capsulotomy. Especially in cases of poor horizontal leveling or overlying trapped gas bubbles during docking, portions of the capsulorhexis can remain uncut.

Observation of the bubble pattern can be helpful to determine whether the capsulorhexis is complete in a region. Round bubbles coalescing at the capsulotomy cut usually indicate a complete cut. If the bubbles are oblong or sausage-shaped, this can indicate an incomplete cut and a very careful examination of this region is warranted to avoid a capsular tear. In this case, the surgeon must tear the uncut section carefully as if performing a capsulorhexis in order to avoid an errant capsular tear. In situations where bubbles overlie and obscure view of the capsulorhexis, a cohesive viscoelastic can be injected to move the bubbles aside.

Hydrodissection

The cavitation bubbles created by lens fragmentation can move posteriorly behind the lens. The trapping of these bubbles, along with a forceful hydrodissection, can create a posterior capsular tear. If posterior bubbles are observed, they can be released by gently tapping on the anterior surface of the lens. In addition, forceful hydrodissection is typically not required in FLACS as the gas helps to "pneumodissect" at the capsular plane (Figs. 33.9 and 33.10).

Nuclear Disassembly

The grooves made by femtosecond laser decrease the amount of energy needed to chop the lens. However, these grooves are often narrower than grooves made with phacoemulsification, and may require special narrow second instruments in order to separate. A standard ball chopper used for horizontal chopping in non-FLACS surgery is not ideal, as the ball may not fit into the laser grooves. Most instrument manufacturers now have femtosecond laser optimized instrumentation available for purchase (Figs. 33.11 and 33.12).

Cortex Removal

Cortex removal can be slightly more challenging in FLACS cases, as the normal cortex tag that extends centrally toward the center of the eye is cleaved by the laser at the capsulorhexis edge. Thus, movements to grasp the cortex at the capsulorhexis edge may be more risky to the anterior capsule. Instead of the standard occlude and central pull technique, the probe can be moved circumferentially underneath the capsulorhexis to grab multiple clock hours of cortex before moving centrally.

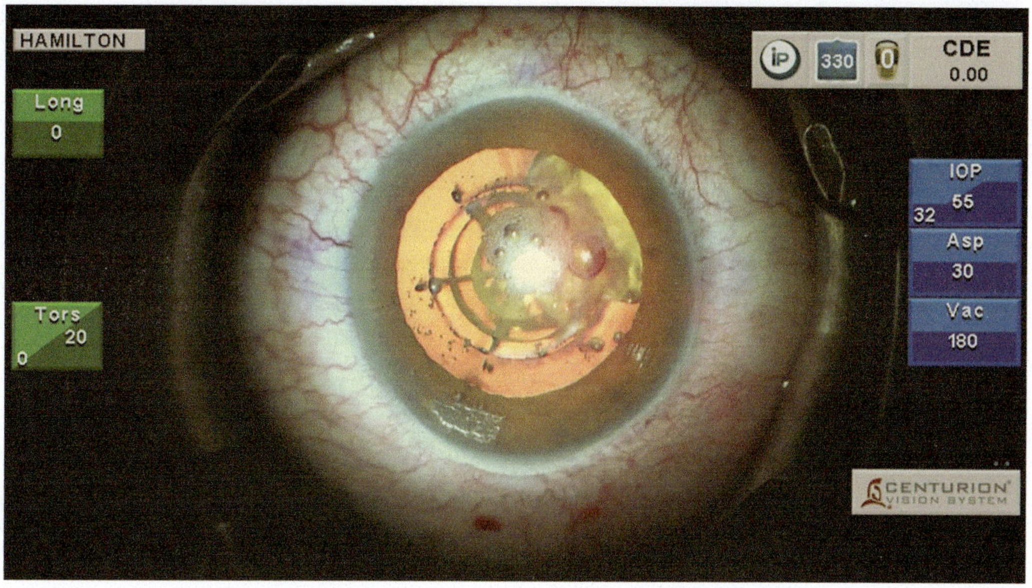

Fig. 33.9: A large gas bubble trapped at 5 o'clock posterior to the lens. Gentle tapping on the anterior surface of the lens after capsule removal allows the gas bubble to escape anteriorly prior to hydrodissection.

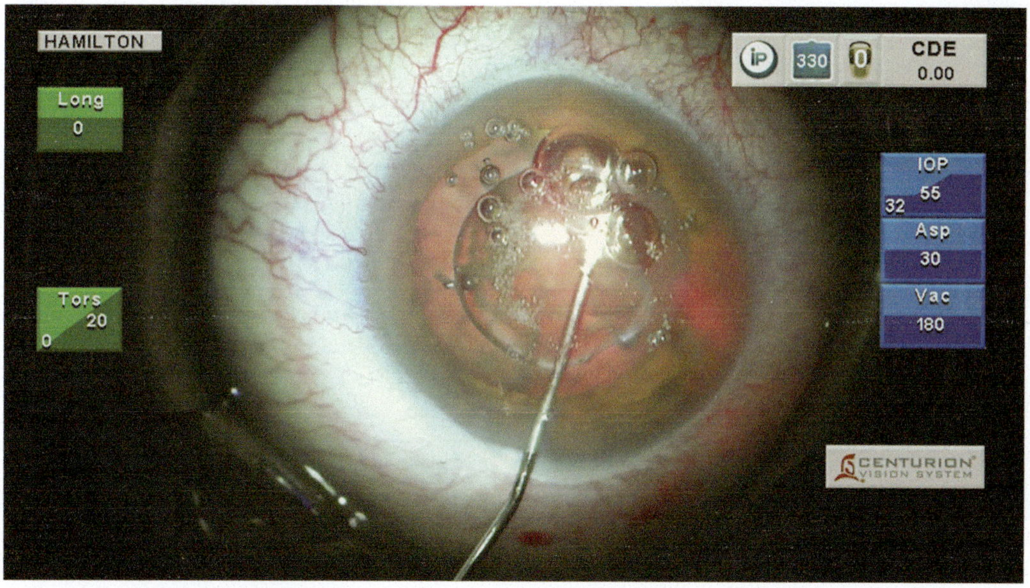

Fig. 33.10: After tapping on the anterior surface, the posteriorly trapped bubble is released.

CONCLUSION AND THE FUTURE

Femtosecond laser has been cautiously adopted in its early phase. In today's market, the femtosecond laser has augmented the value proposition for the cataract surgeon from the offering of goods only (premium lenses) to the offering of goods and services (premium lenses and advanced laser cataract surgery). Femtosecond laser has fervent supporters and opponents, just as phacoemulsification did in the early years of its use. If history is any guide, widespread adoption will likely be driven by complementary technologies.

Consider the history of phacoemulsification. Early phacoemulsification machines were crude, and did not offer clear benefits for the patient. For surgeons, there was little benefit to a small phacoemulsification incision when subsequent incision enlargement was necessary to insert a 6 mm lens. It took more than two decades and the invention

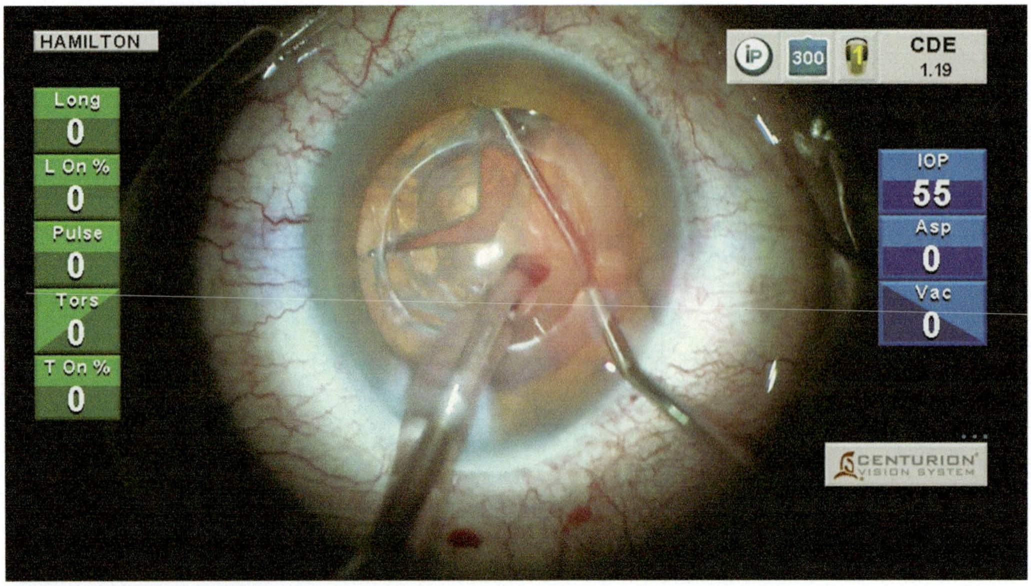

Fig. 33.11: Very minimal phacoemulsification energy is needed to cleave the lens along the laser energy planes.

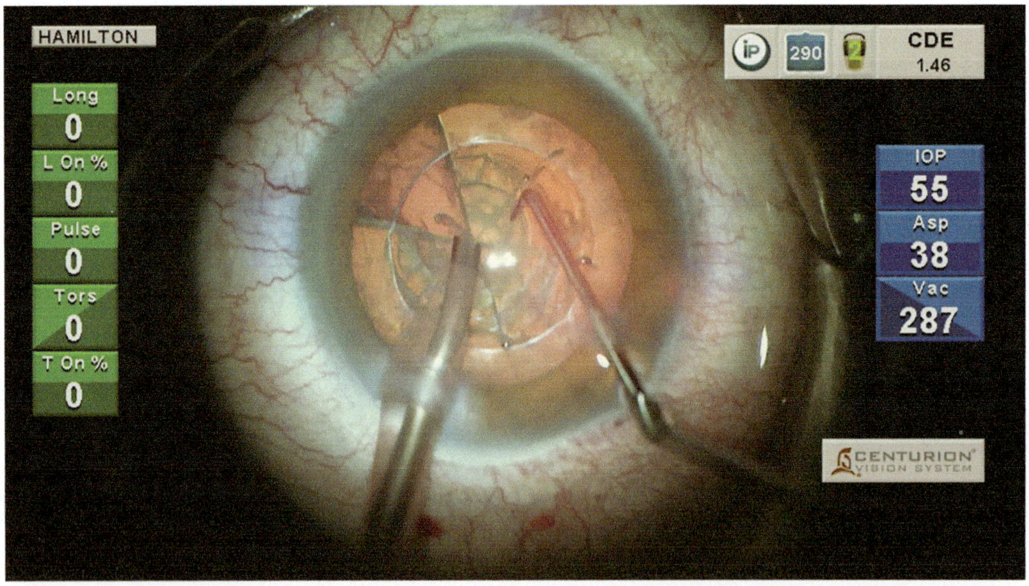

Fig. 33.12: One "slice" is removed at a time, allowing for a well-controlled nuclear disassembly.

of foldable intraocular lenses to create a truly compelling reason to adopt phacoemulsification as the gold standard.

Femtosecond laser adoption may follow a similar trajectory. Although the benefits of precise capsulorhexis and intraocular lens centration are proven, the evidence for improved visual outcomes with femtosecond laser is mixed. Indeed, many surgeons are divided on the utility of the technology in its current state. However, it is likely that complementary technologies will be developed in the coming years to enhance the utility of FLACS.

Imagine if a toric intraocular lens could be designed with pegs to be fit precisely into precut holes in the anterior capsule, eliminating unintended rotation. Or imagine if a new accommodating intraocular lens relied on a precisely cut capsulorhexis in order to work effectively. Perhaps cataract removal in the future could be performed in a minimally invasive fashion through small, precise openings in the capsular bag, with injection of a polymer material to truly restore accommodation. All of these technologies are on the horizon, and would make a compelling case for widespread adoption of the femtosecond laser.

Therefore, femtosecond laser should be thought of as more than a tool for today, but as a platform and launchpad for the ophthalmic innovations of tomorrow.

REFERENCES

1. Erie JC. Rising cataract surgery rates: demand and supply. Ophthalmology. 2014;121:2-4.
2. Bellan L. The evolution of cataract surgery: the most common eye procedure in older adults. Geriatrics and Aging. 2008;11:328-32.
3. Zhao J, Sui R, Jia L, et al. Visual acuity and quality of life outcomes in patients with cataract in Shunyi County, China. Am J Ophthalmol. 1998;9394:515-23.
4. Hayashi K, Hayashi H, Nakao F, et al. Risk factors for corneal endothelial injury during phacoemulsification. J Cataract Refract Surg. 1996;22:1079-84.
5. Park JH, Lee SM, Kwon JW, et al. Ultrasound energy in phacoemulsification: a comparative analysis of phaco-chop and stop-and-chop techniques according to the degree of nuclear density. Ophthalmic Surg Lasers Imaging. 2010;41:236-41.
6. Han YK, Miller KM. Comparison of vacuum rise time, vacuum limit accuracy, and occlusion break surge of 3 new phacoemulsification systems. J Cataract Refract Surg. 2009;35:1424-9.
7. Monaco G, Gari M, Di Censo F, et al. Visual performance after bilateral implantation of 2 new presbyopia-correcting intraocular lenses: Trifocal versus extended range of vision. J Cataract Refract Surg. 2017;43:737-47.
8. Cochener B. Clinical outcomes of a new extended range of vision intraocular lens: International Multicenter Concerto Study. J Cataract Refract Surg. 2016;42:1268-75.
9. Souza CE, Muccioli C, Soriano ES, et al. Visual performance of AcrySof ReSTOR apodized diffractive IOL: a prospective comparative trial. Am J Ophthalmol. 2006;141:827-32.
10. Toto L, Falconio G, Vecchiarino L, et al. Visual performance and biocompatibility of 2 multifocal diffractive IOLs. Six-month comparative study. J Cataract Refract Surg. 2007;33:1419-25.
11. Elhofi AH, Helaly HA. Comparison between digital and manual marking for toric intraocular lenses: a randomized Trial. Medicine (Baltimore). 2015;94:e1618.
12. Chayet A, Sandstedt C, Chang S, et al. Correction of myopia after cataract surgery with a light-adjustable lens. Ophthalmology. 2009;116:1432-5.
13. Chayet A, Sandstedt CA, Chang SH, et al. Correction of residual hyperopia after cataract surgery using the light adjustable intraocular lens technology. Am J Ophthalmol. 2009;147:392-7.e1.
14. Uy HS. Femtosecond laser lens fragmentation for higher grade cataracts. In: Program and Abstracts of the Annual meeting of ISRS. Illinois, USA; 2010.
15. Kullman G, Pineda R 2nd. Alternative applications of the femtosecond laser in ophthalmology. Semin Ophthalmol. 2010;25:256-64.
16. Miháltz K, Knorz MC, Alió JL, et al. Internal aberrations and optical quality after femtosecond laser anterior capsulotomy in cataract surgery. J Refract Surg. 2011;10:711-6.
17. Kránitz K, Mihâltz K, Sándor GL, et al. Intraocular lens tilt and decentration measured by Scheimpflug camera following manual or femtosecond laser-created continuous circular capsulotomy. J Refract Surg. 2012;4:259-63.
18. Szigeti A, Kránitz K, Takacs AI, et al. Comparison of long-term visual outcome and IOL position with a single-optic accommodating IOL after 5.5- or 6.0-mm Femtosecond laser capsulotomy. J Refract Surg. 2012;9:609-13.
19. Mastropasqua L, Toto L, Calienno R, et al. Scanning electron microscopy evaluation of capsulorrhexis in femtosecond laser-assisted cataract surgery. J Cart Refract Surg. 2013;39:1581-6.
20. Kránitz K, Takacs A, Mihâltz K, et al. Femtosecond laser capsulotomy and manual continuous curvilinear capsulorrhexis parameters and their effects on intraocular lens centration. J Refract Surg. 2011;8:558-63.
21. Ali MH, Ullah S, Javaid U, et al. Comparison of characteristics of femtosecond laser-assisted anterior capsulotomy versus manual continuous curvilinear capsulorrhexis: a meta-analysis of 5-year results. J Pak Med Assoc. 2017.pp.1574-9.
22. Conrad-Hengerer I, Hengerer FH, Schultz T et al. Effect of femtosecond laser fragmentation on effective phacoemulsification time in cataract surgery. J Refract Surg. 2012;12:879-83.
23. Abell RG, Kerr NM, Vote BJ. Toward zero effective phacoemulsification time using femtosecond laser pretreatment. Ophthalmology. 2013;120:942-8.
24. Reddy KP, Kandulla J, Auffarth GU. Effectiveness and safety of femtosecond laser-assisted lens fragmentation and anterior capsulotomy versus the manual technique in cataract surgery. J Cataract Refract Surg. 2013;39:1297-306.
25. Takács AI, Kovács I, Mihâltz K, et al. Central corneal volume and endothelial cell count following femtosecond laser-assisted refractive cataract surgery compared to conventional phacoemulsification. J Refract Surg. 2012;6:387-91.
26. Abell RG, Allen PL, Vote BJ. Anterior chamber flare after femtosecond laser-assisted cataract surgery. J Cataract Refract Surg. 2013;39:1321-6.
27. Al-Mohtaseb Z, He X, Yesilirmak N, et al. Comparison of corneal endothelial cell loss between two femtosecond laser platforms and standard phacoemulsification. J Refract Surg. 2017;10:708-12.
28. Ranjini H, Murthy PR, Murthy GJ, et al. Femtosecond laser-assisted cataract surgery versus 2.2 mm clear corneal phacoemulsification. 2017;65:942-8.
29. Filkorn T, Kovács I, Takács A, et al. Comparison of IOL power calculation and refractive outcome after laser refractive cataract surgery with a femtosecond laser versus conventional phacoemulsification. J Refract Surg. 2012;28:540-4.
30. Lawless M, Bali SJ, Hodge C, et al. Outcomes of femtosecond laser cataract surgery with a diffractive multifocal intraocular lens. J Refract Surg. 2012;28:859-64.
31. Khandekar R, Behrens A, Al Towerki AE, et al. Determinants of visual outcomes in femtosecond laser assisted cataract surgery and phacoemulsification: a nested case control study. Middle East Afr J Ophthalmol. 2015;22:356-61.
32. Roberts TV, Lawless M, Chan CC, et al. Femtosecond laser cataract surgery: technology and clinical practice. Clin Exp Ophthalmol. 2013;41:180-6.
33. Donaldson KE, Braga-Mele R, Cabot F, et al. Femtosecond laser-assisted cataract surgery. J Cart Refract Surg. 2013;39:1753-63.

Chapter 34

Choosing the Best Intraocular Lens for the Patient's Needs

Todd Driver, Uday Devgan

INTRODUCTION

Cataract surgery and intraocular lens (IOL) implantation is the most commonly performed surgical procedure worldwide and the demand for this surgery only continues to rise.[1,2] There are numerous IOLs available for cataract surgeons and the choice of IOL can be one of the most important decisions a cataract surgeon makes during surgical planning. Important factors to consider in IOL selection include the following: (1) IOL material; (2) IOL light filtering properties; (3) aspheric versus spherical IOLs; (4) toric IOLs; (5) presbyopia-treating IOLs; and (6) the presence of decreased capsular support.[3-6] This chapter will review the different options for IOLs and special cases for when specific IOLs should be used and avoided.

INTRAOCULAR LENS MATERIAL

A variety of intraocular lens materials are available. The two major groups are acrylic and silicone lenses. Acrylic lenses are further divided into the following: rigid poly (methyl methacrylate) (PMMA); foldable hydrophobic acrylic; and foldable hydrophilic acrylic.[7]

There is no difference between the IOL materials with regard to the development of postoperative inflammation. This is true for patients with preexisting uveitis as well.[8,9] A recent study found that hydrophobic acrylic IOLs had the highest incidence of late foreign-body cell reaction, followed by hydrophilic acrylic IOLs and silicone IOLs. However, this inflammatory reaction was clinically insignificant in all cases.[8]

Anterior capsule opacification was found to be highest in patients implanted with silicone IOLs and the lowest with those implanted with hydrophilic IOLs over a 3-year follow-up period.[10] IOL material does not influence posterior capsule opacification (PCO) formation but the presence of a square posterior optic edge on the IOL can prevent PCO formation by providing a barrier to lens epithelial cell migration.[7]

Interlenticular opacification is an important consideration when implanting piggyback IOLs. There are two methods to avoid interlenticular opacification. The first is to place the two IOLs in the capsular bag with a large capsulorrhexis so the cut edge of the capsulorrhexis can fuse with the posterior capsule and sequester the lens epithelial cells that cause interlenticular opacification. The other recommendation is to implant one IOL in the capsular bag and the other in the ciliary sulcus with a small capsulorrhexis.[11,12] A small capsulorrhexis margin will adhere to the anterior surface of the IOL in the capsular bag and sequester lens epithelial cells. It is also recommended that the IOL fixated in the sulcus have a smooth, rounded anterior optic edge along with thin haptics which minimizes its contact with the posterior iris surface.[13,14] Although there is no proven association between IOL material and interlenticular opacification, it is recommended to use a different IOL material in the ciliary sulcus than the material of the IOL in the capsular bag in order to reduce interface inflammation.

Glistenings are fluid-filled microvacuoles that form within the body of the IOL and are rarely visually significant[15] (Fig. 34.1). They can be present in any IOL type; however, it is most commonly reported in hydrophobic acrylic lenses. Various factors are associated with glistening formation, such as conditions that result in breakdown of the blood-aqueous barrier such as glaucoma and the use of topical glaucoma eye drops.[16]

Rarely, calcification of hydrophilic IOLs can be a complication leading to IOL explantation (Fig. 34.2). The causes of this calcification appear to be multifactorial and include issues with the IOL manufacturing process, packaging, surgical technique, and metabolic conditions present in the patient.[7] There are also several studies that report the appearance of calcium on the surface of silicone IOLs in eyes with asteroid hyalosis. The cause of this remains unknown.[17-20]

Additionally, it is recommended to avoid implantation of silicone IOLs in eyes either filled with silicone oil or eyes

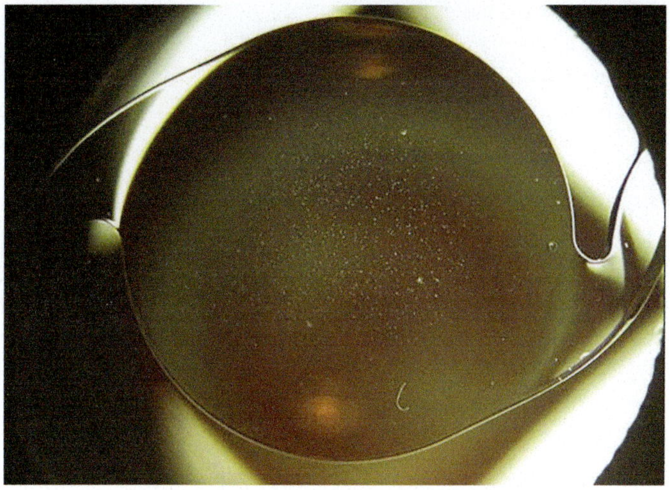

Fig. 34.1: Intraocular lens glistenings.
Source: Dr Madhu Shekar, Aravind Eye Hospital, Madurai.

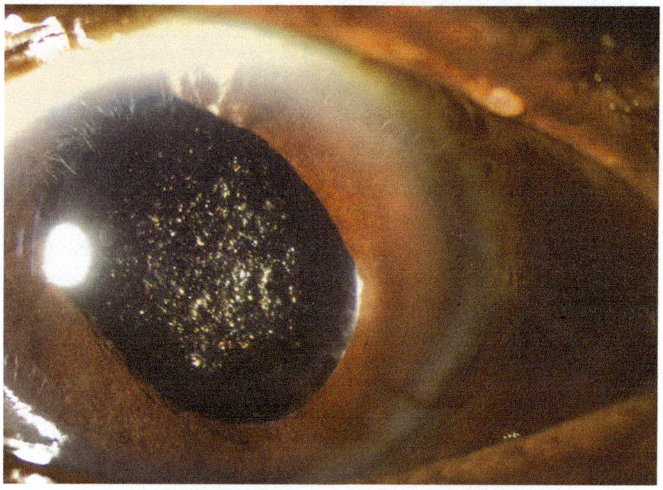

Fig. 34.2: Intraocular lens calcification.
Source: Dr Madhu Shekar, Aravind Eye Hospital, Madurai.

at risk for requiring silicone oil fill in the future (e.g. those at risk of retinal detachment). Several studies have shown that silicone oil is maximally adherent to silicone IOLs and can result in permanent silicone adherence to the IOL, altering its optics.[21,22]

LIGHT-FILTERING INTRAOCULAR LENSES

Recently, IOL manufacturers have promoted IOLs with transmittance properties that filter visible short-wavelength light (blue light), claiming that they provide a macular photoprotective effect. The cornea, vitreous, and aqueous transmit wavelengths in the visible and near-visible spectrum that are greater than 300 nm. The crystalline lens alone absorbs ultraviolet (UV) radiation and its UV absorption increases with age.[23] In addition, IOLs which filter shorter-wavelength light may provide a more natural color temperature compared to IOLs which do not.

Initially, IOLs manufactured from PMMA did not include ultraviolet radiation (UVR)-blocking chromophores. However, after retinal phototoxicity secondary to UVR transmission was recognized in pseudophakic eyes, most IOLs were developed to contain UVR-absorbing chromophores by 1980.[24,25] These UV-only filtering IOLs typically absorb wavelengths up to 420 nm. However, blue-light filtering IOLs additionally block wavelengths between 400 nm and 500 nm[26] (Fig. 34.3). These lenses include the Alcon AcrySof Natural IOLs, the Bausch + Lomb SofPort AO with Violet Shield Technology, and the Hoya Corporation YA-60BBR (Fig. 34.4).

Several studies have been published on the efficacy of blue-light filtering IOLs and central vision. A study of bilaterally pseudophakic patients with UV-only filtering IOLs found that the addition of clip-on short-wavelength, blue-light-filtering lenses improved PhotoStress recovery time and glare disability.[27] Other studies have shown that the use of blue-light-filtering IOLs produce no clinically significant difference in visual outcomes. One study of 93 patients with a blue-light-filtering IOL in one eye and a UV-only filtering IOL in the fellow eye found no differences in visual acuity, contrast sensitivity or color perception between the two eyes.[28] Additionally, another study found no significant lasting difference in cyanopsia between eyes with UV-only filtering IOLs and eyes with blue-light-filtering IOLs. The authors, however, recommended avoiding implanting a blue-light-filtering IOL in one eye and a UV-only filtering IOL in the fellow eye since patients may be able to notice the difference in color temperature.[29]

Oxidative stress from a cumulative lifetime exposure to short-wavelength light is associated with the development of age-related macular degeneration (AMD).[30,31] Therefore, it is thought that a blue-filtering IOL could have a protective effect on the retina. A 2-year prospective observational study comparing fundus autofluorescence photos in 79 eyes with UV-only filtering IOLs and 52 eyes with blue-light-filtering IOLs found that the UV-only filtering IOL group had increased fundus autofluorescence over the 2-year study period, suggesting that the blue-light-filtering IOL had a protective effect on the retina.[32] Another study found that eyes with blue-light-filtering IOLs had a slower rate of

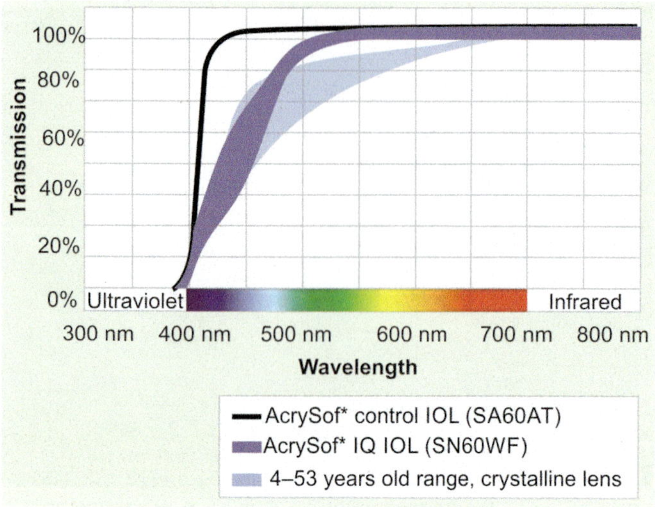

Fig. 34.3: Light transmission of blue-blocking intraocular lens (IOL) versus ultraviolet (UV) only blocking IOL. Both IOLs block light in the UV spectrum. The blue-blocking IOL filters out more light in the shorter wavelengths in the visible spectrum compared to the UV only blocking IOL.

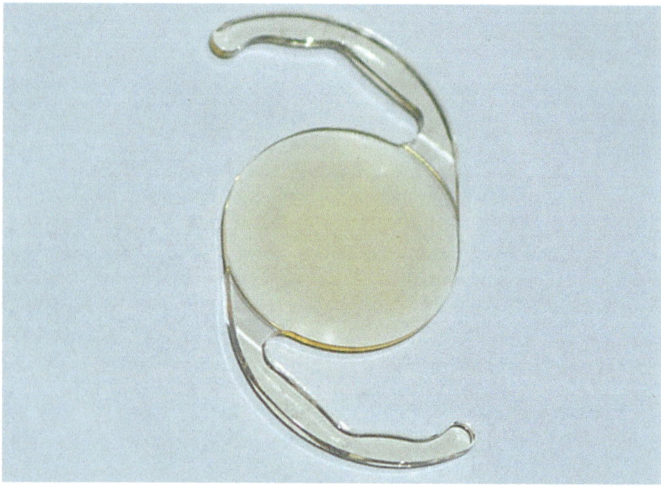

Fig. 34.4: A blue-blocking intraocular lens, notice its yellow tint.
Source: Dr Shivakumar, Aravind Eye Hospital, Tirunelveli.

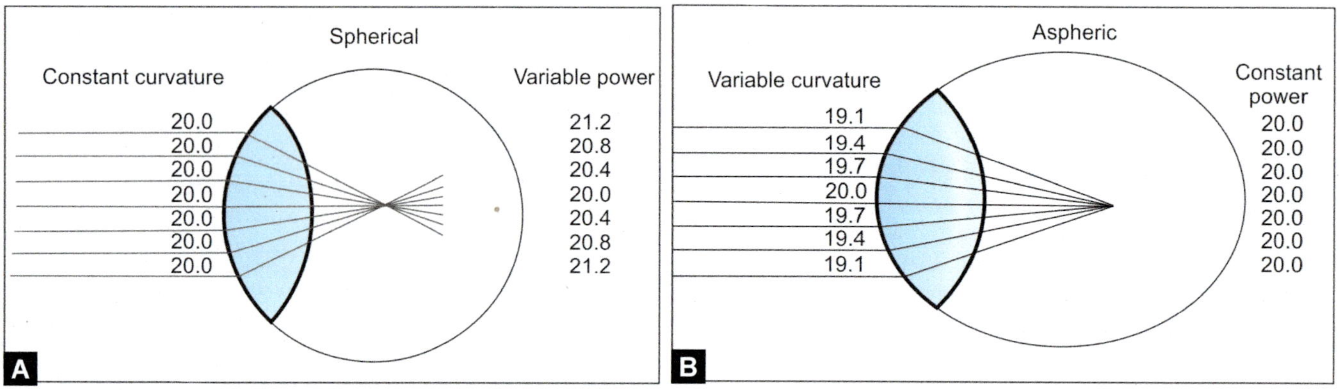

Figs. 34.5A and B: Ray-tracing diagram showing a spherical intraocular lens (IOL) (A) versus an aspheric IOL (B). The aspheric IOL is designed to reduce positive spherical aberration and focus more incoming light rays onto a single point.

progression of geographic atrophy compared to those with UV-only filtering IOLs.[33]

Overall, blue-light-filtering IOLs do not seem to have any significant impact on central vision compared to UV-only filtering IOLs. However, there is some evidence to suggest that blue-filtering-IOLs provide a protective effect on the retina.

ASPHERIC VERSUS SPHERICAL INTRAOCULAR LENSES

Aspheric IOLs were developed to optically compensate for the positive spherical aberration naturally produced by the prolate cornea, optically behaving similar to the young crystalline lens.[34,35] Aspheric lenses are designed to reduce positive spherical aberration and optimize image quality compared to a spherical IOL[36] (Figs 34.5A and B). A recent meta-analysis found that aspheric IOL implantation was associated with improved contrast sensitivity compared to spherical IOL implantation, especially under mesopic conditions.[37] Another recent meta-analysis found that aspheric monofocal IOLs produced less ocular spherical aberration and fewer higher order aberrations than spherical IOLs. For pupil sizes ranging from 4.0 mm to 6.0 mm, the authors found that Abbott TECNIS aspheric IOLs produced approximately zero ocular spherical aberration and Alcon AcrySof aspheric IOLs kept a small amount of positive spherical aberration. These differences, however, were visually insignificant.[38] When using aspheric IOLs with negative spherical aberration, it is important to remember

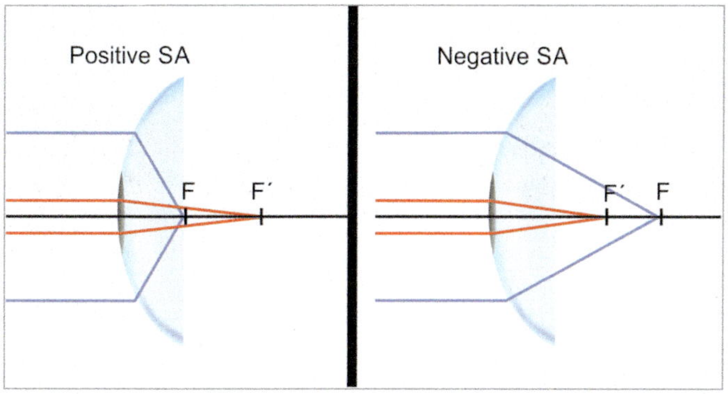

Fig. 34.6: Ray-tracing diagram showing the positive spherical aberration (SA) induced by myopic laser-assisted in situ keratomileusis (LASIK) and the negative spherical aberration induced by hyperopic LASIK. Notice the corneal flattening induced by myopic LASIK and increased corneal steepening induced by hyperopic LASIK.

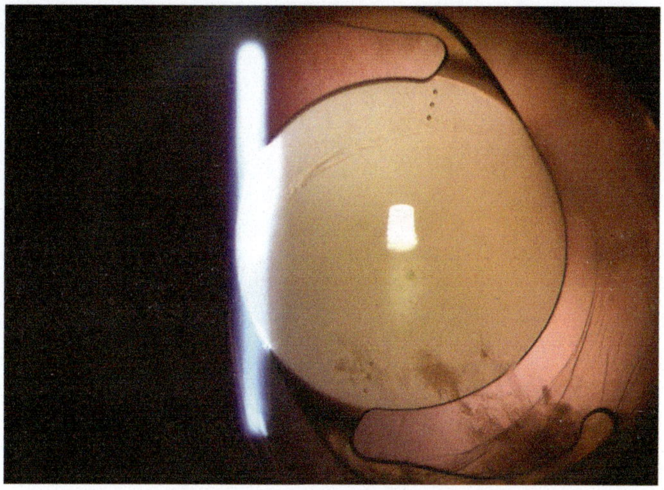

Fig. 34.7: Toric intraocular lens (IOL) implanted in the posterior chamber. Notice the toric marker at the superior and inferior aspect of the IOL.
Source: Dr Madhu Shekar, Aravind Eye Hospital, Madurai.

that they are more sensitive than zero spherical aberration lenses to optical degradation from IOL tilt or decentration and that reducing positive spherical aberration can reduce pseudophakic depth of field.[39,40]

Aspheric IOLs currently FDA-approved include: Abbott ZCB00 and Z9000 series; Alcon AcrySof IQ series; Bausch + Lomb SofPort AO, Akreos AO, Akreos MICS, and Crystalens AO; and STAAR Surgical Afinity and nanoFLEX series.

Given that aspheric IOLs are designed to compensate for the natural positive sphericity of the prolate cornea, it is important to consider the changes brought about by corneal refractive surgery. Myopic laser in situ keratomileusis (LASIK) induces corneal flattening and thus increases positive spherical aberration.[41] In patients who have undergone previous myopic LASIK, aspheric IOLs were shown to provide better optical and visual outcomes compared to spherical IOLs.[42-44] More recent excimer lasers are able to treat the desired refractive error without significantly changing the spherical aberration profile of the cornea.

Hyperopic LASIK and keratoconus increase corneal steepening and negative spherical aberration.[45] Thus, spherical IOLs with positive spherical aberration should theoretically offset this additional negative spherical aberration to produce optimal visual outcomes; however, there is limited evidence in the literature to support this[46] (Fig. 34.6).

TORIC INTRAOCULAR LENSES

Toric IOLs are astigmatism correcting IOLs. Residual postoperative astigmatism is a significant cause of missing planned emmetropia after cataract surgery.[47,48] Correcting residual astigmatism can also result in significantly better visual acuity at all contrast levels.[49] FDA-approved toric IOLs can correct up to four diopters (D) of corneal astigmatism while use of corneal relaxing incisions is best for 1.5 or less diopters of astigmatism.[50] A recent meta-analysis found that in those with preoperative regular corneal astigmatism, patients with toric IOLs had better uncorrected distance visual acuity (UCDVA) and greater distance spectacle independence compared to those with non-toric IOLs. Additionally, residual postoperative astigmatism was lower in those with toric IOLs compared to those who had non-toric IOLs plus relaxing corneal incisions. On average, in the meta-analysis, toric IOLs rotated less than 5°.[51] Misalignment of a toric IOL can lessen the astigmatic benefit with all benefit lost with 30° of rotation (Fig. 34.7).

Food and Drug Administration approved Toric IOLs include the Alcon AcrySof Toric IOL, the Abbot Medical Optics TECNIS Toric IOL, the Staar Surgical Toric IOL, and the Bausch + Lomb Trulign Toric IOL. There are also multifocal toric IOLs and extended depth of field toric IOLs for patients who wish to address both astigmatism and presbyopia concurrently.

PRESBYOPIA-TREATING INTRAOCULAR LENSES

The ultimate goal in cataract surgery is to develop an IOL that matches the ability of the natural crystalline lens to change refractive power in order to provide in-focus vision at different distances. Currently, there are no IOLs available

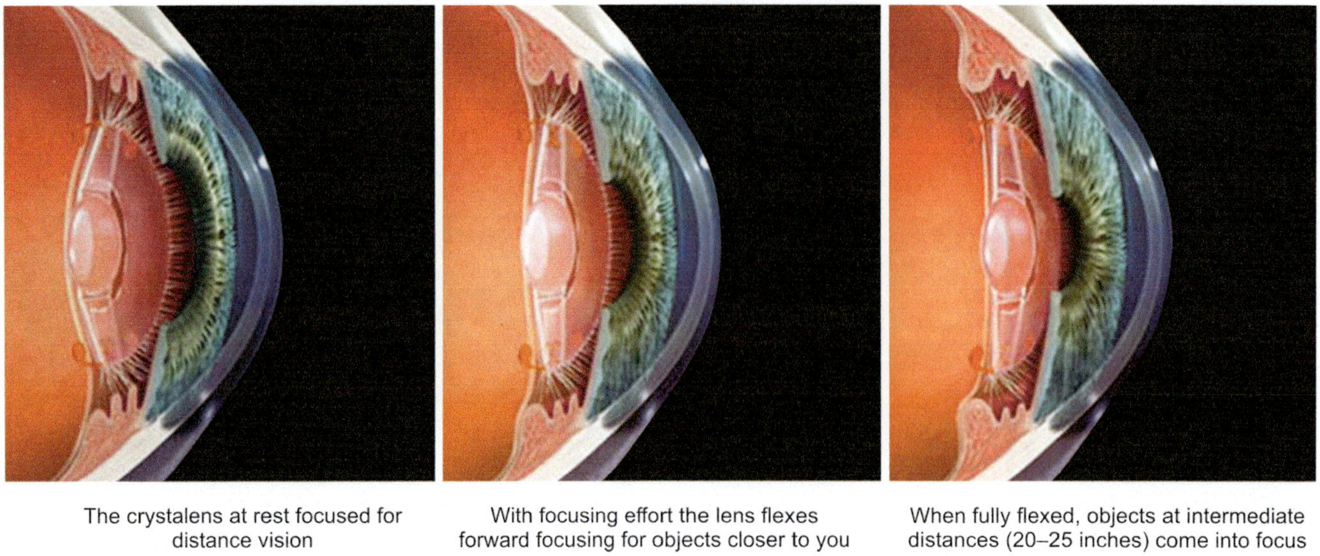

Fig. 34.8: Illustration of a partially accommodative intraocular lens (IOL) implanted into the capsular bag. Notice how the optic moves anteriorly for near vision and posteriorly for distance vision.

that can do this. However, three different IOLs have been developed in order to increase pseudophakic depth of focus: (1) partially-accommodative IOLs; (2) multifocal IOLs; and (3) extended depth of focus (EDOF) IOLs.[52]

Partially-accommodative Intraocular Lenses

Partially-accommodative IOLs are designed to change axial position and optic curvature in the eye during near and distance vision. By forwardly displacing during near vision and posteriorly displacing during distance vision, they are able to provide patients with adequate vision at near and distance. These IOLs include the Bausch + Lomb Crystalens, the HumanOptics 1 CU, and the Lenstec Tetraflex (Fig. 34.8).[53] The evidence in support of partially accommodative IOLs is mixed. One study comparing the Crystalens (Bausch + Lomb), Tek-Clear (Tekia), and the monofocal SA60AT (Alcon) IOLs found that all patients had similar postoperative corrected distance visual acuity but the partially-accommodative IOLs produced modestly better uncorrected near visual acuity and distance corrected near visual acuity compared to the monofocal IOL.[54] Additionally, partially accommodative IOLs have been shown to have better contrast sensitivity under photopic conditions than multifocal IOLs.[55,56] However, the Crystalens was found to have inferior distance-corrected near visual acuity compared to the Alcon ReSTOR multifocal IOL and that the accommodative response of the Crystalens was less than 0.4 D.[57,58] Other studies have also shown that the partially accommodative IOLs produce inferior near visual outcomes to multifocal lenses and also lose their accommodative amplitude over time because of capsular contraction.[59-61] Newer design, truly accommodating IOLs are currently in development and we anticipate that in the future, a few diopters of true accommodation will be achieved.

Multifocal Intraocular Lenses

Multifocal IOLs (MFIOLs) increase accommodative amplitude by simultaneously separating light into different foci and then relying on neuro-adaptation for patients to achieve satisfactory vision at different distances.[62]

Multifocal IOLs can be refractive, diffractive or a combination of the two. Refractive MFIOLs work by providing annular zones of different refractive powers (Fig. 34.9). They are very sensitive to different pupil sizes and decentration. The rough transitions between the refractive zones also can result in glares, halos, and reduced contrast sensitivity. Diffractive MFIOLs work by placing diffractive microstructures in concentric zones and decreasing the distance between the zones as they get further from the center in order to produce multiple optic foci (Fig. 34.10). Diffractive MFIOLs are less pupil size dependent and are more tolerant of decentration than refractive MFIOLs. However, traditional two-foci diffractive MFIOLs produce inferior intermediate vision outcomes compared to refractive MFIOLs and result in more lost light energy secondary to light scatter at the diffractive surfaces, resulting in decreased contrast sensitivity. There are some newer trifocal MFIOLs that provide intermediate

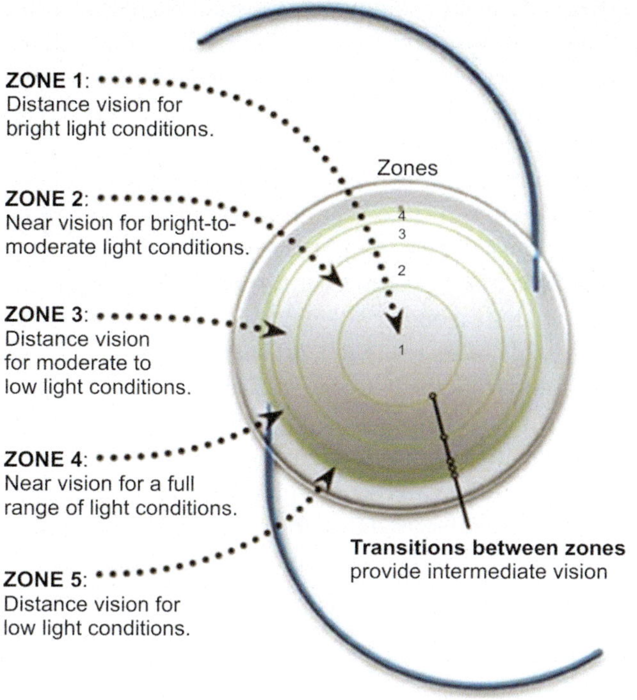

Fig. 34.9: Diagram showing the different annular zones of a refractive multifocal intraocular lens.

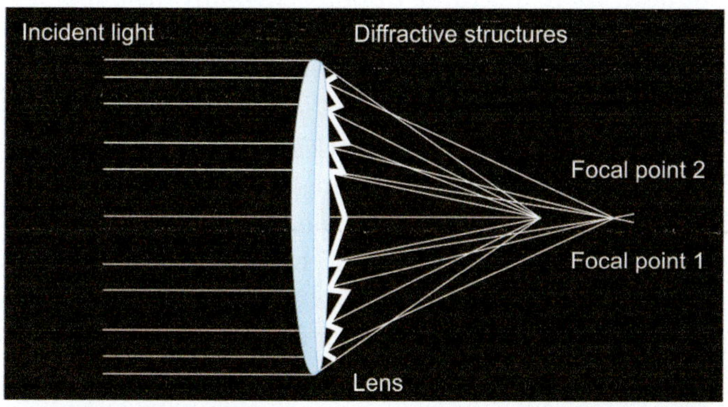

Fig. 34.10: Ray-tracing diagram showing how a diffractive multifocal intraocular lens uses diffractive microstructures in concentric zones to produce multiple optic foci to increase a patient's depth of field.

vision through redistribution of diffracted light to additional foci.[63]

Numerous studies have investigated the outcomes of refractive and diffractive MFIOLs. A recent review found that 57.1% of refractive MFIOL groups and 70.6% of diffractive MFIOL groups achieved UCDVA better than 20/25. Out of total, 19.23% of refractive MFIOL groups and 47.3% of diffractive IOL groups achieved better than 20/25.[64] A recent Cochrane review also found that monofocal IOLs or MFIOLs produced similar postoperative UCDVA but patients with MFIOLs achieved better uncorrected near visual acuity (UCNVA) and spectacle independence. No difference in UCDVA and UCNVA was observed when patients with MFIOLs were compared with those with monovision. Though MFIOLs resulted in a greater degree of spectacle independence, they also produced a higher incidence of postoperative glare and halos compared to monovision.[65] Splitting light into two or more focal points with diffractive optics will always come with a relative compromise in image quality and contrast sensitivity.

When deciding on whether to choose a MFIOL, it is important to evaluate for ocular comorbidities, and select patients wisely.[63,64] Traditionally, MFIOLs were reserved for patients with low amounts of corneal astigmatism as greater than 1.50 diopters of regular corneal astigmatism was shown to produce poorer visual outcomes with MFIOLs.[64] However, the introduction of toric MFIOLs have been shown to produce similar visual outcomes in patients with 0.75–2.82 diopters of corneal astigmatism compared to non-toric MFIOLs in patients with less than 0.75 diopters of corneal astigmatism.[66] Patients with irregular corneal astigmatism or any posterior segment abnormality (such as glaucoma, AMD, diabetic retinopathy) that can cause reduced contrast sensitivity are not recommended for MFIOL implantation. Patients with mild zonular weakness are recommended to have a capsular tension ring implanted at the time of MFIOL implantation. However, MFIOLs are generally not recommended in patients with risk of late decentration due to zonular dehiscence. When selecting candidates for MFIOL implantation, it is important to consider that MFIOLs are better suited for patients with realistic postoperative visual expectations and those who understand that MFIOLs do not produce a guaranteed refractive outcome or absolute freedom from spectacle use.[64]

Refractive MFIOLs include the Abbot ReZoom (no longer made). Diffractive MFIOL models include the following: Abbot TECNIS ZKB00, ZLB00, ZMB00, ZMT; Zeiss Lisa series; Alcon ReSTOR SN6AD1-3, SND1T2-5; PhysIOL FineVision series; Oculentis Lentis Mplus series; and the Hanita SeeLens MF series.

Extended Depth of Focus Intraocular Lenses

A third modality to increase accommodative amplitude in pseudophakic patients is through EDOF IOLs, which work by creating a single elongated focal point to enhance range of vision (Fig. 34.11). The TECNIS Symfony IOL (Abbott Medical Optics) has an anterior aspheric surface and a

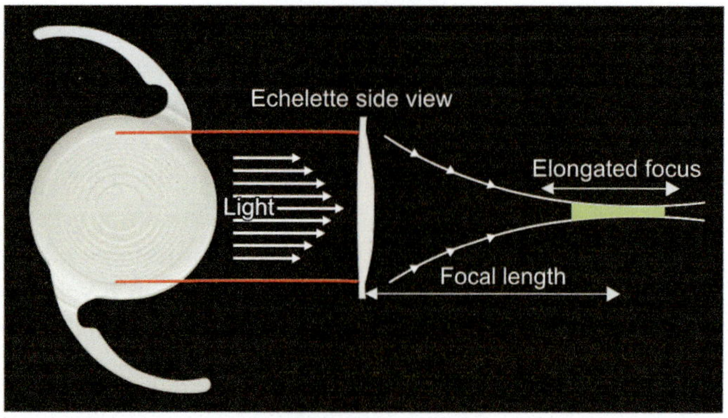

Fig. 34.11: Diagram showing how the anterior aspheric surface and the posterior diffractive surface creates a single elongated focal point for the extended depth of focus (EDOF) intraocular lens.

posterior achromatic diffractive surface which produces an achromatic diffractive pattern that elongates a single focal point and compensates for the chromatic aberration of the cornea. A recent study found that the Symfony IOL produced significantly better uncorrected monocular and binocular distance intermediate and near visual acuities compared to the monofocal TECNIS ZCB00 IOL. There was no significant difference in contrast sensitivity between the EDOF IOL and monofocal IOL groups.[67] A recent randomized controlled study compared the Alcon trifocal PanOptix MFIOL with the Abbott Symfony EDOF IOL found that the trifocal MFIOL produced better uncorrected near and intermediate visual acuities but similar uncorrected distance visual acuities. Higher order aberrations were similar between the two groups.[68] The incidence of night glare and halos with EDOF IOLs is significantly worse than monofocal IOLs.

INTRAOCULAR LENSES IN THE SETTING OF DECREASED CAPSULAR SUPPORT

When there is a tear in the posterior capsule in the presence of adequate anterior capsular support, it may be necessary to implant an IOL in the ciliary sulcus. IOLs implanted in the ciliary sulcus should always be a 3-piece IOL and never a single-piece IOL to avoid iris chafing and uveitis-glaucoma-hyphema (UGH) syndrome. No IOLs in the United States are specifically designed for sulcus placement but some recommend the STAAR AQ2010 and AQ5010 IOLs for sulcus placement as they are the largest lenses available, which helps increase stability in the ciliary sulcus. The disadvantage of the STAAR lenses is that they are made of silicone, which is problematic if the patients require retinal detachment surgery in the future. Other non-silicone 3-piece lenses typically used for ciliary sulcus placement include the acrylic Alcon MA60AC and TECNIS ZA9000 series, and the silicone Bausch & Lomb Li61AO.

When choosing which IOL power to use for ciliary sulcus placement, it is recommended that the surgeon first accounts for the difference in A-constant and then use the rule of 9's to adjust for the more anterior position of the IOL in the ciliary sulcus compared to the capsular bag. The rule of 9's splits IOL powers at 9, 18, and 27, and recommends that the IOL power be reduced by 0.5, 1.0, and 1.5 D, respectively, as shown in Table 34.1. For example, if the surgeon is planning on using a +24.0 D IOL with an A-constant of 119.2 in the capsular bag and is planning on switching to a different IOL with an A-constant of 118.7, the surgeon would first need to account for the difference in A-constant (119.2 - 118.7 = 0.5) and adjust the IOL power to +23.5 D (= 24.0 - 0.5 D). Then, according to Table 34.1, the IOL power should be decreased by an additional 1.0 D for ciliary sulcus placement, making the final selection be a +22.5 IOL with a 118.7 A-constant.

When there is no adequate anterior or posterior capsular support, there are three options currently available: (1) anterior chamber IOLs (ACIOL); (2) sulcus fixated IOLs; and (3) suture fixated IOLs (sutured to the iris or sclera).

Modern 4-point-fixation flexible anterior chamber IOLs (ACIOLs) such as the Alcon MTA-U0 lens series can be used when there is inadequate capsular support. The common practice for ACIOL sizing is to add 1 mm to the horizontal white-to-white distance of the limbus. Scleral sutured IOLs are typically 3-piece IOLs that are transsclerally secured with Prolene sutures or fixated within the sclera using glue.[69] When choosing between an ACIOL and a scleral fixated IOL, the evidence suggests they produce similar visual outcomes and result in a similar incidence

Table 34.1: Rule of 9's for sulcus intraocular lens (IOL) placement.

Original IOL power	Adjustment for IOL power for sulcus placement
0.0–8.5	None
9.0–17.5	– 0.5 D
18.0–26.5	–1.0 D
27.0 or higher	–1.5 D

*Note these conversions assume the same A-constant for the original IOL and the sulcus IOL.

of postoperative complications including pseudophakic bullous keratopathy, elevated IOP, implant malposition, and postoperative cystoid macular edema.[70]

Traditionally, Prolene transscleral sutures have been used for scleral fixation of 3-piece IOLs. However, suture breakage and erosion have been problematic with this technique.[71] Therefore, there is interest in using Gore-Tex suture for scleral fixation of IOLs as it has greater tensile strength and presumably has a lower risk of suture breakage.[72] A recent study found that using Gore-Tex sutures for scleral fixation of either the Bausch + Lomb Akreos AO60 or the Alcon CZ70BD IOL was well tolerated and resulted in no cases of suture erosion or breakage over approximately 1-year of follow-up.[73]

Iris suture fixated IOLs are another option that can produce stable visual outcomes in the setting of inadequate capsular support (Fig. 34.12). A recent study found that iris suture fixated IOLs were well tolerated with 95% of implants being well centered and stable over 1 year of follow-up. The most common complications were transient intraocular hemorrhage and postoperative glaucoma. The authors of this study recommended using a 3-piece IOL with 10-0 Prolene sutures for iris fixation.[74]

Intraocular lens selection is one of the most important decisions a cataract surgeon will make during surgical planning. As IOL technology continues to develop, it is important that cataract surgeons understand how different IOLs will affect the quality of vision patients will experience postoperatively. Choosing the best IOL based on the patient's anatomy and postoperative visual goals will not only result in excellent surgical results but will also result in the best possible visual outcome for the patient.

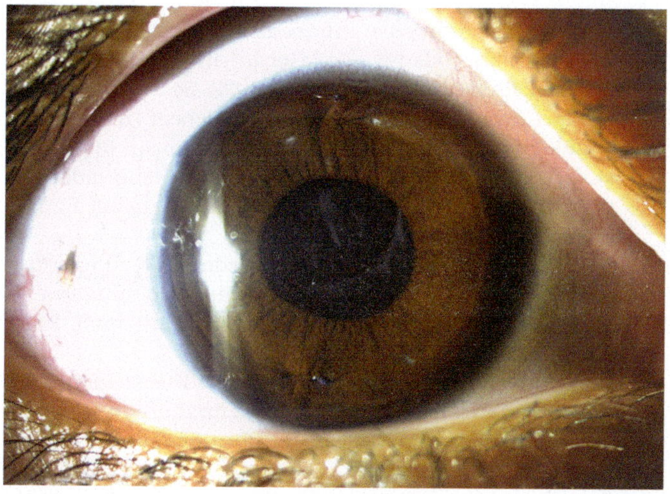

Fig. 34.12: Iris fixated intraocular lens (IOL). Notice the Prolene sutures at 12:00 and 6:00 securing the IOL to the posterior surface of the iris.
Source: Dr Madhu Shekar, Aravind Eye Hospital, Madurai.

REFERENCES

1. Allen D, Vasavada A. Cataract and surgery for cataract. BMJ. 2006;333(7559):128-32.
2. Etzioni DA, Liu JH, Maggard MA, et al. The aging population and its impact on the surgery workforce. Ann Surg. 2003;238(2):170-7.
3. Hayashi H, Hayashi K, Nakao F, et al. Quantitative comparison of posterior capsule opacification after polymethylmethacrylate, silicone, and soft acrylic intraocular lens implantation. Arch Ophthalmol. 1998;116(12):1579-82.
4. Hayashi K, Hayashi H, Nakao F, et al. Changes in posterior capsule opacification after polymethylmethacrylate, silicone, and acrylic intraocular lens implantation. J Cataract Refract Surg. 2001;27(6):817-24.
5. van der Linden JW, van der Meulen IJ, Mourits MP, et al. Comparison of a hydrophilic and a hydrophobic apodized diffractive multifocal intraocular lens. Int Ophthalmol. 2013;33(5):493-500.
6. Koch DD, Wang L. Custom optimization of intraocular lens asphericity. Trans Am Ophthalmol Soc. 2007;105:36-41.
7. Werner L. Biocompatibility of intraocular lens materials. Curr Opin Ophthalmol. 2008;19(1):41-9.
8. Abela-Formanek C, Amon M, Schild G, et al. Uveal and capsular biocompatibility of hydrophilic acrylic, hydrophobic acrylic, and silicone intraocular lenses. J Cataract Refract Surg. 2002;28(1):50-61.
9. Abela-Formanek C, Amon M, Schild G, et al. Inflammation after implantation of hydrophilic acrylic, hydrophobic acrylic, or silicone intraocular lenses in eyes with cataract and uveitis: comparison to a control group. J Cataract Refract Surg. 2002;28(7):1153-9.
10. Abela-Formanek C, Amon M, Kahraman G, et al. Biocompatibility of hydrophilic acrylic, hydrophobic acrylic, and silicone intraocular lenses in eyes with uveitis having cataract surgery: Long-term follow-up. J Cataract Refract Surg. 2011;37(1):104-12.
11. Akaishi L, Tzelikis PF. Primary piggyback implantation using the ReSTOR intraocular lens: case series. J Cataract Refract Surg. 2007;33(5):791-5.
12. Cao KY, Sit M, Braga-Mele R. Primary piggyback implantation of 3 intraocular lenses in nanophthalmos. J Cataract Refract Surg. 2007;33(4):727-30.
13. LeBoyer RM, Werner L, Snyder ME, et al. Acute haptic-induced ciliary sulcus irritation associated with single-piece AcrySof intraocular lenses. J Cataract Refract Surg. 2005;31(7):1421-7.
14. Chang WH, Werner L, Fry LL, et al. Pigmentary dispersion syndrome with a secondary piggyback 3-piece hydrophobic acrylic lens. Case report with clinicopathological correlation. J Cataract Refract Surg. 2007;33(6):1106-9.
15. Chang A, Kugelberg M. Glistenings 9 years after phacoemulsification in hydrophobic and hydrophilic acrylic

intraocular lenses. J Cataract Refract Surg. 2015;41(6):1199-204.

16. Colin J, Orignac I, Touboul D. Glistenings in a large series of hydrophobic acrylic intraocular lenses. J Cataract Refract Surg. 2009;35(12):2121-6.
17. Stringham J, Werner L, Monson B, et al. Calcification of different designs of silicone intraocular lenses in eyes with asteroid hyalosis. Ophthalmology. 2010;117(8):1486-92.
18. Werner L, Kollarits CR, Mamalis N, et al. Surface calcification of a 3-piece silicone intraocular lens in a patient with asteroid hyalosis: a clinicopathologic case report. Ophthalmology. 2005;112(3):447-52.
19. Wackernagel W, Ettinger K, Weitgasser U, et al. Opacification of a silicone intraocular lens caused by calcium deposits on the optic. J Cataract Refract Surg. 2004;30(2):517-20.
20. Foot L, Werner L, Gills JP, et al. Surface calcification of silicone plate intraocular lenses in patients with asteroid hyalosis. Am J Ophthalmol. 2004;137(6):979-87.
21. Apple DJ, Federman JL, Krolicki TJ, et al. Irreversible silicone oil adhesion to silicone intraocular lenses. A clinicopathologic analysis. Ophthalmology. 1996;103(10):1555-61.
22. Stolba U, Binder S, Velikay M, et al. Intraocular silicone lenses in silicone oil: an experimental study. Graefes Arch Clin Exp Ophthalmol. 1996;234(1):55-7.
23. Bron AJ, Vrensen GF, Koretz J, et al. The ageing lens. Ophthalmologica. 2000;214(1):86-104.
24. Mainster MA. Spectral transmittance of intraocular lenses and retinal damage from intense light sources. Am J Ophthalmol. 1978;85(2):167-70.
25. Mainster MA. The spectra, classification, and rationale of ultraviolet-protective intraocular lenses. Am J Ophthalmol. 1986;102(6):727-32.
26. Li X, Kelly D, Nolan JM, et al. The evidence informing the surgeon's selection of intraocular lens on the basis of light transmittance properties. Eye. 2017;31(2):258-72.
27. Hammond BR. Attenuating photostress and glare disability in pseudophakic patients through the addition of a short-wave absorbing filter. J Ophthalmol. 2015;2015:607-35.
28. Landers J, Tan TH, Yuen J, et al. Comparison of visual function following implantation of Acrysof Natural intraocular lenses with conventional intraocular lenses. Clin Exp Ophthalmol. 2007;35(2):152-9.
29. Miyata A. Neutralization method for detecting the incidence of color perception changes after cataract surgery. J Cataract Refract Surg. 2015;41(4):764-70.
30. Age-Related Eye Disease Study 2 Research G. Lutein + zeaxanthin and omega-3 fatty acids for age-related macular degeneration: the Age-Related Eye Disease Study 2 (AREDS2) randomized clinical trial. JAMA. 2013; 309(19):2005-15.
31. Beatty S, Koh H, Phil M, et al. The role of oxidative stress in the pathogenesis of age-related macular degeneration. Surv Ophthalmol. 2000;45(2):115-34.
32. Nagai H, Hirano Y, Yasukawa T, et al. Prevention of increased abnormal fundus autofluorescence with blue light-filtering intraocular lenses. J Cataract Refract Surg. 2015;41(9): 1855-9.
33. Pipis A, Touliou E, Pillunat LE, et al. Effect of the blue filter intraocular lens on the progression of geographic atrophy. Eur J Ophthalmol. 2015;25(2):128-33.
34. Packer M, Fine IH, Hoffman RS. Aspheric intraocular lens selection: the evolution of refractive cataract surgery. Curr Opin Ophthalmol. 2008;19(1):1-4.
35. Glasser A, Campbell MC. Presbyopia and the optical changes in the human crystalline lens with age. Vision Res. 1998;38(2):209-29.
36. Guo H, Goncharov AV, Dainty C. Comparison of retinal image quality with spherical and customized aspheric intraocular lenses. Biomed Opt Express. 2012;3(4):681-91.
37. Schuster AK, Tesarz J, Vossmerbaeumer U. The impact on vision of aspheric to spherical monofocal intraocular lenses in cataract surgery: a systematic review with meta-analysis. Ophthalmology. 2013;120(11):2166-75.
38. Schuster AK, Tesarz J, Vossmerbaeumer U. Ocular wavefront analysis of aspheric compared with spherical monofocal intraocular lenses in cataract surgery: Systematic review with metaanalysis. J Cataract Refract Surg. 2015;41(5):1088-97.
39. Altmann GE, Nichamin LD, Lane SS, et al. Optical performance of 3 intraocular lens designs in the presence of decentration. J Cataract Refract Surg. 2005;31(3):574-85.
40. Rocha KM, Soriano ES, Chamon W, et al. Spherical aberration and depth of focus in eyes implanted with aspheric and spherical intraocular lenses: a prospective randomized study. Ophthalmology. 2007;114(11):2050-4.
41. Oshika T, Miyata K, Tokunaga T, et al. Higher order wavefront aberrations of cornea and magnitude of refractive correction in laser in situ keratomileusis. Ophthalmology. 2002;109(6):1154-8.
42. Fernandez-Vega L, Madrid-Costa D, Alfonso JF, et al. Optical and visual performance of diffractive intraocular lens implantation after myopic laser in situ keratomileusis. J Cataract Refract Surg. 2009;35(5):825-32.
43. Alfonso JF, Madrid-Costa D, Poo-Lopez A, et al. Visual quality after diffractive intraocular lens implantation in eyes with previous myopic laser in situ keratomileusis. J Cataract Refract Surg. 2008;34(11):1848-54.
44. Madrid-Costa D, Perez-Vives C, Ruiz-Alcocer J, et al. Visual simulation through different intraocular lenses in patients with previous myopic corneal ablation using adaptive optics: effect of tilt and decentration. J Cataract Refract Surg. 2012;38(5):774-86.
45. Soler V, Benito A, Soler P, et al. A randomized comparison of pupil-centered versus vertex-centered ablation in LASIK correction of hyperopia. Am J Ophthalmol. 2011; 152(4):591-9.e2.
46. Ruiz-Alcocer J, Perez-Vives C, Madrid-Costa D, et al. Effect of simulated IOL tilt and decentration on spherical aberration after hyperopic LASIK for different intraocular lenses. J Refract Surg. 2012;28(5):327-34.
47. Behndig A, Montan P, Stenevi U, et al. Aiming for emmetropia after cataract surgery: Swedish National Cataract Register study. J Cataract Refract Surg. 2012;38(7):1181-6.
48. Wilkins MR, Allan B, Rubin G, et al. Spectacle use after routine cataract surgery. Br J Ophthalmol. 2009;93(10):1307-12.

49. Lehmann RP, Houtman DM. Visual performance in cataract patients with low levels of postoperative astigmatism: full correction versus spherical equivalent correction. Clin Ophthalmol. 2012;6:333-8.
50. Rubenstein JB, Raciti M. Approaches to corneal astigmatism in cataract surgery. Curr Opin Ophthalmol. 2013;24(1): 30-4.
51. Kessel L, Andresen J, Tendal B, et al. Toric intraocular lenses in the correction of astigmatism during cataract surgery: a systematic review and meta-analysis. Ophthalmology. 2016;123(2):275-86.
52. Leyland M, Zinicola E. Multifocal versus monofocal intraocular lenses after cataract extraction. Cochrane Database Syst Rev. 2003(3):CD003169.
53. Alio JL, Alio Del Barrio JL, Vega-Estrada A. Accommodative intraocular lenses: where are we and where we are going. Eye Vis (Lond). 2017;4:16.
54. Sadoughi MM, Einollahi B, Roshandel D, et al. Visual and refractive outcomes of phacoemulsification with implantation of accommodating versus standard monofocal intraocular lenses. J Ophthalmic Vis Res. 2015;10(4):370-4.
55. Alio JL, Plaza-Puche AB, Montalban R, et al. Visual outcomes with a single-optic accommodating intraocular lens and a low-addition-power rotational asymmetric multifocal intraocular lens. J Cataract Refract Surg. 2012;38(6): 978-85.
56. Alio JL, Plaza-Puche AB, Montalban R, et al. Near visual outcomes with single-optic and dual-optic accommodating intraocular lenses. J Cataract Refract Surg. 2012;38(9): 1568-75.
57. Vilupuru S, Lin L, Pepose JS. Comparison of contrast sensitivity and through focus in small-aperture inlay, accommodating intraocular lens, or multifocal intraocular lens subjects. Am J Ophthalmol. 2015;160(1):150-62.e1.
58. Perez-Merino P, Birkenfeld J, Dorronsoro C, et al. Aberrometry in patients implanted with accommodative intraocular lenses. Am J Ophthalmol. 2014;157(5):1077-89.
59. Uthoff D, Gulati A, Hepper D, et al. Potentially accommodating 1CU intraocular lens: 1-year results in 553 eyes and literature review. Journal of Refractive Surgery. 2007;23(2):159-71.
60. Tan N, Zheng D, Ye J. Comparison of visual performance after implantation of 3 types of intraocular lenses: accommodative, multifocal, and monofocal. Eur J Ophthalmol. 2014;24(5):693-8.
61. Mastropasqua L, Toto L, Falconio G, et al. Long-term results of 1 CU accommodative intraocular lens implantation: 2-year follow-up study. Acta Ophthalmol Scand. 2007;85(4):409-14.
62. Alfonso JF, Fernandez-Vega L, Baamonde MB, et al. Prospective visual evaluation of apodized diffractive intraocular lenses. J Cataract Refract Surg. 2007;33(7):1235-43.
63. Alio JL, Plaza-Puche AB, Fernandez-Buenaga R, et al. Multifocal intraocular lenses: An overview. Surv Ophthalmol. 2017;62(5):611-34.
64. Braga-Mele R, Chang D, Dewey S, et al. Multifocal intraocular lenses: relative indications and contraindications for implantation. J Cataract Refract Surg. 2014;40(2):313-22.
65. de Silva SR, Evans JR, Kirthi V, et al. Multifocal versus monofocal intraocular lenses after cataract extraction. Cochrane Database Syst Rev. 2016;12:CD003169.
66. Lehmann R, Modi S, Fisher B, et al. Bilateral implantation of +3.0 D multifocal toric intraocular lenses: results of a US Food and Drug Administration clinical trial. Clin Ophthalmol. 2017;11:1321-31.
67. Pedrotti E, Bruni E, Bonacci E, et al. Comparative analysis of the clinical outcomes with a monofocal and an extended range of vision intraocular lens. J Refract Surg. 2016;32(7):436-42.
68. Monaco G, Gari M, Di Censo F, et al. Visual performance after bilateral implantation of 2 new presbyopia-correcting intraocular lenses: Trifocal versus extended range of vision. J Cataract Refract Surg. 2017;43(6):737-47.
69. Ganekal S, Venkataratnam S, Dorairaj S, et al. Comparative evaluation of suture-assisted and fibrin glue-assisted scleral fixated intraocular lens implantation. J Refract Surg. 2012;28(4):249-52.
70. Donaldson KE, Gorscak JJ, Budenz DL, et al. Anterior chamber and sutured posterior chamber intraocular lenses in eyes with poor capsular support. J Cataract Refract Surg. 2005;31(5):903-9.
71. Vote BJ, Tranos P, Bunce C, et al. Long-term outcome of combined pars plana vitrectomy and scleral fixated sutured posterior chamber intraocular lens implantation. Am J Ophthalmol. 2006;141(2):308-12.
72. Nottage JM, Bhasin V, Nirankari VS. Long-term safety and visual outcomes of transscleral sutured posterior chamber IOLs and penetrating keratoplasty combined with transscleral sutured posterior chamber IOLs. Trans Am Ophthalmol Soc. 2009;107:242-50.
73. Khan MA, Gupta OP, Smith RG, et al. Scleral fixation of intraocular lenses using Gore-Tex suture: clinical outcomes and safety profile. Br J Ophthalmol. 2016;100(5):638-43.
74. Soiberman U, Pan Q, Daoud Y, et al. Iris suture fixation of subluxated intraocular lenses. Am J Ophthalmol. 2015;159(2):353-9.

Chapter 35

Astigmatism Vectors in Cataract Surgery

Cameron Pole, Uday Devgan

INTRODUCTION

Astigmatism is defined as a deviation of the optical refractive surfaces from spherical curvature. The classic example likens a standard spherical corneal surface to a basketball and an astigmatic surface to a football so that the corneal steepness is greater in one axis than the other. This aberration has the optical effect of distorting and stretching retinal image and the effects on visual acuity can be significant compared with measured refractive error. Office-based refraction has long attempted to approximate the degree of astigmatism using cylindrical equivalents which usually achieve very good refractive outcomes. Lenses that correct astigmatism also known as toric lenses have been developed for both soft contact lenses, rigid gas-permeable contact lenses and as intraocular lenses (IOLs). However in many cases, emmetropia cannot be achieved with traditional spectacles or contact lenses, and surgical approaches may provide definitive treatment, especially when cataract surgery is already an option.

Astigmatism can be further categorized on other parameters. In terms of direction, with-the-rule astigmatism, more typical in younger patients contains the corneal steep axis vertically (±30°), while against-the-rule astigmatism, more typical in older patients contains the steep axis horizontally (±30°). Both have steep axes on the principal meridians, i.e. the x-axis and y-axis of a standard graph. The "rule" in this case refers to the average adult cornea having a vertical diameter of 11 mm and horizontal diameter of 12 mm leading to an ellipsoid shape. Additionally, regular astigmatism is characterized by the steep axes being 180° apart and approximately equal in curvature. This is often represented by the classic "bowetie" shape on corneal topography, and these can often be treated effectively with spectacles or IOLs (Fig. 35.1). Irregular astigmatism refers to deviation from this shape.

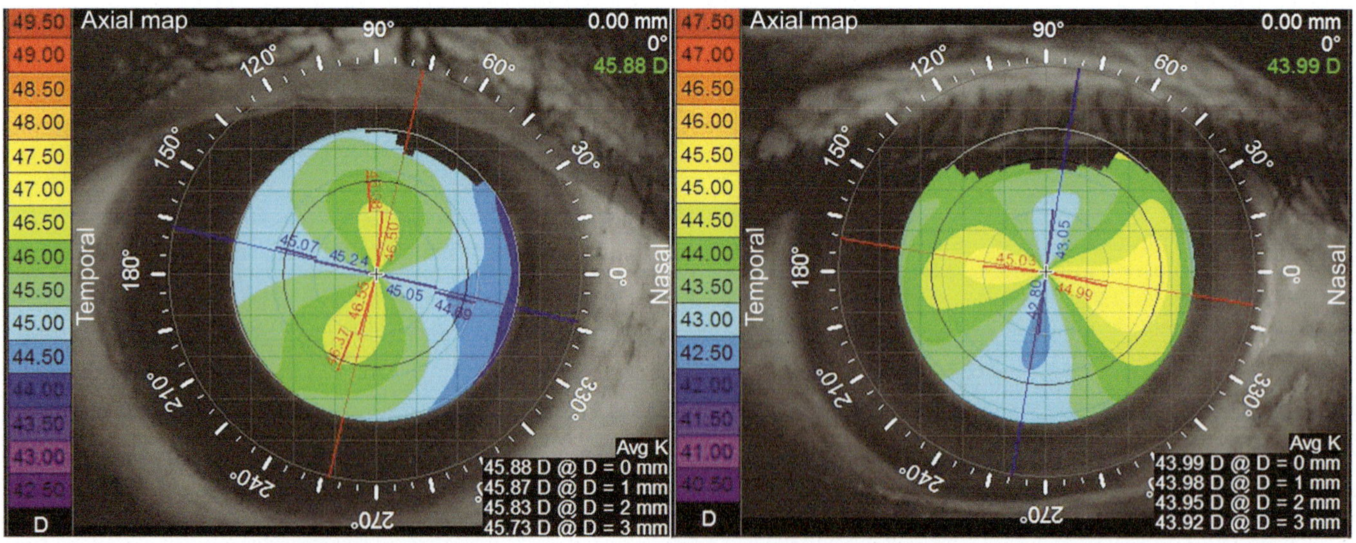

Fig. 35.1: Keratometric displays of typical astigmatisms. Left panel: Keratometric display of typical with-the-rule astigmatism. Note the steepening (yellow) of the vertical axis and relatively flattening along the horizontal axis. Right Panel: Keratometric display of typical against-the-rule astigmatism. Note the steepening of the horizontal axis and relatively flattening along the vertical axis. Keratometric Diopter value references for color gradients are displayed on the left side of each panel.

Source: Dr Madhu Shekar, Aravind Eye Hospital, Madurai.

Although anterior corneal shape is most commonly calculated, both posterior corneal curvature and lenticular aberrations can induce astigmatism and can prove challenging to identify and correct. Therefore, the total astigmatism is equal to the corneal astigmatism plus the lenticular astigmatism. This is why corneal topography prior to surgery is of utmost importance even in the astigmatic eye. A patient may have both corneal and lenticular astigmatismas that combine to give spherical refraction. However, as the lens will be removed during surgery, the corneal astigmatism is the primary factor in calculating postoperative refractive error.[1,2]

SURGICAL PLANNING TO CORRECT ASTIGMATISM

Astigmatism can be thought of as a vector since it has both magnitude and direction. Simple addition and subtraction cannot determine the net result of an incision, and a careful individual patient plan must be constructed that accounts for each surgical step affecting corneal curvature. Traditional surgical approaches for correcting astigmatism include strategically placed primary surgical incisions, secondary incisions or cuts and more recently developed toric IOLs that attempt to offset the astigmatism inherent in the cornea.

Surgical incisions referred to during cataract surgery as clear corneal incisions (CCI), contract during healing and tend to flatten the cornea in the same axis. To determine the surgically-induced astigmatism (SIA) of an incision on the cornea, we need to know three primary sets of data: keratometry both pre- and postoperative and the location of the corneal incision. Traditional office-based manifestation or autorefraction gives cylinder values and axes that indicate the magnitude and axis of cylinder with the tradition of positive cylinder indicating the steeper axis and vice versa for negative cylinder. However, it has become routine to use topographic mapping for preoperative planning in cases of atypical astigmatism. Placido disk-based topography is often used to routinely measure anterior keratometry and astigmatic patterns. Newer Scheimpflug tomographers can measure posterior corneal keratometrics and can be useful to evaluate surprising postoperative aberrations such as postoperative astigmatism even with apparently spherical anterior keratometry.

From these data, we can use vector math to calculate the surgically induced astigmatism of our incision. By placing the cataract incision on either the steep or flat axis, the magnitude of the astigmatism will change but the direction will remain constant (Fig. 35.2). On-axis incisions are most common when the astigmatic axis is on the

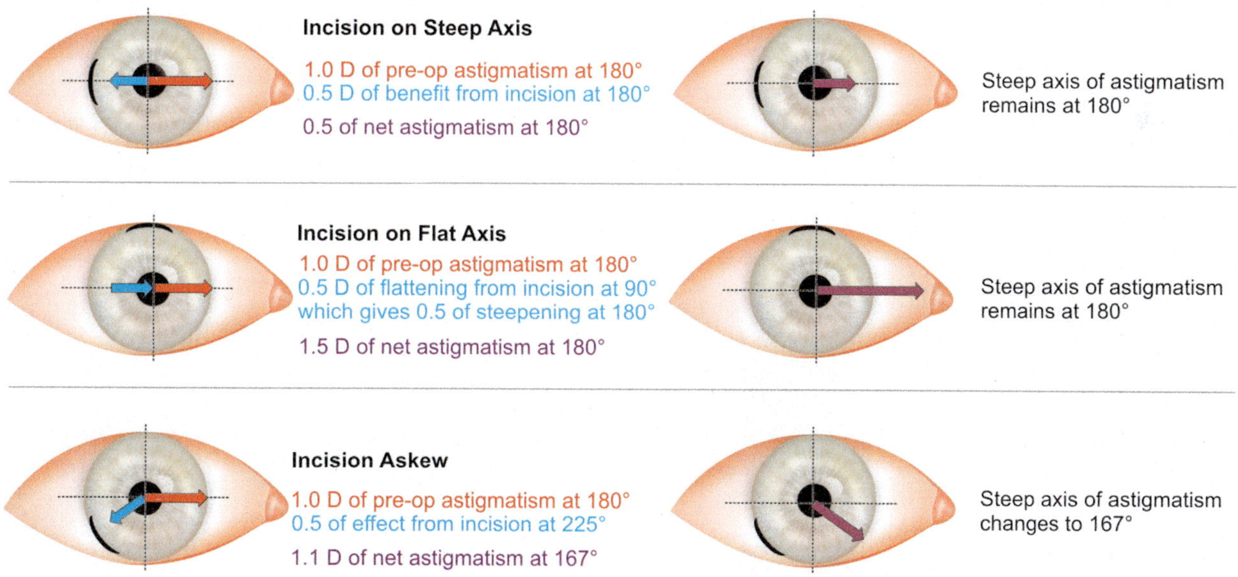

Fig. 35.2: Illustrations of surgical incision options. Placing the phaco incision on the steep axis (top frame) is the best solution since it will decrease the pre-existing astigmatism and keep any residual astigmatism at the same meridian. The second best option is to place the phaco incision on the flat axis (middle frame) since it will not change the direction of the astigmatism, however, it will increase its magnitude which can then be addressed by a toric IOL. The least desirable option (bottom frame) is to make the incision askew from steep and flat axis since this will alter both the amount of astigmatism as well its meridian, thereby making orientation of a toric IOL more challenging. Red arrows: vector of intrinsic corneal astigmatism. Blue arrows: vector of SIA. Purple arrows: additive vector of intrinsic and surgically induced astigmatism.

Source: Devgan A, Joseph A. SIA: a practical plan in cataract surgery. [Webpage]. 2016; *https://www.ophthalmologymanagement.com/issues/2016/september-2016/sia-a-practical-plan-in-cataract-surgery*. [Accessed October, 2017]

principal meridians. This technique has been reported useful for cases with less than 1.0–1.5 D of astigmatism, although in our experience most modern phacoemulsification incisions create around 0.12–0.50 D astigmatism depending on location and size. Moreover, there have been reports of increased net astigmatism following SIA with preoperative astigmatism less than 0.25 D. Superior incisions have been found to have greater SIA than temporal or superotemporal incisions while nasal incisions create more SIA than temporal ones.[1] Making the incision off-axis will induce a change in both the magnitude and direction of the final corneal astigmatism, an option infrequently utilized.

When obtaining preoperative measurements, the patient must be situated carefully in front of the keratometer, topographer or phoropter to ensure visual axes are aligned appropriately. While although the patient is upright during these measurements, intraoperative determinations are usually performed with the patient supine which can induce significant cyclotorsion. Most surgeons prefer marking the eye with a surgical marking pen while the patient is upright prior to the start of surgery. This eliminates positional changes and mass effect of retrobulbar anesthesia on intraoperative marking.

Various aspects of the incision other than location affect SIA including width of the CCI, radius from the central corneal apex and length (depth) of the incision (Figs. 35.3A to D). A more central incision will cause more flattening at that meridian. Peripheral incisions like limbal relaxing incisions (LRIs) cause less flattening but are more forgiving and less likely to induce undesired irregular astigmatism. With penetrating incisions, shorter corneal tunnels produce more flattening than longer ones.[3] For example, with the clear corneal incisions used for cataract surgery, the shorter the tunnel length, the more the

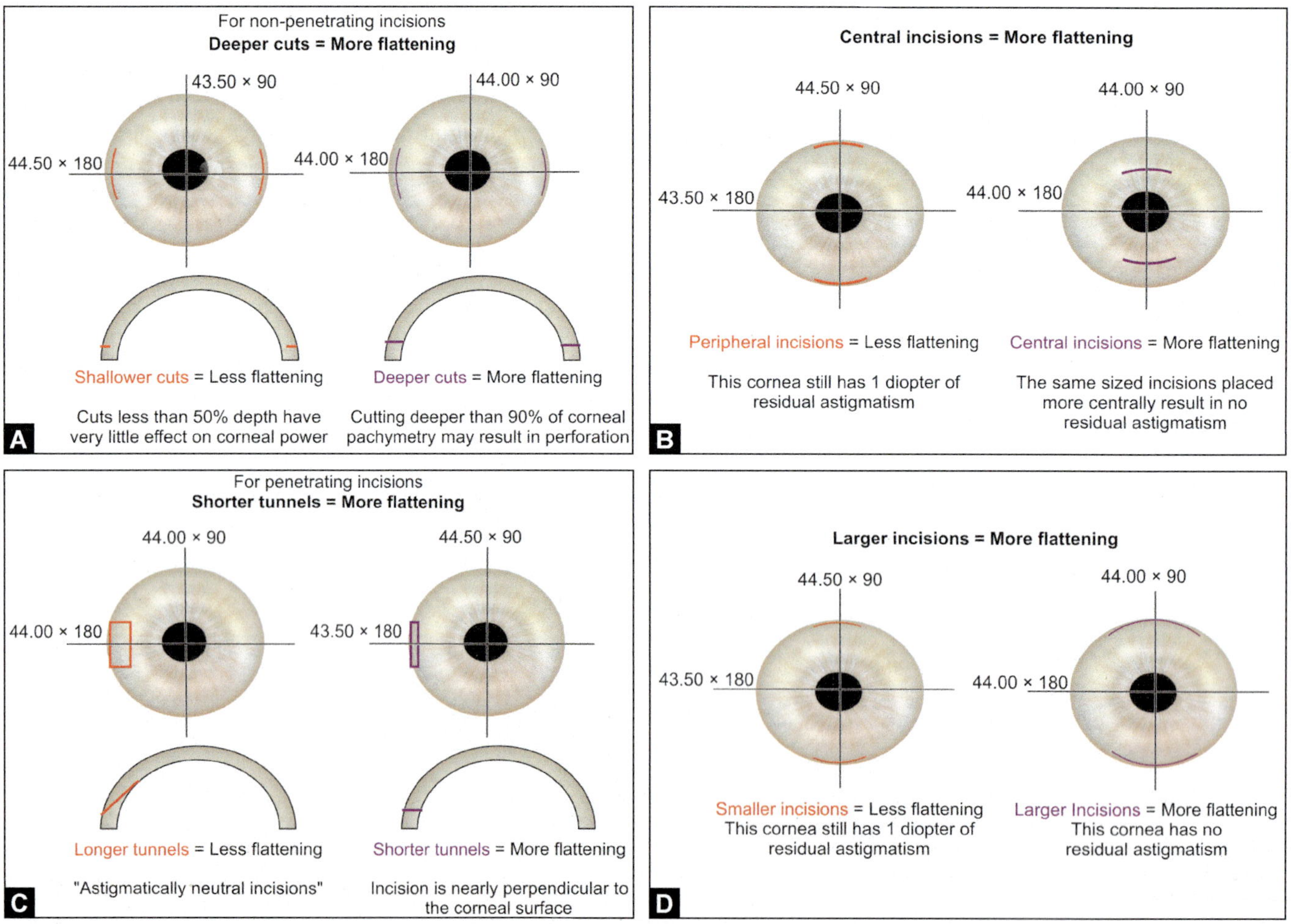

Figs. 35.3A to D: Illustrations demonstrating the effect of variations in incision architecture.

flattening effect at that meridian and the steeper the effect at axis 90° away. A symmetrical and long, square corneal incision will seal well and have little effect on astigmatism. The short tunnels can provide more SIA are more prone to leakage postoperatively. Another important contributing factor is patient age. The same incision on a younger person will have less of an astigmatic effect as compared to its effect on an older patient. Pachymetry can also affect the cornea's reaction to the incision made for the cataract. This is why residents are encouraged to make gray-line incisions barely nicking the limbal vessels instead of making CCIs. With nonpenetrating incisions such as LRIs, deeper incisions cause more flattening. Although surgeons are more protected from unintentional corneal perforation with shallow incisions, they have less ability to correct the astigmatism.

Many of these variables tend to remain relatively constant among individual surgeons. Modern surgery aims for consistently peripheral and increasingly narrow incisions, technology permitting, in order to allow for reliable postoperative refractive outcomes. Furthermore, one study showed no difference in SIA between the results of two surgeons performing similar incisions.[4] Taking into account the corneal diameter, evidence suggests that the smaller the horizontal corneal diameter, the greater the SIA (more significant effects when <12.0 mm).[5] Additionally, a phenomenon called the corneal coupling effect refers to a reduction in corneal curvature along the incision axis and an increase in curvature along the perpendicular axis. This must be considered when judging the degree of SIA desired (Fig. 35.4).

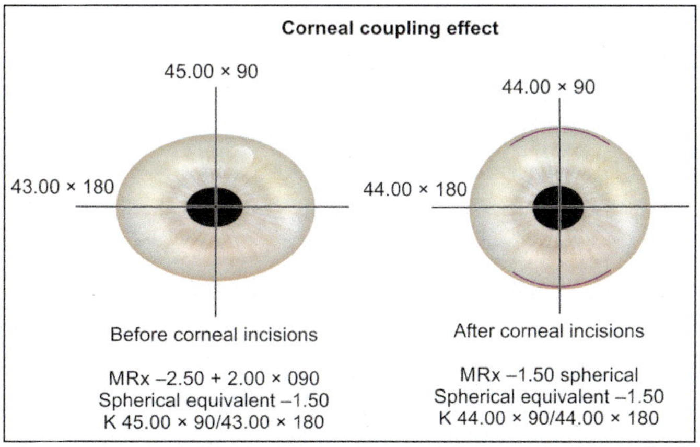

Fig. 35.4: Example of the corneal coupling effect encountered after corneal incisions. The axis 90° to the incision axis (purple lines) steepens in an equal magnitude to the flattening achieved along the incisional axis, leaving the same spherical equivalent. This remains true as long as the incisions lie along the same axis, i.e. are not skew.

Surgical Techniques

The surgeon may opt for additional techniques at the time of cataract surgery to optimize refractive outcome. As described above, for less than about 1.0 D of astigmatism, the CCI should be placed on the steep axis. Adding an additional on-axis opposite CCI can provide more correction in the same meridian and is advocated for 1.0–2.0 D of corneal astigmatism, although this has the disadvantage of creating another perforating corneal wound. For slightly more astigmatism (1.5–2.5 D), techniques such as astigmatic keratotomy (AK) or peripheral corneal relaxing incisions (PCRIs), another name for LRIs may be performed either at the time of surgery or at a later date. AK is an older technique involving paired paracentral arcuate nonpenetrating cornea incisions intended to correct astigmatism in the axis of incision. Due to their central location, they tend to create significant glare and unpredictable results. They have largely been supplanted by adjunctive laser technology or PCRIs. A PCRI is an evolution of AK that moves the incision farther towards the periphery with the benefit of safer, more predictable result. For a bow-tie configuration regular astigmatism, also the most common form, paired incisions are made approximately 450–600 µm in length at ideally 90% of corneal thickness along the steep meridian. Most LRIs are performed with preset depths of 500, 550 or 600 µm, while AK depth is usually a percentage of local corneal thickness. The incisions are as long in clock hours as the cornea is steep in astigmatism, i.e. 2.0 clock hours for 2.0 D of astigmatism. Additionally, the phacoemulsification incision can be placed through one of the PCRIs. Asymmetric bow-ties can be addressed with asymmetric PCRIs. The longer incision is located on the steeper side and the sum of the lengths of the incisions divided by two gives the astigmatic correction in Diopters. We have found the nomograms of Nichamin and Koch to be quite accurate for preoperative PCRI planning.[6,7] For even more astigmatism, toric IOLs are ideal. However, PCRIs can be beneficial if a spherical cornea is desired. This is because although a toric IOL with a toric cornea may create an astigmatism-free eye, this toric combination introduces considerable distortion.

OTHER CONSIDERATIONS

Other ocular surface conditions can present challenges while attempting to plan intraoperative astigmatism correction. Dry eye syndrome can cause corneal irregularities on topographic testing that appear as white spots or dropout. Treatment of dry eye syndrome as well as other ocular surface diseases should be accomplished well in advance of cataract surgery to avoid any postoperative refractive surprises. Once tear film stability and corneal topography consistency has been achieved, the surgeon can reasonably proceed with cataract surgery.

Epithelial basement membrane dystrophy (EBMD) is a rather common cause of irregular, asymmetric and unstable corneal astigmatism. In mild cases, it may minimally change the corneal topography and keratometric values; while in other cases, it can induce a large degree of corneal irregularity, thereby confounding the refractive accuracy and predictability of cataract surgery. In the latter case, the corneal epithelium can be scraped manually or with an excimer laser and then allowed to heal before cataract surgery is scheduled.

With pterygia, elastotic degeneration and fibrotic traction can affect the conjunctiva as well as the cornea and can induce large degrees of irregular astigmatism. While it may be tempting to perform the pterygium removal at the same time as the cataract surgery, this often results in an unpredictable postoperative refraction. The pterygium depending on its extent can make it very difficult to obtain accurate keratometry measurements for use in the lens calculations. The best course of action for refractive accuracy is to first remove the pterygium and smoother the cornea allowing weeks to months for healing and stability. Once the corneal topography is shown to be stable over the serial clinical examinations, accurate keratometry and lens calculations can be done and cataract surgery can be performed.

Corneal incisional techniques whether CCIs or LRIs can take days to weeks to stabilize after surgery. The hydration of CCIs to give sutureless closure at the end of surgery causes temporary stromal edema, which can alter corneal curvature and astigmatism. After the healing is complete, a careful clinical evaluation and refraction can be performed to determine the effectiveness of the astigmatic treatments. Patients should be educated about temporary postoperative refractive aberrations and inflammation that may resolve during the recovery.

The burgeoning environment of multifocal IOLs, premium IOLs and novel refractive surgeries requires the surgeons to maintain the tools to address most forms of corneal astigmatism at the time of cataract surgery. With a minimal investment of instruments and time, most can start with generalized nomograms, track their individual results and hone their personal technique. By simply reducing the patient's astigmatism at the time of cataract surgery, one can deliver good uncorrected visual acuities and high patient satisfaction.

TIPS AND TRICKS

- Double check that the incisions are on the correct axes. The most common mistake is making the incision 90° of, thereby doubling the patient's astigmatism.
- Preoperative corneal topography allows surgeons to understand the extent and location of the corneal astigmatism and to screen out patients who may have subclinical keratoconus.
- Be consistent with your incision architecture and placement with respect to the limbus. With time and more cases completed, the surgeon will develop incisional consistency.
- Use a temporal incision since it is the farthest from the visual axis and it has less astigmatic effect compared to other locations.
- Make the incision on the steep axis if possible or the flat axis if needed but never make the incision askew to these axes. While we prefer to keep the incision on the steep axis, even placing it on the flat axis will not change the direction of the astigmatism though it will increase its magnitude.
- Do not overcorrect the astigmatism as this will reverse the axis and result in unaccustomed astigmatism. Overcorrection of with-the-rule astigmatism will result in new against-the-rule astigmatism and it will be unsatisfactory to the patient. Slight undercorrection is far better than changing the cylinder axis.
- Apply a thin coat of a dispersive viscoelastic to the corneal surface prior to performing the LRI. Doing so will help the blade glide smoothly and prevent abrasions to the epithelium.
- Make all surgical markings, i.e. incision locations while the patient is awake and upright to avoid any effects of anesthesia and supination on mark location. This technique will ensure that any cyclotorsion of the eye does not cause a misplacement of the incisions.
- We feel that the most accurate instruments for PCRIs are diamond knives of which, many are available in preset or adjustable depths.

REFERENCES

1. Hashemi H, Khabazkhoob M, Soroush S, et al. The location of incision in cataract surgery and its impact on induced astigmatism. Curr Opin Opthalmol. 2016;27(1):58-64.
2. Amesbury EC, Miller KM. Correction of astigmatism at the time of cataract surgery. Curr Opin Opthalmol. 2009;20(1):19-24.
3. Kim TG, Noh SR, Jin KH. The effects of distance between the corneal apex and the inner and outer corneal wound edges on corneal astigmatism after cataract surgery. J Refractr Surg. 2017;33(7):460-8.
4. Theodoulidou S, Asproudis I, Athanasiadis A, et al. Comparison of surgically induced astigmatism among different surgeons performing the same incision. Int J Opthalmol. 2017;10(6):1004-7.
5. Theodoulidou S, Asproudis I, Kalogeropoulos C, et al. Corneal diameter as a factor influencing corneal astigmatism after cataract surgery. Cornea. 2016;35(1):132-6.
6. Nichamin LD. Nomogram for limbal relaxing incisions. J Cataract Refractr Surg. 2006;32(9):1408.
7. Wang L, Misra M, Koch DD. Peripheral corneal relaxing incisions combined with cataract surgery. J Cataract Refractr Surg. 2003;29(4):712-22.

Chapter 36 Management of the Small Pupil during Cataract Surgery

Sandip Suresh, Uday Devgan

INTRODUCTION

A persistently miotic pupil during cataract surgery is a common yet major surgical challenge that increases the risk of intraoperative and postoperative complications. The ability to visualize the lens capsule during capsulorhexis or having adequate space to manipulate instruments in the anterior chamber is critical to successful cataract surgery. The consequences of a small pupil are potentially substantial and include increased operative time, iris trauma, capsular tear, vitreous loss or dropped nucleus.

PREOPERATIVE MANAGEMENT

Patients should routinely receive several rounds of 2 mydriatic agents including an adrenergic stimulant such as 2.5% phenylephrine and an antimuscarinic such as 1% tropicamide. Care should also be taken to discontinue any miotics at least 1 day prior to surgery. Alpha-1 antagonists such as tamsulosin contribute to intraoperative floppy iris syndrome (IFIS) and should be discontinued for 1–2 weeks prior to surgery though even this may not be sufficient to reverse the iris atony caused by these medications.[1] Topical non-steroidal anti-inflammatory drugs (NSAIDs) can also be helpful in counteracting the miotic effect of prostaglandins released during manipulation of the iris and improve the postoperative pain and inflammation. Important comorbidities to evaluate prior to surgery include uveitis, posterior synechiae, iridodialysis, pseudoexfoliation, zonular dehiscence, iridoschisis and IFIS. Additional measures should be utilized for patients whose dilated pupil size remains less than 7.0 mm.[2,3]

INTRAOPERATIVE MANAGEMENT

Steps can be taken intraoperatively to improve dilation first with intracameral pharmacological mydriasis then with mechanical dilation such as viscomydriasis, separation of posterior synechiae, manual pupil separation and use of pupil expanders.

Intracameral Mydriatics

The benefits of intracameral mydriatics include rapid onset and minimal systemic side effects though carry risk of endothelial toxicity and anterior segment syndrome. A typical intracameral mydriatic injection consists of 0.1 mL 2.5% phenylephrine and epinephrine diluted to 1:4,000 with balanced salt solution (BSS). Bisulfite-free preparations such as epi-Shugarcaine can help to minimize the endothelial toxicity associated with intracameral medication and includes lidocaine for local anesthesia. Epinephrine can also be added to the BSS irrigation infusion help to maintain mydriasis throughout the surgery. In addition Omidria (Omeros Corp), a combination of 1% phenylephrine and 0.3% ketorolac added to the BSS infusion has recently been approved for intraoperative miosis and pain control during cataract surgery. Early studies have shown it is effective in reducing surgical time, operative costs and use of assistive devices though more studies may be needed to validate its clinical utility.[4,5]

Viscomydriasis

Viscomydriasis entails gentle expansion of the pupil by injecting viscoelastic sodium hyaluronate at the pupillary margin (Fig. 36.1). This not only produces mydriasis but also increases the anterior chamber depth. Viscomydriasis is effective in most patients though to varying degrees and the effect is often temporary as the viscoelastic is displaced through aspiration or through the incision site. Utilization of a viscoadaptive such as Healon 5 (Advanced Medical Optics) is well suited for this purpose, given its dynamic cohesive and dispersive properties. Under low vacuum and aspiration rates, a viscoadaptive acts as dispersive allowing easier positioning of the viscoelastic for mechanical dilation of the pupil. At higher sheer forces, a viscoadaptive becomes more cohesive allowing for easier removal from the anterior chamber at the end of a case. Thus, it is important to maintain low sheer forces intraoperatively for effective viscomydriasis and to

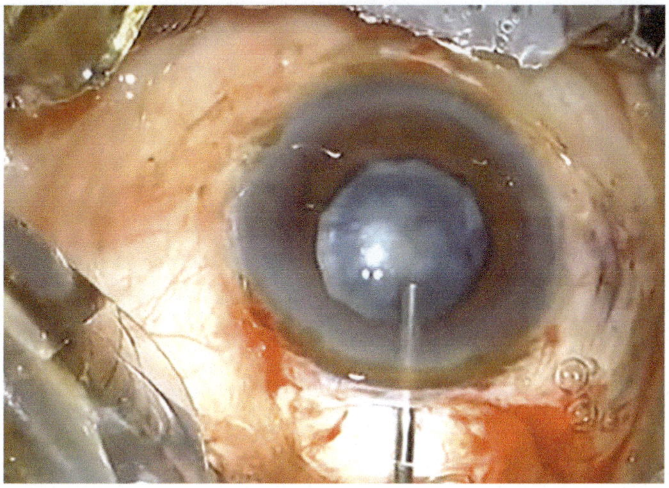

Fig. 36.1: Viscomydriasis. An ophthalmic viscoelastic device is placed at the pupillary margin and viscoelastic is injected to assist in dilation of the pupil.
Source: Dr Madhu Shekar, Aravind Eye Hospital, Madurai, Tamil Nadu, India

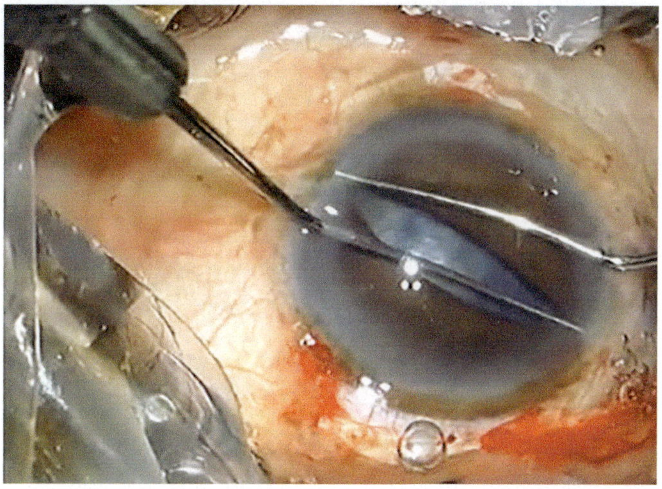

Fig. 36.2: Bimanual pupil stretching. Two hooks are used to grasp the pupillary margin at opposite ends and physically stretch the pupil in opposite directions.
Source: Dr Madhu Shekar, Aravind Eye Hospital, Madurai, Tamil Nadu, India

minimize loss of viscoelastic. Still despite proper technique, reapplication of viscoelastic throughout cataract surgery is usually necessary to maximize pupillary dilation.[6]

Posterior Synechiolysis and Peripupillary Membranectomy

Posterior synechiae can severely limit dilation and often require lysis intraoperatively if they do not respond to pharmacological mydriasis. Synechiolysis is best performed by placing a viscoelastic cannula underneath openings in the pupillary margin and sweeping laterally to free adhesions. If synechiae around the pupillary border have been adequately cleared without resultant improvement in dilation there may also be adhesions more distal from the margin.

In patients with previous uveitis, a thick fibrotic peripupillary membrane can form alongside synechiae and cause adhesions between the iris and lens. This membrane can often be peeled away using intraocular or capsulorhexis forceps.[7]

Pupil Stretching and Sphincterotomy

Bimanual pupil stretching using hooks or choppers to pull the pupillary border in opposite directions is a relatively quick means of mechanically enhancing dilation (Fig. 36.2). Stretching repeatedly in perpendicular directions helps ensure optimal dilation. This technique effectively creates microtears in the sphincter. It tends to preserve more sphincter tissue and is more cosmetically appealing than true sphincterotomies. However, final pupil size may be smaller than other surgical techniques for dilation and the microtears occur in a relatively uncontrolled fashion. Single-handed stretching tools such as the Beehler pupil dilator (Ambler Surgical Corp) are also available and carry an additional benefit of more uniformly stretching the pupil. Reinjection of viscoelastic after pupil stretching often produces improved viscomydriasis.[6]

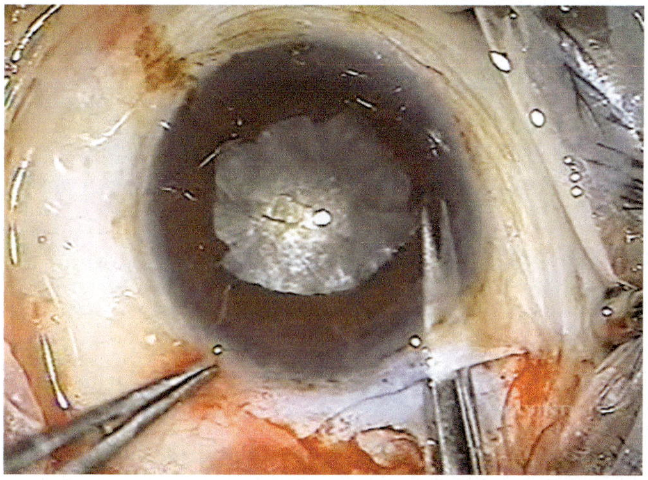

Fig. 36.3: Sphincterotomy. Intraocular scissors are used to make small cuts in the pupillary margin.
Source: Dr Madhu Shekar, Aravind Eye Hospital, Madurai, Tamil Nadu, India

If more definitive mechanical dilation is required, a sphincterotomy can be performed using intraocular scissors to create evenly placed cuts in the sphincter (Fig. 36.3). After the cuts are made, iris hooks should be used to further retract the iris. Benefits over pupil stretching include larger

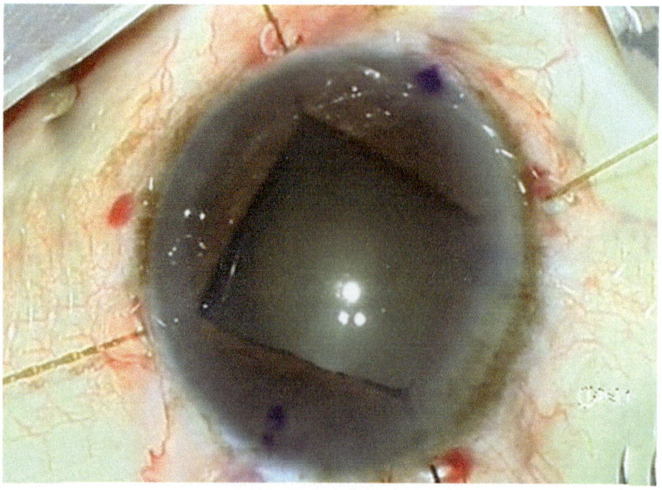

Fig. 36.4: Iris hooks—hooks are attached at the pupillary margin in four quadrants to maintain physical dilation and a square-shaped pupil throughout surgery.
Source: Dr Manas Nath, Aravind Eye Hospital, Puducherry, India.

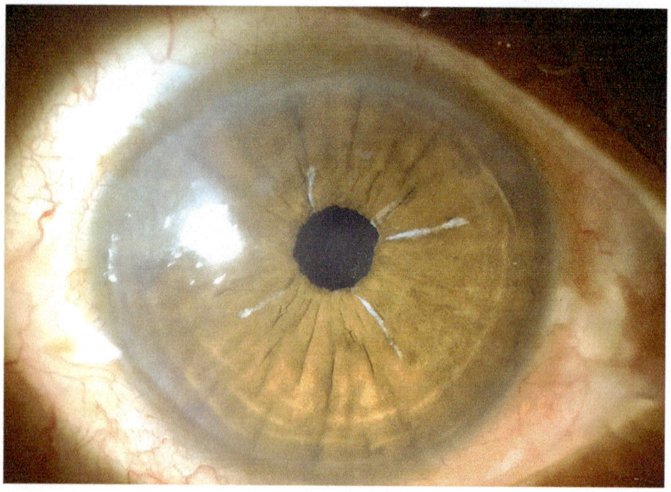

Fig. 36.5: Iris atrophy from intraoperative iris hooks. If used intraoperatively, iris hooks can leave a characteristic pattern of radial lines of iris atrophy extending from the pupil margin.
Source: Dr Manas Nath, Aravind Eye Hospital, Puducherry, India.

end pupil size and more controlled placement of cuts than the microtears created during pupil stretching. It should be noted that both of these techniques permanently weaken the iris sphincter and should be avoided in eyes with floppy iris syndrome or iridoschisis as iris tone will be even further decreased resulting risk of prolapse or aspiration of the iris.

Iris-retracting Hooks

Iris hooks (Fig. 36.4) are an effective tool though time consuming means of producing stable dilation throughout the surgery particularly in patients with IFIS and iridoschisis in which sphincter tearing techniques should be avoided. Multiple side port incisions are created through which the iris hooks are placed. Proper positioning of side ports as posteriorly as possible is critical to prevent the iris bowing forward and causing a narrow anterior chamber. A variable number of side ports can be utilized at the discretion of the surgeon though typically 4 hooks are used. A 5th hook can also be placed subincisionally to prevent iris prolapse into the main incision. Iris hooks can produce characteristic radial postoperative atrophy due to repetitive contact with the iris[6] (Fig. 36.5).

Pupil Expansion Rings

Numerous different pupil expanders exist to aid the surgeon in physically maintaining mydriasis, should if pharmacologic techniques not suffice. All are devices placed on the pupil margin and intended to maintain pupil retraction throughout surgery. Though not an exhaustive list, a handful of potential commercially available devices are discussed later, each with slightly different physical characteristics and pupil expanding properties. The newest of the expansion rings is the Malyugin ring 2.0 (MicroSurgical Technology), a 5-0 polypropylene iris expander consisting of 4 scrolls that engage the pupil margin when properly positioned. It is designed with an injector capable of fitting through a 2 mm clear corneal incision. The injector is used to engage the first scroll of the Malyugin ring with pupil margin opposite the insertion site. As the ring leaves the injector, the 2 scrolls perpendicular to the injection site should engage with the pupil as well. The final scroll must be manipulated into position using a hook. Once in place at the pupil margin, the ring drapes over the iris to create either a 6.25 or 7 mm diameter pupil. Adjustments may be needed to center the pupil and create uniform dilation.

The Visitec I-ring (Beaver Visitec) is a single use polyurethane expander designed to create uniform dilation of the pupil. It is first inserted into the anterior chamber through the main incision and then the 4 outward facing corners are positioned at the pupillary margin using Sinskey hooks. As it engages the pupil margin it expands to 6.3 mm, while also providing some protection from instrumentation.

The Assia pupil expander (APX Ophthalmology) uses a pair of spring loaded retractors inserted in 1.1 mm ports opposite each other to separate the pupil at 4 different points leaving a square or rectangularly- shaped pupil. Its main benefit is providing increased room around the pupil for instrumentation as the majority of the pupil border is left uncovered by the expander.

Femtosecond Laser-assisted Cataract Surgery

The femtosecond laser-assisted cataract surgery is a newer surgical technique that is used to assist in correcting corneal astigmatism, anterior capsulotomy and liquefaction of the lens. Miosis during femtosecond laser-assisted surgery is well-described and thought to be due to intraoperative release of prostaglandins particularly during capsulotomy. As such topical NSAID pretreatment has been shown to be highly effective in minimizing this risk of miosis. Aggressive management of miosis prior to laser pretreatment is also recommended as the degree of postlaser miosis can be severe. Expedited removal of the lens within 15 minutes of laser treatment may also help to avoid potential complications.[2,8]

Fluidics

Miotic pupils are more likely to be damaged during phacoemulsification as irrigation/aspiration takes place closer to the iris. Iris damage can be minimised by reducing flow parameters. Decreasing vacuum and aspiration flow rate increases anterior chamber diameter which can help with dilation and provide more separation between the aspiration tip and the iris.[7]

Alternative Surgical Techniques

Should the aforementioned techniques fail to effectively dilate the pupil or if the necessary tools for mechanical dilation are not readily available, modifications in surgical techniques can help in managing cataract surgery through small pupils.

Creating the Capsulorhexis

The minimum pupil size needed for safe surgery is 4 mm however, limiting the capsulorhexis to this size leads to difficulty with phacoemulsification and may eventually predispose the eye to capsular phimosis, intraocular lens decentration and compromised zonular support. Though more technically challenging, creating a capsulorhexis of 5–5.5 mm that extends beyond the visible pupil margin can help avoid some of these complications.When completing the capsulorhexis in such cases, it is important to guide the leading edge under the iris in a controlled fashion. Injection of viscoelastic can help flatten the anterior lens capsule giving more control. A hook can also be used to lift a sector of the iris to verify the position of the capsulorhexis. Use of a centripetal force while the edge is just beyond pupillary margin can help maintain control even without optimal visualization.

Phacoemulsification and Intraocular Lens Placement

A small pupil can be exploited to grant more room to instrument during hydrodissection and phacoemulsification of the nucleus. Prolapsing the nucleus out of the capsular bag and resting it on the iris, one can use a chopper to cleave the nucleus while simultaneously aspirating. However, care must be taken to avoid endothelial injury as the phaco probe must be placed in closer proximity to the cornea. As such it is important to minimize phaco power and diligently apply dispersive viscoelastic. Circumferentially visualizing the cortex in a marginally dilated pupil is challenging and even more so when attempting to irrigate and aspirate lens contents. Management of fluidics can help such as using bimanual irrigation/aspiration to separate the infusion and aspiration for better control and improved positioning for full circumferential access. Utilizing smaller gauge instruments makes operating at the equator more accessible as well. At the completion of lens removal, a hook should be employed to lift the iris circumferentially to visualize the entirety of the bag. Injecting viscoelastic into the bag will dilate the pupil and the bag to help with cortex visualization, removal of any remaining fragments and insertion of the intraocular lens. Once the lens is adequately positioned bimanual irrigation/aspiration should be used to remove any remaining viscoelastic.

SURGICAL PEARLS FOR CHALLENGING CASES

Hypermature Cataract

A large dense cataract presents numerous surgical challenges, two of which are a difficult capsulotomy with increased risk of posterior capsular rupture compounded by a poorly dilating pupil with inadequate visualization of the capsulorhexis. Though similar measures can be taken to ensure sufficient dilation, the use of a capsular dye such as trypan blue or indocyanine green can be utilized to improve visualization of the capsule against a white or brunescent cataract.

Intraoperative Floppy Iris Syndrome

Patients taking alpha-1 antagonists such as tamsulosin are prone to develop intraoperative miosis with iris atony increasing the risk of iris billowing and prolapse. Though these medications should be discontinued preoperatively, many patients on chronic alpha-1 antagonists develop iris atrophy that does not improve with acute cessation of the offending agent. In such cases, one should avoid iris manipulation with stretching or sphincterotomy as these will further decrease iris tone. Instead pupil expanding rings can be an effective means of maintaining control over the atonic iris. Aggressive use of viscomydriasis will also help to maintain mydriasis as well as displacing the iris and preventing billowing/prolapse.[1,3]

Pseudoexfoliation

Though associated with multiple complications during surgery, poor dilation of the pupil is often the most limiting feature of cataract surgery in a pseudoexfoliation patient. Dilation is often limited by excessive deposition of extracellular matrix inside the iris stroma resulting in a fibrotic, inelastic sphincter. These patients often do well with pupil stretching techniques to break the fibrotic infiltrative material.[9,10]

Uveitis

Though surgery should be avoided until intraocular inflammation is quiet, eyes with previous episodes of anterior uveitis develop sequelae such as posterior synechiae and peripupillary fibrotic membranes that prevent adequate pharmacologic dilation. Careful slit-lamp examination to identify the extent of synechiae and fibrosis will help guide surgical planning. Preoperative steroids and NSAIDs should be considered depending on the level of ongoing inflammation and to prevent a heightened postoperative inflammatory response. Intraoperatively, it is important to attempt viscomydriasis and then lysis of any synechiae with viscoelastic or blunt dissection. Removal of fibrotic membranes may necessitate membrane peeling using intraocular forceps. Pupil stretching or sphincterotomy should then be considered if synechiolysis fails to permit adequate dilation.[6,7]

Iridodialysis

Post-traumatic iris disinsertion can cause an irregular, decentered pupil that fails to dilate and precludes physical manipulation of the iris. Prior to cataract surgery the iris should be reattached to the sclera using nonabsorbable horizontal mattress sutures. Once adequately secured, the iris can be safely manipulated until sufficiently dilated.[6] Though small pupil cataract surgery can pose considerable challenges to safe and effective cataract surgery, the ongoing advancement of small pupil surgical techniques have helped mitigate many of these risks. The surgeon must be familiar with the myriad tools available including pharmacological, mechanical and surgical techniques in order to minimize complications of a small pupil during surgery.

REFERENCES

1. Flach AJ. Intraoperative floppy iris syndrome: pathophysiology, prevention, and treatment. Trans Am Ophthalmol Soc. 2009;107:234-9.
2. Schultz T, Joachim SC, Stellbogen M, et al. Prostaglandin release during femtosecond laser-assisted cataract surgery: main inducer. J Refract Surg. 2015;31(2):78-81.
3. Hashemi H, Seyedian MA, Mohammadpour M. Small pupil and cataract surgery. Curr Opin Ophthalmol. 2015;26(1): 3-9.
4. Lawuyi LE, Gurbaxani A. The clinical utility of new combination phenylephrine/ketorolac injection in cataract surgery. Clin Ophthalmol.2015;9:1249-54.
5. Bucci FP Jr, Michalek B, Fluet AT. Comparison of the frequency of use of a pupil expansion device with and without an intracameral phenylephrine and ketorolac injection 1%/0.3% at the time of routine cataract surgery. Clin Ophthalmol. 2017;11:1039-43.
6. Osher RH, Osher JM. Management of the Small Pupil. In: Colvard M (Ed). Achieving Excellence in Cataract Surgery A Step-by-Step Approach. 2009. pp. 59-66.
7. Ratra V, Lam DSC. Small Pupil—Big Problem: A Management Alogrithm. Asia-Pacific J Ophthalmol. 2015;4(3):131-3.
8. Nagy ZZ, Takacs AI, Filkorn T, et al. Complications of femtosecond laser-assisted cataract surgery. J Cataract Refract Surg. 2014;40(1):20-8.
9. Sangal N, Chen TC. Cataract Surgery in Pseudoexfoliation Syndrome. Semin Ophthalmol. 2014;29(5-6):403-8.
10. Fontana L, Coassin M, Iovieno A, et al. Cataract surgery in patients with pseudoex-foliation syndrome: current updates. Clin Ophthalmol. 2017;11:1377-83.

Chapter 37

IOL Calculations: The Past, the Present and the Future

Aazim A Siddiqui, Uday Devgan, Albert S Jun

INTRODUCTION

Estimated to be responsible for approximately 51%[1] of worldwide sight loss and for bilateral vision loss in more than 20 million individuals, cataract is the leading cause of blindness. This makes cataract surgery the most commonly performed eye surgery. As the average life expectancy continues to increase, the incidence and prevalence of cataract will only rise. In fact, the World Health Organization[2] predicts that by the year 2020, there will be 32 million cataract surgeries performed yearly. These statistics serve to highlight the importance of cataract surgery and place emphasis on a crucial step in the preoperative process: Intraocular lens (IOL) calculations.

Cataract surgery involves the replacement of the opacified natural lens of the eye with a plastic IOL rendering a two-lens system, the cornea and the IOL which forms the basis for IOL power calculations.[3] Calculating the most accurate IOL power is a critical factor in optimizing patient outcomes.[4] Several mathematical formulae have been described over the years to guide the surgeons to pick the most appropriate IOL for a given patient. The ultimate goal of these formulae is to calculate the IOL power value which will correspond to a targeted refraction chosen for a given patient's vision-specific postoperative needs and desires. In most cases, the postoperative target refraction is often chosen to achieve emmetropia or slight myopia.[5-7] These modern formulae are sophisticated and vary in their approach to determining the power of the IOL.

In a general sense, all IOL formulae are composed of a similar structure which includes calculation for vergence and prediction of the postoperative anterior chamber depth (ACD) or estimated lens position (ELP), i.e. the distance between the optical center of the implanted IOL and the anterior surface of the cornea.[3,8] These formulae are essentially centered around 2 primary optical and anatomical parameters of the eye: axial length and corneal power. These two variables play an important role in most formulae for the vergence calculation and the prediction of ELP.[8] Some modern formulae also require additional variables for more accurate results such as preoperative ACD,[9] lens thickness,[10] white-to-white distance[10] and some variation of the A-constant value.

The constant desire to have higher success rates in reaching desired postoperative targets has driven the need for development of new formulae to calculate more accurate results.

THE PAST

The history of IOL calculations is rich and dates as far back as more than a half a century ago when Sir Harold Ridley pioneered the 1st IOL and lens implant surgery for patients with cataract.[11] He implanted his 1st IOLs in 1949 which were made of acrylic plastic called Perspex inspired by the plastic cockpit canopies of British aircrafts from World War II.[12] Prior to his invention, cataract surgery involved lens removal followed by refractive correction with aphakic spectacles. Although this unprecedented attempt yielded a myopia of –21 D and –15 D due to the high index of refraction of the lens material used, Ridley's innovative leap spawned the field of IOL implantation and calculations.[12,13]

In the years following, IOL calculations simply relied on the 'clinical history' method which took into account a patient's preoperative refraction in the following equation:[14]

$$P = 18 + (1.25 \times Ref)$$

Where P is the power of the iris-supported IOL targeting emmetropia and Ref is the patient's preoperative refraction in diopters (D) prior to the development of cataract. This method yielded in refractive surprises greater than 1 D in 50% of the eyes, with some as high as 9 D.[14]

The next major advancement in IOL calculations did not happen until 1967 when Fedorov et al.[15] (also known as Fyodorov) sparked a new generation of IOL formulae when they postulated the use of a vergence formula. In the 1970s, due to improved biometric devices and A-scans, several similar theoretical vergence formulae targeting emmetropia were developed by a number of individuals. Thijssen,[16] Colenbrander,[17] Fyodorov,[18] van der Heijde,[19] and Binkhorst[20] each developed their own IOL formula. These theoretical formulae were based purely on the mathematical and geometric principles involving the optics of the eye.[14] These formulae not only produced similar results but were also mathematically alike, resembling the following equation:

$$P = n \div (L - C) - n \div [(n \div K) - C]$$

Where P is the power in diopters of the implanted IOL targeting emmetropia, n is the index of refraction of the aqueous and vitreous (1.336), L is the axial length in meters, C is the ELP, and K is the corneal power in diopters.[14] Due to the substantial inaccuracies of these formulae, further refinements were made to these formulae by individuals such as Hoffer, Shammas, and Binkhorst in the 1980s to improve their accuracy. This work furthered the ability to predict an accurate ELP as it was found to be related to the axial length value rather than being a static value.[3]

As the 1970s were marked by the advent of vergence formulae, the 1980s were with the regression-based formulae and gave birth to what is now known as the "first generation" of IOL formulae (Table 37.1). The trio of Sanders-Retzlaff-Kraff (SRK) decided to work backwards by way of retrospective regression analysis to empirically generate a formula based on a dataset of actual postoperative outcomes. They came up with the SRK I formula which was a simple linear regression equation:[21]

$$P = A - 0.9K - 2.5L$$

Where P is the IOL power in diopters targeting emmetropia, A is the A-constant value that is a fixed numeric value for each IOL type, K is the corneal power measurement using a refractive index of 1.3375 and L is the axial length in millimeters.

Since the SRK I was based on a regression of a confined sample dataset of eyes, it performed reasonably well for eyes that were of average parameters (i.e. eyes reflective of the sample dataset) but not so for eyes that were extremely short or long. Thus, the SRK II formula[22] was developed in 1988 as a revision to the SRK I to address its limitations for short and long eyes—eventually giving rise to the "second generation" of IOL formulae (Table 37.1):

$$P - A1 - 0.9K - 2.5L$$

The variables here are the same as the SRK I formula except for the A-constant $A1$, which was made to vary with axial length. This methodology created a way for the A-constant value to become a malleable variable to allow for personalization and optimization of these and other formulae to account for differences in surgical technique and biometric instruments.[8]

THE PRESENT

Cataract surgery with IOL implantation is the most commonly performed eye surgery. And indeed IOL calculations have come a long way since the first and second generations of IOL formulae as these methodologies have steadily continued to evolve. The 1990s gave birth to the 'third generation' of IOL formulae (Table 37.1): Holladay I,[23] SRK/T,[24] and Hoffer Q.[25] These formulae remain as the most commonly used ones given their more accurate results and simplicity over predecessors. These formulae reverted to a more theoretical-based approach where the ELP was no longer only associated to the axial length alone but also to the corneal power which resulted in significantly improved accuracy. Each formula also used its own version of the A-constant as part of its calculations with differing order of magnitude. However at their core, these constants are still intimately related to the manufacturer's A-constant.[3]

Later in the decade, a "fourth-generation" of advanced theoretical formulae came about (Table 37.1): Holladay II, Barrett, Olsen and Haigis.[26,27] These formulae focused on further perfecting the ELP prediction by utilizing additional variables in the calculation process. For example, the Holladay II formula relates the ELP estimation with axial

Table 37.1: The five generations of IOL formulae.

Generation	Formula	ELP Prediction Method	Era
First	SRK, Binkhorst	Constant value	1970s
Second	SRK II	Axial length only	1980s
Third	SRK/T, Holladay I, Hoffer Q	Axial length and corneal power	1990s
Fourth	Holladay II, Haigis, Olsen, Barrett	Multi-variate approach	1990s, 2000s
Fifth	Ladas Super Formula, Hill-RBF	Formula-specific for Ladas Super Formula	2010s

length, corneal power, white-to-white measurement, measured ACD, lens thickness and patient age.

Use of a constant modification and personalization was seen with the SRK II formula but this methodology has now become a common practice by ophthalmologists to fine-tune their modern IOL formulae. The surgeon factor for Holladay,[23] A-constant for SRK/T, [24] personalized ACD for Hoffer Q,[25] and ACD for the Holladay II are all in essence the same constant related to the manufacturer's A-constant for each IOL type. The A-constant can be manipulated to optimize the formula performance. A library of optimized A-constants for many of the lenses is provided by the User Group for Laser Interference Biometry (ULIB)—a global group of experts who provide optimized A-constants for a particular IOL based on clinical data.

Several modifications have also been implemented in the process of refining IOL calculations. The Wang-Koch adjustment[28] for example, is essentially a "fudge factor" to the axial length variable of the Holladay formula in order to get more precise ELP predictions in very myopic eyes. As many ophthalmologists have continued to use these formulae, several "rules of thumb" have been noted where it has become a recommended practice to use the Hoffer Q for short eyes, the Holladay I for average eyes, and the SRK/T for longer eyes.

Despite these rules and modifications and the advent of new complex and multivariate IOL formulae, the process of IOL calculations remains an imperfect science. Although the results have significantly improved since the days of the clinical history method, on average 25 out of 100 IOL implantations may deviate from the intended target by 0.5 D or more.[7] The gap in accuracy is in large part due to the complex anatomy of the eye. Eyes can have a variation in the depth of anterior chamber from being shallow to deep in conjunction with an axial length that can also vary from being short to long. These different combinations can therefore, cause large prediction errors in lens calculations.

THE FUTURE

Intraocular lens calculations have indeed come a long way since the days of clinical history method and the original SRK I formula. And as accurate as the modern IOL formulae are, they are in general successful approximately 70–80% of the time in reaching within 0.5 D of the desired outcome. There is not a single perfect IOL formula or solution which can be used for both the "average" eyes and for those that belong to the extremities of keratometry and axial length. Since there is no one formula or framework that is perfect, surgeons have always resorted to using multiple formulae and dedicating a significant portion of their workflow to deciding on their preferred IOL calculation solution and lens implant choice. The constant need and desire for a simple yet supremely accurate form of IOL calculation blueprint has fueled the drive for the next generation of IOL formulae.

Hoffer H-5 formula is one example of the "fifth-generation" of IOL formulae (*see* Table 37.1). It is based on the third generation Hoffer Q and the fourth generation Holladay II formulae. It harnesses these formulae by making them more customizable and personalized for a particular patient with the addition of the gender and race variables. For example, with this methodology, the formula takes into account the slightly longer eye with a flatter cornea and deeper ACD of a male compared to female. This then further customizes the formula for a specific patient and yields better results.

In 2015, Ladas and colleagues[29] described a novel method of representing the modern IOL formulae in three dimensions which then allowed for a seamless amalgamation of these formulae into a single Super Formula. The Ladas Super Formula takes the best portions of each of the modern IOL formulae, combines it into a single formula and acts as a one-stop solution for not only eyes of average length but also for those that fall on the extremities of axial lengths and keratometry. The formula further seeks to incorporate artificial intelligence and advanced mathematical techniques to minimize errors in IOL calculations.

A similar approach was taken by the Hill-RBF formula where the formula is purely a machine-learned algorithm based on a dataset of 600 eyes. Similar to the linear regression of the original SRK I formula, the Hill-RBF formula is based on a certain dataset, lens type and limited to a single biometer.

The future of IOL calculations is bright and exciting. The constant need and desire to want improved outcomes for patients and pursue the ideal goal of spectacle independence is powering the continued progress in the field. These formulae and their calculation frameworks can also then be applied to other relevant areas such as the postrefractive, toric, and pediatric corners of IOL calculations. An improvement in mathematical techniques, incorporation of artificial intelligence, continued precision of biometric instruments, addition of more variables and inclusion of larger and more diverse datasets are just some of the things to look forward to in the future generations of IOL formulae.

CONFLICT OF INTEREST

The authors are principals in Advanced Euclidean Solutions which owns the Ladas Super Formula and Ladas Super Surface and their trademarks, trade secrets, and copyrights.

REFERENCES

1. Pascolini D, Mariotti SP. Global estimates of visual impairment: 2010. Br J Opthalmol. 2011;96(5):614-8.
2. World Health Organization. Blindness: Vision 2020—control of major blinding diseases and disorders. Geneva: World Health Organization; 2016.
3. Colvard M. Achieving Excellence in Cataract Surgery: A Step-by-Step Approach. 2009.
4. Lee AC, Qazi MA, Pepose JS. Biometry and intraocular lens power calculation. Curr Opin Ophthalmol. 2008;19(1):13-7.
5. Beiko GH. Comparison of visual results with accommodating intraocular lenses versus mini-monovision with a monofocal intraocular lens. J Cataract Refractr Surg. 2013;39(1):48-55.
6. Narváez J, Zimmerman G, Stulting RD, et al. Accuracy of intraocular lens power prediction using the Hoffer Q, Holladay I, Holladay II, and SRK/T formulae. J Cataract Refractr Surg. 2006;32(12):2050-3.
7. Aristodemou P, Cartwright NE, Sparrow JM, et al. Formula choice: Hoffer Q, Holladay I, or SRK/T and refractive outcomes in 8108 eyes after cataract surgery with biometry by partial coherence interferometry. J Cataract Refractr Surg. 2011;37(1):63-71.
8. Olsen T. Calculation of intraocular lens power: a review. Act Opthalmol Scand. 2007;85(5):472-85.
9. Olsen T. Prediction of the effective postoperative (intraocular lens) anterior chamber depth. J Cataract Refractr Surg. 2006;32(3):419-24.
10. Fenzl R. Refractive and visual outcome of hyperopic cataract cases operated on before and after implementation of the Holladay II formula. Ophthalmology. 1998;105(9):1759-64.
11. François J, Goes F, Strobel J. Determination of intraocular lenses by ultrasound. In: Ultrasonography in Ophthalmology Proceedings of SIDUO V, 5th Congress of the International Society for Ultrasonic Diagnosis in Ophthalmology, Ghent. Basel: Karger Publishers; 1975. pp. 233-8.
12. Ridley H. Intra-ocular acrylic lenses. Transac Ophthalmol Soc UK. 1951;71:617.
13. Apple DJ, Sims J. Harold Ridley and the invention of the intraocular lens. Surv Ophthalmol. 1996;40(4):279-92.
14. Shammas HJ. Historic overview. In: Shammas HJ (Ed). Intraocular Lens Power Calculations. Thorofare. NJ, USA: Slack Inc; 2003. pp. 7-12.
15. Fedorov SN, Kolinko AI, Kolinko AI. Estimation of optical power of the intraocular lens. Vestn Oftalmal. 1967;80(4):27-31.
16. Thijssen J. The Emmetropic and the iseikonic implant lens: computer calculation of the refractive power and its accuracy. Ophthalmol. 1975;171(6):467-86.
17. Colenbrander MC. Calculation of the power of an iris clip lens for distant vision. Br J Ophthalmol. 1973;57(10):735-40.
18. Fyodorov SN, Galin MA, Linksz A. Calculation of the optical power of intraocular lenses. Invest Ophthalmol. 1975;14(8):625-8.
19. Heijde GL. A nomogram for calculating the power of the prepupillary lens in the aphakic eye. Bibliotheca Ophthalmologica. 1975;(83):273-5.
20. Binkhorst RD. The optical design of intraocular lens implants. Ophthalmic Surg. 1975;6(3):17-31.
21. Retzlaff J. A new intraocular lens calculation formula. J Am Intraocul Implant Soc. 1980;6(2):148-52.
22. Sanders DR, Retzlaff J, Kraff MC. Comparison of the SRK II™ formula and other second generation formulas. J Cataract Refractr Surg. 1988;14(2):136-41.
23. Holladay JT, Musgrove KH, Prager TC, et al. A three-part system for refining intraocular lens power calculations. J Cataract Refractr Surg. 1988;14(1):17-24.
24. Retzlaff JA, Sanders DR, Kraff MC. Development of the SRK/T intraocular lens implant power calculation formula. J Cataract Refractr Surg. 1990;16(3):333-40.
25. Hoffer KJ. The Hoffer Q formula: a comparison of theoretic and regression formulas. J Cataract Refractr Surg. 1993;19(6):700-12.
26. Barrett GD. An improved universal theoretical formula for intraocular lens power prediction. J Cataract Refractr Surg. 1993;19(6):713-20.
27. Haigis W, Lege B, Miller N, et al. Comparison of immersion ultrasound biometry and partial coherence interferometry for intraocular lens calculation according to Haigis. Graefes Arch Clin Exp Opthalmol. 2000;238(9):765-73.
28. Wang L, Shirayama M, Ma XJ, et al. Optimizing intraocular lens power calculations in eyes with axial lengths above 25.0 mm. J Cataract Refractr Surg. 2011;37(11):2018-27.
29. Ladas JG, Siddiqui AA, Devgan U, et al. A 3-D "Super Surface" combining modern intraocular lens formulas to generate a "Super Formula" and maximize accuracy. JAMA Ophthalmol. 2015;133(12):1431.

Chapter 38

Optical Coherence Tomography Abnormalities of the Retina that may Affect the Outcome of Cataract Surgery

David Xu, Juliet Essilfie, David Sarraf

Patients being evaluated for cataract surgery should undergo comprehensive evaluation including dilated funduscopic examination. Macular and peripheral retinal diseases and visually significant cataract are prevalent in the same age group. The posterior segment examination can be limited by concurrent media opacity. With advanced cataract, fine macular details may not be identified and peripheral retinal pathology may be missed. More uncommonly, view of the posterior segment may be lost entirely. In these cases, B-scan ultrasonography is a valuable tool to evaluate for vitreous and retinal pathology that may influence surgical planning and guide preoperative counseling.

Careful preoperative examination of the posterior segment is important for a number of reasons: macular disease may limit postoperative visual outcome after cataract surgery, cataract surgery may adversely affect existing retinal disease, and retinal pathology may influence the preoperative planning, operative management or post-operative course.

Optical coherence tomography (OCT) is a noninvasive imaging technique that has revolutionized retinal care. The technique uses light waves to create a *tomographic* (cross-sectional) view of ocular structures similar to ultrasound. With OCT backscattered light waves rather than sound waves create the image contrast (Fig. 38.1).[1] OCT provides micron-scale, depth-resolved, volumetric imaging of the individual retinal layers in the macula. The technique utilizes interferometry to extract single-backscatter, coherent light and tends to reject noncoherent, scattered light giving it excellent axial image resolution even in the presence of dense cataract or posterior capsular opacification.

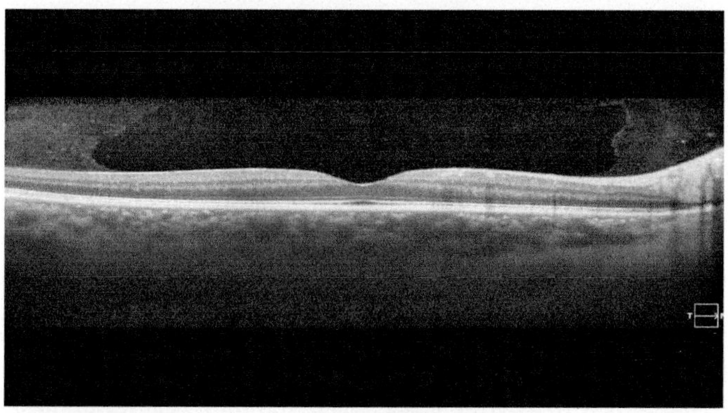

Fig. 38.1: Spectral domain optical coherence tomography cross-section of a normal eye. The retinal layers, photoreceptors, retinal pigment epithelium, and choroid can be clearly visualized.

There are two generations of ophthalmic OCT devices currently available on the market.[2] Time domain OCT utilizes a beam splitter to separate a coherent light source into two independent paths, one of which passes to the sample and another which reflects back from a mechanically translated reference arm mirror. The interference patterns from the two light sources generate the image contrast. Spectral domain OCT (SD-OCT) has replaced the earlier time domain systems and utilizes a broad spectrum light source, a stationary reference arm mirror and a spectrometer to simultaneously capture a full line scan in a single exposure. SD-OCT is comparatively much faster in acquisition speed and provides greater resolution. Swept source OCT (SS-OCT) is a newer device which improves upon existing OCT scanners by utilizing a tunable laser which "sweeps" through a range of frequencies. SS-OCT yields higher acquisition speed and deeper penetration, leading to scans with finer scan spacing and wider field of view. OCT boasts exquisite sensitivity in detecting retinal edema, fluid in various retinal layers, and many other macular abnormalities.

RETINAL DISEASES AFFECTING VISUAL OUTCOME

Precataract surgery OCT screening is routinely performed in some clinics. Patient expectations with cataract surgery outcomes are increasing. Those electing for advanced-technology lenses may incur significant out-of-pocket expense in the United States, so it is important to manage expectations in light of concurrent retinal disease. Retinal disease is a relative contraindication to multifocal intraocular lenses (IOLs) given that they cause a reduction in contrast sensitivity. When OCT is routinely performed preoperatively, one study identified pathology in 13% of patients in a consecutive series while occult funduscopic pathology was identified with OCT in 6% of cases in another study.[3,4] This section reviews common retinal abnormalities that affect the ultimate visual outcome.

Age-related Macular Degeneration

Age-related macular degeneration (AMD) is the leading cause of legal blindness in the developed world and the primary cause of vision loss in persons over the age of 50.[5] AMD has a prevalence of approximately 1 in 3 in persons over the age of 75 and approximately 10% of patients display signs of advanced disease.[6,7] There are two forms of this disorder: the dry or non-neovascular (Fig. 38.2A) and the wet or neovascular form (Fig. 38.2B).[8] Wet AMD accounts for about 15% of all cases but is responsible for 90% of the severe vision loss associated with AMD. Patients with dry AMD generally maintain moderate to good visual function except in the presence of geographic atrophy (GA), which can be associated with severe vision loss. The hallmark features of AMD include macular drusen (subretinal or sub-retinal pigment epithelial [RPE] deposits comprised of lipid-rich extracellular debris), RPE pigmentary changes, and geographic atrophy in the non-neovascular type, and intraretinal fluid, subretinal fluid, pigment epithelial detachment and choroidal (or retinal) neovascularization in the neovascular type. Reticular pseudodrusen (RPD) is a subretinal, interlacing network of discrete deposits that are best visualized on OCT and infra-red reflectance imaging. The presence of RPD is associated with greater risk for development of neovascular AMD and GA. Patients with signs of AMD should be referred to a retinal specialist for further management. The impact of cataract surgery on the progression of AMD is discussed in a later section.

Vitreomacular Traction Syndrome

Vitreomacular traction syndrome (VMT) is a vitreomacular interface disorder caused by vitreous syneresis and persistent vitreofoveal attachment.[9,10] The spectrum of vitreomacular interface disorders ranges from asymptomatic vitreomacular adhesion (VMA), VMT, to full-thickness macular hole (Fig. 38.3). Patients with VMT may be asymptomatic or may have significant metamorphopsia and central vision decline. VMT is often funduscopically occult but can be clearly identified using OCT. The classic OCT presentation is perifoveal posterior vitreous separation with foveal traction with or without intraretinal fluid.

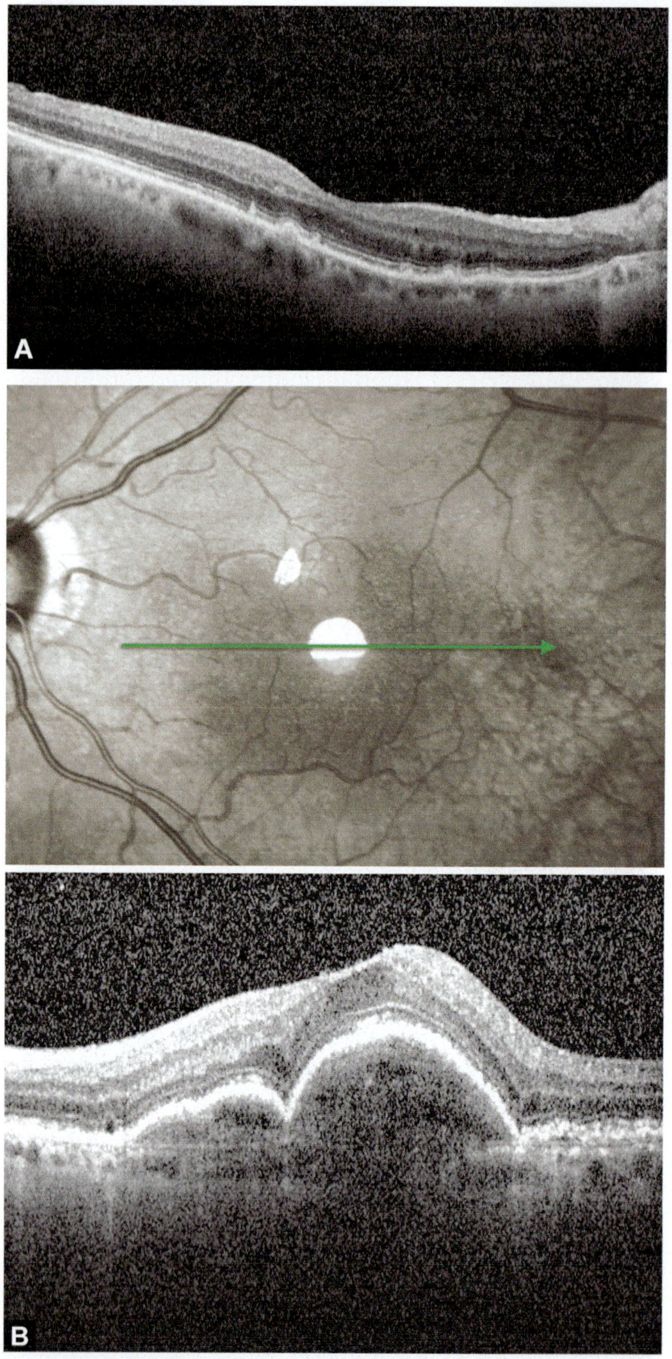

Figs. 38.2A and B: (A) Optical coherence tomography (OCT) of dry age-related macular degeneration demonstrating numerous drusen; (B) Infrared scanning laser ophthalmoscope (middle) and OCT (bottom) of wet age-related macular degeneration with fibrovascular pigment epithelial detachment.

Cataract extraction may promote the development of VMT in patients with existing VMA.[11] Management options include pars plana vitrectomy, pneumatic vitreolysis, enzymatic vitreolysis and observation.[12] Patients with vitreomacular

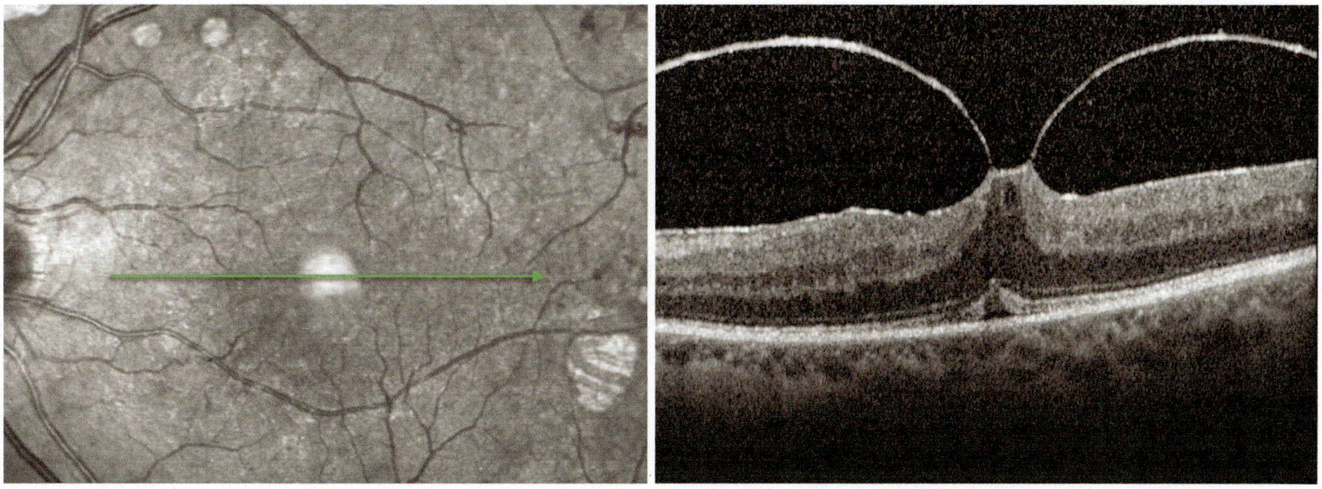

Fig. 38.3: Vitreomacular traction syndrome causing distortion of the normal foveal architecture.

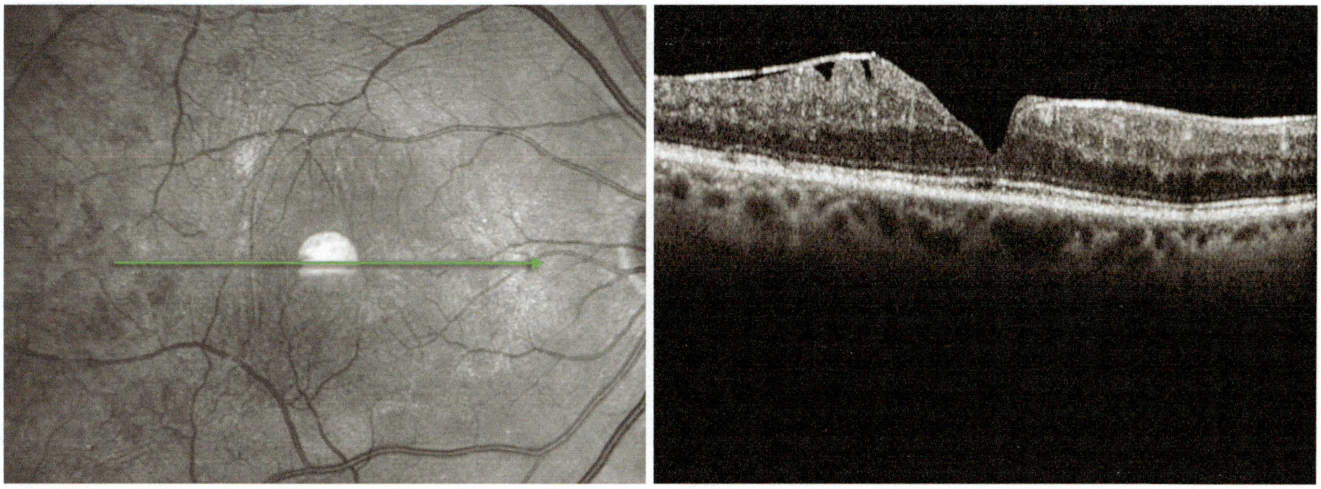

Fig. 38.4: Epiretinal membrane causing retinal wrinkling and distortion of the foveal architecture.

interface disorders should be warned of the possibility of progressive symptoms and the need for further treatment.

Epiretinal Membrane

Epiretinal membrane (ERM), or macular pucker, has a prevalence of 7% in the general population.[13] It is classified as a vitreomacular interface disorder caused by fibrocellular proliferation overlying the inner retina (Fig. 38.4). Visual deficits range from no loss to severe visual loss. The disease can be associated with metamorphopsia, monocular diplopia, or micropsia among other symptoms. A mild or early form of ERM may be funduscopically occult and difficult to detect in the presence of a dense cataract. OCT has been shown to have greater sensitivity than clinical examination in the detection of ERM.[14] The morphologic appearance of ERMs on OCT can also correlate with visual function. Studies have implicated central subfield thickness, ellipsoid band integrity, and the presence of ectopic inner foveal layers as clinically significant correlates of visual function.[14-17] Patients with ERM should undergo evaluation with a retina specialist. The treatment of this disease is primarily surgical, if significant visual decline or distortion is associated with the ERM. If pars plana vitrectomy is deemed appropriate, the timing of vitreoretinal surgery may be before, after, or at the same time as cataract surgery. The order of the surgeries should be determined in a coordinated consultation with the patient, retinal surgeon and cataract surgeon as determined on a case-by-case basis.

Diabetic Macular Edema

Diabetic retinopathy (DR) is the most common cause of vision loss in working age adults.[18,19] Visual decline is most often caused by diabetic macular edema (DME), vitreous hemorrhage due to proliferative retinopathy, and cataract. The 10-year incidence of DME is approximately 20–40%. Treatment of DME is guided by OCT findings of increased central subfield thickness and presence of cystoid macular edema (CME) or subretinal fluid (Fig. 38.5). OCT provides serial quantitative monitoring of macular thickness and can localize macular edema as either center-involving or non-center involving. Antivascular endothelial growth factor (VEGF) intravitreal injections are considered the gold standard of care for DME and are employed much more commonly than local steroid injection, laser therapy or pars plana vitrectomy.[20]

Cataract surgery can cause progression of DME in those with existing DR or edema.[21] Anti-VEGF therapy before or at the time of cataract surgery may decrease the risk of postsurgical DME and should be considered in at-risk patients.[22] Pseudophakic cystoid macular edema (CME), or Irvine-Gass syndrome, can co-exist with DME and may complicate the diagnosis. Patients with existing DR should be evaluated with OCT postoperatively to assess for macular edema and be given appropriate treatment. Patients with prior diabetic macular edema may experience benefit from combined cataract surgery and intraoperative anti-VEGF or steroid injection.[23,24]

High Myopia

High axial myopia can be associated with important macular findings identified with OCT including VMT, ERM, lamellar or full thickness macular hole, macular schisis (Fig. 38.6), retinal atrophy or choroidal neovascularization (CNV).[25-27] Other OCT findings in high myopes include peripapillary atrophy, posterior staphyloma, retinal thinning, and choroidal thinning.[28,29] Posterior staphyloma can complicate proper axial length measurement, and certain IOL calculation formulations require correction in long axial length eyes.[30,31] OCT evaluation is warranted in these patients to detect the aforementioned problems before proceeding with surgery.

MACULAR DISEASE AFFECTING PERIOPERATIVE PLANNING

Choice of Intraocular Lens

In routine phacoemulsification cases, the IOL design and power should be based on the patient and surgeon's refractive preference and the full range of intraoperative findings. However, IOL selection is especially important in patients with significant retinal disease and these critical factors are reviewed in this section.

Multifocal IOLs are pseudoaccomodating lenses comprised of concentric rings that use refractive or diffractive optics to focus light at different focal points. This provides focus at various near and far distances. Because the incoming light is split, contrast sensitivity at any given focal point is decreased. The indication for using multifocal IOL implants with concurrent retinal disease depends on the severity of the retinal abnormalities, the expected progression, and the availability of treatment.[32] Common macular disorders including AMD, diabetic retinopathy, and ERM can decrease central visual acuity and retinal sensitivity. In this setting, OCT evaluation can be very helpful in identifying the presence and severity of any coexisting retinal abnormality.

Additional considerations relate to retinal surgery, which can be more technically difficult through a multifocal IOL due to impaired fundus visualization.[33] Challenges may be encountered during epiretinal membrane peeling, with

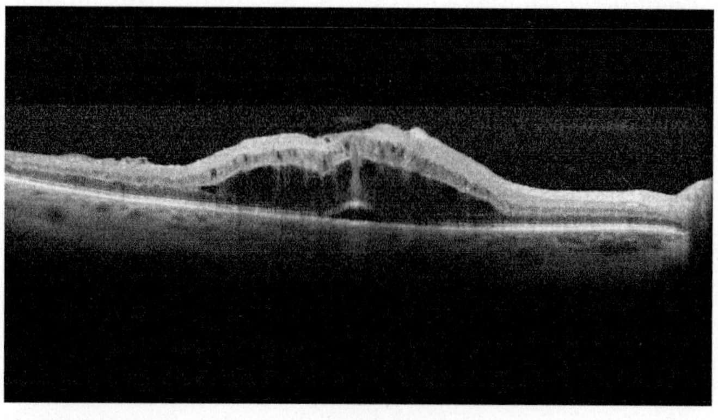

Fig. 38.5: Florid center-involving diabetic macular edema with intraretinal cystoid edema and subretinal fluid.

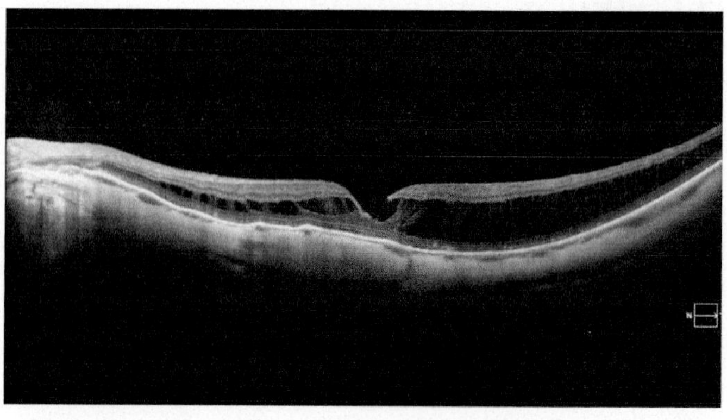

Fig. 38.6: Myopic macular schisis in a patient with pathologic myopia with separation of the outer nuclear layer.

use of triamcinolone acetonide contrast agent for internal limiting membrane peeling, and with retinal detachment repair.[34,35] Scleral buckling produces axial myopia and can compromise focusing through a multifocal lens. Post vitrectomy eyes may undergo a mild myopic shift due to shifting of the lens position or due to anterior chamber shallowing, and there may be a greater risk of decentration of the optic.[36,37] Eyes with existing silicone oil tamponade, prior retinal detachment or other complex retinal disease should not receive silicone IOLs in expectation of the need for silicone oil. Such eyes may suffer silicone oil condensation on the optic. Hydrophilic acrylic lenses may develop lens calcifications with the use of intraocular gas tamponade.

Blue-protective intraocular lens implants that filter out blue and ultraviolet (UV) light may benefit patients with age-related macular degeneration. Examples of blue-protective lenses include the Alcon Acrysof SN60AT and SN60WF IOLs. The Beaver Dam Eye Study implicated cataract extraction and blue light exposure as risk factors for AMD progression. Use of blue-protective IOLs however is controversial as several subsequent studies have found no correlation between blue light exposure and AMD progression.[38] On the other hand, studies have found a measurable decrease in contrast acuity and blue/yellow foveal threshold when blue-protective IOLs are used. When one eye has a blue-protective IOL, it is recommended to implant the same type of IOL in the fellow eye.[39]

Timing of Vitreoretinal and Cataract Surgery

When cataract surgery and vitreoretinal surgery are both indicated, the surgical team must decide the optimal sequence of surgery. Importantly, cataract surgery should be performed before vitreous surgery if there is inadequate visualization due to a mature cataract.

Performing combined phacoemulsification and vitrectomy has the advantages of a single operation, improved visualization during vitrectomy and no return trip to the operating room. It has been shown to have similar success rates compared to staged operations in eyes with epiretinal membrane, macular hole, proliferative diabetic retinopathy and other retinal disorders.[40-43] Reported complications with the combined approach include greater postoperative inflammation, posterior synechiae formation, increased intraocular pressure, and increased rate of posterior capsular opacification. Additionally, use of intraocular gas tamponade may increase the risk of anterior lens dislocation and pupillary capture due to posterior pressure against the capsular bag and IOL.

Cataract typically progresses rapidly after vitrectomy in over 80% of patients after one year.[44,45] Cataract surgery in post-vitrectomy eyes can be technically more difficult due to loss of vitreous support of the posterior capsule leading to a more mobile posterior capsule, zonular weakness and a greater risk of intraoperative posterior capsule rupture. Cataract surgeons should be aware of the increased risk for anterior chamber (AC) shallowing and other surgery-related complications during phacoemulsification.

CATARACT SURGERY IMPACTING MACULAR DISEASE

Age-related Macular Degeneration

The impact of cataract extraction on the progression of AMD is controversial. A number of studies have implicated cataract surgery as a risk factor for the development of neovascular AMD.[46-52] This relationship may be theoretically plausible given that removal of the native crystalline lens leaves the retina more susceptible to light damage. Iatrogenic trauma to Bruchs membrane, intraocular inflammation, and the development of cystoid macular edema may be additional risk factors for neovascular AMD. In contrast, other studies did not find an association between cataract surgery and progression of AMD.[53-55] Overall, cataract surgery in eyes with macular degeneration can lead to significant improvement in visual acuity[56,57] and can be a worthwhile endeavor even in the presence of advanced AMD. However, close vigilance for the development of choroidal neovascularization supplemented with regular OCT evaluation of the macula is critical for the early identification and treatment of CNV in AMD eyes at greatest risk of this complication (i.e. eyes with CNV or high-risk macular drusen in the affected or fellow eye). Early therapy of neovascular AMD can improve anatomical and visual outcomes.[58]

Diabetic Retinopathy

Although cataract extraction leads to a significant visual improvement in diabetic patients,[59-61] growing evidence suggests that diabetic retinopathy may progress at a faster rate after cataract surgery.[62] The main postoperative complications include diabetic macular edema (DME) and proliferative retinopathy.[61,63,64] Other studies however have found no correlation of lens status and diabetic retinopathy, and suggest the progression of retinopathy may be part of the natural progression of the disease.[65,66]

Optical coherence tomography has proven to be an essential tool in monitoring macular edema. Topical nonsteroid anti-inflammatory drops have demonstrated efficacy in reducing postsurgical macular edema.[67,68] In patients with pre-existing DME who are scheduled for cataract surgery, pre-operative intravitreal anti-VEGF or steroid therapy may be important in stabilizing macular edema and optimizing visual outcome.[22] The use of an intravitreal dexamethasone implant has been suggested for longer-term maintenance.[69] Postoperatively, differentiating the etiologic cause of CME, whether from diabetic retinopathy or pseudophakic CME, is challenging although OCT can help distinguish between these entities.[70]

Pseudophakic Cystoid Macular Edema

The incidence of pseudophakic cystoid macular edema (PCME), also known as Irvine-Gass syndrome, in uncomplicated cataract surgery without known risk factors is estimated to be approximately 1–2% (Fig. 38.7).[21] It is thought to arise from increased concentrations of inflammatory mediators in the aqueous and vitreous leading to increased vascular permeability in the retinal capillaries.[70,71] Risk factors include preoperative prostaglandin use, capsular rupture, vitreous loss, vitreomacular traction syndrome, epiretinal membrane formation, retinal vein occlusion and uveitis.[21,72] Postoperative use of topical steroid and nonsteroidal drops has been shown to improve pseudophakic CME.[68]

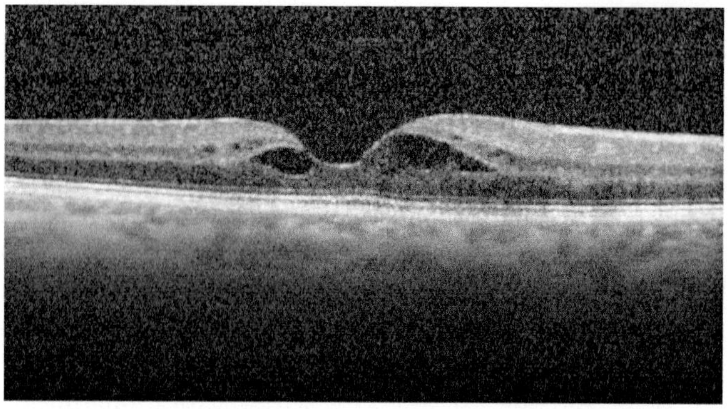

Fig. 38.7: Pseudophakic cystoid macular edema demonstrates parafoveal pockets of intraretinal fluid.

REFERENCES

1. Gabriele ML, Wollstein G, Ishikawa H, et al. Optical coherence tomography: history, current status, and laboratory work. Invest Ophthalmol Vis Sci. 2011;52(5):2425-36.
2. Forte R, Cennamo GL, Finelli ML, et al. Comparison of time domain Stratus OCT and spectral domain SLO/OCT for assessment of macular thickness and volume. Eye. 2008;23(11):2071-8.
3. Klein BR, Brown EN, Casden RS. Preoperative macular spectral-domain optical coherence tomography in patients considering advanced-technology intraocular lenses for cataract surgery. J Cataract Refract Surg. 2016;42(4):537-41.
4. Enright NJ, Catran A, Perera N, et al. Yield of routine pre-cataract surgery macular optical coherence tomography in finding clinically undetected macular pathology: Letter to the Editor. Clin Experiment Ophthalmol. [Internet]. 2017 Jun 15 [cited 2017 Sep 22]; Available from: *http://doi.wiley.com/10.1111/ceo.12973*
5. Klein R, Klein BE, Linton KL. Prevalence of age-related maculopathy. The Beaver Dam Eye Study. Ophthalmology. 1992;99(6):933-43.
6. Friedman DS, O'Colmain BJ, Muñoz B, et al. Prevalence of age-related macular degeneration in the United States. Arch Ophthalmol Chic Ill 1960. 2004;122(4):564-72.
7. van Leeuwen R, Klaver CCW, Vingerling JR, et al. The risk and natural course of age-related maculopathy: follow-up at 6 1/2 years in the Rotterdam study. Arch Ophthalmol Chic Ill 1960. 2003;121(4):519-26.
8. Ferris FL, Davis MD, Clemons TE, et al. A simplified severity scale for age-related macular degeneration: AREDS Report No. 18. Arch Ophthalmol Chic Ill 1960. 2005;123(11):1570-4.
9. Duker JS, Kaiser PK, Binder S, et al. The International Vitreomacular Traction Study Group classification of vitreomacular adhesion, traction, and macular hole. Ophthalmology. 2013;120(12):2611-9.
10. Reichel E, Jaffe GJ, Sadda SR, et al. Prevalence of vitreomacular adhesion: an optical coherence tomography analysis in the retina clinic setting. Clin Ophthalmol Auckl NZ. 2016;10:627-33.
11. Yaman A, Karahan E, Arikan G, et al. Acute vitreomacular traction syndrome after uneventful phacoemulsification. Ann Ophthalmol Skokie Ill. 2008;40(1):15-8.
12. Flynn HW, Relhan N. The Charles Schepens Lecture: Management Options for Vitreomacular Traction: Use an Individualized Approach. Ophthalmol Retina. 2017;1(1):3-7.
13. Stevenson W, Prospero Ponce CM, Agarwal DR, et al. Epiretinal membrane: optical coherence tomography-based diagnosis and classification. Clin Ophthalmol Auckl NZ. 2016;10:527-34.
14. Inoue M, Morita S, Watanabe Y, et al. Preoperative inner segment/outer segment junction in spectral-domain optical coherence tomography as a prognostic factor in epiretinal membrane surgery. Retina Phila Pa. 2011;31(7):1366-72.
15. Suh MH, Seo JM, Park KH, et al. Associations between macular findings by optical coherence tomography and visual outcomes after epiretinal membrane removal. Am J Ophthalmol. 2009;147(3):473-480.e3.

16. Falkner-Radler CI, Glittenberg C, Hagen S, et al. Spectral-domain optical coherence tomography for monitoring epiretinal membrane surgery. Ophthalmology. 2010;117(4):798-805.
17. Govetto A, Lalane RA, Sarraf D, et al. Insights into epiretinal membranes: presence of ectopic inner foveal layers and a new optical coherence tomography staging scheme. Am J Ophthalmol. 2017;175:99-113.
18. Stratton IM, Kohner EM, Aldington SJ, et al. UKPDS 50: risk factors for incidence and progression of retinopathy in Type II diabetes over 6 years from diagnosis. Diabetologia. 2001;44(2):156-63.
19. Klein R, Klein BE, Moss SE, et al. The Wisconsin Epidemiologic Study of Diabetic Retinopathy: XVII. The 14-year incidence and progression of diabetic retinopathy and associated risk factors in type 1 diabetes. Ophthalmology. 1998;105(10):1801-15.
20. Moisseiev E, Loewenstein A. Diabetic macular edema: emerging strategies and treatment algorithms. Dev Ophthalmol. 2017;60:165-74.
21. Chu CJ, Johnston RL, Buscombe C, et al. Risk factors and incidence of macular edema after cataract surgery: A Database Study of 81984 Eyes. Ophthalmology. 2016;123(2):316-23.
22. Boscia F, Giancipoli E, D'Amico Ricci G, et al. Management of macular oedema in diabetic patients undergoing cataract surgery. Curr Opin Ophthalmol. 2017;28(1):23-8.
23. Gallego-Pinazo R, Dolz-Marco R, Berrocal M, et al. Outcomes of cataract surgery in diabetic patients: results of the Pan American Collaborative Retina Study Group. Arq Bras Oftalmol. 2014;77(6):355-9.
24. Salehi A, Beni AN, Razmjoo H, et al. Phacoemulcification with intravitreal bevacizumab injection in patients with cataract and coexisting diabetic retinopathy: prospective randomized study. J Ocul Pharmacol Ther Off J Assoc Ocul Pharmacol Ther. 2012;28(3):212-8.
25. Silva R. Myopic maculopathy: a review. Ophthalmologica. 2012;228(4):197-213.
26. Henaine-Berra A, Zand-Hadas IM, Fromow-Guerra J, et al. Prevalence of macular anatomic abnormalities in high myopia. Ophthalmic Surg Lasers Imaging Retina. 2013;44(2):140-4.
27. Gohil R, Sivaprasad S, Han LT, et al. Myopic foveoschisis: a clinical review. Eye Lond Engl. 2015;29(5):593-601.
28. Ikuno Y, Tano Y. Retinal and choroidal biometry in highly myopic eyes with spectral-domain optical coherence tomography. Invest Ophthalmol Vis Sci. 2009;50(8):3876-80.
29. Gupta P, Cheung CY, Saw S-M, et al. Peripapillary choroidal thickness in young Asians with high myopia. Invest Ophthalmol Vis Sci. 2015;56(3):1475-81.
30. El-Nafees R, Moawad A, Kishk H, et al. Intra-ocular lens power calculation in patients with high axial myopia before cataract surgery. Saudi J Ophthalmol. 2010;24(3):77-80.
31. Haigis W. Intraocular lens calculation in extreme myopia. J Cataract Refract Surg. 2009;35(5):906-11.
32. Braga-Mele R, Chang D, Dewey S, et al. Multifocal intraocular lenses: relative indications and contraindications for implantation. J Cataract Refract Surg. 2014;40(2):313-22.
33. Tewari A, Shah GK. Presbyopia-correcting intraocular lenses: what retinal surgeons should know. Retina Phila Pa. 2008;28(4):535-7.
34. Kawamura R, Inoue M, Shinoda K, et al. Intraoperative findings during vitreous surgery after implantation of diffractive multifocal intraocular lens. J Cataract Refract Surg. 2008;34(6):1048-9.
35. Yoshino M, Inoue M, Kitamura N, et al. Diffractive multifocal intraocular lens interferes with intraoperative view. Clin Ophthalmol Auckl NZ. 2010;4:467-9.
36. Byrne SA, Ng J, Steel D. Changes in refraction pre and post pars plana vitrectomy (PPV) in Pseudophakic eyes. Invest Ophthalmol Vis Sci. 2006;47(13):3675.
37. Hamoudi H, Kofod M, La Cour M. Refractive change after vitrectomy for epiretinal membrane in pseudophakic eyes. Acta Ophthalmol (Copenh). 2013;91(5):434-6.
38. Henderson BA, Grimes KJ. Blue-blocking IOLs: a complete review of the literature. Surv Ophthalmol. 2010;55(3):284-9.
39. Wirtitsch MG, Schmidinger G, Prskavec M, et al. Influence of blue-light-filtering intraocular lenses on color perception and contrast acuity. Ophthalmology. 2009;116(1):39-45.
40. Dugas B, Ouled-Moussa R, Lafontaine P-O, et al. Idiopathic epiretinal macular membrane and cataract extraction: combined versus consecutive surgery. Am J Ophthalmol. 2010;149(2):302-6.
41. Muselier A, Dugas B, Burelle X, et al. Macular hole surgery and cataract extraction: combined vs consecutive surgery. Am J Ophthalmol. 2010;150(3):387-91.
42. Lee DY, Jeong HS, Sohn HJ, et al. Combined 23-gauge sutureless vitrectomy and clear corneal phacoemulsification in patients with proliferative diabetic retinopathy. Retina Phila Pa. 2011;31(9):1753-8.
43. Sisk RA, Murray TG. Combined phacoemulsification and sutureless 23-gauge pars plana vitrectomy for complex vitreoretinal diseases. Br J Ophthalmol. 2010;94(8):1028-32.
44. de Bustros S, Thompson JT, Michels RG, et al. Nuclear sclerosis after vitrectomy for idiopathic epiretinal membranes. Am J Ophthalmol. 1988;105(2):160-4.
45. Hsuan JD, Brown NA, Bron AJ, et al. Posterior subcapsular and nuclear cataract after vitrectomy. J Cataract Refract Surg. 2001;27(3):437-44.
46. Klein R, Klein BEK, Wong TY, et al. The association of cataract and cataract surgery with the long-term incidence of age-related maculopathy: the Beaver Dam eye study. Arch Ophthalmol Chic Ill 1960. 2002;120(11):1551-8.
47. Klein R, Klein BE, Jensen SC, et al. The relationship of ocular factors to the incidence and progression of age-related maculopathy. Arch Ophthalmol Chic Ill 1960. 1998;116(4):506-13.
48. Wang JJ, Klein R, Smith W, et al. Cataract surgery and the 5-year incidence of late-stage age-related maculopathy: pooled findings from the Beaver Dam and Blue Mountains eye studies. Ophthalmology. 2003;110(10):1960-7.

49. Freeman EE, Munoz B, et al. Is there an association between cataract surgery and age-related macular degeneration? Data from three population-based studies. Am J Ophthalmol. 2003;135(6):849-56.
50. Cugati S, Mitchell P, Rochtchina E, et al. Cataract surgery and the 10-year incidence of age-related maculopathy: the Blue Mountains Eye Study. Ophthalmology. 2006;113(11):2020-5.
51. Dong LM, Stark WJ, Jefferys JL, et al. Progression of age-related macular degeneration after cataract surgery. Arch Ophthalmol Chic Ill 1960. 2009;127(11):1412-9.
52. Ho J-D, Xirasagar S, Kao L-T, et al. Neovascular age-related macular degeneration is associated with cataract surgery. Acta Ophthalmol (Copenh). 2018;96(2):e213-7.
53. Baatz H, Darawsha R, Ackermann H, et al. Phacoemulsification does not induce neovascular age-related macular degeneration. Invest Ophthalmol Vis Sci. 2008;49(3):1079-83.
54. Wang JJ, Fong CS-U, Rochtchina E, et al. Risk of age-related macular degeneration 3 years after cataract surgery: paired eye comparisons. Ophthalmology. 2012;119(11):2298-303.
55. Dong LM, Stark WJ, Jefferys JL, et al. Progression of age-related macular degeneration after cataract surgery. Arch Ophthalmol Chic Ill 1960. 2009;127(11):1412-9.
56. Forooghian F, Agrón E, Clemons TE, et al. Age-Related Eye Disease Study Research Group. Visual acuity outcomes after cataract surgery in patients with age-related macular degeneration: age-related eye disease study report no. 27. Ophthalmology. 2009;116(11):2093-100.
57. Stock MV, Vollman DE, Baze EF, et al. Functional visual improvement after cataract surgery in eyes with age-related macular degeneration: results of the ophthalmic surgical outcomes data project. Invest Ophthalmol Vis Sci. 2015;56(4):2536-40.
58. Lim JH, Wickremasinghe SS, Xie J, et al. Delay to treatment and visual outcomes in patients treated with anti-vascular endothelial growth factor for age-related macular degeneration. Am J Ophthalmol. 2012;153(4):678-86, 686.e1-2.
59. Liao S-B, Ku W-C. Progression of diabetic retinopathy after phacoemulsification in diabetic patients: a three-year analysis. Chang Gung Med J. 2003;26(11):829-34.
60. Krepler K, Biowski R, Schrey S, et al. Cataract surgery in patients with diabetic retinopathy: visual outcome, progression of diabetic retinopathy, and incidence of diabetic macular oedema. Graefes Arch Clin Exp Ophthalmol Albrecht Von Graefes Arch Klin Exp Ophthalmol. 2002;240(9):735-8.
61. Chew EY, Benson WE, Remaley NA, et al. Results after lens extraction in patients with diabetic retinopathy: early treatment diabetic retinopathy study report number 25. Arch Ophthalmol Chic Ill 1960. 1999;117(12):1600-6.
62. Hong T, Mitchell P, de Loryn T, et al. Development and progression of diabetic retinopathy 12 months after phacoemulsification cataract surgery. Ophthalmology. 2009;116(8):1510-4.
63. Kim SJ, Equi R, Bressler NM. Analysis of macular edema after cataract surgery in patients with diabetes using optical coherence tomography. Ophthalmology. 2007;114(5):881-9.
64. Squirrell D, Bhola R, Bush J, et al. A prospective, case controlled study of the natural history of diabetic retinopathy and maculopathy after uncomplicated phacoemulsification cataract surgery in patients with type 2 diabetes. Br J Ophthalmol. 2002;86(5):565-71.
65. Krepler K, Biowski R, Schrey S, et al. Cataract surgery in patients with diabetic retinopathy: visual outcome, progression of diabetic retinopathy, and incidence of diabetic macular oedema. Graefes Arch Clin Exp Ophthalmol Albrecht Von Graefes Arch Klin Exp Ophthalmol. 2002;240(9):735-8.
66. Kato S, Fukada Y, Hori S, et al. Influence of phacoemulsification and intraocular lens implantation on the course of diabetic retinopathy. J Cataract Refract Surg. 1999;25(6):788-93.
67. Singh RP, Staurenghi G, Pollack A, et al. Efficacy of nepafenac ophthalmic suspension 0.1% in improving clinical outcomes following cataract surgery in patients with diabetes: an analysis of two randomized studies. Clin Ophthalmol Auckl NZ. 2017;11:1021-9.
68. Wielders LHP, Schouten JSAG, Aberle MR, et al. Treatment of cystoid macular edema after cataract surgery. J Cataract Refract Surg. 2017;43(2):276-84.
69. Furino C, Boscia F, Niro A, et al. Combined phacoemulsification and intravitreal dexamethasone implant (Ozurdex®) in diabetic patients with coexisting cataract and diabetic macular edema. J Ophthalmol. 2017;2017:4896036.
70. Munk MR, Jampol LM, Simader C, et al. Differentiation of diabetic macular edema from pseudophakic cystoid macular edema by spectral-domain optical coherence tomography. Invest Ophthalmol Vis Sci. 2015;56(11):6724-33.
71. Benitah NR, Arroyo JG. Pseudophakic cystoid macular edema. Int Ophthalmol Clin. 2010;50(1):139-53.
72. Henderson BA, Kim JY, Ament CS, et al. Clinical pseudophakic cystoid macular edema. Risk factors for development and duration after treatment. J Cataract Refract Surg. 2007;33(9):1550-8.

Chapter 39 Intraoperative Aberrometry

Shawn R Lin, D Rex Hamilton

INTRODUCTION

In recent years, cataract surgery has rapidly evolved from a procedure designed merely to clear the visual axis into one designed to turn back the clock on eye aging

Success with multifocal, extended depth of focus and toric intraocular lenses all rely on the ability of surgeons to achieve a precise refractive endpoint, often as close to plano as possible.[1,2] Advanced optical biometry and next generation lens power formulas now allow surgeons to more consistently hit a refractive target.[3,4]

However, these methodologies all rely on measurements performed preoperatively on the phakic eye. As patient expectations continue to rise, intraoperative aberrometry provides an additional tool to increase refractive precision by measuring optical aberrations in the aphakic state.[5]

The intraoperative aberrometer can be used to take aphakic measurements after removal of the cataract, and prior to the implantation of the intraocular lens. This allows the surgeon to confirm spherical lens power selection. In the aphakic mode, the system can also measure total astigmatism, including the contribution of the posterior corneal surface, as well as the effects of primary and secondary incisions. If the femtosecond laser is used to place astigmatic keratotomies, the aphakic astigmatic measurements include the effects of these unopened incisions.[6]

The surgeon can evaluate the magnitude and meridian of the residual astigmatism and decide if it makes sense to open the laser-placed astigmatic keratotomies. Following lens placement, the aberrometer can then be utilized in the pseudophakic state to measure astigmatism in real-time while rotating a toric lens into the optimal position.

Used in conjunction with preoperative lens calculations, intraoperative aberrometry can decrease the magnitude of postoperative residual refractive error.[4,6-8] In this chapter, we will discuss intraoperative aberrometry technology, outcomes data, best practices, decision-making, case examples and the future of this technology.

TECHNOLOGY

Sean Ianchulev and Wolfgang Haggis were two early pioneers of intraoperative aberrometry. They described methods to refract a patient without the need for an axial length measurement or keratometry.[5] The first commercially available interoperative aberrometer was the WaveTec Orange Aberrometry System.[4]

WaveTec Orange

The orange aberrometry system uses laser light and principles of Talbot-Moiré interferometry to take measurements of the eyes.[4]

In the first stage of this process, a narrow laser beam is sent into the eye and the reflected wavefront is captured by the aberrometer. In the second stage, the reflected light is passed through a pair of diffractive gratings to generate a fringe pattern. Finally, the system utilizes a proprietary algorithm to analyze the fringe pattern and calculate the final refraction (Fig. 39.1).[4]

Alcon ORA VerifEye+ (Optiwave Refractive Analysis)

WaveTec was subsequently acquired by Alcon and the original system was succeeded by the optiwave refractive analysis system (ORA), which improves visualization of the eye, speeds up data capture and displays streaming real-time measurements.[9]

With VerifEye+, a built-in reticle visible through the operating microscope allows surgeons to visualize real-time streaming information without looking away from the operating field (Figs. 39.2A and B)

Global Database Optimization

De-identified preoperative prediction data and post-operative outcomes data is uploaded into a worldwide database. This data can then be utilized to further optimize

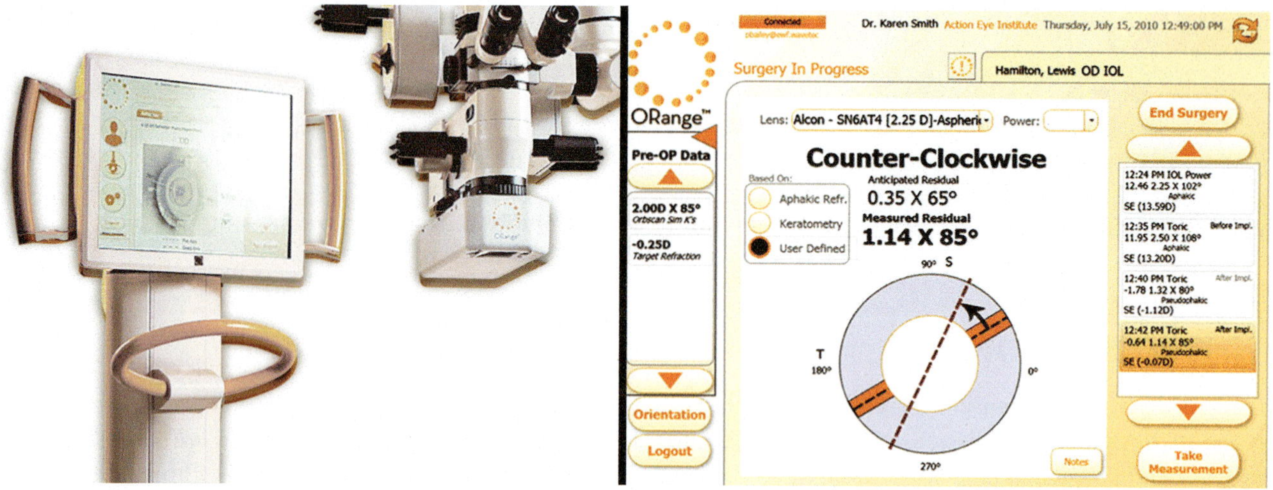

Fig. 39.1: The first generation WaveTec Orange system, showing the control stand and microscope attachment (left). The interface is illustrated in the right figure, demonstrating rotational recommendations during placement of a toric lens.

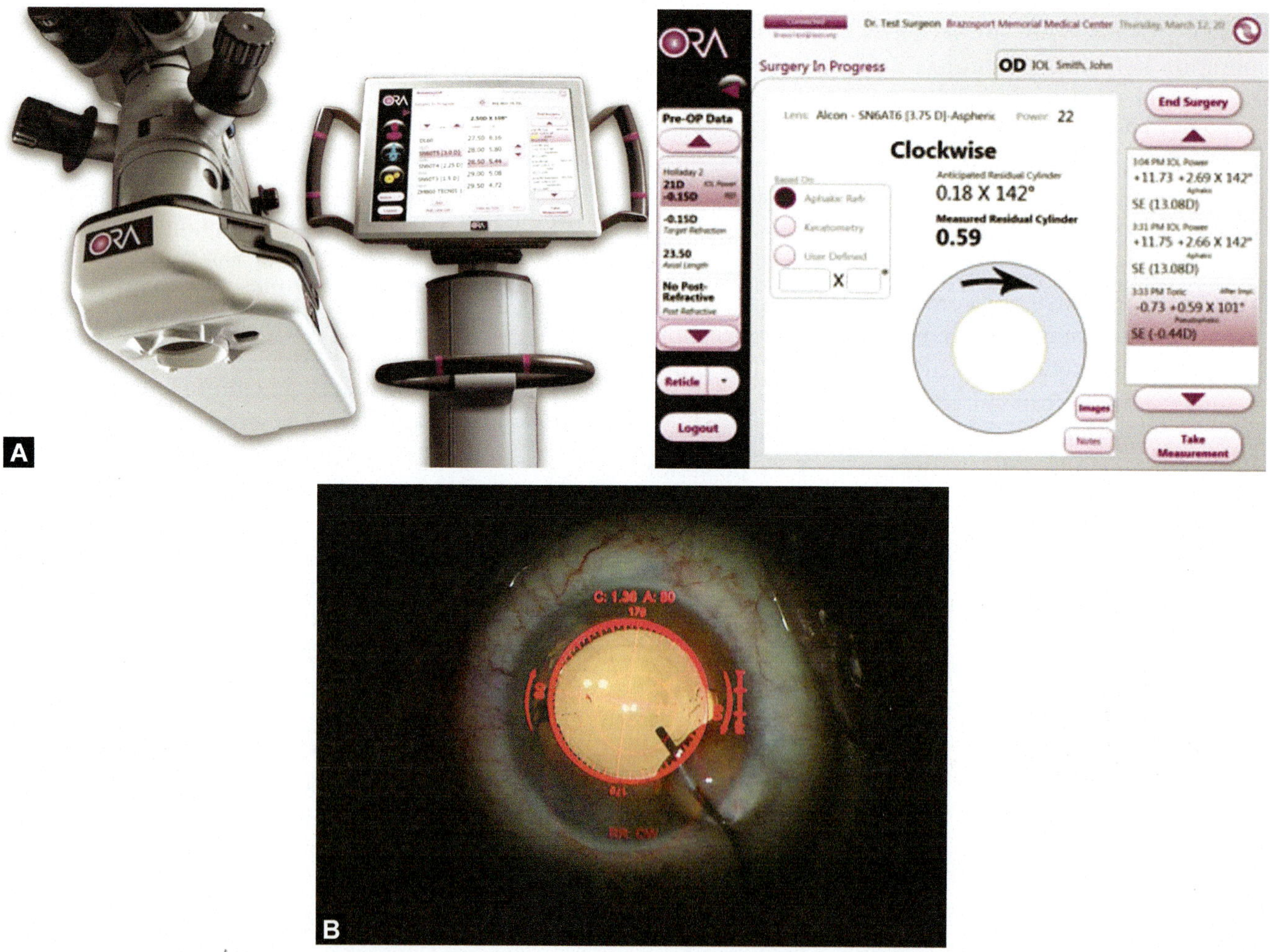

Figs. 39.2A and B: (A) The second-generation Alcon ORA system with an updated control stand, microscope attachment, and interface; (B) Optiwave refractive analysis (ORA) with VerifEye+. A reticle overlay shows real time cylinder (C) and axis (A), along with arrows to show direction of lens rotation necessary to neutralize astigmatism.

the calculation algorithms by specific lens type and patient subtype.

The ORA system updates postoperative data analysis periodically throughout the year and will automatically personalize the calculations for a particular surgeon once the accuracy of the lens power predictions exceeds that available from the global database prediction.

OUTCOMES DATA

The literatures on interoperative aberrometry support the use of the technology in standard cataract surgery with increasing efficacy for cataract surgery in patients with previous refractive surgery.

Routine Cataract Surgery

For standard cataract surgery in eyes without previous refractive surgery, a study of 215 eyes comparing ORA, Holladay I and II, Hoffer Q and SRK/T showed a mean absolute error of 0.36 ± 0.30 D spherical error (SE) with intraoperative aberrometry versus a mean absolute error of 0.53 ± 0.44 D with the aforementioned formulas.[4] The intraoperative aberrometer was significantly more accurate than standard lens formulas.

Cataract Surgery in Eyes with Previous Refractive Surgery

The greatest benefit of intraoperative aberrometry occurs within the subsegment of patients with prior refractive surgery. In this segment, the altered nature of the cornea leads to breakdowns in the accuracy of calculations using standard formulas. For example, in an eye with previous myopic refractive surgery (e.g. RK, LASIK, PRK), the corneal power is overestimated. This leads to an IOL power selection that is too low, resulting in a hyperopic surprise.[10]

Ianchulev showed in a study of 246 eyes that ORA achieves a significantly lower median absolute error of 0.35 D, compared to 0.6 D, 0.53 D, and 0.51 D with other formulas. In addition, 67% of eyes achieved outcomes within 0.5 D of targeted and 94% within 1.0 D of targeted.[6] This study was supported by Fram's study in 2015 showing 0.25 D of median absolute error compared to 0.37 D for Haigis. However, these differences did not reach statistical significance.[7]

Toric Lenses

Studies on the implantation of toric intraocular lenses illustrate the advantages of intraoperative aberrometry. In these patients, malrotation of even 10° results in the loss of 33% of the intended cylindrical correction. Malrotation of 30° results in no reduction of cylinder magnitude and inversion of the cylinder axis.[4]

A primary challenge for the refractive cataract surgeon trying to correctly orient the toric IOL is the induction of cyclotorsion when a patient moves from the upright to the supine position on the operating table. While various methods of preoperative marking have been developed, numerous studies demonstrate the inaccuracy of these measures.[11]

A 2015 study showed a significant improvement in final residual refractive astigmatism in the group using aberrometry-driven toric IOL power selection and placement versus the group using a preoperative toric calculator and traditional marking.[12] A paper presented at American Society of Cataract and Refractive Surgery (ASCRS) found 96% of patients achieved less than or equal to 0.5 D of residual cylinder in the aberrometry group versus 56% in the control group.[13]

Corneal Relaxing Incisions

The ORA system used in conjunction with femtosecond laser created astigmatic keratotomy incisions adds an additional level of precision to the treatment of astigmatism. While the creation of a femtosecond arcuate incision has some effect on corneal astigmatism, the majority of the effect is realized once the incision is opened. Intraoperative measurement of the amount and orientation of corneal astigmatism allows the surgeon to compare the effect of opening those incisions to leaving them unopened.

Even when manual limbal relaxing incisions (LRIs) are employed, assessing corneal astigmatism using the ORA system after clear corneal incisions have been placed can improve precision in reducing cylinder. A 2010 study by Packer et al. shows a 5.7x decrease in the odds ratio of needing post-cataract surgery excimer laser enhancement when astigmatism is treated using aberrometry assisted LRIs versus manual LRIs.[8]

BEST PRACTICES

The following are best practice considerations compiled from published literature, user focus groups, and industry experts. These practices can help a surgeon achieve accurate and consistent intraoperative aberrometry performance and quickly become second-nature. Once perfected, intraoperative aberrometry on routine cases rarely adds more than 2–3 minutes to case duration.

Anesthesia and Patient Fixation

It is important to note that patients undergoing intraoperative aberrometry must undergo surgery under topical anesthesia and should only be minimally sedated. The procedure requires patients to follow directions and gaze at a fixation target. Measurement quality can be suspect if taken when the patient is inattentive, if the patient has a strong intraoperative bells reflex or if the patient is overly sedated and cannot fixate on the target.

In our operating rooms, we direct anesthesiology to administer fentanyl and minimize Versed to improve attentiveness.

Patient Positioning

In order to achieve high accuracy, the patient should lay supine with the operative eye in primary gaze and level to the microscope. This is critical because contraction of the rectus muscles can induce astigmatism and introduce inaccuracy.

Lid Speculum

The lid speculum should be positioned such that only minimal pressure is exerted upon the globe. The eye should be well-centered inside the lid speculum. The margins of the lid speculum should be at least 1–2 mm away from the limbus, as the lid speculum blades can induce astigmatism. If the intraoperative aberrometry device reports unexpected deviation from preoperative measurements, it is prudent to check the lid speculum position.

Intraocular Pressure

To ensure consistent results, the intraocular pressure (IOP) of the eye should be kept at or slightly above physiologic conditions.[14,15] This can be checked with a weighted corneal applanator and by paying attention to visual cues such as corneal and capsular folds in both the infrared and moiré insets displayed on the Alcon ORA device. An excellent way to ensure proper IOP is to fill the anterior chamber and capsular bag with a cohesive viscoelastic. Additional viscoelastic should then be injected through the paracentesis until the slightest amount of viscoelastic is noted to prolapse out of the main wound. There is no need to 'burp' the wound to remove any additional viscoelastic (Figs. 39.3A and B).

Corneal Surface

The corneal surface should be hydrated with a few drops of balanced salt solution (BSS) prior to each formal measurement. This is recommended to ensure a smooth optical surface. The surgeon should avoid excessive irrigation, as significant pooling of BSS in the fornices can lead to erroneous measurements.

Wound Hydration

The surgical incisions should be watertight and hydration should not extend into the visual axis. Excessive corneal hydration increases local corneal intrastromal thickness and can induce transient corneal astigmatism.

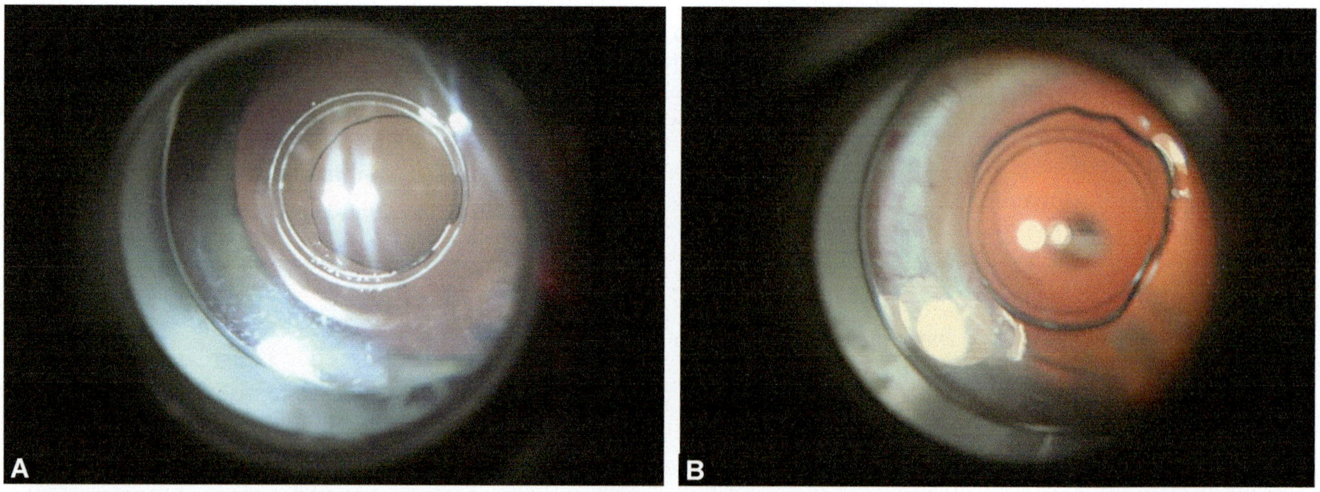

Figs. 39.3A and B: A weighted corneal depression tonometer is placed atop a viscoelastic filled eye. The depressed area on the cornea should be at or slightly within the two imprinted rings on the device. (A) The measured intraocular pressure is too high, and viscoelastic was removed to achieve the correct pressure; (B) Intraocular pressure was too low, and viscoelastic was added.

Vitreous Floaters

The infrared eye display and moiré inset on the ORA allow for evaluation of the clarity of the visual axis for measurement. This is an important display to monitor as vitreous floaters can degrade the quality of the measurement. If a floater remains in the visual axis, the patient should be instructed to initiate a saccade laterally and back, and the capture should be immediately initiated before the floater has a chance to move back across the visual axis.

Measurement Capture

Measurement capture on the VerifEye+ device is streamed into the surgeon's scope in real-time. However, formal sets of measurements must be obtained by clicking on the 'Capture' button on the device. The system rapidly averages 40 measurements in order to make a recommendation. With toric lenses, this process adds an additional rotational recommendation.

For toric lenses, we find it is most helpful to try to decrease real-time measurements to less than 0.5 D of cylinder before taking a formal set of measurements. This avoids excessive time spent making gross adjustments to the lens. With this precapture streaming alignment technique, we are able to achieve the goal of 'No rotation recommended (NRR)' on first attempt in 50–60% of cases.

Reduced Operative Space

Current intraoperative aberrometers attach to the bottom of the operative microscope and take up approximately 3 inches of vertical space underneath the scope. This may require some alteration of surgical technique to deal with the reduced instrument clearance. Many surgical instrument manufacturers now offer shorter instruments that are compatible with the space requirements of intraoperative aberrometers. If necessary, scope oculars can be switched from the usual 175 mm lens to 200 mm lens to offset some lost space.

Case Duration

As with the adoption of any new technology, incorporation of intraoperative aberrometry has a learning curve that will initially change operating room workflow and result in increased case duration. However, this increased case duration decreases rapidly over time with most routine cases ultimately adding only about 2–3 minutes to total case duration.

In toric cases, intraoperative aberrometry adds approximately 4–5 minutes to total case duration, depending on the number of rotation attempts needed to achieve astigmatic neutralization. Operating room staff require adequate training to understand and operate the ORA user interface.

Lens Availability

Intraoperative aberrometry is best utilized in surgical centers with a full consignment of lenses, along with high-quality inventory management. For most cases, the lens power is selected preoperatively and lenses immediately above and below that power should be available (i.e.19.5 D, 20.0 D, 20.5 D).

For toric cases, it is ideal to have full two-dimensional (i.e. 0.5 dioptric steps above and below the preselected spherical lens power and 0.5 cylindrical dioptric steps above and below the preselected cylindrical lens power) consignments of toric IOLs. This adds an additional dimension of inventory complexity (3 spherical combinations × 3 cylindrical combinations = 9 lenses).

COMPLEX DECISION-MAKING

An intraoperative aberrometry recommendation agreeing with preoperative calculations can lend credibility to the accuracy of the preoperative plan.

However, the art of intraoperative aberrometry lies in deciding how to handle disagreements between aberrometry recommendations and preoperative calculations. The decision to trust the aberrometry measurement or not depends on the following factors:

Measurement Accuracy

Both the accuracy of preoperative calculations and intraoperative aberrometry should be considered. Preoperative calculations that were performed in the setting of poor patient cooperation or large measurement standard deviation should be taken into account. In addition, the factors detailed in the last section on use of intraoperative aberrometry should be reviewed. The most common causes of intraoperative aberrometry error are:

- Poor lid speculum positioning
- Improper intraocular pressure
- Improper patient fixation

History of Refractive Surgery

In cases of prior refractive surgery, many studies report intraoperative aberrometry as providing more accurate IOL power recommendations than preoperative power calculations using other techniques (e.g. Haigis-L formula, Modified Maloney method, Clinical History method).[6,7] In these settings, if a difference occurs between the preoperative calculation and the aberrometry recommendation, we prefer to err towards the intraoperative aberrometry measurement, especially if the recommendation would leave the patient more myopic.

New versus Established Lenses

Intraoperative aberrometry systems benefit from continual optimization of algorithms using postoperative data entered by thousands of surgeons worldwide. As of today, the Alcon ORA system has logged more than 880,000 surgeries. When a new IOL is released, the aberrometry power recommendations may not be as accurate because the system has not benefited from thousands of postoperative results to optimize the calculation. Until sufficient postoperative data for the new IOL has been entered into the global ORA database, deviation from preoperative calculations should be made with caution.

Surgeon Personalized Data

Each surgeon will develop his/her own level of trust for intraoperative aberrometry recommendations in each particular case. This is facilitated by a robust ORA postoperative analysis platform which allows a surgeon to finely filter his/her cases to make better preoperative and intraoperative decisions.

As more postoperative data is entered into the database, the ORA system will personalize the calculations for the individual surgeon, improving accuracy of calculations across a wider range of dioptric powers, axial lengths and K-readings.

The gold-colored bar above the lens choice indicates that the values are globally optimized. With enough data for that lens type, the gold bar turns to platinum, indicating that surgeon personalized values are most accurate for that particular lens.

CASE EXAMPLES

Case 1: Extended Depth of Focus Lens

A 63-year-old hyperopic female with uncorrected glare visual acuity of 20/40 and preoperative refraction of +1.75 + 0.50 × 5 underwent femtosecond laser-assisted capsulorhexis, prechop and incision placement. The surgical plan was to place a Symfony extended depth of focus intraocular lens targeted at -0.25 spherical equivalent (Fig. 39.4).

The Hoffer Q formula was utilized given her short axial length, with an estimated intraocular lens power of 21.5 diopters, resulting in an estimated residual refraction of -0.16 D. Intraoperatively, the ORA estimated a residual refraction of -0.36 D with a 21.5 D lens.

The 21.5 D Symfony lens was selected and postoperative week 2 refraction was -0.25 spherical equivalent with a final vision of 20/20-1 distance and J3 near.

In this case, the preoperative lens selection was confirmed by the intraoperative aberrometer with an on-target final result.

Case 2: Extended Depth of Focus Lens with Corneal Relaxing Incisions

A 40-year-old myopic female with uncorrected visual acuity of counting fingers and preoperative refraction of -8.00 +1.00 × 108 underwent femtosecond laser-assisted capsulorhexis, prechop and incision placement. In addition, the preoperative Galilei scan showed 0.65 D

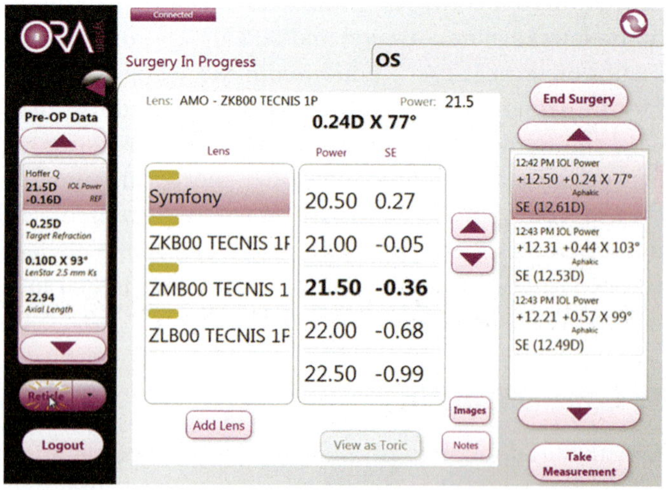

Fig. 39.4: The preoperative lens selection was confirmed by the intraoperative aberrometer with an on-target final result.

of astigmatism at 76° and the femtosecond laser was used to place two 29° long laser arcuates centered at 76 and 256°. These arcuates were cut to 80% corneal depth and were left closed. The surgical plan was to place a Symfony extended depth of focus intraocular lens targeted at –0.25 D (Figs. 39.5 and 39.6).

Holladay I predicted an intraocular lens power of 12.0 D resulting in an estimated residual refraction of –0.34 D. Intraoperatively, the ORA estimated a residual refraction of - 0.32 with a 12.0 D lens, but showed a residual astigmatism of 0.76 at 61°. Given the agreement of the ORA with the preoperative Galilei scans, the decision was made to open up the laser arcuates at 76 and 256°.

Postoperative week 2 refraction was –0.25 with 0 cylinder for a final distance vision of 20/20 and reading vision of J3.

In this case, the intraoperative aberrometer was used to measure the true residual astigmatism following lens removal. The femtosecond laser arcuates were opened to exert their full effect.

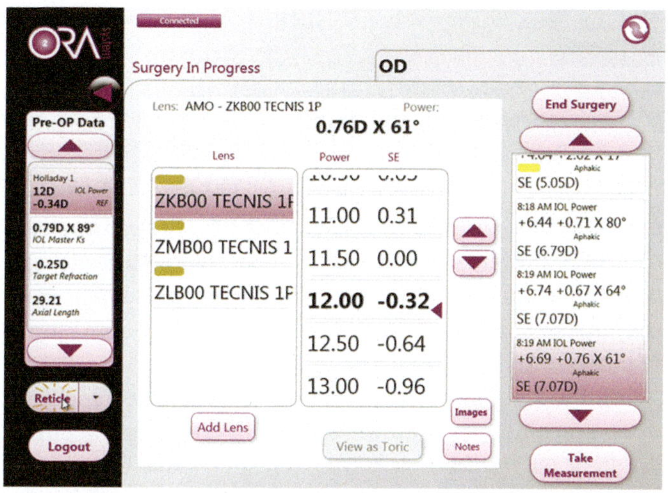

Fig. 39.5: The intraoperative aberrometer was used to measure the true residual astigmatism following lens removal. The femtosecond laser arcuates were opened to exert their full effect.

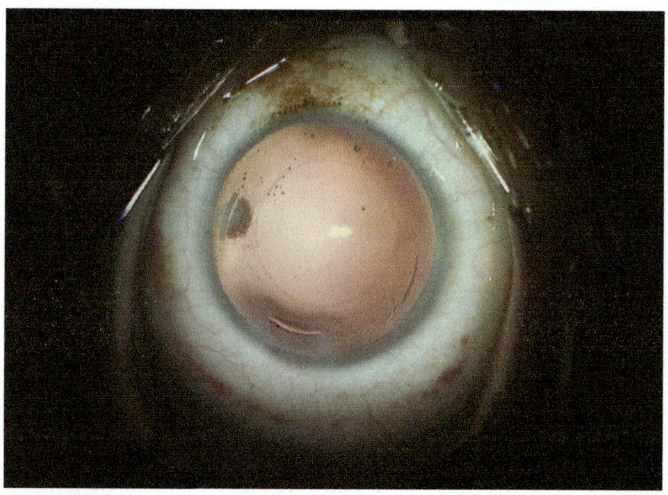

Fig. 39.6: In this view, the temporal incision is at approximately 350° (bottom of image), an opened laser arcuate at 256°, a closed laser arcuate at 76°, and the paracentesis at 60°.

Case 3: Toric Lens in a Post-RK Patient

A 61-year-old post-RK hyperopic male with uncorrected visual acuity of 20/40 and preoperative refraction of +0.25 +1.75 × 3 underwent femtosecond laser-assisted capsulorhexis, prechop and incision placement. The surgical plan was to place a 22.5D SN6AT5 toric intraocular lens targeted at plano.

Holladay I predicted an intraocular lens power of 22.5 D, resulting in an estimated residual refraction of plano. Intraoperatively, the ORA estimated a residual refraction of –0.28 with a 23.0 D lens. Given the difference, the higher power of 23.0 D lens was selected (Figs. 39.7 and 39.8).

On calculation of cylindrical power, an SN6AT4 lens (2.25 D astigmatism correction) left residual astigmatism of 0.05 D at 8, while an SN6AT5 lens (3.0 D astigmatism correction) left residual astigmatism of 0.45 D at a flipped axis of 98. Thus, the cylindrical power was reduced to SN6AT4.

Postoperative week 2 refraction was plano +0.25 × 176 with a final distance vision of 20/20.

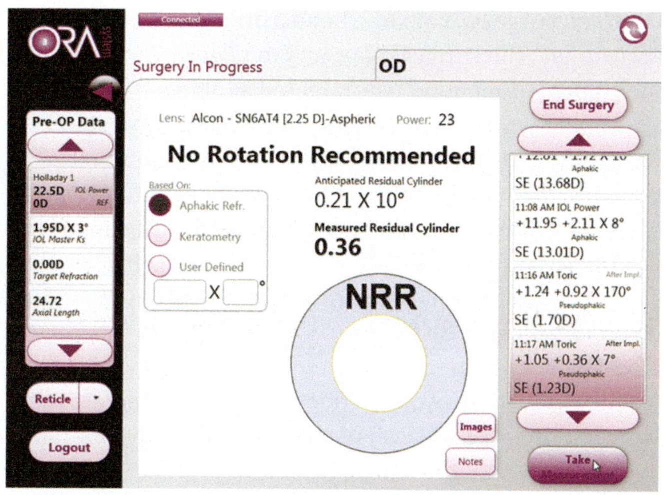

Fig. 39.7: The preoperative lens power and cylinder were changed with ORA. The desired endpoint of lens alignment is "no rotation recommended."

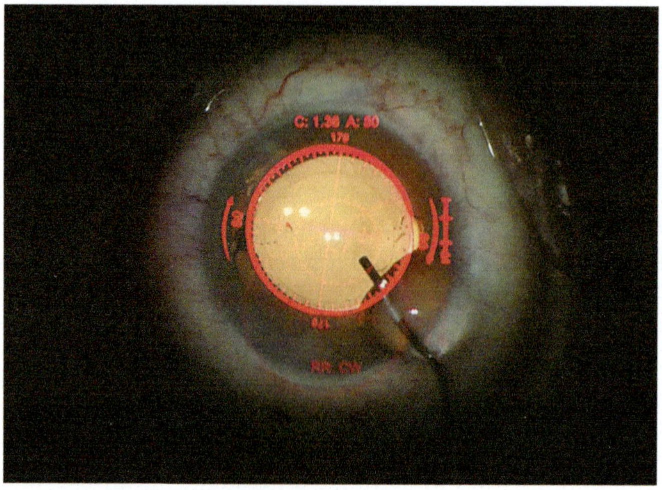

Fig. 39.8: Optiwave refractive analysis (ORA) with VerifEye+, a reticle overlay shows real-time cylinder (C) and axis (A) along with arrows to show direction of lens rotation necessary to neutralize astigmatism.

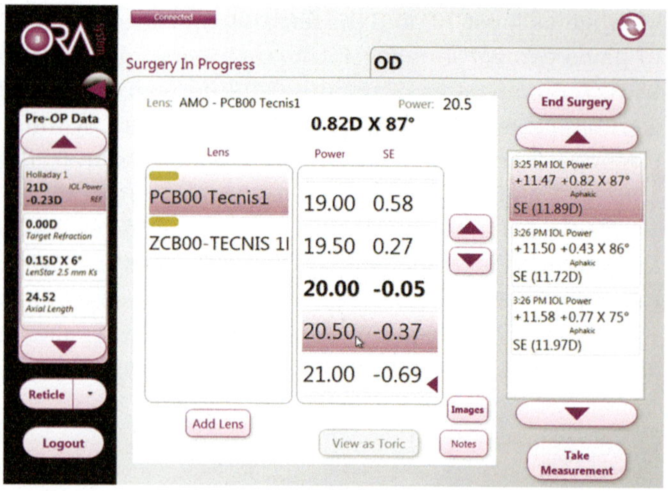

Fig. 39.9: Preoperative lens calculations would have resulted in 0.5 D of myopia. Choosing the intermediate value between preoperative calculations and the intraoperative aberrometer resulted in a plan result.

In this complex post-RK patient, following the preoperative lens calculation plan would have resulted in 0.5 D of hyperopia and flipping of the astigmatic axis. Choosing the ORA lens recommendation gave the patient a result closer to the preoperative goal.

Case 4: Monofocal Lens on Post-LASIK Patient

A 61-year-old post myopic LASIK male with uncorrected visual acuity of 20/60 and preoperative refraction of +1.00 +0.50 × 145. He underwent femtosecond laser-assisted catarect surgery, capsulorhexis, prechop and incision placement. The surgical plan was to place a Tecnis PCB00 monofocal intraocular lens targeted at plano.

Holladay 1 predicted an intraocular lens power of 21.0 D, resulting in an estimated residual refraction of ×0.23 D. Intraoperatively, the ORA estimated a residual refraction of –0.05 with a 20.0 D lens. Given the difference, the intermediate power, 20.5 D lens was selected (Fig. 39.9).

Postoperative week 2 refraction was plano with a final distance vision of 20/15.

In this case, preoperative lens calculations would have resulted in 0.5 D of myopia. Choosing the intermediate value between preoperative calculations and the intraoperative aberrometer resulted in a plano result.

THE FUTURE

It is important for all cataract surgeons to consider the accuracy of their postoperative outcomes as patient expectations continue to rise. With the first generation of LASIK patients now beginning to reach cataract age, traditional methods of predicting intraocular lens power may not be sufficient to account for the unique aberrations of these complex eyes.

Intraoperative aberrometry is an exciting development in cataract surgery technology, and increasingly accurate predictions are possible with each successive generation. In addition, these devices are driving a trend towards easier analysis of postoperative data, and towards the sharing of de-identified data to further improve the outcomes of all surgeons globally.

Furthermore, increasingly integrated solutions are being developed which will allow all devices in the clinic and operating room to communicate with one another. One of these advances is iris registration, embodied in such devices as Alcon's Verion Image Guidance System. These systems match up the iris of a patient undergoing biometry calculations with the same iris landmarks while the patient is undergoing surgery. This feature corrects for cyclotorsional errors, decreases the need for preoperative toric marking and increases the precision of astigmatic treatments. When synced with a femtosecond laser, preplanned main, secondary and astigmatic incisions can be precisely placed based on preoperative iris landmarks.

A fully integrated and synced biometry device, surgical planning platform and intraoperative aberrometer can decrease staff data entry time, minimize transcription errors and further optimize the efficiency of workflow.

Although preoperative calculations will likely always exist, we can envision a future in which we rely more heavily on the precise, customized measurements of an intraoperative aberrometer rather than on today's population-based regression formulas. In the future, we will hope to truly customize lens selection for each individual patient in order to achieve the best possible postoperative results.

REFERENCES

1. Visser N, Nuijts RM, de Vries NE, et al. Visual outcomes and patient satisfaction after cataract surgery with toric multifocal intraocular lens implantation. J Cataract Refract Surg. 2011;37(11):2034-42.
2. Behndig A, Montan P, Stenevi U, et al. Aiming for emmetropia after cataract surgery: Swedish National Cataract Register study. J Cataract Refract Surg. 2012;38(7):1181-6.
3. Sheard R. Optimising biometry for best outcomes in cataract surgery. Eye. 2013;28(2):118-25.
4. Wiley WF, Bafna S. Intra-operative aberrometry guided cataract surgery. Int Opthalmol Clin. 2011;51(2):119-29.
5. Ianchulev T, Salz J, Hoffer K, et al. Intraoperative optical refractive biometry for intraocular lens power estimation without axial length and keratometry measurements. J Cataract Refract Surg. 2005;31(8):1530-6.
6. Ianchulev T, Hoffer KJ, Yoo SH, et al. Intraoperative refractive biometry for predicting intraocular lens power calculation after prior myopic refractive surgery. Ophthalmology. 2014;121(1):56-60.
7. Fram NR, Masket S, Wang L. Comparison of intraoperative aberrometry, OCT-based IOL formula, Haigis-L, and Masket formulae for IOL power calculation after laser vision correction. Ophthalmology. 2015;122(6):1096-101.
8. Packer M. Effect of intraoperative aberrometry on the rate of postoperative enhancement: retrospective study. J Cataract Refract Surg. 2010;36(5):747-55.
9. Woodcock MG, Lehmann R, Cionni RJ, et al. Intraoperative aberrometry versus standard preoperative biometry and a toric IOL calculator for bilateral toric IOL implantation with a femtosecond laser: One-month results. J Cataract Refractr Surg. 2016;42(6):817-25.
10. Kim JH, Shammas A, Labree L, et al. Correcting the corneal power measurements for intraocular lens power calculations after myopic laser in situ keratomileusis. Am J Opthalmol. 2003;136(3):426-32.
11. Igarashi A, Kamiya K, et al. Clinical evaluation of accuracy of horizontal median limbal marking. Optom Vis Sci. 2013;90(6):540-5.
12. Elhofi AH, Helaly HA. Comparison between digital and manual marking for toric intraocular lenses. medicine (Baltimore). 2015;94(38):e/618
13. Wiley WF. Use of real-time refractive measurements to improve outcomes with toric IOL. Virginia: ASCRS; 2011.
14. Huelle JO, Katz T, Druchkiv V, et al. First clinicial results on the feasibility , quality and reproducibility of aberrometry-based intraoperative refraction during cataract surgery. Br J Opthalmol. 2014;98(11):1484-91.
15. Haque M, Jabbour S, Fadlallah A, et al. Integrity of intrastromal arcuate keratotomies performed by femtosecond laser. J Refractr Surg. 2016;32(1):67-8.

Chapter 40

Managing a Ruptured Capsule during Cataract Surgery

Juliet Essilfie, David Xu, Jean Pierre Hubschman

INTRODUCTION

Ruptured lens capsule has long been a feared complication of cataract surgery because it has the potential to cause multiple negative consequences. Risk factors for this complication include: surgeon inexperience, dense white/brunescent cataract, pseudoexfoliation, diabetic retinopathy, glaucoma, phacodonesis, increased age and small-dilated pupil size.[1] One of the most important consequences of a ruptured capsule is a decreased vision potential. Eyes with capsule rupture are 3.8 times more likely to have a best corrected visual acuity (BCVA) of less than 20/40.[2] Factors influencing vision morbidity include retinal detachment, postoperative endophthalmitis and cystoid macular edema (CME).

Compared to eyes with uncomplicated cataract surgery, eyes with posterior capsule rupture have a 10–20% increased incidence of CME.[3] The incidence of retinal detachment following an uncomplicated cataract surgery is less than 1%. Conversely, it is up to 4% in eyes with capsule rupture.[4] There is also an 8-14-fold increased incidence of endophthalmitis in eyes following capsule rupture.[5-7] This greater risk of endophthalmitis can be explained by the decreased bacterial load required to cause an infection in the vitreous. Unlike aqueous humor which has rapid turnover rate (2.4 ± 0.6 μL/min), the vitreous is a denser and less mobile structure that does not regenerate. Therefore, the vitreous tends to be a better environment for the growth of bacteria.

IDENTIFYING A RUPTURED CAPSULE

Mechanisms for ruptured capsule include radialization of an anterior capsule tear, direct puncture by the phacoemulsification probe tip or mechanical trauma to the capsule during manipulation of the native or artificial lens (Figs. 40.1A to C). In addition to direct visualization of the tear, there are other perioperative signs that can aid the surgeon in detecting a broken capsular bag. The surgeon may experience rebound loss in which pieces of the nuclear material become more difficult to move around because they are entangled in vitreous that has prolapsed into the anterior chamber. Another sign is that the depth of the anterior chamber increases thus, decreasing the focus of the microscope. The pupil may also assume an abnormal or peaked shape as vitreous flows into the anterior chamber and out of the incisional corneal wound causing tension along the involved pupil margin. Phacoemulsification also

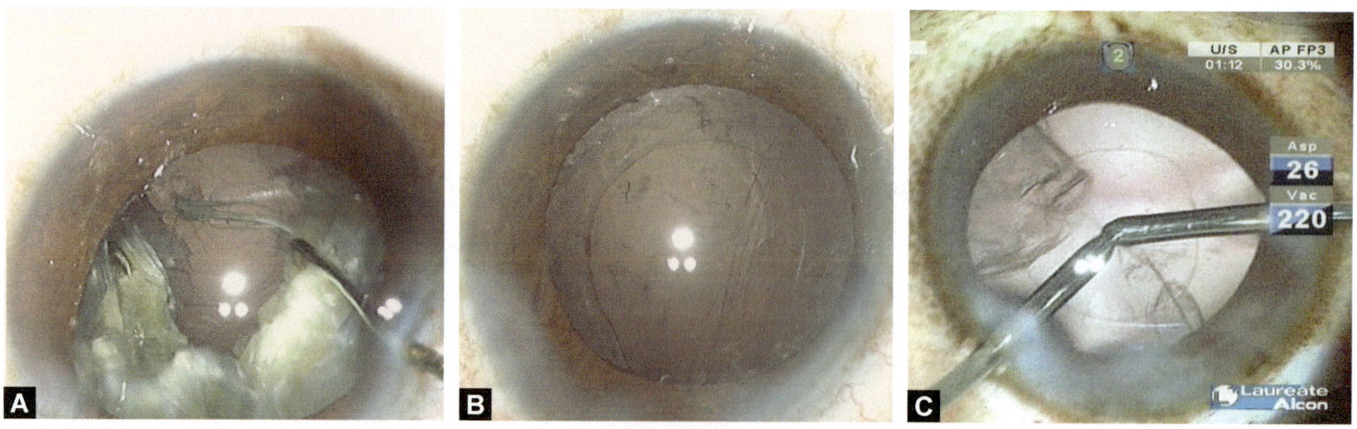

Figs. 40.1A to C: Different mechanisms of posterior capsular rupture. (A) During nucleus cracking with the second instrument; (B) Radialized rhexis tear; (C) Posterior capsule caught in the IA probe during cortex aspiration just before PCR (note the posterior capsule folds).

Source: Dr Manas Nath, Aravind Eye Hospital, Puducherry, India becomes more difficult due to blockage of the probe tip by vitreous. Depending on the amount of lens material remaining in the capsule, the surgeon may also notice a sudden increase in red reflex.[8] Lastly lens material that appears to be fading off into the distance can signal to the presence of a ruptured capsule.

PERIOPERATIVE MANAGEMENT

Though initially daunting it is important for the surgeon to remain calm when a capsule rupture is encountered. Despite the dreaded sequelae of a ruptured capsule, a majority of patients still attain a BCVA of 20/40 or better if no further complications are encountered.[2]

Stabilize the Anterior Chamber

Upon capsule rupture, the phacoemulsification probe should be kept in the anterior chamber with the foot pedal in position one. This allows for continuous irrigation which maintains the volume of the anterior chamber. This relative increase in pressure in the anterior chamber helps keep the vitreous fluid in the vitreous chamber. Alternatively, removing the probe decreases the pressure in the anterior chamber which could encourage vitreous prolapse because the vitreous has a tendency to move from areas of high pressure to low pressure.

Using the second hand, inject a dispersive ophthalmic viscosurgical device (OVD) through a small paracentesis wound. Dispersive OVD is preferred to cohesive OVD because its lower viscosity prevents it from readily escaping the eye via the corneal wound. Its dispersive properties also allows it to stay in place during the dynamic fluidics caused by phacoemulsification.[9] A generous amount of the dispersive OVD should be applied. Gentle injection under the nucleus fragment and directly over the violated posterior capsule creates a desired partition between the vitreous cavity and posterior chamber by pushing the vitreous posteriorly and the lens fragments anteriorly. This also helps maintain the pressure of the anterior chamber so that the phacoemulsification probe can be safely removed without causing a decrease in the anterior chamber pressure. A 10-0 nylon suture should then be placed in the main incision to create a watertight closure.

Preparing for Anterior Vitrectomy

Anterior vitrectomy is not always indicated after a capsule tear. The surgeon may choose to forgo performing an anterior vitrectomy when the posterior capsule tear is very small and there is no vitreous prolapse. The small tear should be visualized in its entirety and without larger linear extensions radiating from it. In such a case, a small 2–3 mm posterior capsulotomy can be performed.[10] The surgical technique of posterior capsulorhexis is more challenging than that of anterior capsulorhexis so if in doubt, the posterior capsulotomy can be deferred to the postoperative period using Nd:YAG laser. Performance of the posterior capsulotomy is the key in avoiding visually significant capsular phimosis in the late postoperative period.

If, however, the capsule rupture is larger or there is evidence of vitreous prolapse, an anterior vitrectomy should be performed. Administration of additional anesthesia is not mandatory but is advisable because performing an anterior vitrectomy will prolong the total operative time. The patient also tends to feel the eye manipulation more with an anterior vitrectomy; so extra anesthetics may help keep the patient still during surgery, reducing the risk of iatrogenic complications. Anesthetic options include intracameral, intravitreal, or retrobulbar block. Preservative-free lidocaine should be used in the case of intraocular anesthesia. Keep in mind that contact of the posterior segment by lidocaine can cause a transient retinal amaurosis.[11] Retrobulbar block should be reserved for cases were pars plana vitrectomy (PPV) is performed. With a retrobulbar block, care must be taken to ensure that the globe has a watertight closure because posterior retrobulbar pressure could potentially lead to extrusion of the intraocular content.

There are additional instruments required to perform an anterior vitrectomy that may not be available in the standard cataract surgery tray (Table 40.1). Familiarity with these instruments is the key to ensuring efficient and prompt management of a ruptured capsule. The surgeon

Table 40.1: Instrument for anterior vitrectomy.

Extra dispersive ophthalmic viscosurgical device
Microvitreoretinal blade
Preservative-free kenalog
Forceps, needle holder, suture, scissors
Sheet's glide
Anterior vitrectomy hand-piece
25-guage J cannula
Extra BSS syringe
Lens retrieval instrument

should consider having a ready made sterile peel-pack specific for anterior vitrectomy to streamline the transition into performing this surgery. The list below describes the additional equipment needed.

- *Extra dispersive OVD:* As described earlier, it helps create a cleavage plane between the lens and the vitreous cavity while maintaining the anterior chamber.
- *Microvitreoretinal (MVR) blade,* to create a pars plana incision when PPV is indicated.
- *Preservative-free triamcinolone acetate* (i.e. Kenalog, Triesence), to aid with visualization of vitreous.
- *Forceps, needle holder, suture, scissors,* to close the main incision and create a watertight wound.
- *Sheet's glide*: This is typically placed under the nucleus and above the posterior capsule to effectively create a pseudoposterior capsule. It facilitates removal of nucleus fragments with the phacoemulsification probe while limiting the risk of dropping lens pieces into the posterior segment. It can also be used to remove epinuclear and cortex material without engaging significant amount of vitreous.
- *Anterior vitrectomy handpiece,* for vitrectomy.
- *25-gauge J-cannula,* for gentle and more controlled removal of cortex material.
- *Extra BSS syringe*
- *Lens retrieval instrument*

Approach to Anterior Vitrectomy

First create an incision for the anterior vitrectomy. Options for location of the incision include the pars plana approach or the limbal approach. The pars plana approach, the preferred approach for retina specialist, has multiple advantages. Its watertight incision allows for a closed working space thus creating less turbulence while facilitating thorough removal of lens fragments and prolapsed vitreous. There is also easier access to the capsular bag fornix for removal of lens material. Lastly it is easier to remove lens pieces that have already fallen into the vitreous cavity via the pars plana approach. Disadvantage of this approach includes potential complications such as a retinal tear or detachment due to surgeon inexperience. Therefore, the pars plana approach should be reserved for trained surgeons. The surgeon should also be confident in his or her ability to perform a 360° peripheral retinal exam to rule out retinal injury upon completion of the surgery.

The limbal approach tends to be the preferred approach for general cataract surgeons because there is less concern for inducing retinal injury (Fig. 40.2). In theory, there is a tendency for vitreous strands to persist in the anterior chamber with this approach. The vitreous strand may track into the incision as it attempts to travel towards a lower pressure gradient. Vitreous to wound can increase the

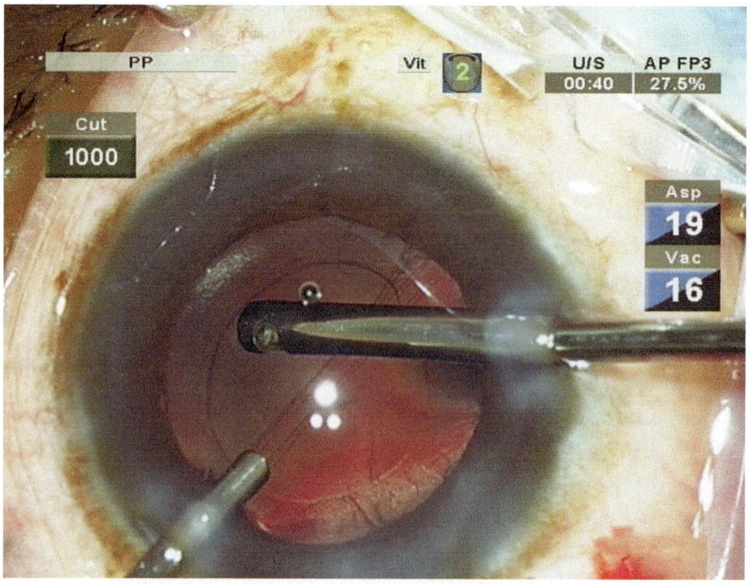

Fig. 40.2: Bimanual anterior vitrectomy via limbal approach. Note a second small side-port wound was created as opposed to using the main incision wound.
Source: Dr Manas Nath, Aravind Eye Hospital, Puducherry, India.

risk of postoperative endophthalmitis.[12] Nevertheless, it is very common to adequately remove any residual vitreous strands with the application of triamcinolone acetate when using the limbal approach.

Performing the Anterior Vitrectomy

The goal when performing the anterior vitrectomy is to safely remove any vitreous that has prolapsed into the anterior chamber and any remaining lens fragments while causing the least amount of damage to the retina. As such it is recommended that lens fragments that have fallen deep into the vitreous chamber be left behind. First, the surgeon must decide whether to use bimanual or coaxial irrigation—the former has a separate vitrector and irrigation while the latter has the irrigation physically attached to the vitrector. The setup for coaxial irrigation is easier. However, it has the disadvantage of causing local turbulence that could worsen capsular tear when the vitrector is working in the anterior vitreous (Fig. 40.3).

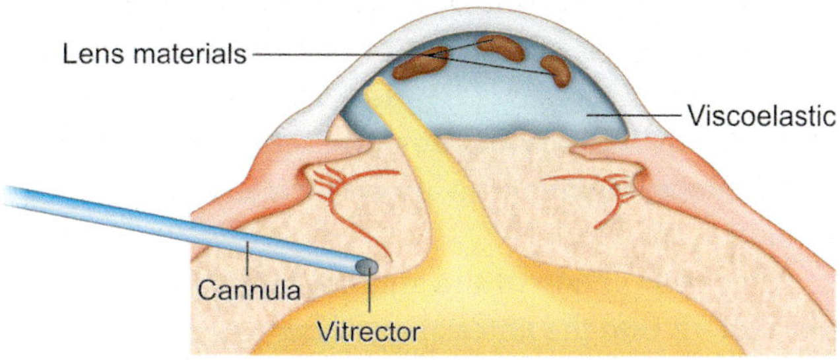

Fig. 40.3: Pars plana vitrectomy approach. Through a sclerotomy 4 mm away from the limbus, a coaxial irrigation and vitrector is used to remove the anterior vitreous, separating it from the remaining vitreous body. The aspiration port of the vitrector should face towards the cornea and always be in clear view of the surgeon during use.

If bimanual irrigation is chosen, introduce a 23-gauge infusion line via a separate sideport (the paracentesis wound created earlier during the cataract surgery can be used as well). This infusion line will help maintain the anterior chamber pressure as you proceed with the surgery. Then use a blade to create a sideport for the anterior vitrector. Apply a small amount of preservative-free triamcinolone into the anterior chamber to help visualize the vitreous (Fig. 40.4). If preservative-free triamcinolone is not available then, simply dilute the non-preserved triamcinolone to decrease toxicity to the retina. Diluted triamcinolone also avoids "over-staining the vitreous" which can cause the entire anterior chamber to look like a shaken snow globe.

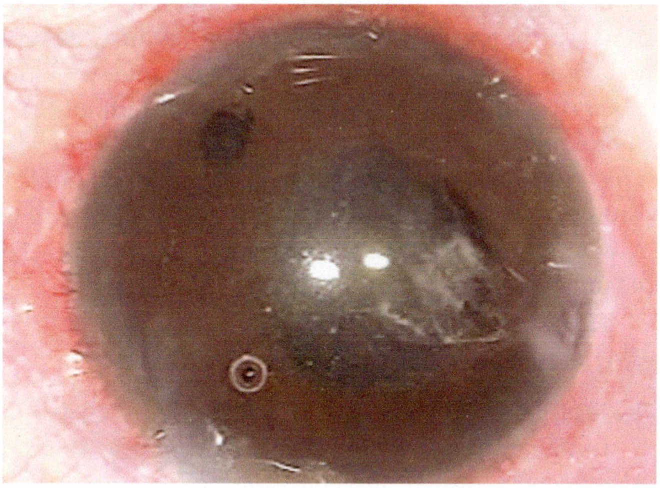

Fig. 40.4: Preservative-free steroid staining vitreous within the anterior chamber. Note the stronger staining close to the main incision wound on the right of the image, as vitreous tends to move towards lower pressure.
Source: Dr Madhu Shekhar, Aravind Eye Hospital, Madurai, Tamil Nadu, India.

The preferred initial vitrector mode is IA-Cut. In this mode, the cut rate is set to the highest setting available while the aspiration and vacuum setting is low. The high cut rate is ideal for vitreous removal because the cut starts immediately after aspiration is initiated. By doing so, it reduces turbulence and traction on the retina. In general, the aspiration port of the cutter should face towards the cornea and maintain a central position while cutting. Avoid working in the far periphery or in any area where there is no visualization (i.e. beyond the iris root). Doing so may cause stress on the vitreous base or an involuntary collision between the cutter and the iris, ciliary body or retina. The goal is to remove just enough vitreous to clear the central anterior vitreous cavity.

Once the vitreous has been cleared from the anterior chamber, the IA-Cut setting should be used for removal of residual nuclear lens fragments. The setting is best for lens fragment removal because there are 3 foot pedal positions to work with. The first pedal position is irrigation only. The second pedal position involves irrigation and aspiration which allows the vitrector to engage the residual fragment and then aspirate it. The third pedal position includes the irrigation, aspiration and cut mode so that the vitrector can chop the lens fragments if it is too stiff to be aspirated. Care should be taken to elevate the nuclear fragments towards the anterior chamber, as this is the safest space in which to work. Residual cortical fragments can be removed by turning off the cutter and using low vacuum or by using the J-cannula to manually aspirate the pieces. Avoid chasing lens fragments that have fallen deep into the vitreous chamber with the vitrector. This can cause pulling of the vitreous which increases the risk of inadvertent collision, bleeding, involuntary traction and retinal tear. Eyes with retained lens fragment can always be referred to the retina surgeon in the future.

After completion of the anterior vitrectomy, consider injecting air into the anterior chamber to identify vitreous remnant. Vitreous and air have a distinct interface that aids in the surgeon's visualization. Sweep the anterior chamber 360° to remove any remnant vitreous strands.

Inject Miochol/acetylcholine (less than equal to 2 mL of 10 mg/mL) into the anterior chamber to constrict the pupil. A peaked iris after injection suggests persistent vitreous strands in the anterior chamber. Miochol has the additional benefit of decreasing postoperative intraocular pressure spikes (IOP spikes). Additional intracameral antibiotic (i.e. gatifloxacin) or subconjunctival antibiotic (i.e. cefuroxime) is recommended to decrease the risk of endophthalmitis.[13] Note that intracameral cefuroxime is contraindicated in eyes with posterior capsule rupture due to concern for potential retinal toxicity.[14]

Intraocular Lens Placement

The decision of where to place the intraocular lens depends on the integrity of the remnant posterior capsule. Options include endocapsular intraocular lens (IOL), sulcus IOL, iris-sutured IOL, scleral-fixated IOL and anterior chamber IOL (ACIOL). Placement of endocapsular, sulcus and scleral-fixated IOL should be done prior to injection of Miochol as described above. Alternatively, placement of iris-sutured and anterior chamber IOL should be done after the injection of Miochol. An endocapsular IOL with a single piece acrylic lens is appropriate for a small anterior or posterior capsular tear that can be seen in its entirety with an intact hyaloid face. The lens should be oriented with its haptics situated 90° away from the tear before it is unfolded in the capsular bag.[15]

For larger capsule tear with good posterior capsular support, the IOL should be placed in the ciliary sulcus. A 3-piece IOL is the lens of choice (Fig. 40.5). Single piece foldable IOL should be avoided because it increases the risk of CME, pigment dispersion, chronic iridocyclitis and ocular hypertension.[16]

For capsule rupture where the capsulozonular integrity is questionable or clearly inadequate, a scleral-fixated IOL can be chosen. This technique allows for the attachment

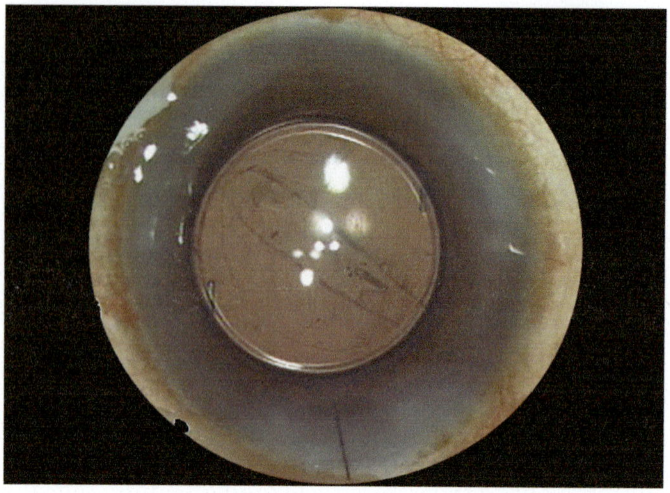

Fig. 40.5: Three-piece IOL placed in the sulcus. Note the posterior capsular tear.
Source: Dr Shivakumar Chandrasekaran, Aravind Eye Hospital, Tirunelveli, Tamil Nadu, India

of the IOL to the sclera within the sulcus using a suture (typically 10-0 polypropylene). An ab interno (passing the needle from inside to outside) or ab externa (passing the needle from outside to inside) approach can be chosen.

The surgeon may alternatively elect to place an ACIOL in the setting of poor capsular support, deep anterior chamber and normal corneal endothelium. The IOL can be inserted into the anterior chamber by enlarging the corneal incision to approximately 6 mm or by creating a new 6 mm scleral tunnel. Unlike an enlarged corneal incision, a scleral tunnel avoids inducing additional astigmatic refractive error. The scleral tunnel can be created adjacent to the superior or temporal limbus. A peripheral iridotomy (PI) can then be made before or after inserting the lens, depending on the surgeon's preference. Note that there is a possibility of bleeding after making the PI which could potentially limit the view for implantation of the lens. The PI can be created using the vitrector or by grasping a piece of iris and excising it with a scissors. If the vitrector is used to create the PI, it is recommended to use the IA-Cut mode. This will cause the aspiration to first engage the iris into the port followed by cutting of the iris. Only one or two cuts are needed to create a PI. The PI should ideally be located away from the IOL haptics. Alternatively, the PI can also be created via laser on postoperative day 1. The purpose of the PI is to avoid postoperative pupillary block and ocular hypertension.

With the anterior chamber filled with dispersive OVD, a Sheet's glide can then be used to facilitate insertion of the ACIOL (Fig. 40.6). Using forceps, the ACIOL can be gently

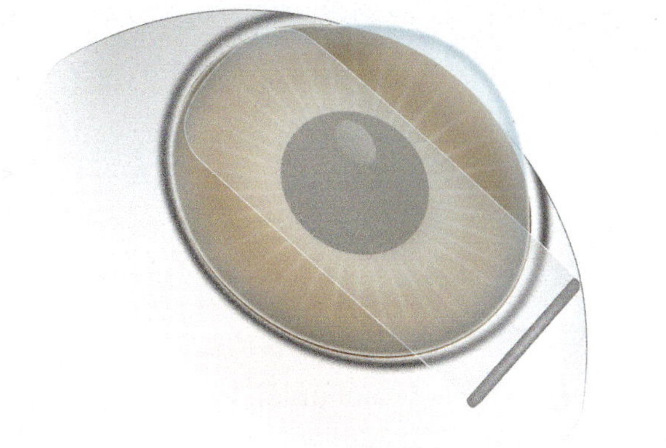

Fig. 40.6: A Sheet's glide is placed into the anterior chamber via a scleral tunnel to facilitate insertion of an anterior chamber IOL.

placed through the scleral tunnel. Care should be taken to ensure both ends of the haptics remain above the iris plane. The diameter of the ACIOL should be equal to the limbal white-to-white diameter plus 1 mm. Once the ACIOL is securely in place, close the scleral tunnel with 10-0 nylon to ensure a watertight wound.

Selection of IOL Power

It is important to remember that the power of the IOL must be adjusted if the decision is made to insert an extracapsular IOL. There are a few general rules for choosing IOL power in the event that the surgeon does not have the lens calculations for alternative IOL positions. The more anterior the IOL, the less power the IOL needs. For sulcus lens, the IOL power should be reduced by 0.5 D, 1 D or 1.5-2 D if the original predicted IOL power was less than 18 D, 18–25 D or more than 25 D respectively. The power of the IOL placed in the anterior chamber typically needs to be decreased by 3–3.5 D.

POSTOPERATIVE MANAGEMENT

It is important to discuss the surgical complication with the patient. Medical jargon can be confusing to the patient so a simple explanation is recommended. The patient should be reassured that the bulk of the cataract was extracted and that the IOL had to be placed in a different location for optimal visual outcome. All patients will need a detailed posterior segment exam to rule out retained lens fragments or a retinal tear. They will also need more frequent follow-up to monitor for intraocular pressure spikes and inflammation. Consider prolonged steroid or nonsteroidal anti-inflammatory drugs (NSAIDs) treatment to decrease the risk of postoperative CME. The surgeon should have a low threshold for referring the patient for an evaluation with a retina specialist, particularly if they are not confident in doing a 360° peripheral retinal exam.[17]

REFERENCES

1. Narendran N, Jaycock P, Johnston RL, et al. The Cataract National Dataset electronic multicentre audit of 55,567 operations: risk stratification for posterior capsule rupture and vitreous loss. Eye (Lond). 2009;23(1):31-7.
2. Ionides A, Minassian D, Tuft S. Visual outcome following posterior capsule rupture during cataract surgery. Br J Ophthalmol. 2001;85(2):222.
3. Blomquist PH, Rugwani RM. Visual outcomes after vitreous loss during cataract surgery performed by residents. J Cataract Refract Surg. 2002;28(5):847-52.
4. Jakobsson G, Montan P, Zetterberg M, et al. Capsule complication during cataract surgery: retinal detachment after cataract surgery with capsule complication. J Cataract Refract Surg. 2009;35(10):1699-705.
5. Wong T, Chee SP. The epidemiology of acute endophthalmitis after cataract surgery in an Asian population. Ophthalmology. 2004;111(4):699-705.
6. Hatch WV, Cernat G, Wong D, et al. Risk factors for acute endophthalmitis after cataract surgery: a population-based study. Ophthalmology. 2009;116(3):425-30.
7. Durand ML. Endophthalmitis. Clin Microbiol Infect. 2013;19(3):227-34.
8. Jacobs PM. Vitreous loss during cataract surgery: prevention and optimal management. Eye. 2008;22(10):1286-9.
9. Devgan U. Understanding and using the full spectrum of OVDs. Rev Ophthalmol; 2009.
10. Ronge L. Posterior capsular rupture during cataract surgery. EyeNet Mag; 2005.
11. Hoffman RS, Fine IH. Transient no light perception visual acuity after intracameral lidocaine injection. J Cataract Refract Surg. 1997;23(6):957-8.
12. Ruiz RS, Teeters VW. The vitreous wick syndrome. Am J Ophthalmol. 1970;70(4):483-90.
13. Shorstein NH, Winthrop KL, Herrinton LJ. Decreased postoperative endophthalmitis rate after institution of intracameral antibiotics in a Northern California eye department. J Cataract Refract Surg. 2013;39(1):8-14.
14. Delyfer MN, Rougier MB, Leoni S, et al. Ocular toxicity after intracameral injection of very high doses of cefuroxime during cataract surgery. J Cataract Refract Surg. 2011;37(2):271-8.
15. Aaron M, Chen S, Davison J, et al. Complex Case management: choice of IOL after an anterior capsular tear. Cataract Refract Surg Today. 2011.
16. Chang DF, Masket S, Miller KM, et al. Complications of sulcus placement of single-piece acrylic intraocular lenses. J Cataract Refract Surg. 2009;35(8):1445-58.
17. Dubey R, Birchall W, Grigg J. Improved refractive outcome for ciliary sulcus-implanted intraocular lenses. Ophthalmology. 2012;119(2):261-5.

Chapter 41

Challenging Cataract Cases: Posterior Polar

Erika Tanaka, Kevin M Miller

INTRODUCTION

Posterior polar cataracts (PPC) are unique, dense white, congenital opacities that are located at the posterior pole of the crystalline lens. They can be a problem for patients and cataract surgeons alike in that they are often associated with an abnormal posterior capsule at the site of this opacity. These types of cataracts pose a unique challenge to the cataract surgeon given their predisposition to posterior capsule rupture, vitreous loss, and dropped lens fragments due to a strong adherence of the opacity to the weak or incompletely formed posterior capsule. Special precautions and modifications to surgical technique during cataract surgery can decrease risk for complications associated with posterior capsule rupture.

The pathogenesis of PPC is currently unknown, although it has been suggested that PPC is caused by persistence of the hyaloid artery or by invasion of the lens by mesoblastic tissue (Fig. 41.1).[1]

Posterior polar cataracts can occur sporadically or be inherited in an autosomal dominant fashion. Autosomal dominant posterior polar cataracts are genetically heterogeneous. Two loci on 1p36 and 20p12 have been associated with PPC. Additionally, mutations in *CRYAB* on 11q21 and *PITX3* on 10q25 have been associated with PPC. Patients with mutations in *PITX3* can have isolated PPC or PPC associated with other anterior segment developmental abnormalities, such as Peter's anomaly, peripheral sclerocornea, iris defects, and zonular abnormalities.[2,3]

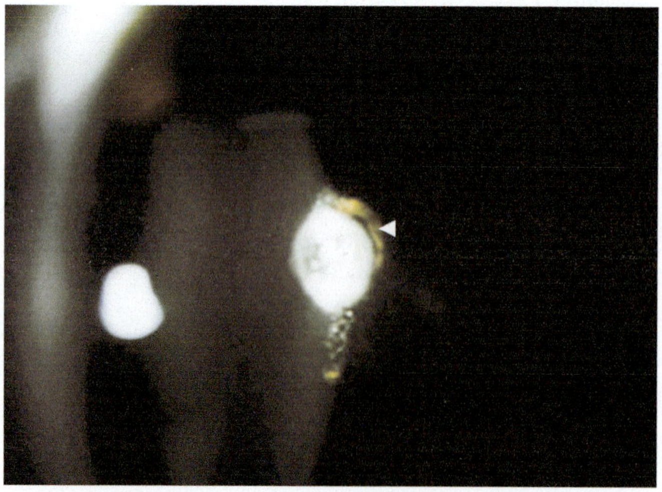

Fig. 41.1: Slit-lamp photograph of a posterior polar cataract with attached remnants of hyaloid vasculature (arrowhead).
Source: Dr Manas Nath, Aravind Eye Hospital, Puducherry, India.

CLINICAL PRESENTATION

Posterior polar cataracts are usually present bilaterally and can be stationary or progressive. Stationary PPC is characterized by a dense, white, disciform plaque opacity located on the central posterior capsule, surrounded by concentric rings in a bull's eye pattern. This opacity has a cone-shaped projection into the subcapsular region and central posterior cortex. It is seldom visually significant (Figs. 41.2A and B). Progressive PPC is associated with progressively expanding subcapsular opacities in the posterior cortex extending peripherally from the central plaque (Fig. 41.3). Progressive PPC is associated with symptomatic glare as the peripheral opacity enlarges. In general, the most common symptoms associated with PPC are glare in photopic illumination conditions and difficulty reading. Despite glare disability, many patients have excellent visual acuity. Most patients do not experience a decrease in visual acuity until the more typical age-related cataract develops.

At presentation, eyes with PPC can be classified into three clinical categories. The first type has an intact posterior capsule that is at risk of dehiscence (Fig. 41.4). The second type has a preexisting posterior capsule defect. A preexisting capsule defect can be detected on slit-lamp biomicroscopy as an elliptically shaped hole that is usually vertically oriented around the central bull's eye opacity. Iridescent lens particles and onion skinning of the central plaque can also be seen (Figs. 41.5A and B). The third type presents with a spontaneous dislocation of the lens through the posterior capsular defect.[4]

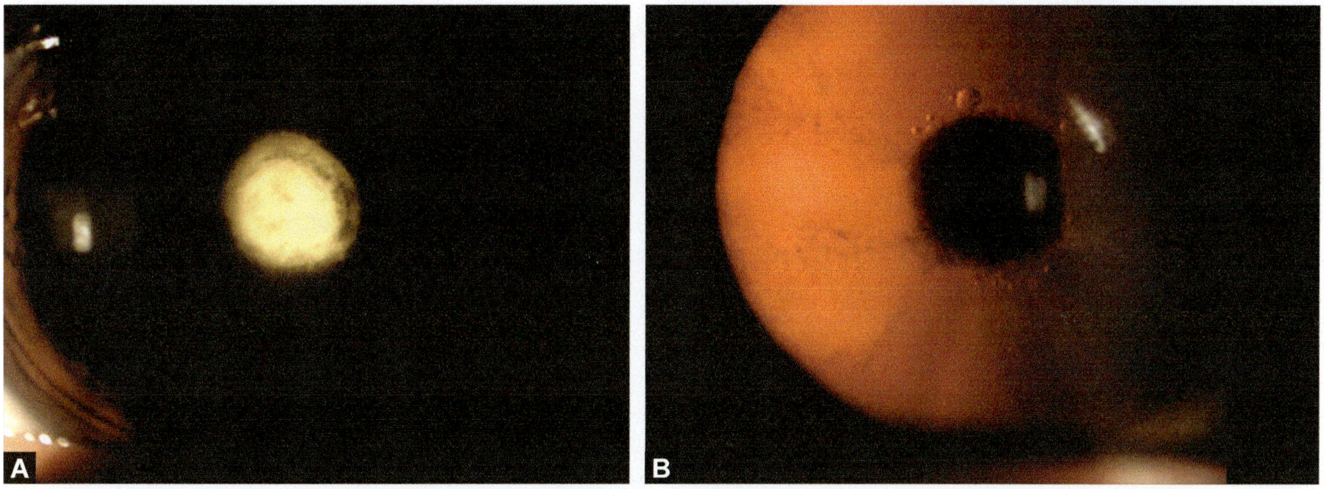

Figs. 41.2A and B: Slit-lamp photographs of stationary PPC with direct (A) and retroillumination (B).
Source: Uday Devgan.

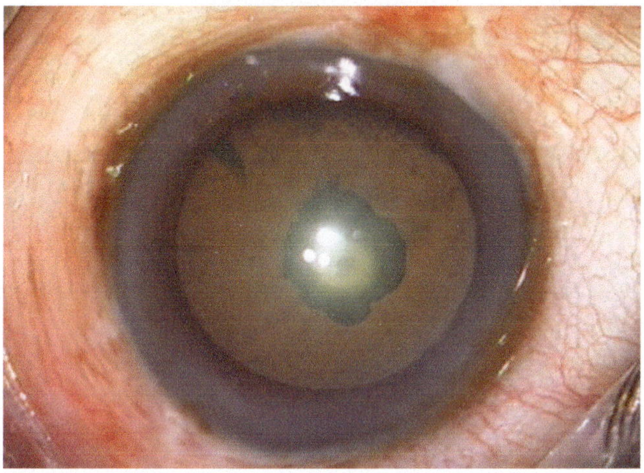

Fig. 41.3: Photograph of progressive type PPC with expanding subcapsular opacities in the posterior cortex extending peripherally from the central plaque.
Source: Dr Shivakumar Chandrasekaran, Aravind Eye Hospital, Tirunelveli, Tamil Nadu, India.

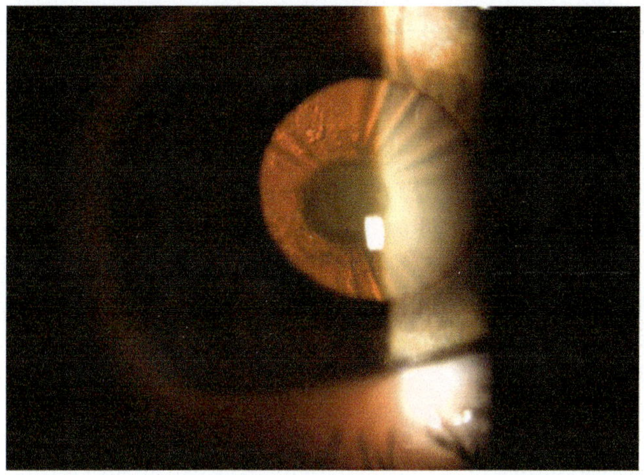

Fig. 41.4: PPC with high risk for capsule rupture. The radial striae in the posterior capsule indicate posterior capsule compromise.
Source: Uday Devgan.

It can be difficult to distinguish a true PPC from a focal, dense posterior subcapsular cataract (PSC). PPCs have well-defined, sharply demarcated borders while PSCs have less defined edges. However, making this distinction can be especially difficult in cases where the posterior opacification is obscured by a dense nucleus. Given the high risk of complications from a PPC, it is best to err on the side of approaching such cataracts as PPCs.

Two systems have been proposed for grading the severity of PPC. [1]

- Schroeder classification:
  - *Grade 1:* A small opacity without any effect on the optical quality of the clear part of the lens.
  - *Grade 2:* A two-thirds obstruction of the red reflex without other effect.
  - *Grade 3:* A disk-like opacity in the posterior capsule surrounded by an area of further optical distortion. Only a dilated pupil shows a clear red reflex surrounding this zone.
  - *Grade 4:* The opacity is totally occlusive. No clear red reflex is obtained by dilation of the pupil.
- Singh's classification:
  - *Type 1:* The posterior polar opacity is associated with a posterior subcapsular cataract.
  - *Type 2:* Sharply defined round or oval opacity with ringed appearance like an onion with or without grayish spots at the edge.

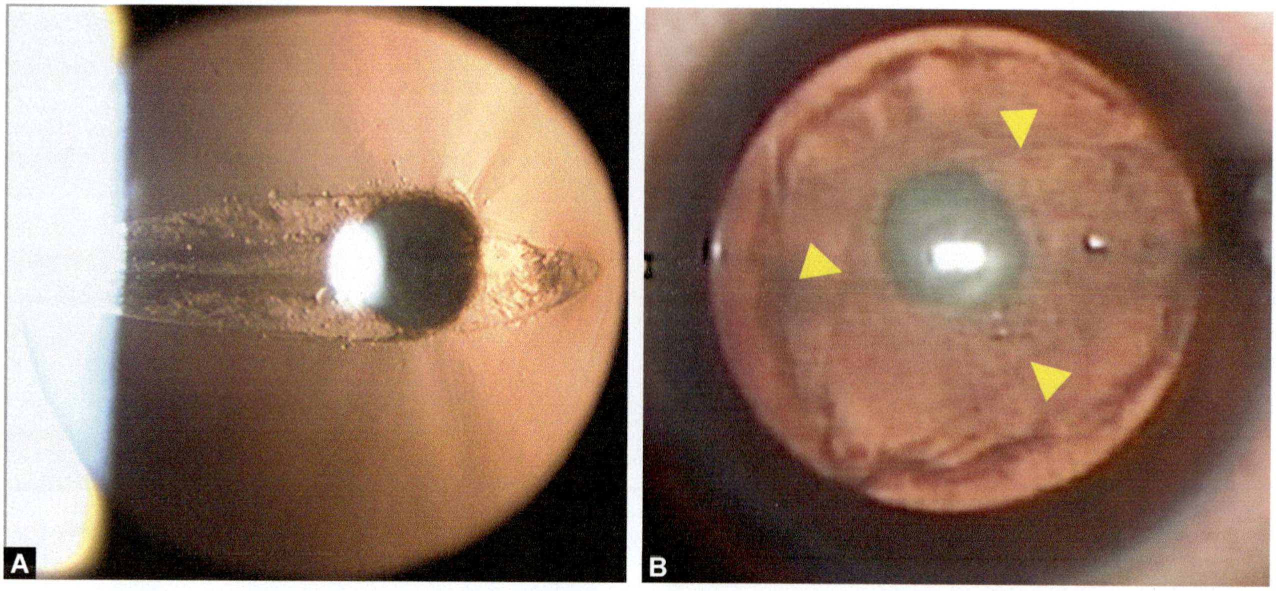

Figs. 41.5A and B: Posterior polar cataracts (PPC) with pre-existing posterior capsular rupture. Slit-lamp photograph (A) and surgical view with posterior capsule defect outlined with yellow arrowheads (B).
Source: Dr Manas Nath, Aravind Eye Hospital, Puducherry, India.

- *Type 3:* Sharply defined round or oval white opacity with dense white spots at the edge often associated with thin or absent posterior capsule.
- *Type 4:* Combination of one of the above 3 types with nuclear sclerosis.

RISK FOR POSTERIOR CAPSULE RUPTURE

The incidence of posterior capsule rupture during removal of PPC has been reported to be as high as 36%.[5] However, with proper precautions and modifications to surgical technique discussed later in this chapter, more recent rates of posterior capsule rupture have decreased to 6–7%.[6]

In some eyes with PPC, disruption of the posterior capsule can be detected preoperatively on slit-lamp examination. For eyes with a seemingly intact capsule, increasing size of the polar opacity has been associated with a higher risk of posterior capsule rupture.[11]

In addition to clinical examination, anterior segment optical coherence tomography (AS-OCT) can be used to identify eyes at highest risk for posterior capsule rupture. In a study by Chan et al., AS-OCT was used to grade PPC with no obvious capsule tear on clinical examination. Their grading system looked at the relationship of the polar opacity to the posterior capsule on high-resolution AS-OCT images. Grade 3 (high risk) cataracts were those with a defect in the posterior capsule or those where the posterior capsule could not be delineated from the polar opacity (Fig. 41.6). Grade 1 or 2 (lower risk) cataract demonstrated a hyporeflective gap between the posterior capsule and the polar opacity.[6]

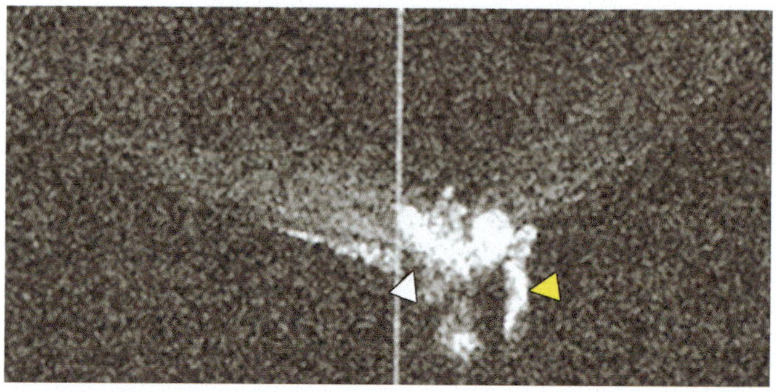

Fig. 41.6: High-resolution anterior segment OCT image of a grade 3 high-risk posterior polar cataract. This image demonstrates a discontinuity of the posterior capsule (white arrowhead) with attached remnants of the hyaloid vasculature (yellow arrowhead).
Source: Dr Manas Nath, Aravind Eye Hospital, Puducherry, India.

SURGICAL TECHNIQUE

Counseling

Before cataract surgery, patients should be counseled regarding the increased risk of intraoperative posterior capsular rupture, vitreous loss, and dropped nucleus. As PPCs are congenital, the possibility of amblyopia limiting visual outcome must also be considered and discussed with them. They should also be prepared for the need to perform an early neodymium: yttrium-aluminum-garnet (Nd:YAG) capsulotomy for residual plaque on the posterior capsule.[4]

Intracapsular and Pars Plana Techniques

Intracapsular cataract extraction and pars plana lensectomy can be used to remove PPC. No modifications are needed to these techniques to address the posterior polar cataract. Pars plana lensectomy eliminates the risk of an unexpected capsular rupture and may be considered in cases where a posterior capsule defect is detected preoperatively.[4]

Phacoemulsification

Phacoemulsification in eyes with PPC can be performed safely with important modifications in surgical technique to maintain the integrity of the barrier between the anterior and posterior segments in the context of a compromised posterior capsule. Great care must be taken during all steps of cataract surgery to avoid large pressure fluctuations and turbulence in the anterior chamber and to minimize pressure against the posterior capsule.

The capsulorhexis should be well centered and slightly smaller than the diameter of the optic with an optimal size of approximately 5 mm. Femtosecond lasers are very helpful in this regard. A capsulorhexis size of less than 4 mm can make it difficult to prolapse the nucleus into the anterior chamber, if needed, while a capsulorhexis larger than 5 mm may not provide adequate support for optic capture of a sulcus fixated intraocular lens (IOL) in the event of posterior capsular rupture.[4]

Cortical cleaving hydrodissection should be avoided in patients with a PPC. The fluid wave can rupture a compromised posterior capsule. Fine et al. described a technique for hydrodissection using small injections of fluid in multiple quadrants, avoiding extension of the fluid wave across the posterior capsule.[7] However, given the high risk for hydraulic rupture of the posterior capsule, many experts advocate simply avoiding the step of hydrodissection in its entirety.

Hydrodelineation can be helpful to create a cushion of epinucleus to protect the posterior capsule during nucleus removal. With the conventional technique for hydrodelineation, the cannula is pierced into the lens mid periphery and fluid is injected from the outside of the lens to the inside (Figs. 41.7A and B). With this technique, there is risk of fluid inadvertently being injected into the subcapsular plane, leading to unwanted hydrodissection. Allen et al. recommends deeply embedding the cannula in the nucleus and taking great care not to inject prior to embedding or after withdrawing the cannula from the nucleus to decrease the probability of inadvertent hydrodissection.[4] An additional risk of hydrodissection is mechanical stress to the capsular bag when embedding the cannula into a firm nucleus. Vasavada AR et al. have suggested an *inside-out* technique for hydrodelineation to avoid both the risk of inadvertent hydrodissection and stressing the capsule. A central trench is sculpted using the phacoemulsification probe with care not to rock the

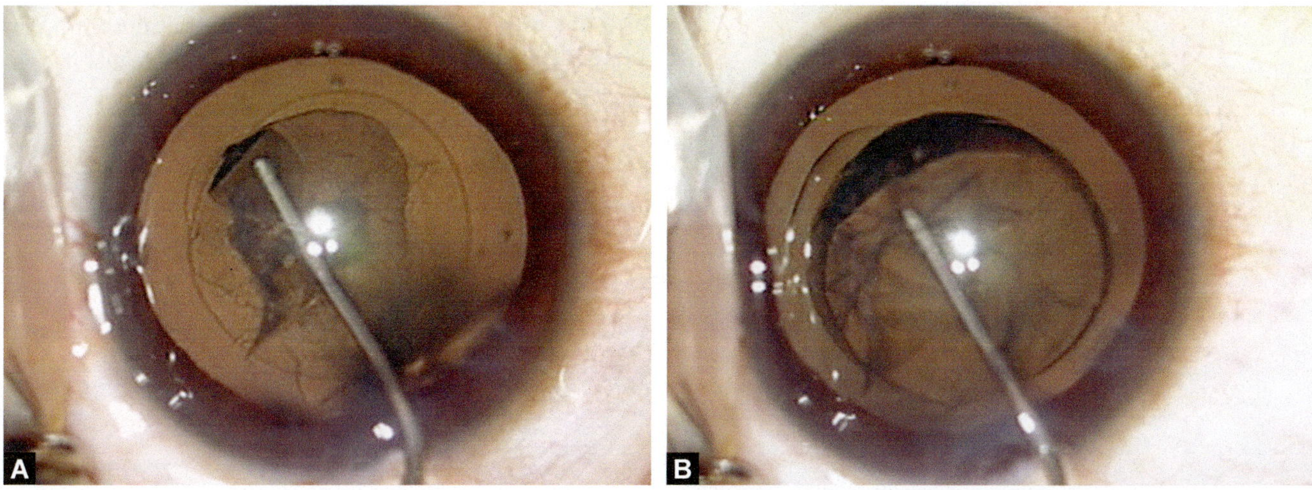

Figs. 41.7A and B: Surgical images of the conventional hydrodelineation technique showing insertion of the cannula into the lens midperiphery with initiation of the hydrodelineation (A) and finished hydrodelineation of the lens nucleus (B).
Source: Dr Shivakumar Chandrasekaran, Aravind Eye Hospital, Tirunelveli, Tamil Nadu, India.

lens mechanically. A right-angled cannula mounted on a 2 cc syringe filled with fluid is introduced through the main incision with the tip placed adjacent to the wall of the trench. The cannula is pushed into the lens material and fluid is injected through the wall of the trench delineating the nucleus from the epinucleus by fluid traversing inside out. This is performed in multiple waves from center to periphery. A golden ring is a sign of successful delineation (Figs. 41.8 and 41.9).[4] The advantages of this technique are reduced stress to the capsule and zonules, precise delineation of the central core of the nucleus, and reduced risk for inadvertent hydrodissection.

Rotation of the nucleus should be avoided as it can lead to posterior capsular rupture. After successful delineation, the nucleus can be aspirated within the cushion of the epinucleus, which protects the posterior capsule by minimizing disruption of the posterior cortex. Bimanual cracking maneuvers should be performed gently and with caution as traction on the already weak capsule can be enough to break the capsule. Low aspiration flow rate and vacuum should be used to minimize turbulence inside the eye and to prevent large postocclusion break surges.[8] Cohesive viscoelastic should be injected to reform the anterior chamber prior to withdrawal of the phacoemulsification probe to avoid sudden collapse of the anterior chamber and forward movement of the vitreous gel that could cause a defect in the posterior capsule to enlarge suddenly.

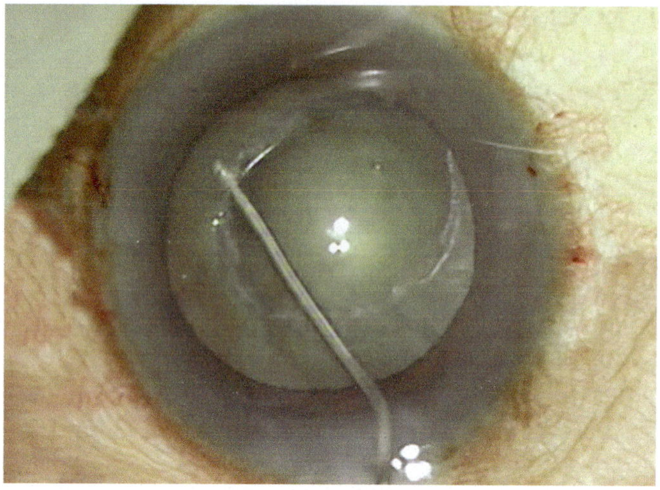

Fig. 41.8: Surgical image demonstrating the cannula position used for *inside-out* hydrodelineation.
Source: Dr Shivakumar Chandrasekaran, Aravind Eye Hospital, Tirunelveli, Tamil Nadu, India.

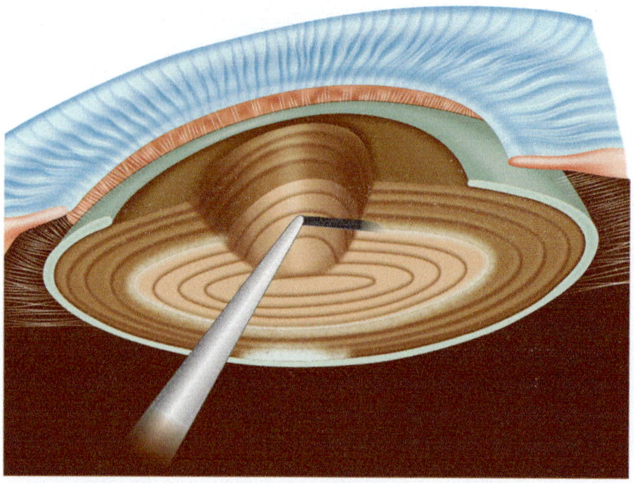

Fig. 41.9: Illustration demonstrating the cannula position used for *inside-out* hydrodelineation.

Multiple techniques have been suggested for epinucleus removal. Vasavada AR et al. suggest a two-step approach. First the epinucleus in the clock hours opposite the main incision is stripped off the capsule with the probe with care to leave the central posterior cortex intact. The sub-incisional epinucleus is separated from the capsule using careful hydrodissection. Risk for damaging the posterior capsule using hydrodissection at this time is slightly safer because the capsular bag is not fully occupied so the hydraulic pressure exerted by the hydrodissection is less likely to rupture the posterior capsule.[4]

An alternate technique for separating the residual epinucleus and cortex from the capsule is viscodissection. A dispersive viscoelastic is injected between the remaining lens material and the capsule to gently separate the two structures (Fig. 41.10). The injection of a dispersive viscoelastic pressurizes the anterior segment and can tamponade any defects in the capsule keeping the capsule and any vitreous back while pushing the remaining lens material forward. The viscoelastic must be injected in a slow

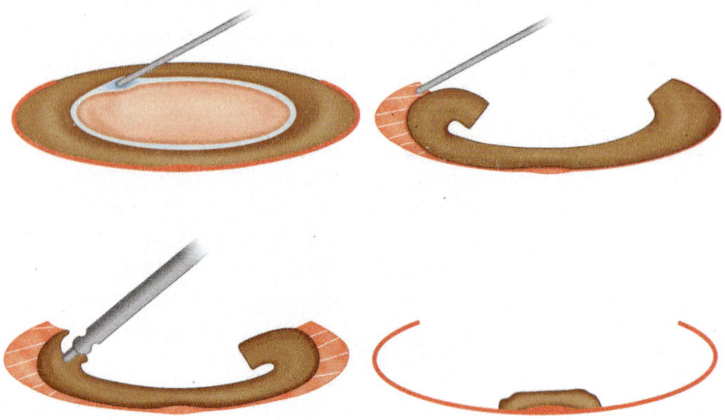

Fig. 41.10: Illustration demonstrating viscodissection by injecting dispersive viscoelastic between the remaining lens material and the capsule to gently separate the two structures.

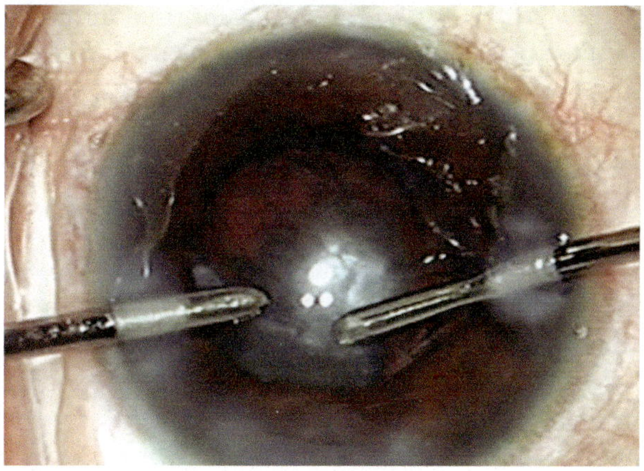

Fig. 41.11: Surgical image demonstrating I/A of the cortex leaving the posterior plaque for last.
Source: Dr Manas Nath, Aravind Eye Hospital, Puducherry, India.

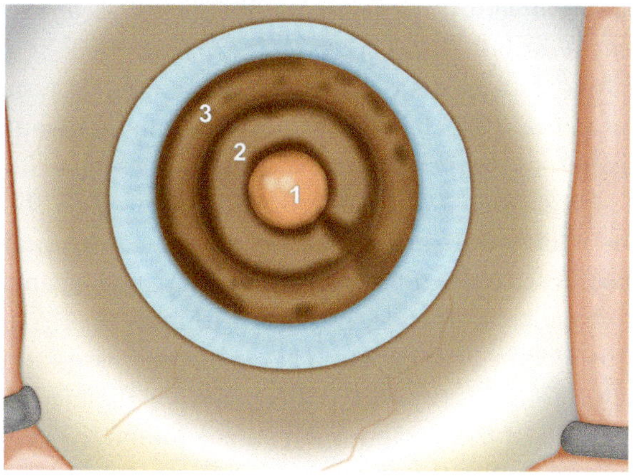

Fig. 41.12: Illustration demonstrating the cylindrical femtosecond laser lens fragmentation pattern.

and controlled manner, as there is still risk for rupturing the posterior capsule.[9]

Regardless of the technique used to separate the epinucleus and cortex from the capsule, this remaining lens material should aspirated with the irrigation/aspiration (I/A) hand piece on a low flow and low vacuum setting quadrant by quadrant, leaving the posterior plaque for last (Fig. 41.11).[4]

The plaque can be peeled gently by aspiration or with viscoelastic. It often looks like a manhole cover. Often times a fibrotic plaque will remain on the posterior capsule. A technique using a Corydon forceps to peel the plaque from the posterior capsule has been described. Alternatively, a posterior curvilinear capsulorhexis can be performed to remove the posterior plaque.[8] However, given the high risk for complications when manipulating the already abnormal posterior capsule, adherent posterior plaques should be left behind and posterior capsule polishing should be avoided. A Nd:YAG capsulotomy can be performed postoperatively if the patient is symptomatic from the remaining opacity. The laser capsulotomy is far safer than attempting to manipulate the posterior capsule.[4]

If a defect in the posterior capsule is discovered, a dispersive viscoelastic material should be injected over the area of the defect before the phacoemulsification or I/A probe is withdrawn from the eye. Careful anterior vitrectomy is followed by I/A of any remaining lens material.[4]

Femtosecond Laser-assisted Cataract Surgery

The femtosecond laser can be used to assist in cataract surgery for PPC. As previously discussed, a small and well centered capsulorhexis is essential. Use of the femtosecond laser allows for very predictable and well-centered capsulorhexis. Vasavada AR et al. described a technique of femtodelineation for use in eyes with PPC. After the laser is docked, the laser is used to make the anterior capsulorhexis, nuclear division, and corneal incisions. A cylindrical pattern of nucleus division is used to create 3 cylinders within the nucleus with the outermost cylinder set at 5.5 mm. An offset of 500–800 microns from the posterior capsule is set to protect the fragile posterior capsule from posterior gas accumulation. This pattern of nuclear division creates three cylinders of demarcation concentrically extending from the center of the nucleus leaving a fourth layer of protective epinuclear shell (Fig. 41.12). Once the patient is under the operating microscope, the incisions are opened, viscoelastic is injected, and the anterior capsule is removed. No hydrodissection or hydrodelineation is needed as the laser has already segmented the nucleus. Starting with the center cylinder of nucleus, each cylinder is gently emulsified within the protective outer epinuclear layer. Each concentric layer of nucleus acts as a shock absorber to protect the posterior cortex from turbulence. Segmentation of the nucleus also eliminates the need for mechanical chopping techniques that can place stress on the capsule and zonules. The epinucleus is then carefully aspirated off the capsule and the rest of the surgery is performed with the modifications previously discussed.[10]

INTRAOCULAR LENS SELECTION AND IMPLANTATION

Preoperative planning should include intraocular lenses (IOL) for the capsular bag, sulcus, and anterior chamber.

Intraoperatively, the integrity of the posterior capsule will dictate IOL choice and placement.

Once all lens material has been adequately removed using an I/A probe, it is very important to maintain anterior chamber and capsular bag volume before inserting an IOL. Irrigation should be continued through the I/A probe while viscoelastic material is injected through the paracentesis. Once the anterior chamber and bag are filled with viscoelastic, it is safe to gently withdraw the I/A probe.

Inspection of the posterior capsule and assessment of the available IOL support at this point will dictate the IOL to be used. If the posterior capsule is intact, the IOL can be placed within the capsular bag. Given the preexisting weakness of the posterior capsule, a defect in the posterior capsule can develop during IOL insertion.

In eyes with a small posterior capsular defect, a posterior continuous curvilinear capsulorhexis (PCCC) can be made to allow in-the-bag implantation by increasing the stability of the tear. The technique for creating a PCCC involves injecting a high viscosity viscoelastic through the defect to separate the posterior capsule from the anterior hyaloid. Microforceps are then used to grasp the edge of the tear and guide it circumferentially, creating a circular opening in the posterior capsule.[4]

In eyes with large posterior capsule defects (or small defects and failed PCCC) a 3-piece IOL can be placed in the sulcus if there is adequate zonular support. If a tear has not extended to involve the anterior capsule, optic capture can also be performed to provide additional stability for the optic. With viscoelastic material maintaining the anterior chamber, the optic is nudged posteriorly to trap it behind the anterior capsulorhexis. Once captured, the opening of the anterior capsulorhexis often assumes a cat eye or elliptical shape.[4] If the short axis of the anterior capsule opening is too small, it means the diameter of the capsulorhexis was too small.

If capsular damage is extensive and capsular bag instability is present, an appropriate IOL can be fixated to the sclera or iris or it can be placed in the anterior chamber without any modifications specific to PPC eyes.

After implanting the IOL, the viscoelastic material must be removed carefully. A bimanual technique that utilizes two small paracenteses is safer than a coaxial technique that utilizes the main incision. The latter technique risks chamber collapse and vitreous pressure against the posterior capsule or forward migration of vitreous gel through a compromised capsule during probe withdrawal. Placing a suture in the main incision may help ensure the integrity of the anterior chamber during the early postoperative period.[4]

PROGNOSIS

Patients with posterior polar cataracts often maintain excellent functional vision into their fourth and fifth decades of life. Once their cataracts become visually significant, cataract surgery can usually be undertaken safely with the necessary precautions to avoid complications due to posterior capsule compromise. Most patients experience significant improvements in vision after surgery. However, if there is vitreous loss, these patients experience the same increased risk of dropped nucleus or lens fragments, retinal detachment, and endophthalmitis experienced by other patients.[8]

REFERENCES

1. Kalantan H. Posterior polar cataract: a review. Saudi J Ophthalmol. 2012;26(1):41-9.
2. Addison PK, Berry V, Ionides AC, et al. Posterior polar cataract is the predominant consequence of a recurrent mutation in the PITX3 gene. Br J Ophthalmol 2005;89(2):138-41.
3. Finzi S, Li Y, Mitchell TN, et al. Posterior polar cataract: genetic analysis of a large family. Ophthalmic Genet. 2005;26(3):125-30.
4. Vasavada AR, Raj SM, Vasavada V, et al. Surgical approaches to posterior polar cataract: a review. Eye (Lond). 2012;26:761-70.
5. Hayashi K, Hayashi H, Nakao F, et al. Outcomes of surgery for posterior polar cataract. J Cataract Refract Surg. 2003;29:45-9.
6. Chan TC, Li EY, Yau JC. Application of anterior segment optical coherence tomography to identify eyes with posterior polar cataract at high risk for posterior capsule rupture. J Cataract Refract Surg. 2014;40(12):2076-81.
7. Fine IH, Packer M, Hoffman RS. Management of posterior polar cataract. J Cataract Refract Surg. 2003;29:16-9.
8. Vasavada A, Singh R. Phacoemulsification in eyes with posterior polar cataract. J Cataract Refract Surg. 1990;16:157-62.
9. Allen D, Wood C. Minimizing risk to the capsule during surgery for posterior polar cataract. J Cataract Refract Surg. 2002;28(5):742-4.
10. Vasavada AR, Vasavada V, Vasavada S, et al. Femtodelineation to enhance safety in posterior polar cataracts. J Cataract Refract Surg. 2015;41:702-7.
11. Kumar S, Ram J, Sukhija J, et al. Phacoemulsification in posterior polar cataract: does size of lens opacity affect surgical outcome? Clin Exp Ophthalmol. 2010;38:857-61.

Chapter 42

Challenging Cataract Cases: Dense Brunescent Cataracts and White Cataracts

Elisha Garg, John Bartlett

INTRODUCTION

Despite the advances in cataract surgery with the development of Kelman phacoemulsification (phaco) and foldable intraocular lens implantation,[1-3] the mature cataract still presents one of the biggest challenges to the cataract surgeon. The dense brunescent nuclear and white cataract each poses its own unique difficulties that can result in unwanted complications even with adequate preparation. A dense brunescent cataract occurs when the central nuclear component of the lens opacifies to the point of browning (Fig. 42.1).[4] A white cataract, on the other hand, can be either dense and hard, or soft and intumescent.[5,6]

Phacoemulsification using small clear corneal incisions has become the standard technique for cataract surgery in developed countries[7] such as the United States. In regions where resources are limited or technology is not available, extracapsular cataract extraction (ECCE) and more recently, manual small incision cataract surgery (MSICS)[8,9] are used for dense cataracts. However, these methods have disadvantages including large incision wounds, greater astigmatism, and longer postoperative recovery time. As such, this chapter will focus on techniques for successful phacoemulsification.

Preoperative evaluation should include a detailed history for possible trauma, particularly in the setting of unilateral cataract, and a review of potential causative medications. Imperative is a careful slit-lamp examination for corneal guttae, anterior chamber depth, zonular laxity or dehiscence, and phacodonesis.[10,11] Management of traumatic cataracts, pseudoexfoliation, and weak zonular support are discussed elsewhere in this section (*see* Chapter 44). Frequently there is a limited view of the fundus. While B-scan ultrasonography can exclude gross retinal detachments and masses, patients should be adequately counseled on the possibility of poor visual potential from undiagnosed retinal pathology (Fig. 42.2). Since dense cataracts can preclude optical biometry for lens calculation, A-scan biometry, preferably immersion, may be needed to select the appropriate lens power (Fig. 42.3).[12-14]

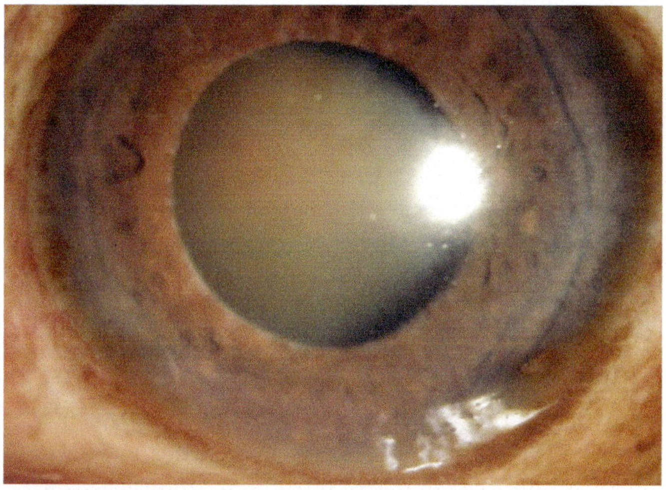

Fig. 42.1: Dense brunescent nuclear cataract. Notice the dark yellowing and browning of the sclerotic nucleus. The lens cortex material is poorly visible.
Source: Dr N Venkatesh Prajna, Aravind Eye Hospital, Madurai.

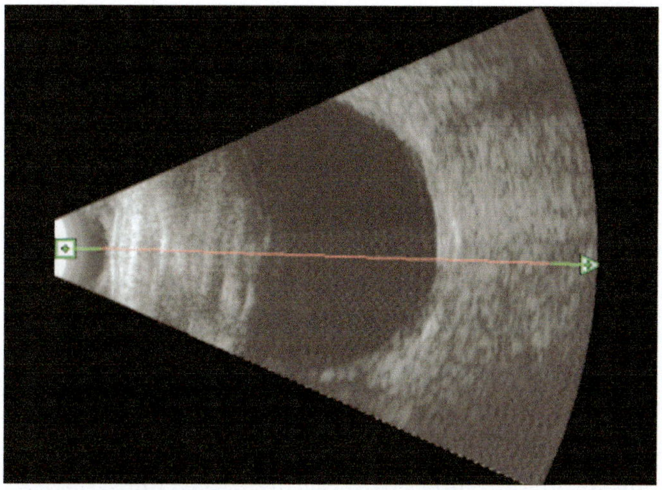

Fig. 42.2: B-scan ultrasonography. A dense lens is visible with no retinal detachment or masses.
Source: Dr N Venkatesh Prajna, Aravind Eye Hospital, Madurai.

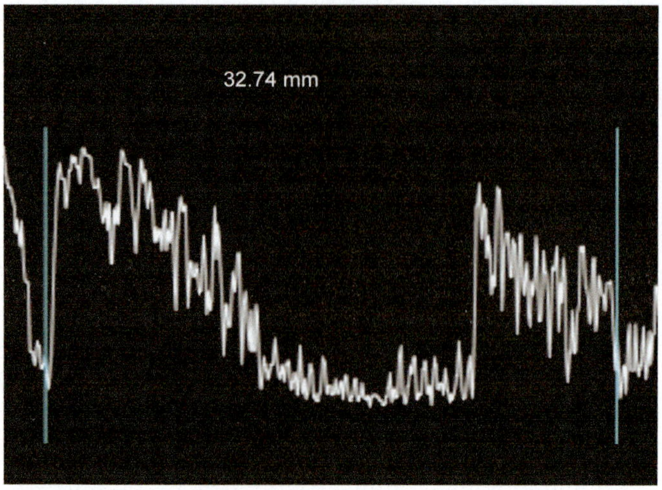

Fig. 42.3: A-scan measurement. This is an A-scan of a very long eye.
Source: Dr N Venkatesh Prajna, Aravind Eye Hospital, Madurai.

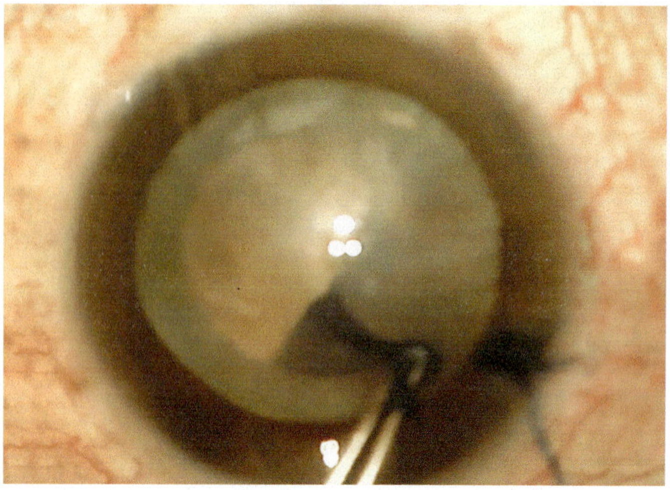

Fig. 42.4: Curvilinear capsulorhexis being created with trypan blue.
Source: Uday Devgan.

DENSE BRUNESCENT CATARACTS

Surgery for dense brunescent cataracts carries increased risk for four main complications: capsulorhexis tear, wound burn, corneal endothelial damage, and posterior capsule rupture (PCR).

Capsulorhexis Tear

A poor red reflex with a dense cataract makes visibility of the anterior capsule difficult. Although a can-opener capsulotomy could be performed, the creation of a continuous curvilinear capsulorhexis (CCC) is still possible under high magnification. The use of 0.1% trypan blue makes successful completion of a CCC much easier (Fig. 42.4).[15,16] It provides visualization of the anterior capsule during phacoemulsification and throughout the remainder of the case.

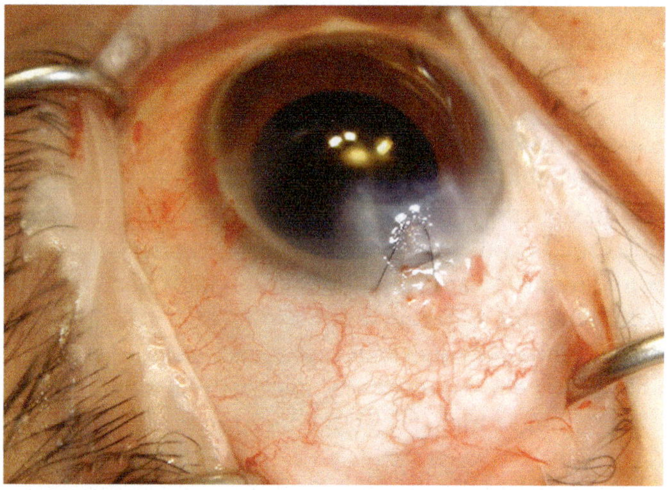

Fig. 42.5: Ultrasound heat-induced wound burn. Notice the characteristic fish-mouth appearance.
Source: Uday Devgan.

Wound Burn

The high phaco power required for the fragmentation of a dense nucleus can result in an ultrasound heat-induced wound burn,[10] as vibrational energy is transferred from the phaco tip to the incision (Fig. 42.5). If the corneal incision temperature rises past 60°C, this can cause stromal whitening with acute tissue contracture, which can result in the loss of the watertight seal and high residual astigmatism.[17,18] Unfortunately, this typically occurs quickly, in the matter of just one to three seconds, before a surgeon has time to react appropriately.[19]

Ophthalmic viscosurgical devices (OVDs) can play a role in wound burn. An eye that is completely filled with viscoelastic will restrict fluid flow. When heat cannot dissipate out of the eye, high heat is generated in the phaco probe and is transmitted to the corneal tissue. Removal of some OVDs just above the nucleus can minimize this risk.[17] Care must also be taken to ensure adequate flow through the irrigation sleeve at all times. Reducing total ultrasound energy by the use of chopping techniques, the use of advanced phaco settings like pulse or hyperpulse, where energy is only delivered for a portion of a duty cycle, or the use of torsional instead of longitudinal phaco power can help to mitigate the increased energy required to dissect a dense nucleus.[10]

Undoubtedly, it is better to prevent thermal wound burn, than to manage it after it occurs. However, should a corneal wound burn occur, interrupted sutures, wound revision, or a patch graft may be required to close the incision.[18] Often multiple sutures are required to close the wound, which can result in significant postoperative corneal astigmatism that may need additional management after the fact. Using conjunctival flaps to minimize residual astigmatism have been described, but if the corneal incision is not completely closed this can result in a filtering bleb and postoperative hypotony.[20] First and foremost, the priority in managing a corneal burn is to close the incision in a watertight fashion. Management of postoperative astigmatism is always secondary.

Corneal Endothelial Damage

Just as high phaco energy can lead to wound burns, it can also cause endothelial damage. Meticulous care must be taken to avoid pseudophakic bullous keratopathy and corneal failure in these patients, for which full or partial-thickness corneal transplant is ultimately the only definitive treatment. Longer phaco times required for dense nuclei can wash out OVD injected in the beginning of the surgery. Dispersive OVDs should be used to coat and protect the corneal endothelium, as they are retained longer.[21,22]

First introduced by Arshinoff, a *soft-shell technique* (SST) with a combination of dispersive and cohesive viscoelastic can be used for hard nuclei, and for those patients at high risk of endothelial decompensation, such as those with Fuchs endothelial corneal dystrophy (FECD).[23] Initially a dispersive OVD (e.g. Viscoat) is injected onto the anterior surface of the lens. Then a cohesive OVD (e.g. Healon GV) is injected into the posterior center of the dispersive OVD, such that the cohesive OVD fills the AC and spreads the dispersive OVD to create a smooth, uniform, and pressurized layer under the corneal endothelium (Fig. 42.6A).[23] A modification to this is the tri-soft shell technique (TSST), which also employs balanced salt solution (BSS) onto the anterior capsule surface to facilitate capsulorhexis creation (Fig. 42.6B).[24]

Increasing the distance from the phaco tip to the cornea will minimize damage to the endothelium. Prolapsing the nucleus into the anterior chamber is not advised; all phacoemulsification should be performed within the capsular bag if possible. Debulking the core nucleus first before emulsification is also a feasible option, since the central nucleus tends to be the hardest. Conventional bevel-up phaco tip is also imperative. The phaco tip should never be pointed downward, as this positioning is associated with a substantially greater risk of endothelial cell loss.[25]

Techniques to reduce phaco time and energy should also be employed. Many different strategies have been reported.

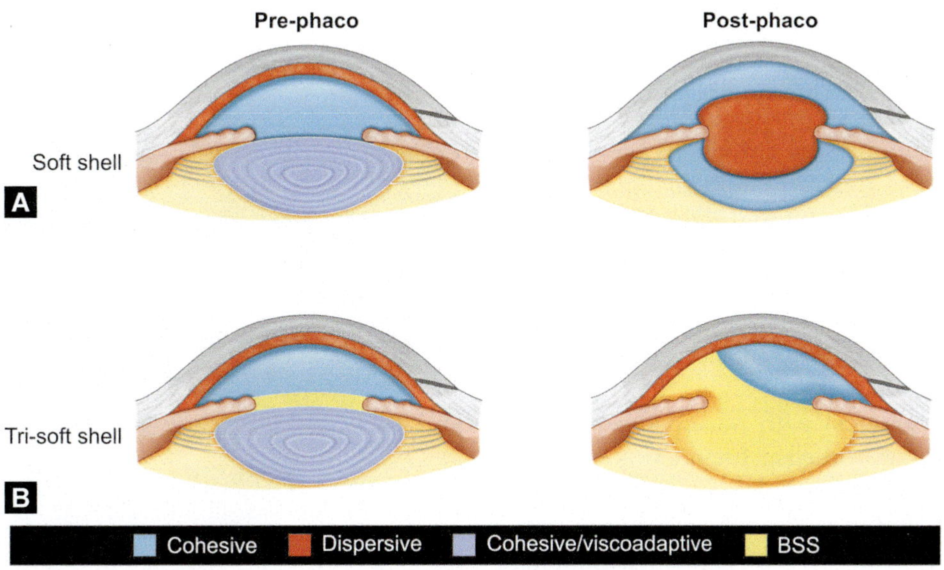

Figs. 42.6A and B: Soft-shell technique and tri-soft shell technique.
(BSS: Balanced salt solution)

Using a pulse or burst mode will minimize total energy to the eye compared with continuous phacoemulsification.[26] Techniques that fracture the lens, such as *stop-and-chop,*[27] *phaco-chop,*[27] and *forward-chop*[28] can all be used effectively in hard nuclei to reduce the total amount of phacosculpting.

Conventional longitudinal modes versus torsional ultrasound have also been debated. With the conventional, longitudinal ultrasound mode, the phaco tip oscillates back and forth in a linear direction, resulting in a jackhammer movement that breaks the lens apart with minimal cavitational energy.[29] With higher energies required for denser cataracts, this jackhammer effect begets a disadvantage, as it produces a repulsion effect. The longitudinal phaco pushes the nucleus away as the tip moves forward, wasting energy with each attempt. With a torsional system on the other hand, side-to-side rotating oscillations are made,[7] reducing repulsion. Torsional phacoemulsification has been reported to have lower ultrasound time and energy, ultimately preserving endothelial cell count.[30,31] Therefore, torsional modes can be beneficial when dealing with a dense cataract. Ultimately the technique and ultrasound modality chosen is best individualized toward the special needs of the patient.

Posterior Capsule Rupture

The dense brunescent nuclear cataract has also been called the *naked-nucleus* cataract, due to the absence of lens cortex material between the sclerotic nucleus and the posterior lens capsule.[32] It is not surprising therefore, that these dense cataracts pose a substantially greater risk for posterior capsule rupture (PCR). Without a layer of cortex protecting it, the posterior capsule can be easily damaged by the sharp phaco tip or secondary instruments. PCR is a known cause for poor visual outcome[33] after cataract surgery, with higher rates of cystoid macular edema, vitreous loss, retinal detachment, and endophthalmitis.[33-36] Only 93.8% versus 98.5% of patients achieve a visual acuity of 20/40 or better after PCR compared to uneventful cases.[37] While the reported incidence of PCR for all cataracts ranges from 1% to 4%,[35,37] PCR in dense brunescent cataracts is considerably greater, thought to be higher than 5%.[32,38,39]

Risk of PCR is greatest with postocclusion surge, particularly after the last nuclear fragment is removed. When the phaco tip is occluded with a nuclear fragment, irrigation continues and pressure in the anterior chamber rises. Meanwhile, vacuum continues to build in the system generating negative pressure which causes the tubing to collapse. After occlusion breaks with the last fragment emulsified, fluid rushes into the tubing and the vacuum previously generated in the aspiration lines is broken from tubing reexpansion. The intraocular pressure plummets, causing the anterior chamber to shallow.[40] The posterior capsule can be easily swung toward the phaco tip and result in PCR.

Dense nuclei are at greater risk of surge given the higher energies and longer phacoemulsification times. Standard methods for preventing surge include using rigid tubing with less compliance, venting the system periodically to equilibrate the pressures between the aspiration tubing lines and the anterior chamber, or reducing vacuum before the last nuclear piece is aspirated.[40]

Understanding the concept of surge has led to the development of procedures to protect the posterior capsule during phacoemulsification. Similar to Arshinoff's soft-shell technique where a layer of OVD is used to protect the corneal endothelium, Sato et al. describe a *visco-shell* technique, where OVD is used to protect the posterior capsule.[41] In this method, a viscoadaptive OVD (e.g. Healon5) is injected to surround a dense cataract, protect both endothelium and posterior capsule before phacoemulsification is utilized (Fig. 42.7). A modification to this, is the *IOL-shell technique,*[32] where the intraocular lens is inserted between the last nuclear fragment and the posterior capsule. After insertion, the final nuclear fragment is removed with phacoemulsification (Fig. 42.8). Both the *visco-shell* and *IOL-shell* techniques help protect against surge and provide a barrier between the dense lens and the posterior capsule, providing a safe environment for emulsification to occur.

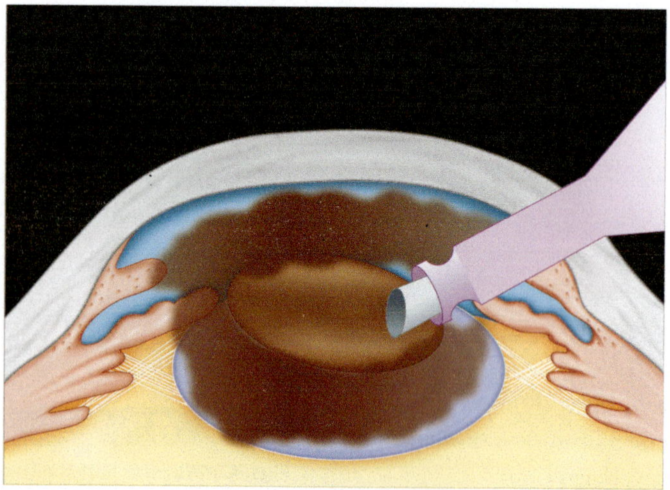

Fig. 42.7: Visco-shell technique.

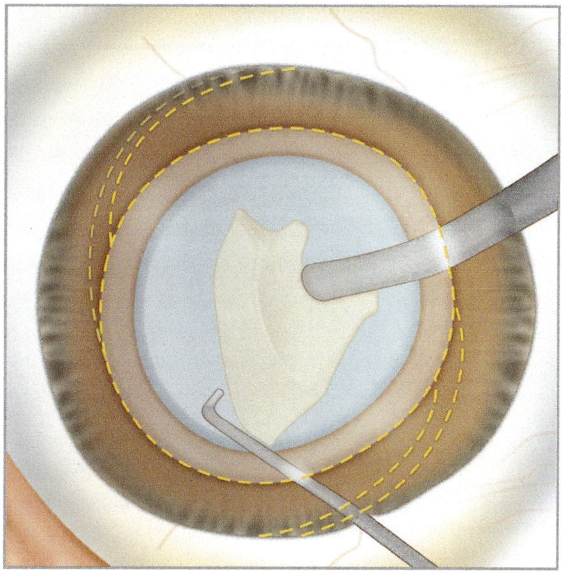

Fig. 42.8: IOL-shell technique.

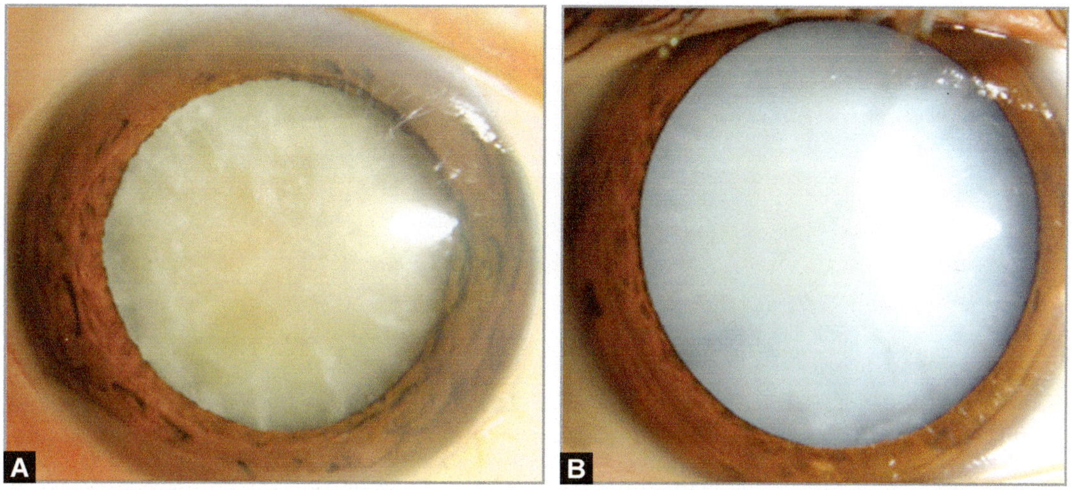

Figs. 42.9A and B: Different subtypes of the white cataract. (A) Hard white cataract with likely a dense nucleus; (B) Soft white intumescent cataract likely to demonstrate egress of fluid.
Source: Uday Devgan.

DENSE WHITE CATARACTS

White cataracts can be just as, if not more difficult to manage surgically, than brunescent cataracts. These white cataracts can be classified into two main subtypes, those which are normotensive and are entirely solid, and those with liquefied cortex material which are pressurized and intumescent (Figs. 42.9A and B).[42] When liquefied cortical material seeps out of the lens, the lens capsule can shrink and become wrinkled and fibrotic, forming a hypermature cataract (Fig. 42.10).[42] When nearly the entire cortex is liquefied, the nucleus can move freely and sink to bottom of the capsular bag, referred to as a Morgagnian cataract (Figs. 42.11A and B).[41,43] Not only do these cataracts provide similar problems with high phacoemulsification energy requirements previously discussed, but they also have a much higher risk of capsulorhexis tear. Rates of capsulorhexis tear or incomplete CCC range from 4% to as high as 28%.[6,44,45] Milky-white liquefied cortical material can leak, blocking visibility in the anterior chamber, the anterior capsule is more fragile, and calcium plaques on both the anterior and posterior capsule can result in unpredictable

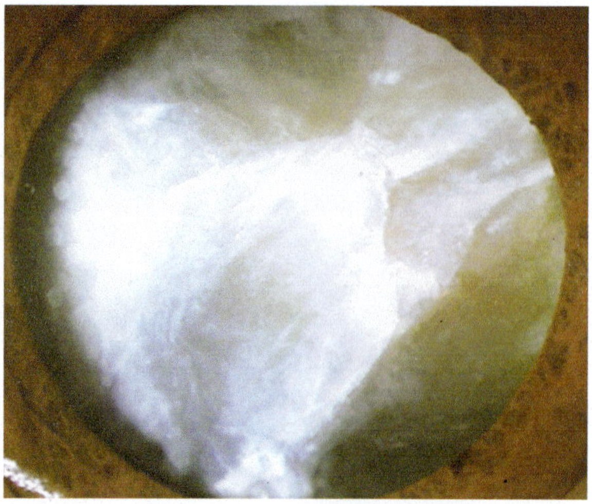

Fig. 42.10: A hypermature cataract. Notice the fibrotic and wrinkled anterior capsule.
Source: Uday Devgan.

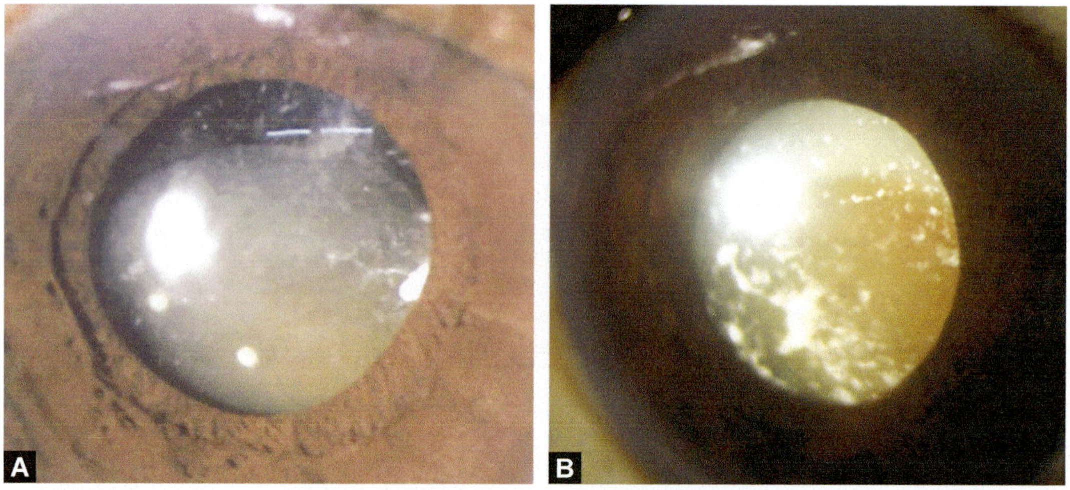

Figs. 42.11A and B: Morgagnian cataract. (A) Notice that the dense nucleus has dropped due to liquefied cortex; (B) This Morgagnian cataract also has a fibrotic capsule.
Source: Dr N Venkatesh Prajna, Aravind Eye Hospital, Madurai.

tears.[46] Finally, removing the opaque cortical material of a white cataract may reveal a hard nucleus, exponentially raising the barrier to a successful outcome.

Capsulorhexis Tear

A white cataract can block the red reflex entirely, so staining the anterior lens capsule with trypan blue is important for promoting adequate visualization of the anterior capsule for capsulorhexis.[15,16,47] Unique to the intumescent white cataract is the elevated intralenticular pressure.[6,48] Sudden equilibration of hydrostatic pressure across the capsule can cause radialization of a trypan blue stained anterior capsule and is responsible for the dreaded *Argentinian Flag Sign* (Fig. 42.12).[6,48] If a tear radializes posteriorly, such that the posterior capsule is violated, subsequent vitreous loss, nucleus drop, and zonular rupture can ensue. Multiple methods have been described to prevent incomplete CCC and the Argentinian flag sign, including anterior capsule puncture with aspiration,[49,50] performing CCC in a closed anterior chamber,[51] a two-stage capsulorhexis,[5,52] and phaco capsulotomy.[53]

Once the anterior capsule is broken, liquefied cortex material can seep into the anterior chamber and block a surgeon's view of the anterior capsule. This is seen in nearly half of all intumescent cataract cases.[52] Anticipating milky fluid egress, anterior capsule puncture and aspiration can equalize lenticular pressure and prevent radialization. A

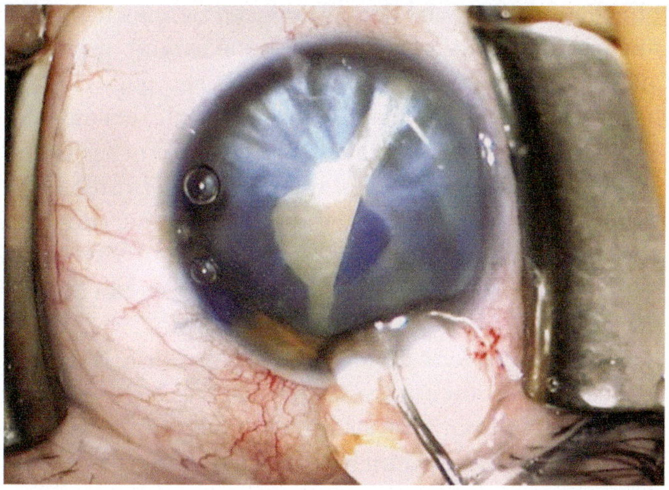

Fig. 42.12: The Argentinian flag sign. A trypan blue stained capsule with a radialized anterior tear in a white cataract resembles the Argentinian flag.
Source: Uday Devgan.

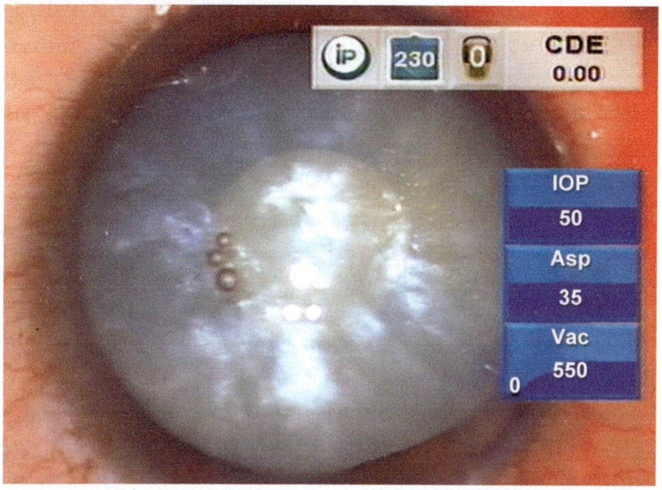

Fig. 42.13: A 3 mm mini-capsulorhexis. Aspiration of milky fluid egress and equilibration of pressure is undertaken before the 6 mm capsulorhexis is made.
Source: Dr N Venkatesh Prajna, Aravind Eye Hospital, Madurai.

small cystotome or 27-gauge needle on a syringe is used to poke a hole in the central anterior capsule. Then fluid is aspirated manually from the needle or through an irrigation/aspiration (I/A) system.

Paramount to a successful surgery is maintaining positive pressure in the anterior chamber throughout the operation.[6] Positive pressure in the anterior chamber slows the pressure equilibration rate after anterior capsule puncture. When a cohesive OVD is used to fill the anterior chamber, it will flatten the anterior capsule and minimally displace the anterior subcapsular cortex, creating a small depressurized area for safe anterior capsule puncture.[6,48] Unfortunately, OVD can easily egress through the clear corneal incision wound, shallowing the anterior chamber and causing uncontrolled anterior capsule tear. Therefore, some perform anterior capsule puncture or CCC in a closed anterior chamber, where these steps are undertaken through the paracentesis incision before the main incision wound is created.[51]

Gimbel described the two-stage CCC.[52] First, a deliberate, small CCC of approximately 3 mm is created (Fig. 42.13). Then liquid cortex material is removed with a small 26 or 30-gauge needle attached to an I/A system. Once completed, a second, larger 5–6 mm CCC can then be made in standard fashion. With this method, a CCC is achieved in 90–95% of cases.[5,54]

The two-stage CCC works because the small round opening lacks corners that can tear as the pressure equalizes. Phaco capsulotomy utilizes the same concept. The phaco probe is placed on the anterior capsule and punches out a circle with ultrasound.[51] This has the added advantage that the entire circle is created instantaneously. Milky cortex material can then be easily aspirated with the phaco probe before completion of the standard CCC.

Despite a two-step rhexis or a round phaco capsulotomy, anterior capsular tears can still occur. It has been recognized that there are two pressurized compartments in the intumescent white cataract. One is located anteriorly, just underneath the anterior lens capsule, and the other, posteriorly. While it was previously believed that the posterior pressure derived from the vitreous,[52] it is now thought to be intralenticularly located, generated from the space between the posterior surface of the nucleus and the posterior capsule. It is theorized that an equatorial barrier is formed by peripheral lens capsule compression against the lens equatorial edge. This separates the anterior and posterior intralenticular compartments, both pressurized with liquefied cortex material.[48] Aspiration of the liquefied cortex material after initial anterior capsule puncture will decompress the anterior compartment, but the posterior pressure can push the lens upward. This can still cause anterior capsular tearing as the larger CCC is attempted.[48]

Therefore, it is important that both compartments are addressed and decompressed to achieve a successful larger sized CCC. After the 3 mm mini-rhexis is made, bimanual irrigation aspiration ports can be brought to the equator to aspirate the liquid cortex material behind the lens, depressurizing the posterior intralenticular compartment.[48] Once decompressed, the capsulorhexis can be safely expanded to the traditional 5–6 mm size. This is cleverly coined the *Brazilian technique* by Figueiredo.[48] Certainly, there are other strategies to tackling the pressure gradient between the two chambers, including anterior vitrectomy, vitreous tap, and peripheral iridotomy.[55,56] However, this strategy appears to be one of the least invasive.

Posterior Capsule Rupture

Hydrodissection should be limited or avoided altogether for risk of the posterior capsule blowout. Often hydrodissection is unnecessary as the central nucleus is already loose from the liquefied cortex. As fluid passes posterior to the equator, even small increase in volume can raise the posterior lenticular pressure and cause the posterior capsule to rupture.[48,52]

After a CCC is successfully made, surgery can proceed with a similar approach to phacoemulsification as with other dense cataracts, paying special attention to preventing corneal wound burn and endothelial damage. A dense nucleus may be revealed under the white cataract, requiring high phaco energy. While the milky liquefied material is easily aspirated, the posterior plate can be fibrous and difficult to dissect.

Even in the hands of an experienced surgeon, PCR can and will occur. Whether from extension of the Argentinian flag anterior capsule tear posteriorly, blowout despite careful hydrodissection, or mechanical tears from a nuclear fragment or the phaco tip, the surgeon must have an armamentarium for managing PCR in the dense white cataract. In simple cataract surgery, PCR usually occurs after phacoemulsification is completed, such as in postocclusion surge discussed previously. In this setting, a standard sulcus IOL is placed. In contrast, PCR in a dense white cataract frequently happens early in the case, before the entire cataract has been removed. Continued phacoemulsification with a PCR can result in a dropped nucleus or vitreous prolapse.

A surgeon must maintain good habits when dealing with a PCR in the presence of nonemulsified nuclear fragments. As soon as it is identified, phacoemuesification should stop but irrigation should continue. A small hole can be plugged with a dispersive viscoelastic agent to prevent vitreous prolapse. Dispersive agents are optimal as they are less likely to wash out.

Next it is important to evaluate for vitreous loss. Injection of triamcinolone can stain the vitreous and aid in visualization.[57] If there is no vitreous loss and depending on the comfort level of the surgeon, the remaining nuclear fragments can be removed either manually or with phacoemulsification. Viscoelastic can be injected under nuclear fragments to float them to the wound or into the anterior chamber for safe removal. A sheets glide can also be used as a barrier to facilitate lens removal,[58] or convert to ECCE if necessary. If vitreous loss is identified or suspected, a thorough anterior vitrectomy should be performed. Any vitreous to the wound or in the anterior chamber should be adequately removed to curtail vitreous traction.[59,60] A sulcus lens with appropriately adjusted lens power can then be placed.

Should any lens fragments drop posteriorly, it is of utmost importance to resist the urge to fish for these fragments. Attempts to chase after a dropped nuclear fragment can be extremely detrimental and harmful to the patient, greatly increasing risks of retinal tears and detachment.[61] Advanced strategies such as posterior-assisted levitation[62] should be left in the hands of only the most experienced surgeon and will not be discussed here.

The surgeon must honestly evaluate his or her capabilities as judicious assessment of one's limit can greatly impact a patient's final visual outcome. In situations of a dropped nucleus or other more serious complications, having the foresight to enlist the assistance of the vitreoretinal surgeon can be just as valuable as the surgical skillset of the techniques described.

ADVANCED TECHNOLOGIES: FEMTOSECOND LASER-ASSISTED CATARACT SURGERY AND INTRAOPERATIVE REFRACTIVE BIOMETRY

Since first described by Nagy et al. in 2009,[63] femtosecond laser-assisted cataract surgery (FLACS) has been increasingly utilized to facilitate three cataract surgery steps: corneal incision creation, capsulorhexis creation, and lens fragmentation.[64-66] It has been advocated by early adopters to provide better CCC centration, reduce ultrasound energy and ultimately improve refractive outcome.[63-65,67] The exact role of FLACS technology in dense nuclear and white cataracts is still not clear.

One purported advantage of FLACS is the reduction of ultrasound energy and theoretically, reduction in endothelial cell loss and postoperative corneal edema. Certainly, FLACS reduces both phacoemulsification time and mean ultrasound energy, reducing the cumulative dissipated energy (CDE). Compared to manual cataract surgery, it can reduce phaco time by approximately 50%

and ultrasound energy by 65%.[67] However, whether this translates to a reduction in corneal endothelial cell loss is unclear. Reports thus far have been inconclusive.[67-69]

For the dense brunescent cataract, advantages for using FLACS appear to be in the reduction of phaco energy from lens fragmentation and implied reduced damage to the corneal endothelium. However, sometimes the lens can be so dense that laser cannot fragment the nucleus and the surgery may still require the use of substantial amounts of ultrasound energy. In the white cataract, a benefit of FLACS is in creation of the CCC as this is created in a closed system, pressure differences between the anterior chamber and lens is minimized. A common cause for incomplete CCC with femtosecond laser is the immediate release of the liquefied cortex. This material clouds the anterior chamber and interferes with subsequent laser pulses.[70,71] Moreover, with dense white cataracts, adequate OCT image acquisition can be challenging, impeding complete lens fragmentation.[70] Even though FLACS can facilitate some surgical steps, it should never serve as a substitute for understanding and mastering the conventional techniques of cataract surgery. The surgeon must develop sufficient competence to troubleshoot any situation if, and when complications arise.

With both the surgeon and the patient now desiring an emmetropic refractive outcome from cataract extraction, mature cataracts become especially problematic. Optical biometry normally deployed in soft and moderate cataracts is of poor utility in the advanced cataract. Patients may not be able to fixate and there may be no optical view posteriorly. Both dense brunescent and white cataracts rely on A-scan ultrasound for lens power calculation. Contact A-scan is variable based on technician skill. Regularly underestimating axial length from corneal indentation of the applanation tip, myopic outcomes are not uncommon. A 1 mm error in axial length can result in 2–3 D of error, depending on the true axial length of the eye.[72] In clinical practice, contact applanation induces a mean shortening of 0.25–0.33 mm compared to immersion, rendering approximately 1 D of potential error into the IOL power.[73] Generally, immersion A-scan is superior to contact applanation A-scan for this reason. Compared to optical biometry, immersion A-scan typically has good correlation and similar refractive outcomes.[13] However, there can be exceptions. A-scans measure the anatomical axial length of the eye, but optical methods measure to the macula, allowing for the true functional axial length. Usually the anatomical and functional axial lengths are the same, but in certain situations, such as patients with a staphyloma, the immersion A-scan measurements will result in an undesired hyperopic outcome.

When emmetropia is desired, intraoperative refractive biometry (IRB) becomes helpful. In IRB, a wavefront aberrometer [e.g. optiwave refractive analysis (ORA) system] measures an aphakic autorefraction before insertion of the IOL.[74,75] This helps to either confirm IOL power or prospectively choose a lens. Given the potential inaccuracies in axial length measurements preoperatively, ORA or other IRB technologies can be a valuable adjunct to IOL calculations in mature cataracts cases.

Ultimately, it is the responsibility of the physician to conduct a thorough preoperative evaluation, provide appropriate counseling, and develop a nuanced surgical plan when presented with a dense brunescent or white mature cataract. Experience and continued education are vital to the care of these patients. With adequate preparation and practice, the ophthalmological surgeon can ensure the best visual outcome possible, leaving patients both satisfied and grateful.

REFERENCES

1. Kelman CD. Phaco-emulsification and aspiration. A new technique of cataract removal. A preliminary report. Am J Ophthalmol. 1967;64(1):23-35.
2. Riaz Y, Mehta JS, Wormald R, et al. Surgical interventions for age-related cataract. Cochrane Database Syst Rev. 2006(4):CD001323.
3. Shah PA, Yoo S. Innovations in phacoemulsification technology. Curr Opin Ophthalmol. 2007;18(1):23-6.
4. Levin ML. Opalescent nuclear cataract. J Cataract Refract Surg. 1989;15(5):576-9.
5. Kara-Junior N, de Santhiago MR, Kawakami A, et al. Mini-rhexis for white intumescent cataracts. Clinics (Sao Paulo). 2009;64(4):309-12.
6. Megur D, Megur B. Capsulorhexis in white intumescent cataracts: the five commandments to follow. J Vis Sci. 2015;1(1):33-6.
7. Fakhry MA, El Shazly MI. Torsional ultrasound mode versus combined torsional and conventional ultrasound mode phacoemulsification for eyes with hard cataract. Clin Ophthalmol. 2011;5:973-8.
8. Khanna R, Pujari S, Sangwan V. Cataract surgery in developing countries. Curr Opin Ophthalmol. 2011;22(1):10-4.
9. Riaz Y, de Silva SR, Evans JR. Manual small incision cataract surgery (MSICS) with posterior chamber intraocular lens versus phacoemulsification with posterior chamber intraocular lens for age-related cataract. Cochrane Database Syst Rev. 2013(10):CD008813.

10. Crispim J JL, Paz L, Allemann N, et al. The surgical challenges dense brunescent cataracts present. Exp Rev Ophthalmol. 2014;10(1):10.
11. Shingleton BJ, Crandall AS, Ahmed, II. Pseudoexfoliation and the cataract surgeon: preoperative, intraoperative, and postoperative issues related to intraocular pressure, cataract, and intraocular lenses. J Cataract Refract Surg. 2009;35(6):1101-20.
12. Haigis W, Lege B, Miller N, Schneider B. Comparison of immersion ultrasound biometry and partial coherence interferometry for intraocular lens calculation according to Haigis. Graefes Arch Clin Exp Ophthalmol. 2000;238(9):765-73.
13. Packer M, Fine IH, Hoffman RS, et al. Immersion A-scan compared with partial coherence interferometry: outcomes analysis. J Cataract Refract Surg. 2002;28(2):239-42.
14. Watson A, Armstrong R. Contact or immersion technique for axial length measurement? Aust N Z J Ophthalmol. 1999;27(1):49 51.
15. Chung CF, Liang CC, Lai JS, et al. Safety of trypan blue 1% and indocyanine green 0.5% in assisting visualization of anterior capsule during phacoemulsification in mature cataract. J Cataract Refract Surg. 2005;31(5):938-42.
16. Melles GR, de Waard PW, Pameyer JH, Houdijn Beekhuis W. Trypan blue capsule staining to visualize the capsulorhexis in cataract surgery. J Cataract Refract Surg. 1999;25(1):7-9.
17. Sorensen T, Chan CC, Bradley M, et al. Ultrasound-induced corneal incision contracture survey in the United States and Canada. J Cataract Refract Surg. 2012;38(2):227-33.
18. Sugar A, Schertzer RM. Clinical course of phacoemulsification wound burns. J Cataract Refract Surg. 1999;25(5):688-92.
19. Khodabakhsh AJ, Zaidman G, Tabin G. Corneal surgery for severe phacoemulsification burns. Ophthalmology. 2004;111(2):332-4.
20. Haldar K, Saraff R. Closure technique for leaking wound resulting from thermal injury during phacoemulsification. J Cataract Refract Surg. 2014;40(9):1412-4.
21. Adina B. The influence of viscoelastic substances on the corneal endothelium during cataract surgery by phacoemulsification. Ophthalmology. 2008;52(1):84-9.
22. Storr-Paulsen A, Norregaard JC, Farik G, et al. The influence of viscoelastic substances on the corneal endothelial cell population during cataract surgery: a prospective study of cohesive and dispersive viscoelastics. Acta Ophthalmol Scand. 2007;85(2):183-7.
23. Arshinoff SA. Dispersive-cohesive viscoelastic soft shell technique. J Cataract Refract Surg. 1999;25(2):167-73.
24. Arshinoff SA, Norman R. Tri-soft shell technique. J Cataract Refract Surg. 2013;39(8):1196-203.
25. Faramarzi A, Javadi MA, Karimian F, et al. Corneal endothelial cell loss during phacoemulsification: bevel-up versus bevel-down phaco tip. J Cataract Refract Surg. 2011;37(11):1971-6.
26. Ozkurt YB, Evciman T, Sengor T, et al. Comparison of burst, pulse, and linear modes used in phacoemulsification surgery. Eur J Ophthalmol. 2010;20(2):353-64.
27. Storr-Paulsen A, Norregaard JC, Ahmed S, et al. Endothelial cell damage after cataract surgery: divide-and-conquer versus phaco-chop technique. J Cataract Refract Surg. 2008;34(6):996-1000.
28. Ram J, Wesendahl TA, Auffarth GU, Apple DJ. Evaluation of in situ fracture versus phaco chop techniques. J Cataract Refract Surg. 1998;24(11):1464-8.
29. Zacharias J. Role of cavitation in the phacoemulsification process. J Cataract Refract surg. 2008;34(5):846-52.
30. Liu Y, Zeng M, Liu X, et al. Torsional mode versus conventional ultrasound mode phacoemulsification: randomized comparative clinical study. J Cataract Refract Surg. 2007;33(2):287-92.
31. Zeng M, Liu X, Liu Y, et al. Torsional ultrasound modality for hard nucleus phacoemulsification cataract extraction. Br J Ophthalmol. 2008;92(8):1092-6.
32. Luo L, Lin H, Chen W, et al. Intraocular lens-shell technique: adjustment of the surgical procedure leads to greater safety when treating dense nuclear cataracts. PLoS One. 2014;9(11):e112663.
33. Sparrow JM, Taylor H, Qureshi K, et al. The Cataract National Dataset electronic multi-centre audit of 55,567 operations: risk indicators for monocular visual acuity outcomes. Eye (Lond). 2012;26(6):821-6.
34. Frost NA, Sparrow JM, Strong NP, et al. Vitreous loss in planned extracapsular cataract extraction does lead to a poorer visual outcome. Eye (Lond). 1995;9(Pt 4):446-51.
35. Ionides A, Minassian D, Tuft S. Visual outcome following posterior capsule rupture during cataract surgery. Br J Ophthalmol. 2001;85(2):222-4.
36. Osher RH, Cionni RJ. The torn posterior capsule: its intraoperative behavior, surgical management, and long-term consequences. J Cataract Refract Surg. 1990;16(4):490-4.
37. Ti SE, Yang YN, Lang SS, et al. A 5-year audit of cataract surgery outcomes after posterior capsule rupture and risk factors affecting visual acuity. Am J Ophthalmol. 2014;157(1):180-5.e1.
38. Hwang HS, Kim EC, Kim MS. Drill-and-crack technique for nuclear disassembly of hard nucleus. J Cataract Refract Surg. 2010;36(10):1627-30.
39. Simanjuntak GW, Tan JF, Mailangkay HH. Double extra sharp chopper increase efficacy of phacoemulsification for hard mature cataract surgery. Semin Ophthalmol. 2010;25(1-2):8-12.
40. Sharif-Kashani P, Fanney D, Injev V. Comparison of occlusion break responses and vacuum rise times of phacoemulsification systems. BMC Ophthalmol. 2014;14:96.
41. Sato M, Mizushima Y, Oshika T. Visco-shell technique with sodium hyaluronate 2.3% in phacoemulsification of Morgagnian cataract. J Cataract Refract Surg. 2008;34(11):1824-7.
42. Brazitikos PD, Tsinopoulos IT, Papadopoulos NT, et al. Ultrasonographic classification and phacoemulsification of white senile cataracts. Ophthalmology. 1999;106(11):2178-83.

43. Sukhija J, Kaur S. Images in clinical medicine. Morgagnian cataract. N Engl J Med. 2014;370(24):2326.
44. Chakrabarti A, Singh S. Phacoemulsification in eyes with white cataract. J Cataract Refract Surg. 2000;26(7):1041-7.
45. Vajpayee RB, Bansal A, Sharma N, et al. Phacoemulsification of white hypermature cataract. J Cataract Refract Surg. 1999;25(8):1157-60.
46. Ermiss SS, Ozturk F, Inan UU. Comparing the efficacy and safety of phacoemulsification in white mature and other types of senile cataracts. Br J Ophthalmol. 2003;87(11):1356-9.
47. Jacob S, Agarwal A, Agarwal A, et al. Trypan blue as an adjunct for safe phacoemulsification in eyes with white cataract. J Cataract Refract Surg. 2002;28(10):1819-25.
48. Figueiredo CG, Figueiredo J, Figueiredo GB. Brazilian technique for prevention of the Argentinean flag sign in white cataract. J Cataract Refract Surg. 2012;38(9):1531-6.
49. Rao SK, Padmanabhan P. Capsulorhexis in eyes with phacomorphic glaucoma. J Cataract Refract Surg. 1998;24(7):882-4.
50. Bhattacharjee K, Bhattacharjee H, Goswami BJ, et al. Capsulorhexis in intumescent cataract. J Cataract Refract Surg. 1999;25(8):1045-7.
51. Chan DD, Ng AC, Leung CK, et al. Continuous curvilinear capsulorhexis in intumescent or hypermature cataract with liquefied cortex. J Cataract Refract Surg. 2003;29(3):431-4.
52. Gimbel HV, Willerscheidt AB. What to do with limited view: the intumescent cataract. J Cataract Refract Surg. 1993;19(5):657-61.
53. Mahalingam P, Sambhav K. Phaco capsulotomy in intumescent cataract. Nepal J Ophthalmol. 2014;6(2):242-3.
54. Vasavada A, Singh R, Desai J. Phacoemulsification of white mature cataracts. J Cataract Refract Surg. 1998;24(2):270-7.
55. Gorovoy IR, Jeng BH. Peripheral iridotomy to prevent Argentinian flag sign during capsulorhexis in the white cataract. J Cataract Refract Surg. 2014;40(2):335-6.
56. Chang DF. Pars plana vitreous tap for phacoemulsification in the crowded eye. J Cataract Refract Surg. 2001;27(12):1911-4.
57. Burk SE, Da Mata AP, Snyder ME, et al. Visualizing vitreous using Kenalog suspension. J Cataract Refract Surg. 2003;29(4):645-51.
58. Michelson MA. Use of a Sheets' Glide as a pseudoposterior capsule in phacoemulsification complicated by posterior capsule rupture. J Cataract. 1993;5(1):70-2.
59. Chalam KV, Shah VA. Successful management of cataract surgery associated vitreous loss with sutureless small-gauge pars plana vitrectomy. Am J Ophthalmol. 2004;138(1):79-84.
60. Jacobs PM. Vitreous loss during cataract surgery: prevention and optimal management. Eye (Lond). 2008;22(10):1286-9.
61. Moore JK, Scott IU, Flynn HW Jr, et al. Retinal detachment in eyes undergoing pars plana vitrectomy for removal of retained lens fragments. Ophthalmology. 2003;110(4):709-13.
62. Chang DF, Packard RB. Posterior assisted levitation for nucleus retrieval using Viscoat after posterior capsule rupture. J Cataract Refract Surg. 2003;29(10):1860-5.
63. Nagy Z, Takacs A, Filkorn T, et al. Initial clinical evaluation of an intraocular femtosecond laser in cataract surgery. J Refract Surg. 2009;25(12):1053-60.
64. Abouzeid H, Ferrini W. Femtosecond-laser assisted cataract surgery: a review. Acta Ophthalmol. 2014;92(7):597-603.
65. Hooshmand J, Vote BJ. Femtosecond laser-assisted cataract surgery, technology, outcome, future directions and modern applications. Asia Pac J Ophthalmol (Phila). 2017;6(4):393-400.
66. Chen X, Xiao W, Ye S, et al. Efficacy and safety of femtosecond laser-assisted cataract surgery versus conventional phacoemulsification for cataract: a meta-analysis of randomized controlled trials. Sci Rep. 2015;5:13123.
67. Kanellopoulos AJ, Asimellis G. Standard manual capsulorhexis/Ultrasound phacoemulsification compared to femtosecond laser-assisted capsulorhexis and lens fragmentation in clear cornea small incision cataract surgery. Eye Vis (Lond). 2016;3:20.
68. Ho JW, Afshari NA. Advances in cataract surgery: preserving the corneal endothelium. Curr Opin Ophthalmol. 2015;26(1):22-7.
69. Takács AI, Kovacs I, Mihaltz K, et al. Central corneal volume and endothelial cell count following femtosecond laser-assisted refractive cataract surgery compared to conventional phacoemulsification. J Refract Surg. 2012;28(6):387-91.
70. Taravella MJ, Meghpara B, Frank G, et al. Femtosecond laser-assisted cataract surgery in complex cases. J Cataract Refract Surg. 2016;42(6):813-6.
71. Titiyal JS, Kaur M, Singh A, et al. Comparative evaluation of femtosecond laser-assisted cataract surgery and conventional phacoemulsification in white cataract. Clin Ophthalmol. 2016;10:1357-64.
72. Ademola-Popoola DS, Nzeh DA, Saka SE, et al. Comparison of ocular biometry measurements by applanation and immersion A-scan techniques. J Curr Ophthalmol. 2015;27(3-4):110-4.
73. Lee AC, Qazi MA, Pepose JS. Biometry and intraocular lens power calculation. Curr opin Ophthalmol. 2008;19(1):13-7.
74. Ianchulev T, Salz J, Hoffer K, et al. Intraoperative optical refractive biometry for intraocular lens power estimation without axial length and keratometry measurements. J Cataract Refract Surg. 2005;31(8):1530-6.
75. Wong AC, Mak ST, Tse RK. Clinical evaluation of the intraoperative refraction technique for intraocular lens power calculation. Ophthalmology. 2010;117(4):711-6.

Chapter 43

Challenging Cataract Cases: Highly Myopic and Hyperopic Eyes

Benjamin C Campbell, Uday Devgan

Cataract surgery in highly myopic and hyperopic eyes can be very rewarding for both the patient and surgeon. In addition to correcting the lenticular opacity, most or all of the preexisting refractive error can be addressed simultaneously. With successful surgery, these patients gain the best vision of their lives after previously being dependent on spectacle correction. For the surgeon, cataract surgery is one of the most effective forms of refractive surgery with the widest range, from –30 to +20 diopters of refractive correction. In order to help these patients, however, it is imperative that the cataract surgeon be familiar with the unique challenges that these very long and short eyes present. Extra diligence and attention are required during the preoperative evaluation, surgical technique, and postoperative management in patients with high myopia and hyperopia.

HIGH MYOPIA

Preoperative Evaluation

A detailed preoperative examination is necessary before proceeding with cataract surgery in highly myopic eyes. The risk of retinal complications that could be vision limiting is higher in myopic eyes. Carefully examine for any retinal breaks, holes, or degeneration prior to surgery. These eyes may also have macular pathology, such as epiretinal membranes or macular degeneration (Fig. 43.1). Consider referral to a retinal specialist prior to cataract surgery if any abnormality is found. These patients have a risk of retinal detachment for their entire life and will need to continue with routine annual ophthalmic examinations. It is also important to establish appropriate expectations for postoperative visual potential if there is macular pathology that could limit the vision post cataract surgery.

One of the most difficult challenges that high axial myopia presents in the preoperative evaluation is in determining the correct intraocular lens (IOL) power required for emmetropia. In general, there is a tendency for conventional formulas to calculate too low of an IOL power, leading to a hyperopic outcome.[1-9] The problem becomes worse as axial length (AL) increases and a lower plus power or even a negative power IOL is required. Accurate biometry is more difficult in long eyes, and the effective lens position (ELP) is less predictable. Third generation formulas indirectly determine the ELP and tend to underestimate necessary IOL power, thus resulting in hyperopic outcomes. Of these formulas, however, the SRK/T has generally been shown to be the most accurate.[1-9] Traditionally, the simplest strategy has been to aim for a myopic refraction using the SRK/T formula. Patients accustomed to high degrees of myopia will be much happier with a small amount of residual myopia rather than a hyperopic surprise. This strategy leads to imperfect postoperative refractions, however, and the desire for more accurate outcomes has inspired significant research to improve results.

Several strategies have involved improving AL measurement and utilization in highly myopic eyes. Measuring AL in these eyes can be challenging and has generally been thought of as a major contributor to hyperopic outcomes. The difficulty in measuring AL

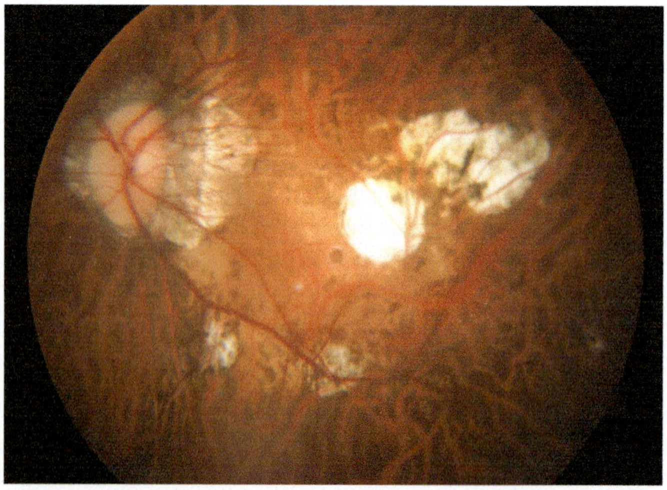

Fig. 43.1: Fundus with myopic degeneration. Preoperative examination is important prior to cataract surgery in myopic patients as retinal pathology may need to be addressed. The postoperative visual acuity may be limited by these retinal findings.
Source: Dr Karthick Srinivasan, Aravind Eye Hospital, Chennai.

depends on the type of biometry employed. The presence of posterior pole staphylomas in myopic eyes can lead to overestimation of axial length if using A-scan biometry to determine the anatomic axial length[1] (Fig. 43.2). B-scan can be used to locate staphylomas and increase accuracy. Theoretically, optical methods of biometry can also more precisely determine the refractive axial length by measuring at the fovea and avoiding the effect of staphylomas to give a falsely long AL (Fig. 43.3). Myopic eyes often have ocular comorbidities, however, that may lead to variable fixation and unpredictable optical biometry results. In fact, studies[2-3] comparing the different biometry techniques (A-scan vs B-scan assisted A-scan vs optical biometry) showed a similar overestimation error across all three methods. This would suggest that minimizing the adverse impact of staphylomas on AL measurement does not completely prevent hyperopic outcomes.

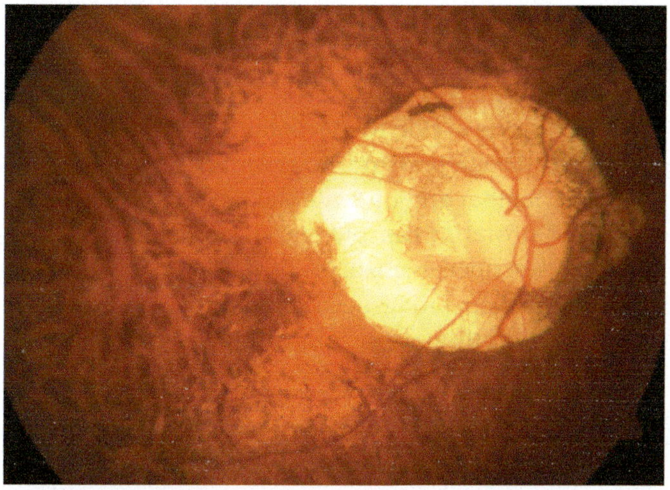

Fig. 43.2: Posterior staphyloma in myopic eye. A-scan biometry can give inaccurate axial length measurements. B-scan can identify the presence of posterior staphylomas as depicted in this fundus photo.
Source: Dr Karthick Srinivasan, Aravind Eye Hospital, Chennai

One theory[4] to explain the non-superiority of optic coherence biometry over ultrasound biometry in long eyes involves the index of refraction for the vitreous body. Standard optic coherence biometry assigns a single, fixed index of refraction for all eyes based on studies from eyes with average axial lengths. In longer eyes, the proportion of vitreous increases and there is a higher degree of liquefaction, which leads to a different refractive index and extrapolation error. The error is large enough that it cannot be fully compensated with lens constant optimization alone. This theory led to the Wang-Koch modification for axial length, which optimizes the measured AL using regression equations. In several studies, the Wang-Koch AL modification has shown improved refractive outcomes in myopic eyes >25 mm long when used in all standard equations, but particularly when used in conjunction with the Holladay 1 and Haigis formulae.[4-6]

Another theory to improve outcomes involves the ELP and the geometry of the lower power and negative power IOLs used in these myopic eyes. The difference in lens geometry affects the position of the principal plane, which is related to the ELP and ultimately calculated using the lens constants. Thus, using plus power constants with minus power IOLs may introduce significant error in determining the ELP. Haigis[7] proposed using different A-constants for

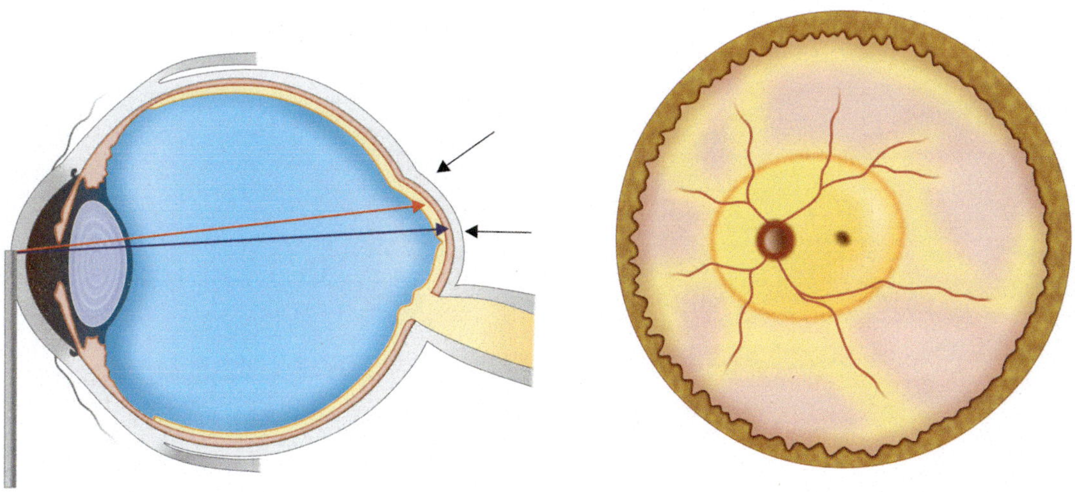

Fig. 43.3: Measuring axial length in a myopic eye with posterior staphyloma. The presence of posterior staphyloma can give a falsely elongated axial length measurement, leading to inaccurate IOL calculations. As depicted, the blue arrow represents the axial length obtained with A-scan ultrasound biometry and gives an overestimation to true axial length. The red arrow represents a more accurate measurement of axial length obtained via optical biometry and centered on the fovea.

positive and negative lenses to correct this error. This approach has been met with some debate, however,[4,9-11] as the ELP may not be as critical in IOL calculations for myopic eyes. This is demonstrated in studies in which zero powered IOLs were placed and yet the myopic eyes still ended up with hyperopic outcomes.[2,12]

Ultimately, there are several formulae that are available and have shown promise in more accurately predicting IOL power in long eyes. As mentioned previously the Holladay I and Haigis formulas using the Wang-Koch AL modification are effective options. Several studies suggest the Barrett Universal II formula is particularly effective.[3-6,9,13] The Hill-RBF has performed as well as 4th generation formulas with long AL.[14,15] The Ladas Super Formula has shown great promise.[15,16] If available, intraoperative wavefront aberrometry (ORA) has also been shown to be as effective as AL-optimized equations in predicting residual refractive error and reducing hyperopic outcomes.[14] Furthermore, many of these patients will have had prior corneal refractive surgery which also must be accounted for in order to prevent additional hyperopic surprise.

The selection of the IOL also must be considered and is based on the patient's ocular status and needs. A toric lens is beneficial to those patients with high degrees of corneal astigmatism in addition to their axial myopia. Other patients may do well with multifocal or accommodating IOLs. It is advisable to always place an IOL when possible, even if it is zero power, to provide a barrier to vitreous prolapse in the event of a future YAG laser capsulotomy, thereby preventing further complications. There are multiple manufacturers who make an extended range of IOLs, including minus power IOLs. It is important to ensure the proper lens is available prior to surgery.

Surgical Technique

Myopic eyes have deep anterior chambers which can be beneficial to allow more room during phacoemulsification. However, it is important to avoid over inflating the anterior chamber and causing excessive deepening during surgery. When this occurs the iris comes in contact with the anterior lens capsule, leading to a reverse pupillary block. With the infusion into the anterior chamber the pressure becomes greater than in the posterior chamber and the entire lens-iris diaphragm is pushed more posteriorly. This excessively deepened chamber makes phacoemulsification more challenging for the surgeon and uncomfortable for the patient. One option to prevent this phenomenon is to lower the infusion pressure, however this can shallow the anterior chamber and increase the risk of post occlusion surge and posterior capsule tear. A surgical technique[17] has been described to break the reverse pupillary block by mechanically separating the iris from the lens capsule with the phacoemulsification tip, irrigation/aspiration probe, or a second instrument (Figs. 43.4A and B). A single nasal hook can be placed for the duration of the surgery to prevent this occurrence entirely. This equalizes the pressure between the two chambers at all times and corrects chamber depth.

There have been conflicting reports[18-22] on whether high axial length increases the risk for surgical complications, such as posterior capsule tears. The differences likely are related to surgeon experience in operating in highly

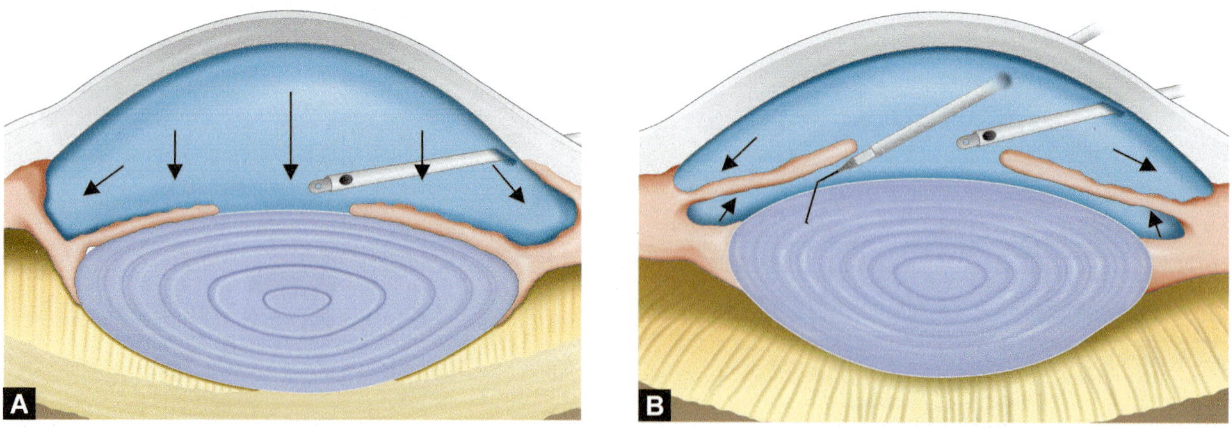

Figs. 43.4A and B: Intraoperative management of reverse pupillary block. (A) Over-inflation of the anterior chamber during cataract surgery causing excessive deepening. The iris is in contact with the anterior lens capsule, leading to reverse pupillary block. The anterior chamber pressure continues to increase and the lens-iris diaphragm is displaced posteriorly; (B) A Sinskey hook is used to lift up the iris edge and disrupt the reverse pupillary block, allowing communication between the anterior and posterior chambers and normalization of anterior chamber depth.

myopic eyes and the technique employed. One strategy to avoid such complications is to avoid anterior chamber collapse. This also helps avoid postoperative retinal tears or detachments in these myopic fundi that are already at risk for such complications. When the anterior chamber collapses, the posterior capsule and vitreous have a tendency to move anteriorly. This can happen rather quickly when removing the phaco probe or irrigation/aspiration probe from the eye, placing tension and traction on the vitreous base which can lead to retinal breaks. This can be avoided by maintaining AC depth with viscoelastic or BSS via the paracentesis when removing the phaco probe or irrigation/aspiration probe.

Postoperative Management

The postoperative refraction can take some time to stabilize in highly myopic eyes due to variation in effective lens position as the capsular bag tightens around the IOL. The patient will likely be left with a large degree of anisometropia between eyes and performing timely surgery in the fellow eye can minimize patient discomfort. These patients also may benefit from further refractive surgery following cataract surgery to fine tune their refractive results. A contact lens can be placed in the fellow eye during the initial postoperative period of the first eye in order to minimize the anisometropia.

It is crucial to perform a repeat dilated fundus exam postoperatively and to continue to follow these patients on a regular basis, as their myopia places them at risk for retinal complications for the rest of their lives. While myopia increases the risk of retinal detachment in general, there are differing reports on whether cataract surgery in myopic patients significantly increases the risk.[18,23-25] The variation likely is related to several factors. It has been noted that leaving a patient aphakic increases the risk of postoperative detachment, while the placement of an IOL, even if it has zero power, is protective.[18] Posterior capsule tear also increases the risk of retinal breaks, and those patients with lattice degeneration or a history of retinal detachment in the fellow eye are at a particularly increased risk.

HIGH HYPEROPIA

Preoperative Evaluation

The patients with high hyperopia typically have small eyes with axial lengths less than 22.0 mm. A detailed preoperative evaluation is important to prepare for the challenging variables that can be associated with operating in these small eyes. There is a spectrum of hyperopic eyes with short axial length (AL) based on anterior chamber depth (ACD) and concomitant ocular comorbidities. Although there is no clear consensus on exact AL values for these definitions,[26,27] it can be helpful to classify them according to the following classification (Figs. 43.5A to C):

- *Microphthalmos:*
  - These are eyes with short AL but normal ACD. This means that the lens is located proportionally closer to the retina than in a normal eye. Microphthalmic eyes can be simple or complex, based on whether there are other ocular malformations. Evaluate for the presence of microcornea, iris colobomas, chorioretinal colobomas, persistent fetal vasculature, or retinal dysplasia. Typically, they have normal scleral thickness.
- *Nanophthalmos:*
  - These are proportionally small eyes with short AL and shallow ACD. They normally have thickened

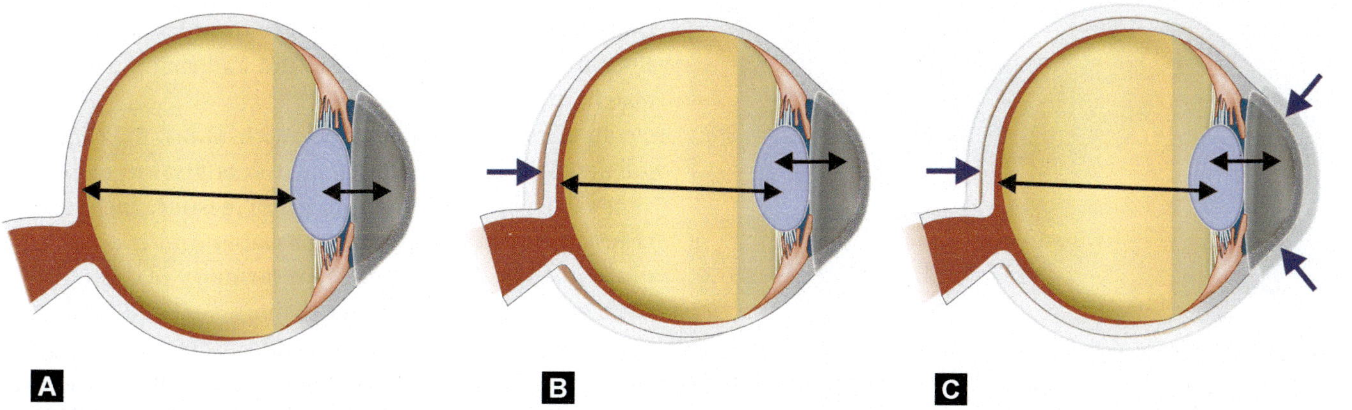

Figs. 43.5A to C: Nanophthalmos versus microphthalmos. (A) Normal sized eye; (B) Microphthalmic eye with a normal sized anterior chamber but shallow vitreous cavity and overall short axial length; (C) Nanophthalmic eye with shallow anterior chamber and vitreous cavity and subsequent short axial length.

choroid and sclera with propensity for uveal effusion. These eyes also have narrow angles and are at risk for angle closure glaucoma. They may also have microcornea. An estimated 20% of eyes with short AL also have shallow ACD.[26,28]

It is important to be aware of ACD for both intraocular lens (IOL) calculations and surgical planning. Ultrasound biomicroscopy or anterior segment OCT may be helpful in assessing anterior segment proportions and anatomic variations. One study[29] suggested a positive correlation between risk for perioperative complication and reducing AL and ACD. Abnormal IOP may also be associated with higher complications overall. Careful examination of the corneal endothelium is vital. There may be an increased incidence of Fuchs endothelial dystrophy with small eyes, and consideration of performing endothelial cell count or central corneal pachymetry should be made to document preexisting corneal disease.[30] This is especially important in eyes with narrow ACD as the endothelium is already at increased risk of intraoperative damage. Small corneal size can also mean that a standard phaco incision may induce more astigmatic change. An advanced cataract in an eye with a small anterior chamber and narrow angles is at further risk for angle closure (Fig. 43.6). It is also possible that a small eye with advanced cataract may have minimal refractive error or even a mild amount of myopia if there has been a myopic shift due to advanced nuclear cataract.

If there are significant differences in visual acuity in the presence of a similar degree of cataract, there may be a component of amblyopia. Even a relatively small amount of anisohyperopia can result in amblyopia.[26,31] This should be discussed with the patient prior to surgery so that there are appropriate expectations for visual outcomes.

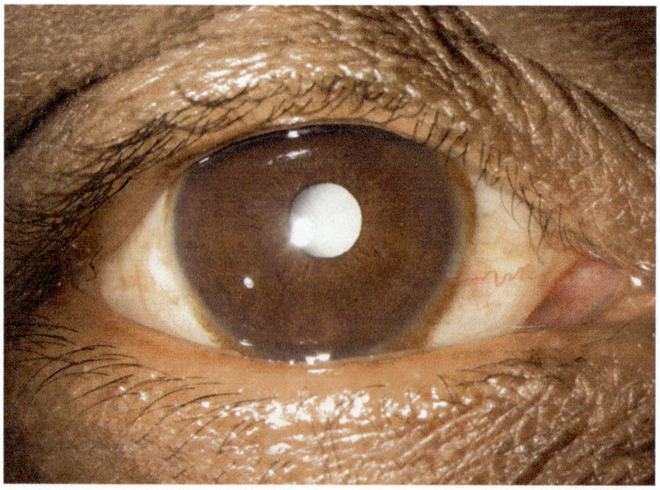

Fig. 43.6: An eye with a very shallow anterior chamber and dense cataract. The advanced cataract puts this patient at an increased risk for angle closure as the anterior chamber was already previously narrow. Cataract surgery requires careful surgical planning in such eyes as the small anterior chamber carries unique challenges.

Source: Dr Sharmila Rajendrababu, Aravind Eye Hospital, Chennai.

Accurate preoperative biometry is imperative as there is little room for error when determining IOL power. A small inaccuracy in AL can result in larger refractive errors in the small eye compared to eyes with normal AL. Thus, it is important to use accurate method for determining AL, such as optical based biometry. Microphthalmic eyes tend to require higher IOL powers than nanophthalmic eyes. As a result, slight changes in effective lens position (ELP) can alter refractive results significantly. The closer the IOL is to the retina, the more ELP affects outcomes as well. For this reason, it is important to optimize A-constants, and consider personalized A-constants that are used separately for small eyes.[26,32]

Certain formulae have been shown to be more accurate in eyes with high hyperopia. The third generation formulas determine the expected ACD to the lens as a function of axial length, thus they predict the position of the lens too far anterior in microphthalmic eyes with normal ACD and short AL.[28] This results in a hyperopic error. They perform better with nanophthalmic eyes where the ACD and AL are proportionately small. The Hoffer Q formula attenuates the scaling of the predicted ACD and is best suited amongst the third generation formulas for small eyes. In general, fourth generation formulas are better suited for short AL. The incorporation of multiple variables, including horizontal white to white diameter, ACD, and lens thickness, in addition to AL and corneal power make the fourth generation formulas more accurate with small eyes. Several studies have proven the superiority of the Hoffer Q formula amongst the third generation formulas, and even more so the Holladay II and Haigis equations, at determining IOL power in these eyes.[26, 29, 33-40] Newer formulas, including the Barrett Universal II, Hill-RBF, and Ladas Super Formula, also have shown promise.[13,15,16]

In some situations, eyes with short AL require a particularly high power IOL. It is advisable to place a single IOL when able for a variety of reasons. There usually is less room in the anterior chamber and it is easier to place a single IOL. In addition, primary placement of 2 IOLs in the capsular bag has been associated with inter-lenticular membranes and opacifications as well as a late hyperopic shift.[26, 41-43] There are many approved IOLs with powers greater than +30.0, and the Acrys of SN60AT (Alcon Laboratories, Inc.) is a single piece acrylic IOL with power up to +40.0 in the United States. The difficulty comes when an even higher refractive power is required. One option is to place the highest powered IOL available and consider corneal refractive surgery, contact lens, or spectacles to correct the remaining refractive error. Another option is to place piggyback IOLs.[28,44] Theoretically using two lenses is optically superior than a single extremely high dioptric power lens as there is less spherical aberration. It is advised to place one IOL in the capsular bag and the second piggyback lens in the ciliary sulcus. Many surgeons use different IOL materials. Due to difficulty with calculating IOL power of the second lens, it may be easier to place the one lens in the bag at the initial surgery, and then place the piggyback lens as a second staged procedure after the eye has healed so that accurate calculations for the second IOL can be made. Other countries may have access to custom made, higher power IOLs in order to allow implantation of a single IOL.

Surgical Technique

Cataract surgery in small eyes is generally more challenging due to a crowded anterior chamber (Fig. 43.7). There are variable complication rates reported, likely dependent on surgeon experience.[29,45] Often these small eyes sit deeper in the orbit and make access challenging. If the cornea is thicker than average, it can complicate wound creation into a shallow anterior chamber. If the tunnel length of the main incision is too long, this may make it difficult to access the lens. Altering the angle of the wound entry can help prevent this. Suboptimal dilation is often present, and iris hooks are preferable to an iris ring as there is less space to maneuver the ring in place and risk damaging corneal endothelium. Small eyes may have a higher frequency of zonular dehiscence as well.[29]

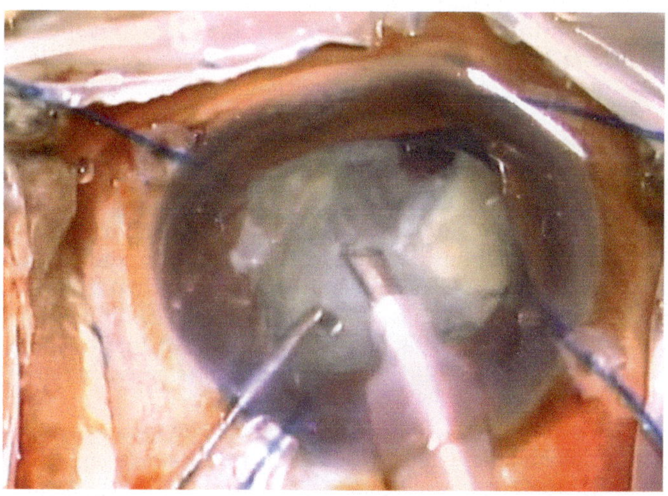

Fig. 43.7: Phacoemulsification in a small nanophthalmic eye with crowded and small anterior chamber. Iris hooks are being used due to poor dilation. Care must be taken to avoid corneal endothelial damage in the shallow anterior chamber. Ophthalmic viscosurgical devices are useful to deepen the chamber.
Source: Dr Sharmila Rajendrababu, Aravind Eye Hospital, Chennai.

The thickened sclera and choroid of nanophthalmic eyes increase the risk of uveal effusion or choroidal hemorrhage, which has been well documented but may not be as common now with modern phacoemulsification.[26,29,46,47] These eyes may have chronic uveal effusions that can be seen preoperatively. Scleral windows can be made to facilitate outflow of choroidal fluid, although this may not be advisable when using phacoemulsification as the pressurized intraocular environment can lead to uveal and vitreous prolpase.[26] If a uveal effusion is noted intraoperatively, sclerectomies may need to be performed, or consider closing all wounds and completing the case at a later date. If possible, retro-orbital blocks should be avoided in cases with very small AL as they may increase the risk of uveal effusion by increasing orbital congestion. Consider topical anesthesia instead. Also limit the pressure fluctuations during surgery to reduce the risk of uveal effusion or suprachoroidal hemorrhage.

One of the biggest challenges is simply the limited space in the anterior chamber in these highly hyperopic eyes. In some eyes the anterior chamber is so shallow to preclude capsulorhexis formation. A cohesive ophthalmic viscosurgical device (OVD) can be used to deepen the chamber. Other strategies involve decreasing posterior pressure to increase ACD. Acetazolamide or IV mannitol given 30 minutes prior to surgery can reduce vitreous volume.[26,48] Alternatively, a vitreous tap or limited pars plana anterior vitrectomy can be done to help deepen the anterior chamber. Care must be taken to avoid taking too much vitreous and making the anterior chamber too deep. Because the volume of the anterior chamber is less, the phaco probe is closer to the cornea. Dispersive OVD can help protect the endothelium, and phaco techniques performed within the capsular bag are generally preferred. It is also important to watch for iris prolapse as the iris sits closer to the wounds.

Postoperative Management

As mentioned previously, there is variation in the actual rate of complications involved with cataract surgery in small eyes. Those complications reported are serious, however, and careful postoperative monitoring is advised.

Complications reported include iris prolapse, postoperative cystoid macular edema, aqueous misdirection, prolonged anterior uveitis, suprachoroidal hemorrhage, persistent corneal edema, retinal detachment, and uveal effusions.[48] Eyes with prior history of angle closure glaucoma may have abnormal blood aqueous barrier than results in prolonged postoperative inflammation.[49] Aqueous misdirection, or malignant glaucoma, is one of the most serious possible complications and can be difficult to manage. The present of a flat or shallow anterior chamber postoperatively should raise suspicion for aqueous misdirection, even if the intraocular pressure is initially normal. Some surgeons suggest a surgical iridectomy be made at the time of surgery to facilitate laser zonulotomy or hyaloidotomy if malignant glaucoma occurs.[29] Although phacoemulsification normally improves anterior chamber anatomy and angle configuration, small eyes are still at risk for angle closure, especially in the setting of peripheral uveal effusions. It can be difficult to differentiate between this and aqueous misdirection, and ultrasound biomicroscopy can be beneficial.

In summary, cataract surgery in patients with high myopia and hyperopia poses many challenges. The anatomic variations present in these eyes makes determining the correct IOL difficult, and often alterations in surgical technique need to be employed. They often have other ocular comorbidities that may limit their vision, and postoperative complications that can be devastating. Yet despite these challenges, successful surgery can be performed and these patients tend to be particularly happy after a lifetime of refractive error and spectacle dependence.

REFERENCES

1. Zaldivar R, Shultz MC, Davidorf JM, et al. Intraocular lens power calculations in patients with extreme myopia. J Cataract Refract Surg. 2000;26:668-74.
2. Maclaren RE, Sagoo MS, Restori M, et al. Biometry accuracy using zero- and negative-powered intraocular lenses. J Cataract Refract Surg. 2005;31:280-90.
3. Wang JK, Hu CY, Chang SW. Intraocular lens power calculation using the IOLMaster and various formulas in eyes with long axial length. J Cataract Refract Surg. 2008; 34:262-7.
4. Wang L, Shirayama M, Ma XJ, et al. Optimizing intraocular lens power calculations in eyes with axial lengths above 25.0 mm. J Cataract Refract Surg. 2011; 37:2018-27.
5. Abulafia A, Barrett GD, Rotenberg M, et al. Intraocular lens power calculation for eyes with an axial length greater than 26.0 mm: comparison of formulas and methods. J Cataract Refract Surg. 2015;41:548-56.
6. Geggel HS. Comparison of formulas and methods for high myopia patients requiring intraocular lens powers less than six diopters. Int Ophthalmol. 2018;38(4):1497-504.
7. Haigis W. Intraocular lens calculation in extreme myopia. J Cataract Refract Surg. 2009;35:906-11.
8. Aristodemou P, Cartwright NEK, Sparrow JM, et al. Formula choice: Hoffer Q, Holladay 1, or SRK/T and refractive outcomes in 8108 eyes after cataract surgery with biometry by partial coherence interferometry. J Cataract Refract Surg. 2011;37:63-71.
9. Petermeier K, Gekeler F, Messias A, et al. Intraocular lens power calculation and optimized constants for highly myopic eyes. J Cataract Refract Surg. 2009;35:1575-81.
10. Preussner PR. Letter in response to Hiaigs "Intraocular lens calculation in extreme myopia." J Cataract Refract Surg. 2010;36:531-2.
11. Yokoi T, Moriuama M, Hayashi K, et al. Evaluation of refractive error after cataract surgery in highly myopic eyes. Int Ophthalmol. 2013;33:343-8.
12. Pomberg ML, Miller KM. Preliminary efficacy and safety of zero diopter lens implantation in highly myopic eyes. Am J Ophthalmol. 2005;139:914-5.
13. Kane JX, Van Heerden AV, Atik A, et al. Intraocular lens power formula accuracy: comparison of 7 formulas. J Cataract Refract Surg. 2016;42:1490-500.
14. Hill DC, Sudhakar S, Hill CS, et al. Intraoperative aberrometry versus preoperative biometry for intraocular lens power selection in axial myopia. J Cataract Refract Surg. 2017;43:505-10.
15. Kane JX, Van Heerden AV, Atik A, et al. Accuracy of 3 new methods for intraocular lens power selection. J Cataract Refract Surg. 2017;43:333-9.
16. Ladas JG, Siddiqui AA, Devgan U, et al. A 3-D "super surface" combining modern intraocular lens formulas to generate a "super formula" and maximize accuracy. JAMA Ophthalmol. 2015;133:1431-6.
17. Cionni RJ, Barros MG, Osher RH. Management of lens-iris diaphragm retropulsion syndrome during phacoemulsification. J Cataract Refract Surg. 2004;30:953-6.
18. Zuberbuhler B, Seyedian M, Tuft S. Phacoemulsification in eyes with extreme axial myopia. J Cataract Refract Surg. 2009;35:335-40.
19. Fesharaki H, Peyman A, Rowshandel M, et al. A comparative study of complications of cataract surgery with phacoemulsification in eyes with high and normal axial length. Advanced Biomedical Research. 2012;1(2):1-4.
20. Fan DSP, Lam DSC, Li KKW. Retinal complications after cataract extraction in patients with high myopia. Ophthalmology. 1999;106:688-91; discussion by M Stirpe, 691-2.
21. Lyle WA, Jin GJC. Phacoemulsification with intraocular lens implantation in high myopia. J Cataract Refract Surg. 1996; 22:238-42.
22. Ochi T, Gon A, Kora Y, et al. Intraocular lens implantation and high myopia. J Cataract Refract Surg. 1988;14:403-8.
23. Cetinkaya S, Acir NO, Cetinyaka YF, et al. Phacoemulsification in eyes with cataract and high myopia. Arq Bras Oftalmol. 2015;78(5):286-9.

24. Lam JKM, Chan TCY, Ng ALK, et al. Outcomes of cataract operations in extreme high axial myopia. Graefes Arch Clin Exp Ophthalmol. 2016;254:1811-7.
25. Bernheim D, Rouberol F, Palombi K, et al. Comparative prospective study of rhegmatogenous retinal detachments in phakic or pseudophakic patients with high myopia. Retina. 2013;33:2039-48.
26. Hoffman RS, Vasavada AR, Allen QB, et al. Cataract surgery in the small eye. J Cataract Refract Surg. 2015;41:2565-75.
27. Srinivasan S. From the editor: Small eyes—big problems. J Cataract Refract Surg. 2015;41:2345-6.
28. Holladay JT, Gills JP, Leidlein J, et al. Achieving emmetropia in extremely short eyes with two piggyback posterior chamber intraocular lenses. Ophthalmology. 1996; 103:1118-23.
29. Day AC, MacLaren RE, Bunce C, et al. Outcomes of phacoemulsification and intraocular lens implantation in microphthalmos and nanophthalmos. J Cataract Refract Surg. 2013;39:87-96.
30. Pitts JF, Jay JL. The association of Fuchs's corneal endothelial dystrophy with axial hypermetropia, shallow anterior chamber, and angle closure glaucoma. Br J Ophthalmol. 1990;74:601-4.
31. Weakley DR. The association between nonstrabismic anisometropia, amblyopia, and subnormal binocularity. Ophthalmology. 2001;108:163-71.
32. Terzi E, Wang L, Kohnen T. Accuracy of modern intraocular lens power calculation formulas in refractive lens exchange for high myopia and high hyperopia. J Cataract Refract Surg. 2009;35:1181-9.
33. Fenzl RE, Gills JP, Cherchio M. Refractive and visual outcome of hyperopic cataract cases operated on before and after implementation of the Holladay II formula. Ophthalmology. 1998;105:1759-64.
34. Bal L, Zhang ZP, Yi GL, et al. Selection of accurate IOL formula in patients with cataract and high hyperopia. Chin J Ophthalmol. 2008;44:1063-5.
35. Day AC, Foster PJ, Stevens JD. Accuracy of intraocular lens power calculations in eyes with axial length <22.00 mm. Clin Exp Ophthalmol. 2012;40:855-62.
36. Carifi G, Aiello F, Zygoura V, et al. Accuracy of the refractive prediction determined by multiple currently available intraocular lens power calculations formulas in small eyes. Am J Ophthalmolo. 2015;159:577-83.
37. Gavin EA, Hammond CJ. Intraocular lens power calculation in short eyes. Eye. 2008;22:935-8.
38. Moschos MM, Chatziralli IP, Koutsandrea C. Intraocular lens power calculation in eyes with short axial length. Indian J Ophthalmol. 2014;62:692-4.
39. Haigis W. IOL-Kalkulation bei hohen Ametropien [IOL calculation for high ametropia]. Ophthalmologe. 2008; 105:999-1004.
40. Hoffer KJ. Clinical results of using the Holladay 2 intraocular lens power formula. J Cataract Refract Surg. 2000;26:1233-7.
41. Werner L, Apple DJ, Pandey SK, et al. Analysis of elements of interlenticular opacification. Am J Ophthalmol. 2002; 133:320-6.
42. Gayton JL, Apple DJ, Peng Q, et al. Interlenticular opacification: clinicopathological correlation of a complication of posterior chamber piggyback intraocular lenses. J Cataract Refract Surg. 2000;26:330-6.
43. Shugar JK, Schwartz T. Interpseudophakos Elschnig pearls associated with late hyperopic shift: a complication of piggyback posterior chamber intraocular lens implantation. J Cataract Refract Surg. 1999;25:863-7.
44. Gayton JL. Implanting two posterior chamber intraocular lenses in microphthalmos. Ocular Surgery News. 1994;64-5.
45. Carifi G, Safa F, Aiello F, et al. Cataract surgery in small adult eyes. Br J Ophthalmol. 2014;98:1261-5.
46. Wu W, Dawson DG, Sugar A, et al. Cataract surgery in patients with nanophthalmos: results and complications. J Cataract Refract Surg. 2004;30:584–90.
47. Faucher A, Hasanee K, Rootman DS. Phacoemulsification and intraocular lens implantation in nanophthalmic eyes; report of a medium-size series. J Cataract Refract Surg. 2002; 28:837-42.
48. Steijns D, Bijlsma WR, Van der Lelij A. Cataract surgery in patients with nanophthalmos. Ophthalmology. 2013; 120:266-70.
49. Higashihara H, Sotozono C, Yokoi N, et al. The blood-aqueous barrier breakdown in eyes with endothelial decompensation after argon laser iridotomy [letter]. Br J Ophthalmol. 2011;95:1032-4.

Chapter 44

Challenging Cataract Cases: Weak Zonules, Pseudoexfoliation, and Traumatic Cataracts

Eric Shieh, Kevin M Miller

INTRODUCTION

Cataract surgery in eyes with weak zonules, pseudoexfoliation (PXF), or prior trauma presents a number of unique challenges for the anterior segment surgeon. Patients with these problems frequently have iris abnormalities, glaucoma, and unstable lenses, which can make phacoemulsification difficult.[1,2] Despite the risks, successful cataract surgery can be accomplished with careful preoperative planning, intraoperative technique, and postoperative care, resulting in a stable, well-centered intraocular lens (IOL) and improved functional vision.

WEAK ZONULES

Preoperative Evaluation

A thorough patient history can identify risk factors for weak zonules. Common predisposing conditions include PXF, trauma, advanced age, mature cataracts, high myopia, uveitis, and prior eye surgery such as vitrectomy or glaucoma filtering surgery.[3] Less common causes of zonular pathology include retinopathy of prematurity, retinitis pigmentosa, Marfan syndrome, homocystinuria, Weill-Marchesani syndrome, Axenfeld-Rieger syndrome, myotonic dystrophy, hyperlysinemia, and sulfite oxidase deficiency.[3]

During slit-lamp biomicroscopy, one must be vigilant for signs of zonular weakness (Figs. 44.1A to C). These include iridodonesis, phacodonesis, anterior chamber depth asymmetry within or between the eyes, a shallow or excessively deep anterior chamber, or vitreous in the anterior chamber.[1] Gonioscopy and ultrasound biomicroscopy can help elicit subtle anterior chamber or angle asymmetry. If severe zonular loss is present, as reflected by lens subluxation or frank areas of zonular dehiscence, alternate approaches to lens extraction and IOL insertion need to be considered (Figs. 44.2A and B). Capsular tension devices, some of which can be sutured to the sclera to create artificial zonules and stabilize the capsular bag, are discussed later in this chapter.[3] If the bag is unsalvageable, the surgeon may choose to implant a sulcus posterior chamber IOL with optic capture, scleral suture or tunnel fixated posterior chamber IOL, or anterior chamber IOL.

Capsulorhexis Creation

It is preferable to identify zonular weakness preoperatively, but it may not be noticed until after the case has already begun. If zonular instability is present, the first sign may be star-shaped striae on the anterior capsule surface during the capsule puncture, a shimmering movement of the lens, or anterior or posterior displacement of the lens relative to the

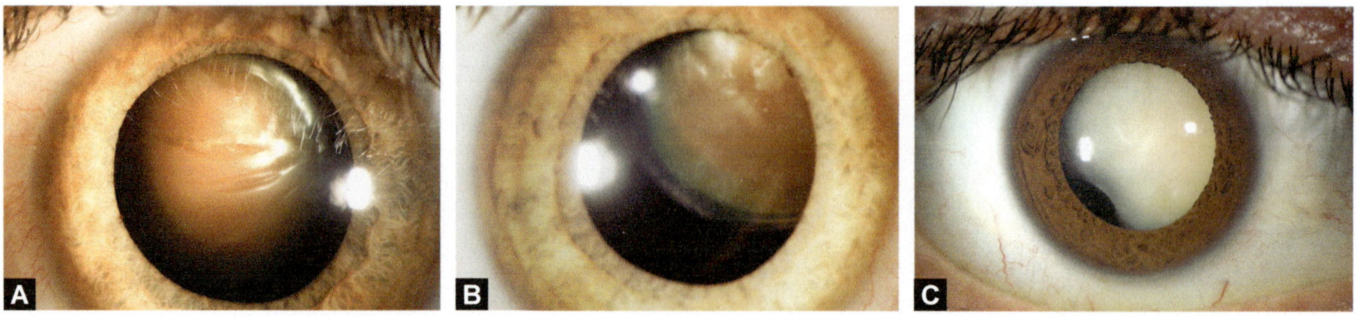

Figs. 44.1A to C: Signs of zonular weakness. (A) Anterior capsular folds in an eye with a dense brunescent cataract; (B) Marked phacodonesis and lens subluxation in the fellow eye; (C) A dense white cataract with a focal notch from zonular dehiscence.

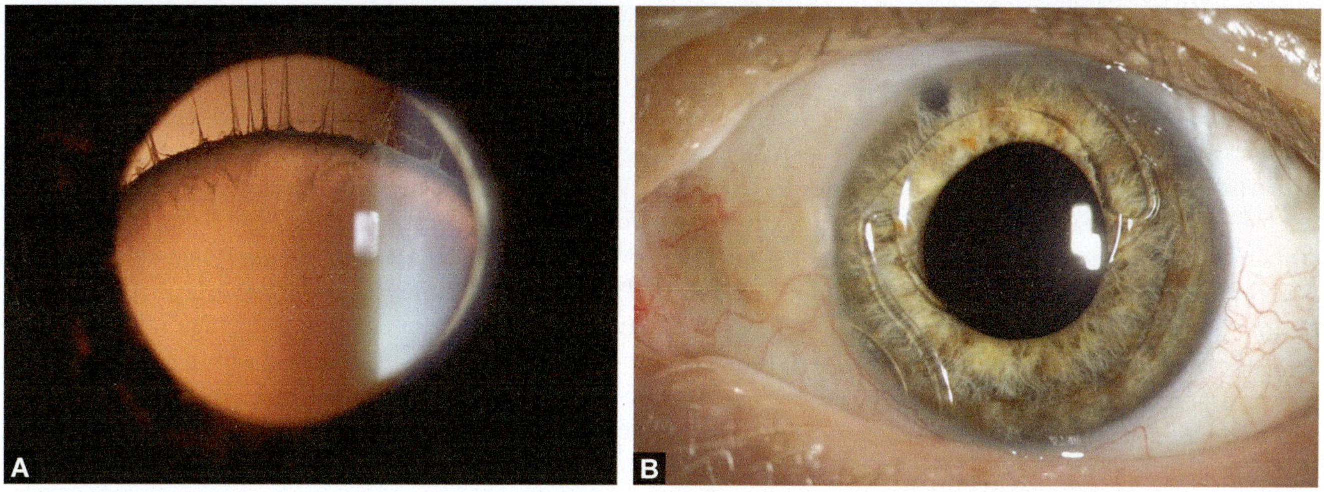

Figs. 44.2A and B: Nontraumatic ectopia lentis of unclear etiology requiring anterior chamber intraocular lens implantation. (A) Inferior lens subluxation indicating significant zonular loss. The cataract was extracted using phacoemulsification. Capsule retractors were used to provide intraoperative capsulorhexis stabilization; (B) After complete capsulectomy, an anterior chamber intraocular lens was implanted.

posterior iris.[1] In the absence of zonular countertraction on the lens capsule, manual countertraction may be required for capsulorhexis creation, with either a second instrument such as a Kuglen Hook or capsular support devices. Generally, one should aim for a continuous curvilinear capsulorhexis of approximately 5–5.5 mm in diameter.[1] A smaller diameter makes phacoemulsification difficult to perform, resulting in increased stress on the zonules. A small capsulorhexis also predisposes to postoperative anterior capsular phimosis, which can cause IOL tilt and decentration and glare with pupil dilation.[4] An oversized capsulorhexis, however, may preclude the use of capsular tension devices.

Hydrodissection

Thorough hydrodissection with balanced salt solution (BSS) and complete rotation of the lens within the capsular bag should be attempted. This will free the lens from the capsule, thereby decreasing zonular stress during the subsequent steps of surgery. Hydrodissection should be performed gently, as aggressive maneuvers can lead to lens dislocation even before phacoemulsification has begun. Care must be taken to avoid overfilling the anterior chamber with fluid, which stresses the zonules.[1] This situation can be avoided by gently burping the paracentesis during hydrodissection.

Phacoemulsification

Favored techniques include zonule-friendly maneuvers like vertical and horizontal chopping for denser nuclei or prolapsing the lens into the center of the pupillary zone for softer nuclei.[4] Sculpting maneuvers such as divide and conquer can also be performed as long as excessive force is not applied to the zonules. One must note that a shallow or collapsed anterior chamber increases the risk of vitreous prolapse through areas of zonular dialysis. Keeping the anterior chamber formed with either BSS or an ophthalmic viscosurgical device (OVD), particularly during insertion and removal of instruments, is therefore essential. Misdirection of irrigation fluid behind the lens capsule complex can occur in areas where the zonules are absent, leading to increased vitreous pressure.[5] Lowering the irrigation rate and sealing areas lacking zonules with a dispersive OVD can help prevent or decrease aqueous misdirection.[1]

Cortex Removal

Zonular dialysis can cause a slack capsule to aspirate into the port on an irrigation and aspiration probe. Removing cortex from a flaccid capsule is therefore difficult. Cortical clean up causes more stress to the zonular apparatus than any step of cataract surgery except nucleus rotation. To minimize the transmission of force to the zonules, most surgeons favor gentle tangential stripping of cortical material rather than radial stripping.[4,6] To prevent excess deepening of the anterior chamber and retropulsion of the capsule, lower flow rate and vacuum settings are recommended during irrigation and aspiration.

Intraocular Lens Insertion

There is debate over whether one- or three-piece foldable IOLs are more appropriate in eyes with zonular weakness.[4]

One piece IOLs unfold gently, can be dialed into the bag with minimal stress on the zonules, and are thought to be less likely to decenter. On the other hand, three-piece IOLs, by virtue of their broad stiff haptics can buttress areas of zonular loss when the IOL rests in the capsular bag.[4] Furthermore, one study demonstrated a lower incidence of capsular phimosis with a three-piece AcrySof IOL as compared to a single-piece AcrySof IOL.[6] If a three-piece IOL is implanted in the sulcus, the haptics should be oriented perpendicular to the area of zonular dehiscence, which tends to move inward due to absence of outward tension. The optic should be captured posteriorly to the capsulorhexis to stabilize the capsular bag.

Hydrophobic, acrylic, square-posterior-edge IOLs are preferred as they decrease the risk of anterior capsular phimosis and posterior capsular opacification.[4,6] Acrylic lenses are also compatible with silicone oil. This is an important consideration in patients with zonular instability who are at increased risk of vitreous loss and retinal detachment, as well as in patients with known retinal disease who may eventually need to undergo vitrectomy and silicone oil tamponade. Premium multifocal and accommodative IOLs are usually avoided in eyes with zonular instability, since these lenses require excellent centration.

Adjusting the intraocular lens power in patients in suspected zonular laxity can help prevent postoperative hyperopic surprise. With zonular laxity the lens-iris diaphragm may be pushed forward, leading to a shallower anterior chamber during the preoperative examination. After the thicker native lens is replaced by a thinner intraocular lens implant, the optic can reside more posteriorly than predicted by the preoperative anterior chamber depth. Adding 0.5 D to intraocular lens power may help decrease the likelihood of postoperative hyperopic surprise.

Capsular Tension Devices

Capsular tension devices are useful adjuncts for managing zonular instability. They are available as standard capsular tension rings (CTR), capsule retractors, modified capsular tension rings, and capsular tension segments (Figs. 44.3A to D).[3,7]

The standard CTR is a C-shaped polymethyl methacrylate (PMMA) ring that is implanted inside the capsular bag to impart an outward centrifugal force.[8,9] The force is equally distributed throughout the bag, redistributing tension between areas with normal zonules and areas with weak or absent zonules. In this way, intraoperative and postoperative complications are reduced.[8,10] The ring is most useful for mild, focal zonular instability with fewer than three or four clock hours of zonular dialysis. Two CTRs are currently approved by the United States Food and Drug Administration (FDA): the Reform Ring (Morcher GmbH, Stuttgart, Germany) and the StabilEyes CTR (Ophtec, Groningen, the Netherlands). Typically, a ring is inserted as late as possible during surgery to prevent it from interfering with removal of nuclear and cortical material, which can become trapped between the device and the capsular wall.[11] However, if needed to improve bag stability, a standard CTR can be implanted any time after the capsulorhexis is constructed.

A CTR can be injected or dialed manually into the bag with forceps. With either technique, the CTR should be gently directed toward the area of focal zonular weakness. A recently described *fishtail* technique does not require dialing and therefore may exert less stress on the zonules.[12] Ideally, a CTR is sized such that the eyelets at each end of the CTR overlap slightly to provide 360° support.[7] White-to-white measurements or axial length can be used to predict the capsular bag diameter so that the CTR is sized appropriately.[13] Most surgeons, however, implant the largest ring available in most eyes. Absolute contraindications include the presence of an anterior or posterior capsular tear or any question of bag compromise. A capsular tear will almost certainly extend due to the outward forces placed on the capsular bag by a ring and lead to advancement of the ring into the posterior segment.

If severe zonular compromise is observed, a standard CTR will not be sufficient and temporary capsule retractors may instead be utilized. Mackool capsule retractors are modified versions of standard iris hooks that are available in reusable and single-use forms.[3] Mackool retractors function by engaging the capsulorhexis edge, supporting the bag, and serving as temporary artificial zonules.

Mackool capsule retractors cannot be left in the eye permanently. If permanent artificial zonules are required, as in eyes with advanced zonular weakness or more than three or four clock hours of zonulolysis, modified CTRs or Cionni rings are indicated to ensure a stable and well-centered IOL.[14] Modified CTRs have either one or two eyelets located anterior to the plane of the ring. Via the eyelet, a modified CTR can be sutured to the sclera, typically with 9-0 polypropylene or CV-8 Gore-Tex. Unlike a standard CTR, these devices can only be implanted after nuclear

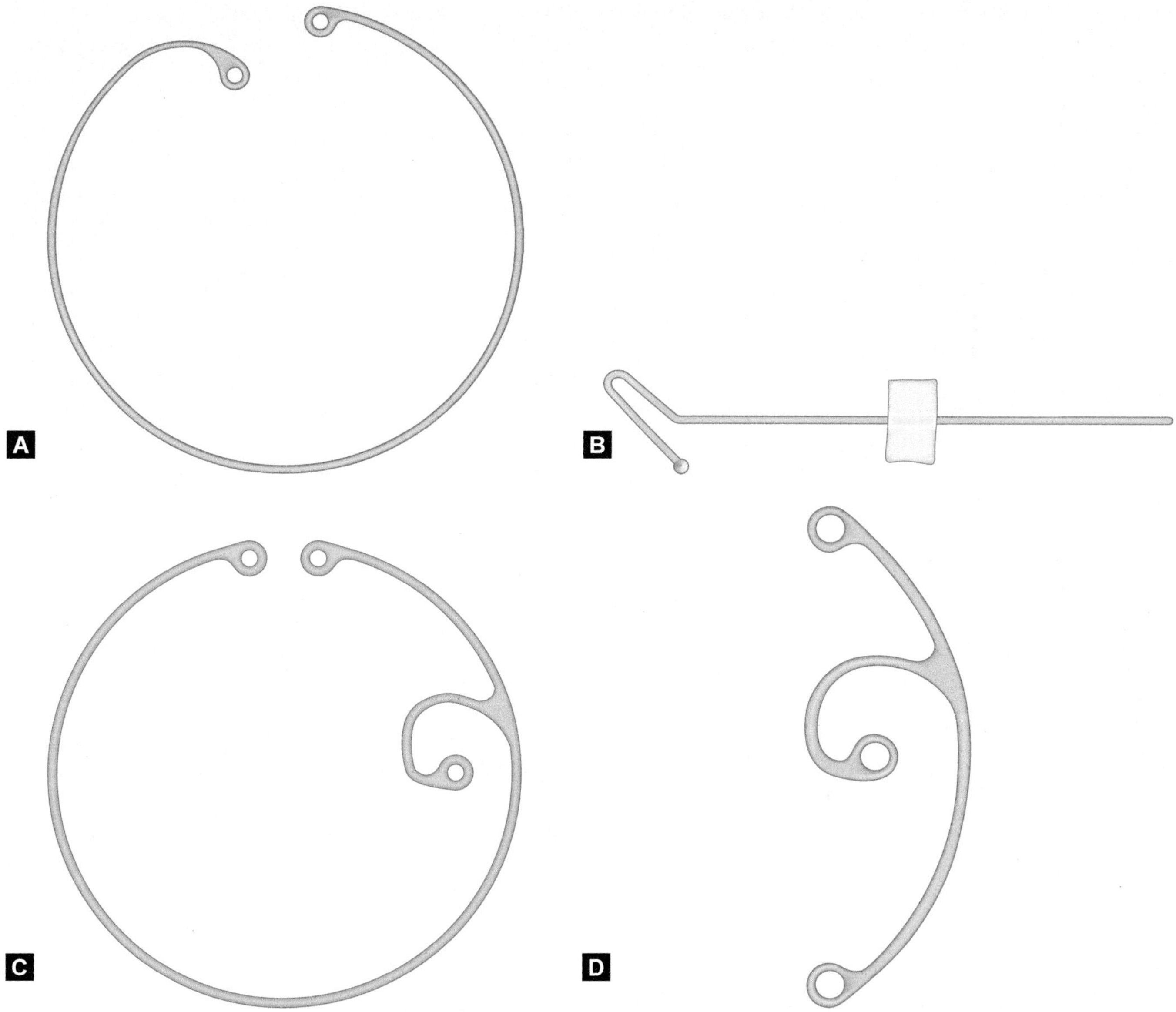

Figs. 44.3A to D: Capsular tension devices. (A) Standard capsular tension ring; (B) Capsule retractor; (C) Modified capsular tension ring; (D) Capsular tension segment.
Source: Morcher GmbH, Stuttgart, Germany.

and cortical material is removed and thus cannot provide zonular support during phacoemulsification. Similar to a standard CTR, these devices must be pushed and dialed into the capsular bag, which may exert tangential shearing forces on the zonules.

In 2002, Ahmed introduced the versatile capsular tension segment.[15] This device offers 90° of capsular support, and more than one segment can be placed in an eye. The capsular tension segment has several distinct advantages. It can be sutured via its one eyelet to the sclera, creating a permanent artificial zonule. By contrast to the standard CTR and modified CTR, the capsular tension segment requires no dialing and can be used even in the presence of capsular tears or a discontinuous capsulorhexis. The segment is also less likely to trap cortical or nuclear material.

More eyes with zonular weakness, which would have previously undergone implantation of an anterior chamber or sutured posterior chamber IOL, are now undergoing CTR implantation.[6] The long-term outcomes of this approach are unknown, and there is concern that with further zonular loss postoperatively, the entire bag-lens-CTR complex could dislocate posteriorly (Fig. 44.4).[16-18] Permanently fixating a CTR to the eye is a consideration, but cataract surgeons also note the need to balance the risk

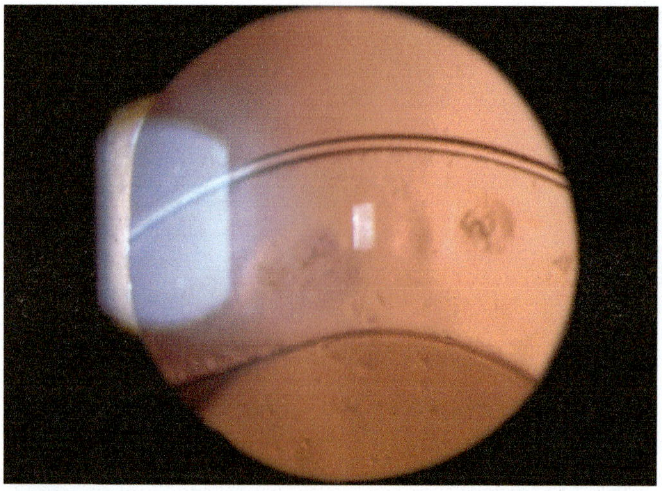

Fig. 44.4: Postoperative dislocation of the capsular bag, intraocular lens, and capsular tension ring in an eye with chronic nongranulomatous iridocyclitis and glaucoma. Intraocular lens and capsular tension ring repositioning with scleral suture fixation was performed.

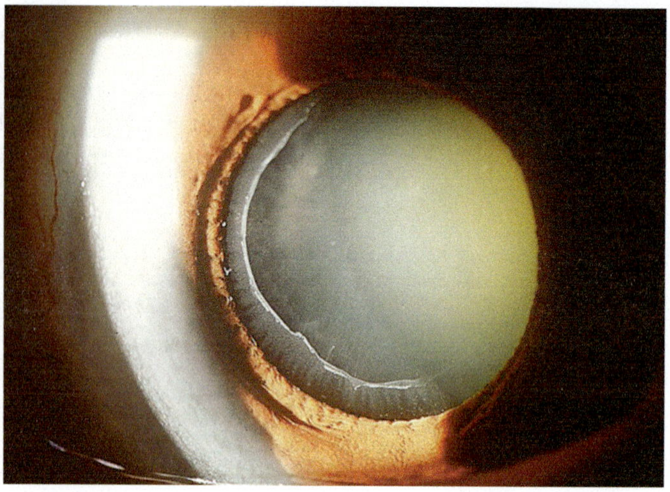

Fig. 44.5: Pseudoexfoliation material on the anterior lens capsule.

of lens dislocation with the risks of increased intraocular manipulation and long-term suture erosion, breakage, or infection.

PSEUDOEXFOLIATION SYNDROME

Eyes with PXF frequently have weak zonules, increasing the risk of vitreous loss, capsule rupture, and late postoperative dislocation of the capsular bag. They are additionally at risk for other complications, including early postoperative intraocular pressure spikes, persistent inflammation, anterior capsular phimosis, and corneal decompensation.[1,19] PXF is an age-related systemic disorder in which fibrillar extracellular material is synthesized and deposited throughout the anterior segment of the eye.[20] The classic clinical presentation is a target-shaped ring of white or gray flaky residue on the anterior lens capsule, though PXF material can also be seen on the iris, angle structures, zonules, and ciliary processes (Fig. 44.5). Pupillary transillumination defects or pigment dispersion may indicate early PXF. However, the degree of PXF deposition visible in the eye may not correlate with the degree of zonular instability.

Complications in Pseudoexfoliation

Elevated intraocular pressure and glaucoma: PXF syndrome is strongly associated with elevated intraocular pressure and glaucoma. The incidence of glaucoma at diagnosis of PXF is approximately 15%, and the cumulative risk of requiring glaucoma treatment is approximately 40–50% at 15 years.[21,22] For this reason, the preoperative evaluation must include treatment of elevated intraocular pressure, if present, and screening for glaucomatous optic nerve damage. While cataract surgery decreases intraocular pressure for eyes with PXF in the long run, eyes with PXF are at higher risk for early postoperative intraocular pressure spikes.[23,24] Complete removal of OVD is therefore critical. One may consider instilling carbachol intracamerally, administering topical glaucoma medication and oral acetazolamide immediately after surgery, or decompressing the eye by burping the paracentesis if the intraocular pressure is elevated.[1] Monitoring intraocular pressure for 4–6 hours postoperatively in patients with advanced glaucoma is recommended by some.[4]

Small pupils: Intraoperative miosis is an important risk factor for surgical complications in PXF.[4] A poorly dilating pupil, which is frequently seen in PXF, is thought to be caused by infiltration of PXF material into the iris stroma. Approximately, 50% of eyes with PXF have poor intraoperative mydriasis as compared to approximately 10% of eyes without PXF.[25] Iris atrophy and pupil margin transillumination defects visualized at the slit-lamp suggest a poorly dilating pupil. If a pupil is small, topical mydriatics and nonsteroidal anti-inflammatory drugs (NSAIDs) should be used preoperatively. If posterior synechiae binding the iris to the lens capsule are seen, they should be released prior to other intraoperative maneuvers. The pupil can be further expanded with a highly cohesive OVD and iris stretching devices such as iris hooks or pupillary rings.[5] However, excess dilation should be avoided.

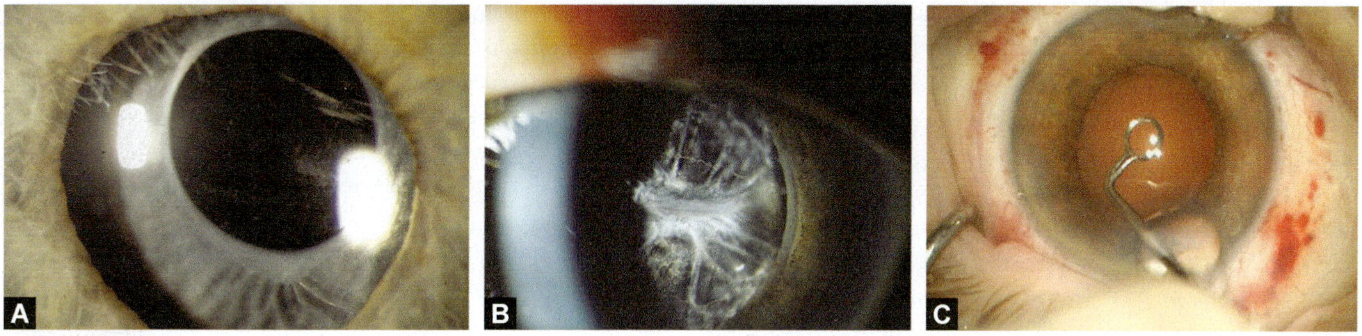

Figs. 44.6A to C: Postoperative anterior capsular phimosis. (A) Moderate capsular fibrosis and phimosis; (B) Complete closure and ectropion of the capsulorhexis; (C) Polishing the undersurface of the anterior capsule to remove lens epithelial cells can decrease the risk of anterior capsular fibrosis and capsulorhexis phimosis.

Overfilling the anterior chamber with viscoelastic exerts posterior pressure on the lens and stresses the zonules, while manipulation of fragile iris tissue can lead to an irregular atonic pupil.[1] If a small pupil is still problematic, bimanual phacoemulsification techniques may be used.

Increased inflammation and postoperative anterior capsular phimosis: The pseudoexfoliative process in PXF syndrome leads to alterations in iris vasculature, dysfunction of the blood-aqueous barrier, and increased oxidative stress.[1,25] For these reasons, eyes with PXF are at increased risk of developing early cataracts, prolonged postoperative intraocular inflammation, cystoid macular edema, anterior capsular phimosis, and posterior capsular opacification.[1,4,19] Thus, one should consider preoperative NSAIDs and a longer course of postoperative topical corticosteroids.[26] Attention must be paid to the development of postoperative anterior capsular phimosis, which can lead to stretching of zonules and IOL decentration or tilt (Figs. 44.6A to C). At the earliest signs of capsular phimosis, relaxing incisions with Nd:YAG laser in areas of anterior capsular contraction at the capsulorhexis margin should be considered.[27] The risk of capsular phimosis and an off-centered IOL can be reduced by creating an appropriately sized, round, and central capsulorhexis; polishing the undersurface of the anterior capsule to remove all lens epithelial cells; and implanting a CTR.[10,28] Posterior capsular opacification, when visually significant, can be routinely treated with Nd:YAG capsulotomy.

Corneal decompensation: PXF eyes are also at increased risk of corneal decompensation. The cause is multifactorial and could be due to the reduced endothelial cell counts in eyes with PXF and the increased operating time required for more complex eyes.[5] To reduce the risk of postoperative corneal edema, the endothelium can be coated with a dispersive OVD.[1]

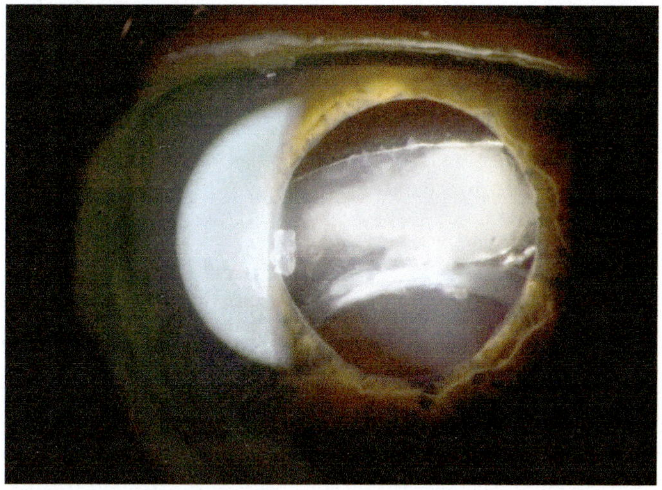

Fig. 44.7: Late postoperative dislocation of an intraocular lens and capsular bag secondary to pseudoexfoliation syndrome. On examination, the lens implant and capsular bag were subluxated inferiorly. In the operating room, the lens implant and capsular bag were completely dislocated posteriorly, requiring a pars plana vitrectomy and implantation of an anterior chamber intraocular lens.

Late spontaneous dislocation of the capsular bag: Late spontaneous postoperative dislocation of the capsular bag is a well-known complication of PXF and occurs at a rate of 8.4–10.6% (Fig. 44.7).[1,4,16,18] This is thought to occur because PXF material is continuously deposited on the zonules even after cataract surgery, leading to proteolysis of the zonules. Anterior capsular phimosis, which likely occurs due to the altered blood-aqueous barrier, may further increase stress on the zonules, eventually resulting in lens subluxation or complete dislocation. The mean interval between cataract surgery and late in-the-bag dislocation is approximately 8.5 years.[19] In younger patients with PXF, one should therefore consider implanting a standard CTR or suturing a modified CTR or capsular tension segment to the sclera. If the IOL has already dislocated, reasonable options include transscleral fixation or anterior chamber IOL implantation, though anterior chamber IOLs should be used in cautiously patients with glaucoma.

Complication rates in eyes with PXF: While some studies find a higher risk of cataract surgery complications in eyes with PXF, other studies report no increased risk.[24,26,29-33] For example, one study demonstrated a statistically significant difference in the incidence of vitreous loss between eyes in PXF and eyes without PXF (4% vs. 0%, $p < 0.001$) but no difference in the risk of corneal edema, iritis, or lens decentration between the two groups.[24] By contrast, another study comparing eyes with and without PXF found no significant differences in the incidence of intraoperative and early postoperative complications or visual outcomes.[31,33] Taken together, these studies suggest that intraoperative complications may be encountered in PXF patients, but that satisfactory postoperative outcomes similar to those seen in eyes without PXF can be achieved with the appropriate care.

TRAUMATIC CATARACTS

As in eyes with PXF, cataract surgery in the setting of ocular trauma is uniquely challenging and may require flexibility and ingenuity on the part of the surgeon. These eyes often have multiple comorbidities and extensive surgical histories. Understanding the mechanism of injury, indications for surgery, choices regarding surgical timing, and different surgical approaches are key to providing excellent care in these difficult cases.

Cataracts are a well-known sequelae of ocular trauma. In the general population, the cumulative lifetime prevalence of any eye trauma is approximately 15%, while the incidence of cataracts caused by ocular trauma ranges from 32% to 60%.[34-36] Cataracts can develop from blunt trauma or penetrating trauma to the globe. No standard morphologic classification exists, as the morphology of the cataract frequently varies depending on the mechanism of injury.[37]

Blunt trauma can occur with or without globe rupture. In blunt trauma, coup and contrecoup forces result in either direct or indirect injury to the lens, capsular bag, and zonular apparatus.[38] This can lead to focal or diffuse cataract, rupture of the anterior, posterior, or equatorial capsule, or zonulolysis with resultant lens subluxation or total dislocation. Metaplasia of lens epithelial cells caused by trauma can lead to a fibrous anterior subcapsular cataract, while intraocular inflammation from trauma can lead to cataract formation even in the absence of capsular damage. Blunt trauma is also associated with posterior subcapsular cataracts and rosette-shaped cataracts, in which focal cortical opacities create a flower-shaped pattern of opacities (Fig. 44.8A).

In penetrating trauma, the size of the cataract usually depends on the extent of the break in the lens capsule created by the foreign object. Focal lens opacities may form adjacent to a small, self-sealing capsular rupture, whereas diffuse white cataracts with flocculent cortical material may ensue from a large capsular opening (Fig. 44.8B). Cataracts may form immediately after trauma, though they may also develop gradually in the weeks and months after the original insult. Damage to the cornea, iris, trabecular meshwork, and posterior segment are common in eyes with a history of penetrating injury.

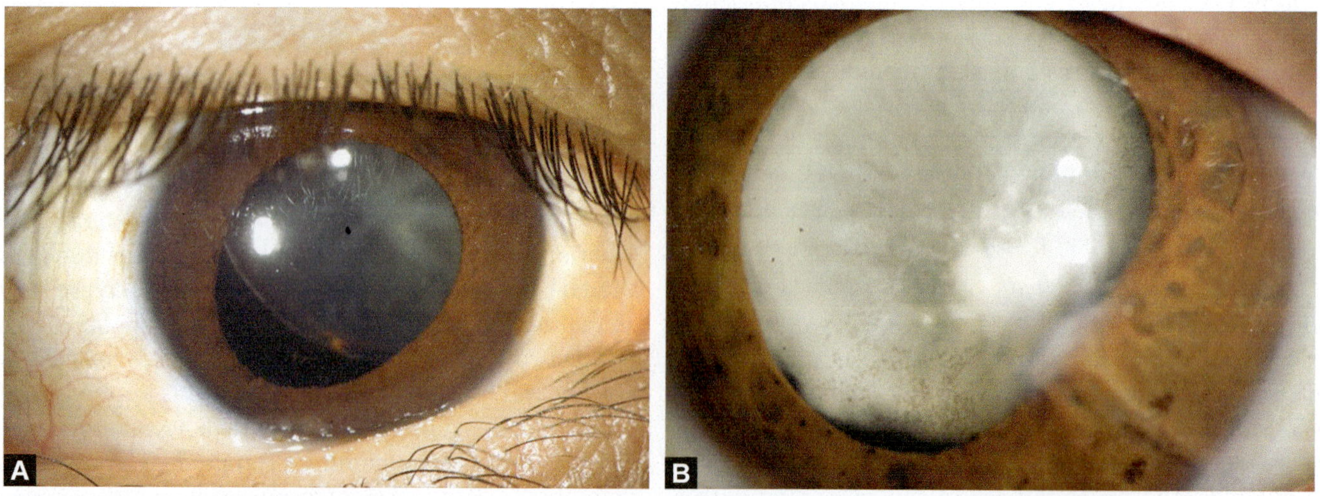

Figs. 44.8A and B: Blunt and penetrating traumatic cataracts. (A) Deep cortical opacities in a rosette pattern secondary to blunt eye trauma. Note that the lens is subluxated superonasally secondary to zonular disruption inferotemporally. The pupil sphincter muscle is also damaged at this location; (B) Dense focal cortical opacities and posterior synechiae secondary to penetrating eye trauma.

Surgical Indications

If a traumatic cataract results in significant loss of functional visual acuity, surgery is indicated. Other indications include lens-induced glaucoma or inflammation, lens swelling from capsular rupture, and a poor view of the posterior segment that hinders management of other ocular conditions.[38] Many traumatic cataracts do not cause a significant loss of visual acuity and may be small, nonprogressive, and located outside the pupil. Some eyes can be treated medically with topical miotics or mydriatics.[38] Miotics can be useful if an opacity nearing the visual axis causes symptoms like glare or monocular diplopia or if a subluxated lens produces astigmatism. On the other hand, mydriatics can enable aphakic correction if a lens is significantly subluxated.

Preoperative Evaluation

Thorough preoperative evaluation guides decisions on the timing and type of surgery required. This evaluation includes visual acuity, refraction, pupils, intraocular pressure measurement, slit-lamp examination, ophthalmoscopy, and potentially other testing such as B-scan or computed tomography (CT) imaging to assess for an intraocular foreign body, ruptured globe, or posterior segment pathology. In the acute setting, an open globe is more likely if the exam shows diffuse chemotic subconjunctival hemorrhage, corectopia, hyphema, an excessively shallow or deep anterior chamber, decreased intraocular pressure, restricted extraocular motility, a frank laceration, or Seidel positivity. Attention should be paid to evidence of corneal damage, intraocular inflammation, and vitreous prolapse into the anterior chamber. Gonioscopy should be performed gently to evaluate for iris and angle deformities; these are common in blunt ocular trauma, with an incidence of angle recession in 80% of eyes and iris abnormalities in 37%.[39]

Care should be taken to ensure that a cataract is truly present and not the illusion of a cataract created by hypotony or fibrin overlying the lens.[38] The extent and type of cataract, the integrity of the capsule, and signs of zonular weakness, such as iridodonesis or lens subluxation, should be noted. B-scan ultrasonography performed at a frequency of 20 MHz, anterior segment OCT, and Scheimpflug imaging may be useful in evaluating for zonular instability or occult posterior capsular rupture.[2]

In acute ocular trauma, accurate IOL power calculation may be difficult to perform. One may attempt measurements from the traumatized eye, use data from the fellow eye, or obtain calculations from the traumatized eye once primary closure of the ruptured globe has been completed. This usually includes refraction, A-scan ultrasonography, and keratometry measurements. Whereas a few smaller studies have shown that data from the fellow eye are generally acceptable, one study with 30 eyes showed that measurements obtained from the traumatized eye after primary closure of the ruptured globe were more accurate than measurements obtained from the fellow eye.[2]

Timing of Surgery

No consensus exists regarding the timing of cataract surgery in the context of a ruptured globe.[37] Cataract surgery can be performed in conjunction with primary ruptured globe repair, early in the weeks after the globe has been repaired, or as a late procedure weeks to years after the eye has been repaired and has become quiet.[40]

Cataract surgery in conjunction with ruptured globe repair is the best approach in some settings. If flocculent lens material is seen in the anterior chamber, early lensectomy with anterior chamber washout can decrease the risk of lens particle-induced uveitis, elevated intraocular pressure, and glaucoma. Likewise, a swollen lens that results in pupillary block should be removed early to prevent glaucoma. Cataract surgery simultaneous with rupture globe repair may also be considered in eyes with simple corneal lacerations and traumatic cataracts. Satisfactory outcomes, including corrected distance visual acuities of 20/40 of better, have been be achieved in eyes with simultaneous corneal laceration repair, cataract extraction, and posterior chamber IOL implantation.[41]

Primary ruptured globe repair followed within a few weeks by early cataract surgery carries the advantage of a stable wound and watertight globe, which allows for safer phacoemulsification.[2] Once the eye has healed and media opacities have cleared, a more accurate assessment of visual potential can be performed. The benefits of cataract surgery may at this time be deemed negligible in eyes with severe traumatic optic nerve or retinal pathology. Further, cataract surgery performed as a secondary procedure tends to be carried out in a more controlled operating room setting with better infrastructure and more experienced supporting staff.

Cataract surgery performed as a late procedure in a quiet eye offers the added advantages of better intraoperative visibility, decreased risk of postoperative inflammation, and more accurate IOL power calculation.[2,37] Whether early or late globe repair results in better visual outcomes is unclear, and the data vary in the literature.[40,42] However, in pediatric patients, early removal of media opacities and cataracts is imperative to prevent stimulus deprivation amblyopia.[2]

Surgical Approach

The surgical approach to traumatic cataracts depends on many factors, including the severity of the cataract, degree of zonular stability and capsule integrity, risk of vitreous loss, and presence of posterior segment pathology. Either an anterior or pars plana approach can be taken.[2,38]

An anterior approach is suitable for cataracts with intact capsules, cataracts with ruptured anterior capsules, and anteriorly subluxated or dislocated lenses (Fig. 44.9).[38] If the anterior capsule is ruptured, hydration and opacification of the lens cortex can result in a poor red reflex. Capsule stains such as trypan blue can improve visualization of the anterior capsule. If possible, a continuous curvilinear capsulorhexis should be made, though a can-opener capsulotomy may be necessary. In some cases of ocular trauma, a femtosecond laser may be used to create a more predictable capsulorhexis and minimize zonular stress.[43]

If a lens is subluxated anteriorly, an anterior approach can be used if the risk of posterior lens dislocation is reduced. Care must be taken to reduce stress on the zonules, using the techniques described previously in the chapter. If vitreous prolapses into the anterior chamber, it must be removed before cataract extraction. If a lens is dislocated anteriorly, miotics may be used to trap the lens in the anterior chamber. At this point, cataract extraction may proceed through irrigation and aspiration of a soft lens or through removal of an entire dense lens using external pressure and an irrigating vectis or cryoprobe.

In the presence of a posterior capsular tear, an anterior approach can still be used in certain situations. Posterior capsular tears whose torn edges are thicker, more fibrotic, and have developed over time are less likely to extend compared to tears whose torn edges are thin and less mature.[2] Smaller tears with a diameter of less than 6 mm are more likely to support an in-the-bag IOL than larger tears. If an anterior approach is taken, caution must be taken to avoid enlarging the tear or hydrating the vitreous.

By contrast, large posterior capsular tears are better suited to the pars plana approach.[38] The pars plana approach is also indicated for intraocular lenses or cataracts that are subluxated or dislocated posteriorly. If one suspects significant zonular laxity, the position of the lens or intraocular lens can be examined with the patient sitting upright at the slit-lamp and with the patient reclined in the supine position under the indirect ophthalmoscope. If the lens is observed to fall posteriorly into the mid-vitreous with the patient in the supine position, the pars plana approach is indicated. Eyes with concomitant posterior segment pathology may be more appropriate for the pars plana approach (Figs. 44.10A and B).

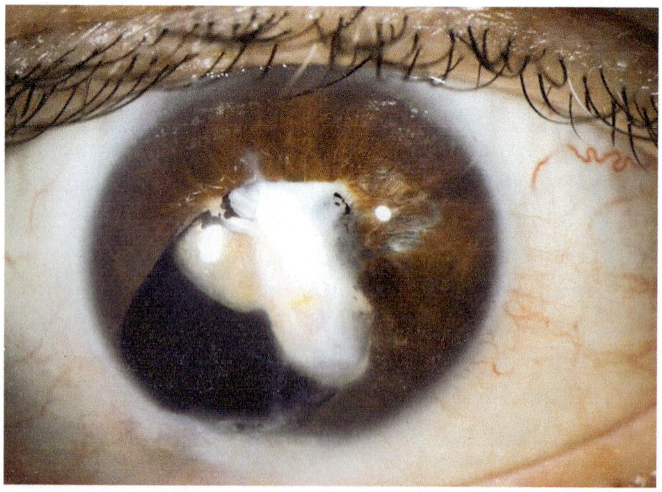

Fig. 44.9: Penetrating ocular trauma resulting in corneal laceration, iris damage, lens capsule rupture, traumatic cataract, zonular rupture, and corectopia. This injury necessitated penetrating keratoplasty, posterior synechialysis, intracapsular cataract extraction, anterior vitrectomy, implantation and suture fixation of a posterior chamber intraocular lens, and implantation and suture fixation of a HumanOptics artificial iris in the right eye.

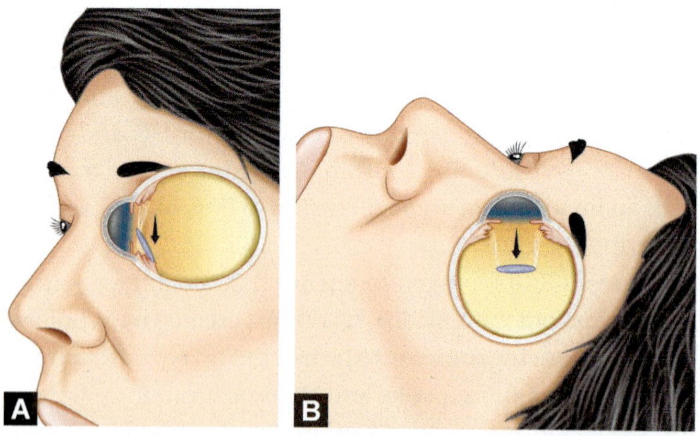

Figs. 44.10A and B: Examining the patient in the supine position can help determine whether a pars plana approach is more appropriate in an eye with severe zonular laxity. (A) When the patient is seated upright at the slit-lamp microscope, the intraocular lens and capsular bag complex appear to sit just behind the iris; (B) When the patient is laying supine under the surgical microscope or indirect ophthalmoscope, the intraocular lens and capsular bag complex can fall posteriorly into the mid-vitreous if there is severe zonular laxity.

SUMMARY

The presence of zonular instability and a history of PXF or prior ocular trauma can complicate many steps of cataract surgery. An understanding of the basic principles and techniques for managing these difficult cases is critical for good outcomes. Meticulous preoperative evaluation can help the anterior segment surgeon plan for potential intraoperative problems, while employing appropriate surgical strategies helps to minimize intraoperative and postoperative complications.

REFERENCES

1. Sangal N, Chen TC. Cataract surgery in pseudoexfoliation syndrome. Semin Ophthalmol. 2014;29(5-6):403-8.
2. Jacobs EJ, Tannen BL. Traumatic cataract: a review. J Ocular Biol. 2016;4(1): 4.
3. Riedel PJ, Samuelson TW. Capsular tension rings. In: DM Colvard (Ed.) Achieving Excellence in Cataract Surgery: A Step-By-Step Approach. Los Angeles: DM Colvard; 2009. pp.115-21.
4. Kastelan S, Tomic M, Kordic R, et al. Cataract surgery in eyes with pseudoexfoliation (PEX) syndrome. Clin Exp Ophthalmol. 2013;S1(9):1-5.
5. Belovay GW, Varma DK, Ahmed II. Cataract surgery in pseudoexfoliation syndrome. Curr Opin Ophthalmol. 2010;21(1):25-34.
6. Ronge L. Weak Zonules: New Tools for Tough Cases: American Academy of Ophthalmology. 2017. [online] Available from: https://www.aao.org/eyenet/article/weak-zonules-new-tools-tough-cases. [Accessed December, 2017].
7. Goldman JM, Karp CL. Adjunct devices for managing challenging cases in cataract surgery: pupil expansion and stabilization of the capsular bag. Curr Opin Ophthalmol. 2007;18(1):44-51.
8. Gimbel HV, Sun R, Heston JP. Management of zonular dialysis in phacoemulsification and IOL implantation using the capsular tension ring. Ophthalmic Surg Lasers. 1997;28(4):273-81.
9. Hara T, Hara T, Yamada Y. "Equator ring" for maintenance of the completely circular contour of the capsular bag equator after cataract removal. Ophthalmic Surg. 1991;22(6):358-9.
10. Bayraktar S, Altan T, Kucuksumer Y, et al. Capsular tension ring implantation after capsulorhexis in phacoemulsification of cataracts associated with pseudoexfoliation syndrome. Intraoperative complications and early postoperative findings. J Cataract Refract Surg. 2001;27(10):1620-8.
11. Ahmed II, Cionni RJ, Kranemann C, et al. Optimal timing of capsular tension ring implantation: Miyake-Apple video analysis. J Cataract Refract Surg. 2005;31(9):1809-13.
12. Angunawela RI, Little B. Fish-tail technique for capsular tension ring insertion. J Cataract Refract Surg. 2007;33(5): 767-9.
13. Vass C, Menapace R, Schmetterer K, et al. Prediction of pseudophakic capsular bag diameter based on biometric variables. J Cataract Refract Surg. 1999;25(10):1376-81.
14. Cionni RJ, Osher RH. Management of profound zonular dialysis or weakness with a new endocapsular ring designed for scleral fixation. J Cataract Refract Surg. 1998;24(10): 1299-306.
15. Hasanee K, Ahmed, II. Capsular tension rings: update on endocapsular support devices. Ophthalmol Clin North Am. 2006;19(4):507-19.
16. Jehan FS, Mamalis N, Crandall AS. Spontaneous late dislocation of intraocular lens within the capsular bag in pseudoexfoliation patients. Ophthalmology. 2001;108(10):1727-31.
17. Scherer M, Bertelmann E, Rieck P. Late spontaneous in-the-bag intraocular lens and capsular tension ring dislocation in pseudoexfoliation syndrome. J Cataract Refract Surg. 2006;32(4):672-5.
18. Oner FH, Kocak N, Saatci AO. Dislocation of capsular bag with intraocular lens and capsular tension ring. J Cataract Refract Surg. 2006;32(10):1756-8.
19. Shingleton BJ, Crandall AS, Ahmed II. Pseudoexfoliation and the cataract surgeon: preoperative, intraoperative, and postoperative issues related to intraocular pressure, cataract, and intraocular lenses. J Cataract Refract Surg. 2009;35(6):1101-20.
20. Schlotzer-Schrehardt U, Naumann GO. Ocular and systemic pseudoexfoliation syndrome. Am J Ophthalmol. 2006;141(5):921-37.
21. Jeng SM, Karger RA, Hodge DO, et al. The risk of glaucoma in pseudoexfoliation syndrome. J Glaucoma. 2007;16(1):117-21.
22. Mitchell P, Wang JJ, Hourihan F. The relationship between glaucoma and pseudoexfoliation: the Blue Mountains Eye Study. Arch Ophthalmol. 1999;117(10):1319-24.
23. Shingleton BJ, Laul A, Nagao K, et al. Effect of phacoemulsification on intraocular pressure in eyes with pseudoexfoliation: single-surgeon series. J Cataract Refract Surg. 2008;34(11):1834-41.
24. Shingleton BJ, Heltzer J, O'Donoghue MW. Outcomes of phacoemulsification in patients with and without pseudoexfoliation syndrome. J Cataract Refract Surg. 2003;29(6):1080-6.
25. Alfaiate M, Leite E, Mira J, et al. Prevalence and surgical complications of pseudoexfoliation syndrome in Portuguese patients with senile cataract. J Cataract Refract Surg. 1996;22(7):972-6.
26. Drolsum L, Ringvold A, Nicolaissen B. Cataract and glaucoma surgery in pseudoexfoliation syndrome: a review. Acta Ophthalmol Scand. 2007;85(8):810-21.
27. Shingleton BJ. How to manage pseudoexfoliation syndrome in cataract surgery. Glaucoma Today. 2013:44-6.
28. Lee DH, Shin SC, Joo CK. Effect of a capsular tension ring on intraocular lens decentration and tilting after cataract surgery. J Cataract Refract Surg. 2002;28(5):843-6.
29. Shastri L, Vasavada A. Phacoemulsification in Indian eyes with pseudoexfoliation syndrome. J Cataract Refract Surg. 2001;27(10):1629-37.

30. Dosso AA, Bonvin ER, Leuenberger PM. Exfoliation syndrome and phacoemulsification. J Cataract Refract Surg. 1997;23(1):122-5.
31. Hyams M, Mathalone N, Herskovitz M, et al. Intraoperative complications of phacoemulsification in eyes with and without pseudoexfoliation. J Cataract Refract Surg. 2005;31(5):1002-5.
32. Scorolli L, Scorolli L, Campos EC, et al. Pseudoexfoliation syndrome: a cohort study on intraoperative complications in cataract surgery. Ophthalmologica. 1998;212(4):278-80.
33. Akinci A, Batman C, Zilelioglu O. Phacoemulsification in pseudoexfoliation syndrome. Ophthalmologica. 2008;222(2):112-6.
34. Katz J, Tielsch JM. Lifetime prevalence of ocular injuries from the Baltimore Eye Survey. Arch Ophthalmol. 1993;111(11): 1564-8.
35. Dannenberg AL, Parver LM, Brechner RJ, et al. Penetration eye injuries in the workplace. The National Eye Trauma System Registry. Arch Ophthalmol. 1992;110(6):843-8.
36. Kazokoglu H, Saatci O. Intraocular foreign bodies: results of 27 cases. Ann Ophthalmol. 1990;22(10):373-6.
37. Shah M, Shah S, Upadhyay P, et al. Controversies in traumatic cataract classification and management: a review. Can J Ophthalmol. 2013;48(4):251-8.
38. Mian SI, Azar DT, Colby K. Management of traumatic cataracts. Int Ophthalmol Clin. 2002;42(3):23-31.
39. Canavan YM, Archer DB. Anterior segment consequences of blunt ocular injury. Br J Ophthalmol. 1982;66(9):549-55.
40. Tabatabaei SA, Rajabi MB, Tabatabaei SM, et al. Early versus late traumatic cataract surgery and intraocular lens implantation. Eye (Lond). 2017;31(8):1199-204.
41. Lamkin JC, Azar DT, Mead MD, et al. Simultaneous corneal laceration repair, cataract removal, and posterior chamber intraocular lens implantation. Am J Ophthalmol. 1992;113(6):626-31.
42. Shah MA, Shah SM, Shah SB, et al. Effect of interval between time of injury and timing of intervention on final visual outcome in cases of traumatic cataract. Eur J Ophthalmol. 2011;21(6):760-5.
43. Nagy ZZ, Kranitz K, Takacs A, et al. Intraocular femtosecond laser use in traumatic cataracts following penetrating and blunt trauma. J Refract Surg. 2012;28(2):151-3.

Part 7 Retina and Vitreous

■ *Srinivas R Sadda*

OUTLINE

Chapter 45 Dye-based Angiography (Fluorescein Angiography and Indocyanine Green) and Polypoidal Choroidal Vasculopathy

Giovanni Staurenghi, Ferdinando Bottoni, Andrea Giani, Marco Pellegrini, Alessandro Invernizzi, Federico Corvi

FLUORESCEIN ANGIOGRAPHY

History

Fluorescein was first used clinically in the late 1950s and early 1960s for visualizing retinal vasculature. Flocks and coworkers obtained fluorescein angiograms in cats but they were not able to apply their technique to humans due to lack of sufficient illumination.[1] In 1959, Bailey and Swan described a special camera used to get cinematography of retinal human vessels.[2] Two years later, Novotny and Alvis published the method to study retinal blood flow by the use of intravascular fluorescein and retinal photography, and they described their preliminary observations.[3] Since they recorded on film the transit of fluorescein, the authors are considered the first authors that executed fluorescein angiography (FA). In the following years, FA increased in popularity and its use was applied to normal clinical practice.[4-7]

Chemical and Pharmacodynamics

The basis of fluorescence is luminescence. It is defined as the absorption and re-emission of the electromagnetic radiation in an energy with another frequency. Free electrons are generated by the absorption of the radiant energy in higher unstable levels of energy and then electrons relapse to their lower levels emitting the absorbed energy. This reemitted radiation has less energy and higher wavelength than the previous.[8] When luminescence is maintained by continuous excitation is called fluorescence. Depending on the chemical substance to be excited, the electromagnetic energy present a particular range of wavelengths called the absorption spectrum.[8]

To perform FA is used the sodium fluorescein, a crystalline substance very water soluble and with low molecular weight (376.27 Da). Its structural formula is $C_{20}H_{12}O_5Na$.[9] After the injection, fluorescein diffuses through most of the body fluids and through the choriocapillaris, but not through the retinal vascular endothelium and the retinal pigment epithelium (RPE). It is eliminated by the liver and kidneys within 24 hours, then retention may increase if renal function is compromised. Sodium fluorescein responds to blue light energy and emits a light that appears green yellow. In particular, the excitation wavelength is between 465 nm and 490 nm and fluoresces at 520–530 nm. The blue light excites only the unbound fluorescein within the blood vessels or the fluorescein that has leaked out of the blood vessels. Approximately, the 80% of fluorescein is bound to protein and only the 20% remains free in the bloodstream and is available for fluorescence.[1,10]

Toxicity

Fluorescein angiography has been extensively used in ophthalmology for the past 50 years, showing a very good safety profile. Life-threatening events related to the dye injection are in fact extremely rare and death incidence has been overall reported to be around 1/220,000.[11] Despite this reassuring safety profile, the intravenous injection of sodium fluorescein can cause a series of side effects, some of them related to the injection procedure (more common) and some others caused by an adverse reaction to the dye (rare).[12] Almost 100% of the patients undergoing FA experience a yellowish tinge of the skin and the mucosae in the hours following the procedure. This happens as a consequence of the physiological free dye leakage from systemic vasculature into the extravascular compartment. The fluorescein is then cleared from the body through the liver and the kidneys, lending an intense yellow-brown color to the urine. Both these events do not represent adverse reactions, should be considered as part of the standard procedure, and disappear within 24 hours in subjects with normal renal function. Nausea and vomiting may occur and seem to be related to the amount of dye and the injection rapidity. Injecting the dye slowly can reduce the rate of this incident. Extravasation of dye can be really painful and cause severe local inflammation due to the highly basic pH of the fluorescein (pH 8–10). Transient loss of consciousness can happen as a vasovagal reaction to the intravenous injection procedure rather than to the dye itself and it is more frequent in young adults. Finally, serious adverse reactions including bronchospasm, laryngeal edema, and anaphylaxis, although rare have been reported and should be treated as life-threatening emergencies.[11] Fluorescein can cross the placenta and is excreted in breast milk.[13,14] Neither teratogenicity (in animals) nor fetal complication in humans have been reported, so far, however, there are not enough data to consider FA as a safe procedure during pregnancy or nursing. Thus, it is generally recommended to avoid the procedure in pregnant or nursing women.

Instrument Comparison

The execution of fluorescein and indocyanine green (ICG) angiography can be performed with two types of instruments: (1) Digital fundus cameras, and (2) Confocal laser ophthalmoscopes. The first type uses a flash with light and specific excitation and barrier filters for selecting the desired imaging modality. The second uses a laser light source with specific wavelength and barrier filter for acquiring only specific range of wavelength. Moreover, laser ophthalmoscopes are confocal systems, meaning that they essentially acquire light from a specific focal plan. This increases the details, while removes information from different confocal planes. The advantages of confocal laser ophthalmoscopes are multiple, and include the possibility to perform simultaneous imaging modalities,[15] reduction of the amount of dye needed to perform angiograms (because of higher sensitivity),[16] and the ability to dynamically analyze vitreous, retina, and vitreoretinal interface.[17]

Injection Technique

The concentration and preparation for intravenous injection of sodium fluorescein and ICG vary with the instrument used. For fundus cameras, characteristically 5 mL of 10% sodium fluorescein are injected into a peripheral vein over a period of a few seconds. For ICG, the standard concentration is 25 mg of ICG dissolved in 5 mL solvent.[18] The dosage may be increased to 50 mg in patients with poorly dilated pupils and heavy pigmentation.[19] For scanning laser ophthalmoscopes (SLOs), combined fluorescein and indocyanine green angiography (ICGA) may be easily performed. The standard dosage is 25 mg of ICG dissolved in 3 mL, and 1 mL of the solution is injected. The solvent may be either saline alone or fluorescein sodium solution at 10–20–25% concentrations. Intravenous ICG injection should be rapid and immediately followed by a 5 mL saline flash. In patients with iodine allergy, infracyanine green is available: this is the iodine-free formula of ICG. The technique of injection is equivalent, but a glucosate solvent should be used for preparation. As a result, combined FA and infracyanine green angiography is not possible.

Imaging Features

Intravenous FA provides excellent spatial and temporal resolution of the retinal circulation, with a high degree of fluorescence efficiency and minimal penetration of the RPE. With up to 80% of the injected dye molecules bound to serum albumin or other protein molecules, the unbound portion can diffuse through small intercellular spaces.[20] In the era of optical coherence tomography (OCT) angiography, three peculiar features of the fluorescein molecule are still extremely useful for retinal imaging: (1) Leakage, (2) Pooling, and (3) Staining. All of them pertain dynamic properties. Fluorescein is normally confined within the retinal vessels by endothelial tight junctions and under the RPE layer by the apical junctions between adjacent cells. Whenever these tight junctions are damaged, we have seen leakage of dye through the vessels or the RPE (Figs. 45.1A to E). Pooling is the progressive accumulation of dye within an anatomic space, either under the neurosensory retina or the RPE. The late hyperfluorescence usually achieved in the late phases of the examination is due to the high concentration of fluorescein molecules within the pool being illuminated by the excitation light (Figs. 45.2A and B). Staining may appear in the normal eye when the unbound fluorescein molecules leak from the choroid determining the late hyperfluorescence of the sclera. Staining can also occur in any disease process characterized by tissues progressively impregnating without abnormal leakage. Commonly used in the past before the advent of OCT, the staining without leakage can still be used for investigating the activity of a choroidal neovascularization (CNV) (to be confirmed by OCT) (Figs. 45.3A to D). Unfortunately, the peculiarities of the fluorescein dye have also disadvantages. In fact, imaging of the choroidal circulation is prevented by secondary poor transmission of fluorescence through ocular media opacities, pathologic manifestations such as serosanguineous fluid or lipid exudation, and fundus pigmentation, including that from the RPE layer.

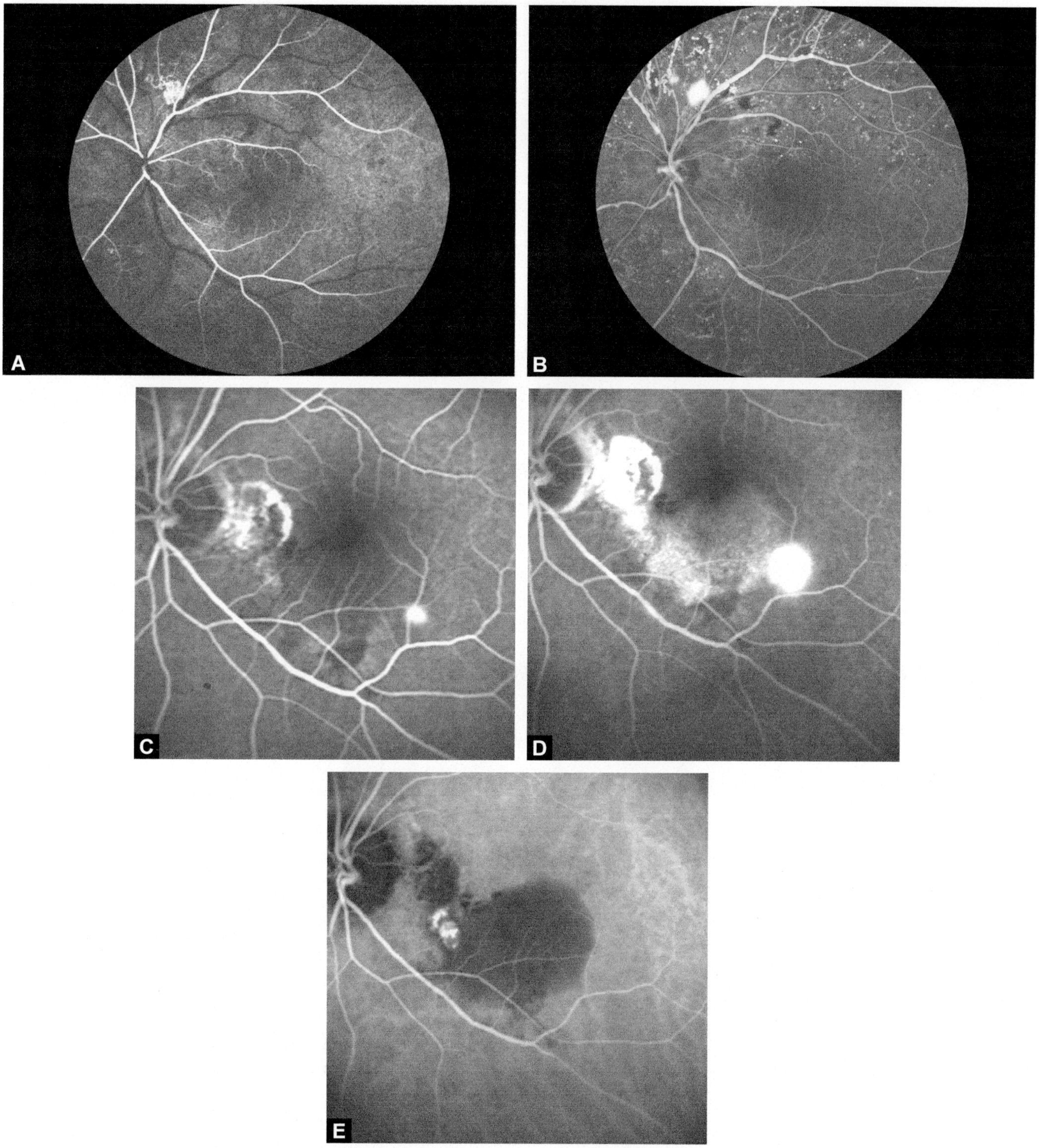

Figs. 45.1A to E: (A) Tuft of new vessels along the superior vascular arcade in a proliferative diabetic retinopathy eye; (B) Diffuse leakage in late phases; (C and D) Increasing leakage of dye along the temporal edge of a retinal pigment epithelium detachment; and (E) That area appeared silent on ICG whereas a type 1 CNV was visible on the nasal side of the detachment.
(CNV: Choroidal neovascularization; ICG: Indocyanine green)

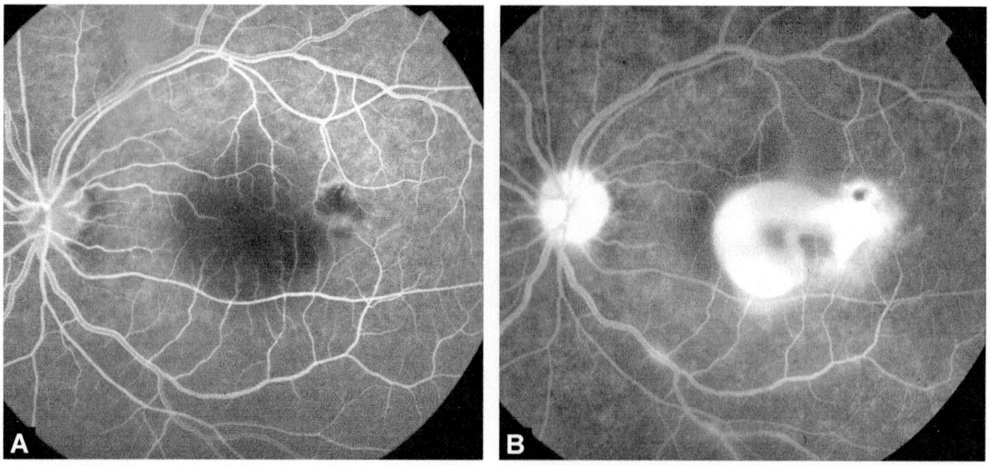

Figs. 45.2A and B: Progressive pooling of dye under the retinal pigment epithelium in active toxoplasmic retinochoroiditis.

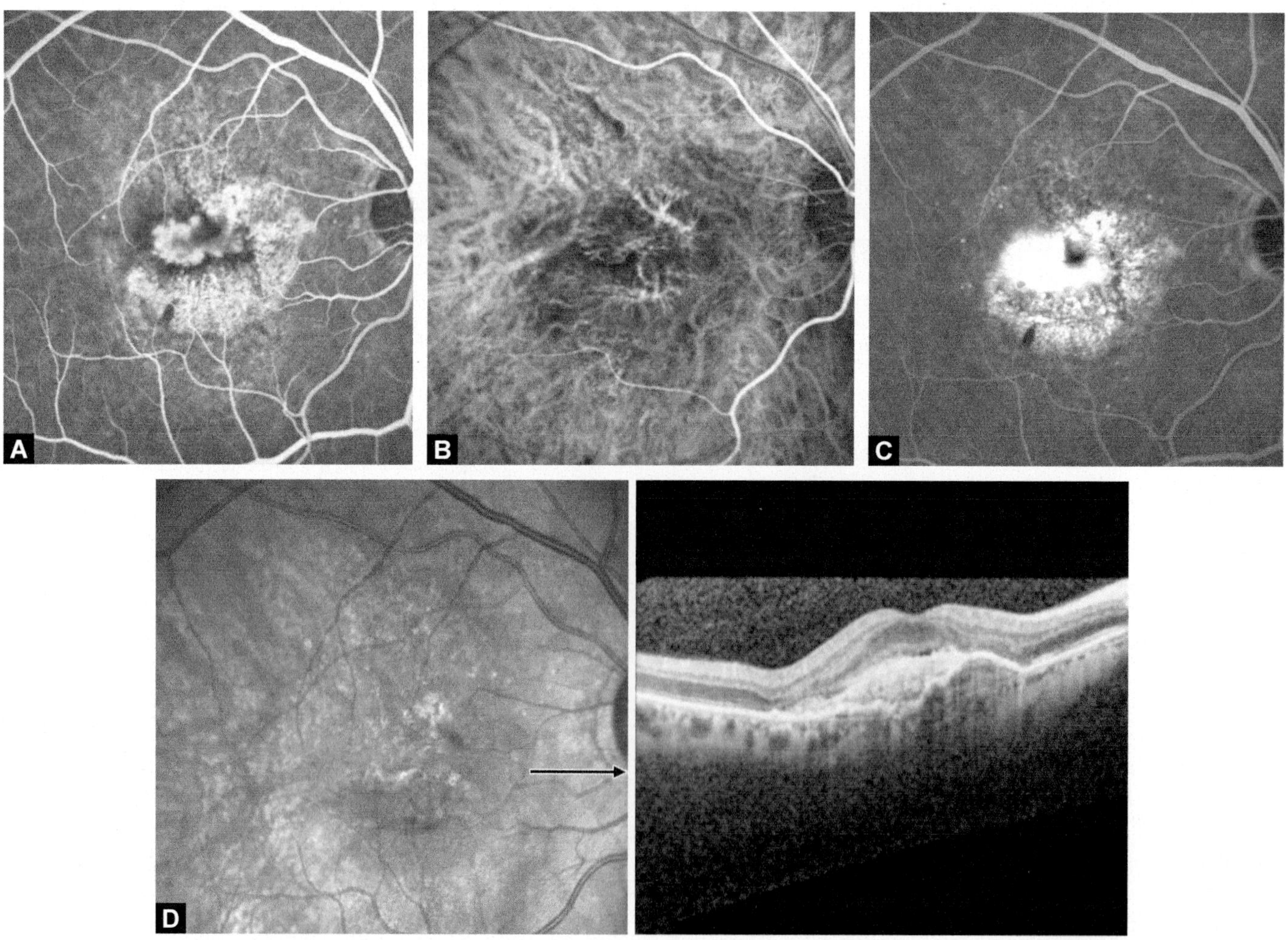

Figs. 45.3A to D: Type 2 CNV in senile macular degeneration. The newvessels are evident in the early phases of either FA (A) and ICG angiography (B). Progressive staining occurs during the late phases of FA (C) without leakage as demonstrated by the corresponding OCT image (D).

(CNV: Choroidal neovascularization; FA: Fluorescein angiography; ICG: Indocyanine green; OCT: Optical coherence tomography)

INDOCYANINE GREEN ANGIOGRAPHY

History

Indocyanine green (ICG) was first employed in cardiology and hepatology.[21-23] In 1972, ICG angiography started to be used to evaluate the human choroid.[24] In the following years, ICG angiography use was assessed in normal and pathologic conditions.[24-26] One of the major limits of ICG angiography, image resolution, was improved by Hayashi and coworkers, who improved filters obtaining images with near-infrared light.[27] Another important development was the introduction of the SLO for ICG videoangiography.[28] The first system that allowed high-resolution and long-duration ICG angiography was developed by Yannuzzi and coworkers.[29]

Chemical and Pharmacodynamics

Indocyanine green is a tricarbocyanine, anionic dye with a molecular weight of 774.96 Da[30] and a structural formula of 2,2'-indo-6,7,6',7'-dibenzocarbocyanine sodium salt.[31] ICG absorbs light in the near-infrared spectrum with a peak at 790 nm.[32] Maximum emission is at 835 nm.[33] This optical properties permits good visualization event through blood, pigment, and melanin.[34] In the circulation about 98% of ICG is bound to proteins, in particular to globulins, such as A1 lipoproteins.[35] ICG is nearly totally excreted by the liver,[36,37] with active mechanism and is strictly dependent on hepatocellular function.[38,39] ICG is excreted into the bile with no metabolic process,[38] ICG removal from vascular compartment is fast, and after 20 minutes no more than 4% remains in plasma.[40] ICG high-molecular weight and bond to plasma proteins reduce leaking through choroid vessels. Thanks to that and to its optical features, ICG is useful for evaluating choroidal vascularization. In angiography, no dye should be visible in late phases (30–40 minutes).[40]

Toxicity

Indocyanine green can be considered safe, with a LD50 of 60 mg × kg^{-1} in mice.[31] ICG is also well tolerated, no effects were reported after 3 hours period of infusion with dosages as high as 50 mg/kg of body weight.[38] Subcutaneous extravasation does not produce effects.[37,41] ICG adverse events rate is modest: 0.15% of mild effects (nausea, vomit, sneezing, and pruritus), 0.2% of moderate effects (urticarial, syncope, pyrexia, and nerve palsy), and 0.05% of severe effects (bronchospasm, laryngospasm, and anaphylaxis).[41] ICG should be avoided in patients with a history of iodine allergy because of a potential danger of anaphylaxis.[41] Also, ICG should be used with attention in patients with liver diseases,[41] and kidney diseases, because in patients in dialysis there was a 9.3% incidence of adverse effects.[35,42] ICG was used to test hemodynamic changes during pregnancy.[43] Nevertheless, Food and Drug Administration (FDA) classified ICG as a pregnancy category C, because of a lack of safety studies.[44]

Imaging Features

In medicine, a core principle for diagnostic imaging is the selection of a technique that best visualizes the disease undergoing investigation. ICG has several advantages over sodium fluorescein in imaging the choroidal vasculature. Its physical characteristics allow for visualization of the dye through overlying melanin, xanthophyll pigment, serosanguineous fluid, or lipid exudates (Figs. 45.4A and B). Additionally, being almost totally bound to plasma proteins, it does not leak into the extravascular space either in the retina (Figs. 45.5A and B) or in the choroid (Figs. 45.6A and B). These two features warrant a better definition for the lesions to be imaged in many chorioretinal diseases. The increase of fluorescence with ICG depends upon the column of dye whereas with sodium fluorescein it depends on the amount of fluorescent dye which is closer to the examining eye. A typical example of such a phenomenon is given in an arteriovenous crossing with the artery lying above the vein. During the venous phase, in FA the crossing will appear less fluorescent than the rest of the vein because of the masking artery (Fig. 45.7). By contrast, in ICGA the crossing will appear more fluorescent than the rest of the vein because of the sum of the residual dye in the artery and the circulating dye in the vein (Fig. 45.7). The use of high-resolution infrared digital fundus cameras and confocal SLOs, specifically designed for ICGA, has reflected a growing awareness and interest in choroidal vascular lesions, and has facilitated the rapid diffusion of ICGA in the ophthalmic community. Even in the era of antivascular endothelial growth factor (anti-VEGF) intravitreal injections, a therapy for which accurate localization of the choroidal neovascular membrane is not as critical, ICGA, among other imaging techniques, is still extremely useful in clinical practice.[45]

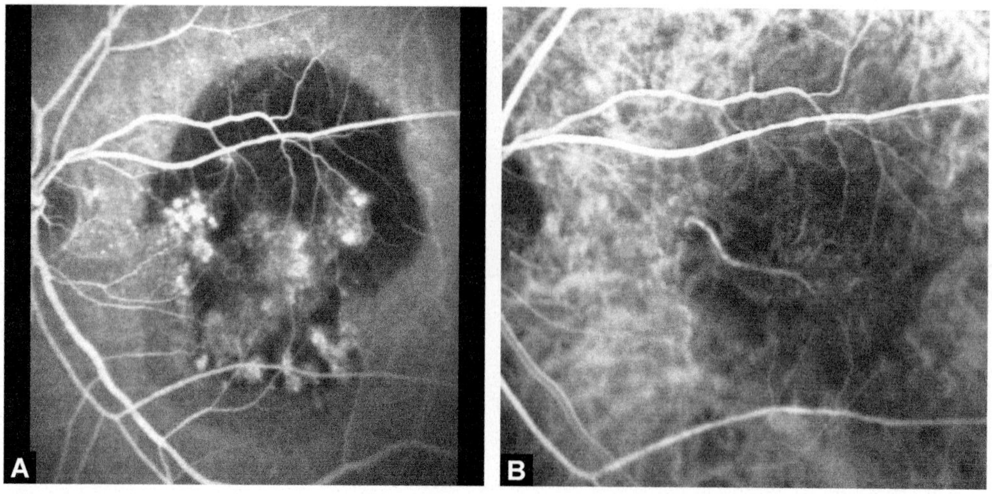

Figs. 45.4A and B: (A) Exudative AMD, type 1 CNV with RPE detachment and subretinal blood masking choroidal details; (B) Early phase ICG image showing a feeder vessel originating outside the area of the RPE detachment and feeding a large neovascular net under the RPE.
(AMD: Age-related macular degeneration; CNV: Choroidal neovascularization; RPE: Retinal pigment epithelium; ICG: Indocyanine green)

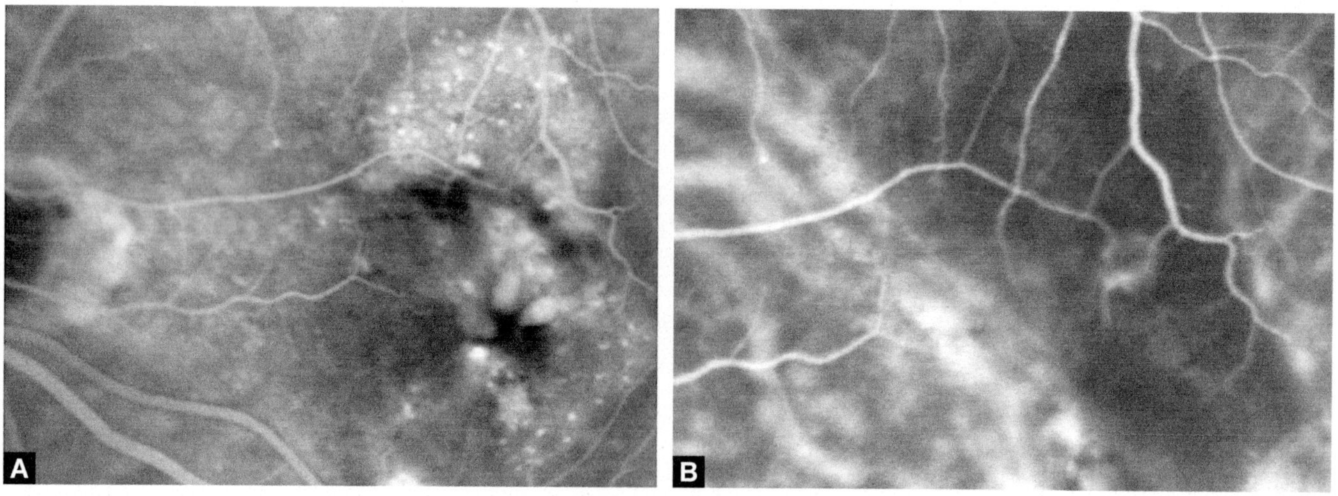

Figs. 45.5A and B: Exudative AMD, type 3 CNV. As compared with FA (A), in ICG angiography (B) RAP does not leak intraretinally and the lesion is readily apparent.
(AMD: Age-related macular degeneration; CNV: Choroidal neovascularization; FA: Fluorescein angiography; ICG: Indocyanine green; RAP: Retinal angiomatous proliferation)

INTERPRETATION

Normal Eye

Fluorescein angiography and ICGA are dynamic examinations in which the characteristic findings are related to the diffusion of the dye in the vascular circulation. Different phases have been recognized according to the time of the injection. In particular, about FA we can distinguish a choroidal phase, arterial retinal phase, an arteriovenous phase, and a venous phase. The choroidal phase is characterized by irregular areas of choroidal filling with adjacent areas of delayed fluorescein filling. The choroidal fluorescence is influenced by the density of the pigment epithelial barrier as more is densely pigmented and greater is the blockage effect. For this reason, a higher concentration of fluorescein is required to overcome an increased density of the pigment epithelial barrier. The macula remains dark due to the high density of xanthophyll at the fovea and due to the RPE cells which are larger and contain more lipofuscin and melanin. Sometimes, a cilioretinal artery may be present. It arises from the peripapillary choroid or directly from one of the short posterior ciliary arteries. Size and area of the retina supplied by a cilioretinal artery vary widely. If present, a

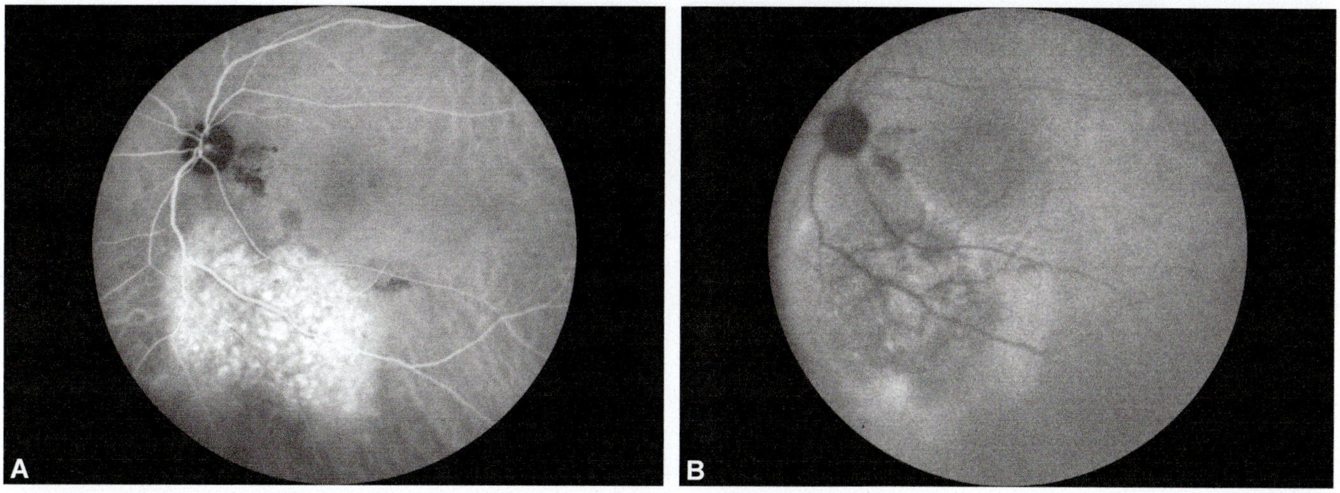

Figs. 45.6A and B: Circumscribed choroidal hemangioma. Late-phase ICGA study demonstrating the choroidal mass (A) and the subsequent hypofluorescence corresponding to the washout effect (B). A halo of minimal hyperfluorescence surrounds the tumor. This may result from staining of the retinal pigment epithelium or leakage of indocyanine green into the subneurosensory retinal space.

(ICGA: Indocyanine green angiography)

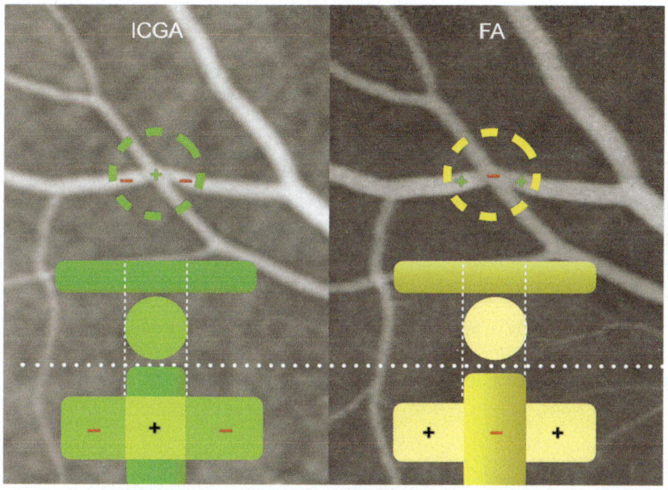

Fig. 45.7: During venous phase in FA the arteriovenous crossing will appear less fluorescent than the rest of the vein because of the masking of the artery. In contrast, in ICGA , the crossing will appear more fluorescent than the rest of the vein because of the residual dye in the artery and the circulating dye in the vein.

cilioretinal artery usually begins to fluoresce as the choroid fluoresces, rather than as the retina fluoresces (Figs. 45.8A to D). In the arterial and arteriovenous phases, the dye diffuses in the retinal arteries and then in the precapillary arterioles, capillaries, and postcapillary venules. The venous phase is characterized by the laminar flow due to the faster flow in the center of the lumen that on the sides. The result is a dark central lamina with fluorescence that starts from the sides. Vessels become dark in approximately 10 minutes, after the injection, as they do not contain more fluorescein. Fluorescence of the choroid and sclera can be appreciated due to the extravasation of the dye from the gaps of the endothelial cells through the choroidal tissue and sclera. Similarly, for ICGA we can find different phases during the examination, as an early phase when the retinal artery is not yet filled, a midphase when both arteries and veins are filled, and a late or recirculation phase more than 10 minutes after injection. In order, the dye diffuses in the deeper Haller's layer then in the intermediate Sattler's layer and next to the choriocapillaris (Figs. 45.9A to C). This is represented as a diffuse indistinct haze due to the low resolution of the cameras in the visualization of the small lobular morphology. Choroidal vortex veins are responsible of the drainage from corresponding segment of the iris, ciliary body, and choroid. These vessels are visible in the late phase of ICGA and are usually four in number (Fig. 45.10). A choriovaginal vein may be found close to the optic disk passing from the choroid through the sclera and draining into the venous plexus of the pial sheath (Figs. 45.11A to C).

Vascular Diseases

Fluorescein angiography is of fundamental importance in the diagnosis and classification of vascular retinal diseases, such as diabetic retinopathy, retinal vein, and artery occlusions. On the other hand, ICG has limited

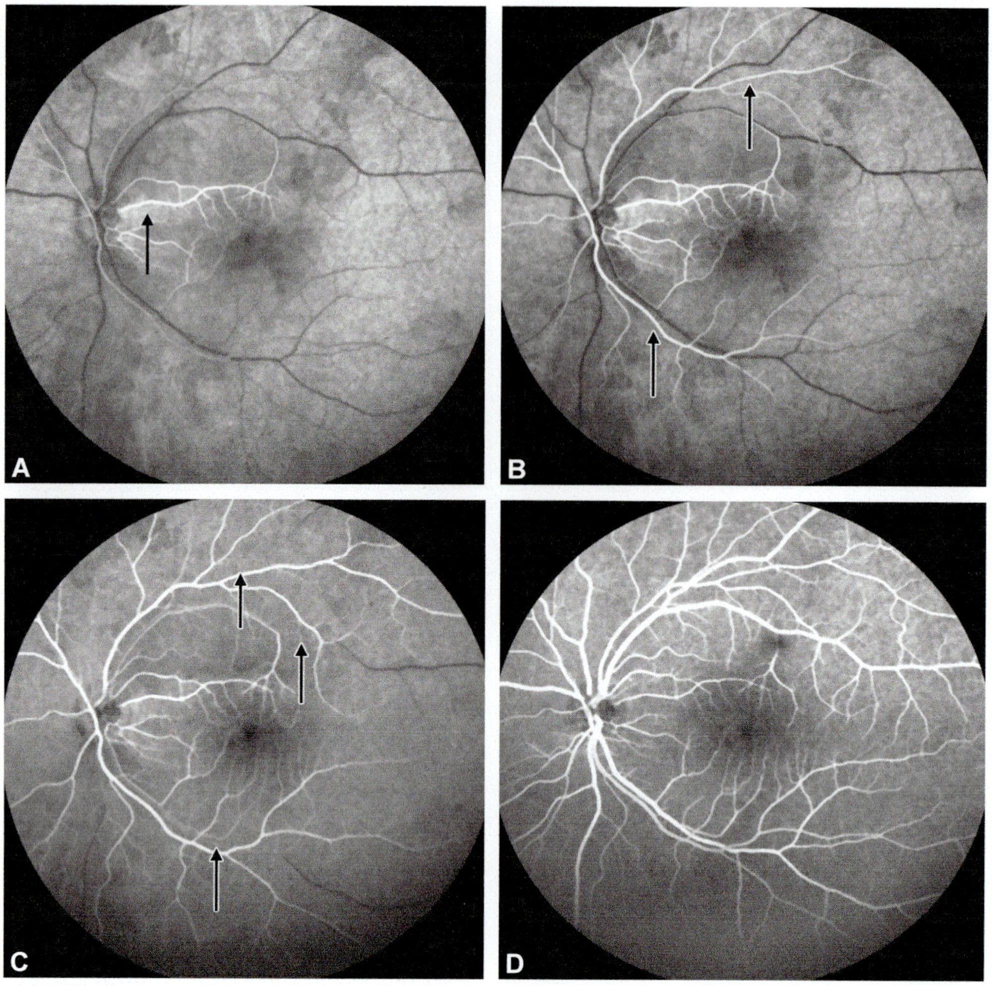

Figs. 45.8A to D: Fluorescein angiography of normal eye. Fluorescein angiogram in the early arterial phase (A) revealing the cilioretinal artery filling (arrow) and the irregular areas of choroidal filling with adjacent areas of delayed fluorescein filling. In the arterial and arteriovenous phases (B), the dye diffuses in the retinal arteries (arrows) and then in the precapillary arterioles, capillaries and postcapillary venules. The venous phase (C) is characterized by the laminar flow in the retinal veins (arrows). In the late venous phase (D) a uniform filling is seen in both arterial and venous circulation.

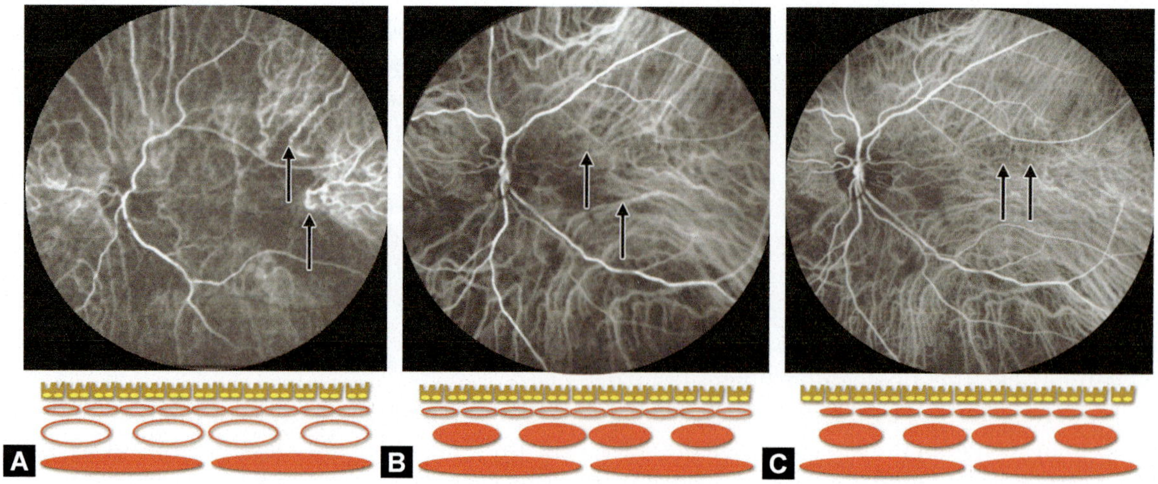

Figs. 45.9A to C: Indocyanine green angiography of normal eye. The dye diffuses in the deeper Haller's layer (A, arrows) then in the intermediate Sattler's layer (B, arrows) and next to the choriocapillaris (C, arrows).

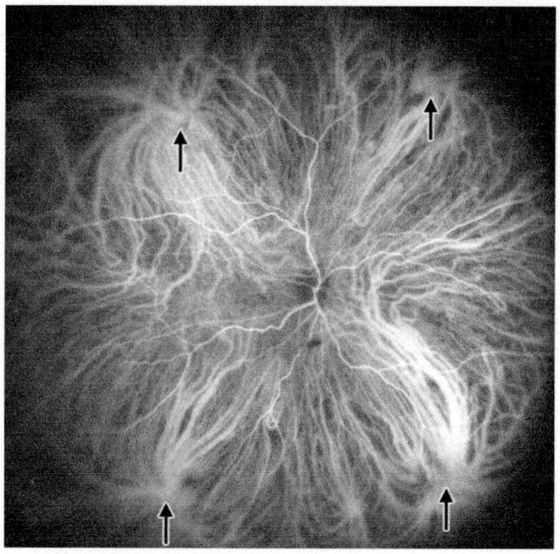

Fig. 45.10: Indocyanine green angiography provides the visualization of the four vortex veins (arrows).

importance in this category of diseases. In diabetic retinopathy, the classification of the severity of retinal alterations is based on fundus stereoscopic photography and FA.[46,47] FA permits to identify microaneurysms, hemorrhages, venous abnormalities, areas of nonperfusion (and enlargement of the foveal avascular zone), and retinal neovascularization. It is useful in assessing the extension of laser photocoagulation. It is also instrumental in detecting and classifying macular cystoid edema.[48,49]

Microaneurysms

Typical of diabetic retinopathy, in FA they appear as spots of hyperfluorescence that shows immediately in the first phases and keep fluorescent throughout the different phases with diffusion of the dye (Figs. 45.12A and B). In ICGA, the microaneurysms appear as white spots, with no leakage in midlate phases of the angiogram (Figs. 45.12C and D).

Retinal Hemorrhages

They appear as black elements in FA, because of blockade effect of the fluorescence (Fig. 45.13). The extension of intraretinal hemorrhages is important to define the grade of severity of diabetic retinopathy. Preretinal hemorrhages are a sign of proliferative diabetic retinopathy or high risk of development of this stage (Fig. 45.14). Also in ICGA hemorrhages block fluorescence but this effect may be limited due to higher penetration of the wavelength used in this angiography technique (Figs. 45.15A and B).

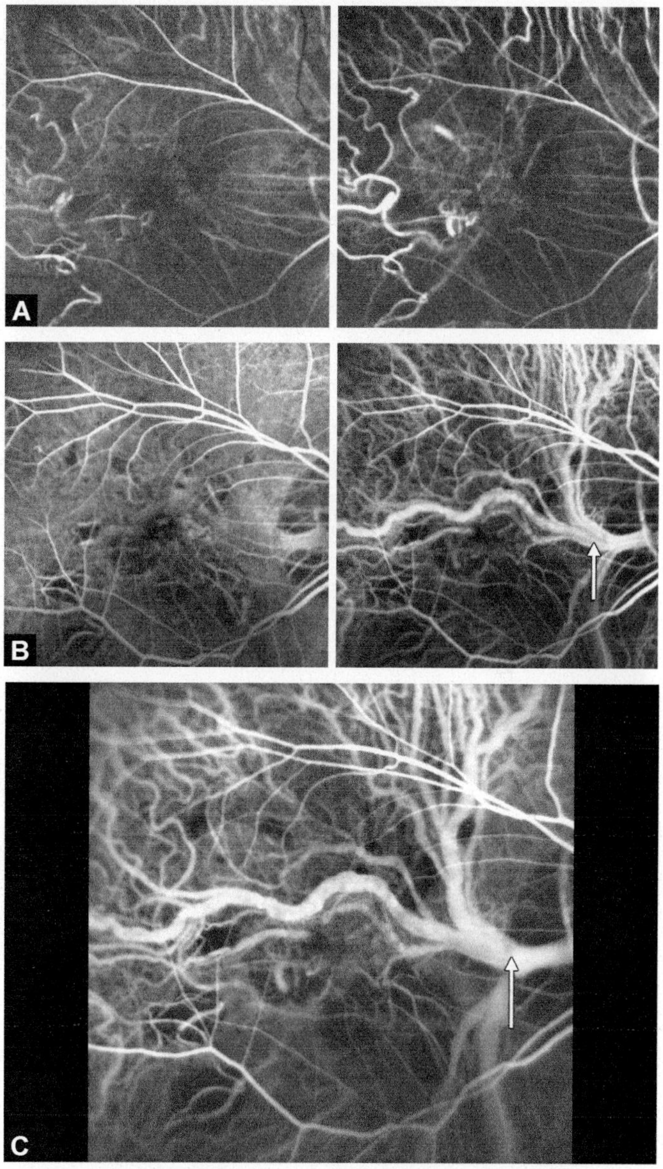

Figs. 45.11A to C: Early arterial phase (A) and venous phase (B) on fluorescein angiography and indocyanine green angiography in a patient with high myopia. ICGA (C) clearly allows the visualization of the choriovaginal vessel (arrow).
(ICGA: Indocyanine green angiography)

Vascular Abnormalities

The identification of these lesions is important because their presence defines the moderate and severe nonproliferative diabetic retinopathy. They are well visualized by FA, as venous beadings (Fig. 45.16) or intraretinal microvascular abnormalities (Fig. 45.17). FA can also show leakage form vessels, in particular in the acute phase of retinal vein occlusion (Fig. 45.18).

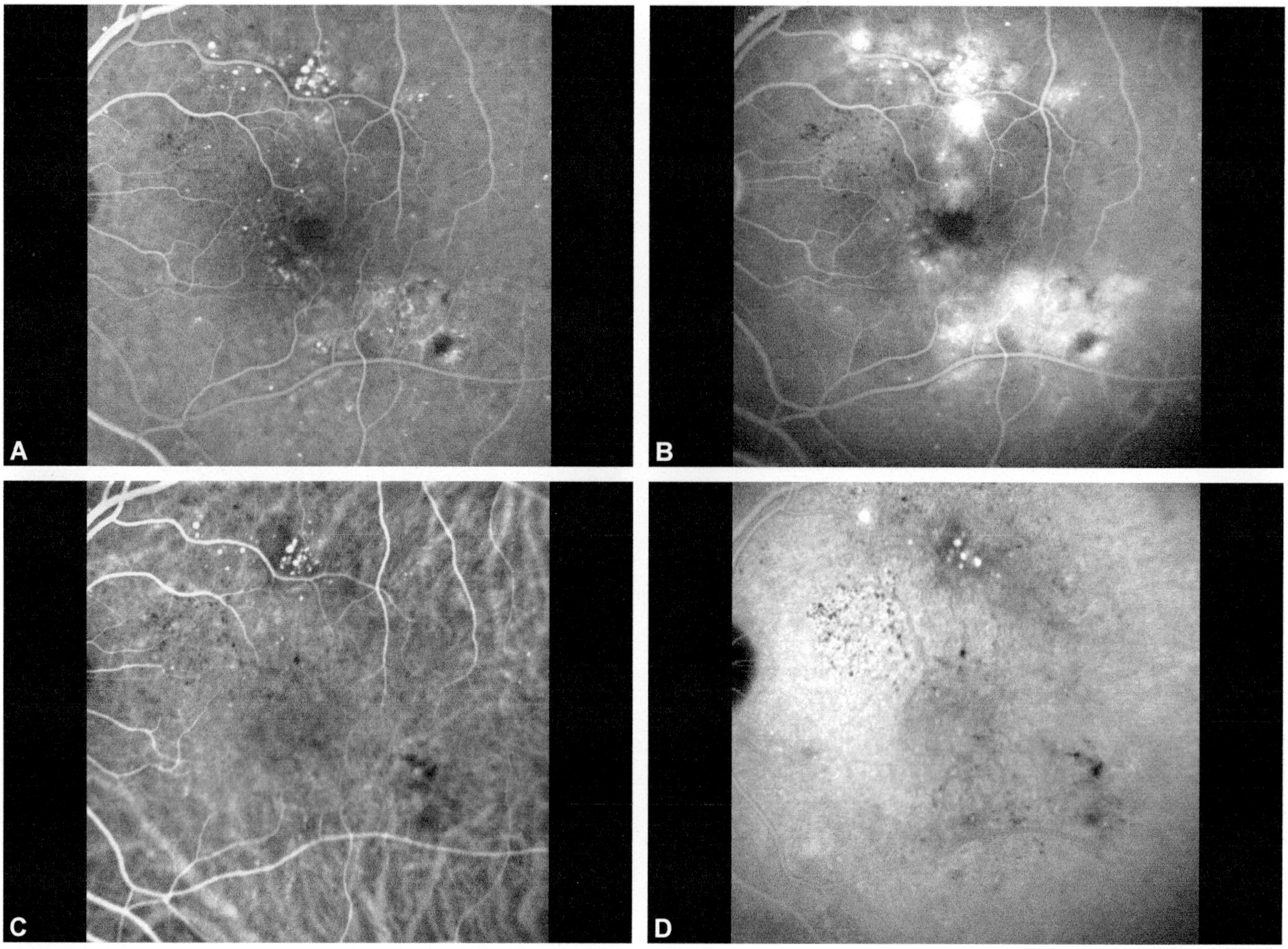

Figs. 45.12A to D: A patient with mild nonproliferative diabetic retinopathy with microaneurysms highly concentrated in proximity of the temporal superior vascular arcade. (A) Fluorescein angiography in the early phase shows the microaneurysms as distinct hyperfluorescent lesions, with progressive leakage in the mid and late phases; and (B to D) Indocyanine green angiography also shows the lesions as hyperfluorescent dots, but without leakage in the later phases of the angiography.

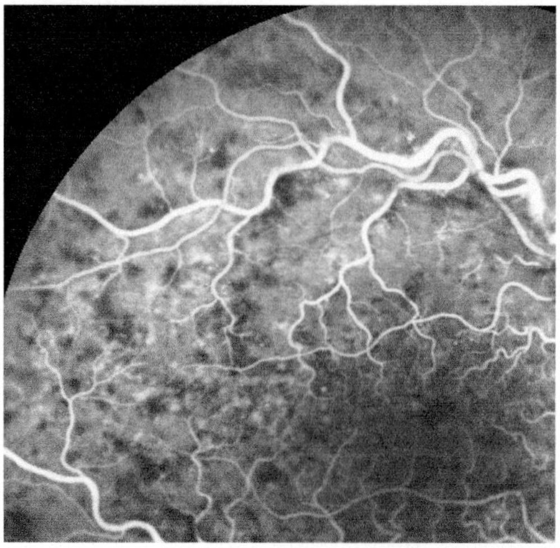

Fig. 45.13: A patient with central vein occlusion with diffuse intraretinal hemorrhages, shown by fluorescein angiography as dark lesions.

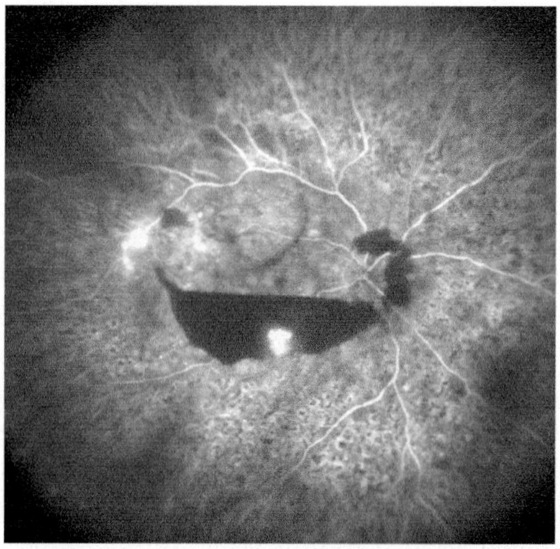

Fig. 45.14: A patient with proliferative diabetic retinopathy and an extensive preretinal hemorrhage at the posterior pole.

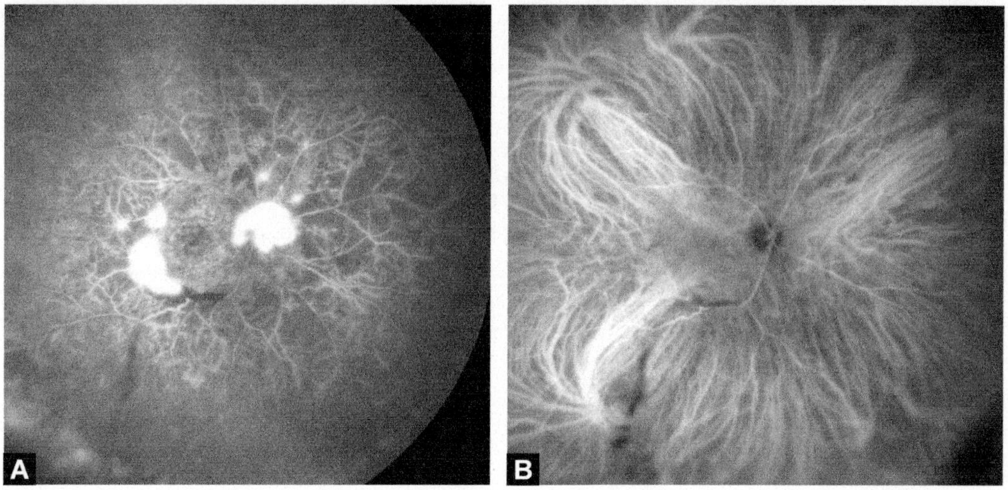

Figs. 45.15A and B: A patient with proliferative diabetic retinopathy. (A) Fluorescein angiography shows new vessels and a preretinal hemorrhage as a black area at the temporal inferior arcade; (B) Indocyanine green angiography only shows the preretinal hemorrhages.

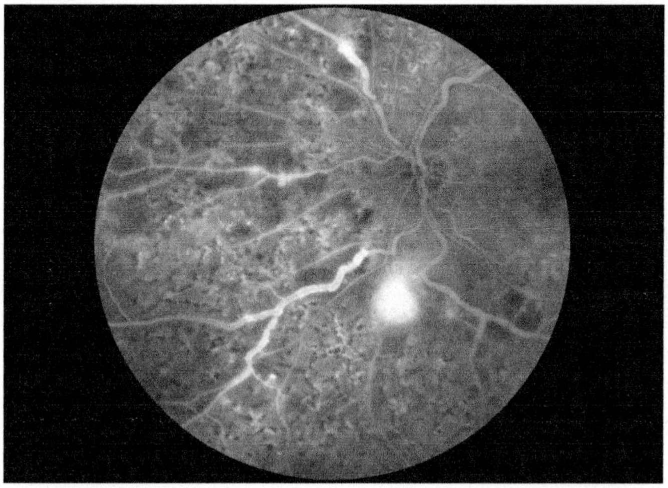

Fig. 45.16: Venous beadings shown by fluorescein angiography.

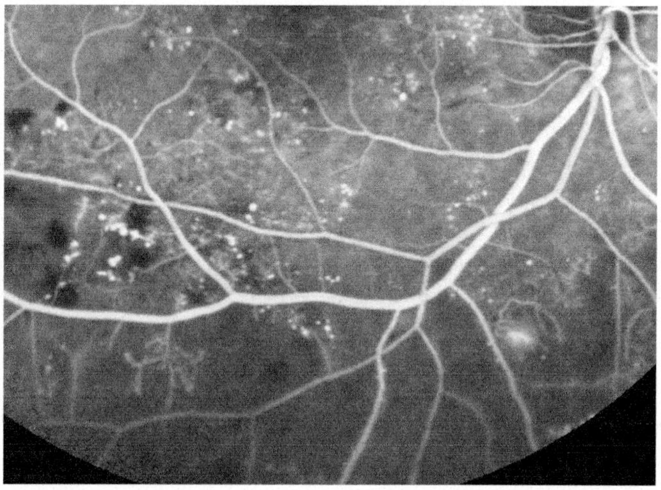

Fig. 45.17: Intraretinal microvascular abnormalities shown by fluorescein angiography. Differently than new vessels, these lesions do not show leakage.

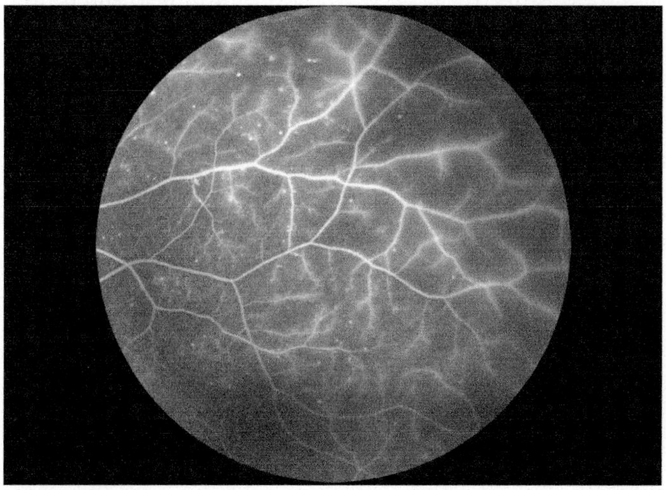

Fig. 45.18: Perivascular leakage in an acute stage of central vein occlusion.

Nonperfusion

The lack of capillary flow is visualized by FA as black areas (Fig. 45.19), in high contrast with surrounding areas of perfusion in which there is evident background fluorescence. FA permits to quantify the extension of areas on nonperfusion which is crucial for treatment decision and follow-up.

Retinal Neovascularization

Retinal new vessels appear early leakage, so that the vascular net can be identified in the very early phases of the angiogram. In the mid and late phases, new vessels appear

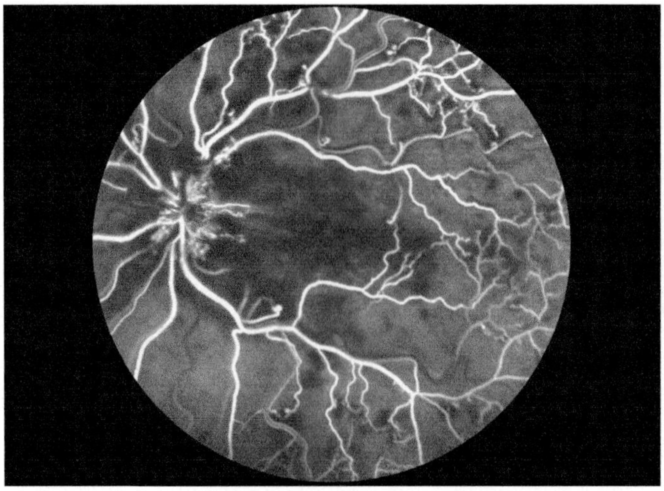

Fig. 45.19: Extensive retinal nonperfusion in an acute stage of ischemic central vein occlusion.

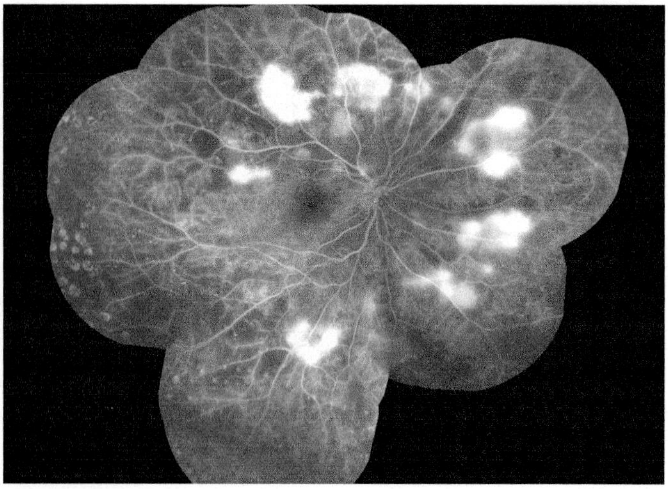

Fig. 45.20: A patient with proliferative diabetic retinopathy with multiple new vessels in midperiphery.

as areas of intense hyperfluorescent with a progressive enlargement loss of contrast with the surrounding areas (Fig. 45.20).

Inflammatory Diseases

Inflammation is a biological response of the body to any harmful stimuli, involving immune cells and molecular mediators with the aim to confine and eventually eliminate the threatening condition. Inflammatory cytokines play a major role in the control of this complex process inducing temporary modifications in the tissues' homeostasis and guiding the immune cells actions. During any inflammatory reaction inflammatory mediators induce several vascular changes including vessels dilation, blood flow modifications, expression of specific surface proteins on the vascular endothelium, and increased vessels permeability. All these changes affect fluorescein and ICG behavior within the eye, creating patterns of signs characterizing different inflammatory diseases.[50,51]

Specific Signs of Inflammation

Intraocular inflammation induces a breakdown of the inner blood retinal barrier regardless of the underlying cause. The resulting sign is the visualization of a certain amount of dye leakage from the retinal vasculature. This phenomenon affects mainly FA images since ICGA cannot exit the retinal vasculature even when the vascular permeability is increased in the majority of the cases. As a result, optic nerve head hyperfluorescence (Fig. 45.21A) is virtually always present in case of inflammation as well as a late leakage from the peripheral retinal vessels. Another area of the retina particularly sensitive to alterations of the vascular permeability is the macula, due to its unique anatomical structure. The detection of leakage from the macular capillaries with dye pooling within cystic spaces causes the commonly detected inflammatory cystoid macular edema (Fig. 45.21B).[52]

Retinal Vasculitis

Specific patterns alterations of the retinal vascular structures can be identified in case of inflammation with some of them being peculiar of certain etiologies. Once again, FA is the gold standard technique to detect such changes since it is more sensitive then ICGA to alterations of the retinal vascular permeability. The inflammation of a retinal vessel can result in an increased plasmatic exudation, detected as leakage on FA (Fig. 45.22A), or in a flow impairment, usually caused by modification of the endothelium surface and visible as nonperfusion on FA images (Fig. 45.22B).[53,54] These two pictures allow to classify the retinal vasculitis into exudative and occlusive and typically occur with a different incidence according to the underlying inflammatory condition.[53,54] Another feature that can help in the classification of retinal vasculitis and consequently in the identification of the causative agent is the kind of affected vessels. Many conditions can in fact involve both veins and arteries, but most of them typically affect mostly ones

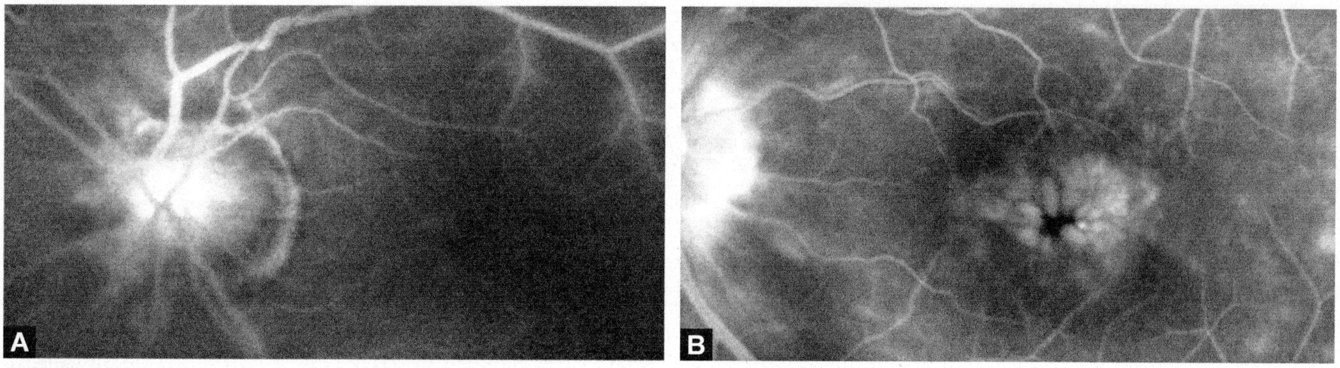

Figs. 45.21A and B: A specific signs of inflammation. (A) Optic nerve head hyperfluorescence increasing overtime is a common sign of inflammation detected on fluorescein angiography (FA) images, regardless of the underlying etiology; (B) Cystoid macular edema often occurs in eyes with inflammatory diseases and is visible on FA images with a typical petaloid pattern.

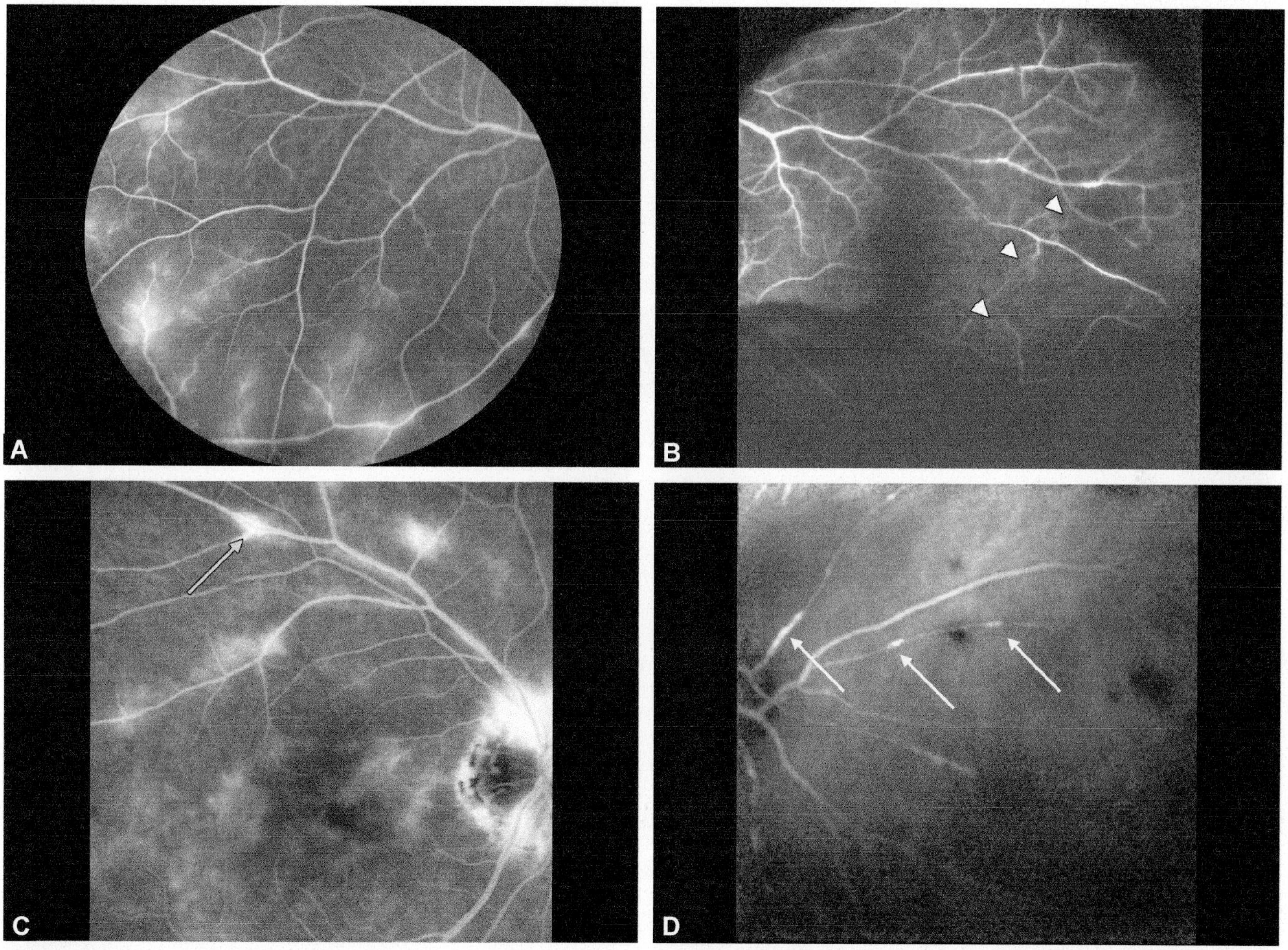

Figs. 45.22A to D: Retinal vasculitis. (A) Exudative vasculitis is visualized on FA images as leakage from retinal vessels; (B) Inflammation of retinal vessels can lead to blood flow impairment ultimately leading to vascular occlusion. Occlusive vasculitis is visualized on FA images as areas of retinal nonperfusion (arrowheads); (C) In case of vasculitis the pattern of leakage on FA images can help in differentiating the underlying etiology. This patient shows a typical segmental pattern, with tracts of vessels leaking (arrow) alternated to segments with normal appearance; (D) Peculiar staining of ICG dye on Kyrieleis plaques (arrows).

(FA: Fluorescein angiography; ICG: Indocyanine green)

or the others. A retinal phlebitis (veins mainly involved) will then suggest certain etiologies whereas an arteritis will direct the diagnosis toward other diseases. Finally, the extent of the vascular involvement allows to distinguish between diffuse and segmental vasculitis (Fig. 45.22C), once again the one or the other being more frequent in specific uveitides.[54] ICG angiography is less useful then FA in the characterization of retinal vasculitis, however, it can help in the identification of specific alterations such as Kyrieleis plaques, a rare vasculitic entity characterizing infectious diseases, particularly toxoplasmosis and viral uveitis, and showing a unique staining on ICG angiography (Fig. 45.22D).[55]

Retinitis

When the entire retina is inflamed a diffuse leakage/staining of fluorescein can be detected.[56] However, focal patches of retinitis are usually necrotic and appear hypofluorescent both on FA and ICGA since the necrotic retina is not perfused. A late staining/leakage can be visualized around the necrotic area on FA due to inflammatory reaction involving the surrounding tissue.[57]

Inflammation of the Choriocapillaris

Both autoimmune (white dots syndromes, sarcoidosis, and serpiginous choroiditis) and infectious (tuberculosis, syphilis) diseases can involve the choriocapillaris leading to inflammation and consequently to vascular disturbances.[58,59] Areas of choriocapillaris with impaired flow usually appear hypofluorescent during the early phases of the FA due to the reduced perfusion, then they disappear over time to ultimately turn hyperfluorescent. This late hyperfluorescence can derive from a staining of dye within the overlying hypoxic retina during the active stages of the disease, or from a window defect resulting from retinal and RPE atrophy in the late stages (Fig. 45.23A). ICGA represents the gold standard technique for the detection and the follow-up of these diseases since it can identify wider areas of impaired flow and it can better assess the disease activity (Fig. 45.23B). In particular, the affected areas appear hypofluorescent on ICGA during the early phases and they gradually become darker overtime due to a progressive increase in contrast between the nonperfused area and the surrounding choroid.[60]

Stromal Choroiditis

When the inflammation involves the deep layers of the choroid (Sattler's and Haller's) it is usually classified as a stromal choroiditis. The gold standard technique to assess choroidal inflammatory changes is ICG angiography.[51,60] When the choroid is inflamed two main signs can be noticed on ICG angiography images: (1) Hypofluorescent round-shaped lesions corresponding to choroidal granulomas, and (2) Hyperfluorescent fuzzy vessels. Choroidal granulomas appear darker than the surrounding tissue in the early phases on the angiogram since the collection of inflammatory cells that forms them prevents the dye from penetrating the area (Figs. 45.24A and B). They usually become less visible overtime due to dye diffusion around

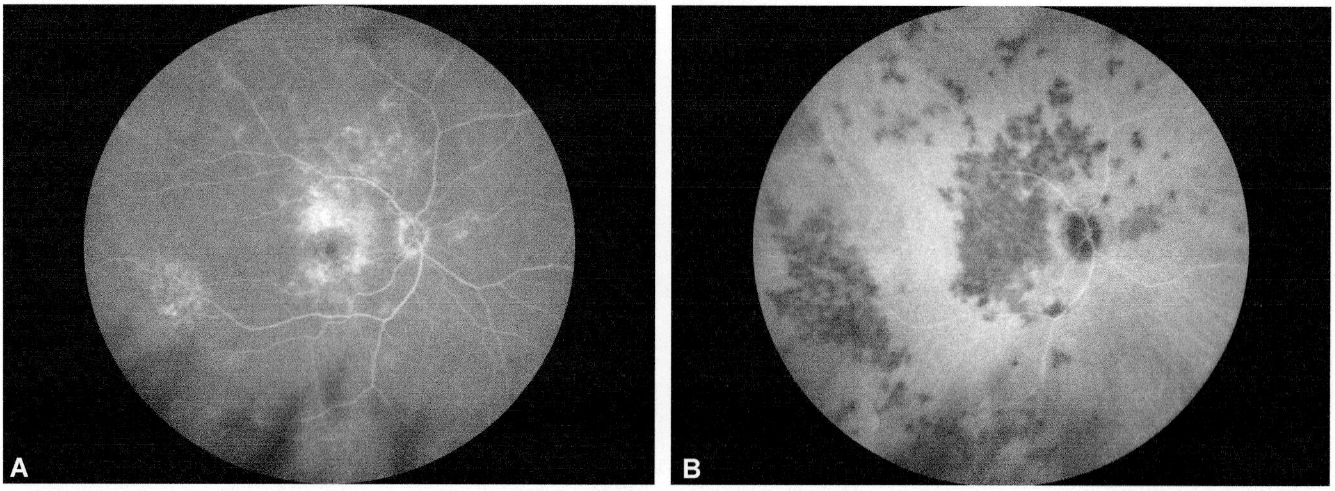

Figs. 45.23A and B: Choriocapillaris. Combined angiography in a patient affected by choriocapillaris. (A) Some lesions can be detected in the late phases of the fluorescein angiogram as hyperfluorescent areas; (B) The simultaneous indocyanine green (ICG) angiogram shows a larger number of affected choriocapillaris appearing as hypofluorescent plaques/dots across the fundus.

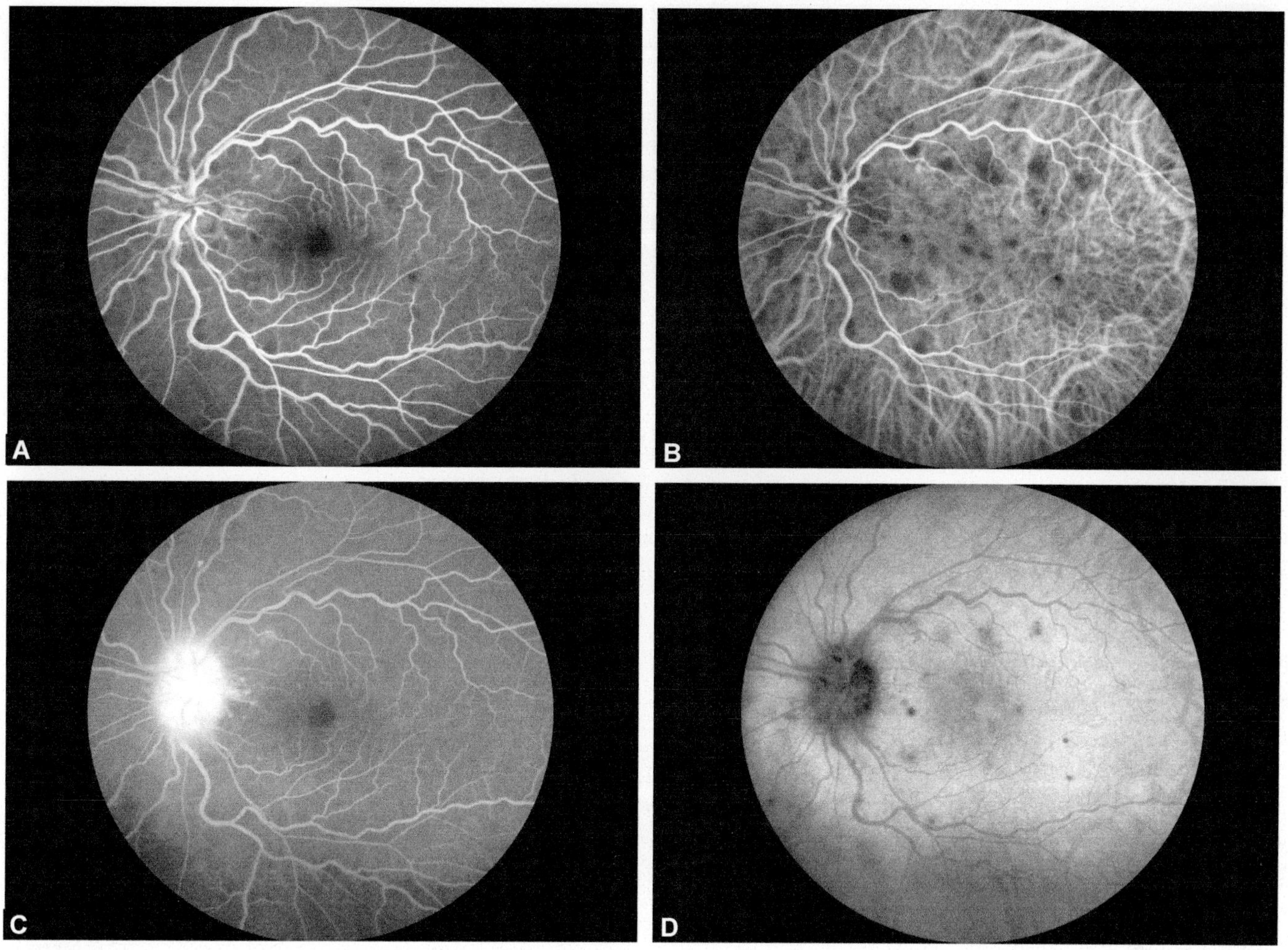

Figs. 45.24A to D: Stromal choroiditis. Combined angiogram in a patient affected by stromal choroiditis. (A) Choroidal granulomas are barely visible as dark round-shaped lesions on early phases of FA; and (C) It become undetectable in the late phases that on the contrary show optic nerve head leakage; (B) A larger number of granulomas is visible on the early phases of the ICG angiogram; and (D) Some of the lesions (full thickness granulomas) remain visible in the late phases of the examination, whereas others (nonfull thickness granulomas) disappear overtime.
(FA: Fluorescein angiography; ICG: Indocyanine green)

them. Large, full thickness lesions may remain visible during the late phases of the examination whereas smaller ones can turn isoreflective hence becoming undetectable (Figs. 45.24C and D).[60] Large choroidal vessels can show blurred margins and hyperfluorescence during the late phases of the angiogram due to ICG leakage.[61,62] Often, when the choroid is seriously inflamed or in case of posterior scleritis, multiple serous retinal detachments (SRDs) can occur due to external blood retinal barrier and choroidal drainage failure. When this happens multiple pinpoints of leakage are visible on FA leading to pooling of dye into the subretinal space (Figs. 45.25A and B).[50]

Neovascular Complications

Inflammatory cytokines have a strong angiogenic effect, thus promoting the formation of new vascular networks. Neovascularizations can occur on the retinal surface driven by the inflammatory stimulus or secondary to VEGF release in case of occlusive vasculitis.[61] When this happens FA show the typical leakage from the neovascular branches. Inflammatory choroidal neovascularization (iCNV) may also occur.[61] They usually develop between the retina and the RPE. The location can be either at the posterior pole or along the edge of a chorioretinal scar. These iCNVs

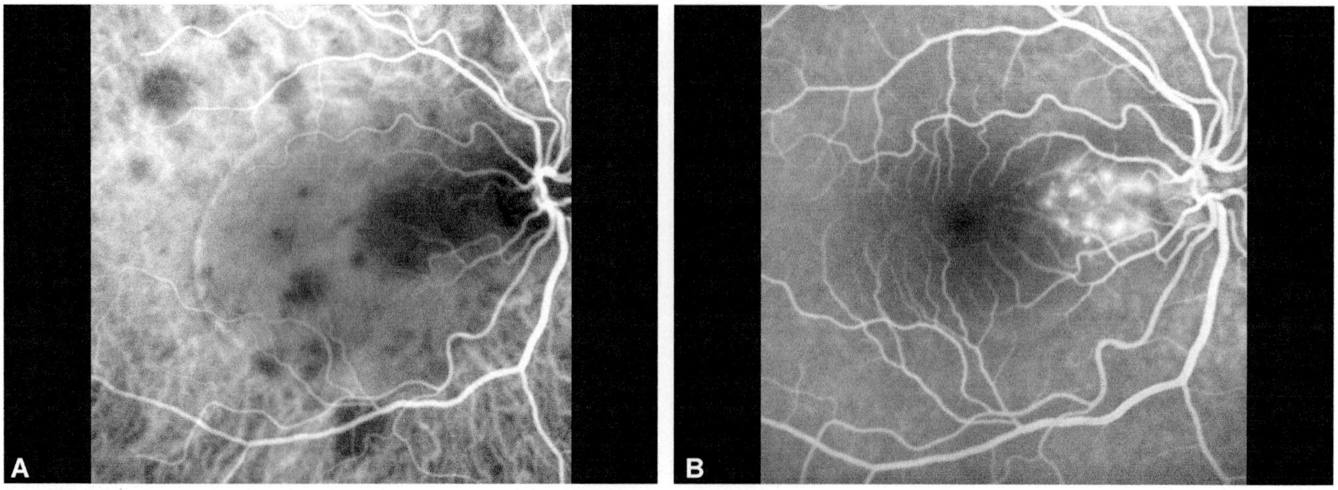

Figs. 45.25A and B: Stromal choroiditis with exudative retinal detachment. (A) ICG angiography clearly shows some choroidal granulomas visible as round-shaped hypofluorescent areas across the posterior pole. The C-shaped border of an exudative retinal detachment is also visible; and (B) On FA, multiple pinpoints of leakage can be visualize along the papillomacular bundle as the dye leaks through the impaired external blood retinal barrier into the subretinal space.

(FA: Fluorescein angiography; ICG: Indocyanine green)

have a classical appearance on FA with dye leakage from the early phases of the angiogram increasing in size and intensity overtime (Figs. 45.26A and B).[63] ICGA can help in these cases in differentiating the neovascular lesions from inflammatory foci.[64]

Exudative Age-related Macular Degeneration

Exudative age-related macular degeneration (AMD) is generally classified based upon the axial location of the CNV. A type 1 CNV is a neovascular membrane that is located under the RPE, whereas a type 2 CNV has passed through the RPE and lies under the neurosensory retina.[65] According to the Macular Photocoagulation Study, type 1 CNV is generally considered to correspond to "occult" CNV on FA (as defined by the Macular Photocoagulation Study), and type 2 CNV generally corresponds to "classic" CNV.[66,67] More recently, type 3 CNV has been defined to be CNV with a definite intraretinal component.[68] The fact that occult CNV accounts for the vast majority of the exudative complications in AMD[69] explains in part why ICGA, with its ability to delineate occult CNV, has become part of standard care in exudative AMD for many clinicians.[70,71] With the advent of anti-VEGF therapy for either classic[72] or occult[73] CNVs, their management has changed from the use of therapy for which accurate localization of the membrane was crucial (i.e. laser photocoagulation, photodynamic therapy) to the nonspecific intravitreal delivery of active and highly effective biologic drugs. Nonetheless, we would still argue that the gold standard diagnostic procedure should be the one which best visualizes the disease (CNV) under investigation.

Type 1 Choroidal Neovascularization

This type of CNV is by definition under the RPE, and corresponds to the occult neovascular network on FA. The Macular Photocoagulation Study recognized two forms of occult CNV: (1) A fibrovascular pigment epithelial detachment (PED); and (2) A late-phase leakage of an undetermined source (LLUS).[66] As for the fibrovascular PED, its prevalence may vary from 22% to 50% of occult CNV lesions,[70,71,74] as opposed to FA, dynamic ICGA may delineate the presence of a neovascular network usually located along the edges of the PED (Figs. 45.27A to C).[71,75,76] Moreover, dynamic ICGA may reveal a feeder vessel that can be successfully treated with laser photocoagulation, when it is located outside the foveal region (*see* Fig. 45.4B).[77,78] In case of LLUS, which may represent 36–78% of occult CNV,[69,70,74] dynamic ICGA may differentiate an occult form of CNV from retinal angiomatous proliferation (RAP) (Figs. 45.28A to C).[74] Considering that one-fourth of patients with an LLUS do have a RAP,[74] and that an early diagnosis of these lesions is crucial for the functional prognosis,[79] the importance of an ICG evaluation for these cases becomes readily apparent. In conclusion, ICG facilitates a better

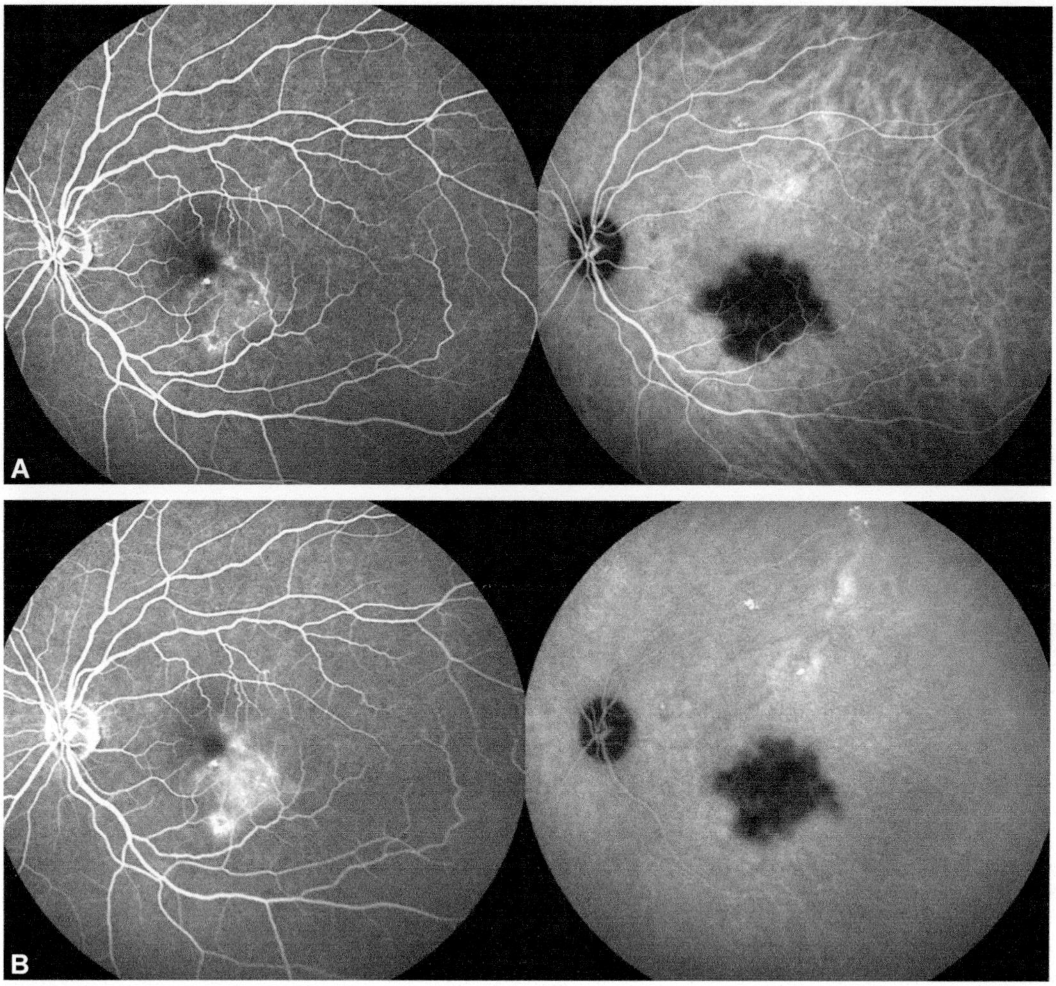

Figs. 45.26A and B: Inflammatory choroidal neovascularization. Combined angiography of a patient affected by serpiginous choroiditis complicated by a choroidal neovascularization. (A and B) The choroidal neovascular membrane is visible in a leaking area along the inferortemporal border of the fovea progressively increasing in size and intesity overtime.

Source: Dr TP Vignesh, Aravind Eye Hospital, Madurai, Tamil Nadu, India.

and more complete classification of occult CNV subtypes, compared to FA. Of note, Yannuzzi et al.[29] found that 39% of lesions classified as poorly demarcated occult lesions by FA were well defined by ICGA.

Type 2 Choroidal Neovascularization

Classic CNV, being localized above the RPE layer, is well outlined by FA. However, leakage of dye from the lesion may obscure the boundaries of the neovascular network. ICGA improves visualization of the fine structure of the neovascular network (Figs. 45.29A to C).[45] This high spatial and temporal resolution permits also the identification of choroidal vessels that feed into the CNV (Figs. 45.30A and B).[80] Watzke et al.[76] showed that 87% of eyes with classic choroidal neovascular membranes were hypercyanescent with distinct edges. This ability to provide a clear delineation of the neovascular network may confer an important advantage in the era of anti-VEGF therapy. It has been reported that VEGF inhibitors were more effective in controlling immature vessels.[81] Mature, larger choroidal vessels may be readily differentiated from immature choroidal capillaries on ICGA. Thus, in patients with chronic AMD or those who did not benefit from previous treatments with anti-VEGF, ICGA might better delineate a more mature stage of CNV.

Type 3 Choroidal Neovascularization

During the past decade, RAP has been labeled with a number of different terms, including "retinal vascular anomalous complex", "retinal choroidal anastomosis",

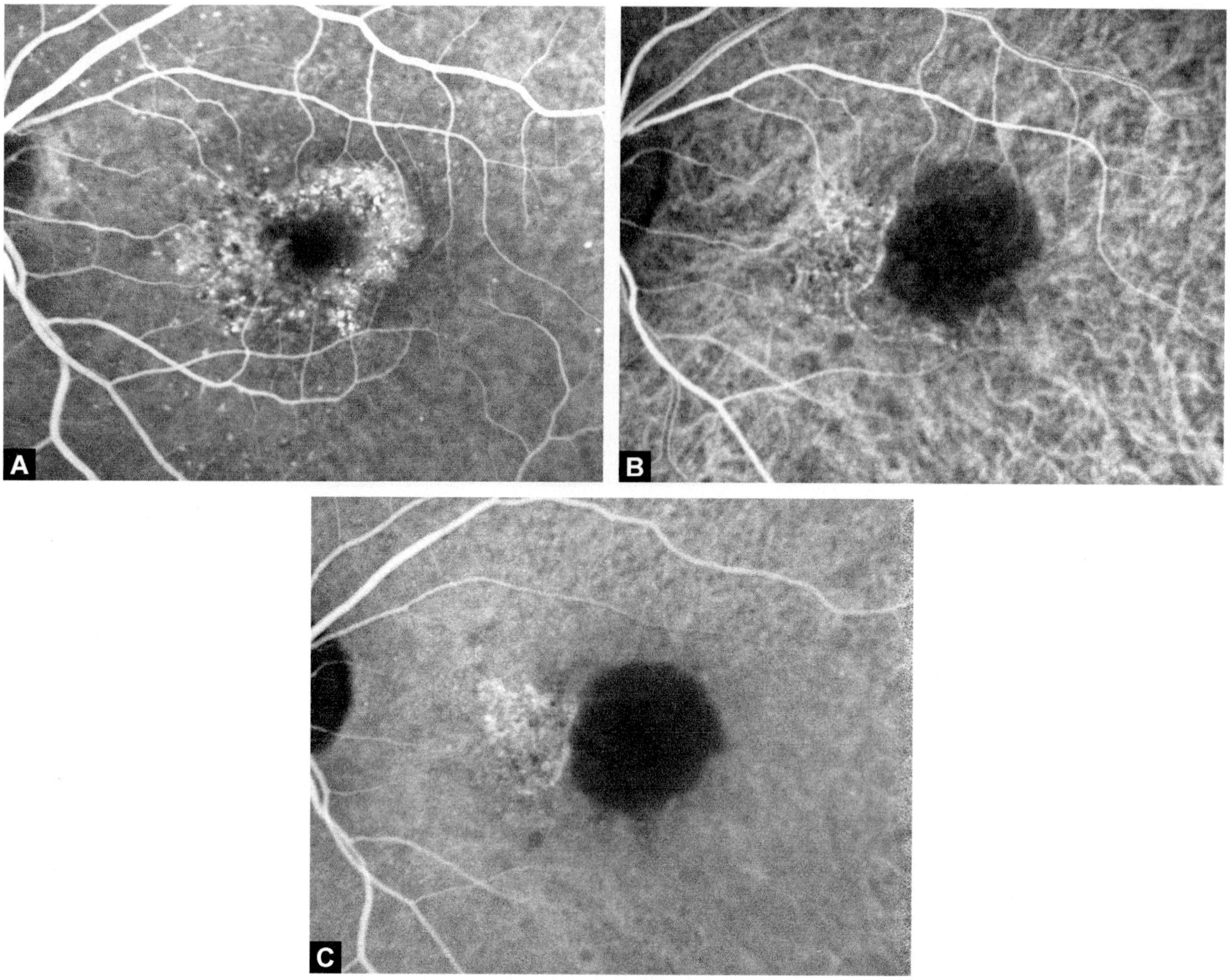

Figs. 45.27A to C: A pigment epithelium detachment (A, fluorescein angiography) with a well-delineated neovascular network located along its edges (B and C, early-late indocyanine green angiography).

"retinal anastomosis to the lesion", and "chorioretinal anastomosis". In a comprehensive article on this entity, Yannuzzi et al.[82] provided evidence to support the original concept of capillaries arising within the inner half of the retina, or Retinal Angiomatous Proliferation, thus suggesting the acronym of RAP as the appropriate descriptor for the disease. Subsequently, Gass et al.[83] suggested a possible choroidal origin for these vessels, emanating from occult CNV and developing into an occult chorioretinal anastomosis. The new category, type 3 neovascularization, has been proposed to harmonize these conflicting theories.[68] Type 3 lesions would encompass the following disease manifestations: (1) Focal neovascular proliferation arising from the deep retinal capillary plexus (the original RAP concept); (2) Intraretinal neovascular extension from an underlying occult/type 1 CNV; and (3) de novo breaks in Bruch's membrane with neovascular infiltration into the retina. Whatever the origin or initial location might be, our understanding of the importance of RAP as a component of neovascular AMD has been enhanced by ICGA. The fluorescein angiographic study generally shows manifestations of occult CNV, either fibrovascular PED (Figs. 45.31A and B) or LLUS (Figs. 45.32A and B) without a characteristic feature to identify and delineate the angiomatous process in the retina (indistinct zone of staining within and beyond the retina). By contrast, ICGA may clearly delineate the vascular structure of the lesion. When associated with PED, the RAP is usually well within the area of detachment and not at the edges, as is typically the case with CNV which vascularizes a serous PED (so-called notched PED configuration on FA). As previously reported, RAP may be present in up to one-fourth of eyes thought to

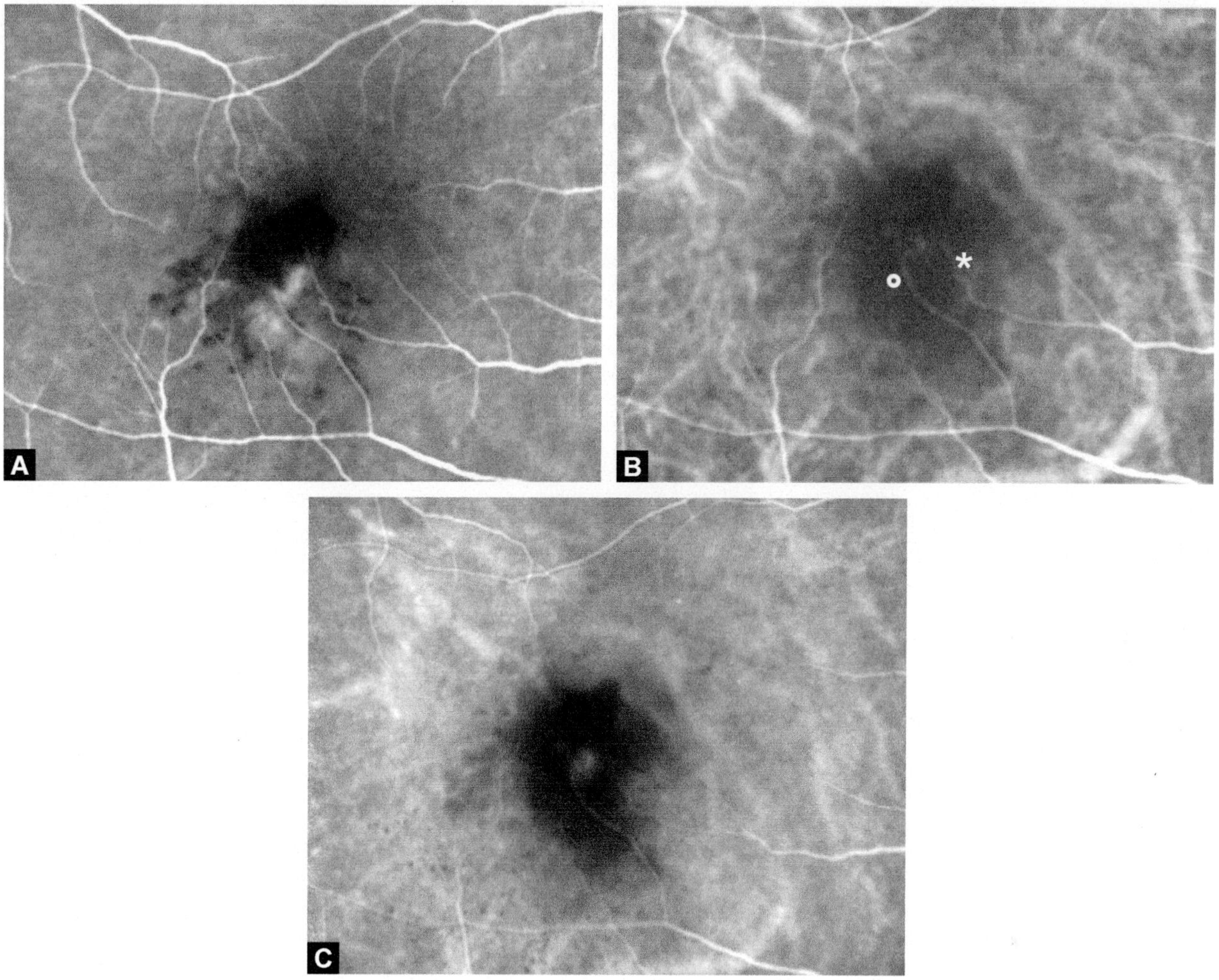

Figs. 45.28A to C: Late leakage of undetermined source (A). In ICG angiography, early images (B) reveal the presence of an RAP with a feeding retinal arteriole (asterisk) and a draining retinal vein (circle). Late phases (C) show late leakage from the lesion which is a typical ICG feature of RAP. (ICG: Indocyanine green; RAP: Retinal angiomatous proliferation)

have occult CNV with LLUS.[74] Dynamic indocyanine green angiography (d-ICGA) has further expanded our capability for an early diagnosis. By definition, a diagnosis of RAP is based upon the temporal evidence of "dye filling of at least one retinal arteriole descending into the deep retinal space to a vascular communication and at least one draining retinal vein" (Figs. 45.31 and 45.32).[84] In conventional angiography, images are usually captured at one frame per second. This makes it virtually impossible to visualize the progression of the dye through the vascular complex, even though images are taken at very early phases. By contrast, d-ICGA takes up to 12 frames per second and captures the progressive filling of the lesion (Figs. 45.33A to E). The possibility of repeated viewing of the dynamic sequence of progression on ICG may further increase our chances of an early diagnosis of RAP (Figs. 45.34A and B). In a series of RAP diagnosed using d-ICGA,[74] the incidence of stage 1 RAP (64.9%) and the mean distance of the lesions from the fovea (682 ± 304 μm) were both consistent with an early-stage disease process, supporting the utility of this imaging procedure. To bring to completion the angiographic diagnostic criteria for RAP definition, two ICGA features seem to be distinctive: (1) Late leakage in ICGA (Fig. 45.28C), and (2) Shunting of blood flow to the neovascular net, defined as a feeding arteriole that shunted a major part of the blood flow from the distal part of the macular arteriole to the neovascular net (Figs. 45.31B and 45.35).[85-87] Late leakage in ICGA has been reported to occur in all RAP cases, while it was found in 7% of other CNVs.[85] Shunting of blood flow was found in 56% of RAP, whereas it was absent in 100% of other CNVs.[85] However, shunting of blood flow to the RAP is a difficult sign to evaluate. The detection of

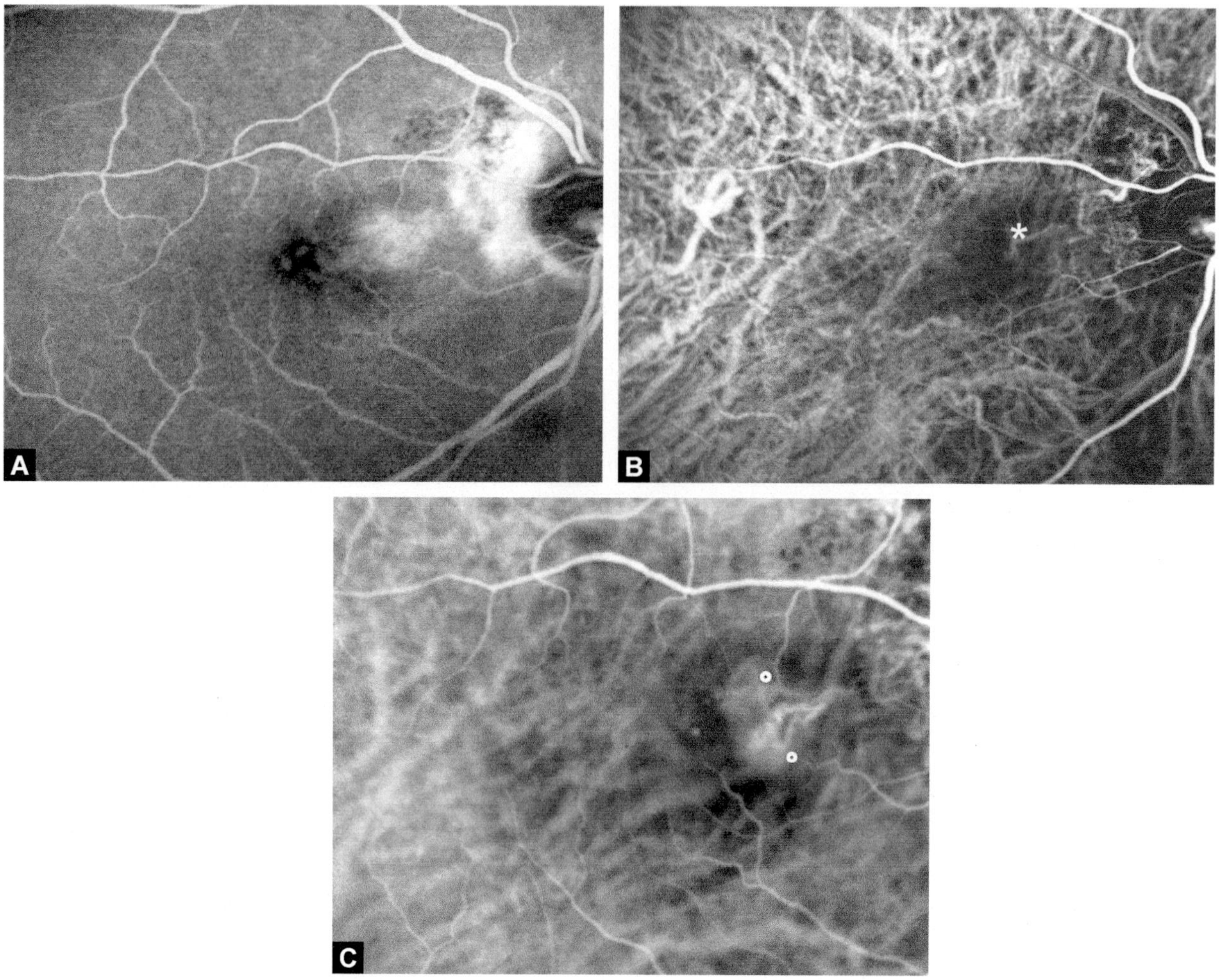

Figs. 45.29A to C: Type 2 CNV. The lesion is well outlined by fluorescein angiography (A). However, leakage of dye may obscure the boundaries of the neovascular network. ICGA improves visualization of the fine structure of the neovascular network showing the feeding artery (B, asterisk) and the draining veins (C, circles).

(CNV: Choroidal neovascularization; ICGA: Indocyanine green angiography)

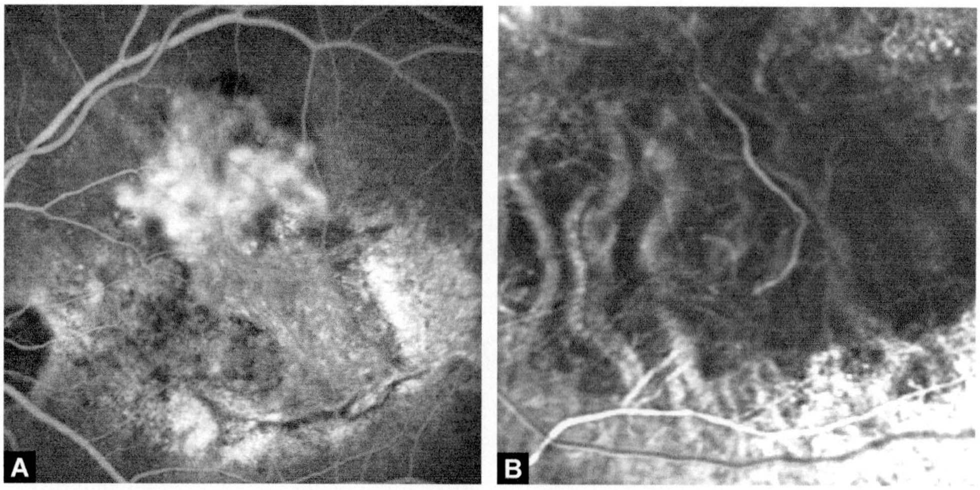

Figs. 45.30A and B: Type 2 CNV. Fluorescein angiography shows the subretinal neovascularization (A) whereas ICGA reveals also a very long feeding vessel (B).

(CNV: Choroidal neovascularization; ICGA: Indocyanine green angiography)

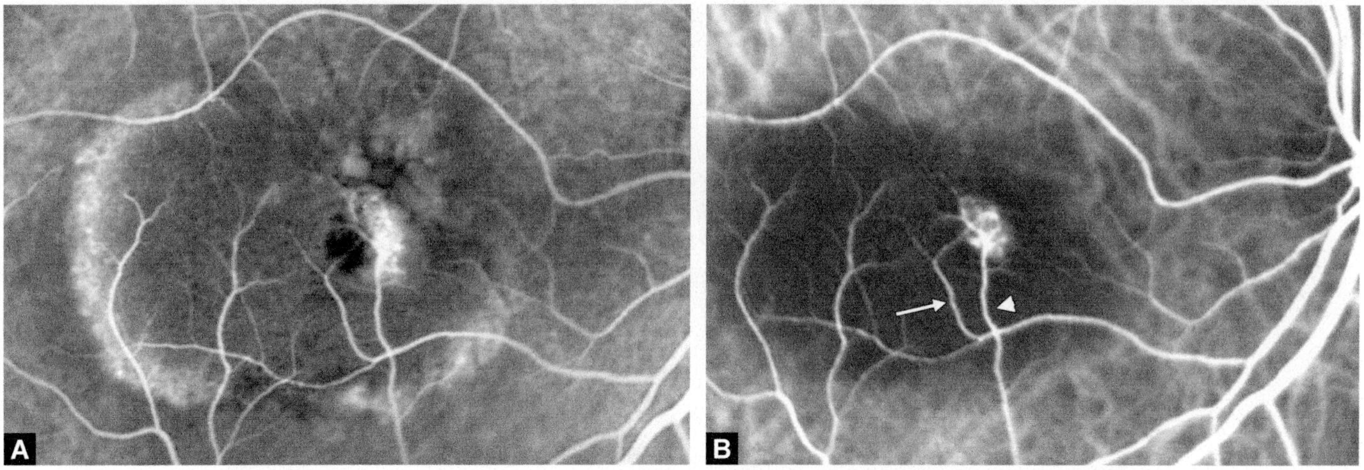

Figs. 45.31A and B: Late-phase fluorescein angiography (A) shows a pigment epithelium detachment (PED) with a "hot spot." Indocyanine green angiography (B) reveals the presence of retinal angiomatous proliferation within the edges of PED. Feeding retinal arteriole (arrow) and draining retinal venule (arrowhead) are clearly visualized. Shunting of blood flow to the neovascular net is also present.

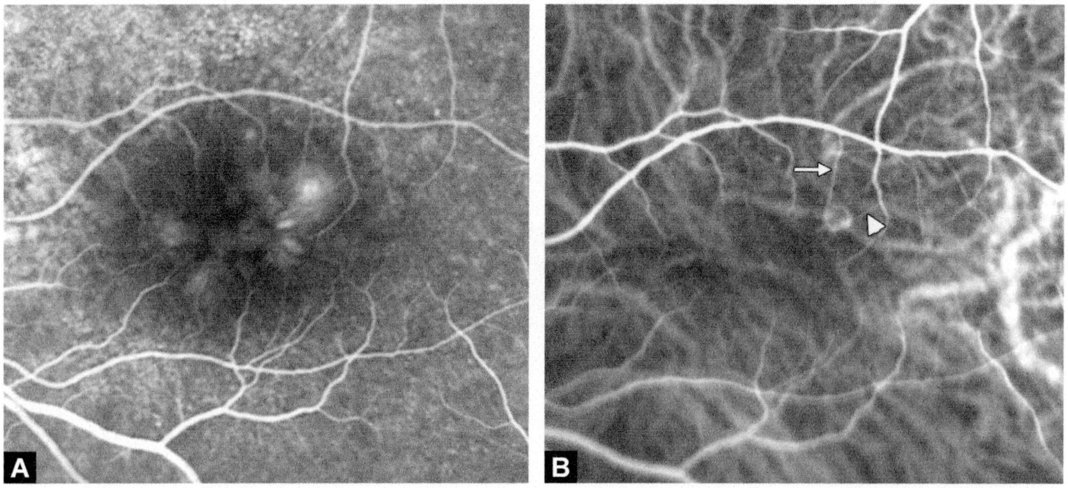

Figs. 45.32A and B: Late-phase fluorescein angiography (A) shows a late leakage of undetermined source. Indocyanine green angiography (B) reveals the presence of retinal angiomatous proliferation. Feeding retinal arteriole (arrow) and draining retinal venule (arrowhead) are clearly visualized.

this feature requires dynamic FA or ICGA, with high-quality images. Moreover, the presence of blood shunting depends on the stage of RAP lesion, being less evident or not present in stage 1. In case of shunting, the increased diameter of the feeding arteriole in respect of the distal end of the original artery is clearly evident (Figs. 45.35A to F). Differences in blood flow between the two vessels (i.e. the feeding retinal arteriole and the distal part of the original arteriole) might explain this phenomenon. In the feeding retinal arteriole, blood flow velocity is likely to be very high because the resistance to flow in the RAP lesion and its venous drainage is low. In the distal part of the original arteriole, the blood flow has to deal with the resistance normally present in the capillary bed. Hence, the blood is shunted toward the RAP. Early and accurate diagnosis of RAP is important because RAP lesions are thought to be more aggressive, with a treatment response that is likely to diminish with more advanced disease stages.[79] Dynamic ICGA is also extremely useful for monitoring the therapeutic effect. A complete remodeling of the vascular structure may be achieved after successful closure and it is clearly highlighted in d-ICGA (Figs. 45.35D to F).[87]

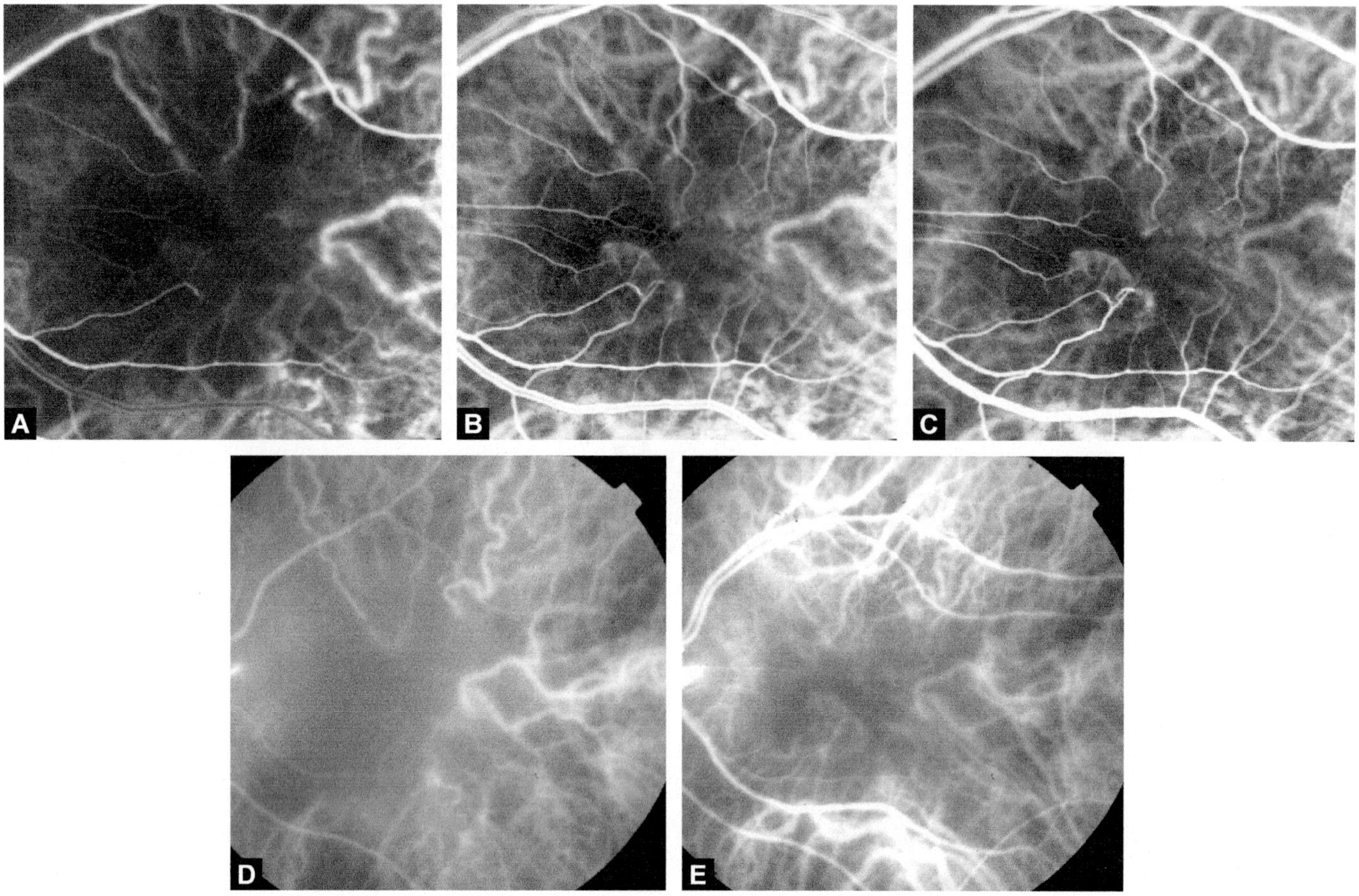

Figs. 45.33A to E: Comparison of dynamic (6 frames per second) and conventional ICG angiography of the same RAP (stage II). Feeding retinal arteriole, filling of the vascular lesion and draining retinal vein are all features visible in the dynamic sequences (A to C). The progression of filling is lost during the first two images captured with a conventional digital system (D and E).
(ICG: Indocyanine green; RAP: Retinal angiomatosus proliferation)

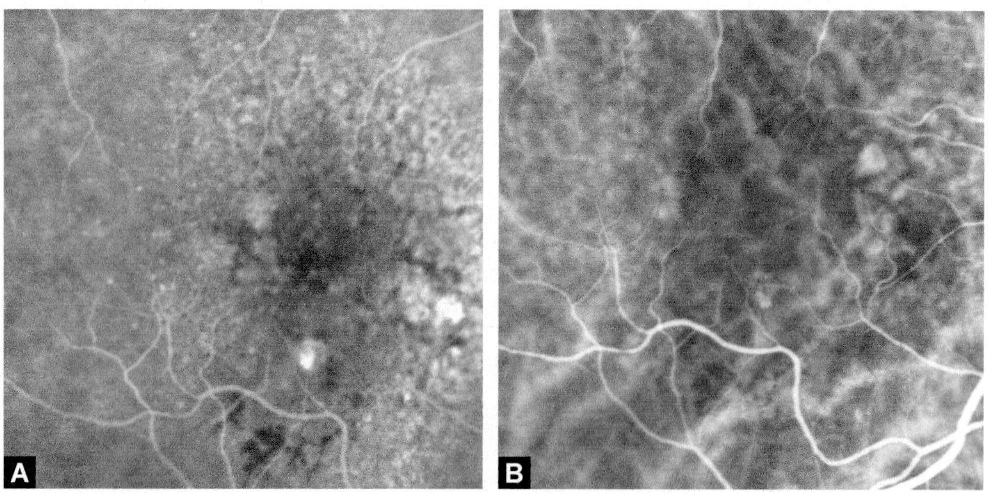

Figs. 45.34A and B: Midphase fluorescein angiography (A) showing a small area of progressive extrafoveal staining at 6 o'clock. Dynamic indocyanine green angiography (B) reveals a well-delineated stage I retinal angiomatous proliferation (RAP) with a feeding retinal arteriole and a draining retinal vein.

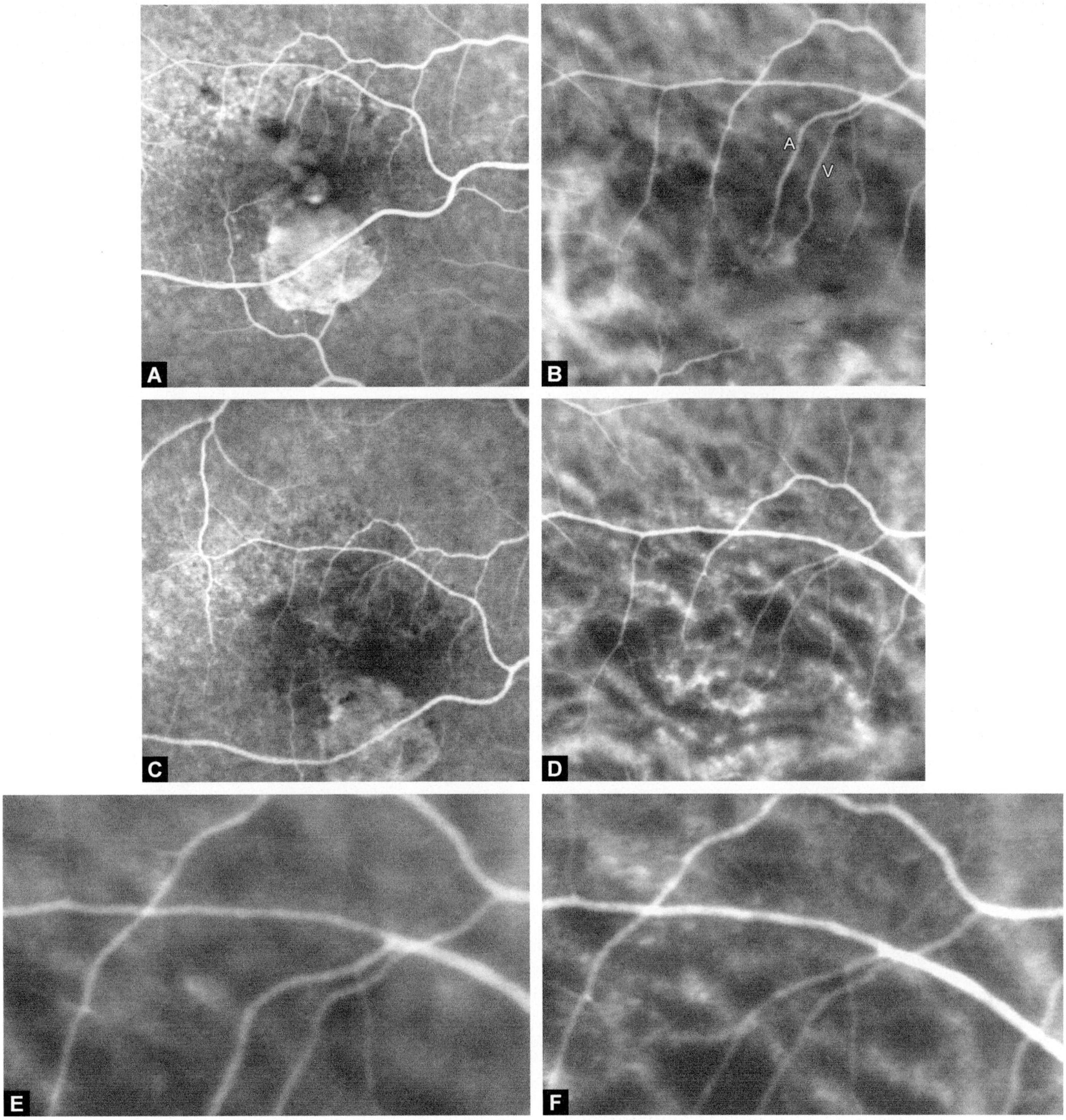

Figs. 45.35A to F: Baseline dynamic (A) FA and (B) ICGA showed a stage II extrafoveal RAP located superotemporal to the fovea. One feeding first-order macular arteriole (A) shunted blood flow from the vascular arcade to the RAP and one draining retinal vein (V). Cystoid macular edema was evident in late fluorescein phases (A). Six months after treatment, the RAP was no longer detectable by either (C) FA or (D) ICGA. Blood flow was again normally directed along the vascular arcade with reduction in size of the first-order macular arteriole (D). The cystoid macular edema resolved (E). After treatment (F), the distal part of the vascular arcade regained its normal appearance (compare E and F) because the first order arteriole decreased in size with the closure of the RAP.
(FA: Fluorescein angiography; ICGA: Indocyanine green angiography; RAP: Retinal angiomatous proliferation)

POLYPOIDAL CHOROIDAL VASCULOPATHY

The term polypoidal choroidal vasculopathy (PCV) was first described by Yannuzzi as a new clinical entity, detected, and defined by its ICGA appearance.[88] Unfortunately, the definition of PCV is controversial as some authors have used the term PCV to identify a distinct clinical entity, whereas others have used it to describe a focal morphological manifestation within a wider neovascular process. It has been known that type 1 neovascularization is characterized by the growth of vessels under the RPE.[89] Focal polypoidal morphological changes are commonly seen within the type 1 lesion. In this contest, polyps should be considered as a structural variant of neovascular tissue rather than signifying a distinct pathogenic mechanism underlying the process of neovascularization. For this reason, the term "polypoidal CNV" would therefore seem appropriate to describe all neovascular complexes that demonstrate polypoidal changes (Figs. 45.36A to C).[90] Such terminology would recognize that polyps are a phenotypic manifestation of CNV rather than a separate entity in itself. On the other side, pachychoroid is a term that encapsulates a constellation of choroidal anatomical manifestations that implicates a structural and/or functional choroidal alteration.[91-93] Pachychoroid has been associated with the development of a spectrum of clinical diseases including pigment epitheliopathy, central serous chorioretinopathy (CSC), and neovascularization. These diseases are not necessarily distinct entities and are likely to represent a continuum of the same pathogenic process. In this contest, Freund proposed that pachychoroid may underlie the development of branching vascular networks (BVNs) and may also influence the biological activity of the neovascular process in PCV.[90] The diagnosis of PCV should be reserved for those eyes that show a paucity of the defining features of AMD, the occurrence of pachychoroid features beneath the neovascular process, and the presence of a BVN with terminating polyps (Figs. 45.37 and 45.38). Polyps are a morphological manifestation of a wide range of proliferative neovascular mechanisms and do not signify a distinct pathogenic process. Different imaging techniques can be

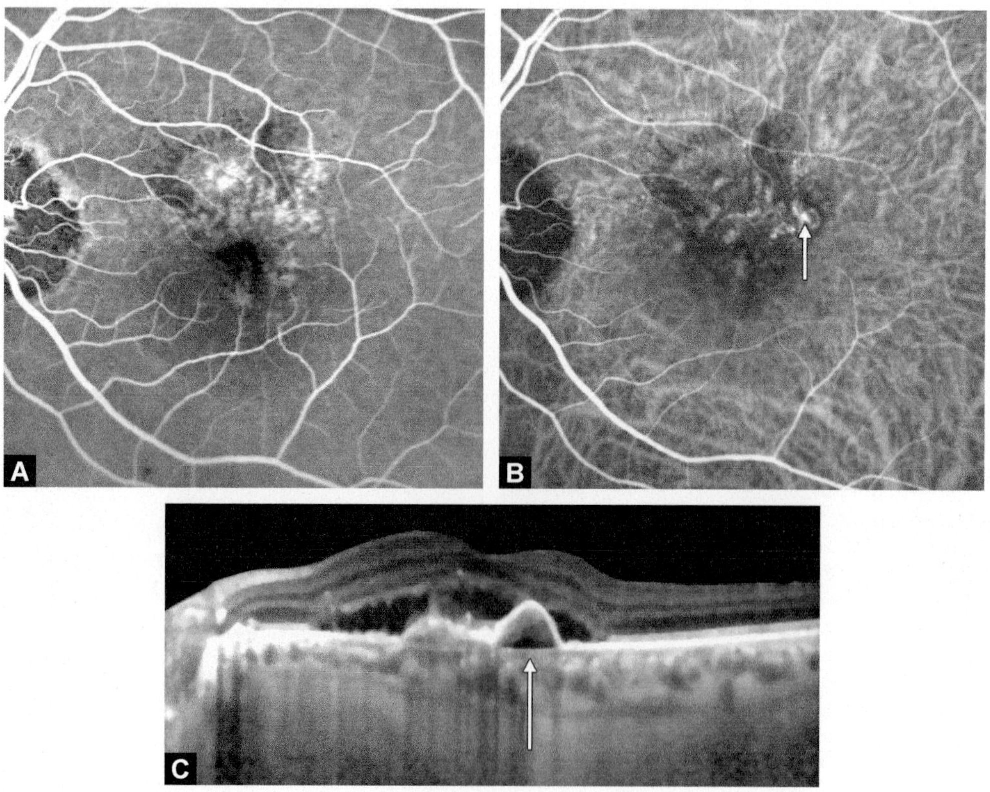

Figs. 45.36A to C: Polypoidal choroidal neovascularization. Fluorescein angiogram (A) revealing a central hypofluorescent area with hyperfluorescence points. Indocyanine green angiogram (B) showing the neovascular network with the polypoidal changes (arrow). Spectral domain optical coherence tomography (C) displaying detachment of retinal pigment epithelium with the enlarged vessel (arrow) and subretinal fluid.

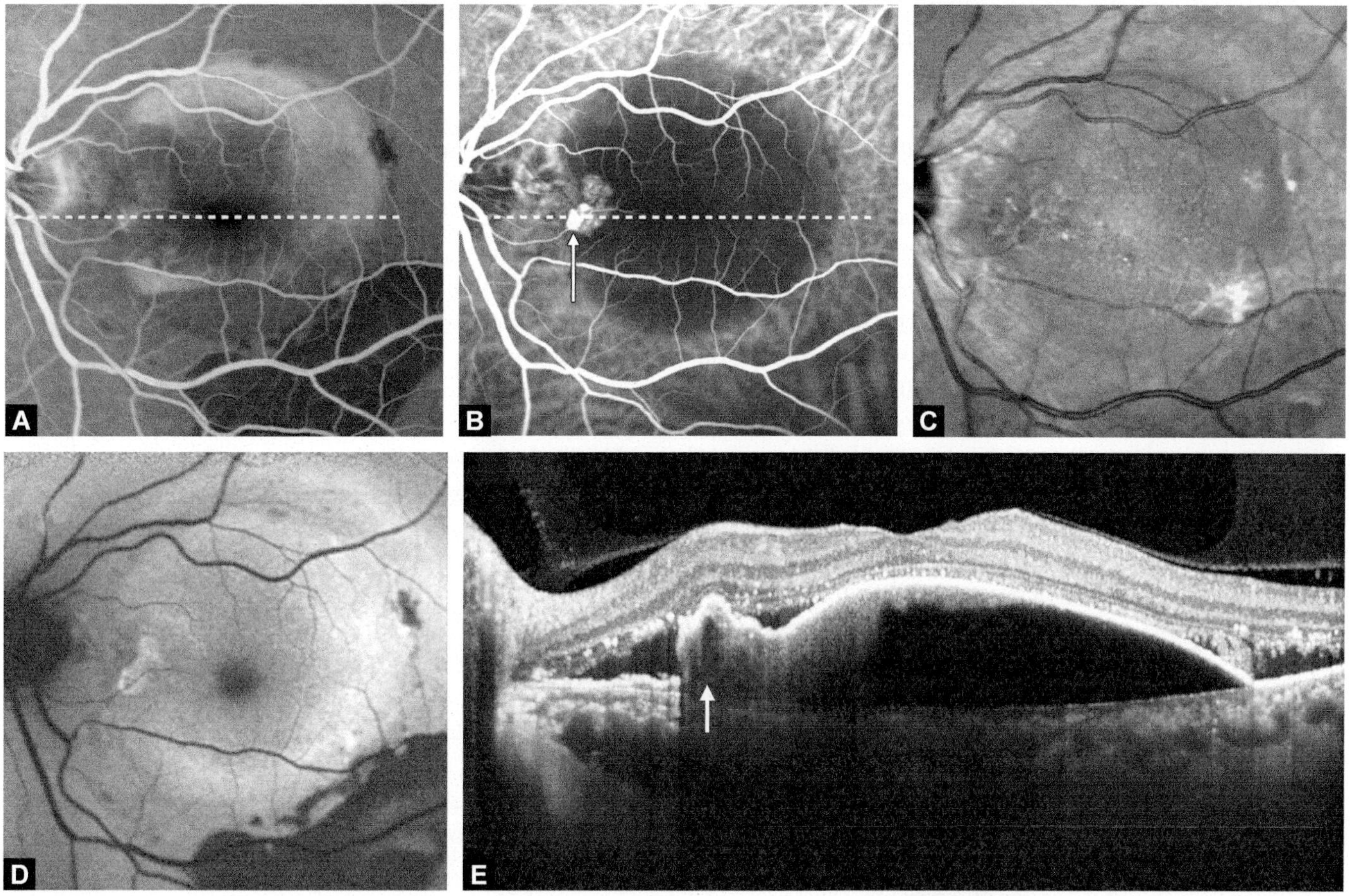

Figs. 45.37A to E: Multimodal imaging of polypoidal choroidal vasculopathy (PCV). Fluorescein angiogram (A) revealing a central hypofluorescent area with peripheral hyperfluorescence corresponding to the detachment of retinal pigment epithelium. Indocyanine green angiogram (B) showing a large hypofluorescence with adjacent focal hyperfluorescence correspoding to the polypoidal lesion (arrow). Infrared reflectance (C) and fundus autofluorescence (D) and optical coherence tomography (E) revealing the polypoidal lesion (arrow) with detachment of retinal pigment epithelium and subretinal fluid.

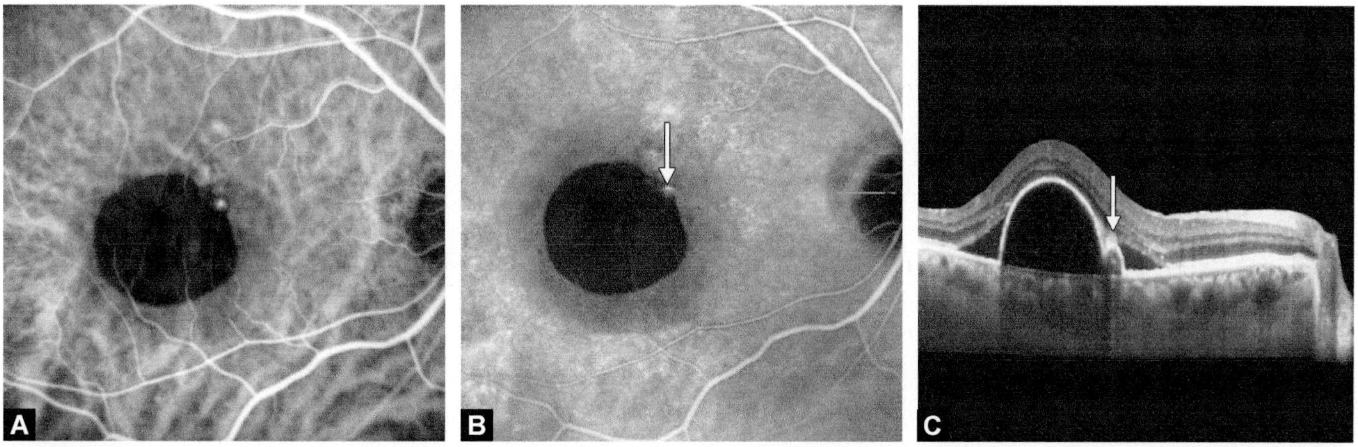

Figs. 45.38A to C: Polypoidal choroidal vasculopathy (PCV). Indocyanine green angiography in the early (A) and late phase (B) revealing a central hypofluorescent area corresponding to retinal pigment detachment with adjacent focal hyperfluorescence correspoding to the polypoidal lesion (arrow). Spectral domain optical coherence tomography (C) showing the detachment of retinal pigment epithelium with the enlarged vessel (arrow) and adjacent subretinal fluid.

used to visualize polyps. Typically, FA is not able to detect the neovascularization as the lesions are located under the RPE. The neovascular network is visible only in cases with large polypoidal lesions and overlying atrophy of the RPE. On the other side, ICGA is the gold standard imaging tool for detect PCV.[94] It presents a longer wavelengths allowing a deeper penetration under the RPE. Based on ICGA findings, PCV is defined as the presence of single or multiple focal nodular areas of hyperfluorescence arising from the choroidal circulation with or without an associated BVN. In particular, EVEREST study is a phase IV, multicenter, randomized, active controlled, double-masked, and exploratory study evaluating the effects of verteporfin photodynamic therapy combined with ranibizumab or alone versus ranibizumab monotherapy in patients with symptomatic macular PCV.[95] The standardized diagnostic criteria used in the EVEREST study to confirm PCV diagnosis consist of the presence of early subretinal focal hyperfluorescence on ICGA (within the first 6 minutes), and at least one of the following criteria: nodular appearance of the polyp on stereoscopic examination, hypofluorescent halo around the nodule, presence of a BVN, pulsation of the polyp on dynamic ICGA, orange subretinal nodules on color fundus photography that correspond to the ICGA nodules, or massive submacular hemorrhage (≥4 disk areas in size).[95]

CENTRAL SEROUS CHORIORETINOPATHY

The hallmark of CSC is the presence of an SRD, usually localized at the posterior pole and accompanied by a serous detachment of the RPE (PED). CSC can develop as a solitary disease or in association with several systemic conditions.[96] Regardless of the etiology the disease is characterized by a disturbance in the choroidal blood flow a dysfunction of the RPE and ultimately a breakdown of the external blood retinal barrier leading to fluid accumulation in the subretinal space. The disease is usually classified into acute CSC (lasting less than 3 months) and chronic CSC (lasting 3+ months).[97] When CSC is complicated by the development of a choroidal neovascular membrane the diagnosis can be challenging and the clinical picture overlaps to the so called "pachychoroid neovasculopathy".[92] Imaging findings may vary among these three entities and will be discussed separately.

The early phases of fundus fluorescein angiography (FFA) are usually characterized by one or more hyperfluorescent dots, caused by the leakage of dye through the RPE, and corresponding to the point of breakdown of the external blood retinal barrier (Figs. 45.39A to C). The identification of leaking point(s) at a safe distance form the foveal region can make the patient eligible for a targeted laser photocoagulation treatment. As time goes by the dye spreads across the subretinal space to ultimately fill the entire SRD (pooling) marking its borders (Figs. 45.39A to C). While the filling is occurring several patterns of dye spreading can be visualized including the classic "smokestack", the inkblot, and the mushroom shaped.[98] A leakage area without pinpoints has also been reported although less frequently. Areas of RPE atrophy and consequent window defect can be detected and usually represent the chronic damage induced by previous episodes of CSC.[97] Early phases of ICGA do not show distinctive features in CSC although a

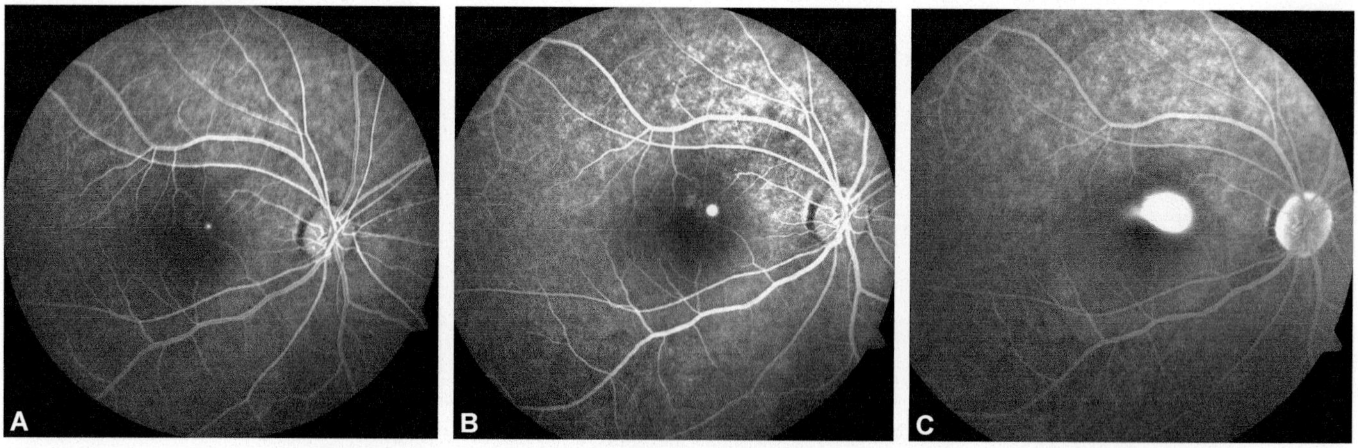

Figs. 45.39A to C: Fundus fluorescein angiography in a case of acute central serous chorioretinopathy. (A) Serial shots from early to; (B) Mid; and (C) Up to late phases of the angiogram demonstrate the progressive enlargement of the hyperfluorescent spot corresponding to the leaking point.
Source: Dr TP Vignesh, Aravind Eye Hospital, Madurai, Tamil Nadu, India.

certain degree of hypofluorescence due to delayed arterial filling has been described. On the contrary in the midphases of the angiogram a peculiar dye leakage from choroidal vessels with increased permeability can be observed.[99] The late phases of the angiogram can be characterized by a dispersion of the dye leading to a negative visualization of large choroidal vessels.[100] The area of RPE damage usually shows persistent leakage.

Chronic Central Serous Chorioretinopathy

Due to chronic damage of the RPE, FFA usually shows several window defects deriving from atrophic areas alternating to multiple leaking points. The resulting increased fluorescence can be alternate to signal blockage deriving from pigment clumps. Finally, areas of diffuse leakage with or without pinpoints slowly filling chronic subretinal fluid pockets can be observed.[101,102] ICGA shows findings similar to the once detected in acute CSC. In addition, areas of diffuse leakage, undetectable through FFA, are often identified in the late phases of the examination[99] and may represent a possible target for photodynamic treatment.

Complicated Central Serous Chorioretinopathy/Pachychoroid Neovasculopathy

This entity is characterized by the presence of thickened choroid with dilatation of the large choroidal vessels compressing the overlying choriocapillaris and Sattler's layer associated with a type 1 choroidal neovascular membrane.[92] On FFA and ICGA, it shows the same findings detected in chronic CSC. In addition, ICGA may show the presence of a discrete plaque of late hyperfluorescence corresponding to type 1 neovascular tissue (Figs. 45.40A and B). PCV can also complicate the clinical picture. In this case the lesion will appear as a hyperfluorescent bulge filled with dye in the early ICGA and then showing a characteristic washout during the late phases of the angiogram.[91]

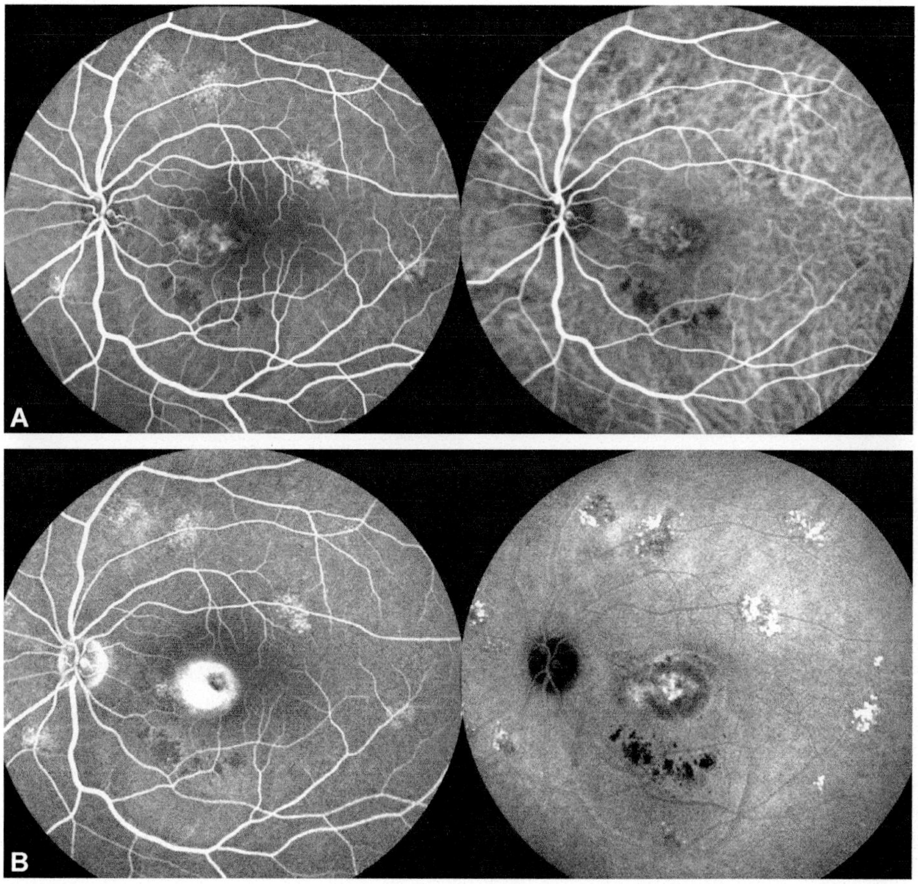

Figs. 45.40A and B: (A) Early and (B) Late. Combined angiography in a case of chronic serous chorioretinopathy complicated by choroidal neovascularization (CNV), shows early hypofluorescence in FFA and a clear vascular network in ICGA and late leakage in both.
Source: Dr TP Vignesh, Aravind Eye Hospital, Madurai, Tamil Nadu, India.

CHOROIDAL TUMORS

The diagnosis and management of a patient affected by a choroidal tumor can be extremely challenging. Despite the diagnosis is typically performed throughout a comprehensive clinical examination by means of biomicroscopy, indirect ophthalmoscopy, and ultrasonography, sometimes a multi-imaging approach can help the clinician to further characterize the lesions. The simultaneous use of fundus autofluorescence (FAF), FA, ICGA, and particularly, enhanced depth imaging-optical coherence tomography (EDI-OCT) has guaranteed in the last decades a better understanding of several conditions. More recently, optical coherence tomography angiography (OCTA) has been used for visualizing retinal and choroidal vasculature with no need for dye injection but its role in ocular oncology remains debated. Also, along with choroidal and retinal tumors, there are many patients referred to an ocular oncology practice presenting with non-neoplastic conditions for whom performing a full set of images and understanding the typical FA and ICGA patterns become crucial for both the diagnostic process and their follow-up.

Choroidal Hemangioma

Choroidal hemangiomas are benign vascular tumors of the choroid.[103] These are nonproliferative lesions with no evidence of cellular proliferation as the results of venous congestion. Histologically, choroidal hemangiomas are classified according to the type of vessels as cavernous type, composed of large vessels separated by limited connective tissue, capillary type, composed of small vessels separated by loose connective tissue, and mixed type, composed of both features.[103] Clinically, they can be differentiated in circumscribed or diffuse lesions.[104] The circumscribed type manifests as an isolated unilateral tumor without systemic associations while the diffuse form occurs frequently in association with Sturge-Weber syndrome.[104] The lesion typically appears as a red-orange mass in the paramacular region and experienced ophthalmologists may be able to diagnose it through an accurate fundus examination.[104] Nevertheless, the lesion may present chronic changes or significant subretinal fluid miming other conditions. On FA, choroidal hemangiomas do not show any pathognomonic features (Figs. 45.41A and B). They can present with early

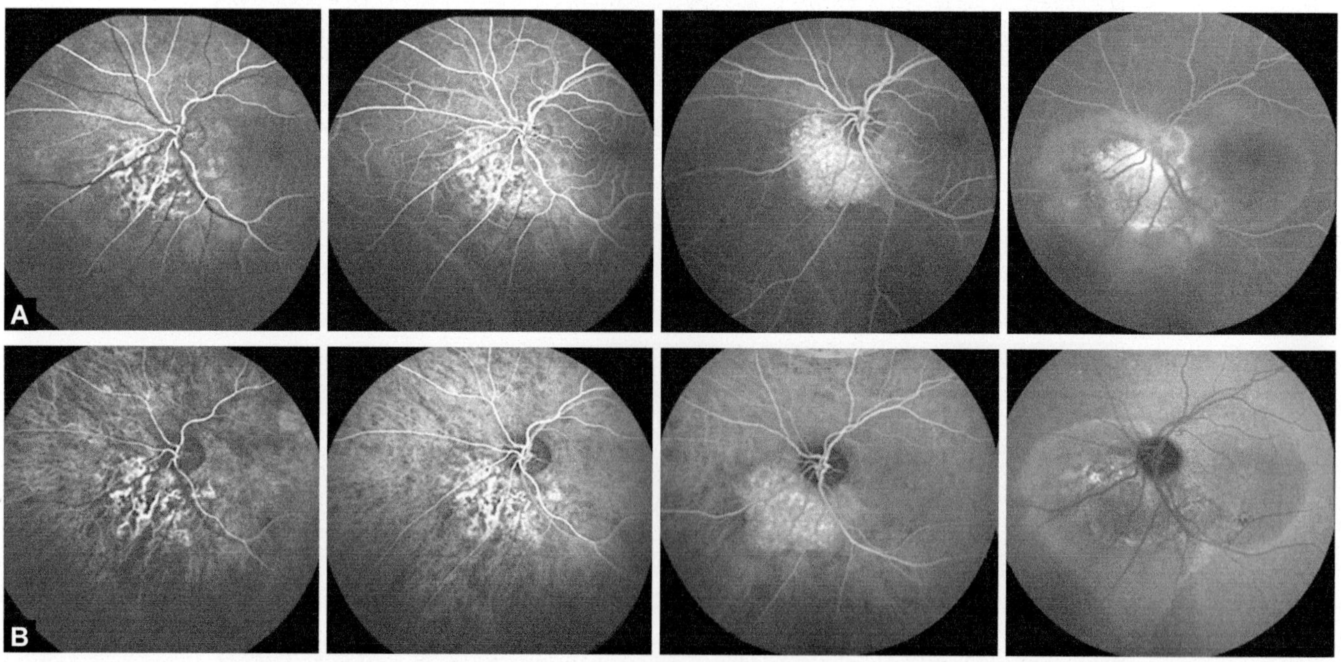

Figs. 45.41A and B: Fluorescein angiography and indocyanine green angiography of choroidal hemangioma. Fluorescein angiography (A) revealing an early lacy hyperfluorescence becoming more intense and with progressive staining and variable leakage in the late phases. Indocyanine green angiography (B) showing a typical rapid and uniform well-defined hyperfluorescence with a lobular aspect in the early phases and with progressive wash out phenomenon in the late phase of the angiogram with a residual hyperfluorescent rim around the lesion.

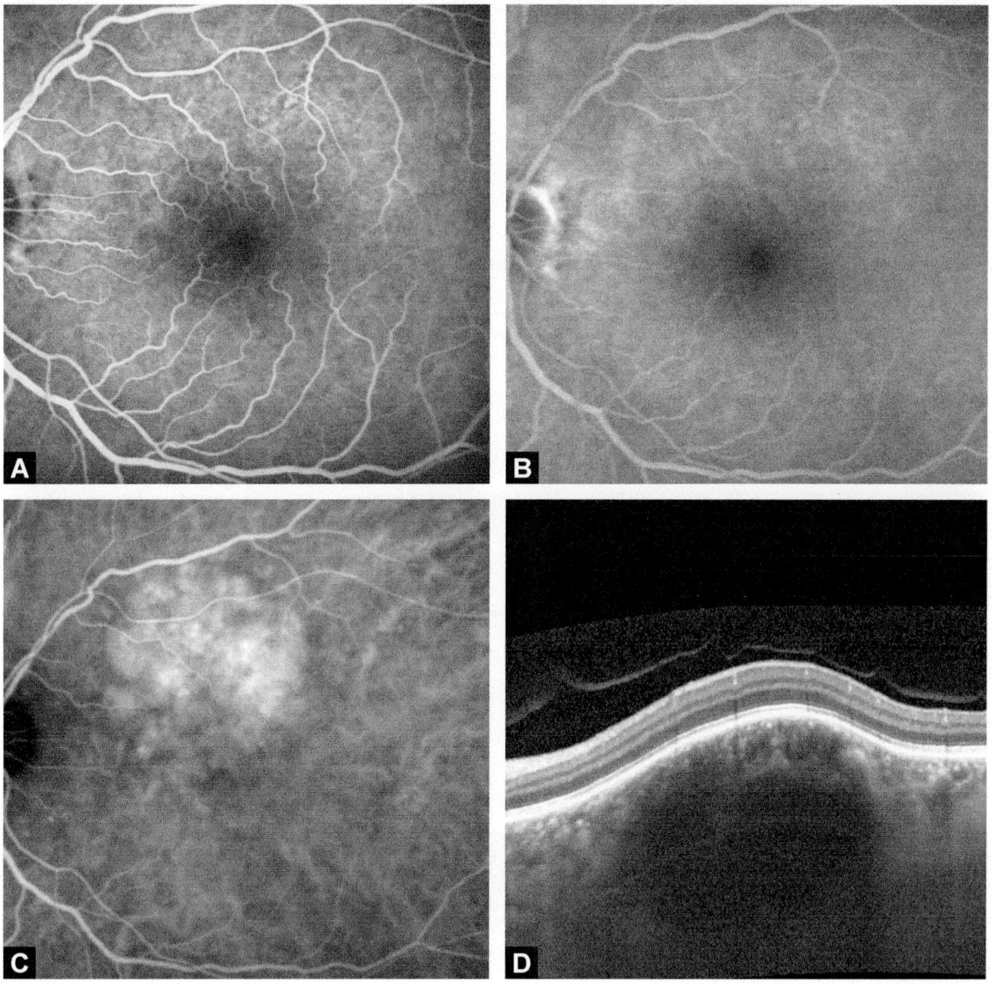

Figs 45.42A to D: Fluorescein angiography, indocyanine green angiography and optical coherence tomography of nonexudative choroidal hemangioma. Fluorescein angiography (FA) (A and B) showing an irregular, mild hyperfluorescence along the superior and inferior vascular arcades. Indocyanine green angiography (ICGA) (C) revealing a well defined hyperfluorescent choroidal lesion. Spectral domain optical coherence tomography displaying the small, smooth dome-shaped surface, expansion of a choroidal hemangioma with no traces of intra or subretinal exudation (D). In this case, the lesion was appreciable only by ICGA and not on FA due to the absence of fluid leakeage or outer retinal alterations

lacy hyperfluorescence that become more intense and with progressive staining of the extravascular tissue of the tumor and with variable leakage in the late phase.[105] The edges of the tumor appear as hypofluorescent due to the blockage of choroidal fluorescence by melanocytes which are pushed to the margins of the tumor. In case of hemangiomas not characterized by subretinal or intraretinal exudation, the lesion may also result completely silent at FA. Differently, ICGA shows a typical rapid and uniform onset of well-defined hyperfluorescence with a lobular aspect in the early phases and filling first peripherally then centrally.[106,107] In the late phases of the angiogram, choroidal hemangiomas show loss of dye, as the characteristic "washout" phenomenon, and a hyperfluorescent rim around the lesion (Figs. 45.42A to D).[106,107]

Choroidal Melanomas

Melanoma is a serious life-threatening malignancy that can involve the skin, the uvea, and other sites.[108] In particular, uveal melanoma is more often found in Caucasians (98%) and primarily involving the choroid (90%), ciliary body (7%), and iris (2%).[24] The early recognition of small choroidal melanomas using characteristic clinical features becomes critical to provide improved patient prognosis.[109] Its diagnosis is mainly based on clinical examination by means of biomicroscopy and indirect ophthalmoscopy and by ultrasonography. Typical clinical findings include the presence of a sessile or dome-shaped lesion with secondary exudative retinal detachment and orange pigment at the level of the RPE. Ancillary tests including FAF and EDI-

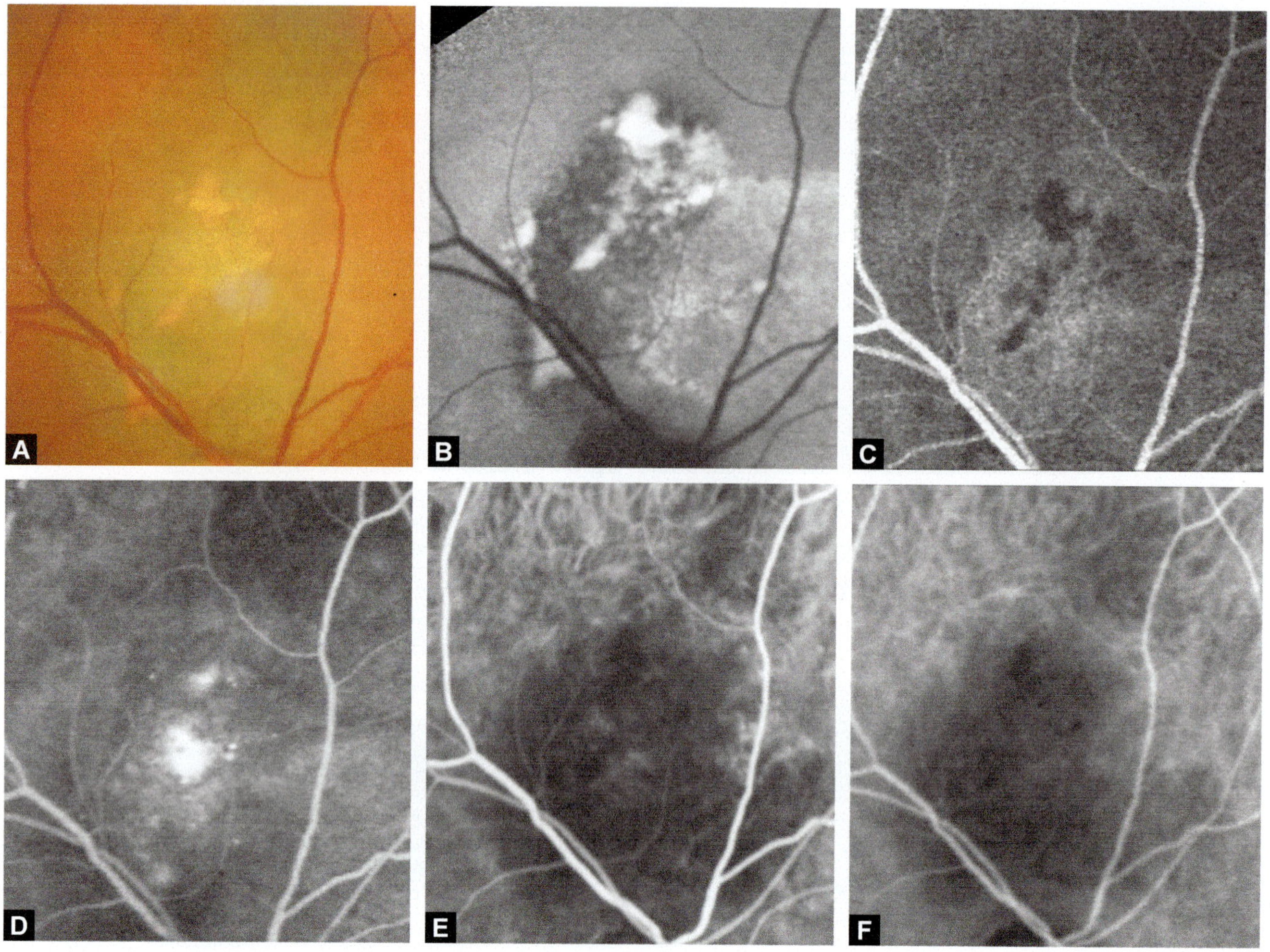

Figs. 45.43A to F: Multimodal imaging of pigmented choroidal melanoma. Color photography (A) revealing a peripapillary pigmented lesion with overlying orange pigment. The lesions appears hypoautofluorescent with hyperautofluorescent flecks in correspondence of the orange pigment by fundus autofluorescence (B). Fluorescein angiography (C and D) showing an iso or mild hyperfluorescence in the early phases (C) with late leakage (C) in correspondence of the lesion. Interestingly, the areas of late leakage do not correspond to the orange pigment which appears hypofluorescent during all the phases of the angiogram. (D) Indocyanine green angiography displaying an hypofluorescent lesion in the early (E) and late phase (F) with a barely visible intrinsic vasculature.

OCT may be used to further characterize the tumor and the adjacent retina. Corresponding to the variability of presentation, the FA features in choroidal melanomas is also variable. FA appearance is considerably influenced by tumor characteristics (size, pigmentation, associated SRD, or hemorrhages) and media transparency. If there is no significant blocking of fluorescence, the filling of the choroidal vessels is accompanied by an irregular hyperfluorescence within the tumor with variable degree of leakage in correspondence of the lesion in the late phases (Figs. 45.43A to F). In contrast, the near-infrared light used for ICGA penetrates the pigmented layers of the fundus more easily than the short-wavelength light used in FA.[110,111] For this reason, ICGA images different microvascular pattern of choroidal melanomas better than FA (Figs. 45.44A to E). Histologically, nine different microvascular pattern have been described with further correlation to in vivo imaging by ICGA.[112] Despite it has been described that these patterns may correlate to systemic prognosis, the utility of these findings and the role of angiography for the differential diagnosis of small melanocytic lesion still remains controversial. Interestingly, the clumps of orange pigment which may be recognized for their classical hyperfluorescence at FAF imaging appear hypofluorescent throughout all the phases of the angiogram on both FA and ICGA imaging.

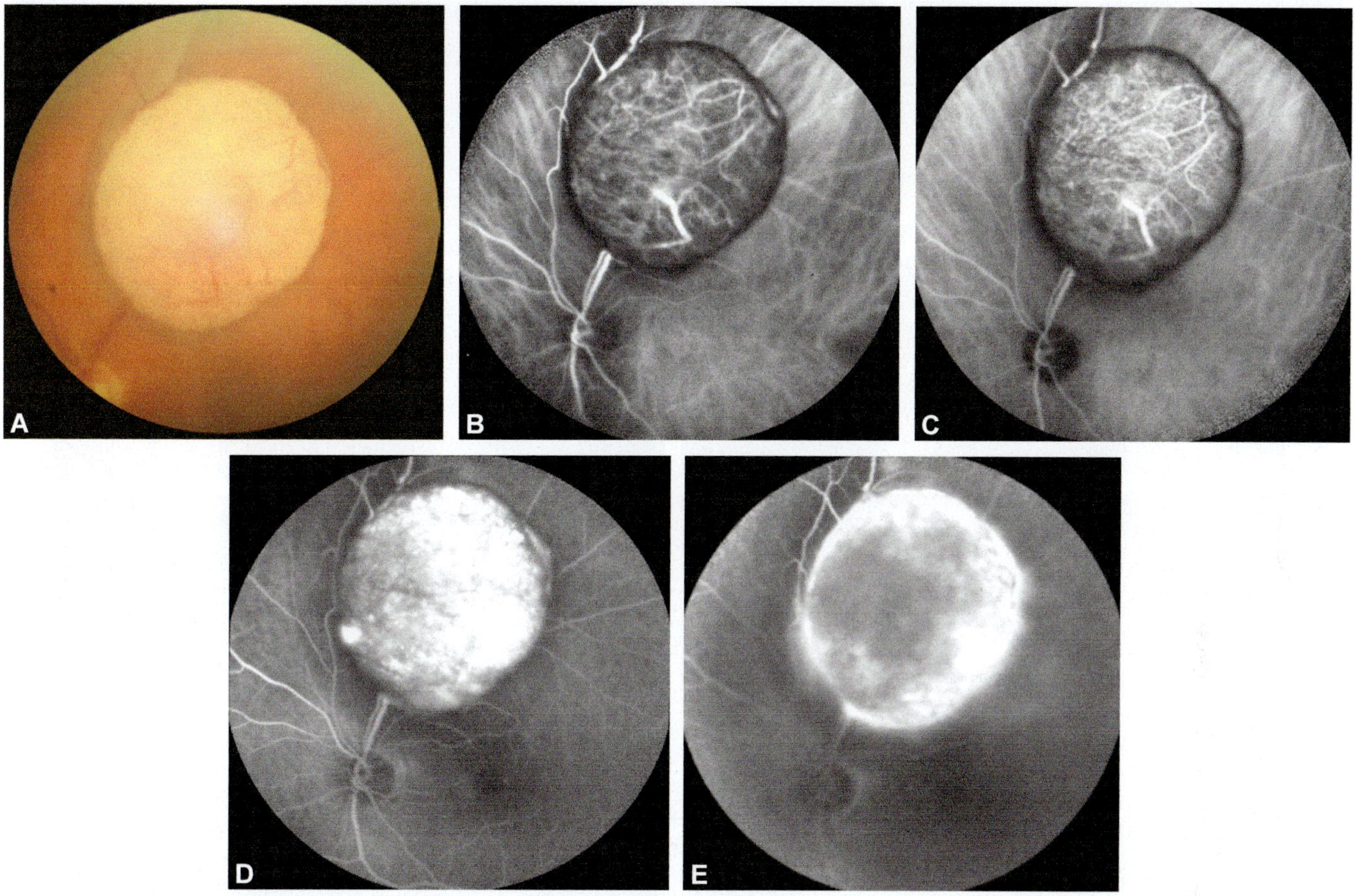

Figs. 45.44A to E: Multimodal imaging of amelanotic choroidal melanoma. Color photography (A) showing an amelanotic, mushroom-shaped lesion with prominent intrinsic vasculature and secondary exudative retinal detachment along the superior vascular arcade. Indocyanine green angiography highlighting the tumor intrinsic vasculature in the early (B) and late phase (C). Fluorescein angiography displaying a hyperfluorescent lesion in the early phase (D) with variable leakage in the late phase of the angiogram (E).

Choroidal metastases likely represent the most frequent form of intraocular malignancy and account for more than the 90% of metastatic occurring in the uveal tract. The most common primary tumors associated to uveal metastases are breast cancer in women and lung carcinoma in men.[113] The clinical features of the lesion and the history of cancer often facilitate the diagnosis; nevertheless, a relevant percentage of the patients presents with uveal metastasis and no history of systemic cancer. For these reasons, FA and ICGA as well as wide-field imaging techniques become essential to document and manage these lesions. FA typically shows blocking of the background fluorescence or mottled hyperfluorescence in correspondence of RPE defects in the early frames whereas in the late phases typically shows irregular areas of hyperfluorescence. ICGA usually reveals the lesions as well-defined areas of hypofluorescence which gradually become more apparent throughout the late phases of the angiogram with a patchy pattern (Figs. 45.45A to F). Occasionally, flecks of hyperfluorescence can be recognized.

Choroidal Osteoma

Choroidal osteoma is a rare, benign tumor of the choroid composed of mature bone with overlying normal retina.[108] Typically, the lesion is unilateral and tends to be located in the juxtapapillary or peripapillary area, often with extension into the macula. The diagnosis is usually clinical and performed in young women within the first 3 decades of life. Choroidal osteoma appears as oval or round lesion with characteristic well-defined scalloped or geographic margins and yellow orange in color, particularly when the tumor is fully calcified and over time, as decalcification occurs, the tumor becomes more pale yellow with visible large choroidal or scleral vessels on the background.[114,115] Ocular ultrasonography shows a pathognomonic high

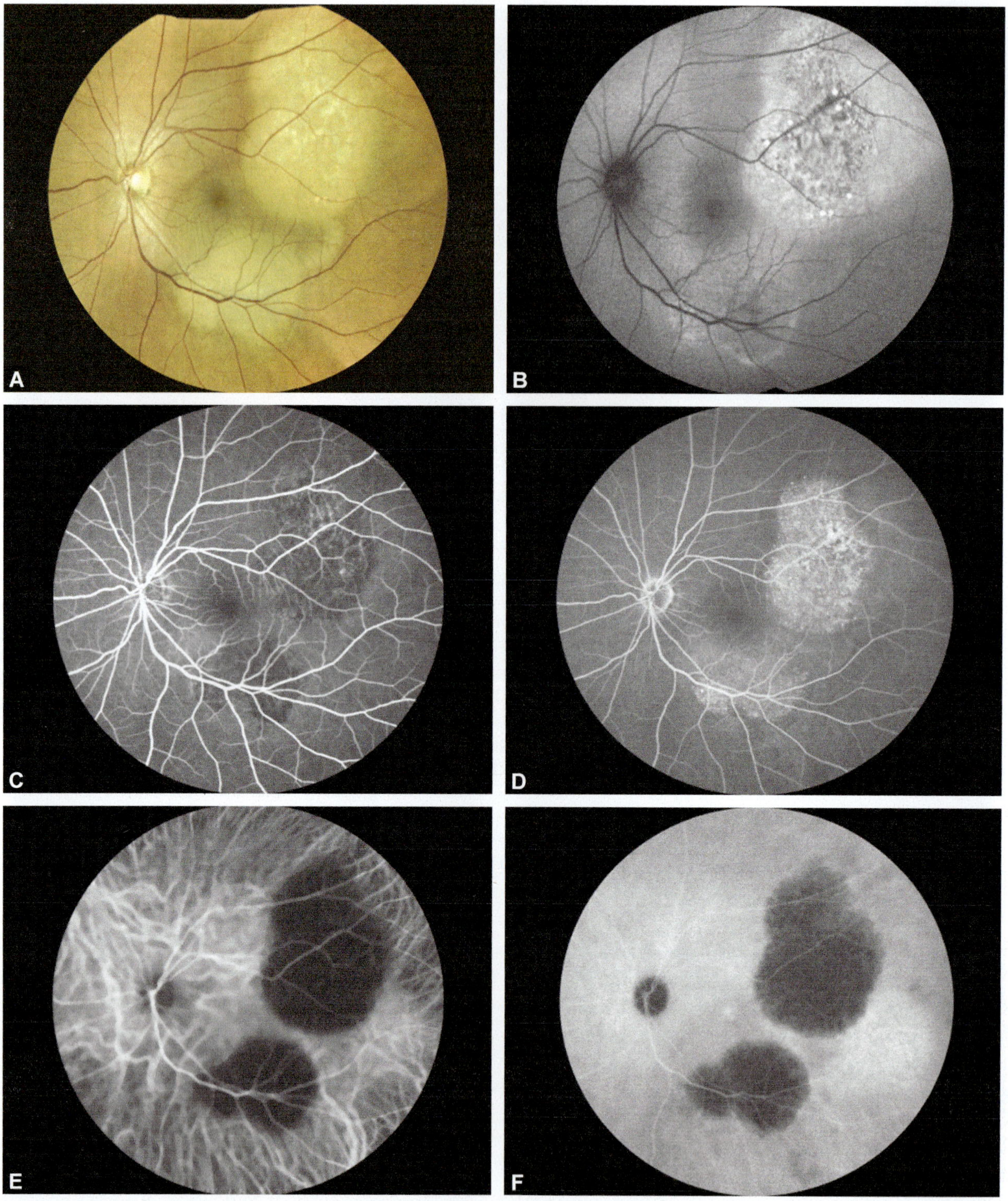

Figs. 45.45A to F: Multimodal imaging of choroidal metastases. Color photography (A) revealing two amelanotic lesions within the vascular arcades and exudative retinal detachment appearing as irregular hyperfluorescent and hypofluorescent areas on fundus autofluorescence (B). Fluorescein angiography displaying a blockage of the background fluorescence with mottled hyperfluorescence in the early phase (C) with irregular dots of hyperfluorescence in the late phase (D). Indocyanine green angiography showing well-defined areas of hypofluorescence in the early phase (E) and more prominent in the late phase (F).

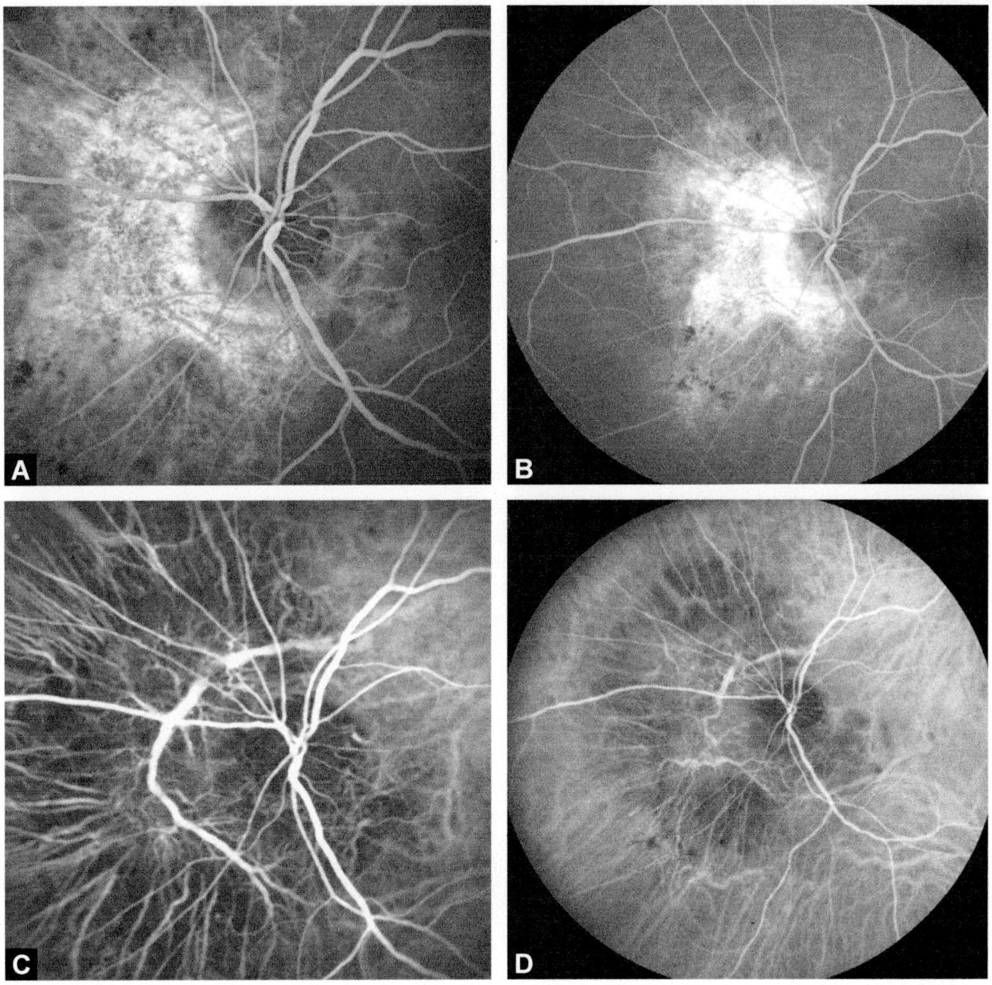

Figs. 45.46A to D: Fluorescein angiography and indocyanine green angiography of choroidal osteoma complicated by choroidal neovascularization. Fluorescein angiography showing an early peripapillary hyperfluorescent choroidal lesion (A) with staining in the late phase (B). Indocyanine green angiography (ICGA) revealing an hypofluorescent area in the early (C) and late phase (D), due to vascular rarefaction and blockage effect, complicated by intralesional neovascular network appreciable only on ICGA.

internal reflectivity persisting at lower sensitivity and decreasing in case of decalcification. Differentials include amelanotic lesions, and in particular, sclerochoroidal calcifications. EDI-OCT may be used to confirm the primary choroidal involvement and displaying a classical multilayer configuration with both spongy pattern and lamellae of compact bone within the mass. On FA, choroidal osteoma shows early patchy hyperfluorescent choroidal filling and diffuse staining in the late phase of the examination, whereas ICGA displays early hypofluorescence secondary to both blockage by the mass and vascular rarefaction, followed by fine diffuse multifocal fluorescence that becomes confluent.[108,116] Occasionally, small intralesional microcirculation may be observed. Despite these description, the diagnosis is typically conducted clinically and by means of ultrasound with both FA and ICGA mainly used to detect the presence of a secondary CNV (Figs. 45.46A to D).[115]

PERIPHERAL EXUDATIVE HEMORRHAGIC CHORIORETINOPATHY

Peripheral exudative hemorrhagic chorioretinopathy (PEHCR) is a relatively uncommon degenerative process of the peripheral retina.[117,118] This condition is characterized by blood in the subretinal or subretinal pigment epithelial space, and typically, spontaneously resolving leaving RPE atrophy, hyperplasia, and fibrosis. According to published series, PEHCR accounts for one of the most frequent

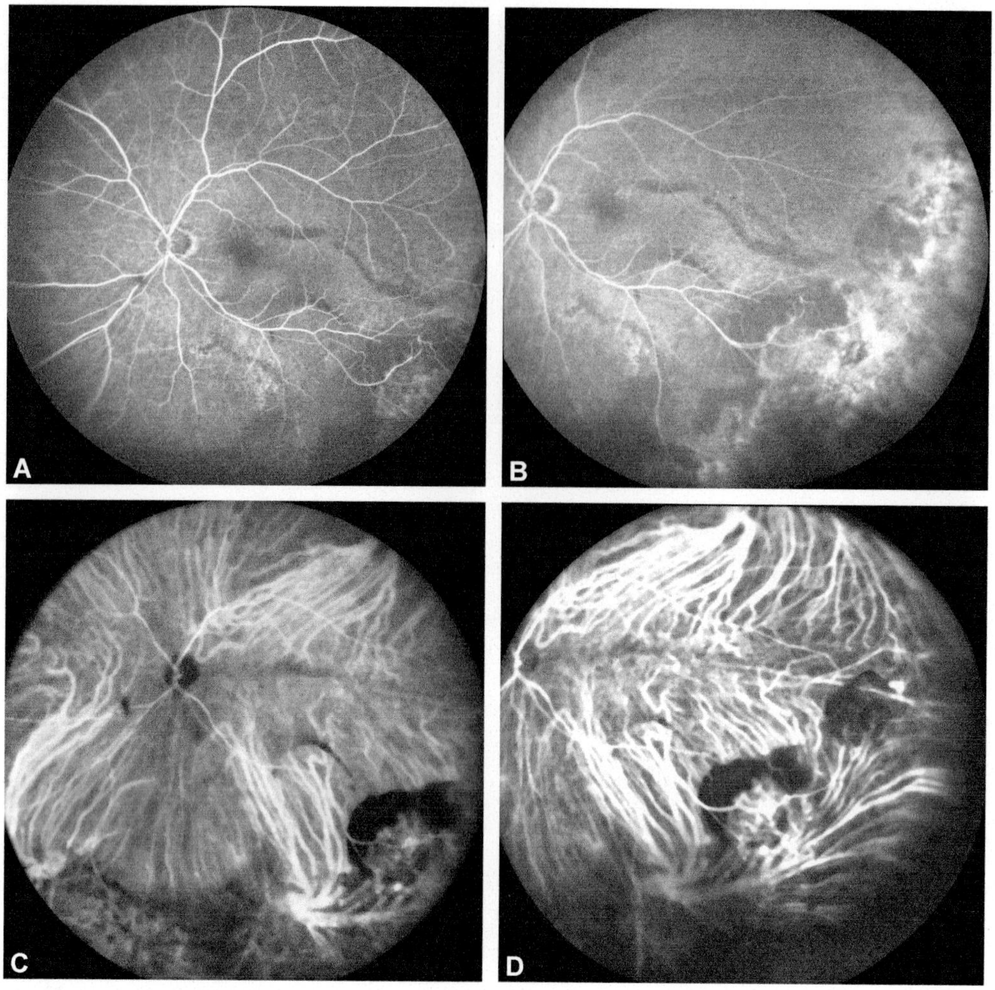

Figs. 45.47A to D: Fluorescein angiography and indocyanine green angiography of peripheral exudative hemorrhagic chorioretinopathy. Fluorescein angiography in the early (A) and late phase (B) showing periperal retinal pigment epithelium alteration with areas of mild blockage of choroidal fluorescence due to subretinal hemorrhage and pigment mottling and hyperfluorecence secondary to leakage occurring from the lesion and fibrosis staining. Indocyanine green angiography in the early (C) and late phase (D) revealing the peripheral choroidal neovascularization as hyperfluorescent dots and nearby vascular network adjacent to subretinal hemmorrhages.

clinical conditions simulating a choroidal melanoma (i.e. pseudomelanomas). In particular, PEHCR is defined by the presence of hemorrhagic and/or exudative lesions in the equatorial region in an older person in the setting of peripheral drusen.[119] Alterations are more frequently bilateral in a person affected by AMD. Any other cause of hemorrhage besides PEHCR and AMD is defined as hemorrhagic detachment of the retina or RPE.[119] Due to its clinical features, PEHCR is often misdiagnosed as an intraocular tumor, especially, as choroidal melanoma. In this contest, an early diagnosis is essential. Angiography examinations are helpful despite there are some technical limitations related to the peripheral location and to blockage of choroidal fluorescence secondary to subretinal or subretinal pigment epithelial hemorrhages, fibrosis, and RPE hyperplasia.[119,120] FA may display an irregular peripheral late hyperfluorescence, homogeneous late hyperfluorescence, or persistent hypofluorescence in case of predominant blood component. In contrast, ICGA may be useful for better displaying the choroidal neovascular processes at the edges of the blood, then FA showing fine or large networks or focal lobular hyperfluorescent lesions; hypofluorescence may be observed for large hemorrhagic components or RPE detachments (Figs. 45.47A to D).

MYOPIA

Choroidal neovascularization occurs in up to 10% of patients with high myopia.[121-124] It is usually located above the RPE (type 2 CNV)[65] and biomicroscopically, it appears

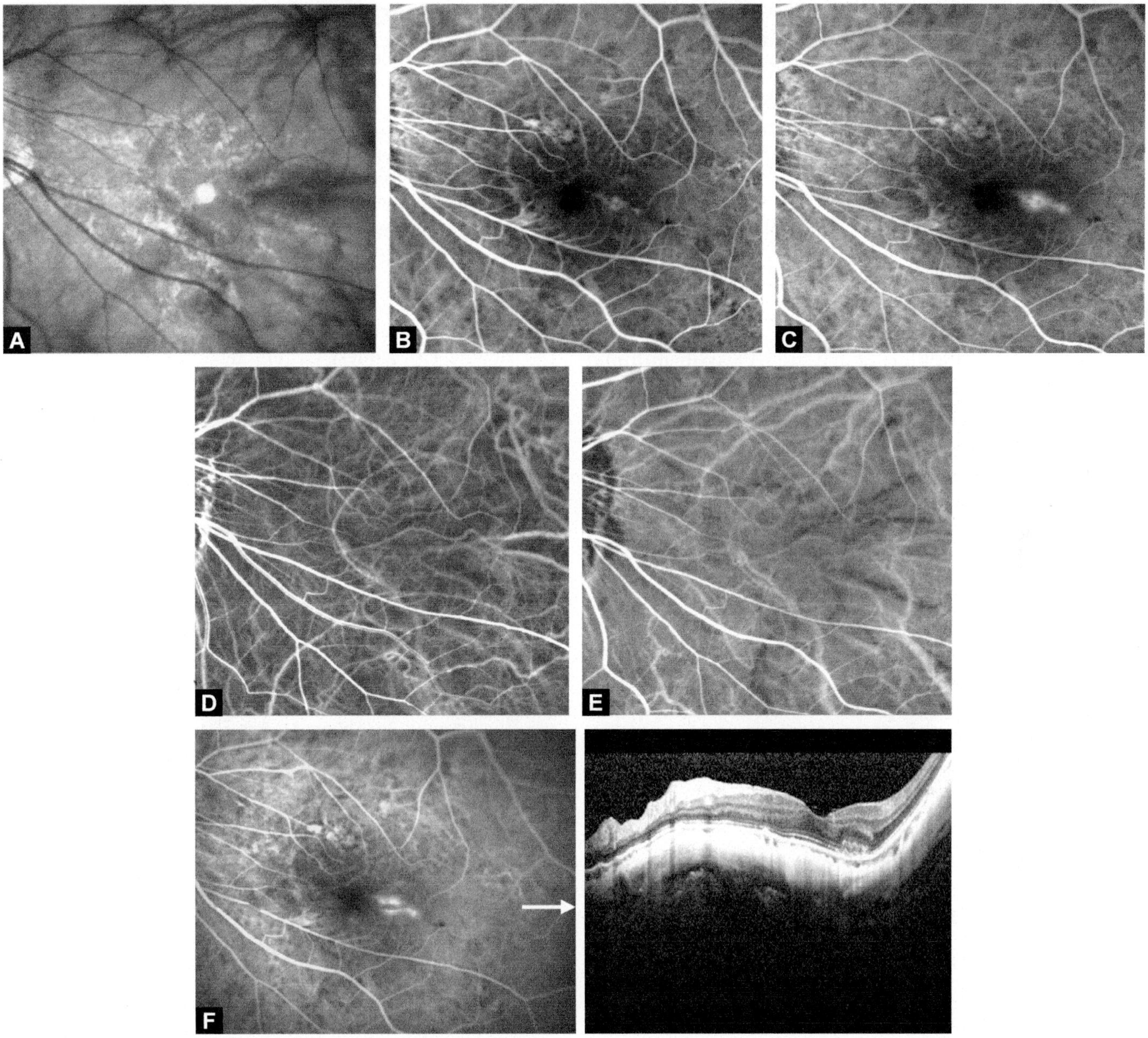

Figs. 45.48A to F: IR imaging (A) depicts hypopigmented posterior pole with radiating lacquer cracks. Hyperfluorescence is evident in the early phase of fluorescein angiography along one of the lacquer cracks (B); a mild leakage can be seen in the late angiograms (C). ICGA does not reveal the neovascular net either in the early (D) or the late (E) phases despite the clear appearance of lacquer cracks (E). The FA/SD-OCT scan (F) shows a corrugated appearance of the outer retina with elevation of the overlying inner retina in correspondence to the suspected lesion, confirming the presence of a small CNV.

as small, flat, and grayish membrane that may have a hyperpigmented border, if chronic or recurrent. However, at early stages, it is generally small and difficult to visualize with fundus biomicroscopy. FA and OCT are generally recommended baseline diagnostic tests in conjunction with color photographs and clinical examination. Being type 2 CNVs, FA may demonstrate its presence, type, and activity with well-demarcated areas of hyperfluorescence in the early phases and subtle leakage of fluorescein dye during the late phases. This late leakage is inferior to the one usually observed in CNV due to AMD. However, this indirect sign may be of great help in the detection of small neovascular nets because it might represent the only feature available for the early detection of active CNV (Figs. 45.48B and C). By contrast, ICGA may reveal the presence of well-structured vascular nets but it may fail to reveal a small, initial neovascularization (Figs. 45.48D and E). ICG angiography may be useful for two purposes: (1) It clearly defines lacquer cracks which are often associated with myopic CNVs (Fig. 45.48E),[125] and (2) Additionally, in case of significant hemorrhage, ICGA can identify the presence of lacquer cracks and/or CNV. It should be noted that OCT alone cannot differentiate myopic CNV from subretinal bleeding due to new lacquer crack formation. That could lead to unnecessary treatment by anti-VEGF therapy for subretinal bleeding without CNV. The advent of instruments that permit two examinations at the same time (FA/OCT, ICGA/OCT) has greatly facilitated the early diagnosis of myopic CNVs (Spectralis system, Heidelberg Engineering, Germany). On OCT, myopic CNV presents as a highly reflective area contiguous above the RPE with minimal subretinal fluid.[126] A B-scan targeted to the leaking area may further confirm the diagnosis (Fig. 45.48F). It has been reported that concordance between different examiners' interpretations of FA features and FA-guided SD-OCT was 70.4% and 94%, respectively.[127] Three main stages of myopic CNV, all of which associated with vision loss, have been described[126] and long-term natural history studies showed almost all patients lose significant vision.[128,129] After 10-year of follow-up of 25 patients with myopic CNV, visual acuity was less than 20/200 in 89% and 96% of patients in 5 and 10 years after onset of CNV, respectively.[129] Therefore, early diagnosis is extremely important, even more important nowadays with the advent of anti-VEGF drugs. Anti-VEGF therapy is recommended due to the superior efficacy of anti-VEGFs over other treatment modalities.[130,131] A prompt treatment with a single intravitreal injection allows promise of substantial visual acuity gain and quality of life.

STARGARDT DISEASE

The two most frequent causes of chorioretinal atrophy are AMD and Stargardt disease. Even if the two pathologies have completely different pathogenesis, it may be difficult to differentiate between them in the late stages. In absence of genetic testing FA and ICG can be useful because of typical signs that characterize Stargardt disease. Typical FA images show reduced background fluorescence, referred as "dark choroid" sign.[132] This may be explained with an increased concentration of lipofuscin in the RPE that blocks the fluorescence from the choroid. In mid and late phases of ICGA, atrophy consequent to Stargardt disease shows hypofluorescence, sign that was described as "dark atrophy". This may be caused by more severe damage of the choriocapillaris in Stargardt disease compared to atrophy secondary to AMD.[133]

REFERENCES

1. Flocks M, Miller J, Chao P. Retinal circulation time with the aid of fundus cinephotography. Am J Ophthalmol. 1959;48:3-10.
2. Bailey P, Swan KC. Cinematography of human retinal vessels: a practical clinical and research technique. J Am Med Assoc. 1959;170:1373-5.
3. Novotny HR, Alvis D. A method of photographing fluorescence in circulating blood of the human eye. Tech Doc Rep SAMTDR USAF Sch Aerosp Med. 1960;60-82:1-4.
4. Alexander A, Sherman J, Horn D. Fundus fluorescein angiography: a summary of theoretical concepts and clinical applications. J Am Optom Assoc. 1979;50:53-63.
5. Kohner EM, Dollery CT. Fluorescein angiography of the fundus in diabetic retinopathy. Br Med Bull. 1970;26:166-70.
6. Schatz H, George T, Liu JH, et al. Color fluorescein angiography: its clinical role. Trans Am Acad Ophthalmol Otolaryngol. 1973;77:254-9.
7. Witmer R. Fluorescent angiography of vascular diseases of the retina. Trans Aust Coll Ophthalmol. 1971;3:42-6.
8. Wolfe DR. Fluorescein angiography basic science and engineering. Ophthalmology. 1986;93:1617-20.
9. Morris PF. Fluorescein sodium and indocyanine green: uses and side effects. In: Saine PJ, Tyler ME (Eds). Ophthalmic Photography: Retinal Photography, Angiography and Electronic Imaging, 2nd edition. Boston: Butterworth-Heinemann; 2002.pp.137-65.
10. Schatz H, Burton TC, Yannuzi LA, et al. History of fluorescein angiography. In: Schatz H, Rabb MF (Eds). Interpretation of Fundus Fluorescein Angiography. Mosby: St Louis; 1978. pp.3-9.
11. Yannuzzi LA, Rohrer KT, Tindel LJ, et al. Fluorescein angiography complication survey. Ophthalmology. 1986;93:611-7.
12. Kwiterovich KA, Maguire MG, Murphy RP, et al. Frequency of adverse systemic reactions after fluorescein angiography. Results of a prospective study. Ophthalmology. 1991;98:1139-42.
13. Mattern J, Mayer PR. Excretion of fluorescein into breast milk. Am J Ophthalmol. 1990;109:598-9.
14. Salem H, Loux JJ, Smith S, et al. Evaluation of the toxicologic and teratogenic potentials of sodium fluorescein in the rat. Toxicology. 1979;12:143-50.
15. Jorzik JJ, Bindewald A, Dithmar S, et al. Digital simultaneous fluorescein and indocyanine green angiography, autofluorescence, and red-free imaging with a solid-state laser-based confocal scanning laser ophthalmoscope. Retina. 2005;25:405-16.
16. Bindewald A, Stuhrmann O, Roth F, et al. Lower limits of fluorescein and indocyanine green dye for digital cSLO fluorescence angiography. Br J Ophthalmol. 2005;89:1609-15.
17. Mainster MA, Timberlake GT, Webb RH, et al. Scanning laser ophthalmoscopy. Clinical applications. Ophthalmology. 1982;89:852-7.
18. Stanga PE, Lim JI, Hamilton P. Indocyanine green angiography in chorioretinal diseases: indications and

interpretation: an evidence-based update. Ophthalmology. 2003;110:15-21.

19. Yannuzzi LA, Flower RW, Slakter JS. Indocyanine Green Angiography. St Louis: Mosby Year Book; 1997.p.46.
20. Gass JD. Pathophysiologic and histopathologic bases for interpretation of fluorescein angiography. In: Gass JD (Ed). Stereoscopic Atlas of Macular Diseases: Diagnosis and Treatment, 3rd edition. St Louis: CV Mosby; 1987.pp.19-41.
21. Fox IJ, Brooker LG, Heseltine DW, et al. A tricarbocyanine dye for continuous recording of dilution curves in whole blood independent of variations in blood oxygen saturation. Proc Staff Meet Mayo Clin. 1957;32:478-84.
22. Fox IJ, Wood EH. Applications of dilution curves recorded from the right side of the heart or venous circulation with the aid of a new indicator dye. Proc Staff Meet Mayo Clin. 1957;32:541-50.
23. Hunton DB, Bollman JL, Hoffman HN. Studies of hepatic function with indocyanine green. Gastroenterology. 1960;39:713-24.
24. Flower RW, Hochheimer BF. Clinical infrared absorption angiography of the choroid. Am J Ophthalmol. 1972;73:458-9.
25. Patz A, Flower RW, Klein ML, et al. Clinical applications of indocyanine green angiography. Doc Ophthalmol Proc Series. 1976;9:245-51.
26. Hyvärinen L, Flower RW. Indocyanine green fluorescence angiography. Acta Ophthalmol (Copenh). 1980;58:528-38.
27. Hayashi K, de Laey JJ. Indocyanine green angiography of submacular choroidal vessels in the human eye. Ophthalmologica. 1985;190:20-9.
28. Scheider A, Schroedel C. High resolution indocyanine green angiography with a scanning laser ophthalmoscope. Am J Ophthalmol. 1989;108:458-9.
29. Yannuzzi LA, Slakter JS, Sorenson JA, et al. Digital indocyanine green videoangiography and choroidal neovascularization. Retina. 1992;12:191-223.
30. Ott P. Hepatic elimination of indocyanine green with special reference to distribution kinetics and the influence of plasma protein binding. Pharmacol Toxicol. 1998;83(Suppl 2):1-48.
31. Lutty GA. The acute intravenous toxicity of biological stains, dyes, and other fluorescent substances. Toxicol Appl Pharmacol. 1978;44:225-49.
32. Bischoff PM, Flower RW. Ten years experience with choroidal angiography using indocyanine green dye: a new routine examination or an epilogue? Doc Ophthalmol. 1985;60:235-91.
33. Flower RW, Hochheimer BF. Indocyanine green dye fluorescence and infrared absorption choroidal angiography performed simultaneously with fluorescein angiography. Johns Hopkins Med J. 1976;138:33-42.
34. Geeraets WJ, Berry ER. Ocular spectral characteristics as related to hazards from lasers and other light sources. Am J Ophthalmol. 1968;66:15-20.
35. Benya R, Quintana J, Brundage B. Adverse reactions to indocyanine green: a case report and a review of the literature. Cathet Cardiovasc Diagn. 1989;17:231-3.
36. Caesar J, Shaldon S, Chiandussi L, et al. The use of indocyanine green in the measurement of hepatic blood flow and as a test of hepatic function. Clin Sci. 1961;21:43-57.
37. Cherrick GR, Stein SW, Leevy CM, et al. Indocyanine green: observations on its physical properties, plasma decay, and hepatic extraction. J Clin Invest. 1960;39:592-600.
38. Leevy CM, Bender J. Physiology of dye extraction by the liver: comparative studies of sulfobromophthalein and indocyanine green. Ann NY Acad Sci. 1963;111:161-76.
39. Stehr A, Ploner F, Traeger K, et al. Plasma disappearance of indocyanine green: a marker for excretory liver function? Intensive Care Med. 2005;31:1719-22.
40. Costa DL, Huang SJ, Orlock DA, et al. Retinal-choroidal indocyanine green dye clearance and liver dysfunction. Retina. 2003;23:557-61.
41. Hope-Ross M, Yannuzzi LA, Gragoudas ES, et al. Adverse reactions due to indocyanine green. Ophthalmology. 199;101:529-33.
42. Iseki K, Onoyama K, Fujimi S, et al. Shock caused by indocyanine green dye in chronic hemodialysis patients. Clin Nephrol. 1980;14:210.
43. Robson SC, Mutch E, Boys RJ, et al. Apparent liver blood flow during pregnancy: a serial study using indocyanine green clearance. Br J Obstet Gynaecol. 1990;97:720-4.
44. Fineman MS, Maguire JI, Fineman SW, et al. Safety of indocyanine green angiography during pregnancy: a survey of the retina, macula, and vitreous societies. Arch Ophthalmol. 2001;119:353-5.
45. Cohen SY, Dubois L, Quentel G, et al. Is indocyanine green angiography still relevant? Retina. 2011;31:209-21.
46. Fundus photographic risk factors for progression of diabetic retinopathy. ETDRS report number 12. Early Treatment Diabetic Retinopathy Study Research Group. Ophthalmology. 1991;98:823-33.
47. The effect of intensive diabetes treatment on the progression of diabetic retinopathy in insulin-dependent diabetes mellitus. The Diabetes Control and Complications Trial. Arch Ophthalmol. 1995;113:36-51.
48. Haj Najeeb B, Simader C, Deak G, et al. The distribution of leakage on fluorescein angiography in diabetic macular edema: a new approach to its etiology. Invest Ophthalmol Vis Sci. 2017;58:3986-90.
49. Staurenghi G, Invernizzi A, de Polo L, et al. Macular edema. Diagnosis and detection. Dev Ophthalmol. 2010;47:27-48.
50. Adi MA, LeHoang P, Bodaghi B. Use of fluorescein angiography in the diagnosis and management of uveitis. Int Ophthalmol Clin. 2012;52:1-12.
51. Herbort CP, Mantovani A, Papadia M. Use of indocyanine green angiography in uveitis. Int Ophthalmol Clin. 2012;52:13-31.
52. Rothova A. Inflammatory cystoid macular edema. Curr Opin Ophthalmol. 2007;18:487-92.
53. Abu El-Asrar AM, Herbort CP, Tabbara KF. Retinal vasculitis. Ocul Immunol Inflamm. 2005;13:415-33.
54. Talat L, Lightman S, Tomkins-Netzer O. Ischemic retinal vasculitis and its management. J Ophthalmol. 2014;2014:197675.

55. Pichi F, Veronese C, Lembo A, et al. New appraisals of Kyrieleis plaques: a multimodal imaging study. Br J Ophthalmol. 2017;101:316-21.
56. Tugal-Tutkun I. Imaging in the diagnosis and management of Behcet disease. Int Ophthalmol Clin. 2012;52:183-90.
57. Atmaca LS, Simsek T, Sonmez PA, et al. Fluorescein and indocyanine green angiography in ocular toxoplasmosis. Graefes Arch Clin Exp Ophthalmol. 2006;244:1688-91.
58. Matsumoto Y, Haen SP, Spaide RF. The white dot syndromes. Compr Ophthalmol Update. 2007;8:179-200.
59. Knecht PB, Papadia M, Herbort CP. Secondary choriocapillaritis in infectious chorioretinitis. Acta Ophthalmol. 2013;91:550-5.
60. Herbort CP, Papadia M, Mantovani A. Classification of choroiditis based on inflammatory lesion process rather than fundus appearance: enhanced comprehension through the ICGA concepts of the iceberg and jellyfish effects. Klin Monbl Augenheilkd. 2012;229:306-13.
61. Kuo IC, Cunningham ET. Ocular neovascularization in patients with uveitis. Int Ophthalmol Clin. 2000;40:111-26.
62. Bouchenaki N, Cimino L, Auer C, et al. Assessment and classification of choroidal vasculitis in posterior uveitis using indocyanine green angiography. Klin Monbl Augenheilkd. 2002;219:243-9.
63. O'Toole L, Tufail A, Pavesio C. Management of choroidal neovascularization in uveitis. Int Ophthalmol Clin. 2005;45:157-77.
64. Yannuzzi LA. Indocyanine green angiography: a perspective on use in the clinical setting. Am J Ophthalmol. 2011;151:745-51.
65. Gass JD. Biomicroscopic and histopathologic considerations regarding the feasibility of surgical excision of subfoveal neovascular membranes. Am J Ophthalmol. 1994;118:285-98.
66. Subfoveal neovascular lesions in age-related macular degeneration. Guidelines for evaluation and treatment in the macular photocoagulation study. Macular Photocoagulation Study Group. Arch Ophthalmol. 1991;109:1242-57.
67. Sadda SR, Liakopoulos S, Keane PA, et al. Relationship between angiographic and optical coherence tomographic (OCT) parameters for quantifying choroidal neovascular lesions. Graefes Arch Clin Exp Ophthalmol. 2010;248:175-84.
68. Freund KB, Ho IV, Barbazetto IA, et al. Type 3 neovascularization: the expanded spectrum of retinal angiomatous proliferation. Retina. 2008;28:201-11.
69. Olsen TW, Feng X, Kasper TJ, et al. Fluorescein angiographic lesion type frequency in neovascular age-related macular degeneration. Ophthalmology. 2004;111:250-5.
70. Guyer DR, Yannuzzi LA, Slakter JS, et al. Classification of choroidal neovascularization by digital indocyanine green videoangiography. Ophthalmology. 1996;103:2054-60.
71. Yannuzzi LA, Hope-Ross M, Slakter JS, et al. Analysis of vascularized pigment epithelial detachments using indocyanine green videoangiography. Retina. 1994;14:99-113.
72. Brown DM, Kaiser PK, Michels M, et al. Ranibizumab versus verteporfin for neovascular age-related macular degeneration. N Engl J Med. 2006;355:1432-44.
73. Rosenfeld PJ, Brown DM, Heier JS, et al. Ranibizumab for neovascular age-related macular degeneration. N Engl J Med. 2006;355:1419-31.
74. Massacesi AL, Sacchi L, Bergamini F, et al. The prevalence of retinal angiomatous proliferation in age-related macular degeneration with occult choroidal neovascularization. Graefes Arch Clin Exp Ophthalmol. 2008;246:89-92.
75. Lim JI, Aaberg TM, Capone AJ, et al. Indocyanine green angiography-guided photocoagulation of choroidal neovascularization associated with retinal pigment epithelial detachment. Am J Ophthalmol. 1997;123:524-32.
76. Watzke RC, Klein ML, Hiner CJ, et al. A comparison of stereoscopic fluorescein angiography with indocyanine green videoangiography in age-related macular degeneration. Ophthalmology. 2000;107:1601-6.
77. Shiraga F, Ojima Y, Matsuo T, et al. Feeder vessel photocoagulation of subfoveal choroidal neovascularization secondary to age-related macular degeneration. Ophthalmology. 1998;105:662-9.
78. Staurenghi G, Orzalesi N, La Capria A, et al. Laser treatment of feeder vessels in subfoveal choroidal neovascular membranes: a revisitation using dynamic indocyanine green angiography. Ophthalmology. 1998;105:2297-305.
79. Viola F, Massacesi A, Orzalesi N, et al. Retinal angiomatous proliferation: natural history and progression of visual loss. Retina. 2009;29:732-9.
80. Flower RW. Optimizing treatment of choroidal neovascularization feeder vessels associated with age-related macular degeneration. Am J Ophthalmol. 2002;134:228-39.
81. Hlushchuk R, Baum O, Gruber G, et al. The synergistic action of a VEGF receptor tyrosine-kinase inhibitor and a sensitizing PDGF-receptor blocker depends upon the stage of vascular maturation. Microcirculation. 2007;14:813-25.
82. Yannuzzi LA, Negrao S, Iida T, et al. Retinal angiomatous proliferation in age-related macular degeneration. Retina. 2001;21:416-34.
83. Gass JD, Agarwal A, Lavina AM, et al. Focal inner retinal hemorrhages in patients with drusen: an early sign of occult choroidal neovascularization and chorioretinal anastomosis. Retina. 2003;23:741-51.
84. Hartnett ME, Weiter JJ, Staurenghi G, et al. Deep retinal vascular anomalous complexes in advanced age-related macular degeneration. Ophthalmology. 1996;103:2042-53.
85. Ravera V, Bottoni F, Giani A, et al. Retinal angiomatous proliferation diagnosis. A multiimaging approach. Retina. 2016;36:2274-81.
86. Kuhn D, Meunier I, Soubrane G, et al. Imaging of chorioretinal anastomoses in vascularized retinal pigment epithelium detachments. Arch Ophthalmol. 1995;113:1392-8.
87. Bottoni F, Romano M, Massacesi A, et al. Remodeling of the vascular channels in retinal angiomatous proliferations treated with intravitreal triamcinolone acetonide and photodynamic therapy. Graefes Arch Clin Exp Ophthalmol. 2006;244:1528-33.
88. Yannuzzi LA, Sorenson J, Spaide RF, et al. Idiopathic polypoidal choroidal vasculopathy (IPCV). Retina. 1990;10:1-8.
89. Jung JJ, Chen CY, Mrejen S, et al. The incidence of neovascular subtypes in newly diagnosed neovascular

age-related macular degeneration. Am J Ophthalmol. 2014;158:769-79.e2.

90. Balaratnasingam C, Lee WK, Koizumi H, et al. Polypoidal choroidal vasculopathy: a distinct disease or manifestation of many? Retina (Philadelphia, Pa). 2016;36:1-8.
91. Gallego-Pinazo R, Dolz-Marco R, Gómez-Ulla F, et al. Pachychoroid diseases of the macula. Med Hypothesis Discov Innov Ophthalmol. 2014;3:111-5.
92. Pang CE, Freund KB. Pachychoroid neovasculopathy. Retina (Philadelphia, Pa). 2015;35:1-9.
93. Warrow DJ, Hoang QV, Freund KB. Pachychoroid pigment epitheliopathy. Retina (Philadelphia, Pa). 2013;33:1659-72.
94. Shiraga F, Matsuo T, Yokoe S, et al. Surgical treatment of submacular hemorrhage associated with idiopathic polypoidal choroidal vasculopathy. Am J Ophthalmol. 1999;128:147-54.
95. Koh A, Lee WK, Chen LJ, et al. EVEREST study: efficacy and safety of verteporfin photodynamic therapy in combination with ranibizumab or alone versus ranibizumab monotherapy in patients with symptomatic macular polypoidal choroidal vasculopathy. Retina (Philadelphia, Pa). 2012;32:1453-64.
96. Tittl MK, Spaide RF, Wong D, et al. Systemic findings associated with central serous chorioretinopathy. Am J Ophthalmol. 1999;128:63-8.
97. Quin G, Liew G, Ho IV, et al. Diagnosis and interventions for central serous chorioretinopathy: review and update. Clin Exp Ophthalmol. 2013;41:187-200.
98. Yamada K, Hayasaka S, Setogawa T. Fluorescein-angiographic patterns in patients with central serous chorioretinopathy at the initial visit. Ophthalmologica. 1992;205:69-76.
99. Guyer DR, Yannuzzi LA, Slakter JS, et al. Digital indocyanine green videoangiography of central serous chorioretinopathy. Arch Ophthalmol. 1994;112:1057-62.
100. Spaide RF, Hall L, Haas A, et al. Indocyanine green videoangiography of older patients with central serous chorioretinopathy. Retina (Philadelphia, Pa). 1996;16:203-13.
101. Daruich A, Matet A, Dirani A, et al. Central serous chorioretinopathy: Recent findings and new physiopathology hypothesis. Prog Retin Eye Res. 2015;48:82-118.
102. Yannuzzi LA, Shakin JL, Fisher YL, et al. Peripheral retinal detachments and retinal pigment epithelial atrophic tracts secondary to central serous pigment epitheliopathy. Ophthalmology. 1984;91:1554-72.
103. Witschel H, Font RL. Hemangioma of the choroid. A clinicopathologic study of 71 cases and a review of the literature. Surv Ophthalmol. 1976;20:415-31.
104. Shields CL, Honavar SG, Shields JA, et al. Circumscribed choroidal hemangioma: clinical manifestations and factors predictive of visual outcome in 200 consecutive cases. Ophthalmology. 2001;108:2237-48.
105. Norton EW, Gutman F. Fluorescein angiography and hemangiomas of the choroid. Arch Ophthalmol. 1967;78:121-5.
106. Shields CL, Shields JA, De Potter P. Patterns of indocyanine green videoangiography of choroidal tumors. Br J Ophthalmol. 1995;79:237-45.
107. Schalenbourg A, Piguet B, Zografos L. Indocyanine green angiographic findings in choroidal hemangiomas: a study of 75 cases. Ophthalmologica. 2000;214:246-52.
108. Shields JA, Shields CL. Intraocular Tumors. Lippincott: Williams & Wilkins; 2008.
109. Shields CL, Kaliki S, Furuta M, et al. Clinical spectrum and prognosis of uveal melanoma based on age at presentation in 8,033 cases. Retina (Philadelphia, Pa). 2012;32:1363-72.
110. Shields CL, Furuta M, Thangappan A, et al. Metastasis of uveal melanoma millimeter-by-millimeter in 8033 consecutive eyes. Arch Ophthalmol. 2009;127:989-98.
111. Mueller AJ, Freeman WR, Folberg R, et al. Evaluation of microvascularization pattern visibility in human choroidal melanomas: comparison of confocal fluorescein with indocyanine green angiography. Graefes Arch Clin Exp Ophthalmol. 1999;237:448-56.
112. Folberg R, Péer J, Gruman LM, et al. The morphologic characteristics of tumor blood vessels as a marker of tumor progression in primary human uveal melanoma: a matched case-control study. Hum Pathol. 1992;23:1298-305.
113. Shields CL, Shields JA, Gross NE, et al. Survey of 520 eyes with uveal metastases. Ophthalmology. 1997;104:1265-76.
114. Aylward GW, Chang TS, Pautler SE, et al. A long-term follow-up of choroidal osteoma. Arch Ophthalmol. 1998;116:1337-41.
115. Shields CL, Sun H, Demirci H, et al. Factors predictive of tumor growth, tumor decalcification, choroidal neovascularization, and visual outcome in 74 eyes with choroidal osteoma. Arch Ophthalmol. 2005;123:1658-66.
116. Lafaut BA, Mestdagh C, Kohno T, et al. Indocyanine green angiography in choroidal osteoma. Graefes Arch Clin Exp Ophthalmol. 1997;235:330-7.
117. Annesley WH. Peripheral exudative hemorrhagic chorio-retinopathy. Trans Am Ophthalmol Soc. 1980;78:321-64.
118. Shields CL, Salazar PF, Mashayekhi A, et al. Peripheral exudative hemorrhagic chorioretinopathy simulating choroidal melanoma in 173 eyes. Ophthalmology. 2009;116:529-35.
119. Shields JA, Mashayekhi A, Ra S, et al. Pseudomelanomas of the posterior uveal tract: the 2006 Taylor R Smith Lecture. Retina (Philadelphia, Pa). 2005;25:767-71.
120. Gonzales JA, Kapoor KG, Gibran SK. Peripheral exudative hemorrhagic chorioretinopathy: a clinical, angiographic, and histologic study. Am J Ophthalmol. 2010;149:1013-4.
121. Hotchkiss ML, Fine SL. Pathologic myopia and choroidal neovascularization. Am J Ophthalmol. 1981;91:177-83.
122. Sperduto RD, Seigel D, Roberts J, et al. Prevalence of myopia in the United States. Arch Ophthalmol. 1983;101:405-7.
123. Grossniklaus HE, Green WR. Pathologic findings in pathologic myopia. Retina (Philadelphia, Pa). 1992;12:127-33.
124. Ohno-Matsui K, Yoshida T, Futagami S, et al. Patchy atrophy and lacquer cracks predispose to the development of choroidal neovascularisation in pathological myopia. Br J Ophthalmol. 2003;87:570-3.
125. Axer-Siegel R, Cotlear D, Priel E, et al. Indocyanine green angiography in high myopia. Ophthalmic Surg Lasers Imaging. 2004;35:139-45.

126. Neelam K, Cheung CM, Ohno-Matsui K, et al. Choroidal neovascularization in pathological myopia. Prog Retin Eye Res. 2012;31:495-525.
127. Milani P, Massacesi A, Setaccioli M, et al. Sensitivity of fluorescein angiography alone or with SD-OCT for the diagnosis of myopic choroidal neovascularization. Graefes Arch Clin Exp Ophthalmol. 2013;251:1891-900.
128. Hampton GR, Kohen D, Bird AC. Visual prognosis of disciform degeneration in myopia. Ophthalmology. 1983;90:923-6.
129. Yoshida T, Ohno-Matsui K, Yasuzumi K, et al. Myopic choroidal neovascularization: a 10-year follow-up. Ophthalmology. 2003;110:1297-305.
130. Wolf S, Balciuniene VJ, Laganovska G, et al. RADIANCE: a randomized controlled study of ranibizumab in patients with choroidal neovascularization secondary to pathologic myopia. Ophthalmology. 2014;121:682-92.e2.
131. Wong TY, Ohno-Matsui K, Leveziel N, et al. Myopic choroidal neovascularisation: current concepts and update on clinical management. Br J Ophthalmol. 2015;99:289-96.
132. Giani A, Pellegrini M, Carini E, et al. The dark atrophy with indocyanine green angiography in Stargardt disease. Invest Ophthalmol Vis Sci. 2012;53:3999-4004.
133. Pellegrini M, Acquistapace A, Oldani M, et al. Dark atrophy: an optical coherence tomography angiography study. Ophthalmology. 2016;123:1879-86.

Chapter 46

Optical Coherence Tomography

A Yasin Alibhai, Eric M Moult, James G Fujimoto, Nadia K Waheed

INTRODUCTION

Over the last decade, optical coherence tomography (OCT) has revolutionized both our understanding of and our treatment paradigms for retinal disease and glaucoma. This chapter will discuss the basics of OCT, its use in retinal disease, and newer advances in the technology.

PRINCIPLES OF OPTICAL COHERENCE TOMOGRAPHY

Optical Coherence Tomography as Low-Coherence Interferometry

Optical coherence tomography generates high-resolution cross-sectional and volumetric images of ocular structures by measuring the magnitude and delay of backscattered light. Because the speed of light is extremely high, these delays cannot be measured directly by electronics; instead OCT uses a technique known as interferometry. Early OCT instruments were based on low-coherence interferometry.[1] Here, "low-coherence" means that OCT uses light consisting of a range of wavelengths rather than a single wavelength; "interferometry" means that OCT obtains measurements by interfering light. While a detailed discussion of the physics underlying low-coherence interferometry is beyond the scope of this text, the general physical concepts are relatively simple. As illustrated in Figure 46.1, an OCT system consists of a light source, an interferometer and scanning optics, a sample arm with a patient interface which scans the OCT beam on the eye, a reference arm, and a detection system. Light emitted from the light source is split between the reference arm and the sample arm. In the reference arm, a mirror reflects light back toward the interferometer; in the sample arm, structures in the eye scatter light back toward the interferometer. The reflected and backscattered light are then interfered, or superposed in the interferometer. This superposition of light is analogous to the superposition that occurs when other types of waves—for example, sound or water waves—are superposed. The output of the interferometer goes to a detection system, which converts the light into electronic signals that can be processed and displayed by a computer. The key idea of OCT is that the interference patterns recorded at the detection system can be used to measure the axial position of the tissue structures (i.e. the layers of the retina) that backscatter the light, relative to that of the reference arm.

Principles of Fourier-Domain OCT

The first OCT systems used time-domain OCT (TD-OCT), in which the reference arm is mechanically scanned and backscattered light with different delays is measured sequentially.[1-4] Current instruments use Fourier-domain (FD) detection methods, which simultaneously measure all of the light from different delays, achieving higher sensitivity and therefore enabling faster A-scan rates.[5-11] FD-OCT works by measuring the interfered light in the so-called "Fourier domain," and then uses a mathematical operation, called the Fourier transformation, to convert these measurements into physical delays or distances. While the details of Fourier detection require sophisticated mathematics, the principle is relatively simple, and the distance-frequency encoding is somewhat analogous to magnetic resonance imaging (MRI). As shown in Figures 46.2A to C, in FD-OCT a single scattering layer at a depth d_1 (Fig. 46.2A.1) creates a sinusoidal interference pattern at the detection system (Fig. 46.2A.2). The key point is that the *frequency* of the sinusoid is proportional to the *depth* of the layer, and that the *amplitude* of the sinusoid is proportional to *how strongly the layer backscatters* light. So, if there is a deeper layer, d_2, that is less backscattering (Fig. 46.2B.1) the measured interferometer signal would have a higher frequency and a smaller amplitude (Fig. 46.2B.2). If both of these layers are present (Fig. 46.2C.1), the measured signal is not a pure sinusoid, but rather the superposition of the two previously discussed sinusoids (Fig. 46.2C.2). The Fourier transformation maps these

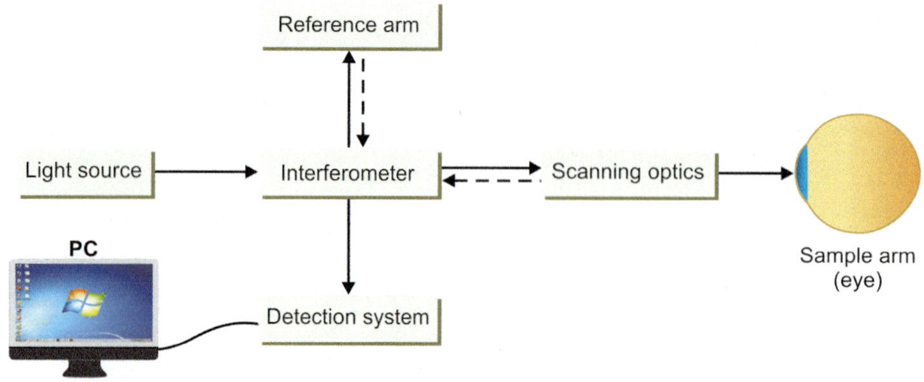

Fig. 46.1: Basic optical coherence tomography configuration. Light from the source is split between a reference arm and a sample arm. The light in the reference arm is reflected (dashed line) from a reference mirror; the light from the sample arm is relayed to the eye using scanning optics where it is then backscattered (dashed line). This reflected and backscattered light is then interfered at an optical interferometer, and is subsequently converted into electrical signals by a detection system. Finally, these electrical signals are sent to a computer (PC) for processing and display.

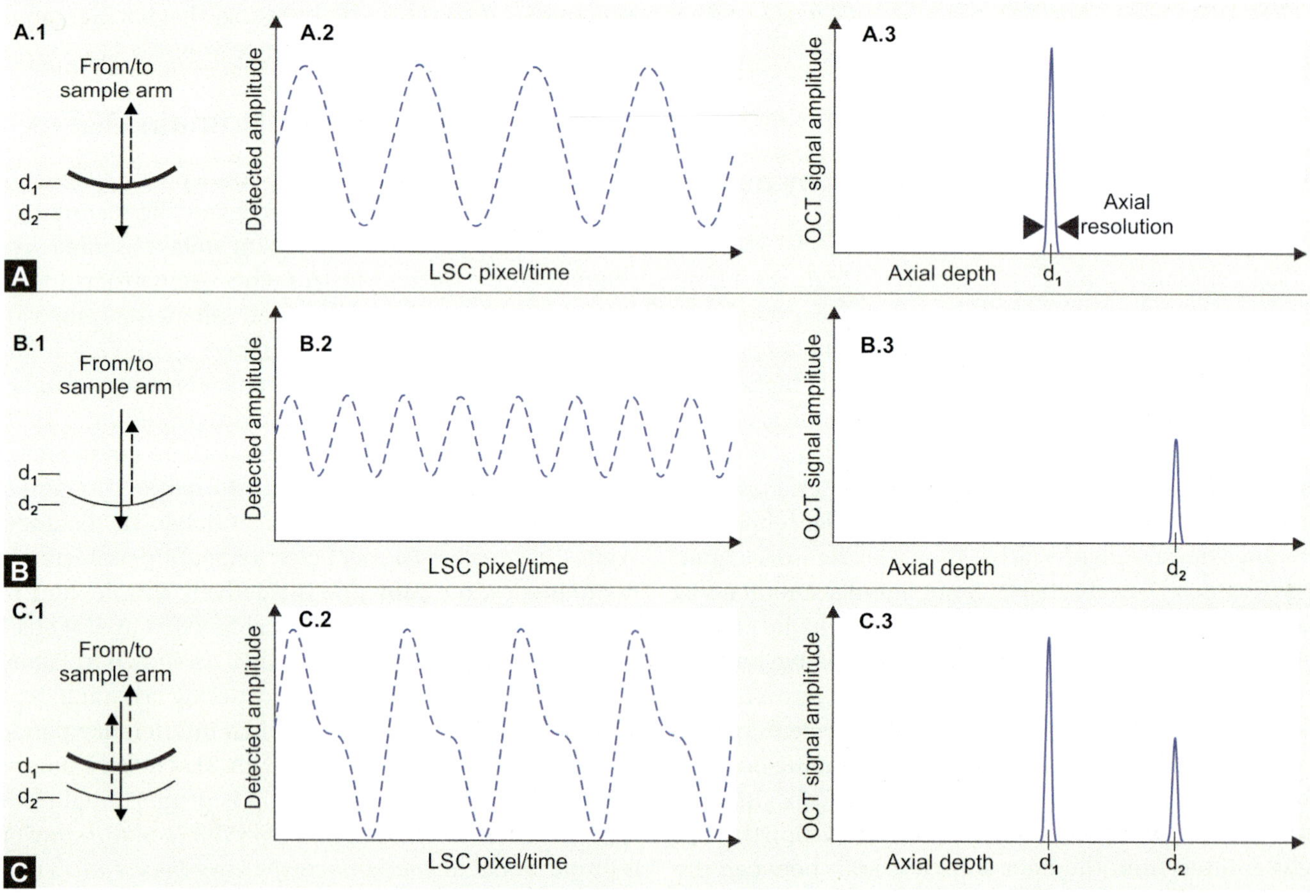

Figs. 46.2A to C: Principles of Fourier-domain OCT (FD-OCT). (A) A single layer positioned at a depth of d_1; (B) a single layer positioned at a depth of $d_2 > d_1$; (C) the two layers are combined. In this example, we assume that the layer at d_1 is more strongly backscattering (indicated by a thicker line) than that at d_2. The first column depicts the depth distribution of the layers, where solid arrows indicate light from the OCT system incident on the eye, and dashed arrows indicate backscattered light. The second column shows the interferometric pattern that would be measured at the detector. The x-coordinate is the pixel index in the case of spectral-domain OCT (SD-OCT; LSC = line scan camera), and time in the case of swept-source OCT (SS-OCT). These two configurations are discussed in section "Spectral-domain OCT versus Swept-source-OCT, and are depicted in Figures 46.3A to D. The third column shows the OCT A-scan resulting from taking the Fourier transformation of the interferometric signals of the second column. The essential feature of FD-OCT is that backscattering layers in the sample arm generate sinusoidal interferometric signals at the detection system; the frequencies of these interferometric signals are proportional to the axial depth of the layer, and their amplitudes are proportional to how strongly the layer backscatters incident light. Note that the width of the OCT peak on an A-scan caused by a single, thin layer corresponds to the axial resolution of the OCT system.

different sinusoids into a physical depth dimension, where the axial distance is proportional to the frequency of the interference fringe and the amplitude is proportional to the amplitude of the interference fringe of that frequency (Figs. 46.2A.3, 46.2B.3, and 46.2C.3). Although not derived here, the axial resolution of OCT is proportional to the square of the central wavelength (shorter wavelengths correspond to better axial resolutions) and inversely proportional to the range of wavelengths output by the source (larger wavelength ranges correspond to better axial resolutions).

Spectral-domain OCT versus Swept-source-OCT

There are two commonly used implementations of FD-OCT: (1) spectral-domain OCT (SD-OCT)[5-8] and swept-source OCT (SS-OCT).[9-11] Like all OCT systems, these two implementations use configurations similar to Figure 46.1. Furthermore, the conceptual operation and data processing for SD-OCT and SS-OCT are very similar; however, the light sources and detection systems are quite different. SD-OCT uses a continuous light source that emits a broad range of wavelengths (Fig. 46.3A). In contrast, SS-OCT uses a swept light source that emits, at any instant in time, a "single" wavelength, which sweeps across a broad range of wavelengths as a function of time (Fig. 46.3B). In SD-OCT, the detection works by separating the interfered light into its different wavelength components using a spectrometer and a line scan camera, a one-dimensional array of detectors which is digitally read at high speed (Fig. 46.3C). In contrast, in SS-OCT the interference spectrum is detected by a single photodetector whose output is digitized as the wavelength is swept (Fig. 46.3D). In SD-OCT, the A-scan rate is set by the exposure and read-time of the line scan camera (how long it takes to digitally read the camera's pixel values), whereas in SS-OCT, the A-scan rate is set by rate at which the light source is swept (Fig. 46.3B).

From this discussion, we can understand that the essential difference between SD-OCT and SS-OCT is that SD-OCT detects the interference *spatially* using a spectrometer, while SS-OCT detects the interference *temporally* using a swept laser. In both configurations, information about the magnitude and delay of the backscattered light is computed by Fourier transforming the interference spectrum.

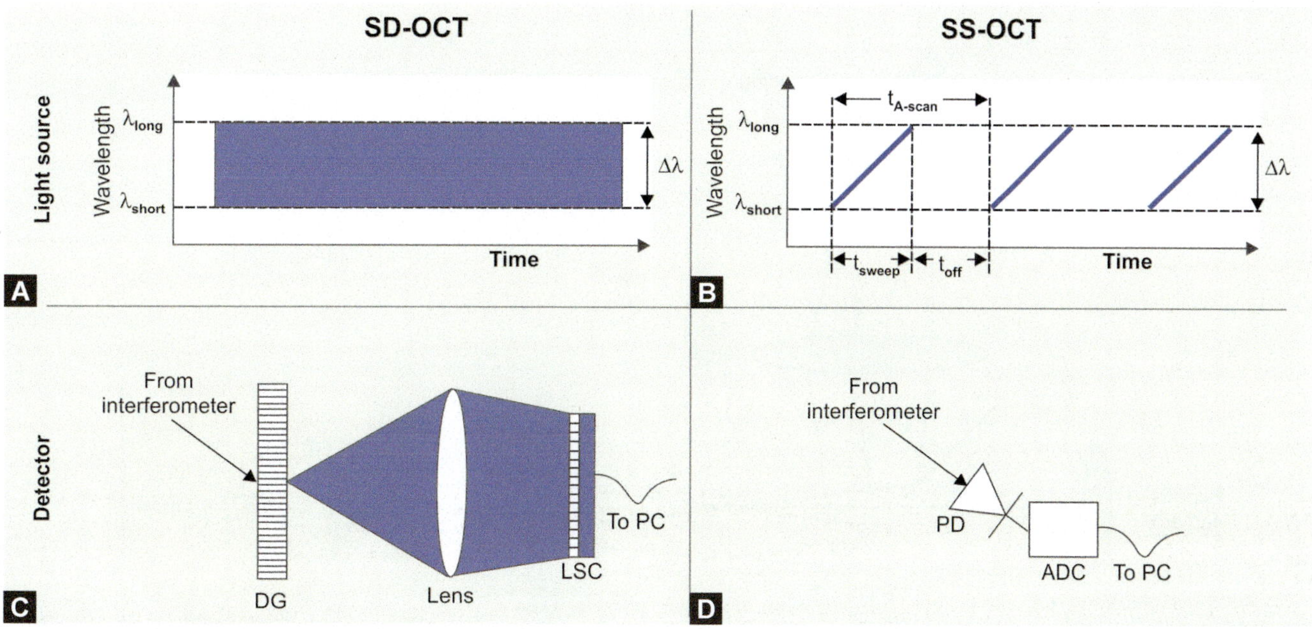

Figs. 46.3A to D: Comparison of the light sources and detectors used in spectral-domain OCT (SD-OCT) and swept-source OCT (SS-OCT). (A) SD-OCT uses a broadband light source that continuously emits light over a broad range of wavelengths; (B) SS-OCT uses a swept laser source which emits, at any instance in time, a narrow range of wavelengths. However, because the wavelength is varied as a function of time, over the period that the light source is swept, t_{sweep}, the light source emits light of a broad range of wavelengths. Depending on the light source used, there is a time, t_{off}, between the end of one sweep and the beginning of the next sweep. The sum of t_{sweep} and t_{off} determines the A-scan time, $t_{A\text{-}scan}$; (C) The detector in the SD-OCT consists of a diffraction grating (DG), which separates the interfered light according to its wavelength. This separated light is then focused by a lens onto an array of camera pixels called a line scan camera (LSC); each pixel in the camera collects light from a small range of wavelengths; (D) In SS-OCT interfered light is converted into an analog electrical signal by a photodetector (PD), and then changed into a digital electrical signal by an analog-to-digital converter (ADC), before being sent to a computer (PC).

A-scans, B-scans, and Volumetric OCT

The previous sections describe how OCT creates depth resolved measurements of the backscattering properties of the eye—these measurements, called "A-scans" are the fundamental unit in OCT. The extension of OCT from 1-D (A-scans), to 2-D (collections of A-scans called "B-scans") to 3-D (collections of B-scans) is achieved by scanning the transverse position of the light beam. Typical ophthalmic OCT systems use two perpendicularly oriented, galvanometer actuated mirrors which scan the beam angle into an optical system that pivots the beam about the pupil and scans the transverse position on the retina (Fig. 46.4). Volumetric OCT data is acquired using a raster scan pattern where the beam is scanned quickly in one transverse direction to acquire a B-scan consisting of many A-scans (this scan axis is commonly called the "fast scan axis"), and the beam is scanned slowly in the perpendicular direction, moving the position of the B-scan (this scan axis is commonly called the "slow scan axis"). The set of B-scans acquires volumetric data over a region of the eye and can be resliced along *en face* planes in postprocessing, rendered volumetrically, or viewed in an orthoplane manner, similar to radiological imaging.

PRINCIPLES OF OPTICAL COHERENCE TOMOGRAPHY ANGIOGRAPHY

How Optical Coherence Tomography Angiography Generates Contrast?

In OCT, the contrast between different ocular structures results from differences in backscattering properties. While larger retinal vessels may be visible in standard OCT images, much of the microvasculature is not well differentiated from surrounding tissues, making it invisible. To visualize the microvasculature, OCT angiography (OCTA) uses a different source of contrast: motion contrast.[12-19] The basic idea of OCTA is to acquire an OCT measurement of a region of tissue and then, a short time later, acquire another OCT measurement of that same region. If the region of tissue contains only static structures (flowing blood cells are *not* present), then the two OCT measurements will be identical. However, if the tissue contains moving elements (flowing blood cells *are* present), the two OCT measurements will be different and these differences can be computationally visualized. In this way, OCTA generates contrast between vasculature and surrounding static tissues.

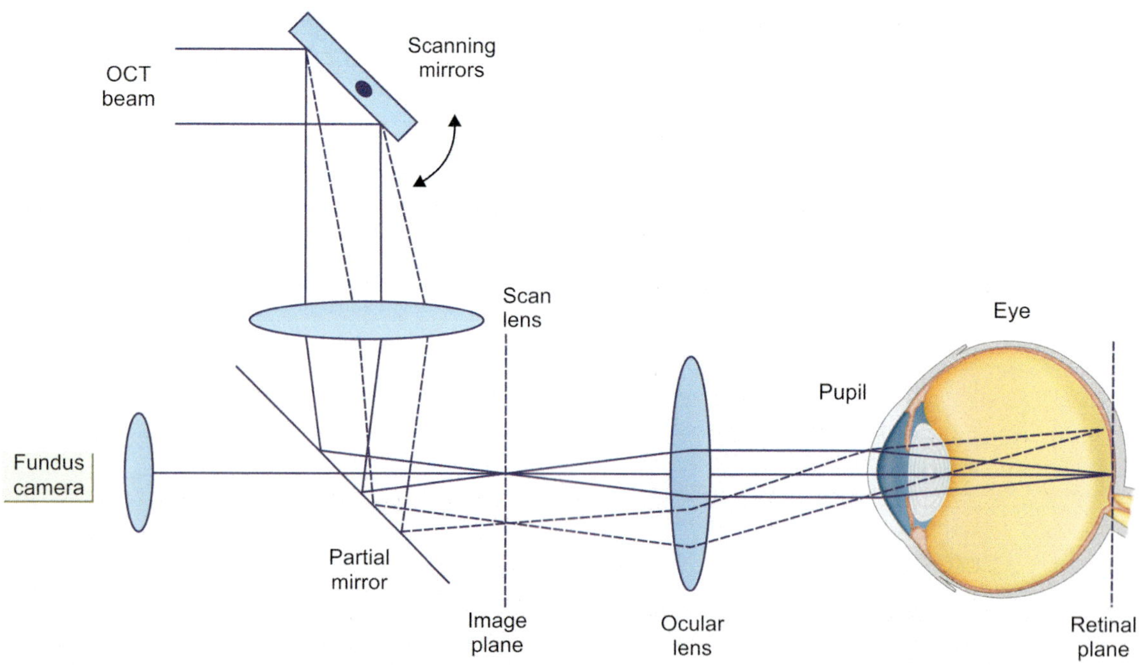

Fig. 46.4: Representative sample arm optics. The OCT beam is reflected by scanning mirrors and then imaged onto the back of the eye. The optics are such that the pivot point of the scanning mirrors is relayed onto the pupil of the eye, which causes changes in mirror rotation to correspond to changes in the angle with which the OCT beam is incident on the pupil. The focusing of the incident OCT beam by the eye transforms angular changes of the incident OCT beam into translations of the focused OCT beam on the retinal plane. Thus, taken together, as the scanning mirrors are rotated, the focused OCT spot is swept across the retinal plane. Using a partially transparent mirror, a fundus camera can also be integrated into the system for alignment.

Factors Affecting the OCTA Signal: Blood Cell Speed and Interscan Time

The two primary determinants of the OCTA signal are: (1) the speed of the blood cells being measured and (2) the time between repeated OCT measurements, the "interscan time." The difference between repeated OCT measurements results from displacement of blood cell(s) in the time between measurements. To a first order approximation, the displacement, $\mathbf{\Delta r}$, of a blood cell is given by the product of the blood cell's speed, *s*, and the interscan time, $\mathbf{\Delta t}$; that is, $\mathbf{\Delta r = s \times \Delta t}$. Changes in either *s* or $\mathbf{\Delta t}$ result in changes in the blood cell's displacement, and thus, in the OCTA signal.[20-23] This dependency is schematically depicted in Figures 46.5 and 46.6.

Implementing OCTA via Repeated B-scans

In principle, it is possible to obtain repeated OCT measurements by acquiring either repeated A-scans, repeated B-scans, or repeated OCT volumes, one after the other. The repeated B-scan acquisition protocol is the most amenable to imaging the eye's microvasculature and is used in all commercial OCTA systems. A sample OCTA scanning protocol is shown in Figures 46.7A to D. The amount of data

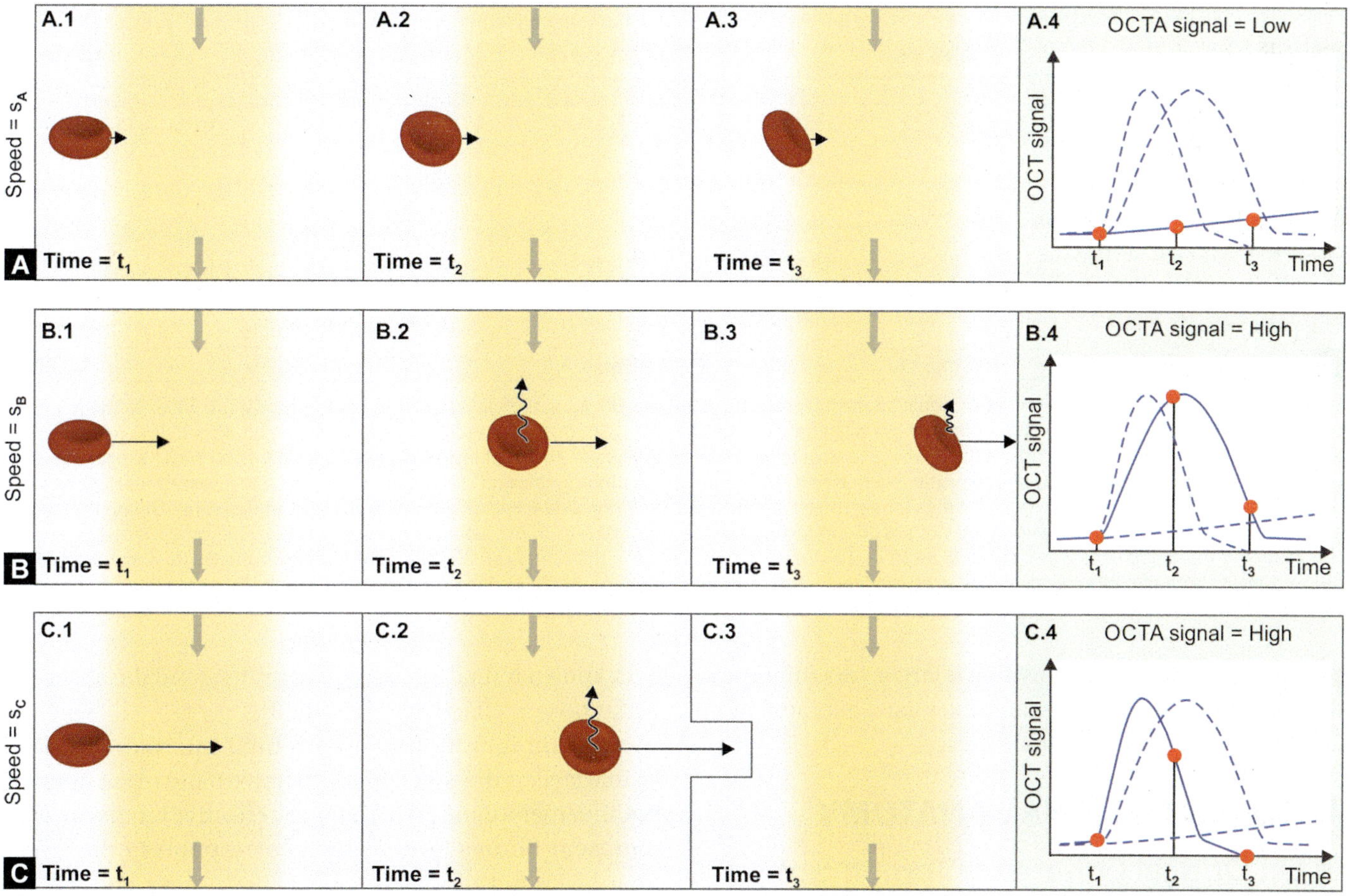

Figs. 46.5A to C: Dependency of the OCTA signal on blood flow speed. Each row corresponds to a different blood cell speed, where $s_A < s_B < s_C$. Columns 1, 2 and 3 correspond to three equally space time points, t_1, t_2, and t_3, respectively. The thick gray arrows point in the direction of the incident OCT beam (yellow). The straight, horizontal black arrows indicate the blood cell velocity, where the length of the arrow is proportional to its speed. The squiggly black arrows indicate the light backscattered from the blood cells, where the length of the arrow indicates the amount of backscattered light; cells without squiggly arrows have generated minimal backscattered light. Column 4 shows the corresponding OCT signal as a function of time (solid curve); the dashed curves show, for reference, the OCT signals corresponding to the other two rows. The circles on the plot indicate the times at which the OCT signal is measured. (A) A slowly moving blood cell displaces minimally between the three measurements, causing only a small variation in OCT signal (A.4). Because the time-variation is small, the OCTA signal will be low; (B) A faster moving blood cell passes through the beam, causing significant variation in OCT signal (B.4). This results in a high OCTA signal; (C) A blood cell moving faster still also causes significant variation in OCT signal (C.4). As in (B), the OCTA signal will be high. In general, it is not possible to distinguish the case of s_B from s_C.

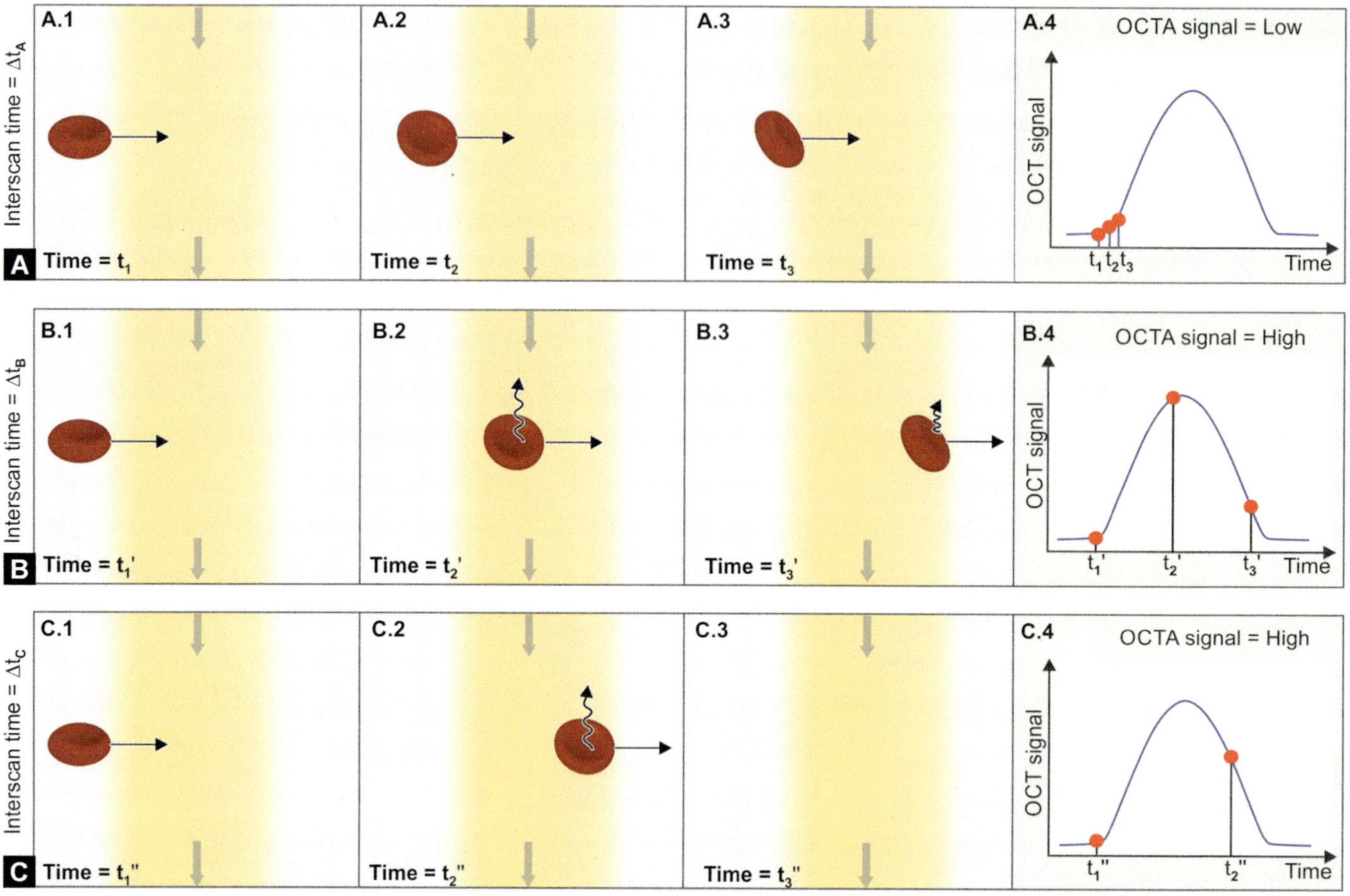

Figs. 46.6A to C: Dependency of the OCTA signal on the interscan time. For this diagram, the blood cell speed is held constant, whereas the interscan time is varied. Each row corresponds to a different interscan time where $\Delta t_A < \Delta t_B < \Delta t_C$. (A) With a short interscan time, the blood cell does not have time to significantly displace. Consequentially, the three OCT measurements are all similar and the resulting OCTA signal is low (A.4); (B) With a longer interscan time, the blood cell has time to traverse the entire width of the OCT beam, generating significant time variation in the OCT measurements (B.4); as such, the resulting OCTA signal will be high; (C) With a longer interscan time still, the blood cell displaces even farther, generating a time-varying OCT signal (C.4), and a high OCTA signal. In general, it is not possible to distinguish the case of Δt_B from Δt_C. Note the parallel between changing the interscan time and changing the blood cell's speed (Figs. 46.5A to C). This parallel exists because the blood cell displacement, on which the OCTA signal depends, is proportional to both the cell's speed and the interscan time—from the point of view of the OCTA signal, doubling/halving the interscan time has the exact same effect as does doubling/halving the cell's speed.

generated in an OCTA acquisition is larger, by a multiple of the number of repeated B-scans, than that generated by an OCT acquisition over the same area.

NORMAL RETINAL ANATOMY

On Optical Coherence Tomography

The OCT images of the retina are generated by light returning from the chorioretinal tissue, where it has undergone varying degrees of reflection, scattering and absorption. The resulting image shows a multilayered structure, with several hyper- and hyporeflective bands. With improved axial resolution from newer ultrahigh-resolution OCT instruments, it is now possible to approximate these bands with known retinal histology and understand the observed variations in reflectivity[24] (Fig. 46.8).

Beginning from the vitreoretinal interface, the first visible layer is the thin hyper-reflective band of the internal limiting membrane (ILM). Hyper-reflective bands on OCT represent fibrous layers which correspond to the nerve fiber layer and plexiform layers (both inner and outer). The hyporeflective bands represent cellular layers made up mostly of neuronal cell bodies. These bands correspond to the ganglion cell layer and nuclear layers (both inner and outer). Retinal blood vessels are seen as well-circumscribed, hyper-reflective circles within the inner retina.

Four hyper-reflective bands are seen within the outer retina[25] (Fig. 46.8). The innermost band represents the

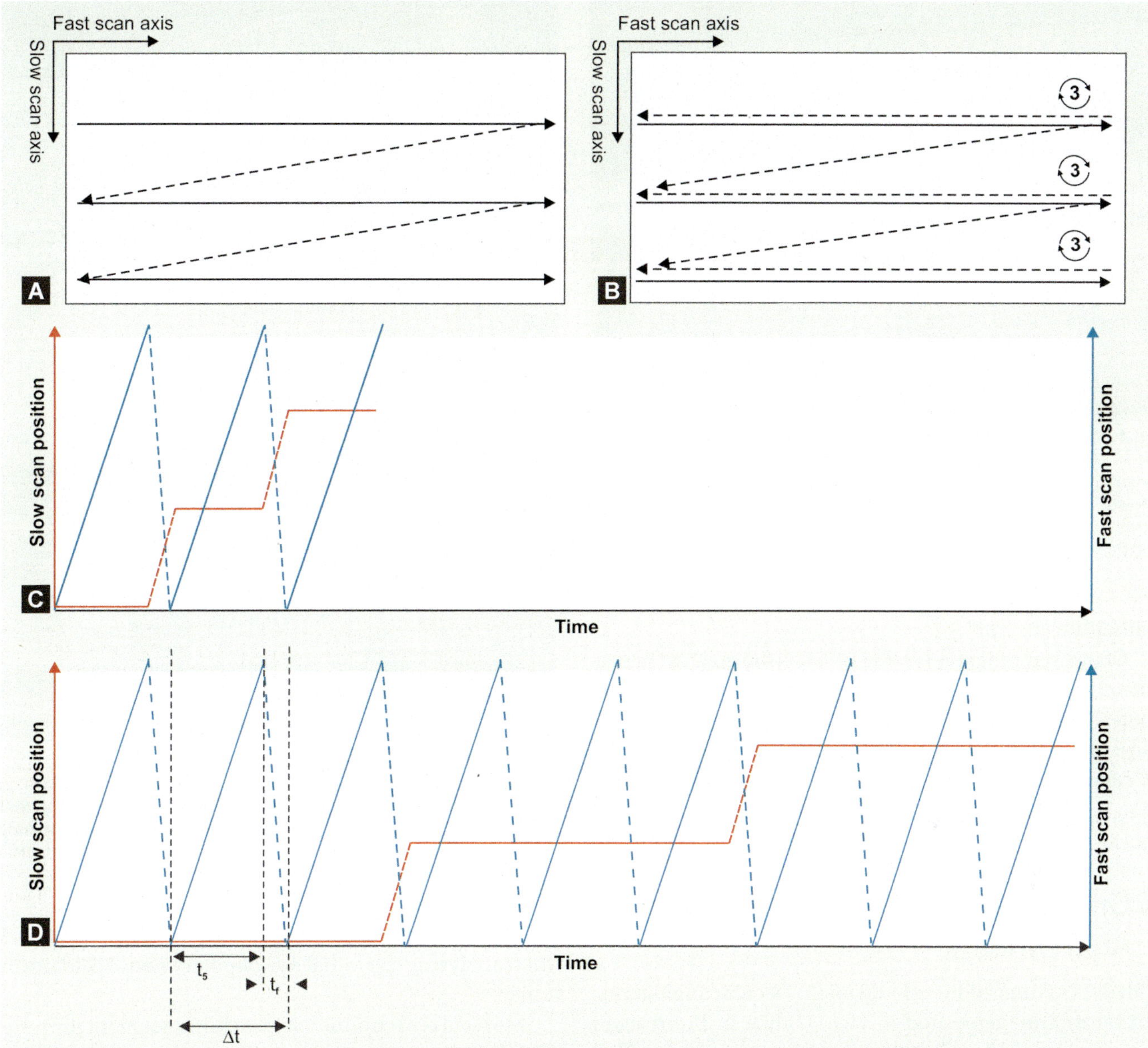

Figs. 46.7A to D: Scanning patterns for volumetric OCT and OCTA. Solid arrows correspond to times at which the A-scans are being recorded. Dashed and dotted lines correspond to times at which the scanning mirrors' positions are being moved but no A-scans are being recorded. (A) Scan pattern for volumetric OCT. A B-scan (solid arrows) is collected by scanning the beam along the fast scan axis. The mirrors are repositioned along the slow and fast scan axes (dashed arrow) to collect the next B-scan. The process then repeats; (B) Scan pattern for volumetric OCTA. At each slow scan position, three repeated OCT B-scans are collected (note that OCTA only requires that more than two repeated B-scans are acquired; current systems typically use between two and five repeated scans). The dotted arrow indicates the return of the mirrors to their starting position (no A-scans are collected during this time). After three repeated OCT B-scans are collected, the mirrors are repositioned along the slow and fast scan axes (dashed arrow) to collect the next set of repeated B-scans; (C and D) The positions of the slow and fast scan mirrors as a function of time for (C) an OCT acquisition, and (D) an OCTA acquisition. Red lines and axis correspond to the slow scan mirror position and blue lines and axis correspond to the fast scan mirror position. Note that the fast scan position has a "sawtooth" shape, whereas the slow scan position has a stepped shape. The time that it takes the scanning mirrors to return to their starting position, after completing a B-scan, is called the "flyback time," denoted here as t_f. The sum of the scanning time, t_s, and the flyback time yields the interscan time, Δt.

external limiting membrane and appears thinner and fainter relative to the others. The second band is commonly referred to as the junction between the inner segment and outer segment (IS/OS) of the photoreceptors. However, some authors believe this second band represents the inner segment ellipsoid zone[26] while others believe this band is the IS/OS.[27] The third visible band is thought to be due to the outer segments from the cone and rod tips.[28]

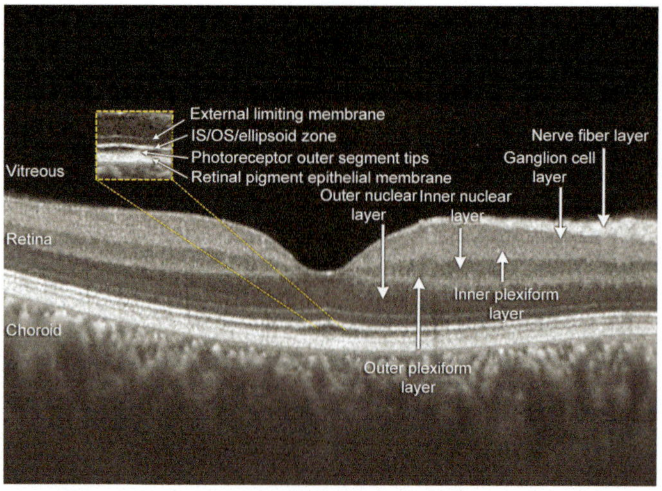

Fig. 46.8: Normal retinal anatomy on SD-OCT imaging. High-resolution image of a normal subject's retina as imaged using SD-OCT. Limited penetration of light past the pigmented RPE and signal drop off results in lower resolution of the choroid. The enlarged area of the outer retina shows the four clearly distinguishable outer retinal bands, each labeled with their histological correlates.

The fourth band is attributed to the retinal pigment epithelium (RPE).[28]

Of the four outer bands, the RPE has the greatest hyperreflectivity because of the melanin pigment within its cell bodies. When imaged by ultrahigh-resolution OCT, the RPE band can be seen as two distinct lines, representing the apical and basal surfaces of the RPE, with contributions from the underlying Bruch's membrane (BM) and choriocapillaris (CC).[28-30]

On Optical Coherence Tomography Angiography

With OCTA, three-dimensional microvascular angiograms can be rapidly generated in vivo. Unlike in fluorescein angiography (FA) and indocyanine green angiography, no intravenous contrast agent is required to visualize either retinal or choroidal blood flow. Furthermore, OCTA is depth-resolved, so segmenting full-thickness retinal scans allows selective viewing and analysis of the different retinal capillary plexuses and choroidal vasculature.[31,32] OCTA images exhibit a level of microvasculature detail that approaches the resolution of histological studies. Estimates of "superficial" and "deep" capillary plexus density on OCTA are similar to those of cadaveric histology.[33] Variations in normal retinal capillary density between the central macula, temporal macula, and peripapillary retina in healthy human eyes have been demonstrated without dye injection using OCTA for the very first time.[12,17,33-35]

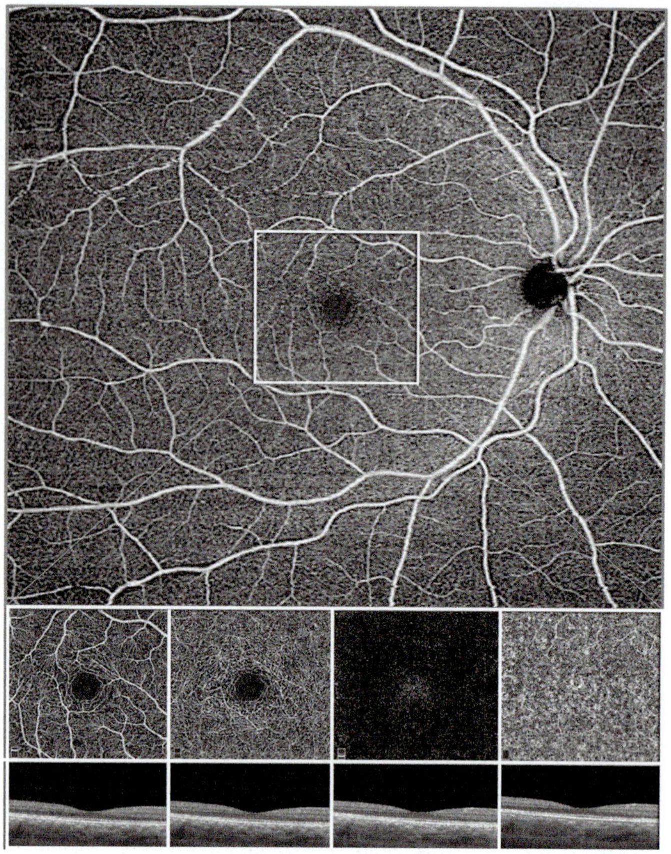

Fig. 46.9: Normal retinal anatomy on OCTA. The preferred method of viewing OCTA images is the en face view. (Top) 12 × 12 mm OCTA scan centered at the macula showing normal retinal vasculature, the foveal avascular zone and optic disc. (Middle row) From L-R with corresponding OCT B-scan (Bottom row) showing the segmentation level: superficial plexus, deep plexus, outer retina and choriocapillaris layer.

OCTA also offers greater vessel detail compared to FA when analyzing the radial peripapillary network in normal subjects.[36]

Most current commercial machines segment the retinal vasculature into the "superficial capillary plexus", which, depending on its location, consists of the retinal vasculature in the peripapillary radial capillary plexus as well as the superficial retinal capillary plexus, and the "deep capillary plexus" which contains the vasculature of the intermediate and deep capillary plexus.[15,32,37] The avascular layer of the retina is separately segmented since this layer may contain abnormal vasculature in pathology. Examples of the "superficial" and "deep capillary plexus" as segmented on commercial OCTA machines are displayed in Figure 46.9.

Another valuable tool in the interpretation of OCTA is the B-scan with flow overlay. The presence of flow overlaid over structural abnormalities is invaluable in identifying abnormal flow patterns on OCTA and differentiating

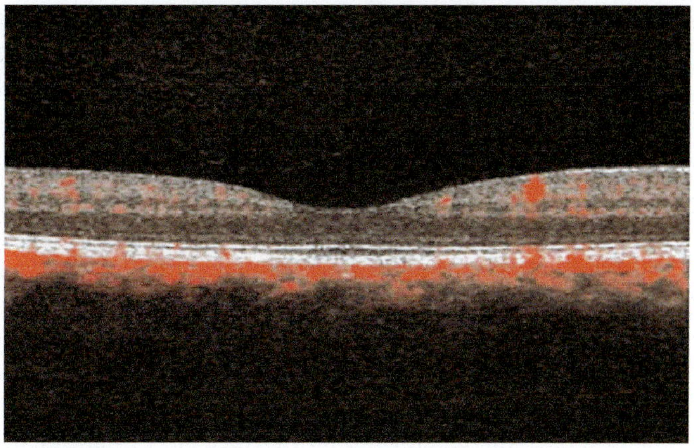

Fig. 46.10: Structural OCT B-scan with OCTA flow signal data overlaid. The false red coloring represents the OCTA flow signal which is very useful when trying to distinguish flow from projection artifact.

projection artifact from true abnormal flow (Fig. 46.10). This is described in more detail below in the artifacts section.

NORMAL CHOROIDAL ANATOMY

On Optical Coherence Tomography

Spectral-domain OCT has a coherence gate or "range" of ~2 mm in which images can be formed from the interference signal. While it is possible to obtain high-resolution images of the retina within this range, there is a marked drop in the SD-OCT's signal strength with increasing range or distance from the zero delay reference position, known as sensitivity roll off. In addition, the choroid is below the RPE which attenuates light and the choroid has vasculature which is also attenuating. This makes visualization of the choroid challenging (Fig. 46.11).

Enhanced depth imaging (EDI) places the choroid, rather than the retina, within the SD-OCT's coherence gate.[38] It does this by moving the OCT's objective lens close to the patient's eye, thereby placing the zero-delay line of the OCT closer to the retina choroidal interface and creating an inverted image. Averaging multiple scans of this inverted image removes background noise and produces improved visualization of the choroid and lamina cribrosa. Consequently, EDI has allowed visualization and measurement of the entire choroid in the majority of subjects, overcoming SD-OCT's inherent technical limitations.

Swept-source OCT instruments offer better visualization of the choroid compared to SD-OCT instruments[39] (Fig. 46.12). The longer wavelength light (1,050 nm) used in SS-OCT is better at penetrating the RPE than that used in

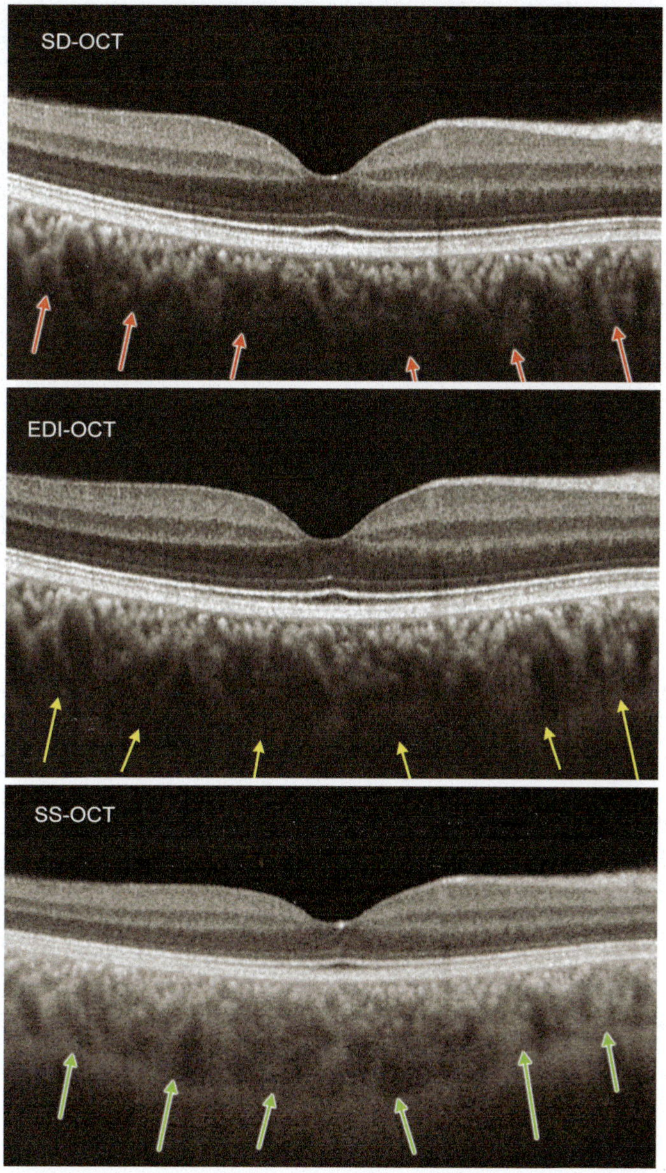

Fig. 46.11: Visualizing the choroid of the same subject using SD-OCT, EDI-OCT and SS-OCT (Top) SD-OCT has limited tissue penetration with increasing depth and struggles to identify the choroidal-scleral border (red arrows). (Middle) EDI-OCT in comparison offers slightly better visualization of the choroid (yellow arrows). (Bottom) SS-OCT uses a longer wavelength light source and is able to penetrate deeper into tissue and undergoes relatively less scattering from the pigmented RPE. The green arrows point to the choroidal-scleral interface which can be clearly visualized.

SD-OCT (840 nm).[40,41] Therefore, more backscattered light is available for imaging the choroid. Furthermore, SS-OCT technology does not suffer from the signal attenuation seen with increasing depth in SD-OCT. As a result, SS-OCT allows dense raster scanning.[42,43] Ultra-widefield imaging of the choroid and measurements of choroidal thickness have been demonstrated using high-speed SS-OCT.[44]

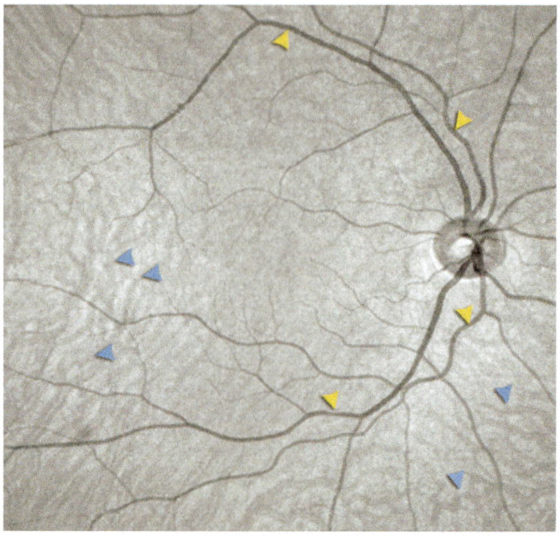

Fig. 46.12: Structural SS-OCT in enface view. The increased signal penetration of the SS-OCT makes visualization of choroidal vasculature easier. The yellow arrowheads to large retinal blood vessels which can be visualized even on structural SD-OCT images. However, the blue arrowheads to clearly visible choroidal vessels which are harder to see on SD-OCT.

Choroidal thickness of normal eyes decreases with age and longer axial length, and with the presence of reticular pseudodrusen.[45-47] Thickening of the choroid, or pachychoroid, has been observed in conditions such as central serous choroidopathy (CSC), polypoidal choroidal vasculopathy, and conditions along the pachychoroid spectrum.[48] Differences in regional thickness have been observed in normal subjects, with thicker choroids being observed temporally, and thinner choroids nasally.[49] The choroid is relatively thinner just inferior to the optic disc.[50] This localized thinning may be caused by the embryonic location of the optic fissure's point of closure.

QUANTITATIVE ANALYSIS

Quantitative Analysis on OCT

Quantification of OCT datasets became possible with the development of image processing software that would allow accurate segmentation of retinal layers. Retinal thickness and retinal nerve fiber layer (RNFL) thickness are two of the early quantitative measurements utilized by researchers and clinicians. Segmentation of retinal thickness and RNFL thickness by automated software enabled false color topographic mapping to assess macular edema or nerve fiber layer atrophy.[51,52] This was possible even in early instruments with limited A-scan rates because the thickness map could be generated using a limited number of B-scans. In addition to total retinal thickness, it is possible to obtain measurements of specific retinal layers, such as the thickness of the ganglion cell layer or the thickness of the photoreceptor outer segments.[53,54] Higher resolution and increased scanning speeds enable quantification and characterization of focal features such as drusen area and volume.[55,56] By comparing a distorted RPE (secondary to the presence of drusen) to a virtual RPE free of deformations, automated measurements of drusen area and volume can be generated and followed up over time.[55,56]

Higher resolution and increased scanning speeds also resulted in the production of large OCT datasets. The impracticality of sequentially analyzing cross-sectional images led to the development of en face OCT imaging. By axial summation of the OCT dataset, en face fundus images are generated, with registration of the cross-sectional image to fundus features becoming possible.[57-60] In this instance, segmentation of retinal layers enables projection OCT fundus imaging for visualizing the OCT dataset.[61] This technique selectively displays specific depth ranges in the retina, thereby enhancing the contrast of retinal structure alterations and allowing rapid assessment of outer retinal pathology. By projecting a sub-RPE slab, regions of geographic atrophy (GA) in eyes with nonexudative age-related macular degeneration (AMD) can be measured and followed up over time (Figs. 46.13A to D). Additionally, areas at risk of developing GA can also be identified.[62]

However, care must be taken when attempting to compare measurements across different instruments.[63,64] Retinal thickness is obtained by segmenting the ILM and a boundary representing extent of the outer retina, e.g. the RPE or the RPE-BM-CC complex (Figs. 46.13A to D). Older TD-OCT instruments suffered from low axial resolution and slower scanning speeds and were unable to delineate the RPE-BM-CC complex.[65] Automated thickness calculations from these instruments used the IS/OS junction as the outer retinal boundary, leading to underestimations of true thickness. While newer SD-OCT instruments can resolve the RPE-BM-CC complex into three separate layers, each device manufacturer employs their own proprietary segmentation algorithm.[66] This further complicates interdevice measurement comparisons as each algorithm follows a different border to denote the outer retina (top of the RPE, on the RPE, lower edge of the RPE). Performance of these algorithms is also highly variable when retinal architecture is distorted due to pathology.

It is also possible to obtain measurements of particular retinal layers, such as the thickness of the ganglion cell layer or the thickness of the photoreceptors' outer segments, as

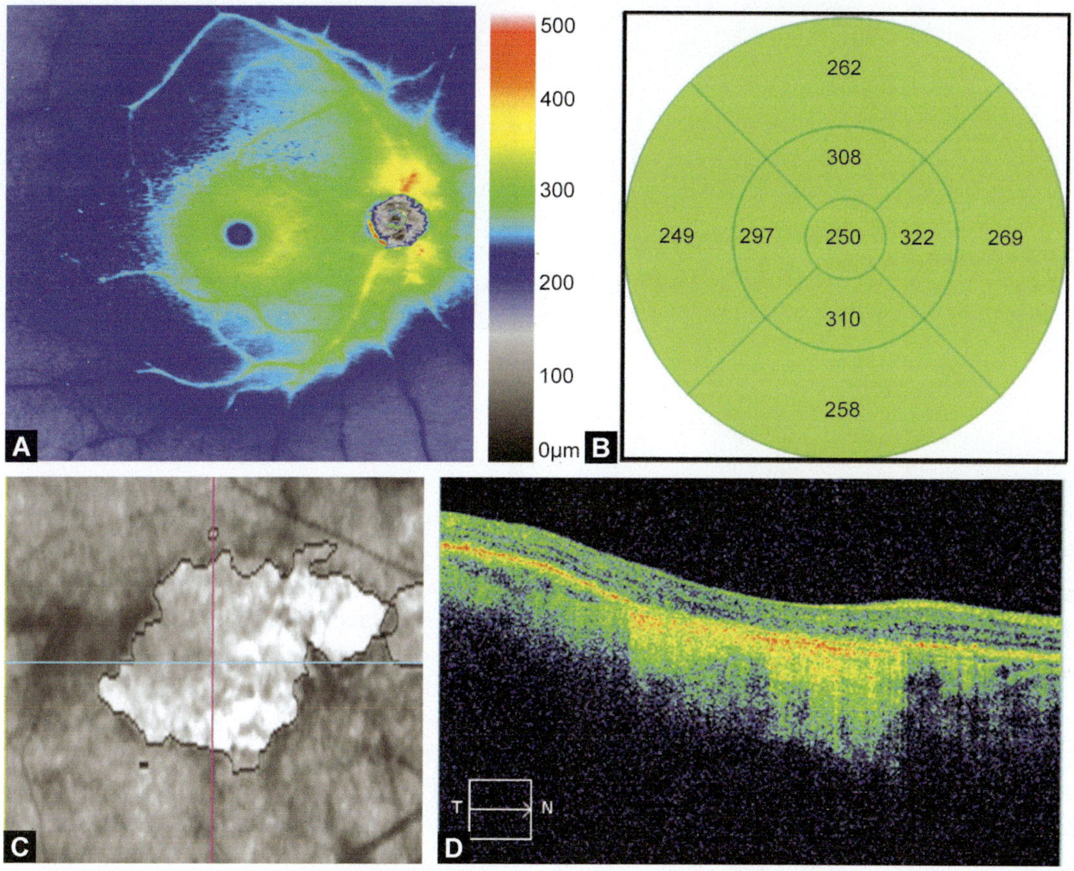

Figs. 46.13A to D: Quantitative OCT analysis. (A and B) Retinal thickness data represented by color-coded scale overlaid onto enface structural OCT image and corresponding macular map showing thickness values in ETDRS subregions. (C and D) Sub-RPE analysis map showing an automated outline of regions with RPE loss, and the OCT B-scan corresponding to the horizontal slice (blue line) showing hypertransmission of OCT signal due to loss of RPE.

well as measurements of retinal lesions, like the area of GA, using different segmentation schemes (Figs. 46.13A to D). This is addressed in greater detail in the section on GA.[50-52]

Measurements of drusen area and volume are also of great interest. Robust, reproducible automated measurements of drusen area and volume can be generated by comparing a distorted RPE (secondary to the presence of drusen) to a virtual RPE free of deformations.[55,56]

Quantitative Analysis of OCTA

Quantifying flow information is of interest to both researchers and clinicians, especially with regard to disease diagnosis and management. Several metrics that derive quantifiable information from en face OCTA projections have been proposed. Measurements of vessel density and foveal avascular zone (FAZ) size have been studied extensively in healthy and diseased eyes.[67-69] Generally speaking, vessel density is the percentage area occupied by vessels and microvasculature within the OCTA scan area. FAZ size refers to area measurements of the avascular region centered at the fovea. Areas of nonperfusion seen on OCTA have also been studied by measuring and mapping the intercapillary area. Automated segmentation of retinal layers allows these measurements to be made for the different retinal capillary plexuses (Fig. 46.14).

Caution must be exercised when trying to compare measurements made using different OCTA instruments. Each OCTA manufacturer employs its own proprietary algorithm to generate OCTA images along with various post-acquisition image processing techniques.[70,71] Consequently, vessel density measurements for the same subject imaged on different OCTA instruments are not the same. Differences in how the manufacturers' software segments retinal layers further complicate matters.[72] What constitutes the "superficial" or "deep" capillary plexus is not standardized across OCTA instruments. Differences between the manufacturers as to what comprises vascular density or flow is also an issue.

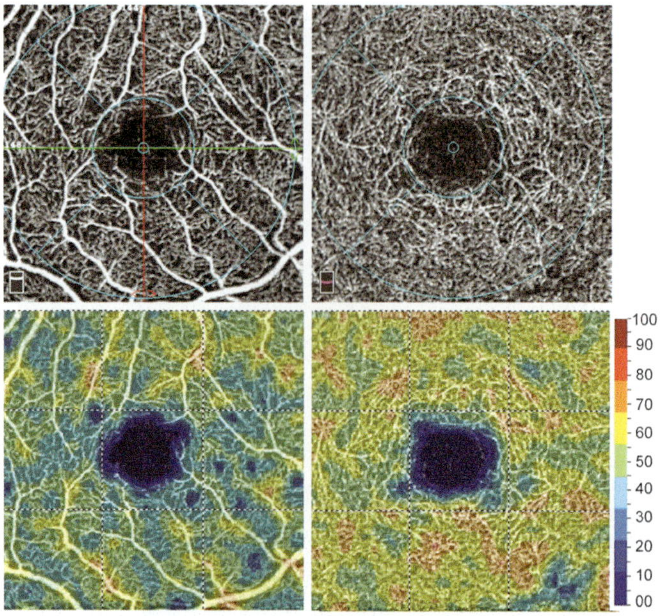

OCT Thickness ILM-RPE & Vessel Density

Density (%)	Section	Thickness (μm)
47.01	Whole Image	N/A
19.69	Fovea	249
49.15	ParaFovea	323
49.86	- Superior-Hemi	323
48.44	- Inferior-Hemi	324
47.37	- Tempo	319
53.15	- Superior	326
46.63	- Nasal	322
49.43	- Inferior	326

Grid-based Vessel Density (%)

49.63	53.87	52.33
45.39	24.19	47.14
48.95	49.99	51.38

OCT Thickness ILM-RPE & Vessel Density

Density (%)	Section	Thickness (μm)
56.38	Whole Image	N/A
20.75	Fovea	249
60.29	ParaFovea	323
60.08	- Superior-Hemi	323
60.50	- Inferior-Hemi	324
57.84	- Tempo	319
61.01	- Superior	326
59.09	- Nasal	322
63.15	- Inferior	326

Grid-based Vessel Density (%)

60.52	61.08	59.73
56.66	27.26	59.64
60.17	63.19	58.28

Fig. 46.14: Quantitative OCTA analysis. (Top row) An en face OCTA of a normal subject demonstrating the (left) superficial retinal plexus and (right) the deep retinal plexus with overlaid circles rings of 1 mm and 3 mm radii overlaid (Middle row). Corresponding enface color-coded OCTA vessel density maps (Bottom row). Corresponding vessel density percentages for the entire image and subregions of the overlaid rings in the top rows. The increased perfusion in the deep retinal plexus compared with the superficial retinal plexus can be appreciated quantitatively with vessel density values and qualitatively with the color maps.

IMAGE ARTIFACTS

Artifacts on Structural OCT

Understanding and interpreting artifacts on OCT imaging is crucial, as failure to do so can result in a wrong diagnosis or incorrect management plan. Artifacts can occur due to software, patient or operator factors.

Specific to FD-OCT instruments is the "mirror" or inverted image artifact. FD-OCT will create an image if the area of interest is placed around the region of the zero-delay line. However, the instrument cannot distinguish between a negative or positive delay. Therefore, if the area being imaged crosses the zero-delay line, an inverted or "mirror" image is formed (Fig. 46.15). These artifacts can occur if the FD-OCT is placed too close to the eye or if ocular pathology such as high myopia requires imaging of an area with a large axial range.

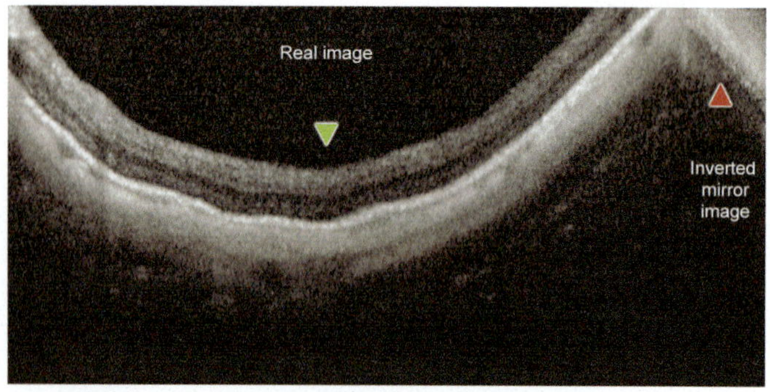

Fig. 46.15: Mirror artifact. The green arrowhead to the regular image of the retina and the red arrowhead to an inverted image caused by the area being imaged placed beyond the zero-delay line.

The presence of blood vessels within the retina and around the optic disc produces a "shadowing" artifact seen on OCT scans (Figs. 46.16A and B). The hyper-reflective vessel wall causes scattering of light. The blood flowing within the vessels can either absorb or randomly scatter the OCT beam. As a result, blood vessels generate shadowing artifacts behind them.

"Vignetting" of the OCT image occurs when the OCT beam is partially obstructed by the iris, resulting in a loss of signal over one side of the image (Fig. 46.17). This can occur when the pupil is not fully dilated.

Patient movements in the axial or transverse direction during OCT acquisition create "motion artifacts" (Fig. 46.18). Common causes include poor fixation, tracking of the light source, heartbeats, respirations or ocular saccades. These lead to either distortion or double scanning of the same area, producing sharp changes in the contour of the B-scan, misalignment of retinal blood vessels, or blurring on fundus images. While manufacturers have tried to limit the effects of motion using software techniques or eye tracking, repeating the scan is sometimes the only option.

Misidentification of the retinal boundaries or sublayers by OCT software can lead to incorrect segmentation (Figs. 46.19A to C). This can cause inaccurate mapping and incorrect quantification of retinal layers within volumetric scans. Misidentification of the inner retinal boundary usually occurs in vitreomacular surface disorders whereas conditions involving the outer retina/RPE such as central

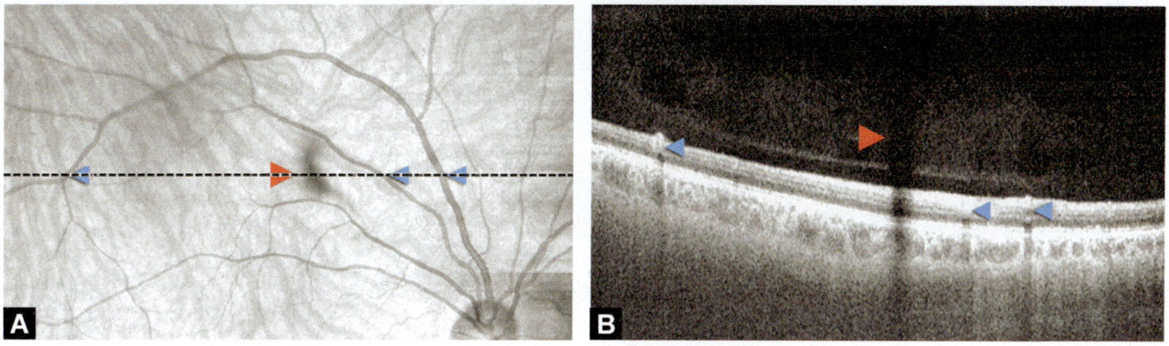

Figs. 46.16A and B: Shadowing artifact. (A) Structural enface OCT of a normal subject. The red arrowhead to a floater in the vitreous and the blue arrowheads to retinal blood vessels. (B) Structural OCT B-scan corresponding to the horizontal black line. The floater is causing a blockage of OCT signal, highlighted by the red arrowhead. The blue arrowheads identify the superficial retinal blood vessels which are causing blockage of OCT signal.

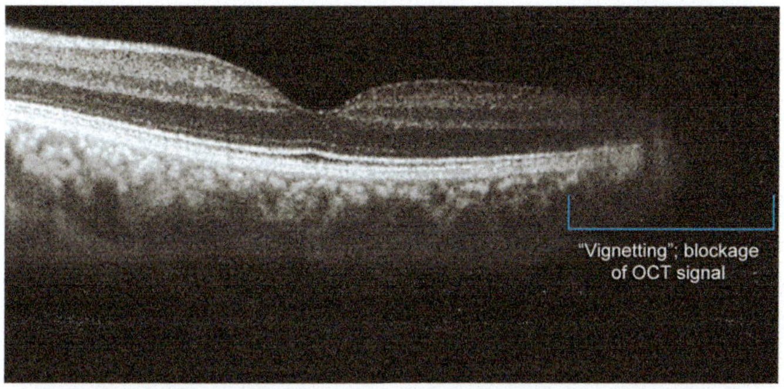

Fig. 46.17: Vignetting artifact. The blue line identifies the area where the OCT beam is obstructed by the iris resulting in reduced signal over one side of the image.

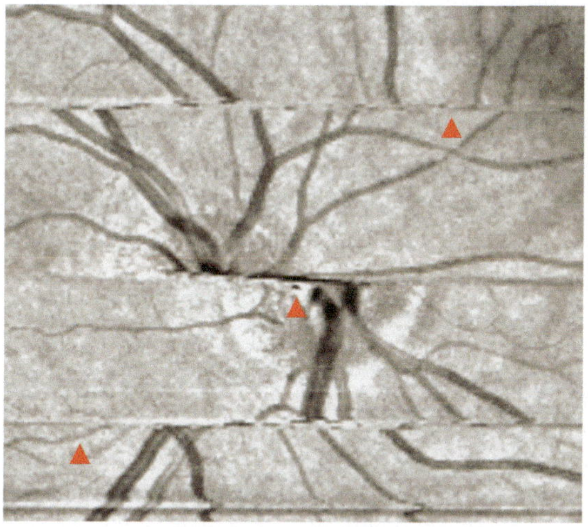

Fig. 46.18: Motion artifact. En face view of optic disc. Eye movements during OCT scanning lead to distortion or double scanning. The red arrowheads to the sharp changes in contour and misalignment of retinal blood vessels.

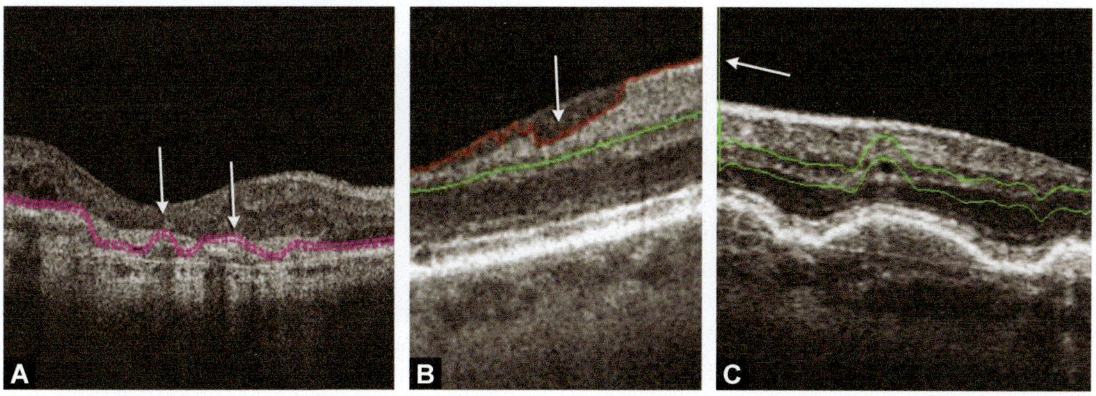

Figs. 46.19A to C: Three examples (white arrows) of automated software segmentation breakdown due to different ocular pathology.

serous chorioretinopathy, age-related macular dystrophy, cystoid macular edema and retinal atrophy commonly cause misidentification of the outer retinal boundaries. Motion artifact is another frequent cause of breakdowns in automated software segmentation. Therefore, caution must be exercised when using OCT imaging and its derivative

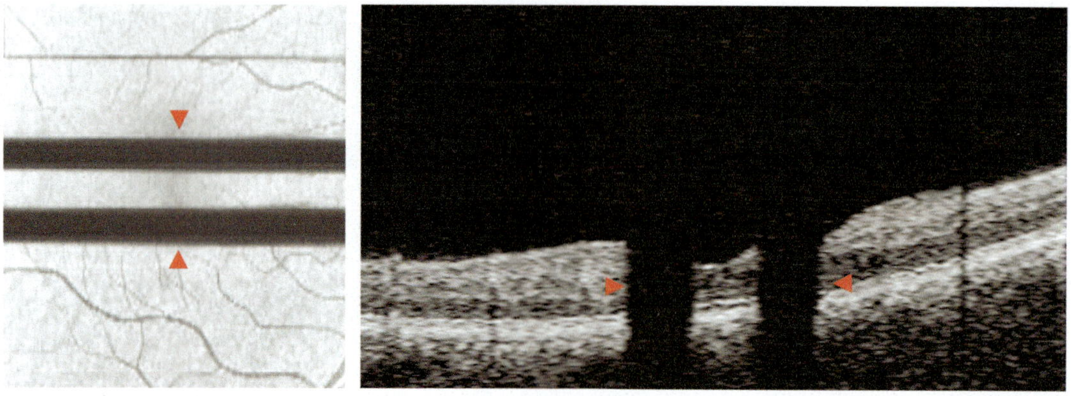

Fig. 46.20: Blink artifacts. Blinking during OCT scan acquisition results in a partial loss of OCT data. Red arrowheads to the black horizontal bars which represent this loss of OCT signal.

quantification for therapeutic decision making in the presence of software breakdowns.

Black horizontal bars on an OCT image occur when the patient blinks during scan acquisition (Fig. 46.20). As the eyelid closes, the momentary loss in OCT signal causes a loss of data. Newer instruments include eye tracking technology that attempts to compensate for blinking by repeat scanning in the area of signal loss.

Artifacts on OCTA

Similar to OCT, OCTA imaging is also prone to the presence of image artifacts. Despite their technical differences, both SD-OCT and SS-OCT offer decreased visualization of blood flow in the choroid relative to the retina. This is caused by the attenuation and scattering of light by the highly pigmented RPE layer and the dense microvasculature of the CC. Both modalities experience relative losses in signal strength in the presence of focal or diffuse media opacities. The larger the drop in signal, the more difficult it becomes to determine the presence or absence of flow in the affected region. An important way of distinguishing shadowing from true flow loss is by looking at structural scans associated with the OCTA image. The en face OCT scans segmented at the level of the OCTA segmentation will show dark areas of signal loss in areas of shadowing. Thus, areas that appear dark on the structural OCT image and on the OCTA image probably reflects a loss of signal (shadowing) rather than a true loss of flow. This is even better visualized when looking at the corresponding OCT B-scans in the area of apparent flow loss. The OCT B-scan in an area of shadowing will show a clear loss of signal or "shadow" (Figs. 46.21A and B). On the other hand, if the flow loss on OCTA is not

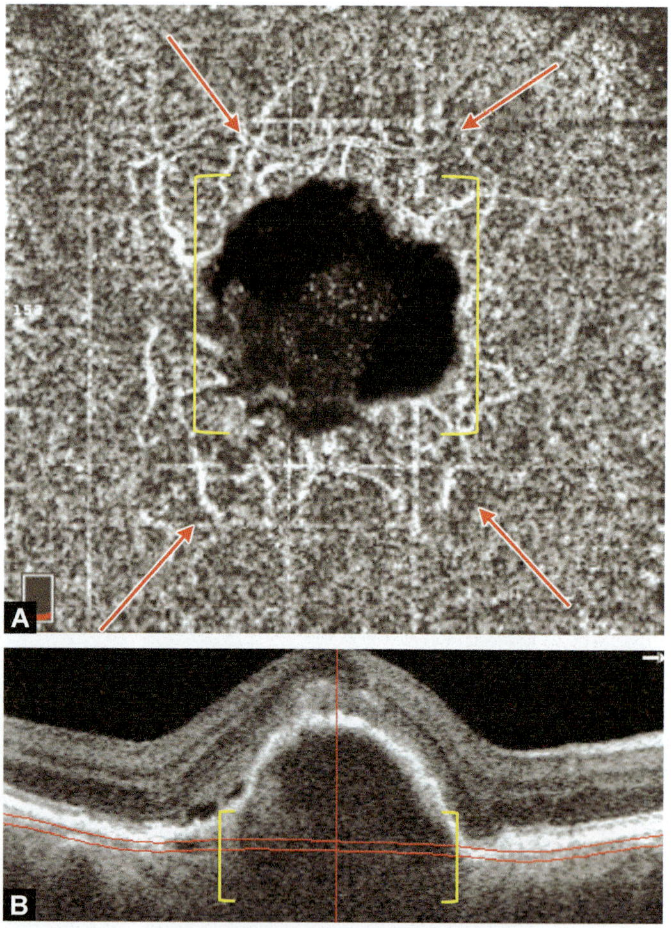

Figs. 46.21A and B: Shadowing from pigment epithelial detachment. (A) En face OCTA segment representing the choriocapillaris (CC). The yellow brackets highlight the apparent loss of blood vessels and the red arrows point to false positive decorrelation signals on the OCTA image; (B) However, the corresponding structural OCT B-scan shows a large PED that is blocking OCT signal resulting in the false appearance of loss of blood vessels in the CC.

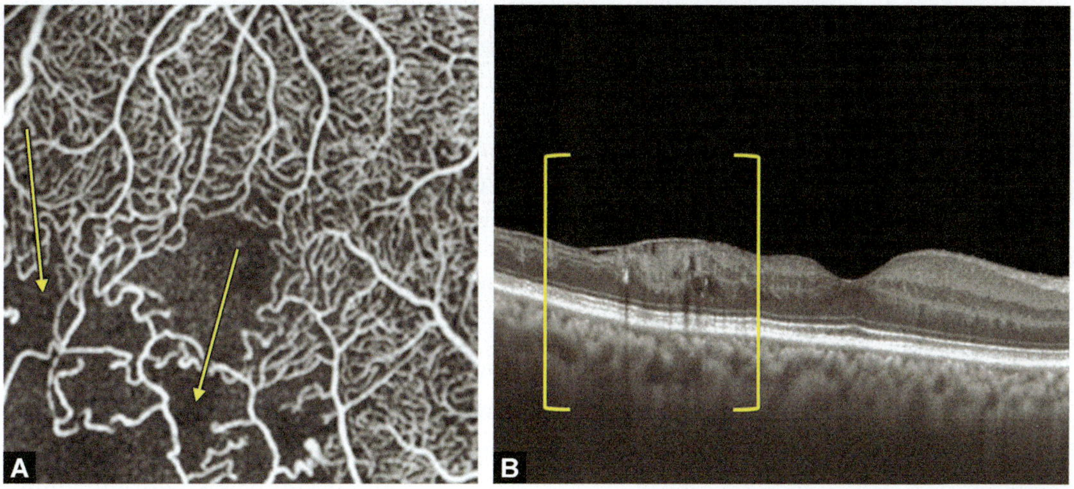

Figs. 46.22A and B: True loss of flow signal. (A) Enface OCTA image of the superficial layer from a patient with a branch retinal vein occlusion. The yellow arrows point to the area of lost blood vessels; (B) The yellow brackets on the structural B-scan highlight the distortion in retinal architecture caused by obstruction of blood flow. By looking at both the enface and structural B-scans, the loss of blood vessels or flow signal is real.

associated with shadowing on the enface image and on the corresponding structural B-scans, it probably represents a true flow loss (Figs. 46.22A and B).

Projection artifact is also common on OCTA. As light encounters a blood vessel, it undergoes variable amounts of reflection, refraction or absorption. Some light will pass through the blood vessel, encounter underlying tissue, and be reflected back to the OCT instrument. As blood continues to flow, the light that passes through will change over time. As a result, the reflection of light from the underlying tissue will also change. Therefore, any reflecting surface under the blood vessels will seem to change over time and will be displayed as having flow. This explains why the hyper-reflective RPE appears to have blood vessels that mimic the pattern of the overlying retinal blood vessels (Fig. 46.23). Understanding OCTA projection artifacts is crucial in deciding whether flow is truly present. Currently available software can remove projection artifacts from OCTA images.[73] As this artifact removal software becomes more sophisticated, the presence of projection artifacts will become less important.

While OCTA projection artifacts are mostly a nuisance, knowledge of their existence can aid in visualization in certain situations. For example, when attempting to visualize the CC, an en face OCTA section through the anatomical location of the CC can show projection artifact from overlying retinal vessels. By moving the section deeper (outside of the true anatomical location of the CC) to the hyporeflective region in the structural OCT where small vessels connecting to the CC are expected, a fine interconnected layer of vessels suggestive of the CC is visualized, without retinal vessel projections. In this instance, the best way to see the CC is not to look directly at it but to look at its projection.[74] However, overlying pathology such as drusen can block the signal resulting in apparent areas of CC loss.

Previously, we discussed the impact of patient movement on OCT images. As OCTA is derived from OCT data, patient movement in either the axial or transverse direction will also result in OCTA image artifacts. Movement in the axial direction would produce a higher decorrelation signal, causing reflective, nonvascular structures to be falsely rendered as having the appearance of flow. Several motion correction methods can compensate for axial movements; but motion in the transverse direction is harder to correct for (Figs. 46.24A and B).

As OCTA images are formed based on signal changes between repeated B-scans, transverse movements during OCTA acquisition will result in scanning of a different area (the initial B-scan would not match the repeat B-scan). This would be detected as a large change in signal, producing a white line artifact on the OCTA image.

As en face viewing of OCTA images is the accepted convention, failures in automated segmentation, secondary to pathological disruption of the retinal architecture, are a major cause of image artifacts. Retinal edema, atrophy, bleeding, and tissue infiltration result in segmentation failure, producing images of the retinal vasculature that do not reflect actual anatomy.[74]

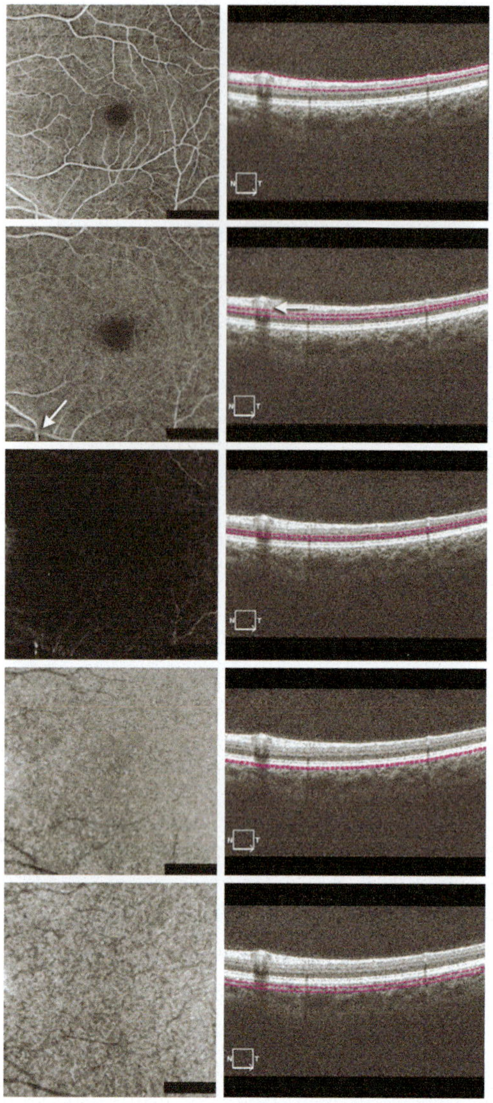

Fig. 46.23: Projection artifacts in OCTA imaging. From top to bottom are different layers of the same eye. The left column is the enface OCTA and the right column is the corresponding B-scan showing the level at which the image was obtained. At the top is the inner retinal circulation. As we lower the slab section, the white arrow points to a blood vessel in the inner retina which can be seen in every subsequent layer.

OPTICAL COHERENCE TOMOGRAPHY IN RETINAL DISEASE

Epiretinal Membrane

An epiretinal membrane (ERM) is a layer of fibrotic tissue that develops on the surface of the retina, most commonly after a posterior vitreous detachment. However, it may occur secondary to uveitis, retinal tears, and retinal detachments.[75] On OCT, an ERM is a highly reflective, thick membrane overlying the ILM. Tractional forces produced by the ERM can generate folds within the inner retinal layer beneath the membrane. Mild ERMs very rarely disrupt retinal architecture or affect visual acuity and thus require no treatment. In more severe cases, disruption in macular contour, loss of the normal foveal depression and changes in the outer retina can cause visual impairment, requiring surgical removal of the ERM.

On OCTA, ERMs may be characterized by tortuosity of the retinal vasculature.

Vitreomacular Traction

With normal aging, liquefaction of the vitreous occurs with complete separation from the macula. Vitreomacular traction (VMT) occurs when there is incomplete separation of the posterior hyaloid from the central macular surface exerting tractional forces on the retina. The extent of vitreous attachment can range from a single point to a broad area. As the vitreous continues to liquefy and separate, tractional forces on the retina result in distortion of retinal architecture, cystoid macular edema formation, and subretinal fluid accumulation. Visual impairment can vary from mild to severe. OCT imaging has proved most useful in the diagnosis and management of VMT disorders. It allows detailed assessment of structural changes in the retina and more accurate prediction of visual function based on analyzing the outer retinal bands and photoreceptors.[76]

Vitreomacular traction will often release spontaneously, therefore an initial period of observation is usually warranted. However, VMT may also worsen or progress to lamellar or full-thickness macular hole. Pharmacologic or surgical interventions should be considered if symptoms become significantly bothersome to the patient.

Diabetic Retinopathy

Diabetic retinopathy is the leading cause of blindness in working age adults in the United States of America, with diabetic macular edema (DME) being the primary cause of vision loss.[77] Diabetic retinopathy can be classified into nonproliferative diabetic retinopathy (NPDR) and proliferative diabetic retinopathy (PDR).

Nonproliferative Diabetic Retinopathy

Nonproliferative diabetic retinopathy represents the earliest stages of retinopathy caused by diabetes. Damage to the small blood vessels of the retina can result in the formation of hard exudates, nerve fiber layer infarcts

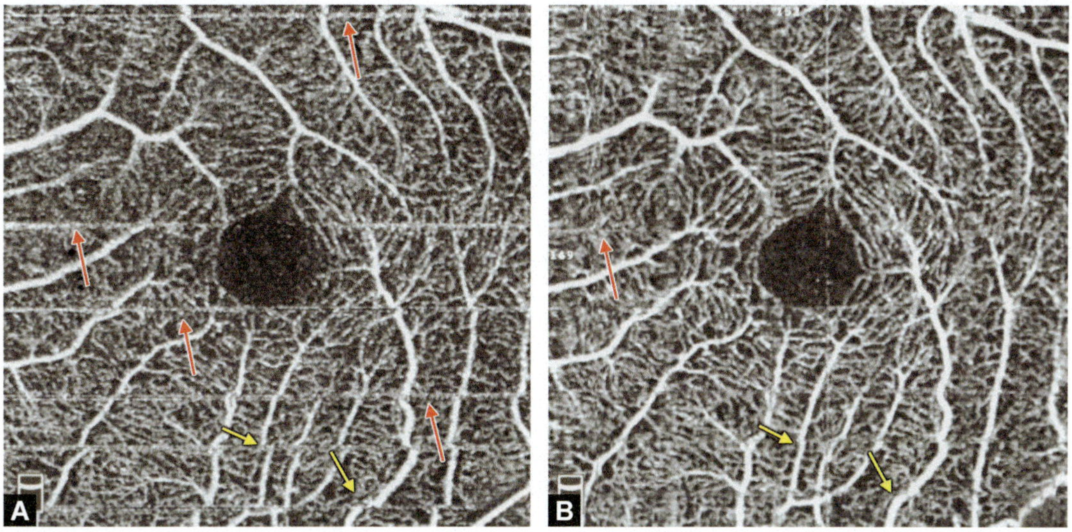

Figs. 46.24A and B: Motion artifact in OCTA imaging. (A) En face OCTA image (without motion correction technology) showing the consequences of eye movements during scan acquisition. The red arrows point to white line defects and the yellow arrows point to "sheared" retinal blood vessels; (B) With motion correction technology employed, the corresponding enface image shows a reduction in motion artifact. However, as the red and yellow arrows show, there is still evidence of white line defects and distorted retinal anatomy.

(cotton wool spots), and intraretinal hemorrhages. On OCT imaging, hard exudates appear as hyper-reflective clusters in the retina, whereas cotton wool spots appear as areas of hyper-reflectivity within the nerve fiber layer.[51] Other microvascular abnormalities, including microaneurysms (MAs) and dilated or tortuous vessels, can also develop. MAs have a characteristic homogenous inner reflectivity with an outer rim of hyper-reflectivity when seen on B-scans. If surrounded by fluid, they may also have a surrounding hyporeflective ring.

On OCTA, NPDR is characterized by tortuosity of the retinal microvasculature, enlargement of the FAZ and capillary dropout in the macular region.[78] Many but not all MAs visible on FA are also visible on OCTA.[74] However, at present, leakage from MAs cannot be visualized on OCTA. Capillary dropout on OCTA can be analyzed and quantified using the various different software packages available on OCT machines, and these may be powerful tools to follow diabetic vascular changes in the future.

Of interest, studies have shown that capillary dropout and FAZ changes in diabetics may happen in advance of clinically visible diabetic retinopathy and that the deep capillary plexus may be the earliest site of such changes.[79]

Diabetic Macular Edema

Diabetic macular edema is characterized by thickening and edema of the macula due to leakage of fluid and lipid-rich exudate from damaged retinal blood vessels. DME can develop at any stage of diabetic retinopathy and results in visual impairment if it involves the fovea. OCT has become the most important ancillary test in DME diagnosis, monitoring treatment and progression.[51] Traditional measures of clinically significant macular edema have largely been replaced by OCT-based parameters such as center-involving macular edema. Moreover, the morphology of the edema on OCT, whether diffuse or cystic, may help predict response to treatment.[80,81] Measurements of retinal thickness using OCT appear more sensitive for detecting mild DME than either biomicroscopy or color fundus imaging.[82,83] Additionally, OCT imaging has enabled accurate monitoring of DME and its response to treatment by intravitreal agents, laser, and vitreoretinal surgery.[84,85]

On OCTA, edema can be easily distinguished from capillary dropout.[86,87] However, the presence of edema may make segmentation of the retinal layers and visualization of the independent capillary plexuses more challenging.[88,89] Studies have shown that the presence of MAs in the deep capillary plexus is more closely associated with the development of DME; that the presence of deep layer ischemia may be associated with a less robust response to anti-vascular endothelial growth factor (VEGF) therapy; that edema occurs in areas of ischemia; and that resolution of the edema does not always result in resolution of the ischemia.[90-95]

Proliferative Diabetic Retinopathy

Proliferative diabetic retinopathy is characterized by neovascularization arising from the optic disc and retina, which may cause preretinal and vitreous hemorrhage. PDR can be visualized with OCT imaging as loops of hyper-reflective blood vessels protruding into the retina that can be visualized as having flow on OCTA.[96] OCTA is particularly invaluable in following these areas of preretinal neovascularization over time and monitoring their response to treatment. Subsequent fibrosis of these new vessels can create tractional forces leading to retinal detachment. OCT imaging is important in determining if the resulting traction impacts the fovea and in guiding decisions regarding the need for surgical intervention.[97]

Branch Retinal Vein Occlusion

Branch retinal vein occlusion (BRVO) is caused by blockage of one of the branches of the central retinal vein. The most common cause involves mechanical compression from an adjacent atherosclerotic artery. Clinical findings include a dilated and tortuous branch retinal vein associated with retinal hemorrhages. OCT imaging is used to detect the presence of macular edema and assess for foveal involvement and to monitor response to treatment.[98] Other OCT findings in BRVO include intraretinal hyper-reflectivity from hemorrhages, shadowing from edema and hemorrhages, and subretinal fluid. On OCTA, BRVO can be seen as a well-demarcated area with usually decreased perfusion, vascular tortuosity and collateral formation between areas with normal vessels and areas that have BRVO. OCTA can be useful to evaluate areas of nonperfusion in patients with retinal vascular occlusion.[99]

Central Retinal Vein Occlusion

Central retinal vein occlusion (CRVO) is caused by blockage of flow at the central retinal vein, at or proximal to the lamina cribrosa. It is the main drainage system for the inner retina and disruption of flow can cause severe visual loss from ischemia, macular edema and/or neovascularization.

Optical coherence tomography is key in diagnosing macular edema and assessing which retinal layers are involved. Discontinuity of the photoreceptors and ellipsoid zone, and increased macular thickness as seen on OCT imaging usually correlates with poor visual outcomes in CRVO.[100] It is also used to monitor response to therapy. Similar to its use in BRVO, OCTA shows the area and extent of ischemia and vascular abnormalities in patients with CRVO.[99]

Branch Retinal Artery Occlusion

Branch retinal artery occlusion (BRAO) results from an obstruction of one of the branches of the central retinal artery. Emboli secondary to either carotid plaques or cardiac thrombi are the most common cause for a BRAO. In the acute phase of a BRAO, OCT imaging shows increased hyper-reflectivity in the affected inner retinal layers with associated retinal thickening. In the chronic phase, atrophy of the nerve fiber layer and the inner retina can be seen with sparing of outer retinal layer architecture and thickness. OCTA shows flow impairment of the affected branch retinal artery. In very subtle BRAOs that present as paracentral acute middle maculopathy, OCT will demonstrate hyper-reflectivity in the middle retina and OCTA will show ischemia confined to the deep capillary plexus.[101]

Central Retinal Artery Occlusion

Central retinal artery occlusion (CRAO) results from obstruction of the central retinal artery, which is a major branch of the ophthalmic artery. Obstruction can be due to thrombotic, inflammatory or traumatic causes. Fundus examination reveals a pale retina with a cherry red spot. Recanalization over time results in resolution of inner retinal edema and associated atrophy. In the acute phase of a CRAO, OCT imaging reveals inner retinal thickening, hyperlucency and loss of distinction between the inner retinal layers. Outer retinal structures comprising the RPE, photoreceptors and outer nuclear layer appear relatively unaffected. In the chronic phase, inner retinal thinning with an intact RPE is visible on OCT imaging.[100]

OCTA imaging demonstrates the profound ischemia, loss of capillaries and attenuation of larger vessels that is also seen on FA in these patients.

Exudative Age-related Macular Degeneration

Choroidal neovascularization (CNV) involves formation of abnormal blood vessels within the macula. A type 1 CNV lies within the sub-RPE space and results in elevation of the overlying RPE-OCT findings include flat, irregular pigment epithelial detachments (PEDs)[102] with occasional thickening of the overlying RPE. Variable reflectivity may be observed within the core of the PED due to the variable nature of its constituents. Intravascular lumens of the CNV complex may be visible, giving the appearance of "stacked" material. Associated subretinal fluid is best seen using the OCT B-scan.[103] OCTA typically shows abnormal vasculature in the subretinal space between the RPE and the BM.[31] The neovascular complexes may have many different appearances but typically consist of thicker central and finer peripheral vessels.[104] There may or may not be a trunk vessel visible on OCTA. OCTA of the CC typically demonstrated loss of CC surrounding the CNV.[105] Type 2 CNVs extend through the subretinal space, sitting between the neurosensory retina and the RPE. On OCT, they typically present as subretinal hyper-reflective material.[106] On OCTA, they can be seen as neovascularization appearing in the "avascular" or deep retinal slab, with many of the qualitative features described above for type 1 CNV.[31] Type 3 CNV, also known as retinal angiomatous proliferation, results from the proliferation of abnormal blood vessels from deep within the retinal tissue. Characteristic OCT findings of these lesions include intraretinal cysts and fluid associated with a PED, with occasional subretinal fluid. Hyper-reflective material below the neurosensory retinal may also be present. If there is a chorioretinal anastomosis, it results in an irregular PED.[107,108] On OCTA, the retinal portion of the neovascular complex may be seen anastomosing with the choroidal vessels in the PED.

Choroidal neovascularization of any type may be seen regressing with treatment on OCTA, with a reduction in lesion size, and these changes may precede resolution of subretinal fluid on the structural OCT.[109-111]

The end stages of CNV lesions produce disciform scars, in which fibrovascular tissue develops within BM, the subretinal space and the sub-RPE space. Disciform scars appear as hyper-reflective tissue with distinct borders on OCT imaging and can be associated with intraretinal cysts overlying the scars caused by retinal degeneration.[112] PED contraction may result in an RPE tear which appears as hyper-reflective tissue rolled up underneath the neurosensory retina. A free edge of "wavy" RPE can be seen at the margins of an area with exposed BM and absent overlying RPE.[113]

Polypoidal choroidal vasculopathy, a variant of type 1 CNV, appears on OCT as multiple, large PEDs with associated subretinal fluid.[114,115] Polyps may be seen adherent to their posterior surface and exudates appear as hyper-reflective intraretinal spots. These are usually associated with a branching vascular network that perfuses the polyp, and that appears on OCT as a shallow separation between the RPE and BM.[116] En face structural OCT is particularly useful in supporting the diagnosis of polypoidal choroidal vasculopathy and detailing the entire extent of the lesion. Although the polyps are variably visualized on OCTA, the branching vascular network is usually well visualized on OCTA.

Dry Age-related Macular Degeneration

Dry AMD is characterized by the presence of drusen and abnormalities of the RPE/BM complex, and underlying CC. Drusen are focal deposits of extracellular debris located between the RPE and BM. Structural OCT imaging has allowed clinicians and researchers to assess the ultrastructure of drusen and study their natural history. They are seen as discrete areas of RPE elevation with variable inner reflectivity, highlighting the variable composition of the underlying material.[117,118] Thinning of photoreceptors overlying drusen has also been observed.[119] Advances in commercial software enable automated quantification of drusen area and volume, allowing these measurements to be followed up over time.[56] OCT imaging has allowed the study of subretinal drusenoid deposits (also known as reticular pseudodrusen), which have been shown to be associated with increased risk of progression to advanced AMD.[120] Characteristics of drusen associated with accelerated progression into advanced AMD include the presence of hyper-reflective foci overlying the drusen, the presence of heterogeneous reflectivity within the surface of the drusen, loss of photoreceptors over drusen and drusen volume.[121,122]

Geographic atrophy, a form of advanced AMD is characterized on structural OCT by loss of the hyper-reflective outer retinal bands, reflecting loss of photoreceptors, RPE and the underlying CC. Loss of the hyper-reflective RPE results in increased OCT signal penetration into the choroid, characterized as a "window defect".[23] Outer retinal tubulations contain degenerating photoreceptors and are identified on cross-sectional OCT scans as a hyper-reflective circular or ovoid structure with a hyporeflective center, located in the outer nuclear layer.[123] En face OCT imaging of the outer retina/IS/OS layer may visualize the areas with IS/OS band disruption and can predict the progression of GA in some eyes.[62,124] Using OCT imaging, researchers have been able to define precursor lesions such as "nascent GA" and "drusen-associated GA" which portend the formation of GA.[125,126]

Central Serous Choroidopathy

Central serous choroidopathy is a disease characterized by serous detachments of the neurosensory retina secondary to the accumulation of fluid which originates from the CC.[127] CSC is characterized by RPE detachments, choroidal thickening and outer retinal granulations on OCT imaging. The presence of serous fluid in the subretinal space and RPE detachments can be followed over time using OCT imaging.[128] OCTA provides the added benefit of being able to visualize flow impairments within the CC and possibly detect for the presence of secondary CNV that may require treatment.[129]

FUTURE DIRECTIONS

Even though the last decade has seen huge advances in OCT technology with the evolution of high-resolution SD-OCT, tracking technology, software and image processing advancements and higher scanning speeds, the true promise of OCT lies in the future. The development of new light sources including longer wavelength light sources, as well as increasing scanning speeds, will allow for better, more detailed, and ultimately higher resolution images. The integration of OCTA into clinical trials will help guide the drug development of the future. Moreover, as the cost decreases and the technology becomes more ubiquitous, it may well be a screening tool used in the clinics of the future.

REFERENCES

1. Huang D, Swanson EA, Lin CP, et al. Optical coherence tomography. Science. 1991;254:1178-81.
2. Izatt JA, Hee MR, Swanson EA, et al. Micrometer-scale resolution imaging of the anterior eye in vivo with optical coherence tomography. Arch Ophthalmol. 1994;112:1584-9.
3. Puliafito CA, Hee MR, Lin CP, et al. Imaging of macular diseases with optical coherence tomography. Ophthalmology. 1995;102:217-29.
4. Schuman JS, Hee MR, Arya AV, et al. Optical coherence tomography: a new tool for glaucoma diagnosis. Curr Opin Ophthalmol. 1995;6:89-95.
5. Wojtkowski M, Leitgeb R, Kowalczyk A, et al. In vivo human retinal imaging by Fourier domain optical coherence tomography. J Biomed Opt. 2002;7:457-63.
6. Leitgeb R, Hitzenberger CK, Fercher AF. Performance of Fourier domain vs. time domain optical coherence tomography. Opt Express. 2003;11:889-94.
7. de Boer JF, Cense B, Park BH, et al. Improved signal-to-noise ratio in spectral-domain compared with time-domain optical coherence tomography. Opt Lett. 2003;28:2067-9.
8. Choma MA, Sarunic M, Yang C, et al. Sensitivity advantage of swept source and Fourier domain optical coherence tomography. Opt Express. 2003;11:2183-9.
9. Chinn SR, Swanson EA, Fujimoto JG. Optical coherence tomography using a frequency-tunable optical source. Opt Lett. 1997;22:340-2.
10. Golubovic B, Bouma BE, Tearney GJ, et al. Optical frequency-domain reflectometry using rapid wavelength tuning of a Cr4+:forsterite laser. Opt Lett. 1997;22:1704-6.
11. Yun S, Tearney G, Bouma B, et al. High-speed spectral-domain optical coherence tomography at 1.3 μm wavelength. Opt Express. 2003;11:3598-604.
12. Makita S, Hong Y, Yamanari M, et al. Optical coherence angiography. Opt Express. 2006;14:7821-40.
13. Fingler J, Schwartz D, Yang C, et al. Mobility and transverse flow visualization using phase variance contrast with spectral domain optical coherence tomography. Opt Express. 2007;15:12636-53.
14. Mariampillai A, Standish BA, Moriyama EH, et al. Speckle variance detection of microvasculature using swept-source optical coherence tomography. Opt Lett. 2008;33:1530-2.
15. Jia Y, Tan O, Tokayer J, et al. Split-spectrum amplitude-decorrelation angiography with optical coherence tomography. Opt Express. 2012;20:4710-25.
16. Wang RK, Jacques SL, Ma Z, et al. Three-dimensional optical angiography. Opt Express. 2007;15:4083-97.
17. An L, Wang RK. In vivo volumetric imaging of vascular perfusion within human retina and choroids with optical micro-angiography. Opt Express. 2008;16:11438-52.
18. Braaf B, Vienola KV, Sheehy CK, et al. Real-time eye motion correction in phase-resolved OCT angiography with tracking SLO. Biomed Opt Express. 2013;4:51-65.
19. Choi W, Mohler KJ, Potsaid B, et al. Choriocapillaris and choroidal microvasculature imaging with ultrahigh speed OCT angiography. PLoS One. 2013;8:e81499.
20. Tokayer J, Jia Y, Dhalla AH, et al. Blood flow velocity quantification using split-spectrum amplitude-decorrelation angiography with optical coherence tomography. Biomed Opt Express. 2013;4:1909-24.
21. Ploner SB, Moult EM, Choi W, et al. Toward quantitative optical coherence tomography angiography: visualizing blood flow speeds in ocular pathology using variable interscan time analysis. Retina. 2016;36 Suppl 1:S118-26.
22. Braaf B, Vermeer KA, Vienola KV, et al. Angiography of the retina and the choroid with phase-resolved OCT using interval-optimized backstitched B-scans. Opt Express. 2012;20:20516-34.
23. Choi W, Moult EM, Waheed NK, et al. Ultrahigh-speed, swept-source optical coherence tomography angiography in nonexudative age-related macular degeneration with geographic atrophy. Ophthalmology. 2015;122:2532-44.
24. Drexler W, Sattmann H, Hermann B, et al. Enhanced visualization of macular pathology with the use of ultrahigh-resolution optical coherence tomography. Arch Ophthalmol. 2003;121:695-706.

25. Anger EM, Unterhuber A, Hermann B, et al. Ultrahigh resolution optical coherence tomography of the monkey fovea. Identification of retinal sublayers by correlation with semithin histology sections. Exp Eye Res. 2004;78(6): 1117-25.
26. Staurenghi G, Sadda S, Chakravarthy U, et al. Proposed lexicon for anatomic landmarks in normal posterior segment spectral-domain optical coherence tomography: the IN*OCT consensus. Ophthalmology. 2014;121:1572-8.
27. Jonnal RS, Kocaoglu OP, Zawadzki RJ, et al. The cellular origins of the outer retinal bands in optical coherence tomography images. Invest Ophthalmol Vis Sci. 2014;55:7904-18.
28. Srinivasan VJ, Monson BK, Wojtkowski M, et al. Characterization of outer retinal morphology with high-speed, ultrahigh-resolution optical coherence tomography. Invest Ophthalmol Vis Sci. 2008;49:1571-9.
29. Gloesmann M, Hermann B, Schubert C, et al. Histologic correlation of pig retina radial stratification with ultrahigh-resolution optical coherence tomography. Invest Ophthalmol Vis Sci. 2003;44:1696-703.
30. Toth CA, Narayan DG, Boppart SA, et al. A comparison of retinal morphology viewed by optical coherence tomography and by light microscopy. Arch Ophthalmol. 1997;115:1425-8.
31. de Carlo TE, Romano A, Waheed NK, et al. A review of optical coherence tomography angiography (OCTA). Int J Retina Vitreous. 2015;1:5.
32. Wang RK, An L, Francis P, et al. Depth-resolved imaging of capillary networks in retina and choroid using ultrahigh sensitive optical microangiography. Opt Lett. 2010;35: 1467-9.
33. Matsunaga D, Y: J, Puliatito CA, et al. OCT angiography in healthy human subjects. Ophthalmic Surg Lasers Imaging Retina. 2014;45(6):510-5.
34. Fingler J, Zawadzki RJ, Werner JS, et al. Volumetric microvascular imaging of human retina using optical coherence tomography with a novel motion contrast technique. Opt Express. 2009;17:22190-200.
35. Kim DY, Fingler J, Werner JS, et al. In vivo volumetric imaging of human retinal circulation with phase-variance optical coherence tomography. Biomed Opt Express. 2011;2:1504-13.
36. Spaide RF, Klancnik JM Jr, Cooney MJ. Retinal vascular layers imaged by fluorescein angiography and optical coherence tomography angiography. JAMA Ophthalmol. 2015;133:45-50.
37. Huang Y, Zhang Q, Thorell MR, et al. Swept-source OCT angiography of the retinal vasculature using intensity differentiation based optical microangiography algorithms. Ophthalmic Surg Lasers Imaging Retina. 2014;45:382-9.
38. Spaide RF, Koizumi H, Pozzoni MC. Enhanced depth imaging spectral-domain optical coherence tomography. Am J Ophthalmol. 2008;146:496-500.
39. Novais EA, Adhi M, Moult EM, et al. Choroidal neovascularization analyzed on ultrahigh-speed swept-source optical coherence tomography angiography compared to spectral-domain optical coherence tomography angiography. Am J Ophthalmol. 2016;164:80-8.
40. Unterhuber A, Povazay B, Hermann B, et al. In vivo retinal optical coherence tomography at 1,040 nm-enhanced penetration into the choroid. Opt Express. 2005;13:3252-8.
41. Povazay B, Hermann B, Unterhuber A, et al. Three-dimensional optical coherence tomography at 1,050 nm versus 800 nm in retinal pathologies: enhanced performance and choroidal penetration in cataract patients. J Biomed Opt. 2007;12:041211.
42. Potsaid B, Baumann B, Huang D, et al. Ultrahigh speed 1,050 nm swept source/Fourier domain OCT retinal and anterior segment imaging at 100,000 to 400,000 axial scans per second. Opt Express. 2010;18:20029-48.
43. Grulkowski I, Liu JJ, Zhang JY, et al. Reproducibility of a long-range swept-source optical coherence tomography ocular biometry system and comparison with clinical biometers. Ophthalmology. 2013;120:2184-90.
44. Mohler KJ, Draxinger W, Klein T, et al. Combined 60 degrees wide-field choroidal thickness maps and high-definition en face vasculature visualization using swept-source megahertz OCT at 1050 nm. Invest Ophthalmol Vis Sci. 2015;56: 6284-93.
45. Branchini LA, Adhi M, Regatieri CV, et al. Analysis of choroidal morphology and vasculature in healthy eyes using spectral-domain optical coherence tomography. Ophthalmology. 2013;120:1901-8.
46. Abbey AM, Kuriyan AE, Modi YS, et al. Optical coherence tomography measurements of choroidal thickness in healthy eyes: correlation with age and axial length. Ophthalmic Surg Lasers Imaging Retina. 2015;46:18-24.
47. Mrejen S, Spaide RF. The relationship between pseudodrusen and choroidal thickness. Retina. 2014;34:1560-6.
48. Gallego-Pinazo R, Dolz-Marco R, Gómez-Ulla F, et al. Pachychoroid diseases of the macula. Med Hypothesis Discov Innov Ophthalmol. 2014;3:111-5.
49. Ouyang Y, Heussen FM, Mokwa N, et al. Spatial distribution of posterior pole choroidal thickness by spectral domain optical coherence tomography. Invest Ophthalmol Vis Sci. 2011;52:7019-26.
50. Margolis R, Spaide RF. A pilot study of enhanced depth imaging optical coherence tomography of the choroid in normal eyes. Am J Ophthalmol. 2009;147:811-5.
51. Hee MR, Puliafito CA, Wong C, et al. Quantitative assessment of macular edema with optical coherence tomography. Arch Ophthalmol. 1995;113:1019-29.
52. Schuman JS, Hee MR, Puliafito CA, et al. Quantification of nerve fiber layer thickness in normal and glaucomatous eyes using optical coherence tomography. Arch Ophthalmol. 1995;113:586-96.
53. Mwanza JC, Oakley JD, Budenz DL, et al. Macular ganglion cell-inner plexiform layer: automated detection and thickness reproducibility with spectral domain-optical coherence tomography in glaucoma. Invest Ophthalmol Vis Sci. 2011;52:8323-9.

54. Lee JE, Lim DW, Bae HY, et al. Photoreceptor layer map using spectral-domain optical coherence tomography. Optom Vis Sci. 2009;86:E1320-7.
55. Gregori G, Wang F, Rosenfeld PJ, et al. Spectral domain optical coherence tomography imaging of drusen in nonexudative age-related macular degeneration. Ophthalmology. 2011;118:1373-9.
56. Yehoshua Z, Wang F, Rosenfeld PJ, et al. Natural history of drusen morphology in age-related macular degeneration using spectral domain optical coherence tomography. Ophthalmology. 2011;118:2434-41.
57. Hitzenberger C, Trost P, Lo PW, et al. Three-dimensional imaging of the human retina by high-speed optical coherence tomography. Opt Express. 2003;11:2753-61.
58. Wojtkowski M, Srinivasan V, Fujimoto JG, et al. Three-dimensional retinal imaging with high-speed ultrahigh-resolution optical coherence tomography. Ophthalmology. 2005;112:1734-46.
59. Jiao S, Knighton R, Huang X, et al. Simultaneous acquisition of sectional and fundus ophthalmic images with spectral-domain optical coherence tomography. Opt Express. 2005;13:444-52.
60. Jiao S, Wu C, Knighton RW, et al. Registration of high-density cross sectional images to the fundus image in spectral-domain ophthalmic optical coherence tomography. Opt Express. 2006;14:3368-76.
61. Gorczynska I, Srinivasan VJ, Vuong LN, et al. Projection OCT fundus imaging for visualising outer retinal pathology in non-exudative age-related macular degeneration. Br J Ophthalmol. 2009;93:603-9.
62. Nunes RP, Gregori G, Yehoshua Z, et al. Predicting the progression of geographic atrophy in age-related macular degeneration with SD-OCT en face imaging of the outer retina. Ophthalmic Surg Lasers Imaging Retina. 2013;44:344-59.
63. Forte R, Cennamo GL, Finelli ML, et al. Comparison of time domain Stratus OCT and spectral domain SLO/OCT for assessment of macular thickness and volume. Eye (Lond). 2009;23:2071-8.
64. Grover S, Murthy RK, Brar VS, et al. Comparison of retinal thickness in normal eyes using Stratus and Spectralis optical coherence tomography. Invest Ophthalmol Vis Sci. 2010;51:2644-7.
65. Pieroni CG, Witkin AJ, Ko TH, et al. Ultrahigh resolution optical coherence tomography in non-exudative age related macular degeneration. Br J Ophthalmol. 2006;90:191-7.
66. Srinivasan VJ, Wojtkowski M, Witkin AJ, et al. High-definition and 3-dimensional imaging of macular pathologies with high-speed ultrahigh-resolution optical coherence tomography. Ophthalmology. 2006;113:2054.e1-14.
67. Hwang TS, Gao SS, Liu L, et al. Automated quantification of capillary nonperfusion using optical coherence tomography angiography in diabetic retinopathy. JAMA Ophthalmol. 2016:134:367-73.
68. Agemy SA, Scripsema NK, Shah CM, et al. Retinal vascular perfusion density mapping using optical coherence tomography angiography in normals and diabetic retinopathy patients. Retina. 2015;35:2353-63.
69. Lupidi M, Coscas F, Cagini C, et al. Automated quantitative analysis of retinal microvasculature in normal eyes on optical coherence tomography angiography. Am J Ophthalmol. 2016;169:9-23.
70. Jia Y, Bailey ST, Hwang TS, et al. Quantitative optical coherence tomography angiography of vascular abnormalities in the living human eye. Proc Natl Acad Sci USA. 2015;112:E2395-402.
71. Chu Z, Lin J, Gao C, et al. Quantitative assessment of the retinal microvasculature using optical coherence tomography angiography. J Biomed Opt. 2016;21:66008.
72. Spaide RF, Curcio CA. Evaluation of segmentation of the superficial and deep vascular layers of the retina by optical coherence tomography angiography instruments in normal eyes. JAMA Ophthalmol. 2017;135:259-62.
73. Zhang A, Zhang Q, Wang RK. Minimizing projection artifacts for accurate presentation of choroidal neovascularization in OCT micro-angiography. Biomed Opt Express. 2015;6:4130-43.
74. Spaide RF, Fujimoto JG, Waheed NK. Image artifacts in optical coherence tomography angiography. Retina. 2015;35:2163-80.
75. Meuer SM, Myers CE, Klein BE, et al. The epidemiology of vitreoretinal interface abnormalities as detected by spectral-domain optical coherence tomography: the Beaver Dam Eye Study. Ophthalmology. 2015;122:787-95.
76. Duker JS, Kaiser PK, Binder S, et al. The International Vitreomacular Traction Study Group classification of vitreomacular adhesion, traction, and macular hole. Ophthalmology. 2013;120:2611-9.
77. World Health Organization. (2016). Global report on diabetes. [online] Available from http://apps.who.int/iris/bitstream/10665/204871/1/9789241565257_eng.pdf. [Accessed December, 2017].
78. Salz DA, de Carlo TE, Adhi M, et al. Select features of diabetic retinopathy on swept-source optical coherence tomographic angiography compared with fluorescein angiography and normal eyes. JAMA Ophthalmol. 2016;1334:644-50.
79. de Carlo TE, Chin AT, Bonini Filho MA, et al. Detection of microvascular changes in eyes of patients with diabetes but not clinical diabetic retinopathy using optical coherence tomography angiography. Retina. 2015;35:2364-70.
80. Otani T, Kishi S, Maruyama Y. Patterns of diabetic macular edema with optical coherence tomography. Am J Ophthalmol. 1999;127:688-93.
81. Kim BY, Smith SD, Kaiser PK. Optical coherence tomographic patterns of diabetic macular edema. Am J Ophthalmol. 2006;142:405-12.
82. Strøm C, Sander B, Larsen N, et al. Diabetic macular edema assessed with optical coherence tomography and stereo fundus photography. Invest Ophthalmol Vis Sci. 2002;43:241-5.
83. Brown JC, Solomon SD, Bressler SB, et al. Detection of diabetic foveal edema: contact lens biomicroscopy

compared with optical coherence tomography. Arch Ophthalmol. 2004;122:330-5.
84. Elman MJ, Bressler NM, Qin H, et al. Expanded 2-year follow-up of ranibizumab plus prompt or deferred laser or triamcinolone plus prompt laser for diabetic macular edema. Ophthalmology. 2011;118:609-14.
85. Michaelides M, Kaines A, Hamilton RD, et al. A prospective randomized trial of intravitreal bevacizumab or laser therapy in the management of diabetic macular edema (BOLT study) 12-month data: report 2. Ophthalmology. 2010;117:1078-86.e2.
86. de Carlo TE, Chin AT, Joseph T, et al. Distinguishing diabetic macular edema from capillary nonperfusion using optical coherence tomography angiography. Ophthalmic Surg Lasers Imaging Retina. 2016;47:108-14.
87. Mané V, Dupas B, Gaudric A, et al. Correlation between cystoid spaces in chronic diabetic macular edema and capillary nonperfusion detected by optical coherence tomography angiography. Retina. 2016;36(Suppl 1):S102-10.
88. Choi W, Waheed NK, Moult EM, et al. Ultrahigh speed swept source optical coherence tomography angiography of retinal and choriocapillaris alterations in diabetic patients with and without retinopathy. Retina. 2017;37:11-21.
89. Couturier A, Mané V, Bonnin S, et al. Capillary plexus anomalies in diabetic retinopathy on optical coherence tomography angiography. Retina. 2015;35:2384-91.
90. Peres MB, Kato RT, Kniggendorf VF, et al. Comparison of optical coherence tomography angiography and fluorescein angiography for the identification of retinal vascular changes in eyes with diabetic macular edema. Ophthalmic Surg Lasers Imaging Retina. 2016;47:1013-9.
91. Hasegawa N, Nozaki M, Takase N, et al. New insights into microaneurysms in the deep capillary plexus detected by optical coherence tomography angiography in diabetic macular edema. Invest Ophthalmol Vis Sci. 2016;57:348-55.
92. Soares M, Neves C, Marques IP, et al. Comparison of diabetic retinopathy classification using fluorescein angiography and optical coherence tomography angiography. Br J Ophthalmol. 2017;101:62-8.
93. Cennamo G, Romano MR, Nicoletti G, et al. Optical coherence tomography angiography versus fluorescein angiography in the diagnosis of ischaemic diabetic maculopathy. Acta Ophthalmol. 2017;95:e36-42.
94. Garcia JM, Lima TT, Louzada RN, et al. Diabetic macular ischemia diagnosis: comparison between optical coherence tomography angiography and fluorescein angiography. J Ophthalmol. 2016;2016:3989310.
95. Coscas G, Lupidi M, Coscas F. Optical coherence tomographic angiography in diabetic macular ischemia: a new step forward. JAMA Ophthalmol. 2016;34:373-4.
96. de Carlo TE, Bonini Filho MA, Baumal CR, et al. Evaluation of preretinal neovascularization in proliferative diabetic retinopathy using optical coherence tomography angiography. Ophthalmic Surg Lasers Imaging Retina. 2016;47:115-9.
97. Hee MR, Fujimoto JG, Ko T, el al. Interpretation of the optical coherence tomography image. In: Schuman JS, Puliafito CA, Fujimoto JG (Eds). Optical Coherence Tomography of Ocular Diseases, 2nd edition. Thorofare, NJ: Slack; 2004. pp. 21-53.
98. Spaide RF, Lee JK, Klancnik JK Jr, et al. Optical coherence tomography of branch retinal vein occlusion. Retina. 2003;23:343-7.
99. Kashani AH, Lee SY, Moshfeghi A, et al. Optical coherence tomography angiography of retinal venous occlusion. Retina. 2015;35:2323-31.
100. Falkenberry SM, Ip MS, Blodi BA, et al. Optical coherence tomography findings in central retinal artery occlusion. Ophthalmic Surg Lasers Imaging. 2006;37:502-5.
101. Chen X, Rahimy E, Sergott RC, et al. Spectrum of retinal vascular diseases associated with paracentral acute middle maculopathy. Am J Ophthalmol. 2015;160:26-34.e1.
102. Freund KB, Zweifel SA, Engelbert M. Do we need a new classification for choroidal neovascularization in age-related macular degeneration? Retina. 2010;30:1333-49.
103. Keane PA, Patel PJ, Liakopoulos S, et al. Evaluation of age-related macular degeneration with optical coherence tomography. Surv Ophthalmol. 2012;57:389-414.
104. Moult E, Choi W, Waheed NK, et al. Ultrahigh-speed swept-source OCT angiography in exudative AMD. Ophthalmic Surg Lasers Imaging Retina. 2014;45:496-505.
105. Coscas GJ, Lupidi M, Coscas F, et al. Optical coherence tomography angiography versus traditional multimodal imaging in assessing the activity of exudative age-related macular degeneration: a new diagnostic challenge. Retina. 2015;35:2219-28.
106. Shah VP, Shah SA, Mrejen S, et al. Subretinal hyperreflective exudation associated with neovascular age-related macular degeneration. Retina. 2014;34:1281-8.
107. Yannuzzi LA, Negrão S, Iida T, et al. Retinal angiomatous proliferation in age-related macular degeneration. Retina. 2001;21:416-34.
108. Freund KB, Ho IV, Barbazetto IA, et al. Type 3 neovascularization: the expanded spectrum of retinal angiomatous proliferation. Retina. 2008;28:201-11.
109. Lumbroso B, Rispoli M, Savastano MC, et al. Optical coherence tomography angiography study of choroidal neovascularization early response after treatment. Dev Ophthalmol. 2016;56:77-85.
110. Lumbroso B, Rispoli M, Savastano MC. Longitudinal optical coherence tomography-angiography study of type 2 naive choroidal neovascularization early response after treatment. Retina. 2015;35:2242-51.
111. Muakkassa NW, Chin AT, de Carlo T, et al. Characterizing the effect of anti-vascular endothelial growth factor therapy on treatment-naive choroidal neovascularization using optical coherence tomography angiography. Retina. 2015;35: 2252-9.
112. Wolf S. Optical coherence tomography. In: Holz FG, Pauleikhoff D, Spaide RF, Bird AC (Eds). Age-related Macular Degeneration, 2nd edition. Berlin-Heidelberg: Springer-Verlag; 2013. pp. 163-72.
113. Chan CK, Abraham P, Meyer CH, et al. Optical coherence tomography-measured pigment epithelial detachment

height as a predictor for retinal pigment epithelial tears associated with intravitreal bevacizumab injections. Retina. 2010;30:203-11.

114. Yannuzzi LA, Sorenson J, Spaide RF, et al. Idiopathic polypoidal choroidal vasculopathy (IPCV). Retina. 1990;10:1-8.
115. Saito M, Iida T, Nagayama D. Cross-sectional and en face optical coherence tomographic features of polypoidal choroidal vasculopathy. Retina. 2008;28:459-64.
116. Alasil T, Ferrara D, Adhi M, et al. En face imaging of the choroid in polypoidal choroidal vasculopathy using swept-source optical coherence tomography. Am J Ophthalmol. 2015;159:634-43.
117. Sikorski BL, Bukowska D, Kaluzny JJ, et al. Drusen with accompanying fluid underneath the sensory retina. Ophthalmology. 2011;118:82-92.
118. Spaide RF, Curcio CA. Drusen characterization with multimodal imaging. Retina. 2010;30:1441-54.
119. Schuman SG, Koreishi AF, Farsiu S, et al. Photoreceptor layer thinning over drusen in eyes with age-related macular degeneration imaged in vivo with spectral-domain optical coherence tomography. Ophthalmology. 2009;116:488-96.e2.
120. Curcio CA, Messinger JD, Sloan KR, et al. Subretinal drusenoid deposits in non-neovascular age-related macular degeneration: morphology, prevalence, topography, and biogenesis model. Retina. 2013;33:265-76.
121. Ouyang Y, Heussen FM, Hariri A, et al. Optical coherence tomography-based observation of the natural history of drusenoid lesion in eyes with dry age-related macular degeneration. Ophthalmology. 2013;120:2656-65.
122. Abdelfattah NS, Zhang H, Boyer DS, et al. Drusen volume as a predictor of disease progression in patients with late age-related macular degeneration in the fellow eye. Invest Ophthalmol Vis Sci. 2016;57:1839-46.
123. Zweifel SA, Engelbert M, Laud K, et al. Outer retinal tubulation: a novel optical coherence tomography finding. Arch Ophthalmol. 2009;127:1596-602.
124. Stetson PF, Yehoshua Z, Garcia Filho CA, et al. OCT minimum intensity as a predictor of geographic atrophy enlargement. Invest Ophthalmol Vis Sci. 2014;55:792-800.
125. Wu Z, Luu CD, Ayton LN, et al. Optical coherence tomography-defined changes preceding the development of drusen-associated atrophy in age-related macular degeneration. Ophthalmology. 2014;121:2415-22.
126. Schaal KB, Gregori G, Rosenfeld PJ. En face optical coherence tomography imaging for the detection of nascent geographic atrophy. Am J Ophthalmol. 2017;174:145-54.
127. Wang M, Munch IC, Hasler PW, et al. Central serous chorioretinopathy. Acta Ophthalmol. 2008;86:126-45.
128. Iida T, Hagimura N, Sato T, et al. Evaluation of central serous chorioretinopathy with optical coherence tomography. Am J Ophthalmol. 2000;129:16-20.
129. Bonini Filho MA, de Carlo TE, Ferrara D, et al. Association of choroidal neovascularization and central serous chorioretinopathy with optical coherence tomography angiography. JAMA Ophthalmol. 2015;133:899-906.

Chapter 47

Fundus Autofluorescence and Multicolor Imaging

Steffen Schmitz-Valckenberg, Monika Fleckenstein, Frank G Holz

INTRODUCTION

Fundus autofluorescence (FAF) and multicolor (MC) imaging are noninvasive diagnostic imaging modalities of the retina. Both have been introduced along with the development and clinical implementation of scanning laser ophthalmoscopy (SLO) and can be consecutively obtained using the same instrument. At the same time, FAF and MC image acquisition requires little time, allowing an easier integration into routine clinical practice.

SCANNING LASER OPHTHALMOSCOPY

The scanning laser ophthalmoscope, introduced in 1980, was first described as the "flying spot television (TV) ophthalmoscope" (Figs. 47.1A to C).[1] A single point of laser light at a specified wavelength, scanning across the retina in a series of parallel lines, provided an alternative method of capturing fundus images.[2,3] Compared to standard fundus cameras, the low-power laser beam of the SLO generates only relatively low amounts of light in both time and space; in contrast, the former uses an intense flash of light, producing a bright cone that illuminates the entire interior part of the eye at once. As a result, SLO imaging is associated with reduced light scatter. When SLO technology is applied in conjunction with confocal optics, the amount of light scatter finally reaching the detector is largely suppressed, allowing for improved image contrast and enhanced detection of signal intensities of the plane of interest (i.e. from the retina), while light originating from the cornea or lens is effectively reduced.

While the acquisition time for fundus camera photography using a single flash is only milliseconds, the frame rate for SLO imaging is longer at approximately 1–8 frames per second and varies between instruments. The longer time required for SLO imaging results in a somewhat greater risk of artifacts caused by eye movements, unstable fixation and lid blinking. However, the sophisticated eye tracking technology used by the modern SLO system allows for automated registration and correction of these potentially interfering factors.[4] As a matter of fact, this can even constitute an advantage for enhancing the signal-to-noise ratio by averaging multiple image frames, which even further increases sensitivity. Finally, it also permits spatial correlation with findings obtained by other imaging modalities, especially spectral domain optical coherence tomography (SD-OCT).

In current systems, SLO imaging typically employs blue, green, and/or near-infrared monochromatic laser light for excitation. Recently, a clinical confocal SLO system was introduced that uses not monochromatic light but a broader spectrum of light for excitation by means of two different light emitting diode (LED) light sources (Eidon, CenterVue SpA; Padova, Italy). SLO reflectance imaging is based on the pure detection of reflected light from the eye. In addition, SLO also allows visualization of fluorescence phenomena by excitation of either exogenous (e.g. fluorescein or indocyanine green angiography) or endogenous (e.g. FAF) fluorophores with specific wavelengths and the subsequent detection of the generated fluorescence. This is achieved by blocking the reflective light in the optical path by means of barrier filters. These filters ensure that mainly the longer wavelength fluorescent light finally is captured by the detector.

FUNDUS AUTOFLUORESCENCE IMAGING

Overview

Fundus autofluorescence imaging allows for metabolic mapping of naturally or pathologically occurring fluorophores of the ocular fundus (Figs. 47.1A to C).[5-8] The physical principle is identical to that of fluorescein or indocyanine green angiography (i.e. molecules are brought to glow by excitation of light within a certain wavelength range). The main difference is that FAF imaging is based

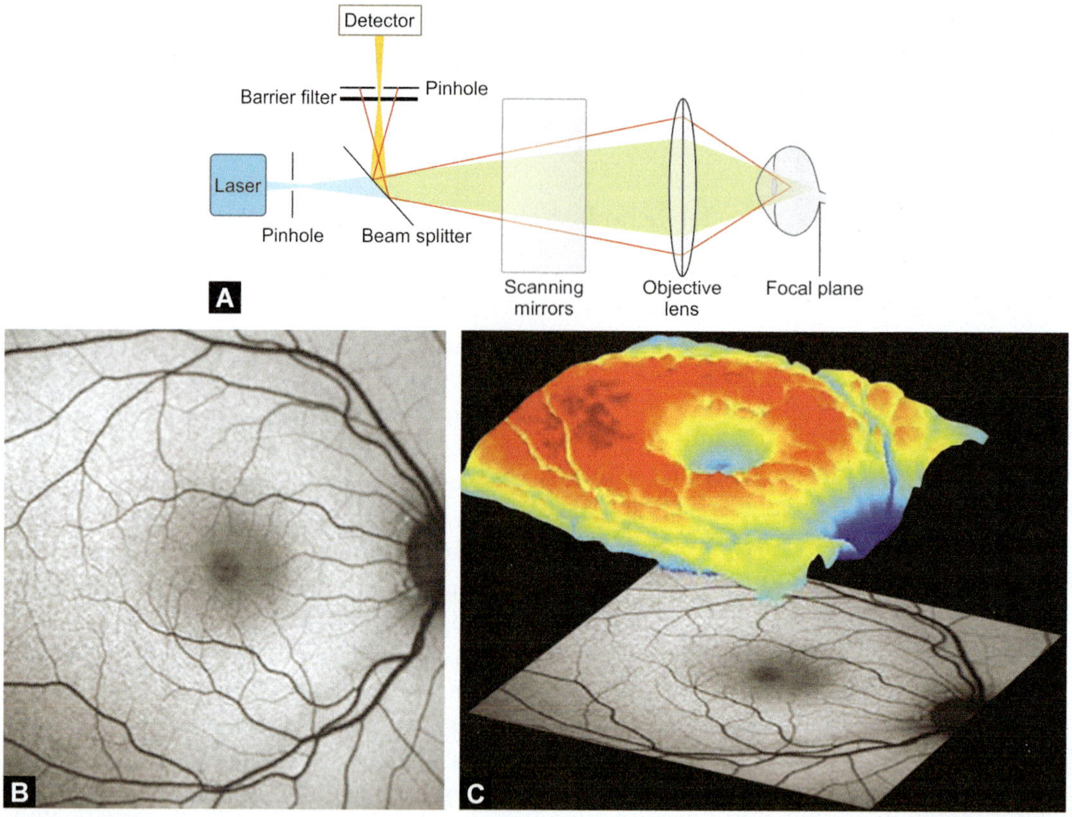

Figs. 47.1A to C: (A) Principle of the confocal scanning laser ophthalmoscope. The laser is focused through a pinhole diaphragm to the focal plane (blue light). The reflected laser light is separated by a beam splitter from the incident laser beam path and is deflected through a second pinhole to reach a photosensitive detector (yellow light). Light originating outside the focal plane is effectively suppressed by the pinhole; (B and C) Normal fundus autofluorescence (FAF) images obtained with a confocal scanning laser ophthalmoscope. The FAF image shows the spatial distribution of the intensity of the FAF signal for each pixel in gray values. By definition, low pixel values (dark portion) illustrate low intensities, and high pixel values (bright) illustrate high intensities. In the normal subject, dark appearing retinal vessels due to absorption from blood contents, a dark optic nerve head due to absence of autofluorescent material, and a relatively decreased signal in the macular area secondary to absorption of luteal pigment can be observed. The relative distribution of FAF intensities can also be illustrated in pseudo three-dimensional reconstruction techniques (C). Areas with low FAF intensities are shown in blue and can be distinguished from the normal background signal (red).

on visualization of endogenous fluorophores, while angiography is based on detection of exogenous molecules. Hence, no intravenously injected agent is required for FAF imaging—the molecules are already available. The second important difference between FAF and angiography is that the FAF signal intensity is much weaker at about two orders of magnitude lower than the background of a fluorescein angiogram at the most intense part of the dye transit. Further, short-wavelength light, which is mainly used as excitation light for FAF imaging, is typically absorbed by nuclear opacities of the crystalline lens. This brownish-yellowing of the lens, which typically occurs with increasing age, can be regarded as a "perfect filter" of blue excitation light, interfering with the detection of autofluorescence intensities at the posterior pole. Overall, the low intensity of the FAF signal and the interference of the crystalline lens require a sensitive imaging system, a perquisite well addressed by the gold standard for FAF imaging—the confocal SLO.

Two important aspects should be considered when applying FAF imaging in the clinical setting. In contrast to OCT, the field of application for FAF is much smaller. Therefore, a prerequisite for using FAF imaging is knowing which situation warrants its use and may even allow identification of key findings for clinical management. Second, FAF imaging should not be regarded as a stand-alone diagnostic tool but should always be used in conjunction with clinical presentation, and particularly with clinical findings by ophthalmoscopy. Additional value is achieved by combining FAF with other imaging modalities, so-called multimodal imaging. In this context, a typical example is the assessment of foveal sparing in geographic atrophy.[9] While FAF imaging is usually very helpful for detecting atrophic areas, the use of FAF imaging alone to assess foveal sparing by atrophy can be challenging because of interference from macular pigment (see later). In this case, the use of corresponding near-infrared reflectance SLO images or OCT is particularly helpful.

Clinical Application

The main application of FAF imaging is to visualize changes at the level of the retinal pigment epithelium (RPE)/photoreceptor complex, because the signal both originates in and is influenced by this retinal layer. While the photopigment of the outer photoreceptor segments acts as a filter of the excitation light, the main source (i.e. the dominant fluorophore) of the FAF signal is lipofuscin, which accumulates as a degradation product of the visual cycle in the lysosomal compartment of RPE cells (Fig. 47.2).[5,10] Lipofuscin is a "biococktail" of different molecules, including retinoid-derived components such as A2E (*N*-retinylidene-*N*-retinylethanolamine) and photo-oxidized derivatives that accumulate in the RPE as byproducts of the visual cycle, increasing both with increasing age and with certain retinal diseases. A2E and its derivatives are chemically characterized by extensive systems of conjugated double bonds, which give them their distinct fluorescent properties.

In accordance to the origin of the signal, FAF imaging is used specifically for retinal diseases associated with changes at the level of the RPE/photoreceptor complex.[6,7] These include age-related macular degeneration (AMD) and other degenerative retinal diseases, such as hereditary retinal dystrophies (e.g. Stargardt disease, variants of retinitis pigmentosa) and acquired maculopathies (e.g. chloroquine maculopathy). Further, FAF imaging may also be used as a screening method for patients with unknown visual impairment in order to gain a rapid and noninvasive overview of the "RPE-Health" status. Before patients are sent to a time-consuming functional test such as electrophysiology or visual field testing, a central FAF scan can be helpful in evaluating for unknown visual loss.

A second clinical application for FAF imaging is the visualization of changes in the distribution of macular pigment deposition. In the physiological state, luteal pigment (i.e. zeaxanthin and lutein) is predominantly located in the inner retinal layers in the fovea and parafoveal area.[11,12] This macular pigment acts as a yellow filter and has been postulated both to improve the optical accuracy of the macula and to reduce damaging photo-oxidative influence on the neurosensory retina. In FAF imaging, macular pigment partially blocks the short-wavelength excitation light. Because less excitation light reaches the

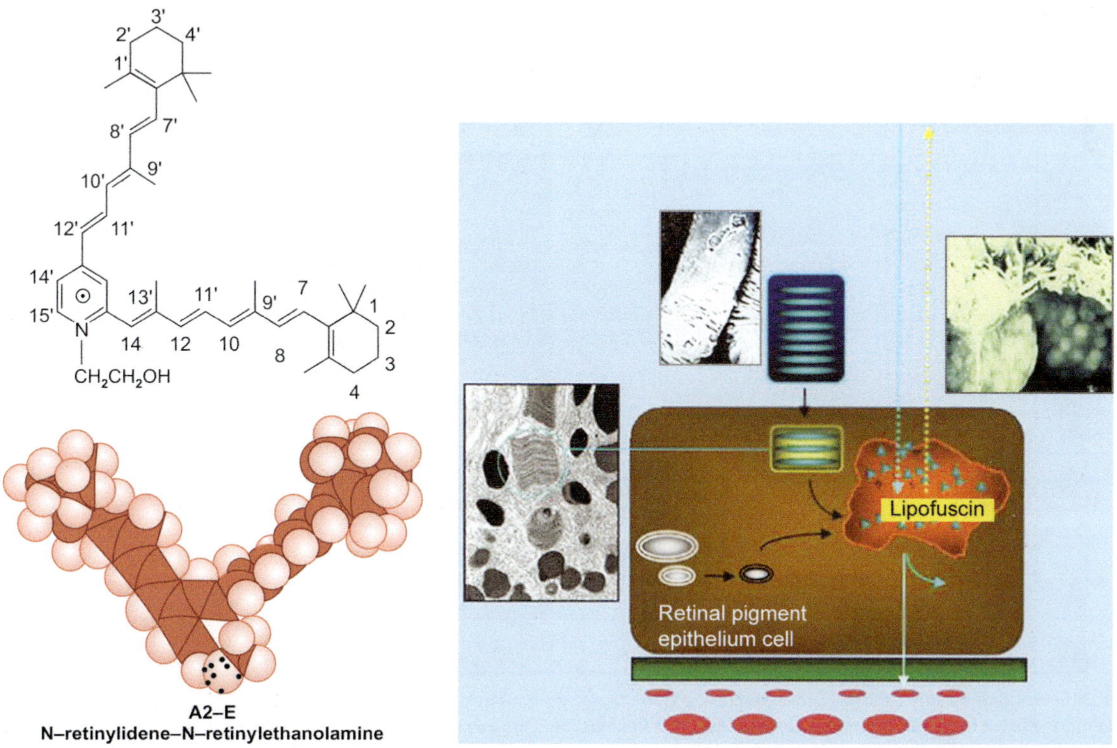

Fig. 47.2: Lipofuscin is considered a "biococktail", consisting of different molecules, including retinoid-derived components such as A2E (*N*-retinylidene-*N*-retinylethanolamine) that accumulate in the retinal pigment epithelium as a byproduct of the visual cycle.

more posterior retinal layers (i.e. outer retina and RPE), less fluorescence light is generated. Finally, a relatively reduced FAF signal is detected in the region of the fovea and parafovea. Macular pigment may condense between intraretinal cystoid cavities in macular edema or schisis, resulting in levels of increased FAF intensities at the site of cystoid cavities. In situations, such as in foveal hypoplasia or macular telangiectasia (MacTel) type 2, there may be a congenital absence or depletion of the macular pigment (Figs. 47.3A to D).[13,14]

A key advantage of FAF imaging is that changes are often more prominent and more visible with a rapidly acquired FAF image than with a clinical examination or with other noninvasive imaging techniques (Figs. 47.3A to D). This may be helpful for establishing a diagnosis, for creating a differential diagnosis, or for refined phenotyping. For example, FAF imaging can help distinguish AMD from late-onset macular dystrophies that mimic the typical age-related changes.

Fundus autofluorescence imaging is mainly a method to visualize changes in the above-mentioned anatomical areas. This also includes monitoring both the natural disease course and the response to therapy over time. In this context, it is noteworthy that the high lateral resolution of confocal scanning laser ophthalmoscope (cSLO) FAF imaging allows precise and ready mapping of the

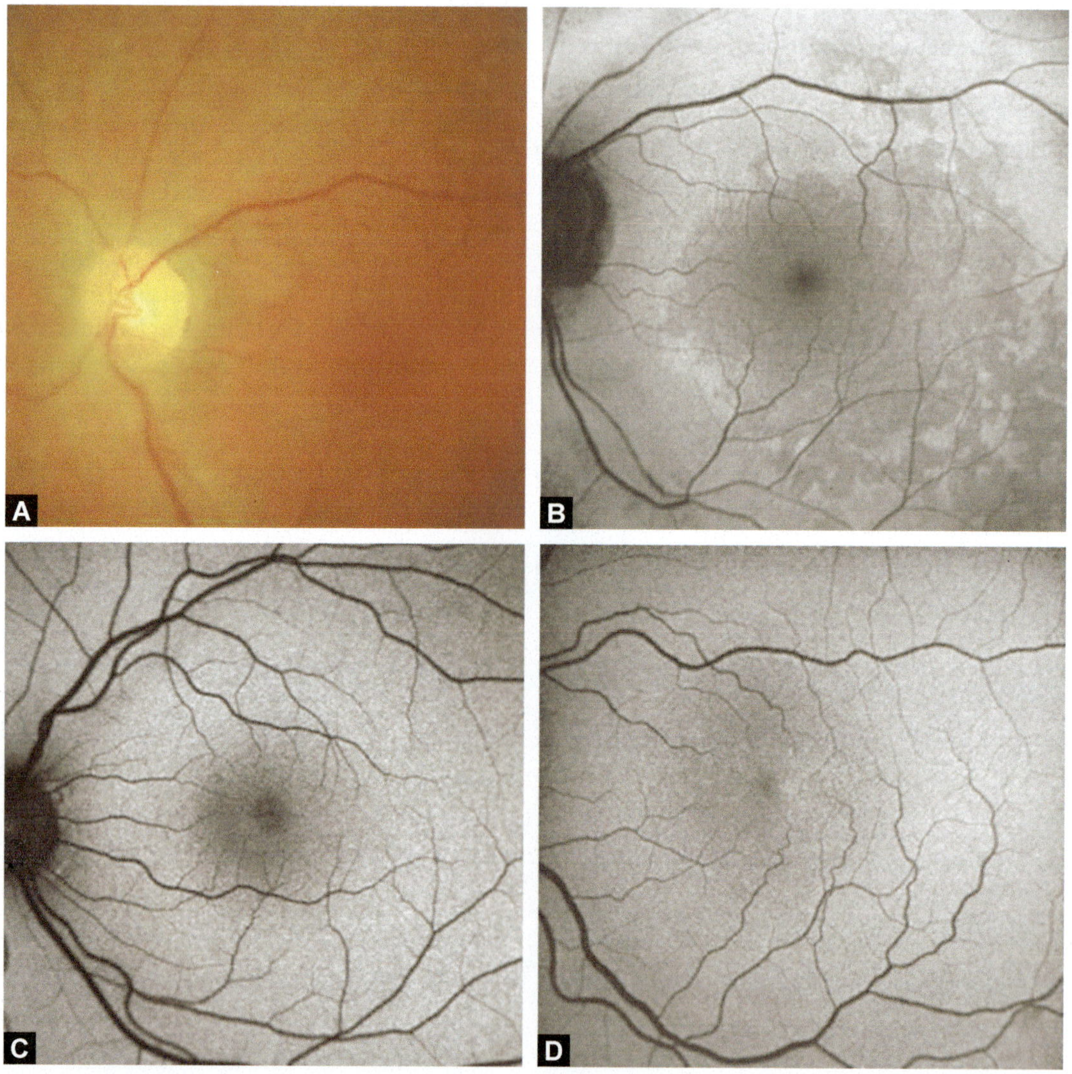

Figs. 47.3A to D: Early diagnosis by fundus autofluorescence (FAF) imaging: Patient with severe retinitis pigmentosa sine pigmento. (A) Color fundus photography is inconclusive (questionable waxy disk, no foveal reflex); (B) FAF shows severe abnormalities. Visual field testing confirms that the central lobular areas demarcated by FAF actually represent the preserved retina. Diagnosis was confirmed by severely reduced scotopic and photopic Ganzfeld-electroretinography; (C) Assessment of macular pigment. In normal subject, relatively decreased intensities are visible by FAF imaging due to macular pigment absorption; (D) In early macular telangiectasia, macular pigment is depleted.

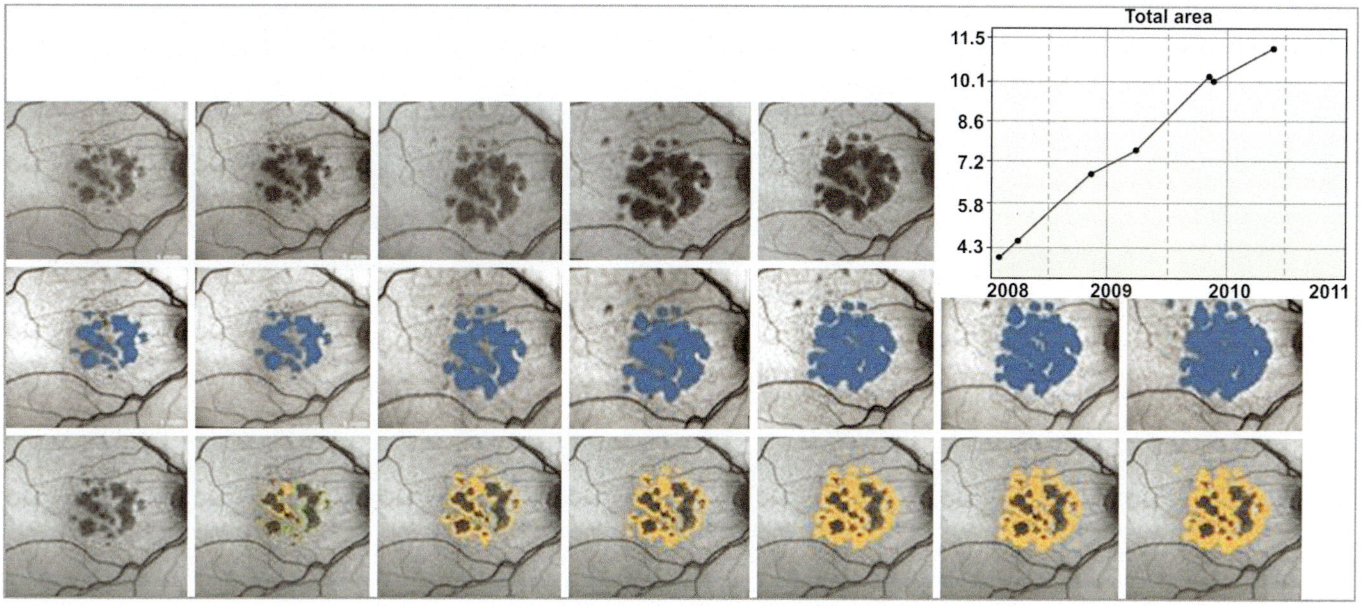

Fig. 47.4: Detection, quantification, and progression of atrophic areas in geographic atrophy secondary to age-related macular degeneration by confocal scanning laser ophthalmoscopy fundus autofluorescence imaging and using customized image analysis software (RegionFinder®; Heidelberg Engineering GmbH, Germany).

planimetric dimensions of retinal lesions. For example, FAF imaging is helpful for detecting and quantifying atrophic areas and for the application of image analysis processing software (Fig. 47.4). Another advantage of FAF imaging is the detection of prognostic markers for the future spread of atrophy. Both a greater extent of areas with abnormal FAF and specific FAF patterns are associated with a more rapid progression of atrophy in following years.[15,16]

Interpretation

The FAF image shows the spatial distribution of the intensity of the FAF signal for each pixel in gray values (arbitrary values from 0 to 255) (*see* Figs. 47.1A and B). Per definition, low pixel values (dark) illustrate low intensities and high pixel values (bright) illustrate high intensities. The topographical distribution of FAF in normal eyes demonstrates a consistent pattern. A diffuse FAF signal can be seen over the posterior pole, while retinal vessels (due to an absorption phenomenon by blood contents, i.e. hemoglobin) and the optic nerve head (absence of autofluorescent material) are characterized by a very low signal and appear dark. When a nonconfocal system is used in patients with nuclear opacities of the lens, the optic nerve head may appear more greyish than black with a more intense diffuse background signal in the surrounding retinal areas (Figs. 47.5A to C). These observations are typical for pseudofluorescence phenomena caused by the generation of secondary long-wavelength reflectance light as the excitation light is partially absorbed within the optical pathway, particularly by the lens. This secondary reflectance light is scattered within the vitreous cavities and again reflected, particularly by the optic nerve head, back through the lens. If a nonconfocal system is used, this confounding signal is not blocked. Therefore, the signal bypasses the barrier filter and finally reaches the detector.

Showing a high degree of interindividual variability, decreased FAF intensities are observed at the macular area with a minimum in the fovea. These decreased intensities are caused by the absorption of short-wavelength light due to luteal pigment (lutein and zeaxanthin). Other contributing factors may be an increased accumulation of melanin and a decreased deposition of lipofuscin granules.[5]

Typical ratios between the intensity of the fovea and perifoveal macula have been established using pixel gray values in normal subjects.[7] Qualitative descriptions of localized FAF changes based on these findings are widely used. Usually, the FAF signal over a certain retinal location is categorized in decreased, normal, or increased intensity in comparison to the background signal of the same image. Table 47.1 shows different causes of an abnormally increased or decreased FAF signal. This systematic overview might be helpful to classify any localized FAF signal alterations, although interpretation of FAF images is usually based mainly on pattern recognition.

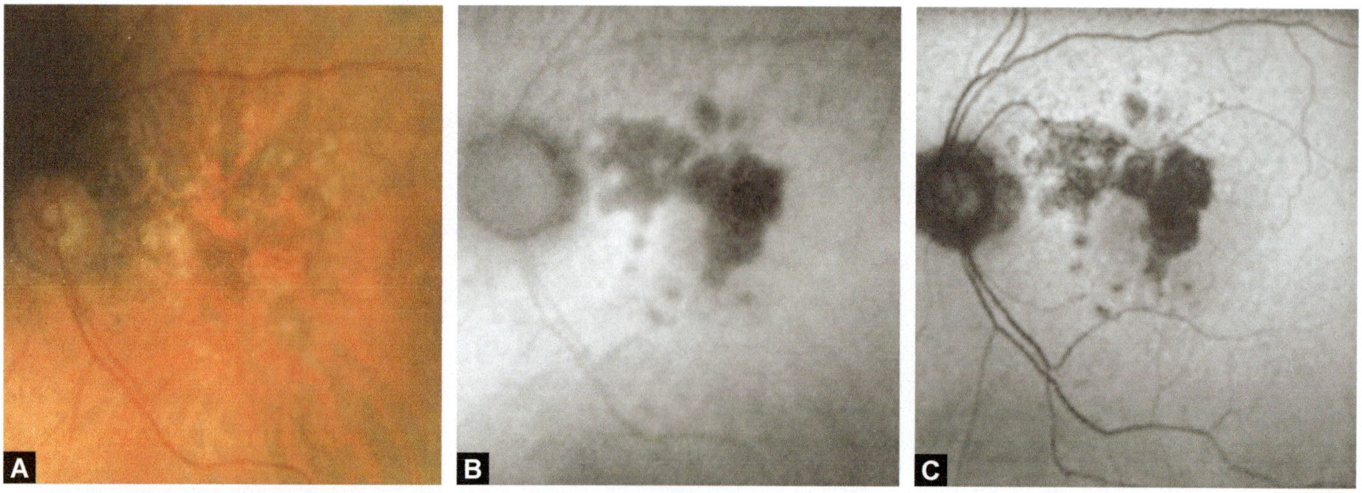

Figs. 47.5A to C: (A) Color fundus camera photograph; (B) Fundus camera autofluorescence photograph; and (C) Confocal scanning laser ophthalmoscopy (cSLO) fundus autofluorescence (FAF) image of the left eye in a patient with geographic atrophy secondary to age-related macular degeneration and an advanced age-related nuclear sclerosis of the lens. The size and configuration of atrophic areas can be better seen with both fundus autofluorescence images as compared to color fundus photography. The signal-to-noise ratio for fundus camera autofluorescence is inferior compared to cSLO FAF imaging. Please note the relatively bright signal of the optic nerve head and a more intense background signal in the surrounding areas of the optic nerve head with fundus camera autofluorescence photography (B). These observations are considered to be artifacts caused by secondary reflectance light generated by partial absorption of the excitation light by the lens.

Table 47.1: Causes of decrease or increase in fundus autofluorescence signal.

Causes for a reduced FAF signal	Causes for an increased FAF signal
Absence/reduction in RPE lipofuscin density • RPE atrophy • Increased RPE melanin content • Local changes in retinal dystrophies	Excessive RPE lipofuscin accumulation • Lipofuscinopathies including Stargardt's disease, Best's disease, and adult vitelliform macular dystrophy • Age-related macular degeneration, e.g. RPE in the junctional zone preceding enlargement of occurrence of geographic atrophy
Absorption from extracellular material/cells/ fluid anterior to the RPE	Lack of absorbing material, loss of photopigment, prolonged exposure to excitation light ("bleaching")
Migrated melanin-containing cells	Occurrence of fluorophores anterior or posterior to the RPE cell monolayer
Intersections of petaloid configuration in macula edema due to macular pigment displacement	Cystoid cavities of the petaloid configuration in macula edema due to displacement of macular pigment
Fresh intra- and subretinal hemorrhages	Subretinal fluid leading to separation of the outer segments of the photoreceptors from the underlying RPE leading to improper outer segment turnover
Intra- and subretinal lipid	Macrophages contained lipofuscin in the subretinal space (choroidal tumors such as nevi and melanomas)
Fibrosis, scar tissue, and borders of laser scars	Drusen in the subpigment epithelial space
Retinal vessels	Migrated RPE cells or macrophages containing lipofuscin or melanolipofuscin (seen as pigment clumping or hyperpigmentation on funduscopy)
Luteal pigment (lutein and zeaxanthin)	Older intra- and subretinal hemorrhages
Media opacities (vitreous, lens, anterior chamber, and cornea)	Choroidal vessel in the presence of RPE and choriocapillaris atrophy, e.g. in the center of laser scars or within patches of RPE atrophy
	Depletion of luteal pigment, e.g. in idiopathic macular telangiectasia type 2 Displacement of luteal pigment, e.g. cystoid macular edema
	Optic nerve head drusen
	Artifacts

(FAF: Fundus autofluorescence; RPE: Retinal pigment epithelium)

In contrast, the quantification of absolute intensities and their comparison, either between subjects or through longitudinal observation in the same subject, are more complicated and remain a challenge in FAF imaging. Of note, as the pixel histogram in the usual available cSLO images is normalized to better visualize the topographic distribution of the FAF intensity, the pixel values are not absolute and these images must not be used for absolute intensity analyses from the outset. Furthermore, when interpreting FAF images, one should take into account that the digital resolution of the detector in current imaging devices exceeds the maximum spatial resolution of ocular media and the optics of the system, mainly due to high-order aberrations. Therefore, single pixel values of a standard FAF image do not reflect the actual anatomical resolution of the image and should not be used to compare intensities between different locations. This also explains why increasing the digital resolution of the detector does not usually improve the resolution of the actual image, but rather results in an artificially high-resolution and posterized image.

When absolute intensities on averaged but non-normalized FAF images are analyzed (after ensuring that the normalization of the pixel histogram is turned off), a great variability of the mean gray value for a certain retinal location is usually noted when FAF images are subsequently acquired from the same subject, directly one after the other, using the same imaging device.[17]

Several confounding factors must be considered when comparing absolute FAF intensities between different examinations and different individuals. This includes standardization not only of settings (laser power, detector sensitivity, correction of refractive errors, and image-processing steps including the number of averaged images), but also of eye movements, position of the patient in the chin rest, orientation of the camera, distance between the camera and the cornea, subtle variations in the illumination of the frame, fluctuations of laser power, and short-term dynamic changes in FAF intensities caused by prolonged exposure to the excitation light or previous dark adaption.[7]

Correlation with Retinal Function

Observations obtained by FAF imaging are also particularly helpful for correlation with retinal function. This includes the lesion boundary discrimination of atrophic areas and thus, detection of scotomata in the presence of geographic atrophy. Further, lines of increased FAF intensities in the form of parafoveal rings in patients with retinitis pigmentosa or cone dystrophy may help demarcate retinal regions with normal function from those with markedly impaired or lost function (Figs. 47.6A and B).[18,19] Additionally, the shrinkage (usually in retinitis pigmentosa) or the enlargement (cone dystrophies and inflammatory diseases) of rings of increased FAF can be monitored over time.

Further Developments

More recently, imaging systems for peripheral FAF visualization (i.e. far beyond the vascular arcades; so-called "wide-angle imaging") have become available.[20,21] Early observations point to advantages similar to those of "central" FAF imaging: pure visualization, detection and monitoring of changes at the level of the RPE/photoreceptor complex, such as retinal atrophy that may be spatially confined to functional impairment (visual field deficits). An interesting aspect is the observation of peripheral FAF signal alterations and longitudinal changes in patients with presumed "macular diseases" (Fig. 47.7). Another development is quantitative autofluorescence (qAF) imaging.[22] Going beyond the mere qualitative description of local signal alterations, this allows for measurement of absolute signal intensities between patients as well as of dynamic longitudinal changes in the same individual. While qAF imaging appears to require high-quality standards for imaging protocols, recent reports have demonstrated that qAF imaging allows reliable detection of both normal age-dependent signal alterations and excessive signal enhancements in patients with retinal degenerations such as Stargardt disease.[23]

Originally, FAF imaging was mainly used with blue excitation light and measured the fluorescence signal in the green-yellow region. Even if this so-called, "blue" FAF imaging with short-wave excitation light is the standard in clinical application. FAF imaging with longer wavelength excitation light and subsequent detection of longer-wave emission spectra (e.g. green or near-infrared FAF imaging) is now easily feasible in the clinical setting. Recently, green excitation FAF has gained interest as it is associated with more patient comfort and is less affected by macular pigment absorption, which is helpful for assessing foveal sparing in atrophic AMD.

Limitations

Several limitations and disadvantages of the use of FAF imaging need to be considered. It represents a separate procedure, which means that time must be allocated in the clinical routine, and funds must be allocated for acquisition and maintenance costs. Pupil dilation is usually necessary to acquire good quality images. The short-wave excitation light

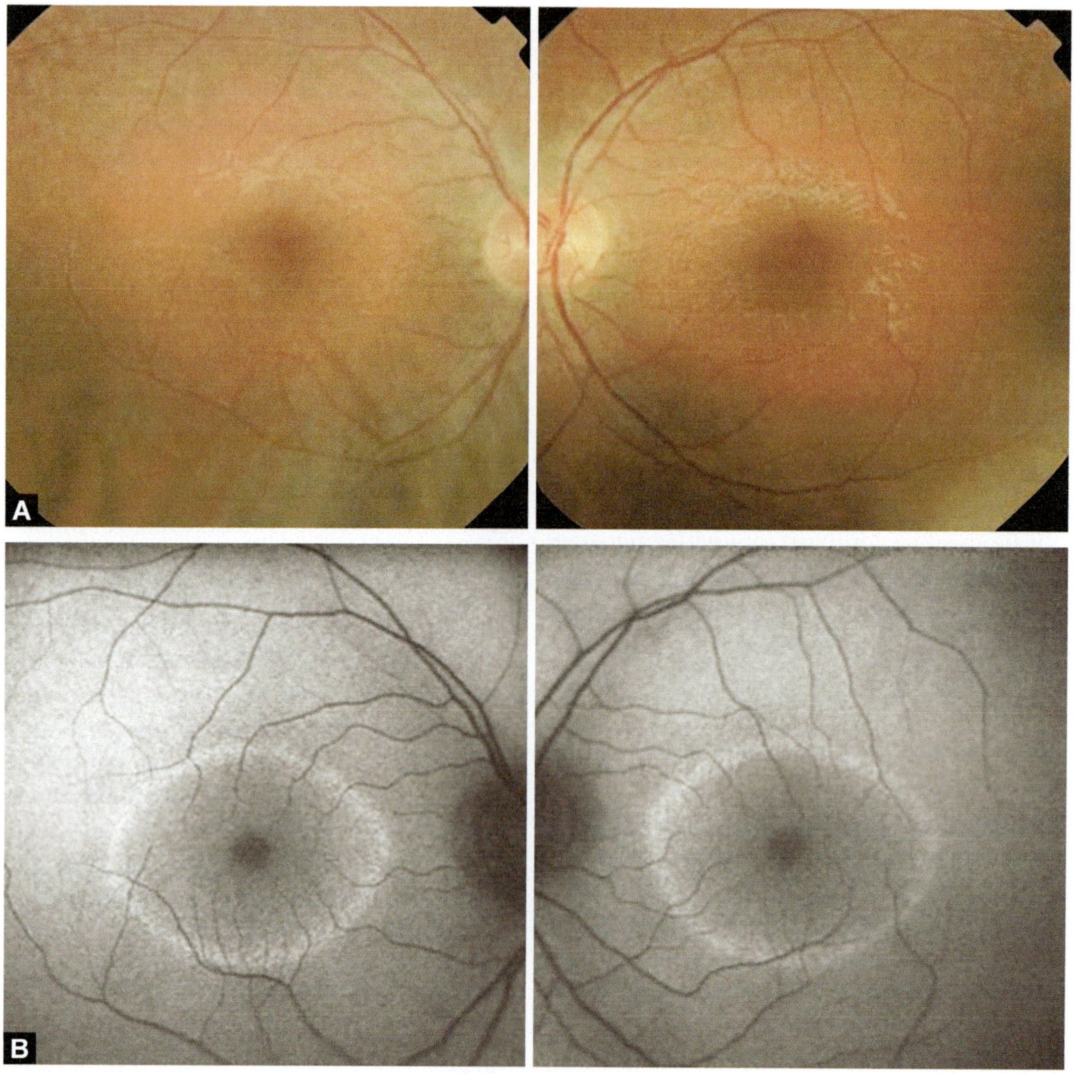

Figs. 47.6A and B: (A) Color fundus photograph and (B) confocal scanning laser ophthalmoscopy fundus autofluorescence (FAF) imaging of both eyes of a patient with retinitis pigmentosa. The detection by a parafoveal ring with increased FAF intensities allows for early diagnosis. Further, the location of the ring demarcates preserved retinal function within the center of the ring.

may be unpleasant for the patient, especially in comparison to the longer-wave excitation light used in OCT imaging. A further challenge in the use of short-wavelength light is the sensitivity to the typical yellow-brownish discoloration of the eye lens (nuclear cataract) with increasing age (as mentioned above). Aside from patient discomfort from the excitation light during acquisition, no detection of toxic light damage after FAF imaging has been reported in humans thus far; and wide application is very possible with modern imaging systems. FAF imaging is a safe procedure for clinical routine, the benefits and advantages of which have been confirmed several times over the past few years. It adds to our armamentarium for diagnosing and managing patients, and has numerous promising future applications.

MULTICOLOR IMAGING

Using monochromatic laser light for SLO imaging allows detection of single-wavelength reflectance light of the ocular fundus, while a typical color fundus camera photograph is based on the full or almost full spectrum of visible light. The inability to obtain an image of the ocular fundus similar to how it is seen during clinical examination is typically regarded as a disadvantage of SLO imaging, particularly when performing multimodal imaging using one instrument and spatially correlating findings from one modality to another. Furthermore, the use of one instrument is also attractive in terms of time savings during diagnostic imaging and improved cost-effectiveness in clinical practice.

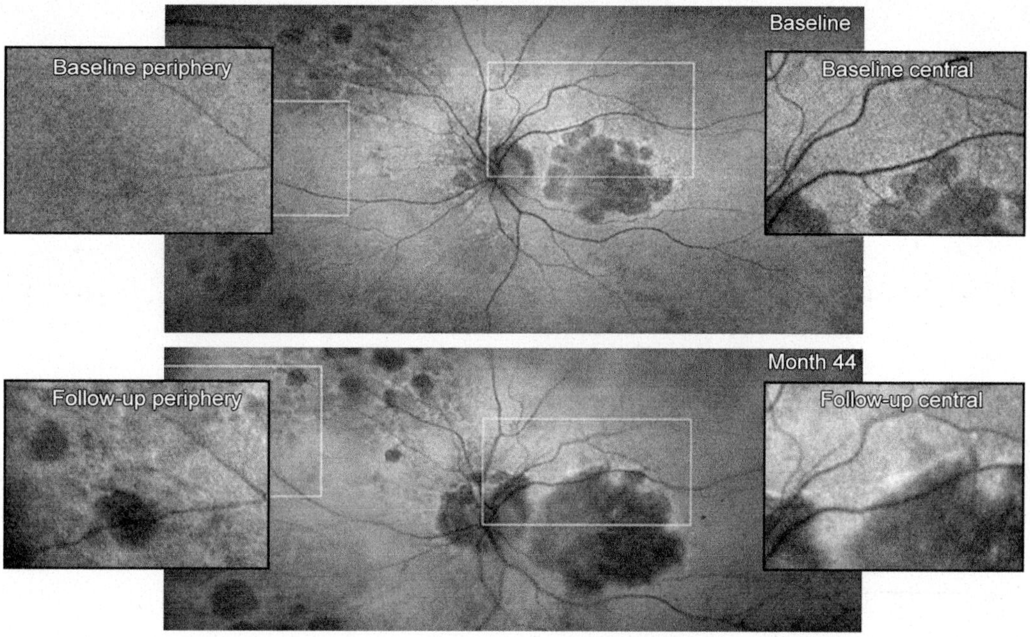

Fig. 47.7: Wide-field autofluorescence imaging in the left eye in a patient with geographic atrophy secondary to age-related macular degeneration. In addition to presence and progression of central atrophy, peripheral areas of atrophy are present at baseline. After approximately 3.5 years (44 months), both development of new as well as spread of existing peripheral atrophic spots is visible.

A combination of different reflectance modes by SLO imaging has been developed to allow the acquisition of so-called "MC", "pseudocolor", or "true-color" images that will better resemble the typical visualization by ophthalmoscopy. The exact technical setup differs between various systems of different manufacturers. For example, for MC imaging, the Spectralis SD-OCT (Heidelberg Engineering GmbH; Heidelberg, Germany) uses three rapidly acquired consecutive reflectance images using three monochromatic laser sources [blue reflectance (488 nm), green reflectance (515 nm), and near-infrared reflectance (820 nm)].[24] The information obtained using these three modalities is then used to generate a MC image. The Optomap (Optos plc; Dunfermline, Scotland) employs two different monochromatic laser sources without the use of confocal optics [green channel (532 nm) and red channel (633–635 nm)]. A bright spectrum of light is used by the Eidon (CenterVue SpA; Padova, Italy), with an LED light source (440–650 nm) rather than a laser used for excitation.

For the clinical application, it is important to consider that short-wavelength light is reflected more on the surface of the retina, while longer wavelength excitation usually achieves deeper tissue penetration. Therefore, blue reflectance particularly allows visualization of the details of the inner retina and the vitreoretinal interface, such as epiretinal membranes, retinal nerve fiber layer thinning, and macular pigment changes. Green reflectance images specifically allow deeper details, such as retinal blood vessels and intraretinal lipid exudation, to be seen. Infrared reflectance predominantly visualizes structures at the level of the outer retina and choroid, including drusen and RPE alterations.[25,26] Due to the laws of optics, the reflectance is reduced at the site of physiological or pathological structures that have a color similar to the excitation light of the reflectance mode applied. For example, small hemorrhages may be missed by near-infrared reflectance light and are better visible with blue reflectance light. Different lesions may appear "artificial" or "not real" by SLO-based MC imaging compared to clinical examination. In the clinical setting, the better visualization of structures may be appreciated. Further, compared to conventional fundus camera photography, visualization of a brownish-dark pigmented lesion might be especially different from SLO-based "multi"-or "pseudocolor" imaging.

The use of SLO-based MC imaging instead of conventional color camera fundus photography offers several advantages. These include the ability to improve the signal-to-noise ratio by averaging multiple frames, reduction of artifacts, and spatial correlation to findings of other modalities. If confocal optics are used, the reduction of scattered light—particularly in eyes with media opacities such as cataracts—can result in "sharper" images with superior discrimination of retinal structures and lesion boundaries.

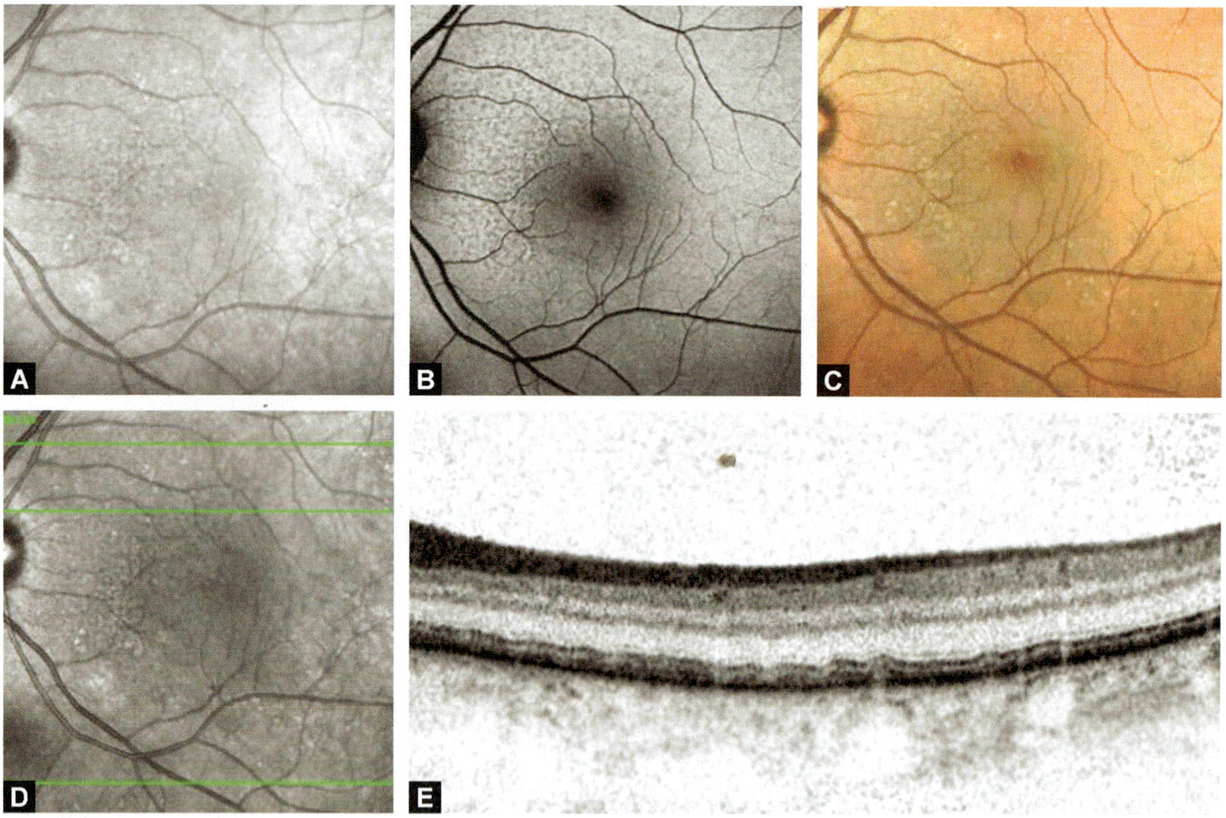

Figs. 47.8A to E: Images of reticular drusen by combined confocal scanning laser ophthalmoscopy and spectral domain optical coherence tomography (SD-OCT). (A to C) Near-infrared reflectance mode, fundus autofluorescence, and multicolor imaging; (D and E) Horizontal SD-OCT B-scan—the green line on the corresponding near-infrared reflectance images indicated the location of the B-scan superior to the fovea.

In eyes with AMD, SLO-based MC imaging is particularly helpful for detecting hemorrhages that might be overlooked when using only near-infrared light (see above). Of note, OCT imaging is also based on near-infrared light and is therefore relatively nonspecific and not sensitive enough to detect small retinal bleeds. Small, subtle lesions that represent a high risk for disease progression, such as reticular pseudodrusen/subretinal drusenoid deposits (SDD), can be imaged more readily and distinctly (Figs. 47.8A to E). The boundaries of atrophic areas are also typically more clearly demarcated compared to conventional color fundus camera photography.

In patients with epiretinal membranes or vitreoretinal interface abnormalities such as macular traction in proliferative diabetic retinopathy, SLO-based MC imaging not only offers the advantage of using the same instrument as for SD-OCT imaging; it also typically gives a superior en face overview of the disease manifestation, including tractional membranes and retinal wrinkling (Fig. 47.9). This visualization can be helpful for monitoring changes over time as well as for decision making, planning, and assessment of surgical success.

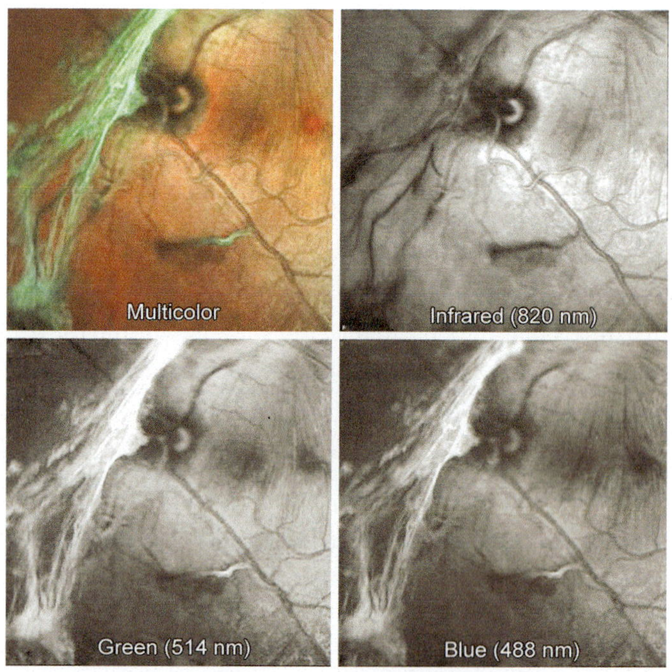

Fig. 47.9: Confocal scanning laser ophthalmoscopy multicolor imaging in the left eye with tractional diabetic retinopathy. With the three different reflectance modes combined, the multicolor image is helpful for assessment of extent and location of epiretinal membranes.

REFERENCES

1. Webb RH, Hughes GW, Pomerantzeff O. Flying spot TV ophthalmoscope. Appl Opt. 1980;19:2991-7.
2. Manivannan A, Van der Hoek J, Vieira P, et al. Clinical investigation of a true color scanning laser ophthalmoscope. Arch Ophthalmol. 2001;119:819-24.
3. Keane PA, Sadda SR. Retinal imaging in the twenty-first century: state of the art and future directions. Ophthalmology. 2014;121:2489-500.
4. Helb HM, Charbel Issa P, Fleckenstein M, et al. Clinical evaluation of simultaneous confocal scanning laser ophthalmoscopy imaging combined with high-resolution, spectral-domain optical coherence tomography. Acta Ophthalmol. 2010;88:842-9.
5. Delori FC, Dorey CK, Staurenghi G, et al. In vivo fluorescence of the ocular fundus exhibits retinal pigment epithelium lipofuscin characteristics. Invest Ophthalmol Vis Sci. 1995;36:718-29.
6. Holz FG, Schmitz-Valckenberg S, Spaide RF, et al. Atlas of Fundus Autofluorescence Imaging. Berlin: Springer; 2007.
7. Schmitz-Valckenberg S, Holz FG, Bird AC, et al. Fundus autofluorescence imaging: review and perspectives. Retina. 2008;28:385-409.
8. von Rückmann A, Fitzke FW, Bird AC. Distribution of fundus autofluorescence with a scanning laser ophthalmoscope. Br J Ophthalmol. 1995;79:407-12.
9. Lindner M, Boker A, Mauschitz MM, et al. Directional kinetics of geographic atrophy progression in age-related macular degeneration with foveal sparing. Ophthalmology. 2015;122:1356-65.
10. Sparrow J. Lipofuscin of the retinal pigment epithelium. In: Holz FG, Schmitz-Valckenberg S, Spaide RF, Bird AC (Eds). Atlas of Fundus Autofluorescence Imaging. Berlin, Heidelberg: Springer; 2007.
11. Wolf-Schnurrbusch UE, Roosli N, Weyermann E, et al. Ethnic differences in macular pigment density and distribution. Invest Ophthalmol Vis Sci. 2007;48:3783-7.
12. Robson AG, Moreland JD, Pauleikhoff D, et al. Macular pigment density and distribution: comparison of fundus autofluorescence with minimum motion photometry. Vision Res. 2003;43:1765-75.
13. Helb HM, Charbel Issa P, Van Der Veen R, et al. Abnormal macular pigment distribution in type 2 idiopathic macular telangiectasia. Retina. 2008;28:808-16.
14. Schmitz-Valckenberg S, Fan K, Nugent A, et al. Correlation of functional impairment and morphological alterations in patients with group 2A idiopathic juxtafoveal retinal telangiectasia. Arch Ophthalmol. 2008;126:330-5.
15. Schmitz-Valckenberg S, Bindewald-Wittich A, Dolar-Szczasny J, et al. Correlation between the area of increased autofluorescence surrounding geographic atrophy and disease progression in patients with AMD. Invest Ophthalmol Vis Sci. 2006;47:2648-54.
16. Holz FG, Bindewald-Wittich A, Fleckenstein M, et al. Progression of geographic atrophy and impact of fundus autofluorescence patterns in age-related macular degeneration. Am J Ophthalmol. 2007;143:463-72.
17. Lois N, Halfyard AS, Bunce C, et al. Reproducibility of fundus autofluorescence measurements obtained using a confocal scanning laser ophthalmoscope. Br J Ophthalmol. 1999;83:276-9.
18. Robson AG, Michaelides M, Saihan Z, et al. Functional characteristics of patients with retinal dystrophy that manifest abnormal parafoveal annuli of high density fundus autofluorescence; a review and update. Doc Ophthalmol. 2007;116:79-89.
19. Fleckenstein M, Charbel Issa P, Helb HM, et al. Correlation of lines of increased autofluorescence in macular dystrophy and pigmented paravenous retinochoroidal atrophy by optical coherence tomography. Arch Ophthalmol. 2008;126:1461-3.
20. Heussen FM, Tan CS, Sadda SR. Prevalence of peripheral abnormalities on ultra-widefield greenlight (532 nm) autofluorescence imaging at a tertiary care center. Invest Ophthalmol Vis Sci. 2012;53:6526-31.
21. Duisdieker V, Fleckenstein M, Zilkens KM, et al. Long-term follow-up of fundus autofluorescence imaging using wide-field scanning laser ophthalmoscopy. Ophthalmologica. 2015;234:218-26.
22. Delori F, Greenberg JP, Woods RL, et al. Quantitative measurements of autofluorescence with the scanning laser ophthalmoscope. Invest Ophthalmol Vis Sci. 2011;52: 9379-90.
23. Duncker T, Lee W, Tsang SH, et al. Distinct characteristics of inferonasal fundus autofluorescence patterns in Stargardt disease and retinitis pigmentosa. Invest Ophthalmol Vis Sci. 2013;54:6820-6.
24. Tan AC, Fleckenstein M, Schmitz-Valckenberg S, et al. Clinical application of multicolor imaging technology. Ophthalmologica. 2016;236:8-18.
25. Pang CE, Freund KB. Ghost maculopathy: an artifact on near-infrared reflectance and multicolor imaging masquerading as chorioretinal pathology. Am J Ophthalmol. 2014;158:171-8.e2.
26. Alten F, Clemens CR, Heiduschka P, et al. Characterisation of reticular pseudodrusen and their central target aspect in multi-spectral, confocal scanning laser ophthalmoscopy. Graefes Arch Clin Exp Ophthalmol. 2014;252:715-21.

Chapter 48 Diabetic Retinopathy and Macular Edema

Marques JP, Cunha-Vaz J

EPIDEMIOLOGY OF DIABETIC RETINOPATHY

Data from the 2015 International Diabetes Federation Atlas report that diabetes mellitus (DM) affects 415 million people worldwide.[1] Fueled by the progressive aging of the population, increased caloric consumption and sedentary lifestyle,[2] this number is projected to ascent to 640 million by 2040,[1] making diabetes as one of the largest global health issues of the 21st century.

Diabetic retinopathy (DR) is among the most frequent microvascular complications of DM.[3] The prevalence of DR is considerably higher in type 1 than in type 2 DM, irrespective of the diabetes duration.[4,5] In fact, after 20 years of disease, more than 60% of patients with type 2 and virtually every patient with type 1 DM show at least some degree of retinopathy.[6] Global prevalence estimates indicate an overall age-standardized prevalence of DR of 34.6%.[4] Fortunately, vision-threatening complications—diabetic macular edema (DME) and proliferative diabetic retinopathy (PDR)—are far less frequent, affecting approximately one-tenth of the diabetic population.[4] Nevertheless, DR is the leading cause of severe vision impairment and blindness in working-age adults in the Western World[3] and DME is the most common cause of vision loss due to diabetes, accounting for 12% of new cases of blindness each year.[7] The relative risk of blindness in diabetic patients is approximately five times the risk of those without diabetes, even after adjusting for potential confounders such as age, sex, race, educational level, blood pressure, smoking, and body mass index.[8] The impact of visual impairment goes far beyond the individual, posing a significant burden in the communities and creating a need for increased social and economic support.[9] The major epidemiologic challenge for the years to come is to combat the spread of obesogenic lifestyles in order to decrease the incidence and prevalence of DM and its inherent complications.

DIAGNOSTIC METHODS

Since diabetes-related vision loss is an undisputable sign of advanced stage retinopathy, visual acuity (VA) alone is not an adequate method to detect or monitor early stages of the disease. At this point, the retinal changes may still be reversible and, therefore, amenable to medical therapy, metabolic control and lifestyle changes. Consequently, a timely diagnosis of DR is vital to avoid its vision-threatening complications.

The diagnosis of DR is usually readily established by fundus examination through slit-lamp biomicroscopy, direct ophthalmoscopy, or indirect ophthalmoscopy. The hallmark lesions are microaneurysms (MAs), hemorrhages, venous beading, hard exudates, cotton wool spots, intraretinal microvascular abnormalities (IRMAs), and new vessels (Fig. 48.1). The fundoscopic findings depend on the severity of the DR, ranging from scarce MAs in mild nonproliferative DR to florid neovascularization, hemovitreous and tractional retinal detachment in PDR.

Although rarely needed to establish the diagnosis, multimodal retinal imaging proves useful to evaluate progression over time, to guide therapeutic decisions, and to monitor treatment response.[10] Ancillary diagnostic tests include color fundus photography (CFP), fluorescein angiography (FA), and optical coherence tomography (OCT).

Color Fundus Photography

Color fundus photography has long been used in clinical trials and screening programs of DR.[11-13] Since regular surveillance by clinical examination of the retina presents a huge challenge to ophthalmology departments, teleophthalmology strategies using CFP were developed to identify sight-threatening DR and to prevent vision loss by promoting a timely referral. Because many of the diabetic clinically significant retinal changes occur around the disk and posterior pole, a single 30–40° field shot encompassing

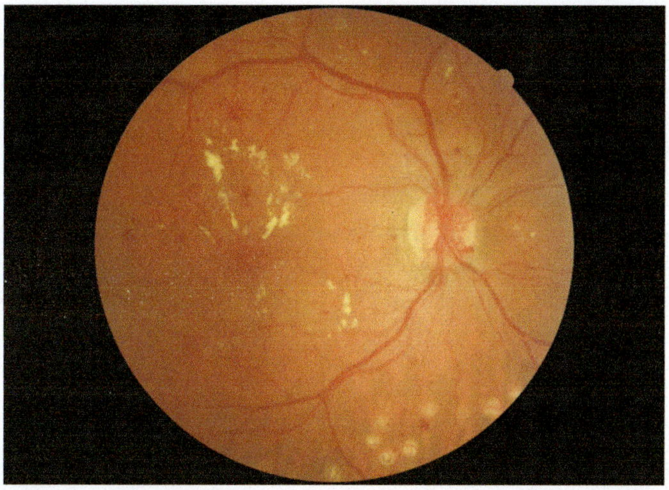

Fig. 48.1: Color fundus photography of a patient with proliferative diabetic retinopathy. Prominent disk neovascularization is seen, as well as microaneurysms, hemorrhages, and hard exudates in the macular region. Outside the inferior temporal vascular arcade, laser photocoagulation marks can be perceived.

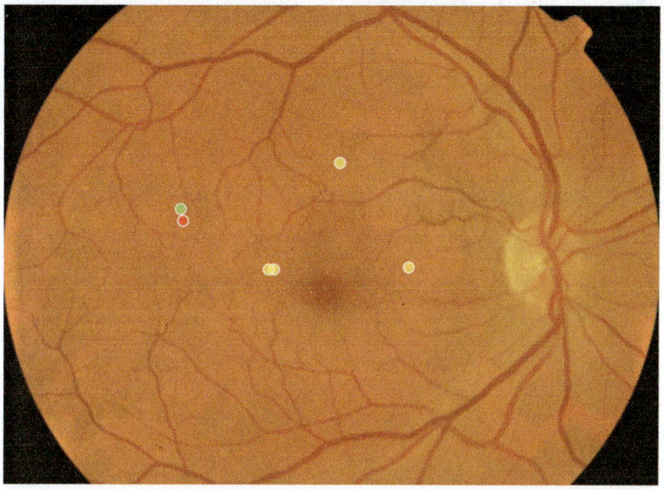

Fig. 48.2: Printscreen of automated diabetic retinopathy (DR) grading using RetmarkerDR® (Retmarker SA; Coimbra, Portugal). The software highlights the number of microaneurysms (MAs) found in a follow-up visit. The colors identify which MAs are new (red), old (green), or no longer visible (yellow) in this visit.

the macula, the optic disk and the major vascular arcades is now the standard for photographic composition [identified as field 2 of the Early Treatment of Diabetic Retinopathy Study (ETDRS) protocol].

National screening programs for DR are effective, but are also labor and economically demanding, as they depend on the availability of trained human graders.[14] This led to the development of automated retinal image analysis systems (ARIAS) (Fig. 48.2). A recent study demonstrated that 2 ARIAS—RetmarkerDR® (Retmarker SA; Coimbra, Portugal) and EyeArt® (Eyenuk Inc; Woodland Hills, CA)—were cost-effective alternatives to a purely manual grading.[14]

Fluorescein Angiography

Fluorescein angiography remains the gold standard for the in vivo evaluation of the retinal circulation as it allows visualization of the vessel architecture, blood flow, and leakage from damaged/diseased retinal capillaries.[15] However, the invasive nature of the procedure limits its repeated use due to possible (although rare) side effects related to the intravenous injection of fluorescein.[16,17]

Fluorescein angiography has historically been used to assess the severity of DR, to determine sites of leakage in macular edema (focal versus diffuse DME), to evaluate the extent of macular and peripheral capillary nonperfusion, and to confirm the presence and extent of neovascularization (Figs. 48.3A to C).[18] Currently, Ultra-Widefield (UWF) FA devices allow capture of a single high-resolution 200° retinal field covering more than 80% of the retinal surface while all vessels are in the same angiographic phase. The nonperfusion identified on UWF FA in diabetic eyes with DR is located primarily in the midperipheral retina, heading posteriorly with increasing severity of the disease. Peripheral nonperfusion likely underlies the development of predominantly peripheral lesions and accounts for the marked increase in retinopathy progression associated with these changes.[19] However, since diabetes is associated with accelerated aging,[20] age-related peripheral poor perfusion should be taken into account, particularly in type 2 DM.

Optical Coherence Tomography and Optical Coherence Tomography Angiography

The advent of OCT revolutionized retinal imaging by providing a fast, simple, and noninvasive method to assess retinal structure at a microscopic level.[21,22] Time-domain (e.g. Stratus OCT) systems were rapidly replaced by spectral-domain (SD) OCT platforms. These systems convey fast scanning speeds and eye tracking, leading to the acquisition of noninvasive, in vivo, high-resolution cross-sectional images that approach histological sections of the retina.[21-23] Refinements included in enhanced depth imaging (EDI) and swept-source (SS) OCT systems brought deeper penetration and improved signal strength in the choroid; thus, facilitating a qualitative and quantitative assessment of this structure.[24] Besides qualitative information on the

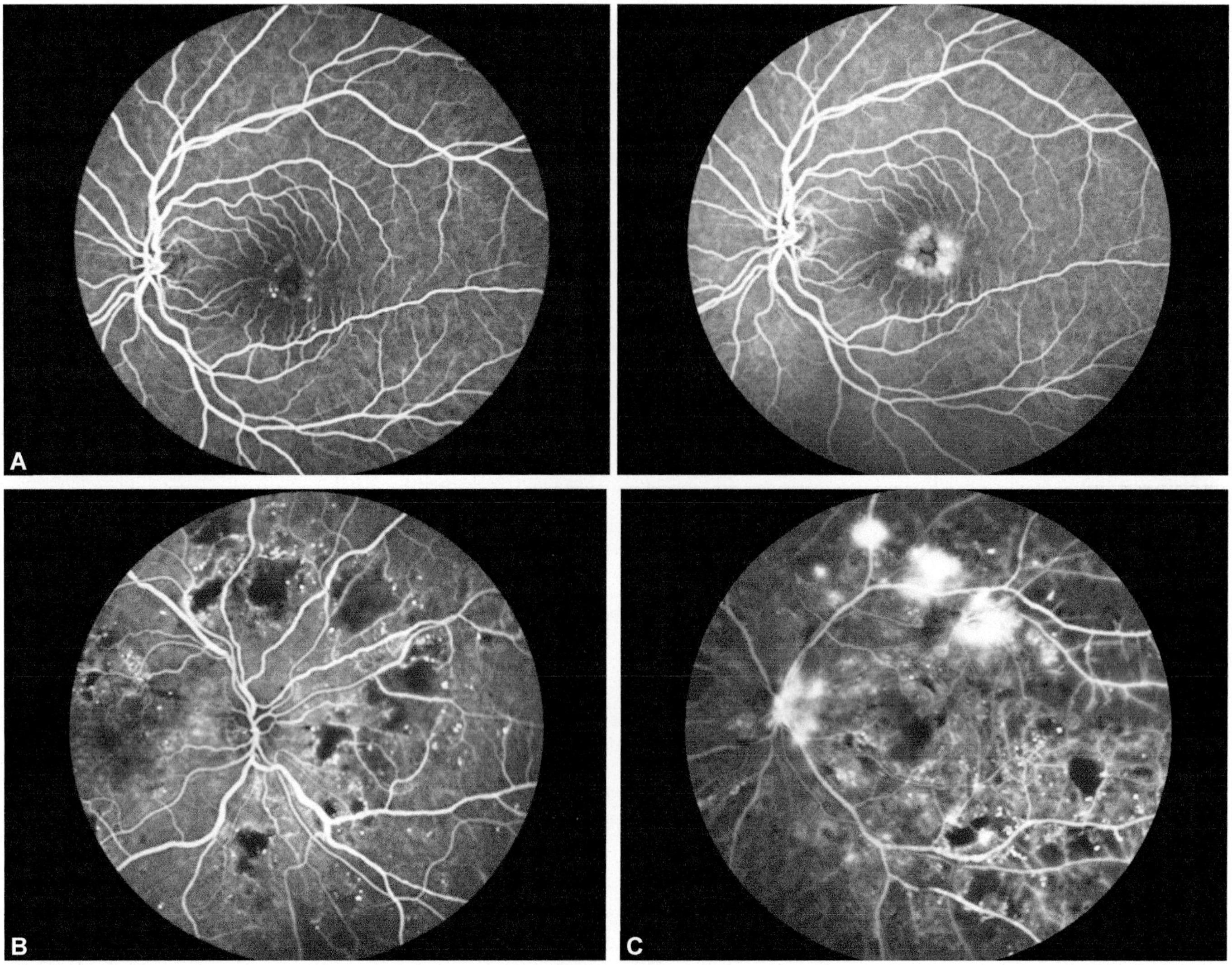

Figs. 48.3A to C: Fluorescein angiography. (A) Early and late frames depicting cystoid diabetic macular edema. Note the petaloid pattern of hyperfluorescence that increases throughout the exam (left to right); (B) A case of severe nonproliferative diabetic retinopathy where several areas of peripheral nonperfusion (black) can be seen; (C) Proliferative diabetic retinopathy with neovascularization in the disk (NVD) and neovascularization elsewhere (NVE), along with severe nonperfusion.

macular architecture and the vitreomacular interface, OCT enables accurate measurement of the retinal thickness and volume and has become indispensable in the management of DME. OCT is used to confirm the presence and identify the morphology of DME, to guide treatment decisions and to monitor treatment effects over time (Fig. 48.4). OCT changes in DME begin with diffuse retinal thickening with a sponge-like appearance of the retinal layers due to retinal extracellular fluid accumulation that further progresses to the typical hyporeflective cystoid spaces.[25] Subretinal fluid accumulation and vitreomacular traction are easily identified with OCT.

The recent introduction of OCT angiography (OCTA) represents a new era of OCT development and a true extension of capabilities from SD-OCT. Eyes with DR show a sparse capillary network with perifoveal areas of capillary nonperfusion surrounded by vascular loops (Figs. 48.5A to F). Vascular density and choroidal flow are decreased when compared to controls, and the foveal avascular zone is large and irregular, with loss of its usual centripetal arrangement.[26] Several studies have shown that the microvascular changes of DR are more obvious in the deep rather than the superficial retinal plexus. Neovascularization at the optic disc or at the posterior pole can also be imaged

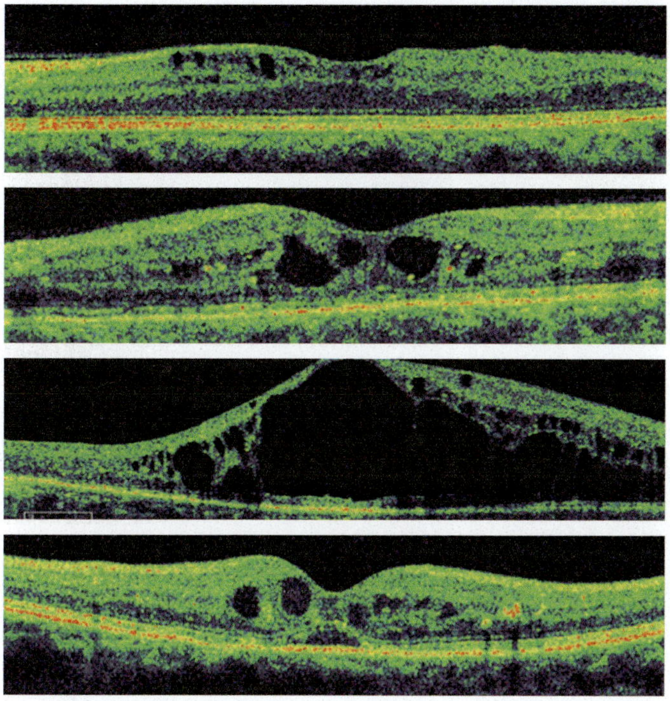

Fig. 48.4: Different examples of spectral-domain optical coherence tomography (SD-OCT) in diabetic macular edema. Note the presence of cysts in the inner retinal layers (top); in the outer retinal layers (top middle tomogram); in both the inner and outer retinal layers (bottom middle tomogram); and subretinal fluid accumulation along with cysts in the outer retinal layers (bottom).

with OCTA. In fact, OCTA is gradually replacing FA as a more sensitive and noninvasive alternative for a detailed evaluation of central macular vascular changes in DR.[27]

A recently developed technology, OCT leakage (OCT-L), was shown to accurately locate and quantitatively evaluate retinal extracellular fluid, in both intra- and subretinal fluid accumulations. OCT-L identifies fluid leakage by recognizing lower than normal optical reflectivity ratios.[28] The complementarity between OCT-L and OCTA is highly promising to achieve a fully noninvasive approach in the management of DR.

NATURAL EVOLUTION OF DIABETIC RETINOPATHY: ETDRS SEVERITY GRADING

Natural History: Severity Grading

Diabetic retinopathy has long been considered a microvascular complication of diabetes. The retinal changes observed in the retina may be associated with progressive cell degeneration and vasoregression or with dysfunction of the blood-retinal barrier (BRB). Abnormalities of the BRB, demonstrated both by FA and vitreous fluorometry, were found to be early evidence of DR, in both human and experimental DR models.[29,30] For a long time, this limited the diagnostic and therapeutic focus to the vascular system. However, recent evidence points towards a neurovascular coupling in DR with significant involvement of both the neuronal and the vascular compartments.[31]

The chronopathology of DR is slow and can be separated into four overlapping clinical stages: (1) retinal damage without any visible microvascular abnormalities in the fundus; (2) nonproliferative retinal microvascular changes (mild and moderate nonproliferative DR with or without DME); (3) more advanced preproliferative changes (severe nonproliferative DR); and (4) PDR and advanced stages of DR. Fundoscopically, the abnormalities seen in DR can conceptually be split into three categories: (1) findings associated with leakage from diseased microvasculature (hemorrhages, lipid exudates, intraretinal, and/or subretinal fluid accumulation); (2) findings associated with structural damage to the microvasculature wall (MA); and (3) findings associated with hypoperfusion and ischemia with subsequent overproduction of cytokines and vascular growth factors (cotton wool spots, IRMAs, preretinal neovascularization, fibrous proliferation, and vitreous hemorrhage).[32] The degree of retinal involvement by each of these findings has been used to quantify the severity of DR using CFP. The original Airlie House classification used five photographic fields. With the Diabetic Retinopathy Study (DRS), a modified Airlie House classification system was developed. The latter uses seven photographic fields and adds more levels of severity, aiming to better evaluate the progression to PDR. Similarly, the ETDRS created a classification to answer whether early treatment with scatter photocoagulation in PDR was beneficial. The ETDRS severity scale became the gold standard for grading the severity of DR in clinical trials. Although laborious and complicated, the DR ETDRS level allows an accurate prediction of the chance of developing high-risk PDR. However, some limitations exist. For instance, a patient presenting with moderate nonproliferative DR (level 47) carries a 1-year risk of developing high-risk PDR of 8.6%, whereas on the next step (level 53), this number rises to 45%. Therefore, a small difference in the numerical level of severity (47–53) results in a substantially higher risk (8.6–45%). When reviewing the ETDRS data, the Global DR Project Group realized that IRMAs and venous beading were significantly better predictors for the progression to

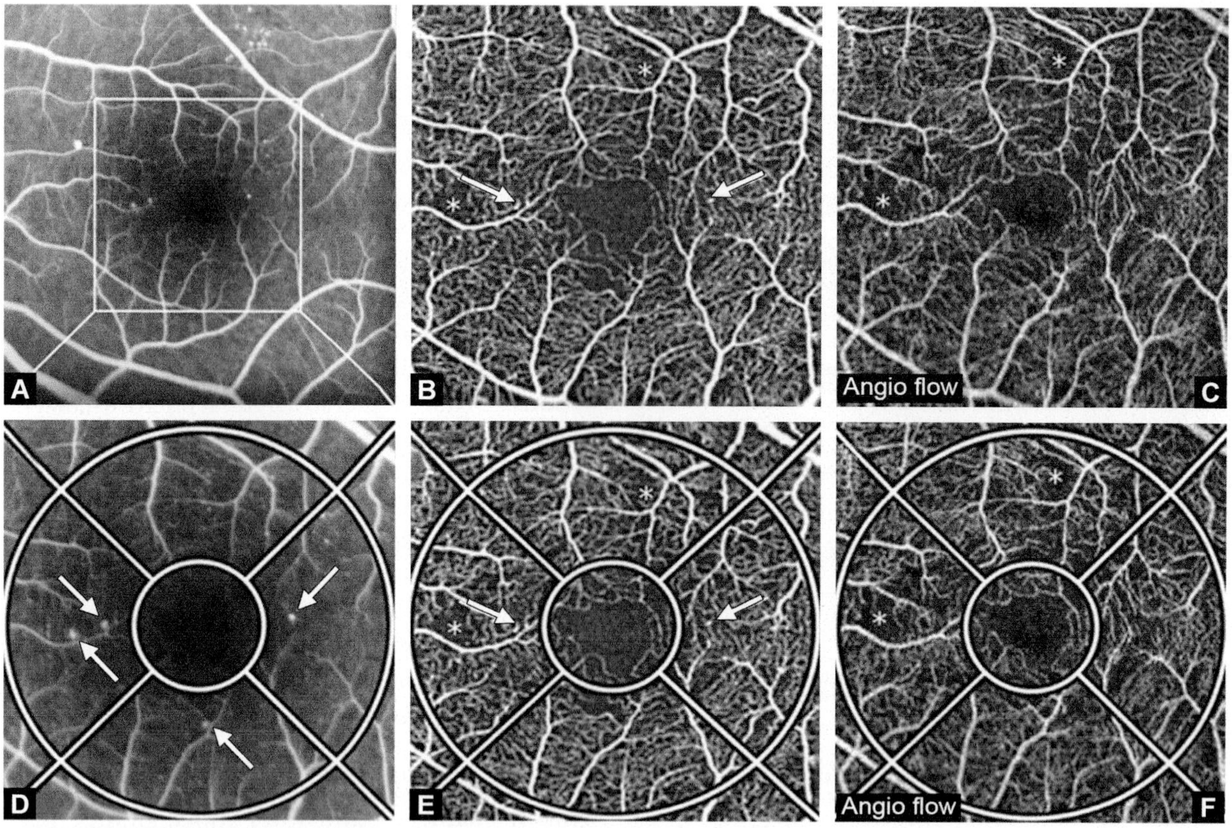

Figs. 48.5A to F: Comparison of fluorescein angiography (FA) with optical coherence tomography angiography (OCTA) images for the superficial retinal layer (AngioPlex—middle column and AngioVue—right column). (A) Early 20° FA image. The white square outlines the area of the 3 × 3 mm graded for this study; (B) 3 × 3 mm OCT angiogram obtained from Zeiss AngioPlex showing areas of nonperfusion (asterisk) and microaneurysms (arrows); (C) 3 × 3 mm OCT angiogram obtained from AngioVue showing the same areas of nonperfusion found for AngioPlex images, but with no evidence of microaneurysms; (D) Magnification of the 3 × 3 mm square with grid overlaid. Arrows show a higher number of microaneurysms seen on FA in comparison with AngioPlex and AngioVue; (E and F) 3 × 3 mm angiograms from AngioPlex and AngioVue are overlaid with grid replicating the central subfield and inner ring of the ETDRS grid.

Source: Used with permission from Soares M, Neves C, Marques IP, et al. Comparison of diabetic retinopathy classification using fluorescein angiography and optical coherence tomography angiography. Br J Ophthalmol. 2017;101(1):62-8.

PDR than MAs and hemorrhages. Another limitation of the ETDRS classification was that macular edema was not considered. A new classification, allegedly easier to use and including macular edema was proposed. However, it did not prove useful due to the increasing availability of OCT, which offers a better characterization of DME. Also, the final result did not translate into clinical practice and lost the advantages of the ETDRS classification to predict progression to proliferative retinopathy.

During the early stages of nonproliferative DR, MAs, small hemorrhages and hard/soft exudates dominate the clinical picture and are the only changes acknowledged in the first four levels (10–43) of the ETDRS classification. MA counting has been suggested as an appropriate marker for the progression of DR.[33] We must, however, realize that MA formation and disappearance is a dynamic process usually referred to as MA turnover. Hellstedt and Immonen[34] observed 395 new MAs and the disappearance of 258 previously identified MAs, using FA in a 2-year follow-up study of 24 type 1 diabetic patients with mild background DR. Several investigators aimed to identify functional retinal changes preceding MA formation and it is now widely accepted that subtle changes in microvascular hemodynamics are one of the earliest findings in DR.[35-38] However, it is still not clear why these changes are sometimes different in eyes of patients with the same level of retinopathy, metabolic control, and duration of the disease.[39] The advent of OCTA has minimized the technical difficulties associated with measuring retinal blood flow in humans and will most certainly contribute to a deeper knowledge of the pathophysiology of DR in the near future.

Vision loss related to DR is associated with the two major complications of DR—DME and PDR, and it does not occur before one of these develops. This is a crucial concept. Thus, DME and PDR are the two most clinically meaningful outcomes in DR. The identification of biomarkers (imaging, genetic, metabolic, etc.) that predict the progression towards these two sight-threatening outcomes remains an unmet medical need.

SYSTEMIC AND OCULAR FACTORS INFLUENCING DIABETIC RETINOPATHY PROGRESSION

Systemic Factors

Identified and widely accepted risk factors for the development and progression of DR include the duration of diabetes, glycemic control, and arterial hypertension.[4]

Glycemic control is a key factor influencing the microvascular changes associated with diabetes, including DR. The effect of poor glycemic control is apparent in both type 1 and type 2 DM, with a sharp increase in the incidence, prevalence, and severity of DR.[40-43] Periods of poor glycemic control have adverse effects on the progression of retinopathy known to persist far beyond the period of poor control. On the other hand, the benefits of intensive control seem to persist even when the intensity of the control is less tight,[44] an effect known as "metabolic memory". The impact of tight blood glucose control on ocular and other microvascular complications of type 1 DM was shown in the Diabetes Control and Complications Trial (DCCT)[45] and in its extension study, the Epidemiology of Diabetes Interventions and Complications (EDIC) Study.[44] The predicted average length of time free of PDR, DME, and blindness would increase by 14.7, 8.2, and 7.7 years, respectively, if tighter control was achieved.[46] The protective effect of tight blood glucose control was also reported for type 2 diabetes in the United Kingdom Prospective Diabetes Study (UKPDS).[47] However, in type 1 diabetes there was no threshold glycated hemoglobin (HbA1c) level below which further normalization of glucose failed to provide additional benefit.[48] In type 2 diabetes, evidence suggests that once glycemic control approaches a target HbA1c of 7.0%, further efforts at intensifying control produce little benefit, at least with regard to DR endpoints.[49] Given the risks associated with hypoglycemic episodes, namely acute cardiovascular events, a target HbA1c of 7.0% seems reasonable, and further tightening, although an individualized decision, may be illadvised.[50] Also, although improved metabolic control is associated with slower progression of DR over extended follow-up periods, a paradoxical worsening of the DR can occur if blood glucose control is achieved over a short period of time, an effect believed to be mediated by concurrent upsurges in insulin-like growth factor 1.[51]

The incidence and severity of DR is increased in patients with systemic hypertension.[44,52,53] In type 1 diabetics included in the Wisconsin Epidemiologic Study of Diabetic Retinopathy, baseline severity of DR and progression to PDR were associated with baseline diastolic blood pressure.[40] Lowering blood pressure was shown to benefit several aspects of DR, both in type 1 and type 2 DM.

The course of DR can also be accelerated during pregnancy.[54] Nonproliferative DR and PDR develop in 18–58% and 5–16%, respectively, of pregnant women with type 1 diabetes.[55]

The reported influence of high total serum cholesterol, anemia, gender, socioeconomic status, and educational level on the prevalence, incidence, and severity of DR has been inconsistent in population-based studies.[56]

Ocular Factors

The main ocular factor associated with progression to PDR is a greater baseline severity of DR. This was shown in the Wisconsin Epidemiologic Study of Diabetic Retinopathy,[57] UKPDS,[58] and ETDRS[12] trials.

Organ-specific biomarkers shown to be predictors for the development of DME include MA turnover[59,60] and subclinical macular edema.[61] In a two-year longitudinal study, MA turnover had a positive predictive value of 20% and a negative predictive value of 96% for the development of DME. The authors concluded that in the presence of a low MA turnover, slow disease progression is to be expected and development of clinically significant macular edema is very improbable.[59] The Diabetic Retinopathy Clinical Research Network (DRCR.net)[61] showed that ¼ to ½ of eyes with subclinical macular edema will progress to clinically significant DME within 2 years after the diagnosis. Accordingly, our group also demonstrated that eyes with subclinical DME at baseline have a 3.686-fold increased risk to progress to clinically significant DME within 2 years.[62]

Optic atrophy, higher intraocular pressure, unilateral glaucoma, and chorioretinal scarring have been considered protective factors for the development of PDR.[51] High myopia has been inconsistently associated with protection from DR.[63]

PATHOPHYSIOLOGY

Changes in blood flow and increased vascular permeability are consequences of intracellular hyperglycemia early in the course of diabetes. This reflects an imbalance between vasodilators (such as nitric oxide) and vasoconstrictors (such as angiotensin II and endothelin-1), along with an increased production of permeability factors such as vascular endothelial growth factor (VEGF).[64] Histopathological studies have revealed that the vascular changes in DR originate in the small vessels, in the form of endothelial proliferation, pericyte damage/loss and MA formation.[65] As the disease progresses, the number of MAs increases and areas of capillary nonperfusion begin to form due to microvascular cell loss. Although capillary obstruction is evident early in the course of DR, precapillary arteriolar and larger arteriolar occlusions are increasingly recognized in later stages of the disease.[66]

Hyperglycemia per se seems to be enough to initiate the changes of DR, as revealed experimentally in animal studies.[67-69] In fact, the hyperglycemia-driven activation of four different biochemical pathways—(1) increased polyol pathway flux; (2) protein kinase C activation; (3) advanced glycation end products; and (4) increased hexosamine pathway flux—explains many aspects of DR.[70] The unified theory of DR recognizes that each of these four pathways reflects a single hyperglycemia-induced process: overproduction of superoxide by the mitochondrial electron-transport chain;[64] thus supporting the concept that the intraocular formation of reactive oxygen species fuels the subsequent pathological and biochemical changes that lead to retinal injury.[64] However, the fact that not all poorly controlled patients develop DR suggests that factors such as genetic predisposition are likely to influence an individual's susceptibility to the disease.[9]

The role of retinal neurodegeneration in the development of early microvascular changes in DR has also been highlighted, namely in the breakdown of the BRB,[9,71] vasoregression,[72] and impairment of neurovascular coupling.[73] Glial dysfunction can contribute to the disruption of the BRB directly or through the upregulation of VEGF,[74] a key element in the pathophysiology of DME and PDR.

Finally, the role of inflammation has recently been supported by a large body of evidence. Macrophage migration, microglia, and complement activation lead to the downstream release of vasoactive cytokines such as tissue growth factor beta and connective tissue growth factor. The mechanism by which these cytokines contribute to neural and vascular apoptosis remains to be elucidated, but it may involve the induction of excitotoxicity, oxidative stress, or mitochondrial dysfunction.[75]

DIABETIC MACULAR EDEMA

Diabetic macular edema is the leading cause of visual loss in DM,[76] affecting approximately one-third of the patients with DR. It is thus a frequent complication of DR, particularly in older type 2 diabetic patients. When involving the central vision, DME poses considerable challenges for the affected individuals, significantly affecting their quality of life.

Diabetic macular edema is mainly extracellular and known to be directly associated with the breakdown of the inner BRB. This is, in fact, one of the first changes observed in the retina of diabetic patients. However, swelling of the Müller cells has also been suggested to play a role.[77]

Fluid accumulation in the retinal extracellular space leads to an increase in retinal tissue volume, easily detected by OCT.[78,79] However, fluorescein leakage in FA or vitreous fluorometry is better to appreciate the breakdown of the BRB.[80] When there is a breakdown of the BRB, the Starling law governing the movements of fluids applies.[81] With an affected BRB, even subtle changes in the equilibrium between hydrostatic, oncotic and osmotic pressure gradients across the retinal vessels contribute to further water movements, ultimately resulting in increased fluid accumulation. In this situation, the "force" driving water across the capillary wall is represented by the result of a hydrostatic pressure ΔP and an effective osmotic pressure difference $\Delta\pi\sigma$. The equation regulating movements across the BRB is, therefore:

$$\text{(driving force)} = Lp\,[(P^{plasma} - P^{tissue}) - \sigma\,(\pi^{plasma} - \pi^{tissue})]$$

where Lp is the hydraulic conductivity or membrane permeability of the BRB; σ, an osmotic reflection coefficient; P^{plasma}, the blood pressure; P^{tissue}, the retinal tissue pressure; π^{plasma}, blood osmotic pressure; and π^{tissue}, the tissue osmotic pressure.

In the advent of a breakdown in the BRB, progression of the edema is directly dependent on the gradient induced by differences between blood pressure and tissue pressure, and the oncotic gradient induced by protein accumulation in the retina.

An increase in ΔP (secondary to an increase in P^{plasma}, a decrease in P^{tissue} or both), leads to increased movement of fluids into the retinal tissue and consequently to retinal extracellular fluid accumulation. The decrease in P^{tissue} is an important component that has been recently given more attention. Changes in the retinal tissue cohesion (i.e. localized cell loss, vitreous traction, etc.), will cause a decrease in P^{tissue}, thus facilitating fluid accumulation in the retina and an increase in retinal thickness, i.e. retinal edema. In fact, diseases of the vitreoretinal interface are now believed to play an important part in chronic DME as vitreous traction avoids fluid reabsorption and thus recovery of a normal retinal architecture.[82] On the other hand, a decrease in $\Delta\pi$ contributes to retinal edema formation due to protein accumulation in the retina. Protein and lipoprotein extravasation (as in hard exudates), increases the osmotic pressure in the retinal tissue, thus drawing more water into the retinal extracellular space. In fact, increased protein leakage is a characteristic feature of the diabetic vasculature and the main factor associated with oncotic-driven fluid movements in the retina, since a reduction in plasma osmolarity severe enough to contribute to retinal edema is an extremely rare event.

The retinal pigment epithelium (RPE) also plays an important role in retinal edema. A capable RPE may compensate fluid accumulation with its pumping mechanisms, drawing fluid out of the retina.[83] Changes in the RPE have been described in diabetes (mostly in experimental models), but their relevance in the initial stages of the disease remains controversial.[84-86]

The ETDRS made an effort to establish guidelines to define "clinically significant macular edema". The main goal was to establish an outcome when designing/conducting clinical trials to test the efficacy of DME treatment. Center-involving macular edema was taken in special consideration due to its influence on visual loss. However, the problems associated with these guidelines are the subjectivity of the evaluation regarding "abnormal" retinal thickening, the presence of "hard exudates" which are not "residual" and the relative involvement of the central 500 μm.

The advent and constant development of OCT radically changed our understanding of the incidence, evolution, and rates of progression of DME.[87] DME can now be fully characterized in a clinical setting, not only regarding its type and distribution, but also its evolution, its pathophysiology and its degree of involvement of the central macular area.[61,62,88]

PROLIFERATIVE DIABETIC RETINOPATHY

Proliferative diabetic retinopathy and its inherent complications represent the end stage in the natural history of DR. Retinal ischemia is considered the main pathogenetic factor behind the development of PDR. It results from severe hypoxia, which leads to an imbalance between angiogenic and antiangiogenic mediators, favoring neovascularization. The first step of new vessel formation is the proteolytic digestion of the basement membrane. This is then followed by the migration and replication of endothelial cells, stimulated by angiogenic factors, especially VEGF.[89] The recently formed vessels are a collection of multiple tortuous and fine capillaries that tend to grow into the vitreous body. They are extremely fragile due to architectural weakness; they lack BRB properties; and they are thus more prone to bleed, causing vitreous hemorrhage and subsequent acute vision loss. As the disease progresses, the new vessels continue to proliferate, with associated connective tissue formation. An important factor affecting the presentation of PDR is the status of the vitreous. In the absence of posterior vitreous detachment, the cortical vitreous provides a scaffold for the proliferation of the new vessels. With sustained neovascular growth, extensive areas of fibrovascular proliferation create firm attachments between the retina and the vitreous cortex. Initial contraction of the fibrous tissue may lead to retinal striae and macular dragging.[56] Further contraction may transmit the vitreous traction to the retina and ultimately lead to a tractional, rhegmatogenous or mixed retinal detachment. This vision threatening complication is usually an indication for vitreoretinal surgery.

When the new vessels arise on or within one disk diameter of the optic nerve head they are referred to as NVD (neovascularization of the disk) (Fig. 48.6). It is now believed that NVD form as VEGF and other growth factors migrate from the peripheral ischemic retina to the disk by means of vitreopapillary drainage.[56] On the other hand, when neovascularization arises one disk diameter or more away from the optic nerve head, it is called NVE (neovascularization elsewhere) (Fig. 48.7). NVE generally arises from retinal veins or postcapillary venules near sites of arteriovenous crossing or venous branching, at the posterior border of capillary nonperfusion sites.[56] Unlike normal retinal vessels, NVD, and NVE leak fluorescein into the vitreous, making them easily identifiable on FA.

Early NVEs may be difficult to distinguish from IRMAs. Actually, some IRMAs may eventually develop into neovascular tissue.[90] A critical distinction is that IRMAs lie exclusively below the level of the internal limiting membrane of the retina, whereas new vessels lie above the internal limiting membrane. In the DRS, NVEs showed little risk for visual loss.[91] This finding supports the clinical

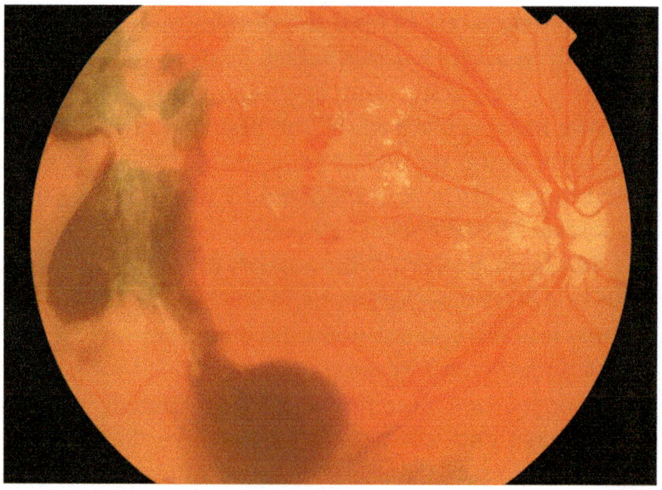

Fig. 48.6: Color fundus photography of proliferative diabetic retinopathy with neovascularization of the disk, along with tractional retinal detachment.

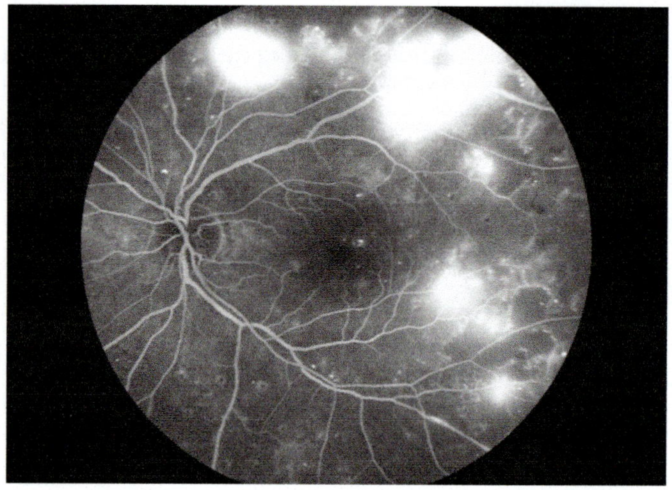

Fig. 48.7: Fluorescein angiography showing proliferative diabetic retinopathy with several foci of neovascularization elsewhere (NVE).

impression that NVEs often proliferate and regress over the years without significant risk for vision loss provided that no NVDs are present.

Anterior ocular neovascularization is a complication of PDR that may ultimately lead to neovascular glaucoma as the new vessels grow into and block aqueous drainage at the iridocorneal angle. Rubeosis frequently starts at the superior pupillary margin and is known to progress more slowly in phakic than aphakic eyes. This difference is presumably due to the effect of the crystalline lens as a barrier to the diffusion of vascular growth factors into the anterior chamber.[56] The presence of rubeotic glaucoma is a poor prognostic indicator for VA and for life expectancy.[92]

MANAGEMENT OF DIABETIC RETINOPATHY

Prevention

Diabetic retinopathy can be prevented by the effective control of glycemia and blood pressure, as demonstrated by the DCCT[93,94] and the UKPDS trial.[47] These studies provided strong evidence that tighter control of glycemia (target HbA1c <7%) reduces the risk of development and progression of DR in both type 1 and type 2 DM. Therefore, the importance of achieving good glycemic control early in the course of diabetes (preferably before the development of DR) cannot be overemphasized. One should realize, however, that even patients with relatively poor metabolic control may remain retinopathy-free or avoid sight-threatening complications, highlighting the effect of other (mostly unidentified) factors. Although dyslipidemia has also been linked to DR, the effects of statin therapy on DR risk have been inconsistent.[18]

Management of Diabetic Macular Edema

For almost three decades, laser photocoagulation has been the standard of care for DME.[95] According to the ETDRS guidelines, laser photocoagulation for clinically significant macular edema decreases the risk of moderate vision loss by 50% over 3 years; but very few patients experience comparable VA gains.[95] Furthermore, laser photocoagulation itself is associated with significant ocular side effects because of its inherent destructive nature. These include induction of scotoma, enlargement of laser scars, and development of secondary neovascularization.[89]

The introduction of intravitreal pharmacotherapy reshaped the management of DME by significantly improving the functional prognosis of these patients.[96] In fact, the use of anti-VEGF agents was shown to be superior to focal and grid laser photocoagulation,[97-99] turning this treatment modality into the new gold standard for diffuse DME. Using a monthly treatment regimen seems to produce the best possible visual results, according to clinical trials.[97] However, the social and economic burden of monthly injections is difficult to maintain in daily clinical practice. To this day, plentiful controversies still exist over the best drug and treatment regimen for the management of DME. The DRCR.net Protocol T[100] gave us the best comparative data for the three available anti-VEGF drugs currently in use: (1) aflibercept, (2) bevacizumab, and (3) ranibizumab. In the first year, the trial showed comparable effects for eyes with baseline VA between 20/32 and 20/40 (+8 letters) but greater gains with aflibercept (+18.9 letters) compared to ranibizumab (+14.2 letters) and bevacizumab (+11.8 letters) for eyes with VA less than and equal to 20/50. Aflibercept also produced a greater decrease in macular thickness (-169 μm) than ranibizumab (-147 μm) or bevacizumab (-101 μm). The differences in response between the licensed drugs (aflibercept and ranibizumab) disappeared after 2 years.[101] Nevertheless, additional trials are needed to validate these data and to identify patient subgroups that respond particularly well or poorly to anti-VEGF treatment. Until then, the choice of which anti-VEGF agent to use for patients with DME should be individualized to healthcare systems, patient preference, and cost.[89]

One of the key mechanisms in the pathogenesis of DME is the activation of inflammatory pathways. Corticosteroids suppress multiple aspects of inflammation, downregulate VEGF expression and reduce the induction of VEGF by proinflammatory mediators.[102] The off-label use of triamcinolone acetonide has been shown to reduce DME and to improve vision in the short term. However, considerable adverse effects (such as cataract and glaucoma) are common. Two sustained-release corticosteroid implants—the dexamethasone delivery system (Ozurdex®) and the fluocinolone acetonide insert (Iluvien®)—are currently approved for the management of DME. Ozurdex® (Allergan, Irvine; California, USA), a biodegradable implant inserted using a 22-gauge applicator, releases 0.7 mg of dexamethasone over the course of 120–180 days. The treatment met the primary efficacy endpoint for improvement in best corrected visual acuity (BCVA) (22.2% of the treated patients had an improvement ≥15 letters vs. 12% in the sham group), with an acceptable safety profile over the course of 3 years.[103] On average, patients received four injections during the study period. Iluvien® (Alimera Sciences, Alpharetta; Georgia, USA) provides a therapeutic effect of up to 36 months by delivering sustained sub-microgram levels of fluocinolone acetonide. The implant can be injected with a 25-gauge needle. The FAME study[104] demonstrated that in chronic DME (≥3 years), significantly more patients treated with Iluvien® had an improvement more than and equal to 15 letters in comparison to the sham group (28.7% versus 18.9%), after 36 months. Unfortunately, neither Ozurdex® nor Illuvien® has been directly compared to anti-VEGF therapy in clearly designed multicenter randomized clinical trials.

Since distinctive pathophysiological features seem to be involved in recent onset and chronic DME, the decision on the adequate therapeutic approach should take into consideration the chronicity of DME, the number of and responses to previous treatment modalities and the pattern of DME (focal vs. diffuse).[96] As DME initially develops, VEGF-associated hyperpermeability, acute inflammation, and vascular dysfunction most likely dominate.[105] In this particular scenario, using an anti-VEGF drug seems to be the best possible strategy. On the other hand, chronic DME is likely associated with a higher non-VEGF cytokine milieu, chronic inflammation, and neuronal damage. This is probably the setting where corticosteroids may be more effective.[105] Focal laser photocoagulation remains a useful mode of treatment for DME not involving the foveal center.

Management of Proliferative Diabetic Retinopathy

The landmark DRS demonstrated that panretinal photocoagulation (PRP) laser reduced the risk of severe vision loss from 33.0% to 13.9% at 5 years in patients with PDR or severe nonproliferative DR.[106] PRP obliterates midperipheral areas of ischemic retina, thus alleviating hypoxia and affecting the hemodynamics of the retinal circulation. Improved retinal oxygenation reduces neovascularization and edema by reducing the production of VEGF and other growth factors.[89] The goal of PRP is to arrest or to cause regression of the neovascularization. Unfortunately, extensive areas of photocoagulation lead to permanently decreased peripheral vision, impaired contrast sensitivity and night vision, and may lead to epiretinal membrane formation or paradoxically increase macular edema.

Intravitreal anti-VEGF therapy has been shown to reduce the level of DR,[107] and its use in PDR is evolving. The results of ranibizumab alone or in combination with PRP in the treatment of high-risk PDR were shown to be comparable or better than PRP alone over the course of 12 months in an exploratory randomized controlled trial (RCT).[108] Later, the DRCR.net conducted a noninferiority RCT (Protocol S) and demonstrated that among eyes with PDR, treatment with ranibizumab resulted in VA gains that were noninferior to (not worse than) PRP treatment at 2 years.[109] Aside from VA, the ranibizumab group experienced less peripheral visual field sensitivity loss, fewer vitrectomies and a lower incidence of DME.[109] Although the number of injections in the first year was high (median of 7), it considerably decreased in year 2 (median 3), suggesting that some disease modulation may occur after 1 year of ranibizumab therapy. These results led to the US Food and Drug Administration (FDA) approval of ranibizumab for the monthly treatment of all forms of DR in April 2017, making ranibizumab the first and only FDA-approved medicine to treat DR in patients either with or without DME.

Vitrectomy plays a vital role in the management of severe complications of PDR. Nowadays, the major indications are nonclearing vitreous hemorrhage, macular-involving or macular-threatening tractional retinal detachment, combined tractional-rhegmatogenous retinal detachment, and severe fibrovascular proliferation with macular architectural changes.[18] Anti-VEGF drugs are able to transiently involute neovascularization and have been used as preoperative adjuvants to facilitate fibrovascular membrane dissection and reduce intra- and postoperative bleeding.[96]

REFERENCES

1. International Diabetes Federation. IDF Diabetes Atlas, 7th edition. Brussels, Belgium: International Diabetes Federation; 2015.
2. Sepulveda J, Murray C. The State of Global Health in 2014. Science. 2014;345(6202):1275-8.
3. Fong DS, Aiello LP, Ferris FL, et al. Diabetic retinopathy. Diabetes Care. 2004;27(10):2540-53.
4. Yau JW, Rogers SL, Kawasaki R, et al. Global prevalence and major risk factors of diabetic retinopathy. Diabetes Care. 2012;35(3):556-64.
5. Tapp RJ, Shaw JE, Harper CA, et al. The prevalence of and factors associated with diabetic retinopathy in the Australian population. Diabetes Care. 2003;26(6):1731-7.
6. Fong DS, Aiello L, Gardner TW, et al. Retinopathy in diabetes. Diabetes Care. 2004;27(Suppl 1):S84-7.
7. Zhang X, Zeng H, Bao S, et al. Diabetic macular edema: new concepts in pathophysiology and treatment. Cell Biosci. 2014;4:27.
8. Bhavsar AR, Emerson GG, Emerson MV, et al. Epidemiology of diabetic retinopathy. In: Browning DJ (Ed). Diabetic Retinopathy: Evidence-based Management. New York, NY: Springer New York; 2010.pp.53-75.
9. Cunha-Vaz J, Ribeiro L, Lobo C. Phenotypes and biomarkers of diabetic retinopathy. Prog Retin Eye Res. 2014;41:90-111.
10. Bernardes R, Lobo C, Cunha-Vaz JG. Multimodal macula mapping: a new approach to study diseases of the macula. Surv Ophthalmol. 2002;47(6):580-9.
11. Tennant MT, Greve MD, Rudnisky CJ, et al. Identification of diabetic retinopathy by stereoscopic digital imaging via teleophthalmology: a comparison to slide film. Can J Ophthalmol. 2001;36(4):187-96.
12. Fundus photographic risk factors for progression of diabetic retinopathy. ETDRS report number 12. Early Treatment Diabetic Retinopathy Study Research Group. Ophthalmology. 1991;98(5 Suppl):823-33.
13. Grading diabetic retinopathy from stereoscopic color fundus photographs—an extension of the modified airlie house classification. ETDRS Report number 10. Early Treatment Diabetic Retinopathy Study Research Group. Ophthalmology. 1991;98(5 Suppl):786-806.
14. Tufail A, Rudisill C, Egan C, et al. Automated diabetic retinopathy image assessment software: diagnostic accuracy and cost-effectiveness compared with human graders. Ophthalmology. 2017;124(3):343-51.
15. Spaide RF, Klancnik JM Jr, Cooney MJ. Retinal vascular layers imaged by fluorescein angiography and optical coherence tomography angiography. JAMA Ophthalmology. 2015;133(1):45-50.
16. Su Z, Ye P, Teng Y, et al. Adverse reaction in patients with drug allergy history after simultaneous intravenous fundus fluorescein angiography and indocyanine green Angiography. J Ocul Pharmacol Ther. 2012;28(4):410-3.
17. Lipson BK, Yannuzzi LA. Complications of intravenous fluorescein injections. Int Ophthalmol Clin. 1989;29(3): 200-5.
18. Lim JI, Rosenblatt BJ, Benson WE. Diabetic retinopathy. In: Yanoff M, Duker JS (Eds). Ophthalmology. London: Elsevier/Saunders; 2013.pp.541-50.
19. Silva PS, Horton MB, Clary D, et al. Identification of diabetic retinopathy and ungradable image rate with ultrawide field imaging in a national teleophthalmology program. Ophthalmology. 2016;123(6):1360-7.
20. Mcdaniel CF. Diabetes: A model of oxidative accelerated aging. Age (Omaha). 1999;22(4):145-8.
21. Huang D, Swanson EA, Lin CP, et al. Optical coherence tomography. Science. 1991;254(5035):1178-81.
22. Swanson EA, Izatt JA, Hee MR, et al. In vivo retinal imaging by optical coherence tomography. Opt Lett. 1993;18(21):1864-6.
23. Marques JP, Silva R. OCT Angiography: redefining standards. Oftalmologia. 2015;39(2):111-4.
24. Alasil T, Ferrara D, Adhi M, et al. En face imaging of the choroid in polypoidal choroidal vasculopathy using swept-source optical coherence tomography. Am J Ophthalmol. 2015;159(4):634-43.
25. Bandello F, Tejerina AN, Vujosevic S, et al. Retinal layer location of increased retinal thickness in eyes with subclinical and clinical macular edema in diabetes type 2. Ophthalmic Res. 2015;54(3):112-7.
26. Ishibazawa A, Nagaoka T, Takahashi A, et al. Optical coherence tomography angiography in diabetic retinopathy: a prospective pilot study. Am J Ophthalmol. 2015;160(1):35-44.
27. Soares M, Neves C, Marques IP, et al. Comparison of diabetic retinopathy classification using fluorescein angiography and optical coherence tomography angiography. Br J Ophthalmol. 2017;101(1):62-8.
28. Cunha-Vaz J, Santos T, Ribeiro L, et al. OCT-leakage: a new method to identify and locate abnormal fluid accumulation in diabetic retinal edema. Invest Ophthalmol Vis Sci. 2016;57(15):6776-83.

29. Cunha-Vaz J, Faria De Abreu JR, Campos AJ. Early breakdown of the blood-retinal barrier in diabetes. Br J Ophthalmol. 1975;59(11):649-56.
30. Waltman S, Krupin T, Hanish S, et al. Alteration of the blood-retinal barrier in experimental diabetes mellitus. Arch Ophthalmol. 1978;96(5):878-9.
31. Antonetti DA, Klein R, Gardner TW. Diabetic retinopathy. N Engl J Med. 2012;366(13):1227-39.
32. Wong KL. Defining diabetic retinopathy severity. In: Browning DJ (Ed). Diabetic Retinopathy: Evidence-based Management. New York, NY: Springer New York; 2010. pp.105-20.
33. Klein R, Meuer SM, Moss SE, et al. The relationship of retinal microaneurysm counts to the 4-year progression of diabetic retinopathy. Arch Ophthalmol. 1989;107(12):1780-5.
34. Hellstedt T, Immonen I. Disappearance and formation rates of microaneurysms in early diabetic retinopathy. Br J Ophthalmol. 1996;80(2):135-9.
35. Dorner GT, Garhofer G, Kiss B, et al. Nitric oxide regulates retinal vascular tone in humans. Am J Physiol Heart Circ Physiol. 2003;285(2):H631-6.
36. Kur J, Newman EA, Chan-Ling T. Cellular and physiological mechanisms underlying blood flow regulation in the retina and choroid in health and disease. Prog Retin Eye Res. 2012;31(5):377-406.
37. Metea MR, Newman EA. Signalling within the neurovascular unit in the mammalian retina. Exp Physiol. 2007;92(4): 635-40.
38. Riva CE, Logean E, Falsini B. Visually evoked hemodynamical response and assessment of neurovascular coupling in the optic nerve and retina. Prog Retin Eye Res. 2005;24(2): 183-215.
39. Ludovico J, Bernardes R, Pires I, et al. Alterations of retinal capillary blood flow in preclinical retinopathy in subjects with type 2 diabetes. Graefes Arch Clin Exp Ophthalmol. 2003;241(3):181-6.
40. Klein R, Klein BE, Moss SE, et al. The Wisconsin epidemiologic study of diabetic retinopathy. II. Prevalence and risk of diabetic retinopathy when age at diagnosis is less than 30 years. Arch Ophthalmol. 1984;102(4):520-6.
41. Klein R, Klein BE, Moss SE, et al. The Wisconsin epidemiologic study of diabetic retinopathy. III. Prevalence and risk of diabetic retinopathy when age at diagnosis is 30 or more years. Arch Ophthalmol. 1984;102(4):527-32.
42. Brown JB, Pedula KL, Summers KH. Diabetic retinopathy: contemporary prevalence in a well-controlled population. Diabetes Care. 2003;26(9):2637-42.
43. Kalesnykiene V, Sorri I, Voutilainen R, et al. The effect of glycaemic control on the quantitative characteristics of retinopathy lesions in patients with type 2 diabetes mellitus: 10-year follow-up study. Graefes Arch Clin Exp Ophthalmol. 2009;247(3):335-41.
44. White NH, Sun W, Cleary PA, et al. Prolonged effect of intensive therapy on the risk of retinopathy complications in patients with type 1 diabetes mellitus: 10 years after the diabetes control and complications trial. Arch Ophthalmol. 2008;126(12):1707-15.
45. The relationship of glycemic exposure (HbA1c) to the risk of development and progression of retinopathy in the diabetes control and complications trial. Diabetes. 1995;44(8): 968-83.
46. Lifetime benefits and costs of intensive therapy as practiced in the diabetes control and complications trial. the diabetes control and complications trial research group. JAMA. 1996;276(17):1409-15.
47. Intensive blood-glucose control with sulphonylureas or insulin compared with conventional treatment and risk of complications in patients with type 2 diabetes (UKPDS 33). UK Prospective Diabetes Study (UKPDS) Group. Lancet. 1998;352(9131):837-53.
48. The absence of a glycemic threshold for the development of long-term complications: the perspective of the diabetes control and complications trial. Diabetes. 1996;45(10): 1289-98.
49. Patel A, Macmahon S, Chalmers J. et al. Intensive blood glucose control and vascular outcomes in patients with type 2 diabetes. N Engl J Med. 2008;358(24):2560-72.
50. Chantelau E, Meyer-Schwickerath R. reversion of 'early worsening' of diabetic retinopathy by deliberate restoration of poor metabolic control. Ophthalmologica. 2003;217(5):373-7.
51. Browning DJ. Systemic and ocular factors influencing diabetic retinopathy. In: Browning DJ (Ed). Diabetic Retinopathy: Evidence-Based Management. New York, NY: Springer New York; 2010.pp.77-103.
52. Leske MC, Wu SY, Hennis A, et al. Incidence of diabetic retinopathy in the Barbados Eye Studies. Ophthalmology. 2003;110(5):941-7.
53. Van Leiden HA, Dekker JM, Moll AC, et al. Risk factors for incident retinopathy in a diabetic and nondiabetic population: the Hoorn study. Arch Ophthalmol. 2003;121(2):245-51.
54. Loukovaara S, Immonen I, Teramo KA, et al. Progression of retinopathy during pregnancy in type 1 diabetic women treated with insulin lispro. Diabetes Care. 2003;26(4):1193-8.
55. Loukovaara S, Harju M, Kaaja R, et al. Retinal capillary blood flow in diabetic and nondiabetic women during pregnancy and postpartum period. Invest Ophthalmol Vis Sci. 2003;44(4):1486-91.
56. Pautler SE. Treatment of Proliferative diabetic retinopathy. In: Browning DJ (Ed). Diabetic Retinopathy: Evidence-based Management. New York, NY: Springer New York; 2010.pp.227-304.
57. Klein R, Knudtson MD, Lee KE, et al. The Wisconsin Epidemiologic Study Of Diabetic Retinopathy: XXII The twenty-five-year progression of retinopathy in persons with type 1 diabetes. Ophthalmology. 2008;115(11):1859-68.
58. Kohner EM, Stratton IM, Aldington SJ, et al. Relationship between the severity of retinopathy and progression to photocoagulation in patients with type 2 diabetes mellitus in the UKPDS (UKPDS 52). Diabet Med. 2001;18(3):178-84.
59. Ribeiro ML, Nunes SG, Cunha-Vaz JG. Microaneurysm turnover at the macula predicts risk of development of clinically significant macular edema in persons with

mild nonproliferative diabetic retinopathy. Diabetes Care. 2013;36(5):1254-9.
60. Nunes S, Pires I, Rosa A, et al. Microaneurysm turnover is a biomarker for diabetic retinopathy progression to clinically significant macular edema: findings for type 2 diabetics with nonproliferative retinopathy. Ophthalmologica. 2009;223(5):292-7.
61. Bressler NM, Miller KM, Beck RW, et al. Observational study of subclinical diabetic macular edema. Eye (Lond). 2012;26(6):833-40.
62. Pires I, Santos AR, Nunes S, et al. Subclinical macular edema as a predictor of progression to clinically significant macular edema in type 2 diabetes. Ophthalmologica. 2013;230(4):201-6.
63. Jain IS, Luthra CL, Das T. Diabetic retinopathy and its relation to errors of refraction. Arch Ophthalmol. 1967;77(1):59-60.
64. Brownlee M. Biochemistry and molecular cell biology of diabetic complications. Nature. 2001;414(6865):813-20.
65. Ashton N. Experimental aspects of diabetic microangiopathy. Trans Opthal Soc UK. 1957;77:127-40.
66. Ashton N. Arteriolar involvement in diabetic retinopathy. Br J Ophthalmol. 1953;37(5):282-92.
67. Kador PF, Akagi Y, Takahashi Y, et al. Prevention of retinal vessel changes associated with diabetic retinopathy in galactose-fed dogs by aldose reductase inhibitors. Arch Ophthalmol. 1990;108(9):1301-9.
68. Engerman RL, Kern TS. Experimental galactosemia produces diabetic-like retinopathy. Diabetes. 1984;33(1): 97-100.
69. Kern TS, Engerman RL. A mouse model of diabetic retinopathy. Arch Ophthalmol. 1996;114(8):986-90.
70. Stuart MW. Pathophysiology of diabetic retinopathy. In: Browning DJ (Ed). Diabetic Retinopathy: Evidence-based Management. New York, NY: Springer New York; 2010. pp.1-30.
71. Silva KC, Rosales MA, Biswas SK, et al. Diabetic retinal neurodegeneration is associated with mitochondrial oxidative stress and is improved by an angiotensin receptor blocker in a model combining hypertension and diabetes. Diabetes. 2009;58(6):1382-90.
72. Feng Y, Wang Y, Stock O, et al. Vasoregression linked to neuronal damage in the rat with defect of polycystin-2. PLoS One. 2009;4(10):e7328.
73. Lecleire-Collet A, Audo I, Aout M, et al. Evaluation of retinal function and flicker light-induced retinal vascular response in normotensive patients with diabetes without retinopathy. Invest Ophthalmol Vis Sci. 2011;52(6):2861-7.
74. Shen W, Li S, Chung SH, et al. Retinal vascular changes after glial disruption in rats. J Neurosci Res. 2010;88(7):1485-99.
75. Barber AJ, Gardner TW, Abcouwer SF. The significance of vascular and neural apoptosis to the pathology of diabetic retinopathy. Invest Ophthalmol Vis Sci. 2011;52(2):1156-63.
76. Aiello LP, Gardner TW, King GL, et al. Diabetic retinopathy. Diabetes Care. 1998;21(1):143-56.
77. Wurm A, Pannicke T, Iandiev I, et al. Purinergic signaling involved in Muller cell function in the mammalian retina. Prog Retin Eye Res. 2011;30(5):324-42.
78. Bolz M, Ritter M, Schneider M, et al. A systematic correlation of angiography and high-resolution optical coherence tomography in diabetic macular edema. Ophthalmology. 2009;116(1):66-72.
79. Soliman W, Sander B, Hasler PW, et al. Correlation between intraretinal changes in diabetic macular oedema seen in fluorescein angiography and optical coherence tomography. Acta Ophthalmol. 2008;86(1):34-9.
80. Lobo CL, Bernardes RC, Figueira JP, et al. Three-year follow-up study of blood-retinal barrier and retinal thickness alterations in patients with type 2 diabetes mellitus and mild nonproliferative diabetic retinopathy. Arch Ophthalmol. 2004;122(2):211-7.
81. Cunha-Vaz JG, Travassos A. Breakdown of the blood-retinal barriers and cystoid macular edema. Surv Ophthalmol. 1984;28 Suppl:485-92.
82. Ghazi NG, Ciralsky JB, Shah SM, et al. Optical coherence tomography findings in persistent diabetic macular edema: the vitreomacular interface. Am J Ophthalmol. 2007;144(5):747-54.
83. Sander B, Larsen M, Moldow B, et al. Diabetic macular edema: passive and active transport of fluorescein through the blood-retina barrier. Invest Ophthalmol Vis Sci. 2001;42(2):433-8.
84. Do Carmo A, Ramos P, Reis A, et al. Breakdown of the inner and outer blood retinal barrier in streptozotocin-induced diabetes. Exp Eye Res. 1998;67(5):569-75.
85. Tso MO, Cunha-Vaz JG, Shih CY, et al. Clinicopathologic study of blood-retinal barrier in experimental diabetes mellitus. Arch Ophthalmol. 1980;98(11):2032-40.
86. Xu HZ, Le YZ. Significance of outer blood-retina barrier breakdown in diabetes and ischemia. Invest Ophthalmol Vis Sci. 2011;52(5):2160-4.
87. Puliafito CA, Hee MR, Lin CP, et al. Imaging of macular diseases with optical coherence tomography. Ophthalmology. 1995;102(2):217-29.
88. Browning DJ, Fraser CM. The predictive value of patient and eye characteristics on the course of subclinical diabetic macular edema. Am J Ophthalmol. 2008;145(1):149-54.
89. Wong TY, Cheung CM, Larsen M, et al. Diabetic retinopathy. Nat Rev Dis Primers. 2016;2:16012.
90. Imesch PD, Bindley CD, Wallow IH. Clinicopathologic correlation of intraretinal microvascular abnormalities. Retina. 1997;17(4):321-9.
91. Rand LI, Prud'homme GJ, Ederer F, et al. Factors influencing the development of visual loss in advanced diabetic retinopathy. Diabetic Retinopathy Study (DRS) Report No. 10. Invest Ophthalmol Vis Sci. 1985;26(7):983-91.
92. Blanc JP, Molteno AC, Fuller JR, et al. Life expectancy of patients with neovascular glaucoma drained by molteno implants. Clin Exp Ophthalmol. 2004;32(4):360-3.
93. Nathan DM, DCCT/EDIC Research Group. The diabetes control and complications trial/epidemiology of diabetes interventions and complications study at 30 years: overview. Diabetes Care. 2014;37(1):9-16.
94. Nathan DM, Genuth S, Lachin J, et al. The effect of intensive treatment of diabetes on the development and progression

of long-term complications in insulin-dependent diabetes mellitus. N Engl J Med. 1993;329(14):977-86.
95. Photocoagulation for diabetic macular edema. early treatment diabetic retinopathy study report number 1. Early Treatment Diabetic Retinopathy Study research group. Arch Ophthalmol. 1985;103(12):1796-806.
96. Stewart MW. Treatment of diabetic retinopathy: Recent advances and unresolved challenges. World J Diabetes. 2016;7(16):333-41.
97. Nguyen QD, Brown DM, Marcus DM, et al Ranibizumab for diabetic macular edema: results from 2 phase III randomized trials: RISE and RIDE. Ophthalmology. 2012;119(4):789-801.
98. Mitchell P, Bandello F, Schmidt-Erfurth U, et al. The RESTORE study: ranibizumab monotherapy or combined with laser versus laser monotherapy for diabetic macular edema. Ophthalmology. 2011;118(4):615-25.
99. Nguyen QD, Shah SM, Khwaja AA, et al. Two-year outcomes of the ranibizumab for edema of the macula in diabetes (READ-2) study. Ophthalmology. 2010;117(11):2146-51.
100. Wells JA, Glassman AR, Ayala AR, et al. Aflibercept, bevacizumab, or ranibizumab for diabetic macular edema. N Engl J Med. 2015;372(13):1193-203.
101. Wells JA, Glassman AR, Ayala AR, et al. Aflibercept, bevacizumab, or ranibizumab for diabetic macular edema: two-year results from a comparative effectiveness randomized clinical trial. Ophthalmology. 2016;123(6):1351-9.
102. Nauck M, Karakiulakis G, Perruchoud AP, et al. Corticosteroids inhibit the expression of the vascular endothelial growth factor gene in human vascular smooth muscle cells. Eur J Pharmacol. 1998;341(2-3):309-15.
103. Boyer DS, Yoon YH, Belfort R Jr, et al. Three-year, randomized, sham-controlled trial of dexamethasone intravitreal implant in patients with diabetic macular edema. Ophthalmology. 2014;121(10):1904-14.
104. Campochiaro PA, Brown DM, Pearson A, et al. Sustained delivery fluocinolone acetonide vitreous inserts provide benefit for at least 3 years in patients with diabetic macular edema. Ophthalmology. 2012;119(10):2125-32.
105. Colucciello M. Current intravitreal pharmacologic therapies for diabetic macular edema. Postgrad Med J. 2015: 1-14.
106. Photocoagulation treatment of proliferative diabetic retinopathy. Clinical application of diabetic retinopathy study (DRS) findings, DRS Report Number 8. The Diabetic Retinopathy Study Research Group. Ophthalmology. 1981;88(7):583-600.
107. Ip MS, Domalpally A, Hopkins JJ, et al. Long-term effects of ranibizumab on diabetic retinopathy severity and progression. Arch Ophthalmol. 2012;130(9):1145-52.
108. Figueira J, Silva R, Henriques J, et al. Ranibizumab for high-risk proliferative diabetic retinopathy: an exploratory randomized controlled trial. Ophthalmologica. 2016;235(1):34-41.
109. Gross JG, Glassman AR, Jampol LM, et al. Panretinal photocoagulation vs intravitreous ranibizumab for proliferative diabetic retinopathy: a randomized clinical trial. JAMA. 2015;314(20):2137-46.

Chapter 49 Retinal Vascular Occlusions

Katrin Fasler, Pearse A Keane

OVERVIEW

Arterial occlusions are mainly caused by thromboembolic mechanisms (e.g. carotid plaques or heart valve calcifications). Less frequent causes are inflammatory conditions (e.g. giant cell arteritis or lupus erythematosus), coagulopathies (e.g. oral contraceptives, sickle cell or antiphospholipid antibodies), ocular abnormalities [e.g. elevated intraocular pressure (IOP), or optic nerve head drusen], or trauma.

Retinal arterial occlusive disease can be classified as occlusion of the ophthalmic artery, central artery, branch artery, or cilioretinal artery or occlusion on a microvascular level [paracentral acute middle maculopathy (PAMM)].

The clinical picture is of a sudden visual loss with scotoma corresponding to the area supplied by the affected vessels along with the typical retinal picture of ischemia: whitening of the inner retinal layers. Depending on the status of the choroidal perfusion, a cherry red spot may be seen. Retinal edema usually takes several hours to develop, and thus, may not be seen at first presentation; but hyper-reflectivity of the inner retinal layers may already be visible on optical coherence tomography (OCT). Fluorescein angiography (FFA) demonstrates delayed, or even absent, filling of the affected vessels. Complications are neovascularization (NV) resulting from ischemia and recurrence in the same or the fellow eye.

The diagnostic workup includes targeted questioning for symptoms of giant cell arteritis, laboratory tests to exclude inflammatory etiology/coagulopathies, and a complete cardiovascular workup, including carotid ultrasound and echocardiography.

The therapeutic approach is mainly addressing the underlying disease and attempting to re-establish ocular blood flow. Thromboembolic arterial occlusion is a form of stroke analogous to cerebral apoplexy and thus should be treated in a multidisciplinary fashion, together with a neurologist/stroke unit. Emergency interventions to restore ocular perfusion have been tried (paracentesis, ocular massage, oral and topical IOP lowering agents), but there is no evidence of efficacy. Panretinal photocoagulation is indicated for neovascular complications.

INTRODUCTION

Occlusion or obstruction of an artery leads to acute loss of vision in the distribution of the affected retina. The first account of such an event in the literature was by von Graefe in 1859, describing central retinal artery occlusion (CRAO) secondary to emboli related to bacterial endocarditis.[1] Since then, our understanding of retinal arterial occlusion has increased dramatically. Although these events are infrequent, not only can they profoundly impact the visual function of the individual, but they can also be the initial indication of a life-threatening systemic disease. An understanding of the basic anatomy and pathologic mechanisms of occlusion is essential in determining the appropriate management and evaluation of patients presenting with acute retinal arterial occlusions.

VASCULAR ANATOMY

Arterial blood supply to the eye is provided by the ophthalmic artery, which is the first intracranial branch of the internal carotid artery. Rarely, the ophthalmic artery may arise from the middle meningeal artery.[2] After entering the orbit, the ophthalmic artery gives off the central retinal artery (CRA), which runs adjacent to the inferior margin of the optic nerve. The CRA penetrates around 10 mm posterior to the globe to course in the center of the nerve to the optic disc to supply the inner retina.[3] Approximately 2–3 posterior ciliary arteries (PCA) arise from the ophthalmic artery, branching into 10–20 short PCAs and two long PCAs that supply the optic disc (via the Circle of Zinn or Haller), the choroid and outer retina, as well as small sectors of the ciliary body and iris.[4]

One or more cilioretinal arteries arise from these short posterior ciliary arteries, or less frequently directly from the choroidal circulation, and are present in 30% of eyes and 50% of individuals.[5-9] In 15% of people, a cilioretinal artery supplies some portion of the macular circulation.[6]

The supply of the optic nerve head is complex and different in its three zones (prelaminar, laminar, and postlaminar). The prelaminar part is supplied by branches of the central and branch retinal arteries. The laminar part of the optic nerve is supplied by branches of the PCAs and pial arteries. The postlaminar optic nerve is supplied by intraneuronal branches from the CRA and recurrent pial branches of the central retinal and ophthalmic artery.[10]

Within the retina, larger branches of the central artery course through the nerve fiber and ganglion cell layers. As the circulation divides into smaller branches and finally into capillaries, vessels distribute vertically to form the capillary retinal plexus. Generally, there are three plexuses (the deep, middle, and superficial); but in the peripapillary region there is an additional, very superficial radial peripapillaryplexus.[10-14] The completely avascular central foveal retina known as the foveal avascular zone (FAZ), is 400–500 mm in diameter in healthy eyes and increases with age (Figs. 49.1 and 49.2).[15,16]

The PCAs are organized into fan-shaped lobules of capillaries that supply localized choroidal areas with watershed zones in between.[17]

Venous drainage from the retina is gathered via the retinal venules and veins to the central retinal vein, which exits the eye within the optic nerve, temporal to the CRA. Leaving the nerve after approximately 10 mm, it drains to the superior ophthalmic vein or directly into the cavernous sinus.[3]

Choroidal blood exits the eye through 1 or 2 vortex veins per quadrant to the superior and inferior ophthalmic veins, which then drain into the cavernous sinus.

Outer Blood-retinal Barrier

The tight cell junctions between the retinal pigment epithelial (RPE) cells form a blood-retinal barrier and prevent leakage of fluid from the choroid to the retina. Breakdown of this barrier occurs when the RPE cells are damaged.[3]

Inner Blood-retinal Barrier

Tight cell junctions between endothelial cells of the retinal vessels form a barrier preventing extravasation of fluid/ macromolecules into the retina. Pericytes, Müller cells and astrocytes also play a role in formation of the barrier.[3]

HISTOPATHOLOGY OF ARTERIAL OCCLUSIONS

The retina has a high oxidative capacity and a high level of glycolytic activity. The decrease or absence of perfusion caused by CRA obstruction leads to decreased delivery of glucose and oxygen to the tissues of the retina.[18] Ischemia leads to edema as neuron cellular membranes burst, producing the associated funduscopic whitening of the retina caused by opacification of the ganglion cell layer.[19,20] The opacification is most prominent in the macular region where the multiple layers of ganglion cells reside. Retinal opacification generally decreases toward the periphery as the ganglion cell population diminishes and is absent from the avascular zone of the foveola where ganglion cells are absent.[21] The classic "cherry red spot" is a result of the visible red reflex of the perfused choroid at this location. Ischemia leads to release of several factors [i.e. vascular endothelial growth factor (VEGF), nitric oxide, glutamate, inflammatory cytokines and reactive oxygen species], which

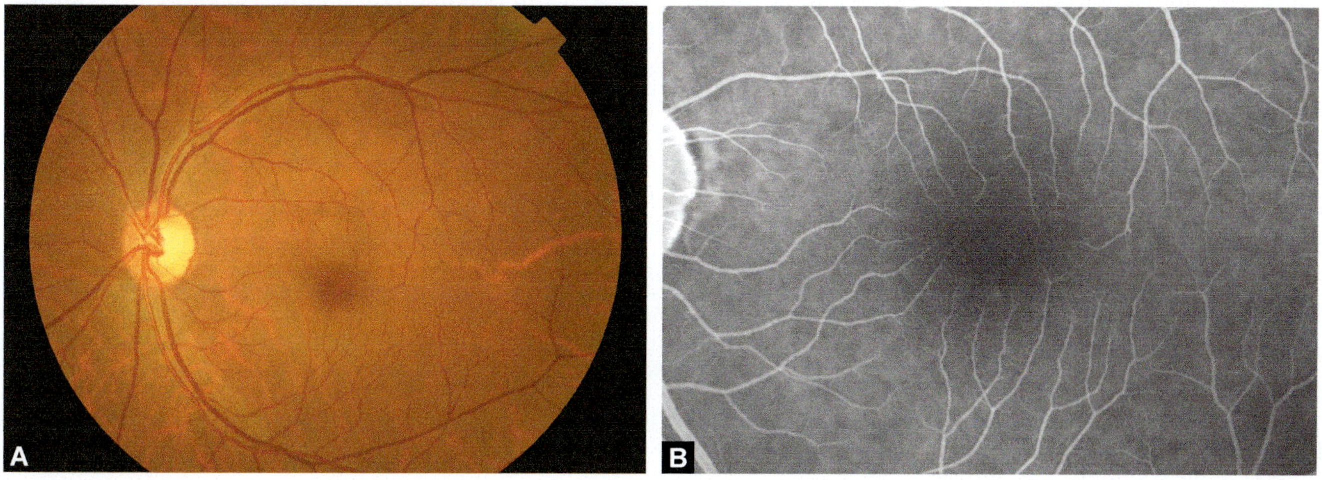

Figs. 49.1A and B: Fundus photography (A) and fluorescein angiogram (B) of right macula showing normal perfusion and foveal avascular zone.

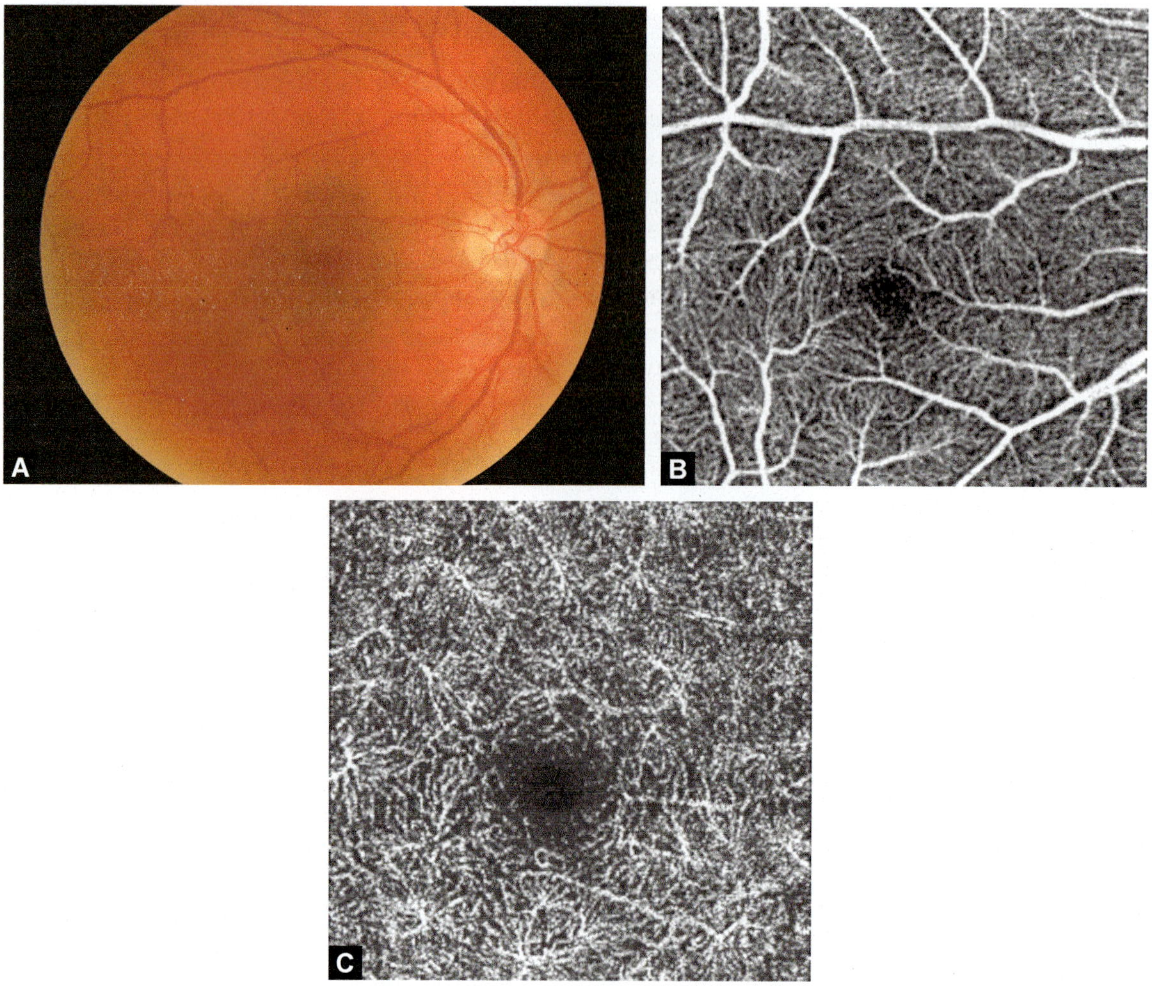

Figs. 49.2A to C: Fundus photography (A) and optical coherence tomography angiography of left macula showing normal perfusion and foveal avascular zone at superficial (B) and deep (C) retinal layers.

contribute to retinal damage and subsequent ganglion cell loss through several pathways.[22]

Animal studies have demonstrated swelling of the organelles that precedes axonal and dendritic rupture with decreased neuronal cell count. Mitochondria, the first organelles affected in the ganglion cells, begin to swell as early as 15 min after CRAO in squirrel monkeys.[18,20] Microtubules and cisternae of the endoplasmic reticulum are also acutely susceptible to ischemia.[18] In Kroll's experimental occlusion of the CRA in squirrel monkeys, swelling of the endoplasmic reticulum had occurred by 3.5 hr.[20] Müller cells were relatively more resistant to ischemia than the ganglion cells in both species, presumably due to their proximity to retinal capillaries and the choriocapillaris and a greater ability to metabolize under anaerobic conditions. These changes are similar to those seen in humans.[20,23,24]

Retinal cellular survival, and thus final visual outcome, in humans is related to duration of ischemia and the presence of residual circulation. However, no controlled data are available in humans. In squirrel monkeys, Kroll observed axonal and dendritic lysis by 3.5 hr and extensive cellular loss by 16 hr.[20] Hayreh and associates found that rhesus monkey retinas could tolerate 97–98 min of total occlusion and that only half of eyes occluded for 102 min recovered vision. However, all eyes occluded 105 min or more suffered irrecoverable ischemia.[18,25,26]

IMAGING

Optical Coherence Tomography

Optical coherence tomography of acute CRAO correlates with these histopathologic features and/or characteristics.

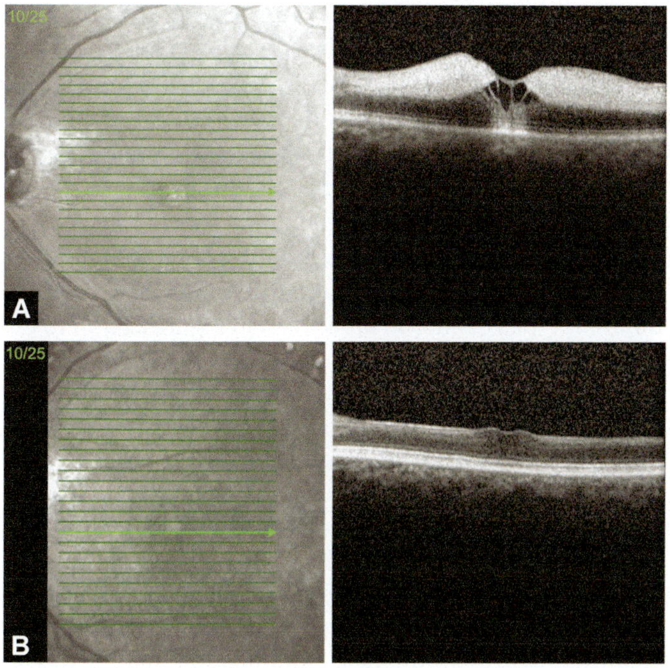

Figs. 49.3A and B: Optical coherence tomography through fovea of left eye showing acute inner retinal whitening (A) and chronic inner retinal atrophy (B) of a central arterial artery occlusion.

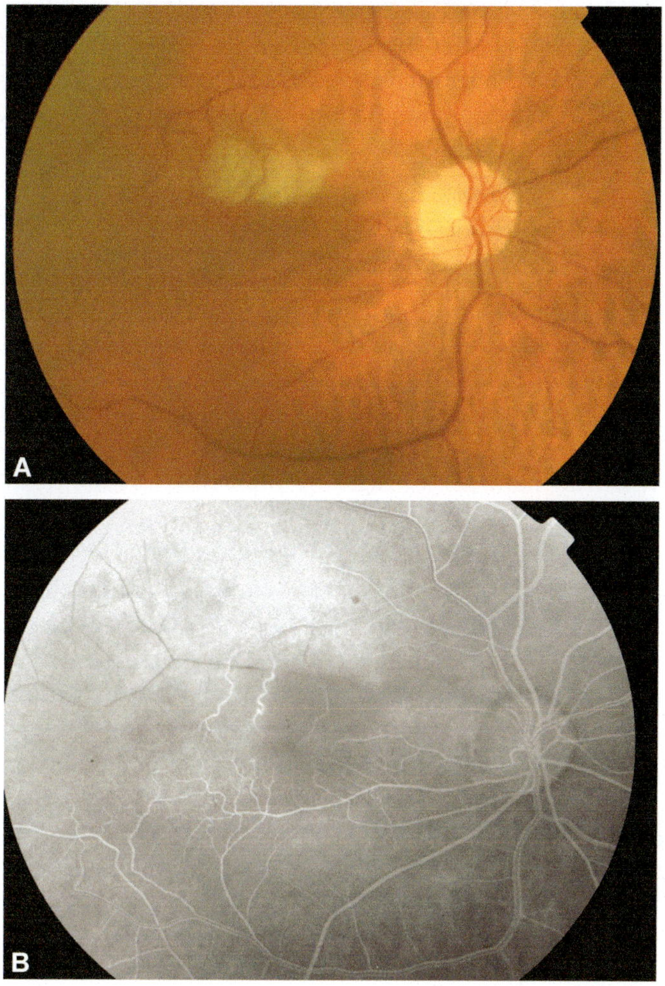

Figs. 49.4A and B: Fundus image (A) and fluorescein angiogram (B) at 34 seconds showing delayed filling of superior macular artery branch after occlusion.

Findings on OCT demonstrate an increase in inner layer reflectivity and muted outer layer reflectivity around the foveola with normal reflectivity of the RPE beneath the foveola.[27] Eventually, cellular debris in the ischemic inner layers of the retina undergoes phagocytosis and gliosis leading to atrophy (Figs. 49.3A and B).[28-30]

Optical Coherence Tomography Angiography

Recent studies suggest that OCT angiography (OCTA) may become a noninvasive alternative imaging technique to characterize macular ischemia and monitor vascular flow changes in ischemia. In contrast to conventional FFA, OCTA can differentiate specific changes in the different retinal capillary plexuses.[31-33]

Fluorescein Angiography

Fluorescein angiography shows delayed or absent flow in the occluded vessel and sometimes retrograde filling in the later phase (Figs. 49.4A and B). Ophthalmic artery occlusion leads to hypoperfusion and thus hypofluorescence of the choroidal background.

EPIDEMIOLOGY

Incidence of retinal arterial occlusions is estimated at 1 or 2 in 100,000 and increases with age.[34,35] Common systemic risk factors for retinal arterial occlusive disease include hypertension, diabetes, lipid disorders, and cardiac and systemic atherosclerotic disease.[36]

MECHANISMS OF OCCLUSION

The principal mechanisms operative in occlusion of the retinal arterial system are embolic, thrombotic, vasospastic, extravascular compressive and vasculitic. Other mechanisms, such as radiation and elevated IOP, occur much less commonly.

In general, age is an important factor in determining the mechanism of occlusion. Patients aged 50 and greater are likely to have occlusions associated with embolic disease while younger patients are more likely to have occlusions secondary to thrombosis.

Embolism/Endogenous

Embolic occlusion arising from the arterial afferent system represents the most common mechanism. Atherosclerosis of the carotid system is the most common source of retinal emboli with 80% being associated with carotid artery disease.[3,37,38] The degree of obstruction of the carotid artery is less important than the presence of ulcerative plaques, which are more likely to lead to emboli than an extensively occluded carotid artery without plaques. Carotid artery disease is evaluated by carotid ultrasonography, arteriography, and computed tomography angiography.

The heart and major vessels are another important source of emboli. Valvular abnormalities, tumors such as atrial myxomas, and thrombus formation in the left atrium secondary to conditions like atrial fibrillation, can lead to emboli formation.[39-41] Additionally, right to left shunts, like a patent foramen ovale, can allow emboli from venous thrombotic disease to reach the arterial circulation.[42] An important technique for evaluating embolic disease originating from the heart is transthoracic/transesophageal echocardiography. Other rare sources of endogenous emboli include fat emboli from long bone fractures or amniotic fluid emboli at the time of delivery.[43-45]

Embolism/Exogenous

Exogenous particles can reach the retinal circulation and cause arterial occlusive events. They are introduced into the arterial blood flow either directly or as venous foreign bodies through an open foramen ovale leading to paradoxical embolism. Examples of exogenous emboli include triamcinolone particles from periorbital/nasal steroid-injections, fragments of catheter tips or artificial heart valves and emboli associated with intravenous drug abuse (e.g. talc retinopathy).[46-51]

Types of Retinal Emboli

Emboli are only visible in 20–30% of all retinal occlusions.[52] Clinically the most common are cholesterol emboli ("Hollenhorst plaques", 74%). Less common are platelet fibrin emboli (15.5%) and calcific emboli (10.5%).[3]

Cholesterol emboli are slim and glistening yellow. They most commonly arise from atherosclerotic plaques of the carotid artery and typically do not occlude the vessel distal to the embolus. Platelet fibrin emboli may appear gray-white, are larger and longer than cholesterol emboli, and may be seen to pass through the retinal vessels.

Calcific emboli are larger and gray-white in color and are associated with more severe local obstructions. They seem to arise more from cardiac valvular disease.[53] The different types of emboli are shown in Figures 49.5A to C.

Thrombosis

Thrombosis is another mechanism causing arterial occlusive disease of the retina, although it is much more common in venous occlusions. Virchow's classic triad concerning the pathogenesis of thrombosis comprises vessel wall abnormalities, stasis of blood flow, and changes in the blood components. While any one of these factors alone may lead to thrombosis, combinations of these factors significantly increase the likelihood of these episodes.

Structural abnormalities in a vessel like a prepapillary arterial loop can contribute to retinal arterial occlusion by thrombosis.[54] Changes in blood coagulability typically cause venous retinal occlusions but may also contribute to arterial vascular occlusion. Hereditary causes of thrombophilia as well as local and systemic factors are shown in Table 49.1.

Antithrombin Deficiency

The plasma protein human antithrombin (AT) is a protease inhibitor that prevents the formation of thrombi.[55] Previously termed ATIII deficiency, AT deficiency was the first described hereditary deficiency of an anticoagulant protein. Inherited as an autosomal dominant trait, AT deficiency is associated with a thrombotic tendency typically manifested as venous thromboembolism. However, retinal arterial occlusions secondary to thrombosis have been reported.[56]

Protein C/S Deficiency

Protein C and protein S are vitamin K-dependent plasma glycoproteins synthesized in the liver. Deficiency in these proteins occurs primarily as a hereditary condition. It is inherited as an autosomal dominant trait but can be an acquired defect associated with advanced severe liver disease. Both protein C and protein S serve as cofactors for the anticoagulant function of activated protein C, a protein

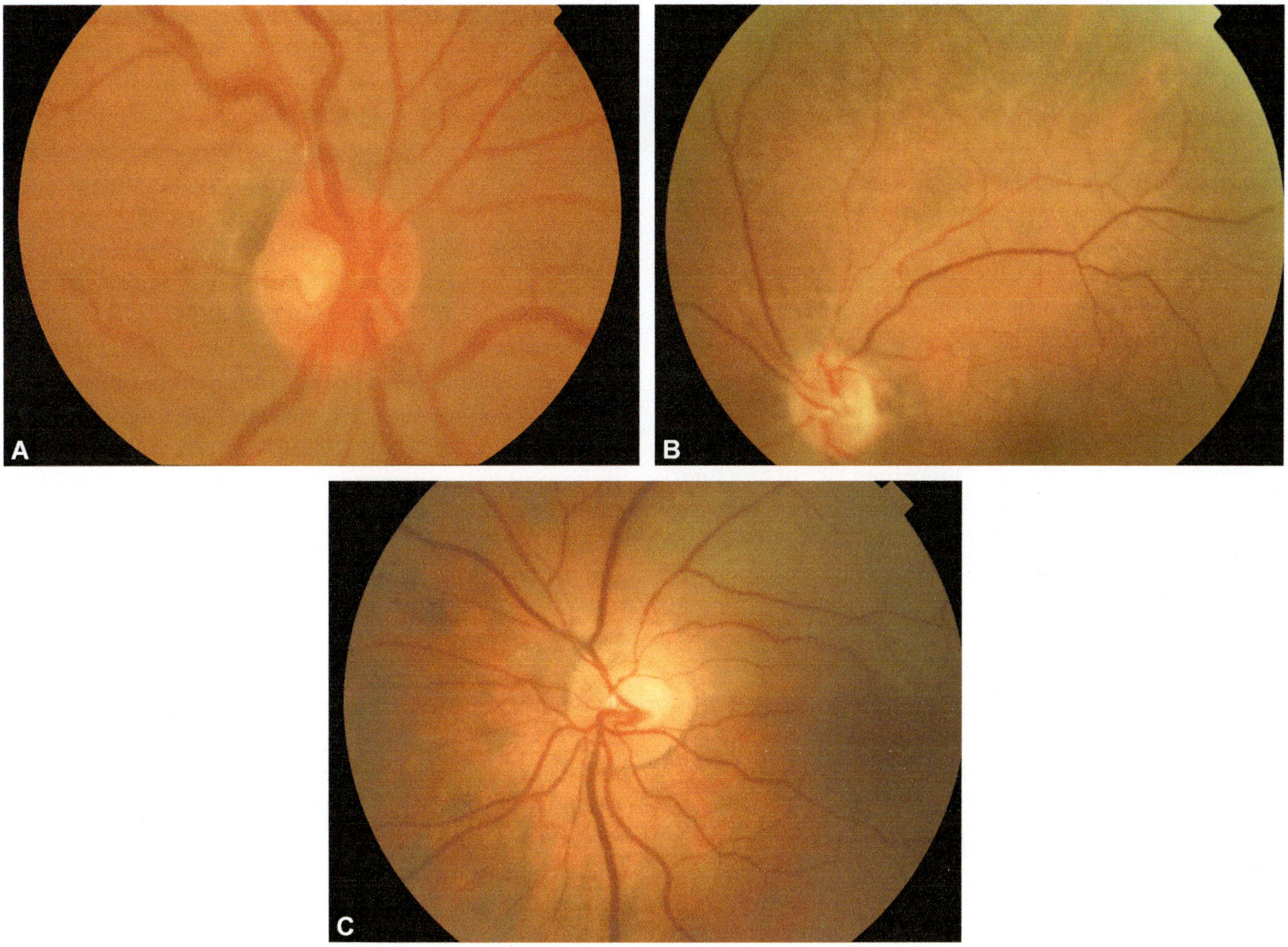

Figs. 49.5A to C: Types of emboli: Hollenhorst (cholesterol) plaque (A), fibrin embolus (B), and calcific embolus (C).

Table 49.1: Factors associated with retinal arterial occlusions.

Thrombophilia (genetic)	Local factors	Systemic factors
Factor V Leiden	Optic nerve head drusen	Trauma
Antithrombin deficiency	Peripapillary arterial loop	Malignancy
Protein C deficiency	Intraocular foreign body	Pregnancy
Protein S deficiency	Elevated intraocular pressure	Oral contraceptives
Hyperhomocysteinemia	External compression of globe	Autoimmune disease
Antiphospholipid antibodies	External compression of central retinal artery/ophthalmic artery	Smoking
Lupus anticoagulant		Sickle cell hemoglobinopathies
Anticardiolipin		Vasculitis
Homozygous C677T polymorphism in methylene tetrahydrofolate reductase		Vasospasm
Prothrombin G20210A		
Dysfibrogenemia		
Elevated factor VIII		
Elevated factor IX		

that inactivates factors V-A and VIII-A and downregulates thrombosis.[55] Deficiencies of either protein C or protein S lead to a thrombotic tendency; and arterial occlusive disease of the retina has been described with each.[57-59]

Activated Protein C Resistance and Factor V Leiden

As mentioned previously, activated protein C inactivates factor V-A and factor VIII-A and downregulates thrombosis. Activated protein C resistance refers to an abnormally reduced anti-coagulant response of a subject's plasma to activated protein C in in-vitro testing. Although any genetic abnormality of the protein C pathway can cause activated protein C resistance, more than 90% of hereditary activated protein C resistant subjects have the same genetic abnormality termed factor V Leiden. Factor V Leiden is an abnormal factor V associated with a point mutation and a single amino acid change. Factor V Leiden is resistant to the proteolytic action of activated protein C, leading to increased thrombin formation.[55] The subsequent hypercoagulable state is a very common hereditary cause of thrombophilia and has been associated with arterial occlusive disease of the retina.[60,61]

Hyperhomocystinemia

Homocysteine is an intermediate in the metabolism of the amino acids methionine and cysteine. Hyperhomocystinemia refers to elevated plasma levels of homocysteine and can be caused by numerous factors. The most common genetic cause of hyperhomocystinemia is a mutation in the enzyme methylene tetrahydrofolate reductase leading to elevated levels of plasma homocysteine. It is present in 10–20% of Caucasians and in 10% of Asians but is rare in blacks. This defect, either alone or in combination with low folate, B_6 or B_{12} levels, or with conditions such as renal failure, hypothyroidism, smoking, excess caffeine consumption, and inflammatory bowel disease, can be associated with increased levels of plasma homocysteine. The exact mechanism of thrombosis associated with hyperhomocystinemia is poorly understood; but endothelial toxicity and smooth muscle proliferation have been proposed. Arterial thrombotic disease of the retina has been reported.[61-63]

Antiphospholipid Syndrome

The antiphospholipid syndrome (previously known as antiphospholipid antibody syndrome, anticardiolipin antibodies syndrome, and lupus anticoagulant) is an acquired disorder associated with thrombotic complications. It can be primary or it can be secondary if associated with conditions such as systemic lupus erythematosus, other autoimmune disorders, viral infections, or malignancies or with some medications. The syndrome is characterized by the presence of antibodies to phospholipid protein complexes (anticardiolipin, antiphosphatidyl serine or anti-β glycoprotein) or by the detection of lupus anticoagulants.[64] The precise mechanism by which these antiphospholipid antibodies promote thrombosis is poorly understood, but it may be related to inhibition of prostacyclin, a platelet inhibitory prostaglandin, or related to impairment of protein C and antithrombin II anticoagulant mechanisms.[65] While venous occlusive disease is most common, arterial occlusive disease of the retina has also been associated with the antiphospholipid syndrome.[61,66]

Vasculitis and Giant Cell Arteritis

Systemic vasculitis leading to arterial occlusions can be associated with collagen vascular diseases such as systemic lupus erythematosus. Behçet disease can also result in arterial occlusions.[67] Localized retinal vasculitis with vessel occlusion can originate from infectious retinitis conditions, such as toxoplasmosis, tuberculosis, syphilis, or Bartonella henselae.[68-70] Susac syndrome, as discussed later, is a presumed autoimmune-mediated, microvascular vasculitis typically associated with branch artery occlusions.

Giant cell arteritis (GCA) is a possible cause for CRAO/cilioretinal artery occlusion in the elderly, with a pathomechanism that is combined vasculitic/thrombotic. Prodromal amaurosis fugax is very common in GCA (40–60%),[71] and ophthalmic manifestations other than retinal arterial occlusion can comprise ocular ischemic syndrome, anterior ischemic optic neuropathy, posterior ischemic optic neuropathy, or oculomotor nerve palsies.[71] Typical symptoms are headache, scalp tenderness, jaw claudication, fever, weight loss, and malaise; however, "occult" GCA (ophthalmic involvement in the absence of systemic signs) occurs in 5–38%.[72]

Diagnostic work-up consists of specific questions and examination regarding its characteristic symptoms and signs, and blood testing for elevated erythrocyte sedimentation rate (ESR), C-reactive protein (CRP) and platelets. The ultimate gold standard for diagnosis is temporal artery biopsy. There is controversy about the length of the biopsy because of the typical skip lesions along the vessel; but a minimum of 2 cm is generally recommended.[73,74] Temporal artery Doppler ultrasound is a newer diagnostic tool that demonstrates the typical dark "halo-sign" around the temporal artery if affected by GCA. Ultrasonography also helps to localize the vessel for biopsy when not palpable.[75] Because of the potential blinding and/or life-threatening consequences of this disease, the suspicion threshold should be low and high dose systemic corticosteroids should be started at an early stage.[71,76,77] In 1990, the American College of Rheumatology proposed diagnostic criteria for GCA, i.e. age at onset more than or equal to 50 years, new headache, temporal artery abnormality (tenderness to palpation, decreased pulsation), elevated erythrocyte sedimentation rate, and abnormal artery biopsy. With more than or equal to 3 out of 5 criteria present, GCA can be diagnosed.[78]

Susac Syndrome

Susac syndrome, first described in 2004, is a rare, presumably autoimmune-mediated, microangiopathy characterized by subacute encephalopathy, branch retinal artery occlusions, and sensorineural hearing loss.[79-81] Susac syndrome mostly affects young women. The typical triad of symptoms is considered pathognomonic; however, only 13% of patients show the complete clinical picture at onset.[82,83] A diagnostic approach using criteria to distinguish between definite, probable, and possible diagnosis of Susac syndrome has been proposed.[83]

The typical clinical picture is retinal involvement with branch retinal artery occlusion (BRAO) (98%); but neuro-ophthalmological pathologies (oculomotor dysfunction with nystagmus, ophthalmoplegia, saccadic eye movements, diplopia) develop in 7% of those affected.[84] Fundoscopy may show signs of BRAO or retinal arterial wall plaques (Gass plaques), which represent lipid extravasations through the defective retinal vessel walls. In contrast to embolic plaques, these are typically not associated with bifurcations (Figs. 49.6A and B).[85,86]

Fluorescein angiography shows the arterial occlusions (which may be small and clinically quiet) and frequently (96%) reveals arterial wall hyperfluorescence (AWH) (Fig. 49.7).[82] These AWHs do not have to be located near the BRAO and can occur in fundoscopically normal arterioles.[84]

Optical coherence tomography has been shown to detect hyper-reflectance in the acute stage of BRAO and subsequent significant atrophy of the outer retinal layers. AWH does not result in any detectable changes in OCT.[87,88]

Vasospasm

Vasospasm is a rare cause of arterial occlusive disease and has been reported in migraine, collagen vascular diseases, and sickle-cell hemoglobinopathies.[89-93]

Other Mechanisms

Local conditions in the eye and orbit may predispose to occlusive events, e.g. peripapillary arterial loop, optic nerve head drusen, intraocular foreign body, elevated IOP, or external compression of the ophthalmic artery or central retinal artery caused by orbital cellulitis, orbital hemorrhage, abscess formation, cavernous sinus thrombosis, or neoplastic disease.[94,95]

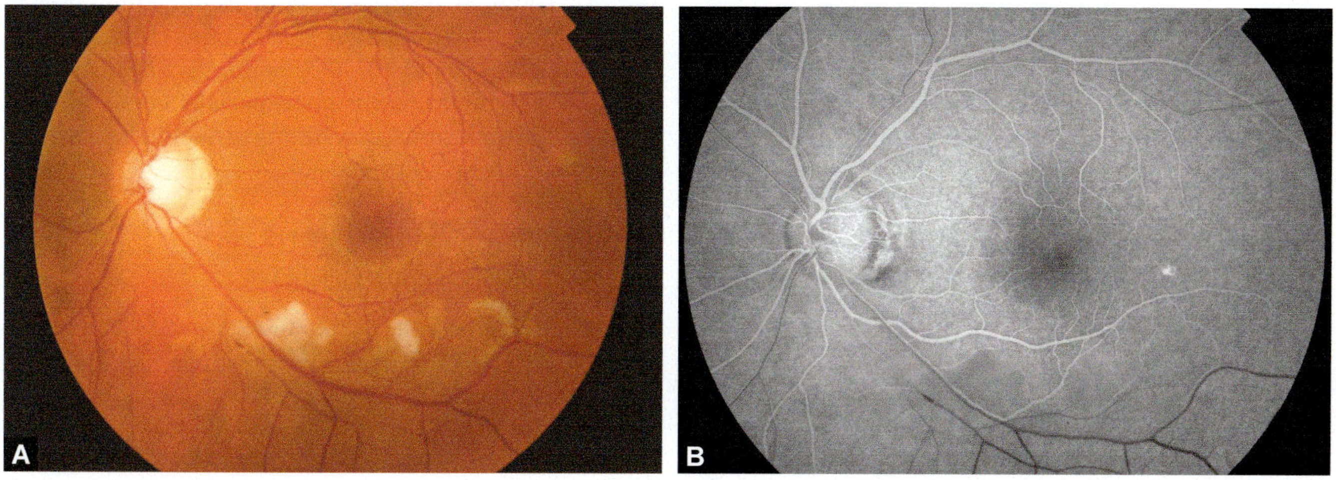

Figs. 49.6A and B: Fundus photography (A) and fluorescein angiogram (B) of inferior branch arterial occlusion in Susac syndrome.

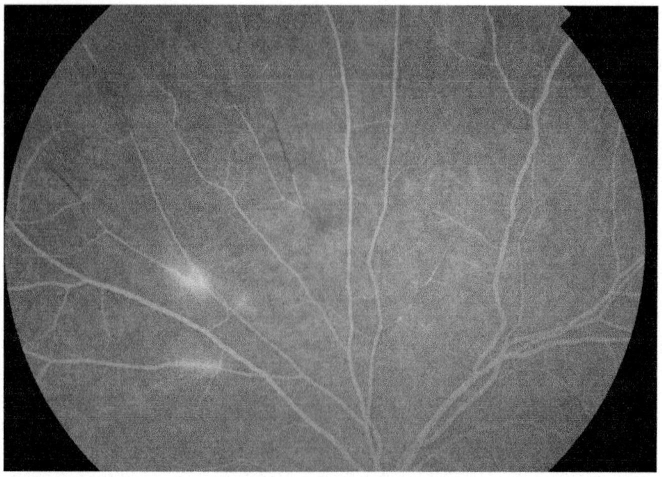

Fig. 49.7: Fluorescein angiogram of arterial wall hyperfluorescence of superior midperipheral arteries in Susac syndrome.

CLINICAL FINDINGS

Amaurosis Fugax

Amaurosis fugax is characterized by transient, painless vision loss in one eye, lasting for up to 20 minutes. Most commonly, it results from carotid or cardiac embolic disease; but it can also occur with giant cell arteritis, migraine, eclampsia, hypotension, hyperviscosity, or vertebrobasilar insufficiency (in which vision loss is bilateral).[96] Management is the same as for arterial occlusion, as there is a 90-day stroke risk of 10% in patients experiencing a transient ischemic attack (TIA).[97-99]

Carotid endarterectomy for amaurosis fugax and carotid stenosis is a controversial topic.[100]

Ophthalmic Artery Occlusion

In ophthalmic artery occlusion, there is ischemia in both retinal and choroidal circulation, resulting in pronounced visual loss (often no light perception) and relative afferent pupillary defect (RAPD). Because choroidal perfusion is absent, funduscopic examination reveals no cherry red spot, but rather extensive retinal whitening. Often, there is a pale disc swelling and box-carring or segmentation of the blood column in retinal vessels. The typical angiographic pictures are shown in Figures 49.8A and B.

Central Retinal Artery Occlusion

Central retinal artery occlusion (CRAO) is a rare disease with an incidence of about 2/100,000.[34] The typical sign of CRAO is a marked, painless visual loss and RAPD. Fundoscopic examination shows a cherry red spot in the macula around retinal whitening from ischemia and box-carring in retinal vessels (Figs. 49.9A and B). If the patient presents very early after closure of the artery, the fundus may appear normal since ischemic signs may be of variable degree depending on the duration of occlusion.[101] The typical angiographic sign is delayed arm-retina time (Figs. 49.10A and B). The acute and chronic changes on OCT are shown in Figures 49.11A and B. Visual outcome is usually guarded except in cases with conserved macular cilioretinal supply. Chronic changes in CRAO include optic disc atrophy, attenuated retinal arteries and veins, atrophic retinal changes, and cilioretinal disc collaterals. Retinal NV, however, seems to be a rare complication and may be caused mainly by concomitant diabetic retinopathy (DR) or ocular ischemia.[101,102]

Branch Retinal Artery Occlusion

In 90% of branch artery occlusions, the etiology is embolic, and the emboli are most likely found at arterial bifurcations. Retinal whitening is restricted to the affected vessel, and visual loss usually is altitudinal, corresponding to the respective area (Figs. 49.12 and 49.13). Depending on foveal involvement, visual acuity (VA) ranges from 20/20 to 20/400, and RAPD may or may not be present.

Ciliary Retinal Artery Occlusion

Since a ciliary artery usually perfuses the central macula, occlusion of the ciliary artery results in sudden loss of central vision (Figs. 49.14A and B). Ciliary artery occlusions seem to be quite rare (estimated at 5% of all arterial occlusions), whereas macular sparing due to an unaffected ciliary artery occurs in about 10% of all CRAOs (Figs. 49.15A and B).[6] Often, no RAPD is present; and the prognosis for an isolated cilioretinal artery occlusion is good, with 90% of cases improving to 20/40 or better. As discussed later, ciliary retinal artery occlusion, especially in combination with venous occlusions, may be due to hemodynamic block rather than to embolic occlusion.

Combined Occlusions (Arterial and Venous)

One relatively frequent combination of arterial and venous occlusions is central retinal vein occlusion (CRVO) and cilioretinal artery occlusion (Figs. 49.16A and B). Cilioretinal ischemia in this context is believed to be a hemodynamic block rather than an embolic occlusion caused by the rise of the intraluminal pressure of the retinal capillary bed.[103]

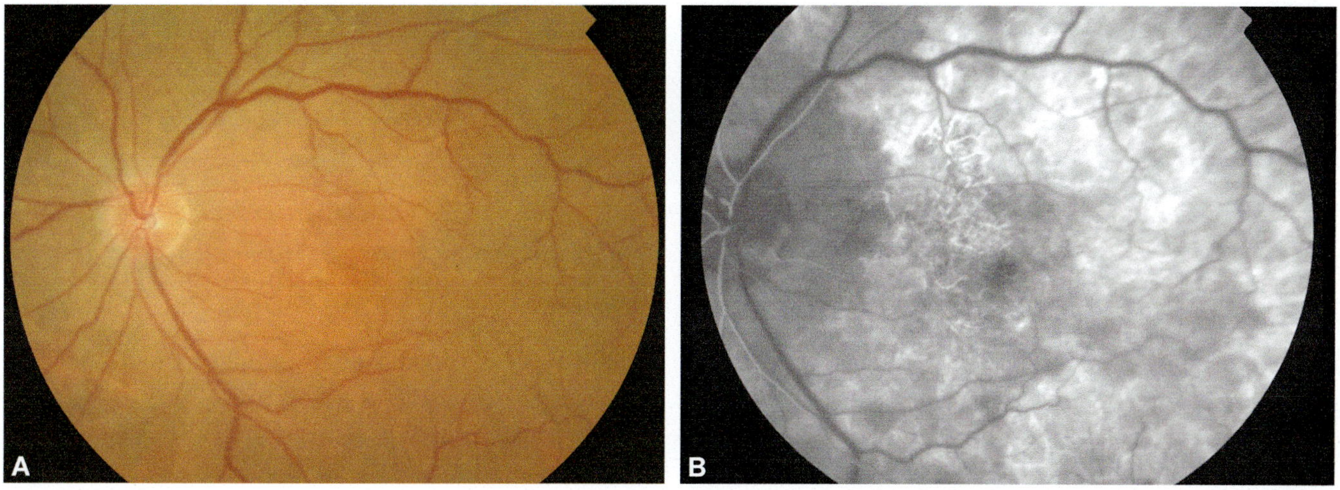

Figs. 49.8A and B: Fundus photography (A) and fluorescein angiogram (B) at 46 seconds showing the absence of a cherry red spot and choroidal non-perfusion after ophthalmic artery occlusion.

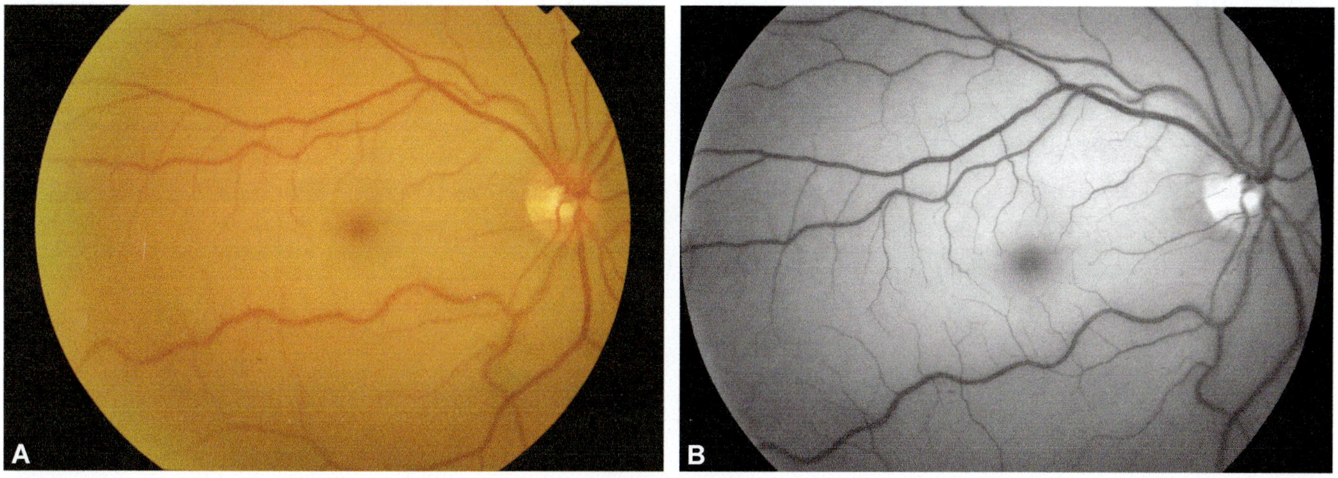

Figs. 49.9A and B: Fundus photography (A) and fundus autofluorescence (B) of acute central artery occlusion showing the typical cherry red spot.

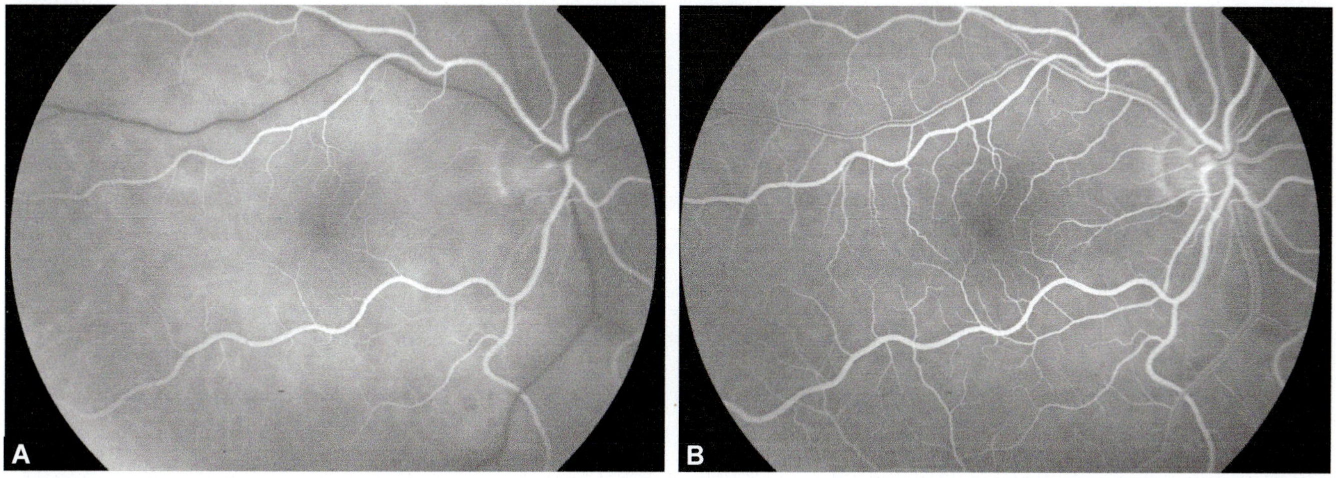

Figs. 49.10A and B: Fluorescein angiograph of acute central retinal artery occlusion at 23 sec (A) and 28 sec; (B) showing delayed arm-retina time.

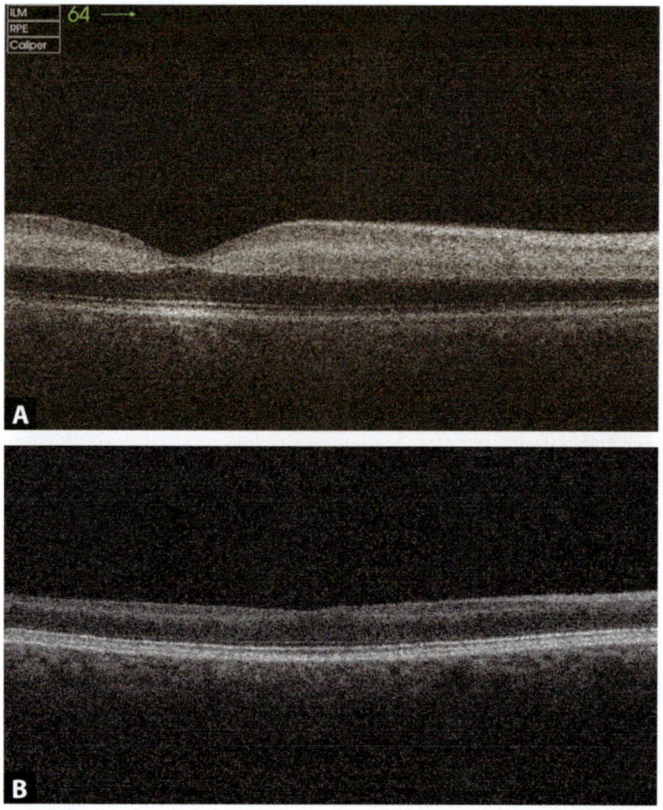

Figs. 49.11A and B: Optical coherence tomography of acute (A) central retinal artery occlusion showing the whitening of the inner retinal layers and of chronic (B) changes with atrophy of the inner retina.

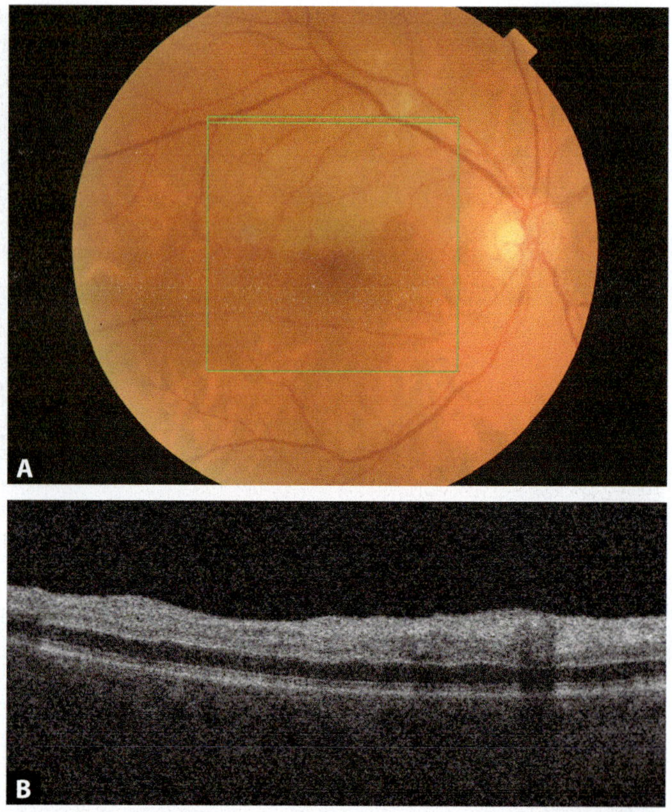

Figs. 49.12A and B: Fundus photography (A) and optical coherence tomography (B) of superior macular branch artery occlusion. The left upper macular region is whitened and corresponds to the whitening of the inner retinal layers in the OCT image.

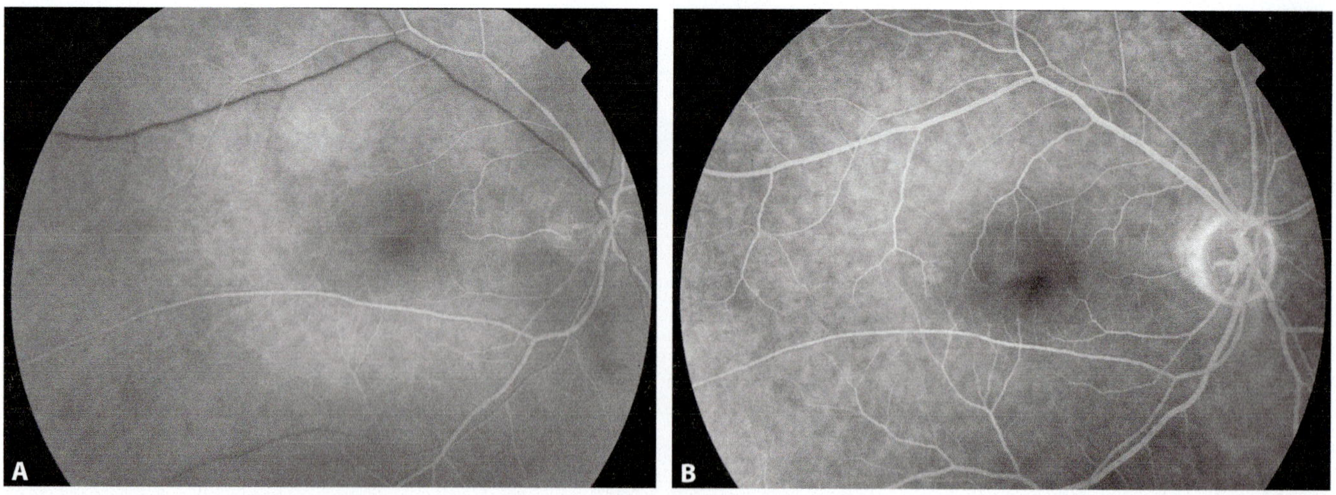

Figs. 49.13A and B: Fluorescein angiogram of the same case as Figure 49.12 at 17 sec (A) and 2 min (B) demonstrating delayed arterial filling time of the affected vessel.

Other combinations (central retinal vein occlusion with central retinal artery occlusion, branch vein occlusion with branch artery occlusion) are rare and are mostly reported in association with systemic factors, i.e. several cardiovascular risk factors, immunological diseases, malignancies, and coagulopathies.[104]

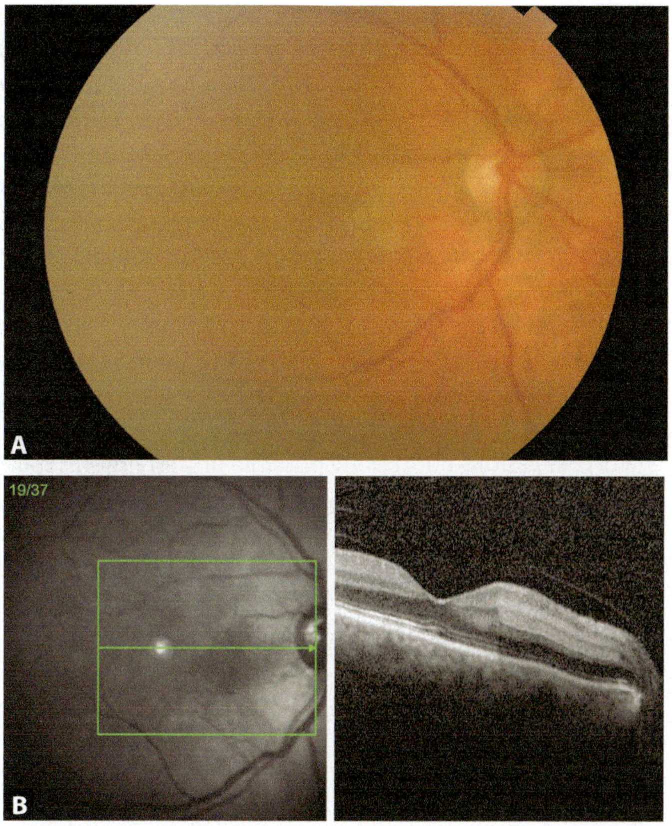

Figs. 49.14A and B: Fundus photography (A) with whitening in the area of supply of the cilioretinal artery and optical coherence tomography (B) demonstrating corresponding inner retinal whitening after cilioretinal artery occlusion.

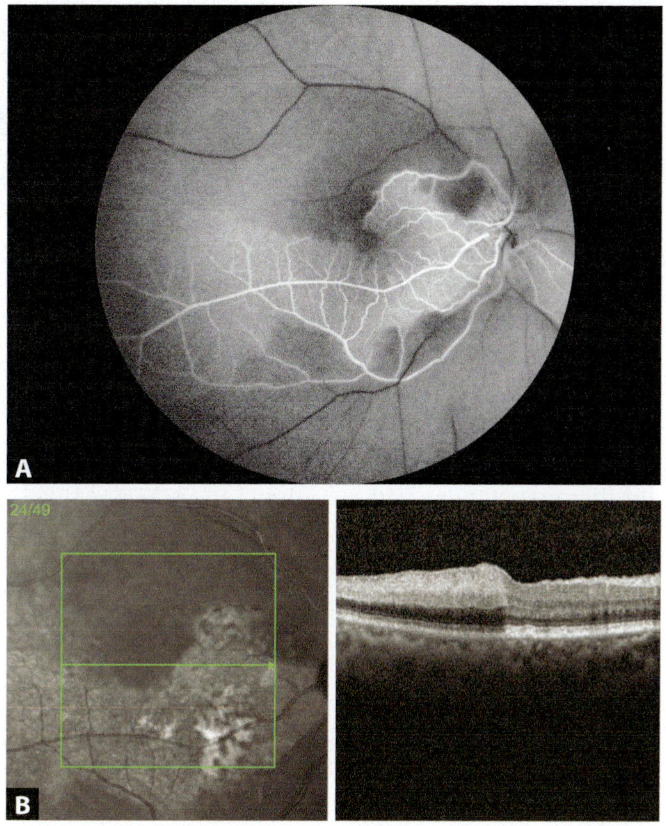

Figs. 49.15A and B: Fluorescein angiogram (A) at 1 min showing cilioretinal artery sparing in the context of central retinal artery occlusion. Corresponding OCT (B) depicts normal retinal architecture in the area of supply of the cilioretinal artery, but whitening of inner retinal layers in the ischemic area of the occluded central retinal artery.

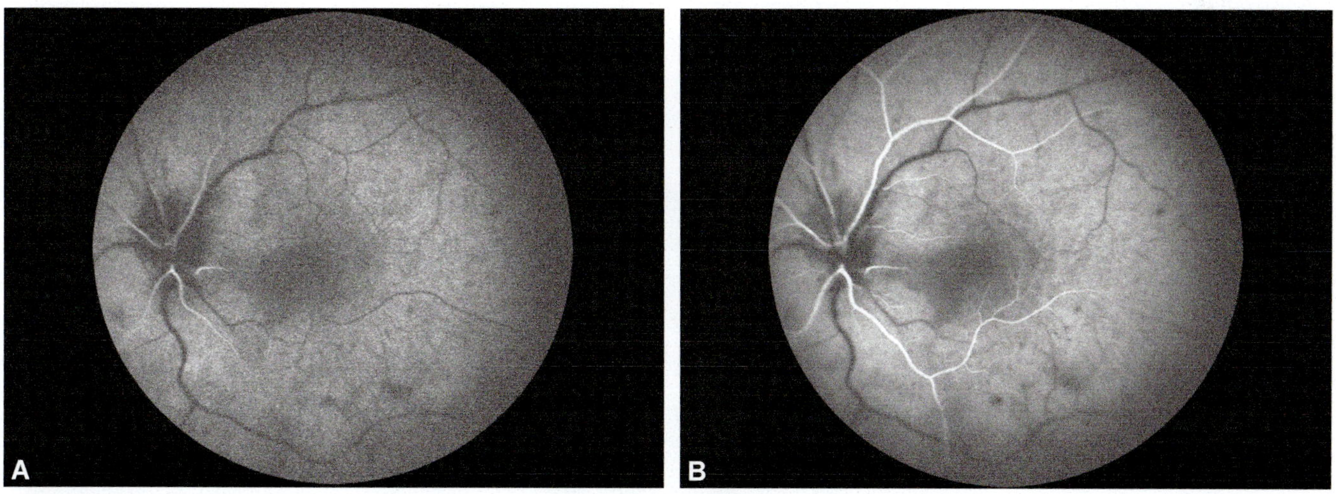

Figs. 49.16A and B: Fluorescein angiogram at 46 sec (A) and 1 min (B) of central retinal vein occlusion and combined hemodynamic blockage of the cilioretinal artery.

Paracentral Acute Middle Maculopathy

Paracentral acute middle maculopathy (PAMM) represents ischemia within the intermediate/deep retinal capillary plexus. The condition was first described by Sarraf in 2013 as a possible variant of acute macular neuroretinopathy (AMN) ("type 1 AMN"); but the distinctive nature of PAMM was demonstrated with the development of diagnostic tools, i.e. spectral domain-OCT (Table 49.2).[105,106]

Patients with PAMM are typically male and in their 50s or 60s. An underlying vascular disease is often found (e.g. hypertensive retinopathy/DR, retinal artery/vein occlusion, sickle cell retinopathy, or Purtscher retinopathy).[107-109] Further associations with migraine, severe hypovolemia, viral illness, or medications (amphetamines, caffeine, vasopressors, oral contraceptives) have been described.[107,108]

The typical clinical presentation is an acute, unilateral, painless paracentral scotoma with possible symptoms from associated disease (e.g. visual loss from vessel occlusion, headache). Funduscopy may reveal the signs of an underlying retinal disease; the wedge-shaped PAMM lesions themselves are slightly whitish or even clinically invisible.[105]

The most important diagnostic tool is the OCT/en face OCT, which demonstrates a hyper-reflective band at the level of the inner nuclear layer (Figs. 49.17A and B). Near infrared image shows corresponding, characteristic dark gray, paracentral, well-circumscribed lesions (Fig. 49.18).[105] Over time, atrophy of the inner nuclear layer results in localized thinning of the area corresponding to the clinically often persistent paracentral scotoma. OCTA has demonstrated attenuation of flow signal at the level of the deep capillary plexus in older lesions while acute lesions may also show inconspicuous flow signal.[110-115] However, definitive interpretation should be made cautiously, bearing in mind that OCTA remains an emerging imaging modality.[113]

Investigations addressing possible underlying vascular disease should be undertaken, especially for younger, otherwise healthy patients where no apparent cause is found. There is no specific therapy for PAMM lesions itself; but depending on the underlying disease, causal therapy is mandated (i.e. addressing carotid artery disease and controlling blood sugar).

MANAGEMENT

Management of arterial occlusions comprises three aspects.

Table 49.2: Typical features of paracentral acute middle maculopathy (PAMM) versus acute macular neuroretinopathy (AMN).

Features	PAMM	AMN
Localization of hyper-reflectivity	Superficial to outer plexiform layer	Deep to outer plexiform layer
Localization of atrophy	Inner nuclear layer	Outer nuclear layer
Epidemiology	Male preponderance, 50/60 years	80% female, 30–40 years, Caucasian
Associations	Vascular disease (vein occlusions, ...)	Nonspecific flu-like illness, contraceptive use, ...
OCT imaging		
Acute: Hyper-reflectivity	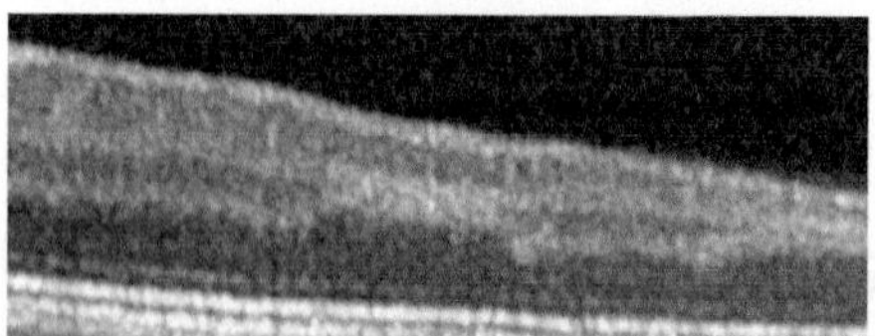	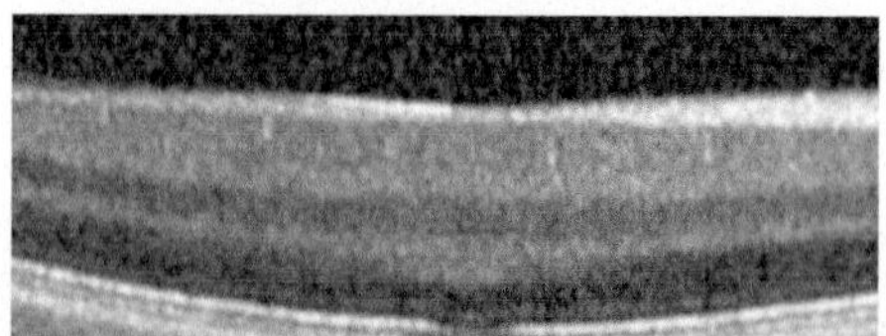
Chronic: Atrophy	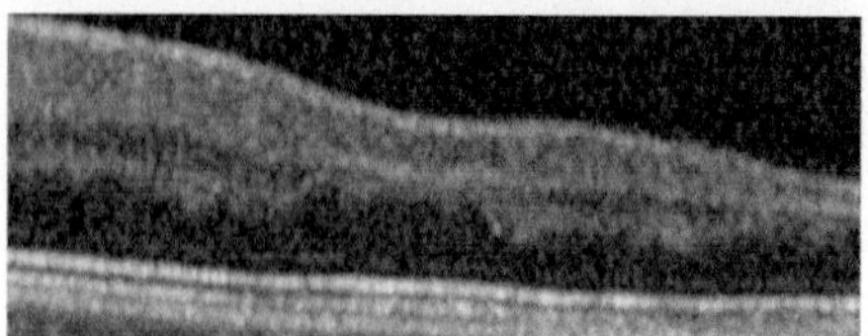	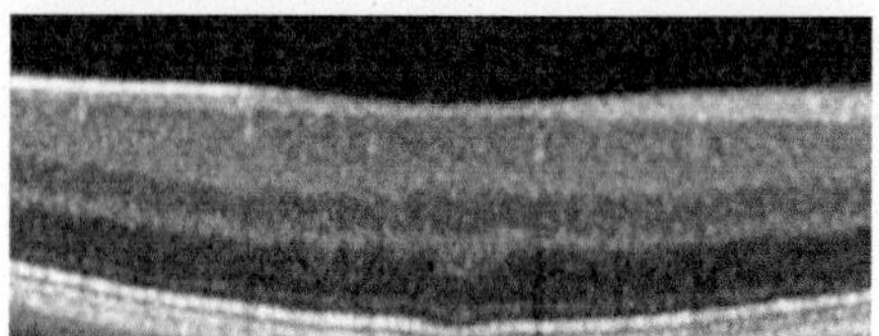

(OCT: Optical coherence tomography)

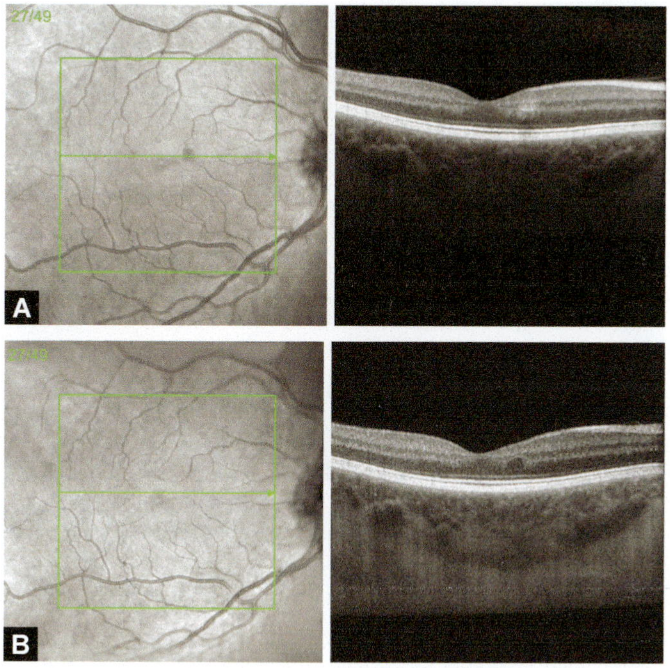

Figs. 49.17A and B: Optical coherence tomography of acute (A) versus chronic (B) changes in paracentral acute middle maculopathy, demonstrating hyper-reflectivity of the inner nuclear layer in the acute phase with subsequent atrophy at the chronic stage.

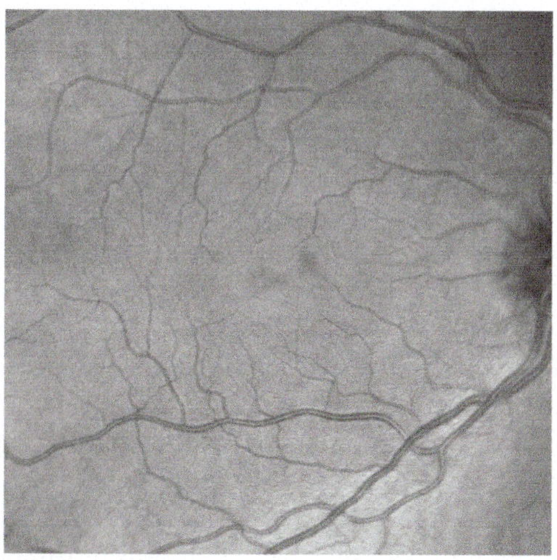

Fig. 49.18: Infrared image of paracentral acute middle maculopathy showing a characteristic dark gray paracentral lesion.

Management of the Acute Occlusive Event, Attempting to Restore Visual Function

The therapeutic goal is to restore ocular perfusion as soon as possible, analogous to treatment of cerebral infarctions. Unfortunately, no treatment has proven beneficial thus far. Treatment options are directed at lowering IOP (local antihypertensive agents, acetazolamide PO/IV, mannitol IV, or anterior chamber paracentesis), increasing vasodilation (sublingual nitroglycerin/isosorbide dinitrate, inhalation of carbogen), and improving retinal perfusion/oxygenation (isovolemic hemodilution, enhanced external counterpulsation, hyperbaric oxygen therapy). Dislodging the thrombus to a more distant site in the vessel through digital ocular massage or Nd:YAG laser embolysis/embolectomy has been tried. There is a lack of clinical evidence that thrombolytic therapy improves visual outcome (EAGLE study), and given the potential systemic side effects (intracranial hemorrhage in about 10%), thrombolytic therapy is generally not recommended today.[97,116-118] However, thrombolysis could have a positive impact if administered early enough, similar to the narrow therapeutic window in cerebral ischemia.[119]

Systemic Work-up/Management

As previously mentioned, an embolic branch or central retinal artery occlusion is a cerebral infarction, and patients accordingly should be emergently referred to the stroke unit/neurologic emergency department for further management.[120]

Systemic management should consider differential etiologies depending on patient age and concurrent risk factors/symptoms. Depending on diagnostic clues pointing to special entities, further investigations should be undertaken (i.e. blood cell count, ESR, and CRP for suspicion of GCA; FFA, contrast-enhanced brain magnetic resonance imaging, lumbar puncture for analysis of cerebral spinal fluid, and audiological assessment for suspected Susac syndrome).

Management of Remote Complications

Neovascular glaucoma is the most devastating long-term complication and has been reported in 2–16% of eyes with arterial occlusive disease. It could, as suggested by Hayreh, be driven more by additional comorbidities than by the arterial occlusion itself, i.e. concomitant DR or ocular ischemia.[101,102]

Generally, panretinal photocoagulation is performed in the presence of retinal/iris/angle NV, with possible bridging off-label use of anti-VEGF to induce regression of NV and lower IOP. There is no definite evidence for this treatment; but anti-VEGF therapy has proven to be of benefit in diabetic neovascular disease (DRCRnet protocol S for ranibizumab, CLARITY study for aflibercept).[121,122]

If neovascular glaucoma is already present, it should be managed appropriately; and if no control can be achieved through panretinal photocoagulation, further options lie with retinal cryotherapy and/or other glaucomatous intervention (cyclophotocoagulation, filtering surgery, aqueous shunt implants).

OCULAR ISCHEMIC SYNDROME

Epidemiology

Ocular ischemic syndrome (OIS)occurs in the elderly with a male preponderance(♂:♀ = 2:1).[123,124] It is associated with cardiovascular diseases such as diabetes, hypertension, coronary artery disease, and stroke/TIA. In 20% of cases, the involvement is bilateral. The estimated incidence is 7.5 per million per year.[123]

Pathogenesis

Ocular ischemia results from high-grade or complete obstruction of the afferent arterial vessels, most commonly the carotid artery, on the involved side.[125] Rarely, the occlusion lies within the ophthalmic artery. Reduction of blood flow to the eye leads to anterior and/or posterior segment ischemia, depending on extent of collateral circulation (mainly via the external carotid artery).

Symptoms

Gradual vision loss is present in 90% of cases, whereas additional acute visual loss may occur in case of embolization of a retinal artery.[126] Transient vision loss (amaurosis fugax) manifests in about 10%.[125] Delayed recovery of visual function after exposure to bright light has also been reported.[123,124]

Visual field defects in OIS can include central/centrocoecal scotoma, nasal defects, and/or pronounced visual field loss with preserved central/peripheral island.[127]

Dull pain in the eye or periorbital area is typical of OIS, occurring in about 40% of cases, and is due to hypoxia of the eyeball or dura mater. The pain usually decreases if the patient is in a supine position.[123]

Findings

Findings of OIS include ischemic changes in both the anterior and posterior segments.[124]

Anteriorly, NV of the iris and angle can be found in 66% of those with OIS. Increased IOP is only present in 50% of patients; and there may even be hypotony due to ischemia of the ciliary body with subsequent shutdown of aqueous production. Anterior chamber flare is present in most cases, and anterior chamber cells (usually few) in 30% of cases. Endothelial precipitates are rare and occur in the context of iridocyclitis. Inflammation may cause posterior synechiae and cataract formation. Pupil reaction may be sluggish, and in cases of severe ischemia, the pupil is fixed and semi-dilated. Dilatation and injection of episcleral and conjunctival vessels may be present.

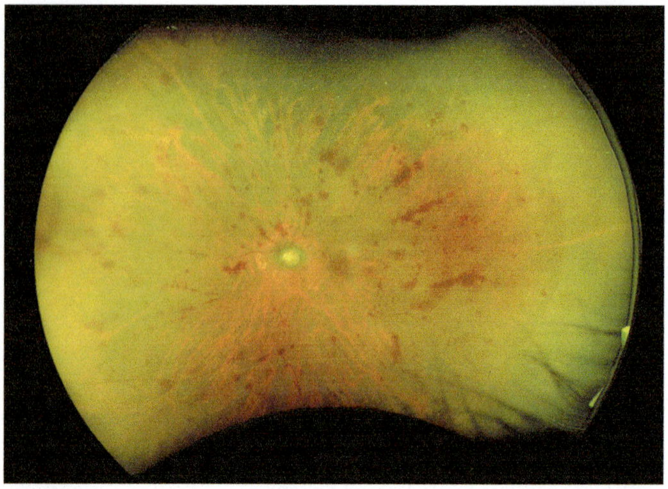

Fig. 49.19: Fundus photography of ocular ischemic syndrome. Typical midperipheral intraretinal hemorrhages and narrowed/attenuated arteries visible.

Posterior ischemic findings are seen more frequently than anterior changes. Retinal arteries appear narrowed and retinal veins typically dilated, even though veins may also be attenuated in some cases. Occasionally, spontaneous retinal arterial pulsations can be observed. In 80% of cases, there are mid-peripheral retinal hemorrhages throughout all quadrants of the fundus (Fig. 49.19). Microaneurysms and macular telangiectatic changes may be present and can cause macular edema (ME). Small arterial branch occlusions may occur and in 12% of cases, a cherry-red spot as a sign of more widespread ischemia is present (i.e. in case of IOP exceeding intraocular perfusion pressure or in case of CRAO). Neovascularization in the posterior segment occurs more frequently on the disc than elsewhere in the retina. Neovascular glaucoma may develop and lead to optic neuropathy. Ischemic changes to the choroid result in areas of chorioretinal atrophy.[124]

ORBITAL INFARCTION SYNDROME

Orbital infarction is a rare syndrome due to ischemia of all intraorbital structures and resulting in orbital pain, ophthalmoplegia, hypotony, ptosis, and corneal hypoesthesia.[123,124]

Imaging

Fluorescein angiography shows prolonged arm-retina time (>20 seconds) and irregular and/or prolonged arteriovenous time (Figs. 49.20A and B).[123,124] Prolonged arteriovenous passage time (normal range within 1–2 seconds) is seen in 95%, making it the most sensitive sign on FFA; but it is not very specific. Delayed choroidal filling on FFA is the most specific sign of OIS and is present in about 60% of cases. Normally, the choroid is filled completely within 5 seconds of the first appearance of dye in the choroidal arteries; but in OIS, choroidal filling can be delayed for over 1 minute. Other signs of OIS on FFA are staining of major retinal vessels in late phase, macular leakage, hyperfluorescence of the optic disc, and retinal capillary non-perfusion.

Indocyanine green angiography shows the most OIS-specific sign, a prolonged arm-choroid circulation time(normally about 10 seconds) as well as prolonged intrachoroidal circulation time (normal timeframe 5–6 seconds from the first appearance of dye in the choroidal arteries to complete choroidal filling) and visible watershed zones ("patchy filling").

Enhanced depth imaging-OCT: Two small retrospective studies have suggested that eyes with OIS may have a decreased subfoveal choroidal thickness; however, there has been no further replication of these results, and the possible pathomechanism remains speculative.[128,129]

Carotid duplex sonography is the method of choice to prove causal stenosis on the involved side in OIS, with a sensitivity of 89% and a specificity of 84% for detecting a high-grade symptomatic carotid artery stenosis.[130] However, duplex sonography can result in incomplete imaging because of a high bifurcation, a long internal carotid artery (ICA) plaque, calcific shadows, borderline severe disease, suspected extracervical disease, ICA near-occlusion, diffuse recurrent stenosis, tortuous vessels, and examiner-dependence.[123]

Color Doppler imaging (CDI) of retrobulbar vessels (ophthalmic artery, central retinal artery, short posterior ciliary arteries) is another helpful imaging method, especially when OIS is suspected but duplex sonography is inconclusive or fails to show significant stenosis.[123] In cases of OIS, CDI demonstrates significantly reduced velocities and pulsatility indices in the ophthalmic and central retinal artery, a normal hemodynamic phenomenon distal to a stenosis.[131] Reversed flow in the ophthalmic artery is highly specific of ipsilateral high-grade ICA stenosis or occlusion.[132] The flow pattern may vary substantially in patients with carotid stenosis, depending on the presence of collateral pathways, the severity of stenosis, and the presence of additional disease (e.g. ischemic heart disease and hypertension).[133] An anterograde flow in the ophthalmic artery on CDI therefore does not rule out OIS.

Diagnosis

Diagnosis is made with the typical clinical and angiographic findings, together with a positive carotid duplex sonography.

Differential Diagnosis

Diabetic retinopathy and central retinal vein occlusion are the most frequent retinal diseases confounded with OIS (*see* Table 49.3). Hyperviscosity syndromes may also cause

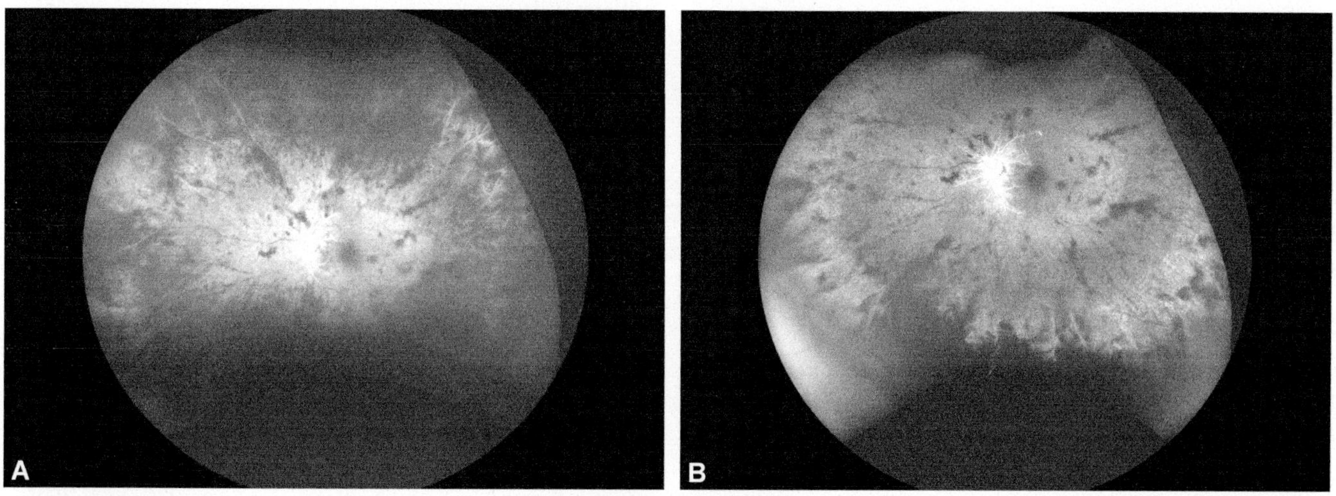

Figs. 49.20A and B: Fluorescence angiography at 33 sec (A) and 52 sec (B) showing delayed arm-retina time, prolonged arteriovenous passage time, and delayed choroidal filling.

Table 49.3: Differential diagnostic signs of ocular ischemic syndrome, central retinal vein occlusion, and diabetic retinopathy.

Features	OIS	CRVO	DR
Hemorrhages	Mid-periphery, dot/blot	Flame-shaped	Dot/blot, posterior pole and mid-periphery
Veins	Dilated, not tortuous	Dilated and tortuous	Dilated, beaded
Microaneurysms	Common, mid-periphery	Uncommon	Common, posterior pole
Microvascular abnormalities	Macular teleangiectasis, a-v communications, capillary dro pout	Optociliary shunts, capillary dropout	Intraretinal microvascular abnormalities, capillary dropout
Hard exudates	No	Rarely	Common
Optic disc	Normal	Commonly swollen	Rarely swollen (diabetic papillopathy)
Central retinal artery perfusion pressure	Decreased	Normal	Normal
FFA—a-v transit time	Prolonged	Prolonged	Normal
FFA—vessel staining	Arteries>veins	Veins>arteries	Usually none
FFA—macular edema	Rare	Common	Common
FFA—choroidal filling	Delayed, patchy	Normal	Normal

(OIS: Ocular ischemic syndrome; CRVO: Central retinal vein occlusion; DR: Diabetic retinopathy; FFA: Fluorescein angiography)

midperipheral hemorrhages, but these do not show the OIS-typical angiographic features.

Etiologies for OIS other than carotid stenosis are rare but important to consider. Aortic arch syndrome (usually bilateral symptoms), giant cell arteritis, and Takayasu disease (uni- or bilateral) can cause the full clinical picture of ocular ischemia.[123]

Therapy

Ocular ischemic syndrome is a systemic disease that demands multidisciplinary treatment from ophthalmologists, vascular surgeons, cardiologists, and neurologists. Because of the cardiovascular comorbidities, mortality is high in patients with OIS.

Systemic/causal treatment for restoring adequate blood supply to the eye in case of carotid stenosis is carotid endarterectomy or carotid arterial stenting. The efficacy of carotid endarterectomy in reducing stroke risk as a primary prevention in patients with carotid stenosis has been demonstrated decades ago, but improvement of ocular signs and symptoms is limited by the chronicity of ocular ischemia.[100,126,134-136] Treatment of the cardiovascular comorbidities includes use of antiplatelets and/or antihypertensive agents, control of diabetes, cessation of smoking, and increasing physical activity.

Local treatment is aimed at treating complications of OIS (neovascular glaucoma). Panretinal photocoagulation (PRP) is usually performed if there is iris and/or retinal NV but is only effective in 36% of cases because choroidal ischemia may be sufficient to induce NV, and there is no evidence-based rationale for PRP.[123] Alternatives are trans-conjunctival cryotherapy and trans-scleral diode laser retinopexy.[123,137] Local treatment of neovascular glaucoma should avoid use of prostaglandins because of their proinflammatory effect and miotics because of possible induction of posterior synechia. Surgical interventions for glaucoma (i.e. trabeculectomy, drainage implants) have a low success rate. If pain in combination with very low vision is predominant, cycloablation can be considered. Retrobulbar alcohol injection or evisceration/enucleation are further treatment options of last resort. Anti-VEGF agents specifically to treat ME are generally not recommended because of insufficient data on efficacy and safety, but these are likely to have a role in treatment of iris and/or retinal NV.[123,138]

RETINAL VENOUS OCCLUSIONS

Introduction

Retinal vein occlusion (RVO) is a common retinal vascular disease.[139] There are three distinct types of RVO: (1) branch retinal vein occlusion (BRVO), (2) CRVO and (3) hemiretinal vein occlusion (HRVO). Retinal venous occlusive disease typically occurs at an arteriovenous crossing in BRVO or at the lamina cribrosa in CRVO and HRVO. Retinal vein occlusions have a characteristic appearance, with intraretinal hemorrhages, cotton-wool spots, tortuous and dilated retinal veins, macular retinal edema, and sometimes disc swelling. Whereas these findings are distributed throughout the whole fundus in CRVO, they are seen just in the affected segment/

superior or inferior hemiretina in BRVO/HRVO. Vision loss is variable, depending on the extent of the occlusion, and ranges from normal vision to complete blindness. Vision loss can be caused by ME and/or nonperfusion, secondary macular epiretinal membrane (ERM), intraretinal hemorrhages, vitreous hemorrhage, neovascular glaucoma, or tractional retinal detachment.[140-144] Timely and adequate treatment can reduce the incidence and severity of possible complications, and adequate workup and management of underlying risk factors can reduce the chance of recurrence and improve general health.

Epidemiology

The overall incidence of RVO in population based-studies varies between 2.14% in patients over 40 years and 4.6% for patients over 80 years, depending on age and study design.[145,146] The risk of developing a second vein occlusion within 4 years after a first event has been estimated at 2.5% in the same eye and 11.9% in the fellow eye.[147] Of all vein occlusions in the Blue Mountain Eye Study (BMES) cohort, 69.5% were BRVO, 25% CRVO, and 5.1% HRVO; 5.1% were bilateral.[148,149]

Central Retinal Vein Occlusion

Introduction

Central retinal vein occlusion (CRVO) is a common retinal pathology in the elderly and can present variably, ranging from an incidental finding to a profound and sudden painless visual loss with RAPD. Due to the association of CRVO with cardiovascular risk factors, a workup by the treating general physician is mandatory. Ocular therapy is mainly directed at treating visually limiting ME and preventing neovascular glaucoma.

Epidemiology

Central retinal vein occlusion is a relatively common cause of vision loss in the elderly. The 15-year cumulative incidence lies at 0.5%, with an increasing incidence with age and no gender predilection.[147-149] Prevalence findings range from 0.1% to1.6%.[145,146,148]

Pathophysiology

The pathogenesis of CRVO is thought to be a complex mechanism caused by—(1) occlusion of the vein by external compression of sclerotic adjacent structures (i.e. central retinal artery and fibrous tissue envelope) and secondary endothelial proliferation; (2) occlusion by primary venous wall degeneration/inflammation; and (3) hemodynamic disturbances caused by a variety of factors (e.g. subendothelial atheromatous lesions in the CRA, arterial spasm, sudden blood pressure reduction, blood dyscrasias). These factors may lead to primary thrombus formation at the level of the lamina cribrosa occluding the central retinal vein with resulting CRVO.[150-152]

Several risk factors for CRVO have been identified, mainly in large population-based surveys. The most important are hypertension, diabetes mellitus, and open-angle glaucoma.[145,146,153] Systemic vasculitis also predisposes to CRVO, i.e. sarcoid, syphilis, and systemic lupus erythematosus. Orbital involvement from thyroid disease or orbital tumor with external globe compression have also been shown to increase risk of CRVO.[154] In women, risk has been shown to be higher with elevated ESR and lower with postmenopausal estrogen substitution.[153] Whether thrombophilia (i.e. hyperhomocysteinemia, factor V Leiden, protein C/S deficiency, antithrombin, deficiency, antiphospholipid antibodies, activated protein C resistance, prothrombin gene mutation, anticardiolipin antibodies, abnormal fibrinogen levels, and lupus anticoagulant) is a risk factor for retinal vein occlusions remains somewhat controversial.[153,155-160]

Clinical Features

Clinical presentation is variable, mostly depending on the state of retinal perfusion: ischemic versus non-ischemic CRVO. About 81% of all CRVO are initially non-ischemic.[147] A summary of the typical features is provided in Box 49.1.

In *ischemic CRVO,* there is typically a marked vision loss, frequently noticed on waking in the morning. Fundus examination shows multiple cotton-wool spots and extensive retinal hemorrhages. Typical findings include a RAPD, visual acuity worse than 30/400, and widespread capillary non-perfusion on FFA (Figs. 49.21A and B).

Box 49.1: Typical features of central retinal vein occlusion.

- Involving all four quadrants
- Dilated, tortuous veins
- Superficial and deep retinal hemorrhages
- Cotton-wool spots
- Optic nerve head swelling/hemorrhages
- Macular edema
- Optociliary shunt vessels on disc
- Neovascularization on the iris (less commonly on optic disc/retina)

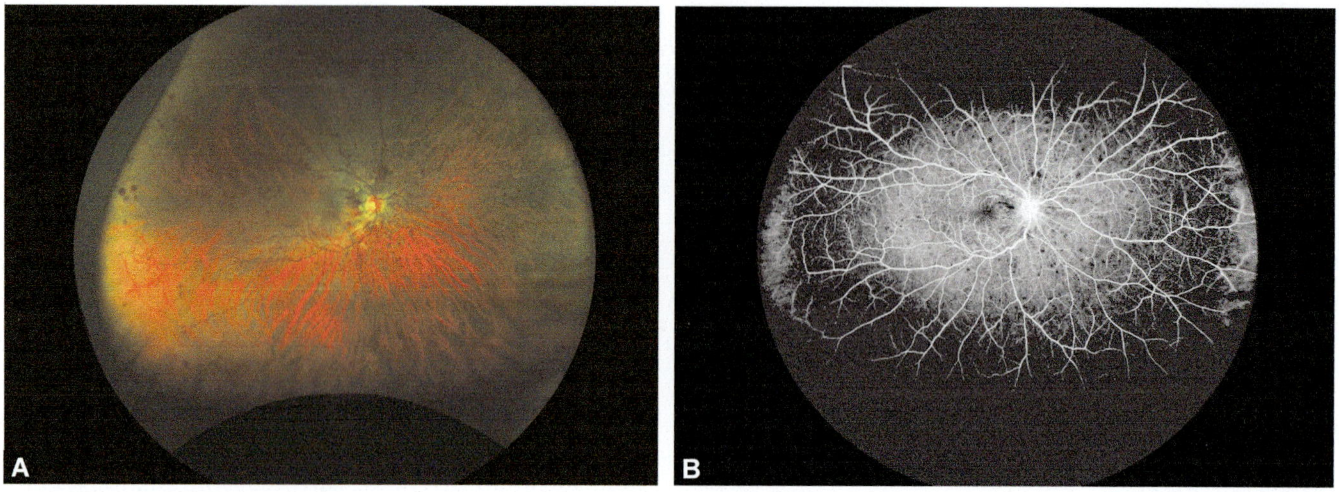

Figs. 49.21A and B: Optos fundus image (A) and fluorescein angiogram (B) of ischemic central retinal vein occlusion. There are extensive retinal hemorrhages in all quadrants and cotton-wool spots close to the optic disc. Fluorescein angiogram shows profound ischemia with complete attenuation of the microvasculature.

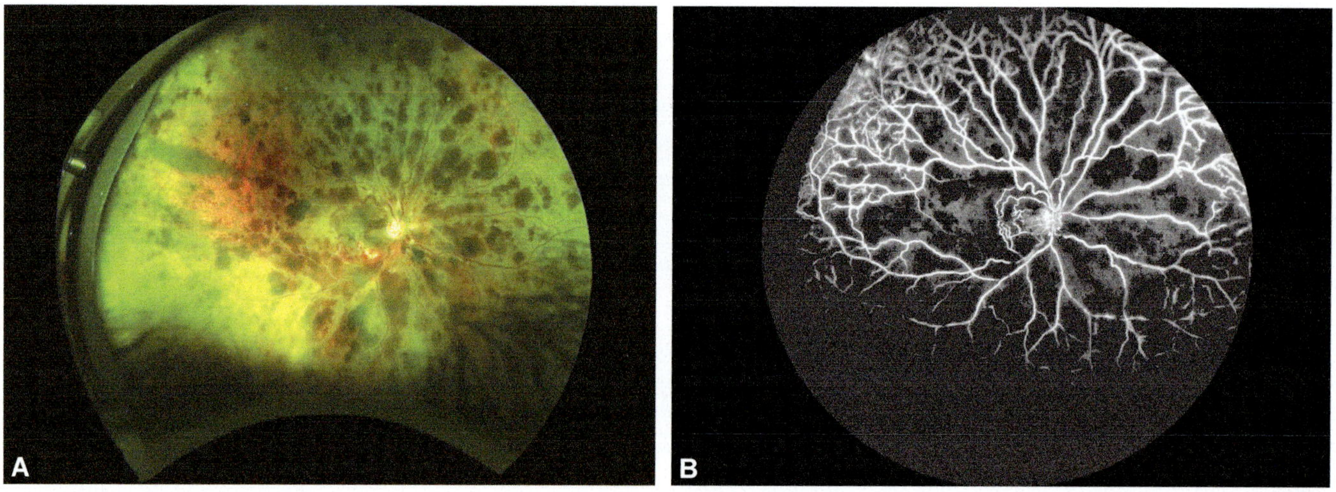

Figs. 49.22A and B: Optos fundus image (A) and fluorescein angiogram (B) of non-ischemic central retinal vein occlusion showing retinal hemorrhages in all quadrants, cotton-wool spots, dilated, slightly tortuous retinal veins without angiographic sign of ischemia (only mild vessel hyperfluorescence and blockages due to hemorrhages).

Non-ischemic CRVO typically has milder fundus changes, no RAPD, VA better than 20/400, and less extensive nonperfusion or no perfusion deficit at all on FFA (Figs. 49.22A and B). Two-thirds of patients with non-ischemic CRVO have a final VA of 20/40 or better; and when there is no associated ischemic retinal disease, non-ischemic CRVO does not lead to neovascular complications.[161] Conversion of the non-ischemic to the ischemic form has been reported to be 18.6% at 18 months for patients over 65 years and 8.1% for patients between 45 years and 64 years.[147]

Fluorescein angiogram shows normal/slightly prolonged arm-retina time, but marked delay of arteriovenous passage time (normal range within 1–2 seconds).[162] Arteriovenous passage time of more than 20 seconds is associated with increased risk of developing neovascular complications.[163] Retinal non-perfusion is seen as patchy areas of hypofluorescence, and there may be staining of retinal venous vessel walls, both of which are indicators of a higher risk of developing iris NV.[163] Historically, CRVO with a non-perfusion area of more than 10 disc areas is considered ischemic; but there is evidence that the threshold for NV-promotion lies much higher, at 30 disc areas of non-perfusion.[140,142,164] Eyes with ischemic CRVO are at higher risk of neovascular complications.[165-168] FFA demonstrates macular changes, i.e. petaloid leakage in ME or increased FAZ in macular ischemia (Figs. 49.23A and B).

Optical coherence tomography shows intra-/subretinal fluid in the presence of ME, as well as hyper-reflective areas at locations with intraretinal hemorrhages or hard exudates in the acute phase (Figs. 49.23A and B). It demonstrates retinal atrophy and ERM as long-standing changes.[169-171]

Optical coherence tomography angiography has been used to analyze the FAZ and the different vascular plexuses. In branch and central vein occlusions, there is an enlarged FAZ, increased parafoveal capillary nonperfusion, and decreased parafoveal vascular density.[172] Macular edema shows as areas with altered inner plexus and absent deep vascular plexus flow. These flow alterations are not reversible with resolution of edema.[173]

Electroretinogram, although not usually performed in a CRVO, has been shown to be the most sensitive method to separate ischemic from non-ischemic forms of CRVO.[174,175] The most sensitive parameter is the reduced b-wave amplitude (sensitivity 80–90%, specificity 70–80%) in photopic and scotopic conditions. Other changes in CRVO seen on ERG are reduced a-wave amplitude and prolonged a- and b-wave implicit time.

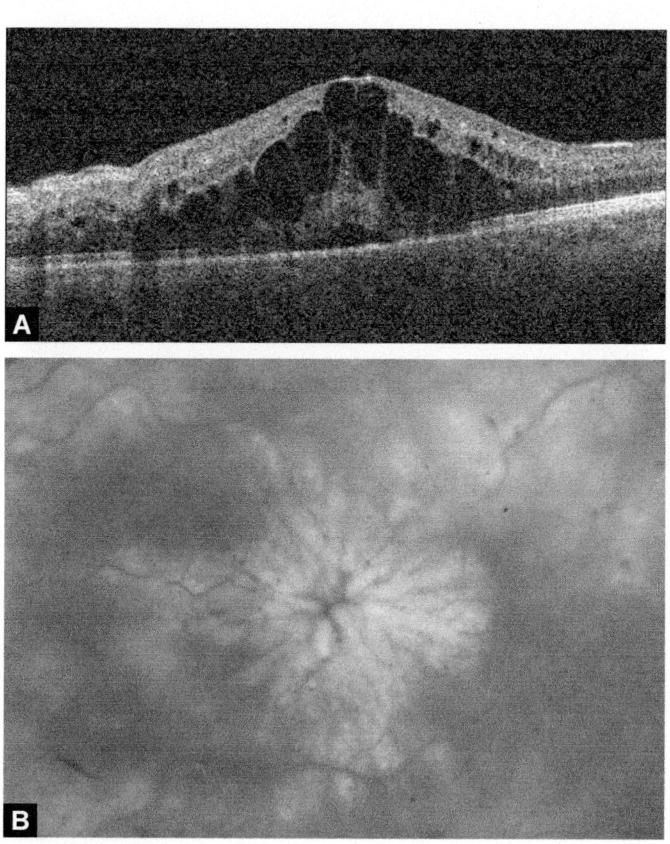

Figs. 49.23A and B: Optical coherence tomography (A) and late frame fluorescein angiogram (B) of macular edema due to central retinal vein occlusion.

Complications

Complications of CRVO are chronic ME and NV within the retina, the angle or the iris with possible development of neovascular glaucoma.

Neovascularization does not occur in non-ischemic CRVO.[142,161] Anterior segment NV is more common than retinal NV and usually develops within the first 6 months (Figs. 49.24A and B). The risk is 63% for iris NV, 49% for angle NV, and 39% for the development of neovascular glaucoma over 5 years.[161] NV of the optic disc should be distinguished from retinociliary collaterals, which develop in 41% of ischemic and 46.5% of non-ischemic CRVOs (Figs. 49.25A to D).[176]

Chronic ME does not have a standardized definition in literature; however, it has been shown that patients with persisting ME despite three months of anti-VEGF treatment have a less favorable long-term outcome than those with resolved ME.[177-179] The appearance of chronic ME is shown in Figures 49.26A and B.

Differential Diagnosis

Diabetic retinopathy can present with similar fundus findings (retinal hemorrhages, microaneurysms); but DR is usually bilateral whereas vein occlusions rarely occur simultaneously in both eyes.

Ocular ischemic syndrome has a similar clinical appearance, but it differs in several aspects: veins are not usually tortuous; retinal hemorrhages are typically mid-peripheral; and there may be a history of amaurosis fugax, TIA, or orbital pain.

For a systematic comparison of differential DR/OIS/CRVO, *see* Table 49.3.

Treatment of Underlying Risk Factors

Identification and treatment of commonly present systemic cardiovascular risk factors in collaboration with the treating general practitioner is most important. Anticoagulation is indicated in cases of concurrent underlying disease but is generally not beneficial for ocular disease. Anticoagulants

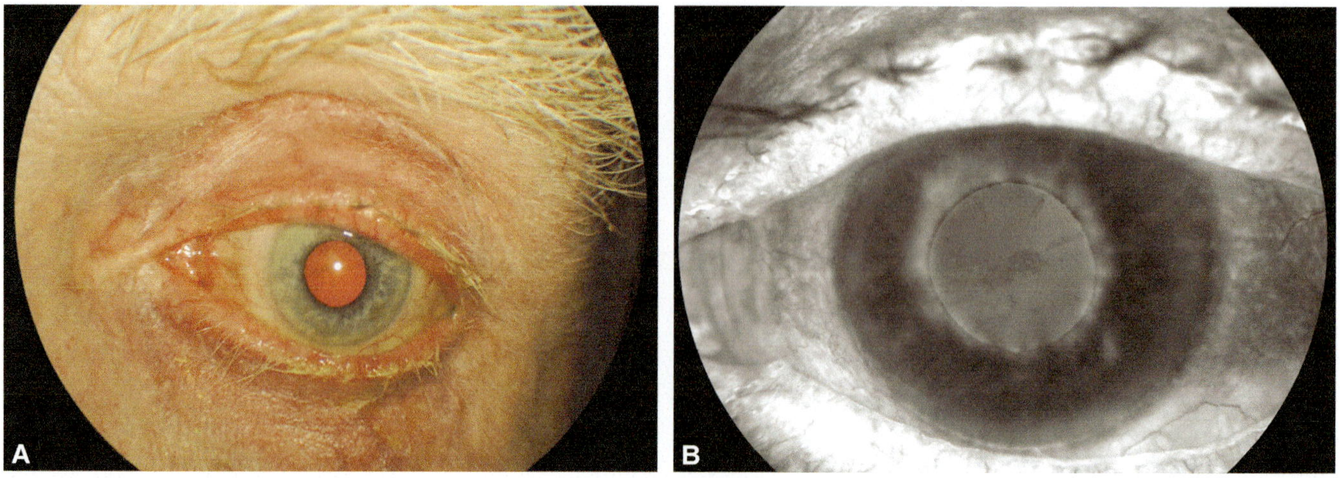

Figs. 49.24A and B: Photograph (A) and fluorescein angiogram (B) of iris neovascularization at the pupillary margin. Neovascular vessels are hyperfluorescent on fluorescein angiogram.

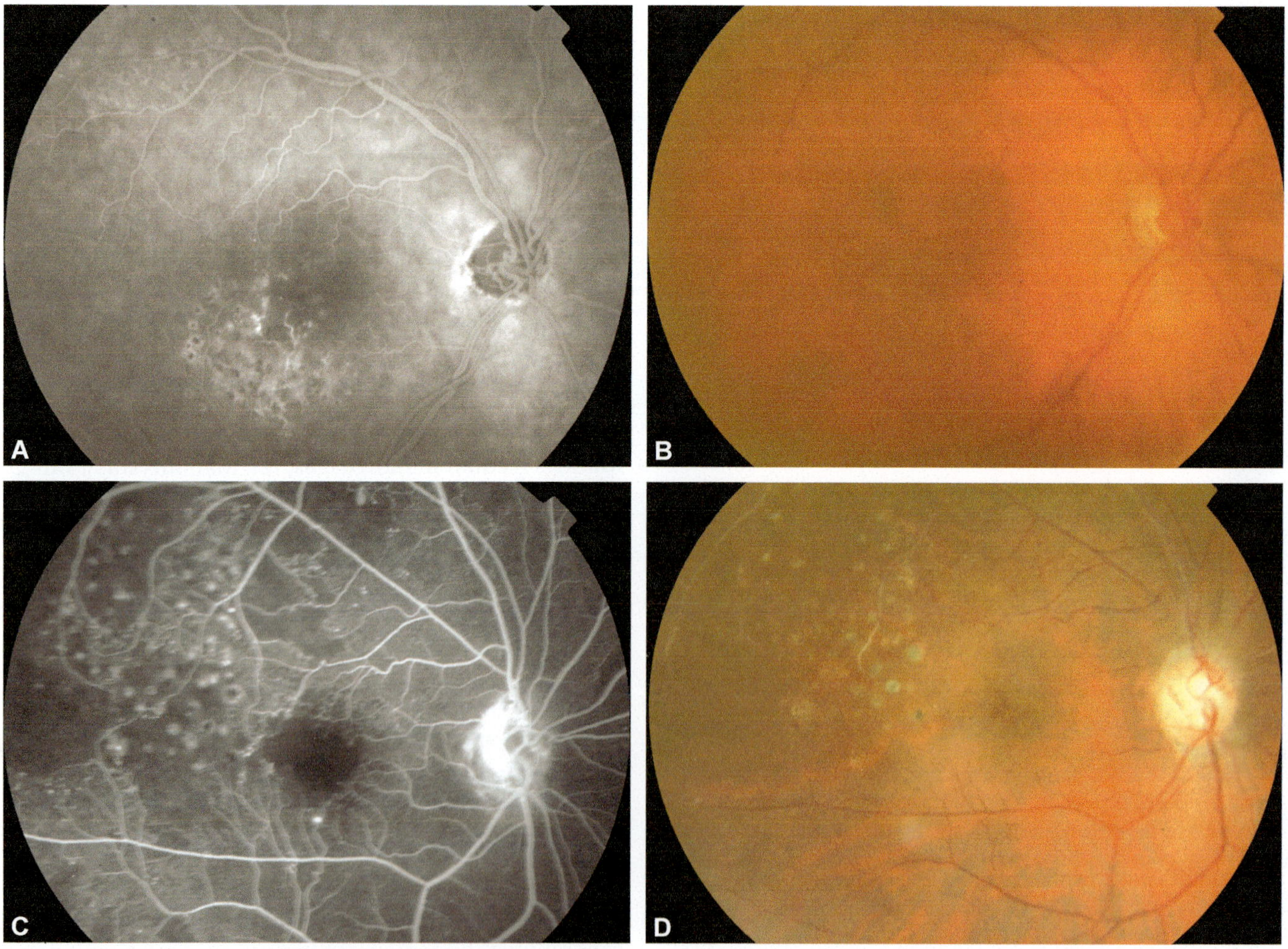

Figs. 49.25A to D: Fundus photography/fluorescein angiogram of disc collaterals (A and B) versus disc neovascularization (C and D). In contrast to collaterals, neovascular vessels show intense hyperfluorescence on fluorescein angiogram.

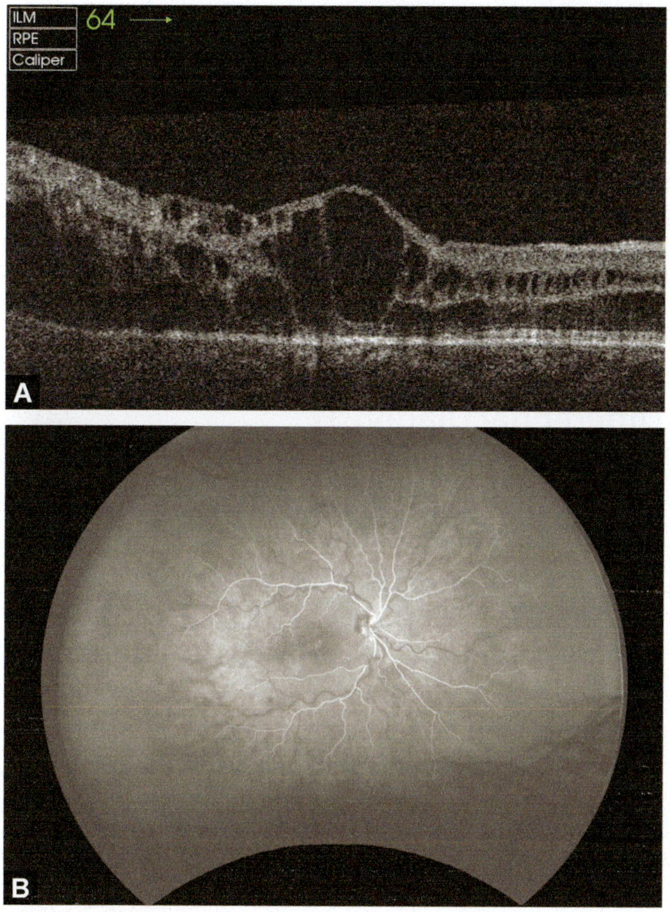

Figs. 49.26A and B: Optical coherence tomography (A) and angiogram (B) of chronic macular edema, unresponsive to anti-vascular endothelial growth factor injections.

may even affect the ophthalmological outcome adversely by increasing retinal hemorrhages.[180-182]

Treatment of Macular Edema

The first-line treatment for ME associated with central vein occlusion is anti-VEGF injections (approval/follow-up studies: CRUISE/RETAIN/HORIZON for ranibizumab, COPERNICUS/GALILEO for aflibercept).[183-187] The injection regimen in those studies was monthly during the first 6 months, then pro re nata (as needed). In several small retrospective studies, a switch from ranibizumab to aflibercept in non-responsive cases resulted in anatomical and visual improvement while prolonging the relapse-free interval between injections.[188,189] Thus, there is a rationale to switch to aflibercept in cases of non-/partial responders if initial therapy was with ranibizumab.

Bevacizumab (not licensed for this condition) has been tested against aflibercept in the SCORE2 study, and aflibercept was shown to have a more favorable outcome on OCT with resolution of edema in 54% versus 29% with bevacizumab; but there was no difference in VA between the two drugs.[190,191]

Intraocular steroids have proven effective in treating ME in two major trials: SCORE and GENEVA.[192,193] The SCORE trial demonstrated efficacy of 1 mg and 4 mg intravitreal triamcinolone; the GENEVA trial, dexamethasone implants. The RANIDEX study has shown equivalent visual and structural outcomes comparing ranibizumab and dexamethasone implant, but given the unfavorable side effects of steroids (mainly IOP rise), they are generally considered second-line or additive treatment in non-/partial responders.[178,194,195] However, the best time point for switching from anti-VEGF to steroid is yet to be determined; current data suggest a switch as early as 3 months for non-/partial responders.[177]

Grid laser therapy as an alternative treatment for ME has not been shown beneficial as monotherapy.[144]

Other/Historical Treatment Modalities

Hemodilution, fibrinolytic/thrombolytic agents, ocular hypotensive therapy, surgical interventions (i.e. radial optic neurotomy), or laser-induced chorioretinal venous anastomosis have not been shown to be beneficial or have even shown to be harmful.[180]

Treatment of Neovascular Complications

Panretinal photocoagulation has been shown to be beneficial in patients with 2 clock hours of iris NV or any angle NV, but not for preventing neovascular complications or for reducing frequency of injections in the presence of ME.[142,196] On the contrary, PRP may exacerbate ME and induce iatrogenic peripheral visual field loss.[196,197] Panretinal photocoagulation is thus only indicated in the presence of ocular NV.

Hemiretinal Vein Occlusion

Introduction

Hemiretinal vein occlusion (HRVO) affects either the inferior or superior hemiretina. It is thought to have two possible pathomechanisms: hemicentral (as variant of CRVO) or hemispheric (as variant of BRVO).[198,199] Clinically, the distinction between those two entities may be difficult or even impossible, and most studies look at HRVO in general. The clinical picture is intermediate between BRVO and CRVO, and the therapy concepts are analogous to those for BRVO/CRVO.[199]

Epidemiology

Hemiretinal vein occlusion is the least common type of venous occlusion. In the BMES, only 5.1% of all vein occlusions were HRVO.[148]

Pathophysiology

Hemicentral retinal vein occlusions occur as a variant of CRVO in cases where the embryonal 2-truncated central retinal vein persists.[200,201] This anomaly is present in about 20% of eyes. Risk factors are similar to those for CRVO.[154,202,203] The occlusion occurs within the optic disc but only affects one of the two central retinal vein trunks. Risk factors are generally identical to those for CRVO.[198,204]

Hemispheric retinal vein occlusions arise from an occlusion of a major branch of the central retinal vein at the level of the disc and, thus, are technically a form of BRVO.[198] Risk factors are thought to be similar to those for BRVO.[164]

Clinical Features

Hemiretinal vein occlusion presents with the same clinical features as CRVO/BRVO with the findings confined to either the upper or lower retinal hemisphere. It can analogously be divided into ischemic (15%) and non-ischemic (85%) HRVO.[198] Collateral vessels may form at the disc or across the median raphe.[205] The typical fundus photograph and corresponding FFA are shown in Figures 49.27A and B for non-ischemic and Figures 49.28A and B for ischemic HRVO.

Complications

Complications are generally the same as for CRVO/BRVO. Patients with ischemic HRVO develop retinal NV more often than anterior segment NV and, thus, have a lower risk of developing neovascular glaucoma compared to those with CRVO.[161,166]

Differential Diagnosis

The possible differential diagnosis is similar to that of CRVO/BRVO, including DR, hypertensive retinopathy, OIS, and radiation retinopathy.

Treatment

Because of the low incidence of HRVO, there are no evidence-based treatment options. Generally, therapy decisions concerning ME or neovascular complications are guided by the existing evidence for CRVO and BRVO with comparable results.[190,199]

Branch Retinal Vein Occlusion

Introduction

Branch retinal vein occlusion (BRVO) is a common vascular pathology resulting from occlusion of a retinal vein. Typically, patients are older and have associated

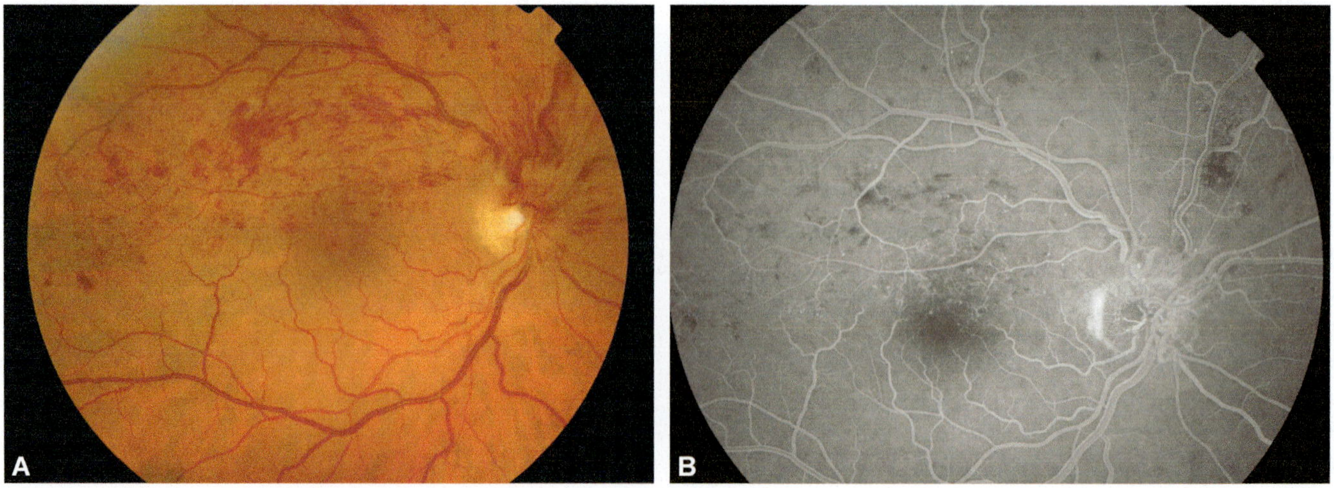

Figs. 49.27A and B: Fundus photography (A) and fluorescein angiogram (B) of non-ischemic superior hemiretinal vein occlusion. Retinal hemorrhages and venous dilation and tortuosity are confined to the superior hemiretina. Angiogram shows no retinal ischemia but blockages due to hemorrhages and microvascular venous abnormalities.

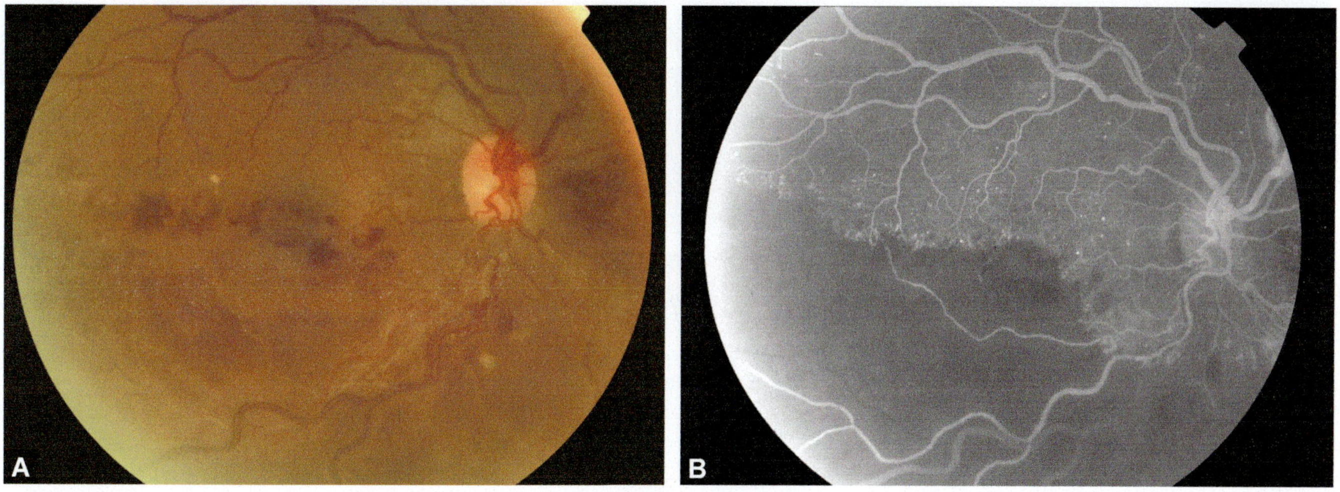

Figs. 49.28A and B: Fundus photography (A) and fluorescein angiogram (B) of ischemic inferior hemiretinal vein occlusion. Retinal hemorrhages and venous dilation and tortuosity as well as sclerosed vessels are seen throughout the inferior hemiretina. Shunt vessels at the optic disc are present. Angiogram shows profound retinal ischemia with a sharp border at the median raphe and profound dropout of vessels.

cardiovascular risk factors. The main reasons for visual loss are ME or ischemia. Symptoms depend on the location and degree of involvement of the macula; typical retinal findings are seen in the area of supply of the occluded vessel. Treatment paradigms have significantly changed with the introduction of anti-VEGF.

Epidemiology

Branch retinal vein occlusion is the most common type of retinal vein occlusion. Prevalence and 5-year incidence were estimated at 0.6% in the Beaver Dam Eye Study.[148] The BMES estimated incidence of BRVO at 1.1% in a population over 49 years.[145] Both studies showed a strong age-related predilection, but no association with gender.

Pathophysiology

Branch retinal vein occlusion results from the focal occlusion of a retinal vein, most frequently at an arteriovenous crossing with the artery overcrossing the vein.[206,207] In contrast to CRVO, BRVO is mainly thought to be the result of compression of the vein through arteriosclerotic changes in the crossing arterial vessel conducted via the common adventitial sheath of both.[207] Well known risk factors are arterial hypertension, smoking, history of cardiovascular disease, increased body mass index, and elevated serum levels of α2-globulin.[208] Rarely, the cause may be a systemic inflammatory disorder, such as sarcoidosis, systemic lupus erythematosus, or Behçet's disease.[68] As in CRVO, the role of hemophilia as contributing factor of BRVO remains controversial.[160] In contrast to CRVO, ocular hypertension and glaucoma are not considered risk factors for BRVO.[164,209]

The most common location for a BRVO is the superotemporal quadrant of the retina; the majority of occlusions involve the area inside the vascular arcades (macular BRVO).[210]

Clinical Features

Findings of BRVO are similar to those of CRVO but are limited to the involved vein and the area of its supply.[211] BRVO can be further differentiated into a major BRVO, affecting one of the four major branches of retinal veins; and a macular BRVO, affecting a branch supplying an area inside of the vascular arcades.[211] In major BRVO, there are ischemic and non-ischemic forms, whereas in macular BRVO the area of possible ischemia is too small to cause neovascular complications.[147,166] Examples of macular BRVO (Figs. 49.29A and B) and ischemic major BRVO (Figs. 49.30A and B) are shown here. Both major and macular BRVOs may cause ME (Figs. 49.31A and B and 49.32).

Complications

In ischemic major BRVO, NV occurs in 9.2% within 12 months.[211] Other complications are chronic ME, visually relevant macular ischemia, collaterals, or ERM formation. Very rarely, fibrovascular proliferation causes tractional retinal detachment.[212] An example of disc NV due to major BRVO is shown in Figures 49.33A and B.

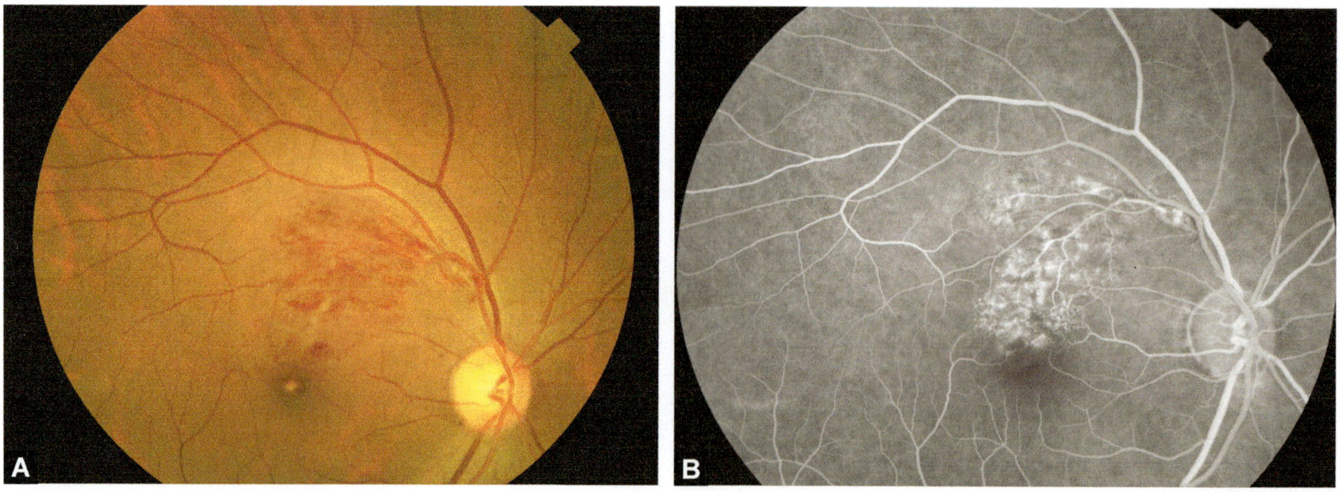

Figs. 49.29A and B: Fundus photography (A) shows a small superior macular branch retinal vein occlusion at an arterio-venous crossing with hemorrhages and few cotton-wool spots in the supply area of the venous branch. Angiogram (B) confirms the absence of ischemia in the presence of blockages due to hemorrhage and microvascular abnormalities with leakage.

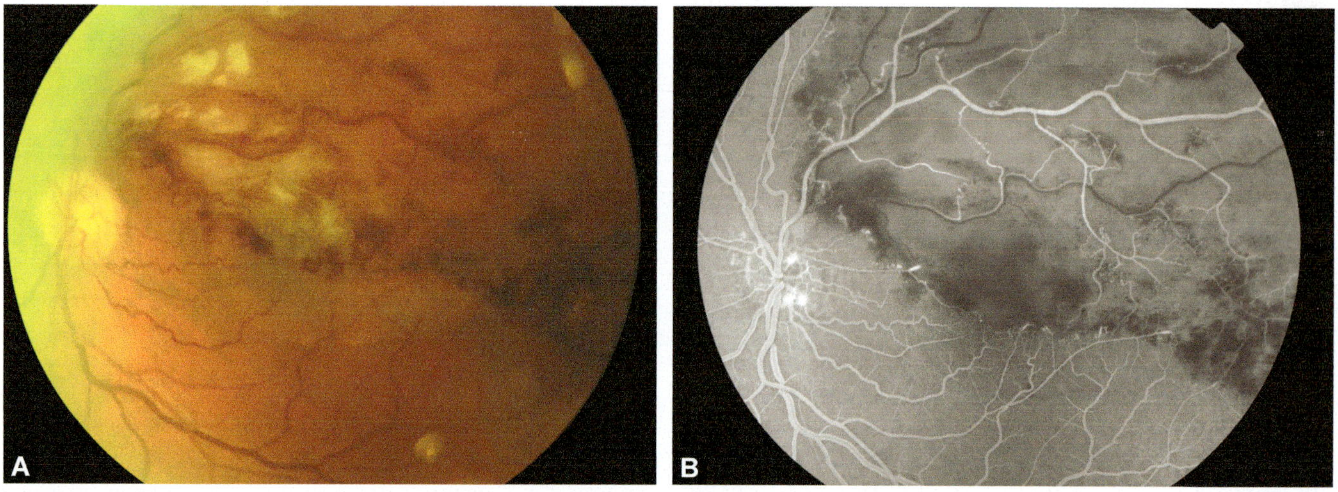

Figs. 49.30A and B: Fundus photography (A) and angiogram (B) of a major superotemporal branch retinal vein occlusion. Severe retinal hemorrhages, vessel tortuosity and dilation and cotton-wool spots are seen in the superotemporal quadrant. Angiogram reveals severe impairment of venous flow in the affected vein and profound ischemia respecting the median horizontal raphe.

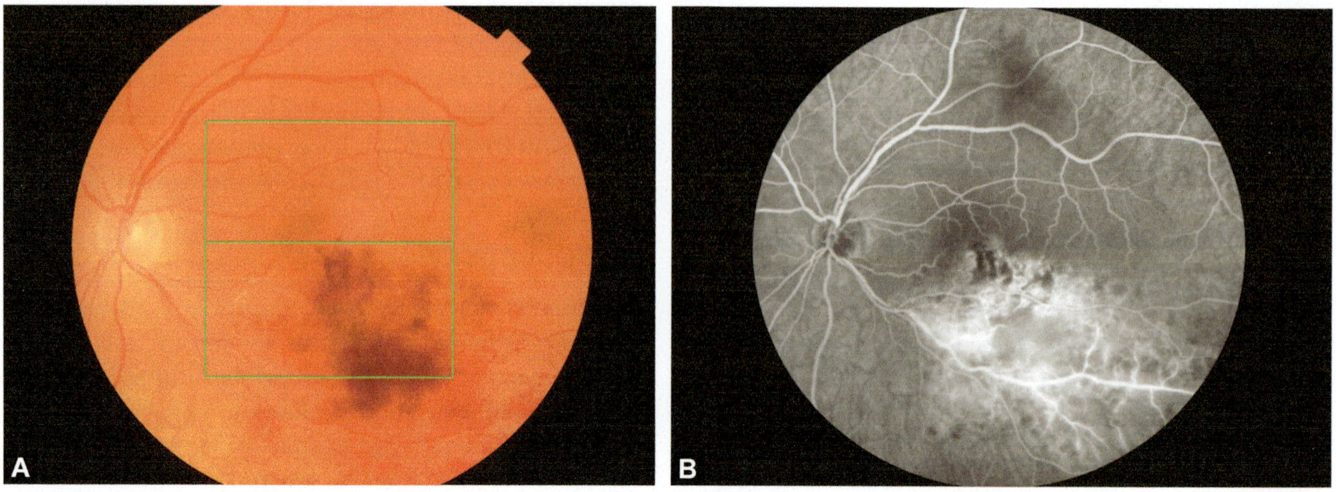

Figs. 49.31A and B: Fundus photography (A) and angiogram (B) of a major inferotemporal branch retinal vein occlusion. The dense hemorrhages seen in photography prevent definite assessment of ischemia in the angiogram at the time of imaging.

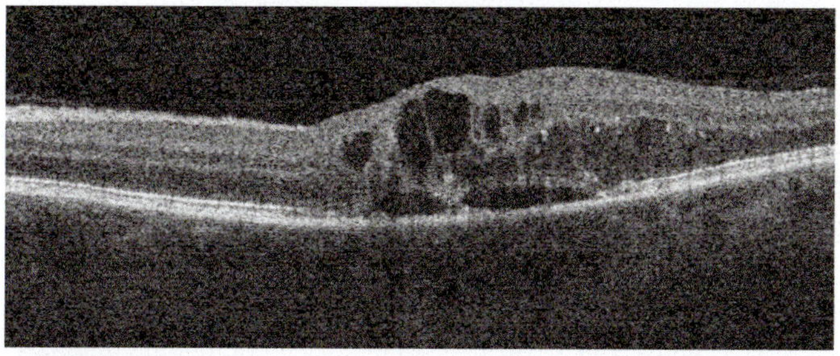

Fig. 49.32: Corresponding optical coherence tomography of Figures 49.33A and B showing cystoid macular edema with small accumulation of subretinal fluid due to the branch retinal vein occlusion.

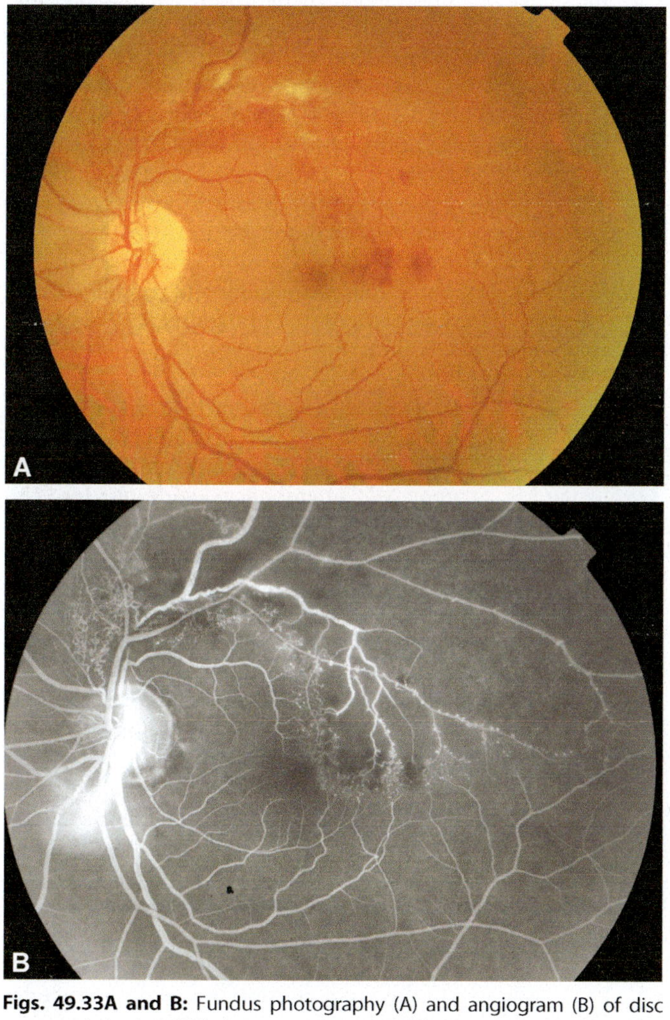

Figs. 49.33A and B: Fundus photography (A) and angiogram (B) of disc neovascularization (NV) due to superotemporal major branch retinal vein occlusion. Angiogram reveals severe capillary dropout, abnormal arterio-venous shunt vessels and an intensively hyperfluorescent NV at the optic disc.

Differential Diagnosis

Diabetic retinopathy and hypertensive retinopathy have features similar to BRVO; but both are generally bilateral and involve all four quadrants of the retina. Radiation retinopathy needs to be considered in the differential.

Treatment

As in CRVO, a general cardiovascular work-up is indicated in BRVO.

Macular edema is treated primarily with intravitreal anti-VEGF injections; but intravitreal corticosteroids are also effective.[213] Laser photocoagulation used to be the gold standard treatment for ME associated with BRVO according to the Branch Vein Occlusion Study; but this treatment has mostly been replaced by anti-VEGF and steroids.[213,214] Panretinal photocoagulation is not beneficial in treating ME.[196]

Neovascular complications are an indication for PRP, reducing the risk of vitreous hemorrhage from 60% to 30%.[214] Preventive treatment of ischemic areas is not recommended.[215]

REFERENCES

1. Graefe A. Ueber Embolie der Arteria centralis retinae als Ursache plötzlicher Erblindung. Albrecht von Graefes Archiv für Ophthalmologie. 1859;5:136-57.
2. Hayreh SS, Dass R. The ophthalmic artery: I. Origin and intra-cranial and intra-canalicular course. Br J Ophthalmol. 1962;46:65-98.
3. Hayreh SS. Acute retinal arterial occlusive disorders. Prog Retin Eye Res. 2011;30:359-94.
4. Hayreh SS. Posterior ciliary artery circulation in health and disease: the Weisenfeld lecture. Invest Ophthalmol Vis Sci. 2004;45:749-57.
5. Awan KJ. Arterial vascular anomalies of the retina. Arch Ophthalmol. 1977;95:1197-202.
6. Brown GC, Shields JA. Cilioretinal arteries and retinal arterial occlusion. Arch Ophthalmol. 1979;97:84-92.
7. Justice J, Lehmann RP. Cilioretinal arteries. A study based on review of stereo fundus photographs and fluorescein angiographic findings. Arch Ophthalmol. 1976;94:1355-8.
8. Hegde V, Deokule S, Matthews T. A case of a cilioretinal artery supplying the entire retina. Clin Anat. 2006;19:645-7.
9. Hayreh SS. The cilio-retinal arteries.Br J Ophthalmol. 1963;47:71-89.
10. Kiel JW. Anatomy. In: The Ocular Circulation. San Rafael, CA: Morgan & Claypool Life; 2010.
11. Henkind P. Radial peripapillary capillaries of the retina. I. Anatomy: human and comparative. Br J Ophthalmol. 1967;51:115-23.
12. Spaide RF, Klancnik JM, Cooney MJ. Retinal vascular layers imaged by fluorescein angiography and optical coherence tomography angiography. JAMA Ophthalmol. 2015;133: 45-50.

13. Park JJ, Soetikno BT, Fawzi AA. Characterization of the middle capillary plexus using optical coherence tomography angiography in healthy and diabetic eyes. Retina. 2016;36:2039-50.
14. Chan G, Balaratnasingam C, Yu PK, et al. Quantitative morphometry of perifoveal capillary networks in the human retina. Invest Ophthalmol Vis Sci. 2012;53:5502-14.
15. Wu LZ, Huang ZS, Wu DZ, et al. Characteristics of the capillary-free zone in the normal human macula. Jpn J Ophthalmol. 1985;29:406-11.
16. Wu LZ, Huang ZS, Wu DZ, et al. Characteristics of the macular microvasculature. Jpn J Ophthalmol. 1985;29:412-6.
17. Hayreh SS. Segmental nature of the choroidal vasculature. Br J Ophthalmol. 1975;59:631-48.
18. Hayreh SS, Weingeist TA. Experimental occlusion of the central artery of the retina. I. Ophthalmoscopic and fluorescein fundus angiographic studies. Br J Ophthalmol.1980;64:896-912.
19. Wise GN, Dollery CT, Henkind P. The retinal circulation. New York: Harper & Row; 1971.pp. 507-15.
20. Kroll AJ. Experimental central retinal artery occlusion. Arch Ophthalmol. 1968;79:453-69.
21. Hayreh SS, Zimmerman MB. Central retinal artery occlusion: visual outcome. Am J Ophthalmol. 2005;140:376-91.
22. Kaur C, Foulds WS, Ling EA. Hypoxia-ischemia and retinal ganglion cell damage. Clin Ophthalmol. 2008;2:879-89.
23. Shakib M, Ashton N. II. Ultrastructural changes in focal retinal ischaemia. Br J Ophthalmol. 1966;50:325-84.
24. Dahrling BE. The histopathology of early central retinal artery occlusion.Arch Ophthalmol. 1965;73:506-10.
25. Hayreh SS, Jonas JB. Optic disk and retinal nerve fiber layer damage after transient central retinal artery occlusion: an experimental study in rhesus monkeys. Am J Ophthalmol. 2000;129:786-95.
26. Hayreh SS, Kolder HE, Weingeist TA. Central retinal artery occlusion and retinal tolerance time. Ophthalmology. 1980;87:75-8.
27. Ozdemir H, Karacorlu S, Karacorlu M. Optical coherence tomography findings in central retinal artery occlusion. Retina. 2006;26:110-2.
28. Kapoor KG, Barkmeier AJ, Bakri SJ. Optical coherence tomography in retinal arterial occlusions: case series and review of the literature. Semin Ophthalmol. 2015;30:74-9.
29. Coady PA, Cunningham ET, Vora RA, et al. Spectral domain optical coherence tomography findings in eyes with acute ischaemic retinal whitening. Br J Ophthalmol. 2015;99: 586-92.
30. Guo J, Zhu W, Shi F, et al. A framework for classification and segmentation of branch retinal artery occlusion in SD-OCT. IEEE Trans Image Process. 2017.
31. Baumal CR. Optical coherence tomography angiography of retinal artery occlusion. Dev Ophthalmol. 2016;56:122-31.
32. Bonini Filho MA, Adhi M, de Carlo TE, et al. Optical coherence tomography angiography in retinal artery occlusion. Retina. 2015;35:2339-46.
33. Mastropasqua R, Di Antonio L, Di Staso S, et al. Optical coherence tomography angiography in retinal vascular diseases and choroidal neovascularization.J Ophthalmol. 2015;2015:343515.
34. Leavitt JA, Larson TA, Hodge DO, et al. The incidence of central retinal artery occlusion in Olmsted County, Minnesota. Am J Ophthalmol. 2011;152:820-3.e2.
35. Park SJ, Choi NK, Seo KH, et al. Nationwide incidence of clinically diagnosed central retinal artery occlusion in Korea, 2008 to 2011. Ophthalmology. 2014;121:1933-8.
36. Callizo J, Feltgen N, Pantenburg S, et al. Cardiovascular risk factors in central retinal artery occlusion: results of a prospective and standardized medical examination. Ophthalmology. 2015;122:1881-8.
37. Kollarits CR, Lubow M, Hissong SL. Retinal strokes. I. Incidence of carotid atheromata. JAMA. 1972;222:1273-5.
38. Shah HG, Brown GC, Goldberg RE. Digital subtraction carotid angiography and retinal arterial obstruction. Ophthalmology. 1985;92:68-72.
39. Jampol LM, Wong AS, Albert DM. Atrial myxoma and central retinal artery occlusion. Am J Ophthalmol. 1973;75:242-9.
40. Zamora RL, Adelberg DA, Berger AS, et al. Branch retinal artery occlusion caused by a mitral valve papillary fibroelastoma. Am J Ophthalmol. 1995;119:325-9.
41. Penner R, Font RL. Retinal embolism from calcified vegetations of aortic valve. Spontaneous complication of rheumatic heart disease. Arch Ophthalmol. 1969;81:565-8.
42. Ho IV, Spaide R. Central retinal artery occlusion associated with a patent foramen ovale. Retina. 2007;27:259-60.
43. Kim IT, Choi JB. Occlusions of branch retinal arterioles following amniotic fluid embolism.Ophthalmologica. 2000;214:305-8.
44. Kwiatt ME, Seamon MJ. Fat embolism syndrome. Int J Crit Illn Inj Sci. 2013;3:64-8.
45. Chuang EL, Miller FS, Kalina RE. Retinal lesions following long bone fractures. Ophthalmology. 1985;92:370-4.
46. Rush JA, Kearns TP, Danielson GK. Cloth-particle retinal emboli from artificial cardiac valves. Am J Ophthalmol. 1980;89:845-50.
47. Nehen AM, Damgaard-Jensen L, Hansen PE. Foreign body embolism of retinal arteries as a complication of carotid angiography. Neuroradiology. 1978;15:85-8.
48. Beiter G, Lerche W, Oberhauser M. Occlusion of a branch of the central retinal artery by a corpus alienum as a rare complication of the carotid arteriography. Dev Ophthalmol. 1987;13:147-50.
49. AtLee WE. Talc and cornstarch emboli in eyes of drug abusers. JAMA. 1972;219:49-51.
50. Tarantola R, Reichstein D, Morrison D, et al. Talc retinopathy presenting as multiple retinal arteriolar occlusions. Retin Cases Brief Rep. 2010;4:120-2.
51. Gaur N, Singh P, Chawla R, et al. Triamcinolone emboli leading to central retinal artery occlusion: a multimodal imaging study. BMJ Case Rep. 2017;2017:bcr2016218908.
52. Brown GC, Magargal LE. Central retinal artery obstruction and visual acuity. Ophthalmology. 1982;89:14-9.
53. Arruga J, Sanders MD. Ophthalmologic findings in 70 patients with evidence of retinal embolism. Ophthalmology. 1982;89:1336-47.

54. Brown GC, Magargal LE, Shields JA, et al. Retinal arterial obstruction in children and young adults. Ophthalmology. 1981;88:18-25.
55. Middeldorp S, Coppens M. Hereditary thrombophilia. In: Kaushansky K, Lichtman MA, Prchal JT(Eds). Williams Hematology, 9th edition. New York: McGraw-Hill; 2016. pp. 2222-3.
56. Bertram B, Remky A, Arend O, et al. Protein C, protein S, and antithrombin III in acute ocular occlusive diseases. Ger J Ophthalmol. 1995;4:332-5.
57. Greven CM, Weaver RG, Owen J, et al. Protein S deficiency and bilateral branch retinal artery occlusion. Ophthalmology. 1991;98:33-4.
58. Greiner K, Hafner G, Dick B, et al. Retinal vascular occlusion and deficiencies in the protein C pathway. Am J Ophthalmol. 1999;128:69-74.
59. Greven CM. Retinal arterial occlusions in the young. Curr Opin Ophthalmol. 1997;8:3-7.
60. Tayyanipour R, Pulido JS, Postel EA, et al. Arterial vascular occlusion associated with factor V Leiden gene mutation. Retina. 1998;18:376.
61. Dixon SG, Bruce CT, Glueck CJ, et al. Retinal vascular occlusion: a window to diagnosis of familial and acquired thrombophilia and hypofibrinolysis, with important ramifications for pregnancy outcomes. Clin Ophthalmol. 2016;10:1479-86.
62. Sottilotta G, Oriana V, Latella C, et al. Role of hyperhomocystinemia in retinal vascular occlusive disease. Clin Appl Thromb Hemost. 2007;13:104-7.
63. Weger M, Stanger O, Deutschmann H, et al. The role of hyperhomocysteinemia and methylenetetrahydrofolate reductase (MTHFR) C677T mutation in patients with retinal artery occlusion. Am J Ophthalmol. 2002;134:57-61.
64. Rand JH. The antiphospholipid syndrome. Hematology. 2007;2007:136-42.
65. Levine JS, Branch DW, Rauch J. The antiphospholipid syndrome. N Engl J Med. 2002;346:752-63.
66. Greven CM, Slusher MM, Weaver RG. Retinal arterial occlusions in young adults.Am J Ophthalmol. 1995;120: 776-83.
67. Ozdal PC, Ortaç S, Taskintuna I, et al. Central retinal artery occlusion associated with ocular Behçet's disease. Eur J Ophthalmol. 2002;12:328-30.
68. Agarwal A, Karkhur S, Aggarwal K, et al. Epidemiology and clinical features of inflammatory retinal vascular occlusions: pooled data from two tertiary-referral institutions. Clin Experiment Ophthalmol. 2017.
69. Williamson TH, Meyer PA. Branch retinal artery occlusion in toxoplasma retinochoroiditis. Br J Ophthalmol. 1991;75:253.
70. Kopsachilis N, Brar M, Marinescu AI, et al. Central nervous system tuberculosis presenting as branch retinal vein occlusion. Clin Exp Optom. 2012;96:121-3.
71. Hayreh SS, Podhajsky PA, Zimmerman B. Ocular manifestations of giant cell arteritis. Am J Ophthalmol. 1998;125:509-20.
72. Chen JJ, Leavitt JA, Fang C, et al. Evaluating the incidence of arteritic ischemic optic neuropathy and other causes of vision loss from giant cell arteritis. Ophthalmology. 2016;123:1999-2003.
73. Frohman L, Wong AB, Matheos K, et al. New developments in giant cell arteritis. Surv Ophthalmol. 2016;61:400-21.
74. Tariq Bhatti M, El-Dairi MA, Cummings TJ, et al. "Diagnostic algorithm for patients with suspected giant cell arteritis" Useful, but no substitute for thorough histopathology: response. J Neuroophthalmol. 2016;36:343-4.
75. Nesher G, Shemesh D, Mates M, et al. The predictive value of the halo sign in color Doppler ultrasonography of the temporal arteries for diagnosing giant cell arteritis. J Rheumatol. 2002;29:1224-6.
76. El-Dairi MA, Chang L, Proia AD, et al. Diagnostic algorithm for patients with suspected giant cell arteritis. J Neuroophthalmol. 2015;35:246-53.
77. Hayreh SS. Diagnostic algorithm for patients with suspected giant cell arteritis: Comment. J Neuroophthalmol. 2016;36:224-5.
78. Hunder GG, Bloch DA, Michel BA, et al. The American College of Rheumatology 1990 criteria for the classification of giant cell arteritis. Arthritis Rheum. 1990;33:1122-8.
79. van der Kooij SM, van Buchem MA, Overbeek OM, et al. Susac syndrome: a report of four cases and a review of the literature. Neth J Med. 2015;73:10-6.
80. Kothari N, Kuriyan AE. Branched retinal artery occlusions and Susac Syndrome. JAMA Neurol. 2016;73:884-5.
81. Susac JO. Susac's syndrome. Am J Neuroradiol. 2004;25: 351-2.
82. Dörr J, Krautwald S, Wildemann B, et al. Characteristics of Susac syndrome: a review of all reported cases. Nat Rev Neurol. 2013;9:307-16.
83. Kleffner I, Dörr J, Ringelstein M, et al. Diagnostic criteria for Susac syndrome. J Neurol Neurosurg Psychiatr. 2016;87:1287-95.
84. Dörr J, Ringelstein M, Duning T, et al. Update on Susac syndrome: new insights in brain and retinal imaging and treatment options. J Alzheimers Dis. 2014;42(Suppl 3): S99-108.
85. Egan RA, Hills WL, Susac JO. Gass plaques and fluorescein leakage in Susac syndrome. J Neurol Sci. 2010;299:97-100.
86. Egan RA, Ha Nguyen T, Gass JDM, et al. Retinal arterial wall plaques in Susac syndrome. Am J Ophthalmol 2003;135:483-6.
87. Brandt AU, Oberwahrenbrock T, Costello F, et al. Retinal lesion evolution in Susac syndrome. Retina. 2016;36:366-74.
88. Ringelstein M, Albrecht P, Kleffner I, et al. Retinal pathology in Susac syndrome detected by spectral-domain optical coherence tomography. Neurology. 2015;85:610-8.
89. Katz B. Migrainous central retinal artery occlusion. J Clin Neuroophthalmol. 1986;6:69-75.
90. Beversdorf D, Stommel E, Allen C, et al. Recurrent branch retinal infarcts in association with migraine. Headache. 1997;37:396-9.
91. Gutteridge IF, McDonald RA, Plenderleith JG. Branch retinal artery occlusion during a migraine attack. Clin Exp Optom. 2007;90:371-5.
92. Gass JD, Tiedeman J, Thomas MA. Idiopathic recurrent branch retinal arterial occlusion.Ophthalmology. 1986;93:1148-57.

93. Al-Abdulla NA, Haddock TA, Kerrison JB, et al. Sickle cell disease presenting with extensive peri-macular arteriolar occlusions in a nine-year-old boy. Am J Ophthalmol. 2001;131:275-6.
94. Brown GC, Magargal L, Augsburger JJ, et al. Preretinal arterial loops and retinal arterial occlusion. Am J Ophthalmol. 1979;87:646-51.
95. Newman NJ, Lessell S, Brandt EM. Bilateral central retinal artery occlusions, disk drusen, and migraine. Am J Ophthalmol. 1989;107:236-40.
96. Hayreh SS, Zimmerman MB. Amaurosis fugax in ocular vascular occlusive disorders: prevalence and pathogeneses. Retina. 2014;34:115-22.
97. Vodopivec I, Cestari DM, Rizzo JF. Management of transient monocular vision loss and retinal artery occlusions. Semin Ophthalmol. 2017;32:125-33.
98. Johnston SC, Gress DR, Browner WS, et al. Short-term prognosis after emergency department diagnosis of TIA. JAMA. 2000;284:2901-6.
99. Johnston SC, Rothwell PM, Nguyen-Huynh MN, et al. Validation and refinement of scores to predict very early stroke risk after transient ischaemic attack. Lancet. 2007;369:283-92.
100. Wolintz RJ. Carotid endarterectomy for ophthalmic manifestations: is it ever indicated? J Neuroophthalmol. 2005;25:299-302.
101. Hayreh SS, Zimmerman MB. Fundus changes in central retinal artery occlusion. Retina. 2007;27:276-89.
102. Hayreh SS, Podhajsky P. Ocular neovascularization with retinal vascular occlusion. II. Occurrence in central and branch retinal artery occlusion. Arch Ophthalmol. 1982;100:1585-96.
103. Hayreh SS, Fraterrigo L, Jonas J. Central retinal vein occlusion associated with cilioretinal artery occlusion. Retina. 2008;28:581-94.
104. Schmidt D. Comorbidities in combined retinal artery and vein occlusions. Eur J Med Res. 2013;18:27.
105. Sarraf D, Rahimy E, Fawzi AA, et al. Paracentral acute middle maculopathy: a new variant of acute macular neuroretinopathy associated with retinal capillary ischemia. JAMA Ophthalmol. 2013;131:1275-87.
106. Bhavsar KV, Lin S, Rahimy E, et al. Acute macular neuroretinopathy: acomprehensive review of the literature. Surv Ophthalmol. 2016;61:538-65.
107. Chen X, Rahimy E, Sergott RC, et al. Spectrum of retinal vascular diseases associated with paracentral acute middle maculopathy. Am J Ophthalmol. 2015;160:26-34.e1.
108. Rahimy E, Kuehlewein L, Sadda SR, et al. Paracentral acute middle maculopathy: what we knew then and what we know now. Retina. 2015;35:1921-30.
109. Yu S, Pang CE, Gong Y, et al. The spectrum of superficial and deep capillary ischemia in retinal artery occlusion. Am J Ophthalmol. 2015;159:53-63.e12.
110. Dansingani KK, Inoue M, Engelbert M, et al. Optical coherence tomographic angiography shows reduced deep capillary flow in paracentral acute middle maculopathy. Eye (Lond) 2015;29:1620-4.
111. Nemiroff J, Phasukkijwatana N, Sarraf D. Optical coherence tomography angiography of deep capillary ischemia. Dev Ophthalmol. 2016;56:139-45.
112. Sridhar J, Shahlaee A, Rahimy E, et al. Optical coherence tomography angiography and en face optical coherence tomography features of paracentral acute middle maculopathy. Am J Ophthalmol. 2015;160:1259-1268.e2.
113. Del Porto L, Petzold A. Optical coherence tomography angiography and retinal microvascular ramification in acute macular neuroretinopathy and paracentral acute middle maculopathy. Surv Ophthalmol. 2017;62:387-9.
114. Nemiroff J, Kuehlewein L, Rahimy E, et al. Assessing deep retinal capillary ischemia in paracentral acute middle maculopathy by optical coherence tomography angiography. Am J Ophthalmol. 2016;162:121-132.e1.
115. Pecen PE, Smith AG, Ehlers JP. Optical coherence tomography angiography of acute macular neuroretinopathy and paracentral acute middle maculopathy. JAMA Ophthalmol. 2015;133:1478-80.
116. Feltgen N, Neubauer A, Jurklies B, et al. Multicenter study of the European Assessment Group for Lysis in the Eye (EAGLE) for the treatment of central retinal artery occlusion: design issues and implications. EAGLE Study report no. 1: EAGLE Study report no. 1. Graefes Arch Clin Exp Ophthalmol. 2006;244:950-6.
117. Schumacher M, Schmidt D, Jurklies B, et al. Central retinal artery occlusion: local intra-arterial fibrinolysis versus conservative treatment, a multicenter randomized trial. Ophthalmology. 2010;117:1367-75.e1.
118. Wolf A, Schumacher M, Neubauer AS, et al. Comparison of superselective intraarterial fibrinolysis with conservative therapy. Use in patients with acute non-arteritic central retinal artery occlusion [In German]. Ophthalmologe. 2010;107:799-805.
119. Dattilo M, Biousse V, Newman NJ. Update on the management of central retinal artery occlusion. Neurol Clin. 2017;35:83-100.
120. Sacco RL, Kasner SE, Broderick JP, et al. An updated definition of stroke for the 21st century: a statement for healthcare professionals from the American Heart Association/ American Stroke Association. Stroke. 2013;44:2064-89.
121. Sivaprasad S, Prevost AT, Vasconcelos JC, et al. Clinical efficacy of intravitreal aflibercept versus panretinal photocoagulation for best corrected visual acuity in patients with proliferative diabetic retinopathy at 52 weeks (CLARITY): a multicentre, single-blinded, randomised, controlled, phase 2b, non-inferiority trial. Lancet. 2017;389:2193-203.
122. Writing Committee for the Diabetic Retinopathy Clinical Research Network, Gross JG, Glassman AR, et al. Panretinal photocoagulation vs intravitreous ranibizumab for proliferative diabetic retinopathy: arandomized clinical trial. JAMA. 2015;314:2137-46.
123. Mendrinos E, Machinis TG, Pournaras CJ. Ocular ischemic syndrome. Surv Ophthalmol. 2010;55:2-34.
124. Terelak-Borys B, Skonieczna K, Grabska-Liberek I. Ocular ischemic syndrome-a systematic review. Med Sci Monit. 2012;18:RA138-44.

125. Brown GC, Magargal LE. The ocular ischemic syndrome. Clinical, fluorescein angiographic and carotid angiographic features. Int Ophthalmol. 1988;11:239-51.
126. Sivalingam A, Brown GC, Magargal LE. The ocular ischemic syndrome. III. Visual prognosis and the effect of treatment. Int Ophthalmol. 1991;15:15-20.
127. Mizener JB, Podhajsky P, Hayreh SS. Ocular ischemic syndrome. Ophthalmology. 1997;104:859-64.
128. Kim DY, Joe SG, Lee JY, et al. Choroidal thickness in eyes with unilateral ocular ischemic syndrome. J Ophthalmol. 2015;2015:620372-5.
129. Kang HM, Lee CS, Lee SC. Thinner subfoveal choroidal thickness in eyes with ocular ischemic syndrome than in unaffected contralateral eyes. Graefes Arch Clin Exp Ophthalmol. 2014;252:851-2.
130. Wardlaw JM, Chappell FM, Best JJ, et al. Non-invasive imaging compared with intra-arterial angiography in the diagnosis of symptomatic carotid stenosis: a meta-analysis. Lancet. 2006;367:1503-12.
131. Costa VP, Kuzniec S, Molnar LJ, et al. Clinical findings and hemodynamic changes associated with severe occlusive carotid artery disease. Ophthalmology. 1997;104:1994-2002.
132. Reynolds PS, Greenberg JP, Lien LM, et al. Ophthalmic artery flow direction on color flow duplex imaging is highly specific for severe carotid stenosis. J Neuroimaging. 2002;12:5-8.
133. Fujioka S, Karashima K, Nakagawa H, et al. Classification of ophthalmic artery flow in patients with occlusive carotid artery disease. Jpn J Ophthalmol. 2006;50:224-8.
134. Dzierwa K, Pieniazek P, Musialek P, et al. Treatment strategies in severe symptomatic carotid and coronary artery disease. Med Sci Monit. 2011;17:RA191-7.
135. Rubin JR, McIntyre KM, Lukens MC, et al. Carotid endarterectomy for chronic retinal ischemia. Surg Gynecol Obstet. 1990;171:497-501.
136. Neroev VV, Kiseleva TN, Vlasov SK, et al. Visual outcomes after carotid reconstructive surgery for ocular ischemia. Eye (Lond). 2012;26:1281-7.
137. Gross R. Neovascular glaucoma and ocular ischemic syndrome. J Glaucoma. 2000;9:409-12.
138. Kofoed PK, Munch IC, Larsen M. Profound retinal ischaemia after ranibizumab administration in an eye with ocular ischaemic syndrome. Acta Ophthalmol. 2010;88:808-10.
139. Orth DH, Patz A. Retinal branch vein occlusion. Surv Ophthalmol. 1978;22:357-76.
140. Natural history and clinical management of central retinal vein occlusion. The Central Vein Occlusion Study Group. Arch Ophthalmol. 1997;115:486-91.
141. Baseline and early natural history report. The Central Vein Occlusion Study. Arch Ophthalmol. 1993;111:1087-95.
142. A randomized clinical trial of early panretinal photocoagulation for ischemic central vein occlusion. The Central Vein Occlusion Study Group N report. Ophthalmology. 1995;102:1434-44.
143. Scott IU, Ip MS, VanVeldhuisen PC, et al. A randomized trial comparing the efficacy and safety of intravitreal triamcinolone with standard care to treat vision loss associated with macular edema secondary to branch retinal vein occlusion: the Standard Care vs Corticosteroid for Retinal Vein Occlusion (SCORE) study report 6. Arch Ophthalmol. 2009;127:1115-28.
144. Evaluation of grid pattern photocoagulation for macular edema in central vein occlusion. The Central Vein Occlusion Study Group M report. Ophthalmology. 1995;102:1425-33.
145. Mitchell P, Smith W, Chang A. Prevalence and associations of retinal vein occlusion in Australia. The Blue Mountains Eye Study. Arch Opththalm. 1996;114:1243-7.
146. Shin YU, Cho H, Kim JM, et al. Prevalence and associated factors of retinal vein occlusion in the Korean National Health and Nutritional Examination Survey. 2008-2012:a cross-sectional observational study. Medicine (Baltimore). 2016;95:e5185.
147. Hayreh SS, Zimmerman MB, Podhajsky P. Incidence of various types of retinal vein occlusion and their recurrence and demographic characteristics. Am J Ophthalmol. 1994;117:429-41.
148. Klein R, Klein BE, Moss SE, et al. The epidemiology of retinal vein occlusion: the Beaver Dam Eye Study. Trans Am Ophthalmol Soc. 2000;98:133-4.
149. Klein R, Moss SE, Meuer SM, et al. The 15-year cumulative incidence of retinal vein occlusion: the Beaver Dam Eye Study. Arch Ophthalmol. 2008;126:513-8.
150. Hayreh SS. Retinal vein occlusion. Indian J Ophthalmol. 1994;42:109-32.
151. Klien BA, Olwin JH. A survey of the pathogenesis of retinal venous occlusion, emphasis upon choice of therapy and an analysis of the therapeutic results in fifty-three patients. AMA Arch Ophthalmol. 1956;56:207-47.
152. Klien BA. Sidelights on retinal venous occlusion. Am J Ophthalmol. 1966;61:25-36.
153. Risk factors for central retinal vein occlusion. The Eye Disease Case-Control Study Group. Arch Opththalmol. 1996;114:545-54.
154. Hayreh SS, Zimmerman B, McCarthy MJ, et al. Systemic diseases associated with various types of retinal vein occlusion. Am J Ophthalmol. 2001;131:61-77.
155. Weger M, Stanger O, Deutschmann H, et al. Hyperhomocyst(e)inemia and MTHFR C677T genotypes in patients with central retinal vein occlusion. Graefes Arch Clin Exp Ophthalmol. 2002;240:286-90.
156. Battaglia Parodi M, Di Crecchio L. Hyperhomocysteinemia and retinal vascular occlusive disease. Eur J Ophthalmol. 2003;13:500-1.
157. Chak M, Wallace GR, Graham EM, et al. Thrombophilia: genetic polymorphisms and their association with retinal vascular occlusive disease. Br J Ophthalmol. 2001;85:883-6.
158. Ahluwalia J, Rao S, Varma S, et al. Thrombophilic risk factors are uncommon in young patients with retinal vein occlusion. Retina. 2015;35:715-9.
159. Liu Q, Lahey JM, Karlen R, et al. Laboratory evaluation of hypercoagulable states in patients with central retinal vein occlusion who are less than 56 years of age. Retina. 2017.
160. Janssen MCH, Heijer den M, Cruysberg JRM, et al. Retinal vein occlusion: A form of venous thrombosis or

a complication of atherosclerosis? A meta-analysis of thrombophilic factors. Thromb Haemost. 2005;93:1021-6.
161. Hayreh SS, Zimmerman MB. Ocular neovascularization associated with central and hemicentral retinal vein occlusion. Retina. 2012;32:1553-65.
162. Gass JD. A fluorescein angiographic study of macular dysfunction secondary to retinal vascular disease. II. Retinal vein obstruction. Arch Ophthalmol.1968;80:550-68.
163. Sinclair SH, Gragoudas ES. Prognosis for rubeosis iridis following central retinal vein occlusion. Br J Ophthalmol. 1979;63:735-43.
164. Hayreh SS. Prevalent misconceptions about acute retinal vascular occlusive disorders. Prog Retin Eye Res. 2005;24:493-519.
165. Magargal LE, Brown GC, Augsburger JJ, et al. Neovascular glaucoma following central retinal vein obstruction. Ophthalmology. 1981;88:1095-101.
166. Hayreh SS, Rojas P, Podhajsky P, et al. Ocular neovascularization with retinal vascular occlusion-III. Incidence of ocular neovascularization with retinal vein occlusion. Ophthalmology. 1983;90:488-506.
167. Laatikainen L, Kohner EM, Khoury D, et al. Panretinal photocoagulation in central retinal vein occlusion: A randomised controlled clinical study. Br J Ophthalmol. 1977;61:741-53.
168. May DR, Klein ML, Peyman GA, et al. Xenon arc panretinal photocoagulation for central retinal vein occlusion: a randomised prospective study. Br J Ophthalmol. 1979;63:725-34.
169. Ogino K, Murakami T, Tsujikawa A, et al. Characteristics of optical coherence tomographic hyperreflective foci in retinal vein occlusion. Retina. 2012;32:77-85.
170. Lerche RC, Schaudig U, Scholz F, et al. Structural changes of the retina in retinal vein occlusion--imaging and quantification with optical coherence tomography. Ophthalmic Surg Lasers. 2001;32:272-80.
171. Ozdemir H, Karacorlu M, Karacorlu S. Serous macular detachment in central retinal vein occlusion. Retina. 2005;25:561-3.
172. Kang JW, Yoo R, Jo YH, et al. Correlation of microvascular structures on optical coherence tomography angiography with visual acuity in retinal vein occlusion. Retina. 2017;37:1700-9.
173. Spaide RF. Volume-rendered optical coherence tomography of retinal vein occlusion pilot study. Am J Ophthalmol. 2016;165:133-44.
174. Hayreh SS, Klugman MR, Podhajsky P, et al. Electroretinography in central retinal vein occlusion. Correlation of electroretinographic changes with pupillary abnormalities. Graefes Arch Clin Exp Ophthalmol. 1989;227:549-61.
175. Hayreh SS, Klugman MR, Beri M, et al. Differentiation of ischemic from non-ischemic central retinal vein occlusion during the early acute phase. Graefes Arch Clin Exp Ophthalmol.1990;228:201-17.
176. Hayreh SS, Zimmerman MB. Fundus changes in central retinal vein occlusion. Retina. 2015;35:29-42.
177. Ashraf M, Souka AA, Singh RP. Central retinal vein occlusion: modifying current treatment protocols. Eye (Lond). 2016;30:505-14.
178. Sharareh B, Gallemore R, Taban M, et al. Recalcitrant macular edema after intravitreal bevacizumab is responsive to an intravitreal dexamethasone implant in retinal vein occlusion. Retina. 2013;33:1227-31.
179. Bhisitkul RB, Campochiaro PA, Shapiro H, et al. Predictive value in retinal vein occlusions of early versus late or incomplete ranibizumab response defined by optical coherence tomography. Ophthalmology. 2013;120:1057-63.
180. Hayreh SS. Management of central retinal vein occlusion. Ophthalmologica. 2003;217:167-88.
181. Hayreh SS, Zimmerman MB, Podhajsky P. Hematologic abnormalities associated with various types of retinal vein occlusion. Graefes Arch Clin Exp Ophthalmol. 2002;240:180-96.
182. Hayreh SS, Podhajsky PA, Zimmerman MB. Central and hemicentral retinal vein occlusion: role of anti-platelet aggregation agents and anticoagulants. Ophthalmology. 2011;118:1603-11.
183. Brown DM, Campochiaro PA, Singh RP, et al. Ranibizumab for macular edema following central retinal vein occlusion: six-month primary end point results of a phase III study. Ophthalmology. 2010;117:1124-1133.e1.
184. Brown DM, Heier JS, Clark WL, et al. Intravitreal aflibercept injection for macular edema secondary to central retinal vein occlusion: 1-year results from the phase 3 COPERNICUS study. Am J Ophthalmol. 2013;155:429-437.e7.
185. Korobelnik JF, Holz FG, Roider J, et al. Intravitreal aflibercept injection for macular edema resulting from central retinal vein occlusion: one-year results of the phase 3 GALILEO Study. Ophthalmology. 2014;121:202-8.
186. Campochiaro PA, Sophie R, Pearlman J, et al. Long-term outcomes in patients with retinal vein occlusion treated with ranibizumab: the RETAIN study. Ophthalmology. 2014;121:209-19.
187. Heier JS, Campochiaro PA, Yau L, et al. Ranibizumab for macular edema due to retinal vein occlusions: long-term follow-up in the HORIZON trial. Ophthalmology. 2012;119:802-9.
188. Papakostas TD, Lim L, van Zyl T, et al. Intravitreal aflibercept for macular oedema secondary to central retinal vein occlusion in patients with prior treatment with bevacizumab or ranibizumab. Eye (Lond). 2016;30:79-84.
189. Eadie JA, Ip MS, Kulkarni AD. Response to aflibercept as secondary therapy in patients with persistent retinal edema due to central retinal vein occlusion initially treated with bevacizumab or ranibizumab. Retina. 2014;34:2439-43.
190. Scott IU, VanVeldhuisen PC, Ip MS, et al. Baseline factors associated with 6-month visual acuity and retinal thickness outcomes in patients with macular edema secondary to central retinal vein occlusion or hemiretinal vein occlusion: SCORE2 Study Report 4. JAMA Ophthalmol. 2017;135:639-49.
191. Sun JK. Comparing anti-vascular endothelial growth factor therapies for central retinal vein occlusion. JAMA Ophthalmol. 2017;135:649-50.

192. Haller JA, Bandello F, Belfort R, et al. Randomized, sham-controlled trial of dexamethasone intravitreal implant in patients with macular edema due to retinal vein occlusion. Ophthalmology. 2010;117:1134-46.e3.
193. Ip MS, Scott IU, VanVeldhuisen PC, et al. A randomized trial comparing the efficacy and safety of intravitreal triamcinolone with observation to treat vision loss associated with macular edema secondary to central retinal vein occlusion: the Standard Care vs Corticosteroid for Retinal Vein Occlusion (SCORE) study report 5. Arch Ophthalmol. 2009;127:1101-14.
194. Ozkok A, Saleh OA, Sigford DK, et al. The OMAR Study: Comparison of ozurdex and triamcinolone acetonide for refractory cystoid macular edema in retinal vein occlusion. Retina. 2015;35:1393-400.
195. Chatziralli I, Theodossiadis G, Kabanarou SA, et al. Ranibizumab versus dexamethasone implant for central retinal vein occlusion: the RANIDEX study. Graefes Arch Clin Exp Ophthalmol. 2017;117:313.
196. Campochiaro PA, Hafiz G, Mir TA, et al. Scatter photocoagulation does not reduce macular edema or treatment burden in patients with retinal vein occlusion: the RELATE Trial. Ophthalmology. 2015;122:1426-37.
197. Hayreh SS, Klugman MR, Podhajsky P, et al. Argon laser panretinal photocoagulation in ischemic central retinal vein occlusion. A 10-year prospective study.Graefes Arch Clin Exp Ophthalmol. 1990;228:281-96.
198. Hayreh SS, Zimmerman MB. Hemicentral retinal vein occlusion: natural history of visual outcome. Retina. 2012;32:68-76.
199. Scott IU, VanVeldhuisen PC, Oden NL, et al. Baseline characteristics and response to treatment of participants with hemiretinal compared with branch retinal or central retinal vein occlusion in the standard care vs corticosteroid for retinal vein occlusion (SCORE) study: SCORE study report 14. Arch Ophthalmol. 2012;130:1517-24.
200. Chopdar A. Dual trunk central retinal vein incidence in clinical practice. Arch Opththalmol. 1984;102:85-7.
201. Chopdar A. Hemi-central retinal vein occlusion. Pathogenesis, clinical features, natural history and incidence of dual trunk central retinal vein. Trans Ophthalmol Soc UK. 1982;102(pt 2):241-8.
202. Appiah AP, Trempe CL. Differences in contributory factors among hemicentral, central, and branch retinal vein occlusions. Ophthalmology. 1989;96:364-6.
203. Hayreh SS, Zimmerman MB, Beri M, et al. Intraocular pressure abnormalities associated with central and hemicentral retinal vein occlusion. Ophthalmology. 2004;111:133-41.
204. Sperduto RD, Hiller R, Chew E, et al. Risk factors for hemiretinal vein occlusion: comparison with risk factors for central and branch retinal vein occlusion: the eye disease case-control study. Ophthalmology. 1998;105: 765-71.
205. Hayreh SS, Hayreh MS. Hemi-central retinal vein occulsion. Pathogenesis, clinical features, and natural history. Arch Opththalmol. 1980;98:1600-9.
206. Christoffersen NL, Larsen M. Pathophysiology and hemodynamics of branch retinal vein occlusion. Ophthalmology. 1999;106:2054-62.
207. Weinberg D, Dodwell DG, Fern SA. Anatomy of arteriovenous crossings in branch retinal vein occlusion. Am J Ophthalmol.1990;109:298-302.
208. O'Mahoney PRA, Wong DT, Ray JG. Retinal vein occlusion and traditional risk factors for atherosclerosis. Arch Ophthalmol. 2008;126:692-9.
209. Appiah AP, Trempe CL. Risk factors associated with branch vs. central retinal vein occlusion. Ann Ophthalmol. 1989;21:153-7.
210. Hayreh SS, Zimmerman MB. Branch retinal vein occlusion: natural history of visual outcome. JAMA Ophthalmol. 2014;132:13-22.
211. Hayreh SS, Zimmerman MB. Fundus changes in branch retinal vein occlusion. Retina. 2015;35:1016-27.
212. Joondeph HC, Joondeph BC. Posterior tractional retinal breaks complicating branch retinal vein occlusion. Retina. 1988;8:136-40.
213. Ehlers JP, Kim SJ, Yeh S, et al. Therapies for macular edema associated with branch retinal vein occlusion: a report by the American Academy of Ophthalmology. Ophthalmology. 2017;124:1412-23.
214. Argon laser photocoagulation for macular edema in branch vein occlusion. The Branch Vein Occlusion Study Group. Am J Ophthalmol. 1984;98:271-82.
215. Hayreh SS, Rubenstein L, Podhajsky P. Argon laser scatter photocoagulation in treatment of branch retinal vein occlusion. A prospective clinical trial. Ophthalmologica. 1993;206:1-14.

Chapter 50

Age-related Macular Degeneration

Tiarnan Keenan, Emily Chew

INTRODUCTION

Age-related macular degeneration (AMD) is a slowly progressive degenerative disease with pathology centered principally in the *macula lutea*. It accounts for approximately 9% of all global blindness. The number of people with AMD worldwide is projected to be 196 million in 2020, rising to 288 million in 2040.[1] AMD is the leading cause of blindness in developed countries. In the United States of America (USA), it was estimated in 2004 to account for 54% of blindness and 23% of low vision in Caucasian people.[2]

The human *macula lutea* (or yellow spot) is the central portion of retina responsible for high acuity central vision. It is defined anatomically as the circular area of retina lying within the vascular arcades, centered on the fovea and with a diameter of approximately 6 mm (Figs. 50.1A to C). Its histological definition is the central portion of retina where the ganglion cell layer contains more than one layer of nuclei. Disturbances in the highly ordered structure of the macula can lead to significant central visual problems, affecting the ability of individuals to read, drive, and recognize faces.

In common with other neurodegenerative conditions such as Alzheimer's disease, AMD is very strongly associated with aging. The prevalence of advanced AMD in Caucasian populations has been estimated at 1.4% at 70 years, rising to 5.6% at 80 years and 20% at 90 years.[3] The onset of clinical features varies between individuals but typically begins at some point after the age of 55 years.[4] In the early course of the disease, visual symptoms may be absent or minimal. However, in advanced cases, AMD leads to severely reduced central vision and loss of visual acuity, often in both eyes. For this reason, AMD has major implications for individuals and for society, as patients with this condition may experience many years of decreased quality of life, reduced independence, and even depression.[5-8]

EARLY EPIDEMIOLOGICAL STUDIES

The foundation for much of our current knowledge regarding the epidemiology and natural history of AMD arose out of several early long-term studies of age-related eye disease, including the Beaver Dam Eye Study and the Blue Mountains Eye Study.

The Beaver Dam Eye Study began in 1987 and consisted of baseline and follow-up examinations of almost 5,000 of the approximately 6,000 people aged 43–86 years in the town of Beaver Dam, Wisconsin. This included fundus photography and standardized macular grading using the Wisconsin age-related maculopathy grading system.[9] Amongst many other findings, the study provided some of the first prevalence and incidence estimates of AMD in Caucasian populations,[10,11] demonstrated increased risk of progression to late AMD in eyes with soft drusen or pigmentary abnormalities[11] (see later), and provided evidence of strong genetic involvement in AMD (see later) through sibling studies.[12] It also examined potential associations between AMD and various long-term environmental risk factors such as cigarette smoking,[13] sunlight exposure,[14] and cardiovascular risk factors.[15]

Similarly, the Blue Mountains Eye Study in Australia consisted of baseline and follow-up examinations of approximately 3,500 people aged 49 years and older in a specified urban area near Sydney from 1992. Again, fundus photography was performed with standardized macular grading using the Wisconsin age-related maculopathy grading system. This study again observed a very strong association between age and AMD;[16] like the Beaver Dam Eye Study, it also reported higher risk of progression to late AMD in eyes with soft drusen or pigmentary abnormalities.[17] Similarly, it provided evidence of associations between AMD and risk factors including smoking,[18] plasma fibrinogen levels,[19] and family history.[20]

CLASSIFICATION OF AGE-RELATED MACULAR DEGENERATION

Several classification systems have been used in recent decades to describe and study the clinical features of AMD, including the Age-Related Eye Disease Study (AREDS) grading system,[21] which was adapted from the more complex Wisconsin age-related maculopathy grading system mentioned above.[9] In 2013, the Beckman Initiative

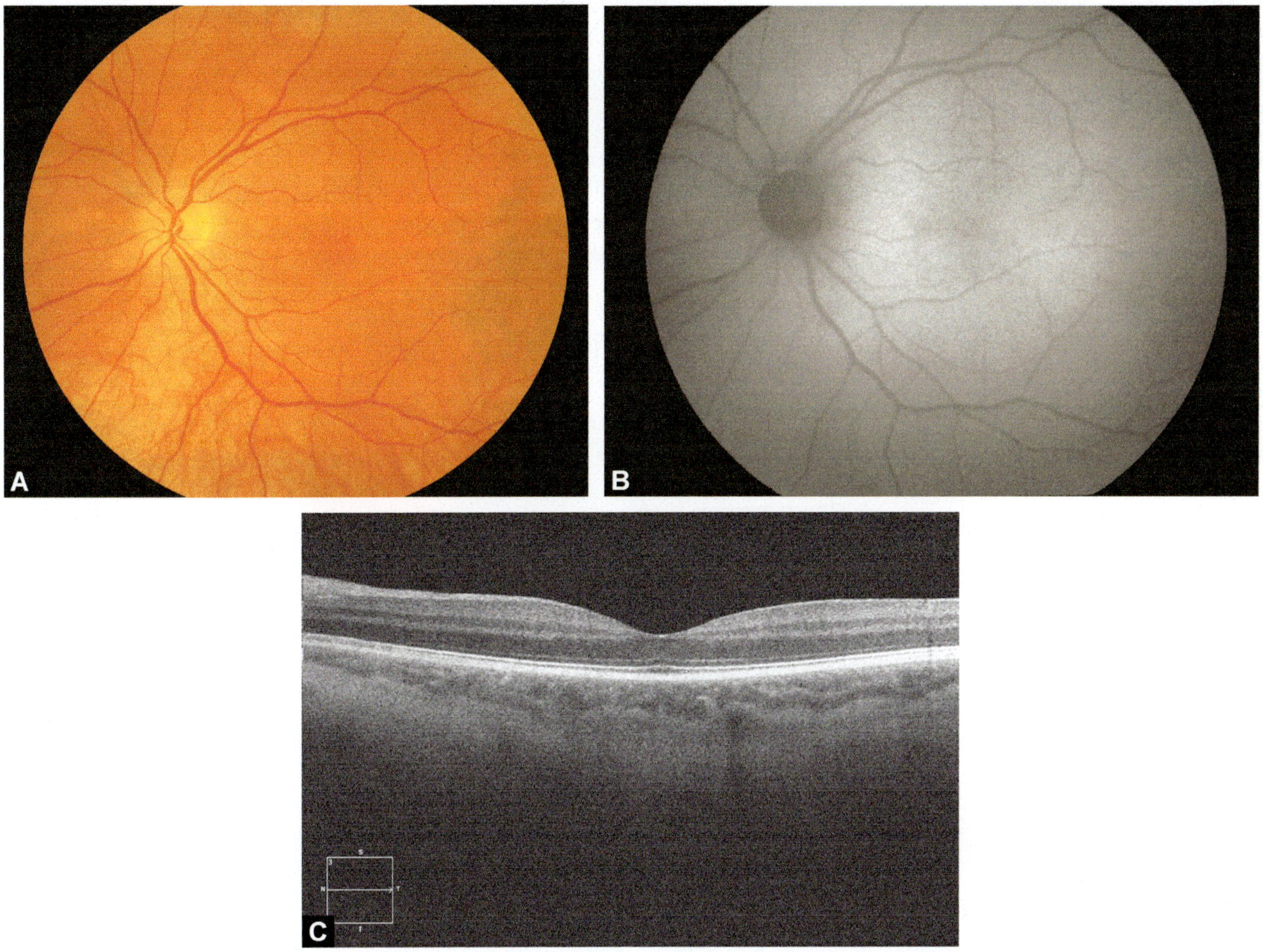

Figs. 50.1A to C: Normal human macula: (A) Color fundus photograph; (B) Fundus autofluorescence; (C) Optical coherence tomography scan.

for Macular Research Classification Committee proposed the integration of previous systems into a new unified AMD clinical classification system (summarized in Table 50.1), following a consensus meeting of experts.[22]

Age-related macular degeneration is classified into three stages—early, intermediate, and late, based on features present on clinical examination or on color fundus photography, though additional imaging modalities (see later) may also be used to aid staging. In the context of early AMD, it is important to make the distinction between normal and pathological aging changes.

CLINICAL AND IMAGING FEATURES OF AMD BY STAGE

Early Age-related Macular Degeneration

Early AMD is characterized clinically by the presence of macular drusen in individuals aged 50 years and above.[21,22] Visual symptoms are typically absent at this stage. Drusen are extracellular deposits of lipid and protein that accumulate between the retinal pigment epithelium (RPE) and Bruch's membrane and are seen clinically as yellowish deposits at the macula (Figs. 50.2A to C).[23-25] In contrast to normal aging changes, where small drusen (diameter ≤ 63 μm, also known as "drupelets") may be observed, early AMD requires the presence of medium-sized drusen (diameter > 63 μm and ≤ 125 μm). Hence, careful assessment of drusen size (and other characteristics) is important in distinguishing between normal and pathological aging.

Indeed, it is important to note that drusen take different forms, some of which are more closely associated with AMD than others, and that drusenoid and other deposits are observed in conditions other than AMD, including monogenic disorders (such as extensive drusen in Doyne honeycomb dystrophy and fleck deposits in Stargardt disease). Subtypes of drusen, their appearance on multimodal imaging, and their relationship with aging and AMD have been reviewed in detail.[26] In particular, soft

Table 50.1: Clinical classification of age-related macular degeneration (AMD), as proposed by the Beckman Initiative for Macular Research Classification Committee.

Classification of AMD	Definition: Lesions assessed within two disc diameters of fovea
No apparent aging changes	(i) No drusen and (ii) No AMD pigmentary abnormalities*
Normal aging changes	(i) Only small drusen and (ii) No AMD pigmentary abnormalities*
Early AMD	(i) Medium drusen and (ii) No AMD pigmentary abnormalities*
Intermediate AMD	(i) Large drusen and/or (ii) Any AMD pigmentary abnormalities*
Late AMD	(i) Neovascular AMD and/or (ii) Any geographic atrophy

**AMD pigmentary abnormalities*: Any definite hyper- or hypopigmentary abnormalities associated with medium or large drusen but not associated with known disease entities; small drusen are ≤ 63 μm; medium drusen > 63 μm and ≤ 125 μm; large drusen > 125 μm.

Source: Reprinted with permission from Elsevier Inc. Ferris FL 3rd, Wilkinson CP, Bird A, et al. Clinical classification of age-related macular degeneration. Ophthalmology. 2013;120:844-51.

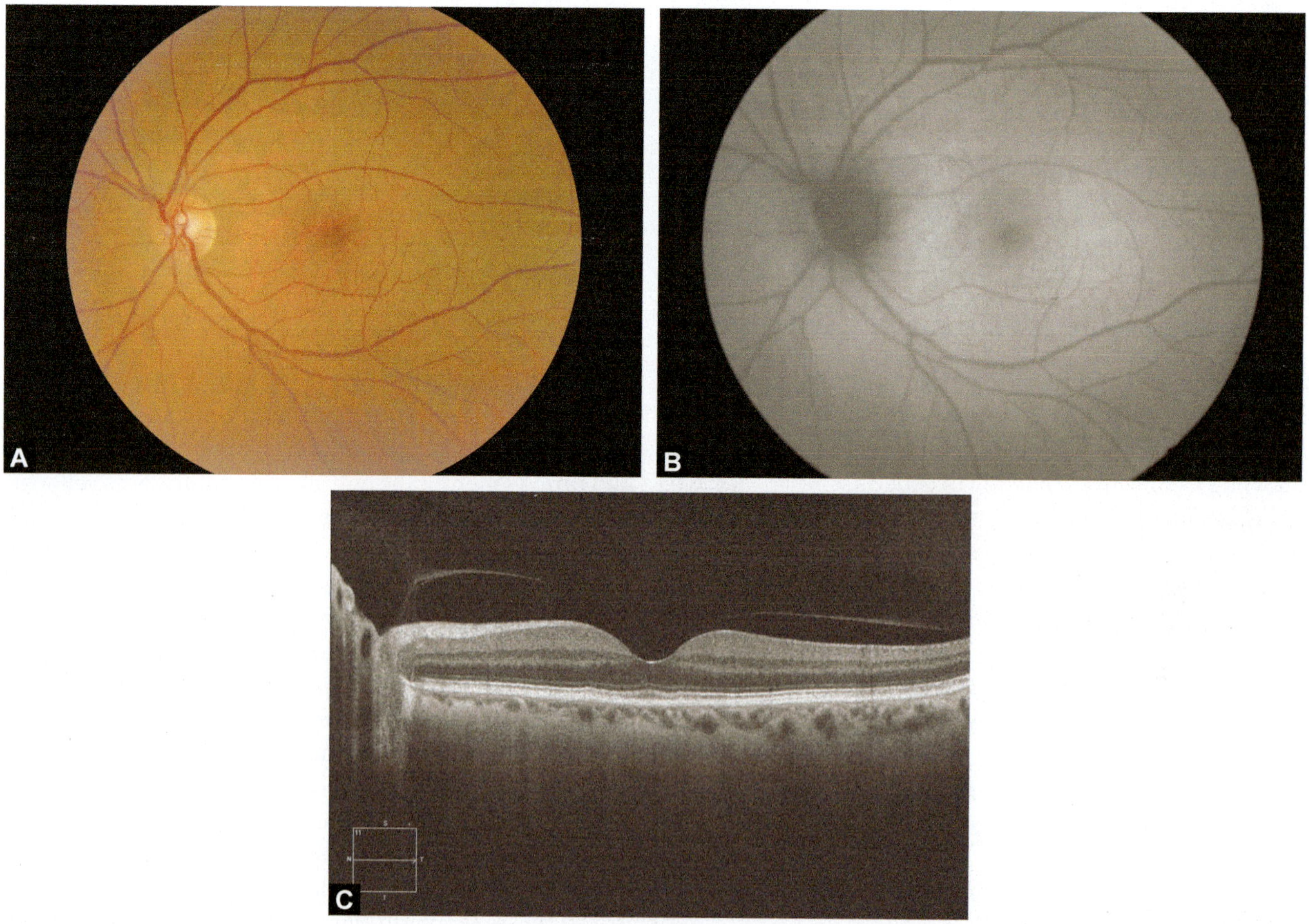

Figs. 50.2A to C: Early age-related macular degeneration: (A) Color fundus photograph; (B) Fundus autofluorescence; (C) Optical coherence tomography (OCT) scan. Medium-sized drusen are present on the color fundus photograph and drusen are observed on the OCT scan as irregular elevations under the retinal pigment epithelium.

drusen are regarded as the hallmark deposit of AMD. In contrast to hard drusen (small discrete deposits that may be found in the macula and peripheral retina with normal aging), soft drusen are large (usually >125 μm diameter) yellow deposits that are less discrete and are found only in the posterior pole (Figs. 50.2A to C). Reticular pseudodrusen (Figs. 50.3A to C) are another important subtype of drusenoid deposit. These deposits were first described clinically as a yellowish interlacing macular pattern seen best in blue light fundus photography;[27] they represent an additional clinical phenotype of AMD and an independent risk factor for progression to late AMD.[28] Further discussion of these and other drusen subtypes (such as cuticular drusen and colloid drusen, together with drusenoid and fleck deposits seen in other conditions) are beyond the scope of this chapter but are discussed in the above review.

The imaging characteristics of early AMD are based primarily on the identification of medium-sized drusen (together with the absence of other features such as pigmentary abnormalities) on color fundus photography and ocular coherence tomography (OCT) imaging (Figs. 50.2A to C). Drusen characteristics on OCT have been reviewed recently;[29] they are seen as sub-RPE hyperreflective deposits but may be distinguished according to morphology and size. Fundus autofluorescence imaging features of early AMD include altered signal (typically moderate hyperautofluorescence) associated with drusen; the absence of pigmentary abnormalities of the RPE means that associated hypo- or hyperautofluorescence features should be absent or minimal.

Intermediate Age-related Macular Degeneration

Intermediate AMD represents an important stage in disease evolution where the macula is at significantly higher risk of progression to late AMD over the following 5 years.[30,31] Risk estimates range from 0.5% for the "normal aging changes" group to 50% for the highest category within the intermediate AMD group (see later for AMD simplified severity scale). Symptoms are typically mild in intermediate AMD and may consist of a small reduction in visual acuity and/or early presence of metamorphopsia. This stage is diagnosed by the presence of large drusen (diameter

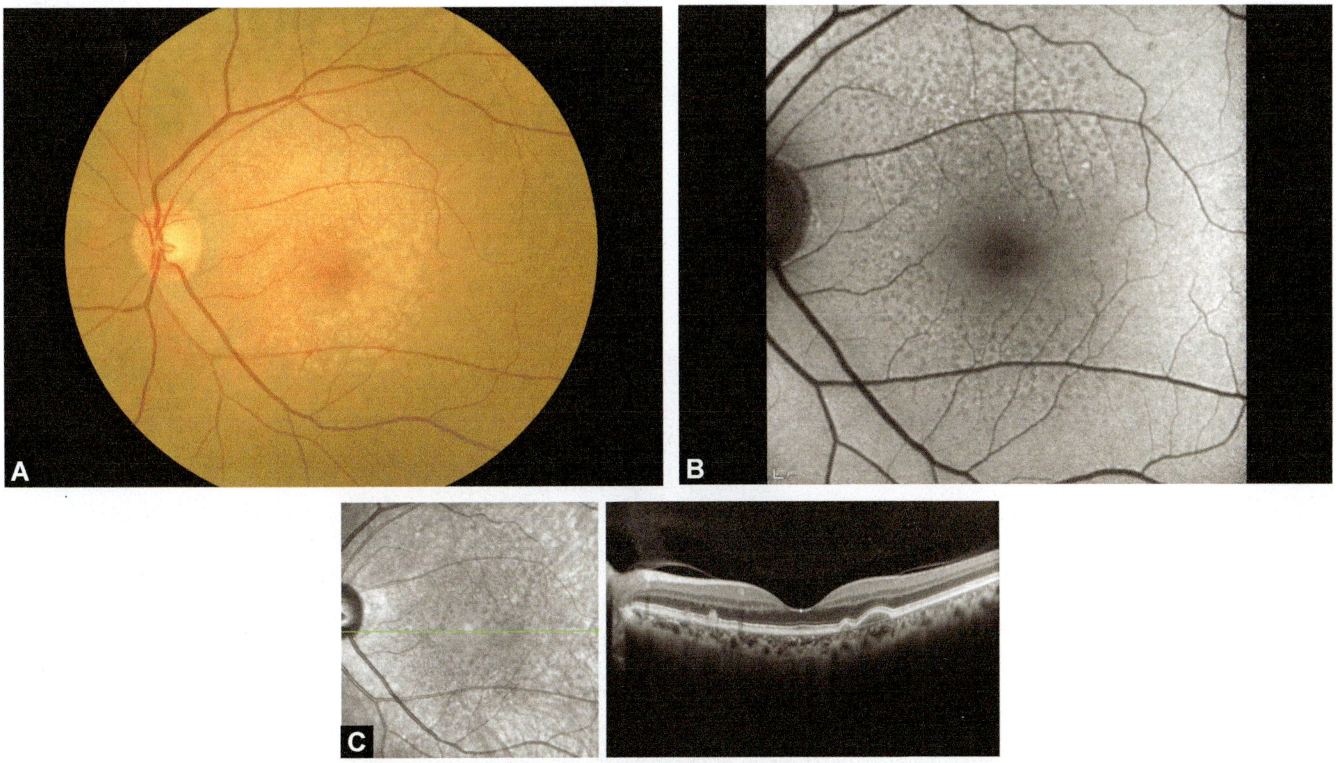

Figs. 50.3A to C: Reticular pseudodrusen and soft drusen: (A) Color fundus photograph; (B) Fundus autofluorescence; (C) Optical coherence tomography (OCT) scan with accompanying infrared reflectance image. Confluent soft drusen (seen on the color fundus photograph and OCT scan) are present temporal to the fovea but reticular pseudodrusen (seen on all four imaging modalities) encircle the fovea in the remaining areas. The cross-sectional appearance of the two distinct types of drusenoid deposit is seen to differ on the OCT scan.

≥125 μm) and/or pigmentary abnormalities at the macula (Figs. 50.4A to C). These pigmentary changes arise from RPE disturbances; for intermediate AMD, they are defined as definite hyper- or hypopigmentary abnormalities associated with medium or large drusen but not associated with other known disease entities.

The imaging characteristics of intermediate AMD on color fundus photography include observation of large drusen and/or pigmentary abnormalities (Figs. 50.4A to C). The large soft drusen are typically yellow with poorly demarcated edges and may become partially confluent over time with increased size. On fundus autofluorescence imaging, large drusen may demonstrate increased or heterogeneous signal, while pigmentary abnormalities of the RPE are associated with small areas of increased signal and/or decreased signal (atrophic RPE) not meeting the criteria for geographic atrophy (see later). OCT imaging of intermediate AMD is characterized by the presence of large sub-RPE hyperreflective deposits and/or intraretinal hyperreflective foci, together with additional features, including loss of integrity of the RPE and ellipsoid zone.[29]

A recent study has also demonstrated a significantly higher prevalence of peripheral retinal changes (including peripheral drusen, pigmentary abnormalities, neovascularization, and geographic atrophy) in the eyes of patients with at least intermediate AMD.[32] Together with other evidence, this suggests that the pathology in AMD may be more widespread than the macula alone.

Late Age-related Macular Degeneration

Late AMD is divided into neovascular disease (exudative or “wet’” AMD) and atrophic disease (“dry” AMD). However, it is important to note that these can coexist in the same eye; atrophic lesions may develop neovascular disease and neovascular disease is frequently followed by outer retinal atrophy.[33] Late AMD is the stage typically associated with severe central visual loss, in the form of a dense central scotoma and/or severe metamorphopsia. Neovascular AMD was previously responsible for over 90% of severe visual loss in AMD,[34-36] since untreated neovascular disease usually leads almost inevitably to extensive macular damage and irreversible visual loss to the level of legal blindness. However, now that treatment of neovascular AMD is possible and typically associated with substantially improved visual outcomes (see later), atrophic AMD represents an important disease burden and research priority, since no treatments are currently available in routine clinical use for this form of advanced disease.

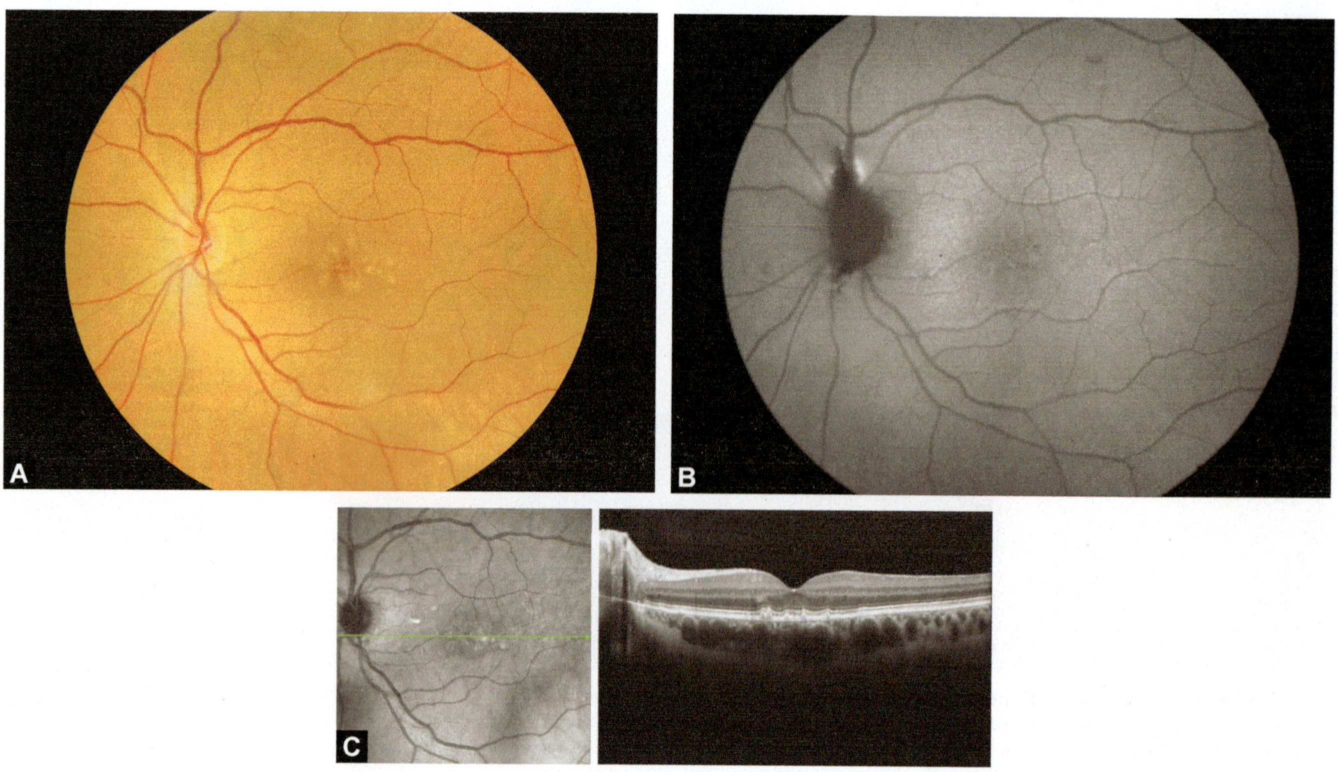

Figs. 50.4A to C: Intermediate age-related macular degeneration: (A) Color fundus photograph; (B) Fundus autofluorescence; (C) Optical coherence tomography (OCT) scan with accompanying infrared reflectance image. Large drusen are observed on the color fundus photograph and the OCT scan.

Neovascular Age-related Macular Degeneration

Neovascular AMD is characterized by the growth of new blood vessels from the choroid into the subretinal or sub-RPE space, in the form of choroidal neovascularization (CNV). The growth of new capillaries from the choriocapillaris is permitted by loss of integrity of Bruch's membrane in association with alterations in the local balance of pro- and antiangiogenic factors. The developing CNV membrane contains proliferating vascular endothelial cells and RPE cells. Its immature capillaries may lead to serous or hemorrhagic detachment of the RPE or neurosensory retina, such that a pigmented epithelial detachment (Figs. 50.5A and B) is a key feature of progression to neovascular disease. If untreated, CNV growth over time is usually accompanied by hemorrhage, lipid exudation, expansion of subretinal fibrous tissue and widespread RPE and photoreceptor atrophy in the form of a disciform scar (Figs. 50.6A and B).[37]

For these reasons, important warning symptoms for the possibility of incident neovascular disease include a relatively rapid increase in metamorphopsia, decrease in visual acuity, and/or central scotoma, ideally noticed quickly by the patient through frequent monocular monitoring using an Amsler grid (or newer devices such as the ForeseeHome AMD Monitoring Program).[38] Similarly, key clinical features to suggest neovascular disease activity

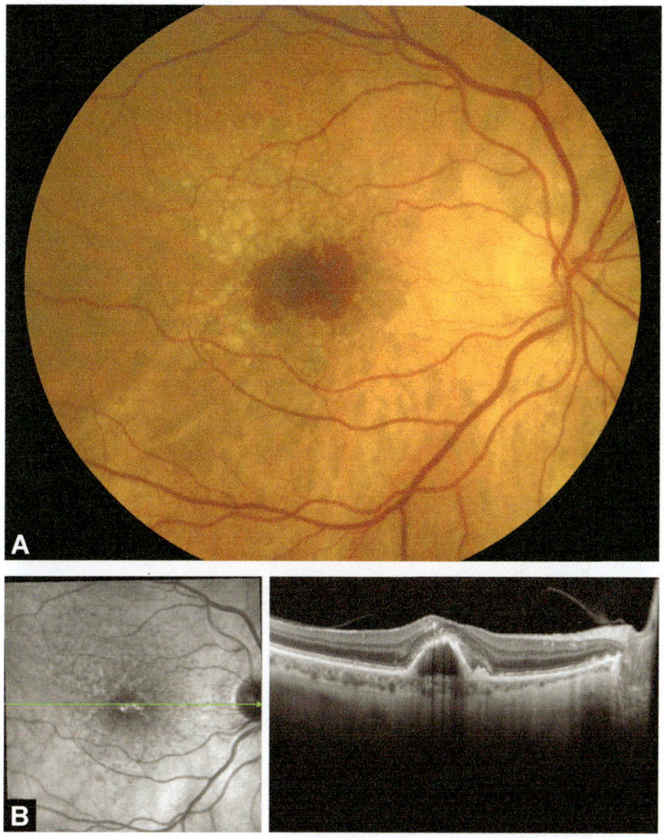

Figs. 50.5A and B: Neovascular age-related macular degeneration (with pigment epithelial detachment from choroidal neovascular membrane): (A) Color fundus photograph; (B) Optical coherence tomography scan with accompanying infrared reflectance image. Subretinal hemorrhage is observed as red material on the color fundus photograph. In this case, soft drusen are present temporal to the fovea but reticular pseudodrusen are observed (on all three imaging modalities) encircling the fovea in the remaining areas.

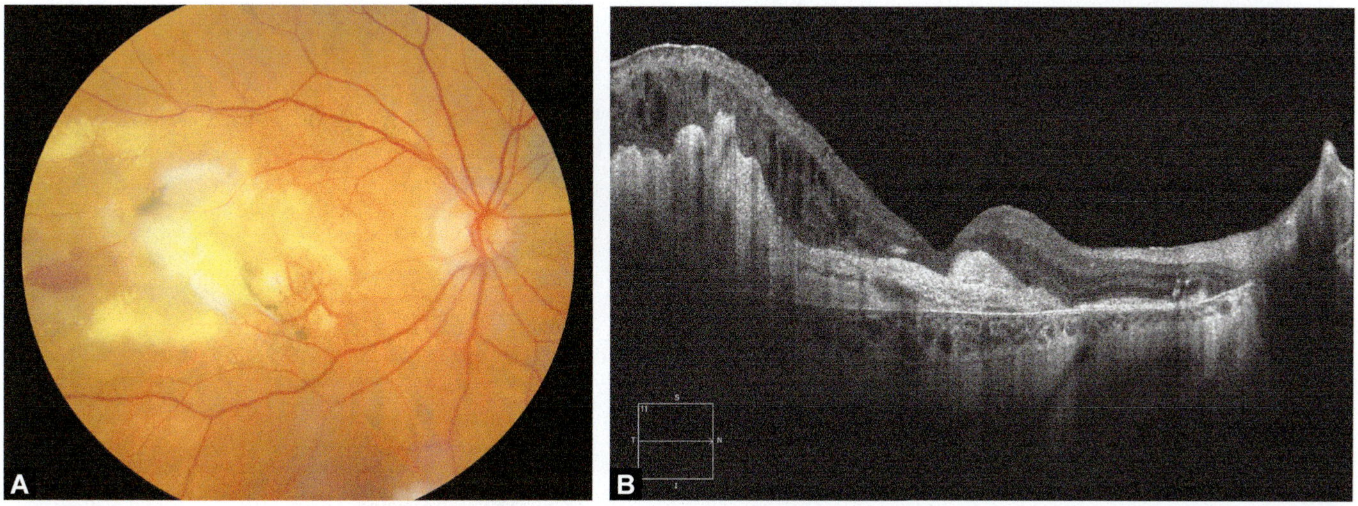

Figs. 50.6A and B: Disciform scar in untreated neovascular age-related macular degeneration: (A) Color fundus photograph; (B) Optical coherence tomography (OCT) scan. Retinal hemorrhage (red), lipid exudate (yellow), and fibrosis (yellow/white) are observed on the color fundus photograph. Fibrosis is observed on the OCT scan as subretinal hyperreflective material, accompanied by cystic intraretinal fluid, atrophy of the retinal pigment epithelium, and disorganized retinal architecture.

include retinal hemorrhage, hard exudate, and subretinal and/or intraretinal fluid, observed clinically and on OCT imaging (Figs. 50.5A and B), which should prompt immediate angiographic evaluation, usually with fundus fluorescein angiography (FFA).

Retinal imaging features in neovascular AMD have recently been reviewed.[39] CNV membranes were traditionally diagnosed and classified on the basis of their location and characteristics on FFA (Table 50.2; Figs. 50.7A to D), though indocyanine green (ICG) angiography

Table 50.2: Characteristic features of choroidal neovascular lesions on fundus fluorescein angiography.

CNV lesion	Hyperfluorescence	Lesion borders	Leakage	Flat or elevated
Classic	Early intense hyperfluorescence; may be lacy	Initially well-defined	Progressive leakage	Flat or minimally elevated
Occult: fibrovascular PED	Hyperfluorescence at 1–2 min; often stippled	Variable	Late staining or leakage	Irregular elevation of RPE
Occult: late leakage of undetermined source	Late hyperfluorescence at 2–5 min; often speckled	Poorly defined	No visible source of leakage	Flat

(CNV: Choroidal neovascularization; PED: Pigment epithelial detachment; RPE: Retinal pigment epithelium)

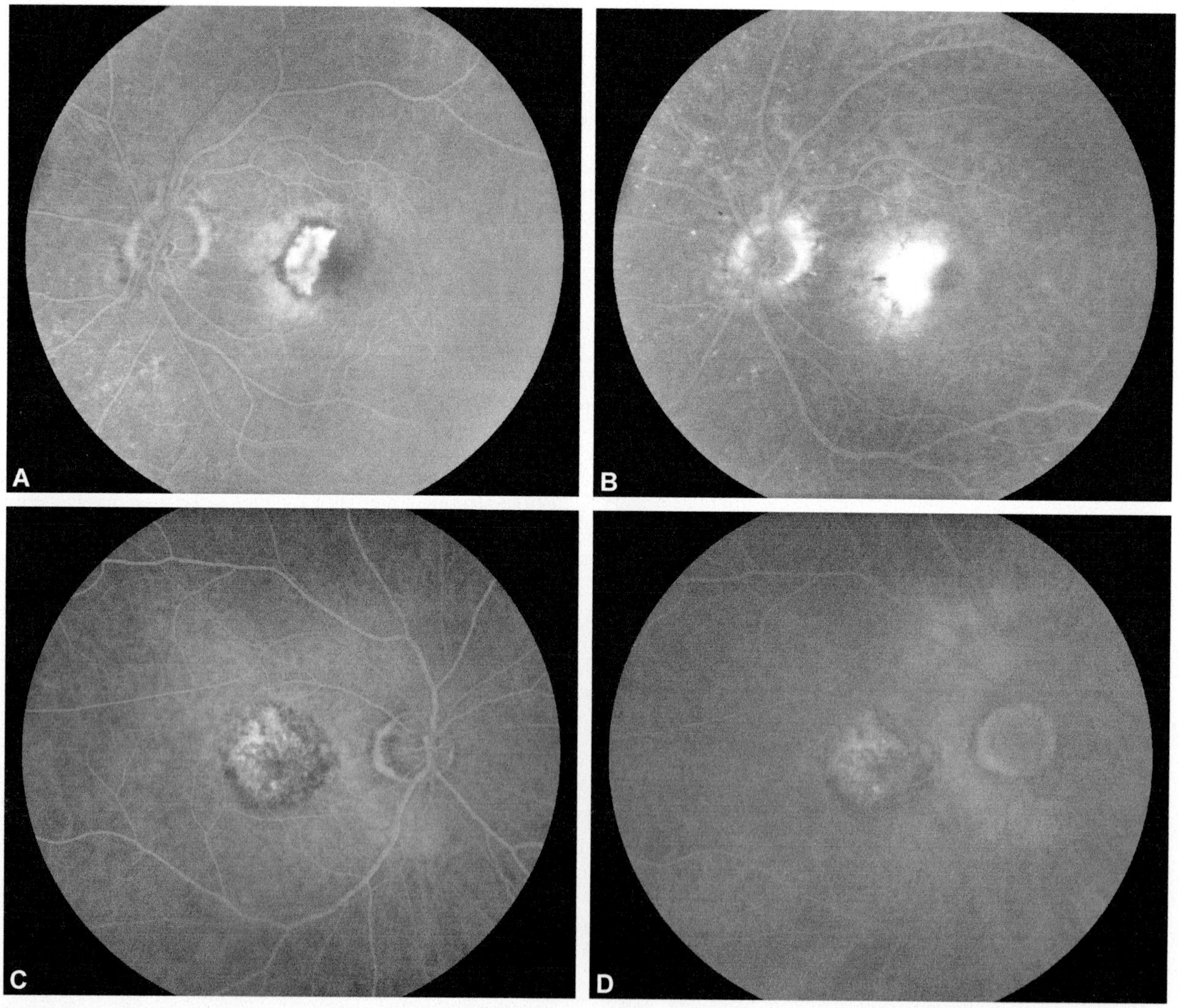

Figs. 50.7A to D: Fundus fluorescein angiography in neovascular age-related macular degeneration: classic choroidal neovscular membrane in (A) early and (B) late phases of the angiogram; occult choroidal neovascular membrane (fibrovascular pigment epithelial detachment) in (C) early and (D) late phases of the angiogram. With the classic membrane, the angiogram reveals early intense lacy hyperfluorescence and lesion borders that are initially well-defined (A), followed by progressive leakage (B). With the occult membrane, the angiogram demonstrates stippled hyperfluorescence at 1 minute and moderately well-defined borders (C), followed by late leakage and staining (D).

and/or OCT angiography (Fig. 50.8) may also be used as complementary imaging modalities. The traditional division of CNV into classic and occult subtypes arose through FFA classification in the Macular Photocoagulation Study.[40] An occult CNV membrane is located in the sub-RPE space, while a classic CNV membrane is present in the subretinal space (i.e. between RPE and retina) (Figs. 50.7A to D). Mixed lesions are frequently found, where CNV is present in both spaces. Retinal angiomatous proliferation represents a distinct subset of CNV lesions; these are characterized in their late stages by anastomosis between proliferating intraretinal capillaries and subretinal CNV.[41] Another important relative of neovascular AMD is polypoidal choroidal vasculopathy (PCV). This condition is more prevalent in Asian and African-American than Caucasian populations and typically has a younger age of onset. Clinical features of this partially distinct AMD phenotype have been reviewed;[42] these comprise polypoidal lesions of the choroidal vasculature (as demonstrated on ICG angiography; Figs. 50.9A and B), typically affecting the extramacular area and often leading to serous and hemorrhagic detachment of the RPE and retina.

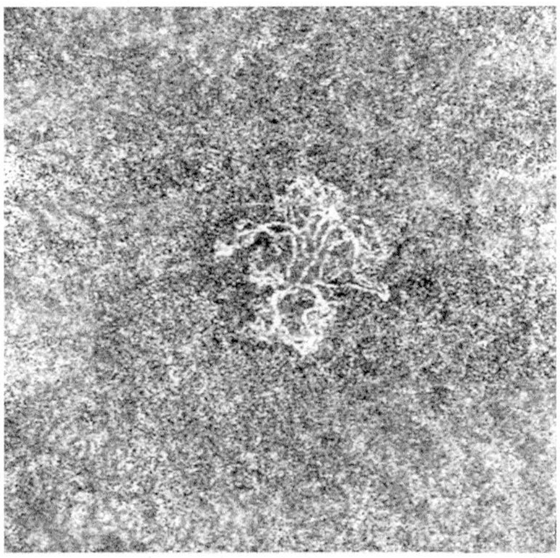

Fig. 50.8: Optical coherence tomography angiography in neovascular age-related macular degeneration: choroidal neovascular membrane visualized without contrast dye injection.

Indocyanine green angiography can be useful alongside FFA in the diagnosis and classification of neovascular AMD. In particular, it allows for imaging of the choroidal circulation and associated pathology, as the near-infrared light emitted is better able to penetrate pigment and blood. In clinical practice, ICG angiography is recommended alongside FFA in AMD for several indications—the identification of PCV, of occult CNV (particularly with a significant vascularized pigmented epithelial detachment), and of recurrent CNV,[43] though clinical practice varies by country and setting.[44]

Optical coherence tomography angiography is a more recent addition to the list of imaging tools in the diagnosis and characterization of neovascular AMD (Fig. 50.8).[45] It uses the principle of motion contrast to visualize retinal vasculature without use of a contrast agent. Although OCT angiography is prone to multiple forms of artifact,[46] a major advantage is the ability to perform noninvasive vascular imaging that is depth-resolved and includes the choroidal circulation. Its clinical use in neovascular AMD is increasing rapidly, though it is recommended as a complementary modality alongside conventional angiography.

One important note is that individuals with presumed intermediate AMD may in some cases have undiagnosed

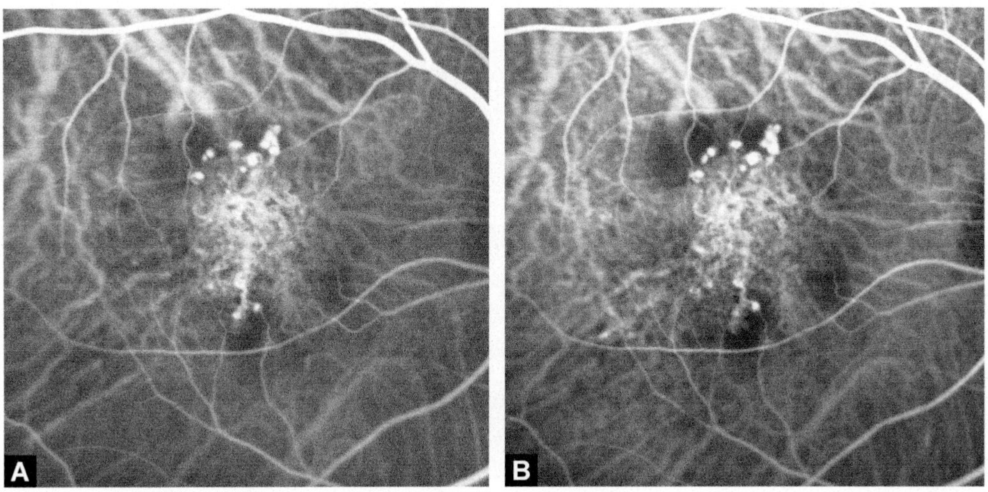

Figs. 50.9A and B: Indocyanine green angiography of polypoidal choroidal vasculopathy: (A) Early; and (B) late frames. Polypoidal vascular abnormalities are observed as multiple hypercyanescent lesions connected by a branching vascular network arising from the choroidal circulation.

neovascular disease, particularly where occult CNV lesions are nonexudative or minimally exudative. In the scenario where the normal clinical and OCT signs of neovascular disease (such as retinal hemorrhage and sub- or intraretinal fluid) have been absent or minimal, FFA is rarely performed so CNV is unlikely to be diagnosed. This phenomenon has been demonstrated recently using frequent OCT angiography on patients with presumed intermediate AMD, with evidence of occult and minimally exudative CNV membranes corroborated by ICG angiography.[47] The natural history and potential response of these lesions to anti-vascular endothelial growth factor (VEGF) therapy is not well-understood.

Atrophic Age-related Macular Degeneration

The definitive lesion in the atrophic form of late AMD is geographic atrophy (Figs. 50.10A to C).[48,49] Gass used this description to refer to one or more circumscribed areas of atrophy in the macula that may gradually enlarge and coalesce.[50] The term relates to confluent loss of the RPE under the retina, usually with a sharply demarcated border between depigmented and apparently normal retina, though the RPE atrophy is usually accompanied by degeneration of the outer retina and choriocapillaris in a similar area (Figs. 50.10A to C).[51]

Geographic atrophy in AMD is thought to affect over 8 million people worldwide.[3] Importantly, unlike the situation for neovascular AMD, no drug therapies are currently available clinically to treat or slow down visual loss from geographic atrophy. It is also important to note that geographic atrophy may arise from other retinal conditions such as inherited retinal dystrophies (e.g. Stargardt disease and maternally inherited diabetes and deafness).

Geographic atrophy usually begins in the parafoveal region and often takes several years to involve the central fovea, though around 15–20% of cases have foveal involvement from the outset.[49] Vision is severely limited in areas of the retina affected by geographic atrophy, such that dense scotomata may be observed in the corresponding visual field. If the fovea is affected by atrophy (so-called central geographic atrophy), visual acuity is likely to be very poor. In the Beaver Dam Eye Study, for example, 42% of participants with geographic atrophy were categorized as blind (i.e. with visual acuity worse than 20/200 in

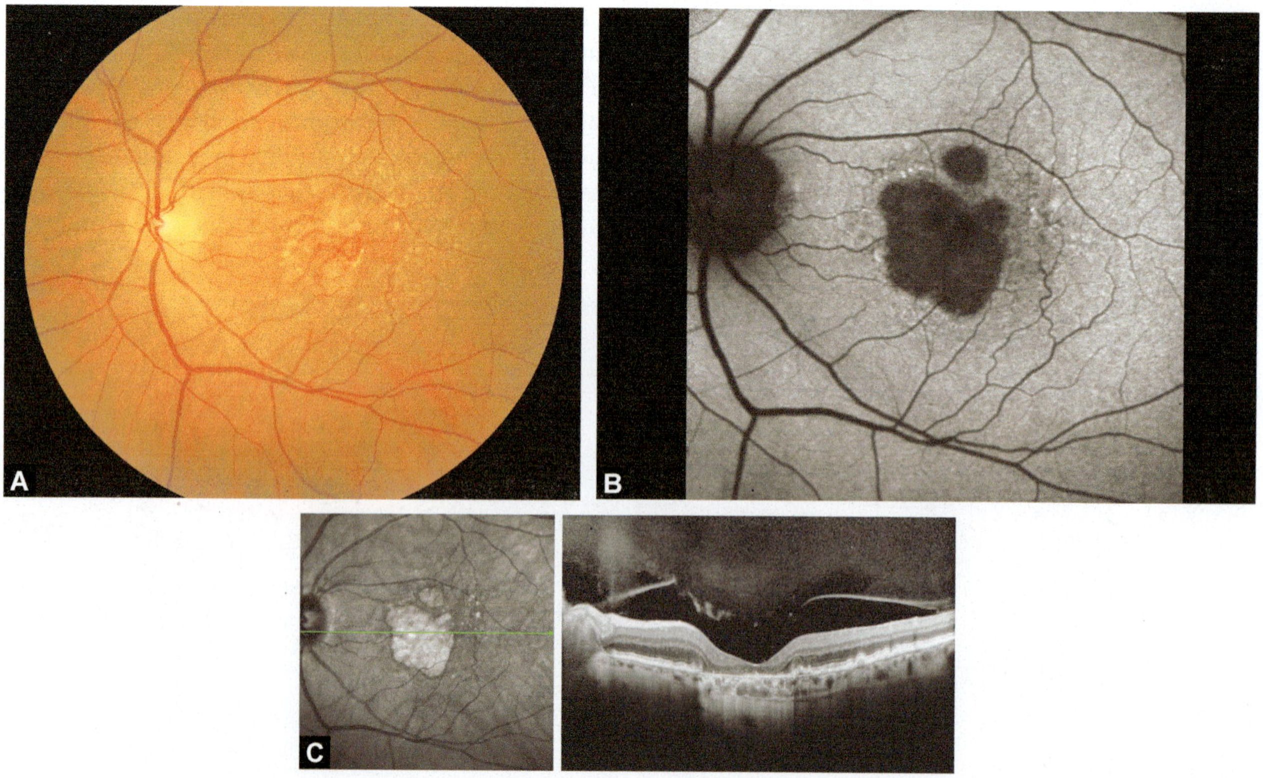

Figs. 50.10A to C: Geographic atrophy: (A) Color fundus photograph; (B) Fundus autofluorescence; (C) Optical coherence tomography scan with accompanying infrared reflectance image. The large central atrophic lesion is accompanied superiorly by a small satellite lesion. Soft drusen are observed temporal to the atrophy.

the worse eye.[52] Even in individuals where geographic atrophy is noncentral, vision is usually highly impaired in the performance of tasks such as reading and facial recognition.[53]

A common clinical definition for geographic atrophy in AMD from the AREDS is a discrete area of retinal depigmentation more than or equal to 175 μm in diameter, with a sharp border and visible choroidal vessels, in the absence of neovascular changes in the same eye (Figs. 50.10A to C).[21] However, different studies have employed varying minimum size requirements in the definition of geographic atrophy, such as 433 μm diameter on color fundus photography in AREDS2.[54] Different imaging modalities also introduce complexity to the definition of geographic atrophy, as discussed below. In addition, it is important to note that some authors [particularly in the Comparison of Age-related macular degeneration Treatments Trial (CATT)] use the term to include atrophic lesions with current or prior neovascular disease in the same eye.[55] A review of conflicting definitions of geographic atrophy has recently been presented, together with historical perspectives.[56]

Traditionally, color fundus photography has been used as the main technique for identifying geographic atrophy (Figs. 50.10A to C), with planimetry of color photographs used to measure atrophic areas and quantify growth over time. More recently, fundus autofluorescence, OCT, and near-infrared imaging have provided additional imaging modalities to identify atrophy and measure progression rates. Imaging characteristics on fundus autofluorescence and OCT have been reviewed.[49,57] Fundus autofluorescence demonstrates a markedly reduced signal in the area of atrophy (Figs. 50.10A to C); patterns of hyperautofluorescence surrounding the atrophic lesion (e.g. banded or diffuse-trickling) have also been used to characterize lesions and help predict growth rates.[58] OCT features include choroidal signal enhancement, thinning of the outer nuclear layer, and loss of the ellipsoid zone and external limiting membrane lines (Figs. 50.10A to C). Early OCT features of so-called "nascent geographic atrophy" have been identified and are thought to predict progression to atrophy.[59]

RISK FACTORS FOR AGE-RELATED MACULAR DEGENERATION

In addition to increased age, susceptibility to AMD can be considered through a combination of genetic and environmental factors.

Increased Age

Age-related macular degeneration is very strongly associated with increased age. Early data from both the Beaver Dam Eye Study[10] and the Blue Mountains Eye Study[16] clearly demonstrated increased prevalence rates according to age. Since then, further studies have demonstrated by meta-analysis that the prevalence of AMD increases exponentially with age (odds ratio 4.2 per decade): in populations of European ancestry, the prevalence of late AMD is reported at 1.4% at 70 years of age, rising to 5.6% at age 80 and 20% at age 90.[3] Analyzed separately, the prevalence of atrophic and neovascular AMD are reported to increase with age: from 0.7% for both at 70 years, to 2.9% and 2.8% at 80 years and to 11.3% and 10.5% at 90 years, respectively.

Genetic Risk Factors for Age-related Macular Degeneration

Early evidence for strong genetic involvement in AMD came from epidemiological reports including sibling and twin studies.[60,61] However, the past decade has seen substantial progress in our understanding of AMD genetics through linkage studies, followed more recently by genome-wide association studies (GWAS). In 2005, a breakthrough occurred when several groups reported a strong association between late AMD and variants at the *complement factor H* (*CFH*) locus on chromosome 1q.[62-65] This was followed closely by the report of an association between late AMD and variants in two tightly linked genes on chromosome 10q26, (*ARMS2/HTRA1*), i.e. *age-related maculopathy susceptibility 2* and *high temperature requirement factor A1* genes.[66,67] Multiple GWAS subsequently expanded the list of genetic variants associated with AMD. The largest GWAS of late AMD to date was achieved through the International AMD Genomics Consortium (IAMDGC). This collaboration analyzed data from 16,000 patients and 18,000 control individuals to identify 52 independently associated genetic variants across 34 loci (Table 50.3).[68]

Hence, in all relevant GWAS, strong associations have consistently been demonstrated with haplotypes at the two major loci mentioned above:

1. Variants associated with genes on chromosome 1 that encode regulators of the complement system, specifically *CFH* and *CFHR1-5*.
2. Variants associated with two tightly linked genes on chromosome 10q26 (*ARMS2/HTRA1*).

Table 50.3: Genome-wide association study of late age-related macular degeneration (AMD) by the International AMD Genomics Consortium. This genome-wide single-variant association analysis identified 34 loci for advanced AMD with genome-wide significance ($p < 5 \times 10^{-8}$) on the basis of logistic regression in 16,144 cases and 17,832 controls of European ancestry. Shown for each locus are the *p* value and effect size (odds ratio) for the variant with the smallest *p* value (lead variant) and the number of independent signals at the locus.

Lead variant	Chr	Position[a]	Major/minor allele	Locus name[b]	Number of signals[c]	MAF		Association	
						Cases	Controls	OR	P
Known (previously reported with genome-wide significance, $p < 5 \times 10^{-8}$)									
rs10922109	1	196,704,632	C/A	*CFH*	8	0.223	0.426	0.38	9.6×10^{-618}
rs62247658	3	64,715,155	T/C	*ADAMTS9-AS2*	1	0.466	0.433	1.14	1.8×10^{-14}
rs140647181	3	99,180,668	T/C	*COL8A1*	2	0.023	0.016	1.59	1.4×10^{-11}
rs10033900	4	110,659,067	C/T	*CFI*	2	0.511	0.477	1.15	5.4×10^{-17}
rs62358361	5	39,327,888	G/T	*C9*	1	0.016	0.009	1.80	1.3×10^{-14}
rs116503776	6	31,930,462	G/A	*C2-CFB-SKIV2L*	4	0.090	0.148	0.57	1.2×10^{-103}
rs943080	6	43,826,627	T/C	*VEGFA*	1	0.465	0.497	0.88	1.1×10^{-14}
rs79037040	8	23,082,971	T/G	*TNFRSF10A*	1	0.451	0.479	0.90	4.5×10^{-11}
rs1626340	9	101,923,372	G/A	*TGFBR1*	1	0.189	0.209	0.88	3.8×10^{-10}
rs3750846	10	124,215,565	T/C	*ARMS2-HTRA1*	1	0.436	0.208	2.81	6.5×10^{-735}
rs9564692	13	31,821,240	C/T	*B3GALTL*	1	0.277	0.299	0.89	3.3×10^{-10}
rs61985136	14	68,769,199	T/C	*RAD51B*	2	0.360	0.384	0.90	1.6×10^{-10}
rs2043085	15	58,680,954	T/C	*LIPC*	2	0.350	0.381	0.87	4.3×10^{-15}
rs5817082	16	56,997,349	C/CA	*CETP*	2	0.232	0.264	0.84	3.6×10^{-19}
rs2230199	19	6,718,387	C/G	*C3*	3	0.266	0.208	1.43	3.8×10^{-69}
rs429358	19	45,411,941	T/C	*APOE*	2	0.099	0.135	0.70	2.4×10^{-42}
rs5754227	22	33,105,817	T/C	*SYN3-TIMP3*	1	0.109	0.137	0.77	1.1×10^{-24}
rs8135665	22	38,476,276	C/T	*SLC16A8*	1	0.217	0.195	1.14	5.5×10^{-11}
New (reported with genome-wide significance, $p < 5 \times 10^{-8}$, for the first time)									
rs11884770	2	228,086,920	C/T	*COL4A3*	1	0.258	0.278	0.90	2.9×10^{-8}
rs114092250	5	35,494,448	G/A	*PRLR-SPEF2*	1	0.016	0.022	0.70	2.1×10^{-8}
rs7803454	7	99,991,548	C/T	*PILRB-PILRA*	1	0.209	0.190	1.13	4.8×10^{-9}
rs1142	7	104,756,326	C/T	*KMT2E-SRPK2*	1	0.370	0.346	1.11	1.4×10^{-9}
rs71507014	9	73,438,605	GC/G	*TRPM3*	1	0.427	0.405	1.10	3.0×10^{-8}
rs10781182	9	76,617,720	G/T	*MIR6130-RORB*	1	0.328	0.306	1.11	2.6×10^{-9}
rs2740488	9	107,661,742	A/C	*ABCA1*	1	0.255	0.275	0.90	1.2×10^{-8}
rs12357257	10	24,999,593	G/A	*ARHGAP21*	1	0.243	0.223	1.11	4.4×10^{-8}
rs3138141	12	56,115,778	C/A	*RDH5-CD63*	1	0.222	0.207	1.16	4.3×10^{-9}
rs61941274	12	112,132,610	G/A	*ACAD10*	1	0.024	0.018	1.51	1.1×10^{-9}
rs72802342	16	75,234,872	C/A	*CTRB2-CTRB1*	1	0.067	0.080	0.79	5.0×10^{-12}
rs11080055	17	26,649,724	C/A	*TMEM97-VTN*	1	0.463	0.486	0.91	1.0×10^{-8}
rs6565597	17	79,526,821	C/T	*NPLOC4-TSPAN10*	1	0.400	0.381	1.13	1.5×10^{-11}
rs67538026	19	1,031,438	C/T	*CNN2*	1	0.460	0.498	0.90	2.6×10^{-8}
rs142450006	20	44,614,991	TTTTC/T	*MMP9*	1	0.124	0.141	0.85	2.4×10^{-10}
rs201459901	20	56,653,724	T/TA	*C20orf85*	1	0.054	0.070	0.76	3.1×10^{-16}

[a]Chromosomal position is given according to the NCBI RefSeq hg19 human genome reference assembly.
[b]The locus name is a label of the region using the nearest gene(s) but does not necessarily state the responsible gene.
[c]Number of independently associated variants in this locus.
(Chr: Chromosome; MAF: Minor allele frequency; OR: Odds ratio)

Source: Reprinted with permission from Macmillan Publishers Ltd. Fritsche LG, Igl W, Bailey JN, et al. A large genome-wide association study of age-related macular degeneration highlights contributions of rare and common variants. Nat Genet. 2016;48:134-43.

Complement Factor H and Complement Factor H Related Proteins

The association between haplotypes at loci encompassing *CFH* and *CFHR1-5* has been consistently observed in multiple studies of European-descended populations in different countries, including recent GWAS.[68-73] The haplotype structure of this genetic region (whereby some of the polymorphisms tend to be inherited in combination) has made it difficult to ascertain with certainty which particular variants are linked most closely with risk of late AMD. However, the Y402H polymorphism in *CFH* has received much attention as a potential pathogenic variant. The frequency of the 402H allele in European-descended populations has been estimated by meta-analysis at 30%, with an odds ratio per 402H allele of 1.9 for any AMD and 2.3 for late AMD.[74] Other common and rare polymorphisms within and nearby the *CFH/CFHR1-5* genes are associated with altered risk of AMD, including the well-characterized haplotype with deletion of *CFHR3/1* associated strongly with protection against late AMD.[75]

Age-related Maculopathy Susceptibility 2 and High Temperature Requirement Factor A1 Genes

Similarly, strong associations with AMD have consistently been demonstrated with variants related to two tightly linked genes on chromosome 10q26: the *ARMS2/HTRA1* locus. These associations have been supported in multiple GWAS. The minor allele frequency of the relevant variants has been estimated by meta-analysis at around 30% (though significantly higher in Asian than Caucasian populations).[76] In the recent IAMDGC GWAS, the minor allele at rs3750846 in *ARMS2* was associated with an odds ratio of 2.8 per allele for late AMD.[68] However, because the variants in *ARMS2* and *HTRA1* are in almost perfect linkage disequilibrium, it has been very difficult to determine which gene carries the disease susceptibility. Controversy surrounding this area has previously been reviewed,[77] including discussion of exonic versus intronic variants, reports of RNA and protein localization, and potential functions of proteins.

Other Genes Related to the Complement System

Even before the discovery of the link between *CFH* genotype and AMD risk, biochemical studies of human macular tissue had already provided evidence that complement dysregulation was likely to be implicated in AMD pathogenesis.[23,78] However, further evidence came from the discovery that variants in multiple other genes in the complement pathway were associated with increased or decreased risk of AMD. Following previous reports, the IAMDGC GWAS also found that variants in *CFI, C9, C2/CFB,* and *C3* were strongly associated with altered risk.[68]

Genes Involved in Other Biological Pathways

Variants in genes other than *ARMS2/HTRA1* and those related to the complement system have been linked with AMD risk in recent GWAS. In particular, variants related to genes involved in several distinct biological pathways have been implicated: lipid transport (e.g. *LIPC*), extracellular matrix remodeling (e.g. *TIMP3*), angiogenesis (e.g. *VEGFA*), and cell survival (e.g. *RAD51B*).[60,68] Common and rare variants in the genes involved in these pathways may provide important insights into disease pathogenesis. However, it is important to emphasize that, compared to the influence of variants in *CFH/CFHR1*-5 and *ARMS2/HTRA1*, the effect exerted by each of these genes appears relatively small.

Further Considerations

Several lines of evidence have suggested particular genotype–phenotype associations in AMD. The IAMDGC GWAS found that the risk variant at *ARMS2/HTRA1* was preferentially associated with neovascular AMD.[68] Similarly, recent evidence from AREDS and AREDS2 has demonstrated that risk variants at *CFH* were strongly associated with macular drusen, whereas those at *ARMS2/HTRA1* were preferentially linked to neovascular AMD (particularly hemorrhagic CNV) (van Asten F, Simmons M, Singhal A, et al. A Deep Phenotype Association Study Reveals Specific Phenotype Associations with Genetic Variants in Age-related Macular Degeneration: Age-related Eye Disease Study 2 (AREDS2) Report No. 14. Ophthalmol. 2018;125:559-68). This might also help explain some important geo-epidemiological differences in the prevalence and characteristics of AMD,[60,79] whereby Caucasian populations are found to have higher prevalence of macular drusen and Asian populations to have higher prevalence of neovascular AMD (including polypoidal disease). This has led some researchers to suggest that AMD may consist of at least two partially distinct entities:[80,81] one caused by genetic variants in chromosome 1, where disease is driven predominantly by the complement system; and another caused by variants in chromosome 10, where individuals are more susceptible to neovascular disease.

Similarly, ongoing research suggests that variants in some genes more than others may be associated with incident disease versus progression from early to late AMD.[60] In this context, the *ARMS2/HTRA1* genotype seems more powerful than the *CFH/CFHR* genotype in influencing progression from early or intermediate to late disease.[82] Finally, considerable interest has arisen in potential genetic influences on response to treatment.

In summary, haplotypes containing variants in the *CFH* and *CFHR* genes, together with variants at the *ARMS2/HTRA1* locus, are a defining feature of genetic susceptibility to AMD, though genetic variants at multiple other loci involved in several biological pathways also contribute to risk. This has led to the development of AMD risk calculators, where various combinations of demographic information, environmental factors, and genotype data are combined to produce predictions of incident and progressive disease.[61]

Environmental Risk Factors for AMD

Susceptibility to AMD arises through a complex interplay between genetics, aging, and other environmental factors.[60] Many potential environmental risk factors have been examined over recent decades in the Beaver Dam Eye Study, the Blue Mountains Eye Study, and multiple other studies in different countries. Some consistent and strong risk factors have emerged, such as cigarette smoking, while results for others factors have been weaker or less consistent.

Systematic review and meta-analysis (of studies comprising 17,000 people with late AMD) have provided estimates of the association between late AMD and 16 potential risk factors.[83] Aside from family history and increased age, the environmental factors that showed strong and consistent associations with late AMD were current cigarette smoking and previous cataract surgery (Table 50.4). Risk factors that had moderate and consistent associations were higher body mass index, history of cardiovascular disease, hypertension, and higher plasma fibrinogen. The pooled estimates of these associations are listed in Table 50.4. Cigarette smoking has consistently been linked to increased risk of AMD in multiple studies in different countries.[84] As for cataract surgery, however, more recent reports have suggested that cataract surgery might not in fact be associated with incident AMD or disease progression.[85-87]

Table 50.4: Summary of pooled relative risks (for prospective studies) and odds ratios (for cross-sectional and case-control studies), by systematic review and meta-analysis: environmental factors with strong or moderate association with late age-related macular degeneration.[83]

Risk factor	Prospective	Cross-sectional	Case-control
Cigarette smoking	1.86 (1.27–2.73)	3.58 (2.68–4.79)	1.78 (1.52–2.09)
Cataract surgery	3.05 (2.05–4.55)	1.59 (1.08–2.34)	1.54 (1.24–1.91)
Body mass index (≥ 25)	1.28 (0.98–1.67)	1.21 (0.97–1.53)	1.52 (1.15–2.00)
Cardiovascular disease	1.22 (0.92–1.63)	1.12 (0.86–1.47)	2.20 (1.49–3.26)
Hypertension	1.02 (0.77–1.35)	1.15 (0.88–1.51)	1.48 (1.22–1.78)
Plasma fibrinogen (per standard deviation increase)	1.03 (0.81–1.32)	1.45 (1.22–1.73)	—

Source: Adapted with permission from BioMed Central Ltd. Chakravarthy U, Wong TY, Fletcher A, et al. Clinical risk factors for age-related macular degeneration: a systematic review and meta-analysis. BMC Ophthalmol. 2010;10:31.

The role of nutrition and diet as potentially modifiable environmental factors has received considerable interest.[88] Dietary factors that may be implicated in disease risk or protective effects include carotenoids (lutein, zeaxanthin and beta-carotene), vitamins (A – E), mineral supplements (zinc, copper and selenium), dietary fatty acids (including omega-3 fatty acids), and carbohydrates.[89] For example, dietary consumption of lutein and zeaxanthin has been linked to decreased risk of intermediate and late AMD.[90] While high total dietary fat and high glycemic index diet are known to increase risk of disease, higher consumption of omega-3 fatty acids (e.g. as found in oily fish and nuts) is suggested in some studies but not others to be linked with reduced risk of AMD.[89]

Dietary supplementation with different combinations of antioxidants, zinc, carotenoids, and fatty acids will be discussed separately below.

Further potential risk factors continue to be examined and reported, such as the role of obstructive sleep apnea in increasing risk of disease and of poor response to treatment.[91,92]

MANAGEMENT OF AMD

Management of Early AMD

No ocular or systemic drugs are known to treat early AMD, in terms of reducing the risk or speed of progression to later disease stages. In particular, there is no evidence from the

AREDS for administration of that formulation of antioxidants and minerals at the stage of early AMD. The mainstay of early AMD management is therefore patient counseling and lifestyle modification. In particular, cessation of cigarette smoking is thought to be the most important modifier of disease risk.[93] Other lifestyle and nutritional interventions have been reviewed.[94,95] Recommendations include regular physical activity, together with low glycemic index diet, low daily intake of sodium, solid fats, added sugars, cholesterol, and refined grain foods, ideally in the form of a healthy dietary pattern like the Mediterranean diet. Advice on seeking regular dilated fundus examinations is given; it may also be helpful to counsel individuals that, based on the AREDS simplified severity score, the risk of progression from early to late AMD is approximately 0.5% over 5 years.

Management of Intermediate AMD

As mentioned above, intermediate AMD represents an important stage in the evolution of AMD where the risk of progression to late disease and visual loss is significantly higher. The AREDS simplified severity score is helpful in stratifying individuals in terms of risk of progression; according to the presence of large drusen and pigmentary abnormalities in one or both eyes, this may range within the intermediate AMD category from 3% to 50% over 5 years.[30,31] Individuals with intermediate AMD are therefore likely to require more frequent and intensive monitoring, ideally using a wider range of retinal imaging, including OCT and fundus autofluorescence. In addition, recommendations include frequent monocular monitoring using an Amsler grid or newer technology such as the ForeseeHome AMD Monitoring Program,[38] where alerts or altered symptoms should prompt immediate retinal evaluation.

The mainstay of interventional treatment at the stage of intermediate AMD has been oral supplementation with a combination of antioxidants and minerals, in order to reduce the risk of progression to late AMD. A commonly used formula derived from the AREDS2 is daily oral supplementation with vitamin C (500 mg), vitamin E (400 IU), zinc (either 80 mg or 25 mg), copper (2 mg), lutein (10 mg), and zeaxanthin (2 mg). Data from AREDS demonstrated approximately 25% reduction in the risk of progression from intermediate to late AMD, and in the risk of progression from unilateral to bilateral late AMD.[96,97] Hence, supplementation is also recommended for individuals with unilateral late AMD.

No strong evidence base exists for other interventional treatments in intermediate AMD. Potential treatment strategies under investigation have included laser photocoagulation of drusen. While meta-analysis of relevant studies has shown that laser treatment can cause drusen regression, this has not so far been associated with reduced risk of neovascular AMD or geographic atrophy.[98]

Management of Neovascular AMD

Neovascular AMD was for many years an untreatable condition that led almost inevitably to disciform scar formation and profound visual loss. Before the anti-VEGF era, treatment was difficult and often associated with poor visual outcomes. The results of the Macular Photocoagulation Study[99] demonstrated that, in a subset of CNV lesions, laser photocoagulation was associated with improved outcomes compared to natural history, though success was measured in terms of reduced loss of visual acuity rather than visual improvement. Importantly, lesion recurrence rates after treatment were high, and laser photocoagulation of subfoveal CNV usually led to an immediate decrease in vision.

Photodynamic therapy was introduced as a novel laser treatment in the late 1990s to help mitigate against these factors. In this modality, a photosensitizing chemical (e.g. verteporfin) is administered by intravenous injection, followed by low fluence (or 'cold') laser to the CNV lesion, leading to photoactivation of the chemical and a local treatment effect. The Treatment of Age-related macular degeneration with Photodynamic therapy (TAP) and Verteporfin in Photodynamic Therapy (VIP) studies demonstrated improved outcomes in a subset of CNV lesions versus natural history; but again, success was usually limited to stabilization of visual loss and some lesion subtypes (especially occult CNV) had poor outcomes.[100,101]

Other treatment modalities attempted before the advent of the anti-VEGF era were transpupillary thermotherapy, intravitreal steroid, radiation, and surgical excision of CNV membranes, all of which generally had poor visual outcomes and significant limitations.

A major breakthrough in the treatment of neovascular AMD occurred with the advent of anti-VEGF therapy.[102,103] For the first time, visual acuity was often improved rather than stabilized with treatment, as demonstrated in landmark clinical trials.[102,103] Another major advantage of anti-VEGF therapy has been broad efficacy across a wide range of CNV lesion subtypes (including occult, classic and mixed), though the need for repeated intravitreal drug injection (with attendant risk of endophthalmitis, intraocular hemorrhage or retinal detachment) has been a limitation. The need for prolonged treatment, together with imaging studies, has demonstrated that intravitreal anti-VEGF therapy may be effective in decreasing exudative and angiogenic activity but does not eliminate CNV membranes.

Three main anti-VEGF drugs are currently in widespread use in the world—bevacizumab (Avastin), ranibizumab (Lucentis) and, more recently, aflibercept (Eylea). Bevacizumab is a humanized murine monoclonal antibody that inhibits VEGFA, but is not approved by the United States Federal Drug Administration for intraocular use. Ranibizumab is a Fab (fragment antigen-binding) derived from the same monoclonal antibody as bevacizumab; it also inhibits VEGFA but is approved for intraocular use. In contrast, aflibercept is a protein made by the fusion of domains from VEGF receptors to a portion of IgG.[104] It thereby inhibits VEGFA, VEGFB, and placental growth factor by "trapping" these factors and preventing them from interacting with their native receptors.

Relative efficacy and associated safety data for the three anti-VEGF drugs have been examined in many studies, along with different regimens for drug dosing and monitoring response, as discussed in recent review papers.[105-107] For example, the CATT study showed non-inferiority of bevacizumab to ranibizumab in neovascular AMD,[108] while the VIEW studies demonstrated non-inferiority of aflibercept to ranibizumab, with similar safety profiles.[109, 110] The ocular and systemic safety profiles for all three drugs appear broadly similar, with an average infective endophthalmitis rate of approximately 1/3000;[111] however, some controversy exists as to whether bevacizumab may be associated with a higher rate of endophthalmitis (perhaps through drug reconstitution) and/or higher systemic risk profile (through longer systemic half-life).

Dosing regimens have been another area of intense interest in recent years. Three main strategies have been adopted: 1. fixed dosing, e.g. at monthly intervals, 2. pro re nata (PRN) dosing, usually comprising fixed monthly assessments, including OCT, with treatment decisions made at each visit, 3. "treat and extend" dosing, where treatment is given at every visit but the interval between visits may be extended or contracted depending on markers of disease activity. It is also worth noting that aflibercept is approved for fixed dosing every 2 months (following three once-monthly injections). The relative merits and disadvantages of these dosing regimens have been analyzed and reviewed.[105,112,113] This includes the observation from both CATT and Inhibit VEGF in Age-related choroidal neovascularization (IVAN) trials that fixed monthly dosing (of ranibizumab and bevacizumab) was associated with slightly improved visual outcomes compared to PRN treatment.[108,114] Others have argued that higher levels of VEGF inhibition may be associated with increased tendency to geographic atrophy.[115]

Despite the great success of anti-VEGF therapy, the substantial burden of monthly visits and repeated intravitral injections on patients and physicians has created interest in new potential treatments and delivery systems. Novel therapies at the clinical trial stage or in development have been reviewed.[105] These include novel delivery systems for anti-VEGF drugs (such as extended-release implants and cell encapsulation devices), novel anti-VEGF agents [such as brolucizumab and designed Ankyrin repeat proteins (DARPins)], anti-platelet-derived growth factor (PDGF) drugs (such as Fovista, recently trialed in combination with anti-VEGF therapy), tyrosine kinase inhibitors (e.g. topical Pazopanib), radiation (including epimacular brachytherapy in combination with anti-VEGF therapy), as well as gene therapy approaches (e.g. RetinoStat delivery of endostatin and angiostatin). In the context of combination treatment, it is worth noting that the most commonly used combination therapy in current practice is photodynamic therapy alongside anti-VEGF therapy in the treatment of PCV.[42]

Management of Atrophic AMD

No evidence-based treatments are currently available for routine clinical use in atrophic AMD. This area therefore represents an important priority in AMD research. Patients are often recommended to adopt the same lifestyle modifications as above, and many continue to take oral AREDS2 supplements; but there is no specific evidence for the role of antioxidant or mineral supplementation in decreasing the growth rate of geographic atrophy.

Clinical trials and investigational therapies for geographic atrophy are underway and have been reviewed.[49,116] One major direction has been an attempt to target the complement pathway, given strong genetic and biochemical evidence of its implication in AMD pathology. The MAHALO phase IB/II trial of lampalizumab (a humanized anti-complement factor D antibody) reported a 20% reduction in geographic atrophy growth rates at 18 months with monthly intravitreal injection, leading to initiation of the phase III studies CHROMA and SPECTRI currently underway. Multiple other drugs targeting the complement system and inflammation are at different stages of development. Other approaches have included targeting the visual cycle (using e.g. fenretinide, a synthetic vitamin A derivative thought to decrease lipofuscin and A2E accumulation, and emixustat, which inhibits the RPE65 enzyme), neuroprotection (using e.g. intravitreal CNTF implants or antioxidants such as OT-551), modulation of amyloid, and cell replacement therapy (using stem cell technology).

Visual Rehabilitation

Finally, visual rehabilitation remains an important therapy for all patients with visual loss,[117] along with liaison with appropriate social services. Low visual aid assessment by specialized optometrists or ophthalmologists is useful in conjunction with optical aids (magnifiers, telescopes and electronic devices). Implantable miniature telescopes have been used in some cases.[118] Retinal prostheses have also been used in some individuals with profound visual loss, including a small number of individuals with AMD.[119] Other important considerations include searching for comorbid conditions alongside AMD, particularly hearing loss, cognitive impairment, and depression. Finally, patients with visual loss may develop visual hallucinations, in the form of Charles-Bonnet syndrome,[120] and should be counseled regarding the benign nature of these experiences.

CONCLUSION

Age-related macular degeneration is a common blinding disease whose frequency continues to increase with the aging population. It arises from a complex interplay of aging, environmental, and genetic factors. Large advances in our understanding of AMD genetics have yet to be followed by a full understanding of biological disease mechanisms. The treatment of neovascular AMD has been revolutionized by the advent of anti-VEGF therapy, though the development of additional drugs and delivery systems may improve outcomes further and reduce the burden of repeated intravitreal administration. The absence of effective treatments for atrophic AMD represents a large clinical problem and research priority. In particular, future treatments should ideally be targeted against the underlying disease process, perhaps even personalized by AMD genotype; visual outcomes would be improved if this were possible at an earlier stage of disease progression, before the onset of irreversible structural damage and visual decline.

REFERENCES

1. Wong WL, Su X, Li X, et al. Global prevalence of age-related macular degeneration and disease burden projection for 2020 and 2040: a systematic review and meta-analysis. Lancet Glob Health. 2014;2:e106-16.
2. Congdon N, O'Colmain B, Klaver CC, et al. Causes and prevalence of visual impairment among adults in the United States. Arch Ophthalmol. 2004;122:477-85.
3. Rudnicka AR, Jarrar Z, Wormald R, et al. Age and gender variations in age-related macular degeneration prevalence in populations of European ancestry: a meta-analysis. Ophthalmology. 2012;119:571-80.
4. Ratnapriya R, Chew EY. Age-related macular degeneration-clinical review and genetics update. Clin Genet. 2013;84: 160-6.
5. Cimarolli VR, Casten RJ, Rovner BW, et al. Anxiety and depression in patients with advanced macular degeneration: current perspectives. Clin Ophthalmol. 2016;10:55-63.
6. Coleman AL, Yu F, Ensrud KE, et al. Impact of age-related macular degeneration on vision-specific quality of life: Follow-up from the 10-year and 15-year visits of the study of osteoporotic fractures. Am J Ophthalmol. 2010;150: 683-91.
7. Bonastre J, Le Pen C, Anderson P, et al. The epidemiology, economics and quality of life burden of age-related macular degeneration in France, Germany, Italy and the United Kingdom. Eur J Health Econ. 2002;3:94-102.
8. Casten RJ, Rovner BW. Update on depression and age-related macular degeneration. Curr Opin Ophthalmol. 2013;24:239-43.
9. Klein R, Davis MD, Magli YL, et al. The Wisconsin age-related maculopathy grading system. Ophthalmology. 1991;98:1128-34.
10. Klein R, Klein BE, Linton KL. Prevalence of age-related maculopathy. The Beaver Dam Eye Study. Ophthalmology. 1992;99:933-43.
11. Klein R, Klein BE, Jensen SC, et al. The five-year incidence and progression of age-related maculopathy: the Beaver Dam Eye Study. Ophthalmology. 1997;104:7-21.
12. Heiba IM, Elston RC, Klein BE, et al. Sibling correlations and segregation analysis of age-related maculopathy: the Beaver Dam Eye Study. Genet Epidemiol. 1994;11:51-67.
13. Klein R, Klein BE, Linton KL, et al. The Beaver Dam Eye Study: the relation of age-related maculopathy to smoking. Am J Epidemiol. 1993;137:190-200.
14. Cruickshanks KJ, Klein R, Klein BE. Sunlight and age-related macular degeneration. The Beaver Dam Eye Study. Arch Ophthalmol. 1993;111:514-8.
15. Klein R, Klein BE, Franke T. The relationship of cardiovascular disease and its risk factors to age-related maculopathy. The Beaver Dam Eye Study. Ophthalmology. 1993;100:406-14.
16. Mitchell P, Smith W, Attebo K, et al. Prevalence of age-related maculopathy in Australia. The Blue Mountains Eye Study. Ophthalmology. 1995;102:1450-60.
17. Wang JJ, Foran S, Smith W, et al. Risk of age-related macular degeneration in eyes with macular drusen or

hyperpigmentation: the Blue Mountains Eye Study cohort. Arch Ophthalmol. 2003;121:658-63.
18. Smith W, Mitchell P, Leeder SR. Smoking and age-related maculopathy. The Blue Mountains Eye Study. Arch Ophthalmol. 1996;114:1518-23.
19. Smith W, Mitchell P, Leeder SR, et al. Plasma fibrinogen levels, other cardiovascular risk factors, and age-related maculopathy: the Blue Mountains Eye Study. Arch Ophthalmol. 1998;116:583-7.
20. Smith W, Mitchell P. Family history and age-related maculopathy: the Blue Mountains Eye Study. Aust N Z J Ophthalmol. 1998;26:203-6.
21. Age-Related Eye Disease Study Research Group. The Age-Related Eye Disease Study system for classifying age-related macular degeneration from stereoscopic color fundus photographs: the Age-Related Eye Disease Study Report Number 6. Am J Ophthalmol. 2001;132:668-81.
22. Ferris FL 3rd, Wilkinson CP, Bird A, et al. Clinical classification of age-related macular degeneration. Ophthalmology. 2013;120:844-51.
23. Hageman GS, Luthert PJ, Victor Chong NH, et al. An integrated hypothesis that considers drusen as biomarkers of immune-mediated processes at the RPE-Bruch's membrane interface in aging and age-related macular degeneration. Prog Retin Eye Res. 2001;20:705-32.
24. Anderson DH, Mullins RF, Hageman GS, et al. A role for local inflammation in the formation of drusen in the aging eye. Am J Ophthalmol. 2002;134:411-31.
25. Anderson DH, Radeke MJ, Gallo NB, et al. The pivotal role of the complement system in aging and age-related macular degeneration: hypothesis re-visited. Prog Retin Eye Res. 2010;29:95-112.
26. Khan KN, Mahroo OA, Khan RS, et al. Differentiating drusen: Drusen and drusen-like appearances associated with aging, age-related macular degeneration, inherited eye disease and other pathological processes. Prog Retin Eye Res. 2016;53:70-106.
27. Mimoun G, Soubrane G, Coscas G. Macular drusen [in French]. J Fr Ophtalmol. 1990;13:511-30.
28. Sivaprasad S, Bird A, Nitiahpapand R, et al. Perspectives on reticular pseudodrusen in age-related macular degeneration. Surv Ophthalmol. 2016;61:521-37.
29. Schmidt-Erfurth U, Klimscha S, Waldstein SM, et al. A view of the current and future role of optical coherence tomography in the management of age-related macular degeneration. Eye (Lond). 2017;31:26-44.
30. Davis MD, Gangnon RE, Lee LY, et al. The Age-Related Eye Disease Study severity scale for age-related macular degeneration: AREDS Report No. 17. Arch Ophthalmol. 2005;123:1484-98.
31. Vitale S, Clemons TE, Agron E, et al. Evaluating the validity of the Age-Related Eye Disease Study Grading Scale for age-related macular degeneration: AREDS2 Report 10. JAMA Ophthalmol. 2016;134:1041-7.
32. Writing Committee for the OPERA Study, Domalpally A, Clemons TE, et al. Peripheral retinal changes associated with age-related macular degeneration in the Age-related Eye Disease Study 2: Age-Related Eye Disease Study 2 Report Number 12 by the Age-Related Eye Disease Study 2 Optos PEripheral RetinA (OPERA) Study Research Group. Ophthalmology. 2017;124:479-87.
33. Kaszubski P, Ben Ami T, Saade C, et al. Geographic atrophy and choroidal neovascularization in the same eye: a review. Ophthalmic Res. 2016;55:185-93.
34. Munoz B, West SK, Rubin GS, et al. Causes of blindness and visual impairment in a population of older Americans: The Salisbury Eye Evaluation Study. Arch Ophthalmol. 2000;118:819-25.
35. Vingerling JR, Dielemans I, Hofman A, et al. The prevalence of age-related maculopathy in the Rotterdam Study. Ophthalmology. 1995;102:205-10.
36. Weih LM, VanNewkirk MR, McCarty CA, et al. Age-specific causes of bilateral visual impairment. Arch Ophthalmol. 2000;118:264-9.
37. Miller JW. Age-related macular degeneration revisited--piecing the puzzle: the LXIX Edward Jackson memorial lecture. Am J Ophthalmol. 2013;155:1-35.
38. Chew EY, Clemons TE, Bressler SB, et al. Randomized trial of the ForeseeHome monitoring device for early detection of neovascular age-related macular degeneration. The HOme Monitoring of the Eye (HOME) study design - HOME Study report number 1. Contemp Clin Trials. 2014;37:294-300.
39. Schmidt-Erfurth U, Waldstein SM. A paradigm shift in imaging biomarkers in neovascular age-related macular degeneration. Prog Retin Eye Res. 2016;50:1-24.
40. Argon laser photocoagulation for senile macular degeneration. Results of a randomized clinical trial. Arch Ophthalmol. 1982;100:912-8.
41. Tsai AS, Cheung N, Gan ATL, et al. Retinal angiomatous proliferation. Surv Ophthalmol. 2017;62:462-92.
42. Koh AH, Expert PCV Panel, Chen LJ, et al. Polypoidal choroidal vasculopathy: evidence-based guidelines for clinical diagnosis and treatment. Retina. 2013;33:686-716.
43. Stanga PE, Lim JI, Hamilton P. Indocyanine green angiography in chorioretinal diseases: indications and interpretation: an evidence-based update. Ophthalmology. 2003;110:15-21.
44. Yannuzzi LA. Indocyanine green angiography: a perspective on use in the clinical setting. Am J Ophthalmol. 2011;151: 745-51.e1.
45. Gao SS, Jia Y, Zhang M, et al. Optical coherence tomography angiography. Invest Ophthalmol Vis Sci. 2016;57:OCT27-36.
46. Spaide RF, Fujimoto JG, Waheed NK. Image artifacts in optical coherence tomography angiography. Retina. 2015;35:2163-80.
47. Roisman L, Zhang Q, Wang RK, et al. Optical coherence tomography angiography of asymptomatic neovascularization in intermediate age-related macular degeneration. Ophthalmology. 2016;123:1309-19.
48. Holz FG, Strauss EC, Schmitz-Valckenberg S, et al. Geographic atrophy: clinical features and potential therapeutic approaches. Ophthalmology. 2014;121:1079-91.
49. Danis RP, Lavine JA, Domalpally A. Geographic atrophy in patients with advanced dry age-related macular

degeneration: current challenges and future prospects. Clin Ophthalmol. 2015;9:2159-74.
50. Gass JD. Drusen and disciform macular detachment and degeneration. Arch Ophthalmol. 1973;90:206-17.
51. Bird AC, Phillips RL, Hageman GS. Geographic atrophy: a histopathological assessment. JAMA Ophthalmol. 2014;132:338-45.
52. Klein R, Wang Q, Klein BE, et al. The relationship of age-related maculopathy, cataract, and glaucoma to visual acuity. Invest Ophthalmol Vis Sci. 1995;36:182-91.
53. Sunness JS. Face fields and microperimetry for estimating the location of fixation in eyes with macular disease. J Vis Impair Blind. 2008;102:679-89.
54. Danis RP, Domalpally A, Chew EY, et al. Methods and reproducibility of grading optimized digital color fundus photographs in the Age-related Eye Disease Study 2 (AREDS2 Report Number 2). Invest Ophthalmol Vis Sci. 2013;54:4548-54.
55. Grunwald JE, Pistilli M, Ying GS, et al. Growth of geographic atrophy in the comparison of age-related macular degeneration treatments trials. Ophthalmology. 2015;122:809-16.
56. Schmitz-Valckenberg S, Sadda S, Staurenghi G, et al. Geographic atrophy: semantic considerations and literature review. Retina. 2016;36:2250-64.
57. Zarbin MA, Casaroli-Marano RP, Rosenfeld PJ. Age-related macular degeneration: clinical findings, histopathology and imaging techniques. Dev Ophthalmol. 2014;53:1-32.
58. Holz FG, Bindewald-Wittich A, Fleckenstein M, et al. Progression of geographic atrophy and impact of fundus autofluorescence patterns in age-related macular degeneration. Am J Ophthalmol. 2007;143:463-72.
59. Wu Z, Luu CD, Ayton LN, et al. Optical coherence tomography-defined changes preceding the development of drusen-associated atrophy in age-related macular degeneration. Ophthalmology. 2014;121:2415-22.
60. Fritsche LG, Fariss RN, Stambolian D, et al. Age-related macular degeneration: genetics and biology coming together. Annu Rev Genomics Hum Genet. 2014;15:151-71.
61. Sobrin L, Seddon JM. Nature and nurture- genes and environment- predict onset and progression of macular degeneration. Prog Retin Eye Res. 2014;40:1-15.
62. Hageman GS, Anderson DH, Johnson LV, et al. A common haplotype in the complement regulatory gene factor H (HF1/CFH) predisposes individuals to age-related macular degeneration. Proc Natl Acad Sci U S A. 2005;102:7227-32.
63. Klein RJ, Zeiss C, Chew EY, et al. Complement factor H polymorphism in age-related macular degeneration. Science. 2005;308:385-9.
64. Haines JL, Hauser MA, Schmidt S, et al. Complement factor H variant increases the risk of age-related macular degeneration. Science. 2005;308:419-21.
65. Edwards AO, Ritter R III, Abel KJ, et al. Complement factor H polymorphism and age-related macular degeneration. Science. 2005;308:421-4.
66. Jakobsdottir J, Conley YP, Weeks DE, et al. Susceptibility genes for age-related maculopathy on chromosome 10q26. Am J Hum Genet. 2005;77:389-407.
67. Rivera A, Fisher SA, Fritsche LG, et al. Hypothetical LOC387715 is a second major susceptibility gene for age-related macular degeneration, contributing independently of complement factor H to disease risk. Hum Mol Genet. 2005;14(21):3227-36.
68. Fritsche LG, Igl W, Bailey JN, et al. A large genome-wide association study of age-related macular degeneration highlights contributions of rare and common variants. Nat Genet. 2016;48:134-43.
69. Yu Y, Bhangale TR, Fagerness J, et al. Common variants near FRK/COL10A1 and VEGFA are associated with advanced age-related macular degeneration. Hum Mol Genet. 2011;20:3699-709.
70. Chen W, Stambolian D, Edwards AO, et al. Genetic variants near TIMP3 and high-density lipoprotein-associated loci influence susceptibility to age-related macular degeneration. Proc Natl Acad Sci U S A. 2010;107:7401-6.
71. Neale BM, Fagerness J, Reynolds R, et al. Genome-wide association study of advanced age-related macular degeneration identifies a role of the hepatic lipase gene (LIPC). Proc Natl Acad Sci U S A. 2010;107:7395-400.
72. Cipriani V, Leung HT, Plagnol V, et al. Genome-wide association study of age-related macular degeneration identifies associated variants in the TNXB-FKBPL-NOTCH4 region of chromosome 6p21.3. Hum Mol Genet. 2012;21:4138-50.
73. Fritsche LG, Chen W, Schu M, et al. Seven new loci associated with age-related macular degeneration. Nat Genet. 2013;45:433-9.
74. Sofat R, Casas JP, Webster AR, et al. Complement factor H genetic variant and age-related macular degeneration: effect size, modifiers and relationship to disease subtype. Int J Epidemiol. 2012;41:250-62.
75. Schramm EC, Clark SJ, Triebwasser MP, et al. Genetic variants in the complement system predisposing to age-related macular degeneration: a review. Mol Immunol. 2014;61:118-25.
76. Tong Y, Liao J, Zhang Y, et al. LOC387715/HTRA1 gene polymorphisms and susceptibility to age-related macular degeneration: A HuGE review and meta-analysis. Mol Vis. 2010;16:1958-81.
77. Wang G. Chromosome 10q26 locus and age-related macular degeneration: a progress update. Exp Eye Res. 2014;119:1-7.
78. Mullins RF, Russell SR, Anderson DH, et al. Drusen associated with aging and age-related macular degeneration contain proteins common to extracellular deposits associated with atherosclerosis, elastosis, amyloidosis, and dense deposit disease. FASEB J. 2000;14:835-46.
79. Reibaldi M, Longo A, Pulvirenti A, et al. Geo-epidemiology of age-related macular degeneration: new clues into the pathogenesis. Am J Ophthalmol. 2016;161:78-93.

80. DeWan A, Bracken MB, Hoh J. Two genetic pathways for age-related macular degeneration. Curr Opin Genet Dev. 2007;17:228-33.
81. Sobrin L, Reynolds R, Yu Y, et al. ARMS2/HTRA1 locus can confer differential susceptibility to the advanced subtypes of age-related macular degeneration. Am J Ophthalmol. 2011;151:345-52.
82. Ding Y, Liu Y, Yan Q, et al. Bivariate analysis of age-related macular degeneration progression using genetic risk scores. Genetics. 2017;206:119-33.
83. Chakravarthy U, Wong TY, Fletcher A, et al. Clinical risk factors for age-related macular degeneration: a systematic review and meta-analysis. BMC Ophthalmol. 2010;10:31.
84. Woodell A, Rohrer B. A mechanistic review of cigarette smoke and age-related macular degeneration. Adv Exp Med Biol. 2014;801:301-7.
85. Ehmann DS, Ho AC. Cataract surgery and age-related macular degeneration. Curr Opin Ophthalmol. 2017;28:58-62.
86. Chew EY, Sperduto RD, Milton RC, et al. Risk of advanced age-related macular degeneration after cataract surgery in the Age-Related Eye Disease Study: AREDS report 25. Ophthalmology. 2009;116:297-303.
87. Hooper CY, Lamoureux EL, Lim L, et al. Cataract surgery in high-risk age-related macular degeneration: a randomized controlled trial. Clin Exp Ophthalmol. 2009;37:570-6.
88. Gorusupudi A, Nelson K, Bernstein PS. The Age-Related Eye Disease 2 Study: Micronutrients in the treatment of macular degeneration. Adv Nutr. 2017;8:40-53.
89. Zampatti S, Ricci F, Cusumano A, et al. Review of nutrient actions on age-related macular degeneration. Nutr Res. 2014;34:95-105.
90. Age-Related Eye Disease Study Research Group, SanGiovanni JP, Chew EY, et al. The relationship of dietary carotenoid and vitamin A, E, and C intake with age-related macular degeneration in a case-control study: AREDS Report No. 22. Arch Ophthalmol. 2007;125:1225-32.
91. Keenan TD, Goldacre R, Goldacre MJ. Associations between obstructive sleep apnoea, primary open angle glaucoma and age-related macular degeneration: record linkage study. Br J Ophthalmol. 2017;101:155-9.
92. Schaal S, Sherman MP, Nesmith B, et al. Untreated obstructive sleep apnea hinders response to bevacizumab in age-related macular degeneration. Retina. 2016;36:791-7.
93. Myers CE, Klein BE, Gangnon R, et al. Cigarette smoking and the natural history of age-related macular degeneration: the Beaver Dam Eye Study. Ophthalmology. 2014;121:1949-55.
94. Cheung LK, Eaton A. Age-related macular degeneration. Pharmacotherapy. 2013;33:838-55.
95. Carneiro A, Andrade JP. Nutritional and lifestyle interventions for age-related macular degeneration: a review. Oxid Med Cell Longev. 2017;2017:6469138.
96. Chew EY, Clemons TE, Agron E, et al. Long-term effects of vitamins C and E, beta-carotene, and zinc on age-related macular degeneration: AREDS report No. 35. Ophthalmology. 2013;120:1604-11.
97. Age-Related Eye Disease Study Research Group. A randomized, placebo-controlled, clinical trial of high-dose supplementation with vitamins C and E, beta carotene, and zinc for age-related macular degeneration and vision loss: AREDS report no. 8. Arch Ophthalmol. 2001;119:1417-36.
98. Virgili G, Michelessi M, Parodi MB, et al. Laser treatment of drusen to prevent progression to advanced age-related macular degeneration. Cochrane Database Syst Rev. 2015:CD006537.
99. Macular Photocoagulation Study Group. Argon laser photocoagulation for neovascular maculopathy. Five-year results from randomized clinical trials. Arch Ophthalmol. 1991;109:1109-14.
100. Bressler NM, Treatment of Age-Related Macular Degeneration with Photodynamic Therapy Study Group. Photodynamic therapy of subfoveal choroidal neovascularization in age-related macular degeneration with verteporfin: two-year results of 2 randomized clinical trials-tap report 2. Arch Ophthalmol. 2001;119:198-207.
101. Verteporfin In Photodynamic Therapy Study Group. Verteporfin therapy of subfoveal choroidal neovascularization in age-related macular degeneration: two-year results of a randomized clinical trial including lesions with occult with no classic choroidal neovascularization--verteporfin in photodynamic therapy report 2. Am J Ophthalmol. 2001;131:541-60.
102. Rosenfeld PJ, Brown DM, Heier JS, et al. Ranibizumab for neovascular age-related macular degeneration. N Engl J Med. 2006;355:1419-31.
103. Brown DM, Michels M, Kaiser PK, et al. Ranibizumab versus verteporfin photodynamic therapy for neovascular age-related macular degeneration: Two-year results of the ANCHOR study. Ophthalmology. 2009;116:57-65.e5.
104. Holash J, Davis S, Papadopoulos N, et al. VEGF-Trap: a VEGF blocker with potent antitumor effects. Proc Natl Acad Sci U S A. 2002;99:11393-8.
105. Villegas VM, Aranguren LA, Kovach JL, et al. Current advances in the treatment of neovascular age-related macular degeneration. Expert Opin Drug Deliv. 2017;14:273-82.
106. Arnold JJ. Age-related macular degeneration: anti-vascular endothelial growth factor treatment. BMJ Clin Evid. 2016;2016.pii:0701.
107. Agarwal A, Aggarwal K, Gupta V. Management of neovascular age-related macular degeneration: a review on landmark randomized controlled trials. Middle East Afr J Ophthalmol. 2016;23:27-37.
108. CATT Research Group, Martin DF, Maguire MG, et al. Ranibizumab and bevacizumab for neovascular age-related macular degeneration. N Engl J Med. 2011;364:1897-908.
109. Sarwar S, Clearfield E, Soliman MK, et al. Aflibercept for neovascular age-related macular degeneration. Cochrane Database Syst Rev. 2016;2:CD011346.
110. Heier JS, Brown DM, Chong V, et al. Intravitreal aflibercept (VEGF trap-eye) in wet age-related macular degeneration. Ophthalmology. 2012;119:2537-48.

111. Gregori NZ, Flynn HW Jr, Schwartz SG, et al. Current infectious endophthalmitis rates after intravitreal injections of anti-vascular endothelial growth factor agents and outcomes of treatment. Ophthalmic Surg Lasers Imaging Retina. 2015;46:643-8.
112. Schmidt-Erfurth U, Chong V, Loewenstein A, et al. Guidelines for the management of neovascular age-related macular degeneration by the European Society of Retina Specialists (EURETINA). Br J Ophthalmol. 2014;98:1144-67.
113. Schmucker CM, Rucker G, Sommer H, et al. Treatment as required versus regular monthly treatment in the management of neovascular age-related macular degeneration: a systematic review and meta-analysis. PLoS One. 2015;10:e0137866.
114. Chakravarthy U, Harding SP, Rogers CA, et al. Alternative treatments to inhibit VEGF in age-related choroidal neovascularisation: 2-year findings of the IVAN randomised controlled trial. Lancet. 2013;382:1258-67.
115. Miller JW. Beyond VEGF-The Weisenfeld Lecture. Invest Ophthalmol Vis Sci. 2016;57:6911-8.
116. Hanus J, Zhao F, Wang S. Current therapeutic developments in atrophic age-related macular degeneration. Br J Ophthalmol. 2016;100:122-7.
117. Hooper P, Jutai JW, Strong G, et al. Age-related macular degeneration and low-vision rehabilitation: a systematic review. Can J Ophthalmol. 2008;43:180-7.
118. Hau VS, London N, Dalton M. The treatment paradigm for the implantable miniature telescope. Ophthalmol Ther. 2016;5:21-30.
119. Humayun MS, de Juan E Jr, Dagnelie G. The bionic eye: a quarter century of retinal prosthesis research and development. Ophthalmology. 2016;123:S89-S97.
120. Pang L. Hallucinations experienced by visually impaired: Charles Bonnet syndrome. Optom Vis Sci. 2016;93:1466-78.

Chapter 51 Central Serous Chorioretinopathy and Pachychoroid Disease

Kunal K Dansingani, Orly Gal-Or, K Bailey Freund

INTRODUCTION

Central serous chorioretinopathy (CSC) is an enigmatic and poorly understood condition which continues to challenge ophthalmologists and retina specialists. It was first described in 1866 by von Graefe, who referred to it as a "relapsing central luetic retinitis."[1] Case reports and small series subsequently appeared in the literature with increasing frequency; in the 1930s, Kitahara described a large cohort of 150 cases, and Horniker performed a qualitative meta-analysis.[2] One of the earliest literature reviews was published in 1955 by Bennett, who referred to the condition as "central serous retinopathy," consolidated the understanding that the etiology was neither infectious nor inflammatory, and suggested that the choroid was the primary site of pathology.[2] This choroidal hypothesis was supported by Maumenee, who demonstrated that central serous *chorio*retinopathy was characterized by fluorescein leakage from the choroidal circulation, visualized at the level of the retinal pigment epithelium (RPE).[3,4] Developments in multimodal imaging have subsequently expanded the spectrum of clinical features recognized in CSC.

The term pachychoroid first appeared in the literature in 2013 as a descriptor for the pachymetric and morphological choroidal features of CSC that were recognized in a broader set of conditions subsequently referred to as pachychoroid disorders. Since then, evidence has shown that the choroidal characteristics defining pachychoroid are likely to represent hemodynamic features that constitute a disease *mechanism*.

The aim of this chapter is to present a pragmatic approach for ophthalmic clinicians to understand the diagnostic features of CSC and pachychoroid disease and to plan and effect treatment, using multimodal imaging to illustrate pathogenesis and treatment response.

CENTRAL SEROUS CHORIORETINOPATHY

Central serous chorioretinopathy is characterized by the appearance of serous neurosensory detachments with or without serous pigment epithelial detachments at the posterior pole in the absence of inflammation or neoplasia.

Most cases are episodic and self-limited but a subset of patients can experience a chronic clinical course featuring cumulative and more widespread damage to the RPE and outer retina, and sequelae such as macular neovascularization and atrophy.

The biggest epidemiologic population based study in the United States documented cases of CSC from 1980–2002 and reported an incidence of 9.9 per 100,000 in men and 1.7 per 100,000 in women, with a male-to-female ratio of approximately 6 to 1.[5] A subsequent study reported a significantly different male-to-female ratio of 2.6 to 1.[6] The age range at diagnosis ranged from 22.2 years to 82.9 years, with a mean age of 49.8 years.

Acute Central Serous Chorioretinopathy

Patients with new onset CSC present with painless, acute or subacute visual disturbance due to a combination of metamorphopsia, micropsia, decreased visual acuity and/or hypermetropic shift. Through diligent inquiry, a history may often be elicited of a life event or other psychological stressor having coincided with the time of peak symptoms, with sleep deprivation, or with a history of exogenous corticosteroid exposure.

Ophthalmoscopy shows serous retinal detachment at the posterior pole, although this may be difficult to detect clinically in subtle cases and often also shows one or more serous pigment epithelial detachments (PEDs). In patients with unilateral symptoms, ophthalmoscopy of the fellow eye may reveal extrafoveal involvement. There may be a prior history of episodes of similar symptoms in one or both eyes.

Diagnosis is usually made clinically and is supported by a number of multimodal imaging findings summarized in Table 51.1. The majority of cases resolve over several weeks or months with gradual resolution of symptoms and recovery of vision, without intervention or with education about the roles of stress and corticosteroids. An illustrative case is presented as Figures 51.1A to H.

Table 51.1: Multimodal imaging findings in acute and chronic central serous chorioretinopathy (CSC), including neovascular findings.

	Acute CSC	Chronic CSC
Color photography	• Reduced fundus tessellation • Serous retinal detachment at the posterior pole • (± subretinal fibrin)	• Reduced fundus tessellation • Neurosensory detachment with increased likelihood of subretinal fibrin • Features of type 1 neovascularization (sub-RPE or subretinal hemorrhage; ± aneurysmal lesions) • Bullous, exudative retinal detachment
FA	Focal leakage at the level of the RPE with a spread pattern reminiscent of *smokestack* discharge or an *expanding ink blot*	• Early phase hyperfluorescence in areas of RPE atrophy • Diffuse leakage at the level of the RPE in the mid-phase angiogram • Features of type 1 neovascularization: occult pattern of mid-phase hyperfluorescence with late leakage; ± aneurysmal (polypoidal) lesions
ICGA	• Regional choroidal hyperpermeability localized to the area of leakage seen on FA • Areas of choroidal hypoperfusion	• Regional choroidal hyperpermeability • Areas of choroidal hypoperfusion • Dilated choroidal veins at the posterior pole and in areas of RPE disease • Features of type 1 neovascularization: mid-phase hyperfluorescent lesion with late stage plaque; ± aneurysmal (polypoidal) lesions
Fundus autofluorescence	• Unaltered or subtly altered isoautofluorescence • Mild granularity	• Nonspecific pigment epitheliopathy with mottled texture • Reticular figures with radial hyperautofluorescent spokes • Gravitating tracks • Annular pigment epitheliopathy • Zonal areas of hyper- and hypoautofluorescence
OCT	• Serous retinal detachment associated with hyperfluorescent focus seen on FA • Variable number of discrete pigment epithelial detachments with smooth, convex contours and uniformly hyporeflective contents • Subretinal fibrin with a central lucency may be seen in the proximity of the active leak	• Subretinal fluid with retained hyper-reflective outer segments • Subretinal hyper-reflective material (fibrin, exudate or hemorrhage) • Features of neovascularization: Shallow irregular pigment epithelial detachment with intermediate reflectivity within; ± peaked pigment epithelial detachments consistent with aneurysmal (polypoidal) lesions • Outer retinal atrophy (outer nuclear layer and ellipsoid zone loss) • Cystoid macular degeneration
Enhanced depth imaging OCT and swept-source OCT	• Thicker subfoveal choroid than expected for age and refraction • Choroidal vascular markings difficult to discern • ± dilated vessels in Haller's layer	• Thicker subfoveal choroid than expected for age and refraction • Choroidal markings better defined than in acute CSC • Dilated vessels in Haller's layer • Reduced combined thickness of choriocapillaris and Sattler's layers in places • In extrafoveal disease, extrafoveal choroidal thickness may exceed subfoveal choroidal thickness
En face OCT	• *En face* distribution of subretinal fluid and PED appreciated • Choroidal markings not well resolved	• *En face* distribution of subretinal fluid, PED and atrophy appreciated. • Morphology, distribution and course of pathologically dilated Haller's layer vessels (pachy vessels) appreciated • Choroidal thickness mapping • Distribution of type 1 aneurysmal (polypoidal) lesions
OCT angiography	Nonspecific alterations in choriocapillaris flow signal possible	• Zones of reduced choriocapillaris flow signal. • Mature "tangled" networks at sites of type 1 neovascularization

(RPE: Retinal pigment epithelium; FA: Fluorescein angiography; ICGA: Indocyanine green angiography; OCT: Optical coherence tomography; PED: Pigment epithelial detachment)

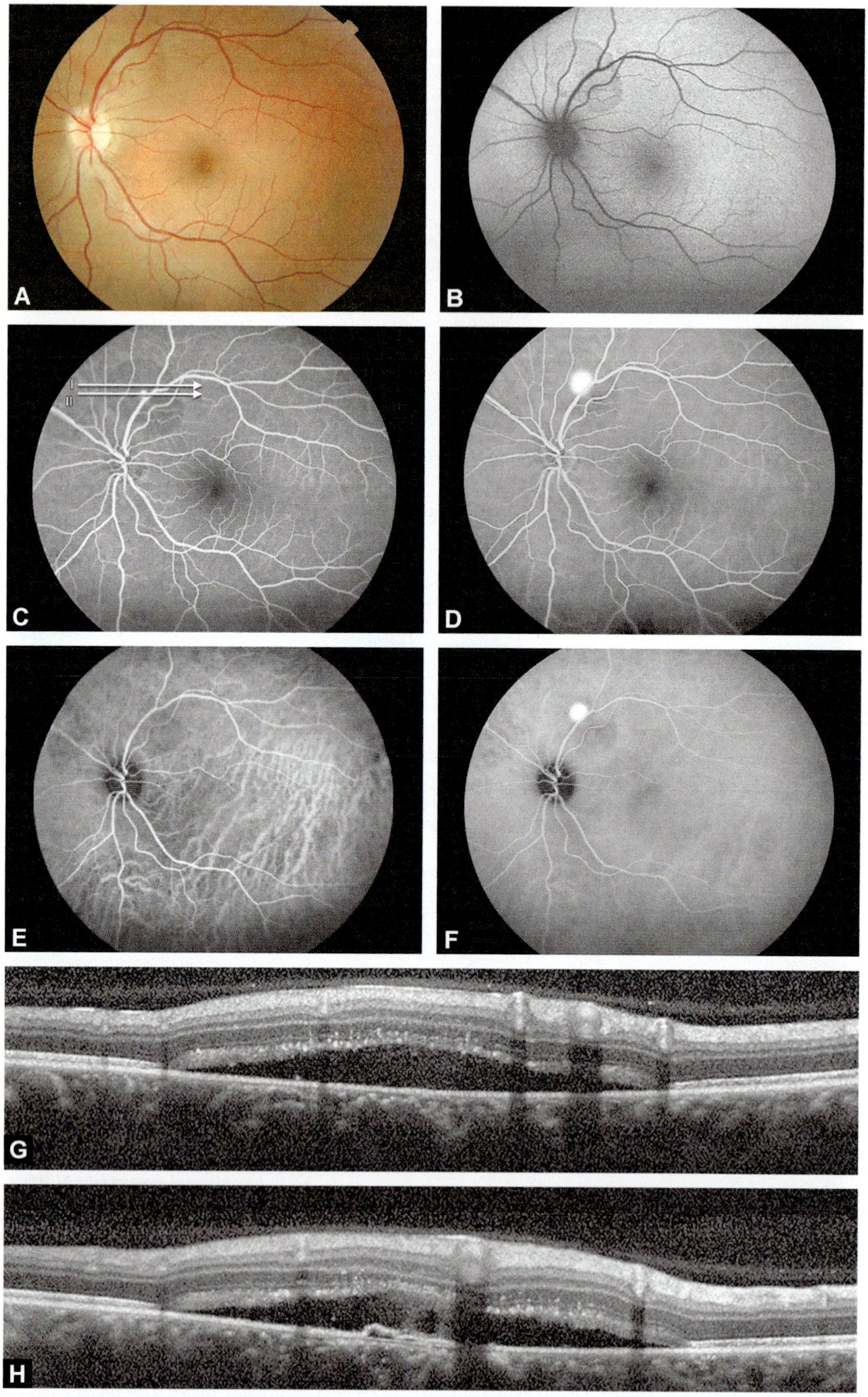

Figs. 51.1A to H: Acute central serous chorioretinopathy. (A) Color photograph shows the outline of a serous retinal detachment superior to the optic nerve; (B) Fundus autofluorescence shows an absence of retinal pigment epithelial changes, and other features of chronicity; (C and D) Arteriovenous phase fluorescein angiography shows focal hyperfluorescence which expands in the late phase simulating the expansion of an "ink blot"; (E and F) Indocyanine green angiography shows subtle choroidal hyperpermeability at the fovea and at the site of the lesion, with late staining at the site of leakage; (G and H) Spectral domain optical coherence tomography shows neurosensory detachment. Some hyper-reflective fibrin is seen in the subretinal space with a hyporeflective lucency within, corresponding to the site of leakage. While some enlargement of Haller's layer vessels is appreciated, the choroidal markings are generally indistinct.

Chronic Central Serous Chorioretinopathy

While the majority of cases of acute CSC resolve within 3–6 months of onset, a subset of patients experience a prolonged or remitting and relapsing course. Central serous chorioretinopathy is considered chronic if single or multiple episodes of neurosensory detachment span 6 months or longer. Chronic CSC is distinguished from acute CSC by the more fibrinous, or exudative subretinal fluid and by cumulative irreversible tissue changes, mainly at the level of the RPE and outer retina.[6]

The appearance of clinically detectable fibrin is accounted for by increased permeability of the RPE component of the blood-ocular barrier to large molecules originating from the choroid. The permeability changes are reflected in the pattern of expanding hyperfluorescence seen on fluorescein angiography (FA) which, in chronic disease, is typically more multifocal or diffuse than in acute CSC (Figs. 51.2A to G). The presence of atrophy is detectable as hyperfluorescence during the early phase of the fluorescein angiogram ('window defect') but is best appreciated by fundus autofluorescence.[7] Atrophy can vary in morphology, distribution and severity; the legacy of chronic CSC on the RPE and outer retina has previously been referred to as "diffuse retinal pigment epitheliopathy."[8] The most frequently seen patterns are listed in Table 51.1 and illustrated in Figures 51.3A to F.[7,9]

On cross-sectional optical coherence tomography (OCT), atrophic lesions feature reduced reflectivity and thinning of the outer hyper-reflective (RPE) band in areas of hypoautofluorescence. Interspersed hyperfluorescent foci may be related to RPE thickening or hyperplasia.[9] Advanced atrophy is characterized by outer retinal disruption, which is detected as outer nuclear layer thinning, loss of the ellipsoid zone and alterations in the external limiting membrane. This may be accompanied by cystoid macular degeneration.

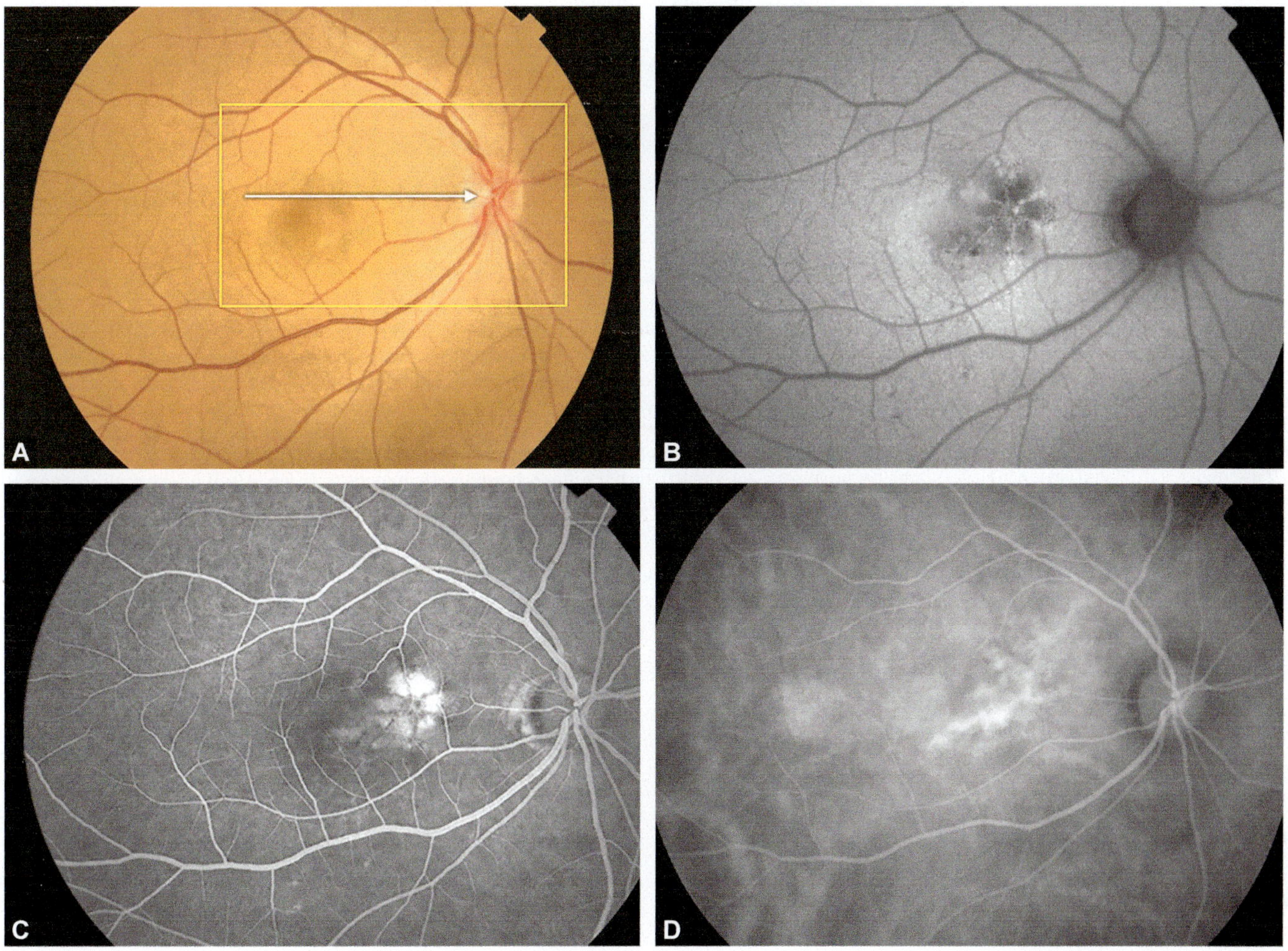

Figs. 51.2A to D

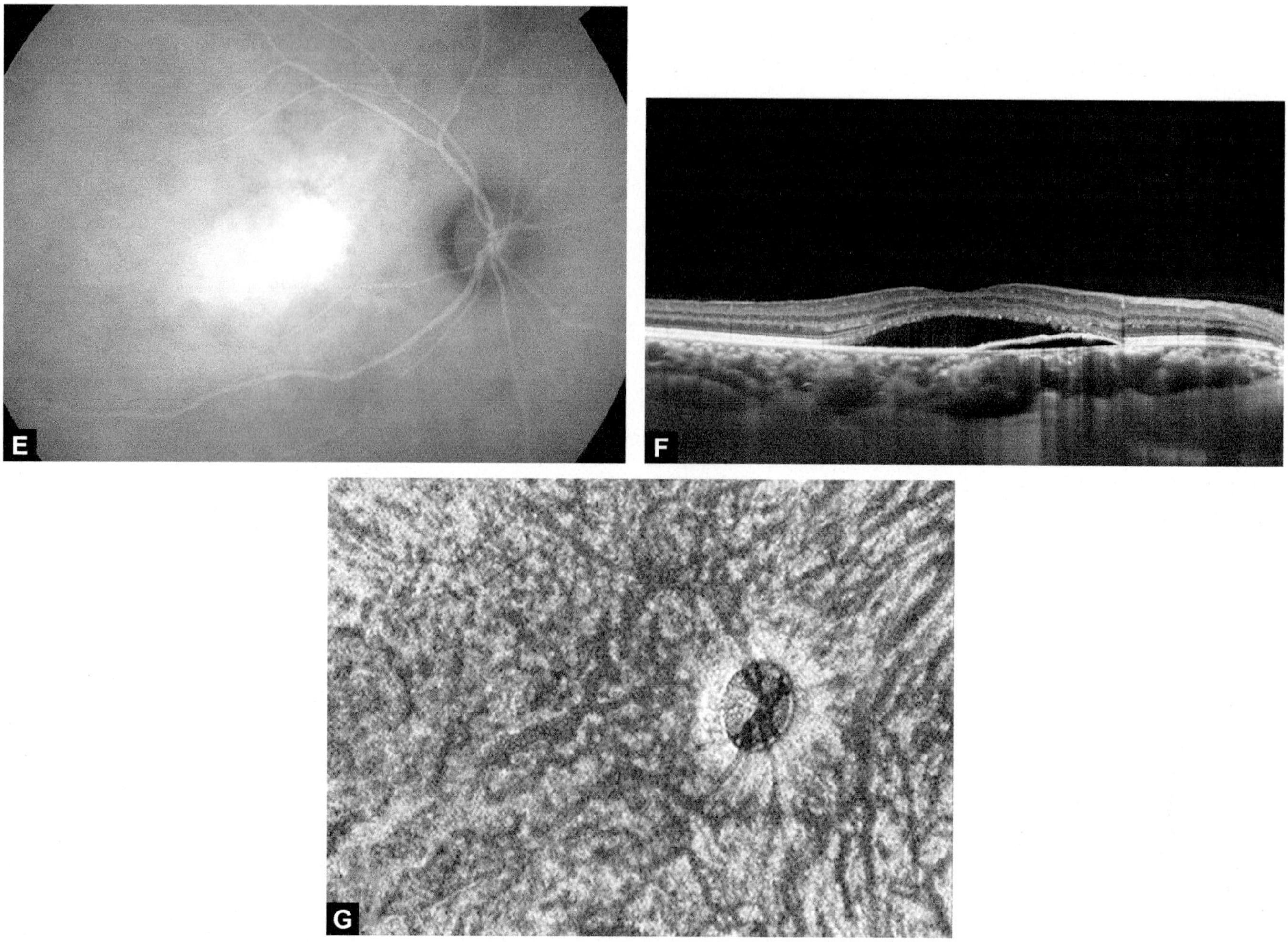

Figs. 51.2E to G

Figs. 51.2A to G: Chronic central serous chorioretinopathy. (A) Color photograph shows reduced fundus tessellation throughout the posterior pole; (B) Fundus autofluorescence shows nonspecific granularity at the foveal center and a stellate, "reticular" lesion consisting of hyperfluorescent spokes at the superonasal border of the fovea; (C) Fluorescein angiography shows pooling of dye beneath a serous pigment epithelial detachment with areas of masked fluorescence due to the spokes of the reticular lesion; (D) Mid-phase indocyanine green angiography shows irregular hyperfluorescence which appears to follow a vascular course, and more generalized choroidal hyperpermeability within the macular area; (E) Staining is seen at the fovea in the late phase; (F) Spectral domain optical coherence tomography shows serous detachment of the neurosensory retina and of the retinal pigment epithelium. The choroid is thickened due to dilated vessels in Haller's layer (pachy vessels), anterior to which the inner choroid is attenuated; (G) *En face* swept source optical coherence tomography at the level of the deep choroid shows the hyporeflective lumina of pachyvessels at the fovea and also nasal to the optic nerve.

The introduction of enhanced depth imaging (EDI) OCT and swept source OCT to the study of CSC has revealed much about the nature and architecture of the choroid and provided clues as to the mechanisms which might link a choroidal etiology with clinical manifestations at the level of the RPE and outer retina.[10] Patients with chronic CSC generally have increased subfoveal choroidal thickness relative to normal subjects. Moreover, in patients with unilateral disease, the subfoveal choroid is also thickened in the unaffected fellow eye, supporting the view that CSC has a systemic or constitutional basis. In eyes with CSC, choroidal thickening may also be observed at *extrafoveal* locations that are correlated spatially with the sites of RPE leakage.[11] This thickening is attributable mainly to pathologically dilated vessels in Haller's layer with focal thinning of the choriocapillaris and Sattler's layers at the site of disease. Choroidal vascular observations in CSC have formed the basis for defining pachychoroid, initially as a family of diseases which share a choroidal phenotype and, more recently, as a more generic disease *mechanism* which operates over a wider disease spectrum to give rise to a common set of manifestations resembling CSC and its related entities (see later in this chapter).

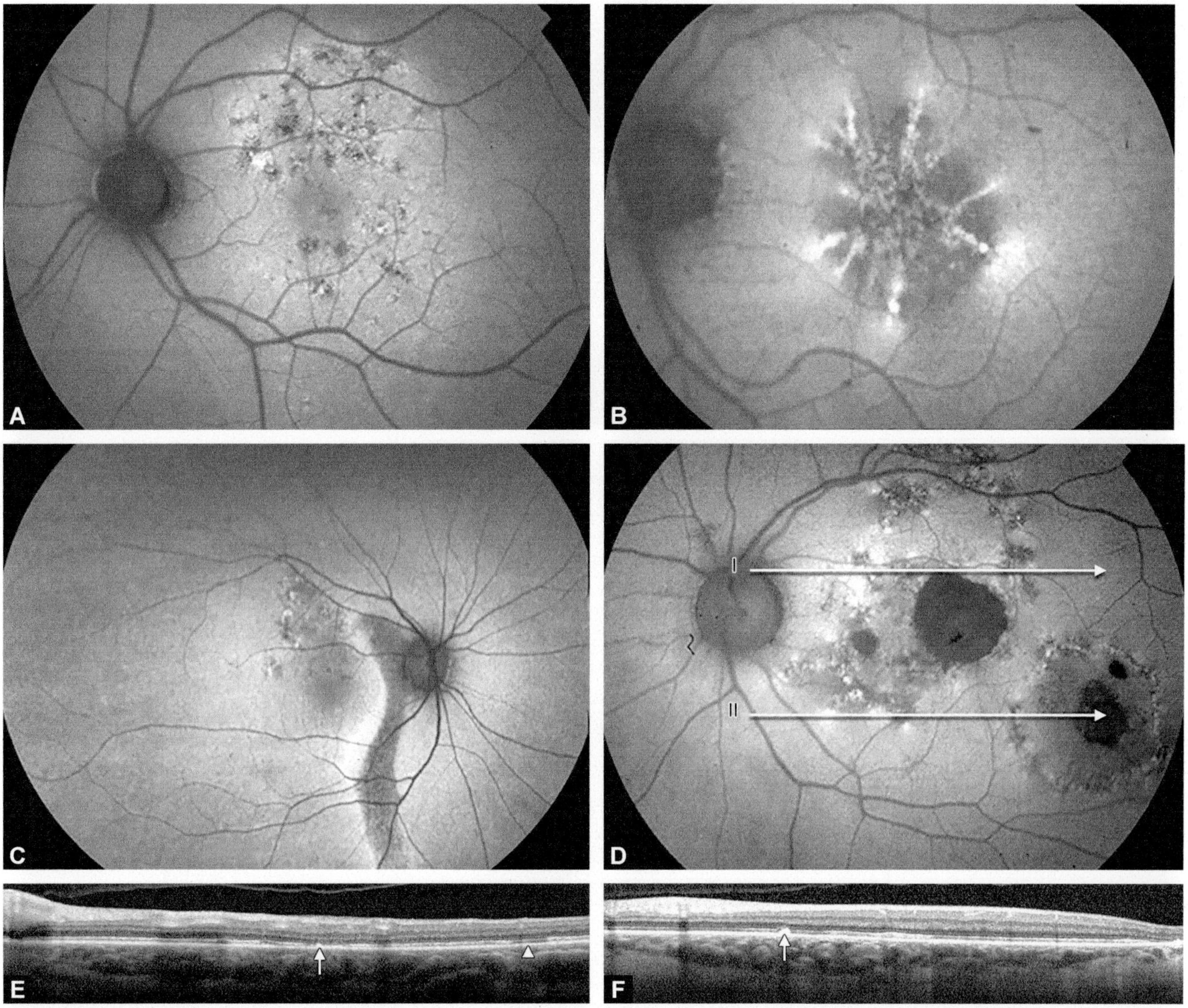

Figs. 51.3A to F: Patterns of retinal pigment epithelium (RPE) disease seen in chronic central serous chorioretinopathy, imaged with fundus autofluorescence. (A) Nonspecific or mottled; (B) Stellate or reticular figure; (C) Nonspecific at the fovea with a descending, or gravitating track originating superior to the papillomacular bundle; (D) Annular lesions composed of nonspecific pigment epitheliopathy arranged in a ring. Also seen are areas of RPE atrophy. Notably, pigment epitheliopathy in central serous chorioretinopathy frequently features hyperautofluorescent foci interspersed with hypoautofluorescent foci; (E and F) Optical coherence tomography performed through hyperautofluorescent foci shows thickening of the outer hyper-reflective band representing the RPE (arrows). More ill-defined and zonal areas of hyperautofluorescence represent unmasking of RPE autofluorescence due to reduced photopigment density in the overlying outer retina (arrowhead). Optical coherence tomography scans E and F correspond to the position of lines I and II, respectively.

Bullous Exudative Retinal Detachment

Neurosensory detachment in CSC is typically localized to the posterior pole and is usually shallow in configuration, even in eyes with multifocal serous retinal detachment or widespread autofluorescence changes. Bullous retinal detachment has been described as a very rare but well characterized complication (Figs. 51.4A to E).

In 2000, Sahu and colleagues described 13 eyes of 11 patients (aged 23–39 years, all male) with bullous exudative retinal detachment complicating CSC, noting that the majority of cases were unilateral, that leaking PEDs were observed on FA in all cases, that resolution of exudative retinal detachment took 12–14 weeks, and that laser photocoagulation did not seem to offer any benefit.[4] Otsuka et al. studied 46 eyes of 25 patients (mean age

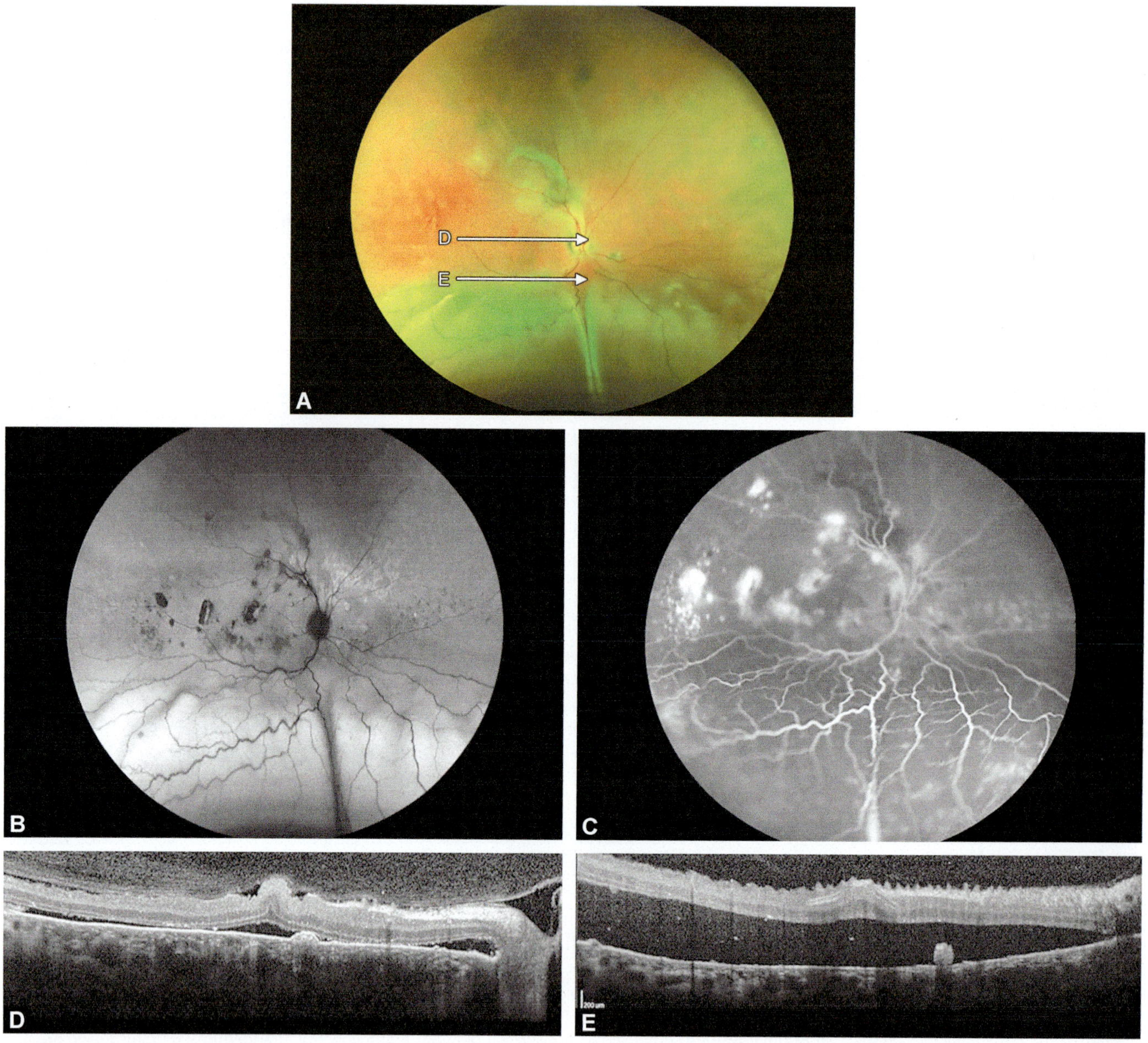

Figs. 51.4A to E: Bullous retinal detachment in central serous chorioretinopathy. (A) Ultra widefield fundus color photograph shows an inferior bullous detachment; (B) Ultra widefield fundus autofluorescence illustrates multiple areas of retinal pigment epithelium disease; (C) Fluorescein angiography demonstrates multifocal areas of active leakage; (D and E) Optical coherence tomography B-scans corresponding to the orange arrows in (A) show subretinal fluid and subretinal fibrin.

43 years, 84% male) with severe bullous retinal detachment complicating CSC.[12] They noted multifocal involvement and discussed the potential role of corticosteroids in the etiology. Seventeen of their patients had undergone laser photocoagulation without apparent benefit.

In 2016, Balaratnasingam and colleagues described 21 eyes of 14 patients (mean age 54, 64% male) with multimodal imaging and compared these patients with a larger cohort of patients without bullous retinal detachment (122 eyes of 84 patients).[13] A history of corticosteroid use had been elicited in 50% of patients with bullous retinal detachment and in only 25% of patients without. Patients with bullous retinal detachment had histories of severe renal disease (1 patient), bone marrow transplantation for chronic lymphocytic leukemia (1 patient), idiopathic thrombocytopenic purpura with systemic lupus erythematosus (1 patient), and hypertension (2 patients). By contrast, none of the patients in the nonbullous cohort had histories of renal disease or organ transplantation.

Eyes with bullous retinal detachments had turbid subretinal fluid. Fibrin was appreciated clinically, and multimodal imaging showed multifocal leakage at the level of the RPE on FA, localized to the vicinity of PEDs. Fibrin was also localized to the vicinity of the sites of leakage and appeared hyperfluorescent on early phase FA, with late staining. Twenty of the 21 eyes in the bullous CSC group also exhibited RPE tears at sites where PEDs had been identified at preceding visits. Enhanced depth imaging OCT of the choroid showed hyper-reflective dots in the inner choroid and hyper-reflective "sheets" in the outer choroid; these were not seen in eyes without bullous retinal detachments.

Neovascularization

Type 1 neovascularization is a relatively common complication of chronic CSC and occurs in approximately 25% of cases (manuscript under peer review). The neovascular tissue gives rise to a pattern of "occult" hyperfluorescence on FA, with ill-defined late leakage. Indocyanine green angiography (ICGA) may show a hyperfluorescent lesion in the mid-phase with a hyperfluorescent "plaque" in the late phase. However, the RPE leakage on FA attributable to the underlying CSC, and the presence of choroidal hyperpermeability on ICGA, can hinder the detection specificity of features of neovascularization and thereby undermine the sensitivity of dye angiography for detecting its presence.[14]

Cross-sectional OCT is helpful in diagnosing neovascularization in CSC and typically shows PED with intermediate or heterogeneous internal reflectivity. In the context of CSC, vascularized PEDs often have a shallow irregular morphology on cross-sectional OCT, quite different from the serous PEDs of acute or uncomplicated CSC. This PED morphology, characterized by a wide base but small height, was first described in patients with aneurysmal (polypoidal) type 1 neovascularization in terms of a "double layer sign" denoting a shallow separation of the RPE from Bruch's membrane.[15]

Phenotypic features which help to distinguish type 1 neovascularization occurring in chronic CSC from that occurring in neovascular age-related macular degeneration (AMD) are summarized in Table 51.2.

Table 51.2: Type 1 neovascularization in chronic central serous chorioretinopathy (CSC) and neovascular age-related macular degeneration.

	Type 1 neovascularization in chronic CSC	Type 1 neovascularization in age-related macular degeneration
Age of onset	50–70	>70 years
Fundus tessellation	Reduced	Increased
Drusen	Minimal or absent. (There may be irregular lesions resembling drusen which have been called "pachydrusen.")[16]	Soft drusen typical
Reticular pseudodrusen (subretinal drusenoid deposits)	Absent	Frequent
Onset of symptoms	Quiescent or insidious	Acute metamorphopsia
Findings at presentation	Subretinal fluid with infrequent hemorrhage	Subretinal fluid with exudate and frequent hemorrhage
Vascularized PED	Shallow and irregular with minimal Bruch's membrane RPE separation ("double layer" sign on OCT)[15]	Fibrovascular PED with subretinal fluid, exudate, hemorrhage and heterogeneous or multilayered contents on OCT
Aneurysmal (polypoidal) lesions	May be present	Rare (see Pachychoroid discussion)
Choroid	Relatively thickened with pachychoroid characteristics (see pachychoroid discussion)	Relatively thinned, often with age-related choroidal atrophy
Response to intravitreal anti-angiogenic treatment	Variable, with some eyes requiring prolonged treatment to maintain an absence of subretinal fluid	More predictable response with resolution of subretinal fluid and exudate in most eyes.
Retinal pigment epithelial tears	Rare	May occur when PEDs are large
Hemorrhage	Unusual unless aneurysmal (polypoidal) lesions present	Frequent hemorrhage at presentation
Subretinal fibrosis	Approximately, 25% of cases	Frequent, especially if history of subretinal hemorrhage

(PED: Pigment epithelial detachment; RPE: Retinal pigment epithelium; OCT: Optical coherence tomography)

Pathogenesis

Systemically, CSC is known to be associated with abnormalities of corticosteroid metabolism and steroid response. Indeed, this is an important feature which, in older literature, distinguished CSC from uveitic disorders that feature serous or exudative retinal detachment. As many as 52% of patients with CSC give a positive history of corticosteroid exposure coinciding temporally with peak visual symptoms; corticosteroid exposure also appears to be associated with more severe clinical manifestations, such as bullous retinal detachment.[17]

Importantly, the patient with CSC may not necessarily be the one being treated primarily with steroids but may be exposed inadvertently, for example, while assisting a child or dependent with topical steroid application for cutaneous indications such as eczema. The association with an anomalous steroid response is also thought to explain the observation that patients with CSC often admit to having experienced a period of undue psychological stress coinciding with peak symptoms, even when they have not been exposed to exogenous steroids.

Multimodal imaging has revealed information about the sequence of events which culminate in the recognizable signs of clinically significant disease and has therefore provided valuable clues about the pathological mechanisms involved. In particular, the choroidal vasculature is implicated as the primary site of disease and as the source of subretinal fluid that defines CSC.[18-20] Recent investigation has also shown that the choroid expresses mineralocorticoid receptors, that stimulation of these receptors by aldosterone in rodents increases choroidal thickness and vascular congestion, and that this effect is reversed by mineralocorticoid receptor antagonists.[21,22] The effects of mineralocorticoid receptor antagonists such as spironolactone and eplerenone have been investigated in humans, but with limited or unpredictable benefit which might be related to tissue bioavailability.[23]

The mechanisms by which fluid traverses tissue boundaries to sequester in the sub-RPE and subretinal spaces remain elusive but it is clear that a breakdown occurs in the barrier function of the RPE. However, the extent to which the clinical heterogeneity seen in CSC is due to variations in choroidal biology versus variations in RPE biology remains undetermined.

Treatment and Prognosis in Central Serous Chorioretinopathy

Most cases of acute CSC resolve without intervention within 3–4 months but up to 50% of patients might experience recurrence within 1 year.[24-27] When fluid and/or symptoms persist for an extended period, various treatment options exist, but none of these are reliably and predictably efficacious, whether for acute or chronic CSC. Moreover, most of the available treatment modalities are at least to some extent invasive and are therefore usually employed in a stepwise escalation for partially responsive or refractory disease.

Patients may benefit in the first instance from education about the nature of CSC and its reported associations with psychological stress, aberrant sleep patterns and sleep deprivation, and corticosteroids. Steroid restriction in patients with a history of exposure is often beneficial.

Thermal Laser

Thermal laser may be used to treat CSC when the site of leakage at the level of the RPE is small and extrafoveal. The principle of thermal laser is to apply a photocoagulative burn to the RPE at the site of leakage. The underlying pathology in the choroidal vasculature therefore remains untreated.

It is presumed that the leak is arrested by scar formation, though it is well-known that high intensity thermal burns applied to the RPE can damage Bruch's membrane, upregulate vascular endothelial growth factor (VEGF) expression and lead to neovascularization. Thermal laser would be impractical and increasingly tissue-destructive if applied in disease with multifocal or diffuse leakage.

Micropulse diode laser photocoagulation is applied in a similar fashion to thermal laser. While micropulse laser has the advantage of not causing visible signs of laser damage and of not causing scotoma, the mode of action is currently unknown. Verma et al. have shown non-inferiority to thermal laser in a pilot randomized trial involving 30 patients with CSC,[28] but many experts feel that further study with longitudinal follow-up of treated cases is needed to assess the potential role of this treatment for the management of acute and chronic CSC.

Photodynamic Therapy

Photodynamic therapy (PDT) with verteporfin treats pathological vasculature with nonthermal laser. Intravenously administered verteporfin is taken up by the abnormal choriocapillaris and releases free radicals when exposed to light in the presence of oxygen, so that treatment is delivered selectively to this target tissue.

Photodynamic therapy may be delivered "conventionally" (normal dose and normal fluence) but half-dose PDT and half-fluence PDT have also been shown effective in reducing subretinal fluid.[29] Lai et al. noted, however, that half-dose PDT may be less definitive as reflected by recurrence rates, particularly in patients with bilateral disease,[30] though not all studies report this. In a survey of retina specialists with a publication record on CSC, Mehta and colleagues found that two-thirds offered PDT as first-line treatment for chronic disease and that the most popular protocol (60.6%) was full dose with half-fluence.[31]

In 2014, Lim et al. published findings from a multicenter retrospective study of patients who had undergone PDT for CSC.[32] Data on 265 eyes of 237 patients were collected by means of a survey administered to members of the Macula Society. The mean age of patients was 52 and one-fourth of patients were female. Patients had received normal fluence or half-fluence PDT (approximately, 50% in each group). The number of treatments administered was 1 in 89% of patients, 2 in 7% and 3 in 3% with a follow-up range from 1 month to more than 1 year. Improvement in visual acuity by 3 or more Snellen lines was seen in less than 1%, 29% and 48% of eyes with baseline visual acuity ≥20/32, 20/40 to 20/80 and ≤20/100, respectively. Resolution of subretinal fluid was achieved in 81% of patients. Retinal pigment epithelial atrophy occurred in 4% of patients, and severe visual loss was seen in 1.5%. Visual outcomes did not appear to be related to the choice of normal or half-fluence therapy, and discrepancies between resolution of subretinal fluid and visual outcome were attributed to irreversible outer retinal damage.

In the same year, Erikitola and associates conducted a meta-analysis of the literature concerning PDT for CSC and examined 31 studies representing 787 eyes.[33] They examined several endpoints, including resolution of subretinal fluid, visual outcome, recurrence, and complications such as neovascularization and choriocapillaris ischemia, and concluded that a half-dose protocol appears to be the safest and most effective, while a half-fluence protocol carried a greater risk of recurrence. The authors also noted that the majority of investigators had selected laser spot sizes based on leakage seen on FA and suggested that spot sizes based on hyperpermeability seen on ICGA might be more appropriate and better tailored to the extent of choriocapillaris disease. Rarely, photodynamic therapy can be complicated by choroidal ischemia and visual loss.

Antivascular Endothelial Growth Factor Therapy

Vascular endothelial growth factor is a potent driver of neovascularization, and inhibiting the effects of VEGF has been effective in treating neovascularization in AMD and in other contexts. However, it is recognized that although anti-VEGF therapy is effective in inducing regression during the early stages of angiogenesis, once the neovascular tissue develops pericytes and other features of "maturity," anti-VEGF has the effect of pruning nascent branches while allowing existing trunk vessels to persist.[34] Anti-VEGF therapy is also effective in reducing capillary permeability in situations in which permeability is VEGF-induced.

The CONTAIN study was a prospective, open-label pilot study which examined the effects of treating chronic CSC with intravitreal aflibercept.[35] Twelve patients with angiographically active CSC were enrolled; half were treated monthly for 6 months and half were treated in months 0, 1, 2 and 4. All patients were male (ages 29–64 years). Benefit to visual acuity was not demonstrated in this study, and a trend toward morphological improvement was interpreted with caution due to the small sample size.

Although a role for anti-VEGF therapy in controlling permeability at the level of the choriocapillaris or the RPE has not been established in the treatment of CSC, intravitreal anti-VEGF therapy is often used to treat exudation associated with type 1 neovascularization related to chronic CSC and in pachychoroid neovasculopathy. However, neovascularization occurring in these entities differs from that occurring in AMD in that it develops in a slow, insidious manner and can be clinically quiescent for months or years. It has been shown in retrospective studies that treating type 1 neovascularization in CSC and pachychoroid neovasculopathy can reduce the elaboration of subretinal fluid, but formal treatment paradigms in this context have yet to be established (Figs. 51.5 and 51.6).

Mineralocorticoid Receptor Antagonists

Endogenous corticosteroids and exogenous therapeutic agents have been linked to aggravation of CSC. Corticosteroids refer to both glucocorticoids and mineralocorticoids. It has recently been demonstrated that both the retina and the choroid express mineralocorticoid receptors and should be considered as target tissue that might play a role in the mechanism of the disease.[21] Spironolactone and eplerenone are competitive inhibitors of mineralocorticoid receptors and are widely used and well tolerated in treating heart failure and hypertension. Both drugs are potassium-sparing diuretics and carry a risk of hyperkalemia if not monitored.

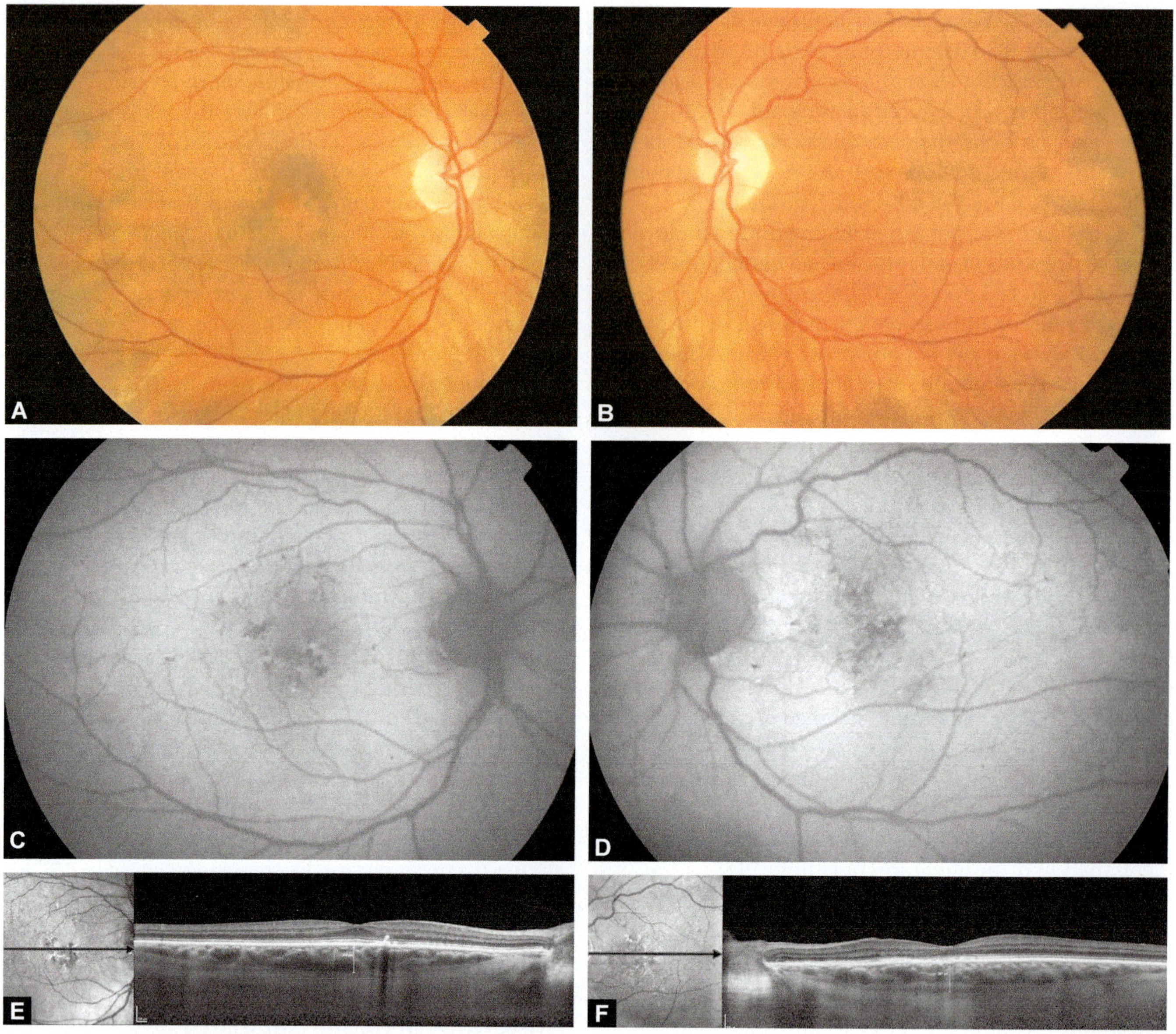

Figs. 51.5A to F: Bilateral pachychoroid pigment epitheliopathy. (A) Color photographs; (B) Fundus autofluorescence; (C) Spectral domain optical coherence tomography of each eye shows choroidal thickening with dilated Haller's layer vessels (pachy vessels) and inner choroidal thinning; (D to F) The outer hyper-reflective band corresponding with the retinal pigment epithelium is altered with foci of thinning and thickening.

No large prospective randomized trials with standard treatment protocol have been performed yet for the use of mineralocorticoid antagonists for patients with chronic CSC. However, several small cohorts and case series have been reported. Thirteen patients with chronic CSC and persistent subretinal fluid for more than 4 months were treated with oral eplerenone (25 mg/day for a week followed by 50 mg/day for 3 months), with significant reduction in central macular thickness and significant improvement in vision.[23] Complete resolution of subretinal fluid occurred in 70% of patients. Another study that included 23 eyes evaluated the effect of mineralocorticoid antagonist (either spironolactone or eplerenone) after 12 months of treatment and follow-up.[36] Both agents were found to improve visual acuity as well as subretinal fluid. This study did not however demonstrate improvement in other anatomical outcomes such as central macular thickness and choroidal thickness. Randomized trials are needed to further understand the benefits of these treatments.

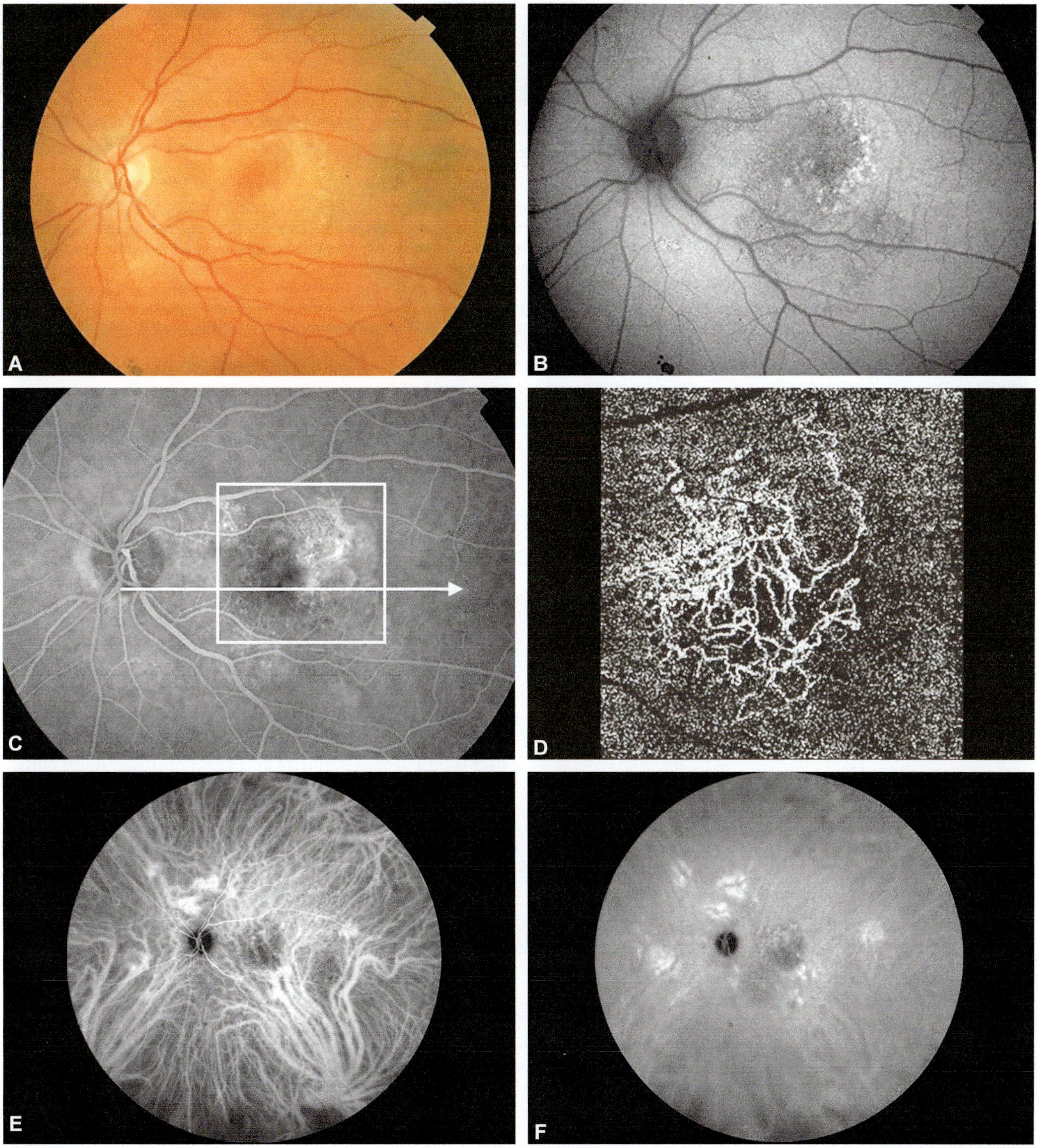

Figs. 51.6A to F

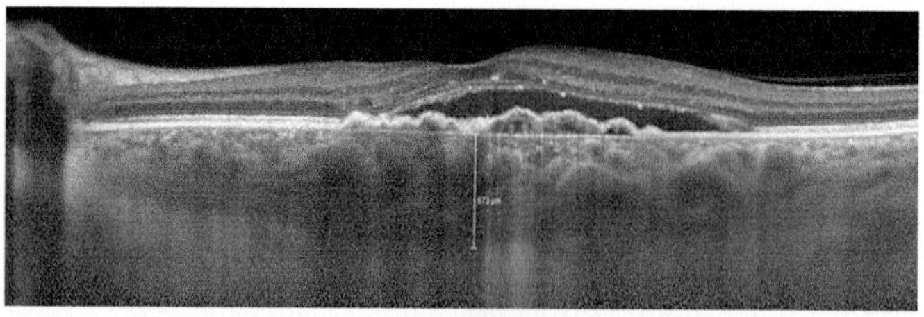

Fig. 51.6G

Figs. 51.6A to G: Pachychoroid neovasculopathy. (A) Color photograph shows reduced fundus tessellation and subtle alteration of the homogeneity of retinal pigment epithelial (RPE) pigmentation at the macula; (B) Fundus autofluorescence shows more clearly the heterogeneity in RPE pigmentation. Notably, hyperautofluorescent foci are seen which are unusual in neovascular age-related macular degeneration but seen frequently in central serous chorioretinopathy and pachychoroid disorders; (C) Fluorescein angiography shows ill-defined hyperfluorescence consistent with "occult choroidal neovascularization"; (D) *En face* optical coherence tomography (OCT) angiography segment at the level of RPE-Bruch's membrane complex reveals the tangled morphology of a type 1 neovascular network at the fovea; (E) Early phase widefield indocyanine green angiography (ICGA) shows pathologically dilated peripapillary and submacular vessels. The macular pachy vessels course toward the inferotemporal vortex vein; (F) Late phase ICGA shows choroidal hyperpermeability and central hyperfluorescent plaque corresponding to type 1 neovascularization; (G) Spectral-domain OCT shows a thick choroid with prominent vascular markings and a shallow irregular pigment epithelial detachment with hyper-reflective contents in the sub-RPE space. A neurosensory detachment overlies the type 1 neovascular lesion.

PACHYCHOROID

The term pachychoroid (Greek: παχυς, thick) was introduced into the literature to refer to a set of choroidal findings, seen on multimodal imaging, which were first described in patients with CSC but subsequently detected in patients with a wider spectrum of manifestations, including pachychoroid pigment epitheliopathy, CSC, pachychoroid neovasculopathy and aneurysmal type 1 neovascularization [polypoidal choroidal vasculopathy (PCV)]. The evolution in understanding of pachychoroid has since occurred in parallel with developments in depth-resolved imaging technologies such as EDI OCT, swept-source OCT with *en face* projection, and OCT angiography.

Pachychoroid pigment epitheliopathy refers to RPE changes at the posterior pole which are reminiscent of CSC but which occur in patients who have not had subretinal fluid to qualify as having CSC.[37] The patients were, however, found to have relatively thick choroids on EDI OCT, especially at the sites of pigment epitheliopathy which could be extrafoveal or peripapillary. They also exhibited regional choroidal hyperpermeability on ICGA. Pachychoroid pigment epitheliopathy was therefore considered to be a *forme fruste* of CSC.

It was noted that patients with pachychoroid pigment epitheliopathy were often asymptomatic and could be referred for putative diagnoses of pigmentary AMD or pattern dystrophy. However, reduced fundus tessellation, the absence of soft drusen, the relatively young age of several of the patients in the initial cohort (18 eyes of 9 patients, age 27–89 years, mean 51 years) and choroidal thickening, all helped to exclude AMD as the cause of the pigment epitheliopathy.

The term pachychoroid neovasculopathy was first used to describe a series of patients who had developed type 1 neovascularization on a background of choroidal thickening and in the absence of drusen.[38] These patients were also noted to have choroidal hyperpermeability on ICGA and one patient also had pachychoroid pigment epitheliopathy in an otherwise unaffected fellow eye. While it is known that type 1 neovascularization can complicate the clinical course of chronic CSC, use of the term pachychoroid neovasculopathy acknowledged that neovascularization could develop from a background of pachychoroid pigment epitheliopathy without the eye first developing CSC. The combination of the relatively young age of these patients (mean 58 years) and the choroidal phenotype also distinguished this form of neovascularization from that seen in AMD.

An additional observation was that all three patients in this series had aneurysmal (polypoidal) lesions on cross-sectional OCT, manifesting as a peaked PEDs with adjacent shallow irregular PEDs as described previously by Sato et al.[15,38] These findings formed the basis for a hypothesis that PCV, considered by many as either a distinct entity or a variant of neovascular AMD, was actually more closely related to CSC, and therefore, more appropriately classified as a pachychoroid entity.

En Face Imaging, Pachy Vessels and Choroidal Sub-segmentation

The introduction of swept source OCT allowed for better depth penetration for imaging the choroid, without the need for averaging. The higher scan speeds also allowed the capture of dense raster scans which could be resegmented to produce depth-resolved *en face* projections.

En face OCT imaging of patients with chronic CSC and other pachychoroid entities demonstrated a number of new findings about the choroidal architecture in these diseases:

- The pathologically dilated vessels seen in Haller's layer on cross-sectional OCT seemed to originate at sites of disease and drain peripherally toward the vortex vein ampullae. For convenience these vessels were referred to as "pachy vessels."
- Pachy vessels were characterized by their dilated caliber, which persisted for most of the length of each vessel, by contrast with the profiles of physiological Haller's layer venules, which arise at the posterior pole with small calibers and increase in diameter as they drain peripherally.
- Areas of manifest disease featured attenuation of the choriocapillaris and Sattler's layer, so that pachyvessels were effectively anteriorized at those foci.
- The thinning of the inner choroid at disease sites was more than negated by the formation of pachy vessels, which therefore formed the basis for the overall *increase* in choroidal thickness at the disease location.

The mechanistic connection between pachy vessels and disease features at the level of the RPE and outer retina is incompletely understood. Hypotheses which have been articulated include—(1) mechanical microtrauma to the RPE from anteriorized pachy vessels, and (2) ischemia of the RPE and outer retina due to atrophic thinning of the inner choroidal layers. The latter is more convincing as a driver for neovascularization and has been quantified in patients with aneurysmal type 1 neovascularization, albeit circumstantially rather than longitudinally.[39]

As the definition of the set of features which constitute the pachychoroid phenotype has matured, the occurrence of this set of features has been detected in a wider spectrum of conditions, some of which are not directly related to CSC and its spectrum. Notable examples of pachy vessels are seen in eyes with myopic staphylomata, dome-shaped maculopathy and choroidal nevi (Figs. 51.7A to E).[40,41] Each of these represent acquired contexts in which choroidal architecture undergoes adaptive changes to conform with the anatomy of the underlying condition, resulting in a zone of abrupt transition in choroidal thickness. At such zones, the inner choroid becomes attenuated and pachyvessels arise. In myopic eyes, pachy vessels are seen at the crest of a dome or at the inflection point of a staphyloma; in eyes with nevi these changes occur in the immediate lateral vicinity of the nevus (manuscript under review). At the level of the RPE and outer retina, a spectrum of changes can occur resembling members of the CSC spectrum described earlier. This resemblance supports the understanding of pachychoroid not so much as an expanded phenotype but as a disease *mechanism* that can underlie CSC as a diffuse manifestation and other entities as focal manifestations (manuscript under review).

Aneurysmal Type 1 Neovascularization (Polypoidal Choroidal Vasculopathy)

The term "(idiopathic) polypoidal choroidal vasculopathy" was introduced by Yannuzzi and associates in 1982 at the annual meeting of the Macula Society and first appeared in the literature in 1990.[42] In the same year, Kleiner et al. described a form of "posterior uveal bleeding syndrome," 5 years after Stern el al. had described a similar phenotype.[43,44] All these reports described a degenerative disease featuring serosanguinous pigment epithelial and retinal detachments with a predilection for middle-aged patients of African ancestry. Over subsequent decades it became apparent that the aneurysmal (polypoidal) lesions are not always confined to the peripapillary region but can also occur at the macula. It has also been shown that this condition is not exclusive to patients of African heritage but also occurs in those of Asian or Caucasian background.

While the older literature on PCV remains somewhat agnostic over whether the pathognomonic lesions lie posterior or anterior to Bruch's membrane, the introduction of OCT and OCT angiography has provided evidence supporting the latter. This in turn has resulted in a re-appraisal of what this disease really is in pathological terms, and a conviction that PCV is really a form of type 1 neovascularization in which saccular aneurysmal lesions arise from the neovascular network. Moreover, the terms "polypoidal" and "polyp" are now understood to be

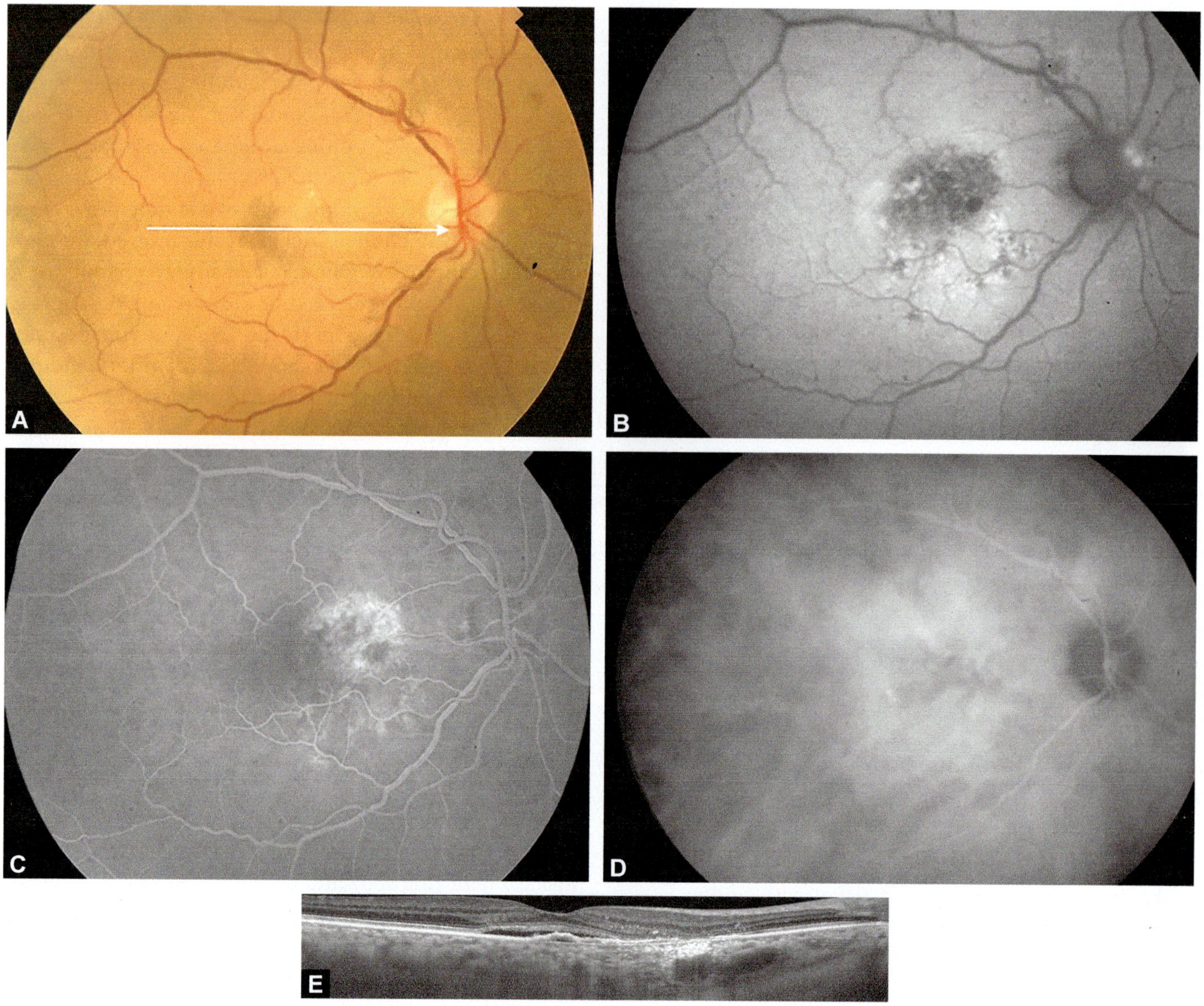

Figs. 51.7A to E: Treatment-naïve pachychoroid neovasculopathy. (A) Color photograph shows reduced fundus tessellation; (B) Fundus autofluorescence shows nonspecific alteration of the autofluorescent pattern at the fovea featuring hyper- and hypoautofluorescent foci. The distribution of autofluorescence changes inferior to the fovea is suggestive of a gravitating influence on the pattern of retinal pigment epithelial disease; (C) Arteriovenous phase fluorescein angiography shows ill-defined hyperfluorescence superonasal to the fovea; (D) Intermediate phase indocyanine green angiography shows choroidal hyperpermeability; (E) Spectral domain optical coherence tomography through the fovea shows subfoveal choroidal thickening which extends nasal to the fovea where the lumina of two large choroidal vessels are seen in Haller's layer. A shallow irregular pigment epithelial detachment is present at the fovea.

misnomers because polyps are fleshy masses of tissue arising from epithelial tissue, usually on mucosal surfaces.

Multimodal imaging of patients with aneurysmal type 1 neovascularization reveals a number of important characteristics (Figs. 51.8A to F). Fluorescein angiography and ICGA show the characteristic lesions to be *perfused*, qualifying them as a form of aneurysm rather than a form of polyp. Indocyanine green angiography also usually reveals an adjacent vascular network or hyperfluorescent "plaque", corresponding to the branching vascular network which feeds the aneurysmal lesion. Cross-sectional OCT localizes the aneurysmal lesions and branching vascular networks to the sub-RPE space but anterior to Bruch's membrane. Additionally, in cases in which the branching vascular networks are not detected by dye angiography, due to the confounding effects of choroidal hyperpermeability, they are frequently detected by OCT angiography, further supporting the contemporary view that aneurysmal

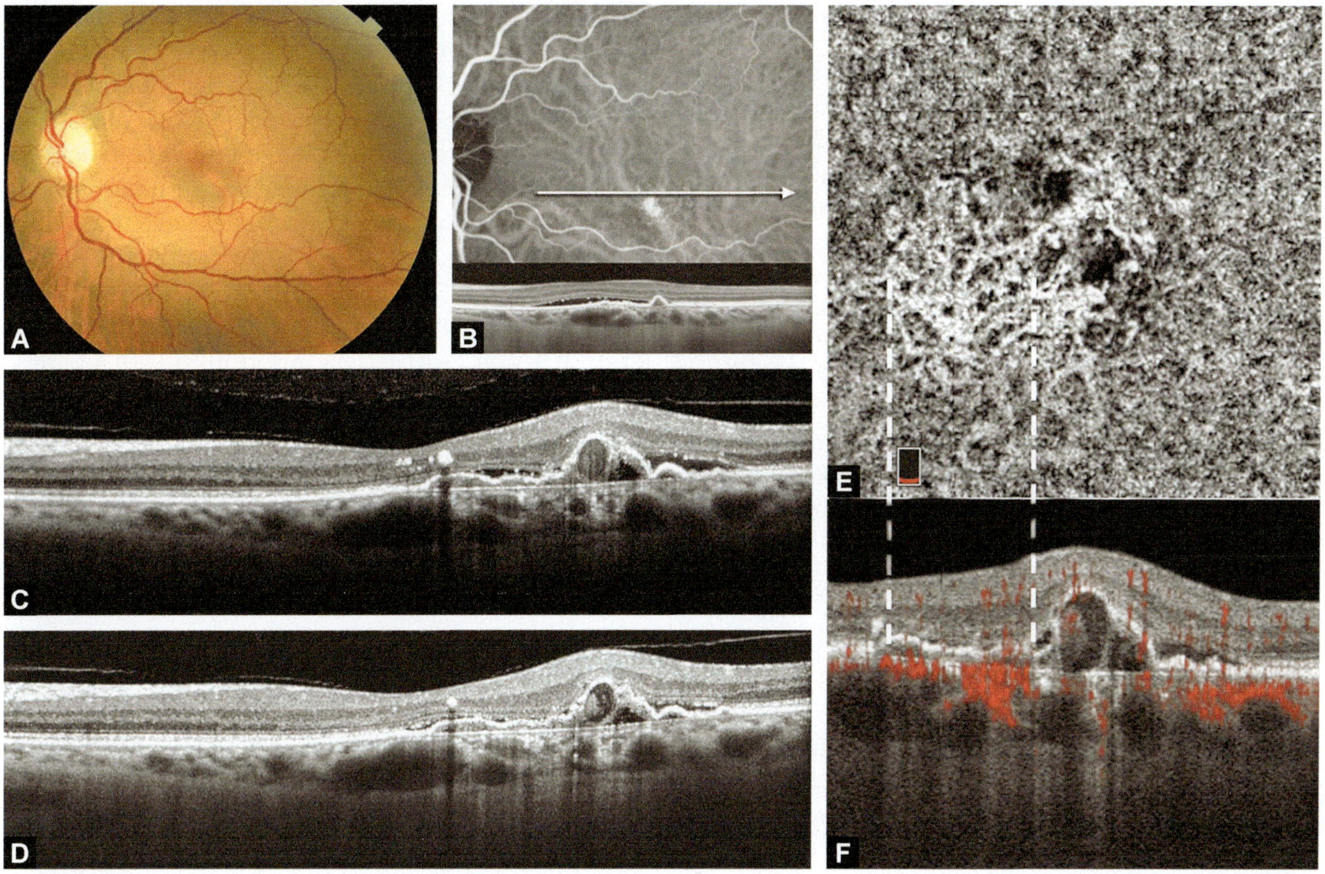

Figs. 51.8A to F: Aneurysmal type 1 neovascularization (polypoidal choroidal vasculopathy). (A) Color photography shows altered retinal pigment epithelial (RPE) pigmentation and blood within the sub-RPE aneurysms; (B) Indocyanine green angiography shows a hyperfluorescent "branching vascular network" originating over large choroidal veins (pachy vessels) with terminal aneurysms at its temporal margin; (C and D) Spectral domain optical coherence tomographies (OCT) show a peaked pigment epithelial detachment (PED) deriving its shape from aneurysmal (polypoidal) lesions in the sub-RPE space. This is contiguous with shallow irregular PED with heterogeneously hyper-reflective contents in the sub-RPE space, corresponding with the type 1 neovascular network from which the aneurysmal lesions originate. The choroid is thickened due to pathologically dilated Haller's vessels (pachy vessels) anterior to which the inner choroid is attenuated; (E) *En face* OCT angiography at the level of the RPE-Bruch's membrane complex shows the morphology of the type 1 neovascular network; (F) Cross-sectional OCT with angiographic flow signal overlay shows flow signal within the shallow irregular PED, confirming the presence of vascularized tissue.

lesions arise from sub-RPE neovascularization and not directly from the choroid. Combined cross-sectional and *en face* OCT imaging demonstrates pachychoroid features.[11,38,45]

The largest expansion in the literature has been seen in papers originating from South-East Asia and the Far East, where the incidence of sub-RPE aneurysms (polypoidal lesions) appears to be particularly high, and where PCV has often been considered and studied as a variant of neovascular AMD, accounting for as much as 22–62% of neovascular AMD.[46-53] More recently, Wong and associates have published a comparative treatise on AMD and PCV and reviewed the evidence from genetic, proteomic and imaging studies to review and update this definition. They have noted from work by Chen et al. and Ma et al. that although several risk-conferring alleles are shared between neovascular AMD and PCV, differential expression is seen at certain loci and might account for an increased tendency for more hemorrhagic phenotypes.[54,55] It is likely, therefore, that many of the alleles considered to predict neovascular AMD might actually determine neovascularization in a more generic sense, as supported by a study from our group examining risk allele expression in patients with pachychoroid disease.[56]

The natural history of aneurysmal type 1 neovascularization is characterized by exudative and hemorrhagic complications if left untreated. Hemorrhage can be of greater volume than that seen in nonaneurysmal type 1 neovascularization and can cause breakthrough vitreous hemorrhage.

Treatment and Prognosis

Although the visual prognosis for PCV is considered better than that of neovascular AMD, the incidence of sub-RPE and subretinal hemorrhage is as high as 30–64%.[52,57] Management aims are early detection, suppression of neovascularization and treatment of aneurysmal (polypoidal) lesions to prevent serosanguinous complications.

Photodynamic therapy is a well-established treatment for aneurysmal type 1 neovascularization (PCV) and has been shown to control the exudative component of the disease and to improve visual acuity in about 50% of treated patients by up to 8 ETDRS letters.[58-65]

The PDT spot size is traditionally determined by the greatest linear dimension of the lesion based on FA, but several authors have reported good results using greatest linear dimensions determined from ICGA.[59,61,65]

Complications of PDT in target tissues include:

- Choriocapillaris ischemia.
- Recurrence of aneurysmal (polypoidal) lesions from surviving branching vascular networks in 5–8% of treated cases.[62,64]
- Hemorrhagic complications in up to a third of patients treated for aneurysmal type 1 neovascularization (PCV).[60,66] Hemorrhage can occasionally be massive and can cause vitreous hemorrhage.[67]
- Recurrent bullous retinal detachment in patients with aneurysmal type 1 neovascularization.[68]
- Chorioretinal anastomosis.[69]
- Upregulation of VEGF expression with accelerated neovascularization.[61,70]

The EVEREST I study was the first randomized controlled trial (RCT) designed to determine the role of anti-VEGF therapy in aneurysmal type 1 neovascularization (PCV).[71] Sixty-one Asian patients were randomized to verteporfin PDT (standard fluence), ranibizumab 0.5%, or a combination. At baseline all patients underwent PDT or placebo, followed by 3 monthly ranibizumab or sham injections. Treatments were to be continued thereafter based on preset criteria, including a minimum 90-day interval before repeat PDT could be considered. The primary outcome measure was regression of aneurysmal (polypoidal) lesions. At 6 months, PDT and combination therapy were more effective (71.4% and 77.8%, respectively) than ranibizumab monotherapy (28.6%). The mean improvement in visual acuity was greatest in the combination arm (10.9 ± 10.9 letters) compared with either PDT monotherapy or (7.5 ± 10.6 letters) or ranibizumab monotherapy (9.2 ± 12.4).

EVEREST II and PLANET were large RCTs reporting on visual outcomes in aneurysmal type 1 neovascularization (PCV) treated with anti-VEGF and combination therapy, and providing level 1 evidence to guide optimal management (Lee et al.,[64] efficacy and safety of intravitreal aflibercept in polypoidal choroidal vasculopathy: 12-month results of the PLANET study, Association for Research in Vision and Ophthalmology, 2017).[72] The mean number of injections was 7.3 (EVEREST-II) and 8.1 (PLANET). Both studies reported significant visual acuity gain in the monotherapy arms at 1 year (+5.1 letters in EVEREST, +10.8 letters in PLANET). The regression rate for aneurysmal (polypoidal) lesions was 34.7% (EVEREST-II) and 38.9% (PLANET). Disease quiescence at 12 months was seen in 51% of eyes in EVEREST II and 81.7% of eyes in PLANET. The DRAGON study was a phase IV randomized, double-masked multicenter study based in China which enrolled 334 patients with aneurysmal type 1 neovascularization (PCV) and compared the efficacy of ranibizumab monotherapy administered by fixed dosing versus a *pro re nata* regimen (Li et al., Ranibizumab 0.5 mg for neovascular age-related macular degeneration: monthly versus as needed dosing in the DRAGON study, American Academy of Ophthalmology, 2016). Both arms achieved visual gains, supporting the results of EVEREST I and II. Visual acuity gains at 12 months were 12.3 letters for monthly dosing and 9.6 letter for *pro re nata* dosing, but this difference was not found to be statistically significant.

Peripapillary Pachychoroid Syndrome

Peripapillary pachychoroid syndrome has been described by Phasukkijwatana and associates as a newly detected disease variant in which the same group of manifestations are seen as in other pachychoroid entities, but in which maximal choroidal thickness occurs close to the optic disk rather than the fovea.[73] The corresponding sequelae at the level of the RPE and outer retina (pigment epitheliopathy, subretinal fluid, gravitating autofluorescence tracks) are localized to the peripapillary region (Fig. 51.9). From a series of 31 study eyes of 16 patients, the authors also noted that 77% had choroidal folds, 39% had axial lengths less than 23 mm and 80% had hyperopic refractive errors. None of the subjects had inflammatory eye disease, and the cluster of findings was felt to be distinct from uveal effusion syndrome by the absence of any detectable choroidal detachment.

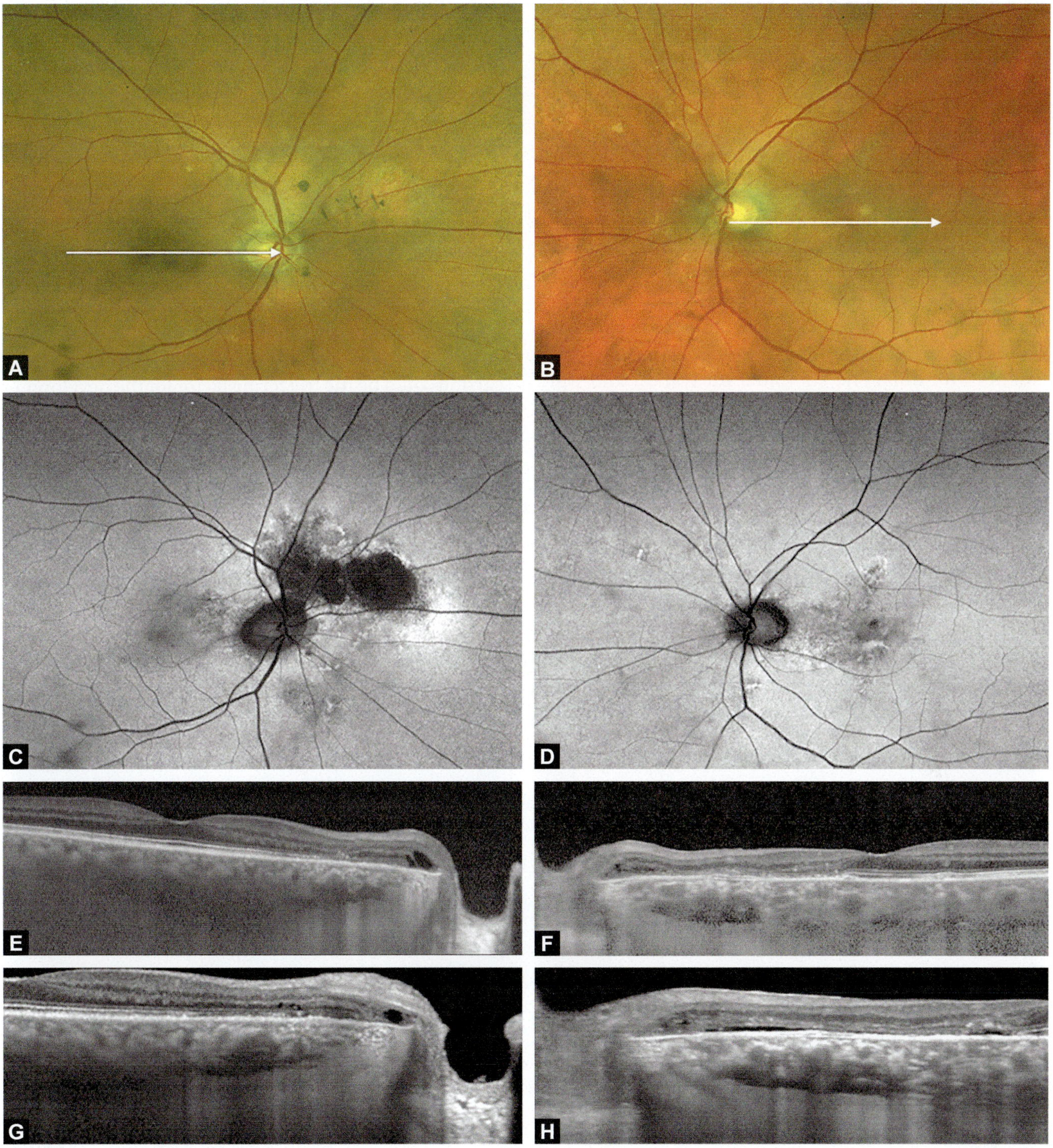

Figs. 51.9A to H: Peripapillary pachychoroid syndrome. (A and B) Color photographs show retinal pigment epithelial (RPE) changes located mainly around the optic disks; (C and D) Fundus autofluorescence shows RPE changes more clearly; (E to H) Spectral domain optical coherence tomographies show diffuse choroidal thickening but also show focal choroidal thickening in the peripapillary region. Atrophic complications at the level of the RPE and outer retina, as well as pathologic dilatation of Haller's layer vessels, is seen in the peripapillary region of both eyes, with some temporal extension in the left eye.

FOCAL CHOROIDAL EXCAVATION

Focal choroidal excavation (FCE) refers to a localized concavity seen in the choroid on cross-sectional OCT, in the absence of staphyloma and scleral ectasia. The choroid is selectively and focally thinned, with tissue loss, but the hyper-reflective band corresponding to the RPE-Bruch's membrane complex and the anterior retina are generally preserved. The retina itself may follow the depressed contour of the RPE (conforming) or may appear suspended (nonconforming), resulting in a hyporeflective subretinal space.

This lesion was first discussed by Jampol and associates in 2006, in the journal Retina, as a diagnostic and therapeutic challenge.[74] In 2010, Wakabayashi et al. described three patients with unilateral choroidal excavation and were the first group to distinguish between the conforming and nonconforming configurations.[75] In 2011, Margolis et al. first used the term FCE to describe the lesion in a wider spectrum of patients.[76] They described 12 patients, all of whom were myopic with thick choroids in the absence of inflammation.

The etiology of FCE remains unknown. Similarly, the natural history is poorly characterized since most reports have not included longitudinal data. In 2017, Chung and colleagues published a review on FCE and of the preceding literature, representing a total of 189 eyes of 168 patients.[75-86] They noted that the majority of patients in the combined meta-analysis were myopic and had thick choroids and that the majority of reports were of FCE detected in the context of CSC, with or without choroidal neovascularization.

Several studies have reported FCE to be associated with inflammatory diseases including multifocal choroiditis/punctate inner choroidopathy (MFC/PIC), which supports the hypothesis that FCE is *acquired*.[87] Kim et al. retrospectively reviewed 54 eyes with MFC/PIC and found FCE in 20%.[88] They hypothesized the focal inflammation of the RPE and inner choroid and subsequent inner choroidal scarring could be the triggering factor for the development of FCE in patients with MFC/PIC. Corbelli and associates described FCE associated with inflammatory choroidal neovascularization, with a favorable course after oral steroid treatment (Fig. 51.10).[89]

The mechanisms which might link FCE with CSC remain elusive. It is unclear whether an acquired form of FCE occurs due to CSC, or whether a localized form CSC might present in the vicinity of FCE. The two possibilities

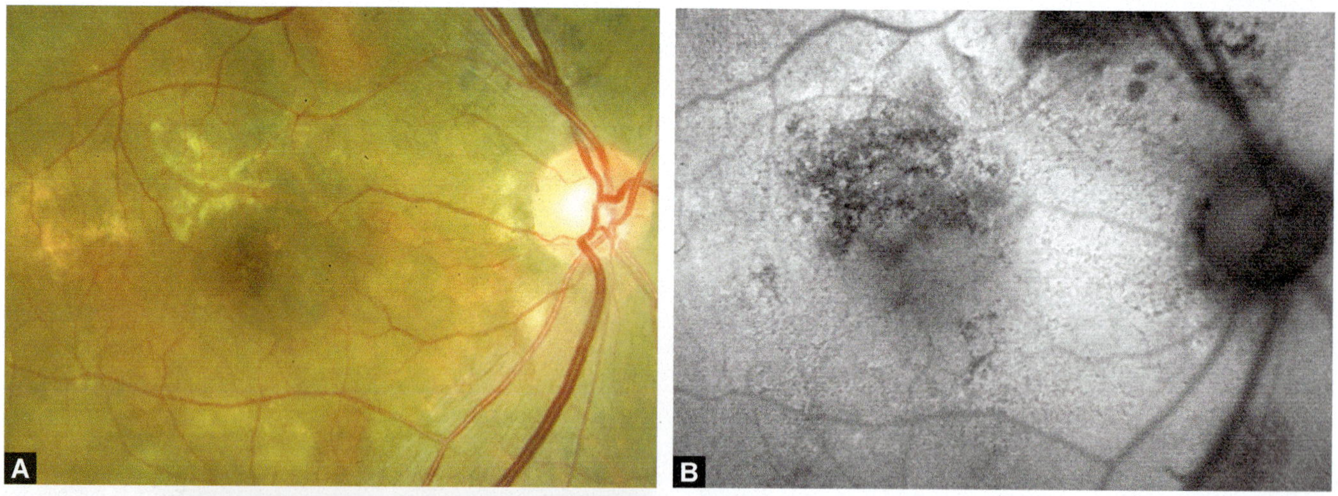

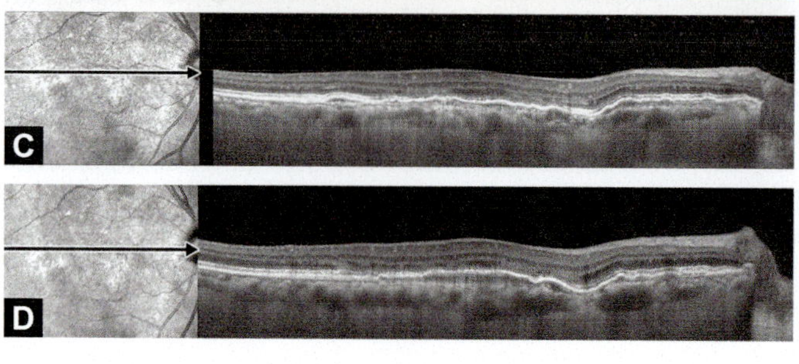

Figs. 51.10A to D: Focal choroidal excavation (FCE). (A and B) Color photography and fundus autofluorescence show extensive retinal pigment epithelial (RPE) changes in the perifoveal region and superior to the papillomacular area; (C and D) Spectral domain optical coherence tomographies show a cavitary lesion of the choroid, into the contour of which the RPE and neurosensory retina conform. Pathologically dilated Haller's layer vessels are seen immediately adjacent to the site of FCE; (D) Shallow RPE detachment from Bruch's membrane is detected.

are not mutually exclusive. In the latter case, it is possible that the inner choroidal thinning at the borders of the excavation results in shunting of blood flow and dilation of neighboring Haller's layer vessels to resemble pachyvessels. It is for this reason that a mechanistic relationship has been proposed between FCE and other pachychoroid disorders.[77]

DIFFERENTIAL DIAGNOSES

Central Serous Chorioretinopathy

- Choroidal hemangioma
- Uveal effusion syndrome
- Cavitary optic disk anomaly (optic disk pit)
- Vogt-Koyanagi-Harada disease
- Chorioretinopathy associated with inhibitors of mitogen-activated protein kinase-kinase (MEK) enzymes
- Bullous rhegmatogenous retinal detachment (mimicking bullous CSC variant).

Pachychoroid Pigment Epitheliopathy

- Age-related macular degeneration
- Pattern dystrophy
- Early stages of cone-rod dystrophy.

Aneurysmal Type 1 Neovascularization (Polypoidal Choroidal Vasculopathy)

- Neovascular AMD
- Causes of fundus obscuring vitreous hemorrhage, such as:
  - Retinal macroaneurysm
  - Branch retinal vein occlusion
  - Hemorrhagic posterior vitreous detachment with or without rhegmatogenous retinal detachment
  - Trauma
- Myopic staphyloma and dome-shaped maculopathy (*see* Chapter 52).

Aneurysmal lesions arising from type 1 neovascular networks have been observed in contexts which are not necessarily subsets of pachychoroid and CSC, but in which the *mechanisms* underlying neovascularization are likely to be related. Examples include myopic staphyloma[40] and dome-shaped maculopathy[41] as well as choroidal nevi. In these contexts, as with pachychoroid, inner choroidal attenuation is seen with associated dilatation of Haller's layer vessels at the site where the neovascular process seems to begin.

CONCLUSION

This composition and layout of this chapter differs from that seen in most of the established textbook literature. This is because it takes into account recent developments in multimodal imaging and recent findings from the last 5–10 years which have necessitated re-examination of the classification schemes for CSC and entities to which it appears to be related.

Advances in imaging have enabled better characterization of the choroid in patients with CSC and have led to discoveries that similar choroidal features are seen in patients with a pigmentary precursor of CSC—pachychoroid pigment epitheliopathy—and with the neovascular variants—pachychoroid neovasculopathy and aneurysmal type 1 neovascularization (formerly polypoidal choroidal neovasculopathy). This family of conditions appears therefore to represent a phenotypic spectrum.

However, the key features of pachychoroid—inner choroidal attenuation and pathologic dilatation of Haller's layer vessels to form "pachy vessels"—have also been observed in patients with conditions which are etiologically unrelated to CSC, namely myopic staphyloma, dome-shaped maculopathy and choroidal nevi. This has opened the discussion further on whether pachychoroid represents a phenotypic spectrum or a step forwards in understanding choroidal hemodynamics and disease mechanisms in a more generic sense. Future research is focused in this direction.

REFERENCES

1. von Graefe A. Ueber centrale recidivierende retinitis. Graefes Arch Clin Exp Ophthalmol. 1866;12:211-5.
2. Bennett G. Central serous retinopathy. Br J Ophthalmol. 1955;39:605-18.
3. Maumenee AE. Serous and hemorrhagic disciform detachment of the macula. Trans Pac Coast Oto Ophthalmol Soc Annu Meet. 1959;40:139-60.
4. Sahu DK, Namperumalsamy P, Hilton GF, et al. Bullous variant of idiopathic central serous chorioretinopathy. Br J Ophthalmol. 2000;84:485-92.
5. Kitzmann AS, Pulido JS, Diehl NN, et al. The incidence of central serous chorioretinopathy in Olmsted County, Minnesota, 1980-2002. Ophthalmology. 2008;115:169-73.
6. Spaide RF, Campeas L, Haas A, et al. Central serous chorioretinopathy in younger and older adults. Ophthalmology. 1996;103:2070-9.
7. Spaide RF, Klancnik JM Jr. Fundus autofluorescence and central serous chorioretinopathy. Ophthalmology. 2005;112:825-33.
8. Yannuzzi LA, Slakter JS, Kaufman SR, et al. Laser treatment of diffuse retinal pigment epitheliopathy. Eur J Ophthalmol. 1992;2:103-14.

9. Dansingani KK, Balaratnasingam C, Mrejen S, et al. Annular lesions and catenary forms in chronic central serous chorioretinopathy. Am J Ophthalmol. 2016;166:60-7.
10. Spaide RF, Koizumi H, Pozzoni MC, et al. Enhanced depth imaging spectral-domain optical coherence tomography. Am J Ophthalmol. 2008;146:496-500.
11. Dansingani KK, Balaratnasingam C, Naysan J, et al. En face imaging of pachychoroid spectrum disorders with swept-source optical coherence tomography. Retina. 2016;36:499-516.
12. Otsuka S, Ohba N, Nakao K. A long-term follow-up study of severe variant of central serous chorioretinopathy. Retina. 2002;22:25-32.
13. Balaratnasingam C, Freund KB, Tan AM, et al. Bullous variant of central serous chorioretinopathy: expansion of phenotypic features using multimethod imaging. Ophthalmology. 2016;123:1541-52.
14. Inoue M, Jung JJ, Balaratnasingam C, et al. A comparison between optical coherence tomography angiography and fluorescein angiography for the imaging of type 1 neovascularization. Invest Ophthalmol Vis Sci. 2016;57:314-23.
15. Sato T, Kishi S, Watanabe G, et al. Tomographic features of branching vascular networks in polypoidal choroidal vasculopathy. Retina. 2007;27:589-94.
16. Spaide RF. Disease expression in nonexudative age-related macular degeneration varies with choroidal thickness. Retina. 2018;38(4):708-16.
17. Carvalho-Recchia CA, Yannuzzi LA, Negrão S, et al. Corticosteroids and central serous chorioretinopathy. Ophthalmology. 2002;109:1834-7.
18. Imamura Y, Fujiwara T, Margolis R, et al. Enhanced depth imaging optical coherence tomography of the choroid in central serous chorioretinopathy. Retina. 2009;29:1469-73.
19. Jirarattanasopa P, Ooto S, Tsujikawa A, et al. Assessment of macular choroidal thickness by optical coherence tomography and angiographic changes in central serous chorioretinopathy. Ophthalmology. 2012;119:1666-78.
20. Maruko I, Iida T, Sugano Y, et al. Subfoveal choroidal thickness in fellow eyes of patients with central serous chorioretinopathy. Retina. 2011;31:1603-8.
21. Zhao M, Valamanesh F, Celerier I, et al. The neuroretina is a novel mineralocorticoid target: aldosterone up-regulates ion and water channels in Müller glial cells. FASEB J. 2010;24:3405-15.
22. Zhao M, Célérier I, Bousquet E, et al. Mineralocorticoid receptor is involved in rat and human ocular chorioretinopathy. J Clin Invest. 2012;122:2672-9.
23. Bousquet E, Beydoun T, Zhao M, et al. Mineralocorticoid receptor antagonism in the treatment of chronic central serous chorioretinopathy: a pilot study. Retina. 2013;33:2096-102.
24. Klein ML, Van Buskirk EM, Friedman E, et al. Experience with nontreatment of central serous choroidopathy. Arch Ophthalmol. 1974;91:247-50.
25. Mudvari SS, Goff MJ, Fu AD, et al. The natural history of pigment epithelial detachment associated with central serous chorioretinopathy. Retina. 2007;27:1168-73.
26. Aggio FB, Roisman L, Melo GB, et al. Clinical factors related to visual outcome in central serous chorioretinopathy. Retina. 2010;30:1128-34.
27. Yannuzzi LA. Central serous chorioretinopathy: a personal perspective. Am J Ophthalmol. 2010;149:361-3.
28. Verma L, Sinha R, Venkatesh P, et al. Comparative evaluation of diode laser versus argon laser photocoagulation in patients with central serous retinopathy: a pilot, randomized controlled trial [ISRCTN84128484]. BMC Ophthalmol. 2004;4:15.
29. Liu HY, Yang CH, Yang CM, et al. Half-dose versus half-time photodynamic therapy for central serous chorioretinopathy. Am J Ophthalmol. 2016;167:57-64.
30. Lai FHP, Ng DS, Bakthavatsalam M, et al. A multicenter study on the long-term outcomes of half-dose photodynamic therapy in chronic central serous chorioretinopathy. Am J Ophthalmol. 2016;170:91-9.
31. Mehta PH, Meyerle C, Sivaprasad S, et al. Preferred practice pattern in central serous chorioretinopathy. Br J Ophthalmol. 2017;101:587-90.
32. Lim JI, Glassman AR, Aiello LP, et al. Collaborative retrospective macula society study of photodynamic therapy for chronic central serous chorioretinopathy. Ophthalmology. 2014;121:1073-8.
33. Erikitola OC, Crosby-Nwaobi R, Lotery AJ, et al. Photodynamic therapy for central serous chorioretinopathy. Eye. 2014;28:944-57.
34. Spaide RF. Optical coherence tomography angiography signs of vascular abnormalization with antiangiogenic therapy for choroidal neovascularization. Am J Ophthalmol. 2015;160(1):6-16.
35. Pitcher JD 3rd, Witkin AJ, DeCroos FC, Ho AC. A prospective pilot study of intravitreal aflibercept for the treatment of chronic central serous chorioretinopathy: the CONTAIN study. Br J Ophthalmol. 2015;99:848-52.
36. Ghadiali Q, Jung JJ, Yu S, et al. Central serous chorioretinopathy treated with mineralocorticoid antagonists: a one-year pilot study. Retina. 2016;36:611-8.
37. Warrow DJ, Hoang QV, Freund KB. Pachychoroid pigment epitheliopathy. Retina. 2013;33:1659-72.
38. Pang CE, Freund KB. Pachychoroid neovasculopathy. Retina. 2015;35:1-9.
39. Lee WK, Baek J, Dansingani KK, et al. Choroidal morphology in eyes with polypoidal choroidal vasculopathy and normal or subnormal subfoveal choroidal thickness. Retina. 2016;36(Suppl 1):S73-82.
40. Tan ACS, Yzer S, Freund KB, et al. Choroidal changes associated with serous macular detachment in eyes with staphyloma, dome-shaped macula or tilted disk syndrome. Retina. 2017;37:1544-54.
41. Naysan J, Dansingani KK, Balaratnasingam C, et al. Type 1 neovascularization with polypoidal lesions complicating dome shaped macula. Int J Retin Vitr. 2015;1:909.
42. Yannuzzi LA, Sorenson J, Spaide RF, et al. Idiopathic polypoidal choroidal vasculopathy (IPCV). Retina. 1990;10:1-8.
43. Kleiner RC, Brucker AJ, Johnston RL. The posterior uveal bleeding syndrome. Retina. 1990;10:9-17.

44. Stern RM, Zakov ZN, Zegarra H, et al. Multiple recurrent serosanguineous retinal pigment epithelial detachments in black women. Am J Ophthalmol. 1985;100:560-9.
45. Dansingani KK, Balaratnasingam C, Klufas MA, et al. Optical coherence tomography angiography of shallow irregular pigment epithelial detachments in pachychoroid spectrum disease. Am J Ophthalmol. 2015;160:1243-54.e2.
46. Byeon SH, Lee SC, Oh HS, et al. Incidence and clinical patterns of polypoidal choroidal vasculopathy in Korean patients. Jpn J Ophthalmol. 2008;52:57-62.
47. Chang YC, Wu WC. Polypoidal choroidal vasculopathy in Taiwanese patients. Ophthalmic Surg Lasers Imaging. 2009;40:576-81.
48. Li Y, You QS, Wei WB, et al. Polypoidal choroidal vasculopathy in adult Chinese: the Beijing Eye Study. Ophthalmology. 2014;121:2290-1.
49. Liu Y, Wen F, Huang S, et al. Subtype lesions of neovascular age-related macular degeneration in Chinese patients. Graefes Arch Clin Exp Ophthalmol. 2007;245:1441-5.
50. Maruko I, Iida T, Saito M, et al. Clinical characteristics of exudative age-related macular degeneration in Japanese patients. Am J Ophthalmol. 2007;144:15-22.
51. Mori K, Horie-Inoue K, Gehlbach PL, et al. Phenotype and genotype characteristics of age-related macular degeneration in a Japanese population. Ophthalmology. 2010;117:928-38.
52. Sho K, Takahashi K, Yamada H, et al. Polypoidal choroidal vasculopathy: incidence, demographic features, and clinical characteristics. Arch Ophthalmol. 2003;121:1392-6.
53. Wen F, Chen C, Wu D, Li H. Polypoidal choroidal vasculopathy in elderly Chinese patients. Graefes Arch Clin Exp Ophthalmol. 2004;242:625-9.
54. Chen H, Liu K, Chen LJ, et al. Genetic associations in polypoidal choroidal vasculopathy: a systematic review and meta-analysis. Mol Vis. 2012;18:816-29.
55. Ma L, Li Z, Liu K, et al. Association of genetic variants with polypoidal choroidal vasculopathy. Ophthalmology. 2015;122:1854-65.
56. Dansingani KK, Perlee LT, Hamon S, et al. Risk alleles associated with neovascularization in a pachychoroid phenotype. Ophthalmology. 2016;123:2628-30.
57. Yoon JS, Lee J, Lee SC, et al. Polypoidal choroidal vasculopathy in Korean patients with large submacular hemorrhage. Yonsei Med J. 2007;48:225-32.
58. Spaide RF, Donsoff I, Lam DL, et al. Treatment of polypoidal choroidal vasculopathy with photodynamic therapy. Retina. 2002;22:529-35.
59. Chan WM, Lam DSC, Lai TYY, et al. Photodynamic therapy with verteporfin for symptomatic polypoidal choroidal vasculopathy: one-year results of a prospective case series. Ophthalmology. 2004;111:1576-84.
60. Akaza E, Mori R, Yuzawa M. Long-term results of photodynamic therapy of polypoidal choroidal vasculopathy. Retina. 2008;28:717-22.
61. Eandi CM, Ober MD, Freund KB, et al. Selective photodynamic therapy for neovascular age-related macular degeneration with polypoidal choroidal neovascularization. Retina. 2007;27:825-31.
62. Gomi F, Ohji M, Sayanagi K, et al. One-year outcomes of photodynamic therapy in age-related macular degeneration and polypoidal choroidal vasculopathy in Japanese patients. Ophthalmology. 2008;115:141-6.
63. Kurashige Y, Otani A, Sasahara M, et al. Two-year results of photodynamic therapy for polypoidal choroidal vasculopathy. Am J Ophthalmol. 2008;146:513-9.
64. Lee WK, Lee PY, Lee SK. Photodynamic therapy for polypoidal choroidal vasculopathy: vaso-occlusive effect on the branching vascular network and origin of recurrence. Jpn J Ophthalmol. 2008;52:108-15.
65. Otani A, Sasahara M, Yodoi Y, et al. Indocyanine green angiography: guided photodynamic therapy for polypoidal choroidal vasculopathy. Am J Ophthalmol. 2007;144:7-14.
66. Hirami Y, Tsujikawa A, Otani A, et al. Hemorrhagic complications after photodynamic therapy for polypoidal choroidal vasculopathy. Retina. 2007;27:335-41.
67. Ojima Y, Tsujikawa A, Otani A, et al. Recurrent bleeding after photodynamic therapy in polypoidal choroidal vasculopathy. Am J Ophthalmol. 2006;141:958-60.
68. Prakash M, Han DP. Recurrent bullous retinal detachments from photodynamic therapy for idiopathic polypoidal choroidal vasculopathy. Am J Ophthalmol. 2006;142:1079-81.
69. Yodoi Y, Tsujikawa A, Otani A, et al. Chorioretinal anastomosis after photodynamic therapy for polypoidal choroidal vasculopathy. Int Ophthalmol. 2008;28:297-9.
70. Schmidt-Erfurth U, Schlötzer-Schrehard U, Cursiefen C, et al. Influence of photodynamic therapy on expression of vascular endothelial growth factor (VEGF), VEGF receptor 3, and pigment epithelium-derived factor. Invest Ophthalmol Vis Sci. 2003;44:4473-80.
71. Koh A, Lee WK, Chen LJ, et al. EVEREST study: efficacy and safety of verteporfin photodynamic therapy in combination with ranibizumab or alone versus ranibizumab monotherapy in patients with symptomatic macular polypoidal choroidal vasculopathy. Retina. 2012;32:1453-64.
72. Koh A, Lai TYY, Takahashi K, et al. Efficacy and safety of ranibizumab with or without verteporfin photodynamic therapy for polypoidal choroidal vasculopathy: a randomized clinical trial. JAMA Ophthalmol. 2017;135(11):1206-13.
73. Phasukkijwatana N, Freund KB, Dolz-Marco R, et al. Peripapillary pachychoroid syndrome. Retina. 2017.
74. Jampol LM, Shankle J, Schroeder R, et al. Diagnostic and therapeutic challenges. Retina. 2006;26:1072-6.
75. Wakabayashi Y, Nishimura A, Higashide T, et al. Unilateral choroidal excavation in the macula detected by spectral-domain optical coherence tomography. Acta Ophthalmol. 2010;88:e87-91.
76. Margolis R, Mukkamala SK, Jampol LM, et al. The expanded spectrum of focal choroidal excavation. Arch Ophthalmol. 2011;129:1320-5.
77. Chung H, Byeon SH, Freund KB. Focal choroidal excavation and its association with pachychoroid spectrum disorders: a review of the literature and multimodal imaging findings. Retina. 2017;37:199-221.
78. Shinojima A, Kawamura A, Mori R, et al. Morphologic features of focal choroidal excavation on spectral domain

optical coherence tomography with simultaneous angiography. Retina. 2014;34:1407-14.
79. Ellabban AA, Tsujikawa A, Ooto S, et al. Focal choroidal excavation in eyes with central serous chorioretinopathy. Am J Ophthalmol. 2013;156:673-83.
80. Lim FPM, Wong CW, Loh BK, et al. Prevalence and clinical correlates of focal choroidal excavation in eyes with age-related macular degeneration, polypoidal choroidal vasculopathy and central serous chorioretinopathy. Br J Ophthalmol. 2016;100:918-23.
81. Obata R, Takahashi H, Ueta T, et al. Tomographic and angiographic characteristics of eyes with macular focal choroidal excavation. Retina. 2013;33:1201-10.
82. Kuroda Y, Tsujikawa A, Ooto S, et al. Association of focal choroidal excavation with age-related macular degeneration. Invest Ophthalmol Vis Sci. 2014;55:6046-54.
83. Lee CS, Woo SJ, Kim YK, et al. Clinical and spectral-domain optical coherence tomography findings in patients with focal choroidal excavation. Ophthalmology. 2014;121:1029-35.
84. Xu H, Zeng F, Shi D, et al. Focal choroidal excavation complicated by choroidal neovascularization. Ophthalmology. 2014;121:246-50.
85. Lee JH, Lee WK. Choroidal neovascularization associated with focal choroidal excavation. Am J Ophthalmol. 2014;157:710-8.e1.
86. Suzuki M, Gomi F, Hara C, et al. Characteristics of central serous chorioretinopathy complicated by focal choroidal excavation. Retina. 2014;34:1216-22.
87. Hashimoto Y, Saito W, Noda K, et al. Acquired focal choroidal excavation associated with multiple evanescent white dot syndrome: observations at onset and a pathogenic hypothesis. BMC Ophthalmol. 2014;14:135.
88. Kim H, Woo SJ, Kim YK, et al. Focal choroidal excavation in multifocal choroiditis and punctate inner choroidopathy. Ophthalmology. 2015;122:1534-5.
89. Corbelli E, Sacconi R, Querques L, et al. Clinical course of inflammatory choroidal neovascularization associated with focal choroidal excavation. Retin Cases Brief Rep. 2017.

Chapter 52 Pathologic Myopia

Colin S Tan, Srinivas R Sadda

EPIDEMIOLOGY

Myopia, also known as *shortsightedness* or *nearsightedness*, is commonly defined as a spherical equivalent of -0.5 diopters or higher. The prevalence of myopia worldwide is estimated to be 22.9%,[1-4] but it varies considerably with geography, ethnicity and age (Table 52.1). It is very high in Asian countries such as Japan, Singapore and Taiwan, where the prevalence of myopia among young adults varies between 41.8% and 90%.[2,5,6]

In contrast, the prevalence of myopia is lower in countries such as Australia and China, where it ranges from 14.0% to 22.9%.

High Myopia

High myopia is defined as a spherical equivalent -6 diopters or higher or an axial length more than or equal to 26.5 mm and occurs in 2.7% of the world's population.[1] While the prevalence of high myopia in the United States was found to be 3.92% among adults aged 18 and older,[7] it was much higher in Taiwan, occurring in 21% of 18-year olds and 40% of college freshmen.[2] A 2015 study reported a prevalence of about 80% for myopia, and about 10% for high myopia, among students aged 16–18 years attending classes of grade 10 and 11 in a Chinese metropolitan region.[6]

Pathologic Myopia

Pathologic myopia (also known as *degenerative myopia*) is defined as high myopia with myopia-specific pathology arising from axial elongation.[8] The frequency of pathologic myopia has been reported as 0.33% in the United States,[7] 1.2% in Australia,[9] and from 0.9% to 3.1% among Asian populations.[10] This was significantly higher than the reported prevalence (<0.2%) among children and adolescents.[11]

Several risk factors have been identified for the development of myopia. These include increased near work, education level and IQ, duration of outdoor activity, exposure to bright light, and genetic factors.

Table 52.1: Prevalence of myopia, high myopia and pathologic myopia among different populations.

	Myopia (%)	High myopia (%)	Pathologic myopia (%)
United States	33.1% (>20 years)	3.92% (>18 years)[7] 11.8% in American Chinese population[12]	0.33%[7]
United Kingdom	49% (>44 years)		
Australia	14% (40–97 years)		
Norway	35% (20–25 years)		
Taiwan	86.1% (18–24 years) 19.4% (>65 years)	21% (18 years) 40% (college freshmen)[2]	
China	22.9% (40–90 years)		
Japan	41.8% (younger adults)		
India	34.6% (>40 years)		
Singapore	38.7% (Chinese >40 years) 26.2% (Malay >40 years) 28.0% (Indian >40 years)		
Indonesia	48.1% (>21 years)		
Overall			0.9–3.1%[10]

Myopia is associated with significant healthcare costs. In the United States, the cost of detection and treatment of refractive error (including glasses, contact lenses or refractive surgery) exceeds US$ 3.8 billion annually.[13] In Singapore, the annual cost of treatment of myopia is estimated to be US$ 755 million per year.[14]

In addition to the economic burden, myopia has been shown to significantly affect a person's quality of life and may have an impact on both professional and leisure activities.

ANATOMIC CHANGES IN THE EYE ASSOCIATED WITH PATHOLOGIC MYOPIA

Retinal Thickness

Studies using optical coherence tomography (OCT) have shown that peripheral retinal thickness decreases with worsening severity of myopia.[15-18] The retina in the parafoveal subfields thins progressively as the spherical equivalent becomes more negative.[15-18] In contrast, the thickness of the central subfield (the 1 mm zone centered on the fovea) does not vary as significantly with myopia.[15,18,19] Myopic axial globe elongation is associated with retinal thinning in the equatorial and pre-equatorial region, while foveal retinal thickness remains mostly unaffected by axial length. This difference suggests that axial elongation takes place predominantly in the equatorial and pre-equatorial region of the eye.[20] Retinal thinning is associated with stretching and wider spacing of the photoreceptors and neurons in the retina.[21,22]

Choroidal Thickness

In contrast to retinal thickness, choroidal thickness throughout the macula has been shown to vary with spherical equivalent and axial length.[23-26] As the severity of myopia worsens, the choroid thins progressively. In one study of young adults, the mean central subfield choroidal thickness varied from 253.8 μm among high myopes to 457.4 μm among emmetropes.[24]

Effects of Retinal Thickness and Choroidal Thickness on Visual Acuity

Several studies have reported significant effects of retinal[18,27] and choroidal thickness[28] on best-corrected visual acuity (BCVA). In a large cohort study of 698 myopes and 148 emmetropes,[18] both spherical equivalent and retinal thickness were found to significantly affect BCVA under normal (photopic) and mesopic lighting conditions. For each diopter increase in myopia, mean BCVA decreased by 0.01 logMAR in photopic conditions and 0.02 logMAR in mesopic conditions (both $p < 0.001$). The mean BCVA was reduced by 0.05 logMAR ($p = 0.003$) and 0.04 logMAR ($p = 0.037$) in photopic and mesopic conditions, respectively, for each 100 μm decrease in retinal thickness.[18]

CLINICAL FEATURES OF PATHOLOGIC MYOPIA INVOLVING THE POSTERIOR POLE

Fundus Tessellation

In any eye with high myopia, the fundus may manifest with a tessellated appearance, due to the increased visibility of the underlying large choroidal vessels (Figs. 52.1A and B).

Chorioretinal Atrophy

Chorioretinal atrophy is defined as an area of atrophy involving both the retina and the underlying choroid. It may be generalized (Figs. 52.2A and B) or it may manifest

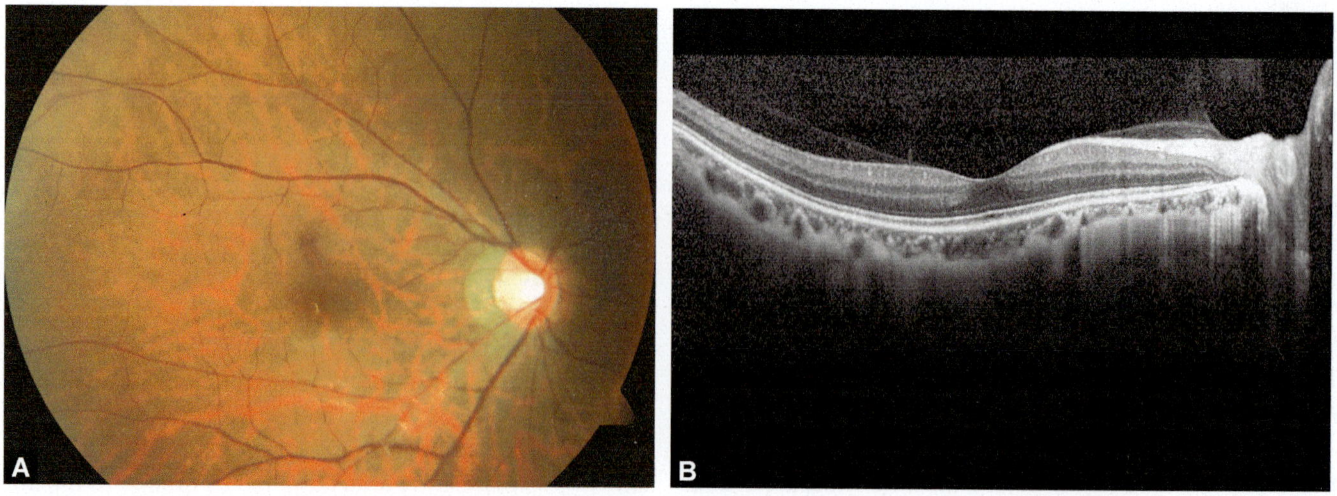

Figs. 52.1A and B: Myopic fundus. (A) Color fundus photograph illustrating a tessellated fundus. The optic disk is slightly tilted and there is surrounding peripapillary atrophy; (B) Optical coherence tomography scan of the same eye showing a normal retina and choroid.

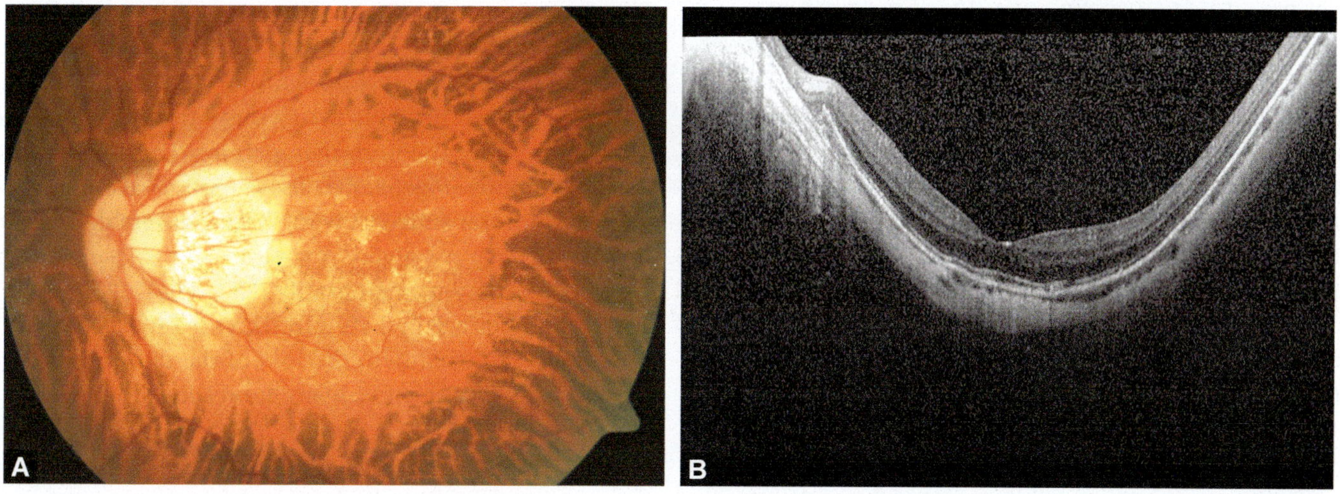

Figs. 52.2A and B: Diffuse atrophy. (A) Color fundus photograph. In addition to a tessellated fundus, there is diffuse atrophy, characterized by a region of hypopigmentation involving the macula. The optic disc is tilted, and there is a large area of peripapillary atrophy; (B) Optical coherence tomography scan showing curvature of the retinal pigment epithelium due to the presence of a staphyloma. While the retina thickness appears normal, the choroid is significantly thinned with loss of the choriocapillaris.

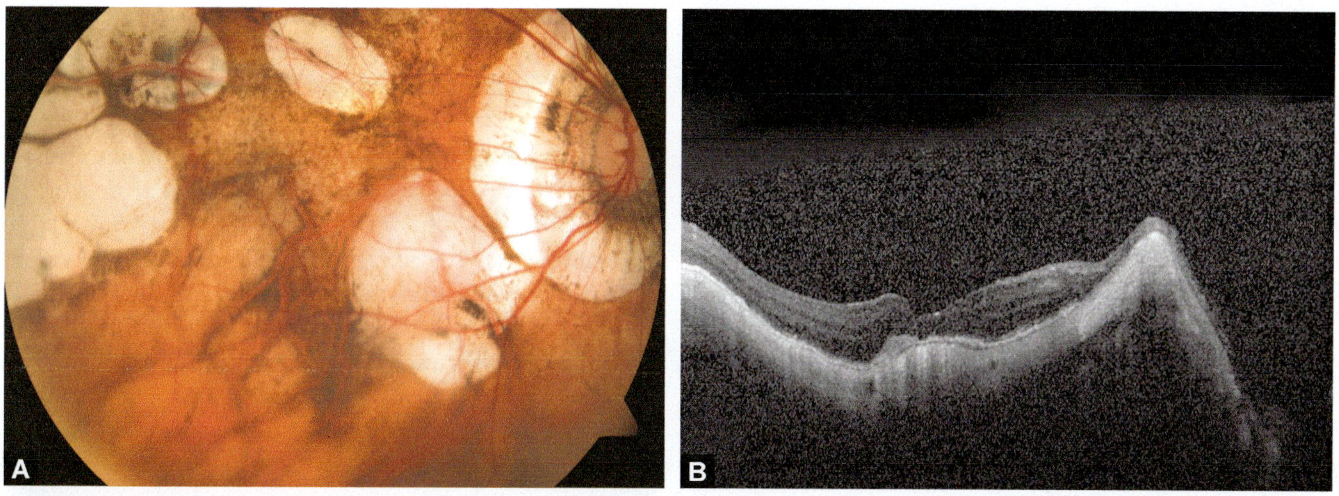

Figs. 52.3A and B: Patchy atrophy. (A) Color fundus photograph showing areas of patchy atrophy, characterized by pale regions with sharp borders. The large choroidal vessels are visible beneath the atrophy; (B) Optical coherence tomography scan showing a very thin choroid, with loss of the ellipsoid zone in some areas. There is also a dome-shaped macula.

as an oval or scallop-shaped region that is relatively pale compared to the surrounding retina and may be surrounded by a hyperpigmented border (Figs. 52.3A and B).

Chorioretinal atrophy is caused by stretching of the retina and choroid as a result of axial elongation of the eye.[29] The atrophy is believed to be due to obstruction of both the large and small choroidal vessels, which results in fibrous tissue formation and leads to photoreceptor cell death.

The frequency of chorioretinal atrophy increases with age[30] and with the prevalence of high myopia. It is among the most common clinical findings in adults with high myopia.[31,32] In a review of young Singaporean males with high myopia (mean age of 21.6 years), the prevalence of chorioretinal atrophy was 6.3%,[33] while among adults with high myopia aged 40 years and above, it was the second most common clinical finding, affecting 19.3% of the cohort.[31]

Classification of Chorioretinal Atrophy

Several classification systems have been devised to describe the clinical features of myopia.

Based on a classification described by Tokoro,[34] chorioretinal atrophy may be *patchy* or *diffuse*. *Patchy* atrophy manifests as gray-white, well-defined lesions. Small areas are termed *spotty atrophy* and may sometimes show slight pigmentary changes around the lesion. When the area of spotty atrophy is more than 0.5 optic disk diameters in size and forms a well-defined, round or oval lesion, it is known as *patchy atrophy* (Fig. 52.3A). Within the area of atrophy, the underlying large choroidal vessels are seen more clearly, due to the loss of the retinal pigment epithelium (RPE). An area of patchy atrophy may occur at the macula region, where it is termed *chorioretinal atrophy of the macula*.

In eyes with *diffuse* chorioretinal atrophy, the atrophy is typically seen as a yellow-white region at the posterior pole, often involving the macula and optic disk (Fig. 52.2).

Another classification scheme for chorioretinal atrophy was described by Steidl and Pruett,[35] with 5 grades of chorioretinal atrophy:

- *Grade 0*: No atrophic changes
- *Grade 1*: Attenuated choroidal vessels, lacquer crack formation, retinal pigment epithelium mottling, or a combination of these features
- *Grade 2*: Total area of chorioretinal atrophy ≤2 optic disk areas
- *Grade 3*: Total area of chorioretinal atrophy >2 disk areas but ≤ 4 disk areas
- *Grade 4*: Total area of chorioretinal atrophy >4 disk areas.

An international photographic classification system for myopic maculopathy was proposed in 2015.[36] The grades of myopic maculopathy are:

- *Category 0*: No myopic retinal degenerative lesion
- *Category 1*: Tessellated fundus
- *Category 2*: Diffuse chorioretinal atrophy
- *Category 3*: Patchy chorioretinal atrophy
- *Category 4*: Macular atrophy.

Imaging Characteristics of Chorioretinal Atrophy

Chorioretinal atrophy can be seen on color fundus photography as pale areas, with distinct borders and possible pigmentary changes occurring within or at the edges of the lesion (Fig. 52.3A).

The borders of the regions of atrophy are sometimes seen more distinctly on fundus autofluorescence (Fig. 52.4). The atrophy typically manifests as regions of hypo-autofluorescence due to the loss of the photoreceptors and RPE.

Optical coherence tomography shows loss of the ellipsoid zone and RPE-Bruch's membrane complex, with thinning of the underlying choroid and loss of the choriocapillaris (Fig. 52.3B). These regions also manifest as increased transmission with sharp borders due to loss of the RPE.

On fluorescein angiography (FA, Figs. 52.5A to C), regions of chorioretinal atrophy often manifest with early hypofluorescence due to the loss of the choriocapillaris (Fig. 52.5A). Subsequently, hyperfluorescence occurs in the late phases of the angiogram as a result of the increased transmission of fluorescence through the RPE window defect (Figs. 52.5B and C). In highly myopic eyes with patchy areas of chorioretinal atrophy, it may be challenging to distinguish whether hyperfluorescence is caused by leakage from choroidal neovascularization (CNV, discussed later), staining of scars or RPE transmission defects. It is important in these cases to correlate these findings with clinical examination or other imaging modalities, such as color fundus photography and OCT.

When indocyanine green angiography (ICGA) is performed (Fig. 52.6), chorioretinal atrophy manifests as regions of hypofluorescence, which appear darker due to the loss of the choriocapillaris and some of the larger choroidal vessels. The remaining large choroidal vessels are seen more clearly and may appear brighter compared to areas without atrophy. Due to the exposure of the choroidal vessels and the configuration of these vessels,

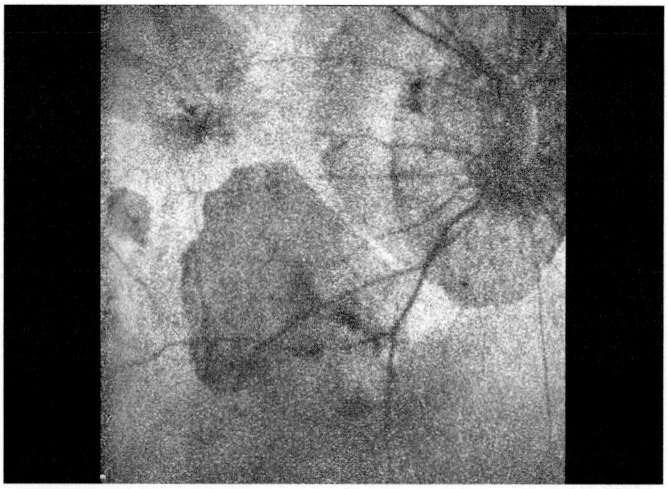

Fig. 52.4: Fundus autofluorescence of an eye with pathologic myopia, illustrating areas of hypoautofluorescence which correspond to regions of chorioretinal atrophy.

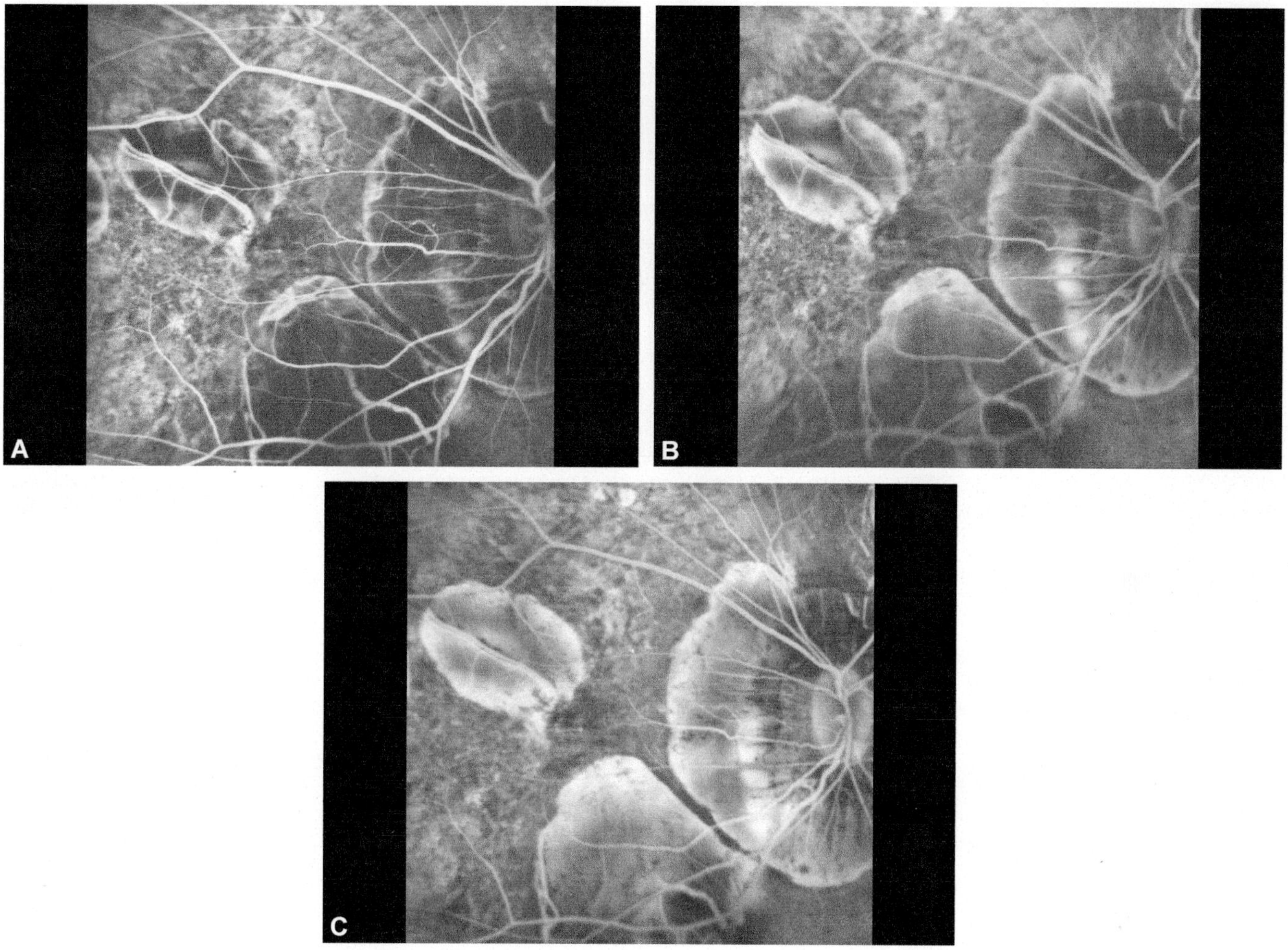

Figs. 52.5A to C: Fluorescein angiography (FA) of an eye with chorioretinal atrophy. (A) Early phase FA, showing areas of hypofluorescence which correspond to regions of patchy chorioretinal atrophy. The background fluorescence also appears irregular due to diffuse atrophy of the retinal pigment epithelium; (B) Mid phase FA. The areas of atrophy appear hyperfluorescent due to staining; (C) Late phase FA. Staining of the areas of atrophy is more pronounced.

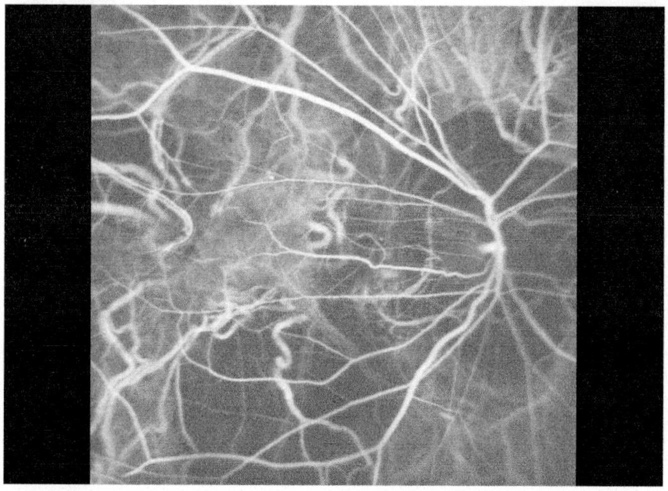

Fig. 52.6: Indocyanine green angiogram of the same eye as Figure 52.5. Some of the large choroidal vessels are visible in this angiogram.

some portions of the choroidal vessels may sometimes be mistaken for pathologic lesions such as polypoidal choroidal vasculopathy.[37]

Sequelae of Chorioretinal Atrophy

Progression of chorioretinal atrophy: Eyes with high myopia have been reported to progress from fundus tessellation to the development of diffuse atrophy and patchy atrophy, which may eventually involve the macula (macular atrophy).[38]

Choroidal neovascularization (Fig. 52.7A): It may develop in the region of breaks in the Bruch's membrane, which results in ischemia and upregulation of vascular endothelial growth factor (VEGF). In Japanese adults with high myopia, the risk of developing CNV was 17.7% among those with

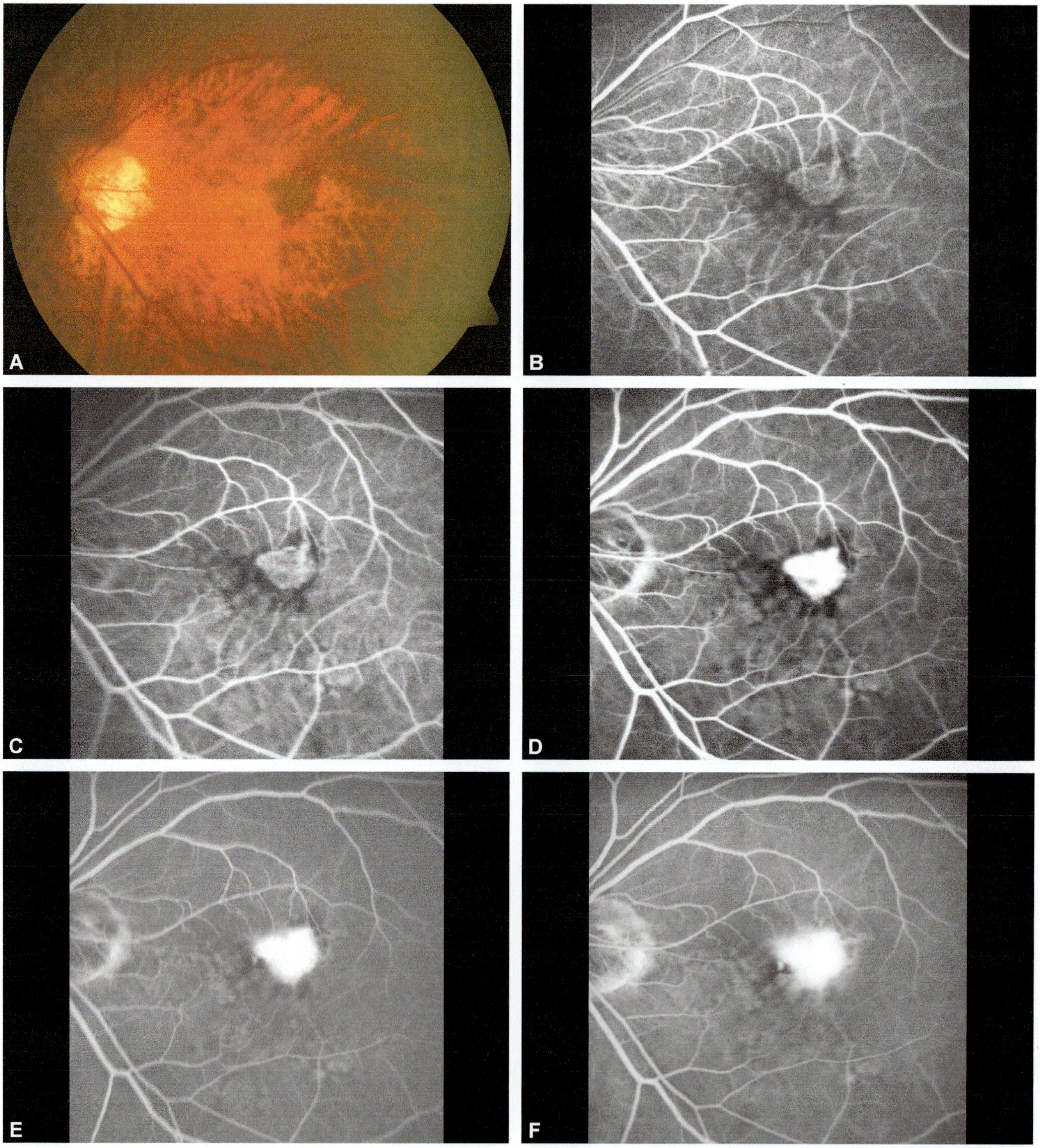

Figs. 52.7A to F: Myopic choroidal neovascularization (mCNV). (A) Color fundus photograph illustrating an area of mCNV involving the fovea; (B) Early fluorescein angiogram (FA) at 17 seconds showing early filling of the CNV lesion; (C) FA at 22 seconds showing a more distinct lesion, with hypofluorescent border; (D) FA at 45 seconds showing early leakage, with hyperfluorescence from the mCNV lesion; (E) Mid phase FA showing leakage from the myopic CNV; (F) Late phase FA. The area of hyperfluorescence has increased in size and the borders of the lesion are less distinct.

diffuse atrophy and 17.2% among those with patchy atrophy.[38] Myopic choroidal neovascularization will be discussed in detail in a later section of this chapter.

Lacquer Cracks

Lacquer cracks are yellowish, branching, linear abnormalities occurring at the macula. These are seen in patients with high myopia (Fig. 52.8A) and are caused by breaks in the Bruch's membrane which result from the associated elongation of the eye.

Although lacquer cracks are frequently associated with high myopia, they are not a common clinical finding. Lacquer cracks were found in 1.8% of Singaporean adults aged 40 and older,[31] while they were reported in only 0.4% of young adults with high myopia.[33]

Imaging Characteristics

Lacquer cracks can be seen on color fundus photography (Fig. 52.8A), although they are often masked by the tessellated appearance of the fundus. On infrared fundus images the lacquer cracks can be visualized as dark branching lines (Fig. 52.8B).

On FA, lacquer cracks are seen as linear hyperfluorescence, which appears in the early phases as a result of the defects in the RPE. These increase gradually during the later phases of the angiogram, although no severe leakage is observed, unless there is associated CNV. In contrast, lacquer cracks are seen as linear, branching areas of hypofluorescence on ICGA (Fig. 52.8C) that are most clearly seen during the late phases of the angiogram.

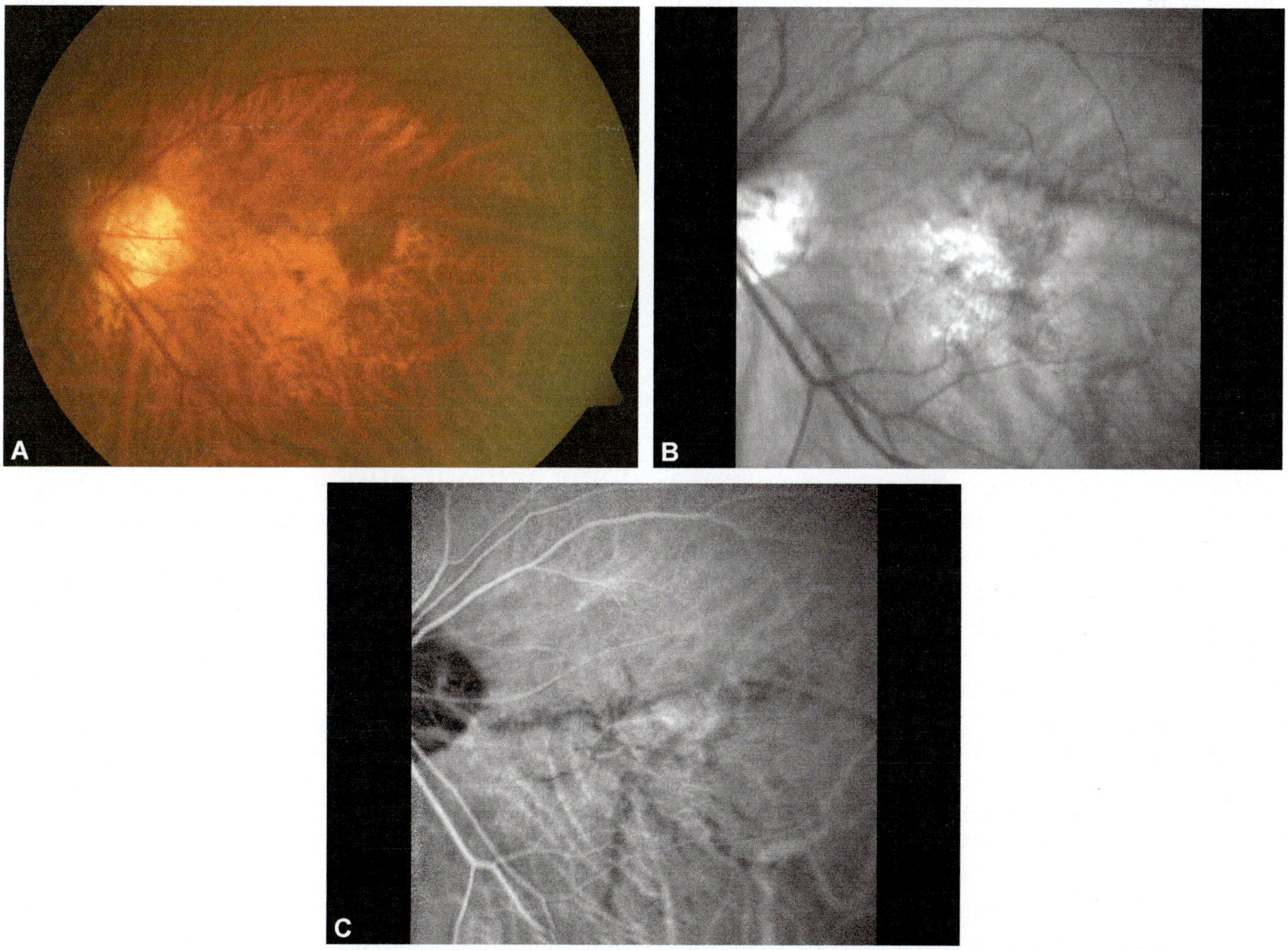

Figs. 52.8A to C: Lacquer cracks. (A) Color fundus photograph illustrating a tessellated fundus with diffuse atrophy. Some lacquer cracks are seen as pale yellow linear streaks; (B) Infrared image showing the lacquer cracks as dark linear streaks; (C) Indocyanine green angiogram at 10 minutes, clearly illustrating the lacquer cracks as distinct, dark linear streaks.

Clinical Sequelae

Progression of lacquer cracks: Lacquer cracks may progress over time. The progress typically occurs slowly. New cracks can form either from the side of an existing lacquer crack or at a location distinct from the original.[39]

Subretinal hemorrhages: Patients with lacquer cracks may develop spontaneous subretinal hemorrhages in the region of the lacquer crack. While these patients may experience visual loss or scotomata, depending on the location of the hemorrhage, these are not associated with CNV lesions. The hemorrhage resolves spontaneously over time, with improvement in visual symptoms.

Myopic CNV: It may develop at the site of lacquer cracks,[39] resulting in subretinal hemorrhage and visual loss. Unlike the spontaneous subretinal hemorrhage described earlier, these eyes have a distinct CNV lesion which can be visualized clinically and on retinal imaging. The manifestations of myopic CNV will be discussed in greater detail in a later section.

Staphyloma

A staphyloma is an abnormal outpouching of scleral tissue that occurs at the posterior pole of the eye. This occurs as a result of axial elongation of the eye in high myopia. Histologic studies have found that the collagen fibers in myopic eyes are smaller in diameter, histologically immature, and have fewer cross-linkages. As a result, these collagen fibers are more elastic and thus more likely to expand and thin out.[40]

Staphylomata are common findings in eyes with high myopia. In a review of 209 eyes of 108 consecutive patients with high myopia, 90% were found to have staphylomata.[41] The prevalence of staphylomata was 80.7% among patients younger than 50 years of age and 72.7% in patients aged 50 and above.[41] Among Singaporean adults with high myopia, the frequency of staphyloma was 23%.

Classification of Staphyloma

Curtin[42] described a classification system for staphyloma. Staphylomata were grouped as primary (Types I to V) and secondary (Types VI to X) as follows:

- *Type I*: Posterior staphyloma
- *Type II*: Macular staphyloma
- *Type III*: Peripapillary staphyloma
- *Type IV*: Nasal staphyloma
- *Type V*: Inferior staphyloma
- *Type VI*: Combination of Type I and Type II staphyloma
- *Type VII*: Combination of Type I and Type III staphyloma
- *Type VIII*: Tiered staphyloma (presence of tiers or steps across the wall of a primary Type I staphyoma)
- *Type IX*: Septal staphyloma
- *Type X*: Plicated staphyloma.

Steidl and Pruett[35] described 5 grades of staphyloma, based on the depth of the staphyloma beneath the RPE on B-scan ultrasonography (Table 52.2).

Table 52.2: Five grades of staphyloma based on the depth of the staphyloma beneath the retinal pigment epithelium (RPE) on B-scan ultrasonography.

S. No.	Grade	Features on B-scan ultrasonography
1.	0	An elongated eye with smooth scleral contour
2.	1	Depth of staphyloma ≤2 mm beneath the RPE
3.	2	Depth of staphyloma between 2 mm and 4 mm beneath the RPE
4.	3	Depth of staphyloma between 4 mm and 6 mm beneath the RPE
5.	4	Depth of staphyloma >6 mm beneath the RPE

Imaging Characteristics

In addition to B-scan ultrasonography described earlier, magnetic resonance imaging has been used to evaluate the shapes of eyes with staphylomata.[43] The shapes described include spheroidal, ellipsoidal, conical, nasally distorted, temporally distorted and barrel shaped.[43]

Clinical Associations

Patients with staphylomata are often asymptomatic. However, they may develop visual field defects secondary to retinal thinning at the edge of the staphyloma.[44] In addition, eyes with staphylomata may develop chorioretinal atrophy, CNV, macular retinoschisis and macular holes.

Dome-shaped Macula

A dome-shaped macula is characterized by an inward bulge of the RPE occurring at the macula (Fig. 52.9).[45,46] It is often, though not always, associated with the presence of a staphyloma.[45,46] A dome-shaped macula is most easily detected using OCT, which clearly shows the inward convexity of the retinal layers and choroid. On stereoscopic examination using slit-lamp biomicroscopy, the posterior pole appears to protrude toward the vitreous. Some eyes

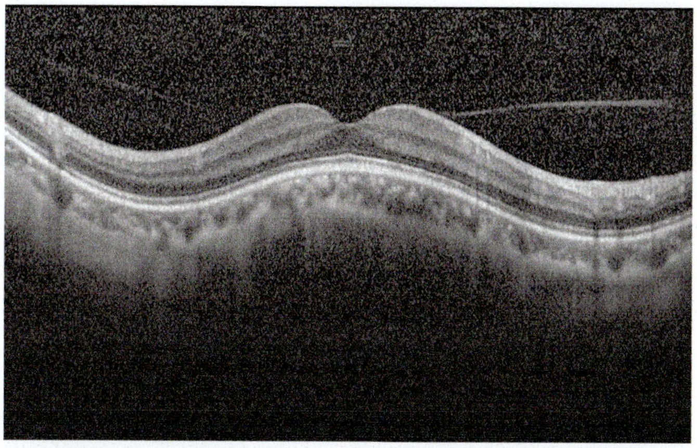

Fig. 52.9: Dome-shaped macula. The retinal pigment epithelium is smoothly elevated beneath the macula, giving a convex, dome-shaped appearance. The underlying choroid is similarly elevated beneath the dome-shaped macula.

with dome-shaped macula may manifest with yellowish-white linear lesions at the posterior pole.[47]

Although dome-shaped maculae may be asymptomatic, they may be associated with other retinal pathologies such as serous retinal detachment, macular hole formation, retinoschisis, and CNV.

Myopic Foveoschisis

Myopic foveoschisis, also known as myopic traction maculopathy, is a thickening of the retina in eyes with high myopia and a posterior staphyloma. It is characterized by intraretinal cleavage of the inner retinal layers from the outer retina. Myopic foveoschisis has a prevalence of between 8% and 34% in individuals with high myopia.[48-50]

Patients with myopic foveoschisis may be asymptomatic or may experience blurring of vision as a result of related complications.[51]

Clinical examination may show a shallow macular elevation with small intraretinal cystic spaces. However, myopic foveoschisis may sometimes be difficult to visualize using slit-lamp biomicroscopy alone.

Imaging Characteristics

Optical coherence tomography is the main investigation technique for the detection of myopic foveoschisis. The retina is split between the inner and outer retina, with bridging columns seen between the layers (Figs. 52.10A and B).[52,53] These are thought to represent the neurons connecting the various retinal cell layers.

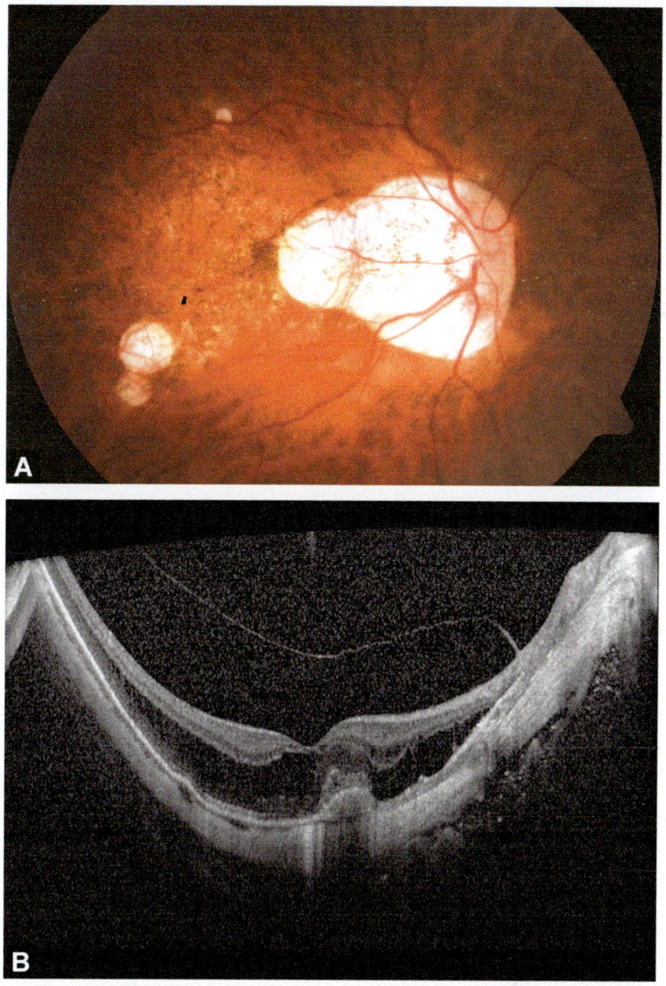

Figs. 52.10A and B: Foveoschisis. (A) Color fundus photograph illustrating diffuse atrophy, especially temporal to the fovea, with areas of patchy atrophy as well. There is a pigmented scar at the temporal border of the patchy atrophy; (B) Optical coherence tomography showing foveoschisis. The layers of the retina are separated, with fine vertical strands connecting them. The choroid is thinned and the underlying sclera is visible.

Clinical Course

Myopic foveoschisis is thought to be slowly progressive, and complications such as foveal detachments and lamellar or full-thickness macular holes may develop. Patients with vision loss as a result of macular holes may require surgical treatment. This may be include vitrectomy and gas tamponade, with or without internal limiting membrane peeling.[54]

Myopic Choroidal Neovascularization

Myopic CNV (mCNV) is a sight-threatening condition that occurs in eyes with myopia. Although mCNV was previously thought to occur more frequently among eyes with high myopia or pathologic myopia, recent expert opinion is that this condition may occur among eyes with any severity of myopia, or even eyes without clinical signs of myopic degeneration.[55]

In population-based studies, the prevalence of mCNV has been reported to range from 0.04% to 0.05%.[9,56] The frequency of mCNV is increased to between 1.5% and 6% among those with pathologic myopia.[9,56] mCNV is the most common type of CNV among people younger than 50 years of age[57] and tends to occur more commonly among females, with a prevalence ranging from 52% to 92%.[10]

The precise pathophysiology of mCNV is uncertain, although several theories have been proposed. The *mechanical theory* postulates that formation of mCNV may develop following release of VEGF as a result of stretching of the retina secondary to axial elongation.[58] In contrast, the *hemodynamic theory* postulates that perfusion changes in the choroid cause the development of mCNV.[59] Yet another possible explanation is a genetic predisposition for mCNV *(the heredodegenerative theory),* which is supported by the association of single nucleotide polymorphisms with progression of mCNV.[60,61]

On clinical examination using slit-lamp microscopy, mCNV appears as a small, grayish-white, subretinal membrane (*see* Fig. 52.7A),[62,63] with surrounding subretinal hemorrhage if the condition is active. It is important to examine the posterior pole carefully as the lesion is usually small and may be masked by the tessellated appearance of the fundus.

The hemorrhage will resolve over time, often forming a scar at the site of the CNV lesion. A chronic lesion appears as a pigmented scar (called a Fuchs' spot or Forster Fuchs' spot) (Fig. 52.11) and may have a surrounding chorioretinal atrophy.[64,65]

Imaging Characteristics

On OCT, mCNV appears as a type 2 CNV, with a hyper-reflective lesion located in the subretinal space (Fig. 52.12A and B). This may be associated with surrounding subretinal or intraretinal fluid.[66] Type 1 CNV (located in the sub-RPE space) is uncommon among eyes with mCNV.[67] Due to the elongation of the eye in high myopia, especially if there is an associated staphyloma, swept-source OCT has been shown to be useful for imaging eyes with pathologic myopia due to the wider scan depth and reduced signal roll-off.

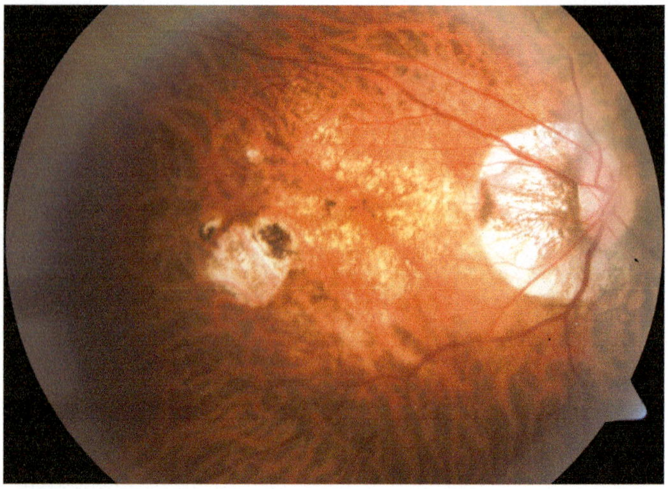

Fig. 52.11: Fuchs' spot. There is diffuse and patchy atrophy, with an area of hyperpigmentation (the Fuchs' spot) at the edge of one of the atrophic patches.

The choroid is usually vary thin in eyes with mCNV and, in some eyes, may barely be discernible (Figs. 52.12A and B).[68,69] Comparing choroidal thickness in eyes with mCNV and in uninvolved fellow eyes, the choroid has been reported to be thinner in the eye with the disease.[68]

Fluorescein angiography is useful for detecting small CNV lesions and for determining whether the lesions are active, based on the presence of leakage (*see* Figs. 52.7A to F). mCNV manifests with a classic pattern of leakage on FA.[66,70,71] Although FA shows early hyperfluorescence that increases in both size and intensity in later phases, mCNV tends to demonstrate less pronounced leakage compared to the classic CNV caused by age-related macular degeneration.[72] This can make it a challenge to differentiate mCNV from staining of surrounding scars in a myopic fundus.

Indocyanine green angiography can demonstrate the CNV lesion (Fig. 52.13), which often appears as a fine network of vessels that seem brighter than the underlying choroidal vessels. ICGA allows better visualization of the CNV lesion than FA because the ICG dye leaks less than fluorescein.

On fundus autofluorescence (Fig. 52.14), abnormal areas usually appear hypo-autofluorescent. These correspond to the mCNV lesion or to areas of subretinal hemorrhage or chorioretinal atrophy.[73]

Optical coherence tomography angiography (OCTA) is a noninvasive method of producing vascular flow maps of the various vascular plexuses in the retina.[23,74] On OCTA, mCNV appears as a hyperintense, vascular anastomotic network, which may be circular or irregular in shape.[75,76]

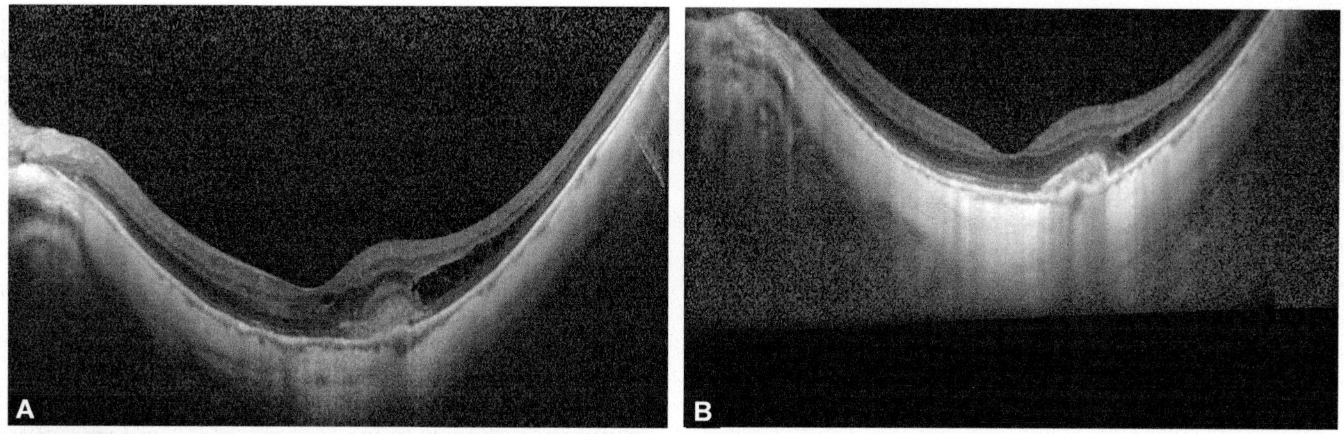

Figs. 52.12A and B: Optical coherence tomography (OCT) of myopic choroidal neovascularization (mCNV). (A) OCT of the mCNV lesion at presentation. The mCNV lesion appears as a subretinal hyper-reflective area temporal to the fovea. The borders of the lesion are less distinct. Note the very thin choroid; (B) OCT of the lesion following successful treatment. The scar is seen as a hyper-reflective lesion at the site of the mCNV. The borders are more distinct, and the lesion is more hyper-reflective. There is shadowing beneath the scar.

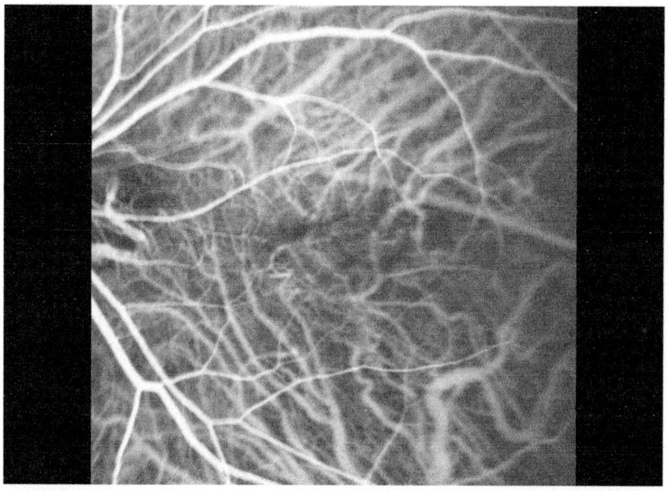

Fig. 52.13: Indocyanine green angiogram of myopic choroidal neovascularization (mCNV). The mCNV lesion is seen as a slightly hyperfluorescent lesion that appears distinct from the underlying choroidal vessels.

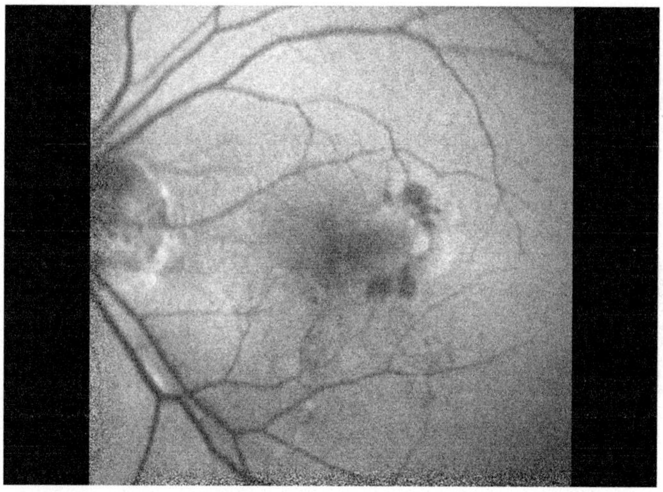

Fig. 52.14: Fundus autofluorescence of myopic choroidal neovascularization (mCNV). The edges of the mCNV lesion appear hyperautofluorescent. Small areas of hypoautofluorescence surrounding the lesion correspond to regions of atrophy or hemorrhage.

Management Options for mCNV

Anti-VEGF agents: Currently, the standard of care for mCNV is anti-VEGF agents. Studies such as **R**anibizumab **A**nd P**D**T [verteporf**I**n] ev**A**luation i**N** myopic **C**horoidal n**E**ovascularization (RADIANCE),[77] REPAIR[78] and MYRROR study[79] have demonstrated the efficacy of intravitreal ranibizumab and aflibercept in the management of mCNV.

Verteprofin photodynamic therapy (vPDT): It allows treatment of CNV lesions occurring at or near the fovea.[55,71,80,81] However, while treatment of mCNV with vPDT does stabilize visual acuity, it usually does not result in improvement. Photodynamic therapy is also believed to result in choroidal ischemia,[82,83] which is of particular concern among highly myopic eyes, in which the choroid is already very thin.

Focal laser photocoagulation: Laser photocoagulation was previously used to treat mCNV. However, scarring occurs at the region of the laser photocoagulation, and new CNV lesions may subsequently develop at the edges of the laser scar. Laser photocoagulation may be an option for lesions located further from the fovea, especially if anti-VEGF agents or PDT is not available.

Posterior Vitreous Detachment

Posterior vitreous detachment consists of separation of the posterior hyaloid face of the vitreous gel from the retinal surface, which may occur anywhere posterior to the vitreous base. This condition increases in frequency with age[84] and with increasing severity of myopia.[84,85] As an individual ages, the vitreous gel undergoes degeneration and normal wear and tear. Portions of the vitreous gel undergo syneresis, wherein the gel liquefies, forming pockets within the remaining solid vitreous. Eventually, the vitreous gel shrinks and collapses, pulling away and separating from the surface of the retina.

People with posterior vitreous detachment commonly experience *floaters,* which may manifest as dark spots, shapes or shadows within the field of vision. The floaters may be single or multiple, and may change gradually over time. They may also experience *flashes of light* (known as *photopsia*), which often occur in the peripheral vision in a dark environment. Photopsia results from traction of the vitreous on the retina, where the mechanical force is perceived as flashes of light. These symptoms may present acutely and then gradually subside over the next few weeks. If the symptoms progress and worsen, however, they may be indicative of more serious pathology, such as retinal tears or retinal detachment.

A posterior vitreous detachment can often be seen clinically, manifesting as a solid vitreous condensation within the clear vitreous cavity. Sometimes, this appears as a Weiss ring, which is a round or oval structure that was originally located at the optic disk. On slit-lamp biomicroscopy, vitreous strands may be seen posterior to the lens, within the anterior vitreous. In some cases, however, the vitreous appears clear and no signs may be observed on clinical examination.

Imaging Characteristics

In cases where clinical examination is inconclusive, OCT can be used to visualize the separation of the posterior hyaloid from the retinal surface. The vitreous separation can be complete, wherein it is separated from the optic nerve, or incomplete, wherein it is still attached to the macula or optic nerve. Optical coherence tomography shows both the vitreomacular interface and changes to the vitreous within the vitreous cavity, where pockets of liquefied vitreous may be seen.[33,86] The use of newer swept-source OCT devices makes this easier due to the increased imaging depth and lower sensitivity roll-off compared to spectral-domain OCT. In addition, a wider horizontal scan length allows a more complete assessment of the vitreous separation at the posterior pole.

Clinical Sequelae

Stable posterior vitreous detachment: A posterior vitreous detachment is benign and typically not sight-threatening, although the symptoms may be disturbing to some patients. In some cases, the symptoms may eventually resolve spontaneously.

Retinal tears: In other cases, however, part of the vitreous gel may be adherent to the retinal surface and may cause a retinal tear (Fig. 52.15) as the gel separates from the retina. A retinal tear typically occurs anteriorly, in the peripheral retina near the ora serrata, and may not be easily visualized without dilated fundus examination with scleral indentation. A retinal tear is a possible cause of vitreous hemorrhage; an ultrasound B-scan may be required to rule out retinal detachments in patients presenting with vitreous hemorrhage.

Rhegmatogenous retinal detachments: Retinal tears may progress to rhegmatogenous retinal detachment (Fig. 52.16) (discussed in a separate section of this chapter).

Lattice Degeneration

Lattice degenerations are linear or oval patches of retinal atrophy located in the peripheral retina. On clinical examination, they appear as sharply demarcated areas of inner retinal thinning, with the long axis usually circumferentially oriented, parallel to the ora serrata. The base of the lesion may appear uneven and moth-eaten, with white lines criss-crossing the lesion. Lattice degeneration may be pigmented or depigmented. As these lesions are located very peripherally, binocular indirect ophthalmoscopy with scleral indentation is often required to properly assess these lesions. Typically, patients with lattice degeneration are asymptomatic.

The prevalence of lattice degeneration in the general population is around 7–10%[87] but increases to between 12.2% and 15% among adults with high myopia.[88,89] A positive correlation has been reported between longer axial length and the presence of lattice degeneration.[90]

Imaging Characteristics

Lattice degeneration can sometimes be imaged using fundus photography if the pupil is well dilated and the

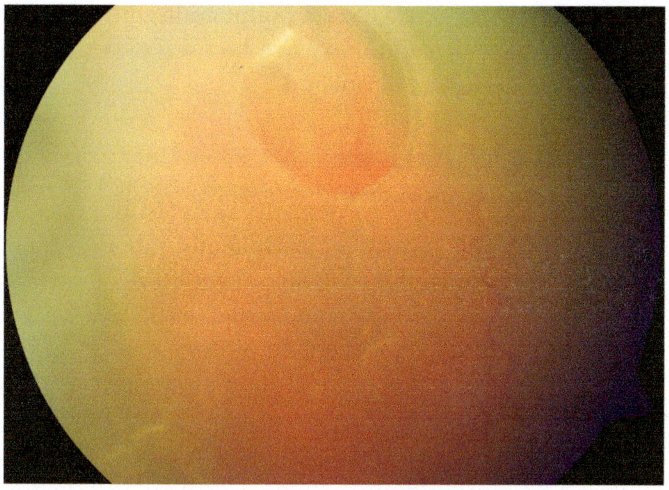

Fig. 52.15: Retinal tear, with a characteristic U-shaped appearance. The surrounding neurosensory retina is detached.

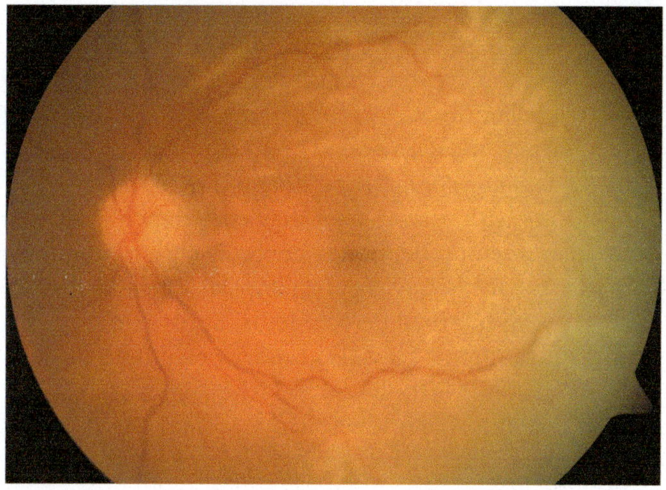

Fig. 52.16: Rhegmatogenous retinal detachment involving the macula (macula-off detachment). The detached neurosensory retina appears paler and irregular.

imaged is steered to the periphery. This can be facilitated by the use of ultra-widefield imaging devices and is useful for documenting peripheral clinical findings.

Optical coherence tomography scans steered to the periphery have demonstrated the presence of retinal thinning without a clear distinction between the inner and outer retinal layers. In addition, as seen on OCT, the vitreous is separated both anterior and posterior to the area of lattice degeneration but remains adherent to the lattice degeneration, resulting in a U-shaped appearance.[91]

Clinical Sequelae

Retinal thinning at sites of lattice degeneration presents a risk of retinal hole or tear formation, with subsequent rhegmatogenous retinal detachment, although the precise risk remains uncertain. Some ophthalmologists have advocated prophylactic laser retinopexy around the area of lattice degeneration to reduce the risk of retinal detachments; but this remains controversial.

White Without Pressure

White without pressure refers to the whitish appearance of a region of the peripheral or equatorial retina which occurs without scleral indentation. This region is sharply demarcated from the surrounding retina and is opposed to the RPE. It is believed to be an optical phenomenon associated with vitreous traction or adhesion to the retinal surface. Patients are commonly asymptomatic. White without pressure occurs in up to 30% of the general population[92] and is among the most common peripheral retinal findings among eyes with high myopia.[88,93]

Imaging Characteristics

On ultra-widefield FA, eyes with white without pressure demonstrated areas of increased peripheral hyperfluorescence, with multiple pinpoint areas of hyperfluorescence in the far periphery.[94] In contrast, eyes without white without pressure demonstrated decreasing amounts of hyperfluorescence toward the periphery.

Clinical Sequelae

While white without pressure is benign, patients with this finding may develop retinal tears, which may progress to rhegmatogenous retinal detachment.

Retinal Tears and Detachments

Retinal tears (Fig. 52.15) may result from posterior vitreous detachments and may occur at areas with retinal thinning, such as lattice degeneration. These often occur in the peripheral retina, near the vitreous base, and may be difficult to visualize clinically unless careful examination is performed with pupils dilated and scleral indentation.

Retinal tears may remain stable, and some patients remain asymptomatic over long periods of time. In these cases, the retinal tears are usually identified incidentally during a dilated fundus examination performed for other indications.

In some eyes, however, fluid from the vitreous cavity may separate the neurosensory retina from the RPE at the site of the retinal tear and then extend from that point, resulting in a rhegmatogenous retinal detachment (Fig. 52.16).

Patients with retinal tears may experience a sudden increase in the number of floaters, as well as a new onset or increase in the frequency of photopsias. These also occur in patients with retinal detachments. Some patients with retinal detachments may also report visual field defects, which correspond to the area of detached retina. A decrease in visual acuity occurs when the retinal detachment involves the macula (a macula-off detachment).

The incidence of retinal tears and detachments varies with population and increases with age. In a study of Taiwanese adults, the incidence of retinal detachments increased with age, with a peak in frequency occurring between 50 years and 69 years of age, and a secondary peak between 20 years and 29 years among women.[95]

High myopia is a risk factor for the occurrence of retinal detachments. Among Taiwanese adults who developed retinal detachments, 10.51% had high myopia.[95] Other causes of rhegmatogenous retinal detachment include trauma or complications of intraocular surgery, such as a posterior capsule rupture with vitreous loss during cataract surgery.

Imaging Characteristics

Retinal tears and detachments can be visualized using fundus photography (Fig. 52.16) if they involve the more posterior portions of the fundus. However, more peripheral or anteriorly located tears and detachments may be difficult to image unless the pupil is widely dilated and the image steered to the periphery. Newer ultra-widefield fundus cameras are able to image up to 200 degrees of the posterior pole in a single field of view and can be further extended by steering the images.[24,96,97] These images are useful for documenting pathology seen on clinical examination. Wide-field spectral domain OCT scans have also been used to image the peripheral retina and are able to visualize retinal tears occurring in the periphery.[98,99]

Clinical Management

Retinal detachments require surgical management to reattach the retina. Currently, retinal detachments may be managed by vitrectomy with gas tamponade and/or scleral buckle. Pneumatic retinopexy can be used if the area of detachment is small and isolated.

CONCLUSION

Pathologic myopia can significantly affect visual performance. The severity of myopia and the associated retinal and choroidal thinning may affect BCVA.

In addition, pathologic myopia may result in a variety of clinical conditions, involving both the macula and the peripheral retina. Some of these, including myopic CNV and retinal detachments, are potentially sight-threatening. It is important for ophthalmologists to recognize the clinical signs and employ the appropriate image modalities to investigate these lesions.

REFERENCES

1. Holden BA, Fricke TR, Wilson DA, et al. Global Prevalence of Myopia and High Myopia and Temporal Trends from 2000 through 2050. Ophthalmology. 2016;123(5):1036-42.
2. Wu PC, Huang HM, Yu HJ, et al. Epidemiology of Myopia. Asia-Pacific J Ophthalmol. 2016;5(6):386-93.
3. Pan CW, Dirani M, Cheng CY, et al. The age-specific prevalence of myopia in Asia: a meta-analysis. Optom Vis Sci. 2015;92(3):258-66.
4. Foster PJ, Jiang Y. Epidemiology of myopia. Eye (Lond). 2014;28(2):202-8.
5. Wong TY, Foster PJ, Hee J, et al. Prevalence and risk factors for refractive errors in adult Chinese in Singapore. Invest Ophthalmol Vis Sci. 2000;41(9):2486-94.
6. Wu LJ, You QS, Duan JL, et al. Prevalence and associated factors of myopia in high-school students in Beijing. PLoS One. 2015;10(3):e0120764.
7. Willis JR, Vitale S, Morse L, et al. The Prevalence of Myopic Choroidal Neovascularization in the United States: analysis of the IRIS (R) Data Registry and NHANES. Ophthalmology. 2016;123(8):1771-82.
8. Adatia FA, Luong M, Munro M, et al. The other CNVM: a review of myopic choroidal neovascularization treatment in the age of anti-vascular endothelial growth factor agents. Surv Ophthalmol. 2015;60(3):204-15.
9. Vongphanit J, Mitchell P, Wang JJ. Prevalence and progression of myopic retinopathy in an older population. Ophthalmology. 2002;109(4):704-11.
10. Wong TY, Ferreira A, Hughes R, et al. Epidemiology and disease burden of pathologic myopia and myopic choroidal neovascularization: an evidence-based systematic review. Am J Ophthalmol. 2014;157(1):9-25.e12.
11. Wong YL, Saw SM. Epidemiology of Pathologic Myopia in Asia and Worldwide. Asia-Pacific J Ophthalmol. 2016;5(6):394-402.

12. Pan CW, Klein BEK, Cotch MF, et al. Racial variations in the prevalence of refractive errors in the United States: the multi-ethnic study of atherosclerosis. Am J Ophthalmol. 2013;155(6):1129-38.e1.
13. Vitale S, Cotch MF, Sperduto R, et al. Costs of refractive correction of distance vision impairment in the United States, 1999-2002. Ophthalmology. 2006;113(12):2163-70.
14. Zheng YF, Pan CW, Chay J, et al. The economic cost of myopia in adults aged over 40 years in Singapore. Invest Ophthalmol Vis Sci. 2013;54(12):7532-7.
15. Othman SF, Kaur S, Manan FA, et al. Macular thickness as determined by optical coherence tomography in relation to degree of myopia, axial length and vitreous chamber depth in Malay subjects. Clin Exp Optom. 2012;95(5):484-91.
16. Cheng SCK, Lam CSY, Yap MKH. Retinal thickness in myopic and non-myopic eyes. Ophthalmic Physiol Opt. 2010;30(6):776-84.
17. Lam DSC, King SL, Mohamed S, et al. Regional variations in the relationship between macular thickness measurements and myopia. Investig Ophthalmol Vis Sci. 2007;48(1):376-82.
18. Tan CS, Li KZ, Tan M, et al. Relationship between Myopia Severity and Macular Retinal Thickness on Visual Performance under Different Lighting Conditions. Ophthalmol Retin. 2017;1(4):339-46.
19. Song WK, Lee SC, Lee ES, et al. Macular thickness variations with sex, age, and axial length in healthy subjects: a spectral domain-optical coherence tomography study. Investig Ophthalmol Vis Sci. 2010;51(8):3913l-8.
20. Jonas JB, Xu L, Bin WW, et al. Retinal Thickness and Axial Length. Investig Opthalmology Vis Sci. 2016;57(4):1791.
21. Chen S, Wang B, Dong N, et al. Macular measurements using spectral-domain optical coherence tomography in Chinese myopic children. Investig Ophthalmol Vis Sci. 2014;55(11):7410-6.
22. Zhang Z, He X, Zhu J, et al. Macular measurements using optical coherence tomography in healthy Chinese school age children. Invest Ophthalmol Vis Sci. 2011;52(9):6377-83.
23. Tan CS, Lim LW, Chow VS, et al. Optical coherence tomography angiography evaluation of the parafoveal vasculature and its relationship with ocular factors. Investig Ophthalmol Vis Sci. 2016;57(9):224-34.
24. Tan CS, Cheong KX, Lim LW, et al. Comparison of macular choroidal thicknesses from swept source and spectral domain optical coherence tomography. Br J Ophthalmol. 2016;100(7):995-9.
25. Shin YU, Kim S, Lee BR, et al. Novel noninvasive detection of the fovea avascular zone using confocal red-free imaging in diabetic retinopathy and retinal vein occlusion. Investig Ophthalmol Vis Sci. 2012;53(1):309-15.
26. Coscas G, Zhou Q, Coscas F, et al. Choroid thickness measurement with RTVue optical coherence tomography in emmetropic eyes, mildly myopic eyes, and highly myopic eyes. Eur J Ophthalmol. 2012;22(6):992-1000.
27. Strang NC, Winn B, Bradley A. The role of neural and optical factors in limiting visual resolution in myopia. Vision Res. 1998;38(11):1713-21.
28. Nishida Y, Fujiwara T, Imamura Y, et al. Choroidal thickness and visual acuity in highly myopic eyes. Retina. 2012;32(7):1229-36.
29. Mcmonnies CW. An examination of the relation between intraocular pressure, fundal stretching and myopic pathology. Clin Exp Opto. 2016;99(2):113-9.
30. Gao LQ. Prevalence and characteristics of myopic retinopathy in a rural chinese adult population. Arch Ophthalmol. 2011;129(9):1199.
31. Chang L, Pan CW, Ohno-Matsui K, et al. Myopia-related fundus changes in Singapore adults with high myopia. Am J Ophthalmol. 2013;155(6).
32. Lichtwitz O, Boissonnot M, Mercié M, et al. Prevalence of macular complications associated with high myopia by multimodal imaging. J Fr Ophtalmol. 2015;39(4):355-63.
33. Gupta P, Cheung CY, Saw SM, et al. Peripapillary choroidal thickness in young Asians with high myopia. Investig Ophthalmol Vis Sci. 2015;56(3):1475-81.
34. Tokoro T. Types of Fundus Changes in the Posterior Pole BT Atlas of Posterior Fundus Changes in Pathologic Myopia. In: Tokoro T (Ed). Tokyo: Springer Japan; 1998.pp.5-22.
35. Steidl SM, Pruett RC. Macular complications associated with posterior staphyloma. Am J Ophthalmol. 1997;123(2):181-7.
36. Ohno-Matsui K, Kawasaki R, Jonas JB, et al. International photographic classification and grading system for myopic maculopathy. Am J Ophthalmol. 2015;159(5):877-83.
37. Tan CS, Ngo WK, Lim LW, et al. EVEREST study report 3: diagnostic challenges of polypoidal choroidal vasculopathy. Lessons learnt from screening failures in the EVEREST study. Graefe's Arch Clin Exp Ophthalmol. 2016;254(10):1923-30.
38. Hayashi K, Ohno-Matsui K, Shimada N, et al. Long-term pattern of progression of myopic maculopathy: a natural history study. Ophthalmology. 2010;117(8):1-5.
39. Kim YM, Yoon JU, Koh HJ. The analysis of lacquer crack in the assessment of myopic choroidal neovascularization. Eye. 2011;25(7):937-46.
40. Curtin BJ, Iwamoto T, Renaldo DP. Normal and staphylomatous sclera of high myopia: An electron microscopic study. Arch Ophthalmol. 1979;97(5):912-5.
41. Hsiang HW, Ohno-Matsui K, Shimada N, et al. Clinical Characteristics of Posterior Staphyloma in Eyes with Pathologic Myopia. Am J Ophthalmol. 2008;146(1):102-10.
42. Curtin BJ, Karlin DB. Axial Length Measurements and Fundus Changes of the Myopic Eye. Am J Ophthalmol. 1971;71(1):42-53.
43. Guo X, Xiao O, Chen Y, et al. Three-dimensional eye shape, myopic maculopathy, and visual acuity: The Zhongshan Ophthalmic Center–Brien Holden Vision Institute High Myopia Cohort Study. Ophthalmology. 2017;124(5):679-87.
44. Tanaka Y, Shimada N, Ohno-Matsui K. Extreme thinning or loss of inner neural retina along the staphyloma edge in eyes with pathologic myopia. Am J Ophthalmol. 2015;159(4):677-82.
45. Gaucher D, Haouchine B, Tadayoni R, et al. Long-term follow-up of high myopic foveoschisis: natural course and surgical outcome. Am J Ophthalmol. 2007;143(3):455-62.

46. Ellabban AA, Tsujikawa A, Matsumoto A, et al. Three-dimensional tomographic features of dome-shaped macula by swept-source optical coherence tomography. Am J Ophthalmol. 2013;155(2):320-8.
47. Liang IC, Shimada N, Tanaka Y, et al. Comparison of Clinical Features in Highly Myopic Eyes with and without a Dome-Shaped Macula. Ophthalmology. 2015;122:1591-600.
48. Henaine-Berra A, Zand-Hadas IM, Fromow-Guerra J, et al. Prevalence of macular anatomic abnormalities in high myopia. Ophthalmic Surg Lasers Imaging Retin. 2013;44(2):140-4.
49. Wu PC, Chen YJ, Chen YH, et al. Factors associated with foveoschisis and foveal detachment without macular hole in high myopia. Eye. 2009;23(2):356-61.
50. Baba T, Ohno-Matsui K, Futagami S, et al. Prevalence and characteristics of foveal retinal detachment without macular hole in high myopia. Am J Ophthalmol. 2003;135(3):338-42.
51. Panozzo G, Mercanti A. Optical coherence tomography findings in myopic traction maculopathy. Arch Ophthalmol. 2004;122(10):1455-60.
52. Takano M, Kishi S. Foveal retinoschisis and retinal detachment in severely myopic eyes with posterior staphyloma. Am J Ophthalmol. 1999;128(4):472-6.
53. Benhamou N, Massin P, Haouchine B, et al. Macular retinoschisis in highly myopic eyes. Am J Ophthalmol. 2002;133(6):794-800.
54. Ikuno Y, Sayanagi K, Ohji M, et al. Vitrectomy and internal limiting membrane peeling for myopic foveoschisis. Am J Ophthalmol. 2004;137(4):719-24.
55. Wong TY, Ohno-Matsui K, Leveziel N, et al. Myopic choroidal neovascularisation: current concepts and update on clinical management. Br J Ophthalmol. 2015;99(3):289-96.
56. Liu HH, Xu L, Wang YX, et al. Prevalence and progression of myopic retinopathy in Chinese adults: the Beijing eye study. Ophthalmology. 2010;117(9):1763-8.
57. Cohen SY, Laroche A, Leguen Y, et al. Etiology of choroidal neovascularization in young patients. Ophthalmology. 1996;103(8):1241-4.
58. Seko Y, Fujikura H, Pang J, et al. Induction of vascular endothelial growth factor after application of mechanical stress to retinal pigment epithelium of the rat in vitro. Invest Ophthalmol Vis Sci. 1999;40:3287-91.
59. Wakabayashi T, Ikuno Y. Choroidal filling delay in choroidal neovascularisation due to pathological myopia. Br J Ophthalmol. 2010;94(5):611-5.
60. Leveziel N, Yu Y, Reynolds R, et al. Genetic factors for choroidal neovascularization associated with high myopia. Invest Ophthalmol Vis Sci. 2012;53(8):5004-9.
61. Akagi-Kurashige Y, Kumagai K, Yamashiro K, et al. Vascular endothelial growth factor gene polymorphisms and choroidal neovascularization in highly myopic eyes. Invest Ophthalmol Vis Sci. 2012;53:2349-53.
62. Avila MP, Weiter JJ, Jalkh AE, et al. Natural history of choroidal neovascularization in degenerative myopia. Ophthalmology. 1984;91(12):1573-81.
63. Neelam K, Cheung CMG, Ohno-Matsui K, et al. Choroidal neovascularization in pathological myopia. Prog Retin Eye Res. 2012;31(5):495-525.
64. Jonas JB, Jonas SB, Jonas RA, et al. Parapapillary atrophy: histological gamma zone and delta zone. PLoS One. 2012;7(10):e47237.
65. Yoshida T, Ohno-Matsui K, Yasuzumi K, et al. Myopic choroidal neovascularization: a 10-year follow-up. Ophthalmology. 2003;110(7):1297-305.
66. Chan WM, Ohji M, Lai TY, et al. Choroidal neovascularisation in pathological myopia: an update in management. Br J Ophthalmol. 2005;89(11):1522-8.
67. Silva R. Myopic maculopathy: a review. Ophthalmologica. 2012;228(4):197-213.
68. Ikuno Y, Jo Y, Hamasaki T, et al. Ocular risk factors for choroidal neovascularization in pathologic myopia. Investig Ophthalmol Vis Sci. 2010;51(7):3721-5.
69. Fujiwara T, Imamura Y, Margolis R, et al. Enhanced depth imaging optical coherence tomography of the choroid in highly myopic eyes. Am J Ophthalmol. 2009;148(3):445-50.
70. Soubrane G. Choroidal neovascularization in pathologic myopia: recent developments in diagnosis and treatment. Surv Ophthalmol. 2008;53(2):121-38.
71. Ruiz-Oliva F, Cortes J. Verteporfin in Photodynamic Therapy (VIP) Study group. Ophthalmology. 2002;109:1043-4.
72. Keane PA, Liakopoulos S, Chang KT, et al. Comparison of the optical coherence tomographic features of choroidal neovascular membranes in pathological myopia versus age-related macular degeneration, using quantitative subanalysis. Br J Ophthalmol. 2008;92(8):1081-5.
73. Sawa M, Gomi F, Tsujikawa M, et al. Abnormal fundus autofluorescence patterns in myopic choroidal neovascularisation. Br J Ophthalmol. 2008;92(9):1236-40.
74. Tan CS, Hariprasad SM, Lim LW, et al. Evaluation of the retinal and choroidal vasculature with OCT angiography versus conventional angiography. Ophthalmic Surg Lasers Imaging Retina. 2016;47(12):1081-5.
75. Querques G, Corvi F, Querques L, et al. Optical coherence tomography angiography of choroidal neovascularization secondary to pathologic myopia. Dev Ophthalmol. 2016;56:101-6.
76. Miyata M, Ooto S, Hata M, et al. Detection of myopic choroidal neovascularization using optical coherence tomography angiography. Am J Ophthalmol. 2016;165:108-14.
77. Wolf S, Balciuniene VJ, Laganovska G, et al. Radiance: a randomized controlled study of ranibizumab in patients with choroidal neovascularization secondary to pathologic myopia. Ophthalmology. 2014;121(3):682-92.
78. Tufail A, Narendran N, Patel PJ, et al. Ranibizumab in myopic choroidal neovascularization: the 12-month results from the repair study. Ophthalmology. 2013;120:1944-5.
79. Ikuno Y, Ohno-Matsui K, Wong TY, et al. Intravitreal aflibercept injection in patients with myopic choroidal neovascularization: The MYRROR study. Ophthalmology. 2015;122(6):1220-7.

80. Blinder KJ, Blumenkranz MS, Bressler NM, et al. Verteporfin therapy of subfoveal choroidal neovascularization in pathologic myopia: 2-year results of a randomized clinical trial--VIP report no. 3. Ophthalmology. 2003;110(4):667-73.
81. Tan CS, Chew MC, Lim TH. Comparison of foveal-sparing with foveal-involving photodynamic therapy for myopic choroidal neovascularization. Eye (Lond). 2014;28(1):17-22.
82. Hayashi K, Ohno-Matsui K, Shimada N, et al. Long-term results of photodynamic therapy for choroidal neovascularization in Japanese patients with pathologic myopia. Am J Ophthalmol. United States; 2011;151(1):137-47.e1.
83. Giansanti F, Virgili G, Donati MC, et al. Long-term results of photodynamic therapy for subfoveal choroidal neovascularization with pathologic myopia. Retina. 2012;32(8):1547-52.
84. Akiba J. Prevalence of posterior vitreous detachment in high myopia. Ophthalmology. 1993;100(9):1384-8.
85. Morita H, Funata M, Tokoro T. A clinical study of the development of posterior vitreous detachment in high myopia. Retina. 1995;15(2):117-24.
86. Ng DSC, Cheung CYL, Luk FO, et al. Advances of optical coherence tomography in myopia and pathologic myopia. Eye. 2016;30(7):901-16.
87. Straatsma BR, Zeegen PD, Foos RY, et al. Lattice degeneration of the retina. XXX Edward Jackson Memorial Lecture. Am J Ophthalmol. 1974;77(5):619-49.
88. Lam DSC, Fan DSP, Chan WM, et al. Prevalence and characteristics of peripheral retinal degeneration in Chinese adults with high myopia: a cross-sectional prevalence survey. Optom Vis Sci. 2005;82(4):235-8.
89. Celorio JM, Pruett RC. Prevalence of lattice degeneration and its relation to axial length in severe myopia. Am J Ophthalmol. 1991;111(1):20-3.
90. Pierro L, Camesasca FI, Mischi M, et al. Peripheral retinal changes and axial myopia. Retina. 1992;12(1):12-7.
91. Manjunath V, Taha M, Fujimoto JG, et al. Posterior lattice degeneration characterized by spectral domain optical coherence tomography. Retina. 2011;31(3):492-6.
92. Shukla M, Ahuja OP. White with pressure (WWP) and white without pressure (WWOP) lesions. Indian J Ophthalmol. 1982;30(3):129-32.
93. Bansal AS, Hubbard GB 3rd. Peripheral retinal findings in highly myopic children < or = 10 years of age. Retina. 2010;30(4 Suppl):S15-9.
94. Orlin A, Fatoo A, Ehrlich J, et al. Ultra-widefield fluorescein angiography of white without pressure. Clin Ophthalmol. 2013;7:959-64.
95. Chen SN, Lian IB, Wei YJ. Epidemiology and clinical characteristics of rhegmatogenous retinal detachment in Taiwan. Br J Ophthalmol. 2016;100(9):1216-20.
96. Tan CS, Heussen F, Sadda SR. Peripheral autofluorescence and clinical findings in neovascular and non-neovascular age-related macular degeneration. Ophthalmology. 2013;120(6):1271-7.
97. Singer M, Sagong M, van Hemert J, et al. Ultra-widefield imaging of the peripheral retinal vasculature in normal subjects. Ophthalmology. 2016;123(5):1053-9.
98. Gregori NZ, Lam BL, Gregori G, et al. Wide-field spectral-domain optical coherence tomography in patients and carriers of X-linked retinoschisis. Ophthalmology. 2013;120(1):169-74.
99. Choudhry N, Golding J, Manry MW, et al. Ultra-widefield steering-based spectral-domain optical coherence tomography imaging of the retinal periphery. Ophthalmology. 2016;123(6):1368-74.

Chapter 53 Hereditary Macular Dystrophies

Etienne M Schönbach, Peter Charbel Issa, Hendrik PN Scholl

INTRODUCTION

Macular dystrophies are a genetically and phenotypically heterogeneous group of diseases with several unifying features. First, they are inherited as Mendelian disorders (i.e. they are monogenic). Second, there is a progressive loss of photoreceptor function in the macula associated with visual loss. In most macular dystrophies, the lesions between the vascular arcades are biomicroscopically visible before symptoms occur. Third, the associated pathology is usually limited to the eye; however, there are exceptions, such as mutations in *CDH3* where macular dystrophies are part of a syndrome. Conditions that are genetically complex and are partly caused by environmental risk factors, such as age-related macular degeneration (AMD), are not considered macular dystrophies. Neither are foveal hypoplasia and ocular albinism, because these conditions are developmental and nonprogressive. The increasing knowledge of the underlying cellular and molecular basis of the conditions has led to clinical trials that may slow photoreceptor degeneration or may even restore vision to some extent. In this chapter a selection of the most prevalent macular dystrophies is being discussed and a more comprehensive list of such diseases and the genes involved in their pathophysiology is provided in Table 53.1.

APPROACH TO A PATIENT WITH A MACULAR DYSTROPHY

Macular dystrophies mainly affect the retinal pigment epithelium (RPE)-photoreceptor complex and the choriocapillaris. Thus, they lead to visual impairment and can affect various dimensions of visual function. With only a few exceptions, macular dystrophies present bilaterally with a high degree of symmetry between the two eyes.

As for all patients with inherited retinal diseases, a careful history may help confirm the presence of a Mendelian condition and the mode of inheritance.

Table 53.1: List of selected macular dystrophies with their respective genetic defects, their prevalences, and their modes of inheritance.

Name	Underlying gene	Chromosome/Locus	Prevalence	Mode of inheritance
Stargardt disease type 1	*ABCA4*	1p22.1	1/8,000–1/10,000	Autosomal recessive
Stargardt disease type 3	*ELOVL4*	6q14.1	Unknown	Autosomal dominant
Stargardt disease type 4	*PROM1*	4p15.32	Unknown	Autosomal dominant
Best macular dystrophy	*BEST1*	11q12.3	1/5,000–1/67,000	Autosomal dominant or autosomal recessive
Adult vitelliform macular dystrophy	*BEST1, PRPH2, IMPG1, IMPG2*	6p21.1 and 11q12.3	Unknown	Autosomal dominant
Pattern dystrophy	*PRPH2*	6p21.1	Unknown	Autosomal dominant
Sorsby fundus dystrophy	*TIMP3*	22q12.3	Unknown	Autosomal dominant
Autosomal dominant drusen	*EFEMP1*	2p16.1	Unknown	Autosomal dominant
North Carolina macular dystrophy	*PRDM13*	6q16.2	<1/1,000,000	Autosomal dominant
Patterned macular dystrophy/Butterfly-shaped pigmentary macular dystrophy	*CTNNA1*	5q31.2	Unknown	Autosomal dominant

Dominant diseases affect all generations but the possibility of incomplete penetrance and variable expressivity must be considered. Autosomal recessive diseases may affect siblings and, in consanguineous families or populations with a high carrier rate, pseudodominance or disease manifestation in more distant relatives may be observed. X-chromosomal recessive diseases usually only affect males, but female carriers can also show signs and symptoms. Possible differential diagnoses such as toxic, infectious, and autoimmune disorders that mimic macular dystrophies must be considered. Conditions like multifocal choroiditis or the presumed ocular histoplasmosis syndrome are less symmetrical. Every patient should be asked about the use of retinotoxic drugs, and especially about the use of medications for rheumatic or autoimmune diseases. Examples of drugs that may mimic macular dystrophies include hydroxychloroquine (Figs. 53.1A to E) for the treatment of systemic lupus erythematosus and Sjögren syndrome, and the breast cancer medication tamoxifen. In addition, antibiotics such as nitrofurantoin,[1] iron-chelating agents like deferoxamine,[2,3] antipsychotic drugs such as chlorpromazine[4] or thioridazine,[5] and the leprosy-treatment drug clofazimine[6] have been reported to cause retinopathy.

INHERITED DYSTROPHIES OF THE MACULA VERSUS PANRETINAL DISEASE

It can be challenging to distinguish macular dystrophies from cone or cone-rod dystrophies using the tools available in a clinical setting. The differentiation between macular dystrophies, cone dystrophies, and cone-rod dystrophies largely depends on electroretinography (ERG) as a key investigation.[7] Accordingly, patients with macular dystrophies show full-field ERG recordings in the (near-) normal range, whereas those with cone and cone-rod dystrophies reveal significantly reduced or extinguished photopic responses and overall reduced (photopic > scotopic) recordings, respectively. This classification may change with disease progression, but few clinicians regularly perform ERGs these days. Also, in Stargardt disease, the peripheral retinal function is often unaffected but there are extended lesions in some cases. Hence, there may be overlap of macular dystrophies with cone dystrophies and cone-rod dystrophies, and macular dystrophies may develop signs of peripheral involvement and become cone or cone-rod dystrophies after several years.[7] For the conditions outlined in this chapter, the most common causative genes have been identified, and it is tempting to classify them solely based on the underlying genes. However, mutations in a single gene may result in a variety of clinical phenotypes, whereas a single phenotype may have a number of different underlying genes. For example, a large proportion of cone-rod dystrophies are caused by *ABCA4*, the causative gene of Stargardt disease type 1.

PURPOSE OF CARE FOR MACULAR DYSTROPHY PATIENTS

Patients with macular dystrophies must be evaluated for several reasons: to provide an accurate diagnosis, in order to counsel the patient about the likely progressive course of the disease and encourage low vision rehabilitation; to counsel the patient on the hereditary nature of the disease and the possible implications for future generations; and to provide the patient with information on current and future treatment trials that may slow the progression of photoreceptor loss or restore vision.

INVESTIGATIONS FOR MACULAR DYSTROPHY PATIENTS

The 2016 AAO Clinical Statement on inherited retinal diseases recommends a number of investigations for assessing patients with macular dystrophies.[8] These procedures, including an ocular history of visual symptoms and medical history on retinotoxic medications, should be performed at baseline and then again regularly at follow-up every 1–2 years. A pedigree should be created and updated on subsequent visits. During every patient encounter, the best-corrected visual acuity (BCVA) and the intraocular pressure should be determined, and slit-lamp and ophthalmoscopic exams should be performed. The extent and progression of macular dystrophies should be documented at each visit with fundus photos, spectral-domain optical coherence tomography (SD-OCT), fundus autofluorescence (FAF), and when available infrared autofluorescence. The recommendations from the American Academy of Ophthalmology on the clinical evaluation of patients with inherited dystrophies involving the macula are presented in Table 53.2. A number of related conditions that may come to light during these examinations, such as cataract formation or the presence of cystoid macular edema, are treatable. The functional extent of vision loss can be documented using kinetic visual

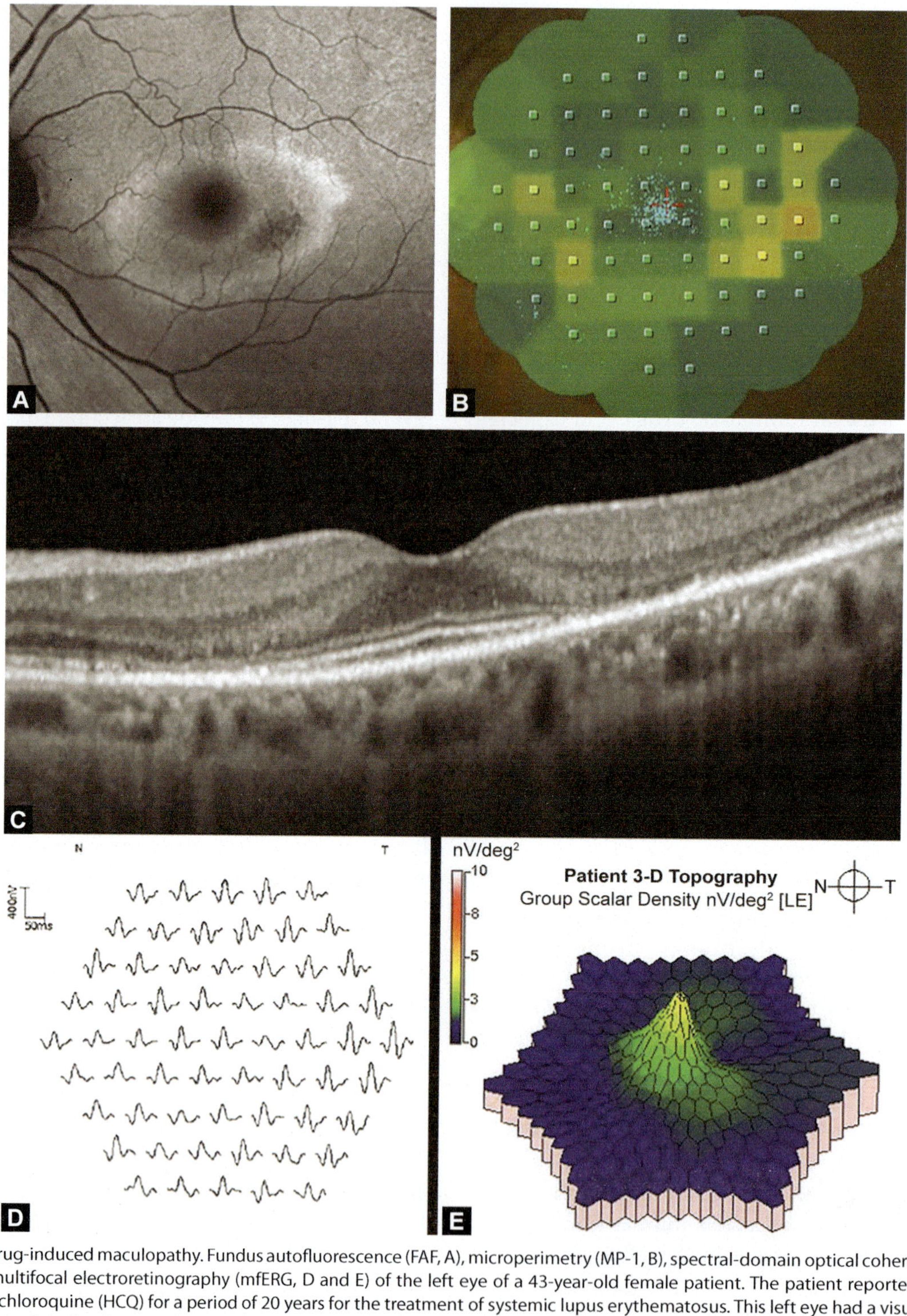

Figs. 53.1A to E: Drug-induced maculopathy. Fundus autofluorescence (FAF, A), microperimetry (MP-1, B), spectral-domain optical coherence tomography (SD-OCT, C), and multifocal electroretinography (mfERG, D and E) of the left eye of a 43-year-old female patient. The patient reported the daily use of 400 mg of hydroxychloroquine (HCQ) for a period of 20 years for the treatment of systemic lupus erythematosus. This left eye had a visual acuity of 20/20 and the examination of the fundus revealed a bull's eye maculopathy. On FAF testing (A), this corresponded to a ring of increased FAF signal and partly reduced signals surrounding the foveal center. The MP-1 (B) exhibited moderately increased light thresholds in the macula surrounding the foveal center. SD-OCT imaging (C) revealed parafoveal thinning and interruption of the outer nuclear layer, the ellipsoid zone, and the interdigitation zone. MfERG testing using the 61-hexagon array according to the ISCEV standards demonstrated parafoveal reduction in response amplitudes (D) and the 3D response density plots revealed parafoveal reductions of responses (E). Drug-induced changes have been reported to phenocopy macular dystrophies, especially those associated with *ABCA4* mutations. Due to the chronic use of HCQ, however, the patient was diagnosed with hydroxychloroquine-associated maculopathy and it is important to consider that the effects of numerous drugs on the retina may imitate the phenotype of macular dystrophies.

Table 53.2: 2016 Recommendations on the clinical evaluation of inherited degenerative diseases of the macula.

Clinical evaluation and assessment for inherited dystrophies that involve the macula	Initial visit	Follow-up visit every 1–2 years
History Ocular (including current needs) Medical (including current medications and history of retinotoxic medication use)	Yes	Yes
Pedigree (family history)	Yes	Yes
Clinical eye examination Best corrected visual acuity: ETDRS (or equivalent) Slit-lamp biomicroscopy Intraocular pressure Indirect ophthalmoscopy	Yes	Yes
Imaging		
Color fundus photos	Yes	No
Spectral-domain optical coherence tomography	Yes	Yes
Fundus autofluorescence: Short wavelength with reduced illumination when possible	Yes	Yes
Infrared autofluorescence (when available)	Yes	Yes
Visual fields		
Kinetic	Yes	Yes
Static	No	No
Microperimetry (when available)	Yes	Yes
Electroretinography		
Full-field ERG (when appropriate)	Yes	No
Multifocal ERG (when appropriate)	Yes	Yes
Genetic diagnostic testing	Yes	No

Source: Reproduced from and modified with permission from the American Academy of Ophthalmology. Clinical Statement. Recommendations on Clinical Assessment of Patients with Inherited Retinal Degenerations. San Francisco, CA: American Academy of Ophthalmology; 2016.

fields and fundus-controlled (micro-) perimetry. The latter is especially useful for eyes that have lost foveal fixation and that must rely on an eccentric location of the retina for fixation. Multifocal electroretinography (mfERG) testing is useful as an objective functional assessment of the macula but is of limited usefulness if fixation is unstable.[9,10] Genetic testing should be performed once at baseline.

GENETIC TESTING FOR MACULAR DYSTROPHIES

Recent advances in genetic diagnostic tools allow identification of the causative mutation in 60–80% of patients with inherited retinal disorders.[11-17] According to the current AAO guidelines, the potential value of genetic testing should be discussed whenever the physician suspects a genetic cause of the clinical phenotype. For the interpretation of the test results, it needs to be considered that specific phenotypes may be caused by multiple different genes and specific mutations may cause multiple different phenotypes in different patients. Genetic testing also allows identification of asymptomatic family members of affected individuals, hence, the implications of a genetic diagnosis without available curative therapies must be discussed with the family member prior to testing.

The primary goals of genetic testing include increased diagnostic and prognostic accuracy and counseling on specific inheritance risks. Genetic testing will also be increasingly necessary to guide therapy since eligibility for gene therapy trials depends on a genetic diagnosis.[18-20] Due to the complexity and sensitivity of the findings, the genetic diagnosis should be disclosed and discussed with the patient by a specialist in inherited retinal diseases or a genetic counselor, and the implications and limitations of the genetic diagnosis should be discussed.

STARGARDT DISEASE (*ABCA4*-ASSOCIATED MACULAR DYSTROPHY)

Pathophysiology and Epidemiology of Stargardt Disease

Autosomal recessive Stargardt disease (STGD1; OMIM, 248200) is the most common inherited disorder of the macula, accounting for about 7% of all retinal dystrophies.[21,22] The condition was first described in 1909 by the German ophthalmologist Karl Stargardt, and the underlying mutation has been identified in the *ABCA4* gene located on chromosome 1p.[21] About 95% of cases are caused by mutations in the *ABCA4* gene (Stargardt disease type 1, STGD1. In this chapter, we are using STGD1 synonymous with *ABCA4*-associated macular dystrophy).[21,23] Genes that cause a similar phenotype include *PRPH2* (Macular pattern dystrophy; OMIM, 169150), *ELOVL4* (Stargardt disease type 3; OMIM, 600110), or *PROM1* (Stargardt disease type 4; OMIM, 603786). The designation Stargardt disease type 2 is no longer used. *ABCA4* encodes a photoreceptor outer segment protein involved in the transportation of retinoids between photoreceptor outer segment disks and the RPE. In the absence of *ABCA4*, retinoid intermediates (NRPE, N-retinylidene-phosphatidylethanolamine) accumulate and form bisretinoids, such as A2E (A2-dihydropyridine-ethanolamine). Bisretinoids and oxidation products are toxic and may lead to cell death.[24,25] Without *ABCA4*, all-transretinal and NRPE cannot be removed and recycled.[23 26] Their concentration increases and toxic bisretinoids form.[26] The photoreceptor inner and outer segments have been shown to be attenuated over intact RPE cells.[27] The *ABCA4* gene was first identified in STGD1[21] but was later shown also to be involved in cone dystrophy, cone-rod dystrophy, and retinitis pigmentosa-like panretinal dystrophy.[28-33] More than 1,000 disease-causing sequence variants in *ABCA4* are known to date,[34] and the residual function of the protein may determine the clinical phenotype and the severity of the disease.

One proposed sequence of events in STGD1 is the accumulation of N-retinylidene-phosphatidylethanolamine in the photoreceptor outer segments. Toxic bisretinoids then accumulate in the RPE and cause death of RPE cells. The photoreceptors then die secondarily, due to the death of their support layer.[35] As the RPE cells endocytose the photoreceptor outer segments, toxic bisretiniods accumulate excessively in the RPE lysosome and result in RPE cell death.[36,37]

Clinical Features of Stargardt Disease

The clinical phenotype of STGD1 is very heterogeneous with a wide range of different clinical presentations, various ages of onset, different progression rates, and various imaging, psychophysical and electrophysiological findings. Before the onset of vision loss, very early stages of the disease may show a normal fundus or mild RPE disturbances with nonspecific mottling and a loss of the foveal light reflex.[38,39] At this stage of the disease, retinal imaging, including FAF, spectral-domain OCT, or psychophysical methods such as microperimetry, may already reveal abnormalities (Figs. 53.2A to C).[38,40-43]

The main complaint at presention is typically progressive BCVA impairment, but patients may also be diagnosed due to an abnormal fundus presentation on a routine eye exam. Color vision may also be affected. The age when the first visual symptoms occur or the age of diagnosis can be as early as within the first decade of life or may be 60 years of age or even later,[38,40,42-45] with the two peaks of highest incidence in childhood and early adulthood.[38,46,47] In the retrospective ProgStar study, half of the enrolled 176 participants reported an age of onset after 30 years of age.[40] An earlier onset of the disease seems to be associated with a more severe disease course, while late-onset patients exhibit relatively resistant cones and foveal sparing.[39,43,46-48]

BCVA may initially be as good as 20/20 or may be reduced to 20/200 or worse.[40] Examination of the posterior pole often reveals bilateral, typically symmetric areas of RPE atrophy.[38] This atrophy is located in the macula and often involves the foveal center. In contrast to geographic atrophy secondary to AMD, the atrophy in STGD1 frequently demonstrates a metallic sheen or "beaten-bronze" appearance. The areas of atrophy are accompanied by numerous yellow-white pisciform (fish tail-shaped) flecks at the posterior pole at the level of the RPE. These flecks may be confined to the vascular arcades or may extend beyond them; they may differ substantially in their number, size, color, and edge definition. In most instances, the flecks are yellow, but the full spectrum is from white to orange. Their number can range from zero to more than 100. They may remain stable for years or become more

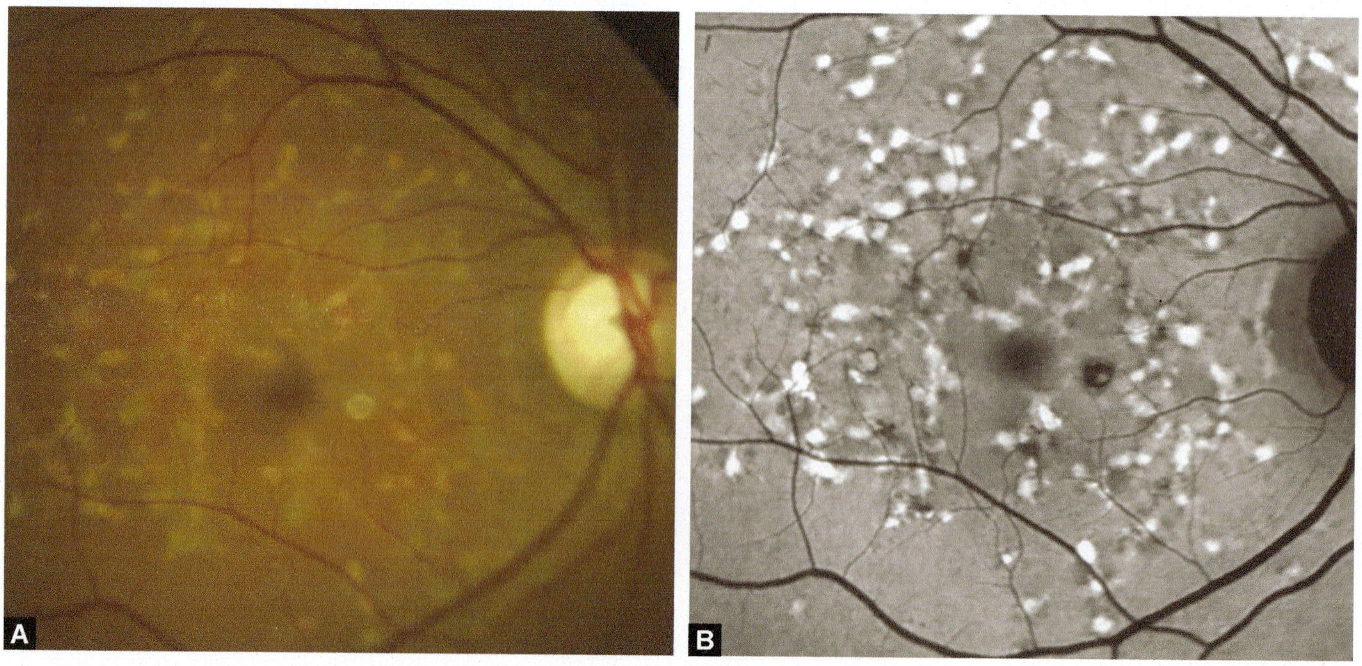

Figs. 53.2A and B

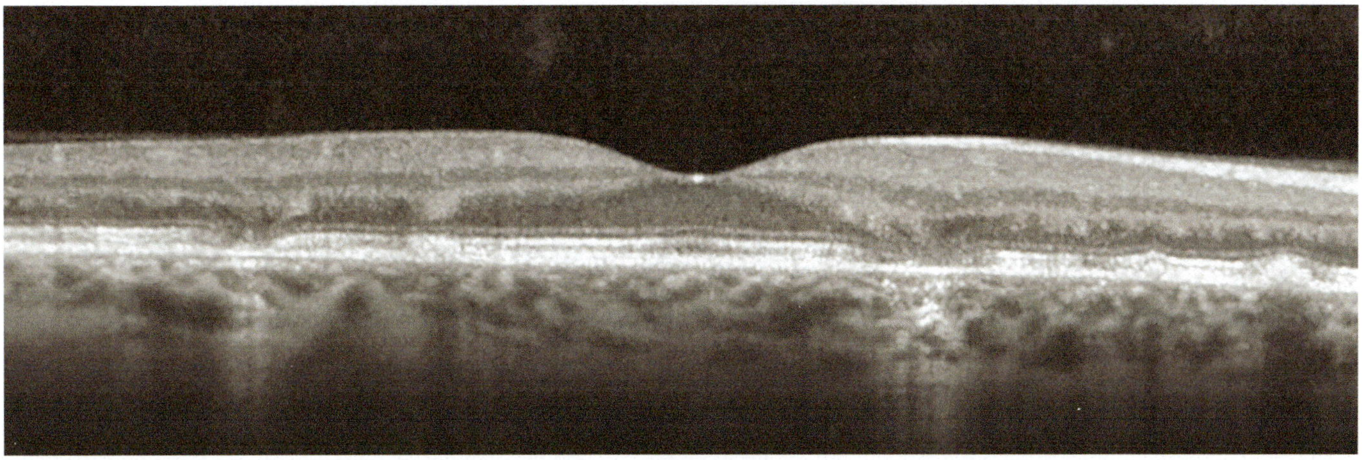

Fig. 53.2C

Figs. 53.2A to C: Multimodal imaging in Stargardt disease. (A) Fundus photograph, fundus autofluorescence (FAF), spectral-domain optical coherence tomography (SD-OCT) of the right eye of a 42-year-old male patient with two mutations in the *ABCA4* gene [Stargardt disease type 1 (STGD1)]. The visual acuity is 20/16. Yellow-white pisciform (fish tail-shaped) flecks at the level of the RPE are a typical finding. In the ProgStar studies, these flecks were found in 82–91% within and in 45% outside the arcades. Compared to drusen, these flecks have a more elongated appearance and a net-like appearance created by their contact to one another. In the ProgStar studies, the prevalence of clinically discernible RPE atrophy was 96%, 67% had flecks within the arcades, 67–81% had RPE pigmentation abnormalities; (B) Changes on FAF imaging are even more obvious and may reveal abnormalities when fundus findings are still normal. Flecks, which represent accumulations of lipofuscin, often exhibit increased FAF signals. As they expand, they leave areas of atrophy of the photoreceptors and RPE which is associated with decreased FAF signals. This is in contrast to age-related macular degeneration where the drusen are typically associated with a decrease in FAF signals; (C) The SD-OCT scan confirms that the outer retinal layers in the foveal region are intact, providing plausibility for the eye's ability to see 20/16. Multiple focal areas of atrophy of the ellipsoid layer can be seen outside of the fovea.

numerous and progress to RPE atrophy (Fig. 53.3). Flecks can be distinguished from drusen by their more elongated appearance and the net-like appearance created by their contact with one another. Franceschetti called the shape of two adjacent flecks "pisciform" (fish tail-shaped). Cases without flecks occur and are occasionally misdiagnosed.[43] Atrophy in *ABCA4*-associated retinal disease typically spares the parapapillary region. This is considered a very reliable sign of the disease and is more easily seen on FAF imaging.[49,50] The largest multicenter study to date of the progression of atrophy secondary to STGD1 investigated the prevalence of the different fundus features (Fig. 53.4).[38] In 1965, Franceschetti and Francois originally described "fundus flavimaculatus" as a condition separate from Stargardt disease,[51,52] but these genetically linked conditions are actually variants of the same disease. Indeed, Stargardt disease can show widespread retinal involvement with flecks diffusely scattered throughout the posterior pole to the midperiphery[53] (Fig. 53.5).

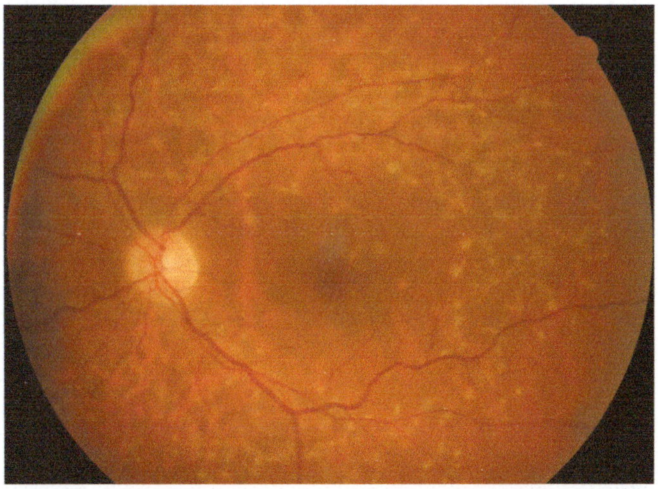

Fig. 53.3: Fundus phenotype in Stargardt disease. Fundus photograph of the left eye of a 51-year-old female with Stargardt disease. This eye has 20/20 visual acuity. Numerous flecks within but mainly outside of the vascular arcades are visible. The flecks have a yellow-white color and a pisciform shape. They seem more elongated than drusen and create a net-like appearance by contacting each other.

Visual Function in Stargardt Disease

Loss of BCVA is the main complaint reported by patients affected with STGD1. In the retrospective ProgStar study (N = 433), 36% of eyes with molecularly confirmed STGD1 had a BCVA of 20/70 or better.[38] About 52% had a BCVA between less than 20/70 and 20/200 and 12% had a BCVA between less than 20/200 and 20/400.[40] Younger symptom onset and longer disease duration have been associated with poorer BCVA readings.[40,54] An overall average loss of 0.3 lines per year was calculated in ProgStar and similar results can be inferred from another study by Rotenstreich et al.[45] For patients with symptom onset before the age of

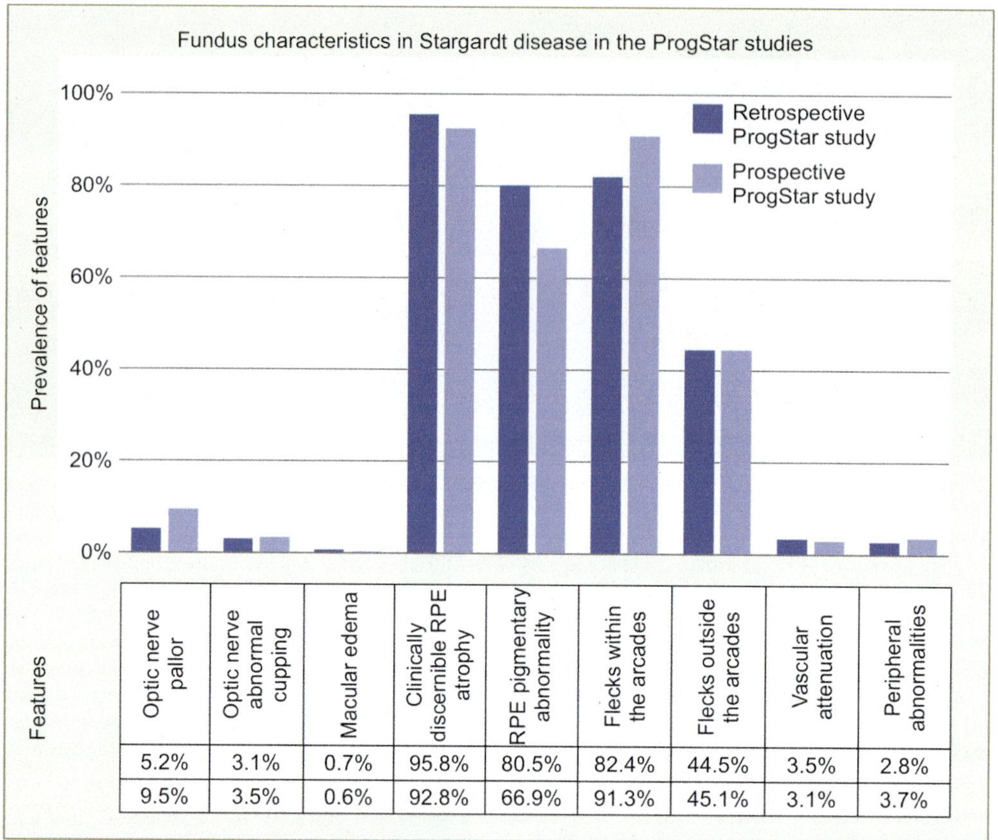

Fig. 53.4: Fundus characteristics of Stargardt disease in the ProgStar studies. Atrophy of the retinal pigment epithelium (RPE), RPE pigmentation abnormalities, and flecks within the arcades were present in most patients in both the retrospective and prospective ProgStar studies. Vascular attenuation, macular edema, or pallor of the optic disk, which are features typical of panretinal diseases such as retinitis pigmentosa, were rarely seen. Flecks located outside of the vascular arcades are present in about half of all eyes.

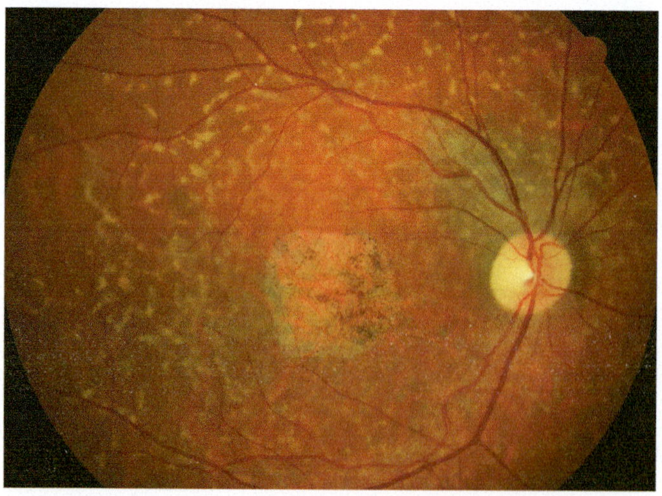

Fig. 53.5: Widespread retinal involvement with flecks extending beyond the vascular arcades (previously known as fundus flavimaculatus). Fundus photograph of the right eye of a 42-year-old male with 2 mutations in the *ABCA4* gene and 20/400 visual acuity shows a variant of Stargardt disease. The appearance of the fundus is characterized by numerous flecks throughout the posterior pole and a central macular area of atrophy and "beaten-bronze" appearance.

30 years, the yearly loss of BCVA was 0.4 lines per year, both in ProgStar[40] and in another cohort.[54] Eyes with extensive extramacular flecks are associated with a poorer visual prognosis in the long-term than eyes that have flecks and atrophy limited to the macula.[53,55] The rate of BCVA loss is also largely dependent on baseline VA, with eyes that have a better BCVA at baseline declining at a higher rate. For a BCVA more than or equal to 20/25, the rate was 1.0 lines per year; for eyes with a BCVA between 20/25 and 20/70, the decline was 0.9 lines per year; for a BCVA between 20/70 and 20/200, the decline was 0.2 lines per year. Eyes with a BCVA worse than 20/200 actually improved by 0.5 lines per year, which may be explained by a change in fixation location and/or by the development of more stable fixation.[42,56-60]

Fundus Autofluorescence in Stargardt Disease

Fundus autofluorescence is a convenient, fast and noninvasive imaging procedure that allows identification

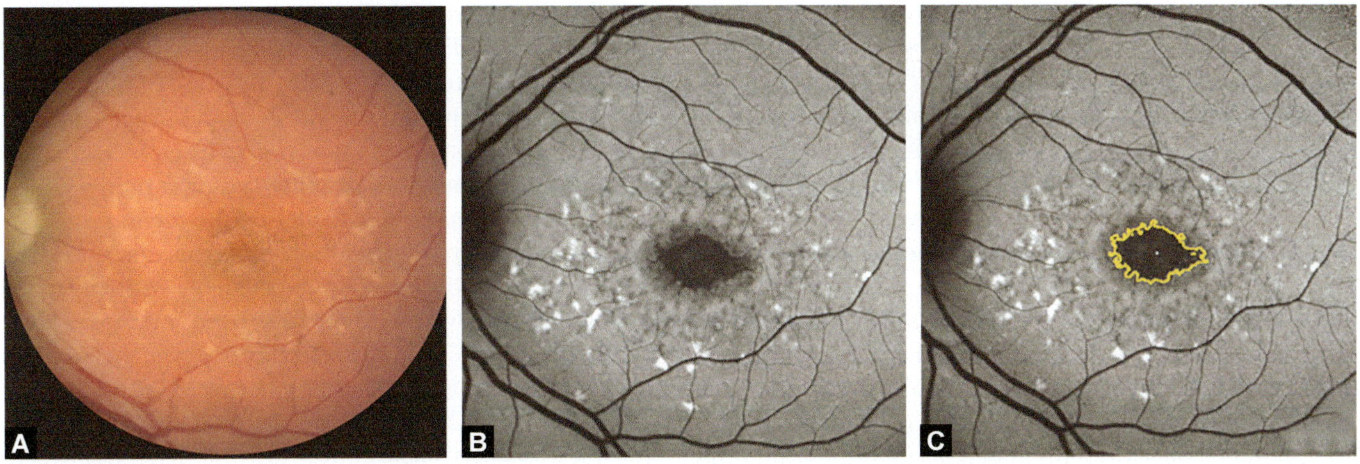

Figs. 53.6A to C: Autofluorescence in the ProgStar studies. Fundus photograph and fundus autofluorescence (FAF) of the left eye of a 26-year-old female with two mutations in the *ABCA4* gene (p.Gly863Ala:c.2588G>C and c.3210_3211insTG). Visual acuity was 20/80. The fundus picture (A) shows a central macular area of atrophy and extensive pisciform flecks surrounding the fovea. In the ProgStar studies, different categories were used for grading of decreased autofluorescence (DAF). Blood vessels and the optic nerve head (ONH) were used as reference points and set as 100% darkness. The normal background autofluorescence was defined as the opposite end of the scale. Areas of more than 90% darkness were defined as definitely decreased autofluorescence (DDAF). Areas of DDAF were delineated and measured using the Region Finder software from Heidelberg Engineering (C). The total area of DDAF at baseline of the prospective study was 4.04 ± 4 mm^2 and the yearly progression rate of DDAF in the retrospective study was 0.51 [95% confidence interval (CI) 0.42–0.61] mm^2/year and that of the total area of DAF was 0.35 (95% CI: 0.28–0.43) mm^2/year.

and quantification of the area of the atrophic retina in STGD1, bull's eye changes in the macula, flecks, and peripapillary sparing.[61] The pathophysiological basis for FAF testing is that lipofuscin, a heterogeneous material with bisretinoids as major components, is known to accumulate in STGD1 at a much higher rate than in normal aging and that STGD1 patients therefore show increased autofluorescence signals.[36,62-64] FAF reflects signals resulting from accumulation of lipofuscin and/or its reduction after RPE cell loss.[65,66] Lipofuscin accumulates early in life, as shown by the case of a 16-month-old child with STGD1 whose eye was enucleated because of retinoblastoma. Histological investigation demonstrated remarkable lipofuscin accumulation within the RPE and substantially increased autofluorescence signal compared to normal aging.[67] As opposed to AMD, in which drusen are rather associated with a decrease in FAF signal,[68,69] the flecks in STGD1 display increased autofluorescence signal. Atrophic areas of the macula show decreased autofluorescence signal. These changes can be detected using FAF before they are visible on ophthalmoscopy.[70,71]

A peripapillary annulus of a few hundred micrometers retains a relatively normal appearance throughout the course of the disease.[72] There is excellent agreement between areas of atrophy quantified by grading of color fundus photos and FAF images. FAF imaging is very helpful for detecting lesions, especially in the early disease stages.[73-75] It is possible to quantitatively delineate regions of accumulated lipofuscin or areas of atrophic or diseased RPE in STGD1 as demonstrated in Figures 53.6A to C.[61,76] Several small studies have used FAF to track the progression of atrophy in STGD1.[77-80] The retrospective ProgStar study analyzed 458 eyes of 251 patients and defined areas of definitely decreased autofluorescence (DDAF) as those areas with a darkness of more than or equal to 90% of the optic disk.[38] The average DDAF lesion area was 2.5 ± 2.9 mm^2 (range, 0.02–16.03 mm^2). Fluorescein angiography with the classical "dark choroid" due to low background fluorescence was used in STGD1 in the past.[81,82] There is some concern that light exposure, and especially exposure to the high-intensity light used in fluorescein angiography or FAF imaging, might accelerate disease progression.

Optical Coherence Tomography in Stargardt Disease

Spectral-domain OCT can visualize the retinal architecture in vivo,[87] making it possible to distinguish single retinal layers and bands.[88] In STGD1, SD-OCT can characterize healthy and affected areas and identify transition zones.[89] Features of STGD1 seen on SD-OCT are a loss of outer retinal tissue, loss of photoreceptors and RPE cells, and retinal thinning. These findings start in the center of the macula and relatively spare the peripheral macula.[38,79,87,90] The earliest feature of STGD1, detected on SD-OCT in children 5 years of age, seems to be thickening of a band corresponding to the external limiting membrane.[67,91-93] The central foveal thickness correlates with BCVA.[48] One study confirmed disorganization or loss of the inner-segment outer-segment junction (IS-OS) in all investigated eyes.[90] The thickness of the peripapillary nerve fiber layer on OCT imaging can be altered, but the significance of this finding is unknown.[94] The structural changes associated with degeneration of photoreceptors on OCT can be detected when FAF testing is still normal or shows only minor changes.[90] These changes are associated with decreased amplitudes on mfERG testing of the central 10 degrees.[95] Comparison of multiple imaging devices has also shown that measuring only the diameter of the area of absent FAF underestimates the extent of ellipsoid loss on SD-OCT.[90] The same authors were able to show a better correlation of the ellipsoid loss measurement with the diameter measured on SD-OCT when including the transition zone on FAF imaging.[90]

Microperimetry in Stargardt Disease

Most retina specialists and clinical studies rely on BCVA as a measure of visual performance.[40,44,96,97] In STGD1, however, the slow rate of BCVA loss makes it less suitable for monitoring disease progression.[40,98] As an alternative psychophysical approach, visual field testing can describe the function of the central retina but conventional visual field testing misses small scotomas and may deliver false results in eyes without central fixation. Accurate structure-function correlation in macular diseases is possible using fundus-controlled (micro-) perimetry.[99,100] The ProgStar studies used the Nidek MP-1 microperimeter (MP-1, Nidek Technologies). The Nidek MP-1 tests retinal sensitivity in predefined regions on a scale from 0 dB (absolute scotoma) to 20 dB where the dimmest light stimulus could be detected by the patient. The mean of the overall microperimetric mean sensitivity (MS) in STGD1 was 11.0 ± 5.0 dB in the ProgStar study,[101] while values in age-matched healthy controls have been reported to be close to 20 dB.[102] Counting the number of absolute scotoma points on the microperimetry grid and calculating the mean sensitivity are two different approaches to quantify macular sensitivity in STGD1, and both showed reduced light sensitivity in the ProgStar study. Overall, the results from microperimetry correlate with BCVA measurements. However, the ProgStar study found a number of cases with low MS results of less than 6 dB and BCVA of 20/40 or better. Functional foveal sparing is a likely explanation for this discrepancy. An additional finding is that microperimetry occasionally underestimates the true BCVA potential in STGD1, whereas BCVA alone does not capture the extensive loss of sensitivity in the rest of the macula.[101] In the ProgStar study the central foveal area had the lowest mean MS of 2.7 ± 4.4 dB. The mean MS in the inner ETDRS ring was 6.8±5.8 dB and in the outer ring was 12.7 ± 5.3 dB. In other words, the functional deficit in STGD1 is most pronounced in the foveal center but is relatively preserved in the peripheral macula (Figs. 53.7A to C), although this may be different in the subgroup of patients with foveal sparing. There were associations between longer duration of STGD1 and worse MS of the macula, lower number of normal test points, and a higher number of absolute scotoma points. In addition, a later age of symptom onset in STGD1 is associated with a milder reduction of sensitivity on microperimetry testing in STGD1.[39,40]

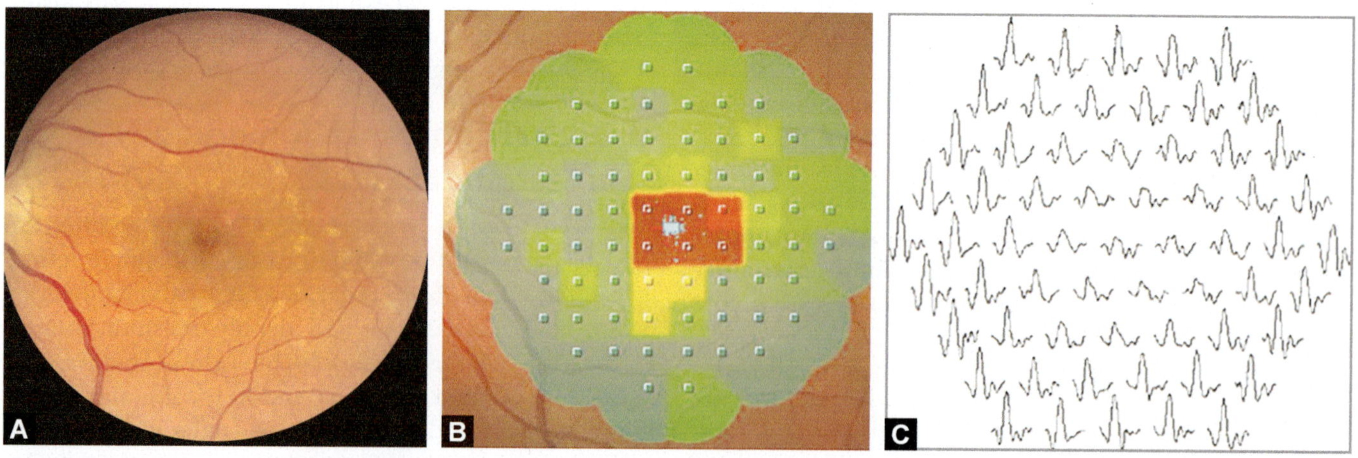

Figs. 53.7A to C: Functional assessment of the macula in Stargardt disease. (A) Fundus photograph of the left eye of a 42-year-old female with Stargardt disease and two identified *ABCA4* mutations. Visual acuity in this eye is 20/32. The macula shows slight pigmentary changes; scattered yellowish flecks can be seen at the level of the retinal pigment epithelium; (B) Microperimetric examination of the same eye shows that foveal light sensitivity is decreased. In the central four test points, the eye was unable to detect the brightest light stimulus the Nidek MP-1 displays. Sensitivity in the peripheral macula, however, was normal. The eye showed central and stable fixation (99% of fixation events within a 2-degree circle), suggesting a small island of at least relatively preserved function within the central absolute scotoma; (C) On testing with the 61-hexagon multifocal electroretinogram according to ISCEV standards, the central hexagons exhibited reduced response amplitudes.

Electrophysiology in Stargardt Disease

Electrophysiologic testing, including full-field electro-retinography (ffERG) and multifocal electro-retinography (mfERG), may be useful in the diagnosis and prognostication of STGD1. The ffERG is typically normal, or at least not measurably abnormal, in conditions confined to the macula such as STGD1. Severe forms of *ABCA4*-related retinal disease may result in abnormal cone- or both abnormal cone- and rod-driven ERG recordings.[55,103-108] In mild forms of STGD1, toxic bisretinoids seem to disturb only the foveal cones, resulting in loss of BCVA but no measurable decrease of the ffERG. Forms with intermediate severity may reduce the cone-driven ERG, and severe forms may affect both the cone and rod recordings.[33,108] To the best of our knowlegde, there is no report of STGD1 patients with electronegative waveforms. Even in patients with only minor fundus abnormalities, the pattern ERG may be abnormal.[103] Lois et al. categorized the ERG abnormalities into three distinct groups.[103] Group 1 is defined as abnormalities exclusively in pattern ERG measurements. The ffERG recordings derived from both rods and cones are normal in group 1.[103] In group 2, there is a reduction of 30 Hz flicker and of photopic wave amplitudes. Rod responses remain normal in group 2.[103] In group 3, there is generalized reduction in 30 Hz flicker and both cone and rod-derived wave amplitudes.[103] When the patients from the original study were followed longitudinally, the authors found a predictive value of such ERG groups. Group 1 has the best prognosis while group 3 has the worst.[79]

Genetics of Stargardt Disease

Stargardt disease can present with a number of different phenotypes and various progression rates.[43,47,79,87,92,109-116] Although it is commonly caused by mutations in *ABCA4*, Stargardt disease is highly heterogeneous from a genetic point of view.[38,46,47,79,112,114,117] Stargardt disease type 3 (OMIM, 600110) is associated with mutations in *ELOVL4* and Stargardt disease type 4 (OMIM, 603786) with mutations in *PROM1*. In addition to Stargardt disease, retinal disease associated with *ABCA4* has also been linked to cone-rod dystrophy and to autosomal recessive retinitis pigmentosa-like retinal dystrophy. The phenotypic variability has several reasons: the disease-causing alleles have variable severity in the population and they interact with environmental modifiers such as smoking, nutrition, or light exposure. In addition, the interaction between the various cells in the retina is very complex. In light of the phenotypic heterogeneity, identifying both disease-causing alleles increases the accuracy of diagnosis and helps in patient counseling. With the help of genetic data, clinicians can give the most accurate information about the patient's prognosis, make decisions about enrollment in clinical trials, and consider factors that might modify the course of the disease.

ABCA4 is a very large gene with 50 exons. The alleles themselves are heterogeneous, and more than 1,000 disease-associated variants in *ABCA4* have been identified.[34,104,118-123] Some of these variations have been associated with different levels of disease severity, and some laboratories offer a pathogenicity score.[124,125] The carrier frequency of disease-causing variations has been estimated to be as high as 5%.[126] In many cases, it is not possible to identify both disease alleles when the mutations lie outside the coding and promotor sequences.

Milder late-onset disease tends to be associated with missense variants, whereas severe early-onset cases are associated with null alleles. However, establishing definite genotype-phenotype correlations has been difficult.[118] Sanger sequencing of the complete *ABCA4* coding region can detect 66–80% of disease-causing alleles.[127,128] However, the procedure is laborious and therefore not suitable for screening. An alternative is screening only for known reported disease-associated alleles. The arrayed primer extension uses this approach to detect 65–75% of reported variants,[129,130] but it misses any novel variations. Next-generation sequencing is able to detect variants, including novel ones, relatively inexpensively in a larger number of patients.[119]

Treatment of Stargardt Disease

There is currently no treatment available for STGD1, but general recommendations used for conditions such as retinitis pigmentosa and other inherited diseases should be discussed with the patient. Affected individuals should be advised to avoid excessive light exposure and to wear protective dark glasses when exposed to sunlight. There is some evidence from animal models that high-energy light may contribute to the disease progression.[83] Patients should also be advised to avoid cigarette smoking and vitamin A supplementation. Gene therapy, pharmacotherapy, and stem cell therapy are currently being investigated in clinical trials. The emerging therapies for inherited macular dystrophies are discussed in the last section of this chapter.

BEST VITELLIFORM MACULAR DYSTROPHY (*BEST1*-ASSOCIATED MACULAR DYSTROPHY)

Genetics and Pathophysiology of Best Disease

Best vitelliform macular dystrophy (OMIM: 153700) is the second most common macular dystrophy after Stargardt disease. It was first described by the German ophthalmologist Friedrich Best in 1905.[131] Its prevalence was determined as 1 in 5,000 in a Swedish population[132] and 1 in 67,000 in a Danish population.[133] Some authors report a prevalence of 1 in 10,000.[134] Best disease is inherited in an autosomal dominant fashion with variable penetrance and expressivity (Figs. 53.8A to F). Modern imaging and genetic testing may yield a higher prevalence.[100] The underlying defect has been identified in the *BEST1* gene (previously known as *VMD2*), located on the long arm of chromosome 11.[135] *BEST1* is expressed in the RPE, and in small amounts in the kidney, brain, spinal cord, and testes.[135,136] It encodes a multifunctional protein, bestrophin-1, localized at the basolateral membrane of the RPE cell[137] and the intracellular compartment.[138,139] Bestrophin-1 functions as a Ca^{2+} activated Cl^- channel.[140,141] The multifunctional bestrophin-1 seems to play a role in the development of the eye as mutations in *BEST1* have been associated with additional conditions that are not discussed in this chapter, such as adult-onset foveomacular vitelliform dystrophy, autosomal dominant vitreoretinochoroidopathy, the "microcornea, rod-cone dystrophy, cataract, posterior staphyloma syndrome", and autosomal recessive bestrophinopathy.[148,149]

Clinical Features of Best Disease

Best vitelliform macular dystrophy has a heterogeneous clinical presentation, with a number of different symptoms and multiple different fundus findings. The age of onset may range from the first decade of life to cases presenting after the sixth decade. The mean age of onset is during the fourth decade.[150-153] The most common presenting complaint is reduced BCVA but metamorphopsia, photophobia, or nyctalopia also occur. Hypermetropia may develop secondary to elevation of the central retina.[154] The fundus may present with manifold different phenotypes in Best vitelliform macular dystrophy. It may present with a normal fundus, with only very discrete RPE alterations, from the classic "fried egg" or "scrambled egg" appearance over fluid accumulation to scarring. A number of different stages have been described. Features of these stages may occur simultaneously and the stages may overlap.[155] The lesions

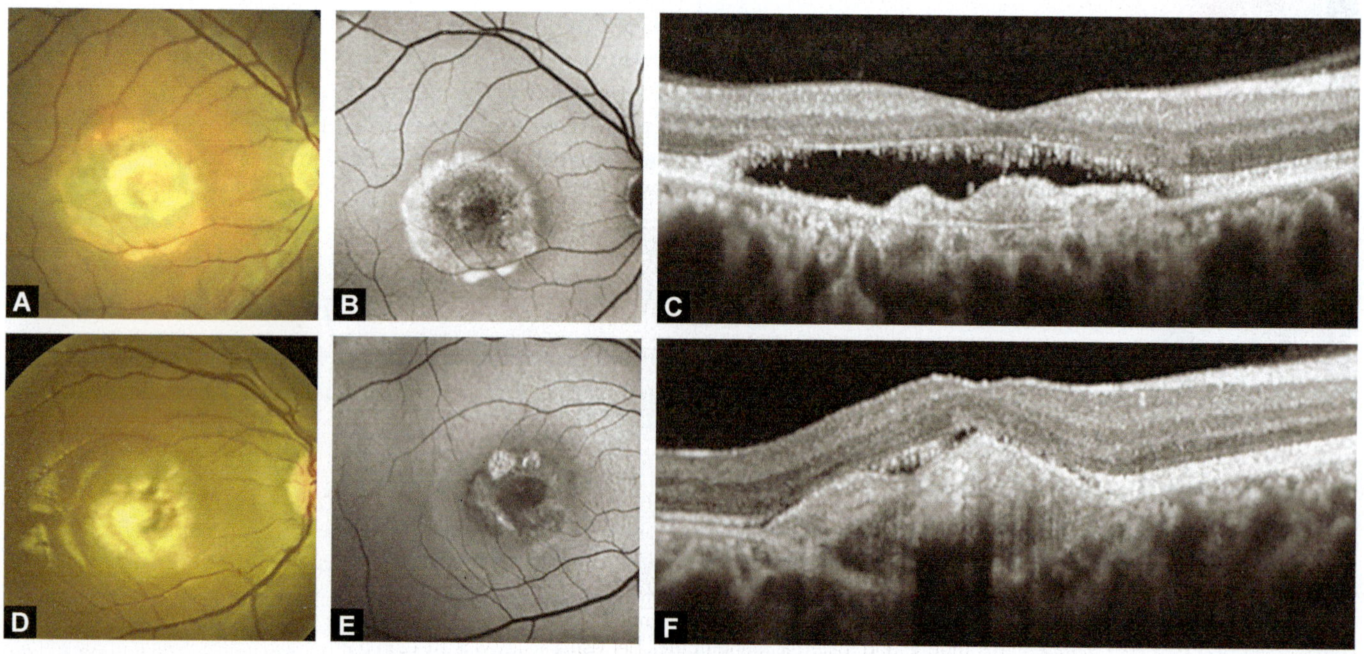

Figs. 53.8A to F: Father and daughter with Best disease—(A) Fundus photograph, (B) fundus autofluorescence, and (C) spectral-domain optical coherence tomography imaging (SD-OCT) of the right eye of a 42-year-old male with Best disease and his daughter at age 16 years (D to F) using the same imaging modalities. Typical for autosomal-dominant disease, each generation shows the disease phenotype. The father's right eye had a visual acuity of 20/40 and the daughter's right eye 20/80. The fundus photographs (A and D) demonstrate the yellow vitelliform lesion which corresponds to areas of increased and decreased autofluorescence signal (B and E). SD-OCT imaging through the fovea demonstrates the hyporeflective space underneath the ellipsoid zone (C) and the hyper-reflective material between the ellipsoid zone and RPE/Bruch's complex (F). Despite the age difference of 26 years the size of the lesions in father and daughter appear similar.

can vary substantially in their appearance and there may be multifocal vitelliform lesions with eccentric or extrafoveal location. Less classic presentations with locations superonasal or superotemporal to the optic disk have been reported.[156] In most reports in the literature, the EOG is abnormal already in the asymptomatic carrier stage of the disease but others indicate that EOG may remain normal in clinically affected mutation carriers (see below).[65,152,153,156,157] A useful way to confirm a clinical suspicion for Best disease is mutation analysis of the *BEST1* gene.

Prognosis of Best Disease

Although vitelliform lesions often develop in the first decade of life, they do not necessarily cause visual impairment. In fact, eyes of mutation carriers with no visible abnormalities or with only mild RPE changes often remain asymptomatic for years;[150,151] and after a follow-up of at least 5 years, up to 88% of patients maintain 20/40 or better BCVA in the better-seeing eye.[150,151] However, BCVA and patient age may correlate;[158] eyes in advanced stages usually rapidly progress to even more advanced stages.[150,151,153] Patients may lose BCVA due to choroidal neovascularization (CNV), scarring or atrophy but may retain 20/50 without treatment.[161] Even cases with central scarring may retain good vision.[150,159] After 50 years of age, many affected individuals have BCVA of 20/40 or worse in the better eye.[151,158]

Fundus Autofluorescence in Best Disease

Fundus autofluorescence is a useful imaging modality for diagnosis and follow-up of inherited retinal diseases in general[38] and allows visualization of changes that are not evident on ophthalmoscopy.[160,161] The yellow subretinal vitelliform material in Best disease has a highly increased autofluorescence signal, which can also be obvious in subclinical cases (Figs. 53.9A to D).[63,147,153,155,156,160,162-164]

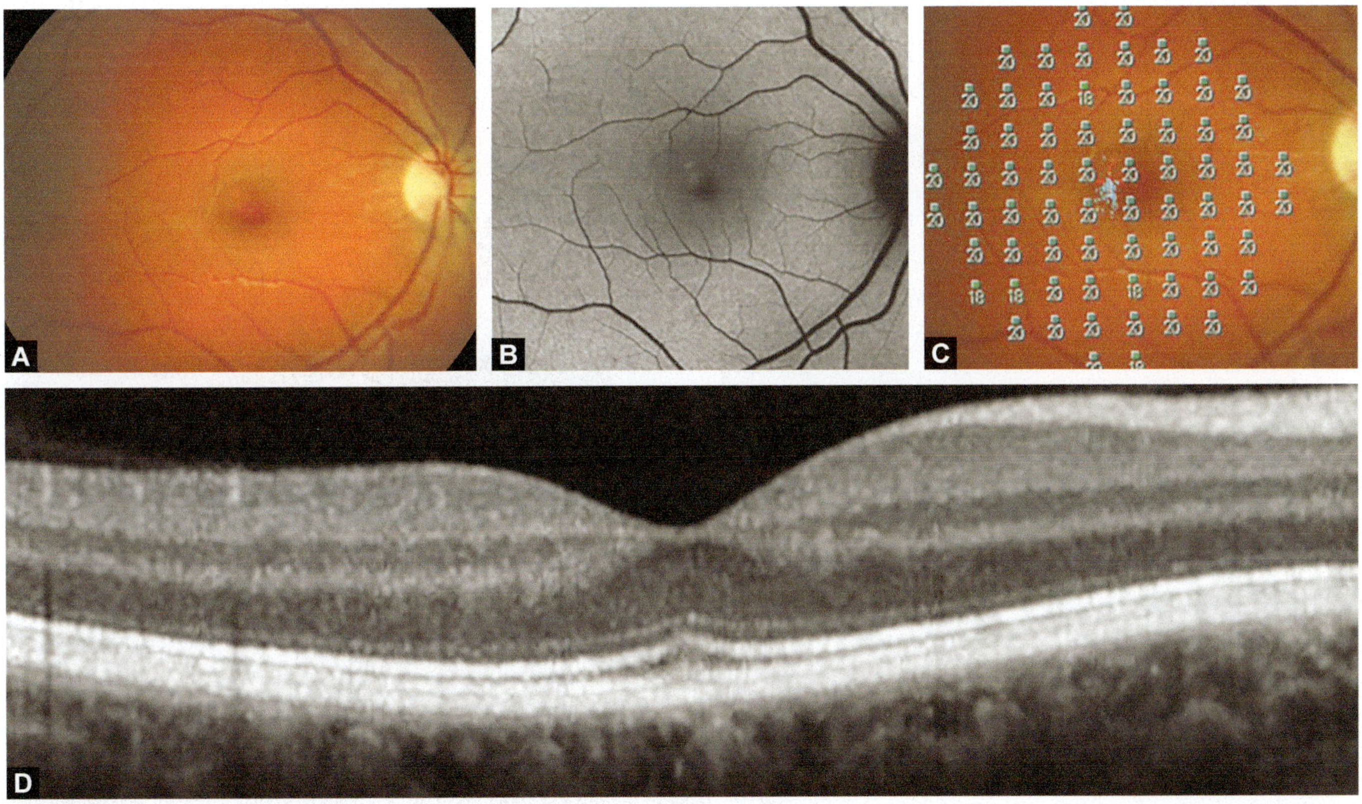

Figs. 53.9A to D: Multimodal imaging in a subclinical case of Best disease. Presented is the right eye of an asymptomatic 27-year-old white female patient with a family history of Best disease in her mother and maternal grandmother. Her visual acuity was 20/12 in both eyes. (A) Examination of the fundus showed very discrete hypopigmented changes in and close to the fovea; (B) Fundus autofluorescence (FAF) demonstrated discrete but clearly visible juxtafoveal regions of increased FAF signal in both eyes; (C) Microperimetric testing using the Nidek MP-1 failed to detect any functional deficits in and around the fovea, although slight decreases in microperimetric sensitivity have been reported in similar subclinical cases of Best disease. Fixation was foveal and stable; (D) Thickening of the hyper-reflective layer corresponding to the photoreceptors' outer segments has been described as the earliest visible change in Best disease using spectral-domain optical coherence tomography imaging. However, this layer was only questionably thickened in this case. Arden ratios were 1.42 in the right and 1.96 in the left eye. PCR amplification and next-generation sequencing revealed a heterozygous mutation in the *BEST1* gene (p.Tyr167Cys:c.500A>G).

Lipofuscin and toxic components (A2E etc.) form the autofluorescent material in Best disease.[70,142,165,166] In more advanced stages, the material with high FAF signal may disperse and a pseudohypopyon may form. In later atrophic and cicatricial stages the same areas demonstrate decreased FAF signal due to RPE atrophy and/or blockage of FAF by scar tissue and loss of autofluorescent material (Figs. 53.10 to 53.12).[146,153,161]

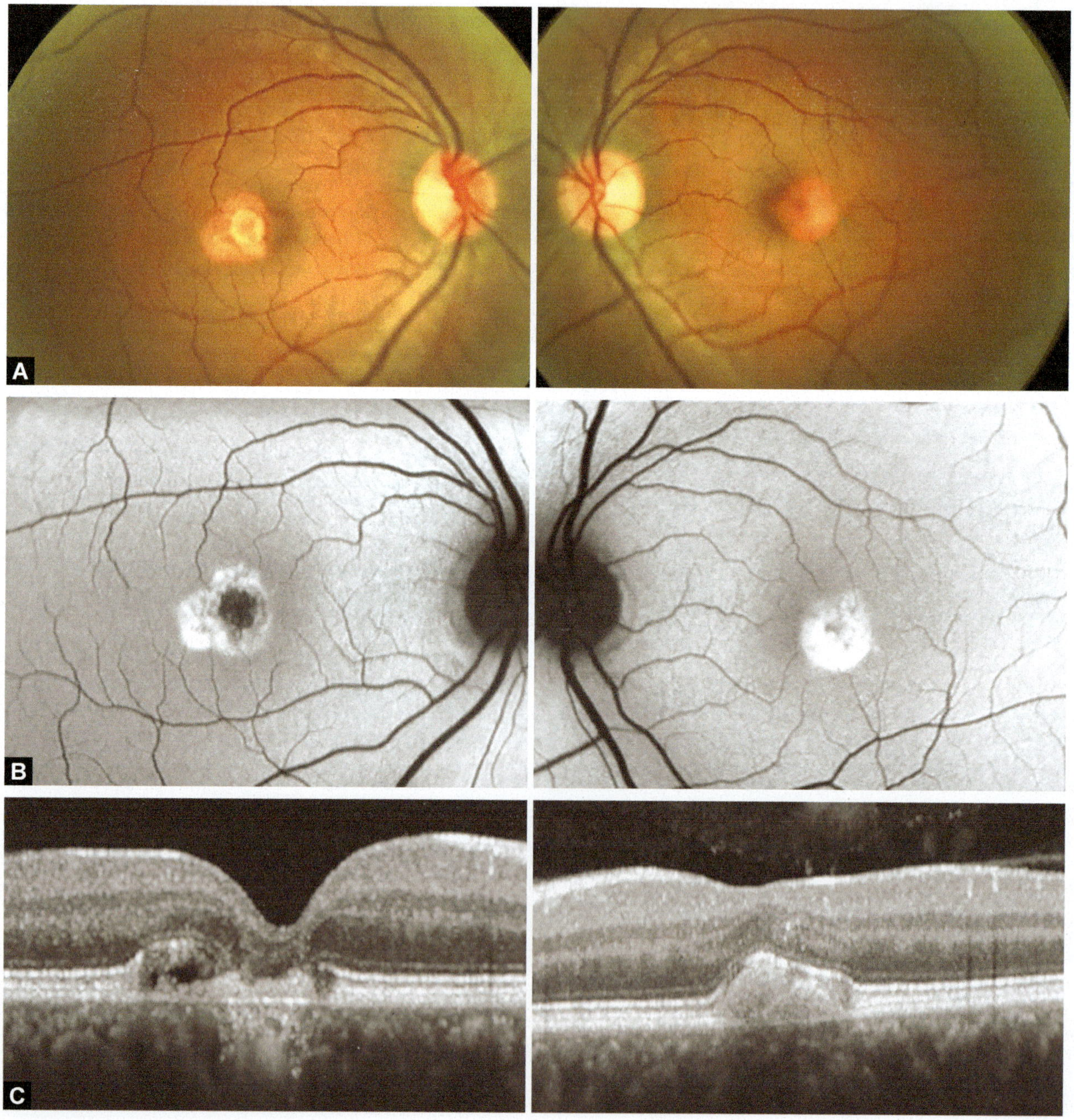

Figs. 53.10A to C: Best disease. (A) Fundus photographs of both eyes of a 38-year-old male patient with Best disease show subfoveal, yellow, and elevated lesions with a surrounding hyperpigmented halo. It is typical for macular dystrophies to show a very similar or even identical phenotype in both eyes. Despite the vitelliform lesions in the fovea, this patient has 20/32 visual acuity in the right and 20/16 in the left eye. The patient reports having a brother with Best disease; (B) Fundus autofluorescence imaging (FAF) reveals that the lesion corresponds to areas of increased FAF signal. Especially the lesion in the right eye shows a central area of decreased FAF signal in a patchy pattern. Otherwise, the distribution of FAF signal appears normal in the central 30 degrees; (C) Imaging with spectral-domain optical coherence tomography exhibits elevation and separation of the neurosensory retina from the outer hyper-reflective layer, i.e. from the RPE/Bruch's membrane complex. Thinning of the outer nuclear layer was evident overlying this area. The elevation appeared to be associated with thickening of the interdigitation zone between the ellipsoid zone and the RPE/Bruch's complex. This thickening corresponds to hyper-reflective material and in the right eye also to hyporeflective spaces. The ellipsoid zone showed focal disruption underneath the material.

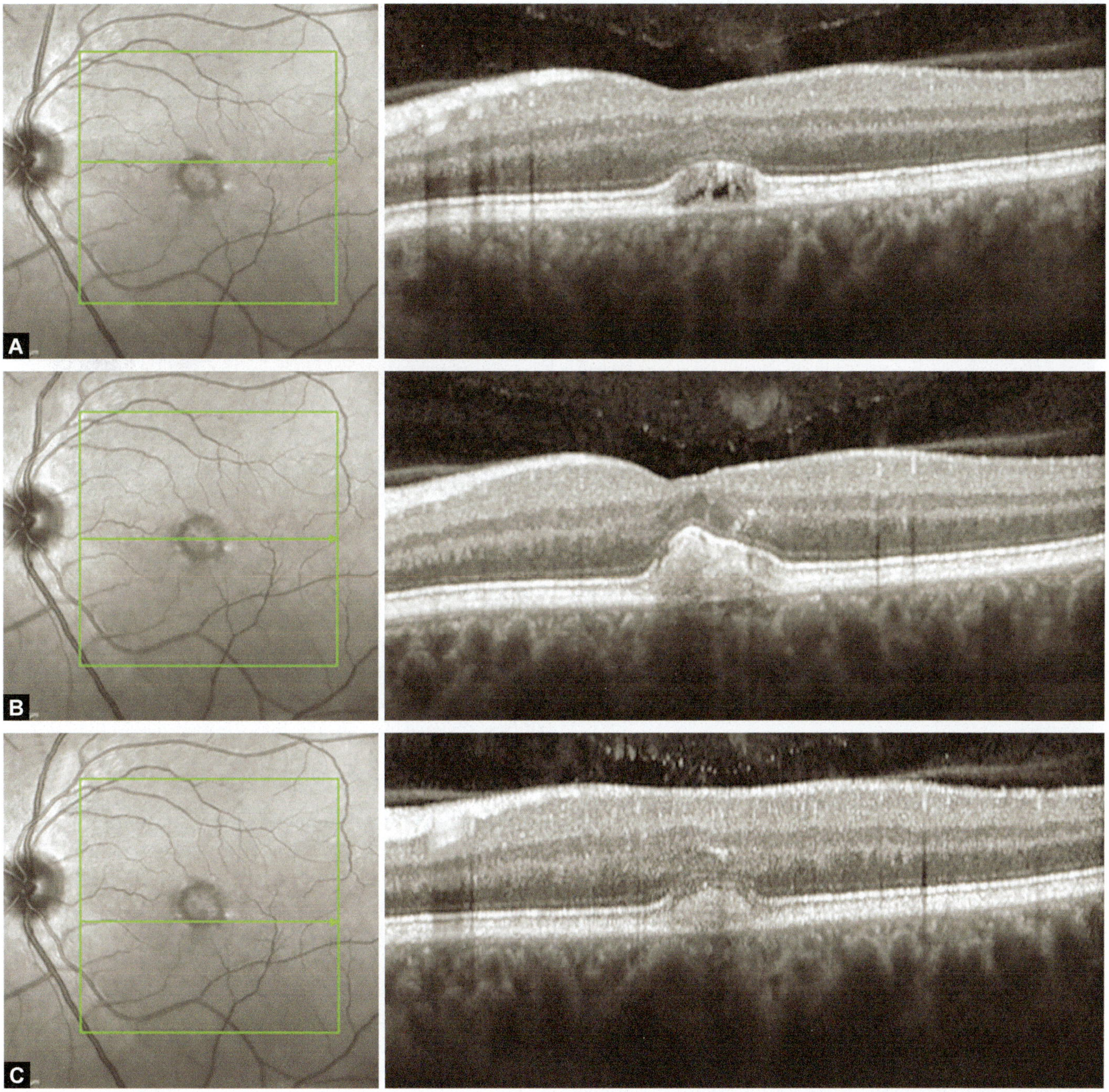

Figs. 53.11A to C: Three sections through the central macular lesion in Best disease obtained using spectral-domain optical coherence tomography in the left eye of a 38-year-old man with 20/16 visual acuity. The typical hyper-reflective material seems to accumulate in and around the interdigitation zone, leading to elevation of the neurosensory retina including the ellipsoid zone and to thinning of the outer nuclear layer on all three sections. As part of the pseudohypopyon, the hyper-reflective material seems to pile up in the inferior sections (B and C) and to create a hyporeflective cyst in the superior portion of the lesion (A). The two hyper-reflective bands surrounding the interdigitation zone are relatively preserved and seem to border the hyper-reflective material.

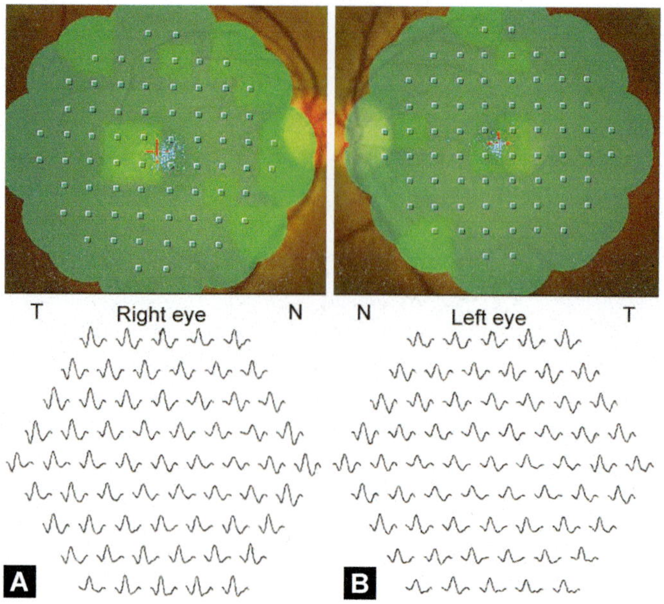

Figs. 53.12A and B: Functional assessment of the retina in Best disease. (A) In the same 38-year-old male patient with Best disease presented in Figures 53.10 and 53.11, light thresholds in the central 20 degrees of the macula were still relatively preserved despite the disruption of the photoreceptors seen on optical coherence tomography testing. Several test locations in the foveal regions had relatively reduced sensitivity measurements when compared to the remainder of the test grid; (B) There are no obvious reductions in amplitudes using multifocal electroretinography according to International Society for Clinical Electrophysiology of Vision (ISCEV) standards. Arden ratios were 0.54 in the right and 1.44 in the left eye (normal, >1.8).

Electrophysiology in Best Disease

Electrophysiologic testing has a central role in evaluating inherited diseases of the retina because it allows an objective assessment of retinal function and can distinguish between disorders that primarily affect the cones or rods.[167] The full-field (also known as Ganzfield) electroretinogram is generally normal in Best disease, whereas the mfERG usually shows abnormalities in the central stimulus rings.[152,153,168,169] The amplitudes are reduced and implicit times increased.[153,168,170] The classic test for Best disease is the electrooculogram (EOG): the Arden ratio is the ratio of the light peak to the dark trough and is regularly reduced both in manifest Best disease[171] and in asymptomatic carriers of the mutation, indicating a global defect in the RPE.[65,152,153,156,157] More recent research shows that the EOG may initially also be normal and remain normal or only slightly abnormal in carriers.[65,102,152,153,156,157]

Microperimetry in Best Disease

Predicting the macular function in Best disease is challenging because similar phenotypes may differ in their ability to detect light stimuli. The central macular lesion in Best disease shows reduced sensitivity.[172] Both lesions of increased and lesions of decreased autofluorescence show decreased light sensitivity in Best disease.[173] Not only the central lesion but also retinal areas beyond the lesion itself and the peripheral retina show detectable loss of function.[174] Although relative scotomas can already be measured in the subclinical stage of Best disease,[174] FAF may detect structural abnormalities in cases where microperimetry is unable to show any functional deficits.[102] The atrophic, most advanced stage of the disease has the most pronounced deficit in macular sensitivity on microperimetry,[175] whereas the lesions in vitelliform, pseudohypopyon, and vitelliruptive stages show similar sensitivity.[175]

Optical Coherence Tomography in Best Disease

Spectral-domain-OCT provides a high-resolution visualization of the retinal lesions in Best disease.[146,176-178] The first change seen on SD-OCT seems to be discrete thickening and hyper-reflectivity of the interdigitation zone.[179] FAF may be more sensitive than SD-OCT for very early retinal changes.[102] In more advanced stages of Best disease, the SD-OCT shows a central macular detachment of the neurosensory retina.[176-178] Scars and CNV in a lesion of Best disease also appear hyper-reflective on SD-OCT.

Treatment of Best Disease

Complications resulting from Best disease include CNV. CNV develops in 2–9% of cases of Best disease[150,151,180,181] and may be more common after ocular trauma. There are reports of cases of CNV treated with argon laser,[182,183] photodynamic therapy,[184] and intravitreal injection of vascular endothelial growth factor-inhibitors such as bevacizumab or ranibizumab.[185,186] However, no treatment is available to treat the underlying disease process. The emerging therapies for inherited macular dystrophies are discussed in the last section of this chapter.

PATTERN DYSTROPHIES AND *PRPH2*-ASSOCIATED MACULAR DYSTROPHY

Pattern Dystrophies and *PRPH2*-associated Retinal Disease

The group of *PRPH2*-associated retinal diseases is both clinically and genetically heterogeneous and affects the cone and rod systems to variable degrees. Conditions such as pattern dystrophies may be associated with mutations in *PRPH2*.[187] The term pattern dystrophy addresses many different phenotypes that have the accumulation of lipofuscin in the RPE in common.[188-191] This lipofuscin accumulation often occurs in distinct "patterns," such as a butterfly shape.[189-192] The atlas by Donald Gass distinguishes five types of pattern dystrophies: the adult-onset foveomacular vitelliform dystrophy, the butterfly-shaped pigment dystrophy, the reticular dystrophy, the multifocal pattern dystrophy simulating STGD1, and the fundus pulverulentus.[193] Results from histopathologic specimens show that the accumulation of lipofuscin occurs within the RPE in areas often directly neighboring distinct areas of photoreceptor and RPE atrophy.[194]

Genetics of Pattern Dystrophies

The most common mutations underlying pattern dystrophies are found in *PRPH2* (previously *RDS*; OMIM #179605).[195-197] *PRPH2* encodes a photoreceptor-specific gene, peripherin-2, which is a transmembrane glycoprotein in the rod and cone photoreceptor outer segments. It has a role in the development and maintenance of outer segments.[198-200] Diseases associated with *PRPH2* mutations include cone-rod dystrophies, retinitis pigmentosa,[201-203] macular dystrophies resembling STGD1, central areolar choroidal dystrophy,[204,205] and pattern dystrophies.[187] At the same time, a number of different mutations in *PRPH2* have been identified in individuals affected by pattern dystrophy.[194,195,197] In one study, families with pattern dystrophy and without *PRPH2* mutations underwent detailed genetic testing and no genetic mutation could be identified.[206] Although autosomal-recessive modes of inheritance have been reported, pattern dystrophies are typically inherited in an autosomal-dominant fashion.[187]

Symptoms of Pattern Dystrophies

Pattern dystrophies can present with various ages of onset, different degrees of severity, and variable penetrance. The main symptom is a very slow decline in BCVA; but vision often remains unaffected. The earliest fundus changes can be seen during the second decade of life, although they usually appear between ages 20 and 30. Another symptom involves macular photostress: after exposure to bright light, it takes minutes for BCVA to recover.

Fundus Changes in Pattern Dystrophies

In the earliest stages of pattern dystrophy, the fundus demonstrates barely visible RPE mottling, followed by progressive and extensive atrophic changes of the macula. The progression of fundus changes occurs very slowly. In the immediate vicinity of the central lesion, pigmentary deposits and irregularities are common. These pigmentary changes may be yellow, whitish, or gray and can be arranged in various "patterns". Those reported in the literature include butterfly patterns,[207] petaloid shapes,[193,208] fundus pulverulentus,[209,210] or the Sjögren reticular dystrophy of the RPE.[207,211,212] Some authors also include adult-vitelliform macular dystrophy as a form of pattern dystrophy.[213]

The butterfly-shaped form of pattern dystrophy has been described by Gass[214] and has a configuration that resembles the arms or wings of a butterfly. This lesion has increased signal on FAF imaging and is smaller in size than vitelliform lesions. It is accompanied by outer retinal loss and decreased BCVA.[215]

Sjögren reticular dystrophy of the RPE presents with pigmented granules in the fovea that progress to a fine network of lines of black pigment at the level of the RPE.[207,211,212] Within the same family of patients with Sjögren reticular dystrophy of the RPE, vitelliform and butterfly-shaped patterns have been reported.[207,216-220] It is possible that a patient's one eye exhibits a vitelliform and the other eye a butterfly pattern of the lesion obviously caused by an identical mutation.[195,196,202] Subretinal neovascularization can complicate cases of pattern dystrophy.[221] A lifetime risk of 18% for developing CNV has been reported for pattern dystrophies associated with *PRPH2*.[222] Cases of spontaneous regression of CNV with stable BCVA and without development of intra- or subretinal fluid after 12 months of follow-up have also been reported.[223]

Investigative Modalities for Pattern Dystrophies

In addition to genetic testing, several functional and structural retinal tests may be useful to confirm or rule out pattern dystrophies of the RPE. Both ffERG and EOG testing yield normal test results.[224] FAF shows areas of increased autofluorescence that spread centrifugally and correspond to the deposition of lipofuscin (Fig. 53.13).[225] The lesion leaves behind areas of decreased autofluorescence that indicate RPE atrophy.[225] OCT imaging reveals focal disruptions of the IS-OS interdigitation zone and hyperreflective deposits.[225]

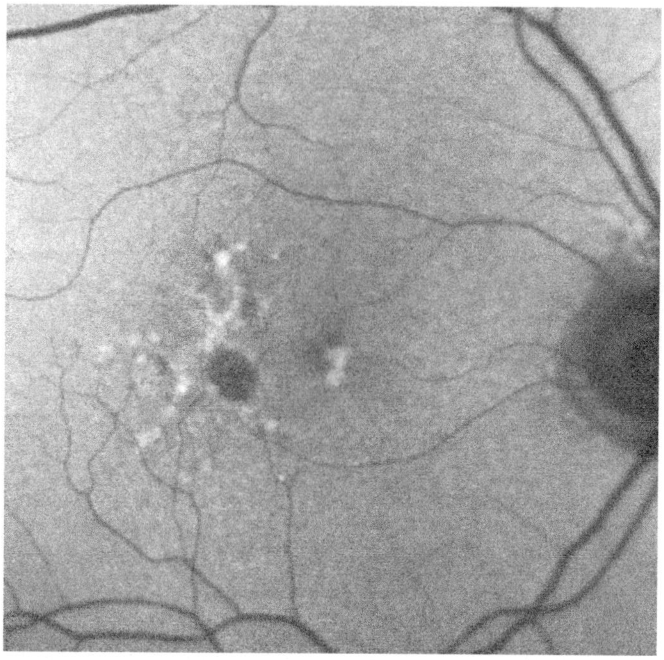

Fig. 53.13: Pattern dystrophy of the retinal pigment epithelium. The fundus in eyes with pattern dystrophy often presents with discrete mottling of the retinal pigment epithelium (RPE) which is followed by progressive and extensive atrophic changes of the macula. Fundus autofluorescence of the right eye shows clearly visible areas of increased signal that correspond to the deposition of lipofuscin. The lesion leaves behind areas of decreased autofluorescence that indicate RPE atrophy.

AUTOSOMAL DOMINANT DRUSEN (*EFEMP1*-ASSOCIATED MACULAR DYSTROPHY)

The term druse refers to extracellular material that is deposited between the RPE and Bruch's membrane.[226] Drusen are the main characteristic of AMD but also belong to the pathology of Sorsby macular dystrophy and autosomal dominant drusen (ADD). ADD is a descriptive term for a rare inherited macular dystrophy, also known as malattia léventinese or Doyne's honeycomb dystrophy. In 1925, Vogt described the disease in a Swiss population in the Leventine valley and introduced the name malattia léventinese.[227] The disease has also been reported in other countries, including the United Kingdom,[228] France,[229] and China.[230] In the 1980s, Gass first described the typical radial distribution of the drusen in the temporal macula.[231]

Histopathology of Autosomal Dominant Drusen

The drusen in ADD and AMD share many features, such as diffuse changes in Bruch's membrane, RPE and photoreceptor atrophy, or basal laminar deposits.[232] However, histopathological studies showed that the drusen in ADD have distinct changes of the extracellular matrix.[233] These include an onion skin-like lamination separating the eosinophilic and sudanophilic layers,[233] the presence of collagen type IV, and nuclei of migrating cells, all of which can exclusively be seen in ADD drusen.[233] While drusen in AMD do not contain molecules of the extracellular matrix, the presence of collagen type IV in Bruch's membrane is suggestive of a possible role of dysgenesis of the extracellular matrix in the pathogenesis of ADD.[233]

Genetics of Autosomal Dominant Drusen

In 1996, ADD were mapped to chromosome 2,[229] and in 1999, a single mutation in *EFEMP1* (for EGF-containing fibrillin-like extracellular matrix protein 1, also known as *fibulin-3*) was identified as the underlying mutation in cases of ADD;[234,235] but additional, presently unknown genes, are thought to be involved in similar diseases with early onset drusen.[236] Mutations in *EFEMP1* do not seem to play a role in AMD.[237] The common *EFEMP1* R345W mutation has been intensively studied, and substantial intrafamilial variability has been described.[69] Cells that express *EFEMP1* involve the neural retina (photoreceptor cells), the RPE and Bruch's membrane, and the choroid.[238] ADD is inherited in an autosomal dominant fashion, and a family history of the condition can often be identified. Nevertheless, normal parents of a patient with juvenile drusen should not exclude the disorder.[69]

Fundus Appearance and Clinical Presentation of Autosomal Dominant Drusen

The diagnosis of ADD is frequently established during a routine examination.[239] Vision is often unimpaired and patients are frequently asymptomatic; but they may occasionally report problems with central vision, especially when driving at night.[239] Even in the presence of extensive macular drusen, BCVA is often excellent unless choroidal neovascularization, central macular atrophy, or pigment proliferation develop at later disease stages.[69,240] A case of a 62-year-old carrier of the R345W mutation in *EFEMP1* with normal BCVA has been reported.[69]

The fundus examination reveals numerous bilateral drusen in the second or third decade of life. Selected patients may exhibit drusen even in early childhood but their BCVA is usually normal or near-normal.[241] Often, a halo of drusen can be seen around the foveal center. Small, elongated basal laminar drusen in the temporal macula are often arranged with a radial distribution and converging towards the fovea.[235,242] The drusen in the central macula and those nasal to the optic disk are often described as large and round with a tendency to coalesce with age. Confluent drusen may resemble a honeycomb (hence, the term Doyne's honeycomb dystrophy). In relation to extent of drusen in the macula, the accumulation of drusen nasal to the optic disk appears striking in ADD.[154,241,243] The phenotype of the disease may vary substantially among members of the same family and even between a patient's two eyes.[69] Figure 53.14 shows an example of the fundus in ADD.

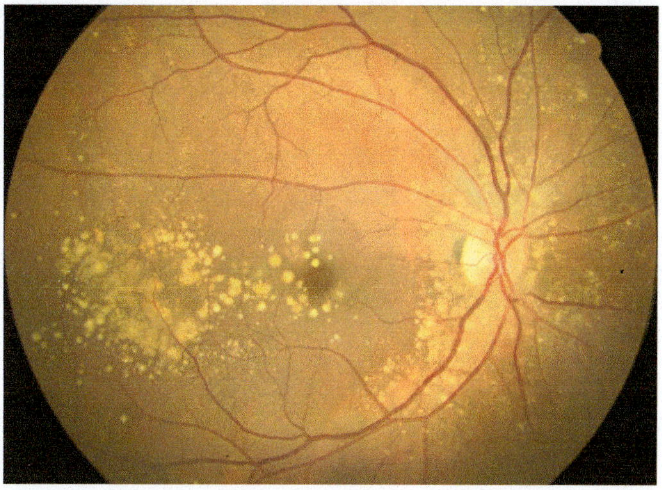

Fig. 53.14: Fundus in an eye with autosomal dominant drusen. Fundus photograph of the right eye of a 46-year-old female with autosomal dominant drusen. This eye has 20/16 visual acuity despite numerous drusen. There is a typical halo of drusen around the foveola as well as a predominance of drusen in the macula and in the peripapillary retina. The presence or even predominance of drusen nasal to the disk has been described as pathognomonic of autosomal dominant drusen.

Complications of Autosomal Dominant Drusen

Progression of the disease may lead to geographic atrophy, subretinal fibrosis, and CNV with loss of BCVA and metamorphopsia.[244] At least for individuals with the *EFEMP1* R345W mutation, CNV appears to be rare.[69] In single reports, CNV secondary to ADD has been treated using anti-VEGF.[240,245]

Structural and Functional Testing for Autosomal Dominant Drusen

In FAF imaging, most drusen in ADD are associated with an increase in FAF signal, and some may display reduced or absent autofluorescence.[69] This is in contrast to the drusen in AMD that usually show decreased FAF signal.[68,69] The drusenoid deposits exhibit early hyperfluorescence on fluorescein angiography.[239] Fluorescein angiography may also be useful to detect formation of CNV. Indocyanine green angiography reveals intense staining reminiscent of cuticular drusen.[239] Features on SD-OCT imaging include loss of the foveal contour, retinal edema, RPE detachments, and prominent, focal and nodular sub-RPE hyperreflective deposits and hyperreflective thickening of the RPE.[240,246,247] These findings are summarized in Figures 53.15A to C. Functional testing can be performed using ERG studies or perimetry. The full-field ERG test is normal in ADD but most eyes with ADD show abnormalities on pattern ERG.[248]

Treatment of Autosomal Dominant Drusen

Patients without CNV formation should be observed. According to some authors, CNV secondary to ADD has been treated using intravitreal anti-VEGF[244] but CNV was not always responsive.[240,245] However, no treatment is available to treat the disease process underlying this inherited macular dystrophy.

EMERGING THERAPIES FOR MACULAR DYSTROPHIES

Emerging Therapies for Inherited Macular and Retinal Diseases

Scientific advances over the last years have shed light on the understanding of the pathophysiological foundation of inherited retinal diseases and the involved molecular and genetic mechanisms, allowing the identification of new therapeutic approaches such as gene therapy or stem cell therapy. Therapies for inherited retinal degenerations must be adapted to the stage of photoreceptor cell degeneration, as some that prevent further cell death such as gene therapy

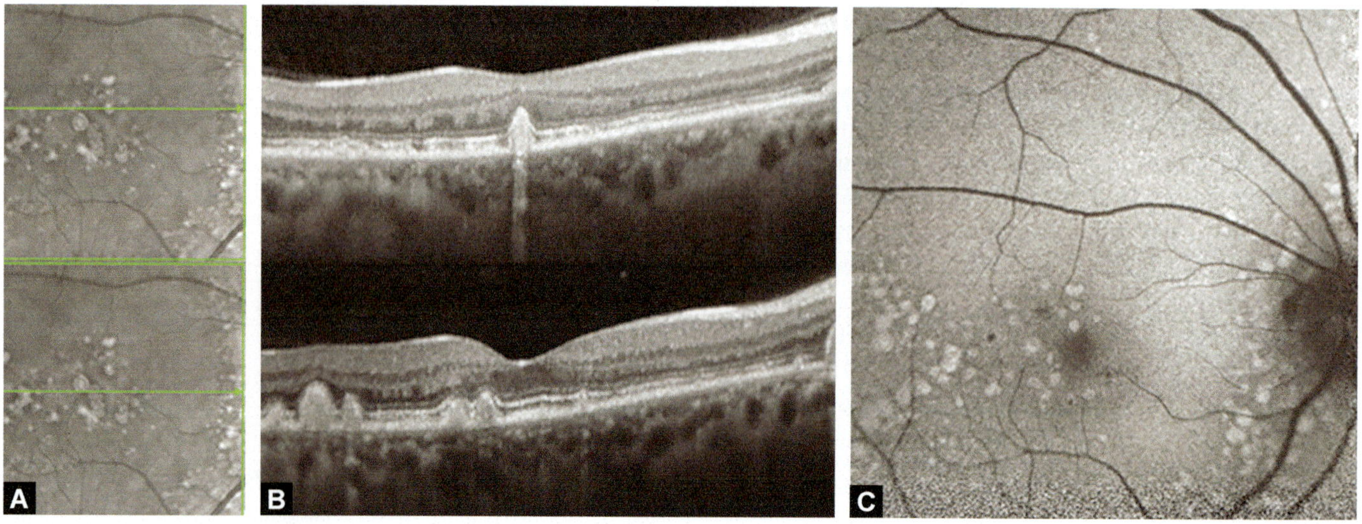

Figs. 53.15A to C: Multimodal imaging in autosomal dominant drusen (ADD). Infrared imaging (IR), spectral-domain optical coherence tomography (SD-OCT), and fundus autofluorescence (FAF) of the right eye of a 46-year-old female with autosomal dominant drusen. This eye has 20/16 visual acuity despite numerous drusen changing the retinal architecture. (A and B) The green line on the IR image (A) shows the position of the two cross-sections displayed on the SD-OCT image (B). The foveal contour in this eye is relatively preserved but asymmetric. Numerous hyper-reflective deposits of various size can be seen and they seem to be located underneath the retinal pigment epithelium (RPE). In some drusen, the material seems to be anterior to the RPE. The hyper-reflective material seems to push up the ellipsoid zone and the external limiting membrane; (C) As opposed to the drusen in age-related macular degeneration with decreased FAF signal, drusen in ADD display increased signal on FAF testing.

or pharmacotherapy are only appropriate when retinal photoreceptors are still intact. Others, such as stem cell therapy or retinal prosthesis, may restore vision in later disease stages (Fig. 53.16). Several of these promising avenues are currently being investigated in clinical trials. These trials benefit from novel technology to accurately image the retina and assess visual function. Retinal prostheses replacing the function of lost photoreceptors have received regulatory approval.

Gene Therapy for Inherited Macular and Retinal Diseases

Figure 53.17 provides an overview of the visual cycle and demonstrates various starting points for different treatments. Gene therapy targets photoreceptor or RPE cells and aims to slow down or prevent further cell death. It requires the cells to be still viable; hence it is best used in relatively early stages of degeneration when the target tissue is still present and in retinal diseases caused by a single recessive gene that can be replaced.[98] A common gene transfer system for human gene therapy including gene augmentation therapy of the retina is the adeno-associated virus (AAV) vector.[249,250] Figure 53.18 illustrates how the AAV vector is being used in a mouse model ($Rs1h^{-/-}$) to introduce the *Rs1* gene. However, the size of certain genes such as

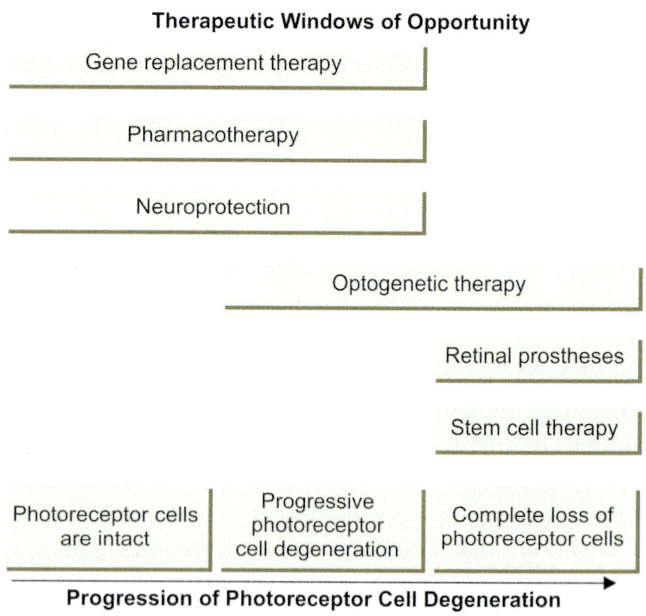

Fig. 53.16: Different strategies for treating retinal degeneration. Therapies for inherited retinal degenerations must be adapted to the stage of photoreceptor cell degeneration. Some approaches, such as gene therapy or pharmacotherapy, aim at prevention of further cell death and seem appropriate only as long as at least some retinal photoreceptors are intact. Others, such as stem cell therapy or retinal prosthesis, may restore vision in later disease stages. Stargardt disease is an example of an inherited disease of the macula where gene therapy, pharmacotherapy, and stem cell therapy are currently being investigated in clinical trials.

Source: Reproduced from Scholl HP, Strauss RW, Singh MS, et al. Emerging therapies for inherited retinal degeneration. Sci Transl Med. 2016;8(368):368rv366; Reprinted with permission from AAAS.

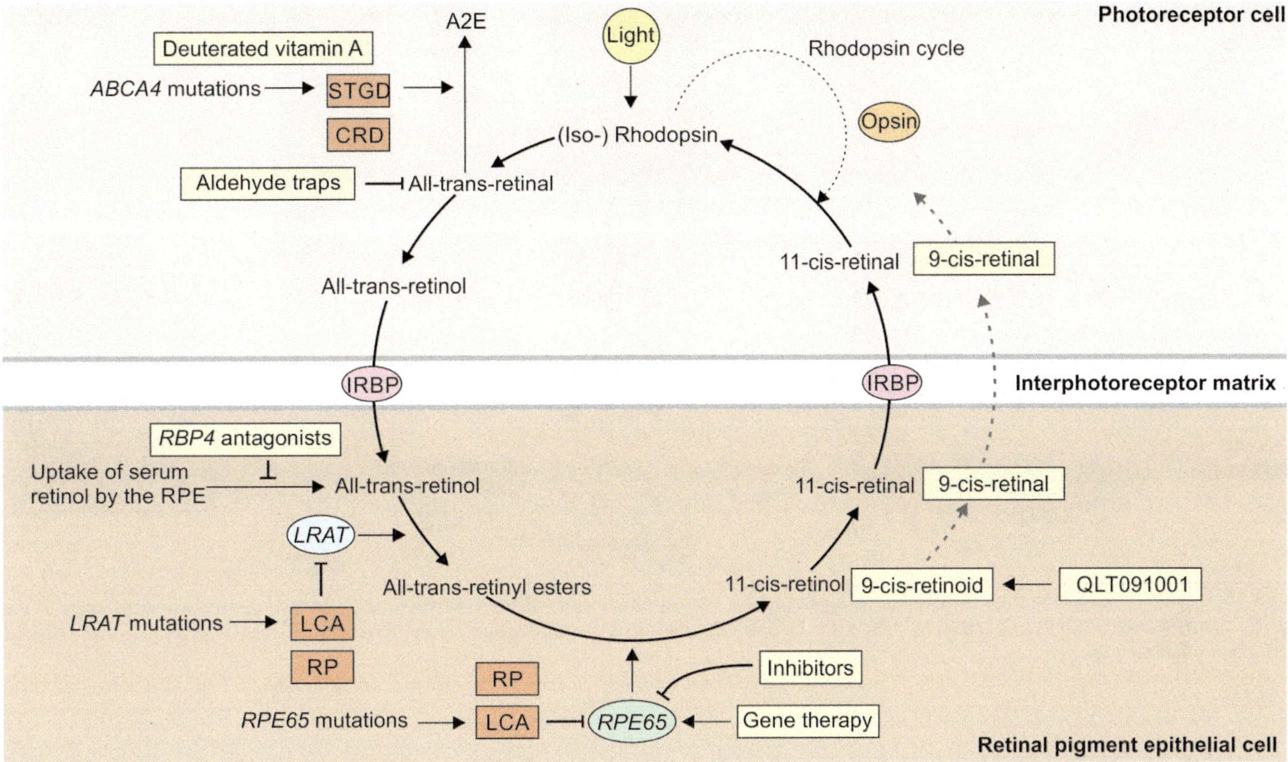

Fig. 53.17: Overview of the visual cycle. The visual cycle allows the conversion of light stimuli into electrical signals. The critical step is the photoisomerization of 11-cis-retinal to all-trans-retinal which initiates the signal transduction via a conformation change of the opsin protein (a G protein) and hyperpolarization of the photoreceptor cell. As an end result of the cycle, all-trans-retinal has to be recycled to 11-cis-retinal. While still in the photoreceptor cell, all-trans-retinal is reduced to all-trans-retinol before the interphotoreceptor binding protein (IRBP) mediates its diffusion into the retinal pigment epithelium (RPE) cell. In the RPE, *LRAT* catalyzes the conversion of all-trans-retinol to all-trans-retinyl esters. The subsequent reaction to 11-cis-retinol is catalyzed by *RPE65*. Both *LRAT* and *RPE65* may not be functional in certain forms of retinitis pigmentosa or Leber congenital amaurosis. As one example for the many points of therapeutic intervention, gene therapy to restore *RPE65* has now been approved by the Food and Drug Administration for confirmed biallelic *RPE65* mutation-associated retinal dystrophy (voretigene neparvovec-rzyl). In *ABCA4*-associated Stargardt disease, the dysfunctional protein leads to accumulation of toxic bisretinoids, such as N-retinylidene-N-retinylethanolamine (A2E). In animal models, deuterated vitamin A which leads to decreased A2E accumulation. *RBP4* antagonists can block the uptake of serum retinol by RPE cells and represent another possible treatment for age-related macular degeneration and Stargardt disease.

Source: Reprinted with permission from AAAS. Scholl HP, Strauss RW, Singh MS, et al. Emerging therapies for inherited retinal degeneration. Sci Transl Med. 2016;8(368): 368rv366.

ABCA4 exceeds the carrier capacity of the AAV vector; and therefore, lentiviral vectors have been developed.[251] One example of successful gene therapy involves the *RPE65* gene. Three different research groups delivered this gene to the retina of patients with Leber congenital amaurosis and were able to restore some visual function with no serious adverse events.[19,20,252] One longitudinal follow-up study reported that 9 of 12 patients with the *RPE65* mutation demonstrated improved visual function in at least one testing modality after a single subretinal injection of a viral vector.[253] For patients with STGD1, an ongoing phase 1/2a clinical trial is investigating the safety and biological activity of ascending doses of a lentiviral vector to replace the defective *ABCA4* gene (NCT01367444). Current challenges to gene therapy for macular dystrophies include gene sequencing, the selection of patients, the identification of the best delivery vectors, and the optimization of surgical techniques. Recent advances in vector development allow lower surgical risks and can deliver genes deep into the retina after intravitreal injection.[254,255] The mouse model of X-linked retinoschisis and *RPE65*-associated Leber congenital amaurosis type 2 showed the efficacy of such vectors.[255] Another approach to restore defective genes is genome editing with CRISPR/Cas9.[256]

Pharmacotherapy for Inherited Macular and Retinal Diseases

Pharmacotherapy addresses biochemical pathways and mechanisms in the photoreceptor and RPE cells. At present,

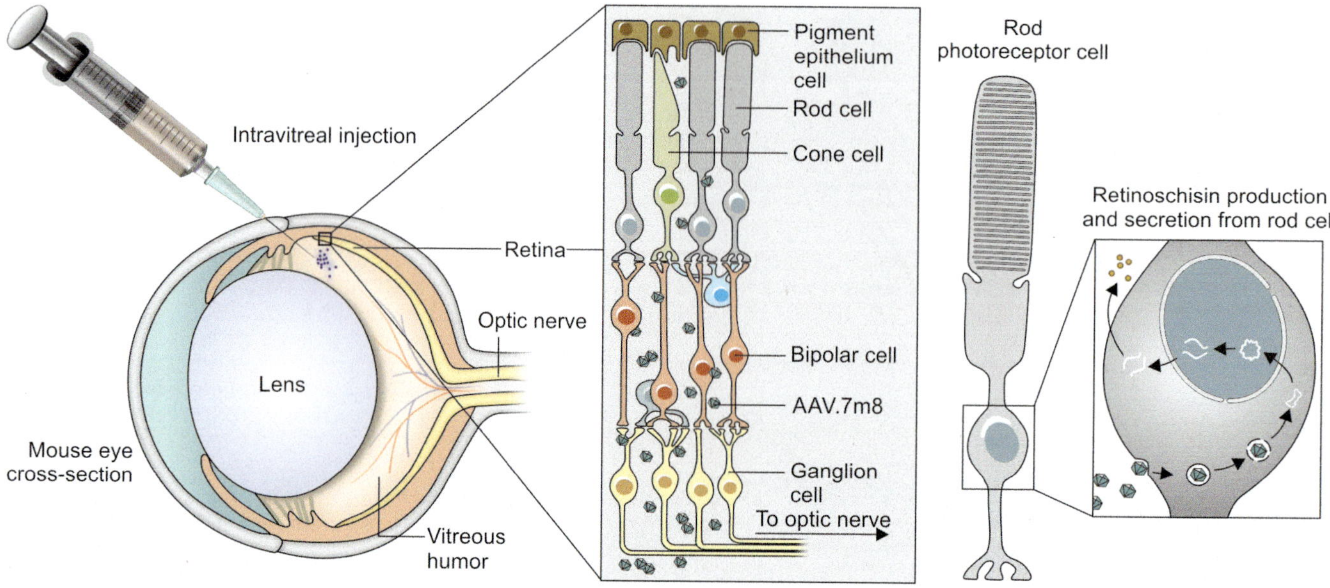

Fig. 53.18: Gene augmentation therapy. The figure illustrates the intravitreal delivery of the AAV vector AAV.7m8 to deliver a healthy copy of the *Rs1* gene in a mouse model (*Rs1h*$^{-/-}$) of X-linked retinoschisis. The desired outcome is the production of functional retinoschisin which provides structural and functional retinal integrity.

Source: Reprinted with permission from AAAS. Scholl HP, Strauss RW, Singh MS, et al. Emerging therapies for inherited retinal degeneration. Sci Transl Med. 2016;8(368):368rv366.

clinical trials using pharmacological compounds are being conducted for retinitis pigmentosa, Leber congenital amaurosis, and *ABCA4*-related retinal disease. Two studies have confirmed the safety and efficacy of an oral dose of a 9-cis-retinyl acetate compound (QLT091001)[257,258] which allows bypass of the genetic defects caused by RPE65 (RPE-specific 65-kDa protein) and *LRAT* (lecithin-retinol acyltransferase) mutations. Both mutations block the visual cycle in humans and are associated with retinitis pigmentosa and Leber congenital amaurosis.[259-262] A consequent impairment of rod photoreceptors and retinal degeneration has been demonstrated in knockout mice.[263] The pathophysiologic basis of Stargardt and *ABCA4*-related retinal diseases involves the formation of toxic bisretinoids and lipofuscin accumulation at an accelerated rate.[264] Inhibiting the dimerization of vitamin A can slow the degeneration of the retina in *ABCA4* knockout mice[265] and the oral delivery of C20-deuterated vitamin A can reduce this dimerization.[265,266] Sequestration of toxic all-trans-retinal with RPE65 inhibitors or retinol-binding protein 4 is another approach.[267]

Stem Cell Therapy for Inherited Macular and Retinal Diseases

In advanced stages of retinal degeneration (Fig. 53.18), cellular targets for gene therapy may no longer be available. Stem cell therapy aims to replace absent photoreceptor and RPE cells and thus to restore vision. The concept of cell replacement may prove to be useful in a number of macular and retinal conditions because it is not gene specific. A current challenge of stem cell therapy is the synaptic integration of the new photoreceptor cells into the visual system. Restoration of RPE cells cannot restore visual function because light exposure does not directly excite them, but they may fulfill their supporting tasks. Using a mouse model, it was shown that it is possible to restore visual function of atrophic retinas using donor-derived rod photoreceptor precursor cells.[268,269] Two recent clinical trials with patients with STGD1 and AMD tried to transplant human embryonic stem cell-derived cells into the transition zone between degenerating and normal retina. The authors reported engraftment of the cells based on visibly increased subretinal pigmentation.[270] Another trial is currently ongoing where a monolayer of RPE cells on a polyester membrane is used to treat patients with exudative AMD (NCT01691261). This trial may establish the safety and efficacy of this method.

REFERENCES

1. Ibanez HE, Williams DF, Boniuk I. Crystalline retinopathy associated with long-term nitrofurantoin therapy. Arch Ophthalmol. 1994;112:304-5.

2. Haimovici R, D'Amico DJ, Gragoudas ES, et al. The expanded clinical spectrum of deferoxamine retinopathy. Ophthalmology. 2002;109:164-71.
3. Gonzales CR, Lin AP, Engstrom RE, et al. Bilateral vitelliform maculopathy and deferoxamine toxicity. Retina. 2004;24:464-7.
4. Delong SL, Poley BJ, McFarlane JR Jr. Ocular changes associated with long-term chlorpromazine therapy. Arch Ophthalmol. 1965;73:611-7.
5. Weekley RD, Potts AM, Reboton J, et al. Pigmentary retinopathy in patients receiving high doses of a new phenothiazine. Arch Ophthalmol. 1960;64:65-76.
6. Craythorn JM, Swartz M, Creel DJ. Clofazimine-induced bull's-eye retinopathy. Retina. 1986;6:50-2.
7. Thiadens AA, Phan TM, Zekveld-Vroon RC, et al. Clinical course, genetic etiology, and visual outcome in cone and cone-rod dystrophy. Ophthalmology. 2012;119:819-26.
8. American Academy of Ophthalmology. Clinical Statement. Recommendations on Clinical Assessment of Patients with Inherited Retinal Degenerations. San Francisco, CA: American Academy of Ophthalmology; 2016.
9. Hood DC, Bach M, Brigell M, et al. ISCEV standard for clinical multifocal electroretinography (mfERG) (2011 edition). Doc Ophthalmol. 2012;124:1-13.
10. Mashayekhi A, Schönbach E, Shields CL, et al. Early subclinical macular edema in eyes with uveal melanoma: association with future cystoid macular edema. Ophthalmology. 2015;122:1923-9.
11. Audo I, Bujakowska KM, Leveillard T, et al. Development and application of a next-generation-sequencing (NGS) approach to detect known and novel gene defects underlying retinal diseases. Orphanet J Rare Dis. 2012;7:8.
12. Consugar MB, Navarro-Gomez D, Place EM, et al. Panel-based genetic diagnostic testing for inherited eye diseases is highly accurate and reproducible, and more sensitive for variant detection, than exome sequencing. Genet Med. 2015;17:253-61.
13. Eisenberger T, Neuhaus C, Khan AO, et al. Increasing the yield in targeted next-generation sequencing by implicating CNV analysis, non-coding exons and the overall variant load: the example of retinal dystrophies. PLoS One. 2013;8:e78496.
14. Song J, Smaoui N, Ayyagari R, et al. High-throughput retina-array for screening 93 genes involved in inherited retinal dystrophy. Invest Ophthalmol Vis Sci. 2011;52:9053-60.
15. Neveling K, Collin RW, Gilissen C, et al. Next-generation genetic testing for retinitis pigmentosa. Hum Mutat. 2012;33:963-72.
16. Wang F, Wang H, Tuan HF, et al. Next generation sequencing-based molecular diagnosis of retinitis pigmentosa: identification of a novel genotype-phenotype correlation and clinical refinements. Hum Genetics. 2014;133:331-45.
17. Capasso JE. The cost of genetic testing for ocular disease: who pays? Curr Opin Ophthalmol. 2014;25:394-9.
18. Bainbridge JW, Smith AJ, Barker SS, et al. Effect of gene therapy on visual function in Leber's congenital amaurosis. New Engl J Med. 2008;358:2231-9.
19. Cideciyan AV, Aleman TS, Boye SL, et al. Human gene therapy for RPE65 isomerase deficiency activates the retinoid cycle of vision but with slow rod kinetics. Proc Natl Acad Sci USA. 2008;105:15112-7.
20. Maguire AM, Simonelli F, Pierce EA, et al. Safety and efficacy of gene transfer for Leber's congenital amaurosis. New Engl J Med. 2008;358:2240-8.
21. Allikmets R, Singh N, Sun H, et al. A photoreceptor cell-specific ATP-binding transporter gene (ABCR) is mutated in recessive Stargardt macular dystrophy. Nat Genet. 1997;15:236-46.
22. Allikmets R, Shroyer NF, Singh N, et al. Mutation of the Stargardt disease gene (ABCR) in age-related macular degeneration. Science. 1997;277:1805-7.
23. Riveiro-Alvarez R, Aguirre-Lamban J, Lopez-Martinez MA, et al. Frequency of ABCA4 mutations in 278 Spanish controls: an insight into the prevalence of autosomal recessive Stargardt disease. Br J Ophthalmol. 2009;93: 1359-64.
24. Sparrow JR, Nakanishi K, Parish CA. The lipofuscin fluorophore A2E mediates blue light-induced damage to retinal pigmented epithelial cells. Invest Ophthalmol Vis Sci. 2000;41:1981-9.
25. Suter M, Reme C, Grimm C, et al. Age-related macular degeneration. The lipofusion component N-retinyl-N-retinylidene ethanolamine detaches proapoptotic proteins from mitochondria and induces apoptosis in mammalian retinal pigment epithelial cells. J Biol Chem. 2000;275: 39625-30.
26. Parish CA, Hashimoto M, Nakanishi K, et al. Isolation and one-step preparation of A2E and iso-A2E, fluorophores from human retinal pigment epithelium. Proc Natl Acad Sci USA. 1998;95:14609-13.
27. Birnbach CD, Jarvelainen M, Possin DE, et al. Histopathology and immunocytochemistry of the neurosensory retina in fundus flavimaculatus. Ophthalmology. 1994;101:1211-9.
28. Cremers FP, van de Pol DJ, van Driel M, et al. Autosomal recessive retinitis pigmentosa and cone-rod dystrophy caused by splice site mutations in the Stargardt's disease gene ABCR. Hum Mol Genet. 1998;7:355-62.
29. Fishman GA, Stone EM, Eliason DA, et al. ABCA4 gene sequence variations in patients with autosomal recessive cone-rod dystrophy. Arch Ophthalmol. 2003;121:851-5.
30. Fishman GA, Stone EM, Grover S, et al. Variation of clinical expression in patients with Stargardt dystrophy and sequence variations in the ABCR gene. Arch Ophthalmol. 1999;117:504-10.
31. Martinez-Mir A, Paloma E, Allikmets R, et al. Retinitis pigmentosa caused by a homozygous mutation in the Stargardt disease gene ABCR. Nat Genet. 1998;18:11-2.
32. Maugeri A, Klevering BJ, Rohrschneider K, et al. Mutations in the ABCA4 (ABCR) gene are the major cause of autosomal recessive cone-rod dystrophy. Am J Hum Genet. 2000;67:960-6.
33. Schindler EI, Nylen EL, Ko AC, et al. Deducing the pathogenic contribution of recessive ABCA4 alleles in an outbred population. Hum Mol Genet. 2010;19:3693-701.

34. Zernant J, Xie YA, Ayuso C, et al. Analysis of the ABCA4 genomic locus in Stargardt disease. Hum Mol Genet. 2014;23:6797-806.
35. Glazer LC, Dryja TP. Understanding the etiology of Stargardt's disease. Ophthalmol Clin North Am. 2002;15:93-100.
36. Cideciyan AV, Aleman TS, Swider M, et al. Mutations in ABCA4 result in accumulation of lipofuscin before slowing of the retinoid cycle: a reappraisal of the human disease sequence. Hum Mol Genet. 2004;13:525-34.
37. Molday RS. ATP-binding cassette transporter ABCA4: molecular properties and role in vision and macular degeneration. J Bioenerg Biomembr. 2007;39:507-17.
38. Strauss RW, Ho A, Munoz B, et al. The Natural History of the Progression of Atrophy Secondary to Stargardt Disease (ProgStar) Studies: Design and Baseline Characteristics: ProgStar Report No. 1. Ophthalmology. 2016;123:817-28.
39. Westeneng-van Haaften SC, Boon CJ, Cremers FP, et al. Clinical and genetic characteristics of late-onset Stargardt's disease. Ophthalmology. 2012;119:1199-210.
40. Kong X, Strauss RW, Michaelides M, et al. Visual acuity loss and associated risk factors in the Retrospective Progression of Stargardt Disease Study (ProgStar Report No. 2). Ophthalmology. 2016;123:1887-97.
41. Kong X, West SK, Strauss RW, et al. Progression of visual acuity and fundus autofluorescence in recent-onset Stargardt disease: ProgStar Study Report #4. Ophthalmol Retina. 2017;1(6):514-23.
42. Schönbach EM, Ibrahim M, Strauss RW, et al. Fixation location and stability using the MP-1 Microperimeter in Stargardt disease: ProgStar Report No. 3. Ophthalmol Retina. 2017;1:68-76.
43. Fujinami K, Zernant J, Chana RK, et al. Clinical and molecular characteristics of childhood-onset Stargardt disease. Ophthalmology. 2015;122:326-34.
44. Rotenstreich Y, Fishman GA, Anderson RJ. Visual acuity loss and clinical observations in a large series of patients with Stargardt disease. Ophthalmology. 2003;110:1151-8.
45. Miraldi Utz V, Coussa RG, Marino MJ, et al. Predictors of visual acuity and genotype-phenotype correlates in a cohort of patients with Stargardt disease. Br J Ophthalmol. 2014;98:513-8.
46. Lambertus S, van Huet RA, Bax NM, et al. Early-onset Stargardt disease: phenotypic and genotypic characteristics. Ophthalmology. 2015;122:335-44.
47. Fujinami K, Sergouniotis PI, Davidson AE, et al. Clinical and molecular analysis of Stargardt disease with preserved foveal structure and function. Am J Ophthalmol. 2013;156:487-501-e1.
48. van Huet RA, Bax NM, Westeneng-van Haaften SC, et al. Foveal sparing in Stargardt disease. Invest Ophthalmol Vis Sci. 2014;55:7467-78.
49. Cideciyan AV, Swider M, Aleman TS, et al. ABCA4-associated retinal degenerations spare structure and function of the human parapapillary retina. Invest Ophthalmol Vis Sci. 2005;46:4739-46.
50. Lois N, Halfyard AS, Bird AC, et al. Fundus autofluorescence in Stargardt macular dystrophy-fundus flavimaculatus. Am J Ophthalmol. 2004;138:55-63.
51. Armstrong JD, Meyer D, Xu S, et al. Long-term follow-up of Stargardt›s disease and fundus flavimaculatus. Ophthalmology. 1998;105:448-58.
52. Franceschetti A, Francois J. Fundus flavimaculatus [In French]. Arch Ophtalmol Rev Gen Ophtalmol. 1965;25:505-30.
53. Hadden OB, Gass JD. Fundus flavimaculatus and Stargardt's disease. Am J Ophthalmol. 1976;82:527-39.
54. Testa F, Melillo P, Di Iorio V, et al. Macular function and morphologic features in juvenile Stargardt disease: longitudinal study. Ophthalmology. 2014;121:2399-405.
55. Oh KT, Weleber RG, Oh DM, et al. Clinical phenotype as a prognostic factor in Stargardt disease. Retina. 2004;24:254-62.
56. Sunness JS, Applegate CA, Gonzalez-Baron J. Improvement of visual acuity over time in patients with bilateral geographic atrophy from age-related macular degeneration. Retina. 2000;20:162-9.
57. Sunness JS, Gonzalez-Baron J, Applegate CA, et al. Enlargement of atrophy and visual acuity loss in the geographic atrophy form of age-related macular degeneration. Ophthalmology. 1999;106:1768-79.
58. Singerman LJ, Wong B, Ai E, et al. Spontaneous visual improvement in the first affected eye of patients with bilateral disciform scars. Retina. 1985;5:135-43.
59. Ishiko S, van de Velde F, Yoshida A. Paradoxical improvement of visual acuity in macular disease. Curr Eye Res. 2010;35:651-6.
60. Sunness JS. Spontaneous improvement in visual acuity in age-related geographic atrophy of the macula. JAMA Ophthalmol. 2014;132:356-7.
61. Fishman GA, Jacobson SG, Alexander KR, et al. Outcome measures and their application in clinical trials for retinal degenerative diseases: outline, review, and perspective. Retina. 2005;25:772-77.
62. Delori FC, Staurenghi G, Arend O, et al. In vivo measurement of lipofuscin in Stargardt's disease--Fundus flavimaculatus. Invest Ophthalmol Vis Sci. 1995;36:2327-31.
63. von Ruckmann A, Fitzke FW, Bird AC. In vivo fundus autofluorescence in macular dystrophies. Arch Ophthalmol. 1997;115:609-15.
64. Burke TR, Duncker T, Woods RL, et al. Quantitative fundus autofluorescence in recessive Stargardt disease. Invest Ophthalmol Vis Sci. 2014;55:2841-52.
65. Pollack K, Kreuz FR, Pillunat LE. Best's disease with normal EOG. Case report of familial macular dystrophy [In German]. Ophthalmologe. 2005;102:891-4.
66. Meunier I, Senechal A, Dhaenens CM, et al. Systematic screening of BEST1 and PRPH2 in juvenile and adult vitelliform macular dystrophies: a rationale for molecular analysis. Ophthalmology. 2011;118:1130-6.
67. Steinmetz RL, Garner A, Maguire JI, Histopathology of incipient fundus flavimaculatus. Ophthalmology. 1991;98:953-6.
68. Evans K, Gregory CY, Wijesuriya SD, et al. Assessment of the phenotypic range seen in Doyne honeycomb retinal dystrophy. Arch Ophthalmol. 1997;115:904-10.
69. Michaelides M, Jenkins SA, Brantley MA Jr, et al. Maculopathy due to the R345W substitution in fibulin-3: distinct clinical features, disease variability, and extent of

retinal dysfunction. Invest Ophthalmol Vis Sci. 2006;47: 3085-97.

70. Bakall B, Radu RA, Stanton JB, et al. Enhanced accumulation of A2E in individuals homozygous or heterozygous for mutations in *BEST1 (VMD2)*. Exp Eye Res. 2007;85:34-43.
71. Weingeist TA, Kobrin JL, Watzke RC. Histopathology of Best's macular dystrophy. Arch Ophthalmol. 1982;100:1108-14.
72. Jayasundera T, Rhoades W, Branham K, et al. Peripapillary dark choroid ring as a helpful diagnostic sign in advanced Stargardt disease. Am J Ophthalmol. 2010;149:656-660 e2.
73. Schmitz-Valckenberg S, Sahel JA, Danis R, et al. Natural history of geographic atrophy progression secondary to age-related macular degeneration (Geographic Atrophy Progression Study). Ophthalmology. 2016;123:361-8.
74. Bearelly S, Khanifar AA, Lederer DE, et al. Use of fundus autofluorescence images to predict geographic atrophy progression. Retina. 2011;31:81-6.
75. Khanifar AA, Lederer DE, Ghodasra JH, et al. Comparison of color fundus photographs and fundus autofluorescence images in measuring geographic atrophy area. Retina. 2012;32:1884-91.
76. Sparrow JR, Gregory-Roberts E, Yamamoto K, et al. The bisretinoids of retinal pigment epithelium. Prog Retin Eye Res. 2012;31:121-35.
77. Cukras CA, Wong WT, Caruso R, et al. Centrifugal expansion of fundus autofluorescence patterns in Stargardt disease over time. Arch Ophthalmol. 2012;130:171-9.
78. McBain VA, Townend J, Lois N. Progression of retinal pigment epithelial atrophy in Stargardt disease. Am J Ophthalmol. 2012;154:146-54.
79. Fujinami K, Lois N, Mukherjee R, et al. A longitudinal study of Stargardt disease: quantitative assessment of fundus autofluorescence, progression, and genotype correlations. Invest Ophthalmol Vis Sci. 2013;54:8181-90.
80. Chen B, Tosha C, Gorin MB, et al. Analysis of autofluorescent retinal images and measurement of atrophic lesion growth in Stargardt disease. Exp Eye Res. 2010;91:143-52.
81. Anmarkrud N. Fundus fluorescein angiography in fundus flavimaculatus and Stargardts disease. Acta Ophthalmol (Copenh). 1979;57:172-82.
82. Ernest JT, Krill AE. Fluorescein studies in fundus flavimaculatus and drusen. Am J Ophthalmol. 1966;62:1-6.
83. Radu RA, Mata NL, Bagla A, et al. Light exposure stimulates formation of A2E oxiranes in a mouse model of Stargardt's macular degeneration. Proc Natl Acad Sci USA. 2004;101:5928-33.
84. Mata NL, Tzekov RT, Liu X, et al. Delayed dark-adaptation and lipofuscin accumulation in abcr+/- mice: implications for involvement of ABCR in age-related macular degeneration. Invest Ophthalmol Vis Sci. 2001;42:1685-90.
85. Mata NL, Weng J, Travis GH. Biosynthesis of a major lipofuscin fluorophore in mice and humans with ABCR-mediated retinal and macular degeneration. Proc Natl Acad Sci USA. 2000;97:7154-9.
86. Boyer NP, Higbee D, Currin MB, et al. Lipofuscin and N-retinylidene-N-retinylethanolamine (A2E) accumulate in retinal pigment epithelium in absence of light exposure: their origin is 11-cis-retinal. J Biol Chem. 2012;287:22276-86.
87. Strauss RW, Munoz B, Wolfson Y, et al. Assessment of estimated retinal atrophy progression in Stargardt macular dystrophy using spectral-domain optical coherence tomography. Br J Ophthalmol. 2016;100:956-62.
88. Staurenghi G, Sadda S, Chakravarthy U, et al. Proposed lexicon for anatomic landmarks in normal posterior segment spectral-domain optical coherence tomography: the IN*OCT consensus. Ophthalmology. 2014;121:1572-8.
89. Lazow MA, Hood DC, Ramachandran R, et al. Transition zones between healthy and diseased retina in choroideremia (CHM) and Stargardt disease (STGD) as compared to retinitis pigmentosa (RP). Invest Ophthalmol Vis Sci. 2011;52:9581-90.
90. Gomes NL, Greenstein VC, Carlson JN, et al. A comparison of fundus autofluorescence and retinal structure in patients with Stargardt disease. Invest Ophthalmol Vis Sci. 2009;50:3953-9.
91. Lee W, Noupuu K, Oll M, et al. The external limiting membrane in early-onset Stargardt disease. Invest Ophthalmol Vis Sci. 2014;55:6139-49.
92. Fujinami K, Singh R, Carroll J, et al. Fine central macular dots associated with childhood-onset Stargardt disease. Acta Ophthalmol. 2014;92:e157-9.
93. Chen Y, Ratnam K, Sundquist SM, et al. Cone photoreceptor abnormalities correlate with vision loss in patients with Stargardt disease. Invest Ophthalmol Vis Sci. 2011;52:3281-92.
94. Genead MA, Fishman GA, Anastasakis A. Spectral-domain OCT peripapillary retinal nerve fibre layer thickness measurements in patients with Stargardt disease. Br J Ophthalmol. 2011;95:689-93.
95. Hood DC, Frishman LJ, Saszik S, et al. Retinal origins of the primate multifocal ERG: implications for the human response. Invest Ophthalmol Vis Sci. 2002;43:1673-85.
96. Walia S, Fishman GA. Natural history of phenotypic changes in Stargardt macular dystrophy. Ophthalmic Genet. 2009;30:63-8.
97. Fishman GA, Farber M, Patel BS, et al. Visual acuity loss in patients with Stargardt's macular dystrophy. Ophthalmology. 1987;94:809-14.
98. Scholl HP, Strauss RW, Singh MS, et al. Emerging therapies for inherited retinal degeneration. Sci Transl Med. 2016;8:368rv6.
99. Charbel Issa P, Helb HM, Rohrschneider K, et al. Microperimetric assessment of patients with type 2 idiopathic macular telangiectasia. Invest Ophthalmol Vis Sci. 2007;48:3788-95.
100. Schönbach EM, Scholl HP. Fundus autofluorescence in a subclinical case of Best disease. Retin Cases Brief Rep. 2017;11(1):S159-62.
101. Schönbach EM, Wolfson Y, Strauss RW, et al. Macular sensitivity measured with microperimetry in Stargardt disease in the Progression of Atrophy Secondary to Stargardt Disease (ProgStar) Study: Report No. 7. JAMA Ophthalmol. 2017;135:696-703.

102. Midena E, Vujosevic S, Cavarzeran F. Normal values for fundus perimetry with the microperimeter MP1. Ophthalmology. 2010;117:1571-76, 1576 e1.
103. Lois N, Holder GE, Bunce C, et al. Phenotypic subtypes of Stargardt macular dystrophy-fundus flavimaculatus. Arch Ophthalmol. 2001;119:359-69.
104. Scholl HP, Besch D, Vonthein R, et al. Alterations of slow and fast rod ERG signals in patients with molecularly confirmed Stargardt disease type 1. Invest Ophthalmol Vis Sci. 2002;43:1248-56.
105. Klevering BJ, Deutman AF, Maugeri A, et al. The spectrum of retinal phenotypes caused by mutations in the *ABCA4* gene. Graefes Arch Clin Exp Ophthalmol. 2005;243:90-100.
106. Fukui T, Yamamoto S, Nakano K, et al. *ABCA4* gene mutations in Japanese patients with Stargardt disease and retinitis pigmentosa. Invest Ophthalmol Vis Sci. 2002;43:2819-24.
107. Gerth C, Andrassi-Darida M, Bock M, et al. Phenotypes of 16 Stargardt macular dystrophy/fundus flavimaculatus patients with known *ABCA4* mutations and evaluation of genotype-phenotype correlation. Graefes Arch Clin Exp Ophthalmol. 2002;240:628-38.
108. Sheffield VC, Stone EM. Genomics and the eye. New Engl J Med. 2011;364:1932-42.
109. Fakin A, Robson AG, Fujinami K, et al. Phenotype and progression of retinal degeneration associated with nullizigosity of *ABCA4*. Invest Ophthalmol Vis Sci. 2016;57:4668-78.
110. Fakin A, Robson AG, Chiang JP, et al. The effect on retinal structure and function of 15 specific *ABCA4* mutations: a detailed examination of 82 hemizygous patients. Invest Ophthalmol Vis Sci. 2016;57:5963-73.
111. Singh R, Fujinami K, Chen LL, et al. Longitudinal follow-up of siblings with a discordant Stargardt disease phenotype. Acta Ophthalmol. 2014;92:e331-2.
112. Fujinami K, Sergouniotis PI, Davidson AE, et al. The clinical effect of homozygous *ABCA4* alleles in 18 patients. Ophthalmology. 2013;120:2324-31.
113. Fujinami K, Lois N, Davidson AE, et al. A longitudinal study of Stargardt disease: clinical and electrophysiologic assessment, progression, and genotype correlations. Am J Ophthalmol. 2013;155:1075-88.e13.
114. Burke TR, Tsang SH. Allelic and phenotypic heterogeneity in ABCA4 mutations. Ophthalmic Genet. 2011;32:165-74.
115. Strauss RW, Munoz B, Jha A, et al. Comparison of short-wavelength reduced-illuminance and conventional autofluorescence imaging in Stargardt macular dystrophy. Am J Ophthalmol. 2016;168:269-78.
116. Kuehlewein L, Hariri AH, Ho A, et al. Comparison of manual and semiautomated fundus autofluorescence analysis of macular atrophy in Stargardt disease phenotype. Retina. 2016;36:1216-21.
117. Michaelides M, Chen LL, Brantley MA Jr, et al. *ABCA4* mutations and discordant *ABCA4* alleles in patients and siblings with bull's-eye maculopathy. Br J Ophthalmol. 2007;91:1650-5.
118. Tanna P, Strauss RW, Fujinami K, et al. Stargardt disease: clinical features, molecular genetics, animal models and therapeutic options. Br J Ophthalmol. 2017;101:25-30.
119. Fujinami K, Zernant J, Chana RK, et al. *ABCA4* gene screening by next-generation sequencing in a British cohort. Invest Ophthalmol Vis Sci. 2013;54:6662-74.
120. Fritsche LG, Fleckenstein M, Fiebig BS, et al. A subgroup of age-related macular degeneration is associated with mono-allelic sequence variants in the *ABCA4* gene. Invest Ophthalmol Vis Sci. 2012;53:2112-8.
121. Rivera A, White K, Stohr H, et al. A comprehensive survey of sequence variation in the *ABCA4 (ABCR)* gene in Stargardt disease and age-related macular degeneration. Am J Hum Genet. 2000;67:800-13.
122. Valverde D, Riveiro-Alvarez R, Bernal S, et al. Microarray-based mutation analysis of the *ABCA4* gene in Spanish patients with Stargardt disease: evidence of a prevalent mutated allele. Mol Vis. 2006;12:902-8.
123. Riveiro-Alvarez R, Lopez-Martinez MA, Zernant J, et al. Outcome of *ABCA4* disease-associated alleles in autosomal recessive retinal dystrophies: retrospective analysis in 420 Spanish families. Ophthalmology. 2013;120:2332-7.
124. Stone EM. Finding and interpreting genetic variations that are important to ophthalmologists. Trans Am Ophthalmol Soc. 2003;101:437-84.
125. Philp AR, Jin M, Li S, et al. Predicting the pathogenicity of RPE65 mutations. Hum Mutat. 2009;30:1183-8.
126. Jaakson K, Zernant J, Kulm M, et al. Genotyping microarray (gene chip) for the ABCR (*ABCA4*) gene. Hum Mutat. 2003;22:395-403.
127. Shroyer NF, Lewis RA, Lupski JR. Analysis of the *ABCR (ABCA4)* gene in 4-aminoquinoline retinopathy: is retinal toxicity by chloroquine and hydroxychloroquine related to Stargardt disease? Am J Ophthalmol. 2001;131:761-6.
128. Yatsenko AN, Shroyer NF, Lewis RA, et al. Late-onset Stargardt disease is associated with missense mutations that map outside known functional regions of *ABCR (ABCA4)*. Hum Genet. 2001;108:346-55.
129. Ernest PJ, Boon CJ, Klevering BJ, et al. Outcome of ABCA4 microarray screening in routine clinical practice. Mol Vis. 2009;15:2841-47.
130. Klevering BJ, Yzer S, Rohrschneider K, et al. Microarray-based mutation analysis of the *ABCA4 (ABCR)* gene in autosomal recessive cone-rod dystrophy and retinitis pigmentosa. Eur J Hum Genet. 2004;12:1024-32.
131. Best F. Über eine hereditäre Maculaffektion. Beitrag zur Vererbungslehre. Z Augenheilk. 1905;13:199-212.
132. Nordstrom S, Holmgren G, Thorburn W. A genetic study of congenital hereditary macular degeneration in the county of Vasterbotten, Sweden. Acta Ophthalmol (Copenh). 1972;50:539-42.
133. Bitner H, Schatz P, Mizrahi-Meissonnier L, et al. Frequency, genotype, and clinical spectrum of Best vitelliform macular dystrophy: data from a national center in Denmark. Am J Ophthalmol. 2012;154:403-12e4.

134. Sohn EH, Mullins RF, Stone EM. Macular Dystrophies. In: Schachat AP, Sadda SR, (Eds). Retina, 5th edition. London: Saunders Elsevier; 2013. pp. 853-90.
135. Marquardt A, Stohr H, Passmore LA, et al. Mutations in a novel gene, VMD2, encoding a protein of unknown properties cause juvenile-onset vitelliform macular dystrophy (Best's disease). Hum Mol Genet. 1998;7:1517-25.
136. Petrukhin K, Koisti MJ, Bakall B, et al. Identification of the gene responsible for Best macular dystrophy. Nat Genet. 1998;19:241-7.
137. Marmorstein AD, Marmorstein LY, Rayborn M, et al. Bestrophin, the product of the Best vitelliform macular dystrophy gene (VMD2), localizes to the basolateral plasma membrane of the retinal pigment epithelium. Proc Natl Acad Sci USA. 2000;97:1275812763.
138. Hartzell C, Putzier I, Arreola J. Calcium-activated chloride channels. Annu Rev Physiol. 2005;67:719-58.
139. Yu K, Qu Z, Cui Y, et al. Chloride channel activity of bestrophin mutants associated with mild or late-onset macular degeneration. Invest Ophthalmol Vis Sci. 2007;48:4694-705.
140. Tsunenari T, Sun H, Williams J, et al. Structure-function analysis of the bestrophin family of anion channels. J Biol Chem. 2003;278:41114-25.
141. Sun H, Tsunenari T, Yau KW, et al. The vitelliform macular dystrophy protein defines a new family of chloride channels. Proc Natl Acad Sci USA. 2002;99:4008-13.
142. Sparrow JR, Boulton M. RPE lipofuscin and its role in retinal pathobiology. Exp Eye Res. 2005;80:595-606.
143. Kraushar MF, Margolis S, Morse PH, et al. Pseudohypopyon in Best's vitelliform macular dystrophy. Am J Ophthalmol. 1982;94:30-7.
144. Liu J, Itagaki Y, Ben-Shabat S, et al. The biosynthesis of A2E, a fluorophore of aging retina, involves the formation of the precursor, A2-PE, in the photoreceptor outer segment membrane. J Biol Chem. 2000;275:29354-60.
145. Fishkin N, Jang YP, Itagaki Y, et al. A2-rhodopsin: a new fluorophore isolated from photoreceptor outer segments. Org Biomol Chem. 2003;1:1101-5.
146. Spaide RF, Noble K, Morgan A, et al. Vitelliform macular dystrophy. Ophthalmology. 2006;113:1392-400.
147. Spaide R. Autofluorescence from the outer retina and subretinal space: hypothesis and review. Retina. 2008;28:5-35.
148. Reddy MA, Francis PJ, Berry V, et al. A clinical and molecular genetic study of a rare dominantly inherited syndrome (MRCS) comprising of microcornea, rod-cone dystrophy, cataract, and posterior staphyloma. Br J Ophthalmol. 2003;87:197-202.
149. Yardley J, Leroy BP, Hart-Holden N, et al. Mutations of VMD2 splicing regulators cause nanophthalmos and autosomal dominant vitreoretinochoroidopathy (ADVIRC). Invest Ophthalmol Vis Sci. 2004;45:3683-9.
150. Mohler CW, Fine SL. Long-term evaluation of patients with Best's vitelliform dystrophy. Ophthalmology. 1981;88: 688-92.
151. Clemett R. Vitelliform dystrophy: long-term observations on New Zealand pedigrees. Aust NZJ Ophthalmol. 1991;19:221-7.
152. Renner AB, Tillack H, Kraus H, et al. Late onset is common in Best macular dystrophy associated with VMD2 gene mutations. Ophthalmology. 2005;112:586-92.
153. Wabbels B, Preising MN, Kretschmann U, et al. Genotype-phenotype correlation and longitudinal course in ten families with Best vitelliform macular dystrophy. Graefes Arch Clin Exp Ophthalmol. 2006;244:1453-66.
154. Deutman A, Jansen LM. The hereditary dystrophies of the posterior pole of the eye. Assen, The Netherlands: Erasmus University Rotterdam/Koninklijke Van Gorcum; 1971.
155. Boon CJ, Theelen T, Hoefsloot EH, et al. Clinical and molecular genetic analysis of Best vitelliform macular dystrophy. Retina. 2009;29:835-47.
156. Boon CJ, Klevering BJ, den Hollander AI, et al. Clinical and genetic heterogeneity in multifocal vitelliform dystrophy. Arch Ophthalmol. 2007;125:1100-6.
157. Testa F, Rossi S, Passerini I, et al. A normal electro-oculography in a family affected by best disease with a novel spontaneous mutation of the BEST1 gene. Br J Ophthalmol. 2008;92:1467-70.
158. Fishman GA, Baca W, Alexander KR, et al. Visual acuity in patients with best vitelliform macular dystrophy. Ophthalmology. 1993;100:1665-70.
159. Chung MM, Oh KT, Streb LM, et al. Visual outcome following subretinal hemorrhage in Best disease. Retina. 2001;21:575-80.
160. Wabbels B, Demmler A, Paunescu K, et al. Fundus autofluorescence in children and teenagers with hereditary retinal diseases. Graefes Arch Clin Exp Ophthalmol. 2006;244:36-45.
161. Boon CJ, Jeroen Klevering B, Keunen JE, et al. Fundus autofluorescence imaging of retinal dystrophies. Vision Res. 2008;48:2569-77.
162. Jarc-Vidmar M, Popovic P, Hawlina M. Mapping of central visual function by microperimetry and autofluorescence in patients with Best's vitelliform dystrophy. Eye (Lond). 2006;20:688-96.
163. Jarc-Vidmar M, Kraut A, Hawlina M. Fundus autofluorescence imaging in Best's vitelliform dystrophy. Klin Monbl Augenheilkd. 2003;220:861-7.
164. Boon CJ, Klevering BJ, Leroy BP, et al. The spectrum of ocular phenotypes caused by mutations in the BEST1 gene. Prog Retin Eye Res. 2009;28:187-205.
165. Delori FC, Dorey CK, Staurenghi G, et al. In vivo fluorescence of the ocular fundus exhibits retinal pigment epithelium lipofuscin characteristics. Invest Ophthalmol Vis Sci. 1995;36:718-29.
166. Boulton M, Rozanowska M, Rozanowski B, et al. The photoreactivity of ocular lipofuscin. Photochem Photobiol Sci. 2004;3:759-64.
167. Schönbach EM, Chaikitmongkol V, Annam R, et al. 7-Hexagon multifocal electroretinography for an objective functional assessment of the macula in 14 seconds. Ophthalmic Res. 2017;58:117-24.

168. Scholl HP, Schuster AM, Vonthein R, et al. Mapping of retinal function in Best macular dystrophy using multifocal electroretinography. Vision Res. 2002;42:1053-61.
169. Glybina IV, Frank RN. Localization of multifocal electroretinogram abnormalities to the lesion site: findings in a family with Best disease. Arch Ophthalmol. 2006;124:1593-600.
170. Scholl HP, Zrenner E. Electrophysiology in the investigation of acquired retinal disorders. Surv Ophthalmol. 2000;45:29-47.
171. Deutman AF. Electro-oculography in families with vitelliform dystrophy of the fovea. Detection of the carrier state. Arch Ophthalmol. 1969;81:305-16.
172. Kay DB, Land ME, Cooper RF, et al. Outer retinal structure in best vitelliform macular dystrophy. JAMA Ophthalmol. 2013;131:1207-15.
173. Parodi MB, Iacono P, Del Turco C, et al. Functional assessment of the fundus autofluorescence pattern in Best vitelliform macular dystrophy. Graefes Arch Clin Exp Ophthalmol. 2016;254:1297-302.
174. Parodi MB, Iacono P, Del Turco C, et al. Near-infrared fundus autofluorescence in subclinical Best vitelliform macular dystrophy. Am J Ophthalmol. 2014;158:1247-52.e2.
175. Battaglia Parodi M, Castellino N, Iacono P, et al. Microperimetry in Best vitelliform macular dystrophy. Retina. 2018;38(4):841-8.
176. Querques G, Regenbogen M, Quijano C, et al. High-definition optical coherence tomography features in vitelliform macular dystrophy. Am J Ophthalmol. 2008;146:501-7.
177. Pianta MJ, Aleman TS, Cideciyan AV, et al. In vivo micropathology of Best macular dystrophy with optical coherence tomography. Exp Eye Res. 2003;76:203-11.
178. Vedantham V, Ramasamy K. Optical coherence tomography in Best's disease: an observational case report. Am J Ophthalmol. 2005;139:351-3.
179. Querques G, Zerbib J, Santacroce R, et al. The spectrum of subclinical Best vitelliform macular dystrophy in subjects with mutations in BEST1 gene. Invest Ophthalmol Vis Sci. 2011;52:4678-84.
180. Miller SA, Bresnick GH, Chandra SR. Choroidal neovascular membrane in Best's vitelliform macular dystrophy. Am J Ophthalmol. 1976;82:252-5.
181. Noble KG, Scher BM, Carr RE. Polymorphous presentations in vitelliform macular dystrophy: subretinal neovascularisation and central choroidal atrophy. Br J Ophthalmol. 1978;62:561-70.
182. Blodi CF, Stone EM. Best's vitelliform dystrophy. Ophthalmic Paediatr Genet. 1990;11:49-59.
183. Andrade RE, Farah ME, Cardillo JA, et al. Optical coherence tomography in choroidal neovascular membrane associated with Best's vitelliform dystrophy. Acta Ophthalmol Scand. 2002;80:216-8.
184. Andrade RE, Farah ME, Costa RA. Photodynamic therapy with verteporfin for subfoveal choroidal neovascularization in Best disease. Am J Ophthalmol. 2003;136:1179-81.
185. Leu J, Schrage NF, Degenring RF. Choroidal neovascularisation secondary to Best's disease in a 13-year-old boy treated by intravitreal bevacizumab. Graefes Arch Clin Exp Ophthalmol. 2007;245:1723-5.
186. Querques G, Bocco MC, Soubrane G, et al. Intravitreal ranibizumab (Lucentis) for choroidal neovascularization associated with vitelliform macular dystrophy. Acta Ophthalmol. 2008;86:694-5.
187. Boon CJ, den Hollander AI, Hoyng CB, et al. The spectrum of retinal dystrophies caused by mutations in the peripherin/RDS gene. Prog Retin Eye Res. 2008;27:213-35.
188. Deutman AF, van Blommestein JD, Henkes HE, et al. Butterfly-shaped pigment dystrophy of the fovea. Arch Ophthalmol. 1970;83:558-69.
189. Hsieh RC, Fine BS, Lyons JS. Patterned dystrophies of the retinal pigment epithelium. Arch Ophthalmol. 1977;95:429-35.
190. Marmor MF, Byers B. Pattern dystrophy of the pigment epithelium. Am J Ophthalmol. 1977;84:32-44.
191. O'Donnell FE, Schatz H, Reid P, et al. Autosomal dominant dystrophy of the retinal pigment epithelium. Arch Ophthalmol. 1979;97:680-3.
192. Prensky JG, Bresnick GH. Butterfly-shaped macular dystrophy in four generations. Arch Ophthalmol. 1983;101:1198-203.
193. Gass JD. Atlas of Macular Diseases: Diagnosis and Treatment. St. Louis: Mosby Co.; 1987.
194. Zhang K, Garibaldi DC, Li Y, et al. Butterfly-shaped pattern dystrophy: a genetic, clinical, and histopathological report. Arch Ophthalmol. 2002;120:485-90.
195. Nichols BE, Sheffield VC, Vandenburgh K, et al. Butterfly-shaped pigment dystrophy of the fovea caused by a point mutation in codon 167 of the RDS gene. Nat Genet. 1993;3:202-7.
196. Gutman I, Walsh JB, Henkind P. Vitelliform macular dystrophy and butterfly-shaped epithelial dystrophy: a continuum? Br J Ophthalmol. 1982;66:170-3.
197. Nichols BE, Drack AV, Vandenburgh K, et al. A 2 base pair deletion in the RDS gene associated with butterfly-shaped pigment dystrophy of the fovea. Hum Mol Genet. 1993;2:601-3.
198. Goldberg AF. Role of peripherin/rds in vertebrate photoreceptor architecture and inherited retinal degenerations. Int Rev Cytol. 2006;253:131-75.
199. Farjo R, Naash MI. The role of Rds in outer segment morphogenesis and human retinal disease. Ophthalmic Genet. 2006;27:117-22.
200. Bok D. Cellular mechanisms of retinal degenerations: RPE65, ABCA4, RDS, and bicarbonate transporter genes as examples. Retina. 2005;25:S18-S20.
201. Kajiwara K, Hahn LB, Mukai S, et al. Mutations in the human retinal degeneration slow gene in autosomal dominant retinitis pigmentosa. Nature. 1991;354:480-3.
202. Weleber RG, Carr RE, Murphey WH, et al. Phenotypic variation including retinitis pigmentosa, pattern dystrophy, and fundus flavimaculatus in a single family with a deletion of codon 153 or 154 of the peripherin/RDS gene. Arch Ophthalmol. 1993;111:1531-42.
203. Farrar GJ, Kenna P, Jordan SA, et al. A three-base-pair deletion in the peripherin-RDS gene in one form of retinitis pigmentosa. Nature. 1991;354:478-80.

204. Hoyng CB, Heutink P, Testers L, et al. Autosomal dominant central areolar choroidal dystrophy caused by a mutation in codon 142 in the peripherin/RDS gene. Am J Ophthalmol. 1996;121:623-9.
205. Keilhauer CN, Meigen T, Weber BH. Clinical findings in a multigeneration family with autosomal dominant central areolar choroidal dystrophy associated with an Arg195Leu mutation in the peripherin/RDS gene. Arch Ophthalmol. 2006;124:1020-7.
206. Daniele S, Restagno G, Daniele C, et al. Analysis of the rhodopsin and peripherin/RDS gene in two families with pattern dystrophy of the retinal pigment epithelium. Eur J Ophthalmol. 1996;6:197-200.
207. Deutman AF, Rumke AM. Reticular dystrophy of the retinal pigment epithelium. Dystrophia reticularis laminae pigmentosa retinae of H. Sjögren. Arch Ophthalmol. 1969;82:4-9.
208. Watzke RC, Folk JC, Lang RM. Pattern dystrophy of the retinal pigment epithelium. Ophthalmology. 1982;89: 1400-6.
209. Slezak H, Hommer K. Fundus pulverulentus. Albrecht Von Graefes Arch Klin Exp Ophthalmol. 1969;178:176-82.
210. de Jong PT, Delleman JW. Pigment epithelial pattern dystrophy. Four different manifestations in a family. Arch Ophthalmol. 1982;100:1416-21.
211. Sjögren H. Dystrophia reticularis laminae pigmentosae retinae, an earlier not described hereditary eye disease. Acta Ophthalmol (Copenh). 1950;28:279-95.
212. Kingham JD, Fenzl RE, Willerson D, et al. Reticular dystrophy of the retinal pigment epithelium. A clinical and electrophysiologic study of three generations. Arch Ophthalmol. 1978;96:1177-84.
213. Giuffre G. Autosomal dominant pattern dystrophy of the retinal pigment epithelium. Intrafamilial variability. Retina. 1988;8:169-73.
214. Gass JD. Stereoscopic Atlas of Macular Disease. Philadelphia: Elsevier; 1997.
215. Querques G, Forte R, Querques L, et al. Natural course of adult-onset foveomacular vitelliform dystrophy: a spectral-domain optical coherence tomography analysis. Am J Ophthalmol. 2011;152:304-13.
216. Fishman GA, Woolf MB, Goldberg MF, et al. Reticular tapeto-retinal dystrophy. As a possible late stage of Sjögren's reticular dystrophy. Br J Ophthalmol. 1976;60:35-40.
217. Chopdar A. Reticular dystrophy of retina. Br J Ophthalmol. 1976;60:342-44.
218. Kempeneers HP, Dewachter A, Kempeneers GM. Pattern dystrophies of the retinal pigment epithelium. The study of three generations in a family. Doc Ophthalmol. 1990;76: 261-72.
219. Cardillo Piccolino F, Zingirian M. Pattern dystrophy of the retinal pigment epithelium with vitelliform macular lesion: evolution in ten years. Int Ophthalmol. 1988;11:207-17.
220. Giuffre G, Lodato G. Vitelliform dystrophy and pattern dystrophy of the retinal pigment epithelium: concomitant presence in a family. Br J Ophthalmol. 1986;70:526-32.
221. Burgess D. Subretinal neovascularization in a pattern dystrophy of the retinal pigment epithelium. Retina. 1981;1: 151-5.
222. Francis PJ, Schultz DW, Gregory AM, et al. Genetic and phenotypic heterogeneity in pattern dystrophy. Br J Ophthalmol. 2005;89:1115-9.
223. Anastasakis A, Goleni F, Livir-Rallatos G, et al. Spontaneous regression of choroidal neovascularization in a patient with pattern dystrophy. Case Rep Ophthalmol Med. 2016;2016:9685290.
224. Theischen M, Schilling H, Steinhorst UH. EOG in adult vitelliform macular degeneration, butterfly-shaped pattern dystrophy and Best disease [In German]. Ophthalmologe. 1997;94:230-3.
225. Kumar V, Kumawat D. Multimodal imaging in a case of butterfly pattern dystrophy of retinal pigment epithelium. Int Ophthalmol. 2017.
226. Gass JD. Drusen and disciform macular detachment and degeneration. Arch Ophthalmol. 1973;90:206-17.
227. Vogt A. Die Ophthalmoskopie im rotfreien Licht. In: Graefe A, Saemisch T (Eds). Handbuch der gesammten Augenheilkunde. Berlin, Leipzig: Verlag von Wilhelm Engelman; 1925. pp. 111-8.
228. Doyne R. Peculiar condition of choroiditis occurring in several members of the same family. Trans Ophthalmol Soc UK. 1899:71.
229. Heon E, Piguet B, Munier F, et al. Linkage of autosomal dominant radial drusen (malattia leventinese) to chromosome 2p16-21. Arch Ophthalmol. 1996;114:193-8.
230. Zhang T, Xie X, Cao G, et al. Malattia leventinese/Doyne honeycomb retinal dystrophy in a chinese family with mutation of the EFEMP1 gene. Retina. 2014;34:2462-71.
231. Gass JD. Diseases causing choroidal exudative and hemorrhagic localized (disciform) detachment of the retina and pigment epithelium. In: Stereoscopic Atlas of Macular Diseases. St Louis: Mosby; 1987. pp. 96-7.
232. Holz FG, Owens SL, Marks J, et al. Ultrastructural findings in autosomal dominant drusen. Arch Ophthalmol. 1997;115: 788-92.
233. Sohn EH, Wang K, Thompson S, et al. Comparison of drusen and modifying genes in autosomal dominant radial drusen and age-related macular degeneration. Retina. 2015;35:48-557.
234. Stone EM, Lotery AJ, Munier FL, et al. A single EFEMP1 mutation associated with both malattia leventinese and Doyne honeycomb retinal dystrophy. Nat Genet. 1999;22:199-202.
235. Querques G, Guigui B, Leveziel N, et al. Multimodal morphological and functional characterization of malattia leventinese. Graefes Arch Clin Exp Ophthalmol. 2013;251:705-14.
236. Narendran N, Guymer RH, Cain M, et al. Analysis of the EFEMP1 gene in individuals and families with early onset drusen. Eye (Lond). 2005;19:11-5.
237. Marmorstein L. Association of EFEMP1 with malattia leventinese and age-related macular degeneration: a mini-review. Ophthalmic Genet. 2004;25:219-26.

238. Marmorstein LY, Munier FL, Arsenijevic Y, et al. Aberrant accumulation of EFEMP1 underlies drusen formation in malattia leventinese and age-related macular degeneration. Proc Natl Acad Sci USA. 2002;99:13067-72.
239. Zweifel SA, Maygar I, Berger W, et al. Multimodal imaging of autosomal dominant drusen. Klin Monbl Augenheilkd. 2012;229:399-402.
240. Sohn EH, Patel PJ, MacLaren RE, et al. Responsiveness of choroidal neovascular membranes in patients with R345W mutation in fibulin 3 (Doyne honeycomb retinal dystrophy) to anti-vascular endothelial growth factor therapy. Arch Ophthalmol. 2011;129:1626-8.
241. Deutman AF, Jansen LM. Dominantly inherited drusen of Bruch's membrane. Br J Ophthalmol. 1970;54:373-82.
242. Piguet B, Haimovici R, Bird AC. Dominantly inherited drusen represent more than one disorder: a historical review. Eye (Lond). 1995;9(Pt 1):34-41.
243. Pearce WG. Doyne's honeycomb retinal degeneration. Clinical and genetic features. Br J Ophthalmol. 1968;52:73-8.
244. Coates H. Autosomal dominant drusen--a case study. J Vis Commun Med. 2013;36:111-6.
245. Ewe SY, Jamieson R, Chang AA. Masquerade macular exudation in mallatia leventinese. Can J Ophthalmol. 2016;51:e27-29.
246. Gaillard MC, Wolfensberger TJ, Uffer S, et al. Optical coherence tomography in malattia leventinese [In French]. Klin Monbl Augenheilkd. 2005;222:180-5.
247. Souied EH, Leveziel N, Letien V, et al. Optical coherent tomography features of malattia leventinese. Am J Ophthalmol. 2006;141:404-7.
248. Haimovici R, Wroblewski J, Piguet B, et al. Symptomatic abnormalities of dark adaptation in patients with EFEMP1 retinal dystrophy (malattia leventinese/Doyne honeycomb retinal dystrophy). Eye (Lond). 2002;16:7-15.
249. Warrington KH Jr, Herzog RW. Treatment of human disease by adeno-associated viral gene transfer. Hum Genet. 2006;119:571-603.
250. Allocca M, Doria M, Petrillo M, et al. Serotype-dependent packaging of large genes in adeno-associated viral vectors results in effective gene delivery in mice. J Clin Invest. 2008;118:1955-64.
251. Byrne LC, Dalkara D, Luna G, et al. Viral-mediated RdCVF and RdCVFL expression protects cone and rod photoreceptors in retinal degeneration. J Clin Invest. 2015; 125:105-16.
252. Bainbridge JW, Mehat MS, Sundaram V, et al. Long-term effect of gene therapy on Leber's congenital amaurosis. New Engl J Med. 2015;372:1887-97.
253. Weleber RG, Pennesi ME, Wilson DJ, et al. Results at 2 years after gene therapy for RPE65-deficient Leber congenital amaurosis and severe early-childhood-onset retinal dystrophy. Ophthalmology. 2016;123:1606-20.
254. Petrs-Silva H, Dinculescu A, Li Q, et al. Novel properties of tyrosine-mutant AAV2 vectors in the mouse retina. Mol Ther. 2011;19:293-301.
255. Dalkara D, Byrne LC, Klimczak RR, et al. In vivo-directed evolution of a new adeno-associated virus for therapeutic outer retinal gene delivery from the vitreous. Sci Transl Med. 2013;5:189ra76.
256. Bakondi B, Lv W, Lu B, et al. In vivo CRISPR/Cas9 gene editing corrects retinal dystrophy in the S334ter-3 rat model of autosomal dominant retinitis pigmentosa. Mol Ther. 2016;24:556-63.
257. Scholl HP, Moore AT, Koenekoop RK, et al. Safety and proof-of-concept study of oral QLT091001 in retinitis pigmentosa due to inherited deficiencies of retinal pigment epithelial 65 protein (RPE65) or lecithin:retinol acyltransferase (LRAT). PLoS One. 2015;10:e0143846.
258. Koenekoop RK, Sui R, Sallum J, et al. Oral 9-cis retinoid for childhood blindness due to Leber congenital amaurosis caused by RPE65 or LRAT mutations: an open-label phase 1b trial. Lancet. 2014;384:1513-20.
259. Kiser PD, Golczak M, Palczewski K. Chemistry of the retinoid (visual) cycle. Chem Rev. 2014;114:194-232.
260. Marlhens F, Bareil C, Griffoin JM, et al. Mutations in RPE65 cause Leber's congenital amaurosis. Nat Genet. 1997;17: 139-41.
261. Gu SM, Thompson DA, Srikumari CR, et al. Mutations in RPE65 cause autosomal recessive childhood-onset severe retinal dystrophy. Nat Genet. 1997;17:194-7.
262. Thompson DA, Li Y, McHenry CL, et al. Mutations in the gene encoding lecithin retinol acyltransferase are associated with early-onset severe retinal dystrophy. Nat Genet. 2001;28:123-4.
263. Redmond TM, Yu S, Lee E, et al. Rpe65 is necessary for production of 11-cis-vitamin A in the retinal visual cycle. Nat Genet. 1998;20:344-51.
264. Travis GH, Golczak M, Moise AR, et al. Diseases caused by defects in the visual cycle: retinoids as potential therapeutic agents. Annu Rev Pharmacol Toxicol. 2007;47:469-512.
265. Charbel Issa P, Barnard AR, Herrmann P, et al. Rescue of the Stargardt phenotype in Abca4 knockout mice through inhibition of vitamin A dimerization. Proc Natl Acad Sci USA. 2015;112:8415-20.
266. Ma L, Kaufman Y, Zhang J, et al. C20-D3-vitamin A slows lipofuscin accumulation and electrophysiological retinal degeneration in a mouse model of Stargardt disease. J Biol Chem. 2011;286:7966-74.
267. Maeda A, Golczak M, Chen Y, et al. Primary amines protect against retinal degeneration in mouse models of retinopathies. Nat Chem Biol. 2011;8:170-8.
268. MacLaren RE, Pearson RA, MacNeil A, et al. Retinal repair by transplantation of photoreceptor precursors. Nature. 2006;444:203-7.
269. Singh MS, Charbel Issa P, Butler R, et al. Reversal of end-stage retinal degeneration and restoration of visual function by photoreceptor transplantation. Proc Natl Acad Sci USA. 2013;110:1101-6.
270. Schwartz SD, Regillo CD, Lam BL, et al. Human embryonic stem cell-derived retinal pigment epithelium in patients with age-related macular degeneration and Stargardt's macular dystrophy: follow-up of two open-label phase 1/2 studies. Lancet. 2015;385:509-16.

Chapter 54 Peripheral Retinal Degenerations

Joseph M Simonett, Mark E Pennesi

INTRODUCTION

This chapter will discuss the heterogeneous group of disorders that involve degeneration of the peripheral retinal. Given the predominance of rod photoreceptors in the periphery, many of these disorders share the phenotype of nyctalopia, or night blindness, in addition to peripheral vision loss; but there is great variance in ocular examination findings, extent of macular involvement, visual prognosis, systemic features, and treatment options. The effects from genetic investigations are seen ubiquitously throughout medicine but are of particular importance to this list of hereditary disorders, where they have led to novel disease classification systems and gene directed therapies, many of which will be discussed here.

RETINITIS PIGMENTOSA AND ALLIED DISORDERS

Inherited pigmentary retinopathies describe a group of hereditary disorders [mostly commonly retinitis pigmentosa (RP)] characterized by progressive photoreceptor dysfunction and death. There is vast heterogeneity among the diseases under the RP umbrella, principally due to the diversity in genetic causes. The age of disease onset ranges from infancy to late adulthood. The final visual burden ranges from regional field loss, which may go unnoticed by the patient, to severe loss of peripheral and central vision. Deterioration of visual acuity can occur at any age but is more frequent in advanced stages of disease. Furthermore, RP can be seen in isolation (typical RP) or in association with a variety of systemic disease presentations (syndromic RP). The diversity in RP makes it difficult to report the true prevalence of disease; but a common estimation is approximately 1 in 4,000 individuals.[1]

Research in RP is extensively documented in the published literature, and the field is rapidly evolving. A Medline literature search performed in February 2017 revealed more than 9,900 relevant articles; therefore, a comprehensive understanding of disease mechanism and potential therapies requires a detailed review of the current literature.

Clinical Features

Nyctalopia

Night blindness, or nyctalopia, is often the earliest hallmark of RP. Patients may first report narrowing of their visual field in low light. Due to impaired dark adaptation, patients also notice a slow recovery of vision after moving from a well-lit to a poorly-lit environment, such as entering a movie theater or stepping inside on a bright day. Difficulties with night-time tasks or becoming accident-prone are also common findings. Symptom onset usually occurs during the first or second decade of life, and onset is often earlier in those with X-linked or autosomal recessive disease compared to those with autosomal dominant disease.[2] Symptoms of night blindness should not be confused with symptoms of night myopia or uncorrected refractive error.

Visual Field Loss

Progressive loss of peripheral vision is the second hallmark symptom in RP. Visual field defects may be evident first under scotopic testing conditions (due to early rod loss) and later under photopic conditions (due to cone loss).[3] As the inferior retina is often involved first, superior visual field deficits are frequently found on initial testing. Visual field deficits coalesce into an annular scotoma, which will usually first extend peripherally then centrally with disease progression.[4]

The reported rate of visual field loss ranges from 4.6% to 14.5% per year.[5,6] One theory, initially proposed by Massof and Finkelstein,[7] suggests that the rate of field loss is nearly identical in all major classes of RP if one corrects for age of symptom onset. With this in mind, the authors described a two-stage hypothesis for RP progression: first, a predisposition for RP, including the wide variety of genetic causes; then the actual retinal degeneration, which follows a physiologically determined timeline common to most, if not all, types of RP.

Importantly, neither nyctalopia nor progressive visual field loss are pathognomonic for RP as both can be seen in a number of other acquired and inherited ocular diseases, including disorders that may be reversible with treatment, such as vitamin A or E deficiency, abetalipoproteinemia, and Refsum disease.[8-11]

Central Vision Loss

Visual acuity in patients with RP is typically preserved until late in the disease; but it can be affected earlier, even when peripheral fields are still intact.[12] It is important to investigate early loss of acuity in RP, as some causes are reversible. Such decline can be secondary to cataract formation, which manifests earlier in RP patients, with posterior subcapsular lens opacities being the most common type (up to 51% of adult patients).[13-16] Additional causes of central vision loss include cystoid macular edema (CME),[17] epiretinal membrane formation,[18] and atrophy of foveal cones.[19] Some genes that cause RP may predispose to early macular atrophy; implicated genes include *IMPG2, C2orf71, CLN3, CDHR1, RDH11, MERTK, CDH3, MFSD8, CERKL*, and Bardet-Biedl syndrome (BBS) gene mutations.[20-28] Importantly, the presence of any pigmentary or atrophic macular lesion has been associated with an increased rate of visual acuity loss.[29]

Fundus Appearance

The fundus appearance of RP can vary throughout the progression of the disease. The earliest changes may only be vascular attenuation and mottling of the retinal pigment epithelium (RPE) in the midperipheral retina. As the disease progresses, atrophy of the outer retina becomes more apparent and intraretinal migration of hyperpigmented RPE cells around inner retinal vessels forms the classic "bone spicules" (Figs. 54.1A to F).[30] Inner retinal gliosis and vascular attenuation result in a waxy pallor of the optic nerves.[31] Drusen involving the optic disk or parapapillary regions can also be seen.[32] Loss of pigment and death of RPE cells result in increased visualization of underlying choroidal structures, although this change may be absent in highly pigmented individuals. In late stages of the disease, atrophy is severe, intraretinal pigmentation can be diffuse, blood vessels may appear gray and thread-like, and optic nerve pallor is common. RP sine pigmento is a term used to describe patients without pigmentary changes; however, this likely represents an early stage in the natural history of RP rather than a specific subtype.[4]

Physiologic Testing

Perimetry

Perimetry testing to assess the distribution and rate of visual field loss is essential for the diagnosis and management of RP. Early testing will commonly reveal small relative scotomas between 20° and 50° from central fixation. These midperipheral areas of decreased retinal sensitivity will enlarge and coalesce into a ring scotoma which progresses outward and then inward, resulting in narrowly restricted tunnel vision. While the macula can become involved at any stage, useful central vision can persist for decades after peripheral vision is lost. Importantly, intersession variability for perimetry testing is higher among RP patients; therefore, large changes over a short-time span should be interpreted cautiously.[33,34]

Dark Adaptation

Testing dark adaptation with an instrument such as the Goldmann-Weekers adaptometer is useful in evaluating nyctalopia. A normal adaptation curve includes two plateaus; the first, reached in about 5 minutes, corresponds to the rapid adaptation of the cone system, and the second, reached in 20–30 minutes, corresponds to the rod system. In classic RP, the curve is elevated and monophasic, and it reaches the normal threshold very late or not at all. Prolonged rod dark adaptation is particularly characteristic of RP caused by *RHO* mutations.[35,36]

Electroretinography

The electroretinogram (ERG) becomes abnormal very early in the disease. As photoreceptors are primarily involved, both a- and b-waves are reduced. The b-waves are prolonged in time and diminished in amplitude. Both rod and cone signals show marked reduction; however, for typical RP, loss of the scotopic response predominates in early disease. Berson et al. reported that the ERG response amplitude decreased by 16–18.5% per year.[6] In another natural history study, RP patients lost an average of 13.3% of their remaining cone 31 Hz flicker response amplitude per year.[37] While the majority of patients with advanced disease have undetectable responses to conventional techniques, signal averaging can often be used to detect

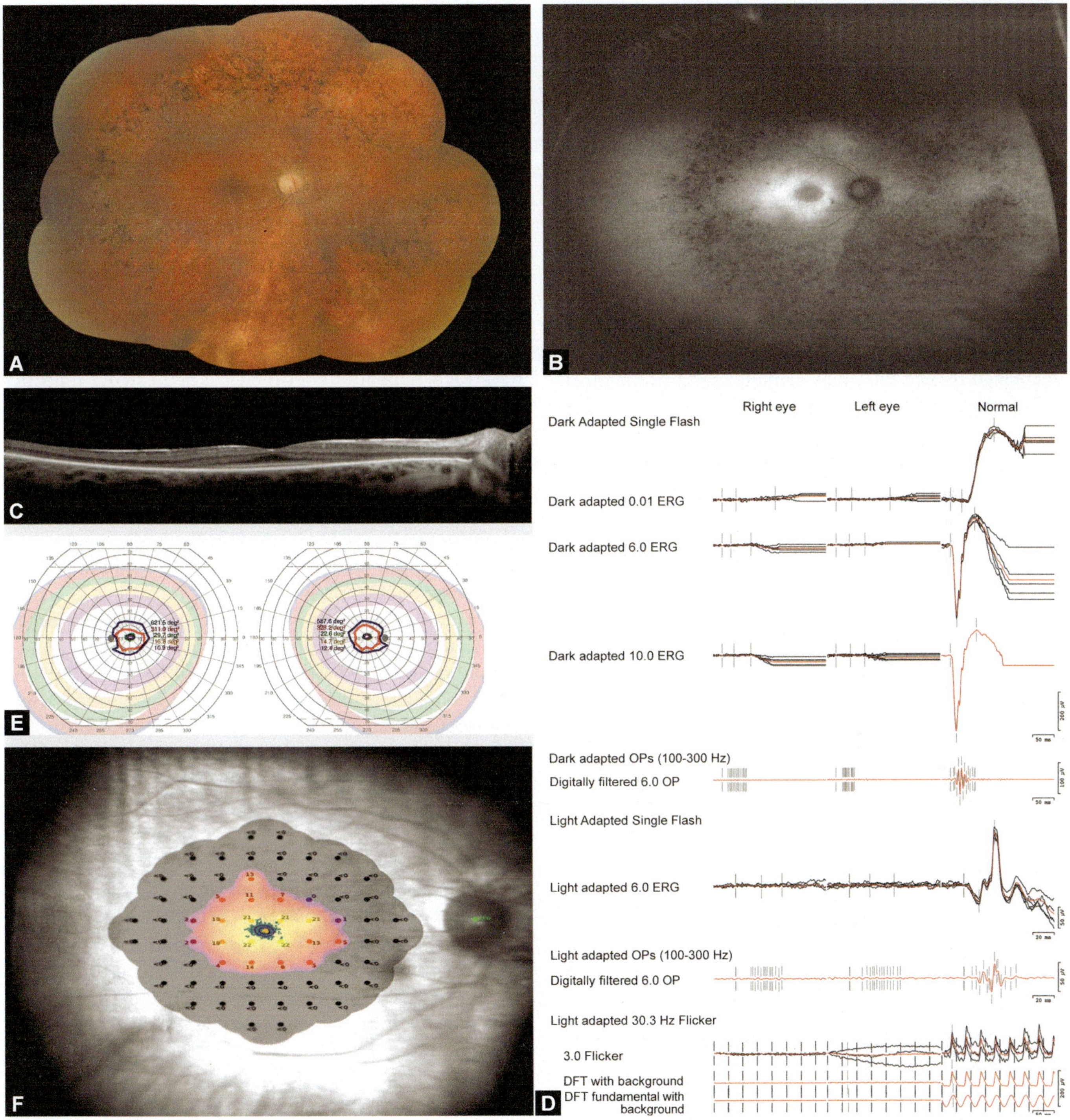

Figs. 54.1A to F: (A) Fundus appearance of the right eye in a 27-year-old female with simplex retinitis pigmentosa; (B) Fundus autofluorescence of the right eye; (C) Note the perifoveal ring of hyperautofluorescence, which correlates with a transition zone from centrally preserved photoreceptors to outer retinal atrophy on OCT; (D) Full-field ERG testing was profoundly abnormal and consistent with a diffuse rod-cone dystrophy; (E) Kinetic visual field; (F) Microperimetry testing demonstrated severely restricted fields with sparing of a small central island of vision. Good visual acuity was retained in both eyes.
(OCT: Optical coherence tomography; ERG: Electroretinogram; OPs: Oscillatory potentials; DFT: Discrete Fourier transform)

small responses.[6,38] Large ERG amplitudes have a positive prognostic value for retaining central visual function.[39]

Imaging Modalities

Fluorescein Angiography

Fluorescein angiography (FA) in RP patients will show hyperfluorescence in areas of RPE atrophy and may demonstrate nonleaking CME. But with the increased use of optical coherence tomography (OCT) and its superior sensitivity for detecting CME, obtaining FA is often unnecessary in RP. Additionally, concerns about light exposure accelerating RP in some animal models have decreased its use.[40] FA may remain useful in diagnostic dilemmas and for identifying vascular or inflammatory complications in RP patients.

Fundus Autofluorescence

Fundus autofluorescence (FAF) takes advantage of retinal fluorophores, primarily those found in lipofuscin granules within the RPE, to obtain clinically useful retinal images.[41] FAF is particularly helpful in pattern recognition for patients with suspected RP and can aid in assessing symmetry between the eyes and differentiating RP from retinal disorders with characteristic FAF patterns such as acute zonal occult outer retinopathy.[42] Bone spicule pigment and punched-out areas of RPE atrophy appear hypoautofluorescent on FAF imaging.[43] Bilateral, symmetric perifoveal rings of increased autofluorescence are seen in most RP patients.[44] These rings demarcate a transition zone between functioning central retina and peripheral degeneration, and have been shown to closely correlate with multifocal ERG and visual field testing.[45,46] Wide-field FAF, which can be used to rapidly obtain 200° views of the fundus, may become a useful tool to quickly document and track retinal atrophy in the mid and far periphery.[47]

The various clinically available FAF imaging systems use different excitation and detection wavelengths. Commonly used systems include short-wave autofluorescence (SW-AF, 488 nm excitation), near-infrared autofluorescence (NIR-AF, 787 nm excitation), and green light wide-field autofluorescence (532 nm). RP-related findings can differ when alternative excitation wavelengths are used, and caution should be applied when comparing imaging from different FAF systems.[48]

Optical Coherence Tomography

Optical coherence tomography has become one of the most informative imaging modalities in RP, as well as in many other retinal disorders, given its high level of resolution and noninvasive technique. The prominent transition zone seen on OCT follows an orderly progression from thinning of the outer segment layer, to thinning of the outer nuclear layer, to complete loss of the inner segment/outer segment junction and outer retinal atrophy when moving from healthy to severely affected peripheral retina.[49] Importantly, macular OCT scans will be normal when degeneration is limited to the periphery; and use of eccentric fixation or wide-field OCT may allow earlier detection.[50] Multiple studies have described correlations between loss of the hyper-reflective photoreceptor bands on OCT and visual function.[51-53] Bone spicules appear as small, hyper-reflective lesions migrating into the retina. OCT is also useful to screen for CME or epiretinal membranes in RP patients with central vision dysfunction.

Optical coherence tomography angiography is a recent imaging advancement that allows noninvasive, 3-dimensional mapping of vascular flow within the retina and choroid.[54] In patients with RP, OCT angiography studies have demonstrated abnormal microvasculature in the deep retinal and choroidal layers.[55,56] Further studies will be required to determine if these vascular changes play a role in disease pathogenesis.

Adaptive Optics Scanning Laser Ophthalmoscopy

Cellular imaging of the retina is typical limited by aberrations of the cornea, lens, or vitreous. Adaptive optics scanning laser ophthalmoscopy (AOSLO) can compensate for these factors, allowing high-resolution imaging of photoreceptor structures, including the photoreceptor mosaic.[57,58] AOSLO imaging has demonstrated decreased cone density in RP patients, even before OCT changes or visual function deficits are evident.[59] Additionally, cone density and spacing data obtained from AOSLO imaging has been used to track RP disease progression over time and may be a useful measurement in therapy trials.[60] Recent advances, such as split-detector AOSLO that can further resolve photoreceptor inner segments, permit cellular quantification even when outer segment structures are affected.[59,61] Due to the expense and intricacy of many AO systems, most devices are relegated to the research setting where they play an important role in clinical trials and in understanding photoreceptor structure and function.[60,62]

Genetic Considerations

Retinitis pigmentosa and allied disorders represent a spectrum of photoreceptor degenerations caused by mutations of more than 100 different genes (Fig. 54.2).[63] Thus, the inheritance pattern of RP can be autosomal recessive, autosomal dominant, X-linked, mitochondrial, or even digenic. The implicated genes are involved in numerous molecular pathways, including the visual cycle, phototransduction, photoreceptor structure, and gene transcription regulation.[64,65] Due to the heterogeneity of genes involved, the phenotypic presentation can vary, depending on the gene involved and even the characteristic of the mutations in a given gene. A further complexity is that multiple genes have been associated with both autosomal dominant and recessive pedigrees. For example, mutations in *RP1* account for approximately 5% of autosomal dominant RP and less than 1% of autosomal recessive RP.[1,66,67] Similarly, mutations in *RPE65*,[68,69] *RHO*,[70,71] and *BEST1*[72] have been reported to cause both autosomal dominant and recessive RP. *RPGR* mutations account for up to 70% of genetically identifiable X-linked RP; dominant-acting mutations have been identified and can be mistaken as having an autosomal mode of inheritance.[73,74]

A careful family history in RP patients will often reveal patterns characteristic of recessive, X-linked, or dominant disease; however, a lack of family history is relatively common. Although such patients are considered to have "simplex" RP and likely have autosomal recessive forms of the disease, dominant or X-linked mutations cannot be ruled out without genetic testing. While the reported percentage of each inheritance pattern is variable, commonly cited values range from 50–60% autosomal recessive, 30–40% autosomal dominant, and 5–15% X-linked.[1]

The reported success rate of identifying a pathologic variant in an RP patient is 50–75% and continues

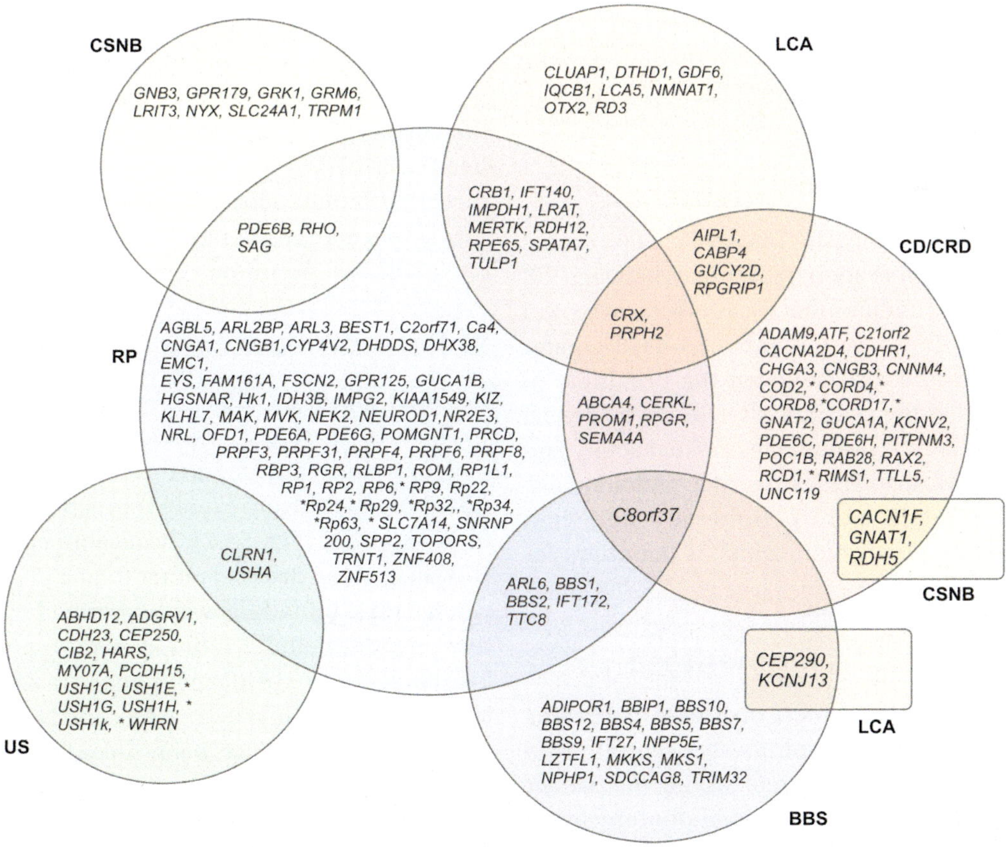

Fig. 54.2: Genes implicated in retinitis pigmentosa (RP) and other photoreceptor diseases including Leber congenital amaurosis (LCA), cone/cone-rod dystrophy (CD/CRD), Bardet-Biedl syndrome (BBS), Usher syndrome (US), and congenital stationary night blindness (CSNB). (*Mapped genetic locus without identified gene)

to improve with advances in molecular diagnostic techniques, including next-generation and whole-exome sequencing.[75-77]

VARIATIONS IN RETINITIS PIGMENTOSA DISTRIBUTION AND FUNDUS APPEARANCE

Nonsyndromic RP is typically symmetrical between the two eyes and involves all quadrants of the retina. Visual field loss starts in the midperiphery, progresses outward to obliterate peripheral visual fields and finally returns centrally to ultimately involve the macula. However, several variations in the pattern of degeneration have been observed.

Sector Retinitis Pigmentosa

Sector RP is characterized by pigmentary changes and visual field defects limited to one or two quadrants (Figs. 54.3A to F).[78] ERG responses are less attenuated and symptoms may be minimal if the macula is not involved. Sector RP has been reported with autosomal dominant or recessive inheritance, and genotype-phenotype correlations have been reported with mutations in the *RHO*[79,80] and *USH1C*[81] genes. Sector RP many not represent a distinct genetic entity but rather early or less severe typical RP that has not yet progressed to diffuse disease.

Pericentral Retinitis Pigmentosa

Pericentral RP is a variation in which visual field loss occurs between 5° and 15° from fixation, rather than between 20° and 50° from fixation (midperipheral), as is seen in typical RP (Figs. 54.4A to E). These patients can have greater disability earlier in the disease given the proximity of the depressed field to the central vision. Some evidence, however, suggests that the overall rate of visual acuity and field loss may be slower in this disease subset.[82] Additionally, these patients maintain more peripheral vision than those with typical RP progression, which is important for navigation skills.

Concentric Retinitis Pigmentosa

Concentric RP is a less severe pattern of disease that begins in the far peripheral retina and progresses centrally at a very slow rate.[83] The macula is spared, leaving the patient with good visual acuity and near normal photoreceptor sensitivity within the preserved visual field.

Unilateral Retinitis Pigmentosa

True unilateral RP has been reported but is exceedingly rare (Figs. 54.5A to D).[84,85] Typically, other affected family members have bilateral RP, suggesting that the unilateral distribution may result from the interplay of other genetic or environmental factors in the affected patient.[85] Noninherited causes of retinopathies, such as trauma, vascular occlusion, and diffuse unilateral subacute neuroretinitis, should be excluded.[86]

X-linked Retinitis Pigmentosa Carriers

Female patients with X-linked RP can present anywhere along a spectrum of disease severity, ranging from asymptomatic to severe retinal degeneration. Visual function can vary significantly between the two eyes.[87] The perimacular area can have a golden metallic-luster appearance, referred to as a tapetal-like reflex (Figs. 54.6A to F).[88] The degree of fundus change may help in determining visual prognosis, as patients with only a tapetal-like reflex at the time of presentation are more likely to retain visual function than those with peripheral pigmentation changes.[89] Both the overall heterogeneity and the tapetal-like reflex in female carriers of X-liked RP have been ascribed to lyonization, the cellular phenomenon in which female carriers create mosaic X-linked gene expression across a tissue through random inactivation of one of the two X chromosomes in each cell.[90,91]

Retinitis Punctata Albescens

Retinitis punctata albescens (RPA), a term first used by Mooren in 1882,[92] is an autosomal recessive retinal degeneration with characteristic glistening white dots distributed relatively evenly throughout the fundus with foveal sparing (Fig. 54.7). It became clear that RPA is a specific genetic disease, rather than a descriptive finding, when causal mutations were described in *RLBP1*, a gene that encodes cellular retinaldehyde-binding protein.[93,94] Two clinical forms of RPA common in restricted geographic areas, Bothnia retinal dystrophy[95] and Newfoundland rod-cone dystrophy,[96] have been linked to specific founder mutations in *RLBP1*. Disease progression is similar to typical RP. Both bone spicule pigment deposits and optic disk pallor can be mild or absent.[96,97]

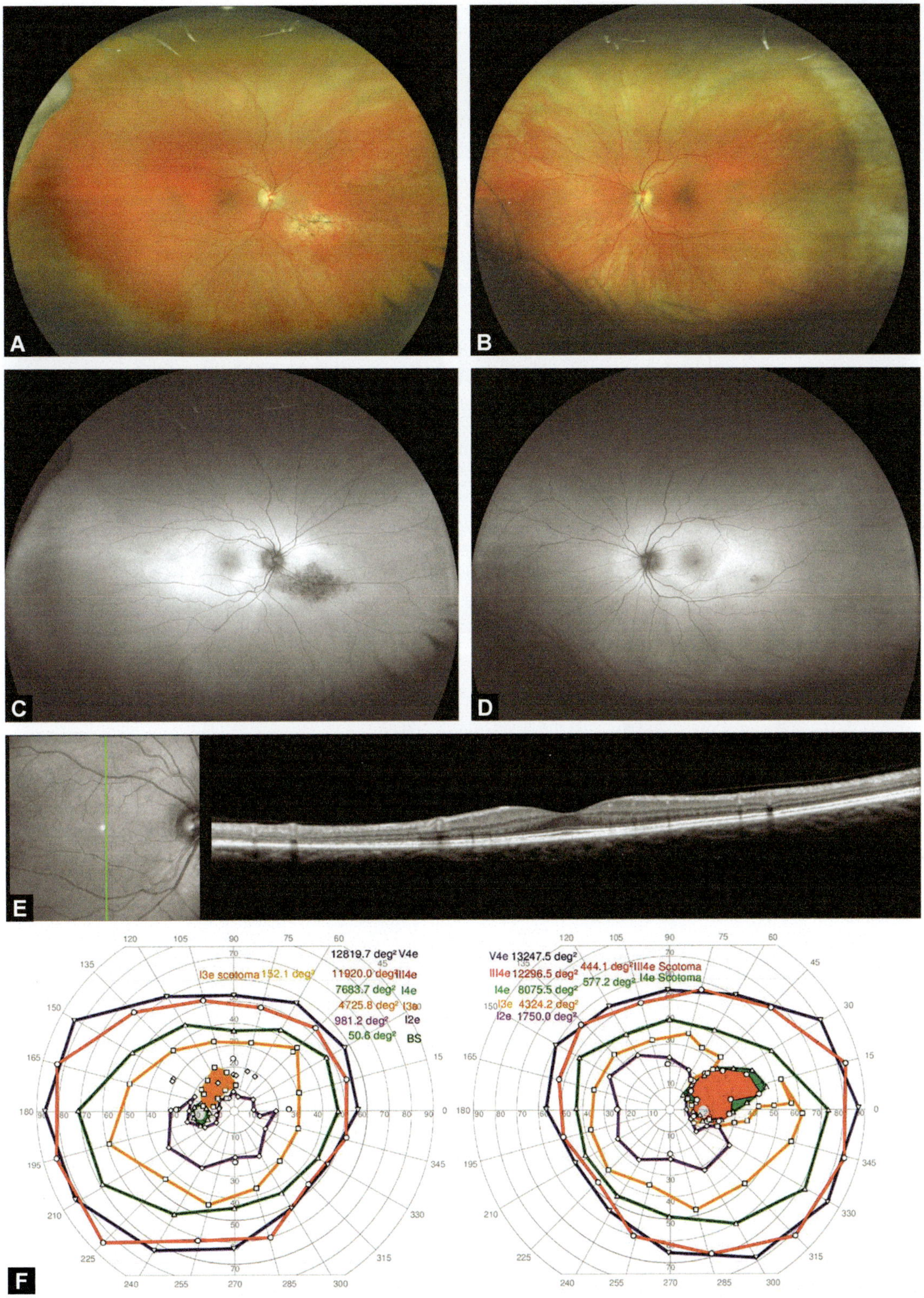

Figs. 54.3A to F: (A and B) Optos wide-field fundus photography in a 57-year-old female with sector retinitis pigmentosa, good visual acuity remained in both eyes. Note the retinal atrophy with pigment clumping isolated to an area inferonasal to the optic nerve head in the right eye and even smaller area inferotemporal to the macula in the left eye; (C and D) Fundus autofluorescence highlight these areas of degeneration; (E) Optical coherence tomography (OCT) shows attenuation of the outer retina and loss of the inner segment/outer segment (IS/OS) junction inferior to the macula; (F) Kinetic visual field testing shows intact peripheral isopters and eccentric scotomas correlating with the location of pigmentary degeneration.

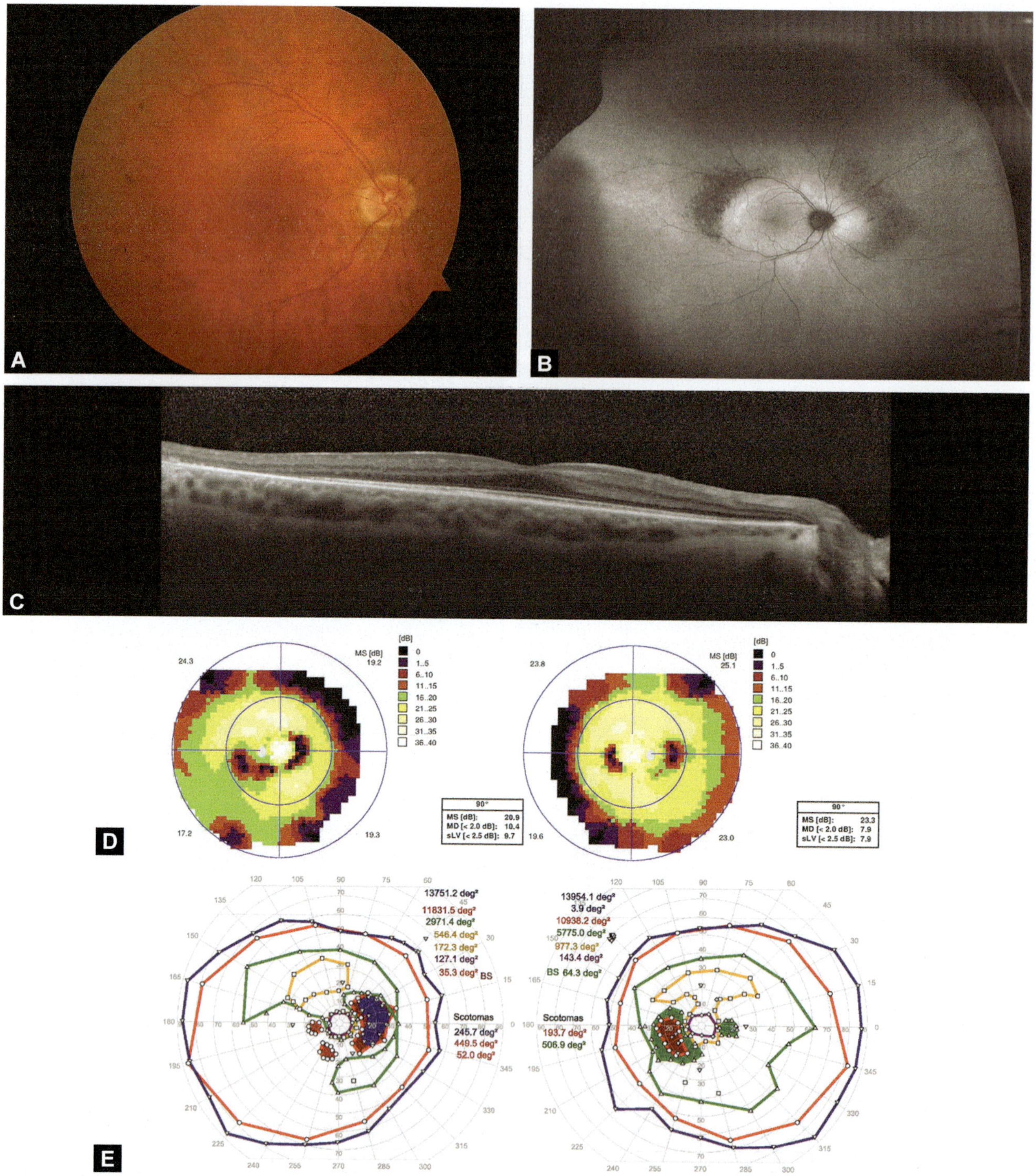

Figs. 54.4A to E: (A) Color fundus photograph of the right eye in a 46-year-old male with pericentral retinitis pigmentosa showing peripheral chorioretinal atrophy and sporadic bone spicule pigmentation; (B) Pericentral ring shaped area of hypoautofluorescence with thin inner ring of hyperautofluorescence is seen on Optos wide-field autofluorescence. Imaging findings were similar in the left eye; (C) Outer retinal atrophy of temporal macula with foveal sparing is seen on optical coherence tomography (OCT); (D) Static and (E) kinetic visual fields demonstrate scattered paracentral scotomas in both eyes aligned on the path of a developing paracentral ring scotoma as well as reduced sensitivity in the far periphery.

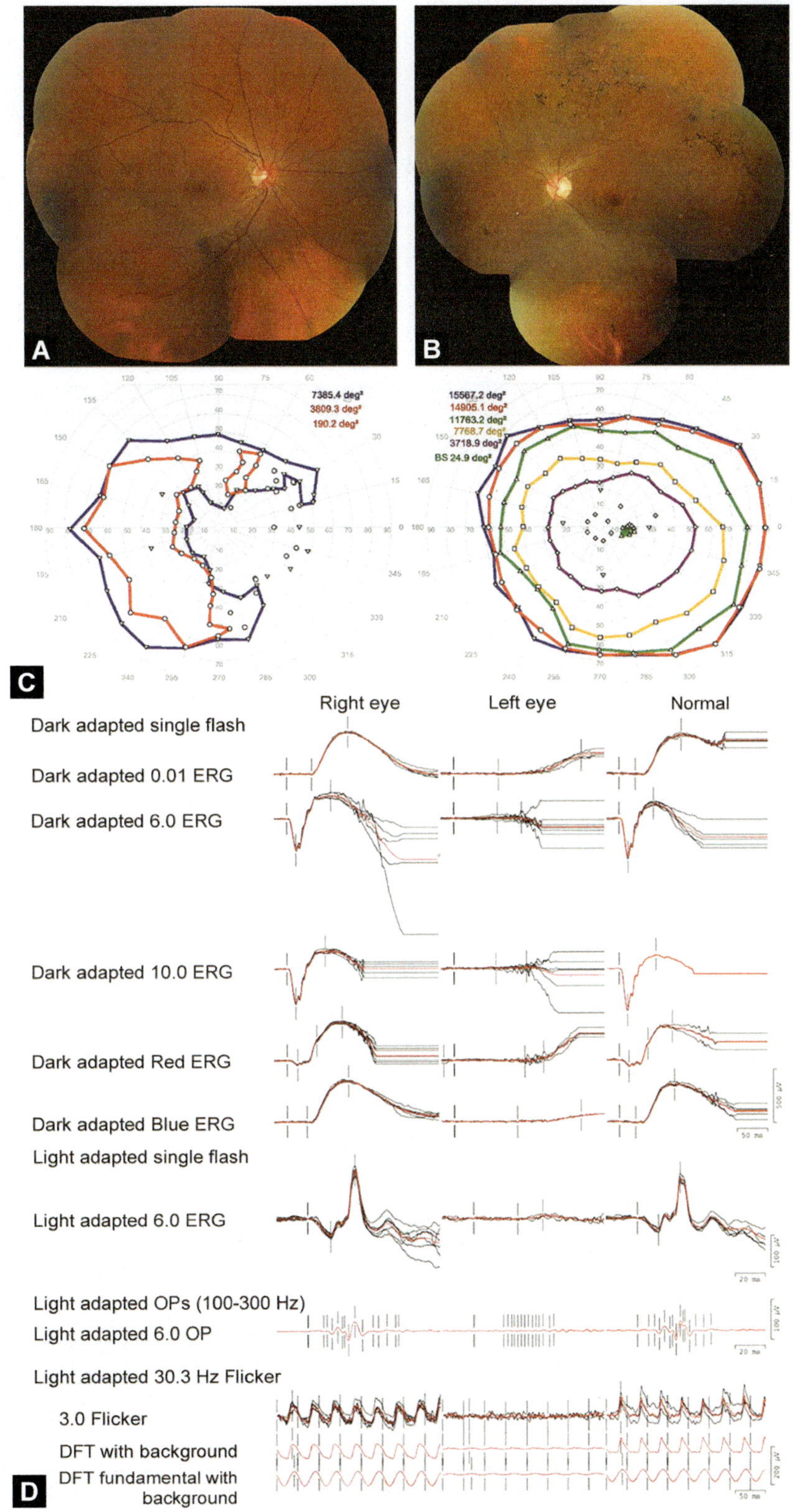

Figs. 54.5A to D: (A and B) Color fundus photographs in a 28-year-old female with unilateral pigmentary changes. Visual acuity was 20/15 in the right eye and 20/600 in the left eye; (C) Kinetic visual field testing showed preserved fields in the right eye and constricted fields with a large central scotoma in the left eye; (D) Scotopic and photopic electroretinogram (ERG).
(DFT: Discrete Fourier transform)

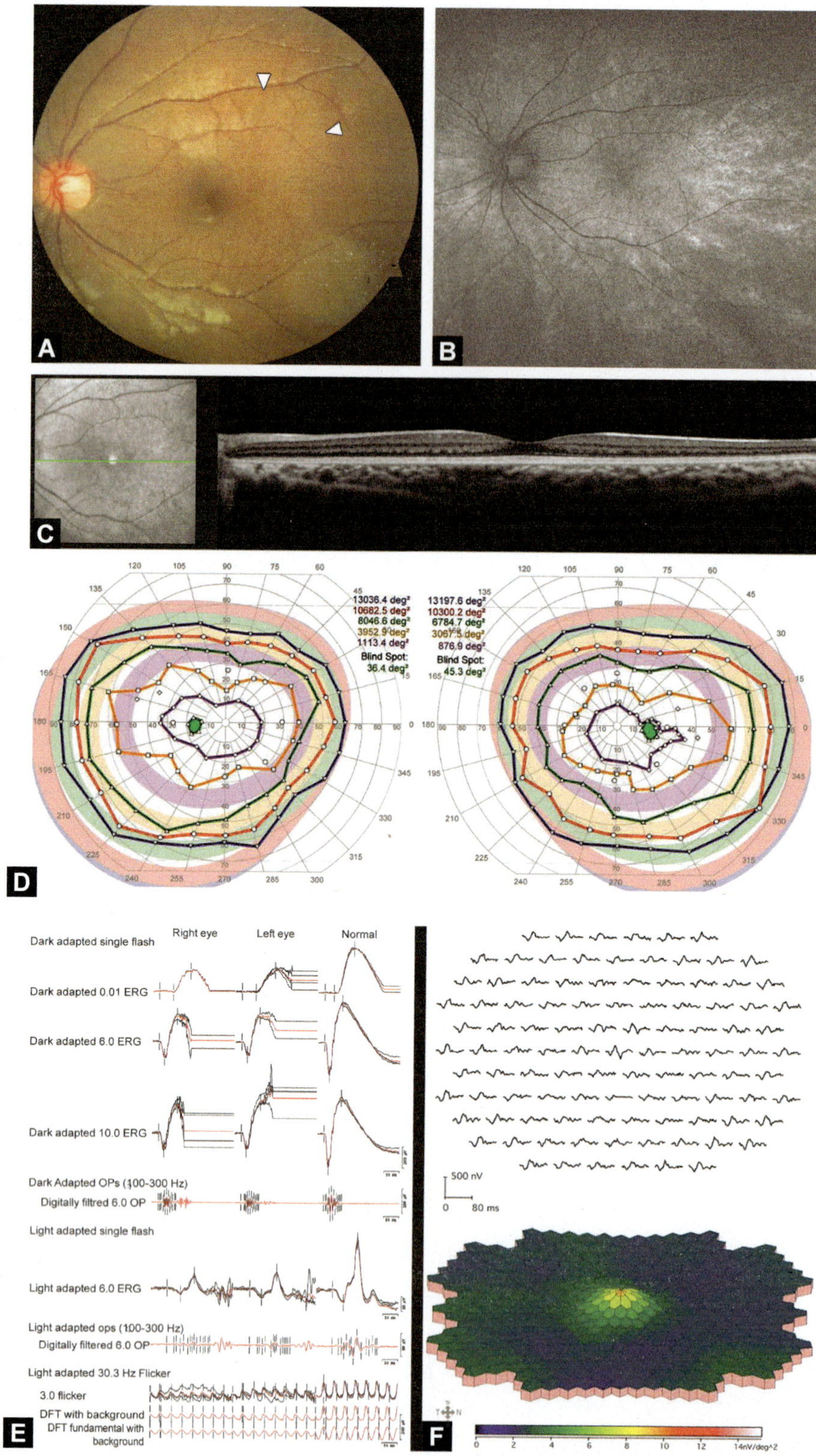

Figs. 54.6A to F: (A) Fundus appearance in an 8-year-old female carrier of X-linked *RPGR* mutation. Note the perifoveal RPE mottling and tapetal sheen (arrowheads) in the posterior pole; (B) Patchy radial streaks of hyperautofluorescence is seen on Optos autofluorescence; (C) OCT shows a preserved IS/OS junction, however the interdigitation zone is difficult to visualize; (D) Mild constriction of peripheral isopters is seen on kinetic visual field testing; (E) Moderate attenuation and implicit time prolongation are seen in both dark and light adapted ERG; (F) Multifocal ERG shows subnormal amplitudes and mildly prolonged latencies in both eyes.

(OCT: Optical coherence tomography; ERG: Electroretinogram; OPs: Oscillatory potentials; RPE: Retinal pigment epithelium; IS/OS: Inner segment/outer segment; DFT: Discrete Fourier transform)

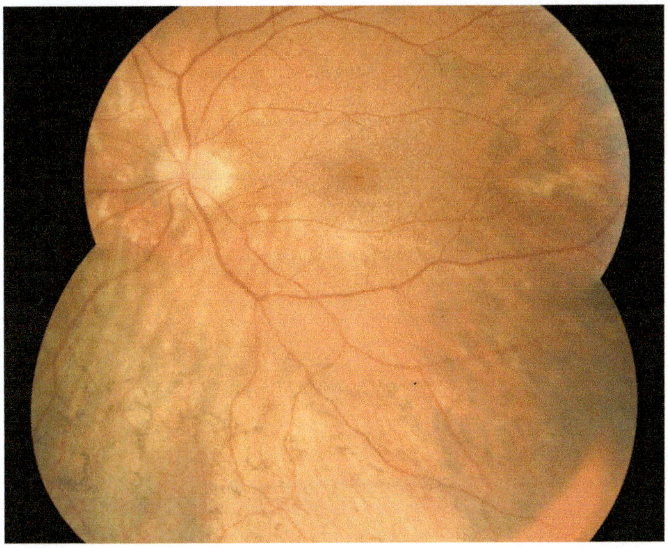

Fig. 54.7: Fundus photograph of retinitis punctata albescens demonstrating white dots throughout the macula with foveal sparing and pigmentary atrophic changes of the inferior peripheral retina.

VARIATIONS IN AGE OF ONSET

Leber Congenital Amaurosis

Leber congenital amaurosis (LCA), first described by Theodore Leber in 1869, is characterized by severe, congenital or infantile-onset retinal dysfunction, nystagmus, and greatly diminished or absent ERG.[98] LCA is no longer considered a single entity, but rather a group of rare disorders caused by mutations in at least 20 different genes. The vast majority of cases are autosomal recessive, but rare families with autosomal dominant inheritance patterns exist.[99,100] Classically, visual symptoms and signs are present at birth or within the first year of life. Different terms, including severe early childhood onset retinal dystrophy and early-onset RP, have been used to describe a milder form of disease, typically with onset between 1 year and 5 years of age.[101-103]

Patients exhibit profound, early visual impairment with best-corrected visual acuity (BCVA) ranging from 20/200 light perception to no light perception. Visual acuity can remain stable (likely due to a floor effect), but progressive declines in BCVA have also been documented.[104,105] Due to severe retinal dysfunction, patients often have poor pupillary reflexes and nystagmus. High hyperopia is also common.[102] Patients may display an oculodigital phenomenon, which consists of a repetitive, deep rubbing of the eyes, probably performed to mechanically induce a visual sensation. Keratoconus is a common finding, with a reported prevalence of 29% among LCA patients;[106] it remains unclear if this association is due to frequent eye rubbing or underlying genetic factors. Other causes of infantile vision deficit and nystagmus, such as albinism, achromatopsia, early infantile neuronal ceroid lipofuscinosis, and congenital stationary night blindness (CSNB) must be carefully excluded. An extinguished ERG response within the first year of life, characteristic of LCA, is helpful for addressing diagnostic dilemmas. The ERG may also be severely depressed or undetectable in patients with severe early childhood onset retinal dystrophy; if the visual acuity deficit is mild, however, night blindness may be the only visual symptom.[101]

Ophthalmoscopy may reveal a normal fundus in infancy; but patients often develop a pigmentary retinopathy with progressive chorioretinal atrophy, retinal vasculature narrowing, and intraretinal pigment migration (Figs. 54.8A to E).[107] Pigment clumping can include nummular or bone spicule shapes and, like typical RP, is often most prominent in the midperiphery.[108] Posterior segment findings are quite variable and genotype-phenotype correlations are present.[109] Prominent macular atrophy with sharply defined, pigmented borders, a finding sometimes referred to as macular coloboma, is most commonly seen with pathogenic variants in *NMNAT1*.[110-112] White retinal dots can also be present and give the fundus a marbleized appearance in patients with mutations in *RPE65* or *CEP290*.[101,113]

Many systemic associations have been made with LCA. Of these, developmental delay is the most common (some studies report a rate of concurrence up to 20%).[114-117] It is important to consider that congenital blindness may result in a child falling behind in-school or failing to meet developmental milestones, which does not necessarily reflect their intellectual capacity. Structural central nervous system (CNS) abnormalities are found in a number of patients with an LCA phenotype. Many of these cases likely represent overlapping syndromic eye disorders, such as neuronal ceroid lipofuscinosis or peroxisomal disorders.[118] Mutations in the *CEP290* gene, which has been recognized as the most common cause of isolated LCA, cause a spectrum of disease ranging from nonsyndromic LCA to Joubert syndrome, which presents a constellation of symptoms, including hypotonia, ataxia, oculomotor apraxia, and cerebellar vermis agenesis.[113]

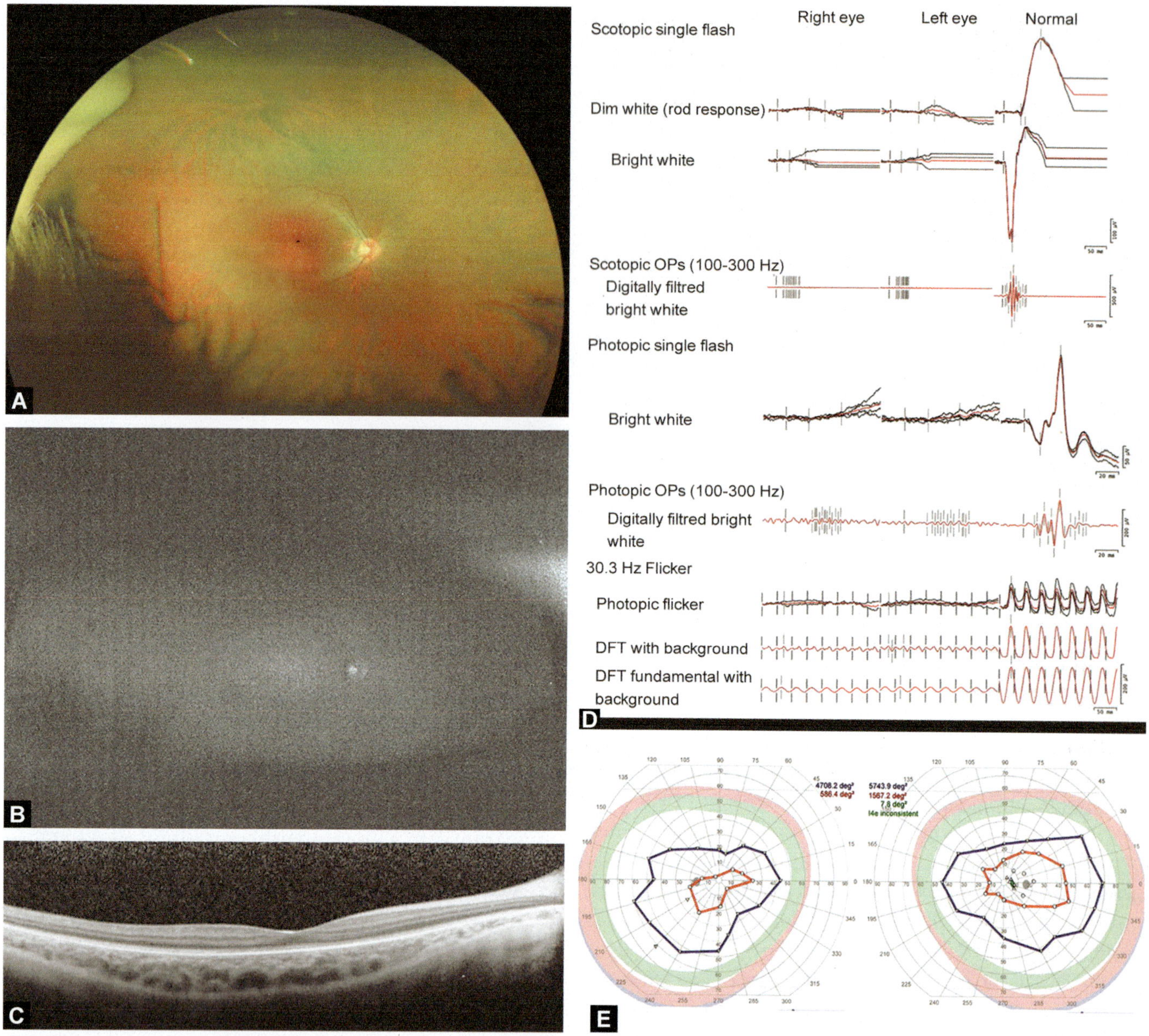

Figs. 54.8A to E: (A) Optos wide-field fundus photograph in a 10-year-old male with Leber congenital amaurosis due to *RPE65* mutation demonstrating vascular attenuation and subtle midperipheral RPE mottling. The patient had congenital nystagmus and severely reduced vision; (B) Fundus autofluorescence shows minimal autofluorescence, typical of *RPE65* mutations; (C) OCT shows mild outer retinal thinning; (D) The ERG was unrecordable in both eyes; (E) Visual fields were constricted to the V4e and III4e targets on kinetic testing.

(OCT: Optical coherence tomography; ERG: Electroretinogram; OPs: Oscillatory potentials; DFT: Discrete Fourier transform)

Late-onset Retinal Degeneration

On the other end of the age spectrum, late-onset retinal degeneration (LORD) is a rare inherited disorder that typically presents as night blindness in the fifth or sixth decade and progresses to severe central and peripheral retinal degeneration. LORD is distinct from age-related macular degeneration in its autosomal dominant inheritance and wider pattern of retinal atrophy.[119] In 2003, Hayward et al. reported on the genetic linkage of LORD to chromosomal region 11q23 and a proposed founder mutation in the *CTRP5* (*C1QTNF5*) gene, which encodes a short-chain collagen that is highly expressed in RPE cells and that is present in 7 of 14 LORD families.[120] Delayed dark adaptation is the first indication of disease in asymptomatic patients who carry the mutation.

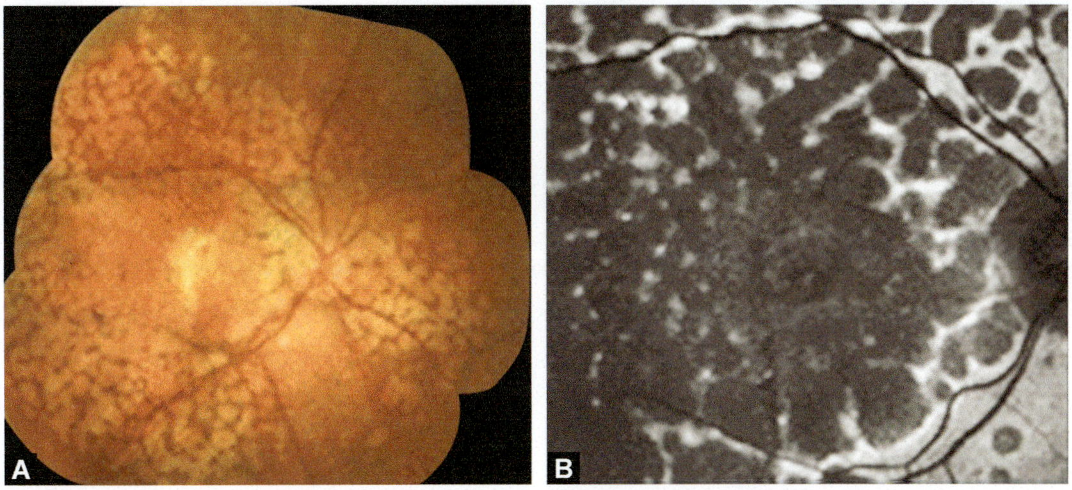

Figs. 54.9A and B: (A) Fundus appearance in a 74-year-old patient with late onset retinal dystrophy; (B) Fundus autofluorescence shows the scalloped areas of retinal pigment epithelium (RPE) atrophy.
Source: Reproduce with permission from soamplis et al. Phenotypic findings in C1QTNF5 retinopathy (late-onset retinal degeneration). Acta ophthalmologica. 2013.

Patients develop extensive drusen-like, sub-RPE deposits that can extend from the central retina into the far periphery.[119] In late stages of disease, fundus examination reveals widespread atrophy in the posterior pole and well-demarcated, scalloped areas of RPE atrophy in the midperiphery (Figs. 54.9A and B). Choroidal neovascularization can also occur. Anterior segment findings include peripapillary iris transillumination defects and abnormally long anterior zonular insertions.[121,122]

Optical coherence tomography imaging demonstrates diffuse photoreceptor loss, outer nuclear layer thinning, and hyper-reflective sub-RPE deposits.[122] If family history is unknown, early cases are often misdiagnosed as age-related macular degeneration, choroideremia, gyrate atrophy, or Sorsby fundus dystrophy.

SYNDROMIC RETINITIS PIGMENTOSA

By definition, typical RP does not affect organ systems outside of the eye. However, there are several inherited syndromes that include both RP-like retinal degeneration and dysfunction of other systems (auditory, olfactory, renal, hepatic, etc.). These diseases typically involve genes that are mutually expressed among different tissues, such as ciliary related proteins.

Usher Syndrome

Usher syndrome is the most common syndromic form of RP. With a reported prevalence as high as 1 in 6,000, Usher syndrome accounts for half of the persons in the United States who are both deaf and blind.[123,124] There are at least 13 causal genes (and 3 additional loci).[63] Usher syndrome is autosomal recessive and manifests with typical RP and congenital sensorineural hearing loss, with or without vestibular involvement.

Usher syndrome has been divided into three major groups based on clinical features. Usher syndrome type 1 is characterized by profound congenital deafness (usually requiring cochlear implants), vestibular areflexia, and an early-onset retinal degeneration (Figs. 54.10A to D).[124] These patients typically demonstrate prolonged time to walk (average age of 24 months compared to less than 18 months in normal children)[125] and may have difficulty with tasks that require vestibular feedback, such as riding a bicycle. Patients with Usher syndrome type 2 have moderate to severe congenital deafness (often requiring hearing aids), no vestibular symptoms, and typical-onset RP (Figs. 54.11A to D). Type 3 is less common and is defined by progressive deafness starting anywhere from the second to forth decade of life and an early onset retinopathy.[126] Atypical presentations can also occur; both environmental factors and modifier genes are thought to influence disease severity.[127] BCVA is generally worse in type 1 Usher syndrome than in type 2, with only 69% of type 1 patients retaining 20/40 visual acuity or better at age 29, compared to 94% in type 2.[128]

The diagnosis of Usher syndrome can be missed in early disease when classic retinal pigmentation has not yet developed, or when pigment clumping is misdiagnosed as rubella retinopathy. ERG is a useful diagnostic tool that can reveal electrophysiological changes (especially in type 1

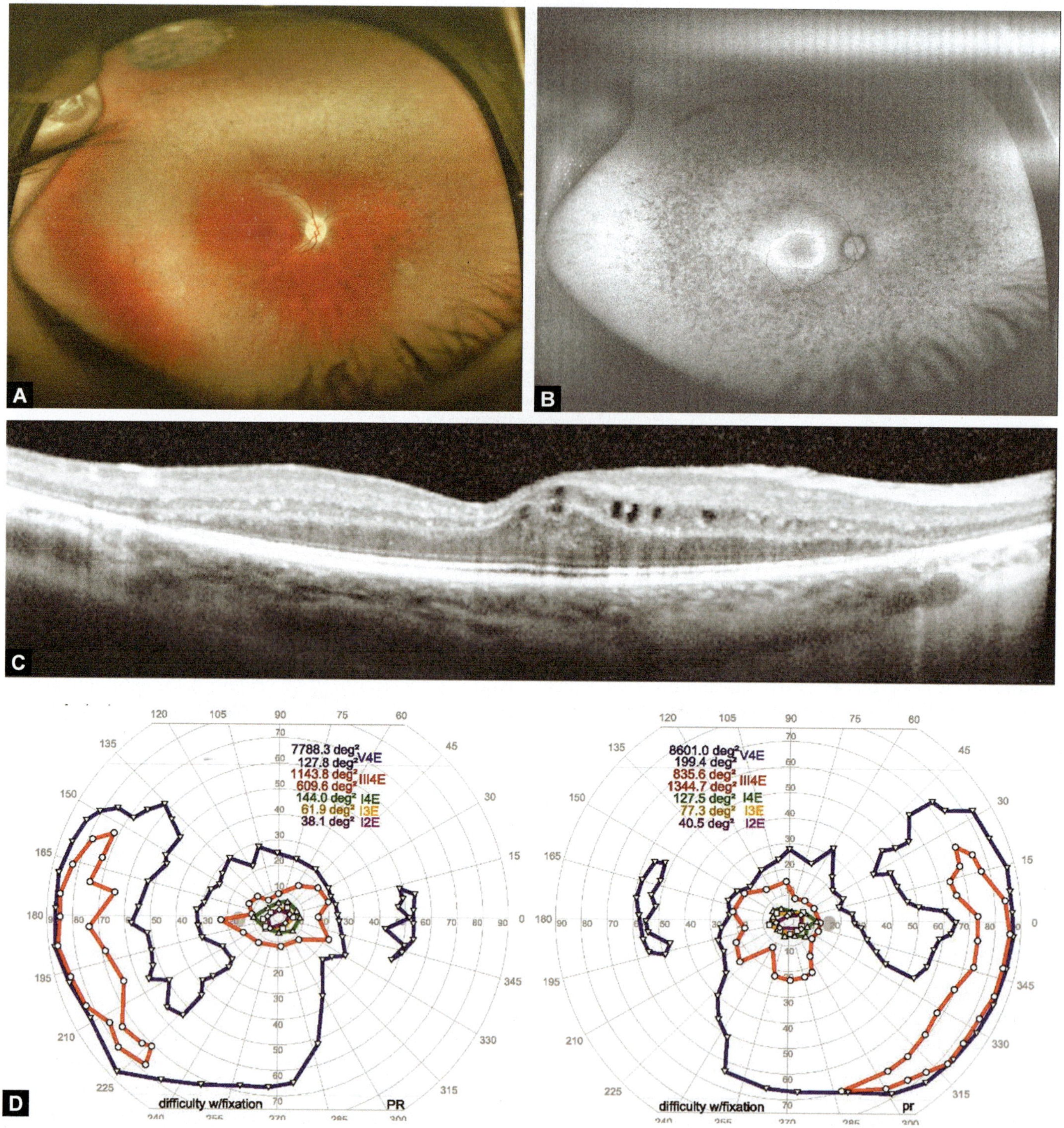

Figs. 54.10A to D: (A) Optos wide-field color fundus photograph in a 23-year-old male with type 1 Usher syndrome due to homozygous mutations of *USH1C*; (B) Optos wide-field autofluorescence additionally shows an oval-shaped ring of hyper-autofluorescence in the macula; (C) Optical coherence tomography (OCT) shows the corresponding transition point at which the inner segment/outer segment junction is lost peripherally as well as cystoid macular edema; (D) Kinetic visual field testing shows large, incomplete midperipheral ring scotomas with symmetric preservation of the temporal periphery in both eyes. This patient received bilateral cochlear implantation early in childhood, which facilitated good development of receptive and expressive language.

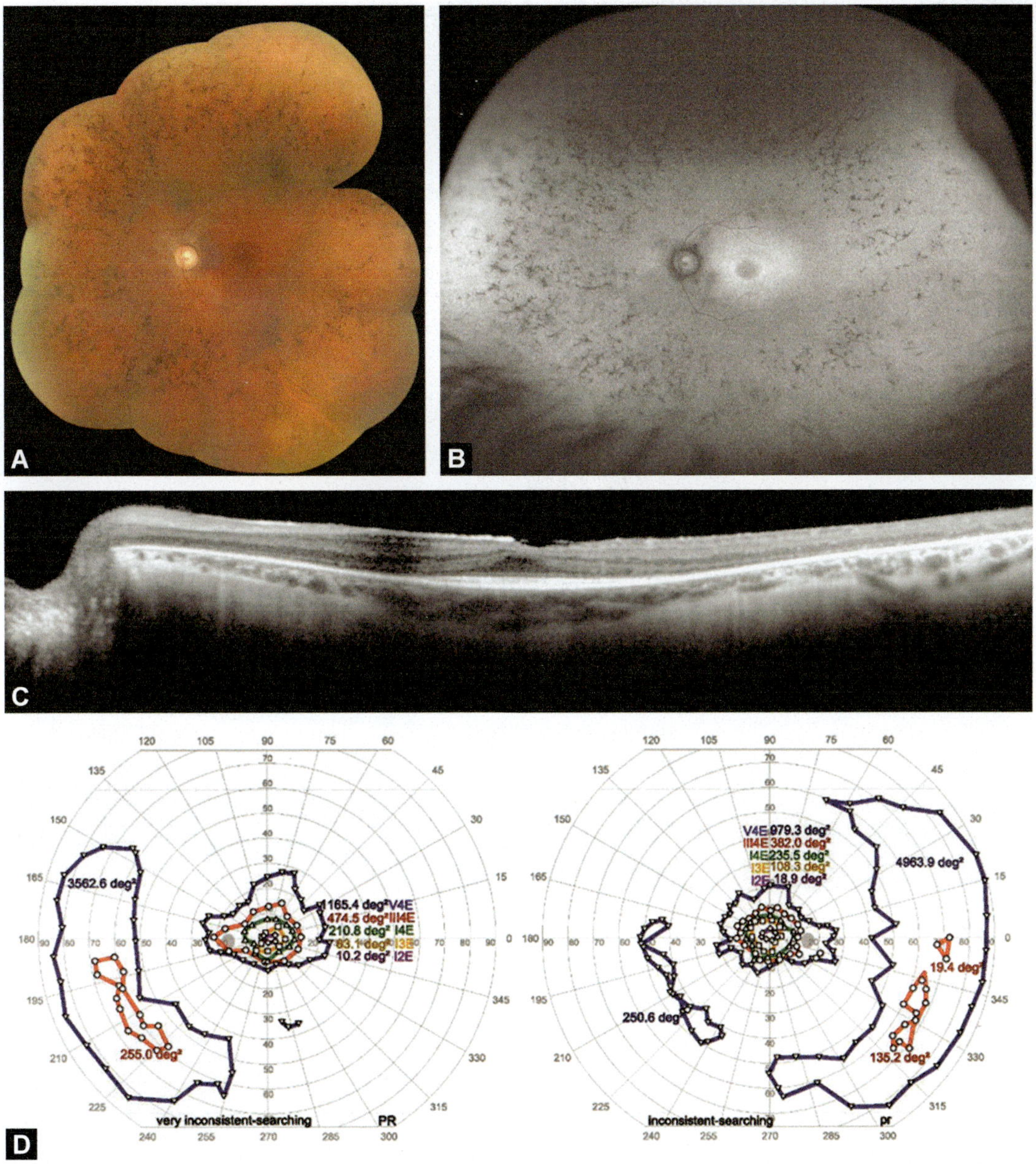

Figs. 54.11A to D: (A) Color fundus photograph montage in a 38-year-old female with type 2 Usher syndrome due to *USH2A* compound heterozygous mutations; (B) Optos wide-field autofluorescence additionally shows a perifoveal ring of hyperautofluorescence, correlating with the transition zone at which the inner segment/outer segment junction is lost peripherally on optical coherence tomography (OCT); (C) OCT also shows a mild epiretinal membrane; (D) Kinetic visual field testing shows severe constriction with some sparing of an inferotemporal island.

Usher) even before visible signs of retinal degeneration are present.[129] Genetic screening in children with congenital hearing loss is also helpful for early diagnosis.[123] Given the involvement of two sensory systems, the diagnosis can feel devastating to patients and families, and a great deal of education and psychosocial support is required.

Bardet-Biedl Syndrome

First described by Bardet in the 1920s, BBS is an autosomal recessive disorder defined by the cardinal features of progressive rod-cone dystrophy, postaxial polydactyly, central obesity, renal dysfunction, cognitive impairment, and genital abnormalities.[130,131] At least 21 disease-causing genes have been identified (*BBS1-BBS21*), many of which are involved in cilia development or function.[132-134] The ocular characteristics in BBS differ from typical RP in that severe visual acuity loss occurs early in the disease course, and peripheral pigmentary lesions may be mild, absent, or atypical (round instead of spicule shaped) (Figs. 54.12A to E).[135,136] Atrophic macular lesions are

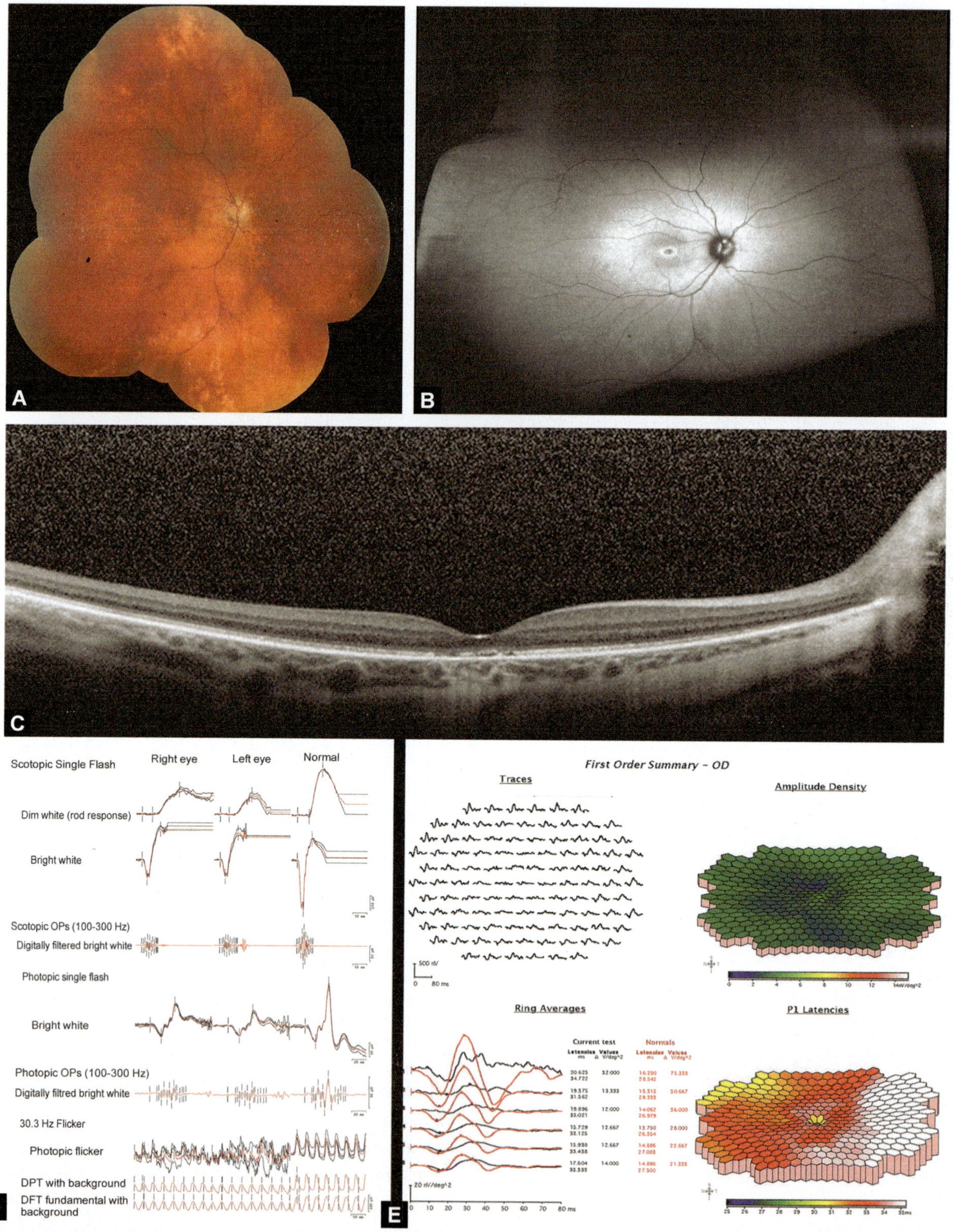

Figs. 54.12A to E: (A) Fundus montage of the right eye in a 26-year-old female with Bardet-Biedl syndrome. In addition to progressive vision loss, she reported being born with extra fingers and toes, which were surgically removed in childhood; (B) Fundus autofluorescence; (C) OCT shows outer nuclear layer thinning and disruption of the inner segment/outer segment junction and RPE within the fovea; (D and E) Full-field and multifocal ERGs are consistent with a diffuse rod-cone dystrophy and macular cone dysfunction.

(OCT: Optical coherence tomography; RPE: Retinal pigment epithelium; ERGs: Electroretinograms; OPs: Oscillatory potentials; DFT: Discrete Fourier transform) common, and approximately three quarters of patients reach legal blindness status by 20 years of age.[137]

While retinal degeneration is the universal finding among BBS patients, manifestation of the systemic features is often incomplete and highly variable.[131] In a large review of BBS patients, postaxial polydactyly was present in 69% of patients and degree of developmental delay varied widely.[131] As extra digits may have been removed in infancy, clinicians should ask specifically about a history of polydactyly and examine the hands and feet for surgical scars. Hypogenitalism is present in roughly half of adult patients and infertility is particularly common in male patients.[131] Renal involvement can progress to end-stage renal failure and is the leading cause of mortality in BBS.[138] Less common features include ataxia, brachydactyly or syndactyly, diabetes mellitus, orodental abnormalities, and cardiovascular involvement.[131,132]

Joubert Syndrome/Senior Loken Syndrome

Joubert syndrome is an autosomal recessive or X-linked congenital cerebellar ataxia with variable RP association (Figs. 54.13A to D). As with BBS, numerous causative genes

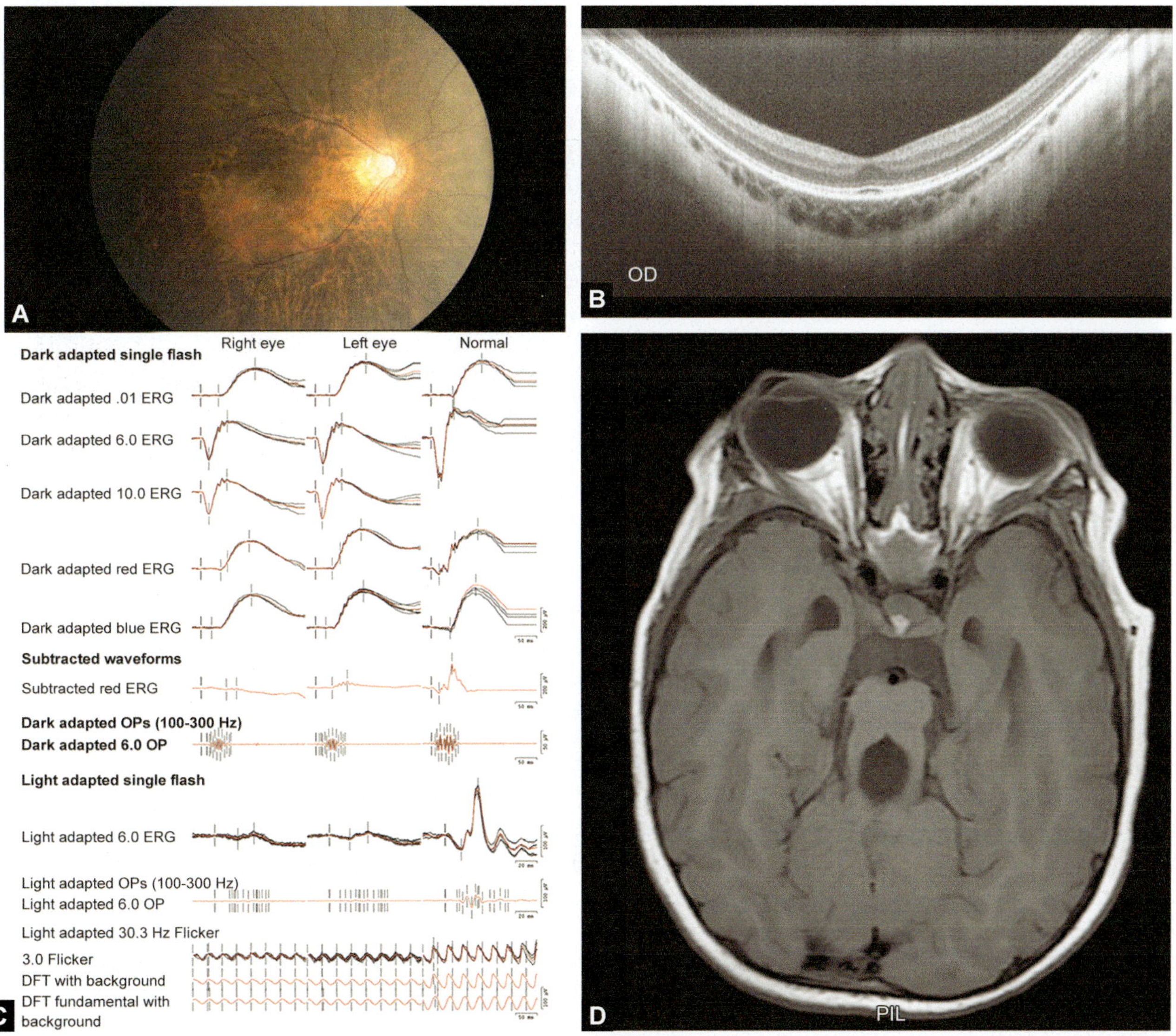

Figs. 54.13A to D: (A) Color fundus photograph in a 9-year-old male with Joubert syndrome. Note the increased cup to disc ratio, small optic nerve coloboma and hypopigmentation in the macula and mid periphery; (B) Optical coherence tomography (OCT) shows intact retinal layers with possible outer nuclear layer thinning and reflects the patient's high myopia; (C) Cone greater than rod dysfunction was seen on electroretinogram (ERG) testing. Examination also revealed intermittent esotropia, and (D) Brain magnetic resonance imaging (MRI) demonstrated the molar tooth sign.
(DFT: Discrete Fourier transform)

have been identified, all of which encode proteins involved in the primary cilium or its apparatus.[139] Neurologic findings are heterogeneous and can include hypotonia, truncal ataxia, breathing dysregulation, and oculomotor or speech apraxia.[140,141] The "molar tooth sign" is a radiographic finding highly suggestive of Joubert syndrome when seen in conjunction with the appropriate clinical context. This term refers to the characteristic resemblance of the midbrain in axial imaging sections to that of a molar tooth, caused by cerebellar vermis hypoplasia and malformation of the superior cerebellar peduncles.[141] Retinal dystrophies are seen in a subset of patients and range in severity from an LCA phenotype to a slowly progressive pigmentary retinopathy with only slightly abnormal ERG responses.[142,143] An association between Joubert syndrome and chorioretinal colobomas has also been reported.[144] Neurologic, ocular, and other systemic manifestations, which can include renal anomalies, liver fibrosis, and polydactyly, are highly genotype dependent.[143,145] Early onset renal failure from a medullary cystic kidney, termed nephronophthisis, can also be associated with Joubert syndrome.

The term "Senior-Loken syndrome" is used to describe autosomal recessive RP and nephronophthisis when other signs of Joubert syndrome are absent.[146] Due to the complicated nosology of the above syndromes, the term "ciliopathies" is sometimes used to describe the growing group of disorders caused by inherited ciliary dysfunction with overlapping clinical features.

Choroidal Dystrophies

Choroideremia

Choroideremia, first described by Austrian ophthalmologist Ludwig Mauthner in 1872 and expanded upon by McCulloch and McCulloch,[147,148] is an X-linked disease resulting in progressive degeneration of the RPE, choriocapillaris and retina. Disease prevalence is approximately 1 in 50,000 in people of European ancestry.[149]

Choroideremia is caused by loss-of-function mutations in the *CHM* gene on the long arm of the X chromosome (Xq21.2).[150] The gene encodes the Rab escort protein-1 (REP-1), a component essential to posttranslational Rab protein modification that is thought to regulate intracellular vesicular transport.[151,152]

In affected males, nyctalopia and concentric peripheral visual field loss become apparent in the first or second decade. Disease progression is gradual, and good central vision is usually preserved until 40 or 50 years of age.[153-155] The initial fundus changes are a "salt-and-pepper" RPE mottling in the mid-periphery, which develops into patchy areas of chorioretinal degeneration that consolidate (Figs. 54.14A to H). Compared to typical RP, the caliber of retinal vessels is relatively preserved and the optic nerves develop less pallor. In late stages of the disease, widespread chorioretinal atrophy occurs with preservation of only larger deep choroidal vessels. This results in exposure of the underlying sclera and a yellowish-white fundus appearance.

Optical coherence tomography imaging demonstrates well-demarcated thinning of the outer nuclear layers and small to medium choroidal vessels. Outer retinal tubulations can be seen at the margins of degeneration, becoming longer and more numerous in advanced disease.[156] OCT can also be used to identify macular changes occasionally associated with choroideremia, including CME,[157] neovascularization,[158] and macular hole formation.[159] FAF imaging will reveal a characteristic speckled pattern over areas of the retina in which RPE is still present.

Structural imaging correlates closely with functional testing. Perimetry testing will show visual field defects that correspond with areas of chorioretinal degeneration. Full-field ERG is reduced early in the disease, in both light- and dark-adapted conditions, and advances to complete signal extinction in most cases.[160] In current practice, establishing the diagnosis typically requires molecular genetic testing in a proband to identify a pathogenic *CHM* variant.

Female carriers often have no visual complaints but may report difficulty with dark adaptation.[161] The fundus appearance is typically milder than that of affected males and may have a spotty distribution of pigmentary mottling and peripheral atrophy, thought to be due to lyonization of the X chromosome.[162] ERG responses can be normal or show subtle changes in amplitude and latency.[160,161] Rare examples of severely affected female heterozygotes have been reported, likely due to highly skewed X-inactivation.[163,164]

Gyrate Atrophy

Gyrate atrophy is a rare chorioretinal degeneration, most common in patients of Finnish descent.[165] It is inherited in an autosomal recessive pattern and is caused by mutations in ornithine delta-aminotransferase (OAT), resulting in an increased serum ornithine concentration.[166]

Visual symptoms, including night blindness and loss of peripheral vision, become apparent in the first to third decade of life. Disease progression can be rapid, resulting

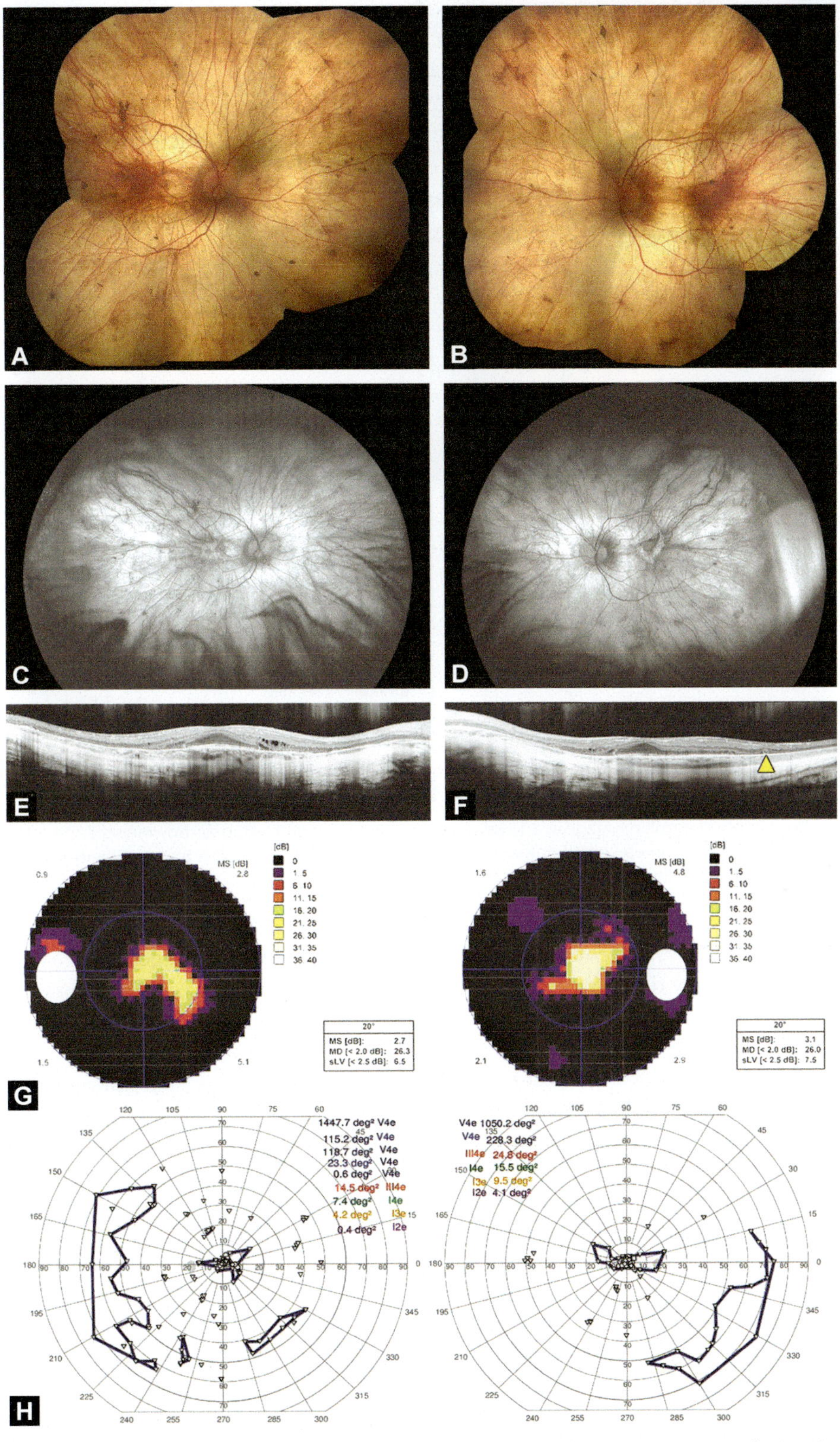

Figs. 54.14A to H: (A and B) Color fundus photography in a patient with choroideremia demonstrates severe chorioretinal atrophy with relative preservation of the retinal vessels in both eyes; (C and D) Small islands of partially preserved retinal pigment epithelium (RPE) can be seen in the central macula of both eyes on Optos wide-field autofluorescence; (E and F) Optical coherence tomography (OCT) demonstrates diffuse outer retinal and choroidal atrophy with foveal sparing as well as outer retinal tabulation (arrowhead) and intraretinal fluid; (G and H) Only small, central islands remain of visual field testing, which correlate to the geographic shape of preserved RPE in each eye.

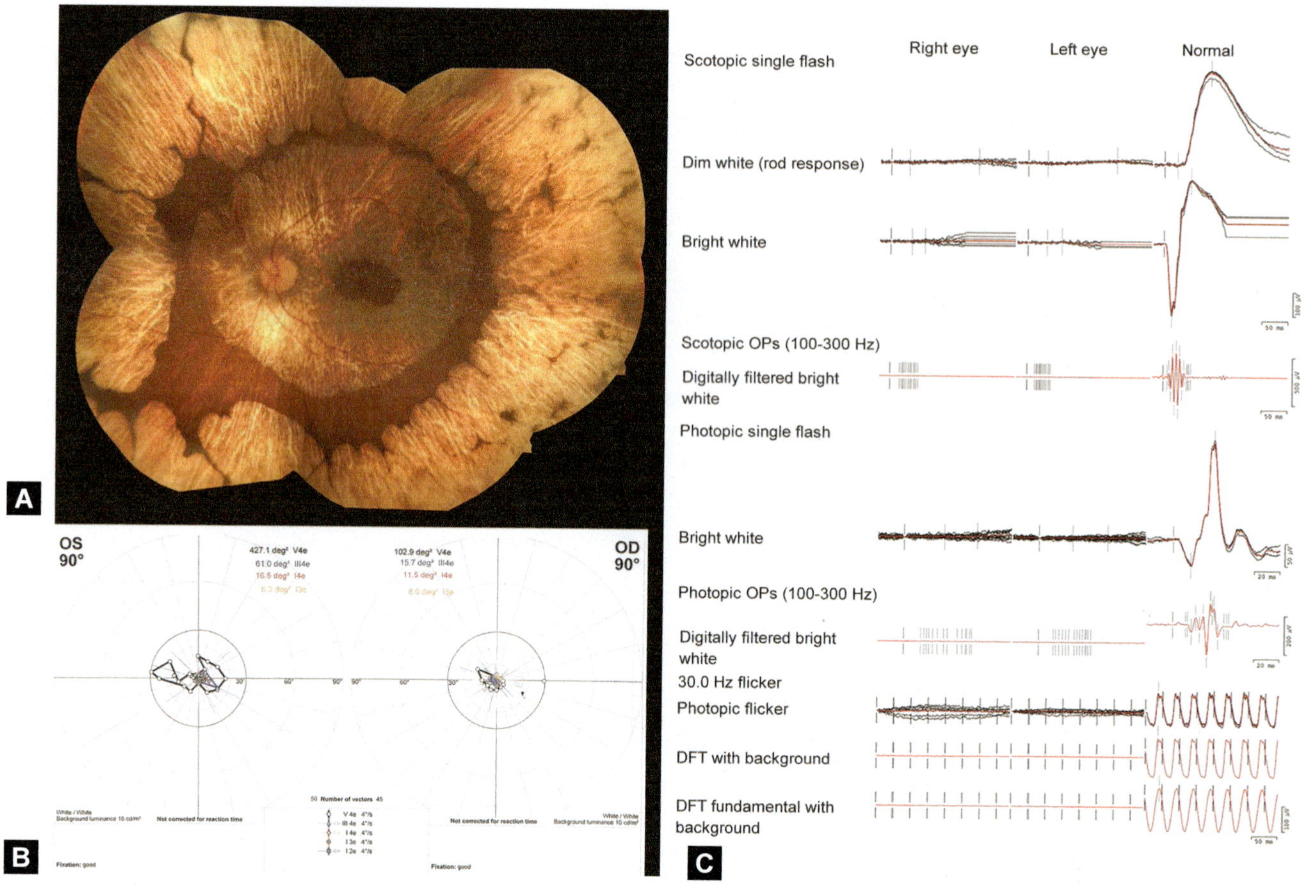

Figs. 54.15A to C: (A) Color fundus photograph montage in a 40-year-old woman with gyrate atrophy showing scalloped chorioretinal atrophy with near-complete coalescence and an island of preserved central retina; (B) A small central area of corresponding sensitivity is preserved on visual field testing; (C) Full field electroretinograms (ERGs) were unrecordable.
(DFT: Discrete Fourier transform)

in severe tunnel vision as early as the second decade. The defining fundus finding is sharply demarcated, scalloped areas of choroidal atrophy that form a circular pattern in the peripheral retina (Figs. 54.15A to C). Atrophy of the overlying retina is also seen. Visual defects often extend beyond the visible areas of atrophy. In late stages, an annular ring of severe atrophy is present with total exposure of the underlying sclera. The retinal vessels usually appear normal but can become attenuated later in disease. Posterior subcapsular cataracts and progressive myopia are frequently seen.[167,168] Foveal thickening with intraretinal cystoid edema can be seen on OCT, even when the central retina appears unaffected on ophthalmoscopic examination.[169] ERGs are usually severely affected or unrecordable, suggestive of widespread rod-cone involvement.[170]

Abnormalities of the muscles and of both the central and peripheral nervous system are also found in patients with gyrate atrophy. Muscle biopsy reveals selective atrophy in type II skeletal muscle fibers.[171] Neurologic studies have found degenerative white matter lesions, EEG abnormalities, and peripheral neurography changes in 50% or more of patients with gyrate atrophy.[172,173]

Given the underlying genetic cause, gyrate atrophy is potentially treatable with the correction of hyperornithinemia. Strict dietary restriction of arginine, the primary precursor used for ornithine synthesis, has been found to reduce ornithine serum levels and, in some cases, slow disease progression in observational studies.[174-176] Arginine restriction requires strict low-protein diets with supplementation of essential amino acids, making adherence quite difficult for many patients. High-dose vitamin B_6 (pyridoxine) supplementation (900 mg daily) has also been studied, as OAT is a B_6-dependent enzyme.[177,178] Unfortunately only 5% of patients are responsive to therapy, which likely represents the proportion of patients with mutations directly affecting the pyridoxal-5'-phosphate binding site of OAT.[179]

Bietti Crystalline Dystrophy

Bietti crystalline dystrophy, first described by Bietti in 1937, is an autosomal recessive, progressive retinal dystrophy that presents with visual impairment in the second to fourth decade of life and with fundus findings including glistening, yellow-white crystalline retinal deposits, progressive RPE atrophy, and choroidal sclerosis (Figs. 54.16A and B). In 2004, Li and colleagues mapped disease causing mutations to the *CYP4V2* gene, a member of the cytochrome *P450* gene family.[180-182] In some patients, small crystalline deposits are also seen in the corneal limbus.[182] Most of the retinal crystalline deposits are located at the level of the RPE/Bruch's membrane complex, but can be seen on OCT anywhere throughout the retina.[182] Disappearance of crystals overtime is associated with expanding RPE and choriocapillaris atrophy.[182] While the precise composition of the crystals remains unknown, complex lipid inclusions have been found in fibroblasts and circulating lymphocytes, suggesting that Bietti crystalline dystrophy may result from a systemic abnormality in fatty acid metabolism.[183-185] Disease prevalence is highest among patients of East Asian descent.[186] With time, vision loss progresses to legal blindness in most patients.

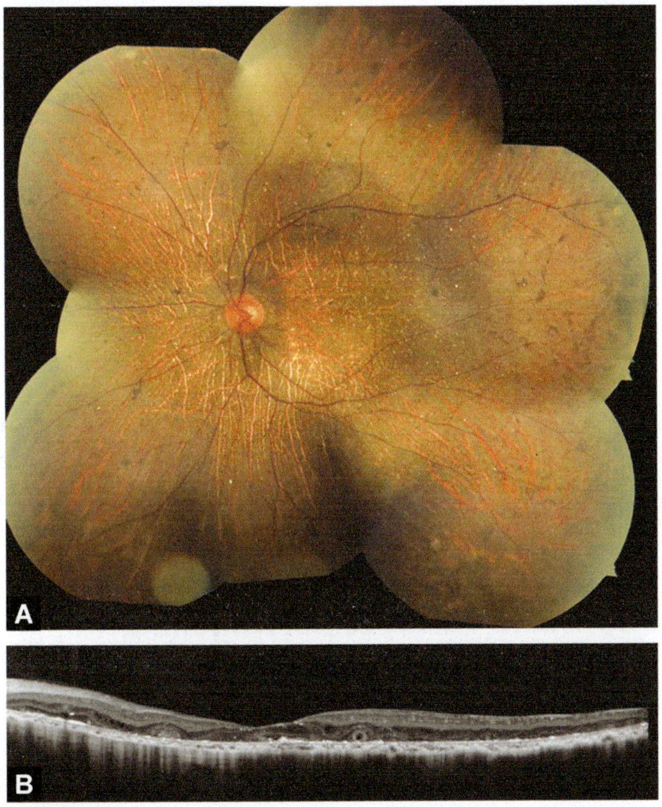

Figs. 54.16A and B: (A) Fundus photograph in a 43-year-old man with Bietti's crystalline dystrophy; (B) Optical coherence tomography (OCT) demonstrates chorioretinal atrophy and highly reflective deposits in the retina and on Bruch's membrane, at some locations these deposits appear to be encapsulated by residual retinal pigment epithelium (RPE).

Vitreoretinopathies

Familial Exudative Vitreoretinopathy

Familial exudative vitreoretinopathy (FEVR) is a rare disorder of retinal angiogenesis that usually presents in childhood, but can cause sight-threatening complications at any age.[187] The diagnosis of FEVR becomes particularly challenging in premature infants given the significant clinical overlap with retinopathy of prematurity (ROP). The hallmark finding of FEVR is avascular zones in the peripheral retina, which often have a V-shaped pattern and are most common in the temporal periphery (Figs. 54.17A and B).[188] The disease may be mild and limited to the periphery in some patients; but moderate to severe retinal ischemia can result in retinal neovascularization, vitreous traction, and retinal detachments. Retinal detachments, which can be rhegmatogenous, exudative or tractional, are a common finding occurring in 21–64% of patients with FEVR. [189,190] Advanced tractional retinal detachments can progress to cause falciform retinal folds, a well-recognized but not pathognomonic feature of FEVR. These radial folds often run temporally and can range from dry, narrow "knife-like" folds to broad folds with underlying exudate.[190]

Fluorescein angiography is the most helpful diagnostic test and can often reveal subtle peripheral avascularity or retinal vascular leakage not readily apparent on clinical exam alone. The differentiation from ROP is based on disease tempo and progression. ROP follows a predictable timeline with neovascularization and retinal detachment occurring around postmenstrual ages of 37 and 41 weeks, respectively.[191] In contrast, disease progression in FEVR is variable, and neovascular, tractional, or exudative findings can appear or evolve at any age.[190]

Mutations in five genes, *LRP5*,[192] *FZD4*,[193] *ZNF408*,[194] *TSPAN12*,[195] and *KIF11*,[196] have been linked to autosomal dominant FEVR. Mutations in *LRP5*, *FZD4*, and *TSPAN12* can also be associated with autosomal recessive disease.[197-199] Patients with FEVR caused by *LRP5* mutations can have associated low bone density, giving this presentation significant clinical overlap with osteoporosis pseudoglioma, a similar but sometimes more severe syndrome also caused by mutations in the *LRP5* gene.[200,201] Mutations in *NDP* result

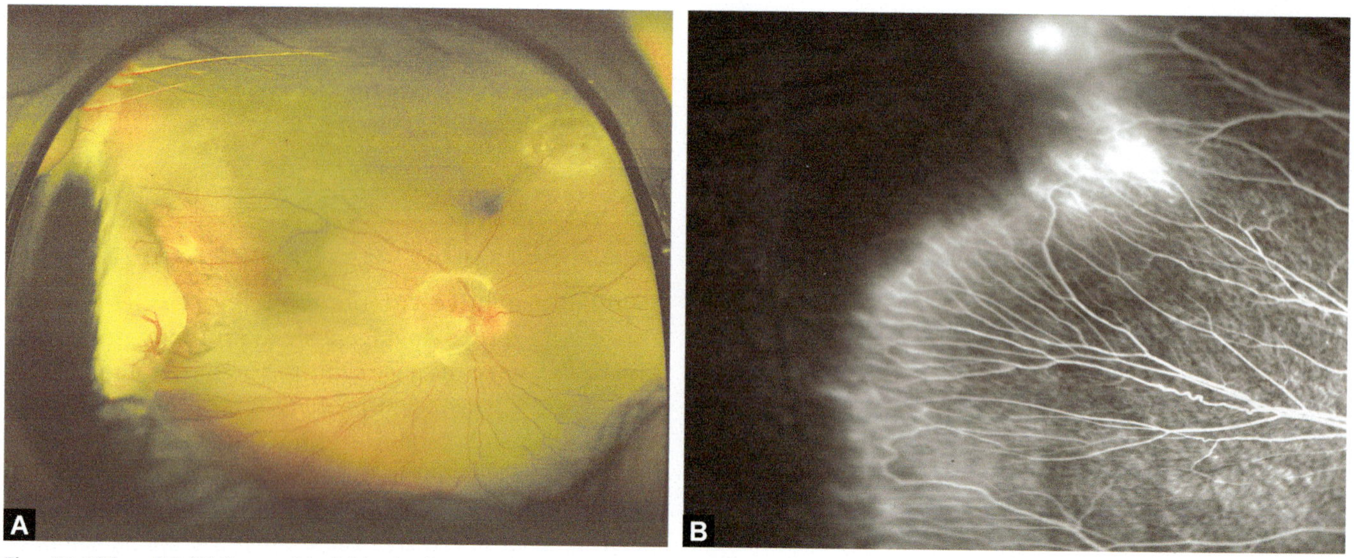

Figs. 54.17A and B: (A) Optos wide-field color fundus photograph in a patient with familial exudative vitreoretinopathy. Note the vitreoretinal traction in the temporal periphery; (B) Fluorescein angiography in another patient highlights the border between perfused and nonperfused retina with vascular leakage at the interface.

in a spectrum of X-linked retinopathies that includes FEVR and the most severe phenotype, Norrie disease. These cases are characterized by congenital blindness, a greyish yellow fibrovascular mass (pseudoglioma) secondary to retinal vascular dysgenesis and detachment, developmental delay and sensorineural hearing loss.[202]

VCAN-related Vitreoretinopathies

Wagner syndrome and erosive vitreoretinopathy are allelic disorders caused by autosomal dominant mutations in the *VCAN* (previously *CSPG2*), which encodes for the versican protein.[203,204] *VCAN*-related retinopathy is characterized by an optically empty vitreous with avascular strand and veil formation; presenile, dot-like cortical cataracts; perivascular pigmentation; and slowly progressive chorioretinal atrophy (Fig. 54.18). Patients have also been reported to have pseudostrabismus from congenital temporal displacement of the fovea.[203] Uveitis can also occur, and intraocular inflammation has rarely been described as the initial disease finding.[205,206] The frequency and severity of retinal detachments is highly family dependent.[207] The ERG can be normal in early life, but diffuse loss of cone and rod responses occurs as chorioretinal atrophy progresses.[208] Visual field loss can be variable, and may include constricted central visual fields or partial midperipheral ring scotomas associated with the chorioretinal atrophy.[205]

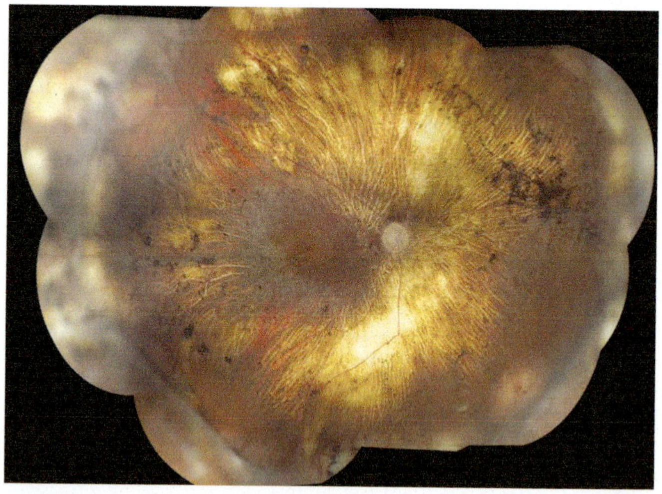

Fig. 54.18: Fundus appearance in a patient with erosive vitreoretinopathy. *Source*: http://webeye.ophth.uiowa.edu/eyeforum/atlas/pages/erosive-vitreoretinopathy2.htm.

Snowflake Vitreoretinal Degeneration

Snowflake vitreoretinal degeneration (SVD) is an autosomal dominant disorder first described by Hirose and colleagues in 1974[209] and later mapped to the *KCNJ13* gene.[210] In addition to the findings shared among hereditary vitreoretinopathies (early onset cataracts, congenital vitreous liquefaction, and an increased predisposition to rhegmatogenous retinal detachments), SVD exhibits a progressive degeneration of the peripheral retina with

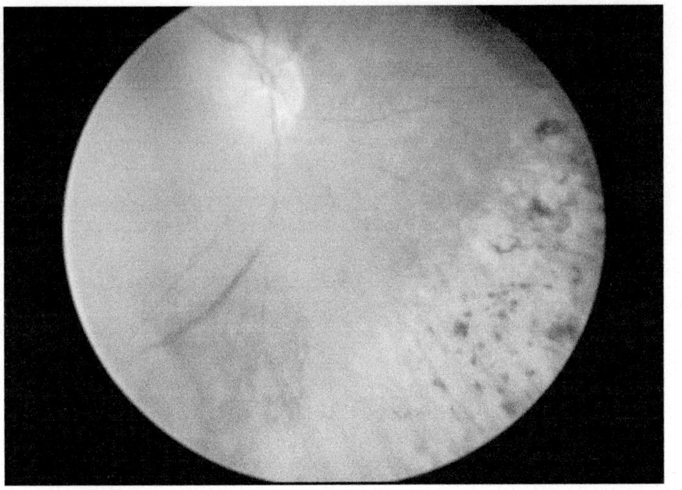

Fig. 54.19: Fundus appearance in a patient with autosomal dominant snowflake vitreoretinal degeneration.

Source: Reproduce with permission from Lee et al. Snowflake vitreoretinal degene ration follow-up of the original family. Ophthalmology; 2013.

retinal vessel sheathing and the unique finding of tiny, snowflake-like crystalline deposits in the inner retina (Fig. 54.19). Other ocular features include a dysmorphic optic nerve head that appears flat and lacks an optic cup as well as corneal guttae that can be identical in appearance to Fuchs' endothelial corneal dystrophy.[211] Poor dark adaptation and reduced scotopic b-wave with dim light are seen in most SVD patients; however, vision typically remains excellent following surgery for visually significant cataracts.[211] Genetic testing for mutations in *KCNJ13* remains the diagnostic gold standard given the significant clinical overlap with other hereditary vitreoretinopathies.

Retinal Nuclear Receptor (NR2E3) Related Diseases: Goldmann-Favre Syndrome and Enhanced S-Cone Syndrome

The *NR2E3* gene codes for a transcription factor expressed only in photoreceptors and is involved in the regulation of cone cell proliferation.[212] Mutations in *NR2E3* account for both Goldmann-Favre syndrome (GFS) and enhanced S-cone syndrome (ESCS), which can variably present with early-onset night blindness, retinal degeneration with nummular pigment clumping along the vascular arcades, macular and peripheral retinoschisis, posterior subcapsular cataract, enhanced S-cone function on ERG and/or fibrillar vitreous degeneration (Figs. 54.20A to F).[213-216] Significant overlap exists between the GFS and ESCS phenotypes, both of which were described before they were determined to be allelic disorders, and identical *NR2E3* mutations have been described in both conditions.[217,218] Mutations in the *NRL* gene, which is upstream of *NR2E3* in a pathway regulating rod versus cone cellular differentiation, can cause overlapping features, including relative S-cone function preservation, and a severe RP.[219-221]

The pathognomonic ERG includes an undetectable rod response, nearly identical photopic and scotopic waveforms, and a 30 Hz flicker ERG amplitude smaller than the single flash cone ERG a-wave.[222] Animal[223] and physiologic[224] studies suggest that these changes may be due to an overabundance of S-cone photoreceptors and reciprocal loss of M cones, L cones, and rod photoreceptors. This theory is further supported by the histologic examination of a postmortem retina from an ESCS patient, which revealed a two-fold increase in cone photoreceptors, of which 92% were S-cones, and complete loss of rod photoreceptors.[225]

Collagenopathies

Stickler Syndrome

Stickler syndrome describes a syndrome of chondrodysplasia and associated vitreoretinal degeneration caused by mutations in multiple different collagen genes. Mutations in *COL2A1* and *COL11A1* typically cause autosomal dominant disease,[226] while pathogenic variants in *COL9A1*,[227] *COL9A2*,[228] and *COL9A3*[229] have more recently been implicated in autosomal recessive Stickler syndrome. A nonocular form of the disease has also been described and is caused by mutations in *COL11A2*.[230] The systemic features are highly variable and can include midface hypoplasia, conductive and sensorineural hearing loss, early-onset arthritis, and some marfanoid features.[226,231,232] Stickler syndrome has also been associated with the Pierre–Robin anomaly, which is defined as micro- or retrognathia, glossoptosis, and a cleft soft palate.[233]

Abnormalities of vitreous gel architecture are the most characteristic feature and have been used to divide Stickler syndrome into two clinical subgroups (retrolenticular membranous versus beaded degeneration); however, these findings are not always reliable and genetic testing is likely the best diagnostic approach.[226] Other ocular features include congenital high myopia, presenile cataracts, and perivascular lattice degeneration (Figs. 54.21A to F).[226] Giant retinal breaks and rhegmatogenous retinal detachments are common; and the most vision-threatening complication, prophylactic retinopexy, has been shown to be beneficial.[234] Unlike in *VCAN*-related retinopathies, the ERG is normal once myopic changes are taken into account.

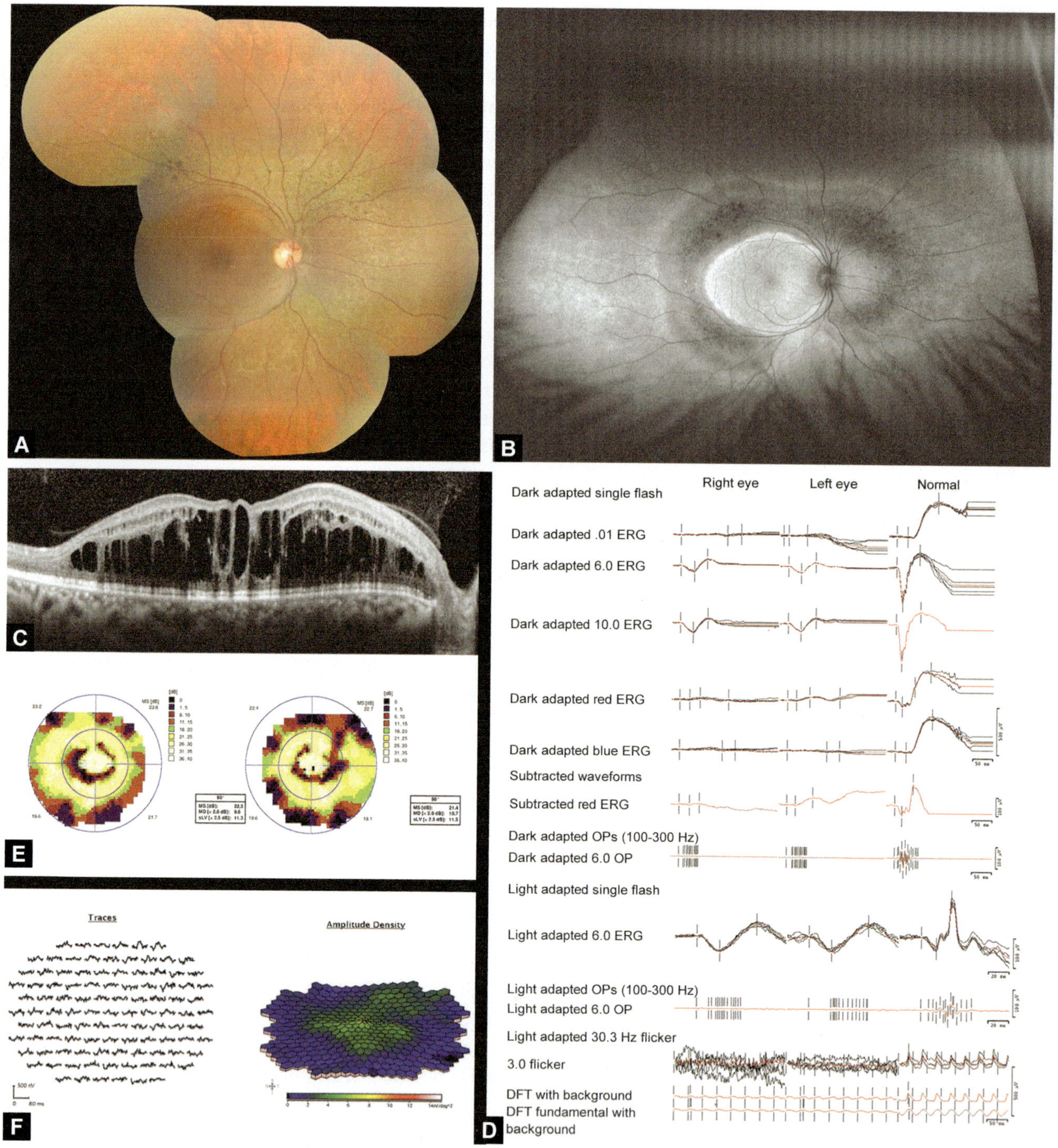

Figs. 54.20A to F: (A) Fundus appearance in a 29-year-old female with *NR2E3* related retinopathy showing cystoid macular edema and midperipheral atrophy with nummular pigmentation; (B) Wide field fundus autofluorescence shows a hyperautofluorescent ring just inside the vascular arcades with surrounding hypoautofluorescence; (C) OCT demonstrates cystoid macular edema; (D) Dark adapted ERG was unrecordable, light adapted ERG showed a slow and simplified waveform lacking oscillatory potential, and 30 Hz flicker amplitude was significantly reduced all consistent with an enhanced S-cone syndrome; (E) Static visual field testing showed decreased sensation in the far periphery and near complete ring scotoma at 30°; (F) Multifocal ERG demonstrated decreased macular cone sensitivity.

(OCT: Optical coherence tomography; ERG: Electroretinogram; OPs: Oscillatory potentials; DFT: Discrete Fourier transform)

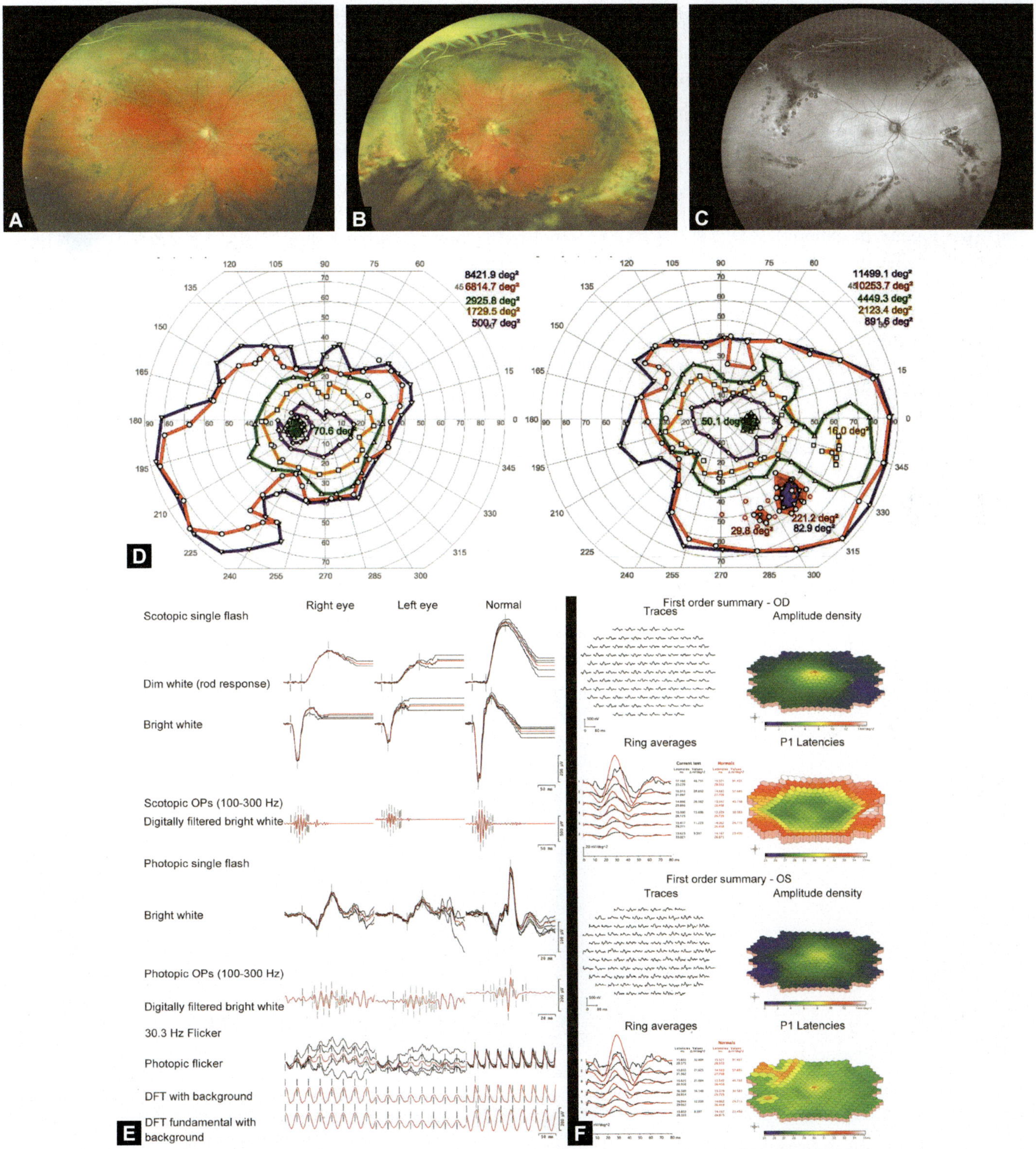

Figs. 54.21A to F: (A and B) Right and left fundus appearance in a 36-year-old male with Stickler syndrome. He had a history of retinal detachment in the left eye repaired with a scleral buckle and bilateral retinopexy; (C) Fundus autofluorescence demonstrates a pattern of radial, perivascular lattice degeneration with surround laser spots; (D) Kinetic visual field testing shows left greater than right constriction to all targets, best corrected visual acuity was 20/20 in each eye; (E and F) Full field and multifold ERG testing demonstrate decreased rod and cone responses, partially due to myopia and retinal detachment in the left eye.

(ERG: Electroretinogram; OPs: Oscillatory potentials; DFT: Discrete Fourier transform)

Alport Syndrome

Alport syndrome is characterized by renal failure secondary to glomerulonephritis, progressive sensorineural hearing loss, and numerous ocular abnormalities, all due to cellular basement membrane dysfunction. 85% of patients have X-linked disease caused by a mutation in the *COL4A5* gene, which codes for the collagen IV α5-chain; the remaining patients have autosomal dominant or recessive inheritance due to pathogenic mutations in *COL4A3* or *COL4A4*, which code for the collagen IV α3 and α4-chains, respectively.[235-237] The clinical findings of Alport syndrome are attributed to the loss of the collagen IV α3α4α5 network and the persistence of the immature collagen IV α1α1α2 network, which has less cross-linking and is more susceptible to biomechanical strain.[238]

Corneal features of Alport syndrome include recurrent corneal erosions from an abnormal Bowman membrane and posterior polymorphous corneal dystrophy.[239,240] Anterior lenticonus has been reported in 22% of cases; this finding is highly suggestive of Alport syndrome when present.[241] The most prominent fundus finding is a perimacular and peripheral dot and fleck retinopathy, thought to be due to defects in the inner limiting membrane (Figs. 54.22A to D).[242] A retinal "lozenge" or dull macular reflex is seen in some patients and corresponds to severe inner retinal defects, which are most obvious on OCT and usually found in the temporal macula.[243] There is also a predilection for giant macular holes.[244,245]

Knobloch Syndrome

Knobloch syndrome is a rare, recessively inherited disorder caused by mutations in *COL18A1*, resulting in changes in collagen XVIII, a basement membrane proteoglycan important to the development and function of structures in the eye, kidney, and nervous system.[246,247] The disorder is characterized by high myopia, early cataract formation, chorioretinal atrophy, and retinal detachments with or without occipital skull deformities; however, there is significant clinical heterogeneity in the ocular and extraocular findings (Figs. 54.23A to C). Patients often present in infancy with nystagmus and high myopia. The chorioretinal atrophy can appear similar to the *VCAN*-related retinopathies and is associated with cone-rod dysfunction on ERG.[248] Retinal detachments are the most common cause of deterioration in visual acuity.[248] Additional ocular findings include glaucoma, persistence of fetal vasculature, and developmental abnormalities of the anterior segment, such

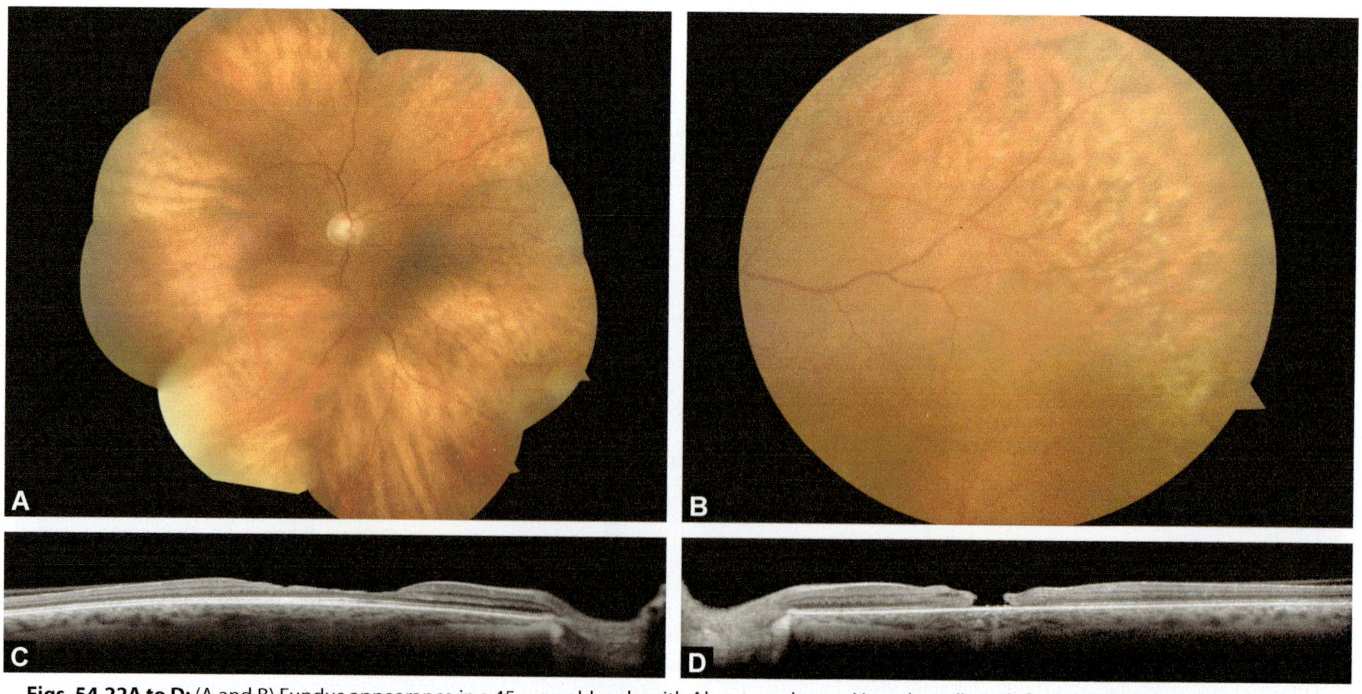

Figs. 54.22A to D: (A and B) Fundus appearance in a 45-year-old male with Alport syndrome. Note the yellowish flecks visible in the mid periphery; (C and D) Inner retinal defects of the macula are seen on optical coherence tomography (OCT), including a full thickness macular hole in the left eye.

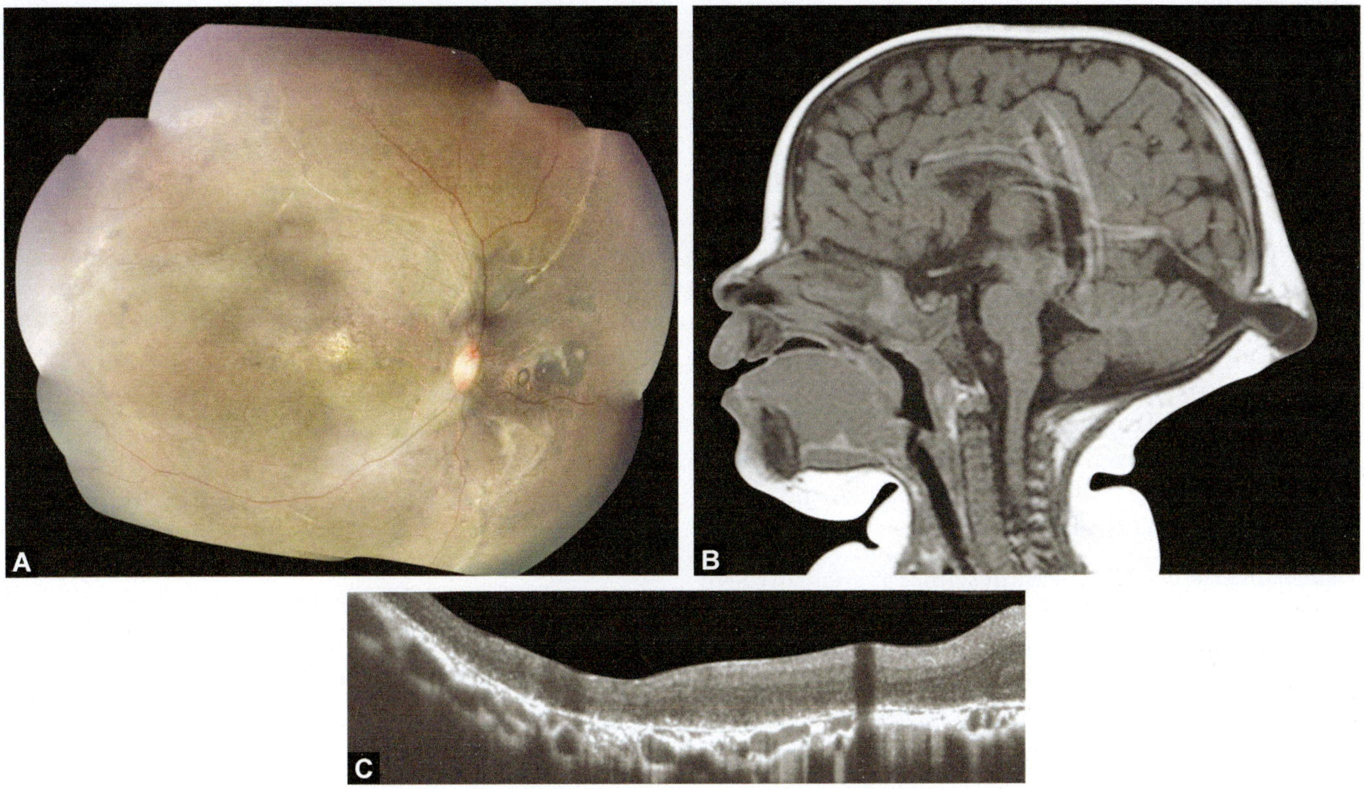

Figs. 54.23A to C: (A) Fundus photography in a 6-year-old female with Knobloch syndrome showing a highly dysplastic retina with elongated and tilted optic nerve, pigmentary changes, and vitreous membranes. The left eye had a macula off retinal detachment, not shown here; (B) An associated occipital cephalocele is demonstrated on sagittal brain magnetic resonance imaging (MRI); (C) Optical coherence tomography (OCT) demonstrates diffuse chorioretinal atrophy with loss of retinal laminations. Visual acuity was count figures in both eyes.

as absent iris crypts and iris transillumination defects.[248,249] Patients with Knobloch syndrome should be screened for structural brain abnormalities, as occipital findings can include any combination of cutaneous scalp abnormalities, encephalocele/meningocele, and polymicrogyria.[250]

Disorders of Rod Function

Congenital Stationary Night Blindness

Congenital stationary night blindness (CSNB) is a nonprogressive disorder of reduced night vision. First described by Cunier in 1838 in an autosomal dominant pedigree, CSNB is now recognized as a variable group of disorders associated with any of the common genetic inheritance patterns.[251] Mutations in genes on the X chromosome, including *NYX* and *CACNA1F*, account for the majority of cases. While visual function is "stationary" by definition, there can be shared genetic etiologies of CSNB and progressive retinal disorders (*see* Fig. 54.2).

Electroretinogram and dark adaptation testing are helpful for the diagnosis and classification of CSNB. X-linked and autosomal recessive CSNB is associated with a "negative" ERG response to maximum bright-field stimulation, where there is a near normal a-wave and markedly reduced b-wave.[252] These patients have been further classified into "complete" or "incomplete" according to the degree of detectable rod function loss on ERG and dark-adaptation curves.[253]

The fundus examination is usually normal, aside from high myopia, in patients with CSNB, however two specific phenotypes with fundus findings have been described: (1) fundus albipunctatus and (2) Oguchi disease.

Fundus albipunctatus: Patients with fundus albipunctatus will present with typical CSNB symptoms and ophthalmoscopy findings significant for yellowish-white dots scattered throughout the fundus with foveal sparing. The disorder is caused by a mutation in the *RDH5* gene, which encodes 11-cis-retinol dehydrogenase, an enzyme utilized in the visual cycle.[254] Likely due to the dysfunction in visual pigment regeneration, scotopic ERG responses are reduced, but can normalize after prolonged dark adaptation.[255] It is important to differentiate fundus albipunctatus from RPA, a progressive retinal degeneration with similar fundus findings. In addition to following visual function over time, Genead et al. described how multimodal imaging could help differentiate the two disorders. On OCT, white spots in RPA correlate with wide based lesions at the level of the RPE with extension up to and elevating the inner segment/outer segment (IS/OS) junction.[256] In contrast, lesions in fundus albipunctatus are dome-shaped and extend through the IS/OS junction into the outer nuclear layer. Additionally, a parafoveal ring of hyperautofluorescence on FAF imaging in RPA and typical RP is absent in fundus albipunctatus.[256,257]

Oguchi disease: Oguchi disease describes a variant of CSNB accompanied by the Mizuo-Nakamura phenomenon, in which there is a golden sheen to the retina following light exposure that disappears after prolonged dark adaptation.[258] Mutations in *SAG* and *GRK1* have been implicated in Oguchi disease. Both produce gene products involved in the regulation of the phototransduction cascade.[259,260]

Cone and Cone-Rod Dystrophies

Cone/cone-rod dystrophies are a collection of inherited retinal dystrophies characterized by progressive, diffuse cone dysfunction, and associated retinal degeneration.[261] These genetically heterogeneous disorders differ from congenital color blindness, which typically has stationary disease with no associated retinal degeneration, and macular dystrophies, where pathology is restricted to the densely packed macular cones. A high index of suspicion and electrophysiologic testing is often needed for diagnosis. There is significant genetic overlap between cone/cone-rod dystrophies, RP, and LCA. Interestingly, mutations of both alleles of some genes implicated in autosomal dominant cone or cone-rod dystrophies (*AIPL1*, *CRX*, *GUCY2D*, and *PRPH2*) have also been found to cause a LCA phenotype.[262-265]

Patients with cone/cone-rod dystrophies usually develop symptoms within the first three decades of life, including visual acuity loss, color vision dysfunction, and photophobia; however, there are reports of patients presenting later in life.[266,267] Some patients will have a pure cone dystrophy, while others develop symptoms of rod dysfunction (cone-rod dystrophy) including night blindness and peripheral vision loss.[261] The fundus appearance in cone/cone-rod dystrophies is variable and is often normal in early stages of disease. When present, macular atrophy is generally symmetric between the two eyes and may appear as bilateral bull's eye lesions. Peripheral pigmentary degeneration and temporal disk atrophy can also be seen in later disease stages.[268-270] Perimetry testing during early stages of disease will show bilateral central scotomas, and patients with cone-rod dystrophies will have progressive peripheral field loss.[261]

The ERG can be dependent on the underlying genetic cause but will usually demonstrate significantly diminished or undetectable amplitude of photopic responses and delayed implicit times.[261] Rod function may also be reduced, particularly in the later stages of cone-rod dystrophies; but overall, it is less affected. Severely diminished scotopic ERG at the time of presentation should strongly suggest an alternative diagnosis, and RP must be considered.

Syndromic Cone-Rod Dystrophies

Alström Syndrome

Alström syndrome is a very rare, autosomal recessive disorder caused by mutations in *ALMS1*, another gene involved in ciliary function.[271,272] Clinical features include a cone-rod dystrophy (present in all patients with Alström syndrome), sensorineural hearing loss, type 2 diabetes mellitus, truncal obesity, and cardiomyopathy.[273] Visual deficits are severe and nearly always present in infancy, vision continues to worsen, and patients reach no light perception by the age of 20 years.[274] Full-field ERG is either undetectable or significantly reduced with a typical cone-rod dystrophy pattern. Bull's eye maculopathy or pigmentary clumping are uncommon findings.[274] A dilated cardiomyopathy is often present in infancy and can result in congestive heart failure at any age.[275]

Jalili Syndrome

Jalili syndrome presents with early onset cone-rod dystrophy and amelogenesis imperfecta, defined as grossly abnormal tooth enamel caused by dental biomineralization defects.[276,277] This recessively inherited syndrome is caused by mutations in *CNNM4*, which is expressed in both the neural retina and ameloblasts, which are cells responsible for enamel deposition during tooth development.[277] Progressive vision loss begins in infancy or early childhood.

TREATMENT

While many of the diseases discussed in this chapter have no definite cure, management and treatment of disease-related complications help patients maintain useful vision. Additionally, recent advances offer hope for future preservation or even restoration of vision. As always, it is essential to consider potentially reversible causes of ocular disease that may mimic RP or the other disorders discussed in this chapter, particularly if the genetic diagnosis is not forthcoming, including vitamin A or E deficiency, abetalipoproteinemia, syphilis, tuberculosis, and Refsum disease.[8-11,278]

Refraction

Refraction is always the initial therapeutic intervention, particularly as many of the inherited retinal degenerations are associated with refractive error. Even when retinal degeneration appears severe, accurate refraction can have a large impact on visual acuity, overall function, and independence.

Cataracts

Presenile, visually significant cataracts are common among patients with peripheral retinal degenerations.[16] Even in patients with a significant retinal disease burden, cataract removal can be beneficial, and surgery should be considered and recommended in appropriate patients. Bastek and colleagues reported a two-line or better visual acuity gain in 83% of RP patients after cataract extraction; however, examination and OCT imaging of the macula should always be performed before surgery to assess the likelihood of improvement in visual function.[15]

Cystoid Macular Edema

Cystoid macular edema is another common treatable source of vision loss in hereditary retinal degenerations that occurs in approximately 25% of the RP population.[279] Suggested mechanisms have included chronic, low-grade inflammation leading to vascular leakage,[280,281] dysfunctional RPE cell fluid transport,[282] and deleterious effects of antiretinal antibodies.[283] OCT is highly sensitive for the detection of intraretinal fluid; however, the direct relationship between central retinal thickness and visual acuity has not always been found in the RP literature.[284,285]

Carbonic anhydrase inhibitors, including topical dorzolamide and oral acetazolamide, are the most established therapies for RP-associated CME, but they do carry the risk of rebound CME with prolonged use.[282,286-288] Intravitreal corticosteroids have been used when CME is refractory to topical and oral therapies; however, studies do not consistently show a visual acuity improvement, and the potential benefit must be balanced with the risk of side effects, including cataract formation and glaucoma.[289-292]

Supplements

The therapeutic effects of a number of supplements have been studied in RP, including vitamins A and E, docosahexaenoic acid (DHA), and lutein.[293-295] Unfortunately, while support of mild ERG response preservation exists in some cases, no strong evidence has been found for the use of any supplement.[293-295] However, most experts recommend diets high in antioxidant compounds.

A large, randomized, and double-masked study started in 1984 investigating the effects of oral vitamin A and vitamin E on RP progression reported a slower rate of cone ERG amplitude decline in the vitamin A supplementation cohort.[293] However, the recommendations from this study remain controversial due to the question of clinical significance of the reported benefit as well as statistical validity of the subgroup analysis employed.[296,297] Therefore, vitamin A is not routinely recommended by many experts in the field. If patients do initiate therapy they should undergo monitoring for hepatic toxicity and osteoporosis, and female patients of child-bearing age should be counseled on the risk of fetal defects.

Neuroprotective Compounds

Neuroprotective compounds or neurotrophic factors are endogenous proteins that protect neurons from degeneration by promoting cellular survival and maintenance, a number of which have been studied in neurodegenerative disorders of the CNS.[298] Ciliary neurotrophic growth factor and nerve growth factor are among those that have been tested in RP.[299,300] Overall, there is no conclusive evidence from human RP trials to support the use of these agents. One particular challenge is that multiple molecular pathways may need to be targeted to achieve a therapeutic effect. However, pursuit of a neuroprotective strategy is still valuable as such treatments would likely be more mutation independent than other gene-directed therapies.

GENETIC TESTING AND COUNSELING

Obtaining a genetic diagnosis is becoming increasingly important in the management of inherited retinal disorders, as this information informs individual and offspring risk assessments and identifies patients who may benefit from novel gene-based therapies or enrollment in gene-directed clinical trials. With this in mind, and with the rapid advancement in genetic sequencing technology, molecular testing should be a routine part of clinical practice in patients with inherited retinal dystrophies. Ensuring that patients and their family members understand the role and significance of genetic testing is essential. Experts agree that a multidisciplinary approach, particularly one that includes team members trained in genetic counseling, leads to improved patient care.[301,302]

Panel-based approaches that target a growing number of implicated genes have been shown to greatly improve clinical sensitivity.[75,303] Occasionally, a specific inheritance pattern, ocular finding or systemic association can implicate a single gene; but this is rare. In most cases, there is a limited role for single gene testing, particularly in presentations such as nonsyndromic RP, where there is both frequent locus heterogeneity (the same phenotype caused by mutations in different genes) and allelic heterogeneity (variable phenotypes caused by different mutations in the same gene).

Gene Therapy

Multiple factors make the retina an ideal target for gene-based therapies. Inherited retinal diseases tend to be symmetric, thus allowing treatment of one eye with comparison to other eye as a control. Additionally, the subretinal space is relatively immunoprivileged due to its location behind the blood-retina barrier and molecules produced by RPE cells, including Fas ligand (FasL), that induce apoptosis in inflammatory cells.[304,305] Furthermore, high-resolution retinal imaging facilitates noninvasive acquisition of near histological level data, and can be correlated with psychophysical functional measurements such as perimetry. As is the case in much of medicine, human gene therapy trials are built on a foundation of preclinical research that unveils underlying mechanisms and supports the potential efficacy of gene-based interventions.

Gene Therapy for Leber Congenital Amaurosis

Patients with LCA due to *RPE65* mutations were the first to undergo human gene therapy trials for an inherited eye disease. Human studies were based on highly successful animal experimentation that showed sustained improvement in visual function and retinal structure after gene transfer in *RPE65* mutant animal models.[306-309] Early results from three independent human clinical trials were published in 2008, demonstrating a favorable safety profile and modest efficacy of injection with recombinant adeno-associated virus (AAV) vectors carrying wild-type *RPE65* into the subretinal space.[310-312] Longer follow-up in one cohort of 15 patients over 3 years demonstrated improved visual acuity and photoreceptor sensitivity in treatment eyes and a sustained safety profile;[313] however, 3-year follow-up in another cohort of 12 treated patients showed attenuation of the retinal sensitivity benefit after 6–12 months, no improvement in ERG measurements and two cases of deterioration in visual acuity.[314] A more recent phase 1 trial, which included 12 patients, showed no serious adverse events and provided preliminary data that suggested the largest visual acuity gains occur in younger patients.[315] In 2017, the results were published from an open-label, randomized, controlled phase 3 trial conducted at the University of Iowa and Children's Hospital of Philadelphia, which led to the first Food and Drug Administration (FDA)-approved gene therapy.[316] This landmark study, including 29 patients with *RPE65*-mediated retinal dystrophy, tested the safety and efficacy of gene replacement therapy using adeno-associated virus type 2 (AAV2)-hRPE65v2 delivered by subretinal injection. The treatment arm was found to have a significant improvement in the study's primary endpoint, which was 1-year change in multi-luminance mobility testing, a functional assessment of vision-based mobility that incorporates aspects of visual acuity, visual field, and contrast sensitivity.

Gene Therapy for Retinitis Pigmentosa due to *MERTK* Mutations

MERTK encodes a membrane-bound tyrosine kinase that mediates RPE cell phagocytosis of photoreceptor outer-segments and is a rare cause of autosomal recessive RP in humans.[317-319] Multiple studies have demonstrated histologic and functional improvements in *MERTK* mutant rats following introduction of the normal gene.[320-322] A phase I trial has been completed in a small cohort of *MERTK*-related RP patients with subretinal administration of an AAV vector carrying a functional copy of human *MERTK*.[323] Initial ocular and systemic safety profiles appear acceptable; but additional trials will be required to determine long-term safety and efficacy.

Gene Therapy for Retinitis Pigmentosa due to *MYO7A* Mutations

MYO7A is a large gene associated with Usher syndrome type 1B.[324] Because the *MYO7A* gene exceeds the AAV packaging capacity of (~5 kb),[325] gene replacement approaches using lentiviral vectors have been studied.[326,327] A recent study in mice and macaque disease models has led to an ongoing phase I/IIa gene replacement trial in Usher syndrome type 1B patients.[327,328]

Gene Therapy for Choroideremia

Similar to the disease above, preclinical studies have laid the groundwork for *CHM* replacement therapy in choroideremia patients. Tolmachova and colleagues demonstrated a dose-dependent improvement in ERG responses in *CHM* mutant mice following transduction with an AAV2 vector encoding the REP-1 protein.[329] Successful transduction and gene expression was also confirmed in human retinal explants obtained from patients undergoing retinectomy for complex retinal detachment surgery.[329]

A phase I-II clinical trial, inclusive of six male choroideremia patients, reported on the safety and initial efficacy of subretinal AAV2/REP-1.[330] Because many young patients with choroideremia will have near normal visual acuity, the effect of preserving visual function may not become apparent until several years after treatment. The two patients in this initial trial who did have low baseline BCVA were found to have sustained visual acuity improvement in the treatment eye 3.5 years after therapy while the untreated contralateral eyes had a loss of visual acuity.[331] Phase III trials are underway.[332,333]

Ribonucleic Acid Modulation to Treat Retinitis Pigmentosa

Autosomal dominant forms of RP present a more complicated problem for genetic rescue, as a solution requires addressing a gain-of-function mutation rather than introducing a functional gene product to cells with homozygous, loss-of-function mutations. Gene-silencing therapies targeting the unique messenger RNA (mRNA) transcript produced by mutant *RHO* genes have had some success in animal models.[334,335] One significant drawback to this approach is that a different mRNA target is required for each specific gene mutation, so that the normal, functional allele is not targeted for silencing. An alternative approach, involving suppression of both the mutant and wild-type allele with RNA interference (RNAi) in parallel with the addition of a replacement gene refractory to the RNAi suppression, could be efficacious for any mutation in a specific gene.[336] This method has been successful in animal models and has the potential to provide one effective gene therapy solution per autosomal dominant RP gene despite any degree of mutational heterogeneity.[337]

Stem Cell Therapy

Most stem cell-based strategies focus on photoreceptor or RPE cell replacement and offer an enormous treatment potential for retinal degenerations. Embryonic stem cells (ESCs) and induced pluripotent stem cells (iPSCs) from human and nonhuman origins can be cultured and differentiated along the retinal lineage.[338] Human iPSC-derived photoreceptors have been cultured to the point of early outer-segment disk formation and photosensitivity, which represents another step toward successful photoreceptor replacement therapy.[339] Preclinical data supported the first FDA-approved clinical trial involving transplantation of human ESC-derived RPE cells to the subretinal space in patients with Stargardt's macular dystrophy and age-related macular degeneration.[340,341] The application of stem cell-based therapies to different inherited retinal dystrophies will continue to grow as the processes involved in the culture, differentiation, and transplantation of ESC and iPSC-derived retinal tissue are further refined.

In addition to cellular replacement strategies, iPSCs derived from patients with inherited retinal dystrophies can be used to model the disease in vitro; this approach has been used to study cellular disease mechanism in cell lines derived from patients with RP, LCA, and Best disease.[342-344]

Retinal Prosthesis

Investigators have tested many electronic prostheses with electrical stimulation at different locations along the visual pathway, including the visual cortex,[345,346] optic nerve,[347] and retina.[348] At this time, only retinal prostheses have undergone clinical trials.

Currently available retinal prosthesis systems include implanted and external components. Patients wear glasses with a small frame-mounted camera, connected to a video-processing unit carried by a shoulder strap or belt. Visual data collected by the camera is converted into a brightness map and transmitted to the surgically implanted components, which include a receiving antenna and electronics case, secured externally to the globe, and an electrode array that sits directly on the macula. In real time, the brightness map data is used to compute the appropriate stimulation amplitude at each electrode, with the goal of triggering ganglion cell action potentials and inducing the perception of light.

The Argus II Retinal Prosthesis System (Second Sight Medical Products Inc.; Sylmar, CA),[349] an epiretinal prosthesis, is the only device to date with United States FDA approval, while a subretinal prosthesis, developed by Retina Implant AG (Reutlingen, Germany), is also approved for use in Europe.[350] Five-year follow-up data suggests that improvements in visually locating objects and determining direction of motion can be maintained if complications are avoided.[351] Close monitoring is required and device explantation has been reported.[351]

REFERENCES

1. Hartong DT, Berson EL, Dryja TP. Retinitis pigmentosa. Lancet. 2006;368:1795-809.
2. Tanino T, Ohba N. Studies on pigmentary retinal dystrophy. II. Recordability of electroretinogram and the mode of inheritance. Jpn J Ophthalmol. 1976;20:482-6.
3. Puech B, De Laey J-J. Retinitis pigmentosa and allied Disorders. In: Puech B, De Laey J-J, Holder GE (Eds). Inherited Chorioretinal Dystrophies: A Textbook and Atlas. Berlin, Heidelberg: Springer Berlin Heidelberg; 2014. pp. 99-120.
4. Gregory-Evans K, Pennesi ME, Weleber RG. Retinitis pigmentosa and allied disorders. In: Sadda SR, Hinton DR, Schachat AP, Wilkinson CP, Wiedemann P, Schachat AP, Saunders WB (Eds). Retina, 5th edition. London: Saunders/Elsevier; 2013. pp. 761-835.
5. Nagy D, Schönfisch B, Zrenner E, et al. Long-term follow-up of retinitis pigmentosa patients with multifocal electroretinography. Invest Ophthalmol Vis Sci. 2008;49:4664-71.
6. Berson EL, Sandberg MA, Rosner B, et al. Natural course of retinitis pigmentosa over a three-year interval. Am J Ophthalmol. 1985;99:240-51.
7. Massof R, Finkelstein D. A two-stage hypothesis for the natural course of retinitis pigmentosa. In: Zrenner E, Krastel H, Goebel HH (Eds). Advances in the Biosciences. Oxford: Pergamon; 1987. pp. 29-58.
8. Kemp CM, Jacobson SG, Faulkner DJ, et al. Visual function and rhodopsin levels in humans with vitamin A deficiency. Exp Eye Res. 1988;46:185-97.
9. Runge P, Muller DP, McAllister J, et al. Oral vitamin E supplements can prevent the retinopathy of abetalipoproteinaemia. Br J Ophthalmol. 1986;70:166-73.
10. Chowers I, Banin E, Merin S, et al. Long-term assessment of combined vitamin A and E treatment for the prevention of retinal degeneration in abetalipoproteinaemia and hypobetalipoproteinaemia patients. Eye (Lond). 2001;15:525-30.
11. Leroy BP, Hogg CR, Rath PR, et al. Clinical features and retinal function in patients with adult Refsum syndrome. Adv Exp Med Biol. 2003;544:57-8.
12. Grover S, Fishman GA, Anderson RJ, et al. Visual acuity impairment in patients with retinitis pigmentosa at age 45 years or older. Ophthalmology. 1999;106:1780-5.
13. Berson EL, Rosner B, Simonoff E. Risk factors for genetic typing and detection in retinitis pigmentosa. Am J Ophthalmol. 1980;89:763-75.
14. Heckenlively J. The frequency of posterior subcapsular cataract in the hereditary retinal degenerations. Am J Ophthalmol. 1982;93:733-8.
15. Bastek JV, Heckenlively JR, Straatsma BR. Cataract surgery in retinitis pigmentosa patients. Ophthalmology. 1982;89:880-4.
16. Fishman GA, Anderson RJ, Lourenco P. Prevalence of posterior subcapsular lens opacities in patients with retinitis pigmentosa. Br J Ophthalmol. 1985;69:263-6.
17. Strong S, Liew G, Michaelides M. Retinitis pigmentosa-associated cystoid macular oedema: pathogenesis and avenues of intervention. Br J Ophthalmol. 2017;101:31-7.
18. Hansen RI, Friedman AH, Gartner S, et al. The association of retinitis pigmentosa with preretinal macular gliosis. Br J Ophthalmol. 1977;61:597-600.
19. Fishman GA, Maggiano JM, Fishman M. Foveal lesions seen in retinitis pigmentosa. Arch Ophthalmol. 1977;95:1993-6.
20. van Huet RA, Collin RW, Siemiatkowska AM, et al. IMPG2-associated retinitis pigmentosa displays relatively early macular involvement. Invest Ophthalmol Vis Sci. 2014;55:3939-53.
21. Collin RW, Safieh C, Littink KW, et al. Mutations in C2ORF71 cause autosomal-recessive retinitis pigmentosa. Am J Hum Genet. 2010;86:783-8.
22. Dulz S, Wagenfeld L, Nickel M, et al. Novel morphological macular findings in juvenile CLN3 disease. Br J Ophthalmol. 2016;100:824-8.
23. Ba-Abbad R, Sergouniotis PI, Plagnol V, et al. Clinical characteristics of early retinal disease due to CDHR1 mutation. Mol Vis. 2013;19:2250-9.
24. Xie YA, Lee W, Cai C, et al. New syndrome with retinitis pigmentosa is caused by nonsense mutations in retinol dehydrogenase RDH11. Hum Mol Genet. 2014;23:5774-80.

25. Ksantini M, Lafont E, Bocquet B, et al. Homozygous mutation in MERTK causes severe autosomal recessive retinitis pigmentosa. Eur J Ophthalmol. 2012;22:647-53.
26. Scheidecker S, Hull S, Perdomo Y, et al. Predominantly cone-system dysfunction as rare form of retinal degeneration in patients with molecularly confirmed Bardet-Biedl syndrome. Am J Ophthalmol. 2015;160:364-72.
27. Khan AO, Bolz HJ. Phenotypic observations in «hypotrichosis with juvenile macular dystrophy» (recessive CDH3 mutations). Ophthalmic Genet. 2016;37:301-6.
28. Aleman TS, Soumittra N, Cideciyan AV, et al. CERKL mutations cause an autosomal recessive cone-rod dystrophy with inner retinopathy. Invest Ophthalmol Vis Sci. 2009;50:5944-54.
29. Flynn MF, Fishman GA, Anderson RJ, et al. Retrospective longitudinal study of visual acuity change in patients with retinitis pigmentosa. Retina. 2001;21:639-46.
30. Gartner S, Henkind P. Pathology of retinitis pigmentosa. Ophthalmology. 1982;89:1425-32.
31. Milam AH, Li ZY, Fariss RN. Histopathology of the human retina in retinitis pigmentosa. Prog Retin Eye Res. 1998;17:175-205.
32. Grover S, Fishman GA, Brown J Jr. Frequency of optic disc or parapapillary nerve fiber layer drusen in retinitis pigmentosa. Ophthalmology. 1997;104:295-8.
33. Ross DF, Fishman GA, Gilbert LD, et al. Variability of visual field measurements in normal subjects and patients with retinitis pigmentosa. Arch Ophthalmol. 1984;102:1004-10.
34. Seiple W, Clemens CJ, Greenstein VC, et al. Test-retest reliability of the multifocal electroretinogram and Humphrey visual fields in patients with retinitis pigmentosa. Doc Ophthalmol. 2004;109:255-72.
35. Jacobson SG, Kemp CM, Sung CH, et al. Retinal function and rhodopsin levels in autosomal dominant retinitis pigmentosa with rhodopsin mutations. Am J Ophthalmol. 1991;112:256-71.
36. Kemp CM, Jacobson SG, Roman AJ, et al. Abnormal rod dark adaptation in autosomal dominant retinitis pigmentosa with proline-23-histidine rhodopsin mutation. Am J Ophthalmol. 1992;113:165-74.
37. Birch DG, Anderson JL, Fish GE. Yearly rates of rod and cone functional loss in retinitis pigmentosa and cone-rod dystrophy. Ophthalmology. 1999;106:258-68.
38. Andreasson SO, Sandberg MA, Berson EL. Narrow-band filtering for monitoring low-amplitude cone electroretinograms in retinitis pigmentosa. Am J Ophthalmol. 1988;105:500-3.
39. Marmor M. The electroretinogram in retinitis pigmentosa. Arch Ophthalmol. 1979;97:1300-4.
40. Cideciyan AV, Jacobson SG, Aleman TS, et al. In vivo dynamics of retinal injury and repair in the rhodopsin mutant dog model of human retinitis pigmentosa. Proc Natl Acad Sci USA. 2005;102:5233-8.
41. Delori FC, Dorey CK, Staurenghi G, et al. In vivo fluorescence of the ocular fundus exhibits retinal pigment epithelium lipofuscin characteristics. Invest Ophthalmol Vis Sci. 1995;36:718-29.
42. Fujiwara T, Imamura Y, Giovinazzo VJ, et al. Fundus autofluorescence and optical coherence tomographic findings in acute zonal occult outer retinopathy. Retina. 2010;30:1206-16.
43. Schuerch K, Marsiglia M, Lee W, et al. Multimodal imaging of disease-associated pigmentary changes in retinitis pigmentosa. Retina. 2016;36(Suppl 1):S147-58.
44. Robson AG, El-Amir A, Bailey C, et al. Pattern ERG correlates of abnormal fundus autofluorescence in patients with retinitis pigmentosa and normal visual acuity. Invest Ophthalmol Vis Sci. 2003;44:3544-50.
45. Robson AG, Saihan Z, Jenkins SA, et al. Functional characterisation and serial imaging of abnormal fundus autofluorescence in patients with retinitis pigmentosa and normal visual acuity. Br J Ophthalmol. 2006;90:472-9.
46. Popović P, Jarc-Vidmar M, Hawlina M. Abnormal fundus autofluorescence in relation to retinal function in patients with retinitis pigmentosa. Graefes Arch Clin Exp Ophthalmol. 2005;243:1018-27.
47. Ogura S, Yasukawa T, Kato A, et al. Wide-field fundus autofluorescence imaging to evaluate retinal function in patients with retinitis pigmentosa. Am J Ophthalmol. 2014;158:1093-8.
48. Duncker T, Tabacaru MR, Lee W, et al. Comparison of near-infrared and short-wavelength autofluorescence in retinitis pigmentosa. Invest Ophthalmol Vis Sci. 2013;54:585-91.
49. Hood DC, Lazow MA, Locke KG, et al. The transition zone between healthy and diseased retina in patients with retinitis pigmentosa. Invest Ophthalmol Vis Sci. 2011;52:101-8.
50. McNabb RP, Grewal DS, Mehta R, et al. Wide field of view swept-source optical coherence tomography for peripheral retinal disease. Br J Ophthalmol. 2016;100:1377-82.
51. Konieczka K, Bojinova RI, Valmaggia C, et al. Preserved functional and structural integrity of the papillomacular area correlates with better visual acuity in retinitis pigmentosa. Eye (Lond). 2016;30:1310-23.
52. Fischer MD, Fleischhauer JC, Gillies MC, et al. A new method to monitor visual field defects caused by photoreceptor degeneration by quantitative optical coherence tomography. Invest Ophthalmol Vis Sci. 2008;49:3617-21.
53. Rangaswamy NV, Patel HM, Locke KG, et al. A comparison of visual field sensitivity to photoreceptor thickness in retinitis pigmentosa. Invest Ophthalmol Vis Sci. 2010;51:4213-9.
54. Jia Y, Tan O, Tokayer J, et al. Split-spectrum amplitude-decorrelation angiography with optical coherence tomography. Opt Express. 2012;20:4710-25.
55. Rezaei KA, Zhang Q, Chen CL, et al. Retinal and choroidal vascular features in patients with retinitis pigmentosa imaged by OCT based microangiography. Graefes Arch Clin Exp Ophthalmol. 2017;255:1287-95.
56. Battaglia Parodi M, Cicinelli MV, Rabiolo A, et al. Vessel density analysis in patients with retinitis pigmentosa by means of optical coherence tomography angiography. Br J Ophthalmol. 2017;101:428-32.

57. Dubra A, Sulai Y, Norris JL, et al. Noninvasive imaging of the human rod photoreceptor mosaic using a confocal adaptive optics scanning ophthalmoscope. Biomed Opt Express. 2011;2:1864-76.
58. Chui TY, Song H, Burns SA. Adaptive-optics imaging of human cone photoreceptor distribution. J Opt Soc Am A Opt Image Sci Vis. 2008;25:3021-9.
59. Sun LW, Johnson RD, Langlo CS, et al. Assessing photoreceptor structure in retinitis pigmentosa and usher syndrome. Invest Ophthalmol Vis Sci. 2016;57:2428-42.
60. Talcott KE, Ratnam K, Sundquist SM, et al. Longitudinal study of cone photoreceptors during retinal degeneration and in response to ciliary neurotrophic factor treatment. Invest Ophthalmol Vis Sci. 2011;52:2219-26.
61. Scoles D, Sulai YN, Langlo CS, et al. In vivo imaging of human cone photoreceptor inner segments. Invest Ophthalmol Vis Sci. 2014;55:4244-51.
62. Wang Q, Tuten WS, Lujan BJ, et al. Adaptive optics microperimetry and OCT images show preserved function and recovery of cone visibility in macular telangiectasia type 2 retinal lesions. Invest Ophthalmol Vis Sci. 2015;56:778-86.
63. RetNet. (2017). The Retinal Information Network. [online]. Available from: *https://sph.uth.edu/retnet/* [Accessed December 2017].
64. Daiger SP, Sullivan LS, Bowne SJ. Genes and mutations causing retinitis pigmentosa. Clin Genet. 2013;84:132-41.
65. Wright AF, Chakarova CF, Abd El-Aziz MM, et al. Photoreceptor degeneration: genetic and mechanistic dissection of a complex trait. Nat Rev Genet. 2010;11:273-84.
66. Bowne SJ, Daiger SP, Hims MM, et al. Mutations in the RP1 gene causing autosomal dominant retinitis pigmentosa. Hum Mol Genet. 1999;8:2121-8.
67. Khaliq S, Abid A, Ismail M, et al. Novel association of RP1 gene mutations with autosomal recessive retinitis pigmentosa. J Med Genet. 2005;42:436-8.
68. Morimura H, Fishman GA, Grover SA, et al. Mutations in the RPE65 gene in patients with autosomal recessive retinitis pigmentosa or Leber congenital amaurosis. Proc Natl Acad Sci USA. 1998;95:3088-93.
69. Bowne SJ, Humphries MM, Sullivan LS, et al. A dominant mutation in RPE65 identified by whole-exome sequencing causes retinitis pigmentosa with choroidal involvement. Eur J Hum Genet. 2011;19:1074-81.
70. Dryja TP, McGee TL, Hahn LB, et al. Mutations within the rhodopsin gene in patients with autosomal dominant retinitis pigmentosa. N Engl J Med. 1990;323:1302-7.
71. Rosenfeld PJ, Cowley GS, McGee TL, et al. A null mutation in the rhodopsin gene causes rod photoreceptor dysfunction and autosomal recessive retinitis pigmentosa. Nat Genet. 1992;1:209-13.
72. Davidson AE, Millar ID, Urquhart JE, et al. Missense mutations in a retinal pigment epithelium protein, bestrophin-1, cause retinitis pigmentosa. Am J Hum Genet. 2009;85:581-92.
73. Breuer DK, Yashar BM, Filippova E, et al. A comprehensive mutation analysis of RP2 and RPGR in a North American cohort of families with X-linked retinitis pigmentosa. Am J Hum Genet. 2002;70:1545-54.
74. Wu DM, Khanna H, Atmaca-Sonmez P, et al. Long-term follow-up of a family with dominant X-linked retinitis pigmentosa. Eye (Lond). 2010;24:764-74.
75. Audo I, Bujakowska KM, Léveillard T, et al. Development and application of a next-generation-sequencing (NGS) approach to detect known and novel gene defects underlying retinal diseases. Orphanet J Rare Dis. 2012;7:8.
76. Corton M, Nishiguchi KM, Avila-Fernandez A, et al. Exome sequencing of index patients with retinal dystrophies as a tool for molecular diagnosis. PLoS One. 2013;8:e65574.
77. Stone EM, Andorf JL, Whitmore SS, et al. Clinically focused molecular investigation of 1000 consecutive families with inherited retinal disease. Ophthalmology. 2017;124:1314-31.
78. Bietti G. Su alcune forme atipiche o rare di degenerazione retinica (degenerazioni tappeto-retiniche e quadri morbosi similari). Boll Oculist. 1937;16:1159-244.
79. Heckenlively JR, Rodriguez JA, Daiger SP. Autosomal dominant sectoral retinitis pigmentosa. Two families with transversion mutation in codon 23 of rhodopsin. Arch Ophthalmol. 1991;109:84-91.
80. Shah SP, Wong F, Sharp DM, et al. A novel rhodopsin point mutation, proline-170-histidine, associated with sectoral retinitis pigmentosa. Ophthalmic Genet. 2014;35:241-7.
81. Saihan Z, Stabej Ple Q, Robson AG, et al. Mutations in the USH1C gene associated with sector retinitis pigmentosa and hearing loss. Retina. 2011;31:1708-16.
82. Sandberg MA, Gaudio AR, Berson EL. Disease course of patients with pericentral retinitis pigmentosa. Am J Ophthalmol. 2005;140:100-6.
83. Milam AH, De Castro EB, Smith JE, et al. Concentric retinitis pigmentosa: clinicopathologic correlations. Exp Eye Res. 2001;73:493-508.
84. Mukhopadhyay R, Holder GE, Moore AT, et al. Unilateral retinitis pigmentosa occurring in an individual with a germline mutation in the RP1 gene. Arch Ophthalmol. 2011;129:954-6.
85. Farrell DF. Unilateral retinitis pigmentosa and cone-rod dystrophy. Clin Ophthalmol. 2009;3:263-70.
86. Fahim AT, Daiger SP, Weleber RG. Nonsyndromic retinitis pigmentosa overview. In: Pagon RA, Adam MP, Ardinger HH (Eds). GeneReviews® [Internet]. Seattle (WA): University of Washington, Seattle; 1993-2017. [online]. Available from: *https://www.ncbi.nlm.nih.gov/books/NBK1417/?report=printable* [Accessed December 2017].
87. Jacobson SG, Yagasaki K, Feuer WJ, et al. Interocular asymmetry of visual function in heterozygotes of X-linked retinitis pigmentosa. Exp Eye Res. 1989;48:679-91.
88. Fishman GA, Weinberg AB, McMahon TT. X-linked recessive retinitis pigmentosa. Clinical characteristics of carriers. Arch Ophthalmol. 1986;104:1329-35.
89. Grover S, Fishman GA, Anderson RJ, et al. A longitudinal study of visual function in carriers of X-linked recessive retinitis pigmentosa. Ophthalmology. 2000;107:386-96.
90. Jay B. X-linked retinal disorders and the Lyon hypothesis. Trans Ophthalmol Soc UK. 1985;104:836-44.

91. Wegscheider E, Preising MN, Lorenz B. Fundus autofluorescence in carriers of X-linked recessive retinitis pigmentosa associated with mutations in RPGR, and correlation with electrophysiological and psychophysical data. Graefes Arch Clin Exp Ophthalmol. 2004;242: 501-11.
92. Mooren A. Fünf Lustren Ophthalmologischer Wirksamkeit. Wiesbaden: Verlag Von J. F. Bergmann; 1882. https://books.google.com/books?id= GO4nAAAAYAAJ&printsec=frontcover& source=gbs_ge_summary_r&cad=0#v=onepage&q&f=false Accessed date: April 1, 2017.
93. Maw MA, Kennedy B, Knight A, et al. Mutation of the gene encoding cellular retinaldehyde-binding protein in autosomal recessive retinitis pigmentosa. Nat Genet. 1997;17:198-200.
94. Morimura H, Berson EL, Dryja TP. Recessive mutations in the RLBP1 gene encoding cellular retinaldehyde-binding protein in a form of retinitis punctata albescens. Invest Ophthalmol Vis Sci. 1999;40:1000-4.
95. Burstedt MS, Sandgren O, Holmgren G, et al. Bothnia dystrophy caused by mutations in the cellular retinaldehyde-binding protein gene (RLBP1) on chromosome 15q26. Invest Ophthalmol Vis Sci. 1999;40:995-1000.
96. Eichers ER, Green JS, Stockton DW, et al. Newfoundland rod-cone dystrophy, an early-onset retinal dystrophy, is caused by splice-junction mutations in RLBP1. Am J Hum Genet. 2002;70:955-64.
97. Burstedt MS, Forsman-Semb K, Golovleva I, et al. Ocular phenotype of Bothnia dystrophy, an autosomal recessive retinitis pigmentosa associated with an R234W mutation in the RLBP1 gene. Arch Ophthalmol. 2001;119:260-7.
98. Leber T. Über Retinitis Pigmentosa und angeborene Amaurose. Albrecht von Graefes Arch Klin Ophthalmol. 1869;15:1-15.
99. Sohocki MM, Sullivan LS, Mintz-Hittner HA, et al. A range of clinical phenotypes associated with mutations in CRX, a photoreceptor transcription-factor gene. Am J Hum Genet. 1998;63:1307-15.
100. Bowne SJ, Sullivan LS, Mortimer SE, et al. Spectrum and frequency of mutations in IMPDH1 associated with autosomal dominant retinitis pigmentosa and Leber congenital amaurosis. Invest Ophthalmol Vis Sci. 2006;47:34-42.
101. Weleber RG, Michaelides M, Trzupek KM, et al. The phenotype of Severe Early Childhood Onset Retinal Dystrophy (SECORD) from mutation of RPE65 and differentiation from Leber congenital amaurosis. Invest Ophthalmol Vis Sci. 2011;52:292-302.
102. Walia S, Fishman GA, Jacobson SG, et al. Visual acuity in patients with Leber's congenital amaurosis and early childhood-onset retinitis pigmentosa. Ophthalmology. 2010;117:1190-8.
103. Foxman SG, Heckenlively JR, Bateman JB, et al. Classification of congenital and early onset retinitis pigmentosa. Arch Ophthalmol. 1985;103:1502-6.
104. Lambert SR, Kriss A, Taylor D, et al. Follow-up and diagnostic reappraisal of 75 patients with Leber›s congenital amaurosis. Am J Ophthalmol. 1989;107:624-31.
105. McAnany JJ, Genead MA, Walia S, et al. Visual acuity changes in patients with leber congenital amaurosis and mutations in CEP290. JAMA Ophthalmol. 2013;131:178-82.
106. Elder MJ. Leber congenital amaurosis and its association with keratoconus and keratoglobus. J Pediatr Ophthalmol Strabismus. 1994;31:38-40.
107. De Laey JJ. Leber's congenital amaurosis. Bull Soc Belge Ophtalmol. 1991;241:41-50.
108. Schroeder R, Mets MB, Maumenee IH. Leber's congenital amaurosis. Retrospective review of 43 cases and a new fundus finding in two cases. Arch Ophthalmol. 1987;105:356-9.
109. Galvin JA, Fishman GA, Stone EM, et al. Evaluation of genotype-phenotype associations in Leber congenital amaurosis. Retina. 2005;25:919-29.
110. Chiang PW, Wang J, Chen Y, et al. Exome sequencing identifies NMNAT1 mutations as a cause of Leber congenital amaurosis. Nat Genet. 2012;44:972-4.
111. Koenekoop RK, Wang H, Majewski J, et al. Mutations in NMNAT1 cause Leber congenital amaurosis and identify a new disease pathway for retinal degeneration. Nat Genet. 2012;44:1035-9.
112. Perrault I, Hanein S, Zanlonghi X, et al. Mutations in NMNAT1 cause Leber congenital amaurosis with early-onset severe macular and optic atrophy. Nat Genet. 2012;44:975-7.
113. Perrault I, Delphin N, Hanein S, et al. Spectrum of NPHP6/CEP290 mutations in Leber congenital amaurosis and delineation of the associated phenotype. Hum Mutat. 2007;28:416.
114. Dekaban AS. Mental retardation and neurologic involvement in patients with congenital retinal blindness. Dev Med Child Neurol. 1972;14:436-44.
115. Vaizey MJ, Sanders MD, Wybar KC, et al. Neurological abnormalities in congenital amaurosis of Leber. Review of 30 cases. Arch Dis Child. 1977;52:399-402.
116. Schuil J, Meire FM, Delleman JW. Mental retardation in amaurosis congenita of Leber. Neuropediatrics. 1998;29: 294-7.
117. Casteels I, Spileers W, Demaerel P, et al. Leber congenital amaurosis—differential diagnosis, ophthalmological and neuroradiological report of 18 patients. Neuropediatrics. 1996;27:189-93.
118. den Hollander AI, Roepman R, Koenekoop RK, et al. Leber congenital amaurosis: genes, proteins and disease mechanisms. Prog Retin Eye Res. 2008;27:391-419.
119. Kuntz CA, Jacobson SG, Cideciyan AV, et al. Sub-retinal pigment epithelial deposits in a dominant late-onset retinal degeneration. Invest Ophthalmol Vis Sci. 1996;37:1772-82.
120. Hayward C, Shu X, Cideciyan AV, et al. Mutation in a short-chain collagen gene, CTRP5, results in extracellular deposit formation in late-onset retinal degeneration: a genetic model for age-related macular degeneration. Hum Mol Genet. 2003;12:2657-67.

121. Ayyagari R, Mandal MN, Karoukis AJ, et al. Late-onset macular degeneration and long anterior lens zonules result from a CTRP5 gene mutation. Invest Ophthalmol Vis Sci. 2005;46:3363-71.
122. Soumplis V, Sergouniotis PI, Robson AG, et al. Phenotypic findings in C1QTNF5 retinopathy (late-onset retinal degeneration). Acta Ophthalmol. 2013;91:e191-5.
123. Kimberling WJ, Hildebrand MS, Shearer AE, et al. Frequency of Usher syndrome in two pediatric populations: Implications for genetic screening of deaf and hard of hearing children. Genet Med. 2010;12:512-6.
124. Smith RJ, Berlin CI, Hejtmancik JF, et al. Clinical diagnosis of the Usher syndromes. Usher Syndrome Consortium. Am J Med Genet. 1994;50:32-8.
125. Dammeyer J. Development and characteristics of children with Usher syndrome and CHARGE syndrome. Int J Pediatr Otorhinolaryngol. 2012;76:1292-6.
126. Pakarinen L, Karjalainen S, Simola KO, et al. Usher's syndrome type 3 in Finland. Laryngoscope. 1995;105: 613-7.
127. Khateb S, Zelinger L, Mizrahi-Meissonnier L, et al. A homozygous nonsense CEP250 mutation combined with a heterozygous nonsense C2orf71 mutation is associated with atypical Usher syndrome. J Med Genet. 2014;51:460-9.
128. Piazza L, Fishman GA, Farber M, et al. Visual acuity loss in patients with Usher's syndrome. Arch Ophthalmol. 1986;104:1336-9.
129. West SK, Hindocha M, Hogg CR, et al. Electroretinogram assessment of children with sensorineural hearing loss: implications for screening. J AAPOS. 2015;19:450-4.
130. Bardet G. Sur un syndrome d'obèsitè infantile avec polydactyly et rètinite pigmentaire (contribution à l'étude des formes cliniques de l'obésité hypophysaire). Paris: Université de Paris; 1920.
131. Beales PL, Elcioglu N, Woolf AS, et al. New criteria for improved diagnosis of Bardet-Biedl syndrome: results of a population survey. J Med Genet. 1999;36:437-46.
132. Forsythe E, Beales PL. Bardet-Biedl syndrome. Eur J Hum Genet. 2013;21:8-13.
133. Schaefer E, Stoetzel C, Scheidecker S, et al. Identification of a novel mutation confirms the implication of IFT172 (BBS20) in Bardet-Biedl syndrome. J Hum Genet. 2016;61:447-50.
134. Heon E, Kim G, Qin S, et al. Mutations in C8ORF37 cause Bardet Biedl syndrome (BBS21). Hum Mol Genet. 2016;25:2283-94.
135. Riise R, Andreasson S, Wright AF, et al. Ocular findings in the Laurence-Moon-Bardet-Biedl syndrome. Acta Ophthalmol Scand. 1996;74:612-7.
136. Iannaccone A, De Propris G, Roncati S, et al. The ocular phenotype of the Bardet-Biedl syndrome. Comparison to non-syndromic retinitis pigmentosa. Ophthalmic Genet. 1997;18:13-26.
137. Klein D, Ammann F. The syndrome of Laurence-Moon-Bardet-Biedl and allied diseases in Switzerland. Clinical, genetic and epidemiological studies. J Neurol Sci. 1969;9:479-513.
138. O'Dea D, Parfrey PS, Harnett JD, et al. The importance of renal impairment in the natural history of Bardet-Biedl syndrome. Am J Kidney Dis. 1996;27:776-83.
139. Valente EM, Dallapiccola B, Bertini E. Joubert syndrome and related disorders. Handb Clin Neurol. 2013;113: 1879-88.
140. Joubert M, Eisenring JJ, Robb JP, et al. Familial agenesis of the cerebellar vermis. A syndrome of episodic hyperpnea, abnormal eye movements, ataxia, and retardation. Neurology. 1969;19:813-25.
141. Romani M, Micalizzi A, Valente EM. Joubert syndrome: congenital cerebellar ataxia with the molar tooth. Lancet Neurol. 2013;12:894-905.
142. Coppieters F, Casteels I, Meire F, et al. Genetic screening of LCA in Belgium: predominance of CEP290 and identification of potential modifier alleles in AHI1 of CEP290-related phenotypes. Hum Mutat. 2010;31:E1709-66.
143. Valente EM, Marsh SE, Castori M, et al. Distinguishing the four genetic causes of Jouberts syndrome-related disorders. Ann Neurol. 2005;57:513-9.
144. Laverda AM, Saia OS, Drigo P, et al. Chorioretinal coloboma and Joubert syndrome: a nonrandom association. J Pediatr. 1984;105:282-4.
145. Brancati F, Barrano G, Silhavy JL, et al. CEP290 mutations are frequently identified in the oculo-renal form of Joubert syndrome-related disorders. Am J Hum Genet. 2007;81: 104-13.
146. Helou J, Otto EA, Attanasio M, et al. Mutation analysis of NPHP6/CEP290 in patients with Joubert syndrome and Senior-Loken syndrome. J Med Genet. 2007;44:657-63.
147. Mauthner L. Ein Fall von Chorioideremie. Berl Natur-med Ver Innsbruck. 1872;2:191.
148. McCulloch C, McCulloch RJ. A hereditary and clinical study of choroideremia. Trans Am Acad Ophthalmol Otolaryngol. 1948;52:160-90.
149. MacDonald IM, Sereda C, McTaggart K, et al. Choroideremia gene testing. Expert Rev Mol Diagn. 2004;4:478-84.
150. Cremers FP, van de Pol DJ, van Kerkhoff LP, et al. Cloning of a gene that is rearranged in patients with choroideraemia. Nature. 1990;347:674-7.
151. Seabra MC, Brown MS, Slaughter CA, et al. Purification of component A of Rab geranylgeranyl transferase: possible identity with the choroideremia gene product. Cell. 1992;70:1049-57.
152. Seabra MC, Brown MS, Goldstein JL. Retinal degeneration in choroideremia: deficiency of rab geranylgeranyl transferase. Science. 1993;259:377-81.
153. Karna J. Choroideremia. A clinical and genetic study of 84 Finnish patients and 126 female carriers. Acta Ophthalmol Suppl. 1986;176:1-68.
154. Coussa RG, Kim J, Traboulsi EI. Choroideremia: effect of age on visual acuity in patients and female carriers. Ophthalmic Genet. 2012;33:66-73.
155. Roberts MF, Fishman GA, Roberts DK, et al. Retrospective, longitudinal, and cross sectional study of visual acuity impairment in choroideraemia. Br J Ophthalmol. 2002;86:658-62.

156. Jain N, Jia Y, Gao SS, et al. Optical coherence tomography angiography in choroideremia: correlating choriocapillaris loss with overlying degeneration. JAMA Ophthalmol. 2016;134:697-702.
157. Genead MA, Fishman GA. Cystic macular oedema on spectral-domain optical coherence tomography in choroideremia patients without cystic changes on fundus examination. Eye (Lond). 2011;25:84-90.
158. Sawa M, Tamaki Y, Klancnik JM Jr, et al. Intraretinal foveal neovascularization in choroideremia. Retina. 2006;26:585-8.
159. Zinkernagel MS, Groppe M, MacLaren RE. Macular hole surgery in patients with end-stage choroideremia. Ophthalmology. 2013;120:1592-6.
160. Sieving PA, Niffenegger JH, Berson EL. Electroretinographic findings in selected pedigrees with choroideremia. Am J Ophthalmol. 1986;101:361-7.
161. Preising MN, Wegscheider E, Friedburg C, et al. Fundus autofluorescence in carriers of choroideremia and correlation with electrophysiologic and psychophysical data. Ophthalmology. 2009;116:1201-9.e1-2.
162. Vajaranant TS, Fishman GA, Szlyk JP, et al. Detection of mosaic retinal dysfunction in choroideremia carriers electroretinographic and psychophysical testing. Ophthalmology. 2008;115:723-9.
163. Harris GS, Miller JR. Choroideremia. Visual defects in a heterozygote. Arch Ophthalmol. 1968;80:423-9.
164. Bonilha VL, Trzupek KM, Li Y, et al. Choroideremia: analysis of the retina from a female symptomatic carrier. Ophthalmic Genet. 2008;29:99-110.
165. Takki KK, Milton RC. The natural history of gyrate atrophy of the choroid and retina. Ophthalmology. 1981;88:292-301.
166. Simell O, Takki K. Raised plasma-ornithine and gyrate atrophy of the choroid and retina. Lancet. 1973;1:1031-3.
167. Kaiser-Kupfer M, Kuwabara T, Uga S, et al. Cataract in gyrate atrophy: clinical and morphologic studies. Invest Ophthalmol Vis Sci. 1983;24:432-6.
168. Peltola KE, Nanto-Salonen K, Heinonen OJ, et al. Ophthalmologic heterogeneity in subjects with gyrate atrophy of choroid and retina harboring the L402P mutation of ornithine aminotransferase. Ophthalmology. 2001;108:721-9.
169. Sergouniotis PI, Davidson AE, Lenassi E, et al. Retinal structure, function, and molecular pathologic features in gyrate atrophy. Ophthalmology. 2012;119:596-605.
170. Raitta C, Carlson S, Vannas-Sulonen K. Gyrate atrophy of the choroid and retina: ERG of the neural retina and the pigment epithelium. Br J Ophthalmol. 1990;74:363-7.
171. Sipila I, Simell O, Rapola J, et al. Gyrate atrophy of the choroid and retina with hyperornithinemia: tubular aggregates and type 2 fiber atrophy in muscle. Neurology. 1979;29:996-1005.
172. Peltola KE, Jaaskelainen S, Heinonen OJ, et al. Peripheral nervous system in gyrate atrophy of the choroid and retina with hyperornithinemia. Neurology. 2002;59:735-40.
173. Valtonen M, Nanto-Salonen K, Jaaskelainen S, et al. Central nervous system involvement in gyrate atrophy of the choroid and retina with hyperornithinaemia. J Inherit Metab Dis. 1999;22:855-66.
174. Valle D, Walser M, Brusilow SW, et al. Gyrate atrophy of the choroid and retina: amino acid metabolism and correction of hyperornithinemia with an arginine-deficient diet. J Clin Invest. 1980;65:371-8.
175. Kaiser-Kupfer MI, Caruso RC, Valle D. Gyrate atrophy of the choroid and retina. Long-term reduction of ornithine slows retinal degeneration. Arch Ophthalmol. 1991;109:1539-48.
176. Kaiser-Kupfer MI, Caruso RC, Valle D, et al. Use of an arginine-restricted diet to slow progression of visual loss in patients with gyrate atrophy. Arch Ophthalmol. 2004;122:982-4.
177. Weleber RG, Kennaway NG. Clinical trial of vitamin B6 for gyrate atrophy of the choroid and retina. Ophthalmology. 1981;88:316-24.
178. Tanzer F, Firat M, Alagoz M, et al. Gyrate atrophy of the choroid and retina with hyperornithinemia, cystinuria and lysinuria responsive to vitamin B6. BMJ Case Rep. 2011;2011.
179. Valle D, Simell O. The Hyperornithinemias. In: Stansbury JB, Wyn-gaarden JB, Fredrickson DS, Goldstein JL, Brown MS (Eds). The Metabolic Basis of Inherited Disease, 5th edition. New York: McGraw-Hill; 1983. pp. 382-401.
180. Li A, Jiao X, Munier FL, et al. Bietti crystalline corneoretinal dystrophy is caused by mutations in the novel gene CYP4V2. Am J Hum Genet. 2004;74:817-26.
181. Rossi S, Testa F, Li A, et al. Clinical and genetic features in Italian Bietti crystalline dystrophy patients. Br J Ophthalmol. 2013;97:174-9.
182. Halford S, Liew G, Mackay DS, et al. Detailed phenotypic and genotypic characterization of Bietti crystalline dystrophy. Ophthalmology. 2014;121:1174-84.
183. Wilson DJ, Weleber RG, Klein ML, et al. Bietti's crystalline dystrophy. A clinicopathologic correlative study. Arch Ophthalmol. 1989;107:213-21.
184. Kaiser-Kupfer MI, Chan CC, Markello TC, et al. Clinical biochemical and pathologic correlations in Bietti's crystalline dystrophy. Am J Ophthalmol. 1994;118:569-82.
185. Lee J, Jiao X, Hejtmancik JF, et al. The metabolism of fatty acids in human Bietti crystalline dystrophy. Invest Ophthalmol Vis Sci. 2001;42:1707-14.
186. Yin X, Yang L, Chen N, et al. Identification of CYP4V2 mutation in 36 Chinese families with Bietti crystalline corneoretinal dystrophy. Exp Eye Res. 2016;146:154-62.
187. Benson WE. Familial exudative vitreoretinopathy. Trans Am Ophthalmol Soc. 1995;93:473-521.
188. Miyakubo H, Hashimoto K, Miyakubo S. Retinal vascular pattern in familial exudative vitreoretinopathy. Ophthalmology. 1984;91:1524-30.
189. van Nouhuys CE. Signs, complications, and platelet aggregation in familial exudative vitreoretinopathy. Am J Ophthalmol. 1991;111:34-41.
190. Ranchod TM, Ho LY, Drenser KA, et al. Clinical presentation of familial exudative vitreoretinopathy. Ophthalmology. 2011;118:2070-5.

191. Repka MX, Tung B, Good WV, et al. Outcome of eyes developing retinal detachment during the Early Treatment for Retinopathy of Prematurity Study (ETROP). Arch Ophthalmol. 2006;124:24-30.
192. Toomes C, Bottomley HM, Jackson RM, et al. Mutations in LRP5 or FZD4 underlie the common familial exudative vitreoretinopathy locus on chromosome 11q. Am J Hum Genet. 2004;74:721-30.
193. Robitaille J, MacDonald ML, Kaykas A, et al. Mutant frizzled-4 disrupts retinal angiogenesis in familial exudative vitreoretinopathy. Nat Genet. 2002;32:326-30.
194. Collin RW, Nikopoulos K, Dona M, et al. ZNF408 is mutated in familial exudative vitreoretinopathy and is crucial for the development of zebrafish retinal vasculature. Proc Natl Acad Sci USA. 2013;110:9856-61.
195. Poulter JA, Ali M, Gilmour DF, et al. Mutations in TSPAN12 cause autosomal-dominant familial exudative vitreoretinopathy. Am J Hum Genet. 2010;86:248-53.
196. Hu H, Xiao X, Li S, et al. KIF11 mutations are a common cause of autosomal dominant familial exudative vitreoretinopathy. Br J Ophthalmol. 2016;100:278-83.
197. Poulter JA, Davidson AE, Ali M, et al. Recessive mutations in TSPAN12 cause retinal dysplasia and severe familial exudative vitreoretinopathy (FEVR). Invest Ophthalmol Vis Sci. 2012;53:2873-9.
198. Jiao X, Ventruto V, Trese MT, et al. Autosomal recessive familial exudative vitreoretinopathy is associated with mutations in LRP5. Am J Hum Genet. 2004;75:878-84.
199. Khan AO, Lenzner S, Bolz HJ. A family harboring homozygous FZD4 deletion supports the existence of recessive FZD4-related familial exudative vitreoretinopathy. Ophthalmic Genet. 2017;38:380-2.
200. Qin M, Hayashi H, Oshima K, et al. Complexity of the genotype-phenotype correlation in familial exudative vitreoretinopathy with mutations in the LRP5 and/or FZD4 genes. Hum Mutat. 2005;26:104-12.
201. Ai M, Heeger S, Bartels CF, et al. Clinical and molecular findings in osteoporosis-pseudoglioma syndrome. Am J Hum Genet. 2005;77:741-53.
202. Sims KB. NDP-related retinopathies. In: Pagon RA, Adam MP, Ardinger HH (Eds). GeneReviews® [Internet]. Seattle (WA): University of Washington, Seattle; 1993-2017. [online]. Available from: *https://www.ncbi.nlm.nih.gov/books/NBK1331/* [Accessed December 2017].
203. Miyamoto T, Inoue H, Sakamoto Y, et al. Identification of a novel splice site mutation of the CSPG2 gene in a Japanese family with Wagner syndrome. Invest Ophthalmol Vis Sci. 2005;46:2726-35.
204. Mukhopadhyay A, Nikopoulos K, Maugeri A, et al. Erosive vitreoretinopathy and Wagner disease are caused by intronic mutations in CSPG2/Versican that result in an imbalance of splice variants. Invest Ophthalmol Vis Sci. 2006;47:3565-72.
205. Thomas AS, Branham K, Van Gelder RN, et al. Multimodal imaging in Wagner syndrome. Ophthalmic Surg Lasers Imaging Retina. 2016;47:574-9.
206. Brezin AP, Nedelec B, Barjol A, et al. A new VCAN/versican splice acceptor site mutation in a French Wagner family associated with vascular and inflammatory ocular features. Mol Vis. 2011;17:1669-78.
207. Brown DM, Kimura AE, Weingeist TA, et al. Erosive vitreoretinopathy. A new clinical entity. Ophthalmology. 1994;101:694-704.
208. Graemiger RA, Niemeyer G, Schneeberger SA, et al. Wagner vitreoretinal degeneration. Follow-up of the original pedigree. Ophthalmology. 1995;102:1830-9.
209. Hirose T, Lee KY, Schepens CL. Snowflake degeneration in hereditary vitreoretinal degeneration. Am J Ophthalmol. 1974;77:143-53.
210. Hejtmancik JF, Jiao X, Li A, et al. Mutations in KCNJ13 cause autosomal-dominant snowflake vitreoretinal degeneration. Am J Hum Genet. 2008;82:174-80.
211. Lee MM, Ritter R 3rd, Hirose T, et al. Snowflake vitreoretinal degeneration: follow-up of the original family. Ophthalmology. 2003;110(12):2418-26.
212. Yanagi Y, Takezawa S, Kato S. Distinct functions of photoreceptor cell-specific nuclear receptor, thyroid hormone receptor beta2 and CRX in one photoreceptor development. Invest Ophthalmol Vis Sci. 2002;43:3489-94.
213. Bernal S, Solans T, Gamundi MJ, et al. Analysis of the involvement of the NR2E3 gene in autosomal recessive retinal dystrophies. Clin Genet. 2008;73:360-6.
214. Schorderet DF, Escher P. NR2E3 mutations in enhanced S-cone sensitivity syndrome (ESCS), Goldmann-Favre syndrome (GFS), clumped pigmentary retinal degeneration (CPRD), and retinitis pigmentosa (RP). Hum Mutat. 2009;30:1475-85.
215. Favre M. Two cases of hyaloid-retinal degeneration. Ophthalmologica. 1958;135:604-9.
216. Jacobson SG, Roman AJ, Roman MI, et al. Relatively enhanced S cone function in the Goldmann-Favre syndrome. Am J Ophthalmol. 1991;111:446-53.
217. Sharon D, Sandberg MA, Caruso RC, et al. Shared mutations in NR2E3 in enhanced S-cone syndrome, Goldmann-Favre syndrome, and many cases of clumped pigmentary retinal degeneration. Arch Ophthalmol. 2003;121:1316-23.
218. Haider NB, Jacobson SG, Cideciyan AV, et al. Mutation of a nuclear receptor gene, NR2E3, causes enhanced S cone syndrome, a disorder of retinal cell fate. Nat Genet 2000;24:127-31.
219. Oh EC, Cheng H, Hao H, et al. Rod differentiation factor NRL activates the expression of nuclear receptor NR2E3 to suppress the development of cone photoreceptors. Brain Res. 2008;1236:16-29.
220. DeAngelis MM, Grimsby JL, Sandberg MA, et al. Novel mutations in the NRL gene and associated clinical findings in patients with dominant retinitis pigmentosa. Arch Ophthalmol. 2002;120:369-75.
221. Nishiguchi KM, Friedman JS, Sandberg MA, et al. Recessive NRL mutations in patients with clumped pigmentary retinal degeneration and relative preservation of blue cone function. Proc Natl Acad Sci USA. 2004;101:17819-24.
222. Vincent A, Robson AG, Holder GE. Pathognomonic (diagnostic) ERGs. A review and update. Retina. 2013; 33:5-12.

223. Haider NB, Naggert JK, Nishina PM. Excess cone cell proliferation due to lack of a functional NR2E3 causes retinal dysplasia and degeneration in rd7/rd7 mice. Hum Mol Genet. 2001;10:1619-26.
224. Hood DC, Cideciyan AV, Roman AJ, et al. Enhanced S cone syndrome: evidence for an abnormally large number of S cones. Vision Res. 1995;35:1473-81.
225. Milam AH, Rose L, Cideciyan AV, et al. The nuclear receptor NR2E3 plays a role in human retinal photoreceptor differentiation and degeneration. Proc Natl Acad Sci USA. 2002;99:473-8.
226. Snead MP, Yates JR. Clinical and molecular genetics of Stickler syndrome. J Med Genet. 1999;36:353-9.
227. Van Camp G, Snoeckx RL, Hilgert N, et al. A new autosomal recessive form of Stickler syndrome is caused by a mutation in the COL9A1 gene. Am J Hum Genet. 2006;79:449-57.
228. Baker S, Booth C, Fillman C, et al. A loss of function mutation in the COL9A2 gene causes autosomal recessive Stickler syndrome. Am J Med Genet A. 2011;155A(7): 1668-72.
229. Faletra F, D'Adamo AP, Bruno I, et al. Autosomal recessive Stickler syndrome due to a loss of function mutation in the COL9A3 gene. Am J Med Genet A. 2014;164A(1):42-7.
230. Sirko-Osadsa DA, Murray MA, Scott JA, et al. Stickler syndrome without eye involvement is caused by mutations in COL11A2, the gene encoding the alpha2 (XI) chain of type XI collagen. J Pediatr. 1998;132:368-71.
231. Couchouron T, Masson C. Early-onset progressive osteoarthritis with hereditary progressive ophtalmopathy or Stickler syndrome. Joint Bone Spine. 2011;78:45-9.
232. Acke FR, Swinnen FK, Malfait F, et al. Auditory phenotype in Stickler syndrome: results of audiometric analysis in 20 patients. Eur Arch Otorhinolaryngol. 2016;273:3025-34.
233. van den Elzen AP, Semmekrot BA, Bongers EM, et al. Diagnosis and treatment of the Pierre Robin sequence: results of a retrospective clinical study and review of the literature. Eur J Pediatr. 2001;160:47-53.
234. Ang A, Poulson AV, Goodburn SF, et al. Retinal detachment and prophylaxis in type 1 Stickler syndrome. Ophthalmology. 2008;115:164-8.
235. Storey H, Savige J, Sivakumar V, et al. COL4A3/COL4A4 mutations and features in individuals with autosomal recessive Alport syndrome. J Am Soc Nephrol. 2013;24: 1945-54.
236. Barker DF, Hostikka SL, Zhou J, et al. Identification of mutations in the COL4A5 collagen gene in Alport syndrome. Science. 1990;248:1224-7.
237. Rosado C, Bueno E, Felipe C, et al. COL4A4 gene study of a European population: description of new mutations causing autosomal dominant Alport syndrome. Int J Mol Epidemiol Genet. 2014;5:177-84.
238. Gunwar S, Ballester F, Noelken ME, et al. Glomerular basement membrane. Identification of a novel disulfide-cross-linked network of alpha3, alpha4, and alpha5 chains of type IV collagen and its implications for the pathogenesis of Alport syndrome. J Biol Chem. 1998;273:8767-75.
239. Burke JP, Clearkin LG, Talbot JF. Recurrent corneal epithelial erosions in Alport's syndrome. Acta Ophthalmol (Copenh). 1991;69:555-7.
240. Teekhasaenee C, Nimmanit S, Wutthiphan S, et al. Posterior polymorphous dystrophy and Alport syndrome. Ophthalmology. 1991;98:1207-15.
241. Pirson Y. Making the diagnosis of Alport's syndrome. Kidney Int. 1999;56:760-75.
242. Savige J, Liu J, DeBuc DC, et al. Retinal basement membrane abnormalities and the retinopathy of Alport syndrome. Invest Ophthalmol Vis Sci. 2010;51:1621-7.
243. Ahmed F, Kamae KK, Jones DJ, et al. Temporal macular thinning associated with X-linked Alport syndrome. JAMA Ophthalmol. 2013;131:777-82.
244. Navarro R, Casaroli-Marano R, Mateo C, et al. Optical coherence tomography findings in Alport syndrome. Retin Cases Brief Rep. 2008;2:47-9.
245. Shah SN, Weinberg DV. Giant macular hole in Alport syndrome. Ophthalmic Genet. 2010;31:94-7.
246. Sertie AL, Sossi V, Camargo AA, et al. Collagen XVIII, containing an endogenous inhibitor of angiogenesis and tumor growth, plays a critical role in the maintenance of retinal structure and in neural tube closure (Knobloch syndrome). Hum Mol Genet. 2000;9:2051-8.
247. Knobloch WH, Layer JM. Retinal detachment and encephalocele. J Pediatr Ophthalmol. 1971:181-4.
248. Hull S, Arno G, Ku CA, et al. Molecular and clinical findings in patients with Knobloch syndrome. JAMA Ophthalmol. 2016;134:753-62.
249. Duh EJ, Yao YG, Dagli M, et al. Persistence of fetal vasculature in a patient with Knobloch syndrome: potential role for endostatin in fetal vascular remodeling of the eye. Ophthalmology. 2004;111:1885-8.
250. Caglayan AO, Baranoski JF, Aktar F, et al. Brain malformations associated with Knobloch syndrome--review of literature, expanding clinical spectrum, and identification of novel mutations. Pediatr Neurol. 2014;51:806-13.e8.
251. Cunier F. Histoire d'une héméralopie héréditaire depuis deux siècles: dans une famille de al commune de Vendémian près Montpellier. Ann Soc Med Gand. 1838;4:385-95.
252. Kim JM, Payne JF, Yan J, et al. Negative electroretinograms in the pediatric and adult population. Doc Ophthalmol. 2012;124:41-8.
253. Miyake Y, Yagasaki K, Horiguchi M, et al. Congenital stationary night blindness with negative electroretinogram. A new classification. Arch Ophthalmol. 1986;104:1013-20.
254. Yamamoto H, Simon A, Eriksson U, et al. Mutations in the gene encoding 11-cis retinol dehydrogenase cause delayed dark adaptation and fundus albipunctatus. Nat Genet. 1999;22:188-91.
255. Sergouniotis PI, Sohn EH, Li Z, et al. Phenotypic variability in RDH5 retinopathy (Fundus Albipunctatus). Ophthalmology. 2011;118:1661-70.
256. Genead MA, Fishman GA, Lindeman M. Spectral-domain optical coherence tomography and fundus autofluorescence characteristics in patients with fundus albipunctatus and

retinitis punctata albescens. Ophthalmic Genet. 2010;31: 66-72.
257. Lima LH, Cella W, Greenstein VC, et al. Structural assessment of hyperautofluorescent ring in patients with retinitis pigmentosa. Retina. 2009;29:1025-31.
258. Oguchi C. Über eine Abart von Hemeralopie. Acta Soc Ophthalmol Jpn. 1907;11:123-34.
259. Codega P, Della Santina L, Gargini C, et al. Prolonged illumination up-regulates arrestin and two guanylate cyclase activating proteins: a novel mechanism for light adaptation. J Physiol. 2009;587:2457-72.
260. Sakurai K, Chen J, Khani SC, et al. Regulation of mammalian cone phototransduction by recoverin and rhodopsin kinase. J Biol Chem. 2015;290:9239-50.
261. Michaelides M, Hardcastle AJ, Hunt DM, et al. Progressive cone and cone-rod dystrophies: phenotypes and underlying molecular genetic basis. Surv Ophthalmol. 2006;51:232-58.
262. Sohocki MM, Perrault I, Leroy BP, et al. Prevalence of AIPL1 mutations in inherited retinal degenerative disease. Mol Genet Metab. 2000;70:142-50.
263. Swaroop A, Wang QL, Wu W, et al. Leber congenital amaurosis caused by a homozygous mutation (R90W) in the homeodomain of the retinal transcription factor CRX: direct evidence for the involvement of CRX in the development of photoreceptor function. Hum Mol Genet. 1999;8:299-305.
264. Lotery AJ, Namperumalsamy P, Jacobson SG, et al. Mutation analysis of 3 genes in patients with Leber congenital amaurosis. Arch Ophthalmol. 2000;118:538-43.
265. Wang X, Wang H, Sun V, et al. Comprehensive molecular diagnosis of 179 Leber congenital amaurosis and juvenile retinitis pigmentosa patients by targeted next generation sequencing. J Med Genet. 2013;50:674-88.
266. Rowe SE, Trobe JD, Sieving PA. Idiopathic photoreceptor dysfunction causes unexplained visual acuity loss in later adulthood. Ophthalmology. 1990;97:1632-7.
267. Sakuramoto H, Kuniyoshi K, Tsunoda K, et al. Two siblings with late-onset cone-rod dystrophy and no visible macular degeneration. Clin Ophthalmol. 2013;7:1703-11.
268. Fishman GA, Stone EM, Eliason DA, et al. ABCA4 gene sequence variations in patients with autosomal recessive cone-rod dystrophy. Arch Ophthalmol. 2003;121:851-5.
269. Nakazawa M, Kikawa E, Chida Y, et al. Autosomal dominant cone-rod dystrophy associated with mutations in codon 244 (Asn244His) and codon 184 (Tyr184Ser) of the peripherin/RDS gene. Arch Ophthalmol. 1996;114:72-8.
270. Heckenlively JR, Martin DA, Rosales TO. Telangiectasia and optic atrophy in cone-rod degenerations. Arch Ophthalmol. 1981;99:1983-91.
271. Collin GB, Marshall JD, Ikeda A, et al. Mutations in ALMS1 cause obesity, type 2 diabetes and neurosensory degeneration in Alstrom syndrome. Nat Genet. 2002;31: 74-8.
272. Li G, Vega R, Nelms K, et al. A role for Alstrom syndrome protein, alms1, in kidney ciliogenesis and cellular quiescence. PLoS Genet. 2007;3:e8.
273. Marshall JD, Maffei P, Collin GB, et al. Alstrom syndrome: genetics and clinical overview. Curr Genomics. 2011;12: 225-35.
274. Russell-Eggitt IM, Clayton PT, Coffey R, et al. Alstrom syndrome. Report of 22 cases and literature review. Ophthalmology. 1998;105:1274-80.
275. Michaud JL, Heon E, Guilbert F, et al. Natural history of Alstrom syndrome in early childhood: onset with dilated cardiomyopathy. J Pediatr. 1996;128:225-9.
276. Jalili IK, Smith NJ. A progressive cone-rod dystrophy and amelogenesis imperfecta: a new syndrome. J Med Genet. 1988;25:738-40.
277. Parry DA, Mighell AJ, El-Sayed W, et al. Mutations in CNNM4 cause Jalili syndrome, consisting of autosomal-recessive cone-rod dystrophy and amelogenesis imperfecta. Am J Hum Genet. 2009;84:266-73.
278. Morgan CM, Webb RM, O›Connor GR. Atypical syphilitic chorioretinitis and vasculitis. Retina. 1984;4:225-31.
279. Huckfeldt RM, Comander J. Management of cystoid macular edema in retinitis pigmentosa. Semin Ophthalmol. 2017;32:43-51.
280. Vinores SA, Kuchle M, Derevjanik NL, et al. Blood-retinal barrier breakdown in retinitis pigmentosa: light and electron microscopic immunolocalization. Histol Histopathol. 1995;10:913-23.
281. Newsome DA. Retinal fluorescein leakage in retinitis pigmentosa. Am J Ophthalmol. 1986;101:354-60.
282. Cox SN, Hay E, Bird AC. Treatment of chronic macular edema with acetazolamide. Arch Ophthalmol. 1988;106:1190-5.
283. Heckenlively JR, Jordan BL, Aptsiauri N. Association of antiretinal antibodies and cystoid macular edema in patients with retinitis pigmentosa. Am J Ophthalmol. 1999;127:565-73.
284. Hirakawa H, Iijima H, Gohdo T, et al. Optical coherence tomography of cystoid macular edema associated with retinitis pigmentosa. Am J Ophthalmol. 1999;128:185-91.
285. Adackapara CA, Sunness JS, Dibernardo CW, et al. Prevalence of cystoid macular edema and stability in oct retinal thickness in eyes with retinitis pigmentosa during a 48-week lutein trial. Retina. 2008;28:103-10.
286. Fishman GA, Gilbert LD, Fiscella RG, et al. Acetazolamide for treatment of chronic macular edema in retinitis pigmentosa. Arch Ophthalmol. 1989;107:1445-52.
287. Genead MA, Fishman GA. Efficacy of sustained topical dorzolamide therapy for cystic macular lesions in patients with retinitis pigmentosa and Usher syndrome. Arch Ophthalmol. 2010;128:1146-50.
288. Apushkin MA, Fishman GA, Grover S, et al. Rebound of cystoid macular edema with continued use of acetazolamide in patients with retinitis pigmentosa. Retina. 2007;27: 1112-8.
289. Ozdemir H, Karacorlu M, Karacorlu S. Intravitreal triamcinolone acetonide for treatment of cystoid macular oedema in patients with retinitis pigmentosa. Acta Ophthalmol Scand. 2005;83:248-51.

290. Scorolli L, Morara M, Meduri A, et al. Treatment of cystoid macular edema in retinitis pigmentosa with intravitreal triamcinolone. Arch Ophthalmol. 2007;125:759-64.
291. Artunay O, Yuzbasioglu E, Rasier R, et al. Intravitreal ranibizumab in the treatment of cystoid macular edema associated with retinitis pigmentosa. J Ocul Pharmacol Ther. 2009;25:545-50.
292. Yuzbasioglu E, Artunay O, Rasier R, et al. Intravitreal bevacizumab (Avastin) injection in retinitis pigmentosa. Curr Eye Res. 2009;34:231-7.
293. Berson EL, Rosner B, Sandberg MA, et al. A randomized trial of vitamin A and vitamin E supplementation for retinitis pigmentosa. Arch Ophthalmol. 1993;111:761-72.
294. Hoffman DR, Locke KG, Wheaton DH, et al. A randomized, placebo-controlled clinical trial of docosahexaenoic acid supplementation for X-linked retinitis pigmentosa. Am J Ophthalmol. 2004;137:704-18.
295. Aleman TS, Duncan JL, Bieber ML, et al. Macular pigment and lutein supplementation in retinitis pigmentosa and Usher syndrome. Invest Ophthalmol Vis Sci. 2001;42:1873-81.
296. Norton EW. A randomized trial of vitamin A and vitamin E supplementation for retinitis pigmentosa. Arch Ophthalmol. 1993;111:761-72.
297. Massof RW, Finkelstein D. Supplemental vitamin A retards loss of ERG amplitude in retinitis pigmentosa. Arch Ophthalmol. 1993;111:751-4.
298. Weissmiller AM, Wu C. Current advances in using neurotrophic factors to treat neurodegenerative disorders. Transl Neurodegener. 2012;1:14.
299. Birch DG, Bennett LD, Duncan JL, et al. Long-term follow-up of patients with retinitis pigmentosa receiving intraocular ciliary neurotrophic factor implants. Am J Ophthalmol. 2016;170:10-4.
300. Ferrari MP, Mantelli F, Sacchetti M, et al. Safety and pharmacokinetics of escalating doses of human recombinant nerve growth factor eye drops in a double-masked, randomized clinical trial. BioDrugs. 2014;28: 275-83.
301. Sutherland JE, Day MA. Genetic counseling and genetic testing in ophthalmology. Curr Opin Ophthalmol. 2009;20:343-50.
302. Branham K, Yashar BM. Providing comprehensive genetic-based ophthalmic care. Clin Genet. 2013;84:183-9.
303. Consugar MB, Navarro-Gomez D, Place EM, et al. Panel-based genetic diagnostic testing for inherited eye diseases is highly accurate and reproducible, and more sensitive for variant detection, than exome sequencing. Genet Med. 2015;17:253-61.
304. Jorgensen A, Wiencke AK, la Cour M, et al. Human retinal pigment epithelial cell-induced apoptosis in activated T cells. Invest Ophthalmol Vis Sci. 1998;39:1590-9.
305. Li Q, Miller R, Han PY, et al. Intraocular route of AAV2 vector administration defines humoral immune response and therapeutic potential. Mol Vis. 2008;14:1760-9.
306. Acland GM, Aguirre GD, Ray J, et al. Gene therapy restores vision in a canine model of childhood blindness. Nat Genet. 2001;28:92-5.
307. Narfstrom K, Katz ML, Bragadottir R, et al. Functional and structural recovery of the retina after gene therapy in the RPE65 null mutation dog. Invest Ophthalmol Vis Sci. 2003;44:1663-72.
308. Acland GM, Aguirre GD, Bennett J, et al. Long-term restoration of rod and cone vision by single dose rAAV-mediated gene transfer to the retina in a canine model of childhood blindness. Mol Ther. 2005;12:1072-82.
309. Bemelmans AP, Kostic C, Crippa SV, et al. Lentiviral gene transfer of RPE65 rescues survival and function of cones in a mouse model of Leber congenital amaurosis. PLoS Med. 2006;3:e347.
310. Maguire AM, Simonelli F, Pierce EA, et al. Safety and efficacy of gene transfer for Leber›s congenital amaurosis. N Engl J Med. 2008;358:2240-8.
311. Bainbridge JW, Smith AJ, Barker SS, et al. Effect of gene therapy on visual function in Leber›s congenital amaurosis. N Engl J Med. 2008;358:2231-9.
312. Hauswirth WW, Aleman TS, Kaushal S, et al. Treatment of Leber congenital amaurosis due to RPE65 mutations by ocular subretinal injection of adeno-associated virus gene vector: short-term results of a phase I trial. Hum Gene Ther. 2008;19:979-90.
313. Jacobson SG, Cideciyan AV, Ratnakaram R, et al. Gene therapy for Leber congenital amaurosis caused by RPE65 mutations: safety and efficacy in 15 children and adults followed up to 3 years. Arch Ophthalmol. 2012;130:9-24.
314. Bainbridge JW, Mehat MS, Sundaram V, et al. Long-term effect of gene therapy on Leber›s congenital amaurosis. N Engl J Med. 2015;372:1887-97.
315. Weleber RG, Pennesi ME, Wilson DJ, et al. Results at 2 years after gene therapy for RPE65-deficient leber congenital amaurosis and severe early-childhood-onset retinal dystrophy. Ophthalmology. 2016;123:1606-20.
316. Russell S, Bennett J, Wellman JA, et al. Efficacy and safety of voretigene neparvovec (AAV2-hRPE65v2) in patients with RPE65-mediated inherited retinal dystrophy: a randomised, controlled, open-label, phase 3 trial. Lancet. 2017;390: 849-60.
317. Graham DK, Dawson TL, Mullaney DL, et al. Cloning and mRNA expression analysis of a novel human protooncogene, c-mer. Cell Growth Differ. 1994;5:647-57.
318. D›Cruz PM, Yasumura D, Weir J, et al. Mutation of the receptor tyrosine kinase gene Mertk in the retinal dystrophic RCS rat. Hum Mol Genet. 2000;9:645-51.
319. Gal A, Li Y, Thompson DA, et al. Mutations in MERTK, the human orthologue of the RCS rat retinal dystrophy gene, cause retinitis pigmentosa. Nat Genet. 2000;26:270-1.
320. Vollrath D, Feng W, Duncan JL, et al. Correction of the retinal dystrophy phenotype of the RCS rat by viral gene transfer of Mertk. Proc Natl Acad Sci USA. 2001;98:12584-9.
321. Smith AJ, Schlichtenbrede FC, Tschernutter M, et al. AAV-Mediated gene transfer slows photoreceptor loss in the RCS rat model of retinitis pigmentosa. Mol Ther. 2003;8:188-95.
322. Tschernutter M, Schlichtenbrede FC, Howe S, et al. Long-term preservation of retinal function in the RCS rat model

of retinitis pigmentosa following lentivirus-mediated gene therapy. Gene Ther. 2005;12:694-701.
323. Ghazi NG, Abboud EB, Nowilaty SR, et al. Treatment of retinitis pigmentosa due to MERTK mutations by ocular subretinal injection of adeno-associated virus gene vector: results of a phase I trial. Hum Genet. 2016;135:327-43.
324. Weston MD, Kelley PM, Overbeck LD, et al. Myosin VIIA mutation screening in 189 Usher syndrome type 1 patients. Am J Hum Genet. 1996;59:1074-83.
325. Grieger JC, Samulski RJ. Packaging capacity of adeno-associated virus serotypes: impact of larger genomes on infectivity and postentry steps. J Virol. 2005;79:9933-44.
326. Hashimoto T, Gibbs D, Lillo C, et al. Lentiviral gene replacement therapy of retinas in a mouse model for Usher syndrome type 1B. Gene Ther. 2007;14:584-94.
327. Zallocchi M, Binley K, Lad Y, et al. EIAV-based retinal gene therapy in the shaker1 mouse model for Usher syndrome type 1B: development of UshStat. PLoS One. 2014;9:e94272.
328. ClinicalTrials.gov Identifier: NCT01505062. (2012). A Phase I/IIa Dose Escalation Safety Study of Subretinally Injected UshStat® Administered to Patients With Retinitis Pigmentosa Associated With Usher Syndrome Type 1B. [online]. Available from: *https://clinicaltrials.gov/ct2/show/NCT01505062* [Accessed December 2017].
329. Tolmachova T, Tolmachov OE, Barnard AR, et al. Functional expression of Rab escort protein 1 following AAV2-mediated gene delivery in the retina of choroideremia mice and human cells ex vivo. J Mol Med (Berl). 2013;91:825-37.
330. MacLaren RE, Groppe M, Barnard AR, et al. Retinal gene therapy in patients with choroideremia: initial findings from a phase 1/2 clinical trial. Lancet. 2014;383:1129-37.
331. Edwards TL, Jolly JK, Groppe M, et al. Visual acuity after retinal gene therapy for choroideremia. N Engl J Med. 2016;374:1996-8.
332. ClinicalTrials.gov identifier: NCT02341807. (2015). A Phase 1/2 Safety Study in Subjects With CHM (Choroideremia) Gene Mutations Using an Adeno-Associated Virus Serotype 2 Vector to Deliver the Normal Human CHM Gene [AAV2-hCHM] to the Retina. [online]. Available from: *https://clinicaltrials.gov/ct2/show/NCT02341807* [Accessed December 2017].
333. ClinicalTrials.gov identifier: NCT02553135. (2015). An Open Label Phase 2 Clinical Trial of Retinal Gene Therapy for Choroideremia Using an Adeno-associated Viral Vector (AAV2) Encoding Rab-escort Protein 1 (REP1). [online]. Avilable from: *\https://clinicaltrials.gov/ct2/show/NCT02553135* [Accessed December 2017].
334. Gorbatyuk M, Justilien V, Liu J, et al. Preservation of photoreceptor morphology and function in P23H rats using an allele independent ribozyme. Exp Eye Res. 2007;84:44-52.
335. Lewin AS, Drenser KA, Hauswirth WW, et al. Ribozyme rescue of photoreceptor cells in a transgenic rat model of autosomal dominant retinitis pigmentosa. Nat Med. 1998;4:967-71.
336. O'Reilly M, Palfi A, Chadderton N, et al. RNA interference-mediated suppression and replacement of human rhodopsin in vivo. Am J Hum Genet. 2007;81:127-35.
337. Mao H, Gorbatyuk MS, Rossmiller B, et al. Long-term rescue of retinal structure and function by rhodopsin RNA replacement with a single adeno-associated viral vector in P23H RHO transgenic mice. Hum Gene Ther. 2012;23:356-66.
338. Ovando-Roche P, Georgiadis A, Smith AJ, et al. Harnessing the potential of human pluripotent stem cells and gene editing for the treatment of retinal degeneration. Curr Stem Cell Rep. 2017;3:112-23.
339. Zhong X, Gutierrez C, Xue T, et al. Generation of three-dimensional retinal tissue with functional photoreceptors from human iPSCs. Nat Commun. 2014;5:4047.
340. Schwartz SD, Hubschman JP, Heilwell G, et al. Embryonic stem cell trials for macular degeneration: a preliminary report. Lancet. 2012;379:713-20.
341. Schwartz SD, Regillo CD, Lam BL, et al. Human embryonic stem cell-derived retinal pigment epithelium in patients with age-related macular degeneration and Stargardt's macular dystrophy: follow-up of two open-label phase 1/2 studies. Lancet. 2015;385:509-16.
342. Tucker BA, Mullins RF, Streb LM, et al. Patient-specific iPSC-derived photoreceptor precursor cells as a means to investigate retinitis pigmentosa. Elife. 2013;2:e00824.
343. Singh R, Shen W, Kuai D, et al. iPS cell modeling of Best disease: insights into the pathophysiology of an inherited macular degeneration. Hum Mol Genet. 2013;22:593-607.
344. Parfitt DA, Lane A, Ramsden CM, et al. Identification and correction of mechanisms underlying inherited blindness in human iPSC-derived optic cups. Cell Stem Cell. 2016;18:769-81.
345. Dobelle WH, Quest DO, Antunes JL, et al. Artificial vision for the blind by electrical stimulation of the visual cortex. Neurosurgery. 1979;5:521-7.
346. Normann RA, Greger B, House P, et al. Toward the development of a cortically based visual neuroprosthesis. J Neural Eng. 2009;6:035001.
347. Veraart C, Raftopoulos C, Mortimer JT, et al. Visual sensations produced by optic nerve stimulation using an implanted self-sizing spiral cuff electrode. Brain Res. 1998;813:181-6.
348. Humayun MS, Dorn JD, da Cruz L, et al. Interim results from the international trial of Second Sight's visual prosthesis. Ophthalmology. 2012;119:779-88.
349. Ho AC, Humayun MS, Dorn JD, et al. Long-term results from an epiretinal prosthesis to restore sight to the blind. Ophthalmology. 2015;122:1547-54.
350. Stingl K, Bartz-Schmidt KU, Besch D, et al. Subretinal visual implant alpha IMS—clinical trial interim report. Vision Res. 2015;111:149-60.
351. da Cruz L, Dorn JD, Humayun MS, et al. Five-year safety and performance results from the Argus II Retinal Prosthesis System Clinical Trial. Ophthalmology. 2016;123:2248-54.

Chapter 55

Tumors and Paraneoplastic Disorders

Tara A McCannel, Vidal Soberon

INTRODUCTION

When faced with an unusual lesion of the anterior or posterior segment, it is helpful to create a comprehensive differential diagnosis. This will allow both vision- and life-threatening disorders to be considered and systematically ruled out. Appropriate clinical investigation and/or imaging may then be instituted to help support the diagnosis and determine the subsequent management strategy.

To consider all categories of disease, a mnemonic such as "CINE-TV" can be used.

C—congenital, hereditary
I—infectious, iatrogenic, idiopathic
N—neoplastic
E—endocrine
T—trauma
V—vascular

A tumor may be benign or malignant, the latter having the ability to metastasize and result in the patient's demise. This chapter will review intraocular tumors according to their location in the eye. Ocular paraneoplastic disease, a result of autoimmune activation in patients with metastatic cancer, may involve multiple ocular structures.

IRIS TUMORS

Iris Nevus

An iris nevus is the most common benign lesion of the iris[1] (Fig. 55.1). A range of clinical presentations exists, from a focal area of increased pigmentation to a solid appearing mass of the iris stroma. Ectropion uveae may occur in lesions that involve the pupillary border. Iris nevi do not usually cause a sector cataract. Finally, iris nevi rarely cause elevated intraocular pressure (IOP). An iris melanoma must be considered in the presence of cataract or elevated IOP.[2] The management of an iris nevus is observation for possible growth with IOP monitoring.

Ultrasound biomicroscopy, photography, including goniophotography, and anterior segment ocular coherence tomography (OCT) may be useful in clinical documentation.

Iris Melanoma

Iris melanomas comprise less than 3% of all uveal malignant melanoma.[3] The prognosis for metastasis is more favorable with iris melanoma than with posterior segment melanoma, with a 3% overall risk for the development of metastasis.[4] The clinical appearance of an iris melanoma may be similar to that of the spectrum of a nevus, often with more signs of physical effect on the iris and anterior chamber: corectopia, ectropion uveae, pigmentation in the angle, involvement of the angle, unilateral elevated IOP and/or hyphema.[3] The clinical diagnosis of iris melanoma is best made with documentation of growth (Figs. 55.2A and B).

Iris melanoma may be treated with either resection or radiotherapy (Figs. 55.3 and 55.4).[4] Focal iris lesions at the pupillary border with a low likelihood of angle

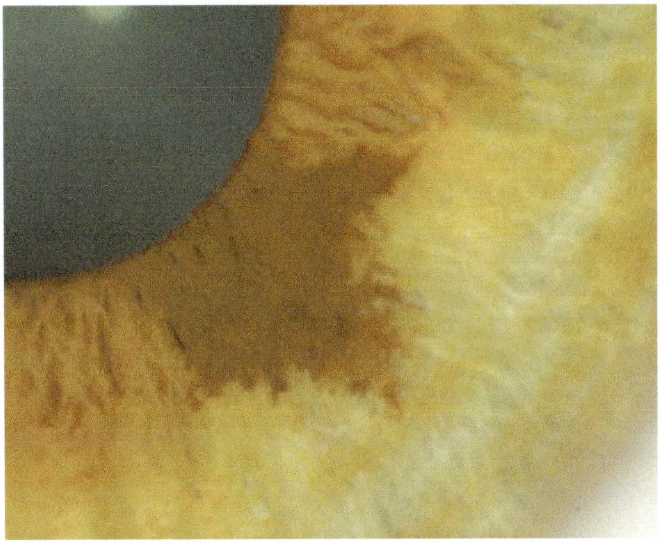

Fig. 55.1: Iris nevus.

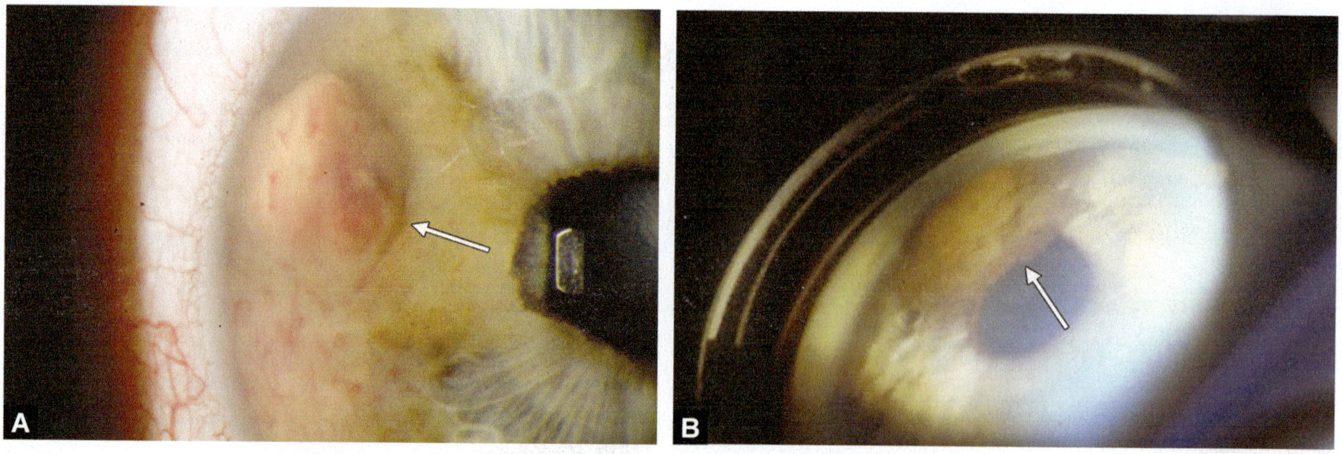

Figs. 55.2A and B: Iris melanoma.

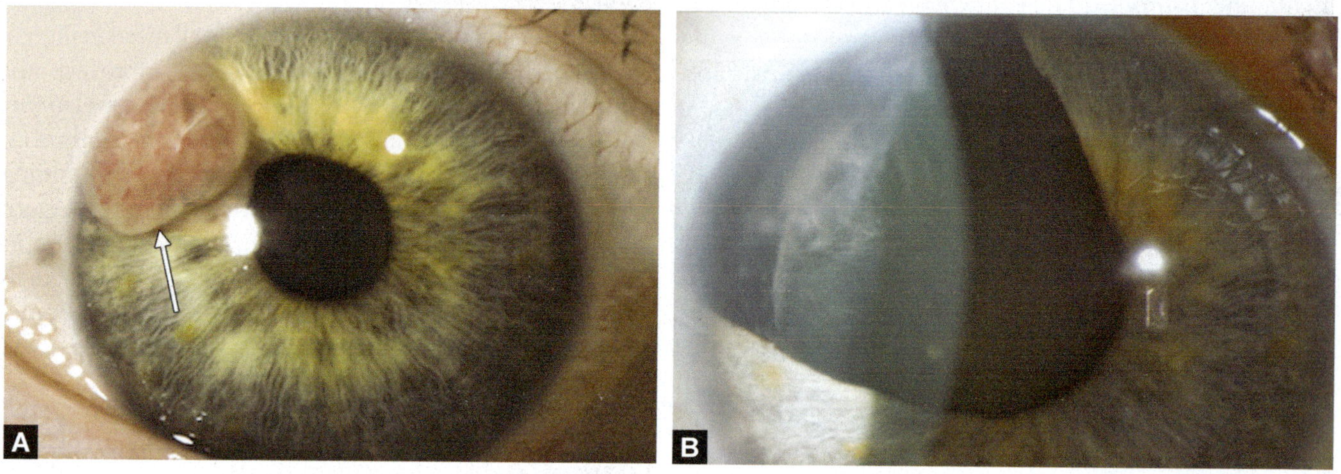

Figs. 55.3A and B: Iris melanoma pre- and postresection.

involvement may be considered for resection. However, most iris melanomas do indeed involve the angle and may also involve the ciliary body. Unless the ciliary body portion of an iris melanoma is elevated, it may not be detected with clinical examination or ultrasonography. Radiotherapy allows for a margin beyond the tumor to receive treatment, thereby reducing the risk of incomplete lesion treatment, particularly in angle-involving iris melanoma.

Radiation treatment of iris melanoma is most commonly performed with iodine-125 brachytherapy.[5] An episcleral plaque may be safely placed directly on the cornea over the iris melanoma and sutured to the adjacent sclera. In cases of diffuse iris melanoma, a "donut-shaped" plaque may be created where the maximal dose is centered at the iris and ciliary body plane. Unlike a conventional plaque for treatment of diffuse iris melanoma, the donut plaque allows for a significant reduction in dose to the cornea. Proton beam radiotherapy may also be used to treat iris melanoma.[6]

Radiation treatment of iris melanoma almost always results in cataract progression, particularly in patients who already have mild nuclear sclerotic changes. Glaucoma is usually secondary open angle and rarely neovascular, due to the low risk of ischemic retinopathy in the treatment of iris melanoma. However, neither resection nor radiation therapy of iris melanoma results in resolution of elevated IOP; treated iris melanoma patients must continue to be monitored and appropriately treated for glaucoma to maintain the best visual outcome.[5,7]

Metastatic Iris Lesions

Primary systemic cancers, including breast, lung and prostate malignancies, may infrequently metastasize to the iris (Fig. 55.5).[8] Renal cell carcinoma and carcinoid tumors may also metastasize to the iris (Figs. 55.6A and B). The appearance of a metastatic tumor to the iris may be chalky, fluffy, or infiltrative. The tumor is usually

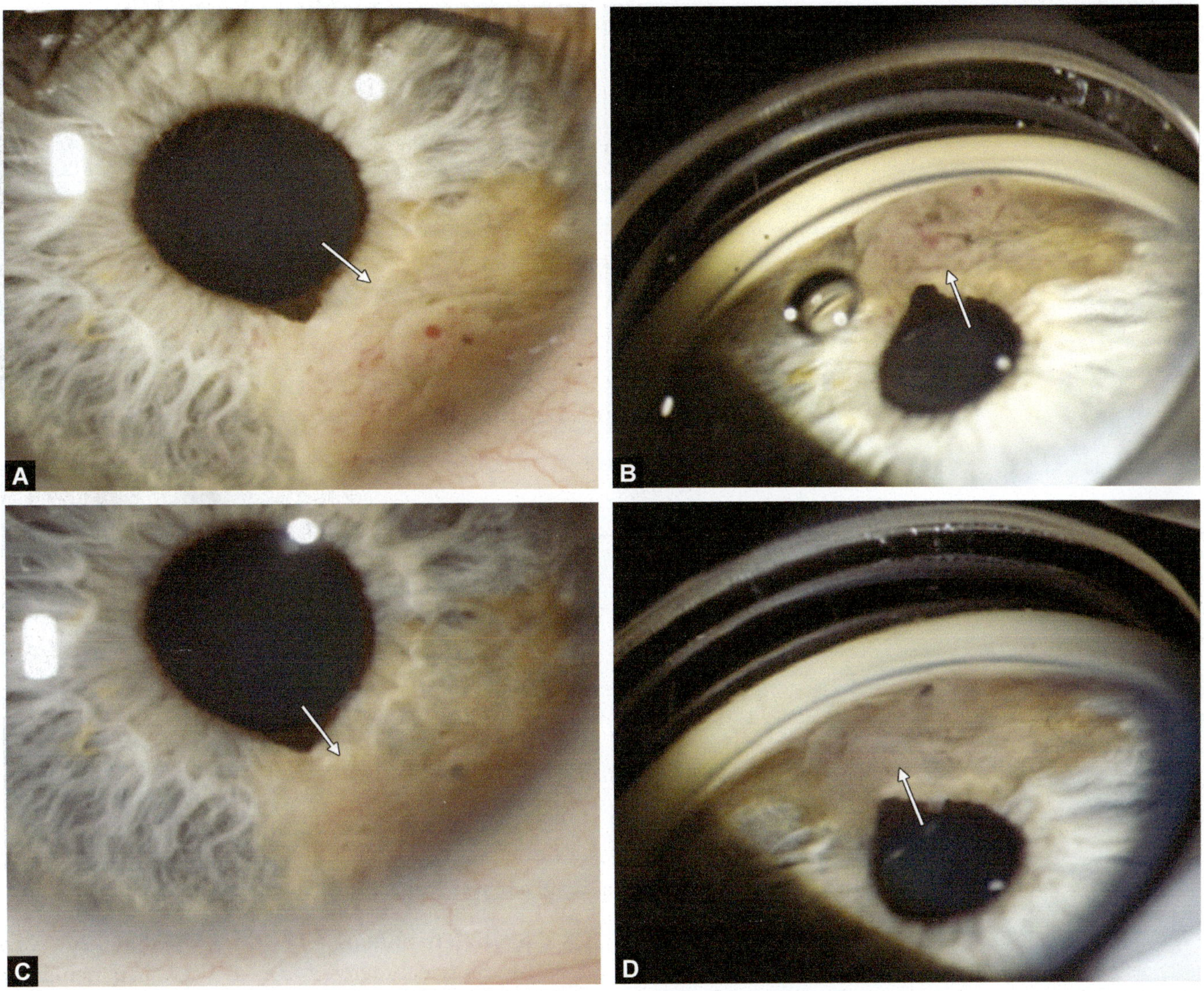

Figs. 55.4A to D: Iris melanoma pre- and postbrachytherapy.

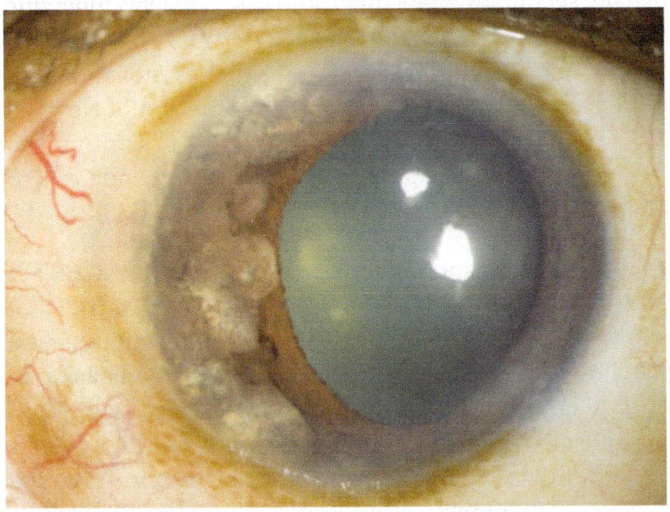

Fig. 55.5: Prostate cancer metastatic to iris.

not as well circumscribed as a primary iris melanoma. Radiation therapy with brachytherapy may be offered for local tumor control.

Iris Cyst

An iris cyst is a frequent, benign configuration of the iris, often shown to involve multiple lesions by ultrasound biomicroscopy. A focal elevation of the iris stroma on undilated examination or the observation of a uniformly pigmented bulge at the pupillary opening upon dilation are the most common clinical presentations of an iris cyst (Fig. 55.7).[9] Ultrasound biomicroscopy is important to confirm the cyst-like nature of the lesion and to evaluate for any more concerning solid component (Fig. 55.8). Rarely, a large iris cyst may cause secondary angle closure (posterior

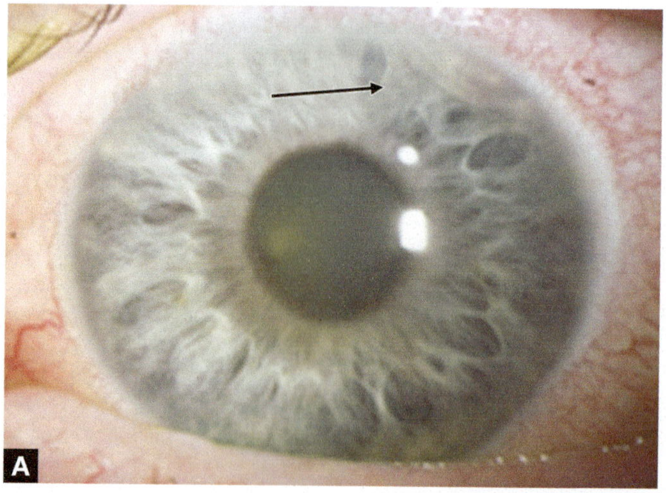

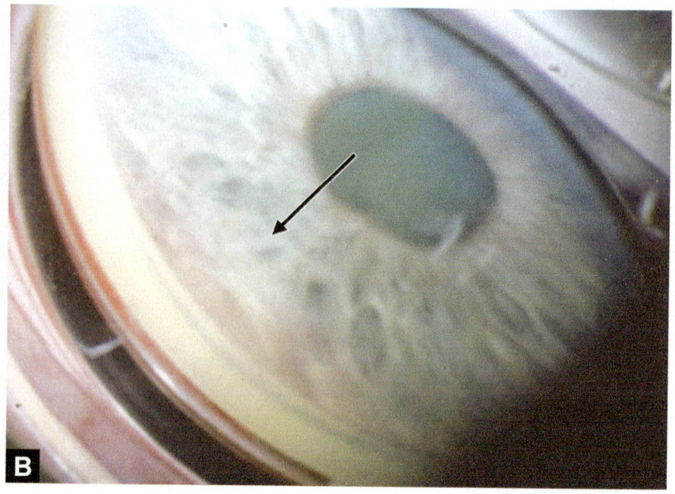

Figs. 55.6A and B: Renal cell cancer metastatic to iris (arrows).

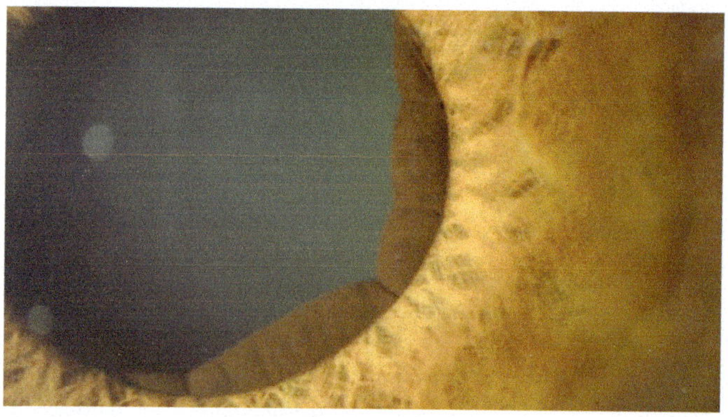

Fig. 55.7: Iris cyst.

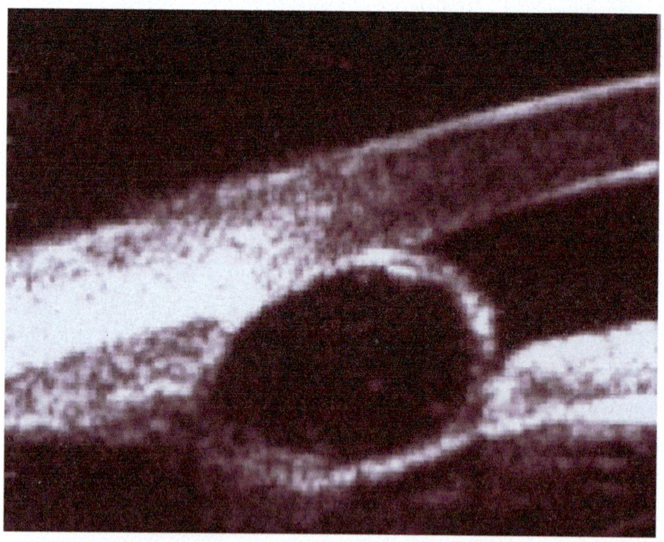

Fig. 55.8: Ultrabiomicroscopy of iris cysts.

pushing mechanism); in such cases, iris cyst drainage may be indicated. Iris cysts have been known to dislodge into the posterior chamber or posterior segment.[10,11] The vast majority of iris cysts will require observation only.

Infectious Iris Lesions

Infectious lesions of the iris are rare and may be bilateral or multifocal in nature. One must consider masquerade etiologies, such as syphilis, tuberculosis, Epstein-Barr virus[12,13] or fungus (Figs. 55.9A and B).

CHOROIDAL TUMORS

Choroidal Nevus

Choroidal nevi are believed to be present in 5% of individuals[14] and are most frequently detected on dilated fundus examination. Nevi are almost always asymptomatic. Occasionally, a nevus may develop a secondary choroidal neovascular membrane, which may need treatment if located in the macula.[15]

Clinical features most commonly associated with a benign nevus include drusen, retinal pigment epithelial atrophic changes inferior to the lesion, absence of subretinal fluid, and high internal reflectivities by A-scan ultrasonography (Fig. 55.10).[16] But keep in mind that choroidal melanoma may also harbor all of these same signs; thus, the presence of these findings does not rule out a diagnosis of choroidal melanoma.

The most concerning aspect of a choroidal nevus is the potential risk of malignant transformation. A benign

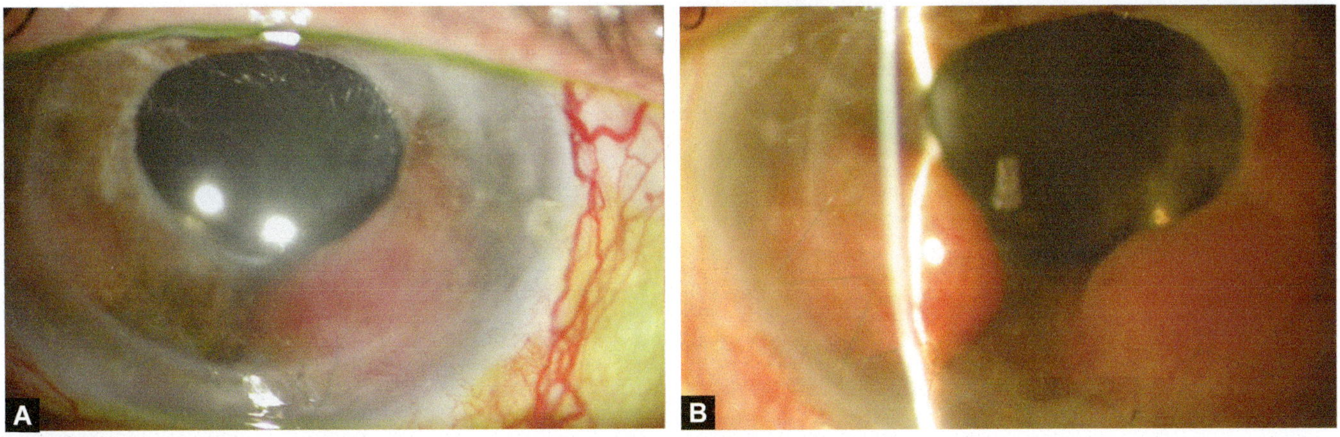

Figs. 55.9A and B: Epstein-Barr virus infection of the iris.

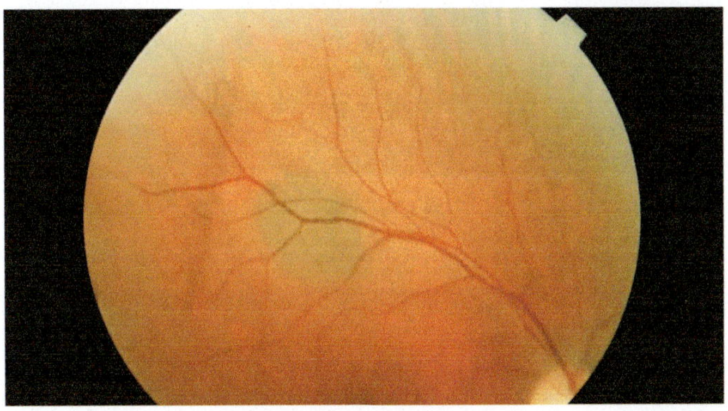

Fig. 55.10: Choroidal nevus.

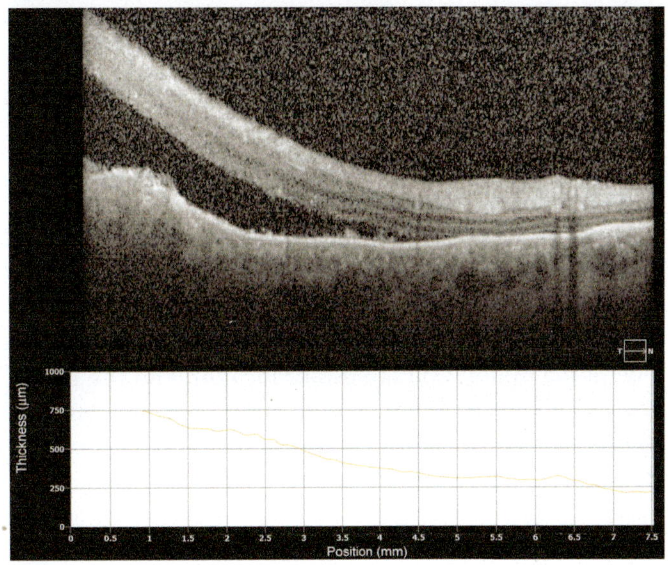

Fig. 55.11: Optical coherence tomography of malignant transformation from nevus to melanoma demonstrating development of serous retinal detachment.

choroidal nevus has a 1 in 5,000 to 1 in 10,000 risk of transforming into a choroidal melanoma.[17] Although observation is necessary for all choroidal nevi, elevated choroidal nevi (>1.0 mm in thickness) must be monitored more closely than flat nevi. Risk factors for malignant transformation, in addition to greater lesion thickness, include the presence of subretinal fluid, visual symptoms (noticing photopsia or blind spot), and the presence of orange pigment.[17]

Diagnostic imaging studies that are useful for observing choroidal nevi include color fundus photography, ultrasonography and OCT. Volume scans through the lesion may detect subtle changes, such as the development of subretinal fluid, which may indicate malignant transformation (Fig. 55.11).

Choroidal Melanoma

Clinical Features

Choroidal melanoma is the most common primary intraocular cancer of adults. The incidence is 3.1 cases per million population per year.[18] Although choroidal melanoma affects mostly people of Caucasian ancestry (97%), cases have been reported among other racial ethnicities.[19,20]

At this time, there are no identifiable causal risk factors for the development of choroidal melanoma. However, several associations have been reported. Individuals with blue or green irides are at greater risk than those with brown irides.[21] Furthermore, patients with oculodermal melanocytosis have a 1 in 400 risk of developing choroidal melanoma.[22] The BRCA1-associated protein-1 (BAP-1) tumor predisposition syndrome has been described where a germline mutation in the tumor suppressor gene BAP-1 results in autosomal dominant transmission of a phenotype

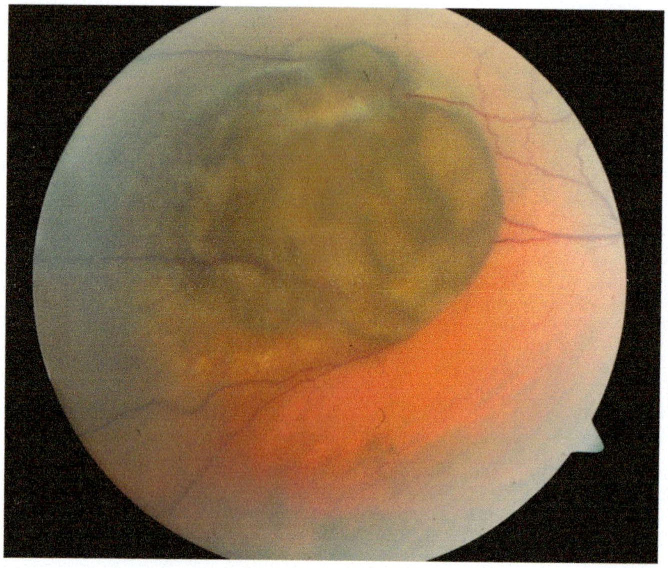

Fig. 55.12: Choroidal melanoma.

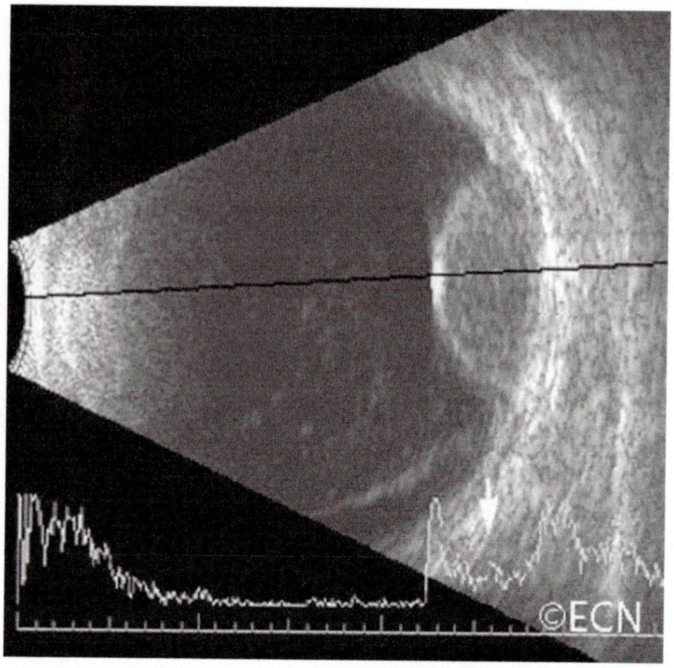

Fig. 55.13: Ultrasonography of choroidal melanoma demonstrating dome shape and low-medium reflectivities.

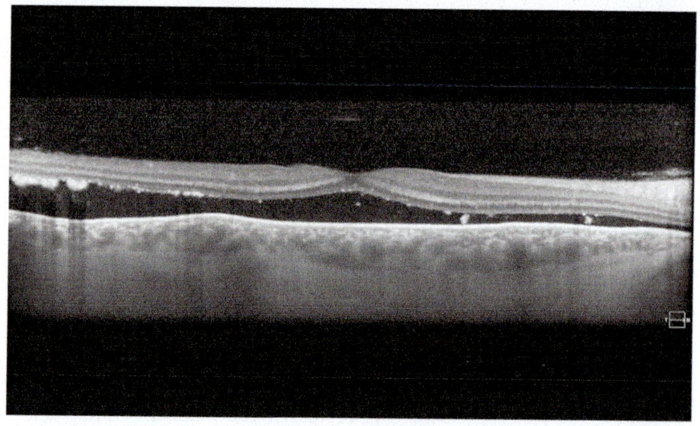

Fig. 55.14: Optical coherence tomography of choroidal melanoma demonstrating photoreceptor alterations and serous retinal detachment.

that may manifest with uveal melanoma, renal carcinoma, and other cancers passed from generation to generation.[23]

Choroidal melanoma may be detected on routine dilated retinal examination, by wide-angle nonmydriatic fundus photography, and following a change in vision or visual symptoms. The visual symptoms of choroidal melanoma depend on the tumor location and the extent of associated serous retinal detachment. Symptoms may include decreased vision, photopsias, and awareness of a blind spot. Occasionally, choroidal melanoma may present with vitreous hemorrhage; or it may be misdiagnosed as age-related macular degeneration, a choroidal hemorrhage[24] or a benign nevus.

The most important component in the evaluation of a patient with a suspected choroidal melanoma is the clinical examination. Although most choroidal melanomas are pigmented and dome-shaped, some may be minimally pigmented, variably pigmented, multilobular, diffuse, or fibrotic-looking (Fig. 55.12). The larger the tumor, the more likely it may be associated with a clinically detectable retinal detachment. It is important to keep in mind the broad spectrum of clinical appearance in choroidal melanoma.

Ultrasonography is a valuable ancillary test because information is obtained from both the B-scan (shape of the tumor) and the A-scan (internal reflectivity). The typical findings of a melanoma with ultrasonography are a dome-shaped lesion with low to medium internal reflectivity (Fig. 55.13). It is important to keep in mind, however, that the absence of these findings does not rule out a choroidal melanoma. Photos and fluorescein angiography (FA) are helpful to evaluate the level of lesion activity. An OCT evaluation of the macula and the tumor provides more subtle information regarding the disruption of the overlying retina and can indicate the presence of subretinal fluid associated with the lesion (Fig. 55.14). Subretinal fluid detected by clinical examination, ultrasonography or OCT is often a sign of tumor activity and may be concerning in a suspected case of choroidal melanoma.

Choroidal Melanoma Metastasis

Less than 5% of patients diagnosed with choroidal melanoma have clinical evidence of metastatic disease.

Among all patients with choroidal melanoma, metastatic disease occurs in at least 50%.[18] The rate of metastasis increases with longer follow-up. The risk of metastatic development is most strongly associated with larger tumor size and tumor cytogenetic profile.[25] Other risk factors associated with a higher metastatic risk are older patient age, ciliary body location, epithelioid cell type and presence of vascular loops (the latter two are determined by evaluation of an enucleated specimen).[26]

The liver is involved in over 90% of patients who develop metastasis.[26] It is believed that the metastasis occurs via hematogenous spread and that the melanoma cells lie dormant in the liver, undetectable by any current imaging modality. The lung is a known, but less common, site for metastatic spread, followed by the bone and skin. Although no systemic therapies have been demonstrated to successfully treat or significantly influence mortality from metastasis,[27] a patient with clinical metastatic disease may have several therapeutic options available, depending upon the extent of metastatic disease. Some treatments involve selective therapies to the liver. Patients must be encouraged to discuss potential therapeutic options with their oncologist, including enrolling in clinical trials.

Choroidal Melanoma Treatment

The Collaborative Ocular Melanoma Study (COMS), a multicentered, prospective, randomized clinical trial conducted in the 1990s and early 2000s, established the use of iodine-125 brachytherapy for the local treatment of choroidal melanoma. The COMS small tumor trial was mostly observational and did not achieve sufficient enrollment.[28] The COMS medium tumor trial randomized patients with tumors sized between 3 mm and 8 mm to iodine-125 plaque brachytherapy compared to enucleation and found no significant difference in mortality.[29] With no mortality benefit demonstrated by enucleating eyes with melanoma, we now recommend globe-sparing therapies when possible. The COMS large tumor trial randomized patients to enucleation alone compared to pre-enucleation radiation and found no survival advantage with the additional radiation.[30] Because of this, most centers offer enucleation alone for eyes with a large tumor (with or without extrascleral extension).

In large tumors where the vision is poor or the greatest basal dimension of the tumor exceeds the greatest plaque size diameter, enucleation is recommended. Although proton beam radiotherapy can technically treat very large melanoma, going beyond the limits possible with plaque brachytherapy, complications from neovascular glaucoma and phthisis are high given the large tumor volume that must be irradiated.[31] Many eyes come to enucleation despite these efforts to salvage the globe; and the high doses of radiation to the orbit may compromise the periorbital tissue and complicate prosthesis fitting.[32,33]

Fortunately, globe-sparing therapy is possible for most patients with choroidal melanoma. The most common and most successful therapies to treat the primary melanoma are radiation-therapy based. Brachytherapy with the radioisotope iodine-125 with intraoperative ultrasonography for optimal plaque positioning has been shown to have the lowest rates of local treatment failure.[34] Brachytherapy may also be performed with the radioisotope palladium-103. Proton beam radiotherapy is the next most common treatment method for choroidal melanoma.

Therapies that involve laser treatments, such as Visudyne photodynamic therapy or transpupillary thermotherapy, may be treatment alternatives; but these are often used as adjunctive treatment or in cases of tumor recurrence. There is a relatively high rate of local treatment failure;[35] therefore, laser treatment is less frequently a consideration for primary tumor treatment.

Several centers have reported on tumor endoresection as a technique for removing the primary tumor. However, results are variable and some centers report relatively high rates of local treatment failure.[36,37] Furthermore, these cases must be performed with hypotensive anesthesia to minimize choroidal bleeding. Hypotensive anesthesia may increase systemic risk to the patient, possibly even resulting in a stroke or a myocardial infarction; therefore, thorough consideration of the pros and cons of this treatment option must be discussed with the patient, particularly when safer and more successful therapies are readily available.

Local treatment failure, otherwise known as tumor recurrence, is a serious complication following an attempt to treat the primary tumor. Tumor recurrence carries an increased risk for subsequent ocular morbidity due to additional treatments to the eye (which often include enucleation). Patients who develop local treatment failure have a higher rate of developing metastatic spread than those whose treatments resulted in excellent local tumor control.[38] Therefore, when considering strategies to treat the primary tumor, excellent tumor control must be the most important priority.

Radiation Complications

Although radiation therapy offers the best local tumor control, radiation may damage other parts of the eye. By 3 years, almost half of those patients who have undergone iodine-125 brachytherapy have vision worse than 20/200 in the treated eye.[39] Keratitis, as well as lid and caruncular abnormalities, is more common with proton beam therapy than with plaque. Cataract, glaucoma, radiation maculopathy and ischemic vasculopathy are seen in both brachytherapy and other radiation-based treatments.[40]

Clinical features of radiation retinopathy include peripapillary cotton wool spots, retinal hemorrhages, exudates and retinal edema (Figs. 55.15A and B). FA may detect the earliest vascular changes in asymptomatic patients. The sequence of abnormality is angiographic macular edema, diffuse leaking peripheral vessels, progressive nonperfusion and proliferative radiation retinopathy (Figs. 55.16A to E).[41] Younger patients tend to have more proliferative retinopathy than older patients;[40] therefore, monitoring young patients closely with ancillary imaging studies is helpful for early detection. Sectoral and full panretinal laser photocoagulation may be considered when there is retinal ischemia.

Radiation maculopathy may be treated by antivascular endothelial growth factor (VEGF) agents; although it is not clear whether there is visual benefit beyond 2 years.[42] This underscores the importance of preventive strategies to reduce the radiation at the time of the initial treatment. Several reports have demonstrated both clinical and visual benefit to using silicone oil 1,000 centistokes (cSt) as a vitreous attenuating substance.[43-45] Vitrectomy with placement of silicone oil 1,000 cSt is performed immediately after ultrasound confirmation of the plaque to “shield” the optic nerve and macula during brachytherapy treatment. The silicone oil may be removed at the time of plaque removal or kept in place longer to tamponade serous retinal detachment while the tumor responds to treatment (Fig. 55.17).

Choroidal Metastatic Tumors

The most common intraocular tumor is a metastatic tumor from a distant primary source.[46] Breast, lung, colon and prostate cancers being common cancers must all be considered in the medical history of the patient with a possible choroidal metastasis. Often a patient will be aware of his or her cancer diagnosis; but the ocular metastatic tumor may also be the first presenting sign of metastatic disease.

Most choroidal metastatic tumors are yellow in color and are associated with mottled pigmentary change at the surface (Fig. 55.18). The borders are diffuse. There may be more than one tumor.[46] Most metastatic tumors present in the posterior pole and are associated with serous retinal detachment. B-scan ultrasonography may reveal a diffuse mass, without

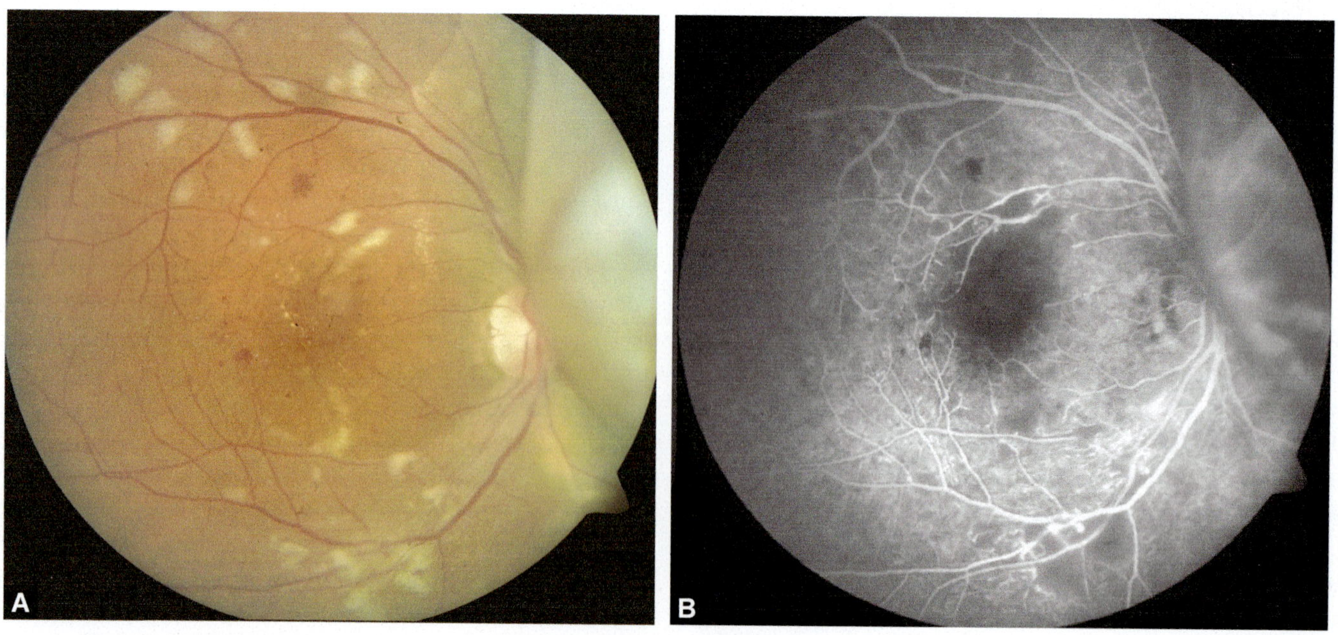

Figs. 55.15A and B: Radiation retinopathy demonstrating cotton-wool spots, retinal hemorrhages, exudates and macular ischemia.

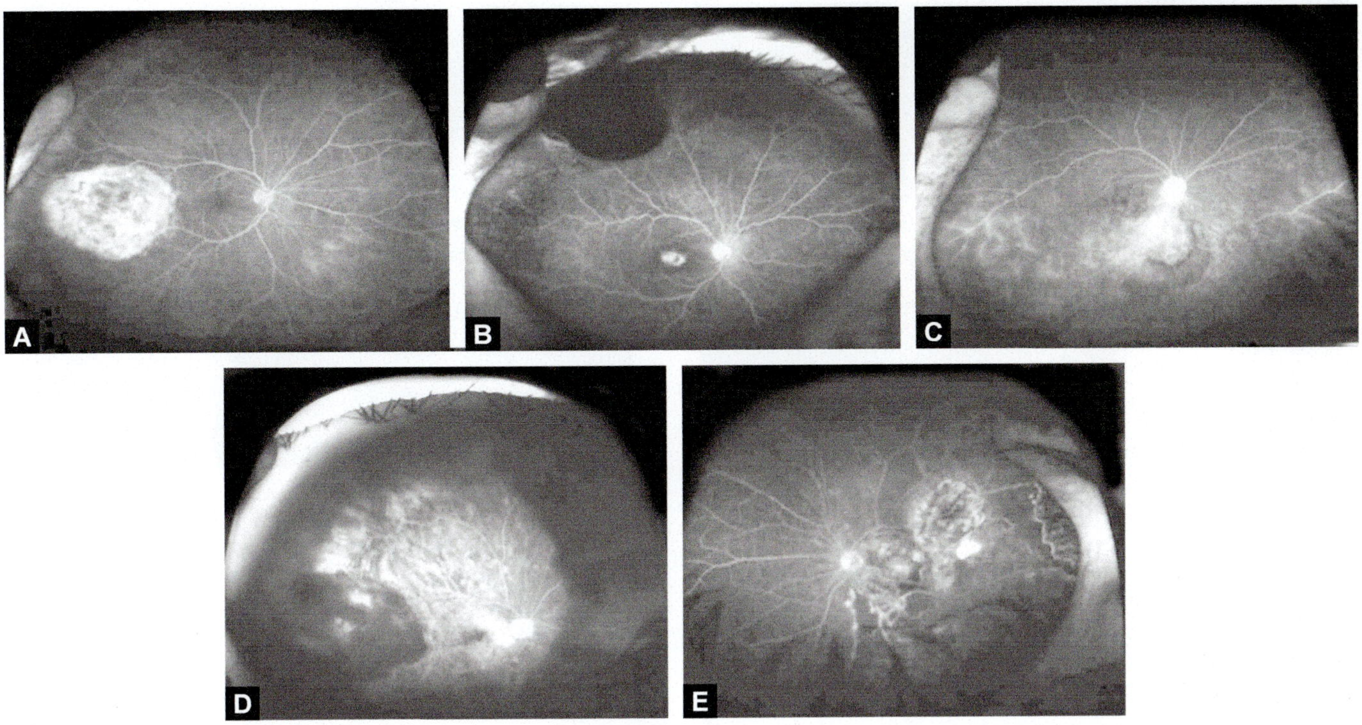

Figs. 55.16A to E: Fluorescein angiographic grading severity photo. (A) Grade 0, no vascular abnormality outside the tumor (mild nonspecific choroidal stain inferonasally, not retinal vascular leakage); (B) Grade 1, foveal leakage; (C) Grade 2, peripheral leakage; (D) Grade 3, nonperfusion; (E) Grade 4, retinal neovascularization.

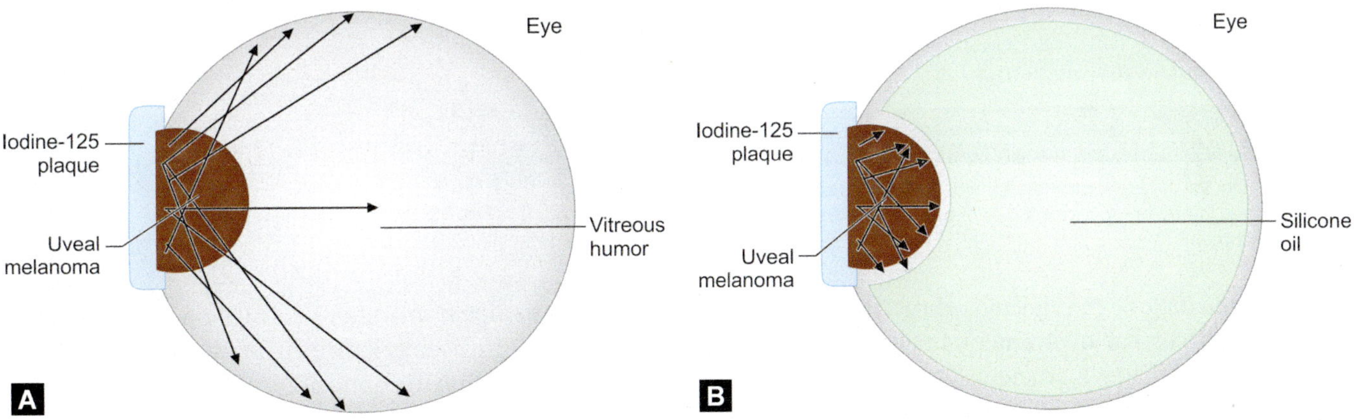

Figs. 55.17A and B: Diagram demonstrating the use of silicone oil 1,000 centistokes (green) as a vitreous substitute to attenuate radiation beyond the plaque and reduce radiation exposure of healthy tissues.

a dome-shaped appearance (Fig. 55.19). A-scan has no typical reflectivity pattern in metastatic tumors. OCT may demonstrate a "lumpy-bumpy" appearance of the choroid on enhanced depth imaging (Fig. 55.20).[47]

Occasionally, it may be difficult to distinguish the metastatic tumor from a primary uveal melanoma. A systemic baseline evaluation, including positron emission tomography-computed tomography (PET-CT) imaging, may be recommended for all diagnoses of uveal melanoma to rule out the possibility of systemic cancer.[46] Fine needle biopsy for cytopathology at the time of brachytherapy can help identify whether the tumor is primary or metastatic.

Radiation for local tumor control and visual preservation is recommended if the metastatic tumor has affected the vision. If the patient has evidence of central nervous system metastasis, external beam radiotherapy may be performed

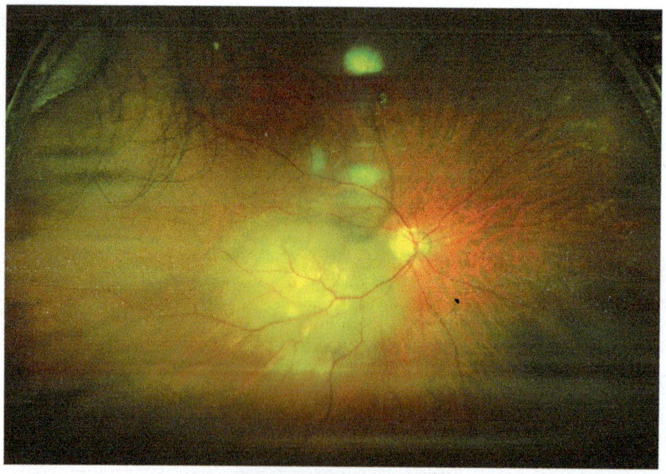

Fig. 55.18: Choroidal metastatic tumor secondary to lung cancer primary.

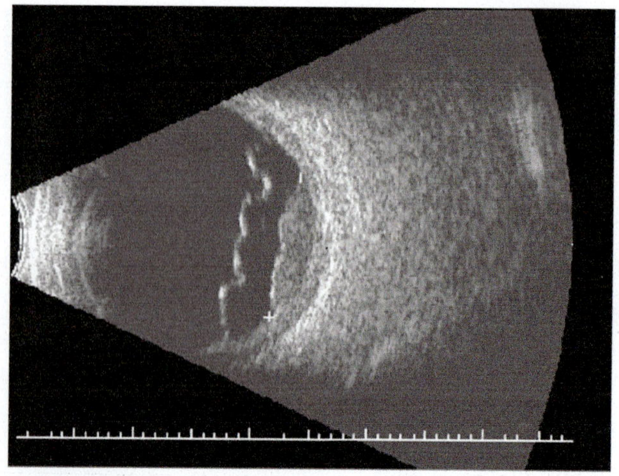

Fig. 55.19: Ultrasonography of a choroidal metastatic tumor demonstrating irregular lesion with variable reflectivities.

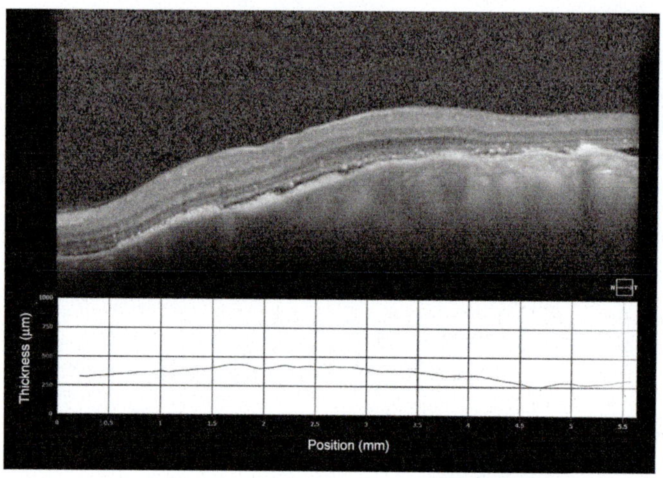

Fig. 55.20: Optical coherence tomography of choroidal metastatic tumor demonstrating lumpy-bumpy appearance of tumor associated with serous retinal detachment.

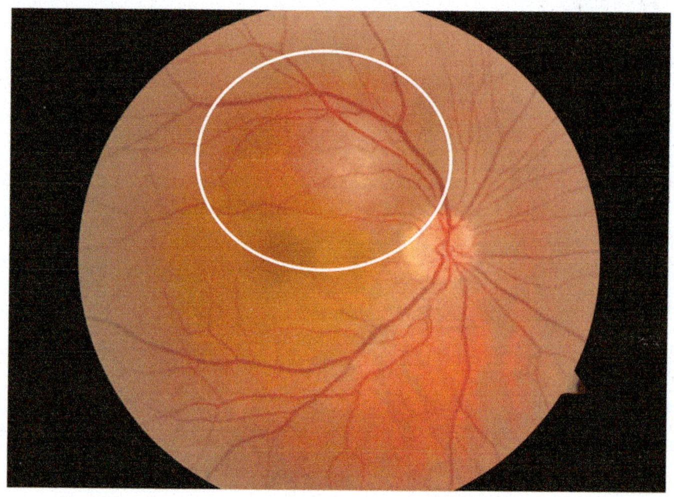

Fig. 55.21: Choroidal hemangioma.

with a plan to include the affected orbit. If the patient does not have neurological involvement, brachytherapy plaque may be able to achieve efficient local tumor control. A biopsy of the lesion is often helpful for the oncology team, particularly in establishing the extent of the cancer and the rationale for altering systemic therapy.[48]

Choroidal Hemangioma

Choroidal hemangioma is a benign vascular tumor of unknown etiology. It is often picked up on a routine dilated examination; or it may be discovered after visual symptoms occur due to the development of subretinal fluid. The distinctive feature of choroidal hemangioma is its typical orange color on fundus examination.[49] However, some choroidal hemangiomas may be pigmented, making clinical distinction from a choroidal melanoma challenging. These tumors are usually located in or near the macula and close to or involving the optic nerve (Fig. 55.21).

Ultrasonography usually reveals a dome-shaped lesion with mostly high reflectivities. OCT reveals hyper-reflective areas on the infrared reflectance image and minimal choroidal compression on enhanced depth imaging.[50]

Asymptomatic choroidal hemangiomas may be observed. Lesions that leak fluid in the macula may be considered for Visudyne photodynamic therapy, theoretically to cause occlusion of the leaking vessels.[51]

Melanocytoma

Melanocytoma is a benign pigmented lesion involving the inner retina that is most frequently found on the optic nerve

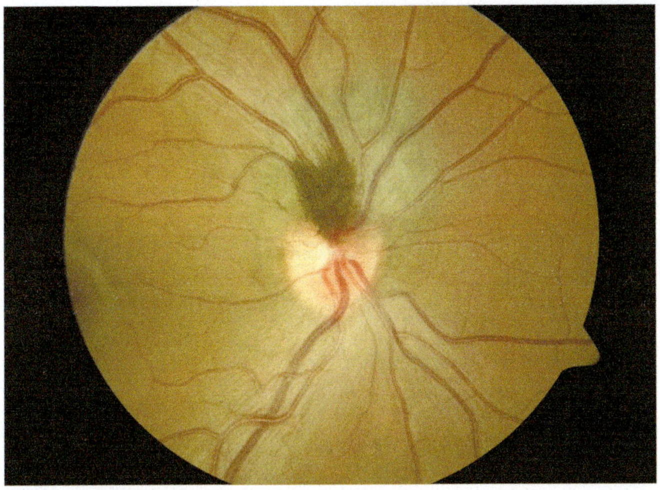

Fig. 55.22: Melanocytoma of the optic nerve head.

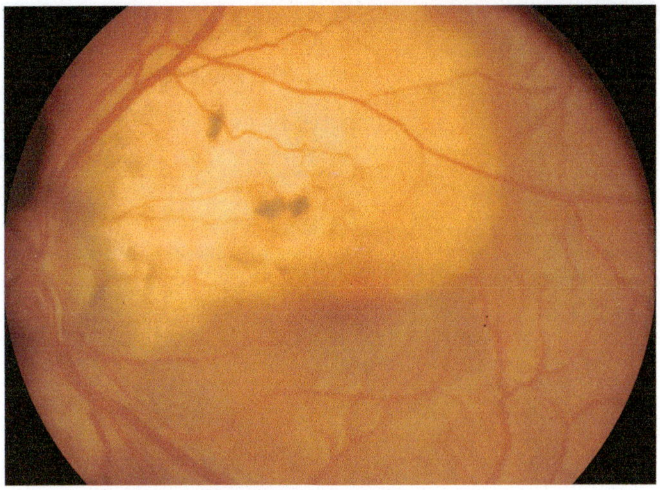

Fig. 55.23: Choroidal osteoma.

head.[52] Over time, these lesions may lose pigmentation. Unlike a melanoma, melanocytomas are rarely associated with subretinal fluid. Visual field defects have been reported in some cases of large melanocytoma. Observation alone is recommended for these lesions (Fig. 55.22).

Choroidal Osteoma

A choroidal osteoma is a benign, calcium-containing tumor often found in the macula or adjacent to the optic nerve. The osteoma demonstrates pseudopodal-type margins and is found more frequently in females (Fig. 55.23).[53] Classically, the calcium within these lesions makes for intense orbital shadowing on B-scan ultrasonography (Fig. 55.24).[54] Although initially asymptomatic, choroidal osteoma may demonstrate growth over time and cause visual decline in cases of foveal involvement. Secondary choroidal neovascularization may be treated with anti-VEGF agents. The use of Visudyne photodynamic therapy is controversial, and treatment near the fovea may result in vision decline. Periodic observation is recommended for these lesions.

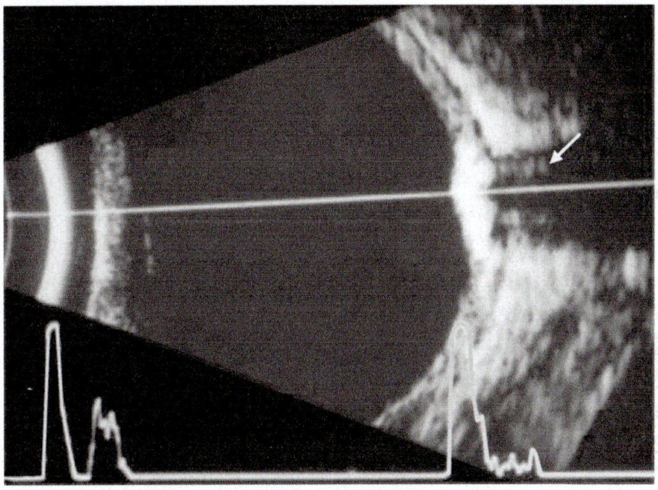

Fig. 55.24: Ultrasonography of choroidal osteoma demonstrating intense orbital shadowing secondary to presence of calcium (arrow).

RETINAL PIGMENT EPITHELIUM TUMORS

Congenital Hypertrophy of the Retinal Pigment Epithelium

Congenital hypertrophy of the retinal pigment epithelium (CHRPE) lesions are relatively common and benign. Presenting more often anterior to the equator than posterior, these lesions are characterized by well-defined borders and often appear entirely flat (Fig. 55.25). In young myopic patients of pigmented ethnicity, the vitreoretinal interface makes CHRPE lesions appear elevated on funduscopy. A white without pressure phenomenon may simulate the clinical appearance of subretinal fluid.[55] With time, CHRPE lesions may form discrete areas of depigmentation called "lacunae". Some CHRPE lesions may lose their pigmentation entirely. CHRPE lesions are almost always flat, and OCT scans through the lesion itself reveal overlying photoreceptor loss (Fig. 55.26).[56] Although most CHPRE lesions do not affect vision, CHRPE lesions in the macula may be associated with decreased vision. Periodic observation is recommended due to the rare possibility of these lesions transforming into retinal pigment epithelium (RPE) adenocarcinoma.[57]

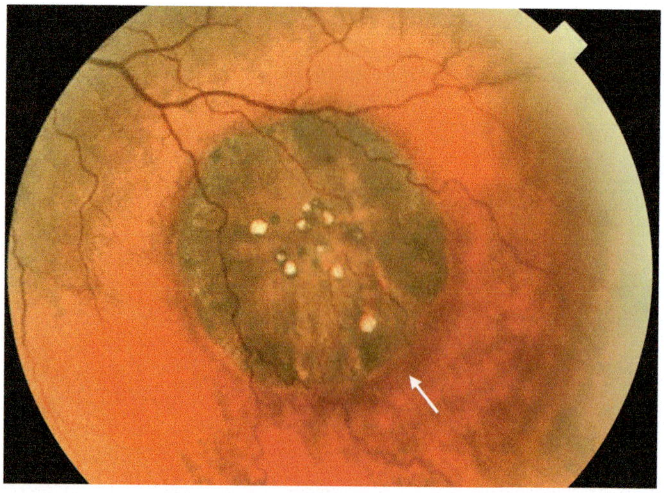

Fig. 55.25: Congenital hypertrophy of the retinal pigment epithelium (arrow).

Combined Hamartoma of the Retinal Pigment Epithelium and Retina

Combined hamartoma of the RPE and retina is often considered a pediatric condition due to the frequent association of amblyopia with the central macula and optic nerve being involved.[58] The pigmented component derives from the RPE, and the retinal component contributes to varying degrees of retinal distortion from epiretinal membrane (ERM) (Fig. 55.27).

In many cases, vitrectomy with peeling of the ERM may improve the visual acuity by reducing the retinal distortion.[59] Vitrectomy with membrane peeling for combined hamartoma of the RPE and retina may be a particularly important consideration in children, due to the greater chance of improving visual acuity with ERM removal followed by aggressive treatment of amblyopia.

Retinal Pigment Epithelium Adenoma

The RPE adenoma is an uncommon, mildly elevated, uniformly pigmented lesion of the retinal periphery with discrete borders (Fig. 55.28). There may be drusen-like deposits in the deep retina at its posterior border and some degree of ERM (often asymptomatic) of the macula may be appreciated by OCT imaging.[60] FA reveals hyperintense late leaking at the site of the lesion that is uncharacteristic of most posterior segment lesions (Figs. 55.29). RPE adenomas may depigment with time and rarely cause visual symptoms other than a mild increase in floaters due to the pigment that may shed from the lesion into the vitreous cavity.

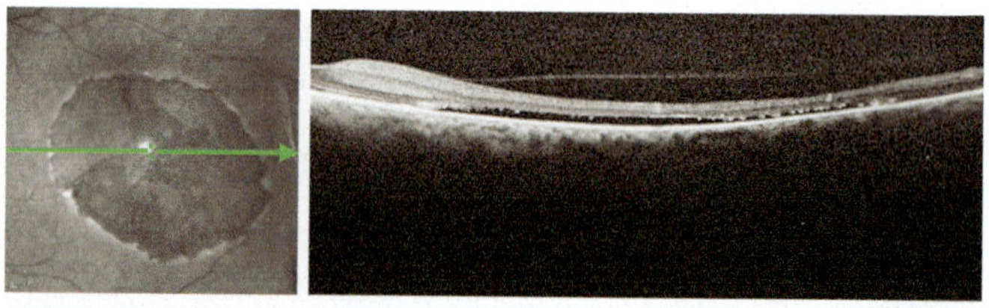

Fig. 55.26: Optical coherence tomography of a congenital hypertrophy of the retinal pigment epithelium lesion demonstrating photoreceptor loss overlying the lesion.

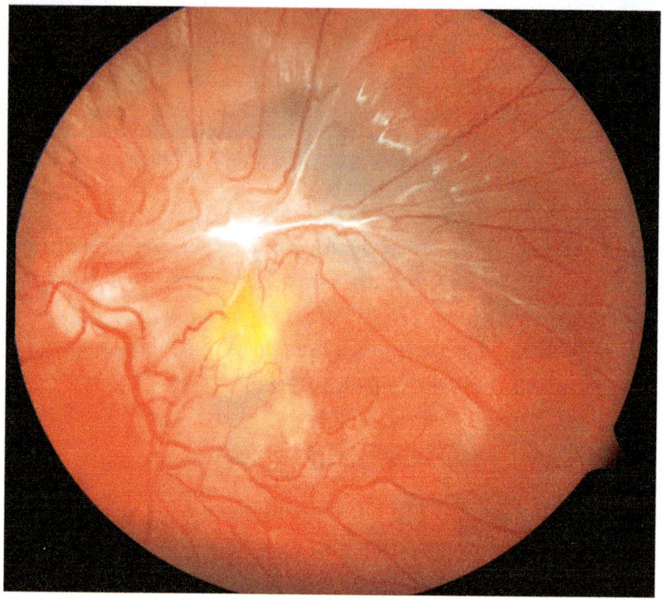

Fig. 55.27: Combined hamartoma of the retinal pigment epithelium and retina.

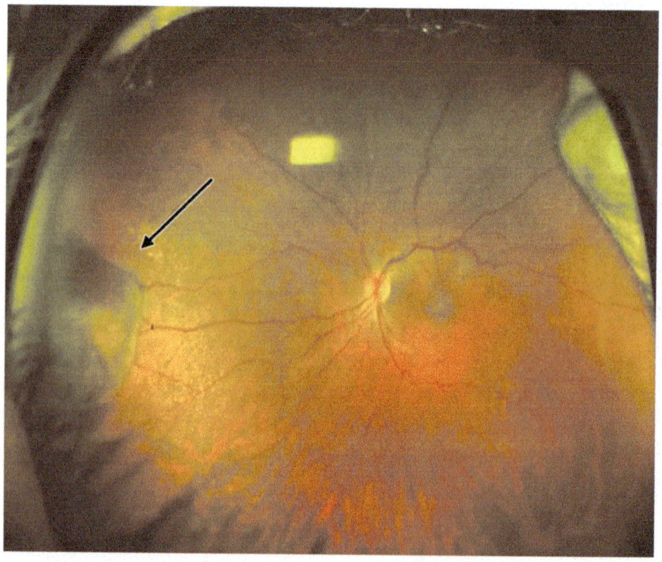

Fig. 55.28: Retinal pigment epithelial adenoma (arrow).

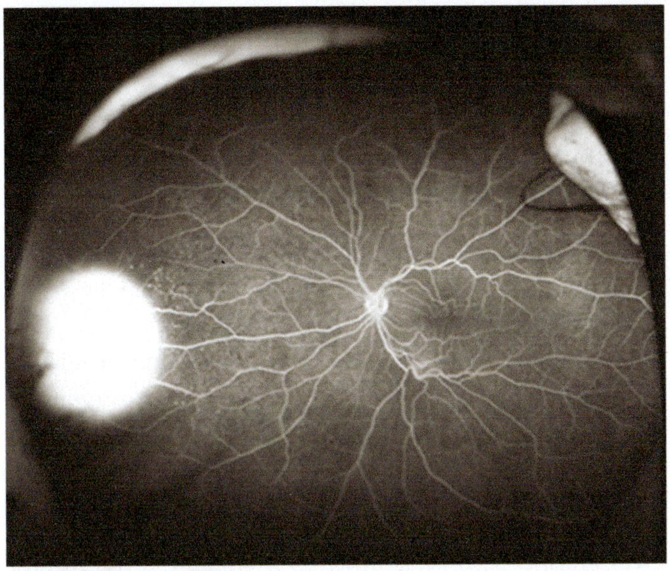

Fig. 55.29: Fluorescein angiogram of retina pigment epithelial adenoma demonstrating late intense hyperfluorescence of the lesion.

There have been rare reports of RPE adenomas transforming to malignant RPE adenocarcinomas. Periodic observation for RPE adenomas is warranted, in addition to vitrectomy with membrane peeling in cases where an ERM is associated with visual decline.[61]

RETINAL TUMORS

Retinoblastoma

Retinoblastoma is the most common intraocular primary malignancy of childhood. The incidence is 1 in 14,000–20,000 live births. The average age of unilateral retinoblastoma is 24 months. The average age of bilateral retinoblastoma is 12 months. Bilateral cases are found in 30% of all retinoblastoma.[62]

Retinoblastoma is the result of a mutation in the RB-1 gene, a tumor suppressor gene. Both alleles must be mutated to manifest the retinoblastoma phenotype (Knudson's two-hit hypothesis). Nonhereditary retinoblastoma is less common and requires mutations in both alleles of the RB-1 gene. In hereditary retinoblastoma, there is already a carrier status, where one of the alleles of the RB-1 gene is mutated. Only one spontaneous mutation of the remaining RB-1 gene is required to manifest the retinoblastoma phenotype.[63]

Retinoblastoma, and particularly nonhereditary retinoblastoma which is not anticipated, may be detected by the presentation of leukocoria (white reflex) upon evaluation of the red reflex by the pediatrician. Other clinical presentations of retinoblastoma are strabismus, red eye, heterochromia, spontaneous hyphema, and pseudohypopyon.[62] Retinoblastoma must be ruled out by a thorough dilated fundus examination, with or without anesthesia, given any of these conditions (Fig. 55.30).

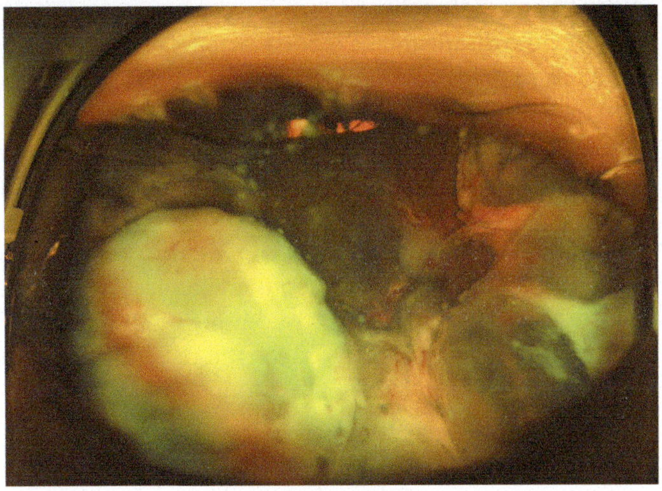

Fig. 55.30: Retinoblastoma.

The management of retinoblastoma is best delivered in a tertiary care setting and involves a team approach, including an experienced pediatric hematologist-oncologist, an ophthalmologist, a genetic counselor, and appropriate social support. Frequent examinations under anesthesia will be the mainstay of follow-up for early detection and treatment of additional tumors until the child is able to cooperate for a dilated fundus examination with scleral depression in the clinic setting.

The size and location of the tumor and the status of the fellow eye are important considerations in treatment decisions. A large tumor in a single poor-vision eye may be definitively treated by enucleation. Moderate-sized tumors may be treated with radiotherapy (external beam, proton beam). Smaller tumors may be treated with laser photocoagulation and cryotherapy. Systemic chemotherapy is frequently administered in conjunction with local ocular therapy to reduce the risk of systemic spread.[64]

Intra-arterial chemotherapy is a relatively newer method of treating the primary tumor wherein a catheter is threaded through a large artery in the inner thigh into the ophthalmic artery.[65] Melphalan is the most commonly administered drug. The advantage of intra-arterial chemotherapy may be a reduction in the systemic side effects of systemic chemotherapy and the possibility of salvaging an eye that may have otherwise been enucleated. However, the disadvantage of intra-arterial chemotherapy is the risk of inadequate primary tumor control, resulting in an increased risk of secondary cancers in a patient's life.

Patients with bilateral retinoblastoma are at a 10% increased risk for developing secondary soft tissue cancers.[66,67] Often poorly responsive to therapy, these secondary malignant cancers are osteogenic sarcomas, pinealomas, cutaneous melanomas and soft tissue sarcomas. Definitive treatment of the primary retinoblastoma is critical to reduce the risk of secondary cancers that may present later in a young patient's life.

Retinal Capillary Hemangioblastoma

Retinal capillary hemangioblastomas are often present in the retinal periphery. Presentation at the posterior fundus may also occur but is less frequent (Fig. 55.31). These vascular tumors are characterized by a red-orange mass with dilated efferent and afferent vessels. Macular exudates (macular star) may be the initial presenting sign. The natural history of retinal capillary hemangioblastomas is one of gradual growth with increasing retinal vascular exudation and serous retinal detachment. Prompt and early treatment of these lesions is recommended for both visual and ocular preservation.[68]

Retinal capillary hemangioblastomas may present as an isolated lesion in an otherwise systemically healthy individual. However, these vascular tumors may be part of von Hippel-Lindau disease, a systemic disease arising from a genetic mutation of a tumor suppressor gene on chromosome 3p.[69] Von Hippel-Lindau disease is inherited in an autosomal dominant fashion, with multiple bilateral retinal capillary hemangioblastomas and vascular tumors of the cerebellum, spine and brainstem. Patients with von Hippel-Lindau disease are also susceptible to renal cell carcinoma and pheochromocytomas and must undergo routine systemic evaluations to detect and treat these associated cancers and vascular tumors.

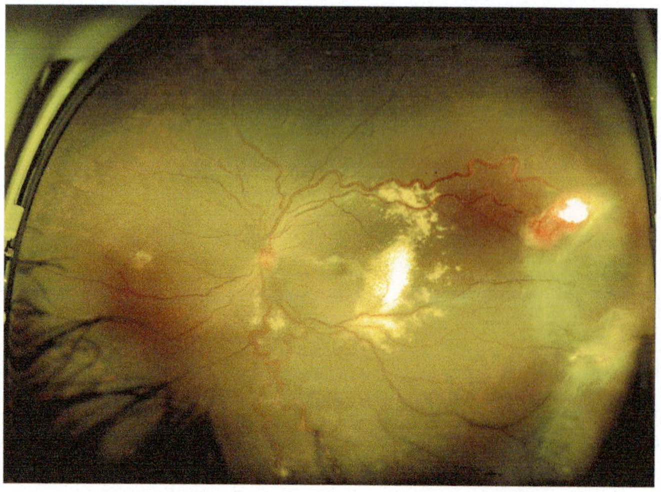

Fig. 55.31: Retinal capillary hemangioblastoma.

The treatment of retinal capillary hemangioblastomas is most successful when the tumors are small.[68] Because the natural history of retinal capillary hemangioblastoma is one of progressive growth and retinal vascular exudation, early detection with prompt treatment is imperative for visual and ocular preservation. The smallest of lesions may be treated with laser photocoagulation or cryotherapy if in the retinal periphery. Larger lesions may be treated with brachytherapy or internal cryotherapy with vitrectomy and repair of retinal detachment. Significant epiretinal proliferation with ERM must be managed at the time of vitrectomy for intraocular treatment and/or repair of retinal detachment. Screening examinations with wide-angle FA may be helpful to detect very small retinal vascular lesions that can be easily treated with laser photocoagulation.[70]

Astrocytic Hamartoma

Retinal astrocytic hamartoma is a rare tumor frequently associated with tuberous sclerosis and neurofibromatosis.[71] The retinal lesions appear white and wispy and may be evanescent in nature in early cases. In long-standing cases, calcification in a mulberry pattern is classically observed (Figs. 55.32A to C).

PARANEOPLASTIC DISORDERS

Paraneoplastic disorders of the fundus are associated with a metastatic cancer, usually previously known, and may be the presenting feature of diffuse metastasis. The exact mechanism is not entirely understood, but paraneoplastic disorders are thought to be secondary to an autoimmune response of the body against cancer antigens that have similarity to ocular tissues. Therefore, steroids are often considered in treatment of paraneoplastic disorders, in addition to management of the underlying cancer and less effective therapies such as plasmapheresis or immunoglobulin G (IgG) therapy.[72]

Vitelliform Maculopathy

Vitelliform maculopathy is almost always present in diffuse metastatic disease. Focal serous detachments with yellow material thought to be lipofuscin are present in the

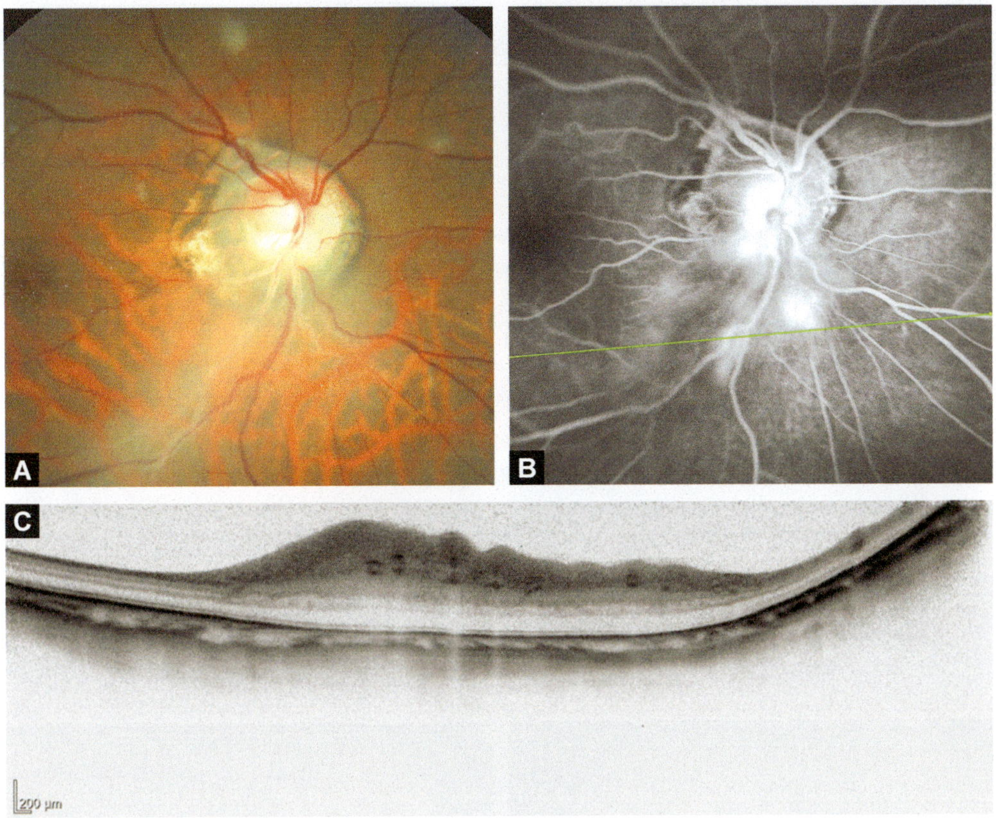

Figs. 55.32A to C: Astrocytic hamartoma.

macula.[73] Often presenting late in the course of metastatic disease, these lesions may reduce vision if there is subfoveal involvement. However, vitelliform findings may be altered by systemic therapies to the underlying cancer (Figs. 55.33A to C).

Bilateral Diffuse Uveal Melanocytic Proliferation

Multiple focal choroidal lesions, often similar in clinical appearance to uveal melanoma, comprise the clinical picture of bilateral diffuse uveal melanocytic proliferation (BDUMP).[74] The condition may be asymmetric or unilateral. However, both eyes usually demonstrate diffuse retinal pigment epitheliopathy with serous pigment epithelial detachments and retinal pigment epithelial alterations that can be observed clinically (Figs. 55.34A and B) with OCT and with FA. Serous retinal detachment may be present in advanced cases. BDUMP may also be associated with premature nuclear sclerosis of the lenses and iris cysts.[75] Management of cataract and serous retinal detachment with vitrectomy may help improve vision. However, management of the underlying cancer remains the ultimate challenge.

Cancer-Associated Retinopathy

Cancer-associated retinopathy (CAR) is frequently associated with underlying metastatic cutaneous melanoma, otherwise known also as melanoma-associated retinopathy (MAR). Unlike vitelliform maculopathy and BDUMP, which involve the RPE and choroid, CAR/MAR is an actual retinal vasculitis.[76] Clinically, patients present with bilateral decreased vision with no clear explanation on clinical examination; vessels may appear attenuated or normal in appearance. FA reveals diffusely leaking vessels and staining of the optic nerve in more clear-cut cases (Fig. 55.35).[77] Electroretinogram classically demonstrates a decrease in the B-wave.[77]

Because systemic steroids are frequently contraindicated in these patients who may be on immunotherapies to boost the immune system, periocular steroid treatment may be attempted. There have been several case reports where periocular and intravitreal steroid resulted in clinical benefit.[78] However, as in other paraneoplastic syndromes, therapies are often ineffective in improving vision for patients.

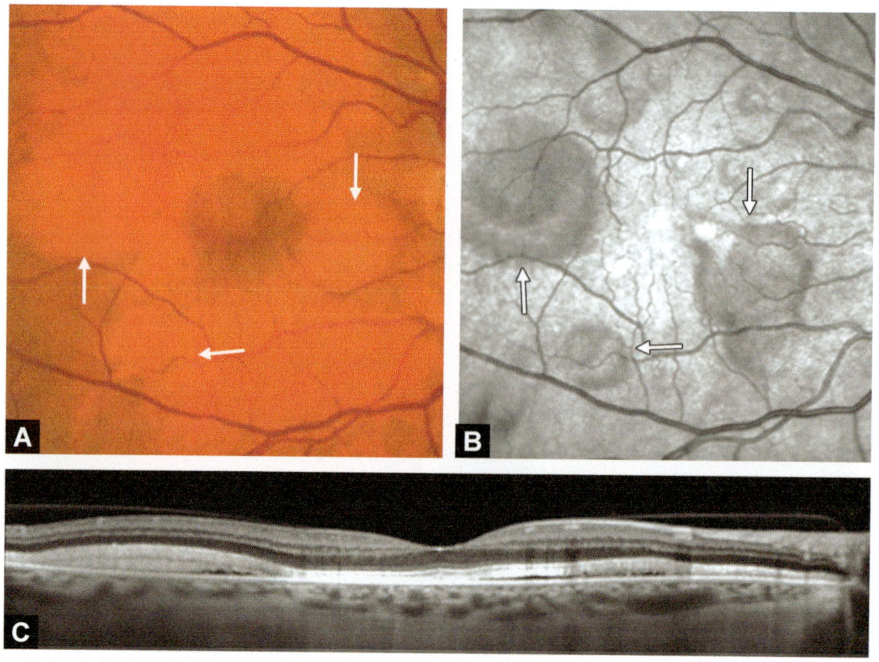

Figs. 55.33A to C: Vitelliform maculopathy. White arrows indicating lesions.

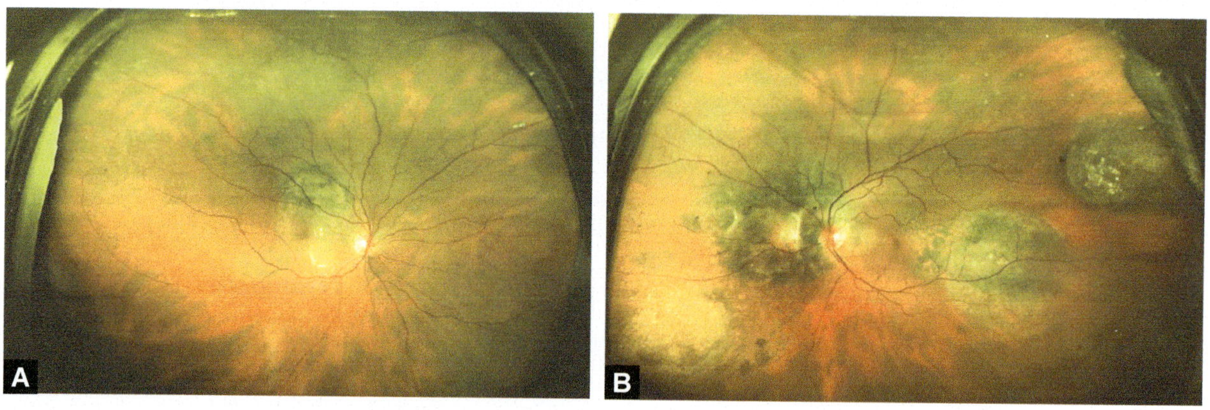

Figs. 55.34A and B: Bilateral diffuse unilateral melanocytic proliferation.

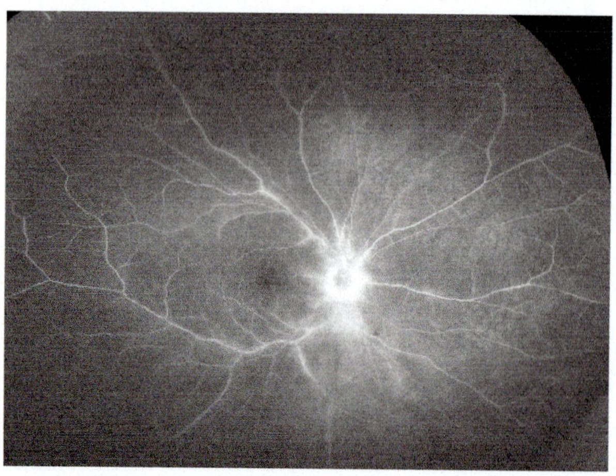

Fig. 55.35: Diffuse retinal vasculitis associated with cancer- or melanoma-associated retinopathy.

REFERENCES

1. Schwab C, Zalaudek I, Mayer C, et al. New insights into oculodermal nevogenesis and proposal for a new iris nevus classification. Br J Ophthalmol. 2015;99:644-9.
2. Shields CL, Kaliki S, Hutchinson A, et al. Iris nevus growth into melanoma: analysis of 1,611 consecutive eyes: the ABCDEF guide. Ophthalmology. 2013;120:766-72.
3. Khan S, Finger PT, Yu GP, et al. Clinical and pathologic characteristics of biopsy-proven iris melanoma: a multicenter international study. Arch Ophthalmol. 2012;130:57-64.
4. Shields CL, Shields JA, Materin M, et al. Iris melanoma: risk factors for metastasis in 169 consecutive patients. Ophthalmology. 2001;108:172-8.
5. Shields CL, Shah SU, Bianciotto CG, et al. Iris melanoma management with iodine-125 plaque radiotherapy in 144 patients: impact of melanoma-related glaucoma on outcomes. Ophthalmology. 2013;120:55-61.

6. Rahmi A, Mammar H, Thariat J, et al. Proton beam therapy for presumed and confirmed iris melanomas: a review of 36 cases. Graefes Arch Clin Exp Ophthalmol. 2014;252:1515-21.
7. Sharkawi E, Oleszczuk JD, Bergin C, et al. Baerveldt shunts in the treatment of glaucoma secondary to anterior uveal melanoma and proton beam radiotherapy. Br J Ophthalmol. 2012;96:1104-7.
8. Shields CL, Kaliki S, Crabtree GS, et al. Iris metastasis from systemic cancer in 104 patients: the 2014 Jerry A. Shields lecture. Cornea. 2015;34:42-8.
9. Georgalas I, Petrou P, Papaconstantinou D, et al. Iris cysts: a comprehensive review on diagnosis and treatment. Surv Ophthalmol. 2017. pii: S0039-6257(17)30102-9.
10. Rotsos T, Bagikos G, Christou S, et al. Free-floating iris pigmented epithelial cyst in the anterior chamber. Case Rep Ophthalmol Med. 2016;2016:4731037.
11. Al-Kahtani E, Alkatan HM. Surgical treatment and histopathology of a symptomatic free-floating primary pigment epithelial iris cyst in the anterior vitreous. Middle East Afr J Ophthalmol. 2011;18:331-2.
12. Gupta A, Bansal R, Gupta V, et al. Ocular signs predictive of tubercular uveitis. Am J Ophthalmol. 2010;149:562-70.
13. Rohrbach JM, Kröber SM, Teufel T, et al. EBV-induced polymorphic lymphoproliferative disorder of the iris after heart transplantation. Graefes Arch Clin Exp Ophthalmol. 2004;242:44-50.
14. Chien JL, Sioufi K, Surakiatchanukul T, et al. Choroidal nevus: a review of prevalence, features, genetics, risks, and outcomes. Curr Opin Ophthalmol. 2017;28:228-37.
15. Chiang A, Bianciotto C, Maguire JI, et al. Intravitreal bevacizumab for choroidal neovascularization associated with choroidal nevus. Retina. 2012;32:60-7.
16. Singh AD, Kalyani P, Topham A. Estimating the risk of malignant transformation of a choroidal nevus. Ophthalmology. 2005;112:1784-9.
17. Shields CL, Furuta M, Berman EL, et al. Choroidal nevus transformation into melanoma: analysis of 2,514 consecutive cases. Arch Ophthalmol. 2009;127:981-7.
18. Singh AD, Turell ME, Topham AK. Uveal melanoma: trends in incidence, treatment, and survival. Ophthalmology. 2011;118:1881-5.
19. Abowd MC, Black EH, Iezzi R, et al. Choroidal melanoma with massive extrascleral extension in a young black man. Ophthal Plast Reconstr Surg. 2005;21:240-2.
20. McCannel TA, Wu MY, Burgess BL. Clinical and cytogenetic characteristics of choroidal melanoma in Vietnamese Asians. Mol Vis. 2011;17:231-6.
21. Singh AD, Bergman L, Seregard S. Uveal melanoma: epidemiologic aspects. Ophthalmol Clin North Am. 2005;18:75-84.
22. Plateroti AM, Scavella V, Abdolrahimzadeh B. An update on oculodermal melanocytosis and rare associated conditions. Semin Ophthalmol. 2017;32:524-8.
23. Rao R, Pointdujour-Lim R, Ganguly A, et al. Multifocal melanoma in a patient with germ line BRCA-associated protein 1 mutation. Retin Cases Brief Rep. 2018;12(1):1-4.
24. Cunliffe IA, Rennie IG. Choroidal melanoma presenting as vitreous haemorrhage. Eye (Lond). 1993;7(Pt 5):711-3.
25. Onken MD, Worley LA, Ehlers JP, et al. Gene expression profiling in uveal melanoma reveals two molecular classes and predicts metastatic death. Cancer Res. 2004;64:7205-9.
26. Kaliki S, Shields CL, Shields JA. Uveal melanoma: estimating prognosis. Indian J Ophthalmol. 2015;63:93-102.
27. Diener-West M, Hawkins BS, Markowitz JA, et al. A review of mortality from choroidal melanoma. II. A meta-analysis of 5-year mortality rates following enucleation, 1966 through 1988. Arch Ophthalmol. 1992;110:245-50.
28. Mortality in patients with small choroidal melanoma: COMS report no. 4. The Collaborative Ocular Melanoma Study Group. Arch Ophthalmol. 1997;115:886-93.
29. Melia BM, Abramson DH, Albert DM, et al. Collaborative Ocular Melanoma Study (COMS) randomized trial of I-125 brachytherapy for medium choroidal melanoma. I. Visual acuity after 3 years. COMS report no. 16. Ophthalmology. 2001;108:348-66.
30. The Collaborative Ocular Melanoma Study (COMS) randomized trial of pre-enucleation radiation of large choroidal melanoma II: initial mortality findings. COMS report no. 10. Am J Ophthalmol. 1998;125:779-96.
31. Bensoussan E, Thariat J, Maschi C, et al. Outcomes after proton beam therapy for large choroidal melanomas in 492 patients. Am J Ophthalmol. 2016;165:78-87.
32. Munzenrider JE, Verhey LJ, Gragoudas ES, et al. Conservative treatment of uveal melanoma: local recurrence after proton beam therapy. Int J Radiat Oncol Biol Phys. 1989;17:493-8.
33. Jeganathan VS, Wirth A, MacManus MP. Ocular risks from orbital and periorbital radiation therapy: a critical review. Int J Radiat Oncol Biol Phys. 2011;79:650-9.
34. Lin AJ, Rao YJ, Acharya S, et al. Patterns of care and outcomes of proton and eye plaque brachytherapy for uveal melanoma: review of the National Cancer Database. Brachytherapy. 2017;16:1225-31.
35. Canal-Fontcuberta I, Salomão DR, Robertson D, et al. Clinical and histopathologic findings after photodynamic therapy of choroidal melanoma. Retina. 2012;32:942-8.
36. Chang MY, McCannel TA. Local treatment failure after globe-conserving therapy for choroidal melanoma. Br J Ophthalmol. 2013;97:804-11.
37. Karkhaneh R, Chams H, Amoli FA, et al. Long-term surgical outcome of posterior choroidal melanoma treated by endoresection. Retina. 2007;27:908-14.
38. Ophthalmic Oncology Task Force. Local recurrence significantly increases the risk of metastatic uveal melanoma. Ophthalmology. 2016;123:86-91.
39. Quinlan-Davidson S, AlMahmoud T, Shenouda G, et al. Intraoperative sonographically assisted radioactive iodine-125 plaque brachytherapy for choroidal melanoma: visual acuity outcome. J Ultrasound Med. 2013;32:995-1001.
40. Mendez CA, Singh AD. Radiation therapy: anterior segment complications. Dev Ophthalmol. 2013;52:102-13.
41. McCannel TA, Kim E, Kamrava M, et al. New ultra-wide-field angiographic grading scheme for radiation retinopathy after iodine-125 brachytherapy for uveal melanoma. Retina. 2017.
42. Wen JC, McCannel TA. Treatment of radiation retinopathy following plaque brachytherapy for choroidal melanoma. Curr Opin Ophthalmol. 2009;20:200-4.

43. McCannel TA, McCannel CA. Iodine 125 brachytherapy with vitrectomy and silicone oil in the treatment of uveal melanoma: 1-to-1 matched case-control series. Int J Radiat Oncol Biol Phys. 2014;89:347-52.
44. Oliver SC, Leu MY, DeMarco JJ, et al. Attenuation of iodine-125 radiation with vitreous substitutes in the treatment of uveal melanoma. Arch Ophthalmol. 2010;128:888-93.
45. Ahuja Y, Kapoor KG, Thomson RM, et al. The effects of intraocular silicone oil placement prior to iodine 125 brachytherapy for uveal melanoma: a clinical case series. Eye (Lond). 2012;26:1487-9.
46. Konstantinidis L, Damato B. Intraocular metastases: a review. Asia Pac J Ophthalmol (Phila). 2017;6:208-14.
47. Al-Dahmash SA, Shields CL, Kaliki S, et al. Enhanced depth imaging optical coherence tomography of choroidal metastasis in 14 eyes. Retina. 2014;34:1588-93.
48. Konstantinidis L, Rospond-Kubiak I, Zeolite I, et al. Management of patients with uveal metastases at the Liverpool Ocular Oncology Centre. Br J Ophthalmol. 2014;98:92-8.
49. Shields CL, Hanaver SG, Shields JA, et al. Circumscribed choroidal hemangioma: clinical manifestations and factors predictive of visual outcome in 200 consecutive cases. Ophthalmology. 2001;108:2237-48.
50. Rojanaporn D, Kaliki S, Ferenczy SR, et al. Enhanced depth imaging optical coherence tomography of circumscribed choroidal hemangioma in 10 consecutive cases. Middle East Afr J Ophthalmol. 2015;22:192-7.
51. Singh AD, Kaiser PK, Sears JE, et al. Photodynamic therapy of circumscribed choroidal haemangioma. Br J Ophthalmol. 2004;88:1414-8.
52. Shields JA, Demirci H, Mashayekhi, et al. Melanocytoma of optic disc in 115 cases: the 2004 Samuel Johnson Memorial Lecture, part 1. Ophthalmology. 2004;111:1739-46.
53. Alameddine RM, Mansour AM, Kahtani E. Review of choroidal osteomas. Middle East Afr J Ophthalmol. 2014;21:244-50.
54. Shields CL, Sun H, Demirci H, et al. Factors predictive of tumor growth, tumor decalcification, choroidal neovascularization, and visual outcome in 74 eyes with choroidal osteoma. Arch Ophthalmol. 2005;123:1658-66.
55. Shields CL, Mashayekhi A, Ho T, et al. Solitary congenital hypertrophy of the retinal pigment epithelium clinical features and frequency of enlargement in 330 patients. Ophthalmology. 2003;110:1968-76.
56. Shields CL, Materin MA, Walker C, et al. Photoreceptor loss overlying congenital hypertrophy of the retinal pigment epithelium by optical coherence tomography. Ophthalmology. 2006;113:661-5.
57. Trichopoulos N, Augsburger JJ, Schneider S. Adenocarcinoma arising from congenital hypertophy of the retinal pigment epithelium. Graefes Arch Clin Exp Ophthalmol. 2006;244:125-8.
58. Shields CL, Manalac J, Das C, et al. Review of spectral domain-enhanced depth imaging optical coherence tomography of tumors of the retina and retinal pigment epithelium in children and adults. Indian J Ophthalmol. 2015;63:128-32.
59. Benhamou N, Massin P, Spolaore R, et al. Surgical management of epiretinal membrane in young patients. Am J Ophthalmol. 2002;133:358-64.
60. Shields JA, Shields CL. Tumors and related lesions of the pigmented epithelium. Asia Pac J Ophthalmol (Phila). 2017;6:215-23.
61. Cupp DG, McCannel TA. Macular pucker in association with RPE adenoma: a report of a case and review of the literature. Semin Ophthalmol. 2014;29:199-201.
62. Pandey AN. Retinoblastoma: an overview. Saudi J Ophthalmol. 2014;28:310-5.
63. Knudson AG Jr. Mutation and cancer: statistical study of retinoblastoma. Proc Natl Acad Sci U S A. 1971;68:820-3.
64. Cassoux N, Lumbroso L, Levy-Gabriel C, et al. Retinoblastoma: update on current management. Asia Pac J Ophthalmol (Phila). 2017;6:290-5.
65. Wyse E, Handa JT, Friedman AD, et al. A review of the literature for intra-arterial chemotherapy used to treat retinoblastoma. Pediatr Radiol. 2016;46:1223-33.
66. Friend SH, Bernards R, Rogelj S, et al. A human DNA segment with properties of the gene that predisposes to retinoblastoma and osteosarcoma. Nature. 1986;323:643-6.
67. Kamihara J, Bourdeaut F, Foulkes WD, et al. Retinoblastoma and neuroblastoma predisposition and surveillance. Clin Cancer Res. 2017;23:e98-106.
68. Lefevre A, Mathis T, Denis P, et al. Retinal hemangioblastoma: treatment strategy and long-term follow-up in a retrospective cohort. J Fr Ophtalmol. 2017. pii: S0181-5512(17)30441-2.
69. Chan CC, Collins AB, Chew EY. Molecular pathology of eyes with von Hippel-Lindau (VHL) disease: a review. Retina. 2007;27:1-7.
70. Shuin T, Yamasaki I, Tamura K, et al. Von Hippel-Lindau disease: molecular pathological basis, clinical criteria, genetic testing, clinical features of tumors and treatment. Jpn J Clin Oncol. 2006;36:337-43.
71. Aronow ME, Nakagawa JA, Gupta A, et al. Tuberous sclerosis complex: genotype/phenotype correlation of retinal findings. Ophthalmology. 2012;119:1917-23.
72. Pelosof LC, Gerber DE. Paraneoplastic syndromes: an approach to diagnosis and treatment. Mayo Clin Proc. 2010;85:838-54.
73. Al-Dahmash SA, Shields CL, Bianciotto CG, et al. Acute exudative paraneoplastic polymorphous vitelliform maculopathy in five cases. Ophthalmic Surg Lasers Imaging. 2012;43:366-73.
74. Rahimy E, Coffee RE, McCannel TA. Bilateral diffuse uveal melanocytic proliferation as a precursor to multiple systemic malignancies. Semin Ophthalmol. 2015;30:206-9.
75. Joseph A, Rahimy E, Sarraf D. Bilateral diffuse uveal melanocytic proliferation with multiple iris cysts. JAMA Ophthalmol. 2014;132:756-60.
76. Grewal DS, Fishman GA, Jampol LM. Autoimmune retinopathy and antiretinal antibodies: a review. Retina. 2014;34:827-45.
77. Shildkrot Y, Sobrin L, Gragoudas ES. Cancer-associated retinopathy: update on pathogenesis and therapy. Semin Ophthalmol. 2011;26:321-8.
78. Javaid Z, Rehan SM, Al-Bermani A, et al. Unilateral cancer-associated retinopathy: a case report. Scott Med J. 2016;61:155-9.

Chapter 56

Vitreoretinal Interface Diseases of the Macula

Alain Gaudric, Elise Philippakis

INTRODUCTION

The vitreoretinal interface consists of vitreous cortex, retinal internal limiting membrane (ILM), and Müller cell footplates. During embryogenesis, the Müller cells are involved in the synthesis of vitreous fibrils of the secondary vitreous and start to form the ILM.

The posterior vitreous cortex (PVC) is attached to the ILM by macromolecules such as laminin, fibronectin, chondroitin, and heparan sulfate proteoglycans, as well as other extracellular matrix proteins. The presence of different types of collagen, including types II, VI, VII, and XVIII has been shown in the vitreoretinal interface. Types VI and XVIII collagens are also widely expressed in the ILM and could thus be involved in the anchoring of the ILM and vitreous cortex. Lastly, the PVC contains a few cells called hyalocytes, the role of which in various vitreoretinal diseases has not been fully elucidated.[1-3] It is therefore not surprising that many retinal diseases involve both the inner retina and the PVC.

NORMAL VITREORETINAL INTERFACE ON OPTICAL COHERENCE TOMOGRAPHY

The posterior vitreous may be analyzed by spectral domain optical coherence tomography (SD-OCT) or swept-source (SwS) OCT,[4] which provides B-scans of 6,12, and even 15 mm long.[5] However, the depth of the window in which the vitreous may be imaged, even with SwS-OCT, does not exceed 2 mm, so most of the vitreous gel cannot be examined.

Structure of the Attached Posterior Vitreous Cortex on Optical Coherence Tomography

In young subjects, the PVC is still completely attached to the retina. It is usually not visible on the central 3 mm OCT B-scan centered on the fovea because it is too thin and too tightly attached to the retinal surface to give a signal independent of the ILM. However, on longer scans, it becomes progressively thicker from the foveal center and gives a faintly hyper-reflective laminated signal. The PVC, later described as the posterior precortical vitreous cortex,[6] constitutes the posterior wall of the premacular bursa,[7] which measures about 7 mm in width on a horizontal B-scan, 9 mm on a vertical scan, and about 0.6 mm in height when measurable.[8] The height of the premacular bursa may vary considerably with the axial length.[9]

Anteriorly, the formed vitreous constitutes the inner wall of the bursa. On a horizontal B-scan, the premacular bursa ends on the wall of the Cloquet's canal, which limits the area of Martegiani in front of the optic nerve. The fact that the PVC is connected to the wall of the Cloquet's canal has surgical implications. After core vitrectomy, pulling on the remnants of the Cloquet's canal is a good technique to detach "en bloc" the Weiss' ring and the PVC. It has also been shown, using multiple scans centered on the macula and the optic disk, that the superior part of the premacular bursa is connected to the Cloquet's canal at a variable distance above the optic disk.[8] However, this interpretation is controversial, and the premacular bursa may connect to another cavity, the canalis ciliobursalis, as described by Worst.[10,11] Both assumptions suggest that the premacular space could be connected to the retrolental space via intravitreal channels (Figs. 56.1A and B).

Steps in the Aging Process of Posterior Vitreous Detachment and Vitreomacular Adhesion

A posterior vitreous detachment (PVD) is a progressive process, which starts in the fifth decade of life and ultimately results, as the eye ages, in complete detachment of the vitreous cortex from the optic disk and retina up to the equator. The process is asymptomatic, taking years to decades before it is complete. Complete PVD is

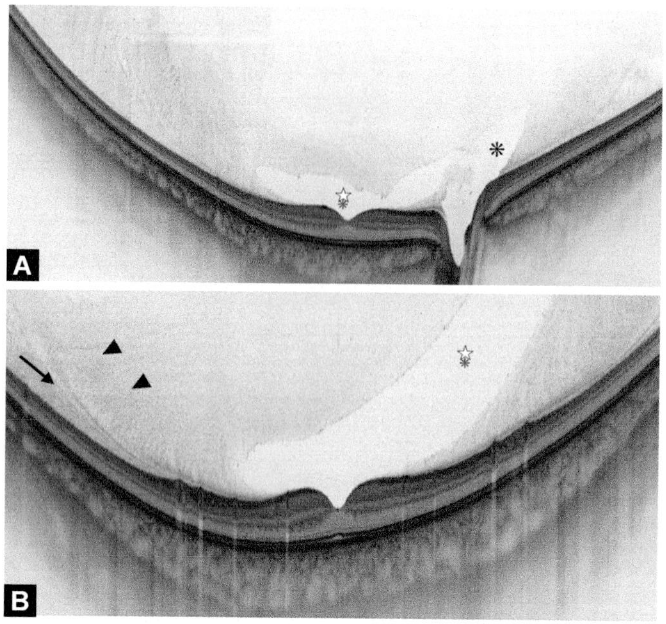

Figs. 56.1A and B: Normal vitreous in a young subject on swept-source OCT B-scan. (A) *Horizontal 12 mm B-scan:* Premacular bursa in front of the macula (star) and Cloquet's canal (asterisk); (B) *Vertical B-scan:* Vertical extension of the premacular bursa (star) that is connected to the Cloquet's canal. Note the laminated posterior vitreous cortex (arrow) to which the fibrils of the vitreous body converge (arrowheads).

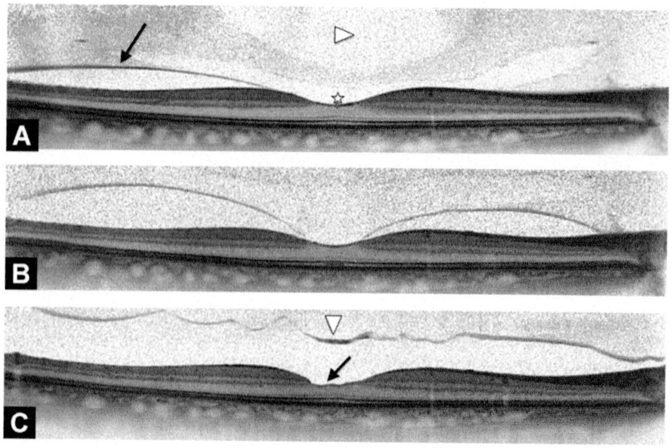

Figs. 56.2A to C: Steps of posterior vitreous detachment in the fellow eye of a 62-year-old woman. (A) Partial detachment of the posterior vitreous cortex on the temporal side of the posterior pole (arrow). The premacular bursa is present in front of the macula (star). Note the presence of a lacuna more centrally in the vitreous body (arrowhead); (B) Perifoveal vitreous detachment with normal foveal surface (vitreomacular adhesion); (C) Macular detachment of the posterior vitreous cortex with persistent attachment to the optic disc. A pseudo-operculum is visible attached to the posterior vitreous cortex (arrowhead), and corresponds to a discrete foveal defect (arrow).

often indicated by the appearance of a Weiss' ring, the symptomatic end of the long and silent process.[12-14]

Why the PVC loses its adhesion to the retina is not really understood. It is usually assumed that a vitreous gel liquefaction and concurrent weakening of the vitreoretinal adhesion result in a nonpathologic PVD.[15] However, the relationship between the vitreous gel liquefaction and the progressive detachment of the PVC remains unclear. Lastly, the origin of the forces exerted on the retina at the sites where the PVC is still attached remains unclear.

Imaging of the vitreomacular interface with OCT reveals that the PVD begins in the perifoveal macula. The vitreoretinal separation is usually asymmetric, starting in a sector of the perimacular area and extending contiguously to other quadrants. The vitreous cortex ultimately detaches from the fovea and then from the optic disk (Figs. 56.2A to C).

The situation in which the PVC still adheres to the fovea but is detached from the rest of the posterior pole is called "perifoveal vitreous detachment" or "vitreomacular adhesion (VMA)".[16] The foveal profile remains normal on OCT; the concavity of the foveal surface is unchanged; and no intrafoveal structural change is visible.

However, the PVC may sometimes remain firmly attached to the retina, mainly at the fovea or along the temporal vascular arcades and around the optic disk. In this situation, the retinal surface may be focally elevated at the site of vitreous adhesion, which defines the vitreomacular traction (VMT).

PRIMARY VITREOMACULAR ADHESION AND VITREOMACULAR TRACTION

Prevalence

Vitreomacular adhesion without traction is relatively common and has been found in 26% of subjects aged 63 years or more. Conversely, VMT is rare and has been reported in only 1.6% of subjects in the same study.[17]

Aspects of Vitreomacular Adhesion

Vitreomacular adhesion is a perifoveal vitreous detachment that has been redefined by anatomical features detected by OCT.[16] This stage, referred to as stage 1 PVD, has been illustrated by various diagrams.[12,14] The concept of VMA refers to two different steps in the evolution of the vitreoretinal adhesion. In young subjects, the vitreous cortex is completely attached to the retinal surface. The PVC is well identified by SD-OCT, and even better SwS-OCT. On the posterior pole, PVC appears as a multilayered structure faintly reflective on the retinal surface. On horizontal scans, the PVC appears symmetrically thicker near the optic disk and in temporal of the macula when it becomes thinner on the margin of the macula and invisible in the foveal pit. The fibrils of the vitreous body are obliquely attached to the vitreous cortex. In front of the macula, the bursa premacularis forms an empty space (Figs. 56.1A and B).

Later in life, the vitreous cortex starts to separate from the macular surface without any anomaly of the retinal structure. The term "VMA" also applies to this specific stage of vitreous separation during which a partial detachment of the vitreous in the perifoveal area has occurred without structural change in the retina.[16]

When the PVC starts to detach from the retina, its posterior surface becomes visible on OCT B-scan as a new interface in front of the retina, including its prefoveal portion, which did not signal on OCT when it was completely attached (*see* Figs. 56.2A to C). On OCT, the posterior surface of the detached vitreous cortex is smooth and hyper-reflective, and it outlines a concave curve toward the retinal surface. It should be noted, however, that while the vitreous cortex appears as a coherent structure, fully detached from the retina, histologically a thin layer of vitreous collagen fibers remains attached to the retinal surface after PVD.[18] This may be the case in particular when the detached PVC is broken in front of the macula (Fig. 56.3).

Vitreomacular adhesion, which is a natural process in healthy eyes, may also be associated with macular abnormalities, including age-related macular degeneration, retinal vein occlusion (RVO), diabetic macular edema, or other disorders, without being the causative agent of these conditions.

This chapter is focused on primary retinal disorders caused by an abnormal PVD at the posterior pole.

Aspects of the Vitreomacular Traction

The difference between VMA and VMT relies on the analysis of OCT B-scans. The characterization of VMA and VMT has evolved with the improvement of OCT resolution with SD- and SwS-OCT devices.

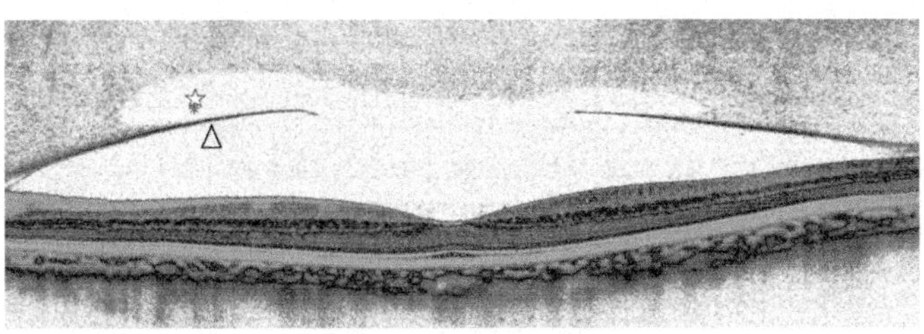

Fig. 56.3: Posterior vitreous detachment with central opening of the posterior vitreous cortex. The hyper-reflective posterior vitreous cortex (arrow) is detached from the retinal surface. The content of the premacular bursa (star) communicates with the retrohyaloidal space. Note that the foveal profile remains normal.

The vitreous is supposed to exert traction on the macula when changes in the foveal contour or intraretinal foveal anomalies occur. High-resolution B-scans and the analysis of tight raster scans allow detection of minute changes, the clinical significance of which is somewhat uncertain. In more advanced stages of traction, the foveal floor may be elevated above the level of the surrounding retinal surface, in association with intraretinal structural anomalies, including pseudocyst formation. Ultimately, the central photoreceptors may detach from the retinal pigment epithelium (RPE).

According to the International VMT Study Group classification of VMA, traction and macular hole (MH),[16] all of the following anatomical criteria should appear on at least one B-mode OCT scan for an eye to be classified as having VMT:

- Evidence of perifoveal vitreous cortex detachment from the retinal surface
- Macular attachment of the vitreous cortex within a 3 mm radius from the fovea
- Attachment associated with distortion of the foveal surface or elevation of the foveal floor (no full-thickness disruption of all macular layers of the RPE).

Vitreomacular traction may be isolated or associated with an epiretinal membrane (ERM) proliferation; or it may occur in the fellow eye of a patient with a MH.

Simple Vitreomacular Traction

Simple VMT refers to the condition in which the distortion of the macular surface or structure is only due to the persistence of an abnormal vitreofoveal attachment without any epiretinal proliferation or posterior hyaloid thickening. The absence of an ERM is confirmed when reading the en-face OCT image of the macula, which shows a smooth retinal surface without any folds (Figs. 56.4A to D). This phenomenon may worsen (Figs. 56.5A and B) or resolve spontaneously[19] and may be more responsive to enzymatic or gas vitreolysis. It may be symptomatic or it may be discovered fortuitously.

Vitreomacular Traction Associated with an Epiretinal Membrane

In other cases, VMT is associated with an ERM. The sequence of events resulting in this association is unknown; it is

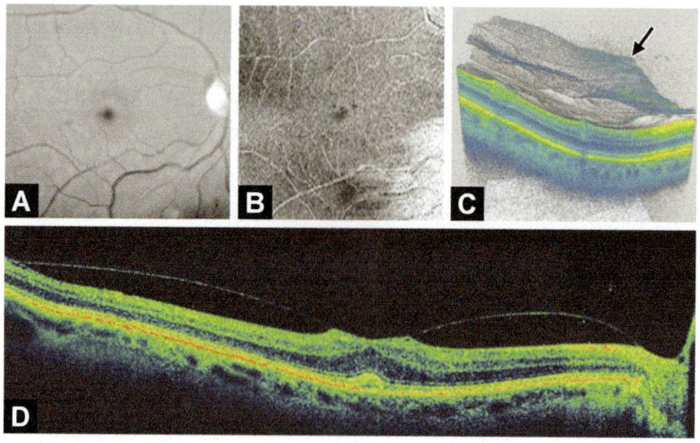

Figs. 56.4A to D: Early vitreomacular traction. (A) Blue reflectance fundus photograph showing the absence of retinal folds; (B) Enface optical coherence tomography (OCT) showing a smooth retinal surface; (C) Three-dimensional OCT showing the cone of the partially detached posterior vitreous cortex (PVC) adhering to the elevated fovea; (D) Horizontal B-scan showing the thin posterior vitreous cortex (PVC) attached to the elevated fovea.

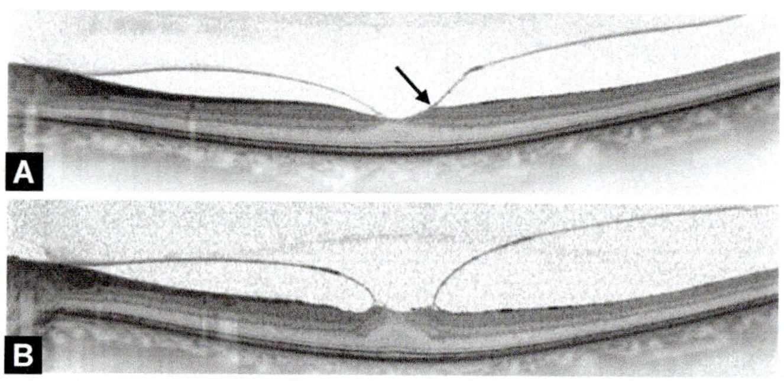

Figs. 56.5A and B: Worsening of a vitreomacular traction (VMT) over 6 months. (A) Discrete irregularity of the foveal edge at an attachment area of the posterior vitreous cortex (arrow); (B) 6 months later, worsening of the VMT with elevation of the fovea.

most likely due to proliferation of the ERM concomitantly with the appearance of a chronic and progressive VMT. The diagnosis is made based on OCT. On the B-scan, an ERM is visible as a hyper-reflective structure at the retina surface, which reflects on the posterior face of the PVC at its junction with the retina, lining the detached vitreous cortex, which appears thickened and hyper-reflective.[20] En-face OCT clearly shows the retinal folds induced by the ERM contraction (Figs. 56.6 and 56.7). VMT may also result in cystoid macular changes, with or without fluorescein leakage (Figs. 56.7 and 56.8). Histologically, this corresponds to proliferation of a fibrocellular ERM on vitreous collagen remnants lying at the retinal surface and along the detached PVC.[20,21] In this situation, a spontaneous resolution is unlikely, and the efficacy of vitreolysis is reduced.[22]

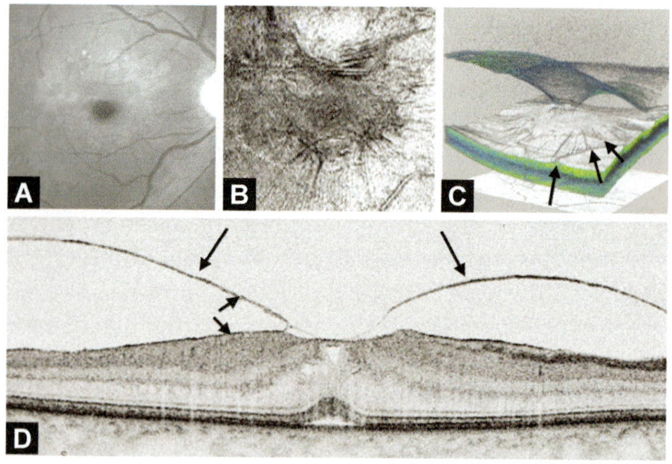

Figs. 56.6A to D: Vitreomacular traction associated with epiretinal membrane (ERM). (A) Blue reflectance fundus photograph showing the hyper-reflectivity of an ERM; (B) En-face optical coherence tomography (OCT) showing the retinal folds induced by the ERM contraction; (C) Three-dimensional OCT showing the cone of vitreous cortex adhering to the elevated fovea. Note the retinal folds induced by the ERM contraction (arrows); (D) Horizontal B-scan showing the posterior vitreous cortex [posterior vitreous cortex (PVC), long arrows] attached to the elevated and thickened fovea. The PVC is abnormally thick and hyper-reflective due to the reflection of the ERM (short arrows) on its posterior face. Note also the presence of small intraretinal cystic spaces and an elevation of the central photoreceptors.

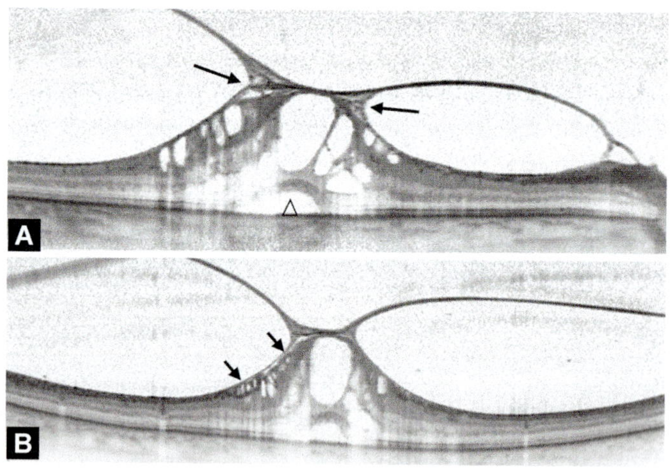

Figs. 56.7A and B: Severe vitreomacular traction associated with epiretinal membrane (ERM), cystoid maculopathy and foveal detachment. (A) Horizontal B-scan showing the connection between the ERM and the posterior vitreous cortex, firmly sealing this adhesion (long arrows). Note also the foveal detachment (arrowhead) induced by the traction, and the large intrafoveal cystic spaces; (B) Vertical B-scan, on which the ERM is better visible on the macular surface (short arrows).

Vitreomacular Traction as a Cause of Impending Macular Hole

The initial stage of impending MH is usually detected by OCT only when it occurs in a patient with a MH in the

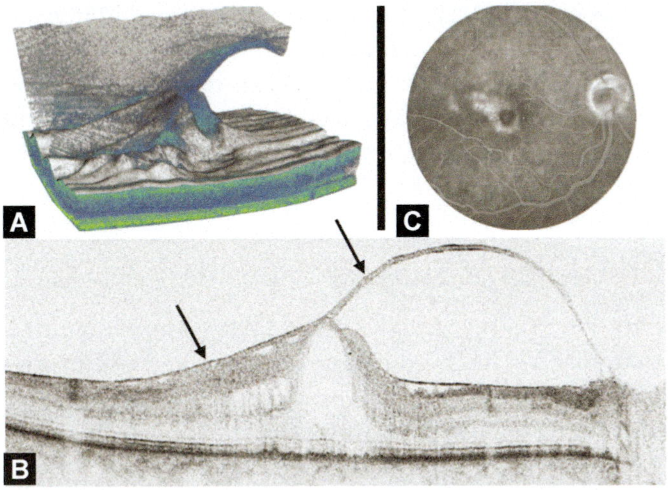

Figs. 56.8A to C: Severe vitreomacular traction associated with epiretinal membrane (ERM) and cystoid macular edema (CME). (A) Three-dimensional optical coherence tomography (OCT) showing the large adherence of the posterior vitreous cortex (PVC) to the temporal part of the macula; (B) Horizontal OCT B-scan showing the adherence of an ERM and the PVC on the temporal part of the macula and detached in front of its nasal part (arrows). Note the large intraretinal cystic spaces. (C) CME on fluorescein angiography.

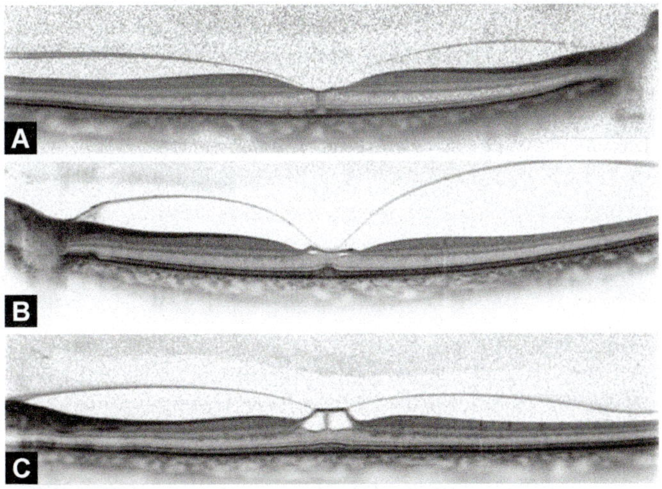

Figs. 56.9A to C: Aspects of vitreomacular traction (VMT) in fellow eyes of macular hole. (A) VMT with narrow adherence of the vitreous cortex in the umbo of the fovea. Note the central disruption of the ellipsoid zone, and the vertical hyper-reflectivity in the foveal center; (B) VMT with cystic changes in the inner fovea; (C) VMT with large foveal cystoid spaces.

other eye. The first signs of VMT are minute changes in the curvature of the foveal pit. More frequently, surface anomalies are already associated with various degrees of foveal microstructural changes, an elevation of the ellipsoid zone (EZ), a change in reflectivity of the foveal center, an inner foveal cyst, a central split in the fovea, an outer foveal cavitation, or a combination of these changes.[23-25] These anomalies may be asymptomatic but may evolve over time. In more advanced cases, the retinal layers are disrupted in the whole thickness of the fovea, except at a very superficial layer containing the ILM, forming an "occult" MH,[23-26] former stage 1B (Figs. 56.9 and 56.10).[27]

At any stage of impending MH, a complete resolution is possible if the VMT decreases or spontaneously releases (Figs. 56.11 and 56.12). However, there is a significant risk of evolution toward a full-thickness MH. Data available on the risk of MH in a fellow eye when a VMT is associated or not with structural intrafoveal anomalies are limited. According to recent publications, the risk could range between 30% and 50%.[26,28]

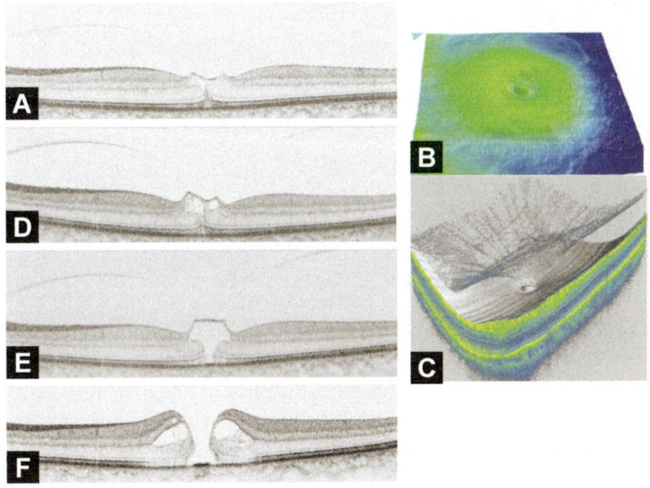

Figs. 56.10A to F: Evolution of vitreomacular traction (VMT) towards full-thickness macular hole (MH). (A to C) Initial examination with VMT, inner cystic spaces, and elevation of the foveal floor and central photoreceptor outer segments; (D) Enlargement of the foveal cystic spaces 6 months later with an impending MH; (E) Disruption of the whole thickness of the fovea except a very superficial layer containing the internal limiting membrane (ILM) forming an "occult" MH. The vitreous cortex remains adherent to the fovea 4 months later; (F) Full-thickness MH with posterior vitreous detachment 14 months after the first examination.

Natural History of Vitreomacular Adhesion/Vitreomacular Traction and Symptoms

The natural history of VMA and VMT is not well known for several reasons. VMA is usually asymptomatic; thus its onset cannot be known precisely. Its evolution to VMT is rare. VMT is uncommon and is often stable over time.[29,30] A spontaneous release may occur in 13–32%[22] of cases[29] studied; but it is difficult to compare these results to the general population due to the selection of cases, VMT severity, whether an ERM is present, and the duration of

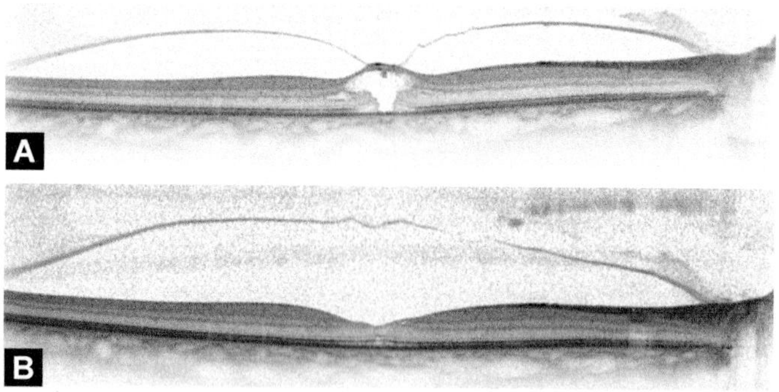

Figs. 56.11A and B: Spontaneous resolution of an impending macular hole (MH). (A) Impending MH with vitreomacular traction (VMT) and "occult" MH; (B) Normalization of the macular profile after spontaneous release of the VMT.

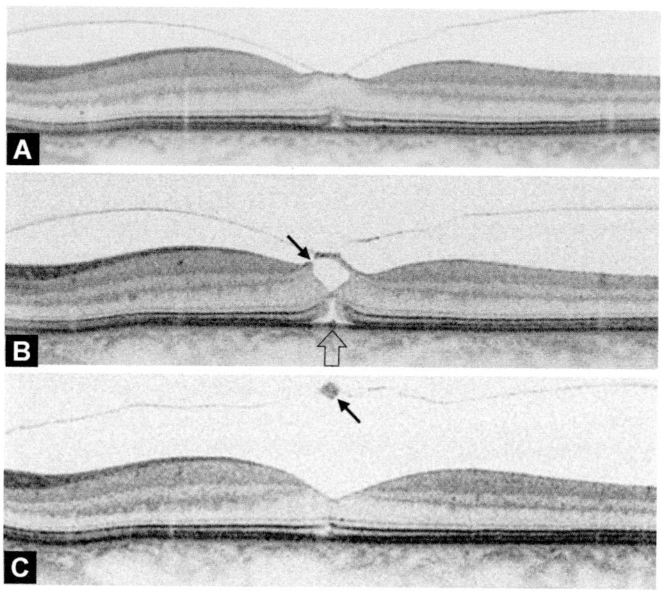

Figs. 56.12A to C: Worsening and spontaneous improvement in an impending macular hole. (A) Vitreomacular traction (VMT) with narrow adherence of the vitreous cortex in the umbo of the fovea and central disruption of the ellipsoid zone; (B) Persistent VMT resulting in an opening of an inner foveal cyst (thin arrow) and elevation and disruption of the foveal photoreceptors (block arrow); (C) Release of the VMT with detachment of an operculum in the plane of the detached posterior vitreous cortex (arrow) and normalization of the foveal profile.

follow-up. In a recent review of the electronic medical records of 1,254 patients, 70.5% of cases did not require vitrectomy over a 10-month follow-up period.[31]

Treatments of Vitreomacular Adhesion/Vitreomacular Traction

In cases of VMA, no treatment or particular monitoring is needed because it is part of the physiological process of PVD aging.

In cases of VMT, treatment may be needed if vision is threatened, knowing that the traction may also spontaneously release.[19] The usual treatment remains vitrectomy; but enzymatic or pneumatic vitreolysis may be used in selected cases.

Vitrectomy

Principles of Surgery

First described by Smiddy et al. in 1988,[32] pars plana vitrectomy for VMT has become simpler, faster, and less invasive with transconjunctival 25- or 27-gauge instrumentation. The PVC is often stained with triamcinolone acetonide or various dyes[33] to improve detection.

In cases of simple VMT, various methods are used to detach the vitreous from the macula or to cut the PVC around the fovea in order to minimize traction forces on the fragile roof of a foveal cyst. In cases of VMT associated with ERM, after the conic insertion of the PVC on the fovea has been cut, the ERM must be peeled of the retina by detaching "en bloc" the membrane and vitreous remnants.

Histologic specimens have shown the reality of this connection between an ERM and the vitreous in these cases of VMT.[20,34]

Visual Outcomes

Vitrectomy usually results in visual acuity (VA) improvement; but the published series are small and the indications for surgery may differ from one publication to another. On average, about 80% of patients with VMT will improve by at least two VA lines after vitrectomy.[35] Various factors are considered favorable to the postoperative outcome, including focal VMT versus broad VMT, a younger age, a short symptom duration,[36] the absence of intrafoveal cleavage[37] or no elongation of the photoreceptor outer segments.[38] Complications mainly include an increased risk of peripheral breaks in these eyes with abnormal vitreous and the occurrence of MH.[31,39]

Enzymatic Vitreolysis

Enzymatic vitreolysis may be proposed to release traction in selected cases of VMT.[40] In a second randomized trial,[22] ocriplasmin (JETREA®, ThromboGenics NV, Leuven; Belgium) has been shown to release VMT in 37.9% of cases (without MH), mainly in cases with focal vitreous adherence (<1500 μm). When an ERM was associated with the VMT, the efficacy of vitreolysis to release traction was only 13.1%.

Pneumatic Vitreolysis

Several small case series treated with pure perfluoropropane injection in the vitreous to release the VMT have been published since the initial work by Chan.[41] This technique has recently regained interest as an alternative to enzymatic vitreolysis, resulting in a VMT release rate of 80% or more in selected cases.[42,43] Complications and adverse events of vitreoretinal surgery are the same for most vitreoretinal interface diseases and will be discussed at the end of the chapter.

MACULAR HOLE

Prevalence

The prevalence of MH was 4 per 1,000 in a population of subjects aged 63–102 years in a 2015 report of the Beaver Dam study[17] based on SD-OCT. The median age at the time of surgery was 70 years, and there was a female predominance (2/3 of cases).[44] When a MH is already present in the fellow eye, the risk for the second eye depends on the persistence or not of a VMT. In eyes with VMT, the risk has been assessed at between 42% in a series examined with time-domain OCT[45] and 11.9% in a series examined with SD-OCT.[25] The risk may be increased when intrafoveal changes are already associated with a VMT in the fellow eye.[25]

Primary Macular Hole

Macular hole is a round, full-thickness opening in the foveal center. In most cases, it is primary, i.e. due to an abnormal vitreofoveal traction. MH symptoms are not very specific. Patients complain of a rapidly progressive vision loss in one eye, especially in near vision, often associated with microscotoma and sometimes metamorphopsia and micropsia.

Macular Hole with Vitreomacular Traction

The role of the vitreous cortex in MH pathogenesis began to be better understood with the biomicroscopic observations by Gass.[27,46] The advent of OCT, showing the partially detached posterior hyaloid, clarified the understanding of MH formation.[23,24,47] SD-OCT subsequently provided more detailed views of the initial foveal changes induced by the vitreofoveal traction. MH classification has been recently updated and is based on both, hole diameter and presence or the absence of a residual vitreous traction on its edge.[16] The success rate for MH surgery, which was initiated by Kelly and Wendel[48] in 1991, gradually increased and is now high.

Macular hole with persistent vitreous traction includes what was previously referred to as stage 2 MH, described as a crescent retinal defect in the fovea with a diameter of less than 400 µm.[27,49] OCT has subsequently shown that the incompletely detached operculum is pulled forward by the traction of the PVC.[23,47] The operculum may contain neuronal elements detected by OCT;[25] this supports the histological findings of Ezra, who has shown the presence of cone components in two-thirds of opercula he examined (Figs. 56.13A to E).[50]

Macular holes with persistent vitreous traction may present various profiles and a large range of diameters, from a very small break to a large foveal opening greater than 400 µm. In a recent study assessing 100 consecutive idiopathic MHs, the mean preoperative hole diameter was not significantly different depending on the presence or the absence of a VMT: 339 ± 134 µm in eyes with VMT and 423 ± 191 µm in eyes without VMT ($p = 0.057$). 22% had VMT; and the MH diameter was 400 µm or less in only 13% of cases and 250 µm or less in 6% of cases.[51]

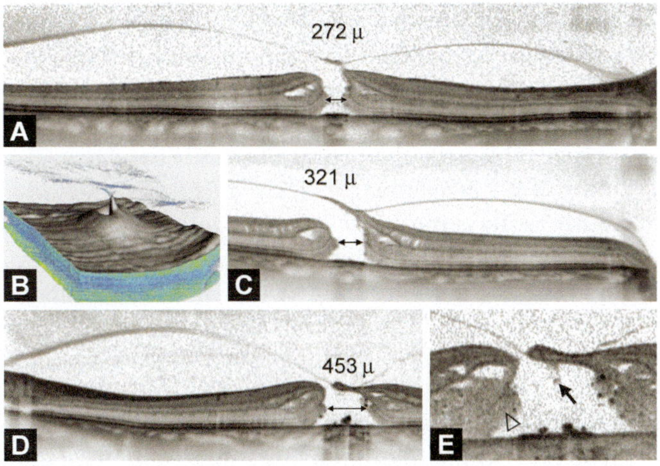

Figs. 56.13A to E: Macular holes (MH) with vitreomacular traction (VMT). (A) Small MH (272 µm) with the vitreous cortex attached to the hole edge; (B) Medium MH (321 µm), three-dimensional view showing the vitreous cortex still attached to the hole edge; (C) *B-scan*: Posterior vitreous cortex still adherent to the undetached operculum; (D and E) Large MH (453 µm), B-scan showing the vitreous attachment to the MH edge. Detail showing the elongation of the detached photoreceptor outer segments (arrowhead) and remnants of cones still attached to the operculum (arrow).

Small MHs may close spontaneously when the VMT spontaneously releases, but this event is rare.[22,52]

Macular Hole Without Vitreomacular Traction

According to the International VMT Study classification,[16] this category includes all cases in which the posterior hyaloid is detached from the hole edge, regardless of whether the vitreous is also detached from the optic disk. In the Gass definition, stage 3 MH was a hole larger than 400 µm with undetached vitreous (Figs. 56.14A and B). The presence of a Weiss ring defined stage 4. Subsequently, OCT has shown that even when the vitreous was not detached from the optic disk, it could be completely detached from the retinal surface on the posterior pole and not connected to the hole edge. The proportion of MH smaller than 400 µm with detached vitreous is the same as for small MH with VMT (Table 56.1).

Lamellar Macular Hole

The term "lamellar MH (LMH)" was coined by Gass in 1976[53] to characterize a macular lesion resulting from the opening of the central cyst of a cystoid macular edema. The term "lamellar hole" has been used to describe both the end stage of a cystoid macular edema[54] and the aborted process of MH formation.[24,55]

The symptoms of LMH are usually mild with a moderate decrease in VA associated or not with microscotoma. There is no reliable information on the natural history of LMH due to the inconsistency of disease description in the literature, and the usual insidious onset of this condition.

Lamellar MHs are characterized on OCT by an irregular thinning of the foveal floor, a cleavage between the inner and outer retina at the lamellar hole edge, and the absence of contractile ERM.[55,56] An epiretinal proliferation occurs at the retina surface, around the lamellar hole in about one-third of cases[56,57] and is well visible on SD-OCT on the ILM. On en-face OCT, this proliferation is smooth, noncontractile, and histologically, it does not contain myofibroblasts, unlike typical ERMs.[57,58]

However, the differential diagnosis with macular pseudoholes (MPH) remains highly controversial because the macular profile on the OCT B-scan may be very similar, whereas there is usually no macular thickening in LMH.[59] The use of en-face images with segmentation at the retina surface allows easily distinguishing of cases with epiretinal contraction (i.e. MPHs) from those with a smooth retinal surface (i.e. LMHs)(Figs. 56.15A to C).[59]

Table 56.1: Classification used for full-thickness MH and International Vitreomacular Traction Study.

Classification commonly used for full-thickness MH	International VMT study
Stage 2: Small hole	Small or medium FTMH with VMT
Stage 3: Large hole	Medium or large FTMH with VMT
Stage 4: FTMH with PVD	Small, medium or large FTMH without VMT

(MH: Macular hole; FTMH: Full-thickness macular hole; VMT: Vitreomacular traction; PVD: Posterior vitreous detachment)
Source: Duker JS, Kaiser PK, Binder S, et al. The International Vitreomacular Traction Study Group classification of vitreomacular adhesion, traction, and macular hole. Ophthalmology. 2013; 120:2611-9.[16]
Small ≤250 µm, Medium >250 µm and ≤400 µm, Large >400 µm.

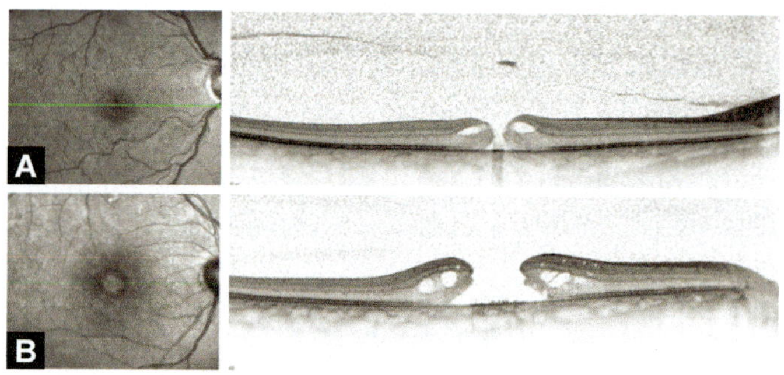

Figs. 56.14A and B: Macular holes (MH) without vitreomacular traction. (A) Small MH with the vitreous cortex detached from the macula, but still attached to the optic disk; (B) Large MH with the vitreous cortex completely detached from the macula and the optic disk.

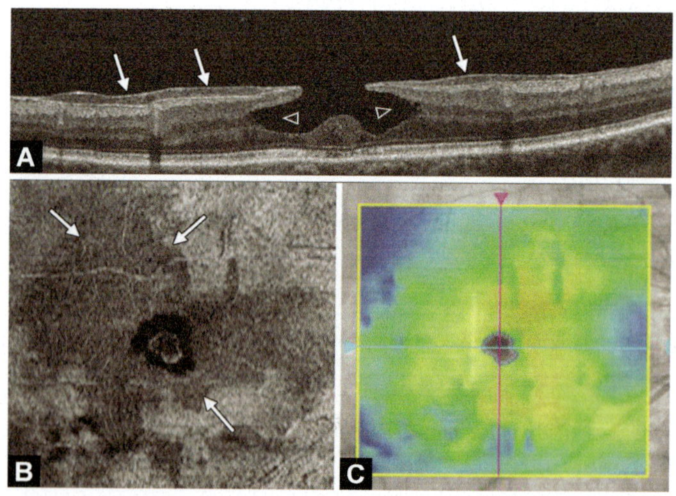

Figs. 56.15A to C: Lamellar macular hole (LMH) with epiretinal proliferation. (A) Horizontal B-scan showing a deep cleavage between the inner and the outer retina (arrowheads). Thick epiretinal proliferation on the retinal surface (arrows); (B) En-face image segmented at the retinal surface showing the smooth hyper-reflectivity of the epiretinal proliferation. Note the absence of retinal folds; (C) Macular thickness map showing the contour of the moderate thickening of the macula around the LMH.

Treatments of Primary Macular Hole and Outcomes

Surgery: MH surgery has greatly benefited from the advent of small gauge transconjunctival sutureless vitrectomy.

Posterior hyaloid detachment: The detachment of the PVC is a crucial step in cases in which MH is associated with VMT, but also in MH in which the vitreous still adheres only to the optic disk. Direct aspiration of the vitreous fibers attached to the Weiss ring with the 25- or 27-gauge vitrectomy probe is a very effective method for lifting the vitreous cortex "en bloc" and progressively extending its detachment to the equator. To improve the visualization of the PVC, it is possible to inject diluted triamcinolone or Brilliant Blue G in front of the posterior pole.

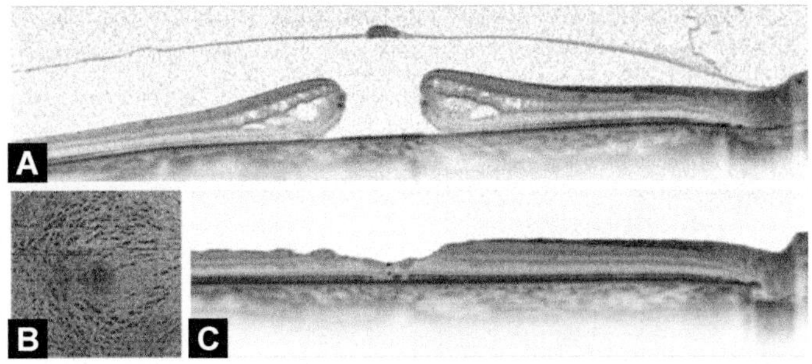

Figs. 56.16A to C: Macular hole (MH) closure after surgery including inner limiting membrane peeling. (A) Preoperative B-scan of a large MH without vitreomacular traction; (B) En-face optical coherence tomography (OCT) image after MH closure showing the aspect of dissociated optic nerve fiber layer (DONFL); (C) Postoperative B-scan showing closure of the MH. Note thinning of the inner retina temporal to the fovea, with dimples in the optic nerve fiber and ganglion cell layers corresponding to the DONFL.

Extensive vitrectomy: Although it is not possible to demonstrate the superiority of extensive vitrectomy over more limited vitrectomy, several arguments support extensive vitreous removal, i.e. removal of the vitreous gel, followed by shaving of the vitreous base. The removal of as much vitreous as possible allows injecting more gas mixture into the eye and subsequently prolongs the effect of the gas tamponade. Shaving the vitreous base, especially in the lower periphery, also reduces the risk of postoperative lower retinal breaks and detachment by preventing the gas bubble from exerting traction on the remaining vitreous fibers.[60,61]

Epiretinal proliferation peeling: When present, an epiretinal proliferation around the hole should be peeled off.[62,63] These epiretinal proliferations are usually yellow, soft, and friable compared to those of LMH. They may be removed by brushing the retinal surface, a method that is better than with forceps. They firmly adhere to the thickness of the hole edge. If a dye such as Brilliant Blue is used to stain the ILM before removal, the epiretinal proliferation is not stained and appears as "negative" at the ILM surface. The epiretinal proliferation may also be removed "en bloc" together with the ILM.

Inner limiting membrane peeling: Peeling of the ILM is greatly facilitated by the use of dyes to improve its visualization. End-gripping forceps are used to pinch and tear an ILM flap without touching the optic nerve fibers. The ILM is then peeled off in a circular movement, thus creating a "maculorrhexis".[64] The optimal size of the peeling area remains debated. Postoperatively, ILM peeling results in a characteristic pattern of the retinal surface referred to as dissociation of the optic nerve fiber layer (DONFL) that is clearly seen on blue reflectance photograph and en-face OCT (Figs. 56.16A to C).[65,66] Recently, an inverted ILM flap technique has been proposed, which consists of maintaining the ILM flap partially attached to the hole edge to cover its surface. This technique may be useful in large MH or in case of failure of an initial surgery.[67]

Use of vital dyes: The use of dyes to stain the ERM and ILM has made peeling of the retinal surface more precise, more complete and less traumatic.

- *Indocyanine green and infracyanine*: Indocyanine green (ICG) dye has a selective affinity for the ILM and was initially used at a concentration of 0.5%; but due to changes in the RPE and visual field defects,[68] this concentration has been reduced to 0.125% or even 0.05%, which makes the staining paler but still useful. Use of a concentration of 0.05%, whose osmolarity is 290 mOsm, combined with a brief contact time not exceeding 30 seconds with the retina, does not seem to be toxic to the RPE.[69] Infracyanine, an iodine-free product, diluted in 5% glucose is an iso-osmolar solution, which might be safer for the retina.[70] Finally, as light exposure seems to increase the risk of damage to the retina, the light should be turned off during the short time of ICG contact with the retina.[71] Vitreoretinal surgeons remain divided on the possible toxicity of ICG to the retina. ICG should therefore be used only at minimal concentrations and for a short time.
- *Trypan blue*: Trypan blue (TB) stains the ERM well, but stains the ILM poorly. To improve TB staining of the ILM, it should be used after fluid gas exchange or after

mixing isovolumetrically the dye in 10% glucose, to create heavy TB, which falls onto the posterior pole and results in acceptable staining after a 2-minute contact.[72] However, it has been suggested that this may also increase its osmolarity to toxic levels.[73] Ready-to-use solutions combining TB with a viscosity- and density-increasing agent are also available in some countries. In most studies, TB has shown no signs of toxicity to the RPE or neuronal tissue.[74]

- *Brilliant blue*: Brilliant blue has a selective affinity for the ILM and provides good staining in an iso-osmolar solution of 0.25 mg/mL (0.025%). The staining is visible after a brief contact with the dye injected onto the retinal surface. In animal experiments, the safety profile of Brilliant Blue was good[75] and it appears to be the best alternative to ICG.[76]

Type of gas to be used in MH surgery: Various gases have been used in MH surgery, including C3F8, C2F6, SF6, and air. The rationale for preferring one gas to another is based on the expected duration of the gas bubble. If we assume that most MH close within 3–7 days of tamponade, a bubble large enough to insulate the macula from intraocular fluid during this period will be sufficient. This is, for instance, the case for a 17% C2F6-air mixture, provided that vitrectomy is large enough to create a large gas bubble. With this mixture, the gas bubble still covers the macula 1 week after surgery if the head is in the upright position, and still fills more than 70% of the vitreous cavity. The essential characteristic of the gas mixture is not so much to persist for a long time in the eye, but to cover the fovea in any position of the head during the first postoperative days.[77,78] If the hole is small and a 3-day tamponade is assumed to be sufficient, 20% SF6-air, or even air alone, might be enough.

Use of silicone oil in MH surgery: Silicone oil has been used to avoid the need for positioning in patients unable to maintain the face-down position, to allow air travel after surgery or to ensure prolonged tamponade in case of failure of the initial surgery. In such cases, some authors stressed the advantages of using silicone oil.[79,80] Others have noted that the anatomical outcomes were not better with silicone oil compared to C3F8 or that the visual outcomes were worse.[81,82] Consequently, silicone oil should be used sparingly in MH surgery.[83]

Surgery outcomes: In the initial series of 52 cases published by Kelly and Wendel in 1990,[48] the closure success rate after MH surgery was 58%. The current closure rate is 90–95% or more.[83,84]

Role of hole size: The concept that the success rate of MH surgery depends on hole diameter emerged in 2002.[85,86] The spontaneous closure of a MH is also more likely to occur if its diameter is less than 200 μm.[52] In the randomized study assessing the efficacy of intravitreal ocriplasmin, the best closure rate was obtained for MH smaller than 250 μm.[22] These findings paved the way for treatments tailored to the initial size of the hole.

Role of ILM peeling: Since the publication by Eckardt[87] showing that the MH closure rate could improve if the ILM is peeled off, many publications, mainly of retrospective studies, have reported closure rates of 87–100% in relatively large case series after ILM peeling.[88-91] Some of these studies have also compared ILM peeling and nonpeeling in large series of eyes and reported success rates of 77–89% without peeling compared to 92–97% with peeling.[91-93] So far, however, only 3 small, prospective, randomized studies comparing ILM peeling and nonpeeling in MH surgery have been published. Success rates in the peeling groups ranged from 84% to 92% compared to only 32–48% in the nonpeeling groups.[94-96] These results for nonpeeling are far below the success rate of 58% initially obtained by Kelly and Wendel in 1991.[48] The discrepancy between the results of the control groups in the above-mentioned randomized studies and those of other retrospective studies seems to indicate that other conditions, in addition to ILM peeling, are needed for a high rate of MH closure.

On the other hand, it appears that the need for ILM peeling may depend on the hole size. In a retrospective study, Tadayoni et al.[97] have shown that ILM peeling improved MH closure in a series of 84 eyes when MHs were larger than 400 μm (100% of MH closure with peeling versus 83.3% without peeling) while MHs smaller than 400 μm closed in all cases regardless of ILM peeling. The need for ILM peeling could then be modulated according to the hole size.[98]

Indeed ILM peeling may lead to various side effects, including to DONFL visible on blue reflectance photographs[65] and on en-face OCT[99] that is seen as arcuate striae of the macular surface in the area of ILM peeling. These correspond to dimples into the retinal nerve fiber layer on OCT B-scan (Fig. 56.16).[100] Several studies have also shown that the thickness of the retinal ganglion cell layer-inner plexiform layer was significantly reduced after ILM peeling even when the ILM was stained with Brilliant

Blue G, a safe dye for ganglion cells, and was associated with decreased retinal sensitivity on microperimetry.[101,102]

Role of postoperative positioning: Since the beginning of MH surgery, a face-down positioning for at least 1 week has been considered essential for MH closure. However, from as early as 1997, Tornambe has obtained a reasonable success rate of 79% for hole closure without any face-down positioning.[103] In a randomized prospective trial comparing face-down and seated positioning, face-down positioning was found to result in a better closure rate, although no difference was found when the MH diameter was smaller than 400 µm.[84] Another prospective randomized study has compared face-down positioning and an alleviated position for MH up to 400 µm in diameter, after surgery without ILM peeling, and found a success rate of greater than 90% for both positions.[104] In MHs larger than 400 µm, ILM peeling and a nonsupine positioning had a success rate of at least 90%, similar to that of face-down positioning.[105] It therefore appears that a face-down positioning after MH surgery is not essential, provided that the gas bubble stays in contact with the macula until the healing process has started to close the hole.[78] For this purpose, various gas mixtures may be used, as long as the volume of the gas bubble remains large enough for 3–5 days to make an effective tamponade of the macula in the upright position. Conversely, holes larger than 600 µm may need a longer face-down positioning and a longer acting gas mixture.

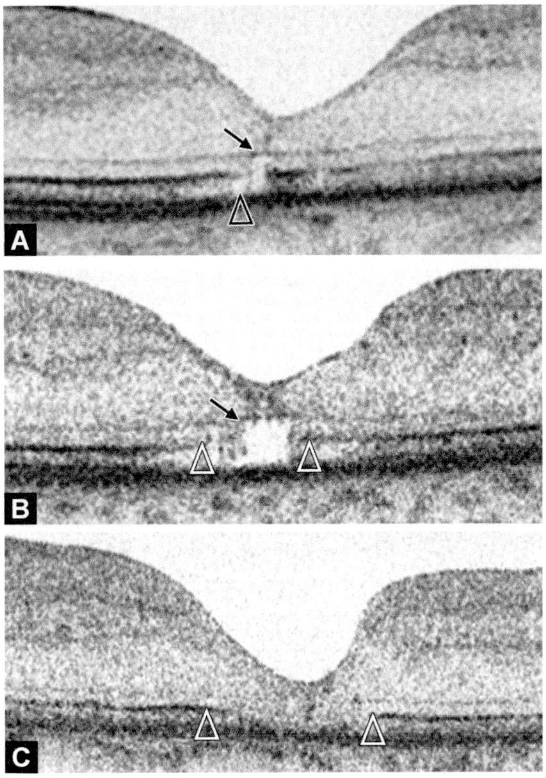

Figs. 56.17A to C: Three different profiles of closed macular holes. (A) Small gap in the interdigitation and ellipsoid zones (EZ, arrowhead). The outer limiting membrane has recovered its continuity; (B) Larger breakdown in the outer retina, with larger disruption in the EZ (arrowheads), but the outer limiting membrane is present (arrow); (C) Atrophy of the outer retina (between arrowheads) with disruption of the EZ and the outer limiting membrane.

Visual outcomes:

- *Overall results*: MH closure usually results in visual improvement. However, due to the high rate of postoperative cataract, a better VA is only achieved once the cataract has been operated on, or after combined cataract and MH surgery. Two recent series have shown that VA improved over time and that the mean VA reached 20/32 or better 1 year after surgery.[106,107] The VA improves mainly because of the improvement in fixation stability,[108] despite the persistence of microscotoma.[109,110]
- *Anatomical and visual correlation*: Large and lasting MH has been considered as associated with a low closure rate and a poor visual outcome.[85,86,111] However, this may not be systematically the case, because ILM peeling has improved the anatomical prognosis of large holes, which is nearly the same as that of smaller ones, and even lasting MH may benefit from surgery.[112] However, the closure of large holes may leave a larger glial scar than that of smaller ones, thus affecting the visual outcome. On OCT, the morphology and thickness of the foveal photoreceptor layer correlate with the final VA (Figs. 56.17A to C).[95,106,113,114]

Enzymatic vitreolysis: In a phase 3 trial, the overall closure rate of MH smaller than 400 µm was 30% in the ocriplasmin group compared to 15.4% in the placebo group.[22] For MH with a diameter of 250 µm or less, the success rate increased to 48.0%; but for holes with a diameter of 250–400 µm, it was only 23.0%. Since the proportion of small holes with persistent VMT is small,[51] the optimum indications of enzymatic vitreolysis remain limited so far to less than 5% of MHs.[115]

Adverse events include photopsia, dyschromatopsia, subretinal fluid, and outer retina changes in the macula.[22,116,117] Foveal detachment occurring after intravitreal ocriplasmin may be due to a direct pharmacological effect of the enzyme on the outer retina.[118]

Secondary Macular Hole

The most common causes of secondary MHs are blunt trauma and high myopia. Traumatic MHs usually occur in children and young adult males following accidents at work or home or during ball games.[119,120] Unlike in idiopathic MH, the vitreous is not detached from the posterior pole. These secondary MHs are due to sudden axial compression of the eye, resulting in an equatorial expansion and retinal rupture of the fovea. The hole may be associated with other fundus lesions, such as choroidal or Bruch membrane disruption, commotion retinae, sclopetaria, or peripheral breaks. The visual prognosis depends not only on hole closure but also on the topography of the other lesions. Surgery is usually successful, but a traumatic MH may also sometimes close spontaneously within the first weeks of occurrence.[121,122] MH is also one of the complications of high myopia together with posterior staphyloma and choroidal atrophy. The pathogenesis may be different from that in nonmyopic eyes because the vitreous cortex often remains adherent to the retinal surface (see later in this chapter). Many other causes have been described but these are anecdotal.[77]

EPIRETINAL MEMBRANE—A COMPLICATION OF VITREOMACULAR SEPARATION

Prevalence

The prevalence of ERMs in a population aged 63 years or over was 34% as detected by SD-OCT. In the Beaver Dam study, 30% of subjects who had an ERM in one eye had bilateral ERMs.[17] The prevalence of ERM increased with age, prevalence was 28% before age 74 years and reached 53% after 85 years. In a previous study based on fundus photographs in a population aged 49 years or more, the prevalence of ERMs was 7%, with only one-third of subjects presenting with retinal folds.[123]

In 80% of cases, ERMs are primary, i.e. they are only related to PVD. In most of the remaining cases, ERMs are secondary, when they complicate the course of other diseases, including diabetic retinopathy, posterior and intermediate uveitis, and retinal detachment (RD).[124] Lastly, in rare cases, ERMs may be present in young adults or even children and are probably congenital.[125]

Primary Epiretinal Membrane

Macular ERMs are formed by the self-limiting proliferation of cells of various origins, including hyalocytes and retinal glial cells. These membranes cover the macular area and posterior pole and result in retinal folding when they contract.[126-128]

Pathogenesis and Histology of Primary Epiretinal Membrane

The temporal relationship between symptomatic PVD and the occurrence of an ERM based on clinical observations was first suggested by Wise in 1975.[128] The histological observation in postmortem eyes by Foos[129] showing that vitreous collagen was present between the ERM and the ILM has also suggested that ERMs had proliferated after vitreoretinal separation, resulting in collagen fiber accumulation at the posterior pole surface. Later, Wiznia[130] has observed that the proportion of ERMs increased from 9 to 41% after an 18-month follow-up for symptomatic PVD in a prospective study of 34 eyes. It is indeed common to observe a high incidence of PVD in eyes with ERM while ERM associated with VMT is rare. However, the mechanism by which the PVD promotes the development of cell proliferation resulting in an ERM remains incompletely understood.

Clinical and histological studies have shown that the spontaneous separation of the vitreous cortex from the retina may result in a thin layer of vitreous collagen fibers at the retinal surface[1,18,131] that may serve as a scaffold for cell proliferation. This splitting of the laminated PVC, also referred to as vitreoschisis,[132,133] contains hyalocytes,[134] cells originating from bone marrow-derived cells that have a slow turnover.[135] These cells could play a role in the recruitment of astrocytes, Müller cells, and RPE cells,[136] which are commonly found in ERM, transdifferentiated into fibroblasts and myofibroblasts. Hyalocytes could also transdifferentiate into myofibroblast-like cells. Along with glial cells, in particular Müller cells, they are the main cells involved in primary ERM.[34] Proliferating cells secrete a more or less abundant extracellular matrix. How glial cells migrate across the ILM is not clearly known, but the anchorage of epiretinal cell proliferation in the inner retina through defects in the ILM may explain the retinal folding due to the ERM contraction and the frequent removal of large pieces of ILM together with the ERM during surgery.[137]

Symptoms and Natural History

Many ERMs are asymptomatic and are often discovered during an OCT examination performed before cataract surgery for instance. In other cases, however, the vision may be affected by various symptoms, including progressive vision loss, blurred vision, macropsia, metamorphopsia, aniseikonia, and binocular diplopia. Macropsia is assumed to be due to the contraction of central photoreceptors in a smaller area and may be responsible for aniseikonia.[138] Binocular diplopia may occur in case of severe macular ectopia due to an asymmetric contraction of an ERM. Usually, the tangential foveal displacement is more moderate and contributes to vision loss and metamorphopsia.[139,140] Metamorphopsia is also assumed to be related to inner nuclear layer thickening.[141,142]

The natural history of ERM is poorly documented due to the usual insidious and progressive vision loss. It appears that, in many cases, the vision decreases very slowly over several years before becoming uncomfortable. However, in some cases, patients report the symptoms of a symptomatic PVD, followed within a few weeks by the occurrence of metamorphopsia and vision loss worsening in a few months (Figs. 56.18A and B). In eyes with good vision at the time of diagnosis, the VA remains stable for 2 years in most cases.[143] The spontaneous resolution of an ERM is rare and is more likely to occur in younger subjects,[144] either through avulsion by the vitreous in case of incomplete PVD or by winding on itself.

Diagnostic Tests

Fundus biomicroscopy and fundus photography remain useful in the diagnosis of ERM. The glistening reflex of cellophane ERM is mainly seen on fundus biomicroscopy. Blue reflectance photography also shows the abnormal reflectivity of the ERM and its limits (Figs. 56.19A to F). SD-OCT can show the presence of an ERM, even when it is very thin, and has the double advantage of showing and quantifying the macular thickening induced by ERM contraction. The ERM appears as a hyper-reflective structure lining the retinal surface, of variable thickness,

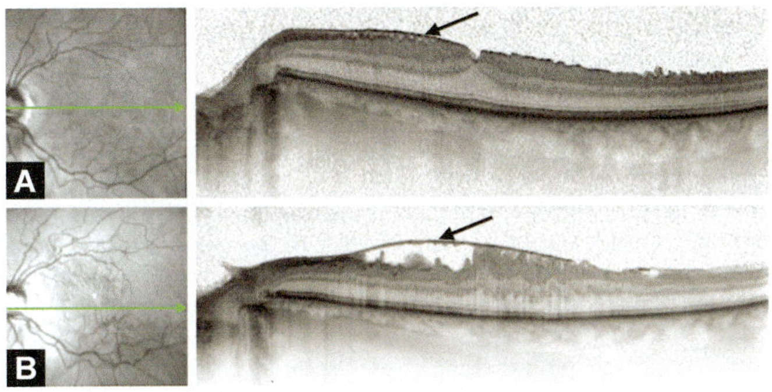

Figs. 56.18A and B: Worsening of an epiretinal membrane (ERM) over 18 months. (A) Moderate thickening of the macula induced by the contraction of an ERM visible at the surface of small superficial retinal folds (arrow). The foveal pit is attenuated but still visible; (B) Worsening of macular folding 18 months later. The ERM (arrow) is thicker, partially detached from the nasal part of the macula, but its contraction induces deep retinal folds involving the fovea.

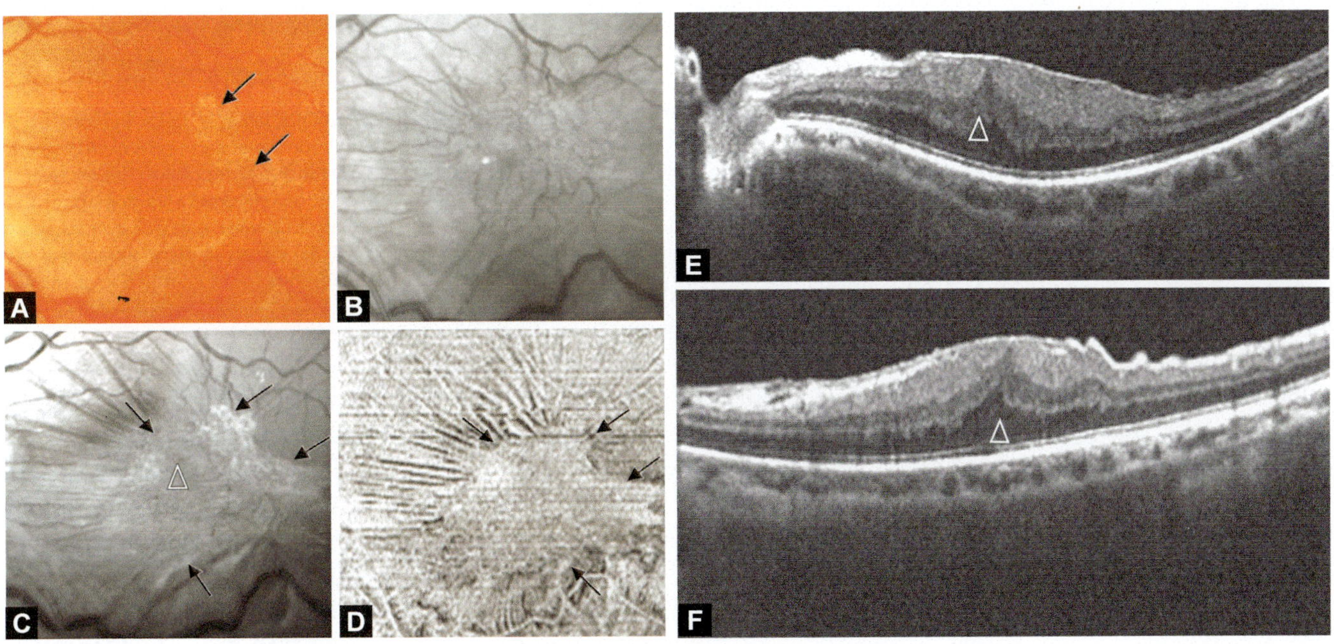

Figs. 56.19A to F: Imaging modalities of an epiretinal membrane (ERM). (A) Color fundus photograph showing distortion of retinal vessels and the faint reflectivity of an ERM in the temporal part of the fovea (arrows); (B) Red-free fundus photograph better showing the retinal vessel distortion, but not the ERM; (C) Blue reflectance fundus photograph showing the reflectivity and contours of the ERM (arrows) as well as the constricted xanthophyll pigment (arrowhead); (D) En-face OCT segmented at the retinal surface showing the contours of the constricted ERM (arrows) and the retinal folds induced by this constriction; (E and F) Horizontal and vertical B-scans passing through the foveal center. Note the overall macular thickening and closure of the foveal pit (arrowheads).

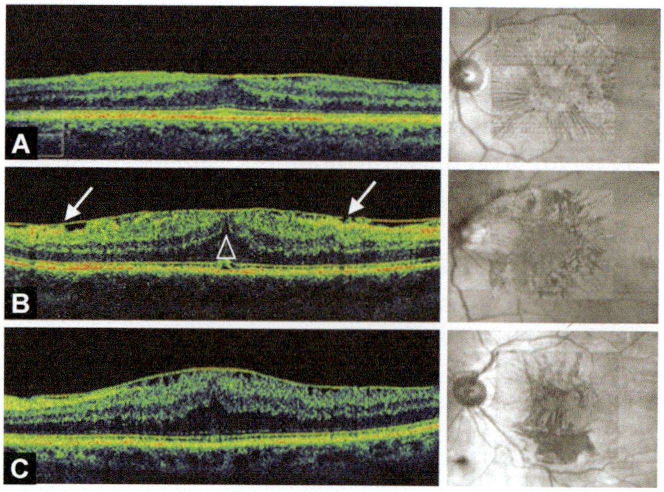

Figs. 56.20A to C: Various degrees of epiretinal membrane (ERM) contraction on horizontal optical coherence tomography (OCT) B-scans on the right and en-face OCT on the left; (A) Flat macular profile, moderate contraction of an ERM firmly adherent to the macular surface; (B) Convex macular thickening with complete closure of the foveal pit (arrowhead). The contracted membrane bridges some retinal folds (arrows); (C) Severe macular contraction with full-thickness macular folds. Note the undulations of the outer plexiform layer.

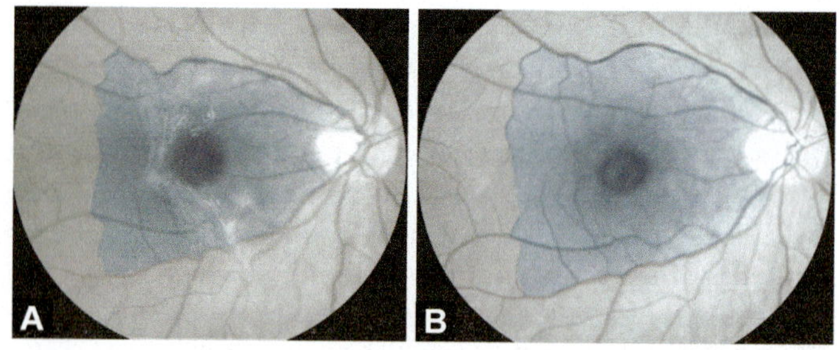

Figs. 56.21A and B: Extent of the posterior pole after epiretinal membrane removal. (A) Before surgery, the apparent surface of the posterior pole is colored in blue; (B) After surgery, the surface of the posterior pole, in blue, follows the same vascular landmarks. Note about 35% extent of the surface.

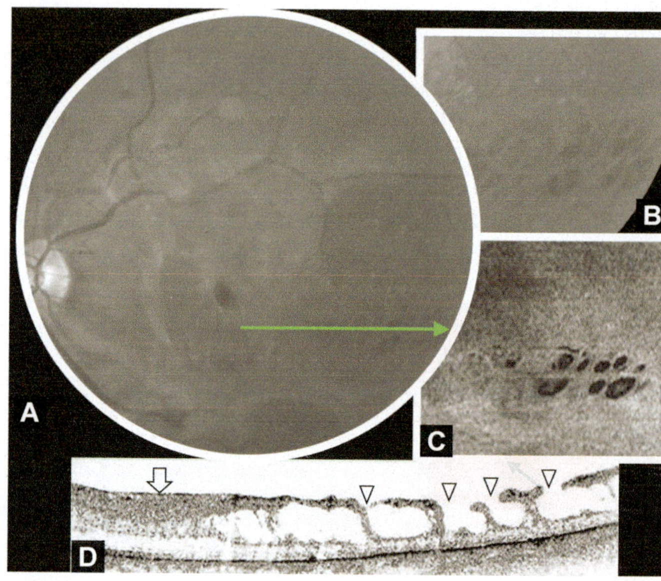

Figs. 56.22A to D: Extramacular retinal lamellar holes induced by the tangential traction exerted by an epiretinal membrane (ERM). (A) Extended contractile ERM on blue reflectance fundus photograph. The green arrow represents the direction of the optical coherence tomography (OCT) B-scan; (B) Detail showing a cluster of lamellar holes or cystoid spaces; (C) Same area seen on en-face OCT; (D) B-scan showing intraretinal cysts and lamellar retinal holes (arrowheads) due to the contraction of an ERM.

more visible when it bridges inner retinal folds. The coronal scans (C-scans) segmented at the vitreoretinal interface provides very suggestive images of the ERM and induced retinal folds (Figs. 56.20A to C). Fluorescein angiography has lost its relevance in the current diagnosis of ERM but may be useful, in case of cystoid spaces present on the OCT B-scan, to detect cases associated with fluorescein leakage.

Patterns of Epiretinal Membrane Contraction and Macular Pseudohole

The most common finding is the macular thickening caused by the constriction of the ERM, resulting in the disappearance of the foveal depression. The anterior profile of the macula may be flat, irregular, or often convex. This thickening is partly due to the macular constriction, which often significantly reduces the apparent surface of the posterior pole (Figs. 56.21A and B).[145,146] In some cases, the ERM contraction is so severe that it results in scattered lamellar microholes along the temporal vessels (Figs. 56.22A to D).[147] The ERM contraction may also cause acute angle, deep retinal folds, resulting in an impairment of the axoplasmic transport, appearing as cotton wool spots (Figs. 56.23A to C).[148]

A subfoveal hyper-reflective deposit is present in about 20% of cases on OCT and associated with a subfoveal yellow spot on fundoscopy. These could be due to the centripetal contraction of the membrane, resulting in an elevation of central photoreceptors (Figs. 56.24A to C).[149]

Microcystic changes have been associated with macular thickening in 7.5% of cases, in the absence of VMT, in the Beaver Dam study.[17] This proportion could be higher in cases eligible for surgery and these changes are inconstantly associated with fluorescein leakage.[150] In such cases, the role of cystoid macular edema as a cause or a consequence of ERM should be discussed (Figs. 56.25A to C).[150,151] In most cases, however, microcystic

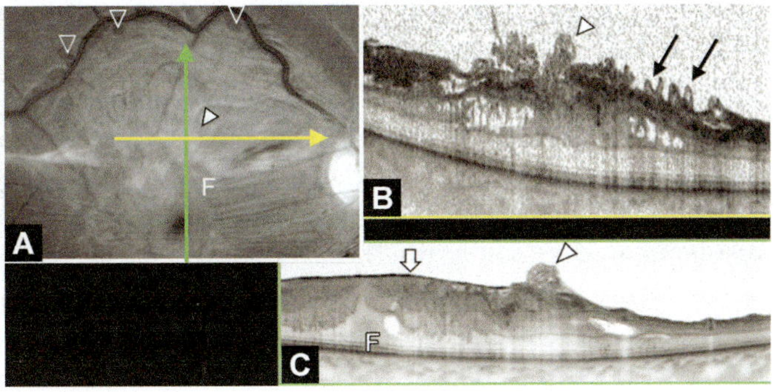

Figs. 56.23A to C: Impairment of the axoplasmic transport due to severe epiretinal membrane (ERM) contraction; (A) Blue reflectance fundus photograph showing the severe ERM contraction resulting in the focal whitening of the optic nerve fibers (white arrowhead) above the fovea (F). Note also the presence of lamellar retinal holes along the temporal retinal vein (empty arrowheads). The green line shows the direction of the vertical optical coherence tomography (OCT) B-scan and the yellow line that of the horizontal B-scan; (B) Horizontal OCT B-scan (magnification) showing the folds of the partially avulsed inner limiting membrane. Swelling of the nerve fibers (arrowhead); (C) Vertical OCT B-scan showing a thick contracted ERM resulting in full-thickness retinal folds and cystoid spaces. Swelling of the optic nerve fibers (white arrowhead) above the fovea.

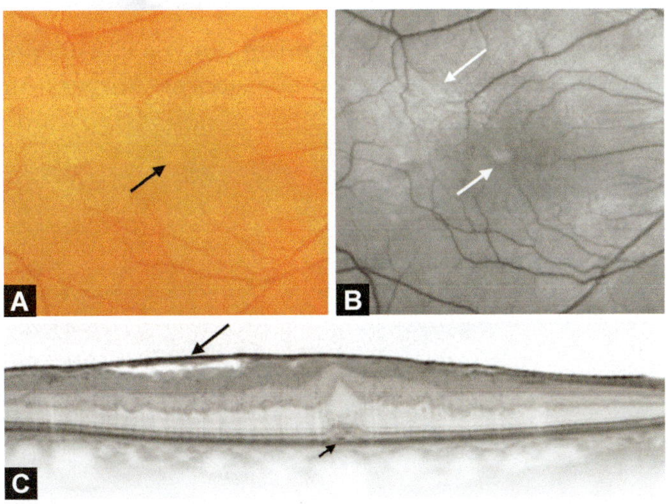

Figs. 56.24A to C: Subfoveal yellow spot due to the contraction of an epiretinal membrane (ERM). (A) Color fundus photograph showing a yellow subfoveal spot (arrow); (B) Red-free fundus photograph showing reflectivity of the ERM (white arrow); (C) OCT B-scan showing that the yellow spot corresponds to a subretinal deposit (arrow). Note the thick contractile ERM (long arrow).

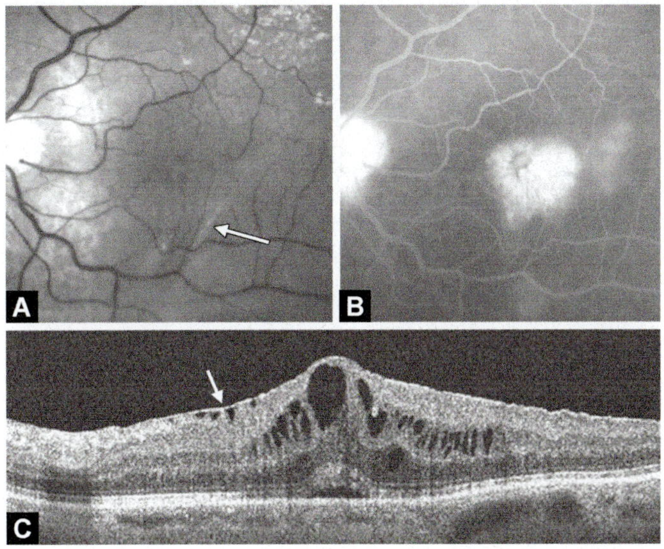

Figs. 56.25A to C: Cystoid macular edema associated with an epiretinal membrane (ERM). (A) Red-free fundus photograph showing reflectivity of the ERM (long arrow); (B) Late phase of fluorescein angiography showing dye pooling in the cystoid cavities; (C) Optical coherence tomography (OCT) B-scan showing the ERM (arrow) associated with the cystoid cavities.

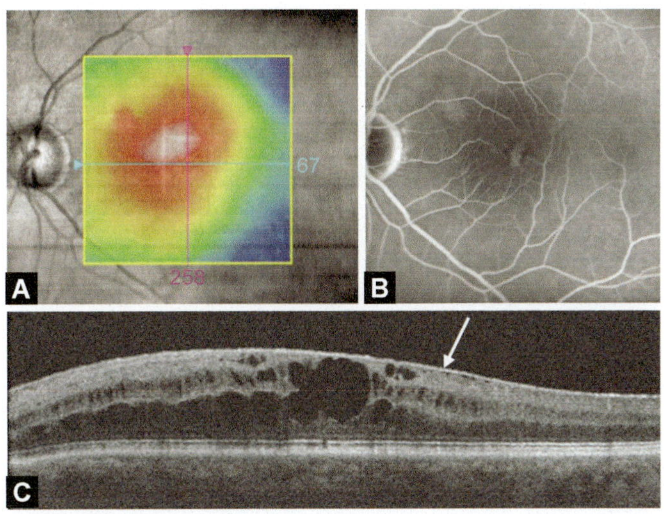

Figs. 56.26A to C: Cystoid maculopathy associated with an epiretinal membrane (ERM). (A) Macular thickness map showing severe macular thickening; (B) No dye leakage is seen on fluorescein angiography; (C) Optical coherence tomography (OCT) B-scan showing the ERM (arrow) associated with the cystoid cavities.

changes are unrelated to fluorescein leakage[150] and their pathogenesis is unknown. They are not related to VA worsening (Figs. 56.26A to C).[151]

In other cases, contraction of the ERM results in formation of a MPH in about 15% of cases.[59] In 1976, Allen and Gass[152] published the first description of an ERM whose contraction simulated a MH by contraction of the foveal pit and coined the term "pseudomacular hole", subsequently redefined as "MPH".[153] Their description was based on biomicroscopic observations. Today, SD-OCT may easily show this typical foveal profile of MPH with a steepened foveal pit combined with thickened foveal edges and a small foveal pit diameter (Figs. 56.27 and 56.28).[55,59] This usually corresponds to a round, reddish foveal image

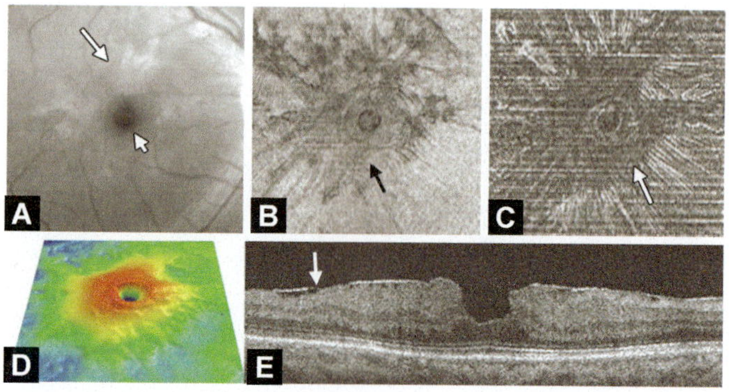

Figs. 56.27A to E: Pseudomacular hole due to contraction of an epiretinal membrane (ERM). (A) Blue reflectance fundus photograph showing reflectivity of the ERM (long arrow). Round aspect of the fovea (short arrow); (B) En-face optical coherence tomography (OCT) scan segmented at the retinal surface showing the attraction of superficial retinal folds to the contracted ERM (arrow); (C) Enface OCT scan segmented just below the retinal surface showing the centripetal inner retinal folding (arrow). (D) Three-dimensional OCT showing the cylindrical shape of the foveal pit in a thickened macula. (E) OCT B-scan showing the verticalization of the foveal edge due to the ERM contraction.

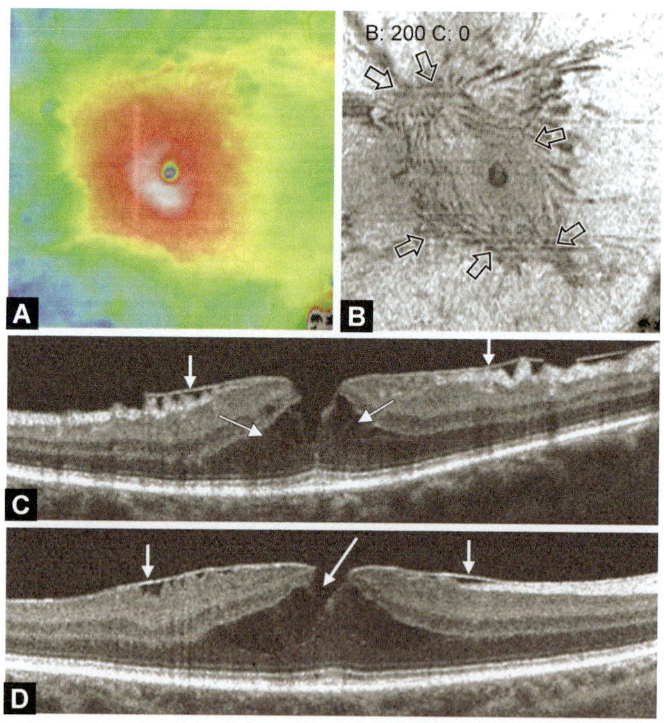

Figs. 56.28A to D: Pseudomacular hole with stretched foveal edge due to contraction of an epiretinal membrane (ERM). (A) Macular thickness map showing a severe macular thickening; (B) En-face optical coherence tomography (OCT) scan segmented at the retinal surface showing multiple eccentric epicenters of the ERM contraction; (C and D) Horizontal (C) and vertical (D) OCT B-scans showing distension of the Henle fiber layer (short arrows) due to the asymmetrical contraction of the ERM (long arrow).

on biomicroscopy. However, OCT also reveals other aspects of MPH with an irregular profile on OCT B-scan, including some degree of intraretinal distension or cleavage in the foveal edge giving rise to controversies[151,154] about the differential diagnosis with LMH.[155]

Indeed, the asymmetrical contraction of some ERM results in an eversion of the foveal edge with a distension of the Henle fiber layer between the inner nuclear layer and the ganglion cell layer, mimicking a cleavage between the outer and inner retina. The difference with LMH may be difficult to appreciate on OCT B-scan; but the OCT C-scan (en-face OCT) pattern is very different. In cases of LMH, the macular surface is smooth, even when a noncontractile epiretinal proliferation is associated,[56] while in MPH the retinal surface is folded by the ERM contraction (Figs. 56.29A to D).[58] Interestingly in MPH with a steeper foveal pit contour, the ERM contraction is centripetal, centered on the fovea with retinal folds converging towards the foveal center, while in MPH with stretched foveal edge, tangential traction forces converge to several eccentric epicenters.[59] In both cases, the macular thickness is globally increased by the ERM contraction.

Although this discussion might only be considered semantic, it has practical consequences. Surgery for

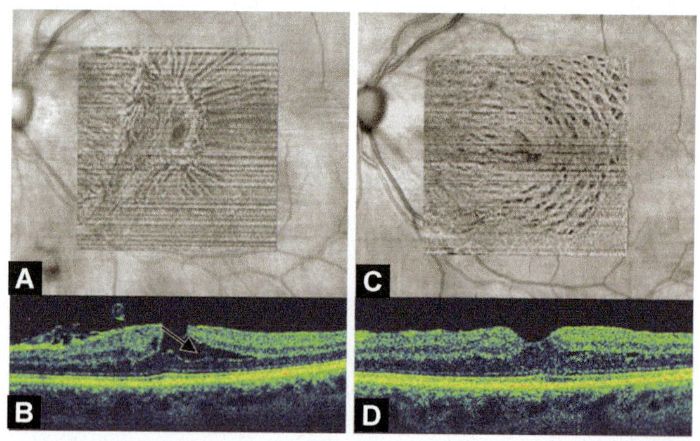

Figs. 56.29A to D: Pseudomacular hole with stretched foveal edge before and after surgery consisting of epiretinal membrane (ERM) and inner limiting membrane peeling without gas injection. (A) En-face optical coherence tomography (OCT) scan segmented at the retinal surface showing the stretching of the fovea between several epicenters of ERM contraction; (B) OCT B-scan showing macular thickening and stretched foveal edge (arrow); (C) Postoperative en-face OCT scan segmented at the retinal surface showing the characteristic image of dissociated optic nerve fiber layer. There is no ERM remnant; (D) Corresponding OCT B-scan showing the recovery of a foveal pit contour with a complete resolution of the foveal cleavage.

MPH only requires peeling of the ERM, and incidentally of the ILM, to improve the macular profile. No fluid gas exchange is needed (Fig. 56.29). Conversely, in true LMH, the indication for surgery is controversial because of the suspicion that some degree of tissue avulsion is preventing visual improvement. If surgery is performed, a fluid gas exchange is recommended.[59]

Lastly, in rare cases, ERM contraction may result not in a closure of the foveal pit, but on the contrary, in a herniation of the fovea through a central defect of a very constrictive membrane (Figs. 56.30A to C).[156]

Determinants of Visual Acuity

The VA is inversely proportional to macular retinal thickness;[157] but this correlation is relatively modest, and there is a wide dispersion of VA values for each degree of macular thickening.[150,158] Other factors have been tested in correlation with preoperative VA or in view of predicting the visual outcome after surgery.

The foveal photoreceptor deformation index[159] or thickness of the outer retina[160] have been found to be related to the preoperative VA, like the thickness of the inner and outer nuclear layers or EZ integrity. Age, symptom duration, and initial VA appear to be valuable predictive factors of visual improvement in patients undergoing ERM surgery.[161]

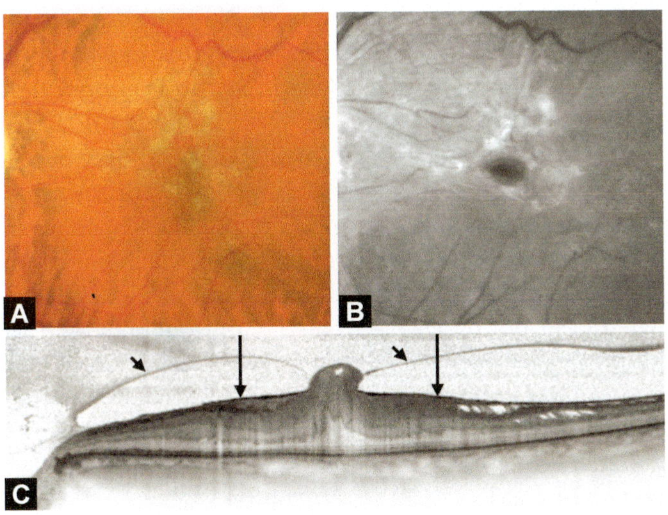

Figs. 56.30A to C: Foveal herniation induced by epiretinal membrane (ERM) contraction. (A and B) Color (A) and blue reflectance (B) fundus photographs showing the severe contraction of the macula by an opaque ERM; (C) Optical coherence tomography (OCT) B-scan showing the macular thickening and the herniation of the fovea above the plane of the retinal surface. Note the thick and hyper-reflective ERM (long arrows) and the persistent adherence of the posterior vitreous cortex to the herniated fovea (short arrows).

But although many studies have attempted to find the best predictive factors for postoperative visual improvement, these factors only help to inform the patient of the potential risk of limited improvement after surgery in some cases.

Surgery for Epiretinal Membrane and Results

As for the other vitreoretinal diseases, surgery has been simplified thanks to the use of small transconjunctival vitrectomy. It is a fast and simple surgery because the vitreous is usually already detached from the posterior retina. The indications for combined cataract surgery and complications of surgery are discussed at the end of the chapter.

Principles of surgery:

- *Vitrectomy*: Core vitrectomy is usually sufficient to enable ERM manipulation, as well as to remove vitreous opacities causing floaters. In a minority of cases, the vitreous is still partially attached to the ERM or to the optic disk. This is especially true for ERM in young subjects. In these cases, triamcinolone acetonide may be used to stain the vitreous cortex and facilitate its detachment.
- *ERM and ILM peeling*: Although many instruments have been developed to facilitate ERM peeling, end-gripping forceps are most often used to initiate and complete the membrane detachment. The dissection is started remote from the fovea and extended progressively. If possible, the membrane is removed in a single piece. The dissection should not be started in front of an axoplasmic transport accumulation. In most cases, large pieces of ILM come off with the ERM,[137] causing a whitening of the retinal surface and sometimes some capillary bleeding. The need to achieve a complete ILM peeling after ERM removal is controversial.
- *Use of dyes*: Staining the ERM with TB facilitates visualization of the membrane limits and makes its removal easier and safer. To visualize whether the ILM has been removed, a second staining with diluted ICG or Brilliant Blue may be made.[137]

Indications and results of surgery:

- *Indications for surgery*: Surgical ablation of an ERM is indicated when the VA decreases to 20/40 or worse or when the binocular vision is impaired by metamorphopsia or aniseikonia, regardless of the VA level.[162,163]

- *Results*:
  - *Anatomical results*: The macular thickness significantly decreases after surgery, although it rarely returns to normal and the foveal pit rarely reappears. Although the macula regains a better appearance on fundus examination, its thickness remains greater than normal in two-thirds of cases on OCT scans; but this does not prevent visual improvement (Fig. 56.29).[150,161]

    In addition, the macular thickness is reduced for several months or years after surgery.[164] The decrease in macular thickness is not affected by ILM peeling.[165,166] It is therefore possible that ERM, as a disorder, is not limited to epiretinal glial cell proliferation but also includes a certain degree of intraretinal gliosis.

    The completion of ERM ablation may be easily controlled by observing the OCT C-scan, which may show membrane remnants. If the remnants remain in the periphery of the macular area, they do not interfere with foveal and visual improvement. The presence of a DONFL on the OCT C-scan or on blue reflectance photographs reflects the extent of ILM peeling (Fig. 56.29).[65,167]

    When a foveal detachment is present, it usually disappears a few months after surgery.[149] Microcystic changes present before surgery have a variable outcome. They may remain unchanged or decrease progressively after surgery. New cystoid spaces may also occur, especially in cases of combined ERM and cataract surgery;[168] but the relationship with fluorescein leakage has not been systematically studied.
  - *Visual results*: The results of ERM surgery are good, overall resulting in a vision improvement by 2 Snellen lines or more in about 60–70% of cases,[150,161] with few complications. However, patients with significant preoperative disturbance often benefit more from surgery than those with lessdisturbance.[169,170] On the other hand, patients with a better initial VA achieve better visual outcomes.[171] Patients with an initial VA of 0.5 LogMAR or less (20/63 or better) are more likely to reach 0.2 LogMAR or less (20/32 or better) after surgery. The endpoint of VA improvement should be assessed after cataract surgery. In a series of operated eyes with a mean initial VA of 20/40, the mean final VA was 20/32 in eyes that were pseudophakic at the final examination.[163] In a recent study including only cases with combined ERM and cataract surgery, 42% of patients achieved a VA of 20/20. These patients had a shorter duration of symptoms and a better initial vision than those with a lower vision improvement.[161] Lastly, the postoperative improvement in metamorphopsia is a quite slow process compared to the postoperative VA improvement.[172] A postoperative loss of vision is rare outside surgical complications.
  - *Results according to ILM peeling*:[35] Two studies have shown no difference between ILM peeling or nonpeeling. No study has reported better results after peeling the ERM alone. Five studies have found that peeling the ILM with the ERM reduced the recurrence rate of ERMs.

Epiretinal Membrane in Young Subjects

Idiopathic ERM are rare in children and young adults. They are more likely to be opaque, to adhere to a retinal temporal vessel and to develop without PVD (Figs. 56.31A and B).[173] Surgical removal may result in a significant and lasting visual improvement, although published series are small.[173,174]

Secondary Epiretinal Membrane

A variety of retinal diseases may result in ERM proliferation. A 2011 study by Yazici et al. looked at 168 secondary ERMs that were surgically treated; among these cases, the etiology was determined to be diabetic retinopathy in 64%, RVO in 16%, uveitis in 7%, RD surgery in 3%, and various other ocular disorders in 10% of cases.[175]

After successful surgery for RD, an ERM may occur, typically within 6–8 weeks after surgery, with a rapid contraction referred to as macular pucker. These types of ERM were the first to be operated by Machemer R in 1978.[176] Symptomatic retinal tears without detachment, whether or not they were treated with laser, may also be found in the recent history of a patient with vision loss due to ERM contraction; or they may be asymptomatic, discovered during examination of the fundus periphery.[177] Cataract surgery is also a known factor for increased risk of secondary ERM.[178]

MYOPIC FOVEOSCHISIS AND ABNORMAL VITREOMACULAR ADHESION

In 1999, Takano and Kishi[179] first described foveal retinoschisis in myopic eyes, using time-domain OCT. The

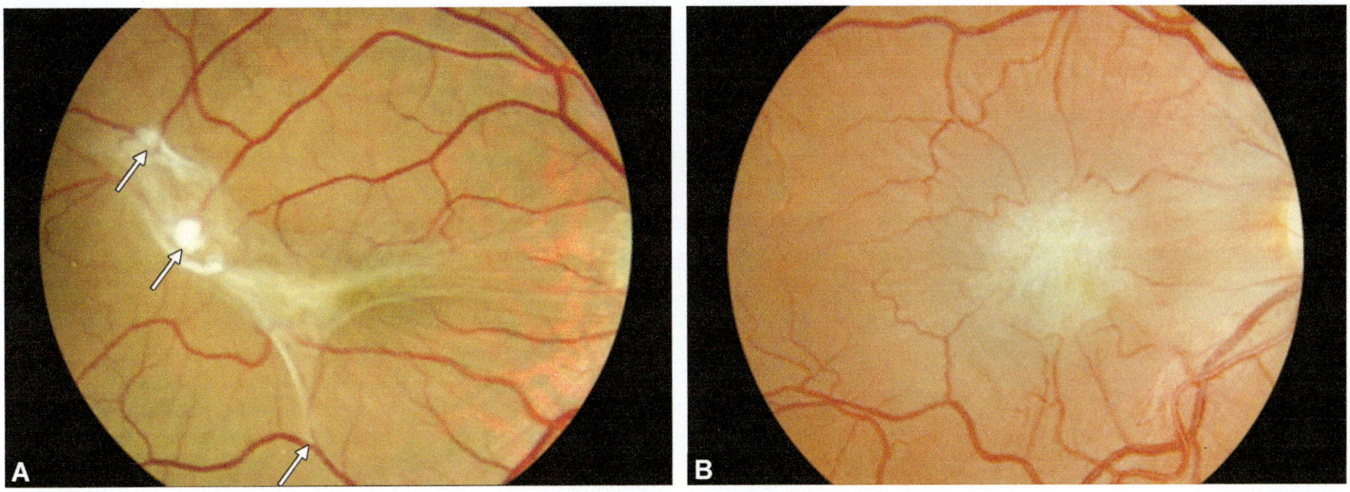

Figs. 56.31A and B: Epiretinal membrane (ERM) in young subjects. (A) A 16-year-old girl with idiopathic ERM and recent vision loss. Note the opacity of the ERM, which is also attached in 3 points to the retinal vessels (arrows); (B) Opaque idiopathic ERM in a 20-year-old man, centered on the fovea.

term "myopic foveoschisis (MF)"[180] is now more often used. Rare clinical and histological observations of this condition have been made in the past.[181-183]

Description and Natural History of Myopic Foveoschisis

Myopic foveoschisis occurs in 9–30% of highly myopic eyes with a refractive error of –8 diopters or more[179,184-186] and is associated with posterior staphyloma. However, MF may be underestimated because of the absence of patient complaints in some cases.

Pathogenesis

Myopic foveoschisis results from stretching of the retina between the RPE following the curve of the posterior staphyloma and epiretinal structures such as the PVC or ERM, that are tense on the retinal surface.[187] In highly myopic eyes, early vitreous liquefaction leads to the formation of a large, fluid-filled pocket in front of the macula that may mimic a complete PVD on biomicroscopic examination,[188] whereas a large remnant of PVC is still present on the retinal surface. This abnormal PVD, also referred to as vitreoschisis,[1,132,133] results in a stiffening of the retinal surface[18] facing the concave deformation of the posterior staphyloma.[187] Remnants of vitreous cortex are present in 75–100% of cases with MF.[51,185,187,189] This pathophysiological hypothesis is confirmed by the reapplication of the retina on the curvature of the staphyloma after surgical peeling of all pathological epiretinal structures.

Symptoms and Diagnosis

Symptoms of MF are not specific. The visual loss seems to occur at a late stage of the evolution, and at least one-third of patients with MF are asymptomatic.[185,190] In a systematic study of myopic patients, eyes with a MF that extended to the whole macula had near normal vision at initial examination.[191]

The diagnosis of MF is mainly made based on OCT, which provides information far superior to that provided by fundus biomicroscopy, which would only show cystic changes in the macula. MF is characterized by a distension between the inner and outer retinal layers, which occurs in the Henle fiber layer and gives an aspect of columns bridging the outer and inner retina, delimiting cystic spaces (Figs. 56.32A and B).[192] Cystic changes may also be present in the distended inner plexiform layer and between the ILM and the ganglion cell layer (Figs. 56.33 and 56.34). The increase in macular retinal thickness is by itself paradoxically not correlated with VA decrease.[190] MF may be associated with lamellar hole, MPH, ERM, and foveal detachment, with or without photoreceptor defects,[190,193,194] which may result in vision impairment (Figs. 56.33 to 56.35).

Natural History

The VA may remain stable for a long time in the absence of MH or foveal detachment.[190] Changes in VA have been reported in a series of 207 eyes with MF with a mean follow-up of 36.2 months.[191] However, as for the anatomical progression, these statistics depend on the time of diagnosis

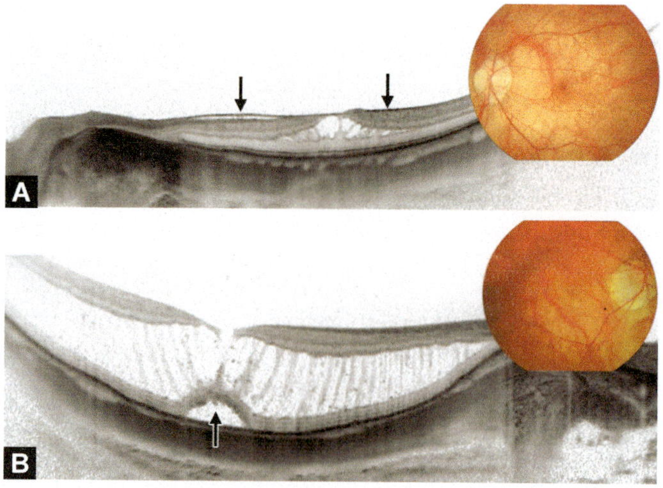

Figs. 56.32A and B: Examples of myopic foveoschisis. (A) Optical coherence tomography (OCT) B-scan. Foveal stretching resulting in cystoid spaces in the Henle fiber layer (foveoschisis). Note the presence of an epiretinal structure (arrows), which could be an epiretinal membrane, a remnant of posterior vitreous cortex or both. *Inset*: Color fundus photograph showing the tessellation of the myopic fundus; (B) OCT B-scan. Extended foveoschisis with severe distension of the Henle fibers in a myopic eye with staphyloma. Foveal detachment (arrow) but no epiretinal structure is visible on OCT. *Inset*: Color fundus photograph showing choroidal atrophy in the staphyloma.

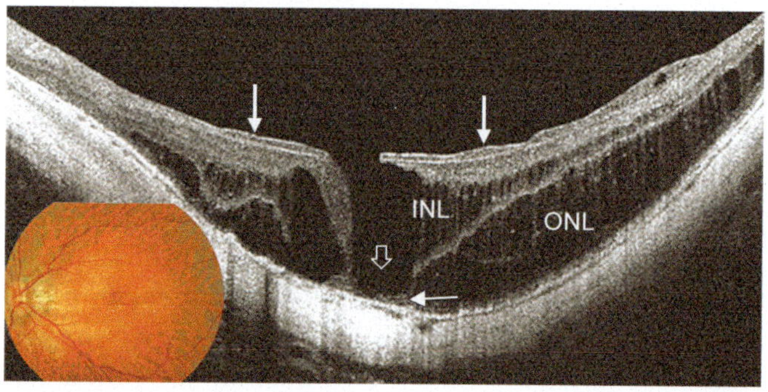

Figs. 56.33: Myopic foveoschisis with lamellar macular hole. Major macular thickening with schisis in the outer nuclear layer, Henle fiber layer and inner nuclear layer. Deep lamellar hole (large empty arrow) with a thin remnant of photoreceptor on the retinal pigment epithelium (thin arrow). Thick epiretinal proliferation (white arrows). *Inset*: Color fundus photograph showing diffuse chorioretinal atrophy in the staphyloma.
(INL: Inner nuclear layer; ONL: Outer nuclear layer)

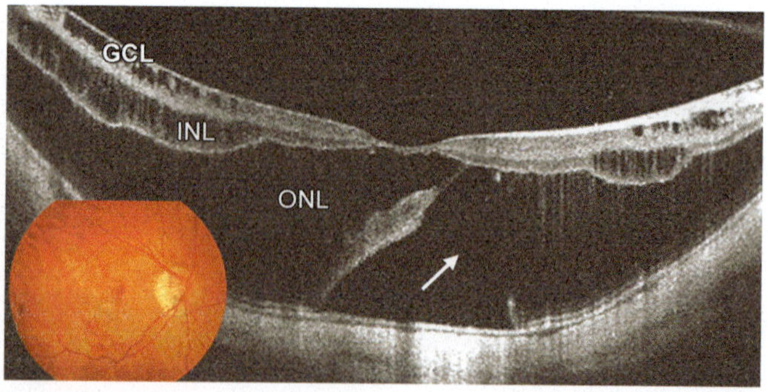

Fig. 56.34: Myopic foveoschisis with foveal detachment and photoreceptor disruption. Major macular thickening with schisis in the outer nuclear layer, Henle fiber layer, inner nuclear layer and ganglion cell layer. Foveal detachment with breakdown in the continuity of the photoreceptor (long arrow). *Inset*: Color fundus photograph showing the myopic foveoschisis with diffuse chorioretinal atrophy in the staphyloma.
(GCL: Ganglion cell layer; INL: Inner nuclear layer; ONL: Outer nuclear layer)

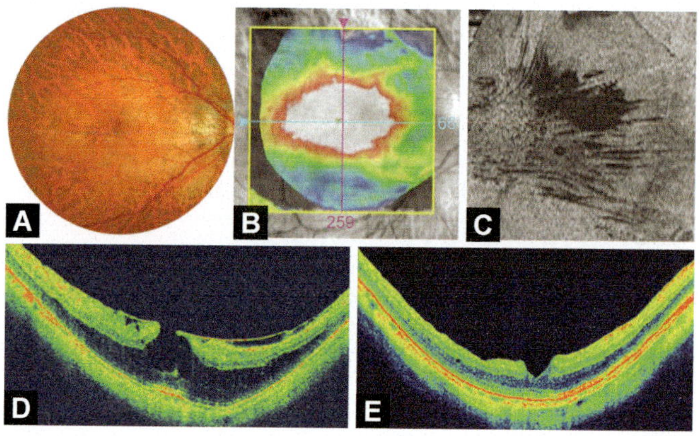

Figs. 56.35A to E: Results of vitreoretinal surgery in a case of myopic foveoschisis. (A) Color fundus photograph showing diffuse chorioretinal atrophy in the staphyloma; (B) Macular thickness map showing the major macular thickening; (C) En-face optical coherence tomography (OCT) showing the inner retinal folds induced by the presence of an epiretinal membrane (ERM); (D) Preoperative B-scan showing the myopic foveoschisis associated with an ERM; (E) Postoperative improvement in macular profile after vitrectomy, vitreous cortex and ERM peeling.

of the disease. When MFs are diagnosed because of visual symptoms, they are more likely to worsen than when the diagnosis is made based solely on OCT.

Anatomically, a small proportion of MFs may improve spontaneously.[191] It has been shown that partial MF sparing the foveal center tends to be stable, whereas MF involving the macular center tends to progress in more than 40% of cases after a 3-year follow-up.[191] Worsening of MF includes a progressive thickening of the macula and a foveal detachment that increases the risk of MH.[190,192,195,196]

Surgery for Myopic Foveoschisis and Results

Indications for Surgery

The indications for surgery are still challenging and the appropriate timing for vitrectomy has not been clearly established.[197] On the one hand, MF may be stable for a long time; on the other hand, when vision decreases along with an increase in macular thickening and the occurrence of a foveal detachment, the risk of postoperative MH also increases.[198] The VA appears to be the best criterion to decide whether surgery should be performed. In these highly myopic eyes, however, the baseline VA is often less than normal because of an imperfect correction of the refractive error or some degree of chorioretinal atrophy and not solely because of the MF. The surgical decision is then based more on the recent VA worsening and especially on the loss of reading acuity. It has indeed been shown that the preoperative VA is the main prognostic factor for postoperative visual recovery, with a cut-off around 20/50.[199]

The presence of a foveal detachment is an ambiguous factor in the surgical decision. While the onset of a foveal detachment exposes the patient to a spontaneous risk of MH as well as a higher risk of postoperative MH,[198] the best VA improvement has been found in eyes with preoperative foveal detachment.[200] When the foveal detachment is associated with a photoreceptor breakdown and foveal thinning, the risk of spontaneous or postoperative MH is high.[201]

Principles of Surgery

The surgical procedure consists of core vitrectomy, which is often done rapidly due to the liquefaction of the vitreous gel, followed by the removal of the PVC. The use of triamcinolone acetonide to stain the vitreous cortex is essential as the cortex often adheres tightly to the retina and cannot be easily removed by simple aspiration, requiring the use of end-gripping forceps. The PVC is still attached to the posterior pole in more than 85% of eyes with MF.[202] After vitreous removal, staining the retinal surface with TB allows detection and removal of a possible ERM proliferation.

The systematic removal of the ILM is still debated. When a significant layer of dense vitreous cortex or an ERM has been removed, this may be sufficient to soften the retinal surface and flatten the foveoschisis. However, it is usually assumed that the rigidity of the ILM could cause a tangential traction and maintain the foveoschisis.[203] This is especially the case when no tissue is found at the retinal surface. ILM removal is a very common maneuver, but when the foveal center is thinned between a foveal detachment and a lamellar hole, it may destabilize the foveal structure and result in a MH.[190,204] Shimada et al.[204] have proposed a technique of "fovea-sparing ILM peeling" to limit the risk of postoperative MH. The detection of a microhole during ILM peeling is not easy in these eyes and may be improved by the use of intraoperative OCT.[205]

The use of gas tamponade at the end of the procedure is disputable in the absence of MH,[206] but is common when the ILM has been peeled off.[207]

Results of Surgery

Complete resolution of the foveoschisis has been achieved in 75–100% of cases,[199,207] or the foveal thickness decreased significantly after surgery (Fig. 56.35).[197,208] VA improved in 62–76% of cases,[198,199] and the visual gain ranged between 0.20 LogMAR and 0.26 LogMAR.[197,207,208] Anatomical and visual improvements are usually progressive and should be assessed at least 6 months after surgery.[208] The main predictive factor for postoperative visual improvement is the preoperative VA.[198,199,208] The presence of a preoperative foveal detachment has been correlated with a better postoperative visual improvement by Ikuno,[200] but not in other studies.[197,198]

The results of surgery may be adversely affected by the occurrence of a MH in 5–11% of cases.[198,201,207] Factors predisposing to a postoperative MH are foveal detachment, lamellar hole, or the conjunction of both, resulting in foveal center thinning and EZ disruption.[198] It should also be noted that a microhole may be present preoperatively and only detected by a thorough OCT examination using multiple tight raster B-scans.[193] The availability of intraoperative OCT also allows detecting microholes during surgery.[205]

COMPLICATIONS OF SURGERY FOR VITREORETINAL INTERFACE DISEASES OF THE MACULA

Vitreoretinal surgery for macular disorders is associated with a low rate of complications, including rhegmatogenous RD, which is common regardless of the etiology of vitreomacular diseases. It should be noted that RD is an important element in macular surgery decision making. The introduction of small gauge transconjunctival vitrectomy systems has reduced RD after macular surgery from about 3% using 20-gauge probes[60,209] to less than 1% using the 25-gauge probes.[210-212] The occurrence of postvitrectomy RD may be due to intraoperative or postoperative retinal breaks. The rate of intraoperative retinal breaks has been assessed at between 1.8% and 13.9%.[210,211,213] Intraoperative retinal breaks may result from different mechanisms, including traction over the vitreous base during insertion of instruments, induction of the PVD, or excessive aspiration level during vitreous base shaving.

The use of small gauge cannulated systems has been shown to reduce the intraoperative rate of retinal breaks.[213]

Vitrectomy fluidics is also still improving with higher cutting rates and lower flow surges due to smaller gauges, acting as a passive flow control. All together, miniaturizing and improving vitrectomy systems reduces retinal traction and thereby reduces the risk of iatrogenic retinal breaks.[214,215] However, the intraoperative induction of PVD may cause equatorial retinal breaks that should be detected by a careful examination of the peripheral retina under scleral depression at the end of surgery.[210,211] If properly treated during surgery, these breaks do not result in postoperative RD.

The rate of residual postoperative RD (about 1%) is then similar to that observed after cataract surgery,[210,216] but RD tends to occur earlier, within the first week after surgery.[210,212]

Of the two other main complications, cataract is benign, appearing as early as 3 months after vitrectomy in most patients over 60 years, and requiring surgery in more than 50% of cases at 1 year.[217] Endophthalmitis, the most serious complication, is exceptional (0.03% or less of cases).[218]

COMBINED CATARACT SURGERY

When the lens opacity is assumed to impair an accurate view of the fundus during surgery, combined phacovitrectomy is a valuable option. However, because of the high rate of cataract progression after pars plana vitrectomy in adults,[217] there is a tendency to operate systematically on the cataract and the retina during the same operation. This option offers a faster visual rehabilitation by avoiding a subsequent cataract surgery and is therefore more cost effective.[219] However, in diseases such as ERM or VMT, when the vision is only moderately impaired, the role of a phacosclerosis may not be ruled out. Starting with cataract surgery may prevent the need for macular surgery in about 15% of cases.[220] Nevertheless, two steps, sequential or combined phacovitrectomy results in functional or anatomical outcomes.[220]

REFERENCES

1. Gupta P, Yee KM, Garcia P, et al. Vitreoschisis in macular diseases. Br J Ophthalmol. 2011;95:376-80.
2. Sebag J. Vitreous: the resplendent enigma. Br J Ophthalmol. 2009;93:989-91.
3. Ponsioen TL, Hooymans JM, Los LI. Remodelling of the human vitreous and vitreoretinal interface—a dynamic process. Prog Retin Eye Res. 2010;29:580-95.
4. Liu JJ, Witkin AJ, Adhi M, et al. Enhanced vitreous imaging in healthy eyes using swept source optical coherence tomography. PLoS One. 2014;9:e102950.
5. Pang CE, Freund KB, Engelbert M. Enhanced vitreous imaging technique with spectral-domain optical coherence tomography for evaluation of posterior vitreous detachment. JAMA Ophthalmol. 2014;132:1148-50.
6. Kishi S, Shimizu K. Posterior precortical vitreous pocket. Arch Ophthalmol. 1990;108:979-82.
7. Worst JGF. The Bursa Intravitrealis Premacularis. In: Deutman AF (Ed). New Developments in Ophthalmology. The Hague: Junk; 1976. pp. 275-9.
8. Schaal KB, Pang CE, Pozzoni MC, et al. The premacular bursa's shape revealed in vivo by swept-source optical coherence tomography. Ophthalmology. 2014;121:1020-8.
9. Itakura H, Kishi S, Li D, et al. Observation of posterior precortical vitreous pocket using swept-source optical coherence tomography. Invest Ophthalmol Vis Sci. 2013;54:3102-7.
10. Spaide RF. Visualization of the posterior vitreous with dynamic focusing and windowed averaging swept source optical coherence tomography. Am J Ophthalmol. 2014;158:1267-4.
11. Worst JG. Cisternal systems of the fully developed vitreous body in the young adult. Trans Ophthalmol Soc UK. 1977;97:550-4.
12. Johnson MW. Posterior vitreous detachment: evolution and complications of its early stages. Am J Ophthalmol. 2010;149:371-82.e1.
13. Ma F, Arcinue CA, Barteselli G, et al. Optical coherence tomography findings of the vitreoretinal interface in asymptomatic fellow eyes of patients with acute posterior vitreous detachment. Retina. 2014;34:4474-54.
14. Uchino E, Uemura A, Ohba N. Initial stages of posterior vitreous detachment in healthy eyes of older persons evaluated by optical coherence tomography. Arch Ophthalmol. 2001;119:1475-79.
15. Sebag J. Anomalous posterior vitreous detachment: a unifying concept in vitreo-retinal disease. Graefes Arch Clin Exp Ophthalmol. 2004;242:690-8.
16. Duker JS, Kaiser PK, Binder S, et al. The International Vitreomacular Traction Study Group classification of vitreomacular adhesion, traction, and macular hole. Ophthalmology. 2013;120:2611-9.
17. Meuer SM, Myers CE, Klein BE, et al. The epidemiology of vitreoretinal interface abnormalities as detected by spectral-domain optical coherence tomography: the Beaver Dam Eye Study. Ophthalmology. 2015;122:787-95.
18. Kishi S, Demaria C, Shimizu K. Vitreous cortex remnants at the fovea after spontaneous vitreous detachment. Int Ophthalmol. 1986;9:253-60.
19. Almeida DR, Chin EK, Rahim K, et al. Factors associated with spontaneous release of vitreomacular traction. Retina. 2015;35:492-7.

20. Chang LK, Fine HF, Spaide RF, et al. Ultrastructural correlation of spectral-domain optical coherence tomographic findings in vitreomacular traction syndrome. Am J Ophthalmol. 2008;146:121-7.
21. Gandorfer A, Rohleder M, Grosselfinger S, et al. Epiretinal pathology of diffuse diabetic macular edema associated with vitreomacular traction. Am J Ophthalmol. 2005;139:638-52.
22. Dugel PU, Tolentino M, Feiner L, et al. Results of the 2-year Ocriplasmin for Treatment for Symptomatic Vitreomacular Adhesion Including Macular Hole (OASIS) randomized trial. Ophthalmology. 2016;123:2232-47.
23. Gaudric A, Haouchine B, Massin P, et al. Macular hole formation: new data provided by optical coherence tomography. Arch Ophthalmol. 1999;117:744-51.
24. Haouchine B, Massin P, Gaudric A. Foveal pseudocyst as the first step in macular hole formation: a prospective study by optical coherence tomography. Ophthalmology. 2001;108:15-22.
25. Takahashi A, Nagaoka T, Yoshida A. STAGE 1-A macular hole: a prospective spectral-domain optical coherence tomography study. Retina. 2011;31:127-47.
26. Takahashi A, Yoshida A, Nagaoka T, et al. Macular hole formation in fellow eyes with a perifoveal posterior vitreous detachment of patients with a unilateral macular hole. Am J Ophthalmol. 2011;151:981-9.
27. Gass JD. Reappraisal of biomicroscopic classification of stages of development of a macular hole. Am J Ophthalmol. 1995;119:752-9.
28. Kumagai K, Hangai M, Larson E, et al. Vitreoretinal interface and foveal deformation in asymptomatic fellow eyes of patients with unilateral macular holes. Ophthalmology. 2011;118:1638-44.
29. Tzu JH, John VJ, Flynn HW Jr, et al. Clinical course of vitreomacular traction managed initially by observation. Ophthalmic Surg Lasers Imaging Retina. 2015;46:571-6.
30. John VJ, Flynn HW Jr, Smiddy WE, et al. Clinical course of vitreomacular adhesion managed by initial observation. Retina. 2014;34:442-6.
31. Jackson TL, Donachie PH, Johnston RL, Vitreomacular Traction Study Group. Electronic medical record database study of vitrectomy and observation for vitreomacular traction. Retina. 2016;36:1897-904.
32. Smiddy WE, Michels RG, Glaser BM, et al. Vitrectomy for macular traction caused by incomplete vitreous separation. Arch Ophthalmol. 1988;106(5):624-8.
33. Toklu Y, Demirel S, Sarac O, et al. Anatomic and functional outcome of triamcinolone-assisted 23-gauge vitrectomy in vitreomacular traction syndrome. Semin Ophthalmol. 2012;27:73-7.
34. Zhao F, Gandorfer A, Haritoglou C, et al. Epiretinal cell proliferation in macular pucker and vitreomacular traction syndrome: analysis of flat-mounted internal limiting membrane specimens. Retina. 2013;33:77-88.
35. Folk JC, Adelman RA, Flaxel CJ, et al. Idiopathic Epiretinal Membrane and Vitreomacular Traction Preferred Practice Pattern(®) Guidelines. Ophthalmology. 2016;123:P152-81.
36. Yang CS, Hsieh MH, Chang YF, et al. Predictive factors of visual outcome for vitreomacular traction syndrome after vitrectomy. Retina. 2017.
37. Witkin AJ, Patron ME, Castro LC, et al. Anatomic and visual outcomes of vitrectomy for vitreomacular traction syndrome. Ophthalmic Surg Lasers Imaging. 2010;41:425-31.
38. Ichiyama Y, Kawamura H, Fujikawa M, et al. Photoreceptor outer segment length and outer foveal thickness as factors associated with visual outcome after vitrectomy for vitreomacular traction syndrome. Retina. 2016;36:1707-12.
39. Gonzalez MA, Flynn HW Jr, Bokman CM, et al. Outcomes of pars plana vitrectomy for patients with vitreomacular traction. Ophthalmic Surg Lasers Imaging Retina. 2015;46:708-14.
40. Stalmans P, Benz MS, Gandorfer A, et al. Enzymatic vitreolysis with ocriplasmin for vitreomacular traction and macular holes. N Engl J Med. 2012;367:606-15.
41. Chan CK, Wessels IF, Friedrichsen EJ. Treatment of idiopathic macular holes by induced posterior vitreous detachment. Ophthalmology. 1995;102:757-67.
42. Rodrigues IA, Stangos AN, McHugh DA, et al. Intravitreal injection of expansile perfluoropropane (c(3)f(8)) for the treatment of vitreomacular traction. Am J Ophthalmol. 2013;155:270-6.e2.
43. Steinle NC, Dhoot DS, Quezada Ruiz C, et al. Treatment of vitreomacular traction with intravitreal perfluoropropane (C3f8) injection. Retina. 2017;37:643-50.
44. Jackson TL, Donachie PH, Sparrow JM, et al. United Kingdom National Ophthalmology Database study of vitreoretinal surgery: report 2, macular hole. Ophthalmology. 2013;120:629-34.
45. Chan A, Duker JS, Schuman JS, et al. Stage 0 macular holes: observations by optical coherence tomography. Ophthalmology. 2004;111:2027-32.
46. Gass JD. Idiopathic senile macular hole. Its early stages and pathogenesis. Arch Ophthalmol. 1988;106:629-39.
47. Hee MR, Puliafito CA, Wong C, et al. Optical coherence tomography of macular holes. Ophthalmology. 1995;102:748-56.
48. Kelly NE, Wendel RT. Vitreous surgery for idiopathic macular holes. Results of a pilot study. Arch Ophthalmol. 1991;109:654-9.
49. Johnson RN, Gass JD. Idiopathic macular holes. Observations, stages of formation, and implications for surgical intervention. Ophthalmology. 1988;95:917-24.
50. Ezra E, Fariss RN, Possin DE, et al. Immunocytochemical characterization of macular hole opercula. Arch Ophthalmol. 2001;119:223-31.
51. Philippakis E, Amouyal F, Couturier A, et al. Size and vitreomacular attachment of primary full-thickness macular holes. Br J Ophthalmol. 2017;101:951-4.
52. Privat E, Tadayoni R, Gaucher D, et al. Residual defect in the foveal photoreceptor layer detected by optical coherence tomography in eyes with spontaneously closed macular holes. Am J Ophthalmol. 2007;143:814-9.

53. Gass JD. Lamellar macular hole: a complication of cystoid macular edema after cataract extraction. Arch Ophthalmol. 1976;94:793-800.
54. Frangieh GT, Green WR, Engel HM. A histopathologic study of macular cysts and holes. Retina. 1981;1:311-36.
55. Haouchine B, Massin P, Tadayoni R, et al. Diagnosis of macular pseudoholes and lamellar macular holes by optical coherence tomography. Am J Ophthalmol. 2004;138:732-9.
56. Pang CE, Spaide RF, Freund KB. Epiretinal proliferation seen in association with lamellar macular holes: a distinct clinical entity. Retina. 2014;34:1513-23.
57. Pang CE, Maberley DA, Freund KB, et al. Lamellar hole-associated epiretinal proliferation: A clinicopathologic correlation. Retina. 2016;36:1408-12.
58. Compera D, Entchev E, Haritoglou C, et al. Lamellar hole-associated epiretinal proliferation in comparison to epiretinal membranes of macular pseudoholes. Am J Ophthalmol. 2015;160:373-84.
59. Gaudric A, Aloulou Y, Tadayoni R, et al. Macular pseudoholes with lamellar cleavage of their edge remain pseudoholes. Am J Ophthalmol. 2013;155:733-42.
60. Guillaubey A, Malvitte L, Lafontaine PO, et al. Incidence of retinal detachment after macular surgery: a retrospective study of 634 cases. Br J Ophthalmol. 2007;91:1327-30.
61. Yagi F, Takagi S, Tomita G. Incidence and causes of iatrogenic retinal breaks in idiopathic macular hole and epiretinal membrane. Semin Ophthalmol. 2014;29:66-9.
62. Blain P, Paques M, Massin P, et al. Epiretinal membranes surrounding idiopathic macular holes. Retina. 1998;18:316-21.
63. Cheng L, Azen SP, El-Bradey MH, et al. Effects of preoperative and postoperative epiretinal membranes on macular hole closure and visual restoration. Ophthalmology. 2002;109:1514-20.
64. Park DW, Lee JH, Min WK. The use of internal limiting membrane maculorrhexis in treatment of idiopathic macular holes. Korean J Ophthalmol. 1998;12:92-7.
65. Tadayoni R, Paques M, Massin P, et al. Dissociated optic nerve fiber layer appearance of the fundus after idiopathic epiretinal membrane removal. Ophthalmology. 2001;108:2279-83.
66. Sabry D, El-Kannishy A, Kamel R, et al. Correlation between en face optical coherence tomography defects of the inner retinal layers and ganglion cell inner plexiform layer analysis after internal limiting membrane peeling for idiopathic full-thickness macular hole. Invest Ophthalmol Vis Sc. 2016;57:OCT444-450.
67. Michalewska Z, Michalewski J, Adelman RA, et al. Inverted internal limiting membrane flap technique for large macular holes. Ophthalmology. 2010;117:2018-25.
68. Rodrigues EB, Meyer CH, Mennel S, et al. Mechanisms of intravitreal toxicity of indocyanine green dye: implications for chromovitrectomy. Retina. 2007;27:958-70.
69. Stalmans P, Van Aken EH, Veckeneer M, et al Toxic effect of indocyanine green on retinal pigment epithelium related to osmotic effects of the solvent. Am J Ophthalmol. 2002;134:282-5.
70. Haritoglou C, Gandorfer A, Gass CA, et al. Histology of the vitreoretinal interface after staining of the internal limiting membrane using glucose 5% diluted indocyanine and infracyanine green. Am J Ophthalmol. 2004;137:345-8.
71. Yip HK, Lai TY, So KF, et al. Retinal ganglion cells toxicity caused by photosensitising effects of intravitreal indocyanine green with illumination in rat eyes. Br J Ophthalmol. 2006;90:99-102.
72. Lesnik Oberstein SY, de Smet MD. Use of heavy Trypan blue in macular hole surgery. Eye. 2010;24:1177-81.
73. Mohr A, Bruinsma M, Oellerich S, et al. Dyes for Eyes: hydrodynamics, biocompatibility and efficacy of 'heavy' (dual) dyes for chromovitrectomy. Ophthalmologica. 2013;230(Suppl 2):51-8.
74. Grisanti S, Szurman P, Tatar O, et al. Histopathological analysis in experimental macular surgery with trypan blue. Br J Ophthalmol. 2004;88:1206-8.
75. Enaida H, Hisatomi T, Hata Y, et al. Brilliant blue G selectively stains the internal limiting membrane/brilliant blue G-assisted membrane peeling. Retina. 2006;26:631-6.
76. Rodrigues EB, Costa EF, Penha FM, et al. The use of vital dyes in ocular surgery. Surv Ophthalmol. 2009;54:576-617.
77. Gaudric A, Tadayoni R. Macular hole. In: Schachat AP Wilkinson CP, Hinton DR, Sadda SR, Wiedemann P (Eds). Ryan's Retina, 6th edition. New York: Elsevier; 2017. pp. 2213-32.
78. Alberti M, la Cour M. Gas-foveal contact: A new approach to evaluating positioning regimens in macular hole surgery. Retina. 2017.
79. Goldbaum MH, McCuen BW, Hanneken AM, et al. Silicone oil tamponade to seal macular holes without position restrictions. Ophthalmology. 1998;105:2140-7.
80. Schurmans A, Van Calster J, Stalmans P. Macular hole surgery with inner limiting membrane peeling, endodrainage, and heavy silicone oil tamponade. Am J Ophthalmol. 2009;147:495-500.
81. Karia N, Laidlaw A, West J, et al. Macular hole surgery using silicone oil tamponade. Br J Ophthalmol. 2001;85:1320-3.
82. Tafoya ME, Lambert HM, Vu L, et al. Visual outcomes of silicone oil versus gas tamponade for macular hole surgery. Semin Ophthalmol. 2003;18:127-31.
83. Gaudric A. Macula hole surgery: simple or complex? Am J Ophthalmol. 2009;147:381-3.
84. Guillaubey A, Malvitte L, Lafontaine PO, et al. Comparison of face-down and seated position after idiopathic macular hole surgery: a randomized clinical trial. Am J Ophthalmol. 2008;146:128-34.
85. Ip MS, Baker BJ, Duker JS, et al. Anatomical outcomes of surgery for idiopathic macular hole as determined by optical coherence tomography. Arch Ophthalmol. 2002;120:29-35.
86. Ullrich S, Haritoglou C, Gass C, et al. Macular hole size as a prognostic factor in macular hole surgery. Br J Ophthalmol. 2002;86:390-3.
87. Eckardt C, Eckardt U, Groos S, et al. Removal of the internal limiting membrane in macular holes. Clinical and morphological findings. Ophthalmologe. 1997;94:545-51.

88. Rice T. Internal limiting membrane removal in surgery for full-thickness macular holes. In: Madreperla SA, McCuen BW (Eds). Macular hole pathogenesis diagnosis and treatment. Boston: Butterworth Heinemann; 1999. pp. 125-46.
89. Brooks HLJ. Macular hole surgery with and without internal limiting membrane peeling. Ophthalmology. 2000;107:1939-48.
90. Haritoglou C, Gass CA, Schaumberger M, et al. Macular changes after peeling of the internal limiting membrane in macular hole surgery. Am J Ophthalmol. 2001;132:363-638.
91. Sheidow TG, Blinder KJ, Holekamp N, et al. Outcome results in macular hole surgery: an evaluation of internal limiting membrane peeling with and without indocyanine green. Ophthalmology. 2003;110:1697-701.
92. Kumagai K, Furukawa M, Ogino N, et al. Vitreous surgery with and without internal limiting membrane peeling for macular hole repair. Retina. 2004;24:721-7.
93. Tognetto D, Grandin R, Sanguinetti G, et al. Internal limiting membrane removal during macular hole surgery: results of a multicenter retrospective study. Ophthalmology. 2006;113:1401-10.
94. Kwok AK, Lai TY, Wong VW. Idiopathic macular hole surgery in Chinese patients: a randomised study to compare indocyanine green-assisted internal limiting membrane peeling with no internal limiting membrane peeling. Hong Kong Med J. 2005;11:259-66.
95. Christensen UC, Kroyer K, Sander B, et al. Value of internal limiting membrane peeling in surgery for idiopathic macular hole stage 2 and 3: a randomised clinical trial. Br J Ophthalmol. 2009;93:1005-15.
96. Lois N, Burr J, Norrie J, et al. Internal limiting membrane peeling versus no peeling for idiopathic full-thickness macular hole: a pragmatic randomized controlled trial. Invest Ophthalmol Vis Sci. 2011;52:1586-92.
97. Tadayoni R, Gaudric A, Haouchine B, et al. Relationship between macular hole size and the potential benefit of internal limiting membrane peeling. Br J Ophthalmol. 2006;90:1239-41.
98. Morescalchi F, Costagliola C, Gambicorti E, et al. Controversies over the role of internal limiting membrane peeling during vitrectomy in macular hole surgery. Surv Ophthalmol. 2017;62:58-69.
99. Kishimoto H, Kusuhara S, Matsumiya W, et al. Retinal surface imaging provided by Cirrus high-definition optical coherence tomography prominently visualizes a dissociated optic nerve fiber layer appearance after macular hole surgery. Int Ophthalmol. 2011;31:385-92.
100. Spaide RF. "Dissociated optic nerve fiber layer appearance" after internal limiting membrane removal is inner retinal dimpling. Retina. 2012;32:1719-26.
101. Baba T, Yamamoto S, Kimoto R, et al. Reduction of thickness of ganglion cell complex after internal limiting membrane peeling during vitrectomy for idiopathic macular hole. Eye (Lond). 2012;26:1173-80.
102. Tadayoni R, Svorenova I, Erginay A, et al Decreased retinal sensitivity after internal limiting membrane peeling for macular hole surgery. Br J Ophthalmol. 2012;96:1513-6.
103. Tornambe PE, Poliner LS, Grote K. Macular hole surgery without face-down positioning. A pilot study. Retina. 1997;17:179-85.
104. Tadayoni R, Vicaut E, Devin F, et al. A randomized controlled trial of alleviated positioning after small macular hole surgery. Ophthalmology. 2011;118:150-5.
105. Alberti M, la Cour M. Face-down positioning versus non-supine positioning in macular hole surgery. Br J Ophthalmol. 2015;99:236-9.
106. Bonnabel A, Bron AM, Isaico R, et al. Long-term anatomical and functional outcomes of idiopathic macular hole surgery. The yield of spectral-domain OCT combined with microperimetry. Graefes Arch Clin Exp Ophthalmol. 2013;251:2505-11.
107. Purtskhvanidze K, Treumer F, Junge O, et al. The long-term course of functional and anatomical recovery after macular hole surgery. Invest Ophthalmol Vis Sci. 2013;54:4882-91.
108. Tarita-Nistor L, Mandelcorn MS, Steinbach MJ, et al. Fixation stability and location in patients with unilateral idiopathic epiretinal membrane. Ophthalmic Surg Lasers Imaging Retina. 2013;44:46-9.
109. Guez JE, Le Gargasson JF, Massin P, et al. Functional assessment of macular hole surgery by scanning laser ophthalmoscopy. Ophthalmology. 1998;105:694-9.
110. Haritoglou C, Ehrt O, Gass CA, et al. Paracentral scotomata: a new finding after vitrectomy for idiopathic macular hole. Br J Ophthalmol. 2001;85:231-3.
111. Ryan EH Jr, Gilbert HD. Results of surgical treatment of recent-onset full-thickness idiopathic macular holes. Arch Ophthalmol. 1994;112:1545-53.
112. Scott RA, Ezra E, West JF, et al. Visual and anatomical results of surgery for long standing macular holes. Br J Ophthalmol. 2000;84:150-3.
113. Itoh Y, Inoue M, Rii T, et al. Correlation between length of foveal cone outer segment tips line defect and visual acuity after macular hole closure. Ophthalmology. 2012;119:1438-46.
114. Ruiz-Moreno JM, Arias L, Araiz J, et al. Spectral-domain optical coherence tomography study of macular structure as prognostic and determining factor for macular hole surgery outcome. Retina. 2013;33:1117-22.
115. Chaudhary K, Mak MY, Gizicki R, et al. Proportion of patients with macular hole surgery who would have been favorable ocriplasmin candidates: A Retrospective Analysis. Retina. 2017;37:76-9.
116. Fahim AT, Khan NW, Johnson MW. Acute panretinal structural and functional abnormalities after intravitreous ocriplasmin injection. JAMA Ophthalmol. 2014;132:484-6.
117. Quezada-Ruiz C, Pieramici DJ, Nasir M, et al. Outer retina reflectivity changes on SD-OCT after intravitreal ocriplasmin for vitreomacular traction and macular hole. Retina. 2015;35:1144-50.
118. Johnson MW, Fahim AT. Understanding the adverse effects of ocriplasmin—reply. JAMA Ophthalmol. 2015;133:230.
119. Atmaca LS, Yilmaz M. Changes in the fundus caused by blunt ocular trauma. Ann Ophthalmol. 1993;25:447-52.

120. Shakin JL, Yannuzzi LA. Posterior segment manifestations of orbital trauma. Adv Ophthalmic Plast Reconstr Surg. 1987;6:115-35.
121. Barreau E, Massin P, Paques M, et al. Surgical treatment of post-traumatic macular holes. J Fr Ophtalmol. 1997;20:423-39.
122. Parmar DN, Stanga PE, Reck AC, et al. Imaging of a traumatic macular hole with spontaneous closure. Retina. 1999;19:470-2.
123. Mitchell P, Smith W, Chey T, et al. Prevalence and associations of epiretinal membranes. The Blue Mountains Eye Study, Australia. Ophthalmology. 1997;104:1033-40.
124. Klein R, Klein B, Wang Q, et al. The epidemiology of epiretinal membranes. Trans Am Ophthalmol Soc. 1994;92:403-29.
125. Barr CC, Michels RG. Idiopathic nonvascularized epiretinal membranes in young patients: report of six cases. Ann Ophthalmol. 1982;14:335-41.
126. Foos R. Vitreoretinal juncture-epiretinal membranes and vitreous. Invest Ophthalmol Vis Sci. 1977;16:416-22.
127. Maumenee AE. Further advances in the study of the macula. Arch Ophthalmol. 1967;78:151-65.
128. Wise GN. Relationship of idiopathic preretinal macular fibrosis to posterior vitreous detachment. Am J Ophthalmol. 1975;79:358-62.
129. Foos RY. Vitreoretinal juncture—simple epiretinal membranes. Albrecht Von Graefes Arch Klin Exp Ophthalmol. 1974;189:231-50.
130. Wiznia RA. Posterior vitreous detachment and idiopathic preretinal macular gliosis. Am J Ophthalmol. 1986;102:196-8.
131. Roth AM, Foos RY. Surface wrinkling retinopathy in eyes enucleated at autopsy. Trans Am Acad Ophthalmol Otolaryngol. 1971;75:1047-58.
132. Kakehashi A, Schepens CL, de Sousa-Neto A, et al. Biomicroscopic findings of posterior vitreoschisis. Ophthalmic Surg. 1993;24:846-50.
133. Sebag J. Vitreoschisis. Graefes Arch Clin Exp Ophthalmol. 2008;246:329-32.
134. Snead MP, Snead DR, Richards AJ, et al. Clinical, histological and ultrastructural studies of the posterior hyaloid membrane. Eye (Lond). 2002;16:447-53.
135. Qiao H, Hisatomi T, Sonoda KH, et al. The characterisation of hyalocytes: the origin, phenotype, and turnover. Br J Ophthalmol. 2005;89:513-7.
136. Lazarus HS, Schoenfeld CL, Fekrat S, et al. Hyalocytes synthesize and secrete inhibitors of retinal pigment epithelial cell proliferation in vitro. Arch Ophthalmol. 1996;114:731-6.
137. Vila Sola D, Nienow C, Jurgens I. Assessment of the internal limiting membrane status when a macular epiretinal membrane is removed in a prospective study. Retina. 2017;37:2310-6.
138. Han J, Han SH, Kim JH, et al. Restoration of retinally induced aniseikonia in patients with epiretinal membrane after early vitrectomy. Retina. 2016;36:311-20.
139. Ichikawa Y, Imamura Y, Ishida M. Metamorphopsia and tangential retinal displacement after epiretinal membrane surgery. Retina. 2017;37:673-9.
140. Lee SM, Pak KY, Kwon HJ, et al. Association between tangential contraction and early vision loss in idiopathic epiretinal membrane. Retina. 2017.
141. Watanabe A, Arimoto S, Nishi O. Correlation between metamorphopsia and epiretinal membrane optical coherence tomography findings. Ophthalmology. 2009;116:1788-93.
142. Okamoto F, Sugiura Y, Okamoto Y, et al. Inner nuclear layer thickness as a prognostic factor for metamorphopsia after epiretinal membrane surgery. Retina. 2015;35:2107-14.
143. Byon IS, Pak GY, Kwon HJ, et al. Natural history of idiopathic epiretinal membrane in eyes with good vision assessed by spectral-domain optical coherence tomography. Ophthalmologica. 2015;234:91-100.
144. Meyer CH, Rodrigues EB, Mennel S, et al. Spontaneous separation of epiretinal membrane in young subjects: personal observations and review of the literature. Graefes Arch Clin Exp Ophthalmol. 2004;242:977-85.
145. Gaudric A, Fardeau C, Goberville M, et al. Ablation of the internal limiting membrane, macular unfolding and visual outcome in surgery of idiopathic epimacular membranes. J Fr Ophtalmol. 1993;16:571-76.
146. Kofod M, la Cour M. Quantification of retinal tangential movement in epiretinal membranes. Ophthalmology. 2012;119:1886-91.
147. Errera MH, Cohen SY, Chahed S, et al. Scattered lamellar microholes as a complication of epiretinal membranes. Ophthalmic Surg Lasers Imaging. 2010;41 Online:e1-4.
148. Arroyo JG, Irvine AR. Retinal distortion and cotton-wool spots associated with epiretinal membrane contraction. Ophthalmology. 1995;102:662-8.
149. Pison A, Dupas B, Couturier A, et al. Evolution of subfoveal detachments secondary to idiopathic epiretinal membranes after surgery. Ophthalmology. 2016;123:583-9.
150. Massin P, Allouch C, Haouchine B, et al. Optical coherence tomography of idiopathic macular epiretinal membranes before and after surgery. Am J Ophthalmol. 2000;130:732-9.
151. Michalewski J, Michalewska Z, Cisiecki S, et al. Morphologically functional correlations of macular pathology connected with epiretinal membrane formation in spectral optical coherence tomography (SOCT). Graefes Arch Clin Exp Ophthalmol. 2007;245:1623-31.
152. Allen AWJ, Gass JMD. Contraction of perifoveal epiretinal membrane simulating a macular hole. Am J Ophthalmol. 1976;82:684-91.
153. Fish RH, Anand R, Izbrand DJ. Macular pseudoholes. Clinical features and accuracy of diagnosis. Ophthalmology. 1992;99:1665-70.
154. Witkin AJ, Ko TH, Fujimoto JG, et al. Redefining lamellar holes and the vitreomacular interface: an ultrahigh-resolution optical coherence tomography study. Ophthalmology. 2006;113:388-97.

155. Govetto A, Dacquay Y, Farajzadeh M, et al. Lamellar macular hole: two distinct clinical entities? Am J Ophthalmol. 2016;164:99-109.
156. Zarbin MA, Michels RG, Green WR. Epiretinal membrane contracture associated with macular prolapse. Am J Ophthalmol. 1990;110:610-8.
157. Wilkins JR, Puliafito CA, Hee MR, et al. Characterization of epiretinal membranes using optical coherence tomography. Ophthalmology. 1996;103:2142-51.
158. Kim J, Rhee KM, Woo SJ, et al. Long-term temporal changes of macular thickness and visual outcome after vitrectomy for idiopathic epiretinal membrane. Am J Ophthalmol. 2010;150:701-9.e1.
159. Hosoda Y, Ooto S, Hangai M, et al. Foveal photoreceptor deformation as a significant predictor of postoperative visual outcome in idiopathic epiretinal membrane surgery. Invest Ophthalmol Vis Sci. 2015;56:6387-93.
160. Arichika S, Hangai M, Yoshimura N. Correlation between thickening of the inner and outer retina and visual acuity in patients with epiretinal membrane. Retina. 2010;30:503-8.
161. Kauffmann Y, Ramel JC, Lefebvre A, et al. Preoperative prognostic factors and predictive score in patients operated on for combined cataract and idiopathic epiretinal membrane. Am J Ophthalmol. 2015;160:185-92.e5.
162. Asaria R, Garnham L, Gregor ZJ, et al. A prospective study of binocular visual function before and after successful surgery to remove a unilateral epiretinal membrane. Ophthalmology. 2008;115:1930-7.
163. Thompson JT. Epiretinal membrane removal in eyes with good visual acuities. Retina. 2005;25:875-82.
164. Fleissig E, Zur D, Moisseiev E, et al. Five-year follow-up after epiretinal membrane surgery: a single-center experience. Retina. 2017.
165. Kumagai K, Ogino N, Furukawa M, et al. Retinal thickness after vitrectomy and internal limiting membrane peeling for macular hole and epiretinal membrane. Clin Ophthalmol. 2012;6:679-88.
166. Schechet SA, DeVience E, Thompson JT. The effect of internal limiting membrane peeling on idiopathic epiretinal membrane surgery, with a review of the literature. Retina. 2017;37:873-80.
167. Ito Y, Terasaki H, Takahashi A, et al. Dissociated optic nerve fiber layer appearance after internal limiting membrane peeling for idiopathic macular holes. Ophthalmology. 2005;112:1415-20.
168. Dolz-Marco R, Hoang QV, Gallego-Pinazo R, et al. Assessment of the significance of cystic changes after epiretinal membrane surgery with internal limiting membrane removal. Retina. 2016;36:727-32.
169. Song SJ, Kuriyan AE, Smiddy WE. Results and prognostic factors for visual improvement after pars plana vitrectomy for idiopathic epiretinal membrane. Retina. 2015;35:866-72.
170. Miliatos I, Lindgren G. Epiretinal membrane surgery evaluated by subjective outcome. Acta Ophthalmol. 2017;95:52-9.
171. Dawson SR, Shunmugam M, Williamson TH. Visual acuity outcomes following surgery for idiopathic epiretinal membrane: an analysis of data from 2001 to 2011. Eye (Lond). 2014;28:219-24.
172. Kim JH, Kang SW, Kong MG, et al. Assessment of retinal layers and visual rehabilitation after epiretinal membrane removal. Graefes Arch Clin Exp Ophthalmol. 2013;251:1055-64.
173. Benhamou N, Massin P, Spolaore R, et al. Surgical management of epiretinal membrane in young patients. Am J Ophthalmol. 2002;133:358-64.
174. Ferrone PJ, Chaudhary KM. Macular epiretinal membrane peeling treatment outcomes in young children. Retina. 2012;32:530-6.
175. Yazici AT, Alagoz N, Celik HU, et al. Idiopathic and secondary epiretinal membranes: do they differ in terms of morphology? An optical coherence tomography-based study. Retina. 2011;31:779-84.
176. Machemer R. The surgical removal of epiretinal macular membranes (macular puckers). Klin Monbl Augenheilkd. 1978;173:36-42.
177. Appiah AP, Hirose T. Secondary causes of premacular fibrosis. Ophthalmology. 1989;96:389-92.
178. Cheung N, Tan SP, Lee SY, et al. Prevalence and risk factors for epiretinal membrane: the Singapore Epidemiology of Eye Disease Study. Br J Ophthalmol. 2017;101:371-6.
179. Takano M, Kishi S. Foveal retinoschisis and retinal detachment in severely myopic eyes with posterior staphyloma. Am J Ophthalmol. 1999;128:472-6.
180. Ikuno Y, Tano Y. Vitrectomy for macular holes associated with myopic foveoschisis. Am J Ophthalmol. 2006;141:774-6.
181. Phillips CI. Retinal detachment at the posterior pole. Br J Ophthalmol. 1958;42:749-53.
182. Rochon-Duvigneaud M. Déformation et lésions de l'oeíl myope. In: Mawas J (Ed). Introduction à l'étude de la myopie et des chorio-rétinites myopiques. Paris: Bull Soc Ophthalmol; 1934. pp. 1-10.
183. Tang J, Rivers MB, Moshfeghi AA, et al. Pathology of macular foveoschisis associated with degenerative myopia. J Ophthalmol. 2010;2010. pii:175613.
184. Baba T, Ohno-Matsui K, Futagami S, et al. Prevalence and characteristics of foveal retinal detachment without macular hole in high myopia. Am J Ophthalmol. 2003;135:338-42.
185. Panozzo G, Mercanti A. Vitrectomy for myopic traction maculopathy. Arch Ophthalmol. 2007;125:767-72.
186. Ripandelli G, Rossi T, Scarinci F, et al. Macular vitreoretinal interface abnormalities in highly myopic eyes with posterior staphyloma: 5-year follow-up. Retina. 2012;32:1531-8.
187. Spaide RF, Fisher Y. Removal of adherent cortical vitreous plaques without removing the internal limiting membrane in the repair of macular detachments in highly myopic eyes. Retina. 2005;25:290-5.
188. Akiba J. Prevalence of posterior vitreous detachment in high myopia. Ophthalmology. 1993;100:1384-8.
189. Kobayashi H, Kishi S. Vitreous surgery for highly myopic eyes with foveal detachment and retinoschisis. Ophthalmology. 2003;110:1702-7.
190. Gaucher D, Haouchine B, Tadayoni R, et al. Long-term follow-up of high myopic foveoschisis: natural course and surgical outcome. Am J Ophthalmol. 2007;143:455-62.

191. Shimada N, Tanaka Y, Tokoro T, et al. Natural course of myopic traction maculopathy and factors associated with progression or resolution. Am J Ophthalmol. 2013;156:948-57.e1.
192. Benhamou N, Massin P, Haouchine B, et al. Macular retinoschisis in highly myopic eyes. Am J Ophthalmol. 2002;133:794-800.
193. Sayanagi K, Morimoto Y, Ikuno Y, et al. Spectral-domain optical coherence tomographic findings in myopic foveoschisis. Retina. 2010;30:623-8.
194. Sayanagi K, Ikuno Y, Soga K, et al. Photoreceptor inner and outer segment defects in myopic foveoschisis. Am J Ophthalmol. 2008;145:902-8.
195. Shimada N, Ohno-Matsui K, Baba T, et al. Natural course of macular retinoschisis in highly myopic eyes without macular hole or retinal detachment. Am J Ophthalmol. 2006;142:497-500.
196. Ikuno Y, Tano Y. Early macular holes with retinoschisis in highly myopic eyes. Am J Ophthalmol. 2003;136:741-4.
197. Lim LS, Ng WY, Wong D, et al. Prognostic factor analysis of vitrectomy for myopic foveoschisis. Br J Ophthalmol. 2015;99:1639-43.
198. Huang Y, Huang W, Ng DSC, et al. Risk factors for development of macular hole retinal detachment after pars plana vitrectomy for pathologic myopic foveoschisis. Retina. 2017;37:1049-54.
199. Kumagai K, Furukawa M, Ogino N, et al. Factors correlated with postoperative visual acuity after vitrectomy and internal limiting membrane peeling for myopic foveoschisis. Retina. 2010;30:874-80.
200. Ikuno Y, Sayanagi K, Soga K, et al. Foveal anatomical status and surgical results in vitrectomy for myopic foveoschisis. Jpn J Ophthalmol. 2008;52:269-76.
201. Gao X, Ikuno Y, Fujimoto S, et al. Risk factors for development of full-thickness macular holes after pars plana vitrectomy for myopic foveoschisis. Am J Ophthalmol. 2013;155:1021-7.e1.
202. Philippakis E, Couturier A, Gaucher D, et al. Posterior vitreous detachment in highly myopic eyes undergoing vitrectomy. Retina. 2016;36:1070-5.
203. Sayanagi K, Ikuno Y, Tano Y. Tractional internal limiting membrane detachment in highly myopic eyes. Am J Ophthalmol. 2006;142:850-2.
204. Shimada N, Sugamoto Y, Ogawa M, et al. Fovea-sparing internal limiting membrane peeling for myopic traction maculopathy. Am J Ophthalmol. 2012;154:693-701.
205. Bruyere E, Philippakis E, Dupas B, et al. Benefit of intraoperative optical coherence tomography for vitreomacular surgery in highly myopic eyes. Retina. 2017.
206. Uchida A, Shinoda H, Koto T, et al. Vitrectomy for myopic foveoschisis with internal limiting membrane peeling and no gas tamponade. Retina. 2014;34:455-60.
207. Kim KS, Lee SB, Lee WK. Vitrectomy and internal limiting membrane peeling with and without gas tamponade for myopic foveoschisis. Am J Ophthalmol. 2012;153:320-6.e1.
208. Fujimoto S, Ikuno Y, Nishida K. Postoperative optical coherence tomographic appearance and relation to visual acuity after vitrectomy for myopic foveoschisis. Am J Ophthalmol. 2013;156:968-73.e1.
209. Gaudric A, Cohen D. Surgery of idiopathic epimacular membranes. Prognostic factors. J Fr Ophtalmol. 1992;15:657-68.
210. Marie-Louise J, Philippakis E, Darugar A, et al. Occurrence rate of retinal detachment after small gauge vitrectomy for idiopathic epiretinal membrane. Eye (Lond). 2017;31:1259-65.
211. Mura M, Barca F, Dell'Omo R, et al. Iatrogenic retinal breaks in ultrahigh-speed 25-gauge vitrectomy: a prospective study of elective cases. Br J Ophthalmol. 2016;100:1383-7.
212. Rizzo S, Belting C, Genovesi-Ebert F, et al. Incidence of retinal detachment after small-incision, sutureless pars plana vitrectomy compared with conventional 20-gauge vitrectomy in macular hole and epiretinal membrane surgery. Retina. 2010;30:1065-71.
213. Tan HS, Mura M, de Smet MD. Iatrogenic retinal breaks in 25-gauge macular surgery. Am J Ophthalmol. 2009;148:427-30.
214. Rizzo S, Genovesi-Ebert F, Belting C. Comparative study between a standard 25-gauge vitrectomy system and a new ultrahigh-speed 25-gauge system with duty cycle control in the treatment of various vitreoretinal diseases. Retina. 2011;31:2007-13.
215. Teixeira A, Chong LP, Matsuoka N, et al. Vitreoretinal traction created by conventional cutters during vitrectomy. Ophthalmology. 2010;117:1387-92.e2.
216. Daien V, Le Pape A, Heve D, et al. Incidence, risk factors, and impact of age on retinal detachment after cataract surgery in France: a national population study. Ophthalmology. 2015;122:2179-85.
217. Jackson TL, Donachie PHJ, Sparrow JM, et al. United Kingdom National Ophthalmology Database Study of Vitreoretinal Surgery: report 1; case mix, complications, and cataract. Eye (Lond.) 2013;27:644-51.
218. Park JC, Ramasamy B, Shaw S, et al. A prospective and nationwide study investigating endophthalmitis following pars plana vitrectomy: incidence and risk factors. Br J Ophthalmol. 2014;98:529-33.
219. Seider MI, Michael Lahey J, Fellenbaum PS. Cost of phacovitrectomy versus vitrectomy and sequential phacoemulsification. Retina. 2014;34:1112-5.
220. Hamoudi H, Correll Christensen U, La Cour M. Epiretinal membrane surgery: an analysis of 2-step sequential- or combined phacovitrectomy surgery on refraction and macular anatomy in a prospective trial. Acta Ophthalmologica. 2017.

Chapter 57

Rhegmatogenous Retinal Detachment

Patrick Oellers, Dean Eliott

INCIDENCE OF RHEGMATOGENOUS RETINAL DETACHMENT

Rhegmatogenous retinal detachment is the most common form of retinal detachment and a leading cause of vision loss worldwide. The overall incidence is approximately 1–2 in 10,000 people. Because of its association with the development of posterior vitreous detachment, it has a peak incidence in 50- to 79-year-old patients, with 2–3 cases per 10,000 and a significantly lower rate in younger individuals.[1,2] The incidence of rhegmatogenous retinal detachment is slightly higher in males than in females. Geographic variations in the incidence of rhegmatogenous retinal detachment exist, and the incidence may be lower in East Asians than in Caucasians, despite the higher prevalence of high myopia in Asians.[3]

PATHOPHYSIOLOGY OF RHEGMATOGENOUS RETINAL DETACHMENT

Rhegmatogenous (rhegma = break; Greek) *retinal detachment* occurs from a full thickness retinal break, usually induced by vitreous traction, that allows liquefied vitreous to enter the subretinal space, thereby lifting the retina from the underlying retinal pigment epithelium (RPE) (Fig. 57.1).[4] The most common type of retinal break is a *retinal tear* (also called a *horseshoe tear*), which is a U-shaped break in the retinal periphery at the posterior edge of the vitreous base (Figs. 57.2A to C). Horseshoe tears are usually formed in the process of posterior vitreous detachment, with the vitreous traction and the flap of the tear pointing toward the vitreous base, where the vitreous remains attached. A less common type of retinal break is a *retinal hole* (with or without an associated operculum), which is often present in myopic eyes with lattice degeneration (Fig. 57.3). Another type of defect that can result in retinal detachment is termed *retinal dialysis*, which describes a dehiscence of the retinal insertion from the ora serrata, a

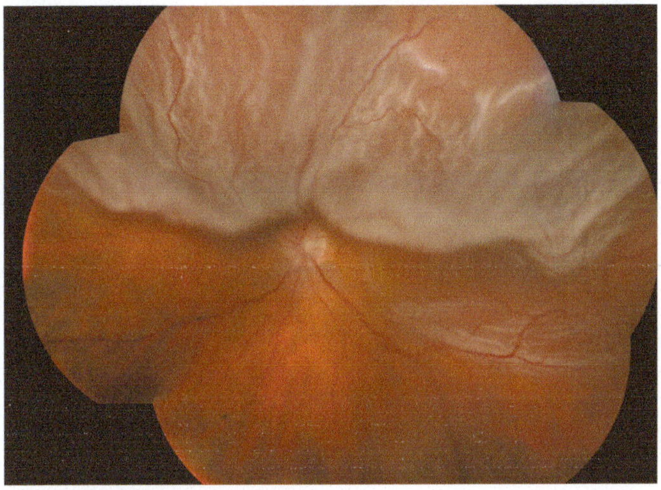

Fig. 57.1: Rhegmatogenous retinal detachment. Superior bullous retinal detachment with hydration lines. The macula is detached with slightly less bullous subretinal fluid.

rare consequence of blunt trauma to the eye (Fig. 57.4). A *giant retinal tear* is a horseshoe-type break that spans over 3 or more clock hours (Fig. 57.5). Rarely, a *macular hole* may result in rhegmatogenous retinal detachment. Risk factors for retinal detachment include age-associated vitreous liquefaction and the acute event of posterior vitreous detachment, myopia, lattice degeneration, inherited vitreoretinopathies (for example, *Stickler syndrome*), aphakia and pseudophakia, degenerative retinoschisis, as well as infectious and noninfectious uveitis and trauma.

DIAGNOSIS AND PREOPERATIVE EVALUATION OF RHEGMATOGENOUS RETINAL DETACHMENT

The classic symptoms reported by patients prior to the onset of rhegmatogenous retinal detachment are photopsias (flashing lights) and floaters. Photopsias are caused by vitreous traction on the retina resulting in neuronal activation by means of mechanical manipulation.

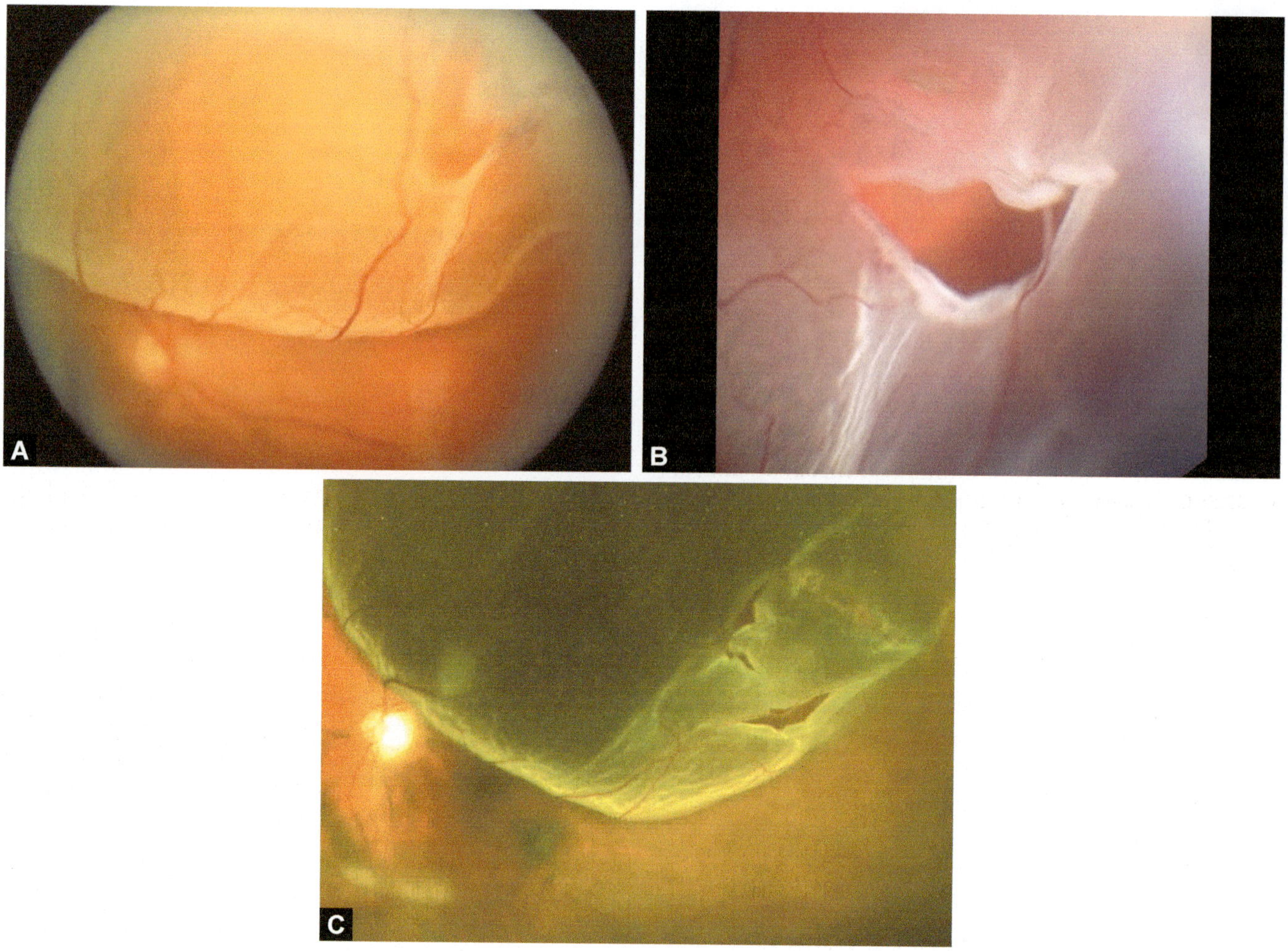

Figs. 57.2A to C: Horseshoe tear-associated rhegmatogenous retinal detachment. (A) Superior bullous rhegmatogenous retinal detachment with temporal horseshoe tear; (B) Close up of a horseshoe tear with a bridging blood vessel; (C) Superior bullous rhegmatogenous retinal detachment with two linear, perivascular horseshoe tears within lattice degeneration.

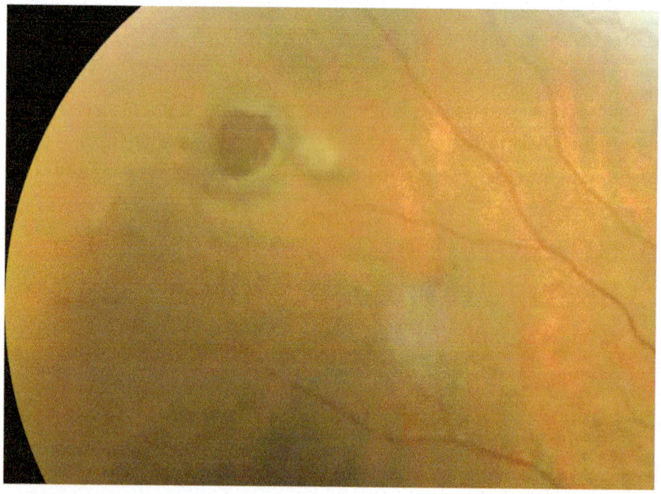

Fig. 57.3: Operculated retinal hole. Fundus photograph demonstrating a retinal hole with retinal operculum. The operculum is suspended in the overlying vitreous gel. There is a small cuff of subretinal fluid surrounding the hole.

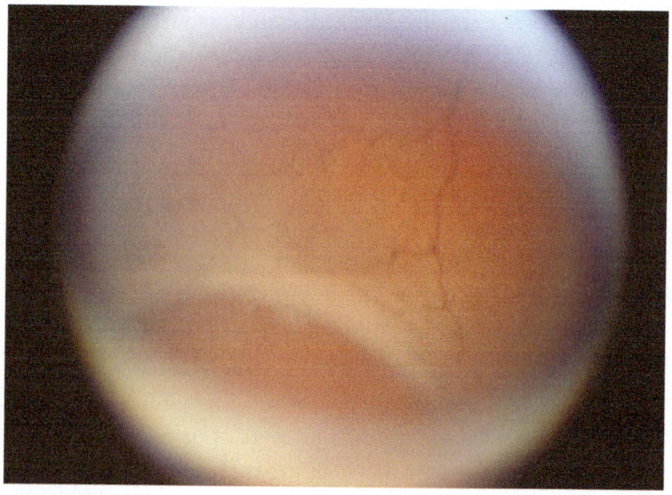

Fig. 57.4: Retinal dialysis associated retinal detachment. There is a shallow inferotemporal retinal detachment with a localized retinal dialysis.

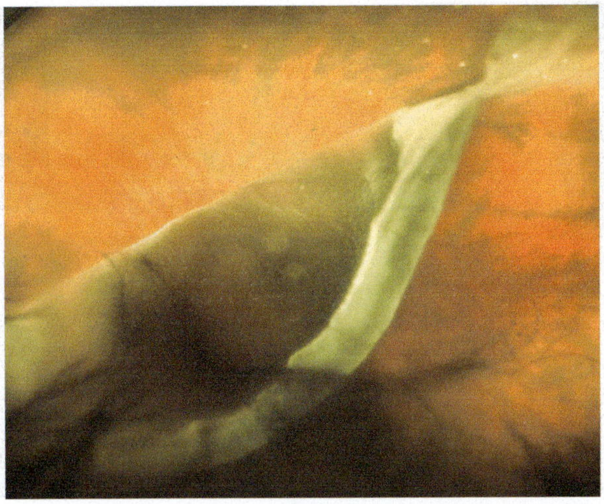

Fig. 57.5: Giant retinal tear associated retinal detachment. Wide-field fundus photograph demonstrating a giant retinal tear from 7 o'clock to 2 o'clock. The posterior retina is flipped over.

Floaters may derive from condensations of vitreous gel, pigment granules or vitreous hemorrhage released in the process of retinal break formation. Many patients describe a sudden shower of floaters with simultaneous photopsias shortly before the advent of peripheral visual field loss, often described as a curtain moving across the field of vision. Eventually, central visual loss results as the retinal detachment progresses to involve the macula.

Evaluation of retinal detachment should involve measurement of visual acuity, visual field, intraocular pressure, slit-lamp biomicroscopy and binocular indirect ophthalmoscopy with scleral depression. Visual acuity usually depends on the status of the macula. In a macula-on detachment, central vision is usually unaffected unless significant media opacity such as a vitreous hemorrhage is present. The visual field defect corresponds to the area of detached retina. Intraocular pressure can be slightly reduced in rhegmatogenous retinal detachment, especially in chronic cases. Rarely, there can be a retinal detachment-induced elevation of intraocular pressure caused by photoreceptor outer segments and other debris clogging the trabecular meshwork (Schwartz-Matsuo syndrome).

Slit-lamp findings may include mild anterior chamber reaction. The presence of pigmented cells in the anterior vitreous (tobacco dust or Shafer's sign) is a common finding and is due to retinal pigment epithelial cells gaining access to the vitreous cavity through the retinal break. It is important to note whether a Weiss-ring is present, as this is a definitive sign of posterior vitreous detachment. Indirect ophthalmoscopy with scleral depression best allows for visualization of the extent of subretinal fluid and the detection of retinal breaks.

Usually rhegmatogenous retinal detachment has a convex configuration and the retina appears slightly opaque, often with linear or arc-shaped ripples known as hydration lines due to retinal edema. More subtle retinal detachments with less subretinal fluid can be detected due to loss of the underlying choroidal pattern. In acute retinal detachment, the retina demonstrates mobility with eye movements. There are several signs that depict more chronic retinal detachment such as decreased mobility of the detached retina, demarcation lines that are formed by migration of retinal pigment epithelial cells at the border of attached and detached retina, retinal thinning due to atrophy, large intraretinal cysts and visible preretinal and/or subretinal membranes [proliferative vitreoretinopathy (PVR)].

Proliferative vitreoretinopathy is characterized by glial and retinal pigment epithelial cell migration. This proliferation causes retinal traction as well as retinal contraction and foreshortening. PVR can occur in primary rhegmatogenous retinal detachment or after any retinal procedure, and it is the most common cause of failure after initially successful retinal detachment surgery. There are ocular, genetic and behavioral risk factors for PVR. Ocular risk factors include prolonged retinal detachment, vitreous hemorrhage, multiple retinal breaks, trauma (especially open globe injury), choroidal detachment, and use of cryopexy among others.[5] Several grading schemes exist, but PVR is most commonly clinically divided into three grades describing increasing intensity of the disease according to the updated Proliferative Vitreoretinopathy Grade Classification from 1991.[6]

Grade A: The earliest stage consists of vitreous haze, vitreous pigment clumps and/or pigment deposits on the inferior retina (Fig. 57.6).

Grade B: The moderate stage consists of wrinkling of the inner retinal surface, retinal stiffness, vessel tortuosity, rolled and irregular edges of a retinal tear, or decreased mobility of the vitreous gel (Fig. 57.7).

Grade C: The most severe stage consists of focal, diffuse or circumferential full thickness retinal folds or subretinal bands, anterior displacement of the retina or condensed vitreous strands. It is either anterior (A) or posterior (P) to the equator of the globe. Its presence is also noted by the number of clock hours affected (1–12), which do not need to be contiguous (Figs. 57.8A to C).

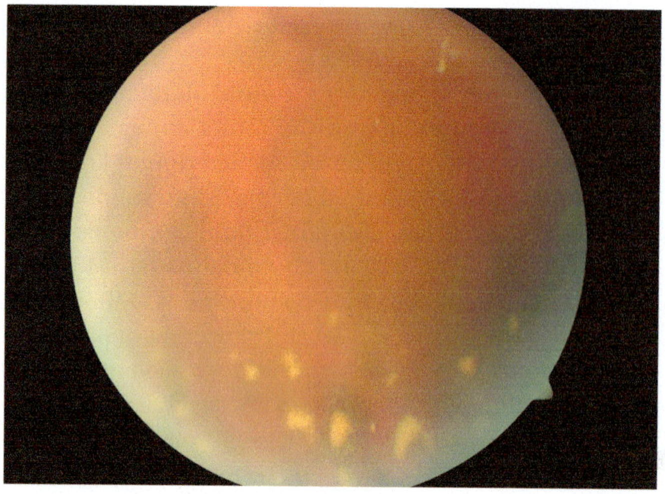

Fig. 57.6: Proliferative vitreoretinopathy Grade A. Fundus photograph showing a retinal detachment with associated inferior pigment clumping, depicting Grade A proliferative vitreoretinopathy.

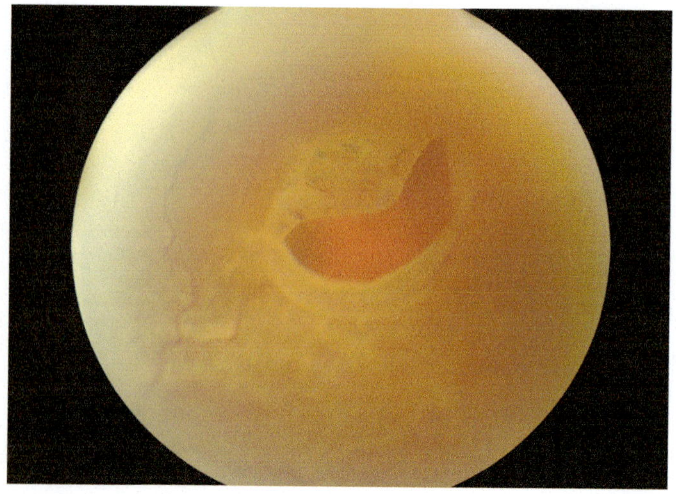

Fig. 57.7: Proliferative vitreoretinopathy Grade B. Fundus photograph of a horseshoe tear with rolled edges, depicting Grade B proliferative vitreoretinopathy.

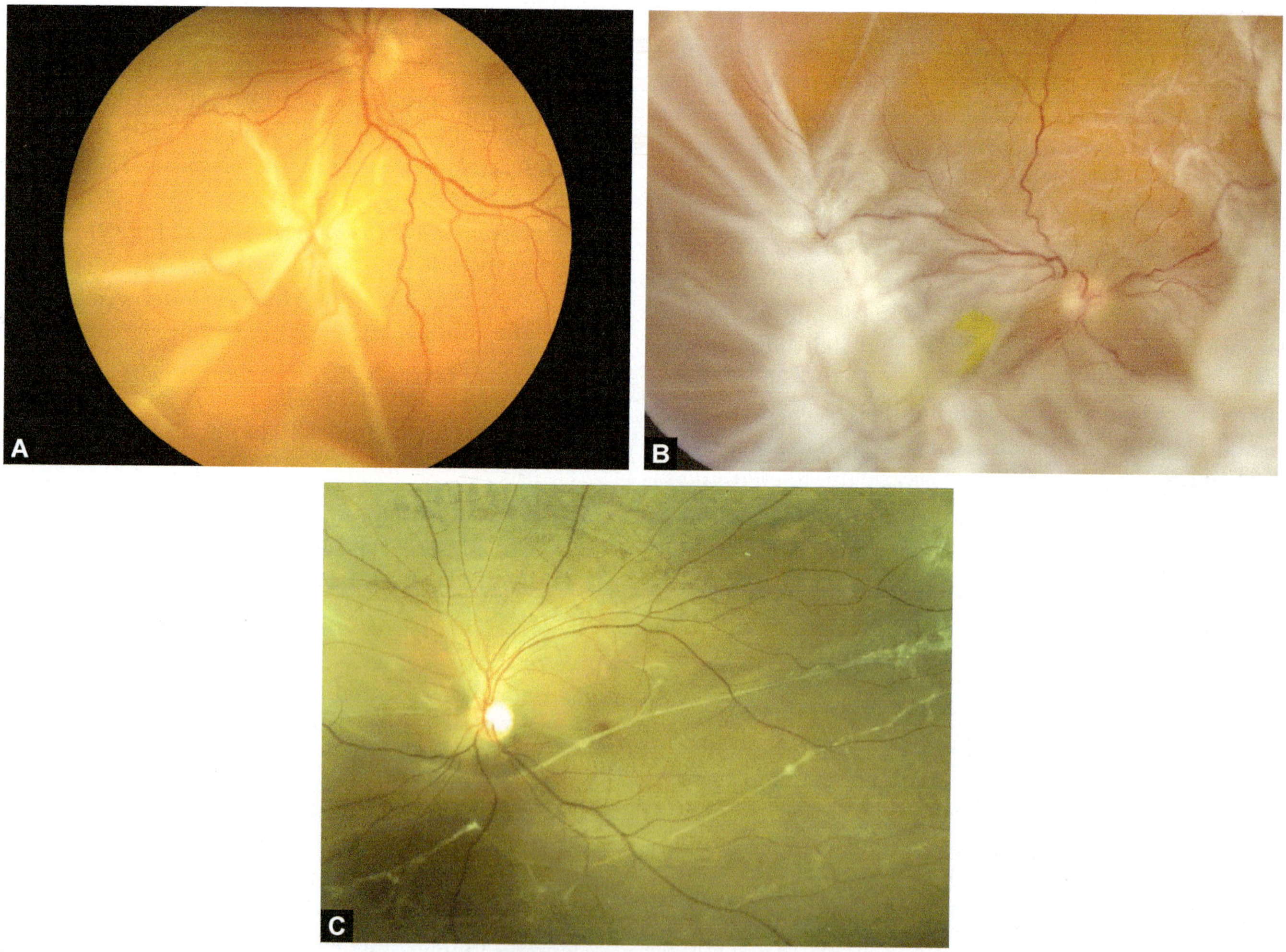

Figs. 57.8A to C: Proliferative vitreoretinopathy Grade C. (A) Fundus photograph demonstrating a starfold, caused by preretinal membrane growth with vitreoretinal traction and retinal contraction; (B) Extensive retinal membranes are present in this proliferative vitreoretinopathy Grade C rhegmatogenous retinal detachment; (C) Localized subretinal bands in macula off rhegmatogenous retinal detachment.

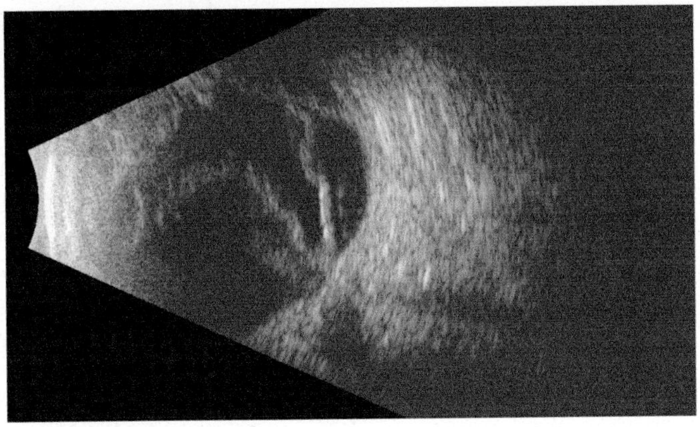

Fig. 57.9: Ultrasound B-scan. Ultrasound B-scan demonstrates retinal detachment in an eye with media opacity without view to the fundus.

When examining a patient with retinal detachment, a meticulous, complete ophthalmic examination is critical. Lens-status (cataract, pseudophakia, aphakia) should be noted, including the status of the capsule in pseudophakia. The status of the macula (macula in this setting refers to the fovea), attached versus detached, in addition to duration of symptoms and vision loss needs to be noted to make adequate plans for timing of the repair. Importantly, the physician should know the extent of the retinal detachment (usually described in clock hours) and the presence and location of all retinal breaks. Finding the break(s) is a crucial task for preoperative planning. By studying patterns of subretinal fluid location in relation to retinal breaks, Lincoff has summarized rules that can be very helpful to find the retinal break.

Ultrasound B-scan

In cases with no view to the fundus (dense cataract, vitreous hemorrhage or vitritis), B-scan ultrasonography is essential and can be used to diagnose retinal detachment (Fig. 57.9).

PREOPERATIVE CONSIDERATIONS

Timing of the Surgery

- *Status of the macula:* Macula-on rhegmatogenous retinal detachment, in general, is usually operated on within a 24-hour time frame to protect the status of the macula. In many cases, however, the risk of progression is low, and surgery can be delayed. In macula-off rhegmatogenous retinal detachment, timing becomes less critical, with most surgeons recommending intervention within a week from presentation. This provides the benefit of being able to operate during routine hours under the best circumstances with the surgeon's standard operating team. Certainly, there are exceptions to these very general guidelines, and decisions must be made individually depending on the particular circumstances.
- *Duration of detachment:* Retinal detachment cases with acute symptoms and rapid progression may undergo prompt surgery, whereas chronic cases, especially those with PVR or other complicating factors, usually undergo surgery during a routine surgical day.
- *Location of the break and status of the vitreous gel:* Due to gravity and fluid currents in the eye, rhegmatogenous retinal detachments with superior retinal breaks usually progress faster than detachments with inferior breaks. Inferior rhegmatogenous retinal detachments without posterior vitreous detachment typically progress very slowly and are usually amenable to routine scheduling.
- *Systemic health considerations:* It is important to factor general health issues into the surgical planning. Cardiovascular, pulmonary and diabetic status should be optimized as much as possible. In certain cases, it may be helpful to pause anticoagulants prior to surgery in close collaboration with the prescribing doctor (usually the cardiologist or primary care physician) if this is deemed systemically safe and if the retinal detachment allows waiting for a few days to normalize pharmacologic coagulopathy. Similarly, patients often need to position face down after the surgery and this can be difficult for many patients, especially those with musculoskeletal disease. Certain cases may benefit from optimization of the position abilities prior to surgery. There are many devices and specialized chairs that assist with postoperative face down requirements, which can be rented by patients.

PRINCIPLES OF SURGICAL RETINAL REATTACHMENT

The overlying principle of any retinal detachment repair is localizing the retinal break and preventing fluid entry into the subretinal space by creation of a chorioretinal adhesion.

The primary procedures available to repair rhegmatogenous retinal detachment are:

- Vitrectomy
- Scleral buckle
- Combination of vitrectomy with scleral buckle
- Pneumatic retinopexy

Each of these techniques has their own advantages and disadvantages and will be discussed in detail here.

RHEGMATOGENOUS RETINAL DETACHMENT REPAIR TECHNIQUES

Pars Plana Vitrectomy

Since the introduction of pars plana vitrectomy by Robert Machemer in 1971,[7] this procedure has gained increasing popularity and is currently the most commonly employed technique for rhegmatogenous retinal detachment repair in most parts of the world.[8] The principle involves localization of any breaks, relieving the vitreous traction by cutting the vitreous gel, endodrainage of subretinal fluid either through the existing break or a especially created drainage retinotomy, creation of a chorioretinal adhesion by endolaser, and tamponade of the retinal break with either gas [perfluoropropane (C_3F_8), sulfur-hexafluoride (SF_6)] or silicone oil. Figure 57.10 demonstrates a partial postoperative gas fill after retinal detachment repair by pars plana vitrectomy with C_3F_8 gas.

Modern Advances in Vitrectomy

Modern techniques and advances in instrumentation have improved the vitrectomy procedure for rhegmatogenous retinal detachment repair.[9]

- *Instrument size:* Most surgeons utilize 23-gauge or 25-gauge microincisional vitrectomy instruments which allow for more rapid healing, less inflammation and reduced postoperative discomfort compared to traditional 20 gauge instrumentation. Newer 27-gauge instruments can be used in certain situations, although some surgeons feel that higher instrument flexibility and lower efficiency of vitreous removal prevent the use of 27-gauge vitrectomy for more complicated cases.
- *Vitrectomy cutter speed:* Current technology allows 7,500–160,000 cuts per minute (cpm), which subsequently allows for very efficient and safe cutting of vitreous, enabling the surgeon to cut closely over mobile retina that would be attracted toward the cutter with lower cutting speeds. This also allows for aggressive shaving of the vitreous base with reduced risk for iatrogenic retinal breaks.
- *Wide-angle viewing systems:* The development of wide-field viewing systems allowed for improved intraoperative visualization of the peripheral retina, ora serrata and pars plana with the abilities to shave anterior vitreous base and treat anterior pathology. Both noncontact and contact viewing systems exist, and their use is primarily dictated by surgeon preference; but contact viewing systems generally require a skilled assistant to hold the lens and may make dynamic vitrectomy with simultaneous external scleral depression more challenging.
- *Illumination:* Handheld fiberoptic light pipes have been developed that allow for widefield, directional and safe endoillumination. Used in conjunction with wide-angle viewing systems and scleral depression, these light pipes allow detection and treatment of subtle pathology and more complete shaving of the vitreous compared to older techniques.
- *Valved cannulas:* The development of valved cannulas has turned vitrectomy into a more closed system surgery that reduces the amount of infusion fluid and allows dynamic control of intraocular pressure.[10]

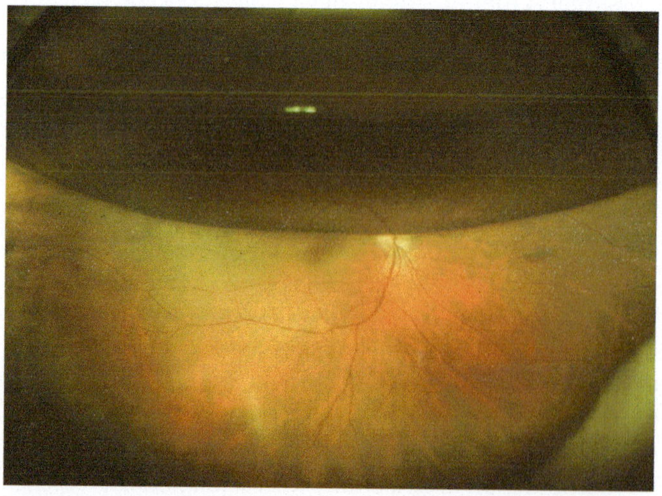

Fig. 57.10: Partially gas filled eye. Postoperative photograph taken 5 weeks after retinal detachment repair by vitrectomy with C_3F_8 gas showing an approximate 45% gas fill superiorly.

Indications for Vitrectomy in Rhegmatogenous Retinal Detachment

The classic indication for primary vitrectomy in rhegmatogenous retinal detachment is superior detachment with one or more superior breaks. Pseudophakic eyes allow for more complete shaving of the vitreous base compared to phakic eyes; and it is important to remove as much peripheral vitreous as possible regardless of the phakic status. Other concerns include extensive lattice degeneration as the vitreous gel is usually adherent to areas of lattice degeneration, and eyes with multiple retinal breaks. In principle, any rhegmatogenous retinal detachment can be treated with vitrectomy alone; however, certain detachments are best treated with an alternative method, such as rhegmatogenous detachment in a young myope with an attached hyaloid, or detachment due to retinal dialysis. These pathologies are best served with scleral buckle alone in the authors' opinion. Please note that surgeon preference and experience are most important when deciding which technique to employ.

Technique and Surgical Steps of Pars Plana Vitrectomy for Rhegmatogenous Retinal Detachment

Anesthesia: It is possible to perform the surgery with either general anesthesia or monitored anesthesia care. The choice depends on comfort of the surgeon, as well as surgical and patient factors. Generally, we prefer monitored anesthesia care when possible due to increased patient safety, shorter turnover between cases, ability of the patient to cooperate, and also cost-effectiveness. However, anticipated longer duration of surgery, patient anxiety, claustrophobia or inability to lie still for a prolonged time often mandates general anesthesia.

Three-port pars plana vitrectomy setup: Generally, we place sclerotomy incisions 3.0 mm posterior to the limbus in pseudo- and aphakic eyes and 3.5 mm from the limbus in phakic eyes. The port for the infusion cannula is placed inferotemporally. The infusion is connected and correct placement within the vitreous cavity is always confirmed with the external light pipe illumination via the cornea. This step is crucial to prevent infusion into the suprachoroidal space, which could result in choroidal effusion and/or hemorrhage, or in very rare instances systemic air embolism during fluid-air exchange. The infusion is turned on, and the subsequent ports are placed superotemporally and superonasally slightly above the midline of the eye. These ports are then used for the vitrectomy cutter and fiberoptic endoilluminator and are interchangeable.

Core vitrectomy: Next, the vitrectomy cutter and light pipe are inserted into the eye, and the retina and vitreous are visualized with the operating microscope in conjunction with the viewing system. Initially, it is preferred to remove vitreous close to the temporal sclerotomy to prevent iatrogenic breaks and vitreous incarceration into the cannula or sclerotomy. Then, the actual core vitrectomy is commenced by removing the central vitreous. This step is repeated for the nasal side, as it is important not to cross instruments too much beyond a line drawn from 12 o'clock to 6 o'clock in phakic eyes to prevent instrument lens touch and subsequent cataract formation. In pseudo- or aphakic eyes, crossing the vertical midline is safe. Next, the status of the posterior hyaloid is examined. If a posterior vitreous detachment is present, peripheral vitrectomy is commenced; otherwise the hyaloid is stripped by active suction with either the vitrectomy cutter or a soft-tip cannula. In most cases of rhegmatogenous retinal detachment with horseshoe-type breaks, the posterior vitreous is already detached and elevated up to the posterior insertion of the vitreous base. In unclear cases, the use of intravitreal triamcinolone can help to check the status of the posterior hyaloid, as the steroid crystals mix and adhere to the vitreous and hence allow for better visualization of the gel.

Peripheral vitrectomy: Next, peripheral vitrectomy and shaving of the vitreous base is performed, usually aided by scleral depression. We believe that shaving of the vitreous base, as much as safely possible, as well as release of any vitreous traction, often by excising the flap of the tear, are key steps to achieve good surgical outcomes. In addition, shaving the vitreous gel adherent to areas of lattice degeneration is also important. Tears can be marked with intraocular diathermy to aid later visualization, as the view under air may be difficult.

Fluid-air exchange: Once all breaks are identified and vitreous traction is relieved, the infusion is turned to air and the subretinal and vitreous cavity fluid are actively removed in exchange for air. Subretinal fluid can be drained through the primary retinal break, or in cases with very anterior breaks, a drainage retinotomy can be created. A soft-tipped cannula is used for drainage, with the tip being placed through the retinal break and carefully positioned so as not to touch the edge of the break or the underlying retinal pigment epithelium. We have learned that subretinal fluid can be drained even through very anterior breaks when the eye and even the patient's head is tilted toward the break, which facilitates shifting of the fluid from posterior toward the anterior break. In many instances, the break is slightly enlarged with the vitreous cutter to enable subretinal fluid drainage in this manner. In select cases, perfluorocarbon liquid (PFO), a heavy liquid, may be used to express subretinal fluid through the break, especially anterior breaks.

Heavy liquids: Perfluorocarbon liquid is a commonly referred to as a "third hand" for retina surgeons. It is a liquid that is heavier than water, has optical clarity and low viscosity and is immiscible with water and oil. It is extremely useful, especially in complex cases, to stabilize the posterior retina, to flatten the retina in cases of giant retinal tear or large relaxing retinectomies, and to express subretinal fluid through an anterior break. Care needs to be taken to avoid intraocular PFO retention. In almost all cases, retained PFO does not cause any problems; however, in rare instances, subretinal PFO can exert toxic effects on the retina,[11] whereas intraocular PFO retention may cause an inflammatory response.[12]

Laser photocoagulation: After subretinal fluid has been removed, retinal tears and other areas of pathology are treated with laser photocoagulation to create a chorioretinal adhesion that prevents influx of fluid through the break. Curved laser probes, optionally lighted, are available that allow for treatment of anterior pathology. This has mostly abolished the need for external cryotherapy. Breaks and any other suspicious areas are typically treated with 2–3 rows of laser spots, usually to the ora serrata.

Tamponade: Air is then exchanged with either isoexpansile SF_6 gas, C_3F_8 gas or silicone oil. SF_6 at isoexpansile concentration remains in the eye for about 2–4 weeks and is often used for noncomplicated rhegmatogenous retinal detachment with superior breaks. Due to the difficulty of tamponading inferior breaks or in cases of breaks in multiple locations, C_3F_8 is preferred for its more complete initial vitreous cavity fill and longer duration. It remains in the eye for about 4–8 weeks. Characteristics of intraocular gases used in retinal detachment surgery are listed in Table 57.1. Alternatively, silicone oil is used in eyes that benefit from long-term tamponade, for example retinal detachment with PVR. Another relative indication for the use of silicone oil is monocular status so that the patient can have some vision during the postoperative recovery.

Table 57.1: Gas types used in retinal detachment surgery.

Gas	Iso-expansile concentration	Expansion of 100% pure gas	Duration
Air	N/A	N/A	3–7 days
Sulfur hexafluoride (SF_6)	18–20%	2×	2–4 weeks
Perfluoropropane (C_3F_8)	12–15%	4×	4–8 weeks

The downsides of silicone oil are less tamponade effect due to the lower interfacial tension between silicone oil and fluid, the need for a second operation to remove the silicone oil, and postoperative emulsification of silicone oil with associated glaucoma and other issues.

Positioning after the surgery: Generally, the patient needs to be positioned face down as early as possible after the surgery to prevent a macular fold that can occur from postoperative fluid shifts. After the patient has completed 12–24 hours of face-down positioning, some surgeons recommend positioning the patient in a way that places the break as the highest point of the body since gas and silicone oil float. Others have their patients remain face down for 3 or more full days. Generally, the location of the break, surgeon experience and the cooperation abilities of the patient dictate postoperative positioning. In most cases, a sufficient chorioretinal adhesion around the break is achieved after 1 week, and position requirements are loosened around that time. It is important that patients avoid face-up positioning at all times while gas is in the eye since such positioning can lead to cataract formation or to pupillary block glaucoma. Patients should wear a gas bracelet at all times as long as gas remains in the eye, which can be detected in emergency situations and can serve to notify other physicians of the presence of intraocular gas (and thereby position requirements and contraindication for N_2O gas anesthesia). Patients need to be counseled that they cannot travel by airplane or visit high elevation mountains due to the expansile properties of the gas.

Combination of Vitrectomy with Scleral Buckle

Cases with inferior retinal breaks (especially phakic eyes), multiple retinal breaks, (extensive) lattice degeneration, conditions with abnormal vitreoretinal interface (e.g. Stickler syndrome), reoperations, or poor outcome of the fellow eye with vitrectomy alone may benefit from combined scleral buckle with vitrectomy. Most commonly, a relatively thin encircling band is chosen to protect the vitreous base for 360°. This is generally placed prior to vitrectomy and should ideally be planned prior to commencing the surgery. Choice of vitrectomy alone versus vitrectomy combined with scleral buckle mostly depends on surgeon preference and experience.

Complications of Pars Plana Vitrectomy

Complications of pars plana vitrectomy include cataract formation with need for subsequent cataract surgery in many phakic patients 6 months to 2 years after the retinal detachment repair, retinal or vitreous incarceration, choroidal effusion due to hypotony, transient elevation of intraocular pressure or development of glaucoma, vitreous hemorrhage and displacement of the lens due to gas pressure. Endophthalmitis rates after vitrectomy are very low. There was some initial concern about higher endophthalmitis rates in sutureless microincisional vitrectomy compared to 20-gauge vitrectomy; but beveling of incisions and placement of sutures in appropriate cases have reduced the discrepancy.[13] Additionally, sympathetic ophthalmia after vitrectomy may be an extremely rare complication.

Scleral Buckle

Scleral buckle was popularized by Charles Schepens in the late 1950s due to his work with the indirect ophthalmoscope[14] and has long been the most commonly employed technique to repair retinal detachment. The principle of scleral buckle is that an exoplant is used to create an indentation or buckle effect of the sclera, thereby moving the detached retina closer to the retinal pigment epithelium. A buckle also alters vitreous vector forces and reduces vitreoretinal traction.

Indications for Scleral Buckle in Rhegmatogenous Retinal Detachment Repair

In general, almost any primary rhegmatogenous retinal detachment is amenable to repair by scleral buckle. Many different variations of scleral buckling surgery exist; as long as the breaks are supported and well treated, in principle, a scleral buckle should work to repair the detachment. With the advent of modern day vitrectomy, the main indication for primary scleral buckle is rhegmatogenous retinal detachment in phakic eyes with high myopia and round holes, and especially inferior holes, without posterior vitreous detachment; as well as retinal detachment due to retinal dialysis. As previously stated, many cases such as retinal detachment with widespread lattice degeneration or other anterior retinal pathology may benefit from combination vitrectomy with scleral buckle. The benefits of scleral buckle over vitrectomy are no or reduced postoperative positioning requirement, maintenance of the natural crystalline lens that remains unaltered after scleral buckling surgery, and permanent protection of the vitreous base which may help to prevent recurrent retinal detachment. The downsides of scleral buckling include the inability to completely drain subretinal fluid, risk for subretinal hemorrhage as a complication in cases of external drainage, increased postoperative discomfort and inflammation, possible postoperative scleral buckle migration or exposure, postoperative double vision, and the risks of general anesthesia since the surgery generally takes longer than vitrectomy and is usually performed under general anesthesia.

Technique and Surgical Steps of Scleral Buckling Surgery for Rhegmatogenous Retinal Detachment

Anesthesia: Most cases of scleral buckling warrant general anesthesia due to intraoperative discomfort, manipulation of external eye muscles and longer duration of the surgery; but selected cases may be amenable to monitored anesthesia care.

Peritomy and isolation of the muscles: Initially, a 360° peritomy is performed with subsequent isolation of the four recti muscles. Muscles are most commonly slung onto temporary 2-0 silk sutures for subsequent manipulation of the globe and placement of the encircling band.

Localization of the break and external cryotherapy: Next, the retina is examined via indirect ophthalmoscopy with scleral depression. The location of break is marked externally on the sclera to plan for the choice and exact placement of the buckle exoplant. External cryotherapy is then applied to the retinal break and possibly to other suspicious appearing lesions.

Placement of the buckle exoplant and sutures: Many variations of buckle exoplants and suture placement exist, and this chapter is not intended to cover all details. Generally, the surgeon choses between a 360° encircling element that protects the posterior edge of the vitreous base all around the eye, versus a segmental buckle that only covers certain clock hours of the eye. Rarely, radial elements can be helpful: for example to treat very posterior breaks that cannot be otherwise reached.

Encircling elements usually induce a myopic shift, whereas segmental or radial elements may be more neutral in terms of refraction. Each element is chosen so that it protects the break and other potential pathology. Exoplants are usually fixated on the sclera by permanent sutures, most commonly nylon, or alternatively by use of so-called *"belt loops,"* which are partial thickness scleral tunnels through which the exoplant can be threaded.

External drainage of subretinal fluid: Certain cases of rhegmatogenous retinal detachment, such as chronic retinal detachment with thick viscous subretinal fluid or highly bullous detachment with substantial subretinal fluid, may benefit from external drainage. However, this step is optional and has some potential complications. If warranted, a scleral cut-down toward the choroid within the anticipated bed of the buckle is performed at a site with high subretinal fluid. Diathermy is applied to both scleral edges to create some gaping of the edges. Then, the choroid is punctured with a 30-gauge needle (or similar) to allow egress of subretinal fluid. Subretinal fluid then emerges through the sclerotomy, and this can be facilitated by gentle scleral massage. Of note, many different variations of this step exist, and the use primarily depends on surgeon preference and experience. Subsequent hypotony can be counteracted by intravitreal injection of air or gas (C_3F_8 vs SF_6). The status of the retina (level of subretinal fluid, retinal incarceration, subretinal hemorrhage) should be checked immediately after the drainage with careful indirect ophthalmoscopy.

Re-examination of the retina: Retinal and optic nerve head perfusion, scleral buckle location and height of indentation, as well as presence of any remaining subretinal fluid and fish-mouthing of the retinal break, should be checked and judged by indirect ophthalmoscopy. Pressure should be lowered immediately for any compromise of retinal perfusion by means of anterior chamber paracentesis. Buckle height and position may be adjusted as needed.

Gas tamponade: Another optional step in scleral buckling surgery is injection of pure, expansile C_3F_8 gas, SF_6 gas or air (in selected cases) to provide internal tamponade facilitating absorption of subretinal fluid. Intravitreal gas can also be used to protect the macula in selected cases. In cases of intravitreal gas injection, care should be taken to lower intraocular pressure to adequate levels by means of anterior chamber paracentesis. Also, the patient needs to be instructed to position toward the break postoperatively or face down depending on circumstances.

Complications

Postoperative complications of scleral buckling surgery include discomfort, increased intraocular pressure, prolonged inflammation, and retinal incarceration or subretinal hemorrhage due to external drainage. Long-term complications include diplopia with a need for prism glasses or strabismus surgery, as well as late migration, exposure and scleral buckle infection.

Pneumatic Retinopexy

Pneumatic retinopexy is the youngest of the three common surgical techniques to repair retinal detachment and was first introduced by Hilton and Grizzard in 1986.[15] The principle of pneumatic retinopexy is the creation of chorioretinal adhesion either by cryotherapy or laser photocoagulation with injection of expansile intraocular gas as tamponade agent. Pneumatic retinopexy does not provide release of vitreoretinal traction like pars plana vitrectomy or alter tractional forces like scleral buckling surgery. Potential benefits are that pneumatic retinopexy can be performed in the office setting without the need for specialized anesthesia care and postoperative preservation of a clear lens in phakic cases contrary to vitrectomy. Potential disadvantages are more narrow criteria for suitable cases, as well as lower reported success rates compared to more definitive vitrectomy and scleral buckling surgery.

Indications for Pneumatic Retinopexy in Rhegmatogenous Retinal Detachment

The classic indication for pneumatic retinopexy is a phakic eye with superior retinal detachment with a single retinal break (located within the superior 6 clock hours), without any other retinal pathology such as lattice degeneration, and the presence of a posterior vitreous detachment. Due to the smaller gas bubble employed in pneumatic retinopexy, inferior retinal breaks cannot be adequately covered, and as such, pneumatic retinopexy may not be used for inferior breaks. Pseudophakia represents a relative contraindication for pneumatic retinopexy due to the higher prevalence of smaller, subtler breaks that can be missed on clinical examination alone. Additionally, the benefit of crystalline lens preservation does not apply to pseudophakia, and as such, vitrectomy may be a more reasonable choice in these cases. We are cautious to perform pneumatic retinopexy in eyes with attached posterior hyaloid due to potential induction of vitreoretinal traction by the gas bubble injection. Cases with very bullous detached retina may be difficult to treat with cryotherapy due to inability to create sufficient required contact between the retina and retinal pigment epithelium. In either way, indications and relative contraindications for pneumatic retinopexy depend on surgeon experience and preferences.

Technique and Surgical Steps of Pneumatic Retinopexy

Anesthesia: Usually, topical anesthesia such as subconjunctival injection of 2–4% lidocaine is sufficient to provide analgesia. Inability of the patient to cooperate in the office setting usually directs the surgeon to perform vitrectomy or scleral buckle in the operating room.

Cryotherapy: Initially, external cryotherapy is performed to the break. Alternatively, some surgeons prefer to use laser photocoagulation after the retina has been flattened by the injection of gas; but this may be challenging due to difficult view with indirect ophthalmoscopy in a partially gas filled eye.

Anterior chamber paracentesis: To prevent extreme elevation of intraocular pressure after the injection of intraocular gas, anterior chamber fluid can be removed before gas injection. Depending on surgeon preference and experience, this step can also be performed after injection of intravitreal gas.

Intravitreal gas injection: Next, either 0.3 mL of C_3F_8 gas or 0.6 mL of SF_6 gas at 100% concentration (each will expand to approximately 1.2 mL in the eye to approximately cover the superior 90° of the retina in most cases) is injected. Care should be taken to avoid subretinal gas migration and "fish eggs". In cases of fish eggs, which represent multiple small gas bubbles, it is advisable to position the patient in such a way that gas is away from the break until the gas has coalesced into a single bubble, usually within 12–24 hours, to prevent subretinal gas migration.

Postoperative Positioning

The patient is then instructed to position in a way that places the break as the highest point of the body (for example sitting upright in case of a superior retinal break) to achieve optimal tamponade effect.

Complications of Pneumatic Retinopexy

The main complications of pneumatic retinopexy are subretinal gas migration and iatrogenic retinal tears that can occur due to intravitreal injection of gas in the vitreous filled eye.[16] Also, the gas can push anterior fluid posteriorly, resulting in an iatrogenic detachment of the previously attached macula. Other complications include intraocular pressure elevation from gas injection, vitreous hemorrhage, and endophthalmitis.

OUTCOMES OF RHEGMATOGENOUS RETINAL DETACHMENT REPAIR

Outcomes are classified by anatomic success and functional visual outcome. Anatomic success is divided into single surgery success (attachment of the retina after a single surgery) and final anatomic success (attachment of the retina after one or more procedures). As visual outcomes are multifactorial and not always influenced by surgical factors (macular detachment and duration, coexisting disease of the macula such as macular degeneration, presence of the lens, and many others), most surgeons place higher weight on anatomic outcome when analyzing surgical success. In general, single anatomic success rates for pars plana vitrectomy and scleral buckle are reported in the 80–90% range, whereas pneumatic retinopexy single anatomic success rates are slightly lower, in the 60–90% range. The greatest reason for failure of vitrectomy surgery for rhegmatogenous retinal detachment is proliferative vitreoretinopathy, followed by missed or iatrogenic retinal breaks. Reasons for failure of scleral buckle include proliferative vitreoretinopathy, missed breaks, inadequate buckle position or height, and inadequate cryotherapy. Reasons for pneumatic retinopexy failure (in appropriately selected cases) are proliferative vitreoretinopathy, missed breaks, iatrogenic breaks, inadequate cryotherapy or subretinal gas migration. Generally, all surgeries that require postoperative internal tamponade by gas or silicone oil may fail if the patient is noncompliant with positioning.

REFERENCES

1. Mowatt L, Shun-Shin G, Price N. Ethnic differences in the demand incidence of retinal detachments in two districts in the West Midlands. Eye (Lond.) 2003;17:63-70.

2. Wilkes SR, Beard CM, Kurland LT, et al. The incidence of retinal detachment in Rochester, Minnesota, 1970-1978. Am J Ophthalmol. 1982;94:670-3.
3. Park SJ, Choi NK, Park KH, et al. Five year nationwide incidence of rhegmatogenous retinal detachment requiring surgery in Korea. PLoS One. 2013;8:e80174.
4. Ghazi NG, Green WR. Pathology and pathogenesis of retinal detachment. Eye (Lond.) 2002;16:411-21.
5. Eliott D, Stryjewski TP, Andreoli MT, et al. Smoking is a risk factor for proliferative vitreoretinopathy after traumatic retinal detachment. Retina. 2017;37:1229-35.
6. Machemer R, Aaberg TM, Freeman HM, et al. An updated classification of retinal detachment with proliferative vitreoretinopathy. Am J Ophthalmol. 1991;112:159-65.
7. Machemer R, Buettner H, Norton EW, et al. Vitrectomy: a pars plana approach. Trans Am Acad Ophthalmol Otolaryngol. 1971;75:8138-20.
8. Day S, Grossman DS, Mruthyunjaya P, et al. One-year outcomes after retinal detachment surgery among medicare beneficiaries. Am J Ophthalmol. 2010;150:338-45.
9. Thompson JT. Advantages and limitations of small gauge vitrectomy. Surv Ophthalmol. 2011;56:162-72.
10. Oellers P, Stinnett S, Mruthyunjaya P, et al. Small-gauge valved versus nonvalved cannula pars plana vitrectomy for retinal detachment repair. Retina 2016;36:744-9.
11. Tewari A, Eliott D, Singh CN,et al. Changes in retinal sensitivity from retained subretinal perfluorocarbon liquid. Retina. 2009;29:248-50.
12. Elsing SH, Fekrat S, Green WR, et al. Clinicopathologic findings in eyes with retained perfluoro-n-octane liquid. Ophthalmology. 2001;108:45-8.
13. Govetto A, Virgili G, Menchini F, et al. A systematic review of endophthalmitis after microincisional versus 20-gauge vitrectomy. Ophthalmology. 2013;120:2286-91.
14. Schepens CL. Scleral buckling procedures. Trans Am Acad Ophthalmol Otolaryngol. 1958;62:206-18.
15. Hilton GF, Grizzard WS. Pneumatic retinopexy. A two-step outpatient operation without conjunctival incision. Ophthalmology. 1986;93:626-41.
16. Chan CK, Lin SG, Nuthi AS, et al. Pneumatic retinopexy for the repair of retinal detachments: a comprehensive review (1986-2007). Surv Ophthalmol. 2008;53:443-78.

Chapter 58 Principles of Vitreoretinal Surgery

Ferenc Kuhn, Agnieszka Kudasiewicz-Kardaszewska

BRIEF HISTORY OF VITREORETINAL SURGERY

As unbelievable as it may sound today, until the late 1960s no real treatment existed for any disease involving the vitreous body—a tissue that makes up 73% (4.4 mL of 6 mL) of the human eye and that is a close neighbor to the retina.[1] In fact, the vitreous gel was long considered a "no-go zone"; when it prolapsed during intracapsular cataract surgery, residents were taught not to touch it to avoid secondary complications. If postextraction retinal detachment developed, the surgeon was accused of violating the gel.

A dramatic reversal took place in 1968 when Kasner suggested that in eyes with a cloudy vitreous (primary amyloidosis) the gel can, and indeed, should be removed because such removal may improve vision, and the risk involved is reasonable.[2]

But, while open-sky vitrectomy effectively removed the opaque gel, it had several drawbacks—the surgery produced a very large wound (including the occasional need for corneal transplantation); the lens had to be removed; the instrumentation used was inadequate; traction could be transmitted to the peripheral retina via the anterior hyaloid, with serious repercussions; and most importantly, the risk of severe intraoperative hemorrhage was measurable.

The next step in the evolution of vitreoretinal (VR) surgery was the introduction of closed pars plana vitrectomy (PPV).[3] The initial instrument used was a full-function probe (a "vitreous infusion suction cutter or VISC"),[4] measuring 1.5 mm in diameter (16 g), with a motor-driven rotary cutter that also provided for infusion (other variants had an additional intraocular light source, a sleeve, and surrounding the probe). In the case of the VISC, there was no fiber optic light; instead, the microscope was equipped with a slit illuminator and the Goldmann contact lens was used to visualize the deeper structures.[5] Interestingly, the slit-lamp illumination option has had a renaissance (albeit limited) in the recent past.[6]

During the early years, the list of indications for VR surgery was pretty much restricted to pathologies of the vitreous itself; the retina was to be avoided ("land-to-sea technique"). The road leading to today's techniques and technology was long and included many milestones,[a] including among others, the "standard 20 g, three-port" approach (separating the infusion, the light, and the vitrectomy cutter, which were now pneumatic and axial-cutting);[7] the removal of newly-developed membranes from the retinal surface;[8] cutting of the retina itself;[9,10] splitting the retina itself [intentional removal of the internal limiting membrane (ILM)];[11-13] intraocular gases;[14,15] silicone oil;[16-18] subretinal surgery;[19] and the development of a huge variety of hand instruments.[20]

ANATOMY, BIOCHEMISTRY, AND (PATHO-) PHYSIOLOGY OF THE VITREOUS AND THEIR CLINICAL IMPLICATIONS FOR THE VITREORETINAL SURGEON

Macroanatomy of the Vitreous

There are several—mostly invisible—landmarks in the vitreous body of which the VR surgeon should be aware. These are listed in Table 58.1.[21-23]

Biochemistry of the Vitreous

Approximately, 98% of the vitreous is made up of water; the remainder consists of collagen fibers (mostly type II), hyaluronan, numerous other molecules such as chondroitin sulfate, and a relatively small number of cells (hyalocytes and fibroblasts).[1,21,22]

---

[a] This is a highly selective list; for a comprehensive account of the development of VR surgery several textbooks are available.

Table 58.1: Anatomical landmarks in the vitreous body and their clinical implications.

Landmark	Remark
Vitreous cortex	The outermost part of the gel, consisting of densely packed collagen fibers. Its anterior aspect (anterior hyaloid membrane or face) is located anterior to the vitreous base (see below); behind the vitreous base the cortex is described by various terms such as posterior cortical vitreous or hyaloid face. While the anterior cortex is only 2 μ thick, the posterior is 100 μ. There is no cortex over the optic disk.
Anterior hyaloid face	It adheres to, but is not interconnected with, the posterior lens capsule. The adherence is strong in young persons (hence the rationale never to remove the posterior lens capsule in people younger than ~30 years of age unless an anterior vitrectomy is performed first); but it weakens with age.
Weigert's ligament	A disk, 8–9 mm in diameter, which connects the gel to the posterior lens capsule. Only in the epicenter does a small space exist between the two tissues (Berger's space).
Posterior hyaloid face	It is adherent to (but typically not interconnected with) the posterior retina; the adherence is via an extracellular matrix. The adherence has more than average strength at certain locations—the margin of the macula or the parafoveal area, along the major blood vessels, in areas of certain retinal degenerations such as lattice, and especially at the margin of the optic disk (Weiss ring, see below). Just as the anterior hyaloid face becomes easier to separate from the posterior lens capsule in older people, the posterior vitreoretinal adherence also weakens with age. But very strong connections between the two tissues can develop in pathologies such as at the site of chorioretinal scars; overly strong laser spots ("black" retina) may appear if the cortical vitreous is "burnt" into the inner retina. In the posterior pole, the vitreous cortex is relatively easy to separate from the retina (surgical PVD) in people beyond ~20 years of age; but how far this separation can be carried anteriorly not only depends on age but varies greatly between individuals. Advancing the PVD too anteriorly is the most common intraoperative cause of RD.
Vitreous base	A several mm thick, 3-dimensional ring, extending up to 2 mm anteriorly and up to 3 mm posteriorly from the ora serrata and separating the posterior and anterior cortices. The collagen fibers of the vitreous are contiguous with those of the peripheral retina, making separation (vitreous detachment) of the two tissues impossible.
Weiss ring	A condensation of the gel's collagen fibers at the margin of the optic disk. If the vitreous detaches, the ring may become visible inside the vitreous cavity as a mobile, truly ring-like structure.
Premacular bursa	An optically empty space measuring 7 mm in width and 0.6 mm axially, containing only fluid. It is connected to the area of Martegiani (cisterna preoptica) in front of the optic disk and its superior extension fuses with Cloquet's canal, which courses through the vitreous and terminates behind the lens.

(PVD: Posterior vitreous detachment; RD: Retinal detachment)

Early in life, the normal vitreous is a perfect and homogenous gel; there is no free water content. For the gel to remain so and to fill the vitreous cavity completely, both the collagen fibers and the hyaluronan are essential. Without the former, the vitreous becomes a viscous fluid; without the latter, it shrinks.

As a person ages, the vitreous gel begins to break down; as early as 4 years of age, the process of syneresis (liquefaction) begins. With the breakdown of the normal collagen-hyaluronan relationship, lacunae, which contain free fluid (aqueous), begin to appear. By the time a person is 18 years old, up to one-fifth of the vitreous has liquefied. Aggregated collagen fragments are "swimming" in the lacunae, casting a mobile shadow on the retina as the eyeball moves. People typically describe them as "flying flies" (floaters and muscae volitantes).[23]

Having such a gel-fluid admixture in the vitreous cavity has important consequences for the VR interface and thus for the retina (attachment vs detachment). While a perfect gel does not allow it to be mobile, the syneretic vitreous does move, exerting a shearing force on the retina.[24,25] The potential outcomes of a spontaneous posterior vitreous detachment (PVD) are described in Table 58.2.

Micro- and Macroanatomy of the Retina

The neuroretina has nine layers, being "glued" on its external surface to a monolayer of ~120 million pigmented cells [retinal pigment epithelium (RPE)], which plays a crucial role in maintaining retinal attachment.[1] The innermost layer of the retina, the ILM consists mostly of the basal lamina of the Müller cells. The ILM gives the retina a smooth inner surface and a shiny light reflex in younger individuals. It is 0.5 μ thick in the periphery and ~1.5 μ thick centrally but is absent over the optic disk and occasionally over the major blood vessels. It is the only rigid component of the retina, justifying ILM removal in several pathological conditions. Being completely transparent, the ILM is invisible during PPV (unless the surgeon holds the

Table 58.2: Spontaneous posterior vitreous detachment: Possibilities and their implications.

Option	Description and implications
No PVD	The cortical vitreous maintains the uniform contact with the opposing retina (ILM). As long as the gel is intact (no syneresis present), there is no risk of VR traction; once the liquefaction process starts, VR traction is possible even if there is no PVD
Complete PVD	The vitreous truly separates from the posterior retina; the risk of VR traction is (close to) zero
Incomplete PVD: vitreoschisis	While this condition is not a PVD, it must be discussed here because the anterior wall of the vitreoschisis cavity almost always appears to the clinician as a true PVD. The misdiagnosis results in the assumption that a PVD exists; the VR surgeon will not seek to complete the vitrectomy and the left-behind posterior cortical vitreous will maintain the potential to exert traction on the posterior retina
Incomplete PVD; anomalous PVD	If liquefaction is present but the VR adherence is at least partially maintained, VR traction is present; the mobile vitreous has a shearing effect on the retina at all areas of adhesion. This can lead to various pathologies such as vitreomacular traction syndrome, edema, retinal tears, and RD

(PVD: Posterior vitreous detachment; ILM: Internal limiting membrane; VR: Vitreoretinal; RD: Retinal detachment)

endoilluminator at a certain angle), explaining the need to use vital stains in VR surgery.[26]

The retina is thinnest in the periphery (~0.1 mm) and becomes progressively thicker posteriorly, reaching 0.23 mm at the periphery of the macula.

The ora serrata ("ora" in everyday usage) is the point (circle) anterior to which the 10-layered retina becomes contiguous with the nonpigmented epithelium of the pars plana ciliaris. The ora is straddled by the vitreous base.

The pars plana is the posterior section of the ciliary body, a ring ~4 mm wide in adults; it is not part of the retina, yet it is crucial for the VR surgeon since it provides the safe "entrance door" to the vitreous cavity.

The macula (lutea) is a horizontally oval area of 2 × 0.9 mm with a center 3.4 mm temporal to, and 0.8 mm inferior to, the margin at the midline (3 o'clock in the left eye and 9 o'clock in the right) of the optic disk. The macula is responsible for ~20° of the visual field.

The central depression in the macula is the fovea, with a diameter of 1.5 mm. The light reflex seen here is explained by its slanted architecture (clivus). The avascular zone inside the fovea is 0.5 mm in diameter; this is the "forbidden zone" when performing laser treatment. The epicenter, called the foveola, has a diameter of 0.35 mm. It has no cells except the outer segment of red and green cones.

The fovea is surrounded by a 0.5 mm wide ring called the parafoveal area, which in turn is encircled by another, 1.5 mm wide ring, the perifoveal area.

The optic disk is the entry point for the arterial system of the eye and the exit point for the veins and axons. The optic disk is an oval area, measuring 1.76 mm horizontally and 1.92 mm vertically in the emmetropic eye, located nasally from the macula, 2.3 mm from the optical axis.

The posterior pole is generally understood as the area bordered by the vascular arcades.

The equator is an important, although rather inconspicuous, landmark. As a general rule, the surgical PVD should not be carried anterior to the equator.[27] The vortex veins and occasionally the different coloration of the fundus help identify it.

The maculopapillary bundle is the area between the fovea and the optic disk. It contains the most crucial nerve fibers, those responsible for central vision; during ILM peeling, the surgeon should try to avoid regrabbing the ILM here.

The peripheral retina is a ring of ~15 mm width, extending from the equator to the ora serrata.

External Anatomy for the Vitreoretinal Surgeon

The external anteroposterior diameter of the eye is ~24 mm; internally it is 22 mm. The sclera is thickest at the insertion of the optic disk (1.2 mm) and thinnest (0.3 mm) at the insertion of the extraocular muscles. The thickness is 0.5 mm at the equator and 0.8 mm at the limbus.[20,28]

The distance between the limbus and the ora serrata varies by quadrant—6.5 mm temporally, 6.1 mm superiorly, 5.7 mm nasally, and 6.2 mm inferiorly. The distances are longer in myopic eyes and shorter in hyperopic eyes. The distance between the limbus and the equator is ~13 mm.[1,20]

The insertion point of the extraocular muscles into the sclera as measured from the limbus also varies—5.5 mm for the medial rectus, 6.6 mm for the inferior, 6.9 mm for the lateral, and 7.5 mm for the superior.[1]

The seven vortex veins (fewer temporally than nasally) penetrate the sclera 3–6 mm posterior to the equator internally and 14–25 mm from the limbus externally.

Physiology—What Keeps the Retina Attached?

Two main forces work against the separation of the neuroretina from the RPE. The most crucial is the RPE pump—active fluid transport ("suction") from the vitreous cavity toward the choriocapillaris. In highly myopic eyes with a posterior staphyloma, reduced pumping by the RPE is assumed to play a role in development of the central retinal detachment. The peripheral retina is easier to detach in diabetic eyes than in nondiabetic eyes, presumably because of the reduced efficiency of the RPE pump in diabetic eyes.[27]

The second most important factor in maintaining retinal attachment is the interphotoreceptor matrix, which acts as a glue between the neuroretina and the RPE (its weakness is another potential contributory factor in the two aforementioned conditions).[29] The interphotoreceptor matrix requires time to regain its adhesive power; once broken intraoperatively, the glue will not regain its full efficacy for a few days postoperatively.

Two additional factors maintain retinal attachment, but these are of much less significance—the presence of the (healthy) vitreous gel, which mechanically prevents retinal detachment as long as it fills the vitreous cavity completely; and the intraocular pressure (IOP), which "pushes" the retina against the RPE.[27]

EQUIPMENT, INSTRUMENTATION, AND MATERIALS

The basic principles and main purpose[b] of the vitrectomy machine are to (1) cut and then aspirate material (gel, proliferative membranes, fluid, etc.) from the vitrectomy cavity; (2) maintain the preset IOP by supplying as much fluid (balanced salt solution and silicone oil) or air (gas) as is needed to instantly compensate for the amount of material removed; and (3) provide intraocular illumination (hand-held fiber optic and/or some type of "chandelier").[20,28]

In a typical set-up for VR surgery today, the surgeon sits at the operating table, viewing the operation through the microscope. The eye is entered with three sharp blades (trocars) that deliver microcannulas (of 23 g, 25 g, or 27 g), which are used intraoperatively to gain access to the vitreous cavity through the pars plana. The cannulas are gateways for the infusion, the vitrectomy probe, and the fiber optic, all of which are connected to the vitrectomy machine (Fig. 58.1). The same cannulas allow the surgeon to introduce all additional tools required (scissors, forceps, etc. see further). There are other, less frequently used, options for performing vitrectomy that are not detailed here.[20]

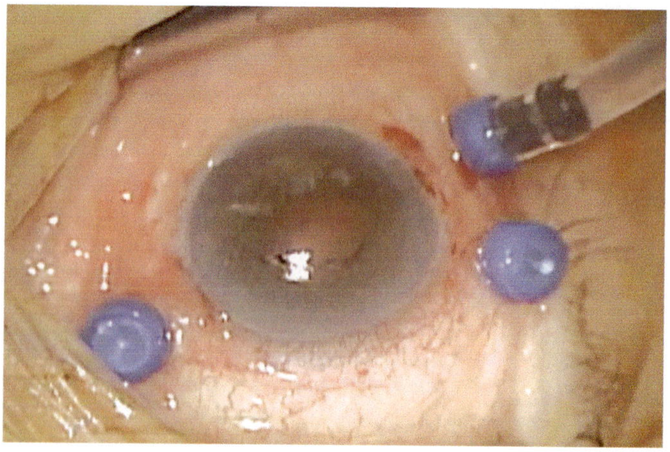

Fig. 58.1: *23 g cannulas in place*: Three valved cannulas have been inserted; the infusion line has been connected to the inferotemporal cannula. The two superior "working" cannulas are placed just above the 3- and 9-o'clock positions to allow access to the vitreous base at 6 o'clock, even in the phakic eye.

The most important characteristics of the vitrectomy machine are reviewed in Table 58.3.

Although not part of the vitrectomy machine itself, the wide-angle viewing systems [such as the binocular indirect ophthalmomicroscope (BIOM)[c]] must be briefly mentioned here (Fig. 58.2). These contact or noncontact systems allow visualization of a field of up to 130° while also providing sufficient resolution for even the most delicate maneuvers (ILM peeling). One of the many benefits of wide-angle viewing is that the system makes it possible to operate on eyes with a small pupil.[20,30]

The list of available hand instruments is long. They can be classified as squeezable (the handle needs to be squeezed to activate the tool's action—forceps, scissors, and certain types of laser probes), nonsqueezable (the handle needs no activation by the surgeon's fingers—bent needle, spatula, etc.), and hybrid (the handle requires minimal action by the surgeon—flute needle, retractable magnet, etc.).

---

[b] The concept and instrumentation for vitrectomy are utilized for a wide variety of non-vitreoretinal conditions, but these are not discussed in this chapter.

[c] Oculus Optikgeräte GmbH, Wetzlar, Germany.

Table 58.3: A brief description of the most important characteristics of the vitrectomy machine and its components.

Variable	Comment
Illumination	The goal is to provide the surgeon with excellent brightness with a minimal risk of light toxicity. The latter also depends on, among other things, the type of the light source [xenon, LED, etc.], the distance of the light pipe from the retina, the time of illumination, and the use and types of filters. In the "standard" setting, the light pipe is held in the vitreous cavity by the surgeon. This allows illumination from either the nasal or temporal side and at various angles. But this setup also prevents true bimanual surgery. Conversely, a chandelier-type of illuminator allows the surgeon to use both hands (e.g. hold a scissors in one hand and a forceps in the other) but creates shadows that are cast by the instrument and severely limits adjustment of the illumination angle. The light pipe should be shielded (mechanically blocking light emission on one side so that the surgeon's eyes do not receive direct illumination). The light emission should be wide angle. The vitrectomy machine must have two bulbs; if one burns out, the spare can instantly be switched on
Pump	The goal is to provide the most precise control of material-movement in front of the vitrectomy probe's port without a noticeable loss of speed. In general, a flow-control pump is preferable to a vacuum-driven one (Venturi). Hybrid systems also exist, offering the advantages of both systems and providing individualized options while maximizing safety.
Infusion	The IOP should be continually monitored by the machine to allow immediate adjustments of the infusion pressure, independent of the position (height as measured from the floor) of the patient's head, to maintain the IOP exactly as set.
Cannula or size	Transconjunctival surgery (23/25/27 g) is more convenient to the patient than the "traditional", cannula-free 20 g surgery; but the presence of the cannula also limits both the type and size of the tools that can be inserted. The ideal cannula has a valve (and one that "survives" the full duration of the operation without breaking down) that prevents leakage and therefore allows precise maintenance of the IOP throughout. The insertion of the cannula with the trocar should be a one-step procedure.
Vitrectomy probe: Size	In principle, the smaller, the better since a smaller probe means less morbidity for the patient and allows faster wound healing. In reality, a smaller size involves compromises such as increased bending of the instrument/s, slower material-removal (despite industry claims to the contrary), and lack of the full armamentarium (such as silicone oil injection).
Vitrectomy probe: Length	The probe should be long enough to reach the posterior pole, even in a highly myopic eye (axial length exceeding ~32 mm). Sadly, most probes do not allow this—the surgeon is forced to indent the eyewall to reach the back of the eye.
Vitrectomy probe: Cut rate	In general, the higher the cut rate (cps), the less tissue movement and traction in front of the vitrectomy probe's port and the safer the surgery. Today's machines are capable of achieving 16,000 cps.
Vitrectomy probe: Duty cycle	Until recently, most probes allowed the port to be open only 50% of the time; today the "ideal" has been reached, with certain machines allowing the port to be open during the entire time (continuous flow). This dramatically reduces the risk of undesirable tissue movement (causing traction or even inadvertent "biting" into a mobile and detached retina) in front of the port.
Vitrectomy probe: Port location	The closer the port to the tip of the probe, the higher the potential for a more complete the removal of the material—not just the vitreous gel but also proliferative membranes in front of or on top of the retina. In general, the smaller the gauge, the closer the port is to the tip.
Foot pedal	Ideally, the pedal is wireless and programmable yet simple; it should also incorporate the laser function.
Endodiathermy probe	This should have a non-sticky surface, and both a pointed tip and a flat tip should be available.

(IOP: Intraocular pressure; cps: Cuts per second)
Source: EVA, DORC, Zuidland, The Netherlands.

One additional, crucially important tool is the endolaser probe, which may be straight or bent (preferred) or a combination—memory material (a curved probe housed in a straight tube) or a tip that bends as the surgeon squeezes the handle (see above).

There are many different materials that the surgeon uses intraoperatively and/or leaves in the vitreous cavity postoperatively.[30-36] A brief summary of these is provided in Table 58.4.

CAVEATS FOR THE VITREORETINAL SURGEON

Who should and Who should not be a Vitreoretinal Surgeon?

Vitreoretinal surgery is dramatically different from cataract surgery. The latter is a refined, highly standardized operation where the deviation in technique between two

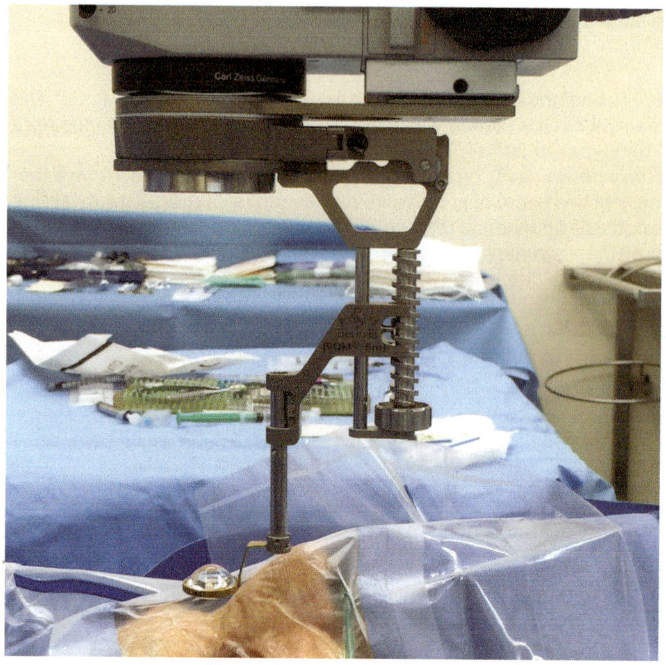

Fig. 58.2: *The binocular indirect ophthalmomicroscope*: The patient has been prepped and the binocular indirect ophthalmomicroscope (BIOM) with the wide-angle, high-resolution "gold" lens is about to be lowered over the cornea. Its distance when finally *in situ* will be approximately 3 mm from the eye.

cases is typically minimal. In VR surgery, the exact opposite is true; in addition, the surgeon's efforts, however, complex and difficult, are quite often not rewarded by success.[20] Any ophthalmologist who is not willing to accept or to be content with, living such a life should not choose to become a VR surgeon.

Vitreoretinal Surgery: A Team Effort

To be successful the VR surgeon needs constant attention, active contribution, and unwavering support from several people. The anesthesiologist must ensure that the patient does not have pain, which would increase the risk for movement of the head (even a small repositioning of the leg may lead to significant head movement). A circulatory nurse must always be presented in case some not-yet-prepared material, equipment, or tool is needed (because the original has run out or broken down or because the item was not expected to become necessary). Presence of an assistant (typically a resident or fellow) is not mandatory but such assistance can be of immense help. The most important person of the team; however, is the nurse. The quality of the surgeon's job cannot exceed that of the nurse—if the nurse does not do a good job preparing for the

Table 58.4: Materials commonly used in vitreoretinal surgery.

Material[1]	Comment
Air	Air is mainly employed intraoperatively to determine whether VR traction still persists, as a tool to force the subretinal fluid into the vitreous cavity, and to help with the collection of silicone oil bubbles. A less commonly utilized function of air is to allow visualization of the peripheral vitreous while also keeping the retina attached during PPV here ("pneumovitrectomy"). Acting as a lens, air is useful when performing endolaser photocoagulation in the peripheral retina. Additional uses include demonstration of vitreous presence in the anterior chamber or behind the lens capsule. It is rarely used today as a postoperative tamponade.
Gases	Gases of different type and concentration are used as postoperative tamponade to cover a retinal break, including a macular hole. They can be expansile or nonexpansile.
Heavy liquids	These are used as an intraoperative tool, almost never left behind postoperatively (at least not intentionally). They can force the subretinal fluid to exit into the vitreous cavity through a peripheral break, "uncurl" the inverted retina in a giant-tear RD, and maintain retinal attachment while the surgeon is performing other tasks such as endolaser photocoagulation during surgery for RD. Less commonly used is the heavier-than-water fluid for tamponading intraoperative bleeding, keeping the retina away from the surgeon's tools during subretinal work (the heavy liquid is injected subretinally), bringing lens remnants or nonmetallic IOFBs anteriorly, or pushing liquefied blood out of the suprachoroidal space.
Silicone oil	Available in various viscosities and molecular weights, silicone oil ("oil") is a long-term tamponade after surgery for conditions with a proliferative element (PVR and PDR) and to prevent postoperative RD. Oil is an option after failed macular-hole surgery. It is a last resort in preventing phthisis.
Stains ("vital dyes" and "chromovitrectomy")	Both the normal vitreous and the ILM are basically invisible; the edge (extent) of an ERM is often impossible to determine. Various stains (ICG, trypan blue, brilliant blue, etc.) are available to allow visualization of these tissues; in addition, triamcinolone acetonide is used to mark (not "stain") the vitreous, whether in the periphery or on the retinal surface (lack of PVD).
Viscoelastics	These can be used as a tool to open a closed funnel in eyes with RD or to separate epiretinal proliferative tissue from the retina (delamination). They are also used in the anterior chamber to keep the pupil wide or to force out the prolapsed silicone oil.
Exchange of materials	Various VR surgery books provide detailed descriptions of what material can or should not be exchanged for what other material.

(VR: Vitreoretinal; PPV: Pars plana vitrectomy; RD: Retinal detachment; IOFB: Intraocular foreign body; PVR: Proliferative vitreoretinopathy; PDR: Proliferative diabetic retinopathy; ILM: Internal limiting membrane; ERM: Epiretinal membrane; ICG: Indocyanine green; PVD: Posterior vitreous detachment) case or is not attentive during the operation, the surgeon's concentration will unnecessarily deviate from the task ahead, which risks iatrogenic complications.

The Vitreoretinal Surgeon at the Operating Table

The VR surgery can be very long, and most surgeons do several cases a day. It is therefore of utmost importance that the surgeon sits comfortably (i.e. the height of the chair, the operating table, and the microscope should be adjusted so that he sits comfortably, instead of, as is often the case with beginners, the other way around). Poor posture results in acute pain and risks longer-term complications such as a herniated disk in the surgeon's neck or lower back.

The patient must also be in a comfortable position to reduce the risk of movement under local anesthesia. The patient's head (face) should be parallel to the floor.

The pedals should be arranged in a logical way, not simply ensuring easy, comfortable access to them. Since during vitrectomy, the microscope pedal is worked much more than that of the vitrectomy machine, the former should be under the surgeon's dominant foot.

Even though some surgeons look down on those who use one type or another of arm or hand support, such a mechanical support is highly recommended to reduce any avoidable tremor. Perhaps the best option is a U-shaped, padded bar around the patient's head. The "U" is fixed to the operating table, but its vertical position is adjustable.

VITREORETINAL SURGERY: GENERAL CONSIDERATIONS

Diagnostics

A good history is crucial and should be taken by the ophthalmologist, not a technician or a nurse.[20] The rest of examination will then be guided by the history with this notion in mind: If the outcome of a test does not change the management plan, the test is unnecessary (the only exception is if the test is beneficial for medicolegal purposes). A thorough external inspection is next, followed by obtaining visual acuity for both eyes. Other useful functional examinations may include Amsler tests and reading ability.[37]

The slit-lamp examination is crucially important, first with the "naked eye" and then using a 60–90 D lens. If the reason for the evaluation is other than an open globe injury, the IOP should also be measured. Unless the media are opaque, indirect ophthalmoscopy is mandatory.

If a macular condition is encountered, optical coherence tomography (OCT)[38-41] is a uniquely important tool. Ultrasonography[42,43] is also very useful in many cases, although it should never be the final word in determining whether a PVD[44-46] is present. Conversely, both electrophysiology and fluorescein angiography are rarely indicated for the VR surgeon.

Indicating versus Declining Surgery and Counseling

Once a pathology amenable to surgery is identified, the VR surgeon may immediately be tempted to indicate it. This is understandable since few such pathologies will improve spontaneously, and delaying the repair may carry a risk of irreversible damage. Indeed, most VR pathologies worsen with time, some within "minutes" (endophthalmitis),[47] others over several months (macular edema).[48]

On the other hand, the VR surgeon may recognize that a surgery should not have been done only after a severe intra- or postoperative complication has occurred.[20,49] The surgeon must constantly navigate between Scylla and Charybdis to achieve the best possible outcome in each case.

One purpose of proper counseling is to share the decision-making with the patient–the goal is not to avoid the burden of making the decision but to make the patient a partner in the entire treatment process. The surgeon must inform the patient about the condition (comparing it to the "normal"), offer options, and describe the likely or possible outcomes with each option, being as specific (percentages) as possible. If the counseling is properly done, almost all reasonable persons will be able to make a decision regarding the treatment, which the surgeon should then follow.

If, after receiving counseling, the patient answers with a question, such as, "And what would you do if you yourself had this condition?" the surgeon needs to readdress the issue. The information-sharing process must be repeated until the person truly understands the condition and the treatment options and is then able to make the choice.

The surgeon should never promise success (even in an "easy" case serious complications may occur intraoperatively or postoperatively). The patient must also understand that the goal of surgery is to restore the anatomy (e.g. reattach the retina). Whether and to what extent functional improvement follows can be difficult to predict. Even if the anatomy is restored, the vision may simply be preserved at its preoperative state or its deterioration may be simply slowed rather than stopped.[d] In the latter two situations, the surgeon may have to convince the patient to seriously consider ("agree to") surgery since choosing to undergo an operation that does not lead to a tangible benefit (functional improvement), and that does not do so quickly, is not intuitive.

The Management Plan

If the person's choice is to elect surgery because the potential benefits exceed the possible risks, the surgeon must design a plan.[20,49] The plan involves strategic issues such as how many surgeries are optimal to achieve the desired outcome (especially in cases of severe trauma, multiple operations, rather than a single procedure, may be preferable), the timing of the intervention, or whether the surgery will be combined with cataract or glaucoma surgery. These decisions are made preoperatively. The plan is a roadmap that describes how to get from the current condition of the eyeball to the desired one; and just as a driver may use a map to design the route but change the original plan if a roadblock is encountered, the surgeon must be willing to change his plan based on the individual circumstances.

The other part of planning is tactical—details such as how a membrane is attacked, how the ILM is peeled, the type of gas used, how much laser is used (Fig. 58.3) and numerous other issues. These decisions are made intraoperatively, and they are often changed based on the tissue's reaction to the surgical maneuvers.[20]

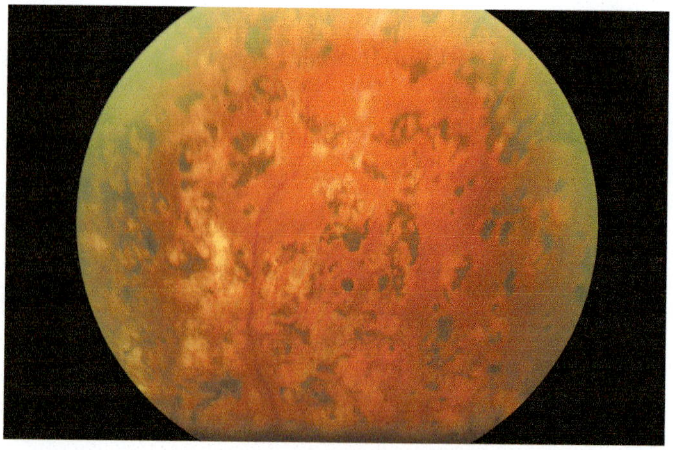

Fig. 58.3: *Heavy laser in a patient with diabetic retinopathy*: The treatment was not only too strong but also almost contiguous; such laser treatment may prevent the development of proliferative disease; but the patient loses the visual field, and macular complications (scar-formation and edema) may still occur.

Anesthesia

At certain institutions, there is a set policy to always use either general or some type of local anesthesia, unless there is an overriding issue such as the patient being too young or otherwise uncooperative. Both options have certain advantages and disadvantages; whenever local policies allow, it is best to make an individualized decision which one to use. One less commonly mentioned criterion in the decision-making process is the potential need to discuss an issue with the patient during surgery (see above, counseling) if an unforeseen circumstance arises.

Before Entering the Eye

The surgeon must rethink the preoperative plan and ensure that all major "components" are in place—surgical team, equipment, and instruments; the pedals are properly positioned, etc. The vitrectomy machine's settings must be preprogrammed and the actual surgeon's preferences selected.

It is also important that the surgeon has no outside issues (divorce, child's death, etc.) that could interfere with his concentration during the case; while the existence of such issues may be outside the surgeon's control, if any such issue would remain on the surgeon's mind during the operation, it is best to defer the surgery or to have it done by a colleague.

The Basic Rules of Vitreoretinal Surgery

Depending upon how "basic" is defined, the number of "rules" can vary from a few to the infinite. Table 58.5 provides an overview of a selected few.

Complications and Side Effects

If the eye is phakic, cataract development is unavoidable (i.e. the surgeon need not injure the posterior capsule for cataract to form)—it is a side effect, not a complication.

The list of possible complications is very long. A selected few are listed in Table 58.6.

[d] This is a good example showing the difference between being a VR and being a cataract surgeon: for the latter, an outcome that does not result in visual improvement in a patient with age-related lens opacity is typically appreciated as a failure.

Table 58.5: Selected basic rules of vitreoretinal surgery.

Variable	Rule—comment
Phacovitrectomy	If accommodation is not an issue, it makes sense to combine the PPV with lens removal (and typically intraocular lens implantation). A nonmedical factor in the decision-making is whether both procedures would be reimbursed by the insurance company.
Draping	Even if the draping is done by the nurse, the surgeon is responsible for ensuring the drape is firmly adhered to the skin and does not separate—as it often does on the nasal side. This is especially dangerous (endophthalmitis risk!) if the patient has a running nose or if there is a removable prosthetic device on the other side.
Speculum selection	It may appear to be an insignificant issue preoperatively yet become a source of frustration during the operation. The ideal speculum is self-tightening, has a wire-type blade, and has no outcroppings or unlooped endings.
Cannula placement	It is all too common to see surgical videos with the two working cannulas placed too superiorly; the ideal positions are at just above the horizontal meridian. This ensures access to the inferior vitreous base, even in the phakic eye.
The infusion cannula	If the infusion line is pulled partially out, the infusion can become subretinal or choroidal; if the infusion is air, it can also get into the bloodstream and cause death. The surgeon or nurse must monitor the correct position of the infusion cannula or line during the entire procedure.
Angle of instrument insertion or removal	Especially in eyes with a thin sclera (high myopia, reoperation, rheumatoid arthritis, etc.), the cannulas can easily be pulled out during instrument withdrawal. This inconvenience is less likely to occur if the instruments are inserted or removed at the same angle at which the cannula was inserted (~15º); it also reduces the risk of delayed wound closure with leakage and hypotony. If the PPV is long, the cannulas are more prone to be inadvertently pulled out since the cannula is extensively rotated during surgery.
Holding instruments	No matter what type of tool is in the surgeon's hand, it must be supported at all times by at least three, not two, fingers; in addition, the surgeon's little finger should be rested on the patient's forehead for added stability.
Rotating the eyeball	Since two instruments are inserted into the vitreous cavity, both must be moved simultaneously and covering the same distance to avoid wrinkling the sclera or cornea.
Syringe-injection	The safest method is to push the plunger with the palm of the hand, not with the thumb or index finger. This reduces the risk of a jet, which could damage the retina or inadvertently inject the material subretinally.
Capsulectomy	If the eye is pseudophakic, a judicious central capsulectomy should nearly always be performed, with only a few exceptions. The capsule is likely to opacify later, and while YAG capsulectomy is possible subsequently, it is not as accurate as one done with the vitrectomy probe and it leaves a large floater behind.
PVD	Unless it is impossible or very dangerous (young patient and extremely adherent posterior cortical vitreous), no gel should be left on the posterior retina
The direction of vitreous removal	Typically, posterior-anterior; except in cases of vitreoretinal (macular) traction, or hazy vitreous (hemorrhage).
The amount of vitreous to be removed	In certain etiologies (RD, PVR, PDR, endophthalmitis, trauma, etc.), the gel should be removed as much as possible (consistent with safety). Conversely, in macular cases the gel removal may be much more limited.
Scleral indentation	In a phakic eye this must be done by the nurse or assistant; in aphakic or pseudophakic eyes the surgeon can also self-indent. Both techniques have advantages and disadvantages: an individual decision must be made, and the criteria should include the expertise of the nurse or assistant.
Removal of subretinal strands	In transconjunctival surgery, forceps with long blades cannot be inserted into the vitreous; it may therefore be necessary to create several retinotomies. The angle at which the strand is approached is also important, unless a multipurpose forceps is used.
Feedback during surgery	It is practically always visual, not tactile or audible; this is one reason for using vital dyes.
Loss of visualization	The causes can range from the microscope or BIOM to vitreous hemorrhage. It must be identified and dealt with, rather than "operating in the dark".
Video recording of the surgery	Following these simple steps helps to achieve the most optimal recording—adjusting the microscope focus to the camera first and to the surgeon's eyes second; having the camera's auto-iris function on; keeping the target area in the center of the visual field (the camera's visual field is smaller than the area viewed by the surgeon); avoiding shining light onto white surfaces; using the minimal amount of light from the endoilluminator; and having a designated person in the operating room who constantly directs the surgeon ("focus" and "center").

(PPV: Pars plana vitrectomy; RD: Retinal detachment; PVR: Proliferative vitreoretinopathy; PDR: Proliferative diabetic retinopathy; BIOM: Binocular indirect ophthalmomicroscope)

Source: FC23.R06, Vitreq, Vierpolders, The Netherlands.

Table 58.6: Selected intra- and postoperative complications of vitreoretinal surgery.

Complication	Comment
Intraoperative	
Hemorrhage	A truly "expulsive" type of bleeding is very rare; most hemorrhages are self-limiting (e.g. during ILM peeling). The most common indication associated with severe bleeding used to be PDR; however, the preoperative injection of Avastin largely eliminated this issue.
Retinal tear	Typically caused by the surgeon extending the PVD too anteriorly.
Lens damage	Breaking the posterior capsule with the vitrectomy probe or, less commonly, the light pipe.
Postoperative	
Deterioration or loss of vision	The list is very long, ranging from tight scleral sutures and corneal edema to RD, extreme IOP elevation, and orbital hemorrhage. The patient must be made aware that there is virtually no vision while a large gas bubble is in the vitreous cavity.
Endophthalmitis	The most severe of the (relatively) common complications, requiring immediate and appropriate intervention (see later in this chapter); it appears within the first few days.
Hypotony	Common causes include a scleral wound that is not closed, and choroidal or retinal detachment. Rarely a true ciliary body shutdown is the cause.
Glaucoma	Typically, an expanding gas bubble is responsible. Longer-term, the glaucoma is typically neovascular, especially in diabetics.
Vitreous hemorrhage	Most commonly diabetes is in the background; all such patients undergoing PPV must be informed that there is no guaranty against (re)bleeding. It is crucial to control the patient's systemic blood pressure.
EMP	While most of the cases with this "mini-PVR" are idiopathic, PPV or extensive panretinal laser can also be causative.
RD	Retinal breaks may occur not just intraoperatively (see above) but also weeks to months after surgery due to residual or newly developed traction.
PVR	A truly sight-threatening chronic complication, occurring weeks to months after the PPV. The most common original etiologies include RD, trauma, and recurrence of previous PVR; the most difficult to treat is PVR that occurs in an eye with PDR.

(ILM: Internal limiting membrane; PDR: Proliferative diabetic retinopathy; PVD: Posterior vitreous detachment; RD: Retinal detachment; IOP: Intraocular pressure; PPV: Pars plana vitrectomy; EMP: Epimacular proliferation; PVR: Proliferative vitreoretinopathy)

MAJOR INDICATIONS FOR VITREORETINAL SURGERY[e]

Endophthalmitis (Postoperative)

The diagnosis is usually straightforward—the eye is painful and red, the vision deteriorates, and there is a hypopyon (Fig. 58.4).[47,50] Once the diagnosis is made, one of the possible treatment options (Flowchart 58.1) must immediately be initiated. The most important question is whether the ophthalmologist chooses to follow the recommendations of the Endophthalmitis Vitrectomy Study (EVS)[51]—perform PPV only if the visual acuity drops to light perception. In all other cases, the choice is injection of intravitreal antibiotics (and a corticosteroid).[f]

Most ophthalmologists today question the validity of the EVS recommendations and opt for surgery much

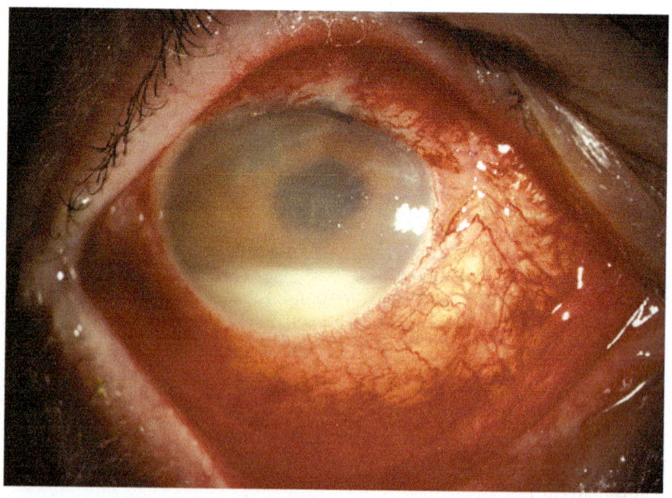

Fig. 58.4: *Hypopyon*: The eye is red; the cornea edematous; there is pus in the anterior chamber; and the pupil is small. These are the typical signs of (postoperative) endophthalmitis.

[e] In alphabetic order.

[f] E.g. Vancomycin 2 mg, Ceftazidime 2.25 mg, Dexamethasone 0.4 mg.

Flowchart 58.1: Treatment options for eyes with postoperative endophthalmitis.

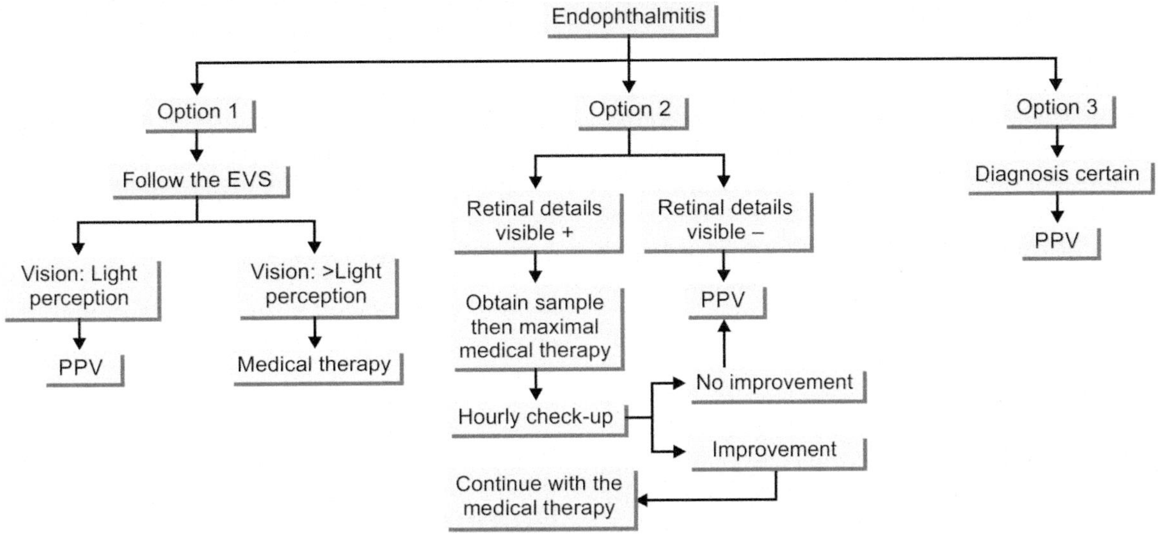

(EVS: Endophthalmitis vitrectomy study; PPV: Pars plana vitrectomy)

Table 58.7: Selected technical issues in vitrectomy for postoperative endophthalmitis.

Variable	Comment
Cornea	The epithelium needs to be scraped
Anterior chamber	The hypopyon must be irrigated and the fibrinous membrane removed (from the pupillary area, iris surface, and angle)
Pupil	Maximum dilatation is to be achieved, using iris retractors if necessary
Lens	Removal is rarely necessary; however, if it interferes with visualization or the completion of gel removal, the lens must be sacrificed
IOL	It is very uncommon that the implant needs to be removed, but the capsular bag must be thoroughly irrigated —a large capsulectomy is therefore unavoidable. If cataract surgery is done during the case, IOL implantation is acceptable in early cases of endophthalmitis but is best avoided in advanced cases
Vitreous gel	Unless the visualization is very poor, an almost complete vitrectomy is the goal; this involves a PVD and careful shaving of the vitreous base. The latter; however, involves a less than close shaving to reduce the risk of retinal injury. The anterior hyaloid face is to be detached and completely removed
Retinal surface	It should be vacuumed, especially in the macular area. In principle, the best tool is a soft-tipped flute needle; passive aspiration is to be employed
Silicone oil use	Oil is not for routine use, but it does have several advantages: it tamponades the retina and keeps it attached (fear of RD was the main concern in the EVS); it provides a clear postoperative view of the retina early on; organisms do not live inside the oil; medications can be injected into the oil (the recommended dose is 1/3–1/2 of the normal)

(IOL: Intraocular lens; PVD: Posterior vitreous detachment; RD: Retinal detachment; EVS: Endophthalmitis vitrectomy study)

earlier.[47,52] As a general rule, the later PPV is performed for endophthalmitis, the more technically difficult the surgery becomes and the worse the prognosis. In advanced cases, only very experienced surgeons should perform the intervention. At the conclusion of surgery, antibiotics and a corticosteroid must be injected into the vitreous cavity. Table 58.7 provides an overview of the surgery, which must be conducted in a step-by-step fashion.

In eyes with endogenous endophthalmitis, the justification for performing surgery is even more pronounced, but the prognosis is poorer. Systemic therapy, according to the general conditions, is mandatory.[50,53] In a trauma setting, these recommendations are even more true;[49] this is discussed later in this chapter.

Hyphema

The VR surgeon typically does not get involved in the management of patients with a hyphema unless the anterior chamber is full of blood and/or it is clotted.[49] The presence of a large amount of blood in the anterior chamber in eyes with even mildly elevated IOP represents a considerable risk for corneal "blood staining", which is a misnomer since the blood actually enters the stroma (imbibition). It may take many months for the hemorrhage to spontaneously absorb, during which period the deeper structures cannot be visualized. The bar to surgically remove the hyphema must therefore not be high—the risk of the procedure is extremely low.

Irrigation of the blood when it is in fluidic form is straightforward, whether a bimanual or monomanual technique is used. If the blood is clotted; however, an anterior chamber maintainer should be inserted first, typically on the nasal side; in the phakic eye, the tip is best kept over the iris to avoid inadvertent lens damage since the surgeon rotates the eye a lot during clot removal and his attention will be focused on maneuvering with the vitrectomy probe, not on the infusion cannula's position.

The vitrectomy probe should be introduced from the temporal side, even if doing so requires use of the surgeon's nondominant hand. The port should be kept horizontal (i.e. not turned downwards or upwards) and inside the clot (so as to constantly be occluded by the clot), and the vacuum or flow should be kept at relatively low levels.

Lens- and Intraocular Lens-related Phacovitrectomy

As mentioned earlier, it makes sense to perform combined surgery in persons who do not have useful accommodation or in eyes with incipient cataract.[54-57] Certain elements of combined procedures are discussed in Table 58.8.

Lensectomy

If there is significant vitreous prolapse into the anterior chamber, or if the lens is soft and both capsules are to be removed, use of the vitrectomy probe is preferred to phacoemulsification.[58] Table 58.9 provides an overview of certain technical aspects of lensectomy.

Dropped Nucleus

This term, used extensively in clinical practice, is misleading—often almost the entire lens (Fig. 58.5) is lost or at least substantial amounts of cortical material are also found in the vitreous.[59,60]

The most crucial element in the management of this complication of phacoemulsification (although the

Table 58.8: Phacovitrectomy—suggestions for the surgeon.*

Variable	Suggestions
Infusion cannula	Place the pars plana cannula before the cataract operation begins; it is much harder to do this after the completion of the cataract surgery since the eye is soft. The infusion line need not be connected before the actual PPV starts.
Presence of vitreous in anterior chamber	Perform intracameral vitrectomy first (an infusion line is necessary), then decide whether lensectomy or "standard" phacoemulsification is to be done. The prolapsed vitreous may be impossible to detect through the microscope; use triamcinolone to verify its presence.
Capsulorhexis	Do not make it larger than 5 mm; the pressure in the vitreous cavity may be high during PPV, pushing the optic of the IOL out of the bag.
Viscoleastic in the anterior chamber	Consider keeping it there until the completion of the PPV in the following cases—consistently shallow anterior chamber or "prolapsing IOL"; floppy iris; constricting pupil; intravitreal blood seeping into the anterior chamber; and silicone oil prolapsing.
Preserving the (posterior) capsule	As a general rule, do not remove the capsule. Exceptions include young patients with lens trauma (to reduce the risk of phthisis due to capsular contraction); prolapse of silicone oil into the anterior chamber through the zonules; or weak zonules extending over at least one quadrant. If IOL will not be implanted (no functional need for it; the refraction of the eyeball does not require one), consider the benefit of retaining the capsule.**
Posterior capsulectomy	Always perform a judicious one
IOL implantation	As a general rule, implant the IOL before the PPV is started. Exceptions include an eye that will not benefit because the IOL will improve neither the central nor the peripheral vision; the eye's refractive power does not require it—in these cases, as mentioned above, no implant is indicated. If extensive manipulations in the retinal periphery are required, consider holding off with the implantation until the PPV is completed—the edge of the IOL may be rather bothersome here, often causing "double vision" or constant adjustments in how the peripheral retina is visualized.

(PPV: Pars plana vitrectomy; IOL: Intraocular lens)

*Assuming that it is the VR surgeon who performs both parts of the operation. If an anterior segment specialist does the cataract surgery, the VR surgeon should negotiate about the relevant issues listed below.

**The old adage of "compartmentalizing the eye" does not hold true anymore.

Table 58.9: Selected technical issues during lensectomy.

Variable	Comment
Infusion	Some type of infusion is always necessary; typically, it is introduced through the pars plana.
Access to the lens	The superotemporal pars plana incision is the preferred route of approaching to the lens (not a limbal incision).
Breaching the lens capsule	The surgeon should first puncture the capsule at the equator with a sharp tool [such as the (largest possible size) needle] to avoid injuring the zonules by pushing the lens with the blunt vitrectomy port.
Port position	It is best to turn the vitrectomy probe's port sideways, thus avoiding injury to the anterior capsule.
Posterior capsule	It is almost impossible to preserve the posterior capsule; it is invisible and the lens is collapsing as the lens material is being reduced. (One method to possibly avoid this is to introduce the infusion into the lens itself.) Conversely, the integrity of the anterior capsule is easy to maintain.
Removal of the lens material	The surgeon should take small bites of the lens cortex or nucleus—as opposed to the longer passages when the phaco probe is used. Usually, the cutting option of the vitrectomy probe is also utilized—the size of the probe's inner tube is small and the probe may get clogged by even the soft cortex.

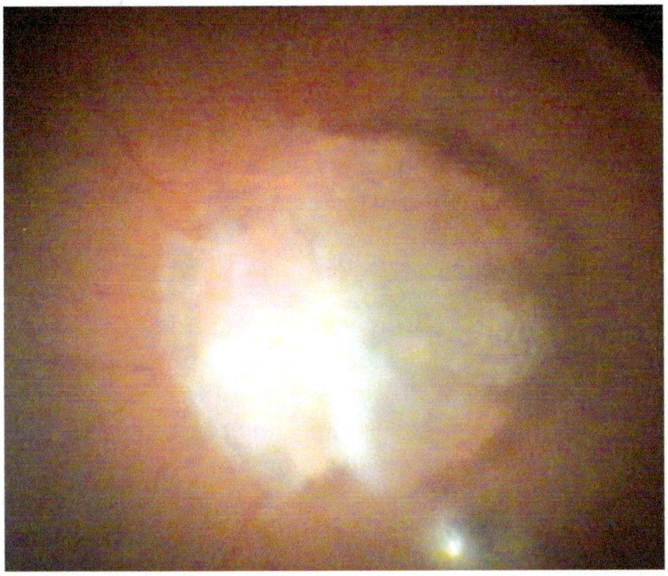

Fig. 58.5: *Dislocated crystalline lens*: Almost the entire lens is lying on the posterior retina (see the text for more details).

condition may also occur in certain diseases such as Marfan's syndrome or as a result of trauma) is to convince the cataract surgeon to refer the case to the VR surgeon instead of going "fishing" himself for the lost lens particles.

The second crucial issue is the timing of surgery. The literature is divided as to whether doing the PPV immediately or early brings better results than delaying it for a few weeks.[61-64] This is, however, an unacceptably phrased dilemma as it completely takes out of the equation the most important "part" of the question—the patient. To reduce the anxiety the patient undergoes until the resolution of this potentially sight-threatening complication, the sooner the PPV is performed the better.

The removal of the vitreous should be completed (including the PVD, visually confirmed with triamcinolone use) before the lens material is tackled; in these cases the vitreous base should also be shaved. The lens is then approached first with the vitrectomy probe and as much of the cortex (possibly the nucleus) removed as the hardness of the lens and the characteristics of the vitrectomy system allow. When attacking the nucleus (which, unlike the cortex, will not change its configuration to conform upon presenting to the port), the flow or aspiration must be very high and the cut rate low. If the latter recommendation is not obeyed, the surgeon will see the lens particle constantly being pushed away from the port. The light pipe can be used to feed parts of the nucleus into the port or to crush larger pieces into smaller ones.

If the lens material is too hard or the vitrectomy probe is repeatedly clogged by it, the surgeon should switch to phacofragmentation.[20] The lowest possible power is to be used —not exceeding 20%, and even that only once the lens particle has been lifted and brought into the midvitreous. The light pipe should be used to help keep the lens at the fragmentor's tip. While phacofragmentation is not technically demanding, it can be time-consuming as multiple trips will have to be made to pick up all the pieces from the retinal surface. One caveat is the IOP—if the (large) port of the phacofragmentor is not kept occluded and the aspiration or flow is high, the eye can instantly collapse.

Some surgeons prefer not to use either of the steps described above but use instead some type of heavy liquid, filling the vitreous cavity completely and thus floating the lens toward the anterior chamber, then removing it through a limbal incision. (obviously this method cannot be used if an intraocular lens (IOL) has already been implanted.)

Whatever technique is used to remove lens particles from the vitreous cavity, the risk of causing an iatrogenic retinal break is greater than during an "average" PPV; before the cannulas are withdrawn, the retinal periphery should be checked by scleral indentation.

Intraocular Lens Luxation

The surgeon has several options (Table 58.10); whichever option is chosen, the vitrectomy must always be completed first (see above).[65-67]

Macular Diseases—Diseases with Significant Traction in the Etiology

The conditions listed here have varying degrees of traction,[68,69] which either is their essence or is at least a contributory factor in their pathophysiology. In all cases, the surgeon must ask the patient not only about the drop in visual acuity but also about metamorphopsia; the OCT image is also crucial in determining the anatomical consequences of the pathology and in following its course. Below are specific remarks about each condition; Table 58.11 lists selected practical suggestions about the surgery itself. The technique of peeling the ILM is discussed later in this chapter, under macular edema.

Table 58.10: Surgical options in eyes with the intraocular lens luxated into the vitreous.

Option	Comment
Retain the IOL and place it back into the bag	This is advisable only if the lesion in the posterior capsule is small—and does not enlarge during the manipulations
Retain the IOL and place it in the sulcus	The haptics may be sutured to the iris or sclera, or buried (glued) into a scleral tunnel
Remove the IOL and do not implant a new one	If the IOL does not bring functional improvement
Remove the IOL and implant a new one in the sulcus over the existing capsule	The haptics may be sutured to iris or sclera, or buried (glued) into a scleral tunnel
Remove the IOL and the capsule/s and implant an IOL	The haptics may be sutured to iris or sclera, or buried (glued) into a scleral tunnel. If the capsule serves no support function for the IOL and/or its contraction threatens to lead to phthisis, it is best removed
Remove the IOL and the capsule/s and implant an iris-claw IOL	Implanting such an IOL is a very easy and fast procedure
Retain the IOL and implant a second one	This should never be done

(IOL: Intraocular lens)

Vitreomacular Traction Syndrome

The anterioposterior traction results from a vitreous that has lost its uniform gel structure but maintains rather strong adherence to the central retina.[39,40,70,71] The pathology, however, is not restricted to the posterior pole. The sheet-like cortical vitreous may exert severe traction on the peripheral retina—something the surgeon must keep in mind, both when indicating (or declining) surgery and while performing it.

Enzymatic vitreolysis with the use of hyaluronidase,[72] recombinant microplasminogen and tissue plasminogen activator,[73] and ocriplasmin[74,75] have shown some success in dealing with vitreomacular traction syndrome (VMTS), but this success remains rather unpredictable and the price tag high.

Cellophane Maculopathy

The condition is observed by the ophthalmologist as a wrinkling of the macular surface (i.e. the folds are superficial, not full-thickness); there is no visible scar tissue on the macular surface. Some consider it the early stage of an epimacular proliferation (EMP).[71] It is especially crucial in this pathology for the ophthalmologist not to dismiss the patient's complaints as exaggeration—the anatomical findings may indeed be discreet, apparently disproportional to the visual acuity, hence the need to ask about metamorphopsia and reading ability.[76]

Epimacular Proliferation (Epiretinal Membrane) (Fig. 58.6)

A true scar (proliferative tissue) is found over the macular surface, causing full-thickness retinal folds in its advanced stage (Fig. 58.7)—this is the origin of the often used term "macular pucker".[68] As the scar contracts, it causes additional anatomical abnormalities (edema, hemorrhages, macular ectopia, and corkscrew-like coursing of the perifoveal blood vessels). In most cases, the proliferation is idiopathic.[77-80]

Even though some ophthalmologists "treat" the EMP with intravitreal antivascular endothelial growth factor (VEGF) injections, such medications address only the secondary edema, not the heart of the problem.

Table 58.11: Vitrectomy for diseases with vitreomacular traction.

Disease	Comments for the VR surgeon
Vitreomacular traction syndrome	To avoid exerting additional traction on the fovea, the surgeon should, after removing a small amount of gel in front of the macula, inject triamcinolone to highlight the exact anatomy. Before proceeding, an individualized plan regarding tactics must be developed, based on the now-visible condition of the vitreomacular interface. If the vitreous forms a solid sheet as it inserts onto the retina surface, which is quite often the case, scissors rather than the vitrectomy probe may have to be used to sever the connection between the two tissues. The PVD should be completed only after these connections have been cut. This may require very delicate maneuvering on the surgeon's part. Because of the potentially strong vitreoretinal connections toward the retinal periphery, the surgeon should proceed with extreme caution with the rest of the vitrectomy. Peeling the ILM is often done because this ensures that no vitreous is left on the macula and may also help treat the edema. The macula is often convex, not concave, in which case the peeling technique needs to be similar to that done in eyes with true macular edema (see later in this chapter). At the conclusion of the vitrectomy, the surgeon should consider performing a prophylactic laser cerclage.
Cellophane maculopathy	Once a small amount of vitreous has been removed from above the macula, the surgeon should stain the ILM; the microfolds will become much more visible than before as the dye pools in the "valleys" of the wrinkled surface. When grabbing the ILM with forceps, the surgeon must hold the jaws of the instrument so that it is perpendicular with, never parallel to, and the direction of the folds.
Epimacular proliferation	Despite the removal of the epimacular scar being a seemingly easier task than removing the much thinner ILM, it is not the case—dexterity may indeed be more demanding with the latter, but the decision-making regarding tissue tactics is much more complex for EMP removal. The surgeon should consider, among others, the proliferative membrane's extent, thickness, elasticity, "multilayerness", and traction potential—the latter can be very different at different locations within the same membrane, and this is not obvious until the membrane is actually lifted. In the vast majority of eyes with EMP a PVD is present, but the surgeon should still use triamcinolone to be certain. The EMP may be stained (or the ILM alone be stained to show a negative staining of the EMP). As a general rule, the EMP occupies a larger surface than it first appears to. Even if no stain is used, changing the angle at which the light pipe is held can be very helpful, enhancing the view of the scar. The membrane may be multilayered; if the surgeon is not at the correct plane, the procedure becomes much more difficult. An elastic membrane (increased cellular content) presents a higher degree of challenge than a nonelastic one. Once the EMP has been removed, the surgeon should decide whether to also remove the ILM. Removing the latter has two main advantages—it ensures that no scar tissue is left behind, and that the 5–10% recurrence risk is eliminated.
Macular hole	The surgeon should, as described above, create a PVD and then stain the ILM; even if the peeling can be accomplished without staining, it makes the procedure technically easier and less traumatic. The direction of the peeling should never be away from (centrifugal) but either toward (centripetal) or around the hole; this is important to avoid enlarging the hole. The question of how far to extend the peeling has no scientific answer; the reason why many surgeons do it up to the arcades is to not feel "guilty" if the surgery failed. A variation of the technique is called "inverted flap": part of the ILM is not removed but turned onto the hole. Typically, the surgery is completed by using a gas tamponade, although some surgeons use silicone oil primarily.

(VR: Vitreoretinal; PVD: Posterior vitreous detachment; ILM: Internal limiting membrane; EMP: Epimacular proliferation)

Macular Hole

There are two potential traction forces at play—(1) vitreomacular (sagittal) and (2) tangential (surface-parallel).[12,13,81-85] The condition is often accompanied by an EMP. OCT is very important in the differential diagnosis, If the EMP spares the fovea, only a "pseudohole" is present, even if this clinically resembles a macular hole. OCT also enables the ophthalmologist to distinguish a full-thickness hole from a partial thickness one.[40]

Macular Diseases: Edema

Performing vitrectomy for macular edema has two rationales. First, it eliminates any VR traction that is either the cause (*see* Table 58.11) or a contributory factor in the pathology. Second, if the ILM is also removed, the resulting intraretinal gliosis acts as a preventive element against recurrence; this is crucial if the underlying disease (e.g. diabetes) cannot be cured. In addition, the increased intravitreal oxygen tension may improve the retinal function postoperatively.[21,48,86-89]

It is very important that the surgeon creates a PVD (its presence proven by triamcinolone) and does a rather complete vitreous removal, followed by ILM peeling.

Unlike in the previously discussed macular conditions, where the macula is completely or mostly healthy (reducing the risk of iatrogenic injury as long as the surgeon is properly attentive during ILM peeling), the edematous

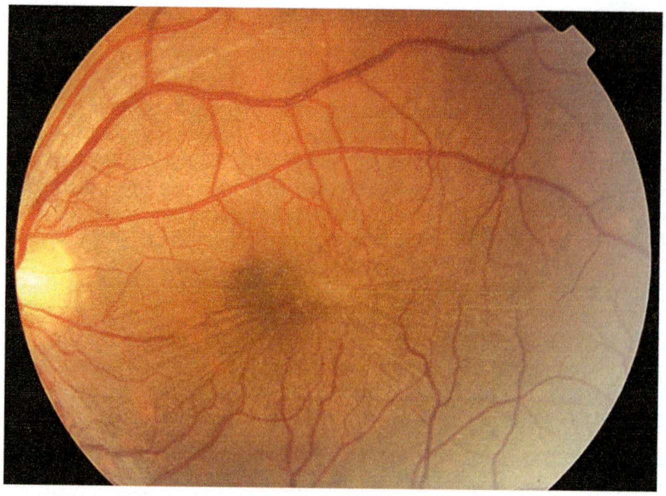

Fig. 58.6: *Epimacular proliferation*: The scar tissue over the center of the macula is relatively small, but it causes radiating, full-thickness retinal folds. Some of the vessels surrounding the area have a crooked course.

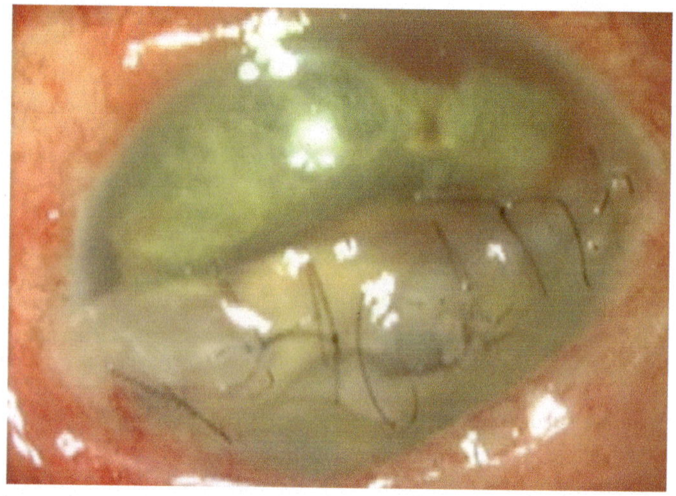

Fig. 58.7: *Post-traumatic endophthalmitis without hypopyon*: The patient suffered a car accident 3 weeks earlier; he was not wearing the seatbelt and exited his vehicle through the windshield. The corneal wound was sutured; but even though the need for reconstructive surgery was obvious, it was not done. Just prior to the vitrectomy, the patient had no pain; no sign of endophthalmitis was detected at the slit lamp; and the visual acuity was light perception. During temporary keratoprosthesis vitrectomy, the eye was found to be full of pus, and still there was no posterior vitreous detachment. The culture yielded three different kinds of bacteria.

macula is a "sick" tissue with a diminished tolerance for surgical trauma. It also has a convex configuration, often forcing the surgeon to peel "uphill", rather than "downhill". Consequently, staining the ILM is much more crucial in eyes with edema than in those with the tractional conditions described above.

The angle of peeling in these eyes should also be different from that done over a healthy retina. To avoid putting undue traction on the already damaged tissue, and especially, to prevent the unroofing of an intraretinal cyst, the angle at which the ILM is separated from the retina should be as closed to parallel as possible. The caveat is for the surgeon to closely monitor not only the site where the ILM is being lifted but also the actual location of the tip of the forceps. The fact that the eyewall has a concave configuration is obvious to the brain but is not readily visible intraoperatively—there is a danger of "bumping" into the retina if the surgeon is not mindful.

As opposed to the vastly more commonly employed intravitreal drug therapy, which is effective but requires multiple injections[90]—vitrectomy offers a good chance as a single-intervention success. In the authors' own series, 91% of eyes with diabetic macular edema maintained permanent dryness at 36 months postoperatively (unpublished data).

Proliferative Vitreoretinopathy and Proliferative Diabetic Retinopathy

There are similarities (newly-formed, collagen-rich, contractile membranes pulling the retina off) and differences (etiology; the condition of the retina—typically healthy in the former and moderately to dramatically fragile in the latter) between the two conditions;[34,91,92] but the surgical treatments for both have many similarities and are therefore discussed together in this chapter.

The goal is in principle the same—reattaching the retina by removing all of the traction-exerting forces, preferably without creating iatrogenic retinal breaks.[92] Table 58.12 provides an overview of the most important features of the surgery for both conditions.

Retinal Detachment

The surgeon must address both the underlying dynamic VR traction and the consequent retinal break to achieve permanent reattachment of the retina.[27,54,56,91,93] If scleral buckling is the chosen method, the surgeon must have assumed that the traction is only moderate and that there is no vitreous opacity (hemorrhage) to interfere with visualization.[27,91] The buckle can be limbus-parallel—either segmental or encircling or radial. In either case, it should be sufficiently high to counteract the traction (but not so high as to cause anterior segment ischemia). The buckle is placed so that the break rests either directly on top or just a bit peripheral to the crest of the indentation. If the detachment is very high (bullous), drainage is unavoidable

Table 58.12: Surgery for the two most important proliferative vitreoretinal diseases.

Variable	PDR	PVR
Condition of the retina	Damaged by the underlying diabetic disease and causing significant fragility	Mostly healthy, certainly much more resistant to surgical trauma than the retina in an eye with PDR
Presence of RD	Commonly	Almost always, but its extent is highly variable
Additional retinal pathology	Typically, macular edema	Typically, none
Contour of the detached retina	Concave; does not change shape with eye movement	
Presence of retinal breaks	Possible but not necessary	Usually; may be primary (causing the original RD) but also secondary (the traction forces tearing the retina apart; these breaks are usually characteristically oval in shape and fairly large)
The indication to operate	The progression may be very slow; if the macula is not threatened and the patient is satisfied with the current vision, close observation may be preferable	Untreated, the condition can very quickly involve the entire retina. Conversely, if a recurrence occurs and the eye contains silicone oil, it may be preferable to wait until the macula is threatened; the progression of the RD is much slower and may even be halted under oil. Another argument in favor of not operating early for a recurrent PVR-RD is to wait until the proliferation cycle ends (~3 months): removal of the already visible membranes will not prevent the development of those that are not yet visible or mature
Risk of intraoperative bleeding	Very high, due to the diabetes; giving an intravitreal Avastin injection 2–3 days preoperatively greatly reduces the risk	Not more than in most indications for VR surgery
Presence of vitreous hemorrhage preoperatively	Rather common	Extremely rare
Presence of PVD	Almost never; typically, a vitreoschisis is found, and the surgeon must make sure that both the obvious, visible anterior membrane (anterior wall of the vitreoschisis cavity), and the invisible, posterior cortical membrane (posterior wall), which is not only not detached but is extremely adherent to the ILM, are removed	Partial (incomplete)
Disk involvement in the proliferation	Typically yes. The surgeon should consider leaving the stump behind, after cauterizing it—if it is removed and there is a bleeding, this is difficult to stop (endodiathermy is no longer an option)	Never
Surgical technique	A truly complete vitreous removal is mandatory. The goal then is to separate the proliferative membrane/s from the retina and remove them until the traction forces are gone and the retina can be reattached without being stretched. Whether the surgeon chooses to progress in a centripetal or centrifugal direction is partially dependent on the individual situation but also on the surgeon's preference. The separation between retina and membranes can be delamination (separating the two tissues while keeping the proliferative membrane in a single sheet; typical in PVR surgery, less so in PDR cases) or segmentation (cutting the proliferative membrane 360° around areas of strong VR connections; typical in PDR surgery, uncommon in PVR cases). Again, the choice is up to the surgeon. Bimanual surgery has both advantages and disadvantages. The membranes can be "attacked" with the vitrectomy probe, especially if a small gauge-probe is used, but using scissors offers greater control over what happens—this, though, requires increased dexterity on the surgeon's part. In eyes with PDR, islands of proliferative tissue may be left behind, but they should be cauterized—just as should sites of retinal bleeding—to prevent a postoperative hemorrhage. In general, it is fair to say that scissors are much more commonly employed in PDR than in PVR surgery; in the latter, forceps play a much more significant role If subretinal membranes are present (quite common in both conditions), they may be left behind if they are not strong enough to cause RD, this is easily tested by a fluid-air exchange. If significant amounts of subretinal fluid are present, drainage is unavoidable, especially if oil is to be used. Should a retinal break already be present, this should be utilized for drainage; otherwise a retinotomy is required, preferably in the midperiphery superonasally. If a PVD cannot be created or if the membranes are inseparable from the retina, a retinectomy may be necessary so that the remaining central retina has a surface devoid of any tissue. The edge of the retina must then be lasered	

Contd...

Contd...

Variable	PDR	PVR
ILM removal	It should be seriously considered in both conditions, for different reasons. In eyes with PDR, the main reasons are to be absolutely certain no proliferative tissue (cortical vitreous) is left on the retinal surface and to fight the edema in eyes with PVR, removal of the macular ILM ensures that if reproliferation occurs, the central retina will be spared	
Intraoperative panretinal laser treatment	Almost always	No; the breaks are to be surrounded and a laser cerclage should also be carried out
Tamponade	The most reassuring is silicone oil. If the fill is truly 100%, this may prevent PVR by not allowing the postoperative accumulation of proliferative cells in the vitreous cavity, and it certainly prevents rapid detachment of the retina even if RD occurs. The oil also acts as a prophylactic weapon against postoperative bleeding. An argument can also be made against using oil in diabetic eyes with poor circulation, possibly making it worse	
Postoperative hemorrhage	Rather common, unless silicone oil has been implanted (which is, indeed, the only "guaranty" against it)	No
Recurrence rate	Usually very low; occasionally true PVR occurs, making the reoperation one of the toughest indications in VR surgery	Rather common, especially if trauma is the original etiology. The chance of success diminishes with each surgery

(PDR: Proliferative diabetic retinopathy; PVR: Proliferative vitreoretinopathy; RD: Retinal detachment; PVD: Posterior vitreous detachment; ILM: Internal limiting membrane)

since it is impossible to predict exactly where the break will settle. Laser or cryopexy needs to be performed as well. The "pexy" is aimed at creating a strong chorioretinal adhesion at the edge (not inside!) of the break. Although cryopexy does create a stronger bond, it is less preferred because of the increased risk of developing proliferative vitreoretinopathy (PVR).[20]

If the tractional component is very limited, the media are clear, the detachment is not too high, and the retinal breaks are superior and close together, pneumatic retinopexy[94] is another treatment option—cryopexy or laser, combined with an expanding gas bubble injected into the vitreous. The "pexy" may precede or follow the gas injection. The procedure has a lower success rate than either of the other two options discussed here, but its failure does not worsen the prognosis of the subsequent surgery.

Vitrectomy, unlike the other two options mentioned above, offers a viable treatment modality regardless of the condition of the media, the extent of the VR traction, the presence of subretinal proliferations, the location or number or size of the break/s, or the configuration of the detached retina. If PPV is the chosen option, the surgeon must ensure that all vitreous is removed—contrary to common belief, there is no PVD present in more than half of the eyes.[27] The VR traction can be eliminated and the subretinal fluid almost always drained through the existing break, which is much more likely to be identified during PPV than during the preoperative examination preceding either a buckling procedure or a pneumatic retinopexy; this is especially important in pseudophakic eyes with an opaque posterior capsule. Peeling of the ILM[11] should also be considered, especially if the macula has been detached; this reduces the risk of macular involvement should PVR subsequently develop. With the gel removed, the surgeon can also employ silicone oil, rather than gas, as a tamponade.

Trauma

If the trauma has caused endophthalmitis (which may be masked by other consequences of the injury, Fig. 58.8), immediate and complete vitrectomy is strongly indicated, combined with the full armamentarium of anti-infectious therapy. With today's technology, PPV carries a very low risk of complications. In fact, the patient's risk of losing vision due to traumatic endophthalmitis is much lower if PPV is performed early than if the surgery is delayed or not performed at all.[49,95]

Vitreous hemorrhage in an eye with open globe injury represents another indication for very early vitrectomy; the risk of PVR is very high, especially in young patients. Even if the trauma is a contusion (i.e. closed-globe injury), early vitrectomy to remove the blood is preferred to waiting for spontaneous clearance.

If an intraocular foreign body (IOFB) is present, it may be removed without PPV if there is no additional pathology. Otherwise, it is best to extract the IOFB as part of a complete vitrectomy.

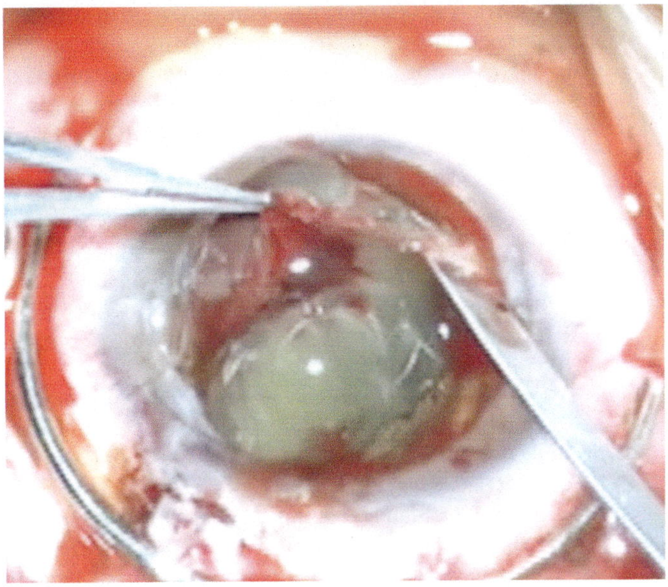

Fig. 58.8: *Temporary keratoprosthesis vitrectomy following severe open-globe trauma*: A Flieringa ring has been sutured to the sclera and the central corneal button removed. A disorganized mass is visible. A forceps and a spatula are shown here as tools in an attempt to identify what is present. Once it is determined that retinal prolapse has not occurred, the procedure will continue beyond the open-sky approach; the temporary keratoprosthesis will be placed, and a "funnel" will be created on the nasal side to identify the position (location) of the retina. The hemorrhagic intravitreal mass will be removed and the (posterior) retina reattached. Silicone oil will be implanted and a corneal graft placed.

If there is direct retinal injury (an impact site is identifiable) that also involves the choroid (IOFB injury with a deep impact; an exit wound in perforating trauma, or incarceration in case of a rupture), prophylactic chorioretinectomy[96,97] should be done to reduce the risk of PVR development.

The operation on an eye with severe trauma, especially if the patient is young and there is substantial vitreous hemorrhage, should always be done by a very experienced surgeon. It is difficult to distinguish between various structures such as a normal but dislocated tissue and abnormal tissues such as vitreous layers suffused by blood or newly-formed material such as fibrin (*see* Fig. 58.3). The bar for silicone oil use should be low[98] and the oil removal should not be hurried (keeping it in the eye for at 4-6 months to prevent PVR development).

Vitreous Opacities

There are several types of opacities; in addition to that which is part of the normal aging process (muscae volitantes), the surgeon often sees patients with synchysis scintillans.[42,99] In the latter, cholesterol crystals are found attached to the collagen fibers—even if, shockingly, many patients are not bothered by them, they may be so numerous as to block the view of the retina or prevent laser treatment.

Conversely, certain people are extremely bothered by even a few floaters—some of which are so small that the surgeon has difficulty visualizing them. The real question is not how to remove them—a simple vitrectomy is what needs to be done, but whether the ophthalmologist accepts that the eyeball is "owned by the patient", who has the right to decide whether he accepts the risk of surgery in order to have the unhealthy gel removed (see earlier in this chapter under counseling).

In summary, VR surgery is a relatively new subspecialty within ophthalmology, able to offer definite treatment in numerous conditions, many of which not very long ago would have led to blindness. The road that the ophthalmology resident needs to travel to become a competent VR surgeon is as difficult and long as it is intellectually rewarding.

REFERENCES

1. Forrester J. Anatomy of the eye and orbit. In: Forrester J (Ed). The Eye Basic Sciences in Practice, 1st edition. London: Elsevier; 1996; pp. 19-48.
2. Kasner D, Miller GR, Taylor WH, et al. Surgical treatment of amyloidosis of the vitreous. Trans Am Acad Ophthalmol Otolaryngol. 1968;72(3):410-8.
3. Machemer R, Buettner H, Norton EW, et al. Vitrectomy: a pars plana approach. Trans Am Acad Ophthalmol Otolaryngol. 1971;75(4):813-20.
4. Machemer R. The development of pars plana vitrectomy: a personal account. Graefes Arch Clin Exp Ophthalmol. 1995;233(8):453-68.
5. Machemer R, Buettner H, Parel JM. Vitrectomy, a pars plana approach. Instrumentation. Mod Probl Ophthalmol. 1972;10:172-7.
6. Tavolato M, Lo Giudice G, Cian R, et al. Outcomes of 195 consecutive patients undergoing 2-port pars plana vitrectomy with slit-lamp illumination system for posterior segment disease: a retrospective study. Retina. 2013;33(4):785-90.
7. O›Malley C, Heintz Sr RM. Vitrectomy with an alternative instrument system. Ann Ophthalmol. 1975;7(4):585-8, 591-4.
8. Machemer R. Pars plana vitrectomy. Removal of preretinal membranes. Trans Sec Ophthalmol Am Acad Ophthalmol Otolaryngol. 1976;81(3 Pt 1):420-5.
9. Machemer R. Retinotomy. Am J Ophthalmol. 1981;92(6): 768-74.
10. Odrobina D, Bednarski M, Cisiecki S, et al. Internal limiting membrane peeling as prophylaxis of macular pucker formation in eyes undergoing retinectomy for severe proliferative vitreoretinopathy. Retina. 2012;32(2):226-31.

11. Kuhn F. Internal limiting membrane removal for macular detachment in highly myopic eyes. Am J Ophthalmol. 2003;135(4):547-9.
12. Mester V, Kuhn F. Internal limiting membrane removal in the management of full-thickness macular holes. Am J Ophthalmol. 2000;129(6):769-77.
13. Ando F, Sasano K, Ohba N, et al. Anatomic and visual outcomes after indocyanine green-assisted peeling of the retinal internal limiting membrane in idiopathic macular hole surgery. Am J Ophthalmol. 2004;137(4):609-14.
14. Briggs M, Wong D, Groenewald C, et al. The effect of anaesthesia on the intraocular volume of the C3F8 gas bubble. Eye (Lond). 1997;11(Pt 1):47-52.
15. Casini G, Loiudice P, De Cilla S, et al. Sulfur hexafluoride (SF6) versus perfluoropropane (C3F8) tamponade and short term face-down position for macular hole repair: a randomized prospective study. Int J Retina Vitreous. 2016;2:10.
16. Momirov D, van Lith GH, Zivojnović R. Electroretinogram and electrooculogram of eyes with intravitreously injected silicone oil. Ophthalmologica. 1983;186(4):183-8.
17. Scott IU, Flynn HW, Lai M, et al. First operation anatomic success and other predictors of postoperative vision after complex retinal detachment repair with vitrectomy and silicone oil tamponade. Am J Ophthalmol. 2000;130(6): 745-50.
18. Scott JD. Fluorosilicone oil for retinal detachment. Br J Ophthalmol. 1990;74(11):641-2.
19. Lambert HM, Capone A, Aaberg TM, et al. Surgical excision of subfoveal neovascular membranes in age-related macular degeneration. Am J Ophthalmol. 1992;113(3):257-62.
20. Kuhn F. Vitreoretinal Surgery Strategy and Tactics, 1st edition. New York: Springer International Publishing; 2016. p. 95
21. Sebag J, Balazs EA. Morphology and ultrastructure of human vitreous fibers. Invest Ophthalmol Vis Sci. 1989;30(8): 1867-71.
22. Sebag J. Classifying posterior vitreous detachment: a new way to look at the invisible. Br J Ophthalmol. 1997;81(7):521.
23. Sebag J. Ageing of the vitreous. Eye (Lond). 1987;1(Pt 2): 254-62.
24. Sebag J. Vitreoschisis in diabetic macular edema. Invest Ophthalmol Vis Sci. 2011;52(11):8455-6.
25. Sebag J. Anatomy and pathology of the vitreo-retinal interface. Eye (Lond). 1992;6(Pt 6):541-52.
26. Hernandez F, Alpizar-Alvarez N, Wu L. Chromovitrectomy: an update. J Ophthalmic Vis Res. 2014;9(2):251-9.
27. Kuhn F, Aylward B. Rhegmatogenous retinal detachment: a reappraisal of its pathophysiology and treatment. Ophthalmic Res. 2014;51(1):15-31.
28. Williamson TH. Vitreoretinal Surgery, 1st edition. New York: Springer; 2008. p. 230.
29. Hageman GS, Marmor MF, Yao XY, et al. The interphotoreceptor matrix mediates primate retinal adhesion. Arch Ophthalmol. 1995;113(5):655-60.
30. de Oliveira PR, Berger AR, Chow DR. Vitreoretinal instruments: vitrectomy cutters, endoillumination and wide-angle viewing systems. Int J Retina Vitreous. 2016;2:28.
31. Burk SE, Da Mata AP, Snyder ME, et al. Indocyanine green-assisted peeling of the retinal internal limiting membrane. Ophthalmology. 2000;107(11):2010-4.
32. Luke M, Grisanti S, Luke J. International Chromovitrectomy C. The retinal biocompatibility of dyes in the ex vivo model of the isolated superfused vertebrate retina. Ophthalmologica. 2013;230 Suppl 2:21-6.
33. Scott IU, Flynn HW, Murray TG, et al. Outcomes of complex retinal detachment repair using 1000- vs 5000-centistoke silicone oil. Arch Ophthalmol. 2005;123(4):473-8.
34. Schwartz SG, Flynn HW Jr, Lee WH, et al. Tamponade in surgery for retinal detachment associated with proliferative vitreoretinopathy. Cochrane Database Syst Rev. 2014;(2):Cd006126.
35. Cheema RA, Mushtaq J, Al-Khars W, et al. Role of intravitreal bevacizumab (Avastin) injected at the end of diabetic vitrectomy in preventing postoperative recurrent vitreous hemorrhage. Retina. 2010;30(10):1646-50.
36. Mohr A, Bruinsma M, Oellerich S, et al. Dyes for eyes: hydrodynamics, biocompatibility and efficacy of ‹heavy› (dual) dyes for chromovitrectomy. Ophthalmologica. 2013;230 Suppl 2:51-8.
37. Nguyen JH, Yee KM, Sadun AA, et al. Quantifying visual dysfunction and the response to surgery in macular pucker. Ophthalmology. 2016;123(7):1500-10.
38. Machado LM, Furlani BA, Navarro RM, et al. Preoperative and intraoperative prognostic factors of epiretinal membranes using chromovitrectomy and internal limiting membrane peeling. Ophthalmic Surg Lasers Imaging Retina. 2015;46(4):457-62.
39. Martins TG, Martins TG, Rodriguez EE, et al. Vitreomacular traction syndrome. Einstein (Sao Paulo, Brazil). 2015;13(2):334-5.
40. Duker JS, Kaiser PK, Binder S, et al. The International Vitreomacular Traction Study Group classification of vitreomacular adhesion, traction, and macular hole. Ophthalmology. 2013;120(12):2611-9.
41. Henrich PB, Haritoglou C, Meyer P, et al. Anatomical and functional outcome in brilliant blue G assisted chromovitrectomy. Acta Ophthalmol. 2010;88(5):588-93.
42. Mamou J, Wa CA, Yee KM, et al. Ultrasound-based quantification of vitreous floaters correlates with contrast sensitivity and quality of life. Invest Ophthalmol Vis Sci. 2015;56(3):1611-7.
43. Sebag J. Imaging vitreous. Eye (Lond). 2002;16(4):429-39.
44. Gupta P, Yee KM, Garcia P, et al. Vitreoschisis in macular diseases. Br J Ophthalmol. 2011;95(3):376-80.
45. Sebag J. Anomalous posterior vitreous detachment: a unifying concept in vitreoretinal disease. Graefes Arch Clin Exp Ophthalmol. 2004;242(8):690-8.
46. Sebag J, Buzney SM, Belyea DA, et al. Posterior vitreous detachment following panretinal laser photocoagulation. Graefes Arch Clin Exp Ophthalmol. 1990;228(1):5-8.

47. Kuhn F, Gini G. Vitrectomy for endophthalmitis. Ophthalmology. 2006;113(4):714.
48. Adelman R, Parnes A, Michalewska Z, et al. Strategy for the management of diabetic macular edema: the European Vitreoretinal Society Macular Edema Study. Biomed Res Int. 2015;352-487.
49. Kuhn F. Ocular Traumatology, 1st edition. Heidelberg Germany: Spinger; 2008.
50. Durand ML. Bacterial and fungal endophthalmitis. Clin Microbiol Rev. 2017;30(3):597-613.
51. Results of the Endophthalmitis Vitrectomy Study. A randomized trial of immediate vitrectomy and of intravenous antibiotics for the treatment of postoperative bacterial endophthalmitis. Endophthalmitis Vitrectomy Study Group. Arch Ophthalmol. 1995;113(12):1479-96.
52. Kuhn F, Gini G. Ten years after... are findings of the Endophthalmitis Vitrectomy Study still relevant today? Graefes Arch Clin Exp Ophthalmol. 2005;243(12):1197-9.
53. Odouard C, Ong D, Shah PR, et al. Rising trends of endogenous Klebsiella pneumoniae endophthalmitis in Australia. Clin Exp Ophthalmol. 2017;45(2):135-42.
54. Tosi GM, Balestrazzi A, Baiocchi S, et al. Complex retinal detachment in phakic patients: Previtrectomy phacoemulsification versus combined phacovitrectomy. Retina. 2017;37(4):630-6.
55. Krishnan R, Tossounis C, Fung Yang Y. 20-gauge and 23-gauge phacovitrectomy for idiopathic macular holes: comparison of complications and long-term outcomes. Eye (Lond). 2013;27(1):72-7.
56. Smith M, Raman SV, Pappas G, et al. Phacovitrectomy for primary retinal detachment repair in presbyopes. Retina. 2007;27(4):462-7.
57. Ling R, Simcock P, McCoombes J, et al. Presbyopic phacovitrectomy. Br J Ophthalmol. 2003;87(11):1333-5.
58. Singh MS, Casswell EJ, Boukouvala S, et al. Pars plana vitrectomy and lensectomy for ectopia lentis with and without the induction of a posterior vitreous detachment. Retina. 2018;38(2):325-30. .
59. Zafar S, Kamil Z, Bokhari SA, et al. Visual outcome of pars plana vitrectomy for dropped nucleus after phacoemulsification. J Coll Physicians Surg Pak. 2012;22(6):367-70.
60. Koh KM, Kim HS, Cho HJ, et al. Surgical outcomes of 23-gauge vitrectomy for the management of lens fragments dropped into the vitreous cavity during cataract surgery. Saudi J Ophthalmol. 2014;28(4):253-6.
61. Modi YS, Epstein A, Smiddy WE, et al. Retained lens fragments after cataract surgery: outcomes of same-day versus later pars plana vitrectomy. Am J Ophthalmol. 2013;156(3):454-9.e1.
62. Vanner EA, Stewart MW. Vitrectomy timing for retained lens fragments after surgery for age-related cataracts: a systematic review and meta-analysis. Am J Ophthalmol. 2011;152(3):345-57.e3.
63. Colyer MH, Berinstein DM, Khan NJ, et al. Same-day versus delayed vitrectomy with lensectomy for the management of retained lens fragments. Retina. 2011;31(8):1534-40.
64. Stefaniotou M, Aspiotis M, Pappa C, et al. Timing of dislocated nuclear fragment management after cataract surgery. J Cataract Refract Surg. 2003;29(10):1985-8.
65. Schallenberg M, Dekowski D, Hahn A, et al. Aphakia correction with retropupillary fixated iris-claw lens (Artisan) - long-term results. Clin Ophthalmol. 2014;8:137-41.
66. Forlini M, Soliman W, Bratu A, et al. Long-term follow-up of retropupillary iris-claw intraocular lens implantation: a retrospective analysis. BMC Ophthalmol. 2015;15:143.
67. Gabor SG, Pavlidis MM. Sutureless intrascleral posterior chamber intraocular lens fixation. J Cataract Refract Surg. 2007;33(11):1851-4.
68. Sebag J, Gupta P, Rosen RR, et al. Macular holes and macular pucker: the role of vitreoschisis as imaged by optical coherence tomography/scanning laser ophthalmoscopy. Trans Am Ophthalmol Soc. 2007;105:121-9.
69. Krebs I, Brannath W, Glittenberg C, et al. Posterior vitreomacular adhesion: a potential risk factor for exudative age-related macular degeneration? Am J Ophthalmol. 2007;144(5):741-6.
70. Azuma K, Ueta T, Eguchi S, et al. Effects of internal limiting membrane peeling combined with removal of idiopathic epiretinal membrane: A Systematic Review of Literature and Meta-Analysis. Retina. 2017;37(10):1813-9.
71. Bottos JM, Elizalde J, Rodrigues EB, et al. Current concepts in vitreomacular traction syndrome. Curr Opin Ophthalmol. 2012;23(3):195-201.
72. Gottlieb JL, Antoszyk AN, Hatchell DL, et al. The safety of intravitreal hyaluronidase. A clinical and histologic study. Invest Ophthalmol Vis Sci. 1990;31(11):2345-52.
73. Chen W, Huang X, Ma XW, et al. Enzymatic vitreolysis with recombinant microplasminogen and tissue plasminogen activator. Eye (Lond). 2008;22(2):300-7.
74. Stalmans P, Delaey C, de Smet MD, et al. Intravitreal injection of microplasmin for treatment of vitreomacular adhesion: results of a prospective, randomized, sham-controlled phase II trial (the MIVI-IIT trial). Retina. 2010;30(7):1122-7.
75. Stalmans P, Duker JS, Kaiser PK, et al. OCT-based interpretation of the vitreomacular interface and indications for pharmacologic vitreolysis. Retina. 2013;33(10):2003-11.
76. Stevenson W, Prospero Ponce CM, Agarwal DR, et al. Epiretinal membrane: optical coherence tomography-based diagnosis and classification. Clin Ophthalmol. 2016;10:527-34.
77. Miguel AI, Legris A. Prognostic factors of epiretinal membranes: a systematic review. J Fr Ophtalmol. 2017; 40(1):61-79.
78. Schechet SA, DeVience E, Thompson JT. The effect of internal limiting membrane peeling on idiopathic epiretinal membrane surgery, with a review of the literature. Retina. 2017;37(5):873-80.
79. Liu H, Zuo S, Ding C, et al. Comparison of the effectiveness of pars plana vitrectomy with and without internal limiting

membrane peeling for idiopathic retinal membrane removal: a meta-analysis. J Ophthalmol. 2015;2015:974568.
80. Garcia-Fernandez M, Castro Navarro J, Gonzalez Castano C, et al. Epiretinal membrane surgery: anatomic and functional outcomes. Arch Soc Esp Oftalmol. 2013;88(4):139-44.
81. Wendel RT, Patel AC, Kelly NE, et al. Vitreous surgery for macular holes. Ophthalmology. 1993;100(11):1671-6.
82. Kelly NE, Wendel RT. Vitreous surgery for idiopathic macular holes. Results of a pilot study. Arch Ophthalmol. 1991;109(5):654-9.
83. Kuhn F, Morris R, Mester V, et al. Internal limiting membrane removal for traumatic macular holes. Ophthalmic Surg Lasers. 2001;32(4):308-15.
84. Madi HA, Masri I, Steel DH. Optimal management of idiopathic macular holes. Clin Ophthalmol. 2016;10:97-116.
85. Michalewska Z, Michalewski J, Adelman RA, et al. Inverted internal limiting membrane flap technique for large macular holes. Ophthalmology. 2010;117(10):2018-25.
86. Adelman RA, Parnes AJ, Bopp S, et al. Strategy for the management of macular edema in retinal vein occlusion: the European VitreoRetinal Society macular edema study. Biomed Res Int. 2015;2015:870987.
87. Shirakata Y, Fujita T, Nakano Y, et al. Pars plana vitrectomy combined with internal limiting membrane peeling to treat persistent macular edema after anti-vascular endothelial growth factor treatment in cases of ischemic central retinal vein occlusion. Case Rep Ophthalmol. 2016;7(1):1-8.
88. Shirakata Y, Fukuda K, Fujita T, et al. Pars plana vitrectomy combined with internal limiting membrane peeling for recurrent macular edema due to branch retinal vein occlusion after antivascular endothelial growth factor treatments. Clin Ophthalmol. 2016;10:277-83.
89. Jackson TL, Nicod E, Angelis A, et al. Pars plana vitrectomy for diabetic macular edema: A Systematic Review, Meta-Analysis, and Synthesis of Safety Literature. Retina. 2017;37(5):886-95.
90. Sivaprasad S, Oyetunde S. Impact of injection therapy on retinal patients with diabetic macular edema or retinal vein occlusion. Clin Ophthalmol. 2016;10:939-46.
91. Adelman RA, Parnes AJ, Sipperley JO, et al. Strategy for the management of complex retinal detachments: the European Vitreo-Retinal Society retinal detachment study report 2. Ophthalmology. 2013;120(9):1809-13.
92. Sternfeld A, Axer-Siegel R, Stiebel-Kalish H, et al. Advantages of diabetic tractional retinal detachment repair. Clin Ophthalmol. 2015;9:1989-94.
93. Scott IU, Flynn HW, Murray TG, et al. Outcomes of surgery for retinal detachment associated with proliferative vitreoretinopathy using perfluoro-n-octane: a multicenter study. Am J Ophthalmol. 2003;136(3):454-63.
94. Sebag J, Tang M. Pneumatic retinopexy using only air. Retina. 1993;13(1):8-12.
95. Kuhn F, Morris R, Witherspoon CD, et al. Epidemiology of blinding trauma in the United States Eye Injury Registry. Ophthalmic Epidemiol. 2006;13(3):209-16.
96. Ozdek S, Hasanreisoglu M, Yuksel E. Chorioretinectomy for perforating eye injuries. Eye (Lond). 2013;27(6):722-7.
97. Kuhn F, Teixeira S, Pelayes DE. Late versus prophylactic chorioretinectomy for the prevention of trauma-related proliferative vitreoretinopathy. Ophthalmic Res. 2012;48 Suppl 1:32-7.
98. Kuhn F, Mester V, Morris R. A proactive treatment approach for eyes with perforating injury. Klin Monbl Augenheilkd. 2004;221(8):622-8.
99. Ivanova T, Jalil A, Antoniou Y, et al. Vitrectomy for primary symptomatic vitreous opacities: an evidence-based review. Eye (Lond). 2016;30(5):645-55.

Peyman's
Principles and Practice of
OPHTHALMOLOGY

Peyman's Principles and Practice of OPHTHALMOLOGY

SECOND EDITION

VOLUME 2

Editor-in-Chief

N Venkatesh Prajna DNB FRCOphth
Academic Director
Aravind Eye Care System
Madurai, Tamil Nadu, India

Foreword

Morton F Goldberg

JAYPEE

JAYPEE BROTHERS MEDICAL PUBLISHERS
The Health Sciences Publisher
New Delhi | London | Panama

Jaypee Brothers Medical Publishers (P) Ltd.

Headquarters
Jaypee Brothers Medical Publishers (P) Ltd.
4838/24, Ansari Road, Daryaganj
New Delhi 110 002, India
Phone: +91-11-43574357
Fax: +91-11-43574314
Email: jaypee@jaypeebrothers.com

Overseas Offices

JP Medical Ltd.
83, Victoria Street, London
SW1H 0HW (UK)
Phone: +44 20 3170 8910
Fax: +44 (0)20 3008 6180
E-mail: info@jpmedpub.com

Jaypee-Highlights Medical Publishers Inc.
City of Knowledge, Bld. 235, 2nd Floor, Clayton
Panama City, Panama
Phone: +1 507-301-0496
Fax: +1 507-301-0499
E-mail: cservice@jphmedical.com

Jaypee Brothers Medical Publishers (P) Ltd.
Bhotahity, Kathmandu, Nepal
Phone: +977-9741283608
E-mail: kathmandu@jaypeebrothers.com

Website: www.jaypeebrothers.com
Website: www.jaypeedigital.com

Inquiries for bulk sales may be solicited at: jaypee@jaypeebrothers.com

Peyman's Principles and Practice of Ophthalmology (Vols 1 and 2)

First Edition: 1987
Second Edition: **2019**

ISBN: 978-93-5270-291-6

Printed at: Replika Press Pvt. Ltd.

Dedicated to

The Founders of the Aravind Eye Care System
for creating one of the largest, efficient, compassionate and equitable eye care delivery system of global standards.

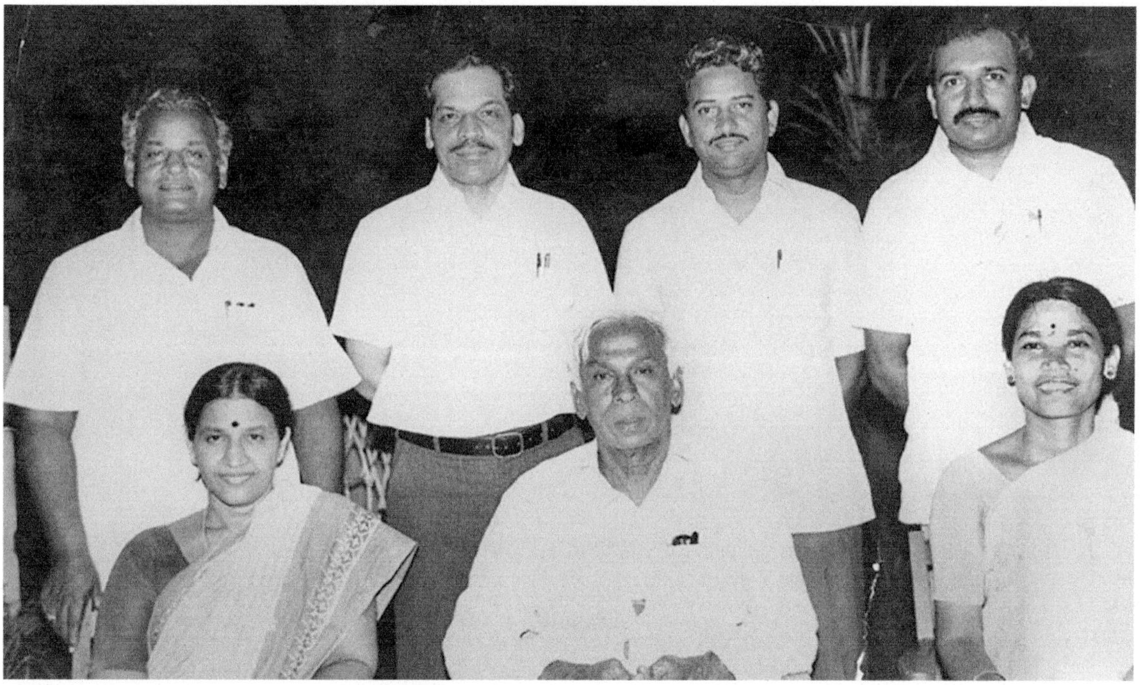

Standing from left to right
Mr G Srinivasan, Dr P Namperumalsamy, Dr M Srinivasan and Mr RD Thulasiraj

Sitting from left to right
Dr G Natchiar, Dr G Venkataswamy and Dr P Vijayalakshmi

Section Editors

Vision Rehabilitation

August Colenbrander MD PhD
Affiliate Senior Scientist
Smith-Kettlewell Eye Research Institute
San Francisco, USA

The Lens, Cataract and its Management

Uday Devgan MD FACS FRCS (Glasg)
Cataract and Refractive Surgeon
Devgan Eye Surgery, Los Angeles, California, USA
Partner, Speciality Surgical Center, Beverly Hills, California, USA
Chief of Ophthalmology, Olive View—UCLA Medical Center
Professor of Ophthalmology, Jules Stein Eye Institute
UCLA School of Medicine, Los Angeles, California, USA

Ocular Pathology

Deepak P Edward MD FACS FARVO
Professor (Ophthalmology and Pathology)
Department of Ophthalmology and Visual Sciences
University of Illinois Eye and Ear Infirmary
UIC College of Medicine
Chicago, Illinois, USA
King Khaled Eye Specialist Hospital
Riyadh, Kingdom of Saudi Arabia

Orbit and Oculoplasty

Shannon S Joseph MD
Assistant Professor
Department of Ophthalmology
Division of Oculoplastic Surgery
WK Kellogg Eye Center
University of Michigan
Ann Arbor, Michigan, USA

Optics and Rehabilitation

Joseph M Miller MD MPH
Professor of Ophthalmology
Optical Sciences and Public Health
University of Arizona College of Medicine
Tucson, Arizona, USA

Pediatric Ophthalmology and Strabismus

Michael O'Keeffe FRCS
Consultant Ophthalmic Surgeon
Mater Private Hospital and Beacon Hospital
Dublin, Ireland

Conjunctiva and Cornea

N Venkatesh Prajna DNB FRCOphth
Academic Director
Aravind Eye Care System
Madurai, Tamil Nadu, India

Glaucoma

Pradeep Ramulu MD PhD MHS
Professor of Ophthalmology (Glaucoma)
Wilmer Eye Institute
Johns Hopkins Hospital
Baltimore, Maryland, USA

Scleritis and Uveitis

SR Rathinam FAMS PhD
Professor of Ophthalmology and Head of Uveitis Service
Aravind Eye Hospital and Postgraduate Institute
of Ophthalmology
Madurai, Tamil Nadu, India

Retina and Vitreous

Srinivas R Sadda MD
President and Chief Scientific Officer
Doheny Eye Institute
Professor of Ophthalmology
University of California-Los Angeles
Los Angeles, California, USA

Neuro-ophthalmology

Prem S Subramanian MD PhD
Professor of Ophthalmology, Neurology and Neurosurgery
and Vice Chair for Academic Affairs
UC Health/Sue Anschutz-Rodgers Eye Center
Department of Ophthalmology
University of Colorado School of Medicine
Aurora, Colorado, USA

Contributors

Tushar Agarwal
Professor (Ophthalmology)
Dr Rajendra Prasad Centre for Ophthalmic Sciences
All India Institute of Medical Sciences (AIIMS)
New Delhi, India

Shweta Agarwal MD
Consultant
CJ Shah Cornea Services
Dr G Sitalakshmi Memorial Clinic for Ocular Surface Disorders
Sankara Nethralaya
Chennai, Tamil Nadu, India

Aniruddha Agarwal MS
Clinical Fellow in Vitreoretinal and Uveitis
Postgraduate Institute of Medical Education and Research (PGIMER)
Chandigarh, India

Kanika Aggarwal MS
Senior Research Associate
Postgraduate Institute of Medical Education and Research (PGIMER)
Chandigarh, India

Md Shahid Alam MS
Consultant Ophthalmologist
Orbit, Oculoplasty, Reconstructive and Aesthetic Services
Sankara Nethralaya
Kolkata, West Bengal, India

Mohammad Javed Ali FRCS PhD
Head
Govindram Seksaria Institute of Dacryology
LV Prasad Eye Institute (LVPEI)
Hyderabad, Telangana, India

A Yasin Alibhai MD
OCT Research Fellow
New England Eye Center
Tufts Medical Center
Boston, Massachusetts, USA

Hind Alkatan MD
Assistant Professor and Consultant
Director, Ophthalmology Training Programs
College of Medicine
Associate Director for External Accreditation Unit
Departments of Ophthalmology/ Pathology and Postgraduate Medical Education (PGME)
King Saud University-Medical City
Riyadh, Saudi Arabia

Eleftherios Anastasopoulos MD PhD
Consultant in Ophthalmology
2nd Department of Ophthalmology
Papageorgiou General Hospital
Aristotle University of Thessaloniki
Greece

Pamela Anketell PhD
Lead in Pediatric Orthoptics
Belfast Health and Social Care Trust (BHSCT)
Eye and Ear Clinic
Royal Victoria Hospital
Belfast, Ireland

Amreen Aslam MD
Senior Resident (Cornea)
Cataract and Refractive Surgery Services
Dr Rajendra Prasad Centre for Ophthalmic Sciences
All India Institute of Medical Sciences (AIIMS)
New Delhi, India

Ariana Austin MS
Study Coordinator
Francis I Proctor Foundation
University of California
San Francisco, California, USA

James T Banta MD
Bascom Palmer Eye Institute
Miami, Florida, USA

John Bartlett MD
Assistant Clinical Professor (Ophthalmology)
Jules Stein Eye Institute
UCLA School of Medicine
Los Angeles, California, USA

Rodanthi Christina Bartzoulianou MD
1st Department of Ophthalmology
AHEPA Hospital
Aristotle University of Thessaloniki
Greece

M Tariq Bhatti MD
Professor
Departments of Ophthalmology Neurology and Neurosurgery
Duke Eye Center
Duke University Hospital
Durham, North Carolina, USA

Ferdinando Bottoni MD FEBO
Department of Biomedical and Clinical Science "Luigi Sacco"
Luigi Sacco Hospital, University of Milan
Milan, Italy

Marc A Bouffard MD
Instructor
Department of Neurology
Beth Israel Deaconess Medical Center
Boston, Massachusetts, USA

Richard Bowman MA MD FRCOphth
Consultant Ophthalmologist
Great Ormond Street Hospital
London, UK

Anthony Brune
Clinical Lecturer
Department of Ophthalmology and Visual Sciences
University of Michigan
Ann Arbor, Michigan, USA

Matthew J Burton PhD FRCOphth
Professor
International Eye Health
London School of Hygiene and Tropical Medicine
London, UK

Stathopoulos C MD
Ocular Oncology, Pathology and Genetics
Jules-Gonin Eye Hospital
Switzerland

Benjamin C Campbell MD
Resident (Physician Ophthalmology)
Jules Stein Eye Institute
UCLA School of Medicine
Los Angeles, California, USA

Jayne E Camuglia MBBS BSc FRANZCO
Visiting Medical Officer
Department of Ophthalmology
Children's Health Queensland
South Brisbane, Queensland, Australia

Dean Cestari MD
Associate Professor of Ophthalmology, Neuro-ophthalmology and Adult Strabismus
Harvard Medical School
Boston, Massachusetts, USA
Director, Adult Strabismus Service
Director, Ophthalmology Fellowship Education
Co-Director, Center for Thyroid Eye Disease and Orbital Surgery

Tiffany Chan OD
Associate
Drs Chan, Moon and Associates
Family Vision Care
Clinical Faculty
Frank Stein and Paul S May Center for Low Vision Rehabilitation
Department of Ophthalmology
California Pacific Medical Center
San Francisco, California, USA

Jessica R Chang MD
Assistant Professor of Ophthalmology
University of Southern California
Roski Eye Institute
Keck School of Medicine of USC
Los Angeles, California, USA

Ta Chen Peter Chang MD
Associate Professor of Clinical Ophthalmology and Pediatrics
Bascom Palmer Eye Institute
University of Miami
Miller School of Medicine
Miami, Florida, USA

Yanjun Chen MD PhD
Assistant Professor
Department of Ophthalmology and Visual Sciences
University of Wisconsin School of Medicine and Public Health
Madison, Wisconsin, USA

Emily Chew MD
Deputy Director
Division of Epidemiology and Clinical Research at NIH
Washington DC Metro Area Research NIH

Catherine J Choi MD MS
Department of Ophthalmology
University of Miami, Miller School of Medicine
Miami, Florida, USA

Natalie N Chung MD
Research Scholar (Ophthalmology)
Shiley Eye Institute
University of California
San Diego, California, USA

August Colenbrander MD PhD
Affiliate Senior Scientist
Smith-Kettlewell Eye Research Institute
San Francisco, USA

Federico Corvi MD
Resident (Ophthalmology)
Eye Clinic
Department of Biomedical and Clinical Science "Luigi Sacco"
Luigi Sacco Hospital, University of Milan
Milan, Italy

Roberta Dalley MD
Associate Professor
Department of Radiology
University of Washington
Seattle, Washington, USA

Kunal K Dansingani MA FRCOphth
Associate Professor (Ophthalmology)
Department of Ophthalmology
University of Pittsburgh Medical Center
Pittsburgh, Pennsylvania, USA

Manoranjan Das DNB
Professor
Department of Cornea and Refractive Surgery
Aravind Eye Hospital
Madurai, Tamil Nadu, India

Shilpa Das MBBS MS
Cornea Consultant
Cornea and Cataract Services
Nethradhama Superspecialty Eye Hospital
Bengaluru, Karnataka, India
Fellow-Cornea/Anterior Segment
LV Prasad Eye Institute (LVPEI)
Hyderabad, Telangana, India

Janet L Davis MD
Leach Distinguished Professor of Ophthalmology
Bascom Palmer Eye Institute
University of Miami, Miller School of Medicine
Miami, Florida, USA

Hakan Demirci MD
Associate Professor
Richard N and Marilyn K Witham Professor
WK Kellogg Eye Center
University of Michigan
Ann Arbor, Michigan, USA

Uday Devgan MD FACS FRCS (Glasg)
Cataract and Refractive Surgeon
Devgan Eye Surgery, Los Angeles
California, USA
Partner, Speciality Surgical Center
Beverly Hills, California, USA
Chief of Ophthalmology
Olive View—UCLA Medical Center
Professor of Ophthalmology
Jules Stein Eye Institute
UCLA School of Medicine, Los Angeles
California, USA

K Dharmalingam MSc PhD
Director (Research)
Aravind Medical Research Foundation
Madurai, Tamil Nadu, India

Stephanie Ding BA
Orbital Oncology and Ophthalmic Plastic Surgery
Department of Plastic Surgery
The University of Texas
MD Anderson Cancer Center
Houston, Texas, USA

Raymond S Douglas MD PhD
Department of Surgery
Cedars-Sinai Medical Center
Los Angeles, California, USA

Todd Driver MD
PGY-4, UCLA Stein Eye Institute
University of California, San Francisco
San Francisco, California, USA

Vikram Durairaj MD
Oculoplastic Surgeon
TOC Eye and Face
Austin, Texas, USA

Deepak P Edward MD FACS FARVO
Professor
(Ophthalmology and Pathology)
Department of Ophthalmology and Visual Sciences
University of Illinois Eye and Ear Infirmary
UIC College of Medicine
Chicago, Illinois, USA
King Khaled Eye Specialist Hospital
Riyadh, Kingdom of Saudi Arabia

Dean Eliott MD
Stelios Evangelos Gragoudas Associate Professor
Department of Ophthalmology
Harvard Medical School
Associate Director
Retina Service
Massachusetts Eye and Ear
Boston, Massachusetts, USA

Zachary P Elkin MD MPH
Assistant Professor of Ophthalmology
New York University Langone Eye Center
New York, USA

Monica Ertel MD PhD
Resident
Department of Ophthalmology
Weil Cornell Medical College
New York, USA

Bita Esmaeli MD
Orbital Oncology and Ophthalmic Plastic Surgery
Department of Plastic Surgery
The University of Texas
MD Anderson Cancer Center
Houston, Texas, USA

Juliet Essilfie MD
Ophthalmology
Jules Stein Eye Institute
UCLA School of Medicine
Los Angeles, California, USA

Nina M Farivari MD
Ophthalmology Resident, PGY-4
Vanderbilt University Medical Center
Nashville, Tennessee, USA

Katrin Fasler MD
Honorary Fellow
Moorfields Eye Clinic
London, UK

Munier FL MD
Professor
Head of Ocular Oncology, Pathology and Genetics
Jules-Gonin Eye Hospital
Switzerland

Monika Fleckenstein MD
Consultant
Department of Ophthalmology
University of Bonn
Bonn, Germany

David Fleischman MD MS FACS
Assistant Professor
Department of Ophthalmology
University of North Carolina
Chapel Hill, North Carolina, USA

Donald C Fletcher MD
Envision Center for Low Vision Rehabilitation
Wichita, Kansas, USA

Allen Foster
MB ChB (Hons) FRCS FRCOphth FHEA
Professor of International Eye Health
International Centre of Eye Health
London School of Hygiene and Tropical Medicine
London, UK

Courtney Francis MD
Associate Professor
Department of Ophthalmology
University of Washington
Seattle, Washington, USA

Suzanne K Freitag MD
Director
Ophthalmic Plastic Surgery
Massachusetts Eye and Ear Infirmary
Harvard Medical School
Boston, Massachusetts, USA

K Bailey Freund MD
Clinical Professor
Department of Ophthalmology
The New York University School of Medicine
Vitreous Retina Macula Consultants
New York, USA

Scott J Fudemberg MD
Assistant Professor
Wills Eye Hospital
Philadelphia, Pennsylvania, USA

James G Fujimoto PhD
Elihu Thomson Professor of Electrical Engineering
Department of Electrical Engineering and Computer Science
Massachusetts Institute of Technology
Cambridge, Massachusetts, USA

Orly Gal-Or MD
Medical Retina Consultant
Department of Ophthalmology
Rabin Medical Center
Petah-Tikva, Israel

Elisha Garg MD
Resident (Ophthalmology)
Jules Stein Eye Institute
UCLA School of Medicine
Los Angeles, California, USA

Prashant Garg MS (Ophthalmology)
Consultant
Cornea and Anterior Segment Services
Tej Kohli Cornea Service, KAR Campus
LV Prasad Eye Institute (LVPEI)
Hyderabad, Telangana, India

Alain Gaudric MD
Emeritus Professor
Department of Ophthalmology
Lariboisière Hospital
University of Paris 7-Denis Diderot
Paris, France

Andrea Giani MD
Assistant Professor
Eye Clinic
Department of Biomedical and Clinical Science "Luigi Sacco"
Luigi Sacco Hospital, University of Milan
Milan, Italy

Dimitrios Giannoulis MD MSc
1st Department of Ophthalmology
AHEPA Hospital
Aristotle University of Thessaloniki
Greece

Kimberly K Gokoffski MD PhD
Assistant Professor
University of Southern California
Roski Eye Institute
Los Angeles, California, USA

Daniel Gold DO
Assistant Professor of Neurology
Division of Neuro-Visual and Vestibular Disorders
Ophthalmology, Neurosurgery, Otolaryngology—Head and Neck Surgery
Emergency Medicine
Director, Vestibular and Ocular Motor Oto-Neurology Fellowship
Director, Urgent Neurology
The Johns Hopkins Hospital
Baltimore, Maryland, USA

Glen A Gole
MBBS MD (NSW) FRANZCO FRACS FRCOphth
Professor/Director of Ophthalmology
Department of Ophthalmology
Lady Cilento Children's Hospital (LCCH)
South Brisbane, Queensland, Australia

John A Gonzales MD
Associate Professor
Francis I Proctor Foundation
University of California
San Francisco, California, USA

Rameshkumar Gunasekaran MSc
Microbiologist
Department of Ocular Microbiology
Aravind Eye Hospital
Madurai, Tamil Nadu, India

Noopur Gupta MS (Ophthalmology) PhD
Assistant Professor (Cornea, Cataract and Refractive Surgery Services)
Dr Rajendra Prasad Centre for Ophthalmic Sciences
All India Institute of Medical Sciences (AIIMS)
New Delhi, India

Vishali Gupta MS
Professor
Postgraduate Institute of Medical Education and Research (PGIMER)
Chandigarh, India

Samer Hamada
MD MSc DO (Hons) FRCSEd FRCOphth
Consultant Ophthalmic Surgeon (Adults and Children)
Corneoplastic Unit and Eye Bank
Queen Victoria Hospital NHS Trust
East Grinstead, Sussex, UK

D Rex Hamilton MD MS
Ophthalmology
Jules Stein Eye Institute
UCLA School of Medicine
Los Angeles, California, USA

B Hansen MD
Ophthalmology
UT Southwestern Medical Center
Dallas, Texas, USA

Manali Hazarika MBBS MS (Ophthalmology)
Fellow
Department of Cornea and Anterior Segment Services
Aravind Eye Hospital
Madurai, Tamil Nadu, India

Paul R Healey
BMedSc MBBS (Hons) MMed PhD FRANZCO
Clinical Associate Professor
Sydney Medical School
University of Sydney
Sydney, NSW, Australia

Martina C Herwig-Carl MD
Consultant
Department of Ophthalmology
University Clinic Bonn
Bonn, NRW, Germany

Jeremy JSL Hoffman FRCOphth
Clinical Research Fellow
London School of Hygiene and Tropical Medicine
London, UK

Frank G Holz MD
Chairman and Professor
Department of Ophthalmology
University of Bonn
Bonn, Germany

Jean Pierre Hubschman MD
Ophthalmology
Jules Stein Eye Institute
UCLA School of Medicine
Los Angeles, California, USA

Sarah Hull MBBS MA FRCOphth PhD
Specialist Registrar
Moorfields Eye Hospital NHS Foundation Trust
Honorary Research Associate
UCL Institute of Ophthalmology
London, UK

Alessandro Invernizzi MD
Assistant Professor
Eye Clinic
Department of Biomedical and Clinical Science "Luigi Sacco"
Luigi Sacco Hospital, University of Milan
Milan, Italy

Peter Charbel Issa MD DPhil
Oxford Eye Hospital and Nuffield Laboratory of Ophthalmology
Department of Clinical Neurosciences
University of Oxford
Oxford, UK

Sabita M Ittoop MD MS
Inova Fair Oaks Hospital
Herndon, Virginia, USA

Geetha Iyer MD FRCS
Senior Consultant
CJ Shah Cornea Services
Dr G Sitalakshmi Memorial Clinic for Ocular Surface Disorders
Sankara Nethralaya
Chennai, Tamil Nadu, India

Cunha-Vaz J MD PhD
Association for Innovation and Biomedical Research on Light and Image (AIBILI)
Faculty of Medicine
University of Coimbra (FMUC)
Coimbra, Portugal

Divya Janakiraman
MBBS MD (Ophthalmology)
Clinical Fellow
Department of Cornea and Anterior Segment Services
Aravind Eye Hospital
Madurai, Tamil Nadu, India

Pimkwan Jaru-ampornpan MD
Clinical Instructor
Department of Ophthalmology
Faculty of Medicine
Siriraj Hospital
Mahidol University
Bangkok, Thailand

Bennie H Jeng MD
Professor and Chair
Department of Ophthalmology and Visual Sciences
University of Maryland School of Medicine
Baltimore, Maryland, USA

Imran Jivraj MD
Neuro-ophthalmologist
Department of Ophthalmology
University of Alberta
Edmonton, Alberta, USA

Chris A Johnson PhD DSc
Professor
Department of Ophthalmology and Visual Sciences
University of Iowa Hospitals and Clinics
Iowa City, Iowa, USA

Michael Jordan MD MS
University of Minnesota
Department of Ophthalmology and Visual Sciences
Minneapolis, Minnesota, USA

Shannon S Joseph MD
Assistant Professor
Department of Ophthalmology
Division of Oculoplastic Surgery
WK Kellogg Eye Center
University of Michigan
Ann Arbor, Michigan, USA

Marques JP MD MSc FEBO
Association for Innovation and Biomedical Research on Light and Image (AIBILI)
Faculty of Medicine
University of Coimbra (FMUC)
Coimbra, Portugal

Albert S Jun MD PhD
Wilmer Eye Institute
Johns Hopkins Medical Institutions
Baltimore, Maryland, USA

Malik Y Kahook MD
Professor
Department of Ophthalmology
University of Colorado School of Medicine
Aurora, Colorado, USA

Paavan Kalra MS (Ophthalmology)
Consultant
Cornea and Anterior Segment Services
Tej Kohli Cornea Service, KAR Campus
LV Prasad Eye Institute (LVPEI)
Hyderabad, Telangana, India

Thomas J Kandl MD
Orbital Oncology and Ophthalmic Plastic Surgery
Department of Plastic Surgery
The University of Texas
MD Anderson Cancer Center
Houston, Texas, USA

L Jay Katz MD
Professor
Department of Ophthalmology
Wills Eye Hospital
Thomas Jefferson University
Philadelphia, Pennsylvania, USA

Srinivasan Kavitha MD PhD MS
Consultant
Glaucoma Services
Aravind Eye Hospital and Postgraduate Institute of Ophthalmology
Puducherry, India

Aki Kawasaki MD PhD
Professor
Hôpital Ophtalmique
University of Lausanne
Lausanne, Switzerland

Pearse A Keane MD
Consultant Ophthalmologist
Moorfields Eye Hospital
NIHR Clinician Scientist
University College London
Institute of Ophthalmology
London, UK

Jeremy Keenan MD MPH
Professor of Ophthalmology
Francis I Proctor Foundation and
Department of Ophthalmology
San Francisco, California, USA

Tiarnan Kennan MD PhD
Staff Clinician
Division of Epidemiology and Clinical Applications
National Eye Institute
National Institutes of Health
Bethesda, Maryland, USA

Christina Keskini MD MSc
Laboratory of Research and Clinical Applications in Ophthalmology (LaRCAO)
1st Department of Ophthalmology
AHEPA Hospital
Aristotle University of Thessaloniki
Greece

Peng Tee Khaw PhD FRCS FRCP FRCOphth FRCPath FRSB FCOptom Hon DSc FARVO FMedSci
Director
NIHR Biomedical Research Centre
Moorfields Eye Hospital and UCL
Institute of Ophthalmology
Research and Development
Eyes and Vision Programme
UCL Partners Academic Health Science Centre
Emeritus NIHR Senior Investigator

Kay T Khine MD
Voluntary Assistant Professor
Bascom Palmer Eye Institute
University of Miami
Miami, Florida, USA

Don O Kikkawa MD FACS
Professor of Ophthalmology and Plastic Surgery
Chief, Division of Oculofacial Plastic Surgery and Vice Chairman
UC San Diego Department of Ophthalmology
Shiley Eye Institute
La Jolla, California, USA

Caitriona Kirwan FRCS
Consultant Ophthalmic Surgeon and Pediatric Ophthalmologist
Mater Private Hospital
Dublin, Ireland

Natasha Nayak Kolomeyer MD
Clinical Instructor
Wills Eye Hospital
Philadelphia, Pennsylvania, USA

Bobby S Korn MD PhD
Professor of Ophthalmology and Plastic Surgery
Department of Ophthalmology
UC San Diego School of Medicine
Shiley Eye Institute
La Jolla, California, USA

Agnieszka Kudasiewicz-Kardaszewska MD PhD
Ophthalmology Consultant and Surgeon
Zagorski Eye Surgery Centers
Nałęczów, Poland

Ferenc Kuhn MD PhD
President
International Society of Ocular Trauma
Associate Professor of Ophthalmology
University of Alabama, Birmingham, UK
Vice President for Clinical Research
Helen Keller Foundation for Research and Education
Consultant and Chief
Vitreoretinal Surgeon
Milos Eye Clinic
Belgrade, Serbia
Consultant and Vitreoretinal Surgeon
Zagorski Eye Surgery Center
Nałęczów, Poland

Ashish Kumar DNB
Consultant
Department of Cornea and Refractive Surgery
Aravind Eye Hospital
Madurai, Tamil Nadu, India

Nathan Kung MD
Neuro-ophthalmologist
Blue Sky Neurology
Denver, Colorado, USA

Pallak Kusumgar MS FAICO
Cornea, Refractive Surgeon
Narayana Nethralaya
Bengaluru, Karnataka, India

Jocelyn Lam MD
Department of Ophthalmology
University of Washington
Seattle, Washington, USA

Scott R Lambert MD
Professor of Ophthalmology and Pediatrics
Department of Ophthalmology
Stanford University School of Medicine
Chief of Pediatric Ophthalmology
Lucile Packard Children's Hospital
Palo Alto, California, USA

Suzanne W van Landingham MD
University of Wisconsin
Department of Ophthalmology and Vision Sciences
Madison, Wisconsin, USA

Michael S Lee MD
Department of Ophthalmology and Visual Neurosciences
University of Minnesota
Minneapolis, Minnesota, USA

Gary J Lelli MD
Vice Chair and Associate Professor of Ophthalmology
Director of Ophthalmic Plastic and Reconstructive Surgery
Department of Ophthalmology
Weil Cornell Medical College
New York, USA

S Fabian Lerner MD
Professor of Ophthalmology
University Favaloro
School of Medical Sciences
Buenos Aires, Argentina

Vaitheeswaran LG MBBS MD FICO
Cataract, Cornea and Refractive Surgeon
Narayana Nethralaya
Bengaluru, Karnataka, India

Edward P Lin MD MBA
Assistant Professor
Department of Imaging Sciences
University of Rochester Medical Center
Rochester, New York, USA

Shawn R Lin MD MS MBA
UCLA Jules Stein Eye Institute
UCLA School of Medicine
Los Angeles, California, USA

Katy C Liu MD PhD
Clinical Associate (Ophthalmology)
Duke Eye Center
Duke University Hospital
Durham, North Carolina, USA

James Liu MD
Resident in Ophthalmology
Department of Ophthalmology and Visual Sciences
Washington University
St Louis School of Medicine
St Louis, Missouri, USA

Karin U Loeffler MD
Consultant
Department of Ophthalmology
University Clinic Bonn
Bonn, NRW, Germany

Eibhlín Mc Loone MB BCh BAO FRCOphth
Consultant Pediatric Ophthalmologist
Belfast Health and Social Care Trust (BHSCT)
Eye and Ear Clinic
Royal Victoria Hospital
Belfast, Ireland

Mark J Lucarelli MD FACS
Dortzbach Professor of Ophthalmic Facial Plastic Surgery
Director, Oculoplastic, Facial Cosmetic and Orbital Surgery
University of Wisconsin-Madison
Madison, Wisconsin, USA

Rajeswari Mahadevan PhD
Head of Contact Lens Clinic
Assistant Professor
Elite School of Optometry
Sankara Nethralaya
Chennai, Tamil Nadu, India

Prafulla K Maharana MD DNB
Assistant Professor (Ophthalmology)
Dr Rajendra Prasad Centre for Ophthalmic Sciences
All India Institute of Medical Sciences (AIIMS)
New Delhi, India

Nicholas R Mahoney MD
Wilmer Eye Institute
Johns Hopkins University School of Medicine
Baltimore, Maryland, USA

Siddharth Malaiya MBBS MS
Comprehensive Clinical Fellow
LV Prasad Eye Institute (LVPEI)
KAR Campus
Hyderabad, Telangana, India

Sundas Maqsood MBBS
Consultant Ophthalmic Surgeon (Adults and Children)
Corneoplastic Unit and Eye Bank
Queen Victoria Hospital NHS Trust
East Grinstead, Sussex, UK

Ian Marsh
MD PhD MB ChB FRCS (Ed) FRCOphth
Consultant Ophthalmologist
Department of Ophthalmology
Aintree University Hospitals NHS Foundation Trust
Liverpool, UK

Louise A Mawn MD
Professor of Ophthalmology and Neurological Surgery
Vanderbilt Medical Centre
Nashville, Tennessee, USA

Tara A McCannel MD PhD
Ophthalmic Oncology Center
Stein Eye and Doheny Eye Institutes
Department of Ophthalmology
University of California
Los Angeles, California, USA

Collin M McClelland MD
Associate Professor
Department of Ophthalmology and Visual Neurosciences
University of Minnesota
Minneapolis, Minnesota, USA

John McSoley OD
Bascom Palmer Eye Institute
Miami, Florida, USA

Joseph M Miller MD MPH
Professor of Ophthalmology
Optical Sciences and Public Health
University of Arizona College of Medicine
Tucson, Arizona, USA

Kevin M Miller MD
Professor of Clinical Ophthalmology
Jules Stein Eye Institute
UCLA School of Medicine
Los Angeles, California, USA
Kolokotrones Chair in Ophthalmology
Chief, Cataract and Refractive Surgery Division
Director, Anterior Segment Diagnostic Laboratory

Anthony T Moore
MA FRCS FRCOphth FMedSci
Michael Vilensky Endowed Chair in Ophthalmology
The University of California, San Francisco (UCSF) School of Medicine
Koret Vision Center
San Francisco, California, USA

VV Mootha MD
Ophthalmology
UT Southwestern Medical Center
Dallas, Texas, USA

Eric M Moult BSc
Research Assistant
Department of Electrical Engineering and Computer Science
Massachusetts Institute of Technology
Cambridge, Massachusetts, USA

Bipasha Mukherjee MS DNB
Consultant Ophthalmologist
Orbit, Oculoplasty, Reconstructive and Aesthetic Services
Sankara Nethralaya
Medical Research Foundation
Chennai, Tamil Nadu, India

Harsha Nagaraja MBBS MS
Consultant Ophthalmolgist
Cornea and External Eye Diseases
Narayana Nethralaya
Bengaluru, Karnataka, India

Paolo Nucci PROF
Director
Department of Ophthalmology
San Giuseppe Hospital
University of Milan
Milan, Italy

Michael O'Keeffe FRCS
Consultant Ophthalmic Surgeon
Mater Private Hospital and Beacon Hospital
Dublin, Ireland

Patrick Oellers MD
Thomas J Madden Fellow in Vitreoretinal Surgery
Massachusetts Eye and Ear
Harvard Medical School
Boston, Massachusetts, USA

Hilal Eser Ozturk MD
Assistant Professor (Ophthalmology)
Faculty of Medicine
Ondokuz Mayis University
Samsun, Turkey

Srikanta Kumar Padhy MD
Resident (Ophthalmology)
Dr Rajendra Prasad Centre for Ophthalmic Sciences
All India Institute of Medical Sciences (AIIMS)
New Delhi, India

Prema Padmanabhan MD
Head
Department of Cornea Services and Refractive Surgery
Medical Research Foundation
Chennai, Tamil Nadu, India

Arun Kumar Panigrahi MS
Consultant
Department of Cornea and Refractive Surgery
Aravind Eye Hospital
Madurai, Tamil Nadu, India

Maria Papadopoulos MB BS FRACO
Consultant Ophthalmic Surgeon
Glaucoma Service
Moorfields Eye Hospital NHS Foundation Trust
London, UK

Vivek R Patel MD
Associate Professor
University of Southern California
Roski Eye Institute
Los Angeles, California, USA

Marco Pellegrini MD
Eye Clinic
Department of Biomedical and Clinical Science "Luigi Sacco"
Luigi Sacco Hospital, University of Milan
Milan, Italy

Mark E Pennesi MD PhD
Associate Professor (Ophthalmology)
Casey Eye Institute
Oregon Health and Science University
Portland, Oregon, USA

Monica S Perlmutter OTD OTR/L SCLV FAOTA
Associate Professor
Occupational Therapy and Ophthalmology
Lead OT (Low Vision in Home and Community Services)
Washington University Program in Occupational Therapy
St Louis, Missouri, USA

Chee Soon Phaik MBBS FRCS(G) MMed(Ophth) FRCS(Ed) FRCOphth
Head of Department and Senior Consultant
Cataract Subspecialty Service and Ocular Inflammation and Immunology Service
Singapore National Eye Centre
Singapore

Elise Philippakis MD
Consultant
Department of Ophthalmology
Lariboisière Hospital
University of Paris 7-Denis Diderot
Paris, France

Cameron Pole MD
Jules Stein Eye Institute
UCLA School of Medicine
Los Angeles, California, USA

Zia S Pradhan DNB FRCOphth
Consultant
Glaucoma Services
Narayana Nethralaya
Bengaluru, Karnataka, India

N Venkatesh Prajna DNB FRCOphth
Academic Director
Aravind Eye Care System
Madurai, Tamil Nadu, India

Lalitha Prajna MD (Microbiology)
Chief Microbiologist
Department of Ocular Microbiology
Aravind Eye Hospital and Postgraduate Institute of Ophthalmology
Madurai, Tamil Nadu, India

Narendra K Puttaiah DNB
Consultant
Glaucoma Services
Narayana Nethralaya
Bengaluru, Karnataka, India

Naveen Radhakrishnan MS FICO
Consultant
Department of Cornea and Refractive Surgery
Aravind Eye Care System
Madurai, Tamil Nadu, India

Pradeep Ramulu MD PhD MHS
Professor of Ophthalmology (Glaucoma)
Wilmer Eye Institute
Johns Hopkins Hospital
Baltimore, Maryland, USA

Harsha L Rao MD DNB PhD
Consultant
Glaucoma Services
Narayana Nethralaya
Bengaluru, Karnataka, India

SR Rathinam FAMS PhD
Professor of Ophthalmology and Head of Uveitis Service
Aravind Eye Hospital and Postgraduate Institute of Ophthalmology
Madurai, Tamil Nadu, India

Thulasiraj Ravilla MBA
Executive Director
Lions Aravind Institute of Community Ophthalmology (LAICO)
Madurai, Tamil Nadu, India

Sathya T Ravilla MS (Ophthalmology)
Consultant
Pediatric Ophthalmology and Strabismus Clinic
Aravind Eye Hospital
Madurai, Tamil Nadu, India

Hasika Ravula MS FICO
Cornea and Refractive Surgeon
Department of Cornea
Nayana Eye Care
Kakinada, Andhra Pradesh, India

Michael X Repka MD MBA
David L Guyton, MD, and Feduniak Family
Professor of Ophthalmology
Wilmer Eye Institute
Johns Hopkins University School of Medicine
Baltimore, Maryland, USA

Rajaraman Revathi MS
Professor
Department of Cornea and Refractive Surgery Services
Aravind Eye Hospital
Coimbatore, Tamil Nadu, India

Alan L Robin MD
Professor
Department of Ophthalmology and Visual Sciences
University of Michigan
Ann Arbor, Michigan, USA

V Romano MD
Consultant Ophthalmic Surgeon
Royal Liverpool University Hospital
Liverpool, UK

James T Rosenbaum MD
Professor of Ophthalmology, Medicine and Cell Biology
Edward E Rosenbaum Professor of Inflammation Research
Oregon Health and Science University
Portland, Oregon, USA

Jennifer Rose-Nussbaumer MD (Medical Doctor)
Assistant Professor
Francis I Proctor Foundation
University of California
San Francisco, California, USA

Aravind Roy MS (Ophthalmology)
Consultant
Cornea and Anterior Segment Services
Tej Kohli Cornea Service, KVC Campus
LV Prasad Eye Institute (LVPEI)
Vijayawada, Andhra Pradesh, India

Srinivas R Sadda MD
President and Chief Scientific Officer
Doheny Eye Institute
Professor of Ophthalmology
University of California-Los Angeles
Los Angeles, California, USA

Oded Sagiv MD
Orbital Oncology and Ophthalmic Plastic Surgery
Department of Plastic Surgery
The University of Texas
MD Anderson Cancer Center
Houston, Texas, USA

Pranita Sahay MD
Senior Resident
Dr Rajendra Prasad Centre for Ophthalmic Sciences
All India Institute of Medical Sciences (AIIMS)
New Delhi, India

Sherveen S Salek BS MD
Vitreoretinal Fellow
Department of Ophthalmology
Emory University School of Medicine
Atlanta, Georgia, USA

Gunjan Saluja MD
Senior Resident
Dr Rajendra Prasad Centre for Ophthalmic Sciences
All India Institute of Medical Sciences (AIIMS)
New Delhi, India

Virender S Sangwan MS
Dr Paul Dubord Chair in Cornea
Tej Kohli Cornea Institute
Director, Center for Ocular Regeneration (CORE)
Director, Srujana-Center for Innovation
LV Prasad Eye Institute, KAR Campus
Hyderabad, Telangana, India

Steven S Saraf MD
Instructor
Bascom Palmer Eye Institute
University of Miami
Miller School of Medicine
Miami, Florida USA

VR Saravanan DNB
Consultant
Department of Retina and Vitreous
Aravind Eye Hospital and Postgraduate Institute of Ophthalmology
Coimbatore, Tamil Nadu, India

David Sarraf MD
Ophthalmology
Jules Stein Eye Institute
UCLA School of Medicine
Los Angeles, California, USA

Matteo Scaramuzzi MD
Resident
Department of Ophthalmology
San Giuseppe Hospital
University of Milan
Milan, Italy

Emily M Schehlein MD
Department of Ophthalmology and Visual Sciences
University of Michigan
Ann Arbor, Michigan, USA

Steffen Schmitz-Valckenberg MD
Consultant
Department of Ophthalmology
University of Bonn
Bonn, Germany

Hendrik PN Scholl MD MA
Director
Institute of Molecular and Clinical Ophthalmology Basel (IOB)
Professor and Chairman
Department of Ophthalmology
University of Basel, Switzerland
Adjunct Professor of Ophthalmology
Wilmer Eye Institute
Johns Hopkins University, USA

Etienne M Schönbach MD
Resident (Ophthalmology)
Department of Ophthalmology and Visual Sciences
Case Western Reserve University
Cleveland, Ohio, USA

Leonard K Seibold MD
Associate Professor
Department of Ophthalmology
University of Colorado School of Medicine
Aurora, Colorado, USA

Juan Carlos Serna-Ojeda MD MSc
Cornea, Refractive Surgery and Ocular Surface Specialist
Banco de Ojos de Aguascalientes
Aguascalientes, Mexico

Ayad Shafiq
FRCOphth MRCPPaeds DCH MA BM & BCh
Consultant Ophthalmologist
Royal Victoria Infirmary
Newcastle Upon Tyne, UK

Parag K Shah DNB
Consultant
Department of Retina and Vitreous
Aravind Eye Hospital and Postgraduate Institute of Ophthalmology
Coimbatore, Tamil Nadu, India

Namrata Sharma
Professor of Ophthalmology
Dr Rajendra Prasad Centre for Ophthalmic Sciences
All India Institute of Medical Sciences (AIIMS)
New Delhi, India

Sankalp Singh Sharma DO DNB
Medical Consultant (Ophthalmology)
Aravind Eye Hospital and Postgraduate Institute of Ophthalmology
Madurai, Tamil Nadu, India

Rohit Shetty FRCS PhD
Vice Chair and Translational Scientist
Narayana Nethralaya
Bengaluru, Karnataka, India

Eric Shieh MD
Physician
Jules Stein Eye Institute
UCLA School of Medicine
Los Angeles, California, USA

Aazim A Siddiqui MD
Resident Physician
Department of Ophthalmology and Visual Sciences
Montefiore Medical Center
Albert Einstein College of Medicine
New York, USA

Joseph M Simonett MD
Resident (Ophthalmology)
Casey Eye Institute
Oregon Health and Science University
Portland, Oregon, USA

Rashmi Singh MD (Ophthalmology)
Senior Resident (Cornea, Cataract and Refractive Surgery Services)
Dr Rajendra Prasad Centre for Ophthalmic Sciences
All India Institute of Medical Sciences (AIIMS)
New Delhi, India

Vidal Soberon
Retina and Oncology Fellow
Jules Stein Eye Institute
University of California-Los Angeles
Los Angeles, USA

Marie Somogyi MD
Oculoplastic Surgeon
TOC Eye and Face
Austin, Texas, USA

Bhaskar Srinivasan MD
Senior Consultant
CJ Shah Cornea Services
Dr G Sitalakshmi Memorial Clinic for Ocular Surface Disorders
Sankara Nethralaya
Chennai, Tamil Nadu, India

K Srinivasarao MS
Resident
Postgraduate Institute of Medical Education and Research (PGIMER)
Chandigarh, India

Giovanni Staurenghi MD FARVO FEBO
Chairman–Director
Eye Clinic
Department of Biomedical and Clinical Science "Luigi Sacco"
Luigi Sacco Hospital, University of Milan
Milan, Italy

Greg Van Stavern MD
Professor of Ophthalmology and Visual Sciences and Neurology
Department of Ophthalmology and Visual Sciences
Washington University in St Louis School of Medicine
St Louis, Missouri, USA

B Steger MD
Assistant Professor (Ophthalmology)
Department of Ophthalmology
Innsbruck, Austria

Prem S Subramanian MD PhD
Professor of Ophthalmology, Neurology and Neurosurgery and Vice Chair for Academic Affairs
UC Health/Sue Anschutz-Rodgers Eye Center
Department of Ophthalmology
University of Colorado School of Medicine
Aurora, Colorado, USA

Sandip Suresh MD
Jules Stein Eye Institute
UCLA School of Medicine
Los Angeles, California, USA

Colin S Tan
MBBS MMed (Ophth) FRCSEd (Ophth)
Associate Professor and Senior Consultant (Ophthalmology)
National Healthcare Group Eye Institute
Singapore

Erika Tanaka MD
Ophthalmology
Jules Stein Eye Institute
UCLA School of Medicine
Los Angeles, California, USA

Radhika Tandon
MD DNB FRCSEd FRCOphth
Professor of Ophthalmology
Faculty In-charge
Unit 6—Cornea and External Diseases Cataract and Refractive, Ocular Oncology and Low Vision Services
Co-Chairperson National Eye Bank
Dr Rajendra Prasad Centre for Ophthalmic Sciences
All India Institute of Medical Sciences (AIIMS)
New Delhi, India

David Taylor FRCOphth DSc (Med)
Professor Emeritus
The UCL Great Ormond Street Institute of Child Health
London, UK

Honeylen Maryl T Teo MD
Fellow (Ocular Oncology)
WK Kellogg Eye Center
University of Michigan
Ann Arbor, Michigan, USA

Sudip D Thakar MD
Orbital Oncology and Ophthalmic Plastic Surgery
Department of Plastic Surgery
The University of Texas
MD Anderson Cancer Center
Houston, Texas, USA

Fotis Topouzis MD MSc PhD
Professor of Ophthalmology
Chair 1st Department of Ophthalmology
AHEPA Hospital
Aristotle University of Thessaloniki
Greece

Roksolyana Tourkevich MD
Instructor of Neurology
Division of Neuro-Visual and Vestibular Disorders
Departments of Neurology, Otolaryngology—Head and Neck Surgery
The Johns Hopkins Hospital
Baltimore, Maryland, USA

David T Tse MD
Bascom Palmer Eye Institute
University of Miami,
Miller School of Medicine
Miami, Florida, USA

Ilknur Tugal-Tutkun MD
Professor (Ophthalmology)
Istanbul University
Istanbul Faculty of Medicine
Istanbul, Turkey

Mayjane Joan Tumulak Diplomate, Philippine Board of Ophthalmology
Consultant in Ocular Inflammation and Immunology
Maria Reyna-Xavier University Hospital
Cagayan de Oro City, Misamis Oriental
Philippines

Swati Upadhyaya MD PhD DNB
Consultant
Glaucoma Services
Aravind Eye Hospital and Postgraduate Institute of Ophthalmology
Puducherry, India

Prabhu V MS FICO
Consultant
Department of Cornea and Refractive Surgery Services
Aravind Eye Hospital
Coimbatore, Tamil Nadu, India

Saujanya Vadoothker MD
Clinical Fellow
Department of Ophthalmology and Visual Sciences
University of Maryland School of Medicine
Baltimore, Maryland, USA

Vikram Vaidee DNB FRCS (Glasg)
Consultant
Department of Cornea and Refractive Surgery Services
Aravind Eye Hospital
Coimbatore, Tamil Nadu, India

M Vanathi MD
Professor
Department of Ophthalmology
All India Institute of Medical Sciences (AIIMS)
New Delhi, India

Nithya Vijayakumar BS
Department of Ophthalmology and Visual Sciences
WK Kellogg Eye Center
University of Michigan
Ann Arbor, Michigan, USA

Perumalsamy Vijayalakshmi
MS (Ophthalmology)
Professor of Ophthalmology
Pediatric Ophthalmology and Strabismus Clinic
Aravind Eye Hospital
Madurai, Tamil Nadu, India

Suneetha Viswanathaiah
MBBS MD (Medical Microbiology)
Consultant Microbiologist
Department of Ocular Microbiology
Aravind Eye Hospital
Salem, Tamil Nadu, India

Ivan Vrcek MD
Oculoplastic Surgeon
Texas Eye Plastics
Dallas, Texas, USA

Nadia K Waheed MD MPH
Tufts Medical Center
Boston, Massachusetts, USA

Orli Weisser-Pike
Doctor of Occupational Therapy
OTD, OTR/L, CLVT, SCLV, CAPS
Department of Occupational Therapy
University of Tennessee Health Science Center
Memphis, Tennessee, USA

Zoë R Williams MD
Associate Professor
Departments of Ophthalmology, Neurology and Neurosurgery
Flaum Eye Institute
University of Rochester Medical Center
Rochester, New York, USA

CE Willoughby BSc MD FRCOphth
Professor
Department of Ophthalmology
Ulster University
Northern Ireland, UK

Kimberly M Winges MD
Assistant Professor (Neuro-ophthalmology)
Casey Eye Institute
Oregon Health and Science University and VA Portland Health Care System
Portland, Oregon, USA

Natalie Wolkow MD PhD
Ophthalmic Plastic Surgery Service
Massachusetts Eye and Ear Infirmary
Harvard Medical School
Boston, Massachusetts, USA

Maria A Woodward MD MS
Assistant Professor
Ophthalmology and Visual Sciences
WK Kellogg Eye Center,
University of Michigan
Ann Arbor, Michigan, USA

Fasika A Woreta MD MPH
Assistant Professor of Ophthalmology
Associate Residency Program Director
Director, Eye Trauma Center
Wilmer Ophthalmological Institute
Johns Hopkins University School of
Medicine, Baltimore, Maryland, USA

David Xu MD
Ophthalmology
Jules Stein Eye Institute
UCLA School of Medicine
Los Angeles, California, USA

Sung Jae Yang MD PhD
Associate Professor
Department of Ophthalmology
Gangneung Asan Hospital
University of Ulsan
College of Medicine
South Korea

Tamara Zompa MD
Glaucoma Service
Centro Oftalmológico Charles
Buenos Aires, Argentina

Foreword

Four decades have elapsed since the writing of the first edition, *Principles and Practice of Ophthalmology*. Quite a bit has happened since then! The time has clearly come for a reincarnation.

When Gholam A Peyman, Donald R Sanders and I compiled and edited the initial version of this multi-volume book in 1980, we utilized the considerable talents of our colleagues and students, all of whom were based in North America. Many of them were affiliated with the University of Illinois in Chicago (our academic home at the time). Now, the Editor-in-Chief is Dr N Venkatesh Prajna, the Chief, Department of Education, and the Director of Academics at the justifiably famous Aravind Eye System (*www.aravind.org*), headquartered in Madurai, Tamil Nadu, India. He has obtained 116 totally new chapters (almost 3 times as many as in the 1980 version).

These chapters have been written by experts from 10 countries, not just the USA. The results reflect the latest opinions from international authorities on diagnostic and therapeutic principles and techniques. Indeed, many of the subjects represent knowledge that did not even exist at all in 1980, such as the following: innovative techniques of cataract surgery; imaging modalities including OCT, for both retinal disease and glaucoma; pharmacotherapy for retinal and macular diseases; new forms of medical and surgical therapy for glaucoma; immunosuppression for uveitis; and many others.

Interestingly, reviews of the original book could equally well apply to this latest version. For example, Professor David Cogan of Harvard University and the National Eye Institute said the following in the New England Journal of Medicine: the book has "a high order of excellence for readers who want a modern and relatively complete thesaurus of ophthalmology…". In the Archives of Ophthalmology, reviewers concluded that "this is a comprehensive…textbook…for residents and practicing physicians…with well-written (chapters)…excellent photographs, drawings, and tables, (that) are well referenced…these volumes fill a need for a comprehensive review of general ophthalmology…and various subspecialty areas."

Our 1987's preface stated: "This book is intended to be a readable and comprehensive textbook for residents and practicing ophthalmologists. It is also meant to be a current, practical guide to a variety of diagnostic and therapeutic approaches to ophthalmic diseases". Dr Prajna and his highly experienced contributors have more than fulfilled our original attempt.

Congratulations!

Morton F Goldberg
MD FAOS FACS Dr Hon Causa (Univ Coimbra)

Director Emeritus
Wilmer Eye Institute
Johns Hopkins University School of Medicine (JHUSOM)

Advisory Board Member
Aravind Eye Foundation

Preface to the Second Edition

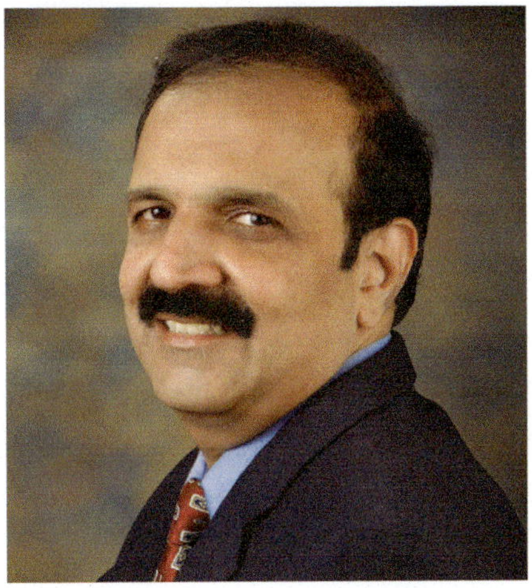

It is very rare to get an opportunity to become the Editor-in-Chief of the same book that one studied during the residency years I consider myself immensely fortunate to have got this chance to edit the book, which was my guiding force during my postgraduation career. The close personal and professional association of one of the previous editors, namely, Dr Morton F Goldberg , who has been a tremendous source of inspiration for all of us at Aravind Eye Care System, made this job an even more memorable one.

The previous edition of *Principles and Practice of Ophthalmology* was a comprehensive book for ophthalmologists in the 1980s. It was one of the most sought after books to get contemporary knowledge of the whole ophthalmology of those times and was presented with great lucidity. During these three decades ever since, ophthalmology has grown in leaps and bounds, and hence there was an urgent need to bring out a current edition of the book to reflect all these advances. The current edition has been designed to concentrate on the relevant practical details of all the advancements in the field and has been generously adorned with illustrations and photographs.

I am very thankful to all the esteemed Section Editors namely, Drs August Colenbrander (Vision Rehabilitation), Uday Devgan (Cataract), Deepak P Edward (Ocular Pathology), Shannon S Joseph (Orbit and Oculoplasty), Joseph M Miller (Optics and Refraction), Michael O'Keeffe (Pediatric Ophthalmology and Strabismus), Pradeep Ramulu (Glaucoma), Srinivas R Sadda (Retina and Vitreous), SR Rathinam (Scleritis and Uveitis) and Prem S Subramanian (Neuro-ophthalmology). All of them are well-respected doyens in their fields and the book has benefitted immensely due to their expertise. They have toiled hard to work with individual authors to produce excellent chapters.

It is always a challenge to mesh the basic concepts and the current advances straddling the entire specialty of ophthalmology in just two volumes. The expertise of heading a world class teaching program at Aravind Eye Hospitals for the past two decades, has helped me to understand the needs of the ophthalmology residents, and I do sincerely hope that this book would be a guiding force for them as well. The book would not have been possible without the blessings of my parents, Dr P Namperumalsamy and Dr G Natchiar; unwavering support of my wife, Dr Lalitha; and my children, Dr Meera Lakshmi and Aravind Krishna and I am very grateful for their love and affection. It is also a unique coincidence that my parents did their fellowships with Drs Gholam A Peyman and Morton F Goldberg in the 1970s in the University of Illinois, Chicago, USA. I am also extremely thankful for the management of the entire Aravind Eye Care System, which gave me all the support during this period.

N Venkatesh Prajna
Academic Director
Aravind Eye Care System
Madurai, Tamil Nadu, India

Preface to the First Edition

This book is intended to be a readable and comprehensive textbook for residents and practicing ophthalmologists. It is also meant to be a current, practical guide to a variety of diagnostic and therapeutic approaches to ophthalmic diseases.

Material is divided into large, well-defined subject areas: To maximize its practicality, the basic chapter style is standardized, containing, when applicable, (1) introduction, (2) basic anatomy and physiology, (3) techniques of examination, and (4) clinical entities with diagnostic procedures and medical and surgical therapies. Theoretical material is added only when it applies specifically to the clinical material under consideration.

Surgical techniques are presented in great detail and are extensively illustrated, so that the reader can easily visualize the recommended approaches. Most chapters are also liberally illustrated with clinical photographs and additional artists' drawings. Color plates are used for further clarity.

Contributors of chapters, while presenting their own approaches, do not neglect others' viewpoints. Alternatives are discussed in detail, or appropriate source material is referenced.

Completion of a project of the size required the cooperation of a great many people. We wish to thank all of the contributors for their time, effort, and patience, not only for composing their chapters initially, but also, in many cases, for revising them to conform to the standards and format of the book. Three talented medical Illustrators—Jean McConnell, Linda Warren, and Leonard Morgan, provided both valuable information and considerable beauty. Special thanks are due our Medical Editors—Maxine Gere and Jane Lantz, who did for the words of this book what our artists did for its illustrations. We appreciate the secretarial assistance of Diann Robinson, who helped bring order out of chaos. Finally, the painstaking efforts and, at times, almost daily cooperation of the WB Saunders Company are gratefully acknowledged.

Gholam A Peyman MD
Donald R Sanders MD
Morton F Goldberg MD

Acknowledgments

I have received tremendous support from all the section editors of this book and the entire Aravind Eye Care System (AECS) in bringing out this book. Without their help and insights, it would not have been possible to bring out a revised edition of this magnitude. I would also like to sincerely acknowledge and thank the disciplinary secretarial help rendered to me by Mrs S Kalyani, from the Department of Medical Education, Aravind Eye Care System, who patiently helped in coordinating with all the authors, section editors and the publishers. I am very grateful for the management of the Aravind Eye Care System for giving me unlimited time and support for making this exercise possible. I would also like to acknowledge the tremendous support of my immediate family for patiently supporting my professional career. My parents Dr P Namperumalsamy and Dr G Natchiar were excellent teachers in their own right and I have learnt a lot from them. My wife, Dr Lalitha and my children Dr Meera Lakshmi and Aravind Krishna have been a source of joy and pride in my professional journey. I do sincerely hope that the book becomes one of the widely used textbooks in ophthalmology globally.

Contents

VOLUME 1

VOLUME 2

Part 8: Glaucoma

Pradeep Ramulu

Part 12: Orbit and Oculoplasty

Shannon S Joseph

Part 8 Glaucoma

Pradeep Ramulu

OUTLINE

Chapter 59 Examining the Eye for Glaucoma

Ta Chen Peter Chang, John McSoley

INTRODUCTION

An adult patient may require glaucoma evaluation in one of several scenarios. The patient may present with sudden onset of symptoms suggestive of very high intraocular pressure (IOP), such as blurriness, halos, and/or pain, or, more commonly, the patient may be asymptomatic and be suspicious of having glaucoma due to a combination of factors, such as elevated IOP, a suspicious optic disk, an abnormal visual field, knowledge of a family history, or an abnormal anterior segment appearance. The levels of detail and goals of the examinations differ between initial and follow-up evaluations.[1] In general, the evaluation consists of taking a history, performing a slit-lamp examination and ancillary tests.

INITIAL EVALUATION

This section applies to the evaluation of a patient who is new to the physician and/or has not had prior glaucoma evaluation. The goals of the initial evaluation are to determine whether there are any treatable causes of elevated IOP to be addressed, and to establish a baseline structural and functional status of the optic nerve. Furthermore, the initial evaluation may help in determining whether the patient has manifest glaucoma, or remains a glaucoma suspect, i.e. if some or most of the findings are too ambiguous for the physician to make a definitive glaucoma diagnosis.

History

Elicit any history of corticosteroid use and/or ocular injury, which aids in evaluating a patient with elevated IOP. Corticosteroid use may include topical use of prescribed or over-the-counter agents. It is possible that topical agents may not be recognized by the patient as containing a corticosteroid product. Ask about a family history of glaucoma and its severity. A family history of severe glaucoma increases the suspicion that a patient may have a similarly severe course. Obtain a detailed past medical history. Any history of sulfa allergy may make sulfa-based IOP-lowering medications contraindicated, while cardiac and/or respiratory problems make the patient a relatively poor candidate for nonselective beta-blockers. A history of vasospasm (Reynaud's phenomenon and migraine) and low blood pressure may increase the patient's risk to glaucomatous damage, whereas a past hypotensive crisis (such as significant blood loss during major surgeries) increase the suspicion that the optic nerve damage may be due to changes in perfusion rather than the present IOP. If the IOP is reported to have been elevated, try to identify to what level and when this was first recognized. The timing and rapidity of onset of glaucomatous damage may give insight to risk of future progression and guide treatment. Record any history of IOP-lowering medication use and intolerances.

Vision and Refraction

Test both the distant and near visual acuities of each eye, and perform a manifest refraction. This aids in establishing the baseline function and in risk stratification (hyperopic eyes are more likely to have angle closure, whereas axial myopia makes the eye more susceptible to pressure-induced damage). The eye's best corrected visual acuity and refraction also helps in choosing and properly performing the appropriate automated visual field test.

Slit-lamp Examination

In the initial evaluation of an asymptomatic patient, the slit-lamp examination is most useful in ruling out the presence of pigment dispersion syndrome, pseudoexfoliation syndrome, forgotten trauma, and asymptomatic inflammation. By convention, the examination proceeds outside-in, starting with external and slit-lamp examination of the ocular adnexa, noting any periocular scarring that might indicate prior trauma. Examine the lid for increased laxity or inflammatory changes, which may make the patient a poor candidate for a filtering procedure (if needed in the future). Note the integrity and vascularity of the conjunctiva, and rule out the presence of blebs or implants; some patients may not volunteer a history of glaucoma surgery if it were performed concurrent with cataract extraction. Under high magnification, examine the corneal endothelium with an oblique light beam for inflammatory cells (Fig. 59.1) or Krukenberg spindles (Fig. 59.2). Examine the anterior chamber for inflammatory cells and/or pigment, and note its depth both centrally and peripherally. With low-to-medium magnification and using a bright and focused light beam, look carefully at the iris for transillumination defects (Fig. 59.3), sphincter tears or pseudoexfoliation material (Fig. 59.4), and note any posterior bowing configuration that may be present in pigment dispersion syndrome (Figs. 59.5A and B). Note the positions and numbers of iridotomies, if present. Both iridotomies and transillumination defects are best observed via retroillumination, wherein a bright beam of

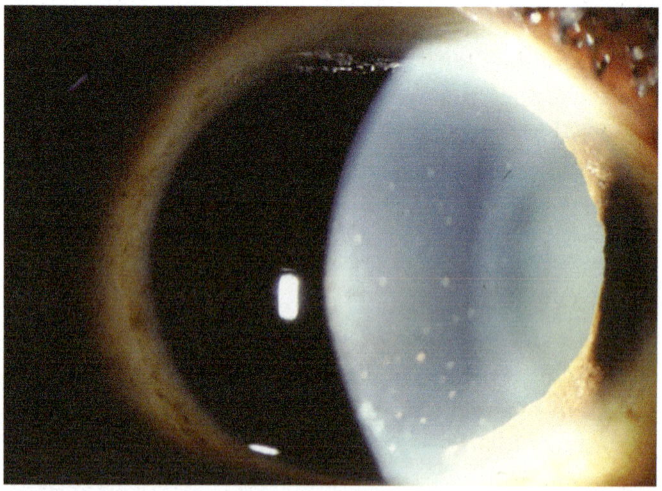

Fig. 59.1: Inflammatory cells on the corneal endothelium.

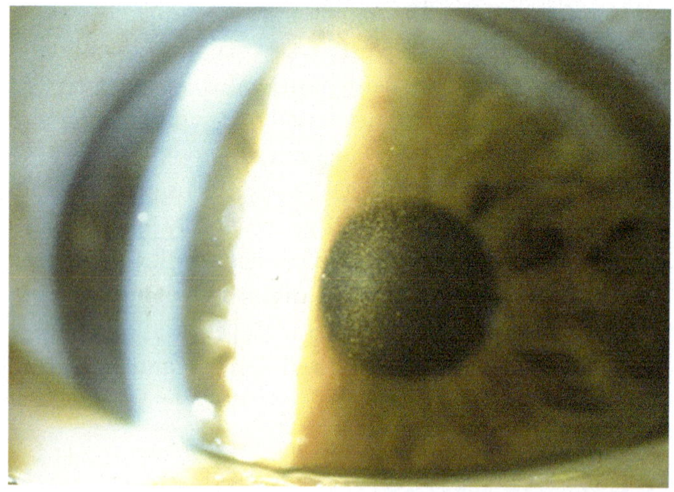

Fig. 59.2: Pigment on the corneal endothelium (Krukenberg spindle) in a patient with pigment dispersion syndrome

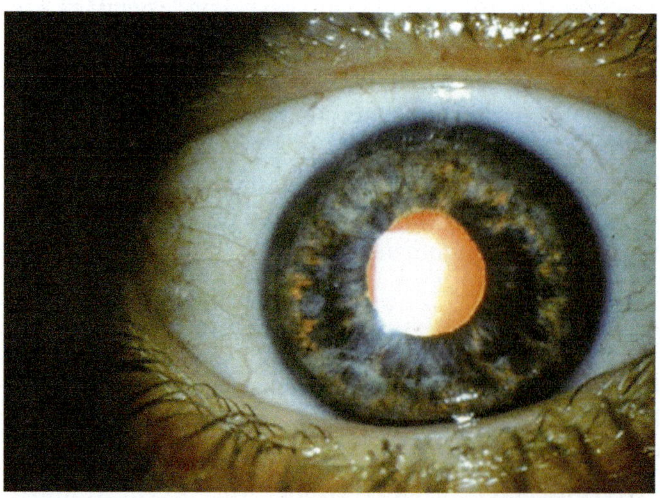

Fig. 59.3: Iris transillumination defect in pigment dispersion syndrome. Note that the low-to-medium magnification as to allow the entire iris to be examined at once.

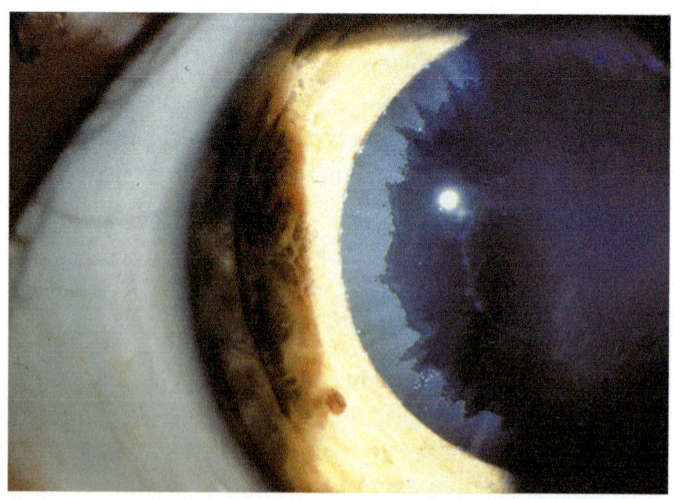

Fig. 59.4: Pseudoexfoliation material on the iris border. Note that the pseudoexfoliation material on the anterior lens capsule can be very difficult to detect without a dilated examination.

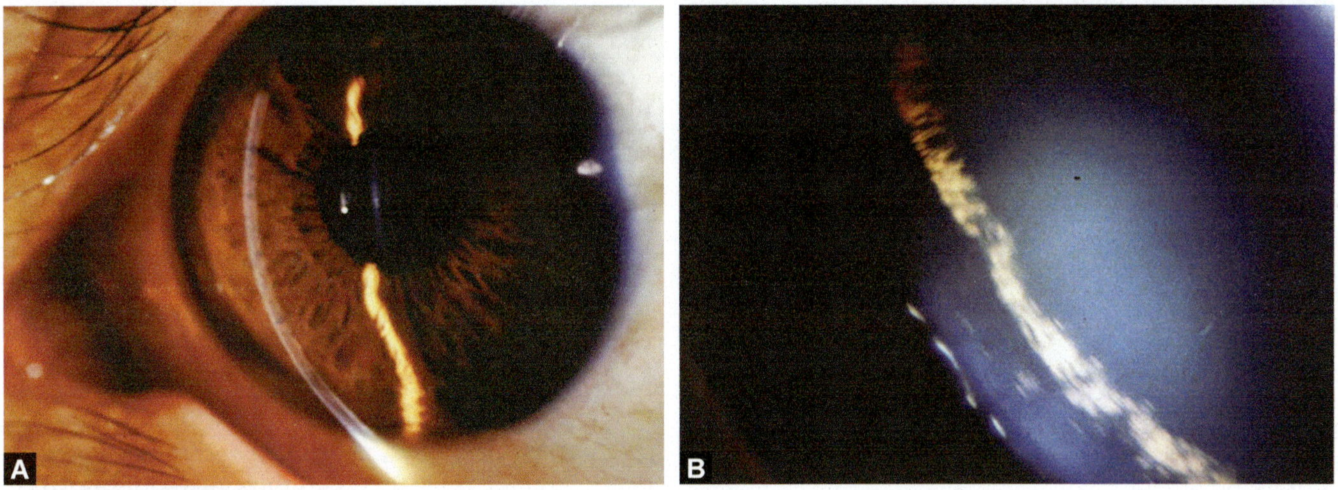

Figs. 59.5A and B: Posterior iris bowing in pigment dispersion syndrome.

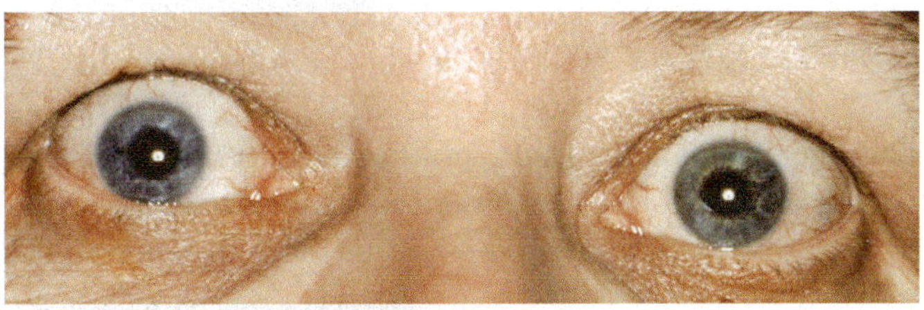

Fig. 59.6: Subtle heterochromia in Fuchs heterochromic iridocyclitis. The lighter-color right eye has elevated pressure.

light not contacting the iris is shined into the pupil while looking for reflected light coming through the iris. Also examine for subtle heterochromia between the eyes (Fig. 59.6). Deliberate slit-lamp examination of the iris and anterior lens capsule with a dilated pupil is worthwhile. Atrophic peripupillary iris changes and transillumination defects may indicate past inflammation or injury as well as iridocapsular contact, such as with pseudoexfoliation or relative pupillary block. Pseudoexfoliation may also demonstrate whitish material at the pupillary margin, and this might be the only sign of the disease in pseudophakic eyes. Examine the anterior lens capsule carefully for pseudoexfoliation material (Figs. 59.7A and B). If the patient is pseudophakic, estimate the position of the haptics and note the presence of any residual cortical material. Note the stability of the lens. Phacodonesis suggests zonular instability and would reasonably prompt attention to the possibility of pseudoexfoliation or past injury. If an anterior chamber intraocular lens (IOL) is present, note whether an iridotomy or iridectomy is present. Also inspect and record the position of the IOL to allow future comparison,

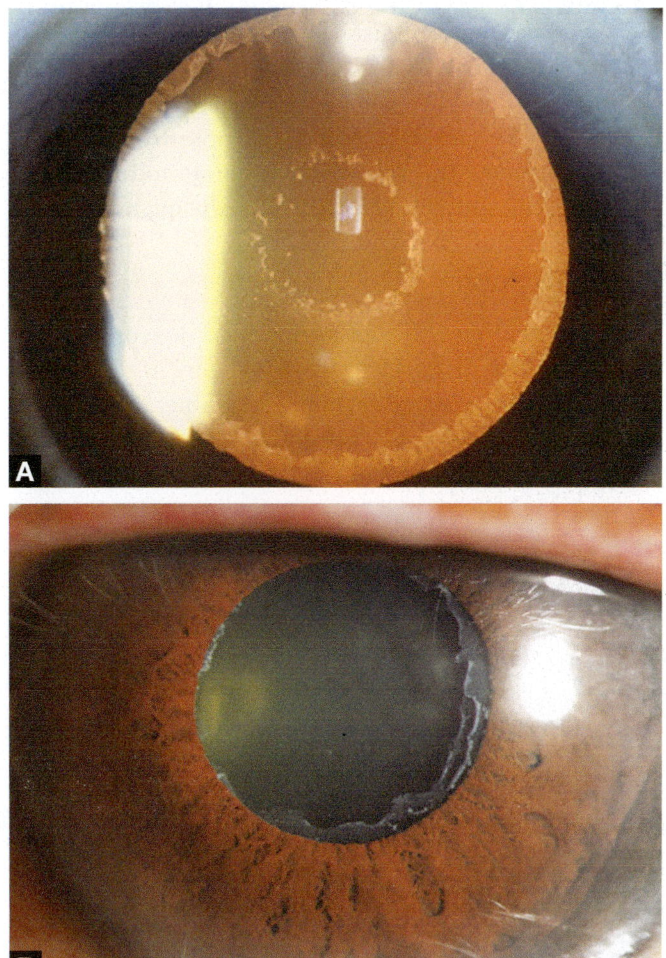

Figs. 59.7A and B: (A) Pseudoexfoliation material on the anterior lens capsule; (B) Scrolled pseudoexfoliative material on the anterior lens capsule that was only visible with a dilated pupil. Note the poor dilation despite multiple drops of dilating agents.

as a poorly positioned and mobile IOL can cause both inflammation and elevated IOP.

Pachymetry

Measure and record the patient's central corneal thickness. In a glaucoma suspect with elevated IOP, the central corneal thickness is useful in calculating the patient's risk of developing glaucoma.[2] Glaucoma patients with thin corneas may also be at a greater risk for disease worsening.

Tonometry

Goldmann applanation tonometry is preferred as it is the method of IOP measurement in numerous prospective clinical trials that yield diagnostic and prognostic information in glaucoma. Record the time and method of measurement and note any disparate readings between the two eyes. Do not adjust the IOP based on the patient's central corneal thickness.[3] If Goldmann applanation tonometry is not available or impractical, measure the IOP using another established method and note to use the same method on follow-up evaluations. Calibrate and service the machineries regularly as instructed by the manufacturer.

Gonioscopy

Under topical anesthesia, perform gonioscopy with a gonioprism using a narrow, focal light beam in a darkroom avoiding illumination of the pupil if possible. A broad light beam and/or bright ambient lighting may cause pupillary constriction and yield a false impression of an open angle. Start by examining the inferior angle and note the position of the Schwalbe's line using oblique lighting and finding the corneoscleral light wedge (Fig. 59.8). A thin, sharply focused obliquely directed light will remain single across the iris and up the angle wall. but split into 2 less intense curved lines of light at Schwalbe's line. Identification of this anterior structure in the angle is helpful in localizing the remainder of the angle structures particularly in eyes with narrow angles, poorly defined structures, areas of broad peripheral anterior synechiae, multiple pigment lines, or a nonpigmented trabecular meshwork. Note the visible anatomy of the angle with and without compression in all quadrants. First, determine whether the angle is open (greater than 6 clock hours of visible posterior trabecular meshwork). In an open angle, look for heavy pigmentation (Fig. 59.9), angle recession (Figs. 59.10A and B), neovascularization (Fig. 59.11), developmental anomalies, such as Axenfeld-Rieger phenotype (Fig. 59.12), or blood in Schlemm's canal (Fig. 59.13). Areas of increased trabecular meshwork pigmentation in a narrow angle may indicate intermittent apposition. If the angle is closed or very narrow, determine whether there are peripheral anterior synechiae with compression (Figs. 59.14A and B).

Funduscopy

Examine the optic disk with the patient's pupils dilated. A narrow, optical section beam can delineate the disk contour better than does diffuse illumination. Direct lenses, such as the Hruby lens or the fundus contact lens provide exquisite

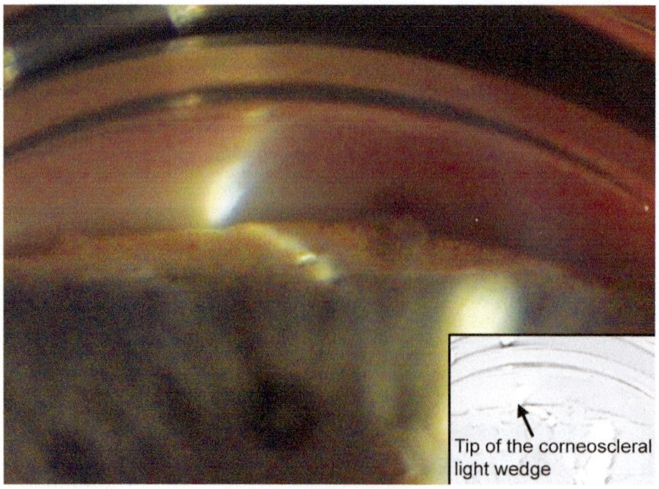

Fig. 59.8: A closed angle in which the tip of the corneoscleral light wedge coincides with the iris. There is no visible trabecular meshwork.

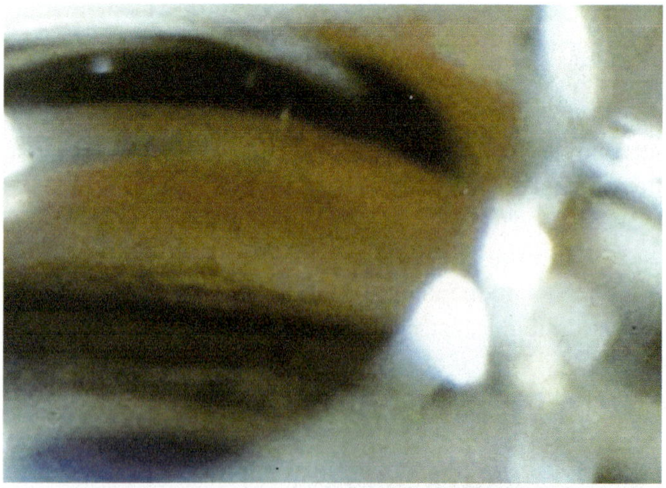

Fig. 59.9: Heavy trabecular meshwork pigmentation in a patient with pigment dispersion syndrome.

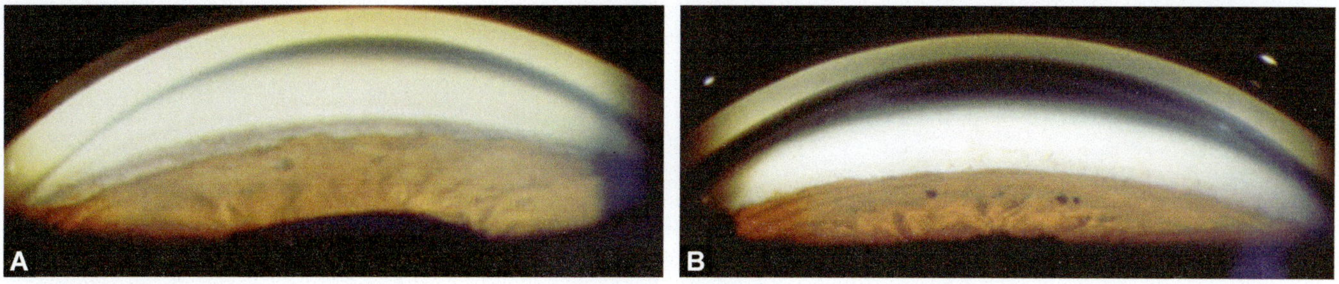

Figs. 59.10A and B: Angle recession. (A) Angle recession in an eye with previous trauma. Note the very lightly pigmented trabecular meshwork and the broadened ciliary body band; (B) Normal fellow eye for comparison.

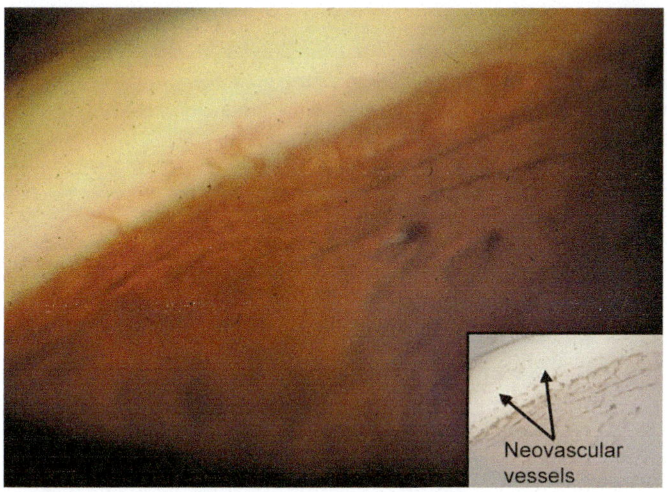

Fig. 59.11: Neovascularization of the angle. Note the branching vessels in the trabecular meshwork as part of a larger fibrovascular membrane. When the membrane contracts, the iris is pulled anteriorly, which results in angle closure and elevated pressure.

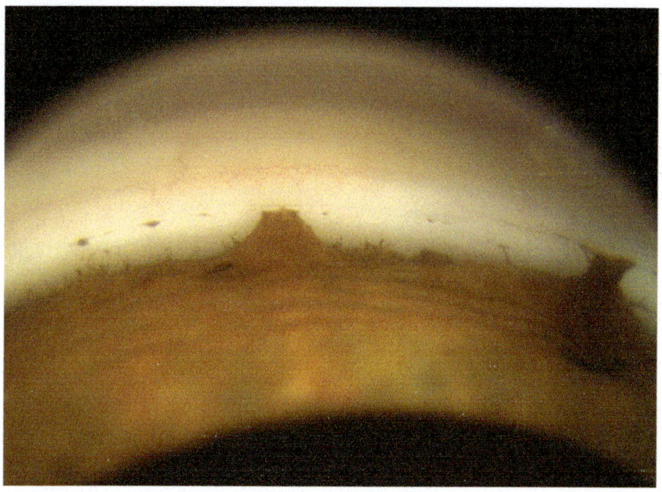

Fig. 59.12: Axenfeld-Rieger syndrome. There is iris tissue adherent to the prominent Schwalbe's ring.

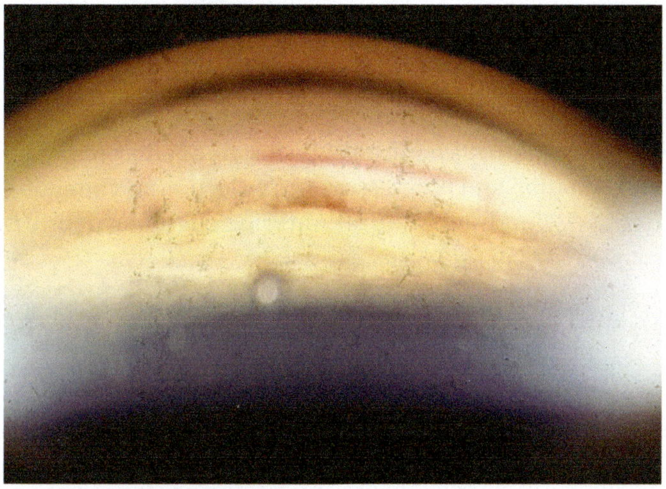

Fig. 59.13: Blood in Schlemm's canal.

stereopsis, though indirect lenses (66 D, 78 D, or 90 D) provide adequate details without sacrificing efficiency. An appreciation of the disks size and shape can provide insight to significance of the size and shape of the cup. Attention to the width and pattern of the neuroretinal rim is helpful. Note the presence or absence of notches and hemorrhages; assess the color of the rim and the size/contour of the cup. Express to the nearest one-hundredth the ratio of the vertical diameter of the cup to the vertical diameter of the disk. Note the presence or absence of venous pulsation. Any clinically evident alterations of the nerve fiber layer should be noted. Examine the fundus for evidence of other diseases, such as old branch retinal vessel occlusions or other retinal lesions that may correspond to visual defects.

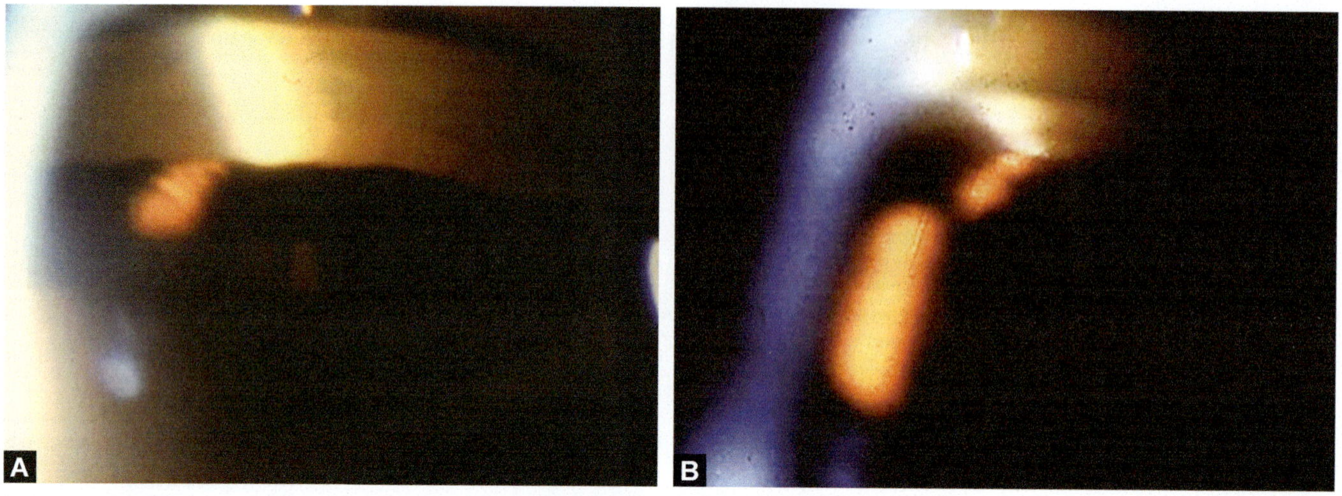

Figs. 59.14A and B: Angle anatomy as revealed by dynamic gonioscopy. (A) A closed angle; (B) Compression with gonioprism revealed pigmented trabecular meshwork without peripheral anterior synechiae. Note the contour of the iris based on the light as well as the continuity of the beam of light across the angle structures when compression is performed.

Ancillary Testing

Supplement the initial examination by performing and interpreting baseline automated visual field testing and optic nerve imaging. These topics will be discussed in the subsequent chapters. Any patient with unilaterally heavy pigmentation on the trabecular meshwork or an angle which is very narrow in one area only will require echography to rule out intraocular tumors (B-scan) and melanomalytic process and/or iris cysts (ultrasound biomicroscopy) which can result in sectoral angle closure. Also obtain an echographic (B-scan) examination on any eye with sufficient media opacity such that precludes a detailed fundus examination.

At the conclusion of the initial evaluation, treatable causes of elevated IOP should be addressed, e.g. performing an iridotomy in an eye suspected to have primary angle closure IOP elevation. Based on the amount of glaucomatous damage present, the likely rate of progression (based on the diagnosis) and the patient's life expectancy, treatment is considered or initiated, and a follow-up schedule is set.

FOLLOW-UP EVALUATION

The goals of the follow-up evaluation are to determine whether the patient is stable both anatomically and functionally, to rule out subtle findings that may not have been apparent on the initial examination, and to determine whether the current therapy, if initiated, is both effective and well-tolerated.

History

Ask the patient about any interim changes in their vision, their general health, and when applicable, whether there are any side effects of ocular medications. Update the medication list, paying special attention to new systemic or topical steroids, sulfa medications or bronchodilators, even the infrequent use of an inhaler. Have the patient described the ocular medication schedule that he or she is using, which may not correspond to the schedule prescribed. If the patient has difficulties adhering to the prescribed regimen, sort out the cause of the difficulties (medication cost, lack of insight, forgetfulness, etc.).

Vision and Refraction

Check the vision with the most recent refraction. Repeat manifest refraction if the vision declines by more than one line. A myopic shift may be a sign of anterior ciliary body rotation and progressive angle closure, and attention the peripheral and central anterior chamber depth is warranted.

Slit-lamp Examination

Examine the ocular adnexa and anterior segment and note any interim changes from the baseline examination. Periocular skin changes, conjunctival injection, and follicles or papillae may indicate some poor tolerance to mediation. Specifically, note any changes in these external structures.

Look at the iris carefully for subtle transillumination defects or pseudoexfoliation material that might not have been apparent during the initial evaluation. If previously recorded, note the patency of iridotomy. If the patient is pseudophakic, note the position of the IOL. A shifting or rotation IOL (in the sulcus or in the anterior chamber) may result in occult, intermittent IOP spikes.

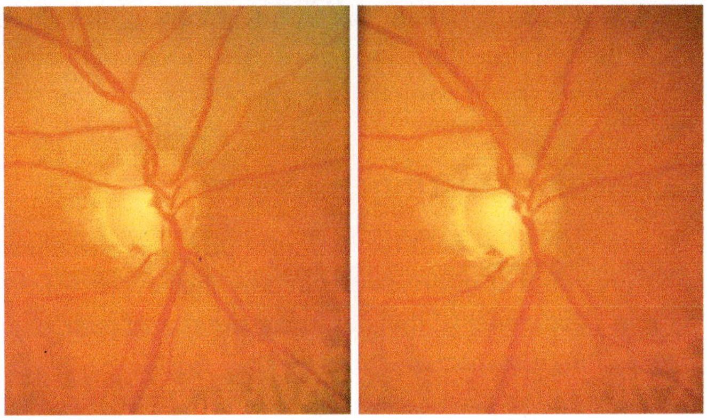

Fig. 59.15: Stereophotograph demonstrating a vertically oval cup with focal thinning of the rim inferiorly and an adjacent disk hemorrhage at ~ 7:30.

Tonometry

Check the IOP in both eyes, record the time of measurement, and time of last medication usage. An IOP at or below the patient's target pressure in the clinic does not mean the pressure is always low, but an IOP above the target in the clinic usually means that the pressure is not well-controlled.

Funduscopy

Examine the optic disk for hemorrhage at every visit, with or without dilation. Disk hemorrhages may be subtle or obvious. Often a deliberate binary decision as to the presence or absence of a hemorrhage is more productive than a casual view of the disk. A dilated fundus examination is usually performed yearly in a patient without concurrent retinal pathology. However, if there is a change that suggests possible progression, such as presence of disk hemorrhage (Fig. 59.15), possible increased cupping compared to baseline photos (Figs. 59.16A and B), or the presence of a new onset visual field defect, a dilated exam is performed to rule out retinal vascular events mimicking glaucomatous visual field changes, and to allow optic disk imaging for comparison to baseline studies. Dilation may also be performed if subjective or objective changes in acuity suggest the presence of new or worsening retinal disease.

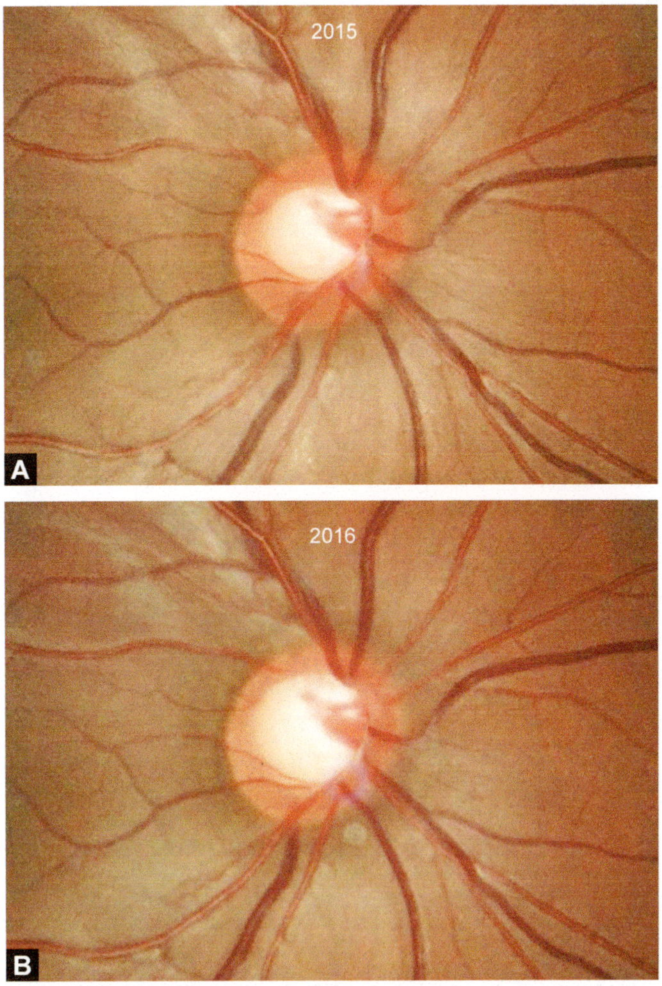

Figs. 59.16A and B: Progressive cupping as evidence of pre-perimetric glaucoma. The patient has pigment dispersion syndrome with intermittently elevated pressures. Sequential photographs showed concentric enlargement of the optic nerves.

Gonioscopy

Routine gonioscopy is performed every 1–2 years in a phakic patient to monitor progressive angle closure due to age-related lens growth. If the patient presents with an unexpected myopic shift, elevated IOP or both, gonioscopy is performed to rule out progressive angle closure.

Pachymetry

Pachymetry is performed on follow-up visits if there are corneal changes on slit-lamp examination (e.g. edema and opacity) and if the patient has undergone procedures that may change corneal thickness since the initial evaluation (e.g. corneal ablation refractive surgery).

Ancillary Testing

Automated visual field testing and optic nerve imaging are performed at intervals dictated by the severity of the patient's glaucoma (if diagnosed) or the risk of glaucoma conversion (if suspected).

REFERENCES

1. Chang TC, Ramulu PY, Hodapp EA. Clinical Decisions in Glaucoma, 2nd edition. Miami, FL/Charleston SC: Createspace Publishing; 2016.
2. Gordon MO, Beiser JA, Brandt JD, et al. The Ocular Hypertension Treatment Study: baseline factors that predict the onset of primary open-angle glaucoma. Arch Ophthalmol. 2002;120(6):714-20.
3. Brandt JD, Gordon MO, Gao F, et al. Adjusting intraocular pressure for central corneal thickness does not improve prediction models for primary open-angle glaucoma. Ophthalmology. 2012;119(3):437-42.

Chapter 60 Visual Testing for the Diagnosis and Monitoring of Glaucoma

Chris A Johnson

INTRODUCTION

Evaluation of the peripheral field of view has been a diagnostic test procedure for more than 2,000 years, dating back to the time before Hippocrates.[1] Perimetry and visual field testing are able to provide an evaluation of visual function for the range of locations that a person can see, and have been critical components of the clinical monitoring of individuals with glaucoma. With the development of new diagnostic test procedures for structural analysis of the optic nerve and retinal nerve fiber layer, the question arises as to whether or not visual field testing is needed for the management of glaucoma. However, a recent publication indicates that perimetry and visual field testing remain as a vital portion of the clinical glaucoma examination procedure, and that structural and functional assessment of individuals with glaucoma or at risk of developing glaucoma are both necessary and provide complementary information to the practitioner.[2]

Perhaps the most important benefit of visual field testing is that many individuals are accustomed to using their central vision (macula and fovea) for tasks involving detection and recognition of fine details (e.g. reading, object identification, face recognition) and are unaware of progressive changes to peripheral vision, particularly if they are gradual changes that occur only in one eye, as is often the case with glaucoma. Testing the field of view can thus provide information about visual function loss that the person may not be aware of, even though it may be responsible for impairment of activities of daily living and quality of life.[3-6] Visual field testing can also be useful in detection of visual pathologic changes, assist in determining the locus of involvement along the visual pathways (using the pattern, shape and location of areas of visual sensitivity loss), and monitor the status of visual impairment over time to determine when additional medical or surgical intervention is needed.

This chapter will present an overview of the various forms of perimetry and visual field testing, the types of visual field loss that occur with glaucoma, methods for interpretation of results, a description of artifactual test results, new visual field test procedures, and other psychophysical tests that can be used for detecting and monitoring glaucoma.

VISUAL FIELD TESTING PROCEDURES

There are several different types of perimetry and visual field testing that are available, depending on the equipment and resources that can be utilized and the specific question that is being asked. Confrontation visual field testing is rapid and easy to perform[7] (Fig. 60.1). It can be conducted when the patient is seated in the examination chair, at the bedside for inpatients or any other suitable location. The examiner faces the patient, and presents targets (hands, fingers, colored balls, finger puppets for children, etc.) to different locations in the visual field while looking for areas of poor detection sensitivity, or differences by comparing their visual field to the patient's, or evaluating asymmetries across the vertical and horizontal midlines. It is a technique that is able to detect moderate to advanced sensitivity losses, but is not sensitive for detecting small, subtle deficits. Similar to this, suprathreshold static perimetry presents targets on a uniform background that can be readily detected by a high percentage (95–99%) of the population with normal vision because their intensity is well above the threshold for detection. The stimuli are presented at key locations that are likely to be affected by pathologic changes to the visual pathways.[8,9] Stimuli at each location are then graded as "seen" or "unseen". There are many different procedures that have been developed for suprathreshold static perimetry, which results in a variety of performance characteristics (sensitivity and specificity) and different testing times. Both confrontation visual field testing and suprathreshold static perimetry can be regarded as screening procedures designed to distinguish normal from abnormal visual fields. An example of results obtained by a typical visual field screening procedure is presented in Figure 60.2.

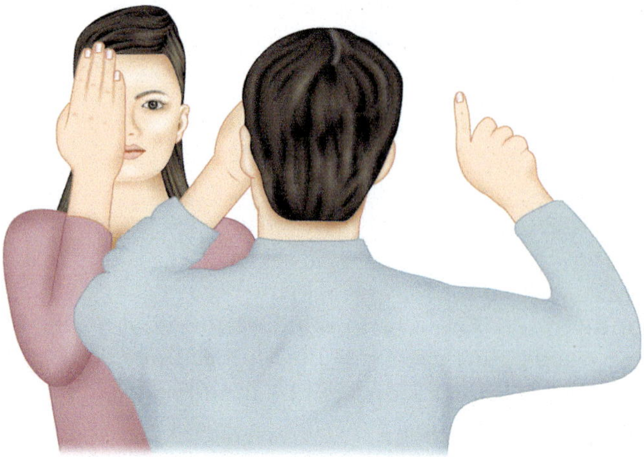

Fig. 60.1: An example of confrontation visual field testing.

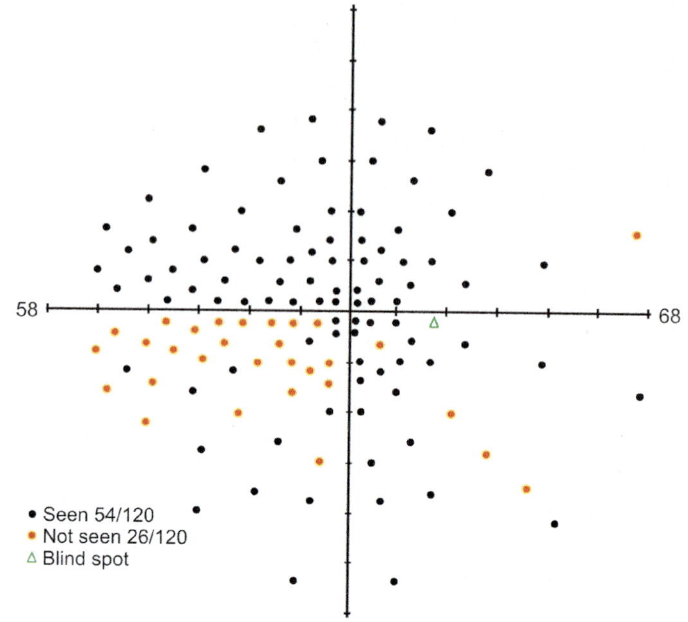

Fig. 60.2: Results of a visual field screening procedure for the right eye of a patient with glaucoma that was obtained on the Humphrey field analyzer.

There are two major forms of visual field testing that provide quantitative measurement of sensitivity to light in the periphery, referred to as kinetic and static perimetry. Kinetic perimetry, as the name implies, evaluates the ability of a patient to detect a moving target of a specific size and intensity that is superimposed on a uniform background luminance. At photopic (daylight) levels, sensitivity to detecting light is highest at fixation (the fovea) and progressively decreases at greater eccentricities, and the mapping of sensitivity to light resembles an island in a sea of blindness, as indicated in Figure 60.3. Targets of a specific size and intensity are moved at a constant rate of speed (2–4° per second) along various meridians to determine locations of equal sensitivity which are connected and are referred to as isopters (Fig. 60.4). By using targets of varying size and intensity, a mapping of the visual field's sensitivity to light can be obtained, and different target sizes and intensities are color coded. The shape of isopters is determined by redirecting moving target scans toward the expected boundary of the visual field. Regions of sensitivity loss within isopters (scotomas) are also identified and are indicated by filled shapes, using the color coding for that specific target (Fig. 60.4). Kinetic perimetry is used sparingly for glaucoma, with manual procedures being limited by the lack of available devices for performing this procedure, and an automated version of this procedure only becoming available recently. The performance of kinetic perimetry varies with the skill level of the examiner, and it is most efficient for assessing the far periphery beyond 30° radius.

Static perimetry, as the name implies, presents stationary targets at key locations in the visual field (Fig. 60.5). It is the most common form of automated visual

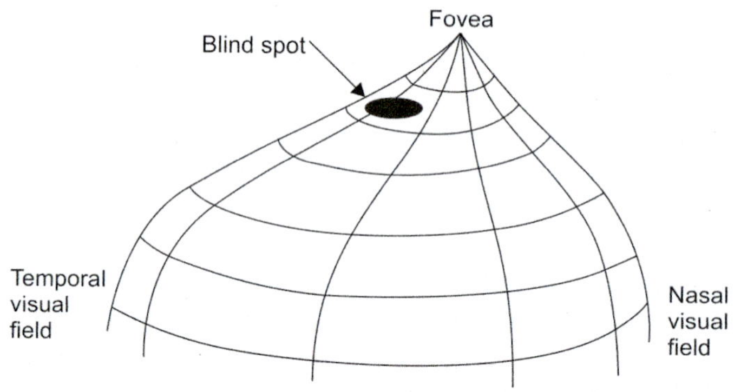

Fig. 60.3: A three-dimensional representation of the visual field sensitivity to light (the "hill of vision in the sea of blindness").

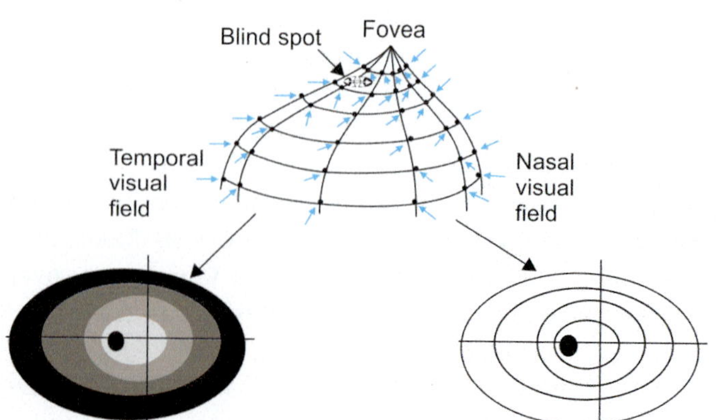

Fig. 60.4: Mapping of the "hill of vision" through kinetic perimetry.

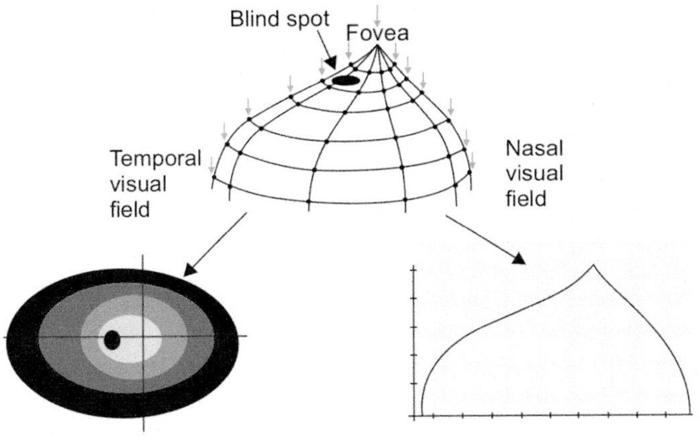

Fig. 60.5: Mapping of the "hill of vision" through static perimetry.

field testing. When a target is presented, the patient is asked to press a response button if it is seen. If the target is seen, the stimulus is next presented at a lower intensity and if it is not seen the stimulus is then presented at a higher intensity. Once an acceptable boundary between seeing and not seeing the stimulus is determined, the minimum intensity threshold for detecting the stimulus on a uniform background is obtained. There are a number of advantages of static perimetry, including: (1) a standardized procedure that can be applied to all patients, (2) a normative age-adjusted database that can be used to compare the patient's responses on a location by location basis, (3) the availability of a statistical analysis package, (4) the ability for practitioners to exchange information, and (5) the ability to electronically store and retrieve visual field information to follow and manage the patient's visual field status. Details concerning these procedures are available in other publications.[10-13]

INTERPRETATION OF VISUAL FIELD INFORMATION

There are a variety of statistical and mathematical procedures that are available for assisting the practitioner to properly interpret visual fields for automated and manual perimeters.[13-18] In addition, it is also critical for the practitioner to make a clinical assessment of visual field results and to make this determination within the context of other clinical and diagnostic test findings. It is important to keep in mind that a patient that is seen in a glaucoma clinic may have a visual impairment other than glaucoma, or may have more than one visual problem affecting different components of the visual pathways. In this view, Box 60.1 presents a brief "cookbook" for evaluating a single visual field. A more extensive evaluation can be found in other publications.[19,20] Not only is the detection of glaucomatous visual field loss important, but the ability to determine the status of the visual field over time (progression, stability or improvement) is a vital component of monitoring the glaucoma patient or the individual that is suspected of developing glaucoma. Unfortunately, there is no consensus as to the best and most sensitive procedure for evaluating multiple glaucomatous visual fields, but there are some techniques that are helpful and are widely used. Finally, one must be aware that a patient's reliability for performing the test is important, and that artifactual findings (not reflecting pathologic changes to the visual pathways) can also occur. Single visual field interpretation, longitudinal perimetry assessment, patterns of glaucomatous visual field loss and artifactual findings will all be included in the following section.

Figure 60.6 contains a single visual field printout for the 30-2 test procedure obtained on the Humphrey field analyzer (left panel) and the Octopus® 900 perimeter (right panel). All of the information that is presented on the

Box 60.1: A "cookbook" for visual field interpretation.

1. Place the left eye results on the left and the right eye results on the right.
2. For each eye, is the visual field normal or are there departures from normal sensitivity?
3. If both eyes are normal, you are done. If abnormal, is it in one eye or both eyes?
4. If in one eye only, the deficit has to be prior to the optic chiasm, where the information from the two eyes is combined.
5. If it is in both eyes, where is the deficit? (binasal is likely to be glaucoma, retina or optic nerve, bitemporal is likely to be chiasm, nasal in one eye and temporal in the other eye is likely to be postchiasm, and central or centrocecal is likely to be retinal or optic neuropathy other than glaucoma). If the deficit is extensive, where is the majority of the loss? Use general locations (superior, inferior nasal temporal) rather than specific details.
6. Now look at the features of the deficit:
   i. Does it "respect" the nasal horizontal meridian (abrupt transition from seeing to nonseeing indicative of glaucoma, branch retinal artery occlusion, anterior ischemic optic neuropathy, etc.)?
   ii. Does it "respect" the vertical meridian (chiasm or postchiasm)?
   iii. Is it a central or centrocecal (candle flame appearance between the blind spot and fixation—retinal or optic neuropathy)?
   iv. Does the defect point to the blind spot (optic nerve)?
   v. Does the defect point to fixation? (chiasm, postchiasm)?
   vi. Is the postchiasm defect congruous (optic tract and occipital lobe lesions are highly congruous, temporal lobe lesions are incongruous, and parietal lobe lesions are partially congruous)?
   vii. Is the defect hemianopic (postchiasm) or a partial hemianopsia (temporal lobe lesions usually create a "pie in the sky" superior visual field deficit, and parietal lobe lesions usually produce an "pie on the floor" inferior visual field defect, while occipital lobe lesions produce cookie-cutter, punched out lesions that appear nearly identical between the two eyes. (Note that one must pay attention and consider the location of the blind spot for this determination).

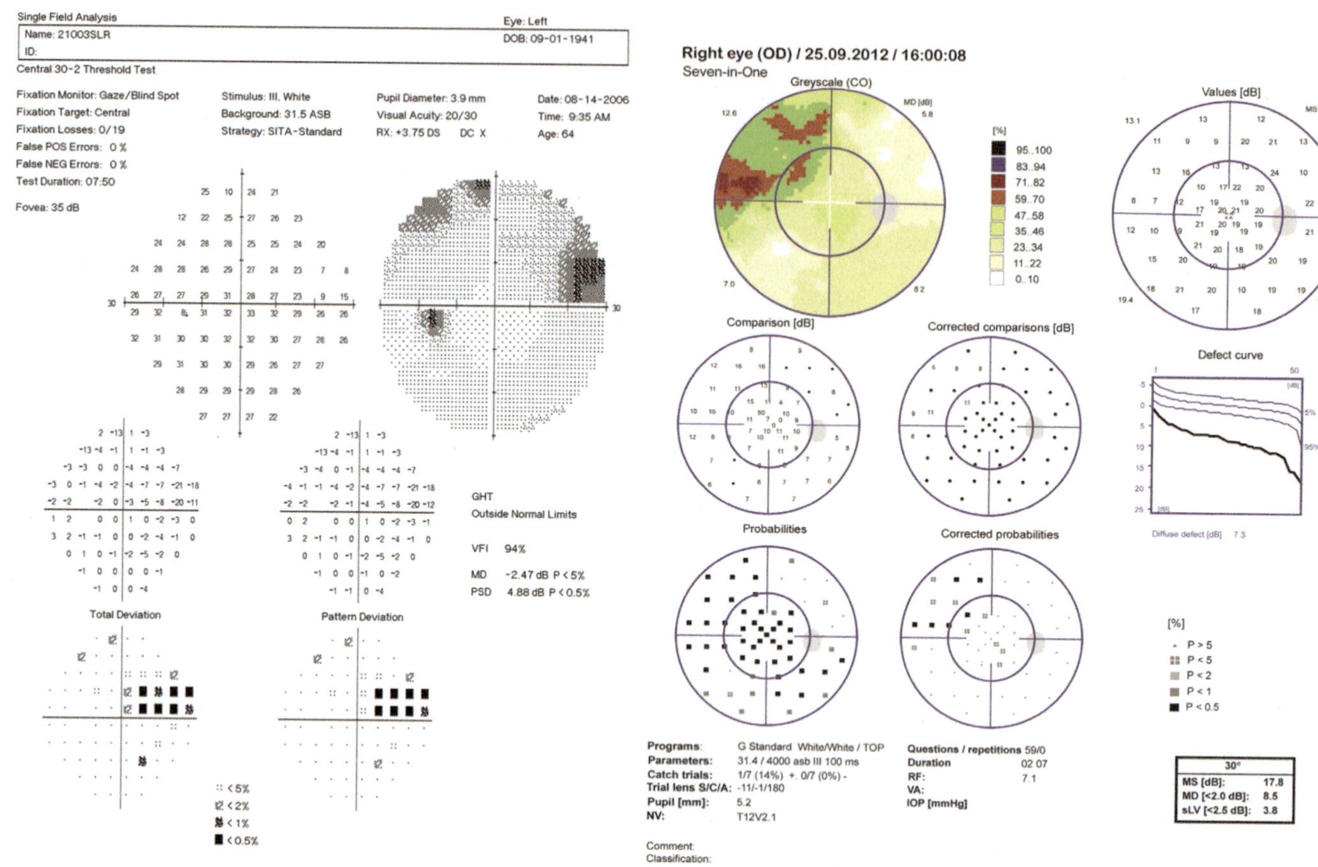

Fig. 60.6: Single visual field printout of results for the Humphrey field analyzer (left panel) and the Octopus® 900 perimeter (right panel).

printed output is important. The text contains information about the patient's eye (pupil size, visual acuity, refraction, etc.), reliability performance (false positives, false negatives, fixation losses, etc.), alignment (gaze tracking, eye movement monitoring), and other relevant information (date of birth, test procedure, test date and time, etc.). Reliability criteria (fixation losses, false-positive and false-negative rates for the Humphrey field analyzer and false positives and false negatives for the Octopus® 900) are also listed. Summary statistics for overall generalized and local sensitivity deficits [mean deviation (MD), pattern standard deviation (PSD) and glaucoma hemifield test (GHT) for the Humphrey field analyzer and mean sensitivity (MS), mean defect (MD) and square root of loss variance (sLV) for the Octopus 900] are also presented. Both perimeters provide numeric sensitivity values and a graphic display (gray or color scale) of visual field sensitivity, along with comparisons of test results to an average person of the same age [total and pattern deviation for the Humphrey field analyzer and comparison, corrected comparison and Bebie (cumulative defect) plots for the Octopus® 900], as well as analyses that evaluate the pattern of glaucomatous

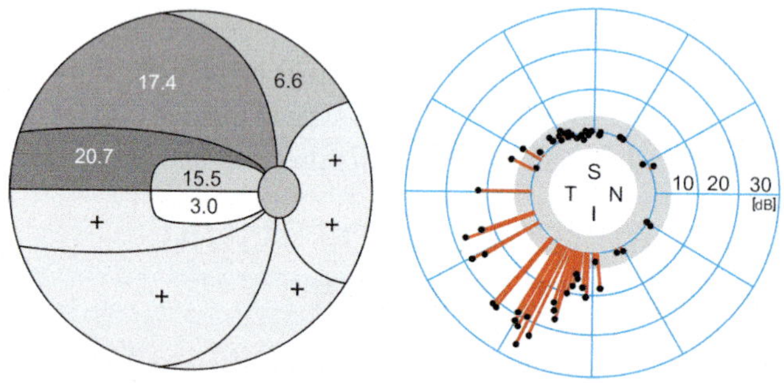

Fig. 60.7: The retinal nerve fiber layer cluster analysis (left panel) revealing a superior arcuate visual field deficit and the polar plot (right panel) indicating the corresponding portion of the optic nerve head that is damaged for the Octopus® 900.

visual field loss (GHT for the Humphrey field analyzer and Cluster and Polar plots for the Octopus® 900, as shown in Figure 60.7, left and right panels, respectively). A detailed description of these procedures can be found in the user manuals of these devices as well as designated source books.[10-13,21]

Interpretation of the pattern and shape of visual field deficits is challenging, and practitioners often concentrate on detailed information before determining the overall general characteristics of visual field results from both eyes (cannot see the forest for the trees), which can lead to an inappropriate diagnosis. A "cookbook" for interpretation of visual field information has been published previously[19,20] which is a valuable resource for those wishing to adopt a consistent procedure for evaluating visual fields. Box 60.1 presents a brief summary of this cookbook. By using these guidelines, it is possible to properly interpret the vast majority of visual fields, although one should also be aware that there are occasionally exceptions to these guidelines.

The patterns of visual field loss that are typically encountered for glaucoma adhere to the shape of the retinal nerve fiber bundles that enter the optic nerve head. It is important to keep in mind that nerve fibers from the temporal retina receive light projections from the nasal visual field and vice versa, while the superior retina receives input from the inferior visual field and vice versa. The majority of nerve fibers enter the temporal portion of the optic nerve, subserving the macula and the region between the macula and the optic nerve head in a candle flame type of shape (the papillomacular bundle, which when damaged, produces a centrocecal visual field deficit). Optic nerve fibers enter the superior and inferior portions of the optic nerve in a fan-shaped or arcing pattern, which produce arcuate visual field defects. The superior and inferior fan-shaped patterns terminate abruptly along the horizontal midline in the temporal retina (nasal visual field) along a distinct raphe, which results in a horizontal nasal step visual field deficit when there is asymmetry in the amount of damage to the superior and inferior fibers. Finally, there is a group of fibers in a radial pattern that enter the nasal part of the optic nerve head (temporal visual field), and temporal wedge visual field losses can occur when these fibers are damaged. Figure 60.8 presents an illustration of the nerve fiber bundle patterns and the deficits that occur when they are damaged.

We have previously classified glaucomatous visual field deficits into various shapes and patterns, have devised specific guidelines for interpreting and classifying glaucomatous visual field loss, and have performed inter-reader agreement (97% for 2 out of 3 readers) and reader consistency over time (88% agreement) for a large number of visual fields in the Ocular Hypertension Treatment Study (OHTS).[22] Details concerning this classification system are available in the publication, but briefly there were eight glaucomatous patterns that were identified that could be applied to the superior and inferior hemifields (nasal step, temporal wedge, paracentral defect, widespread or diffuse loss, partial arcuate, arcuate, altitudinal, total loss) and additional nonglaucomatous patterns that were related to optical, retinal, nonglaucomatous optic neuropathies, chiasmal and postchiasmal deficits, as well as artifactual findings. Figure 60.9 presents representative examples of glaucomatous visual field deficits (nasal step, temporal wedge, paracentral defect, widespread or diffuse loss, partial arcuate, arcuate, altitudinal, total loss).

In addition to detecting visual field loss related to pathologic changes to visual mechanisms, there are also abnormalities that can occur as a result of incorrect information provided to the perimeter, errors in the testing procedure, or patient attributes that are not conducive to proper testing procedures. Examples are presented in

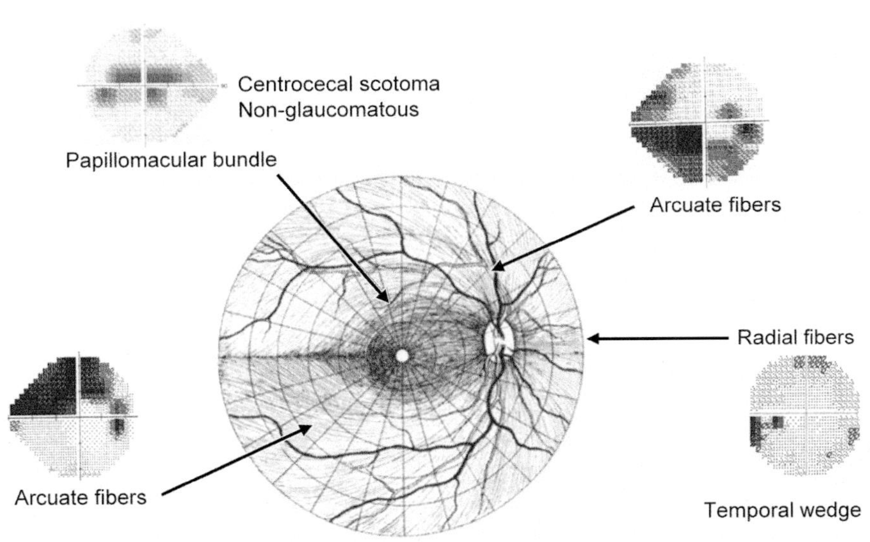

Fig. 60.8: A representation of the visual field deficits that correspond to damage to various nerve fiber bundles entering the optic nerve head.

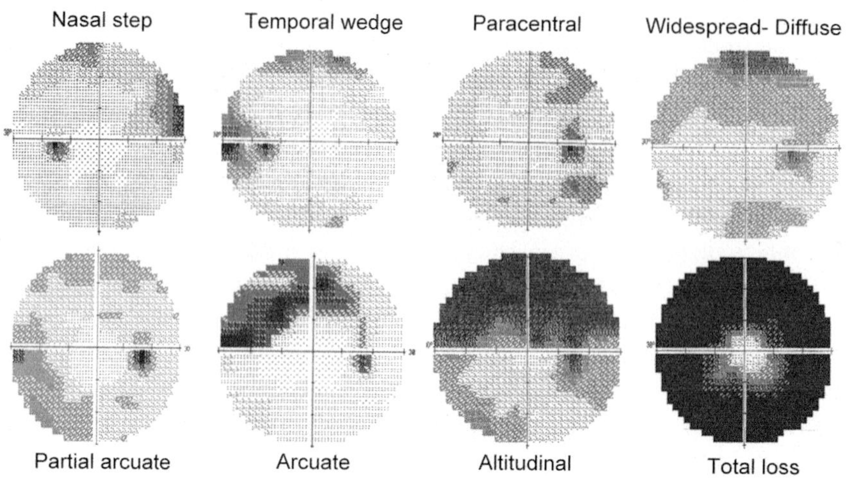

Fig. 60.9: Examples of eight gray scale representations of visual field losses that are commonly seen for glaucomatous damage.

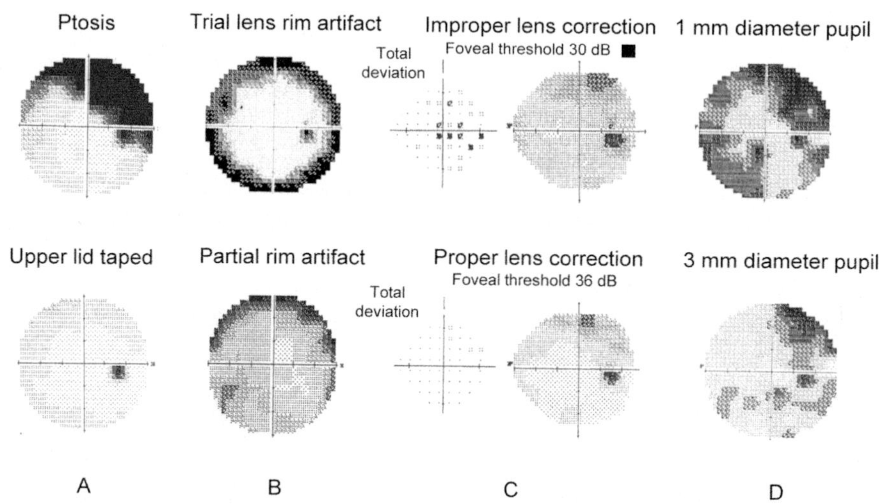

Figs. 60.10A to D: Examples of artifactual visual field results.

Figures 60.10 and 60.11. Some patients, particularly elderly individuals, may have droopy upper eye lids (ptosis) that obstruct the superior portion of the visual field. This can be remedied by using surgical tape to raise the upper lid while still allowing the patient to blink. Visual field results for ptosis (upper figure) and a taped upper lid (lower figure) are presented (Fig. 60.10, panel A). Often, patients have a tendency to back out of the perimeter bowl during testing, and a complete (upper figure) or partial (lower figure) trial lens rim artifact (Fig. 60.10, panel B) will occur because the lens holder now obstructs part of the visual field being evaluated. Figure 60.10, panel C, presents results for a visual field in which an incorrect lens correction was used (upper figure) and when a proper lens was used (lower figure). Small pupils (<3 mm diameter) create a test condition that is not stable and produces visual fields that reveal a greater amount of abnormality. Figure 60.10, panel D, presents the visual field obtained with a 1 mm diameter pupil (upper figure), and when the pupil was dilated to 3 mm diameter (lower figure).

It is important to enter the correct date of birth so that the device can compare the results obtained to an average person of the same age. Figure 60.11, panel A, presents the results for a patient whose birthdate was entered as 40 years younger than his actual age (upper figure), and the same visual field test with the proper date of birth (lower figure). Note the difference in the total deviation probability plot below and to the left of the gray scale output. A person who will respond inappropriately when there is no target presented, or the response is too early

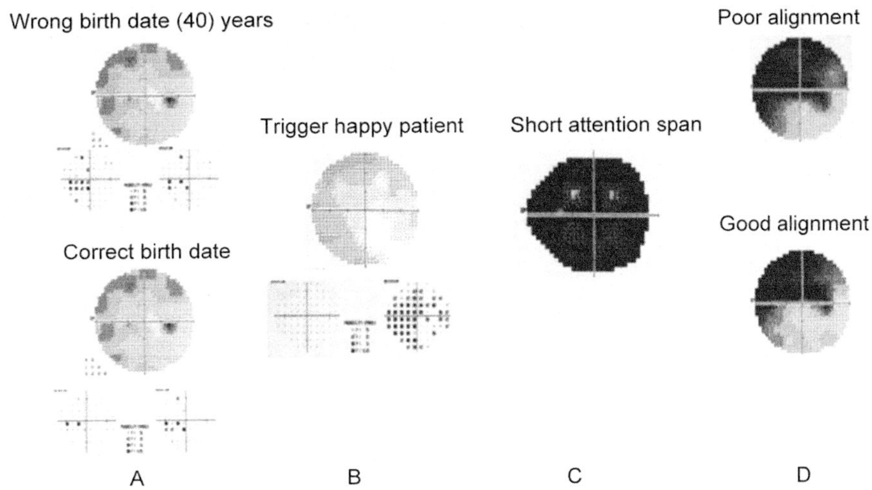

Figs. 60.11A to D: Additional examples of artifactual visual field results.

or too late relative to the stimulus presentation duration (false positives). In these cases, the total deviation plot may be normal or nearly normal but the pattern deviation plot may be quite abnormal, as shown in Figure 60.11, panel B. In this instance, the patient is "trigger happy", responding even when the target is not presented. Often false-positive responses and fixation losses will exceed the normal range of values as well. Figure 60.11, panel C, presents an example of a cloverleaf visual field pattern. The four diagonal locations in the midperiphery have the highest sensitivity and are the first locations to be tested, while the other locations are tested at a later time. This is characteristic of a patient with a 20- to 30-second attention span or cognitive impairment where the patient is able to perform well at first and then becomes distracted. Instructions are also important. To test the fovea, the fixation targets are initially displaced to an eccentric location. Once the fovea is tested, fixation moves back to the center of the bowl and the technician is supposed to direct the patient to redirect their gaze to the central fixation target. However, if this is not done, then fixation will be inferior to the center of the bowl. Figure 60.11, panel D, presents the visual field obtained with improper (upper figure) and proper (lower figure) fixation.

LONGITUDINAL VISUAL FIELD INTERPRETATION

To properly monitor the status of an eye with glaucoma or at risk of developing glaucoma, periodic visual field testing is vital for understanding whether visual status is stable or is undergoing progressive change. Figure 60.12 presents a summary of visual field results obtained on the Humphrey field analyzer. The top panel demonstrates results for two visual field examinations that were obtained at an established baseline (the Humphrey field analyzer uses the average of the two baseline tests to improve reliability). The lower visual field presents the results of the most recent visual field test, which in this case appears to show progressive change. The middle panel presents a linear plot of the visual field index (VFI), which is an eccentricity-weighted mean of pattern deviation scores [normal is 100% and 0 decibels (dB) is to produce a value of between 100% and 0% for the visual field for many tests that have been obtained, and for these cases it reveals a systematic gradual worsening of visual field sensitivity in this eye over time].

Figure 60.13 presents a similar longitudinal presentation of visual field results obtained for the left and right eyes over time with the Octopus® 900 perimeter. The top panels present the cluster analysis results over time for the right and left eyes, with the red solid triangles and V characters representing significant changes in sensitivity for those regions. Below are color-coded sensitivity maps of individual visual field results over time.

It is important to keep in mind that both the sensitivity change over time and the variability of results from successive visual fields are important for determining whether or not the longitudinal visual field results are clinically meaningful. Also, it is important to review all of the visual field results. If one only views a small portion of the findings, it is difficult to appreciate the overall results because one is sampling only a portion of the overall result, and interpretation of improvement, stability or worsening can be incorrect.

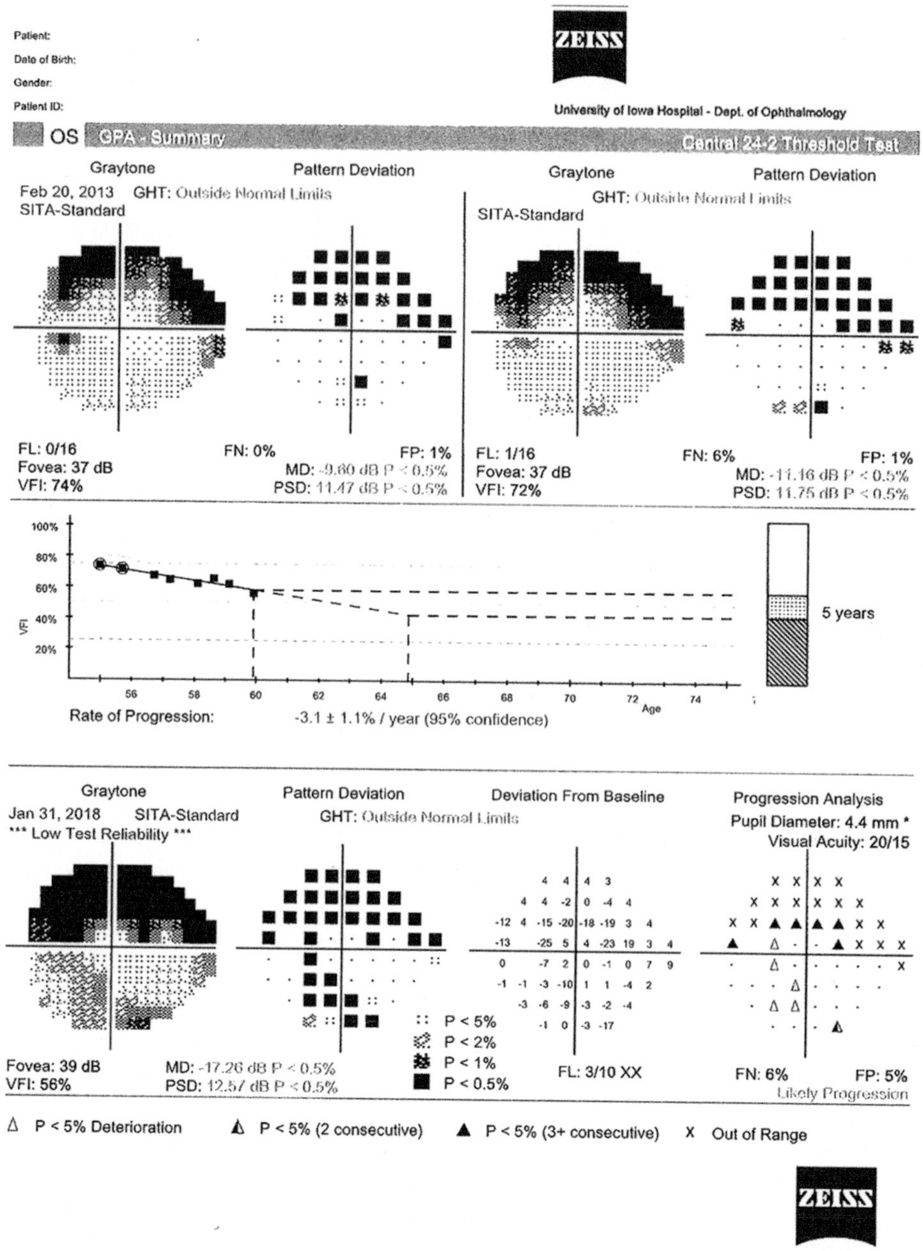

Fig. 60.12: Longitudinal evaluation of multiple visual field examinations that were obtained on the Humphrey field analyzer.

SPECIALIZED VISUAL FIELD TESTING

Although standard automated perimetry (SAP) (white target superimposed on a white background) is the most common form of visual field testing, there are also other visual field test procedures that are available. These tests were designed to isolate and measure the status of specific subgroups of ganglion cells, to assess visual functions that may be more susceptible to glaucomatous pathology, or to produce techniques that are most suitable for visual screening.

SHORT-WAVELENGTH AUTOMATED PERIMETRY

The procedure known as short-wavelength automated perimetry (SWAP) utilizes a high-intensity yellow

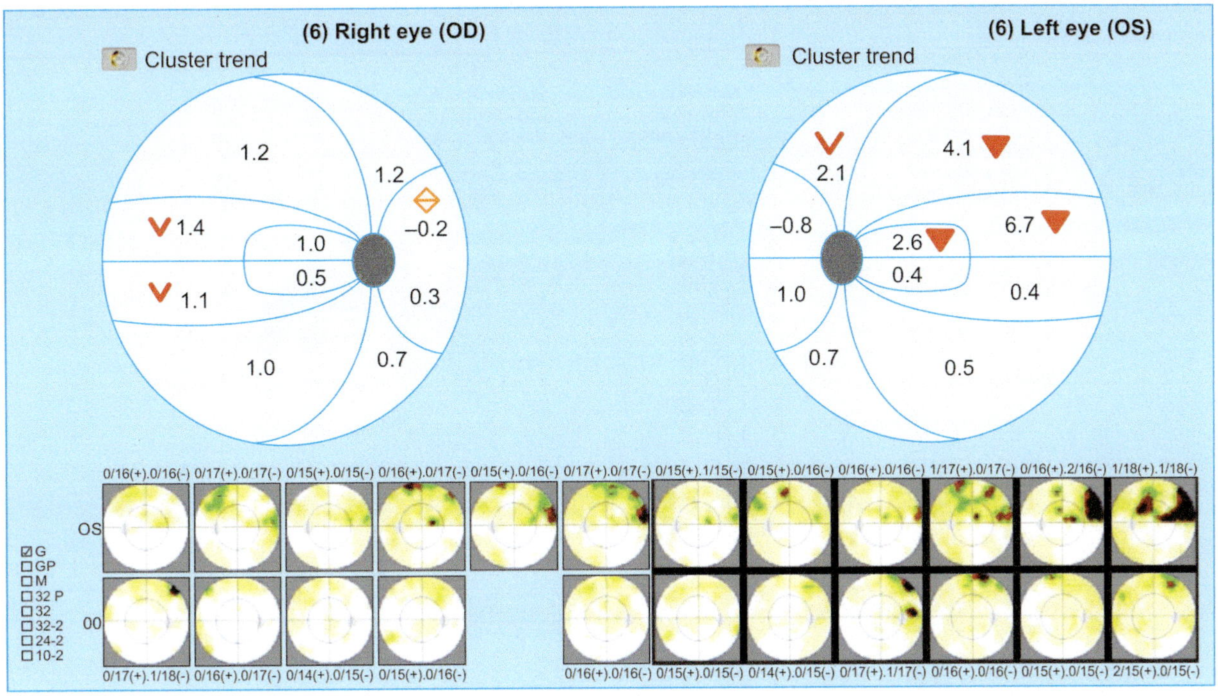

Fig. 60.13: Longitudinal evaluation of multiple visual field examinations that were obtained on the Octopus® 900 perimeter.

background that reduces the sensitivity of middle (green) and long (red) wavelength mechanisms, and a large (size V) blue stimulus to isolate and measure the sensitivity of short-wavelength mechanisms.[23] The ganglion cells that are most sensitive to the short-wavelength stimulus project to the intralaminar koniocellular layers of the lateral geniculate nucleus and represent a distinct short-wavelength sensitive pathway.[23] A number of previous investigations have reported that SWAP is able to detect visual field loss between 3 years and 10 years prior to its appearance with SAP testing.[23-26] Although two recent studies have indicated that SWAP and SAP have equivalent performance in the detection of early glaucomatous visual field loss.[27,28] SWAP is a more difficult test procedure for many patients, but it may be a useful procedure to use when other clinical information is uncertain or equivocal. An example of a glaucomatous visual field deficit with SWAP is presented in Figure 60.14.

FREQUENCY DOUBLING TECHNOLOGY PERIMETRY

When a low spatial frequency sinusoidal grating (below 1 cycle per degree) is counter phase flickered at a high temporal frequency (more than 15 Hz), the sinusoidal grating appears to have approximately twice as many light and dark bars than are physically present. By determining the amount of contrast needed to detect the sinusoidal pattern from a uniform background at different visual field locations, it is possible to determine contrast sensitivity threshold sensitivities throughout the visual field, a procedure referred to as frequency doubling technology (FDT) perimetry. The original FDT device conducted measurements with a 10° by 10° diameter target at 19 locations throughout the central 30° radius visual field, while the second-generation device (the Humphrey Matrix) used smaller targets to perform more detailed assessment of the central 30° visual field, using a 30-2 pattern (69 targets separated by 5°) for the central 30°, and a denser pattern (44 targets separated by 2°) for evaluation of the macular region. Both procedures have been reported to be useful for detection of glaucomatous visual field loss as well as other ocular and neurologic disorders,[29-32] and the Matrix has been reported to be useful for early detection of glaucomatous visual field loss and for monitoring glaucomatous visual field progression.[33] Additionally, FDT testing has been useful successfully for testing children,[34] and it has a rapid and effective screening procedure that requires less than 30 seconds per eye for a normal visual field, and 1–1.5 minutes per eye for a visual field containing pathologic changes. An example of glaucomatous visual field loss for the original FDT device (Fig. 60.15, right panel) and the Humphrey Matrix (Fig. 60.15, left panel) is presented in for the same left eye.

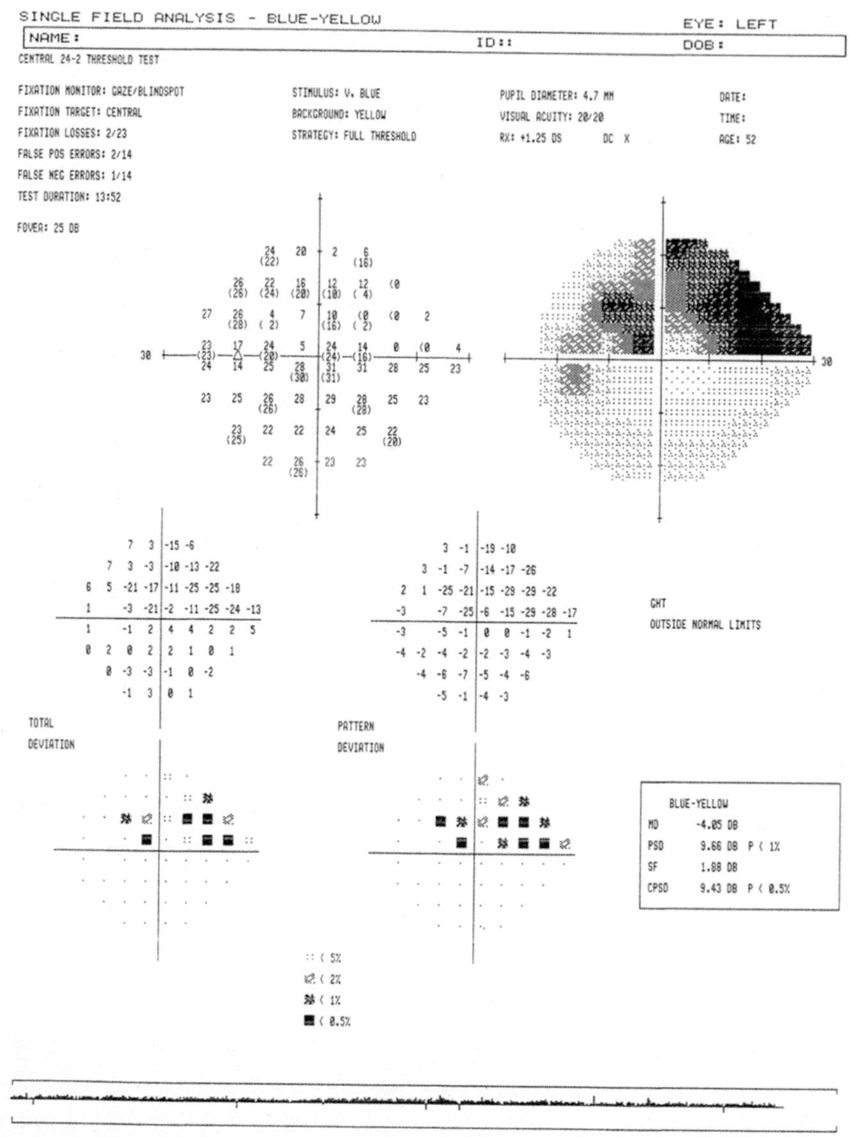

Fig. 60.14: An example of a superior arcuate visual field defect that was obtained for short-wavelength automated perimetry (SWAP).

PULSAR PERIMETRY

Pulsar perimetry uses a two-dimensional sinusoidal grating stimulus that has the appearance of a bull's eye arrangement, and presents stimuli of various combinations of low spatial frequencies and high temporal frequencies. In this view, it is highly similar to FDT testing. The appearance of the stimulus not only has a flickering component, but also the impression of a centrifugal motion flow pattern that assists in its conspicuity. Previous investigations indicate that Pulsar perimetry performs as well as or slightly better than SAP for detection of visual field loss, and has a negligible learning effect.[35,36] Figure 60.16 presents an example of a glaucomatous visual field deficit for Pulsar perimetry.

FLICKER PERIMETRY

There are several methods that have been used to perform flicker perimetry: (1) determining the highest flicker frequency that can be detected from a uniform background, known as critical flicker fusion (CFF), (2) assessing the amount of flicker amplitude (contrast) needed to detect a target of constant flicker rate from a uniform background, referred to as temporal modulation perimetry (TMP), and (3) evaluation of the amount of flicker amplitude that can be detected on an increment of light referred to as luminance-pedestal flicker.[37,38] Each procedure has its own performance characteristics, as well as advantages and disadvantages. It has previously been reported that TMP is

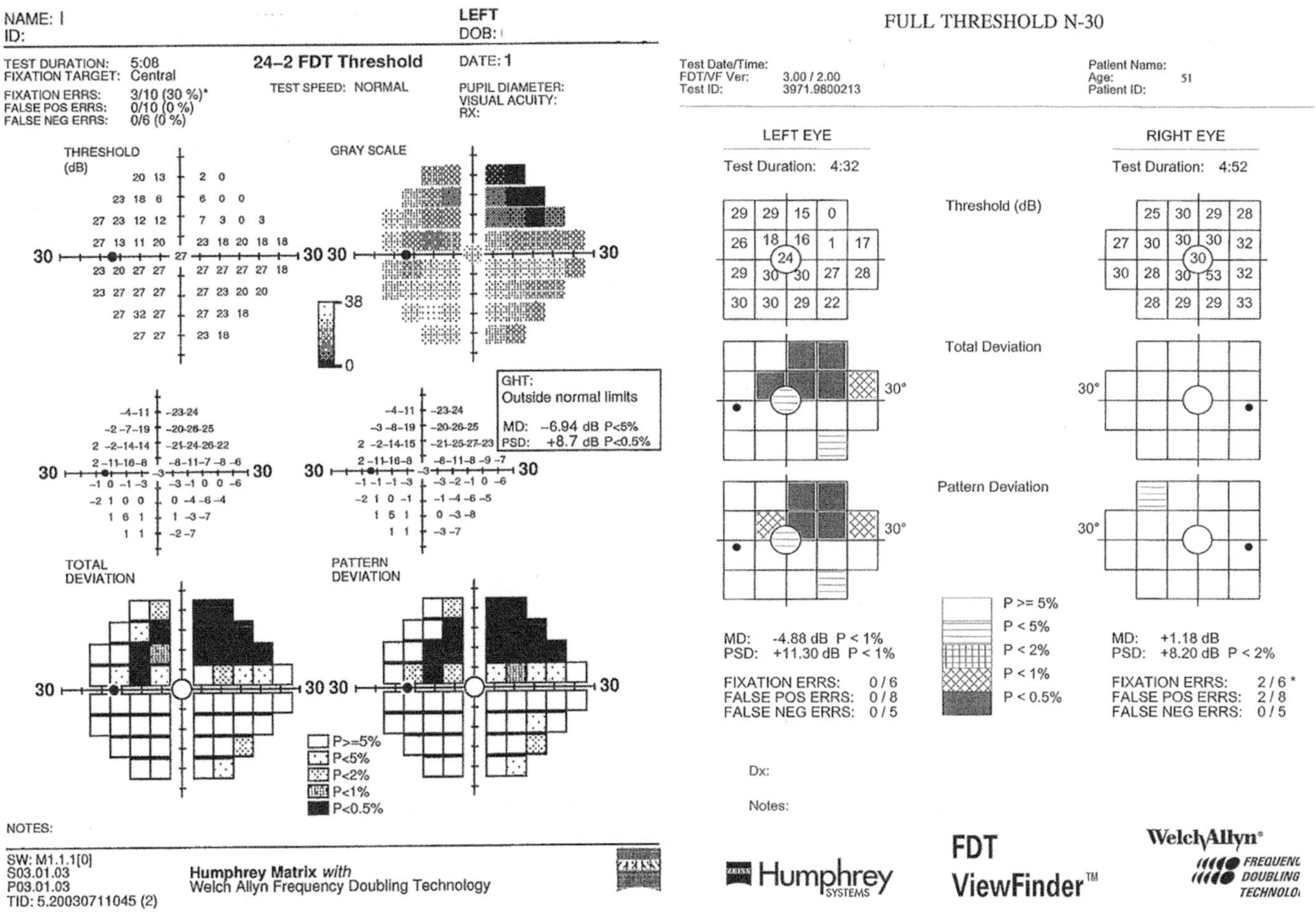

Fig. 60.15: An example of a superior arcuate deficit obtained on the Humphrey matrix frequency doubling perimeter (left panel) and the original frequency doubling technology device (right panel). Results are for the same eye that is shown in Figure 60.14.

better able to detect and characterize glaucomatous loss than CFF perimetry[37] and some patients find luminance-pedestal flicker confusing because it is difficult to dissociate the ability to detect flicker from detection of the increment of light. TMP perimetry has been reported to detect glaucomatous visual field progression earlier than SAP.[39] Figure 60.17 presents an example of a glaucomatous visual field loss with TMP. Unfortunately, there has not been consensus as to the proper method of performing flicker testing, there are limited options for commercial devices that can perform flicker perimetry.

RAREBIT PERIMETRY

Rarebit perimetry presents small targets (pixels) on a computer monitor to perform fine mapping of the central visual field, with both central 30° radius and macula tests available.[40,41] The targets are of relatively high intensity and are easily detectable by individuals with normal visual field sensitivity. The test presents 0, 1 or 2 pixel targets, and the person being examined is asked to press a response button 0, 1 or 2 times. By presenting stimuli in key locations in predetermined localized regions, the test evaluates the "hit rate", or number of stimuli correctly detected in that location. An example of a glaucomatous visual field deficit obtained with Rarebit perimetry is presented in Figure 60.18.

TABLET-BASED VISUAL FIELD TESTING

Current automated perimeters are generally quite large and expensive, making it difficult to use them for rapid testing, particularly in developing countries, facilities with limited testing space, and frequent home testing. Recently, there have been several investigators that have developed and evaluated screening and quantitative methods of visual

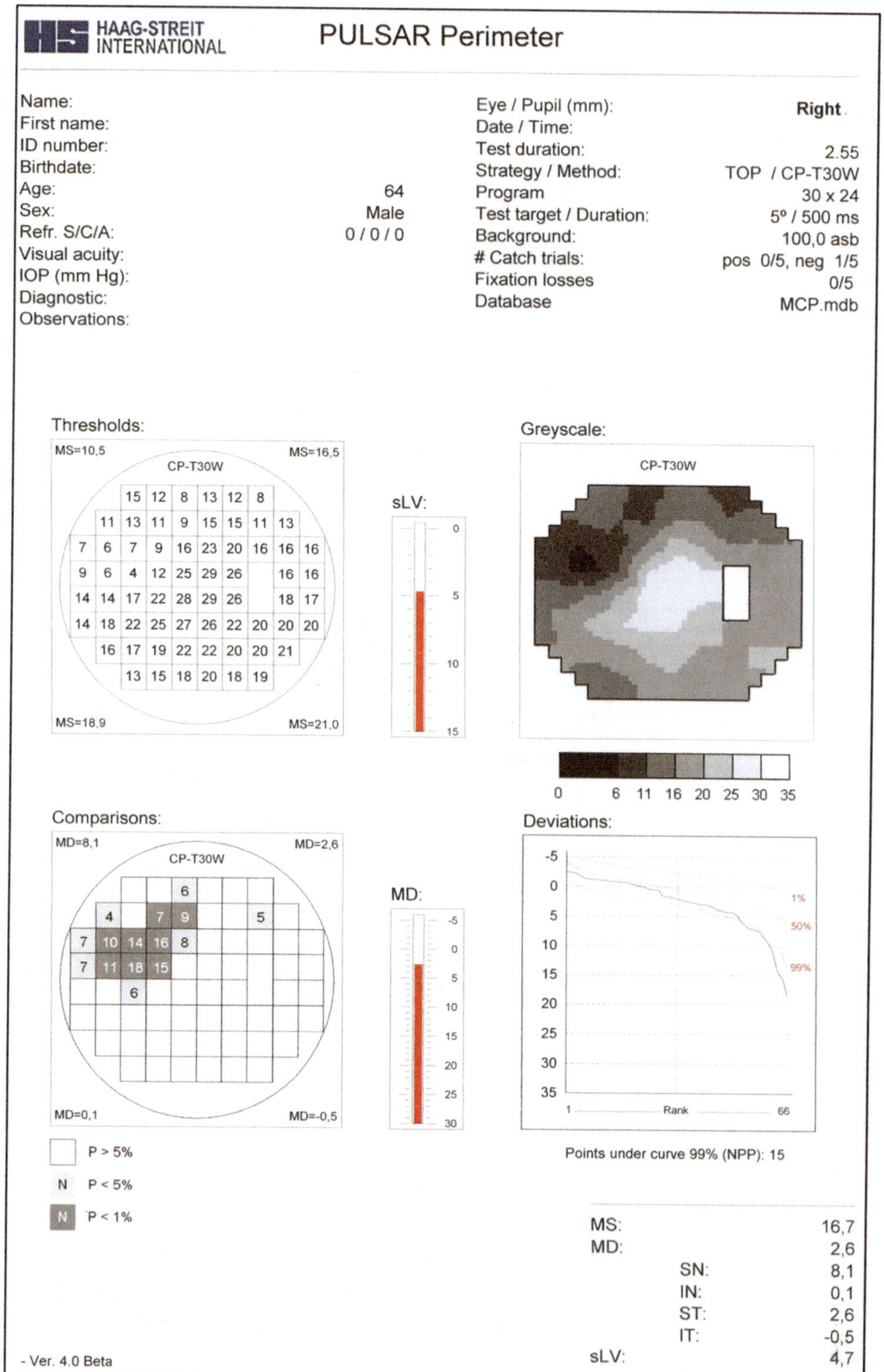

Fig. 60.16: An example of a superior partial arcuate deficit that was obtained with pulsar perimetry.

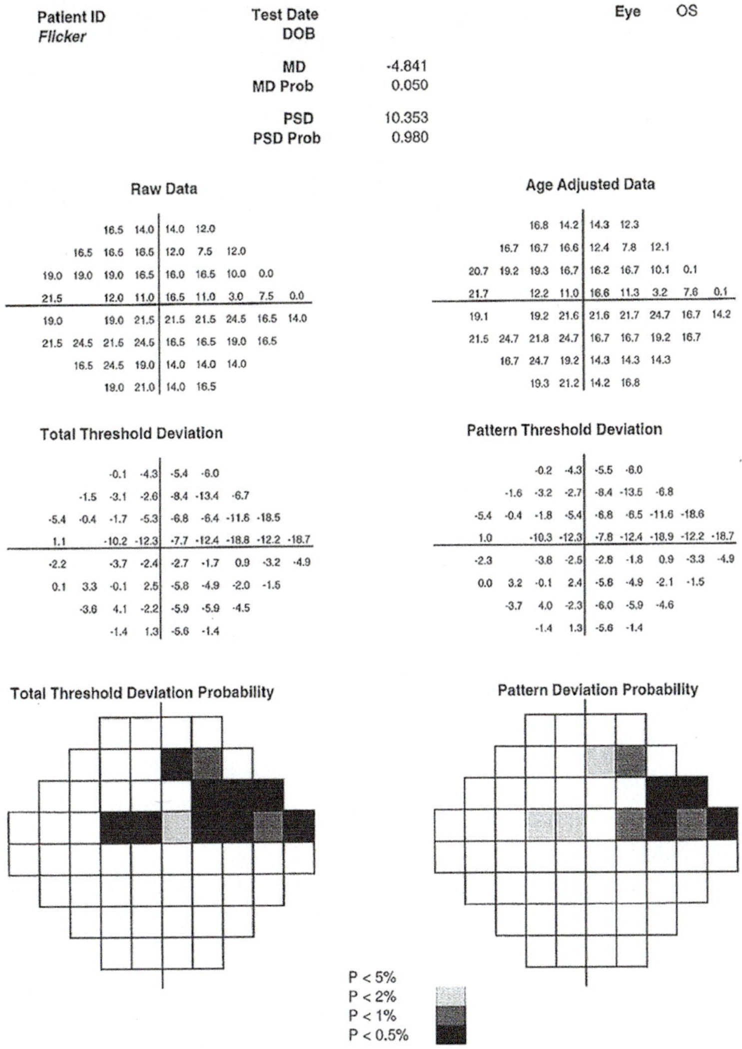

Fig. 60.17: An example of a superior arcuate visual field deficit (same eye as in Figures 60.14 and 60.15) that was obtained with temporal modulation perimetry, a form of flicker perimetry.

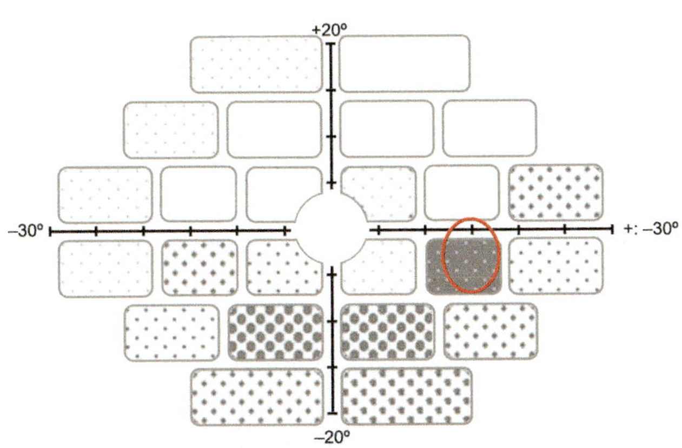

Fig. 60.18: An example of an inferior arcuate deficit that was obtained with Rarebit perimetry testing.

field testing that can be utilized on a tablet or with virtual reality goggles.[42-45] The initial results of these approaches have been quite promising and suggest that this innovative approach may represent a shift in the manner in which this diagnostic test procedure will be used in the near future. The possibility of testing multiple individuals at the same time prior to being seen by a practitioner, storing and retrieving test results from a server, and performing automated analysis and interpretation of results appears to be a viable alternative. Moreover, the portability and use of battery operated instruments opens up the opportunity for accessing a much greater population of individuals who may have limited access to health care and eye examinations. Figure 60.19 presents an example of a glaucomatous visual field deficit for a tablet-based visual field screening test.

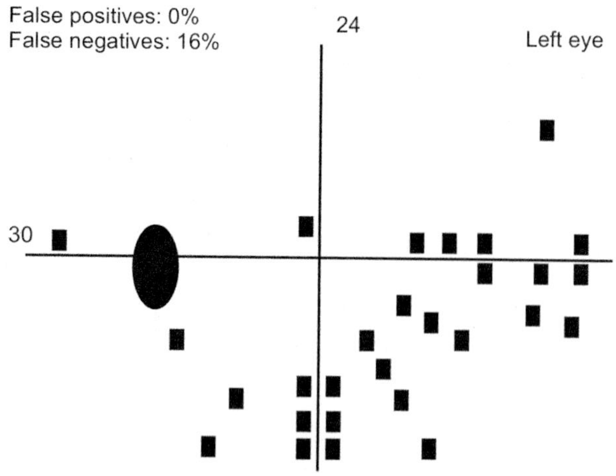

Fig. 60.19: An example of an inferior arcuate visual field deficit that was obtained in a patient with glaucoma who was evaluated with the visual fields easy test on an Apple iPad tablet.

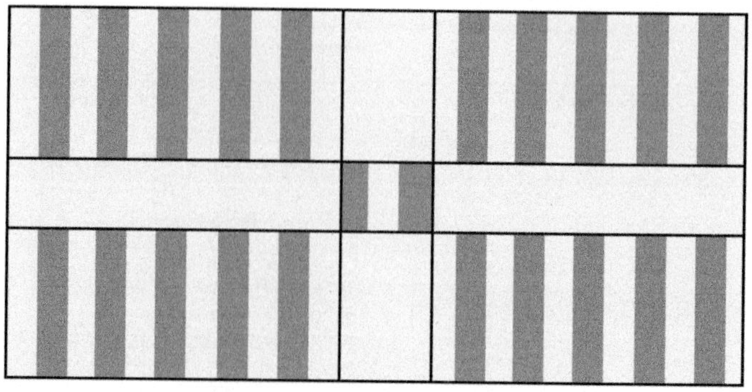

Fig. 60.20: A representation of the patterns used to test contrast sensitivity for the computer-based Spaeth/Richman Contrast Sensitivity (SPARCS) test.

CONTRAST SENSITIVITY

Recently, there has been interest in the measurement of central and peripheral contrast sensitivity in glaucoma patients. Several different procedures for assessing contrast sensitivity have been employed, including variable contrast letters, gray bars of varying contrast, and sinusoidal gratings. In general, contrast sensitivity has been found to be a useful diagnostic procedure for evaluation of glaucoma in that it is correlates with structural deficits, is an important component of face recognition and other object identification tasks related to quality of life and activities of daily living.[46-48] Recently, Gupta and colleagues[48] have performed contrast sensitivity measures for vertical stripes at five locations in the central visual field (Fig. 60.20) and have determined that it is a useful procedure for detecting glaucomatous visual field damage.

ELECTROPHYSIOLOGY

Visual fields and other psychophysical tests are subjective and require proper attention, cooperation and reliability on the part of the patient. A more objective assessment of the integrity of the visual pathways can be attained through evaluating the electrical properties of the visual system. Assessment of the photoreceptors, inner retinal layers and retinal ganglion cells can be achieved through various forms of the electroretinogram (ERG), while the optic nerve and more central portions of the visual pathways can be evaluated with the visual evoked potential (VEP). Localized visual field regions can be assessed through the use of multifocal procedures for the ERG [multifocal ERG (mfERG)] and VEP (multifocal VEP (mfVEP)].[49,50]

The ERG is recorded from the surface of the eye by means of a piggyback contact lens (Burian-Allen) electrode or by skin electrodes placed near the eye, in response to multiple flashes of light or a rapidly alternating black and white pattern (checkerboard or stripes).[49] The normal dark-adapted ERG consists of a negative deflection of the electrical potential known as the A-wave (rod photoreceptors activity), followed by a positive deflection known as the B-wave (inner retinal activity). A higher frequency of alterations on the B-wave are called oscillatory potentials (OPs) and reflect the activity of inner retinal amacrine cells. The photopic ERG is similar and reflects the activity of the cone-dominated system, with faster and more peaked A- and B-waves. Several variations of the ERG are of importance to glaucoma assessment:

- The photopic negative response (PhNR), which is a slow negative component of the ERG that occurs after the B-wave. The PhNR reflects the activity of the retinal ganglion cells which receive input from the cone receptors connecting to cone bipolar cells that project the retinal ganglion cells. The PhNR has been reported to be degraded by early glaucomatous damage.[49]
- The pattern ERG (PERG), which measures retinal electrical activity in response to a rapidly alternating light and dark checkerboard or stripe pattern. The PERG has been reported to be sensitive to early glaucomatous damage and to be able to detect abnormalities up to 4 years before a visual field deficit is present.[49]
- The mfERG, which records the response to a rapidly alternating checkerboard pattern that alters its appearance according to a modified M-sequence that produces a delay in the stimulus alternation pattern

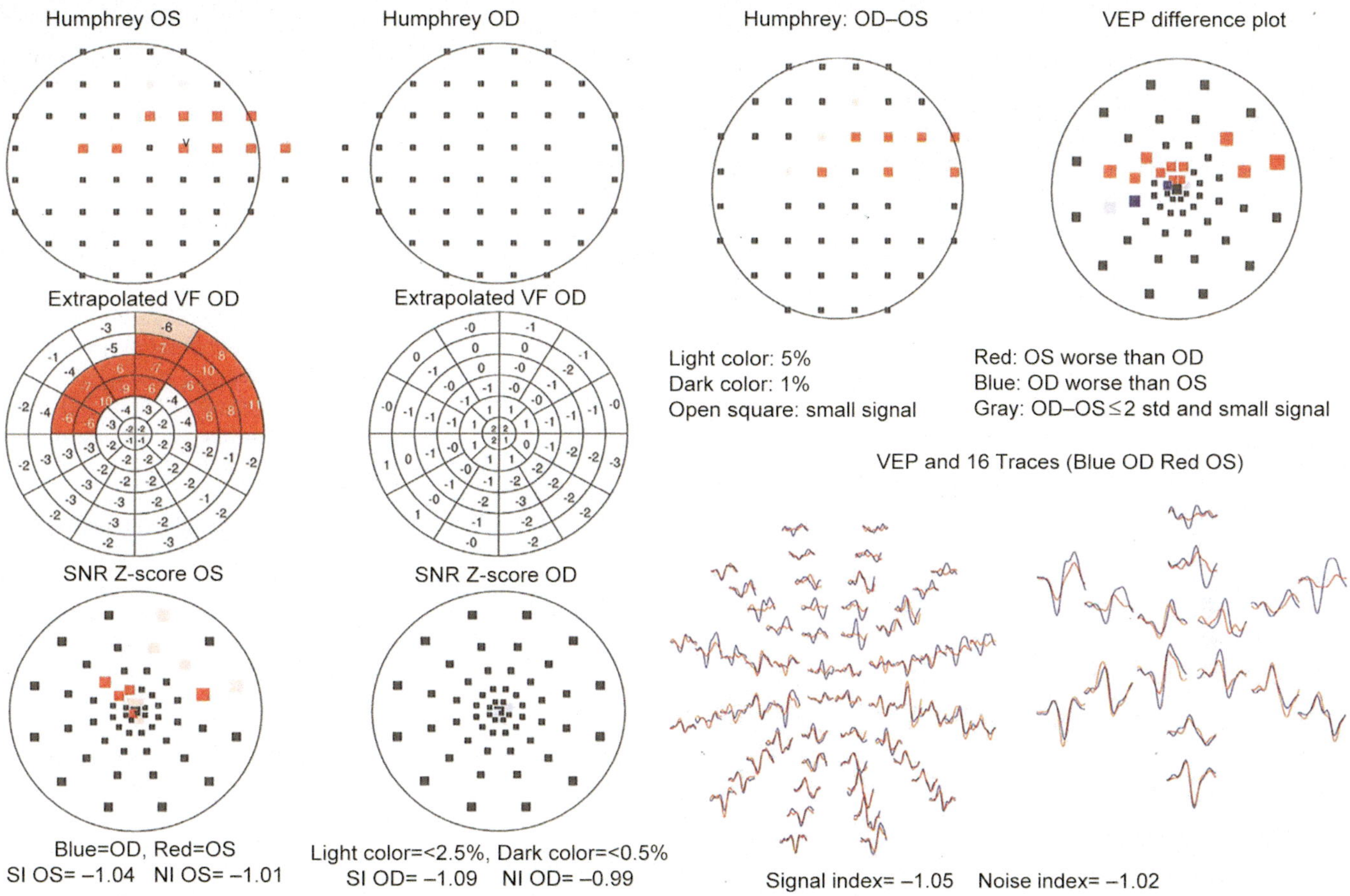

Fig. 60.21: Multifocal visual evoked potential (mfVEP) results for the left and right eyes of a patient with a superior arcuate visual field loss in the left eye.

for various visual field locations. By mathematically deconstructing the resulting continuous ERG waveform, it is possible to obtain the nonlinear components of the ERG to obtain individual waveforms for a number of visual field locations. The current version of the mfERG is time-consuming and difficult to extract and quantify, which limits its diagnostic value,[49] but refinement of this procedure may yield useful diagnostic information in the future.

The VEP is recorded with electrodes placed at the back of the head at or slightly above or below the inion to obtain the electrical activity of the occipital cortex in response to flashes of light or a rapidly alternating pattern (checkerboard or stripes).[50] The main components of the normal VEP consist of a negative deflection at about 70 ms (N70) and a positive deflection at about 100 ms (P100). The amplitude and latency of the N70 and P1000 waveforms are the primary components that are evaluated. The mfVEP is similar to the mfERG, except that the checkerboard stimulus pattern is scaled to account for the cortical magnification factor (i.e. central checks are small and peripheral checks are progressively larger). The mfVEP correlates well with conventional automated perimetry results, but it is not quite as sensitive and it is difficult to obtain signals from visual field areas with large amounts of visual field loss.[50] Figure 60.21 presents an example of mfVEP results for the left and right eyes of a patient with glaucoma in the left eye, as well as the asymmetry in response between corresponding visual field areas of the right and left eyes.

CONCLUSION

It is difficult to present a thorough and comprehensive overview of visual field interpretation within a limited space, but it is hoped that this chapter will provide you with the appropriate tools to allow you to select proper visual field test procedures, assess the quality and reliability of the results, and properly interpret them. The “cookbook” for visual field interpretation will provide you with guidelines that can be successfully applied for the vast majority of cases, but also keep in mind that there will always be exceptions to the rule. Also, it is very important to remember that perimetry and visual field testing are but a portion of the many pieces that comprise a comprehensive clinical examination, and the findings should be incorporated into the composite assessment of the patient, including a thorough patient history and an interactive communication with the individual. It is most important to be a good listener and ask appropriate questions. Finally, we realize that this diagnostic test procedure is a moving target, and what is the standard of care for perimetry today may change in the future.

ACKNOWLEDGMENT

I am deeply indebted to Mrs Patricia Duffel for her wonderful assistance in preparing the figures for this chapter.

REFERENCES

1. Johnson CA, Wall M, Thompson HS. A history of perimetry and visual field testing. Optom Vis Sci. 2011;88:E8-15.
2. Camp AS, Weinreb RN. Will perimetry be performed to monitor glaucoma in 2025? Ophthalmology. 2017;124(12S):S71-5.
3. Abe RY, Diniz-Filho A, Costa VP, et al. Predicting vision-related disability in glaucoma. Ophthalmology. 2018;125: 22-30.
4. Kasneci E, Black AA, Wood JM. Eye-tracking as a tool to evaluate functional ability in everyday tasks in glaucoma. J Ophthalmol. 2017;2017:6425913.
5. Ramulu PY, Hochberg C, Maul EA, et al. Glaucomatous visual field loss associated with less travel from home. Optom Vis Sci. 2014;91:187-93.
6. Kulkarni KM, Mayer JR, Lorenzana LL, et al. Visual field staging systems in glaucoma and the activities of daily living. Am J Ophthalmol. 2012;154:445-51.
7. Wall M, Johnson CA. Principles and techniques of the examination of the visual sensory system. In: Miller NR, Newman NJ, Walsh FB, Hoyt WF (Eds). Walsh and Hoyt's Clinical Neuro-Ophthalmology. Philadelphia: Lippincott, Williams and Wilkins; 2005. pp. 83-149.
8. Artes PH, Henson DB, Harper R, et al. Multisampling suprathreshold perimetry: a comparison with conventional suprathreshold and full threshold strategies by computer simulation. Invest Ophthalmol Vis Sci. 2003;44(6):2582-7.
9. Henson DB. Visual field screening and the development of a new screening program. J Am Optom Assoc. 1989;60:893-8.
10. Anderson DR. Perimetry With and Without Automation. St. Louis: CV Mosby; 1987.
11. Anderson DR. Testing the Field of Vision. St. Louis: CV Mosby; 1982.
12. Anderson DR, Patella VM. Automated Static Perimetry. St. Louis: CV Mosby; 1998.
13. Racette L, Fischer M, Bebie H, et al. Visual Field Digest: A Guide to Perimetry and the Octopus Perimeter. Switzerland: Haag-Streit AG; 2016.
14. Brusini P, Johnson CA. Staging functional damage in glaucoma: review of different classification methods. Surv Ophthalmol. 2007;52:156-79.
15. Spry PG, Johnson CA. Identification of progressive glaucomatous visual field loss. Surv Ophthalmol. 2002;47:158-73.
16. Vesti E, Johnson CA, Chauhan BC. Comparison of different methods for detecting glaucomatous visual field progression. Invest Ophthalmol Vis Sci. 2003;44:3873-9.
17. Hollo G. Influence of test strategy on Octopus perimeter cluster mean defect values: adaptive bracketing normal strategy versus tendency-oriented perimetry. J Glaucoma. 2016;25:830-4.
18. Bryan SR, Eilers PH, Rosmalen JV, et al. Bayesian hierarchical modeling of longitudinal glaucomatous visual fields using a two-stage approach. Statist Med. 2017;36:1735-53.
19. Johnson CA. Psychophysical and electrophysiological testing in glaucoma: visual fields and other functional tests. In: Choplin N, Traverso C (Eds). Atlas of Glaucoma, 3rd edition. London: CRC Press; 2014. pp. 87-112.
20. Johnson CA. Detecting functional changes in the patient's vision: visual field analysis. In: Samples JR, Schacknow PN (Eds). Clinical Glaucoma Care: The Essentials. New York, NY: Springer; 2013. pp. 117-59.
21. Humphrey Field Analyzer 2i55 User Manual. Dublin, California: Carl Zeiss Meditec; 2010.
22. Keltner JL, Johnson CA, Cello KE, et al. Classification of visual field abnormalities in the ocular hypertension treatment study. Arch Ophthalmol. 2003;121:643-50.
23. Johnson CA. Diagnostic value of short wavelength automated perimetry. Curr Opin Ophthalmol. 1996;7:54-8.
24. Johnson, CA, Adams AJ, Casson EJ, et al. Progression of early glaucomatous visual field loss for blue-on-yellow and standard white-on-white automated perimetry. Arch Ophthalmol. 1993;111:651-6.
25. Racette L, Sample PA. Short-wavelength automated perimetry. Ophthalmol Clin North Am. 2003;16:227-36.
26. Sit AJ, Medeiros FA, Weinreb RN. Short-wavelength automated perimetry can predict glaucomatous standard visual field loss by ten years. Semin Ophthalmol. 2004;19:122-4.
27. Bengtsson B, Heijl A. Diagnostic sensitivity of fast blue-yellow and standard automated perimetry in early glaucoma: a comparison between different algorithms. Ophthalmology. 2006;113(7):1092-7.
28. van der Schoot J, Reus NJ, Colen TP, et al. The ability of short-wavelength automated perimetry to predict conversion to glaucoma. Ophthalmology. 2010;117(1):30-4.
29. Anderson AJ, Johnson CA. Frequency doubling technology perimetry. In: Sample PA, Girkin CA (Eds). Ophthalmology Clinics of North America. Philadelphia: WB Saunders; 2003. pp. 213-25.

30. Anderson AJ, Johnson CA, Fingeret M, et al. Characteristics of the normative database for the Humphrey Matrix perimeter. Invest Ophthalmol Vis Sci. 2005;46:1540-8.
31. Huang, C, Carolan J, Redline D, et al. Humphrey Matrix frequency doubling perimetry for neuro-ophthalmic disorders of the optic nerve and chiasm: comparison with Humphrey SITA Standard 24-2. Invest Ophthalmol Vis Sci. 2008;49:917-23.
32. Tavarati P, Woodward K, Keltner J, et al. Sensitivity and specificity of the Humphrey Matrix to detect homonymous hemianopsias. Invest Ophthalmol Vis Sci. 2008;49:924-8.
33. Meira-Freitas D, Tatham AJ, Lisboa R, et al. Predicting progression of glaucoma from rates of frequency doubling technology perimetry change. Ophthalmology. 2014;121:498-507.
34. Quinn LM, Wheeler DT, Gardiner SK, et al. Frequency doubling technology (FDT) perimetry in normal children. Am J Ophthalmol. 2006;142:983-9.
35. Zeppieri M, Brusini P, Parisi L, et al. Pulsar perimetry in the diagnosis of early glaucoma. Am J Ophthalmol. 2010;149:102-12.
36. Salvatet ML, Zeppieri M, Parisi L, et al. Learning effect and test-retest variability of Pulsar perimetry. J Glaucoma. 2013;22:230-7.
37. Yoshiyama KK, Johnson CA. Which method of flicker perimetry is most effective for detection of glaucomatous visual field loss? Invest Ophthalmol Vis Sci. 1997;38:2270-7.
38. Anderson AJ, Vingrys AJ. Effect of eccentricity on luminance-pedestal flicker thresholds. Vision Res. 2002;42(9):1149-56.
39. Casson E, Johnson CA, Shapiro LR. A longitudinal comparison of temporal modulation perimetry to white-on-white and blue-on-yellow perimetry in ocular hypertension and early glaucoma. J Opt Soc Am. 1993;10:1792-806.
40. Frisen L. New, sensitive window on abnormal spatial vision: Rarebit probing. Vision Res. 2002;42:1931-99.
41. Hackett DA, Anderson AJ. Determining mechanisms of visual loss in glaucoma using Rarebit perimetry. Optom Vision Sci. 2011;88:48-55.
42. Johnson CA, Thapa S, George Kong YX, et al. Visual field screening in Nepal using an iPad application to detect moderate and advanced visual impairment. Am J Ophthalmol. 2017;182:147-54.
43. Vingrys AJ, Healey JL, Liew S, et al. Validation of a tablet as a tangent perimeter. Transl Vis Sci Technol. 2016;5(4):3.
44. Kong YX, He M, Crowston JG, et al. A comparison of perimetric results from a tablet perimeter and Humphrey field analyzer in glaucoma patients. Transl Vis Sci Technol. 2016;5(6):2.
45. Wroblewski D, Francis BA, Sadun A, et al. Testing of visual field with virtual reality goggles in manual and visual grasp modes. Biomed Res Int. 2014;2014:206082.
46. Richman J, Zangalli C, Lu L, et al. The Spaeth/Richman contrast sensitivity test (SPARCS): design, reproducibility and ability to identify patients with glaucoma. Br J Ophthalmol. 2015;99:16-20.
47. Ekici F, Loh R, Waisbourd M, et al. Relationships between measures of the ability to perform vision-related activities, vision-related quality of life, and clinical findings in patients with glaucoma. JAMA Ophthalmol. 2015;133:1377-85.
48. Gupta L, Cvintal V, Delvadia R, et al. SPARCS and Pelli-Robson contrast sensitivity testing in normal controls and patients with cataract. Eye (Lond). 2017;31:753-61.
49. Wilsey LJ, Fortune B. Electroretinography in glaucoma diagnosis. Curr Opin Ophthalmol. 2016;27(2):118-24.
50. Hood DC, Greenstein VC. Multifocal VEP and ganglion cell damage: applications and limitations for the study of glaucoma. Prog Retin Eye Res. 2003;22:201-51.

Chapter 61

Optic Nerve Head and Retinal Nerve Fiber Layer Imaging in the Diagnosis and Management of Glaucoma

Harsha L Rao, Zia S Pradhan, Narendra K Puttaiah

INTRODUCTION

Glaucoma is a chronic progressive optic neuropathy with characteristic optic nerve head (ONH) and retinal nerve fiber layer (RNFL) changes. Clinical examination of the ONH and RNFL is routinely done using a slit-lamp biomicroscope and a high-powered convex lens. Although detecting glaucoma by this method is fairly simple in moderate and severe stages of the disease, identification of subtle ONH and RNFL changes in early glaucoma requires training and experience. Another method of detecting glaucoma is evaluation of optic disk stereophotographs. Both these methods, however, are subjective, and the agreement even among glaucoma experts in detecting glaucomatous changes is far from excellent. The other major drawback of these methods is that changes can only be qualitatively assessed but cannot be quantified. These limitations are overcome by ONH and RNFL imaging which is objective and reproducibly quantifies certain parameters that are used to inform the management decisions.

The three imaging technologies that are commercially available for detecting glaucomatous damage are the confocal scanning laser ophthalmoscopy (CSLO), scanning laser polarimetry (SLP), and the optical coherence tomography (OCT).

1. CSLO utilizes confocal optics to obtain multiple sections of the ONH, from the anterior retinal surface to the lamina cribrosa, which are then reconstructed in three dimensions to provide several optic cup- and neuroretinal rim-based measurements.
2. SLP utilizes the birefringent property of the RNFL and measures the retardation of a polarized light beam as it traverses the RNFL, which is then mathematically converted to thickness.
3. OCT uses low-coherence interferometry to determine the echo time delay and the magnitude of backscattered light reflected off the ONH and retinal layers to generate cross-sectional scans through the tissue layers. OCT technology has evolved from time-domain OCT (TD-OCT) to spectral-domain OCT (SD-OCT) which is faster and provides greater resolution (axial resolution of 5 μm). Also, TD-OCT imaging was two-dimensional (line scans for the ONH and circle scans for the RNFL) while SD-OCT scans a 3-dimension cube over a large area covering the ONH. This leads to acquisition of more data and hence less interpolation, resulting in better accuracy and reproducibility.

The wide variability of the optic disk size and neuroretinal rim contour in the normal population limits the usefulness of ONH parameters alone in glaucoma diagnosis and clinical studies have shown these (as measured with CSLO) to have lower sensitivities as compared to RNFL parameters (measured with SLP).[1] Hypothetically, disruption of axonal microtubules (measured as RNFL retardance using SLP) can precede axonal loss (measured as RNFL thickness using OCT); however, longitudinal clinical studies have not shown SLP to bear this advantage and OCT was found to be superior at identification of glaucomatous change.[2] Therefore, for all these reasons, CSLO (which primarily evaluates the ONH) and SLP (which evaluates the RNFL) have been superseded by OCT which has the ability to image both, the ONH and the RNFL, in a single scan. All discussions in this chapter will be restricted to SD-OCT imaging of the ONH and RNFL. The three more commonly used SD-OCT devices include the RTVue (Optovue Inc; Fremont, CA), the Cirrus high-definition OCT (HD-OCT) (Zeiss Meditec; Dublin, CA), and the Spectralis SD-OCT (Heidelberg Engineering; Heidelberg, Germany).

OPTIC NERVE HEAD IMAGING

Optic nerve head analysis with SD-OCT is performed by automated software. Different manufacturers of SD-OCT devices have their own proprietary softwares for ONH analysis, which vary slightly from each other. A brief description of the automated ONH analysis performed in commonly used SD-OCT devices is important to understand the differences between the reported measurements.

The software in Cirrus HD-OCT identifies the termination of Bruch's membrane as the disk margin

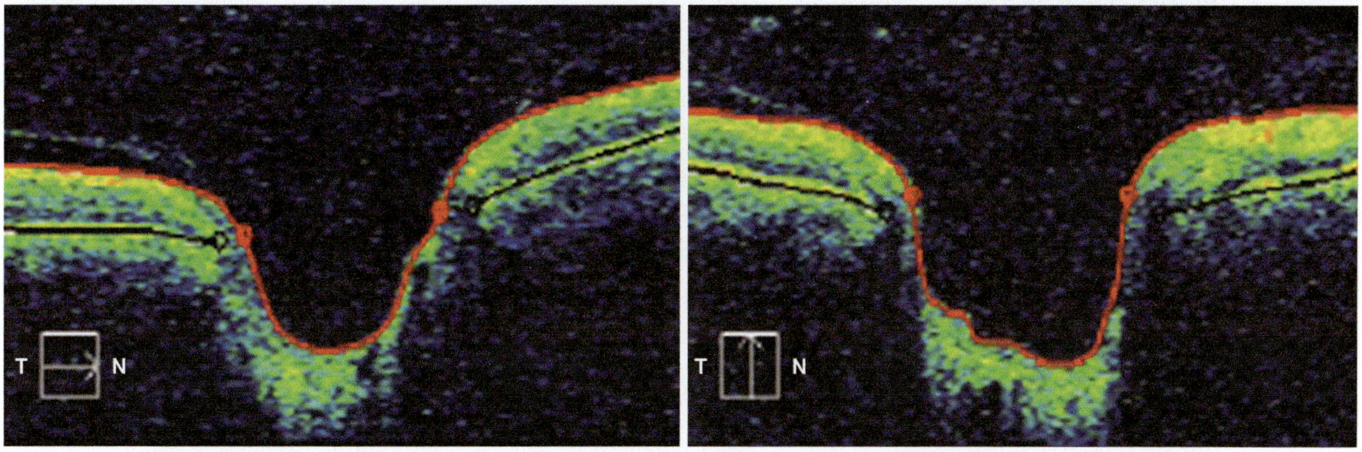

Fig. 61.1: Segmentation of the optic nerve head on Cirrus high-definition optical coherence tomography (HD-OCT) software. Open black circles represent the termination of Bruch's membrane and the red circles represent the demarcation between rim and cup.

from the three-dimensional data set. The software then generates a set of vectors from the disk margin to points on the vitreoretinal interface for each radial direction and calculates a trapezoidal, cross-sectional area associated with each vector. For each point on the disk margin, the vector that produces the minimum cross-sectional area is identified and each of these vectors is geometrically transformed into the plane of the optic disk to provide a two-dimensional representation of the three-dimensional data acquired by the imaging software. In this manner, the cup margin is defined by a set of optimal vectors and the neuroretinal rim area is calculated as a piecewise sum of the corresponding minimum trapezoidal, cross-sectional areas. One of the difficulties in clinical assessment of the ONH is when the viewing angle of the ophthalmologist is not the same as the ONH axis, for example in tilted disks, where the neuroretinal rim appears foreshortened. The two-dimensional representation of the ONH provided by the Cirrus software is as though the viewing angle is parallel to the ONH axis which minimizes the problem of foreshortening (Fig. 61.1).[3]

The ONH protocol of RTVue consists of 12 radial scans, 3.4 mm in length and 6 concentric ring scans ranging from 2.5 mm to 4.0 mm in diameter all centered on the optic disk. Retinal pigment epithelium (RPE) tips are automatically detected by the software. The RTVue software then delineates the optic disk margin by joining the RPE tips. The optic cup is automatically defined by the software by fitting a plane 150 μm parallel to and above the plane that fits the coordinates of the RPE tips. ONH tissue above the cup line and within the perpendicular lines drawn from the RPE tips to the surface of the retina is considered as the neuroretinal rim (Fig. 61.2).

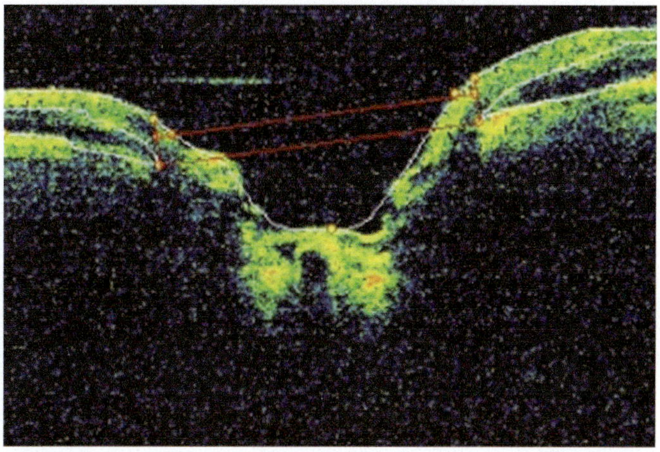

Fig. 61.2: Segmentation of the optic nerve head with RTVue spectral-domain optical coherence tomography (SD-OCT) software. The lower red straight line represents the line connecting the retinal pigment epithelium (RPE) tips and another red line is drawn 150 μm above and parallel to this plane. The optic nerve head (ONH) tissue above the upper red line (between the 3 yellow-colored circles) is defined as the neuroretinal rim tissue.

The software in Spectralis SD-OCT identifies the termination of the Bruch's membrane and delineates the Bruch's membrane opening (BMO) which acts as a surrogate for the disk margin. It subsequently calculates a parameter called minimum rim width (MRW) which is the minimum distance between the BMO line and the surface of the rim tissue (Fig. 61.3).

It is important to remember that the disk parameters of different imaging technologies are dependent on the segmentation performed by the proprietary software and are not necessarily interchangeable with each other. It is also important to note that the OCT-derived ONH parameters are not analogous to those determined by a clinician on the slit-lamp biomicroscopy.

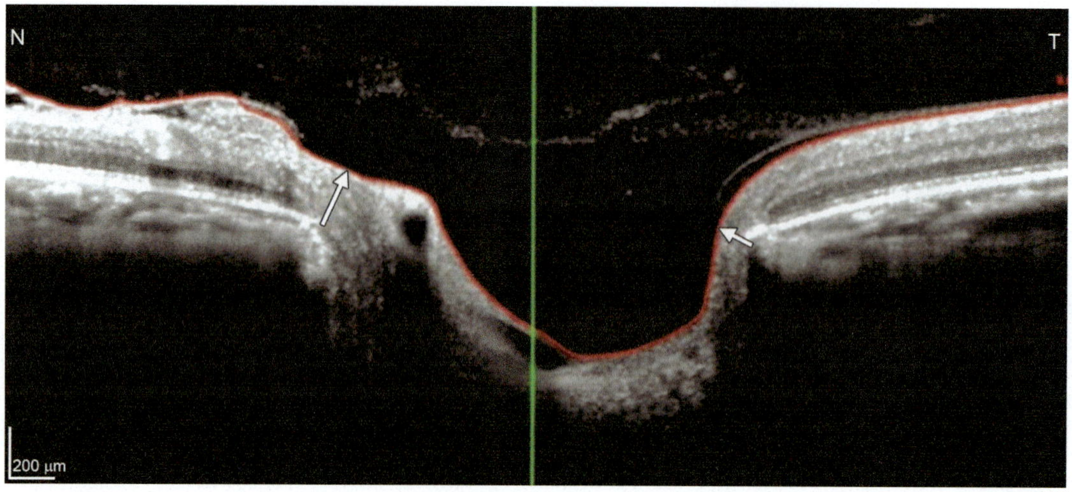

Fig. 61.3: The software in Spectralis spectral-domain optical coherence tomography (SD-OCT) identifies the termination of Bruch's membrane [Bruch's membrane opening (BMO)] as the disk margin. The white arrows represents the minimum rim width (MRW), which is the shortest distance between the BMO and the surface of the rim tissue.

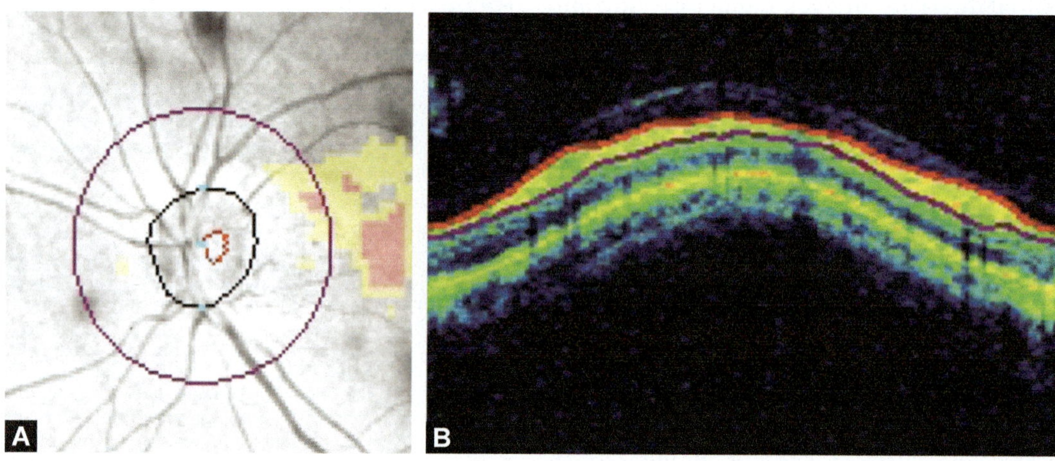

Figs. 61.4A and B: (A) The circle scan along which retinal nerve fiber layer (RNFL) thickness is measured on Cirrus high-definition optical coherence tomography (HD-OCT); (B) The segmentation of RNFL; red line marks the internal limiting membrane and purple line marks the lower border of the RNFL.

RETINAL NERVE FIBER LAYER IMAGING

Like for the ONH, different manufacturers of SD-OCT devices have their own proprietary automated softwares for segmenting the RNFL and measuring its thickness.

Retinal nerve fiber layer thickness on Cirrus HD-OCT is calculated along a circle 3.46 mm in diameter positioned evenly around the center of the optic disk. The calculation circle and the segmentation of RNFL on Cirrus HD-OCT are shown in Figures 61.4A and B. Peripapillary RNFL thickness on RTVue is calculated along a 3.45 mm diameter circle centered on the optic disk. The calculation circle and the segmentation of RNFL on RTVue are shown in Figures 61.5A and B. Spectralis uses fovea-to-disk alignment technology that automatically tracks and aligns circle scans of 3.45 mm diameter to overcome measurement errors due to changing head and/or eye position during scanning. This alignment technology allows accurate comparisons with the normative database to improve the reproducibility of RNFL measurements. The calculation circle and the segmentation of RNFL on Spectralis are shown in Figures 61.6A and B.

Studies have shown that the RNFL thickness values vary between different SD-OCT devices and cannot be used interchangeably.[4,5]

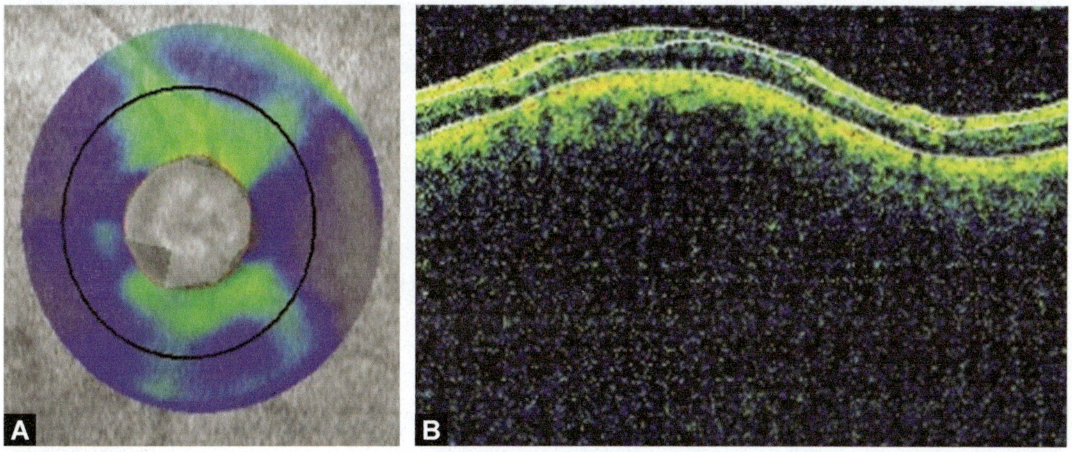

Figs. 61.5A and B: (A) The circle scan along which retinal nerve fiber layer (RNFL) thickness is measured on RTVue spectral-domain optical coherence tomography (SD-OCT); (B) The segmentation of RNFL displayed by the upper two white lines on the B-scan image.

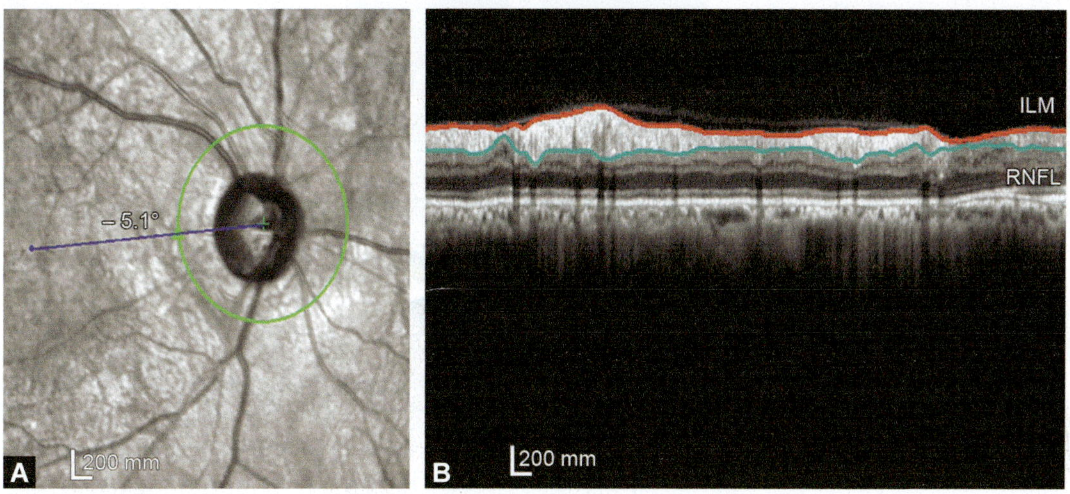

Figs. 61.6A and B: (A) The circle scan (green) along which retinal nerve fiber layer (RNFL) thickness is measured on Spectralis spectral-domain optical coherence tomography (SD-OCT). Note that Spectralis uses FoDi (fovea-to-disk) alignment technology (blue line) to overcome the effect of eye rotation and head tilt on RNFL measurements and to match with alignment of the normative database; (B) The segmentation of RNFL; red line marks the internal limiting membrane (ILM) and blue line marks the lower border of the RNFL.

INTERPRETING THE ONH AND RNFL MEASUREMENTS ON SD-OCT IMAGING IN NORMAL AND GLAUCOMA EYES

Once the ONH and RNFL images are acquired and segmentation performed, the software of the SD-OCT calculates certain ONH and RNFL parameters. All these measurements are then compared with an age-matched reference database within the device to quantify glaucomatous damage and are interpreted either as "within normal limits (color-coded as green)" or "borderline (coded as yellow)" or "outside normal limits (coded as red)". The parameter is coded in green if the subject's measurement falls between the 5th and the 95th percentile values of the reference database (p >5%). The parameter is flagged in yellow if the measurement falls between the 5th percentile and the 1st percentile values (p <5% and p >1%) and "red" if the measurement falls below the lowest one percentile value (p <1%) of the reference database. The following discussion explains the ONH and RNFL imaging results of three of the most commonly used SD-OCT devices.

Figures 61.7A and B show the results of ONH and RNFL imaging performed with Cirrus HD-OCT device in a normal subject (Fig. 61.7A) and a glaucoma patient (Fig. 61.7B). Cirrus HD-OCT provides the following maps that evaluate the RNFL thickness:

1. RNFL thickness map
2. RNFL deviation map

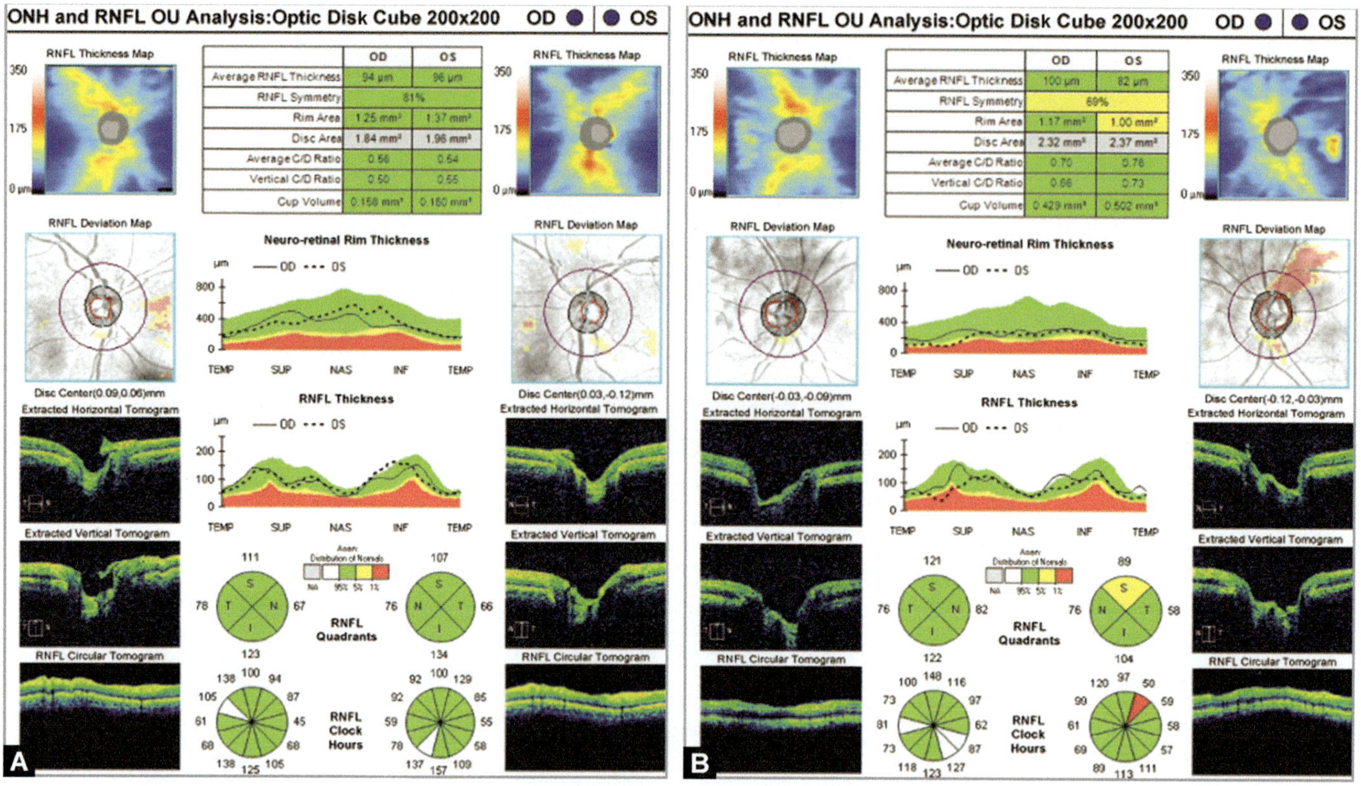

Figs. 61.7A and B: (A) Cirrus HD-OCT printouts of a normal subject; (B) Cirrus HD-OCT printouts of a glaucoma patient.
(RNFL: Retinal nerve fiber layer; OCT: Optical coherence tomography; ONH: Optic nerve head; HD-OCT: High-definition optical coherence tomography)

3. RNFL quadrant/clock hour sector map
4. Temporal-superior-nasal-inferior-temporal (TSNIT) profile map.

The RNFL thickness map is derived from average thickness measurements at pixels (each pixel is a 30 µm square along an A-scan) and reports the RNFL thickness using a color pattern, where cool colors (blues and greens) represent thinner measurements and warm colors (yellows and reds) represent thicker measurements.

The RNFL deviation map is derived from a statistical comparison between the measured average RNFL thickness and the age-matched normal thickness range from the reference database for each superpixel (16 pixels are combined in a 4 × 4 square to form a superpixel), over the entire scanned area. These maps apply the yellow and red colors to superpixels whose average thickness falls in the 1st to 5th percentile and less than 1st percentile of the normal reference database respectively.

The RNFL quadrant and clock hour map reports average thickness along the RNFL calculation circle by quadrants (90° sector) and clock hours (30° sector). Each measurement is color-coded according to its comparison to the age-matched RNFL reference database.

The TSNIT thickness profile displays RNFL thickness at each A-scan location along the calculation circle. TSNIT profile is also compared to the age-matched RNFL reference database and color-coded. Another TSNIT thickness profile displays the neuroretinal rim thickness of the optic disk. The left and right eye RNFL and neuroretinal rim thickness profiles are also showed together to enable comparison of symmetry in specific regions.

In addition to the above maps, the printout of Cirrus HD-OCT also shows a few summary parameters of RNFL and ONH measurements in the tabular form (as shown in Figs. 61.7A and B). These summary parameters are also color-coded according to the reference database classification.

Compared to a normal eye, glaucomatous eye imaged on Cirrus HD-OCT shows:

- Cool colors on the RNFL thickness map showing thinning of RNFL
- Red and yellow regions on the deviation map corresponding to the regions of RNFL thinning
- Reduction of RNFL thickness measurements in quadrant and clock hour maps which are color-coded in red or yellow

- TSNIT profile map showing the RNFL and neuroretinal rim thickness graph falling in the red or yellow shaded region at corresponding locations around the disk
- Reduction in the parameter measurements in the summary table, which is color coded in yellow or red.

With Cirrus HD-OCT, RNFL thickness maps are reported to provide better ability to detect abnormalities in RNFL compared to the deviation and the clock hour maps in early glaucoma.[6]

Figures 61.8A and B show the results of ONH and RNFL imaging performed with the RTVue SD-OCT device in a normal subject (Fig. 61.8A) and a glaucoma patient (Fig. 61.8B). The printout, in addition to the B-scans at the disk, RNFL thickness calculation circle and the RNFL segmentation at the calculation circle, shows:

- RNFL thickness map with RNFL thickness in eight sectors
- RNFL quadrant map
- TSNIT profile graph
- Table with a few summary parameters.

All thickness parameters, similar to that seen in Cirrus HD-OCT, are color-coded according to the reference database classification.

Compared to a normal eye, glaucomatous eye imaged on RTVue SD-OCT shows:

- Cool colors (blue) on the RNFL thickness map showing thinning of RNFL
- Reduction of RNFL thickness in quadrant maps and the eight sectors around the thickness map which are color-coded in red or yellow
- TSNIT profile map showing the RNFL thickness falling in the red- or yellow-shaded region at corresponding locations around the disk
- Reduction in the summary parameters in the tables which are color-coded in yellow or red.

Figures 61.9A and B show the results of RNFL imaging performed with the Spectralis SD-OCT device in a normal subject (Fig. 61.9A) and a glaucoma subject (Fig. 61.9B). The printout, in addition to the RNFL thickness calculation circle and the RNFL segmentation around the calculation circle, shows:

- TSNIT profile graph
- RNFL quadrant/six, sector map.

The TSNIT profile graph displays the RNFL thickness profile measured along the circular scan and, as in other SD-OCT devices, is color-coded after comparing with the age-matched reference database.

The calculation circle is divided into four quadrants and six sectors separately, and average RNFL thickness is reported for each of these zones. Each value is compared against the reference database and color-coded as in the other SD-OCT devices. The color-coding of the bar below the sector map indicates the overall classification.

Compared to a normal eye, glaucomatous eye imaged on Spectralis SD-OCT shows:

1. Reduction of RNFL thickness in quadrant and sector maps which are color-coded in red or yellow
2. TSNIT profile map showing the RNFL thickness falling in the red- or yellow-shaded region at the corresponding locations around the disk.

Figures 61.10A and B show the results of ONH imaging performed with the Spectralis SD-OCT device in a normal subject (Fig. 61.10A) and a glaucoma patient (Fig. 61.10B).

The printout, in addition to the BMO and MRW at 16 locations on the ONH, shows:

- MRW sector map
- TSNIT profile graph of MRW.

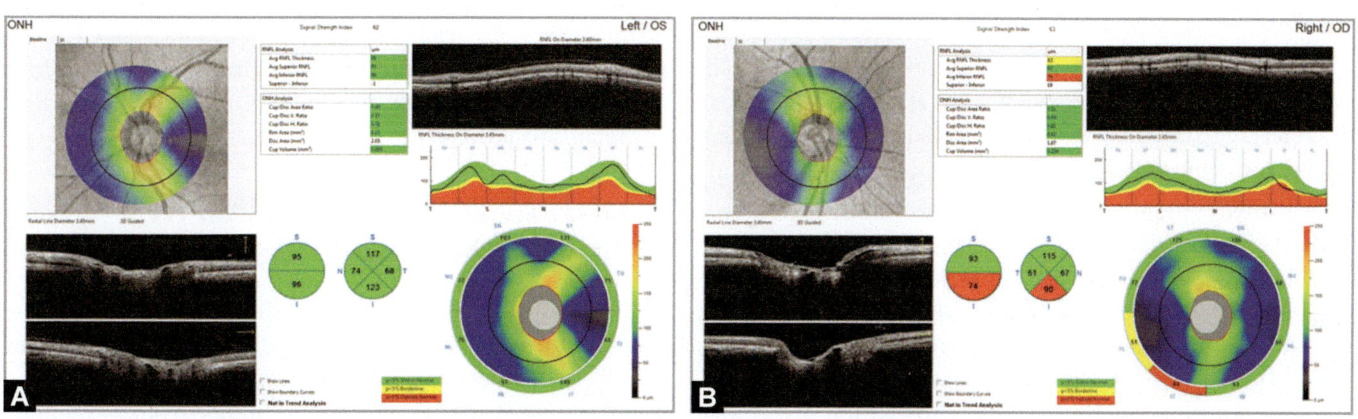

Figs. 61.8A and B: (A) RTVue SD-OCT printouts of a normal subject; (B) RTVue SD-OCT printouts of a glaucoma patient.
(SD-OCT: Spectral-domain optical coherence tomography; ONH: Optic nerve head)

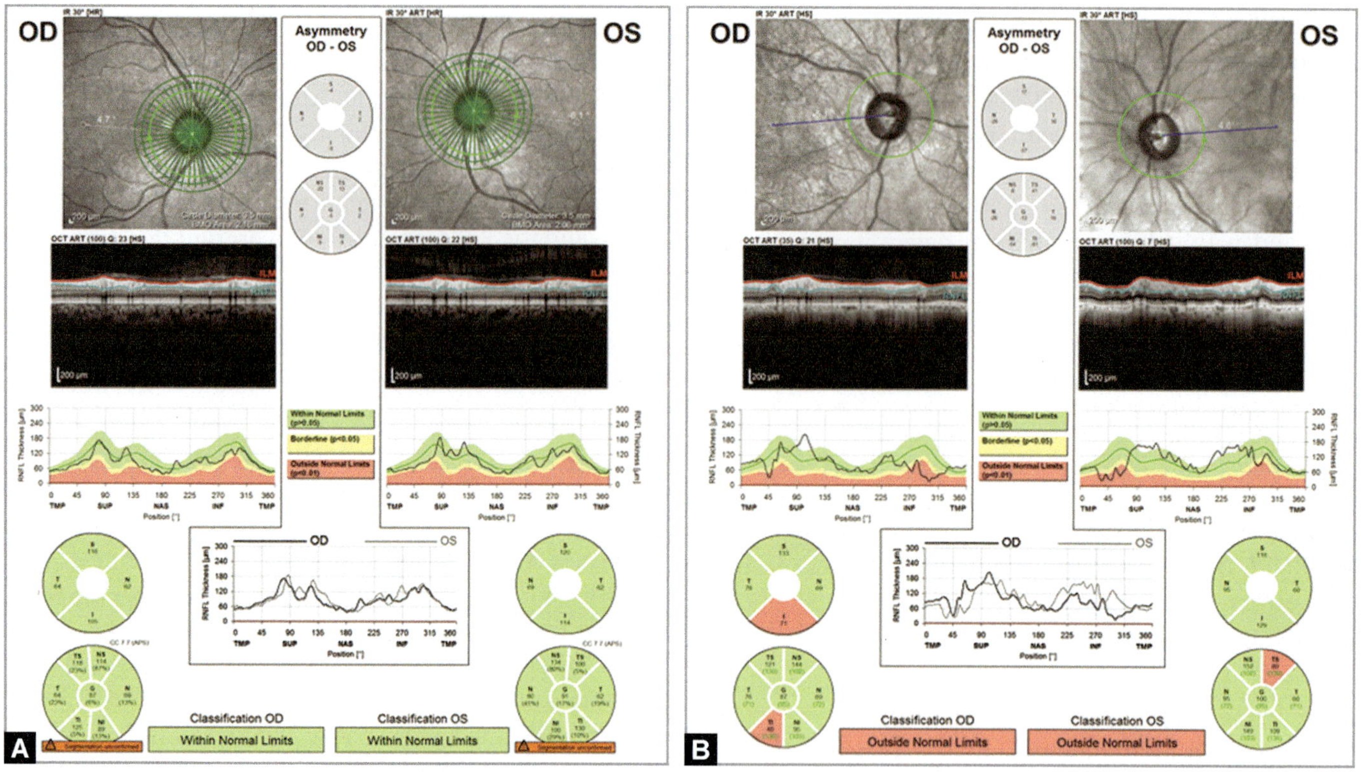

Figs. 61.9A and B: Spectralis spectral-domain optical coherence tomography (SD-OCT) retinal nerve fiber layer (RNFL) printouts (A) of a normal subject; and (B) of a glaucoma patient.

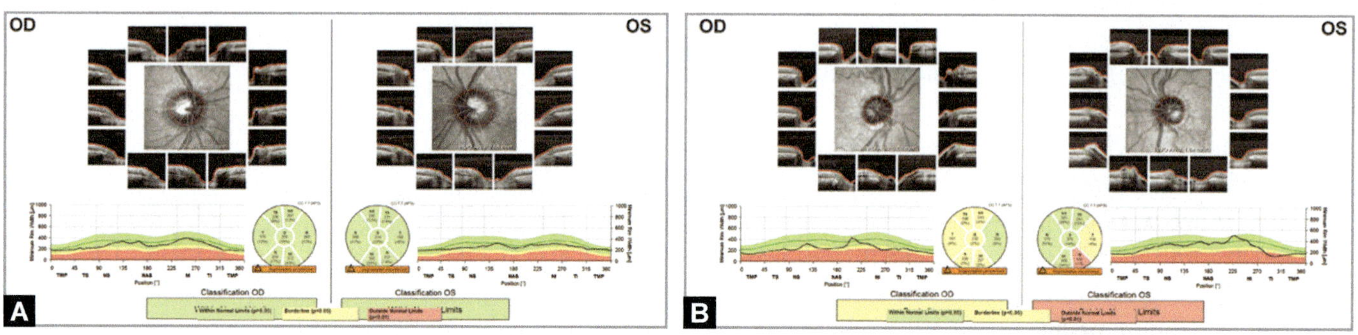

Figs. 61.10A and B: Spectralis spectral-domain optical coherence tomography (SD-OCT) optic nerve head (ONH) printouts (A) of a normal subject; and (B) of a glaucoma patient.

The MRW sector map reports the average MRW in six sectors of ONH separately. Each value is compared against the reference database and color-coded. The color-coding of the bar below the sector map indicates the overall classification.

The TSNIT profile graph displays the MRW profile measured around the ONH and is color-coded after comparing with age-matched reference database.

Compared to a normal eye, glaucomatous eye imaged on Spectralis SD-OCT, shows:

- Reduction of MRW in sector maps which are color-coded in red or yellow
- MRW TSNIT profile map showing the MRW falling in the red- or yellow-shaded region at corresponding locations around the disk.

ONH AND RNFL IMAGING IN GLAUCOMA DIAGNOSIS

Multiple studies have evaluated the ability of ONH and RNFL parameters of SD-OCT in differentiating glaucoma eyes from normal eyes. A Cochrane review of these studies found the ONH and RNFL measurements to have excellent abilities to diagnose glaucoma.[7] It is this ability of imaging modalities to quantify early structural glaucomatous defects prior to the development of visual field defects that led to the term "preperimetric glaucoma".

The RNFL imaging has been found to be especially useful in eyes with suspicious optic disks and normal visual fields. Figures 61.11A to C show an eye with a glaucomatous optic disk (showing neuroretinal rim thinning and the presence of a RNFL defect inferiorly) and normal visual fields. OCT confirms the presence of RNFL thinning and quantifies it which enables monitoring the patient over time for progression. Figures 61.12A to D show an eye with a suspicious optic disk and a probable nasal defect on visual fields. OCT confirms the presence of RNFL thinning inferiorly which aids in the diagnosis and monitoring of this patient.

ONH AND RNFL IMAGING IN MONITORING GLAUCOMA PROGRESSION

One of the most challenging aspects in the management of glaucoma is to diagnose progression early and accurately. Most clinicians believe that structural progression occurs before functional progression in glaucoma. Although this is debatable, ONH and RNFL imaging provide a useful means for the evaluation of glaucoma progression. Like for visual fields, softwares to detect progression in ONH and RNFL measurements also employ trend and event-based analyses. A trend-based analysis estimates the rate of change (slope) of the parameter over time and provides the

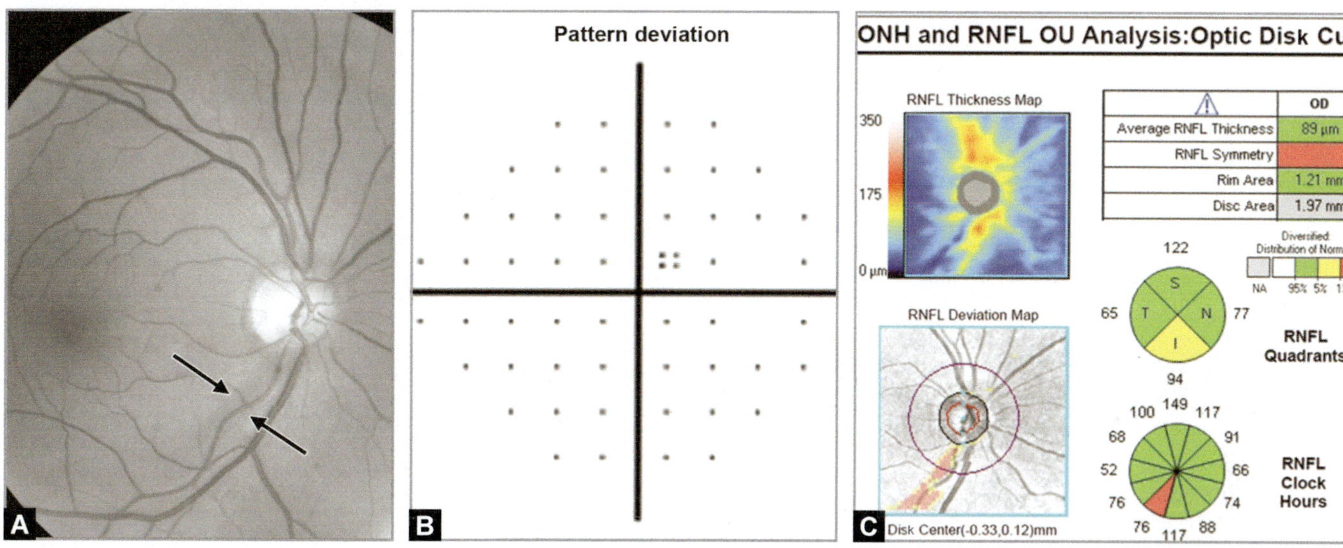

Figs. 61.11A to C: (A) An example of a right eye showing neuroretinal rim thinning and the presence of an RNFL defect inferiorly on the optic disk photograph but (B) normal visual field; (C) OCT confirms the presence of RNFL thinning on RNFL thickness map, deviation map, and clock-hour map. (RNFL: Retinal nerve fiber layer; OCT: Optical coherence tomography; ONH: Optic nerve head)

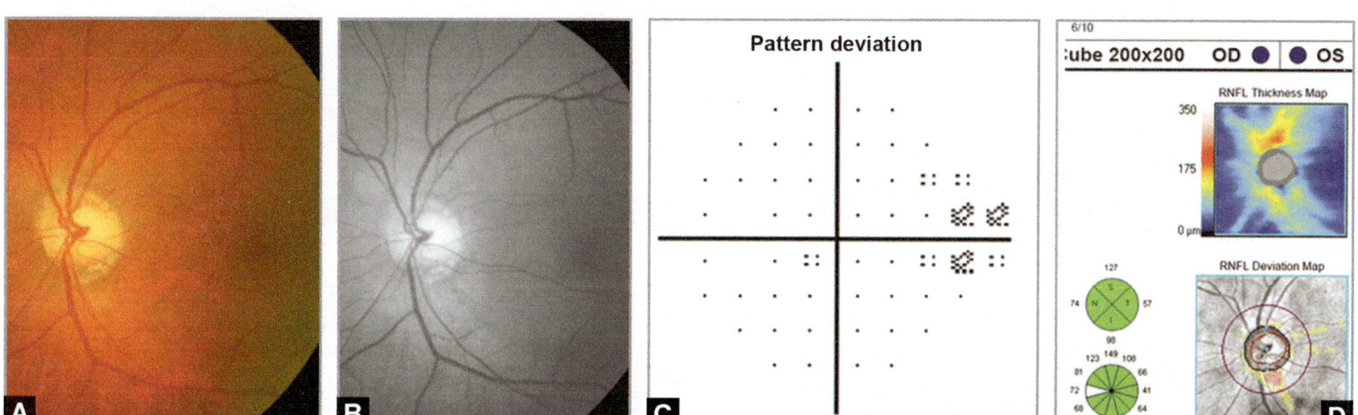

Figs. 61.12A to D: (A) An example of a left eye showing suspicious optic disk; (B) A possible inferotemporal retinal nerve fiber layer (RNFL) defect on red-free photograph; (C) A probable nasal defect on visual fields; (D) Optical coherence tomography (OCT) confirms the presence of inferotemporal RNFL thinning on the thickness map and deviation map. It should be noted that the clock-hour and quadrant maps do not show any abnormal RNFL values and these maps are known to have a poorer diagnostic ability as compared to the thickness and deviation maps.

statistical significance of the slope. An event-based analysis determines progression to have occurred if the amount of change crosses a particular preset value (threshold).

Figure 61.13 shows the progression analysis on Cirrus HD-OCT which employs both trend-based and event-based methods. This is called guided progression analysis (GPA), like the GPA of the Humphrey field analyzer, and currently provides one of the most elaborative automated assessments of progression on imaging. The printout of GPA includes three analyses:

1. A chronological display of RNFL thickness maps and RNFL thickness change maps
2. Average cup to disk ratio (CDR), superior, inferior, and average RNFL thickness graphs representing rate of change, and
3. RNFL thickness profiles comparing the current exam to the baseline exams.

Two good-quality baseline exams are required for all analyses and two good-quality follow-up exams are required to confirm likely change in the ONH and RNFL parameters. Statistically significant changes are summarized with color-codes for possible or likely RNFL thickness loss (or possible RNFL thickness increase).

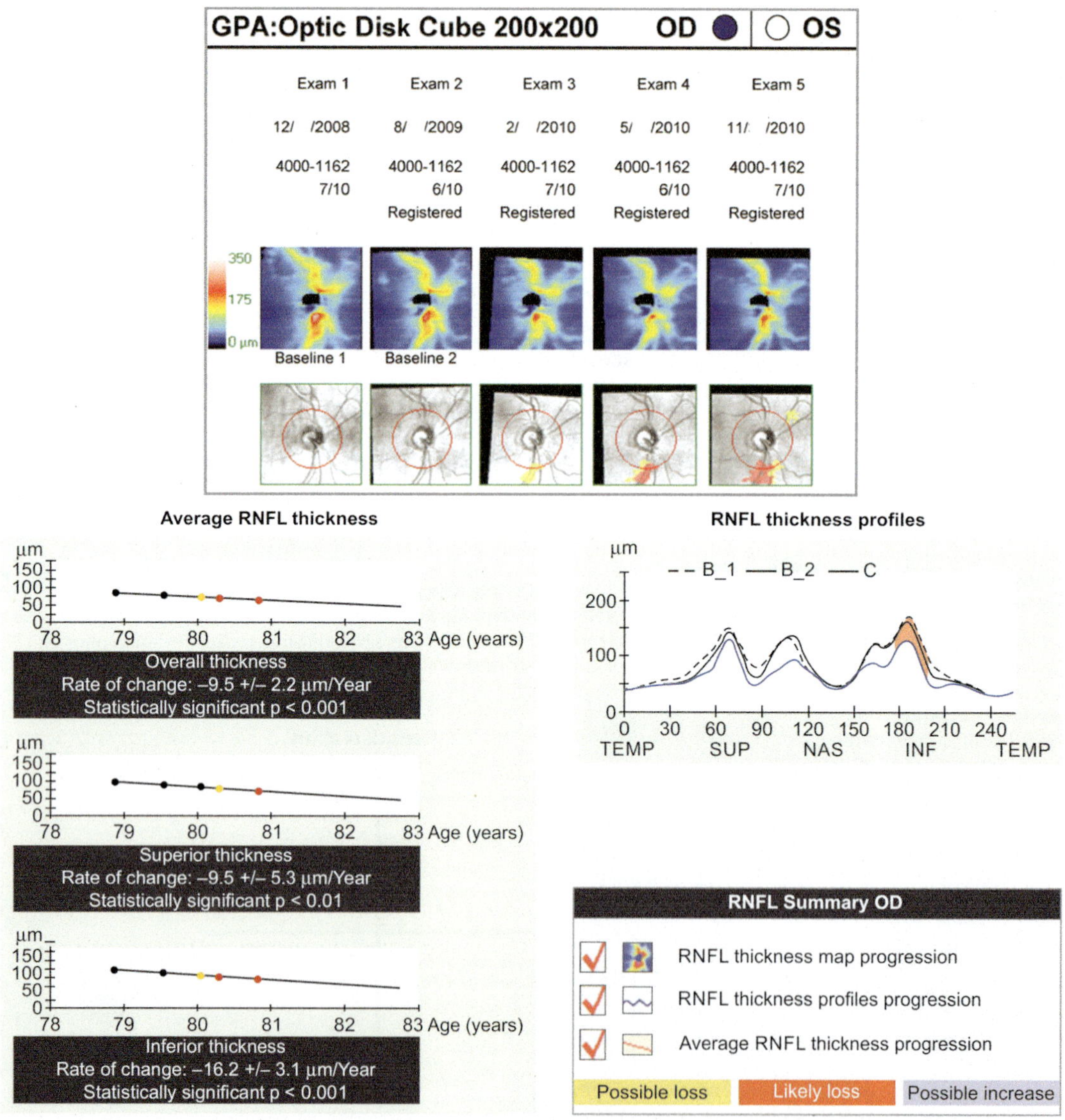

Fig. 61.13: ONH/RNFL progression analysis of Cirrus HD-OCT showing disease progression on both event and trend-based methods. (ONH: Optic nerve head; RNFL: Retinal nerve fiber layer; HD-OCT: High-definition optical coherence tomography; GPA: Guided progression analysis)
Source: www.zeiss.com

Retinal nerve fiber layer thickness map and thickness change map is an event-based analysis, which compares the follow-up exams with the baseline exams and marks out the RNFL regions which have changed by an amount greater than the test-retest variability. When a particular region (20 or more superpixels in a cluster) exceeded the test-retest variability for the first time, it is flagged as a "possible loss" and coded in yellow. When the same region shows a change beyond the test-retest variability in a subsequent exam, it is flagged as a "likely loss" and coded in red. When a particular region shows an increase in RNFL thickness beyond the test-retest variability, it is flagged as a "possible increase" and coded in lavender. In the absence of concurrent retinal pathologies, "possible increase" generally occurs if the baseline exams include poor quality scans with an improvement in scan quality subsequently. RNFL thickness change map is preferred to detect focal changes.

Retinal nerve fiber layer thickness profile analysis is also an event-based analysis, which compares the RNFL profile of the current examination with that of the baseline exams. It detects the regions on the RNFL profile graph that have decreased beyond the expected test-retest variability. A change is considered significant if the change is seen on at least 14 adjacent A-scans (corresponding to 20° over the TSNIT profile). The regions showing the change are flagged as "possible loss", "likely loss", or "possible increase" as mentioned above. RNFL thickness profile analysis, like the RNFL thickness and change map, is preferred to detect focal changes.

Average CDR and RNFL thickness graphs use a trend-based analysis to evaluate the rate of change of average CDR, superior, inferior, and average RNFL thickness measurements over time. Rate of change in these trend-based analyses is estimated using linear regression. The individual data points (from each examination) are highlighted (color-coded) to indicate when the parameter value changed by an amount greater than the test-retest variability. The result shows up as "possible loss" when the rate of loss is statistically significant for only a single visit and is indicated by a yellow symbol. The result shows up as "likely loss" when the rate of loss is statistically significant for two visits in a row and is indicated by a red symbol. The result shows up as "possible increase" when the rate of gain is statistically significant and is indicated by a lavender symbol. Average thickness graphs are preferred to detect diffuse changes unlike the previous two maps.

Figure 61.14 shows the progression analysis on RTVue which employs a trend-based method to evaluate the rate of change of RNFL thickness (average, superior, and inferior sector) over time. The rate of change is color-coded (as represented in Figure 61.14) according to the p value of the slope. In the example, RNFL thickness is decreasing at a magnitude which is significant.

Spectralis OCT also employs both an event and a trend-based method to analyze for progression, like in Cirrus HD-OCT. Figures 61.15A and B show the trend-based analysis of the global RNFL thickness (Fig. 61.15A) and the global MRW (Fig. 61.15B) of Spectralis. The analysis shows the magnitude of slope associated with the change in the parameters with time and also the p value associated with the slope.

It is important to note that the progression analyses, be it from any SD-OCT device, give us statistically significant change, but not clinically significant change. Therefore, the results of the progression analyses should not be interpreted independently but in the context of the entire clinical picture. It is important to consider the results of the clinical evaluation (intraocular pressure, disease stage, occurrence of disk hemorrhage, increase in beta peripapillary atrophic region, etc.) and the standard automated perimetry along with the ONH/RNFL progression analyses while determining glaucoma progression.

LIMITATIONS OF ONH AND RNFL IMAGING

There are a few limitations of imaging which need to be considered. ONH and RNFL imaging requires clear media for good quality scans. Imaging in eyes with media opacities like cataract often leads to poor quality images (poor signal to noise ratio) which can cause misinterpretations and need to be disregarded. Similarly, imaging in high myopic eyes is also challenging as a result of poor image quality as well as issues regarding interpretation due to comparisons drawn using a dissimilar reference database.

The reference databases of the devices include "super-normal subjects" with no evidence of any ocular morbidities and with a limited range of refractive errors. Therefore, caution must be exercised when interpreting the reference database classifications provided by the devices in common "real life" situations like in subjects with coexisting diabetic retinopathy, age-related macular degeneration, high myopia, etc.

Structural measurements, especially the RNFL thickness, are known to level off in more advanced stages of glaucoma, i.e. when the corresponding functional loss on automated perimetry reaches a severity of –10 to –15 dB.[8,9] Further deterioration in the glaucoma severity causes little

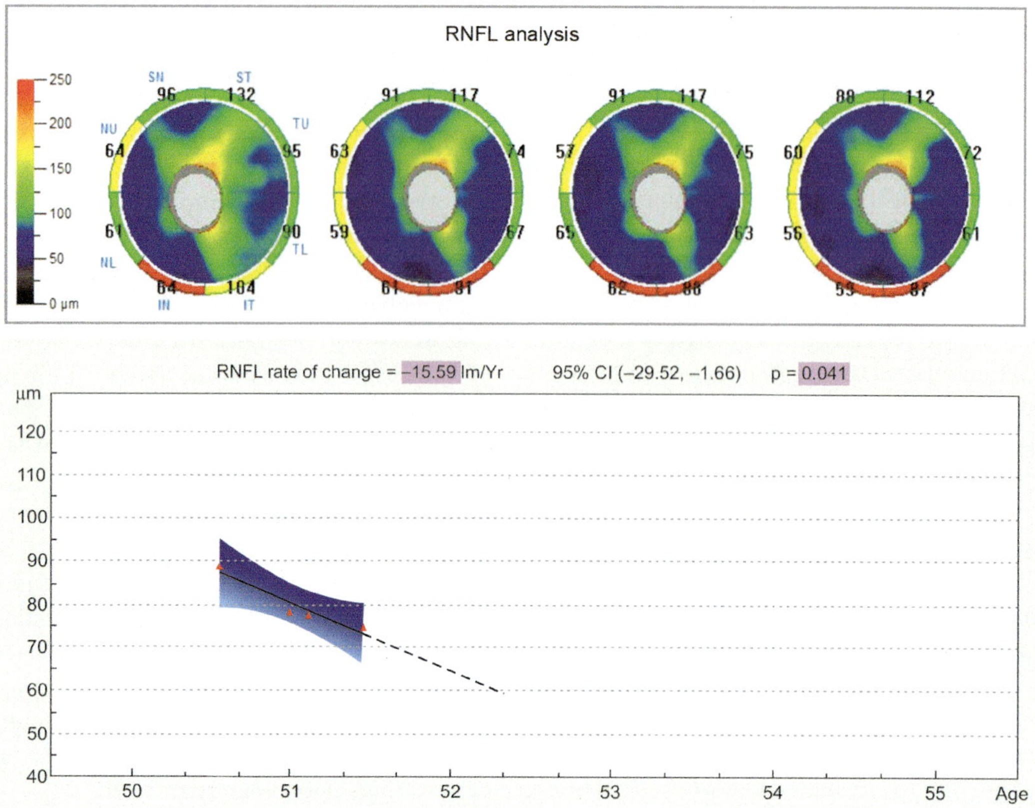

Fig. 61.14: Retinal nerve fiber layer (RNFL) progression analysis of RTVue spectral-domain optical coherence tomography (SD-OCT) showing significant deterioration of average RNFL thickness on the trend-based analysis.

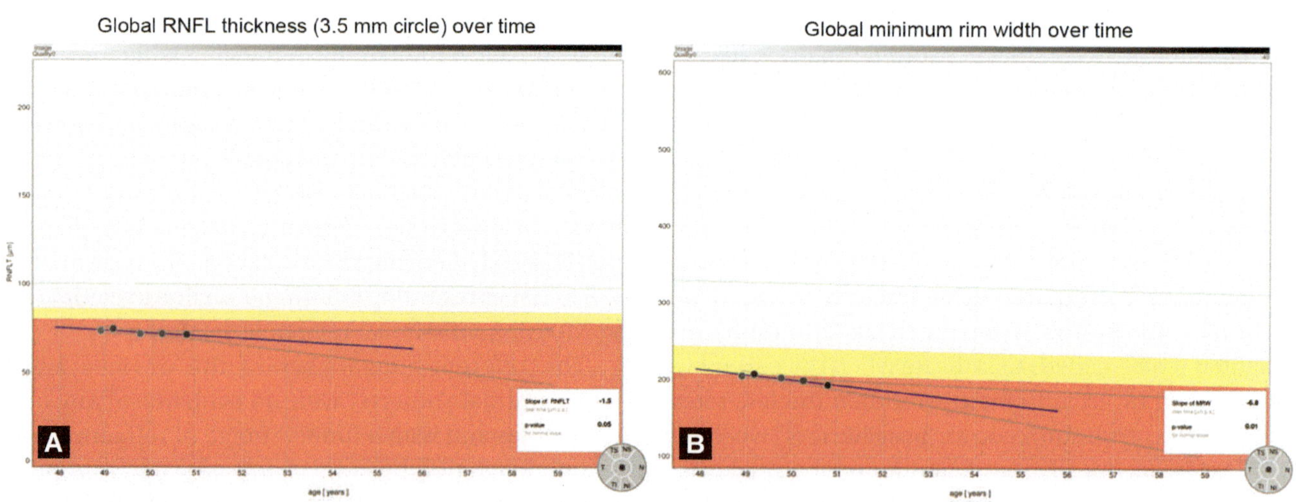

Figs. 61.15A and B: Trend-based progression analysis of global retinal nerve fiber layer (RNFL) thickness and minimum rim width (MRW) of Spectralis spectral-domain optical coherence tomography (SD-OCT).
Source: Dr Sebastian Rausch, Heidelberg Engineering.

change in the RNFL thickness and this has been attributed to the structural tissues other than retinal ganglion cell axons which contribute to the RNFL thickness, resulting in a floor effect. Figures 61.16A and B show an example of a glaucomatous eye showing obvious progression on standard automated perimetry. However, GPA fails to show progression on the RNFL analysis.

Certain clinical findings that are crucial in decision making, like neuroretinal rim pallor and disk hemorrhages, are not picked up by the imaging methods. It is, therefore,

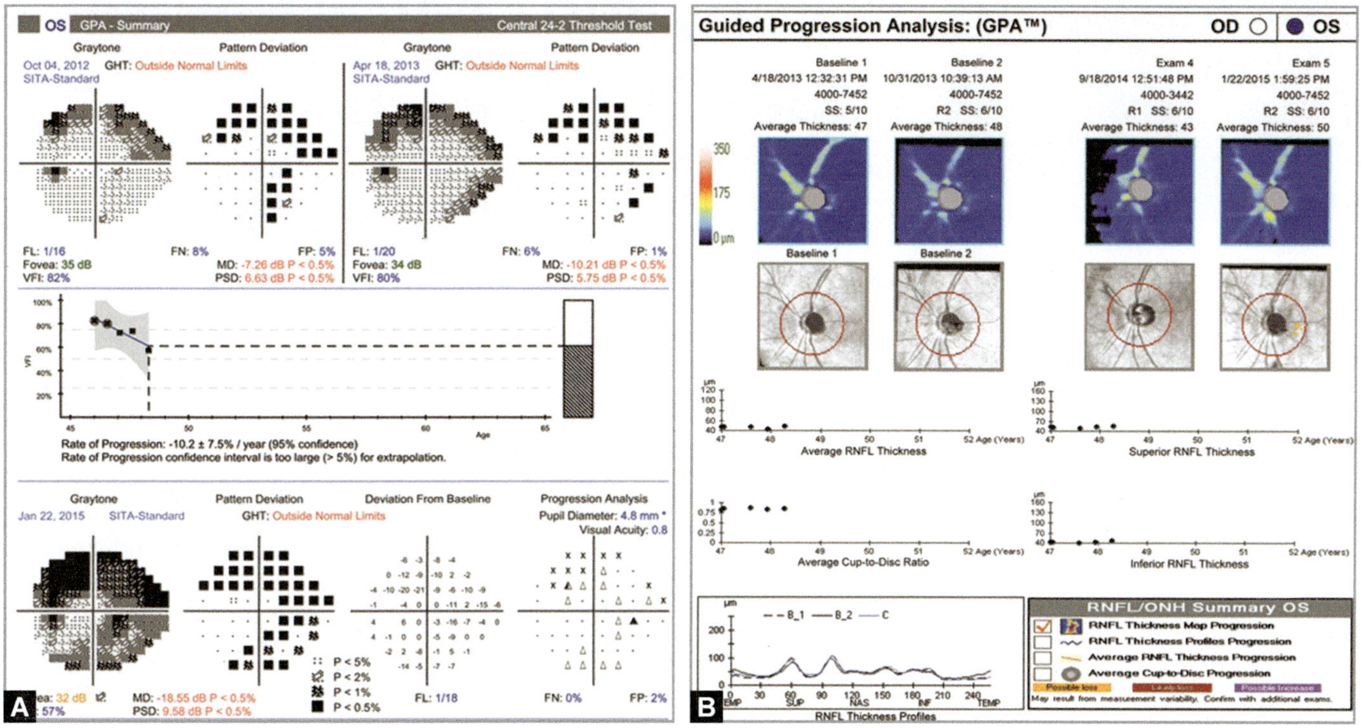

Figs. 61.16A and B: An example of a left eye showing obvious progression on visual fields (A) but showing no progression on guided progression analysis of cirrus high-definition optical coherence tomography (HD-OCT) due to the "floor effect".

imperative to use ONH and RNFL imaging as a complement to a thorough clinical evaluation and visual field examination during the process of decision making.

SUMMARY

Optic nerve head and RNFL imaging, especially after the introduction of SD-OCT, have caused a paradigm shift in the way glaucoma is diagnosed and monitored. SD-OCT imaging of ONH and RNFL has become a part of the routine glaucoma workup in current-day practice. The information derived from ONH and RNFL imaging complements the information derived from the clinical examination and visual field assessment in detecting glaucoma or its progression.

REFERENCES

1. Medeiros FA, Vizzeri G, Zangwill LM, et al. Comparison of retinal nerve fiber layer and optic disc imaging for diagnosing glaucoma in patients suspected of having the disease. Ophthalmology. 2008;115:1340-6.
2. Xu G, Weinreb RN, Leung CK. Retinal nerve fiber layer progression in glaucoma: a comparison between retinal nerve fiber layer thickness and retardance. Ophthalmology. 2013;120(12):2493-500.
3. Mwanza JC, Oakley JD, Budenz DL, et al. Ability of cirrus HD-OCT optic nerve head parameters to discriminate normal from glaucomatous eyes. Ophthalmology. 2011;118(2):241-8.e1.
4. Leite MT, Rao HL, Weinreb RN, et al. Agreement among spectral-domain optical coherence tomography instruments for assessing retinal nerve fiber layer thickness. Am J Ophthalmol. 2011;151:85-92.e1.
5. Pierro L, Gagliardi M, Iuliano L, et al. Retinal nerve fiber layer thickness reproducibility using seven different OCT instruments. Invest Ophthalmol Vis Sci. 2012;53:5912-20.
6. Hwang YH, Kim YY, Kim HK, et al. Ability of cirrus high-definition spectral-domain optical coherence tomography clock-hour, deviation, and thickness maps in detecting photographic retinal nerve fiber layer abnormalities. Ophthalmology. 2013;120:1380-7.
7. Michelessi M, Lucenteforte E, Oddone F, et al. Optic nerve head and fibre layer imaging for diagnosing glaucoma. Cochrane Database Syst Rev. 2015:CD008803.
8. Hood DC, Kardon RH. A framework for comparing structural and functional measures of glaucomatous damage. Prog Retin Eye Res. 2007;26:688-710.
9. Rao HL, Zangwill LM, Weinreb RN, et al. Structure-function relationship in glaucoma using spectral-domain optical coherence tomography. Arch Ophthalmol. 2011;129:864-71.

Chapter 62

Open-angle Glaucoma: Epidemiology, Natural History, and Clinical Course under Optimal Care

Christina Keskini, Dimitrios Giannoulis, Rodanthi Christina Bartzoulianou, Eleftherios Anastasopoulos, Fotis Topouzis

EPIDEMIOLOGY

Glaucoma is considered a major public health problem since it is the second leading cause of global blindness and the most common cause of irreversible blindness.[1] It has been estimated that approximately 8.4 million people would be bilaterally blind from glaucoma in 2010.[2] A recent meta-analysis estimated the total number of people with glaucoma to be 64.3 million in 2013.[3] Open-angle glaucoma (OAG) accounted for most of these individuals, affecting approximately 44 million people. By 2020, the number of glaucoma patients is expected to be 76 million and by 2040 this number will increase to 112 million (53 and 80 million, respectively for OAG).[3]

Data on epidemiology of glaucoma have changed in recent years as a significant number of new population based studies, particularly from Asia, has been conducted providing new information. Global prevalence of OAG varies from 2.2% to 3.05% according to the most recent meta-analyses.[3,4] Black populations (Africans and Afro-Caribbeans) are at higher risk as the prevalence of OAG in these racial groups is approximately 7%, while African-Americans seem to be less affected (4.7%).[5-7] Caucasians and non-Hispanic Whites are the most studied populations with prevalence rates ranging from 1.1% to 5.5%.[7-12] Slightly higher rates appear in Latinos and Hispanic races (2–4.7%).[13,14] Asians seem to be the least affected (1–2.5%), although recent data have revealed increasing prevalence rates of OAG, particularly for certain populations in East Asia (4–4.5%). Moreover, Asia is expected to have approximately 53 million patients with OAG in 2040, bearing the greatest burden worldwide.[15-20] Data from major population based studies are presented in Table 62.1.

Incidence of OAG has also been adequately studied among different racial groups. The duration of the studies varies, however most of them have presented results for at least 4-year incidence of OAG. Average annual rates range from 0.1% to 0.5% with Latinos and Afro-Caribbeans presenting the highest numbers of new glaucoma cases, particularly in older age groups.[21-25]

Despite the large amount of information on the epidemiology of glaucoma, there is poor progress in ensuring proper detection of the disease. This is a challenging issue even for the developed countries as approximately 50% of OAG patients remain undiagnosed, and thus untreated.[9,11,12] Undetected rates are higher in Asia and Africa, rising to as high as 97% for some populations.[6,26] The main factors for undiagnosed glaucoma are younger age[26,27] and lack of regular ophthalmologic examination.[28] Moreover, it has been suggested that patients with POAG are four times more likely to be undiagnosed than patients with pseudoexfoliative glaucoma (PEXG).[28]

Table 62.1: Prevalence of open-angle glaucoma (OAG) in major population based studies.

Prevalence of Open-angle Glaucoma			
Study	**Racial group**	**Age range (years)**	**Prevalence (%)**
Barbados Eye Study	Afro-Caribbeans	40+	6.8
Blue Mountains Eye Study	Caucasians	49+	3
Beaver Dam Eye Study	Caucasians	43–84	2.1
Thessaloniki Eye Study	Caucasians	60+	5.5
Visual Impairment Project	Caucasians	40+	3.4
Rotterdam Study	Caucasians	55+	1.1
Tema Eye Study	Africans	40+	6.8
Proyecto VER	Latinos	40+	2
LALES	Latinos	40+	4.7
Beijing Eye Study	Chinese	40+	2.6
Chan et al. (meta-analysis)	Chinese	40–80	2.3
KNHANES	Korean	40+	4.7
Tham et al. (meta-analysis)	Global	40–80	3

RISK FACTORS FOR PREVALENT AND INCIDENT OPEN-ANGLE GLAUCOMA

Intraocular Pressure

Several studies have indicated an association between elevated intraocular pressure (IOP) and a higher risk of both prevalent and incident OAG. There is an approximately 10–20% additional risk per 1 mm Hg of IOP increase as suggested by cross-sectional and longitudinal studies involving various populations.[20,29-33] Although high IOP is not essential for the diagnosis of glaucoma and not included in the current glaucoma definition, it is the most important independent risk factor and the only one to date that could be modified as part of glaucoma management. Moreover, data from two large randomized controlled trials (RCTs) provide evidence that decreasing IOP in patients with ocular hypertension (OH) could be beneficial for the prevention of OAG.[33,34]

Age

Older age is another factor that has been consistently associated with increased prevalence and incidence of OAG. Prevalence rates range from 0.5% to 1.5% for individuals under 50 years of age and rise over 10% for elderly over 80 years of age.[6,7,10,11,14] Older Latinos and Afro-Caribbeans are more affected since over 20% of these groups have OAG.[5,13] Incidence rates of OAG tend to be also higher as people get older.[21-24] Additionally, multivariate analysis in some prevalence and incidence studies has indicated that older age is an independent risk factor for having OAG as the risk increases approximately 5% for every year of age.[20,29,30]

Race or Ethnicity

Race is an important risk factor since population-based studies have indicated that the prevalence of OAG is significantly higher among individuals with African or Afro-Caribbean origin.[5,6] Moreover, a study in US has revealed that the prevalence of OAG is approximately 4–5 times higher for African Americans compared to White Americans.[7] Caucasians, non-Hispanic Whites and Latinos are at lower risk as they present lower prevalence rates than African populations.[8-10,12,13] Asians are generally considered even less affected, although data from new studies indicate that the rates of OAG are not much lower than those of Whites. South and East Asian populations (especially Koreans and Japanese) present the highest rates among Asians.[15-20] Results from a recent meta-analysis suggest that the risk of OAG when the results were adjusted for several factors including age and gender, was 2.8 times higher in people of African ancestry compared to Europeans. Additionally, the risk was higher but not significantly different for Asians or Hispanics when compared to Europeans.[3]

Family History

Several studies have indicated the association of family history and the development of OAG as the risk increases for those who have relatives (especially of first-degree) with OAG.[29,31,33,35] The risk ratio varies among studies since in most of them data about family history of glaucoma were collected through personal interview which involves limitations including recall bias. In one study that first-degree relatives of glaucoma patients and healthy controls were examined, results revealed that the risk of the development of OAG is 9.2 times higher in individuals with positive family history compared to those with healthy relatives.[36]

Central Corneal Thickness

Thinner corneas have also been associated with the development of OAG.[33,34] Moreover, it has been suggested that the biomechanical properties of the cornea including CCT are confounders for the accuracy of Goldmann applanation tonometry (which is still the gold standard for IOP measurement), potentially resulting in unreliable IOP measurements in case of extreme CCTs.[37] However, using IOP adjusted for CCT in prediction models for OAG development does not provide significantly more accurate predictions.[38] OAG seems to be more prevalent among individuals who have thin CCT (≤510 μm) compared to those with normal or thicker CCT in a Latino population.[32] Additionally, results from an incidence study indicate that there is 40% higher likelihood of developing OAG per 40 μm thinner CCT.[29]

Pseudoexfoliation

There is a considerable number of studies indicating that pseudoexfoliation (PEX) syndrome is related to glaucoma. However, only a few of them provide epidemiological data on PEXG. Prevalence of PEX varies depending on the ethnicity and the age of the population that was studied. PEX rates have been reported to be approximately 23% in northern Sweden, 11.9% in northern Greece, 3.8% in South India and

2.3% in Australia.[9,39-41] These rates tend to be higher for older age groups. Up to 15% of the individuals with PEX syndrome may present glaucomatous damage.[30,31,39-41] Moreover, PEX has been reported to independently increase the risk of glaucoma development approximately 2–3 times in some studies[30,40] or 9–10 times according to others.[31,42] Finally, a prevalence study has shown that when screening IOP was over 20 mm Hg the likelihood of glaucoma was four times higher among patients with PEX compared to those without PEX.[43]

Myopia

Myopia is another risk factor for the development of OAG as many studies have suggested. Moderate to high myopia (≥ -3 D) is associated with higher risk of OAG (2–3.5 times increased likelihood), while results for low myopia remain conflicting.[19,30,44-46] Moreover, individuals with increased axial length are at greater risk compared to those with normal-sized eyes, as prevalence of OAG increases by 26% per every 1 mm of longer axial length.[47]

Ocular Perfusion Pressure

Several studies have indicated the association of low ocular perfusion pressure (OPP) and OAG occurrence.[29,48,49] Diastolic OPP (defined as the difference between diastolic blood pressure and IOP) seems to be of greater importance and results from one study have suggested that the risk could be higher for patients with low OPP status who are under treatment for systemic hypertension.[50] These data could provide evidence for the role of OPP and the possible vascular mechanism in glaucoma pathogenesis.

Other Factors

Sex has been sometimes associated with the prevalence of OAG but findings from studies are conflicting. Males are at higher risk in many studies while others suggest no association.[7,11,29,30] Blood pressure is another factor that has been related to OAG however results are inconsistent. Some of them show positive association between systemic hypertension and glaucoma development while others suggest negative association.[29,51] Migraine and vasospasm have been identified as possible risk factors, relating particularly to normal tension glaucoma.[52] Diabetes mellitus has been weakly associated with OAG since findings from studies are controversial.[30,53] Research in genetic associations is flourishing currently as the technology evolves and the cost of genetic analysis drops. New data on the genetic architecture of glaucoma are expected in near future and this information could provide evidence for new therapeutic targets.

Predictive Factors for the Conversion of Ocular Hypertension to OAG

Two RCTs [the Ocular Hypertension Treatment Study (OHTS) and European Glaucoma Prevention Study (EGPS)] have greatly contributed in providing data regarding the risk factors for the conversion of OHT to OAG. According to the pooled data of these studies the main factors are presented in Table 62.2.

Taking the data in Table 62.2 into consideration, a calculator was developed to estimate the 5-year risk of a person with OH to develop OAG. This is a useful tool in the hands of ophthalmologists helping them to address a more personalized treatment for their patients. However, there are certain limitations in the use of the calculator since it should be applied only to patients with similar characteristics to the population of these studies, meaning patients over 40 years of age, Caucasian or African American and having baseline mean IOP over 22 mm Hg but less than 32 mm Hg. Additionally, some other important factors like PEX and family history of OAG are missing from the model despite that they have been consistently associated with higher risk for the development of OAG.[34,54,55]

NATURAL HISTORY

Glaucoma is an irreversible, progressive neuropathy that can lead to blindness. The beneficial effect of IOP lowering treatment has been evidenced by multiple studies in the past. Consequently, any effort to demonstrate its natural history, by exposing glaucoma patients to no treatment would be reasonably criticized as potentially unethical.

Table 62.2: Risk factors for the conversion of OHT to open-angle glaucoma (OAG) according to OHTS and EGPS.

Risk factors for the conversion of OHT to OAG	
IOP	9% risk increase per 1 mm Hg
Age	26% risk increase per decade
CCT	Two times higher risk per 40 μm thinner
Vertical cup to disk ratio	19% risk increase per 0.1 larger
Pattern standard deviation	13% risk increase per 0.2 dB greater

(OHT: Ocular hypertension; IOP: Intraocular pressure; CCT: Central corneal thickness; OAG: Open-angle glaucoma; OHTS: Ocular Hypertension Treatment Study; EGPS: European Glaucoma Prevention Study)

The small number of studies that primarily aimed to show a benefit to intervention included a group of untreated individuals who were closely monitored in order to satisfy ethical issues. Data analysis of the control arm offered an insight into the clinical course of untreated glaucoma. Progression was defined by the amount of visual field loss or optic disk changes detected, based on prespecified criteria. Similarly, time to event and rate of deterioration contributed substantially in illustrating the natural history of glaucoma.

The Early Manifest Glaucoma Trial (EMGT) was the first large randomized, clinical trial to study the progression of glaucoma among patients with newly detected primary open-angle glaucoma (POAG), normal-tension glaucoma (NTG) and pseudoexfoliation glaucoma (PEXG) that received either IOP lowering treatment or no treatment.[56] Data from the latter study arm provided a unique opportunity to chart the natural history of glaucoma. A succeeding study among the patients of the control group showed that 68% of individuals, followed for at least 6 years without treatment or progressed within 6 years, had definite visual field progression.[57] There was significant difference in proportions between the three groups. More specifically, 74% of high-tension glaucoma (HTG) eyes, 56% of NTG eyes and 93% of PEXG eyes progressed. A large variability could similarly be noted in the progression rate, and therefore in time to progression, among patients not only between the three groups but also within each group. The median time to progression was 42.8 months in the overall control arm, 44.8 months in HTG, 61.1 months in NTG and 19.5 months in PEXG. Their respective mean progression rates were 1.08 dB/year in overall, 1.31 dB/year in HTG, 0.36 dB/year in NTG and 3.13 dB/year in PEXG. The visual field of untreated NTG patients deteriorated rather slowly, at approximately one-fourth of the corresponding speed in the HTG group, whilst individuals with PEXG lost vision relatively rapidly. It should be noted that patients who reached an endpoint received treatment and were no longer followed in the control group. According to a subsequent global trend analysis, the course of glaucoma progression in the long-term is linear.[58] Moreover, linear extrapolation of the first five visual field tests can predict future visual field loss with considerable accuracy, using the visual field index. This is particularly true, when the baseline test of the analysis has visual field defects present.

Another study that shed light on the natural history of glaucoma was a follow-up cohort from St. Lucia, which evaluated visual field progression in untreated black glaucoma patients and suspects over a 10-year period.[59] The estimation of visual field deterioration was based on two scoring algorithms developed for two multicenter clinical trials, the Advanced Glaucoma Intervention Study (AGIS) and the Collaborative Initial Glaucoma Treatment Study (CIGTS). According to those criteria, by 10 years, 52–73% of the eyes identified with glaucoma or glaucoma suspect status showed visual field deterioration, with 14.9–16.4% progressing to end stage glaucoma. Both percentages were higher compared to those reported in studies of visual field loss in treated eyes. More than half of the eyes that reached an end-stage visual field loss had no or minimal field loss at baseline. Even though the study methodology prohibits any investigation of the visual field progression rate, it can be assumed that it is relatively high.

Variable rate of progression was also documented in patients with normal-tension glaucoma in the Collaborative Normal Tension Glaucoma Study (CNTGS), the first prospective study to quantify the effect of IOP on the natural course of this clinical subentity of OAG.[60] As far as progression is concerned, 12% of treated individuals, whose IOP was lowered up to 30%, reached an endpoint compared to 35% in the untreated arm. The mean time to progression was 7.4 and 4.6 years, respectively. In a subsequent data analysis of the untreated cohort, the mean estimated slope of MD deterioration was 0.41 dB/year.[61] Approximately one-third of patients presented localized deterioration within 3 years, and a half within 5–7 years. No statistically significant progression was found in 62 of 109 subjects that were followed for more than 3 years. On the contrary, variable rates of progression were observed in the remaining subjects, including values from 0.2 to 2 dB/year, which is further interpreted in patients with slow, almost nonthreatening, progress and patients with rapid and potentially detrimental course. Faster rate was associated to female sex, history of migraine headaches and optic disk hemorrhages but not to IOP levels. Although the initial intention-to-treat analysis showed no difference between the two groups, eliminating the effect of cataract formation on visual field affirmed the positive role of treatment.

Despite the contribution of the aforementioned studies, various limitations of methodology prohibit a precise estimate of the deterioration rate of glaucoma. Nevertheless, knowledge of its natural history provides many assets to a clinician and raises challenges, both scientific and clinical. Comprehending the nature of this progressive disease helps identify the optimal way to manage it. Differences not only between but also within diverse diagnostic groups enhance the common belief that glaucoma patients should be monitored and treated each time individually.

CLINICAL COURSE UNDER OPTIMAL CARE

Optimal Treatment

Currently, glaucoma treatment is focused on medically or surgically lowering IOP, as IOP is the only known modifiable risk factor for OAG development and progression. Optimal glaucoma treatment aims to maintain the patient's visual function and related quality of life, at a sustainable cost, according to EGS Guidelines.[62] As defined by the American Academy of Ophthalmology (AAO) Preferred Practice Pattern (PPP) Guidelines for the treatment of POAG, the goals of managing patients with POAG are the control of IOP in the target range, the stability of the optic nerve (ON)/ retinal nerve fiber layer (RNFL) status and of the visual fields, while the effects of treatment, the patients' quality of life, and the patients' life expectancy are to be considered in the decision-making process about therapy.[63] Clinicians should document the status of optic nerve structure and function on presentation and estimate the IOP below which further optic nerve damage is unlike to occur. Educating and involving the patient in the management of the disease while minimizing treatment side effects and negative impact on the patient's vision, general health, and quality of life, should be part of the clinician's objectives in order to offer the optimal glaucoma management.[63]

Currently, a widespread approach for an optimal and individualized treatment is the concept of target IOP. Target IOP is the upper limit of the IOP estimated to be compatible with a rate of progression sufficiently slow to maintain vision-related quality of life in the expected lifetime of the patient.[62] Factors considered when setting the target IOP are presented in Table 62.3.

Table 62.3: Factors considered in setting the target IOP according to EGS guidelines, 4th edition.

• Glaucomatous damage stage
• Baseline IOP
• Age and life expectancy
• Rate of progression
• Prognostic factors for progression
• Treatment side effects
• Patient's preferences

(IOP: Intraocular pressure; EGS: European Glaucoma Society)

Glaucoma and Blindness

Despite optimal treatment 'patterns' and 'goals' being specified by updated guidelines, the number of people being visually impaired due to glaucoma remains rather significant. According to World Health Organization (WHO) data published in 2010, glaucoma is responsible for 2% of visual impairment globally, while being the second leading cause of blindness, comprising 8% of the cases.[64] A meta-analysis that assessed the number of individuals visually impaired or blind due to glaucoma reported that from 1990 to 2010, the number of blind or visually impaired due to glaucoma increased by 0.8 million and by 2.3 million, respectively.[65] According to a recently published retrospective study aiming to determine the lifetime risk and duration of blindness in 592 patients with OAG, at the last follow-up visit 42.2% of the patients were blind due to glaucoma in at least one eye and 16.4% in both eyes,[66] with the risk of blindness increasing with higher baseline IOP, worse baseline visual field and older age.[67] The aforementioned data imply that since the global burden of glaucoma increases, glaucoma patients may not be diagnosed early enough in the course of the disease or may not be optimally treated.

Glaucoma Onset in Ocular Hypertensive Patients

Ocular hypertension may be defined as IOP in the highest 97.5% percentile for the population that does not have optic disk or visual field damage.[68] The role of IOP reduction in glaucoma onset among patients with OH and the necessity of treating them with IOP-lowering interventions were mainly investigated in two large RCTs: the OHTS and the EGPS.

Ocular Hypertension Treatment Study

The OHTS is an RCT aiming to evaluate the safety and efficacy of topical ocular hypotensive medication in preventing or delaying the onset of visual field loss and/or optic nerve damage in OH subjects, randomized between medical treatment and no treatment. The treatment goal was to lower IOP to less than 24 mm Hg and at least 20% from baseline.[69] During the study course mean IOP reduction for the treated group and for the control group was 22.5% and 4%, respectively. After 5 years of follow-up the OHTS reported that 4.4% of the treated OH patients had developed OAG versus 9.5% in the control group

($p < 0.0001$), thus suggesting that IOP-lowering treatment results in halving of the risk for conversion to POAG.[70] Quite notably, however, more than 90% of the untreated patients had not converted to POAG, questioning the necessity of early treatment of OH patients.

The same treatment groups were followed-up for a long-term period of 13 years, aiming to compare the safety and efficacy of earlier versus later treatment in preventing POAG in OH individuals. The medical intervention group remained under the same treatment while the control group received medication after 7.5 years of observation. The cumulative proportion of OH patients that have progressed to POAG remained significantly higher for the later treated group compared to the early treated patients (22% vs 16% respectively, $p = 0.009$). However, when evaluating POAG onset, it was made clear that the benefit of early treatment was most evident among individuals at a higher baseline risk of developing POAG (>13%), while the benefit of early treatment was small in individuals with OH at low baseline risk of developing POAG.[71]

European Glaucoma Prevention Study

The EGPS is an RCT designed to evaluate the efficacy of IOP lowering treatment with dorzolamide in preventing OAG onset in patients with OH in comparison with placebo-treated OH subjects. Open-angle glaucoma diagnosis was evaluated based on visual field changes, optic disk changes or both.[72] IOP reduction after 5 years of follow-up was 22% for the dorzolamide-treated patients whereas for the placebo-treated the reported IOP reduction was 16%, not reaching a statistically significant difference. Similarly, the difference in cumulative probability of developing OAG between the two groups failed to reach the level of statistical significance.[73]

The OHTS has clearly demonstrated the protective role of IOP-lowering therapy, while conversely the EGPS failed to prove significantly lower risk for OAG development in dorzolamide-treated OH patients versus those that were in the placebo group. Those discrepancies could be adequately explained by three fundamental differences outlined by Quigley in 2005: (1) the commitment of EGPS to dorzolamide therapy alone, regardless of IOP lowering with placebo control; (2) a major regression to the mean in IOP at 6 months in EGPS; and (3) selective loss to follow-up of persons with higher IOP in EGPS, thus decreasing the mean IOP of the remaining persons, but clearly not because the IOP fell in each retained study subject.[74] Considering IOP and other predictive factors for conversion of OH to OAG, each OH patient should be individually assessed when deciding whether to be treated or not. A useful tool to evaluate the necessity of medical treatment commencement could be the risk calculator as designed by the pooled OHTS-EGPS predictive model. However, the decision to begin IOP-lowering treatment in the glaucoma suspect patient is rather complex and should be based on examination results, risk assessment and patient's preferences.[75]

Open-angle Glaucoma Progression

As mentioned earlier, large population based studies have consistently associated higher IOP levels with glaucoma prevalence[8,9,11-14,17,76-78] and incidence.[31,46,79,80] Given this evidence several RCTs have investigated the role of IOP lowering treatment, mean follow-up IOP values and long-term (inter-visit) IOP fluctuation in preventing OAG progression [defined with visual field and/or optic disk (OD) criteria]. Most of these RCTs have reported that lower mean IOP at follow-up is associated with decreased risk of progression while the role of IOP fluctuation is still under debate. However, the proportion of patients that demonstrated disease progression was variable among those studies.

Early Manifest Glaucoma Trial

The EMGT is a randomized, prospective trial comparing progression as measured with VF and/or optic nerve progression in newly detected treated OAG patients and untreated OAG subjects. All participants in the treatment arm received standardized IOP-lowering therapy, including laser trabeculoplasty and topical betaxolol. After a median follow up of 6 years, mean IOP value was reduced by 25% for the treated group, while it remained unchanged for the untreated. Progression was less frequent in the treated arm as compared to the untreated (45% vs 62% respectively, $p = 0.007$), with progression occurring later in the treated group (median time: 18 months later). Of note, every mm Hg IOP reduction from baseline IOP lowered the risk by 10%.[57]

The EMGT treatment protocol protective effects were maintained even after a longer 8-year follow-up, almost halving progression risk for both high and low baseline IOP patients. However, the proportion of glaucoma patients that have progressed was reported to be 67% overall, with 59% of the treated and 76% of the untreated patients presenting visual field signs of glaucomatous damage deterioration.[81] In addition, each mm Hg of higher mean IOP was associated with an 11% increased risk of deterioration, whilst long-term IOP fluctuation did not reach the level of statistical significance as a risk factor to progression.[82]

Collaborative Normal Tension Glaucoma Study

The CNTGS is a clinical trial evaluating the effect of medically or surgically 30% IOP reduction in normal-tension glaucoma (NTG) patients compared to non-treated NTG subjects. Progression endpoints were verified by visual field or optic nerve worsening. According to endpoint definition analysis, evaluating the patients' clinical course only after IOP reduction goal was achieved, 12% of the treated and 35% of the untreated had progressed, with the overall survival analysis suggesting a statistically significant favorable effect of the intervention. However, only 50% of the patients managed to reach the 30% reduction.[83] When an intention-to-treat analysis was performed significant benefit of the treatment was revealed only after censoring the data for cataract effect on visual field examination.[84]

Advanced Glaucoma Intervention Study

Advanced Glaucoma Intervention Study investigated the efficacy of two different treatment protocols in subjects with advanced open-angle glaucoma damage. One group underwent argon laser trabeculoplasty (ALT) followed if needed by trabeculectomy and then by a second trabeculectomy (1:ATT) while the other group followed an initial trabeculectomy treatment and then if needed an ALT and then a second trabeculectomy (2: TAT). With regards to IOP and progression, results in a post-hoc analysis after at least 6 years of follow-up indicate that eyes with IOP more than 17.5 mm Hg in the first three biannual visits showed significantly higher visual field deterioration as compared to those with IOP less than 14 mm Hg for the same period. Furthermore, eyes presenting constantly with IOP less than 18 mm Hg throughout all visits had no visual field progression, while inadequate IOP control below this level was associated with visual field worsening.[85] IOP fluctuation seemed to be a significant factor only for patients with low mean IOP.[86]

Collaborative Initial Glaucoma Treatment Study

The CIGTS is an RCT comparing medical treatment versus initial filtration surgery in patients with newly diagnosed OAG. A target IOP algorithm was used for every participant and glaucomatous damage deterioration was defined by visual field progression.[87] After 8 years of follow-up, IOP reduction was 35% for the medically treated patients and 45% for the surgically treated.[88] Although mean perimetric progression was small in both groups for many years, after 8 years 21.3% of the surgically managed subjects and 25.5% of the medically treated ones showed perimetric progression[88,89] though the surgical group experienced more frequent progression of cataract.

United Kingdom Glaucoma Treatment Study

The United Kingdom Glaucoma Treatment Study (UKGTS) is the first RCT comparing a specific IOP-lowering medication (latanoprost) to placebo in newly diagnosed OAG patients with regards to visual field preservation. After 24 months of follow-up mean IOP reduction for the medically treated was 19.4% (reduced from 19.6 mm Hg to 15.8 mm Hg) and for the placebo group 4.5% (reduced from 20.1 mm Hg to 19.2 mm Hg). Perimetric progression due to glaucomatous visual field loss was significantly higher for the placebo group (25.6% for placebo group vs 15.2% for the latanoprost group, $p = 0.006$), while visual field preservation was also significantly longer in the latanoprost group than in the placebo group (adjusted hazard ratio 0.44, $p = 0.0003$).[90]

The IOP lowering rates and progression frequencies varied significantly among trials. Those differences can be explained by different study designs, including treatment regimens and interventions, different study populations and different follow-up periods.

The EMGT and UKGTS both recruited patients with newly detected OAG and randomized their patients either to a standard treatment protocol or to no treatment/placebo treatment. Glaucoma progression in the EMGT was detected in 45% of the treated subjects after a 25% IOP reduction whereas in the UKGTS glaucoma progression was detected in 15.2% of the treated subjects after a 19.4% IOP reduction. A greater IOP reduction was achieved in the EMGT as a combined betaxolol/ALT treatment protocol was applied, while UKGTS included only latanoprost treatment. Nevertheless, this greater IOP reduction did not result in a lower proportion of OAG progression. This could be explained by both higher mean baseline IOP in the EMGT treated group, which is known to be a risk factor for progression, (EMGT: 20.6 mm Hg, UKGTS: 19.6 mm Hg) and by mainly longer follow-up time in EMGT (EMGT: 6 years, UKGTS: 2 years). The considerable proportion of progressing patients under treatment in both studies implies that a uniform treatment protocol cannot be effective in all patients, thus highlighting the necessity of individualized treatment including a target IOP for every patient.

The only large RCT that designed participants' therapeutic scheme based on a target IOP was the CIGTS. Of note, there was no difference in the proportion of individuals showing progression between medically and surgically treated subjects with a high overall visual field stability during 5 years of follow-up[91] and a minimal average MD change from baseline in both groups' average.[88] Even after 8 years of follow-up, progression occurred in 21.3% of the surgically treated and in 25.5% of the medically treated patients, significantly lower rates than those reported by the EMGT after 8 years of follow-up. The main reason for those differences may be the fact that in CIGTS each patient was individually treated using a target IOP, thus approaching an optimal treatment pattern, although they could be partially explained by the more strict visual field progression criteria used in the EMGT. Overall IOP reduction was greater in CIGTS compared to EMGT (35% for the medically treated CIGTS patients, 45% for the surgically treated CIGTS patients and 25% for the treated EMGT patients). However, it should be highlighted that in CIGTS although IOP reduction was lower for the surgically treated group compared to the medically treated, this did not add any further prevention of glaucoma damage progression to the patients that underwent filtration surgery. This fact contradicts the perception that the lower the IOP, the better for the patient and introduces the possibility of overtreatment. It may be that, beyond a certain level of IOP lowering, further reduction of IOP does not add any significant benefit. This again highlights the importance of individualized management. Although in CIGTS an individualized target IOP strategy was used, it is possible that the specific target IOP used needs further refinement.

In addition, one could argue that IOP lowering treatment reduced the rate of progression even in progressing patients in both EMGT and UKGTS, thus implying a beneficial treatment outcome. Taking into account that the goal of glaucoma treatment is to maintain the patient's visual function and related quality of life, at a sustainable cost,[62] the statement above highlights the importance of individualized treatment, while introducing the aspect of tolerable rate of progression to prevent visual impairment that could affect patients' quality of life during his/her expected lifetime.

Prognostic Factors for Progression of OAG

As mentioned earlier, when setting the target IOP below which the rate of glaucoma progression will be sufficiently slow to maintain vision-related quality of life in the expected lifetime of the patient, there are certain factors that should be considered. Those factors are: glaucomatous damage stage, baseline IOP, age and life expectancy, rate of progression, patient's preferences, treatment side effects, and prognostic factors for progression. Apart from the positive effect of IOP reduction in glaucoma progression, which has been confirmed from most of the aforementioned RCTs, other prognostic factors have been evaluated and determined mostly by the EMGT. The following having been reported by EMGT as risk factors for OAG progression: older age, IOP lowering, PEX, CCT, disk hemorrhages, bilateral disease, worse baseline MD and cardiovascular disease history.[81,92-94] Increasing age has also been associated with an increased risk of glaucomatous damage progression in the AGIS[95] and the CIGTS,[88] while disk hemorrhages were also reported as a significant prognostic factor of glaucoma progression in the CNTGS.[93]

Target IOP Limitations

Although the concept of target IOP is currently a widespread approach to optimally treat glaucoma patients, there are still some limitations to be considered. While IOP measurements and intervisit differences can be recorded, information on diurnal IOP fluctuation is usually limited, thus questioning whether target IOP is achieved. Additionally, there is no study showing that if a particular target IOP is reached in an individual patient, one can be assured of halting glaucoma progression, even if such progression is defined as a statistical change on perimetry.[96] Finally, there is lack of evidence based on RCTs confirming that the use of a target IOP approach is advantageous to any other approach.[97]

OAG Rate of Progression

Many patients with OAG despite years of treatment and follow-up show no or only small deterioration[60,84] while others may show rapid progression.[84] Therefore, although IOP reduction is an important factor to take into account, measuring disease's rate of progression should be considered for sufficient monitoring and optimal treatment. There are two approaches to computer-assisted visual field progression analysis: (1) the event analysis, designed to define whether progression has occurred, and (2) the trend analysis, quantifying the rate of progression. Rates of progression differ among glaucoma patients from rapid to very slow.[58,98-101] Therefore, the rate of progression of the patient is a key determinant of the necessity of intensifying each patient's treatment. There is limited information regarding risk factors for rate of progression. Older age, PEXG, worse baseline MD, large baseline vertical C/D ratio and disk hemorrhages have been reported as prognostic factors for rapid visual field deterioration.[58,102,103]

Vision-related Quality of Life

The goal of glaucoma treatment is to maintain the patient's visual function and related quality of life, at a sustainable cost.[62] Only few of the aforementioned glaucoma RCTs have reported results associated with vision-related quality of life (VRQOL) providing information that should be considered when treating an OAG patient.

According to EMGT after 6 years of follow-up, VRQOL did not differ between treated and untreated patients while low composite scores were correlated with low visual acuity (VA) and worse perimetric MD,[104] a finding confirmed even after 15 years after initial glaucoma diagnosis.[105] Moreover, visual field index worse than 50% or MD worse than –18 dB was significantly associated with low VRQOL scores.[105] The CIGTS showed that after 5 years of follow-up VRQOL differed among surgically and medically treated patients only with regards to the impact of local eye symptoms that were consistently higher for subjects that underwent immediate filtration surgery.[106] The question of whether rate of visual field progression was associated with VRQOL in patients with similar degrees of integrated binocular visual field was examined by Lisboa et al.[107] They suggest that patients with faster rates of binocular visual field change were at higher risk of reporting abnormal VRQOL.

Finally, when questioning the difference between better-eye visual field mean deviation and integrated visual field (IVF MD) in determining the impact of glaucoma in objective and subjective measures of ability/performance, Ramulu et al. concluded that IVF MD rarely (derived from a combination of right and left eye visual field data) differs from better-eye MD, and similar associations between visual field loss and visual disability are obtained using either MD.[108] Consequently, information from studies using better-eye visual field MD can be more easily integrated into clinical decision-making, making better-eye MD a robust and meaningful method for reporting visual field loss severity.[108]

CONCLUSION

Optimal glaucoma treatment aims to maintain the patient's visual function and related quality of life, at a sustainable cost. Despite guidelines' leading physicians to a more individualized treatment approach, including the concept of target IOP, the global burden of glaucoma seems to enlarge, highlighting the necessity of further treatment patterns' refinement ideally corresponding to each patient's specific needs.

REFERENCES

1. Resnikoff S, Pascolini D, Etya'Ale D, et al. Global data on visual impairment in the year 2002. Bull World Health Organ. 2004;82(11):844-51.
2. Quigley HA, Broman AT. The number of people with glaucoma worldwide in 2010 and 2020. Br J Ophthalmol. 2006;90(3):262-7.
3. Tham YC, Li X, Wong TY, et al. Global prevalence of glaucoma and projections of glaucoma burden through 2040: a systematic review and meta-analysis. Ophthalmology. 2014;121(11):2081-90.
4. Kapetanakis VV, Chan MP, Foster PJ, et al. Global variations and time trends in the prevalence of primary open angle glaucoma (POAG): a systematic review and meta-analysis. Br J Ophthalmol. 2016;100(1):86-93.
5. Leske MC, Connell AM, Schachat AP, et al. The Barbados Eye Study. Prevalence of open angle glaucoma. Arch Ophthalmol. 1994;112(6):821-9.
6. Budenz DL, Barton K, Whiteside-de Vos J, et al. Prevalence of glaucoma in an urban West African population: the Tema Eye Survey. JAMA Ophthalmology. 2013;131(5):651-8.
7. Tielsch JM, Sommer A, Katz J, et al. Racial variations in the prevalence of primary open-angle glaucoma. The Baltimore Eye Survey. JAMA. 1991;266(3):369-74.
8. Klein BE, Klein R, Sponsel WE, et al. Prevalence of glaucoma. The Beaver Dam Eye Study. Ophthalmology. 1992;99(10):1499-504.
9. Topouzis F, Wilson MR, Harris A, et al. Prevalence of open-angle glaucoma in Greece: the Thessaloniki Eye Study. Am J Ophthalmol. 2007;144(4):511-9.
10. Wensor MD, McCarty CA, Stanislavsky YL, et al. The prevalence of glaucoma in the Melbourne Visual Impairment Project. Ophthalmology. 1998;105(4):733-9.
11. Mitchell P, Smith W, Attebo K, Healey PR. Prevalence of open-angle glaucoma in Australia. The Blue Mountains Eye Study. Ophthalmology. 1996;103(10):1661-9.
12. Dielemans I, Vingerling JR, Wolfs RC, et al. The prevalence of primary open-angle glaucoma in a population-based study in The Netherlands. The Rotterdam Study. Ophthalmology. 1994;101(11):1851-5.

13. Varma R, Ying-Lai M, Francis BA, et al. Prevalence of open-angle glaucoma and ocular hypertension in Latinos: the Los Angeles Latino Eye Study. Ophthalmology. 2004;111(8):1439-48.
14. Quigley HA, West SK, Rodriguez J, et al. The prevalence of glaucoma in a population-based study of Hispanic subjects: Proyecto VER. Arch Ophthalmol. 2001;119(12):1819-26.
15. Chan EW, Li X, Tham YC, et al. Glaucoma in Asia: regional prevalence variations and future projections. Br J Ophthalmol. 2016;100(1):78-85.
16. Wang YX, Xu L, Yang H, et al. Prevalence of glaucoma in North China: the Beijing Eye Study. Am J Ophthalmol. 2010;150(6):917-24.
17. Shen SY, Wong TY, Foster PJ, et al. The prevalence and types of glaucoma in malay people: the Singapore Malay eye study. Invest Ophthalmol Vis Sci. 2008;49(9):3846-51.
18. He M, Foster PJ, Ge J et al. Prevalence and clinical characteristics of glaucoma in adult Chinese: a population-based study in Liwan District, Guangzhou. Invest Ophthalmol Vis Sci. 2006;47(7):2782-8.
19. Kim KE, Kim MJ, Park KH, et al. Prevalence, awareness, and risk factors of primary open-angle glaucoma: Korea National Health and Nutrition Examination Survey 2008-2011. Ophthalmology. 2016;123(3):532-41.
20. Suzuki Y, Iwase A, Araie M, et al. Risk factors for open-angle glaucoma in a Japanese population: the Tajimi Study. Ophthalmology. 2006;113(9):1613-7.
21. De Voogd S, Ikram MK, Wolfs RCW, et al. Incidence of open-angle glaucoma in a general elderly population: the Rotterdam Study. Ophthalmology. 2005;112(9):1487-93.
22. Mukesh BN, McCarty CA, Rait JL, Taylor HR. Five-year incidence of open-angle glaucoma: the visual impairment project. Ophthalmology. 2002;109(6):1047-51.
23. Varma R, Wang D, Wu C, et al. Four-year incidence of open-angle glaucoma and ocular hypertension: the Los Angeles Latino Eye Study. Am J Ophthalmol. 2012;154(2):315-25.e1.
24. Cedrone C, Mancino R, Ricci F, et al. The 12-year incidence of glaucoma and glaucoma-related visual field loss in Italy: the Ponza eye study. J Glaucoma. 2012;21(1):1-6.
25. Pan CW, Yang WY, Hu DN, et al. Longitudinal Cohort Study on the Incidence of Primary Open-Angle Glaucoma in Bai Chinese. Am J Ophthalmol. 2017;176:127-33.
26. Chua J, Baskaran M, Ong PG, et al. Prevalence, risk factors, and visual features of undiagnosed glaucoma: The Singapore Epidemiology of Eye Diseases Study. JAMA Ophthalmol. 2015;133(8):938-46.
27. Shaikh Y, Yu F, Coleman AL. Burden of undetected and untreated glaucoma in the United States. Am J Ophthalmol. 2014;158(6):1121-9.e1.
28. Topouzis F, Coleman AL, Harris A, et al. Factors associated with undiagnosed open-angle glaucoma: the Thessaloniki Eye Study. Am J Ophthalmol. 2008;145(2):327-35.
29. Leske MC, Wu SY, Hennis A, et al. Risk factors for incident open-angle glaucoma: the Barbados Eye Studies. Ophthalmology. 2008;115(1):85-93.
30. Topouzis F, Wilson MR, Harris A, et al. Risk factors for primary open-angle glaucoma and pseudoexfoliative glaucoma in the Thessaloniki eye study. Am J Ophthalmol. 2011;152(2):219-28.e1.
31. Le A, Mukesh BN, McCarty CA, et al. Risk factors associated with the incidence of open-angle glaucoma: the visual impairment project. Invest Ophthalmol Vis Sci. 2003;44(9):3783-9.
32. Francis BA, Varma R, Chopra V, et al. Intraocular pressure, central corneal thickness, and prevalence of open-angle glaucoma: the Los Angeles Latino Eye Study. Am J Ophthalmol. 2008;146(5):741-6.
33. Miglior S, Torri V, Zeyen T, et al. Intercurrent factors associated with the development of open-angle glaucoma in the European glaucoma prevention study. Am J Ophthalmol. 2007;144(2):266-75.
34. Gordon MO, Beiser JA, Brandt JD, et al. The Ocular Hypertension Treatment Study: baseline factors that predict the onset of primary open-angle glaucoma. Arch Ophthalmol. 2002;120(6):714-20; discussion 829-30.
35. Tielsch JM, Katz J, Sommer A, et al. Family history and risk of primary open angle glaucoma. The Baltimore Eye Survey. Arch Ophthalmology. 1994;112(1):69-73.
36. Wolfs RC, Klaver CC, Ramrattan RS, et al. Genetic risk of primary open-angle glaucoma. Population-based familial aggregation study. Arch Ophthalmol. 1998;116(12):1640-5.
37. Kohlhaas M, Boehm AG, Spoerl E, et al. Effect of central corneal thickness, corneal curvature, and axial length on applanation tonometry. Arch Ophthalmol. 2006;124(4):471-6.
38. Brandt JD, Gordon MO, Gao F, et al. Adjusting intraocular pressure for central corneal thickness does not improve prediction models for primary open-angle glaucoma. Ophthalmology. 2012;119(3):437-42.
39. Astrom S, Linden C. Incidence and prevalence of pseudoexfoliation and open-angle glaucoma in northern Sweden: I. Baseline report. Acta ophthalmologica Scandinavica. 2007;85(8):828-31.
40. Mitchell P, Wang JJ, Hourihan F. The relationship between glaucoma and pseudoexfoliation: the Blue Mountains Eye Study. Arch Ophthalmol. 1999;117(10):1319-24.
41. Arvind H, Raju P, Paul PG, et al. Pseudoexfoliation in south India. Br J Ophthalmol. 2003;87:1321-3.
42. Curt E. Elevated intraocular pressure and pseudoexfoliation of the lens capsule as risk factors for chronic open-angle glaucoma. A population-based five-year follow-up study. Acta Ophthalmologica. 1993;71:189-95.
43. Topouzis F, Harris A, Wilson MR, et al. Increased likelihood of glaucoma at the same screening intraocular pressure in subjects with pseudoexfoliation: the Thessaloniki Eye Study. Am J Ophthalmol. 2009;148(4):606-13.e1.
44. Mitchell P, Hourihan F, Sandbach J, et al. The relationship between glaucoma and myopia: the Blue Mountains Eye Study. Ophthalmology. 1999;106(10):2010-5.
45. Xu L, Wang Y, Wang S, et al. High myopia and glaucoma susceptibility the Beijing Eye Study. Ophthalmology. 2007;114(2):216-20.
46. Czudowska MA, Ramdas WD, Wolfs RC, et al. Incidence of glaucomatous visual field loss: a ten-year follow-up from the Rotterdam Study. Ophthalmology. 2010;117(9):1705-12.

47. Kuzin AA, Varma R, Reddy HS, et al. Ocular biometry and open-angle glaucoma: the Los Angeles Latino Eye Study. Ophthalmology. 2010;117(9):1713-9.
48. Zheng Y, Wong TY, Mitchell P, et al. Distribution of ocular perfusion pressure and its relationship with open-angle glaucoma: the Singapore Malay Eye Study. Invest Ophthalmol Vis Sci. 2010;51(7):3399-404.
49. Ramdas WD, Wolfs RC, Hofman A, et al. Ocular perfusion pressure and the incidence of glaucoma: real effect or artifact? The Rotterdam Study. Invest Ophthalmol Vis Sci. 2011;52(9):6875-81.
50. Topouzis F, Wilson MR, Harris A, et al. Association of open-angle glaucoma with perfusion pressure status in the Thessaloniki Eye Study. Am J Ophthalmol. 2013;155(5):843-51.
51. Bae HW, Lee N, Lee HS, et al. Systemic hypertension as a risk factor for open-angle glaucoma: a meta-analysis of population-based studies. PLoS One. 2014;9(9):e108226.
52. Gramer G, Weber BH, Gramer E. Migraine and vasospasm in glaucoma: age-related evaluation of 2027 patients with glaucoma or ocular hypertension. Invest Ophthalmol Vis Sci. 2015;56(13):7999-8007.
53. Ko F, Boland MV, Gupta P, et al. Diabetes, triglyceride levels, and other risk factors for glaucoma in the national health and nutrition examination survey 2005-2008. Invest Ophthalmol Vis Sci. 2016;57(4):2152-7.
54. Gordon MO, Torri V, Miglior S, et al. Validated prediction model for the development of primary open-angle glaucoma in individuals with ocular hypertension. Ophthalmology. 2007;114(1):10-9.
55. Miglior S, Pfeiffer N, Torri V, et al. Predictive factors for open-angle glaucoma among patients with ocular hypertension in the European Glaucoma Prevention Study. Ophthalmology. 2007;114(1):3-9.
56. Leske MC, Heijl A, Hyman L, et al. Early Manifest Glaucoma Trial: design and baseline data. Ophthalmology. 1999;106(11):2144-53.
57. Heijl A, Bengtsson B, Hyman L, et al. Natural history of open-angle glaucoma. Ophthalmology. 2009;116(12):2271-6.
58. Bengtsson B. Prediction of glaucomatous visual field loss by extrapolation of linear trends. Arch Ophthalmol. 2009;127(12):1610.
59. Wilson MR, Kosoko O, Cowan CL, et al. Progression of visual field loss in untreated glaucoma patients and glaucoma suspects in St. Lucia, West Indies. Am J Ophthalmol. 2002;134(3):399-405.
60. Anderson DR, Drance SM, Schulzer M. Comparison of glaucomatous progression between untreated patients with normal-tension glaucoma and patients with therapeutically reduced intraocular pressures. Collaborative Normal-Tension Glaucoma Study Group. Am J Ophthalmol. 1998;126(4):487-97.
61. Anderson DR, Drance SM, Schulzer M. Natural history of normal-tension glaucoma. Ophthalmology. 2001;108(2):247-53.
62. European Glaucoma Society. Terminology and Guidelines for Glaucoma, 4th edition. Savona, Italy: Publicomm; 2014.
63. Prum BE, Rosenberg LF, Gedde SJ, et al. Primary Open-Angle Glaucoma Preferred Practice Pattern® Guidelines. Ophthalmology. 2016;123(1):P41-P111.
64. Pascolini D, Mariotti SP. Global estimates of visual impairment: 2010. Br J Ophthalmol. 2012;96(5):614-8.
65. Bourne RR, Taylor HR, Flaxman SR, et al. Number of People Blind or Visually Impaired by Glaucoma Worldwide and in World Regions 1990-2010: a meta-analysis. PloS One. 2016;11(10):e0162229.
66. Peters D, Bengtsson B, Heijl A. Lifetime risk of blindness in open-angle glaucoma. Am J Ophthalmol. 2013;156(4):724-30.
67. Peters D, Bengtsson B, Heijl A. Factors associated with lifetime risk of open-angle glaucoma blindness. Acta Ophthalmologica. 2014;92(5):421-5.
68. Foster PJ, Buhrmann R, Quigley HA, et al. The definition and classification of glaucoma in prevalence surveys. Br J Ophthalmol. 2002;86(2):238-42.
69. Gordon MO, Kass MA. The Ocular Hypertension Treatment Study: design and baseline description of the participants. Arch Ophthalmol. 1999;117(5):573-83.
70. Kass MA, Heuer DK, Higginbotham EJ, et al. The Ocular Hypertension Treatment Study: a randomized trial determines that topical ocular hypotensive medication delays or prevents the onset of primary open-angle glaucoma. Arch Ophthalmol. 2002;120(6):701-13; discussion 829-30.
71. Kass MA, Gordon MO, Gao F, et al. Delaying treatment of ocular hypertension: the ocular hypertension treatment study. Arch Ophthalmol. 2010;128(3):276.
72. European glaucoma prevention study. The European glaucoma prevention study design and baseline description of the participants. Ophthalmology. 2002;109(9):1612-21.
73. European glaucoma prevention study. Results of the European glaucoma prevention study. Ophthalmology. 2005;112(3):366-75.
74. Quigley HA. European Glaucoma Prevention Study. Ophthalmology. 2005;112(9):1642-3; author reply 3-5.
75. Prum BE, Lim MC, Mansberger SL, et al. Primary open-angle glaucoma suspect preferred practice Pattern® Guidelines. Ophthalmology. 2016;123(1):P112-P51.
76. Tielsch JM, Katz J, Singh K, et al. A population-based evaluation of glaucoma screening: the Baltimore Eye Survey. Am J Epidemiol. 1991;134(10):1102-10.
77. Weih LM, Nanjan M, McCarty CA, Taylor HR. Prevalence and predictors of open-angle glaucoma: results from the visual impairment project. Ophthalmology. 2001;108(11):1966-72.
78. Leske MC, Connell A, Wu S-Y, et al. Risk factors for open-angle glaucoma: the Barbados Eye Study. Arch Ophthalmol. 1995;113(7):918-24.
79. Jiang X, Varma R, Wu S et al. Baseline risk factors that predict the development of open-angle glaucoma in a population: the Los Angeles Latino Eye Study. Ophthalmology. 2012;119(11):2245-53.

80. Nemesure B, Honkanen R, Hennis A, et al. Incident open-angle glaucoma and intraocular pressure. Ophthalmology. 2007;114(10):1810-5.
81. Leske MC, Heijl A, Hyman L et al. Predictors of long-term progression in the early manifest glaucoma trial. Ophthalmology. 2007;114(11):1965-72.
82. Bengtsson B, Leske MC, Hyman L, et al. Fluctuation of intraocular pressure and glaucoma progression in the early manifest glaucoma trial. Ophthalmology. 2007;114(2):205-9.
83. Collaborative Normal-Tension Glaucoma Study Group. Comparison of glaucomatous progression between untreated patients with normal-tension glaucoma and patients with therapeutically reduced intraocular pressures. Am J Ophthalmol. 1998;126(4):487-97.
84. Collaborative Normal-Tension Glaucoma Study Group. The effectiveness of intraocular pressure reduction in the treatment of normal-tension glaucoma. Am J Ophthalmol. 1998;126(4):498-505.
85. The AGIS Investigators. The Advanced Glaucoma Intervention Study (AGIS): 7. The relationship between control of intraocular pressure and visual field deterioration. Am J Ophthalmol. 2000;130:429-40.
86. Caprioli J, Coleman AL. Intraocular pressure fluctuation: a risk factor for visual field progression at low intraocular pressures in the Advanced Glaucoma Intervention Study. Ophthalmology. 2008;115(7):1123-9.e3.
87. Musch DC, Lichter PR, Guire KE, et al. The Collaborative Initial Glaucoma Treatment Study: study design, methods, and baseline characteristics of enrolled patients. Ophthalmology. 1999;106(4):653-62.
88. Musch DC, Gillespie BW, Lichter PR, et al. Visual field progression in the Collaborative Initial Glaucoma Treatment Study the impact of treatment and other baseline factors. Ophthalmology. 2009;116(2):200-7.
89. Lichter PR, Musch DC, Gillespie BW, et al. Interim clinical outcomes in the Collaborative Initial Glaucoma Treatment Study comparing initial treatment randomized to medications or surgery. Ophthalmology. 2001;108(11): 1943-53.
90. Garway-Heath DF, Crabb DP, Bunce C, et al. Latanoprost for open-angle glaucoma (UKGTS): a randomised, multicentre, placebo-controlled trial. The Lancet. 2015;385(9975): 1295-304.
91. Musch DC, Gillespie BW, Palmberg PF, et al. Visual field improvement in the collaborative initial glaucoma treatment study. Am J Ophthalmol. 2014;158(1):96-104.e2.
92. Bengtsson B, Leske MC, Yang Z, et al. Disc hemorrhages and treatment in the early manifest glaucoma trial. Ophthalmology. 2008;115(11):2044-8.
93. Anderson DR, Drance SM, Schulzer M. Factors that predict the benefit of lowering intraocular pressure in normal tension glaucoma. Am J Ophthalmol. 2003;136(5):820-9.
94. Leske MC, Heijl A, Hussein M, et al. Factors for glaucoma progression and the effect of treatment: the early manifest glaucoma trial. Arch Ophthalmol. 2003;121(1):48-56.
95. Nouri-Mahdavi K, Hoffman D, Coleman AL, et al. Predictive factors for glaucomatous visual field progression in the Advanced Glaucoma Intervention Study. Ophthalmology. 2004;111(9):1627-35.
96. Singh K, Shrivastava A. Early aggressive intraocular pressure lowering, target intraocular pressure, and a novel concept for glaucoma care. Surv Ophthalmol. 2008;53(Suppl 1):S33-8.
97. Singh K, Shrivastava A. Medical management of glaucoma: principles and practice. Ind J Ophthalmol. 2011;59(Suppl):S88-92.
98. Heijl A, Buchholz P, Norrgren G, et al. Rates of visual field progression in clinical glaucoma care. Acta Ophthalmologica. 2013;91(5):406-12.
99. Chauhan BC, Garway-Heath DF, Goni FJ, et al. Practical recommendations for measuring rates of visual field change in glaucoma. Br J Ophthalmol. 2008;92(4):569-73.
100. Chauhan BC, Mikelberg FS, Artes PH, et al. Canadian Glaucoma Study: 3. Impact of risk factors and intraocular pressure reduction on the rates of visual field change. Arch Ophthalmol. 2010;128(10):1249-55.
101. Ahrlich KG, De Moraes CG, Teng CC, et al. Visual field progression differences between normal-tension and exfoliative high-tension glaucoma. Invest Ophthalmol Vis Sci. 2010;51(3):1458-63.
102. Medeiros FA, Alencar LM, Sample PA, et al. The relationship between intraocular pressure reduction and rates of progressive visual field loss in eyes with optic disc hemorrhage. Ophthalmology. 2010;117(11):2061-6.
103. Lee JM, Caprioli J, Nouri-Mahdavi K, et al. Baseline prognostic factors predict rapid visual field deterioration in glaucoma. Invest Ophthalmol Vis Sci. 2014;55(4):2228-36.
104. Hyman LG, Komaroff E, Heijl A, et al. Treatment and vision-related quality of life in the early manifest glaucoma trial. Ophthalmology. 2005;112(9):1505-13.
105. Peters D, Heijl A, Brenner L, et al. Visual impairment and vision-related quality of life in the Early Manifest Glaucoma Trial after 20 years of follow-up. Acta ophthalmologica. 2015;93(8):745-52.
106. Janz NK, Wren PA, Lichter PR, et al. The Collaborative Initial Glaucoma Treatment Study: interim quality of life findings after initial medical or surgical treatment of glaucoma. Ophthalmology. 2001;108(11):1954-65.
107. Lisboa R, Chun YS, Zangwill LM, et al. Association between rates of binocular visual field loss and vision-related quality of life in patients with glaucoma. JAMA Ophthalmol. 2013;131(4):486-94.
108. Arora KS, Boland MV, Friedman DS, et al. The relationship between better eye and integrated visual field mean deviation and visual disability. Ophthalmology. 2013;120(12):2476-84.

Chapter 63

Primary Angle-closure Glaucoma: Epidemiology, Natural History, and Clinical Course under Optimal Care

Srinivasan Kavitha, Swati Upadhyaya

INTRODUCTION

Glaucoma is the most common cause of irreversible blindness in the world. Primary angle-closure glaucoma (PACG) is a more visually destructive form of disease than primary open-angle glaucoma (POAG). Despite being less prevalent than POAG, PACG is responsible for half of the glaucoma-related blindness in the world. Most of the angle closure, however, is asymptomatic. In some instances, it progresses, leading to an increased intraocular pressure (IOP) resulting in damage to the optic nerve head. It is an ideal condition to take a preventive approach as early diagnosis and appropriate intervention may prevent progression to more advanced stages of the disease.

EPIDEMIOLOGY

Epidemiological studies (Table 63.1) in glaucoma provide us with insights into the prevalence of the disease and its risk factors. According to the recently published meta-analysis by Tham et al.[1] for the population aged 40–80 years, the global prevalence of POAG is 3.05% and PACG is 0.5%. PACG is more common in Asians than in any other ethnic group[2] with a prevalence of 1.09%.[1] By 2020, Asia will have largest number of persons affected by PACG, with approximately 21 million cases, and more than 5.3 million bilaterally blind individuals as a result of PACG.[3] This is due to the population growth as well as the increasing longevity in the Asian region.

Primary angle closure glaucoma, despite being less prevalent than POAG, is responsible for most of the blindness in India.[4] In most of the population-based studies in India, PACG was observed to cause one to four times the proportion of blindness as POAG.[4,5] It is also responsible for most of the uncorrectable bilateral glaucoma blindness in Mongolia and Singapore. Based on the estimates from China, the proportion of those blind with PACG is 25%, twice more than POAG blindness, which is 10%.[6]

Table 63.1: Prevalence of angle closure.

Study	Primary angle-closure glaucoma (PACG) (%)
Blue mountain eye study	0.3
Baltimore eye study	0.9
Aravind comprehensive eye survey	0.5
Vellore eye study	4.32

DEFINITION

Primary angle closure (PAC) has been defined as appositional or synechial closure of anterior chamber (AC) angle caused by pupillary block[7] by the normal lens without any other complicating factors (such as posterior synechiae). The most common mechanism leading to angle closure is relative pupillary block, wherein there is increased resistance to aqueous flow from posterior chamber to anterior chamber. The resultant pressure gradient between the posterior chamber and anterior chamber causes a forward bowing of the peripheral iris so that it covers all or part of the filtering portion of the trabecular meshwork (TM) causing appositional angle closure. Prolonged or repeated contact of peripheral iris with TM leads to peripheral anterior synechiae (PAS) and residual damage to TM.[8]

CLASSIFICATION

The best method of classifying the various types of angle-closure glaucoma continues to be debated. Foster and associates have published a classification of angle closure that has been widely used in prevalence studies and epidemiological research.[9] This system is known as the International Society of Geographical and Epidemiological Ophthalmology (ISGEO) classification (Table 63.2).

It specifies three stages of angle closure:

1. Primary angle-closure suspect (PACS)
2. Primary angle closure (PAC)
3. Primary angle-closure glaucoma (PACG).

This classification is based on the presumed natural history of angle closure glaucoma, constituting a spectrum

Table 63.2: International Society of Geographical and Epidemiological Ophthalmology (ISGEO) classification.

	≥270° of the posterior trabecular meshwork not seen	Raised IOP or PAS	Disc and field changes
PACS	+	-	-
PAC	+	+	-
PACG	+	+	+

(PACS: Primary angle-closure suspect; PAC: Primary angle closure; PACG: Primary angle-closure glaucoma; IOP: Intraocular pressure; PAS: Peripheral anterior synechiae)

ranging from anatomical narrowing (PACS) to evidence of structural trabecular damage (PAC) and finally functional damage in the form of optic neuropathy (PACG).

Primary angle-closure disease (PACD) is the common terminology employed to cover the entire spectrum of disease, from PACS to PACG.

Primary Angle-closure Suspect

The individual with an anatomically narrow angle can be classified as PACS when gonioscopy reveals a shallow peripheral angle recess with the iris reversibly apposing the TM (Figs. 63.1A and B). A diagnosis of PACS is made in the context of:

- Iridotrabecular contact (ITC) precluding the view of TM in three or more quadrants (270°)
- No PAS on indentation
- Normal IOP, optic nerve, and visual field (VF)
- In some of the prevalent surveys, instead of 270°, 180° of ITC is used as a cutoff to diagnose PACS. In essence, these are anatomically narrow angles without any signs of glaucoma. At the same time, it has to be understood that these eyes are at increased risk of progression to PAC or PACG.

Primary Angle Closure

A diagnosis of PAC is made in the following context:

- The individual has ITC in three or more quadrants in which no pigmented TM is visualized
- There may be either elevated IOP (disorder of function) and/or primary PAS (abnormality of structure) (Figs. 63.2A and B), but with a normal optic nerve and VF. The other clinical signs which may be present include iris whorling/atrophic patches, glaucomflecken in the lens and excess pigment deposition in the TM, all of which indicate previous episodes of angle closure (Fig. 63.3).

Primary Angle-closure Glaucoma

In PACG, the individual has the features of PAC along with glaucomatous optic neuropathy and a corresponding VF defect compatible with glaucoma. These eyes are abnormal in structure and function, with characteristic glaucomatous optic nerve head changes.

ETIOLOGY AND MECHANISM OF PRIMARY ANGLE-CLOSURE GLAUCOMA

Angle closure may occur by forces acting at any one of the four successive anatomic levels, as proposed by Ritch et al:[10] (1) block *at the level of iris* results in *pupillary block*

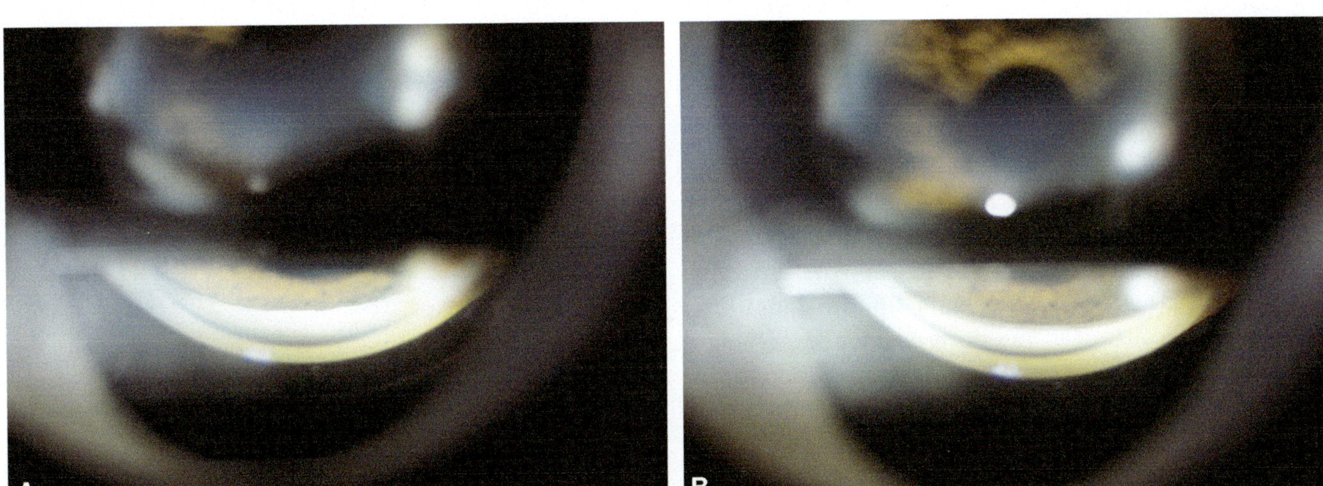

Figs. 63.1A and B: Gonioscopy of occludable angle—(A) No angle structure is made out in primary gaze; (B) Angle opens up to scleral spur on indentation, no peripheral anterior synechiae (PAS) noted.

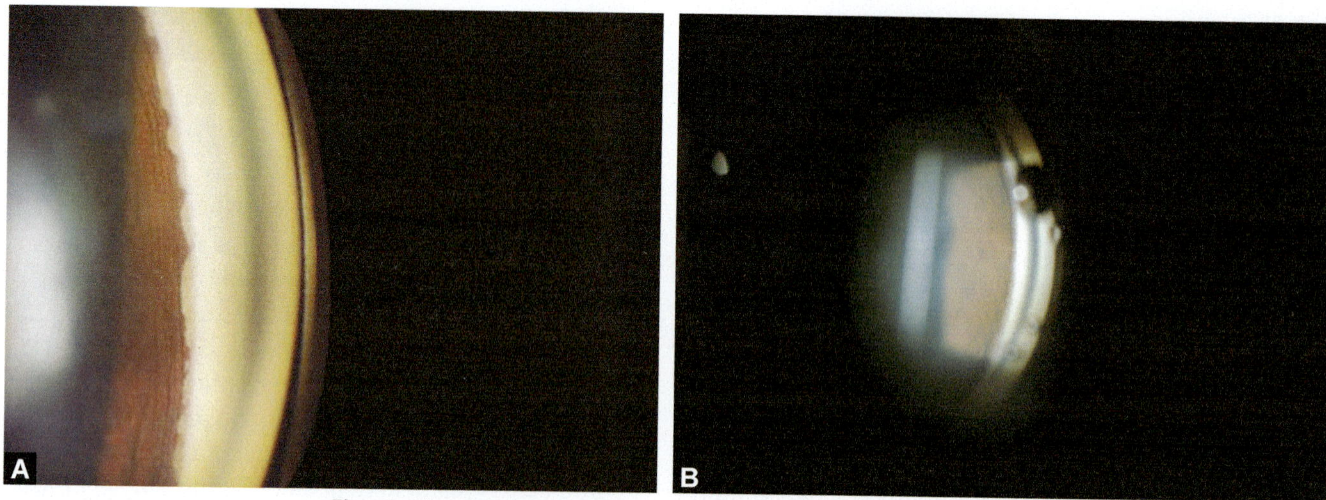

Figs. 63.2A and B: (A) Peripheral anterior synechiae (PAS); (B) Iris processes.
Note: Iris processes are fine, lacy structure, do not cross trabecular meshwork (TM), whereas PAS are broad, crosses the TM and bridge the underlying structures.

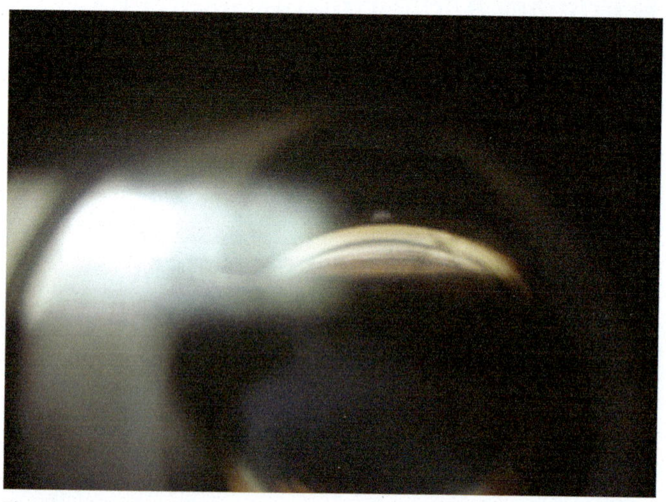

Fig. 63.3: Gonioscopy showing localized hyperpigmentation of trabecular meshwork and Schwalbe's line, indicating a possible prior angle closure attack.

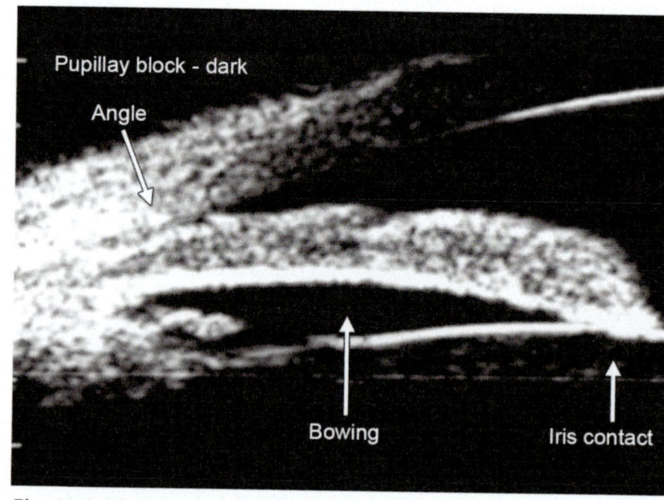

Fig. 63.4: Ultrasound biomicroscopy (UBM) showing pupillary block, note the bowing of the peripheral iris, due to raised pressure in the posterior chamber.

glaucoma, (2) block *at the level of ciliary body* results in *plateau iris configuration/syndrome*, (3) block *at the level of lens* causes *phacogenic mechanism or lens-induced glaucoma,* and (4) block due to *retrolenticular forces* results in *malignant glaucoma.*

The most common mechanism seen in PACG is pupillary block (Fig. 63.4),[11] as detailed in the definition. This happens because of an anteriorly positioned lens, high lens vault (Fig. 63.5) (with or without associated increase in thickness of the lens) resulting in a narrow channel between the iris and the lens. Quigley et al. proposed choroidal expansion as a contributing risk factor for PACG and acute primary angle closure (APAC).[12] The degree to which choroidal expansion occurs depends on many variables including choroidal elasticity and vascular permeability.

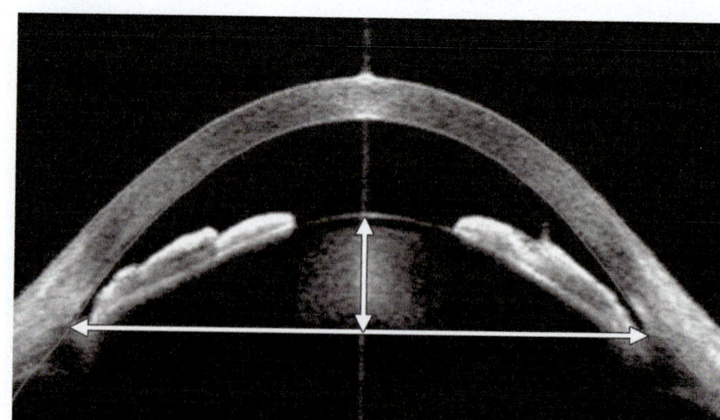

Fig. 63.5: Anterior segment optical coherence tomography (ASOCT) showing lens vault, vertical arrow is the lens vault, defined as the perpendicular distance between the anterior pole of lens and horizontal line connecting the scleral spur on either side.

Primary angle closure not only results from predisposing anterior segment anatomy, but also unfavorable physiological behavior of iris.[12] Quigley demonstrated that in normal eyes, the iris acts as a "sponge" which loses volume on dilatation by egressing fluid to the aqueous. However, in angle-closure glaucoma, the iris does not lose volume and hence blocks the angle. Further evidence to support the concept of abnormal physiological behavior of iris comes from an optical coherence tomography study where iris volume was found to increase significantly following pharmacological dilation of the pupil, a phenomenon most salient in the contralateral eyes of patients with previous APAC.[13] Hence, physiologic pupillary dilation is considered as a possible risk factor for angle closure.

RISK FACTORS FOR ANGLE CLOSURE

There are certain anatomical, physiological, demographic, and genetic risk factors, which predispose an eye to develop angle closure (Box 63.1).

Anatomical Risk Factors

Cross sectional and clinical studies consistently find that eyes with following features are at a greater risk for angle closure:[14]

- Short axial lengths
- Shallow AC, both centrally and peripherally
- Small corneal diameters
- Hyperopic refractive errors
- Thick, relatively anteriorly positioned lens.[14]

The proximity of peripheral iris to the TM is considered a precondition for developing PAC and hence, the width of angle is a commonly used parameter to grade the risk of angle closure. Gonioscopic examination remains the most important method for grading the angle width and describing other signs of angle closure. Several gonioscopic grading methods have been devised, which include Scheie, Shaffer, and Spaeth systems. All these systems are based either on estimation of the width of the angle in degrees and/or visibility of angle land marks.

Gonioscopic grading is a subjective measurement that usually depends on examiner's experience and skill. Objective quantifiable grading of the angle is obtained by anterior segment imaging (or) biometric technologies, such as ultrasound biomicroscopy (UBM), A-scan ultrasound biometry, IOLMaster, scanning peripheral anterior chamber depth analyzer (SPAC), and anterior segment optical coherence tomography (ASOCT). Of these modalities, SPAC, ASOCT and the IOLMaster are fast, noncontact methods, and therefore may be more suitable for large scale screening if sufficient screening algorithms can be validated.

Box 63.1: Risk factors for angle-closure glaucoma.

Anatomical factors
- Short axial length
- Smaller corneal diameter
- Shallow anterior chamber
- Increased lens thickness
- Anterior position of lens
- Increased curvature of anterior lens surface

Physiological factors
- Mid-dilated pupil/emotional stress
- Dim illumination
- Near work
- Prone position

Demographic factors
- Gender: Common in females
- Race: Indians, Eskimos, Chinese, and other Asian groups

Psychosomatic factors
- Type-I personality

Age, Gender and Ethnicity

Increasing age is a risk factor for angle closure. The thickening and anterior movement of lens[15] in older individuals causes shallowing of the AC resulting in pupillary block.

Female gender is also a major predisposing factor for PACD. The prevalence of all categories of angle closure is 2–5 times higher in women than in men, which may in part be due to the presence of shallow AC in women.[16]

Ethnic differences have been well recognized in angle closure. The prevalence and incidence of angle closure is higher in East Asian populations than Europeans.[17] These differences may be attributed to variations in AC and angle anatomy. Indeed, majority of the evidence suggest an inverse association between AC depth and frequency of angle closure in various ethnic groups.

Genetic Predisposition

A genetic etiology for PACG is supported by several epidemiological and clinical studies which showed familial aggregation and higher risk of disease in family members[18,19] as well as heritability of risk factors such as AC depth.[20] All these factors strongly suggests that genetic factors are involved in the pathogenesis of PACG.[21] Vithana et al. conducted a two-stage genome-wide association study (GWAS) to assess the genetic determinants of PACD and found genome wide significant association between PACG and three genetic markers namely: rs11024102 in

PLEKHA7, rs3753841 in COL11A1, and rs1015213 located between PCMTD1 and ST18 on chromosome 8q.[21] A study by Duvesh et al.[22] in a South Indian population replicated findings of this large GWAS, again implicating rs1015213 in the pathogenesis of PACG.

While all the three genes are expressed in tissues of the iridocorneal angle, the exact mechanism by which they cause PACD is not completely understood. The successful identification of novel PACG associated genes has provided insights into the genetic mechanisms underlying the disease susceptibility, though further work is required to understand the structural/physiologic consequences of alterations in these genetic loci.

Family History

A positive family history has long been recognized as a significant predisposing factor to angle closure.[23] The similarities of ocular biometry in the first degree relatives of angle closure indicate that the angle closure-related anatomical characteristics are heritable.

Sihota et al. examined the first degree relatives of Indian PACG patients and reported a prevalence of 36.9% of PACG among their siblings.[18]

We compared the prevalence of angle closure among the siblings of patients with open angles (OA), PACS, and either PAC or PACG, in a South Indian population. Angle closure was more prevalent in both PACS siblings (35%) and PAC/PACG siblings (36.71%) when compared with OA siblings (3.7%).[19] The study showed that the siblings of patients with angle closure are at an 8.8 times greater risk of angle closure. The risk was also greater in women and older siblings.

EVALUATION

The following elements should be performed as part of the evaluation of persons with possible PACD.

History

- Family history, with a positive history suggesting a higher likelihood of disease.
- Medication history, with certain medications increasing the risk of medication-induced angle closure (Box 63.2).
- History suggesting previous subacute episodes marked by pain, redness, haloes, brow ache, and headache.

Ocular Examination

- Refractive status should be determined, with hyperopic eyes at greater risk of PACD.
- Cornea, iris, pupil, and lens should be assessed for the signs of previous angle-closure attack (Box 63.3) including PAS, iris atrophy (Fig. 63.6), glaucomflecken, pupillary dysfunction, or an irregular pupil (Fig. 63.7).
- Intraocular pressure with Goldmann applanation tonometry (gold standard) should be performed before gonioscopy, to avoid false lowering of IOP after gonioscopy, especially with indentation.
- Optic nerve head evaluation should be performed.

Box 63.2: Drugs that can precipitate angle closure in susceptible eyes.

- Antipsychotics—e.g. phenothiazines
- Antidepressants—tricyclic and nontricyclic agents
- Anticonvulsants—e.g. topiramate
- Monoamine oxidase inhibitors
- Antihistamines
- Antiparkinsonian agents—e.g. trihexyphenidyl
- Antibiotics—e.g. sulfa drugs
- Sympathomimetic agents—e.g. adrenaline and naphazoline
- Mydriatic agents—e.g. atropine, homatropine, and tropicamide
- Miotics—e.g. pilocarpine and echothiophate
- Cardiac agents—e.g. disopyramide

Box 63.3: Signs of previous angle-closure attack.

- Pigments back of cornea
- Peripheral anterior synechiae
- Iris atrophic patches
- Posterior synechiae
- Mid-dilated, sluggishly reacting pupil
- Glaukomflecken
- Patchy hyperpigmentation of trabecular meshwork
- Visual field loss
- Optic nerve cupping/pallor

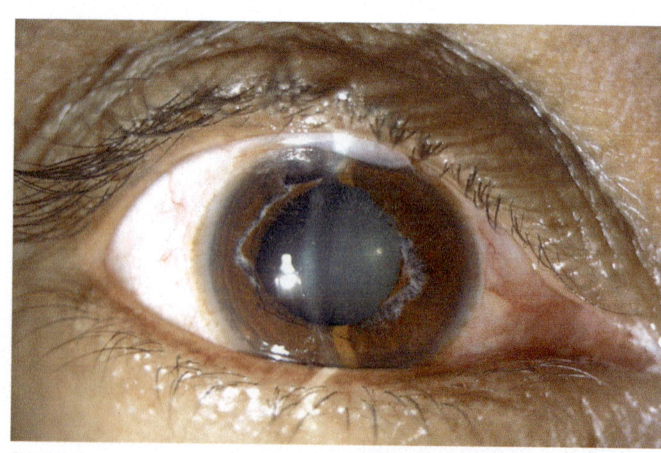

Fig. 63.6: Slit-lamp biomicroscopy showing iris atrophic patches, eye which had acute primary angle closure (APAC), post-trabeculectomy, note surgical peripheral iridectomy (PI) at 11 o'clock.

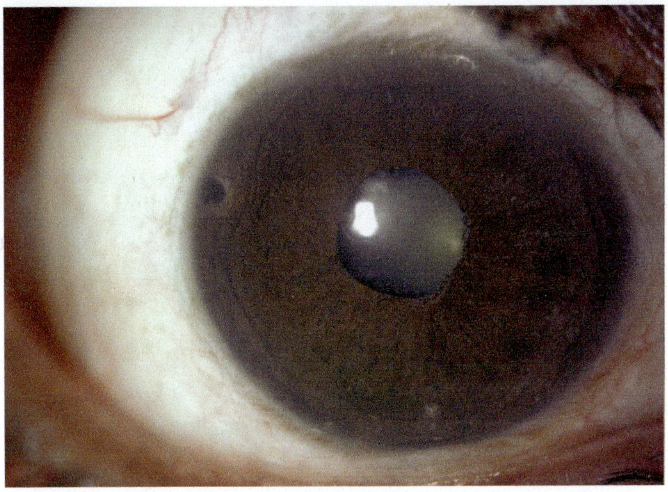

Fig. 63.7: Slit-lamp biomicroscopy showing loss of pupillary ruff, which is a sign of angle closure.

Clinical Evaluation of Anterior Chamber Depth

Oblique Flashlight Test

This test gives cursory information about the depth of the AC. In the presence of a forward bowing of the iris, a light shown from the temporal side of an eye casts a shadow on the nasal side (eclipse sign) (Fig. 63.8).

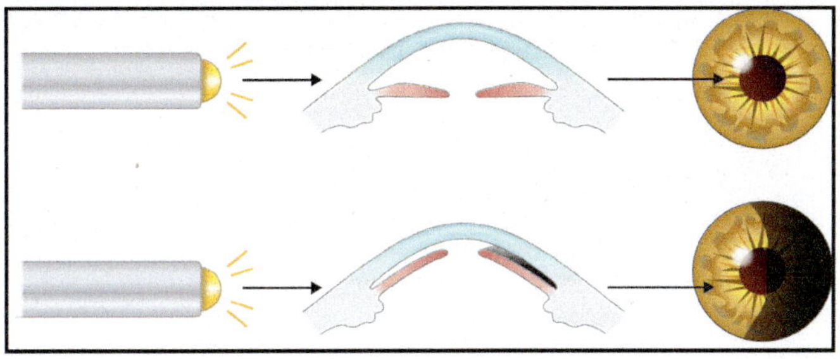

Fig. 63.8: Oblique flashlight test: Shine torchlight from temporal limbus and look for iris shadow. More the iris shadow, shallower the anterior chamber.

Van Herick's Grading

This technique of using the slit lamp to indirectly assess the width of the AC, has a sensitivity of 62–80% and specificity of 89–92%.[24] The optical section of slit lamp, must be placed just inside the limbus and peripheral AC depth (PAC-D) is compared with corneal thickness (CT) and graded as given here:

- Grade 4: PAC-D > ½ CT, wide OA
- Grade 3: PAC-D = ¼ to ½ CT, mild narrow
- Grade 2: PAC-D = ¼ CT, moderate narrow
- Grade 1: PAC-D < ¼ CT, extremely narrow

One should not stop with oblique flash light test or Van Herick's grading, as these tests can only act as preliminary screening measures, and the findings should be confirmed with gonioscopy.

Gonioscopy

A competent gonioscopy technique is compulsory to diagnose angle closure (Flowchart 63.1). Gonioscopy should be performed in a dark room, using 1 mm^2 light with the brightest possible slit lamp beam lighting the eye, away from the pupil, to avoid miosis and false opening up of the angle. One needs to identify the anterior point of iris angle contact, without inadvertent compression. After assessing in primary gaze, indentation gonioscopy should always be performed, with a 4-mirror goniolens. Since this lens diameter is smaller than the corneal diameter, it can indent the cornea. Indentation gonioscopy reveals the angle structures in instances of appositional closure, but not in instances of synechial closure and thus can be used to differentiate these two conditions (Fig. 63.9).

Imaging Techniques

Imaging techniques such as those discussed below help us to understand the pathogenesis and mechanisms of angle closure, but need more validation. Both ASOCT and UBM showed excellent performance in identifying eyes with narrow angles[25] and hence they are good screening tools. They do have certain advantages and disadvantages (Table 63.3). It is important to remember that *these imaging modalities can complement gonioscopy but cannot replace it.*

Ultrasound Biomicroscopy

Ultrasound biomicroscopy allows dynamic high-resolution imaging of the anterior segment structures. Features of UBM include:

- The use of high-frequency ultrasound (50 MHz)
- A high axial resolution (25 μm) and lateral resolution (50 μm)
- Tissue penetration of 4–5 mm
- Use of sound waves which can capture images even through opaque media
- Useful in identifying plateau iris configuration.

Flowchart 63.1: Evaluation of angle, SEAGIG guidelines.

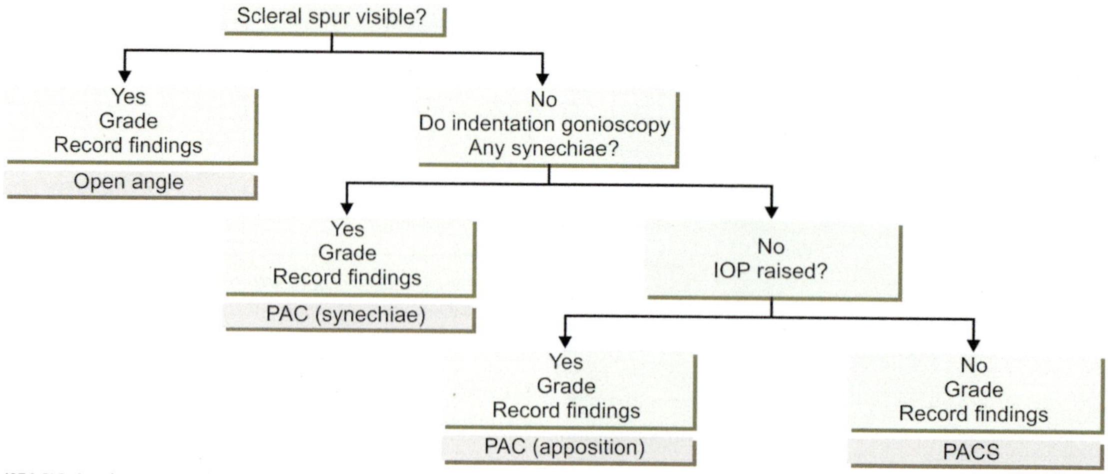

(SEAGIG: South East Asia Glaucoma Interest Group; IOP: Intraocular pressure; PAC: Primary angle closure; PACS: Primary angle-closure suspect)

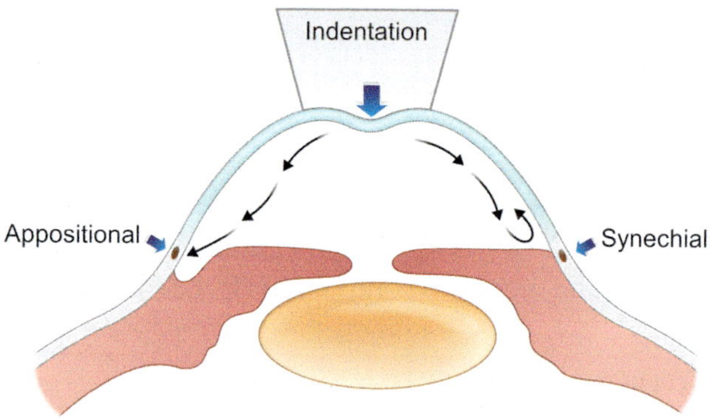

Fig. 63.9: Indentation gonioscopy: Indentation gonioscopy, done with 4-mirror goniolens, forces the aqueous to the angle, pushes the iris away and opens the angle in appositional closure, while it remains closed in synechial closure.

Table 63.3: Comparison of ASOCT and UBM.

ASOCT	UBM
Important landmarks like scleral spur more distinct	Less distinct visualization of structures
Patient has to be seated, more physiological	Patient must lie down, causing lens-iris diaphragm to fall back
All four angle quadrants can be measured simultaneously	One angle at a time
Limited visualization of structures posterior to iris, poor visualization of ciliary body	Detection of ciliary body is better

(ASOCT: Anterior segment optical coherence tomography, UBM: Ultrasound biomicroscopy)

Anterior Segment Optical Coherence Tomography

The ASOCT is a noncontact technique providing high speed imaging of the anterior segment structures. Features of ASOCT include:

- Use of 1310 nm super luminescent light-emitting diode (LED) light source providing high axial resolution (18–25 µm).
- Penetration depth of 6 mm. The posterior pigmented iris and ciliary epithelium blocks the passage of infrared light, preventing visualization of more posterior structures. Its use is limited to angle and iris, and cannot reliably image the ciliary processes and lens. Hence, it is not helpful in identifying plateau iris.
- Suitable only in cases with clear media.
- Ability to provide detailed calculations such as angle opening distance (AOD), angle recess area (ARA), and trabecular iris space area (TISA).
- Superior to UBM for imaging blebs.

ACUTE PRIMARY ANGLE CLOSURE

Acute primary angle closure is often referred to as acute congestive glaucoma or an acute angle closure attack. It is an ophthalmic emergency. The most common mechanism leading to APAC is relative pupillary block. Relative pupillary block often happens when the pupil is in mid-dilated position (5–6 mm), as the iridolenticular contact is maximum in this position. There is increased resistance for aqueous flow from the posterior chamber to AC, leading to a pressure gradient between the posterior chamber and

ACs. This pressure gradient causes forward bowing of the peripheral iris. If the entire circumference of the angle is obstructed suddenly, acute pupillary block happens, raising the IOP rapidly to high levels.

Symptoms

The most common symptom is severe ocular pain associated with a red eye. There may be a profound decrease in vision. Colored haloes may be reported by the patients and are due to scattering of light as a result of corneal epithelial edema, caused by a sudden spike in the IOP. There may be associated headache, nausea, and vomiting. These attacks are usually precipitated by conditions causing pupillary dilation such as watching a movie in the dark, sitting in a dim illuminated room, or emotional stress (mydriasis secondary to increased sympathetic tone). These symptoms may abate if the pupillary block spontaneously resolves especially if circumstances initiating the attack reverse (example conditions causing miosis when the patient goes into brightly lit environment or by falling asleep).

Signs

The conjunctiva will reveal circumcorneal congestion. The cornea is usually steamy with the edema predominantly in the epithelium. The AC will be shallow and may reveal signs of inflammation such as minimal flare/cells. The pupil is typically mid-dilated, vertically oval (Fig. 63.10), and is either fixed or sluggishly reacts to light. There is marked rise in IOP. The markedly elevated IOP can result in focal lens opacities called glaucomflecken (Fig. 63.11), which are localized infarctions of the anterior lens capsule, iris atrophy, and reduced pupillary reactivity. Fundus evaluation is often not possible because of corneal edema. In some instances however, it might reveal hyperemic disc/disc edema. Prolonged appositional touch of the peripheral iris to the cornea often leads to PAS. The fellow eye often reveals narrow/occludable angles.

Differential Diagnosis

The conditions which should be considered in the differential for acutely elevated IOP producing symptoms are detailed in Box 63.4.

Box 63.4: Differential diagnosis for acute primary angle closure.

- Neovascular glaucoma
- Inflammatory/uveitic angle closure
- Iridocorneal endothelial syndrome
- Suprachoroidal effusion caused by systemic medications like topiramate, sulfonamides and phenothiazines
- Ciliary body engorgement associated with retinal vascular occlusion or pan retinal photocoagulation
- Malignant glaucoma
- Lens-induced glaucoma—phacomorphic or subluxated
- Developmental disorders like nanophthalmos
- Iris or ciliary body mass lesions
- Other secondary causes of pupillary block (pupillary block by vitreous, silicone oil)

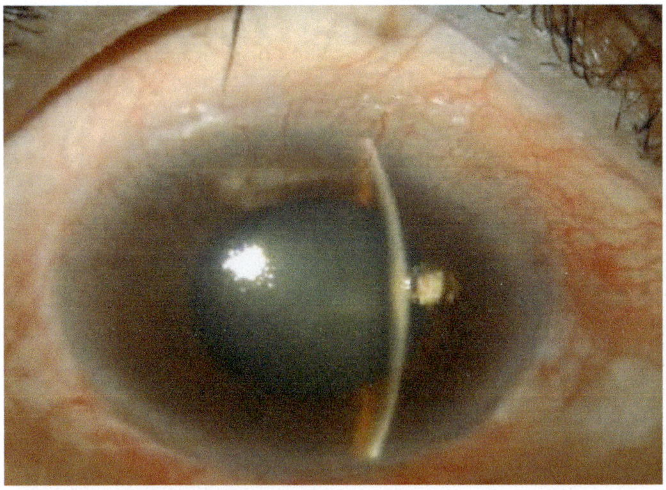

Fig. 63.10: Eye with acute primary angle closure (APAC) showing ciliary congestion, corneal edema and dilated and fixed pupil.

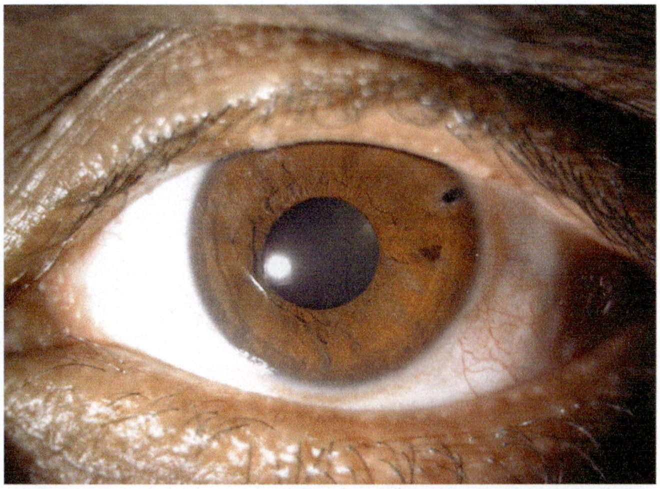

Fig. 63.11: Slit-lamp biomicroscopy showing, Glaukomflecken, grayish white opacities on anterior lens capsule, a sign of acute primary angle closure (APAC), laser peripheral iridotomy (LPI) at 2 o'clock, mid dilated pupil, iris atrophic patches.

PLATEAU IRIS CONFIGURATION AND SYNDROME

These clinical entities are often difficult to distinguish from PACG resulting from pupillary block. Plateau iris configuration occurs due to crowding of the angle with anteriorly placed ciliary process, displacing the peripheral iris anteriorly. When this configuration progresses to a closure of the AC angle, resulting in elevated IOP, it is termed as plateau iris syndrome. In this condition, performing peripheral iridotomy does not eliminate the pupillary block. IOP typically raises after dilation due to greater occlusion of angle. UBM is helpful in diagnosing plateau iris.

MANAGEMENT

Management goals in PACD include:
- Reversal or prevention of the angle closure process
- Controlling the IOP with laser, medicines, or surgery
- Preventing damage to optic nerve.

Laser Therapy

Laser Peripheral Iridotomy

Laser peripheral iridotomy (LPI), using neodymium: yttrium-aluminum-garnet (Nd:YAG-1064 nm) is the current standard approach to relieve pupillary block. It eliminates pressure differences between anterior and posterior chambers thereby alleviates pupillary block (Figs. 63.12A and B). The indications for LPI in PACD include:
- PAC
- PACG
- APAC
- Fellow eyes of APAC

Evidence has shown that about 22% of PACS progress to PAC, during a period of 5 years.[26] In PACS, LPI should be considered especially if:
- There is a need for frequent dilation, for fundus evaluation
- Strong family history of PACD
- Poor access to eye care
- Presence of PAC/PACG/APAC in the fellow eye.

Procedure: Laser peripheral iridotomy is done under topical anesthesia. Topical pilocarpine 2% is used to induce miosis and stretch (and thereby thin) the iris stroma, so that it can be penetrated easily. LPI can be performed with or without contact lenses like Abraham (66 D) or Wise lens (103 D). The advantages of using contact lens are detailed in Box 63.5. A peripherally located iris crypt is selected and penetrated with laser. The energy employed ranges from 3 to 7 mJ. Endpoint includes posterior iris movement and deepening of AC, cloud of pigment billowing forward, transillumination, and visibility of lens edge/zonules/ciliary process depending upon the position of the LPI. The ideal size of LPI is around 150–250 µm. The indications for LPI other than PACD are detailed in Box 63.6.

Alpha agonist like topical brimonidine is applied before and after procedure to tackle laser-induced IOP spikes. Topical steroids are usually given for a week or two, to control the post-LPI inflammation. The complications of LPI are listed in Box 63.7.

Laser peripheral iridotomy is not fully protective against the development of chronic angle closure in all patients, though such cases are rare. A week or two after LPI, a detailed evaluation should be performed, including IOP, gonioscopy, and dilated anterior and posterior segment examination, to decide on further medical and surgical management.

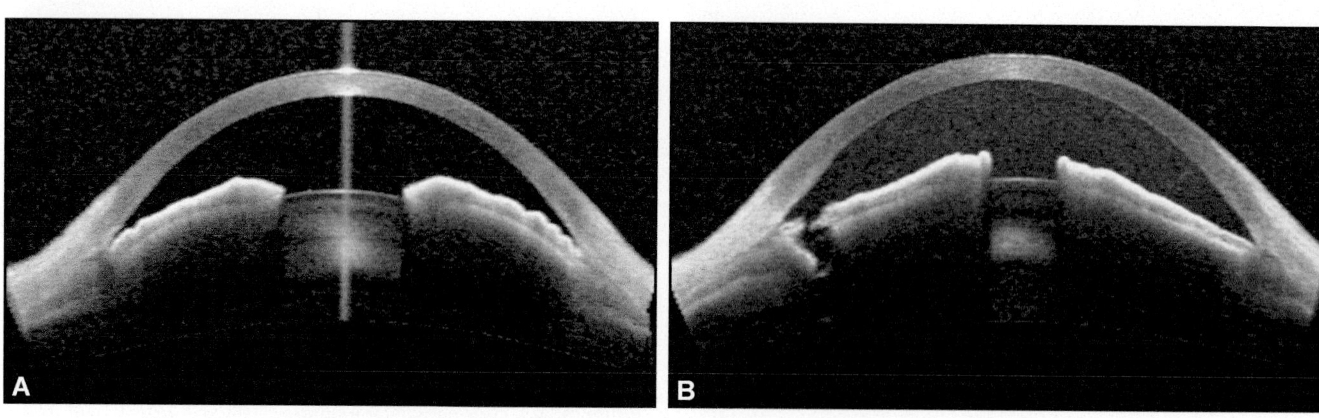

Figs. 63.12A and B: (A) Anterior segment optical coherence tomography (ASOCT) pre-laser peripheral iridotomy (LPI); (B) ASOCT post-LPI, in eye with angle closure, note the widening of angle post-LPI.

Box 63.5: Advantages of using contact lens during laser peripheral iridotomy.

- Separates the lids and fixes the eye
- Improves visualization, provides magnification
- Minimizes corneal burn by acting as heat sink
- Concentrates the energy into a smaller space, and focuses the laser beam
- Helps to apply pressure and control bleeding

Box 63.6: Indications for laser peripheral iridotomy other than PACD.

- Plateau iris syndrome
- Aqueous misdirection/malignant glaucoma
- Spherophakia
- Nanophthalmos
- Pigmentary glaucoma
- ACIOL, phakic IOL
- Aphakic or pseudophakic pupillary block
- Pupillary block by vitreous/silicone oil/subluxated lens
- Open angles with narrow inlets

(PACD: Primary angle-closure disease; ACIOL: Anterior chamber intraocular lens; IOL: Intraocular lens)

Box 63.7: Complications of laser peripheral iridotomy.

- Transient rise in intraocular pressure (IOP)
- Iritis
- Corneal epithelial, stromal, and endothelial damage
- Hyphema
- Damage to lens/zonules
- Failure to perforate/closure of iridotomy
- Retinal burn
- Diplopia/glare/dysphotopsia

Argon Laser Peripheral Iridoplasty

Argon laser peripheral iridoplasty (ALPI) is a procedure to induce immediate focal iris stromal contraction to pull the iris root away from the angle wall thus widening it. In the long-term, it produces thinning and contraction of peripheral iris, giving it a flat contour. The indications for ALPI include:[27]

- Plateau iris syndrome
- Appositional angle closure with or without PAS or elevated IOP
- When angle remains closed after LPI
- In APAC to help break the attack where medical therapy and LPI have failed or contraindicated
- To facilitate access to TM for laser trabeculoplasty.

Procedure: Argon laser peripheral iridoplasty is done under topical anesthesia. Abraham/Wise/Goldmann 3-mirror lens can be used. Argon green or blue green or diode laser is employed. Parameters include 100–200 μm spot size, power of 200–500 mW, duration of 0.2–0.5 seconds and single row of about 25 burns over 360°. Peripheral iris, as peripheral as possible, usually outside the arcus senilis should be aimed. End point is iris stromal contraction with progressive deepening of AC.

Randomized controlled trial comparing ALPI against conventional systemic IOP lowering medications as the first-line treatment of APAC, revealed that ALPI treated group had significantly lower IOP than medically treated group at 15 minutes, 30 minutes, and 1 hour, after the initiation of treatment.[28]

Selective Laser Trabeculoplasty

Selective laser trabeculoplasty (SLT) can be considered as a viable, safe and effective alternative to medications for lowering the IOP in PAC and PACG after LPI, where at least 90° of TM is visible.[29] IOP lowering efficacy of SLT over 6 months was observed to be similar to prostaglandin analogues in eyes with PAC and PACG.

Diode Laser Cyclophotocoagulation

Transscleral diode laser (810 nm) cycloablation can be considered when an eye with PACD goes for an absolute stage, a painful blind eye. It causes coagulative necrosis of ciliary epithelium, damages the source of aqueous production, reduces IOP, and hence relieves pain.

Medical Management

Medical therapy is usually employed to control the residual, elevated IOP post-LPI. Chronically raised IOP in eyes with PAC and PACG is to be managed similar to POAG.

- Beta-blockers, alpha agonist, carbonic anhydrase inhibitors (CAIs), and prostaglandin analogues can be employed depending upon the ocular and systemic profile of the patients.
- Recent studies have demonstrated that prostaglandin analogues such as latanoprost, bimatoprost, and travoprost are effective in lowering IOP in PAC and PACG eyes, even in the presence of 360° PAS.[27]
- Chronic use of pilocarpine is not favored owing to its ocular and systemic side effect profile. Also, pilocarpine therapy cannot substitute LPI, as it can aggravate angle closure as a result of miosis-induced iridolenticular contact.
- In PACS, there is no role for medical therapy, and they should be followed up, 6–12 monthly to assess progression.

Flowchart 63.2: Management of acute primary angle closure.

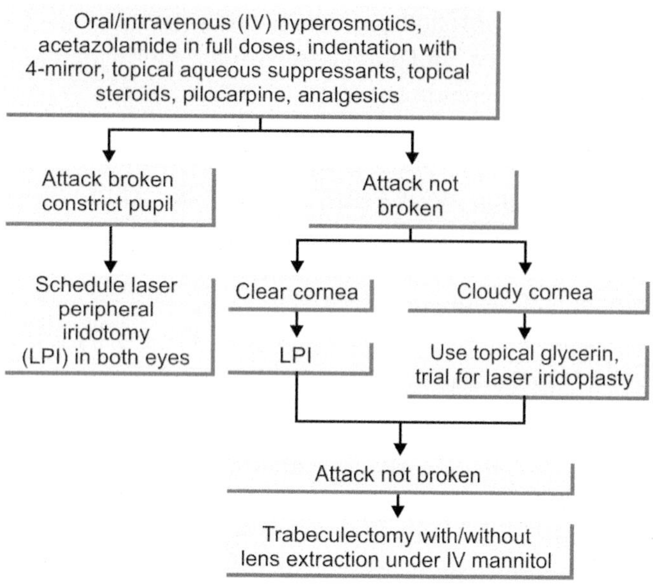

In APAC, the initial treatment is to lower the IOP and relieve the pupillary block (Flowchart 63.2). Medical treatment is initiated with topical miotics, beta blockers, alpha adrenergic agents, and CAI. Oral CAIs can be given if the patient is not allergic to sulfa drugs.

It is best to use intermediate strength miotic drops (pilocarpine 2%) as stronger concentrations can shift the lens iris diaphragm forward, exaggerating the pupillary block. Pupillary response to miotics may be blunted until the IOP drops below 40 mm Hg. Iris ischemia occurs with high IOP and therefore muscles cannot respond to the cholinergic agents.

In those patients where IOP has not come down substantially by the above regimen and threatens optic nerve perfusion, oral hyperosmotic (50% glycerol) or intravenous mannitol (20%, 1–2 g/kg) may be required.

If the pupillary block is not abated, one can use 4-mirror goniolens to indent the cornea, forcing aqueous into the peripheral angle, open it, and break the attack. If cornea is very hazy, topical glycerin eye drops can be used. This will improve the media clarity and helps in identifying angle structures more precisely.

Topical steroids help to reduce the inflammation, while analgesics and antiemetics will make the patient comfortable until LPI.

Surgical Management

Surgical management is indicated:

- When the IOP control is not achieved with medical and laser therapy, especially when there is progression of optic nerve/VF damage
- In case of poor compliance or intolerance to medical therapy
- When the patient develops a significant cataract.

The following are the commonly employed surgeries in PACD.

Paracentesis

In APAC, when there is markedly elevated IOP threatening the optic nerve, emergency paracentesis may be considered. It can be done either on slit lamp or under the microscope. A small risk of injury to the lens is present due to shallow AC. This procedure reduces IOP and clears the cornea, making LPI easier.

Lens Extraction

- In PACS, there is no role for clear lens extraction (CLE), and hence lens extraction should be considered only if the patient develops or has a coexistent cataract.
- For PAC, CLE is considered only if conventional treatment (LPI, ALPI, and medications) does not control the IOP and a significant portion of the angle could be opened on indentation gonioscopy.[30] In the presence of cataract, primary phacoemulsification with option of future trabeculectomy should be considered in patients with persistent appositional angle closure and uncontrolled IOP.[31]
- In APAC, once the attack has been aborted, CLE can be considered when conventional treatment does not adequately reduce IOP. Acute intervention with lens extraction as primary treatment in APAC remains less appealing except in resistant cases due to potential surgical complications that can be avoided by conventional treatment. An elective approach to the lens can be considered, if indicated later.[30]
- After LPI, it is important to treat the patients with PACG aggressively as they have glaucomatous optic neuropathy (Flowchart 63.3). Medically controlled PACG without cataract does not require further intervention. In the presence of significant cataract and

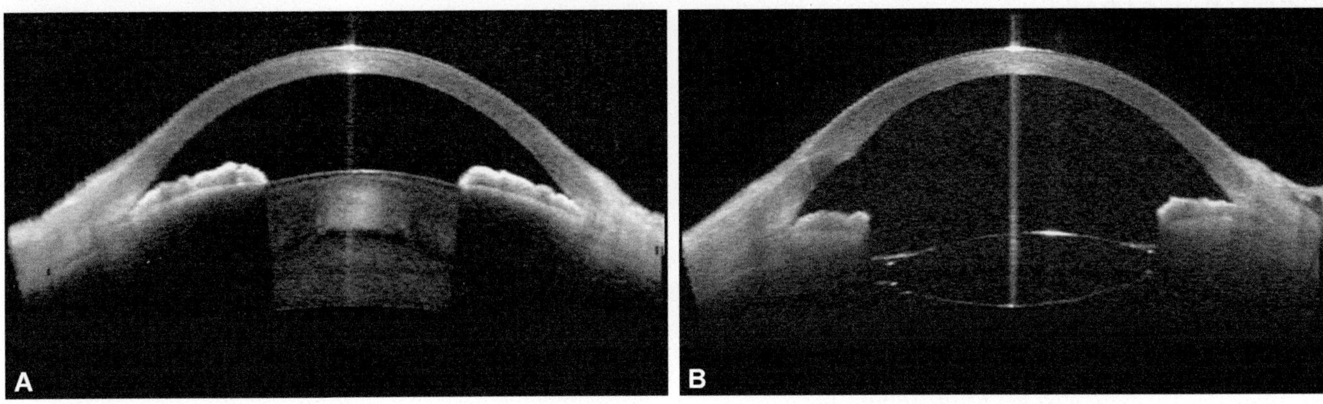

Figs. 63.13A and B: (A) Anterior segment optical coherence tomography (ASOCT) pre-cataract surgery; (B) ASOCT post-cataract surgery in eye with primary angle-closure glaucoma (PACG), note the deepening of chamber, widening of the angle, and change in iris contour after phacoemulsification with intraocular lens (IOL) implantation.

Flowchart 63.3: Management of primary angle-closure glaucoma.

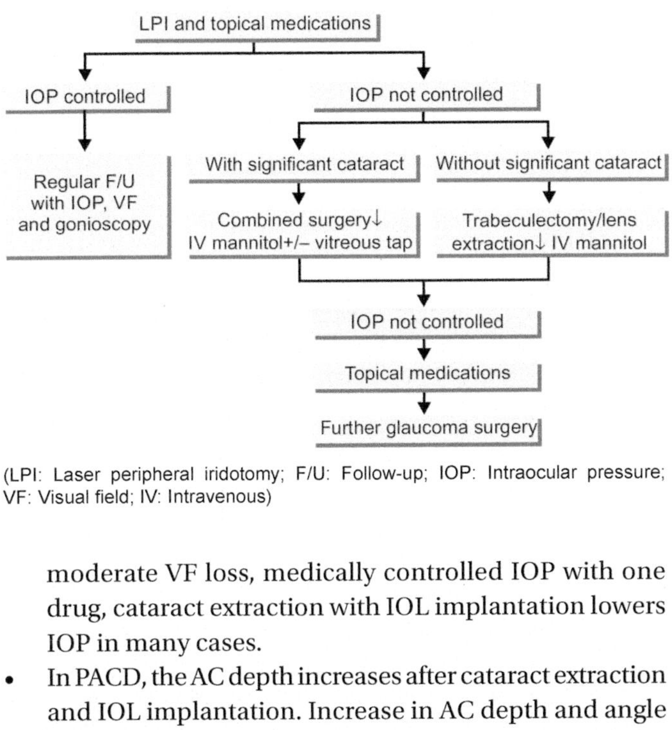

(LPI: Laser peripheral iridotomy; F/U: Follow-up; IOP: Intraocular pressure; VF: Visual field; IV: Intravenous)

moderate VF loss, medically controlled IOP with one drug, cataract extraction with IOL implantation lowers IOP in many cases.

- In PACD, the AC depth increases after cataract extraction and IOL implantation. Increase in AC depth and angle width (Figs. 63.13A and B) relates to the exchange of thick cataractous lens (average 5 mm) with a thin IOL (average 1 mm).
- In the presence of cataract with moderate to severe VF loss, and/or poorly controlled IOP, combined trabeculectomy with cataract extraction can be considered.
- Effectiveness of early lens extraction for the treatment of primary angle-closure glaucoma (EAGLE)[32] study randomized PAC and PACG patients to LPI versus CLE. CLE showed greater efficacy and was cost effective than LPI. CLE can be considered in uncontrolled PACG despite conventional laser and medical treatment especially if "significant" angle opening is possible on indentation gonioscopy.[30]

Goniosynechialysis

This is usually performed in combination with lens extraction. It involves mechanical stripping of PAS from TM, using viscoelastics or cyclodialysis spatula.

Trabeculectomy

- In APAC, trabeculectomy is considered either alone or in combination with lens extraction if the IOP control is not achieved with conventional medical and laser therapy (Flowchart 63.2). It has a poor prognosis, for long-term function in acutely inflamed eyes.[33]
- In PACG, eyes with uncontrolled IOP and moderate VF loss trabeculectomy alone can be considered, especially if there is no cataract (Flowchart 63.3).
- Surgical iridectomy should always be performed while doing trabeculectomy in PACD.
- Trabeculectomy is done in the same way as in POAG, however there is a risk of shallow AC postsurgery with associated risk of PAS formation and aqueous misdirection.

Glaucoma Drainage Implant

This is usually considered when trabeculectomy fails and there is a danger of disease progression.

CONCLUSION

No currently available treatment modalities can, in all cases, reverse or arrest the progression of angle closure to PAS formation in some eyes. Thus, an optimal strategy to address PACG would be, to create awareness about the disease in the community, screen patients at risk, and catch and treat the disease early. Along with sound screening protocols, advances in the imaging and therapeutics can help to reduce the visual morbidity caused by PACG.

REFERENCES

1. Tham YC, Li X, Wong TY, et al. Global prevalence of glaucoma and projections of glaucoma burden through 2040: a systematic review and meta-analysis. Ophthalmology. 2014;121(11):2081-90.
2. Foster PJ. Epidemiology, classification and mechanism. In: Weinreb R, Friedman D (Eds). Angle Closure and Angle Closure Glaucoma. The Hague: Kuegler; 2006. pp. 1-20.
3. Quigley HA, Broman AT. The number of people with glaucoma worldwide in 2010 and 2020. Br J Ophthalmol. 2006;90(3):262-7.
4. Dandona L, Dandona R, Mandal P, et al. Angle-closure glaucoma in an urban population in southern India: the Andhra Pradesh Eye Disease Study. Ophthalmology. 2000;107(9):1710-6.
5. Vijaya L, George R, Arvind H, et al. Prevalence of primary angle-closure disease in an urban south Indian population and comparison with a rural population: the Chennai Glaucoma Study. Ophthalmology. 2008;115(4):655-60.
6. Foster PJ, Johnson GJ. Glaucoma in China: how big is the problem? Br J Ophthalmol. 2001;85(11):1277-82.
7. American Academy of Ophthalmology. Preferred Practice Patterns. San Francisco, CA: American Academy of Ophthalmology; 2005.
8. Chandler PA, Trotter RR. Angle-closure glaucoma: Subacute types. AMA Arch Ophthalmol. 1955;53(3):305-17.
9. Foster PJ, Buhrmann R, Quigley HA, et al. The definition and classification of glaucoma in prevalence surveys. Br J Ophthalmol. 2002;86(2):238-42.
10. Ritch R, Lowe RF. Angle-closure glaucoma: epidemiology and mechanisms. In: Ritch R, Shields MB, Krupin T (Eds). The Glaucomas, 2nd edition. St Louis: CV Mosby; 1996. pp. 801-19.
11. Nolan WP, Foster PJ, Devereux JG, et al. YAG laser iridotomy treatment for primary angle closure in East Asian eyes. Br J Ophthalmol. 2000;84(11):1255-9.
12. Quigley HA, Friedman DS, Congdon NG. Possible mechanisms of primary angle-closure and malignant glaucoma. J Glaucoma. 2003;12(2):167-80.
13. Aptel F, Denis P. Optical coherence tomography quantitative analysis of iris volume changes after pharmacologic mydriasis. Ophthalmology. 2010;117(1):3-10.
14. Lowe RF. Primary angle closure glaucoma: a review of ocular biometry. Clin Experiment Ophthalmol. 1977;5(1):9-17.
15. Lowe RF. Anterior lens displacement with age. Br J Ophthalmol. 1970;54(2):117.
16. He M, Foster PJ, Friedman DS, et al. Gonioscopy in adult Chinese: the Liwan eye study. Invest Ophthalmol Vis Sci. 2006;47(11):4772-9.
17. He M, Foster PJ, Johnson GJ, et al. Angle-closure glaucoma in East Asian and European people. Different diseases? Eye (Lond). 2006;20(1):3-12.
18. Sihota R, Mohan S, Dada T, et al. An evaluation of the darkroom prone provocative test in family members of primary angle closure glaucoma patients. Eye (Lond). 2007;21(7):984-9.
19. Kavitha S, Zebardast N, Palaniswamy K, et al. Family history is a strong risk factor for prevalent angle closure in a South Indian population. Ophthalmology. 2014;121(11):2091-7.
20. He M, Wang D, Zheng Y, et al. Heritability of anterior chamber depth as an intermediate phenotype of angle-closure in Chinese: the Guangzhou Twin Eye Study. Invest Ophthalmol Vis Sci. 2008;49(1):81-6.
21. Vithana EN, Khor CC, Qiao, et al. Genome-wide association analyses identify three new susceptibility loci for primary angle closure glaucoma. Nat Genet. 2012;44(10):1142-6.
22. Duvesh R, Verma A, Venkatesh R, et al. Association Study in a South Indian Population Supports rs1015213 as a Risk Factor for Primary Angle. Invest Ophthalmol Vis Sci. 2013;54(8):5624-8.
23. Lowe RF. Primary angle-closure glaucoma. Inheritance and environment. Br J Ophthalmol. 1972;56(1):13.
24. Thomas R, George T, Braganza A, et al. The flashlight test and van Herick's test are poor predictors for occludable angles. Clin Experiment Ophthalmol. 1996;24(3):251-6.
25. Radhakrishnan S, Goldsmith J, Huang D, et al. Comparison of optical coherence tomography and ultrasound biomicroscopy for detection of narrow anterior chamber angles. Arch Ophthalmol. 2005;123(8):1053-9.
26. Thomas R, George R, Parikh R, et al. Five-year risk of progression of primary angle closure suspects to primary angle closure: a population based study. Br J Ophthalmol. 2003;87(4):450-4.
27. See JL, Aquino MC, Aduan J, et al. Management of angle closure glaucoma. Indian J Ophthalmol. 2011;59(Suppl 1): S82-7.
28. Lam DS, Lai JS, Tham CC, et al. Argon laser peripheral iridoplasty versus conventional systemic medical therapy in treatment of acute primary angle-closure glaucoma: a prospective, randomized, controlled trial. Ophthalmology. 2002;109(9):1591-6.
29. Ho CL, Lai JS, Aquino MV, et al. Selective laser trabeculoplasty for primary angle closure with persistently elevated intraocular pressure after iridotomy. J Glaucoma. 2009;18(7):563-6.
30. Thomas R, Walland MJ, Parikh RS. Clear lens extraction in angle closure glaucoma. Curr Opin Ophthalmol. 2011;22(2):110-4.
31. Roberts TV, Francis IC, Lertsumitkul S, et al. Primary phacoemulsification for uncontrolled angle-closure glaucoma. J Cataract Refract Surg. 2000;26(7):1012-6.
32. Azuara-Blanco A, Foster PJ, Friedman DS, et al. Effectiveness of early lens extraction for the treatment of primary angle-closure glaucoma (EAGLE): a randomised controlled trial. Lancet. 2016;388(10052):1389-97.
33. Aung T, Tow SL, Yap EY, et al. Trabeculectomy for acute primary angle closure. Ophthalmology. 2000;107(7):1298-302.

Chapter 64 Medical Treatment of Glaucoma

Emily M Schehlein, Alan L Robin

INTRODUCTION

The American Academy of Ophthalmology's preferred practice pattern[1] suggests that all newly diagnosed patients with primary open-angle glaucoma (POAG) be given the option of medical, laser, or surgical therapy as their initial therapy for glaucoma. Both the Glaucoma Laser Trial[2] and the Advanced Glaucoma Intervention Study (AGIS)[3] suggest that either laser trabeculoplasty or surgical therapy might be equivalent or superior to medical therapy, respectively. Despite these guidelines and well-controlled multicentered studies, medical therapy continues to be the first-line treatment for POAG in almost all patients. The intraocular pressure-lowering (IOP) achieved by topical medical therapy allows most patients to control their disease with medications alone. It should be noted that in a real world situation, adherence to medical therapy might diminish the potential effect of therapy. Also it should be noted that the US Food and Drug Administration has currently not approved any medications for the treatment of glaucoma, an optic neuropathy. All medications used to treat glaucoma are approved only for the lowering of intraocular pressure. Because it is customary to discuss "glaucoma" medications rather than "intraocular pressure lowering" medications, we will adhere to this convention in this chapter.

Before the turn of the 21st century, multiple medical therapies for glaucoma were developed that are commonly used in current practice. Since then, many fixed-dose combinations, preservative-free formulations, and new chemical additions to current drug classes exist on the market. However, only one new class of glaucoma topical therapy has been developed since latanoprost (Xalatan©) in 1996 (Fig. 64.1). A new class of medications, the rho kinase inhibitors was approved by the US FDA in December, 2017 and became available to patients in April, 2018. Recent work has suggested that this class of medications might also be helpful in maintaining the health of the corneal endothelium.

While medical therapy continues to be the most widely used and common treatment for glaucoma, cost, adverse events, and difficulties with adherence remain barriers to treatment. A working knowledge of the drug classes and their efficacy, cost, and adverse events is important, particularly because the majority of glaucoma patients require multiple classes of medications to control their disease.[4,5]

This chapter outlines the option for, and use of, medical therapy in clinical settings with an emphasis on available topical glaucoma treatments.

WHEN TO PURSUE MEDICAL THERAPY

The majority of clinicians utilize medical therapy to treat glaucoma as the first line of defense against the disease,

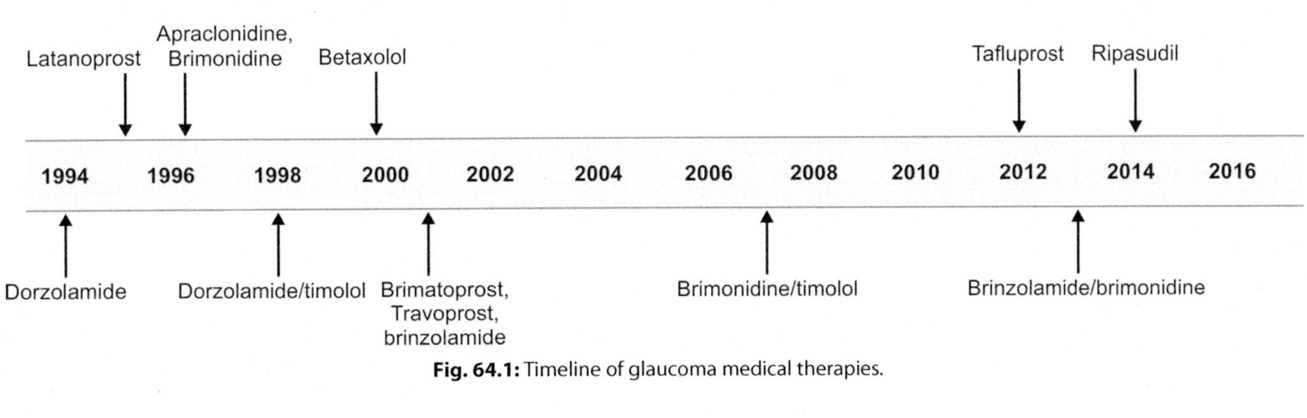

Fig. 64.1: Timeline of glaucoma medical therapies.

given the relative safety, efficacy, and lack of invasiveness as compared to other forms of treatment. While medical therapy would be the first choice for most patients, several factors must be assessed when deciding whether and when to pursue medical therapy.

Ability to Administer an Eye Drop

About 17% of patients are unable to self-administer their own eye drops.[6] When establishing a therapeutic plan, it is imperative to assess a patient's physical and mental ability to follow the prescribed pathway. Additionally, more than one-half of patients who have been on topical therapy for over 6 months, have problems successfully administering an eye drop to their eyes.[7] If a patient is on other systemic medical therapies, it may be helpful to assess their adherence to these other therapies, as this might offer clues regarding a patient's ability to adhere long-term.

Cost

Cost of care is an extremely important issue when considering an action plan for a patient with glaucoma. The costs to the patient and healthcare system of treatment for a chronic disease, such as glaucoma are well documented and are increased in patients with more severe disease.[8] Direct medical costs are estimated to be close to 3 billion dollars annually in the United States (US).[9] Nonmedical costs (e.g. cost of transportation and child care) and indirect costs (e.g. leisure time and lost wages) related to office and pharmacy visits are a much smaller portion of costs but are borne by the patient alone without other means of supplementation.[10] Patients face the highest burden of cost within 6 months of their initial diagnoses, and after 1 year these costs remain constant over time.[11]

Medication costs range from a quarter to over half of the contributory cost of disease in the US.[8] While current implementations in the US allow more patients to cover the cost of their medication through insurance, disparities continue to exist, particularly among those of lower socioeconomic strata.[12] Among patients who are covered, cost continues to be a limiting factor in treatment, with many patients remaining nonadherent to their prescriptions due to the cost of medications.[13] Even a relatively small amount of money per prescription can cause a huge difference in adherence as the degree of cost sensitivity can vary greatly.[14,15]

When comparing the cost of medical therapy to other commonly used glaucoma therapies, such as the American Glaucoma Society; Zhao PY, Rahmathullah R, Stagg BC, Almobarak F, Edward DP, Robin AL, Stein JD. A worldwide price comparison of glaucoma medications, laser trabeculoplasty, and incisional glaucoma surgery. JAMA Ophthalmol. 2018. Sadly, the authors found that glaucoma therapies are not affordable in many nations, especially in developing areas, and there is a great variability in costs. For example, prostaglandin analogs were found to be potentially a more cost-effective treatment option compared to laser trabeculoplasty when patients used the drug with optimal adherence.[16] Several studies have shown the cost-effectiveness of medical therapy when compared to surgical therapy[17] and projected costs of medical therapy compared to the developing microinvasive glaucoma surgeries (MIGS).[18] More research is needed to determine whether medical or surgical therapy has a higher cost burden to patients and healthcare systems in various nations given the decreased adherence levels that glaucoma patients often have with topical therapy, especially when on multiple different IOP-lowering medications.

The subject of cost becomes even more complex in some less developed nations. Both India and China, which account for close to half of the world's population, have multiple generic drugs that are significantly cheaper than brand name products, often by a factor of 10. Regrettably, depending upon the states or districts in which these generics are manufactured, there may be little regulation. Although the savings can be attractive, it is difficult to know if the quality and content of these generic medications are preserved in the context of lower costs.[19,20.]

Adverse Events

Varied local and systemic adverse events may occur with both topical and oral medical treatment for glaucoma. While specific adverse events will be discussed with respect to individual drugs and classes, many patients will experience ocular and/or systemic adverse events that could limit their willingness to use the drug and their adherence. Potential adverse events must be discussed with the patient before and during initiation of a new drug regimen.

Comorbidities

Patients with medical comorbidities, such as renal lithiasis, Stevens-Johnson syndrome, depression, asthma, chronic obstructive pulmonary disease (COPD), or arrhythmias must be carefully evaluated for initiation of treatment with glaucoma medical therapy. Many medications used in the therapy of glaucoma can exacerbate these problems and may be relatively or absolutely contraindicated in these individuals. Also, some topical medications may cause unsightly cosmetic changes that may not be acceptable for many individuals. A careful medical and social history is needed for each patient both before initiating any topical or systemic medical therapy as well as before changing or adding medical therapies. For example, before starting a topical nonselective beta-blocker, it might be advisable to listen for wheezing or stertorous breathing, check for pedal edema, and assess resting heart rates.

The demonstrated potential for exacerbation of these comorbidities is due to the systemic and topical absorption of these eye drops. Patients should be counseled on methods for reducing systemic absorption, such as punctal occlusion, or forced eyelid closure.

Some systemic medications have been shown to minimize the prevalence of open angle glaucoma.[21] Additionally, it has been suggested that the use of topical glaucoma medications can reduce mortality. While the definite reason for this is unknown, the effect is likely multifactorial with absorption of topical medications into systemic circulation, increased health of individuals using medications, and increased access to care.[22]

Pregnancy and Breastfeeding

Although not common, patients who are pregnant or breastfeeding deserve special consideration when determining optimal treatment for glaucoma. Currently, brimonidine is the only glaucoma drug that is classified by the Food and Drug Administration (FDA) as a category B drug (animal studies show no fetal risk and no human studies) but all other glaucoma medications are classified as category C (animal studies showed adverse effects, no human studies). Beta-blockers are most commonly used in pregnancy given the longevity of use with this drug class. With the lack of consensus about the risk status of using these medications in pregnancy, treatment of pregnant, or lactating women should be individualized based on the safety of the mother, the stage of the pre-existing glaucoma damage, the degree of IOP control prior to the pregnancy, the rate of the glaucomatous progression, trimester of pregnancy, risk to the fetus, and the patient's preferences.

TARGET PRESSURE

When treating glaucoma, the initial pretreatment range of IOP is assumed to be at a level that could contribute to the patient's progressive optic nerve damage. Lowering IOP is the only known therapy that prevents or retards optic nerve damage as exemplified by visual field deterioration.[3] It is important to note that the goal in reducing IOP with topical medications is to preserve vision rather than decrease the pressure to a specific millimeter of mercury. The initial IOP goal or "target pressure" must be individualized based on the patient's stage of disease, age and potential life expectancy, pretreatment IOP, visual field deterioration or lack thereof, central corneal thickness, and race, among other risk factors and may change with the evolution of the latter factors.[23]

Landmark multicentered glaucoma trials sponsored by the National Institutes of Health (NIH) have each had different target IOPs and methods of assessing perimetric progression: The Early Manifest Glaucoma Trial (EMGT) lowered IOP by 20%,[24,25] the AGIS targeted an IOP less than 18 mm Hg,[3,26] the Collaborative Initial Glaucoma Treatment Study (CIGTS) was individualized but averaged IOP-lowering of approximately 38%,[27] and the Ocular Hypertension Treatment Study (OHTS) targeted a 20% decrease,[5] all with slowed optic nerve damage and/or slowed visual field deterioration. Both the AGIS[3] and CIGTS[27] found that more stringent IOP-lowering, by at least one-half of the pretreatment baseline, resulted in minimal mean visual field progression. Based on these clinical trials, the discerning clinician will aim to lower pretreatment IOP in patients with definite glaucoma (as judged by coexisting structural measures and visual field loss) by greater than or equal to 30% in most cases to minimize progression.

Unless in an emergent situation with severe disease and threat to vision, patients should complete all pretreatment and diagnostic testing before starting a topical glaucoma drug. Additionally, it is always helpful to have an additional IOP measurement ideally on a different date at a different time of day. The majority of patients should start treatment with monotherapy and allow several weeks for the drug to take effect. The one-eye therapeutic trial, treating just one eye and observing the fellow eye, is usually helpful in determining the actual IOP-lowering of a specific medication[28] and this helps a physician determine whether the IOP-lowering one sees is due to diurnal variation. Since there can be quite a bit of IOP diurnal variation in patients with glaucoma as well as asymmetry of variation, this can be a very helpful tool.[29]

When the goal of IOP is unable to be achieved with the patient's initial therapeutic choice, it is appropriate to switch to another medication class rather than simply adding a medication. Although we may know the "mean" IOP-lowering of a specific class of medications, there is often quite a bit of individual variation in response to that medication. Switching to a different medication within the same class is often unsuccessful if one accounts for diurnal variation. Increasing the patient's medication burden leads to a confluence of difficulties already present in glaucoma topical medication therapy: problems with medication regimens, cost, and adverse events. Additionally, since most (but not all) medications use benzalkonium chloride (BAK) as a preservative, an additional drop can cause corneal epithelial problems due to preservatives.[30] The more medications used, the less likely adherence.[31,32]

However, it is quite common that patients will require more than one ocular hypotensive drug to control their glaucoma: the CIGTS found that at least 75% of study participants required more than one medication to reach the target IOP,[27] while the OHTS found that almost 50% of study participants required two or more medications to reach the target IOP (20% reduction from baseline IOP).[5]

Treatments that target IOP-lowering are important and desired as the increase of each millimeter of mercury increases the likelihood of glaucomatous progression by 11%.[33] However, the goal pressure is a moving target and must be reevaluated at follow-up visits upon review of the optic nerve through direct observation and/or optical coherence tomography (OCT) and visual field testing. The target IOP may also be lowered if a patient can no longer comply with or tolerate therapy or if the patient's disease progresses quickly.

QUALITY OF LIFE AND ADHERENCE

The impact of implementing glaucoma topical therapy on a patient's quality of life is important to consider. One must remember that before blindness or visual disability, glaucoma effects one's quality of life by decreasing daily activity, resulting in one giving up her driver's license, having less physical activity, difficulty with reading, and decreasing facial recognition, among others.[34-39] Quality of life is not demonstrably different with medical therapy as compared to surgical therapy, aside from an increase in local eye symptoms in those undergoing surgery.[40] However, patients and clinicians alike should know that administering drops with topical therapy is very different from swallowing pills or giving injections. Despite the development of drop bottles with a variety of aids and techniques,[41] varied dosing schedules and the threat to vision, nonadherence among glaucoma patients is reported to be as high as almost 60%.[42] This becomes even more important with generics, which may pose problems of their own given issues with squeezing bottles and variable eye drop sizes.[43]

The most common barriers to adherence are forgetfulness, difficulty administering drops, problems following a medication schedule, decreased understanding of the disease, and cost of medications.[44] Additionally, as glaucoma is a disease that disproportionately affects the elderly, these barriers to adherence become more pronounced as the patient population ages, or develops handicaps. They often prove difficult to remedy, but studies have shown that educating patients on correct techniques in self-administration may improve their technique,[45] adherence,[46] and self-efficacy.[47]

Novel drug delivery systems are hopefully on the horizon in glaucoma medical therapy and have the potential to prove important in combating some barriers to adherence in addition to providing IOP-lowering that is sustained over a longer period of time. Delivery systems currently in development include prostaglandins delivered via a punctal plug,[48] intracameral injection,[49] or a ring inserted into the conjunctival fornices.[50]

FIVE MAIN CLASSES OF DRUGS

To summarize, the goal of treatment in POAG is to maintain control of the patient's IOP for 24 hours per day. When choosing therapy, clinicians must keep in mind the patient's preference, stage of disease, IOP-lowering required, safety and adverse events profile of the drug, cost, and dosing schedule. Patients will have different responses to IOP-lowering with each drug class and often will have differing experiences with adverse events. Most commonly, medications will be trialed for 2–6 weeks in order for the drug to take effect. If the patient experiences intolerable side effects, she should be encouraged to communicate these difficulties to the clinician immediately and then, after communication, to stop the drug and come to the office for revaluation of the current regimen.

Current drug classes modulate IOP primarily by three mechanisms: suppressing production of aqueous humor, increasing outflow of aqueous humor via the conventional pathway, and/or increasing aqueous humor outflow via the uveoscleral outflow pathway (Table 64.1).

Increase Aqueous Humor Outflow

Prostaglandin Analogs

Prostaglandin analogs, such as latanoprost (Xalatan®, Pfizer, Inc., New York, NY, USA; generic), bimatoprost (Lumigan®, Allergan, Inc., Irvine, CA, USA), travoprost

Table 64.1: Topical glaucoma medications.

Drug class	Method(s) of action	IOP reduction*	Adverse events	Contraindications	Dosing schedule
Prostaglandin analogs	Increase uveoscleral and trabecular outflow	25–35%	*Local:* Conjunctival injection, hypertrichosis, disorganization of lashes, increased iris pigmentation, periocular hyperpigmentation, uveitis, keratitis, CME, itching, and burning, stinging *Systemic*: Headaches, muscle/back pain	Active uveitis, CME, and history of herpetic keratitis	Once per day (at night)
Cholinergic agonists	Increase trabecular outflow	20–25%	*Local:* Dim vision, conjunctival injection, retinal detachment, and angle-closure glaucoma *Systemic:* Headache, brow ache, sweating, nausea, salivation, and bronchospasm	Uveitic glaucoma, neovascular glaucoma, arrhythmia, hypertension, and recent postoperative inflammation	Up to 4 times per day
Beta-blockers: Nonselective	Suppression of aqueous humor production	20–25%	*Local:* Conjunctival injection, burning, stinging, dry eyes, exacerbation of ocular myasthenia gravis, and keratitis *Systemic:* Bradycardia, arrhythmia, bronchospasm, masked hypoglycemia, sexual dysfunction, and depression	Asthma, COPD, existing arrhythmia, congestive heart failure, and heart block (greater than first-degree)	Twice per day
Beta-blockers: Beta-1 selective	Suppression of aqueous humor production	20%	*Local:* Burning, stinging (may be more pronounced) *Systemic:* Bradycardia, arrhythmia, bronchospasm (may be less pronounced), sexual dysfunction, and depression	Asthma, COPD, existing arrhythmia, congestive heart failure, and heart block	Twice per day
Alpha-adrenergic agonists: Nonselective (epinephrine-like drugs)	Suppression of aqueous humor production	15–20%	*Local:* Conjunctival injection, conjunctival pigmentation, pain, stinging, and macular edema *Systemic:* Hypertension, anxiety, sweating, tachycardia, tachypnea, and headache	Aphakic patients and occludable angles	2–3 times per day
Alpha-adrenergic agonists: Alpha-2 relatively selective	Suppression of aqueous humor production	18–35%	*Local:* Allergic conjunctivitis, conjunctival injection, blurry vision, contact dermatitis, follicular conjunctivitis, eyelid retraction, miosis, and conjunctival blanching *Systemic:* Hypotension, dyspnea, depression, dry nose and mouth, and fatigue	Children, adults with low body weight, and patients using oral MAOIs	2–3 times per day
Carbonic anhydrase inhibitors	Suppression of aqueous humor production	20%	*Local:* Bitter taste, burning, stinging, and superficial punctate keratitis *Systemic:* Headache, paresthesias, transient myopia, dizziness, urticaria, and angioedema	Patients with endothelial dysfunction	2–3 times per day

(IOP: Intraocular pressure; CME: Cystoid macular edema; COPD: Chronic obstructive pulmonary disease; MAOI: Monoamine oxidase inhibitors)

Source: *European Glaucoma Society. Terminology and Guidelines for Glaucoma [Internet], 4th edition. Heijl A, Traverso C (Eds). PubliComm; 2014. 146-151 p. Available from: *www.eugs.org/eng/EGS_guidelines4.asp*

(Travatan®, Travatan® Z, Alcon Laboratories, Inc., Fort Worth, TX, USA), tafluprost (Zioptan™, Merck Sharp and Dohme Corp., North Wales, PA and Vyzulta, latanoprostene bunod, Bausch + Lomb, Bridgewater, NJ), primarily increase aqueous humor outflow via the uveoscleral pathway. Recently, it has been postulated that prostaglandins may also act on the traditional ourflow pathway.[51]

These drugs are most frequently used as the initial therapy for glaucoma given their systemic safety, excellent systemic side effect profile, and once-daily administration. They are particularly important if the patient needs a higher initial level of IOP-lowering as prostaglandins can provide a substantial decrease in IOP for most patients (25–35%).[52] Additionally, prostaglandin analogs have been shown to reduce aqueous flow during sleep, resulting in a more consistent nocturnal IOP-lowering,[53] and they are usually taken once per day, at nighttime.

On the whole, prostaglandins lack systemic side effects, as compared to another commonly used class of glaucoma medications: beta-blockers. Patients most often experience conjunctival injection, hypertrichosis and disorganization of eyelashes, increased iris pigmentation, and periocular hyperpigmentation that should be disclosed to the patient before starting therapy. The increase in iris pigmentation most commonly affects patients with heterochromic or hazel iris color,[54] and is due to an increased number of melanosomes within melanocytes. There is no evidence that this iris color change is permanent.[55] Prostaglandin analogs may also cause periorbital fat atrophy which may give an eye a deep and sunken appearance. Additionally, prostaglandin analog use should be carefully considered in patients with active uveitis or cystoid macular edema due to the potential risk for worsening of inflammation or in patients with any history of herpetic keratitis. Other less common adverse events include uveitis, keratitis, and cystoid macular edema. Pregnant or breastfeeding patients should exercise caution before using this drug.

Cholinergic Agonists

Cholinergic agonists are one of our oldest classes of medications. They act via the traditional outflow pathway via stimulation of the ciliary muscle to contract and increase trabecular outflow. Direct-acting cholinergic agonists in this class include pilocarpine (Isopto® Carpine, Alcon Laboratories, Inc., Fort Worth, TX, USA; Pilocarpine HCL Ophthalmic Solution, Bausch + Lomb, Bridgewater, New Jersey, USA and Alcon Laboratories, Inc., Fort Worth, TX, USA) and carbachol (Isopto® Carbachol, Alcon Laboratories, Inc., Fort Worth, TX, USA), with pilocarpine being most commonly used. However, use of this class of medications is limited in current clinical practice given its multiple-daily dosing and robust ocular adverse event/effect profile, although they are commonly inexpensive. These medications must be dosed up to 4 times per day and have an IOP-lowering effect of 20–25%.[52]

Patients most commonly note ocular side effects of dim vision (due to pupillary constriction) which can be exacerbated in patients with cataracts, along with headache or brow ache. Additionally, pilocarpine should be used with caution in patients who are high myopes given the risk of retinal detachment.[56] Systemic toxicity while rare, also exists with these medications and includes sweating, nausea, and salivation, among other characteristic cholinergic responses. Other, indirect-acting agonists include echothiophate iodide and demecarium bromide, which are not commonly commercially available for treatment.

Suppression of Aqueous Humor Production

Beta-adrenoceptor Antagonists (Beta-blockers)

Beta-adrenoceptor antagonists or beta-blockers, along with prostaglandin analogs, are a mainstay of glaucoma medical therapy. This class of medications decreases IOP by suppressing the production of aqueous humor in the ciliary body via a resulting increase in cyclic adenosine monophosphate (cAMP) production from beta-blockade. These commonly lower IOP by 20–25%,[52] and are relatively inexpensive as the preserved versions of this class are generic. They are most commonly dosed once daily.[57] This class consists of both nonselective beta-blockers and relatively selective beta-blockers. The nonselective beta-blockers block both beta-1 and beta-2 receptors while the selective beta-blockers block only beta-1 receptors. It is interesting that some have suggested that there are no beta-1 sites in the ciliary body.[58] The nonselective beta-blockers are timolol maleate (Istalol®, Bausch + Lomb, Bridgewater, New Jersey, USA; Timoptic®, Timoptic-XE®, Merck Sharp and Dohme Corp., North Wales, PA, USA; generic), timolol hemihydrate (Betimol®, Vistakon Pharmaceuticals, LLC, Jacksonville, FL, USA), levobunolol (Betagan®, Allergan, Inc., Irvine, CA, USA; generic), carteolol (Ocupress, CIBA Vision Sterile Mfg., Mississauga, ON, Canada; generic), and metipranolol (OptiPranolol®, Bausch + Lomb, Bridgewater, New Jersey, USA; generic). The most commonly used drug is twice-daily timolol. Notably, it has been suggested that carteolol has intrinsic sympathomimetic activity (ISA) which may decrease its systemic effects on multiple organ systems, such as plasma lipids.[59] The currently marketed beta-1 selective beta-blocker is betaxolol (Betoptic®, Betoptic® S, Alcon Laboratories, Inc., Fort Worth, TX, USA; generic).

The predominant ocular adverse events associated with topical beta-blockers are ocular dryness and corneal anesthesia, though this is rarely clinically significant. Patients may also experience ocular adverse events of conjunctival hyperemia, irritation including burning or stinging, dry eyes, and potential exacerbation of ocular myasthenia gravis in affected patients. The systemic adverse events attributed to beta-blockers have been widely reported in the literature given the widespread use of topical beta-blockers in glaucoma treatment and oral beta-blockers for other diseases.[60] Systemic adverse events include bradycardia, potential for arrhythmia, bronchospasm, masked hypoglycemia, sexual dysfunction, and depression. The nonselective beta-blockers should not be used in patients with asthma, chronic COPD, congestive heart failure (CHF), second- or third-degree atrioventricular block, syncope, and bradycardia. The patient's medication list should be carefully monitored as drug interactions may occur with multiple medications, including oral beta-blockers, calcium channel blockers, and quinidine. Punctal occlusion and forced eyelid closure as methods of decreasing systemic absorption should be strongly considered for patients using this class of medication given the life-threatening potential of side effects in specific patients. These techniques have been shown to reduce systemic absorption up to 60% of patients.[61]

Although short-term "escape" (an increase in IOP after the initial IOP-lowering when starting a topical beta-blocker) has been described in the literature,[62] it is unclear whether tachyphylaxis commonly occurs with topical beta-blockers as it does with its oral counterparts[63] and whether this phenomenon is due to diurnal variation of IOP.

Topical beta-1 selective beta-blockers are not strictly contraindicated in asthma and COPD and in general have less systemic adverse events[64] (and likewise lower IOP less effectively), making them potentially useful for patients with multiple comorbidities and severe glaucomatous disease. However, many patients using beta-1 selective beta-blockers experience local ocular adverse events (burning and stinging) after administration.[65] The betaxolol 0.5% suspension causes burning and stinging while the 0.25% suspension causes temporary blurred vision.[66]

Alpha-adrenergic Agonists

Adrenergic agonists similarly act on the sympathetic nervous system primarily by decreasing production of aqueous humor via their action on alpha-receptors. Nonselective alpha-agonists, such as epinephrine and dipivefrin hydrochloride (Propine, Allergan Laboratories, Inc., Irvine California, USA) act on alpha-1 and alpha-2 receptors but are no longer commercially available within the US. However, relatively selective alpha-agonists apraclonidine hydrochloride (primarily alpha-1) (Iopidine®; Alcon Laboratories, Inc., Fort Worth, TX, USA, generic) and brimonidine tartrate (primarily alpha-2) (Alphagan®, Alphagan® P; Allergan, Inc., Irvine, CA, USA, 0.1%, generic both 0.15%, and 0.2%) have a greater affinity for the alpha-2 receptors.

Apraclonidine and brimonidine, both relatively selective alpha-agonists, can be dosed twice per day or three times per day. Apraclonidine lowers IOP by 25–35% while brimonidine lowers IOP by 18–25%.[52] Apraclonidine 1% is approved for the prevention of IOP increases following laser surgery for glaucoma and for neodymium-doped yttrium aluminum garnet (Nd:YAG) laser capsulotomies. Apraclonidine 0.5% is less likely to be used in long-term management of POAG as its ocular adverse event profile is robust and a large percentage of patients experience allergic side effects, such as itching of the eyelids, chemosis, and redness after relatively short-term use.[67,68] Brimonidine is a relatively selective alpha-2 agonist and is more commonly used in chronic glaucoma medical therapy.[69] Patients often experience side effects of ocular allergy (less commonly and later in the course of treatment than with apraclonidine,[70] conjunctival hyperemia, and blurry vision.[71] Common ocular adverse events for these selective alpha-agonists include contact dermatitis (more common with apraclonidine), follicular conjunctivitis, eyelid retraction (apraclonidine), miosis (brimonidine), and conjunctival blanching. Similar to beta-blockers, oral forms of these medications are used to treat hypertension (clonidine) or sedate (dexmedetomidine), thus both topical medications can cause systemic adverse events, such as hypotension, dyspnea, sedation, and depression. Specifically, patients taking apraclonidine may note dry nose and mouth while patients using brimonidine may experience fatigue and sleepiness. These drugs are contraindicated in young children or those with very low body weight due to the increased risk of fatal side effects from the drug penetrating the blood–brain barrier. The drugs are also contraindicated in patients taking monoamine oxidase inhibitors (MAOIs).

Carbonic Anhydrase Inhibitors

Carbonic anhydrase inhibitors (CAIs) (one of the most ubiquitous enzymes in the body) work to antagonize carbonic anhydrase in the ciliary epithelium to decrease the production of aqueous humor. Both systemic and topical CAIs are used to treat glaucoma patients. Systemic CAIs are rarely used for long-term treatment as they are difficult to tolerate due to their systemic adverse event profiles.

Systemic therapy includes acetazolamide (Diamox®, Teva Pharmaceuticals, North Wales, PA, USA, generic) and methazolamide (Neptazane®, Fera Pharmaceuticals, Locust Valley, NY, USA, generic). These drugs are used widely in medicine for a variety of illnesses in addition to glaucoma: idiopathic intracranial hypertension, altitude sickness, licorice toxicity, and drug-induced edema. They are very effective for IOP-lowering (up to 30–40%), but are usually used orally or intravenously in urgent situations to decrease the IOP.[52] Their adverse event profiles limit their use for many patients. As diuretics, these drugs cause urinary frequency and electrolyte imbalances (most commonly potassium depletion), and can also cause paresthesias in fingers and toes, taste alteration, kidney stones, blood dyscrasias, Stevens–Johnson syndrome, and metabolic acidosis, in part due to hypokalemia. They should not be used in patients with existing electrolyte imbalances or acidosis, liver disease, or adrenal gland failure. These drugs are sulfonamide derivatives and despite prior concern for causing potentially life-threatening allergic reactions for patients with self-reported allergies to sulfonamide antibiotics, these drugs are chemically and pharmacologically distinct from sulfonamide antibiotics and there is little evidence to show that these cross-reactions exist.[72]

Topical therapy includes dorzolamide (Trusopt®, Merck Sharp & Dohme Corp., North Wales, PA, USA, generic) and brinzolamide (Azopt®, Alcon Laboratories, Inc., Fort Worth, TX, USA). These agents are less effective than their oral counterparts, but can lower IOP by 20% and are used twice or three times per day.[52] Patients most frequently report a bitter taste when using these medications in addition to blurred vision (brinzolamide) and burning and stinging, which is more common with dorzolamide.[73] These medications should not be used in patients with endothelial dysfunction given patients' increased risk of corneal edema.[74,75] Systemically, patients may experience headache, paresthesias, transient myopia, and dizziness.

Hyperosmotic Agents

Hyperosmotic agents work to decrease IOP by acting to reduce vitreous volume via oncotic pressure, also resulting in a deeper anterior chamber. Commonly used oral osmotic agents include glycerol and isosorbide which can lower IOP by 15–20%.[52] Mannitol may also be given intravenously, lowering IOP from 15–30%.[52] Not commonly used in routine medical treatment for glaucoma, these drugs have many side effects which limit their use. Similar to oral CAIs, these are commonly employed in urgent situations or prior to surgery to lower IOP. Patients often complain of nausea, vomiting, increased urination, may develop electrolyte imbalances and metabolic acidosis, and in cases of overdose, lethargy, coma, and seizure. These drugs are relatively infrequently used and should not be given to patients with major organ system failure, such as the heart or renal failure, and they can cause oliguric renal failure in susceptible patients.[76]

NEW MEDICATIONS

Over 2 decades have passed since any new classes of IOP-lowering drugs have been approved in the US, most recently latanoprost (Xalatan®) prior to the turn of the century. Rho kinase inhibitors are currently of great interest in medical treatment of glaucoma given the new rho kinase inhibitor, Ripasudil (Glanatec, Kowa Company, Ltd, Nagoya, Aichi, Japan) approved for use in Japan for glaucoma and ocular hypertension when applied twice daily. Also, Rhopressa (Netarsudil, Aerie Pharmaceuticals, Raleigh, Durham, North Carolina) is now available in the United States as a once daily medication.

This class of drugs acts on rho kinases expressed in the trabecular meshwork to decrease IOP. To date, the approved drug has a favorable safety profile,[77,78] shows increased IOP-lowering when combined with timolol and latanoprost,[79] and may have some neuroprotection benefits.[80] This new class of drugs may serve an important role in glaucoma medical treatment in the future.

COMBINATION THERAPY

Many patients will not be controlled on a singular ocular hypotensive medication and fixed-dose combination therapies have been shown to decrease IOP with greater efficacy than either of their single counterparts alone.[81] This is crucial for patients with difficulties with drop administration, adherence, and low self-efficacy. There are multiple fixed-dose combination drugs available to patients, including dorzolamide-timolol (Cosopt®, Merck Sharp and Dohme Corp., North Wales, PA, USA), brimonidine-timolol (Combigan™, Allergan, Inc., Irvine, CA, USA), Cosopt®PF (Akorn Pharmaceuticals) and brinzolamide-brimonidine (Simbrinza®, Alcon Laboratories, Inc., Fort Worth, TX, USA). Globally, several prostaglandin analog and beta-blocker fixed-dose combinations are available.

While fixed-dose combination drugs have been shown to increase adherence,[82] they are often very costly compared to the component medications, which may be limiting for some patients.[83]

PRESERVATIVE-FREE MEDICATIONS

Ocular symptoms are a challenge to many glaucoma patients. In general, these symptoms of stinging, burning, dry eye, and foreign body sensation increase with age, and their causality (the medications themselves, preservatives, or other reasons) is difficult to determine.[84] Ocular surface toxicity is a clearly documented result of use, especially long-term, of glaucoma medications with preservatives.[85] The most commonly used preservative is BAK, but both BAK-free and preservative-free formulations have been developed across classes of medications.

There are several commercially available BAK-free drugs in the Unites States. Brimonidine (Alphagan-P®), travoprost (Travatan-Z®), and timolol maleate (Timoptic XE®) are available in BAK-free formulations. Other formulations without any preservatives include tafluprost (Zioptan®), timolol in Ocudose (Timoptic®), and dorzolamide-timolol (Cosopt PF®). Other completely preservative-free formulations of prostaglandin analogs are available in other parts of the world, but not currently in the US. While these symptoms may be linked to decreased quality of life and adherence,[86] these drugs are also often costly to the patient, as patients frequently must try and fail the more commonly used preserved option. If not covered by insurance, the cost is high and thus may be limiting to patients who need them the most.

FOLLOW-UP

While there is no evidence-base to guide frequency of follow-up, patients should visit the office often after the initial diagnosis to get a second visual field and to determine efficacy of medication use. Follow-up visits should be based on the patients anticipated life expectancy, extent of damage, level of IOP with prior progression, perceived adherence, and length of stability. We would urge that patients with advanced disease, those with unstable IOP, and those with longer life expectancies be followed more closely. After stabilization of disease, if the patient is controlled on medical therapy, they may follow-up less frequently, even yearly (Table 64.2).

The error we have frequently seen is that IOP alone is used as method of follow-up. IOP is a surrogate endpoint and a target IOP is a construct that may always need refining. Frequent perimetry and optic nerve evaluations are necessary as we are evaluating an optic nerve disease, not an IOP.

Table 64.2: Consensus-based guidelines for follow-up glaucoma status evaluations with optic nerve and visual field assessment.*

Target IOP achieved	Progression of damage	Duration of control (mos)	Approximate follow-up interval (mos)†
Yes	No	≤6	6
Yes	No	>6	12
Yes	Yes	NA	1–2
No	Yes	NA	1–2
No	No	NA	3–6

*Evaluations consist of clinical examination of the patient, including optic nerve head assessment (with periodic color) stereophotography or computerized imaging of the optic nerve and retinal nerve fiber layer structure) and visual field assessment.

†Patients with more-advanced damage or greater lifetime risk from primary open-angle glaucoma may require more frequent evaluations. These intervals as the maximum recommended time between evaluations.

(IOP: Intraocular pressure; NA: Not applicable)

Source: Reproduced with permission from the American Academy of Ophthalmology.

SUCCESS

Success of glaucoma medical therapy is defined by meeting the patient's target IOP while additionally maintaining stable visual field testing and avoiding progressive damage to the optic disk. If a patient is unable to meet these specifications, the clinician should discuss alternative forms of treatment (such as laser and surgical therapies), their efficacies, adverse events, and impacts on patients' quality of life.

OCULAR HYPERTENSION

Determining when and whether to treat patients with ocular hypertension has been extensively studied. The OHTS found that after a 5-year follow-up, 9.5% of patients with untreated ocular hypertension developed glaucoma.[5] In general, these patients should be seen in the office annually or biannually with monitoring of their IOP and testing. Treatment of ocular hypertension should be based on the individual patient and their existing risk factors. Several studies have assessed the cost-effectiveness of treating patients with ocular hypertension. Results of these studies determined that it is not cost-effective to treat all patients with ocular hypertension[87] but that treating patients at high risk of developing glaucoma with higher IOP is cost-effective.[88] Additionally, recent work for phase II of OHTS suggest that it does not hurt to withhold treatment initially as long as the patient is carefully monitored.[89]

MEDICAL TREATMENT OF ANGLE-CLOSURE GLAUCOMA

The optimal treatment for acute angle-closure glaucoma (ACG) is laser peripheral iridotomy (LPI) or perhaps cataract surgery.[90] Medical therapy is commonly used in acute attack management of ACG to decrease IOP, pain, and corneal edema. The goal in medical therapy is to open the angle, reduce vitreous volume to deepen the anterior chamber, and reduce production of aqueous humor. Cholinergic agonists, such as pilocarpine are often used to constrict the pupil, which make iridotomy easier. Topical beta-blockers, alpha-agonists, and CAIs are commonly used in acute ACG to lower the IOP urgently by decreasing aqueous production, in addition to oral CAIs. Oral and/or intravenous hyperosmotic agents dehydrate the vitreous. Interestingly, while medical therapy may be used prior to or in the short-term after definitive laser treatment of ACG, the majority of patients will not have future medical treatment intervention for glaucoma following LPI, especially when the LPIs are bilateral.[91]

CONCLUSION

Although numerous options for glaucoma treatment exist with surgery and lasers, medical therapy remains the first choice of most patients and physicians alike. Well-established classes of medications have been the mainstay of glaucoma treatment for decades, and likely will be for years to come. While medications decrease IOP and slow the progression of glaucoma, the afore-mentioned barriers make adherence difficult for patients and put them in danger of worsening disease. New classes and new administration methods on the horizon for glaucoma medical treatment may be helpful to increase adherence and to increase patient and physician satisfaction.

REFERENCES

1. Prum Jr. BE, Rosenberg LF, Gedde SJ, et al. Primary Open-Angle Glaucoma Preferred Practice Pattern® Guidelines. Ophthalmology. 2017;123(1):41-111.
2. The Glaucoma Laser Trial Research Group. The Glaucoma Laser Trial (GLT) and glaucoma laser trial follow-up study: 7. Results. Glaucoma Laser Trial Research Group. Am J Ophthalmol. 1995;120(6):718-31.
3. The AGIS Investigators. The Advanced Glaucoma Intervention Study (AGIS): 7. The relationship between control of intraocular pressure and visual field deterioration. Am J Ophthalmol. 2000;130(4):429-40.
4. Musch DC, Lichter PR, Guire KE, et al. The Collaborative Initial Glaucoma Treatment Study: study design, methods, and baseline characteristics of enrolled patients. Ophthalmology. 1999;106(4):653-62.
5. Kass MA, Heuer DK, Higginbotham EJ, et al. The Ocular Hypertension Treatment Study: a randomized trial determines that topical ocular hypotensive medication delays or prevents the onset of primary open-angle glaucoma. Arch Ophthalmol. 2002;120(6):701-30.
6. Tsai T, Robin AL, Smith JP 3rd. An evaluation of how glaucoma patients use topical medications: a pilot study. Trans Am Ophthalmol Soc. 2007;105:25-9.
7. Stone JL, Robin AL, Novack GD, et al. An objective evaluation of eyedrop instillation in patients with glaucoma. Arch Ophthalmol. 2009;127(6):732-6.
8. Lee PP, Walt JG, Doyle JJ, et al. A multicenter, retrospective pilot study of resource use and costs associated with severity of disease in glaucoma. Arch Ophthalmol. 2006;124(1):12-9.
9. Rein DB, Zhang P, Wirth KE, et al. The economic burden of major adult visual disorders in the United States. Arch Ophthalmol. 2006;124(12):1754-60.
10. Schehlein EM, Im LT, Robin AL, et al. Nonmedical Out-of-Pocket Patient and Companion Expenditures Associated With Glaucoma Care. J Glaucoma. 2017;26(4):343-8.
11. Stein JD, Niziol LM, Musch DC, et al. Longitudinal trends in resource use in an incident cohort of open-angle glaucoma patients: resource use in open-angle glaucoma. Am J Ophthalmol. 2012;154(3):452-9.
12. Blumberg DM, Prager AJ, Liebmann JM. Variation in Prescription Drug Coverage Enrollment Among Vulnerable Beneficiaries With Glaucoma Before and After the Implementation of Medicare Part D. JAMA Ophthalmol. 2016;134(2):212-20.
13. Blumberg DM, Prager AJ, Liebmann JM, et al. Cost-Related Medication Nonadherence and Cost-Saving Behaviors Among Patients With Glaucoma Before and After the Implementation of Medicare Part D. JAMA Ophthalmol. 2015;133(9):985-96.
14. Choudhry NK. Copayment Levels and Medication Adherence. Circulation. 2009;119(3):365-7.
15. Doshi JA, Zhu J, Lee BY, et al. Impact of a prescription copayment increase on lipid-lowering medication adherence in veterans. Circulation. 2009;119(3):390-7.
16. Stein JD, Kim DD, Peck WW, et al. Cost-effectiveness of medications compared with laser trabeculoplasty in patients with newly diagnosed open-angle glaucoma. Arch Ophthalmol. 2012;130(4):497-505.
17. Kaplan RI, De Moraes CG, Cioffi GA, et al. Comparative Cost-effectiveness of the Baerveldt Implant, Trabeculectomy With Mitomycin, and Medical Treatment. JAMA Ophthalmol. 2015;133(5):560-7.
18. Iordanous Y, Kent JS, Hutnik CML, et al. Projected cost comparison of Trabectome, iStent, and endoscopic cyclophotocoagulation versus glaucoma medication in the Ontario Health Insurance Plan. J Glaucoma. 2014;23(2):e112-8.

19. Aboshiha J, Weir R, Singh P, et al. To what extent does a lack of refrigeration of generic chloramphenicol eye-drops used in India decrease their purity and what are the implications for Europe? Br J Ophthalmol. 2008;92(5):609-11.
20. Weir RE, Zaidi FH, Charteris DG, et al. Variability in the content of Indian generic ciprofloxacin eye drops. Br J Ophthalmol. 2005;89(9):1094-6.
21. Stein JD, Newman-Casey PA, Talwar N, et al. The relationship between statin use and open-angle glaucoma. Ophthalmology. 2012;119(10):2074-81.
22. Stein JD, Newman-Casey PA, Niziol LM, et al. Association between the use of glaucoma medications and mortality. Arch Ophthalmol 2010;128(2):235-40.
23. Jampel HD. Target pressure in glaucoma therapy. J Glaucoma. 1997;6(2):133-8.
24. Leske MC, Heijl A, Hussein M, et al. Factors for glaucoma progression and the effect of treatment: the early manifest glaucoma trial. Arch Ophthalmol. 2003;121(1):48-56.
25. Heijl A, Leske MC, Bengtsson B, et al. Reduction of intraocular pressure and glaucoma progression: results from the Early Manifest Glaucoma Trial. Arch Ophthalmol. 2002;120(10):1268-79.
26. Nouri-Mahdavi K, Hoffman D, Coleman AL, et al. Predictive factors for glaucomatous visual field progression in the Advanced Glaucoma Intervention Study. Ophthalmology. 2004;111(9):1627-35.
27. Lichter PR, Musch DC, Gillespie BW, et al. Interim clinical outcomes in the Collaborative Initial Glaucoma Treatment Study comparing initial treatment randomized to medications or surgery. Ophthalmology. 2001;108(11):1943-53.
28. AJ K, AP R. Validity of the monocular trial of intraocular pressure-lowering at different time points in patients starting topical glaucoma medication. JAMA Ophthalmol. 2016;134(7):742-7.
29. Liu JHK, Realini T, Weinreb RN. Asymmetry of 24-hour intraocular pressure reduction by topical ocular hypotensive medications in fellow eyes. Ophthalmology. 2011;118(10):1995-2000.
30. Raizman MB, Hamrah P, Holland EJ, et al. Drug-induced corneal epithelial changes. Surv Ophthalmol. 2017;62(3):286-301.
31. Robin AL, Covert D. Does adjunctive glaucoma therapy affect adherence to the initial primary therapy? Ophthalmology. 2005;112(5):863-8.
32. Robin AL, Novack GD, Covert DW, et al. Adherence in glaucoma: objective measurements of once-daily and adjunctive medication use. Am J Ophthalmol. 2007;144(4):533-40.
33. Bengtsson B, Leske MC, Hyman L, et al. Fluctuation of intraocular pressure and glaucoma progression in the early manifest glaucoma trial. Ophthalmology. 2007;114(2):205-9.
34. Sherrod CE, Vitale S, Frick KD, et al. Association of vision loss and work status in the United States. JAMA Ophthalmol. 2014;132(10):1236-9.
35. Nguyen AM, van Landingham SW, Massof RW, et al. Reading ability and reading engagement in older adults with glaucoma. Invest Ophthalmol Vis Sci. 2014;55(8):5284-90.
36. Yonge A V, Swenor BK, Miller R, et al. Quantifying fall-related hazards in the homes of persons with glaucoma. Ophthalmology. 2017;124(4):562-71.
37. Ramulu PY, West SK, Munoz B, et al. Driving cessation and driving limitation in glaucoma: the Salisbury Eye Evaluation Project. Ophthalmology. 2009;116(10):1846-53.
38. Ramulu PY, Hochberg C, Maul EA, et al. Glaucomatous visual field loss associated with less travel from home. Optom Vis Sci. 2014;91(2):187-93.
39. Ramulu PY, Swenor BK, Jefferys JL, et al. Difficulty with out-loud and silent reading in glaucoma. Invest Ophthalmol Vis Sci. 2013;54(1):666-72.
40. Janz NK, Wren PA, Lichter PR, et al. The Collaborative Initial Glaucoma Treatment Study: interim quality of life findings after initial medical or surgical treatment of glaucoma. Ophthalmology. 2001;108(11):1954-65.
41. Davies I, Williams AM, Muir KW. Aids for eye drop administration. Surv Ophthalmol. 2017;62(3):332-45.
42. Schwartz GF, Quigley HA. Adherence and persistence with glaucoma therapy. Surv Ophthalmol. 2008;53(Suppl 1):S57-68.
43. Drew T, Wolffsohn JS. Usability of prostaglandin monotherapy eye droppers. Br J Ophthalmol. 2015;99(9):1251-4.
44. Newman-Casey PA, Robin AL, Blachley T, et al. The most common barriers to glaucoma medication adherence: a cross-sectional survey. Ophthalmology. 2015;122(7):1308-16.
45. Carpenter DM, Sayner R, Blalock SJ, et al. The effect of eye drop technique education in patients with glaucoma. Health Commun. 2016;31(8):1036-42.
46. Sleath B, Blalock SJ, Carpenter DM, et al. Ophthalmologist-patient communication, self-efficacy, and glaucoma medication adherence. Ophthalmology. 2015;122(4):748-54.
47. Carpenter DM, Blalock SJ, Sayner R, et al. Communication predicts medication self-efficacy in glaucoma patients. Optom Vis Sci. 2016;93(7):731-7.
48. Perera SA, Ting DS, Nongpiur ME, et al. Feasibility study of sustained-release travoprost punctum plug for intraocular pressure reduction in an Asian population. Clin Ophthalmol. 2016;10:757-64.
49. Lewis RA, Christie WC, Day DG, et al. Bimatoprost Sustained-Release Implants for Glaucoma Therapy: 6-Month Results From a Phase I/II Clinical Trial. Am J Ophthalmol. 2017;175:137-47.
50. Brandt JD, Sall K, DuBiner H, et al. Six-Month Intraocular Pressure Reduction with a Topical Bimatoprost Ocular Insert: Results of a Phase II Randomized Controlled Study. Ophthalmology. 2016;123(8):1685-94.
51. Bahler CK, Howell KG, Hann CR, et al. Prostaglandins increase trabecular meshwork outflow facility in

cultured human anterior segments. Am J Ophthalmol. 2008;145(1):114-9.

52. European Glaucoma Society. Terminology and Guidelines for Glaucoma [Internet], 4th edition. Heijl A, Traverso C (Eds). PubliComm; 2014. 146-151 p. Available from: *www.eugs.org/eng/EGS_guidelines4.asp*
53. Gulati V, Fan S, Zhao M, et al. Diurnal and nocturnal variations in aqueous humor dynamics of patients with ocular hypertension undergoing medical therapy. Arch Ophthalmol. 2012;130(6):677-84.
54. Teus MA, Arranz-Márquez E, Lucea-Suescun P. Incidence of iris colour change in latanoprost treated eyes. Br J Ophthalmol. 2002;86(10):1085-8.
55. Stjernschantz JW, Albert DM, Hu D-N, et al. Mechanism and clinical significance of prostaglandin-induced iris pigmentation. Surv Ophthalmol.; 2002;47 Suppl 1:S162-75.
56. Zimmerman TJ, Wheeler TM. Miotics: side effects and ways to avoid them. Ophthalmology. 1982;89(1):76-80.
57. Derick RJ, Robin AL, Tielsch J, et al. Once-daily versus twice-daily levobunolol (0.5%) therapy. A crossover study. Ophthalmology. 1992;99(3):424-9.
58. Jampel HD, Lynch MG, Brown RH. Beta-adrenergic receptors in human trabecular meshwork. Arch Ophthalmol. 1987;105(1):22.
59. Bartlett JD, Olivier M, Richardson T, et al. Central nervous system and plasma lipid profiles associated with carteolol and timolol in postmenopausal black women. J Glaucoma. 1999;8(6):388-95.
60. Vander Zanden JA, Valuck RJ, Bunch CL, et al. Systemic adverse effects of ophthalmic beta-blockers. Ann Pharmacother. 2001;35(12):1633-7.
61. Zimmerman TJ, Kooner KS, Kandarakis AS, et al. Improving the therapeutic index of topically applied ocular drugs. Arch Ophthalmol. 1984;102(4):551-3.
62. Boger WP 3rd. Short-term "escape" and long-term "drift." The dissipation effects of the beta adrenergic blocking agents. Surv Ophthalmol. 1983;28 Suppl:235-42.
63. Schuman JS, Horwitz B, Choplin NT, et al. A 1-year study of brimonidine twice daily in glaucoma and ocular hypertension. A controlled, randomized, multicenter clinical trial. Chronic Brimonidine Study Group. Arch Ophthalmol. 1997;115(7):847-52.
64. Schoene RB, Abuan T, Ward RL, et al. Effects of topical betaxolol, timolol, and placebo on pulmonary function in asthmatic bronchitis. Am J Ophthalmol. 1984;97(1):86-92.
65. Buckley MM, Goa KL, Clissold SP. Ocular betaxolol. A review of its pharmacological properties, and therapeutic efficacy in glaucoma and ocular hypertension. Drugs.;1990;40(1):75-90.
66. Weinreb RN, Caldwell DR, Goode SM, et al. A double-masked three-month comparison between 0.25% betaxolol suspension and 0.5% betaxolol ophthalmic solution. Am J Ophthalmol. 1990;110(2):189-92.
67. Stewart WC, Laibovitz R, Horwitz B, et al. A 90-day study of the efficacy and side effects of 0.25% and 0.5% apraclonidine vs 0.5% timolol. Apraclonidine Primary Therapy Study Group. Arch Ophthalmol. 1996;114(8):938-42.
68. Butler P, Mannschreck M, Lin S, et al. Clinical experience with the long-term use of 1% apraclonidine. Incidence of allergic reactions. Arch Ophthalmol. 1995;113(3):293-6.
69. Wilensky JT. The role of brimonidine in the treatment of open-angle glaucoma. Surv Ophthalmol. 1996;41(Suppl 1): S3-7.
70. Shin DH, Glover BK, Cha SC, et al. Long-term brimonidine therapy in glaucoma patients with apraclonidine allergy. Am J Ophthalmol. 1999;127(5):511-5.
71. Katz LJ. Brimonidine tartrate 0.2% twice daily vs timolol 0.5% twice daily: 1-year results in glaucoma patients. Brimonidine Study Group. Am J Ophthalmol. 1999;127(1):20-6.
72. Lee AG, Anderson R, Kardon RH, et al. Presumed "sulfa allergy" in patients with intracranial hypertension treated with acetazolamide or furosemide: cross-reactivity, myth or reality? Am J Ophthalmol. 2004;138(1):114-8.
73. Sall K. The efficacy and safety of brinzolamide 1% ophthalmic suspension (Azopt) as a primary therapy in patients with open-angle glaucoma or ocular hypertension. Brinzolamide Primary Therapy Study Group. Surv Ophthalmol. 2000;44 (Suppl 2):S155-62.
74. Tanimura H, Minamoto A, Narai A, et al. Corneal edema in glaucoma patients after the addition of brinzolamide 1% ophthalmic suspension. Jpn J Ophthalmol. 2005;49(4):332-3.
75. Konowal A, Morrison JC, Brown SV, et al. Irreversible corneal decompensation in patients treated with topical dorzolamide. Am J Ophthalmol. 1999;127(4):403-6.
76. Tsai SF, Shu KH. Mannitol-induced acute renal failure. Clin Nephrol. 2010;74(1):70-3.
77. Tanihara H, Inoue T, Yamamoto T, et al. Phase 1 clinical trials of a selective Rho kinase inhibitor, K-115. JAMA Ophthalmol. 2013;131(10):1288-95.
78. Tanihara H, Inoue T, Yamamoto T, et al. Phase 2 randomized clinical study of a Rho kinase inhibitor, K-115, in primary open-angle glaucoma and ocular hypertension. Am J Ophthalmol. 2013;156(4):731-6.
79. Tanihara H, Inoue T, Yamamoto T, et al. Additive Intraocular Pressure-Lowering Effects of the Rho Kinase Inhibitor Ripasudil (K-115) Combined With Timolol or Latanoprost: A Report of 2 Randomized Clinical Trials. JAMA Ophthalmol. 2015;133(7):755-61.
80. Yamamoto K, Maruyama K, Himori N, et al. The novel Rho kinase (ROCK) inhibitor K-115: a new candidate drug for neuroprotective treatment in glaucoma. Invest Ophthalmol Vis Sci. 2014;55(11):7126-36.
81. Higginbotham EJ. Considerations in glaucoma therapy: fixed combinations versus their component medications. Clin Ophthalmol. 2010;4:1-9.
82. Barnebey HS, Robin AL. Adherence to Fixed-Combination Versus Unfixed Travoprost 0.004%/Timolol 0.5% for Glaucoma or Ocular Hypertension: a Randomized Trial. Am J Ophthalmol. 2017;176:61-9.

83. Vold SD, Riggs WL, Jackimiec J. Cost analysis of glaucoma medications: a 3-year review. J Glaucoma. 2002;11(4):354-8.
84. Pisella PJ, Pouliquen P, Baudouin C. Prevalence of ocular symptoms and signs with preserved and preservative free glaucoma medication. Br J Ophthalmol. 2002;86(4):418-23.
85. Okahara A, Tanioka H, Takada K, et al. Ocular toxicity of benzalkonium chloride homologs compared with their mixtures. J Toxicol Pathol. 2013;26(4):343-9.
86. Zimmerman TJ, Hahn SR, Gelb L,. The impact of ocular adverse effects in patients treated with topical prostaglandin analogs: changes in prescription patterns and patient persistence. J Ocul Pharmacol Ther. 2009;25(2):145-52.
87. Stewart WC, Stewart JA, Nasser QJ, et al. Cost-effectiveness of treating ocular hypertension. Ophthalmology. 2008;115(1):94-8.
88. Kymes SM, Kass MA, Anderson DR, et al. Management of ocular hypertension: a cost-effectiveness approach from the Ocular Hypertension Treatment Study. Am J Ophthalmol. 2006;141(6):997-1008.
89. Kass MA, Gordon MO, Gao F, et al. Delaying treatment of ocular hypertension: the ocular hypertension treatment study. Arch Ophthalmol. 2010;128(3):276-87.
90. Azuara-Blanco A, Burr J, Ramsay C, et al. Effectiveness of early lens extraction for the treatment of primary angle-closure glaucoma (EAGLE): a randomised controlled trial. Lancet. 2016;388(10052):1389-97.
91. Bansal S, Balakrishnan SA, Blachley T, et al. Subsequent Receipt of Interventions for Glaucoma Among a Nationwide Sample of Patients Who Underwent Laser Peripheral Iridotomy. Am J Ophthalmol. 2015;160(2):275-82.

Chapter 65

Office-based Laser Treatments for Glaucoma

Natasha Nayak Kolomeyer, Scott J Fudemberg, L Jay Katz

BASICS OF LASER PROCEDURES

Laser procedures have an important role in glaucoma management. Before proceeding into the more clinically relevant material, it is important to step back and understand the basics of the two major lasers we will discuss in this chapter.[1,2]

Argon laser utilizes thermal energy to photocoagulate tissue. At high temperatures, the laser induces chemical changes that cause local inflammation and scarring. Lower energy photocoagulation may cause contraction of collagen, and this is part of the mechanism of pupilloplasty, iridoplasty, and possibly of laser trabeculoplasty. Melanin is the pigment in most target tissues. Blue (488 nm) and green (514 nm) wavelength argon lasers are optimal for absorption by melanin.

Neodymium:yttrium-aluminum-garnet (Nd:YAG) is a laser with near infrared wavelength (1,064 nm) and an ionizing effect. With continuous wave mode, it has a photocoagulative effect; however, with pulsed delivery, Nd:YAG has a photodisruptive effect. A short duration of intense laser energy generates an instantaneous electric field that creates shock and pressure waves that can disrupt both pigmented and nonpigmented tissues. Selective laser trabeculoplasty (SLT) is performed using a Q-switched, frequency-doubled (532 nm) Nd:YAG laser that uses selective thermolysis; it is preferentially absorbed by pigmented, melanin-containing trabecular meshwork cells, while sparing nonpigmented trabecular meshwork.

Variables of laser treatment include spot size (microns), number of applications, exposure duration, energy (joules or millijoules), and power (watts or milliwatts). Lasers, especially argon lasers, can cause retinal or lens injury. The physician performing the laser is theoretically protected due to filters built into the slit lamp. It is important that all bystanders wear safety glasses made specifically for the wavelength of the laser being utilized.

LASER TRABECULOPLASTY

Indications

Laser trabeculoplasty is performed to lower intraocular pressure (IOP) in pseudoexfoliation, pigment dispersion, and primary open-angle glaucoma (POAG). It is less effective in juvenile open-angle glaucoma and inflammatory glaucoma. If there are significant open segments of the angle, laser trabeculoplasty can be considered in patients with chronic angle closure. There are two major lasers that can be used to perform laser trabeculoplasty: argon laser trabeculoplasty (ALT) or SLT. Other lasers can be used to perform laser trabeculoplasty, including micropulse diode, titanium sapphire, and pattern scan laser. Depending on physician and patient preference, laser trabeculoplasty may be considered as initial therapy or after initiating medical therapy.

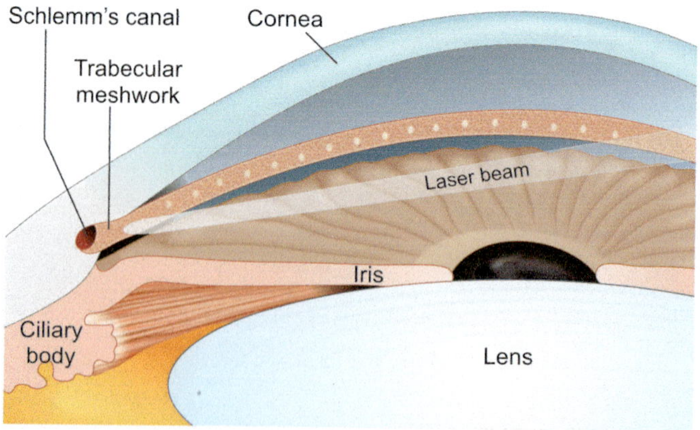

Fig. 65.1: Laser trabeculoplasty. The laser beam is aimed at the trabecular meshwork for SLT. ALT has a smaller laser spot size and is aimed more specifically at the junction between the anterior one-third and posterior two-thirds of the trabecular meshwork.

Mechanism of Argon Laser Trabeculoplasty

There are several theories regarding the mechanism of action of ALT.[1,2] Histological studies show coagulative damage and damage of the structure of trabecular meshwork post-ALT in cadaveric eyes. It has been proposed that this can result in collagen shrinkage and scarring of the inner trabecular ring that subsequently causes widening of the intertrabecular spaces and improvement in aqueous outflow. However, there is limited evidence of this mechanical theory. The biologic theory suggests coagulative necrosis induced by the laser may induce macrophage migration and eventually phagocytosis and clearance of the trabecular meshwork. Recent studies suggest the lasers downstream effects may cause inflammatory release of cytokines which can then induce matrix metalloproteinase expression. ALT also induced increased trabecular cell division in animal studies and organ-cultured human eyes. Tomographic studies have demonstrated an increase in outflow facility with laser trabeculoplasty that suggests improved aqueous flow through the trabecular meshwork.

Mechanism of Selective Laser Trabeculoplasty

Although histological studies of SLT-treated human autopsy eyes did not reveal coagulative damage, there was visible disruption of trabecular beams, cellular debris, and fragmentation of the endothelium.[1,2] Multiple biologic effects of SLT have been suggested, which include increased monocyte recruitment, tight junction disassembly and increased conductivity in Schlemm's canal, and significant change in gene expression.

Procedure

- Obtain informed consent, discussing the most relevant risks, including inflammation, failure to lower IOP, and corneal edema
- Pretreatment 15–30 minutes prior with alpha-2 adrenergic agonist (brimonidine or apraclonidine) to minimize post-laser IOP elevation
- Administer topical anesthesia (proparacaine, tetracaine or lidocaine jelly)
- Apply goniosolution to lens
- A 16–25× magnification in the slit lamp can be a good balance between field of view and details
- *For ALT*:
  - Goldmann 3-mirror lens (Ocular Instruments Inc.; Bellevue, WA) for ALT
  - Treatment area of 180–360° per session
  - Laser settings may vary. Suggestions include 50 um (spot size), 600–800 mW (power) to begin, 0.1 second (duration), 50–100 spot treatments over 180–360°
  - Aim laser to the junction of the anterior one-third and posterior two-thirds of the trabecular meshwork. This is a significantly smaller spot size than SLT and therefore, requires more precision. Aim to have an interval of 3 laser spot sizes between treatment areas
  - Titrate the power to visualize blanching of the tissue and minimal to no bubbles
- *For SLT*:
  - Latina SLT lens or Goldmann 3-mirror lens (Ocular Instruments Inc.; Bellevue, WA)
  - Treatment area of 180–360° per session
  - 400 um (spot size fixed) and 3 ns (duration fixed). Start with 0.5–0.8 mJ (energy). Approximately 50–100 spots per 180–360° of treatment
  - Aim the laser on the entire trabecular meshwork. Try not to overlap treatment spots
  - Titrate to just below or at the threshold energy needed to visualize fine champagne bubbles (without bursts)
- Administer another drop of an alpha-2 adrenergic agonist immediately after laser treatment
- Recheck IOP 30–60 minutes post-laser treatment
- *Tips/tricks*:
  - If you are having difficulty viewing the nasal or temporal angle, ask the patient to look in that direction of the mirror to improve the angle view. If the angle still appears narrow, can consider laser iridotomy (LI) prior to laser trabeculoplasty (with at least one week interval)
  - The superior mirror visualizes the inferior angle. However, the temporal part of the superior mirror is reflecting the temporal part of the inferior angle
  - Rotate and readjust the angle of the goniolens until the laser aiming beam is round and sharp
  - It is important to have a preplanned pattern so that you can restart the laser treatment if interrupted. This includes choosing which quadrant you will start with, and which way you are going to rotate your goniolens. You will rotate your goniolens in the opposite direction that you are applying your spots, i.e. if your treatments are moving clockwise, your goniolens rotation should be counterclockwise

- Avoid laser applications that are too posterior as they can increase the chance of post-laser inflammation
- More pigmented areas require less laser energy.

Management

Post-laser management for ALT and SLT can vary. It may include a short course (4–7 days) of topical steroids or nonsteroidal anti-inflammatory medications, four times a day. Most patients do not require any postlaser anti-inflammatory drops. Follow-up is typically at 1–2 weeks, and then 4–6 weeks. Post-laser IOP spikes require careful management and close follow-up to confirm its resolution. IOP-lowering agents may be administered to blunt the spike.

Complications

- The most common complication is an acute elevation in IOP. This usually occurs within the first two hours after laser treatment. There is a reported 30% incidence of IOP elevation more than 5 mm Hg in ALT, compared to 10% incidence after SLT.[3,4] Increased trabecular meshwork pigmentation is associated with greater chance of transient IOP rise. IOP spike is less likely if treatment is split into smaller groups or if alpha-2 adrenergic agonists are used 15 minutes before or immediately after treatment. Note that alpha-2 adrenergic agonists may be less effective if patient has been using them long term.
- Post-laser iritis is often transient, mild, and self-limited or easily controlled with topical corticosteroids or nonsteroidal anti-inflammatory medications.
- Corneal epithelial defects or opacities usually improve in a few days.
- Hyphema is uncommon and less likely with SLT. If it does occur, it often decreases with gentle application of pressure with goniolens.
- Peripheral anterior synechiae formation can occur in up to 33% of ALT patients, however, is rare with SLT.
- ALT histologically destroys parts of the trabecular meshwork. It is controversial whether ALT may predispose patients to encapsulated blebs during subsequent filtering surgeries.
- Rare cases of corneal edema/decompensation have been observed after SLT. Some cases were noted to resolve, though others did not.

Argon Laser Trabeculoplasty Results

The IOP is usually lowered by 20–30% in 75–85% of patients who received ALT treatment.[5] Studies suggest the IOP lowering effect persists for 1 year in 80% of eyes, for 5 years in 50% of eyes, and for 10 years in 30% of eyes. The full effect usually takes 4 weeks.

The Glaucoma Laser Trial[4] was a randomized clinical trial that enrolled 271 newly diagnosed POAG patients. One eye was randomized to receive initial ALT treatment whereas the fellow eye received 0.5% timolol. ALT was administered in two sessions (each with 45–50 burns over 180°) and spaced 4 weeks apart. At the 2-year follow-up mark, eyes that initially received ALT (1) had a mean improvement in IOP 1.5 mm Hg greater than eyes initially treated with timolol (9.8 vs 8.4 mm improvement from baseline, respectively), and (2) were less likely to require simultaneous prescription of two or more medications to control IOP (56% vs 70%). At 3.5-year follow-up of visual field data, the mean threshold for eyes initially treated with ALT was 0.3 dB higher than for eyes treated with timolol. These differences were not clinically significant however, and primarily demonstrate that both medication and ALT are reasonable initial treatments for POAG patients.

Selective Laser Trabeculoplasty Results

The SLT/Med study[6] was a prospective randomized clinical trial that enrolled 127 eyes, that were randomized to SLT (360°, 100 spots) or medical therapy with a prostaglandin analog. If further treatment was required, the study outlined subsequent steps; in the SLT group patients received repeat 180° SLT; and, in the medication group, additional medication was added. At 1 year follow-up, mean IOP reduction was not statistically different between the SLT and medication groups (6.3 vs 7 mm Hg reduction, respectively). The need for additional treatment rate due to failure was higher in the medical treatment group compared to SLT (24% vs 11%) although this was not statistically significant.

Argon Laser Trabeculoplasty versus Selective Laser Trabeculoplasty

Several randomized-controlled trials have not shown any statistically significant difference in IOP lowering, although a majority had small sample size. As SLT utilizes less energy per pulse than ALT (0.9 mJ vs 50 mJ), post-laser IOP spike is less likely and less severe.

Repeat Laser Trabeculoplasty

Repeat laser trabeculoplasty is more likely to be successful in patients who have responded in the past, even if it was short-lasting. Repeat ALT success rates vary from 5% to 70%, and further decrease over time, though there may be a risk of the IOP rising with ALT. SLT may be repeated safely often as there is less thermal damage to the trabecular meshwork compared to ALT, and concerns over IOP rises after repeat treatment have not been reported. Some consider repeat SLT to be as safe and effective as the initial SLT.[5]

LASER PERIPHERAL IRIDOTOMY

Indications

During laser peripheral iridotomy (LPI), laser energy is used to create a hole in the peripheral iris that allows equalization of the anterior and posterior chambers and deepening of the peripheral anterior chamber and angle. Indications include acute or chronic angle closure, ruling out aqueous misdirection, nanophthalmos, narrow or occludable angles, and acute angle closure in the contralateral eye. LPI is contraindicated in patients who would not tolerate a procedure at the slit lamp, in that case surgical iridotomy or cataract extraction would be required under anesthesia. Additionally, be cautious in patients with iridocorneal touch and those with corneal opacities or dystrophies.

Procedure

- Informed consent; important to mention the risks of linear dysphotopsia (vertical line in vision which can be disturbing to some), glare, ghost imaging, along with the usual risks of bleeding, inflammation, and IOP spike.
- Pretreatment 15–30 minutes prior with pilocarpine (1% or 2%) to cause pupillary constriction and immobility.
- Pretreatment 15–30 minutes prior with alpha-2 adrenergic agonists (apraclonidine or brimonidine) to decrease chance of post-laser IOP spike.
- Administer topical anesthesia (proparacaine, tetracaine or lidocaine jelly).
- Apply viscous coupling solution.
- *Lens choice:* Abraham lens or Wise lens. Applied to eye with goniosolution. This allows control over eye position and focuses the power at a target site.
- *Location:* Avoid 12 o'clock because if and when bubbles form, they often block the view at 12 o'clock. Note that bubbles are more likely with argon laser treatment. Avoid placement in an area that is intermittently covered by the eyelid. The most common locations are likely 11 or 1 o'clock or 3 or 9 o'clock.
- Aim for a crypt or area of thinner iris.
- There are three major options for performing LPI: Argon alone, argon pretreatment then Nd:YAG, or Nd:YAG alone.
  - *Argon treatment alone:* Cases in which pretreatment with argon is particularly recommended include darker pigmented irises without crypts, acute angle closure, and patients on anticoagulation. 50 um (spot size), 500–1,000 mW (power), 0.02–0.2 seconds (shorter bursts are more effective for darker eyes). Up to 100 spots (usually require less than 30 if lighter iris with longer duration).
  - *Nd:YAG alone:* Laser settings may vary with machine and iris pigment. We typically use 6 mJ/pulse and 3 pulse/burst, but also use 11 mJ as a single shot (no burst). Titration is important.
  - *Argon and Nd:YAG combination:* Goal is to use argon to thin the tissue with the above argon settings

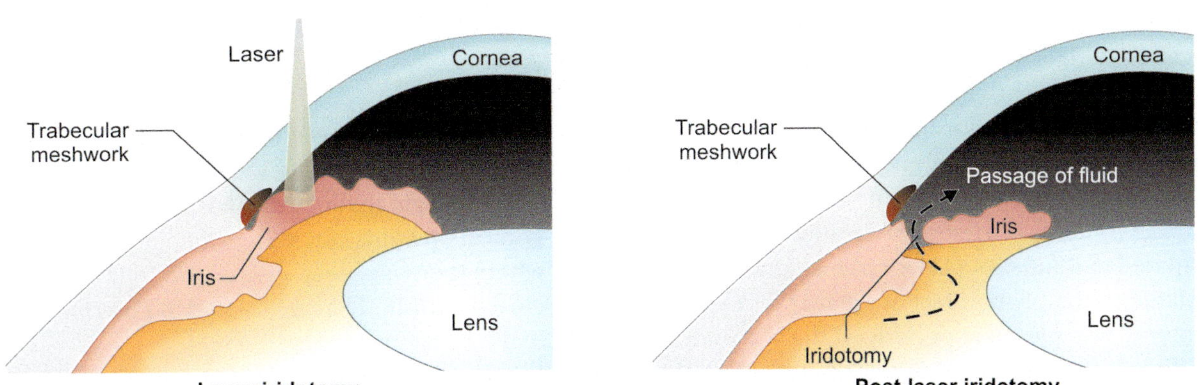

Fig. 65.2: Peripheral laser iridotomy. The laser beam is aimed at the peripheral iris. The hole in the peripheral iris allows equalization of the anterior and posterior chambers and deepening of the peripheral anterior chamber and angle.

and a time of 0.02–0.05 seconds. This often takes 5–30 shots. This is followed by Nd:YAG laser focused on the deepest layer of tissue.
- Pause laser treatment once you see a smoke signal (pigmented debris coming forward). However as the debris clears, it is important to check for significant iris strands through the iridotomy before terminating the procedure.
- Administer another drop of an alpha-2 adrenergic agonist immediately after laser treatment.
- Recheck IOP 30–60 minutes post-laser treatment.

Management

- Postoperative management usually includes using a topical steroid four times a day for 1 week. Postoperative visit is usually at week 1–2 (unless there is an IOP spike). If the LPI is patent and no adverse reaction, can consider LPI in contralateral eye if necessary.
- If the LPIs are patent initial dilation of the pupil may be performed with a weak mydriatic. IOP should be checked before and after dilation. Persistent narrowing of the angle may be present despite patent LPI, especially in eyes with a plateau iris configuration. IOP spikes are uncommon but may occur even in the presence of patent iridotomy (suggesting plateau iris syndrome). Eyes that are at higher risk for LPI closure could be seen again in 1–2 months. These include patients with silicone oil, inflammatory conditions, or a small LPI.

Complications

- Complications include post-laser IOP spike, inflammation, corneal injury, and lens injury. Most lens injuries are self-limited, however, if it results in lens rupture (very rare), it may cause change in fluidics of lens and, therefore, progression of cataract.
- Visual disturbances such as dysphotopsia, glare or ghost imaging can occur in 5–10% of patients. These disturbances are more likely if there is partial coverage of the LPI by the eyelids. A recent study suggested there are less symptoms in a temporal location (3 or 9 o'clock) compared to a superior (11 or 1 o'clock) location.[7] This is related to the prism effect of the tear film when the iridotomy was placed superiorly. If the symptoms are significant, patients can wear a cosmetic contact lens.
- Bleeding is more likely when using Nd:YAG alone as it causes photodisruption, whereas argon causes photocoagulation. Bleeding can be treated with gentle pressure on the eye through the goniolens, and usually resolves.
- Ciliochoroidal effusion or aqueous misdirection (both rare).
- An LPI can close at an unspecified time. Nd:YAG creates a larger zone of iris pigment epithelial loss around the area of iridotomy compared to argon laser. The most common cause of closure of an iridotomy is pigment migration, and therefore Nd:YAG is less likely to result in late closure of LPI.

Laser Peripheral Iridotomy versus Cataract Surgery

The EAGLE[8] (effectiveness of early lens extraction for the treatment of primary angle-closure glaucoma) study enrolled 419 participants who did not have cataracts and were at least 50 years of age (155 with primary angle closure and 263 with primary angle closure glaucoma). They were randomized to receive clear lens extraction or standard care (LPI and topical medical treatment). Clear lens extraction was more cost-effective and resulted in lower mean IOP reduction [–1.99 to –0.38, 95% confidence interval (CI), $p = 0.004$] compared to standard care. Thus, lens extraction may be considered as an alternative to LPI, especially in eyes with cataract, and when IOP-lowering is a goal (eyes with primary angle closure and primary angle closure glaucoma).

LASER PERIPHERAL IRIDOPLASTY

Mechanism

Thermal energy from the argon laser is applied to the peripheral iris, causing the iris stroma to contract and deepen the angle.

Indications

- *Plateau iris:* The clinical presentation is usually a patient with a patent LPI, however, a persistently narrow angle that causes IOP spike after dilation. On gonioscopy, it is often identified as a "double hump" where there is a deep central anterior chamber and a closed peripheral angle related to anterior orientation of the ciliary processes.
- Primary acute angle-closure glaucoma that is resistant to medical therapy to break the attack, although LPI will eventually be the definitive treatment.

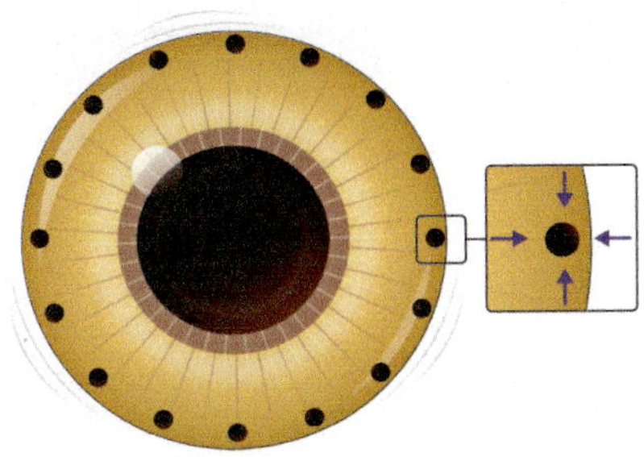

Fig. 65.3: Laser peripheral iridoplasty. Thermal energy from the argon laser is applied to the peripheral iris, causing the iris stroma to contract and deepen the angle. The interval between treatments should be about 1–1.5 times the width of treatment areas.

- Chronic angle closure patients with iridotrabecular contact and residual angle closure. Iridoplasty is more likely to be successful if PAS have been present for less than 6 months.
- Angle closure or narrowing related to size of lens. For example in phacomorphic glaucoma, anterior subluxation of the lens, and nanophthalmos.

Procedure

- Informed consent.
- Pretreatment 15–30 minutes prior with pilocarpine (1% or 2%) to cause pupillary constriction and immobility.
- Pretreatment 15–30 minutes prior with alpha-2 adrenergic agonist (brimonidine or apraclonidine) to minimize post-laser IOP elevation.
- Administer topical anesthesia (proparacaine, tetracaine or lidocaine jelly).
- *Lens choice:* Abraham lens. Applied to eye with goniosolution. This allows control over eye position and focuses the power at a target site.
- *Argon laser settings:* 200–500 µm (spot size), 0.2–0.5 seconds (duration), 300–500 mW (power).
- Aim for the peripheral part of iris. It may be important to overlap your aiming beam with the limbus to a degree to achieve this. Titrate power until there is visible contraction of the iris. However, lower the power if there are visible burns, bubble formation, or burst of pigment. The interval between treatments should be about 1–1.5 times the width of treatment areas.
- Place another drop of brimonidine or apraclonidine after laser treatment.
- Check IOP in 30–60 minutes.

Management

Patient is often given a steroid drop to use four times a day for 1 week and is followed up in 1–2 weeks.

Complications

Can include elevation of IOP, iris atrophy (and therefore change in iris appearance), atonic pupils, mild inflammation, anterior or posterior synechiae, and corneal injury.

Results

A long-term study suggested that 85–90% of angles remained open after receiving laser peripheral iridoplasty to treat residual appositional angle closure after LPI. In previous studies, laser peripheral iridoplasty had similar efficacy as medical therapy in lowering IOP in acute angle-closure glaucoma and phacomorphic glaucoma patients.

REFERENCES

1. Allingham RR, Damji KF, Freedman SF, et al. Shields Textbook of Glaucoma, 6th edition. Pennsylvania: Lippincott Williams & Wilkins; 2011. pp. 448-82.
2. Kahook MY, Schuman JS. Chandler and Grant's Glaucoma, 5th edition. New Jersey: Slack Incorporated; 2013. pp. 469-528.
3. Barkana Y, Belkin M. Selective laser trabeculoplasty. Surv Ophthalmol. 2007;52(6):634-54.
4. Glaucoma Laser Trial Research Group. The Glaucoma Laser Trial (GLT) and glaucoma laser trial follow-up study: 7. Results. Am J Ophthalmol. 1995;120(6):718-31.
5. Ekici F, Waisbourd M, Katz LJ. Current and Future of Laser Therapy in the Management of Glaucoma. Open Ophthalmol J. 2016;10:56-67.
6. Katz LJ, Steinmann WC, Kabir A, et al. Selective laser trabeculoplasty versus medical therapy as initial treatment of glaucoma: a prospective, randomized trial. J Glaucoma. 2012;21(7):460-8.
7. Vera V, Naqi A, Belovay GW, et al. Dysphotopsia after temporal versus superior laser peripheral iridotomy: a prospective randomized paired eye trial. Am J Ophthalmol. 2014;157(5):929-35.
8. Azuara-Blanco A, Burr J, Ramsay C, et al. Effectiveness of early lens extraction for the treatment of primary angle-closure glaucoma (EAGLE): a randomised controlled trial. Lancet. 2016;388(10052):1389-97.

Chapter 66

Secondary Glaucomas: Modification of Treatment Algorithms to Maximize Outcomes

Tamara Zompa, S Fabian Lerner

INTRODUCTION

Secondary glaucomas are an important cause of ocular comorbidities and vision loss. Management must be tailored for each glaucoma subtype, including assessment of contributing chronic disease (i.e. diabetes), treating the underlying causes, as well as medical and surgical treatments, which may differ from the treatment of primary glaucoma.

PSEUDOEXFOLIATIVE GLAUCOMA

Pseudoexfoliation syndrome (XFS) is an age-related disease in which abnormal fibrillar extracellular material is produced and found in the anterior segment structures [endothelium of the iris, cornea, trabecular meshwork (TM) and epithelium of lens and ciliary body]. When associated with characteristic changes in the optic nerve and/or visual field, usually with ocular hypertension, it leads to pseudoexfoliative glaucoma. It is the most common identifiable cause of glaucoma.[1]

Epidemiology and Prognosis

The XFS occurs worldwide in all populations, though it is more prevalent in Caucasian populations in Scandinavian countries, Ireland, Greece, Turkey, and other specific regions. It may account for about 20–25% of open-angle glaucomas worldwide,[2] and its prevalence increases significantly with age (especially >50 years old).

Among patients with XFS, the risk of developing glaucoma is cumulative over time. Twenty-five percent of XFS patients develop ocular hypertension, and nearly 30% of them can develop glaucoma.[2,3] Compared with primary open-angle glaucoma (POAG) eyes, XFG more frequently has these characteristics:

- Bilateral, but asymmetric level of damage.
- Worse clinical course and prognosis.
- Greater glaucomatous damage at the time of diagnosis.
- Poor response to medical treatment.
- Increased need for surgical intervention.
- Faster progression of visual field (VF) damage.
- Greater intraocular pressure (IOP) fluctuations.

Etiopathogenesis

The exact composition of the pseudoexfoliative material (XFM) is unknown. There is an abnormal metabolism of glycosaminoglycans. The protein components of XFM include noncollagenous basement membrane components and epitopes of the elastic fibers system such as fibrillium.[1]

The etiology by which XFM is produced is likely multifactorial, and includes:

- *Genetic factors, defined by*:
  - Familial transmission, with an increased risk in relatives of affected patients.
  - Autosomal dominant, mitochondrial and X-linked inheritance patterns.[3]
  - HLA patterns, with strong associations with 4 antigens.[4]
  - Strong associations with specific variations in the *LOXL1* gene.[5]
- *Nongenetic and environmental factors, including:*
  - Dietary habits
  - Solar exposition
  - Living at lower latitudes and higher altitudes
  - Autoimmunity
  - Infection
  - Anterior segment trauma.

Presentation of glaucoma is most often in the form of:[1-3]

- Chronic open angle glaucoma, defined by:
  - Trabecular cell dysfunction resulting from obstruction of the TM by XFM.
  - Obstruction of the TM by iris pigment.[6]
  - Concomitant chronic open angle glaucoma.
- Acute glaucoma:
  - *With open angle:* Sudden and severe ocular hypertension. The patient can present with red eye, corneal edema and very high IOP.
  - *With closed angle secondary to*:
    - Zonular weakness, with anterior displacement of the iridolenticular diaphragm.
    - Posterior synechiae.

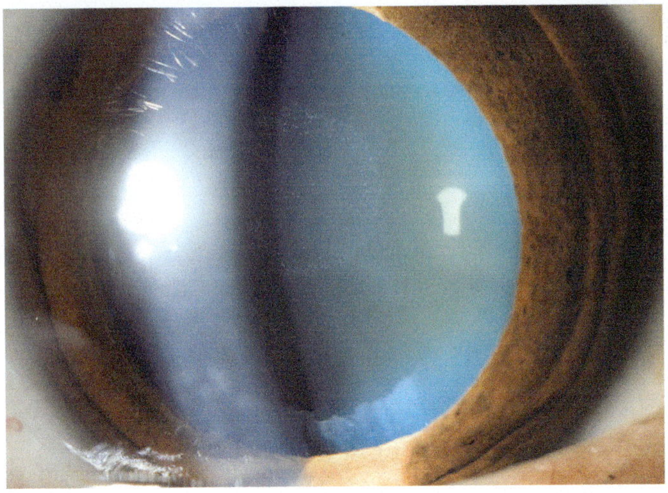

Fig. 66.1: Pseudoexfoliative material on anterior lens capsule in a concentric rings pattern.

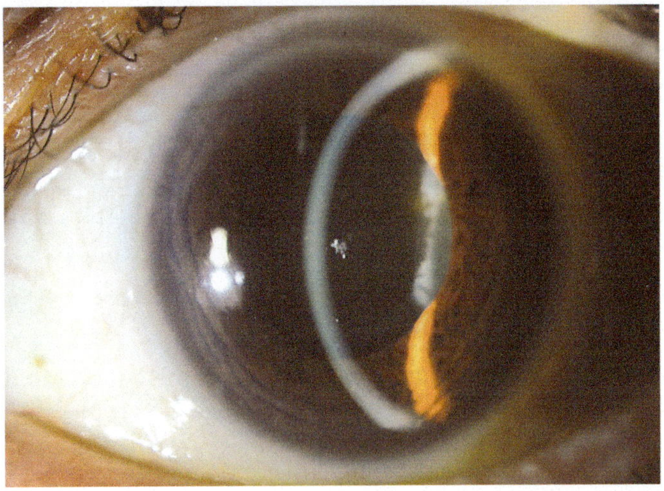

Fig. 66.2: Pseudoexfoliative material deposit on corneal endothelium.

Ocular Manifestations and Diagnosis

Biomicroscopy provides the strongest clues to the presence of pseudoexfoliation. Findings include:

- Pseudoexfoliative white deposits on anterior lens capsule in a three concentric rings pattern, seen under full mydriasis (Fig. 66.1).
- Deposits of XFM at the pupil's edge, iris, angle structures.
- Pigment loss from the iris sphincter and its deposition on anterior chamber structures. This can also be described as peripupillary iris atrophy.
- Phacodonesis/iridodonesis.
- Poor mydriasis.
- Pigment and XFM on the corneal endothelium (Fig. 66.2).
- Association with cataract.

Gonioscopy can also present findings supporting the diagnosis, including:

- Patchy or irregular pigmentation of the TM, with large and dark pigment particles. These findings may appear even before the XFM is seen.[2]
- Sampaolesi's line—a wavy pigmented line anterior to Schwalbe's line.[6]

Management

Clinical treatment is similar to POAG and typically begins with *IOP lowering*. Prostaglandin analogs are usually first line.[7] Pilocarpine can lower the IOP, increase the outflow and may slow the progressive TM damage by limiting pupillary movements and pigment liberation.[1] However, it can lead to more hemato-ocular barrier dysfunction and also induce posterior synechiae formation.

Laser treatment, particularly laser trabeculoplasty can be very effective, and more so when it is performed early in the disease. Lower energies are indicated to reduce the risk of pressure spikes. Trabeculoplasty may be used as primary treatment.

Laser iridotomy is indicated when PXF occurs concurrently with angle closure.

Surgical treatment most often consists of trabeculectomy. Surgical complications with trabeculectomy are more common, particularly choroidal hemorrhage or effusion, hypotony, inflammation and hyphema. Nonpenetrating surgery such as deep sclerectomy and deroofing of Schlemm's canal, is another option. Likewise, minimally invasive glaucoma surgery (MIGS) may also be considered.

PIGMENTARY GLAUCOMA

Pigment dispersion syndrome (PDS) is a condition that can lead to a secondary open angle glaucoma called pigmentary glaucoma (PG).[8]

Epidemiology

The PDS is more common in 30–50-year-old myopic males.[9] It occurs almost exclusively in Caucasian population. Degrees of refractive myopic error are associated with earlier disease onset.[10]

Risk Factors and Natural History

The clinical course of PG can be divided into three phases.[8]

Active Pigment Dispersion

This process can start as early as the teenage years, when pigment is actively liberated and accumulates in the anterior segment. Patients are usually asymptomatic at this stage, with normal IOP. Pigment dispersion can be accelerated by physical exercise, emotional stress and mydriasis (natural or drug-induced).

Conversion to Glaucoma

About 10% of patients in phase 1 may evolve to PG in 5 years, and 15% in 15 years.[11] At this stage, IOP is elevated and there may be glaucomatous damage.

Regression or Burn Out Phase

The pigment starts clearing from the TM. The IOP is normal, but there is still optic nerve and/or visual field defects (pigment reversal sign).[8]

Etiopathogenesis

Etiology of PDS is multifactorial, with each of the following factors are prominent.

Mechanical

Backward bowing of the iris is observed with rubbing between the iris pigment epithelium and lens zonules releasing pigment into the anterior chamber (AC). The pigment granules accumulate in the trabecular meshwork (TM), with denudation, collapse and sclerosis of the trabecular beams, leading to aqueous outflow obstruction. Backward bowing results from reverse pupillary block, where the pressure in the AC is greater than in the posterior chamber, closing the iris-lens diaphragm.

Genetic Abnormalities

The PDS demonstrates strong hereditary associations, with possible mutations at the locus 7q35-q36 and 18q.

Environmental

Mild subclinical inflammation and abnormal ocular immunity may contribute to PDS[1] with elevated expression of IL-8.

Ocular Manifestations and Diagnosis

Patients often report a history of myopia, and may have a family history of glaucoma.[12] Some patients may get what is called *pigment storm* with vigorous physical exercise, shedding large amounts of pigment and developing a markedly elevated intraocular pressure with corneal edema and blurred vision.

Biomicroscopy findings include:

- The triad of Krukenberg spindle (Fig. 66.3) (deposit of pigment) on corneal endothelium, peripheral transillumination defects of the iris and pigment in the anterior trabecular meshwork (only 42% show all 3 signs) (Fig. 66.4).
- A very deep AC with or without pigment showers.

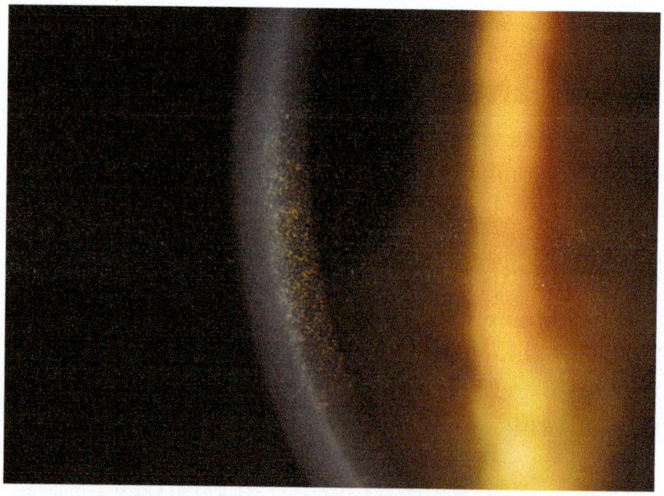

Fig. 66.3: Krukenberg spindle in pigmentary glaucoma.

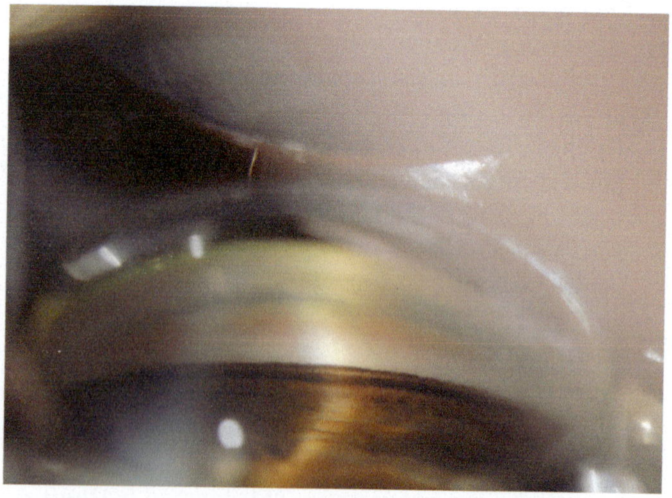

Fig. 66.4: Heavily pigmented angle in pigmentary glaucoma.

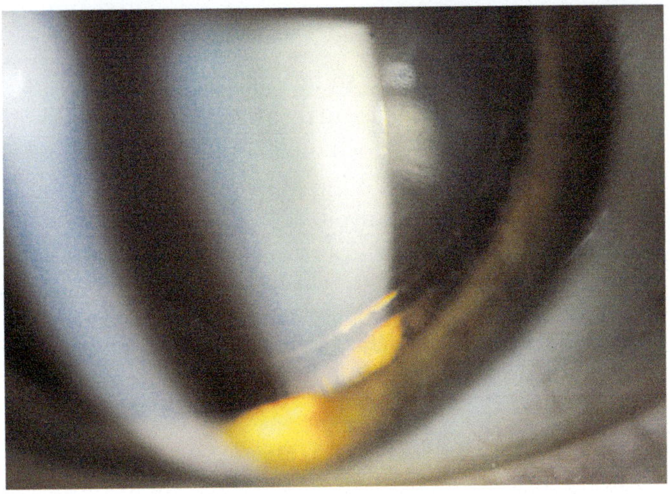

Fig. 66.5: Zentmayer ring in pigmentary glaucoma.

- Subtle pigment in anterior capsule and at junction of zonules with the posterior capsule (Zentmayer ring) (Fig. 66.5) or as a line (Scheie's line) seen with full mydriasis.
- Heterochromia and anisocoria (the pupil of the more affected eye may be more dilated in basal conditions) when the disease is asymmetric.
- On gonioscopy, a band of dark brown pigment on the TM that can cover the entire angle up to the Schwalbe's line.
- Unlike pseudoexfoliation syndrome, the degree of pigment dispersion tends to correspond to severity of glaucoma.

Posterior segment findings have also been associated with PDS including degenerative changes/retinal tears in the peripheral retina. Retinal detachment can occur in 6% of affected eyes with no relation to the degree of myopia.[13]

Management

Initial treatment is typically medical. Cholinergic agents reduce pigment liberation, relieve the reverse pupillary block and decrease the IOP, but may increase the risk of retinal detachment. These agents also make monitoring the retinal periphery more difficult. As a result, treatment with prostaglandin analogs, alpha adrenergic agents and beta-blockers is more typical.

Laser trabeculoplasty is more effective in PG than POAG. Laser energy settings should be lowered. Laser peripheral iridotomy (PI) reduces the iris-lens contact and the chance of reverse pupillary block; and decreases the melanin granules in the aqueous.[14] It may be effective prior to the development of glaucoma.

Filtration surgery may be the best option in eyes that fail medical/laser therapy, but one must be careful using MMC due to the higher risk of hypotony maculopathy in young myopic eyes.

STEROID-INDUCED GLAUCOMA

Steroid glaucoma is defined as elevated IOP and subsequent ON damage triggered by the use of local or systemic corticoids in predisposed patients.[15]

Epidemiology

Significant IOP elevation in response to topical steroids has been reported in 50–90% of glaucoma patients and 5–10% of patients with normal IOP.[12]

The incidence of the steroid response is related to dose, type and route of administration.[12,15]

The risk of steroid-related IOP elevation is greater with topical administration as compared to systemic therapies. Even higher rates are observed with intravitreal corticosteroid injection, after which 50% experience an elevation of the IOP, though only a low number of patients require surgical intervention.[12] With regards to topical therapy, the higher the steroid potency, the greater the ocular hypertensive effect. Potent agents include dexamethasone 0.1% and prednisolone 1%.[16] Even higher rates of IOP elevation are noted with difluprednate, while lower rates are noted with 0.2% loteprednol.

Etiopathogenesis

IOP elevation results from:

- Glucocorticoid-induced changes marked by high deposition of glycosaminoglycans, elastin and fibronectin in the TM, decreasing outflow.[17,18]
- Alteration of the TM cell morphology.[17]
- Upregulation of several genes in the TM cells including the *myocilin* gene.[17]

Risk Factors for Corticosteroid Response

Proven risk factors include:

- Prior history of glaucoma.
- A first-degree relative with POAG.
- High myopia.
- Previous steroid response.
- Older age.
- Connective tissue disease.
- Type 1 diabetes.

Clinical Aspects

Clinical features are similar to those of POAG, with the exception that patients with corticosteroid glaucoma have a history significant for steroid use. It is important to ask for history of asthma, allergies and autoimmune disorders, which might require steroid use. Irreversible steroid-induced ocular hypertension or glaucoma (3% of cases) is most common when there is a history of glaucoma or chronic use of steroid.[16]

Management

Stepwise protocol for management includes:

- Stopping the steroid treatment. In most cases, this alone is effective, decreasing the IOP back to baseline over a variable time period. In cases of intraocular steroid deposits, it may be necessary to remove them surgically.[16,17]
- Switching to milder corticosteroids or to nonsteroidal anti-inflammatory drugs.[16]
- *Hypotensive therapy:* Miotics are avoided since they can exacerbate inflammation and form posterior *synechiae*. Beta-blockers and carbonic anhydrase inhibitors are the first choice of treatment. Prostaglandin analogs may be used with caution; they are relatively contraindicated in eyes with uveitic glaucoma. Alpha-agonists are also useful.
- Laser trabeculoplasty is less effective in these cases, but may be considered when steroids are not used in the context of uveitis.
- *Filtering surgery:* Results are similar to those obtained in POAG (Fig. 66.6).

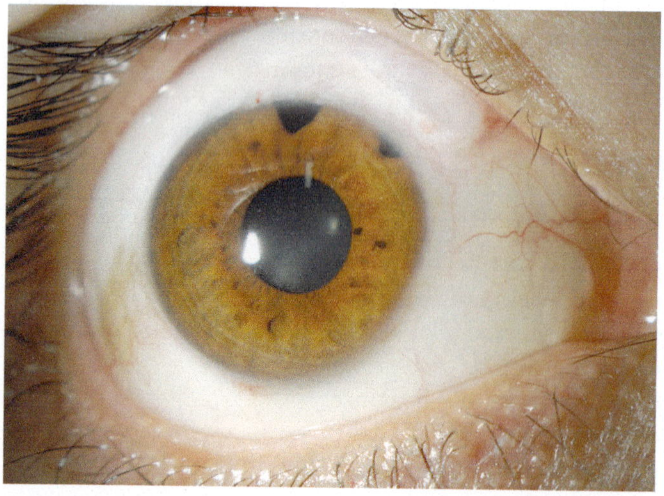

Fig. 66.6: Two trabeculectomies in an eye with steroid-induced glaucoma.

UVEITIC GLAUCOMA

Patients with uveitis have an increased risk of developing glaucoma, not only because of the uveitis, but also as a side effect of the use of corticosteroids. Approximately 20% of uveitis patients in the United States develop glaucoma, most commonly chronic uveitis.[19]

Pathogenesis[20]

Uveitic glaucoma may occur with an open or closed angle through the following mechanisms:

Open-angle Mechanisms

- Increased resistance as a result of mechanical obstruction of the TM, which can be blocked by inflammatory cells, debris, proteins, or fibrin.
- Mediators such as Rho kinases causing a constriction of trabecular endothelium, increasing the outflow resistance.
- Trabeculitis.
- Steroid-induced ocular hypertension.

Closed-angle Mechanisms

- Peripheral anterior *synechiae* (PAS).
- Posterior *synechiae* (PS) leading to pupillary block secondary to iris bombe.
- Forward rotation of the ciliary body secondary to edema and inflammation, causing a nonpupillary block angle closure.

Risk Factors for Elevated IOP

Specific types of uveitis more likely to produce an increased IOP include:

- Anterior uveitis and panuveitis.
- Granulomatous uveitis (mutton fat keratic precipitates and iris nodules).
- Other types of uveitis—Posner-Schlossman syndrome, Fuchs's heterochromy, herpes simplex keratouveitis, Juvenile idiopathic arthritis.[3]
- Chronic and recurrent uveitis.
- Uveitis treated with long-term corticosteroids.

Ocular Manifestations and Diagnosis

Patients with uveitic glaucoma can have blurred vision, and may have severely elevated IOP producing ocular pain, brow ache, redness, nausea, photophobia, and halos.

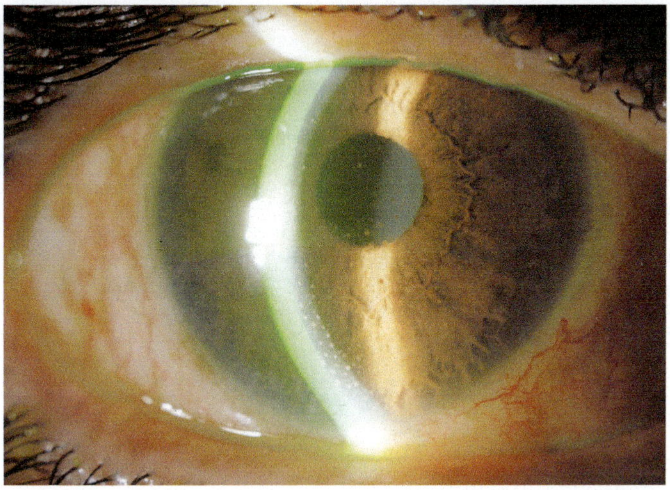

Fig. 66.7: Keratic precipitates in an eye with uveitic glaucoma.

Biomicroscopy findings include AC white cells, flare, keratic precipitates, hypopyon, iris nodules, posterior *synechiae*, iris atrophy, iris heterochromia, corneal edema, and band keratopathy (Fig. 66.7).

Gonioscopy findings include inflammatory material, PAS, and neovascularization in the angle. Topical glycerol may clear the corneal edema. Ultrasound biomicroscopy (UBM) and anterior segment optical coherence tomography (AS-OCT) are useful tools for evaluating the angle.[21]

Management

Management typically begins with medical therapy, but may require surgery in recalcitrant cases.

Medical Management

- Treatment of the systemic inflammatory condition (i.e. with steroids and/or immunosuppressive).
- Mydriatic and cycloplegic agents in the presence of AC cells.
- Topical corticosteroids (steroid responders: 18–30%, occur 2–6 weeks after starting).
- Topical ocular hypotensive treatments, including:
  - Brimonidine (used with caution as granulomatous anterior uveitis has been reported as a late adverse effect.[22]
  - Beta-blockers.
  - Carbonic anhydrase inhibitors.
  - Prostaglandin analogs (although have been reported to induce inflammation, they may be used with caution when the inflammation is controlled.[23,24]
  - Avoidance of cholinergic agents.[25]
- In the rare cases of forward rotation of the ciliary body, with angle closure without pupillary block, the best treatment is immunosuppressive therapy and aqueous humor suppressants. Laser iridoplasty may also be considered in these cases.

Surgical Management

- Laser peripheral iridotomy in cases of iris bombe. Generally more than one iridotomies are placed as they are prone to closure by inflammation.[21] About 40% of these cases require repeated procedures.
- Surgical iridectomy is indicated in cases where laser iridotomy is not possible.
- Goniosynechialysis if angle closure is extensive and PAS are recent.
- Trabeculodialysis or goniotomy in children or young adults, particularly those with juvenile idiopathic arthritis.
- Avoidance of Argon laser trabeculoplasty (ALT), though selective laser trabeculoplasty (SLT), which induces less inflammation, can be used in eyes with quiescent uveitis.[21]
- Trabeculectomy (though future inflammatory episodes can lead to failure).
- Glaucoma drainage devices, particular devices such as the Ahmed valve designed to protect against hypotony.
- Ciliary body destructive procedures (though there is a 10% risk of developing *phthisis bulbi*).[26]

All surgical procedures in these patients carry a risk of postoperative uveitis reactivation in up to 31% of cases. The risk is decreased if the eyes remain quiet for at least 3 months prior to surgery. Flares can be prevented by starting aggressive topical or systemic immunosuppressive agents 1 week before the planned surgery.[25]

NEOVASCULAR GLAUCOMA

Neovascular glaucoma (NVG) is an aggressive form of glaucoma secondary to retinal ischemia, characterized by the development of neovascularization of the iris (NVI) and angle (NVA), elevated IOP and, in many cases, a poor visual prognosis.[27]

Epidemiology

The NVG occurs secondary to numerous systemic and ocular diseases sharing one common etiology: ocular ischemia and hypoxia (Table 66.1).[28]

Table 66.1: Predisposing factors for neovascularization.

Retinal diseases	Inflammatory diseases	Tumors	Systemic diseases	Other procedures
• Central and branch retinal vein occlusion • Diabetic retinopathy • Coats exudative retinopathy • Sickle cell retinopathy • Central and branch retinal artery occlusion • Eales' disease • Retinal vasculitis • Retinal detachment • Retinopathy of prematurity	• Behçet's disease • Sympathetic ophthalmia • Chronic iridocyclitis • Sarcoidosis • Vogt-Koyanagi-Harada syndrome • Crohn's disease	• Iris melanoma • Ciliary body melanoma • Choroidal melanoma • Retinoblastoma • Metastasis • Medulloepithelioma	• Carotid artery obstructive disease • Carotid-cavernous fistula embolization • Takayasu syndrome • Temporal arteritis • Wyburn-Mason syndrome	• Scleral buckle • External beam, proton beam, and plaques radiation • Cataract extraction • Pars plana vitrectomy • Scleral buckling

Pathophysiology

Proangiogenic factors (i.e. vascular endothelial growth factor, VEGF) are upregulated by the ischemic retina producing rubeotic vessels visible in the pupillary border and later the anterior chamber (AC) angle. Angles are initially open, but later a fibrovascular membrane (FVM) starts to grow over the TM obstructing the outflow and elevating the IOP. This FVM eventually grows and contracts causing progressive synechial angle closure and ectropion uveae. These abnormal vessels can bleed (hyphema) and inflammation can develop during any stage, exacerbating IOP elevation.

The most common diseases associated with NVG are:

Central Retinal Vein Occlusion

- 20% can develop NVG.[29] More common in the ischemic type of CRVO.
- In eyes with extensive retinal ischemia, the risk of NVG is 60% over the first 3 months.
- 15% of nonischemic CRVO can evolve to ischemic CRVO in the first 4 months.
- The most important factor predictive of rubeosis iridis is poor visual acuity.[27,28]

Proliferative Diabetic Retinopathy

- One-third of patients with rubeosis iridis have diabetic retinopathy.
- The prevalence of NVG is 2% in diabetic retinopathy, but increases to 21% in PDR.

Ocular Ischemic Syndrome

- About 66% have rubeosis iridis but the IOP may be normal or low, due to impaired ciliary body perfusion.
- Is necessary to achieve at least 90% of carotid occlusion to get the syndrome.[28]

Ocular Manifestation and Diagnosis

Neovascular glaucoma can present without symptoms, or with visual loss sometimes accompanied by pain, photophobia and nausea, vomiting.

Biomicroscopic findings can include:

- Rubeosis iridis *(all cases)* (Fig. 66.8)
- Mild anterior chamber (AC) reaction.
- Corneal edema in cases of very high IOP.
- Ciliary injection (Fig. 66.9)
- Ectropion uveae (Fig. 66.10)
- Hyphema

Gonioscopy can show NVA even when the border of the pupil is not involved. Initially the angle can be open with evidence of vessels crossing the scleral spur, but then evolves to a closed angle with PAS at later stages.

The IOP can be normal in early stages, but is elevated when significant PAS have formed.

Diagnosis can be aided by retinal angiography to identify areas of poor perfusion, or carotid artery Doppler ultrasound to rule in ocular ischemic syndrome.

Management

The treatment depends on the stage of the disease (Table 66.2) and has two principal components: management of IOP and reduction of the ischemic tissue (Flowchart 66.1).[30]

Treatment of Neovascularization or Stage 1

Aim is to reduce the ischemic load, reduce VEGF levels and promote vessel regression.

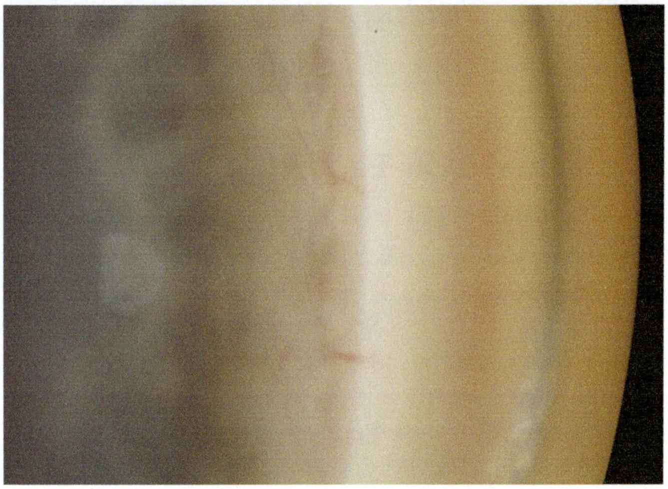

Fig. 66.8: Neovessels in the angle.

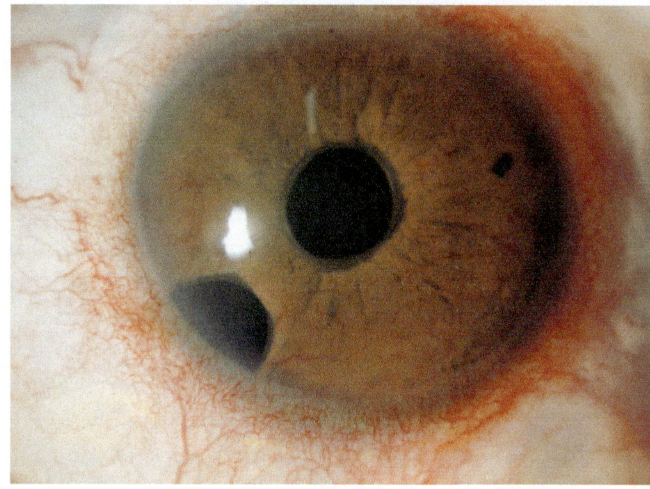

Fig. 66.9: Neovascular glaucoma.

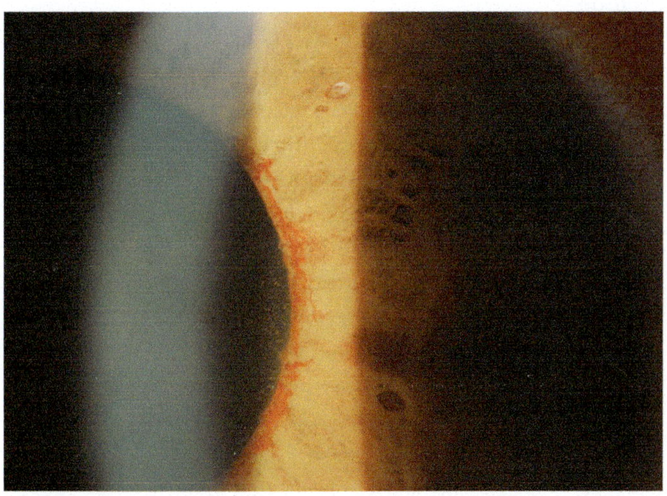

Fig. 66.10: Ectropion uveae and neovessels at the pupillary margin.

Flowchart 66.1: Treatment algorithm for neovascular glaucoma.

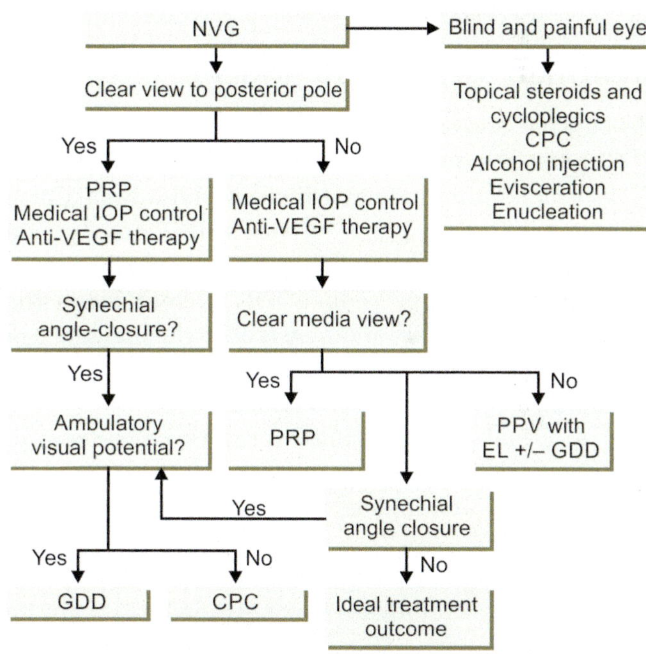

(NVG: Neovascular glaucoma; PRP: Panretinal photocoagulation; GDD: Glaucoma drainage device; PPV: Pars-plana vitrectomy; EL: Endolaser; CPC: Cyclophotocoagulation)

Table 66.2: Stages of neovascular glaucoma.

Stage	Characteristic	Ocular examination	Intraocular pressure	Clinical examination
1	Rubeosis iridis	• Tufts of rubeotic vessels in pupillary margin • NVA (sometimes can precede rubeosis)	Normal	Asymptomatic or decreased VA secondary to vitreous hemorrhage
2	Open-angle glaucoma	• More prominent rubeosis • Mild AC inflammation • Growth of FVM that extends over TM	High	Can have decreased VA by vitreous hemorrhage, or visual field loss
3	Closed-angle glaucoma	• Severe NVI and NVA • Contraction of the FVM • Ectropion uveae • PAS • Moderate AC inflammation	Very high (60–70 mm Hg)	Headache, nausea, vomiting and red eye, acute severe pain, decreased VA and photophobia secondary to hyphema, corneal edema, optic nerve cupping

(FVM: Fibrovascular membrane)

- PRP is effective in inducing regression of NVI and preventing development of NVG if administered before the development of IOP elevation and if the amount of NVA is minimal. Effects are longstanding, and can delay or obviate the need for glaucoma surgery.[30]
- Endolaser and pars plana vitrectomy can be considered when cloudy media is present, particularly when other retinal surgery (laser, repair of tractional RD, etc.) is indicated.
- Intravitreal antiangiogenic factors including off-label bevacizumab, ranibizumab or aflibercept. They induce rapid regression of NVI within 3 days, though recurrence should be expected because of their short duration of action. This treatment is best performed at the time of NVG diagnosis or before PRP/surgery. Repeated intravitreal bevacizumab injections in combination to PRP reduce the rate of surgical interventions in eyes with open angles.[31]

Treatment of Stages 2 and 3

Elevated IOP and significant angle closure:

- Topical hypotensive medications can be started. Prostaglandin analogs, which promote breakdown of the blood-aqueous barrier with worsening of inflammation, should be avoided. Atropine induces cycloplegia, helps reduce IOP by increasing the uveoscleral outflow and may reduce the incidence of hyphema.[27,28]
- Topical steroids can help inflamed eyes.
- Pan-retinal photocoagulation can be considered to destroy anoxic areas.
- Intravitreal antiangiogenic factors to reduce VEGF levels.
- *Surgery:* Trabeculectomy, glaucoma drainage devices (GDD), or cyclodestructive procedures can be considered, with GDDs generally considered a first-line procedure, except in eyes with poor visual acuity. In eyes with poor visual acuity cyclodestruction can be considered primarily.

POST-TRAUMATIC GLAUCOMA

Epidemiology

This glaucoma is most common in young adults with age associated with the environmental cause of the injury.[32] Almost 30% of patients with post-traumatic hyphema have been reported to have high IOP.[33]

Pathophysiology (Table 66.3)[34]

Mechanisms of glaucoma vary with regards to time from injury.

Glaucoma in the Early Post-traumatic Period

Initially low IOP is possible secondary to inflammation, and/or disruption in the angle structures, retinal tear or occult globe rupture. Patients can also present with a transient elevated IOP secondary to AC red blood cells, inflammatory cells and debris obstructing the trabecular meshwork (TM). Hyphema is the most common complication; the likelihood of future glaucoma is proportional to the severity of the hyphema. When hyphemas persist more than 7 days, they can damage the TM or result in rebleeding, which often leads to glaucoma, corneal bloodstaining and synechiae.[35]

Other reasons for early trauma-related glaucoma include:

- Hemolytic glaucoma: An open-angle glaucoma that develops days or weeks after a large intraocular hemorrhage.
- Ghost-cell glaucoma, resulting from traumatic vitreous hemorrhage, where the red blood cells degenerate to spherical forms (the cells appear empty) and migrate forward through a disrupted hyaloid face. Due to the rigidity of the cells, they cannot pass through the TM, resulting in obstruction of the TM. Usually, IOP elevation responds to medical treatment. If not, AC washout with pars plana vitrectomy (PPV) should be performed.

Table 66.3: Seven rings of anterior segment tissue that can become damaged by ocular contusion injury as the anterior-posterior forces are translated into an equatorial stretching.[3]

Tissue affected	Result
Sphincter pupillae	Irregular pupil with decreased light reaction or traumatic mydriasis
Iris base	Iridodialysis (Fig. 66.11)
Anterior ciliary body	Angle recession or tear in the ciliary body muscles (Fig. 66.12)
Attachment of the ciliary body muscle fibers to the scleral spur	Cyclodialysis cleft
Trabecular meshwork	Tear on the anterior portion of the TM
Zonular attachments	Subluxation or dislocation of the lens
Attachment of the retina at the ora serrata	Retinal dialysis and detachment

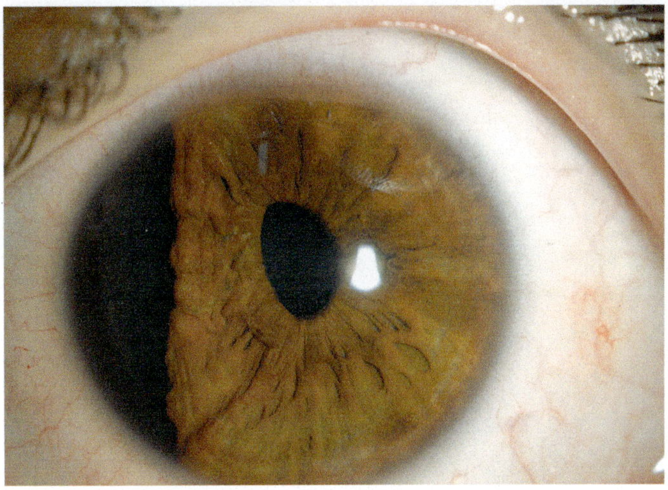

Fig. 66.11: Traumatic glaucoma with important iridodialysis.

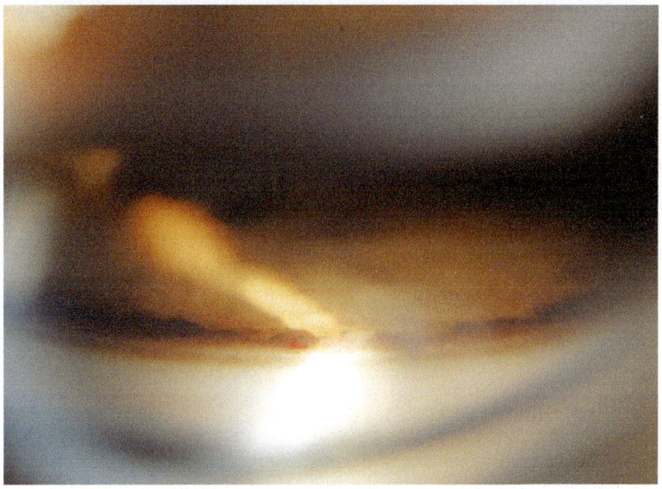

Fig. 66.12: Traumatic angle recession.

- Lens subluxation with pupillary block
  - Lens particle glaucoma can result in IOP elevation due to mechanical obstruction of the TM with lens particles. Peripheral anterior and posterior *synechiae* can form with chronic inflammation. Treatment consists of AC washout and lens removal.
- Shallowing of the AC due to anterior rotation of the lens-iris diaphragm secondary to uveal effusion.
- Vitreous prolapse in the AC.
- Schwartz-Matsuo syndrome[36] resulting from fluctuation of high IOP associated with retinal detachment and a tear in the nonpigmented epithelium of the ciliary body. Photoreceptor outer segments clog the TM, and can be mistaken for uveitis.

Glaucoma in Late Post-traumatic Period

Late post-traumatic glaucoma may develop weeks to years after, with an incidence of 0–20%. Contributing features include:[37]

- Peripheral anterior synechiae formation.
- Increased outflow resistance.
- Fibrosis of the TM.
- Siderosis of the trabecular endothelium.

Patients with angle recession greater than 180 grades may develop a chronic glaucoma, often many years later. Recession is associated with degenerative changes in the TM tissue after the trauma and inflammation, causing obstruction to outflow.[38]

Ocular Manifestations and Diagnosis

In the presence of hyphemas, the extent of the hemorrhage in the AC is evaluated carefully to guide future glaucoma risk. Gonioscopy is performed after the blood has cleared and may reveal an angle recession as an irregular widened ciliary body (CB). Histologically, this represents a separation between the longitudinal and circular muscle fibers of the CB. This can occur in 60–94% of eyes with a traumatic hyphema,[32] and eyes with recession should be followed annually for possible glaucoma. Other features capable of increasing IOP should be noted, including inflammation, lens subluxation/dislocation, anterior capsule disruption, and protruded vitreous through ruptured zonules.

Management

- *Medical:* IOP lowering medications.
- Evacuation of hyphema should be considered according to duration and amount of hyphema, and IOP.[39]
- Trabeculectomy or glaucoma drainage devices (GDD) should be reserved for medically intractable glaucoma; surgery may be associated with complications such as hypotony, choroidal effusion and secondary hemorrhages.

AQUEOUS MISDIRECTION SYNDROME

Aqueous misdirection syndrome (AMS) or malignant glaucoma occurs after intraocular surgery in patients with a history of narrow or closed angle glaucoma.

It is characterized by elevated IOP in the presence of central and peripheral AC shallowing, with a patent peripheral iridotomy and the absence of other posterior segment abnormalities.

Epidemiology

It is more common after incisional surgery for primary angle-closure glaucoma with an incidence of 0.6–4%,[38,40] though it can occur after any other surgery or laser procedure.

Pathophysiology

Although the exact mechanisms are not known, these eyes have defined biometric characteristics: smaller anteroposterior diameter, smaller radius of corneal curvature, flatter anterior chamber and anterior lens insertion.[41]

Mechanism includes posterior diversion of aqueous flow into the vitreous cavity, diminishing the fluid conductivity.[41] Other causative factors include acute choroidal expansion decreasing the ability to transmit aqueous freely from behind the collapsed vitreous across it, diminishing its conductivity,[41] anterior rotation of the ciliary processes against the lens equator in phakic eyes or the anterior hyaloid face in aphakic eyes.

Ocular Manifestations and Diagnosis

Cases should be suspected after a detailed history which reveals recent surgery, particularly for angle-closure glaucoma. Signs include a flat AC, iridolenticular diaphragm anteriorization with secondary angle-closure, conjunctival hyperemia, corneal edema, photophobia, and decreased visual acuity (Fig. 66.13).[42]

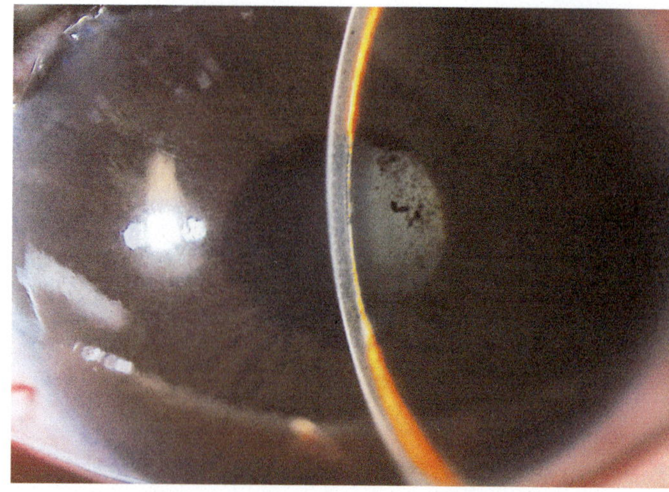

Fig. 66.13: Misdirection syndrome in a patient with angle-closure glaucoma.

B-scan ultrasound should rule out posterior segment tumors, choroidal hemorrhages or effusions if no view is present. UBM and/or AS-OCT may also be useful for diagnosis and monitoring of treatment (i.e. the degree of AC narrowing.[43]

Differential Diagnosis (Table 66.4)

Differential diagnosis includes:

- *Pupillary block glaucoma:* The presence of a patent peripheral iridotomy rules out a pupillary block
- Choroidal detachments (note that IOP for this malignant glaucoma can be in the normal range)
- Suprachoroidal hemorrhage
- Posterior scleritis

Table 66.4: Differential diagnosis of malignant glaucoma.

Diagnosis	Onset of symptoms	Intraocular pressure	Ocular fundus and B-scan ultrasound	Iridotomy
Aqueous misdirection syndrome	During surgery, days, months	Normal or high	Normal	Patent
Pupillary block	During surgery or first days post	Normal or high	Normal	Not patent
Choroidal detachment	During surgery or first 5 days	Low, usually painless	Light brown CD, dome-shaped, hypoechoic	Patent
Choroidal hemorrhage	During surgery or first 5 days	High, with sudden throbbing pain	Dark CD, hyperechoic	Patent

Management

Treatment nearly always requires surgery, but may proceed in a stepwise fashion.

Medical Therapy

Its goal is to dehydrate the vitreous humor, diminish the aqueous humor production and relax the ciliary processes through cycloplegics (1% atropine qid), mydriatics (10% phenylephrine qid), aqueous suppressants and hyperosmolar solutions over the first 3–5 days. Miotics can exacerbate the AC shallowing and should be avoided. Intravenous mannitol (20%; 1.5–2 g/kg weight), given over 45 minutes can temporarily reduce IOP.

Laser

- Peripheral iridotomy (PI)—is performed if it is not already present.
- Hyaloidectomy—disruption of the anterior vitreous face with Nd:YAG laser. This can be performed trough a PI in phakic patients, but extreme care should be taken in order not to damage the lens.
- Posterior capsulotomy with anterior hyaloidectomy—in pseudophakic and aphakic cases.
- Argon cyclophotocoagulation to 4–10 ciliary processes, through a goniolens or an iridectomy—to shrink them and correct the anterior rotation.
- Trans-scleral cyclophotocoagulation.

Surgical

- Pars-plana vitrectomy (PPV) with surgical removal of the anterior hyaloid face and disruption of the posterior capsule.
- In phakic cases—PPV, iridectomy and lensectomy should be considered.
- In pseudophakic eyes—PPV, hyaloido-zonulectomy or hyaloidoposterior capsulotomy and iridectomy.[44]

PENETRATING KERATOPLASTY AND GLAUCOMA

Glaucoma is one of the most important causes of irreversible visual loss after penetrating keratoplasty (PKP).[45]

Incidence

The incidence of ocular hypertension after PKP is 11% to 50%[46] and, after Descemet's stripping endothelial keratoplasty (DSEK) ranges from 0% to 54%.[47] Patients with pre-existing glaucoma have two or three times greater risk of having this complication,[48] and previous glaucoma surgery increases the risk seven times.[49] The causes of post-PKP elevated IOP are listed in Box 66.1.

The initial indications for grafting are important risk factors (Table 66.5).

Pathophysiology

Although the etiology is probably multifactorial, it is related to distortion of the angle from:

- Tight suturing
- Long suture bites
- More compressed tissue
- Large trephine sizes
- Increased peripheral corneal thickness
- Donor cornea smaller than the recipient
- Smaller overall corneal diameter.

Other contributing factors include altered function of the TM by inflammation, mechanical collapse of the TM, particularly in aphakic grafts,[50] development of PAS, and corticosteroid use.[47]

Box 66.1: Causes of elevated IOP after PK.

- Previously diagnosed glaucoma
- Aphakia
- Inflammation, hyphema
- *Surgical technique:* Tight suturing, long bites, same size donor button, viscoelastic substances, wound leak
- PKP combined with cataract surgery or vitrectomy
- Pupillary block glaucoma
- Chronic angle closure glaucoma
- Ghost cell glaucoma
- Aqueous misdirection syndrome
- Steroid-induced glaucoma

Table 66.5: Indications for grafting and related risk of glaucoma post-penetrating keratoplasty.

Low risk	Moderate risk	High risk
• Keratoconus • Stromal corneal dystrophies	• Fuchs' dystrophy • Herpetic infection	• Aphakic or pseudophakic bullous keratopathy • Trauma • Corneal ulcers • Perforation • Iridocorneal endothelial syndrome

Clinical Manifestations and Diagnosis

Patients may be asymptomatic or show symptoms of high IOP. Blurred vision is often not noticed since patients may already have irregular astigmatism. In eyes with a PKP, it is difficult to measure the IOP with accuracy, because of the irregularity of the corneal surface. The IOP can be measured with Tono-pen or pneumatic applanation tonometry.[45] Frequency doubling perimetry (FDT) is independent of mild topographic changes, and may be useful to detect early glaucomatous changes after PKP.[51,52]

Ultrasound biomicroscopy: It is used for evaluation and management when there is inadequate view at the slit-lamp.[53] This helps to evaluate the presence and site of the anterior synechiae formation when cornea is opaque, helping to plan the site for glaucoma filtering surgery and drainage devices.

Management

- Chronic elevated IOP can alter endothelial function of grafts and should be treated aggressively by:
- *Trying to prevent* IOP rise with optimal surgical technique or surgical IOP control prior to or concurrent with PKP.
- *Medical treatment*:
  Although medical treatment is still the first-line of treatment, its side effects may be significant risk factors for graft failure:[45,53]
  - Beta-blockers side effects include superficial keratitis, corneal anesthesia and damage of the ocular surface, leading to a dry eye state.
  - Alpha-2 adrenergic agonists can cause allergic reactions, superficial keratitis and dry eye.
  - Miotics can induce uveitis or posterior *synechiae.*
  - Topical carbonic anhydrase inhibitors should be used with caution, as they cause corneal decompensation in some cases.[53]
  - Systemic carbonic anhydrase inhibitors may be used.
  - Prostaglandin analogs should be used with caution in cases of history of herpes simplex keratitis and history of uveitis.
  - In steroid-responsive glaucoma, taper the steroid drops to the minimum.
- *Laser and surgical treatment*:
  - Laser Trabeculoplasty may be used in open angles, clear grafts and moderately elevated IOP (25–30 mm Hg), even while on glaucoma medications.[45]
  - Trabeculectomy can be considered, but use 5-FU with caution because of corneal toxicity.
  - Glaucoma drainage device (GDD) appears to be preferred over the other options. Tubes are best inserted through the pars plana (in vitrectomized eyes) or posterior chamber (in pseudophakic eyes), and prior to/concurrent with PKP (Fig. 66.14).
  - Cyclodestructive procedures can be considered, particularly in phakic eyes, or in pseudophakic eyes after a GDD. New less aggressive techniques, like micropulse transcleral cyclophotocoagulation may be useful in an earlier state.

GLAUCOMA AFTER VITREORETINAL SURGERY

Types of Glaucoma

This form of glaucoma occurs for many reasons, and treatment should be based on the mechanism responsible for the high IOP.

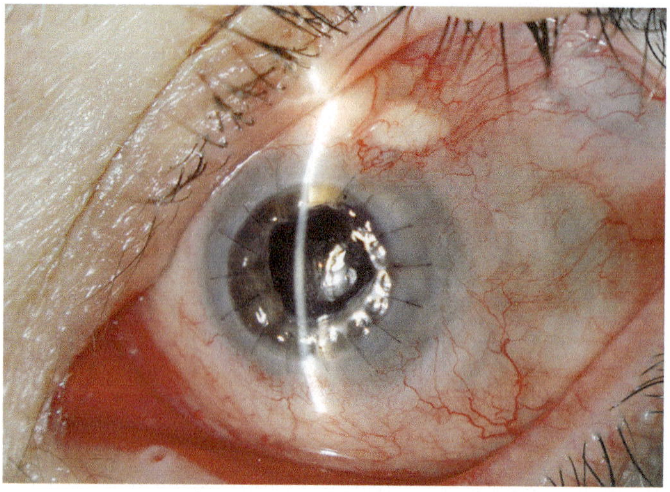

Fig. 66.14: Glaucoma drainage device in an eye with a PKP.

- Glaucoma with open-angles can result from:
  - Gas expansion without angle-closure (the most common mechanism of acute postvitrectomy ocular hypertension
  - Inflammation
  - Silicon oil bubbles in AC
  - Corticosteroid-induced glaucoma (approximately 20% of cases)
  - Ghost-cell glaucoma.
- Pupillary block glaucoma:
  - Ciliary body edema
  - Fibrin
  - Gas
  - Silicon oil.

Scleral Buckling Procedures

Encircling bands may shallow the anterior chamber (AC) and temporary interfere with the venous drainage causing congestion and swelling of the ciliary body.[54]

Risk factors for elevated IOP after scleral buckling include: anterior placement of the buckle, older age, myopia, duration of the retinal detachment, and history of previous narrow angle or choroidal detachments.[55]

Temporary Management

- Medical treatment includes:
  - Topical and/or systemic anti-inflammatory agents if inflammation is present.
  - *Cycloplegics:* To relax the ciliary body muscle and displace the iris-lens diaphragm posteriorly.
  - Aqueous humor suppressants.

- Surgical treatments can be considered if medical treatment is not effective, and include drainage of suprachoroidal fluid or adjustment of the buckle. Glaucoma drainage devices may be used. It has to be remembered that the conjunctiva may be scarred down because of previous surgery, so trabeculectomy may not be effective.

Silicon Oil

- Used in complex retinal detachments, the prevalence of elevated IOP is 6–9% at 36 months after silicon oil injection.[56] Glaucoma can develop with or without the presence of silicon oil in the AC.
- Risk factors include silicon oil in the AC (Fig. 66.15), pre-existing glaucoma, aphakia, early postoperative pressure spike, trauma, diabetes, and postoperative neovascularization of the iris.[55]

Mechanisms

Mechanisms are multiple and include:

- Acute angle closure with pupillary block. This is more frequent in aphakic eyes. Glaucoma can develop in approximately 40% of patients with AC silicon oil[57] and only in 10% of cases with emulsified silicon oil in the angle.[58] Pupillary block may be avoided with a prophylactic inferior peripheral iridectomy, as the silicon oil floats above aqueous humor and can obstruct a superior iridectomy.[55] These inferior iridectomies can close spontaneously.
- OAG with silicon oil in the AC (emulsified or not).
- Iris Rubeosis with secondary angle-closure.

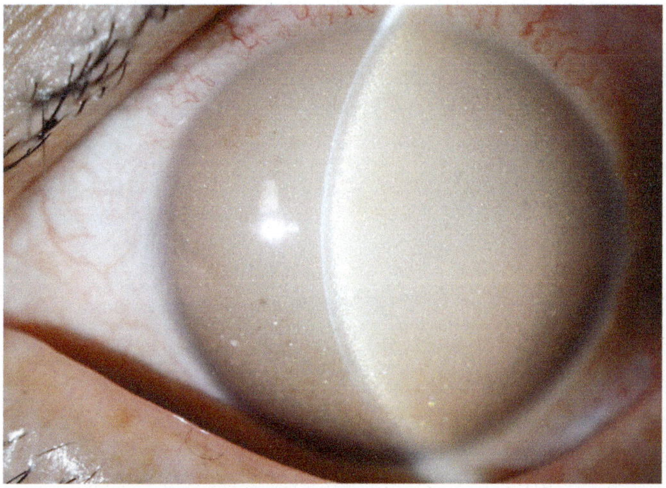

Fig. 66.15: Silicone oil in the anterior chamber.

Management

It is very important to discuss case management with the retina specialist.

- Removal of the silicon oil may not be enough to solve the problem. If done too prematurely, it may be associated with redetachment of the retina.
- Medications control IOP only in 25%.
- Silicon oil removal and glaucoma surgery achieve higher rates of IOP control.
- Glaucoma drainage device (GDD) can control the IOP in the majority of eyes after pars plana vitrectomy and silicon oil injection.[59]
- If the oil needs to remain in the eye, GDD implanted in the inferior quadrants or transscleral laser cycloablation are good options.

Intravitreal Gas Injection

Gas is usually used for retinal tears in the superior quadrants. The increase in the IOP is related to the properties of the gas (i.e. expansive capacity) and final volume of the intraocular bubble (Table 66.6).

Following pneumatic retinopexy, transient elevation in IOP is common. The central retinal artery may collapse, though the IOP usually drops within one hour.[56]

Risk Factors

- Concentration of the gas
- Older age
- Fibrin in the anterior chamber
- Concurrent use of scleral buckle
- Intraoperative endophotocoagulation

Management

- *Tonometry:* The expansive gas can alter the scleral rigidity, so measure the IOP with Goldmann tonometer or the Perkins tonometer. The Tono-pen can be used but it tends to underestimate the IOP when it is over 30 mm Hg.

Table 66.6: Types of gases used in retinal surgery.

	Air	SF_6 20%	C_3F_8 12%
Dose	0.8 mL	0.5 mL	0.3 mL
Duration	4 days	10–14 days	55–65 days
Time to largest size	Immediate	36 hours	3 days
Expansion	No expansion	2 X	4 X

- Aqueous suppressants can lower IOP medically.
- The patient with gas tamponade cannot travel by air or be at 2500 feet high, as they can suffer severe elevation of the IOP.[60]
- Removal of the gas bubble may be necessary in some cases.

LENS-INDUCED GLAUCOMA

These include a number of different glaucomatous processes that share one common mechanism: the lens glaucomas may be:

- Open-angle glaucoma (OAG) (Table 66.7), with obstruction of the trabecular meshwork (TM) from:
  - Phacolytic glaucoma or lens protein glaucoma.
  - Lens particle glaucoma.
  - Phacoanaphylactic glaucoma.
- Closed-angle glaucoma (CAG) from:
  - Phacomorphic glaucoma (acutely swollen lens).
  - Phacotopic glaucoma (anterior lens displacement) or ectopia lentis.

PHACOLYTIC GLAUCOMA

This acute/subacute OAG occurs in the presence of a mature or hypermature cataract, when soluble lens proteins leak through small microscopic defects in the capsule to the AC.

Pathophysiology

Heavy-molecular-weight proteins (HMWP) obstruct the TM. These proteins increase in concentration as the cataract matures.[61,62] HMWP can induce the migration of peripheral blood monocytes and macrophages, probably to remove soluble lens proteins and fragments from AC and TM.

Clinical Examination and Diagnosis

Findings include pain and conjunctival injection and reduced visual acuity:

- *Slit-lamp findings include*:
  - Diffuse corneal edema.
  - Mature (white) or hypermature (small compact nucleus floating in liquefied cortex) cataract (Fig. 66.16).[17]
  - AC with intensive flare (soluble proteins) and a cellular response composed mostly of macrophages.
  - White patches on the lens.
- Gonioscopy (when possible) demonstrates open angles.

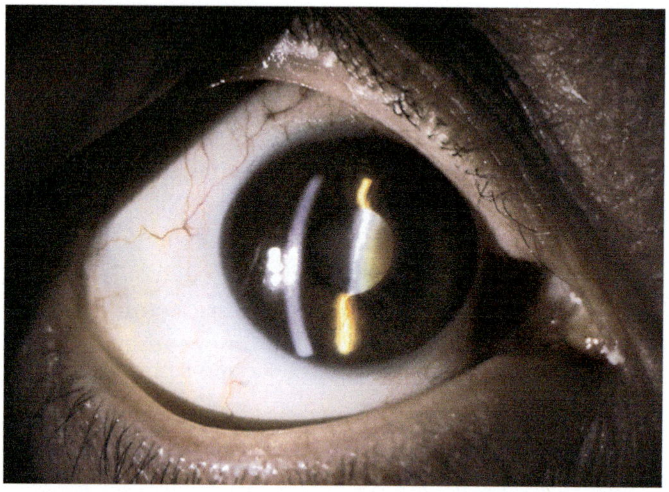

Fig. 66.16: Phacolytic glaucoma in a patient with hypermature cataract.

Table 66.7: Lens-induced open-angle glaucoma.

Types of lens-induced glaucoma	Clinical	Mechanism and TM	Gonioscopy	Intraocular pressure	Capsule status	Management
Phacolytic (lens protein)	Hypermature or mature cataract, white floating material in AC	HMWP obstructing the TM and macrophages Filled with lens material	Open angle	High	Intact but permeable	Antiglaucoma medication, topical steroids, cataract extraction
Lens particle	History of trauma, cataract surgery or laser capsulotomy	Lens material obstructing TM	Generally open angle; closed angle when PAS secondary to inflammation	High	Disrupted	Antiglaucoma medication, steroids, surgical removal of lens material
Phacoanaphylactic	After cataract extraction or trauma	Loss of immune tolerance	Open angle	Low or high	Disrupted, exposure of large lens materials	Removal of lens fragments

Management

Surgical treatment with cataract extraction is the definitive treatment. Capsular stain with trypan blue facilitates the capsulorhexis. In most cases, the situation reverses rapidly after cataract extraction.[17] However, medical therapy is initially used to reduce the IOP, prior to surgery.

Prostaglandin analogs should be used with caution due to the inflammatory nature of the situation. Topical steroids and cycloplegic agents can stabilize the blood-aqueous barrier and reduce pain.

LENS PARTICLE GLAUCOMA OR GLAUCOMA DUE TO RETAINED LENS FRAGMENT

These glaucomas occur when the lens capsule is disrupted and lens cortex and/or proteins are released into the AC.

Pathophysiology

Retained lens particles obstruct the TM, while inflammation can produce PAS and angle closure or pupillary block from posterior *synechiae* (PS). After Nd:YAG laser capsulotomy, lens capsule and cortex fragments can be seen in the AC, though within days, the outflow facility may become normal.[63]

Clinical Examination and Diagnosis

Patients typically have decreased vision and pain after recent trauma, cataract surgery or laser.

- Biomicroscopy shows
  - Lens particles and/or small fragments of lens cortex in AC or corneal endothelium.
  - Corneal edema, cells and flare in the AC.
  - Hypopyon can be present.
- Gonioscopy shows open angle at early stages, though PAS may develop later.

Management

- *Medical therapy* with topical IOP-lowering medication, anti-inflammatory agents and cycloplegic agents.
- *Surgical aspiration* of the lens material is the definitive treatment and should not be delayed to avoid PAS, pupillary block, and inflammatory membranes.

PHACOANAPHYLACTIC GLAUCOMA

This is a rare granulomatous uveitis secondary to traumatic or surgical lens disruption,[17] with an immune complex formation due to loss of normal tolerance to the lens protein.

Pathogenesis

Usually the IOP is normal, but may be high when inflammatory cells and high molecular weight proteins obstruct the TM. Eyes may develop PAS with chronic ACG or pupillary block.

Clinical Examination and Diagnosis

Findings include corneal edema, red eye, and mild or severe granulomatous uveitis days to years after the initial event, with vitreous inflammation. Hypopyon, keratic precipitates, and retained lens material may be seen.

Management

Treatment is primarily surgical, with removal of all residual material including the lens capsule and the intraocular lens. Material should be sent for pathologic evaluation. Topical steroids have little effect on this uveitis and can lead to a corticosteroid-induced glaucoma.

PHACOMORPHIC GLAUCOMA

This is a secondary ACG from a mature/hypermature lens.

Pathophysiology

A mature or hypermature lens that has become intumescent, often acutely or subacutely causes shallowing of the anterior chamber resulting in secondary angle-closure glaucoma (SACG).

Clinical Examination and Diagnosis

Examine both eyes looking for differences in the AC depth or cataract disparities.

Patients often describe chronic or acutely decreased vision, ocular pain, headache and photophobia. Corneal edema may be present along with a mid-dilated pupil and/or iris bombe and shallow AC. A hypermature intumescent cataract is present.

Gonioscopy (when possible) shows a closed-angle, sometimes with PAS. The degree of PAS may be related to the need of glaucoma surgery. There is a rate of 20% of glaucoma progression in 2 years, so these cases need to be closely controlled.[63,64]

Management

- Medical treatment, primarily with aqueous humor suppressants (do not use miotics).
- Laser peripheral iridotomy may open the angle, lower the IOP and allow the eye to be quiet before cataract extraction.
- Definitive treatment involves removal of the intumescent lens. Because of the dense lens, the capsulorhexis may be facilitated using trypan blue staining of the anterior capsule.[65]

PHACOTOPIC GLAUCOMA OR ECTOPIA LENTIS

Represents an anteriorly displaced crystalline lens.

Epidemiology

Some of the causes are:[66]

- Hereditary lens ectopiae from:
  - Marfan syndrome
  - Homocystinuria
  - Weill-Marchesani syndrome (microspherophakia)
  - Ectopia lentis pupillae
  - Isolated ectopia lentis
  - Late spontaneous lens subluxation
  - Isolated microspherophakia.

There are sporadic hereditary causes and secondary causes for lens ectopiae. Among secondary causes, are traumatic, surgical complications and exfoliation syndrome.

Mechanisms

- Attenuation or rupture of the zonules leading to a dislocation of the lens into the pupil or AC, resulting in pupillary block glaucoma (trauma, Marfan syndrome)
- Small and spherical lens that can move anteriorly causing pupillary block glaucoma (Microspherophakia as an isolated disorder or associated with Weill-Marchesani syndrome).

Management

Laser peripheral iridotomy can break pupillary block, as can pupillary dilation in cases of microspherophakia. Definitive treatment involves lens extraction, followed by implantation with scleral fixated intraocular lens (IOL) or ACIOL.

REFERENCES

1. Ritch R, Schlotzer-Schrehardt U. Exfoliation syndrome. Surv Ophthalmol. 2001;45:265-315.
2. Ritch R, Konstas AGP, Sclotzer-Schrehardt U. Exfoliation syndrome and exfoliative glaucoma. In: Shaarawy TM, Sherwood MB, Hitchings RA, Crowston JG (Eds). Glaucoma: Medical Diagnosis and Therapy. Saunders Ed. United States. 2009.pp.339-47.
3. Susanna R, Murad Vessani R. Pseudo-exfoliacao capsular. In: de Almeida HG, Cohen R (Eds). Glaucomas Secondarios. Roca Ed. Sao Pablo, Brasil. 2006.pp.175-92.
4. Fitzsimon JS, Mulvihill A, Kennedy S, et al. Association of HLA type with pseudoexfoliation of the lens capsule. Br J Ophthalmol. 1996;80(5):402-4.
5. Thorleifsson G, Magnusson KP, Sulem P, et al. Common sequence variants in the *LOXL1* gene confer susceptibility to exfoliation glaucoma. Science. 2007;317:1397-400.
6. Sampaolesi R, Zarate J, Croxato O. The chamber angle in exfoliation syndrome. Clinical and pathological findings. Acta Ophthalmol Suppl. 1988;184:48-53.
7. Weinreb RN, Araie M, Susanna R, et al. Medical Treatment of Glaucoma The 7th Consensus Report of the World Glaucoma Association. Section 5: Medical treatments of other types of open-angle glaucomas. 2010. Kugler Publications.
8. Gandolfi SA, Ungaro N, Mora P, Sangermani C. Pigmentary glaucoma. In: Shaarawy TM, Sherwood MB, Hitchings RA, Crowston JG (Eds). Glaucoma: Medical Diagnosis and Therapy. Saunders Ed. United States. 2009.pp.349-60.
9. Farrar SM, Shields MB. Current concepts in pigmentary glaucoma. Surv Ophthalmol. 1993;37:233-52.
10. Gramer E, Thiele H, Ritch R. Family history of glaucoma and risk factors in pigmentary glaucoma. A new clinical study. Klin Monbl Augenheilkd. 1998;212:454-64.
11. Siddiqui Y, Hulzen RDT, Cameron D, et al. What is the risk of developing pigmentary glaucoma from pigment dispersion syndrome? Am J Ophthalmol. 2003;135:794-9.
12. Meyers JS. Secondary open-angle glaucoma. In: Rhee DJ, Rapuano CJ (Eds). Glaucoma, Color Atlas and Synopsis of Clinical Ophthalmology. Williams and Wilkins Ed. Philadelphia, United States; 2012.pp.196-207.
13. Scheie HG, Cameron JD. Pigment dispersion syndrome: a clinical study. Br J Ophthalmol. 1981;65:264-9.
14. Kuchle MK, Nguyen NX, Mardin CY, et al. Effect of neodinium:YAG laser iridotomy on number of aqueous

melanin granules in primary pigment dispersion syndrome. Graefes Arch Clin Exp Ophthalmol. 2001;239:411-5.
15. De Carvalho CA. Glaucoma cortisonico. In: de Almeida HG, Cohen R (Eds). Glaucomas Secondarios, 2nd edition. Roca ed. Sao Pablo: Brasil; 2006.pp.245-9.
16. Kersey JP, Broadway DC. Corticosteroid-induced glaucoma: a review or the literature. Eye (Lond). 2006;20:407-16.
17. Piltz-Seymour J, Uhler TA. Other secondary glaucomas. In: Shaarawy TM, Sherwood MB, Hitchings RA, Crowston JG (Eds). Glaucoma: Medical Diagnosis and Therapy. Saunders Ed. United States. 2009.pp.419-30.
18. Shirato S, Bloom E, Polansky JR, et al. Phagocytic properties of confluent human trabecular meshwork cells. Invest Ophthalmol Vis Sci. 1988;29:125.
19. Gritz DC, Wong IG. Incidence and prevalence of uveitis in Northern California Epidemiology of Uveitis Study. Ophthalmology. 2004;111:491-500.
20. Netland PA, Denton NC. Uveitic glaucoma. Contemp Ophtahlmol. 2006;5:1-26.
21. Siddique SS, Suelves AM, Baheti U, et al. Glaucoma and uveitis. Surv Ophthalmol. 2013;58:1-10.
22. Kuchtey RW, Lowder CY, Smith SD. Glaucoma in patients with ocular inflammatory disease. Ophthalmol Clin North Am. 2005;18(3):421-30.
23. Sallam A, Sheth HG, Habot-Wilner Z, et al. Outcome of raised intraocular pressure in uveitic eyes with and without a corticosteroid-induced hypertensive response. Am J Ophthalmol. 2009;148(2):207-13.
24. Neri P, Azuara-Blanco A, Forrester JV. Incidence of glaucoma in patients with uveitis. J Glaucoma. 2004;13(6):461-5.
25. Benitah N, Bugagge R, Papaliodis GN. Uveitic glaucomas. In: Rhee D, Rapuano CJ (Eds). Glaucoma: Color Atlas and Synopsis of Clinical Ophthalmology. Wills Eye Hospital, 2nd edition. Philadelphia, United States, 2012.pp.208-24.
26. Schuman JS, Bellows AR, Shingleton BJ, et al. Contact transscleral Nd:YAG laser cyclophotocoagulation. Midterms results. Ophthalmology. 1992;99(7):1089-94.
27. Rodrigues GB, Abe RY, Zangalli C, Sodre SL, et al. Neovascular glaucoma: a review. Int J Retina Vitreous. 2016;2:26-35.
28. Kim D, Singh AD, Singh A. Neovascular glaucoma. In: Shaarawy TM, Sherwood MB, Hitchings RA, Crowston JG (Eds). Glaucoma: Medical Diagnosis and Therapy. Saunders Ed. United States. 2009.pp.409-17.
29. Magargal LE, Brown GC, Augsburger JJ, et al. Neovascular glaucoma following central retinal vein obstruction. Ophthalmology. 1981;8:1095-101.
30. Olmos LC, Sayed MS, Moraczewski AL, et al. Long-term outcomes of neovascular glaucoma treated with and without intavitreal bevacizumab. Eye (Lond). 2016;30(3):463-72.
31. Wakabayashi T, Oshima Y, Sakaguchi H, et al. Intravitreal bevacizumab to treat iris neovascularization and neovascular glaucoma secondary to ischemic retinal diseases in 41 consecutive cases. Ophthalmology. 2008;115(9):1571-80.
32. Bazzaz S, Katz LJ, Myers JS. Post-traumatic glaucoma. In: Shaarawy TM, Sherwood MB, Hitchings RA, Crowston JG (Eds). Glaucoma: Medical Diagnosis and Therapy. Volume One. Saunders Ed. United States. 2009.pp.431-9.
33. Crouch WR, Williams PB. Trauma: ruptures and bleeding. In: Tasmani W, Jager E (Eds). Duane's Clinical Ophthalmology. Lippincott Williams. Philadelphia PA, United States; 1953. pp. 1-18.
34. Campbell D. Traumatic glaucoma. In: Schingleton B, Hersh P, Kenyon K (Eds). Eye Trauma. St. Louis: Mosby Year Book. Saint Louis, United States; 1991.pp.117-25.
35. Tesluk GC, Spaeth GL. The occurrence of primary open-angle glaucoma in the fellow eye of patients with unilateral angle-cleavage glaucoma. Ophthalmology. 1985;92:904-11.
36. Matsuo T, Muraoka N, Shiraga F, et al. Schwartz-Matsuo syndrome in retinal detachment with tears of the nonpigmented epithelium of the ciliary body. Acta Ophthalmol Scand. 1998;76:481-5.
37. Bansal S, Gunasekeran DV, Ang B, et al. Controversies in the pathophysiology and management of hyphema. Surv Ophthalmol. 2016;61:297-308.
38. Byrnes GA, Leen MM, Wong TP, et al. Vitrectomy for ciliary block (malignant) glaucoma. Ophthalmology. 1995;102(9):1308-11.
39. Ng DS, Ching RH, Chan CW. Angle recession glaucoma: long-term clinical outcomes over a 10 years period in traumatic mycrohyphèma. Int Ophthalmol. 2015;35:107-3.
40. Paaraj D, Sirisha S, Harsha L R, et al. Treatment outcomes in malignant glaucoma. Ophthalmology. 2013;120:984-90.
41. Quigley HA. Angle-closure glaucoma-simpler answers to complex mechanism: LXVI Edward Jackson Memorial Lecture. Am J Ophthalmol. 2009;148:657-69.
42. Santiago Malta SR, Santiago Malta JBN, Fares Ramalho MA. Glaucoma maligno. In: De Almeida HG, Cohen R (Eds). Glaucomas Secondarios. Roca ed. Sao Pablo, Brasil. 2006. pp.339-50.
43. Wirbelauer C, Karandish A, Haberle H, et al. Optical coherence tomography in malignant glaucoma following filtration surgery. Br J Ophthalmol. 2003;87(8):952-5.
44. Bitrian E, Caprioli J. Pars plana vitrectomy, hyaloido-zonulectomy and iridectomy for aqueous humor misdirection. Am J Ophthalmol. 2010;150:82-7.
45. Ayyala RS. Penetrating keratoplasty and glaucoma. Surv Ophthalmol. 2000;45(2):91-105.
46. Orucoglu F, Blumenthal EZ, Frucht-Pery J, et al. Risk factors and incidence of ocular hypertension after penetrating keratoplasty. J Glaucoma. 2014;23(9):599-605.
47. Anshu A, Price MO, Tan DT, et al. Endothelial keratoplasty: a revolution in evolution. Surv Ophtalmol. 2012;57(3): 236-52.
48. Rahman I, Carley F, Hillarby C, et al. Penetrating keratoplasty: Indications, outcomes and complications. Eye (Lond). 2009;23:1288-94.
49. Tuppin P, Poinard C, Loty B, et al. Risk factors for corneal regraft in patients on the French waiting list. Cornea. 2004;23(7):704-11.
50. Zimmerman TJ, Krupin T, Grodzki W, et al. The effect of suture depth on outflow facility in penetrating keratoplasty. Arch Ophthalmol. 1978;96(3):505-6.

51. Nguyen NX, Horn FK, Seitz B, et al. Frequency-doubling perimetry in patients following penetrating keratoplasty. Cornea. 2008;27:402-5.
52. Haddadin RI, Chodosh J. Corneal transplantation and glaucoma. Semin Ophthalmol. 2014;29(5-6):380-96.
53. Konowal A, Morrison JC, Brown SV, et al. Irreversible corneal decompensation in patients treated with topical dorzolamide. Am J Ophthalmol. 1999;127(4):403-6.
54. Plitz-Seymour J, Uhler TA. Other secondary glaucomas. Glaucoma: medical diagnosis and Therapy. Saunders Ed. Unites States, 2009:419-430
55. Jamil AL, Lawrence SD, Saperstein DA, et al. Glaucoma after retinal surgery. In: Schacknow PN, Samples JR (Eds). Springer. 2104.pp.918-20.
56. Barr CC, Lai MY, Lean JS, et al. The Silicon Study Group. Postoperative intraocular pressure abnormalities in the silicone study. Ophthalomolgy. 1993;100(11):1629-35.
57. Haut J, Ullern M, Chermet M, et al. Complications of intraocular injections of silicone combined with vitrectomy. Ophthalmologica. 1980;180(1):29-35.
58. Valone J Jr, McCarthy M. Emulsified anterior chamber silicone oil and glaucoma. Ophthalmology. 1994;101(12):1908-12.
59. Ishida K, Ahmed II, Netland PA. Ahmed Glaucoma Valve surgicaloutcomes in eyes with and without silicone oil endotamponade. J Glaucoma. 2009;18:325-30.
60. Mills MD, Devenyi RG, Lam WC, et al. An assessment of intraocular pressure rise in patients with gas-filled eyes during simulated air flight. Ophthalmology. 2001;108(1):40-4.
61. Epstein DL, Jedziniak JA, Grant WM. Identification of heavy-molecular-weight soluble protein in aqueous humor in human phacolytic glaucoma. Invest Ophthalmol Vis Sci. 1978;17(5):398-402.
62. Epstein D, Jedziniak JA, Grant WM. Obstruction of aqueous outflow by lens particles and by heavy- molecule-weight soluble lens protein. Invest Ophthalmol Vis Sci. 1978;17(3):272-7.
63. Lim MC and Lesley AG. Lens-associated Open-angle glaucomas. In: Rhee DJ, Rapuano CJ (Eds). Glaucoma: Color Atlas and Synopsis of Clinical Ophthalmology. Wills Eye Institute, Second edn. Philadelphia, United States. 2012. pp.246-57.
64. Lee JW, Lai JS, Yick DW, et al. Retrospective case series on the long-term visual and intraocular pressure outcomes of phacomorphic glaucoma. Eye (Lond). 2010;21(11):1675-80.
65. Lee SJ, Lee CK, Kim WS. Long-term therapeutic efficacy of phacoemulsification with intraocular lens implantation in patients with phacomorphic glaucoma. J Cataract Refract Surg. 2010;36(5):783-9.
66. Cohen R, de Almeida GV, Waiswol M, Della Paolera M. Ectopia e Intumescencia does Cristalino. In: de Almeida HG, Cohen R (Eds). Glaucomas Secondarios. Roca Ed. Sao Pablo, Brasil; 2006.pp.149-62.

Chapter 67

Trabeculectomy: Benefits, Techniques, and Management of Complications

Paul R Healey

TRABECULECTOMY: BENEFITS (AND CAVEATS)

Trabeculectomy is a surgical technique to lower intraocular pressure (IOP) by draining aqueous humor via a tensioned scleral flap into the suprascleral space and from there to the lymphatics and capillaries principally of the conjunctiva. However, its name and description given by the English ophthalmologist JE Cairns in the American Journal of Ophthalmology in October 1968 refers to completely different operation.

As Cairns pointed out in his paper, numerous operations already existed to "create channels for subconjunctival drainage of aqueous humor" but were all subject to high rates of complications. These complications were principally due to the fact that the lymphatics and capillaries of the conjunctiva have a pressure close to atmospheric, leading to profound early hypotony and its many sequelae.

The operation Cairns actually described was a variation of the *trabeculotomy*, an ab externo operation to incise the trabecular meshwork and canal of Schlemm. Concerned about visualization of an ab interno approach and unconvinced that drainage would be maintained without excision of tissue, he described the excision of a small section of trabecular meshwork (2 mm × 2 mm from clear cornea to scleral spur) from beneath a limbus-based partial thickness 3 mm × 3 mm scleral flap. The intention was to close the flap tightly to prevent external drainage. Instead, the outcome was frequently a slow leak of aqueous into the subconjunctival space. The effect of the flap was to limit the flow of aqueous through the sclerostomy and maintain a higher IOP in the early postoperative period. Careful postoperative assessment by many surgeons subsequently lead to the realization that successful trabeculectomies were associated with external drainage and (usually) a clinically identifiable bleb.

This story highlights three important benefits of trabeculectomy:

1. An ab externo approach allows surgery to be performed irrespective of the corneal clarity or angle visualization.
2. Drainage into a large area of very low pressure subconjunctival vessels distal to the usual site of obstruction in glaucoma creates a very large potential pressure gradient and a high flow capacity irrespective of the proximal cause of elevated IOP.
3. A tensioned scleral flap acts as a valve to control flow and pressure in a relatively predictable way.

Glaucoma is not a single entity. It is a final common pathway for optic nerves susceptible to the ravages of intraocular pressure and other predisposing pathologies. Lowering IOP is best thought of as a generic neuroprotective strategy.

Medical therapy and laser trabeculoplasty are dependent on specific receptor or tissue interactions to facilitate their IOP lowering effects. Genetic variations in receptor morphology or biological processes such as tachyphylaxis lead to loss of effect of medical treatments. Furthermore, these treatments are only effective if conventional outflow is relatively normal and usually become ineffective when outflow is extremely low, such as complete angle closure, or advanced pseudoexfoliation, pigment dispersion or myocilin glaucoma. While most patients with open-angle glaucoma can be well-managed with medical and laser therapy, the independence of the IOP lowering mechanism in trabeculectomy is a very useful tool in glaucoma management.

Were there only benefits to trabeculectomy surgery, it would probably be the first choice to treat glaucoma. The risks and complications of trabeculectomy are serious and, like its benefits, unique to external drainage surgery.

There are three fundamental considerations in trabeculectomy surgery:

1. Surgical technique is critical, particularly conjunctival handling, scleral flap construction and suturing. But despite this, poorly understood variations in anatomy and physiology can lead to unexpected IOP outcomes.
2. The presence of a permanent fistula substantially increases the risk of endophthalmitis. This is greatly increased by late thinning of the conjunctiva overlying the bleb.

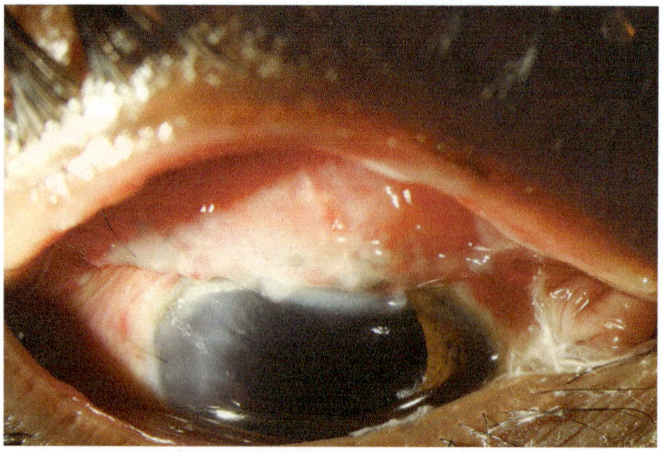

Fig. 67.1: Blebitis often associated with a very thin bleb.
Source: Dr George Varghese Puthuran, Aravind Eye Hospital, Madurai, Tamil Nadu, India.

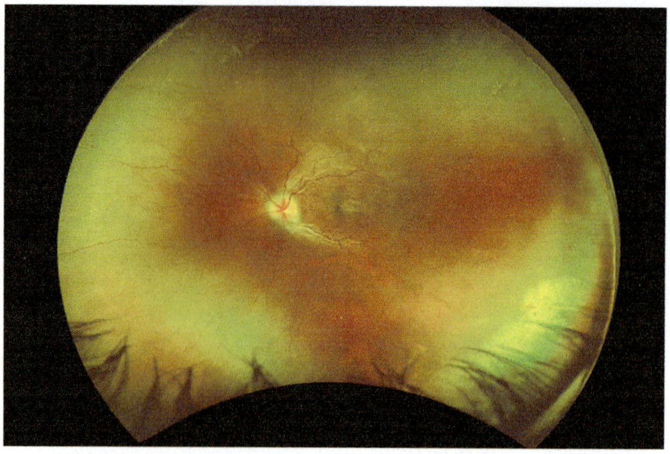

Fig. 67.2: Choroidal folds and maculopathy due to hypotony.
Source: Dr Kim Ramasamy, Aravind Eye Hospital, Madurai, Tamil Nadu, India.

3. The site of drainage contains large amounts of tenon's fascia which exhibits a profound scarring response in the acute, subacute and chronic postoperative wound-healing phases. Closure or walling off of the scleral flap by fibrosis is the most common cause of trabeculectomy failure.

Surgical technique can be improved with training and tips for good techniques will be discussed in the section "Trabeculectomy Techniques". However, it is important to understand not only the template for good surgery, but also the many variations in anatomy and biomechanical properties of the eye that can affect surgery.

Blebitis (Fig. 67.1) and bleb-related endophthalmitis is perhaps the most feared late complication of trabeculectomy. Its risk is critically dependent on the state of the conjunctiva as well as the bacterial environment. While surgical technique can help to minimize the conjunctival risk, long-term changes in bleb morphology and the patient's physical environment play major roles and need to be regularly re-evaluated over the life of the bleb.

The subconjunctival wound-healing response is the major determinant of trabeculectomy outcome and is the reason why antifibrotic therapy is an integral part of trabeculectomy. Fibrosis is variable, poorly predictable and continues through the life of the bleb. The tools available to ameliorate it are limited and their effects are also variable and poorly predictable. After surgical technique, wound-healing is the single most important factor in determining outcome and all glaucoma surgeons need to be intimately familiar with it and its management. Detailed prevention and management strategies will be discussed in the section "Trabeculectomy: Management of Complications".

Even successful IOP lowering from trabeculectomy comes at a price. Achieving a single digit target pressure sufficient to guarantee prevention of blindness from glaucoma carries risks associated with hypotony. While often defined as an IOP less than 5 mm Hg, hypotony is a syndrome, not a number. It can be absent in an eye with no measurable IOP and be severe with an IOP measured at 10 mm Hg. Its three important features are:

1. Choroidal folds and/or macular edema (Fig. 67.2).
2. Choroidal effusions
3. Increased risk of cataract and corneal endothelial failure.

In the absence of signs of hypotony, eyes with low IOPs can suffer visual impairment from irregular astigmatism and refractive instability. Additionally, the physical presence of a bleb can disturb the normal tear flow leading to dellen, epiphora and dysesthesia. Surgical trauma and chemical toxicity can cause limbal stem cell failure as a late complication of trabeculectomy. Lastly, trabecular outflow diminishes substantially in a well-functioning trabeculectomy. Rapid failure (over weeks or months) of the trabeculectomy even after many years of excellent pressure control can lead to very high intraocular pressures and precipitous progression of glaucoma. A single trabeculectomy requires a lifetime of vigilance from both doctor and patient.

TRABECULECTOMY: PLANNING AND TIMING

In glaucoma, surgical decision making for external drainage is always binary and consequential. This means that one always has to choose to do one operation over another and the outcome of the surgery has consequences irrespective of its success or failure which influence subsequent surgery. In contrast to an ineffective medication which has little or no impact on the success of a subsequent agent, anatomical and physiological changes from surgery and the wound healing response often have a profound effect on subsequent surgery in the same area or by the same mechanism. The wound healing response irreversibly changes the suprascleral environment after peritomy even when antifibrotic agents are used. It is also altered by the presence of a drainage bleb or foreign bodies. While generally considered more resistant to failure, Molteno type long drainage tubes actually incite a greater degree of fibrosis due to the seton (and thus require the seton to function). Newer medium length tubes attempt to minimize fibrosis by an ab interno approach obviating the need for a peritomy or more biologically inert material.

These factors lead to some general rules about planning trabeculectomies. A trabeculectomy is less likely to succeed:

- After a prior peritomy at the (superior) surgical site such as in scleral cataract surgery or scleral buckling, superior ocular muscle surgery, a previous trabeculectomy or a long tube to the posterior subconjunctival space. [Thus, trabeculectomy should generally precede rather than follow long tube (e.g. Molteno) surgery.]
- If the eye is or is likely to be inflamed or to produce proinflammatory or fibrotic cytokines such as is found in uveitis or neovascularization or after cataract surgery.
- If the conjunctiva is damaged, inflamed or scarred from such things as trauma, chemical burns or cicatrizing diseases. Chronic use of topical agents including miotics and sympathomimetics can also induce a fibrosis response in the supra-scleral space and reduce success.

Unfortunately, the relative contraindications above are also associated with glaucomas for which trabeculectomy is often required. Additionally, trabeculectomy doubles the rate of cataract formation which makes it an operation that sets itself up for failure. Conversely, the eye which would most probably do best from a trabeculectomy is also the one likely to respond very well to drug monotherapy or laser trabeculoplasty with a much lower risk of treatment induced harm.

Thus, trabeculectomy planning requires some very careful considerations of benefit versus harm, not just for the glaucoma, but for the patient's health over their lifetime. It has the potential to greatly improve or greatly diminish health. Every surgeon must know their own rates, risks and outcomes for intervention along with the natural history of the disease they are treating.

Given the higher safety profile of alternative therapies, trabeculectomy should be undertaken when the patient has a high risk of blindness or poor health with alternative treatment, is likely to benefit from it more than a long tube and where that benefit is higher than the sum or the risk of the operation and the risk of not operating. The decision is best made in partnership with the patient.

TRABECULECTOMY: TECHNIQUES

Trabeculectomy aims to create a scleral valve to control aqueous flow into a suprascleral space from where it returns to the bloodstream via capillaries and lymphatics primarily in the conjunctiva. Whilst surgery is structural, the desired outcome is to create a new dynamic physiology which is maintained for many years without harming the tissues or inciting a prolonged or aggressive wound healing response. We must ensure that we change the anatomy in a way that maximizes the chance of creating the new physiology. To do this we must do the following:

- *Preoperatively*:
  - *Assess the physiology of the eye*:
    - Set the postoperative target IOP range
      - ▷ Target pressures below 10 mm Hg increase risk of hypotony-related complications.
    - Estimate aqueous production and drainage rates
      - ▷ Normal aqueous output states need more flow to achieve the same IOP level. Hypotony risk is higher for low aqueous output states such as ischemia, uveitis and for open-angle glaucoma with low pretreatment IOP.
    - Determine the ability of the sclera, tenons and conjunctiva to support aqueous flow
      - ▷ The hydraulic conductivity of the tenons and conjunctiva determines the rate of aqueous egress from the suprascleral space. If this is lower than that of the scleral flap it determines the IOP. Thicker tissue and a smaller area reduce the total potential flow and therefore lowest IOP achievable.
    - Determine the individual patient's wound healing physiology including the presence of profibrotic factors in the aqueous or conjunctiva
      - ▷ A history of rapid or hypertrophic wound healing, keloid or inflammatory disease of the skin or mucous membranes suggests

a higher risk of excessive fibrosis. In diseases of immune dysregulation such as rheumatoid arthritis, lupus erythematosus and scleroderma the wound healing response is often prolonged, increasing this risk of late fibrosis. Genetic ancestry can inform local variations in wound healing in otherwise normal patients. Direct observation of conjunctival tethering from fibrosis is a high risk sign. A history of long-term topical treatment especially miotics, sympathomimetics is also a risk factor.

- Determine the individual patient's likely response to drugs used in trabeculectomy (antifibrotics, steroids, antibiotics)
  - ▹ A steroid response can substantially reduce trabecular outflow in the early postoperative period and cause an unexpected fall in IOP when reduced. Up to 8% of eyes may be resistant to the antifibrotic effects of Mitomycin-C (MMC). There is no commercially available test for this.
- Determine the individual patient's bacterial conjunctivitis risk
  - ▹ Very thin conjunctiva and a lack of tenons tissue can predispose to conjunctival thinning and avascularity postoperatively. A dirty environment or habits that introduce bacteria to the ocular surface increase the risk of blebitis. Immunosuppression can predispose to and mask early signs of infection.

- *Assess the anatomy of the eye*:
  - Determine the eye's likely anatomical response to IOP reduction including the risks of hypotony and aqueous misdirection
    - ▹ Young patients and large eyes or thin sclera are more at risk of hypotony. Small eyes with thick sclera are at increased risk of choroidal effusions and aqueous misdirection.
  - Determine scleral thickness and rigidity, and plan flap construction
    - ▹ It is difficult to close a very thin scleral flap tightly enough to control flow. High myopes and eyes with buphthalmos tend to have very thin sclera and may need larger scleral flaps with small, very anterior "sclerostomies" (actually keratectomies) to maximize closing forces. The same flap construction in an eye with very thick sclera and high rigidity can maintain a high IOP without any flap closure (Fig. 67.7).
  - Determine the thickness and extent of tenons fascia and plan intraoperative antifibrosis treatment
    - ▹ All other risk equal, thicker tenons in younger patients is more reactive and will need more aggressive antifibrotic treatment. Elderly patients may have very thin conjunctiva. But tissues changes induced by many years of topical therapy can still cause aggressive fibrosis.
  - Determine the state (and presence) of the conjunctiva including signs of previous surgery or fibrosis and plan intraoperative conjunctival handling
    - ▹ Trabeculectomy is impractical when conjunctiva is absent or extensively damaged or scarred. In these circumstances, a Molteno type tube is usually required for external drainage.
- Obtain informed consent for the entire surgical journey including later outcomes and treatments
  - Adherence to postoperative management and follow-up instructions, a good understanding of the surgical journey and good relationship with the surgeon is essential for successful trabeculectomy.
- *Treat risk factors for failure/complications*:
  - Ocular inflammation
  - Infection
  - Anticoagulation
  - Intraocular proinflammatory or fibrotic cytokines
    - ▹ Topical steroids used for several weeks preoperatively can reduce conjunctival inflammatory cells as well as intraocular inflammation. Preoperative systemic, orbital floor or intravitreal steroids may be required for some inflammatory diseases. Anti-VEGF therapy can reduce bleeding and inflammation in eyes with high aqueous VEGF levels.

- *Intraoperatively*:
  - *Protect bystander tissues*:
    - Preventing retinal phototoxicity, corneal drying and intraocular, corneal, conjunctival or

epidermal chemotoxicity improves outcomes but is often forgotten by a surgeon focused on the mechanics of the operation
  - A wet corneal shield is effective but should be removed during antifibrotic use to prevent inadvertent absorption
  - Trypan Blue dye colors antifibrotics without diminishing their effectiveness, making visualization of treatment area and prevention of bystander tissue damage much easier.
- Choose a surgical site that will minimize risk of infection, dysesthesia or exposure
  - Inferior blebs have much higher infection rates and are no longer performed. Dellen formation is more likely when blebs extend to the limbus within the palpebral aperture. The best location for a bleb is usually superior and covered by the upper lid.
- Provide for adequate exposure without traumatizing the bleb site
  - A corneal traction suture avoids the trauma risk of a superior rectus suture.
- Perform a peritomy in such a way as to avoid placing a wound in the bleb
  - Posterior conjunctival wounds tend to migrate anteriorly with fibrosis. If they are tethered to the sclera, they limit posterior aqueous flow
  - Limbal conjunctival wounds tend to become tethered to the sclera. Excessive retraction will cause a wound leak. A limbal conjunctival approach must avoid damaging limbal stem cells.
  - Radial side incisions will limit the bleb extent and increase wound healing
  - When handling the conjunctiva use non-toothed forceps parallel to the tissues with the lower blade under the tenons fascia and as posterior as dissection makes possible (Fig. 67.3). This helps protect the conjunctiva from damage. Once in the subtenons plane, direct visualization is not necessary and retraction or reflection of the tissue risks tearing or button-holing the conjunctiva. When lifting tissues, it is always better to pull toward the incision as this reduces tension on the thin limbal conjunctival edge. Use blunt dissection with Westcott style scissors to break the superior check ligaments between 10 o'clock and 2 o'clock. A squint hook passed flat under the tissues ensures that a continuous space has been made. It is also very useful to blunt dissect with a squint hook over the superior rectus as the tenons tends to tear above the muscle capsule and anterior muscular arteries. In contrast, even blunt dissection with Westcott scissors in a suprascleral plane tends to engage both capsule and associated vessels.

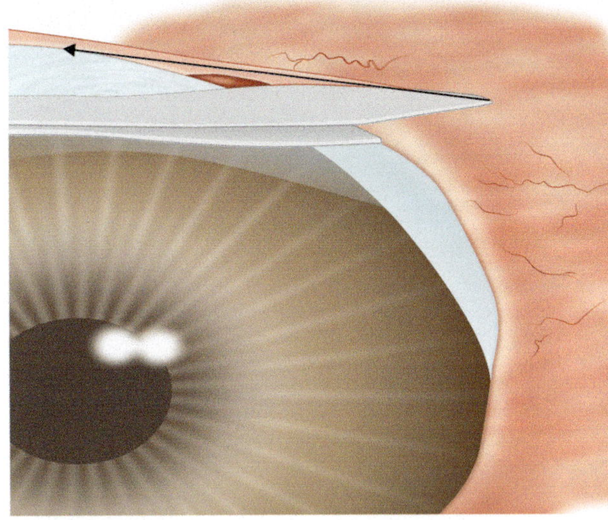

Fig. 67.3: Handling the conjunctiva in trabeculectomy. Use nontoothed forceps parallel to the tissues. Lift up and forward (arrow) when dissecting or placing sponges. This makes room for instruments without creating tension on the conjunctival edge.

- *Perform adequate diathermy*:
  - Plasma has a powerful antifibrotic effect but diathermy causes scleral shrinkage which can prevent adequate scleral flap closure. Furthermore many episcleral veins collect aqueous and should not be arbitrarily destroyed. Light diathermy should be applied only to staunch bleeding and to close vessels that will be perforated during scleral flap construction or closure
  - Diathermy causes tissue shrinkage and can cause gaping of the flap or the edges of its bed.
- *Construct a scleral flap that fulfills its tectonic requirements (Figs. 67.4 and 67.7)*:
  - Large enough perimeter to provide a high flow of aqueous at low velocity
  - Thick enough to be able to close off flow completely if sutured tightly. Thin enough to allow high flow rates if unsutured

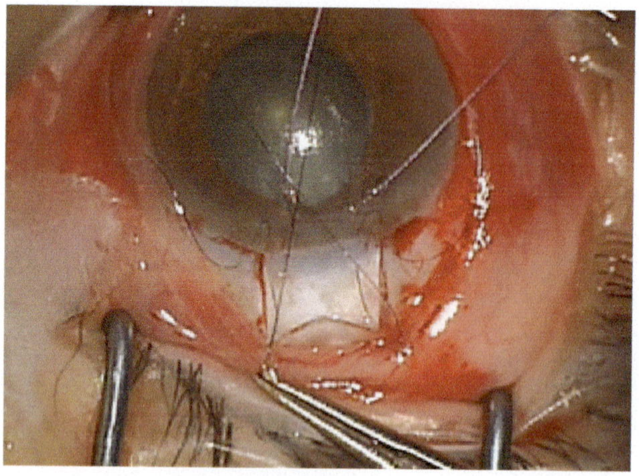

Fig. 67.4: Scleral flap.

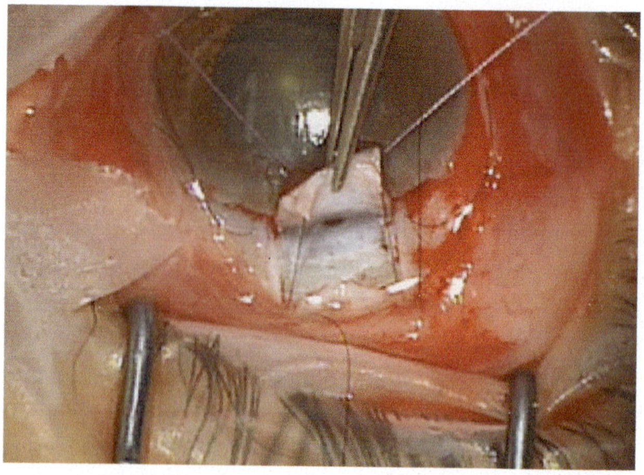

Fig. 67.5: Anterior sclerostomy. A clear corneal/corneal-limbal entry of 500 μm size, perpendicular to the wall of the eye, keeps away from the iris root and its vessels and allows the flap to create more leverage for a tighter closure.

- The flap shape should promote aqueous to flow posteriorly. This can be facilitated by having the shortest distance from the sclerostomy to the posterior edge of the flap
- Historically flaps were made either supertemporally or superonasally in the expectation that the other site would be used for a new flap when the first failed. With modern antifibrotic and revision techniques a single flap at 12 o'clock can last a patient's lifetime and minimize the risk of oblique astigmatism, dysesthesia or exposure.

- *Preplace flap sutures to rapidly restore pressure*:
  - With the eye open, intraocular pressure rapidly falls exposing it to all the complications of hypotony. The aim should be to close the flap and restore IOP (at least to high single digits) as soon as flow is established. Preplacing sutures allows for rapid closure
  - Care must be taken not to cut the sutures when making the sclerostomy.
- Make a small anterior sclerostomy (Fig. 67.5) (actually it is a keratectomy) perpendicular to the wall of the eye
  - A 2 mm × 2 mm block sclerostomy over the trabecular meshwork and canal of Schlem is not necessary to form a bleb
  - A clear corneal/corneolimbal entry keeps away from the iris root and its vessels and allows the flap to create more leverage for a tighter closure
  - 500 μm is usually an adequate sclerostomy size. If there is not copious flow under the unsutured trapdoor then enlargement posteriorly rapidly reduces the mechanical advantage of the trapdoor.
- *Prevent iris incarceration*:
  - Usually aqueous pushes the iris into a newly formed sclerostomy. Full thickness excision of this tissue creates a small iridotomy under the sclerostomy and prevents later incarceration (Fig. 67.6)
  - A thick or rigid iris may need to be grasped through the sclerostomy. Care needs to be taken not to pull on the vessels of the iris root and to ensure the iridotomy overlies the (anteriorly placed) sclerostomy
  - In a pseudophakic eye with a very deep anterior chamber the iris may be so far below the sclerostomy it is difficult to grasp. In this situation iris incarceration is rare even without an iridotomy.
- *Establish the tension/flow properties of the flap (Fig. 67.7)*:
  - The flap tension is the critical factor that determines early postoperative IOP. The relationship between suture tension and flow (and between flow and IOP) differs for each person and should be established by adjusting suture tension and observing flow patterns. Two key pressures can be established by injecting BSS through a paracentesis (or adjusting the flow of an AC maintainer):
    - ▷ The IOP at which flow stops (this should be at or a little below target pressure)

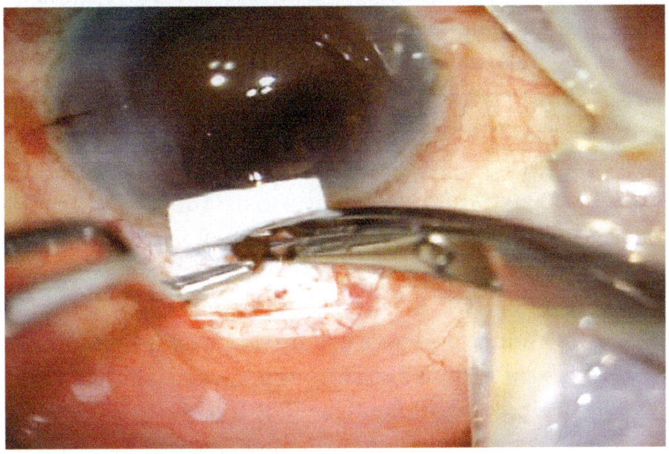

Fig. 67.6: Iridotomy to prevent later incarceration.
Source: Dr George Varghese Puthuran, Aravind Eye Hospital, Madurai, Tamil Nadu, India.

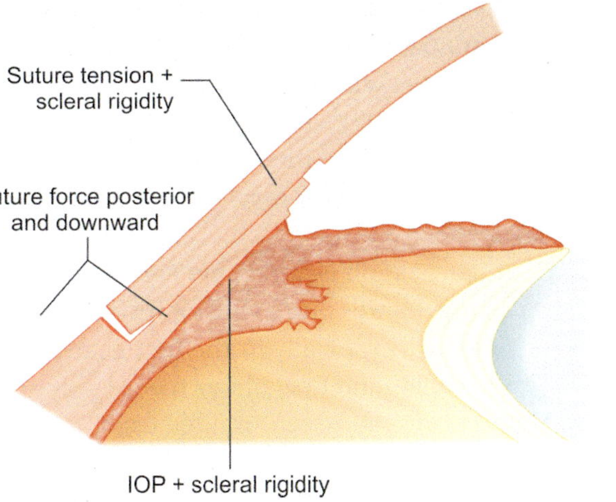

Fig. 67.7: Flow properties of the scleral flap. Adequate thickness of the scleral flap at the limbus creates mechanical advantage when the scleral flap is closed posteriorly. This is enhanced by a more anterior sclerostomy. Both adequate IOP (pushing outward) and suture tension (pushing inward) is required for a watertight seal. The more rigid/thick the sclera, the less important the IOP becomes. The "sclerostomy" is actually through clear cornea avoiding the iris root.
(IOP: Intraocular pressure)

- ▷ The IOP at which flow spontaneously starts (this is the highest pressure the eye can develop in the early postoperative period).
- Some surgeons use an AC maintainer to reduce the risk of hypotony. Its flow rate will always be much greater than aqueous production rate, causing flaps to be left too loose at steady-state IOP. It is useful to turn it off before establishing the flap tension. Patients on aqueous suppressants will have lower spontaneous aqueous flow until their effects wear off in the postoperative period. This tends to cause flaps to be left too tight on the table.
- It is wise to err on the side of overly tight sutures and they can be loosened postoperatively in the clinic.

- *Close the conjunctiva and tenon's fascia in a water tight fashion to its original insertion point (Fig. 67.8)*:
  - Circumferential tension in the conjunctiva and an adequate pressure in the eye are the most important factors in good apposition of these tissues. The conjunctiva is usually elastic. Anteriorly placed drawstring sutures at either end of the incision will create a chord-like tension line between the anchor points. Box sutures between these points reinforce apposition and resist dehiscence from the pull of postoperative bleb fibrosis. Suturing into a groove in the limbus beneath the tension line enhances this effect
  - The anterior tenon's fascia can play an important postoperative role in preventing anterior flow and protecting the conjunctiva from thinning. If it retracts it can contribute to fibrosis at the posterior flap edge. It should be returned to its normal insertion point with the conjunctival drawstring sutures

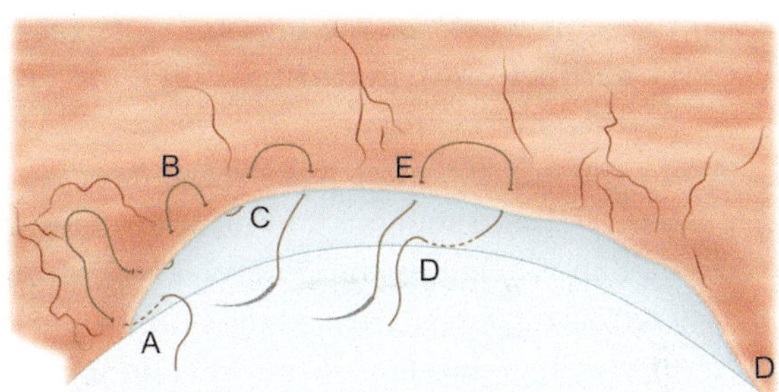

A- Episcleral bite a limbus
B- Purse-string
C- Exit subconjunctival to buy the knot
D- Nasal wing suture closed first

Fig. 67.8: Closing the conjunctiva and tenons. The draw string and box suture technique of conjunctival closure. Draw string (left): The initial bite (A) must anchor the suture laterally and anteriorly. Bite B causes lateral contraction of the conjunctiva. Bite C should be a little more posterior and include tenons facia to restore the limbal anatomy without the risk of cheese-wiring. Box suture (right): Bite D through the limbus along the wound. Alternatively, the bite can run in a premade groove thus suturing the conjunctiva into a groove for a better seal. Bite E should include tenons where present. If the tension from the draw string sutures is inadequate, making bite E larger than D will also contract the conjunctiva. In general, a larger number of smaller suture bites will generate more force of closure with less risk of cheese-wiring.

    - Wound leaks through suture holes can be minimized by the incorporation of tenon's facia, ensuring tissue posterior to the suture is apposed firmly and by using round-bodied needles of the same size as the thread.
  - *Give long-acting anti-inflammatory medicines and antibiotics*:
    - Inflammation is rapid after surgery. Depot long acting steroids play a vital role in dampening this response especially in the first 2 postoperative weeks. Betamethasone or triamcinolone given inferiorly sub-tenons is often used.
- *Postoperatively*:
  - *Assess the speed and severity of the wound healing response*:
    - Regular review is essential to gauge the healing response and adjust antifibrosis therapy in the early postoperative period. For most eyes a cellular response characterizes the first two weeks, causing induction of fibroblasts which migrate and begin making collagen around week three. By week six, the inflammatory response is settling and maturing collagen creates permanent scar tissue.
  - *Assess and adjust the flap tension and aqueous flow*:
    - Early IOP and aqueous flow rates are determined by flap tension as the potential bleb drainage area is very large. Tight sutures can be loosened in the clinic but loose sutures cannot easily be tightened
    - Fibrosis reduces the bleb area and its hydraulic conductivity. Prior to collagen maturation, loosening or removing trapdoor sutures can lower IOP by increasing bleb area. But once the collagen has matured the force of aqueous will not be able to overcome the tissue resistance and suture adjustments will be ineffective
    - The most effective window for intervention is prior to collagen maturation (usually the first 4–6 weeks). However, after exposure to MMC, fibroblasts may produce abnormal collagen which does not mature normally. In such cases, late suture adjustment can lower IOP
    - Low flow rates for the first week or two encourage watertight healing of the conjunctival wound. High and anterior trapdoor flow increases the risk of wound leak.
  - *Titrate postoperative antifibrosis interventions in anticipation of the next phase of fibrosis*:
    - The morphology of the bleb and the IOP at any time are always a consequence of the pathophysiological events that preceded it. There is currently no way to reverse fibrosis
    - Postoperative antifibrosis therapy must be titrated to meet the long term IOP target. But this should be on the basis of bleb assessment rather than IOP. Severe inflammation can transiently reduce aqueous production and IOP. Similarly, overly tight flap sutures in an eye with very little fibrosis will increase IOP. It is the evaluation of the bleb rather than the IOP that will differentiate the cause and therefore the best action
    - Even in a longstanding mature bleb, fibrosis can occur. Patients with blebs need regular long-term review especially during periods of ocular inflammation or trauma.

TRABECULECTOMY: MANAGEMENT OF COMPLICATIONS (INCLUDING FIBROSIS)

Causes of surgical complications fall into three broad categories:

1. Breakdown in normal procedures
2. Abnormal/unexpected anatomy complicating standard surgical techniques
3. Abnormal/unexpected physiological responses during or after surgery.

The best way to manage complications is by preventing them. To do this it is essential that all normal procedures for the entire surgical journey are optimal and regularly reviewed and analyzed. This is not limited to the medical staffs' training and dexterity. It applies equally to servicing of equipment, admission, discharge and follow-up procedures and patient adherence and persistence with their own management advice. During surgery, patient comfort and cooperation is essential.

For trabeculectomy, anatomical variations contribute most to intraoperative complications and unexpected physiological responses in the form of postoperative subconjunctival fibrosis is the cause of the vast majority of postoperative complications. However, complications associated with low aqueous output and low IOP are also important.

- *Abnormal/unexpected anatomy complicating standard surgical techniques*:
  - *Conjunctival fragility and elasticity*:
    - Conjunctival tears and button-holes must be closed. The risk of cheese-wiring and leaking can be minimized by closing from the underside, closing over a piece of tenon's fascia and using a small round-bodied needle of the same size as the thread. Tears and holes where a bleb is not wanted can be closed directly onto the deeper tissues. At the completion of surgery, topical 2% fluorescein or 5% aqueous iodine can be useful to identify areas of leak. A dense viscoelastic (e.g. Healon5™) injected under the conjunctiva via the limbal wound is antifibrotic, will pre-form the bleb, and will egress through any conjunctival tears as well as the limbal wound if not sealed adequately.
    - Where fibrosis has already occurred, the conjunctiva can have no elasticity making closure to the limbus difficult. A very posterior horizontal conjunctival (but not tenon's) incision can relieve anterior tension without causing a leak.
  - *Scleral thickness and rigidity*:
    - Scleral trapdoors of the same dimensions will function very differently when scleral rigidity or thickness is very high or very low. Low rigidity requires a thicker flap and high rigidity a thinner one. While the latter is surgically possible as higher rigidity usually follows thicker sclera in smaller eyes, the converse in not the case. Low scleral rigidity is often associated with high myopia and buphthalmos which are characterized by thin sclera. A less effective flap can be mitigated by a larger size, a smaller, more anterior sclerostomy and more flap sutures.
    - Previous scleral incisions (e.g. intra/extra-capsular cataract surgery) never regain their strength and a flap through these will easily dehisce.
  - *Postoperative management*:
    - Early postoperative wound leaks may have been present intraoperatively or may be caused by tissue retraction around a suture or at the wound edge. They should be searched for with 2% fluorescein drops under a cobalt blue light. Diversion of aqueous through the leaking area reduces bleb area and the presence of the leak makes the surgeon reluctant to be aggressive with antifibrosis therapy. Both of these increase the risk of bleb fibrosis. But as the bleb shrinks and scars, its pressure increases and more aqueous is forced through the leaking area which inhibits epithelialization. It is essential to tamponade the leak immediately. For smaller, more anterior leaks this can often be achieved with a contact lens that can apply adequate pressure to the area. Once flow is stopped, if the conjunctiva is healthy it will cover the defect if small. Antifibrosis measures should not be stopped but if there are signs of epithelial toxicity, preservatives should be removed. Large and nonhealing conjunctival defects usually need surgical repair.
    - Late postoperative wound leaks occur in thin walled blebs due to trauma, conjunctival dryness and the effects of the aqueous pressure and its constituents. The first two causes can often be managed conservatively with copious lubrication and a bandage contact lens. Where leaks recur, surgical repair is necessary to reduce the risk of infection. The specific technique depends on the location and size, but it is important to be aware that the thinned tissue is usually stretched and much smaller once tension is removed by dissection. Where high aqueous pressure in a small bleb causes thinning and avascularity, enlarging the area of the bleb by puncturing the cyst wall subconjunctivally often dramatically improves the state of the conjunctiva, especially if the avascularity is recent.
    - Postoperative underfiltration from a rigid scleral flap despite suture removal can be increased by lifting the flap mechanically, i.e. with bleb needling. Care must be taken to make the minimum necessary anatomical change as hypertension can rapidly become hypotony which has particular risks in a small eye. Postoperative hypotony from overfiltration in an eye with low scleral rigidity presents a challenge and irregular folding of the flap bed worsens apposition over the sclerostomy. Occasionally increasing local tension with a contact lens externally and an anterior chamber fill internally can increase apposition sufficiently to reach target pressure. Viscoelastic in the eye, however,

tends to increase pressure dramatically, forcing itself out through the flap, loosening adjustable sutures on the way and leaving the eye hypotonous again. Relying on fibrosis to raise the IOP is suitably conservative but sets the eye up for trabeculectomy failure and so should be managed closely. Ultimately more flap sutures may be necessary. But placing them through the conjunctiva removes the need for another peritomy.

- *Dysesthetic blebs*:
  - High, anterior or nasal blebs (Fig. 67.9) can be very uncomfortable and are often associated with dryness of the adjacent cornea. Treatment consists initially of lubrication (including ointments overnight). But if the anatomical position of the bleb is not manageable medically, the bleb should be moved more posteriorly by dissecting any posterior cyst walls and compressing or delimiting the anterior part of the bleb with a compression suture or a full thickness conjunctiva/tenons cut-down with resuturing/gluing to the sclera.

- *Abnormal/unexpected physiological responses during or after surgery*:
  - *Subconjunctival fibrosis*: Management of subconjunctival fibrosis begins before surgery with risk assessment and prevention, continues during surgery with antifibrosis treatment and after surgery with postoperative fibrosis management
    - Fibrosis risk assessment and prevention
    - The patient and their eye should be assessed for scarring risk. Risk factors for greater scarring include:
      - ▷ Younger age
      - ▷ Ethnogenetic background
      - ▷ Personal history of rapid or excessive healing (including keloid formation)
      - ▷ Systemic inflammatory diseases which prolong the wound healing response (e.g. rheumatoid arthritis, SLE or scleroderma)
      - ▷ Prior subconjunctival fibrosis from previous surgery (especially superior peritomy), trauma (including alkali injury), inflammation (including cicatricial diseases) or eye drops (especially pilocarpine and phenylephrine)
      - ▷ Intraocular inflammation or cytokines (uveitis, aphakia, neovascularization, pseudoexfoliation syndrome).
  - Preoperative management of neovascularization, and inflammation improve postoperative results. In eyes with conjunctival inflammation including that caused by eye drops, preoperative topical steroids can be beneficial.
  - *Intraoperative antifibrosis therapy (Fig. 67.10)*:
    - 5-fluorouracil (5-FU) and mitomycin-C (MMC) induce fibroblast apoptosis and render living cells defective in collagen production. They are frequently used intraoperatively to reduce postoperative fibrosis. The effect of 5-FU is linear between 25 mg/mL and 50 mg/mL. MMC at

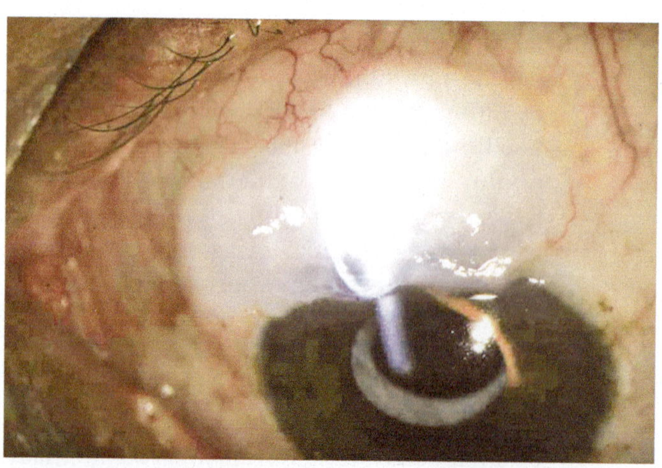

Fig. 67.9: Dysesthetic bleb may cause improper corneal wetting.
Source: Dr George Varghese Puthuran, Aravind Eye Hospital, Madurai, Tamil Nadu, India.

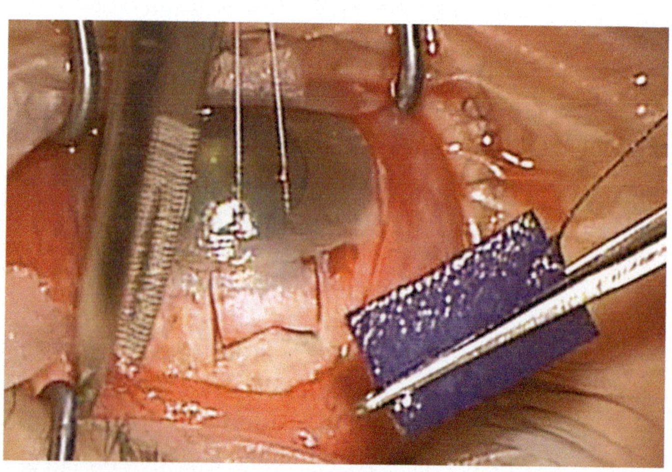

Fig. 67.10: Intraoperative antifibrotic therapy with mitomycin-C (MMC) colored with a few drops of trypan blue.

0.2 mg/mL is at least as effective as 5-FU 50 mg/mL and has a linear dose response up to 0.5 mg/mL. In vitro MMC effects are linearly time dependent up to at least 5 minutes. In vivo, MMC effects can be blunted by serum factors and tissue binding is usually complete by about 3 minutes.

- 5-FU and MMC can be applied to the subtenons space by an oversaturated sponge (such as a surgical instrument wipe) after peritomy or injected into the subtenons space prior to peritomy. 5FU has a very high pH which makes it toxic to epithelial cells. But MMC can be also applied trans-conjunctivally using an oversaturated sponge. Sponge application relies on contact time to titrate effect, injection assumes maximal time and relies on total dosage. As MMC is toxic to vascular endothelium at high doses, a larger volume at lower concentrations is safer when injecting MMC.
- MMC in particular is extremely toxic inside the eye. The eye should be thoroughly washed after application to remove antifibrotic from all epidermal, conjunctival and corneal surfaces.
- When using sponge application, the following should be considered:
  - ▷ Sponges must be placed under, not in, tenons fascia. Gentle scleral depression during insertion using a forceps helps placement
  - ▷ Spaces between sponges will have lower antifibrotic exposure
  - ▷ Sponges should be placed posteriorly, where tenons are thickest and from where the largest number of fibroblast migrate. This maximizes bleb area. Avoid placing sponges on the superior rectus insertion
  - ▷ The anterior extent need only be over the posterior trapdoor as wound healing of the limbal conjunctiva prevents wound leaks, anterior drainage and bleb dysesthesia
  - ▷ Fewer larger sponges, especially if tied with a 6-0 silk thread are easier to retrieve and reduce the risk of inadvertent sponge retention.
- When injecting antifibrotics, the following should be considered:
  - ▷ It is important that the needle tip is visualized in the subtenons space prior to injection. This is easier to achieve posteriorly
  - ▷ Inject slowly, so that the fluid travels throughout the subtenons space rather than being forced up into the subconjunctival space
  - ▷ A bent 30 g needle bevel down helps minimize trauma and bleeding
  - ▷ The antifibrotic often needs to be pushed into the posterior subtenons space through pressure over conjunctiva
  - ▷ After about 3 minutes tissue binding reduces further distribution.
- *Management of postoperative fibrosis*:
  - Fibrosis is an expected part of the wound healing process. If pro and anti-fibrosis factors are well matched, postoperative fibrosis should signal maturation of the bleb, stabilization of the IOP (preventing hypotony) and a reduction in inflammation.
  - Excessive fibrosis (Fig. 67.11) is usually managed medically by increasing steroids (usually topically but also by injection behind the bleb) and giving adjunctive 5-FU behind the bleb. An oral combination of diclofenac, prednisone and colchicine can be very effective where fibrosis is association with excessive inflammation.
  - Surgical management of excessive fibrosis depends on the stage. Prior to collagen maturation, suture loosening and massage over the trapdoor forces aqueous to enlarge the bleb. Once collagen has cross-linked these measures will be less effective. A bleb needle-sweep can divide the fibrotic tissue and

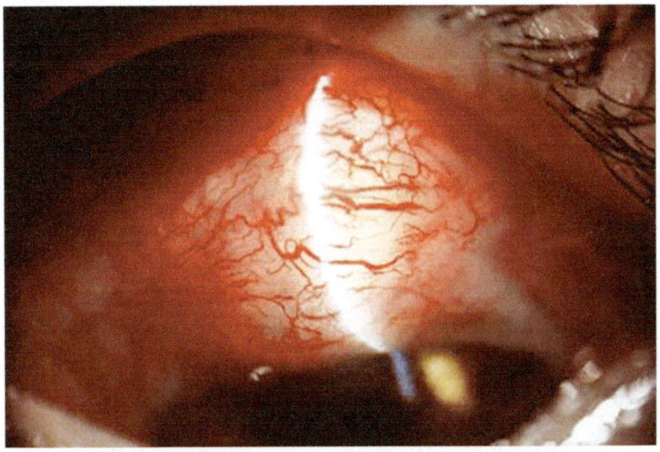

Fig. 67.11: Bleb fibrosis, which needs aggressive management.
Source: Dr George Varghese Puthuran, Aravind Eye Hospital, Madurai, Tamil Nadu, India.

re-establish drainage. If fibrosis has caused the bleb to encyst, multiple punctures through the cyst wall are usually enough. If fibrosis over the flap is the problem, careful lifting of the flap may be necessary. Anterior flap fibrosis may require needle entry into the anterior chamber to facilitate side to side sweeping under the flap edges. There is usually little fibrosis under the flap itself unless uveal tissue has been retained there.

- If fibrosis is unexpectedly mild, steroids are usually reduced. This is also the treatment by many surgeons for overfiltration caused intraoperatively. While effective, it is important to monitor closely as too much fibrosis is much more common than too little and antifibrotic therapy should be ready to be reintroduced.
- Monitoring fibrosis usually requires weekly visits for the first 6 weeks, then tapering as the wound healing response subsides. Additional visits will be required for stronger healers and fewer for more modest healers. Most phakic patients can cease steroids completely by 3 months. In some predisposed patients, the wound healing and inflammatory responses can be prolonged. In these cases, cessation of steroids causes rapid fibrosis and indefinite topical steroid therapy is necessary.

- *Choroidal effusions and hypotony*:
  - A rapid fall in IOP to less than 5 mm Hg is usually required to induce choroidal effusions. But in susceptible eyes it can occur with IOPs in the low teens. Small peripheral effusions need no treatment other than topical cycloplegia and usually resolve spontaneously. Very large effusions that either reduce vision due to macula obstruction (especially in an only-seeing eye) or flatten the anterior chamber need more aggressive treatment, first with raising of a very low pressure to initially above then down to target level. If sight threatening choroidal effusions occur at target pressure, drainage through one or two radial scleral incisions 5–7 mm from the limbus will also deepen the anterior chamber. Small eyes with thick sclera and younger patients are at greater risk of choroidal effusions.
  - Hypotony maculopathy or a choroidal fold through the macula causing vision loss needs to be treated by increasing the IOP to flatten the retina and move the fold elsewhere.
- *Aqueous misdirection*:
  - In small eyes with thick sclera, anterior rotation of the ciliary body, sometimes associated with small supraciliary effusions may cause a severe angle closure characterized by marked axial shallowing of the anterior chamber (Fig. 67.12). While it is usually associated with a high IOP this is not always the case in a functioning trabeculectomy. Treatment requires rotating the ciliary body posteriorly and usually breaking the anterior vitreous face peripherally. The former can be accomplished with intensive (QID) atropine 1% and aqueous suppression. The latter can sometimes be achieved with a YAG laser peripheral capsulotomy/vitreolysis in a pseudophake, but often requires a peripheral vitrectomy with a clear passage for aqueous flow into the anterior chamber.
- *Suprachoroidal hemorrhage*:
  - Suprachoroidal hemorrhage is a differential diagnosis of aqueous misdirection but usually has a sudden painful onset often with severe loss of vision. It is usually associated with a sudden fall in IOP, ocular trauma or a Valsalva maneuver when the IOP is low. The suprachoroidal blood is best seen on ultrasound. While small hemorrhages may resolve spontaneously, larger ones require surgical drainage once the blood has liquefied.
- *Infection*:
  - Early post-trabeculectomy infections are rare and usually associated with a suture abscess and occasionally a bleb leak.

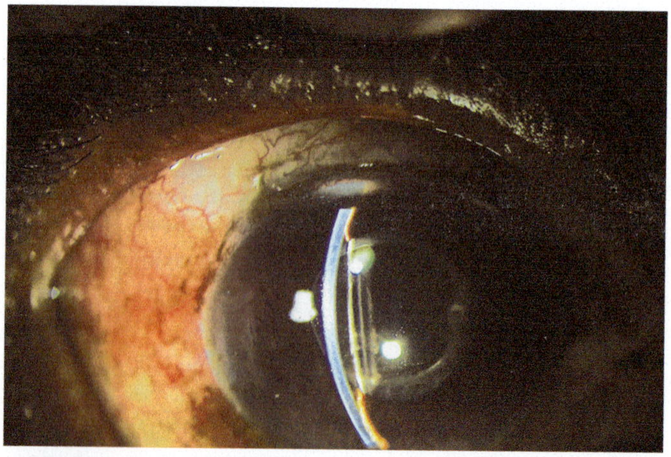

Fig. 67.12: Aqueous misdirection causing a shallow anterior chamber.
Source: Dr George Varghese Puthuran, Aravind Eye Hospital, Madurai, Tamil Nadu, India.

- Late infections are an important complication and always associated with a very thin bleb with or without a macroscopic leak. This is a requirement for bacteria to penetrate the conjunctival tissue. The blebitis that results need to be treated very aggressively to prevent the bacteria traveling through the sclerotomy and causing endophthalmitis (*see* Fig. 67.1). Unlike postcataract endophthalmitis, endophthalmitis secondary to blebitis is usually more aggressive and requires vitrectomy in addition to intravitreal antibiotics.

ACKNOWLEDGMENT

Dr Hamish Dunn [B Lib Stud, MBBS (Hons), FRANZCO] Clinical Lecturer, Sydney Medical School, University of Sydney, Sydney, NSW, Australia (for providing illustrations of this chapter).

SUGGESTED READING

1. Broadway DC, Chang LP. Trabeculectomy, risk factors for failure and the preoperative state of the conjunctiva. J Glaucoma. 2001;10(3):237-49.
2. Cairns JE. Trabeculectomy. Preliminary report of a new method. Am J Ophthalmol. 1968;66(4):673-9.
3. Dunn HP, Zheng L, White AJ, et al. Intraoperative transconjunctival mitomycin-C application for needle revision of trabeculectomy. Clin Exp Ophthalmol. 2016;44(7):640-2.
4. Fuller JR, Bevin TH, Molteno AC, et al. Anti-inflammatory fibrosis suppression in threatened trabeculectomy bleb failure produces good long term control of intraocular pressure without risk of sight threatening complications. Br J Ophthalmol. 2002;86(12):1352-4.
5. Healey PR, Crowston JG. Trypan blue identifies antimetabolite treatment area in trabeculectomy. Br J Ophthalmol. 2005;89(9):1152-6.
6. Pakravan M, Esfandiari H, Yazdani S, et al. Mitomycin C-augmented trabeculectomy: subtenon injection versus soaked sponges: a randomised clinical trial. Br J Ophthalmol. 2017;101(9):1275-80.
7. Wells AP, Ashraff NN, Hall RC, Purdie G. Comparison of two clinical Bleb grading systems. Ophthalmology. 2006 Jan;113(1):77-83.
8. Wells AP, Cordeiro MF, Bunce C, et al. Cystic bleb formation and related complications in limbus-versus fornix-based conjunctival flaps in pediatric and young adult trabeculectomy with mitomycin C. Ophthalmology. 2003;110(11):2192-7.

Chapter 68

Surgical Alternatives to Trabeculectomy in the Management of Glaucoma

Sabita M Ittoop, Leonard K Seibold, Malik Y Kahook

INTRODUCTION

Historically, the standard surgical options for lowering the intraocular pressure (IOP) in glaucomatous eyes involved the creation of filtration pathways to the sub-Tenon's space of the eye. These options include traditional trabeculectomy or guarded filtration surgery with implantation of an Ex-PRESS shunt (Alcon. Fort Worth, TX),[1] with or without antimetabolites, and a range of glaucoma drainage devices (GDD). Filtration procedures are sometimes associated with severe early and late complications that include bleb dysesthesia, hypotony, choroidal effusions, choroidal and retinal detachments, suprachoroidal hemorrhage, corneal decompensation, diplopia, and endophthalmitis. This has encouraged innovation and development of surgical alternatives that optimize physiologic outflow pathways with minimal disruption to the normal anatomy. These more recent options are associated with a shorter postoperative recovery, a lower rate of complications, and less severity of complications. This chapter is intended to be a concise overview of these newer procedures.

TRABECULAR MESHWORK BYPASS DEVICES

iStent Trabecular Micro-bypass Stent

The iStent (Glaukos Corp. San Clemente, CA)[2] is inserted through the trabecular meshwork and into the canal of Schlemm to bypass the focal resistance of the juxtacanalicular meshwork at the site of implantation (Fig. 68.1). This facilitates conventional aqueous outflow into Schlemm's canal and creates a pressure gradient that allows for increased outflow to the collector channels and the downstream episcleral veins.[2]

As the smallest device to be implanted in the human body, the iStent is an L-shaped stent comprised of surgical grade nonferromagnetic titanium that is heparin coated to facilitate self-priming. It is 1 mm in length, 0.33 mm in height, and weighs 60 µg. The footplate includes a self-trephining tip and three retention arches that facilitate entry and stability within Schlemm's canal. The snorkel portion is 0.25 mm long, with a 120 µm diameter, and resides in the anterior chamber. The trabecular meshwork is visualized with intraoperative gonioscopy and the device is deployed from a preloaded, handheld insertion device, using an ab interno approach.[2]

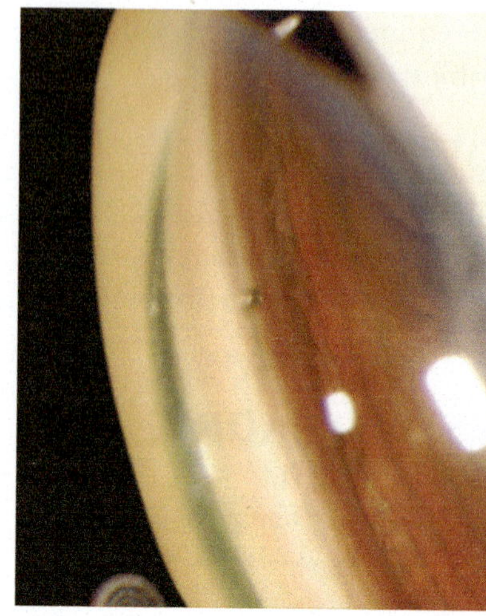

Fig. 68.1: Gonioscopic view of the first-generation iStent seated within Schlemm's canal.

In the Pivotal US Investigational Device Exemption (IDE) clinical trial, patients classified as having mild to moderate stage primary open-angle glaucoma (POAG) were randomized to cataract surgery plus one iStent versus cataract surgery alone. At 12 months, the number of patients with an IOP ≤ 21 mm Hg without glaucoma medications was significantly greater in the treatment group (72% vs. 50%, $p < 0.001$)[3] and remained statistically different at 24 months (61% vs. 50%, $p = 0.036$).[4] The number of patients with an IOP reduction more than or equal to 20% without glaucoma medications was also significantly higher in the treatment group at one year (66% vs. 48%, $p = 0.003$)[3] but not at 2 years of follow-up (61% vs. 54%, $p = 0.09$).[4] In addition, there was a significant delay in initiating postoperative glaucoma medications for patients in the iStent group ($p < 0.001$).

Only 15% of patients in the iStent group required glaucoma medications versus 35% of patients who underwent cataract surgery alone.[3]

Since the iStent is a focal bypass tract, the risk of hypotony is greatly reduced by the remaining, intact trabecular meshwork as well as the inherent resistance of episcleral venous pressure. No cases of hypotony were reported in the IDE trial. The most common adverse events observed for joint iStent implantation and cataract removal included early postoperative corneal edema (8%), BCVA loss of ≥ 1 line at or after the 3 months visit (7%), posterior capsular opacification (6%), stent malposition (2.6%), stent obstruction (4.3%), early postoperative anterior chamber cells (3%), and early postoperative corneal abrasion (3%).[3,4]

In June 2012, the US Food and Drug Administration (FDA) approved the placement of one iStent in conjunction with cataract surgery for the treatment of mild-to-moderate stage POAG.[2] However, studies have demonstrated a benefit to patients with secondary open-angle glaucoma (OAG) including pigmentary, pseudoexfoliative, steroid-induced, and traumatic glaucoma.[5] The iStent, as a stand-alone surgical procedure, and the placement of multiple iStents have shown a therapeutic effect, with the potential for increased efficacy with each additional implant.[6]

The iStent is not recommended in patients with corneal abnormalities that would inhibit a gonioscopic view of the angle and any alterations to the normal angle anatomy. Examples include primary or secondary angle closure glaucoma, neovascular glaucoma, Peters' anomaly, ICE syndrome, posterior polymorphous corneal dystrophy, or previous surgeries such as trabectome or canaloplasty.[2]

Also, it is contraindicated for patients with glaucoma secondary to elevated episcleral venous pressure (EVP), since outflow resistance at the trabecular meshwork is not the root cause of disease. Examples include active thyroid-related orbitopathy, retrobulbar tumors, carotid cavernous fistulas, or Sturge-Weber syndrome.[2]

The iStent is not recommended for Uveitic patients, since inflammatory cells, fibrin, and debris can obstruct the stent.[2]

iStent Inject

The iStent inject (Glaukos Corp. San Clemente, CA)[2] is the second-generation model of the original iStent. The injector is preloaded with two modified iStents to facilitate implantation during surgery. Each stent is a focal bypass tract through the trabecular meshwork that facilitates conventional outflow. The iStent inject, as a stand-alone procedure, has demonstrated equivalence to treatment with two glaucoma medications. Compared to baseline IOP, 94.7% in the iStent inject group maintained an unmedicated IOP reduction of ≥ 20% at 12 months compared to 91.8% in the medical therapy group.[7] Patient selection for the iStent inject, the risk profile, and contraindications to surgery are similar to that of the first-generation iStent. Currently, this model is not yet FDA approved, but clinical trials are going on to assess the safety and efficacy.[2]

Hydrus Microstent

The Hydrus Microstent (Ivantis Inc. Irvine, CA)[8] is a crescent-shaped trabecular bypass device that is made from nitinol, which is a nickel-titanium alloy with shape memory. It is 8 mm long with an open posterior surface and three windows on the anterior surface. The stent is threaded into Schlemm's canal from an ab interno approach such that the 1 mm inlet resides in the anterior chamber and the 7 mm scaffold segment resides within Schlemm's canal and spans 3 clock hours to facilitate canal dilation and allow access to multiple collector channels (Fig. 68.2).[8,9]

In the HYDRUS II study, patients with POAG were randomized to cataract surgery plus Hydrus implantation versus cataract surgery alone. At 24 months, the Hydrus treatment group demonstrated a greater proportion of patients with an IOP reduction ≥ 20% without ocular hypotensive medications (80% vs. 46%, p = 0.0008). In addition, the mean unmedicated IOP in the Hydrus group was significantly lower (16.9 ± 3.3 mm Hg vs. 19.2 ± 4.7 mm Hg, p = 0.0093) and the proportion of patients not treated with additional glaucoma medications was

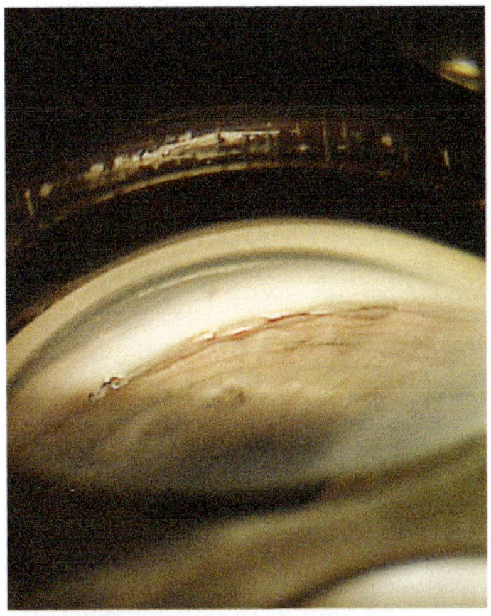

Fig. 68.2: Gonioscopic view of the Hydrus Microstent threaded into Schlemm's canal.[8]

significantly higher (73% vs. 38%, p = 0.0008). At 24 months, 18.8% of patients were noted to have focal iris adhesions to the device or angle structures at or near the anterior chamber inlet. Otherwise, the overall incidence of adverse events was nominal and comparable between the two groups. No cases of hypotony were reported.[9]

The guidelines for patient selection, risk profile, and contraindications for Hydrus implantation are similar to alternative trabecular meshwork bypass tract devices, as described above.

VISCODILATION AND STENTING OF SCHLEMM'S CANAL

Ab externo canaloplasty was introduced over 15 years ago as a nonpenetrating surgical treatment for POAG. The surgical procedure involves 360° circumferential catheterization and viscodilation of Schlemm's canal to reestablish and facilitate the natural trabecular-canalicular outflow of aqueous humor. After performing a conjunctival peritomy, two scleral flaps are constructed to unroof Schlemm's canal and to allow cannulation with the iTrack microcatheter (Ellex).[10] As the catheter is withdrawn, viscoelastic is injected to dilate the canal and a prolene suture is threaded back through the canal and tied with sufficient tension to stent open the canal.

Lewis et al. initially demonstrated the efficacy of the procedure. POAG patients with baseline IOP of 23.6 ± 4.8 mm Hg on 1.9 ± 0.8 glaucoma medications underwent canaloplasty or canaloplasty with cataract surgery. At 24 months, the mean postoperative IOP was 16.0 ± 4.2 mm Hg and mean glaucoma medications was 0.5 ± 0.8. Postoperative complications included hyphema (16.6%), transient IOP spike ≥ 30 mm Hg during the immediate postoperative period (7.9%), and hypotony (0.8%). There were no cases of choroidal detachment and corneal edema.[11]

Ab Interno Canaloplasty

Ab interno canaloplasty (AbiC) is a modification of the original surgery where the canal is viscodilated using the same microcatheter but performed under intraoperative gonioscopy and with an ab interno approach. The iTrack microcatheter is introduced into the eye through a small clear corneal incision and then threaded into the Schlemm's canal through a 1 mm goniotomy incision at the trabecular meshwork. The iTrack is slowly removed during viscodilation of Schlemm's canal. No tension suture is used in this approach.[10]

In a meta-analysis of two recent case series, the preliminary data demonstrated favorable results. A total of 228 patients with POAG underwent AbiC, with or without cataract surgery, with a preoperative mean IOP of 19.0 ± 6.5 mm Hg on an average of 2 glaucoma medications.[10] At 12 months, 48 patients had a mean IOP of 13.3 ± 2.0 mm Hg on an average of 1 glaucoma medication, suggesting a 30% decrease in IOP and 50% reduction in glaucoma medications.[12]

Candidates for AbiC include patients with open-angle glaucoma, a reliable gonioscopic view of the angle structures, and a normal angle anatomy. This category includes POAG, secondary OAG, juvenile glaucoma, patients with a previous history of selective laser trabeculoplasty or modest treatment with argon laser trabeculoplasty, and select patients with a previous history of trabeculectomy or glaucoma implant surgery. However, AbiC is not recommended in neovascular glaucoma, primary and secondary chronic angle closure glaucoma, traumatic glaucoma, and patients with elevated EVP.[10]

VISCO360

VISCO360 (Sight Sciences. Menlo Park, CA)[13] is a device that facilitates viscodilation of Schlemm's canal from an ab interno approach. The angle structures are visualized with intraoperative gonioscopy and the surgery is performed through a limbal, clear corneal incision. The stainless steel cannula is introduced into the anterior chamber and pierces the trabecular meshwork to create a goniotomy incision site. Then the 40 mm polymer microcatheter is threaded into Schlemm's canal. As the microcatheter is retracted, viscoelastic is dispensed to treat 180°. By rotation of the cannula, the device is primed to treat the remaining 2 quadrants. The company is currently participating in clinical trials to evaluate the safety and efficacy of the device.[13]

In one case-control study, 20 patients with POAG underwent ab interno canaloplasty using the VISCO360 and 10 POAG patients underwent trabecular meshwork excision with the Kahook Dual Blade (New World Medical. Rancho Cucamonga, CA).[14] The mean preoperative IOP and glaucoma medications for the VISCO360 group was 17.3 ± 3.2 mm Hg and 1.25 ± 0.79 medications compared to 18.1 ± 4.7 mm Hg and 1.7 ± 1.06 medications in the KDB cohort. At 6 months, the postoperative mean IOP was reduced to 15.6 ± 2.6 mm Hg with a mean of 0.94 ± 0.77 medications in the VISCO360 group and 12.0 ± 3.4 mm Hg on 0.7 ± 1.25 medications in the KDB group. Both groups demonstrated a noteworthy reduction in IOP and glaucoma medication usage that warrants further evaluation through clinical trials.[15]

Ab Interno Treatment of the Trabecular Meshwork

Single incision goniotomy and trabeculotomy have been the established choices for surgical management of pediatric glaucoma.[16] Both surgeries focus on the disruption and opening of the trabecular meshwork, which allows aqueous humor to have direct access to the collector channels and the venous system. While historically used for pediatric glaucoma, goniotomy has also been extensively used to treat adult glaucomas for decades, with variable success. Scarring of the residual trabecular meshwork leaflets is one of the obstacles to success in adults. Over the past decade, new minimally invasive, ab interno strategies have emerged to surgically open, and in some cases, remove the diseased trabecular meshwork to treat adult glaucoma, with noteworthy results.

Trabectome

The Trabectome (NeoMedix. Tustin, CA)[17] is a surgical instrument that performs ab interno, electrocautery of the trabecular meshwork and was approved by the FDA in 2004 for treatment of glaucoma. The handpiece consists of three main components: an insulated polymer footplate to prevent damage to adjacent tissues, a 19.5 gauge tip that allows for tissue ablation, and an irrigation aspiration port to stabilize the anterior chamber, dissipate heat, and aspirate debris. The handpiece is connected to an external console that contains the electrocautery generator and irrigation aspiration unit. A foot pedal allows the surgeon to navigate between 3 functions: irrigation, aspiration, and electrocautery.[17,18]

During surgery, the angle structures are visualized with intraoperative gonioscopy and the handpiece is introduced into the eye through a clear corneal incision. As the instrument approaches the nasal quadrant, the tip of the footplate pierces the trabecular meshwork to enter Schlemm's canal and the target tissues are treated using short bursts of high-frequency electrocautery. The recommended power setting range is 0.5–1.5 W, which can be titrated by 0.1 W units to reach a maximum of 10 W.[17,18]

Numerous studies have demonstrated the safety and efficacy of trabectome as a minimally invasive ab interno procedure. Minckler et al. published one of the largest retrospective case series involving 1,127 patients with POAG or secondary OAG that were treated with trabectome alone or trabectome with phacoemulsification. A subset of patients had a prior ocular history that included laser trabeculoplasty, trabeculectomy, GDD, as well as other corneal and retinal surgeries. The trabectome alone cohort, with a mean preoperative IOP of 25.7 ± 7.7 mm Hg, demonstrated a 40% decrease in IOP at 24 months (n = 46), 41% at 36 months (n = 35), and 32% at 60 months (n = 2). The number of glaucoma medications was reduced from 2.9 ± 1.3 preoperatively to 1.8 ± 1.4 at final follow-up. Patients that underwent trabectome with phacoemulsification had a mean preoperative IOP of 20.0 ± 6.2 mm Hg. This cohort demonstrated a 21% decrease at 6 months (n = 143) and 18% at 12 months (n = 45).[18]

In the trabectome alone cohort, 14% of patients needed additional glaucoma laser and/or surgery to maintain IOP control, with a majority of patients undergoing additional treatment during the first postoperative year. The most common adverse events among all cases included transient elevation of IOP defined as IOP > 10 mm Hg above baseline on postoperative day 1 (5.8%) and intraoperative blood reflux (78%). No cases of postoperative endophthalmitis or choroidal hemorrhage have been reported.[18]

In another retrospective study comparing Trabectome alone to trabeculectomy, much better success was observed in the trabeculectomy group, where Trabectome alone demonstrated a 22.4% versus 76.1% success rate at 2 years ($p < 0.001$). Younger age and lower baseline IOP were significant risk factors for long-term failure for trabectome.[19]

Gonioscopy-assisted Transluminal Trabeculotomy

The gonioscopy-assisted transluminal trabeculotomy (GATT) procedure was first reported in 2011 as a novel means of achieving a 360° trabeculotomy. Similar to other angle procedures, the angle structures are visualized with intraoperative gonioscopy and the surgery is performed through a limbal, clear corneal incision. A goniotomy incision site is created and a suture or the iTrack illuminated microcatheter is threaded into Schlemm's canal for 360°, then it is manually pulled through the trabecular meshwork into the anterior chamber, thus creating a 360° goniotomy.[20,21]

In a preliminary study, 85 patients with POAG underwent GATT, with or without combined cataract surgery. At 6 months, the IOP decreased by 7.7 mm Hg ± 6.2 mm Hg (30%, p < 0.001) with an average decrease of 0.9 ± 1.3 glaucoma medications, from baseline. The 12 months data revealed an IOP decrease of 11.1 ± 6.1 mm Hg (39.8%, p < 0.001) with an average decrease of 1.1 glaucoma medications, from baseline. For secondary OAG patients,

IOP decreased by 19.9 ± 10.2 mm Hg (56.8% $p < 0.001$) with an average of 1.9 fewer glaucoma medications, at 12 months. The most common complication was transient hyphema (30%), which persisted past postoperative week 1, and 9% of patients needed additional glaucoma surgery to maintain IOP control.[20]

It has been previously suggested that successful incisional surgery results in a collapse or decrease in the size of Schlemm's canal that results in an underperfusion of the trabecular meshwork and accumulation of extracellular material leading to an increased resistance of conventional outflow. Grover et al. demonstrated that GATT goniotomy has a role in the surgical management of patients with OAG and prior incisional surgery. By removing the resistance at the trabecular meshwork, there is additional egress of aqueous humor to the downstream collector channels. In one report, 35 patients with POAG and prior incisional surgery including trabeculectomy, GDD, prior trabectome and endocyclophotocoagulation (ECP) underwent GATT to treat 270° or more. The mean preoperative IOP was 25.7 ± 6.5 mm Hg on 3.2 ± 1.0 medications. At 24 months, the mean IOP was reduced to 15.4 ± 4.9 mm Hg on 2.0 ± 1.4 medications ($p < 0.001$).[21]

Gonioscopy-assisted transluminal trabeculotomy is associated with several intraoperative and postoperative complications, including Descemet's membrane detachment, corneal edema, iridodialysis, and cystoid macular edema. Hyphema is the most commonly occurring complication.[20]

Recommended absolute contraindications for the GATT procedure include an inability to stop anticoagulation medication, a bleeding diathesis, and an unstable intraocular lens, inability to clearly identify the angle structures, angle-closure glaucoma, and severe corneal endothelial compromise. Relative contraindications include prior corneal transplant surgery and an inability to maintain head elevation ≥30° for the first 2 weeks, postoperatively.[21]

Kahook Dual Blade Goniotomy

The Kahook Dual Blade (New World Medical. Rancho Cucamonga, CA)[14] is an ophthalmic knife that facilitates the sectoral incision and removal of the trabecular meshwork through a small clear corneal incision under intraoperative gonioscopy. This modified goniotomy is offered as a minimally invasive ab interno procedure for the surgical management of a wide range of glaucomas. While designed as a standalone treatment of glaucoma, the device can also be combined with other procedures including cataract extraction. The surgical grade stainless steel body has a pointed tip that facilitates entry through the trabecular meshwork and a ramp that lifts and stretches the trabecular meshwork tissue as the device is advanced while seated against the anterior wall of Schlemm's canal. There are two parallel blades that create paired incisions to achieve excision of a precise strip of trabecular meshwork (Figs. 68.3 and 68.4). The footplate is microengineered to prevent damage to the outer wall of the canal and enables smooth advancement during treatment.[14,22]

Greenwood et al. reported a case series that included 71 eyes that underwent cataract surgery and goniotomy with the Kahook dual blade. At 6 months, the preoperative mean IOP decreased from 17.4 ± 5.2 mm Hg to 12.8 ±

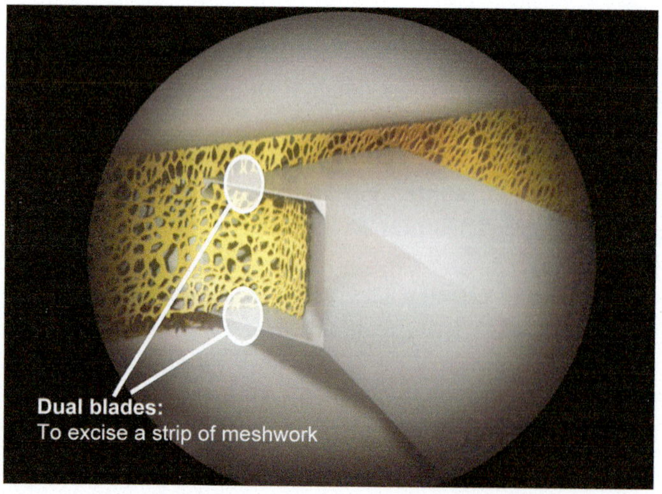

Fig. 68.3: Kahook dual blade ophthalmic knife creating parallel and paired incisions.[14]

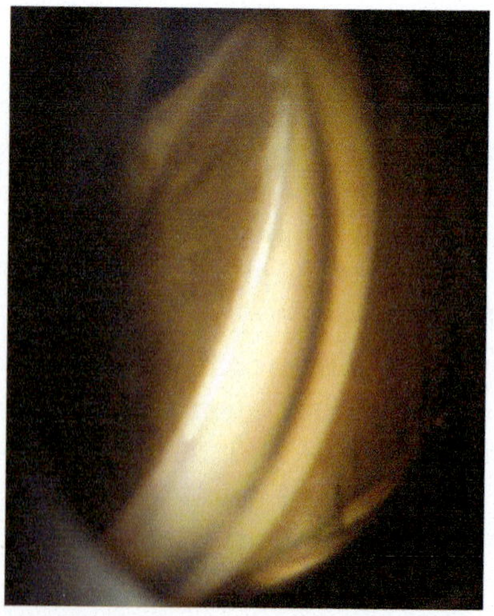

Fig. 68.4: Gonioscopic view of the angle structures after the excision of a precise strip of trabecular meshwork with Kahook dual blade. *Source:* Leonard K Seibold.

2.6 mm Hg ($p < 0.001$) with a decrease in the average glaucoma medication usage from 1.6 ± 1.3 to 0.9 ± 1.0 ($p = 0.005$). The most common observation was reflux of blood at the site of trabecular meshwork removal that allowed exposure of the collector channels (39.4%).[23]

Radcliffe et al. reported a prospective case series that included 122 patients with POAG, angle-closure glaucoma, pigmentary, and pseduoexfoliation glaucoma that underwent goniotomy with the Kahook dual blade, with or without phacoemulsification. Disease severity ranged from mild to end stage. For all patients, the preoperative mean IOP was 18.7 ± 6.7 mm Hg with a mean glaucoma medication usage of 1.8 ± 1.3. At 12 months, there was a significant and sustained reduction in IOP of 30% (-5.7 mm Hg) and 70% of eyes had a reduction of at least one medication. Postoperative mean IOP was reduced to 13.0 ± 2.6 mm Hg while mean glaucoma medication usage fell to 1.0 ± 1.2.[24]

TRAB360

TRAB360 (Sight Sciences. Menlo Park, CA)[13] is a disposable trabeculotome that facilitates removal of the trabecular meshwork. Manufacturing of the handheld device is similar to the VISCO360 device, with similar surgical steps. The angle structures are visualized with intraoperative gonioscopy and the stainless steel cannula is introduced into the anterior chamber and pierces the trabecular meshwork to create a goniotomy incision site. The 40 mm polymer probe is threaded 180° into Schlemm's canal. The device is then maneuvered so that the probe incises the trabecular meshwork for 180° while being manually withdrawn. After the device is reset, rotation of the cannula allows for treatment of the remaining 2 quadrants.[13]

Sarkisian et al. reported a retrospective review of 26 eyes that underwent ab interno trabeculotomy using the TRAB360 device. The preoperative IOP was reduced from 19.8 ± 6.4 mm Hg to 13.5 ± 4.6 mm Hg, at the end of follow-up. Use of glaucoma medications was reduced from a mean of 1.1 ± 1.2 to 0.2 ± 0.5 with 73% of patients requiring no medications. The most frequent complication was transient hyphema.[25]

Supraciliary Bypass Devices

The lack of epithelium at the ciliary body face and iris root allows aqueous humor to passively flow into the space between the choroid and sclera known as the suprachoroidal space, where it is eventually removed by the venous and lymphatic system. This uveoscleral outflow is also known as the unconventional pathway and is driven by the hydrostatic pressure gradient between the anterior chamber and suprachoroidal space.

CyPass

The CyPass device (Alcon. Fort Worth, TX) is a supraciliary microshunt designed to facilitate controlled aqueous outflow from the anterior chamber into the suprachoroidal space. The 6.35 mm, flexible implant is constructed from a biocompatible polyimide material. The main body has a 300 μm inner lumen diameter, a 430 μm outer lumen diameter, and 64 fenestrations that allow for controlled egress of aqueous humor into the suprachoroidal space. Three retention rings that are 510 μm in diameter, provide stability of the shunt once inserted (Fig. 68.5).[1]

During surgery, the angle is visualized with intraoperative gonioscopy and the inserter is introduced into the eye through a clear corneal incision. A blunt-tipped guidewire creates a controlled disinsertion of the ciliary body from the sclera then the CyPass microshunt is threaded along the guidewire and into the cyclodialysis cleft. Then the guidewire is retracted and the inserter is removed from the anterior chamber.[1]

In the CyPass Clinical Experience (cyCLE) study, 167 eyes with POAG underwent cataract surgery with CyPass placement. For all eyes, the preoperative mean baseline IOP of 20.2 ± 6.0 mm Hg was reduced to 15.9 ± 3.1 mm Hg, at 12 months. Patients with IOP ≥ 21 mm Hg demonstrated a 35% decrease in mean IOP and a 49% reduction in mean glaucoma medication usage, whereas patients with an IOP < 21 mm Hg demonstrated a 75% reduction in mean

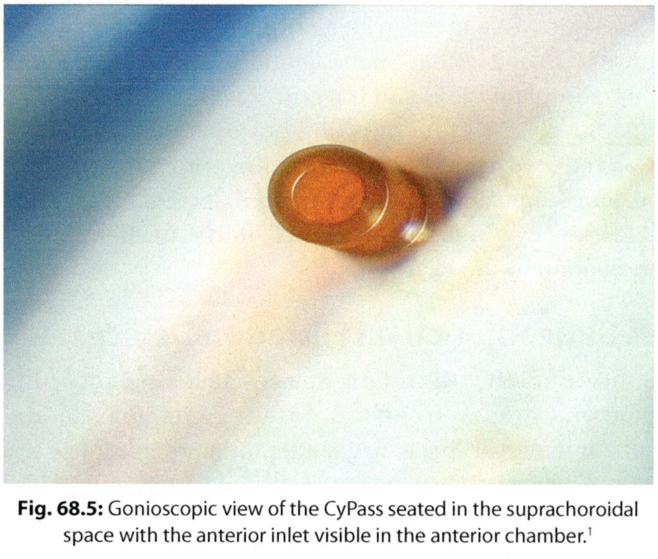

Fig. 68.5: Gonioscopic view of the CyPass seated in the suprachoroidal space with the anterior inlet visible in the anterior chamber.[1]

medication usage while maintaining a mean IOP < 21 mm Hg. At 12 months, the most common adverse event was transient hypotony (IOP ≤ 6 mm Hg, 13.8%) that resolved after 4 weeks and did not require additional surgical intervention. Other adverse events included elevated IOP (>30 mm Hg or increase from baseline IOP of >10 mm Hg, 3%), transient postoperative hyphema (1.2%) that resolved at postoperative week 1, and stent obstruction due to malposition (5.4%) with 1 patient needing stent repositioning. There were no cases of suprachoroidal hemorrhage or effusion, retinal detachment, or hyptony resulting in a flat anterior chamber.[26]

The FDA approved the CyPass in July 2016.[1] In the FDA COMPASS trial, 505 patients with POAG were randomized to cataract surgery alone (control) or cataract surgery with CyPass placement. At 24 months, 77% of CyPass patients versus 60% of controls achieved the primary outcome of a 20% or greater reduction in unmedicated IOP (p = 0.001). The secondary outcome evaluated the proportion of subjects that maintained an unmedicated IOP between 6 and 18 mm Hg, at follow-up. At 12 months, 67% of CyPass patients versus 59% of controls did not require IOP medications, which was maintained at 24 months (65% versus. 44%). Adverse events include elevated IOP > 10 mm Hg above baseline (4.3%), hypotony (2.9%), transient hyphema (2.7%), stent obstruction (2.1%) and cyclodialysis cleft > 2 mm (1.9%).[27]

iStent Supra® Suprachoroidal Micro-bypass Stent

The iStent Supra® (Glaukos Corp. San Clemente, CA) is a 4 mm supraciliary shunt made of polyethersulfone and titanium. Similar to the CyPass shunt, it is implanted into the suprachoroidal space from an ab interno approach.[2] In one case series, 73 patients with an unmedicated preoperative mean IOP of 24.8 ± 1.7 mm Hg underwent a single iStent Supra implantation, and travoprost was prescribed post-operatively. At 12 months, the postoperative mean IOP was reduced to 13.2 mm Hg on travoprost therapy. No major complications were reported.[28] Currently, the safety and efficacy of the iStent Supra is under further clinical evaluation by the FDA.[2]

Subconjunctival Filtration Devices

Subconjunctival filtration devices focus on diverting aqueous humor from the anterior chamber to the subconjunctival space, while attempting to minimize the complications associated with trabeculectomy and GDDs.

Xen Gel Stent

The fundamental design of the XEN Gel Stent (Allergan. Dublin, Ireland) is based on the Hagen-Poiseuille equation that calculates the resistance to flow through a cylindrical tube. Based on this equation, a longer thinner tube will provide more resistance to outflow and therefore, reduce the risk of hypotony. The XEN Gel Stent is a hydrophilic tube composed of a porcine gelatin cross-linked with glutaraldehyde, with an inner lumen diameter of 45 μm, outer lumen diameter of 150 μm, and a length of 6 mm that allows an estimated aqueous filtration rate of 2–2.5 μL/min.[29]

Using intraoperative gonioscopy and an ab interno approach, the preloaded 27-gauge inserter is introduced into the eye through an inferotemporal, clear corneal incision. The XEN Gel Stent is then inserted at the scleral spur and tracked 3.0 mm posterior to the limbus to exit the sclera into the subconjunctival space, to create a shallow bleb (Figs. 68.6 and 68.7).[29] Although the procedure creates a filtration bleb, the ab interno creation of the filtration pathway obviates the need for conjunctival or scleral dissection and suturing. The procedure is often augmented with the application of subconjunctival MMC, typically by injection, at the beginning of the procedure.

In the IDE clinical trial, 65 patients were implanted with the XEN45 Gel Stent. At 12 months, 76.3% of patients obtained an IOP reduction of ≥ 20% from baseline on the same or fewer glaucoma medications, with a mean

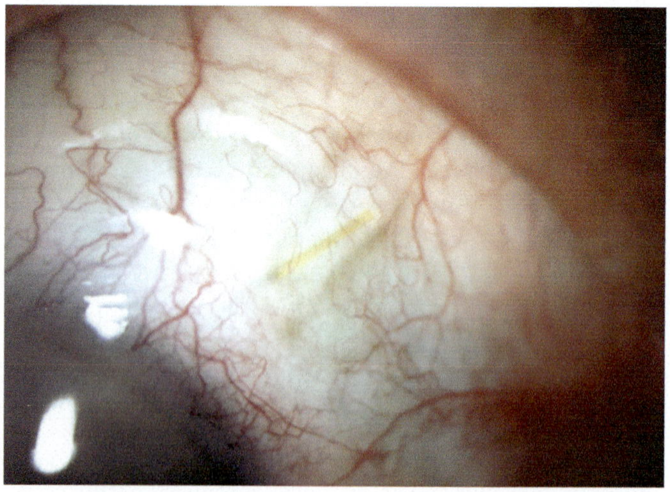

Fig. 68.6: Slit-lamp photograph of the posterior segment of the XEN Gel stent seated in the subconjunctival space.
Source: Leonard K Seibold.

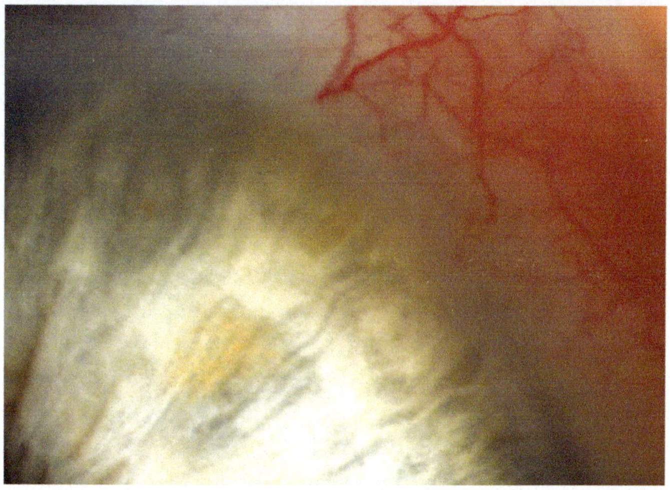

Fig. 68.7: Slit-lamp photograph of the anterior segment of the XEN Gel stent seated in the anterior chamber.
Source: Leonard K Seibold.

IOP reduction of 6.4 ± 1.1 mm Hg. The mean number of glaucoma medications at baseline was 3.5 ± 1.0 compared to 1.7 ± 1.5 at 12 months. The need for additional glaucoma surgery, hypotony defined as IOP < 6 mm Hg, IOP increase ≥ 10 mm Hg from baseline, and needling procedures were cited as the most common adverse events.[30] Other complications include choroidal effusion, hyphema, hypotony, implant migration or exposure, and wound leak.[29]

In November 2016, the FDA approved the XEN Gel Stent for patients with refractory glaucoma despite previous surgical treatment and maximum tolerated medical therapy. It is contraindicated in primary and secondary angle closure glaucoma, patients with conjunctival scarring from prior surgery or trauma in the targeted quadrant of implantation, active neovascular glaucoma, in patients with an anterior chamber IOL, patients with intraocular silicone oil, and the presence of vitreous in the anterior chamber.[29,30]

InnFocus MicroShunt

The InnFocus Microshunt (Santen. Miami, FL) is a 8.5 mm shunt, with a 70 μm lumen, that is made of a nonreactive, non-erodible material known as SIBS.[31] Similar to the insertion of other GDDs, the InnFocus Microshunt is implanted into a sub-Tenon's pocket that is dissected from a limbal peritomy and placed beneath a 1 × 1 mm scleral flap. Subconjunctival mitomycin C is typically applied, by injection or sponges, before insertion to minimize fibrosis. A 25 or 27 gauge needle is used to create a sclerotomy beneath the scleral flap just above the iris plane, which is then used for insertion of the InnFocus Microshunt. A triangular fin on the shaft helps to lock the implant into place and prevent migration into the anterior chamber.[32]

One case series includes 23 patients with refractory OAG glaucoma that were treated with intraoperative, sub-Tenon's mitomycin C and implantation of the InnFocus Microshunt, with or without cataract surgery. Success was defined as an IOP ≤ 14 mm Hg and IOP reduction ≥ 20% from baseline, which was achieved in 100% (year 1), 91% (year 2), and 95% (year 3) of patients. The mean preoperative baseline IOP was 23.8 ± 5.3 mm Hg. Patients demonstrated a mean reduction of 10.7 ± 2.8 mm Hg (55%, year 1), 11.9 ± 3.7 mm Hg (50%, year 2), and 10.7± 3.5 mm Hg (55%, year 3). The mean number of glaucoma medications was reduced from 2.4 ± 0.9 to 0.3± 0.8 (year 1), 0.4± 1.0 (year 2) and 0.7 ± 1.1 (year 3). The most common adverse events reported were shallow chamber, hypotony, hyphema, and choroidal effusions that were transient and did not require further intervention.[32]

Cycloablative Procedures

Traditional glaucoma surgeries focus on the creation of novel pathways for aqueous drainage, while the more modern, minimally invasive, ab interno procedures seek to improve IOP through augmentation of physiologic aqueous outflow pathways. An alternative method of IOP reduction is through aqueous suppression through cycloablative procedures that destroy the aqueous producing ciliary epithelium. Historically, these procedures have been reserved for eyes with poor visual potential or glaucoma refractory to incisional outflow surgeries due to the severity of its associated complications that include hypotony and phthisis from overtreatment. Newer methods for cycloablation have been developed for a more precise ablation of the ciliary epithelium with minimal collateral damage.

Continuous Transscleral Cyclophotocoagulation

Transscleral cyclophotocoagulation (TSCPC) is a non-incisional procedure by which energy from an 810 nm diode laser is transmitted through direct contact with the ocular surface and is absorbed by the pigmented ciliary body tissues as thermal energy to induce coagulative damage to the ciliary epithelium. This results in a reduction of aqueous humor production to lower IOP. Collateral damage to the ciliary muscle and blood vessels may also occur. The treatment is delivered through the wedge shaped, polished tip of a G-probe handle (IRIDEX. Mountain View, CA) that is designed to center treatment 1.2 mm posterior to the surgical limbus.[33] A foot pedal controls laser delivery while the probe is positioned by the surgeon. Due to its noninvasive nature, the procedure can be performed in the office setting or operating room; however, a retrobulbar or peribulbar block is required for pain control.

Kosoko et al. reported the long-term outcomes of TSCPC treatment, with a continuous 810 nm diode laser for refractory, severe stage glaucoma (BCVA 20/400 or worse). A total of 27 patients underwent a standardized laser treatment with a power range of 1.75–2.0 W, 2 second duration, and 17–19 applications to treat 270° of the limbal circumference. The mean baseline IOP was 36.4 ± 12.4 mm Hg with a range of 20–70 mm Hg and was significantly reduced to 20.3 ± 8.7 mm Hg at last follow-up. The most common adverse events include patient discomfort that lasted more than 1 week (48%), anterior chamber inflammation that lasted more than 6 weeks (48%), and the need for repeat TSCPC treatment (7%).[34]

Micropulse Transscleral Cyclophotocoagulation

Historically, direct contact, continuous TSCPC is known to be a painful procedure that is associated with a high risk of hypotony, chronic uveitis, and phthisis bulbi. To mitigate these complications, the micropulse diode laser delivers 810 nm infrared diode laser radiation in a series of repetitive short pulses of energy alternating between rest periods. The curved tip of the MicroPulse P3 probe (IRIDEX. Mountain view, CA) is designed to allow the surgeon to move the probe in a fluid, continuous motion and to center treatment 3 mm posterior to the surgical limbus to allow for transscleral cyclophotocoagulation of the pars plana.[35]

Initial clinical studies have shown positive results. In a randomized, exploratory study, 48 patients with refractory glaucoma received either micropulse or continuous TSCPC.

The primary outcome was defined as an IOP between 6 and 21 mm Hg and at least a 30% reduction in IOP. At 12 months, 75% of the micropulse TSCPC patients and 29% of the continuous TSCPC patients achieved the primary outcome ($p < 0.01$). At 18 months, the success rates fell to 52% versus 30%, respectively ($p = 0.13$). Prolonged anterior chamber inflammation (4% vs. 30%) and phthisis bulbi (0% vs. 4%) were less prominent in the micropulse TSCPC diode cohort.[35]

Endoscopic Cyclophotocoagulation

The TSCPC is performed without direct visualization of the target tissues. This can lead to inadequate treatment or excessive treatment with collateral tissue damage, which is associated with an increased risk of vision-threatening complications. Endoscopic cyclophotocoagulation (ECP) is an ab interno approach to ciliary body ablation that optimizes treatment by direct visualization.[36]

The handheld endoscope (Beaver-Visitec Inc, Waltham, MA) couples a 175 W xenon light source for illumination, 810 nm diode laser for photocoagulation, helium-neon laser aiming beam, and video imaging for intraocular visualization.[37] Initially, the laser is set on continuous duration at 0.25 W and an aiming beam setting of 20–30, then titrated depending on response to treatment. The curved or straight endoscope is then introduced into the anterior chamber or pars plana through a 2 mm incision and up to 270° of the ciliary processes are treated under direct visualization (Fig. 68.8).[36] A second incision opposite the first can allow a full 360° of treatment for further IOP reduction.

Several studies have demonstrated the efficacy and safety of ECP in mild-to-moderate glaucoma, pediatric glaucoma, neovascular glaucoma, and refractory glaucoma despite previous TSCPC and/or surgical intervention. It has demonstrated equivalence to trabeculectomy and Ahmed glaucoma implant surgery, in limited clinical trials. Complications associated with ECP are chronic uveitis, hyphema, cystoid macular edema, and choroidal detachment.[36]

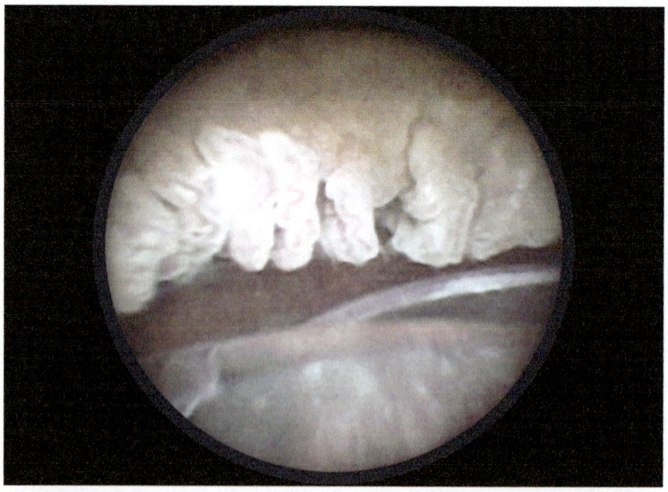

Fig. 68.8: Endoscopic cyclophotocoagulation of the ciliary processes under direct, intraocular visualization using the Endo Optiks Laser Endoscopy. *Source:* Malik Y Kahook.

Francis et al. compared combined ECP and cataract surgery versus cataract surgery alone in 80 patients with medically controlled OAG. The baseline mean IOP was 18.1 ± 3.0 mm Hg and decreased in both groups, however the ECP group achieved a lower IOP (16.0 ± 2.8 vs. 17.5 ± 3.6 mm Hg at 1 year, 16.0 ± 3.3 vs. 17.3 ± 3.2 mm Hg at 2 years) with a lower mean number of glaucoma medications (1.5 ± 0.8 vs. 1.8 ± 1.2 at 1 year, 0.4 ± 0.7 vs. 2.0 ± 1.0 at 2 years). The difference in IOP and medication reduction between the 2 groups was statistically significant across all time points.[38]

Kahook et al. compared outcomes of cataract surgery with ECP from 1 corneal incision site (n = 15, preoperative IOP 23.60 ± 3.89 mm Hg) that left 60 to 120° of untreated ciliary processes with 2 corneal incision sites (n = 25, preoperative IOP 24.48 ± 8.99 mm Hg) that allowed access to the subincisional ciliary processes and a more complete 360° treatment. At 3 months, IOP decreased to 17.93 ± 4.38 mm Hg for patients with one-site versus 13.88 ± 3.22 mm Hg that underwent a two-site approach. At 6 months, the postoperative IOP was 16 ± 2.77 mm Hg for 1-site and 13 ± 3.09 mm Hg for two-site with a lower glaucoma medication requirement in the two-site group (1.93 ± 0.88 vs. 0.52 ± 0.59, respectively). This study suggests that ECP treatment can be titrated and that a two-site approach allows for a greater IOP reduction and less dependence on glaucoma medications.[39]

CONCLUSION

There has been a substantial increase in the number of devices and procedures for the surgical management of glaucoma. These added options allow physicians to contemplate multiple alternatives to trabeculectomy and GDDs that tailor treatment based on a patient's individual needs and existing pathology. Although these surgeries are associated with an improved safety profile and faster postoperative recovery, most have consistently demonstrated a more moderate IOP reduction, as compared to traditional filtration surgeries for glaucoma management. Perhaps these newer procedures will allow for a paradigm shift towards earlier intervention for less advanced glaucoma patients, where modest IOP reductions may be adequate to stabilize their glaucomatous optic neuropathy. Future prospective and comparative studies will help to define the role that these surgeries hold in our practice patterns.

REFERENCES

1. My ALCON. GLAUCOMA SURGERY.[online] Available from: *https://www.myalconstore.com/glaucoma-surgery/*. [Accessed December 2017].
2. GLAUKOS. The iStent Procedure.[online] Available from: *http://www.glaukos.com/istent-procedure/*. [Accessed December 2017].
3. Samuelson TW, Katz LJ, Wells JM, et al. Randomized evaluation of the trabecular micro-bypass stent with phacoemulsification in patients with glaucoma and cataract. Ophthalmology. 2011;118(3):459-67.
4. Craven ER, Katz LJ, Wells JM, et al. Cataract surgery with trabecular micro-bypass stent implantation in patients with mild-to-moderate open-angle glaucoma and cataract: Two-year follow-up. J Cataract Refract Surg. 2012;38(8):1339-45.
5. Buchacra O, Duch S, Milla E, et al. One-year analysis of the istent trabecular microbypass in secondary glaucoma. Clin Ophthalmol. 2011;5(1):321-6.
6. Donnenfeld ED, Solomon KD, Voskanyan L, et al. A prospective 3-year follow-up trial of implantation of two trabecular microbypass stents in open-angle glaucoma. Clin Ophthalmol. 2015;9:2057-65.
7. Fea AM, Belda JI, Rekas M, et al. Prospective unmasked randomized evaluation of the iStent inject® versus two ocular hypotensive agents in patients with primary open-angle glaucoma. Clin Ophthalmol. 2014;8:875-82.
8. IVANTIS. Developmemt of new and innovative solutions for glaucoma. [online]. Available from: *http://www.ivantisinc.com/*. [Accessed December 2017].
9. Pfeiffer N, Garcia-Feijoo J, Martinez-de-la-Casa JM, et al. A randomized trial of a Schlemm's canal microstent with phacoemulsification for reducing intraocular pressure in open-angle glaucoma. Ophthalmology. 2015;122(7):1283-93.
10. ELLEX. Selective laser Trabeculoplasty.[online] Available from: *http://www.ellex.com/physicians/product-portfolio/*. [Accessed December 2017].
11. Lewis RA, von Wolff K, Tetz M, et al. Canaloplasty: circumferential viscodilation and tensioning of Schlemm's canal using a flexible microcatheter for the treatment of open-angle glaucoma in adults: interim clinical study analysis. J Cataract Refract Surg. 2007;33(7):1217-26.
12. Khaimi M. Ab Interno Canaloplasty for Open-Angle Glaucoma. Abstr ASCR, 2016.
13. SIGHT SCIENCES. A vision in Mind. [online]. Available from: *http://sightsciences.com/us/sightsciences/*. [Accessed December 2017].
14. KAHOOK DUAL BLADE (New World Medical). Kahook Dual Blade. [online]. Available from: *http://www.kdbcert.com/*. [Accessed December 2017].
15. Tracer N, Ayoub S, Alvarez D, et al. Comparison of Outcomes between Kahook Dual Blade and VISCO360 in the Treatment of Primary Open-angle Glaucoma. Poster ARVO, 2017.

16. Morales J, Al Shahwan S, Al Odhayb S, et al. Current surgical options for the management of pediatric glaucoma. J Ophthalmol. 2013;2013:763-5.
17. NEOMEDIX. Trabectome. [online]. Available from: *https://www.neomedix.net/Home.* [Accessed December 2017].
18. Minckler D, Mosaed S, Dustin L, et al. Trabectome (trabeculectomy-internal approach): additional experience and extended follow-up. Trans Am Ophthalmol Soc. 2008;106:149-60.
19. Jea SY, Francis BA, Vakili G, et al. Ab interno trabeculectomy versus trabeculectomy for open-angle glaucoma. Ophthalmology. 2012;119(1):36-42.
20. Grover DS, Godfrey DG, Smith O, et al. Gonioscopy-assisted transluminal trabeculotomy, Ab interno trabeculotomy: Technique report and preliminary results. Ophthalmology. 2014;121(4):855-61.
21. Grover DS, Godfrey DG, Smith O, et al. Outcomes of gonioscopy-assisted transluminal trabeculotomy (GATT) in eyes with prior incisional glaucoma surgery. J Glaucoma. 2017;26(1):41-5.
22. SooHoo JR, Seibold LK, Kahook MY. Ab Interno trabeculectomy in the adult patient. Middle East Afr J Ophthalmol. 2015;22(1):25-9.
23. Greenwood MD, Seibold LK, Radcliffe NM, et al. Goniotomy with a single-use dual blade: short-term results. J Cataract Refract Surg. 2017;43(9):1197-201.
24. Radcliffe MN, Abdullah S, Jasek MC, et al. A Novel Dual Blade Device for Goniotomy: 12 Month Follow-up. Poster AGS, 2017.
25. Sarkisian S, Allan EJ, Ding K, et al. New Way for Ab Interno Trabeculotomy: Initial Results. Poster ASCRS 2015.
26. Hoeh H, Vold S, Ahmed IK, et al. Initial clinical experience with the CyPass Micro-stent: safety and surgical outcomes of a novel supraciliary microstent. J Glaucoma. 2016;25(1):106-12.
27. Vold S, Ahmed II, Craven ER, et al. Two-year COMPASS trial results: supraciliary microstenting with phacoemulsification in patients with open-angle glaucoma and cataracts. Ophthalmology. 2016;123(10):2103-12.
28. Jünemann A. Twelve-month Outcomes Following Ab Interno Implantation of Suprachoroidal Stent and Postoperative Administration of Travoprost to treat Open Angle Glaucoma. Poster ESCRS, 2013.
29. XEN GEL STENT (Allergan). The XEN Gel Stent. [online] Available from: *https://www.xengelstent.com/.* [Accessed December 2017].
30. Food and Drug Administration. FDA 510(k) Summary: XEN Glaucoma Treatment System.[online] Available from: *https://www.accessdata.fda.gov/cdrh_docs/pdf16/K161457.pdf.* [Accessed December 2017].
31. INNFOCUS (santen). InnFocus Microshunt. [online] Available from: *http://innfocusinc.com/.* [Accessed December 2017].
32. Batlle JF, Fantes F, Riss I, et al. Three-year follow-up of a novel Aqueous Humor MicroShunt. J Glaucoma. 2016;25(2):e58-65.
33. IRIDEX. MicroPulse Technology. [online] Available from: *http://iridex.com/.* [Accessed December 2017].
34. Kosoko O, Gaasterland DE, Pollack IP, et al. Long-term outcome of initial ciliary ablation with contact diode laser transscleral cyclophotocoagulation for severe glaucoma. Ophthalmology. 1996;103(8):1294-302.
35. Aquino MC, Barton K, Tan AM, et al. Micropulse versus continuous wave transscleral diode cyclophotocoagulation in refractory glaucoma: a randomized exploratory study. Clin Exp Ophthalmol. 2015;43(1):40-6.
36. Seibold LK, SooHoo JR, Kahook MY. Endoscopic cyclophotocoagulation. Middle East Afr J Ophthalmol. 2015;22(1):18-24.
37. BEAVER-VISITEC INC. Endo Optiks Laser Endoscopy. [online] Available from: *http://www.beaver-visitec.com/products/endoscopy/.* [Accessed December 2017].
38. Francis BA, Berke SJ, Dustin L, Noecker R. Endoscopic cyclophotocoagulation combined with phacoemulsification versus phacoemulsification alone in medically controlled glaucoma. J Cataract Refract Surg. 2014;40(8):1313-21.
39. Kahook MY, Lathrop KL, Noecker RJ. One-site versus two-site endoscopic cyclophotocoagulation. J Glaucoma. 2007;16(6):527-30.

Part 9 Pediatric Ophthalmology and Strabismus

■ *Michael O'Keeffe*

OUTLINE

Chapter 69 Corneal Disorders in Children

Samer Hamada, Sundas Maqsood

CONGENITAL CORNEAL OPACITIES

Corneal opacification in children whether congenital or acquired could result in devastating consequences on visual development of a child. It can result in amblyopia or in the worst case scenario blindness. Younger children with central corneal opacities are the most challenging to manage. While management can be conservative, often these children will require surgical intervention to clear the cornea to allow restoring visual development that might be already delayed. We should not underestimate the social and emotional impacts of corneal opacities on the overall development of a child. The management of a child with poor vision requires active involvement of various professionals including healthcare providers, social services and educational institutions. Early diagnosis is essential to avoid delay in treatment and minimize the consequences of corneal damage.

In a large epidemiological study in Spain, congenital corneal opacities prevalence was 6 in 100,000 new live births; half of those were children born with congenital glaucoma; and corneal opacities accounted for 3.11% of congenital eye malformation.[1]

In another study by Hovlykke et al., they found that congenital corneal anomalies accounted for 4% of pediatric keratoplasties in Denmark.[2]

The mnemonic "STUMPED" is helpful for remembering the differential diagnosis for congenital corneal opacities: sclerocornea, tears in Descemet's membrane (usually forceps or congenital glaucoma), ulcers, metabolic [e.g. mucopolysaccharidosis (MPS)], Peters' anomaly, edema [congenital hereditary endothelial dystrophy (CHED), posterior polymorphous dystrophy (PPMD), glaucoma], and dermoid [American Academy of Ophthalmology (AAO), 2017].

Some of the main causes of congenital corneal opacities are described here.

Anterior Segment Developmental Delay

Failure of anterior segment normal development leads to varieties of anterior segment anomalies.[3-6]

Peters' Anomaly

Peters' anomaly is the most common congenital corneal opacity where the most posterior layers of the cornea is missing mainly Descemet's membrane, endothelial cells and often posterior stroma with scarring of the remaining central cornea. There is often an adhesion between the iris and the cornea (iridocorneal adhesions) and/or between the crystalline lens and the cornea (keratolenticular adhesions). Peters' anomaly is normally bilateral and asymmetrical. The management is normally surgical and include unilateral or bilateral keratoplasties with or without lensectomy.[3,7-9]

Sclerocornea

Sclerocornea is normally a bilateral cornea condition that appears like extension of sclera and blood vessels in the cornea obscuring the details of the corneal limbus. Corneal limbal stem cell deficiency might be present. The management is surgical with penetrating keratoplasty with or without limbal epithelial stem cell transplantation.[3]

Cornea Plana

Cornea plana is essentially a flat cornea with central corneal curvature of less than 35 diopters (D). Around 80% of sclerocornea cases have cornea plana. Microphthalmia is an association (Fig. 69.1).[7]

Corneal Dermoid

It is a benign congenital tumor that contain choristomatous tissue (tissue not found normally at that site). It might have hair follicles, fibrous tissue, fat, sweat glands, and sebaceous glands. It is usually raised and covers the inferotemporal part of the limbus and the cornea. However, it can be flat, central, or multiple. Peripheral lesions are less likely to cause significant visual loss but astigmatism is often found and must be treated to avoid refractive amblyopia. Central or larger peripheral dermoid might need excision to improve the vision and/or due to symptoms resulting from

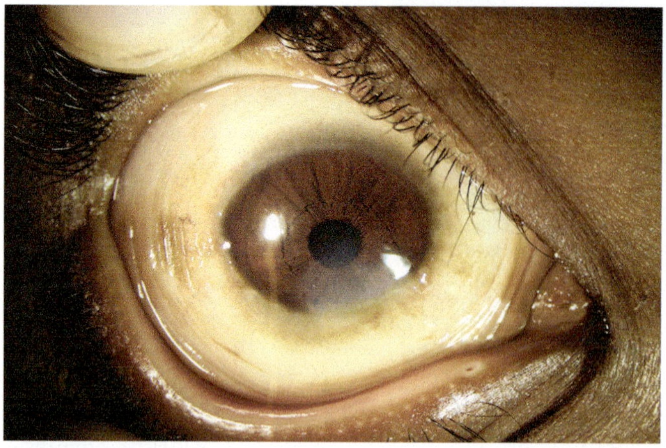

Fig. 69.1: Cornea plana. Small cornea that is horizontally oval due to superior and inferior peripheral corneal scarring. There is also faint superficial corneal opacity in the lower half of the cornea.
Source: Dr N Venkatesh Prajna, Aravind Eye Hospital, India.

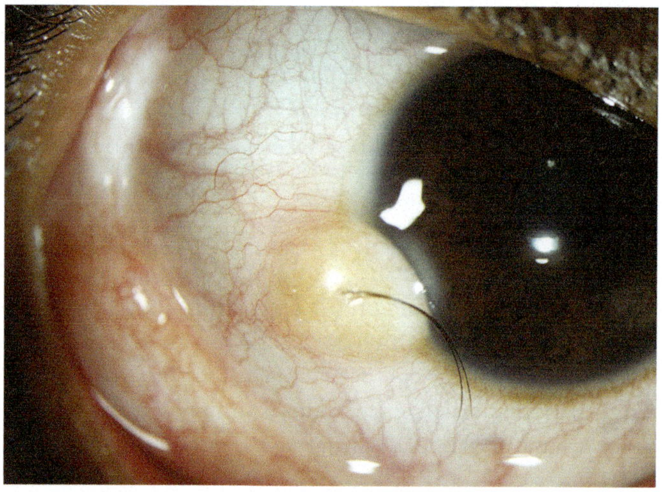

Fig. 69.2: Limbal dermoid. It was present from birth as small smooth and painless mass in the inferotemporal cornea at the limbus. Couple of hairs are seen and could lead to eye irritation. Growth is generally very slow and excision is not always necessary unless the mass is approaching visual axis. However, refractive error should be regularly checked and corrected in indicated.
Source: Dr N Venkatesh Prajna, Aravind Eye Hospital, India.

the large size of the dermoid. Goldenhar's syndrome must be excluded in every case of corneal and ocular surface dermoid (Fig. 69.2).[3]

Congenital Infections

Congenital infections can lead to corneal opacities, which are discussed here.

Viral Infections

Various eye infections can affect the cornea such as rubella, herpes simplex, cytomegalovirus, human influenza, and human parvovirus. It is usually unilateral except Rubella which is bilateral and can lead to cataract, glaucoma, iritis, salt-and-pepper retinopathy, and microphthalmia.

Bacterial Infections

Bacterial infections mainly *Neisseria gonorrhoeae* and *Staphylococcus*. These can be serious and lead to corneal scarring or thinning and perforation. Positive maternal history can aid diagnosis in addition to conjunctival and corneal swabs and culture.

Congenital Syphilis Keratitis

It starts late around age 5 years. Initially it manifests as iritis in the first 6 months and then chorioretinitis. Interstitial keratitis could last for few months before its remission.

Congenital Glaucoma

Congenital glaucoma accounts for almost half of children presenting with congenital cloudy cornea. While it is bilateral in most cases, unilateral cases do exist. The newborn will be tearing excessively and sensitive to light with frequent eye rubbing. The cornea appears large and edematous. The intraocular pressure (IOP) will be high. Early management results in IOP control and cornea clearance, however, delay in treatment could leave the cornea with permanent scarring. Haab's striae remains evident in the cornea during adulthood.[1,10]

Congenital Trauma

Corneal opacities after birth can occur from tears in Descemet's membrane from the use of forceps during delivery. Bruises on the eyelids and presence of localized corneal edema around the breaks in Descemet's membrane can aid diagnosis. Most cases clear without the need for any intervention. But rarely corneal scarring develops and further management might be required.

Other causes of trauma are amniocentesis with sharp needle injury to the eye or accidental knife injury during cesarian section delivery (Fig. 69.3).

Congenital Corneal Dystrophies

CHED and PPMD are the prime examples of congenital corneal dystrophies. The clinical picture of both is very similar to congenital glaucoma. The cornea is cloudy and edematous, however, there is no increase in the size of the cornea. Intraocular pressure is within normal limits

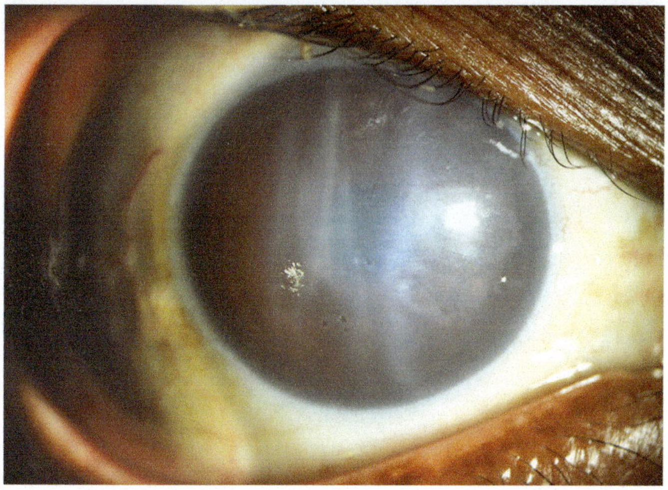

Fig. 69.3: Birth trauma. Birth trauma leads to breaks in Descemet's membrane with corresponding deep corneal scarring.
Source: Dr N Venkatesh Prajna, Aravind Eye Hospital, India.

although it might measure slightly higher due to increased corneal thickness. Hypertonic solutions like sodium chloride 5% might help corneal clarity until definite corneal transplant surgery. Another congenital dystrophy is the congenital hereditary stromal dystrophy (CHSD), which manifests from birth with feathery stromal opacities, but it is not progressive and treatment rarely needed. Finally, a careful examination can confirm fleck corneal dytrophy which is very rare and present without corneal opacification. It is not visually significant and treatment might not be necessary.[11-17]

Congenital Opacities in Systemic Metabolic Disease

Cloudy corneas are seen in mucopolysaccharidosis and mucolipidosis. Other rare metabolic diseases are cystinosis, tyrosinemia, gangliosidosis, congenital porphyria, and Zellweger syndrome. Corneal cloudiness is rarely seen at birth. The exception is MPS 1H (Hurler disease) and gangliosidosis.[3]

CORNEAL ANOMALIES

Microcornea

A cornea with horizontal diameter smaller than 10 mm. The normal corneal diameter at birth is 9.50–10.0 mm, and reaches its normal adult size (>11.75 mm) by age 2. Microcornea refers to cornea involvement only. However, if the entire eye is small but otherwise normal eye then this is called nanophthalmos, and if the anterior segment of the eye is small but the rest is normal then it is called microphthalmos.

The cornea is flat and children are hyperopic. It is normally a bilateral anomaly. Associated ocular findings are: iris coloboma, corectopias, cataract, microphakia, angle closure glaucoma or infantile glaucoma, chromic open angle glaucoma, persistent hyperplastic primary vitreous (PHPV), and retinopathy of prematurity (ROP). Associated systemic conditions are—Ehlers-Danlos syndrome, Marfan's syndrome, Rieger's syndrome, Norries' syndrome, trisomy 21, Turner's syndrome, Weil-Marchesani syndrome, Warburg micro syndrome, cataract-microcornea syndrome, and acroreno-ocular syndrome. The inheritance can be autosomal dominant, autosomal recessive, or sporadic.

Cornea Plana

A cornea with curvature less than 43 D (generally 20–40 D). Reduced corneal curvature leads in most cases to hyperopia, hazy corneal limbus, and arcus lipoides at an early age. It can be inherited as autosomal dominant or recessive anomaly. Sclerocornea is one of the associations. If the cornea is flat and small then it could be a case of microcornea. Other associations include: infantile glaucoma, open or closed angle glaucoma, anterior synechiae, aniridia, retinal aplasia, blue sclera, choroidal coloboma, iris coloboma, and microphthalmia. Systemic associations include: osteogenesis imperfect and epidermolysis bullosa (*see* Fig. 69.1).[18,19]

Megalocornea

A corneal diameter of above 13 mm is categorized as megalocornea (Fig. 69.4). This is a large but clear cornea with increase in corneal steepness. If the anterior segment is also enlarged then it is called megalophthalmos. The most common refractive error is myopia. It is unilateral or bilateral disease, which is inherited as an X-linked recessive trait. About 90% of affected children are male. Females are carriers but could have a slight enlargement of their corneas. Ocular associations include: anterior embryotoxon, mosaic corneal dystrophy, glaucoma, iris hypoplasia, and ectopic lentis. Associated systemic conditions include: Alport's syndrome, craniosynostosis, Down's syndrome, and Marfan syndrome.[20]

Sclerocornea

Discussed elsewhere in this chapter.

Keratoconus

Discussed elsewhere in this chapter.

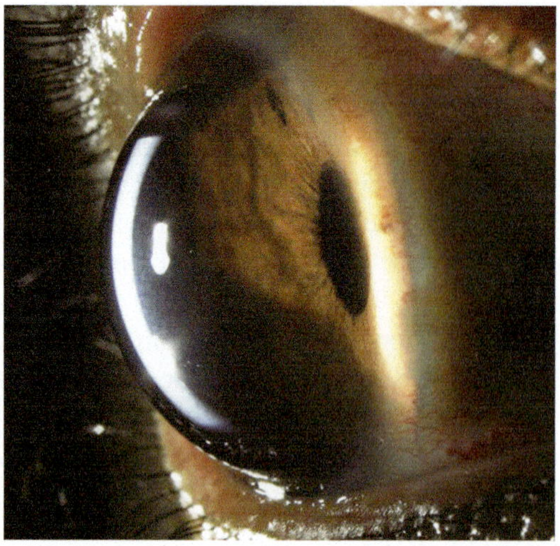

Fig. 69.4: Megalocornea. The cornea is very large (diameter >13 mm) but it has normal thickness as opposite to keratoglobus where the cornea is very thin but of normal size. Here it is part of anterior megalophthalmos that is enlarged anterior segment of the globe.
Source: Dr N Venkatesh Prajna, Aravind Eye Hospital, India.

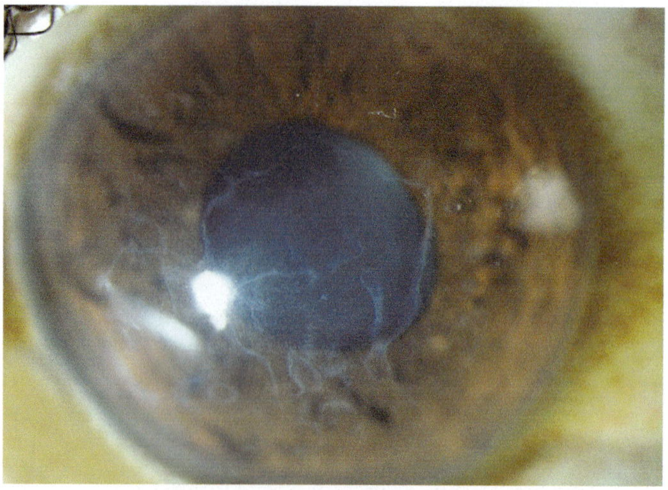

Fig. 69.5: Abnormal basement membrane dystrophy (ABMD). Map, finger print and dots patterns are seen in this advanced ABMD. There is a faint anterior corneal scarring in the center from chronic inflammation and recurrent corneal erosions.
Source: Dr N Venkatesh Prajna, Aravind Eye Hospital, India.

CORNEAL DYSTROPHIES

Meesmann's Epithelial Corneal Dystrophy (Hereditary Juvenile Epithelial Dystrophy)

It is also called Stocker-Holt dystrophy or Meesmann-Wilke syndrome. It is an autosomal dominant condition with a mutation in the gene keratin K3 (KRT3) at locus 12q13. It manifests very early in life. Clinically, there are multiple, tiny epithelial vesicles that are diffusely distributed and extend all the way to the limbus. They are more numerous in the interpalpebral area and are best visualized with retroillumination. The epithelium adjacent to the cysts is clear. The vesicles are the results of accumulation of Periodic Acid-Schiff (PAS) positive material which is called peculiar substance. Normally, the vesicles are not visually significant unless they coalesce and occupy the central part of the cornea. The main symptoms are gritty eyes, light sensitivity, and irritation. Topical eye lubricants can be used and children are advised to use tinted glasses to reduce photophobia.[21-25]

Abnormal Basement Membrane Dystrophy

This is the most frequently seen anterior corneal dystrophy in children. It is also called map-dot fingerprint corneal dystrophy, anterior membrane dystrophy, and Cogan's microcytic dystrophy. A fibrillar protein will deposit between the basement membrane and Bowman's layer. The poor adhesions result in recurrent corneal erosions (Fig. 69.5).

It is normally a bilateral disease and although inheritance is unclear, there is an autosomal dominant form of the disease. Clinically, the lesions can be seen in both eyes and take the shape of dots, maps, or fingerprints. Hypertonic solutions like sodium chloride 5% is useful in these cases, but if it fails to control symptoms then bandage contact lenses could be tried. If conservative measures fails then surgical options include: alcohol delamination, stromal puncture, and phototherapeutic keratectomy (PTK). Corneal scarring can happen in the long-term when Bowman's membrane is breached.[26]

Reis-Buckler's Corneal Dystrophy

There are four autosomal corneal dystrophies mapped to 5q31 where there are mutations in the gene coding for keratoepithelin:

- Granular corneal dystrophy of Groenouw type 1 (CDGG1)
- Reis-Buckler's corneal dystrophy type 1 (CDRB1)
- Lattice corneal dystrophy type 1 (LCD1)
- Avellino corneal dystrophy (ACD).

The inheritance is autosomal dominant with high penetrance.

In Reis-Buckler's, the lesions appear as white gray reticular pacifications at level of Bowman's layer.

The lesions appear early in life and symptoms start when the child starts to develop recurrent corneal epithelial erosions. The lesions appear dense in central to mid-peripheral cornea while the involving the peripheral cornea. The management is corneal erosions is similar to that described in managing abnormal basement membrane dystrophy. Anterior corneal scarring can be reduced or removed using excimer lasers or if deeper lesions then superficial anterior lamellar keratoplasty. This is best achieved using femtosecond lasers for more precise cuts within the cornea.[26,27]

Thiel-Behnke (Corneal Dystrophy of Bowman's Layer II, CDB II)

Clinical picture is very similar to Reis-Buckler's corneal dystrophy but has a less severe course. Visual loss is significantly greater in CDRB I, and recurrences after corneal transplantation seem to be earlier and more extensive in CDRB I compared with CDB II.

Clinically, it might be difficult to distinguish various types of anterior corneal dystrophy and histology is required for a definitive diagnosis.[26]

Anterior Membrane Dystrophy (Grayson-Willbrandt Dystrophy)

It has milder manifestations than Reis-Buckler's corneal dystrophy with later onset, less corneal erosions, normal corneal sensation, sparing of the peripheral cornea, and the nonreticular mount-like corneal opacities.

Granular Corneal Dystrophy (Groenouw Type 1, CDGG1)

This is another autosomal dominant corneal dystrophy where mutated keratoepithelin form amyloidogenic intermediates that precipitate in the corneal stroma. Clinically as it appears white-gray deposits in the anterior stroma usually centrally with clear spaces between them (Fig. 69.6). It is present from the first decade of life but rarely symptomatic until it develops further in the mid-twenties or thirties. The vision is reduced gradually and corneal erosion occurs very infrequently. Histopathologically, hyaline stains well with Mason's trichrome and less with PAS. The deposits are denser in the anterior stroma. Treatment options depend on depth of corneal deposits and include: phototherapeutic keratoplasty (PTK), superficial anterior lamellar keratoplasty (SALK), deep anterior lamellar keratoplasty (DALK), or penetrating keratoplasty (PKP).[26,28]

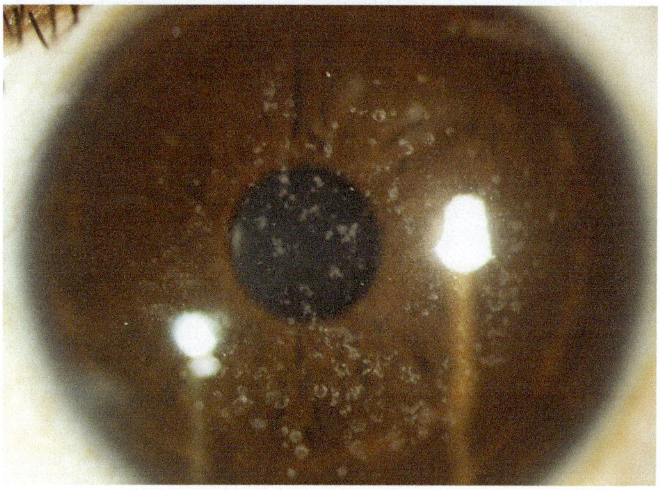

Fig. 69.6: Granular dystrophy. Opacities seen as small, discrete gray and irregular granules located in the anterior corneal stroma. The lesions are mainly in the center of the cornea sparing the periphery. The deep layer of the cornea remains clear until very late stages of the disease. In most cases, anterior lamellar keratoplasty is the treatment of choice. In milder cases, phototherapeutic keratectomy (PTK) might be a good and less invasive option.
Source: Dr N Venkatesh Prajna, Aravind Eye Hospital, India.

Avellino Corneal Dystrophy

It is a rare autosomal dominant dystrophy but with high penetrance. The disease is a mixture of granular and lattice dystrophies and this is evident clinically and on histopathological assessment.

Granular deposits appear earlier in the anterior stroma while lattice deposits appear later and deeper in the cornea. Corneal erosions are more likely to happen than in granular dystrophy. Treatment is with lamellar or full thickness keratoplasty. There is also a role for PTK in recurrent corneal erosions or in early cases of the disease.[26,29]

Lattice Cornea Dystrophy

It is autosomal dominant corneal dystrophy. There are three types of lattice corneal dystrophy (LCD). But only type one is seen in children with abnormal amyloid deposits (abnormal fibrillar protein). Spaces between lesions are clear at start but with age it starts to become hazy with a ground glass appearance. The disease spares posterior cornea. Deposits between epithelium and Bowman's layer can lead to recurrent cornea erosions (Fig. 69.7). Amyloid

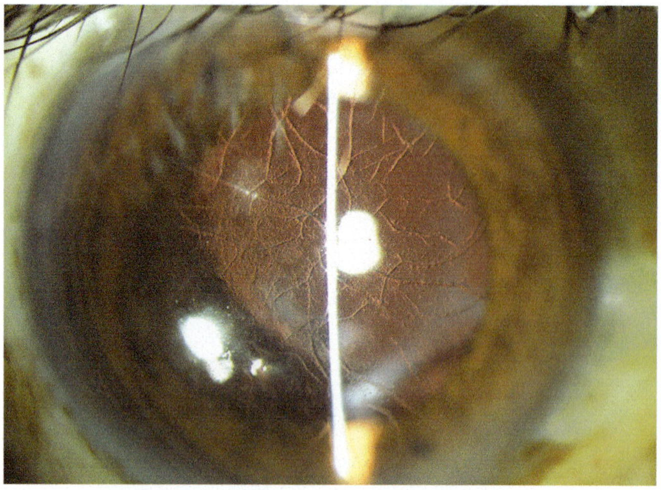

Fig. 69.7: Lattice corneal dystrophy. This is type 1 Lattice corneal dystrophy. Filamentous lesions occupy the center of the cornea and are denser than those seen in type 2 where the disease predominantly presents in the peripheral cornea. Most lesions are located in the anterior stroma.
Source: Dr N Venkatesh Prajna, Aravind Eye Hospital, India.

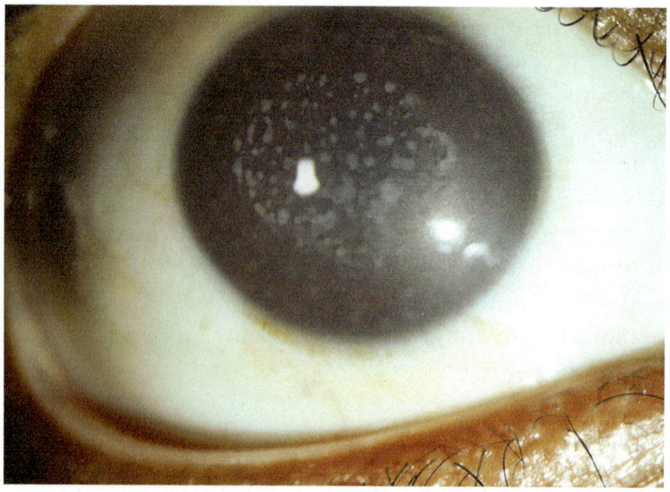

Fig. 69.8: Macular dystrophy. Multiple irregular gray-white opacities in the cornea stroma that are denser in the center but extends to the periphery if the cornea. Unlike granular dystrophy, there are no clear spaces between the opacities.
Source: Dr N Venkatesh Prajna, Aravind Eye Hospital, India.

stains with Congo red and Masson trichrome. Alcohol delamination and/or PTK can help reducing incidence of recurrent cornel erosions. Keratoplasty might be necessary and the disease could recur in the graft in 50% of cases within 3–5 years.[26]

Gelatinous Drop-like Dystrophy

Rare condition where amyloid is deposited in the basal epithelial cells and lead to destruction of Bowman's layer. Treatment is mostly surgical.

Macular Dystrophy

It is the rarest but most severe form of corneal dystrophies, but very common in Iceland. It is inherited as autosomal recessive. It progresses early in life and vision deteriorates quickly. Recurrent corneal erosions are not common. It has two types where abnormal keratin sulfate is deposited in the cornea stroma.

It is seen as white gray lesions with indistinct margins and no intervening clear areas. The lesions are seen centrally at start but gradually it involves the whole cornea (Fig. 69.8). Rarely, it can involve Descemet's membrane and the endothelium layer. Lesions stain with Alcian blue, PAS, and colloidal iron. Penetrating or lamellar keratoplasty is the only treatment of advanced cases but recurrence on the new graft do occur.[26]

Schnyder's Central Corneal Dystrophy

A rare autosomal dominant disorder that is associated with hypercholesterolemia. It is seen as needle-shaped shinny crystals occupying the corneal center but gradually extending to the peripheral cornea without reaching the limbus. Because of the deposition of these material is the anterior corneal stroma, PTK could be a treatment option.

Congenital Hereditary Stromal Dystrophy

It is probably very rare; only a few affected families have been reported in the medical literature. This condition has autosomal dominant inheritance. Slit-lamp examination shows numerous opaque flaky or feathery areas of clouding in the corneal stroma which increase with age, eventually affecting the vision. The corneal endothelium and Descemet's membrane are not affected. The cornea keeps it normal thickness. Corneal transplantation whether lamellar or full thickness is essential to prevent visual loss, amblyopia, strabismus, and nystagmus.

Posterior Polymorphous Dystrophy

Posterior polymorphous dystrophy and CHED are both endothelial corneal dystrophies that affect children and share similar genetic locations on chromosome 20 (Fig. 69.9).

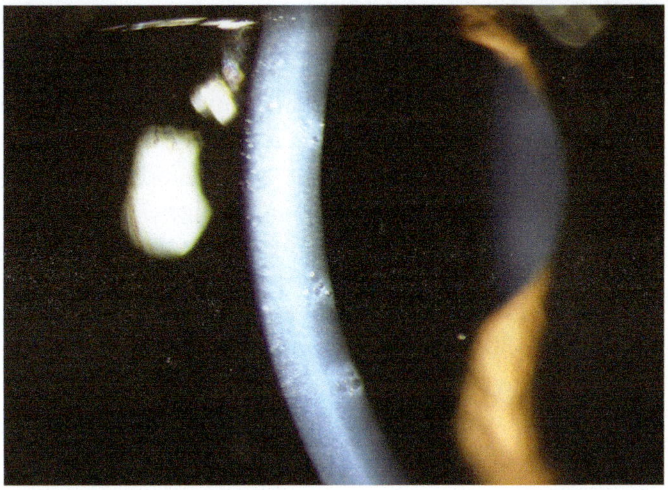

Fig. 69.9: Posterior polymorphous cornea dystrophy (PPMD). Vesicle-like transparent lesions surrounded by grey halos at the level of Descemet's membrane and the endothelium. The cornea is clear in the spaces between the lesions.
Source: Dr N Venkatesh Prajna, Aravind Eye Hospital, India.

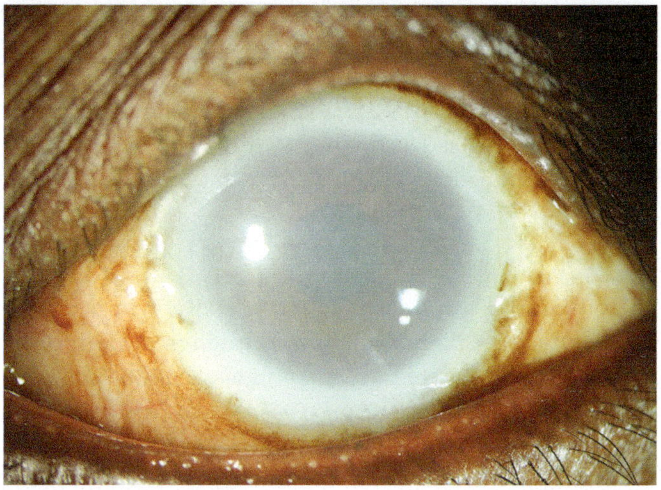

Fig. 69.10: Congenital hereditary endothelial dystrophy (CHED). This is an advanced case of CHED. The cornea is totally cloudy with difficulty to see anterior chamber and iris details.
Source: Dr N Venkatesh Prajna, Aravind Eye Hospital, India.

Posterior polymorphous dystrophy is an autosomal dominant endothelial corneal dystrophy where defective endothelial cells differentiate into epithelial cells rather than endothelial cells. Abnormal cells spread on the posterior cornea forming localized geographical areas of gray-white scarring as well as shedding in the anterior chamber leading to iridocorneal adhesions, corectopia, and even glaucoma.[11,30] It is normally a bilateral disease that manifests in young children, or even cloudy cornea in a newborn baby. Treatment is only indicated if the lesions spread on large part of the cornea leading to total corneal decompensation and visual loss. Recurrences of PPMD in the corneal graft can occur.[11,26]

Congenital Hereditary Endothelial Dystrophy

It is bilateral corneal endothelial dystrophy that is present at birth and leads to corneal edema, thickening, and cloudiness (Fig. 69.10). The corneal clouding in CHED ranges from a mild haze to a ground glass, milky appearance. Corneal sensation and the IOP remain normal. There is no photophobia or eye tearing. It has two types:

1. *CHED I:* It is an autosomal dominant, mild endothelial corneal dystrophy that develops in the first years of life so total corneal cloudiness is delayed allowing for visual maturation and hence nystagmus does not develop.
2. *CHED II:* It is an autosomal recessive, a more severe form of CHED. The cornea is cloudy from birth and hence nystagmus is often present.

Topical hypertonic solutions and IOP lowering agents can help in reducing corneal edema and allow some clarity of the cornea, but ultimately surgical intervention by means of corneal transplantation (penetrating keratoplasty or endothelial keratoplasty) would be necessary.[14,26]

INFECTIOUS KERATITIS

Infectious keratitis in children is uncommon but has greater magnitude of morbidity. It accounts up to 13% of all keratitis.[31] The diagnosis and treatment in children is particularly difficult due to challenging clinical examination, microbial sample collection and lack of compliance to treatment protocols.[32]

Even with good therapeutic control, the eye might end up with poor visual outcomes due to scarring and resultant amblyopia in this age group.[33]

The risk factors and etiology for infectious keratitis in pediatric population vary according to the geographical location. Additionally, the risk factors do alter due to the socioeconomic status and changes in these geographic areas.[34]

The diagnosis of infectious keratitis is mainly clinical and is usually treated empirically with topical antimicrobial agents until the etiological agents are identified.

The predisposing factors vary with presenting age of the infectious keratitis. In neonates, maternal genital tract infections, prematurity and congenital eyelid abnormalities are recognized risk factors to develop infectious keratitis.[35]

In younger children, the prominent predisposing factors are trauma, ocular disease, systemic disease particularly vitamin A deficiency and prior ocular surgery.[33]

In children who are 12 years and above, contact lens use has been recognized as the most prominent risk factor for developing infectious keratitis.[36]

Microbial/Bacterial

Various studies on microbiological analysis in pediatric infectious keratitis has shown prevalence of both gram positive and negative bacteria and less commonly fungi and Acanthamoeba.[36]

However, the spectrum of causative bacteria varies according to the risk factor, gram negative bacteria being the most commonly isolated microorganism in contact lens wearers compared to both gram positive and negative isolates in the rest.[36] Moreover, the prevalence of causative organisms also varies in different geographical locations of the world. Staphylococcal and streptococcal infections tend to occur more in the northern latitude compared to Psuedomonal and fungal infections affecting the southern hemisphere (Fig. 69.11).[37,38]

Like adults, identification of the causative pathogen in children is through microbiological analysis of corneal scraping which may necessitate examination under general anesthesia. The treatment is through topical antibiotics according to the antimicrobial sensitivity. The outcomes are poorer in the presence of ocular and systemic diseases, which are usually associated with polymicrobial infection.[36]

Fungal

Fungal keratitis in children is more common in tropical countries owing to a favorable humid climate and agricultural population.[39] The incidence of fungal keratitis is noticed to be increased during autumn and early winter months due to more humid climate changes.[39,40]

Trauma with vegetable matter is the most common predisposing factor for fungal keratitis in children. Severe systemic illness that can lead to an immunocompromised state also predispose to fungal infection. Other factors include ocular surgery, lid abnormality and exposure and contact lens use.[34] Most commonly isolated species is *Aspergillus* worldwide (Fig. 69.12).[41,42]

Congenital Syphilis

Congenital syphilis can present with interstitial keratitis in the first decade of life. In 10% of older children, it classically presents with bilateral interstitial keratitis. It is usually accompanied by stromal edema followed by deep stromal neovascularization which later transform to ghost vessels. Uveitis, chorioretinitis, arthritis and hearing loss can also be associated with keratitis. The Combination of widely spaced peg-shaped teeth, neuronal deafness and interstitial keratitis in suspected cases of congenital syphilis is known as "Hutchinson triad". Congenital syphilis is diagnosed by dark field microscopy or fluorescent antibody (IgM) detection against *Treponema pallidum*. Neonatal treatment is with intravenous penicillin G. The follow-up

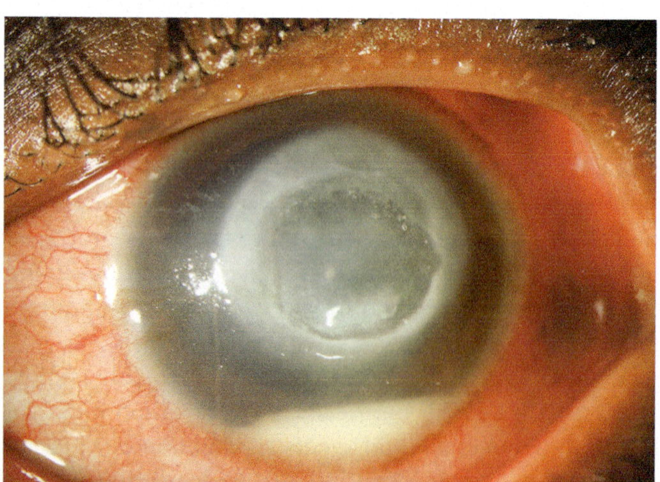

Fig. 69.11: *Pseudomonas keratitis.* This is an aggressive infection of the cornea where ring infiltrate can be seen. The central cornea is thin and necrotic.
Source: Dr N Venkatesh Prajna, Aravind Eye Hospital, India.

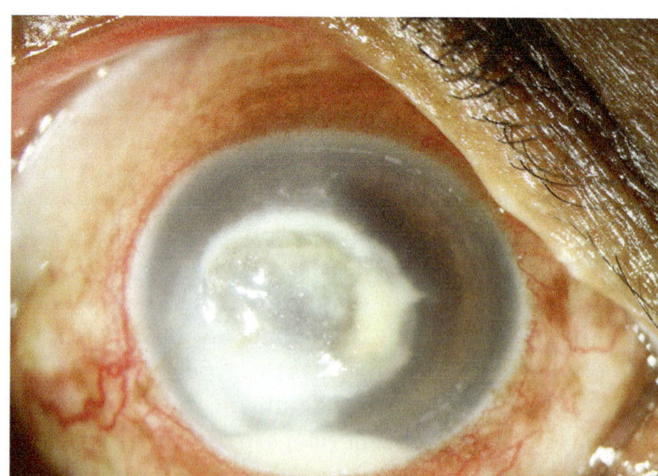

Fig. 69.12: Fungal keratitis. Large central corneal abscess that appears to be deep with hypopyon. The condition was responding to treatment and the center of the abscess started to clear.
Source: Dr N Venkatesh Prajna, Aravind Eye Hospital, India.

is completed with repeat antibody titers at 2, 4, 6 and 12 months. Retreatment is suggested if titers remain persistent or high. Immunosuppression is often necessary to improve the overall sequelae of the disease.

Herpes Simplex Infection

Neonatal herpes simplex virus (HSV) infection is usually caused by HSV-2 virus and occurs in 1 in 3,000–20,000 births. It is typically associated with venereal transmission secondary to genital infection. Eye involvement is usually in the form of the conjunctivitis, keratitis, cataracts and retinochoroiditis. Keratitis can affect either epithelium or stroma. Usual treatment is with systemic acyclovir.

Adenovirus

There are 47 serotypes of adenovirus and several of which cause ocular infection. The typical adenoviral keratitis usually starts as punctate epithelial disease which can progress to multifocal subepithelial keratitis reflecting immune complex deposition. The keratitis is responsible for symptoms of pain, glare, photophobia and visual loss. The diagnosis is usually clinical. The adenoviral infection in older children with contact lens use must be differentiated with punctate epitheliopathy and early stromal infiltrates seen in Acanthamoeba keratitis.

INFLAMMATORY CORNEAL DISEASE

Keratitis or inflammation of the cornea can be mild and transient or most commonly an ongoing inflammatory eye disease with periods of disease remission. The etiology is not always understood. While hereditary keratitis is a rare disease, it can be a localized eye disease or part of systemic disease.

Hereditary Inflammatory Cornea and Ocular Surface Disease

Epidermolysis Bullosa

The eye is almost always affected in epidermolysis bullosa (EB). The conjunctiva, eyelids and cornea are involved. Corneal erosions are the main corneal manifestation and corneal scarring can occur in central corneal lesions. Shortening of fornices results from chronic conjunctiva blistering and inflammation. There are three main subtypes: (1) dystrophic, (2) junctional, and (3) simplex. Ocular involvement is more likely to happen in the autosomal recessive dystrophic and junctional types. Ocular lubricants are essential to treat and prevent cornea erosions.

Ectodermal Dysplasia

It refers to a group of syndromes all deriving from abnormalities of the ectodermal structures. So it can affect hair, skin, teeth, sweat glands, and salivary glands. Lacrimal glands hypoplasia and keratitis occur in types 1 and 3 (anhydrosis and hypohydrosis). Severe keratitis can lead to corneal limbal stem cells failure. Corneal opacification and poor vision requires keratoplasty which is normally a high risk keratoplasty.

Keratitis-Ichthyosis-Deafness Syndrome

It is inherited as autosomal recessive. Chronic keratitis can lead to corneal scarring and possibly limbal stem cell failure. It is very rare and should be suspected in children with sensorineural deafness.

Ectrodactyly-Ectodermal Dysplasia-Clefting Syndrome

It is inherited as autosomal dominant. There might be a partial or full absence insert of one digit to the full cleft and or foot deformity. The child will have cleft lip/palate and ectodermal dysplasia manifestations. Ocular manifestations include lacrimal ducts hypoplasia, chronic keratitis, and rarely absence of meibomian glands. In severe cases, corneal limbal stem cell deficiency and corneal scarring can occur requiring keratoplasty with corneal limbal stem cells transplantation.

Riley-Day Syndromes (Familial Dysautonomia)

Rare autosomal recessive syndrome that occurs exclusively in Ashkenazi Jews. It is caused by genetic mutation of the gene responsible for regulating different kinases involved in proinflammatory signaling. Corneal sensation is normally reduced and there is poor production of tear film leading to chronic irritation to the cornea and keratitis and scarring. Clinical diagnosis is made by finding the following signs: lack of axon flare after intradermal injection of histamine, absence of fungiform papillae in the tongue, miosis of pupil after instillation of pilocarpine 0.125% or methacholine chloride 2.5%, absent deep tendon reflexes, and reduced tear production. Intensive lubrication and narrowing palpebral aperture to reduce ocular exposure (like tarsorrhaphy, or other eye protecting procedures). Induced ptosis is not advised because it might cause amblyopia. Intensive lubrications are required and surgical intervention might be required with corneal scarring but success rate is poor due to corneal neurotrophic status.

Keratoendotheliitis Fugax Hereditaria

It is rare and present between the age 4 and 12 years. Clinically, it manifests as recurrent acute keratoendotheliitis. Steroids can shorten the attack but it is self-limiting and can last from few days to few weeks. Corneal stromal opacities can develop. Prognosis depends on frequency of attack and corneal damage and is not improved by the use of topical corticosteroids. The etiology and pathology are unknown.

Autosomal Dominant Keratitis

This is a variant of PAX6 mutation like aniridia without the full manifestations of aniridia (Figs. 69.13 and 69.14). It is an autosomal dominant disease which starts in the peripheral cornea as anterior stromal corneal opacities with corneal vascularization that is continuous with the limbus. The eyes become red with recurrent anterior stromal keratitis and vascularization which might replace Bowman's membrane. There are no corneal erosions. The child is normally very photophobic. Other findings include iris stromal defects, ectropion uveae, foveal hypoplasia and corneal limbal stem cell deficiency. There are no associated systemic abnormalities. The treatment aims to control inflammation and lubricate the cornea. The prognosis is variable and depends on the disease severity. Penetrating keratoplasty with or without limbal corneal epithelial stem cells transplantation might be necessary and disease recurrence on the graft is possible.[43-45]

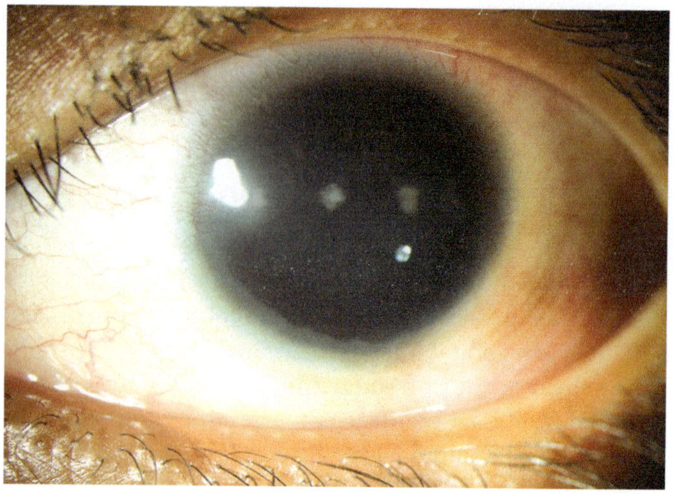

Fig. 69.13: A patient with aniridia and corneal limbal stem cell deficiency. The clinical features of normal limbus had disappeared and replaced by peripheral corneal vascularization and scarring. The cornea started to lose its clarity in the peripheral area first. There is diffuse subepithelial scarring that is worse nasally and temporally. There is also a change in the appearance of corneal surface due to conjunctivalization of the upper half of the cornea.
Source: Dr N Venkatesh Prajna, Aravind Eye Hospital, India.

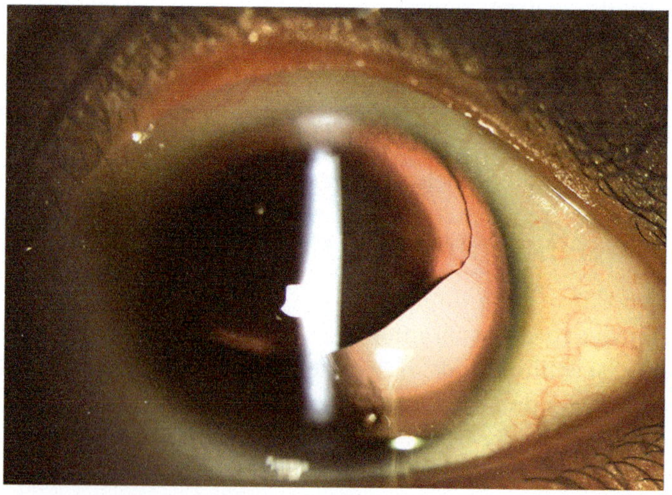

Fig. 69.14: Aniridia with lens coloboma. Only a remnant of rudimentary iris is seen. The natural lens has lost its inferior part and the zonules appear to be intact but stretched.
Source: Dr N Venkatesh Prajna, Aravind Eye Hospital, India

Acquired Keratitis

Dry Eye Disease

The new definition of dry eye disease according to the International Dry Eye Workshop is "a multifactorial disease of the ocular surface characterized by a loss of homeostasis of the tear film, and accompanied by ocular symptoms, in which tear film instability and hyperosmolarity, ocular surface inflammation and damage, and neurosensory abnormalities play etiological roles".[46] The loss of tear film hemostats due to evaporative dry eye such as in meibomian gland dysfunction (MGD), aqueous deficiency dry eye (ADDE) such as in Sjögren syndrome whether primary or secondary, loss of goblet cells and lack of mucin in tear film, or a combination of any would result in dry eye disease (Fig. 69.15). There is an important role for chronic inflammation in damaging ocular surface. Blepharokeratoconjunctivitis (BKC) is one of the most common causes of evaporative dry eye disease and will be discuss later in the chapter.

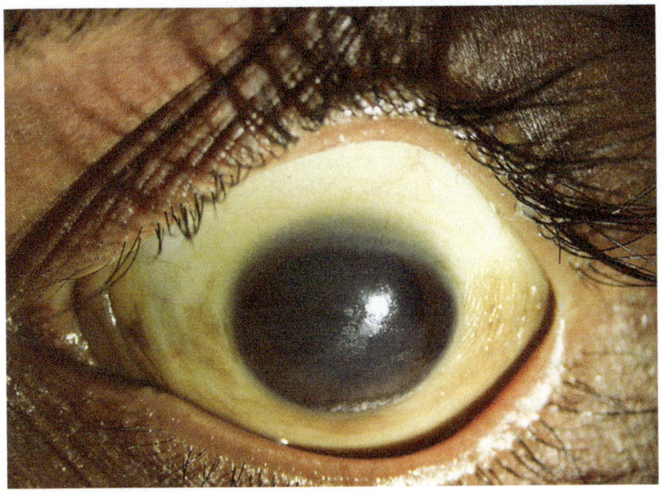

Fig. 69.15: Xerophthalmia. Vitamin A deficiency can lead to pathological dryness of the ocular surface including conjunctiva and cornea. Poor and scattered light reflex indicates irregular cornea surface and possible damage to corneal epithelium. Also keratin started to develop on the bulbar conjunctiva in the exposed areas of conjunctiva.
Source: Dr N Venkatesh Prajna, Aravind Eye Hospital, India.

Exposure Keratopathy

Abnormal anatomy or functions of eyelids could result in exposure keratopathy. Rarely, it happens from corneal exposure during surgery under general anesthesia or during recovery when eyes were not protected during or after surgery. The most frequently encountered causes are lid colobomas, lagophthalmos, and proptosis. Treatment aims to improve eyelid closure and cornea protection. Topical eye lubrications and tarsorrhaphies are frequently needed.

Limbal Stem Cell Deficiency

Corneal limbal stem cell deficiency can be part of congenital eye disease like aniridia or acquired as after corneal burn or trauma, or secondary to ocular surface inflammatory disease such as Stevens-Johnson syndrome.

Vernal Keratoconjunctivitis

Vernal keratoconjunctivitis (VKC) is a bilateral, chronic allergic inflammatory disease of ocular surface affecting children and young adults.[47]

It predominantly affects the male population at boyhood and resolves after puberty.[48] It is prevalent in temperate climates of the Mediterranean region, Central and West Africa, India, the Middle East and South America.

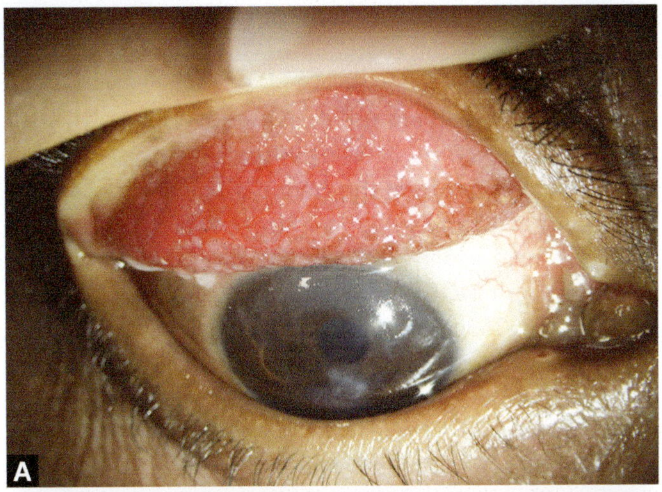

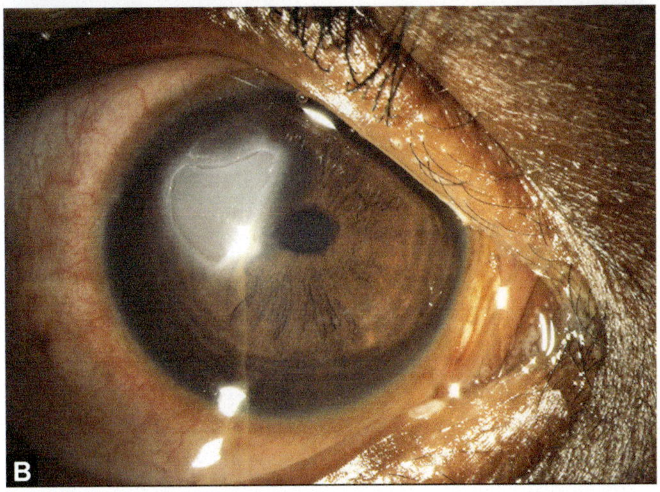

Figs. 69.16A and B: Vernal keratoconjunctivitis. (A) Giant papillary reaction involving the upper tarsal conjunctiva. This is a severe disease and corneal periphery appears to be inflamed with corneal neovascularization and corneal scarring from previous corneal ulceration; (B) Shield ulcers are not unusual and results from mechanical and inflammatory irritation to the cornea. Because its proximity to visual axis, the vision is reduced. Shield ulcers can be complicated with infectious keratitis or lead to corneal scarring or even perforation.
Source: Dr N Venkatesh Prajna, Aravind Eye Hospital, India.

Clinical presentation is with constant ocular irritation, eye rubbing, tearing, mucous discharge and photophobia. The disease prominently causes conjunctival inflammation resulting in giant papillary reaction of tarsal conjunctiva, limbal infiltrates, nodules and hypertrophy. Corneal involvement is only seen in severe disease which can be complicated to permanent loss of vision (Figs. 69.16A and B).

A complex allergic and inflammatory response between the conjunctiva and cornea is responsible for the pathophysiology of VKC. The inflammatory mediators cause structural changes in both these tissues and their reciprocal interaction augments the inflammatory cascade leading to tissue damage.[49]

Corneal involvement starts with the disruption of barrier function of epithelium through repeated mechanical injury from the giant papillae in the superior tarsal conjunctiva. In addition, it also suffers chemical insult form the inflammatory mediators (major basic protein and eosinophil cationic protein) secreted by activated eosinophils. These two granule proteins are cytotoxic in nature and has shown to affect the epithelial wound healing in vitro.[50] Additionally, eosinophils have shown to secrete matrix metalloproteinase (MMP)-9 causing breakdown of epithelial basement membrane and stroma. The exposed stromal fibroblasts get activated by the inflammatory mediators and secrete chemokines which stimulate Th2 cells to augment the allergic inflammation.[49,51] Thus, this vicious cycle continues to produce a prolong inflammatory response which is responsible for various corneal complications of the disease.

Shield ulcers and plaques are significant complications in 3–11% of VKC patients leading to permanent visual loss in 6% of cases.[1] They can further lead to complications like amblyopia, keratitis and corneal perforation.[52-54]

Plaque is formed due to accumulated granule proteins at the base of the shield ulcer and prevent epithelialization.[55] The shield ulcers are reported to evolve from punctate erosions progressing to coarse erosions which coalesce to form macroerosions. These macroerosions in the presence of background chronic inflammation and poor epithelial healing form shield ulcers.[56] Shield ulcers can be divided into three grades.[56] Grade 1 ulcer has transparent base and re-epithelialize with medical treatment leaving minimal scarring. Grade 2 ulcer has translucent base with or without opaque white or yellow deposit. Grade 3 ulcer has elevated plaque with a dense opaque deposit. Grade 2 and 3 ulcers epithelialize very slowly and can develop microbial keratitis in 9–10% cases. They are usually treated with surgical debridement and superficial keratectomy (Excimer laser photorefractive keratectomy and amniotic membrane transplant)[57,58] in advance cases. Medical treatment includes topical antihistamines, mast cell stabilizers, corticosteroids, antibiotics and preservative free lubricants. Recurrence of ulcers following treatment can occur in 14.5%.[56]

There is a well-known association of keratoconus with VKC.[47,59] This is thought to be due to combination of frequent eye rubbing and the biomechanical changes in corneal stroma secondary to chronic inflammation which leads to thinning and ectasia. The incidence of keratoconus in VKC population is reported to be quite variable and can range from 2.1% to 11.3%.[48,60] This difference in incidence is attributed to topographic parameters used to diagnose the disease. Corneal cross-linking is the treatment of choice in pediatric keratoconus as the disease is more aggressive than in adults. The abnormal and slow wound healing in VKC can make crosslinking more challenging. An aggressive preprocedure anti-inflammatory treatment regimen is recommended in these cases to produce good outcomes.[61]

Chronic inflammation and mechanical trauma due to frequent eye rubbing can cause damage to limbal epithelial progenitor cells resulting in limbal stem cell deficiency (LSCD). The incidence of LSCD is reported to be 1.2% in VKC patients and was present in older patients with longer disease duration.[62,63]

Corneal scarring is the major cause of visual loss in VKC population with incidence of 11%.[64] It occurs due to recurrent poor healing of shield and bacterial ulcers and limbal stem cell deficiency.

Some children develop an early cataract. This is blamed to the long-term use to topical corticosteroids.

VKC is primarily an inflammatory disease of conjunctiva which can involve cornea contributing to a significant ocular and visual morbidity. Effective topical anti-inflammatory treatment regimen is recommended to reduce the morbidity associated with complications. The treatment can be challenging and while topical steroids are needed in acute flare-ups of the disease, the use of nonsteroidal immunosuppressants such as cyclosporine and tacrolimus has shown good success in long-term disease control and preventing further disease complications.

Blepharokeratoconjunctivitis

Blepharokeratoconjunctivitis is one of the main causes of cornea and ocular surface inflammatory disease in children. Although the signs and symptoms are similar to those seen in adults but the disease course varies in children. BKC in children can cause significant symptoms including irritation, watering, photophobia and loss of vision from corneal opacity, refractive error or amblyopia.

Chronic inflammation of the cornea can lead to scarring, vascularization and opacity.

Meibomian gland dysfunction is a common finding in BKC. MGD was recently defined as the “chronic, diffuse abnormality of the meibomian glands, commonly characterized by terminal duct obstruction and/or qualitative/quantitative changes in the glandular secretion" (definition of the International Workshop in MGD published in 2011).[65]

Treatment of BKC is directed towards modification of meibomian gland disease and the bacterial flora of lid margin and conjunctiva, and control of ocular surface inflammation.

While prevalent and aggressive among Indo-Pakistani/Middle-Eastern populations, a recalcitrant destructive phenotype in white children/adolescents that persists into early adulthood and may require systemic immunosuppression.[66-69]

Various treatment regimens have been implemented in BKC including regular lid hygiene, topical antibiotics, topical glucocorticoids, topical calcineurin inhibitors and systemic antibiotic usually in combination. Lid hygiene is a key in the management of BKC. The recommendations of the International Workshop on Meibomian Gland Dysfunction, instituting eyelid hygiene with eyelid warming (a minimum of 4 min, once or twice daily) followed by moderate to firm massage and expression of meibomian gland secretions.[65]

Topical corticosteroids have a number of well-recognized potential side-effects like cataract and ocular hypertension, but are a key therapeutic tool to controlling ocular surface inflammation such as is seen in BKC. Systemic tetracyclines are useful as anti-inflammatories as well as antibiotics. There is a growing evidence that omega-3 dietary supplementation improves the clinical picture in patients with blepharitis due to MGD.

In childhood BKC the treatment protocols generally need to be more aggressive and prolonged in light of the frequent recurrence of the disease and the potential for reducing visual acuity.[67]

Pediatric Keratoconus

Keratoconus is defined as a bilateral, asymmetrical, noninflammatory corneal disorder resulting in stromal thinning and cone formation.[70,71] It typically presents in puberty with no race and sex predilection and progress over the period of 10–20 years. Although, recent evidence in literature confirms the progression of the disease can be beyond 30 years of age.[72-76]

The incidence of keratoconus is 1:2,000 with a reported prevalence of 54.5 cases per 100,000 individuals.[77] Various epidemiological studies estimate the annual incidence ranging from 1:3,000 to 1:80,000 per year.[78,79] This variability is likely to be attributed to different study design, increasing modern diagnostic sensitivity and regional differences related to accessibility to healthcare. The regional differences could be related to climate, inducing allergic eye disease and eye rubbing but marked variation has been noticed in the incidence in populations of different ethnic backgrounds living within a single country. In United Kingdom, South Asian population is 7.5 times more likely to have keratoconus compared to Caucasians.[74,80-82]

Genetic factors have shown to play role here which is supported by a growing incidence of disease in patients of consanguineous descent.[74,81,83] A genome-wide association analysis has identified multiple loci conferring susceptibility to low central corneal thickness (CCT) and progression of keratoconus.[84] FOXO1and FNDC3B nuclear polymorphisms have been identified to be associated with development of KC.[85]

Keratoconus may present as an isolated finding or may have associations with other systemic disorders or syndromes, e.g. Down syndrome, atopy, Apert syndrome, brachydactyly, Crouzon's, Ehlers-Danlos syndrome type IV and VI, Marfan syndrome, Laurence-Moon-Biedl syndrome, Noonan's syndrome, Raynaud's syndrome, mitral valve prolapse, chordae tendineae, syndactyly, osteogenesis imperfecta, xeroderma pigmentosum and other connective tissue disorders. A strong association has been found with atopy, where elevated serum IgE levels have been noticed in keratoconic patients.[86] Other associated ocular conditions include aniridia, blue sclera, congenital cataracts, ectopia lentis, microcornea, Leber's congenital amaurosis, retinitis pigmentosa, ROP and VKC.

The clinical features of keratoconus are characterized by central and paracentral thinning and loss of structural integrity of corneal stroma causing bulging and typical cone-shaped appearance. This results in myopic shift and irregular astigmatism causing significant impairment in vision that may not be corrected by spectacles (Fig. 69.17).

The keratoconic cornea has been studied widely and has demonstrated both morphological and molecular changes compared to controls. It is suggested that keratoconus results from atypical tissue response to one or more unidentified stimuli leading to keratocyte dysfunction and depletion, collagen loss and disintegrated extracellular matrix. Morphologically, all corneal layers can be affected in keratoconus. On histology and confocal microscopy, the epithelial and wing cell layer are found to be spindle shaped and enlarged while Bowman's layer shows disruption and protrusion of keratocytes or epithelial cells.[87,88] The stromal layer is found to be having low density keratocytes with

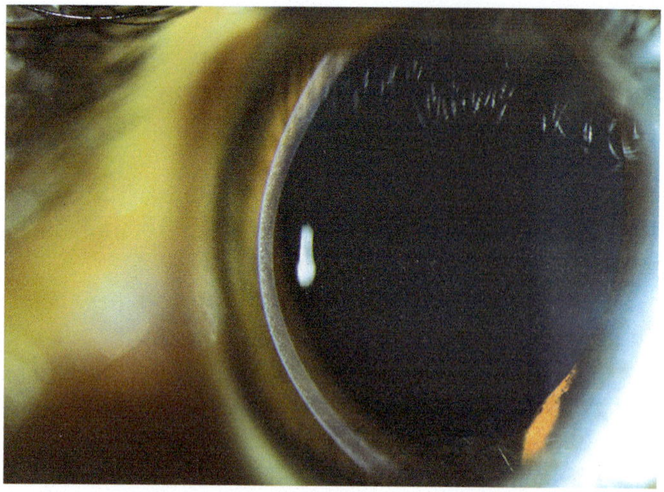

Fig. 69.17: Keratoconus. There is a localized thinning and steepening of the cornea as observed on the slit-lamp examination.
Source: Dr N Venkatesh Prajna, Aravind Eye Hospital, India.

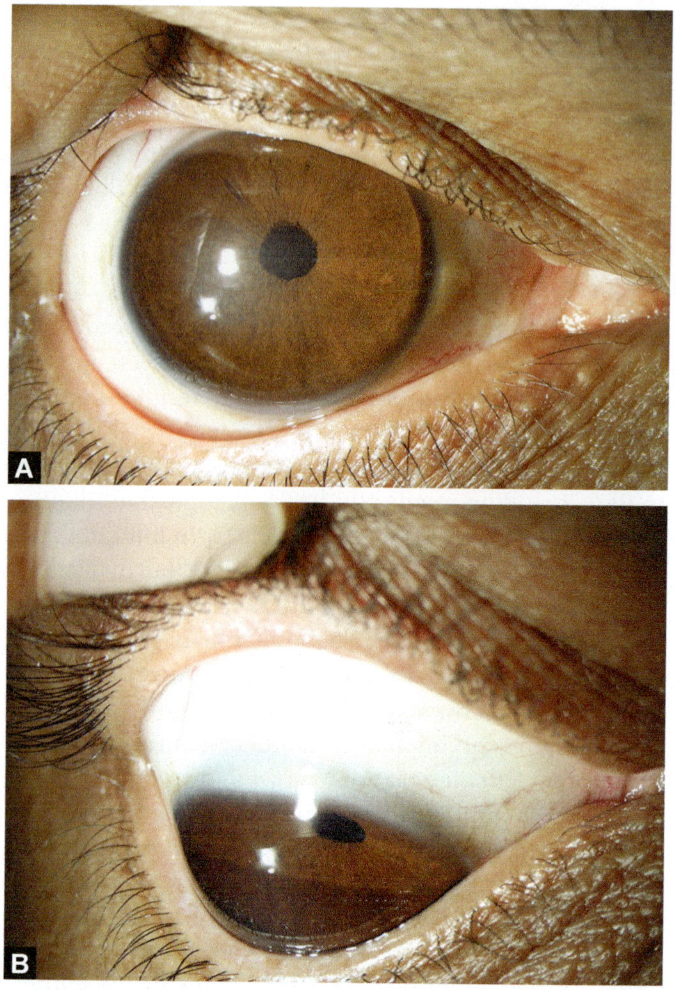

Figs. 69.18A and B: Keratoglobus. This is a global protrusion of the cornea with diffuse corneal thinning. The cornea here is clear but breaks in Descemet's membrane could lead to corneal swelling (acute hydrops) and corneal scarring.
Source: Dr N Venkatesh Prajna, Aravind Eye Hospital, India.

poorly differentiated nuclei.[89] Electron microscopy has also confirmed the scanty proteoglycan with abnormal proteoglycan-collagen network.[90] These changes attribute to biomechanical instability and weakening of the cornea. Protein studies on keratoconus has shown decrease in stromal collagen type XII, I, V[91,92] due to collagen degradation by the overexpression of gelatinases, such as catalase and decrease in tissue inhibitor of matrix metalloproteinase (TIMP).[93-96] Various molecular studies have also suggested the role of inflammation in KC, this is demonstrated by elevated levels of IL-4-8, TNF-alpha, MMP-1.[97,98] Other proteomic studies have suggested a generalized loss of the normal quiescent keratocyte phenotype combined with an elevation in abnormal protein expression (reduced extracellular matrix proteins, such as decorin, lumican and keratocan and elevated cell regulator and apoptotic proteins) found in would healing phenotype.[92]

Various theories that can hypothesize the pathogenesis of keratoconus includes cytokine dysregulation,[99,100] oxidative stress[101-104] or the altered extracellular matrix due to abnormal TGF-beta signaling pathway.[105-107]

Keratoconus in Children

The presentation of keratoconus, especially early onset in children signifies a management dilemma. There are various factors like amblyopia, schooling, developmental milestones and behavior issues to consider compared to when dealing with adults. The management objectives are not only the visual rehabilitation, progression prevention but also educating the parents and school to minimize the impact of the implications of the disease on life.

When dealing with high astigmatism in children, it is important to rule to differential diagnosis when suspecting KC, e.g. Descemet's membrane breaks following traumatic forceps obstetric deliveries leading to development of corneal hydrops.[108,109] Full ocular and systemic examination is essential as other conditions like keratoglobus and congenital glaucoma can present with similar findings (Figs. 69.18A and B).

Diagnostic techniques in childhood keratoconus include clinical examination looking for a scissoring pattern of retinoscopy light. Slit-lamp examination can show Vogt striae (thin parallel striation in Descemet's membrane in the area of cone), Fleisher's ring (brown iron deposition in epithelium at the cone base best visualized with cobalt blue light), prominent corneal nerves, endothelial guttata and posterior shagreen. Other clinical signs include Rizutti's sign (nasal conical reflection when light is shown temporally across the cornea) and Munson's sign (anterior bulging of lower eyelid on down-gaze). Anterior segment optical coherence tomography (AS-OCT) and epithelial imaging can show thicker epithelium superiorly compared to inferior cone epithelium in KC.[110] It is useful in screening children but does not confirm whether epithelial thickness variability is useful in detecting early cases of keratoconus. Corneal topography remains the gold standard diagnostic tools but can be unreliable and challenging due to lack of cooperation in children.

Acute corneal hydrops can occur as a complication of the disease, when aqueous enters the stroma through Descemet's breaks. It is usually treated with hypertonic saline solution, soft contact lenses and patching. It usually resolves in 6–10 weeks and does not warrant surgical treatment. After an attack, the cornea usually clears up with some stromal scarring that can lead to reduction in visual acuity. Protective lenses are recommended in such cases as the cornea is prone to perforation if met with blunt trauma.

A rapidly progressive keratoconus in a child points out at the failure of natural cross-linking process in the corneal collagen fibers primarily affected by transglutaminase and lysyl oxidase enzyme pathways.[111] Therefore, missing genetic makeup, systemic or ocular conditions (Atopy, VKC) and environmental factors play significant role in early manifestation of the keratoconus. An interesting association has also been noticed between chronic eye rubbers and keratoconus.[112]

Eyes under the age of 12 years have different properties compared to adults as they are undergoing visual maturation. This can be depicted by the different behavior of tissues to diseases and surgical interventions noticed in pediatric cases. It has been reported that age play an important factor in maturing corneal biomechanics.[113,114] With age, the viscoelastic cornea stiffens through what is believed to a natural cross-linking process which actually slows down in adulthood. The transition between these two age groups could provide a vulnerable gap for the cornea to develop keratoconus when cornea is about to reach the rigidness but still has significant elasticity.

Although the true mechanism of KC affecting the cornea is unknown, but the susceptible subjects are noticed to have reduced corneal hysteresis (CH) and corneal resistance factor (CRF).[115] KC can affect the normal elastic behavior of cornea to stress and strain which is defined as Young's modulus. It tends to affect the corneal biomechanics in a way that it behaves more plastic, where the original shape regain is not achieved after usually resisted external forces on the cornea. This idea can be strengthened by the fact that diabetics are less likely to develop severe keratoconus.[108,116,117]

The Collaborative Longitudinal Evaluation of Keratoconus (CLEK) study was a multicenter natural history study of 1,209 patients lasted for 8 years and with a minimum age of 12.[118]

The study provided a strong evidence regarding the age being a major factor in assessing the severity of the disease and its future outcomes, particularly scarring. The study also found association between atopy and eye rubbers with aggressive disease.

The first-line treatment for disease stabilization in keratoconus is through corneal cross-linking (CXL). Riboflavin-UVA induced CXL, has been shown to enhance biomechanical rigidity and biochemical resistance,[119-124] thus allowing to slow the keratoconus progression at medium to long-term follow ups.[125,126] Dresden protocol (epithelium off) remains the "gold standard" for CXL with majority of the reported studies on children using this technique.

Microbial keratitis,[127-130] corneal melting, endothelial failure,[131,132] sterile infiltrates/noninfectious keratitis,[72,110] reactivation of herpetic keratitis and corneal haze has been reported as the complications of CXL. Despite all the best efforts to achieve good visual rehabilitation in children with CXL, 10–25% do end up undergoing keratoplasty. It has been noticed that the younger the patients the higher the risk of having keratoplasty.[133,134] Complication of KC like acute hydrops can affect the chances of these patients having successful lamellar grafts in future. Therefore, treating with Epi-On cross-linking even with these thinnest corneas can build enough cross-links to prevent further thinning and hydrops. Magli et al. demonstrated equal efficacy of Epi-On and Epi-Off CXL at 1 year in pediatric population.[135]

In adult studies, corneal haze, sterile infiltrates and microbial keratitis are the main complications noticed with persisted corneal haze up to 12 months.[127-129] These complications are of concern in children with more aggressive disease and in the presence of other associated conditions like VKC and atopy.

REFERENCES

1. Bermejo E, Martinez-Frias ML. Congenital eye malformations: clinical-epidemiological analysis of 1,124,654 consecutive births in Spain. Am J Med Genet. 1998;75(5):497-504.
2. Hovlykke M, Ehlers N, Nielsen K, et al. Clinical results of 40 years of paediatric keratoplasty in a single university eye clinic. Acta Ophthalmol. 2014;92(4):370-7.
3. Sowden JC. Molecular and developmental mechanisms of anterior segment dysgenesis. Eye (Lond). 2007;21(10): 1310-8.
4. Reis LM, Semina EV. Genetics of anterior segment dysgenesis disorders. Curr Opin Ophthalmol. 2011;22(5):314-24.
5. Shigeyasu C, Yamada M, Mizuno Y, et al. Clinical features of anterior segment dysgenesis associated with congenital corneal opacities. Cornea. 2012;31(3):293-8.
6. Stahl ED. Anterior segment dysgenesis. Int Ophthalmol Clin. 2014;54(3):95-104.
7. Kenyon KR. Mesenchymal dysgenesis in Peter's anomaly, sclerocornea and congenital endothelial dystrophy. Exp Eye Res. 1975;21(2):125-42.
8. Parmley VC, Stonecipher KG, Rowsey JJ. Peters' anomaly: a review of 26 penetrating keratoplasties in infants. Ophthalmic Surg. 1993;24(1):31-5.
9. Bhandari R, Ferri S, Whittaker B, et al. Peters anomaly: review of the literature. Cornea, 2011;30(8):939-44.
10. Ratzan RM. Congenital glaucoma. Med Humanit. 2017;43(4):e36.
11. Strachan IM, Maclean H. Posterior polymorphous dystrophy of the cornea. Br J Ophthalmol. 1968;52(3):270-2.
12. Tsuru T, Hori S, Tanishima T. Clinical and histopathological study of congenital hereditary endothelial dystrophy of the cornea (author's transl). Nippon Ganka Gakkai Zasshi. 1981;85(8):144-56.
13. al-Rajhi AA, Wagoner MD. Penetrating keratoplasty in congenital hereditary endothelial dystrophy. Ophthalmology. 1997;104(6):956-61.
14. Ehlers N, Modis L, Moller-Pedersen T. A morphological and functional study of Congenital Hereditary Endothelial Dystrophy. Acta Ophthalmol Scand. 1998;76(3):314-8.
15. Anwar HM, El Danasoury A, Hashem A. Descemet's stripping automated endothelial keratoplasty for congenital hereditary endothelial dystrophy. Clin Ophthalmol. 2012;6:159-63.
16. AlArrayedh H, Collum L, Murphy CC. Outcomes of penetrating keratoplasty in congenital hereditary endothelial dystrophy. Br J Ophthalmol. 2018;102(1):19-25.
17. Chaurasia S, Ramappa M, Kannabiran C. Parents of patients with congenital hereditary endothelial dystrophy should be evaluated for Fuchs endothelial corneal dystrophy. Cornea. 2017;36(12):e34-e35.
18. Forsius H, Damsten M, Eriksson AW, et al. Autosomal recessive cornea plana. A clinical and genetic study of 78 cases in Finland. Acta Ophthalmol Scand. 1998;76(2): 196-203.
19. Jaja Z, Lezrek O, Daoudi R, et al. Cornea plana: Case report and review of the literature. J Fr Ophtalmol. 2017;40(2):e45-e47.
20. Roche O, Uteza Y, Dufier JL, et al. Congenital megalocornea. J Fr Ophtalmol. 2002;25(3):312-8.
21. Kuwabara T, Ciccarelli EC. Meesmann's Corneal Dystrophy. A Pathological Study. Arch Ophthalmol. 1964;71:672-82.
22. Roca PD. Meesmann's hereditary epithelial dystrophy (differential diagnosis). Eye Ear Nose Throat Mon. 1969;48(7):424-5.
23. Tremblay M, Dube I. Meesmann's corneal dystrophy: ultrastructural features. Can J Ophthalmol. 1982;17(1):24-8.
24. Wittebol-Post D, van Bijsterveld OP, Delleman JW. Meesmann's epithelial dystrophy of the cornea. Biometrics and a hypothesis. Ophthalmologica. 1987;194(1):44-9.
25. Yeung JY, Hodge WG. Recurrent Meesmann's corneal dystrophy: treatment with keratectomy and mitomycin C. Can J Ophthalmol. 2009;44(1):103-4.
26. Weiss JS. Corneal dystrophy classification. Ophthalmology. 2009;116(5):1013-4.
27. el Aouni A, Briat B, Mayer F, et al. Reis-Buckler dystrophy: therapeutic photo-ablation with the excimer laser. J Fr Ophtalmol. 1998;21(1):23-7.
28. Roncone DP. Granular corneal dystrophy: a novel approach to classification and treatment. Optom Vis Sci. 2014;91(3):e63-71.
29. Weidle EG. Differential diagnosis of corneal dystrophies of the Groenouw I, Reis-Buckler and Thiel-Behnke type. Fortschr Ophthalmol. 1989;86(4):265-71.
30. Boruchoff SA, Kuwabara T. Electron microscopy of posterior polymorphous degeneration. Am J Ophthalmol. 1971;72(5):879-87.
31. Panda A, Kumar S, Kumar A, et al. Demographic pattern, predisposing factors and management of ulcerative keratitis: evaluation of one thousand unilateral cases at a tertiary care centre. Clin Exp Ophthalmol. 2007;35(1):44-50.
32. Oliva MS, Schottman T, Gulati M. Turning the tide of corneal blindness. Indian J Ophthalmol. 2012;60(5):423-7.
33. Kunimoto DY, Miller D, Rao GN, et al. Microbial keratitis in children. Ophthalmology. 1998;105(2):252-7.
34. Panda, A, Miller D, Rao GN, et al. Mycotic keratitis in children: epidemiologic and microbiologic evaluation. Cornea. 1997;16(3):295-9.
35. Chaurasia S, Ramappa M, Ashar J, et al. Neonatal infectious keratitis. Cornea. 2014;33(7):673-6.
36. Hsiao CH, Yeung L, Ma DH, et al. Pediatric microbial keratitis in Taiwanese children: a review of hospital cases. Arch Ophthalmol. 2007;125(5):603-9.
37. Liesegang TJ, Forster RK. Spectrum of microbial keratitis in South Florida. Am J Ophthalmol. 1980;90(1):38-47.
38. Asbell P, Stenson S. Ulcerative keratitis. Survey of 30 years' laboratory experience. Arch Ophthalmol. 1982;100(1):77-80.
39. Polack FM, Kaufman HE, Newmark E. Keratomycosis. Medical and surgical treatment. Arch Ophthalmol. 1971;85(4):410-6.
40. Cruz OA, Capo H, Alfonso EC, et al. Microbial keratitis in childhood. Ophthalmology. 1993;100(2):192-6.

41. Kulshrestha OP, Bhargava S, Dube MK. Keratomycosis: a report of 23 cases. Indian J Ophthalmol. 1973;21(2):51-5.
42. Jones BR. Principles in the management of oculomycosis. XXXI Edward Jackson memorial lecture. Am J Ophthalmol. 1975;79(5):719-51.
43. Kivlin JD, Apple DJ, Olson RJ, et al. Dominantly inherited keratitis. Arch Ophthalmol. 1986;104(11):1621-3.
44. Mirzayans F, Pearce WG, MacDonald IM, et al. Mutation of the PAX6 gene in patients with autosomal dominant keratitis. Am J Hum Genet. 1995;57(3):539-48.
45. Pearce WG, Mielke BW, Hassard DT, et al. Autosomal dominant keratitis: a possible aniridia variant. Can J Ophthalmol. 1995;30(3):131-7.
46. Craig JP, Nichols KK, Akpek EK, et al. TFOS DEWS II Definition and Classification Report. Ocul Surf. 2017;15(3):276-83.
47. Kumar S. Vernal keratoconjunctivitis: a major review. Acta Ophthalmol. 2009;87(2):133-47.
48. Bonini S, Lambiase A, Marchi S, et al. Vernal keratoconjunctivitis revisited: a case series of 195 patients with long-term followup. Ophthalmology. 2000;107(6): 1157-63.
49. Fukuda K, Nishida T. Ocular allergic inflammation: interaction between the cornea and conjunctiva. Cornea. 2010;29:S62-7.
50. Trocme SD, Gleich GJ, Kephart GM, et al. Eosinophil granule major basic protein inhibition of corneal epithelial wound healing. Invest Ophthalmol Vis Sci. 1994;35(7):3051-6.
51. Fukuda K, Nishida T. Reciprocal interaction of the conjunctiva and cornea in ocular allergy. J Allergy Clin Immunol. 2010;125(2):493-6.e2.
52. Buckley RJ. Vernal keratopathy and its management. Trans Ophthalmol Soc UK. 1981;101(Pt 2):234-8.
53. Kerr N, Stern GA. Bacterial keratitis associated with vernal keratoconjunctivitis. Cornea. 1992;11(4):355-9.
54. Cameron JA, Mullaney PB. Amblyopia resulting from shield ulcers and plaques of the cornea in vernal keratoconjunctivitis. J Pediatr Ophthalmol Strabismus. 1997;34(4):261-2.
55. Trocme SD, Kephart GM, Bourne WM, et al. Eosinophil granule major basic protein deposition in corneal ulcers associated with vernal keratoconjunctivitis. Am J Ophthalmol. 1993;115(5):640-3.
56. Cameron JA. Shield ulcers and plaques of the cornea in vernal keratoconjunctivitis. Ophthalmology. 1995;102(6):985-93.
57. Cameron JA, Antonios SR, Badr IA. Excimer laser phototherapeutic keratectomy for shield ulcers and corneal plaques in vernal keratoconjunctivitis. J Refract Surg. 1995;11(1):31-5.
58. Reddy JC, Basu S, Saboo US, et al. Management, clinical outcomes, and complications of shield ulcers in vernal keratoconjunctivitis. Am J Ophthalmol. 2013;155(3): 550-9.e1.
59. Cameron JA, Al-Rajhi AA, Badr IA. Corneal ectasia in vernal keratoconjunctivitis. Ophthalmology. 1989;96(11):1615-23.
60. Gautam V, Shrestha GS, Rai PG, et al. Topographic corneal changes in children with vernal keratoconjunctivitis: a report from Kathmandu, Nepal. Cont Lens Anterior Eye. 2015;38(6):461-5.
61. Kankariya VP, Shrestha GS, Rai PG, et al. Management of pediatric keratoconus-evolving role of corneal collagen cross-linking: an update. Indian J Ophthalmol. 2013;61(8):435-40.
62. Sangwan VS, Vemuganti GK, Murthy SI, et al. Vernal keratoconjunctivitis with limbal stem cell deficiency. Cornea. 2011;30(5):491-6.
63. Saboo US, Basu S, Tiwari S, et al. Clinical and cytologic evidence of limbal stem cell deficiency in eyes with long-standing vernal keratoconjunctivitis. Asia Pac J Ophthalmol (Phila). 2013;2(2):88-93.
64. Saboo US, Jain M, Reddy JC, et al. Demographic and clinical profile of vernal keratoconjunctivitis at a tertiary eye care center in India. Indian J Ophthalmol. 2013;61(9):486-9.
65. Schaumberg DA, Nichols JJ, Papaset EB, et al. The international workshop on meibomian gland dysfunction: report of the subcommittee on the epidemiology of, and associated risk factors for, MGD. Invest Ophthalmol Vis Sci. 2011;52(4):1994-2005.
66. Viswalingam M, Morlet N, Dart JK, et al. Blepharokeratoconjunctivitis in children: diagnosis and treatment. Br J Ophthalmol. 2005;89(4):400-3.
67. Hamada S, Denniston AK, Rauz S, et al. Childhood blepharokeratoconjunctivitis: characterising a severe phenotype in white adolescents. Br J Ophthalmol. 2012;96(7):949-55.
68. O'Gallagher M, Bunce C, Larkin F, et al. Systemic treatment for blepharokeratoconjunctivitis in children. Cochrane Database Syst Rev. 2016;(5):CD011750.
69. O'Gallagher M, Bunce C, Hingorani M, et al. Topical treatments for blepharokeratoconjunctivitis in children. Cochrane Database Syst Rev. 2017;2:CD011965.
70. Nishida T. Cornea. In: Krachmer JH, Mannis MJ, Holland EJ (Eds). Cornea: fundamentals, diagnosis and management 2nd edition. Philadelphia: Elsevier Mosby; 2005. pp. 3-26.
71. Rabinowitz YS. Keratoconus. Surv Ophthalmol. 1997;42: 97-119.
72. Barbara A. Textbook on keratoconus: new insights. New Delhi: Jaypee-Highlights Medical Publishers; 2012.
73. Gordon-Shaag A, Millodot M, Shneor E. The epidemiology and etiology of keratoconus. Epidemiology. 2012;70:1.
74. Gokhale NS. Epidemiology of keratoconus. Indian J Ophthalmol. 2013;61(8):382-3.
75. Gomes JA, Tan D, Rapuano CJ, et al. Global consensus on keratoconus and ectatic diseases. Cornea. 2015;34(4): 359-69.
76. Sinjab MM. Keratoconus: when, why and why not. A step by step systematic approach, 1st edition. New Delhi: JP Medical Ltd.; 2012.
77. Kennedy RH, Bourne WM, Dyer JA. A 48-year clinical and epidemiologic study of keratoconus. Am J Ophthalmol. 1986;101:267-73.
78. Cozma I, Atherley C, James NJ. Influence of ethnic origin on the incidence of keratoconus and associated atopic disease in Asian and white patients. Eye (Lond). 2005;19:924-5.

79. Ihalainen A. Clinical and epidemiological features of keratoconus genetic and external factors in the pathogenesis of the disease. Acta Ophthalmol Suppl (Oxf). 1986;178:1-64.
80. OBrart DP. Corneal collagen cross-linking: a review. J Optom. 2014;7(3):113-24.
81. Sorkin N, Varssano D. Corneal collagen crosslinking: a systematic review. Ophthalmologica. 2014;232(1):10-27.
82. Sykakis E, Karim R, Evans JR, et al. Corneal collagen cross-linking for treating keratoconus. Cochrane Database Syst Rev. 2015;3:CD010621.
83. Millodot M, Shneor E, Albou S, et al. Prevalence and associated factors of keratoconus in Jerusalem: a cross-sectional study. Ophthalmic Epidemiol. 2011;18(2):91-7.
84. Lu Y, Vitart V, Burdon KP, et al. Genome-wide association analyses identify multiple loci associated with central corneal thickness and keratoconus. Nat Genet. 2013;45(2):155-63.
85. Hameedaldeen A, Liu J, Batres A, et al. FOXO1, TGF-β regulation and wound healing. Int J Mol Sci. 2014;15(9):16257-69.
86. Rahi A, Davies P, Ruben M, et al. Keratoconus and coexisting atopic disease. Br J Ophthalmol. 1977;61(12):761-4.
87. Hollingsworth J G, Bonshek RE, Efron N. Correlation of the appearance of the keratoconic cornea in vivo by confocal microscopy and in vitro by light microscopy. Cornea. 2005;24:397-405.
88. Hollingsworth JG, Efron N. Observations of banding patterns (Vogt striae) in keratoconus: a confocal microscopy study. Cornea. 2005;24:162-6.
89. Hollingsworth JG, Efron N, Tullo AB. In vivo corneal confocal microscopy in keratoconus. Ophthalmic Physiol Opt. 2005;25:254-60.
90. Fullwood NJ, Meek KM, Malik NS, et al. A comparison of proteoglycan arrangement in normal and keratoconus human corneas. Biochem Soc Trans. 1990;18(5):961-2.
91. Cheng EL, Maruyama I, Sundar Raj N, et al. Expression of type XII collagen and hemidesmosome-associated proteins in keratoconus corneas. Curr Eye Res. 2001;22(5):333-40.
92. Chaerkady R, Shao H, Scott SG, et al. The keratoconus corneal proteome: loss of epithelial integrity and stromal degeneration. J Proteomics. 2013;87:122-31.
93. Fini ME, Yue BY, Sugar J. Collagenolytic/gelatinolytic metalloproteinases in normal and keratoconus corneas. Curr Eye Res. 1992;11(9):849-62.
94. Kao WW, Vergnes JP, Ebert J, et al. Increased collagenase and gelatinase activities in keratoconus. Biochem Biophys Res Commun. 1982;107:929-36.
95. Halainen A, Salo T, Forsius H, et al. Increase in type I and type IV collagenolytic activity in primary cultures of keratoconus cornea. Eur J Clin Invest. 1986;16(1):78-84.
96. Kenney MC, Chwa M, Atilano SR, et al. Increased levels of catalase and cathepsin V/L2 but decreased TIMP-1 in keratoconus corneas: evidence that oxidative stress plays a role in this disorder. Invest Ophthalmol Vis Sci. 2005;46(3):823-32.
97. Balasubramanian SA, Mohan S, Pye DC, et al. Proteases, proteolysis and inflammatory molecules in the tears of people with keratoconus. Acta Ophthalmol. 2012;90(4):e303-9.
98. Pannebaker C, Chandler HL, Nichols JJ. Tear proteomics in keratoconus. Mol Vis. 2010;16:1949-57.
99. Jun AS, Cope L, Speck C, et al. Subnormal cytokine profile in the tear fluid of keratoconus patients. PLoS One. 2011;6(1):e16437.
100. Soria J, Villarrubia A, Merayo-Lloves J, et al. Label-free LC-MS/MS quantitative analysis of aqueous humor from keratoconic and normal eyes. Mol Vis. 2015;21:451-60.
101. Behndig A, Karlsson K, Johansson BO, et al. Superoxide dismutase isoenzymes in the normal and diseased human cornea. Invest Ophthalmol Vis Sci. 2001;42(10):2293-6.
102. Buddi R, Lin B, Atilano SR, et al. Evidence of oxidative stress in human corneal diseases. J Histochem Cytochem. 2002;50(3):341-51.
103. Gondhowiardjo TD, van Haeringen NJ. Corneal aldehyde dehydrogenase, glutathione reductase, and glutathione S-transferase in pathologic corneas. Cornea. 1993;12(4):310-4.
104. Gondhowiardjo TD, van Haeringen NJ, Völker-Dieben HJ, et al. Analysis of corneal aldehyde dehydrogenase patterns in pathologic corneas. Cornea. 1993;12(2):146-54.
105. Akhurst RJ. TGF beta signaling in health and disease. Nat Genet. 2004;36:790-630.
106. Dietz HC. TGF-beta in the pathogenesis and prevention of disease: a matter of aneurysmic proportions. J Clin Invest. 2010;120:403-7.
107. Priyadarsini S, McKay TB, Sarker-Nag A, et al. Keratoconus in vitro and the key players of the TGF-β pathway. Mol Vis. 2015;21:577-88.
108. Haney WP, Falls HF. The occurrence of congenital keratoconus posticus. Am J Ophthalmol.1961;52:53-7.
109. Noyes HD. Traumatic keratitis caused by forceps delivery of an infant. Trans Am Ophthalmol Soc. 1895;7:454.
110. Taneri S, Jarade E, Kanellopoulos JA, et al. Current concepts and future developments of corneal cross-linking. J Ophthalmol. 2015;302983:1-2.
111. Barbara R, Pikkel J, Garzozi H, et al. Collagen cross-linking and keratoconus in pediatric patients. Int J Keratoconus Ectatic Corn Dis. 2012. pp. 57-60.
112. McMonnies CW. Abnormal rubbing and keratectasia. Eye Contact Lens. 2007;33(6 Pt 1):265-71.
113. Knox Cartwright NE, Tyrer JR, Marshall J. Age-related differences in the elasticity of the human cornea. Invest Ophthalmol Vis Sci. 2011;52(7):4324-9.
114. Daxer A, Misof K, Grabner B, et al. Collagen fibrils in the human corneal stroma: structure and aging. Invest Ophthalmol Vis Sci. 1998;39(3):644-8.
115. Ortiz D, Shabayek MH, Arnalich-Montiel F, et al. Corneal biomechanical properties in normal, post-laser in situ keratomileusis, and keratoconic eyes. J Cataract Refract Surg. 2007;33(8):1371-5.
116. Kuo IC, Broman A, Pirouzmanesh A, et al. Is there an association between diabetes and keratoconus? Ophthalmology. 2006;113(2):184-90.

117. Wollensak G, Spoerl E, Seiler T. Stress-strain measurements of human and porcine corneas after riboflavin-ultraviolet-a-induced cross-linking. J Cataract Refract Surg. 2003;29(9):1780-5.
118. Wagner H, Barr JT, Zadnik K, Group CLEOKS. Collaborative longitudinal evaluation of keratoconus (CLEK) study: methods and findings to date. Cont Lens Anterior Eye. 2007;30(4):223-32.
119. Wollensak G, Iomdina E. Biomechanical and histological changes after corneal crosslinking with and without epithelial debridement. J Cataract Refract Surg. 2009;35:540-6.
120. Spoerl E, Wollwnsak G, Seiler T. Increased resistance of crosslinked cornea against enzymatic digestion. Curr Eye Res. 2004;29:35-40.
121. Wollensak G, Wilsch M, Spoerl E, et al. Collagen fiber diameter in the rabbit cornea after collagen crosslinking by riboflavin/UVA. Cornea. 2004;23:503-7.
122. Mazzotta C, Balestrazzi A, Traversi C, et al. Treatment of progressive keratoconus by riboflavin-UVA induced cross-linking of corneal collagen: ultrastructural analysis by Heidelberg retinal tomography II in vivo confocal microscopy in humans. Cornea. 2007;26:390-7.
123. Mazzotta C, Traversi C, Baiocchi S, et al. Corneal healing after riboflavin ultraviolet-A collagen cross-linking determined by confocal laser scanning microscopy in vivo: early and late modifications. Am J Ophthalmol. 2008;146:527-33.
124. Wollensak G, Redl B. Gel electrophoretic analysis of corneal collagen after photodynamic cross-linking treatment. Cornea. 2008;27:353-6.
125. Witting- Silva C, Whiting M, Lamoreux E, et al. A randomized controlled trial of corneal collagen cross-linking in progressive keratoconus: preliminary results. J Refract Surg. 2008;24:720-5.
126. Raiskup-Wolf F, Hoyer A, Spoerl E, et al. Collagen crosslinking with riboflavin and ultraviolet-A light in keratoconus: long-term results. J Cataract Refract Surg. 2008;34:796-801.
127. Artola A, Javaloy J, Ali JL, et al. Microbial keratitis after corneal collagen crosslinking. J Cataract Refract Surg. 2009;35(6):1138-40.
128. Pollhammer M, Cursiefen C. Bacterial keratitis early after corneal crosslinking with riboflavin and ultraviolet-a. J Cataract Refract Surg. 2009;35(3):588-9.
129. Raiskup F, Theuring A, Pillunat LE, et al. Corneal collagen crosslinking with riboflavin and ultraviolet-a light in progressive keratoconus: ten-year results. J Cataract Refract Surg. 2015;41(1):41-6.
130. Rana M, Lau A, Aralikatti A, et al. Severe microbial keratitis and associated perforation after corneal crosslinking for keratoconus. Cont Lens Anterior Eye. 2015;38(2):134-7.
131. Rabinowitz YS. Keratoconus. Surv Ophthalmol. 1998;42(4):297-319.
132. Galvis V, Sherwin T, Tello A, et al. Keratoconus: an inflammatory disorder? Eye (Lond). 2015;29(7):843-59.
133. Reeves SW, Stinnett S, Adelman RA, et al. Risk factors for progression to penetrating keratoplasty in patients with keratoconus. Am J Ophthalmol. 2005;140:607-11.
134. Wollensak G. Crosslinking treatment of progressive keratoconus: new hope. Curr Opin Ophthalmol. 2006;17:356-60.
135. Magli A, Forte R, Tortori A, et al. Epithelium-off corneal collagen cross-linking versus transepithelial cross-linking for pediatric keratoconus. Cornea. 2013;32(5):597-601.

Chapter 70 Refractive Error in Childhood

Zachary P Elkin, Scott R Lambert

INTRODUCTION

A major component of clear vision is the ability of light rays entering the eye to form a focused image on the retina. Emmetropia is the state when light is perfectly focused, a complex interaction of the corneal and lenticular refraction and length of the eye. Any deviation from this state results in a refractive error. Refractive errors can be broadly characterized into 3 groups: hyperopia/hypermetropia when light focuses behind the retina; myopia when light focuses in front of the retina; and astigmatism when there are different refractive powers at different axes of the optical system. The amount of correction needed to treat refractive error is measured in diopters (D). Hyperopia is treated with positive lenses, whereas myopia is treated with minus lenses. Unlike adults, however, diagnosing and appropriately treating refractive errors in children is not only important for a child to see clearly, but also allows for appropriate development of the entire visual system. In this chapter, we will explore the epidemiology of refractive error in the growing eye, how to measure refractive errors in children, when to screen, when and how to treat, and the growing epidemic of progressive myopia.

EMMETROPIZATION: NORMAL CHANGES IN REFRACTIVE ERROR

The most straightforward way to understand and remember the normal changes in refractive error is through the process of emmetropization. As described above, the combination of the focusing power of the cornea and lens as well as the length of the eye dictate the overall refraction of an eye. Table 70.1 lists the comparative changes in refractive power of the lens and cornea and length of the eye from birth to early childhood to adulthood. Not surprisingly the short axial length at birth leads to a mild to moderate hyperopic refractive error as a newborn. During the first year of life, there is a rapid increase in the axial length of the eye, leading to a corresponding decrease in hyperopia from approximately +2.00 D to +0.75 D.[1] It is estimated that by age 3, the average axial length increases from 18 mm to 23 mm, with a 2–3 D shift in refraction for each millimeter.[2] Axial elongation continues until approximately 6 years of age at a much slower pace.[1,3] Also during this time, the variation of refractive errors among children decreases, resulting in a more unified distribution with decreases in both hyperopia and myopia.[1]

The process of emmetropization and subsequent myopic shift continues until puberty when it tends to slow down. However, this rate varies largely among populations, particularly with high levels of myopic shift in East Asian populations into the late teenage years. Myopia may become manifest even into early adulthood. This resulting myopia epidemic will be discussed later in this chapter.

Refractive Errors in Children: A Failure in Emmetropization

Refractive errors in children can be considered a failure in the normal process of emmetropization. Eyes can fail to complete

Table 70.1: Refracting power and axial length by age.

	Newborn	3-year-old	Adult
Average refraction (D)	+0.50 to +2.60	+0.60 to +3.00	Plano to –0.50
Corneal power (D)	51–55	43–44	43–43.5
Lens power (D)	25–34	22	19–20
Axial length (mm)	16.7–17.5	22	22.8–23.5

Source: Whitmore WG. Congenital and developmental myopia. Eye (Lond). 1992;6:361-5.

the transition to emmetropia and remain hyperopic or can continue to progress to myopia. Population studies have demonstrated variation in refractive errors by race/ethnicity, geographic location, and gestational age. However, any direct comparison between studies needs to take into consideration the different techniques used for measuring refractive errors, screening methodology, and definitions for cutoffs.

Hyperopia

Hyperopia is most prevalent in young children, particularly under 6 years of age. Most studies have demonstrated no differences in the rate of hyperopia between sexes and socioeconomic classes. Some studies, however, have found a higher prevalence of hyperopia in rural children, children who spend more time outdoors, children with younger mothers and maternal smoking during pregnancy.[4-6]

Figures 70.1 and 70.2 summarize the prevalence of hyperopia in several cross-sectional studies.[6-12] In children 1 year and younger, 40–80% have at least 1 D of hyperopia in these population studies, with 1–7% having greater than 4 D of hyperopia. In general, African American children have the lowest prevalence of hyperopia compared to Caucasian and Hispanic children. The Strabismus, Amblyopia, and Refractive Error in Young Singaporean Children (STARS) study found a lower prevalence of hyperopia than all the United States studies and a study conducted in Shanghai, China.[8,12] Among children aged 3–5 years of varying ethnicity in the United States, Caucasian children have the highest prevalence of hyperopia (greater than 3.00 D) and Asian children the lowest.[10]

After the preschool years, hyperopia becomes less common. A meta-analysis of multiple smaller studies throughout the world showed the prevalence of hyperopia drops to 5% by age 7 and 1% by age 15 years.[4] In Australia, moderate hyperopia decreases from 13.2% to 5.0% from age 6 to 12 years.[5] The decrease is more evident in Asia. In Malaysia, a study of multi-ethnic groups found the prevalence of hyperopia greater than 2.00 D decreased from 3.8–5% in 7 year olds, to 1% in 15-year-olds. It was higher in non-Chinese ethnicities.[13] In rural southern China, hyperopia greater than +2.00 D was less than 1% by age 13.[14]

Myopia

Figures 70.1 and 70.2 demonstrate that even mild myopia is rare in children up to 6 years of age. The highest prevalence of myopia in these studies was in African American children. However, most other populations, including East Asian populations have only 1–2% prevalence of myopia by age 6. As children get older, however, myopia becomes more common. The number of new myopic cases increases the most from ages 9 to 14 years, peaking around age 11 years.[15] Between the ages of 6 and 16 years, myopia progresses on

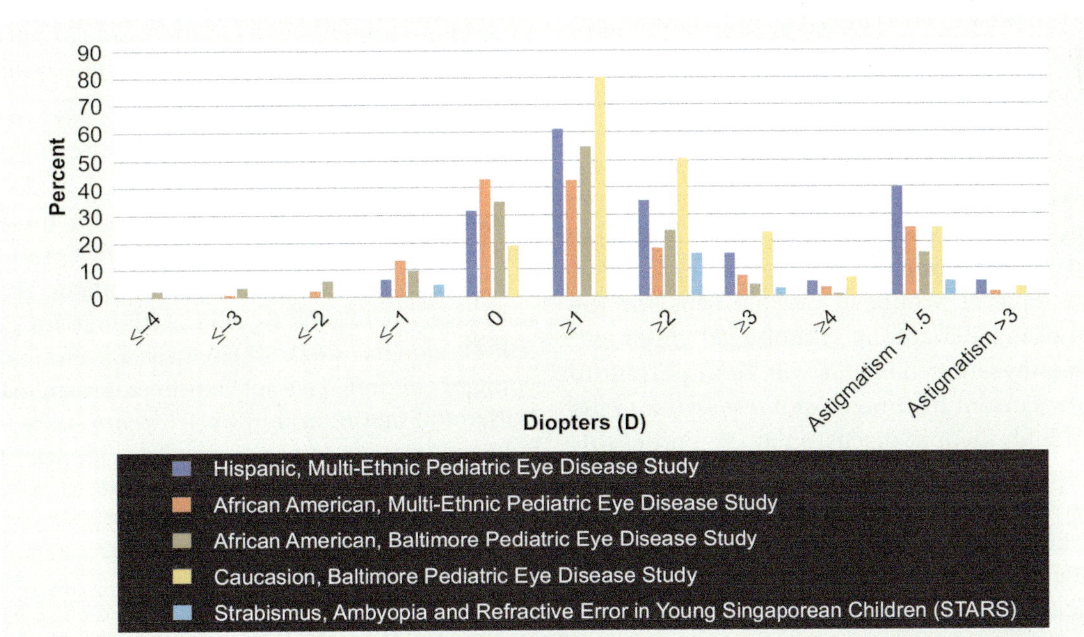

Fig. 70.1: Distribution of refractive errors in the first year of life. The majority of children under the age of 1 have at least 1.00 D of hyperopia in population-based studies in the United States and Asia. Up to 40% have at least 1.50 D of astigmatism. Myopia is uncommon.

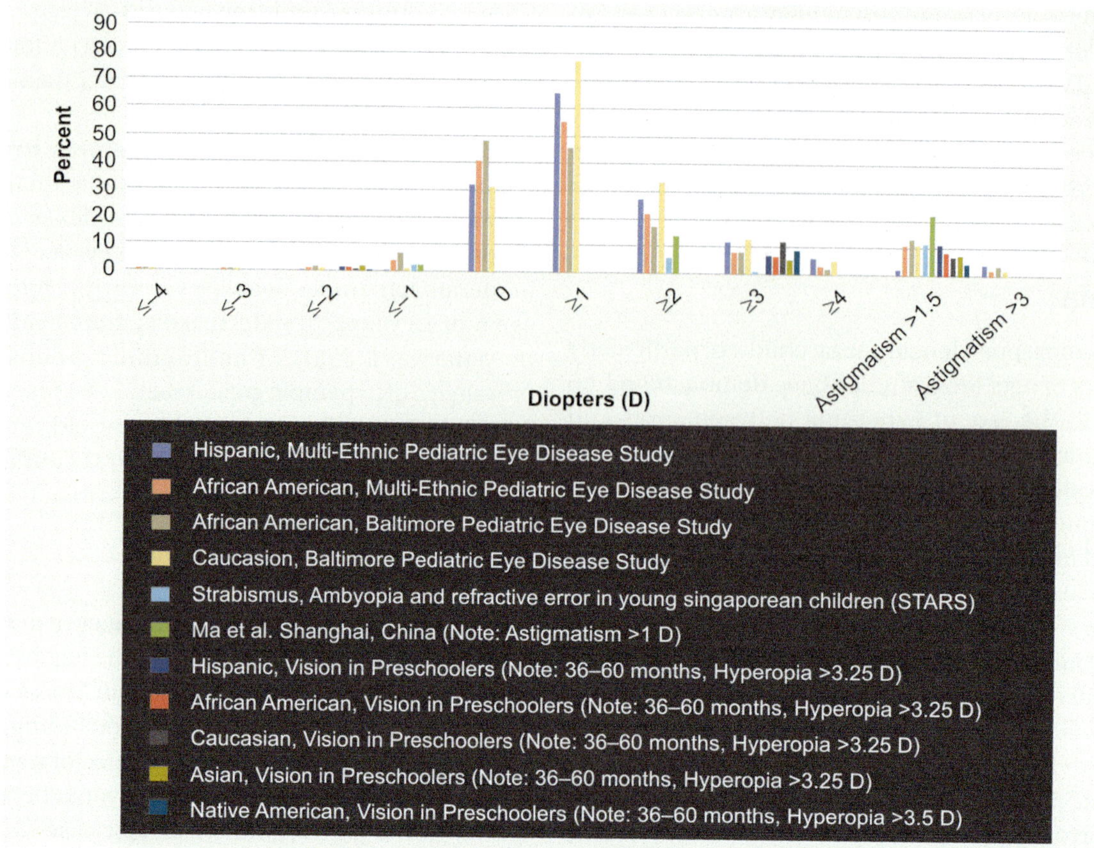

Fig. 70.2: Distribution of refractive errors by age 6. Hyperopia remains the most common refractive error through the preschool age. Compared to 1 year olds, there is a trend towards emmetropia and decreased astigmatism by this age.

average 0.50 D per year.[16] It also occurs more commonly in Asian populations compared to other ethnicities. In Malaysia, for example, myopia of at least 0.50 D increases from 9.8% in 7-year-olds to 34.4% in 15-year-olds, and was most common in children of Chinese ethnicity.[13] In rural China, myopia has a prevalence of 53.9%.[14] This trend is seen in other ethnic groups as well. By age 12, 46% of Australian children need myopic spectacle correction.[17]

There are several proposed mechanisms for the development of myopia among school-aged children.[16] Understanding these mechanisms will be important to understand the current treatments and research into the prevention of high myopia discussed at the end of this chapter. There is likely a genetic component, whereby children with two myopic parents tend to have longer axial lengths. Environmental factors are also likely at play. It has been hypothesized that hyperopic blur, or a slight defocus of light behind the retina, causes the increase in growth factors leading to elongation of the sclera and axial length. This is particularly evident in hyperopic blur of the peripheral retina. Additionally, myopic children have delayed accommodation compared to emmetropes. It has been proposed that delayed focus when doing near work causes blur triggering axial length growth.

Astigmatism

Astigmatism has a high prevalence in the first few years of life. Figure 70.1 demonstrates that 5–40% of children at age 1 year have at least 1.50 D of astigmatism. That generally decreases to 10% by 6 years. Astigmatism greater than 3.00 D remains rare (< 5%) in these age groups. In general, younger children have against-the-rule astigmatism (steep horizontal meridian) but by 4–5 years shifts to with-the-rule astigmatism (steep vertical meridian).[18] It has been proposed that the weight of the eyelids as the child grows causes this shift.

Refractive Errors and Systemic Conditions

Lastly, there are some congenital and systemic conditions that are associated with refractive errors. These include

Down syndrome with hyperopia, Stickler syndrome, X-linked congenital stationary nightblindness and laser treated retinopathy of prematurity with myopia, and albinism with astigmatism.[11,19] Extremely preterm children are more likely to have myopia, hyperopia, and astigmatism.[20]

Measuring Refractive Errors

The act of measuring refractive errors in young, uncooperative children is a skill that requires patience and often combining a variety of techniques to determine the correct refractive error.

Cycloplegic Refraction

Unlike measuring refractive errors in adults, a full cycloplegic refraction is needed in children. Cycloplegia means accommodation, or the ability of the eye to change its focus from distance to near, is paralyzed. Children have such strong accommodation that they can easily change their refractive error while being tested. Over the age of 6 months, cycloplegia is usually achieved in the office with cylopentolate 1% and waiting at least 45 minutes. Phenylephrine 2.5% or tropicamide (0.5% or 1%) may be used to dilate the pupil but are insufficient to achieve cycloplegia. For younger children, drops that combine cyclopentolate 0.2% and phenylephrine 1% can be used. Atropine 1% can also be administered at home by parents one to several days prior to their clinic appointment since it takes longer to work. Atropine is the most effective agent for cycloplegia. However, it is associated with a variety of anticholinergic side effects (e.g. fever, tachycardia, nausea, vomiting, flushing, hyperactivity, etc.) that should be reviewed with parents.[19]

Manifest Refraction

The gold standard for measuring refractive errors is to perform a manifest refraction using a phoropter and a vision chart at the end of the room (Fig. 70.3). A phoropter uses spherical and cylindrical lenses with a Jackson cross cylinder to refine both the spherical and cylindrical components of the prescription. The general process of using the phoropter is to give a patient two choices of lenses and ask them which is clearer and sharper, and continue to show them comparisons until they reach a point that they do not appreciate any differences in clarity. These comparisons are generally done first to refine the spherical power, then the cylinder axis, and finally the cylinder power. Phoropter come with both positive and negative cylinder lenses. Checking refractive errors with a phoropter is often only possible for older children because it requires a significant amount of patient cooperation to understand the concept of comparing two images and to communicate these preferences. It can also be time consuming, especially for beginners, and children will lose patience.

Retinoscopy

Retinoscopy, on the other hand, requires little patient cooperation, and therefore, it is the technique of choice for very young, uncooperative, or nonverbal patients (Fig. 70.4). Retinoscopy uses a retinoscope to shine a slit of

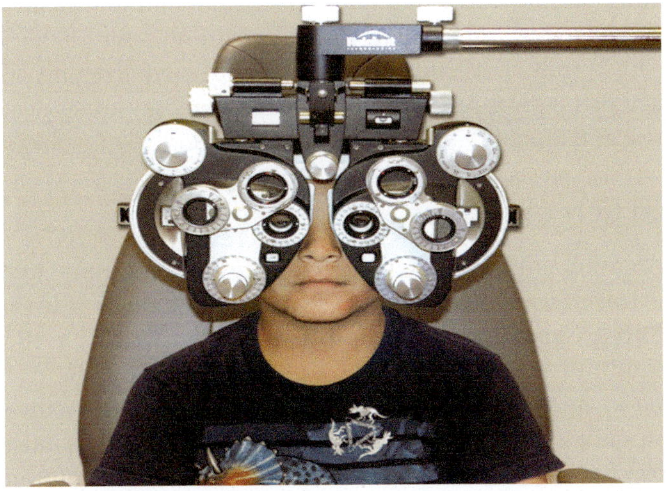

Fig. 70.3: Manifest refraction with phoropter. A child sitting behind a phoropter undergoing manifest cycloplegic refraction.

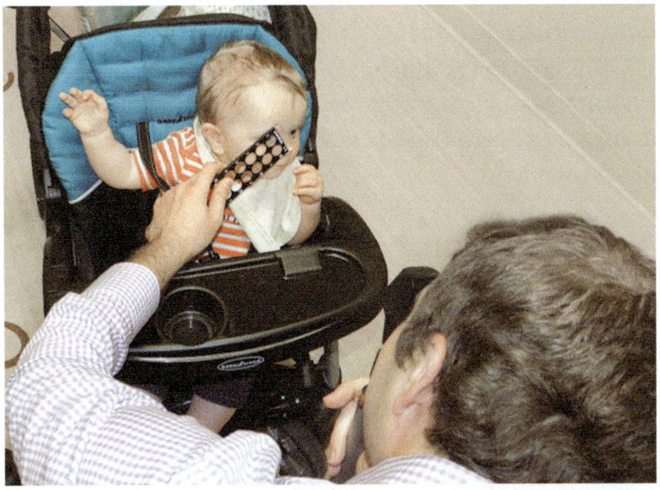

Fig. 70.4: Retinoscopy. Retinoscopy performed with lens bar at a working distance equivalent to 1.50 D (approximately 0.67 meters).

light into the eye and then evaluating the movement of the red reflex to measure the refractive error. When a slit of light is focused directly on the retina (e.g. emmetropia), the red reflex will be uniform and take up the entire pupil. This is called neutralization. When a slit of light focuses behind the retina (e.g. hyperopia) as it moves across the pupil, there will be a linear red reflex that moves in the same direction. This is called *with motion*. When the light focuses in front of the retina (e.g. myopia), the linear red reflex will move in the opposite direction. This is called *against motion*. The goal of retinoscopy is to place different powered lenses, either free lenses or through the phoropter, until the light from the retinocope is neutralized. The prescription for the refractive error is the lenses needed to neutralize the red reflex. Both the horizontal and vertical axes need to be neutralized to check for astigmatism. If the patient has an oblique red reflex, the axis of the reflex represents the axis of astigmatism. The general steps for retinoscopy are:

- Streak the light in both the horizontal and vertical axes, with progressively more minus lenses until with motion is achieved in both axes.
- Progressively add plus power to the lenses until one (or both axes) are neutralized.
- If needed, add additional plus power until the second axis is neutralized.
- The prescription, in plus cylinder notation, will be the lower power lens with the cylinder power as the difference between the two lenses at the axis of the second lens.
- Since you are not checking the retinoscopy at infinite distance, you must subtract your working distance from the sphere to account for the divergence of the light rays as they enter the patient's eyes. For an average sized adult, that is 1.50 D.

This concept is difficult to explain in text, but a simple internet search for online retinoscopy tutorials provides many free tutorials to practice this test prior to performing it on real patients.

Autorefraction

Autorefractors are optical devices that automatically estimate the spherical and cylindrical refractive error (Fig. 70.5). The advantage of autorefractors is the ease of use, speed, and patients' acceptance. Many autorefractors have built in fogging mechanisms that reduce accommodation without cycloplegia, but studies have found that non-cycloplegic autorefractions overminus children.[21] When prescribing glasses, autorefraction should still be done after cycloplegia and then confirmed with retinoscopy or a manifest refraction using a phoropter.

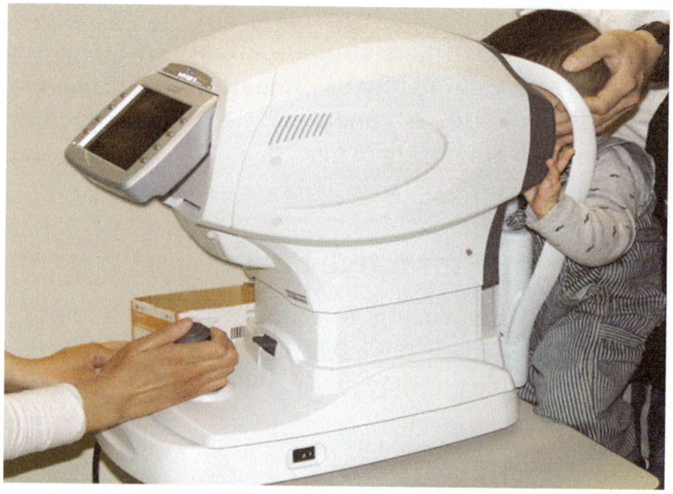

Fig. 70.5: Autorefraction. A 10-month-old child undergoing cycloplegic autorefraction with a table mounted unit.

Photoscreeners

Photoscreeners have become increasingly popular to assess for amblyogenic risk factors including high hyperopia or myopia, astigmatism, and anisometropia (unequal refractive error between the eyes). Photoscreeners use infrared light or a camera flash to capture a red reflex. The brightness and symmetry of the red reflex in the two eyes can be analyzed by practitioners or using algorithms to detect potentially amblyogenic refractive errors.[22] Photoscreeners can be table mounted, handheld, or even smartphone based. They have sensitivities and specificities for detecting amblyogenic risk factors from 70% to 100%.[22] These tools have become popular for pediatricians to screen children for refractive errors since they are easy to use and do not require patient participation.[19]

Screening for Refractive Errors

An adult will know that she needs to have her refractive error checked when she notices her vision is blurry. The prescription she would be provided would be the minimum needed to achieve clear vision, and she can be treated with glasses, contact lenses, or even refractive surgery. For children, knowing when refractive errors must be checked and treated is more complex. Often children are too young to know or communicate that they have blurry vision. Furthermore, they often have sufficient accommodation to overcome their hyperopia and do not do fine tasks that require emmetropia. On the other hand, untreated refractive errors can lead to amblyopia and strabismus.[5,19] In older children, untreated high hyperopia may also be associated with learning difficulties and eye strain.[5] Therefore, a general rule for screening and treating refractive errors is only to do so to prevent amblyopia, improve ocular alignment and binocularity, or reduce eye strain.[19]

As such, the evidence to screen and treat for refractive errors is closely related to screening and treating for amblyopia. Several professional groups, including the United States Preventive Services Task Force (USPSTF) and the American Academy of Ophthalmology (AAO) have described guidelines for screening and treating amblyopia risk factors, including refractive errors. For children under 3 years old, there is currently insufficient evidence to comment on the need for vision screening.[23] Children 3–5 years of age should be screened for amblyopia risk factors at least once, and every 1–2 years thereafter.[19,23] Screening would entail an age appropriate assessment of visual acuity, alignment and motility measurements, and external examination. This is typically completed during a well-child examination in a pediatrician's office. As previously noted, photoscreeners are becoming an increasingly popular vision screening tool and are recommended after 6 months of age.[19] A failed vision screening would warrant referral to an eye care professional for a comprehensive examination, including cycloplegic refraction.

Treating Refractive Errors

Treating refractive errors is a much debated topic because there is still uncertainty whether early correction of refractive error can prevent amblyopia or strabismus, or improve the visual outcome.[19,24] Table 70.2 demonstrates the current AAO recommendations regarding when to treat refractive errors by age based on consensus among experts. In general, hyperopia of +4.50 to +6.00, myopia of -3.00 to -5.00, and astigmatism of 2.00 to 3.00 D are treated. Lesser refractive error is treated in children with strabismus or anisometropia, since they are at higher risk of developing amblyopia. Children with moderate hyperopia (+3.00 to +4.50 D) may still be at increased risk of decreased visual acuity or binocular vision, and should be followed closely;[25] however, there is currently insufficient evidence that spectacles should be prescribed to this population.[26] When prescribing a correction, the associated costs including direct costs of frames and lenses, as well as indirect costs for time lost from work purchasing glasses and going to doctors visits, and psychosocial costs of wearing glasses must be factored.[26]

Furthermore, these recommendations do not necessarily apply to children at high risk for amblyopia including preterm infants, children with Down syndrome, cerebral palsy, and seizure disorders, or children who are less likely to return for follow-up (e.g. children in lower socioeconomic classes who have difficulty accessing care).[19] Children up to 10-year-old with amblyopia due to refractive errors should be counseled to wear their glasses or contact lenses.[27,28]

Glasses

The oldest and mainstay form of treatment is a prescription for glasses. There are many companies now that make glasses specifically for children, and that take into consideration the different anatomy and activity level of children compared to adults. Frames should be made of flexible and durable material (Fig. 70.6). They should be secured either with a strap around the head or flexible ear pieces, may include silicon nose pads for comfort.[29] Children with poor vision should be fit with polycarbonate or Trivex lenses to reduce the risk of shattering. If a child spends a significant amount of time outside or lives in an area with high UV exposure, lenses should block 99% of UVA/B spectrum light. Often polarized lenses are more comfortable in bright light. Finally, children requiring bifocals should be fit in an optician's office to ensure that

Table 70.2: American Academy of Ophthalmology 2012 guidelines for refractive correction.

	<1-year-old	**1–2-year-old**	**2–3-year-old**
Myopia	–5.00 D or more	–4.00 D or more	–3.00 D or more
Hyperopia without strabismus	+6.00 D or more	+5.00 D or more	+4.50 D or more
Hyperopia with strabismus	+2.50 D or more	+2.00 D or more	+1.50 D or more
Astigmatism	3.00 D or more	2.50 D or more	2.00 D or more

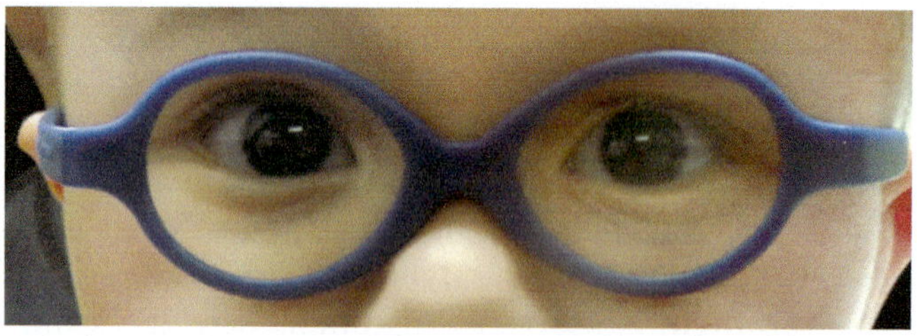

Fig. 70.6: Pediatric spectacles. The durable and flexible materials in the frames protect the spectacles from breaking. The frames should be secured to the back of the head and a silicon nasal bridge can be used for support on the nose if needed.

an executive style bifocal is dispensed that splits the child's pupil.

Adherence to wearing glasses is often the biggest problem for children. Optical problems like induced prism causing double vision can occur with large refractive errors. Surveys have looked at ways to improve glasses' adherence in children.[30] Females and children that have higher refractive errors are more likely to wear their glasses. Style also plays a big role in the acceptance of glasses. Children must like the glasses they wear, and parents should understand that their preferences may change with time. Styles will also vary by culture, so opticians should be prepared with the most up-to-date frames, especially for older children.

Contact Lenses

The Contact Lenses in Pediatrics (CLIP) studies in both the United States and Asia demonstrated that children as young as 8 years can use daily soft contact lenses, without a marked increase in serious adverse events.[16] Younger children, however, often require more time to be trained in using them. Similar to adults, qualitative studies show that for some children, wearing contact lenses has positive benefits on self-esteem and performance in certain activities. Children should work with their provider to make sure that their contact lenses are fit appropriately and that they know how to care for their lenses. Daily disposable lenses are the easiest to maintain, but can be too costly of an option. Children must be educated not to shower, swim, or sleep in their contact lenses, as this increases the risk of infection. Contact lenses are often used in infants who have their lenses removed for congenital cataracts, in children with very large differences in prescriptions between the eyes, or children with irregular astigmatism that cannot be corrected with glasses.

Orthokeratology

Orthokeratology is a specially engineered lens to be worn at night, which provides temporary central corneal thinning and peripheral corneal thickening during the day.[31] The change in the shape of the cornea allows for myopic correction without wearing contact lenses or glasses during the day. Many providers, however, are hesitant to recommend orthokeratology given the increased risk of corneal infections associated with wearing contact lenses while a child sleeps.

Refractive Surgery

Increasingly, laser refractive procedures like laser in situ keratomileusis (LASIK) and photorefractive keratectomy (PRK) are being performed on specific pediatric populations.[32] The first populations studied were children with developmental delay or behavioral problems who were intolerant of contact lenses or glasses. More recently it is also being performed on children with amblyopia arising from anisometropia (different prescription between each eye) or high myopia or hyperopia. Since the eyes are still growing, studies have found 50% of patients will have return of myopia of over 1D per year, and there is a higher proportion of children who will develop corneal haze. Special protocols must also be developed to accommodate general anesthesia and uncooperative children who cannot focus on a target.

MYOPIA EPIDEMIC

Beyond the preschool years, however, there is a growing epidemic of myopia. Myopia is not only a simple refractive error requiring spectacle correction. High myopia also increases the risk of retinal detachments, early-onset cataracts, and glaucoma. In some areas of the world it, is becoming a leading cause of blindness.

Much of the attention of the myopia epidemic is focused in East Asia, where some population-based studies have demonstrated a myopia prevalence of up to 85% by age 18 years.[2] Levels of high myopia (<6.00 D) have reached 20%. The prevalence of myopia in these populations not only increases with age but has increased significantly over the past few decades. In 7-year-olds in Taiwan, the prevalence increased from 5.8% in 1983 to 21.0% in 2000. While not as high as in East Asian populations, the increase in prevalence of myopia is occurring in all ethnicities.[15]

Table. 70.3: Treatment modalities for the prevention of myopic progression.

Strong evidence • Anticholinergic drops: Atropine 0.5%, 0.1%, or 0.01% daily – ATOM2 study showed the least rebound myopia after 2 years of use and 1 year washout with atropine 0.01% daily
Moderate evidence • Peripheral retinal defocus – Orthokeratology or specially designed lenses • Increased outdoor time
Poor evidence • Bifocals or progressive addition lenses
No evidence • Undercorrection of myopia

The increasing prevalence of myopia has been attributed to genetics, prolonged near work, accommodative lag, or other biochemical mediators. The interventions proposed to prevent myopic progression all aim to target these mechanisms. There have been several meta-analyses and reviews summarizing the effects of the different treatment modalities (Table 70.3).[16,29,33]

Undercorrection of Myopia

It has been proposed that if myopia is undercorrected, then less accommodation would be used for near work (eyes would be left a little myopic so they would not need to accommodate as much to read) and this would decrease the myopic drive of accommodation. However, clinical studies have not provided convincing evidence to support this theory.

Bifocal or Progressive Addition Lenses

Similar to undercorrection of myopia, the use of bifocal or transition lenses is hypothesized to decrease the accommodate lag in myopes. Most studies, including the Correction of Myopia Evaluation Trial (COMET) study, demonstrated a small reduction in the progression of myopia after a 3-year follow-up.[34] However, this effect was not deemed to be clinically significant.

Peripheral Retinal Defocus

It has been theorized that hyperopic defocus of the peripheral retina results in axial elongation and progressive myopia. Mechanisms to reduce peripheral retinal defocus either by orthokeratology or specially designed contact lenses or glasses, have mixed results in terms of decreasing myopic progression, but may have a moderate effect.[31,33] Orthokeratology lenses are commercially available.

Time Outdoors

Increased time outdoors have been shown to decrease myopic progression. The mechanism is unknown, but it has been proposed that sunlight releases retinal dopamine which inhibits axial elongation, outdoor activities require less accommodation, or pupillary constriction from intense sunlight increases the depth of focus thereby reduce retinal blur. A meta-analysis of studies found a pooled 2% decrease in the odds of myopia with each additional hour of time spent outdoors in a week. However, there was significant heterogeneity of these studies limiting the direct applicability of these results.[35]

Anticholinergic Agents

Anticholinergic agents have also been shown to slow the rate of myopic progression.[36]

The Atropine for the Treatment of Myopia (ATOM) 1 and 2 trials evaluated the use of varying strengths of daily atropine drops on myopic progression.[37] ATOM 1 showed that compared to placebo, daily use of atropine 1% was associated with an 80% reduction in myopia at 2 years. ATOM 2, similarly showed reductions of myopia, albeit less significant, with 0.5%, 0.1%, and 0.01%. There was a dose-dependent reduction with atropine 0.01% resulting in a 60% reduction in the progression of myopia. Interestingly, after a 1 year washout, the higher doses of atropine had larger rebounds in the progression of myopia. Therefore, after 36 months, the atropine 0.01% had the slowest progression of myopia. Retreatment in children who progressed in all groups for another 2 years with atropine 0.01% resulted in further decreases in myopic progression. The adverse effects for pupil dilation and decreased accommodation were also smallest for the lowest dose group. The mechanism of action of anticholinergic agents on myopia is unclear, but they are believed to inhibit the growth and thinning or the retina and sclera through biochemical changes in muscarinic receptors or dilation causing increased UVA exposure.[36] It is therefore not surprising that higher doses would have a greater effect, but also more chance for rebound axial elongation when the suppression is stopped. It should be cautioned; however, most of the studies on atropine have been limited to the Asian populations and may not be applicable to all population groups.[36]

REFERENCES

1. Flitcroft DI. Emmetropisation and the aetiology of refractive errors. Eye (Lond). 2014;28(2):169-79.
2. Wu PC, Huang HM, Yu HJ, et al. Epidemiology of Myopia. Asia Pac J Ophthalmol (Phila). 2016;5(6):386-93.
3. Whitmore WG. Congenital and developmental myopia. Eye (Lond). 1992;6(Pt 4):361-5.
4. Castagno VD, Fassa AG, Carret ML, et al. Hyperopia: a meta-analysis of prevalence and a review of associated factors among school-aged children. BMC Ophthalmol. 2014;14(1):163.
5. Ip JM, Robaei D, Kifley A, et al. Prevalence of hyperopia and associations with eye findings in 6- and 12-year-olds. Ophthalmology. 2008;115(4):678-85.
6. The Multi-Ethnic Pediatric Eye Disease Study. Prevalence of myopia and hyperopia in 6- to 72-month-old African American and Hispanic children. Ophthalmology. 2010; 117(1):140-3.
7. Fozailoff A, Tarczy-Hornoch K, Cotter S, et al. Prevalence of astigmatism in 6- to 72-month-old African American and Hispanic children: The Multi-Ethnic Pediatric Eye Disease Study. Ophthalmology. 2011;118(2):284-93.
8. Ma Y, Qu X, Zhu X, et al. Age-specific prevalence of visual impairment and refractive error in children aged 3-10 years in Shanghai, China. Invest Ophthalmol Vis Sci. 20161;57(14):6188-96.
9. Giordano L, Friedman DS, Repka MX, et al. Prevalence of refractive error among preschool children in an urban population: the Baltimore Pediatric Eye Disease Study. Ophthalmology. 2009;116(4):739-46,746.
10. Ying GS, Maguire MG, Cyert LA, et al. Prevalence of vision disorders by racial and ethnic group among children participating in head start. Ophthalmology. 2014;121(3): 630-6.
11. Quinn GE, Dobson V, Kivlin J, et al. Prevalence of myopia between 3 months and 5½ years in preterm infants with and without retinopathy of prematurity. Cryotherapy for Retinopathy of Prematurity Cooperative Group. Ophthalmology. 1998;105(7):1292-300.
12. Dirani M, Chan YH, Gazzard G, et al. Prevalence of refractive error in Singaporean Chinese children: the strabismus, amblyopia, and refractive error in young Singaporean Children (STARS) study. Invest Ophthalmol Vis Sci. 2010;51(3):1348-55.
13. Goh PP, Abqariyah Y, Pokharel GP, et al. Refractive error and visual impairment in school-age children in Gombak District, Malaysia. Ophthalmology. 2005;112(4):678-85.
14. He M, Xiang F, Zeng Y, et al. Effect of time spent outdoors at school on the development of myopia among children in China: a randomized clinical trial. JAMA. 2015;314(11): 1142-8.
15. Kleinstein RN, Sinnott LT, Jones-Jordan LA, et al.Collaborative longitudinal evaluation of ethnicity and refractive error study group. New cases of myopia in children. Arch Ophthalmol. 2012;130(10):1274-9.
16. Walline JJ, Jones LA, Rah MJ, et al. Contact Lenses in Pediatrics (CLIP) Study: chair time and ocular health. Optom Vis Sci. 2007;84(9):896-902.
17. Robaei D, Kifley A, Rose KA, et al. Refractive error and patterns of spectacle use in 12-year-old Australian children. Ophthalmology. 2006;113(9):1567-73.
18. Gwiazda J, Scheiman M, Mohindra I, et al. Astigmatism in children: changes in axis and amount from birth to six years. Invest Ophthalmol Vis Sci. 1984;25(1):88-92.
19. Preferred Practice Pattern Guidelines. American Academy of Ophthalmology. 2012. [online] Available from: *www.aao.org/ppp*.[Accessed December 2017].
20. Hellgren KM, Tornqvist K, Jakobsson PG, et al. Ophthalmologic outcome of extremely preterm infants at 6.5 years of age: Extremely Preterm Infants in Sweden Study (EXPRESS). JAMA Ophthalmol. American Medical Association; 2016;134(5):555-62.
21. Choong YF, Chen AH, Goh PP. A comparison of autorefraction and subjective refraction with and without cycloplegia in primary school children. Am J Ophthalmol. 2006;142(1):68-74.
22. Sánchez I, Ortiz-Toquero S, Martin R, et al. Advantages, limitations, and diagnostic accuracy of photoscreeners in early detection of amblyopia: a review. Clin Ophthalmol. 2016;10:1365-73.
23. US Preventive Services (TASK FORCE). (2017).Draft Recommendation Statement: Vision in Children Ages 6 Months to 5 Years: Screening. U.S. Preventive Services Task Force. [online] Available from: *https://www.uspreventiveservicestaskforce.org/Page/Document/draft-recommendation-statement/vision-in-children-ages-6-months-to-5-years-screening*.[Accessed December 2017].
24. Jones-Jordan L, Wang X, Scherer RW, Mutti DO. Spectacle correction versus no spectacles for prevention of strabismus in hyperopic children. Jones-Jordan L, editor. Cochrane Database Syst Rev. Chichester, UK: John Wiley & Sons, Ltd; 2014;41(8):CD007738.
25. Ciner EB, Kulp MT, Maguire MG, et al. Visual function of moderately hyperopic 4- and 5-year-old children in the vision in preschoolers - Hyperopia in Preschoolers Study. Am J Ophthalmol. 2016;170:143-52.
26. Lambert SR. Should glasses be prescribed for all children with moderate hyperopia? Ophthalmology. 2016;123(4): 676-8.
27. Cotter SA, Pediatric Eye Disease Investigator Group, Edwards AR, et al. Treatment of anisometropic amblyopia in children with refractive correction. Ophthalmology. 2006;113(6):895-903.
28. Wallace DK, Chandler DL, Beck RW, et al. Treatment of bilateral refractive amblyopia in children three to less than 10 years of age. Am J Ophthalmol. 2007;144(4):487-96.

29. WSPOS (2017). World Society of Paediatric Ophthalmology & Strabismus Consensus Statement on: Spectacle Frames for Children. [online] Available from: *http://wspos.org/wp-content/uploads/2017/01/WSPOS_Consensus-Statement_SPECTACLES.pdf*.[Accessed December 2017].
30. Keay L, Zeng Y, Munoz B, et al. Predictors of early acceptance of free spectacles provided to junior high school students in China. Arch Ophthalmol. 2010;128(10):1328-34.
31. WSOS.(2017).World Society of Paediatric Ophthalmology & Strabismus Myopia Consensus Statement. [online] Available from: *http://wspos.org/wp-content/uploads/2017/01/WSPOS_Consensus-Statement_Myopia.pdf*.[Accessed December 2017].
32. Daoud YJ, Hutchinson A, Wallace DK, et al. Refractive surgery in children: treatment options, outcomes, and controversies. Am J Ophthalmol. 2009;147(4):573-82.
33. Huang J, Wen D, Wang Q, et al. Efficacy comparison of 16 interventions for myopia control in children: a network meta-analysis. Ophthalmology. 2016;123(4):697-708.
34. Gwiazda J, Hyman L, Hussein M, et al. A randomized clinical trial of progressive addition lenses versus single vision lenses on the progression of myopia in children. Invest Ophthalmol Vis Sci. 2003;44(4):1492-500.
35. Sherwin JC, Reacher MH, Keogh RH. The association between time spent outdoors and myopia in children and adolescents: a systematic review and meta-analysis. Ophthalmology. 2012;119(10):2141-51.
36. Pineles SL. Ophthalmic Technology Assessment Committee Pediatric Ophthalmology/Strabismus Panel. American Academy of Ophthalmology (2017). In Press.
37. Chia A, Lu Q-S, Tan D. Five-year clinical trial on atropine for the treatment of myopia 2: myopia control with atropine 0.01% eyedrops. Ophthalmology. 2016;123(2):391-9.

Chapter 71 Amblyopia

Eibhlín Mc Loone, Pamela Anketell

INTRODUCTION

Amblyopia is a unilateral, or occasionally bilateral, reduction of best-corrected visual acuity which occurs:

- In an otherwise healthy eye or
- In an eye with a structural abnormality where the reduction in vision cannot be attributed solely to the abnormality.[1]

The Pediatric Eye Disease Investigator Group (PEDIG)[2] has further defined amblyopia as 'two or more logMAR lines of interocular difference measured in best correction' with two caveats:

1. An interocular difference of 0.1 logMAR is normal for older children
2. An interocular difference of 0.3 logMAR may be normal for children aged 3–4 years.[2]

The prevalence of amblyopia is reported to be between 1.8% and 5.3% in developing populations.[3-5]

Amblyopia develops due to abnormal input to the binocular visual system during early visual development or the critical period when neural plasticity exists. During this time, abnormal input caused by optical blur, for example in anisometropia, or abnormal binocular development in the presence of strabismus results in reduction/suppression of the binocularly driven ocular dominance columns. The visual system is effectively then a monocular system rather than binocular.[6] Early research suggested that the critical period lasts until the age of 8–9 years with improvement in vision noted with the use of appropriate treatment. However, recent research has reported improvement in visual acuity in young adolescents, who had previously not undergone amblyopia treatment, and in adults suggesting that neural plasticity may be present for longer than previously reported.[7,8]

CLASSIFICATION

Amblyopia can be classified as in Table 71.1 with specific characteristics associated with each category.

Table 71.1: Amblyopia classification.

Classification	Laterality	Causative factor
Strabismic	Unilateral	Presence of a childhood-onset manifest strabismus
Anisometropic	Unilateral	Significant interocular difference in spherical refractive error
Meridional	Unilateral	Significant interocular difference in astigmatic refractive error
Stimulus deprivation	Unilateral or bilateral	Blockage of light and/or form stimulus in early life, e.g congenital cataract or ptosis
Ametropic	Bilateral	Uncorrected bilateral high refractive error (myopia or hyperopia)

CLINICAL ASSESSMENT

- *Case history:* The presence of a constant strabismus, an ocular anomaly such as congenital cataract or family history of amblyopia should be queried.
- *Refractive error:* Cycloplegic refraction should be conducted to identify the presence of any significant refractive error.
- *Ophthalmoscopy:* Normal eye structure should be present in isolated amblyopia.
- *Visual acuity:* While the assessment of visual acuity will be determined by the age and ability of the patient, a linear acuity test type is preferable. In amblyopia, individuals may demonstrate the crowding phenomenon; i.e. a reduction in visual acuity when a target is flanked by a visible object such as a letter or crowding bar.[9] No improvement in visual acuity will be noted when visual acuity is assessed with a pinhole in the amblyopic eye.
- *Cover test:* Observation for the presence of strabismus and the accuracy and speed of fixation.
- *Binocular functions:* In the presence of strabismus, suppression may be present. Higher thresholds of stereopsis are described in the presence of amblyopia.[9,10]

- *Neutral density filter:* Under reduced illumination the visual acuity of the amblyopic eye will remain stable or potentially improve while that of the non-amblyopic eye will further reduce.[11] In the presence of an organic defect in the amblyopic eye, a significant reduction in visual acuity will be seen.[12]

MANAGEMENT

As far back as 900 AD, occlusion has been recommended as the primary treatment for amblyopia.[12] However; it has only been in the last decade or so that robust clinical trials have been conducted to explore the optimal management for amblyopia. The PEDIG Group, in particular, have reported on several studies which have significantly impacted on current practice. Table 71.2 provides a summary of the PEDIG studies to date.

While amblyopia treatment response is noted to be better in children under the age of 7 years, some improvement has been noted in older children, particularly if they are treatment-naive.[13,14]

Flowchart 71.1 summarizes the general principles in managing a child with amblyopia.

Correction of Refractive Error

In the presence of reduced vision, any significant refractive error should be corrected. Optical correction alone

Flowchart 71.1: Management of a child with reduced vision due to amblyopia.

Reduced visual acuity in a child (following age-appropriate testing)

↓

Careful history to include family history of childhood eye problems

↓

Cover test/extraocular movement/stereopsis testing to detect any associated strabismus and to exclude nerve palsies

↓

Check for normal pupillary reactions, color vision, fundus and media to exclude an organic lesion. (Amblyopia can cause a mild RAPD but the presence of a significant RAPD should prompt further investigation)

↓

Cycloplegic refraction to detect any significant refractive error. If present, prescribe glasses and review every 6–12 weeks until vision stable. (Period of refractive adaptation)

↓

Persistent reduction of vision following refractive adaptation indicates presence of amblyopia. Commence patching or atropine or bangerter occlusion foil following discussion with parents and review every 6–12 weeks until no further improvement

↓

If residual amblyopia, consider increasing patching dosage to 6 hours daily or atropine with optical penalization or switching treatment modality*

↓

If maximum vision achieved, taper therapy and monitor for amblyopia recurrence

(RAPD: Relative afferent pupillary defect)

*Evidence for switching treatment modalities in residual amblyopia is limited.

Table 71.2: Summary of the Pediatric Eye Disease Investigator Group (PEDIG) Amblyopia Treatment Studies (ATS).[13]

PEDIG Study	Objective	No. of patients (age range) Initial vision (Follow-up)	Conclusion
ATS 1 (2005)	≥6 hours patching versus daily atropine in young children	419 (3 to <7 years) 20/40 – 20/100 (2 years)	Patching or Atropine for an initial 6 months period produced similar improvement 2 years after treatment
ATS 1 Extended (2014)		188 had long-term follow-up and assessed at 15 years of age	Improvement occurring with amblyopia treatment was maintained until at least 15 years of age
ATS 2A (2003)	Part-time (6 hours) versus full-time patching each combined with ≥1 hour near visual activities.	175 (3 to <7 years) 20/100 – 20/400 (4 months)	Vision improvement similar for 6 hours and full-time patching
ATS 2B (2003)	2 hours versus 6 hours patching each combined with ≥1 hour near visual activities	189 (3 to <7 years) 20/40 – 20/80 (4 months)	Vision improvement similar for 2 hours and 6 hours of patching
ATS 2C (2004)	Risk of recurrence in successfully treated amblyopic children after cessation of treatment with patching or atropine	156 (<8 years) (52 weeks)	25% experienced a recurrence within the first year post-treatment. For patients treated with ≥6 hours of patching the risk of recurrence was greater when patching was stopped abruptly rather than a reduction to 2 hours per day prior to cessation
ATS 2C sub-analysis (2007)	Factors associated with recurrence after cessation of patching in subgroup with clearly recorded patching history	96 (<8 years) (52 weeks)	Recurrence was associated with better visual acuity at time of cessation, greater improvement of amblyopic eye during treatment and previous recurrence

Contd...

Contd...

PEDIG Study	Objective	No. of patients (age range) Initial vision (Follow-up)	Conclusion
ATS 3 (2005)	Evaluate effectiveness of amblyopia treatment in older children 2–6 hours patching and atropine with ≥1 hour near visual activities for children aged 7–12 years 2–6 hours patching alone with ≥1 hour near visual activities for children aged 13–17 years	507 (7–17 years) 20/40 – 20/400 (24 weeks)	• In children aged 7–12 years – Optical correction with patching and atropine treatment was superior to optical correction alone even if the amblyopia had been previously treated • In children aged 13–17 years – Optical correction with patching of little benefit if amblyopia was previously treated but may improve visual outcomes in those not previously treated for amblyopia
ATS 4 (2004)	Daily atropine versus weekend atropine in moderate amblyopia	168 (3 to <7 years) 20/40 – 20/80 (4 months)	Vision improvement similar for daily versus weekend atropine
ATS 5A (2006)	Evaluate effectiveness of optical correction alone for the treatment of anisometropic amblyopia	84 (3 to <7 years) 20/40 – 20/250 (≤ 30 weeks)	Optical correction alone improved visual acuity in many cases and resulted in resolution of amblyopia in at least one third. 83% of patients stopped improving before 15 weeks
ATS 5B (2006)	Optical correction + 2 hours patching with ≥1 hour near visual activities versus optical correction alone following an initial period of refractive adaptation	180 (3 to <7 years) 20/40 – 20/400 (5 weeks)	After a period of refractive adaptation, 2 hours patching with ≥1 hour near visual activities modestly improved visual outcomes
ATS 6 (2008)	2 hours patching with near activities (e.g. crafts, reading, writing, computer games) versus 2 hours patching with distance activities (e.g. supervised outdoor play, watching television)	425 (3 to <7 years) 20/40 – 20/400 (17 weeks)	Performing common near activities with patching did not improve visual acuity outcome
ATS 7 (2007)	Evaluate amount and time course of binocular visual acuity improvement in bilateral refractive amblyopia with optical correction	113 (3 to <10 years) 20/40 – 20/400 (1 year)	73% of children achieved visual acuity of 20/25 or better after one year
ATS 8 (2009)	Weekend atropine + plano lens for sound eye versus weekend atropine alone	180 (3 to <7 years) 20/40 – 20/100 (18 weeks)	Prescribing weekend atropine augmented with a plano lens over the sound eye was not substantially better than prescribing weekend atropine alone
ATS 9 (2008)	2 hours patching versus weekend atropine in older children	193 (7 to <13 years) 20/40 – 20/100 (17 weeks)	Vision improvement similar for atropine and patching. About 20% achieved 20/25 or better vision in the amblyopic eye
ATS 10 (2010)	Bangerter filters versus patching	186 (3 to <10 years) 20/40 – 20/80 (24 weeks)	Vision improvement similar for Bangerter filters and patching.
ATS 11 (2011)	Intensive group (6 hours patching and daily atropine) versus weaning group (4 weeks of reduced treatment of 2 hours patching or once weekly atropine, then stopped) for mild residual amblyopia after treatment with 6 hours patching or daily atropine	55 (3 to <10 years) 20/32 – 20/63 (10 weeks)	An intensive final push of combined treatment of patching and atropine did not produce a better visual acuity outcome compared with a gradual discontinuation of treatment
ATS 12 (2013)	2 hours patching with active vision therapy versus 2 hours patching with placebo vision therapy. (Pilot study)	19 (7 to <13 years) 20/40 – 20/100 (16 weeks)	Recruitment and the ability to monitor adherence objectively with computerized home therapy were problematic

Contd...

Contd...

PEDIG Study	Objective	No. of patients (age range) Initial vision (Follow-up)	Conclusion
ATS 13 (2011)	To assess visual acuity improvement in strabismic and combined strabismic-anisometropic amblyopes treated with optical treatment alone	146 (3 to <7 years) 20/50 – 20/400 (18 weeks)	Optical treatment alone resulted in clinically meaningful improvement in amblyopia for most children, resolving in at least 25% without the need for additional treatment
ATS 14 (2010)	Evaluate efficacy and safety of low dose versus higher dose levodopa for 9 weeks combined with daily ocular occlusion therapy in children with residual amblyopia (Pilot study)	33 (8 to <18 years) 20/50 – 20/400 (19 weeks)	Levodopa therapy for residual amblyopia in older children was well tolerated. Both dosage regimens may improve visual acuity. No serious adverse effects were noted
ATS 15 (2013)	Evaluate the effectiveness of increasing prescribed daily patching from 2 to 6 hours for residual amblyopia when vision stops improving with 2 hours of patching	169 (3 to <8 years) 20/32 – 20/160 (10 weeks)	Increasing patching to 6 hours resulted in more improvement in vision compared with continuing 2 hours daily
ATS 16 (2015)	Evaluate the effectiveness of a plano lens with atropine for residual amblyopia when vision stops improving after atropine treatment alone	73 (3 to <8 years) 20/32 – 20/160 (10 weeks)	There may be a small benefit to augmenting atropine therapy with a plano lens; however, it was not statistically significant. A larger study required
ATS 17 (2015)	Sixteen weeks of oral levodopa or placebo 3 times daily with 2 hours patching for residual amblyopia	139 (7 to <13 years) 20/50 – 20/400 (18 weeks)	Oral levodopa while continuing to patch 2 hours daily did not produce a statistically meaningful improvement in VA compared with placebo and patching
ATS 18 (2016)	Binocular iPad game for 1 hour a day versus 2 hours of patching	385 (5 to <13 years) 20/40 – 20/200 (16 weeks)	Although vision improved with binocular game play, particularly in younger children without prior amblyopia treatment, improvement was not as good as with 2 hours of daily patching

improves visual acuity in many patients and, given time, can lead to resolution of amblyopia in about one third of cases.[15-17] The time taken to reach maximal improvement in visual acuity with optimal optical correction (i.e. the refractive adaptation period) is reported to be less than 15–18 weeks for most patients.[18,19]

Treatment Modalities

Following refractive adaptation, the presence of any significant interocular visual acuity difference should prompt discussion with the child and parents regarding amblyopia therapies. As already mentioned, an interocular visual acuity difference of two or more lines is required to diagnose amblyopia.[2]

Occlusion

Occlusion therapy involves the removal of light and/or form sense to the non-amblyopic eye for a defined amount of time dependent on the level of vision of the amblyopic eye. This can be achieved by several methods including adhesive patch, material extension patch or Bangerter occlusion foil (Figs. 71.1A to C). Although conventionally an adhesive patch has been used to occlude the eye, for children with allergies, alternative methods of occlusion are now more readily available including extension patches and Bangerter occlusion foils both of which fit to the child's glasses. The Bangerter occlusion foil is a useful alternative when children are non-compliant with adhesive patches with PEDIG identifying no significant difference in visual acuity outcome between those using conventional occlusion and those using the foil.[20] However, care must be taken with both the extension patch and foil to ensure the child does not look over or around the occlusion.

In recent years, the daily dosage of occlusion prescribed for amblyopia therapy has been investigated to determine the optimal amount of occlusion required to improve vision.[18,21-24] Following a large randomized control trial, the PEDIG group have recommended initial occlusion of 2 hours daily or 6 hours daily for moderate amblyopia (20/40-20/80) and severe amblyopia (20/100–20/400) respectively.[21,22] In those with moderate amblyopia, where

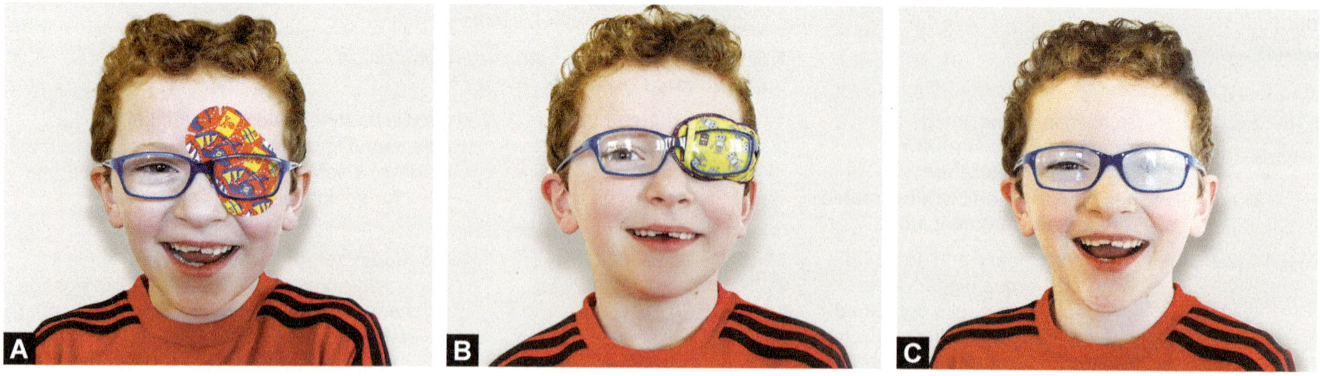

Figs. 71.1A to C: Occlusive treatment modalities in amblyopia. (A) Adhesive patch; (B) Material extension patch; (C) Bangerter occlusion foil.

Table 71.3: Comparison of amblyopia treatment modalities.

Modality	Patching	Bangerter occlusion foil	Atropine
Dose	2–6 hours daily to better seeing eye	Opaque filter of varying densities fitted to back of glasses lens in front of better seeing eye. The foil is worn on the glasses full time.	One drop twice weekly to better seeing eye
Compliance	Variable as child can easily remove patch if resisting treatment	Dependent upon compliance with glasses wear. Filter is not readily apparent to casual observers which aids compliance	Good compliance as effect lasts 1–2 weeks once drop instilled
Potential risks	Skin irritation and allergy (Alternative cloth patches are available)	Poorly fitted glasses can lead to peeking around the filters	Systemic side effects can rarely occur
Amblyopia treatment index*	Less favorable scores compared to atropine	A lower treatment burden compared to patching	More favorable scores compared to patching

* The amblyopia treatment index was developed by the PEDIG group to determine the impact of specific amblyopia treatments on children age 3–6 years.[35]

visual acuity fails to improve after 12 weeks of treatment, increasing the occlusion time to 6 hours from 2 hours daily may result in further visual improvement.[23]

Over the course of treatment, the average number of hours required to achieve optimum visual acuity has been reported to be between 120 and 400 hours of occlusion.[18,25,26] However, when counseling parents, it must be remembered that the duration of treatment will be influenced by the type of amblyopia, the visual acuity deficit and the age at the start of treatment.[25]

Atropine

Atropine sulfate 1% eye drops have historically been offered as a second line treatment in patients with poor compliance using conventional occlusion therapy. However, studies comparing the visual acuity outcomes between individuals using atropine or conventional occlusion as a first line treatment have identified no significant difference in outcomes.[27-31]

Atropine is instilled into the non-amblyopic eye. Once instilled, atropine paralyzes the ciliary muscle thus suspending accommodation and the circular pupillary sphincter muscle thus preventing constriction of the pupil both of which lead to reduced vision in that eye. Specific considerations including the age of the patient, ability to conduct robust crowded visual acuity testing at near and distance fixation distances, the density of amblyopia and the individual's medical history should be taken into account prior to commencing atropine.[32,33]

As with conventional occlusion therapy, a proportion of amblyopes fail to improve on atropine. Although a small improvement in visual acuity in the amblyopic eye was noted by PEDIG with the further penalization of the atropinised eye using a plano lens, it did not reach statistical significance.[34] Refractive penalization could be considered as a supplement to atropine treatment in those with residual amblyopia but, as always, careful monitoring of visual acuity in both eyes should be undertaken to ensure reversal amblyopia does not occur in the non-amblyopic eye.

Table 71.3 provides a comparison of occlusion and atropine treatment modalities.[35]

Recurrence of Amblyopia

The PEDIG reported that 24% of children with successful amblyopia treatment had a recurrence of their amblyopia on cessation of treatment.[36] Risk factors for recurrence included better visual acuity at point of cessation of treatment in the amblyopic eye, greater improvement in vision during treatment and previous recurrence.[37] Those children using 6–8 hours of occlusion had a four-fold risk of recurrence if patching was stopped abruptly compared to those with reduction to 2 hours prior to stopping occlusion; with an absence of orthophoria and stereoacuity being significant risk factors.[37] Therefore, monitoring of visual acuity following cessation of treatment is essential.

Compliance

Compliance with conventional patching is often a significant barrier to treatment success.[38] This can be for a number of reasons including the psychosocial impact on the child, adverse reactions from peers, the strain put on family relationships to comply with treatment and belief in the treatment if little or no visual improvement is noted.[39,40] Various methods have been employed in an effort to improve compliance including provision of educational leaflets, reward charts and, in some instances, physical supports, such as elbow splints, have been proposed.[41-46] However, methods used to aid compliance must be considered in the context of each individual patient and with full parental understanding and consent.

Evolving Treatments

In recent times, it has become apparent that the window of neural plasticity may be greater than previously thought and that older children/young adults may be candidates for newer treatments for amblyopia.[47] As amblyopia results from an abnormal binocular input, there is evolving research into binocular rather than monocular treatments for this *older* population.[48,49]

Dichoptic Binocular Training

During dichoptic binocular training, a visual stimulus is presented to both eyes with the stimulus to the non-amblyopic eye being of reduced signal therefore preventing suppression of the amblyopic eye.[49,50] With time, both eyes will perceive approximately the same image of similar contrast.[50] This field of treatment appears promising with a report of up two logMAR line improvements in visual acuity in a short timescale following movie viewing using this method, but without direct comparison to conventional occlusive therapy, and a report of better visual acuity outcomes after two weeks in patients using a binocular iPAD treatment in comparison to 2 hours of conventional occlusion therapy.[49,51] The PEDIG group identified a visual acuity improvement in the amblyopic eye with both binocular iPAD treatment and conventional patching, but reported a greater improvement with conventional occlusion therapy based on 16 weeks follow-up.[52] Further work is needed in this evolving and exciting area which shows promise as an alternative therapy for amblyopia in the coming years.

Medical Treatment, e.g. Levodopa

Levodopa, when converted to dopamine, has been reported to be important in retinal functioning and visual processing.[53] As previous reports on the beneficial effects of levodopa in amblyopia were conflicting, the PEDIG group assessed its effects on children with residual amblyopia as an adjunct to conventional 2 hours daily occlusion. Oral levodopa, while continuing to patch 2 hours daily, did not produce a statistically meaningful improvement in vision compared with placebo and patching.[53]

Over the last few decades, the treatment of amblyopia has been extensively investigated resulting in significant changes in how this patient population is managed. Future studies will hopefully continue to add to the increasing evidence base for optimal management strategies for amblyopia not just in children but also perhaps in adults with previously failed treatment or who were not diagnosed in childhood.

REFERENCES

1. Braverman RS. (2015). Introduction to Amblyopia. [online] Available from: *https://www.aao.org/pediatric-center-detail/amblyopia-introduction* [Accessed December 2017].
2. Holmes JM, Repka MX, Kraker RT, et al. The treatment of amblyopia. Strabismus. 2006;14:37-42.
3. Friedman DS, Repka MX, Katz J, et al. Prevalence of amblyopia and strabismus in White and African American children aged 6 through 71 months. The Baltimore Pediatric Eye Disease Study. Ophthalmology. 2009;116:2128-34.
4. Pai AS, Rose KA, Leone JF, et al. Amblyopia prevalence and risk factors in Australian preschool children. Ophthalmology. 2012;119:138–44.
5. Preslan MW, Novak A. Baltimore vision screening project. Ophthalmology. 1996;103:105–9.
6. Mansouri B, Thompson B, Hess RF. Measurement of suprathreshold binocular interactions in amblyopia. Vision Res. 2008;48(28):2775-84.

7. Holmes JM, Lazar EL, Melia BM, et al. Effect of age on response to amblyopia treatment in children. Arch Ophthalmol. 2011;129(11):1451-7.
8. Tailor VK, Glaze S, Khandelwal P, et al. Prescribed computer games in addition to occlusion versus standard occlusion treatment for childhood amblyopia: a pilot randomised controlled trial. Pilot Feasibility Stud. 2015;1:23.
9. Greenwood JA, Tailor VK, Sloper JJ, et al. Visual acuity, crowding, and stereo-vision are linked in children with and without Amblyopia. Invest Ophthalmol Vis Sci. 2012;53:7655–65.
10. Levi DM, McKee SP, Movshon JA. Visual deficits in anisometropia. Vision Res. 2011;51:48–57.
11. Rowe F. Clinical Orthoptics. Oxford, England: Blackwell Science;1997.
12. von Noorden GK. Binocular Vision and Ocular Motiliy. Theory and Management of Strabismus., 5th edition. St Louis: Mosby;1996.
13. Pediatric Eye Disease Investigator Group; 2017 *http://pedig.jaeb.org/Publications.aspx*, (Last accessed 01 June 2017).
14. Scheiman MM, Hertle RW, Beck RW et al. The Pediatric Eye Disease Investigator Group. Randomized trial of treatment of amblyopia in children aged 7 to 17 years. Arch Ophthalmol. 2005;123(4):437-47.
15. Moseley MJ, Neufeld M, McCarry B, et al. Remediation of refractive amblyopia by optical correction alone. Ophthalmic Physiol Opt. 2003;22:296-9.
16. Stewart CE, MoseleyMJ, Fielder AR, et al. Refractive adaption in amblyopia: quantification of effect and implications for practice. Br J Ophthalmol. 2004;88:1552-6.
17. Writing Committee for the Pediatric Eye Disease Investigator Group, Cotter SA, Foster NC, Holmes JM et al. Optical treatment of strabismic and combined strabismic-anisometropic amblyopia. Ophthalmology. 2012;119(1):150-8.
18. Stewart CE, Stephens D, Fielder AR, et al. Objectively monitored patching regimens for treatment of amblyopia: randomised trial. BMJ 2007;335(7622):707.
19. The Pediatric Eye Disease Investigator Group. Treatment of Anisometropic Amblyopia in Children with Refractive Correction. Ophthalmology. 2006;113(6):895-903.
20. The Pediatric Eye Disease Investigator Group Writing Committee. A randomized trial comparing Bangerter Filters and Patching for the treatment of moderate amblyopia in children. Ophthalmology. 2010;117(5):998-1004.
21. The Pediatric Eye Disease Investigator Group. A randomized trial of patching regimens for treatment of moderate amblyopia in children. Arch Ophthalmol. 2003;121(5):603-11.
22. Holmes JM, Kraker RT, Beck RW, et al. A randomized trial of patching for treatment of severe amblyopia in children. Ophthalmology. 2003;110(11):2075-87.
23. The Pediatric Eye Disease Investigator Group, Wallace DK, Lazar EL, Crouch III ER et al. A randomized control trial of increasing patching for amblyopia. Ophthalmology. 2013;120:2270-7.
24. Holmes JM, Lazar EL, Melia BM, et al. Effect of age on response to amblyopia treatment in children. Arch Ophthalmol. 2011;129(11):1451-7.
25. Wallace MP, Stewart CE, Moseley MJ, et al. Treatment of amblyopia using personalized dosing strategies: statistical modelling and clinical implementation. Strabismus. 2016;24(4):161-8.
26. Cleary M. Efficacy of occlusion for strabismic amblyopia: can an optimal duration be identified? Br J Ophthalmol. 2000;84(6):572-8.
27. Repka MX, Kraker RT, Holmes JM et al. A randomized Trial of atropine versus patching for treatment of moderate amblyopia: follow-up at 15 years of age. JAMA Ophthalmol. 2014;132(7):799–805.
28. Repka MX, Kraker RT, Beck RW et al. Treatment of severe amblyopia with weekend atropine: results from two randomized clinical trials. J AAPOS. 2009;13(3):258-63.
29. Scheiman M, Hertle RW, Kraker RT, et al The Pediatric Eye Disease Investigator Group. Patching vs atropine to treat amblyopia in children ages 7-12 years: a randomised trial. Arch Ophthalmol. 2008;126(12):1634-42.
30. Li T, Shotton K. Conventional occlusion versus pharmacologic penalization for amblyopia. Cochrane Database Syst Rev. 20097;(4):CD006460.
31. The Pediatric Eye Disease Investigator Group. A randomized trial of atropine vs. patching for treatment of moderate amblyopia in children. Arch Ophthalmol. 2002;120(3):268-78.
32. Taylor K, Hudson C, Merchant K. An audit of atropine penalization as a primary treatment for amblyopia. Br Ir Orthopt J. 2010;7:20-6.
33. Taylor K, Bryant S. Twice weekly atropine as a primary treatment for amblyopia: How does it compare with daily atropine? Br Ir Orthopt J. 2012;9:30-5.
34. The Pediatric Eye Disease Investigator Group. A randomized trial of adding a plano lens to atropine for amblyopia. J AAPOS. 2015;19(1):42–8.
35. Cole SR, Beck RW, Moke PS, et al. The amblyopia treatment index. J AAPOS. 2001;5:250-4.
36. Holmes JM, Beck RW, Kraker RT, et al. Pediatric Eye Disease Investigator Group. Risk of amblyopia recurrence after cessation of treatment. J AAPOS. 2004;8:420-8.
37. Holmes JM, Melia M, Bradfield YS, et al. Factors associated with recurrence of amblyopia on cessation of patching. Ophthalmology 2007;114(8):1427-32.
38. Loudon SE, Polling JR, Simonsz HJ. A preliminary report about the relation between visual acuity increase and compliance in patching therapy for amblyopia. Strabismus. 2002;10(2):79-82. [online] Available from: *http://www.tandfonline.com/toc/istr20/current.*
39. Dixon-Woods M, Awan M, Gottlob I. Why is compliance with occlusion therapy for amblyopia so hard? A qualitative study. Arch Dis Child. 2006;91(6):491-4.
40. Searle A, Norman P, Harrad R, et al. Psychosocial and clinical determinants of compliance with occlusion therapy for amblyopic children. Eye(Lond). 2002;16(2):150-5.
41. Newsham D. A randomised controlled trial of written information: the effect on parental non-concordance with occlusion therapy. Br J Ophthalmol. 2002;86(7):787-91.
42. Loudon SE, Fronius M, Looman CW, et al. Predictors and a remedy for non-compliance with amblyopia therapy in

children measured with the occlusion dose monitor. Invest Ophthalmol Vis Sci. 2006;47(10):4393-400.
43. Tjiam AM, Holtstag G, Vukovic E, et al. An educational cartoon accelerates amblyopia therapy and improves compliance, especially among children of immigrants. Ophthalmology 2012;119(11):2393-401.
44. Tjiam AM, Holtslag G, Van Minderhout HM et al. Randomised comparison of three tools for improving compliance with occlusion therapy: An educational cartoon story, a reward calendar, and an information leaflet for parents. Graefes Arch for Clin Exp Ophthalmol. 2013;251(1):321-9.
45. Sabri K, Easterbrook B, Wakeman B, et al. Elbow splinting as a method to increase patching compliance in amblyopia therapy. Eye(Lond). 2016;31(3):406-10.
46. Dean SE, Povey RC, Reeves J. Assessing interventions to increase compliance to patching treatment in children with amblyopia: a systematic review and meta-analysis. Br J Ophthalmol. 2016;100:159-65.
47. Li J, Thompson B, Deng D, et al. Dichoptic training enables the adult amblyopic brain to learn. Curr Biol. 2013;23(8);R308-9.
48. Hess RF, Thompson B. Amblyopia and the binocular approach to its therapy. Vision Res. 2015;114:4-16.
49. Kelly KR, Jost RM, Dao L, et al. Binocular iPad game vs patching for treatment of amblyopia in children. A randomized clinical trial. JAMA Ophthalmol. 2016;134(12):1402-8.
50. Oltra E (2015). Amblyopia Emerging Treatments. American Academy of Ophthalmology. [Online]Available from: *https://www.aao.org/pediatric-center-detail/amblyopia-emerging-treatments* [Accessed December 2017].
51. Li SL, Reynaud A, Hess RF et al. Dichoptic movie viewing treats childhood amblyopia. J AAPOS. 2015;19(5):401-5.
52. Holmes JM, Manh VM, Lazar EL, et al. Effect of a binocular iPad game vs part-time patching in children aged 5 to 12 years with amblyopia: a randomized clinical trial. JAMA Ophthalmol. 2016;134(12):1391-400.
53. The Pediatric Eye Disease Investigator Group, Repka MX, Kraker RT, Dean TW, et al. A randomized trial of levodopa as treatment for residual amblyopia in older children. Ophthalmology. 2015;122(5):874-81.

Chapter 72 Pediatric Cataract Surgery

Michael O'Keeffe, Caitriona Kirwan

INTRODUCTION

A cataract causes opacification in the eye's natural lens. It is a significant cause of childhood blindness. It results in thousands of children going blind from cataracts in the world.[1] Bilateral cataracts are more common than unilateral and successful management requires early detection and treatment. The red reflex is the most important eye check in the newborn and pupillary dilation may be needed to detect them in some newborns.

The timing of surgery, surgical technique, aphakic correction and management of amblyopia determine the visual prognosis.[2,3] The child's eye is different to the adults. It is smaller, more elastic and the inflammatory response of surgery is more aggressive. Most of the eye growth takes place in the first three years of life. Advances in adult cataract surgery and improved technology have attributed to better outcomes. Postoperative management with aggressive use of steroids and amblyopic treatment has significantly improved the visual prognosis.

ETIOLOGY AND MORPHOLOGY

A careful history is important in determining the etiology. Complications during pregnancy, infections, exposure to drugs, toxins or radiation are sometimes involved. Family history of cataracts is often present. The most common etiology is autosomal dominant inheritance in bilateral cataracts. Other causes of bilateral cataract include trisomy 21 and Aniridia, Lowe syndrome, Hallermann-Streiff syndrome. All of these children will have associated facial and systemic abnormalities (Box 72.1).

Box 72.1: Etiology of cataracts.

- Intrauterine infection
- Drug induced
- Metabolic
- Radiation
- Trauma
- Persistent hyperplastic primary vitreous
- Aneridia
- Retinopathy of prematurity (ROP)
- Inherited
- Chromosomal
- Craniofacial syndrome
- Neurometabolic
- Dermatological GT6

Unilateral cataracts are less frequently associated with systemic disorders. Persistent hyperplastic primary vitreous is sometimes present and this manifests itself with a microphthalmic eye or prominent blood vessels in the iris and lens. The anterior chamber may be shallow with prominent ciliary processes and the retrolental plaque may extend to the retina. Acquired cataracts may arise secondary to corticosteroids, radiation laser photocoagulation for retinopathy of prematurity or other intraocular surgery. It is possible to identify cataracts by their morphology be it nuclear, lamellar polar or lentiglobus. In nuclear cataract, the lens material is opaque and sometimes there is a posterior capsular plaque. Lamellar cataracts involve opacity of the anterior and posterior cortex. Anterior and posterior polar cataracts show a central opacity in the anterior and or posterior capsules. In posterior lentiglobus, there is a posterior bowing of the posterior capsule with posterior capsular defects. Anterior polar lamellar posterior lentiglobus cataracts have a better visual prognosis in contrast to nuclear posterior polar that have a poorer prognosis.[4]

INVESTIGATIONS

A careful history assists the surgeon in selecting the investigations to determine the cataracts etiology. Most unilateral cataracts are idiopathic and do not warrant exhaustive investigations. Laboratory tests in children with bilateral nonhereditary cataracts are listed in Box 72.2.

The ophthalmic examination starts with a complete eye examination to assess the visual fixation, pupillary response and eye movements. Indirect fundus examinations with dilated pupil are helpful unless there is a complete cataract. A B-scan is useful to determine any posterior segment abnormality.

ALTERNATIVE TO SURGERY

Metabolic cataracts such as those caused by galactosemia can be reversed if they are diagnosed early. Elimination of

Box 72.2: Laboratory test for bilateral nonhereditary cataracts.

- Full blood count
- Serum calcium
- Urinary—amino acids
- Red blood cell transferase acid
- Galactokinase
- Toxoplasma titer
- Rubella titer
- Cytomegalo titer
- Herpes simplex titer

galactose from the diet the oil droplets in the lens can be reversed.[5]

Dilation of the pupil with cyclopentolate 1% twice a day can improve the vision and eliminate the need for surgery in the short-term. If localized opacities are confined to the center of the anterior capsule or anterior cortex.

Anesthesia

General anesthesia is the preferred option in pediatric cataracts. A useful marker for anesthetic depth is the position of the eye during surgery.[6] If the cornea moves upwards or downwards, the anesthesia should be deepened. Children's sclera is elastic and any tension on the extra ocular muscles results in loss of the anterior chamber and an increased intraocular pressure.

Surgery

Pediatric cataracts are usually soft. Therefore, the lens material can be aspirated through a 2 mm long incision at the limbus or by lensectomy through the pars plana. When the intraocular lens (IOL) implantation is intended, the limbal wound is enlarged to introduce the intraocular lens. With use of foldable implants the incision is not more than 3 mm. A scleral tunnel is better than a clear corneal incision. The wound should be securely sutured with 10.0 absorbable vicryl sutures to prevent wound dehiscence and iris incarceration.[7]

The pars plana approach was developed with the introduction of vitrectomy machines in the late 1970s.[8] With advances in adult cataract surgery the pars plana approach is being abandoned in favor of the limbal approach because the latter allows preservation of the capsular bag for in bag placement of the IOL. Most surgeons wait until the child is 4 weeks of age and before 8 weeks before performing cataract surgery.[9]

In the premature infant, cataract surgery is performed when the child is 40 weeks postmenstrual age. Other factors that play a part are comorbidities, such as the safety of general anesthesia. In children with bilateral cataracts where there is an anesthetic risk due to unstable medical status two eyes can be operated on sequentially at the same surgery but treating both eyes as separate operations. This is now a practice even when there is no anesthetic risk.[10] It has the additional advantages of reducing the risk of relative amblyopia, frees up the operating room time, reduces exposure to general anesthesia and allows rehabilitation of both eyes simultaneously.[11] However, parents should be informed that this increases the risk of the bilateral endophthalmitis.

The pars plana approach is performed in infants under 2 years of age. The technique requires a guillotine type 23-gauge or 25-gauge vitrectomy and balanced salt solution containing epinephrine (adrenaline) in a concentration of 1 in 500,000. The location of the pars plana in infants is 1.5–3.5 mm from the limbus. The anterior vitrectomy is completed sparing the 2–3 mm peripheral rim of the posterior capsule. This remnant is used to create a shelf of support for a posterior chamber IOL that may be implanted in later life. Turning off the infusion before withdrawing the vitrectomy cutter from the eye avoids vitreous incarceration in the wound. This precaution may reduce the chances of a retinal detachment later in life.[12]

The corneal limbal approach is a widely performed surgical technique. A long tunnel incision reduces the risk of iris prolapse. Sometimes the pupil is meiosed and will not dilate well. This requires intracameral phenylephrine 2.5% and or iris hooks and viscoelastic materials to maintain the anterior chamber depth. These involve either the use of Viscoat or Healon. An anterior chamber maintainer (ACM) is an alternative to maintain the anterior chamber depth and provide a stable intraoperative pressure. Limbal incisions are made with a 23-gauge microvitreoretinal blade (MVR Alcon Laboratories Incorporated, Fort Worth, Texas). These allow for a bimanual technique with one cannula infusing fluid to the anterior chamber and the opposite one aspirating the lens material (Fig. 72.1).

Various techniques have developed to open the anterior capsule. In younger infants, it is more difficult to perform a capsulorhexis as the infants, eye has a very elastic capsule which can easily undergo a radial tear. A manual capsulorhexis using a push-pull technique has been described.[13] A popular alternative is to use the vitrectomy probe to create a small central opening of the anterior capsule. The opening can be enlarged by biting into the anterior capsule with the vitrector until the desired 4–5 mm opening is achieved. An alternative technique is to use the oertli diathermy system which has the oertli system effect of creating a controlled central 5 mm round capsulotomy (Fig. 72.2).[14] Gentle hydrodissection

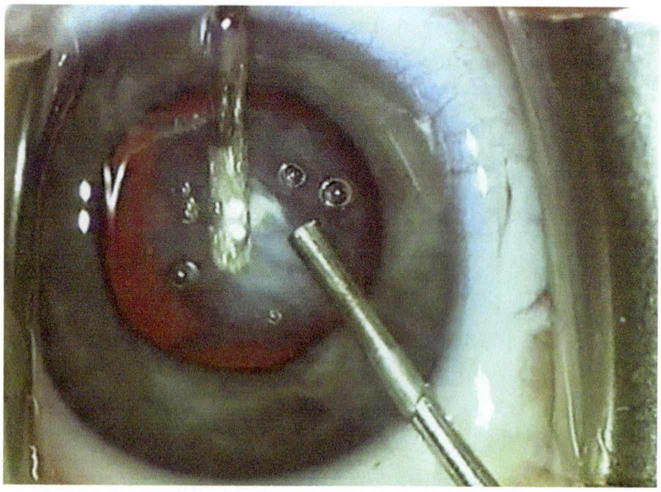

Fig. 72.1: Bimanual aspiration technique.

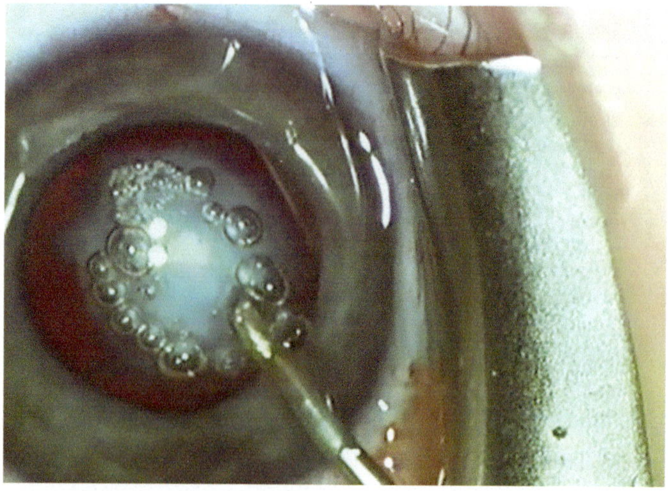

Fig. 72.2: Oertli diathermy creates central 5 mm capsulotomy.

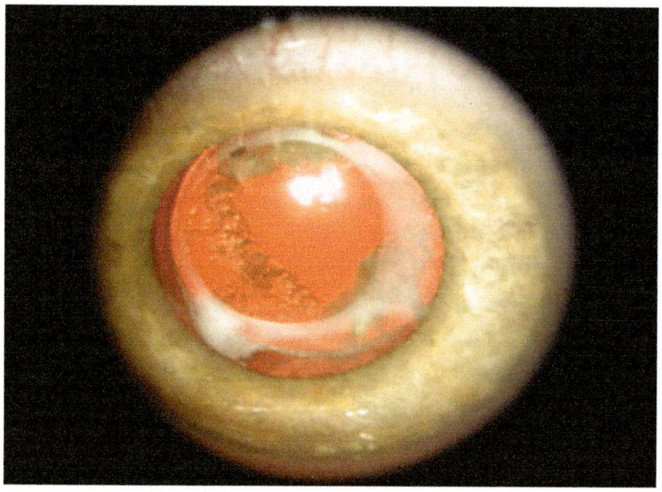

Fig. 72.3: Regrowth of lens epithelial cells.

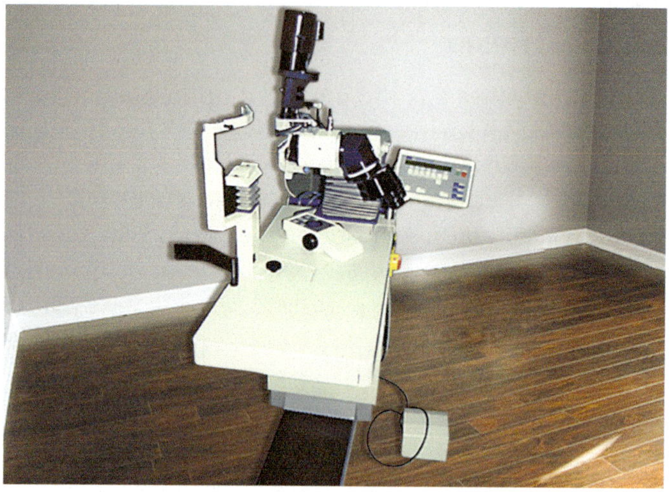

Fig. 72.4: Micropter III horizontal YAG.

and hydrodelineation free the lens material and this can be aspirated using a bimanual technique or with the use of a vitrector.

The management of the posterior capsule is dictated by the age of the patient. Children under 6 years of age should receive an elective posterior capsulotomy and an anterior vitrectomy.[15] The posterior capsulorhexis can be performed manually or with a vitrector and its diameter should be at least 4 mm. The anterior vitrectomy should be generous moving a third of the vitreous to insure a permanent clear visual axis. Smaller posterior capsulotomies and shallow anterior vitrectomy may result in reopacification. Posterior capsulotomies either alone or combined with shallow anterior vitrectomy does not guarantee a clear visual axis because the lens epithelial cells regrow and can form a new membrane (Fig. 72.3).

A modification of the technique includes a translimbal approach with capsulorhexis and lens aspiration using a bimanual technique. The IOL is inserted into the capsular bag. The wound is closed and the anterior chamber is maintained either with viscoelastic or an anterior chamber maintainer. A pars plana approach is used to perform a posterior capsulorhexis and an anterior vitrectomy using a vitrector. An intact posterior capsule in a neonate and young children results in early posterior capsule opacification. The use of yttrium aluminium garnet (YAG) either immediately after surgery or later has limited success particularly in infants or young children.[16] In addition, the logistics of performing it is impossible unless the surgeon has a Micropter III horizontal YAG laser which is not widely available (Fig. 72.4).

CHOICE OF APHAKIC CORRECTION: SPECTACLES, CONTACT LENSES AND INTRAOCULAR LENSES

Aphakic Spectacles

Aphakic spectacles provide a satisfactory correction in children with bilateral aphakia (Fig. 72.5).[2] Most children who wear them develop good visual acuity and they are often better tolerated than contact lenses. The disadvantages include; restriction of peripheral vision, poor cosmetic appearance.

Contact Lenses

During the 1980s contact lenses were the method of choice. They provide a superior optical correction than spectacles and their diopter power can be adjusted.[17] They are expensive and can be difficult to use. Frequent loss, recurrent infection, poor compliance can make them an impractical option.

The Infant Aphakia Treatment Study (IATS) was the first multicenter randomized clinical trial comparing cataract surgery with or without IOLs in infants aged 1–6 months with congenital cataracts.[18] They concluded that primary IOLs should be preserved where the use of contact lenses would result in significant periods of uncorrected aphakia. Many technical problems have been overcome. The introduction of extended wear silicone and custom rigid gas permeable contact lenses is a significant advance.[19] Problems still exist such as compliance, parent and child cooperation, the lenses must be changed on a regular basis. There is also the cost of purchasing them and parents should always have a spare contact lens in case of loss.

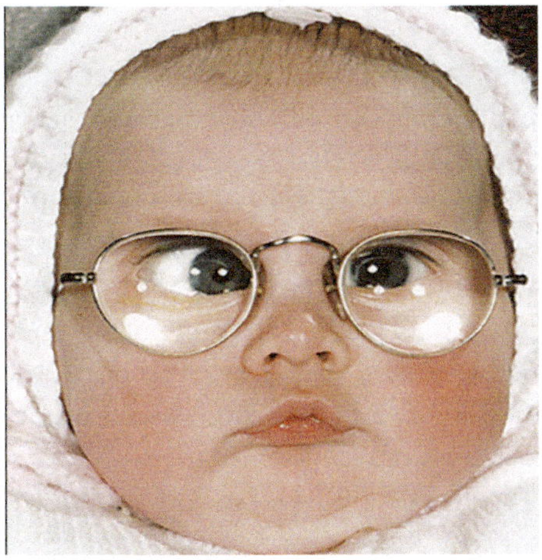

Fig. 72.5: Aphakic spectacles in infant after bilateral cataract surgery.

Intraocular Lenses

The IOL option was originally used in children with congenital cataracts because it resulted in early amblyopia management and provided a more stable correction. Implanting an IOL into a growing eye has problems. The aim is to correct most but not all aphakia and the residual refractive error is corrected by spectacles or contact lenses. The use of an anterior chamber angle supported IOL in children was discontinued in the mid 1980s due to secondary glaucoma, uveitis and corneal decomposition.[20] Posterior chamber IOL implantation is the method of choice. Poly Methyl Methacrylate (PMMA) has been used for more than 50 years. Many surgeons have now switched to the use of foldable hydrophobic IOLs. In young children, an IOL power is chosen to undercorrect the eye and allow for the myopic shift. No IOL formula has been specifically developed for infant eyes.[21] The SRK/T and Holladay IOL calculation formula are the most popular. But all of these formulas do not eliminate the large prediction error. Biometry and the age of the child determine the IOL diopter power. In children under a year the axial length and keratometry (K readings) changes rapidly. Those under one year of age should receive 80% of the power needed for emmetropia. The K readings change rapidly during the first 18 months of life. Therefore, it is more accurate to rely on the axial length only when calculating the IOL diopter power.

Infants and young children can tolerate up to 6 diopters of anisometropia. For children 2–4 years of age the dioptric power should be 90% of that needed for emmetropia at the time of surgery. From 4 years of age the dioptric power should be close to emmetropia (Box 72.3). IOL implantation is controversial in infants. Implantation beyond six months is practiced widely, particularly in unilateral cataracts. In the IAT study, infants with unilateral cataracts younger than six months of age were randomized having lensectomy to either contact lens correction or IOL implantation. The result was a significant number of intraocular procedures

Box 72.3: Guidelines for intraocular lenses dioptric power.

- Children less than one year
- Do biometry and undercorrect by 20%
- Children 1–2 years
- Undercorrect by 10%
- 2–4 years undercorrect by 5%
- Axial Length to calculate IOL power
  - 17 mm 25 D
  - 18 mm 24 D
  - 19 mm 23 D
  - 20 mm 21 D
  - 21 mm 19 D

performed in the IOL group.[18] Gimbel described a special IOL implantation technique. The IOL haptics are placed in the bag fornices, with the optic protruded through the capsulorhexis to be captured beneath the posterior capsule remnants known as IOL capture.[22] This has claimed to have the advantage of reduced risk of after cataract formation. Tassignon developed a technique for a special IOL called the bag-in-the-lens. The technique consists of creating an anterior and posterior capsulorhexis. Although it is technically difficult promising earlier results with this technique suggests it may alleviate the need for an elective anterior vitrectomy.[23]

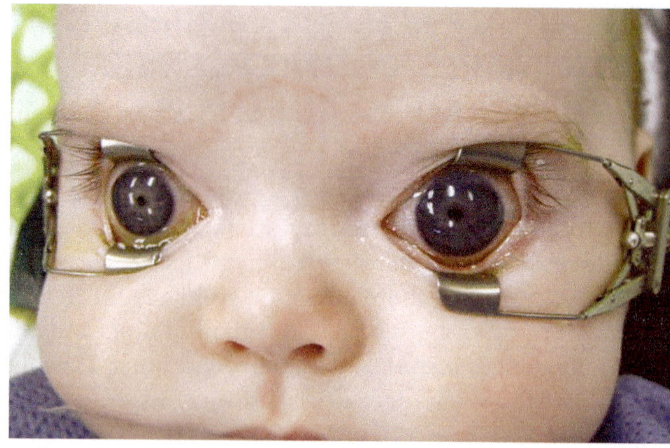

Fig. 72.6: Glaucoma after infant cataract surgery.

POSTOPERATIVE TREATMENT

Infants and younger children eyes are very reactive to surgery. They produce excessive fibrin and as a result, there is an intense inflammatory response soon after surgery. The pupil remains meiosed and there is corneal edema. A combination of intense topical and systemic steroids is used for the first few weeks with the use of atropine or cyclopentolate to dilate the pupils. The medications are tapered off over a period of 4–6 weeks. More recently the use of intracameral triesence 4 mg in 0.1 mL have significantly reduced the inflammation and lessened the need for intensive topical and in particular systemic steroids.[24]

COMPLICATIONS

Intraoperative complications are related to the age of the child at surgery. The anterior chamber may collapse, there may be iris prolapsed and the pupil constricts. Early complications include fibrinous uveitis, high intraocular pressure, iris incarceration in the wound and endophthalmitis. Glaucoma after infant cataract surgery is a major problem (Fig. 72.6).[25] The risk of glaucoma or suspected glaucoma doubles from 12% at one year after surgery to 30% at 5 years with no difference between the two groups. Many reasons have been put forward as a cause for glaucoma such as early surgery, microphthalmic eyes, postoperative uveitis, persistent hyperplastic primary vitreous (PHPV), fetal nuclear cataract, retained lens material and reoperations. The single biggest risk is early surgery.[10] The risk of surgery increases two-fold by performing surgery at one month compared to two months. The rate of additional intraocular procedures to clear the visual axis is particularly high in the first year. This is increased many times when an IOL is implanted at the time of surgery. In addition, the IOL may become subluxated and there is increased inflammation. There may be a large myopic shift. These usually occur in the first year after surgery. The pupil may be distorted secondary to posterior synechiae between the iris and the residual lens material or secondary to iris trauma. Vitreous strands can extend to the wound causing a peaked pupil. Bacterial endophthalmitis is rare but it is a disastrous complication. It is especially important now particularly when sequential bilateral cataract surgery is performed that both eyes should be treated as separate surgeries and intracameral antibiotics should be used. Flame-shaped retinal hemorrhages can develop on the posterior pole that is transient but occasionally the hemorrhage may develop at the fovea causing amblyopia.[26] Retinal detachment is rare but sometimes occurs many years later.

AMBLYOPIA MANAGEMENT

The child's parent need to know that visual rehabilitation only starts after surgery when patching becomes the mainstay of treatment. This must start soon after surgery and unilateral cataracts are the most difficult to manage. Occlusion of the sound eye is for half the waking day of the first year and then this should be increased to at least 80–90% of the waking day after that. Soon after surgery bilateral aphakic spectacles are prescribed and the bifocal lens of +2 or +3 should be prescribed at 2 years of ages. Unilateral aphakic children should have contact lens fitting within 2 weeks of the surgery and patching commenced rapidly. The patching continues until the age of 4 or 5 and in many cases, patching is continued up until the age of about 8 years.

OPTIONS TO CORRECT MYOPIC SHIFT

The growth of the eye is unpredictable and a myopic shift of 7 diopter is not uncommon. IOL exchange in children where the implant has been in place for more than a year or many years, is difficult and carries risk of severe complications. However, in more recent times other options such as contact lenses, refractive surgery secondary IOL to correct the myopia are now readily available and safer.[27] They offer the prospect of good visual outcomes and low risk of complications.

Many years ago the treatment, in particular of monocular congenital cataract was not worth the effort. The outcome of the IAT group are interesting and they reported half of the children had visual acuity better than 20–100 and 20% were better than 20–30 with 20% orthophoric.[18] Binocularity is usually poor after congenital cataract but coarse stereopsis can be expected. The visual outcome largely depends on the type of cataract, timing of intervention, quality of surgery, associated ocular and systemic problems and optical and occlusion management. Pediatric surgery has advanced in the last ten years to the point where outcomes have dramatically improved.

REFERENCES

1. Rahi JS, Dezateux C. Measuring and interpreting the incidence of congenital ocular anomalies, lessons from a study of congenital cataracts in the UK. Invest Ophthalmol Vis Sci. 2001;42(7):1444-8.
2. Elston JS, Timms C. Clinical evidence for the onset of the sensitive period in infancy. Br J Ophthalmol. 1992;76(6): 327-8.
3. Lambert SR, Drack AV. Infantile cataracts surgery of ophthalmology. 1996;40(6): 427-58.
4. Amaya L, Taylor D, Russell-Eggitt I, et al. The morphology and natural history of childhood cataracts. Survey ophthalmology. 2003;48(2):125-44.
5. Burke JP, O Keefe M, Bowell R, et al. Ophthalmic fundus in classical galactosaemia—a population. J Pediatr Ophthalmol Strabismus. 1989;26(4):165-8.
6. Dahan E, Salmenson BD. Pseudophakia in children: precautions, techniques and feasibility. J Cataract Refract Surg. 1990;16(1):75-82.
7. Ahmadiel H, Javadi MA, Ahmadi M, et al. Primary capsulotomy anterior vitrectomy lensectomy and posterior chamber lens implantation in children fundal versus pars plano. J Cataract Refract Surg. 1999;25:768-75.
8. Vishwanath M, Cheong-Leen R, TAylor D, et al. Is early surgery for congenital cataract a risk factor for glaucoma. Br J Ophthalmol. 2010;128:1050-4.
9. Scott R. Lambert MD. The timing of surgery for congenital cataracts minimising the risk of glaucoma following cataract surgery while optimising the visual outcome. J AAPOS. 2016;20(3): 191-2.
10. Dave H, Phoenix V, Becker ER, et al. Simultaneous versus sequential bilateral cataract surgery for infants with congenital cataracts, visual outcomes, adverse events and economic costs. Arch Ophthalmoly 2010;128:1050-4.
11. McLeod D. Congenital cataract surgeries; a retinal surgeons's viewpoint. Aust N Z J Ophthalmol. 1986;14(1):79-84.
12. Nishchal KK. Two incision push-pull capsulorhexis for pediatric cataract surgery. J Cataract Refract Surg. 2002;28:(4) 593-5.
13. Comber RM, Abdulla N, O Keefe M. Radiofrequency diathermy capsulorhexis of the anterior and posterior capsules preliminary results. J Cataract Refract Surg. 1997:23(1);841-4.
14. Vasavada A, Desai J. Primary posterior capsulorhexis with and without anterior vitrectomy in congenital cataracts. J Cataract Refract Surg. 1997;2(1):645-51.
15. Stager DR Jr, Weakley DR Jr, Hunter JS. Long term rates of PC following small incision foldable acrylic intraocular lens implantation in children. J pediatr Ophthalmol Strabismus. 2002;39(2):73-6.
16. Neumann D, Weissman BA, Isenberg SJ, et al. The effectiveness of daily wear contact lenses for the correction of infantile aphakia. Arch Ophthalmol. 1993;111(7):927-30.
17. Infant Aphakia Treatment Study Group. Comparison of contact lens and intraocular lens correction of monocular aphakia during infancy: A randomized Clinical Trial of HOTV Optotype Acuity at Age 4.5 Years and Clinical Findings at Age 5 Years. JAMA Ophthalmol. 2014;132(6):676-82.
18. Repka MX[1]. Treatment outcomes of monocular infantile cataract at 5-year follow-up: work in progress. JAMA Ophthalmol. 2014;132(6):683-4.
19. Hiles DA. Intraocular lens implantation in children with monocular cataracts. 1974-1983. Ophthalmology. 1984;91(10):1231-7.
20. Wilson ME, Apple DJ, Bluestein EC, et al. Intraocular lenses for pediatric implantation: biomaterials, designs, and sizing. J Cataract Refract Surg. 1994;20(6):584-91.
21. Gimbel HV, DeBroff BM. Posterior capsulorhexis with optic capture: maintaining a clear visual axis after pediatric cataract surgery. J Cataract Refract Surg. 1994;20(6):658-64.
22. Tassignon MJ, De Veuster I, Godts D, et al. Bag-in-the-lens intraocular lens implantation in the pediatric eye. J Cataract Refract Surg. 2007;33(4):611-7.
23. Cleary CA[1], Lanigan B, O'Keeffe M. Intracameral triamcinolone acetonide after pediatric cataract surgery. J Cataract Refract Surg. 2010;36(10):1676-81.
24. Lambert SR. The timing of surgery for congenital cataracts: Minimizing the risk of glaucoma following cataract surgery while optimizing the visual outcome. J AAPOS. 2016;20(3):191-2.
25. Vishwanath M, Cheong-Leen R, Taylor D, et al. Is early surgery for congenital cataract a risk for glaucoma? Br J Ophthalmol. 2004;88(7):905-10.
26. Christiansen SP[1], Muñoz M, Capó H. Retinal hemorrhage following lensectomy and anterior virectomy in children. J Pediatr Ophthalmol Strabismus. 1993;30(1):24-7.
27. O'Keeffe M, Kirwan C. Pediatric refractive surgery. J Pediatr Ophthalmol Strabismus. 2006;43(6):333-6.

Chapter 73 Childhood Glaucoma

Maria Papadopoulos, Peng Tee Khaw

INTRODUCTION

Childhood glaucoma is a rare, potentially blinding condition characterized by elevated intraocular pressure (IOP) related damage to the eye and characteristic optic disc cupping. As opposed to adults, the clinical presentation of children with glaucoma varies depending on the age at which the IOP starts to rise. Elevated IOP in infancy can affect the whole eye and not just the optic nerve with cupping. Controlling IOP is essential in managing children with glaucoma but can be challenging. Medical therapy plays an important role but the mainstay of treatment is surgery, which often needs to be repeated in a child's lifetime. Maximizing lifelong visual function relies not only on controlled IOP but also on the correction of ametropia and amblyopia therapy, where indicated. Lifelong follow-up to ensure IOP control and to detect complications is mandatory.

CLINICAL PRESENTATION

A child with glaucoma can present in many ways which include clinical signs of elevated IOP as occurs in infancy; screening because of a family history of childhood glaucoma; with conditions that predispose to glaucoma, e.g. uveitis; having failed routine school vision testing and rarely with progressive myopia or strabismus.

Glaucoma in neonates and infants usually presents with the triad of photophobia, blepharospasm and epiphora which are not entirely specific but very suggestive of glaucoma. Buphthalmos (ox eye) refers to generalized ocular enlargement caused by elevated IOP from any cause in infancy and is due to corneal and scleral collagen immaturity (Fig. 73.1). Continued IOP elevation results in Descemet's membrane eventually rupturing with one edge retracting as a scroll to form a ridge known as Haab's striae (Fig. 73.2). Subsequent aqueous influx into the stroma leads to sudden localized or diffuse corneal edema (Fig. 73.3). Photophobia may persist even with normal IOP due to the Haab's striae.

Many conditions can mimic glaucoma and must be excluded before diagnosing glaucoma in a child. The signs of glaucoma are usually asymmetrical (if bilateral), progressive and associated with ocular enlargement in infancy if untreated. If doubt exists about the diagnosis, then further follow-up, which may include examination under anesthesia (EUA) for a more complete examination, is advisable (Box 73.1).

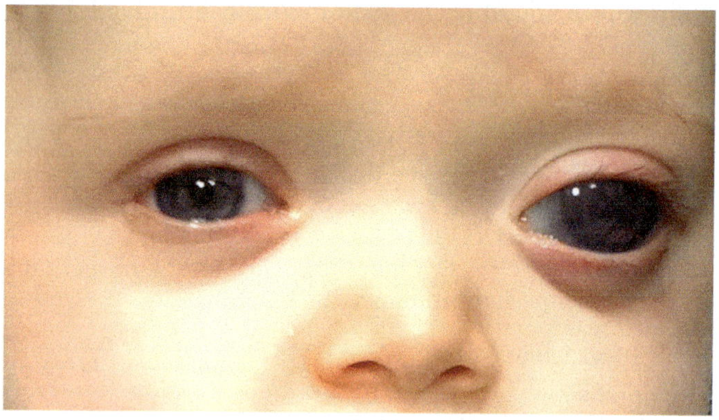

Fig. 73.1: Infant with left buphthalmos.

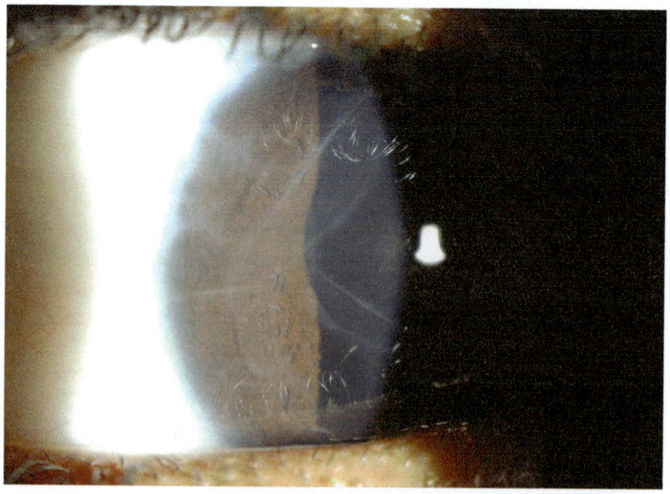

Fig. 73.2: Haab's striae pathognomonic of glaucoma in infancy in the presence of enlarged cornea

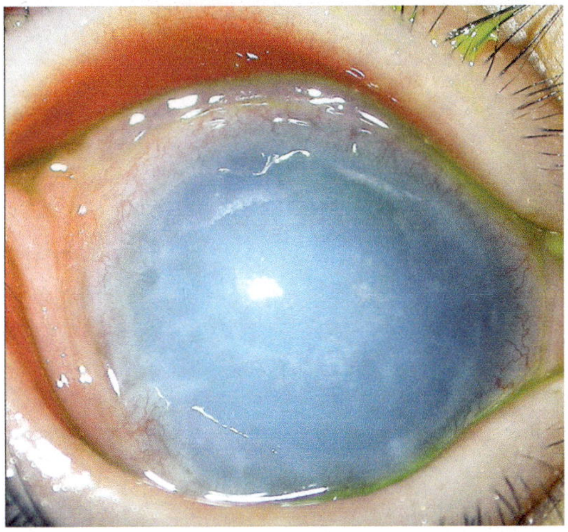

Fig. 73.3: Severe stromal edema from ruptured Descemet's membrane due to elevated IOP and anterior segment dysgenesis.

CLASSIFICATION

Childhood glaucoma is caused by diverse conditions. The World Glaucoma Association recently proposed a definition and simple classification of primary and secondary childhood glaucoma.[1] In primary childhood glaucoma only an abnormality of the anterior chamber (AC) angle exists which is responsible for reduced aqueous outflow. It is further subclassified depending on the age of onset of signs. In secondary childhood glaucoma, reduced aqueous outflow occurs by a non-acquired (congenital) or acquired ocular disease or systemic disorder and syndrome (Boxes 73.2 and 73.3).

Box 73.1: Differential diagnosis of childhood glaucoma in infancy.
Cornea Enlargement **Symmetrical, no Descemet's membrane splits or corneal edema**
• X-linked megalocornea (nonprogressive, optic disc normal, very deep AC with shortened vitreous length)
• Connective tissue disorders (e.g. Osteogenesis imperfecta, Marfan's syndrome)
• Congenital high myopia (physiological cupping with tilted disc, peripapillary scleral crescent)
• LTBP2 mutations (primary congenital megalocornea, spherophakia, ectopia lentis and secondary lens-related pupil block glaucoma)
Corneal Splits **No corneal enlargement, normal optic nerve**
• Trauma (obstetric with forceps use, non-accidental)
• Hydrops (history important)
Corneal Edema or Opacity **Usually no corneal enlargement unless associated with glaucoma which is rare**
• Trauma (obstetric with forceps use, non-accidental)
• Congenital corneal dystrophies (e.g. Congenital hereditary endothelial dystrophy)
• Metabolic disorders (e.g. Mucopolysaccharidoses, mucolipidoses, cystinosis)
• Infection (e.g. Congenital rubella, Herpes simplex keratitis)
Watering and 'Red Eye' **No Descemet's membrane splits, corneal or ocular enlargement, normal optic nerve and IOP**
• Conjunctivitis (often discharge, red eye)
• Nasolacrimal duct obstruction (purulent discharge, no photophobia, no 'runny nose')
• Corneal epithelial defect/keratitis (history and examination important)
• Ocular inflammation
Congenital Optic Nerve Cupping **No corneal enlargement or edema, normal intraocular pressure**
• Physiological cupping in large optic nerves (sometimes family history of large optic nerve heads)
• Congenital optic nerve anomalies (optic nerve pits, optic nerve coloboma)
• Papillorenal syndrome
• Optic nerve hypoplasia with periventricular leukomalacia

Source: Papadopoulos M, Khaw PT. Children Glaucoma. In: Lambert SR, Lyon (Eds). Pediatric Ophthalmology and Strabismus. China: Elsevier Publication. 2017. pp. 362-77.

Box 73.2: Definition of childhood glaucoma and childhood glaucoma suspect.

Definition of childhood glaucoma: 2 or more required

- IOP > 21 mmHg (investigator discretion, if examination under anesthesia data alone due to the variable effects of anesthesia on all methods of IOP assessment)
- *Optic disc cupping*: A progressive increase in cup-disc ratio, cup-disc asymmetry of ≥ 0.2 when the optic discs are of similar size, or focal rim thinning
- *Corneal findings*: Haab's striae/corneal edema or diameter ≥ 11mm in newborn, >12 mm in child <1 year of age, >13 mm any age
- Progressive myopia or myopic shift coupled with an increase in ocular dimensions out of keeping with normal growth
- A reproducible visual field defect that is consistent with glaucomatous optic neuropathy with no other observable reason for the visual field defect

Definition of childhood glaucoma suspect: at least 1 required

- IOP > 21 mm Hg on two separate occasions, or
- Suspicious optic disc appearance for glaucoma, i.e. increased cup-disc ratio for size of optic disc, or
- Suspicious visual field for glaucoma, or
- Increased corneal diameter or axial length in setting of normal IOP

(IOP: Intraocular pressure)
Based on national criteria: <18 years of age (USA); ≤16 years of age (UK, Europe, UNICEF).

Box 73.3: Classification of childhood glaucoma.[1]

Primary childhood glaucoma

1. *Primary congenital glaucoma (isolated trabeculodysgenesis)*

- Neonatal or newborn onset (0–1 month)
- Infantile onset (>1 month 2 years)
- Late onset or late recognized (>2 years)
- Spontaneously arrested (nonprogressive buphthalmos, Haab's striae, normal IOP and optic nerves)

2. *Juvenile open-angle glaucoma*

Secondary childhood glaucoma

1. *Glaucoma Associated with nonacquired ocular anomalies*
   Conditions with predominantly ocular anomalies present at birth which may or may not be associated with systemic signs

- Axenfeld-Rieger anomaly (Syndrome if systemic associations)
- Peters anomaly (Syndrome if systemic associations)
- Congenital ectropion uveae
- Congenital iris hypoplasia
- Aniridia
- Persistent fetal vasculature (if glaucoma present before cataract surgery)
- Oculodermal melanocytosis (Nevus of Ota)
- Microphthalmos/Microcornea
- *Ectopia lentis*:
  - Simple ectopia lentis (no systemic associations)
  - Ectopia lentis et pupillae

2. *Glaucoma associated with nonacquired systemic disease or syndrome*
   Conditions predominantly with known syndromes, systemic anomalies or systemic disease present at birth which may be associated with ocular signs.

- *Phacomatoses*:
  - Sturge-Weber syndrome
  - Neurofibromatosis 1 (NF-1)
  - Klippel-Trenaunay-Weber syndrome

Contd...

Contd...

• Chromosomal disorders such as trisomy 21 (Down's syndrome)
• *Connective tissue disorders*:
– Marfan syndrome
– Weill-Marchesani syndrome
– Stickler syndrome
• *Metabolic disorders*:
– Homocystinuria
– Lowe syndrome
– Mucopolysaccharidoses
• Rubinstein-Taybi syndrome
• Congenital rubella
3. *Glaucoma associated with acquired condition* Conditions which are not inherited or present at birth but which develop after birth
• Uveitis
• Trauma (hyphema, angle recession, ectopia lentis)
• Steroid induced
• Tumors (benign/malignant, ocular/orbital)
• Retinopathy of prematurity (ROP)
• Postsurgery other than cataract surgery
4. *Glaucoma following cataract surgery* Meets glaucoma definition only after cataract surgery performed. Sub-divided into three categories based upon cataract type
• Congenital idiopathic cataract
• Congenital cataract associated with ocular anomalies/systemic disease or syndrome
• Acquired cataract

Primary Childhood Glaucoma

Primary Congenital Glaucoma

Primary congenital glaucoma (PCG) is the most common glaucoma in infancy and is characterized by an immature angle, i.e. isolated trabeculodysgenesis. The immature angle is thought to occur as a result of developmental arrest of angle tissues derived from the cranial neural crest. Obstruction to outflow is now thought to be due to thick, compacted trabecular sheets which also act to prevent the normal posterior migration of the uveal tract (iris and ciliary body), rather than an impermeable membrane (Barkan's membrane).[2] PCG is typically bilateral (70–80%), asymmetric and usually manifests in the first year of life. It occurs more frequently in males than females. The incidence of PCG is about 1 in 10,000–20,000 live births in Western countries.[3] Parental consanguinity is thought to be responsible for the higher prevalence in certain ethnic groups such as the Slovakian Romani who have the highest incidence 1:1250.

Primary congenital glaucoma is usually sporadic but a family history of glaucoma is reported in 10–40% of cases associated with autosomal recessive inheritance and variable penetrance ranging from 40% to 100%. To date four of loci have been associated with PCG with the main one being the *GCL3A* gene which has been mapped to the short arm of chromosome 2 (2p21). Mutations of the *CYP1B1* gene at the *GLC3A* locus have been associated with the majority of PCG cases. It encodes for enzyme cytochrome P4501B1 proposed to participate in the development and function of the trabecular meshwork (TM). Mice deficient in *CYP1B1* develop structural abnormalities in the iridocorneal angle, with decreased amounts of collagen and increased endothelial cells in the trabecular meshwork.[4] *CYP1B1* mutations are associated with variable expressivity.[5] The risk of PCG in siblings and offspring of affected Caucasian patients is low (<5%). Despite this, it is advisable to examine the siblings and offspring of patients, especially in the first 6 months of life. However, if there is a history of consanguinity, the risk is higher making screening of siblings essential.

Primary congenital glaucoma is a surgical condition with angle surgery, goniotomy and trabeculotomy, usually being the procedure of choice. The prognosis of angle surgery is influenced by the timing of the onset of signs, with 3–12 months of age having the most favorable prognosis. The options after failed angle surgery followed by medical therapy are either trabeculectomy with anti-scarring agents or glaucoma drainage device (GDD) surgery.

Juvenile Open-angle Glaucoma

Juvenile open-angle glaucoma is characterized by an open angle, which is normal in appearance. It presents late in childhood up to the age of 35 typically with high pressures. It is not associated with ocular enlargement, ocular anomalies or systemic features. Often there is a strong family history of glaucoma with autosomal dominant inheritance. Up to 20% of patients have mutations of the *MYOC* gene at the *GLC1A* locus on chromosome 1q23. These patients usually respond well to prostaglandin analogues. If medical treatment fails, a trabeculectomy with antiscarring agents can be considered.

Secondary Childhood Glaucoma

With conditions that predispose to secondary glaucoma it is important to remember the potential lifelong risk of glaucoma and so the need for regular IOP review. Consistently elevated IOP should be treated medically before glaucoma develops. Patients with conditions known to be associated with systemic findings should be referred to a pediatrician for assessment. Family screening and genetic counseling is indicated for inherited conditions.

Glaucoma Associated with Nonacquired Ocular Anomalies

Aniridia is a bilateral condition characterized by a variable congenital absence of iris secondary to *PAX6* gene mutations at chromosome 11p13. Inheritance is usually autosomal dominant with high penetrance and variable expressivity.[6] Sporadic aniridia is associated in 30% of cases with WARG syndrome associated with large deletions of 11p13 (Fig. 73.4). Glaucoma occurs in over 50% of cases usually presenting in preadolescence or early adulthood. The angle is usually open but progressive angle closure by the iris stump can occur. When medical therapy fails, surgery should be considered. Angle surgery (goniotomy) is not widely practiced due to the potential risk of intraocular trauma. Trabeculectomy with antiscarring agents is usually first line. If significant cataract is present or trabeculectomy fails, then GDD surgery is indicated.[7] Hypotony should be avoided due to the danger of lens-corneal touch. Symptomatic relief of photophobia can be achieved with lubricants and tinted spectacles. Children with sporadic aniridia should be referred for regular renal assessment.

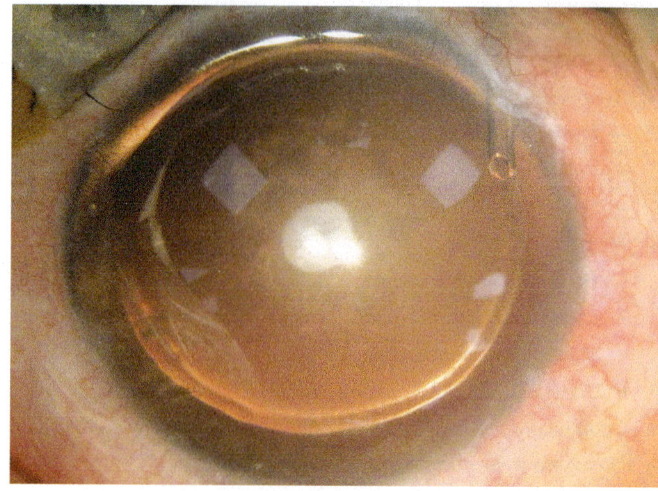

Fig. 73.4: Aniridic eye and superotemporal Baerveldt implant with oblique tube.

Axenfeld-Rieger (AR) anomaly covers a spectrum of disease with overlapping clinical features which include, posterior embryotoxon (anteriorly displaced, prominent Schwalbe's line) with attached iris strands, and iris changes such as corectopia or iris hypoplasia (Figs. 73.5A to C). In association with systemic anomalies such as hypertelorism, periumbilical skin tags, dental and cardiac abnormalities it is referred to as Axenfeld-Rieger syndrome. It is usually bilateral, asymmetrical and autosomal dominantly inherited. Two major genes have been identified, *PITX2* gene at chromosome 4q25 and *FOXC1* at 6p25.[8] Examination of family members, including gonioscopy, is essential to determine sporadic from familial cases, and to occasionally identify undiagnosed cases. Peters anomaly is characterized by a congenital, central corneal opacity with underlying defects in stroma, Descemet's membrane and endothelium. It may be an isolated finding or have iris and lens involvement. Associated with systemic features it is called Peters plus syndrome and carries a higher risk of glaucoma. It is usually bilateral (80%) and sporadic and may result from abnormalities of the *PITX2, FOXC1, CYP1B1* and *PAX6 genes*. The risk of glaucoma for AR and Peters anomaly is 50%. Glaucoma usually occurs in childhood or young adulthood and the IOP is often labile. Medical therapy is

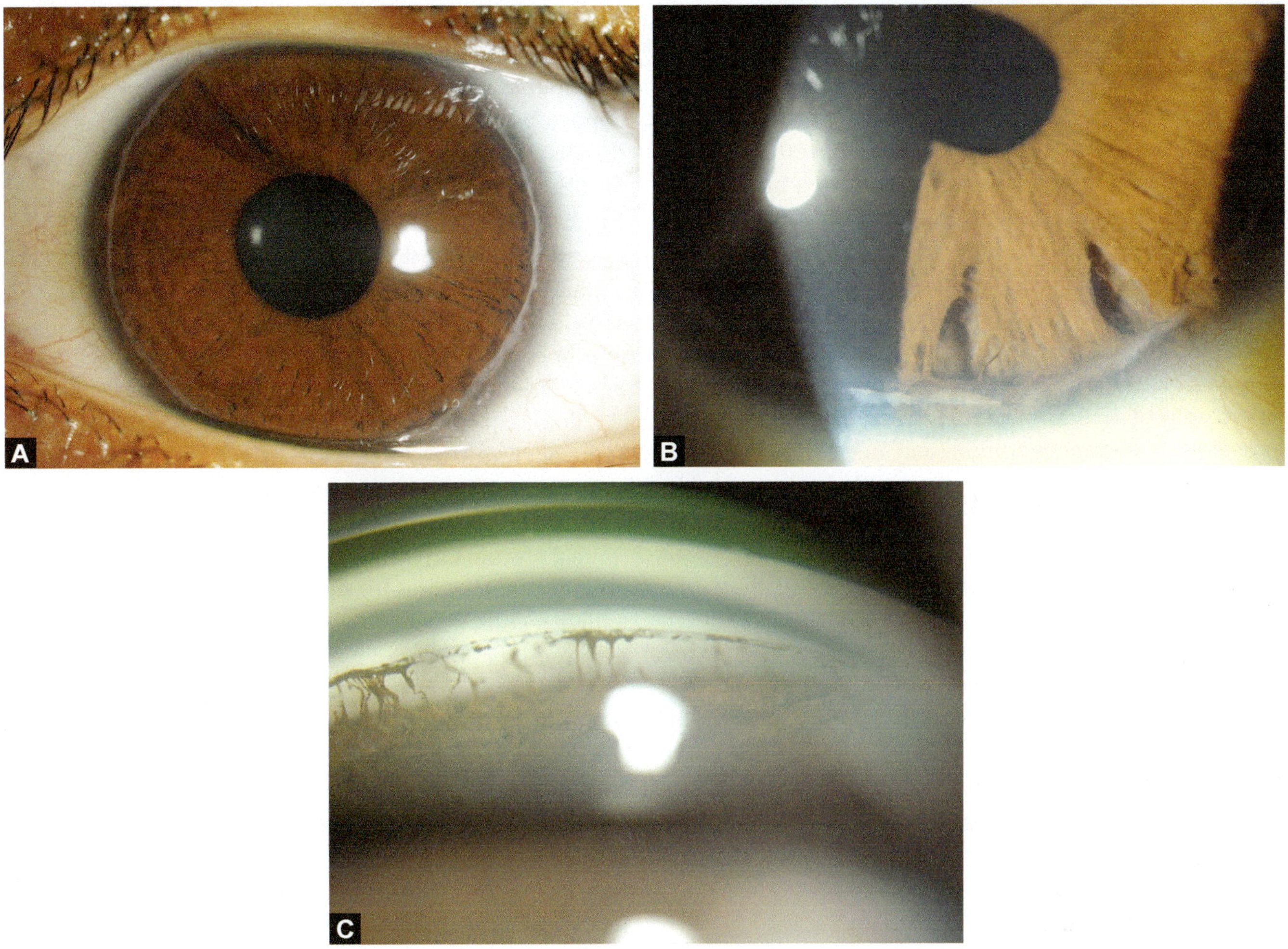

Figs. 73.5A to C: (A) *Axenfeld-Rieger anomaly*: Prominent posterior embryotoxon with iris attachments; (B) *Axenfeld-Rieger anomaly*: Prominent posterior embryotoxon with iris attachments magnified; (C) Gonioscopic appearance of Axenfeld-Rieger anomaly with iris stands to posterior embryotoxon.

first line. Angle surgery is less successful than in PCG and potentially more challenging. Often trabeculectomy with antiscarring agents is necessary to control the IOP. Primary GDD surgery may be indicated in the most severe cases. In cases of Peters anomaly with dense corneal opacities and a clear lens, pupil dilation or a broad optical iridectomy can be performed at the site of maximum corneal clarity. Penetrating keratoplasty is associated with disappointing results, especially in infants.[9,10]

Glaucoma Associated with Nonacquired Systemic Diseases or Syndromes

Sturge-Weber syndrome (encephalotrigeminal angiomatosis) is the most common phakomatosis associated with glaucoma. It is a sporadic, congenital condition characterized by a facial cutaneous vascular malformation (port wine stain) and ocular vascular lesions (episcleral and choroidal hemangioma).[11] It is associated with a somatic mutation in the *GNAQ* gene on chromosome 9q21. Glaucoma occurs in around 30–50% of cases from birth to adulthood. Elevated episcleral venous pressure is thought to cause glaucoma and goniodysgenesis play a role in infantile presentations. Port wine stains involving the ophthalmic division of V1 (especially upper lid and bilateral involvement), and the presence of an episcleral vascular malformation or choroidal hemangioma (40%) increase the risk of glaucoma. When medical treatment fails, surgery is considered based on the age of onset. Congenital or infantile presentations may respond to angle surgery. After failed angle surgery or in older children, either trabeculectomy with antiscarring agents or GDD surgery is indicated. The presence of a choroidal hemangioma significantly increases the potential for serious complications such as suprachoroidal hemorrhage or choroidal effusions. All surgery in these patients must be coupled with measures to minimize hypotony. Smaller surface area implants to reduce the risk of hypotony, e.g. Baerveldt 250 mm^2 with measures to restrict flow should be considered especially in infants. Other phakomatoses are associated with a lower incidence of glaucoma. Klippel-Trenaunay-Weber syndrome, characterized by a triad of cutaneous vascular malformations and varicosities involving one limb and hypertrophy of bone and soft tissue. Neurofibromatosis,[1] an autosomal dominant condition, may first present with iris abnormalities, e.g. ectropion uveae and glaucoma before the systemic disease is apparent.

For rare systemic conditions associated with childhood glaucoma, determining the mechanism of the glaucoma by a thorough history and examination is the best treatment plan. For example, connective tissue and metabolic disorders such as Marfan's syndrome, Weil Marchesani syndrome and homocystinuria may cause childhood glaucoma by lens displacement, secondary pupil block and angle closure. In this context, prophylactic iridectomy and chronic miosis may be required to prevent pupil block glaucoma or dislocation of the lens into the AC.

Glaucoma Associated with Acquired Conditions

Uveitic glaucoma is most commonly seen in juvenile idiopathic arthritis (30%), usually 2–3 years after presentation. It is multifactorial due to chronic cellular trabecular obstruction, trabeculitis, peripheral anterior synechiae (PAS), secondary pupil block, lensectomy and following chronic topical steroid usage. Children with uveitis tend to develop more severe glaucoma than adults. Management of uveitic glaucoma is firstly to aggressively treat the uveitis with topical ± systemic steroids and steroid-sparing therapy, and secondly to control the IOP. The uveitis and glaucoma specialist often need to work closely to maximize outcomes. Glaucoma is often refractory to treatment, especially medical treatment which is first line. Angle surgery often requires medical treatment to control IOP. Trabeculectomy with antiscarring agents may be considered but has been associated with a high rate of reoperation for IOP control.[12] Primary GDD surgery, especially if future lensectomy is contemplated or if aphakia is present, can be considered. Perioperative systemic immunosuppression, particularly with steroids is essential to optimize invasive surgical outcomes. The risk of postoperative hypotony is high in these patients even in the absence of overdrainage, due to compromised aqueous production. Therefore, a GDD with a smaller surface area, e.g. Baerveldt implant 250 mm^2 with measures to restrict flow or an Ahmed implant (184 mm^2) are advisable. Cyclodiode treatment is associated with poor success rates as primary treatment[13] and should be avoided as it aims to reduce the function of an already compromised ciliary body, potentially leading to chronic hypotony.

Trauma, whether blunt or penetrating, can lead to an acute or chronic rise in IOP occurring many years after the original injury. The pathogenesis of traumatic glaucoma is multifactorial due to uveitis which is common, topical steroids, hyphema (the greater the hyphema the greater the potential for raised IOP) and angle recession which results in glaucoma in 5–20% of cases.[14] The risk of glaucoma is related to the extent of angle recession, especially if greater than 180° of recession exists. Medical treatment is first line. Even though children with sickle cell disease are more likely to develop glaucoma, systemic carbonic anhydrase inhibitors should be avoided as they can precipitate a sickle crisis. The risk of corneal staining and of glaucoma determines when to intervene surgically. AC washout of hyphema is recommended with a sustained IOP of greater than 30 mm Hg on maximum tolerated medical therapy or with corneal staining. There is no consensus as to the most appropriate glaucoma operation although GDD surgery is recommended as these eyes are usually very inflamed.

Rarely, childhood tumors such as leukemia, retinoblastoma or medulloepithelioma may cause glaucoma from outflow obstruction by tumor cells or secondary hemorrhage. The treatment of glaucoma in these circumstances is conservative. The primary disorder is treated, along with topical medical treatment and cyclodestruction. Incisional surgery should be avoided to prevent the risk of tumor seeding.

Glaucoma Following Cataract Surgery

Glaucoma following congenital cataract surgery is one of the most common secondary childhood glaucomas. It can occur at any time in either aphakic or pseudophakic eyes. Both chemical (inflammatory cells, lens remnants and vitreous derived factors) and mechanical theories (lack of ciliary body tension and TM collapse) have been proposed combined with developmental reasons, i.e. arrest of postnatal angle maturation due to surgical insult. The incidence of glaucoma following childhood cataract surgery has been variably reported in the literature. The Infant Aphakia Treatment Study reported an incidence of 14% for ocular hypertension and 18% for glaucoma after 5 years of follow-up. Risk factors included younger age (less than 48 days old) and smaller corneal diameters (≤10 mm) which increased the risk of glaucoma by 3 times, but not primary IOL implantation.[15] The angle is usually open. Acute angle closure from secondary pupil block is rare but usually results in glaucoma despite surgery for pupil block. Contact lens intolerance or excessive loss of hyperopia may be useful signs of elevated IOP. Managing glaucoma following congenital cataract surgery is challenging and the visual prognosis tends to be worse in these children compared to those with PCG.[16] Medical treatment is first line but only controls IOP in around 50% cases. Angle surgery is associated with variable success and recent results for circumferential (360°) trabeculotomy suggest modest outcomes.[17] Trabeculectomy with MMC has a poor success rate,[18] and if associated with a thin, avascular bleb excludes postoperative contact lens use due to the risk of bleb-related infection. Cyclodiode laser usually provides limited success with continuation of medications and often has to be repeated.[19] Marked inflammation, retinal detachment and phthisis are possible especially in microphthalmic eyes.[19,20] GDD surgery probably has the highest chance of long-term success and allows contact lens use.[21,22] The tube can be placed in either the AC or behind the iris depending on the anatomy of the anterior chamber.

MANAGEMENT

Assessment

Any suspicion of glaucoma in a child should always be treated seriously and with urgency to minimize visual impairment. This requires examination in either the clinic, office or under anesthesia depending on the child's age and ability to cooperate. Children should be encouraged onto the slit-lamp for more accurate assessment of the IOP with applanation tonometry, and of the optic disc with a magnified, binocular view whenever this becomes possible. It is important in an infant to enquire about a history of epiphora, photophobia, blepharospasm and any change in ocular appearance. Determine the age of clinical onset for prognosis, associated systemic problems for anesthetic risk, problems during pregnancy (rubella) or labor (use of forceps), a family history of childhood glaucoma and parental consanguinity. In older children, a history of trauma, ocular inflammation or surgery and corticosteroid use may be relevant. Assess the child's overall appearance, visual behavior including the presence or absence or nystagmus or strabismus and visual acuity. Sometimes it is important to examine the parents as the presence of subtle signs such as Axenfeld-Rieger anomaly may alter genetic counseling and the management of siblings.

Tonometry

Intraocular pressure in normal neonates is reported to be lower than the adult mean.[23] Measuring IOP in children can be difficult as its accuracy is influenced by many factors which makes it potentially unreliable such as, cooperation, dilation, anesthetic type, tonometer and corneal characteristics (edema, opacities, thickness and biomechanical properties). Hence, avoid measuring the IOP with lid squeezing and crying as they falsely elevate the IOP. Preferably, the eyes should be in the primary position and motionless. Avoid the use of a lid speculum and pressure on the eye.

The reference standard for measuring IOP is with Goldmann applanation tonometry. Tono-pen® and pneumotonometry overestimate the IOP compared to applanation tonometry in both normal children and those with glaucoma.[24,25] Similarly with Icare, a portable rebound tonometer, but the fact it does not require topical anesthesia and can be used in both supine and upright positions, has led to its gaining popularity. The disagreement between the Goldmann tonometer and Icare was found in one study to be greater with increasing IOP and corneal thickness.[26] However, measurements within the normal range were likely to be accurate, therefore likely sparing the child an unnecessary EUA.[26] It is advisable to use the same tonometer for serial examinations. In children undergoing EUA, the reference standard for tonometry is the Perkins handheld tonometer with a blue filter after instillation of fluorescein. As the type of anesthetic influences IOP measurement (e.g. inhalational anesthetics reduce IOP), tonometry under anesthesia generally provides only with an approximation of the true IOP.

In light of the above, IOP should never be the sole finding by which the presence or control of glaucoma is assessed. If IOP measurement is inconsistent with other clinical findings it may be inaccurate and tactile estimation of the IOP may be useful.

Corneal Diameter Measurement

In newborns the horizontal diameter is around 10.5 mm increasing by about 1 mm in the first year of life. A corneal diameter greater than 11 mm in a newborn and 12 mm in an infant less than 1 year is very suggestive of raised IOP but with Haab's striae it is diagnostic. A measurement of greater than 13 mm in a child of any age and asymmetrical corneal diameters is abnormal. During EUA, the horizontal corneal diameter is measured with calipers from limbus to limbus and checked with a graduated ruler with estimation to the nearest 0.25 mm. Serial corneal diameter measurements are useful in establishing the diagnosis and monitoring glaucoma progression until the age of 3 after which the potential for corneal enlargement usually ceases.

Central Corneal Thickness

Patients with PCG and JOAG have thinner corneas and conversely increased corneal thickness is found in patients with aphakia and aniridia. Central corneal thickness (CTT) is known to influence the accuracy of tonometry but its exact effect in children is unknown. Altered biomechanical properties in children with glaucoma may be important.[27] The role of pachymetry in childhood glaucoma remains to be determined and CCT should not be used to correct IOP measurements.

Anterior Segment Examination

Apart from horizontal diameter and thickness, the cornea must be examined for the presence of edema, opacities, posterior embryotoxon and Haab's striae. A portable slit-lamp allows detailed examination. Oblique or retroillumination and magnification are necessary as the signs may be subtle. Persistent corneal edema may be a sign of poorly controlled glaucoma. The presence of corneal enlargement with splits with or without edema indicates raised IOP at some stage in infancy. It is important to exclude primary corneal pathology, with the absence of corneal or ocular enlargement being a useful finding. Detecting iris, pupil abnormalities or coexisting lens opacities is useful as they may influence the choice of glaucoma surgery.

Gonioscopy

Gonioscopy is crucial in determining the correct diagnosis and the most appropriate operation. It should be performed at least once when possible. In a EUA, direct gonioscopy can be performed with a variety of lenses including a Koeppe lens with a portable slit-lamp (Fig. 73.6). In PCG, the characteristic gonioscopic appearance includes a flat anterior, iris insertion, no angle recess and a thin, hypopigmented iris stroma with peripheral scalloping of the posterior pigmented iris layer (Fig. 73.7).

Posterior Segment Examination

The optic disc appearance is the most important and sensitive parameter for both diagnosis and glaucoma progression. A cup-to-disc ratio (CDR) more than 0.3 is rare in normal Caucasian newborn eyes[28] and common in infants less than one year with congenital glaucoma.[29] A cup:disc ratio greater than 0.3 in a Caucasian neonate or infant less than 1 year and disc asymmetry of more than or equal to 0.2 is suggestive of glaucoma. Following dilation,

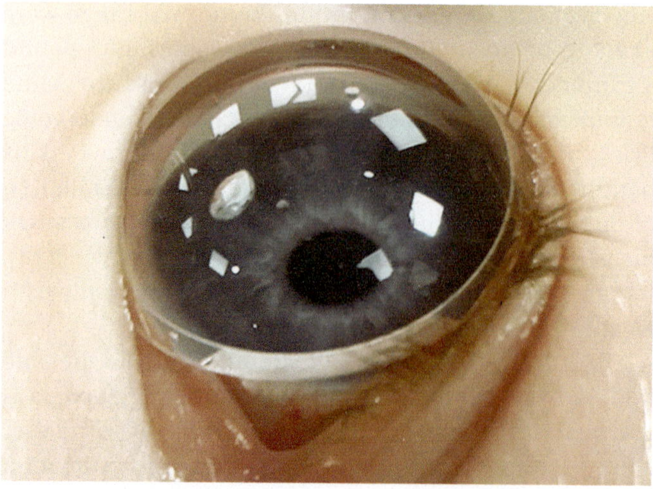

Fig. 73.6: Direct gonioscopy with Koeppe lens.

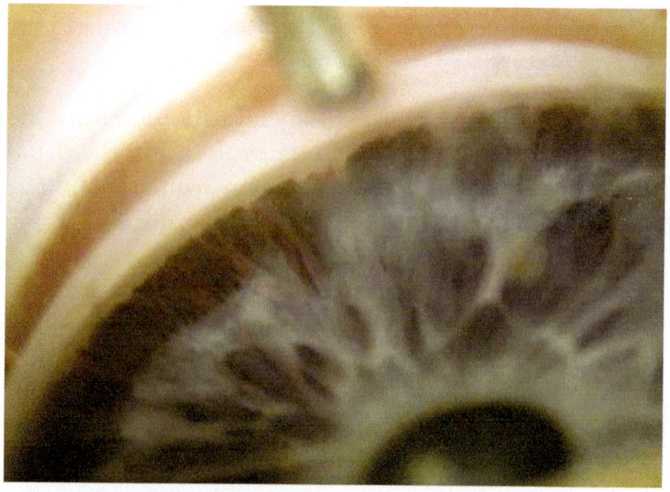

Fig. 73.7: Classic immature primary congenital glaucoma (PCG) angle appearance.

the optic disc size, CDR, focal rim loss and nerve fiber layer defects should be carefully recorded with a drawing and if possible a photograph as a baseline for future comparison. An indirect ophthalmoscope with a small pupil facility can be very useful in obtaining a view of the disc in infants whose pupils dilate poorly. An increase in disc cupping is definite evidence of poorly controlled glaucoma and the need for further treatment, regardless of IOP measurement obtained.

Disc cupping reversal is possible in children following IOP reduction if it occurs before irreversible nerve atrophy. Once the IOP is normalized, compression of the prelaminar neural tissue is relieved allowing the laminar to move anteriorly filling in the cup. However, retinal nerve fiber layer thinning may persist postoperatively despite disc cupping reversal.[30]

The remainder of the fundus should be examined for any associated abnormalities such as foveal hypoplasia associated with aniridia, choroidal hemangiomas in Sturge-Weber syndrome and pigmentary retinopathy associated with rubella.

REFRACTION

Refraction plays an important role both in the diagnosis and monitoring of glaucoma. A significant loss of hypermetropia or the presence of myopia in a neonate or infant is often evidence of glaucoma. Progressive myopia or a myopic shift in aphakic patients suggests inadequate IOP control, especially in the context of progressively increasing axial lengths.

EXAMINATION UNDER ANESTHESIA

As a general rule, all anesthetics lower the IOP with the exceptions of ketamine and chloral hydrate. Inhalation anesthetics, such as sevoflurane, may substantially lower the IOP and cause progressive lowering of IOP with time from induction. It follows that the finding of a normal IOP with the use of agents known to reduce IOP does not exclude glaucoma. Whichever agent is used, it is important to have a consistent approach using the same agent for serial examinations and to measure the IOP first. Ketamine hydrochloride is associated with IOP measurements similar to those taken in awake infants.[31] While the patient is under anesthesia, a general examination and venesection for laboratory investigation (e.g. screening for infective agents and chromosome studies) can also be performed.

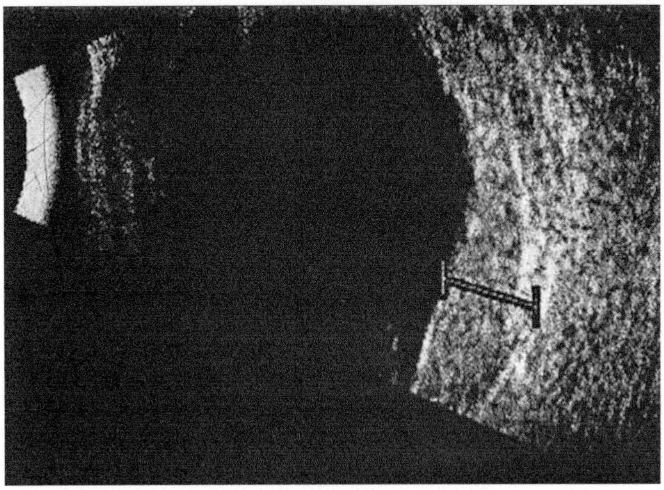

Fig. 73.8: B-scan revealing a large choroidal hemangioma in Sturge-Weber syndrome.

INVESTIGATIONS

Axial length (AL) measurement is useful for diagnosing glaucoma (if it is outside normal limits) and for detecting progression with serial AL when the eye is still distensible. In glaucoma, AL measurements are usually asymmetrical in contrast to X-linked megalocornea and normal eyes. Ultrasound may be critical in detecting lesions like tumors associated with secondary glaucoma or choroidal hemangiomas (Fig. 73.8) which if very large may require radiotherapy before surgery.

Visual fields are usually possible around the age of 7–8 but there is a learning curve. Visual field defects must be reproducible and correspond to the optic disc appearance. The role of automated optic disc imaging in children with glaucomas is being evaluated but is limited by the lack of a normative pediatric database. A prospective, observational study in children with glaucoma revealed retinal nerve fiber layer and macular thickness measurements declined with increasing severity of glaucomatous disc damage as seen in stereophotographs.[32]

TREATMENT

Medical Therapy

Medications are an important part of management.[33] They are usually first-line treatment for most glaucomas, they temporize IOP control prior to surgery, e.g. PCG, and are often required as adjunctive therapy after partially successful surgery for IOP control. Great care must be taken when prescribing in children, as they are at a higher risk of systemic, potentially fatal side effects from topical administration which parents must be warned about. Use the lowest concentration and lowest frequency of an agent where possible to minimize side effects. Surgery must be considered when medications fail to control glaucoma.

Beta-blockers should be avoided in premature or newborn infants and in children with asthma or cardiac problems including arrhythmias. It is important to inquire about asthma symptoms, which may manifest with nocturnal cough in children rather than wheezing. Timolol 0.1%, Timolol gellan 0.25% are the beta-blockers of choice as first-line treatment due to their superior risk profile and efficacy. The prostaglandin analog, Latanoprost, is the first agent to be approved for use in children.[34] It is thought to be at least as effective as Timolol. Patients with JOAG may respond particularly well and it should be considered first line in these patients. The sympathomimetic Brimonidine crosses the blood brain barrier causing drowsiness to the point of coma and apnea in infants. It should be avoided in children less than the age of 6 years or less than 20 kilograms.[35] The use of Apraclonidine in children is theoretically safer as it is less lipophilic and this appears to be the case clinically. The topical carbonic anhydrase inhibitor Brinzolamide is less irritating than Dorzolamide and both are useful as second line drugs. The use of oral acetazolamide in children is limited by serious systemic side effects such as failure to thrive, disturbed behavior and bedwetting. Therefore, it should usually be considered only on a very short-term basis prior to surgery. Parasympathomimetic agents, e.g. Pilocarpine have a limited role in selective cases such as following angle surgery as it may enhance aqueous outflow and prevent peripheral anterior synechiae formation. They may also be highly effective in cases of glaucoma following congenital cataract surgery and with ectopia lentis to prevent anterior lens dislocation.

SURGICAL THERAPY

The surgical procedure of choice is largely determined by the type of glaucoma and may be further influenced by age of onset, corneal clarity, degree of optic nerve damage, associated ocular disease, history of previous surgery and the surgeon's experience.[36]

Angle Surgery

During goniotomy a blade or needle is introduced into the temporal cornea and an incision made in the nasal angle. Adequate visualization of the angle and a deep AC are the keys to safely and successfully performing goniotomy (Fig. 73.9). Its main advantage is that it spares the conjunctiva for future surgery. During trabeculotomy, Schlemm's canal is identified and cannulated by an external approach and the internal wall of Schlemm's canal (SC), including the TM, incised. Trabeculotomy relies on the accurate localization of Schlemm's canal. Its main advantage is that it can be performed irrespective of corneal clarity so has greater application than goniotomy. However, it is more invasive resulting in conjunctival scarring so a temporal incision is preferable. Both goniotomy and conventional trabeculotomy with a trabeculotomy probe incise up to a third of the angle. The introduction of circumferential (360°) trabeculotomy with a blunted 6/0 polypropylene suture [37] or an illuminated microcatheter, for improved safety,[38,39] (Fig. 73.10) threaded into SC has been a significant

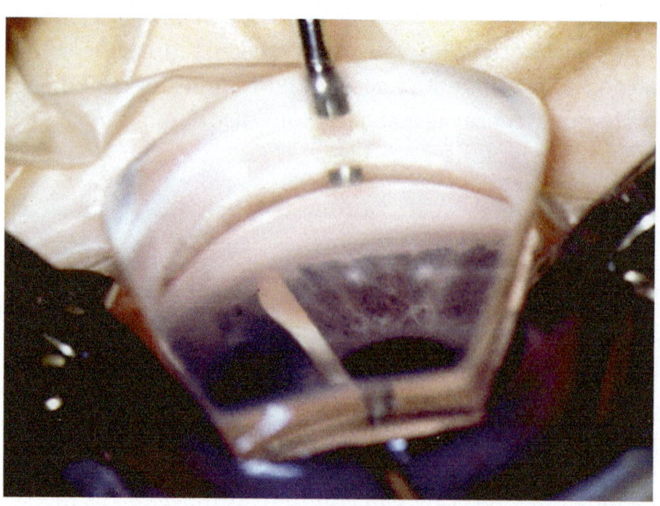

Fig. 73.9: Goniotomy.

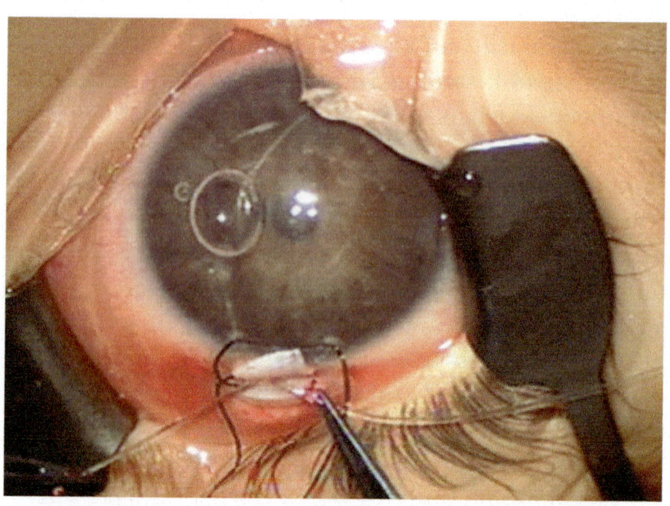

Fig. 73.10: Left ab externo circumferential trabeculotomy with an illuminated microcatheter.

advance in angle surgery as it potentially incises the whole angle in one operation minimizing anesthetic exposure. An ab interno trabeculotomy approach, which is quicker, has also been described. The best outcomes for angle surgery are in PCG usually after multiple goniotomies or probe trabeculotomies of around 90% with medium term follow-up.[40,41] However, results of circumferential trabeculotomy suggest greater success than a single goniotomy, probe trabeculotomy and combined trabeculotomy-trabeculectomy (CTT).[42,43,22] Success rates for secondary childhood glaucomas are generally not as good as for PCG.

Trabeculotomy Combined with Trabeculectomy

Trabeculotomy has the added advantage of being combined with trabeculectomy to provide in theory two major outflow pathways and so improve results but in practice the clinical benefit is unclear.[45-46] Technically, it is a more complex procedure with potentially significant complications especially with the use of antiscarring agents.

Trabeculectomy

Trabeculectomy is indicated after failed angle surgery and for most phakic secondary glaucomas. Technically, it is a more demanding procedure and more likely to fail in children due to a vigorous wound healing response. This necessitates the use of MMC which is associated with higher complication rates. However, with recent simple modifications to the surgical technique (Moorfields Safer Surgery System) [47] and to the intraoperative application of MMC, trabeculectomy can be associated with favorable bleb morphology, reduced complications and satisfactory outcomes in appropriate cases, even infants. (Figs. 73.11 and 73.12).[48,49] Cumulative success rates of MMC trabeculectomy of 59–90% at 2 years reducing to 51–67% at 5 years have been reported.[49-52] Reported risk factors for failure include aphakia[18] and age less than one [51,53] although a recent publication suggests infancy is not associated with an increased risk of failure.[49] When trabeculectomy fails to control IOP, bleb needling may be attempted with an antiscarring agent if the sclerostomy is patent. Another trabeculectomy with a higher dose of MMC or GDD surgery can be considered.

Glaucoma Drainage Devices

Glaucoma drainage devices play a vital role for children with refractory glaucoma. As primary surgery indications include children: who develop glaucoma following cataract surgery; with uveitis who are aphakic or pseudophakic; who have a cataract that will need future imminent removal and those with very severe disease with onset at birth as these cases have a very high failure rate even with MMC trabeculectomy. Buphthalmic eyes have a much higher rate of complication if hypotony occurs and appropriate measures need to be taken to avoid this complication such as vicryl tube occlusion in the early postoperative period. Success rates vary between around 50–80% with success reducing the longer the follow-up with most children

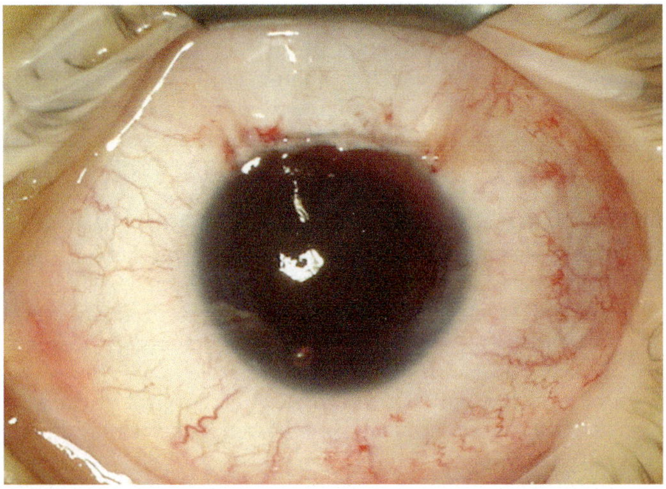

Fig. 73.11: Infantile pediatric trabeculectomy with Moorfields Safer Surgery System 2 months following surgery.

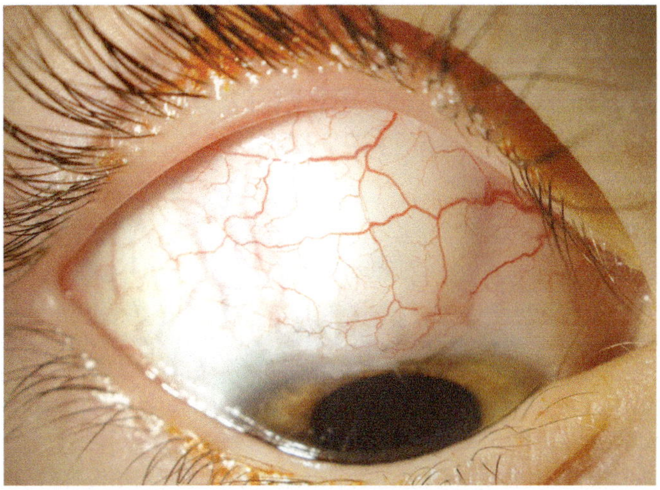

Fig. 73.12: Pediatric trabeculectomy 5 years following surgery.

remaining on medications for IOP control.[54-58] There is no clear superiority of one GDD over another. Plate encapsulation is a major cause of late failure.

Once failure has occurred, the options are either cyclodiode laser or a second GDD.[59] GDDs have a significant complication profile. Consistently reported more commonly in children compared to adults is tube malposition with migration anteriorly causing tube corneal touch or posteriorly leading to retraction (requiring surgical revision in 33% of cases) along with tube erosion and endophthalmitis in up to 10% of cases.[60] Hypotony is another major complication which buphthalmic eyes are especially prone to and occurs even with the use of valved implants.

CYCLODESTRUCTION

The indications for cyclodestruction include: a blind painful eye; poor visual and surgical prognosis; when surgery is technically impossible and when other treatments have failed.

Contact transscleral semiconductor diode laser (810 nm) is the most common method of ciliary body destruction. As buphthalmic eyes often have distorted anatomical landmarks, transillumination of the eye is essential to ensure accurate placement of the laser burns. Care must be taken to avoid areas of pigmentation, hemorrhage and scleral thinning as scleral perforation in a buphthalmic eye has been reported.[61] Transscleral diode laser has limited success (50%) in the short-term, often requires retreatment and the continuation of medications.[19,62] Endoscopic diode has similar results with a lower retreatment rate. Overall visual loss rates of up to 18% have been reported, usually in eyes with pre-existing poor vision.[63]

REFRACTIVE CORRECTION AND AMBLYOPIA THERAPY

The ultimate aim of preserving lifelong vision in children with glaucoma is dependent not only on IOP control but also on several interrelated factors such as the treatment of ametropia and amblyopia. All children with glaucoma within the vulnerable age range should be examined regularly for the presence of amblyopia. Refraction should be part of the periodic examination with glasses prescribed as appropriate when the cornea clears and is practical. Occlusion therapy for amblyopia should be attempted in all children in whom there is potential for visual improvement. Furthermore, parents and later patients should be warned that minor blunt trauma in buphthalmic eyes may result in severe visual loss. Protective eyewear should be recommended, especially in monocular patients.

ACKNOWLEDGMENTS

Peng Tee Khaw and Maria Papadopoulos have received support from the National Institute for Health Research (NIHR), Biomedical Research Centre at Moorfields Eye Hospital NHS Foundation Trust and UCL Institute of Ophthalmology, Medical Research Council, Moorfields Eye Charity, Helen Hamlyn Trust in memory of Paul Hamlyn, Michael and Ilse Katz Foundation, Ron and Liora Moskovitz, Richard Desmond Foundation, and Fight for Sight.

REFERENCES

1. Beck A, Chang TCP, Freedman S. Definition, Classification and differential diagnosis. In: Weinreb RN, Grajewski A, Papadopoulos M, Grigg J, Freedman S. (Eds). Childhood Glaucoma. Amsterdam: Kugler Publications. 2013. pp. 3-10.
2. Anderson DR. The development of the trabecular meshwork and its abnormality in primary infantile glaucoma. Trans Am Ophthalmol Soc. 1981;79:458-85.
3. Papadopoulos M, Cable N, Rahi J, et al. The British Infantile and Childhood Glaucoma (BIG) Eye Study. Invest Ophthalmol Vis Sci. 2007;48(9):4100-6.
4. Teixeira LB, Zhao Y, Dubielzig RR, et al. Ultrastructural abnormalities of the trabecular meshwork extracellular matrix in Cyp1b1-deficient mice. Vet Pathol. 2015;52(2): 397-403.
5. Suri F, Yazdani S, Narooie-Nejhad M, et al. Variable expressivity and high penetrance of CYP1B1 mutations associated with primary congenital glaucoma. Ophthalmology. 2009;116(11):2101-9.
6. Hingorani M, Moore T. In: Pagon RA, Adam MP, Ardinger HH, et al (Eds). Gene Reviews. University of Washington:Seattle; 1993-2017. 2003 May 20 [updated. 2013 Nov 14].
7. Arroyave CP, Scott IU, Gedde SJ, et al. Use of glaucoma drainage devices in the management of glaucoma associated with aniridia. Am J Ophthalmol. 2003;135(2):155-9.
8. Strungaru MH, Dinu I, Walter MA. Genotype-phenotype correlations in Axenfeld-Rieger malformation and glaucoma patients with FOXC1 and PITX2 mutations. Invest Ophthalmol Vis Sci. 2007;48(1):228-37.
9. Rao KV, Fernandes M, Gangopadhyay N, et al. Outcome of penetrating keratoplasty for Peter's anomaly. Cornea. 2008;27(7):749-53.
10. Karadaq R, Chan TC, Azari AA, et al. Survival of primary penetrating keratoplasty in children. Am J Ophthalmol. 2016;171:95-100.
11. Comi A. Current therapeutic options in Sturge-Weber syndrome. Semin Pediatr Neurol. 2015;22(4):295-301.

12. Salmon J, Mermoud A, Ivey A, et al. The detection of post-traumatic angle recession by gonioscopy in a population-based glaucoma survey. Ophthalmology. 1994;101(11):1844-50.
13. Wiese K, Heiligenhaus A, Heinz C. Trabeculectomy in uveitis associated with juvenile idiopathic arthritis: long-term results in pediatric secondary glaucoma. Ophthalmology. 2014;111(4):330-8.
14. Heinz C, Koch JM, Heiligenhaus A. Transscleral diode laser cyclophotocoagulation as primary surgical treatment for secondary glaucoma in juvenile idiopathic arthritis: high failure rate after short term follow up. Br J Ophthalmol. 2006;90(6):737-40.
15. Freedman SF, Lynn MJ, Beck AD, et al. Infant Aphakia Treatment Study Group. Glaucoma-related adverse events in the first 5 years after unilateral cataract removal in the infant aphakia treatment Study. JAMA Ophthalmol. 2015;33(80):907-14.
16. Neustein RF, Bruce BB, Beck AD. Primary congenital glaucoma versus glaucoma following congenital cataract surgery: comparative clinical features and long-term Outcomes. Am J Ophthalmol. 2016;170:214-22.
17. Lim ME, Dao JB, Freedman SF. 360-Degree trabeculotomy for medically refractory glaucoma following cataract surgery and juvenile open-angle glaucoma. Am J Ophthalmol. 2017;175:1-7.
18. Mandal AK, Bagga H, Nutheti R, et al. Trabeculectomy with or without mitomycin-C for paediatric glaucoma in aphakia and pseudophakia following congenital cataract surgery. Eye(Lond). 2003;17(1):53-62.
19. Kirwan JF, Shah P, Khaw PT. Diode laser cyclophotocoagulation: role in the management of refractory pediatric glaucomas. Ophthalmol. 2002;109(2):316-23.
20. Neely D, Plager D. Endocyclophotocoagulation for management of difficult pediatric glaucomas. J AAPOS. 2001; 5(4):221-9.
21. O'Malley Schotthoefer E, Yanovitch TL, Freedman SF. Aqueous shunt device surgery in refractory pediatric glaucomas. I. Long-term outcomes. J AAPOS. 2008;12(1): 33-9.
22. Chen TC, Bhatia LS, Walton DS. Ahmed valve surgery for refractory pediatric glaucoma: a report of 52 eyes. J Pediatr Ophthalmol Strabismus. 2005;42(5):274-83.
23. Radtke ND, Cohan BE. Intraocular pressure measurement in the newborn. Am J Ophthalmol 1974;78(3):501-4.
24. Levy J, Lifshitz T, Rosen S, et al. Is the tono-pen accurate for measuring intraocular pressure in young children with congenital glaucoma? J AAPOS. 2005;9(4):321-5.
25. Bradfield YS, Kaminski BM, Repka MX, et al. Comparison of Tono-Pen and Goldmann applanation tonometers for measurement of intraocular pressure in healthy children. J AAPOS. 2012;16(3):242-8.
26. Dahlmann-Noor AH, Puertas R, Tabasa-Lim S, et al. Comparison of handheld rebound tonometry with Goldmann applanation tonometry in children with glaucoma: a cohort study. BMJ Open. 2013;3(4).
27. Doozandeh A, Yazdani S, Ansari S, et al. Corneal profile in primary congenital glaucoma. Acta Ophthalmol. 2017;95(7):e575-81.
28. Richardson KT. Optic cup symmetry in normal newborn infants. Invest Ophthalmol. 1968;7(2):137-40.
29. Shaffer RN. New concepts in infantile glaucoma. Can J Ophthalmol. 1967;2(4):243-8.
30. Ely AL, El-Dairi MA, Freedman SF. Cupping reversal in pediätric glaucoma—evaluation of the retinal nerve fiber layer and visual field. Am J Ophthalmol. 2014;158(50):905-15.
31. Blumberg D, Congdon N, Jampel H, et al. The effects of sevoflurane and ketamine on intraocular pressure in children during examination under anesthesia. Am J Ophthalmol. 2007;143(3):494-9.
32. El-Dairi MA, Holgado S, Asrani SG, et al. Correlation between optical coherence tomography and glaucomatous optic nerve head damage in children. Br J Ophthalmol. 2009;93(10):1325-30.
33. Albis-Donado O, Bitrian E, Anilkumar M et al. Medications. In: Weinreb RN, Grajewski A, Papadopoulos M, Grigg J, Freedman S. (Eds). Childhood Glaucoma. Amsterdam: Kugler Publications; 2013.pp.63-90.
34. Maeda-Chubachi T, Chi-Burris K, Simons BD, et al. Comparison of latanoprost and timolol in pediatric glaucoma: a phase 3, 12-week, randomized, double-masked multicenter study. Ophthalmology. 2011;118(10):2014-21.
35. Al-Shahwan S, Al-Torbak AA, Turkmani S, et al. Side-effect profile of brimonidine tartrate in children. Ophthalmology. 2005;112(12):2143.
36. Papadopoulos M, Edmunds B, Chiang M, Mandal A, Grajewski AL, Khaw PT. Glaucoma surgery in children. In: Weinreb RN, Grajewski A, Papadopoulos M, Grigg J, Freedman S (Eds). Childhood Glaucoma. Amsterdam: Kugler Publications; 2013.pp.95-134.
37. Beck AD, Lynch MG. 360 trabeculotomy for primary congenital glaucoma. Arch Ophthalmol. 1995;113(9):1200-2.
38. Sarkisian SR Jr. An illuminated microcatheter for 360-degree trabeculotomy [corrected] in congenital glaucoma: a retrospective case series. J AAPOS. 2010;14(5):412-6.
39. Girkin CA, Rhodes L, McGwin G, et al. Goniotomy versus circumferential trabeculotomy with an illuminated microcatheter in congenital glaucoma. J AAPOS. 2012;16(5):424-7.
40. Russell-Eggitt IM, Rice NSC, Jay B, et al. Relapse following goniotomy for congenital glaucoma due to trabecular dysgenesis. Eye (Lond). 1992;6(2):197-200.
41. Akimoto M, Tanihara H, Negi A, et al. Surgical results of trabeculotomy ab externo for developmental glaucoma. Arch Ophthalmol. 1994;112(12):1540-4.
42. Mendicino ME, Lynch MG, Drack A, et al. Long-term surgical and visual outcomes in primary congenital glaucoma: 360 degrees trabeculotomy versus goniotomy. J AAPOS. 2000;4(4):205-10.
43. Shakrawal J, Bali S, Sidhu T, et al. Randomized Trial on Illuminated-Microcatheter Circumferential Trabeculotomy Versus Conventional Trabeculotomy in Congenital Glaucoma. Am J Ophthalmol. 2017;180:158-64.

44. Temkar S, Gupta S, Sihota R, et al. Illuminated microcatheter circumferential trabeculotomy versus combined trabeculotomy-trabeculectomy for primary congenital glaucoma: a randomized controlled trial. Am J Ophthalmol. 2015;159(3):490-7.
45. Al-Hazmi A, Awad A, Zwaan J, et al. Correlation between surgical success rate and severity of congenital glaucoma. Br J Ophthalmol. 2005;89(4):449-53.
46. Dietlein TS, Jacobi PC, Krieglstein GK. Prognosis of primary ab externo surgery for primary congenital glaucoma. Br J Ophthalmol. 1999;83(3):317-22.
47. Khaw PT, Chiang M, Shah P, et al. Enhanced Trabeculectomy - The Moorfields Safer Surgery System. In: Bettin P, Khaw PT (Eds). Glaucoma Surgery. Dev Ophthalmol. Basel: Karger; 2012.pp.1-28.
48. Wells AP, Cordeiro MF, Bunce CV, et al. Cystic bleb formation and related complications in limbus-versus fornix-based conjunctival flaps in pediatric and young adult trabeculectomy with mitomycin C. Ophthalmol. 2003;110(11):2192-7.
49. Jayaram H, Scawn R, Pooley F, et al. Long term outcomes of trabeculectomy augmented with mitomycin-C undertaken within the first two years of life. Ophthalmology. 2015;122(11):2216-22.
50. Sidoti PA, Belmonte SJ, Liebmann JM, et al. Trabeculectomy with mitomycin-C in the treatment of pediatric glaucomas. Ophthalmology. 2000;107(3):422-9.
51. Beck AD, Wilson WR, Lynch MG, et al. Trabeculectomy with adjunctive mitomycin C in pediatric glaucoma. Am J Ophthalmol. 1998;126(5):648-57.
52. Giampani J Jr, Borges-Giampani AS, Carani JC, et al. Efficacy and safety of trabeculectomy with mitomycin C for childhood glaucoma: a study of results with long-term follow-up. Clinics (Sao Paulo). 2008;63(40):421-6.
53. Freedman SF, McCormick K, Cox TA. Mitomycin C-augmented trabeculectomy with postoperative wound modulation in pediatric glaucoma. J AAPOS. 1999;3(2):117-24.
54. Fellenbaum PS, Sidoti PA, Heuer DK, et al. Experience with the Baerveldt implant in young patients with complicated glaucomas. J Glaucoma. 1995;4(2):91-7.
55. El Sayed Y, Awadein A. Polypropylene vs silicone Ahmed valve with adjunctive mitomycin C in paediatric age group: a prospective controlled study. Eye (Lond). 2013;27(6): 728-34.
56. Ishida K, Mandal AK, Netland PA. Glaucoma drainage implants in pediatric patients. Ophthalmol Clin North Am. 2005;18(3):431-42.
57. van Overdam KA, de Faber JT, Lemij HG, et al. Baerveldt glaucoma implant in paediatric patients. Br J Ophthalmol. 2006;90(3):382-32.
58. Budenz DL, Gedde SJ, Brandt JD, et al. Baerveldt glaucoma implant in the management of refractory childhood glaucomas. Ophthalmology. 2004;111(12):2204-10.
59. Shah AA, WuDunn D, Cantor LB. Shunt revision versus additional tube shunt implantation after failed tube shunt surgery in refractory glaucoma. Am J Ophthalmol. 2000;129(4):455-60.
60. Chen TC, Chen PP, Francis BA, et al. Pediatric glaucoma surgery: a report by the American Academy Of Ophthalmology. Ophthalmology. 2014;121(11):2107-15.
61. Sabri K, Vernon SA. Scleral perforation following trans-scleral cyclodiode. Br J Ophthalmol. 1999;83(4):502-3.
62. Hamard P, May F, Quesnot S, Hamard H. Trans-scleral diode laser cyclophotocoagulation for the treatment of refractory pediatric glaucoma. J Fr Ophthalmol. 2000;23(8):773-80.
63. Bock CJ, Freedman SF, Buckley EG, Shields MB. Transscleral diode laser cyclophotocoagulation for refractory pediatric glaucomas. J Ped Ophthalmol Strabismus. 1997;34(4):235-9.

Chapter 74 Congenital Abnormalities of the Retina

Sarah Hull, Anthony T Moore

INTRODUCTION

Congenital abnormalities of the retina result from disordered development of the eye occurring prenatally. They may occur as a result of genetic mutations, chromosomal abnormalities, prenatal infection or occur by chance. Genetic disorders predominate and may lead to abnormalities confined to the retina or associated with other systemic abnormalities. Some retinal disorders are associated with other eye developmental abnormalities and so are detected at birth but the majority present in early infancy with poor vision and nystagmus or strabismus. Congenital abnormalities of the retina can be usefully divided into those that affect retinovascular development and those that affect other aspects of retinal structure and function.

DISORDERS OF RETINAL VASCULAR DEVELOPMENT

The retinal vessels start developing from the optic disc at around 14 weeks gestation towards the retinal periphery reaching the nasal ora serrata at 36 weeks and the temporal ora at term. This process of retinal vessel development may be disturbed in preterm infants causing retinopathy of prematurity but is also seen in children born at term in association with a number of genetic disorders including Norrie disease and familial exudative vitreoretinopathy.[1]

Norrie Disease

Norrie disease is an X-linked disorder in which affected males typically have bilateral retinal detachments at birth.[2] Not all cases have a family history of similarly affected males. The usual presentation is in infancy with poor vision, nystagmus and leukocoria; rarely cases have been identified on prenatal ultrasound.[3] In some infants, there may be retinal folds and vitreous hemorrhage at birth, which soon progress to total retinal detachment. Although most children with Norrie disease show normal development a significant proportion have developmental delay and cognitive impairment. About 30% of affected males develop sensorineural hearing loss in their teens.[4] Female carriers are usually normal but there are a number of reports of peripheral retinal vascular changes in female heterozygotes; this may reflect skewed X-inactivation. The causative gene *Norrin* has been identified and is known to play a key role in Wnt signaling, which is a key biological pathway influencing retinal vascular development.[5,6] Most affected individuals have mutations within the gene but some have chromosomal deletions which results in deletion of the whole gene and adjacent areas of the X-chromosome. Such children are more likely to have developmental delay.

There is no effective treatment for Norrie disease. Most affected males are blind and ultimately develop phthisis bulbi. Lensectomy may be necessary in infancy if there is evidence of pupil block glaucoma. Genetic counseling is an important part of the overall management. Molecular genetic testing of affected males will identify the causative gene in the majority of cases and then females within the family can be offered genetic testing to determine their carrier status. Prenatal and preimplantation diagnosis is possible once the causative mutation is identified. When parents have had prenatal diagnosis and the male fetus carries the mutation some may opt to continue with the pregnancy. If prenatal ultrasound shows an attached retina at 34 weeks early delivery may be considered to allow early photocoagulation; such an approach has been reported to prevent retinal detachment and allow reasonable vision to develop.[7]

Patients with a less severe phenotype characterized by bilateral retinal folds or incomplete peripheral retinal vascularization were found to harbor missense mutations in *Norrin.*[8] Affected males in these families have a form of X-linked familial exudative vitreoretinopathy (FEVR) (Fig. 74.1). They may benefit from laser photocoagulation and generally have a better visual prognosis than Norrie disease. Male children born to carrier females should have a retinal exam soon after birth to determine whether they are affected and whether laser treatment is indicated.

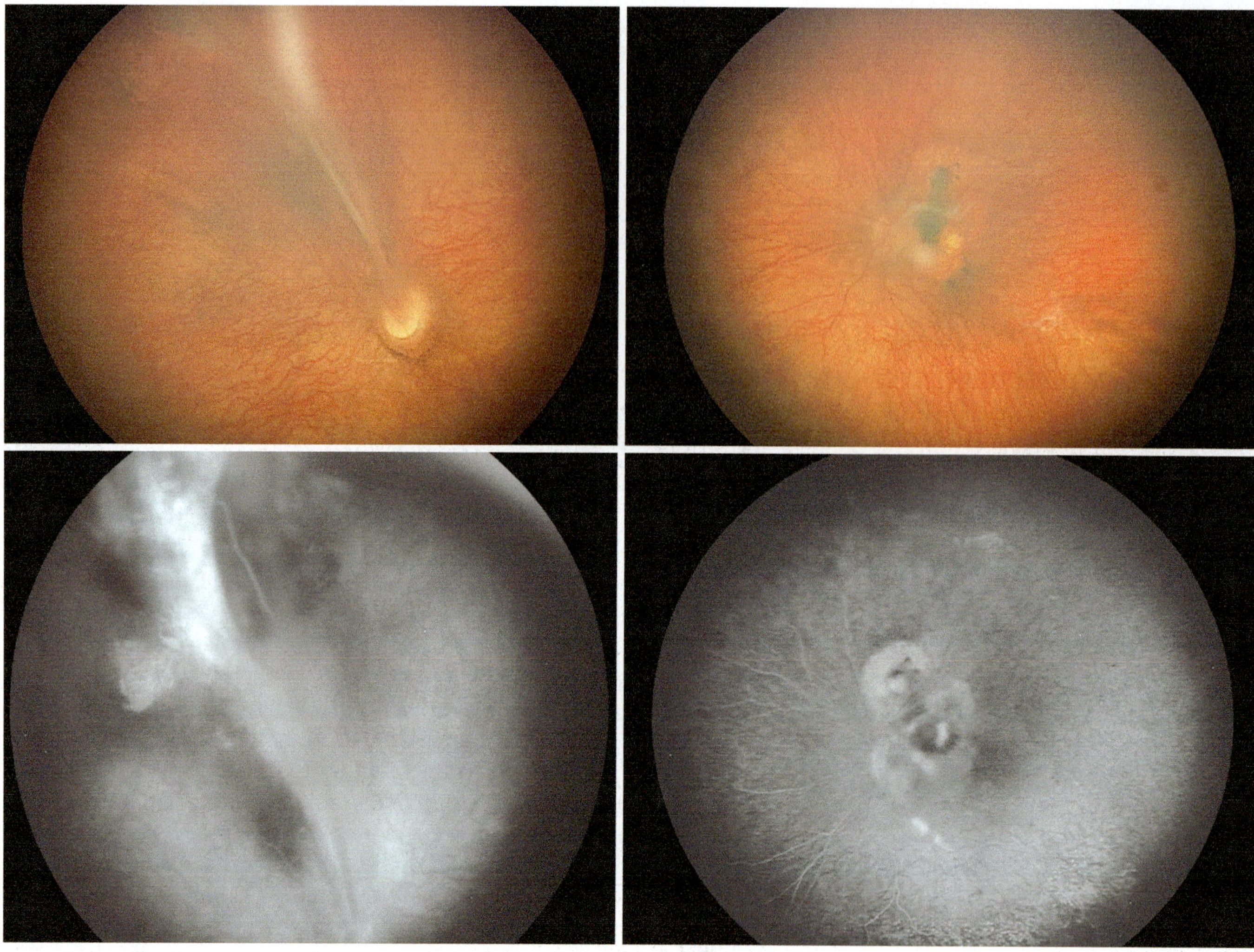

Fig. 74.1: RetCam color fundus photographs and fluorescein angiography of 10-month-old boy with X-linked FEVR showing a retinal fold in the right eye with persistent fetal vasculature in both eyes and reduced temporal retinal blood vessels on the left.

Other Causes of Retinal Detachment in Early Infancy

Other causes of bilateral retinal detachment at birth or early infancy are very rare. They include, various chromosomal abnormalities, osteoporosis-pseudoglioma syndrome, Knobloch syndrome and Walker-Warburg syndrome.[9-11] The infantile bullous form of X-linked retinoschisis may have extensive retinoschisis in early infancy that may be misdiagnosed as retinal detachment.[12]

Familial Exudative Vitreoretinopathy

Familial exudative vitreoretinopathy is characterized by disordered development of the retinal vasculature leading to incomplete retinal vascularization and other retinal abnormalities including retinal folds (Fig. 74.2), retinal exudates and hemorrhage and peripheral retinal neovascularization.[1] Untreated there may be severe visual loss from macular exudation or retinal detachment. Severely affected individuals usually present with nystagmus or strabismus in infancy and often have macular ectopia, severe retinal folds or retinal detachment at first examination. Mildly affected individuals may be asymptomatic and not require treatment; their retinal phenotype may be confined to mild peripheral retinal nonperfusion (Fig. 74.3). Such individuals are more commonly found in families showing autosomal dominant inheritance.

Familial exudative vitreoretinopathy may be X-linked (associated with mutations in *Norrin*) or show autosomal

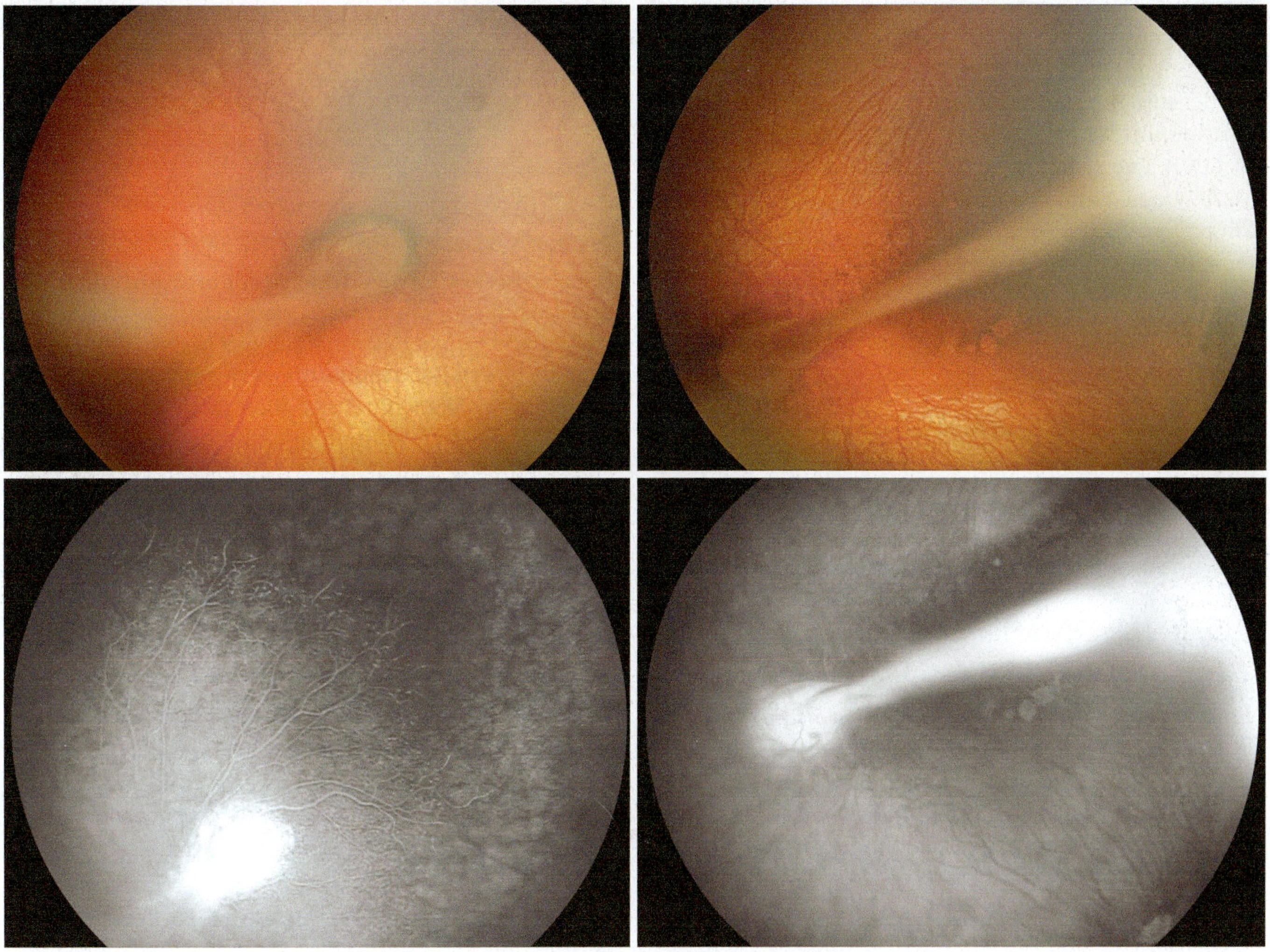

Fig. 74.2: RetCam color fundus photographs and fluorescein angiography of the right and left eye of a 9-month-old infant with *LRP5*-related recessive FEVR demonstrating bilateral retinal folds and incomplete retinal vascularization.

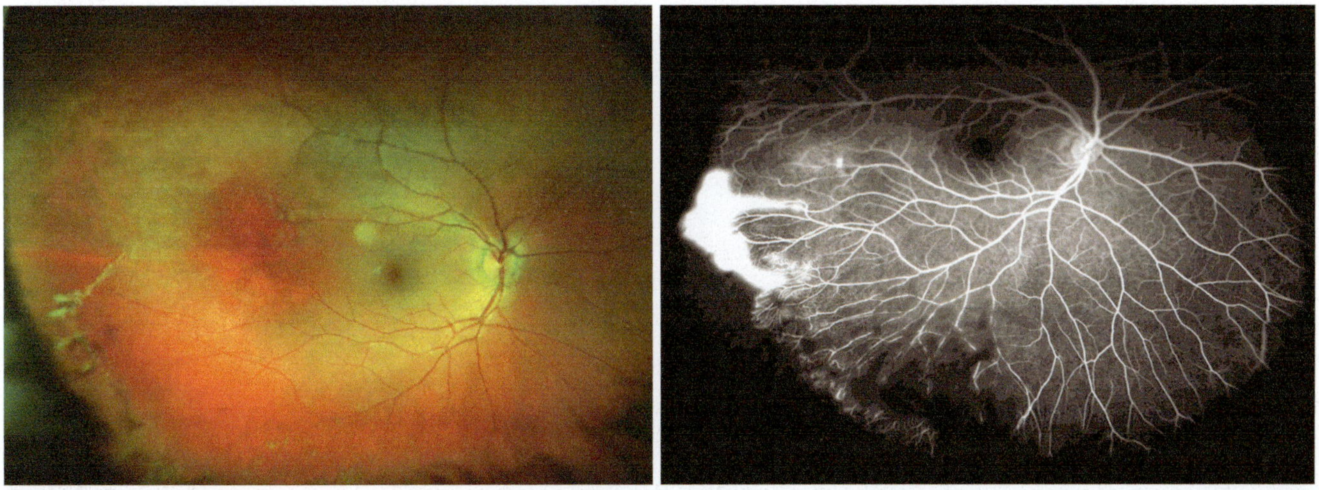

Fig. 74.3: Optos color fundus photographs and fluorescein angiography of the right eye of a 20-year-old female with AD FEVR which shows incomplete temporal retinal vascularization and associated neovascularization.

dominant (AD) or autosomal recessive (AR) inheritance.[13,14] There is considerable genetic heterogeneity. Mutations in *FZD4* (encoding the Frizzled-4 receptor), *LRP5* (encoding low-density lipoprotein receptor 5) and *TSPAN12* (encoding Tetraspanin 12) have been implicated in both AD and AR FEVR. Each of these genes is involved in the Norrin/Frizzle-4 signaling complex which is a key component of the Wnt pathway influencing retinal vascular development.[1,15] Recently mutations in *ZNF408* encoding a zinc finger protein and *CTNNB1* (encoding beta-catenin) have also been implicated in AD FEVR.

Other Ocular Disorders Associated with an FEVR like Phenotype

Abnormal peripheral retinal vascularization has been reported in association with a number of congenital disorders of the optic nerve including Morning Glory Disc and optic nerve hypoplasia.[16] However, such changes are uncommon.

Systemic Disorders Associated with Abnormal Retinal Vascular Development

A number of inherited syndromic disorders have an associated FEVR like phenotype (Box 74.1). The most important of these from the ophthalmological point of view is incontinentia pigmenti (IP). IP is an X-linked dominant disorder, which is associated with abnormalities of skin, teeth, central nervous system and eyes.[17] Ocular involvement may lead to an FEVR like phenotype with incomplete retinal vascularization. The causative gene, *IKBKG* on Xq28 has been identified and molecular diagnosis is possible. IP predominantly affects females; affected male infants usually die *in utero*. Affected infants develop a characteristic bullous

Box 74.1: Systemic disorders with incomplete retinal vascularization.

- Incontinentia pigmenti
- Facioscapulohumeral dystrophy
- Microcephaly chorioretinopathy syndrome
- Walker-Warburg syndrome
- Hemifacial hypoplasia
- Fanconi anemia
- Coats plus syndrome
- Dyskeratosis congenita

skin rash in early infancy, which leads to an early diagnosis. This provides an opportunity for prompt ophthalmology referral and retinal examination and treatment if there is significant peripheral retinal nonperfusion. Although some ophthalmologists will review such infants regularly and only carry out an examination under anesthesia when an abnormality is detected there is strong argument to be made for an examination under anesthesia combined with wide field fluorescein angiography at diagnosis. This will allow a more complete evaluation of retinal vascularization and treatment can be performed if necessary. In those infants whose retinal vasculature is normal no further retinal examinations will be necessary.

Early retinal examinations are also advisable for infants with dyskeratosis congenita where incomplete retinal vascularization may lead to vitreous hemorrhage, retinal exudation and detachment in early childhood.[18] Such complications are prevented by early photocoagulation.

Coats' Disease

Coats' disease is an uncommon disorder in which there is unilateral peripheral retinal telangiectasia and nonperfusion associated with retinal exudation, which with time leads to macular edema and exudation (Fig. 74.4).[19] Most affected patients are male. The usual presentation

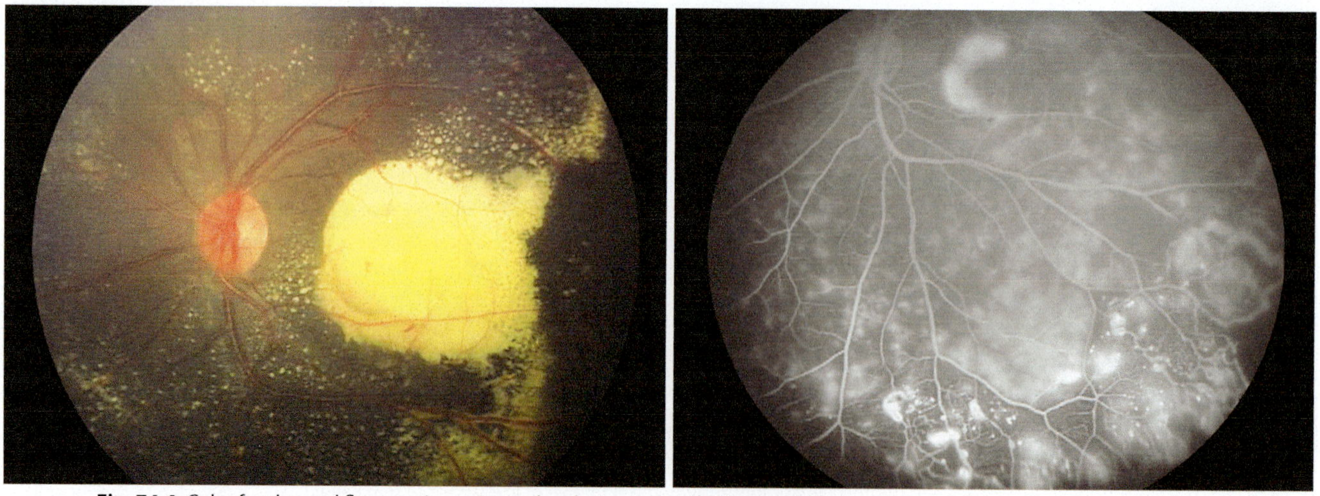

Fig. 74.4: Color fundus and fluorescein angiography photographs of a 3-year-old boy with Coats' disease demonstrating dense macular exudates and peripheral telangiectasia.

Box 74.2: Classification of Coats' disease.[19]

Stage 1: Telangiectasia only
Stage 2: Telangiectasia with exudate in periphery (a) or involving macula (b)
Stage 3: Total (a) or subtotal (b) retinal detachment
Stage 4: RD and secondary glaucoma
Stage 5: Advanced end stage disease

is with unilateral visual loss, strabismus or leukocoria but some patients with early disease may be identified on routine examination. Some children have advanced disease at presentation with total retinal detachment and this may, untreated, lead to neovascular glaucoma. Shields et al[19] have developed a classification of disease based on the severity of involvement (Box 74.2). The aim of treatment is to prevent further vascular leakage and maximize the visual outcome. In most cases, this will involve wide field fluorescein angiography and laser of the peripheral telangiectasia and areas of nonperfusion.[20] In infants and young children this will need to be performed under general anesthesia. Cryotherapy may be needed in areas where there is significant exudation or subretinal fluid. In stage 4 disease, a more complex procedure is needed with drainage of subretinal fluid and treatment of the peripheral telangiectasia with laser or cryotherapy. In such cases visual outcome is poor but treatment will avoid progression to neovascular glaucoma. There are anecdotal reports of successful use of anti-VEGF agents in Coats' disease but in most cases their use has formed part of combination therapy with other treatment modalities.[21]

Persistent Fetal Vasculature

In this congenital abnormality there is a failure of the hyaloid system to regress.[22] The condition is almost always unilateral and there is a wide range of severity. At the mildest end of the spectrum there is a persistent hyaloid artery running forward from the optic disc into the vitreous or a hyaloid remnant on the optic nerve head (Bergmeister's papilla). A minor remnant on the posterior aspect of the lens, a Mittendorf dot is visually asymptomatic and of no clinical significance. At the more severe end of the spectrum the eye is microphthalmic with cataract and retrolental membrane, which may give rise to traction on the ciliary processes. There may be shallowing of the anterior chamber and angle-closure glaucoma. This anterior form of persistent fetal vasculature (PFV), often termed posterior hyperplastic primary vitreous, may be treated with lensectomy and vitrectomy, followed by optical rehabilitation, but generally the visual results are poor. The posterior form of PFV is rare. It is characterized by remnants of the hyaloid system on the retinal surface with epiretinal membrane formation and often an anomalous or dysplastic optic nerve head. There may be associated retinal detachment and generally there is a poor visual prognosis.

PFV may rarely be bilateral when it may have a genetic basis. A mutation in *ATOH7* has been identified in a single family with AR bilateral PFV.[23]

Other Congenital Disorders of the Retinal Vasculature

Other uncommon congenital abnormalities of the retinal vasculature include prepapillary vascular loops and congenital retinal macrovessels (racemose hemangioma). Prepapillary loops are usually seen as an abnormal retinal arteriole which has a looped appearance running forwards off the surface of the optic nerve head into the posterior vitreous (Fig. 74.5).[24] They may be unilateral or bilateral and are usually asymptomatic and found on routine examination. Rarely they may develop a thrombosis which results in a branch retinal artery occlusion.

Congenital retinal macrovessels is a rare unilateral disorder where there is retinal arteriovenous communication associated with dilated and tortuous retinal vessels (Fig. 74.6).[25] They are usually found on routine examination or when vision is found to be reduced in one eye. They are usually nonprogressive but rarely they may be complicated by retinal exudation or vitreous hemorrhage. Although most patients have no other abnormalities intracranial vascular malformations may coexist in the Wyburn-Mason syndrome.

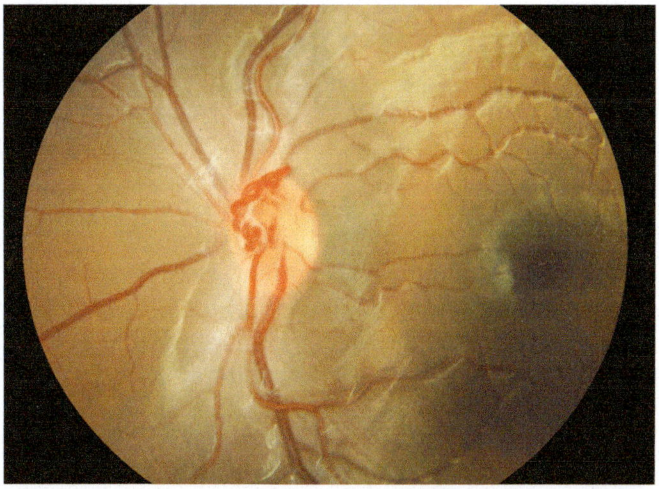

Fig. 74.5: Color fundus photograph of an 8-year-old patient demonstrating prepapillary arterial loop from the left optic disc.

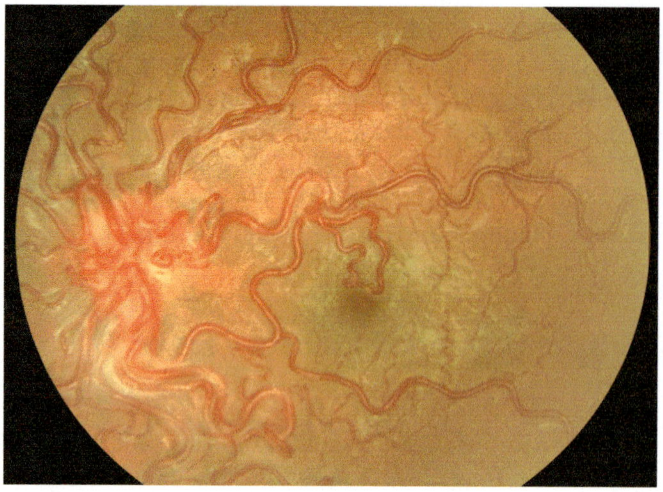

Fig. 74.6: Color fundus photograph of a left fundus demonstrating grossly dilated arteries and veins in an arteriovenous malformation (racemose angioma).

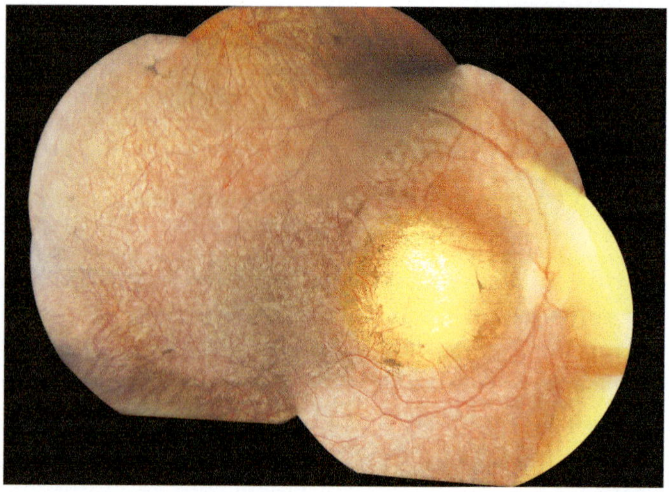

Fig. 74.7: Color fundus photograph of the right eye in a child with LCA due to mutations in the *NMNAT1* gene. There is optic disc pallor, narrowing of the retinal vessels and macular dysplasia.

Retinal arteriolar tortuosity is a rare retinal phenotype which uncommonly has systemic associations.[26] Familial retinal arteriolar tortuosity is a rare autosomal dominant disorder in which there is tortuosity of the small and medium retinal arterioles in each eye—more prominent in the macular region. There may be visual symptoms related to retinal or vitreous hemorrhages. The disorder may be associated with mutations in the *COL4A1* gene. Other mutations in this gene result in infantile onset cerebrovascular disease associated with retinal arteriolar tortuosity. Cerebrovascular disease and retinal arteriolar tortuosity are also seen in patients which are heterozygous mutations in *ACTA2* where there are also dilated pupils which are unresponsive to light. Other causes of retinal vascular tortuosity include regressed retinopathy of prematurity and Fabry disease.[27]

INFANTILE ONSET GENERALIZED RETINAL DYSTROPHIES

There are three broad groups of generalized retinal dystrophies that present in infancy: Leber congenital amaurosis, a severe form of rod cone dystrophy, the cone dysfunction syndromes and the various forms of congenital stationary night blindness. All present in early infancy with poor vision and nystagmus and electroretinography is the key to arriving at the correct diagnosis, although it is likely that molecular genetic testing may be the preferred primary investigation in the future.

Leber Congenital Amaurosis

Leber congenital amaurosis (LCA) is a rare disorder affecting around 1 in 60,000 live births. Infants usually present in the first few months of life with severe visual impairment and nystagmus.[28] Fundus examination may be normal in some infants but in others there may be optic disc pallor, vascular attenuation, macular atrophy or peripheral retinal changes such as pigmentary retinopathy or white flecks at the level of the retinal pigment epithelium (RPE) (Figs. 74.7 and 74.8). High, usually hyperopic, refractive errors are common. The electroretinogram (ERG), is usually non-recordable but occasionally there are small residual responses usually originating from the cone photoreceptors. The inheritance is generally autosomal recessive except for *CRX* which is dominant with a high rate of *de novo* mutations and 3 reports of sporadic heterozygous *IMPDH1* related LCA.[29,30] The disorder although very rare is remarkably genetically

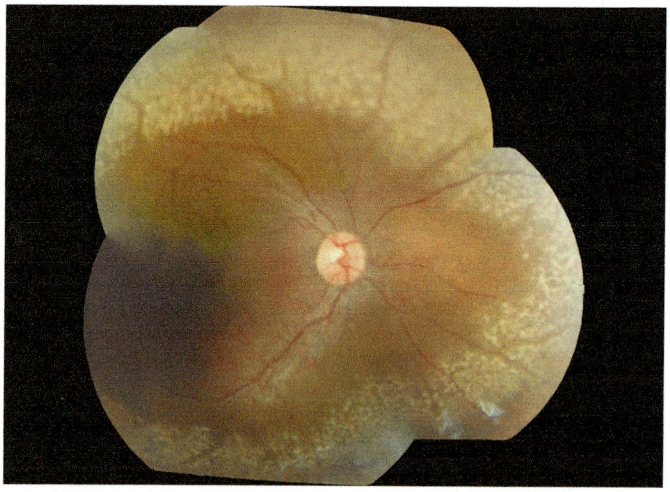

Fig. 74.8: Color fundus photograph of the right eye in a child with LCA due to mutations in *CEP290*. There are white flecks in the peripheral retina but a normal appearance to the posterior pole.

heterogeneous with 17 causative genes identified to date.[28] These genes encode proteins with a variety of functions including those involved with retinal development, the visual cycle, phototransduction, molecular chaperoning and cilia structure and function. Next generation sequencing genetic testing will now identify the molecular cause of disease in more than 70% of patients.[31] Many of these genes are also associated with less severe forms of childhood onset rod cone dystrophy; the cause for the variation in phenotype is for the most part unclear.[28]

Some infants with syndromic disease may develop similar retinal findings in infancy. These syndromic disorders include the peroxisomal disorders, Joubert syndrome, Alstrom syndrome and cobalamin C deficiency but they can generally be distinguished from isolated LCA by the presence of associated systemic abnormalities or by molecular genetic testing.

There is unfortunately no treatment for the various forms of LCA although clinical trials of gene replacement therapy for retinal disease associated with mutations in the *RPE65* gene have shown great promise and may well soon move into clinical practice.[32]

Cone Dysfunction Syndromes

The cone dysfunction syndromes comprise a genetically heterogeneous group of disorders in which there is isolated cone photoreceptor function which is present from birth and generally nonprogressive. Most present in infancy with reduced vision, nystagmus and sensitivity to light.[33]

Achromatopsia

Achromatopsia is an autosomal recessive disorder characterized by a lack of functioning cones in the retina. The clinical presentation is in infancy with marked sensitivity to light, fine rapid nystagmus and poor vision. The nystagmus often becomes less marked with time. Parents often report that vision is much better in dim illumination. Fundus examination is usually normal and high hyperopic refractive errors are common. The diagnosis is made by the finding of absent cone function and normal rod function on electroretinography. When the child is old enough to be formally tested the visual acuity is usually around the level of 6/60 Snellen (1.0 logMAR) and there is a complete lack of color vision. Less commonly there may be incomplete forms of achromatopsia where the vision is somewhat better and there may be residual but abnormal color vision.

Although fundus examination is usually normal, OCT imaging may identify structural abnormalities of the fovea. The condition is genetically heterogeneous and most causative genes encode proteins in the cone phototransduction pathways. These include *CNGB3, CNGA3, GNAT2, PDE6C* and *PDE6H.* The majority of patents have mutations in *CNGA3* and *CNGB3.*[33] Recently mutations in the ubiquitously expressed gene *ATF6* encoding a transcription factor which controls genes involved in endoplasmic reticulum stress have been identified as a rare cause of achromatopsia.

There is no specific treatment for this group of disorders although clinical trials of gene replace therapy for *CNGB3* and *CNGA3* related disease are underway. Children with achromatopsia benefit from low light transmission tinted spectacles, low vision aids and educational support.

X-linked S-cone Monochromatism

S-cone monochromatism (BCM) is a rare X-linked disorder in which affected males have normal rod and S-cone function but lack all L- and M- cone function. The usual presentation is with nystagmus and photophobia in infancy. The ERG in infancy shows absent or severely abnormal cone function but normal rod responses. The clinical features are similar to infants with achromatopsia but the light sensitivity is less severe and visual function is better. A key finding, which is helpful in distinguishing the two conditions, is that in BCM the refractive error is almost always myopic. When the children are older and can be formally tested the visual acuity varies from 6/60 Snellen (1.0 logMAR) to 6/18 Snellen (0.48 logMAR) and color vision testing reveals normal tritan function in contrast to achromatopsia where there is none. Specialized ERG testing may be able to demonstrate normal S-cone responses.

The underlying molecular genetic basis of BCM has been identified. It is an X-linked disorder associated with mutations resulting in loss of function of the L- and M- pigment genes. The mutations are of two main types. Firstly there may be mutations in the locus control region (LCR) upstream of the L- and M- pigment genes; inactivation of the LCR leads to lack of function of both L- and M- pigment genes. Alternatively, the LCR region is unaffected but changes within the pigment genes themselves result in loss of function.[33]

Congenital Stationary Night Blindness

There are a number of different forms of congenital stationary night blindness (CSNB) but not all present in infancy. Those that do usually present with reduced vision and nystagmus with a myopic refractive error. Strabismus is a variable feature. Night blindness does not usually become evident until the child is older. Fundus examination is typically normal but there may be myopic tilted discs and other fundus changes associated with myopia. The diagnosis can be confirmed with an ERG which shows reduced or absent rod specific ERG responses with a profoundly negative ERG to a bright flash indicative of inner retinal dysfunction.[34] Complete and incomplete forms of CSNB can be identified through ERG testing. CSNB which presents in infancy may be inherited as an X-linked or AR disorder and is again very genetically heterogeneous.[35]

DEVELOPMENTAL MACULAR DYSTROPHIES

Most macular dystrophies become symptomatic in later childhood after a period of normal vision. There are however a rare group of disorders where there is disordered development of the macula and structural abnormalities are present from birth or early infancy.[36] There are three broad groups of disorders: (1) foveal hypoplasia, (2) macular abnormalities associated with posterior microphthalmos/nanophthalmos, and (3) North Carolina macular dystrophy and related phenotypes.

Foveal Hypoplasia

In this group of disorders there is a failure of foveal development which results in poor vision and nystagmus. On fundus examination, there is no discernable foveal structure and often retinal blood vessels course across the central retina where the fovea is expected to be. The diagnosis can be confirmed on OCT where there is a lack of normal foveal architecture (Fig. 74.9). Foveal hypoplasia is generally bilateral and has a genetic basis. It is seen in all forms of albinism, in aniridia and in some patients with achromatopsia. It is also seen as an isolated ocular abnormality when the inheritance is usually autosomal recessive.

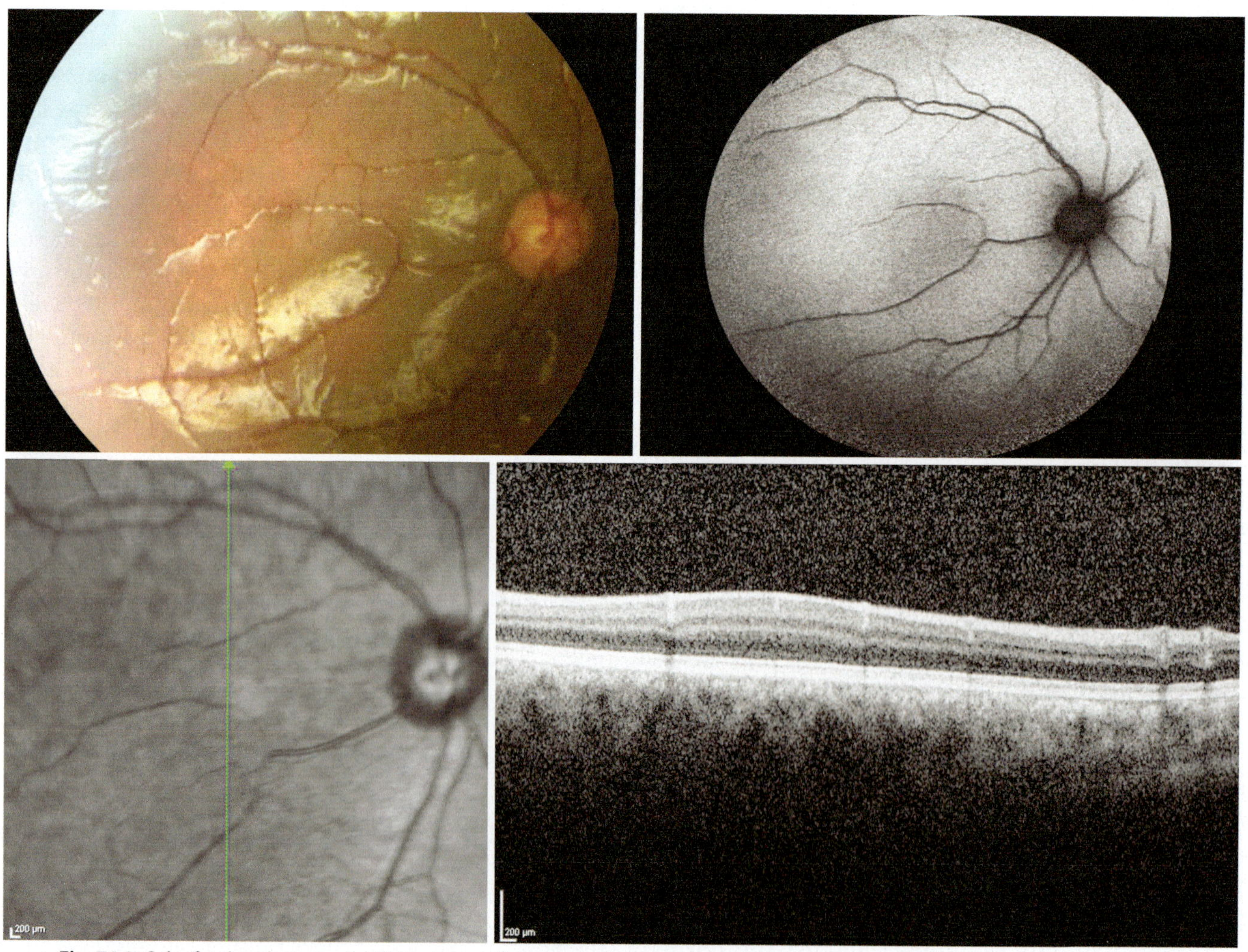

Fig. 74.9: Color fundus photograph, 55° fundus autofluorescence image and optical coherence tomography (OCT) of the right eye in a child with foveal hypoplasia.

Maculopathy Associated with Posterior Microphthalmos

Posterior microphthalmos is a rare developmental eye disorder in which there is high hyperopia, a relatively normal anterior segment, but shortened posterior segment and characteristic maculopathy.[36] Ultrasound biometry shows a very reduced axial length (generally <18 mm). There may be papillomacular folds and a thickened central macula (Fig. 74.10). On OCT the neural retina is thickened at the central macula and projects forward into the vitreous (Fig. 74.10). With time a pigmentary retinopathy may develop in the periphery and the ERG may show reduced rod and cone responses. Posterior microphthalmos is inherited as an autosomal recessive trait and two different causative genes *MFRP and PRSS56* have been identified to date.

North Carolina Macular Dystrophy

North Carolina macular dystrophy (NCMD) (MCDR1) is a fully penetrant autosomal dominant disorder where there is disordered macular development. The clinical phenotype is very variable with some family members having extensive macular atrophy from birth (Fig. 74.11), whilst others have normal visual acuity with yellow drusen like deposits in the central macula (Fig. 74.12 and Box 74.3).[37] The full field ERG and EOG are normal. The condition is nonprogressive but may be occasionally complicated by the development of choroidal neovascularization. NCMD was initially mapped to chromosome 6q and subsequently families with an identical phenotype (MCDR3) were mapped to chromosome 5p. Recently it has been demonstrated that each condition is due to rare variants in nonprotein coding DNA which are thought to disrupt regulatory elements of neighboring genes.[38,39] The exact mechanism by which these variants result in the abnormal macular development is still unknown. Other rare developmental macular phenotypes are reviewed by Michaelides et al.[36]

OTHER DEVELOPMENTAL ANOMALIES

Ocular Coloboma

Ocular coloboma occurs as a result of failure of closure of the fetal fissure during the prenatal period. It may be

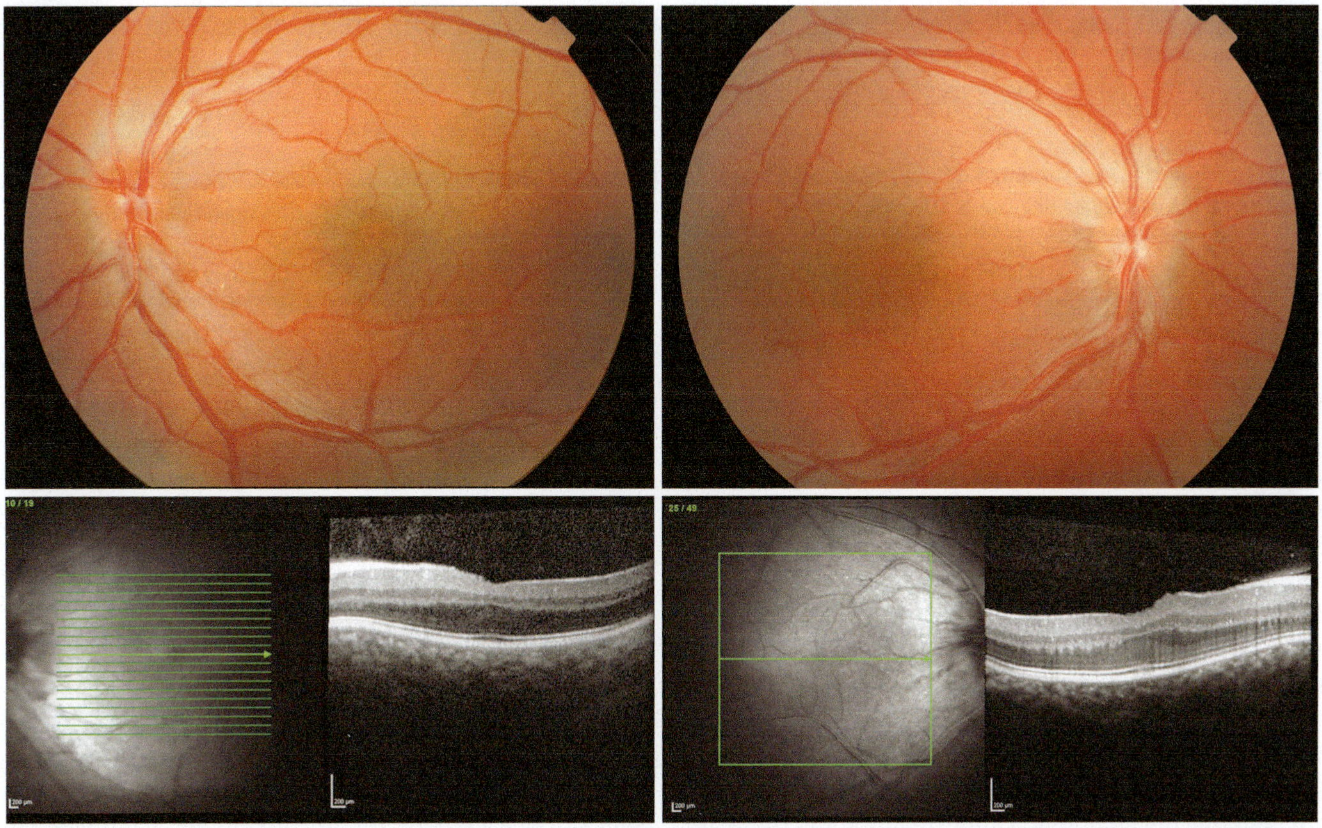

Fig. 74.10: Color fundus photographs and optical coherence tomography (OCT) of both eyes of a patient with posterior microphthalmos. The optic discs are crowded, there are macular striae and OCT shows an abnormal macula appearance with thickening of the central macula.

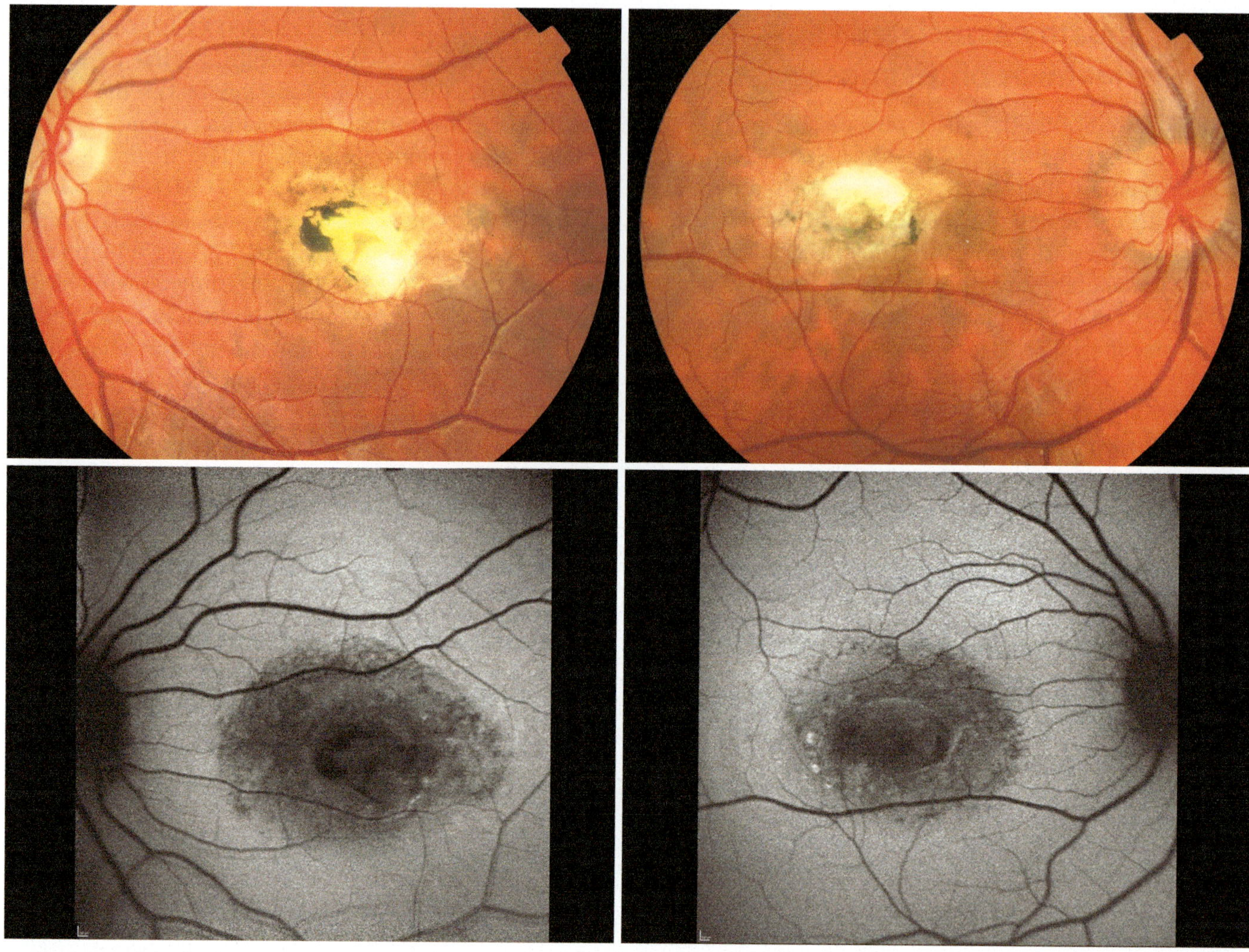

Fig. 74.11: Color fundus photograph and fundus autofluorescence imaging in a 6-year-old child with Stage 3 North Carolina macular dystrophy.

Box 74.3: North Carolina macular dystrophy: Classification.[37]

Grade 1: Small yellow drusen-like deposits in central macula
Grade 2: Confluent macular drusen
Grade 3: Chorioretinal atrophy at macula

unilateral or bilateral and may involve the eyelid, iris, lens, choroid and optic nerve. When there is retinal and optic nerve involvement there may be associated microphthalmos.[40,41] Retinal colobomas are seen as focal defects of choroid and RPE lying below the optic disc at the 6 o'clock position (Figs. 74.13A to C). Coloboma may be associated with chromosomal abnormalities or be inherited as an X-linked, autosomal recessive or autosomal dominant trait. Even within each subgroup there is considerable genetic heterogeneity.[41] It may be isolated or associated with systemic developmental abnormalities and there are many different associated syndromes. Ocular involvement has a wide range of severity. Isolated iris colobomas and small retinal colobomas are asymptomatic and do not affect vision, whereas large optic nerve and retinal colobomas may result in poor vision and nystagmus. Although optic nerve and retinal colobomas remain unchanged throughout life there is a significant risk of developing retinal detachment. All children with coloboma should be referred to a clinical geneticist for investigation and parents and siblings should be examined to exclude small asymptomatic coloboma; such a finding may influence genetic counseling.

Myelinated Nerve Fibers

Normally the optic nerve fibers within the eye are unmyelinated to maintain transparency of the nerve fiber layer but occasionally the myelin sheath extends within

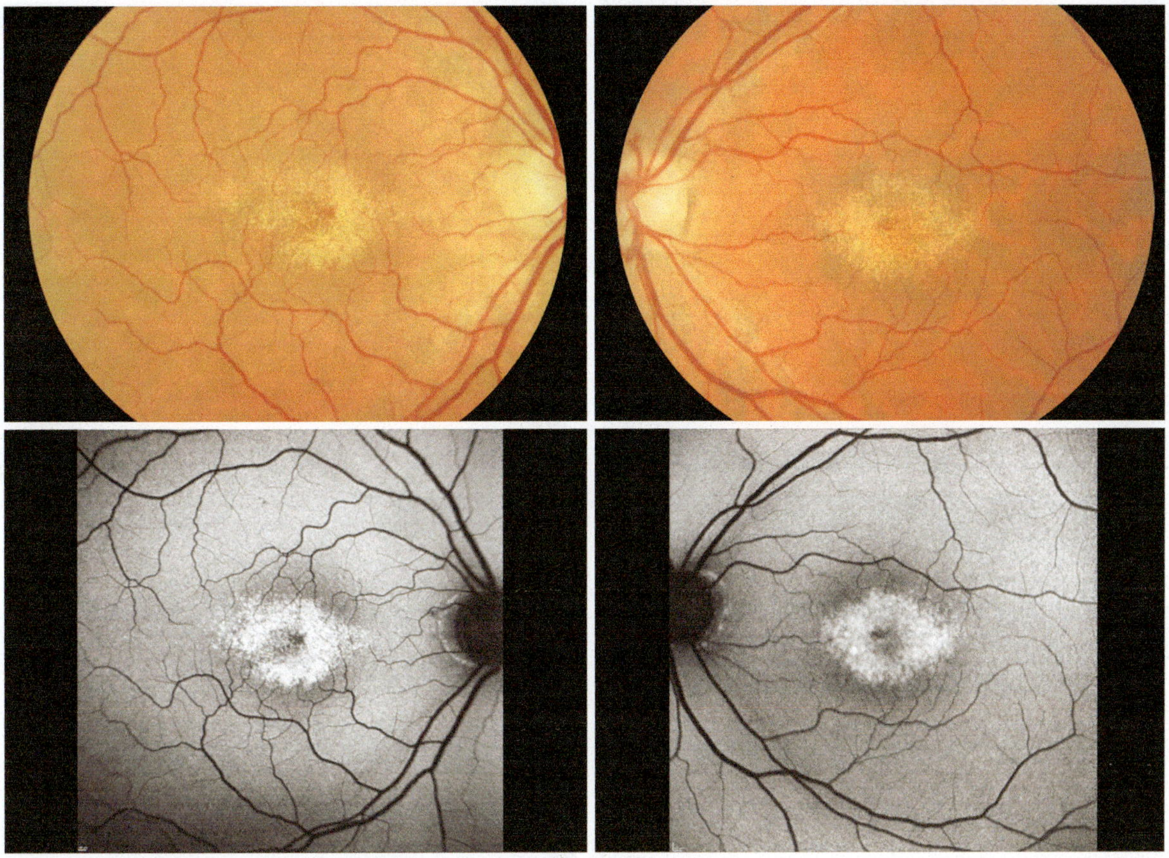

Fig. 74.12: Color fundus photograph and fundus autofluorescence imaging in an asymptomatic individual with Stage 2 NCMD and normal visual acuity.

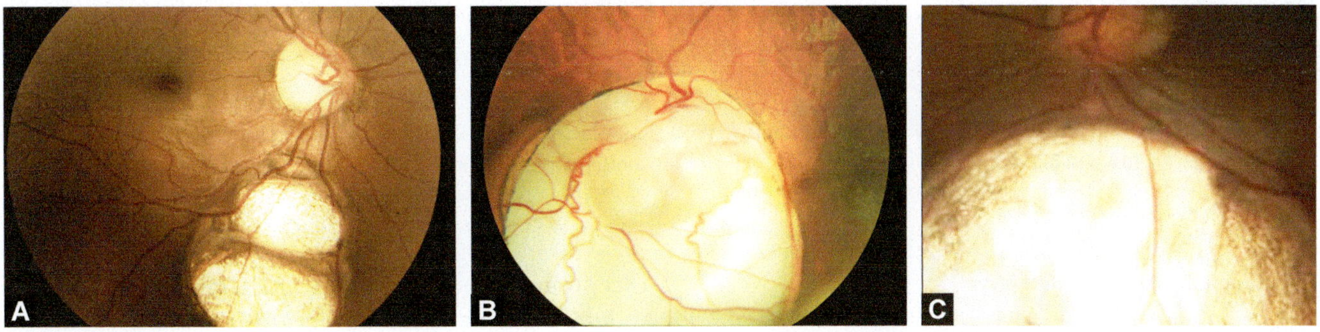

Figs. 74.13A to C: Color fundus photographs of patients with retinal colobomas; (A) Mild optic nerve coloboma and inferior retinal coloboma; (B) Extensive optic nerve and retinal coloboma; (C) Large inferior retinal coloboma.

the eye. Myelinated nerve fibers (MNF) are seen as well demarcated white areas of retina that follow the path of the nerve fiber layer from the disc towards the periphery (Fig. 74.14). They are usually seen in otherwise normal eyes although in some cases of unilateral disease there may be associated high myopia and amblyopia.[42] MNF are usually nonprogressive although rarely there may be associated retinovascular abnormalities that may lead to vitreous hemorrhage. MNF have also been reported to lose their myelin in various forms of optic neuropathy including glaucoma. Most patients with myelinated nerve fibers are otherwise normal but they have been reported in association with a number of syndromes including craniofacial anomalies, Gorlin syndrome and Neurofibromatosis type 1.[42] A few familial cases have also been reported.

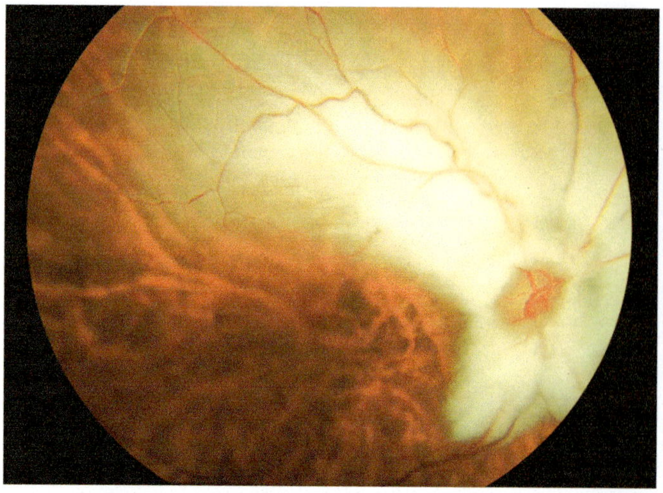

Fig. 74.14: Color fundus photograph of the right eye with extensive myelinated nerve fibers.

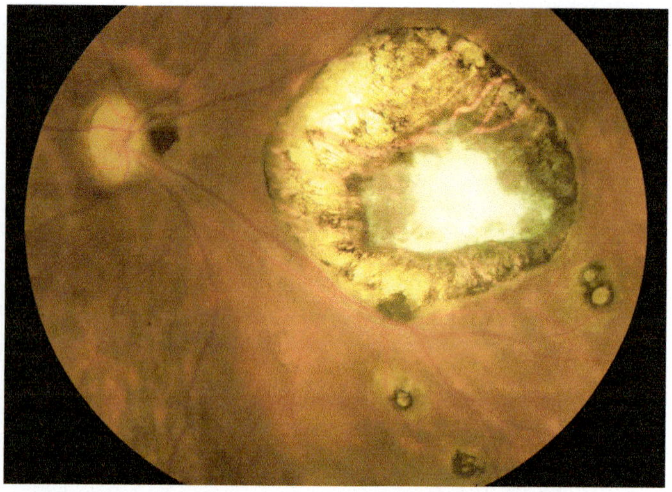

Fig. 74.15: Color fundus photograph of the left eye demonstrating chorioretinal scarring secondary to congenital toxoplasmosis.

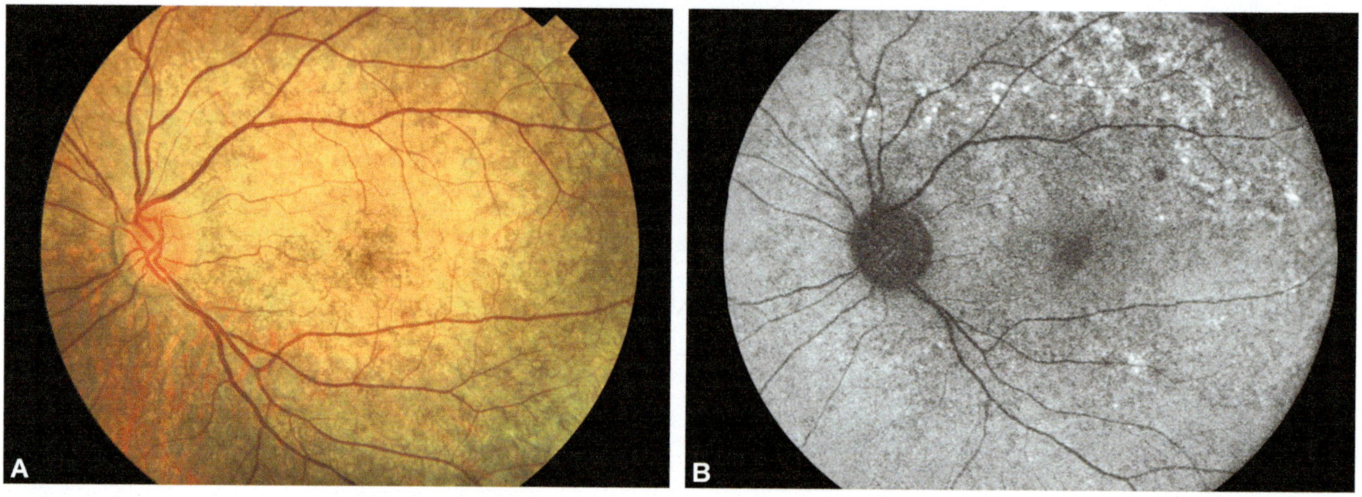

Figs. 74.16A and B: Left fundus photograph (A) showing diffuse mottling of the RPE in a deaf child with rubella embryopathy. Fundus autofluorescence imaging (B) shows patchy increased autofluorescence.

Congenital Infections

Infection of the mother in pregnancy can be transmitted to the fetus and result in loss of the pregnancy or still birth. In infants that survive ocular involvement may lead to significant inflammation and scarring. Organisms that may lead to ocular involvement include *Toxoplasma gondii*, rubella, syphilis, cytomegalovirus, herpes simplex, varicella zoster and zika virus.[43] These disorders may give rise to widespread ocular abnormalities including involvement of the choroid, retinal pigment epithelium and retina which usually leads to chororetinal scarring (Fig. 74.15). The exception is rubella infection which gives rise to a diffuse retinal pigment epithelial mottling without significant scarring (Figs. 74.16A and B). The literature related to ophthalmic manifestations of congenital infections has recently been reviewed by Amaya.[44]

REFERENCES

1. Gilmour DF. Familial exudative vitreoretinopathy and related retinopathies. Eye (Lond). 2015;29(1):1-14.
2. Walsh MK, Drenser KA, Capone A Jr, et al. Early vitrectomy effective for Norrie disease. Arch Ophthalmol. 2010;128(4):456-60.

3. Wu LH, Chen LH, Xie H, et al. Prenatal diagnosis of a case of norrie disease with late development of bilateral ocular malformation. Fetal Pediatr Pathol. 2017;36(3):240-5.
4. Royer G, Hanein S, Raclin V, et al. *NDP* gene mutations in 14 French families with Norrie disease. Hum Mutat. 2003;22(6):499.
5. Chen ZY, Hendriks RW, Jobling MA, et al. Isolation and characterization of a candidate gene for Norrie disease. Nat Genet. 1992;1(3):204-8.
6. Berger W, Meindl A, van de Pol TJ, et al. Isolation of a candidate gene for Norrie disease by positional cloning. Nat Genet. 1992;1(3):199-203.
7. Chow CC, Kiernan DF, Chau FY, et al. Laser photocoagulation at birth prevents blindness in Norrie's disease diagnosed using amniocentesis. Ophthalmology. 2010;117(12): 2402-6.
8. Chen ZY, Battinelli EM, Fielder A, et al. A mutation in the Norrie disease gene (NDP) associated with X-linked familial exudative vitreoretinopathy. Nat Genet. 1993;5(2):180-3.
9. Wilson G, Moore A, Allgrove J. Bilateral retinal detachments at birth: the osteoporosis pseudoglioma syndrome. Br J Ophthalmol. 2001;85(9):1139.
10. Knobloch WH, Layer JM. Retinal detachment and encephalocele. J Pediatr Ophthalmol. 1971;8:181-4.
11. Dobyns WB, Pagon RA, Armstrong D, et al. Diagnostic criteria for Walker-Warburg syndrome. Am J Med Genet. 1989;32(2):195-210.
12. Hinds AM, Fahim A, Moore AT, Wong SC, Michaelides M. Bullous X-linked retinoschisis: clinical features and prognosis. Br J Ophthalmol. 2017;28.
13. Salvo J, Lyubasyuk V, Xu M, et al. Next-generation sequencing and novel variant determination in a cohort of 92 familial exudative vitreoretinopathy patients. Invest Ophthalmol Vis Sci. 2015;56(3):1937-46.
14. Panagiotou ES, Sanjuro Soriano C, Poulter JA, et al. Defects in the cell signalling mediator β-catenin cause the retinal vascular condition FEVR. Am J Hum Genet. 2017;100(6): 960-8.
15. Warden SM, Andreoli CM, Mukai S. The Wnt signalling pathway in familial exudative retinopathy. Semin Ophthalmol. 2007;22(4):211-7.
16. Shapiro MJ, Chow CC, Blair MP, et al. Peripheral nonperfusion and tractional retinal detachment associated with congenital optic nerve anomalies. Ophthalmology. 2013;120(3):607-15.
17. Holmström G1, Thorén K. Ocular manifestations of incontinentia pigmenti. Acta Ophthalmol Scand. 2000;78(3):348-53.
18. Allingham MJ. Bilateral proliferative retinopathy associated with Hoyeraal-Hreidarsson syndrome, a severe form of dyskeratosis congenita. Ophthalmic Surg Lasers Imaging Retina. 2016;47(4):366-8.
19. Shields JA, Shields CL, Honavar SG, et al. Classification and management of Coats disease: the 2000 Proctor Lecture. Am J Ophthalmol. 2001;131(5):572-83.
20. Suzani M, Moore AT. Intraoperative fluorescein angiography-guided treatment in children with early Coats' disease. Ophthalmology. 2015;122(6):1195-202.
21. Park S, Cho HJ, Lee DW, et al. Intravitreal bevacizumab injections combined with laser photocoagulation for adult-onset Coats' disease. Graefes Arch Clin Exp Ophthalmol. 2016;254(8):1511-7.
22. Goldberg MF. Persistent fetal vasculature (PFV): an integrated interpretation of signs and symptoms associated with persistent hyperplastic primary vitreous (PHPV). LIV Edward Jackson Memorial Lecture. Am J Ophthalmol. 1997;124(5):587-626.
23. Prasov L[1], Masud T, Khaliq S, et al. ATOH7 mutations cause autosomal recessive persistent hyperplasia of the primary vitreous. Hum Mol Genet. 2012;21(16):3681-94.
24. Degenhart W, Brown GC, Augsburger JJ, et al. Prepapillary vascular loops. Ophthalmology. 1981;88(11):1126-31.
25. Materin MA, Shields CL, Marr BP, et al. Retinal racemose hemangioma. Retina. 2005;25(7):936-7.
26. Zenteno JC, Crespí J, Buentello-Volante B, et al. Next generation sequencing uncovers a missense mutation in *COL4A1* as the cause of familial retinal arteriolar tortuosity. Graefes Arch Clin Exp Ophthalmol. 2014;252(11):1789-94.
27. Sodi A, Ioannidis AS, Mehta A, et al. Ocular manifestations of Fabry's disease: data from the Fabry Outcome Survey. Br J Ophthalmol. 2007;91(2):210-4.
28. Kumaran N, Moore AT, Weleber RG, et al. Leber congenital amaurosis/early-onset severe retinal dystrophy: clinical features, molecular genetics and therapeutic interventions. Br J Ophthalmol. 2017;101(9):1147-54.
29. Stone EM. Leber congenital amaurosis - a model for efficient genetic testing of heterogeneous disorders: LXIV Edward Jackson Memorial Lecture. Am J Ophthalmol. 2007;144(6):791-811.
30. Bowne SJ, Sullivan LS, Mortimer SE, et al. Spectrum and frequency of mutations in IMPDH1 associated with autosomal dominant retinitis pigmentosa and leber congenital amaurosis. Invest Ophthalmol Vis Sci. 2006;47(1):34-42.
31. Taylor RL, Parry NRA, Barton SJ, et al. Panel-based clinical genetic testing in 85 children with inherited retinal disease. Ophthalmology. 2017;124(7):985-91.
32. Russell S, Bennett J, Wellman JA, et al. Efficacy and safety of voretigene neparvovec (AAV2-hRPE65v2) in patients with RPE65-mediated inherited retinal dystrophy: a randomised, controlled, open-label, phase 3 trial. Lancet. 2017;390(10097):849-60.
33. Aboshiha J, Dubis AM, Carroll J, et al. The cone dysfunction syndromes. Br J Ophthalmol. 2016;100(1):115-21.
34. Audo I, Robson AG, Holder GE, et al. The negative ERG: clinical phenotypes and disease mechanisms of inner retinal dysfunction. Surv Ophthalmol. 2008;53(1):16-40.
35. Zeitz C, Robson AG, Audo I. Congenital stationary night blindness: an analysis and update of genotype-phenotype

correlations and pathogenic mechanisms. Prog Retin Eye Res. 2015;45:58-110.
36. Michaelides M, Jeffery G, Moore AT. Developmental macular disorders: phenotypes and underlying molecular genetic basis. Br J Ophthalmol. 2012;96(7):917-24.
37. Small KW. North Carolina macular dystrophy: clinical features, geneolagy and genetic linkage analysis. Trans Am Ophthalmol Soc. 1998;96:925-61.
38. Small KW, DeLuca AP, Whitmore SS, et al. North Carolina macular dystrophy is caused by dysregulation of the retinal transcription factor PRDM13. Ophthalmology. 2016;123(1):9-18.
39. Cipriani V, Silva RS, Arno G, et al. Duplication events downstream of IRX1 cause North Carolina macular dystrophy at the MCDR3 locus. Sci Rep. 2017;7(1):7512.
40. Gregory-Evans CY, Williams MJ, Halford S, et al. Ocular coloboma: a reassessment in the age of molecular neuroscience. J Med Genet. 2004;41(12):881-91.
41. Williamson KA, FitzPatrick DR. The genetic architecture of microphthalmia, anophthalmia and coloboma. Eur J Med Genet. 2014;57(8):369-80.
42. Tarabishy AB[1], Alexandrou TJ, Traboulsi EI. Syndrome of myelinated retinal nerve fibers, myopia, and amblyopia: a review. Surv Ophthalmol. 2007;52(6):588-96.
43. Fernandez MP, Parra Saad E, Ospina Martinez M, et al. Ocular Histopathologic Features of Congenital Zika Syndrome. JAMA Ophthalmol. 2017;135(11):1163-9.
44. Amaya L. Congenital infections of the eye in pediatric ophthalmology and Strabismus edit Lyons C. and Lambert SR. Elsevier; 2017.pp.102-7.

Chapter 75 Retinopathy of Prematurity

Ayad Shafiq

INTRODUCTION

Retinopathy of prematurity (ROP) is a term used to describe the abnormal vascular proliferative disease of retinal blood vessels which only affects premature infants, leading to various degrees of tractional retinal detachment, and hence visual loss, if left untreated.

In this chapter, the various aspects of ROP will be discussed from background through to treatment outcome and future research, so that the reader has a good understanding of the current knowledge of the disease process.

HISTORY

Retinopathy of prematurity is truly a 20th century disease. Since, without technological advances that led to resuscitation of infants born with extremely immature lungs incapable of self-ventilation, the disease could not have existed.

In 1942, Terry described the first infant who had gray, blood vessel-covered membranes behind the pupil. As more cases were described, the name retrolental fibroplasia (RLF) was coined.[1] It became common around the world in specialist units for preterm infants.

The retrolental tissue was, in fact, the result of total retinal detachment caused by circumferential fibrovascular contraction of the ridge that develops in ROP.

This could be visualized just posterior to the lens in the eye. It was realized that this membrane developed after birth, and over time, causation in these preterm infants became linked to artificial ventilation and oxygen dependency.

Over the ensuing years, it became clearer that this new disease was partially dependent upon the oxygen saturation of blood, leading to current attempts to prevent over-saturation by maintaining saturation between 90% and 95% saturated.

Little in the way of treatment was developed until the 1980s when the theory that ablation of anterior hypoxic avascular peripheral retina with cryotherapy might be effective in halting the tractional changes and detachment.

The landmark and birth of the treatment of the condition was due almost entirely to the CRYO-ROP study published in 1987. This led on to establish the natural history and treatment of ROP and laid the foundations for all research and management to date.[2]

NOMENCLATURE AND STANDARDIZATION

In the 1980s, a group of experts developed the International Classification of ROP (ICROP).[3]

This allowed examiners to describe the eye signs seen in ROP by allocating them a grade and stage, as well as describe how far vessels had vascularized anterior to the optic disk into the retinal periphery.

Zones

Three concentric zones, centered on the fovea define the anteroposterior location of retinopathy.

- *Zone I:* With optic disk as the center, and twice the distance from the disk to fovea, the circle formed is zone I. Using a 25 or 28 diopter (D)—condensing lens, when the nasal edge of the optic disk is kept at one edge, the temporal field of view is zone I extent.
- *Zone II:* It starts from the edge of zone I and extends till the ora serrata nasally, with a corresponding area temporally.
- *Zone III:* Zone III is the remaining crescent of retina temporally.

Extent of Retinopathy

The extent of the ROP is documented by the number of clock hours involved.

Stages of Retinopathy of Prematurity

It denotes the degree of vascular changes. There are five stages:

Stage 1: Demarcation line: A demarcation line is seen between the vascular and avascular retina. It is a thin structure that lies in the plane of the retina.

Stage 2: Ridge: The demarcation line grows to occupy a volume and has a height and width to form a ridge above the plane of retina. Small tufts of new vessels also called *popcorn* vessels, may be seen posterior to the ridge.

Stage 3: Ridge with extraretinal fibrovascular proliferation: In this stage, extraretinal fibrovascular tissue is seen arising from the ridge into the vitreous. It may be continuous or noncontinuous and is posterior to the demarcation of vascularized with nonvascularized retina.

Stage 4: Subtotal retinal detachment: Here a partial detachment of the retina is seen which may be exudative or tractional. It is subdivided into the following:

- 4a: Partial retinal detachment not involving the fovea, but often leading to macular drag with visual impairment, and
- 4b: Partial retinal detachment involving the fovea.

Stage 5: Total retinal detachment.

Plus Disease

It is an indicator of severity of the disease and is defined as venous dilation and arterial tortuosity of the posterior pole vessels.

Pre-Plus Disease

It is defined as posterior pole vascular dilation and tortuosity which is more than normal but less than plus disease.

Aggressive Posterior Retinopathy of Prematurity

This refers to an uncommon, rapidly progressive, form of ROP previously referred to as *rush disease.* It is characterized by a posterior location, severe plus disease, and flat intraretinal neovascularization. It can progress very fast to stage 5 ROP and blindness, if not intervened early. The flat neovascularization can be quite subtle and can easily confuse less experienced examiners.[4]

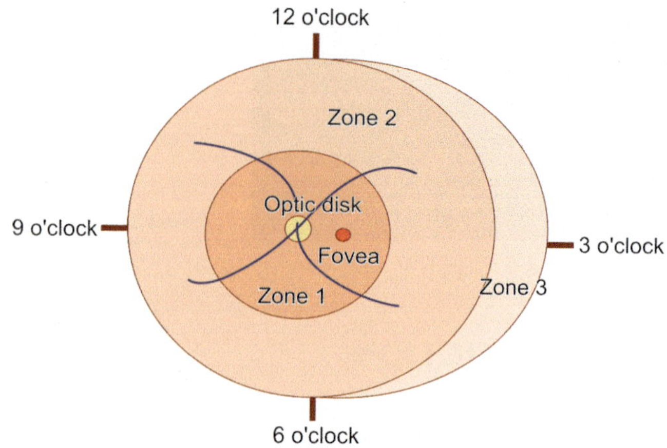

Fig. 75.1: Left eye vascularization towards ore serrate diagrammatically represented in zones and clock hours.

The image (Fig. 75.1), associated with ICROP, shows that how the zones and stages of ROP are typically denoted in handwritten notes or on a pre-printed proforma used for standardization between screeners.

SCREENING AND SCREENING GUIDELINES

The aim of screening is to detect sight-threatening ROP in the early part of the sight-threatening phase. Early detection at *threshold* provides the optimal timing for successful treatment. However, screening examinations are stressful and painful to some extent. Therefore, screeners attempt to minimize the frequency of screening if retinal vessels develop normally. Regular screening detects ROP and the rate of development of ROP becomes a key factor in predicting the timing of repeat examinations. Generally, if ROP starts to develop under 34 weeks' gestational age, the baby is much more likely to reach the 'threshold' for treatment. The speed of ROP change once it develops also is a key factor in predicting need for earlier repeat examination.

The profile of babies born in different countries that develop ROP varies slightly in terms of gestational age and weight. This may be multifactorial with ethnicity playing a role, but is thought mainly to be due to the standards of neonatal care of premature babies.

It is known that early gestational age is the single most important factor for ROP development, closely associated with low birth weight. The earlier gestational ages being most likely to develop ROP.

Therefore, screening for babies for sight-threatening ROP occurs in the USA and Canada for all babies born under 1501 grams or less than or equal to 30 weeks gestational age.[5]

In the UK, screening currently occurs for all babies born less than or equal to 31 weeks gestational age, and less than 1501 grams.[6]

In other nations, guidelines take account of the natural history of ROP in their particular region. Ethnicity as well as factors such as the standards of neonatal and prenatal care available significantly affect the development of ROP. In many nations, ROP occurs in older babies than those who typically develop ROP in the USA, Canada and the developed European nations.

Threshold ROP requires a few weeks to develop, being extremely uncommon below 32 weeks gestational age. Pathologically, the reason for this delay is that the immature retinal vessels undergo a vasoconstrictive phase, with delayed vascularization of the retina and arrest of normal vascularization (Stage 1). This is followed by the vasoproliferative phase (characterized by stage 3 and increased posterior pole engorgement) which leads to the fibrosis causing tractional retinal detachment. The early weeks after birth are consumed with vasoconstriction and delayed vascularization. Therefore, screening starts not earlier than at 30–31 weeks for the extremely early group (depending on screening in the USA or UK) and at 4–5 weeks after birth for the babies whose first screening examination would be older than or equal to 30–31 weeks corrected gestational age at 4–5 weeks of age.

However, the babies most at risk of developing ROP will be those born earliest.

In Newcastle upon Tyne from 2000 to 2013, 24 of 36 (66%) surviving 23 weeks gestational age babies were treated for threshold ROP. Of the babies surviving 24 weeks, 50 of 101 (50%) were treated. Whilst these rates of treatment for gestational age are slightly higher compared to those in other reported cohorts, the majority of babies requiring treatment belong to the earliest gestational ages. These figures also suggest the trend is for decreasing rates of treatment with older gestational age. The largest group of babies surviving prematurity are the oldest babies. Therefore, most screening resources currently are directed towards screening the oldest babies, who are least likely to develop ROP. Table. 75.1 demonstrates the screening criteria of the Royal College of Ophthalmologists, UK.

Table 75.1: Timing of first screen by gestational age.

	Timing of first ROP screen	
Gestational age (weeks)	**Postnatal weeks**	**Postmenstrual weeks**
22	8	30
23	7	30
24	6	30
25	5	30
26	4	30
27	4	31
28	4	32
29	4	33
30	4	34
31	4	35

(ROP: Retinopathy of prematurity)

After the first screening examination, repeated examinations are required at weekly or two weekly intervals. Screening continues until vessels are no longer able to develop ROP, usually having vascularized to zone 3, or where treatment has occurred and there can be no further vascular development following successful laser treatment.

DIGITAL IMAGING AND TELEMEDICINE

Screening of babies by trained ophthalmologists is time-consuming and requires specialist training and knowledge. The RetCam wide angle imaging digital camera (Massie Research Laboratories, 5775 West Las Positas Boulevard, Pleasanton, California) has revolutionized screening and research as well as follow-up of babies. Since 1997, the camera has gained popularity for ROP screening and imaging, mainly as it produces a high quality 130° image. This digital image in ROP means that images of temporal retina, nasal retina and optic disk with arcade vessels, can be captured by a trained user using three images. These can be stored for comparison at next screening examination. The uses of Telemedicine, where very large distances between centers exist, allows effective use of medical personnel to analyze images and provide a treatment service for those babies who develop sight-threatening ROP.

Digital photography has meant that fundal images can be compared objectively and by different observers for research in ROP. This has made multicenter trials much more feasible in ROP.

TREATMENT AS PER THE EVIDENCE-BASED STUDIES

There are three major trials that have shaped the current management of ROP. This is unique in that no other disease management could be summarized in this brevity.

1. Cryotherapy for Retinopathy of Prematurity (CRYO-ROP).[2]
2. The Early Treatment for Retinopathy of Prematurity (ETROP).[7]
3. The Bevacizumab Eliminates the Angiogenic Threat of Retinopathy of Prematurity (BEAT-ROP).[8]

Cryotherapy

Although laser therapy is the mainstay of treatment, cryotherapy was used to ablate the peripheral avascular retina prior to the development of laser therapy. The CRYO-ROP study included the use of cryotherapy and laser but is important in that it set established the evidence base for the treatment.

This multicenter study, with follow-up evidence over 10 years, backing up the initial cohort study findings, led to the development of screening and treatment criteria in ROP. The trial randomly initially assigned one eye of a baby with bilateral threshold ROP to cryotherapy treatment and designated the second eye *a control eye*, receiving no treatment.

From this study, the following concepts developed:

A treatment threshold, whereby the option of no treatment had a greater than 50% risk of adverse structural changes leading to blindness, described as acuity less than 20/200.

The importance of a fibrovascular ridge, called stage 3, which would herald the start of the fibrotic process leading to tractional detachment.

The concept of dilatation and tortuosity of blood vessels at the optic disk, both venous and arterial, signaling a large vascular shunt to supply the fibrovascular ridge. This was termed *PLUS*. A standard photograph of this concept was used in the study for treaters to compare screened eyes for randomization into treatment or observation arms (Fig. 75.2).

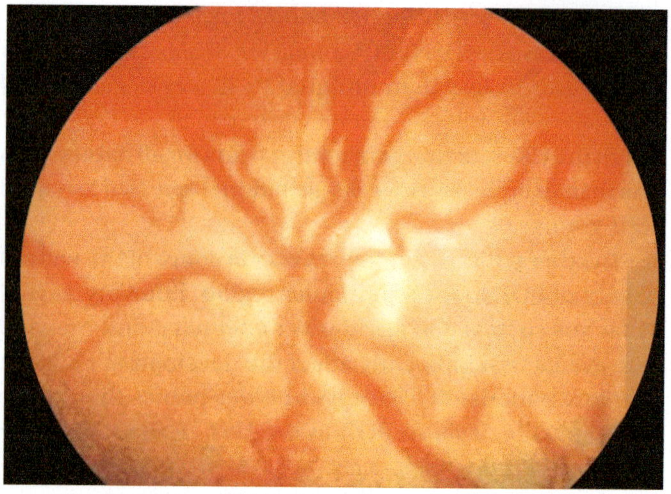

Fig. 75.2: Image of PLUS disease used in the CRYO-ROP trial.

The study concluded that babies of birth weight below 1251 g should be screened for development of ROP, and that treatment should commence with peripheral retinal ablation of avascular retina if the following conditions were met: 5 continuous hours of stage 3, or 8 total interrupted hours, in the presence of PLUS. This was termed 'Threshold disease'.

Laser

Laser treatment is based on the results of the ETROP trial.

The 10-year-follow-up data of the CRYO-ROP cohort found that for both functional and structural primary outcomes, there were fewer unfavorable outcomes in treated versus control eyes: 44.4% versus 62.1% ($p < 0.001$) for distance visual acuity. Meanwhile, indirect laser pan retinal ablation had almost totally replaced cryotherapy as a treatment modality.

Practitioners started implementing treatment at earlier time points, with case series evidence of improved structural outcomes. As well as this, a posterior rapidly evolving variant of ROP was recognized in the lowest gestational age and low-birth-weight babies. This rapidly evolving variant did not go through the typical stages of ROP to stage 3, and responded poorly to laser treatment at threshold. This was described initially as RUSH disease, and then as APROP (Aggressive Posterior ROP).

The ETROP trial compared the results of earlier treatment of randomized eyes to the CRYO-ROP threshold for second eyes. Its aim was to establish if prethreshold treatment (based on the CRYO-ROP standard of threshold) could be shown to improve the structural and hence visual outcomes of treatment.

The results demonstrated that earlier intervention for *high-risk prethreshold disease*, particularly for posterior ROP, produced better structural results. This was at a cost of a small increase in total numbers of eyes treated, that might have not progressed to CRYO-ROP threshold.

These findings form the basis of the current guidelines on which most national evidence-based treatment criteria are based.

The summary findings are below:

Unfavorable structural outcomes were reduced from 15.6% to 9.0% ($p < 0.001$) at 9 months. Further analysis supported retinal ablative therapy for eyes with type I ROP, or *high-risk prethreshold disease*, defined as zone I, any stage ROP with plus disease; zone I, stage 3 ROP without plus disease; or zone II, stage 2 or 3 with plus disease.

The analysis supported a *wait and watch* approach to type II ROP, defined as zone I, stage 1 and 2 without plus disease, or zone II, stage 3 without plus disease.

Plus disease is defined as two quadrants of posterior pole dilatation and tortuosity of retinal veins and arterioles, when using the *Standard CRYO-ROP photo of Plus* which shows all four quadrants as dilated and tortuous (Fig. 75.2).

Laser treatment is the mainstay of ROP treatment, using an infrared diode laser (1018 nm wavelength) to avoid uptake of laser energy by blood vessels around the infantile developing lens (tunica vasculosa lentis) and hemorrhage of ridge vessels in the retina. Laser is effective by destroying hypoxic avascular retina and hence stops VEGF production and stimulation of neovascularization.

The aim of laser treatment is to prevent the fibrous tractional changes caused by the fibrovascular proliferation of the retinal vessels.

Inadequate timing, laser application or delayed treatment, can all result in retinal detachment and loss of sight.

Figure 75.3 shows a left eye prior treatment with signs of posterior zone II APROP, with Plus disease, while Figure 75.4, which is taken three weeks later, shows peripheral laser scars and at the edge of the retinal demarcation, the curved elevated line of fibrotic traction that will continue to cause traction on the retina causing a total retinal tractional detachment.

Laser Treatment Application

- Typical laser treatment which is effective for most ROP at threshold with zone II, stage 3 disease.

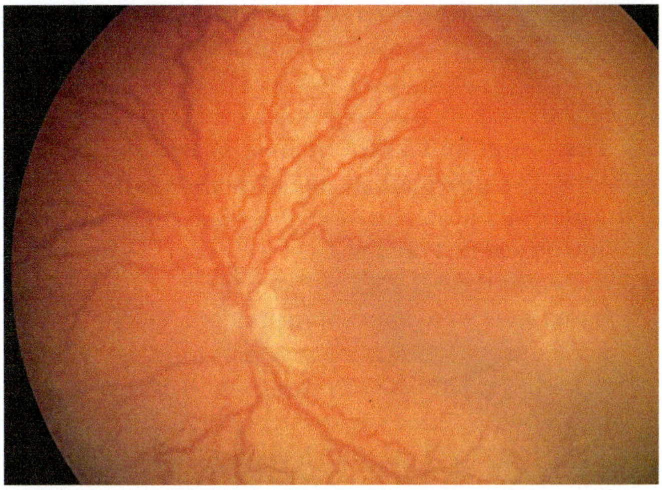

Fig. 75.3: A left eye prior to treatment with signs of posterior zone 2 APROP.

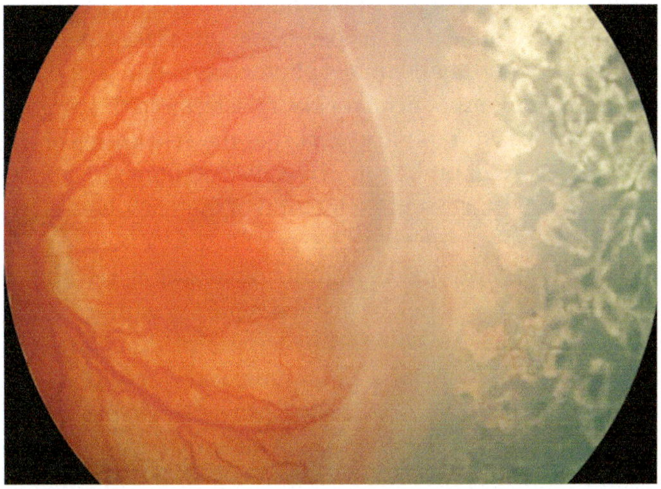

Fig. 75.4: Three weeks after (of the same patient as in Fig. 75.3) peripheral laser scars and at the edge of the retinal demarcation, the curved elevated line of fibrotic traction that will continue to cause traction on the retina causing a total retinal tractional detachment.

- Primary application of posterior to the ridge treatment, used where there is a high ridge (so the stage 3 has presented nearer to the fibrotic phase of the process), as well as anterior retinal ablation.
- Posterior to the ridge rescue treatment.

Laser photocoagulation, if applied densely in the early phase of threshold ROP, is extremely effective in treatment of ROP.

In the ETROP trial, laser alone was effective in preventing retinal detachment in 91% of treated eyes, with the majority of failures being in the posterior ROP or zone I group.

Case series data, from centers with high success rates above this have employed early treatment protocols and dense laser treatment, as well as laser posterior to the vascular demarcation or ridge to achieve even better results.

The use of anti-VEGF treatment, injected into the vitreous, has provided an effective alternative to laser particularly for posterior, APROP, or zone I disease.

1. The typical ROP at threshold with stage 3 in zone II is shown in Figures 75.5 to 75.7 with dense white laser burns anterior to the treatment ridge.
   Laser in zone I APROP treatment: Figure 75.8A is taken at the laser sitting, with threshold ROP, zone I with Plus disease. Three weeks later (Fig. 75.8B) the ROP is completely resolved, with loss of vessel tortuosity and typical laser scars at the level of the retinal pigment epithelium anterior to the demarcation of vascularized retina. This child, age 14 in 2007, has a refractive error of -10 with acuity of 6/6 in this eye.
2. Primary application of posterior to ridge laser, as well as anterior peripheral retinal photocoagulation (Fig. 75.9).
   Proponents of primary laser posterior to the ridge in vascularized retina suggest that the resolution of the fibrovascular proliferation is walled off from the macula by the laser preventing traction of the macular vessels by fibrosis at the ridge. Laser of the area posterior to the ridge, also treats ischemic retina aiding resolution of ROP. Case series have been reported with excellent results, but no comparative trials of this posterior laser plus anterior PRP versus anterior PRP alone have occurred. The author provides examples for the application of this type of laser from cases where resolution of ROP leads to traction on the macula, or macular dragging. This arose in the absence of posterior laser, or secondary *Rescue* treatment where initial treatment has not prevented the fibrotic sequelae of ROP. Posterior to the ridge, laser creates a mechanical barrier to retinal detachment and traction on the macula (Figs. 75.10A and B).
3. 'Rescue' laser treatment, following primary anterior photocoagulation which fails to halt progression.
   An example of progressive traction at the ridge after primary anterior to ridge laser is shown in Figure 75.11, which resolves with *rescue* laser posterior to the ridge, isolating the fibrous tissue at the ridge from the macula (Fig. 75.12). At age 14 the acuity is now -10 Diopters with acuity 6/18 in this eye.
   Macular drag after primary anterior peripheral photocoagulation, with resolution of ROP but tractional changes at ridge, leading to macular dragging. Visual acuity is 6/60 with nystagmus (Figs. 75.13A to C).

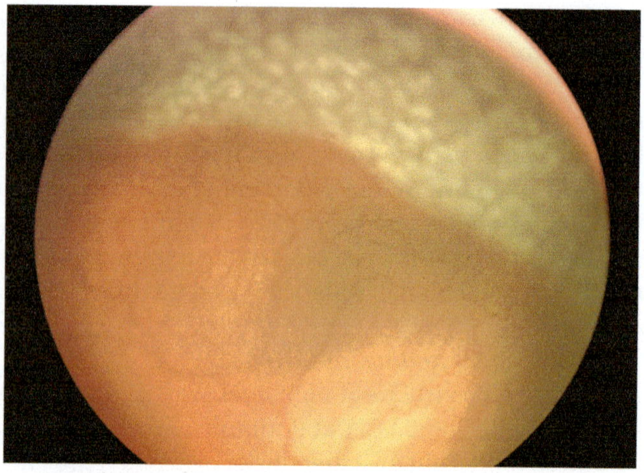

Fig. 75.5: A typical stage 3 ridge with laser white spot burns in avascular anterior retina.

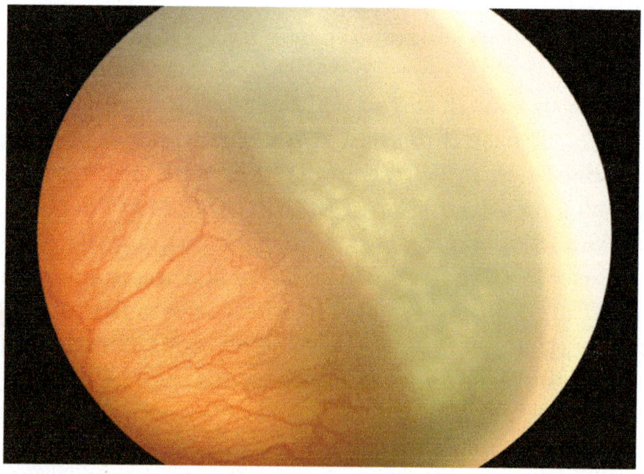

Fig. 75.6: Fibrovascular stage 3 ridge with a typical 'snail' appearance. Vascular tortuosity of vessels leading to ridge.

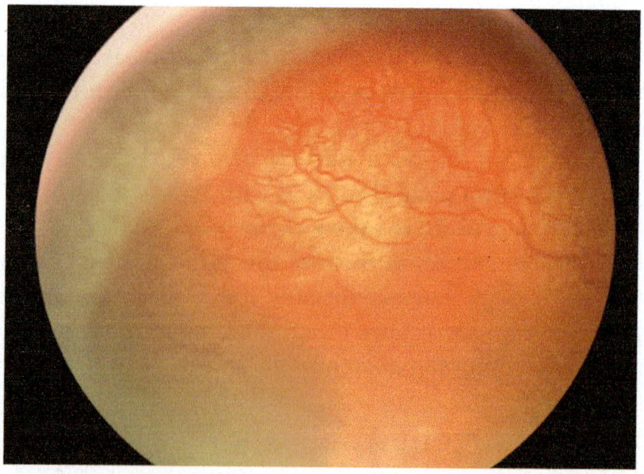

Fig. 75.7: Laser burns anterior to stage 3 ridge, with typical density of burns being separated by less than a half-burn width. Note burns are adjacent to the ridge and most dense at the demarcation of vascular retina with avascular retina.

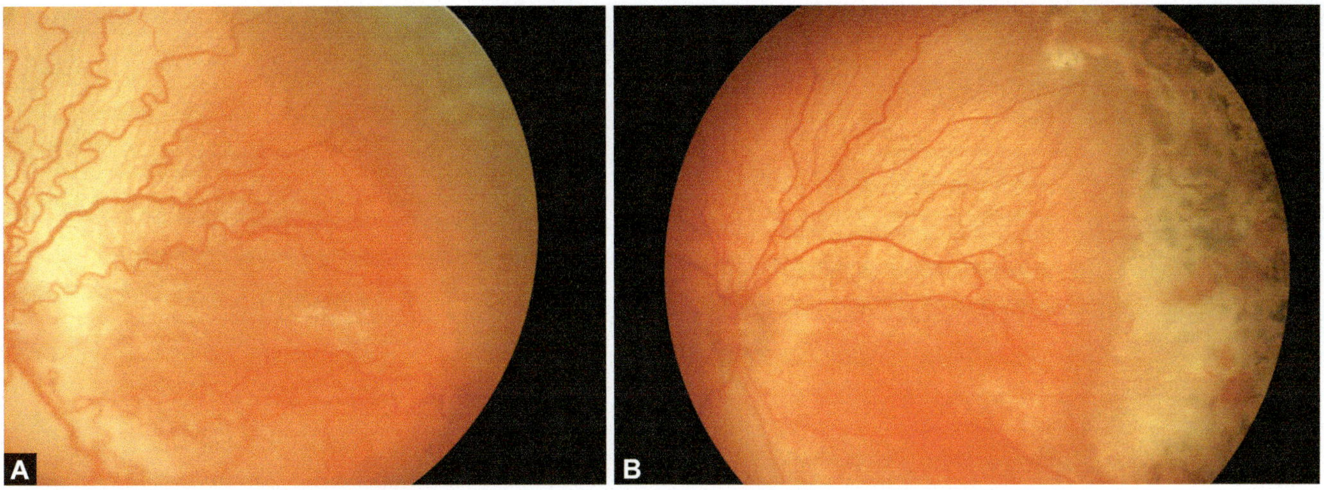

Figs. 75.8A and B: Resolution of ROP (B), 3 weeks after treatment of Zone I, APROP (A).

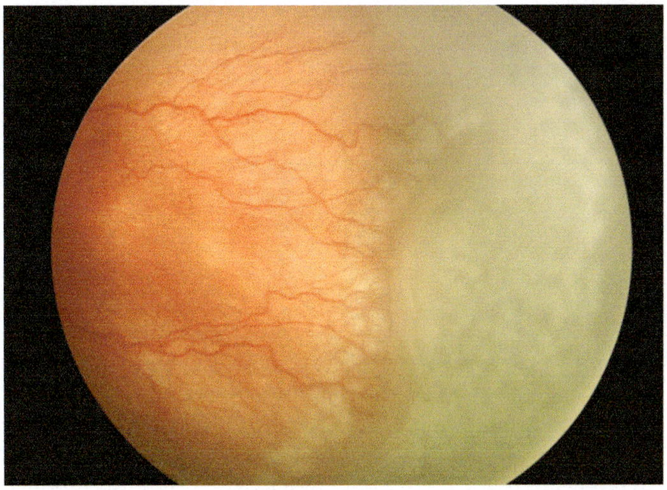

Fig. 75.9: Primary application of posterior to ridge laser, as well as anterior peripheral retinal photocoagulation.

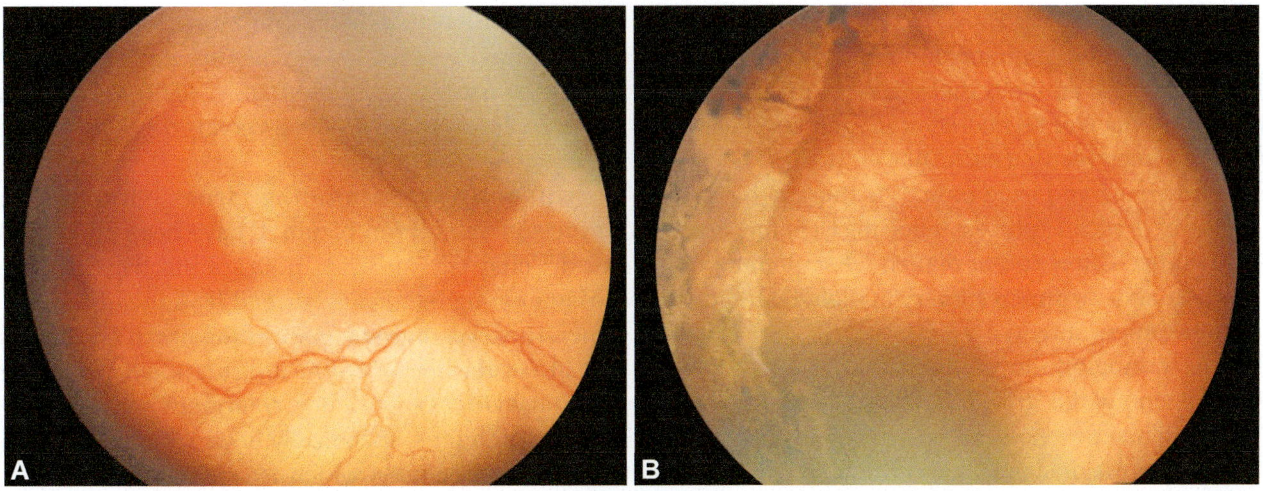

Figs. 75.10A and B: An example of advanced ROP, with high stage 3 ridge and hemorrhages treated with posterior to ridge and anterior laser, resulting in resolution of ROP, without macular drag and an isolated fibrous ridge.

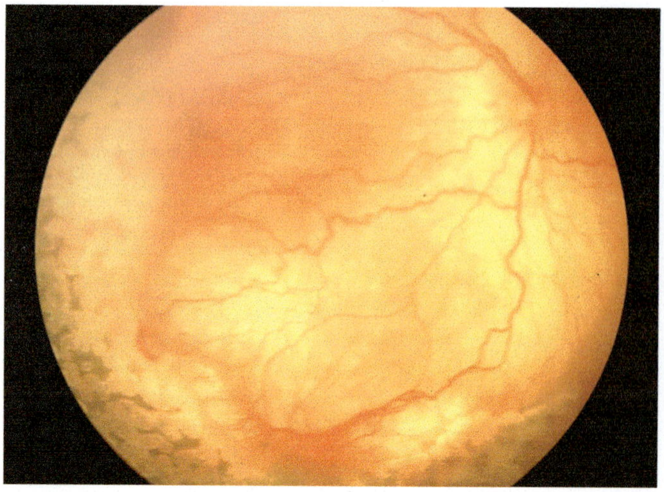

Fig. 75.11: Progressive traction at the ridge seen 3 weeks after primary anterior to ridge laser treatment.

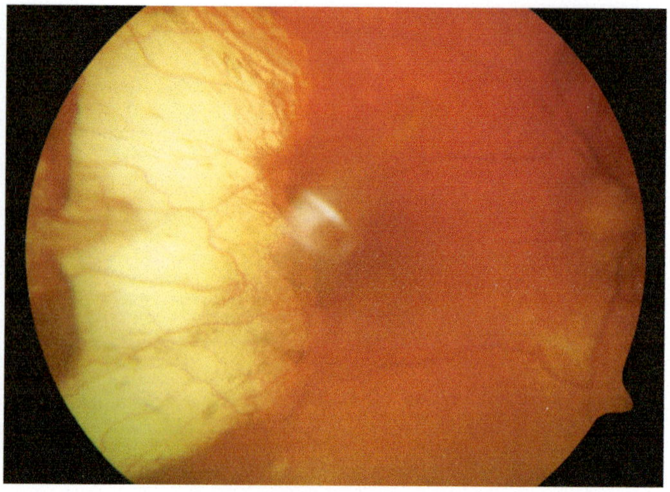

Fig. 75.12: 'Rescue laser' posterior to the ridge, isolating the fibrous tissue at the ridge from the macula, and preventing macula drag.

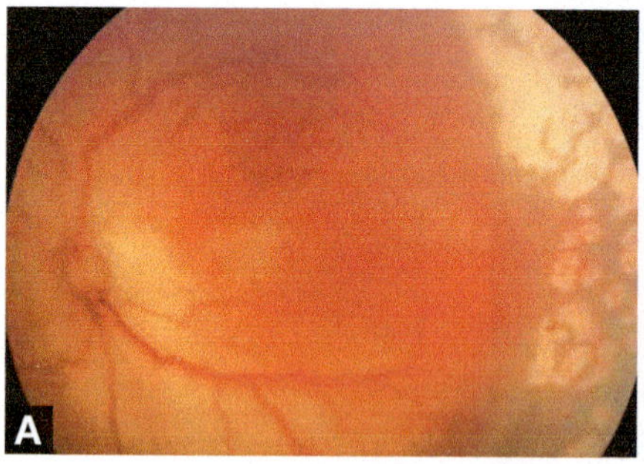

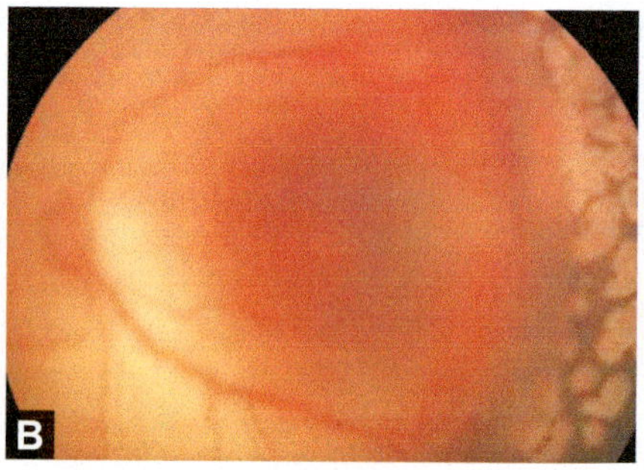

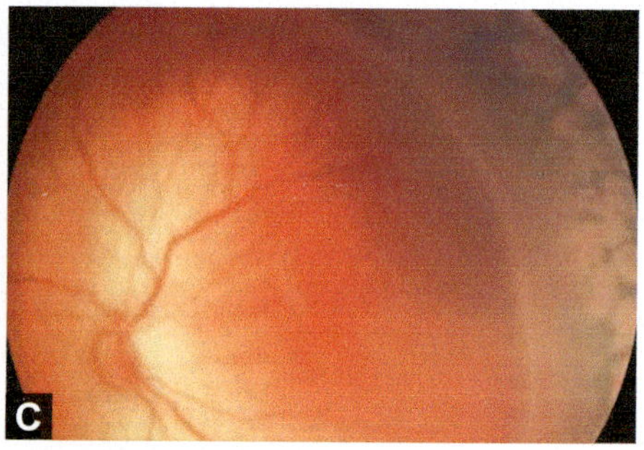

Figs. 75.13A to C: Macular drag (B), after primary anterior peripheral photocoagulation (A), with resolution of ROP but tractional changes at ridge, leading to macular dragging (C).

Inhibition of Vascular Endothelial Growth Factor Treatment (Anti-VEGF Treatment)

The use of anti-VEGF immunoglobulins, in the form of a humanized murine antibody that binds to VEGF, was tried in eyes to treat macular degeneration at an earlier stage, and to limit the damage caused by the fibrotic process resulting from hemorrhage and exudation. The therapy has been used in the neovascular process following ischemic central retinal vein occlusion and in diabetic maculopathy and prior to retinal detachment surgery in diabetic tractional retinal detachment surgery.

The immunoglobulin binds to the VEGF and then limits the action of this growth factor in hemorrhagic and ischemic vascular processes.

In ROP, the major signaling growth factor stimulating neovascularization is VEGF. Thus, when bound by the injected immunoglobulin, the process of neovascularization is halted temporarily, and reversed in practice. Case reports of the efficacy of anti-VEGF began to appear in 2006. Over the years, there has been one multicenter prospective randomized trial of its efficacy as a monotherapy in comparison to laser treatment (BEAT-ROP), as well as many published case series utilizing varying doses and with and without laser treatment.

Different VEGF-binding drugs, predominantly bevacizumab and ranibizumab have been compared for relative efficacy (Fig. 75.14). Both are effective and there are no large enough studies to currently commend one over the other. However, bevacizumab is the much cheaper drug, and in a worldwide sense, the drug that has been most used.

The evidence base for treatment with anti-VEGF immunoglobulins, specifically bevacizumab, comes from the BEAT-ROP study, which is explained in more detail below.

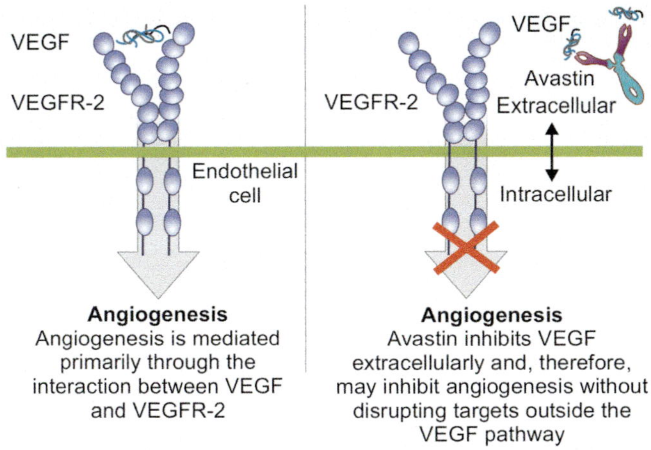

Fig. 75.14: Mechanism of action of bevacizumab and ranibizumab in angiogenesis.

BEAT-ROP Study

This was a multicenter trial that attempted to compare the efficacy of anti-VEGF injection against laser treatment for ROP.

The stated end point of the study was the rate of recurrence of ROP after treatment. In conventional laser therapy, a failure of treatment does not result in resolution of the stage 3 ridge. In fact, the blood vessels may become less tortuous and dilated but there is a persistent fibrovascular remnant at the ridge which undergoes a fibrotic change leading to degrees of tractional retinal detachment. However, treatment with anti-VEGF immunoglobulins leads to rapid initial total resolution of dilatation and tortuosity of blood vessels and dissolution of the fibrovascular ridge. The recurrence of ROP can occur as the drug effects wear off, with progression to stage 3 and subsequent retinal detachment. Thus, although laser treatment does not lead to recurrence of ROP, failure of either treatment leads to tractional retinal detachment, which was measured in this study.

It demonstrated that resolution of ROP occurred with a single dose of avastin 0.65 mg injection into the vitreous at ETROP threshold for treatment, and that this prevented ROP recurrence in the vast majority of eyes requiring treatment.

It showed a benefit over laser particularly in zone I ROP requiring treatment, whereas laser treatment for zone II disease was statistically as effective at preventing recurrence and subsequent tractional changes as avastin.

The BEAT-ROP study showed a significantly higher rate of recurrence in zone I disease with conventional laser therapy compared with intravitreal bevacizumab monotherapy [42% (14 of 33 infants) vs 6% (2 of 31 infants), $p = 0.003$]. However, the rate of recurrence in zone II posterior disease did not differ significantly between the 2 groups [12% (5 of 40 infants) vs 5% (2 of 39 infants), $p = 0.27$].

The study observed a difference in the timeline of recurrence between the 2 groups (16.0 ± 4.6 weeks for intravitreal bevacizumab vs 6.2 ± 5.7 weeks for conventional laser therapy). The authors cautioned clinicians that careful follow-up is required for infants treated with bevacizumab monotherapy and that safety in neonates is an important issue for intravitreal bevacizumab. This study did not observe systemic or local toxicity and the investigators noted that the size of the BEAT-ROP study (150 infants) was not large enough to assess safety.

Laser therapy resulted in permanent destruction of vessels and areas of treated retina. However, eyes treated with intravitreal bevacizumab had continued vessel growth into the peripheral retina.

This is the paper most cited when practitioners are discussing the benefit of injection over laser in treatment of zone I disease. Controversy over the use of avastin exists over the dose and unknown potential side effects of vascular growth factor inhibition in the systemic circulation, because of absorption of the drug from the eye.

The current state of knowledge regarding treatment of ROP using anti-VEGF injections into vitreous is advancing such that by the time of publication, further advances will have been made.

However, the following is now well established:

1. Anti-VEGF injected into the vitreous is an effective treatment for posterior rapidly progressive ROP, and zone I ROP. Injection of the drug is not associated commonly with any immediately recognized systemic side effect.
2. The actual effective dose required to treat ROP at the point of *threshold* is much lower than is currently used. Doses of bevacizumab (avastin) from the standard most commonly utilized dose of 0.65 to 0.06 mg are able to halt progression of ROP for at least one month.

   There are several case series describing longer term structural retinal outcomes with lower doses, although less information on the rate of ROP recurrence is available with lower doses.
3. Significant restriction of visual field caused by laser treatment does not occur following anti-VEGF injection. The vascularization of the retina is significantly delayed but progresses at a slower rate towards the peripheral

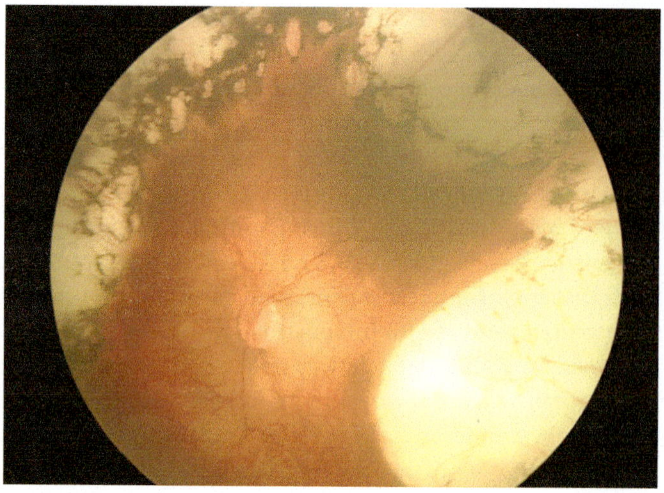

Fig. 75.15: Effective laser for zone I aggressive ROP results in significant visual field constriction, as well as high myopia, as in this infant, an ex 22 weeker whose refraction is currently-19, age 9.

retina. Laser treatment in comparison totally ablates the peripheral retina anterior to the ridge or demarcation treated at the time of *threshold*.

4. High myopia is a common side effect of laser treatment for posterior retinopathy of prematurity (Fig. 75.15). It does not commonly occur in babies treated with anti-VEGF injections.
5. Recurrence of ROP can occasionally occur and can be sight-threatening. It usually occurs at some time between 40 weeks and 50 weeks corrected gestational age. When ROP recurs, it may progress extremely rapidly. Recurrence occurs in zone II with *classical* stage 3. Treatment of recurrent ROP is effective with laser treatment.
6. Systemic absorption of anti-VEGF has been demonstrated. The drug appears to suppress circulating serum VEGF for several weeks. The significance of such an effect on organogenesis, neurodevelopment or other significant side effects has yet to be elucidated. This is a cause of concern for neonatologists and ophthalmologists, and the source of much debate.
7. Anti-VEGF treatment is becoming increasingly popular throughout the world. In countries where the resources required for effective laser treatment do not exist in all areas, anti-VEGF treatment provides a cheap and easily available alternative. It can be administered without the significant technical skills required to perform indirect ophthalmoscopy and laser treatment in babies who do not require sedation or anesthesia.

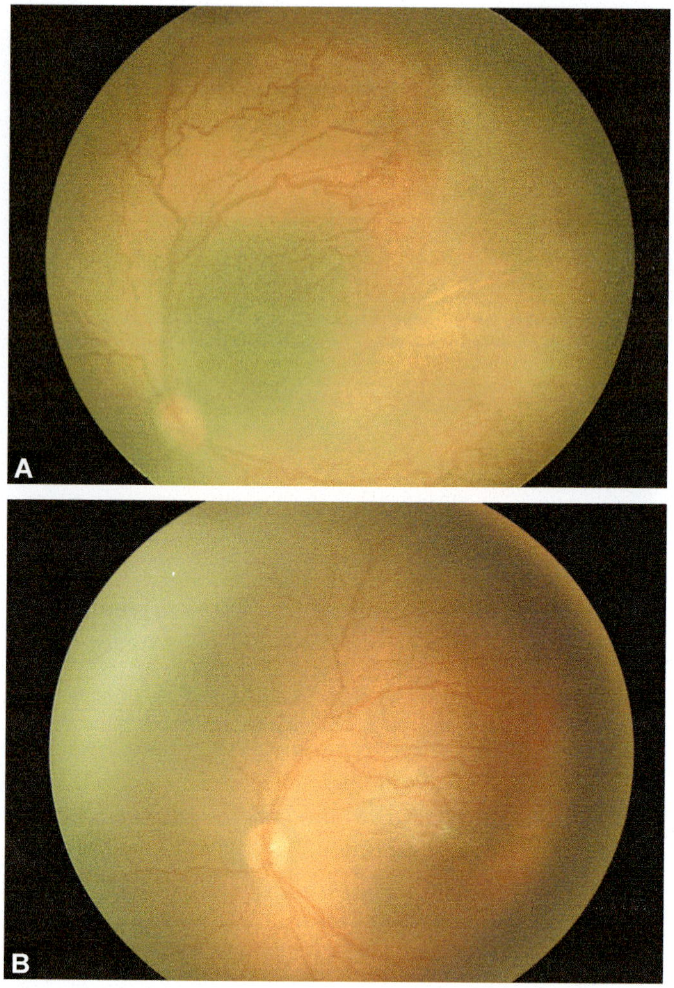

Figs. 75.16 and B: Before and after injection at 6 days. Vasoconstriction and marked straightening of arteries and veins are the early signs of effective treatment.

Practicalities of Anti-VEGF Treatment

In posterior aggressive ROP, and particularly zone I ROP, a small volume of anti-VEGF (0.025 mL or less) is injected into the vitreous cavity at or just posterior to the pars plana (avoiding the lens with the needle track).

The effect of the drug, usually bevacizumab or ranibizumab, can be witnessed within 48 hours (Fig. 75.16A). There is an initial effect of vasoconstriction. Both arteries and veins look constricted as well as less tortuous (Fig. 75.16B). This effect is sustained for several weeks. The progressive vascularization of anterior retina is significantly delayed, gradual, and can be observed with serial images. This can continue until the baby is much older than its projected term date (40 weeks), even over 50 weeks corrected gestational age, and ceases usually into zone III. For this reason, screening continues until there is full vascularization or the vascularization remains static around the 52 weeks age before and after injection at 6 days. Vasoconstriction and marked straightening of arteries and veins are the early signs of effective treatment.

SURGERY FOR RETINOPATHY OF PREMATURITY

Stage 5 ROP is the end stage of the fibrovascular process in ROP. In the event of tractional retinal detachment affecting the macula, the vision is not only lost but the eye develops secondary angle closure glaucoma and eventually becomes phthisical.

Lens-sparing vitrectomy, with or without scleral buckling, can replace anatomical retinal attachment by releasing vitreous and fibrotic traction.

As a result, some vision can be salvaged. Once the macular has detached, however (stage 4b or 5) the chance of a *favorable visual outcome* is low (defined as better than 20/200 in the ETROP follow-up study of children with detached retinas). In the ETROP study follow-up, 6 of the 70 eyes (9%) had an acuity better than 20/200. Of these, 5 were stage 4A.[9]

CONCLUSION

Retinopathy of prematurity is a modern disease that could not have existed without the intensive care technologies that have aided the survival of extremely low gestational age premature babies. It is a biphasic condition which means that there is a variable delay to the point when fibrovascular proliferation arises in some babies which can lead to tractional retinal detachment. The smallest and earliest gestational age babies are most at risk.

Currently, screening guidelines exist for all babies at risk, and is performed to detect those who begin to develop neovascular proliferation. Treatment thresholds have developed based on clinical trials, which provide a visual guide for screeners to instigate treatment that reduces the growth factors responsible for stimulating neovascularization. Cryotherapy and laser treatment are both destructive therapies which reduce the stimulus for avascular proliferation by destroying the hypoxic avascular retinal cells that produce vascular endothelial growth factor (VEGF). Laser treatment is known to be extremely effective in over 90% of all treated eyes in preventing structural retinal detachment and saving sight. Its side effect profile is well known and understood. Since 2006, VEGF-negating immunoglobulins have been injected directly into the vitreous and bind VEGF directly, preventing its action. The use of anti-VEGF treatment has found its place in the most aggressive posterior form of ROP, where laser treatment is least effective. These drugs signify the most significant advance in ROP management since the CRYO-ROP trial was published. They show promising outcomes in the first decade of their use, but have unanswered questions regarding dosing, follow-up screening and treatment and longer term potential side effects.

Currently, in 2017, a baby who develops sight-threatening ROP has a better than 95% chance of successful treatment. The significant advances over the years since the 1980s have been multifactorial. In future, screening and treatment can be refined to best identify the babies at risk and to minimize the potential iatrogenic side effects of treatment.

REFERENCES

1. Terry TL. Fibroblastic Overgrowth of Persistent Tunica Vasculosa Lentis in Infants Born Prematurely: II. Report of Cases-Clinical Aspects. Trans Am Ophthalmol Soc. 1942;40:262-84.
2. Multicenter trial of cryotherapy for retinopathy of prematurity. Preliminary results. Cryotherapy for Retinopathy of Prematurity Cooperative Group. Arch Ophthalmol. 1988;106(4):471-9.
3. An International Classification of Retinopathy of Prematurity. The Committee for the Classification of Retinopathy of Prematurity. Arch Ophthalmol. 1984;102(8):1130-4.
4. International Committee for the Classification of Retinopathy of Prematurity. The International Classification of Retinopathy of Prematurity revisited. Arch Ophthalmol. 2005;123(7):991-9.
5. Fierson WM, American Academy of Pediatrics Section on Ophthalmology, American Academy of Ophthalmology, et al. Screening examination of premature infants for retinopathy of prematurity. Pediatrics. 2013;131(1):189-95.
6. Wilkinson AR, Haines L, Head K, et al. UK retinopathy of prematurity guideline. Eye (Lond). 2009;23(11):2137-9.
7. Early Treatment for Retinopathy of Prematurity Cooperative Group. Revised indications for the treatment of retinopathy of prematurity: results of the early treatment for retinopathy of prematurity randomized trial. Arch Ophthalmol. 2003; 121(12):1684-94.
8. Mintz-Hittner HA, Kennedy KA, Chuang AZ, et al. Efficacy of intravitreal bevacizumab for stage 3+ retinopathy of prematurity. N Engl J Med. 2011;364(7):603-15.
9. Repka MX, Tung B, Good WV, et al. Outcome of Eyes Developing Retinal Detachment During the Early Treatment for Retinopathy of Prematurity Study. Arch Ophthalmol. 2011;129(9):1175-9.

Chapter 76 Retinoblastoma

Stathopoulos C, Munier FL

EPIDEMIOLOGY

Retinoblastoma is not only the most common intraocular malignancy in children with an incidence ranging from 1:15,000 to 20,000 live births (close to 10,000 cases per year worldwide), but is also credited as the most frequent eye cancer in general surpassing uveal melanoma.[1] Untreated, it can lead to death within 1–2 years, but with current treatment modalities the disease is generally well controlled with an impressive overall survival of more than 95% in high-income countries and 40–60% in developing countries.[2] There is no racial or sex predilection. The disease is bilateral in 30–40% of the cases and unilateral in 60–70%. The mean age at diagnosis depends on any family history, the laterality of the disease and the socioeconomic response to symptoms. Patients with a known family history of retinoblastoma and bilateral retinoblastoma are usually diagnosed earlier than unilateral forms (mean age at diagnosis respectively of 4 months and 12 months versus 24 months).[2,3] Overall, most of the cases (90%) are, however, diagnosed before the age of 3 years. Adult onset retinoblastoma has been reported in around 45 cases in patients aged between 20 years and 75 years.[4]

GENETICS

Retinoblastoma is a genetic disease caused by a somatic or a germline mutation in the *RB1* gene, a tumor suppressor gene located on the long arm of chromosome 13 (13q14). Loss or inactivation of both *RB1* copies is required in order for the disease to develop (Knudson's two hit hypothesis).[5] In heritable retinoblastoma, the first mutation occurs in a germ cell (germline mutation), mostly in spermatocytes. After fecundation the mutation is thus carried in all cells of the body, putting the patient at risk not only for retinoblastoma, but also lifelong risk for the development of other second cancers (most commonly osteosarcoma of the long bones, soft tissue sarcomas, cutaneous melanoma, and carcinomas). The causing retinoblastoma occurs in retinal progenitors of red/green cones during the retinal development (up to 4 years of age).[6] Individuals with heritable retinoblastoma have either a heterozygous de novo mutation, or carry the germline mutation of one of the parents (familial retinoblastoma) in an autosomal-dominant manner. In non-heritable retinoblastoma, both mutations occur in the retinoblast where its confined, explaining why these patients have the same risk for developing secondary cancers as the general population.[7]

Nearly 90% of retinoblastoma cases are sporadic (with no positive family history). In two-thirds of these patients the mutation is somatic and results in an isolated unilateral unifocal (only one tumor in one eye) disease, whereas in one-third it is due to a new germline mutation. In the sporadic cases with a germline mutation, as well as in all familial cases, the disease is typically bilateral and multifocal (multiple tumors in both eyes), although approximatively 15% of the sporadic unilateral patients carry a germline *RB1* mutation.[7]

Different types of mutations can affect the *RB1* gene, most of them being nonsense codons or frame shifts. In some instances retinoblastoma is caused by an interstitial deletion of the long arm of chromosome 13, a condition known as 13q-syndrome and characterized by varying degrees of dysmorphic features (low-set ears, wide nasal bridge, bulbous tip of the nose, and thin upper lip) and neurodevelopmental delays.[8] Finally, a rare form of unilateral non-hereditary retinoblastoma (1.4% of the cases) is caused by a *MYCN* oncogene amplification, the *RB1* gene remaining wild type. The disease manifests typically early in these cases (before 6 months), and in a very aggressive manner, usually resulting in enucleation.[9]

All children with retinoblastoma should undergo genetic molecular analysis to determine or confirm a germline mutation, in order to assess the risk for developing pinealoblastoma and second cancers as well as for appropriate genetic counseling. The detection of the mutation is performed on peripheral blood lymphocytes or tumor tissue when available. Nowadays, with the use of a combination of genetic testing (DNA sequencing, polymerase chain reaction amplification and multiplex ligation-dependent probe amplification) over 95% of the mutations can be detected.[10] Genetic counseling can be complex and the family should be referred to a geneticist. Germline mutations carry a 90% penetrance, meaning that 90% of carriers of a mutant allele will develop retinoblastoma. Thus, a bilateral retinoblastoma survivor has a 45% risk of having an affected child, compared to a 7% risk for the unilateral survivor. Normal parents of a child with bilateral involvement have less than a 5% risk of having another child with retinoblastoma. However, if two or more siblings are affected, the risk that another child will be affected increases to 45%.[11]

Options for prenatal testing in pregnancies at increased risk include first trimester molecular analysis of DNA through chorionic villus sampling, amniocentesis or percutaneous umbilical blood sampling at birth. Preimplantation genetic testing with identification of *RB1* mutation in a blastomere (8-cell embryo) obtained by in vitro fertilization technique is also available.[11]

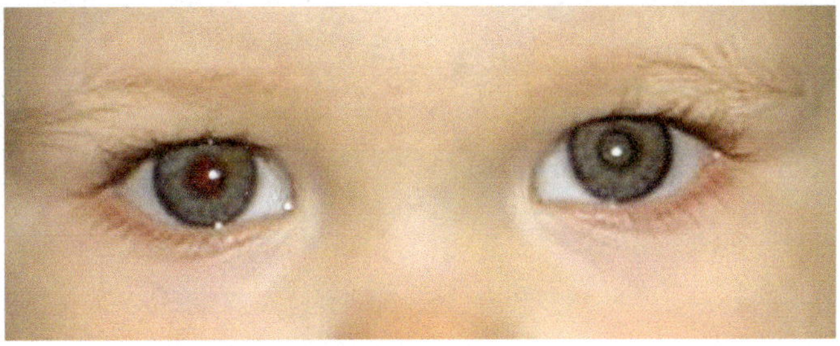

Fig. 76.1: Mild leukocoria in the left eye of a 15-month-old boy with unilateral retinoblastoma.

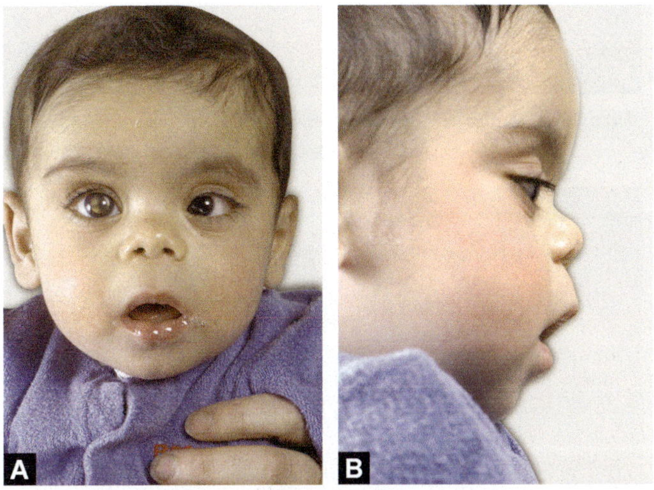

Figs. 76.2A and B: Retinoblastoma presenting with leukocoria and strabismus in the right eye of a child with 13q deletion syndrome. (A) Face appearance shows low-set ears with large lobules, broad nasal bridge and bulbous tip of the nose; (B) Profile appearance with frontal bossing, depressed nasal bridge, long philtrum, and micrognathia.

CLINICAL FEATURES, DIAGNOSIS, AND CLASSIFICATION

Clinical Features of Retinoblastoma at Presentation

The clinical signs of retinoblastoma depend on the extent and location of the tumor(s). The most frequent sign in the developed countries is the leukocoria (60%) (white pupil in Greek) (Fig. 76.1), followed by strabismus (20%) (Figs. 76.2A and B), which occurs in the case of a macular location of the tumor.[12] Associated signs include glaucoma (either secondary to iris neovascularization, tumor seeding in the trabecular meshwork or angle closure due to anterior displacement of the lens iris diaphragma), buphthalmia, heterochromia, cataract or subluxated lens, pseudohypopyon, hyphema, posterior segment neovascularization, and vitreous hemorrhage (Figs. 76.3A and B; Figs. 76.4A and B). Advanced retinoblastoma can manifest further with phthisis, orbital cellulitis from necrotic intraocular retinoblastoma, or proptosis in the case of extraocular extension (orbital retinoblastoma) (Fig. 76.5).[12] Small lesions may be detected on a routine eye examination or screening in at-risk individuals. Rarely will retinoblastoma induce visual complaints, as most of the patients are preschool-age children.

Retinoblastoma originates from a cone precursor and can already develop in the fetus. Initially it appears as a transluscent intraretinal tumor (Figs. 76.6A and B). Chalky-white foci of calcification within the tumor can be sometimes seen ophthalmoscopically (Fig. 76.7). As the tumor develops it can grow toward the vitreous (endophytic growth), toward the subretinal space, producing an overlying retinal detachment (exophytic growth), or in both directions (Figs. 76.8A and B).[13] Retinoblastoma cells can spread from the solid tumor and give rise to secondary tumor implants (seeds) that can invade all eye compartments, namely the subretinal space, retrohyaloid space, the vitreous cavity, as well as the posterior and the anterior chambers (Fig. 76.9).[14] Vitreous seeding can appear as dust, spheres or cloud.[14] Anterior chamber seeding can aggregate on the iris to form nodules and/or settle inferiorly to form a pseudohypopyon. Other rare variants of retinoblastoma are the diffuse infiltrating (Fig. 76.10) (<2%),

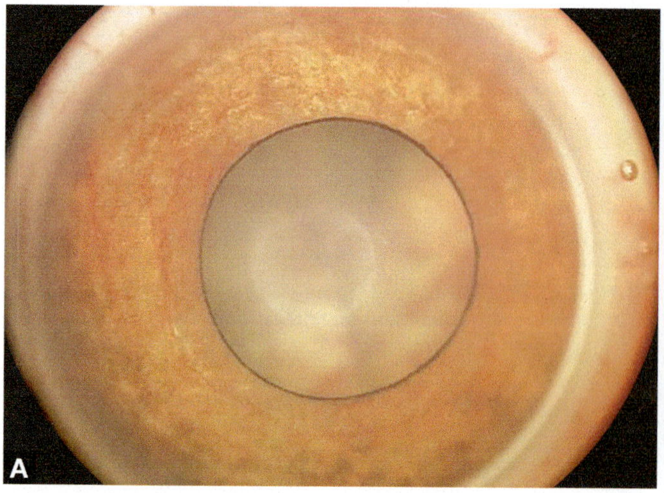

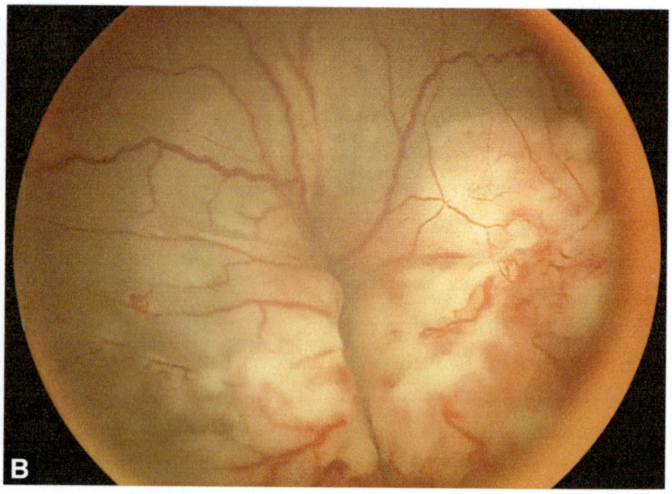

Figs. 76.3A and B: Unilateral retinoblastoma in a 4-year-old girl presenting with leukocoria. (A) Iris neovascularization causing secondary glaucoma; (B) Large retrolental exophytic tumor with secondary total retinal detachment and subretinal seeds.

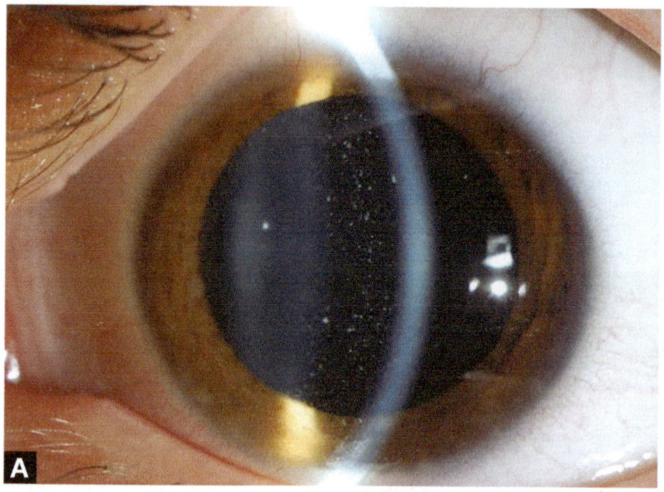

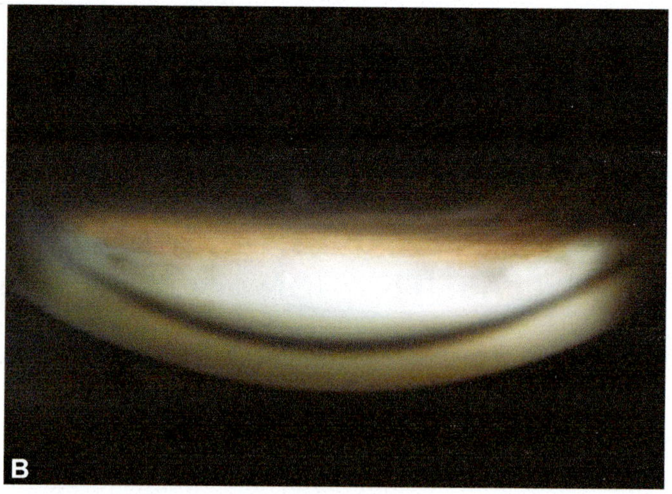

Figs. 76.4A and B: Unilateral retinoblastoma in the left eye of a 10-year-old girl presenting with pseudouveitis and glaucoma. (A) Anterior chamber seeding with free-floating cells and tumoral nodules on the iris; (B) Mild inferior pseudohypopyon.

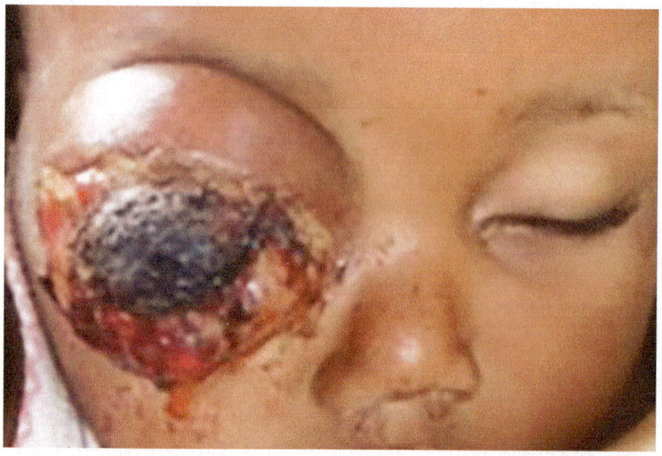

Fig. 76.5: Extraocular retinoblastoma (orbitary retinoblastoma) due to unavailable medical care.

an aggressive form, typically unilateral, without calcification and characterized by a flat infiltrating intraretinal growth and the diffuse anterior retionoblastoma (<1%).[15] Finally, cavitary retinoblastoma (2–7%) is characterized by intratumoral cysts, a low-grade tumor that usually shows poor response to chemotherapy (Figs. 76.11A and B).[16] If left untreated, the retinoblastoma will spread outside the eye via the optic nerve where it can invade the central nervous system (CNS) and/or through the sclera where it can invade the orbit (orbital retinoblastoma). Invasion of the choroid can lead to hematogenous metastasis, whereas invasion of the orbit can lead to both hematogenous and lymphatic metastases.[17]

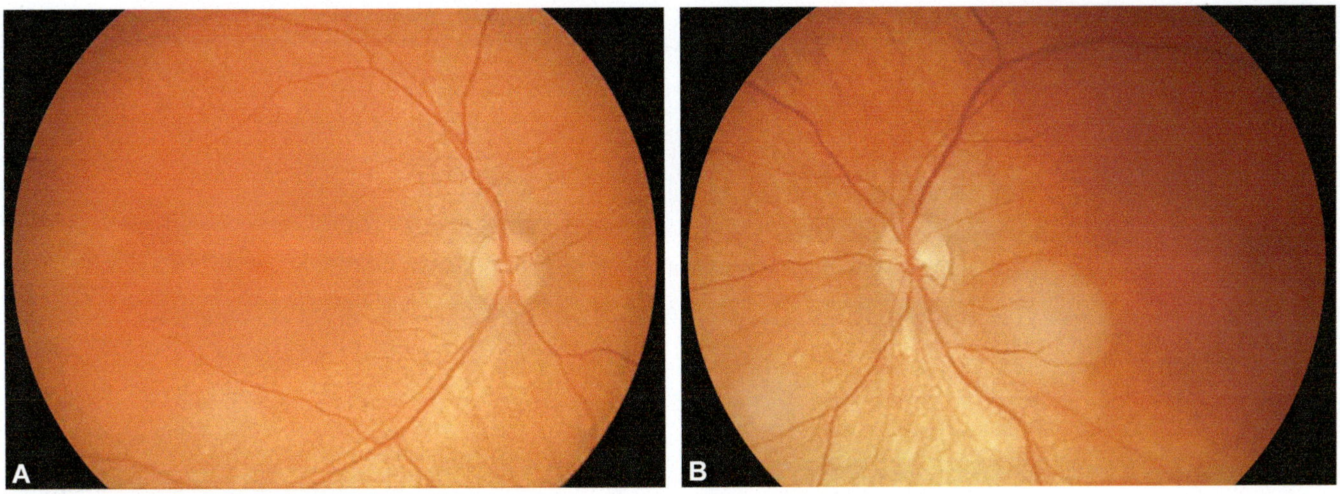

Figs. 76.6A and B: Seven-week-old neonate with bilateral familial retinoblastoma. (A) Right eye with a small tumor confined to the retina located inferiorly to the fovea (group A); (B) Left eye with a larger parafoveal tumor and a small tumor inferonasally to the optic disk (group B).

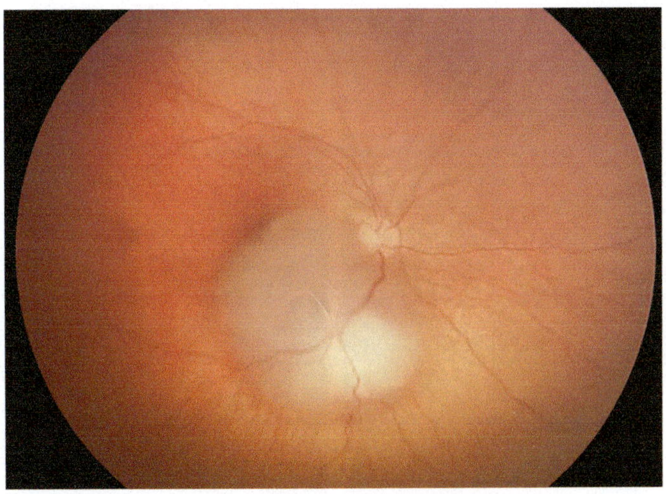

Fig. 76.7: Retinoblastoma in the macular region of the right eye with chalky-white calcification (group B).

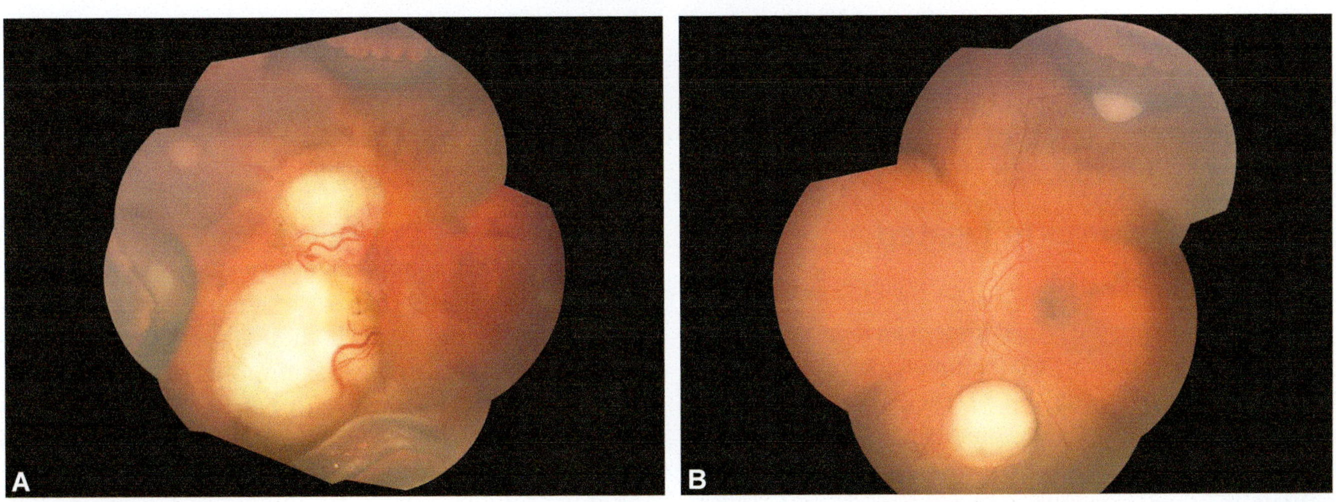

Figs. 76.8A and B: Bilateral retinoblastoma. (A) Right eye. Two large confluent tumors at the posterior pole with exophytic growth causing a secondary retinal detachment and diffuse subretinal seeding inferiorly. Note the presence of two other small primary tumors at 9 and 10 o'clock; (B) Left eye has two tumors with endophytic growth.

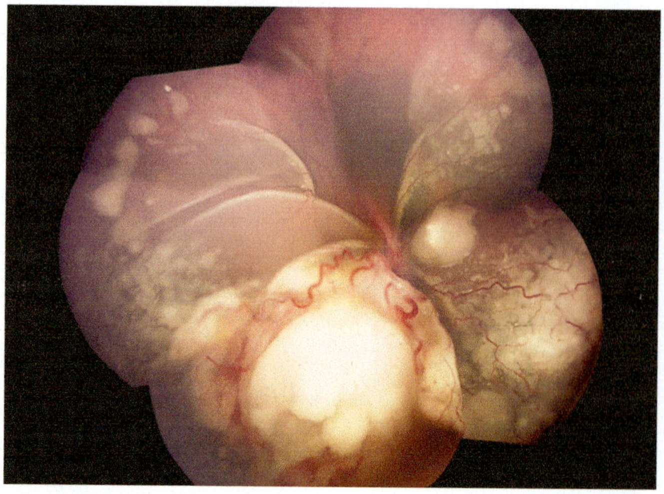

Fig. 76.9: Retinoblastoma showing both exophytic and endophytic growth. The inferior solid tumor grew in the subretinal space causing a secondary total retinal detachment as well as toward the vitreous cavity causing a disruption of the internal limiting membrane and posterior hyaloid. Note the numerous subretinal seeds as well as the intravitreal dispersion of the tumor at the apex.

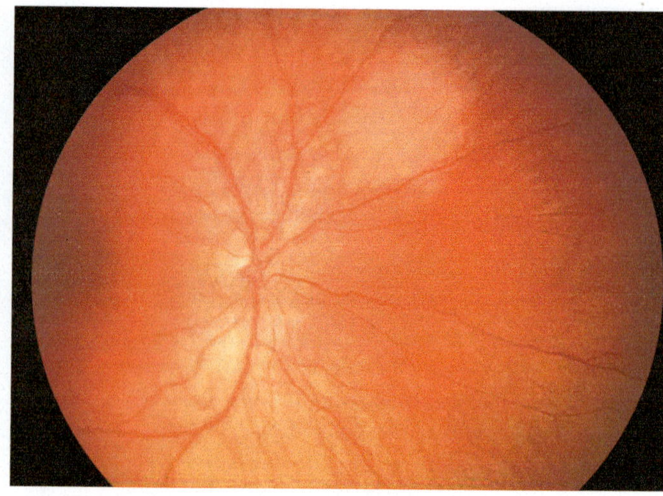

Fig. 76.10: Diffuse infiltrating retinoblastoma in the right eye. Note the minimally elevated flat lesion. The contralateral eye had been enucleated for advanced retinoblastoma.

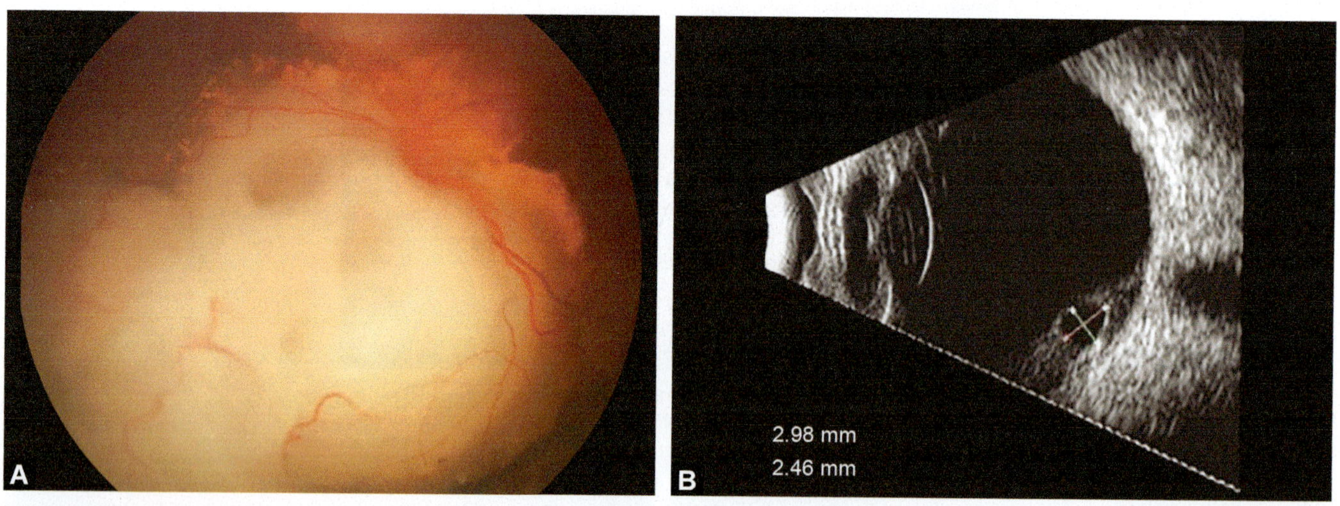

Figs. 76.11A and B: Retinoblastoma in a 17-month-old boy with trisomy 21 after systemic chemotherapy. (A) Left eye with large cavitary tumor partially obscuring the optic disk. Note the thin peritumoral alteration of the retinal pigment epithelium suggesting poor regression after chemotherapy; (B) B-scan ultrasonography shows one of the intratumoral cavities and no invasion of the optic nerve.

Clinical Features in Treated Retinoblastoma

Following treatment, the retinal tumor can regress in one of the following patterns: type 0 (complete disappearance of the tumor with no residual retinal scar), type 1 (completely calcified mass), type 2 (completely noncalcified mass, appearing as a fish flesh or translucent mass), type 3 (partially calcified scar with fish flesh remnant, combination of types 1 and 2) or type 4 (atrophic scar of chorioretinal atrophy).[13] Similar regression patterns have been described to characterized the vitreous and anterior chamber seeds in response to intravitreal chemotherapy, namely vitreous seeding regression type 0 (complete disappearance), regression type 1 (refringent or calcified residues), type 2 (amorphous often nonspherical inactive residues with or without pigment) or type 3 (combination of types 1 and 2).[14]

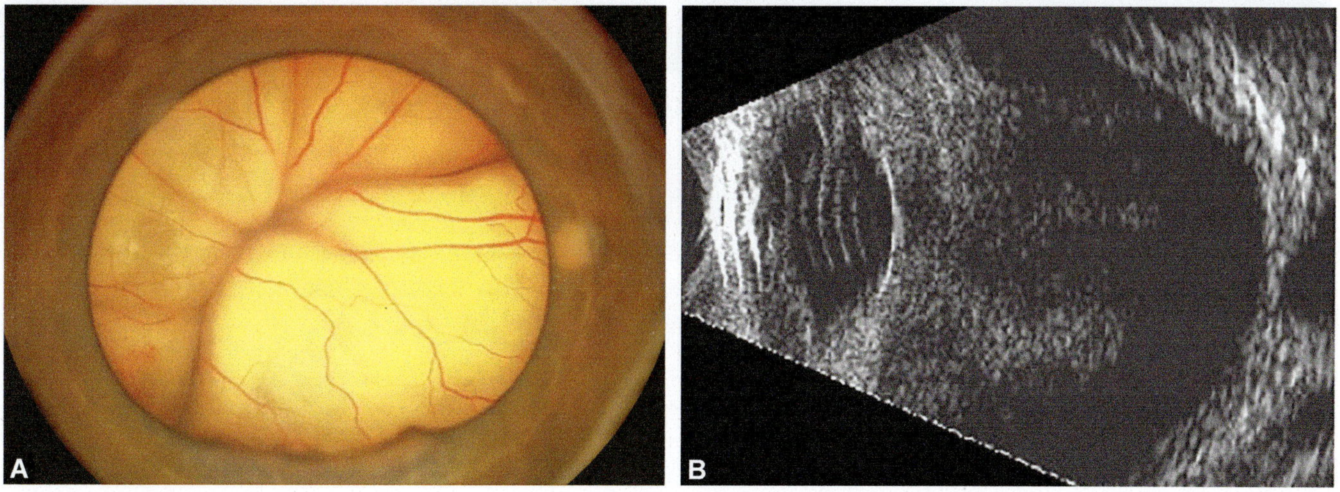

Figs. 76.12A and B: Coats disease in the right eye of 22-month-old child. (A) Xanthocoria (yellow pupillary reflex) secondary to the subretinal exudative material accumulated under the detached retina. Note the telangiectasias of the retinal vessels inferotemporally; (B) B-scan ultrasonography shows absence of intraocular mass.

Associated Diseases

Retinoblastoma may be associated with a 13q-syndrome (*see* Figs. 76.2A and B) and Down's syndrome, both characterized with typical dysmorphic features. Other coincidental associations (Lowe syndrome, microphthalmia, persistent fetal vasculature (PFV), optic nerve hypoplasia, retinopathy of prematurity, Coats disease, and cataract) have been reported.[18]

Differential Diagnosis

Several conditions known as pseudoretinoblastoma can simulate retinoblastoma by presenting a white fundus lesion and/or leukocoria. The most frequent and clinically close differential diagnosis is Coats disease (Figs. 76.12A and B). The main conditions that resemble retinoblastoma are listed in Box 76.1.[19] Comprehensive history with thorough clinical examination and appropriate ancillary tests usually enable misdiagnosis and undesirable treatments to be avoided. Fine-needle aspiration biopsy is rarely needed to establish a diagnosis.

Box 76.1: Pseudoretinoblastoma.

A. *Developmental abnormalities*: • Persistent hyperplastic primary vitreous (PHPV), persistent fetal vasculature • Posterior coloboma • Congenital retinal folds • Myelinated nerve fibers • Morning glory syndrome • Retinal dysplasia • Congenital cataract • Congenital retinoschisis • Incontinentia pigmenti • Norrie disease	C. *Vascular abnormalities*: • Coats disease • Retinopathy of prematurity • Familial exudative vitreoretinopathy D. *Tumors*: • Retinal astrocytic hamartoma • Medulloepithelioma • Glioneuroma • Choroidal hemangioma • Retinal capillary hemangioma • Combined retinal hamartoma • Leukemia • Juvenile xanthogranuloma • Melanoma
B. *Inflammatory disorders*: • Ocular toxocariasis • Congenital toxoplasmosis • Congenital cytomegalovirus retinitis • Herpes simplex retinitis • Endogenous or metastatic endophthalmitis • Orbital cellulitis	E. *Miscellaneous*: • Rhegmatogenous retinal detachment • Vitreous hemorrhage • Trauma • Other

Clinical Examination and Imaging

Children with retinoblastoma should be referred to a specialized ocular and pediatric oncology center. Examination under anesthesia (EUA) is mandatory for a proper assessment of the extent of the tumor. Refraction, corneal diameters, intraocular pressure, anterior chamber slit-lamp examination and dilated fundus examination of both eyes with indentation should be performed at initial diagnosis and every follow-up. RetCam photography is useful in documenting clinical findings and monitoring treatment response. Fluorescein angiography shows characteristic features of the tumor which can vary with the growth pattern of the tumor (Figs. 76.13A and B).[13] It is also performed for both posterior and anterior segment to determine any treatment-related complications such as retinal ischemia or neovascularization. Ultrasound may confirm the presence of a calcified tumor and evaluate

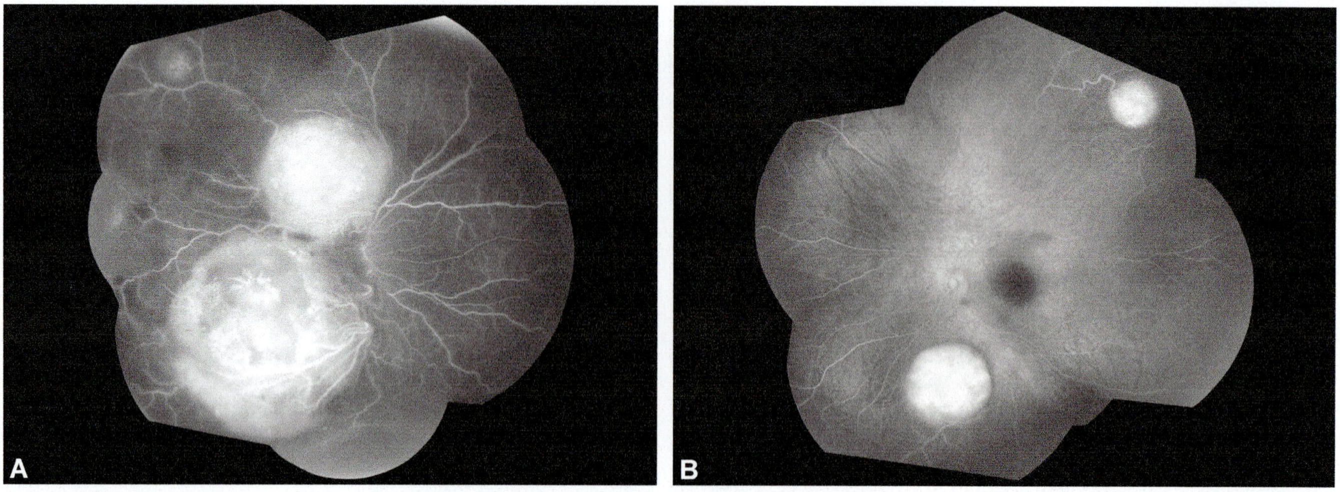

Figs. 76.13A and B: Fluorescein angiography. (A) Venous phase of the tumors shown in Figure 76.8A. Enlarged feeding and drainage vessels of the two tumors located at the posterior pole. The central hypofluorescence in the macular tumor represents areas of ischemia. Note that all four tumors have intrinsic vascularization with early leakage; (B) Venous phase of the tumors shown in Figure 76.8B.

any optic nerve invasion. Handheld optic coherence tomography can be used to assess the fovea status, detect subclinical tumor or recurrence and monitor treatment response (Figs. 76.14A and B).[20] Ultrasonographic biomicroscopy (UBM) is useful for the assessment of the ciliary body and both anterior and posterior chamber (Fig. 76.15).[21] Although the diagnosis of retinoblastoma is clinical, orbito-cerebral MRI [ideally 1.5 or 3-Tesla (T)] is usually performed at diagnosis in order to evaluate any extraocular involvement, especially if the tumor covers the optic nerve and assess the pineal gland (trilateral retinoblastoma) (Fig. 76.16). Systemic metastatic evaluation (typically bone marrow and lumbar puncture) is usually not indicated in children without neurologic abnormalities or evidence of extraocular extension. However, lumbar puncture is recommended in the case of obscured optic nerve head. Parents and siblings should be evaluated for untreated retinoblastoma or spontaneously arrested or regressed retinoblastoma (retinoma), as this would provide evidence for a hereditary predisposition to the disease.

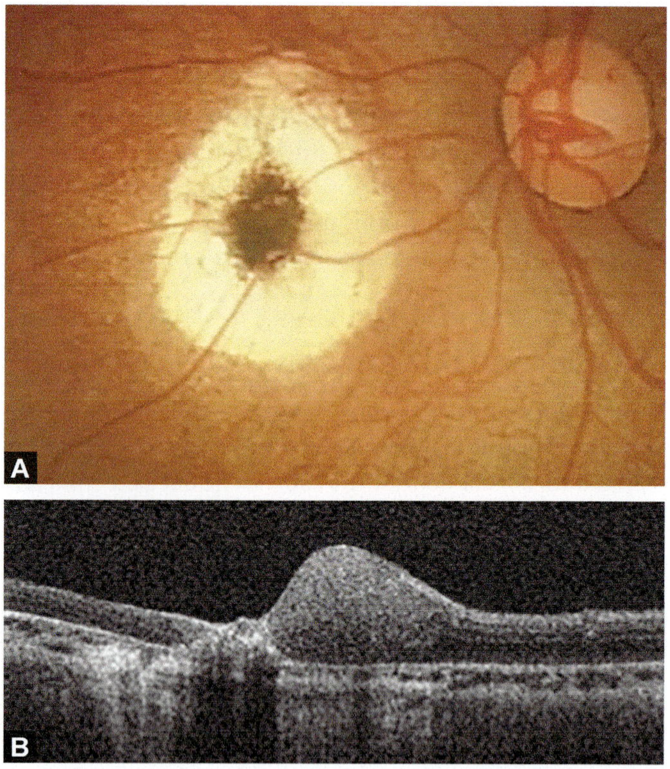

Figs. 76.14A and B: Subclinical detection of retinoblastoma relapse. (A) Follow-up of clinically regressed tumor type 4 (atrophic scar) after transpupillary thermotherapy; (B) Hand-held spectral domain optical coherence tomography showing a homogeneous elevated lesion corresponding to tumor recurrence.

Classification

The classification of intraocular retinoblastoma (grouping) for globe salvage prognosis has known a steady evolution over time parallel to the prevalent modalities of available treatment options. Currently the International Intraocular Retinoblastoma Classification (IIRC)[22] provides a correlation of the natural history of intraocular tumor and likelihood of success with chemoreduction and is the system used in most major retinoblastoma center (Table 76.1). The International Retinoblastoma Staging System (IRSS) [23] proposed in 2006 stratifies extraocular disease for survival prognosis (Table 76.2). Recently the

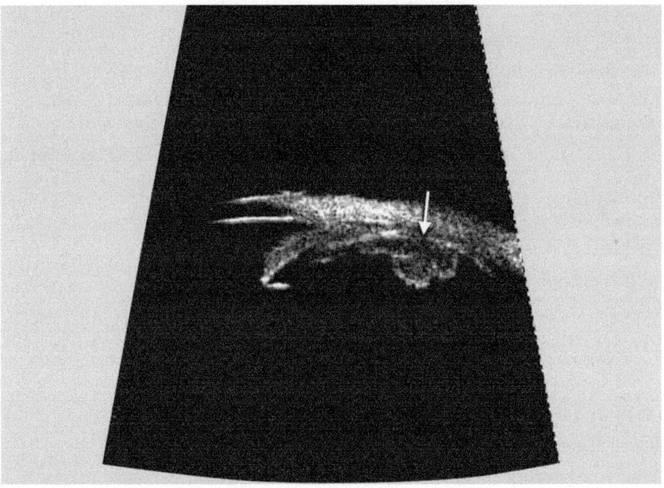

Fig. 76.15: Ultrasound biomicroscopy (UBM) showing the presence of a parietal tumor (arrow). Note that identification of a tumor-free pars plana entry site is mandatory to prevent active mechanisms of tumor spread when performing intravitreal injection of chemotherapy.

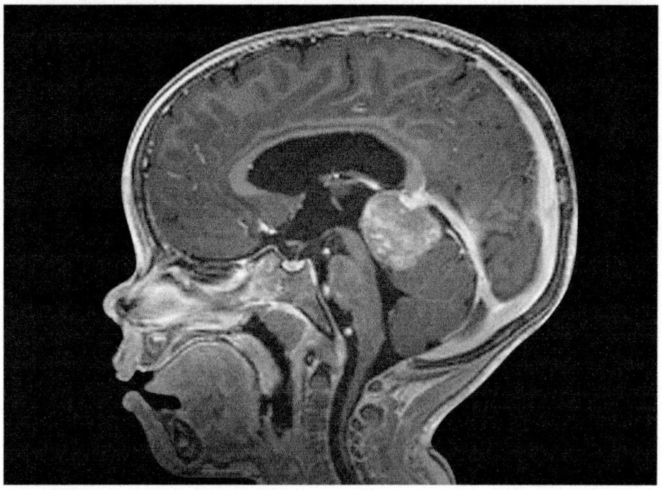

Fig. 76.16: Sagittal magnetic resonance imaging (MRI) in a child with bilateral retinoblastoma showing pinealoblastoma (trilateral retinoblastoma).

Table 76.1: International Intraocular Retinoblastoma Classification (IIRC).

Group A	Small tumors (≤3 mm) confined to the retina (no seeding), at least 3 mm from the fovea and 1.5 mm from optic nerve
Group B	Tumors (>3 mm) confined to the retina in any location, with clear subretinal fluid ≤5 mm from the tumor margin
Group C	Localized vitreous and/or subretinal seeding (<5 mm in total from tumor margin). Up to 1 quadrant subretinal fluid may be present
Group D	Diffuse vitreous and/or subretinal seeding (≥5 mm in total from tumor margin) and/or massive, nondiscrete endophytic or exophytic disease
Group E	Massive retinoblastoma with anatomic or functional destruction of the eye with one or more of the following: • Neovascular glaucoma • Massive intravitreal hemorrhage • Aseptic orbital cellulitis • Tumor anterior to anterior vitreous face • Tumor touching the lens • Diffuse infiltrating tumor • Phthisis or pre-phthisis

Source: Linn Murphree A. Intraocular retinoblastoma: the case for a new group classification. Ophthalmol Clin North Am. 2005;18(1):41-54, viii.

8th edition of "Tumor, Node, Metastasis, and Heritability" cancer staging system for retinoblastoma,[24] making the first system to include heritability (HX, H0, H1), has been proposed to most accurately predict the salvage of the eye(s), metastasis, and death and aims to replace the IIRC (Table 76.3).

PATHOLOGY

Macroscopically, retinoblastoma is a white tumor that arises from the sensory retina, often with chalky-white foci of calcification. Areas of tumor necrosis and hemorrhage are sometimes seen. The endophytic, exophytic or diffuse pattern can usually be recognized on gross examination of the sectioned eye (Fig. 76.17).[13]

Microscopically, retinoblastoma cells have round, oval, or spindle-shaped nuclei of approximately twice the size of a lymphocyte and stain blue with hematoxylin and eosin (H&E) stain. Their nuclei are hyperchromatic with a usually high mitotic activity and are surrounded by an almost imperceptible amount of cytoplasm. Zones of viable tumor cells can coexist with areas of necrosis (pink on H&E stain) and calcification (blue-red on H&E stain) (Fig. 76.18). DNA released from necrotic cells and distinguished as basophilic material may be detected surrounding the tumor vessels.[25]

Retinoblastoma can present various degrees of differentiation, however this is not considered an important prognostic factor.[26] Characteristic features of well-differentiated retinoblastoma are the Flexner-Wintersteiner rosettes and fleurettes, structures that represent attempts of the tumor toward photoreceptor differentiation (Fig. 76.19). Flexner-Wintersteiner rosettes are composed of a ring of columnar cells with eosinophilic cytoplasm and peripheral situated nuclei surrounding an empty lumen, whereas

Table 76.2: International Retinoblastoma Staging System (IRSS).

Stage 0	Stage I	Stage II	Stage III: Regional extension	Stage IV: Metastatic disease	
Conservative treatment	Eye enucleated Completely resected histologically	Eye enucleated Microscopic residual tumor	A. Overt orbital disease B. Preauricular or cervical lymph node extension	A. Hematogenous metastases 1. Single lesion 2. Multiple lesions	B. CNS extension 1. Prechiasmatic lesion 2. CNS mass 3. Leptomeningeal disease

(CNS: Central nervous system)
NB: In cases of bilateral disease, the staging depends on the eye with more advanced disease.
Source: Chantada G Doz F, Antoneli CB, et al. A proposal for an international retinoblastoma staging system. Pediatric Blood Cancer. 2006;47(6):801-5.

Table 76.3: American Joint Committee on Cancer (AJCC) Clinical Staging, 8th edition 2017.

Clinical definitions (cTNM)		
Category	**Subcategory**	**Description**
cT1		*Intra-retinal tumor(s)* with subretinal fluid ≤ 5 mm from base of any tumor
	cT1a	Tumors ≤ 3 mm and further than 1.5 mm from disk and fovea
	cT1b	Tumors > 3 mm or closer than 1.5 mm from disk or fovea
cT2		*Intraocular tumor(s)* with retinal detachment, vitreous seeding, or subretinal seeding
	cT2a	Subretinal fluid > 5 mm from the base of any tumor
	cT2b	Vitreous seeding and/or subretinal seeding
cT3		*Advanced intraocular tumor(s)*
	cT3a	Phthisis or pre-phthisis bulbi
	cT3b	Tumor invasion of choroid, pars plana, ciliary body, lens, zonules, iris, or anterior chamber
	cT3c	Raised intraocular pressure with neovascularization and/or buphthalmos
	cT3d	Hyphema and/or massive vitreous hemorrhage
	cT3e	Aseptic orbital cellulitis
cT4		*Extraocular tumor(s)* involving orbit, including optic nerve
	cT4a	Radiologic evidence of retrobulbar optic nerve involvement or thickening of optic nerve
	cT4b	Extraocular tumor clinically evident with proptosis and/or an orbital mass
N1		Evidence of preauricular, submandibular, and *cervical lymph node involvement*
cM1		Clinical signs of *distant metastasis*
	cM1a	Tumor(s) involving any distant site (e.g. bone marrow and liver) on clinical or radiologic tests
	cM1b	Tumor involving the CNS on radiologic imaging (not including trilateral retinoblastoma)
H		*Hereditary trait*
	HX	Unknown or insufficient evidence of a constitutional *RB1* gene mutation
	H0	Normal *RB1* alleles in blood tested with demonstrated high-sensitivity assays
	H1	Bilateral retinoblastoma, retinoblastoma with an intracranial primitive neuroectodermal tumor (i.e. trilateral retino-blastoma), patient with family history of retinoblastoma, or molecular definition of a constitutional *RB1* gene mutation
Pathological definitions (pTNM)		
Category	**Subcategory**	**Description**
pT1		Intraocular tumor(s) without any *local invasion*, or with focal choroidal invasion, or pre- or intralaminar involvement of the optic nerve
pT2		Intraocular tumor(s) with *local invasion*
	pT2a	Concomitant focal choroidal invasion and pre- or intralaminar involvement of the optic nerve head
	pT2b	Tumor invasion of stroma of iris and/or trabecular meshwork and/or Schlemm's canal
pT3		Intraocular tumor(s) with *significant local invasion*
	pT3a	Massive choroidal invasion (>3 mm in largest diameter, or multiple foci of focal choroidal involvement totalling >3 mm, or any full-thickness choroidal involvement)
	pT3b	Retrolaminar invasion of the optic nerve head, not involving the transected end of the optic nerve
	pT3c	Any partial-thickness involvement of the sclera within the inner two-thirds
	pT3d	Full-thickness invasion into outer third of the sclera and/or invasion into or around emissary channels
cT4		*Extraocular tumor(s)* involving orbit, including optic nerve
	cT4a	Evidence of extraocular tumor: tumor at the transected end of the optic nerve, tumor in the meningeal spaces around the optic nerve, full thickness invasion of the sclera with invasion of the episclera, adjacent adipose tissue, extraocular muscle, bone, conjunctiva, or eyelids

(CNS: Central nervous system)

Source: Mallipatna AC, Gallie BL, Chévez-Barrios P, et al. Retinoblastoma. In: Amin MB, Edge SB, Greene FL, Byrd DR, Brookland RK, Washington MK (Eds). AJCC Cancer Staging Manual, 8th edition. New York: Springer; 2017. pp. 819-31

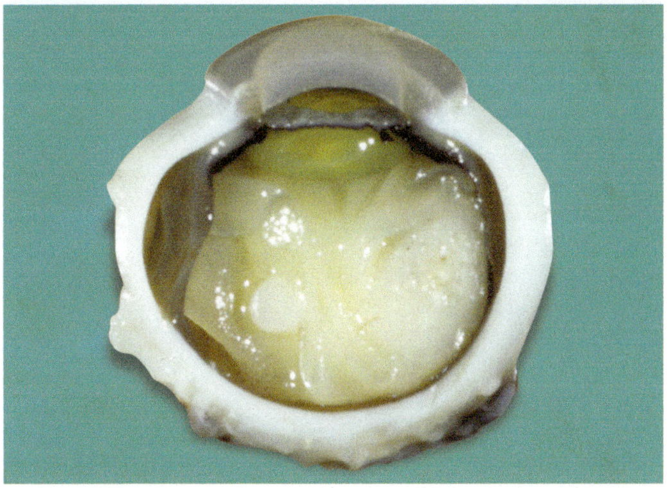

Fig. 76.17: Section of an enucleated eye showing total retinal detachment and voluminous exophytic retinoblastoma touching the lens (group E).
Source: Dr S Uffer.

fleurettes have undergone an even greater photoreceptor differentiation and are composed of curvilinear clusters of cells composed of photoreceptor inner segments (Fig. 76.20). A less common form of rosettes, the Homer-Wright rosettes (sometimes referred as pseudorosettes), are found in other neuroblastic tumors such as neuroblastoma, but can also be found in retinoblastoma. Homer-Wright rosettes consist of a ring of cells with an eosinophilic fibrillary center without lumen (Fig. 76.21). The less differentiated retinoblastoma tumor comprises mostly anaplastic cells without rosette or fleurette formation and have more nuclear pleomorphism and mitotic figures.[13,25]

Finally, retinoma (or retinocytoma) is considered a benign precursor of retinoblastoma that can nevertheless undergo malignant transformation (see below). It is characterized by numerous fleurettes admixed with individual cells that demonstrate varying degrees of photoreceptor differentiation. Retinoma differs from retinoblastoma in having more cytoplasm and more evenly dispersed nuclear chromatin than do retinoblastoma cells, with no mitoses.[25]

OTHER FORMS OF RETINOBLASTOMA

Retinoma (Retinocytoma)

Retinoma or retinocytoma is a spontaneously arrested or regressed retinoblastoma. Its incidence in the general population is unknown but ranges from 1.8% to 10% among first-degree relatives of individuals diagnosed with or

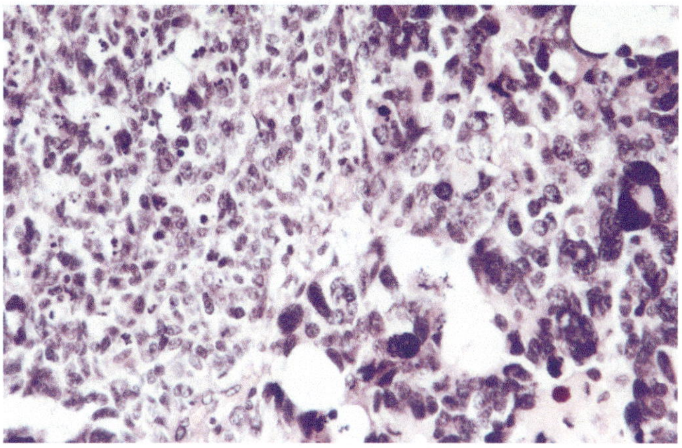

Fig. 76.18: Poorly differentiated retinoblastoma.
Source: Dr S Uffer.

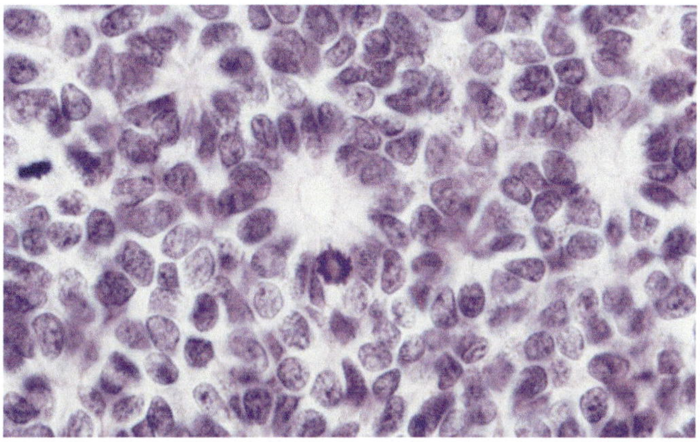

Fig. 76.19: Differentiated retinoblastoma. Typical Flexner–Wintersteiner rosettes. Note the empty lumen of the rosette (hematoxylin-eosin).
Source: Dr A Moulin.

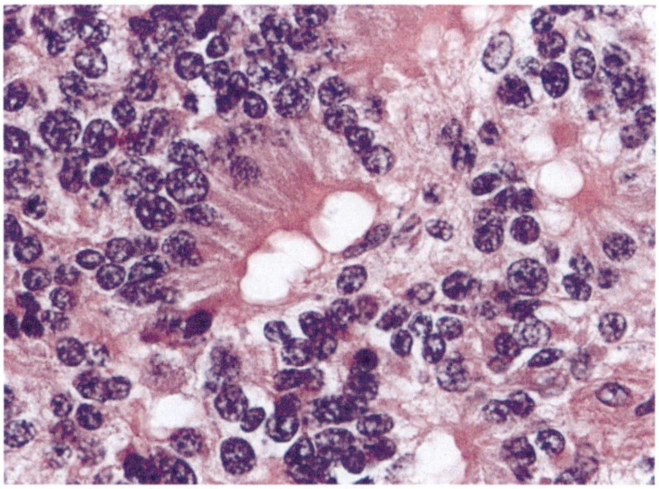

Fig. 76.20: High magnification of fleurettes. The bulbous cellular extension of retinoblastoma cells represents differentiation along the lines of photoreceptor inner segments (hematoxylin-eosin).
Source: Dr A Moulin

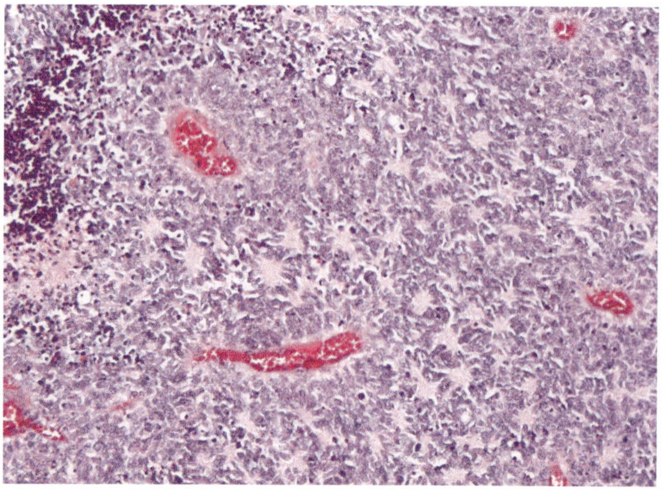

Fig. 76.21: Homer-Wright rosettes typical for neuroblastic differentiation (seen also in neuroblastoma and medulloblastoma) (hematoxylin-eosin). *Source:* Dr A Moulin.

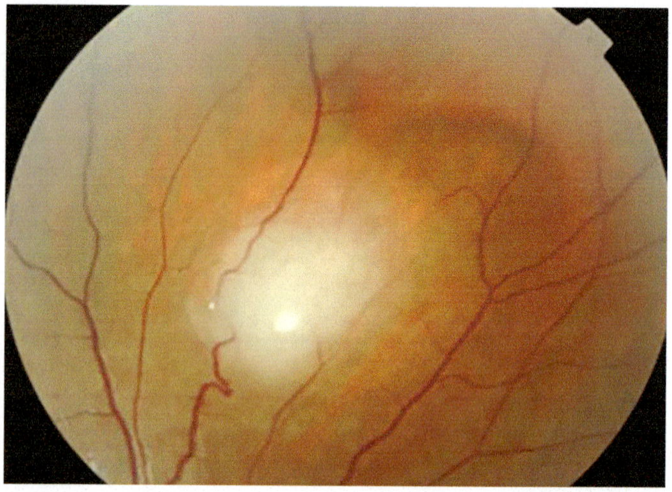

Fig. 76.22: Spontaneously arrested retinoblastoma (retinoma) in a 6-year-old boy. Note the fish-flesh lesion with a central calcification (type 3 pattern) and absence of surrounding alteration of the retinal pigment epithelium. The lesion has remained stable for 12 years.

having a family history of retinoblastoma.[18,27] Spontaneously arrested retinoblastoma appears clinically to have reached a certain size and remain stable despite no treatment (Fig. 76.22). Spontaneously regressed retinoblastoma is characterized by perilesional alterations of the retinal pigment epithelium, similar to a tumor that would have shrunk after a successful treatment (Figs. 76.23A and B).[13,27] Retinoma and retinoblastoma can coexist in the same eye, individual or family (Fig. 76.24). Most of these lesions are diagnosed incidentally on routine eye examination or when a retinoblastoma is found in another family member. Sometimes the diagnosis is made retrospectively when the retinoblastoma shows a poor response to treatment. Retinoma necessitates a lifelong follow-up it can undergo spontaneously malignant transformation into retinoblastoma. Finally, it should be noted that retinoma carries the same genetic implications as retinoblastoma.[28]

Orbital Retinoblastoma

Orbital retinoblastoma is an advanced form of retinoblastoma mostly seen in developing countries. Orbital retinoblastoma generally manifests later than intraocular retinoblastoma, at around 3 years of age.[29] Primary orbital retinoblastoma is the orbital extension of the disease which is evident at presentation clinically or radiologically. Most of the patients with primary orbital retinoblastoma will present with proptosis or a large fungating mass (*see* Fig. 76.5). Secondary orbital retinoblastoma occurs in an enucleated socket after an uncomplicated surgery. Clinically it may present as a palpable mass or an unexplained displacement of the intraorbital implant. The term overt orbital retinoblastoma refers to previously unrecognized extrascleral or optic nerve extension during enucleation. Microscopic orbital retinoblastoma is identified on histopathologic examination of the enucleated eye ball only as a full thickness scleral infiltration, extrascleral extension or optic nerve sheath infiltration. Orbital disease increases the risk of systemic metastasis by 10–27 times and the mortality range from 25% to 100%.[29] In case of orbital retinoblastoma, the current preferred management is multimodal with a combination of chemotherapy, surgery, and external beam radiotherapy (EBRT).

Metastatic Retinoblastoma

Metastatic retinoblastoma occurs in less than 5% of all cases in high income countries, where it occurs usually as a relapse a few months following enucleation. In developing countries, metastatic disease is the major cause of death associated with retinoblastoma. The retinoblastoma can give rise to systemic metastasis after invading the choroid or after extension to the orbit and the lymph nodes followed by hematogenous dissemination. The most frequent locations of metastatic retinoblastoma are bones, bone marrow, and CNS, other organs such as the liver being less frequently involved. Note that CNS dissemination can also occur by direct extension through the optic nerve. Orbito-cerebral MRI, cerebrospinal fluid examination, bone

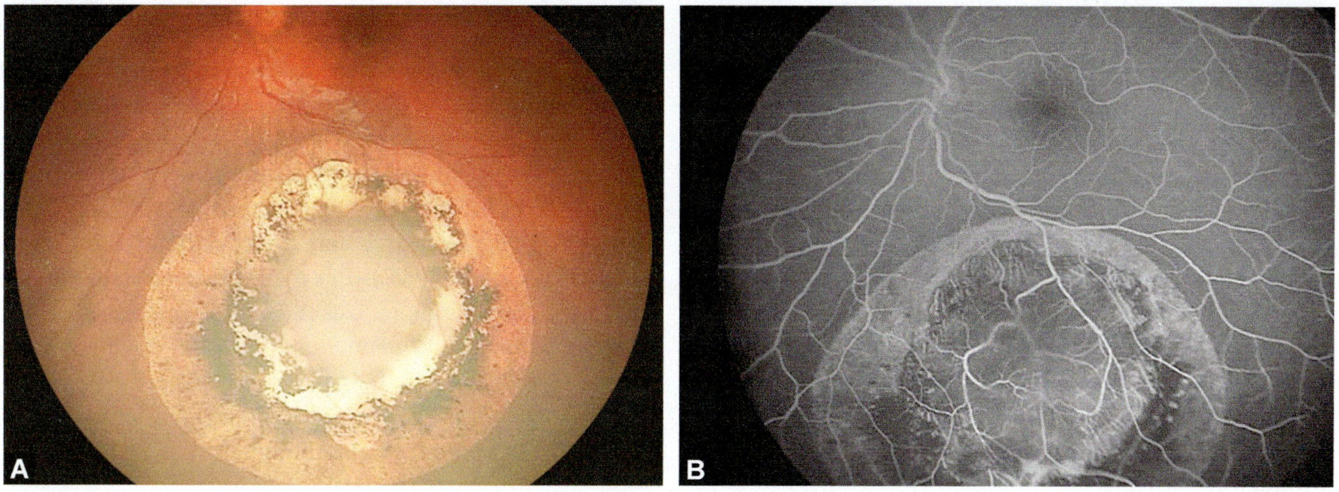

Figs. 76.23A and B: (A) Spontaneously regressed retinoblastoma (retinoma) seen on a routine examination in a 5-year-old boy. Note the fish-flesh appearance of the lesion (type 2 pattern) surrounded by atrophic alterations of the retinal pigment epithelium suggesting that the lesion had grown to a certain size and then regressed; (B) Fluorescein angiography with no signs of tumoral activity. The lesion has remained stable for 6 years.

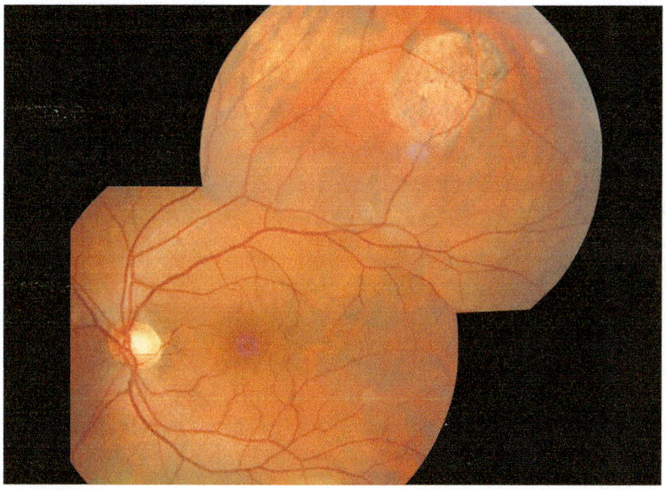

Fig. 76.24: Spontaneously regressed retinoblastoma (retinoma) in the father of a child with bilateral retinoblastoma (type 4 pattern).

marrow evaluation, bone scintigraphy, and abdominal ultrasonography are performed in all cases of metastatic retinoblastoma for staging the disease.[17] Treatment with high dose chemotherapy and autologous stem cell rescue is the only curative treatment currently available for non-CNS metastatic retinoblastoma.[30]

Trilateral Retinoblastoma

The term trilateral retinoblastoma (*see* Fig. 76.16) refers to the presence of a bilateral retinoblastoma associated with intracranial midline primitive neuroectodermal tumor usually located in the pineal gland (pinealoblastoma) or the suprasellar and parasellar region.[31] These intracranial lesions, which are similar to retinoblastoma from embryologic, immunologic and phylogenic standpoints, are true primary tumors (not metastases). Patients with germline *RB1* mutations carry a risk of about 5% of developing trilateral retinoblastoma and should undergo serial imaging of the CNS (minimum once a year), for early detection (ideally 1.5- or 3-T MRI with and without contrast which is most sensitive for CNS involvement and does not expose the patient to radiation) until 6 years of age.[31]

TREATMENTS

Introduction

The management of retinoblastoma is complex and multidisciplinary by nature and should thus be referred to a specialized retinoblastoma team consisting of the ocular and pediatric oncologists, assisted by ocular pathologist, radiologist, interventional neuroradiologist, and geneticist. The primary aim of retinoblastoma treatment is patient survival, followed by globe salvage and ultimately vision rehabilitation. The choice of treatment is based on tumor extent, laterality, IIRC grouping, IRSS staging, and any prior treatments. Conservative management of intraocular retinoblastoma is often achieved by a combination of treatment modalities.

Over the last century, the management of retinoblastoma has known tremendous changes. Initially the only therapeutic option was enucleation. Since the early 1900s, EBRT became for many years the main alternative to enucleation. Although credited with excellent tumor control, EBRT increased the incidence of second cancers, mainly in the field of irradiation, and was also associated with mid-facial hypoplasia (Fig. 76.27) and radiation-induced ocular complications such as cataract, retinopathy, and neuropathy.[11] In the mid-1990s, the use of EBRT was drastically reduced by the introduction of intravenous chemotherapy (IVC), commonly referred to as chemoreduction, associated with focal treatments (cryotherapy, thermotherapy, and laser photocoagulation).[2] Two decades later, the introduction of intra-arterial chemotherapy (IAC) and intravitreal chemotherapy enabled high tumoricidal drug concentrations to be targeted, thus radically transforming the management of retinoblastoma and allowing globe salvage of even advanced retinoblastoma, eliminating definitively the use of EBRT at least as first-line treatment.[32]

Intravenous Chemotherapy

Intravenous chemotherapy aims at decreasing tumor size (chemoreduction), allowing subsequent consolidation with focal therapy such as laser, cryotherapy or brachytherapy. The main agents used for chemoreduction are vincristine, etoposide, and carboplatin in appropriate doses.[2]

Intravenous chemotherapy is still the most widely used conservative treatment worldwide. In centers that could provide IAC as an alternative, IVC is currently performed in cases of bilateral diseases or in unilateral diseases in very young patients (< 3 months old and/or with low body weight < 5 kg) as bridge therapy until vascular maturation allows the child to undergo the IAC safely.[32]

The main reasons for failure of conservative treatment with IVC were subretinal seeding and intravitreous seeding, these nowadays better controlled with intra-arterial and intravitreal chemotherapy respectively.[2]

Chemothermotherapy

Chemothermotherapy (CTT) consists of a combination of transpupillary thermotherapy (TTT, see focal treatments) delivered 1–2 hours after intravenous injection of a single dose of carboplatin. With this sequence, the cytotoxic effect of TTT is raised by virtue of a synergetic effect between heat and drug at the time of its plasmatic peak. Two cycles of chemoreduction are generally administered before CTT in order to decrease the tumor volume first. Typically, a mean of 2 cycles of CTT are required to obtain satisfactory tumor control.[33] The advantage of this therapy is that the chemotherapy is reduced to one drug, and local control is comparable to multiagent regimens. In centers where IAC is available, however, CTT is now only rarely used.

Intra-arterial Chemotherapy

Intra-arterial chemotherapy allows the delivery of high-dose concentrations of chemotherapy agents directly into the eye and with minimal systemic exposure by direct catheterization of the ophthalmic artery. The modern injection technique was described by Abramson and Gobin in 2008.[34] In cases where direct catheterization of the ophthalmic artery fails, other techniques are still possible via various collaterals such as the middle meningeal artery, or by using a balloon transiently inflated downstream to the ostium of the ophthalmic artery.[35] The injected drug of choice is melphalan, with the dosage based on patient weight. Melphalan can also be used in association with topotecan and/or carboplatin.

Intra-arterial chemotherapy can be used as first-line treatment (Figs. 76.25A and B) or in case of recurrence in pretreated eyes (rescue or salvage IAC). Nowadays, IAC is considered as the first-line choice of naïve unilateral group C or D, as well as the preferred salvage treatment for eyes with retinal or subretinal relapse.[32] In cases of bilateral advanced disease, some groups use sequential IAC (tandem IAC). This technique involves retracting the catheter after the first injection, followed by advancing it to the ostium of the contralateral ophthalmic artery.[36]

Compared to IVC, IAC has been shown to provide significantly superior globe salvage (91% vs. 48%, $p = 0.004$) as well as better control for solid tumors (92% vs. 62%, $p = 0.002$), subretinal seeds (86% vs. 31%, $p = 0.006$), and vitreous seeds (74% vs. 25%, $p = 0.006$).[37] Moreover, the use of IAC in group D eyes allowed the time to success to be significantly reduced by half.[38]

The most frequent systemic side effect of IAC is neutropenia, although only affecting 12% versus 80% when patients are treated with IVC. Most local adverse effects include transient lid or periocular edema or redness (29%), ptosis (6%), and thinning or loss of eyelashes (5%).[2] Intraocular toxicity (particularly occlusive choroidopathy and retinal ischemia) is to date poorly understood. Multicentric data collection over a 10-year period of time showed less than 1% risk for metastatic deaths after primary or secondary (salvage) IAC.[39]

Intravitreal and Intracameral Chemotherapy

Treatment of vitreous seeding was challenging because of lack of vasculature in the vitreous, resulting in the inability to achieve tumoricidal concentrations with IVC or IAC.

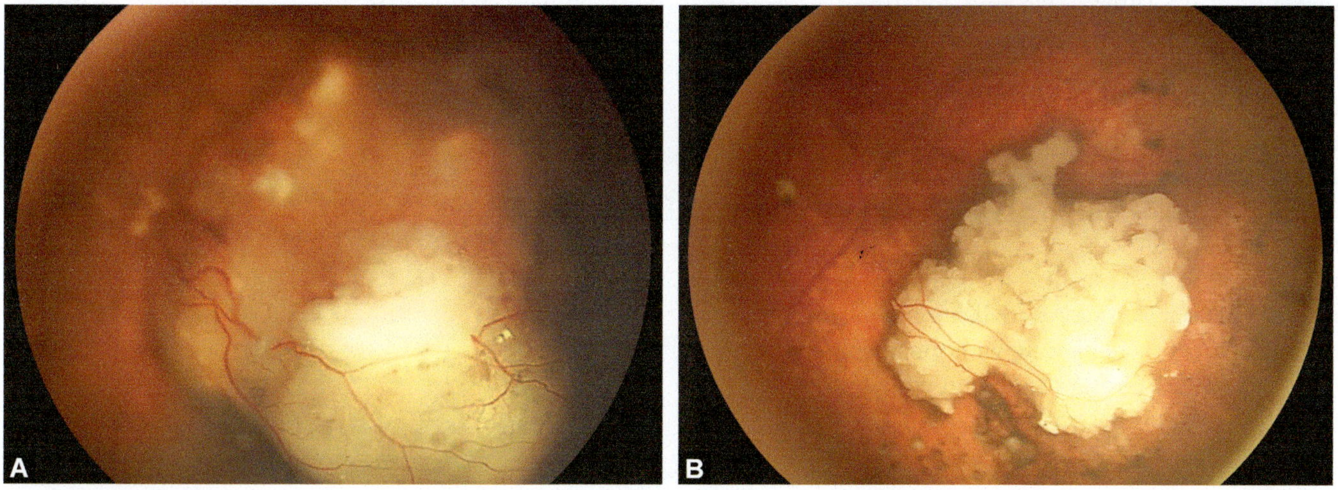

Figs. 76.25A and B: Unilateral retinoblastoma group D in a 3.5-year-old boy. (A) At diagnosis, large exophytic nasal mass partially covering the optic disk. Note the rupture of the internal limiting membrane at the apex with vitreous seeds (spheres); (B) After only two cycles of intra-arterial chemotherapy, lesion showing a type 1 regression pattern. The tumor has remained stable for 4.5 years without further treatment.

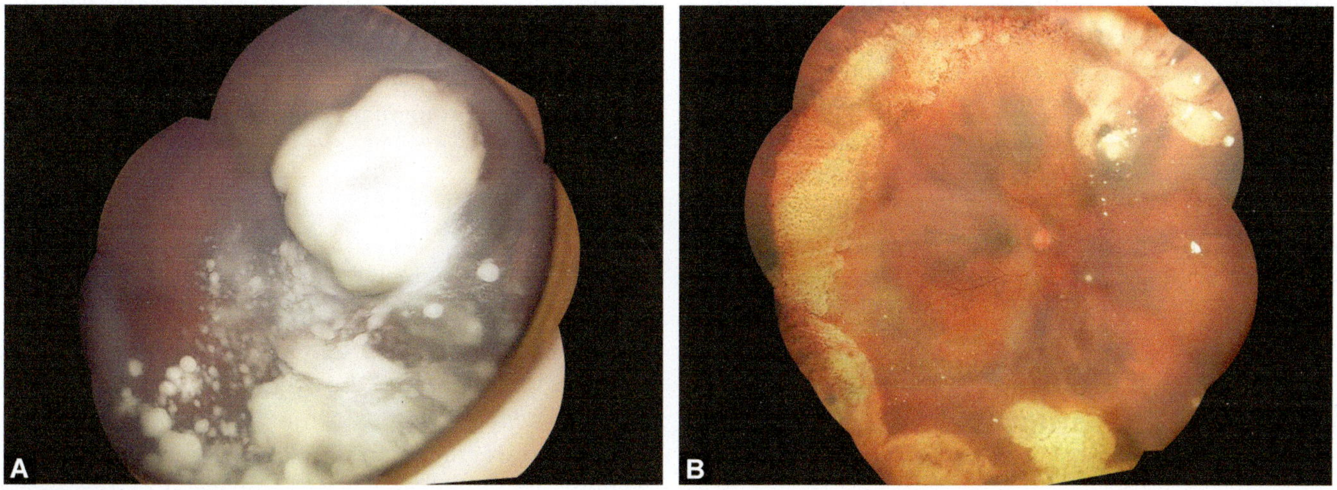

Figs. 76.26A and B: Unilateral endophytic retinoblastoma group D in a 22-month-old boy. (A) At presentation, massive vitreous seeding (dust, spheres, and cloud) obscuring the optic disk view; (B) After one cycle of intra-arterial melphalan chemotherapy, eight intravitreal injections of melphalan and focal treatments. Note the completely regressed vitreous seeding (type 1, refringent calcified seeds). The superonasal primary tumor shows a type 3 (90% calcified) regression pattern. Peripheral cryocoagulation scars.

Fear of extraocular tumor spread prohibited for a long time the use of intravitreal injection of chemotherapy in retinoblastoma patients. In 2012, Munier et al. introduced the modern injection technique through the pars plana (lacking seeds or tumor) with a 32-G needle, using small volume (0.1–0.15 mL) doses of 20–30 μg melphalan, lowering the intraocular pressure with a paracentesis before the injection and sealing the site during removal of the needle with cryotherapy. This technique has since proven to be safe and efficient (68–100% success in vitreous seeds across multiples studies) and is now widely adopted (Figs. 76.26A and B).[2,40,41] The most common side effect is a localized RPE mottling at the site of the injection, this observed in 43% of the cases.[14] Promising results have recently been published with intracameral melphalan for anterior chamber seeding.[42]

Focal Treatments

Focal treatments can be used to treat primary small tumors or recurrence as well as in combination with chemotherapy or plaque brachytherapy for consolidation.[2,40] The treatments are repeated as necessary, the choice of therapy depending on tumor size and location. Transscleral cryotherapy is applied under visualization using indirect ophthalmoscopy with a triple freeze-thaw technique and is typically considered for small lesions located between the equator and the ora serrata. Lesions posterior to the equator are commonly treated with diode laser (810 nm) TTT, which delivers thermal heat directly to the surface of the tumor (45–60° Celsius range).[40] Transscleral diopexy uses a diode laser probe to heat peripheral lesions through the sclera under visualization in a similar way as transscleral cryocoagulation, with the advantage of being less destructive. Photocoagulation with argon laser (532 nm) represents an option to treat small posteriorly located lesions.[40]

Plaque Radiotherapy (Brachytherapy)

Plaque radiotherapy is usually used to treat relapse of a tumor having previously undergone other treatments. The two commonly used radioisotopes are iodine 125 (I^{125}) and ruthenium 106 (Ru^{106}).[43,44] The plaque is secured on the episclera adjacent to the tumor and allows a reduced dose delivery to normal ocular structures and greater irradiation to the tumor base. The dose delivered is usually 45 Gy to the apex of the tumor. Radiation-related complications become manifest usually after the first year. These are, however, less frequent with Ru^{106} because of its limited lateral dosimetry compared to I^{125}.[44]

Periocular Chemotherapy

Periocular chemotherapy (POC) with topotecan or carboplatin enables a tumoricidal dose to be achieved rapidly at 6–10 times the level within the vitreous than that achieved by IVC, and was commonly used for advanced retinoblastoma with diffuse seeding before the introduction of intra-arterial and intravitreal chemotherapy.[45]

External Beam Radiotherapy

External beam radiotherapy was the most popular globe-salvage therapy in retinoblastoma before the introduction of chemotherapy in the 1990s. Side effects of the treatment on the bony orbit included radiation-induced secondary cancer (mainly osteosarcoma) and cosmetic deformity, especially when given before 1 year of age (Fig. 76.27). More sophisticated radiation techniques such as stereotactic conformal or proton beam irradiation were developed to minimize dose to bone and soft tissues.[46] In the era of intra-arterial and intravitreal chemotherapy however, external irradiation for intraocular retinoblastoma has now been virtually eradicated.[32]

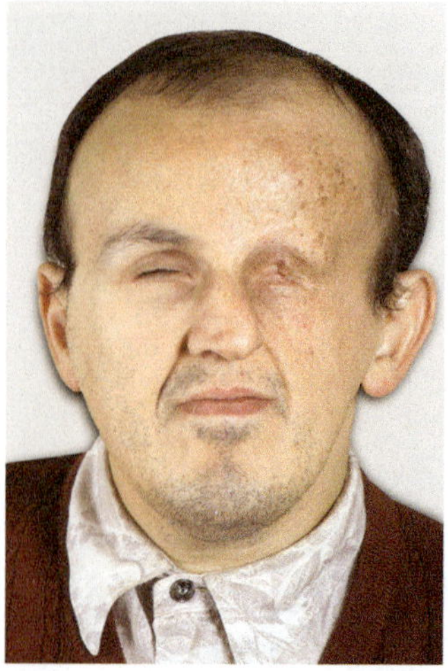

Fig. 76.27: Radiation-induced osseous deformity and eyebrows loss following external beam radiotherapy and bilateral enucleation in early childhood in a patient with bilateral retinoblastoma.

Enucleation

Enucleation consists of the removal of the eye. Replacement of the volume of the eye with an implant deep within the orbit and provision of a prosthetic eye worn in the conjunctival sac behind the eyelids generally provides a good cosmetic outcome. Current indications for primary enucleation are group E and group D (especially in unilateral retinoblastoma) with no visual potential and/or suspicion of retrolaminar invasion. Secondary enucleation is indicated in case of conservative therapy failure, or for eyes developing complications such as untreatable retinal detachment, neovascular complications, intravitreal hemorrhage or phthisis. Histopathologic examination of enucleated eyes is important in order to rule out exteriorization (extrascleral extension, positive optic nerve section) of the disease or higher risk factors for metastasis (choroidal invasion of ≥ 3 mm in largest diameter and/or retrolaminar optic nerve invasion) and evaluate the indication for adjuvant systemic chemotherapy (Fig. 76.28).[47] Recent studies showed that anterior chamber seeding, as well as anterior uveal invasion (iris and/or corpus ciliaris), are no longer considered a risk for metastasis by some centers.[48]

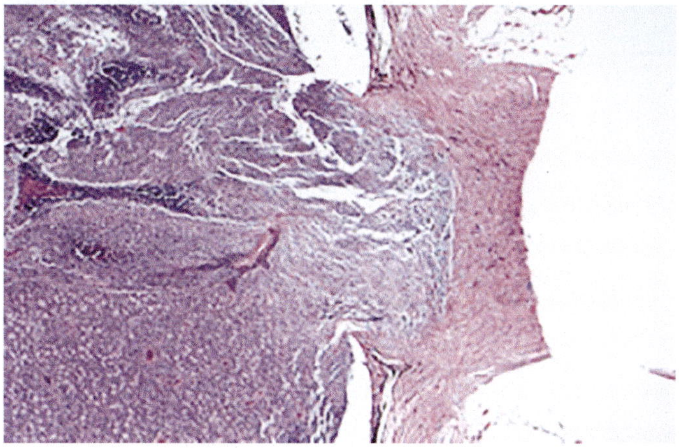

Fig. 76.28: Retinoblastoma covering and invading the optic nerve posterior to the lamina cribrosa (220 μm).
Source: Dr A Moulin.

FOLLOW-UP/PROGNOSIS

The management of retinoblastoma involves life concerns as well as salvage of the eye and vision. Advances in the treatment of retinoblastoma, with more targeted therapies (intra-arterial, intravitreal, and recently intracameral chemotherapy), has improved survival and globe salvage rates. Patients treated for retinoblastoma need lifelong ophthalmic follow-up for early management of late recurrence (rare) and side effects of the treatment (cataract, retinal ischemia associated complications, etc.). Those carrying a germline mutation and/or treated with ERBT and/or IVC are at risk for secondary primary cancers and require lifelong oncologic follow-up. Future trends in retinoblastoma include focus on developing treatments with less toxicity and new innovative delivery systems (episcleral implants, nanoparticles), gene therapy and management of treatment complications. New biomarkers for molecular dissemination of retinoblastoma outside the eye may lead to earlier diagnosis of metastasis and targeted treatments.[2]

REFERENCES

1. Kivela T. The epidemiological challenge of the most frequent eye cancer: retinoblastoma, an issue of birth and death. Br J Ophthalmol. 2009;93:1129-31.
2. Dimaras H, Corson TW, Cobrinik D, et al. Retinoblastoma. Nat Rev Dis Primers. 2015;1:15021.
3. Augsburger JJ, Oehlschlager U, Manzitti JE. Multinational clinical and pathologic registry of retinoblastoma. Retinoblastoma International Collaborative Study report 2. Graefes Arch Clin Exp Ophthalmol. 1995;233:469-75.
4. Sengupta S, Pan U, Khetan V. Adult onset retinoblastoma. Indian J Ophthalmol. 2016;64:485-91.
5. Knudson AG. Two genetic hits (more or less) to cancer. Nat Rev Cancer. 2001;1:157-62.
6. Xu XL, Fang Y, Lee TC, et al. Retinoblastoma has properties of a cone precursor tumor and depends upon cone-specific MDM2 signaling. Cell. 2009;137:1018-31.
7. Dimaras H, Kimani K, Dimba EA, et al. Retinoblastoma. Lancet. 2012;379:1436-46.
8. Mitter D, Ullmann R, Muradyan A, et al. Genotype-phenotype correlations in patients with retinoblastoma and interstitial 13q deletions. Eur J Hum Genet. 2011;19:947-58.
9. Rushlow DE, Mol BM, Kennett JY, et al. Characterisation of retinoblastomas without RB1 mutations: genomic, gene expression, and clinical studies. Lancet Oncol. 2013;14:327-34.
10. Skalet AH, Gombos DS, Gallie BL, et al. Screening children at risk for retinoblastoma: Consensus Report from the American Association of Ophthalmic Oncologists and Pathologists. Ophthalmology. 2017;pii: S0161-6420(17)31784-0.
11. Abramson DH, Schefler AC. Update on retinoblastoma. Retina. 2004;24:828-48.
12. Abramson DH, Frank CM, Susman M, et al. Presenting signs of retinoblastoma. J Pediatr. 1998;132:505-8.
13. Shields J, Shields C. Atlas of Intraocular Tumors, 3rd edition. Philadelphia: Wolters Kluwer; 2016.
14. Munier FL. Classification and management of seeds in retinoblastoma. Ellsworth Lecture Ghent August 24th 2013. Ophthalmic Genet. 2014;35:193-207.
15. Shields CL, Ghassemi F, Tuncer S, et al. Clinical spectrum of diffuse infiltrating retinoblastoma in 34 consecutive eyes. Ophthalmology. 2008;115:2253-8.
16. Chaudhry S, Onadim Z, Sagoo MS, et al. The recognition of cavitary retinoblastoma tumors: implications for management and genetic analysis. Retina. 2017;doi: 10.1097/IAE.0000000000001597. [Epub ahead of print].
17. Rodriguez-Galindo C, Chantada GL, Haik BG, et al. Treatment of retinoblastoma: current status and future perspectives. Curr Treat Options Neurol. 2007;9:294-307.
18. Zografos L. Tumeurs Intraoculaires. 2002. p. 489.
19. Shields CL, Schoenberg E, Kocher K, et al. Lesions simulating retinoblastoma (pseudoretinoblastoma) in 604 cases: results based on age at presentation. Ophthalmology. 2013;120:311-6.
20. Fabian ID, Puccinelli F, Gaillard MC, et al. Diagnosis and management of secondary epipapillary retinoblastoma. Br J Ophthalmol. 2017;101:1412-8.
21. Moulin AP, Gaillard MC, Balmer A, et al. Ultrasound biomicroscopy evaluation of anterior extension in retinoblastoma: a clinicopathological study. Br J Ophthalmol. 2012;96:337-40.
22. Linn Murphree A. Intraocular retinoblastoma: the case for a new group classification. Ophthalmol Clin North Am. 2005;18:41-53, viii.
23. Chantada G, Doz F, Antoneli CB, et al. A proposal for an international retinoblastoma staging system. Pediatr Blood Cancer. 2006;47:801-5.

24. Mallipatna AC, Gallie BL, Chévez-Barrios P, et al. Retinoblastoma. In: Amin MB, Edge SB, Greene FL, Byrd DR, Brookland RK, Washington MK, (Eds). AJCC Cancer Staging Manual, 8th edition. New York: Springer; 2017. pp. 819-31.
25. Spencer WH. Ophthalmic Pathology: An Atlas and Textbook, 4th edition. Philadelphia: WB Saunders Co.;1997.
26. Eagle RC Jr. High-risk features and tumor differentiation in retinoblastoma: a retrospective histopathologic study. Arch Pathol Lab Med. 2009;133:1203-9.
27. Singh AD, Santos CM, Shields CL, et al. Observations on 17 patients with retinocytoma. Arch Ophthalmol. 2000;118: 199-205.
28. Abouzeid H, Schorderet DF, Balmer A, et al. Germline mutations in retinoma patients: relevance to low-penetrance and low-expressivity molecular basis. Mol Vis. 2009;15:771-7.
29. Honavar SG, Manjandavida FP, Reddy VAP. Orbital retinoblastoma: An update. Indian J Ophthalmol. 2017;65:435-42.
30. Palma J, Sasso DF, Dufort G, et al. Successful treatment of metastatic retinoblastoma with high-dose chemotherapy and autologous stem cell rescue in South America. Bone Marrow Transplant. 2012;47:522-7.
31. Yamanaka R, Hayano A, Takashima Y. Trilateral retinoblastoma: A systematic review of 211 cases. Neurosurg Rev. 2017;doi: 10.1007/s10143-017-0890-4. [Epub ahead of print].
32. Abramson DH, Shields CL, Munier FL, et al. Treatment of retinoblastoma in 2015: agreement and disagreement. JAMA Ophthalmol. 2015;133:1341-7.
33. Lumbroso-Le Rouic L, Aerts I, Levy-Gabriel C, et al. Conservative treatments of intraocular retinoblastoma. Ophthalmology. 2008;115:1405-10, 10 e1-2.
34. Abramson DH, Dunkel IJ, Brodie SE, et al. A phase I/II study of direct intra-arterial (ophthalmic artery) chemotherapy with melphalan for intraocular retinoblastoma initial results. Ophthalmology. 2008;115:1398-404, 404 e1.
35. Klufas MA, Gobin YP, Marr B, et al. Intra-arterial chemotherapy as a treatment for intraocular retinoblastoma: alternatives to direct ophthalmic artery catheterization. Am J Neuroradiol. 2012;33:1608-14.
36. Abramson DH, Marr BP, Francis JH, et al. Simultaneous bilateral ophthalmic artery chemosurgery for bilateral retinoblastoma (Tandem Therapy). PLoS One. 2016; 11:e0156806.
37. Shields CL, Jorge R, Say EA, et al. Unilateral retinoblastoma managed with intravenous chemotherapy versus intra-arterial chemotherapy. Outcomes Based on the International Classification of Retinoblastoma. Asia Pac J Ophthalmol (Phila). 2016;5:97-103.
38. Munier FL, Mosimann P, Puccinelli F, et al. First-line intra-arterial versus intravenous chemotherapy in unilateral sporadic group D retinoblastoma: evidence of better visual outcomes, ocular survival and shorter time to success with intra-arterial delivery from retrospective review of 20 years of treatment. Br J Ophthalmol. 2017;101:1086-93.
39. Abramson DH, Shields CL, Jabbour P, et al. Metastatic deaths in retinoblastoma patients treated with intraarterial chemotherapy (ophthalmic artery chemosurgery) worldwide. Int J Retina Vitreous. 2017;3:40.
40. Mendoza PR, Grossniklaus HE. Therapeutic options for retinoblastoma. Cancer Control. 2016;23:99-109.
41. Smith SJ, Smith BD, Mohney BG. Ocular side effects following intravitreal injection therapy for retinoblastoma: a systematic review. Br J Ophthalmol. 2014;98:292-7.
42. Munier FL, Moulin A, Gaillard MC, et al. Intracameral chemotherapy for globe salvage in retinoblastoma with Ssecondary anterior chamber invasion. Ophthalmology. 2017;pii:S0161-6420(17)33341-9.
43. Shields CL, Shields JA, De Potter P, et al. Plaque radiotherapy in the management of retinoblastoma. Use as a primary and secondary treatment. Ophthalmology. 1993;100:216-24.
44. Abouzeid H, Moeckli R, Gaillard MC, et al. (106)Ruthenium brachytherapy for retinoblastoma. Int J Radiat Oncol Biol Phys. 2008;71:821-8.
45. Abramson DH, Frank CM, Dunkel IJ. A phase I/II study of subconjunctival carboplatin for intraocular retinoblastoma. Ophthalmology. 1999;106:1947-50.
46. Munier FL, Verwey J, Pica A, et al. New developments in external beam radiotherapy for retinoblastoma: from lens to normal tissue-sparing techniques. Clin Exp Ophthalmol. 2008;36:78-89.
47. Sastre X, Chantada GL, Doz F, et al. Proceedings of the consensus meetings from the International Retinoblastoma Staging Working Group on the pathology guidelines for the examination of enucleated eyes and evaluation of prognostic risk factors in retinoblastoma. Arch Pathol Lab Med. 2009;133:1199-202.
48. Sreelakshmi KV, Chandra A, Krishnakumar S, et al. Anterior chamber invasion in retinoblastoma: Not an indication for adjuvant chemotherapy. Invest Ophthalmol Vis Sci. 2017;58:4654-61.

Chapter 77 The Chiasm in Childhood

Richard Bowman, David Taylor

GENETICS, EMBRYOLOGY AND DEVELOPMENTAL CHANGES THROUGH CHILDHOOD

Retinal ganglion cells (RGCs) are the first to differentiate from the progenitor cells which ultimately form all of the cellular elements of the retina. At first developing around the future optic disk, they are guided at their tips by specialized "growth cones" which have motile actin-containing filopodia which expand differentially attracted to genetically determined, time-linked, growth cues along the whole length of the pathway to the lateral geniculate body (LGB). When they reach the floor of the third ventricle, at first they all decussate crossing to the other side, right eye fibers go towards the left LGB and left eye fibers to the right. Subsequently approximately equal numbers end ipsilateral and contralateral to their origin. We have recently reported four hemispherectomy patients with better acuity in the contralateral eye (in addition to the expected homonymous hemianopia) suggesting possible greater representation of the macular pathway in the crossed pathway though this has not been substantiated in other studies as yet.[1] The accuracy of their trajectory which is about 95% is determined by an array of growth protein cues which they follow as a gradient as attractants or repellents and are bundled under the influence of others. There is a remarkable over-production of RGCs during gestation: at 16–17 weeks gestation, there are about 3.7 million RGC fibers and by 29–30 weeks, the number has decreased by programmed cell death (apoptosis) to the term number of 1.1 million.[2] This remarkable adjustment may be explained by the survival of those axons which successfully connect with the functionally appropriate LGB neurons.

ANATOMY AND RELATIONS

The axons of the RGCs run posteriorly and upwards 45° from the optic canals to form the intracranial optic nerves, chiasm and optic tracts. The chiasm lies in the suprasellar cistern above the coverings of the pituitary fossa, the diaphragma sellae. Since the intracranial optic nerves vary in length, the position of the chiasm varies: "pre-fixed" when the optic nerves are short and the chiasm anterior and "post-fixed" when posterior. The human optic nerve grows by 80% in the first 3 years of life, reaching adult proportions by 15 years of age,[3] but the anatomical relations are basically similar at all ages. The anterior cerebral arteries, the anterior communicating arteries lie anteriorly above the chiasm and the optic nerves and the carotid arteries lie laterally, the posterior communicating arteries passing below the optic tracts. The chiasm lies in the floor of the anterior end of the third ventricle and posteriorly lie the hypothalamus and the pituitary stalk, the tuber cinereum and the mammillary bodies.

PRESENTATIONS, SYMPTOMS AND SIGNS: THE EASILY MISTAKEN DIAGNOSIS IN CHILDHOOD

It is easy to over or underdiagnose chiasmal disease in children because significant signs are often hidden by the child's propensity for compensation, leading to symptoms or signs being absent until the visual loss becomes both bilateral and significant. They may give a misleading history or their examination may be compromised by their naturally poor cooperation. Thus, cardinal signs such as bitemporal hemianopia can be mistakenly found in relation to disk anomalies or familial optic atrophy or not found (or not adequately tested for) in young children with tumors of or around the chiasm. Preverbal children commonly present late as the signs and symptoms are only detectable when the second eye develops poor acuity. It is remarkable how normally a small child can navigate and behave with one blind eye and the other eye with a complete hemianopia but reasonable acuity. With craniopharyngiomas, this is a common presentation and one which must be acted upon swiftly if blindness is to be avoided. If only more clinicians would get used to testing young children with age-appropriate tests! Confrontation testing if done well is enough in this situation to suggest the correct clinical diagnosis. For verbal and cooperative children are best tested by formal visual field studies and in young children non-automated field studies may be the best, given a skilled tester. Figures 77.1A to F show a typical bitemporal hemianopia in a child with a craniopharyngioma. If a bitemporal hemianopia is associated with at least reasonable acuity in each eye, the child may develop seemingly non-organic symptoms: the intact nasal fields inadequately overlap so they "slide" vertically or horizontally giving confusing symptoms of parts of sentences shifting or letters or even words overlapping or being duplicated.

Color vision must be tested in each eye individually as with optic nerve involvement, color deficits are common. Evidence of a relative afferent pupil defect may provide positive evidence of underlying pathology.

Testing stereoacuity can be done successfully in young children: it can be an important but not a specific clinical clue because stereoacuity can be significantly abnormal in chiasmal diseases even in the presence of good acuity.

Most nystagmus in small children is congenital and idiopathic but if there is a history of it starting after 2–3 months of age or if it is asymmetric or unilateral then magnetic resonance imaging (MRI) is indicated. The classic type of nystagmus associated with chiasmal disease is see-saw nystagmus which might indicate achiasmia if congenital and acquired chiasmal pathology such as a glioma or a craniopharyngioma if the nystagmus is of later onset. Another type of nystagmus traditionally associated with optic pathway, glioma is spasmus nutans (a triad of acquired nystagmus, often dysconjugate, head nodding and torticollis) though a recent large series has challenged this association.[4]

Nevertheless, the late onset of the nystagmus and its asymmetry would prompt MRI which is often abnormal. Examination of the optic disks is essential in all cases suspected of chiasmal disease and it helps to examine them at higher magnification or by direct ophthalmoscopy. Most commonly in affected cases, the optic disks appear evenly pale and the nerve fiber layer evenly reduced but especially in cases with well-preserved nasal visual fields, there appears a horizontal band of optic atrophy (Figs. 77.2A to E). This is caused by the loss of the fibers subserving the defective temporal field being inserted circumferentially around the optic disk but the intact nasal field-related fibers inserting themselves above and below the disk leaving exposed as pale only the horizontal band of atrophy. This can also be shown with OCT (*see* Figs. 77.1A to E). If there is raised intracranial pressure, the intact fibers (above and below the optic disk) subserving the intact nasal field become swollen in a bilobed "twin peaks" pattern (Figs. 77.3A to D).

Visual evoked potentials can be very useful in detecting chiasmal disorders especially in younger children where visual field testing is difficult. Figures 77.4A to C show the normal distribution of cortical signals on each side of the brain and the changes associated with too much crossing as occurs in albinism and too little crossing as may occur in chiasmal compression/infiltration or achiasmia.

The pituitary gland and hypothalamus lie near to the chiasm so growth and other endocrine defects are common in these cases. Infants with hypothalamus-involving tumors may develop the diencephalic syndrome "Russell-Silver dwarfism" rapid weight change with subcutaneous fat loss and behavioral changes which may alert the clinician. Craniopharyngiomas conversely often present with weight gain and sleepiness also due to hypothalamic involvement.

DEVELOPMENTAL DISORDERS

Chiasmal Aplasia and Hypoplasia

Most early cases were based on postmortem studies and studies in mice.[5] Even now, there are only a few cases reported, most are associated with bilateral optic nerve aplasia or optic nerve hypoplasia.

Achiasmia

Achiasmia was originally described as the "non-decussating retinal fugal fiber syndrome"[6] but is now more frequently known as achiasmia.[7,8] In achiasmia, the chiasm is not just hypoplastic, whether or not associated with optic nerve hypoplasia—it has the essential absence or relative lack of crossing fibers—the isolated relative or complete absence of the chiasmal decussation. The proportion of decussating fibers that are missing or defective varies.

Clinically, they often have horizontal and/or see-saw nystagmus: variable, sometimes normal vision, optic nerve hypoplasia or other optic disk anomalies such as Morning Glory Disk Anomaly and a variable degree of developmental delay. Generally except with Septo-optic dysplasia associated cases, endocrine abnormalities are absent but all require endocrinological surveillance or management. There is a typical achiasmic visually evoked potentials (VEP) pattern (Figs. 77.4A to C) and neuroimaging

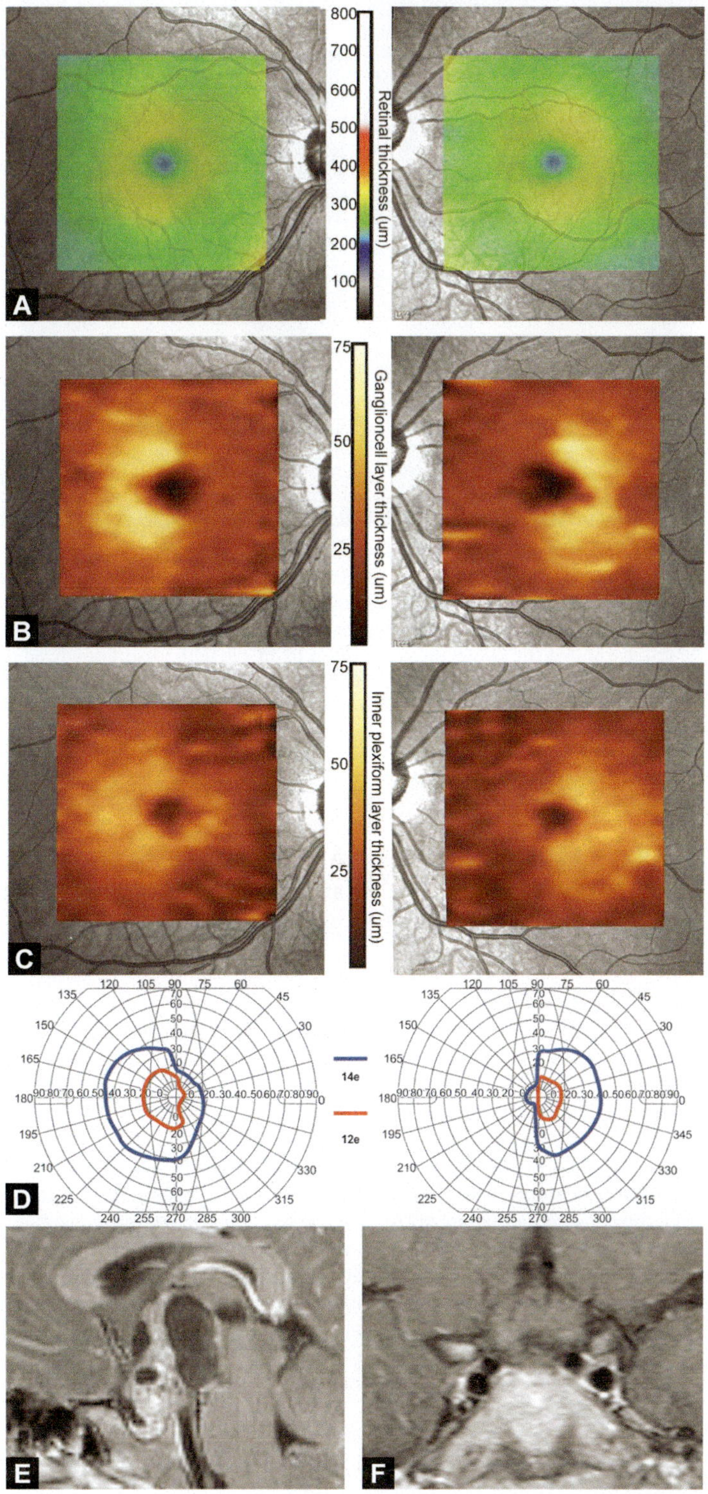

Figs. 77.1A to F: (A to C) Optical coherence tomography (OCT), and (D) Goldman visual fields in a 14-year-old female with long-standing bitemporal hemianopia greater in the left eye (ii) than right eye (i) due to a craniopharyngioma with 0.000 LogMAR in each eye. The hemianopia can be seen at the macula subtly in the total retinal thickness maps (A) and more obviously in the ganglion cell layer (B) and Inner plexiform layer (C) thickness maps which show relative thinning of the retinal layers nasal to the fovea compared to temporal to the fovea. (E and F) Postcontrast enhancement of craniopharyngioma showing heterogeneous consistency and cystic change.

Source (OCT images and visual fields): Dr Sian Handley and Dr Alki Liasis. Visual Electrophysiology, Great Ormond Street Hospital, London.

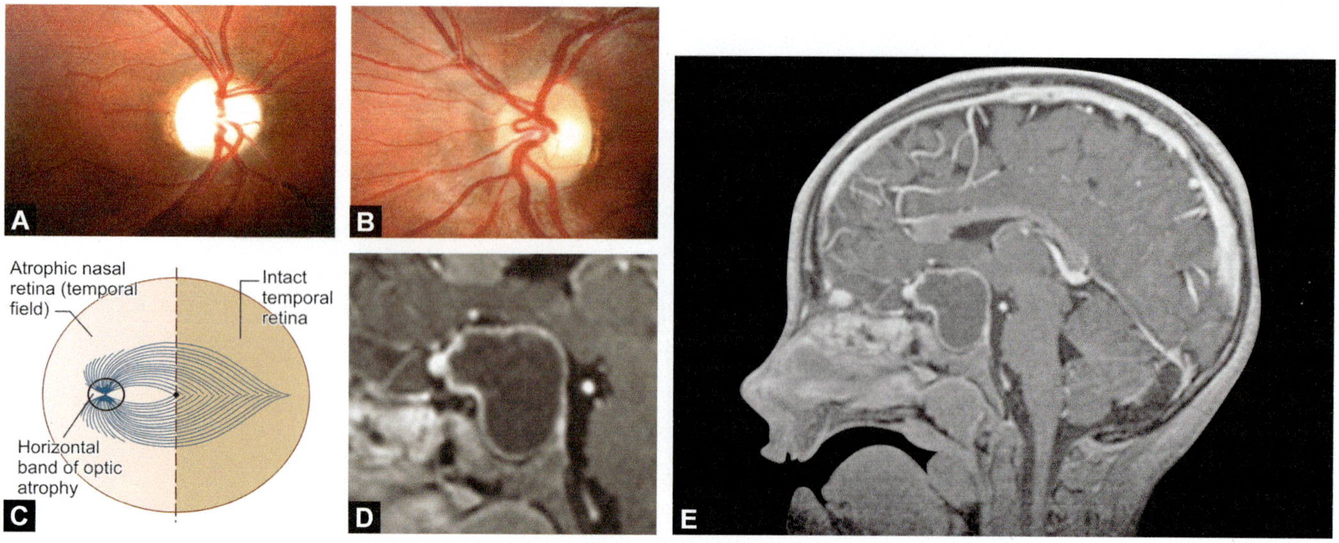

Figs. 77.2A to E: Horizontal band optic atrophy associated with a temporal visual field defect. This 8-year-old child was thought to be dyslexic at school because of difficulties when reading from the right end of a line being read to the next line below on the left. The child was found to have no perception of light in the right eye, a right afferent pupil defect and the left eye had a total temporal hemianopia and a visual acuity of LogMAR 0.0 (6/6, 20/20, 1.0). (A) In the right eye, there is "total" optic atrophy associated with complete loss of all or nearly all the optic nerve axons (ONAs) associated with both the nasal and temporal visual fields; (B) The left eye shows the characteristic findings in an eye with loss of nearly all the optic nerve axons associated with the temporal visual field (nasal retina) which are inserted all around the circumference of the optic disk. The intact nasal field fibers (temporal retina) are inserted into the superior and inferior poles of the optic disk, leaving visible a horizontal band of the atrophic temporal field-associated ONAs (C). D and E show the causative tumor, a slow-growing craniopharyngioma.

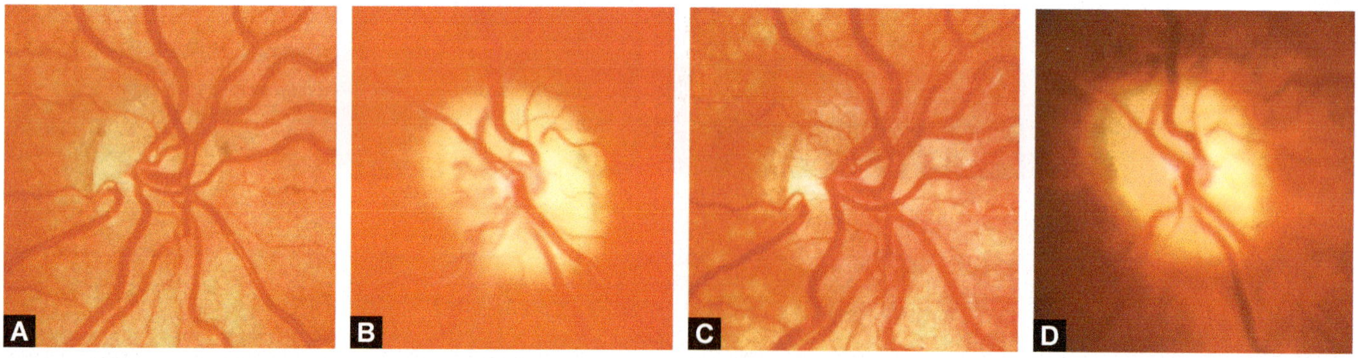

Figs. 77.3A to D: "Twin-peaks" papilledema. (A) Right optic disk of an 8-year-old child with left optic nerve and chiasmal glioma. The right optic disk shows slightly swollen optic nerve fibers above and below the optic disk and a pale horizontal band of mild optic atrophy. Her acuity was LogMAR 0.0 (6/6, 20/20, 1.0) and there was a temporal visual field defect on confrontation; (B) The left eye has "hand movements only" vision, optic atrophy and marked shunt vessels especially inferonasally. Shunt vessels in this situation are mostly seen with chronic compression by tumor, the most common of which in children is optic glioma; (C) 6 months after the images in Figure 77.3A, the patient developed hydrocephalus and the remaining nerve fibers, thickest above and below the optic disk, where the fibers of the intact nasal field, temporal retina are inserted. This 'bilobed' swelling is known as twin-peaks papilledema; (D) 6 months after the image in Figure 77.3B, the shunt vessels have atrophied along with the remaining optic nerve fibers and there is no perception of light.

studies which reveal a normal to small chiasm and in some cases, the radiological signs of a basal encephalocele. Despite the abnormal chiasm, there is usually no evidence of a bitemporal hemianopia, perhaps this is evidence of an adaptive anomalous retinotopic projection. The sophistication of visual electrophysiology in a recent paper has shown that VEPs can identify a functioning chiasm even when not seen on MRI in cases with holoprosencephaly.[9]

Albinism

The general features of albinism are given elsewhere in this book. Of great interest in albinism, are the visual pathway and central connections and whether they are visual pathway-only defects or whether they are more whole-brain and perhaps compensatory anomalies.[10] The neuroophthalmological findings result from a smaller than

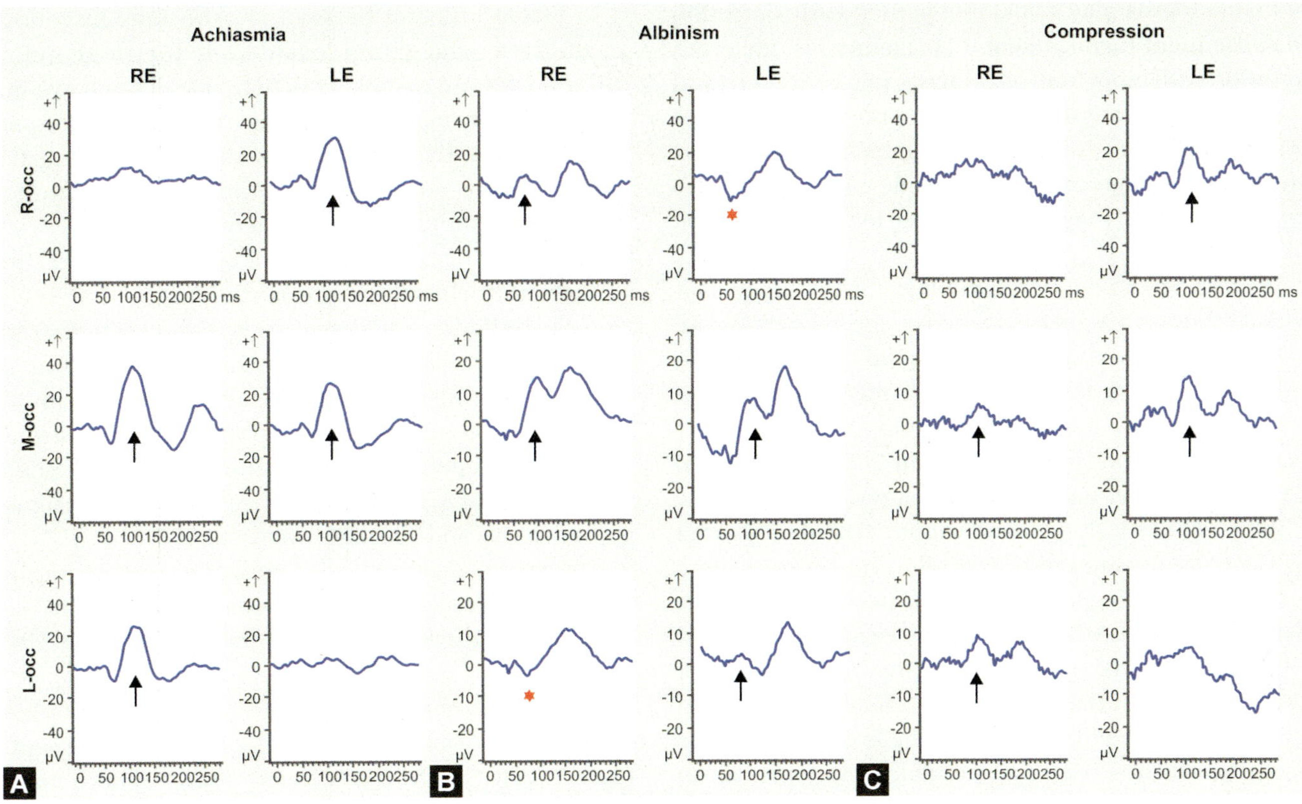

Figs. 77.4A to C: Achiasmia/compression/albinism. Crossed laterality. Flash visual evoked potentials from (A) a patient with achiasmia, (B) albinism, and (C) a craniopharyngioma causing compression of the chiasm. Due to paradoxical lateralization, the major positivity evoked by one hemisphere is recorded over the contralateral hemisphere (↑). For example, stimulating the right eye of a patient with achiasmia will result in right hemisphere activation that is recorded over the left occiput. In comparison, in a patient with albinism, stimulation of the right eye will result in a greater activation of the left hemisphere that is recorded over the right occiput. In addition to the positivity in albinism recorded over the occiput ipsilateral to the eye stimulated, there is a negativity recorded over the occiput contralateral to the eye being stimulated (★). A patient with chiasmal compression has a similar distribution to that observed in achiasmia but there may be an interocular difference.

(RE: Right eye; LE: Left eye; R-occ: Right occipital electrode; M-occ: Mid-occipital electrode; L-occ: Left occipital electrode)

Source: Dr Alki Liassis, Visual Electrophysiologist at Great Ormond Street Hospital, London.

normal anterior visual pathway, a greater decussation of nerve fibers at the optic chiasm (Figs. 77.4A to C), foveal hypoplasia and nystagmus. Visual perception however, is largely preserved perhaps attributable to reorganization among cerebral networks including an increased interhemispheric connectivity of the primary visual areas. In albinism in humans, each brain hemisphere receives inputs primarily from the contralateral eye instead of an almost equal distribution from both eyes,[11] which may be the mechanism for the reduced visual acuity and binocular vision suggested by mouse studies and also functional MRI in humans.

Despite there being no curative treatment for albinism, there is a lot that the ophthalmologist can do to help-starting with making the clinical diagnosis, confirming any involvement of the parents (especially looking for subtle signs in possible X-linked cases), genetic testing where necessary, counseling of the parents from the first visit and ongoing with educational advice and support. Most affected persons need spectacles not least for reducing ambient light and many have significant refractive errors. Regular not frequent refractions are appropriate. They may need advice and management of strabismus. Affected children should be encouraged to wear sun-protective hats and clothing and to use ultraviolet A and ultraviolet B (UVA and UVB) sunscreens.

DEVELOPMENTAL TUMORS

Chiasmal Optic Gliomas

Optic pathway gliomas (OPGs) are rare tumors mostly noninvasive pilocytic or pilomyxoid astrocytomas. Malignant OPGs are extremely rare in children.

Ophthalmologists play a vital role in their early detection and subsequent management. Management is ideally a team effort with input from oncologists, neurosurgeons and radiologists and many other patient support services. Since the tumors are rare and the management often complex, centralizing management to a few centers in each country is an approach that may be beneficial to long-term survival and morbidity.

The first role of an ophthalmologist is in diagnosis—chiasmal gliomas are present to them in the following ways:

1. As the result of a screening program of patients with Neurofibromatosis type 1 (NF1) or the examination of NF1 presenting in non-ophthalmological ways.

   Optic pathway gliomas occur in 5–25% of children with NF1. Over half do not develop visual problems. Thus, regular vision testing cannot exclude a glioma or accurately monitor progression. However in some centers, if the diagnosis of NF1 is suspected, the patients have a baseline MRI including the visual pathway and then clinical vision tests at varying intervals—often every 6–12 months until say, 8 years of age[12] if there is no evidence of OPGs, screening is ceased and the parents warned regarding possible symptoms. There may be some benefit of MRI scanning again late in adolescence.

   NF1-associated OPGs seem to have a more benign prognosis than non-NF1 cases in which a majority of children with sporadic OPGs have significant long-term visual impairment in spite of treatment and in whom tumor progression is common.[13]

2. Some present as a child with suspected poor vision and nystagmus.

   Visual loss can be severe especially in younger children who compensate well for their deficit, both eyes are usually affected, usually one eye first. Accompanying the visual loss, nystagmus is frequent and is usually compound with horizontal, vertical and rotary components which often amount to characteristic "see-saw" nystagmus.

3. As a result of the development of hydrocephalus from third ventricle outflow obstruction.

   Such children may have headache and early morning vomiting, visual loss, nystagmus and head nodding. The "bobble-headed doll" phenomenon is an uncommon but characteristic presentation in which there are episodes repetitive anteroposterior head movements in groups of 3–5 nods. There are usually other signs—nystagmus and vision loss particularly.

4. On account of the chiasmal tumor being extending into the orbital optic nerve and causing proptosis.
5. With the diencephalic syndrome—"Russell-Silver dwarfism."

Many OPGs remain static and do not significantly grow and there is clear evidence that some spontaneously regress (Figs. 77.5A to C).[14] NF1-associated cases may have smaller tumors, less propensity to progress and extend outside the visual pathway to more frequently affect only the optic nerve and to have many fewer cystic changes. The prognosis at diagnosis however, is difficult to predict because of the wide range of behaviors seen in these tumors. Whilst most OPGs behave like relatively benign hamartomas, many especially those younger at presentation and with larger and cystic chiasmal tumors behave in a more aggressive way.

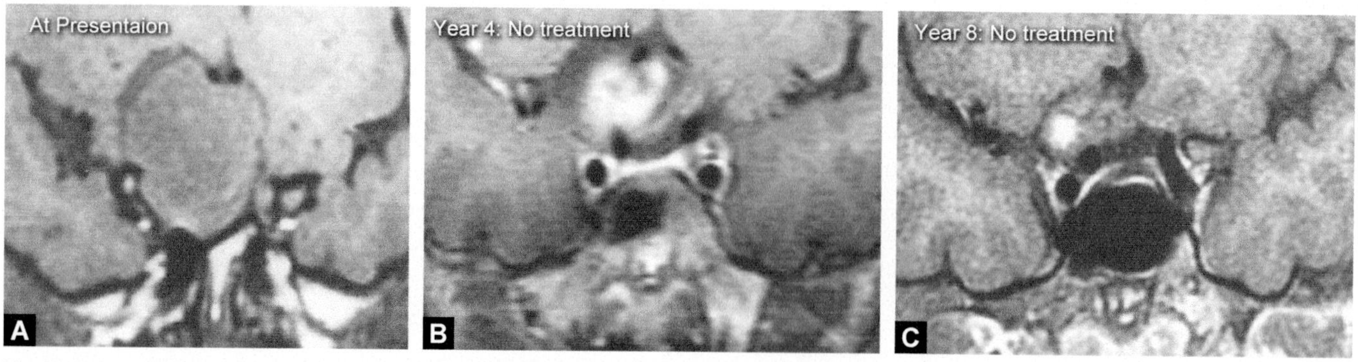

Figs. 77.5A to C: ONG with spontaneous regression. A 4-year-old child with neurofibromatosis type 1 (NF1) presented with a radiologically diagnosed optic chiasmal glioma. One cycle of chemotherapy was carried out at the overseas referring hospital with no response in the size of the tumor: no further treatment was given. Over the subsequent 8 years, there was a steady decline in the size of the tumor.

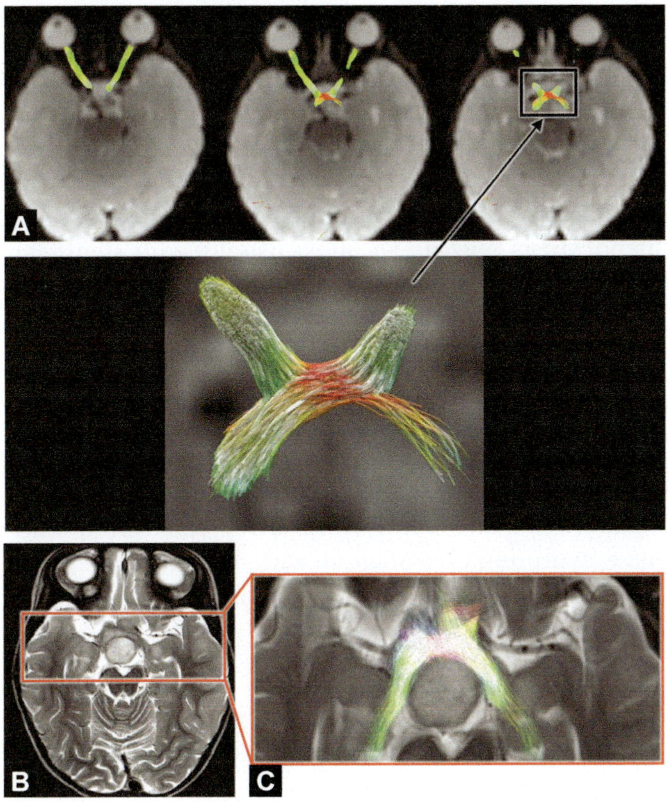

Figs. 77.6A to C: (A and B) Normal chiasmal anatomy, the crossing fibers are colored red; (C) Conventional MRI (left) shows infiltration of the chiasm and hypothalamus by glioma, and (right) tractography shows reduced connectivity in and an anterior displacement of the chiasm.

Diagnosis can usually be made by neuroradiology alone: MRI studies under anesthetic or sedation can demonstrate that the tumor is confined to the optic chiasm but often extends into the optic nerves or the optic tract often involving the hypothalamus. Diffusion tensor imaging which measures water conductivity in white matter tracts may prove a useful adjunct to conventional MRI (Figs. 77.6A to C).[15] In older children visual field studies can be helpful but are often not classically "chiasmal". Pattern visually evoked potentials, performed by experts used to studying young children may be helpful to estimate vision and to detect chiasmal features: they may be a useful tool in assessing possible changes in vision. A few cases mostly with atypical features or cystic changes may require biopsy to establish the diagnosis before management interventions.

Treatment is not universally effective so judicious waiting after diagnosis, where possible, is the best way to achieve some idea of the biological behavior of the tumor. Radiotherapy is generally avoided, most especially in young children as it is damaging to the visual pathway, the developing brain and neuroendocrine system as well as bone in therapeutic doses. Radiosurgery (the "Gamma Knife") may have a role.[16] However, it may sometimes be the preferred treatment for cases associated with the diencephalic syndrome and it has been shown to be effective in extensive cases not responding to chemotherapy. The role of chemotherapy with combinations of actinomycin D, vincristine, etoposide, bevacizumab being most often used together with other agents is not yet fully determined for OPGs. The mitogen activated kinase pathway is activated in low-grade glioma and mitogen activated kinase inhibitor (MEK) such as selumetinib have shown promise particularly in tumors with BRAF mutations.[17] Surgery because of the difficulties arising from the intermingling of tumor with visual fibers is risky and usually confined to biopsy and draining or removal of clearly cystic areas. "Debulking" of large areas is now not often advocated.

Craniopharyngiomas

Craniopharyngiomas are unusual (6% of all intracranial tumors) in children, slowly developing, congenital tumors arising from Rathke's cleft or other embryonal epithelium remnants but they can present at any age and most variably and subtly in the first years of life. This subtlety demands superior awareness and diagnostic skills from ophthalmologists as many are diagnosed late and only when visual loss is advanced.[18]

Craniopharyngiomas occur in the region of the pituitary stalk and grow slowly compressing the chiasm, optic nerves and pituitary fossa from above: endocrine function is frequently affected. Obstructive hydrocephalus may be caused by tumor growth into the third ventricle or more posteriorly into the posterior fossa with resulting headache, diplopia, ataxia and hearing loss.

In young children, the visual loss caused by compressive optic atrophy, is frequently significant. The typical presentation occurs only when the second eye is affected in that it has a temporal hemianopia and the presentation arises because central vision is compromised. Typically, there is diffuse optic atrophy in the first affected eye and band atrophy or twin peaks papilloedema (if there is raised intracranial pressure) in the second affected eye (*see* Fig. 77.3)

Although plain X-rays of the head may reveal flattening of the pituitary fossa and intratumoral calcification, MRI is the most useful modality (*see* Fig. 77.2) and avoids the irradiation of computerized tomographic (CT) scanning which is reserved for older children or when the detection of calcification is otherwise necessary but difficult. Endocrine and visual assessments are mandatory and demand follow up unless the surgical removal is complete without residual damage.

Adamantinomatous craniopharyngiomas is the most frequent type in children: there is a solid portion of epithelial calcified tumor cells and a cystic component filled with a dark, oily fluid. Their capsule is adherent to surrounding structures, including major vessels. They are more locally aggressive and recurrent than the "papillary" tumors seen in adults. Both are histologically nonmalignant but are adherent and placed in surgically challenging areas.

Treatment is difficult and demanding in many cases as the tumor may be large and adherent. Total removal is the aim but the risks demand caution although the cystic component can be drained and much of the solid component and the capsule be safely removed, the removal is often incomplete and radiotherapy or radiosurgery may be indicated with extra caution in young children. Intracystic injection via a reservoir of radioactive phosphorus P^{32} antineoplastics or interferon-alpha are also used.

Although 5 and 10-year overall survival rates are higher than 90%, the visual and endocrine morbidity may be significant.

OTHER TUMORS AND SPACE-OCCUPYING LESIONS

Pituitary Adenomas

Pituitary adenomas are rare until late adolescence but their endocrine abnormalities and sometimes their mass effect can compromise both quality and length of life.[19] They are more frequent in females either macroadenomas or microadenomas and present with oligomenorrhea and galactorrhea in females and headaches in males. Pubertal development can be abnormal in macroadenomas. Growth failure is rare. Secreting tumors are mostly associated with hyperprolactinemia, Cushing's syndrome and acromegaly. Pituitary apoplexy (Sheehan's syndrome) denotes the occurrence of sudden large hemorrhages into a pituitary enlarged from pregnancy or tumor: it is only occasionally seen in children with pituitary adenomas.[20]

Granulomas and Dysgerminomas

Granulomas (xanthomatous hypophysitis and xanthogranuloma) and germinomas are rare but may occasionally present to ophthalmologists. Juvenile Xanthogranulomas very rarely involve this area but Eosinophilic granulomas and Langerhans cell histiocytosis may do so, most usually with significant systemic involvement demanding multidisciplinary services. Occasionally, visual system involvement requires ophthalmological attention.

Dysgerminomas although rare, may present in an interesting fashion. The patients are often adolescents to young adult females with visual symptoms and signs of chiasmal involvement such as bitemporal hemianopia, color vision and acuity loss. They not infrequently have symptoms associated with diabetes insipidus. Neuroradiology shows a small tumor around the chiasm and pituitary fossa.

Sphenoid Sinus Disease

Casteels[21] presented the case of a 10-year-old girl with no nasal or respiratory symptoms who developed a headache. The next day she became totally blind in the right eye and over 5 days vision in the left eye deteriorated to bare light perception. The diagnosis of a sphenoid sinus mucocoele was made radiologically (Figs. 77.7A and B) and drainage via an endonasal sphenoidectomy produced 12 mL of brownish fluid. Endoscopic biopsy of the wall confirmed the diagnosis of a mucocoele. Steroid treatment was given postoperatively but vision recovered to 6/12 in the left eye only. Such cases are rare but are a treatable cause of chiasmal compression.

Third Ventricle Distension and Visual Loss

In hydrocephalus especially from Sylvian Aqueduct Obstruction, the third ventricle may become distended sometimes severely and acutely. The ballooning ventricle may cause stretching of the optic nerves and chiasm with resulting acuity and visual field loss. Unilateral visual defects may occur from optic nerve damage.

Trauma

Trauma severe enough to damage the chiasm is usually substantial and most frequently it is associated with damage

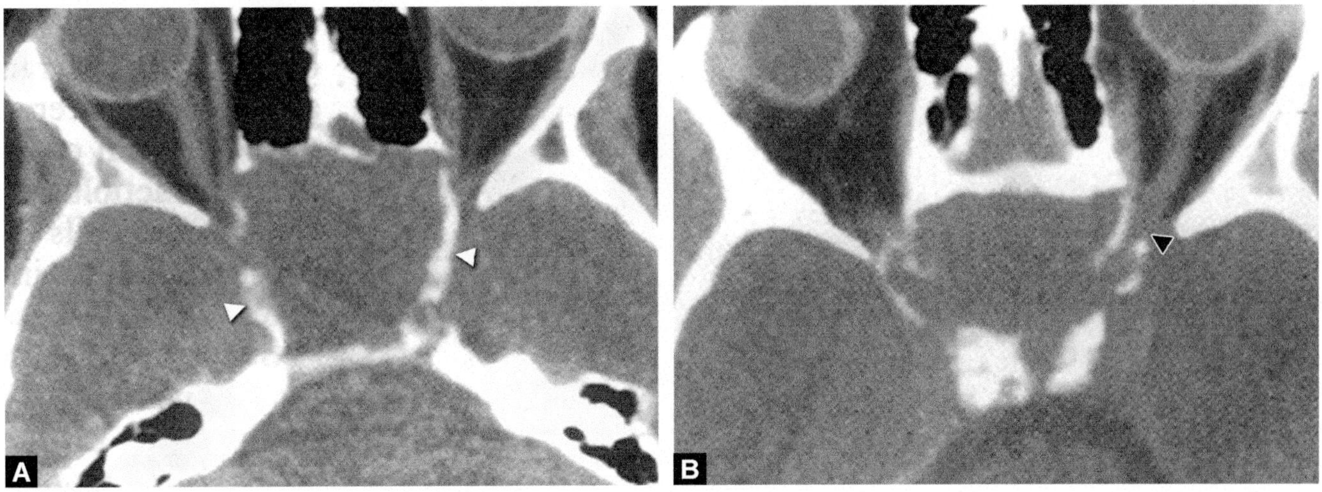

Figs. 77.7A and B: Sphenoid sinus expansion compressing ONs. (A) Axial CT scan showing an expanded sphenoid sinus with thinning and erosion of the walls (white arrowheads) and ballooning of the sella turcica floor in a 10-year-old child; (B) Axial CT scan showing bilateral optic nerve compression (black arrowhead) giving rise to bilateral severe visual loss. Prompt diagnosis is essential for timely treatment to avoid damage to the optic nerves and chiasm by the expanded sphenoid sinus.

Source: Dr Ingele Casteels, University Hospital KU Leuven. Also see Casteels I, DeLoof E, Brock P, et al. Brit J Ophthalmol. 1992;76:502-4.

to surrounding neural and endocrine structures which may obscure the chiasmal element of the damage. Occasionally however, forces are set up which serve the chiasm more or less completely and may even divide it in two resulting in a complete loss of both sets of decussating fibers and an "absolute" bitemporal hemianopia. As in optic nerve trauma, there is mixed evidence as to whether interventional treatment of any sort is effective but systemic steroids have been used when safe from the point of view of systemic effects, in the hope of limiting secondary damage from swelling especially if the damage to the chiasm is partial.

INFLAMMATIONS AND VASCULAR DISEASE

Chiasmal Neuritis

Chiasmal neuritis has become defined by modern MRI imaging (Figs. 77.8A to C) of chiasmal inflammation.[22] The various symptoms, causes and management are similar to that of optic neuritis.

Vascular Disease and Malformations

Intracranial aneurysms in small children may be large or very large so called "giant aneurysms". They rarely affect the chiasm specifically but can occur in relation to the Circle of Willis vessels and thus affect the chiasm. They may be present for many years but do leak or rupture presenting with sudden headache and sometimes visual loss from chiasm or tract damage. A similar presentation may occur from arteriovenous malformations "berry" or dissecting aneurysms also occur in association with Ehlers-Danlos syndrome (especially type IV), Marfan's syndrome amongst other rare diseases and small aneurysms occur with subacute bacterial endocarditis and Moyamoya disease more usually affecting the hemispheres.

Radionecrosis

Injury to the optic chiasm can be a serious complication of radiation treatment of diseases of or around the optic chiasm especially in conditions requiring higher doses, even if fractionated such as chiasmal gliomas and recurrent craniopharyngiomas. Enhancement of chiasmal MRIs after gadolinium and thickening of the chiasm suggests inflammation following damage to capillaries. It is found especially when vision is reduced but even before it. The radiation damage may not become apparent symptomatically or on clinical examination until many months following the end of the course of treatment. In babies and small children, the greater sensitivity of surrounding tissues and the sensitivity of the developing germinal matrix and neuropil is associated with a greater predisposition to damage. The result is a usually slow and relentless loss of acuity and colour vision and visual field constriction. Typical "chiasmal" features are unusual.

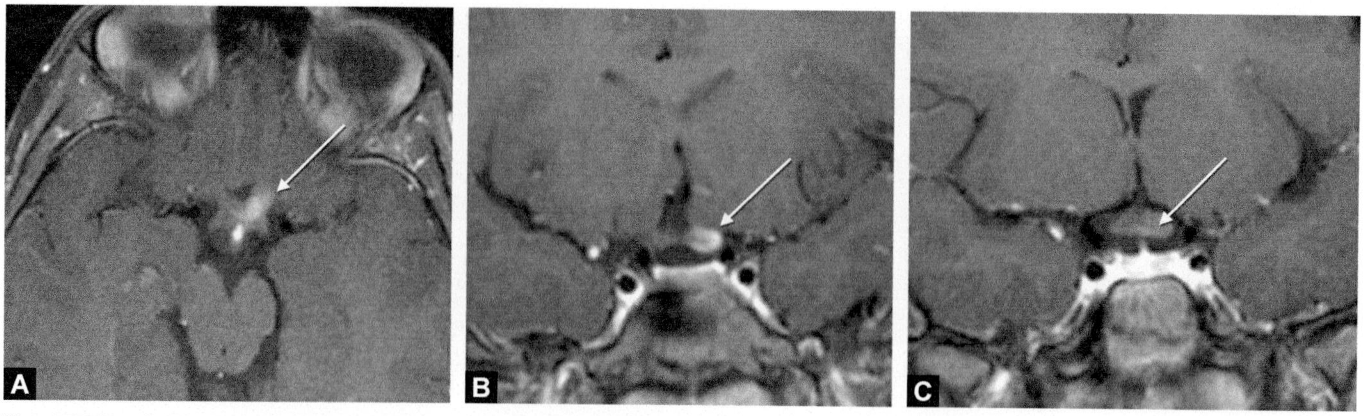

Figs. 77.8A to C: A patient with recurrent optic and chiasmal neuritis without myelitis but with IgA deficiency and coeliac disease. In chiasmal neuritis, vision is often reduced in both eyes and the visual fields show evanescent defects with features that are sometimes not clearly "chiasmal". (A) Axial MRI post-contrast, showing involvement of the left optic nerve and the left side of the chiasm; (B and C) Coronal MRIs showing left optic nerve and chiasmal involvement.

Source: Dr Philippe Demaerel, Neuroradiology, University Hospital KU Leuven.

Extrinsic Chiasmal Disease

Opticochiasmatic arachnoiditis was a name given to cases where the suprasellar cistern and the chiasm became affected by a "blanket" of adhesive tissue which was associated with damage to these structures. The logic of the commonly used surgical treatment was probably misdirected as it is likely that the underlying cause was infections such as meningitis, TB, fungal disease, cysticercosis, hydatid disease or many other conditions. Such basically chronic infective diseases are probably now better diagnosed and treated.

The Empty Sella Syndrome

Extension of the subarachnoid space through a deficient sellar diaphragm, partly or completely filling the sella turcica with CSF comprises an "empty sella". It was once thought not to exist in children but is more commonly recognised today with MRI scanning and greater awareness of the signs. Females are more affected than males. It may occur following surgery in the region of the pituitary fossa or in association with Septo-optic dysplasia when the anterior pituitary is small and the posterior is ectopic. Most commonly however, it occurs in children who have had prolonged raised intracranial pressure, particularly in association with Idiopathic Intracranial Hypertension. Some have hyperprolactinemia and other endocrine disturbances including precocious puberty.

REFERENCES

1. Handley SE, Vargha-Khadem F, Bowman RJC, et al. Visual function 20 years after childhood hemispherectomy for intractable epilepsy. Am J Ophthalmol. 2017;177:81-9.
2. Provis J, van Driel P, Billson FA, et.al. Human fetal optic nerve: overproduction and elimination of retinal axons during development. J Comp Neurol. 1985;238:92-100.
3. Bernstein SL, Meister M, Zhuo J, et al. Postnatal growth of the human optic nerve. Eye. 2016;30:1378-80.
4. Bowen M, Peragallo JH, Kralik SF, et al. Magnetic resonance imaging findings in children with spasmus nutans. J AAPOS. 2017;21(2):127-30.
5. Bein HJ. Ueber vererbliche Aplasie des Sehnerven bei der Maus. Ophthalmologica, 1947; 113(1):12-36.
6. Apkarian P, Bour LJ, Barth PG, et.al. Non-decussating retinal-fugal fibre syndrome. An inborn achiasmatic malformation associated with visuotopic misrouting, visual evoked potential ipsilateral asymmetry and nystagmus. Brain. 1995;118(pt 5):1195-216.
7. Leitch RJ, Thompson D, Harris CM, et al. Achiasmia in a case of midline craniofacial cleft with seesaw nystagmus. Br J Ophthalmol. 1996;80(11):1023-4.
8. Sami DA, Saunders D, Thompson DA, et al. The Achiasmia spectrum:congenitally reduced chiasmal decussation. BrJ Ophthalmol. 2005;89(10):1311-7.
9. Handley SE, Liasis A. Multichannel Visual Evoked Potentials in the evaluation of visual pathways of children with marked brain abnormalities. J AAPOS. 2017;21(1):52-6.
10. Welton T, Ather S, Proudlock FA, et.al. Altered whole-brain connectivity in albinism. Hum Brain Mapp. 2017;38(2): 740-52.
11. Prieur DS, Rebsam A. Retinal axon guidance at the midline: chiasmatic misrouting and consequences. Dev Neurobiol. 2017;77(7):844-60.

12. Evans DGR, Salvador H, Chang VY. Cancer and Central Nervous System Tumor Surveillance in Pediatric Neurofibromatosis 1. Clin Cancer Res. 2017;23(12): e46-e53.
13. Wan MJ, Ullrich NJ, Manley PE. Long-term visual outcomes of optic pathway gliomas in pediatric patients without neurofibromatosis type 1. J Neuro Oncol. 2016;129(1):173-8.
14. Parsa CF, Hoyt CS, Lesser RL, et al. Spontaneous regression of optic Gliomas. Arch Ophthalmol. 2001;119(4): 516-29.
15. de Blank PM, Berman JI, Liu GT, et al. Fractional anisotropy of the optic radiations is associated with visual acuity loss in optic pathway gliomas of neurofibromatosis type 1. Neuro Oncol. 2013;15(8):1088-95.
16. El-Shehaby AM, Reda WA, Abdel Karim KM, et al. Single-session Gamma Knife radiosurgery for optic pathway/ hypothalamic gliomas. J Neurosurg. 2016;125(Suppl1):50-7.
17. Banerjee A, Jakacki RI, Onar-Thomas A, et al. A phase I trial of the MEK inhibitor selumetinib (AZD6244) in pediatric patients with recurrent or refractory low-grade glioma: a Pediatric Brain Tumor Consortium (PBTC) study. Neuro Oncol. 2017;19(8):1135-34.
18. PDQ Pediatric Treatment Editorial Board. Childhood Craniopharyngioma Treatment (PDQ®): Health Professional Version. 2017.
19. Cannavò S, Venturino M, Curtò L, et al. Clinical presentation and outcome of pituitary adenomas in teenagers. Clin Endocrinol. 2003;58(4):519-27.
20. Kinoshita Y, Tominaga A, Usui S, et al. Pituitary adenomas in childhood and adolescence with a focus on intratumoral hemorrhage. Pituitary. 2014;17(1):1-6.
21. Casteels I, De Loof E, Brock P. Sudden blindness in a child: presenting symptom of a sphenoid sinus mucocele. Br J Ophthalmol. 1992;76:502-4.
22. Caluwaerts E, De Waele L, Buyse G. Chiasmal optic neuritis in a 4-year-old girl: a case report and review of the literature. Bull Soc Belge Ophtalmol. 2012;320:5-10.

Chapter 78 Nystagmus

Paolo Nucci, Matteo Scaramuzzi

INTRODUCTION

The aim of this chapter is to offer a brief but complete and modern insight to this often considered a obscure field. Unfortunately, it suffers for the demand of conciseness of this volume. Much of what is reported in this book comes from our understanding of reading and listening of two mentors: Larry Dell'Osso and Richard Hertle, whose views are not necessarily concordant with our synthetic approach and this is also the result of an extensive clinical practice in the field.

Nystagmus is an unintentional and uncontrolled, often purposeless rhythmic see-sawing, that can involve one or both eyes. Estimates of prevalence and incidence of nystagmus vary: the prevalence in young children has been reported between 0.16% and 0.35%, but it is higher in subgroup of patients like in children with Down syndrome (≈16%), with intellectual disability (≈5%) or in children with strabismus (≈50%).[1]

A unique and convincing explanation of the nature of nystagmus has not been accepted yet, but different models attempted to explain the mechanisms behind it. Three major supranuclear systems (pursuit system, the vestibular system and neural integrator) are crucial in stabilizing eye movements. The pursuit system provides major inputs to fixation stability; right and left vestibular apparatus provides neural charges that drive the eyes contralaterally (diseases that affect this system can cause different manifestations of acquired nystagmus); neural integrator is a hypothesized neuronal system that plans the firing rate and the muscle tone of the extraocular muscles in order to overcome the elastic forces of the orbit and/or maintain an eccentric position of gaze.[2]

It is important to differentiate nystagmus from other abnormal movements such as saccadic intrusions or saccadic oscillations that affect fixation: clinically, they are arrhythmic involuntary movements with chaotic nature and a slow phase is not recognizable, which is a key feature to conform to the definition of nystagmus.

The jerk nystagmus is characterized by two phases: the first one drifts from the visual target ("slow-phase") followed by a corrective one that comes back to the target ("fast-phase"). By convention, the jerk nystagmus direction is reported as its fast-phase orientation.

Slow-phase movements that oscillate equally in both directions without a fast phase, characterize pendular nystagmus (Fig. 78.1).

In acquired nystagmus, patients may often report oscillopsia, a disturbing sensation of a jelly-like movement of the environment which is absent in children with congenital nystagmus. Associate neurologic symptoms like vertigo, ataxia, motor or sensory weakness should be investigated too. It is important to differentiate between congenital and acquired nystagmus in order to consider the greater implications related to neuropathology.

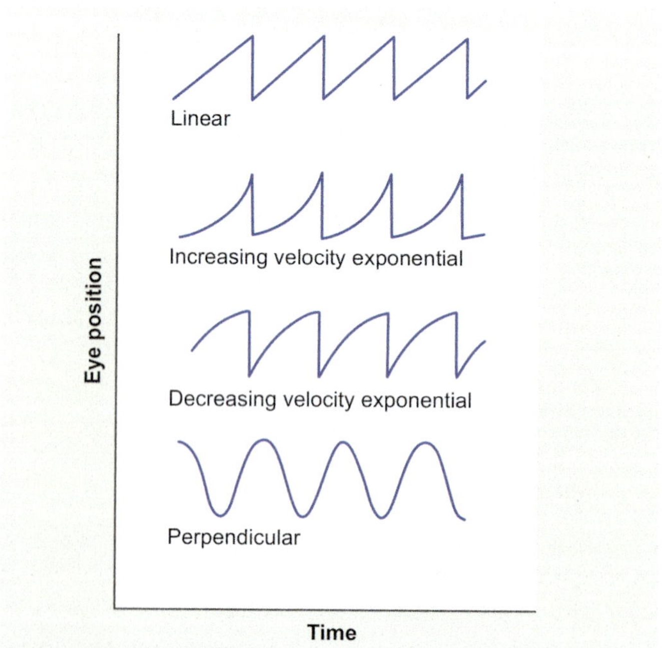

Fig. 78.1: Nystagmus waveforms, named for their slow-phase velocity profile.

Box 78.1: Types of common nystagmus.

- *Early onset (Jerk and/or Pendular):*
  - Infantile nystagmus syndrome (Congenital nystagmus)
  - Fusion maldevelopment nystagmus syndrome
  - Spasmus nutans
- *Acquired jerk:*
  - Vestibular
  - Gaze-evoked
  - Periodic alternating
  - Downbeat
  - Upbeat
  - Convergence retraction
- *Acquired pendular:*
  - Oculopalatal myoclonus
  - See-saw

Most common forms of nystagmus can be grouped primarily on the basis of the predominant waveform and secondarily on the age of onset (Box 78.1). In this chapter, we have classified the different forms of nystagmus following the indication of the Committee for the Classification of Eye Movement Abnormalities and Strabismus (CEMAS).[3]

EVALUATION

History

Primarily, the clinician needs to detect the outset of the disease if the patient has been afflicted from childbirth or if it appeared in the first months of life or if it was an acquired one.The history should also include questions about perinatal events (labor, delivery, infections, prematurity, etc.).

Inheritance should also be investigated. Many forms of nystagmus are inherited as direct genetic defect or associated with other ocular conditions (Box 78.2). The majority of early forms of nystagmus is sporadic, but inheritance has been described. The most common inheritance pattern is the X-linked one while the autosomal cases are more rare, both dominant or recessive. Examination of affected family members can provide useful information.

OCULAR EXAMINATION

Visual Acuity

Quality of vision is the most important prognostic information to offer to the parents and although difficult to obtain, every effort should be undertaken in order to provide as early as possible information about the visual function and all the possible limitation for the patient's future life.

Box 78.2: Ocular conditions associated with nystagmus.

- *Anterior segment abnormalities:*
  - Congenital cataract
  - Congenital glaucoma
  - Iridocorneal dysgenesis
- *Retinal abnormalities:*
  - Leber congenital amaurosis
  - Achromatopsia
  - Congenital stationary night blindness
  - Foveal hypoplasia (albinism, aniridia)
- *Vitreoretinal abnormalities:*
  - Retinopathy of prematurity
  - Coloboma involving macula
  - Familial exudative vitreoretinopathy
  - Congenital retinoschisis
  - Retinoblastoma
- *Optic nerve disorders:*
  - Optic nerve hypoplasia
  - Optic nerve coloboma
  - Optic atrophy
- *Infectious diseases:*
  - Congenital toxoplasmosis
  - Cytomegalovirus
  - Rubella
  - Lymphocytic choriomeningitis virus
  - Syphilis

Binocular VA should be measured first, evaluating distance and near vision with any desired head position to assess the best corrected visual acuity (BCVA) in the real life. Near VA is often better. Any anomalous head posture (AHP) needs to be confirmed observing the patient for several minutes, looking for a possible change in head posture (it can happen in patients with congenital nystagmus, see later).

Monocular VA should be tested fogging the contralateral eye because occlusion may increase oscillations further reducing the foveation period.

A significant decrease during monocular testing is expected and it is considered normal.

The most accurate test is the early treatment diabetic retinopathy study (ETDRS) chart in older and co-operative children while in nonverbal patients you can simply use fixation behavior, Teller acuity cards, LEA symbols or hot vision test (HOTV).

The cover/uncover test and the alternate cover test are fundamental to analyze the ocular alignment.

Binocular function for distance and near (worth four dot test and Lang stereotest or random dot test in older children) should always be tested at this time.

In order to calculate the foveation periods in this kind of patients, the expanded nystagmus acuity function (NAFX) algorithm has been developed. With the help of the NAFX algorithm, it is now possible to determine with a greater accuracy the best corrected potential visual acuity in the majority of nystagmus forms.[4] Thanks to the NAFX reliability, the most important recent clinical studies considering potential therapies in humans or animal models assessment had used this mathematical method as biomarker for ocular motor outcome measure.[5]

Psychological factors (as anxiety, agitation) need to be taken into account in the evaluation of these patients as intensity of nystagmus may significantly vary. Patients with nystagmus and nearly normal VA probably have a benign entity. Conversely marked decreased VA suggests retinal or optic nerve abnormalities.

Refraction

Refractive errors compensation therapy should be attempted in all cases.

Complete cycloplegic refraction is a fundamental and useful tool for the clinician, considering that many older children or even adults could present uncorrected hyperopia or astigmatism, which are not disclosed with subjective refraction.

Pupils

The examiner should investigate direct reaction to light, afferent defect, reaction to darkness and anatomical structure. Optic nerve or retinal abnormalities are the major causes of an impaired response to light, or of the presence of an afferent pupillary defect. Responses can be normal in mild abnormalities, as foveal hypoplasia, incomplete achromatopsia or primary motor nystagmus.

Paradoxical pupillary response can be a sign of congenital stationary night blindness and complete achromatopsia.

Irregular pupil can disclose an embryological defect suggesting an optic nerve or retinal coloboma.

We suggest that the first sign to be investigated in nystagmus patients is iris transillumination, a pathognomonic sign of albinism although a positive test is very specific, its absence cannot rule out this diagnosis. In the everyday practice, transillumination in nystagmus makes genetic testing clinically redundant.

Ocular Motility

The examination of ocular motility begins assessing alignment and ocular stability in primary gaze, then it is crucial to differentiate the type of nystagmus, characterizing it with specific attributes capable to classify the form:

- Monocular or binocular
- Conjugate or disconjugate (same direction or not)
- Associated or dissociated (eyes behave similarly or not)
- Horizontal, vertical, torsional or multiplanar
- Slow-phase only (pendular) or with fast-slow phases (jerk)
- Gaze-evoked
- Reduced at null point (field gaze at which the nystagmus is minimal or absent)

Other features are frequency (oscillations per unit of time), amplitude (angular distance) and intensity (product with the frequency and the amplitude). Gaze position can affect amplitude and frequency. This is particularly true for jerk nystagmus, which can have a null point or decreased intensity of oscillations. A manifestation of this condition is the head posture that patients assume in order to reduce nystagmus.

Ocular motor recording (electro- or video-oculography, infra-red tracking, and electromagnetic techniques) provides a precise measure, but they are rarely needed in clinical practice. Video recording is a useful way to analyze eye movements characteristics.

Strabismus could be an independent manifestation or else the result of poor vision caused by nystagmus; on the other hand, strabismus could cause nystagmus as in fusion maldevelopment nystagmus syndrome (FMNS). Patients affected by manifestation of latent nystagmus often fixate with the preferred eye in adduction and their head turned to maximize their VA.

Fundus

Certain forms of nystagmus can be associated with retinal disorders that show detectable peculiarities but in others fundus appears normal or with aspecific signs such as an abnormal distribution of pigment epithelium anomalous distribution, vascular pattern abnormalities and uncommon macular region appearance. Electrophysiologic testing may be necessary to identify the cause. We suggest to early document with retinography and optical coherence tomography (OCT), the fundus appearance (Figs. 78.2 and 78.3).

EARLY-ONSET (CHILDHOOD) NYSTAGMUS

Infantile Nystagmus Syndrome (Congenital Nystagmus)

Infantile nystagmus syndrome (INS) previously named congenital nystagmus (CN) is usually recognized during first week of life.

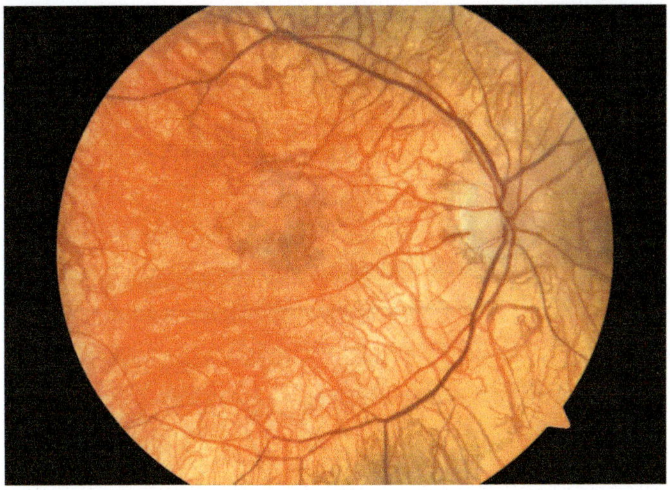

Fig. 78.2: Fundus hypopigmentation in patient with albinism with visible deep choroidal vasculature.

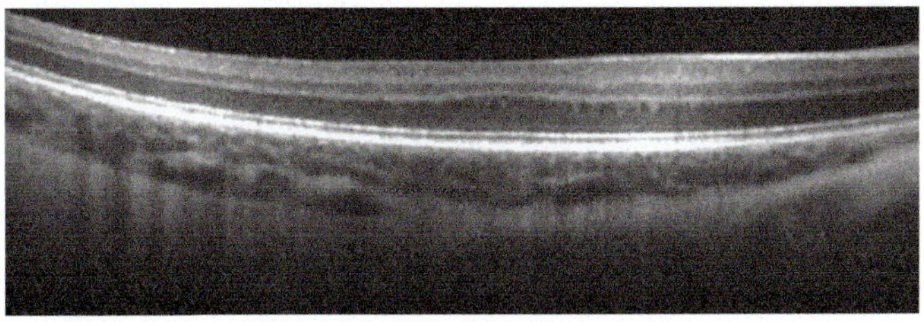

Fig. 78.3: Optical coherence tomography (OCT) macula in patient with albinism with absence of foveal pit.

Parents may be affected too. The transmission could be autosomal or X-linked. The most frequent mutation is over *FRMD7 protein* as a dominant X-linked trait with incomplete penetrance.[6]

The etiology is unknown nowadays. It can be isolated and named as idiopathic and may be associated with afferent pathway diseases or other pathologies that compromise visual development in the early period such as albinism, achromatopsia, optic nerve hypoplasia, aniridia, foveal hypoplasia, congenital stationary night blindness.

The cause of INS is still unknown. The previous definition described CN as "sensorial" or "motor" but it has now been overtaken. A misunderstanding over David Cogan's article[7] has falsely accorded him the paternity of the relationship pendular nystagmus-sensorial deficit and jerk nystagmus-motility disorder. Years of motility recordings didn't prove any association between waveforms and presence or absence of visual deficit.[8] This old definition assumes that two different pathophysiological mechanisms exist, but no scientific evidences have been shown.

The most likely scenario is that the slow-phase speed is due to a high-gain instability of the smooth pursuit system (an amplification of the relation between output and input) whereas fast-phase is a corrective mechanism.[9] Infantile nystagmus syndrome is a binocular conjugate horizontal nystagmus, even in up- and down-gaze. It may be continuous or intermittent and appears as jerk or pendular in different gaze positions. The jerk waveform shows an exponential increase in velocity of slow-phase. In INS, it is possible to identify a "neutral zone", an area of the vision in which are present pendular waves (or bi-directional jerks) that lie between area of right jerk and left jerk waves.

INS often has a null point with an associated AHP (between 20% and 70% of cases) that becomes more pronounced as the child approaches school age, increasing his/her visual demand for far tasks. The AHP can also change over time cyclically or more than one position can be disclosed during observation in the same setting. This particular form of nystagmus is called asymmetric periodic alternating nystagmus (APAN) characterized by regular or irregular amplitude and directional change over time. APAN occurs in about 17% of INS, more frequently associated with albinism.[10] During the examination, it is very important to observe for several consecutive minutes, the posture to avoid missing the diagnosis of APAN.

In INS, amplitude and velocity are amplified by visual attention and fixation, whereas amplitude damps with convergence called "convergence damping" and it is abolished in sleep or in darkness.

When combined with esotropia at distance in the attempt to damp it, it is classified as "nystagmus blockage syndrome". If one eye is adducted the nystagmus damps, if the fixating eye is abducted it gets worse. Moreover, an inconstant angle of esotropia is present that increases if the clinician places a base-out prism in front of the fixating eye.

Two-thirds of patients with INS show a characteristic feature: a paradoxical inversion of the optokinetic response. Normally, if a patient with right jerk nystagmus views an optokinetic drum rotating left, the nystagmus intensity increases. But in INS patients the intensity decreases or even it appears at left jerk nystagmus.[11]

Oscillopsia, typical of acquired nystagmus is usually not present.

The VA is related to the foveation period between involuntary movements as well as to a possible afferent disease but invariably the near performance is better than at distance.

Fusion Maldevelopment Nystagmus Syndrome

Fusion maldevelopment nystagmus syndrome (FMNS), formerly known as latent nystagmus (LN) or manifest latent nystagmus (MLN), is an early-onset, horizontal conjugate jerk nystagmus that is accentuated by monocular viewing. The current name FMNS arises from the fact that it always occurs in patients with altered fusion resulted by early-onset strabismus or decreased vision in one or both eyes with an immaturity of optokinetic system that persists for the missed development of binocular vision.[2]

If the patient's gaze has the same orientation of the fast-phase, that is always headed toward the fixating eye, there is an augmentation in the amplitude of the nystagmus as described by Alexander law. Consequently, patients rotate their head toward the fixating eye (we called this "the "hunter position") to reach the point in which the nystagmus is minimum (the "adduction null"), obtaining an AHP.[12]

The fast-phase is oriented in the opposite direction of the covered eye (the slow-phase toward the nose) hence, it reverses direction alternating the covered eye. This nystagmus is the only form that reverses direction toward the uncovered eye. Therefore, VA is better in binocular and it decreases if measured with the use of a standard occluder. To obtain a better VA in fellow eye, avoiding nystagmus, positive lens (approximately +5.00 D) or filters is used on one eye to create a fogging effect. FMNS is almost always associated with essential infantile esotropia and frequently with dissociated vertical deviation (DVD), strabismus is considered a necessary insufficient requisite to develop FMNS.[13]

FMNS is usually evoked after occluding one eye but could be also present in monocular viewing with both eyes open and this was originally called manifest LN. Because most patients have esotropia, manifest LN is initiated when the esotropic eye is suppressed and the patient is concentrated on the fixating eye.

As for INS, even in FMNS the most important information are given by the analysis of the slow-phase. In FMNS the waveform raises sharply, meanwhile in LN the slow-phase speed is regular (Figs. 78.4A and B).

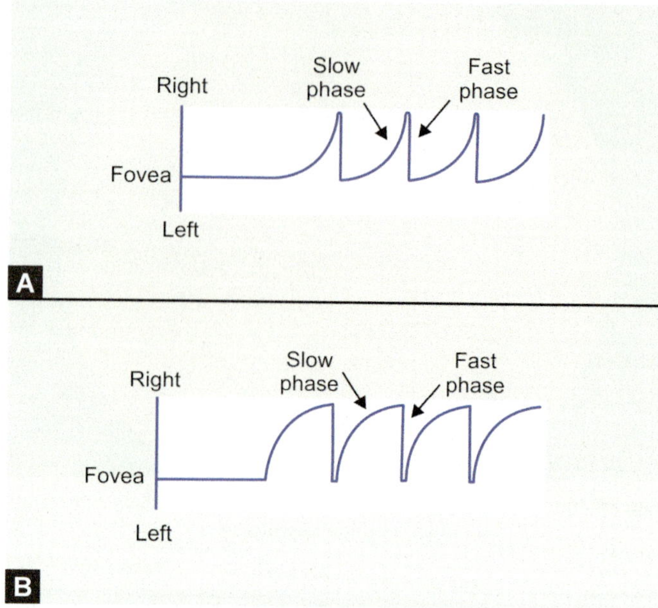

Figs. 78.4A and B: Left jerk nystagmus. (A) Congenital motor nystagmus; (B) Manifest latent nystagmus.

Spasmus Nutans

Spasmus nutans (SN) syndrome is an idiopathic acquired binocular but dissociated nystagmus that manifests during the first 2 years of life and clinically disappeared in 2 years presenting as a triad of:

- Generally small-amplitude, high frequency (shimmering) pendular nystagmus.
- Head nodding, continuous oscillations on sagittal line.
- Torticollis.

The nystagmus is often asymmetric (it could appear monocular) and can vary with gaze position. Movement can be horizontal, vertical or torsional, occasionally intermittent. Head nodding and torticollis are possibly compensatory movements in order to maximize the acuity.[14] Usually abnormal head and eye movements diminish by 3–4 years of age. Possible consequences could frequently be strabismus and amblyopia.[15]

In general, SN is distinguished from INS by abnormal head movements and head posture, the intermittent and variable nature of nystagmus and the relatively high frequency of eye movements. It could be difficult to differentiate SN from other monocular nystagmus of childhood.

Spasmus nutans is a benign disorder in majority of cases but it has been seen with chiasmal or suprachiasmal tumors and retinal dystrophies. Neuroimaging is, therefore, warranted if any manifestation of optic nerve dysfunction or any sign of neurologic abnormality is found to exclude anterior visual pathways or parasellar hypothalamic tumors. If SN appears after the 3rd year of age, a solid cerebral tumor must be ruled out with magnetic resonance imaging (MRI).

Table 78.1: Types of early-onset nystagmus.

	INS	FMNS	SN
Early onset	Yes	Yes	Yes
Possible visual deficit alone	Yes	Yes	Yes
Possible disease association	Yes (albinism, achromatopsia, aniridia, optic nerve hypoplasia)	Yes (strabismic amblyopia)	Yes (optic pathway glioma or retinal dystrophy)
Characteristics	Bilateral, conjugate, symmetrical, jerk, pendular, or mixed	Bilateral, conjugate, symmetrical, jerk, beats toward unoccluded eye	Low amplitude, high frequency, disconjugate, asymmetrical, pendular
Fixation/Stress worsening	Yes	No	No
Convergence/Rest improvement	Yes	Yes	–
AHP	≈20% eccentric point	5–10% "adduction null"	multiplanar
Strabismus	≈50%	≈100%	≈10–20%
Latent component	Occasionally	Yes	No
History	Amplitude decreases, but persists	Amplitude decreases, but persists	Disappears by 2–4 years of age
Oculography	Increasing velocity in slow phase	Decreasing or linear velocity in slow phase	>10 Hz, disconjugate, multiplanar, pendular
Other features	Maintains horizontal directionality in upgaze	Alternating direction of fast phase with alternate eye occlusion	Neuroimaging evaluation

(AHP: Anomalous head posture; FMNS: Fusion maldevelopment nystagmus syndrome; INS: Infantile nystagmus syndrome; SN: Spasmus nutans)

In Table 78.1, the most characteristics features of these three early-onset types of nystagmus are summarized to allow an immediate comparison.[16]

Anomalous Head Posture in Patients with Strabismus and Nystagmus

As seen above, AHP, strabismus and nystagmus are frequently associated. When these three signs are present at the same time, it is very important to understand the etiology of the AHP. For this purpose, it's extremely useful the diagnostic algorithms proposed by Hertle in 2000[17] divided in four steps (Flowchart 78.1):

1. The first step consists of the realignment of the patient's head and then observe which sign changes, if nystagmus or strabismus. Usually, you observe an exacerbation of the cause of AHP.
2. In the second step, we observe how the responsible condition changes. Is there a worsening or an improvement? For example, if the strabismus improves with the head realignment, it is not very likely that strabismus is the causing condition. Conversely, if the nystagmus gets worse, this is the most probable cause of AHP and it remains to understand if we are dealing with INS or with FMNS.
3. The third step answers to this question. The clinician must observe how the fixating eye changes during the head realignment. If this eye is aligned with respect to the socket with the head and chin-up or chin-down, there is a CN. If the fixating eye is in abduction, it can never be a FMNS because these patients are characterized by the "adduction null" position and FMNS gets worse in abduction.
4. The forth step analyzes, the hypothesis of fixating eye in adduction, a condition that can be present both in INS and FMNS and it is the most frequent. Although electronystagmography is the best examination to reveal with high levels of confidence a decreasing or increasing slow-phase, respectively typical of FMNS or INS, this examination is not available in the office setting so we can observe the nonfixating eye conduct:
    - A decrease of nystagmus intensity in non-fixating eye in abduction suggests an INS whereas a decrease in adduction suggests majorly a FMNS (even if APAN can simulate this aspect).
    - Perform the cover-uncover test in far adduction of the fixating eye and observe the nonfixating eye's nystagmus: if it reverses again, it is an APAN.[18,19]

Flowchart 78.1: Etiology of abnormal head position in patients with strabismus and nystagmus.

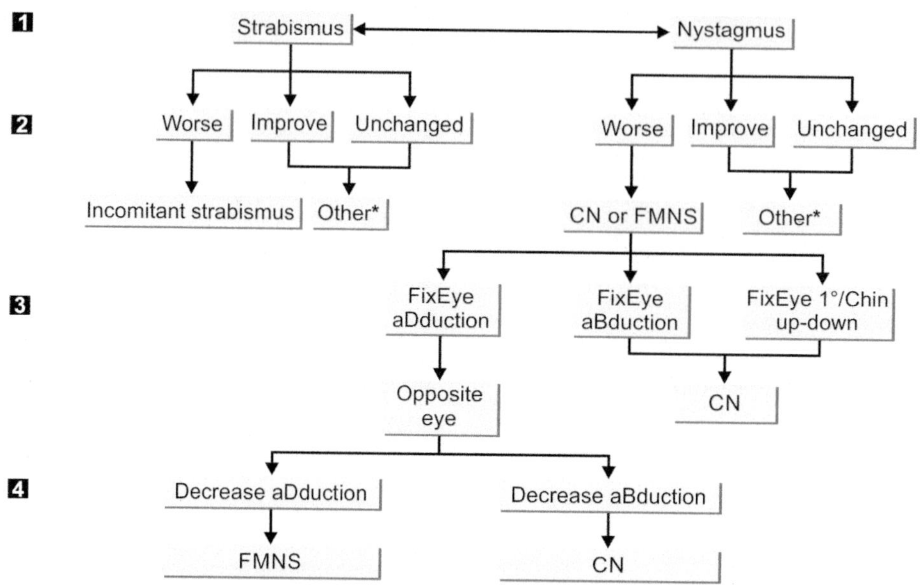

(CN: Congenital nystagmus; FMNS: Fusion maldevelopment nystagmus syndrome)

*Refractive errors, lid anomalies, media opacities, central nervous system diseases, head-neck-face-shoulder-back anomalies.

TREATMENT

The treatment is chosen among many depending on the clinical features (Table 78.2).

Prism

Use of the prisms can normalize an anomalous head position by shifting the retinal image toward the null point or improve vision by inducing artificial divergence. They can be used as the sole treatment or as a method to predict surgical success.

The Fresnel press-on prisms can be used if power of less than 20 D is required. They are thin inexpensive transparent plastic membranes that can be cut and applied to framed glasses.

Built-in prisms cause less distortion and are preferred for patients who require permanent, but smaller amount of correction, but often a big amount of prism diopters is necessary to correct AHP in nystagmus.

To correct head position, the prism is mounted with the apex pointing the null point, i.e. if the patient has a left head turn with a null point in right gaze, the prism before the right eye should be oriented base-in and the one before left eye should be oriented base-out. This shift images to the right and decreases the amount of head turn.[20] If this technique improves head position, it is also likely that nystagmus surgery will be effective.

Prisms base-in can also improve VA by stimulating fusional convergence, which damps the nystagmus. They are placed in front of both eyes in amounts determined by trial and error.

Pharmacologic Therapy

Drugs are used in forms of vestibular, congenital or acquired nystagmus or additional eye movement disorders.

A $GABA_B$ receptor agonist (baclofen) is used in certain acquired form of periodic alternating nystagmus.[21]

Carbamazepine derivatives and beta-blockers are frequently effective in superior oblique myokymia.[22]

Downbeat and other central vestibular forms of nystagmus can be helped by $GABA_A$ receptor agonist (clonazepam).

Other GABAnergic drugs (like Memantine or Gabapentin) may reduce nystagmus severity and improve patients' visual acuity.[23]

Unilateral retrobulbar injection of Botulinum toxin type A was investigated to decrease amplitude of nystagmus and to produce improvements for those who are willing to have a one-eyed sight.[24]

Table 78.2: Possibilities of nystagmus treatment.

	Drugs/Procedures	Surgery
AHP	Prisms (base-out in adducting eye and base-in in abducting eye)	"Anderson-Kestenbaum" resection-recession both eyes
Strabismus	Prisms	Recess/Resect procedures
Oscillopsia	Optical retinal image stabilization *Medications (off-label use)*: Baclofen Gabapentin Clonazepam Memantine Carbamazepine	Botulinum toxin injection Retroequatorial rectus recession
Blockage Nystagmus syndrome	Prism spectacles (base-out in both eyes)	Bimedial rectus recession
Decreased vision	Contact lens Bioptics	Retroequatorial rectus recession Horizontal rectus tenotomy

(AHP: Anomalous head position)

SURGERY

In Patients with Abnormal Head Position

Extraocular muscle surgery for nystagmus is indicated for correction of an AHP which is achieved by shifting the null point closer to the primary position. It may also improve visual acuity by decreasing nystagmus intensity and consequently improving foveation time.

The types of surgery typically recommended are:

- Anderson procedure, a conjugate recession in each eye.[25]
- Kestenbaum procedure, a recession-resection on both eyes.[26]
- A recession of all four horizontal rectus muscles.[27]

In horizontal AHP, the eyes are surgically rotated following the orientation of the head turn, opposite from the null point or preferred gaze position.[28] For instance, in INS, left head turn and null point in right gaze, eyes are surgically rotated to the left by recession of the right lateral and left medial rectus muscles and by resection of right medial and left lateral rectus muscles (Kestenbaum procedure) shifting the null point in primary position. The amounts of recession-resection modified by Parks[29] performed are listed in Table 78.3. For head turns of 30°, a 40% augmentation is recommended and for turns of 45°, augmentation of 60% is recommended. Augmented procedures often cause limitation of motility which is usually necessary to achieve a satisfactory result.

If vertical torticollis is present with INS, prisms or surgery may ameliorate chin-up or chin-down posturing. As for horizontal nystagmus, the eyes need to be rotated away from the null point.

If there is a chin-down eyes-up head position is present, superior rectus muscles are recessed with or without inferior recti resection. Another possibility is to weak agonist vertical muscles (recti and oblique muscles) in both eyes, i.e. in a chin-up position, inferior rectus and superior oblique muscles are weakened.

In torsional head posture, the approach is the horizontal transposition of vertical recti: take the vertical recti off, move the eyes in the direction of the head posture and reattach them.

In multiplanar head posture the approach considers three-muscle each eye: the surgeon combines respective oblique muscle plus vertical rectus (considering chin-up or chin-down presence) with recession of lateral rectus of abducting eye and recession of medial rectus of adducting eye for head turn or recess/resect one horizontal rectus on each eye for strabismus with no head turn.[30]

When there is no eccentric null point and the Kestenbaum procedure is not indicated, a recession of all horizontal rectus muscles has been offered as alternative (8–10 mm recession for both medial rectus and 10–12 for both lateral rectus).[27]

Recent studies demonstrate that simply disinserting and reattaching horizontal rectus muscles, without any resection or recession, produces similar results with less adverse effects (inducing new strabismus). This procedure has modest effect on VA, even if the foveation time is appreciably longer.[31]

Table 78.3: Amount of surgery for Kestenbaum procedure and modification.

Procedure	Kestenbaum (mm)	40% augmented (mm)	60% augmented (mm)
Eye adducted in null point			
Recess medial rectus	5.0	7.0	8.0
Resect lateral rectus	8.0	11.0	12.5
Eye abducted in null point			
Recess lateral rectus	7.0	10.0	11.0
Resect medial rectus	6.0	8.5	9.5

In Patients with Strabismus

The surgical procedure aims to shift the null point and must be performed on the dominant fixating eye, a two steps procedure can be considered on non-dominant eye to adjust the residual strabismus. For example, a patient who is right-eye dominant, with a right head turn and a null point in left gaze would recess right medial rectus and resect right lateral rectus in amounts indicated in Table 78.3. This procedure reduces esotropia, a remaining deviation can be corrected with a second surgery on the unoperated eye.

In Patients without Strabismus and Anomalous Head Position

Surgical approach needs to be considered even in some patients without AHP or strabismus.

In patients with convergence damping, an artificial divergence could be considered. Surgically, this goal can be achieved with a bilateral recession of medial rectus muscles.[30]

In nystagmus alone a bilateral horizontal recti tenotomy with reattachment has been proposed.[31]

REFERENCES

1. Sarvananthan N, Surendran M, Roberts EO, et al. The Prevalence of Nystagmus: the Leicestershire Nystagmus Survey. Invest Opthalmol Vis Sci. 2009;50(11):5201-6.
2. Hertle RW. Nystagmus in infancy and childhood. Semin Ophthalmol. 2008;23(5):307-17.
3. CEMAS Working Group. A National Eye Institute-Sponsored Workshop and Publication on the Classification of Eye Movement Abnormalities and Strabismus; 2001.
4. Dell'Osso LF, Jacobs JB. An expanded nystagmus acuity function: intra- and intersubject prediction of best-corrected visual acuity. Doc Ophthalmol. 2002;104(3):249-76.
5. Felius J, Fu VL, Birch EE, et al. Quantifying nystagmus in infants and young children: relation between foveation and visual acuity deficit. Invest Opthalmol Vis Sci. 2011;52(12):8724-31.
6. Tarpey P, Thomas S, Sarvananthan N, et al. Mutations in FRMD7, a newly identified member of the FERM family, cause X-linked idiopathic congenital nystagmus. Nat Genet. 2006;38(11):1242-4.
7. Cogan DG. Congenital nystagmus. Can J Ophthalmol. 1967;2(1):4-10.
8. Hertle RW, Dell'Osso LF. Clinical and ocular motor analysis of congenital nystagmus in infancy. J AAPOS Off Publ Am Assoc Pediatr Ophthalmol Strabismus. 1999;3(2):70-9.
9. Dell'Osso L, Gauthier G, Liberman G, et al. Eye movement recordings as a diagnostic tool in a case of congenital nystagmus. Am J Optom Arch Am Acad Optom. 1972;49(1):3-13.
10. Hertle RW, Yang D, Kelly K, et al. X-Linked Infantile Periodic Alternating Nystagmus. Ophthalmic Genet. 2005;26(2):77-84.
11. Dell'Osso LF, van der Steen J, Steinman RM, et al. Foveation dynamics in congenital nystagmus. I: Fixation. Doc Ophthalmol. 1992;79(1):1-23.
12. Dell'Osso LF, Schmidt D, Daroff RB. Latent, manifest latent, and congenital nystagmus. Arch Ophthalmol. 1979;97(10):1877-85.
13. Dell'osso LF, Traccis S, Abel LA. Strabismus–a necessary condition for latent and manifest latent nystagmus. Neuro-ophthalmology. 1983;3(4):247-57.
14. Gottlob I, Zubcov AA, Wizov SS, Reinecke RD. Head nodding is compensatory in spasmus nutans. Ophthalmology. 1992;99(7):1024-31.
15. Gottlob I, Wizov SS, Reinecke RD. Spasmus nutans. A long-term follow-up. Invest Ophthalmol Vis Sci. 1995;36(13):2768-71.
16. Hertle RW. Nystagmus in Infancy and Childhood. In: Pediatric Ophthalmology. Philadelphia: Springer. 2009. pp. 243-54.
17. Hertle RW, Zhu X. Oculographic and clinical characterization of thirty-seven children with anomalous head postures, nystagmus, and strabismus: the basis of a clinical algorithm. J AAPOS. 2000;4(1):25-32.
18. Nucci P, Hertle RW. Anomalous head posturing in essential infantile esotropia: a hypothesis. Eur J Ophthalmol. 2012;22(3):297-300.

19. Nucci P, Curiel B, Lembo A, et al. Anomalous head posture related to visual problems. Int Ophthalmol. 2015;35(2):241-8.
20. Ansons AM, Davis H. Diagnosis and Management of Ocular Motility Disorders. Oxford: John Wiley & Sons; 2013.
21. Comer RM, Dawson ELM, Lee JP. Baclofen for Patients with Congenital Periodic Alternating Nystagmus. Strabismus. 2006;14(4):205-9.
22. Riva R, Contin M, Albani F, et al. Lateral gaze nystagmus in carbamazepine-treated epileptic patients: correlation with total and free plasma concentrations of parent drug and its 10,11-epoxide metabolite. Ther Drug Monit. 1985;7(3): 277-82.
23. Shery T, Proudlock FA, Sarvananthan N, et al. The effects of gabapentin and memantine in acquired and congenital nystagmus: a retrospective study. Br J Ophthalmol. 2006;90(7):839-43.
24. Lennerstrand G, Nordbø OA, Tian S, et al. Treatment of strabismus and nystagmus with botulinum toxin type A. An evaluation of effects and complications. Acta Ophthalmol Scand. 1998;76(1):27-7.
25. Anderson JR. Causes and treatment of congenital eccentric nystagmus. Br J Ophthalmol. 1953;37(5):267-81.
26. Kestenbaum A. Nouvelle opération du nystagmus. Br J Opthalmol. 1963;47(6):339-45.
27. Helveston EM, Ellis FD, Plager DA. Large recession of the horizontal recti for treatment of nystagmus. Ophthalmology. 1991;98(8):1302-5.
28. Traboulsi E, Utz V. Practical Management of Pediatric Ocular Disorders and Strabismus. Springer, New York; 2016; pp. 822.
29. Parks MM. Symposium: nystagmus. Congenital nystagmus surgery. Am Orthopt J. 1973;23:35-9.
30. Hertle RW, Dell'Osso LF. Nystagmus in infancy and childhood: current concepts in mechanisms, diagnoses, and management. Oxford University Press; 2013. pp. 323.
31. ElKamshoushy A, Shawky D, ElMassry A, et al. Improved visual acuity and recognition time in nystagmus patients following four-muscle recession or Kestenbaum-Anderson procedures. J AAPOS. 2012;16(1):36-40.

Chapter 79

Examination of a Child with Concomitant Strabismus

Perumalsamy Vijayalakshmi, Sathya T Ravilla

INTRODUCTION

Strabismus or misalignment of the eyes causes disruption of the normal binocular vision. There are many natural compensatory mechanisms that take place to alleviate the bothersome visual disturbances that result due to this disruption. It is important to have some basic understanding of binocular vision and the adaptive mechanisms in strabismus before proceeding to evaluation.

EFFECTS OF STRABISMUS

Binocular single vision refers to the perception of a single image through coordinated movements of the two eyes and cortical fusion. It occurs when corresponding retinal elements in both eyes are stimulated giving a common subjective visual direction (Fig. 79.1A).

In the presence of strabismus, the two foveae are stimulated by different objects; the object of fixation is projected on the fovea of the straight eye and an image of an object along the line of deviation is projected on the fovea of the deviating eye (Fig. 79.1B). These dissimilar images are transmitted to a single cortical perceptual area and results in a transient phenomenon of *confusion* as there is a patchy superimposition of two different images.[1] This cortical/retinal rivalry is easily overcome and the brain settles immediately for the single image projected by the fovea of the straight eye and hence, confusion is not a common complaint.

Alternately, the object of fixation would stimulate the fovea in the straight eye and an extrafoveal point in the misaligned eye causing the subject to view the object as two resulting in *diplopia*. The distance between the two objects visualized would be directly proportional to the amount of deviation.

The phenomenon of diplopia causes poor judgment of depth and can be alarming. There are various motor and sensory adaptations that occur to overcome this. But the sensory adaptations are only possible during the first few years of life usually before 6 years of age. After that there is minimal visual-neurological plasticity.[2]

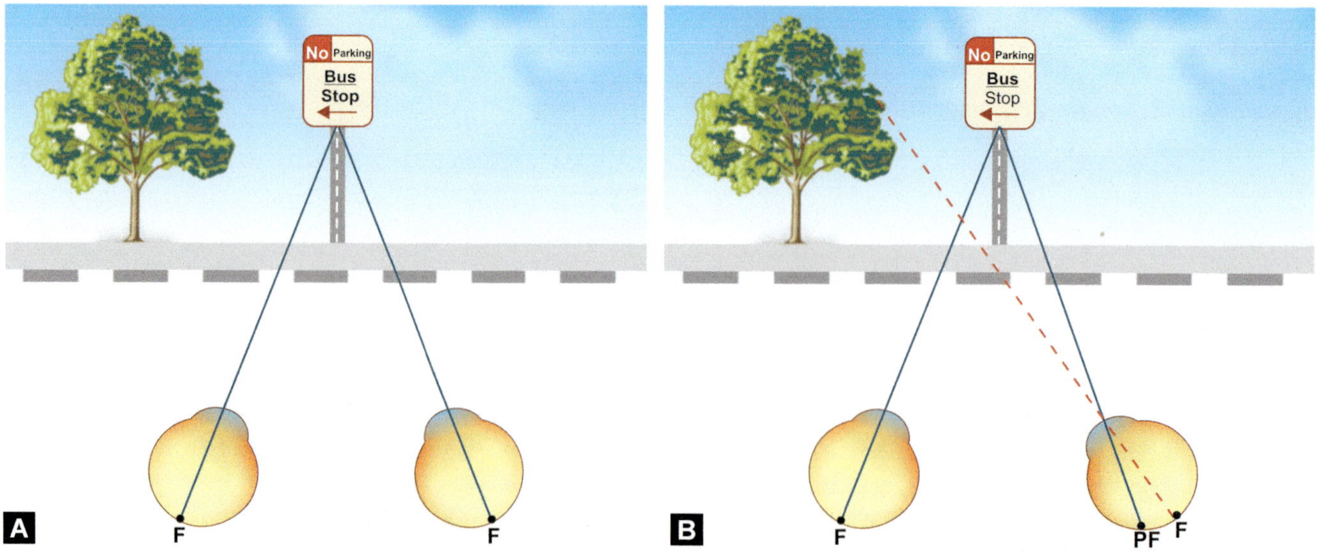

Figs. 79.1A and B: (A) Normal binocular vision on stimulation of corresponding retinal elements in the two eyes; (B) Stimulation of an extra-foveal point by the object of fixation in a left eye esotropia. This can result in confusion or diplopia.

Motor Adaptations

Fusion is the innate ability to join the two similar images perceived in the macula of each eye and see them as one fused image. This is made possible by both convergence and divergence movements. In a normal viewing state, both the eyes lie parallel to each other due to a tonic convergence. When an object moves closer to the face, both eyes need to converge further so as to ensure that the image is perceived in the fovea of both eyes constantly. A strong ability to converge could ensure that an exophoria remains latent and prevents it from becoming manifest. Similarly, the ability to diverge would help in controlling an esophoria but is less strong than the ability to converge. In incomitant strabismus, there are certain positions of gaze where the eyes would be orthophoric and hence, free of diplopia. It is therefore common to notice a compensatory head posture (CHP) adopted in a paralytic or restrictive strabismus to ensure that the image of the object focuses on both the foveae. This is also noticed in vertically incomitant and comitant strabismus such as in A and V pattern. For instance, a child with a V pattern exotropia would prefer to view objects with his chin elevated and one with V-esotropia would prefer chin depression. When evaluating such patients, it is important to examine for binocular vision in their preferred head posture.

One should also be aware that there are other reasons of adopting a head posture. Patients with nystagmus irrespective of the presence of strabismus might adopt a head posture to bring the eyes to the null zone. Occasionally patients with deep amblyopia in one eye would adopt a CHP to have a larger field of vision.

Blind spot mechanism has been described mostly in moderate esotropias of 30–35 prisms of deviation (PD) where the image of fixation would fall on the retina closer to the optic disc. In this motor response, the esotropic eye is further deviated such that the image seen by the deviating eye is focused inside the blind spot. However, this theory is controversial.[3]

Sensory Adaptations

Suppression is a cortical mechanism where there is an active inhibition of the image received from the deviating eye. Suppression could occur only in the deviated eye or can be alternating as fixation changes from one eye to the other.

Foveal suppression in the deviated eye will overcome confusion; suppression of the extrafoveal part of the retina that is stimulated by the fixation object will overcome diplopia (Fig. 79.2A). The suppressed area is described as a scotoma, meaning a blind spot. In esotropes, the suppression scotoma becomes D-shaped with the straight line coinciding with the fovea and in exotropes it encompasses the entire temporal hemi-retina of the deviating eye.

Suppression can also be defined as facultative or obligatory. Facultative suppression is present only when the eyes are in the deviated state and absent in all other states. Obligatory suppression is present at all times and can lead onto amblyopia in children. Younger the child, more rapidly the suppression develops. It is unusual for children over 8 years of age to suppress and even rarer to find suppression in strabismus of adult onset.

Abnormal Retinal Correspondence

Alternately, abnormal retinal correspondence (ARC) develops in some forms of manifest strabismus wherein the fovea of the straight eye forms a correspondence with the nonfoveal area of the deviating eye that received the image of object of fixation (Fig. 79.2B). This coordinated function of the fovea of the fixing eye and the nonfoveal area of the deviating eye results in an abnormal form of binocular single vision and may even have stereopsis though subnormal. Commonly this occurs in strabismus of angles between 15 PD and 30 PD.[2]

When the deviation is fully neutralized sensorially, it is termed harmonious ARC and when the shift in visual directions does not fully compensate for the deviation, it is referred to as unharmonious ARC.

Monofixation Syndrome

In small angle strabismus (less than or equal to 10 PD), the suppression scotoma would be small and will allow for peripheral fusion. This sensory adaptation has been termed the monofixation syndrome. These patients often have amblyopia but may also demonstrate low levels of stereopsis.[2]

Other Adaptations

In the presence of a manifest strabismus, true depth perception is lost. In time, people with strabismus learn to use other monocular clues such as the known size of objects, shadows, etc. to appreciate the depth.

In subjects with alternate squint, the deviating eye contributes to the overall binocular field of vision, this being smaller in esotropes and wider in exotropes.

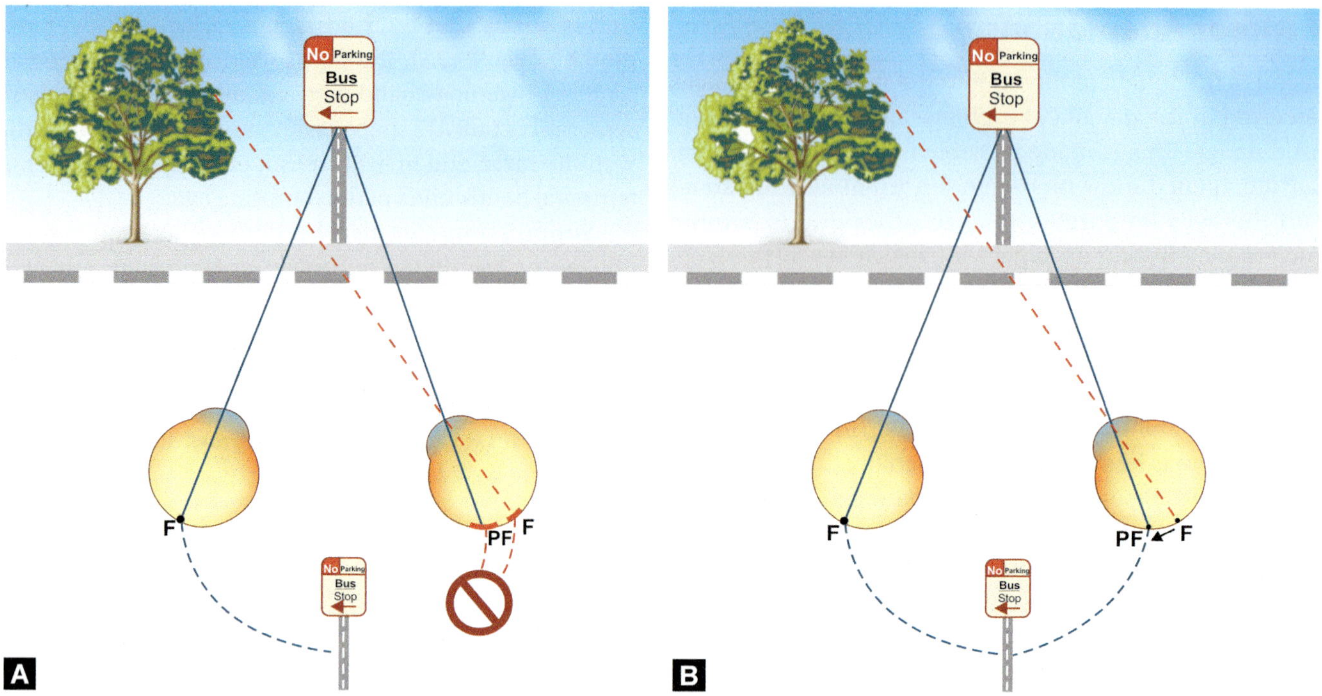

Figs. 79.2A and B: Sensory Adaptations. (A) *Suppression*: Scotoma is seen over the fovea and the extra-foveal point; (B) *Anomalous retinal correspondence*: the parafoveal point (PF) in the esotropic eye is considered as the corresponding point to the fovea (F) of the straight eye.

EVALUATION OF STRABISMUS

The purpose of evaluating a patient with strabismus is to diagnose the type of strabismus, measure the amount of deviation, the potential for binocularity and to determine the muscles that need to be tackled at surgery. A thorough evaluation ensures better planning and surgical results and reduces the likelihood of undesirable postoperative results.

History

Although most of the children presenting with strabismus will be of concomitant etiology, a congenital or an early acquired neurologic defect of ocular movement is not uncommon. It is important to obtain history from a reliable source and from one who spends most time with the child.

History should be obtained like when the squint was noticed, whether it is unilateral or alternating, if the onset was acute or gradual, the constancy and progression of squint. When available, examine photographs of the child at various stages to roughly ascertain the onset of squint. In a squint of acute onset, ask for history of head or eye trauma, recent illness or vaccination.

Younger children most often do not complain of diplopia. It is therefore important to ask for history of any abnormal head posture while looking at the blackboard or watching television. A history of closing one eye in sunlight could be suggestive of diplopia experienced in an intermittent exotropia.

It is also important to obtain information on family history of strabismus, the birth of the child, developmental milestones and other systemic illness. Document information on previous surgeries, occlusion therapy, and spectacle use.

Inspection

Observe a child as they walk into your cubicle for any altered head posture, gait disturbances and general behavior as a child with a CHP would become conscious of it while being examined and hence, mask it. It is pertinent to document the presence of any skull or facial asymmetry.

The palpebral fissures should be inspected for symmetry, ptosis, epicanthal folds, telecanthus and the presence of a mongoloid or anti-mongoloid slant. The interpupillary distance (IPD) should also be measured. A wide IPD or epicanthal folds could give a picture of a pseudoexotropia or a pseudoesotropia respectively. Look for any anisocoria or pupillary abnormalities as most of the methods employed in strabismus evaluation rely on the relation of the corneal light reflex to the pupil. Evaluation in a dilated pupil will be less reliable due to variations in accommodation and blurry vision. The presence of nystagmus and its amplitude, frequency and direction should be noted.

Estimation of Visual Acuity

In general, the deviating eye may exhibit significant vision loss when the onset of the strabismus was at a younger age and is more constant. Estimating the exact visual acuity in infants, toddlers and in children with delayed mentation is challenging. Hence, vision is roughly estimated objectively by comparing the child's response between both eyes to some of the tests described. However, in older children and in a subgroup of younger children who are cooperative, the standardized vision charts are ideal.

Complete occlusion of one eye is mandatory for monocular assessment of visual acuity. Beyond 6 months, the phrase "central, steady and maintained (CSM)" is preferred to describe the fixation ability. Central refers to the corneal reflex from a fixation light falling at the center of the pupil. Steadiness of the fixation is assessed while moving the light source; nystagmus or oscillations denote unsteady fixation. Maintenance of fixation refers to the ability to keep the eye fixed on a target when either eye is covered (Table 79.1).

Table 79.1: Visual acuity estimation by assessing fixation of light.

Fixation	Rough estimate of visual acuity
Holds fixation well with both eyes, alternates spontaneously, cross-fixes	6/6 each eye
Central fixation can hold fixation with both eyes, but strongly prefers other eye	6/9 to 6/18
Central fixation demonstrable with squinting eye but does not hold fixation	6/24 to 6/60
Unsteady central fixation	6/60 or less
Absent fixation to gross eccentric fixation	1/60 or less

Forced preferential looking charts (Fig. 79.3A) are useful in toddlers, however, they need a trained observer and a cooperative child. In preverbal children, recognition acuity tests can be used. There are a variety of matching cards available such as the HOTV vision chart, Sheridan Gardiner, Cambridge crowding cards and Snellen optotypes (Fig. 79.3B).

Corneal Reflex Test

In this test, the patient fixes on a spot light held centrally at eye level at 33 cm. The reflection of the light in both corneae are noted and compared. If a manifest deviation is present, the reflection on the deviating eye will be displaced nasally in exotropia and temporally in esotropia. The corneal reflex is displaced inferiorly and superiorly in hypertropia and hypotropia respectively (Figs. 79.4A to D). At this stage, it is important to differentiate this from a pseudostrabismus due to angle kappa and an eccentric fixation that might be present in macular pathologies.

Angle Kappa

The visual axis refers to a line connecting the fovea with the fixation point and the pupillary axis refers to a line passing through the center of the pupil perpendicular to the cornea. When these two lines do not coincide, angle kappa results (Fig. 79.5A).[4] A positive angle kappa (Fig. 79.5B) is said to be present, when the corneal light reflex is displaced nasally giving the appearance of exotropia. Emmetropes and hyperopes tend to have this type of angle kappa. A negative angle kappa (Fig. 79.5C) is said to be present, when the light reflex is displaced temporally giving the appearance of esotropia. This is common in patients with high myopia. The angle kappa can be unilateral or bilateral and can be

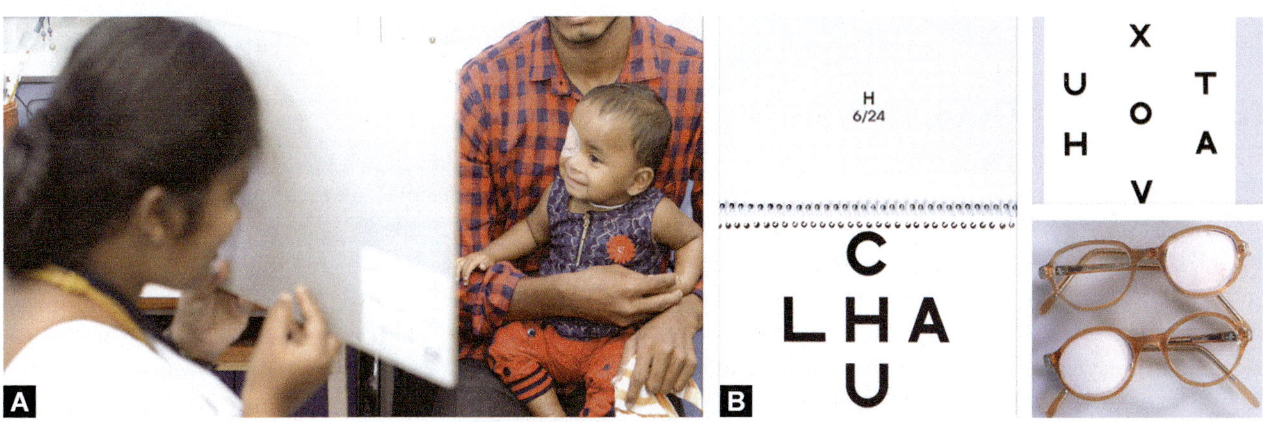

Figs. 79.3A and B: Estimation of visual acuity. (A) Teller's forced preferential looking test; (B) Cambridge crowded matching card with spectacles designed to occlude each eye.

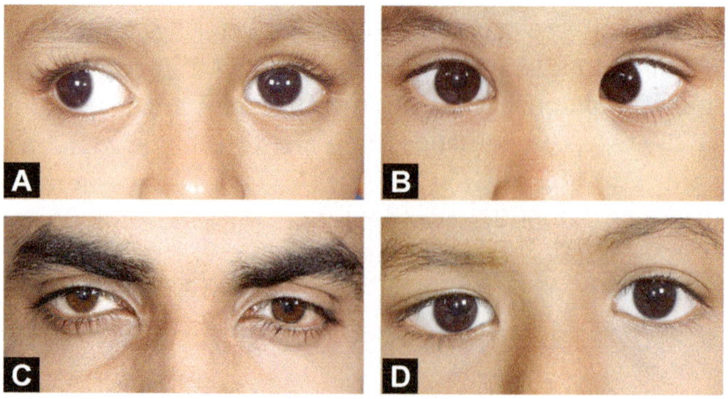

Figs. 79.4A to D: (A) Corneal reflex moved nasally in exotropia; (B) Temporally in esotropia; (C) Inferiorly in hypertropia; (D) Superiorly in hypotropia.

measured by the synoptophore, but this is rarely needed as the absence of deviation is readily revealed on a cover test.

Sensory Evaluation

In a patient with strabismus, it is important to assess the binocular status and the binocular potential. Various methods have been described to test for binocular vision, fusional ability and stereopsis. Diplopia tests use one fixation target seen by both eyes that are dissociated by colored or polarized glasses. Haploscopic test has two fixation targets, one for each eye and is the principle used in a synoptophore. Before commencing a sensory evaluation, one should ensure that the patient wears appropriate refractive correction; contact lenses are preferred in cases of anisometropia and in high myopia.

All tests are tainted by the inability to reproduce patient's casual seeing. The more dissociative the test, the less the test simulates everyday use of the eyes. The afterimage test is considered most dissociating and the Bagolini striated glasses is least dissociating. These tests should ideally be done before doing the cover test as this would dissociate the eyes and convert a phoria to a tropia and could induce facultative suppression.

TESTS FOR BINOCULAR VISION

Worth's Four Dot Test

This test is easier to perform on younger children who would find it difficult to comprehend the Bagolini test. The red and green glasses provide dissociation. The test should be done both at near (Fig. 79.6A) and distance. Patients with the monofixation syndrome would fuse the near W4DT as it subtends at 6° or 12Δ allowing for peripheral fusion but demonstrate suppression of the microtropic eye at distance

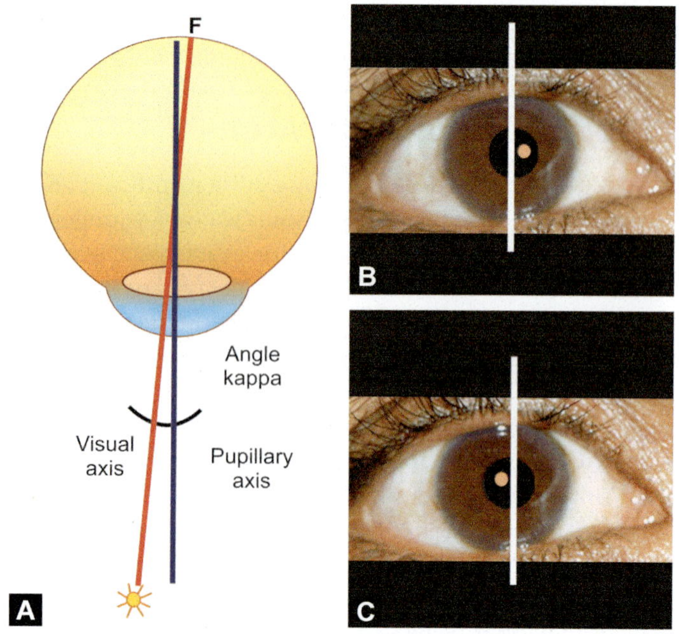

Figs. 79.5A to C: (A) Angle kappa refers to the angle between the visual axis and pupillary axis; (B) Positive angle kappa; (C) Negative angle kappa

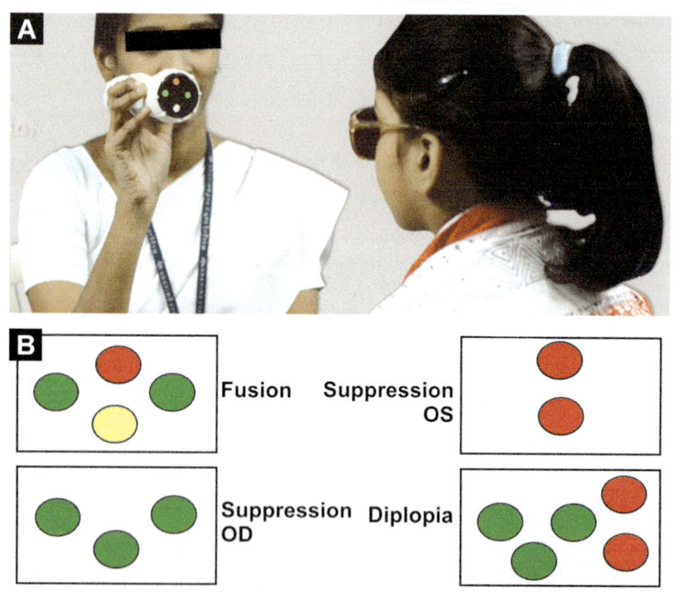

Figs. 79.6A and B: (A) Testing for W4DT at near with red before right eye and green before left eye; (B) *Results*: When all four lights are seen this indicates normal or abnormal retinal correspondence; two red or three green lights indicate suppression; five lights signify diplopia.

as it would subtend at 1.25°, falling within the suppression scotoma. Interpretation of the test is described in Figure 79.6B. The W4DT test can also be done with the room lights dimmed or turned off but this makes it extremely dissociating.

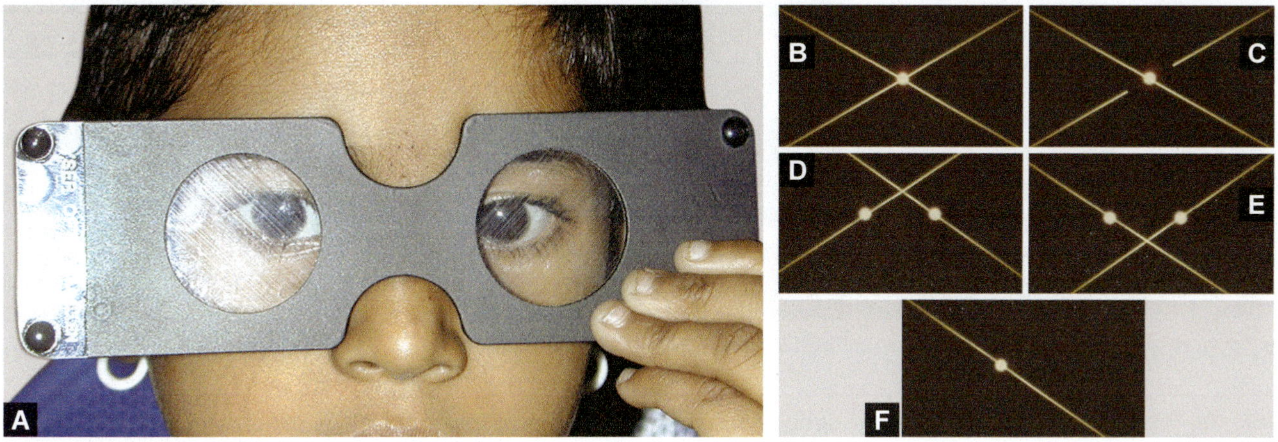

Figs. 79.7A to F: (A) Testing with Bagolini striated glasses. Interpretation of responses; (B) Binocular single vision-orthophoria or intermittent XT; (C) Small central suppression scotoma (Microtopia); (D) NRC with diplopia (no suppression)—Esotropia; (E) NRC with diplopia (no suppression)—Exotropia; (F) Total suppression of the image from OD-ET\XT with preference to fix with LE.

Bagolini Striated Glasses

Bagolini striated glasses are used to diagnose whether retinal correspondence is normal or abnormal and to confirm the presence of binocular single vision. This is particularly useful in small angle strabismus.

Bagolini glasses are available both in the form of single lenses which can be used over a trial frame or as a mounted one (Fig. 79.7A). They consist of fine parallel lines or striations at 45 and 135°. The striations are oriented obliquely giving a better chance of picking up scotomas in microtropia that are most often horizontal. When a spot light is viewed through the glass, a cross-like image would be observed across the center of the spot light.

The test is performed in normal clinic lighting with the striated glasses held in front of the patient›s eyes and the spot light held at 33 cm and then repeated with the light held at 6 m. The possible responses are depicted (Figs. 79.7B to F).

Measuring the Range of Fusion

It is important to measure the patients' range of fusion especially in those with an intermittent strabismus. It assesses the ability to control a deviation and maintain it as a phoria. This can be done using the prism bar (Fig. 79.8) or the synoptophore.

A target is first viewed through smallest base-in prism of the prism bar and then gradually stepped up through higher strengths until the patient is unable to diverge and maintain fusion. It is then repeated with the prism bar base-out to assess convergence. Subjectively, patient will complain of blurring of the target followed by diplopia. Make a note of the blur point, breakpoint and the recovery of fusion.

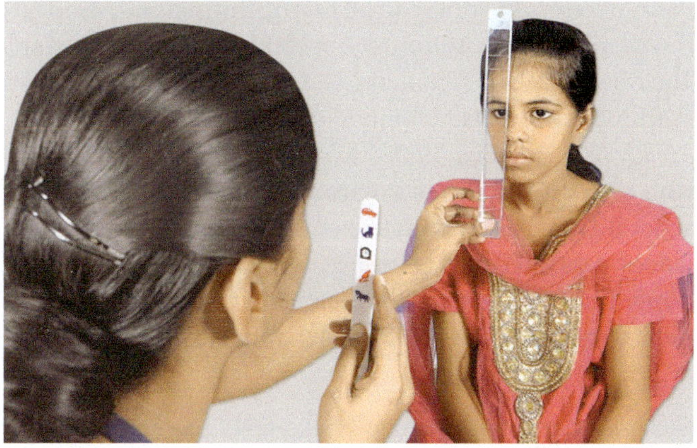

Fig. 79.8: Checking prism fusion amplitude (convergence and divergence) with prism bar.

Fusion is maximal in convergence almost greater than 25 PD and smaller in divergence rarely surpassing 10 PD and is still smaller in vertical vergences within 3–4 PD.[3]

TESTS TO MEASURE STEREOACUITY

Stereoacuity measures the smallest disparity that produces depth perception just as visual acuity measures the smallest image that can be recognized. A number of tests are available:

Random dot stereoacuity test: This test uses two identical set of spots that are horizontally displaced and placed amongst randomly scattered spots. In the TNO test, the spots in the identical sets are red and green and designed

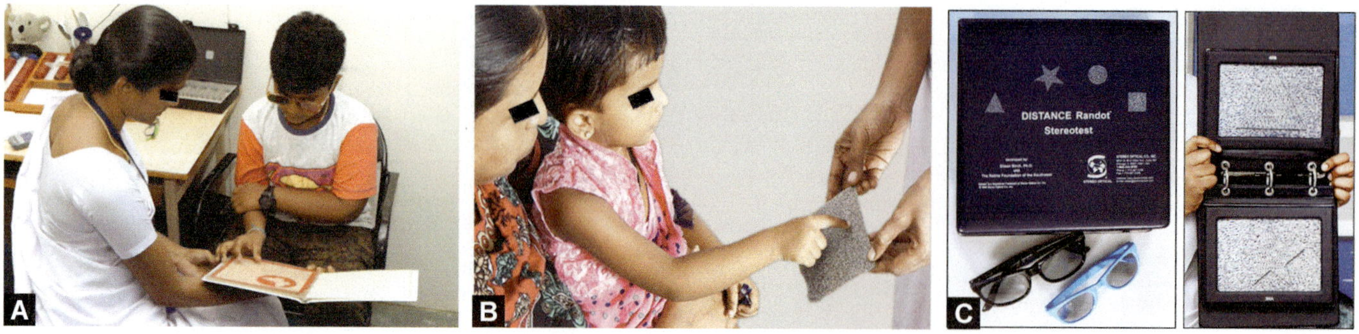

Figs. 79.9A to C: (A) Stereoacuity tests: TNO test through red green glasses; (B) Langs test in naked eye; (C) Distance stereotest with polarized glasses.

to take the form of a recognizable shape such as a circle. When viewed through red and green glasses at a distance of 40 cm (Fig. 79.9A), the matched dots can be identified, implying that binocular single vision (BSV) is present and because they stimulate disparate retinal elements within Panum's area, the dots can be fused. The plates in the TNO test range in disparity from 480 seconds to 15 seconds of arc. The random dot stereoacuity tests are more advantageous as they have almost no monocular clues.

Lang's test (Fig. 79.9B) is useful in younger children who refuse to wear the Polaroid or red-green glasses.[4] A separate image is provided to each eye through cylindrical lenses imprinted on the surface lamination of the test card. When held at a testing distance of 40 cm, the disparity of the cat, car and star is 1,200, 600 and 550 seconds of arc, respectively.

Contour stereoacuity tests: These tests use stereoscopic figures with a continuous contoured edge placed amongst flat figures. The *Titmus or wirt test* comprises of 3 sets of pictures—a fly, rows of animals and groups of circles. The image seen by one eye is polarized at 90° to the image seen by the other eye when the pictures are viewed through the polarized spectacles provided. The range of disparity is from approximately 3,000 seconds (the fly) to 40 seconds at the testing distance of 40 cm. As each stereoscopic figure is made of two drawings horizontally shifted off center, it is disadvantageous as it can be identified monocularly.

Distance stereopsis: It can be measured at 3 m with distance Randot Stereotest (Fig. 79.9C) and the measured stereopsis is between 400 seconds and 60 seconds of arc.

Assessing Binocular Potential

In a patient with strabismus, repeating the binocular tests after placing prisms to neutralize the deviation can assess binocular potential. This should ideally be done in all patients preoperatively as it helps in judging functional outcomes, long-term stability and to explain the prognosis to the patient.

The patient should also be questioned about diplopia and when in doubt, allow the patient to adapt to the prisms for 15–30 minutes while performing normal routine activities. Assess whether the diplopia is crossed or uncrossed and variation in diplopia with the change in prism strengths. This gives a rough assessment of the area of scotoma and is essential in preventing postoperative diplopia by aligning the eyes such that the image in the deviated eye would still fall within the scotoma.

MOTOR EVALUATION

Cover Test

Cover test is one of the most important steps in evaluation of strabismus. The observations are highly reliable in the presence of central fixation, good vision in both eyes and a reasonably good range of ocular movements.

The cover test is performed in two ways, the cover/uncover test and the alternate cover test. Both are mandatory and give different inferences. The tests should be done both with and without refractive correction and for distance and near. Best results will be obtained by using specific fixation targets both for near and distance to control the accommodation. Any single letter in a vision chart can be used as a fixation target at 6 m. A fixation target for use beyond 6 m can usually be found through a window or down the corridor. A light source of comfortable brightness could be used as a fixation target when vision is poor.

Cover test is also crucial in differentiating a pseudostrabismus. The absence of any movement in an apparently squinting eye when the other eye is covered could indicate an angle kappa or an eccentric fixation. This can be differentiated by assessing the fixation status.

Cover test also will be helpful in differentiating ocular torticollis wherein the abnormal head posture will be abolished on occluding one eye.

Cover/Uncover test

The cover/uncover test is of significance both in a manifest and a latent deviation. Head posture if any has to be corrected before commencing the cover test. If the patient has ptosis, the lid has to be manually lifted up for cover test. In this test when one eye is covered, observations are made both in the uncovered eye and in the covered eye on removal of the cover.

In a manifest deviation, the cover-uncover test helps in identifying the dominant eye.

- The apparently fixing eye is covered, for instance the right eye in a left eye esotropia; and the behavior of the uncovered eye (left) is observed. If there is considerably good vision in the left eye, it will move to take up the primary position to fixate on the target.
- Continue observing the left eye while uncovering the right eye to assess dominance. If it is the less dominant eye, it might return to its squinting position. If there is equal dominance, the patient will continue to maintain fixation in the left eye.
- The test must be repeated by covering the left eye and watching for movement of the right eye. Throughout the test, the examiner must make sure that the patient is fixing at the light source.
- The test is repeated using an accommodative target instead of the light. The movement of the deviating eye may increase or decrease as a result of accommodation and this should be recorded. In general, esotropia increases and exotropia decreases due to accommodative convergence.
- The test is repeated using a target at 6 m, and the response compared.

While performing the cover/uncover test in the absence of a manifest strabismus (Fig. 79.10), one should observe for a latent deviation and the speed of recovery.

- One eye is covered and then uncovered as described above, but here the behavior of the eye behind the cover is observed as the cover is taken away. In heterophoria, the eye behind the cover deviates, then straightens as the cover is removed. This happens irrespective of which eye is covered. The test should be performed at 33 cm and 6 m, comparing the amount of deviation seen and particularly the type of recovery movement to realign.
- The speed of recovery indicates the patient's ability to keep the heterophoria under control. A rapid recovery indicates good control whereas a slow or delayed recovery after a blink suggests that the heterophoria could cause symptoms or could become a manifest squint.

Alternate Cover Test

The alternate cover (cross cover) test is done after the cover/uncover test to identify the maximum deviation. In this test, the occluder is switched back and forth between the two eyes ensuring that one of the eyes is covered at all times. By preventing binocular vision, progressive dissociation of the eyes occurs and the total deviation can be measured.

Heterophoria and intermittent type of heterotropia can increase on alternate cover test. The direction and amount

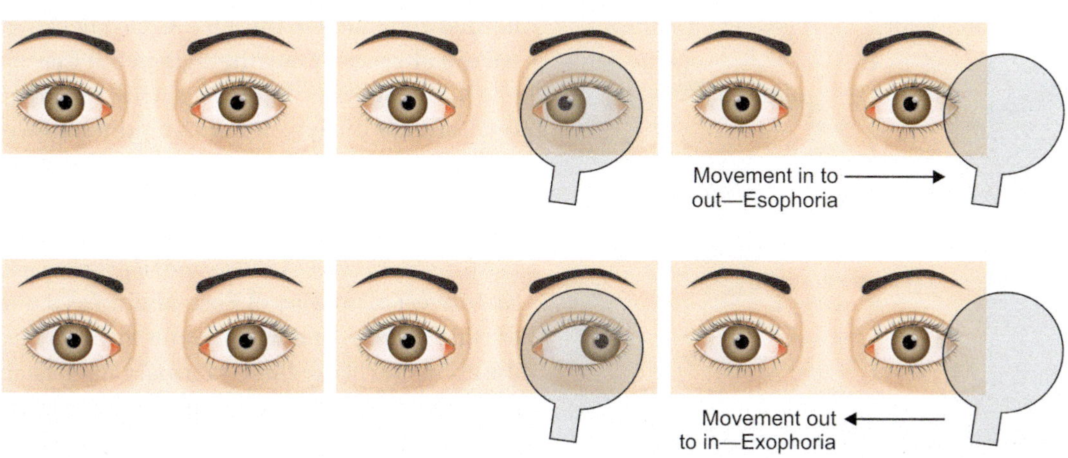

Fig. 79.10: Cover/uncover test in a latent strabismus demonstrating esophoria and exophoria with good recovery.

of movement of each eye will reveal the type of deviation (Fig. 79.11)

When indicated, cover/uncover test should be repeated after the alternate cover test in order to see whether there is any recovery and whether the result is the same as it was before the alternate cover test. For example, a poorly controlled phoria may become manifest for a short time after an alternate cover test. If a shift is noted on alternate cover test one should allow the patient to be binocular, observe if patient immediately shifts to recover (phoria) or stays manifest (Intermittent heterotropia).

From the above cover tests, we get the information on the presence of strabismus, type of deviation, whether it is constant or intermittent, dominance, patients' control over the deviation and whether it is influenced by accommodation. Other signs which may be seen on cover testing are incomitance, where the squint is larger when fixing with one eye than with the other; presence of nystagmus, which may have a latent component with an increase in the amount or speed of movement when either eye is covered. The test results should be recorded as type of squint, fixing eye, estimated size of the deviation as small/medium/large with the distance at fixation, difference in the deviations at near and distance, with or without spectacle, etc. In cases of latent squint, the type and the speed of its recovery should be recorded, giving an estimation of its size at near (33 cm) and at distance (6 m).

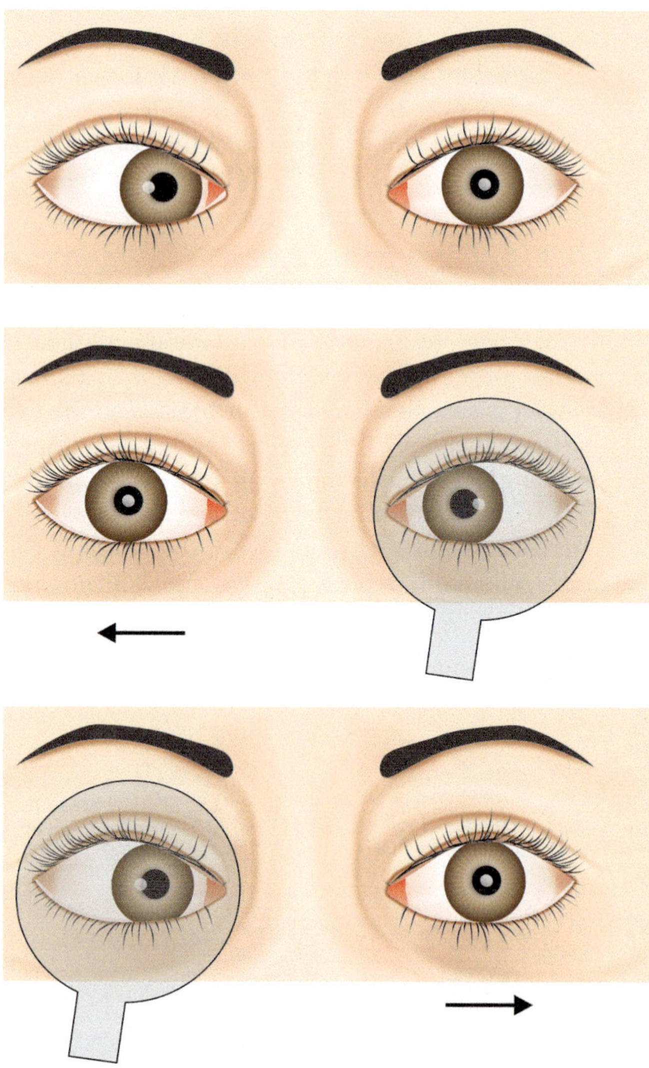

Fig. 79.11: Alternate cover test showing alternate esotropia.

Clinical Assessment of Range of Ocular Movements

Versions refer to binocular eye movements and ductions refer to uniocular movements (Figs. 79.12A and B). With the head kept straight using a light source or a target, versions are first tested in all diagnostic positions of gaze. Horizontal movements are always tested first followed by vertical movements. During examination one should observe whether movements are full; the presence of any over/under actions of extraocular muscles and grade the same if present; whether there is an increase in the horizontal deviation on up or downgaze (Figs. 79.13A and B); change in the palpebral fissures width on horizontal movements, position of the eyeballs (enophthalmos, prominence) any abnormal lid movements.

Whenever a limitation of movement is noted on versions, this should be confirmed by checking the movement on duction (Fig. 79.12C). In infantile esotropia, a child may have cross-fixation and would use the right eye to fix an object in the left gaze giving an appearance of limited abduction in the left eye. On checking abduction of left eye after occluding the right eye, it may appear full.

Normally in maximum adduction, an imaginary vertical line through the lower lacrimal punctum would coincide with a boundary line between the inner-third and outer-two-thirds of the cornea. In normal maximum abduction, the temporal corneal limbus should just touch the outer canthus (Fig. 79.14).[4] The most precise measure is the limbus test of motility of Kestenbaum as it does not rely on the lids for assessment but relates to direct measurement of the excursion of the globe. Normal values established are 10 mm for adduction, abduction and depression and 5–7 mm for elevation.[4]

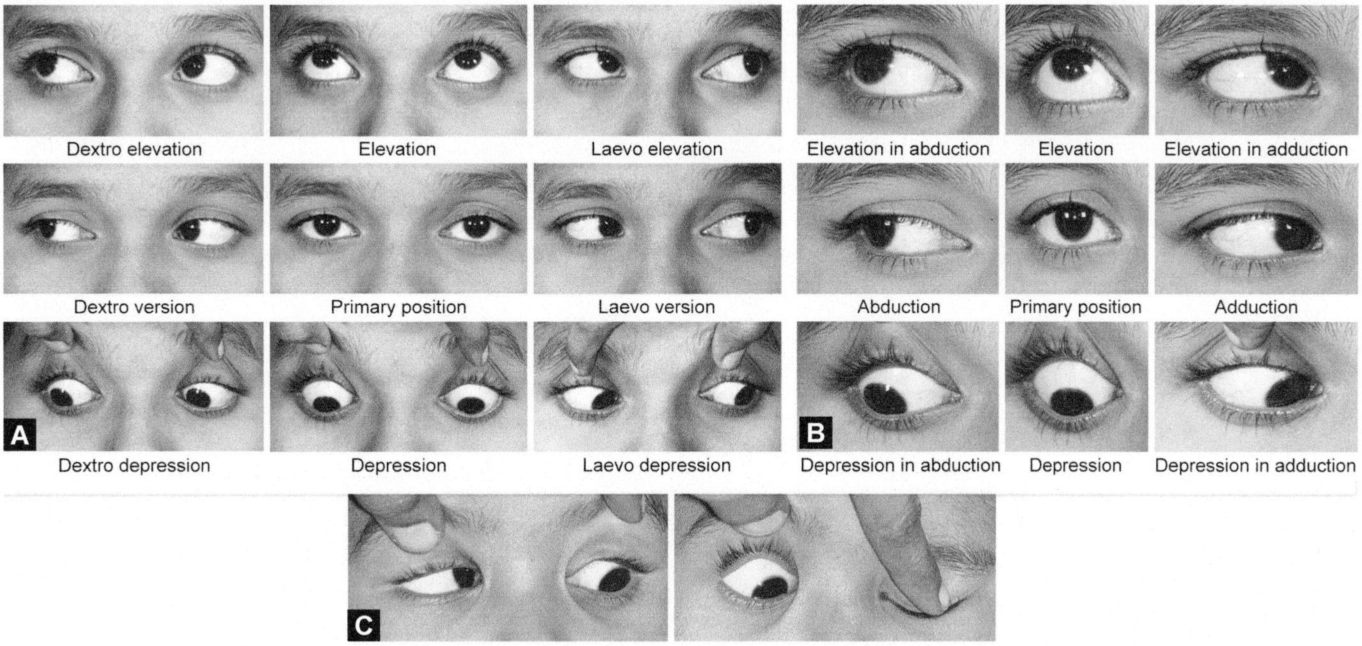

Figs. 79.12A to C: (A) Version movements; (B) Right eye duction movements; (C) Note the limitation in right eye on laevo depression; and the same improving on duction.

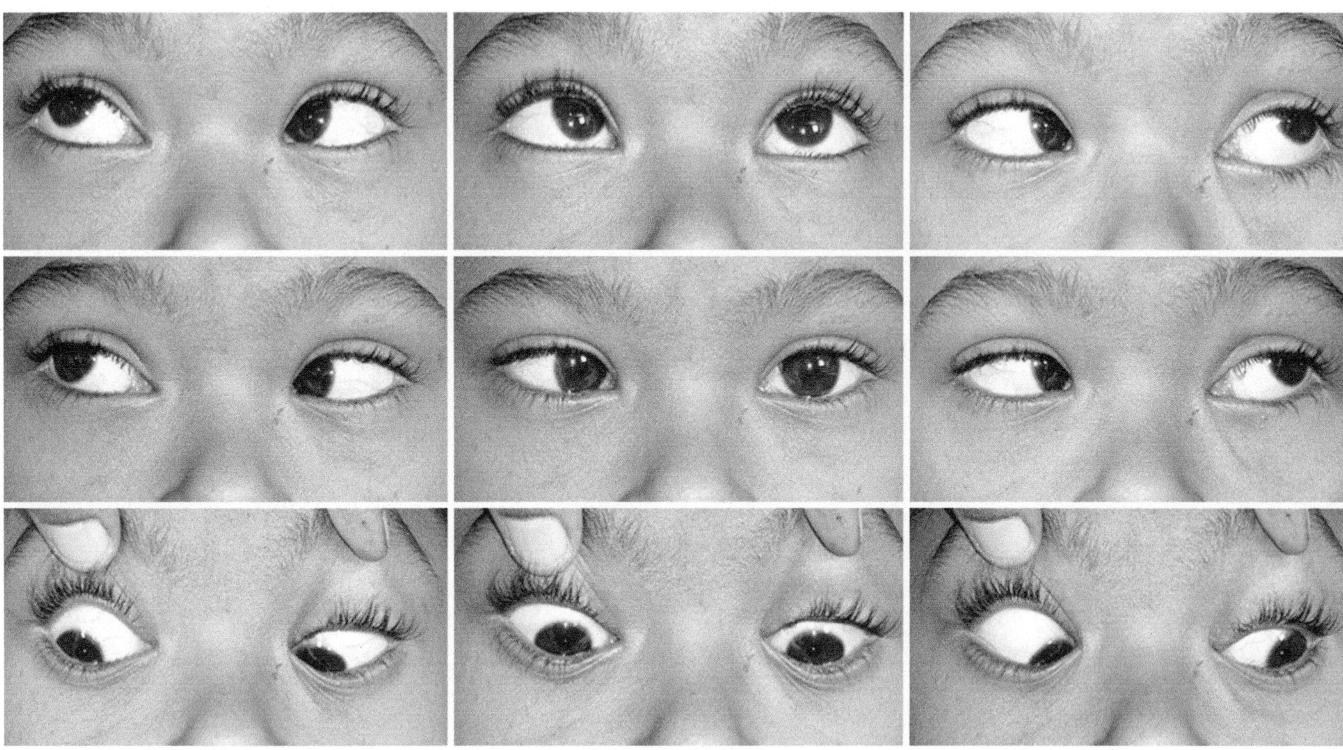

Fig. 79.13A

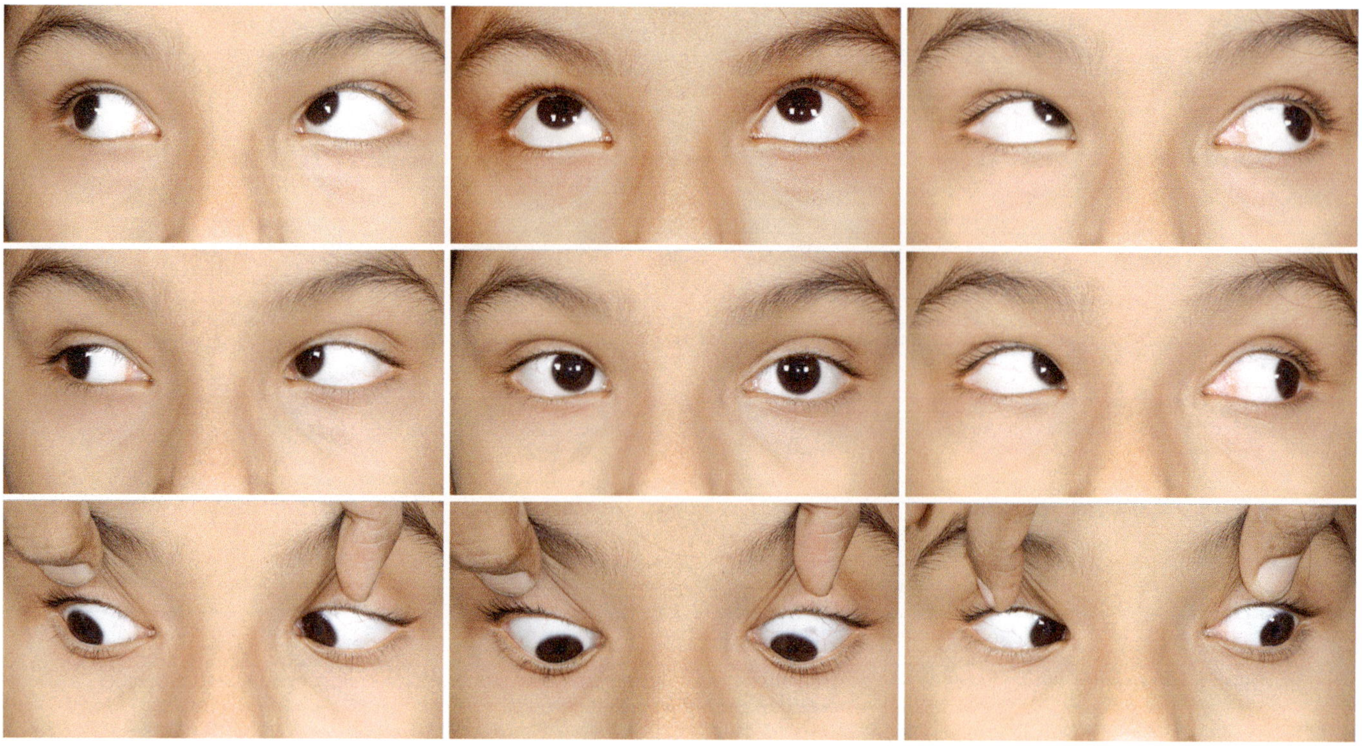

Fig. 79.13B

Figs. 79.13A and B: (A) Note the pattern esotropia with overaction of superior oblique in both eyes; (B) Note the V pattern esotropia with overaction of inferior oblique in both eyes and mild underaction of superior oblique.

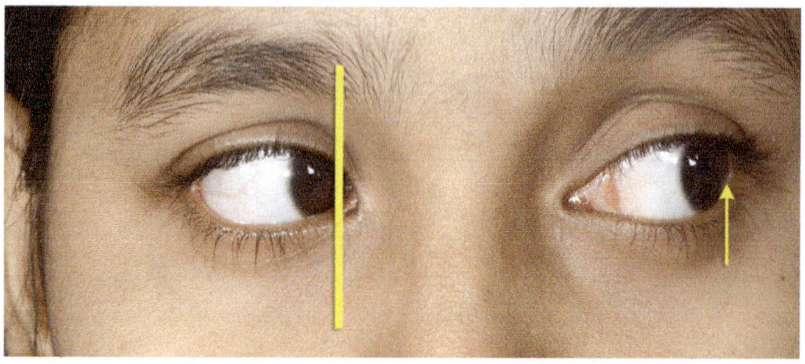

Fig. 79.14: In normal adduction, an imaginary vertical line through the lower larcimal punctum would coincide with a boundary line between the inner third and outer two-thirds of the cornea. In normal abduction, the temporal corneal limbus will just touch the outer canthus.

Grading of Over Actions and Under Actions

If sclera is just visible on maximum adduction and abduction, the limitation is graded as –1 and an inability to abduct or adduct the eye more than half-way into the field of action of the muscle is graded –2. Inability to abduct or adduct an eye more than a quarter-way into the field of action of the muscle is graded –3 and if the eye is unable to move at all from the primary position into the field of action of that muscle, the limitation is graded –4 (Figs. 79.15A to E). Horizontal rectus over action is graded according to the amount of cornea covered by the canthus. In extreme over action, half of the cornea is buried which is graded +4.[5]

Oblique over actions and under actions are graded by comparing the height of the inferior limbus of each eye. Over actions are graded from +1 representing a slight over action to +4 characterized by abduction of the eye in extreme oblique position (splaying out). Under actions of the obliques are graded from –1 representing the smallest under action to –4 denoting an inability of the eye to move vertically from the midline in the field of action of the oblique being tested (Figs. 79.16A to E).

Findings of extraocular movements can be represented in a simple drawing as shown in Figure 79.17.

Measurement of the Angle of Squint

Hirschberg Test

The corneal reflex test gives a rough measure of the amount of deviation. Depending on where the light reflex falls in relation to the pupil and limbus, a rough assessment of the amount of deviation can be made. The Hirschberg method

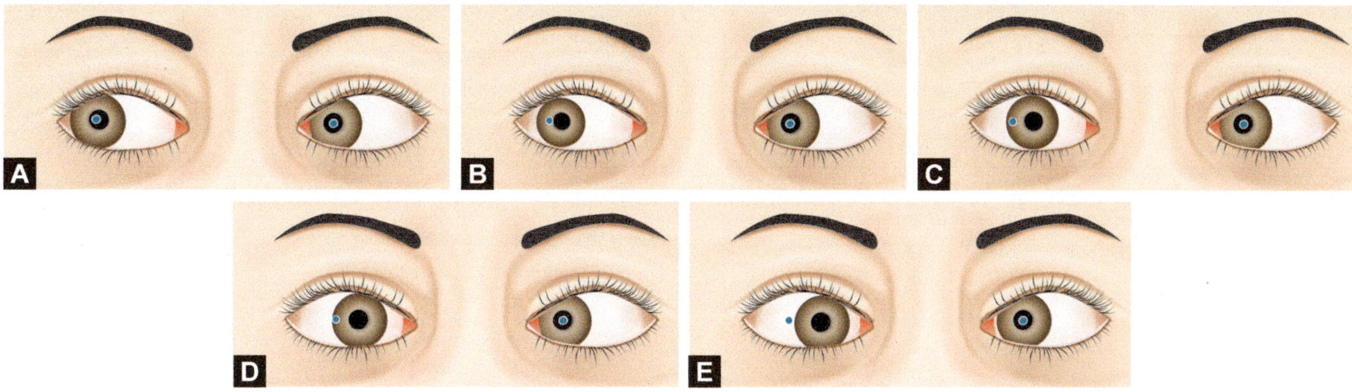

Figs. 79.15A to E: Underaction of abduction in right eye graded from –1 to –5 as depicted from (A) to (E) in the figure. In –5 underaction (E), the eyeball cannot cross the midline.

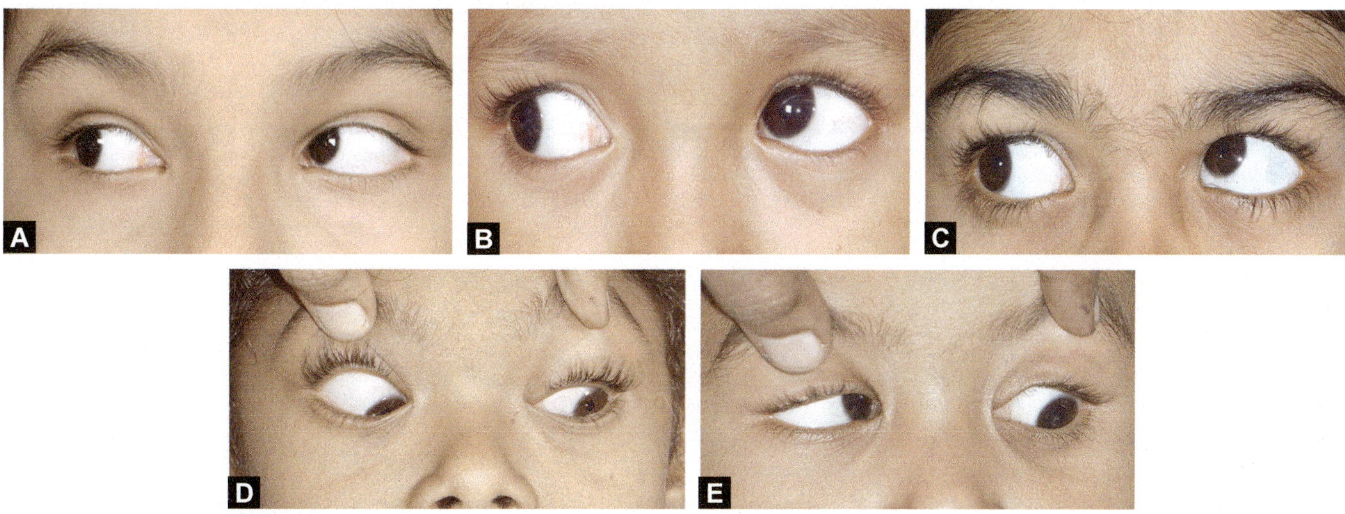

Figs. 79.16A to E: Diffrerent grades of overaction of inferior oblique is seen in the left eye on dextroversion. 1+ (A); 2+(B); 3+(C). Figure (D) and (E) shows overaction and underaction respectively of the right superior oblique in laevo depression.

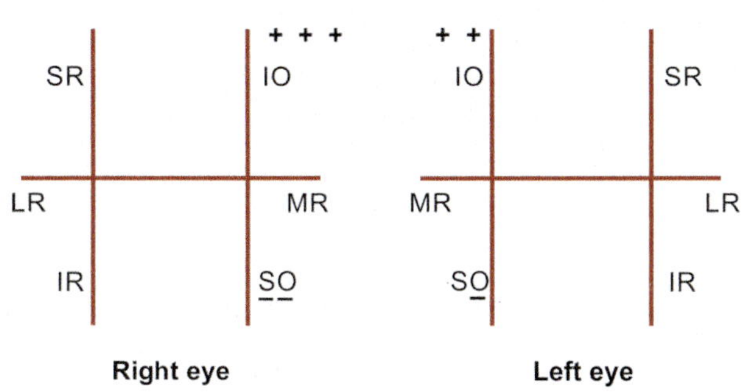

Fig. 79.17: Depiction of over/under actions of extraocular muscles.

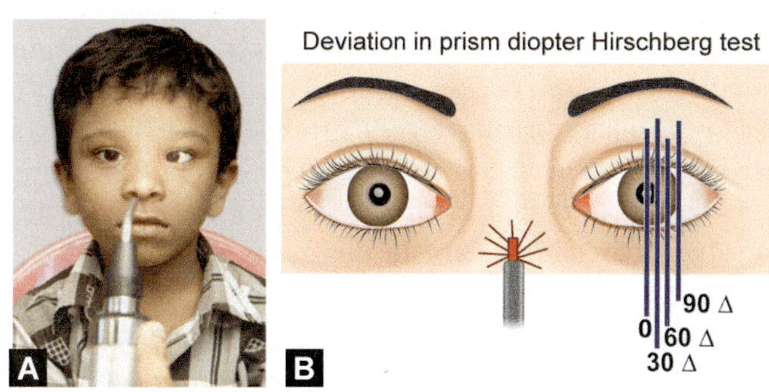

Figs. 79.18A and B: (A) Corneal light reflex test showing left esotropia; (B) A rough measure of the deviation is assessed by the location of the corneal light reflex in relation to the pupil and limbus.

is based on the principle that 1 mm of decentration of the corneal light reflection corresponds to approximately 7° or 15 D, of deviation of the visual axis.[6] Therefore, a light reflex at the pupillary margin is about 2 mm from the pupillary center (in a 4 mm pupil) which corresponds to 15° or approximately 30D. A reflex in the mid-iris is roughly 30° and that at the limbus is 45° (Figs. 79.18A and B). This method is useful when the angle cannot be measured by prism cover test (PCT) or prism reflex test. However, this test is less accurate for vertical measurements.

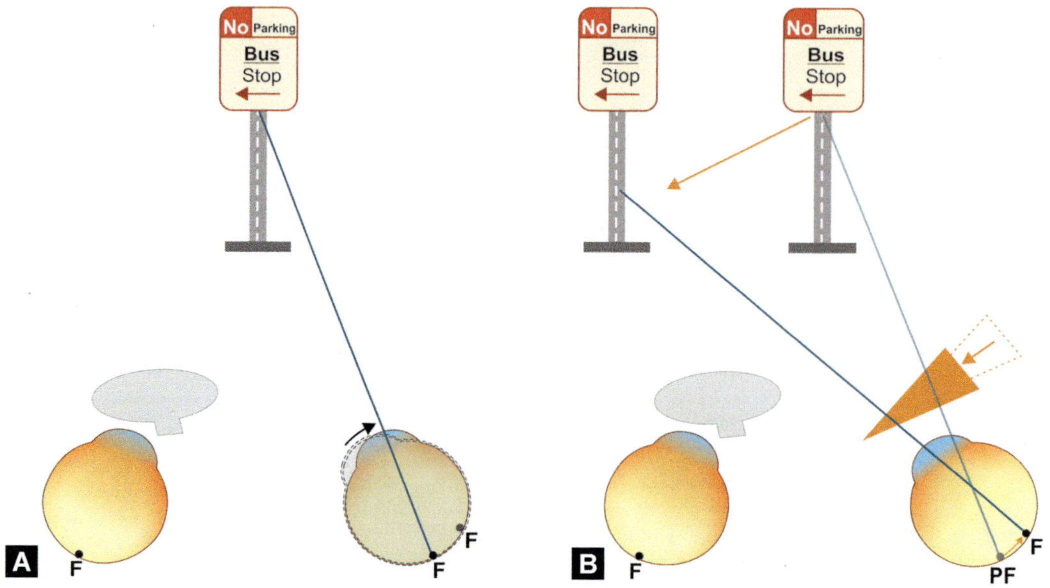

Figs. 79.19A and B: (A) On occluding the left eye, the esotropic right eye will make a movement to fix with the right eye; (B) When a prism of sufficient strength is placed in front of the deviating eye to make the image fall on the fovea (F), there will be no movement on the cover test. The strength of the prism required to neutralize this movement signifies the amount of deviation.
(PF: Parafoveal point)

Prism Cover Test

Prisms cause the image of an object visualized through it to be displaced towards the apex. To measure the deviation, we assess how much prisms is required to move the image of fixation from the extrafoveal point in the retina of a strabismic eye to its fovea. For instance, a right eye esotropia can be neutralized by placing a base-out prism in front of it (Figs. 79.19A and B).

The PCT is the most preferred method to measure strabismus. The prerequisites for the PCT are good central fixation in both eyes, sufficient cooperation to maintain steady fixation and reasonably good ocular motility.

Loose plastic prisms (Fig. 79.20) are easier to use than a prism bar and are placed in the frontal position. The prisms must be held upright parallel to the infraorbital margin with the apex in the direction of the deviation.

The patient is asked to fixate on an easily seen picture or letter at 33 cm (Fig. 79.21A) and the prisms are placed in front of the squinting eye in manifest deviation or in either eye in a latent deviation. The prism is placed base-in for exodeviations, base-out for esodeviations and base-down in hypertropia.

An alternate cover test is then performed while observing the movement of each eye as the cover is changed (Fig. 79.22). Sufficient time must be given for the patient to fix through the prism. The final point of neutralization occurs when there is no re-fixation movement. The strength of the prisms is increased or decreased until this occurs. The strength of deviation inferred by the PCT can be verified by placing a prism greater than that calculated and observe for a reversal of deviation.

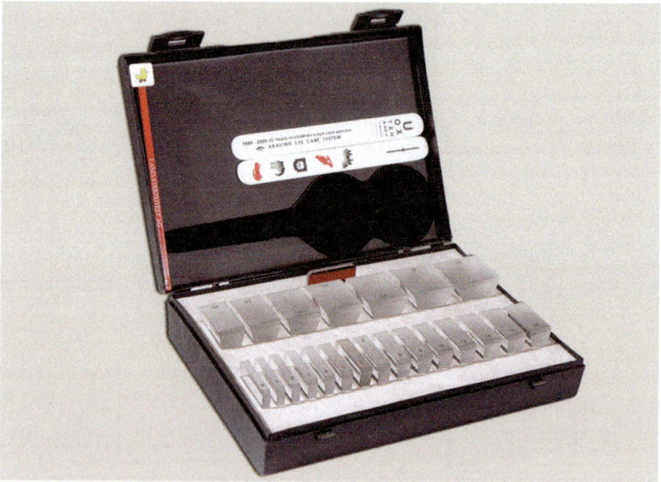

Fig. 79.20: Requirements for the prism cover test: Loose plastic prisms, occluder, Lang's and accommodative target.

In cases of combined horizontal and vertical squint, the larger angle is measured first. A vertical prism is then introduced keeping the horizontal prism in place, placing the prism base-down for hypertropia, base-up for hypotropia. The strength is adjusted until the vertical movement is neutralized. Alternately, the second prism can be placed in front of the other eye.

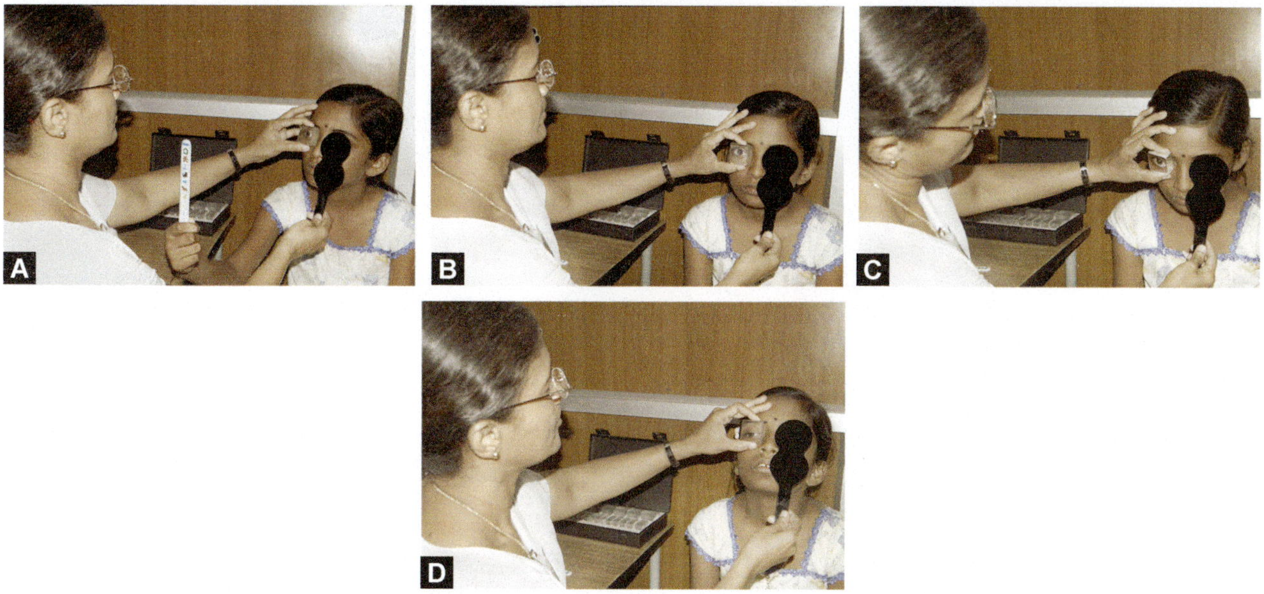

Figs. 79.21A to D: (A) Prism cover test for near; (B) For distance; (C) In up-gaze; (D) In down-gaze.

The test is repeated using a distant target (Fig. 79.21B). To measure deviation in the diagnostic nine gazes, the patient fixates on a distant target and the head is moved so that the eyes take up the required positions of extreme gaze (Figs. 79.21C and D). It is important that the eyes are in extreme gaze positions when performing the prism cover tests to ensure reproducibility.[5] This helps in detecting lateral incomitance and measuring the angle variations in pattern deviation.

Prism Reflection Test/Krimsky test

When a prism is placed base-in in front of the fixing eye, that eye will move out to regain foveal fixation. At the same time, the squinting eye will make a conjugate and equal inward movement (Hering's law of equal innervation). The strength of the prism placed is increased until the corneal reflection appears to fall centrally in the deviated eye (Figs. 79.23A and B). The strength of prism is taken as the measurement of the angle of squint at the distance tested. This test is employed in very young and uncooperative children, and when there is poor vision in one of the eyes.

The Krimsky test was originally described by placing prisms in front of squinting eye. However, for an easy and more objective determination, prisms are placed in front of the fixing eye and this is termed as the modified Krimsky test. The limitations of this test include that it can be used only for near, cannot measure variable angles or very large angles and could yield false results when performed in eyes with good visual acuity.

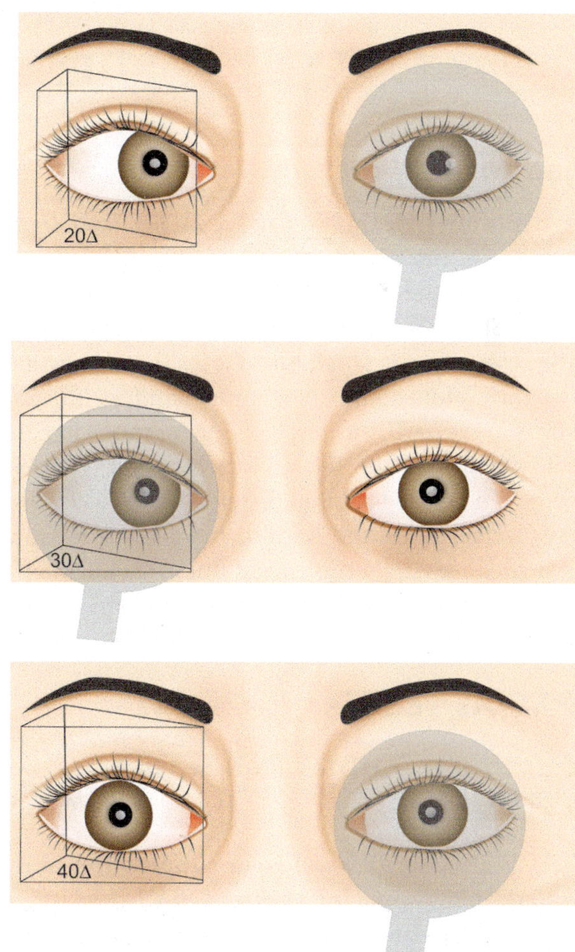

Fig. 79.22: Alternate prism cover test. Note the right esotropia being neutralized with prisms.

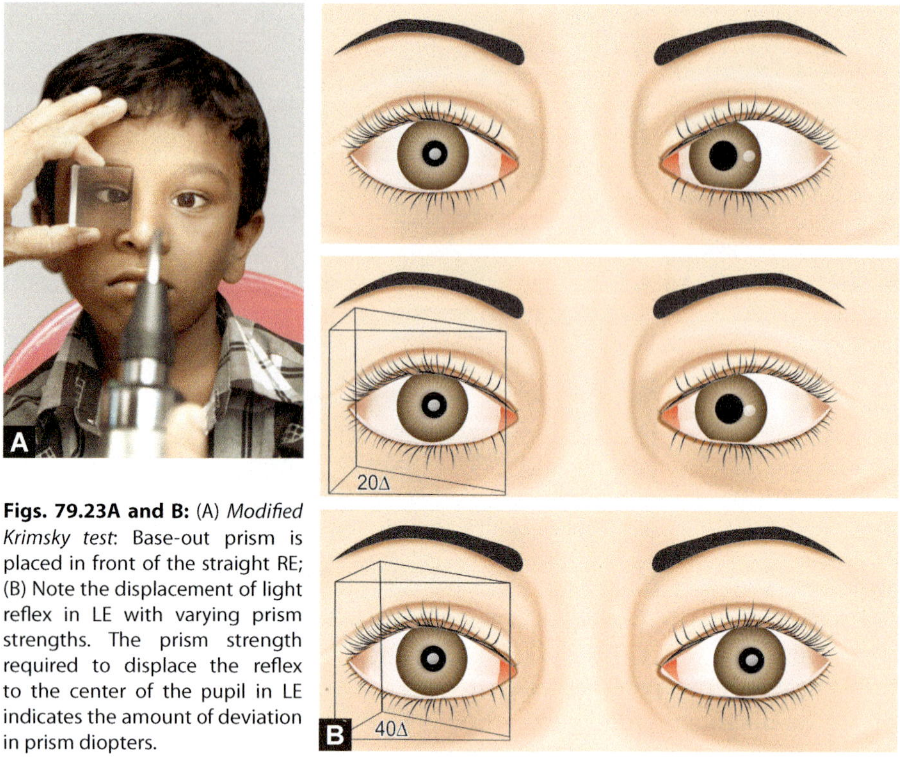

Figs. 79.23A and B: (A) *Modified Krimsky test*: Base-out prism is placed in front of the straight RE; (B) Note the displacement of light reflex in LE with varying prism strengths. The prism strength required to displace the reflex to the center of the pupil in LE indicates the amount of deviation in prism diopters.

Maddox Rod

Either white or red Maddox rod can be used in this subjective test. The rod is placed in front of one eye in a trial frame with the ridges horizontally for a horizontal deviation. This eye will see a vertical red line whereas the other eye sees the spotlight as it is. This dissociation facilitates any latent squint to become manifest. The angle of squint is measured by using prisms to move the line until it coincides with the light. The Maddox rod is generally used at 6 m but can be used at other distances also. To measure the vertical deviations, the Maddox rod is placed with the ridges vertical, giving a horizontal line. It is particularly useful in hyperphoria and in small amounts of hypertropia which can be difficult to measure accurately using the PCT.

SPECIAL TESTS

Four Prism Diopter Reflex Test (4 PD test)

This test is used to detect foveal suppression and to differentiate microtropia from bifoveal BSV.

The patient fixes on a small fixation target at 6 m, e.g. a Snellen letter. A 4 diopter prism is placed base-out in front of one eye and the behavior of both eyes is observed both as the prism is placed in position and when it is removed. The test is then repeated with the prism in front of the other eye. Normal and abnormal responses are depicted (Figs. 79.24A to D).

Measuring the Accommodative Convergence/Accommodation Ratio

While viewing an object at close quarters, the near vision triad of accommodation, convergence and miosis comes into play. Thus for every diopter of accommodation, a certain amount of convergence occurs. As children have greater reserve of accommodation, they also have a higher tendency to converge. It is postulated that this could explain the higher incidence of sensory ET in children than XT when there is disruption of binocularity.

Normally for every diopter of accommodation, 2–5 PD of convergence occurs.[2] When this is greater, the child would have the tendency to develop an accommodative esotropia. Testing of AC/A ratio is indicated when there is a variation in deviation of more than 10 prisms between measurement at distance and near. The AC/A ratio can be determined by measuring the variation in convergence on creating

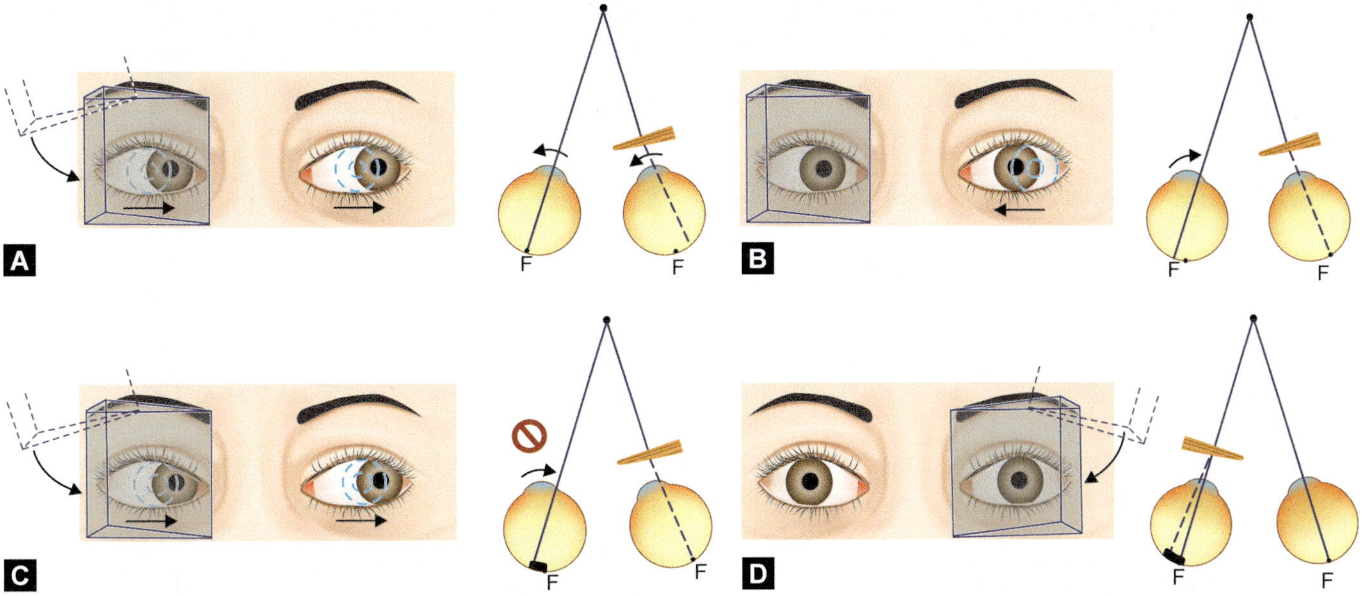

Figs. 79.24A to D: *Normal response*: (A) On placing 4 prism base-out in right eye, the right eye moves in and there is an equal outward movement in the left eye; (B) An immediate recovery movement (adduction) is seen in the left eye indicating a normal response. *Responses in left microtropia*: (C) On placing the 4 prism in front of right eye, left eye deviates out, but shows no recovery movement as the image falls within the scotoma; (D) On placing the prism in front of the microtropic eye (left), neither eye shows any movement.

variation in accommodation. The accommodation is varied by changing the fixation distance in the *heterophoria* method and by ophthalmic lenses in the *gradient* method.

An AC/A ratio of greater than 5:1 is considered high and would indicate an accommodative etiology. If the esotropia is greater at near than distance, but with a low AC/A ratio; this could be attributed to an excessive tonic convergence.[4]

Gradient Method

At a fixed distance, introducing a minus lens would stimulate an accommodation and a plus lens would relax accommodation. The PCT is repeated with addition of +3 DS lenses for near or with –3 DS lenses for distance. The AC/A ratio can be determined by the formula

AC/A = Original deviation – Deviation with added lens/ Power of lens introduced

Heterophoria Method

In this method, deviation is measured at distance on the assumption that no accommodation is exerted at optical infinity and then at near (33 cm). The amount of accommodation required to focus at a certain distance is determined by the reciprocal of the distance in meters. Thus, at 33 cm or one-third of a meter, 3D of accommodation would be required. The heterophoria method also takes into account interpupillary distance (IPD) as a larger convergence would be required, the wider the IPD. The AC/A ratio is determined by the formula

AC/A = IPD + Deviation at near – Deviation at distance/ fixation distance in diopter

The gradient method is considered to be more accurate than the heterophoria method.[4] The heterophoria method has the tendency to overestimate the AC/A ratio as the tonic convergence also comes into play at near.

Patch Test

The Marlow patch test involves occluding of one eye for longer periods of time to attain maximum dissociation and to abolish tonic convergence. When the deviation is more at distance than at near in a patient with intermittent exotropia (IXT), the patch test helps in differentiating a pseudo and true divergence excess IXT.

One eye is occluded for 60 minutes and the PCT is repeated in all gazes while taking precautions to ensure that one of the eyes is occluded until completion of evaluation (Fig. 79.25). Longer durations of occlusion is required when the patient has stronger fusional ability to control deviation.

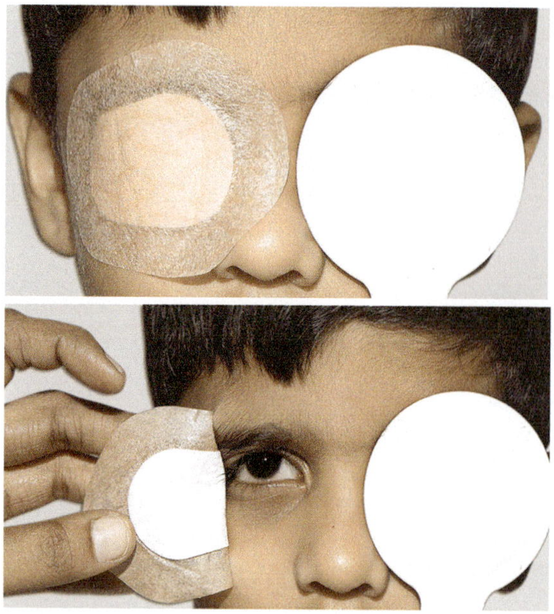

Fig. 79.25: *Patch test*: Ensure that the other eye is well covered before removing the patch.

Cycloplegic Refraction

Full cycloplegic refraction is mandatory for all children with strabismus since the presence of uncorrected refractive errors will have a great influence on the deviation. Hence, even a small refractive correction should be prescribed before deciding on any surgical correction. As children have high accommodation, atropine is recommended especially in esodeviations. Other drugs used are cyclopentolate, homide and tropicamide.

Fundus Evaluation

Detailed fundus evaluation is done to rule out any sensory (pathological) cause for strabismus, fixation status, to check for the presence of torsion and if present to measure the same. Eccentric fixation means the patient is viewing from an extrafoveal part of the retina. The fixation target in the direct ophthalmoscope can be used to assess the fixation (Fig. 79.26). After projecting the image on the central retina, the patient is asked to look at the image uniocularly. With central fixation, the patient will re-fixate to place the image on the fovea. With eccentric fixation, the patient will view with his preferred extrafoveal area and may show a wandering or unsteady fixation. The more peripheral the eccentric fixation, lesser will be the visual potential.

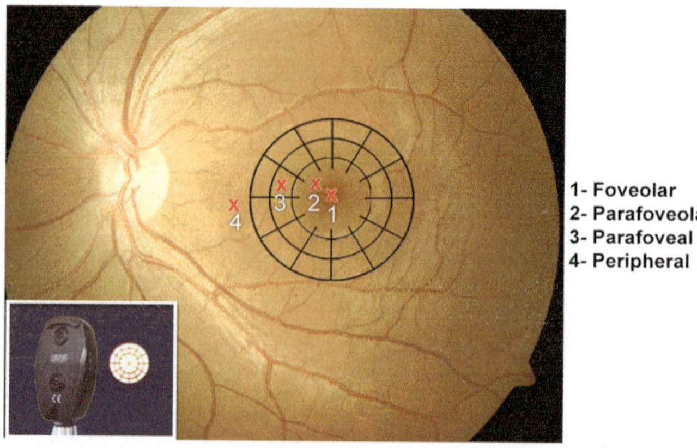

Fig. 79.26: Patient is asked to fixate at the light in the visuoscope to assess fixation. The fixation status is described as depicted in the picture.

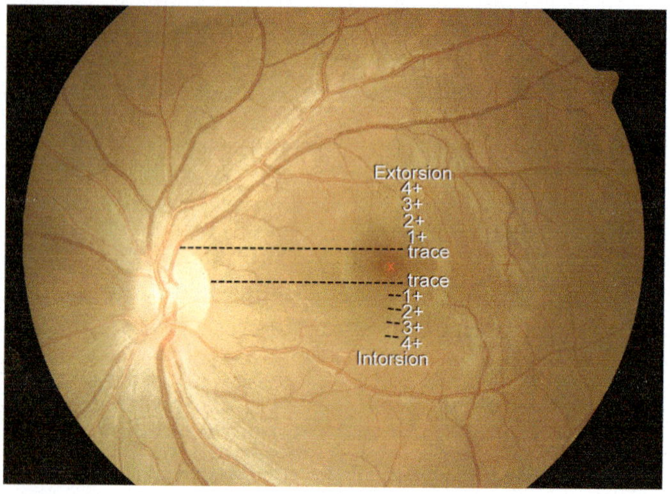

Fig. 79.27: Grading of abnormal torsion on indirect ophthalmoscopic view of a right eye fundus.

Torsion of the eye can be assessed objectively using an indirect ophthalmoscope. The patient is seated and is told to look into the dimly illuminated light of the indirect ophthalmoscope with the eye that is being tested. Normally, an imaginary horizontal line through the fovea will pass through the superior-half of the disk in the 'indirect ophthalmoscope view.' The line will be above the disk when extorted and below the superior-half of disk when intorted. A grading system proposed by Guyton is depicted in Figure 79.27.[7]

Synoptophore

No chapter on evaluation of strabismus is complete without a mention of the synoptophore (Fig. 79.28) also referred to as the major amblyoscope. It is still popular

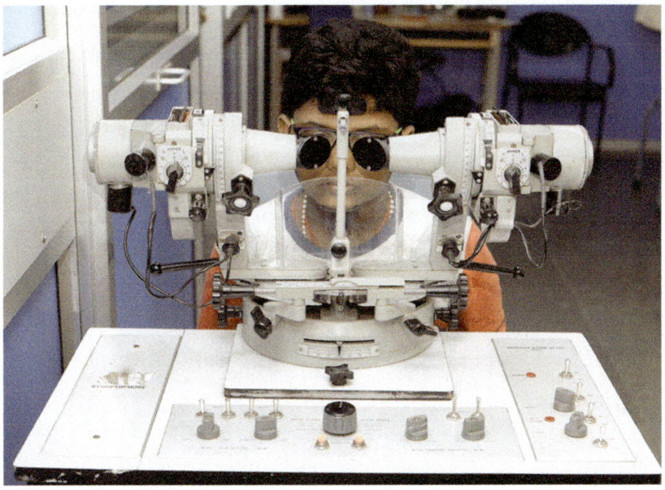

Fig. 79.28: Synoptophore.

Table 79.2: A synopsis of evaluation of concomitant strabismus.

Steps	Significance
History	Throws light on etiology of squint and past treatment
Inspection Head posture Orbital adnexa Anterior segment	 CHP could suggest potential for binocularity Rules out pseudostrabismus Anisocoria could interfere with measurement; cause of sensory strabismus identified
Vision assessment	Rules out associated amblyopia
Corneal reflex	Assessment of type of manifest squint, angle kappa
Sensory tests Binocular vision Stereopsis	Binocular vision and stereopsis is directly proportional to better long-term outcomes
Cover/Uncover test	Identifying a latent squint and the dominant eye
Alternate cover test	Unmasks total deviation (manifest and latent)
Hirschberg test	Rough measure of deviation with only torch light
Prism cover test 9–gaze measurement	Measurement of deviation in different gazes Detects lateral incomitance and pattern deviation
Modified Krimsky	Rough measure of deviation when uncooperative or poor fixation in one eye
Ocular movements	To identify any over actions or under actions
Special tests Maddox rod Four prism test Patch test AC/A ratio	 Subjective measure of phorias To diagnose microtropia To measure total deviation in an intermittent exotropia To classify accommodative esotropia
Cycloplegic refraction	Ideal in children to rule out any refractive errors
Fundus evaluation	Rules out retinal pathology; assessment of torsion

in some practices and does have some added benefits. It works on the haploscopic principle and the grades of binocular vision can be individually analyzed. Some of the superior advantages of the synoptophore are its use in assessing the deviation in all nine gazes, distance stereopsis, measuring angle kappa, and the assessment of torsional fusion.

CONCLUSION

Though comitant strabismus is commonly encountered in the pediatric population, restrictive or paralytic strabismus is not rare and may be misleading if not carefully sought for. This mandates the importance of a step-by-step approach in evaluating every case of strabismus (Table 79.2). One

Table 79.3: Differentiating comitant and incomitant strabismus.

Sl. No.	Characteristics	Concomitant strabismus	Restrictive strabismus	Paralytic strabismus
1.	Type of onset	Congenital or shortly after birth; rarely sudden	Could be present at birth or following trauma	Often sudden and acquired but may be congenital
2.	Age of onset	Infancy/childhood	Infancy/childhood	Any age, more common in elderly
3.	Difference between primary and secondary deviation	Usually absent	Secondary deviation will be greater than primary	Secondary deviation will be greater than primary
4.	Diplopia	Uncommon	Not uncommon	Common
5.	Comitance	Common	Incomitant	Tends to become comitant over time
6.	Compensatory head posture	Rarely seen	Commonly seen	Commonly seen
7.	Ocular movement	Usually full; may be limited adduction or abduction in large exotropia and esotropia respectively. Over action of oblique muscles are not uncommon	Limitation usually on entire gaze rather than in direction of muscle action. Duction = Version. Restriction of ocular motility that is out of proportion to deviation in primary position Muscle sequelae do not develop Fissure changes on movement are common	Maximum limitation of movement in field of main action of affected muscle. Duction usually exceeds version. Abnormal smooth pursuit movements. Muscle sequelae likely to develop
8.	Deviation in primary position	Often obvious	Little or no deviation	Present
9.	Forced duction test	Usually negative; longstanding large deviation can cause contracture	Positive	Usually negative

should pay attention to head posture, fissure changes, motility changes, globe changes and binocularity which will aid in differentiating comitant and incomitant strabismus (Table 79.3). In general, one can be successful in getting the required information from a child to formulate a management plan in the initial visits with confidence when the examiner is patient, attentive enough and willing to adopt the methodology to suit the child's age and mentation.

REFERENCES

1. Tychsen L. Binocular Vision. In: Hart WM (Ed). Adler's physiology of the eye: clinical application, 9th edition. St. Louis: Mosby; 1992. pp. 888.
2. Wright KW, Spiegel PH. Pediatric ophthalmology and strabismus, 2nd edition. New York: Springer-Verlag; 2013. pp. 1087.
3. Prieto-Diaz J, Souza-Dias C, Lydia G. Strabismus, 4th edition. Boston: Butterworth-Heinemann; 2000. pp. 528.
4. Von Noorden GK, Campos EC, Gunter K. Binocular vision and ocular motility: theory and management of strabismus, 6th edition. St. Louis: Mosby; 2002.
5. Vivian AJ, Morris RJ. Diagrammatic representation of strabismus. Eye (Lond). 1993;7(Pt 4):565-71.
6. Pratt-Johnson JA, Tillson G. Motor evaluation of strabismus. In: Pratt-Johnson JA, Tillson G (Eds). Management of strabismus and amblyopia: a practical guide. New York: Thieme Medical Publishers; 1994. pp. 50-65.
7. Rosenbaum AL, Santiago AP. Clinical strabismus management: principles and surgical techniques. Philadelphia: Saunders; 1999. pp. 569.

Chapter 80 Congenital Esotropia

Ian Marsh

INTRODUCTION

The term congenital esotropia is probably an incorrect term used to describe an onset of a convergent deviation early in a child's life. The correct term to use would be early-onset esotropia as this deviation appears not at birth but usually after 3 months of life.[1,2]

HISTORY

It is quite normal in the first 3–4 months of a child's life to have ocular instability often manifested by an intermittent deviation of the eyes. This deviation is often divergent. When the primitive visual system matures in the postnatal period, these ocular misalignments disappear. Any deviation which remains constant and is present after this initial period is pathological and parents should not be advised that their child will "grow out of it". In early-onset esotropia the history is that the deviation begins intermittently and then becomes constant often increasing in size/angle from 3 months of age. It is important to obtain an accurate birth history with particular reference to any maternal problems during the pregnancy particularly in the first trimester. The mode of delivery of the baby may be relevant especially the utilization of any instrumentation. In the postnatal period, any history of head injury or other concerns about milestone development might be relevant. Other associated history might include the parent's observation of head position or abnormal oscillations of the eyes particularly if the child is viewing monocularly.

A family history may reveal other related members of the close family with strabismus or amblyopia.

EXAMINATION

- Observation of head posture
- Visual acuity
- Cover test
- Ocular deviation including measurement of size
- Extraocular movements both versions and ductions
- Cycloplegic refraction
- Disk, macular and retinal assessment
- Observation of the lids and palpebral aperture
- Systemic examination.

Observation of Head Posture

Some varieties of early-onset esotropia will have an anomalous head position using a face turn to fixate with the eye in adduction. This may be present in patients with nystagmus as part of their syndrome. The head posture can also be present in cases of sixth nerve palsy where abduction is deficient. This may direct further systemic examination appropriately.

Visual Acuity

The assessment of visual function or acuity in a child can be divided into two methods:

1. Subjective
2. Objective

Subjective acuity assessment is more often used in older individuals by asking them to identify decreasing size letters, pictures or symbols until a threshold is reached. This may not be relevant or achievable in the infants.

The usual technique for assessment of vision in children is objective where the examiner makes an assessment of the child's response to a stimulus delivered sometimes in a masked manner to the observer. The stability of fixation during a cover test or objection to occlusion of the fixating eye might give important information about acuity. Assessment of fixation preference and ability to hold fixation following removal of occlusion may give an indication of whether vision is equal between the eyes although an objective measurement will not be possible.[3]

Vision assessment: This is best assessed using objective measurements. The commonest method is preferential looking (PL). In the experimental situation this is often performed by two observers where one presents the gratings and makes a masked choice as to which direction the infant is looking while the second observer notes the actual direction of the grating. Observer bias is therefore eliminated. This process is known as forced choice preferential looking; however, due to the need for two observers this is not usually used in the clinical situation. One examiner presenting the stimulus and observing the reaction may introduce bias but works in busy clinical practice. Other different stimuli can be used but the same principle holds for all of these.[4,5]

If it is difficult or impossible to undertake visual assessment then the use of electrodiagnostic testing can give a measure of visual potential. This however, is rarely used as most infants can participate in some external form of visual assessment.

Cover Test

Important information can be gained through a simple cover test. In a cooperative child, covering the better seeing eye can cause a variety of reactions ranging from crying through to an attempt to remove the occlusion. In patients with minimal amblyopia or equal vision, no objection to occlusion is likely. Observation of the speed of fixation of the nonfixing eye following occlusion of the fixing eye will give an idea of the level of vision. A rapid foveal fixation movement can be compared to a "searching" motion. Similarly if the patient shows no preference for fixation with one eye, it can be inferred that the level of vision is equal in each eye. Other information which can be gained from the cover test is the presence of any vertical deviation in either the primary position or eccentric gaze positions. Observation of the covered eye on recovery will help to diagnose dissociated vertical deviation (DVD).

Ocular Deviation Measurement

The conventional way of measuring the ocular deviation is by the use of prisms to neutralize the deviation and is recorded as an alternate prism cover test. This can only be measured for near fixation in young children. It is vital to ensure that the prisms are held in the correctly calibrated position to ensure that an accurate measurement is achieved. There is however considerable intraobserver error. The particular issues that allow for the difference in measurements include the position at which the reading is taken, the distance away from the eyes and the observation of the point of reversal of the deviation. Accurate measurements are difficult in small children. Because some of these patients also have vertical dysfunctions then recordings undertaken in all nine positions of gaze might be important but probably not achievable. It might be important to observe whether stability is present but because of the intraobserver error this might not be reliable. If an accurate prism cover test is not possible then estimation of the deviation using the light reflex on the cornea might be the only way of measurement. This is the so-called Krimsky technique. Again there is considerable intra-observer error.

The use of the synoptophore to measure the angle is not possible below age 3 years.

Extraocular Movements

It is important to ensure that there is a full range of ocular movements in these children particularly as they may appear to show a significant reduction of lateral movement. Making the distinction between congenital esotropia and bilateral sixth nerve palsies is vital to ensure that any required investigation is not missed or is applied appropriately. A significant number will show apparent underaction of the lateral rectus muscles and may also have a face turn to fix with the eye in adduction. There are two techniques used to differentiate between these two conditions:

1. Occlusion of one eye will show that the congenital squint has full abduction; however, the sixth nerve palsy will not.
2. The swinging baby test: In this situation, the child is rotated so inducing the vestibulo-ocular reflex (VOR). In the congenital squint, abduction will become complete unlike the sixth nerve palsy.

It is often difficult to get a child to fixate on a target to perform this examination and sometimes using a noisy toy may help. Children of this age might not be interested in looking at a light. Examination of the vertical gaze directions is also important so that the presence or absence of inferior oblique overactions is documented. It can be very difficult to differentiate between an inferior oblique overaction and a DVD. It is important to observe a light reflex on the cornea. In patients with inferior oblique problems, the light reflex is still visible on the cornea as the eye starts to elevate whereas in DVD the torch beam may be blocked by the nose in side gaze and elevation occurs at that point.

Ductions (monocular movements) may be difficult to elicit particularly when the child objects to occlusion. It is important at some point during the child's care to evaluate their responses to an opticokinetic nystagmus drum.[8] The use of this stimulus when presented monocularly can be helpful in the diagnosis of DVD. Patients who are potentially going to develop this condition will have an abnormal response when the stimulus is presented moving from nasal to temporal. The eye will have a normal following and re-fixation movement when this is presented from the temporal field to the nasal area.

Cycloplegic Refraction

All children with an ocular deviation should have refraction with cycloplegia. The use of the appropriate strength of this agent should be considered. There is a balance between effective cycloplegia and possible toxicity. The use of these drops will also allow an examination of the fundus. The difficult decision in these patients is when to prescribe spectacles. Some may have an accommodative element and provision of glasses may reduce the angle, however, if the prescription is similar in each eye and amblyopia is not present then the dispensing of glasses may halt the process of emmetropization.[6,7] Glasses should only be prescribed when there is significant astigmatism, anisometropia or excessive hypermetropia. The fitting of glasses is also difficult in this age range. Astigmatism of greater than one diopter or with differing axes in each eye should be corrected. If this is not undertaken then these children will be at risk of meridional amblyopia. Patients who have greater than two diopters of hypermetropic difference between the two eyes should also be prescribed. These children will not be focusing on distant objects so refractive errors of less than four diopters of symmetrical hypermetropia should not be corrected. The presence of myopia is unlikely in this condition.

Disk Macula and Retinal Assessment

The examination of the retinal fundus is likely to be normal; however, should be undertaken so that no gross abnormalities are missed. Binocular indirect ophthalmoscopy is probably the gold standard here. Any anomalies should be investigated with the appropriate modality.

Lid and Palpebral Fissure Observation

It is important to ensure that Duane's syndrome is not present and so direct observation of the position of the eyelids in various horizontal gaze positions is vital. The movement and closure of the eyelids should also be assessed so that cases of Moebius syndrome are correctly diagnosed.

Flowchart 80.1: Diagnostic decision tree.

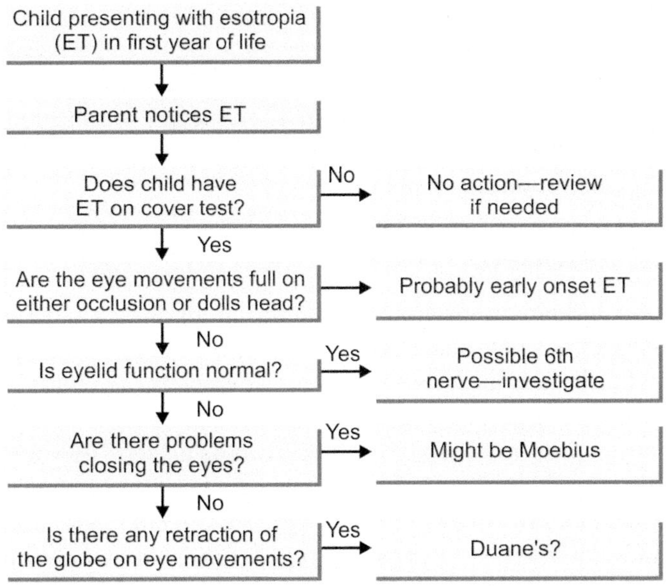

Systemic Examination

If the ocular examination is atypical or the parents express concerns regarding the general condition of their child or there are concerns that the diagnosis is a bilateral sixth nerve palsy then systemic examination should be performed and referral to the appropriate specialist be undertaken. This is beyond the remit of the ophthalmologist) (Flowchart 80.1).

MANAGEMENT OF EARLY ONSET ESOTROPIA

The first and most important part of management is to ensure that correct diagnosis has been made. Once Duane's retraction syndrome, Moebius syndrome and sixth nerve palsy have been excluded then the patient can be classified as either having:

- Early-onset esotropia
- Ciancia syndrome
- Nystagmus blocking syndrome.

Ciancia syndrome is manifested by a large angle strabismus with a face turn to fix in adduction. Manifest latent nystagmus is present and is worsened in abduction. It can sometimes be difficult to differentiate this condition from nystagmus blocking syndrome. In this condition, the patient will converge to slow or eliminate the nystagmus movements; however, they are still often present even with the large angle strabismus. They do worsen with monocular occlusion making their differentiation between the two difficult conditions.

There is still a significant amount of controversy regarding the management of early-onset esotropia. In particular, these can range from when surgery is indicated, preoperative evaluation and care, operation type and the use of botulinum toxin.

Preoperative Evaluation and Care

The decision as to whether to prescribe spectacles in these cases has been discussed previously; however, there are other factors important to be considered. These children often have very small faces with no real bridge to their nose upon which a pair of glasses can be placed. They will also tend to irritate behind the ears and may not be well-tolerated. If a definite indication such as unequal refraction or significant astigmatism is present then the provision of glasses through well-qualified pediatric optometrist would be best for the child. The spectacles should be able to withstand falling to the ground and being sat upon. A strong sturdy pair of glasses should be preferred rather than flimsy designer wear.

A number of practitioners whilst waiting for stability of the deviation, practice alternate patching where one eye is covered in turn. The evidence for the use of this regime is limited; however, it might be sensible to use this technique if the child prefers fixing with one eye over the other so that true alternation occurs. Amblyopia is unlikely as these patients cross-fixate using their left eye to look right and their right eye to look left whilst using each eye in turn in the primary position. The deviation starts usually quite small and increases over time and so, therefore, measurement will change as well. When planning surgical intervention some clinicians opt to wait until stability occurs.

Timing of Surgery

There is still controversy regarding when surgical intervention is required for these children.[9,10] The proponents of "early surgery" suggest that early alignment may be associated with the development of either rudimentary or good binocular responses. The advocates of "late surgery" feel that good accurate measurements are then possible and that all the component parts of the early-onset esotropia can be dealt with in a single surgical episode. They also suggest that binocularity is unlikely and all that surgery is offering is to improve the appearance of the child's eyes.

The timing is also dependent upon other associated colleague's support as these children require experienced practitioners who are comfortable with anesthetizing such small patients.

Types of Surgery

The deviation is often larger for near fixation so consequently weakening or recession of the medial rectus muscles is often used.[11,12] To enhance this surgical intervention in the past, recession of the conjunctiva over the muscles was undertaken—the so-called en-bloc recession.

Some clinicians prefer a unilateral recession of the medial rectus and resection of the lateral rectus. In larger deviations, spreading the surgery between three and four horizontal rectus muscles may allow smaller amounts of movement and not produce an incomitant deviation. There are a number of surgical nomograms available within the literature. Experience will show the surgeon what works best in their hands.

Apart from the horizontal deviation there are often vertical elements. The management of these is often related to appearance. There are two types of vertical deviation that might require surgical management. These are:

- Dissociated vertical deviation
- Inferior oblique overaction.

The timing of intervention for these conditions is usually later in the child's life. This can range from 5 years to 15 years of age.[13]

If these both coexist then a single operation may well solve both problems. Anteriorization of the inferior oblique muscle to the lateral side of the inferior rectus will reduce the overaction of this muscle and also create an anti-elevation situation so helping the DVD. These conditions are usually bilateral and therefore surgery to both sides is likely.

If the only pathology present is inferior oblique overaction then surgical weakening of this muscle is indicated. This can either be by recession or myectomy. There is little to choose between these techniques. If DVD is present without inferior oblique overaction then usually weakening of the superior rectus is undertaken. This can be in the form of a recession or Faden operation. Some authors recommend asymmetrical surgery if the DVD is different between the two eyes. Others feel that symmetrical surgery should be offered to all. Superior rectus recession is a much easier surgical technique than Faden surgery. Suturing the superior rectus to the globe behind the equator with a nonabsorbable suture requires adequate exposure of the operative site. However, anatomically in the area where the stitch is to be placed is the superior oblique muscle. Some newer surgical techniques have been suggested such as the Scott procedure where a simultaneous resection of a rectus muscle is combined with recession of the proximal stump so creating a gaze deficit in the direction of action of the muscle. This can also be combined with an adjustable technique though this may not be appropriate in this age range.

Botulinum Toxin

One of the most controversial areas is the role of botulinum toxin in the management of early-onset esotropia. One group of authors showed that a significant percentage of these children achieved high grades of binocular function following injections of botulinum toxin to both medial rectus muscles. This tends to suggest that early intervention in this condition could potentially produce a better outcome than waiting until later to act. The problems that could arise from this advice include, early identification of the condition, early presentation to the ophthalmologist and finally finding an anesthetist who will be willing to administer anesthesia below the age of 12 months as recommended in the publication. To ensure accurate placement of botulinum toxin, electromyography has to be used and a normal anesthetic technique abolishes the vestibulo-ocular reflex (VOR) or "doll's head response" required to administer this treatment. The VOR ensures that rotating the head while the patient is awake causes the eyes to deviate to the opposite side. The type of anesthetic required uses ketamine which allows preservation of these brainstem reflexes; however, this has now become a drug of abuse and is not within the normal anesthetists' armamentarium. Other authors have suggested open access to the medial rectus muscles by opening the conjunctiva and injecting botulinum toxin under direct vision. This approach negates the benefit of botulinum toxin which would normally be delivered transconjunctivally without subsequent scarring. The short duration of the effect of this drug probably means that it is unlikely to be used above the age of 12 months where the likelihood of "cure" is greatly reduced (Flowchart 80.2).[21-26]

RISKS AND BENEFITS OF TREATMENT

Early intervention whether by botulinum toxin or surgical intervention has the potential for the development of binocularity which although crude may allow the maintenance of parallel visual axis in the longer term. It has been shown; however, that early intervention leads to a greater number of surgical operations over the life of the child to achieve a good appearance. The other risk from intervening early is that once the angle of deviation is small and the parents may consider that treatment is complete and default. These patients are at greater risk of developing amblyopia as they no longer have any visual drive to alternate fixation. Close monitoring of their visual performance is vital until the connections between eye and the visual cortex are complete.[14-20] Accurate examination is not achievable below 12 months of age and so the vertical deviations, inferior oblique overactions or the presence of DVD may well be missed and might require further intervention in the future. Inferior oblique overactions are associated with a V pattern which may not be clinically

Flowchart 80.2: Treatment options for early-onset esotropia (ET).

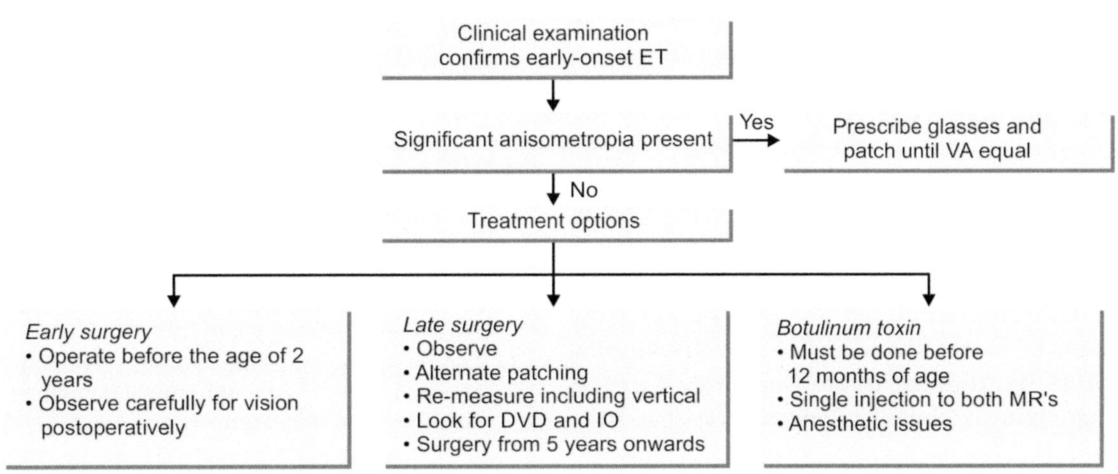

relevant in the infant becomes much more important at school age. The one major benefit from intervening at an early stage is the improvement in ocular alignment and the consequent improvement in psychosocial functioning of the child. It is well recognised that children can identify differences between themselves and the presence of a strabismus which might be large when they enter school might lead to them being excluded from their peer group. There is also parental pressure to intervene early to make their child look more normal. The parents themselves may well be pressurized by their close family or friends to get their child operated upon. In the longer term, a child operated on early may not remember the procedure; however, those who have surgery later in their lives can recall the process.

Surgical interventions at a later age aim to correct all deviations, patterns and complications in one operation. These are obviously larger procedures and take longer in the operating theater and are more likely to be remembered long term by the patients. There is no information available regarding psychosocial functioning between those having an earlier operation against those having a later operation. If the child is able to cooperate then, these later procedures may well be performed using adjustable sutures.

Follow-up Required

It is usually advised that these patients should continue under follow-up until they have reached the age of visual maturity at approximately 7–8 years of life. At that stage, they can be discharged back to the care of their local optometrist. During the follow-up period, they should have refraction undertaken intermittently as some of them may develop at later stages a hypermetropic prescription that might require provision of spectacles. It is not unknown for a congenital/early-onset esotropia to develop an accommodative esotropia later in life.

OUTCOME MEASURES

It is difficult sometimes to assess the success of a surgical procedure for strabismus. The aim of any intervention in these children is to produce a stable binocular alignment hopefully within 10 prism diopters of straight. Some will develop microtropia with rudimentary binocularity. Other outcome measures which might be worth analyzing would include the number of surgical procedures to produce alignment, any complications associated with the operations and final deviation at discharge. Any induced amblyopia might be considered a significant complication.

COMPLICATIONS

The most common complication from management of early-onset esotropia is inadequate ocular alignment. This can range from an undercorrection to an overcorrection where the patient has a divergence postoperatively. An undercorrection is likely to be due to either an incorrect diagnosis or inadequate amount of surgery. Patients with undetected sixth nerve palsies may have a good correction initially and then, recur because of the weak lateral rectus.

Overcorrection in the early postoperative period can be due to excessive surgical intervention or slipped/lost muscle. Late divergence may be due to the development of a pseudotendon. Either of these complications will require further surgical intervention to be corrected.

Postoperative infection is rare along with perforation of the globe causing endophthalmitis.

PRACTICE POINTS

1. Ensure that the correct diagnosis has been made and other mimicking conditions have been excluded or investigated.
2. Prescribe glasses if significant anisometropia is found, either spherical or cylindrical.
3. Decide whether early or late surgery is indicated in conjunction with the parents.
4. Pick the operation that works for you.
5. Maintain good follow-up until visual maturity. Ensure that the parents understand that surgery is not the end of the process.
6. Monitor refraction to ensure accommodative element is not missed.
7. Ensure that parents and you both work toward the some possible outcome if straight eyes and rudimentary binocularity.

REFERENCES

1. Nelson LB, Wagner RS, Simon JW, et al. Congenital esotropia. Surv Ophthalmol. 1987;31(6):363-83.
2. Helveston EM. 19th annual Frank Costenbader Lecture—the origins of congenital esotropia. J Pediatr Ophthalmol Strabismus. 1993;30(4):215-32.
3. Lennerstrand G, Andersson G, Axelsson A. Clinical assessment of visual functions in infants and young children. Acta Ophthalmol Suppl. 1983;157:63-7.

4. Teller DY, McDonald MA, Preston K, et al. Assessment of visual acuity in infants and children: the acuity card procedure. Dev Med Child Neurol. 1986;28(6):779-89.
5. Gwiazda J, Wolfe JM, Brill S, et al. Quick assessment of preferential looking acuity in infants. Am J Optom Physiol Opt. 1980;57(7):420-7.
6. Ingram RM, Gill LE, Lambert TW. Emmetropisation in normal and strabismic children and the associated changes of anisometropia. Strabismus. 2003;11(2):71-84.
7. Birch EE, Stager DR Sr, Wang J, et al. Longitudinal changes in refractive error of children with infantile esotropia. Eye (Lond). 2010;24(12):1814-21
8. Wright KW. Clinical optokinetic nystagmus asymmetry in treated esotropes. J Pediatr Ophthalmol Strabismus. 1996;33(3):153-5.
9. Helveston EM, Neely DF, Stidham DB, et al. Results of early alignment of congenital esotropia. Ophthalmology. 1999;106(9):1716-26.
10. Ing MR. The timing of surgical alignment for congenital (infantile) esotropia. J Pediatr Ophthalmol Strabismus. 1999;36(2):61-8.
11. Keskinbora KH, Pulur NK. Long-term results of bilateral medial rectus recession for congenital esotropia. J Pediatr Ophthalmol Strabismus. 2004;41(6):351-5.
12. Keskinbora KH, Gonen T, Horozoglu F. Outcome of surgery in long-standing infantile esotropia with cross fixation. J Pediatr Ophthalmol Strabismus. 2011;48(2):77-83.
13. Neely DE, Helveston EM, Thuente DD, et al. Relationship of dissociated vertical deviation and the timing of initial surgery for congenital esotropia. Ophthalmology. 2001;108(3):487-90.
14. Wright KW, Edelman PM, McVey JH, et al. High-grade stereo-acuity after early surgery for congenital esotropia. Arch Ophthalmol. 1994;112(7):913-9.
15. Uretmen O, Pamukçu K, Köse S, et al. Binocular visual function in congenital esotropia after bilateral medial rectus recession with loop suture. Strabismus. 2002;10(3):215-24.
16. Ing MR, Okino LM. Outcome study of stereopsis in relation to duration of misalignment in congenital esotropia. J AAPOS. 2002;6(1):3-8.
17. Louwagie CR, Diehl NN, Greenberg AE, et al. Long-term follow-up of congenital esotropia in a population-based cohort. J AAPOS. 2009;13(1):8-12.
18. Ing MR. Stability of the Functional Cure in Congenital Esotropia. J Pediatr Ophthalmol Strabismus. 2015;52(6): 335-8.
19. Simonsz HJ, Kolling GH, Unnebrink K. Final report of the early vs. late infantile strabismus surgery study (ELISSS), a controlled, prospective, multicenter study. Strabismus. 2005;13(4):169-99.
20. Simonsz HJ, Kolling GH. Best age for surgery for infantile esotropia. Eur J Paediatr Neurol. 2011;15(3):205-8.
21. de Alba Campomanes AG1, Binenbaum G, Campomanes Eguiarte G. Comparison of botulinum toxin with surgery as primary treatment for infantile esotropia. J AAPOS. 2010;14(2):111-6.
22. Baggesen K, Arnljot HM. Treatment of congenital esotropia with botulinum toxin type A. Acta Ophthalmol. 2011;89(5):484-8.
23. McNeer KW, Spencer RF, Tucker MG. Observations on Bilateral Simultaneous Botulinum Toxin Injection in Infantile Esotropia. J Pediatr Ophthalmol Strabismus. 1994;31(4):214-9.
24. Campos EC, Schiavi C, Bellusci C. Critical age of botulinum toxin treatment in essential infantile esotropia. J Pediatr Ophthalmol Strabismus. 2000;37(6):328-32.
25. McNeer KW, Tucker MG, Spencer RF. Management of essential infantile esotropia with botulinum toxin A: review and recommendations. J Pediatr Ophthalmol Strabismus. 2000;37(2):63-7.
26. McNeer KW, Tucker MG, Guerry CH, et al. Incidence of stereopsis after treatment of infantile esotropia with botulinum toxin A. J Pediatr Ophthalmol Strabismus. 2003;40(5):288-92.

Chapter 81 Accommodative Esotropia

Glen A Gole, Jayne E Camuglia

INTRODUCTION

Accommodative esotropia (AET) is a convergent deviation of the eyes associated with activation of the accommodative reflex.[1] There are two causative factors: one is moderate to high hyperopia and the other is a high accommodative convergence/accommodation (AC/A) ratio even in the presence of emmetropia;[2] uncommonly both may act in the one patient. As a result, the term accommodative esotropia really encompasses two different entities: refractive esotropia where a normal physiologic response (accommodation) is matched to an abnormal clinical situation (high hyperopia) and nonrefractive esotropia where an abnormal response (excessive accommodative convergence) is linked to a normal clinical situation (low to moderate hyperopia).[3]

Refractive esotropia is usually managed by spectacles alone which often need to be worn beyond childhood. If surgery is required for partially corrected AET, glasses may still need to be worn after surgery for optical reasons. Nonrefractive esotropia is usually managed by bifocal glasses which can be replaced by surgery particularly if there is a small esotropia at distance. Long term, patients with nonrefractive esotropia may be able to dispense with glasses altogether.

EPIDEMIOLOGY/RISK FACTORS

Accommodative esotropia was first described by Donders.[4] It is the most common strabismus entity in Western countries with an overall prevalence of about 1% of the population in the United States. In a population-based cohort of 385 US children with esotropia, 36.4% were fully accommodative, and 10.1% partially accommodative[5] so about half of all children with esotropia will have AET. The onset of AET is generally between 18 months and 4 years of age although it can occur much earlier in infancy (early-onset AET) and even up to teenage years if the child is unwell.[6] In the largest population study reported to date (nearly 100,000 Danish children), AET accounted for 32.8% of all strabismus; the mean age of onset of refractive AET was 32.0 months and for partially AET, it was 26.1 months.[7]

The risk factors leading to AET include one and/or many of the following: uncorrected hypermetropic refractive error, high AC/A ratio, poor binocularity/subnormal stereopsis and fusion, anisometropia, family history and monocular occlusion.[8,9] Anisometropia greater than 1 diopter (D) has relative risk of 1.68 that a hypermetropic patient will become esotropic (paradoxically, this effect is most at lower levels of hypermetropia where anisometropia and a spherical equivalent of +2 D to +3 D has a RR of 7.8) and that the patient will have poorer control of the strabismus in spectacles.[9] Infantile esotropia is a well-known risk factor because following surgical correction, 60% of patients will later develop AET. This is thought to occur due to the disrupted binocularity from the duration of the initial misalignment (>3 months of duration) and allows AET to occur with low levels of hypermetropia in this population.[10]

The onset of AET may occur after a period of illness and/or fatigue, and becomes more constant over weeks/months[11] or the condition can present acutely causing diagnostic confusion with a neurologic condition. Trauma to the eye and head injuries have also been reported as causal event with the trauma causing a loss of motor fusion.[12]

There is a genetic component in AET; Ziakas et al. reported a history of strabismus in 26% of first-degree relatives in children with AET; a higher figure than for other types of strabismus.[13] Birch et al. also reported 25% of first-degree relatives, 12% of second-degree relatives and 2–3% of third- and fourth-degree relatives of children with AET were affected.[14]

Binocularity/Stereopsis

Since the 1980s, with the ability to test stereopsis in younger children, we know that the onset of stereopsis occurs at 3–4 months of age with a rapid development to 12 months

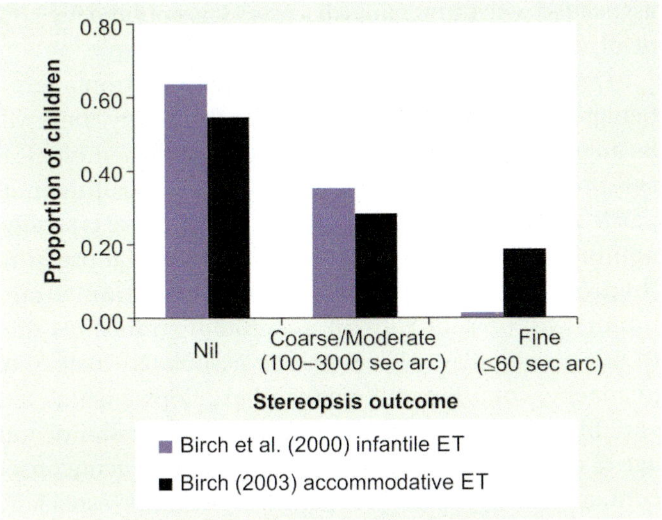

Fig. 81.1: Stereoacuity outcomes at age greater than 5 years after treatment for infantile or accommodative esotropia (ET).
Source: Reprinted with permission from Reference 15.

of age. Stereopsis then continues to improve slowly until 24 months of age.[15] In children with esotropia, despite early treatment with glasses and/or surgery, defective stereopsis is still the rule; only 0.5% of children with infantile esotropia and 18% of children with AET achieve normal stereopsis[14,15] (Fig. 81.1).

Because maturation of binocular fusion and stereopsis occurs mostly in the first year of life, and AET does not usually develop later until the age of 18–48 months, we would not expect that stereopsis would be severely affected in AET or that stereopsis should not often recover with treatment. However, the low rates of stereopsis in children with treated AET at follow-up indicate that while the critical period of maturation of stereopsis is complete by the time of the AET onset, the critical period of susceptibility to loss of stereopsis is much longer (at least to age 5).[14] If the duration of misalignment in AET exceeds 4 months, children are much more likely to have abnormal binocularity [poorer stereopsis, fusional vergences, absent sensory foveal fusion and asymmetric motion visual-evoked potential (VEP) responses] than children with misalignment of 0–3 months.[16] Fine random dot stereopsis is only possible if the duration of misalignment is less than 4 months.[17] There may also be a primary defect in stereopsis (that drives AET to occur in the first place) because 40% of patients with AET will have poor stereopsis at presentation even when the misalignment is still intermittent.[14] Abnormal retinal correspondence was found in nearly 50% of patients in a Japanese study, further supporting the idea of a pre-existing anomaly in some cases of AET.[18] There is also an association between AET and hyperopic anisometropia.[9]

We should therefore, aim for prompt treatment to re-establish orthophoria (within 4 months of onset) as a priority for patients with AET.[17] The benefit of even subnormal stereopsis is worth trying to achieve as improved stereoacuity is associated with stability of the alignment, reduced amblyopia, improved sensorimotor developmental milestones, better reading and quality of life.[15]

DIAGNOSIS

The diagnosis of AET can often be suspected if there is a history of variable intermittent esotropia, especially when associated with accommodative effort. During the initial examination, variable esotropia can also be a feature. The diagnosis is confirmed when the patient is given their full hyperopic prescription and after a period of glasses wear, the squint is either fully or partially controlled when wearing the glasses.

CLASSIFICATION

There are various classification systems in place, many of which have overlapping terminology which can lead to confusion. Von Noorden[19] described four entities:

1. Refractive AET where the alignment is completely corrected by wearing spectacles containing the full hypermetropic correction
2. Nonrefractive esotropia (with a high AC/A ratio) where a near esotropia persists despite full distance optical correction
3. Hypoaccommodative esotropia (very rare-treated with bifocal glasses)
4. Partially AET where the wearing of the full cycloplegic refraction does not result in complete resolution of the misalignment.

Convergence excess esotropia occurs when there is a large angle of esotropia at near fixation in the presence of orthotropia or a small angle esophoria or esotropia at distance [Duane A (1896)[20]]. Convergence excess esotropia has been variously defined by others as normal binocular single vision for distance (with glasses if required) but esotropia on accommodation for near fixation[21] or an esotropia at near greater than at distance by 10 prism diopters (PD, Δ) or more.[22] Because of the widely differing definitions of convergence excess esotropia, comparing outcomes of treatment by either surgery or bifocals by different investigators is very difficult.[23] The term convergence excess esotropia also encompasses "nonaccommodative convergence excess", i.e. patients with esotropia greater at near than distance but with a normal or low AC/A ratio unrelated to an uncorrected refractive error with a normal near point of accommodation. This strabismus entity does not respond to refractive correction and requires surgical correction.[20]

A practical way to manage patients with AET is to consider it in the following ways:

- Fully accommodative (refractive) esotropia
- Partially AET
- Convergence excess esotropia
  - With high AC/A ratio (nonrefractive esotropia)
  - With normal or low AC/A ratio (nonaccommodative convergence excess)
- Infantile-onset AET.

Infantile-onset AET affects about 15% of patients with onset of esotropia below 6 months of age; 40% of these patients will be fully corrected by spectacles alone if the refractive error is greater than or equal to +2.25 D.[24] However, many will ultimately require surgery.

DIFFERENTIAL DIAGNOSIS

The differential diagnosis of AET includes pseudoesotropia, infantile esotropia, myasthenia gravis, sensory esotropia, syndromes (Duane, Möbius) and 6th nerve palsy. There is also a group of patients with what was described as "acute acquired comitant esotropia" which develops in older children or even adults.[25]

Acute acquired comitant esotropia may occur:

- Following monocular occlusion (e.g. patching for amblyopia or corneal abrasion).
- With no apparent cause (or may follow illness, physical or psychological trauma/shock) where there is typically a large angle esodeviation and diplopia in a low hypermetrope. There is full abduction with usually good binocularity.

  Patients in the above two groups either have a past history of normal binocular vision (with a good prognosis for treatment, usually surgery) and those with pre-existing microtropia.
- Associated with myopia. This is an esodeviation occurring where the uncorrected myopic patient develops increased tone in the medial recti either through prolonged near work, convergence excess or paralysis of divergence.

Acquired non-AET can also occur in children aged 1–5 with a prevalence greater than infantile esotropia; it responds well to conventional surgery and is infrequently associated with intracranial disease.[26] It accounted for 5.0% of all cases of strabismus in a large Danish sample.[7]

Over 99% of acute acquired comitant esotropia has a benign cause, but in the remaining small minority, there will be an underlying neurological cause.[27] Subtle neurological symptoms and signs should prompt neuroimaging, particularly for a Chiari I malformation.[27] More typically, neurological disease due to raised intracranial pressure (hydrocephalus, Arnold-Chiari malformation, brain tumor) will present with an incomitant strabismus due to 6th nerve palsy. There may be associated history of headache, vomiting, diplopia, and oscillopsia which are variably reported depending on the patient's ability and age to describe symptoms. In the patient with acute onset comitant esotropia, the presence of nystagmus (especially abducting nystagmus), (and of course papilledema) are important features of the examination which would warrant neuroimaging.[27,28] In patients with acute onset esotropia, the lack of fusion potential (which can be tested preoperatively by prisms or synoptophore) is another clue to an underlying neurologic cause.[29]

ASSESSMENT

The initial assessment should proceed along standard lines, i.e. measure the visual acuity using an age appropriate test (or at least determine if there is a fixation preference present), measure the angle of squint, particularly at near and distance in the straight ahead position, as well as measurement in the standard nine positions of gaze and an assessment of ductions and versions. It is important to do near measurements with the patient looking straight ahead because patients with a V pattern will be more convergent in downgaze, i.e. when reading; this can lead to a misdiagnosis of convergence excess. Use of a standard squint measurement diagram is recommended to enable you to organize your thoughts[30] and decide management. Accommodative targets are essential when assessing children where the diagnosis of AET is suspected so should be used for all new patients. Fixation sticks with some detail are useful as near targets; toys held by a relative or screen-based cartoons almost always attract a child's attention sufficiently to stimulate accommodation. We would now recommend measuring the accommodative near point (and or use dynamic retinoscopy) and the gradient AC/A ratio (if possible) so patients with nonaccommodative convergence excess or hypoaccommodative AET are diagnosed at the outset.

A dilated fundus examination should always be carried out at the first visit. In particular, papilledema and optic atrophy should be excluded and the macula should appear normal.

In amblyopia is present, particularly if severe, an OCT scan of the macula should be performed to exclude subtle pathology.

Measuring Refraction

Accurate (and frequent) refraction is the key to successful management of AET. We use cyclopentolate because it enables measurement of refractive error at the first visit with the aim being to prescribe glasses, i.e. begin management, at the initial office visit. Cyclopentolate undercorrects the full refractive error by about 0.5 D when compared to full atropine refraction[31] so we generally recheck the refraction after a few months of glasses wear to unmask any latent hypermetropia. In children with dark irides, tropicamide can be added about 15 minutes after the cyclopentolate after so both drugs are exerting their maximum effect at the same time (30 minutes after instillation). Using this regimen, we rarely find it necessary to do an atropine refraction which is reserved for children with really dark irides who do not respond to cyclopentolate. We repeat the refraction within 6 months of the first visit and then at least yearly. If a previously well-controlled esotropia starts to recur, the first thing to do is to recheck the refraction as hypermetropia might have increased.[32]

Measurement of AC/A Ratio

The AC/A ratio is measured either by the gradient or heterophoria methods.[33] The distance/near disparity method makes the assumption that the AC/A ratio is high if the difference between the distance and near esotropia is at least 10 PD. It does not actually measure the AC/A ratio but is widely used clinically for management purposes, especially in the United States.[34] The heterophoria method diagnoses a high AC/A ratio more frequently than the gradient method which itself has some variability according to whether the testing method is applied at near or distance.[35] The normal AC/A ratio is 4 ± 2 (Δ/D), low is less than 2 (Δ/D) and high is greater than 6 (Δ/D).

- *Gradient method*: This determines the AC/A ratio by dividing the change in deviation in PD by the change in lens power. This is known as the stimulus AC/A as distinct from the response AC/A which is not in clinical use and which measures the accommodative response. An accommodative target must be used, the full distance correction must be worn and the working distance is held constant (typically at 1/3 and 6 m). Plus or minus lenses (e.g. +1, +2, +3 at near and –1, –2, –3 at distance) are used to vary the accommodative requirement. In clinical practice only –3 lenses are used for distance and +3 lenses for near. The change in measurement at a fixed distance divided by the test lens used is the AC/A ratio, i.e. AC/A = (deviation with lens – original deviation)/lens power. The AC/A ratio measured by the gradient method can vary according to whether it is measured at distance or near[35] so the clinician should decide which test distance they will use in order to ensure consistency of measurements.[36] Most clinicians use the near measurement.[20]
- *Heterophoria method*: The angle of strabismus is measured at distance and near and the following formula applied AC/A = interpupillary distance (IPD) (cm) + near distance (m) × (near-distance deviation-PD). Note eso = +, exo = – for these calculations. This method does not account for proximal convergence so it is rarely used clinically.
- *Distance/near disparity method*: This is in widespread clinical use because it requires much less cooperation than the gradient method which may not be possible in the younger patient. If there is more than 10 PD difference between the distance and near measurements, a high AC/A ratio is assumed so bifocals are usually prescribed if the full distance correction does not work initially.

However, many patients with an increased esotropia at near do not have a high AC/A ratio when actually measured; Von Noorden reported that 17% of patients with convergence excess had a normal AC/A ratio.[20] Havertape et al. reported that only 36% of their patients with a high AC/A ratio by the distance/near disparity method had a high AC/A ratio by the gradient method when measured at both near and distance (some had an abnormal AC/A at either near or distance, while 13% had a normal AC/A ratio at both near and distance; this overdiagnosis effect was most noticeable for deviations at near between 10 and 19 Δ.[35] Arnoldi et al. reported that of 77 patients with convergence excess esotropia, only 51% had a high AC/A ratio measured by the gradient method and 48% had a normal AC/A ratio.[37]

TREATMENT

The aims of treatment are to: (1) maintain or develop good vision in both eyes, (2) restore ocular alignment into the normal range, and (3) restore binocularity.

The mainstay of treatment is full-time spectacles which correct the full hyperopic refractive error. Bifocals are added for those with a high AC/A ratio. Other nonsurgical options such as miotics, contact lenses and laser refractive surgery in older children are collectively rarely used. Surgery is considered for the partially accommodative group where there is residual esotropia despite appropriate spectacle wear.

The treatment of refractive AET is spectacles. Full strength spectacles based on a cycloplegic refraction need to be prescribed in order to treat any accommodative component that is present. Anything less than full strength spectacles can result in significant undercorrection which can lead to deterioration of the squint and predispose to unnecessary surgery.[38] The elimination of a factor for "ciliary body tonus" and the prescription of full strength spectacles was thought to be a major factor leading to a 63% fall in the number of children undergoing esotropia surgery in Scotland between 1986 and 2001.[39]

Single vision lenses should be prescribed in the first instance for all cases (Figs. 81.2A and B) because even when there is an apparent high AC/A ratio at the first visit, full strength single vision lenses will occasionally correct the extra near deviation.[32] There are differences in the clinical findings at presentation which will predict whether or not single vision glasses, bifocals or surgery will be required; Reddy et al. reported that early age at presentation, higher refractive error, uncorrected distance and near deviation together were predictive of failure of single lens wear; they supplied an algorithm to predict failure.[40] In a series of 21 patients, Semmlow et al.[41] predicted that glasses would be necessary if the AC/A ratio exceeded 4 Δ/D and/or there was a distance esophoria of more than 16 PD with "poor control". After a period of single lens wear of weeks to months, if the deviation is not corrected at distance, we rerefract the patient before considering surgery. If the misalignment is satisfactory at distance but not at near, then bifocals are prescribed (Figs. 81.3A to C). Note that Von Noorden reported that this delay in the ordering of bifocals is unnecessary and that they can be reliably prescribed at the first visit[20] but this is not universal practice.[32] We order flat top bifocals with the upper edge at the pupil margin (this should be specified in writing on the glasses prescription otherwise a presbyopic type low segment bifocal will be dispensed) although practically, if they are at least 3 mm above the 6 o'clock position on the limbus,[1] this is satisfactory. Executive type bifocals are preferred by some but they are bulkier than flat top bifocals. In order to maintain the bifocal segment at pupil height, frequent visits to the optician are necessary (Fig. 81.4). The spectacles are correct if the child does not have to adopt a chin-down posture for distance in order to see over the near segment not do they have to adopt a chin-up posture to use the bifocals. Some authors recommend titrating the bifocal strength to the lowest power needed to restore esophoria at near[20,42] but we generally start at +3.00[43] and begin to reduce the bifocal power by 0.75 D per year when the child is 10 or so with the aim to be out of the bifocal segment at least by age 12 although Kushner reported that only 77% of his cohort had outgrown bifocals by age 13 but 99% had done so by age 18.[44] During early adolescence, the onset of teenage myopia often enables spectacles to

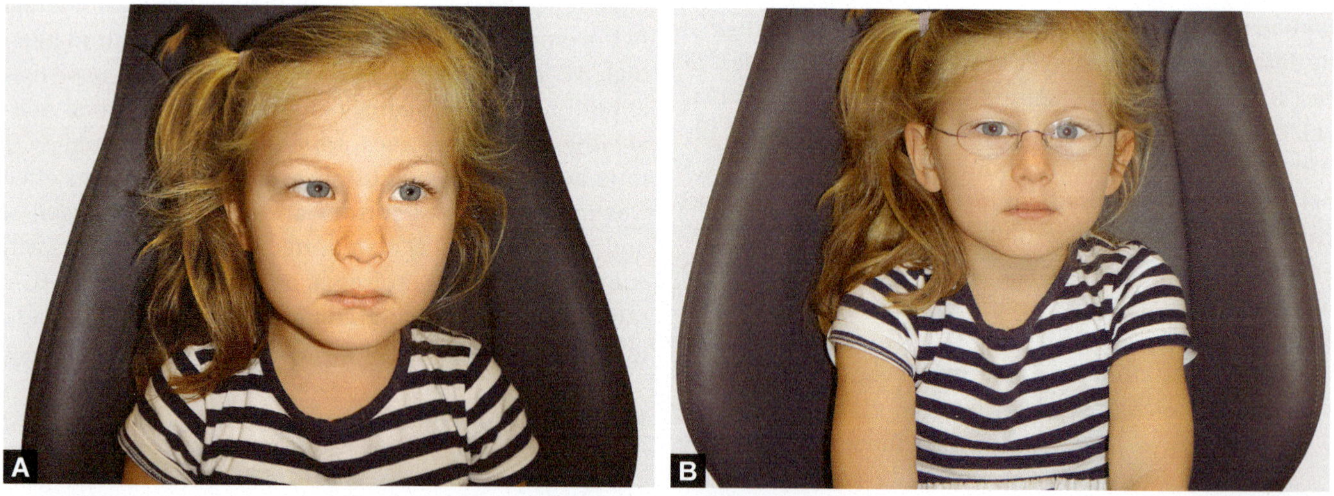

Figs. 81.2A and B: Refractive accommodative esotropia. Right +8.25/–1.00 × 180. Left +8.25/–0.25 × 90. (A) 30 PD esotropia at distance and near without spectacles; (B) 8 PD esophoria at distance and near on cover test when wearing spectacles.

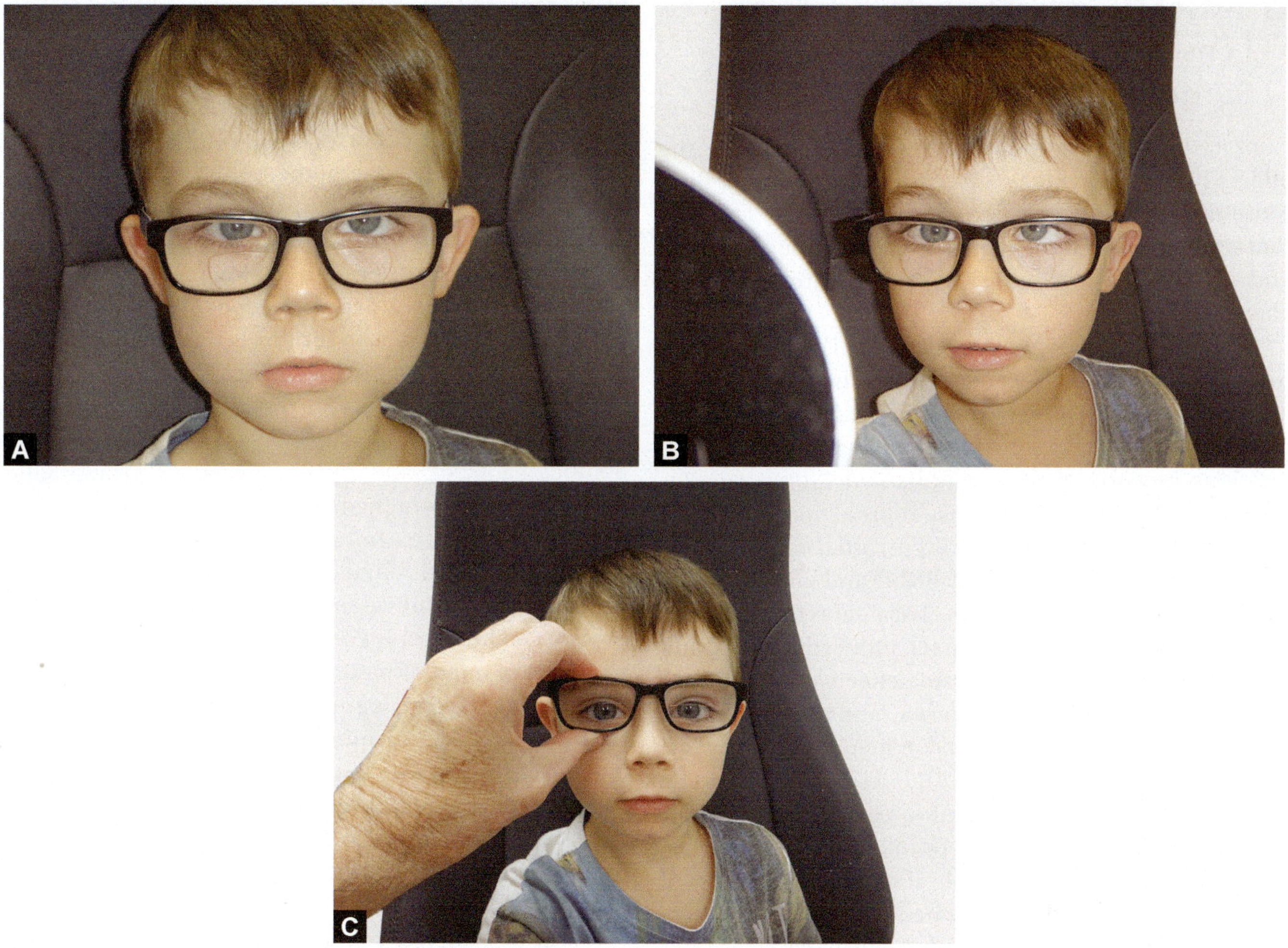

Figs. 81.3A to C: Convergence excess esotropia with prescription bifocals. Right +5.50/–0.75 × 105. Left +5.50/–0.75 × 60 with near add +3.00. (A) 8 PD esotropia at distance when looking through the distance prescription; (B) 18 PD esotropia at near when looking through the distance prescription; (C) 8 PD esotropia at near when looking through the bifocal.

Note: Near testing done with patient looking straight ahead, not in downgaze.

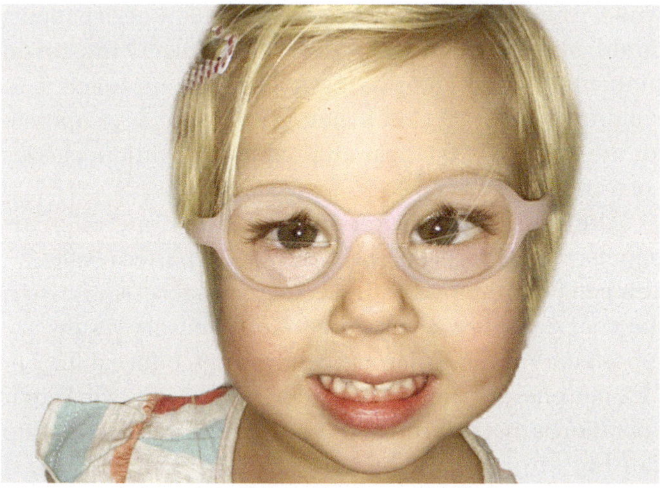

Fig. 81.4: Poorly fitting bifocals. The frames are too small for her face, the right bifocal segment could be higher and the left lens is rotated in the spectacle frame.

be discarded altogether. Should this not occur, then single vision glasses can continue to be worn and supplemented by contact lenses for sport or full-time wear.

Progressive addition lenses are thought not to be as efficacious as flat top type bifocals but, in a retrospective study, good sensory and motor outcomes were reported for progressive addition lenses which were equivalent to the outcomes with conventional flat top bifocals.[45] However, progressive addition lenses are expensive, difficult to center accurately and their design for presbyopes means the full near add at the bottom of the lens might be too low for good near control in a child. They might, however, have a role in teenagers who find bifocals no longer cosmetically acceptable.

Lesser Used Treatments: Contact Lenses, Miotics and Laser Refractive Surgery

Contact lenses have limited use possibly because the effectivity of contact lenses is less than spectacles. Both Morton et al.[46] and Gonzalez et al. (n = 1 study) reported that contact lenses did not produce acceptable alignment and stability in a previously successful wearers of bifocal glasses.[47]

Miotics (e.g. phospholine iodide—PI) are no longer freely available in most countries and they have serious side effects so their use has become very limited and largely abandoned. The 0.125% strength is still available in some locations; its main use is in diagnosis of AET (once a day for several weeks) but sustained use is problematic because weaker strength (0.06%, 0.03%) drops, often used for long-term treatment, are no longer available and side effects are related to the drop concentration. Local side effects include ocular irritation, iris cysts, cataract, induced myopia, and retinal detachment. Systemic side effects of cholinergic drugs include "salivation, nausea, abdominal cramps lacrimation, urinary and fecal incontinence".[48]

There has been a great deal of interest in laser refractive surgery for AET. It can be used to correct up to 5 D of hypermetropia; it is generally performed after the refractive components of the eye are stable at around 10–12 years of age, with the youngest child treated to date being 9 years old.[49,50] Treatment of adults with refractive AET using laser in situ keratomileusis (LASIK) to produce emmetropia ±1.0 D has been reported to produce good alignment.[51-53] Treatment of residual esotropia after laser refractive surgery in adults should still be performed for the near angle.[54]

Surgery

Surgery is indicated if the misalignment is fully not corrected by wearing of spectacles (including bifocals) containing the full cycloplegic refraction. Surgery for fully corrected refractive AET in childhood has some advocates (who are in the minority) mostly in Europe[41] but the overwhelming opinion is that such surgery is unnecessary.[55]

Partially corrected esotropia is managed surgically. If there is a normal AC/A ratio where the distance and near deviation are basically the same, surgery can be carried out using standard tables of surgical amounts for the distance deviation[56] or for mean of the deviation with and without glasses. In patients with partially corrected AET, Hwang et al. reported no difference between outcomes in an augmented surgery (mean of near angle with and without glasses) group and a prism adapted group.[57]

In convergence excess esotropia, surgery for the distance angle not corrected by spectacles (i.e. the nonaccommodative component only) was conventional management[34] for many decades but which resulted in frequent undercorrections[3] so surgery for the near angle is now commonly performed. Operating for the near angle produces few distance overcorrections.[22] Brodsky and Jung suggested that the reason for this is that the preoperative distance deviation is possibly being underestimated due to the presence of "tenacious distance fusion" controlling a larger esophoria at distance.[58,59] Garretty had proposed a subcategory of convergence excess esotropia called "simulated convergence excess"[59] where the distance deviation increases following a period of monocular occlusion. This "simulated convergence excess" may be physiologically equivalent to the simulated divergence excess seen in intermittent exotropia.[58]

Bilateral medial rectus surgery (rather than recess/resect procedures) using a variety of approaches is the preferred option but the common theme is to do enhanced surgery for the near, not the distance angle. An early approach was to add a fixed amount to the standard recession amount for the corrected distance angle[1,60] but this was modified by Kushner according to the size of the distance near disparity with excellent motor and sensory results over a 15-year period of follow-up (19/22 patients have between 0 Δ and 10 Δ of esotropia).[61]

Good results are reported for surgery for the near angle with full hyperopic correction worn; West and Repka reported reduced the need for glasses including bifocals[62] while Arnoldi and Tychsen reported that 96% of 23 patients could eliminate bifocals and 70% showed improved binocularity or stereopsis.[63] An alternate approach is in children with +3.00 D of hyperopia or more, is to operate for the average of the near angle with and without glasses correction.[57,64]

The posterior fixation suture (Faden operation) is popular, especially in Europe[65] with good reported results.[66,67] This can be combined with medial rectus recessions when the near deviation is very large. Good sensory results are reported after the Faden procedure (16% bifoveal fusion, 71% peripheral fusion).[21] The main objection to the Faden operation is that it permanently affects the muscle structure causing atrophy and postoperative scarring which, if required, makes it very difficult and unpredictable to reverse. In a randomized, masked trial of patients with partly AET with a high AC/A ratio, Kushner reported better outcomes with augmented medial rectus recessions rather than medial rectus recessions of a standard amount supplemented by posterior fixation sutures.[3]

Other strabismus procedures such as slanting insertions, pulley sutures, Y splitting of the medial rectus muscle[68] and marginal myotomy are used but much less commonly reported.

The results of surgery for convergence excess are basically similar regardless whether graded recessions for the near angle or the Faden operation is used;[69] each technique has its adherents.

The results of surgery for the near angle are good with success (commonly reported at residual angle of <10 PD at near) reported in 96% of a series; cessation of bifocals with improvement in binocularity in 70% by Arnoldi and Tychsen[63] and 86% by Peterseim and Buckley.[67]

Preoperative prism adaptation has been advocated in order to improve outcomes[70] and can lead to elimination of the need for bifocals and the elimination of glasses in 50% of patients.[70] Hwang et al. found no difference with preoperative prism adaptation for near angle versus augmented surgery but curiously this study excluded patients with a distance near of greater than 10 PD[57] so his patients did not have convergence excess. Responders to prism adaptation have a better surgical outcome than nonresponders so a positive response to prism adaptation is a good predictor of surgical success.[71]

Ludwig et al. reported (n = 119 patients) that deterioration of AET correlated with the severity grade of the AC/A ratio but not time to deterioration, treatment delay, age of onset or amblyopia;[72] these latter risk factors were found to be significant in their later paper based on a larger number of patients (n = 354).[73] In another study by the same authors, they reported on a long follow-up study (at least 5 years) of 65 children who required bifocals to maintain their near alignment; 40 (61%) were able to discontinue bifocals after an average of 5.5 years of wear but of these 20 (50%) required surgery to do so.[42] A high AC/A ratio was the only factor that predicted long-term bifocal wear.

Operating to eliminate bifocals alone when the eyes are straight at distance can be deferred until late teenage years because most children (99% of a series of 252 patients controlled with bifocals alone in childhood) will normalize their AC/A ratio by this time and no longer require bifocals.[44]

LONG-TERM OUTCOMES

Angle Stability

Long-term follow-up studies have been performed to observe the stability of the ocular alignment after treatment of AET. Mohan and Sharma observed orthophoria or less than 10 PD esotropia in 75% of their patients with mean follow-up of nearly 12 years;[74] other outcomes reported were consecutive exotropia 5–15% (requiring reduction in hyperopic correction or surgery) or decompensation/deterioration of the esotropia (5%).[74,75]

Deterioration defined as a worsening of distance esotropia by 10 PD has been identified in 13–16.8% patients in follow-up studies.[75,76] Risk factors for deterioration in AET have been reported in some studies (and not in others) to be earlier age at onset of esotropia, delayed treatment, increased hyperopia, breakdown of sensory binocularity, high AC/A ratio, incomplete treatment or poor compliance.[72,74-76] In the largest series reported to date (n = 354 patients), deterioration of control was correlated with increasing distance near disparity, earlier age of onset, inferior oblique overaction and amblyopia.[73]

In Dickey and Scott's series, the average age of children who deteriorated was 7.6 years (3.8–13.3) while the average period of time between first glasses prescription and deterioration was 3.8 years (1.3–8.8).[76] This illustrates the need for long-term follow-up in children with AET.

Many of these long-term studies combine all children with AET together, but it appears that hyperopic children with a low AC/A ratio rarely deteriorate while children with low hyperopia and a high AC/A ratio are the group most likely to deteriorate and require surgery.

Weaning of Spectacles Over Time

Emmetropization and a reduction in hypermetropia in children without strabismus provides hope for accommodative esotropes to wean out of glasses with time. Both infantile-onset accommodative esotropes and later-onset AET children remain hyperopic until age 7. A myopic shift of –0.43 D per year commences in infantile-onset accommodative esotropes but not in children with later-onset AET who remain hyperopic at least until age 12.[77] The prevalence and magnitude of astigmatism increases with age and amblyopia and anisometropia are associated with deficient emmetropization in AET overall.[77]

Parents often ask at the time of diagnosis about the likelihood of "growing out" of glasses so it is important to give advice on natural history so that they have realistic expectations.

Many patients will often remain in spectacles for their high levels of hypermetropia, myopia and/or astigmatism. For those patients with AET who are wearing glasses purely for their strabismus control, weaning out of spectacles is often attempted after age 7 years because emmetropization does not generally commence in children with AET until after that age.[77] Weaning the prescription down by 0.50 D every 6 months if control is reasonable is a guide with the aim to avoid inducing recurrent esotropia or blurred vision.[78] Hutcheson et al. reported that the mean weaning time till patients were successfully spectacle free was 17.3 ± 8.4 months (range 6.0–31.7). Weaning was completed by a median age of 9.0 years.[78]

Children with lower hypermetropia (<+3.0 D) had 91% probability of becoming spectacle free but for those children with moderate hyperopia (+3–5 D) only 20% were spectacle free by age 10 years (Fig. 81.5).[79] Mohney reported only 37% of 306 patients with AET were spectacle free by 20 years after diagnosis.[80] In one study of 39 optometrically managed (older) patients, only 4 patients (10.2%) were free of optical correction at average age 16.8 years.[81] In the Mulvihill et al. series of 103 children with AET, none were able to dispense with glasses over time possibly due to a failure of emmetropization.[82]

The general conclusion is that the ability of children with AET to outgrow their spectacles is dependent on their refractive error; children with greater than +3 D of hypermetropia usually remain in their glasses.

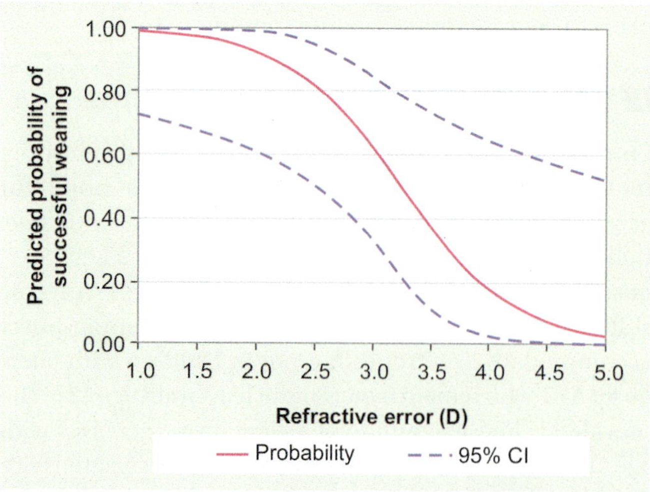

Fig. 81.5: Probability of successfully weaning a child with AET versus the initial spherical equivalent refractive error in the least hyperopic eye. *Source:* Reprinted with permission from Reference 79.

CONTROVERSY

Bifocals versus Single Vision Lenses versus Surgery

The use of bifocals for convergence excess esotropia has formed the mainstay of ophthalmic treatment for over 50 years, particularly in North America. The rationale for their use has been to help restore binocularity at near and so give better sensory and motor outcomes long term. However, Pratt-Johnson and Tillson reported on the outcome of 99 patients allocated to either bifocals (n = 45) or single vision lenses and followed for an average of 8 years; there was no difference in sensory outcomes between the two groups.[43] Gerling and Arnoldi reported that treatment of a group of children (n = 22) with high AC/A esotropia with single vision lenses alone did produce adverse sensory outcomes; all children either retained their level of stereopsis or remained stable.[83] Whitman et al. reported on a nonrandomized cohort study of 180 patients who were either treated using bifocal or single vision lenses; in both groups the stereopsis outcomes were the same but in the bifocal group there was a 3.6-fold higher rate of strabismus surgery. However, the two groups were not randomized; the bifocal group had statistically significantly lower hyperopia and larger near angle than the single vision group so the study groups could have been biased at entry with the bifocal group more likely to have convergence excess esotropia (with a predictably worse outcome requiring surgery) than the single vision group.[84] Nonetheless, the notion that bifocals produce better sensory outcomes than single vision lenses does not appear to be supported by the available literature. The arguments against routine use of bifocals were recently summarized in detail by Olitsky.[85] Surgery may be an acceptable alternative to the use of bifocals but there is insufficient high-level evidence to support one modality over the other.

CONCLUSION

1. The treatment of AET needs to be undertaken with 4 months of onset to achieve best binocular outcomes.
2. The management of refractive AET requires accurate (and repeated) refraction. Surgery for partially corrected esotropia is managed using standard tables of surgical amounts.
3. The management of convergence excess esotropia is controversial[23] because of the lack of high-quality evidence but the cornerstone is correct diagnosis of

type; in particular we should differentiate nonrefractive (high AC/A ratio) esotropia (usually managed initially by bifocals) from nonaccommodative convergence excess which is best managed by surgery. It is therefore important to not only measure refraction and the distance and near alignment in these patients but to measure their AC/A ratio directly if this is possible.

4. It is now generally accepted that surgery for convergence excess esotropia should be based on measurement of the near angle with and without glasses.

ACKNOWLEDGMENTS

Many thanks to Cassie Raynor, Built Amporndanai and Kevin Blais for background support. Glen A Gole continues to be grateful to his teachers, Graham Pittar FRANZCO, G Frank Judisch MD and William E Scott MD.

REFERENCES

1. Parks MM, Mitchell PR, Wheeler MB. Concomitant esodeviations. In: Tasman W, Jaeger EA (Eds). Duane's Ophthalmology. Hagerstown, MD: Lippincott, Williams and Wilkins; 2009.
2. Breinin GM. Accommodative strabismus and the AC-A ratio. Am J Ophthalmol. 1971;71(1 Pt 2):303-11.
3. Kushner BJ, Preslan MW, Morton GV. Treatment of partly accommodative esotropia with a high accommodative convergence-accommodation ratio. Arch Ophthalmol. 1987;105(6):815-8.
4. Donders FC. Strabismus convergens, the result of hypermetropia. In: Donders FC (Ed). On the Anomalies of Accommodation and Refraction of the Eye. London: The New Sydenham Society; 1864. pp. 291-309.
5. Greenberg AE, Mohney BG, Diehl NN, et al. Incidence and types of childhood esotropia: a population-based study. Ophthalmology. 2007;114(1):170-4.
6. Pollard ZF, Greenberg MF. Unusual presentations of accommodative esotropia. Trans Am Ophthalmol Soc. 2000;98:119-24.
7. Torp-Pedersen T, Boyd HA, Skotte L, et al. Strabismus incidence in a Danish population-based cohort of children. JAMA Ophthalmol. 2017;135(10):1047-53.
8. Birch EE, Fawcett SL, Morale SE, et al. Risk factors for accommodative esotropia among hypermetropic children. Invest Ophthalmol Vis Sci. 2005;46(2):526-9.
9. Weakley DR Jr, Birch E, Kip K. The role of anisometropia in the development of accommodative esotropia. J AAPOS. 2001;5(3):153-7.
10. Birch EE, Fawcett SL, Stager DR Sr. Risk factors for the development of accommodative esotropia following treatment for infantile esotropia. J AAPOS. 2002;6(3):174-81.
11. Lambert SR. Accommodative esotropia. Ophthalmol Clin North Am. 2001;14(3):425-32.
12. Pollard ZF. Accommodative esotropia after ocular and head injury. Am J Ophthalmol. 1990;109(2):195-8.
13. Ziakas NG, Woodruff G, Smith LK, et al. A study of heredity as a risk factor in strabismus. Eye (Lond). 2002;16(5):519-21.
14. Birch EE. Marshall Parks lecture. Binocular sensory outcomes in accommodative ET. J AAPOS. 2003;7(6):369-73.
15. Birch EE, Wang J. Stereoacuity outcomes after treatment of infantile and accommodative esotropia. Optom Vis Sci. 2009;86(6):647-52.
16. Fawcett SL, Birch EE. Risk factors for abnormal binocular vision after successful alignment of accommodative esotropia. J AAPOS. 2003;7(4):256-62.
17. Fawcett S, Leffler J, Birch EE. Factors influencing stereoacuity in accommodative esotropia. J AAPOS. 2000;4(1):15-20.
18. Inatomi A. Retinal correspondence in typical accommodative esotropia. Graefes Arch Clin Exp Ophthalmol. 1988;226(2):165-7.
19. Von Noorden G. Binocular Vision and Ocular Motility, 5th edition. St. Louis: Mosby-Year Book; 1996. p. 300.
20. Von Noorden GK, Morris J, Edelman P. Efficacy of bifocals in the treatment of accommodative esotropia. Am J Ophthalmol. 1978;85(6):830-4.
21. Leitch RJ, Burke JP, Strachan IM. Convergence excess esotropia treated surgically with Faden operation and medical rectus muscle recessions. Br J Ophthalmol. 1990;74(5):278-9.
22. Wygnanski-Jaffe T, Trotter J, Watts P, et al. Preoperative prism adaptation in acquired esotropia with convergence excess. J AAPOS. 2003;7(1):28-33.
23. Vivian AJ, Lyons CJ, Burke J. Controversy in the management of convergence excess esotropia. Br J Ophthalmol. 2002;86(8):923-9.
24. Havertape SA, Whitfill CR, Cruz OA. Early-onset accommodative esotropia. J Pediatr Ophthalmol Strabismus. 1999;36(2):69-73.
25. Burian HM, Miller JE. Comitant convergent strabismus with acute onset. Am J Ophthalmol. 1958;45(4):55-64.
26. Mohney BG. Acquired nonaccommodative esotropia in childhood. J AAPOS. 2001;5(2):85-9.
27. Hentschel SJ, Yen KG, Lang FF. Chiari I malformation and acute acquired comitant esotropia: case report and review of the literature. J Neurosurg. 2005;102(4 Suppl):407-12.
28. Williams AS. Acute comitant esotropia in children with brain tumors. Arch Ophthalmol. 1989;107(3):376.
29. Hoyt CS, Good WV. Acute onset concomitant esotropia: when is it a sign of serious neurological disease? Br J Ophthalmol. 1995;79(5):498-501.
30. Vivian AJ, Morris RJ. Diagrammatic representation of strabismus. Eye (Lond). 1993;7(Pt 4):565-71.
31. Rosenbaum AL, Bateman JB, Bremer DL, et al. Cycloplegic refraction in esotropic children. Cyclopentolate versus atropine. Ophthalmology. 1981;88(10):1031-4.
32. Black BC. The influence of refractive error management on the natural history and treatment outcome of accommodative esotropia (an American Ophthalmological Society thesis). Trans Am Ophthalmol Soc. 2006;104:303-21.

33. Von Noorden GK. Binocular Vision and Ocular Motility. St. Louis: Mosby-Year Book; 1996. pp. 90-2.
34. Parks MM. Abnormal accommodative convergence in squint. AMA Arch Ophthalmol. 1958;59(3):364-80.
35. Havertape SA, Cruz OA, Miyazaki EA. Comparison of methods for determining the AC/A ratio in accommodative esotropia. J Pediatr Ophthalmol Strabismus. 1999;36(4): 178-83.
36. Garretty T. Convergence excess accommodative esotropia: a descriptive review of patients presenting over a period of 10 years. Br Ir Orthopt J. 2015;8:23-8.
37. Arnoldi K. Convergence excess:characteristics and treatment. Am Orthop J. 1999;49:37-47.
38. MacEwen CJ, Lymburn EG, Ho WO. Is the maximum hypermetropic correction necessary in children with fully accommodative esotropia? Br J Ophthalmol. 2008;92(10):1329-32.
39. MacEwen CJ, Chakrabarti HS. Why is squint surgery in children in decline? Br J Ophthalmol. 2004;88(4):509-11.
40. Reddy AK, Freeman CH, Paysse EA, et al. A data-driven approach to the management of accommodative esotropia. Am J Ophthalmol. 2009;148(3):466-70.
41. Semmlow J, Putteman A, Vercher JL, et al. Surgical modification of the AC/A ratio and the binocular alignment ("Phoria") at distance; its influence on accommodative esotropia: a study of 21 cases. Binocul Vis Strabismus Q. 2000;15(2):121-30.
42. Ludwig IH, Parks MM, Getson PR. Long-term results of bifocal therapy for accommodative esotropia. J Pediatr Ophthalmol Strabismus. 1989;26(6):264-70.
43. Pratt-Johnson JA, Tillson G. The management of esotropia with high AC/A ratio (convergence excess). J Pediatr Ophthalmol Strabismus. 1985;22(6):238-42.
44. Kushner BJ. Surgical treatment of teenagers with high AC/A ratios. Am Orthopt J. 2014;64:37-42.
45. Mezer E, Wygnanski-Jaffe T, Stolovich C. Progressive addition lenses for accommodative esotropia with a high accomodative element. Strabismus. 2015;23(4):170-5.
46. Morton GV, Kushner BJ, Lucchese NJ, et al. The efficacy of SimulVue and Unilens RGP aspheric bifocal contact lenses in the treatment of esotropia associated with a high accommodative convergence/accommodation ratio. J AAPOS. 1998;2(2):108-12.
47. Gonzalez E, Barra F, Sanchez I, et al. High AC/A accommodative esotropia strabismus treated with contact lenses: a single case design (N = 1) study. Binocul Vis Strabismus Q. 2007;22(2):90-5.
48. Hiatt RL. Medical management of accommodative esotropia. J Pediatr Ophthalmol Strabismus. 1983;20(5):199-201.
49. Phillips CB, Prager TC, McClellan G, et al. Laser in situ keratomileusis for high hyperopia in awake, autofixating pediatric and adolescent patients with fully or partially accommodative esotropia. J Cataract Refract Surg. 2004;30(10):2124-9.
50. Brugnoli de Pagano OM, Pagano GL. Laser in situ keratomileusis for the treatment of refractive accommodative esotropia. Ophthalmology. 2012;119(1):159-63.
51. Hoyos JE, Cigales M, Hoyos-Chacon J, et al. Hyperopic laser in situ keratomileusis for refractive accommodative esotropia. J Cataract Refract Surg. 2002;28(9):1522-9.
52. Magli A, Forte R, Gallo F, et al. Refractive surgery for accommodative esotropia: 5-year follow-up. J Refract Surg. 2014;30(2):116-20.
53. Nucci P, Serafino M, Hutchinson AK. Photorefractive keratectomy for the treatment of purely refractive accommodative esotropia. J Cataract Refract Surg. 2003;29(5):889-94.
54. Nucci P, Serafino M, Hutchinson AK. Photorefractive keratectomy followed by strabismus surgery for the treatment of partly accommodative esotropia. J AAPOS. 2004;8(6):555-9.
55. Jampolsky A, Von Noorden GK, Spiritus M. Unnecessary surgery in fully refractive accommodative esotropia. Int Ophthalmol. 1992;16(2):129-30; discussion 30-1.
56. Sami D. Comitant strabismus. In: Albert D, Miller J, Azar D, Blodi B (Eds). Albert and Jakobiec's Principles and Practice of Ophthalmology, 3rd edition. Philadelphia: Saunders; 2008.
57. Hwang JM, Min BM, Park SC, et al. A randomized comparison of prism adaptation and augmented surgery in the surgical management of esotropia associated with hypermetropia. J Pediatr Ophthalmol Strabismus. 1999;36(4):196-200.
58. Brodsky MC, Jung J. Intermittent exotropia and accommodative esotropia: distinct disorders or two ends of a spectrum? Ophthalmology. 2015;122(8):1543-6.
59. Garretty T. Convergence excess esotropia: a proposed new classification and the effect of monocular occlusion on the AC/A ratio. J Pediatr Ophthalmol Strabismus. 2010;47(5):308-12.
60. Rosenbaum AL, Jampolsky A, Scott AB. Bimedial recession in high AC/A esotropia. A long-term follow-up. Arch Ophthalmol. 1974;91(4):251-3.
61. Kushner BJ. Fifteen-year outcome of surgery for the near angle in patients with accommodative esotropia and a high accommodative convergence to accommodation ratio. Arch Ophthalmol. 2001;119(8):1150-3.
62. West CE, Repka MX. A comparison of surgical techniques for the treatment of acquired esotropia with increased accommodative convergence/accommodation ratio. J Pediatr Ophthalmol Strabismus. 1994;31(4):232-7.
63. Arnoldi KA, Tychsen L. Surgery for esotropia with a high accommodative convergence/accommodation ratio: effects on accommodative vergence and binocularity. Ophthalmic Surg Lasers. 1996;27(5):342-8.
64. Wright KW, Bruce-Lyle L. Augmented surgery for esotropia associated with high hypermetropia. J Pediatr Ophthalmol Strabismus. 1993;30(3):167-70.
65. De Decker W. The Faden operation. When and how to do it. Trans Ophthalmol Soc U K. 1981;101(Pt 2):264-70.
66. Akar S, Gokyigit B, Sayin N, et al. Medial rectus Faden operations with or without recession for partially accommodative esotropia associated with a high accommodative convergence to accommodation ratio. Br J Ophthalmol. 2013;97(1):83-7.

67. Millicent M, Peterseim W, Buckley EG. Medial rectus fadenoperation for esotropia only at near fixation. J AAPOS. 1997;1(3):129-33.
68. Akar S, Gokyigit B, Aygit ED, et al. Is y-split recession of the medial rectus muscle as effective as scleral retroequatorial myopexy of the medial rectus muscle for partially accommodative esotropia with convertgence? A report of results in 61 cases. Binocul Vis Strabolog Q Simms Romano. 2013;28(3):167-75.
69. Akar S. Surgical treatment for partially accommodative esotropia associated with a high accommodative convergence/accommodation ratio. EMJ Ophth. 2013; 1:27-33.
70. Lueder GT, Norman AA. Strabismus surgery for elimination of bifocals in accommodative esotropia. Am J Ophthalmol. 2006;142(4):632-5.
71. Kutschke PJ, Keech RV. Surgical outcome after prism adaptation for esotropia with a distance-near disparity. J AAPOS. 2001;5(3):189-92.
72. Ludwig IH, Parks MM, Getson PR, et al. Rate of deterioration in accommodative esotropia correlated to the AC/A relationship. J Pediatr Ophthalmol Strabismus. 1988;25(1):8-12.
73. Ludwig IH, Imberman SP, Thompson HW, et al. Long-term study of accommodative esotropia. Trans Am Ophthalmol Soc. 2003;101:155-60; discussion 60-1.
74. Mohan K, Sharma A. Long-term treatment results of accommodative esotropia. J AAPOS. 2014;18(3):261-5.
75. Jianhua Y, Shaomei Y, Yimin W. The deterioration of refractive accommodative esotropia. Yan Ke Xue Bao. 1997;13(3):144-7.
76. Dickey CF, Scott WE. The deterioration of accommodative esotropia: frequency, characteristics, and predictive factors. J Pediatr Ophthalmol Strabismus. 1988;25(4):172-5.
77. Wang J, Morale SE, Ren X, et al. Longitudinal development of refractive error in children with accommodative esotropia: onset, amblyopia, and anisometropia. Invest Ophthalmol Vis Sci. 2016;57(4):2203-12.
78. Hutcheson KA, Ellish NJ, Lambert SR. Weaning children with accommodative esotropia out of spectacles: a pilot study. Br J Ophthalmol. 2003;87(1):4-7.
79. Lambert SR, Lynn M, Sramek J, et al. Clinical features predictive of successfully weaning from spectacles those children with accommodative esotropia. J AAPOS. 2003;7(1):7-13.
80. Mohney BG, Lilley CC, Green-Simms AE, et al. The long-term follow-up of accommodative esotropia in a population-based cohort of children. Ophthalmology. 2011;118(3): 581-5.
81. Rutstein RP, Marsh-Tootle W. Clinical course of accommodative esotropia. Optom Vis Sci. 1998;75(2):97-102.
82. Mulvihill A. Outcome in refractive accommodative esotropia. Br J Ophthalmol. 2000;84(7):746-9.
83. Gerling A, Arnoldi K. Single-vision lenses: a comparison of management of high AC/A esotropia and refractive esotropia. Strabismus. 2013;21(2):106-9.
84. Whitman MC, MacNeill K, Hunter DG. Bifocals fail to improve stereopsis outcomes in high AC/A accommodative esotropia. Ophthalmology. 2016;123(4):690-6.
85. Olitsky SE. High AC/A ratio esotropia: do we really need to be using bifocals? Am Orthopt J. 2016;66(1):5-9.

Chapter 82 Paralytic Strabismus in Childhood

Michael X Repka

INTRODUCTION

A justifiable concern for patients of all ages is the onset of diplopia or eye movement disturbances, but these feelings are intensified among parents when their previously well child is affected. Some of these situations are emergent and serious while others are much less so. The role of an ophthalmologist is to successfully triage these with a careful ophthalmologic exam in emergency ward or the office. The differential diagnosis of paralytic strabismus differs substantially from that seen in adults where microvascular disease from diabetes mellitus and hypertension are very commonly associated with paralytic strabismus. This difference changes the clinical approach. Throughout this chapter to simplify wording, I will use the term "paresis" to represent a partial deficit, as well as the complete functional deficit, "palsy".

The clinical evaluation begins with a thorough medical and ophthalmological history. The examiner should assess whether the child is comfortable, irritable or bothered with a headache, whether the vision is affected, whether the diplopia remains with one eye covered and the direction in which diplopic image is displaced. These questions are supplemented with observations from the parents and the clinician about the drifting eye's direction: inwards, outwards or vertically and whether there are unusual head movements or postures. Exploring the duration of the deviation can be very helpful in determining the need for and the rapidity for obtaining any necessary work up. Photos can be very helpful in documenting this important issue. Review of the family history for strabismus of any type. Medical history including recent viral infections and vaccinations should be elicited. The presence, duration and type of headache is important along with any personal or family history of migraine.

The eye examination needs to include assessment of lid height and symmetry, pupil size, symmetry and reactivity, visual acuity of each eye and a critical assessment of the optic disc appearance. Assessment of the completeness of ductions is important but will only detect substantial to complete deficits. Critical inspection of eye movement, comitance of extraocular muscles and the measurements in primary position as well as each of the diagnostic positions of gaze can help with minor deficits. For esotropic deviations, a cycloplegic refraction is highly recommended or even mandatory to explore the issue of onset of accommodative esotropia.

When examining a child who is noticing diplopia or an extraocular muscle disturbance, the examiner must consider several circumstances that can be associated with paretic strabismus. Non-accidental head trauma needs to be considered in every case as this can be associated with strabismus, comitant and incomitant. Other common imitators in the differential diagnosis of abducens nerve paresis are acute acquired comitant esotropia and Duane syndrome. Of the acute acquired esotropias, accommodative esotropia is the most common and of course, benign in character. Although, it is typically insidious with periodically deviating eyes interspersed with normal alignment, the esotropia may also develop rapidly over a few days and thus, appears to have been of sudden onset. Accommodative esotropia seems to occur most often in early childhood with some cases developing much later on, even after 5 years of age. Acquired comitant esotropia may also be associated with seemingly minor stress, trauma, decompensated phoria and central nervous system (CNS) disease. The proportion of children with CNS disease as their etiology increases with age as the number with comitant or refractive strabismus onset declines. Therefore, it is common to clinically monitor children with normal optic discs and full ductions if younger than 6 years of age especially when moderately or highly hyperopic but order imaging for older children in the same circumstances when there is no clear cause of the strabismus such as high hyperopia. Beyond imaging the laboratory work up of these children will need to be individualized.

While some children with paralytic strabismus are congenital, most cases are acquired from trauma, tumor and inflammatory etiologies. Rarely, the strabismus is due to autoimmune etiologies such as myasthenia gravis and Guillain-Barré syndrome. Additional conditions to include in the differential diagnosis are Duane syndrome, Moebius syndrome, orbital disease and orbital and head trauma. A prevalence study of paralytic strabismus among children in the Rochester, Minnesota region of the United States found a rate of 7.6 per 100,000.[1] The proportions of cranial neuropathies found were fourth in 36%, sixth in 33%, third in 22% and multiple nerve palsies in 9%. Reassuringly in this cohort, only 3 of 36 cases were associated with neoplasm. This is in marked contrast with the retrospective case series of etiologies cited in the individual nerve sections below which are from institutions and this selection bias likely increases the relative proportion of children with more serious abnormalities representing worse case scenarios than would be seen in the general population.

OCULOMOTOR NERVE PALSY/PARESIS (THIRD CRANIAL NERVE)

Oculomotor nerve paresis is the least common ocular motor nerve palsy in childhood according to a prevalence study.[1] It is arguably the most difficult form of paralytic strabismus to manage because of involvement of 4 out of 6 extraocular muscles. An oculomotor nerve paresis may be present at birth or may develop at any time during childhood. In one study of 41 children from a tertiary care facility 8 years of age and younger, they had an average at onset of 25 months.[2] In terms of etiology, congenital was determined in 39%, trauma in 37%, neoplasm in 17%, ophthalmoplegic migraine in 2% and CNS inflammation in 2%. A similar study from the Hospital for Sick Children in Toronto found the cause to be trauma in 40%, congenital in 30%, infection in 20% and the remainder divided among migraine, neoplasm and unknown. Some of the undiagnosed cases in the past are likely caused by schwannomas of the intracranial portion of the cranial nerve, which have escaped detection on imaging (Figs. 82.1A and B). Typically, these produce a slowly progressive ocular motor neuropathy. There has been unresolved debate about whether such a lesion could cause episodic paresis with pain, termed ophthalmoplegic migraine in the past because some of the patients would develop migraine in later years. However, other authors have found inflammatory thickening of the nerve that can respond to steroids in some cases with functional improvement. Given the uncertainty of causation, recent publications are suggesting a new term for such an entity, recurrent painful ophthalmoplegic neuropathy.[3] In adults, the presence of an oculomotor nerve paresis must always suggest the possibility of cerebral aneurysm. In children, cerebral aneurysm producing an oculomotor nerve paresis is very rare but do occur and are usually associated with signs of a subarachnoid hemorrhage. As with other acquired oculomotor nerve paresis, MRI and MRA are required along with careful follow-up.

Given these data on causation of oculomotor nerve paresis, a reasonable clinical approach is to determine if the process is congenital or post-traumatic with adequate documentation. If so then, additional work up would

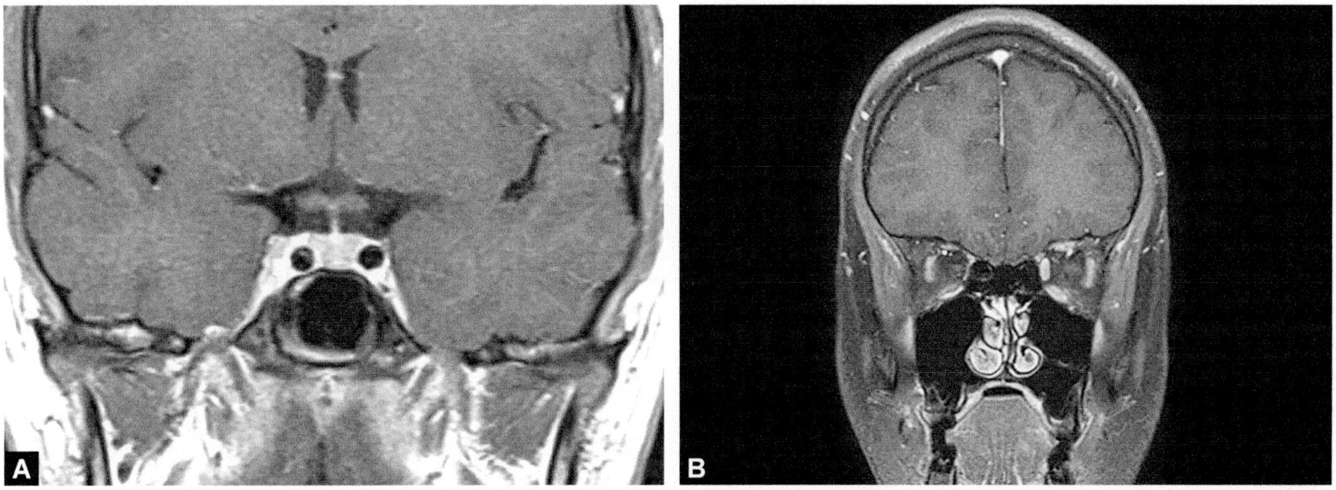

Figs. 82.1A and B: A 15-year-old male with an oculomotor nerve palsy that was slowly progressive on the right side. (A) Coronal section MRI through the cavernous sinus shows thickening of the oculomotor nerve in the superior aspect of the right cavernous sinus which increased in size with time. Highlighted on its medial and inferior margins by bright signals adjacent to the internal carotid artery; (B) Coronal section MRI through the orbit showing atrophy of the medial, inferior, and superior rectus muscles on the right side compared with normal caliber on the left side.

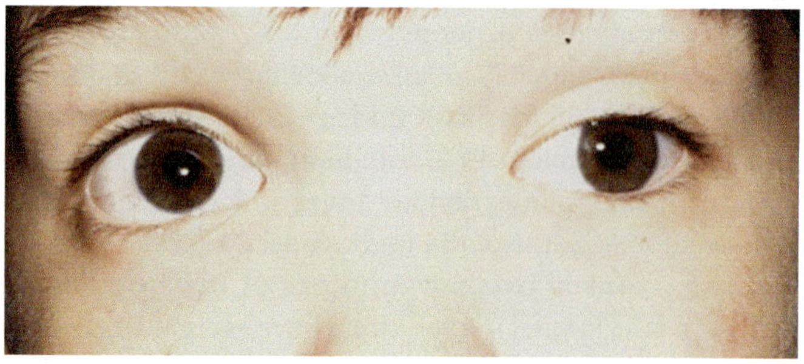

Fig. 82.2: A 10-year-old boy with primary position exotropia due to a paresis of the left oculomotor nerve. Note the ptosis on the side of the exotropia and the mydriasis.

not be needed in most of those cases where follow up is possible. On the other hand, the new onset of oculomotor nerve paresis implies a high chance for serious intracranial pathology and the need for brain imaging. In adults, there is always urgency because of the possibility of an aneurysm while this risk is much lower in children but it is not absent. Thus, imaging should have good quality with high spatial resolution images to evaluate the child for tumor in the brainstem, cavernous sinus and posterior orbit.

The clinical signs of oculomotor nerve dysfunction include deficits of elevation, depression, adduction, ptosis and mydriasis (Fig. 82.2). The relative involvement of each muscle's function will vary based on the particular situation and the portion of the nerve involved. Involvement of both superior and inferior divisions creates an exotropia but usually no vertical deviation is observed because of balanced deficits. Inferior division paresis affects the inferior oblique and inferior rectus muscles producing difficulty with upgaze and thus, a hypertropia of the affected eye with or without pupillary involvement. Involvement of the superior division affecting levator muscle and superior rectus muscle produces a hypotropia with ptosis.

Isolated palsies of the inferior rectus and inferior oblique muscles have been identified in rare instances. Some cases can be correctly identified with the Parks-Bielschowsky 3-step test (described in most clinical exam texts of strabismus) but when the results do not make sense, the examiner needs to consider other options (see trochlear nerve paresis section later).[4,5] Isolated inferior oblique palsy has not typically been associated with other medical or neurological problems simply because a troublesome lesion would affect other brainstem structures.[6] In all cases, follow up is mandatory to assure no progression and if so imaging of the brainstem and the cavernous sinus.

Pupillary dilation tends to closely follow the level of extraocular muscle involvement in children affected with an oculomotor nerve paresis rather than be spared as frequently is reported for microvascular lesions in adults. Pupil-only lesions of the third nerve would be extremely rare, if ever. Much more often if mydriasis is seen without extraocular muscle weakness, these are instances of tonic pupil. However in each case where there is pupillary mydriasis, the clinician should examine the child searching for signs of extraocular muscle dysfunction, ptosis and an exotropia that could represent a very early oculomotor nerve paresis.

Another sign associated with some cases of oculomotor nerve paresis is aberrant re-innervation (regeneration) in which some oculomotor nerve fibers are rerouted to the wrong muscles. Clinically, this usually is seen as an eye lid that elevates on attempted adduction or even a pupil that constricts with eye movement into the field of one of the extraocular muscles. This phenomenon can occur with both congenital and acquired lesions, so it is not useful as a clue to time of onset or whether the lesion is benign or serious. Acquired aberrant re-innervation is typically associated with compressive lesions. Although, the prevalence of the phenomenon varies widely, one study found aberrant re-innervation in 33% of congenital lesions and 50% of acquired lesions.[2]

Amblyopia is very common even at presentation unlike the lower rates seen with trochlear and abducens nerve paresis. Presumably this is due to the lack of binocularity in any position of gaze, the ptosis and the lack of accommodation. We found median visual acuity was already substantially reduced to a median of 20/100 (6/30) at presentation with only 30% in the normal range.[2] Even with treatment there was substantial morbidity persisting after longer term follow up. In terms of visual acuity, there was no change. However based on subgroups, the congenital cases improved, the traumatic cases were stable while those with neoplasm worsened. These outcomes likely are caused by the relative ease of treatment of the congenital cases and difficulty to treat children with neoplasm. While amblyopia management is hard in many cases, it should be attempted when possible but the child's overall prognosis should be considered in how and when to intervene.

Amblyopia treatment employs the traditional methods of glasses for refractive error, occlusion with an adhesive patch or spectacle mounted patch and atropine eye drops. In addition, the ability of the amblyopic or paretic eye to accommodate should be evaluated, typically done with dynamic retinoscopy.[7] In most cases, use of bifocal is required but the segment needs to be placed fairly high in the frame because of the inability of the affected eye to make large vertical eye movements. Where there is no vertical movement and some position of binocularity, children should be offered two pair of glasses and chosen depending on the near or distance activity. For children with serious associated medical conditions such as a child undergoing treatment for a brain tumor, the ophthalmic treatment other than glasses for vision and occlusion for diplopia are typically deferred.

Surgery

Once the oculomotor nerve paresis has been followed for about 1 year and there is no further worsening or improvement, strabismus surgery can be considered. The goal is to place and keep the eye in primary position; normal movements will not usually be possible. The most successful patients have had some recovery of ocular motor nerve function. While patients with a large neoplasm usually do not worsen after surgery and chemotherapy, patients with cryptic lesions or schwannomas often continue to progress and the surgery fails or needs to be repeated in the future (Figs. 82.1A and B). The outcomes are certainly better for children with divisional paresis and incomplete paresis as more muscles have some function which can be utilized for the repair. More so than with trochlear and abducens nerve palsies, the management of oculomotor nerve paresis is varied and highly individualized.

General principles suggest that if there is some adduction (medial rectus muscle is functioning), recession of the lateral rectus and a maximal resection of the paretic medial rectus muscle can be performed. This can be combined with minor vertical transpositions depending on the vertical deviation with movement down if there is a hypotropia and movement up if there is a hypertropia. The addition of a large recession of the contralateral lateral rectus muscle initially or as a second step can enhance the effect by utilizing Hering's law to generate a stronger abduction impulse in the fellow eye and the same for adduction in the affected eye.

For a complete oculomotor nerve paresis, horizontal nasally-directed transpositions of the vertical rectus muscles are not usually helpful long term as the vertical rectus muscles have little tone to maintain the adduction and the correction generally fails. Performing this surgery will make future strabismus surgery more difficult with fewer choices as the transposition procedure has destroyed the anterior segment circulation from the vertical recuts muscles. There other specific surgeries. For a hypotropia, Gottlob and her coworkers described disinserting the superior oblique tendon to eliminate the unbalanced infraduction, reattaching the superior oblique tendon near the superior border of the medial rectus muscle which might even add some adduction force.[8] Alternatively, disinsertion of the lateral rectus muscle was described with direct attachment of the lateral rectus muscle tendon to the lateral orbital wall with permanent suture.[9] This has become popular because other options are poor but little follow-up information is available. Alternatively, a patient could undergo serial botulinum toxin injections to the lateral rectus muscle for years. Such an approach is not typically well-tolerated in children. For isolated inferior oblique palsy, a guarded weakening of the ipsilateral superior oblique muscle using a silicone spacer or suture to prevent significant superior oblique underaction is recommended.

TROCHLEAR NERVE PALSY/PARESIS

Trochlear nerve palsy (also commonly called superior oblique paresis) is suspected when there is an incomitant hypertropia and/or vertical diplopia often associated with a head-tilt toward the opposite side as the hypertropia. The diagnosis is trochlear nerve palsy, and is typically confirmed in the clinic with the use of the Parks-Bielschowsky 3-step test. In this 3-step test, the examiner determines which eye is hypertropic and in which direction of lateral gaze the hypertropia is greater and lastly in which direction of head-tilt the deviation is greater. As an example, a 14-year-old boy presents after a fall from a step ladder with a 6 prism diopter (PD) hypertropia of the left eye (Figs. 82.3A to C). The deviation increases to 20 PD in right gaze but decreases to orthotropia in left gaze. Lastly, the deviation increases in right head-tilt to 14 PD but decreases to 8 PD in left head-tilt. This pattern is diagnostic of a right superior oblique palsy. The 3-step test can also suggest a problem with each of the vertical rectus muscles or the inferior oblique muscles depending on the observations. However, this test is valid only with recent ocular motor mononeuropathies and not orbital disease, myasthenia or thyroid eye disease in which cases it can be misleading. The results are best corroborated with additional examination details and often repeated measurements.[5]

Additional findings that support the diagnosis of trochlear nerve paresis include incomplete depression of the eye in adduction along with fundus excyclotorsion with indirect ophthalmoscopy, inferior oblique overaction and a head-tilt toward the affected side. The latter is

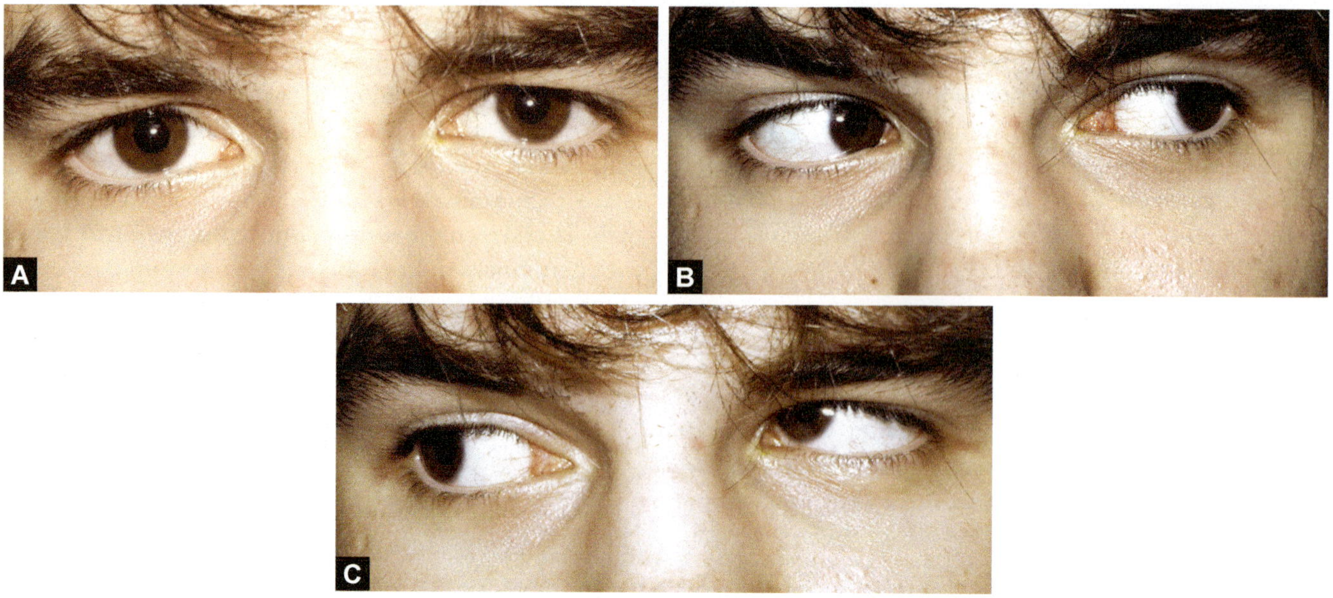

Figs. 82.3A to C: A 14-year-old boy with a hypertropia of the left eye after a fall. (A) Primary position with a small deviation; (B) No deviation seen in left gaze; (C) Large left hypertropia seen in right gaze.

typically evident after the deviation has been present for many months. The presence of alternating hypertropias, left in right gaze and right in left gaze with minimal or no primary position deviation suggests bilateral involvement. A Vpattern and excyclotorsion greater than 8°, also suggest bilateral involvement.

In those children with trochlear nerve palsy or any hypertropia who have had imaging, coronal images of the orbital MRI should be reviewed. If imaging is being ordered, be certain to obtain orbital images with coronal views along with brainstem images to carefully examine the course of trochlear nerve from the dorsum of the brainstem through the cavernous sinus.[4] Visible asymmetry with a smaller cross-sectional diameter of the superior oblique muscle on the hypertropic side can be viewed as confirmatory evidence of the paresis. Also suggestive of a long-standing superior oblique palsy are large vertical fusional amplitudes, far exceeding the 1–2 PD found in normal individuals.

In a population-based series of children with paralytic strabismus from the Mayo Clinic, trochlear nerve paresis represented 36% of paretic ocular motility deficits.[10] An earlier Mayo case series, found about 50% of cases to be congenital/idiopathic with most of the rest related to trauma (37%).[11] Rare associations have been reported with hydrocephalus, pseudotumor cerebri, neoplasm, orbital and CNS inflammatory disease.[12] A subsequent Johns Hopkins review of 92 children younger than 8 years of age at presentation found 50 to be boys and 82 to be unilateral.[13] In this case, series more than half of the paresis were congenital (56%), with idiopathic (18%) and craniofacial anomalies (13%) accounting for most of the rest of the cases.

An important long-standing clinical consideration is whether tumor can be associated with an isolated superior oblique palsy in children. There were no cases of newly detected intracranial pathology in the Johns Hopkins series of isolated superior oblique paresis, although three cases developed after neurosurgery.[13] Similarly, there was no tumor in the Mayo population-based prevalence study[10] and there was a single case in the Mayo cohort study which also developed after neurosurgery.[11] At this time, it is reasonable to conclude that isolated trochlear nerve palsy in children and teens is typically associated with a benign etiology when present childhood. Therefore, when isolated and follow-up reasonably assured, no immediate work-up is required.

Unlike the other causes of paralytic strabismus, amblyopia is very uncommon with trochlear palsy.[13] This is likely due to the ability of the child to maintain binocularity in some position of gaze at least for some of the time. Periodic monitoring of visual acuity and stereoacuity is recommended during the first 8–10 years of life and appropriate treatment if detected.

Most patients with superior oblique paresis have substantial vertical fusional amplitudes, which help control their symptoms and delays the need for intervention for many years. Treatment may include observation, prism and surgery. When the head-tilt is minimal and the diplopia is not present or not bothersome, the child can be followed. Some authors have suggested that early surgery even for minor symptoms may prevent the development of facial asymmetry; there are no prospective studies that convincingly prove that outcome can be averted. A small and symptomatic palsy can be treated with ground-in prism glasses, although this is much more often used in adults than in children because of the need to use these throughout life and many children do not require glasses. Some deviations may progress in size with time. When the symptoms of diplopia, asthenopia, difficulty reading, worsening stereoacuity or size of angle becomes bothersome to the child or teens, strabismus surgery is required.

Surgery

The choice of strabismus surgery for superior oblique paresis depends on a number of factors including the size of the angle, the direction of greatest deviation, any torsion and the amount to inferior oblique overaction. Typically for most cases with small to moderate deficits and some inferior oblique overaction, weakening of the ipsilateral inferior oblique muscle will solve the problem. My preferred surgery is a myectomy which seems to have much less tendency to produce a hypotropia compared with an inferior oblique recession. In the past, this outcome was considered representative of a masked bilateral paresis but the explanation of Ellis and colleagues of the limitation of upgaze produced by the inferior oblique muscle recession seems correct.[14,15] In the absence of inferior oblique overaction, recession of the contralateral inferior rectus muscle (yoke muscle) when the deviation is greater in down gaze or recession of the ipsilateral superior rectus muscle, when the deviation is worse in upgaze should be performed. A superior oblique tendon tuck is reserved for children with congenital deficits. These superior oblique muscles typically have tendon laxity on forced traction testing.[16] The problem is that this is often an intraoperative determination so consent should include the possibility of a mild ipsilateral Brown syndrome resulting. If there is excyclotorsion that is affecting fusion and the inferior oblique muscle has already been weakened, the use of a torsion correcting surgery is recommended.[17] Most surgeons will recommend a variant of a tendon advancement or tucking procedure to incyclorotate the eye first proposed by Harada and Ito to reduce the extorsion.

ABDUCENS NERVE PALSY/PARESIS (SIXTH CRANIAL NERVE)

Abducens nerve paresis is the second most common form of paralytic strabismus reported in children in a prevalence study from the United States accounting for slightly more than 1/3rd of cases.[1] In addition, abducens nerve paresis represented 6.5% of all childhood esotropias.[18] It may be unilateral or bilateral at presentation. The history of onset is important (e.g. sudden or insidious) and a review of photos to show the prior ocular alignment can be helpful in determining the urgency of any evaluation. A key consideration in the photo album review is exclusion of pre-existing esotropic Duane syndrome and Moebius syndrome which often look like an abducens paresis, particularly hard to examine in a preschool child.

If the deviation is new, the diagnosis of an abducens nerve paresis should be based on key clinical findings:

1. Are there new abduction deficits in one or both eyes (Figs. 82.4A and B)?
2. The abduction deficit can be verified by demonstration of incomitance on prism and alternate cover measurements. Lateral incomitance is an esodeviation which increases in lateral gaze with a smaller deviation in primary position. In addition, the deviation usually measures less to no deviation at near fixation compared with an esotropia at distance fixation. These two findings would not be found in typical accommodative and non-accommodative strabismus. In infants and young children, these measurements are often not possible and demonstration of limitation of ductions can be very difficult. Infants with early-onset esotropia often appear to have incomplete ductions masquerading as an abducens nerve paresis. Having the examiner spin on a stool while holding the child facing her or him may demonstrate the presence or absence of a normal duction as the eyes move in the direction of the rotation. This maneuver is especially important to perform with early-onset esotropia with a large angle as cross-fixation inhibits the need for the child to look in the direction desired for the examination.
3. Rule out an acquired accommodative or partially-accommodative esotropia. A cycloplegic refraction needs to be performed to explore the possibility of a refractive comitant esotropia.
4. Family history review is helpful as many children with strabismus have a positive family history; much less often with paralytic abducens nerve paresis.

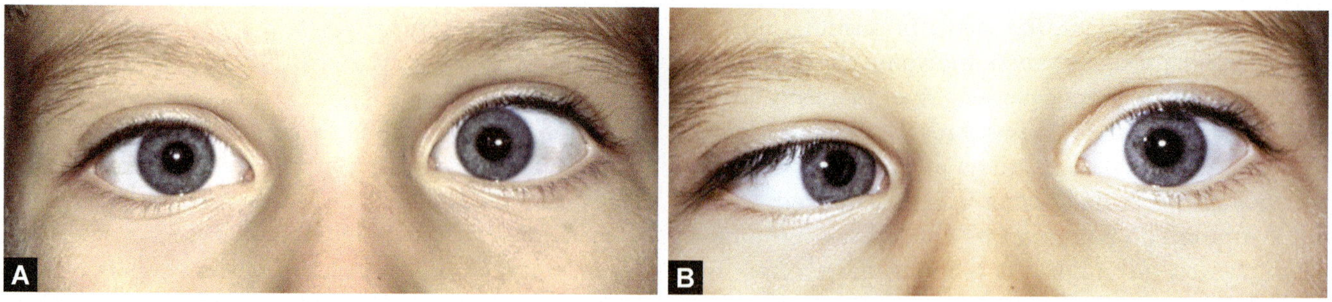

Figs. 82.4A and B: An 8-year-old girl with left abducens nerve paresis after a viral infection. (A) Small angle left esotropia in primary position; (B) Large abduction deficit of the left eye in left lateral gaze. Neuroimaging was normal and the deficit cleared in 6 months.

5. A dilated fundus examination including the optic nerve and macula is mandatory to evaluate the possibility of optic disk swelling and increased intracranial pressure as well as a retinal lesion that has led to a sensory esotropia.

The most frequent cause of abducens nerve paresis in children appears to be tumor, followed closely by non tumor increased intracranial pressure. In one study of 64 children younger than 8 years at presentation with an abducens palsy, 59% were male and 67% unilateral.[19] These children were a mean of 3.3 years of age (range: birth to 8 years) at presentation. Tumor was found in 33%, nontumor increased intracranial pressure (ICP) in 23% and trauma in 19%. Another report found tumor to be even more frequent accounting for 45%[20] with similar rates for causation by non tumor increased ICP and trauma. Congenital onset was noted in about 10%. Both studies found idiopathic or isolated deficits in about 5%. Isolated abducens nerve palsies are thought to be most often post-viral. Vincristine and some other chemotherapeutic agents have been associated with abducens nerve paresis.

These data on etiology are important to consider in planning a work up. The clinician needs to review the case for trauma or congenital timing of onset. If these are not present, nearly all of the remaining diagnoses are serious involving tumor or inflammation of the brain or increased intracranial pressure, all of which require imaging.

Recovery rates for abducens nerve paresis other than congenital are varied. In one series we found that if recovery occurred, it was after a mean of 0.6 years.[19] The recovery rate varied widely, from 5% for tumor to 67% for idiopathic but the sample was small and there could be substantial variance from these rates. Care should be used in communicating these rates to parents. These rates are much lower than seen with adult lesions, many of which are microvascular and often improve. Recovery can easily require a year or more. While monitoring for recovery, the use of prism, botulinum toxin and patching for amblyopia have specific indications. Where the deviation is sufficiently small it can be corrected with prism. Parents need to know these prisms may change often and are most effective in a small range of horizontal movement but this could improve the child's quality of life, provide single vision in some directions and possibly prevent amblyopia. The value of botulinum toxin injections into the antagonist medial rectus muscle remains uncertain in these age groups. While certainly the injection will straighten or improve the alignment temporarily and this may make the child more comfortable and able to treat their amblyopia; it is not known if these injections help long-term as had originally been suggested after the introduction of the medication.[21] Insufficient data are available in children to routinely recommend chemodenervation with botulinum neurotoxin although, a case can be made for its routine use for a severely esotropic eye that cannot be effectively used for vision during patching of the fellow eye. Occlusion therapy for management of amblyopia, just as with oculomotor and trochlear nerve paresis needs to be done if there is a visual acuity deficit and the clinical setting makes this therapy reasonable in overall patient management. In our study, the initial visual acuity was normal in 73% with a mean of 20/35; after follow up 67% were normal with a mean visual acuity of 20/30.[19] Most improvement was seen in trauma or idiopathic cases and least improvement in cases with with brain tumor.

Surgery

There are two basic approaches to surgical correction: (1) Operate on the affected lateral rectus or (2) avoid surgery on the affected lateral rectus muscle to preserve its anterior ciliary vessels. If there is some abduction force from the lateral rectus muscle seen on ductions or with force generation testing, the preferred surgical approach is an ipsilateral medial rectus muscle recession with a large lateral rectus resection. The weaker the lateral rectus muscle, the larger the resection that is needed. Surgical tables are not particularly helpful and will often produce an undercorrection. A second operation can be to weaken the contralateral medial rectus muscle. This procedure on the fellow eye activates Hering's Law, causing the operated medical recuts muscle of the fellow eye and the lateral rectus muscle of the affected eye to receive additional innervational tonus enhancing gaze into the paretic field of the lateral rectus muscle.

For the child with no or very minimal abduction, the surgeon should avoid operating on the lateral rectus muscle thereby, preserving its vasculature to protect the anterior segment from ischemia when the other rectus muscles requires surgery (Fig. 82.5). The classic surgery for a substantial paresis or palsy is a full-tendon transposition of both the superior and inferior rectus muscles. Commonly known as vertical rectus muscle transposition (VRT), the muscles are detached and then re-attached along the spiral of Tillaux adjacent to the lateral rectus muscle. Many patients were undercorrected or required simultaneous medial rectus muscle recession surgery or chemodenervation with botulinum toxin to treat the undercorrections. Innumerable surgical variations on this approach have been promoted to improve on under correction rate. One of the most popular has been the "Foster" modification of VRT.[22] In that surgery, a suture is placed 9 mm posterior to the lateral rectus muscle insertion, fixing about ¼ of the transposed muscle to the sclera at the edge of the lateral rectus muscle. While other types of transpositions have been suggested in the past including partial muscle VRT or a procedure binding the vertical muscles to the lateral rectus muscles, each of these causes substantial muscle scarring reducing ocular rotations to some extent and making re-operations difficult.

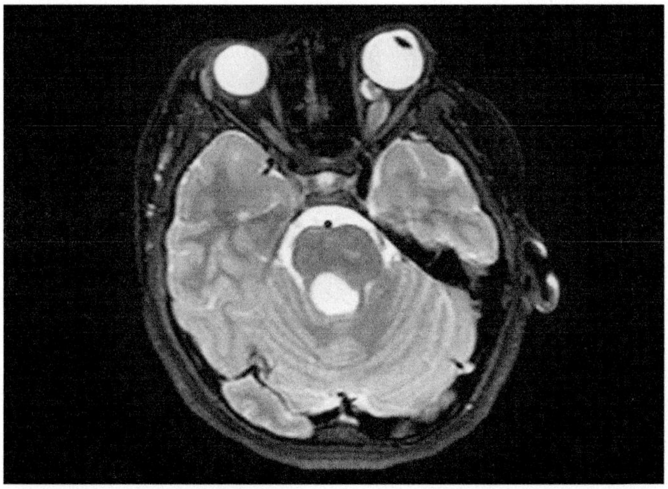

Fig. 82.5: An 11-year-old girl with hydrocephalus and bilateral abduction deficiencies with marked enlargement of the fourth ventricle.

Recognizing the difficulty of obtaining a good outcome in surgery for abducens nerve palsy, novel approaches are continually being introduced. Recently popularized is a technique disinserting and transposing the superior rectus muscle laterally to the border of the lateral rectus muscle and adding a medial rectus muscle recession, with or without an adjustable suture technique.[23] Intuitively, it would seem to not be sufficiently powerful but has had published results similar to VRT of both vertical muscles. It is remarkable that torsional and vertical changes have not been observed as had been with conventional VRT inferior.[24]

MULTIPLE OCULAR MOTOR NEUROPATHIES

The presence of deficits of ocular motor function beyond that consistent with a single ocular motor neuropathy suggests myasthenia, a lesion of the cavernous sinus or orbital apex or progressive external ophthalmoplegia. If this situation is newly acquired or the clinician is uncertain, the child needs neuroimaging of the orbit, cavernous sinus and the brainstem. If the imaging does not have a finding that could cause the ocular motor problem, evaluation for myasthenia gravis along with neurology consultation is undertaken. Multiple ocular motor neuropathies represented 9% of cases in a prevalence study.[1]

MYASTHENIA GRAVIS IN CHILDREN

Myasthenia gravis rarely affects children. It is typically subdivided into three types based on time of onset: transient neonatal, congenital and acquired. The vast majority of cases are acquired, caused by autoantibodies targeting the acetylcholine receptor within the neuromuscular junction of skeletal muscles. About 90% of childhood cases will have ocular findings. The typical signs of childhood-onset myasthenia are ptosis (90%) and ophthalmoplegia (about 75%), typically exotropia and rarely esotropia.[25-29] About 50% are diagnosed with antibody testing while the remainder are detected with endrophonium testing. Combining these case series into a general concept, onset is typically between 2 and 5 years of age, signs are extremely variable and the clinical course fluctuates greatly. Diplopia is not a typical complaint but amblyopia occurs in about

10%. About 50% of children respond to pyridostigmine. The children may also have weakness and failure to thrive. In one retrospective study of 39 children, about one-quarter resolved while one-quarter developed generalized disease. While strabismus surgery is not a first line treatment, if a deficit has become static then strabismus surgery can be performed with improvement in the eye alignment.[30] However, multiple surgeries were often required probably because of residual unbalanced muscular weakness rather than a recurrence of the myasthenia. The techniques would be the same except that the surgeon should not follow the traditional surgical dosing tables but rather use maximum resections and recessions, often one eye at a time. I prefer adjustable suture surgery for these children, given the unpredictable nature of the correction. Additional surgery is often needed.

REFERENCES

1. Holmes JM, Mutyala S, Maus TL, et al. Pediatric third, fourth, and sixth nerve palsies: a population-based study. Am J Ophthalmol. 1999;127(4):388-92.
2. Mudgil A, Repka MX. Ophthalmological outcome following third cranial nerve palsy or paresis in childhood. J AAPOS. 1999;3(1):2-8.
3. Gelfand AA, Gelfand JM, Prabakhar P, et al. Ophthalmoplegic "migraine" or recurrent ophthalmoplegic cranial neuropathy: new cases and a systematic review. J Child Neurol. 2012;26(6):759-66.
4. Parks MM. Isolated cyclovertical muscle palsy. AMA Arch Ophthalmol. 1958;60(6):1027-35.
5. Kushner BJ. Errors in the three-step test in the diagnosis of vertical strabismus. Ophthalmology 1989;96(1):127-32.
6. Pollard ZF. Diagnosis and treatment of inferior oblique palsy. J Pediatr Ophthalmol Strabismus. 1993;30(1):15-8.
7. Guyton DL, O'Connor GM. Dynamic retinoscopy. Curr Opin Ophthalmol. 1991;2(1):78-80.
8. Gottlob I, Catalono RA, Reinecke RD. Surgical management of oculomotor nerve palsy. Am J Ophthalmol. 1991;111(1):71-6.
9. Morad Y, Kowal L, Scott AB. Lateral rectus muscle disinsertion and reattachment to the lateral orbital wall. Br J Ophthalmol. 2005;89(8):983-5.
10. Holmes JM, Mutyala S, Maus TL, et al. Pediatric third, fourth, and sixth nerve palsies: a population-based study. Am J Ophthalmol. 1999;127(4):388-92.
11. Kodsi SR, Younge BR. Acquired oculomotor, trochlear, and abducent cranial nerve palsies in pediatric patients. Am J Ophthalmol. 1992;114(5):568-74.
12. Phillips PH, Repka MX, Lambert SR. Pseudotumor Cerebri in Children. J AAPOS. 1998;2(1):33-8.
13. Tarczy-Hornoch K, Repka MX. Superior oblique palsy or paresis in pediatric patients. J AAPOS. 2004;8(2):133-40.
14. Stein LA, Ellis FJ. Apparent contralateral inferior oblique muscle overaction after unilateral inferior oblique muscle weakening procedures. J AAPOS. 1997;1(1):2-7.
15. Ellis FJ, Stein LA, Guyton DL. Masked bilateral superior oblique muscle paresis. A simple overcorrection phenomenon? Ophthalmology. 1998;105(3):544-51.
16. Plager DA. Tendon laxity in superior oblique palsy. Ophthalmology. 1992;99(7):1032-8.
17. Helveston EM, Mora JS, Lipsky SN, et al. Surgical treatment of superior oblique palsy. Trans Am Ophthalmol Soc. 1996;94:315-28.
18. Greenberg AE, Mohney BG, Diehl NN, et al. Incidence and types of childhood esotropia: a population-based study. Ophthalmology. 2007;114(1):170-4.
19. Ariochane M, Repka MX. Outcome of sixth nerve palsy or paresis in young children. J Pediatr Ophthalmol Strabismus. 1995;32(3):152-6.
20. Lee MS, Galetta SL, Volpe NJ, et al. Sixth nerve palsies in children. Pediatr Neurol. 1999;20(1):49-52.
21. Holmes JM, Beck RW, Kip KE, et al. Botulinum toxin treatment versus conservative management in acute traumatic sixth nerve palsy or paresis. J AAPOS. 2000;4(3):145-9.
22. Foster RS. Vertical muscle transposition augmented with lateral fixation. J AAPOS. 1997;1(1):20-30.
23. Mehendale RA, Dagi LR, Wu C, et al. Superior rectus transposition and medial rectus recession for Duane syndrome and sixth nerve palsy. Arch Ophthalmol. 2012;130(2):195-201.
24. Lee YH, Lambert SR. Outcomes after superior rectus transposition and medial rectus recession versus vertical recti transposition for sixth nerve palsy. Am J Ophthalmol. 2017;177:100-5.
25. Mullaney P, Vajsar J, Smith R, et al. The natural history and ophthalmic involvement in childhood myasthenia gravis at the hospital for sick children. Ophthalmology. 2000;107(3):504-10.
26. Kim JH, Hwang JM, Hwang YS, et al. Childhood ocular myasthenia gravis. Ophthalmology. 2003;110(7):1458-62.
27. Ortiz S, Borchert M. Long-term outcomes of pediatric ocular myasthenia gravis. Ophthalmology. 2008;115(7):1245-8.
28. McCreery KM, Hussein MA, Lee AG, et al. Major review: the clinical spectrum of pediatric myasthenia gravis: blepharoptosis, ophthalmoplegia and strabismus. A report of 14 cases. Binocul Vis Strabismus Q. 2002;17(3):181-6.
29. Pineles SL, Avery RA, Moss HE, et al. Visual and systemic outcomes in pediatric ocular myasthenia gravis. Am J Ophthalmol. 2010;150(4):453-9.
30. Peragallo JH, Velez FG, Demer JL, et al. Long-term follow-up of strabismus surgery for patients with ocular myasthenia gravis. J Neurophthalmol. 2013;33:40-4.

Part 10 Scleritis and Uveitis

■ *SR Rathinam*

OUTLINE

Chapter 83

Uveitis Nomenclature, Classification and Clinical Work-up in Uveitis

SR Rathinam

INTRODUCTION

Uveitis refers to the inflammatory process that predominantly affects the uveal tissues with or without subsequent damage to the cornea, lens, retina, vitreous and optic nerve. In several instances, the occurrence of uveitis represents systemic diseases that primarily affects other parts of the body and may even be the first evidence of underlying systemic disease. Hence, the ophthalmologists have a crucial role in not only to treat the ophthalmic condition but also help in the early diagnosis of systemic disease.[1-4]

Causes of uveitis vary because of variations in climatic, socioeconomic, demographic, genetic and systemic morbidity patterns of each study population.[5] The prevalence and severity of diseases in developing and developed countries may also vary because of lack of primary healthcare screening, lack of insurance or high health care cost and/or poor compliance. Uveitis experts need to master not only the clinical skills but also sharpen their knowledge on epidemiological, geographic, socioeconomic factors and systemic diseases of their patients, so that a proper list of differential diagnosis (DD) can be formed.[1-4]

AN ALGORITHMIC APPROACH IN THE CLINICAL WORK-UP FOR UVEITIS

Uveitis is caused by diverse etiologies including infectious and noninfectious causes. While a number of entities may share a common clinical picture, it might also happen that a single etiology may be present with varying clinical pictures in different patients. The work up has to start with an elaborate history followed by a thorough examination including the systemic and ocular study. A step-wise algorithmic approach leads to a reliable DD, which helps to order relevant laboratory investigations. These tailored investigations guide the clinician towards final diagnosis to institute an appropriate treatment (Flowchart 83.1).

Flowchart 83.1: Algorithmic approach in uveitis.

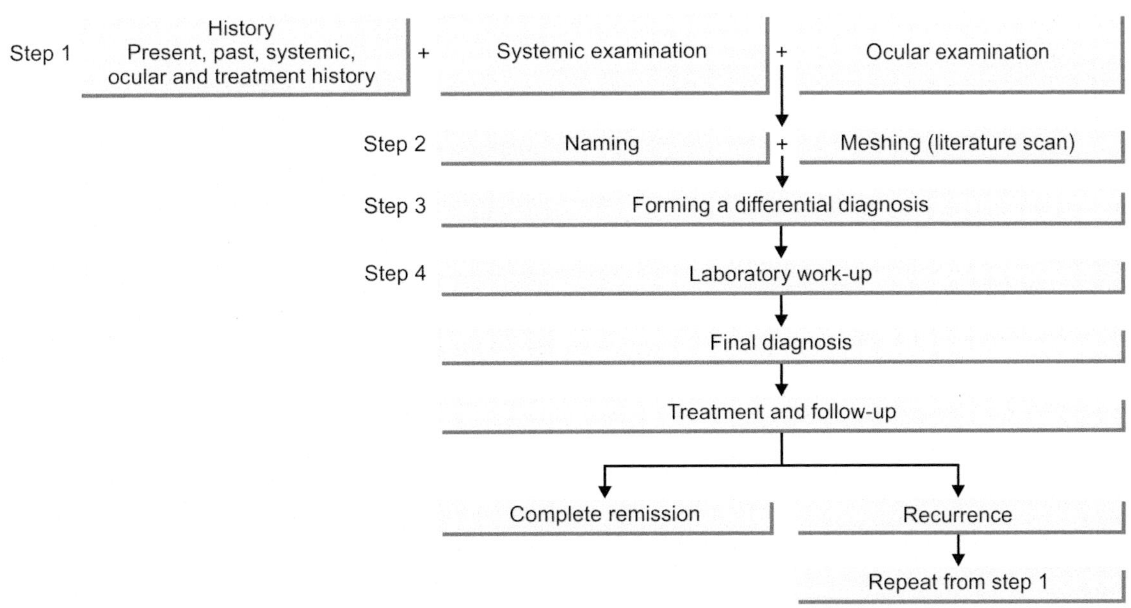

HISTORY IN UVEITIS

Adequate time should be spent on an elaborate history taking which includes demographic details, the relevant present and past ocular history, systemic history and treatment history (Box 83.1).[2] It has been our experience that when this process is done methodically, 70% of diagnosis can be made on this basis and unnecessary expensive investigations can be avoided. The importance of demography cannot be over emphasized. A bilateral chorioretinitis scar in a patient from Sub-Saharan Africa might be due to onchocerciasis, while the same presentation in a patient from South East Asia should raise the suspicion of tuberculosis. The social history or an occupational history alerts the physician on exposure to risk factors while a positive family history suggests a contagious disease or genetic disorder. Likewise histories of associated systemic symptoms act as diagnostic predictors in some patients. A choroidal granuloma in a patient with established pulmonary tuberculosis should be treated as a tubercular etiology, unless proven otherwise.

CLINICAL EXAMINATION

A comprehensive systemic examination should precede the ocular examination. In a patient with bilateral chronic granulomatous uveitis, in the presence of integumentary signs such as poliosis and vitiligo may indicate a possibility of Vogt-Koyanagi-Harada (VKH) syndrome, while associated erythematous skin lesions may indicate sarcoidosis (Figs. 83.1 and 83.2).[6,7] Important systemic clinical signs that are relevant in a uveitis patient are depicted in Table 83.1 (Figs. 83.1 to 83.4).

Often uveitis patients may require additional assessment by neurologists, rheumatologists, dermatologists and pediatricians depending upon the system involved.

Ocular examination starts from the forehead to optic disk. Before going to the slit-lamp examination, a simple torch light examination may reveal absence of eye lashes, poliosis, vitiligo, which may otherwise be missed. A detailed slit-lamp and gonioscopic examination followed by indirect ophthalmoscopy with scleral indentation are very important in every case of uveitis irrespective of anatomical or etiological classification. Important ocular signs in uveitis are given with clinical examples in Table 83.2 (Figs. 83.5 to 83.25).

Box 83.1: History in uveitis.

Demography
- Age
- Gender
- Socioeconomic history
  - Race
  - Residence
  - Occupation

Ocular present and past history
- Primary symptom
  - Onset
  - Duration
  - Laterality
  - Severity
  - Course
- Associated events
- Ocular treatment history

Systemic history
- Systemic symptoms associated with present eye disease
- Other systemic ailments

Treatment history

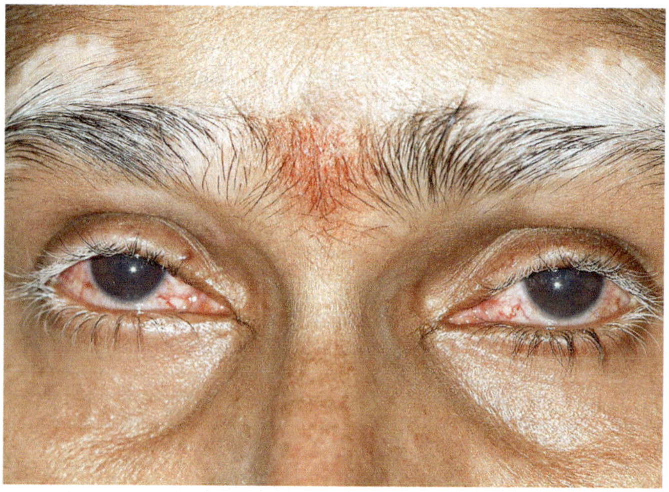

Fig. 83.1: Vitiligo and poliosis in a patient with Vogt-Koyanagi-Harada (VKH) syndrome. Bilateral granulomatous uveitis in its chronic recurrent stage.

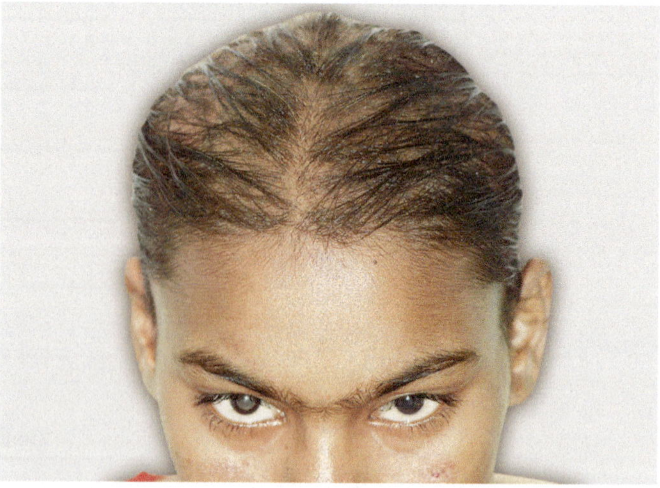

Fig. 83.2: Alopecia and butterfly rashes in a young girl with systemic lupus erythematosus.

Table 83.1: Systemic signs in uveitis with clinical examples.

System	Sign	Disease
The integumentary system	Poliosis	Vogt-Koyanagi-Harada syndrome, sympathetic ophthalmia
	Loss of hair	Systemic lupus erythematosus, syphilis, Vogt-Koyanagi-Harada syndrome
	Vitiligo	Leprosy, sympathetic ophthalmia and Vogt-Koyanagi-Harada syndrome
	Rash	Vasculitic disease, systemic lupus erythematosus, Behçet's disease, syphilis
	Erythema nodosum	Inflammatory bowel disease, sarcoidosis, tuberculosis, and Behçet's disease
	Scaling of the skin	Systemic lupus erythematosus, psoriatic arthritis, syphilis and Reiter's syndrome
	Discoid lesions	Systemic lupus erythmatosus, sarcoidosis, leprosy and tuberculosis.
	Nail abnormalities	Psoriatic arthritis, Reiter's syndrome and vasculitis
Mucosal involvement	Oral and genital lesions	Behçet's disease, Reiter's syndrome and syphilis
	Oral ulcers alone	Systemic lupus erythematosus and inflammatory bowel disease
	Nasopharyngeal manifestations including sinusitis	Wegener's granulomatosis, sarcoidosis, Whipple's disease and mucormycosis
Musculoskeletal system	Arthralgias and arthritis	*Autoimmune diseases* Seronegative spondyloarthropathies, rheumatoid arthritis, Behçet's, sarcoidosis, collagen vascular diseases *Postinfectious inflammation* Chikungunya, West Nile virus infection Leptospirosis, syphilis, Lyme's disease Tuberculosis, lepromatous leprosy
	Cartilage loss	Relapsing polychondritis, syphilis, gonococcal disease, leprosy and Wegener's granulomatosis
Respiratory system	Respiratory symptoms	Tuberculosis, sarcoidosis, Wegener's granulomatosis
Circulatory system and lymphatic system	Lymph nodes	Tuberculosis, sarcoidosis, lymphoma
	Vasculitis	Behçet's disease, sarcoidosis, tuberculosis, toxoplasmosis, acute retinal necrosis
Digestive system	Bowel disease	Ulcerative colitis, Whipple's disease, Crohn's disease
Nervous system	Neuropathy	Leprosy, herpes zoster, sarcoidosis, multiple sclerosis, syphilis and sarcoidosis, collagen vascular disease
	Hearing loss	Vogt-Koyanagi-Harada syndrome, sympathetic ophthalmia, sarcoidosis.
Genitourinary system	Urethral discharge	Reiter's syndrome, syphilis, herpes simplex and gonococcal urethritis
	Epididymitis	Behçet's disease, tuberculosis
	Prostatitis	Reiter's syndrome, ankylosing spondylitis and gonococcal disease
	Bladder (cystitis)	Whipple's disease and Reiter's disease
	Nephritis	Vasculitis in Wegener's granulomatosis, tubulointerstitial nephritis and uveitis syndrome (TINU), systemic lupus erythematosus (SLE), Behçet's disease, sarcoidosis, tuberculosis
General	Fever, fatigue, myalgia	Collagen vascular disease, tuberculosis, leptospirosis

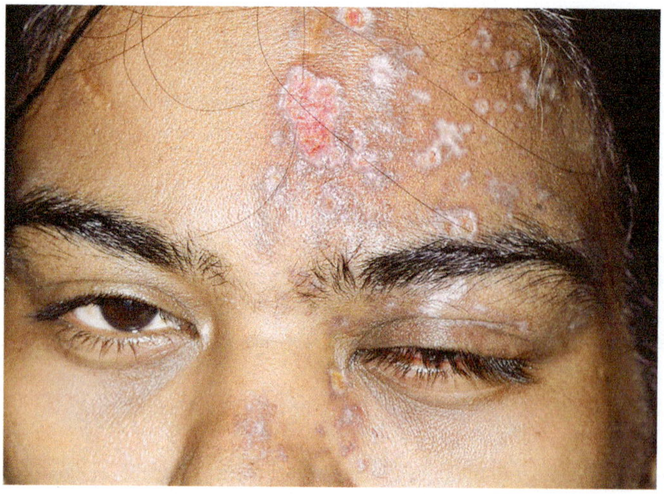

Fig. 83.3: Herpes zoster ophthalmicus involving left upper trigeminal branch.

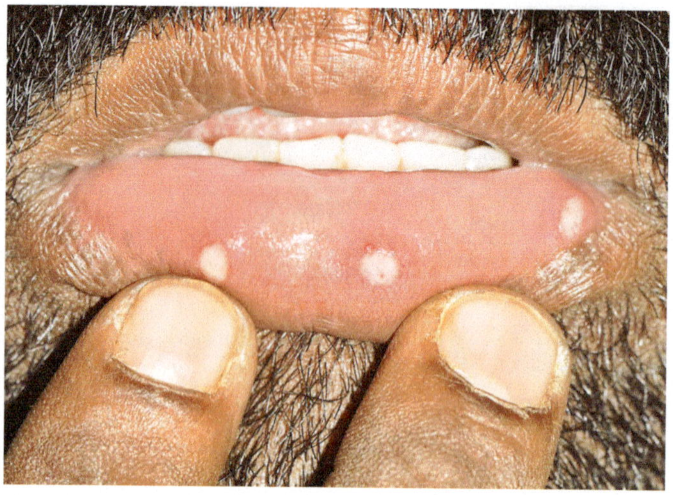

Fig. 83.4: Recurrent mouth ulcers in Behçet's disease.

Table 83.2: Ocular signs in uveitis with clinical examples.

Anatomical location	Examples
Forehead and adnexa	
Vitiligo	VKH, scleroderma
Vesicles	Herpes zoster ophthalmicus
Poliosis	VKH
Nodules	Sarcoidosis, leprosy
Madarosis	Leprosy
Conjunctiva	
Cyst	Cysticercosis
Granulomas	Foreign body granulomas, sarcoid, tuberculosis, trematode granuloma
Leproma	Leprosy
Sclera/episclera	
Scleritis and episcleritis	Collagen vascular disorders, Syphilis, tuberculosis, leprosy, viral
Cornea	
Band keratopathy	Juvenile rheumatoid arthritis, sarcoidosis
Dendritic keratitis	Viral uveitis
Superficial punctate keratitis	Viral uveitis
Sclerokeratouveitis	Syphilis, tuberculosis, leprosy and viral
Exposure keratitis	Leprosy
Iris/pupil	
Miotic and irregular pupils	Any uveitis except Fuch's uveitis
Posterior synechiae	Any uveitis except Fuch's uveitis
Busacca Nodules	Tuberculosis, sarcoidosis, syphilis
Relative afferent pupillary defect	Herpetic uveitis, neurosyphilis
Iris atrophy	Viral uveitis, leprosy, traumatic uveitis
Anterior segment	
Hypopyon	Behçet's disease, leptospirosis, HLA B27 related diseases
Hyphema	Viral uveitis, Masquerade syndrome
Gonioscopic evaluation	
Peripheral anterior synechiae	Sarcoidosis, tuberculosis
Iris nodules	Sarcoidosis, tuberculosis
Hyphema	Herpetic uveitis
Foreign body	Traumatic uveitis

(VKH: Vogt-Koyanagi-Harada syndrome)

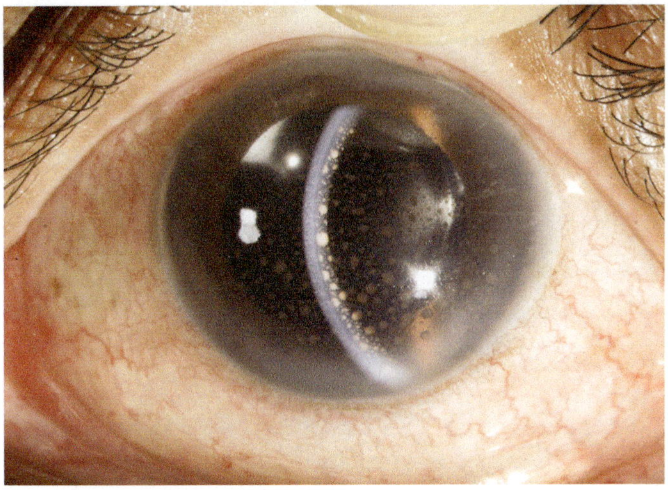

Fig. 83.5: Granulomatous keratic precipitates.

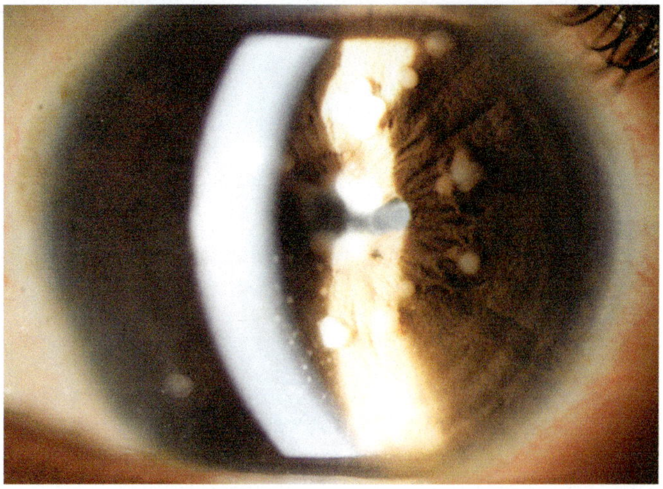

Fig. 83.6: Multiple busacca nodules in a patient with granulomatous uveitis.

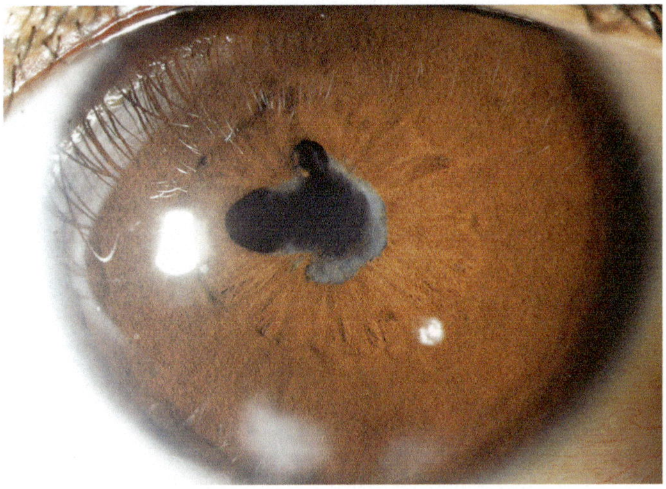

Fig. 83.7: Posterior synechiae with festooned pupil.

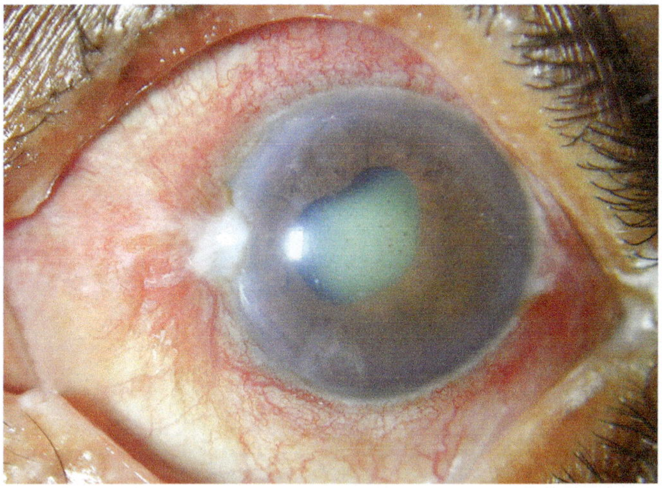

Fig. 83.8: Pigmented keratic precipitates with festooned pupil in viral uveitis.

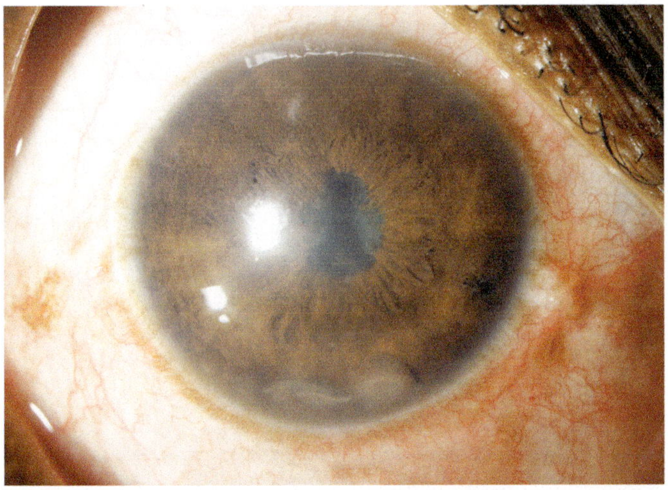

Fig. 83.9: Annular synechiae, iris bombe and peripheral anterior synechiae in a patient with uveitic glaucoma. Patient has undergone YAG-laser peripheral iridotomy at 4 o'clock position.

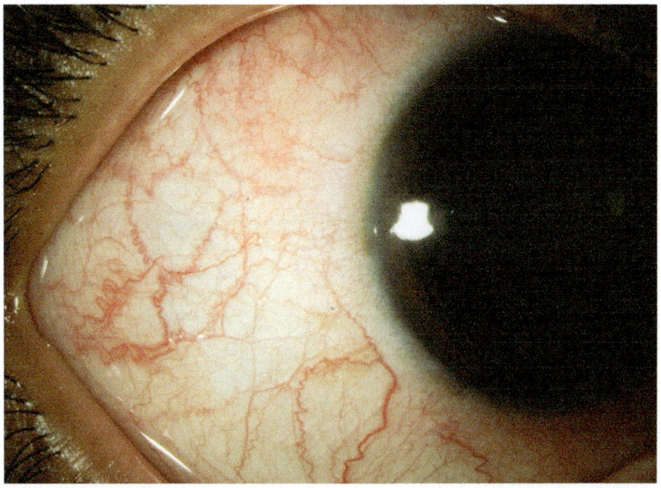

Fig. 83.10: Diffuse episcleritis in rheumatoid arthritis.

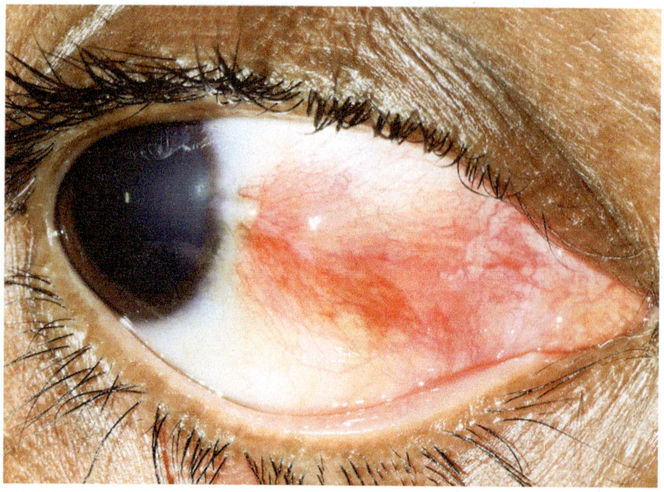

Fig. 83.11: Nodular scleritis in rheumatoid arthritis.

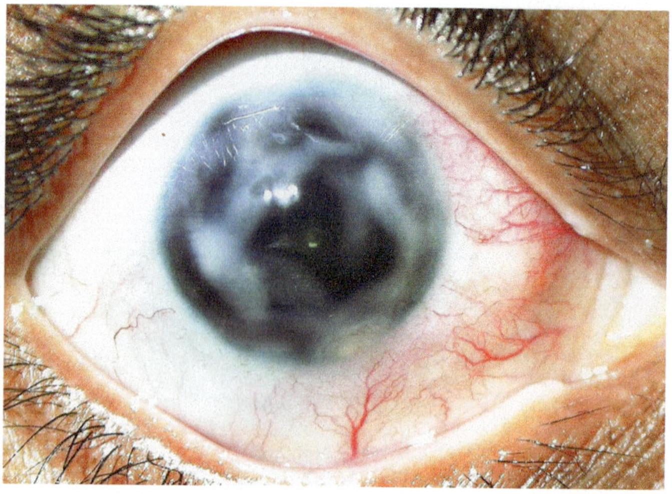

Fig. 83.12: Recurrent sclerokeratitis in a patient with tuberculosis.

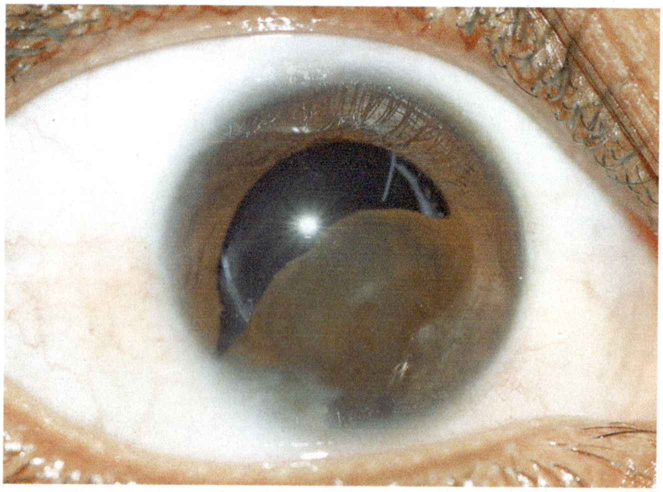

Fig. 83.13: Iris cyst after a thorn injury at 7 o'clock position. Patient has undergone intraocular lens implantation for traumatic cataract.

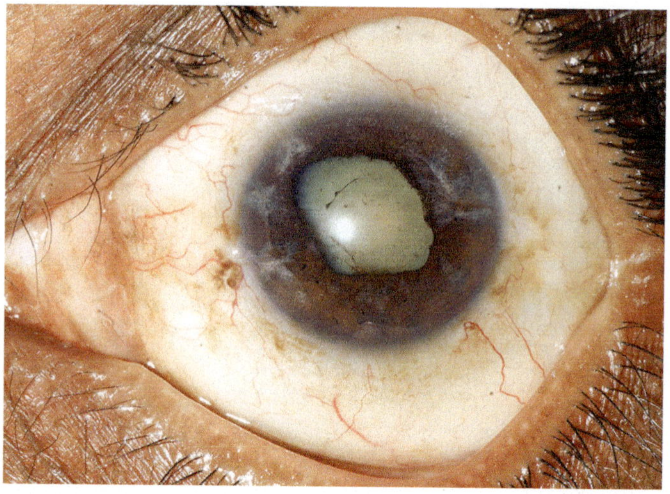

Fig. 83.14: Iris atrophic patches after viral uveitis in an elderly patient. Patient also has senile cataract.

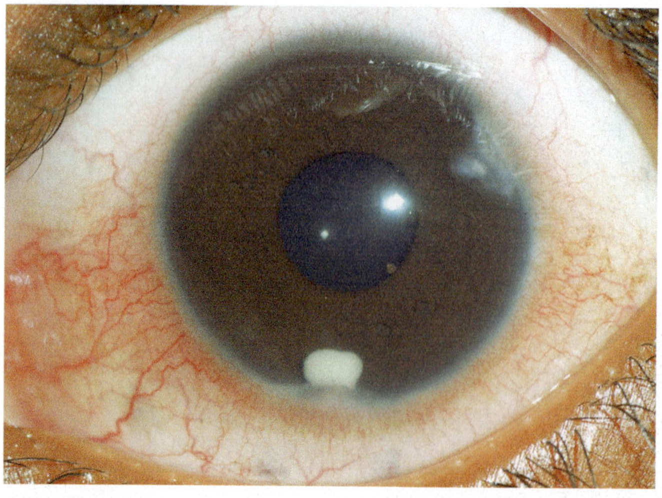

Fig. 83.15: Trematode granuloma at 2 and 6 o'clock positions in a child.

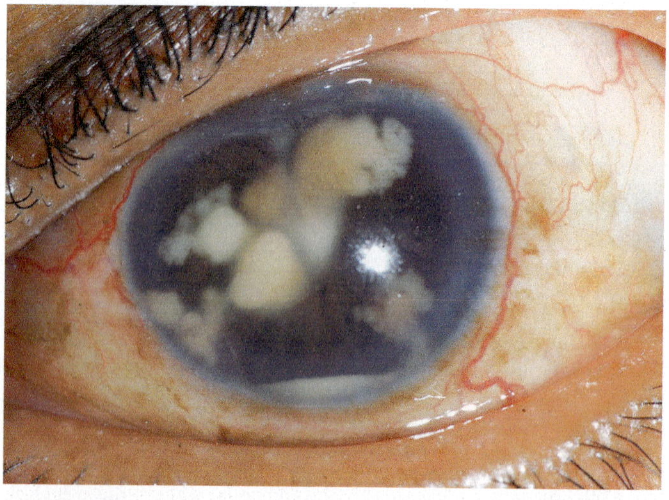

Fig. 83.16: Post-traumatic fungal granulomas with hypopyon.

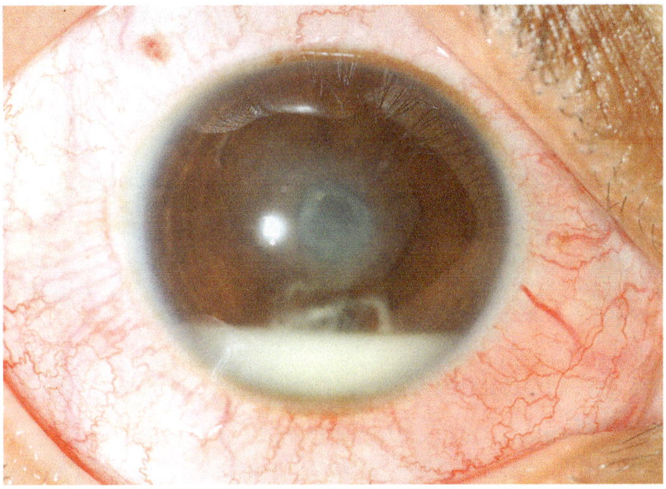

Fig. 83.17: Acute nongranulomatous anterior uveitis with fibrinous exudates and hypopyon in a patient with ankylosing spondylitis.

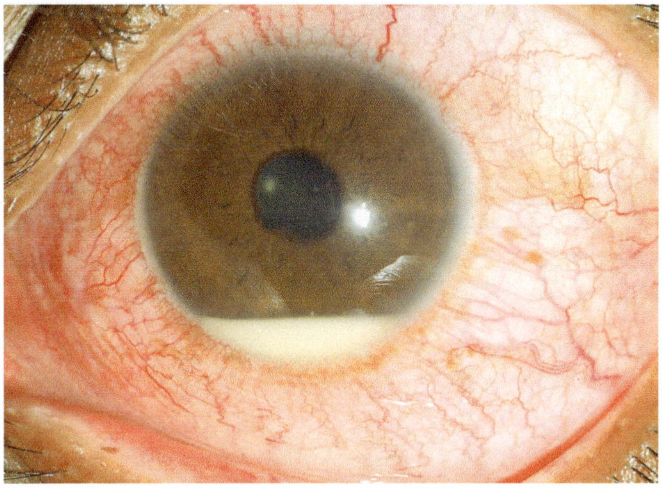

Fig. 83.18: Chronic nongranulomatous anterior uveitis with fluid level hypopyon in a patient with Behçet's disease. Note the absence of fibrinous reaction.

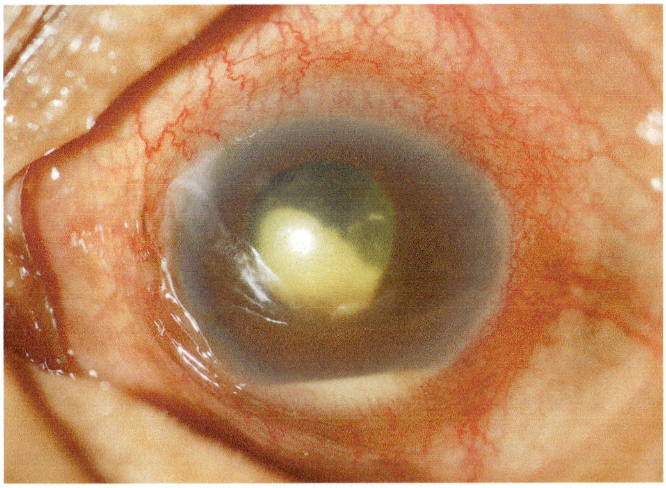

Fig. 83.19: Leaking morgagnian cataract with hypopyon in an elderly patient. Lens is partially absorbed.

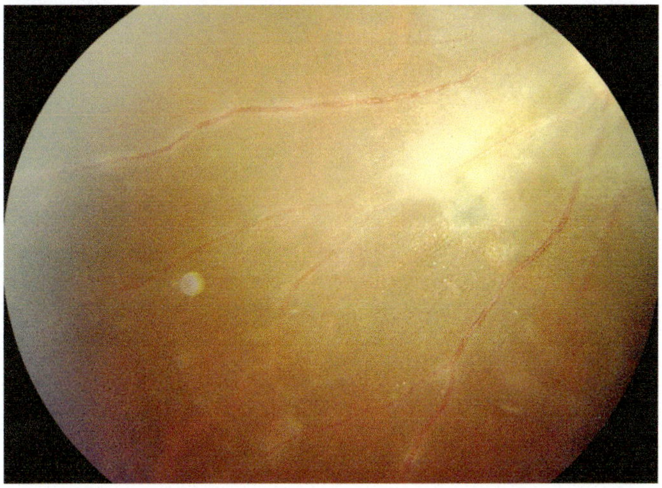

Fig. 83.20: Acute posterior uveitis with active retinitis and healed pigmented scar suggestive of toxoplasmosis. Note the phlebitis and arteritis.

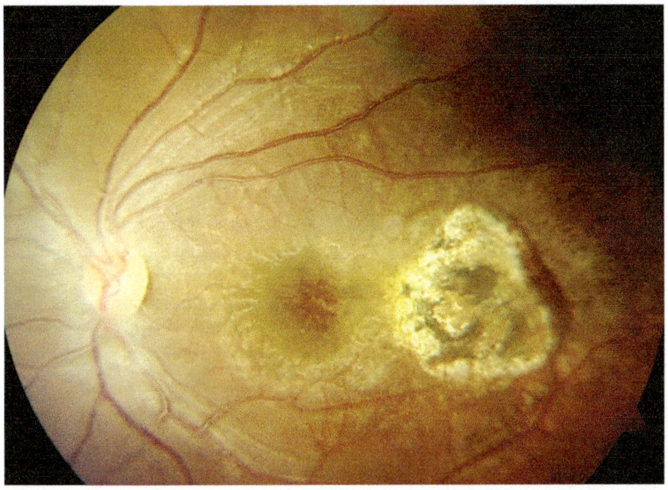

Fig. 83.21: Healed focal toxoplasmic retinochoroiditis.

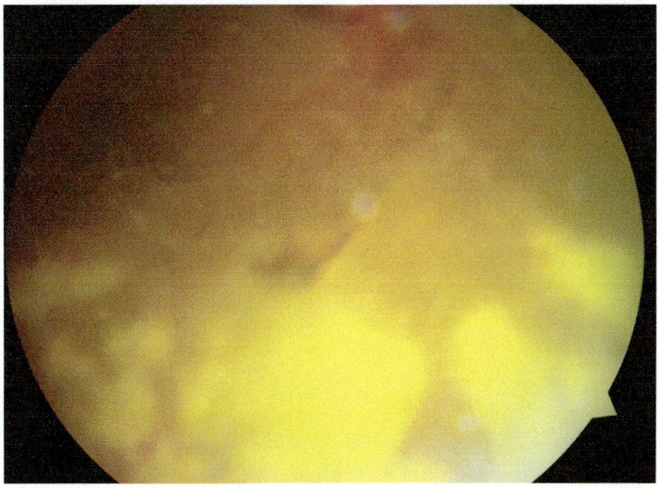

Fig. 83.22: Multifocal retinitis, vasculitis with hemorrhage and intense vitreous inflammatory reaction in acute retinal necrosis (ARN).

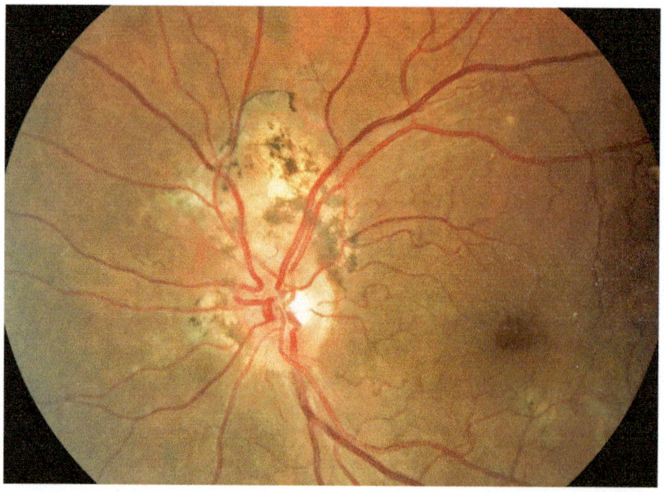

Fig. 83.23: Healed juxtapapillary chorioretinal scar in a patient with treated tubercular posterior uveitis.

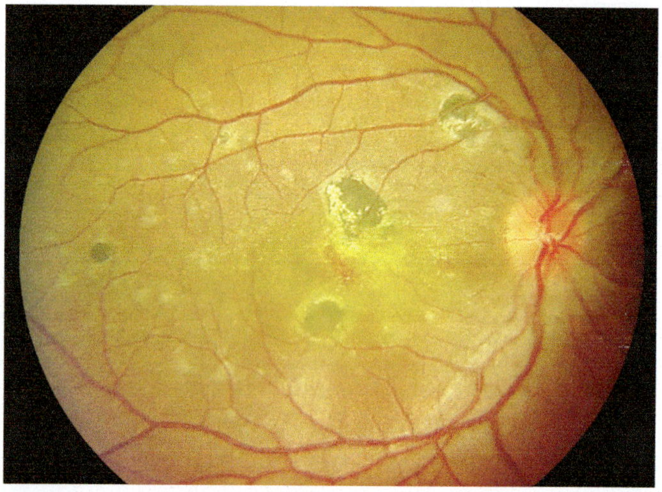

Fig. 83.24: Healed multifocal chorioretinal scars in a patient with treated tubercular posterior uveitis.

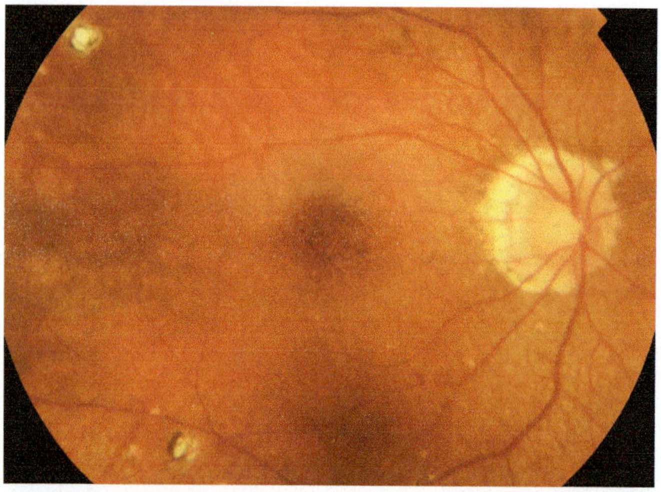

Fig. 83.25: Sunset glow fundus in a patient with Vogt-Koyanagi-Harada (VKH) syndrome. Peripapillary atrophy is seen with resolved peripheral Dalen Fuch's nodules.

CLASSIFICATION OF UVEITIS

To assist in collecting and understanding all fundamental information on demographics, anatomical location of inflammation, onset and other characteristics, the following classification systems and terminologies are used in this subspeciality. They greatly contribute in construction of clinical diagnosis. In addition, standardization enhances comparability among reports from different groups.

Anatomical Classification

Incorporating International Uveitis Study Group (IUSG) classification scheme, the Standardization of Uveitis Nomenclature (SUN) study group developed an anatomic classification (Table 83.3).[8-10] It comprises of four distinct anatomic types such as anterior, intermediate, pan- and posterior uveitis. This classification is based on the primary site of inflammation. When the primary site of inflammation is in the anterior chamber, even with minimal spill over cells in posterior segment, the uveitis is named as anterior uveitis. Likewise intermediate, posterior and pan-uveitis are named after considering the primary location of inflammation. It is important to note that the presence of secondary complications such as macular edema, peripheral vascular sheathing or neovascularization will not change this classification. Clinical examples of anterior, intermediate, posterior and panuveitis are given in Tables 83.4 to 83.6.

Table 83.3: Anatomic classification of uveitis.

Type	Primary site of inflammation	Includes
Anterior uveitis	Anterior chamber	Iritis Iridocyclitis Anterior cyclitis
Intermediate uveitis	Vitreous	Pars planitis Posterior cyclitis Hyalitis
Posterior uveitis	Retina or choroid	Focal, multifocal, or diffuse choroiditis Chorioretinitis Retinochoroiditis Retinitis Neuroretinitis
Panuveitis	Anterior chamber, vitreous, and retina or choroid	

Source: Jabs DA, Nussenblatt RB, Rosenbaum JT. Standardization of uveitis nomenclature for reporting clinical data: results of the first international workshop. Am J Ophthalmol 2005;140:509-16.

Table 83.4: Clinical examples of anterior uveitis.

Nongranulomatous anterior uveitis	Granulomatous anterior uveitis	Noninfectious anterior uveitis	Infectious anterior uveitis
HLA B27 uveitis*	Tuberculosis	Seronegative arthropathy*	Herpetic
Traumatic	Sarcoidosis	Sarcoidosis	Tuberculosis
Behçet's syndrome	Syphilis	Traumatic	Syphilis
Leptospirosis	Leprosy	Lens induced	Leprosy
Early sarcoidosis	Herpetic	Fuch's heterochromic uveitis	Leptospirosis
Early tuberculosis	VKH/sympathetic ophthalmia	Postoperative	Parasitic
Early syphilis	Lens-induced uveitis	Juvenile rheumatoid arthritis	Fungal infection

*HLA-B27 related uveitis includes ankylosing spondylitis, Reiter's syndrome, psoriatic arthropathy, inflammatory bowel syndrome.
(VKH: Vogt-Koyanagi-Harada syndrome)

Table 83.5: Clinical examples of intermediate uveitis.

Intermediate uveitis	Common complications
Idiopathic	Cystoid macular edema
Sarcoidosis	Cataract
Tuberculosis	Retinal vasculitis
Lyme disease	Ciliary atrophy
Syphilis	Cyclitic membrane
Leptospirosis	Cataract
Multiple Sclerosis	Opaque vitreous

Onset Characteristics

The SUN working study group has defined the terminologies for onset, duration and course of the disease (Table 83.7).[10] Onset is described as either "sudden" or "insidious". The typical example of sudden onset is HLA B27 associated anterior uveitis characterized by acute pain, redness and photophobia. The best example of "insidious" onset is anterior uveitis of juvenile idiopathic arthritis characterized by a painless, white eye with minimal symptoms.

Severity and Activity of Uveitis

Activity of uveitis is measured with cells and flare in anterior chamber and cells and haze in posterior segment. Previously, there were different systems for measuring flare and cells, making it difficult to compare. This has been rectified by a standardized set of criteria for grading as proposed by SUN working group.[10] The accurate grading of the inflammatory signs of the anterior chamber as evidenced by the presence of flare and cells are given in Table 83.8. Inactive anterior uveitis is defined as rare cells or less. According to this classification, the presence or absence of a hypopyon is recorded separately its presence will not grade as 4 cells.

Table 83.6: Clinical examples of posterior and panuveitis.

Noninfectious	
	Sarcoidosis Vogt-Koyanagi-Harada syndrome
	Sympathetic ophthalmia
	Behçet's disease
	Serpiginous choroidopathy
Infectious	
Bacterial	Tuberculosis
	Syphilis
	Lyme's disease
	Leptospirosis
	Brucellosis
	Septic retinitis
Fungal	*Nocardia asteroides*
	Candidiasis
	Histoplasmosis
	Cryptococcus neoformans
	Aspergillosis
Viral	CMV retinitis
	Herpes simplex
	Herpes zoster
	Chikungunya
	West Nile virus
Parasitic	Toxoplasmosis
	Toxocara canis
	Cysticercosis
	Onchocerca volvulus

(CMV: Cytomegalovirus)

Course Characteristics

The course of the uveitis may be acute or chronic. Acute uveitis is characterized by limited duration of less than 3 months. Any prompt relapse in less than 3 months on

Table 83.7: Descriptors of uveitis—standardization of uveitis nomenclature.

Category	Descriptor	Comment
Onset	Sudden Insidious	
Duration	Limited Persistent	≤3 months duration >3 months duration
Course	Acute	Episode characterized by sudden onset and limited duration
	Recurrent	Repeated episodes separated by periods of inactivity without treatment ≥3 months in duration
	Chronic	Persistent uveitis with relapse in <3 months after discontinuing treatment

Source: Jabs DA, Nussenblatt RB, Rosenbaum JT. Standardization of uveitis nomenclature for reporting clinical data: results of the first international workshop. Am J Ophthalmol. 2005;140:509-16.

Table 83.8: Grading scheme for anterior chamber cells and flare.

Grade-cells	Cells in field†	Grade flare	Description
0	<1	0	None
0.5+	1–5	1+	Faint
1+	6–15	2+	Moderate (iris and lens details clear)
2+	16–25	3+	Marked (iris and lens details hazy)
3+	26–50	4+	Intense (fibrin or plastic aqueous)
4+	>50		

†Field size is a 1 mm by 1 mm slit beam.
Source: Jabs DA, Nussenblatt RB, Rosenbaum JT. Standardization of uveitis nomenclature for reporting clinical data: results of the first international workshop. Am J Ophthalmol. 2005;140:509-16.

Table 83.9: The SUN working group—activity of uveitis terminology.

Term	Definition
Inactive	Grade 0 cells†
Worsening activity	Two step increase in level of inflammation (e.g. anterior chamber cells, vitreous haze) or increase from grade 3+ to 4+
Improved activity	Two step decrease in level of inflammation (e.g. anterior chamber cells, vitreous haze) or decrease to grade 0
Remission	Inactive disease for ≥3 months after discontinuing all treatments for eye disease

†Applies to anterior chamber inflammation.
Source: Jabs DA, Nussenblatt RB, Rosenbaum JT. Standardization of uveitis nomenclature for reporting clinical data: results of the first international workshop. Am J Ophthalmol. 2005;140:509-16.

cessation of therapy will be considered as chronic uveitis. Recurrent uveitis is characterized by repeated episodes of active inflammation, interspersed by periods of inactivity. The term remission refers to inactive disease for at least 3 months after discontinuing all treatments for eye disease (Table 83.9).

Pathological Classification

Pathologically, uveitis may be classified as granulomatous or nongranulomatous. However, it has to be understood that this pathological classification is not based on any histopathological evidence but purely from a clinical presentation. Mutton fat KPs or Busacca nodules on the iris implies a diagnosis of granulomatous uveitis.

Laterality, Age and Gender

Uveitis can be either unilateral or bilateral. The bilaterality may be symmetrically equal as in VKH or sympathetic ophthalmia or asymmetric as in Behçet's or sarcoidosis.[11-13] Other parameters such as age, gender also give a clue towards the etiology.[14,15] Certain entities are known to be active only in children such as juvenile idiopathic uveitis while Behçet's or VKH syndrome is seen more commonly in middle age. Leprosy and masquerade syndrome occur often in elderly. Certain entities are known to show a gender predilection. For example, sarcoidosis is common in women and ankylosing spondylitis is common in men. Table 83.10 gives some clinical examples to describe the uveitis patient under examination.

Etiological Classification

The final classification and the most important one is the etiological classification of uveitis.

Etiological classification is often challenging because several infectious and noninfectious uveitis entities may not present with a specific clinical picture. The same disease may have varying manifestations with respect to the onset, severity and course in different patients. Similarly, several uveitis entities of varying causes can present with virtually

Table 83.10: Descriptive terminologies in uveitis with common clinical examples.

Onset	Examples	Age	Examples
Sudden	HLA B27 uveitis	Pediatric uveitis	JRA, parsplanitis
Insidious	Sarcoidosis	Middle age	Collagen vascular disorders, sarcoidosis
Duration		Geriatric	Viral, masquerade
Limited	Traumatic	**Gender**	
Persistent	Sarcoidosis	Male	HLA B27 uveitis
Course		Female	Sarcoidosis
Acute	Acute retinal necrosis	**Pathology**	
Recurrent	HLA B27 uveitis	Nongranulomatous	HLA B27 uveitis
Chronic	Sarcoidosis	Granulomatous	Tuberculosis, sarcoidosis
Anatomical		**Severity**	
Anterior	HLA B27 uveitis	Mild	Fuch's uveitis
Intermediate	Pars planitis	Moderate	Sarcoidosis
Posterior	Toxoplasmosis	Severe	Acute retinal necrosis
Panuveitis	VKH syndrome	**Etiological**	
Laterality		Infectious	Tuberculosis
Unilateral	Fuch's uveitis	Immunological	Sarcoidosis
Unilateral alternating	HLA B27 uveitis	Masquerade	Lymphoma
Bilateral	VKH syndrome	Idiopathic	

(VKH: Vogt-Koyanagi-Harada syndrome; JRA: Juvenile rheumatoid arthritis)

identical clinical features.[1-4] Uveitis can happen in nearly 100 specific diseases. While infectious and noninfectious uveitis encompass a majority of uveitis cases, masquerade syndromes should be kept in mind as well. This latter group consists of malignancy, degenerative disorders, metabolic diseases and others (Table 83.11). Comprehensive history, ocular and systemic examination, laboratory work up and meticulous follow up will greatly enhance the chance of deriving an accurate etiological diagnosis.

Table 83.11: Disorders masquerading as uveitis.

Nonmalignant cells in vitreous	Malignant cells
RBCs in vitreous hemorrhage	Lymphomas
Pigments in vitreous—retinitis pigmentosa	Leukemia
Intraocular foreign body	Retinoblastoma
Retinal detachment	Medulloepithelioma
Drug adverse reactions—moxifloxacin	Secondaries
Myopic degeneration	Juvenile xanthogranuloma
Multiple sclerosis	Metastatic carcinoma
Post-vaccination reaction	Diffuse uveal melanocytic proliferation
Metabolic diseases—amyloidosis	

(RBCs: Red blood cells)

Naming and Meshing

Finally a specific name is assigned to the clinical entity by using a set of descriptive terminologies in uveitis (Table 83.10 and Box 83.1). This descriptive name can then be compared to the known uveitis patterns. The above two steps are known as "naming and meshing step".

DIFFERENTIAL DIAGNOSIS

Uveitis specialists need to have a thorough knowledge of all entities (Tables 83.12 and 83.13). With that background knowledge, probable list of etiologies or causes are listed as differential diagnosis (DD). After arriving at a DD, tailored investigations are performed to arrive at a specific diagnosis. Table 83.14 is an algorithm showing systematic workup in uveitis.

Laboratory Diagnosis

The laboratory diagnosis of uveitis, comes after the clinical diagnosis and offers a supportive evidence. A tailored laboratory work up is always preferred than a nonselective elaborate approach. A general laboratory investigation like

Table 83.12: Differential diagnosis of various anterior segment clinical signs.

Hypopyon	Iris atrophy
HLA B27 uveitis	Viral uveitis—herpes zoster
Behçet's disease	Viral uveitis—herpes simplex
Leptospirosis	Traumatic
Phacolysis	Post-laser atrophy
Endophthalmitis	Postoperative uveitis
Postoperative uveitis	Hansen's uveitis
Leukemia	Fuch's heterochromic uveitis
Retinoblastoma	Anterior segment ischemia
Neuroblastoma	Essential Iris atrophy
Drug induced	ICE syndrome
Hyphema	**Irregular anterior chamber depth**
Fuch's heterochromic uveitis	Iris cyst
Viral uveitis	Subluxated lens
Syphilis	Leaking Morgagnian cataract
Gonococcal uveitis	Ciliary body tumor
Leukemia	Peripheral anterior synechiae
Glaucoma in the absence of synechiae	**Low tension in uveitis**
Sarcoidosis	Bilateral exudative retinal detachment
Toxoplasmosis	Ciliary body detachment
Viral uveitis	Retinal detachment induced uveitis
Fuch's heterochromic uveitis	Ciliary shock in acute uveitis
Lens protein uveitis	Traumatic and perforated globe

Table 83.13: Differential diagnosis of various posterior segment clinical signs.

Vitreous cells and opacities	Retinal vasculitis and Infectious causes
Inflammatory cells	Acute retinal necrosis
Red blood cells	CMV retinitis
Degenerated old cells	Measles (SSPE)
Pigments	Chikungunya
Amyloidosis	West Nile virus
Asteroid hyalosis	Tuberculosis
Malignant cells: Leukemia lymphoma	Syphilis
Lens cortical material	Leptospirosis
Parasitic cyst	Lyme's disease
Macular edema	Toxoplasmosis
Pars planitis	Candidiasis
HLA B27 related uveitis	Rickettsia
Postoperative uveitis	**Retinal vasculitis and Noninfectious causes**
Vogt-Koyanagi-Harada syndrome	Behçet's syndrome
Sympathetic ophthalmia	Systemic lupus erythematosus
Traumatic uveitis	Polyarteritis nodosa
Rarely Behçet's syndrome	Wegener's granulomatosis
Posterior scleritis	Giant cell arteritis
Optic disk edema in uveitis	Takayasu's arteritis
Vogt-Koyanagi-Harada syndrome	Relapsing polychondritis
Sympathetic ophthalmia	Leukemia
Leptospirosis	**Exudative retinal detachment**
Pars planitis	Vogt-Koyanagi-Harada syndrome
Juxtapapillary choroiditis	Sympathetic ophthalmia
Multiple sclerosis	Posterior scleritis
Neuroretinitis	Post-steroid treatment in CSR

(SSPE: Subacute sclerosing pan-encephalitis; CSR: Central serous retinopathy; CMV: Cytomegalovirus)

complete blood count is performed to know the general status of the patient at the onset of treatment and during the follow up. Specific investigations are done for confirmation of the diagnosis or for assessment after treatment (Table 83.14). Serological investigations are useful in syphilis, toxoplasmosis, leptospirosis and for autoimmune disorders.[16] Microbiological evaluation is needed to confirm the infectious etiology in case of tuberculosis, nocardiosis, endogenous endophthalmitis and others. Histopathological studies are highly useful in tuberculosis, sarcoidosis, parasitic ocular diseases and foreign body granulomas.[17,18] Image analysis or radiographic studies are useful in tuberculosis, sarcoidosis, metastatic infiltration and intraocular foreign bodies. MRI may be informative in multiple sclerosis associated uveitis.

Ancillary ophthalmologic investigations like fundus fluorescein angiography (FFA) is highly useful in papillitis, retinal vasculitis, retinal nonperfusion, retinal neovascularization, macular ischemia, cystoid macular edema, pigment epithelium leak, subretinal pooling and retinal detachment.[19] Indocyanine green angiography (ICGA) is the preferred investigation for identifying choroidal inflammatory involvement. Ultrasonography is a valuable tool in studying the anatomical integrity of the ocular structures especially when the media is opaque and ultrasound biomicroscope (UBM) assists in studying the ciliary body atrophy/detachment/mass lesion or foreign bodies. Optical coherence tomography (OCT) is a non invasive high resolution high speed imaging modality and helps to provide cross-sectional views (tomography) of

Table 83.14: General and specific investigations in uveitis.

General investigations	Indication (Examples)
• Complete blood count	Base line evaluation
• Blood sugar	Patients on steroids
• Renal function tests	Patients on cyclosporin
• Liver function tests	Patients on methotrexate, antitubercular drugs
• Urine sugar	Patients on steroids
• RBCs in urine	Patients on cyclophosphamide
• ESR, CRP	Autoimmune disorders, Bacterial sepsis
• Purified protein derivative (PPD)	Screening for tuberculosis
Specific investigations	
• Serology	VDRL, FTA-ABS-Syphilis ELISA—HIV Western blot—HIV ELISA—toxoplasmosis ELISA for leptospirosis Microagglutination test for leptospirosis Rheumatoid factor—rheumatoid arthritis ANA, ANCA—SLE and Wegener's granulomatosis
• Microbiological	Smear and Culture—endogenous endophthalmitis Traumatic scleral abscess
• Histopathological	Sympathetic ophthalmia, tubercular lymph node biopsy
• Biochemical test	Angiotensin converting enzyme (ACE)—sarcoidosis
• Molecular diagnostics	RT PCR—tuberculosis HIV, herpetic group of viruses
Ocular imaging	FFA—VKH syndrome, sympathetic ophthalmia, retinal vasculitis, Behçet's disease, white dot syndromes and parsplanitis USG—VKH syndrome, sympathetic ophthalmia UBM— Ciliary body detachment, atrophy, OCT—CME
Radiological investigations	X-ray chest—tuberculosis, sarcoidosis X-ray orbit—intraocular foreign bodies
	CT chest—tuberculosis, sarcoidosis, masquerade syndrome, CT brain in cysticercosis
	MRI-—multiple sclerosis, masquerade syndrome In primary central nervous system lymphoma MRI studies show hypodense lesions on T1-weighted and hyperdense on T2-weighted images

(ELISA: Enzyme-linked immunosorbent assay; HIV: Human immunodeficiency virus; FFA: Fundus fluorescein angiography; FTA-ABS: Fluorescent treponemal antibody absorption; RT PCR: Real-time polymerase chain reaction; USG: Ultrasonography; UBM: Ultrasound biomicroscopy; OCT: Optical coherence tomography; CME: Cystoid macular edema; VDRL: Venereal disease research laboratory test; VKH: Vogt-Koyanagi-Harada syndrome)

internal tissue structures such as vitreoretinal interface, cystoid macular edema and retinal thickness in a wide variety of etiologies.[20]

Diagnostic vitrectomy plays a major role in the confirmatory diagnosis of infectious uveitis specifically in endophthalmitis, parasitic disease, masquerade syndromes such as intraocular lymphoma and metastatic diseases.[21-23] Direct detection of the pathogen relies on either positive culture of the aqueous or vitreous fluid or on staining procedures. However, except for bacterial endophthalmitis, most intraocular pathogens are difficult to culture from the ocular fluid. Other diagnostic modalities that are highly useful include polymerase chain reaction (PCR), reverse transcriptase PCR, real-time PCR and quantitative PCR. Diagnosis of masquerade syndrome requires special processing such as use of cytospin, a rapid histopathology staining, hematopathology work up and special tissue culture media.

TREATMENT

Uveitis is comprised of infectious and noninfectious causes and the treatment is based on etiological diagnosis whenever possible. Specific goal is the treatment of infectious cause if any; otherwise, it is adequate control of inflammation (Boxes 83.2 and 83.3). Some of the inflammatory disorders also have systemic manifestations. Necrotizing scleritis may indicate the onset of a potentially life- threatening systemic vasculitis. Accurate treatment of such severe systemic inflammation preserves vision as well as prevents systemic morbidity and mortality.[24]

Corticosteroids are the mainstay of therapy for ocular inflammatory disease of noninfectious nature. They are used as eye drops, periocular injections, oral preparations and intravenous injections (Table 83.15).[25,26] Immunosuppressives and Newer Biologic agents, used in refractory cases are becoming important and are dealt in separate chapters.

Uveitis work-up may appear challenging, however, it is highly rewarding to bring back vision in conditions which otherwise have high morbidity. An appropriate knowledge of the relevant systemic disease, a comprehensive systemic and local examination, a targeted approach towards investigation and treatment and more importantly the compliance of the patient are determinants of the ultimate success.

Table 83.15: Use of steroids in uveitis.

Steroids	Suggested guidelines
Topical steroids • Initial dose • Maintenance dose • Monitoring	 • Hourly—in severe uveitis • 6–8 hourly—in mild forms • Depending upon the severity tapered over a month • To look for increased IOP and cataract
Periocular steroid injection • Initial dose • Frequency	 • 0.5–1 mL (20–40 mg) posterior subtenon injection of triamcinolone acetonide • Once in a month • Monitor for glaucoma and cataract
Oral steroids	• Prednisolone 1–1.5 mg/kg body weight • Tapered slowly—depending on the etiology, severity and course of uveitis
Intravenous steroids • Drug • Dose • Monitor	 • Intravenous methyl prednisolone • 500–1,000 mg once a day for 3 days • To look for anaphylactic reaction while starting the intravenous treatment • Regular monitoring for blood pressure and blood sugar

Box 83.2: Goals of treatment.

- Treatment of infectious cause if any
  - Example: Antitubercular treatment for tubercular uveitis
- Otherwise proper control of inflammation
  - Example: Timely control of macular edema
- Right selection of drug and appropriate duration of treatment
  - Example: Corticosteroids/immunosuppressives/newer biologicals
- Prevention/treatment of complications
  - Example: Cataract and glaucoma
- Measurement and management of sequelae
  - Example: Photocoagulation for retinal vascular occlusion and neovascularization

Box 83.3: Naming and meshing technique in uveitis—clinical examples.

The relevant points from the history are combined with findings of ocular and systemic examination to derive a name for the uveitis.

Example 1:

A 55 years old lady gives history of on and off eye pain, defective vision and redness in both eyes for 5 years with history of small joints pain. Examination reveals bilateral granulomatous panuveitis, retinal vasculitis and vitreous snow balls. Radiological examination shows evidence of hilar lymphadenopathy and her angiotensin converting enzyme (ACE) is elevated. Her purified protein derivative (PPD) is negative and she never had any history suggestive of systemic tuberculosis. She has previously improved with oral steroids, however, she presently suffers from uncontrolled diabetes mellitus and hypertension.

Naming of this patient in nutshell is "Chronic bilateral granulomatous panuveitis with small joints pain, high ACE and hilar lymphadenopathy in a middle aged female patient".

Meshing step compares this clinical picture with existing literature and derives a differential diagnosis (DD). The above example of bilateral granulomatous panuveitis can have DD of Sarcoidosis, Vogt-Koyanagi syndrome, sympathetic ophthalmia and tuberculosis for example. There is no history of trauma or surgery, no vitiligo or poliosis inspite of its chronicity. The work-up shows high ACE and hilar lymphadenopathy with a negative PPD. Final diagnosis of sarcoidosis is made and treatment is planned accordingly.

Example 2:

A 30 years old man presents with history of right eye severe pain, redness and defective vision for 2 days. Past history reveals two similar episodes in left eye few years back. He also has early morning low back pain and neck rigidity for past 6 years on and off. Examination reveals unilateral non-granulomatous anterior uveitis with fibrinous hypopyon and posterior synechiae. Radiological examination shows evidence of ankylosing spondylitis.

Naming of this second patient is, "acute unilateral recurrent alternating anterior uveitis in a young male patient with ankylosing spondylitis."

Meshing step clearly points out a possibility of a final diagnosis HLA-B27 related uveitis and treatment is planned accordingly.

REFERENCES

1. Smith RE, Nozik RA. Uveitis: a clinical approach to diagnosis and management, 2nd edition. Baltimore: Williams and Wilkins; 1989. pp. 27-41.
2. Whitcup SM. Examination of the patient with uveitis. In: Nussenblatt RB, Whitcup SM (Eds). Uveitis: fundamentals and clinical practice, 4th edition. St. Louis: Mosby; 2010. pp. 41-50.
3. Rao NA, Forster DJ, Aigsburger JJ. General approach to the uveitis patient. In: The Uvea: uveitis and intraocular neoplasms. New York: Gower Medical Publishing; 1992. pp. 2.1-2.18.
4. Harper SL, Chorich III LJ, Foster CS. Diagnosis of uveitis. In: Foster CS, Vitale AT (Eds). Diagnosis and Treatment of Uveitis. Philadelphia: WB Saunders Co; 2002. pp. 79-103.
5. Rathinam SR, Namperumalsamy P. Global variation and pattern changes in epidemiology of uveitis. Ind J Ophthalmol. 2007;55(3):173.
6. Zierhut M, Oréfice F, Clovis A, et al. Evaluation. In: Zierhut M, Pavesio C, Ohno S, Oréfice F, Rao NA (Eds). Intraocular Inflammation. Berlin Heidelberg: Springer-Verlag; 2016. pp. 93-113.
7. Rao NA, Sukavatcharin S, Tsai JH. Vogt–Koyanagi–Harada disease diagnostic criteria. Intophthalmol. 2007;27(2-3):195-9.
8. Bloch-Michel E, Nussenblatt RB. International Uveitis Study Group recommendations for the evaluation of intraocular inflammatory disease. Am J Ophthalmol. 1987;103(2):234-5.
9. Deschenes J, Murray PI, Rao NA, et al. International Uveitis Study Group. International Uveitis Study Group (IUSG): clinical classification of uveitis. OculImmunol Inflamm. 2008;16(1):12.
10. Jabs DA, Nussenblatt RB, Rosenbaum JT. Standardization of uveitis nomenclature for reporting clinical data: results of the first international workshop. Am J Ophthalmol. 2005;140:509-16.
11. Damico FM, Marin ML, Goldberg AC, et al. Revised diagnostic criteria for Vogt-Koyanagi-Harada disease: considerations on the different disease categories. Am J Ophthalmol. 2009;147(2):339-45.
12. Cunningham ET Jr, Lowder CY, Miserocchi E, et al. Sarcoid uveitis. Ocul Immunol Inflamm. 2014;22(4):253-6.
13. International Study Group for Behçet's Disease. Criteria for diagnosis of Behçet's disease. Lancet. 1990;335(8697): 1078-8.
14. Holland GN, Denove CS, Yu F. Chronic anterior uveitis in children: clinical characteristics and complications. Am J Ophthalmol. 2009;147(4):667-78.
15. Reeves SW, Sloan FA, Lee PP, et al. Uveitis in the elderly: epidemiological data from the National Long-term Care Survey Medicare Cohort. Ophthalmology. 2006;113(2): 307.e1.
16. De Groot-Mijnes JD, Rothova A, Van Loon AM, et al. Serology, Anterior Chamber and Vitreous Diagnostics. In: Zierhut M, Pavesio C, Ohno S, Oréfice F, Rao NA (Eds). Intraocular Inflammation. Berlin Heidelberg: Springer-Verlag; 2016. pp. 149-58.
17. Rathinam SR, Arya LK, Usha KR, et al. Novel etiological agent: molecular evidence for trematode-induced anterior uveitis in children. Arch Ophthalmol. 2012;130(11):1481-4.
18. Rathinam SR, Kamath Y. Ocular Parasitic Infections. In: Biswas J, Majumder PD (Eds). Uveitis: An Update. New Delhi: Springer India; 2016. pp. 119-32.
19. Herbort CP. Fundus ICG, angiography. In: Gupta A, Gupta V, Herbort CP, Khairallah M (Eds). Uveitis text and imaging. New Delhi: Jaypee Brothers Medical publishers; 2009. pp. 88-143.
20. Gupta V, Gupta P, Singh R, et al. Spectral-domain Cirrus high-definition optical coherence tomography is better than time-domain Stratus optical coherence tomography for evaluation of macular pathologic features in uveitis. Am J Ophthalmol. 2008;145(6):1018-22.
21. Davis JL, Mandelcorn ED. Ocular Biopsy, Diagnostic Vitrectomy. In: Zierhut M, Pavesio C, Ohno S, Oréfice F, Rao NA (Eds). Intraocular Inflammation. Berlin Heidelberg: Springer-Verlag; 2016. pp. 217-25.
22. Coupland SE. The pathologist's perspective on vitreous opacities. Eye (Lond). 2008;22(10):1318-29.
23. Cole CJ, Kwan AS, Laidlaw DH, et al. A new technique of combined retinal and choroidal biopsy. Br J Ophthalmol. 2008;92(10):1357-60.
24. Bianka Sobolewska B, Doycheva D, Deuter C, et al. Biologicals in Uveitis. In: Biswas J, Majumder PD (Eds). Uveitis: An Update. New Delhi: Springer India; 2016. pp. 119-32.
25. Agarwal M, Zierhut M. Corticosteroids. In: Zierhut M, Pavesio C, Ohno S, Oréfice F, Rao NA (Eds). Intraocular Inflammation. Berlin Heidelberg: Springer-Verlag; 2016. pp. 273-84.
26. Nozik RA. Periocular injection of steroids. Trans Am Acad Ophth Otol. 1972;76(3):695-704.

Chapter 84 Infectious Uveitis

Mayjane Joan Tumulak, Chee Soon Phaik

OVERVIEW

Uveitis can be infectious or noninfectious in origin. While immune-mediated uveitis remains the major etiology of uveitis in developed countries around the world, there is evidence of a large number of infectious organisms that have been shown to cause infectious uveitis. Demographics, genetics and environmental factors significantly affect the distribution of the different etiologies.

This chapter describes the manifestations of the major bacterial, viral, parasitic and fungal infections causing uveitis and outlines the treatment.

INTRODUCTION

Infectious uveitis accounts for majority of cases in developing countries. Epidemiology varies considerably by geographic location and can be attributed to the difference in regional distribution of various microorganisms. It could be caused by bacteria, virus, parasite or fungi.

VIRAL UVEITIS

Several different herpes virus have been described but so far eight are found in humans. Herpes simplex virus-1 (HSV-1), herpes simplex virus-2 (HSV-2), varicella-zoster virus (VZV), cytomegalovirus (CMV), Epstein-Barr virus (EBV) and human herpes virus 6, 7, 8. Three members of the *Herpesviridae* family—herpes simplex virus (HSV), VZV and most recently, CMV—have been cornered as causes of acute, recurrent and chronic anterior uveitis. Along with VZV, HSV (HSV-1 and HSV-2) can cause acute retinal necrosis (ARN) in otherwise healthy individuals of both sexes and of any age but may occur in immunocompromised patients in the form a progressive outer retinal necrosis (PORN).

Herpes Simplex Virus

Diagnosis of herpetic anterior uveitis is straight forward when the patient has typical features such as crops of vesicles on the eyelid or keratitis but can be more challenging in patients without evidence of previous corneal or dermal involvement (Fig. 84.1).

Ocular Manifestations

- Corneal scar
- Reduced corneal sensation
- Mostly granulomatous but may manifest as fine stellate keratic precipitates (KPs), diffusely distributed on the corneal endothelium beyond Arlt's triangle
- Iris transillumination defects involving the posterior iris pigment epithelium mostly sector but may be spiral in pattern
- Raised intraocular pressure (IOP).

Treatment

Oral acyclovir 400 mg five times daily with intensive topical corticosteroid (in the absence of active epithelial lesion) and a cycloplegic/mydriatic agent should be started on diagnosis. Systemic antivirals—acyclovir, famciclovir or valacyclovir should be prescribed because they protect the cornea as well as treat the uveitis.

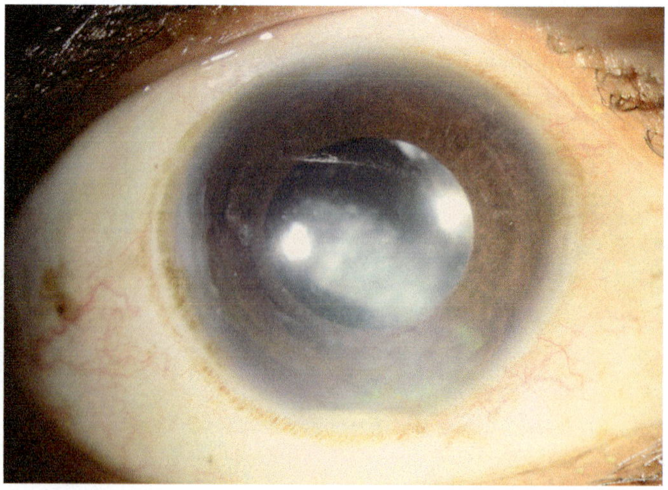

Fig. 84.1: Herpetic keratouveitis with hypopyon and iris atrophy.

Varicella-Zoster Virus

History and other systemic manifestations such as history of chickenpox and dermatome distribution of skin lesions may help in the diagnosis of VZV. Cutaneous vesicles at the tip of the nose (Hutchinson sign) indicate nasociliary nerve involvement and a greater likelihood of ocular involvement (Figs. 84.2 and 84.3).

Ocular Manifestations

- Pseudodendrites
- Reduced corneal sensation
- Sectoral iris atrophy
- Granulomatous anterior uveitis
- Raised IOP.

Treatment

Oral acyclovir 800 mg five times daily along with topical corticosteroids and a cycloplegic/mydriatic agent should be given for 2–3 weeks or until the inflammation subsides. In chronic or recurrent disease, acyclovir 400 mg thrice a day (dose should be reduced in renal impairment) can be given on the long-term to maintain remission. Other than acyclovir, other antivirals such as valacyclovir which has better bioavailability can also be used.

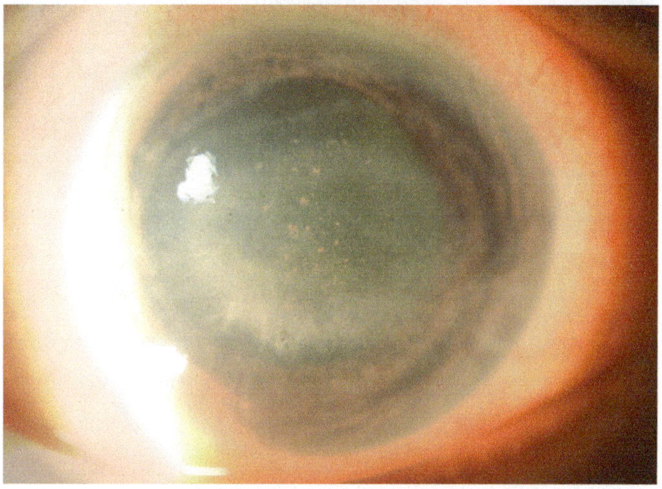

Fig. 84.2: Varicella-zoster virus (VZV) endotheliitis.

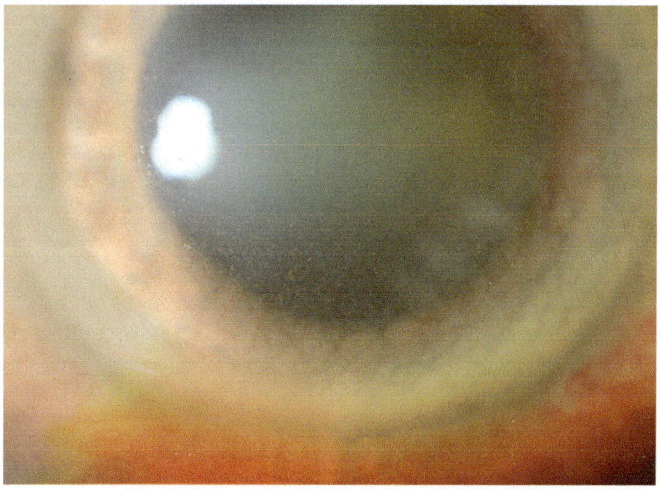

Fig. 84.3: Varicella-zoster virus keratouveitis.

Cytomegalovirus

Cytomegalovirus is a double-stranded DNA virus in the *Herpesviridae* family. Anterior uveitis is the hallmark of CMV infection in immunocompetent individuals. This may present either as an acute recurrent uveitis or a chronic form.

Ocular Manifestations

Usually presents as a unilateral acute recurrent hypertensive uveitis, with only few fine to large KPs located in Arlt's triangle. Sometimes the KPs may be linear or arranged in a circular manner (coin-shaped lesions). The IOP elevation exceeds 45 mm Hg in 65% of eyes. White or pigmented nodular endothelial lesions may be seen. Cystoid macular edema is not a feature.

The KPs in the chronic form of CMV uveitis are fine or stellate and tend to be evenly distributed over the corneal endothelial surface resembling Fuchs heterochromic uveitis and may be associated with diffuse or patchy iris atrophy and ocular hypertension (Figs. 84.4 and 84.5). Posterior synechiae is not a feature.[1]

Both CMV phenotypes are associated with the development of glaucomatous optic neuropathy and cataract.

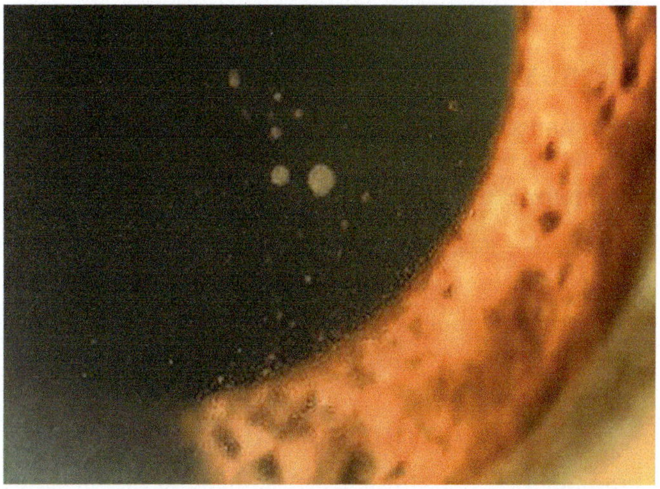

Fig. 84.4: CMV anterior uveitis showing a few fine to large keratic precipitates with diffuse atrophy.

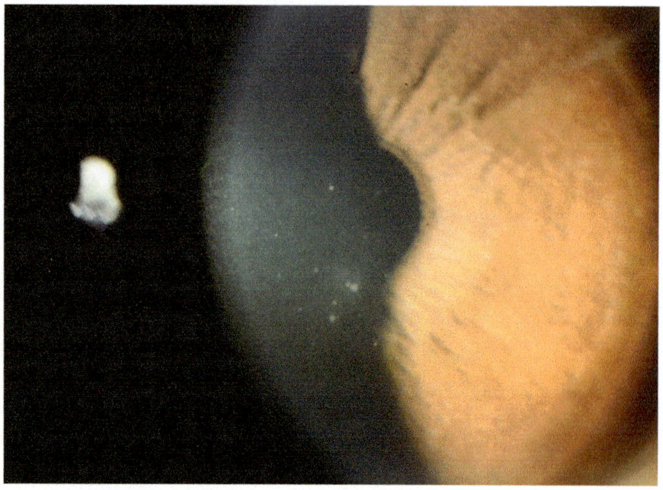

Fig. 84.5: CMV fine to medium-sized keratic precipitates.

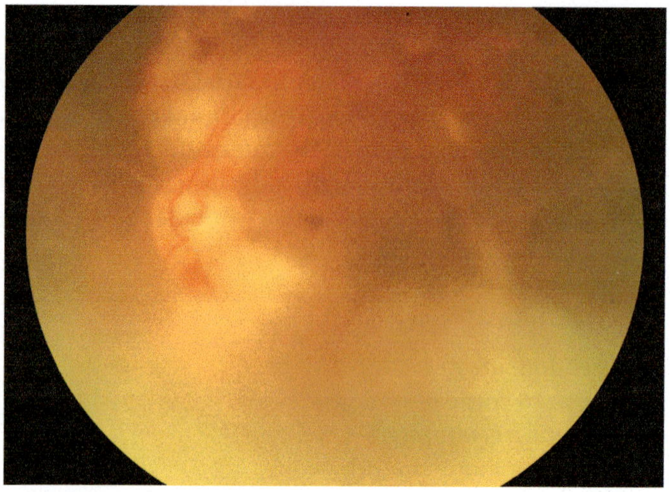

Fig. 84.6: CMV retinitis edematous type with papillary involvement in a 38-year-old male with HIV.

Table 84.1: Comparison of clinical features of herpes viral uveitis.

Clinical features	HSV	VZV	CMV
Onset	Acute	Acute	Acute recurrent
Keratic precipitates (KP)	Granulomatous or nongranulomatous	Granulomatous or nongranulomatous	KP granulomatous and few in acute recurrent uveitis, fine and diffuse in chronic uveitis. Nodular endothelial lesions may be present
Fibrin formation	–	–	–
Iris changes	Focal atrophy	Sectoral or focal atrophy	Diffuse or patchy stromal atrophy
Posterior synechiae	+	+	Nil
Pupil	May be eccentric	May be eccentric	Round
Mean maximum IOP (mm Hg)	30	35	50 (28–80)
Corneal changes	Dendritic keratitis; endotheliitis	Dendritic keratitis; endotheliitis	Coin-shaped endothelial lesions in chronic cases
Vitritis	+	±	Mild

(HSV: Herpes simplex virus; VZV: Varicella-zoster virus; CMV: Cytomegalovirus; IOP: Intraocular pressure)

The endothelial cell count is reduced in many of the infected eyes. Indeed, this may be a surrogate marker for CMV.

Diagnosis

Confirmation with aqueous polymerase chain reaction (PCR) is necessary. CMV real-time PCR analysis is useful for monitoring the response to therapy.

Treatment

Oral or topical ganciclovir are effective but disease may relapse if treatment is discontinued (Table 84.1).

Cytomegalovirus Retinitis

Cytomegalovirus retinitis (CMVR) usually results from a reactivation of a latent CMV infection secondary to immunodeficiency and accounts for 90% of the infectious retinopathies in acquired immunodeficiency syndrome (AIDS) patients. It usually occurs in the late stages of the disease in patients with a CD4 count of less than 50/mm^3.

Three clinical forms:

1. Typical form, edematous—small white lesions in the periphery and a central zone of atrophic retina with vessels of white cords appearance (Fig. 84.6).
2. Atypical form, indolent—granulomatous lesion with small dots infiltrates without hemorrhages. It may appear as a scar lesion but continues to progress slowly (Fig. 84.7).
3. Perivascular form—"Frosted branch angiitis"—diffuse vascular retinal sheathing, retinal hemorrhages, retinal necrosis, active retinitis progressing from the borders of the lesion sometimes with hemorrhagic papillitis.[2] The vitreous is typically devoid of haze.

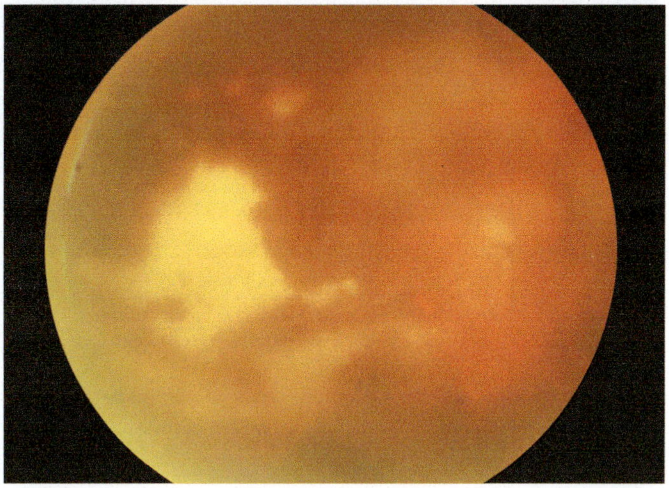

Fig. 84.7: CMV retinitis granular type. Fundus photograph of a 34-year-old male with HIV, presenting as zonal retinitis that looks like a scar.

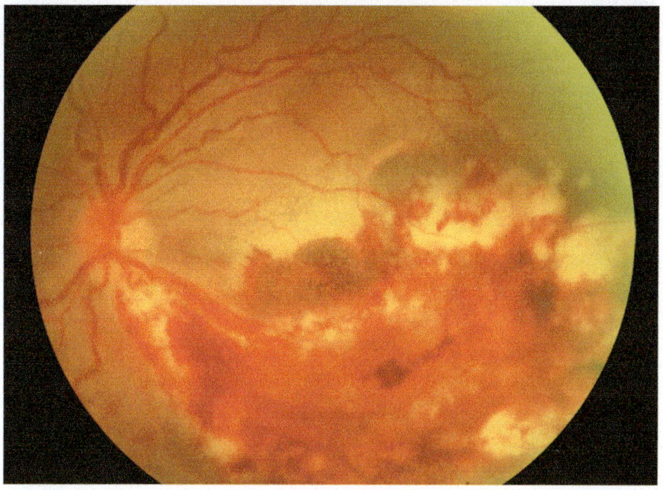

Fig. 84.8: Cytomegalovirus (CMV) retinitis. Patch of hemorrhage over the inferior arcade bordering the infected tissue resembling a brush fire appearance.

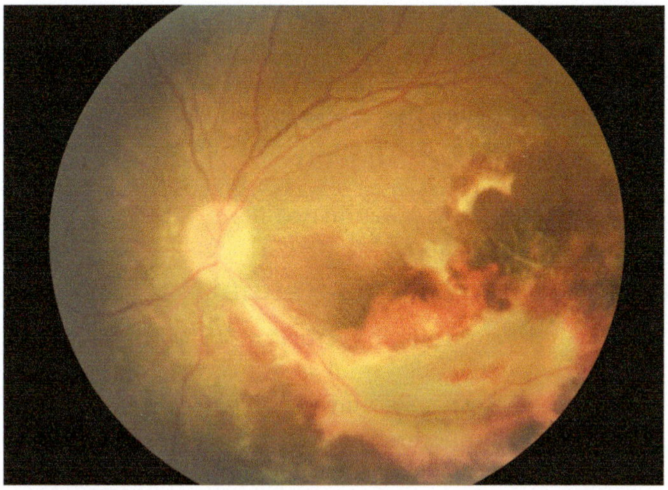

Fig. 84.9: Cytomegalovirus (CMV) retinitis hemorrhagic. Fundus photograph after receiving IVT ganciclovir and intravenous ganciclovir.

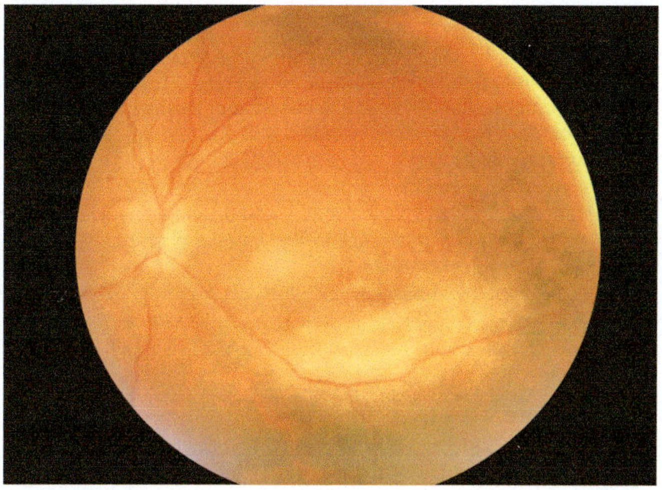

Fig. 84.10: Cytomegalovirus (CMV) retinitis after IVT Cidofovir. Retinal atrophy consistent with healing in areas with previously active infection.

Diagnosis is of CMVR is usually clinical. In atypical patients, PCR from vitreous or aqueous tap provides high sensitivity and specificity.

Treatment

The principal antiviral drugs are ganciclovir, foscarnet and cidofovir. All three are virostatic DNA polymerase inhibitors. Control of CMVR may occur with intravitreal injections of either ganciclovir or foscarnet. Injections are not directly retinotoxic even though intravitreal levels of these agents are within the toxic range for the drug.[2] In one study, treatment with oral valganciclovir 900 mg twice a day for 21 days followed by a maintenance dose of 900 mg/daily was similarly effective to initial intravenous ganciclovir. However, regular monitoring of complete blood count should be done because this drug causes myelosuppression (Figs. 84.8 to 84.10).

Acute Retinal Necrosis

The etiology of acute retinal necrosis (ARN) is due to the herpes group of viruses that affect all layers of the retina. HSV-1 and 2, VZV and CMV are the most common causes of ARN. The American Uveitis Society has established a criteria for making the diagnosis of ARN on the basis of the following clinical characteristics (Box 84.1, Figs. 84.11 and 84.12).

Visual outcomes are generally poor despite appropriate treatment. Retinal detachment occurs in half to three-quarters of eyes and is the most common cause of decreased

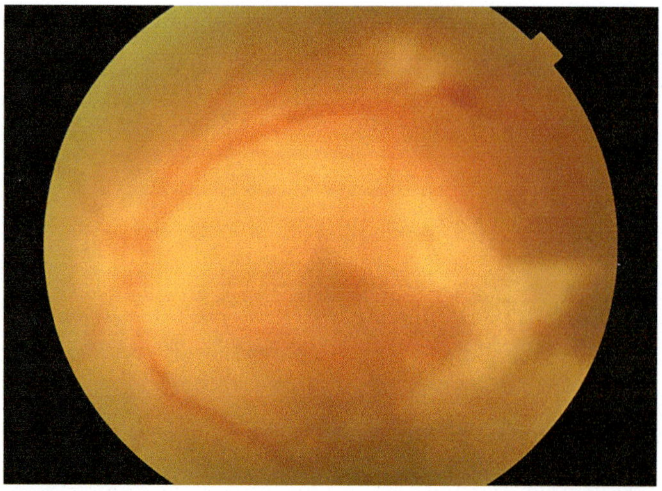

Fig. 84.11: Diffuse peripheral retinal necrosis in a concentric pattern with vitritis. Note absence of retinal hemorrhage which is characteristic.

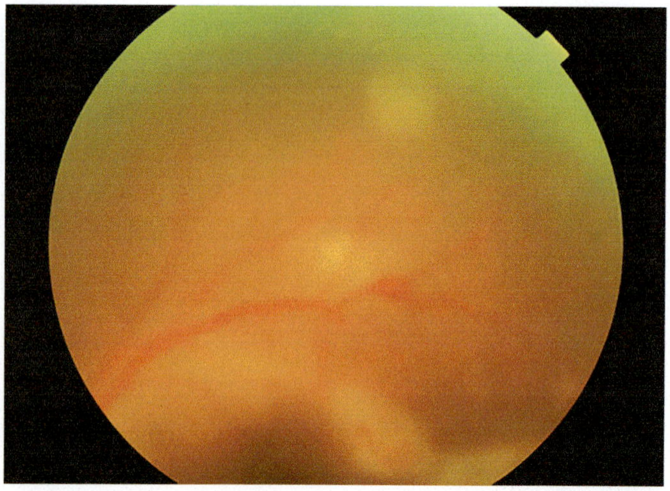

Fig. 84.12: Acute retinal necrosis showing multiple foci of retinitis with discrete folders in the peripheral retinal and obliterative vasculopathy.

Box 84.1: American Uveitis Society criteria for diagnosing acute retinal necrosis (ARN) syndrome.

Required clinical criteria

1. Rapid progression of disease in absence of therapy
2. One or more foci of retinal necrosis with discrete borders in peripheral retina
3. Circumferential spread
4. Evidence of occlusive vasculopathy and arteriolar involvement
5. Prominent vitreous inflammation and anterior chamber reaction
6. Supporting clinical criteria
7. Optic neuropathy/atrophy
8. Scleritis
9. Pain

vision. Bilateral ARN occurs in up to 70% of untreated patients.[3] Contralateral involvement usually occurs within a few months but may occur years later.

Diagnosis

Serum or intraocular fluid antibody testing using the Goldmann Witmer coefficient, retinal biopsy, immunocytochemistry and PCR is warranted.[4,5] PCR of aqueous and vitreous specimens are both sensitive and specific.[6] Diagnostic testing is important when the patient is immunocompromised. Differential diagnosis includes toxoplasmosis and syphilis.

Treatment

Intravitreal therapy of foscarnet immediately following diagnostic sampling of vitreous fluid can be given. Intravenous acyclovir 10 mg/kg every 8 hours or 1500 mg/m^2 per day divided into 3 doses for 7–10 days followed by an oral valaciclovir is the most established treatment regimen.[6] In cases of severe inflammation, administration of oral corticosteroids can be considered. However, caution should be taken because this may promote untreated viral replication.

Adjuvant local therapy such as early pars plana vitrectomy before retinal detachment and laser retinopexy around areas of necrosis may be initiated soon after the initiation of systemic antiviral treatment.[7]

Progressive Outer Retinal Necrosis

Progressive outer retinal necrosis also known as rapidly progressive herpetic retinal necrosis (RPHRN) causes devastating vision loss and is difficult to treat. PORN occurs in immunocompromised patients such as those co-infected with HIV-1. VZV is usually the causative agent. PORN resembles ARN but is distinguished from it clinically by the following four features (Fig. 84.13):

1. Full thickness involvement of the outer retina taking on a "cracked-mud" appearance.
2. Absence of any significant inflammation in the vitreous or aqueous humor.
3. Absence of involvement of the retinal vasculature.
4. Rapid progression.

Optic neuropathy may precede PORN in rare cases.[8] Severe visual loss from the diffuse retinal necrosis, optic atrophy and retinal detachment occurs in up to 70% of patients. In these patients, the onset of pain with vision loss may be a key finding.

Treatment

A combination of intravitreal foscarnet and ganciclovir as well as intravenous administration of both drugs is

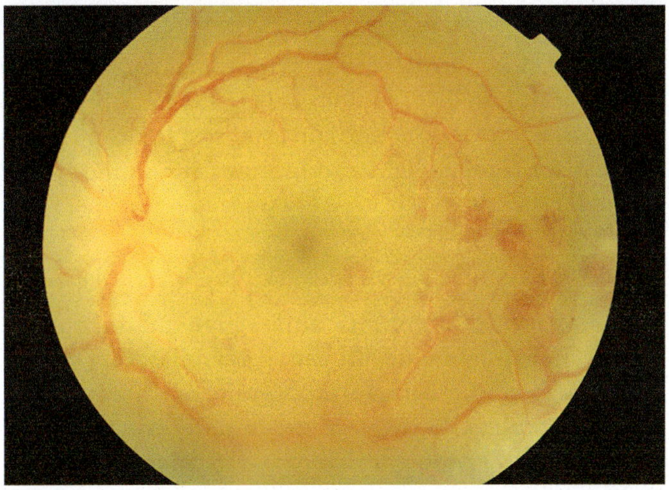

Figs. 84.13: Fundus photograph of left eye showing full thickness retinal edema with tortuous dilated veins with vasculitis, hemorrhage and small patches of retinitis in a patient with HIV.

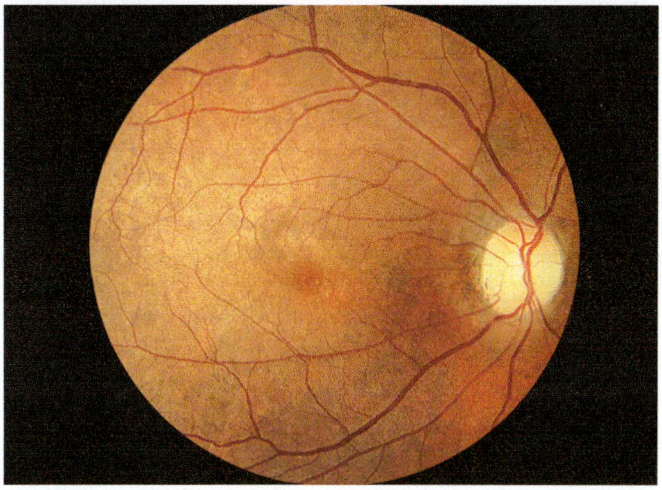

Fig. 84.14: Acquired rubella. Salt-and-pepper retinopathy without optic disk pallor and serous retinal detachment.

associated with better outcomes.[9] Indefinite maintenance therapy with valacyclovir is necessary in patients with persistent immunosuppression.

Epstein-Barr Virus

Is a double-stranded DNA virus of *gamma-herpesviridae* family commonly associated with infectious mononucleosis and has been implicated in Burkitt's lymphoma, nasopharyngeal carninoma, Hodgkin's and Sjogrens' syndrome.[10] Antibodies against EBV can be detected in approximately 90% of the population but only a few suffer from ocular disease.[11] EBV transmission can be via direct contact with saliva or by blood transfusion or rarely by airborne route.

Ocular Manifestations

It may present with uveitis, conjunctivitis, multifocal chorioretinitis characterized by punch-out areas of pigment epithelial changes and vitritis.[12]

Diagnosis

Serum IgG and IgM antibodies, EBV-related antigen and PCR viral DNA in ocular fluids have been successful.[13]

Treatment

In general, EBV-related chorioretinitis appears to be self-limiting. Uveitis sometimes requires corticosteroid therapy. Severe cases especially those rare instances where the posterior segment is affected may require similar antiviral agents as those used in acute retinal necrosis syndrome: intravenous aciclovir, ganciclovir, brivudine, valganciclovir and foscarnet.[20]

Rubella

Rubella is a single-stranded RNA from the *togaviridae* family. It is a prototypical teratogenic viral agent. The fetus is infected with the rubella virus transplacentally, secondary to maternal viremia during the course of primary infection. Incidence is highest during the first 10 weeks of gestation and during the final month of pregnancy.

However, rubella may also be acquired and although the systemic infection is mild self-limiting febrile exanthem, the virus may remain within the ocular tissues for an indefinite period of time. Local intraocular antibody production to rubella has been demonstrated in over 90% of eyes manifesting as Fuchs uveitis syndrome in Europe.

The classical features of Congenital Rubella Syndrome (CRS) include cardiac malformations, deafness and ocular findings (cataract, corneal clouding, microophthalmia, strabismus, chorioretinitis and glaucoma).

Ocular Manifestations

Congenital:

Most common ocular manifestation of CRS is a unilateral or bilateral pigment retinopathy often described as "salt-and-pepper" fundus showing finely stippled, bone spicule-like, small black irregular mass with coarse mottling (Fig. 84.14).[15,16]

Acquired:

Conjunctivitis is the most frequent ocular complication of acquired rubella infection followed by keratitis and retinitis. Fuch's heterochromic irdiocyclitis in association with rubella infection has also been reported.

Diagnosis

Pathognomonic retinal findings with associated systemic findings and a history of maternal exposure to rubella suggest a diagnosis of CRS. Four-fold increase of rubella-specific IgG in serum after 1–2 weeks or appearance of rubella-specific IgM. Specific IgM or IgA antibodies to rubella in the fetal blood cord confirms the diagnosis. Detection of rubella RNA and intraocular antibody production by using Goldmann-Witmer coefficient is helpful in diagnosis.

Treatment

No specific antiviral therapy and treatment is supportive. Treatment of Fuchs heterochromic uveitis includes control of glaucoma and removal of cataract. Topical corticosteroids are often not effective in treating inflammation.

Measles/Subacute Sclerosing Panencephalitis

A single-stranded RNA of the genus *Morbillivirus* in the *Paramyxoviridae* family that is highly contagious and is transmitted by air droplets to the mucous membranes of the conjunctiva or respiratory tract or from a pregnant woman to her fetus transplacentally.

Measles retinopathy is more common in acquired disease and may present with profound visual loss 6–12 days after the appearance of characteristic exanthem and may or may not be accompanied by encephalitis.

Ocular Manifestations

Most common ocular complications of measles are keratitis, mild papillary non-purulent conjunctivitis, chorioretinitis, pigmentary retinopathy (salt-and-pepper) that may or may not be accompanied by encephalitis, vasculitis and optic neuropathy.[14] It may occur concomitantly with measles encephalitis also known as subacute sclerosing panencephalitis (SSPE).[15-20]

Diagnosis

Systemic along with ocular symptoms and serology by enzyme linked immunoassay (ELISA) confirms the diagnosis. Lumbar puncture and cerebrospinal fluid (CSF) analysis for serology IgM and IgG measles antibody and globulin is helpful.

Treatment

Mainstay of treatment is supportive management. Prophylactic treatment with gamma globulin 0.25 mL/kg administered within 5 days of exposure for pregnant women, children younger than 1 year and immunocompromised patients. Topical antibiotics to prevent secondary infections and use of systemic corticosteroids should be considered for cases of acute measles retinopathy. Prognosis of measles (rubeola) in vaccinated population is good. There is no definitive treatment for SSPE.

West Nile Virus

The West Nile virus (WNV) is a single-stranded RNA *Flavivirus* from the *Flaviviridae* family that is transmitted by infected mosquitoes. WNV can be found in North America, Europe, Africa, Asia and Australia. WNV infections are asymptomatic or present with a mild, self-limited febrile illness with fever, headache, myalgia, vomiting and chills. Posterior uveitis is associated with WNV meningoencephalitis.[16-17]

Ocular Manifestations

Vitritis, bilateral or rarely unilateral multifocal chorioretinitis in the midzone to periphery, supported by angiographic features of early hypofluorescence and late staining, is the most common finding in acute west nile virus associated illness. Optic neuritis, ocular nerve palsy, and retinal vasculitis may be present.[18,19]

Diagnosis

High index of suspicion with positive WNV-specific IGM antibody in the serum, CSF or both is diagnostic.[30]

Treatment

Supportive management as chorioretinitis is self-limiting with good visual prognosis. Topical prednisolone may be given to reduce the inflammation. There is no proven treatment. Complications of WNV may be managed with panretinal photocoagulation for neovascularization, vitrectomy for vitreous hemorrhage or retinal detachment and intravitreal injection of antivascular endothelial growth factor agent for macular edema.[20]

Rift Valley Virus

Rift Valley virus is a zoonotic disease which belongs to the family *Bunyraviridae* and genus *Pheloboviridae*. This is a self-limiting disease in humans with influenza-like symptoms with a biphasic pattern of fever and life-threatening hemorrhagic fever.

Ocular Manifestations

Patients may develop unilateral or bilateral macular or paramacular necrotizing retinitis associated with vitritis and optic nerve swelling.[21] Non-granulomatous anterior uveitis may be present but this may resolve spontaneously within 2 weeks from onset of systemic symptoms and retinitis usually recovers within 10–12 weeks.[34] Permanent visual loss is common mainly due to macular or paramacular scarring, retinal vascular occlusion and optic atrophy.

Diagnosis

Primarily based on epidemiologic data, systemic symptoms and serologic testing by PCR.[22,23,34]

Treatment

There is no effective and proven antiviral therapy yet. Supportive management with intravenous fluid resuscitation is warranted.

Chikungunya

Chikungunya virus is a single-stranded RNA virus of genus *Alphavirus* in the family *Togaviridae*. It is transmitted to humans by the bite of infected mosquitoes, *Aedes aegypti* and *Aedes albopictus*. Chikungunya epidemics have been reported from several parts of the world especially South-east Asia and India.

Bite of the infected mosquito transmits the virus causing a self-limiting illness characterized by sudden onset of fever, chills, headache, malaise, arthritis or arthralgia, skin rash and low back pain.[37]

The exact mechanism of ocular involvement followed by Chikungunya infection is not yet studied in detail.

Ocular Manifestations

At the time of fever, numerous ocular features may occur including conjunctivitis, episcleritis, anterior uveitis, retinitis, choroiditis, neuroretinitis, panuveitis, exudative retinal detachment, optic neuritis or cranial nerve palsies.[29-31,41] Anterior uveitis can be granulomatous or non-granulomatous which can be associated with high intraocular pressure. Fuch's heterochromic iridocyclitis in association with chikungunya infection has also been reported (Figs. 84.15A and B).

Diagnosis

The gold standard in diagnosis of chikungunya is a viral culture inoculation of mosquito cell cultures or mammalian cell cultures.[37] Real-time polymerase reaction (qPCR) and virus isolation during acute viremic phase and estimation

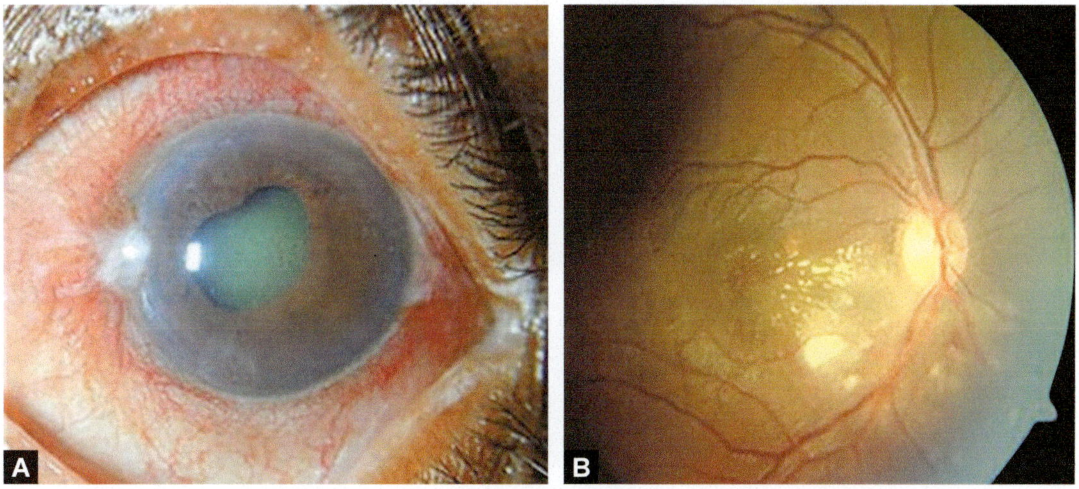

Fig. 84.15: Chikungunya, anterior segment and fundus of patient with chikungunya virus infection showing panuveitis and peripapillary retinal vasculitis resembling neuroretinitis.
Source: SR Rathinam.

of chikungunya IgM and IgG antibodies titers in the serum during the later phase aids in diagnosis.[38,39] PCR of the aqueous has been reported to be positive in cases of anterior uveitis.

Treatment

Mainstay of treatment is supportive management. Topical steroids in anterior uveitis and systemic steroids in posterior uveitis, panuveitis and optic neuritis are required to control inflammation.[24]

Dengue-related Ocular Disease

Single-stranded RNA virus from *Flaviviridae* transmitted by *Aedes* species. Dengue fever is endemic in Asia and South America. There is wide spectrum of systemic manifestations, of which, the most severe and fatal is dengue hemorrhagic fever. Ocular symptoms generally develop 7 days (1–28 days) after onset of dengue symptoms corresponding to nadir of thrombocytopenia. Patient may present with anterior uveitis, petechial subconjunctival hemorrhage, ciliary congestion, retinal hemorrhages, retinal vasculitis, maculopathy (foveolitis, edema) and optic neuropathy (Figs. 84.16A to C).

Diagnosis

Confirmation by means of PCR, viral RNA, ELISA particularly nonstructural protein 1 (NS1) antigen which is highest during the first week of onset of the disease. As the fever settles, serology IgM or a rise in serum IgG is preferred.

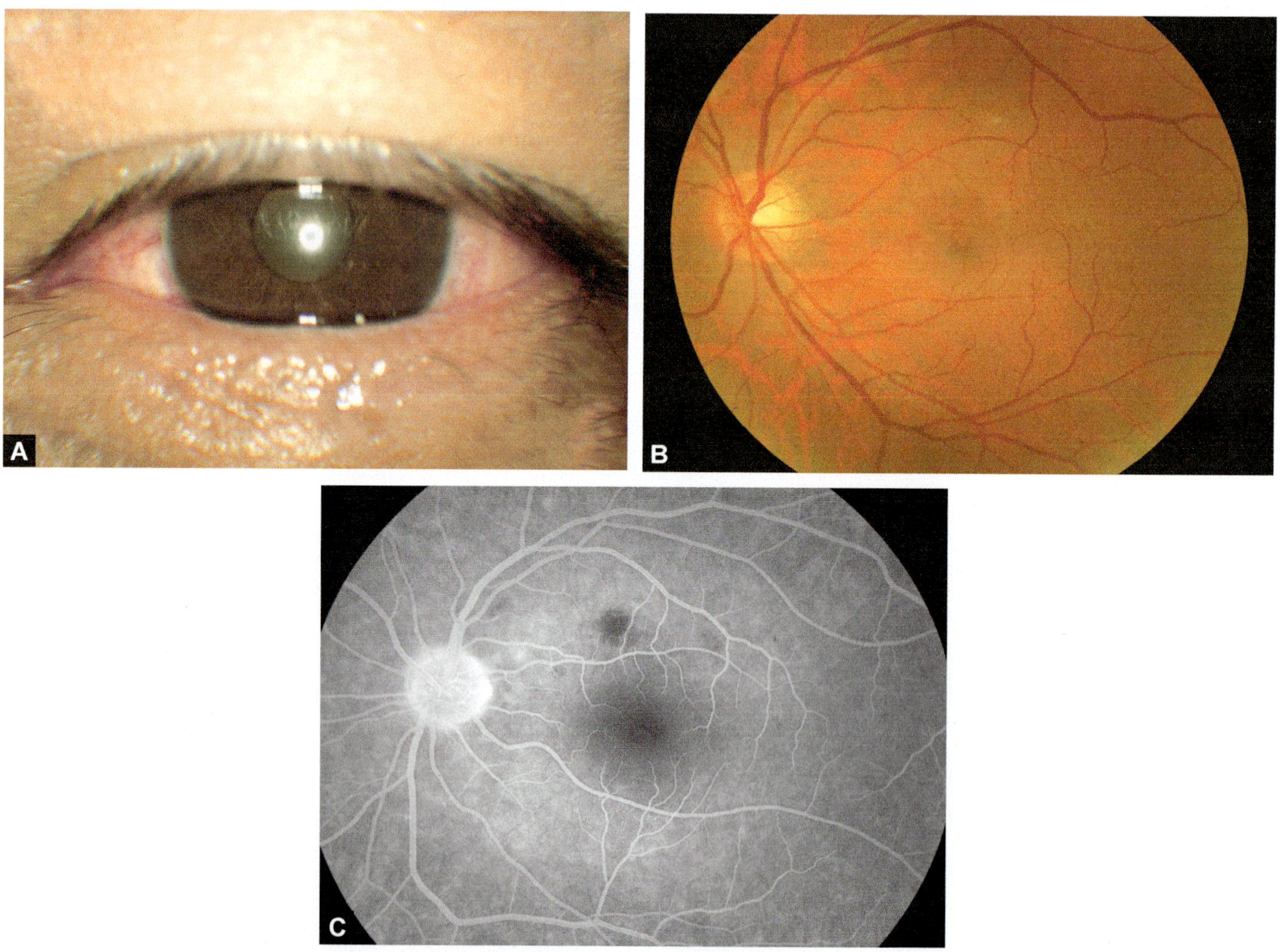

Figs. 84.16A to C: (A) Anterior segment photograph with subconjunctival hemorrhage; (B) Fundus photograph of left eye showing swelling of the macula with few cotton wool spot; (C) FFA showing leakage in the disk in mid-phase.

Treatment

Supportive measures such as intravenous fluid resuscitation and platelet transfusion in dengue hemorrhagic fever. Use of corticosteroids systemically is controversial.

Zika Virus

Zika virus (ZIKV) is from the family *Flaviviridae* and is transmitted by mosquitoes from *Culicidae* family and *Aedes aegypti* mosquito. In 2007, the first ZIKV outbreak outside of Africa and Asia was reported in Micronesia and caused a relatively mild disease. In 2015, the first local transmission of the ZIKV was reported in Brazil. In 2016, World Health Organization announced that the ZIKV outbreak constitutes a "Public Health Emergency of International Concern". Maternal infection during first trimester has been associated with microcephalic births.[42]

Ocular Manifestations

Macular pigment mottling, chorioretinal atrophy and optic disk hypoplasia may develop in presumed ZIKV congenital infection.[25] Recently, anterior uveitis has been reported as a manifestation of acute ZIKV infection in adults.[26]

Diagnosis

A diagnosis of Zika during pregnancy should be considered after the appearance of symptoms of fever, arthralgia, rash and conjunctivitis in people living in endemic areas. Evidence of the presence of ZIKV infection relies on molecular detection by reverse transcriptase PCR and also estimation of serum IgG and IgM specific to Zika antibodies.

Treatment

There is no proven treatment yet.

Ebola Virus

It is a single-stranded RNA from family of *Flaviviridae* of genus *Ebola* virus. In 2014, an outbreak in West Africa was reported.[27,28] Nonspecific systemic manifestations such as fever, severe headache, arthralgia, diarrhea and unexplained hemorrhage appear after an average of 10 days incubation period. Uveitis may develop as an immune response to the Ebola virus.[29]

Ocular Manifestations

Bilateral, asymptomatic and non-icteric conjunctivitis is a key sign with good prognostic value. Hemorrhagic conjunctivitis is predictive of death within a few days. An analysis of Ebola virus survivors in West Africa reports that patients who contract the virus are at higher risk of developing uveitis. They manifest in the form of anterior, posterior and panuveitis. Some developed Ebola virus disease (EVD)-associated optic neuropathy.

Diagnosis

Ebola virus is detected by ELISA, reverse transcriptase PCR assay or by viral culture from the serum, semen, conjunctival swab or aqueous samples.

Treatment

Corticosteroids may be used to suppress inflammation. There are currently no licensed vaccines for preventing Ebola virus infection.

Bacterial Syphilis

Syphilis is caused by a spirochete, *Treponema pallidum* that is sexually transmitted when organisms enter through a skin or mucous membrane abrasion; its transmission can also occur by kissing, blood transfusion or percutaneous injury or by transplacental route to the fetus from an infected mother.

Ocular Manifestations

Presentation of syphilis is protean and thus, the disease acquired the nickname, "the great masquerader". Ocular manifestations when present are typically associated with neurosyphilis which can occur early or late in the course of infection. CSF lumbar puncture should be done to confirm presence of spirochetes in the meninges.

Uveitis is the most common sign (anterior uveitis, chorioretinitis, vitritis and panuveitis), optic neuritis and neuroretinitis in 2–5% of patients with secondary or tertiary syphilis (Figs. 84.17A and B).[38,39,48] Anterior uveitis accounts for more than 70% of the eye findings.[30] A specific type of focal chorioretinitis, acute posterior placoid chorioretinitis, characterized by large, often solitary yellow lesions that occur typically in the macula is pathognomonic of syphilis.[31]

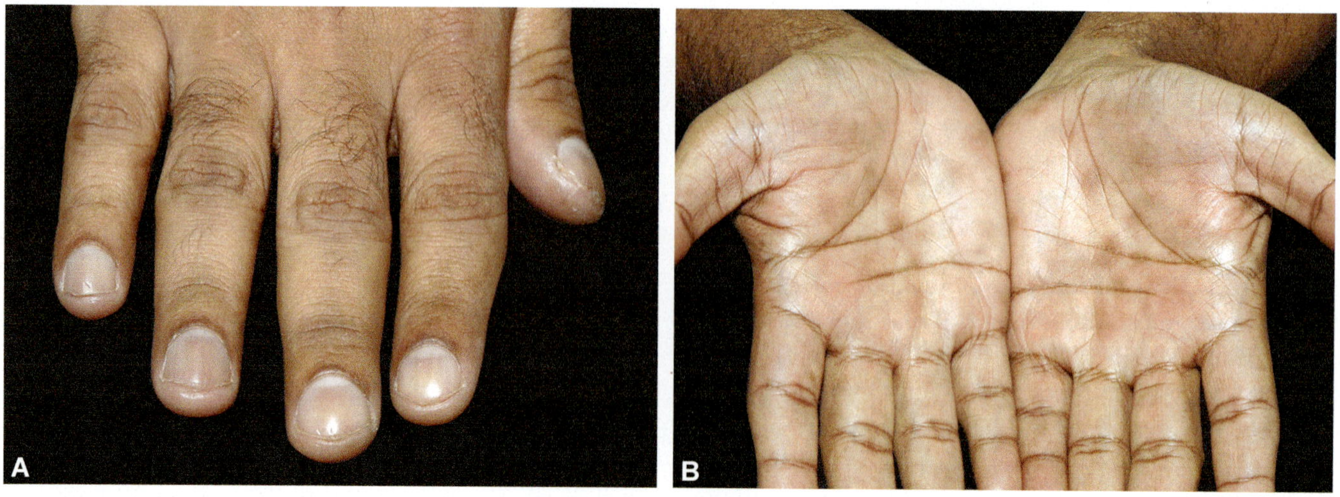

Figs. 84.17A and B: (A) Secondary syphilis showing nail pitting; (B) Non-painful maculopapular rash in palms and soles of secondary syphilis.

Diagnosis

All patients with presumed ocular syphilis should have a lumbar puncture to exclude concomitant neurosyphilis which may be present in 40% of patients.[32,33] All patients with ocular syphilis should be tested for human immunodeficiency virus (HIV).[34] A high index of suspicion is required and appropriate laboratory studies are necessary to confirm and rule out other disease entities (Table 84.2).

Table 84.2: Laboratory test for diagnosis of syphilis.

Dark field microscopy/Immunofluorescent staining (early phase)	
Nontreponemal tests	• Venereal Disease Research Laboratory • Rapid plasma reagin
Treponemal tests	• Fluorescent treponemal antibody absorption tests (FTA-ABS) • Hemagglutination treponemal test for syphilis • Hemagglutination assay for *Treponema pallidum* • Microhemagglutination tests

Treatment

This should be under the supervision of an infectious diseases specialist but generally consists of an extended course of parenteral penicillin for all forms and stages of syphilis. Center for disease Control has set guidelines for treatment of syphilis as shown on Table 84.3.

Topical and systemic steroids may be given in conjunction with antibiotics to ameliorate inflammatory damage. The Jarisch-Herxheimer reaction is a systemic response to treponemal antigens released on commencement of therapy and may include progression of ocular signs.[35]

Lyme Disease

Lyme disease (borreliosis) like syphilis is caused by a spirochete. The responsible organism *Borrelia burgdorferi* is transmitted through tick bites, deer are important vectors. The disease is endemic in regions of North America, Europe and Asia but can be difficult to diagnose. Lyme disease is classified into three stages (Table 84.4).

Ocular Manifestations

Like syphilis, Lyme has protean manifestations. Ocular features tend to occur in established *stage 2* and *stage 3* (late) disease.[36,53] Uveitis is relatively uncommon but can be granulomatous or non-granulomatous anterior uveitis, intermediate or posterior uveitis including multifocal choroiditis, vasculitis and neuroretinitis.[37,38,54]

Diagnosis

The PCR of CSF or synovial fluid is performed in appropriate cases. Diagnosis relies on a combination of clinical features with the pathognomonic rash of erythema migrans and positive serology if results are equivocal, it can be followed with a more confirmatory test such as the western blot.[39]

Treatment

Oral doxycycline 100 mg twice daily for 14 days is the antibiotic of choice in nonpregnant adults and children

Table 84.3: Guidelines for the treatment of syphilis based on current CDC recommendations.

Stage of syphilis	Penicillin treatment	Penicillin-allergic patients
Primary, secondary, and early latent syphilis, no neurologic involvement	Benzathine penicillin G 2.4 million units IM, single dose	Doxycycline 100 mg PO BID for 2 weeks Tetracycline 500 mg PO QID for 2 weeks
Late latent or latent syphilis of unknown duration, no neurologic involvement	Benzathine penicillin G 2.4 million units IM, once per week for 3 weeks	Doxycycline 100 mg PO BD for 28 days Tetracycline 500 mg PO QID for 28 days
Tertiary (late) syphilis without neurologic involvement	Benzathine penicillin G 2.4 million units IM, once per week for 3 weeks	Consult infectious disease specialist
Neurosyphilis Alternative regimen	Aqueous crystalline penicillin G 3–4 million units IV Q4H, or continuous IV infusion for total 18–24 million units per day, for 10–14 days Procaine penicillin 2.4 million units IM daily plus probenecid 500 mg PO QID, both for 10–14 days	

Table 84.4: Stages of Lyme disease.

Stage 1	Appearance of erythema migrans rash 3–30 days after tick bite
Stage 2	Multiorgan involvement
Stage 3	Chronic arthritis and neurologic syndromes

aged 8 years and older.[40] Keratitis and uveitis may need steroid treatment, however, systemic steroids should not be given without concomitant antibiotics.[41] Appropriate personal protection (clothing, insect repellent) should be adopted in endemic areas to reduce the risk of tick bite. Lyme disease vaccine is available but does not offer complete or prolonged protection.[42]

Brucellosis

Brucellosis is one of the most common zoonotic diseases worldwide. The disease is caused by Brucella species and is transmitted from animals to humans by direct contact with infected animals or consumption of raw animal products such as unpasteurized milk or cheese.[55-59] It is a multisystemic disease that may present with a broad spectrum of clinical manifestations and its complications can affect almost all organs and systems with varying incidence.[55,56]

Ocular Manifestations

Manifestations of brucellosis in the eye are myriad. It can present as uveitis, dacryoadenitis, episcleritis, nummular keratitis, optic neuritis, optic neuropathy, papillitis, papilledema, retinal detachment, retinal hemorrhage or extraocular muscle palsies.[43,44,58-60] Anterior uveitis and chorioretinitis are the most frequent ocular manifestations.[69] Panuveitis, in which nearly all patients had lost their vision is reported in one-fifth of all uveitis cases.[45]

Diagnosis

A diagnosis of brucellosis is based on the presence of clinical as well as a positive reaction to a serologic test such as standard agglutination test, ELISA, IgM and IgG for Brucella and a positive blood culture for Brucella species.

Treatment

Standard treatment with administration of rifampin and doxycycline and in case of eye involvement with local and systemic corticosteroids for 2–4 weeks leads to considerable improvement.[46,47]

Tuberculosis

Tuberculosis (TB) is a major public health issue worldwide and is one of the common causes of infectious uveitis in developing countries. Intraocular tuberculosis caused by the acid-fast bacilli *Mycobacterium tuberculosis* (MTB) is one of the rare forms of extrapulmonary TB.

Ocular Manifestations

It is either unilateral or asymmetrically bilateral characterized by a chronic and insidious course. It can affect any part of the eye with protean manifestations. Tubercular uveitis may present as anterior, intermediate, posterior and panuveitis. It often presents more as a granulomatous than nongranulomatous uveitis.[48]

Anterior uveitis is usually granulomatous with mutton fat-KPs which could be unilateral or bilateral. Iris nodules are less frequent. Chronic recurrent inflammation produces synechiae and is usually broad-based.[61]

Intermediate uveitis presents as vitritis, snowballs, phlebitis with cystoid macular edema as the cause of

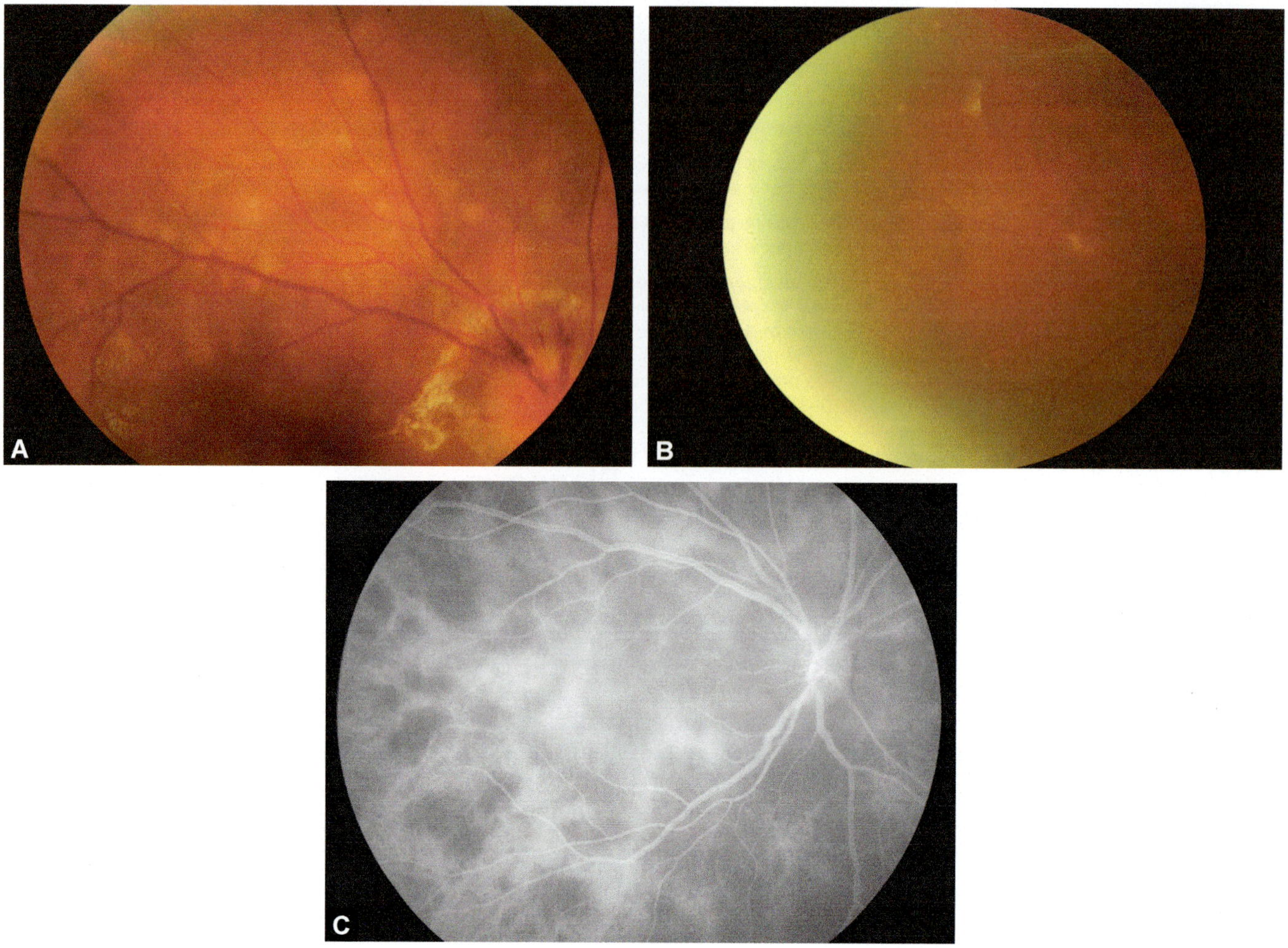

Figs. 84.18A to C: (A) Multiple yellowish choroiditis associated with optic disk hyperemia, swelling and hemorrhages; (B) Peripheral vasculitis in ocular tuberculosis; (C) ICG showing multiple hypofluorescent dark spots corresponding to the choroidal lesions seen in the fundus photograph.

visual loss. It is most commonly associated with latent TB infection.

Choroiditis is characterized by deep, multiple, discrete, yellowish lesions which is usually diagnostic of disseminated TB and indicates a hematogenous spread of tubercle bacilli. Multifocal serpiginoid choroiditis is highly specific for tubercular uveitis. It presents as vitritis with multifocal lesions which are not contiguous to optic disk and spread in a serpiginoid pattern. They respond very well to anti-TB treatment and oral corticosteroids. Retinal vasculitis affects males more than females and is previously called Eales' disease (Figs. 84.18A to C).

Tubercular endophthalmitis and panophthalmitis can mimic as ocular tumors. Diagnosis in these cases is confirmed by microbiologic or histopathologic evidence of MTB.

Optic nerve involvement results from direct infection or a hypersensitivity reaction and can present as neuroretinitis, optic neuritis, retrobulbar neuritis and papillitis.

Diagnosis

The screening process for active tuberculosis requires a combination of a detailed medical history, chest radiology and microbiologic analysis of sputum or abnormal radiology suggestive of pulmonary tuberculosis. Positive Mantoux Test or Quantiferon-TB Gold test is indicative of prior exposure to TB but not necessarily of active systemic infection.[78]

Diagnosis of intraocular tuberculosis (IOTB) is classified as Confirmed, Probable and Possible IOTB as suggested by Gupta et al. (Table 84.5).

Table 84.5: Classification of intraocular tuberculosis (IOTB).

Clinical diagnostic group	Case definition criteria
Confirmed IOTB (both 1 and 2)	1. At least one clinical sign suggestive of IOTB 2. Microbiological confirmation of *Mycobacterium tuberculosis* (MTB) from ocular fluids/tissues
Probable IOTB (1, 2, and 3 together)	1. At least one clinical sign suggestive of IOTB (and other etiologies excluded) 2. Evidence of chest X-ray consistent with TB infection or clinical evidence of extraocular TB or microbiological confirmation from sputum or extraocular sites 3. *At least one of the following*: a. Documented exposure to TB b. Immunological evidence TB infection
Possible IOTB (1, 2, and 3 together) (or 1 and 4)	1. At least one clinical sign suggestive of IOTB (and other etiologies excluded) 2. Chest X-ray not consistent with TB infection and no clinical evidence of extraocular TB 3. *At least one of the following*: a. Documented exposure to TB b. Immunological evidence TB infection 4. Evidence of chest X-ray consistent with TB infection or clinical evidence of extraocular TB but none of the characteristics given in 3

Diagnosis is considered as definitive TB only when the bacilli are isolated from the ocular tissues. The criterion for presumed tuberculous uveitis is reported to be presence of any one of the following clinical signs such as choroidal granuloma, broad-based posterior synechiae, retinal vasculitis with or without choroiditis or serpiginous-like choroiditis with a positive tuberculin skin test or Quantiferon-TB Gold test or any other relevant tests such as chest radiograph and computed tomography.[49,50] Good response to antitubercular treatment and absence of recurrence further, supports the diagnosis of presumed ocular tuberculosis.

Histopathological evidence of TB is the gold standard for diagnosing IOTB but is never used as first-line diagnostic tool. PCR has low sensitivity and high specificity while multi-targeted PCR has emerged as a novel method which shows improved sensitivity.

Treatment

There are no specific guidelines yet, on the treatment protocol of IOTB. Anti-TB treatment (ATT) administered for 9 months with an anti-inflammatory therapy has been associated with an elevenfold reduction of recurrence of uveitis. Corticosteroid is given with ATT and is tapered depending on the patient's clinical response. The conventional four-drug ATT comprises of isoniazid, rifampicin, ethambutol and pyrazinamide for 2 months followed by isoniazid and rifampicin for another 9–10 months, along with pyridoxine supplementation.

Bartonella

Cat-scratch disease (CSD) is a worldwide distributed self-limiting systemic illness caused by gram-negative bacillus, *Bartonella henselae*. It is characterized by regional lymphadenopathy with associated febrile illness. The eye can be involved either by primary inoculation complex resulting in Parinaud's oculoglandular syndrome or by hematogenous spread leading to an array of ocular manifestations.

Ocular Manifestations

The most common posterior manifestation of CSD is a unilateral or bilateral neuroretinitis. Unifocal or multifocal white areas of retinitis or chorioretinitis may accompany neuroretinitis or in the absence of optic disk involvement.

Diagnosis

The gold standard for diagnosis is serology. Positive IgG for *Bartonella henselae* indicates previous contact with the bacteria and a titer greater than 1:256 indicates an acute infection. PCR presents high specificity but low sensitivity for cases of ocular disease.

Treatment

Doxycylcine 100 mg every 12 hours for 1 month is recommended to treat secondary ocular symptoms of CSD. In cases of severe infection, intravenous doxycycline with rifampicin 300 mg twice daily is effective. Use of ciprofloxacin and azithromycin has shown good response.

Leptospirosis

Leptospirosis is caused by the gram-negative spirochete *Leptospira interrogans*.[51] Humans contract the disease upon exposure of contaminated soil, water and tissues of infected animals. The organism gains systemic access through mucous membrane or abraded skin surfaces. It is a common cause of uveitis in tropical countries and generally occurs during the immune phase of this biphasic illness.

Ocular Manifestations

It may present as a non-granulomatous hypopyon uveitis or panuveitis with marked vitritis and retinal vasculitis primarily affecting the retinal veins. It may manifest within 2 months to 1 year after infection. Retinitis and choroiditis are never seen in leptospiral uveitis (Figs. 84.19A and B).

Diagnosis

Definitive diagnosis requires isolation of organism from bodily fluids during the first week of infection which can be seen under dark-field microscopy. Microagglutination is considered to be the gold standard. A presumptive diagnosis is made on the basis of serology or on a fourfold rise in paired serum samples in the appropriate clinical context. Other serological tests include ELISA, LEPTO dipstick, macroscopic agglutination test and molecular diagnostics such as PCR and real-time PCR.

Treatment

Corticosteroids are the mainstay of treatment for leptospiral uveitis. The role of intravenous antibiotics during the systemic phase of leptospirosis is not yet known to prevent long-term complications such as uveitis.

PROTOZOAN UVEITIS

Toxoplasma gondii is a ubiquitous coccidian protozoan that usually causes asymptomatic infection in humans but can cause significant disease in congenitally infected infants and immunocompromised patients and occasionally in immunocompetent individuals.

Transmission to humans is mainly by ingestion of viable tissue cysts in uncooked meat or of food or water contaminated with oocysts. Less commonly, there is congenital transmission or transplantation of an infected organism.

Ocular toxoplasmosis is the most common infectious cause of posterior uveitis in the United States. It is a worldwide infection that may cause a majority of posterior uveitis cases in highly endemic areas such as Brazil and France.

Ocular Manifestations

The characteristic funduscopic findings in ocular toxoplasmosis include a creamy yellow retinochoroidal lesion adjacent to an old scar and marked vitreous inflammation (headlight in the fog) (Figs. 84.20A to C). These lesions occur commonly in the posterior pole or near the optic disk. Retinal vessels near the active lesions may show perivasculitis with diffuse venous sheathing and adjacent periarterial lipidic exudates (Kyrieleis arteriolitis). There may be cystoid macular edema, serous retinal detachment, choroidal neovascular membrane arising from a previous retinochoroidal scar and optic neuritis.

In 80% of infected newborns, congenital toxoplasmosis is associated with bilateral retinochoroidal lesions in the macula (wagon-wheel scar).[64,66]

Diagnosis

The diagnosis of ocular toxoplasmosis is essentially clinical. Serologic serum toxoplasma-IgM and IgG assays can help distinguish acute from chronic infection and can identify

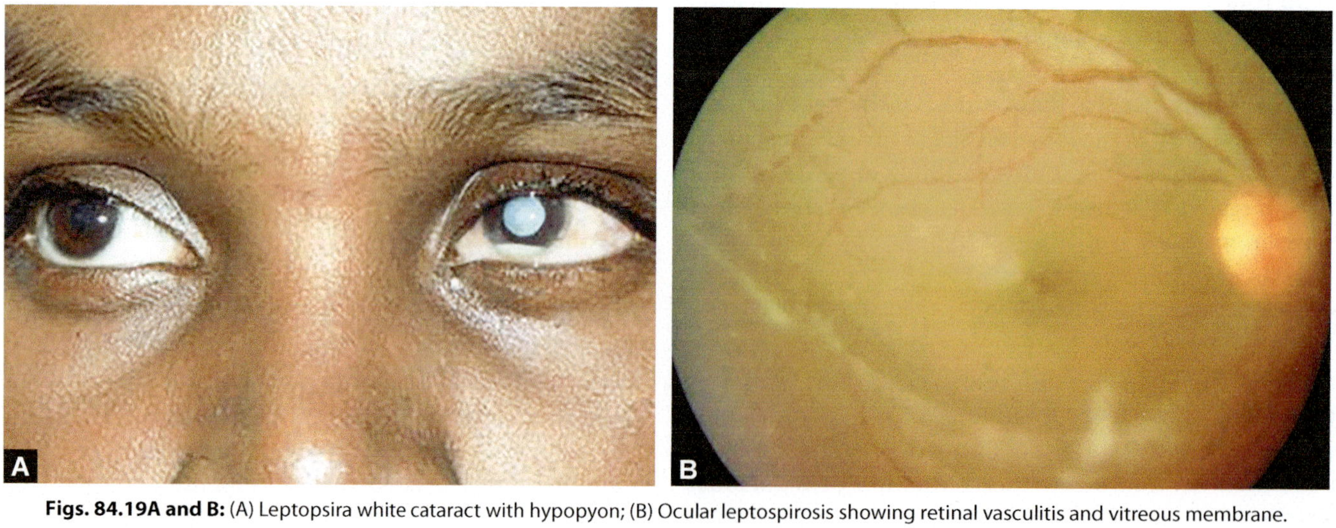

Figs. 84.19A and B: (A) Leptopsira white cataract with hypopyon; (B) Ocular leptospirosis showing retinal vasculitis and vitreous membrane.
Source: SR Rathinam.

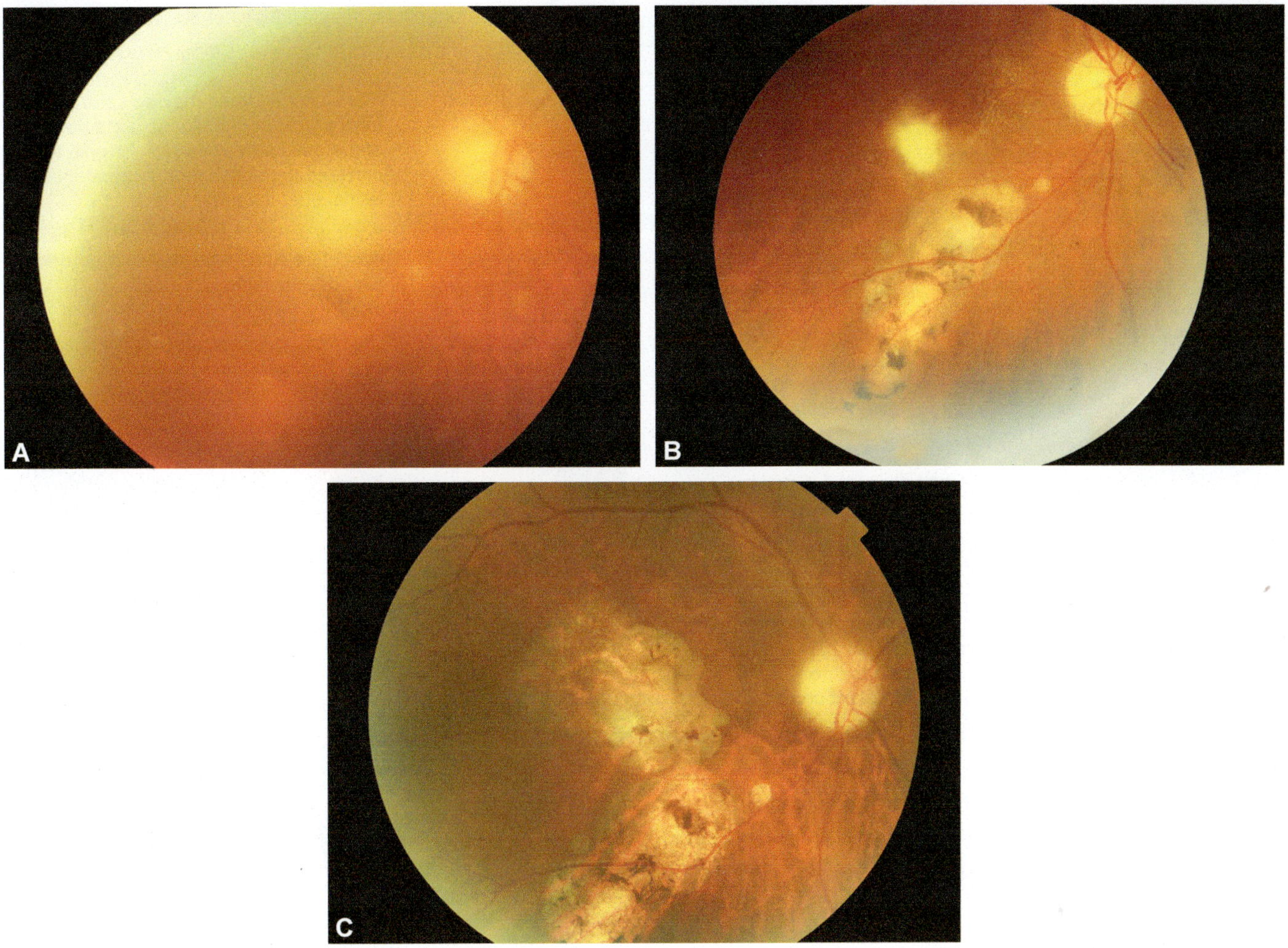

Figs. 84.20A to C: (A) Fluffy yellow retinitis adjacent to a pigmented scar with overlying vitritis typically described as headlight in the fog; (B) Fluffy yellow retinitis in the macular area adjacent to a pigmented scar with kyrieleis arteriolitis; (C) Typical resolved ocular toxoplamosis after treatment.

patients at risk for reactivation. Maternal infection is often asymptomatic. IgM positive test results are a marker of acute infection. Congenital infection may be asymptomatic or appear with neurologic or ocular manifestations and this form is diagnosed in utero by PCR of amniotic fluid or after birth by serology or PCR.[80] In cases of less typical presentation, the former is possible through calculation of the Goldmann-Witmer or Witmer-Desmonts coefficient based on the correlation between titers of specific antibodies to *Toxoplasma gondii* in aqueous humor or serum versus the globulin titers in the same fluids.[62]

In yet uncertain cases, PCR of aqueous humor/ vitreous can be a valuable tool for a definitive diagnosis of toxoplasmosis and other infectious etiologies. The positivity of vitreous samples often exceeds that of aqueous humor samples.[80]

Management

Toxoplasmic retinochoroiditis may be self-limited in some patients. The decision to treat should thus, be based on several factors including individual immune status as well as location, size and local repercussion of the active lesion.[64] Treatment is almost always indicated in immunocompromised patients, patients with congenital toxoplasmosis and pregnant women with acquired disease.[63,82]

A recent report from the American Academy of Ophthalmology highlighted the limited data that are available from randomized controlled trials with well-defined endpoints demonstrating the benefits of therapy. Box 84.2 and Table 84.6 show the indications of treatment and treatment therapy for ocular toxoplasmosis.

Box 84.2: Indications for treatment of ocular toxoplasmosis.

Lesions threatening the optic nerve or fovea
- Decreased visual acuity
- Lesions associated with moderate-to-severe vitreous inflammation
- Lesions greater than 1 disk diameter in size
- Presence of multiple active lesions for more than 1 month

Table 84.6: Medical management of ocular toxoplasmosis.

Classic therapy: Pyrimethamine (100 mg loading dose given over 24 hours for 2 days, followed by 25–50 mg daily + Folinic acid (PO) 10–20 mg daily (during and 1 week after therapy with pyrimethamine) + Sulfadiazine (1 g given four times daily for 4–6 weeks)
Alternatives: Pyrimethamine–folinic acid (same as above dose) + Clindamycin (PO or IV) 300 mg Q6H or Atovaquone (PO) 1500 mg PO twice daily or Trimethoprim-sulfamethoxazole (PO or IV) 10 mg/kg/day (trimethoprim component) divided in two to three doses or Clarithromycin (PO) 500 mg Q12H or Azithromycin (PO) 900–1200 mg/day

Folinic acid (leucovorin) should always be given with pyrimethamine to prevent leukopenia and thrombocytopenia. Folic acid must not be used as a substitute for folinic acid.

Systemic corticosteroids are generally started either at the time of antimicrobial therapy or within 48 hours in immunocompromised patients. Use of long-acting periocular or intraocular corticosteroid such as triamcinolone is contraindicated because of potential severe uncontrollable inflammation and loss of the eye. The use of photocoagulation is controversial.

HELMINTHIC UVEITIS

Toxocara

Ocular toxocariasis (OT) is transmitted in humans by accidentally ingesting eggs of a roundworm from soil or eating food contaminated with dog (*Toxocara canis*) or cat (*Toxocara cati*) feces.

Ocular toxocariasis usually occurs in children older than 3 years and in young adults. They present with strabismus, decreased vision and leukocoria which is an important differential diagnosis for retinoblastoma.[64,67,68] It has three different ocular manifestations as seen in Table 84.7 (Fig. 84.21).

Table 84.7: Different ocular manifestations of ocular toxocariasis.

Types	Characteristic lesion
Peripheral granuloma	Fibrovascular band may be seen running from a whitish granuloma in the periphery of the optic nerve or posterior pole which can lead to tractional or rhegmatogenous retinal detachment
Posterior pole chorioretinal granuloma	Solitary well-defined mass of 1–2 disk diameters size in the posterior pole with associated vitritis
Chronic endophthalmitis/ diffuse panuveitis (most common)	Mutton fat KPs, hypopyon yellowish whitish mass may be faintly seen through vitreous haze, sometimes with dense vitreous hemorrhage

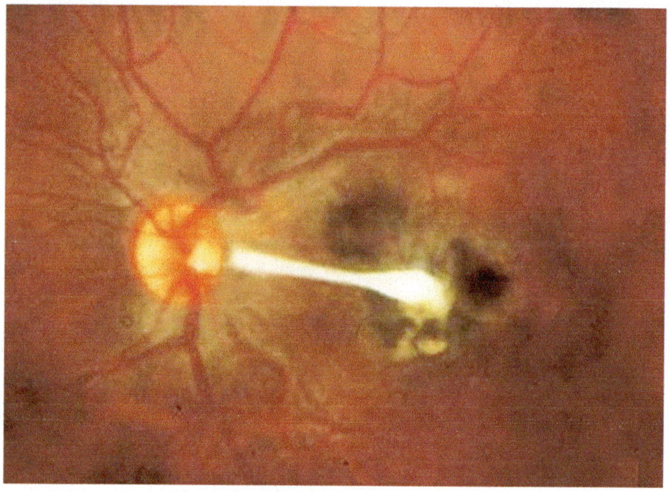

Fig. 84.21: Toxocara showing a fibrovascular band leading to a tractional retinal detachment.

Diagnosis

Eosinophilia is noted in blood with systemic toxocariasis while eosinophil count is normal in patients with OT. Serum indirect ELISA for *Toxocara canis* can help to support the diagnosis by detecting the immunogenic proteins known as *Toxocara* excretory-secretory (TES) antigens (Ag) that are shed from the larvae. Increased titer of anti-TES-Ag immunoglobulin E (IgE) antibody indicate acute toxocariasis. Increased Toxo-IgG titers confirm past or present infection without significant inflammation. Ultrasonography is important to differentiate retinoblastoma.

Treatment

Topical, periocular and systemic corticosteroid are indicated for treatment of uveitis. Antihelminthic agents such as mebendazole and thiabendazole are effective in killing the worm. However, death of the worms may promote even more severe inflammation.[65,80] Vitrectomy is helpful for sight-threatening tractional retinal detachments.

Diffuse Unilateral Subacute Neuroretinitis

The diffuse unilateral subacute neuroretinitis (DUSN) is a clinical syndrome due to the presence of a single motile sub-retinal nematode such as *Toxocara canis, Baylisascaris procyonis* and *Ancylostoma caninum*. It should be considered among otherwise healthy young patients presenting with posterior uveitis. Misdiagnosis is common because the worm is too small to be recognized.

Ocular Manifestations

The DUSN is characterized by insidious monocular visual loss from recurrent episodes of focal, multifocal and diffuse inflammation of the retina, retinal pigment epithelium (RPE) and optic nerve. In acute stage, crops of grey-white outer retinal lesions, vitritis, papillitis with overlying retinal detachment is seen. It is at this stage that the worms are easily visualized in the sub-retinal space (Figs. 84.22A and B).[73]

Diagnosis

Based on clinical setting and observation of worm in the sub-retinal space.

Treatment

Photocoagulation (200 µm, 0.2–0.5 s, 150–300 mW) is the treatment of choice when a worm can be visualized (less than 50%).[52,70] Systemic albendazole (400 mg for 30 days) or vitrectomy may be appropriate in some cases. Steroid cover may be prudent with all treatment modalities.

Onchocerciasis

It is one of the leading causes of blindness worldwide. It is endemic in Africa and in isolated Central and South America. Humans are the only host for the filarial onchocerca volvulus.[75] It is transmitted through the bite of female black flies of the *Simulium* genus. They thrive in flowing streams, hence the disease is commonly called river blindness. Microfilariae migrate through the skin and eye either from direct invasion of the eye, penetration through vascular bundles or through hematogenous spread.

Ocular Manifestations

Presence of live microfilariae in the cornea or anterior chamber.[71] It could range from mild to severe anterior uveitis, chorioretinal changes and disk atrophy.

Diagnosis

Diagnosis is based on clinical findings and history of pathogen exposure in endemic areas demonstrating microfilaria in skin biopsies or in the eye.

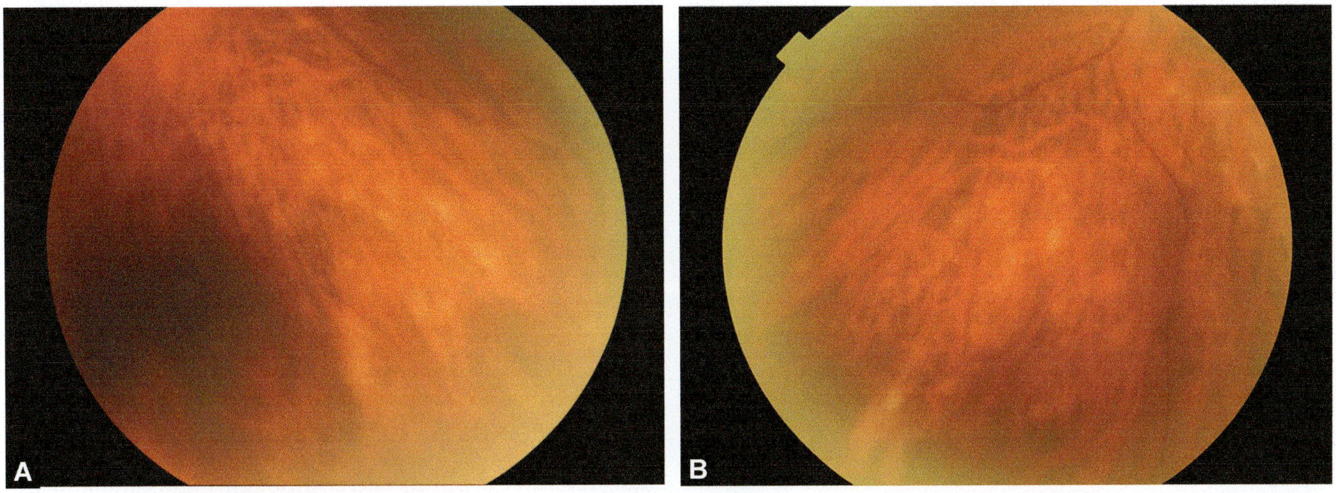

Figs. 84.22A and B: (A) Focal retinal hyperplasia of the retinal pigment epithelium; (B) A subretinal track with some degree of focal alteration of the RPE in the inferior temporal region with subretinal worm in the vicinity of these lesions.

Treatment

Ivermectin, a macrolytic lactone is the treatment of choice.

Endophthalmitis

Endophthalmitis is a rare but potentially blinding complication caused predominantly by bacteria or fungi that can occur after ocular surgery or trauma (exogenous) or as a consequence of a systemic infection (endogenous).

Acute Postoperative Endophthalmitis

Endophthalmitis after ocular surgery is the most common form of the condition. Approximately 90% of postoperative endophthalmitis cases develop after cataract surgery. It can also occur after glaucoma filtration surgery, vitrectomy and corneal transplantation. Presentation within 6 weeks of surgery is termed acute and beyond 6 weeks as chronic endophthalmitis.

The median time to diagnosis is 5.5 days following surgery with more than two-thirds of patients presenting within the first 7 days after surgery. Only 30–50% of these post-cataract surgery cases achieve a final best-corrected visual acuity of 20/40 or better.[76]

The most common organisms causing acute cataract postoperative endophthalmitis are predominantly gram-positive especially coagulase-negative *Staphylococcus, Streptococci* and less commonly gram-negative *Enterococcus* and *Pseudomonas* species.[72,75,76]

Ocular Manifestations

Symptoms include eye pain and redness with reduced visual acuity in 75–95% of cases. An afferent pupillary defect may be present in 12% and eyelid edema, conjunctival injection and chemosis, corneal edema, anterior chamber inflammation and fibrin accumulation can be observed. A hypopyon is present in up to 86% of cases and the red reflex is absent in 67% (Fig. 84.23).

Treatment

The Endophthalmitis-Vitrectomy Study evaluated the role of pars plana virtrectomy versus intraocular antibiotic injection and systemic antibiotics in the treatment of acute postoperative endophthalmitis. The results demonstrated that eyes with presenting visual acuity of counting fingers (CF) or better and eyes that do not require pars plana vitrectomy are more likely to have a final visual acuity of

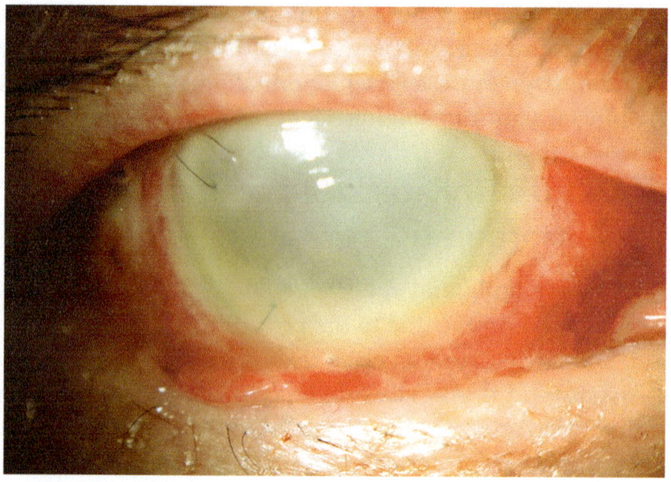

Fig. 84.23: Postoperative endophthalmitis. Group B *Streptococcus*—corneal edema, and sliding hypopyon.

20/40 or better. Intravenous antibiotics have no additional benefit but in cases of rapid deterioration of vision, the use of appropriate systemic antibiotics may be considered. Intravitreal vancomycin has been shown to be effective against more than 99% of gram-positive endophthalmitis isolates. Amikacin (0.4 mg in 0.1 mL) is useful for gram-negative coverage. Ceftazidime demonstrates similar gram-negative sensitivity as amikacin and is not associated with retinal toxicity.

Prophylaxis

European society of cataract and refractive surgeons multicentre study (ESCRS Study) has identified multiple risk factors predisposing to endophthalmitis. These include diabetes mellitus, chronic blepharitis, infected lacrimal drainage, prolonged surgery, posterior capsule rupture, vitreous loss, wound leak and vitreous incarceration.[74-78] Povidone-iodine has been reported to effectively decrease conjunctival flora in several studies by up to 91%.[77] The use of intracameral cefazolin (1.0 mg/0.1 mL) or cefuroxime (1.0 mg/0.1 mL) have been reported to decrease the rate of endophthalmitis and the incidence has also been lowered with prophylactic use of intracameral vancomycin (0.1 mg in 0.1 mL of normal saline) and tobramycin (16 mg/L of irrigation solution).[75,78]

Bleb-related Endophthalmitis

Bleb-related infections can complicate glaucoma filtration surgery, especially following filtering surgeries with adjunctive mitomycin C with a reported incidence of 1.5%

at 2.5 years of follow up. The most common pathogens identified in bleb-related infections are *Streptococcus* species, coagulase-negative *Staphylococcus*, *Haemophilus influenzae* and *Enterococcus* species.[79-82] It may present early within 15 days following surgery or delayed for up to 30 years following filtering surgery.

Risk Factors

- Leaking bleb
- Inferior quadrant positioned trabeculectomy
- Use of 5-fluorouracil and mitomycin C
- Thin avascular bleb
- Pseudophakia
- Repeated filtering surgery
- High bleb and coexisting blepharitis.

Endophthalmitis after Intravitreal Injections

Intravitreal injections are now commonly performed for patients with vitreoretinal pathology such as age-related macular degeneration, diabetic maculopathy and retinal vein occlusion. The incidence of acute endophthalmitis after intravitreal injections (both in the West as well as in Asia) ranges from 0.01% to 0.10%.[83-85]

Post-traumatic Endophthalmitis

Post-traumatic endophthalmitis may complicate open globe eye injury. The incidence ranges from 2.1% to 5.1%. The risk of endophthalmitis is significantly higher among eyes with pure corneal injuries, intraocular foreign bodies, traumatic lens rupture and trauma resulting from needles. Infection by *Bacillus* species (in approximately 25%) can result in rapidly progressive endophthalmitis with a high risk of visual loss due to the destruction caused by cytolysins and enzymes produced by the bacteria.[86-88] Other commonly isolated bacteria include coagulase-negative staphylococcal species such as *Staphylococcus epidermidis* and *Staphylococcus saprophyticus*, *Pseudomonas aeruginosa* and *Escherichia coli*. The most commonly isolated fungus is *Aspergillus*.

Chronic Postoperative Endophthalmitis

Chronic postoperative endophthalmitis (CPE) is a rare complication and occurs more than 6 weeks to years after the initial event. The patient typically presents with persistent low-grade anterior chamber inflammation with a characteristic white plaque on the posterior lens capsule and decreased visual acuity in the affected eye. Some patients may experience mild pain and anterior vitreous inflammation is common.

The most common isolated organism in CPE cases is *Propionibacterium acnes* but there are reports of other rare causative indolent organisms such as *Ochrobactrum anthropic*, *Massilia timonae*, *Mycobacterium manitobense*, *Acinetobacter calcoaceticus*, *Torulopsis candida*, *Corynebacterium minutissimum* and *Alcaligens xylosoxidans*.

With the advent of PCR sequencing based pathogen identification in addition to routine culture methods help in identifying the microorganisms. Scanning electron microscopy and PCR techniques have demonstrated the adherence of bacteria on the surface of explanted intraocular lens and capsular bag.

Endogenous Endophthalmitis

Endogenous endophthalmitis is a rare metastatic ocular infection which can affect immunocompromised individuals. The medical conditions commonly associated with this are diabetes mellitus, hepatobiliary disease, liver cirrhosis and malignancy. Other underlying associated conditions include renal failure, indwelling catheters, immunosuppressive diseases, recent surgery, endocarditis and intravenous drug abuse. In Asia, pyogenic liver abscess (PLA) is the most common source and other sources include pneumonia, osteomyelitis, urinary tract infection, soft tissue infection, peritonitis, septic arthritis, catheter-related infection, infective endocarditis and meningitis. However, the source may remain unidentifiable in up to 7.4–35% of patients despite extensive systemic investigations.[89-90]

Causative Organisms

Gram-positive bacteria such as *Staphylococcus aureus* and *Streptococcus pneumoniae* have been reported to be the most common causative organisms of endogenous endophthalmitis in the West. However, the gram-negative bacteria such as *Klebsiella pneumoniae*, *Escherichia coli* and *Pseudomonas aeruginosa* are reported to be responsible for the majority of endogenous endophthalmitis in many case series from Asia.[90,91]

Other causative organisms such as *Bacillus cereus* endophthalmitis among intravenous drug abusers,

Haemophilus influenzae and *Neisseria meningitides* endophthalmitis among pediatric individuals and *Nocardia-asteroids* and *Mycobacterium tuberculosis* endophthalmitis are also reported as rare cases in Asia.[88-90]

Hepatobiliary tract infection is a major source of *Klebsiella* bacteremia (45–62%); there is a 3.0–7.8% risk of developing endophthalmitis among patients with liver abscess. Other reported risk factors include disseminated intravascular coagulation and delayed diagnosis and treatment. The interval between the diagnosis of liver abscess and endophthalmitis was approximately 3.12 days to 4.4 days; 4.9–19% of patients presented with ocular symptoms before the diagnosis of sepsis and liver abscess were confirmed (Figs. 84.24A and B).

Pseudomonas aeruginosa infection can also present as endogenous endophthalmitis although it is more commonly related to infective keratitis, scleritis or postsurgical endophthalmitis.

Besides gram-negative organisms, gram-positive organisms such as *Staphylococcus aureus*, *Streptococcus pneumoniae*, group B *Streptococcus* and *Staphylococcus epidermidis* are most frequently spread from infective endocarditis, skin, bone and joint infections.

One-third of the patients may have an underlying chronic disease such as diabetes mellitus, underlying malignancy or *AIDS* but group B *Streptococcus* endophthalmitis can also affect healthy individuals.

Serratia marcescens has been reported to cause irido-lenticular abscess from endogenous endophthalmitis as a result of nosocomial infections in susceptible immunocompromised individuals.[92]

Patients can present with intractable pain and angle closure. High-frequency ultrasound biomicroscopy is needed to detect ciliary body abscesses that may be missed by B-scan ultrasonography. This is an aerobic, gram-negative bacillus that is commonly associated with respiratory and catheter-related bacteremia in susceptible individuals.

Clinical Features

Presenting symptoms of endogenous endophthalmitis are similar to that of postoperative endophthalmitis: ocular pain, reduction of vision and eye redness.

However, certain features have been reported to be characteristic of certain causative organisms such as a "pupillary hypopyon" with fibrous obscuring the pupil among cases with *Klebsiella pneumoniae*, a "sliding hypopyon"[92] among cases with Group B *Streptococcus* and a pink or dark hypopyon with *Serratia* infection.[93,94] The majority was unilateral although 14–25% of cases may have bilateral involvement. Most patients (up to 87%) had poor visual acuity at presentation (worse than 4/200) and septicemia or an extraocular focus of infection was often present before the presentation of visual symptoms.

Gram-negative organisms commonly presents with focal whitish nodules within the choroid or choroidal abscess with rapid involvement of the retina. Intense vitritis is often seen in diffuse severe disease with poor fundal view. Perivascular hemorrhages, inflammatory infiltrates and arterial emboli may be observed. Frank retinal necrosis and globe perforation at the site of an abscess may also occur. In

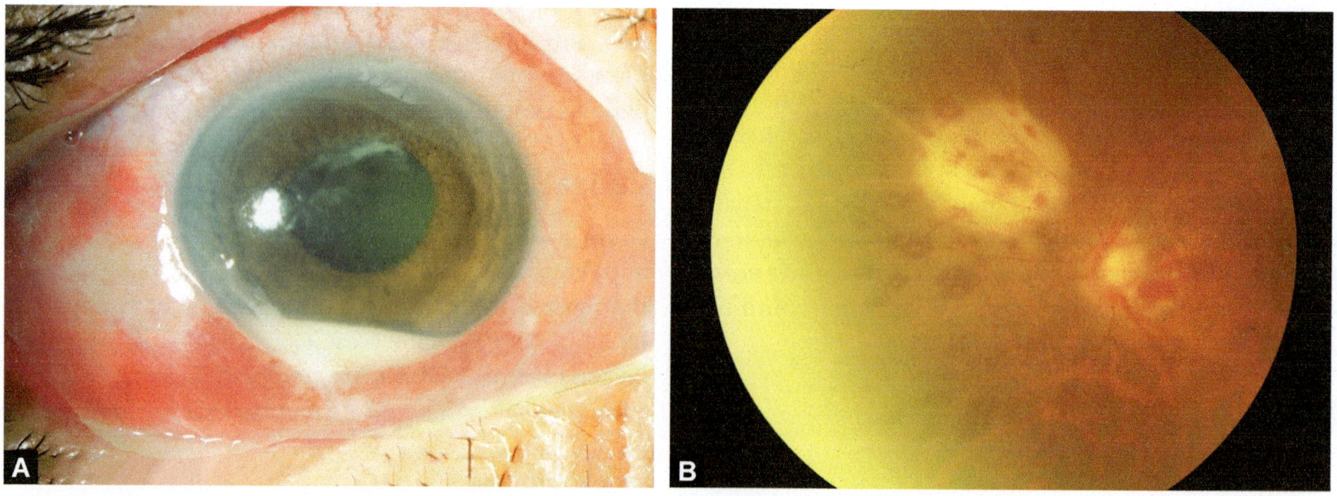

Figs. 84.24A and B: (A) Conjunctival injection with chemosis and hypopyon in patient with *Klebsiella* liver abscess; (B) *Klebsiella endophthalmitis*. Solitary early choroidal abscess with multiple roth spots and arteritis.

contrast, gram-positive organisms may be multifocal with Roth's spots and retinal vasculitis.

The infection can sometimes spread to the orbital tissues and result in panophthalmitis with lid edema, chemosis, proptosis and limited ocular motility, especially if the infection is caused by *Klebsiella* or *Pseudomonas* species. Another rare presentation is anterior focal disease with discrete foci as iris nodules or microabscesses and mild to moderate anterior segment inflammation.

Fungal Endophthalmitis

Fungal endophthalmitis is a sight-threatening disease most commonly caused by *Candida* species followed by *Aspergillus* species. It can result from hematogenous dissemination and rarely from direct inoculation following penetrating trauma, eye surgery and intraocular extension of ocular surface infections. Risk factors include immunosuppression, intravenous drug abuse, bacterial sepsis, prolonged hyperalimentation, systemic antibiotics, corticosteroid therapy, recent abdominal surgery, malignancy, diabetes mellitus and hemodialysis.

Candida Endophthalmitis

Candida species is the most common cause of invasive fungal infections in humans. Candida exists predominantly as unicellular yeasts with small, thin-walled ovoid cells that reproduce by budding.

Ocular Manifestations

Chorioretinitis typically with several, small, creamy-white circumscribed chorioretinal lesions with overlying vitritis. Vitreous opacities resemble fluffy balls that may be linked together by strands giving them the so-called "string of pearl appearance". This may lead to vitreoretinal traction and retinal detachment (Fig. 84.25).

The anterior segment may develop ciliary injection, non-granulomatous KPs and hypopyon.

Aspergillus Endophthalmitis

Aspergillus is a ubiquitous saprophytic fungi found in soil, decaying vegetables and water. Inhalation of the conidia or asexual spore of *Aspergillus* is an important route of entry into humans.

Aspergillus endogenous endophthalmitis tends to present more acutely than *Candida* endophthalmitis and progresses more rapidly. Thorough respiratory and cardiac workup is necessary because it usually involves these areas.

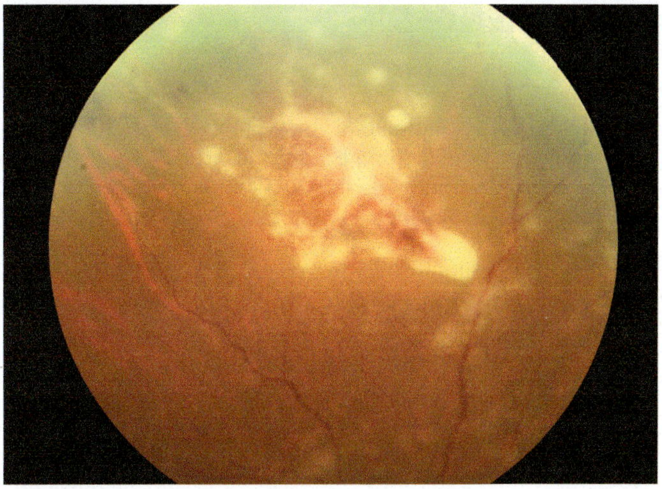

Fig. 84.25: Endogenous candida endophthalmitis showing multiple satellite lesions with overlying snowballs superiorly.

Ocular Manifestations

It presents as an iridocyclitis with or without a hypopyon, with a characteristic confluent central yellowish macular infiltrate in the choroid and subretinal space. They have a propensity for vascular invasion leading to thrombosis, necrosis and eventually retinal detachment.

Diagnosis

Clinical findings in high-risk patients and isolation of Candida or *Aspergillus* in colonized sites and blood aids in the diagnosis. Vitreous biopsy can help to confirm the diagnosis of endophthalmitis but the yield of positive cultures is varied ranging from 26% to 68% in the literature. PCR has been shown to be of high specificity for fungal detection in vitreous and may allow rapid diagnosis.

Treatment

Systemic treatment with an alternative antifungal such as azole (fluconazole and voriconazole) or in combination with an intravitreal antifungal is now the preferred management option because of their greater bioavailability, excellent ocular penetration and broad spectrum activity. Systemic amphotericin has a broad-spectrum coverage but its penetration of the vitreous cavity is poor. Doses of 5–10 mg intravitreal amphotericin have been used but have been associated with a higher incidence of retinal toxicity.

REFERENCES

1. Chee SP, Bacsal K, Jap A, et al. Clinical features of cytomegalovirus anterior uveitis in immunocompetent patients. Am J Opthalmol. 2008;145(5):834-40.
2. Studies of Ocular Complications of AIDS Research Group in collaboration with the AIDS Clinical Trials Group: Foscarnet-ganciclovir cytomegalovirus Retinitis Trial 5. Clinical features of cytomegalovirus retinitis at diagnosis. Am J Ophthalmol. 1997;124:141-1.
3. Forrester JV, Dick AD, McMenamin PG, et al. General and ocular pharmacology. The Eye: Basic Sciences in Practice. Philadelphia: Saunders; 2001:338-69.
4. Paylay DA, Sternberg P, Davis J, et al. Decrease in the risk of bilateral acute retinal necrosis by acyclovir therapy. Am J Ophthalmol. 1991;112(3):250-5.
5. Scott D, Schoenberger MD, Kim SJ, et al. Diagnosis and Treatment of Acute Retinal Necrosis. Ophthalmology. 2017;124(3):382-92.
6. Lau CH, Missotten T, Slazmann J, et al. Acute retinal necrosis: features, management, and outcomes. Ophthalmology. 2007;114:756-62.
7. Tibbetts MD, Shah CP, Young LH, et al. Treatment of acute retinal necrosis. Ophthalmology. 2010;117:818-24.
8. Hillenkamp J, Nolle B, Bruns C, et al. Acute retinal necrosis: clinical features, early vitrectomy, and outcomes. Ophthalmology. 2009;116:1971-5.
9. Nakamoto BK, Dorotheo EU, Biousse V, et al. Progressive outer retinal necrosis presenting with isolated optic neuropathy. Neurology. 2004;63:2423-2.
10. Roig-Melo EA, Macky TA, Heredia-Elizondo ML, et al. Progressive outer retinal necrosis syndrome: successful treatment with a new combination of antiviral drugs. Eur J Ophthalmol. 2001;11(2);200-2.
11. Matoba AY. Ocular disease associated with Epstein-Barr virus infection. Surv Ophthalmol. 1990;35:145-50.
12. Heilingenhaus A, Helbig H, Fiedler M. Herpesviruses In: Foster CS, and Vitale AT (Eds). Diagnosis and Treatment of Uveitis. Philadelphia: Saunders; 2002.pp.315-32.
13. Tideman JS. Epstein-Barr viral antibodies in multifocal choroiditis and panuveitis. Am J Ophthalmol. 1987; 103(5):659-63.
14. Khurana RN, Sadda SR. Images in clinical medicine. Salt-and-Pepper retinopathy of rubella. N Engl J Med. 2006;355(5):499.
15. Yoser SL, Forster DJ, Rao NA. Systemic viral infections and their retinal and choroidal manifestations. Surv Ophthalmol. 1993;37:313-52.
16. Scheie HG, Morse PH. Rubeola retinopathy. Arch Ophthalmol. 1972;88:341-4.
17. Serdaroglu A, Gücüyener K, Dursun I, et al. Macular retinitis as a first sign of subacute sclerosing panencephalitis: the importance of early diagnosis. Ocul Immunol Inflamm. 2005;13(5):405-10.
18. Baillif S, Tieulie N, Queyrel V, et al. New aspects of viral necrotizing retinitis in subacute sclerosing panencephalitis with spectral-domain optical coherence tomography. Retina Cases Brief Rep. 2012;6:235-41.
19. Yimenicioglu S, Yakut A, Erol N, et al. Chorioretinitis as a first sign of SSPE. Neuropediatrics. 2012;43:149-51.
20. Hasbun R, Garcia MN, Kellaway J, et al. West Nile Virus retinopathy and associations with long term neurological and neurocognitive sequelae. PLoS One. 2016;11(3):e0148898.
21. Khairallah M, Yahia SB, Letaief M, et al. A prospective evaluation of factors associated with chorioretinitis in patients with West Nile Virus infection. Ocul Immunol Inflamm. 2007;15:435-39.
22. Garg S, Jampol LM, Wilson JF, et al. Ischemic and hemorrhagic retinal vasculitis associated with West Nile Virus infection. Retina. 2006;26:365-67.
23. Anninger WV, Lomeo MD, Dingle J, et al. West Nile virus-associated optic neuritis and chorioretinitis. Am J Ophthalmol. 2003;136:1183-5.
24. Afshar AR, Hariprasad SM, Jampol LM. Use of intravitreous bevacizumab to treat macular edema in West Nile Virus chorioretinitis. Arch Ophthalmol. 2012;130(3):396-8.
25. Al-Hazmi A, Al-Rajhi AA, Abboud EB, et al. Ocular complications of Rift Valley fever outbreak in Saudi Arabia. Ophthalmology. 2005;112:313-8.
26. Shawky S. Rift Valley fever. Saudi Med J. 2000;21:1109-5.
27. Himeidan YE, Kweka EJ, Mahgoub MM, et al. Recent outbreaks of rift valley Fever in East Africa and the Middle East. Front Public Health. 2014;2:169.
28. Lalitha P, Rathinam S, Banushree K, et al. Ocular involvement associated with an epidemic outbreak of chikungunya virus infection. Am J Ophthalmol. 2007;144:552-6.
29. Chanana B, Azad RV, Nair S. Bilateral macular choroiditis following Chikungunya virus infection. Eye. 2007;21:1020-1.
30. Mahendradas P, Ranganna SK, Shetty R, et al. Ocular Manifestations Associated with Chikungunya. Ophthalmology. 2008;115:287-1.
31. Ventura CV, Maia M, Travassos SB, et al. Risk factors associated with the ophthalmoscopic findings identified in infants with presumed Zika virus congenital infection. JAMA Ophthalmol. 2016;134(8):912-8.
32. Furtado JM, Espósito DL, Klein TM, et al. Uveitis associated with Zika virus infection. N Engl J Med. 2016;375:394-96.
33. Mattia JG, Vandy MJ, Chang JC, et al. Early clinical sequelae of Ebola virus disease in Sierra Leone: a cross-sectional study. Lancet Infect Dis. 2016;16:331-8.
34. Vingolo EM, Messano GA, Fragiotta S, et al. Ocular manifestations of Ebola virus disease: an ophthalmologist's guide to prevent infection and panic. Biomed Res Int. 2015.
35. Chancellor RJ, Sriranjani P, Thomas GC, et al. Uveitis and Systemic Inflammatory Markers in Convalescnt phase of Ebola Virus disease, Emerging Infectious Disease. 2016;22(2):295-7.
36. Becerra LI, Ksiazek SM, Savino PJ, et al. Syphilis uveitis in human immunodeficiency virus-infected and noninfected patients. Ophthalmology. 1989;96:1727-30.
37. Halperin LS, Berger AS, Grand MG. Syphilitic disc edema and periphlebitis. Retina. 1990;10(3):223-5.

38. Tamesis RR, Foster CS. Ocular syphilis. Ophthalmology. 1990;97(10):1281-7.
39. Eandi CM, Neri P, Adelman RA, et al. Acute syphilitic posterior placoid chorioretinitis: report of a case series and comprehensive review of the literature. Retina. 2012;32:1915-41.
40. Rush JA, Ryan EJ. Syphilitic optic perineuritis. Am J Ophthalmol. 1981;91(3):404-6.
41. TOshniwal P. Optic perineuritis with secondary syphilis. J Clin Neuroophthalmol. 1987;7(1):6-10.
42. Kunkel J, Schurmann D, Pleyer U, et al. Ocular syphilis—indicator of previously unknown HIV infection. J Infect. 2008;58:32-6.
43. Putkonen T, Salo OP, Mustakallio KK. Febrile Herxheimer reaction in different phases of primary and secondary syphilis. Br J Vener Dis. 1966;42:181-4.
44. Brown ST. Adverse reactions in syphilis therapy. J Am Vener Dis Assoc. 1976;3:172-6.
45. Mikkila HO, Seppala IJ, Viljanen MK, et al. The expanding clinical spectrum of ocular Lyme borreliosis. Ophthalmology. 2000;107:581-7.
46. Breeveld J, Rothova A, Kuiper H. Intermediate uveitis and Lyme borreliosis. Br J Ophthalmol. 1992;76:181-2.
47. Rothermel H, Hedges TR, Steere AC. Optic neuropathy in children with Lyme disease. Pediatrics. 2001;108:477-81.
48. Balcer LJ, Winterkorn JM, Galetta SL. Neuro-ophthalmic manifestations of Lyme disease. J Neuroophthalmol. 1997;17:108-21.
49. Murillo G, Ramirez B, Romo LA, et al. Oculopalpebral borreliosis as an unusual manifestation of Lyme disease. Cornea. 2013;32:87-90.
50. DePietropaolo DL, Powers JH, Gill JM, et al. Diagnosis of Lyme disease. Am Fam Physician. 2005;72(2):297-304.
51. Wormser GP, Dattwyler RJ, Shapiro ED, et al. The clinical assessment, treatment, and prevention of Lyme disease, human granulocytic anaplasmosis, and babesiosis: clinical practice guidelines by the Infectious Diseases Society of America. Clin Infect Dis. 2006;43(9):1089-134.
52. Baum J, Barza M, Weinstein P, et al. Bilateral keratitis as a manifestation of Lyme disease. Am J Ophthalmol. 1988;105:75-7.
53. Hamelin A. Ocular Lyme borreliosis. Am J Ophthalmol. 1989;108:651-7.
54. Stanek G, Strle F. Lyme borreliosis. Lancet. 2003;362:1639-7.
55. Güngür K, Bekir NA, Namiduru M. Ocular Complications associated with brucellosis in an endemic area. Eur J Ophthalmol. 2002;12:232-7.
56. Al-Kaff AS. Ocular brucellosis. Int Ophthalmol Clin. 1995;35(3):139-45.
57. Rolando I, Olarte L, Vilchez G, et al. Ocular manifestations associated with brucellosis: a 26-year experience in Peru. Clin Infect Dis. 2008;46:1338-45.
58. Al Faran MF. Brucella melitensis endogenous endophthalmitis. Ophthalmologica. 1990;201:19-22.
59. Rabinowitz R, Schneck M, Levy J, et al. Bilateral multifocal choroiditis with serous retinal detachment in a patient with. Arch Ophthalmol. 2005;123:116-8.
60. R Ghasemi Barghi,H Meraat, AA Pahlevan. A Review on Ophthalmic Manifestations of Brucellosis and Reporting a Case of Ophthalmic Brucellosis. Iran Red Crescent Med J. 2011;13(5):352-3.
61. Gupta A, Bansal R, Gupta V, et al. Ocular signs predictive of tubercular uveitis. Am J Ophthalmol. 2010;149:562-70.
62. Palmer MF. Laboratory diagnosis of leptospirosis. Med Lab Sci. 1988;45:174-8.
63. Kodjikian L, Wallon M, Fleury J, et al. Ocular manifestations in congenital toxoplasmosis. Graefes Arch Clin Exp Ophthalmol. 2006;244:14-21.
64. Orefice F, Vasconcelos-Santos DV, Cordeiro CA, et al. Toxoplasmosis. In: Foster CS, Vitale AT (Eds). Diagnosis and Treatment of Uveitis, 2nd edition. New Delhi: Jaypee-Highlights, 2013. pp. 671-7.
65. Silveira C, Belfort R, Muccioli C, et al. A follow-up study of. Am J Ophthalmol. 2001;131:351-4.
66. Holland GN, Lewis KG. An update on current practices in the management of ocular toxoplasmosis. Am J Ophthalmol. 2002;134:102-14.
67. Lightman, Susan, Towler, Hamish. Uveitis. London, United Kingdom: BMJ Books; 1998.
68. Despommier D. Toxocariasis: clinical aspects, epidemiology, medical ecology, and molecular aspects. Clin Microbiol. Rev. 2003;16:265-27.
69. Gass JD, Gilbert WR, Guerry RK, et al. Diffuse unilateral subacute neuroretinitis. Ophthalmology. 1978;85:521-45.
70. Raymond LA, Gutierrez Y, Strong LE, et al. Living retinal nematode (filarial-like) destroyed with photocoagulation. Ophthalmology. 1978;85:944-9.
71. D Scott Smith. Onchocerciasis (River Blindness) Treatment and Management. October 29,2013.
72. Hughes DS, Hill RJ. Infectious endophthalmitis after cataract surgery. Br J Ophthalmol. 1994;78:227-32.
73. Javitt JC, Street DA, Tielsch JM, et al. National outcomes of cataract extraction. retinal detachment and endophthalmitis after outpatient cataract surgery. Cataract Patient Outcomes Research Team. Ophthalmology. 1994;101:100-5.
74. Wong TY, Chee SP. The epidemiology of acute endophthalmitis after cataract surgery in an Asian population. Ophthalmology. 2004;111:699-705.
75. Ravindran RD, Venkatesh R, Chang DF, et al. Incidence of post-cataract endophthalmitis at Aravind Eye Hospital: outcomes of more than 42,000 consecutive cases using standardized sterilization and prophylaxis protocols. J Cataract Refractr Surg. 2009;35:629-36.
76. Results of the Endophthalmitis Vitrectomy Study. A randomized trial of immediate vitrectomy and of intravenous antibiotics for the treatment of postoperative bacterial endophthalmitis. Endophthalmitis Vitrectomy Study Group. Arch Ophthalmol. 1995;113:1479-96.
77. Endophthalmitis Study Group European Society of Cataract and Refractive Surgery. Prophylaxis of postoperative endophthalmitis following cataract surgery: results of the ESCRS multicenter study and identification of risk factors. J Cataract Refractr Surg. 2007;33:978-88.

78. Barry P. Adoption of intracameral antibiotic prophylaxis of endophthalmitis following cataract surgery: update on the ESCRS Endophthalmitis Study. J Cataract Refractr Surg. 2014;40(1):138-42.
79. Hori N, Mochizuki K, Ishida K, et al. Clinical characteristics and risk factors of glaucoma filtering bleb infections. Nippon Ganka Gakkai Zasshi. 2009;113:951-63.
80. Jampel HD, Quigley HA, Kerrigan-Baumrind LA, et al. Risk factors for late-onset infection following glaucoma filtration surgery. Arch Ophthalmol. 2001;119:1001-8.
81. Poulsen EJ, Allingham RR. Characteristics and risk factors of infections after glaucoma filtering surgery. J Glaucoma. 2000;9:438-43.
82. Ashkenazi I, Melamed S, Avni I, et al. Risk factors associated with late infection of filtering blebs and endophthalmitis. Ophthalmic Surg. 1991;22(10):570-4.
83. Falavarjani KG, Aghamirsalim M, Modarres M, et al. Endophthalmitis after resident-performed intravitreal bevacizumab injection. Can J Ophthalmol. 2015;50:33-6.
84. Falavarjani KG, Modarres M, Hashemi M, et al. Incidence of acute endophthalmitis after intravitreal bevacizumab injection in a single clinical center. Retina. 2013;33:971-74.
85. Mithal K, Mathai A, Pathengay A, et al. Endophthalmitis following intravitreal anti-VEGF injections in ambulatory surgical centre facility: Incidence, management and outcome. Br J Ophthalmol. 2013;97:1609-12.
86. David DB, Kirkby GR, Noble BA. Bacillus cereus endophthalmitis. Br J Ophthalmol. 1994;78:577-80.
87. Long C, Liu B, Xu C, et al. Causative organisms of post-traumatic endophthalmitis: a 20-year retrospective study. BMC Ophthalmol. 2014;14:34.
88. Das T, Chowdhury K, Sharma S, et al and the Endophhtlmitis Research Group. Clinical profile and outcome in Bacillus endophthalmitis. Ophthalmology. 2001;108:1819-25.
89. Okada AA, Johnson RP, Liles WC, et al. Endogenous bacterial endophthalmitis. Report of a ten-year retrospective study. Ophthalmology. 1994;101:832-38.
90. Chee SP, Jap A. Endogenous endophthalmitis. Current Opinion Ophthalmol. 2001;12(6):464-70.
91. Chen YJ, Kuo HK, Wu PC, et al. A 10-year comparison of endogenous endophthalmitis outcomes: an east Asian experience with *Klebsiella pneumoniae* infection. Retina. 2004;24:383-90.
92. Lee SY, Chee SP. Group B *Streptococcus* endogenous endophthalmitis : case reports and review of the literature. Ophthalmology. 2002;109:1879-86.
93. Tan N, Galvante PR, Chee SP. Endogenous *Serratia marcescens* endophthalmitis: an atypical presentation. Eye (Lond). 2014;28:108-9.
94. Equi RA, Green WR. Endogenous *Serratia marcescens* endophthalmitis with dark hypopyon: case report and review. Surv Opthalmol. 2001;46:259-68.

Chapter 85 Noninfectious Uveitis

Ilknur Tugal-Tutkun, Hilal Eser Ozturk

INTRODUCTION

Uveitis is classified as noninfectious when there is no known ocular or systemic infectious etiology. Then, the pathogenesis is presumed to be immune-mediated that may involve autoimmune and autoinflammatory mechanisms where the adaptive and innate arms of the immune system play the predominant role respectively.[1]

The diagnostic approach to a patient with uveitis is based on consideration of epidemiologic and demographic features, careful history and review of systems (Table 85.1) and characterization of intraocular inflammation along several dimensions including laterality, duration of onset and course, anatomic classification, identification of clinical features by ophthalmic examination and imaging studies and response to a previous therapy (Fig. 85.1). A differential diagnosis is thus, formulated and further systemic investigations are carried out when required for a definitive diagnosis (Table 85.2). All infectious etiologies and masquerading conditions should be ruled out for the diagnosis of non-infectious uveitis; which may be a specific uveitis entity without any systemic association, uveitis associated with a systemic noninfectious disease or an undefined presumably autoimmune, intraocular inflammation which is frequently labeled as "idiopathic".

Noninfectious uveitis accounts for a majority of cases reported in large surveys from the developed world whereas infectious uveitis is relatively more common in developing countries.[2] This chapter focuses on specific non-infectious uveitic entities with or without systemic disease associations.

ANTERIOR UVEITIS

Anterior uveitis is characterized by inflammation of the iris and anterior part of the ciliary body. It accounts for up to 90% of uveitis cases seen at community-based practices but 40–60% of cases at referral centers.[3] Almost 50% of patients with anterior uveitis have no identifiable cause or do not fit in any defined clinical syndrome.

Table 85.1: Systemic signs and symptoms associated with noninfectious uveitis.

Signs and/or symptoms	Disease association
Sacroiliitis	AS, reactive arthritis, IBD
Arthritis	RA, JIA, reactive arthritis, psoriatic arthritis, Behçet's disease, sarcoidosis
Oral ulcers	Behçet's disease, reactive arthritis, IBD
Genital ulcers	Behçet's disease, reactive arthritis, IBD
Skin rash	Behçet's disease, reactive arthritis, psoriatic arthritis, sarcoidosis, SLE
Skin nodules	Sarcoidosis
Erythema nodosum	Behçet's disease, sarcoidosis
Vitiligo, poliosis, alopecia	VKH
Headache	VKH, sarcoidosis, Behçet's disease
Pleocytosis in CSF	VKH, sarcoidosis, Behçet's disease, APMPPE
Paresthesia	MS, Behçet's disease
Psychosis	VKH, Behçet's disease, sarcoidosis
Neurosensory deafness	VKH, sarcoidosis
Pulmonary symptoms	Sarcoidosis, Wegener
Diarrhea	IBD
Salivary and/or lacrimal gland swelling	Sarcoidosis
Sinusitis	Sarcoidosis, Wegener
Nephritis	TINU, PAN, Wegener
Epididymitis	Behçet's disease, reactive arthritis, PAN
Circinate balanitis	AS, reactive arthritis
Keratoderma blennorrhagicum	AS, reactive arthritis
Urethral discharge	Reactive arthritis
Hematuria	Wegener, PAN, SLE
Fever	Behçet's disease, PAN, reactive arthritis, IBD
Flu-like symptoms	APMPPE, MEWDS, VKH

(AS: Ankylosing spondylitis; IBD: Inflammatory bowel disease; RA: Rheumatoid arthritis; JIA: Juvenile idiopathic arthritis; VKH: Vogt-Koyanagi-Harada disease; CSF: Cerebrospinal fluid; TINU: Tubulointerstitial nephritis and uveitis; APMPPE: Acute posterior multifocal placoid pigment epitheliopathy; MEWDS: Multiple evanescent white dot syndrome; SLE: Systemic lupus erythematosus; PAN: Polyarteritis nodosa)

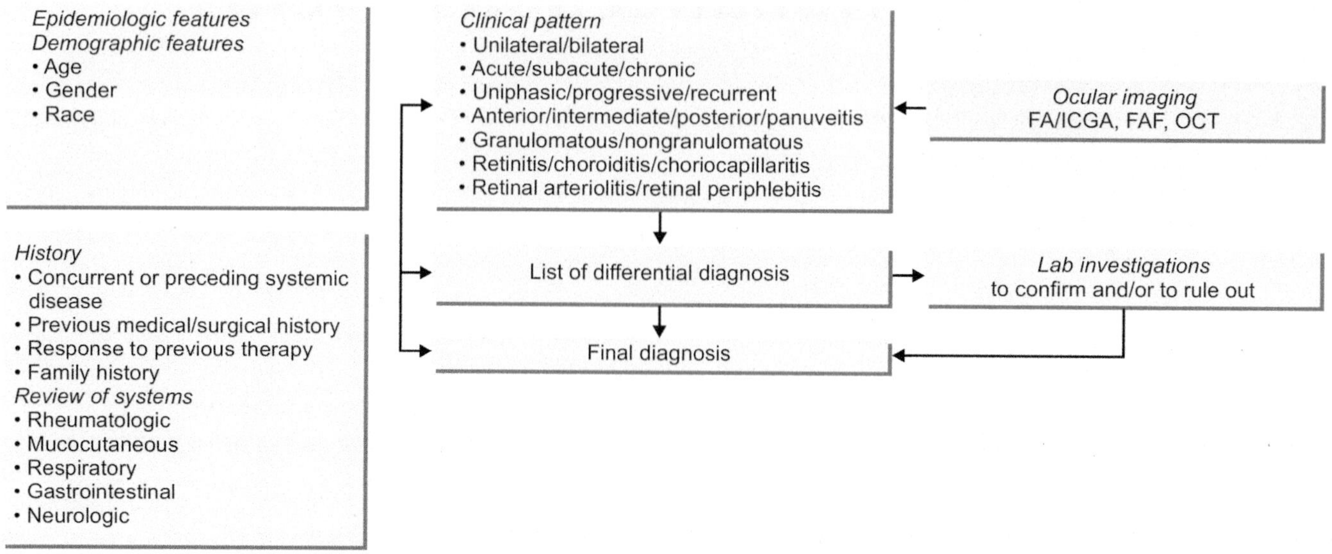

Fig. 85.1: Diagnostic approach to a patient with uveitis.
(FA: Fluorescein angiography; ICGA: Indocyanine green angiography; FAF: Fundus autofluorescence; OCT: Optical coherence tomography)

Table 85.2: Systemic investigations that should be considered in noninfectious uveitis.

Disease	Investigations
Ankylosing spondylitis	Imaging of sacroiliac joints, HLA-B27
Juvenile idiopathic arthritis	ANA, RF
Tubulointerstitial nephritis and uveitis	Renal function tests, urinalysis, β_2 microglobulin in urine, CBC, ESR, CRP, HLA-DQA1, HLA-DQB1, HLA-DRB1
Multiple sclerosis	Brain MRI, CSF analysis
Birdshot retinochoroiditis	HLA-A29
Sarcoidosis	Chest imaging, serum ACE, serum lysozyme, PPD, liver enzymes, serum and urinary calcium, bronchoalveolar lavage, tissue biopsy
Vogt-Koyanagi-Harada disease	CSF analysis, audiogram, HLA-DR4
Behçet's disease	Pathergy test, HLA-B51

(HLA: Human leukocyte antigen; ANA: Antinuclear antibody; RF: Rheumatoid factor; CBC: Complete blood count; ESR: Erythrocyte sedimentation rate; CRP: C-reactive protein; ACE: Angiotensin converting enzyme; MRI: Magnetic resonance imaging; CSF: Cerebrospinal fluid; PPD: Purified protein derivative)

Acute anterior uveitis (AAU) is more common than the chronic type. Patients with AAU typically present with sudden onset of redness, ocular pain, photophobia and the inflammation which has a limited duration. Chronic anterior uveitis typically has a more insidious onset, becomes symptomatic after development of significant complications and is characterized by persistent inflammation and/or relapses upon tapering or discontinuation of treatment.

HLA-B27 Associated Acute Anterior Uveitis

The AAU associated with the *HLA-B27* gene is the most common, well-defined anterior uveitic entity. Although intraocular inflammation may occur alone, 50–75% of HLA-B27 positive patients with uveitis also have spondyloarthropathies (SpA), most commonly ankylosing spondylitis (AS), or less frequently reactive arthritis (RA), psoriatic arthritis (PA), or inflammatory bowel disease (IBD).[4] There are also HLA-B27 negative patients with spondyloarthropathies and the distinct phenotype of acute anterior uveitis.

The HLA-B27 associated AAU is characterized by unilateral episodes of symptomatic, sudden onset non-granulomatous anterior uveitis. Recurrences may alternate between the two eyes. A marked ciliary injection, endothelial dusting, high-grade anterior chamber cells and flare are the typical clinical features. There may be spill-over of anterior vitreous cells. Prodromal symptoms such as ocular pain and photophobia often precede the development of clinical findings. If not adequately treated, the inflammation can get severe with an intense anterior chamber fibrin exudation, hypopyon, gluing of the pupil, and even diffuse cellular infiltration of the vitreous (Figs. 85.2A to D). The intraocular pressure (IOP) is typically low.[3,5,6] Clinically detectable macular edema is not an early finding however, cystoid macular edema (CME) may develop after a few weeks. Therefore, careful examination of the fundus and monitoring of macular thickness by optical coherence tomography (OCT) imaging may be required even when anterior segment inflammation seems to subside with treatment. Measurement of anterior chamber flare by laser flare photometry (LFP) has been reported to be a more reliable parameter than grading of anterior chamber cells for the timely administration of additional therapeutic measures in order to prevent complications.[7] The most frequent complication is permanent posterior synechiae. Steroid-induced cataract, ocular hypertension or glaucoma may develop. A minority of patients may go on to develop chronic un-remitting inflammation. An insidious-onset chronic bilateral uveitis involving the posterior segment may also develop in patients with HLA-B27-negative psoriatic arthritis or inflammatory bowel disease.[8]

In a prospective study that used a novel practical algorithm, the Dublin Uveitis Evaluation Tool (DUET), 40% of patients presenting with acute anterior uveitis were found to have previously undiagnosed SpA.[9] Patients with AAU especially those who are HLA-B27 positive, should be carefully questioned about lower back pain that improves by exercise, symptoms of arthritis, enthesitis, dactylitis and colitis as well as family history of SpA (Fig. 85.3).[10]

Early and effective treatment of acute anterior uveitis with frequent application of potent topical corticosteroids and diligent use of mydriatic and cycloplegic agents will lead to resolution of inflammation and minimize complications. Initiation of treatment at the onset of prodromal symptoms may prevent development of severe episodes. The prognosis is good with adequate treatment of inflammatory episodes.

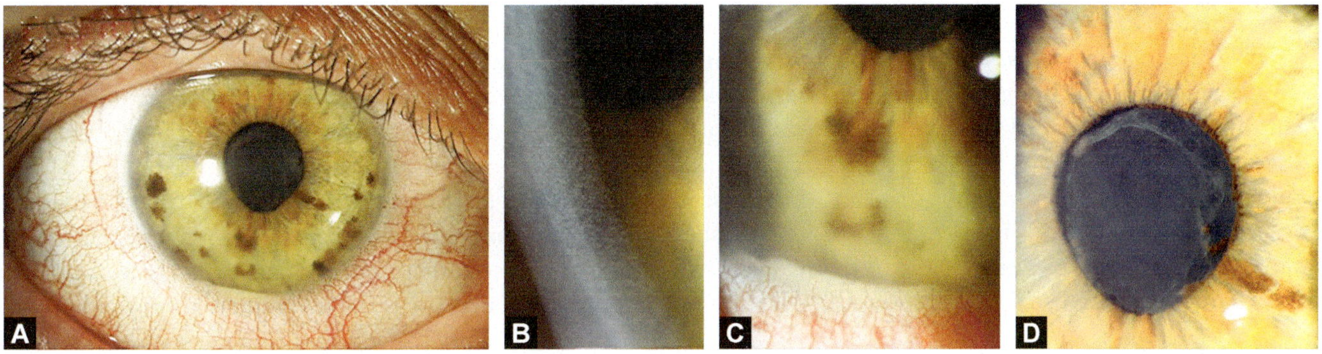

Figs. 85.2A to D: (A) Slit-lamp photograph of the right eye of a patient with HLA-B27-associated acute anterior uveitis show ciliary injection. (B) Corneal endothelial dusting; (C) Sticky hypopyon; (D) Fibrinous membrane in the pupillary area.

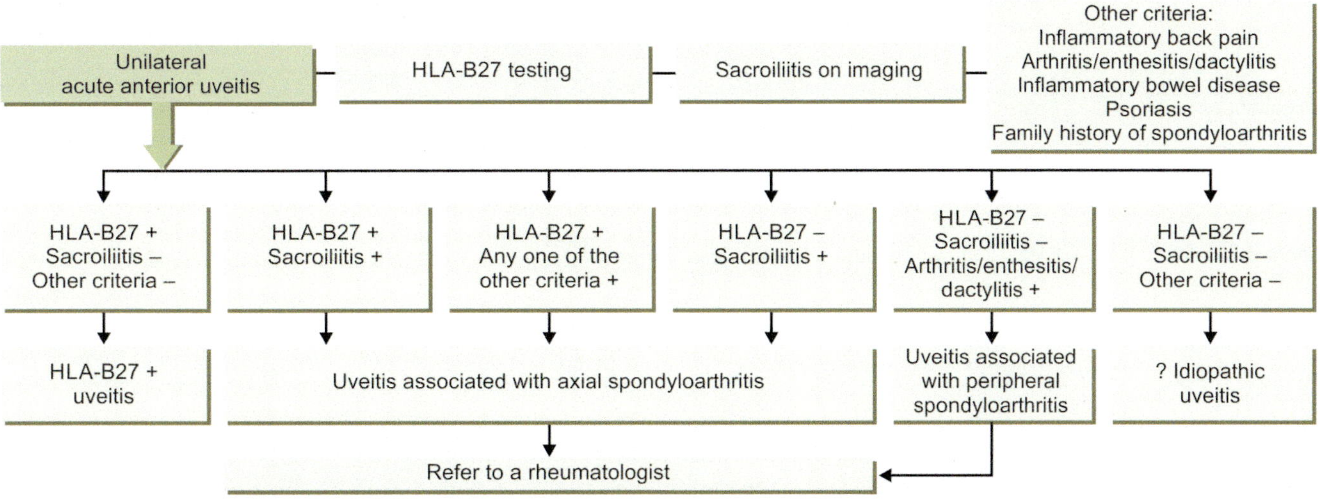

Fig. 85.3: Diagnostic approach to a patient with unilateral (may be alternating) acute anterior uveitis based on the classification criteria suggested by the Assessment of Spondyloarthritis International Society (ASAS). Note that the combination of inflammatory back pain, anterior uveitis, and positivity for HLA-B27 is sufficient to classify a patient as having axial spondyloarthritis.

In patients with frequent recurrences, sulfasalazine, methotrexate and oral nonsteroidal anti-inflammatory agents may be used in order to reduce the frequency and severity of the attacks. Monoclonal anti-TNF alpha antibodies may be needed in a minority.[5]

Juvenile Idiopathic Arthritis Associated Chronic Anterior Uveitis

Juvenile idiopathic arthritis (JIA) is the most common systemic association of uveitis in childhood. It is defined as chronic arthritis of unknown cause affecting at least one joint, persisting for at least 6 weeks in a child younger than 16 years of age. According to the International League of Association for Rheumatology (ILAR) criteria, JIA has seven subtypes (Table 85.3).[11] Uveitis is most common in the oligoarthritis subtype. Young age at the onset of arthritis, female gender, antinuclear antibody (ANA) positivity and rheumatoid factor negativity are risk factors for development of uveitis.[12]

The JIA-associated uveitis is characterized by insidious-onset, chronic, bilateral, nongranulomatous inflammation in the anterior segment of the eye.[13] Arthritis usually precedes the onset of uveitis and the majority of cases are diagnosed within 4 years from the onset of arthritis. Most of the cases have simultaneous involvement of both eyes and in patients with unilateral uveitis at diagnosis, involvement of the second eye is unusual after 12 months. Because of the asymptomatic onset and course of uveitis, periodic screening by slit-lamp examination is recommended depending on the JIA subtype and the presence of additional risk factors (Table 85.3).[14] In around 10% of the patients who develop uveitis before arthritis, the prognosis is worse because of delayed diagnosis and treatment.

Although the disease has a chronic course with persistent low-grade cells and perceptible flare in the anterior chamber, exacerbations may occur with numerous fine and sometimes medium sized keratic precipitates. Spill-over anterior vitreous cells may be seen with prolonged or severe inflammation. Elevated aqueous flare values as measured by LFP have been shown to be associated with complications at baseline and also indicate an increased risk of new complications. The most common complications are band keratopathy, posterior synechiae, cataract and ocular hypertension. Recent OCT studies have shown that macular edema is also a common complication (Figs. 85.4A to D). Glaucoma or phthisis may develop in most severe cases and cause irreversible blindness. A poorer prognosis has been associated with the presence of ocular complications at presentation, positive ANA, male gender, younger age at disease onset, a short period between onset of arthritis and uveitis and delayed diagnosis and treatment.[12,15]

Topical corticosteroids along with short-acting mydriatics and cycloplegic agents should be started at an adequate dose and tapered properly with close monitoring of the intraocular pressure. Inadequate response to topical

Table 85.3: Subtypes of juvenile idiopathic arthritis and recommended screening.

	Gender	Frequency of uveitis	Type of uveitis		ANA	Age at onset of JIA (years)	Duration of JIA (years)	Recommended frequency (months)
Oligoarthritis	F>M	25–30%	Chronic		+	≤6	≤4	3
					+	≤6	>4	6
Polyarthritis RF–	F>M	5–15%	Chronic		+	≤6	≥7	12
					+	>6	≤2	6
Psoriatic arthritis	F>M	10–20%	Chronic	Screening Guidelines	+	>6	>2	12
					–	≤6	≤4	6
Undifferentiated arthritis	F>M	%	Chronic		–	≤6	>4	12
					–	>6	N/A	12
Enthesis-related arthritis	M>F	10–15%	Acute		N/A	N/A	N/A	12
Polyarthritis RF+	F>M	< 5%	Chronic		N/A	N/A	N/A	12
Systemic arthritis	F=M	Rare			N/A	N/A	N/A	12

(JIA: Juvenile idiopathic arthritis; ANA: Antinuclear antibody; RF: Rheumatoid factor; N/A: Not applicable)

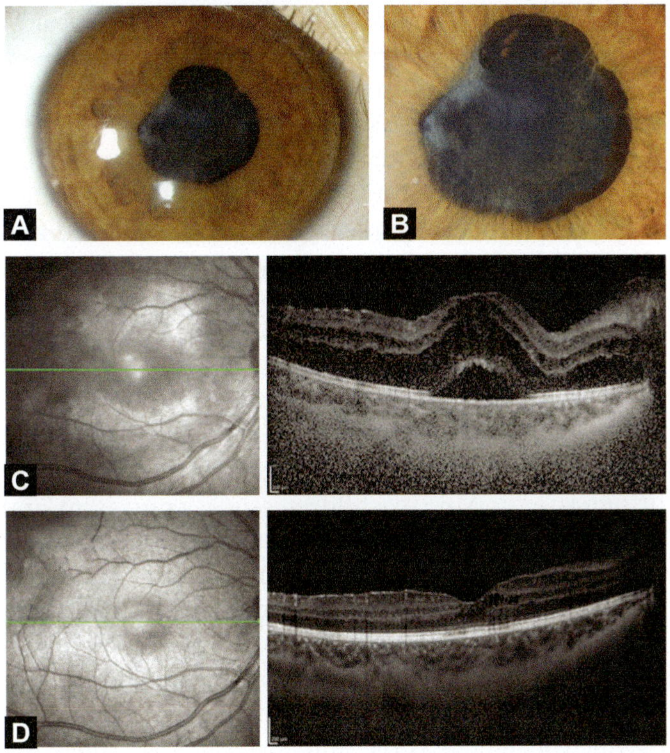

Figs. 85.4A to D: Slit-lamp photographs and OCT images of the right eye of a 10-year-old girl with JIA-associated chronic anterior uveitis resistant to conventional and anti-TNF therapy. (A) Slit-lamp photograph shows band keratopathy and extensive posterior synechiae; (B) Pupillary membrane; (C) OCT images show cystoid macular edema and its resolution; (D) After intravenous tocilizumab infusion.

treatment may be managed by a short course of systemic corticosteroids. Early immunomodulatory therapy with less tolerance for even low-grade inflammation decreases the risk of complications and improves visual prognosis. Methotrexate is generally used as first choice. In case of inefficacy or intolerance, other immunosuppressive agents such azathioprine or mycophenolate may be tried. Anti-TNF alpha therapy can be used upon failure of conventional treatment. The efficacy of adalimumab has been proven in a randomized controlled trial.[16] In case of anti-TNF failure, other biologic agents may be tried.

When surgical intervention is needed for the treatment of ocular complications, maximum suppression of intraocular inflammation with medical therapy is mandatory.[12] Due to a better control of intraocular inflammation with an earlier and increased use of immunomodulatory and biologic therapies, the need for cataract surgery has decreased, the age at surgery has been delayed and good outcomes can be obtained with intraocular lens implantation.

Tubulointerstitial Nephritis and Uveitis

Tubulointerstitial nephritis and uveitis (TINU) is a rare entity that typically affects young people with more female predominance. Patients have bilateral, sudden onset and non-granulomatous anterior uveitis. Posterior uveitis is rare. Uveitis may precede, occur simultaneously or follow the renal symptoms. A definite diagnosis can be made in the presence of a positive renal biopsy for tubulointerstitial nephritis. The presence of abnormal renal function and systemic symptoms such as fever, weight loss, fatigue, weakness and anorexia may suggest the diagnosis.[17] Urinary beta-2 microglobulin is highly sensitive to detect tubular function and may remain elevated for a long time in TINU patients.[18]

Renal disease may resolve spontaneously or may need corticosteroid therapy. Because of high recurrence rate and chronicity of uveitis in some TINU patients, ocular complications such as posterior synechiae, optic disk edema and/or macular edema may develop. Periocular or oral corticosteroids and/or immunomodulatory therapy may be required for long-term management.[17,19]

INTERMEDIATE UVEITIS

In intermediate uveitis (IU), the inflammation predominantly affects the vitreous, ciliary body and the peripheral retina. It may or may not be associated with systemic diseases such as sarcoidosis and multiple sclerosis (Table 85.4). Pars planitis is a subset of idiopathic intermediate uveitis characterized by formation of snowbanks and snowballs.[20]

Table 85.4: Noninfectious systemic diseases that may present with intermediate uveitis, and masquerading conditions that may mimic intermediate uveitis.

Noninfectious causes	Masquerade syndromes
Multiple sclerosis	Primary intraocular lymphoma
Sarcoidosis	Leukemia
Tubulointerstitial nephritis and uveitis	Retinoblastoma
Inflammatory bowel disease	Intravitreal hemorrhage
Reactive arthritis	Retinal detachment
Behçet's disease	Intraocular foreign body
ANCA-associated vasculitis	Synchysis scintillans/asteroid hyalosis
Systemic lupus erythematous	Retinitis pigmentosa
Autoimmune hepatitis	Amyloidosis

(ANCA: Antineutrophil cytoplasmic antibody)

Idiopathic IU most commonly affects patients of 5–35 years of age and does not show any gender predilection. The majority of patients have bilateral involvement.[21] Patients commonly present with floaters and blurred vision. The most typical findings at presentation include minimal or no anterior chamber inflammation, diffuse vitreous cells, moderate to high grade vitreous haze, bands, veils and condensations of especially inferior vitreous, optic disk inflammation, cystoid macular edema, peripheral retinal vascular sheathing and snowballs which are aggregates of inflammatory cells in the mid-vitreous and inferior vitreous (Figs. 85.5A to F). Snowbanks are inflammatory exudates over the pars plana region composed of inflammatory cells, fibroblasts and organized collagen.[21,22]

In children, pars planitis is the most common form of IU. Anterior chamber inflammation is also more pronounced without causing red or painful eyes. Early onset in childhood is related to more severity of disease. Peripheral corneal endotheliopathy is a common finding in children presenting as edema of the inferior peripheral cornea with underlying medium sized keratic precipitates. Band keratopathy, extensive posterior synechiae, high grade anterior chamber cells and flare and condensed anterior vitreous adherent to the posterior lens capsule may be seen at presentation. Children may also first present with vitreous hemorrhage resulting from NVD and/or NVE associated with snowbanks. Peripheral retinoschisis and/or exudative retinal detachment are also more common in children (Figs. 85.5A to F). CME is the most common cause of visual loss in all age groups.[22]

Treatment of uncomplicated intermediate uveitis is controversial. Treatment is required in the presence of vitreous haze causing visual blurring, CME or other complications caused by ongoing active inflammation. Periocular corticosteroid injections are preferentially applied in unilateral or asymmetrical involvement and in the management of CME. Systemic corticosteroids may be reserved for patients with bilateral involvement or recalcitrant unilateral uveitis. Intravitreal corticosteroid injections or implants may be used for the treatment of persistent CME. In children, short courses of oral corticosteroids may be preferred because of the high risk of glaucoma and cataract with local corticosteroid injections. Steroid-sparing immunosuppressive agents should be considered in patients who need prolonged treatment. When the conventional immunosuppressive agents are not sufficient to control the inflammation, biologic agents may be considered as the third step. Cryotherapy of the pars plana region and peripheral retina is not as widely employed as in the past because of the potential severe complications. Laser photocoagulation is mostly performed

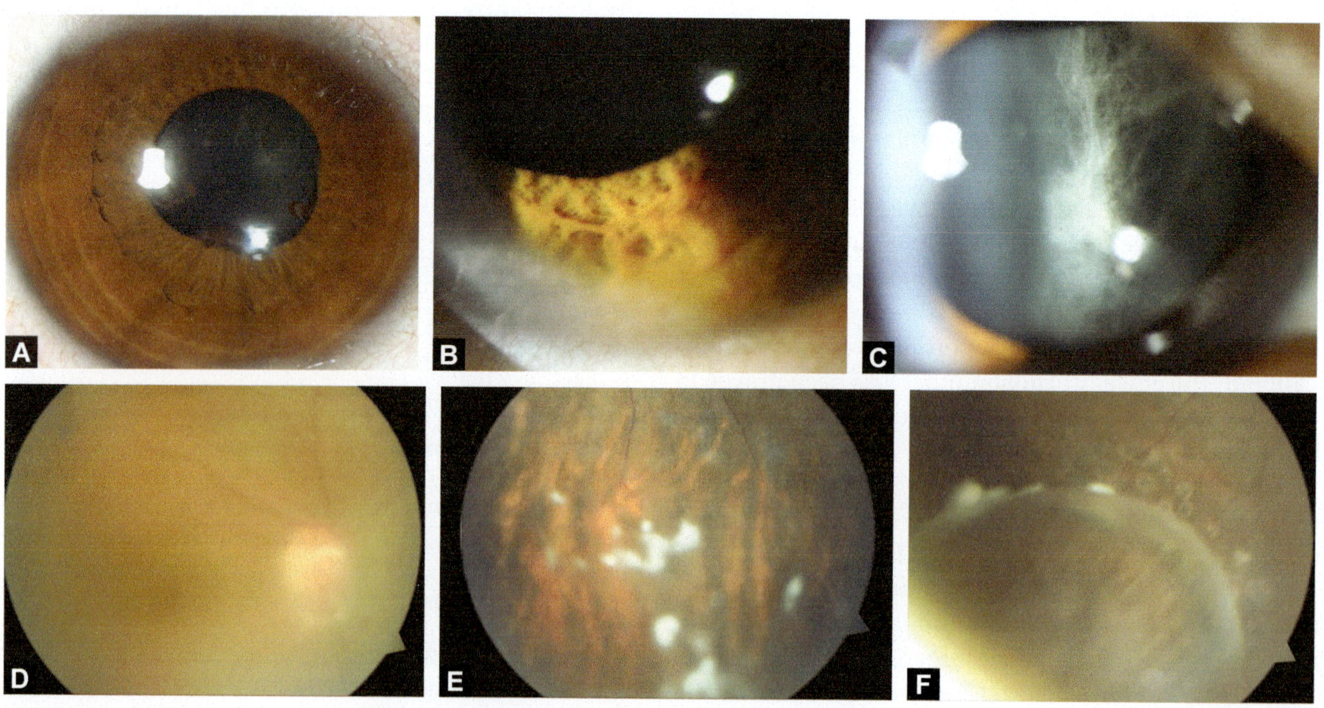

Figs. 85.5A to F: Slit-lamp and fundus photographs of children with pars planitis. (A) Slit-lamp photograph shows posterior synechiae; (B) Inferior peripheral corneal endotheliopathy; (C) Condensed anterior vitreous adherent to the posterior lens capsule; (D) Fundus photograph shows high-grade vitreous haze; (E) Snowballs in the inferior vitreous; (F) Inferior peripheral retinoschisis.

in eyes with peripheral neovascularizations and also to create a barrier in eyes with peripheral retinoschisis and/or exudative retinal detachments.[22] Pars plana vitrectomy (PPV) may be needed for posterior segment complications such as epiretinal membranes, vitreous tractions, persistent or recurrent vitreous hemorrhages or rhegmatogenous retinal detachments. Even though PPV was found to be associated with an increased probability of remission in a large retrospective cohort,[23] therapeutic vitrectomy is advocated by some but not all centers.

A complete remission can be observed in more than 40% of cases after several years of follow up.[24]

Multiple Sclerosis

While intermediate uveitis is the most common form of uveitis associated with multiple sclerosis (MS), the routine screening for MS is not generally recommended. On the other hand, patients with any current or past neurological symptoms suggestive of MS should be properly investigated. Patients with intermediate uveitis should also be informed about the risk of developing MS after several years. Bilaterality, female gender and the presence of peripheral retinal periphlebitis have been reported as risk factors for the development of MS.[25]

POSTERIOR UVEITIS

In posterior uveitis, the primary site of inflammation is the retina/choroid however, adjacent structures such as the vitreous body, optic nerve head and retinal vessels are frequently involved.[20] It may present in the form of focal, multifocal or diffuse choroiditis, chorioretinitis, retinochoroiditis, retinitis or neuroretinitis. Multimodal posterior imaging modalities are used for accurate localization as well as for assessment of the distribution of inflammatory lesions in the fundus. Color fundus photography, fundus autofluorescence imaging (FAF), fluorescein angiography (FA), indocyanine green angiography (ICGA), spectral domain (SD) retinal and choroidal OCT help in the differential diagnosis and monitoring of posterior uveitides. There are also an increasing number of reports describing features of different entities on OCT angiography, a new noninvasive imaging modality. Table 85.5 shows posterior uveitis that are collectively called white dot syndromes.[26-28] The choriocapillaris and outer retinal layers are primarily or exclusively affected in all of them except in birdshot retinochoroiditis. Anterior chamber inflammation is mild or absent in all except in multifocal choroiditis (MFC) and panuveitis.

Birdshot Retinochoroiditis

Birdshot retinochoroiditis is a chronic, slowly progressive, bilateral posterior uveitis characterized by involvement of the retinal vessels and the choroid. It is strongly associated with the HLA-A29 antigen, which is more prevalent in the Northern European populations. The average age at diagnosis is 50 years and patients often present with blurred vision, floaters, nyctalopia and photopsia. Although the characteristic fundus picture includes multiple yellow-white ovoid lesions, measuring 500–1500 μm diameter at the level of deep retina radiating from the disk throughout the post-equatorial fundus, these lesions are absent in early stages and mild-to-moderate vitritis, optic nerve head inflammation and CME may be the only clinical findings.[26-29]

Dual FA and ICGA confirm involvement of both the retina and the choroid, even in patients without birdshot lesions by showing retinal vascular and capillary leakage on FA and widespread hypofluorescent dots on ICGA (Figs. 85.6A to E). FAF displays hypoautofluorescent areas indicating RPE atrophy not exactly corresponding to the birdshot lesions. Although FA may show early hyperfluorescence with subtle late staining in early birdshot lesions, they are generally silent on FA. CME or perifoveal retinal thickening may be found on OCT. Subsequently, patchy or generalized disruption in ellipsoid zone (EZ) and generalized retinal thinning may be observed. Progressive choroidal thinning is seen in later stages. Both rod and cone functions may be disrupted in electroretinogram (ERG) and 30 Hz flicker response is most sensitive. Visual field examination may reveal enlarged blind spot, central/paracentral scotoma and/or peripheral constriction.[27,29] Both ERG and visual field are useful in monitoring sub-clinical functional impairment. However, ICGA is most useful in monitoring occult choroidal inflammation.

Because of the chronic progressive course of the disease and the risk of legal blindness reported in up to 9.8% of patients, early treatment is recommended. Local and systemic corticosteroids are used to suppress active inflammation. Steroid-sparing immunomodulatory treatment is required for the long-term disease control. Recently, TNF inhibitors and IL-2 receptor blocking agents have been employed successfully.[29,30]

Table 85.5: White dot syndromes.

	Birdshot Retinochoroiditis	Serpiginous choroiditis	MEWDS	APMPPE	MCP	PIC	SFU	AZOOR
Age	40s–60s	30s–60s	20s–50s	20s–30s	20s–60s	Young (<40)	10s–30s	Young woman
Gender	F > M	M = F	F > M	M = F	F > M	F > M	F > M	F > M
Laterality	Bilateral	Bilateral asymmetric	Unilateral	Bilateral	Bilateral	Bilateral	Bilateral	Variable (75% Bilateral)
Onset	Insidious	Variable	Acute	Acute	Insidious	Insidious	Insidious	Insidious
Prodrome	None	None	Variable	Variable	Variable	None	None	Variable
Symptoms	Blurred vision, floaters, photopsia, nyctalopia	Blurred vision, scotoma, photopsia, metamorphopsia	Blurred vision, scotomas, photopsia	Blurred vision, scotoma, photopsia	Blurred vision, scotoma, photopsia, floaters	Decreased visual acuity, scotoma, photopsia, metamorphopsia	Decreased visual acuity	Visual field defect, blurred vision, photopsia
Findings	Multiple, ill-defined, cream colored oval, postequatorial lesions, (500–1500 m)	Geographic zone of gray-yellow discoloration of RPE in peripapillary/ macular area with centripedal extension with active peripheral edge	Yellowish-white dots (100–200 m) in perimacular area and macular granularity	Multiple, flat, creamy colored, placoid lesions in different stages in posterior pole	Yellow-white lesions (50–100 m) which evolve into punch-out scars with pigmented borders	White-yellow chorioretinal lesions; punch-out scars deeper than those of MCP	Yellow-white lesions (50–500 m) posterior pole to midperiphery, subretinal fibrosis zones	Normal appearance or late pigment migration
Course	Chronic	Chronic	Self-limited	Self-limited	Chronic	Self-limited	Chronic	Self-limited or chronic
Anterior chamber/ vitreous inflammation	Moderate inflammation	No or mild inflammation	No inflammation	No inflammation	Moderate inflammation	No inflammation	Moderate inflammation	No or mild inflammation
FA	Vascular leakage; optic disk staining	Active: early hypo late hyperfluorescent Healing: staining of borders Scars: window defects	Early hyperfluorescent lesions in wreathlike configuration with late staining; optic disk staining	Early blockage with late staining in acute phase; window defects in later stage	Early hypofluorescent, late staining in acute phase; window defects of atrophic lesions	Early hypofluorescent, late staining in acute phase; window defects of atrophic lesions	Multiple areas of alternating hypo/ hyperfluorescent	Normal or changes such as hyperfluorescence, window defect and optic disk staining
ICG	Hypofluorescent dots in midphase more numerous than fundus exam or FA	Hypofluorescence of both active lesions and scars throughout the angiography	More hypofluorescent dots than detected on fundus exam or FA	More hypofluorescent plaques than detected on fundus exam or FA	More hypofluorescent lesions than detected on fundus exam or FA	Hypofluorescent spots corresponding to those seen on fundus exam or FA		Hypofluorescence corresponding to the zone of RPE change

Contd..

Contd..

	Birdshot Retinochoroiditis	Serpiginous choroiditis	MEWDS	APMPPE	MCP	PIC	SFU	AZOOR
FAF	Hypoautofluorescent of atrophic lesions	Hyperautofluorescent of active lesions and hypoautofluoresce of scars	Hypoautofluorescent dots	Hypoautofluorescent lesions	Hypoautofluorescent lesions	Hypoautofluorescent lesions with hyperautofluorescent margins		Normal or hyperautofluorescent
OCT	CME; EZ disruption; possible appearance of generalized atrophy of the choroid	Hyperreflectivity of outer retina; EZ disruption; increased reflectance of choroid	EZ disruption, hyperreflective material on RPE	Hyperreflective outer retinal layers in early period; EZ and outer retinal disruption; RPE atrophy	Deposition of material in sub-RPE area; choroidal thickening beneath lesions; vitreous cells	Focal elevation of RPE with hyporeflective space and focal thickening of choroid in acute stage; focal atrophy of the outer retina and RPE and focal thinning of choroid in chronic stage	Subretinal fibrosis and fluid	Loss or irregularity of outer retinal layers
ERG/EOG	Abnormal rod and cone ERG	Normal	Abnormal ERG	Abnormal ERG and EOG, improves with disease resolution	Normal or abnormal ERG	Normal	Abnormal ERG/EOG	Abnormal ERG
Treatment	CS, IMT, IVIG, anti-TNF alpha	CS, IMT, anti-VEGF for CNV	Observation	Observation	CS; IMT, anti-VEGF for CNV	Observation or CS; anti-VEGF for CNV	CS, IMT, anti-TNF alpha, rituximab	Observation
Structural complications	Disk edema, CME, retinal and choroidal thinning, CNV	CNV, RPE mottling, scarring	Optic disk edema, rarely CNV	Mild scarring	Optic disk edema; peripapillary atrophy, CME, CNV	CNV, serous detachment over confluent lesions	Neurosensory retinal detachment, subretinal fibrosis, CME, CNV	RPE mottling, occasional CME
Prognosis	Guarded	Guarded	Very good	Good	Guarded	Good	Poor	Guarded

(MEWDS: Multiple evanescent white dot syndrome; APMPPE: Acute posterior multifocal placoid pigment epitheliopathy; MCP: Multifocal choroditis and panuveitis; PIC: Punctate inner choroidopathy; SFU: Subretinal fibrosis and uveitis; AZOOR: Acute zonal occult outer rethinopathy; F: Female; M: Male; VA: Visual acuity; AC: Anterior chamber; FA: Fluorescein angiography; ICG: Indocyanine green angiography; FAF: Fundus autofluorescence; OCT: Optical coherence tomography; ERG: Electroretinography; EOG: Electrooculography; EZ: Ellipsoid zone; CME: Cystoid macular edema; CNV: Choroidal neovascularization; RPE: Retina pigment epithelium; CS: Corticosteroid; IMT: Imunomodulatory treatment; TNF: Tumor necrosis factor; VEGF: Vascular endothelial growth factor)

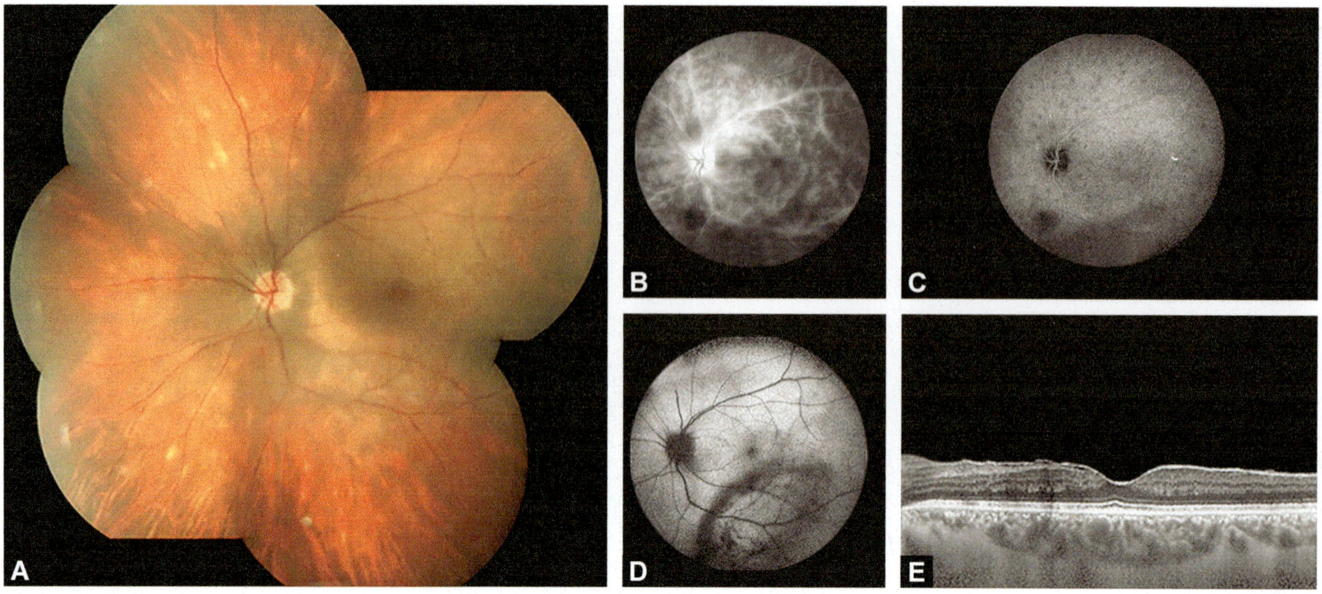

Figs. 85.6A to E: Multimodal imaging of the left eye of a 37-year-old man with HLA-A29-positive birdshot retinochoroiditis involving both eyes symmetrically. (A) Composite color fundus photograph shows faint birdshot lesions radiating from around the optic disk; (B) Dual fluorescein and indocyanine green frames at 11 minutes of the angiogram show disk staining and diffuse retinal vascular leakage on FA; (C) Numerous dark dots on ICGA; (D) FAF image only shows shadowing by posterior vitreous opacity; (E) OCT shows an epiretinal membrane and mild retinal thinning.

Serpiginous Choroiditis

Serpiginous choroiditis is a rare, bilateral, chronic recurrent inflammation of the inner choroid and outer retina that is typically seen in middle-aged patients. Presenting symptoms are blurred vision, central/paracentral scotoma, photopsia and metamorphopsia. Fundus examination reveals retinochoroidal lesions originating in the peripapillary area spreading outwards in an irregular serpentine fashion with finger-like projections and leaving prominent chorioretinal scarring. Recurrent inflammation typically develops at the border of the scars and is seen as a gray-white extension at the level of the RPE (Figs. 85.7A to D). Choroidal neovascularization (CNV) develops in 13–35% of the patients.[31]

The FA displays early hypo- and late diffuse hyperfluorescence of acute lesions and hyperfluorescent border of subacute lesions. Both active lesions and inactive scars appear hypofluorescent on ICGA and the full extent of involved area is better perceived. On FAF imaging, scars are hypoautofluorescent and active lesions may present as a hyperautofluorescent halo. However, ICGA is the earliest to detect inner choroidal inflammation. Active lesions demonstrate hyper-reflectivity of the outer retina with disruption of EZ on OCT imaging. Enhanced-depth imaging (EDI)-OCT may show focal choroidal thickening and loss of inner choroidal reflectivity. Loss of outer retinal layers and thinning and hyper-reflectivity of the underlying choroid are seen with the formation of scars (Fig. 85.8).[27,31,32]

Active inflammation should be controlled rapidly with corticosteroids to limit scarring, protect the fovea and prevent formation of CNV. Several lines of immunomodulatory agents singly or in combination have been used with variable success.

Although latent tuberculosis is more typically associated with serpiginous-like or multifocal serpiginoid choroiditis that may first involve the macula, it should also be ruled out in all patients with classical serpiginous choroiditis, as described here.

Multiple Evanescent White Dot Syndrome

Multiple evanescent white dot syndrome (MEWDS) is a unilateral, acute, self-limiting posterior uveitis that affects mostly young and healthy females. Patients present with acute onset of blurred vision, temporal and/or paracentral scotoma, dyschromatopsia and photopsia. Antecedent viral illness is reported in about one-third of the cases. Fundus picture is characterized by multiple, faint, yellowish-white spots (100–200 μ) in the peripapillary and perimacular area and complete resolution of these lesions occurs spontaneously within 6–12 weeks. Foveal granularity is a

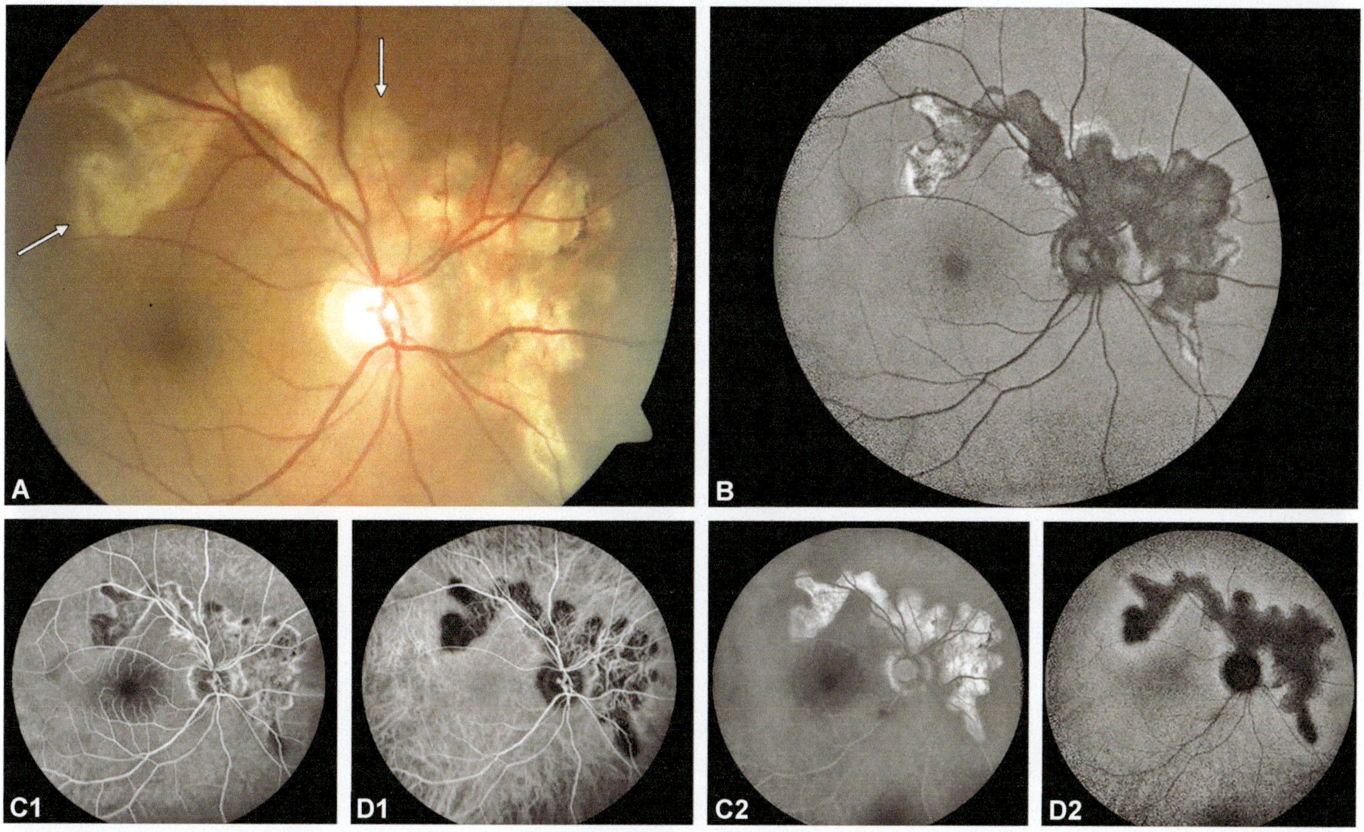

Figs. 85.7A to D: Color fundus photographs, FAF, FA and ICGA imaging of the right eye of a 53-year-old man with serpiginous choroiditis. (A) Fundus photograph shows chorioretinal scar with a serpentine pattern radiating from the peripapillary area and faint grayish active inflammation at the edges indicated by arrows; (B) FAF shows hypoautofluorescence of old scars, bright hyperautofluorescence of subacute areas, and hyperautofluorescent halo of active fronds; (C) Active fronds appear early hypo- and late diffuse hyperfluorescent on FA; (D) The whole lesion is hypofluorescent on ICGA.

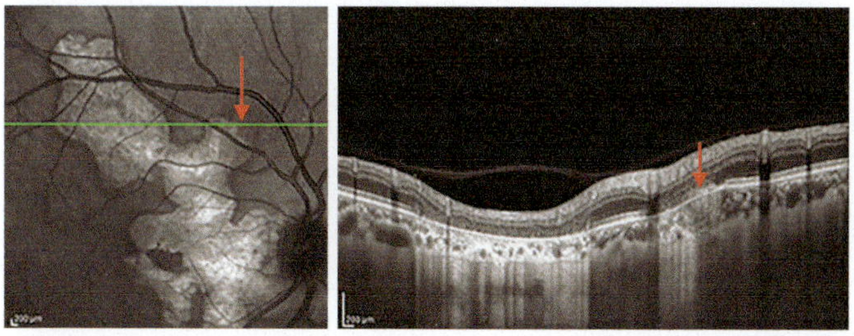

Fig. 85.8: Ocular coherence tomography (OCT) section through the active frond (arrows) in the right eye of a patient with serpiginous choroiditis shows disruption of the outer retinal layers and mild choroidal thickening with loss of choroidal vascular lumens beneath the active region; and loss of outer retinal layers, hyper-reflectivity and thinning of the underlying choroid in the scarred areas, causing an increased transmission effect.

pathognomonic sign and may persist after resolution of the white dots.[26,27]

The FA shows late hyperfluorescent dots in a wreath-like configuration and ICGA exhibits more hypofluorescent lesions than those detected on fundus examination or FA. Hyperautofluorescence is seen on FAF in the acute period. Foveal granularity may cause hypoautofluorescence. OCT reveals a disrupted EZ and accumulated hyper-reflective debris on the RPE and then, normalization of outer retinal layers with resolution of white dots (Figs. 85.9A to H). ERG and EOG show abnormalities in the acute stage that are also normalized with resolution of the disease.[27]

Because of self-limiting character of the disease and good visual prognosis, no treatment is required.

Acute Posterior Multifocal Placoid Pigment Epitheliopathy

Acute posterior multifocal placoid pigment epitheliopathy (APMPPE) is a bilateral, acute onset, self-limiting posterior uveitis that is seen in young adults of both genders. Patients present with a sudden onset of blurred vision and central and paracentral scotomas, typically in both eyes. Flu-like symptoms precede in about one-third of the cases and an associated cerebral vasculitis may rarely develop within a few weeks after the onset. Ophthalmoscopy shows multifocal, yellowish-white placoid lesions at the level of

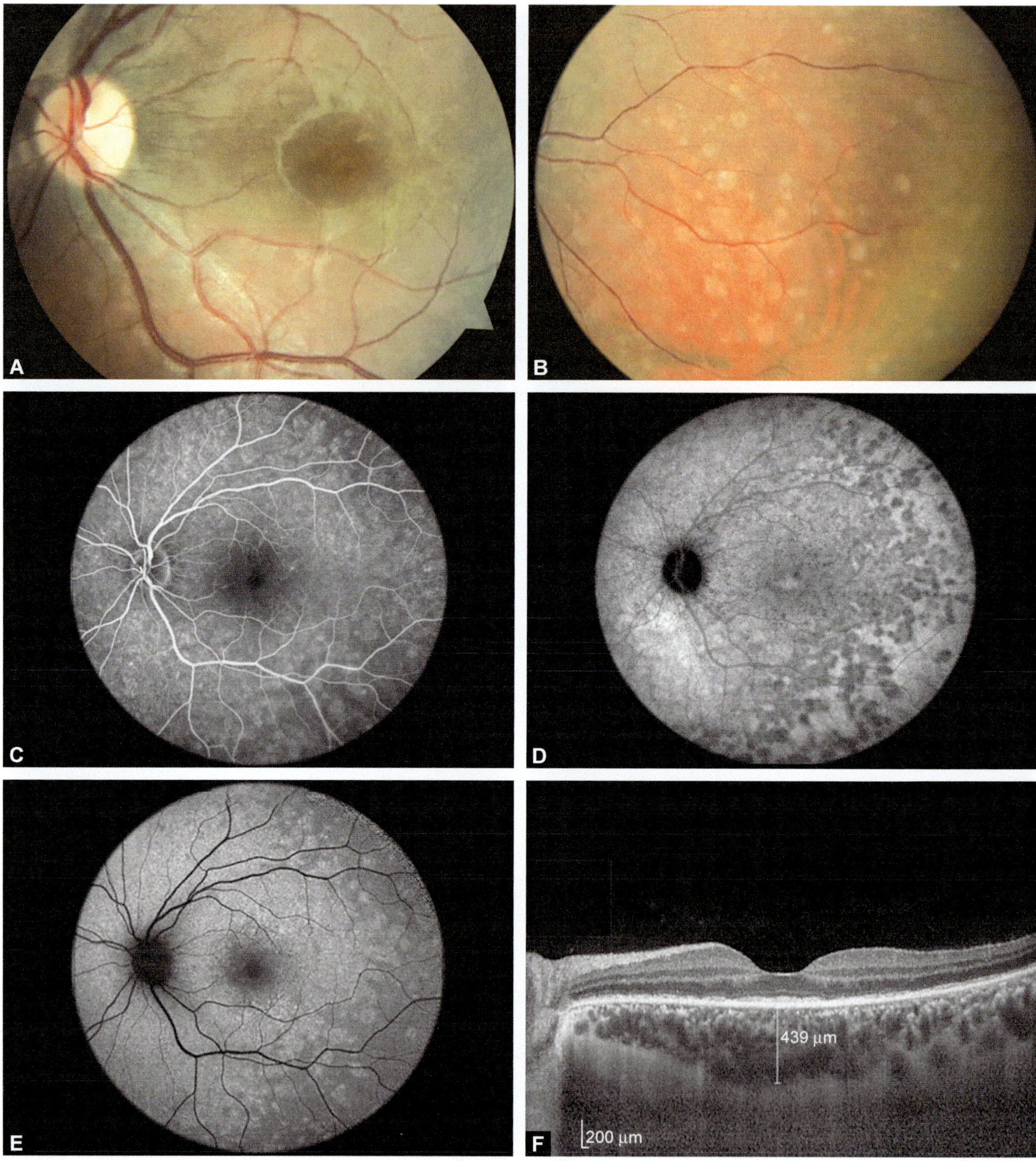

Figs. 85.9A to F

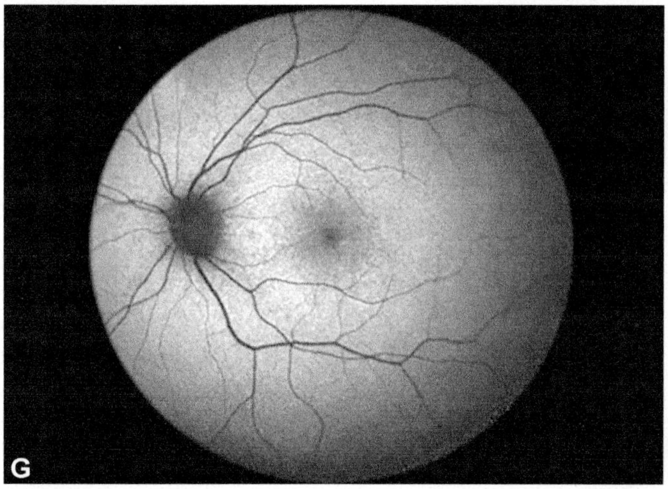

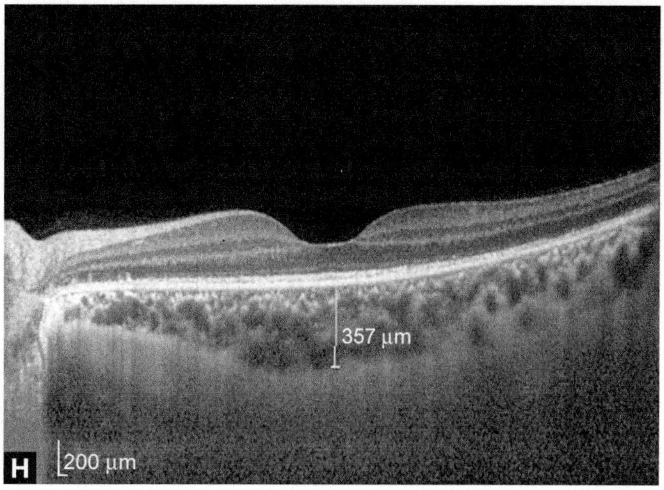

Figs. 85.9G and H

Figs. 85.9A to H: Multimodal imaging of the left eye of a 26-year-old woman with multiple evanescent white dot syndrome (MEWDS). (A) Color fundus photograph shows foveal granularity; (B) Faint white dots; (C) Dots are hyperfluorescent on FA; (D) Hypofluorescent on ICGA. (E) Hyperautofluorescent on FAF; (F) EDI-OCT shows disruption of the ellipsoid zone; (G) 1 month later, dots have mostly disappeared on FAF; (H) The ellipsoid zone has been mostly restored.

the RPE at the posterior pole and scattered posterior to the equator. New lesions may appear during the first few weeks after the onset. Placoid lesions fade gradually within a few weeks with minimal scarring.[26,28]

The characteristic FA pattern of APMPPE is early hypofluorescence and late hyperfluorescent staining. ICGA reveals hypofluorescent lesions more numerous than seen on ophthalmoscopy or FA. Hyper-reflective outer retinal layers, disruption of EZ and RPE atrophy are seen in OCT images. A focal serous retinal detachment may be seen in some lesions. Abnormal ERG and EOG findings that are seen in acute phase normalize with the resolution of the disease suggesting that APMPPE may be a transient RPE problem.[27]

The APMPPE is generally a self-limiting disease with a good visual prognosis. Corticosteroid treatment is suggested only in patients with foveal involvement causing profound visual loss or in cases of CNS vasculitis.[26]

Multifocal Choroiditis and Panuveitis, Punctate Inner Choroiditis, Subretinal Fibrosis and Uveitis

These entities may represent variants of a bilateral chronic recurrent posterior uveitis predominantly affecting myopic women. Patients may present with blurred vision, photopsia, scotoma or metamorphopsia with the emergence of new lesions that appear as discrete deep yellow-white spots or the development of CNV at the posterior pole, usually in an eye with numerous small (50–100 μm in size) randomly distributed chorioretinal scars. Curvilinear chorioretinal streaks (Schlaegel lines) may be seen in the far periphery. Anterior uveitis and vitritis may accompany active lesions in multifocal choroiditis and panuveitis (MCP) and subretinal fibrosis and uveitis (SFU) whereas intraocular inflammation is absent in punctate inner choroiditis (PIC), where punch-out atrophic and pigmented scars are confined to the posterior pole and rarely spread out to the periphery. While peripapillary subretinal fibrosis may develop in MCP, progressive diffuse subretinal fibrosis in the posterior pole and mid-periphery is a characteristic feature of SFU.[26]

New lesions show early hypofluorescence with late staining and old scars show window defects on FA. More hypofluorescent lesions can be identified on ICGA than on fundus examination. FAF demonstrates diffuse peripapillary and perimacular hyperautofluorescent areas that fade with treatment and the hypoautofluorescent scars. A ring of hyperautofluorescence has been described in PIC lesions. OCT demonstrates disruption of photoreceptor-RPE complex. Active lesions show a consistent appearance of RPE elevation with deposition of homogenous material of medium reflectivity. Subsequent infiltration of the sub-retinal space and outer retina leads to loss of the outer retinal architecture. There may be slight thickening of the choroid beneath the active lesions.

Visual field examination may reveal an enlarged blind spot and sometimes peripheral loss of field. Electrophysiological tests show variable results. Multifocal ERGs generally demonstrate loss of function.[27]

Systemic corticosteroid therapy has been shown to reduce outer retinal inflammation and subsequent damage. There is no standard long-term therapy that is uniformly effective. Intravitreal anti-VEGF treatment is considered in case of CNV formation.[28] The prognosis is especially poor in SFU. There are only a few publications in the literature reporting successful results with infliximab or rituximab therapy.[33,34]

Acute Zonal Occult Outer Retinopathy

The acute zonal occult outer retinopathy (AZOOR) is a unilateral or bilateral condition that occurs mostly in young and myopic women. Presenting symptoms include chronic photopsia and visual field loss. Ocular examination reveals mild vitritis with no or minimal retinal findings at presentation. Pigment clumping and RPE atrophy may develop in the affected zone with time.[26]

Visual field testing demonstrates loss of temporal visual field including the blind spot. This defect may expand with time. ERG is abnormal.[26] FA may be completely normal while FAF mostly shows hyperautofluorescence[35] and OCT reveals loss or irregularity of outer retinal layers in the affected zone.

Visual prognosis is quite good.[36] Most of the patients stabilize without any recurrence however, one-third experience recurrences. No efficient treatment has yet been found for AZOOR. [28]

PANUVEITIS

Panuveitis is a generalized intraocular inflammation involving both the anterior and posterior segments of the eye. There is usually an underlying systemic disease that needs to be treated and the risk of vision threatening complications is higher compared to the other anatomic forms.

Sarcoidosis

Sarcoidosis is a multisystem inflammatory disease characterized by non-caseating granulomas in lymph nodes, lung, and various other organs including the eyes and periocular structures. Intraocular inflammation occurs in around 20% of patients and may present in any anatomic form. Sarcoid uveitis is more common in women and majority of the patients have bilateral involvement. A chronic granulomatous panuveitis is seen in one-third of the patients.

Signs of granulomatous inflammation in the anterior segment include mutton-fat keratic precipitates, iris nodules (sticky Koeppe nodules at the pupillary margin and Busacca nodules in iris stroma), trabecular meshwork nodules and tent-shaped peripheral anterior synechia (PAS). Snowballs may be seen forming a string configuration named "string of pearls". Multiple small, round, yellowish-white chorioretinal lesions are found especially in the inferior peripheral fundus. Active lesions have faint borders whereas scars have sharp margins. Solitary choroidal granuloma and nodules or granulomas at the optic disk are rare but highly suggestive findings for sarcoidosis. Periphlebitis is a common finding characterized by segmental or extensive sheathing and perivenous exudates described as "candle wax drippings" (Figs. 85.10A to D). The presence of macroaneurisms in an inflamed eye is also considered typical for sarcoid uveitis.[37-39] Angiographic imaging reveals perivascular leakage, optic disk staining, early blockage with late staining of active chorioretinal lesions on FA. Manifest or occult choroidal granulomas appear as hypofluorescent dots in the mid-phase becoming isofluorescent in the late phase of ICGA.[27] Late diffuse choroidal hyperfluorescence and peripheral pin-point hyperfluorescence may also be present.[39]

A definitive diagnosis of sarcoidosis requires biopsy confirmation. A presumed or probable diagnosis can be made in patients with suggestive ocular findings and systemic investigations such as bilateral hilar lymphadenopathy, elevated serum angiotensin converting enzyme (ACE) and serum lysozyme levels and a negative tuberculin skin test. Syphilis and tuberculosis must be excluded in all patients.[39]

The CME is a common complication of chronic sarcoid uveitis. Cataract caused by severe inflammation and/or long-term use of steroids and glaucoma caused by trabecular obstruction with inflammatory cells, trabecular nodules or PAS are other serious ocular complications of sarcoid uveitis.[38]

Sarcoid uveitis usually responds well to corticosteroids. Immunosuppressive treatment may be required in chronic cases. In refractory patients, treatment with TNF-alpha inhibitors may be an alternative.[38,40]

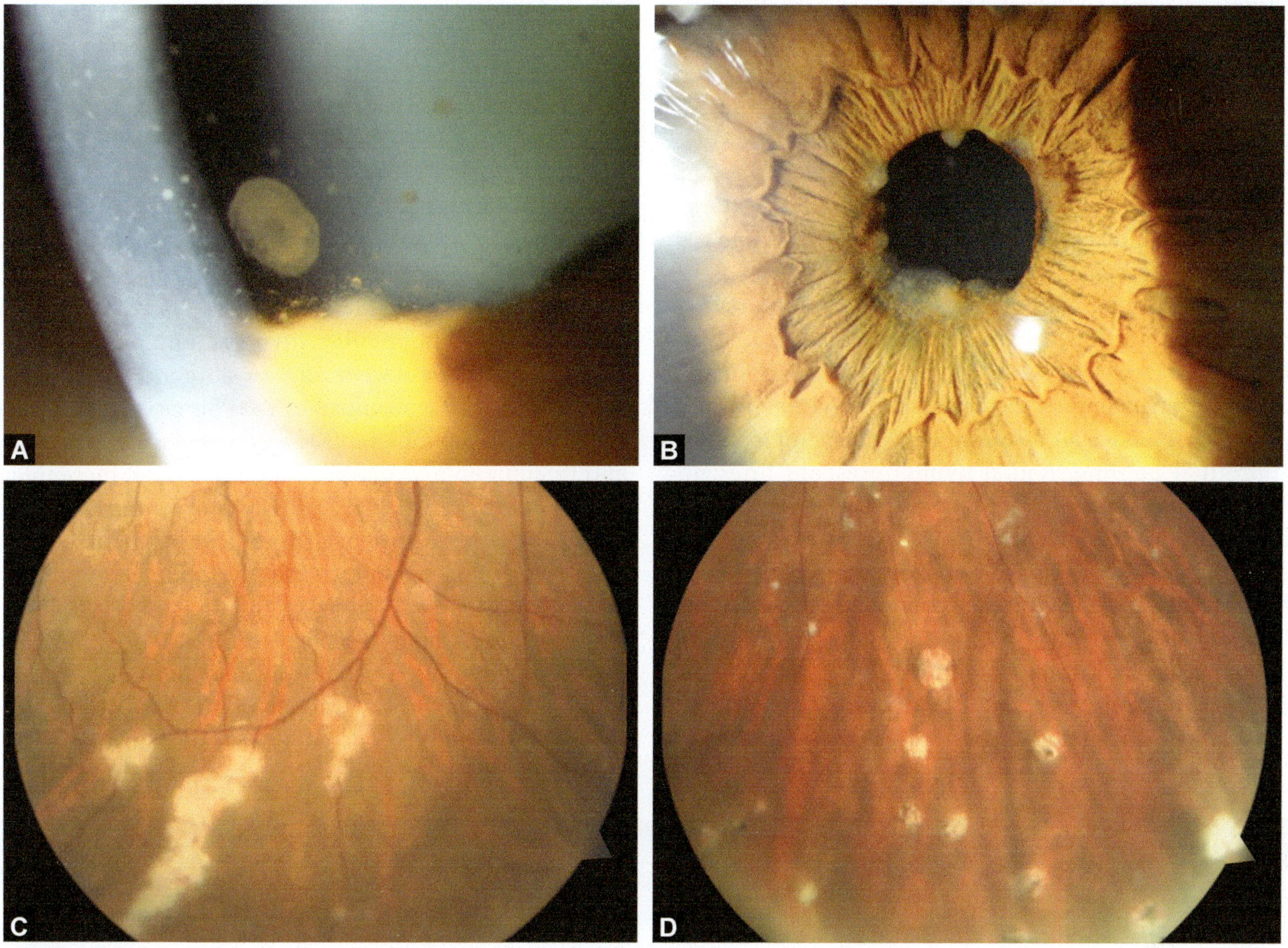

Figs. 85.10A to D: Slit-lamp and fundus photographs of patients with sarcoidosis. (A) Slit-lamp photograph shows mutton-fat keratic precipitates; (B) Sticky Koeppe nodules; (C) Fundus photograph shows periphlebitis that looks like candle wax drippings; (D) Inferior peripheral chorioretinal scars.

Vogt-Koyanagi-Harada Disease

Vogt-Koyanagi-Harada (VKH) disease is an autoimmune inflammatory disease characterized by bilateral, granulomatous panuveitis associated with central nervous system (CNS), auditory and integumentary manifestations. Environmental factors are thought to trigger a T-lymphocyte mediated autoimmunity against melanocytes in genetically susceptible individuals. It is more prevalent in Asians, Native Americans, Hispanics, Asian Indians, and Middle Easterners. It is more common in women. Typical age of onset is 30–40 years but it is also seen in children and less commonly in elderly patients.[41]

The course of VKH disease has four stages. In the *prodromal stage*, patients may have CNS and auditory symptoms such as headache, meningismus, nausea, vertigo, fever, orbital pain, tinnitus, and hearing loss lasting for a few days or weeks. Cerebrospinal fluid pleocytosis may be found at this stage. *Acute uveitic stage* starts with sudden onset of blurred vision. Although the primary site of inflammation is the choroid, patients may first present with optic disk inflammation. Swelling of the ciliary body and forward displacement of the iris-lens diaphragm may cause myopization and acute angle closure. Bilateral exudative retinal detachment will develop as a result of diffuse severe choroiditis. In the *convalescent stage*, resolution of inflammation is observed with pigment clumping and depigmentation in the fundus. Choroidal depigmentation results in "sunset glow" fundus which is characterized by a bright orange-red discoloration of the fundus in inadequately treated patients. Small atrophic lesions which are named Dallen-Fuchs nodules may be seen. Integumentary findings may develop at this stage. *Chronic recurrent stage* is characterized by granulomatous anterior uveitis however, there is usually occult choroiditis that may occasionally result in recurrent exudative retinal detachments. Ocular complications such as cataract, glaucoma, band keratopathy, subretinal fibrosis and CNV develop at this stage.[41,42]

Multimodal imaging helps in the diagnosis and monitoring of VKH disease. In the *acute uveitic stage*, B-scan ultrasonography shows a diffuse, low to medium reflective thickening of the choroid; FA reveals optic disk hyperfluorescence and "starry night" pin-point leaks with subretinal pooling. Radial hypofluorescent lines may also be seen. There is no retinal vascular leakage. Typical findings on ICGA include delayed choroidal perfusion, early hyperfluorescence of choroidal stromal vessels, hypofluorescent dots in the intermediate phase that fade in the late phase. OCT/EDI-OCT shows multilobular exudative retinal detachments with subretinal septae, RPE undulations and inward bowing, diffuse choroidal thickening with homogenous hyporeflectivity, loss of inner choroidal hyperreflectivity and reduction of choroidal vessel lumens (Figs. 85.11A to I).[41,42]

With an effective treatment of acute disease, subretinal fluid resolves and choroidal thickness decreases gradually both of which can be monitored non-invasively by OCT/EDI-OCT imaging. However, ICGA is the most reliable imaging method to monitor resolution of choroidal inflammation and to detect occult relapses in the posterior segment during the chronic stage of VKH disease.[41,42]

The diagnosis of VKH disease is based on clinical findings. Bilateral ocular involvement and absence of a history of ocular trauma or surgery are absolute requirements for a diagnosis of VKH disease which can be categorized as complete VKH when ocular CNS/auditory and integumentary manifestations are seen; incomplete when ocular and CNS/auditory or integumentary manifestations are present and probable when there are no extraocular manifestations.[43] The development of complete disease can be prevented by treatment.

High dose systemic corticosteroids are administered to control acute VKH usually given as pulse intravenous treatment, followed by oral corticosteroids with a slow taper over 6–9 months. Concurrent immunosuppressive

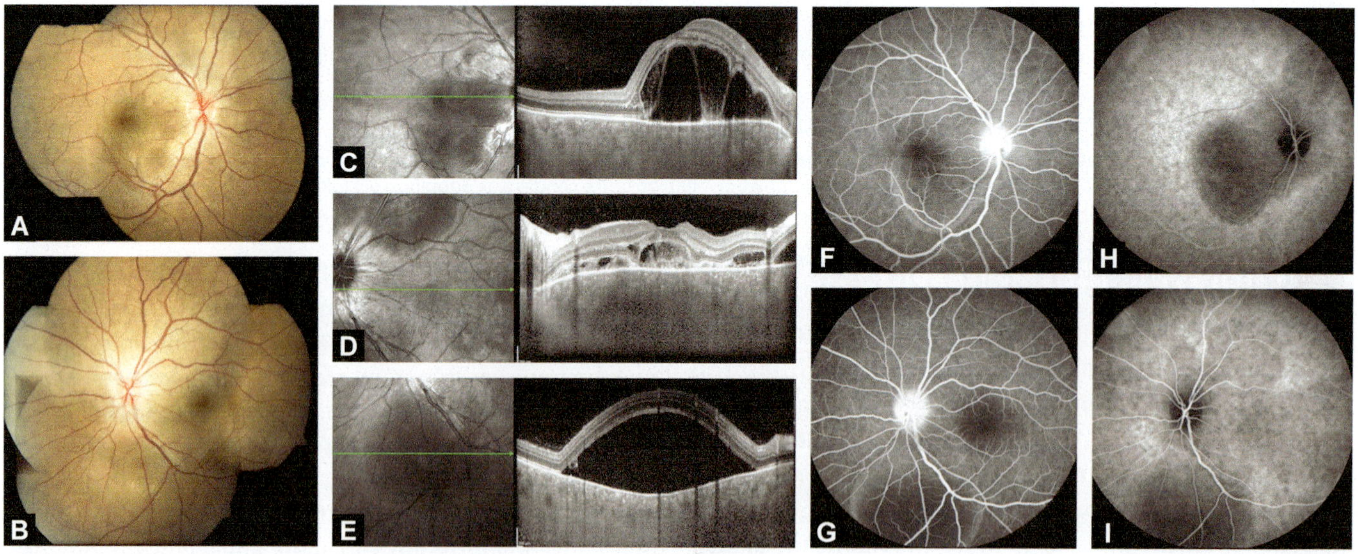

Figs. 85.11A to I: Color fundus photographs, OCT and angiographic images of both eyes of a 30-year-old woman with Vogt-Koyanagi-Harada disease. (A and B) Color fundus photographs of the right and the left eye show hyperemic optic disks and pockets of subretinal fluid at the posterior pole and peripapillary region; (C) OCT section through the fovea shows a high exudative retinal detachment with thin septae in the right eye; (D) Hyper-reflective subretinal fluid with thick septae in the left eye as well as thickening and hyporeflectivity of the choroid with reduced large vessel lumens in both eyes. (E) A high detachment with clear subretinal fluid is seen on OCT section of the pocket inferior to the optic disk in the left eye; (F and G) Late phase FA shows optic disk staining and faint marking of the borders of retinal detachment by pooling of the dye in the right and the left eye; (H and I) Mid-phase ICGA shows diffuse hypofluorescent dots and hypofluorescence corresponding to the pockets of subretinal fluid in the right and the left eye.

treatment has been reported to provide a better prognosis. There is an absolute indication for immunomodulatory therapy in patients presenting at the chronic recurrent stage. Anti-TNF or other biologic agents should be considered in patients refractory to conventional therapy.[41,42,44]

Sympathetic Ophthalmia

Sympathetic opthalmia (SO) is a rare, bilateral, granulomatous uveitis which develops after an ocular trauma or surgery. Its incidence is 0.2–0.5% after trauma and 0.01% after surgery. A non-perforating procedure such as irradiation of the eye, plaque brachytherapy and cyclodestructive therapy may rarely cause SO. The eye which is exposed to the trauma or surgery is named the "exciting" eye and the fellow eye is referred as the "sympathizing" eye. The time between the trauma or surgery and the onset of SO varies from 5 days to 50 years however, most of them occur within the first year. The role of primary enucleation for the prevention of SO is controversial and it is only suggested for an eye that is considered impossible to reconstruct. Early enucleation after the onset of SO is also debatable because the final visual acuity in the exciting eye may be better than the sympathizing eye.[45-47]

The SO has a clinical and pathological picture similar to VKH disease, both in the acute and chronic phase. Moreover, patients with SO may rarely demonstrate similar extraocular findings. The history of ocular injury or surgery is the main differentiating feature.[48] The treatment of SO shares the same principles as VKH.

Behçet's Disease

Behçet's disease (BD) is a multisystem inflammatory disorder that affects primarily the young adults. It has a high prevalence in populations along the ancient Silk Road. Both autoinflammatory and autoimmune mechanisms are involved in the pathogenesis. It has a strong association with the HLA-B51 antigen.[49]

The diagnosis is based on clinical criteria including recurrent oral ulcers, genital ulcers, skin lesions, uveitis and a positive skin pathergy test.[50] Other manifestations can be seen as well such as arthritis, epididymitis, thrombophlebitis, gastrointestinal and central nervous system lesions. Uveitis is the initial manifestation in 10–15% of patients. Men have more severe disease than women.[51]

Ocular involvement is characterized by bilateral non-granulomatous panuveitis and retinal vasculitis with a relapsing and remitting course. Severe episodes may be associated with a smooth-layered shifting hypopyon. Diffuse vitreous cells and haze, papillitis, retinal infiltrates and hemorrhages, occlusive periphlebitis and diffuse retinal edema are seen at acute episodes.[52] Retinal infiltrates resolve rapidly without visible scarring however, may lead to retinal nerve fiber layer defects when located at the posterior pole.[53] During resolution of vitritis,

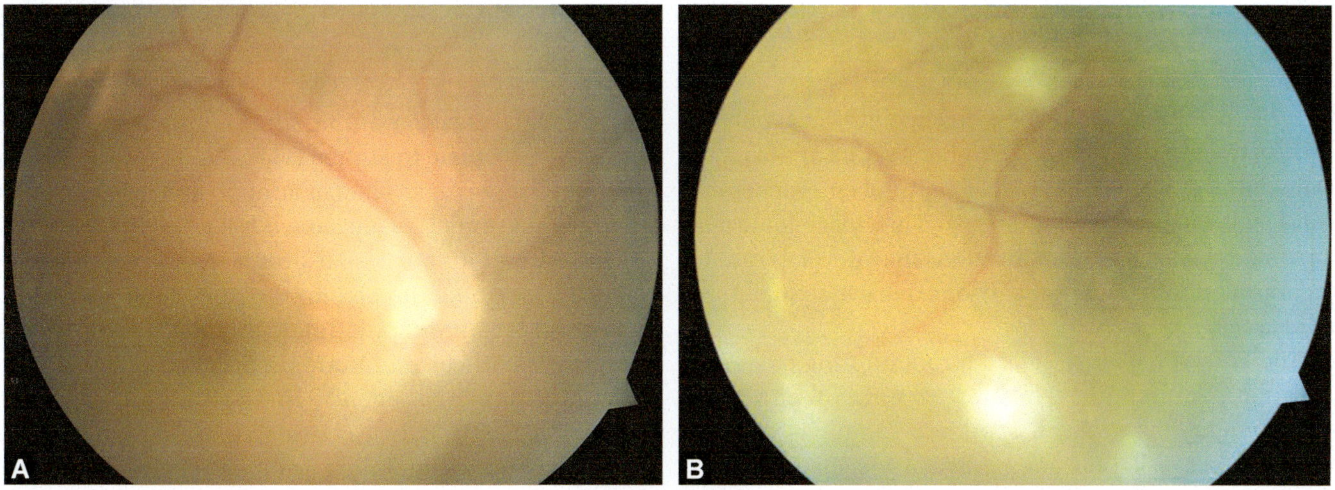

Figs. 85.12A and B

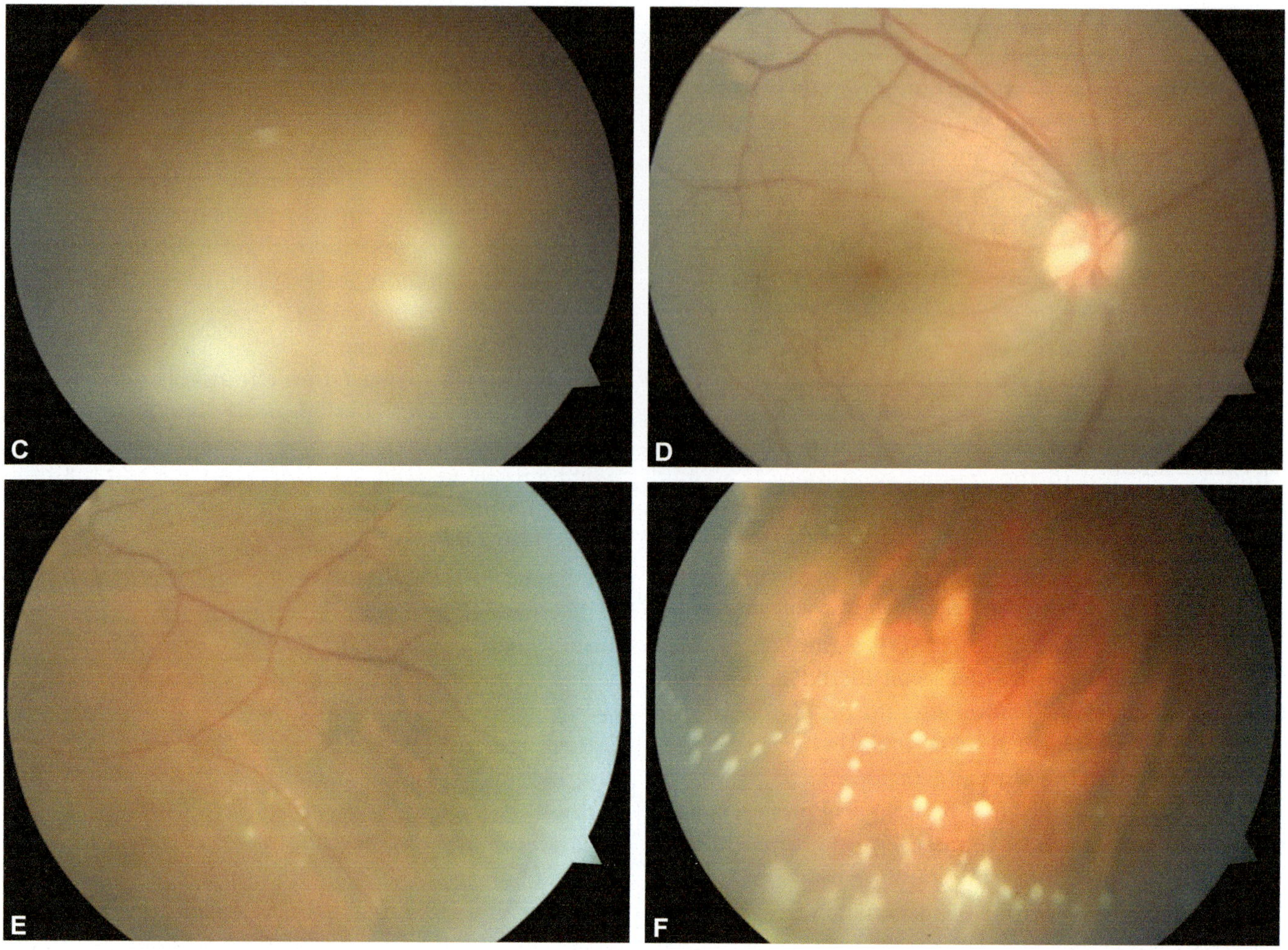

Figs. 85.12C to F

Figs. 85.12A to F: (A to C) Color fundus photographs of the right eye of a 25-year-old man with Behçet's disease show vitreous haze and peripheral retinal infiltrates; (D and E) Decreased vitreous haze, resolution of infiltrates, and appearance of inferior pearl-like precipitates; (F) 9 days later.

pearl-like precipitates may appear usually in a linear pattern on the surface of the inferior peripheral retina or posterior hyaloidal face (Figs. 85.12A to F). Recurrent episodes result in diffuse retinal and optic atrophy and macular edema and scarring. Neovascular complications may develop due to uncontrolled inflammation and/or extensive retinal non-perfusion.[52]

The FA is the gold standard for monitoring posterior segment inflammation. The most common FA findings are staining of the optic disk and fern-like diffuse retinal capillary leakage. Retinal non-perfusion, macular edema or ischemia, NVE and/or NVD can be detected by FA. Persistent retinal capillary leakage during clinically quiescent periods suggests inadequate treatment (Figs. 85.13A to D). Macular complications such as edema, atrophy and vitreomacular interface abnormalities are shown by OCT.[54,55]

Because of a poor visual prognosis in patients with posterior segment involvement, there is an absolute indication for immunomodulatory therapy. High doses of systemic corticosteroids are used in combination with immunosuppressive agents. Interferon-alpha or anti-TNF-alpha agents may be considered as first-line therapy for severe disease or more frequently after failure of conventional therapy.[56]

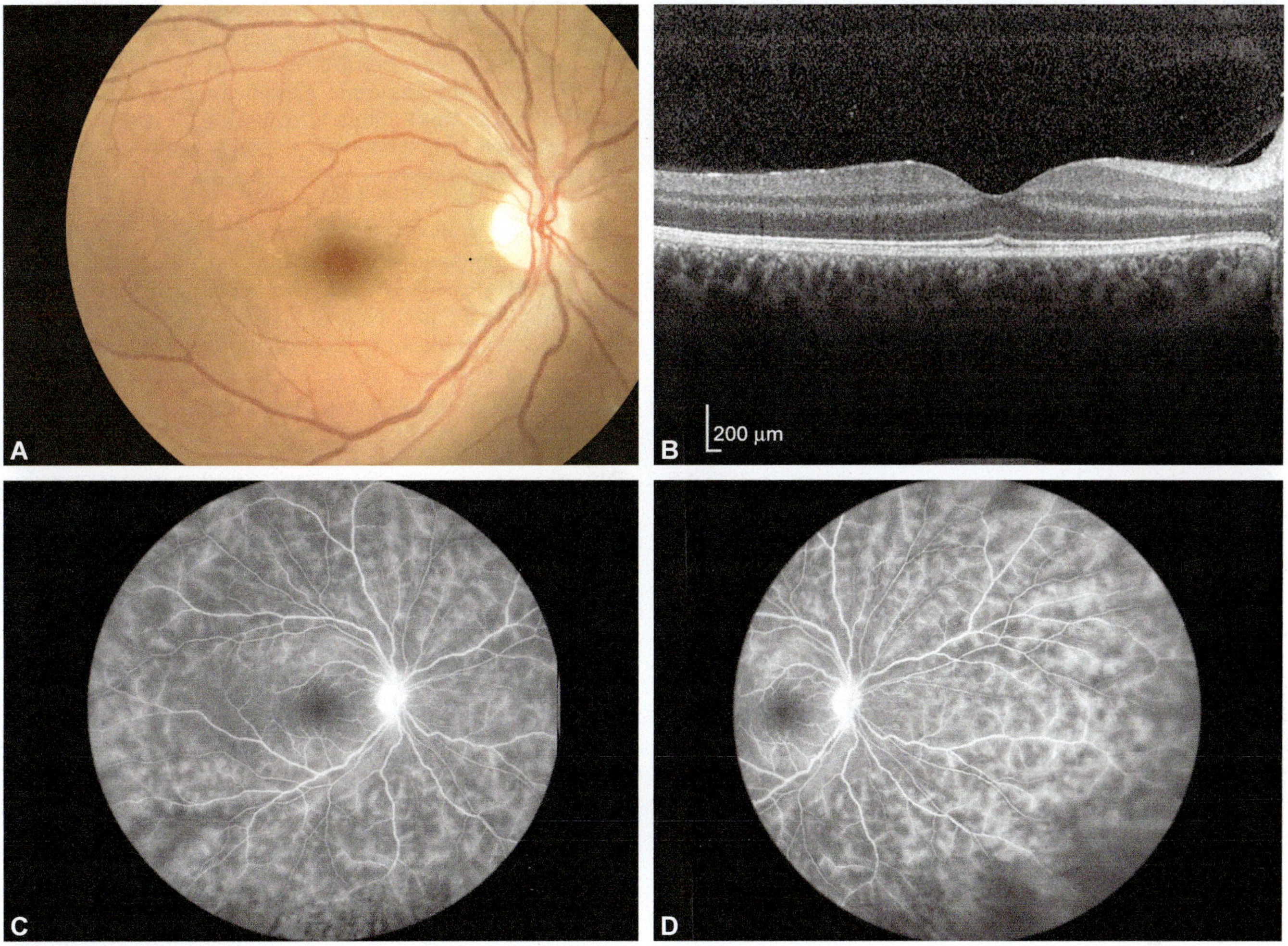

Figs. 85.13A to D: (A) Color fundus photograph, OCT, and FA of the right eye of a 21-year-old woman with Behçet's disease in clinical remission show no sign of active inflammation on (A) fundus photograph or (B) OCT; (C and D) However, there is persistent fern-like retinal capillary leakage on FA indicating that her disease is not effectively controlled.

REFERENCES

1. Willermain F, Rosenbaum JT, Bodaghi B, et al. Interplay between innate and adaptive immunity in the development of non-infectious uveitis. Prog Retin Eye Res. 2012;31(2):182-94.
2. Rathinam SR, Namperumalsamy P. Global variation and pattern changes in epidemiology of uveitis. Indian J Ophthalmol. 2007;55(3):173-83.
3. Rosenbaum JT. New developments in uveitis associated with HLA B27. Curr Opin Rheumatol. 2017;29(4):298-303.
4. Kopplin LJ, Mount G, Suhler EB. Review for disease of the year: epidemiology of HLA-B27 associated ocular disorders. Ocul Immunol Inflamm. 2016;24(4):470-5.
5. Khan MA, Haroon M, Rosenbaum JT. Acute anterior uveitis and spondyloarthritis: more than meets the eye. Curr Rheumatol Rep. 2015;17(9):59.
6. Wakefield D, Yates W, Amjadi S, et al. HLA-B27 anterior uveitis: immunology and immunopathology. Ocul Immunol Inflamm. 2016;24(4):450-9.
7. Bernasconi O, Papadia M, Herbort CP. Sensitivity of laser flare photometry compared to slit-lamp cell evaluation in monitoring anterior chamber inflammation in uveitis. Int Ophthalmol. 2010;30(5):495-500.
8. Rosenbaum JT. Uveitis in spondyloarthritis including psoriatic arthritis, ankylosing spondylitis, and inflammatory bowel disease. Clin Rheumatol. 2015;34(6):999-1002.

9. Haroon M, O'Rourke M, Ramasamy P, et al. A novel evidence-based detection of undiagnosed spondyloarthritis in patients presenting with acute anterior uveitis: the DUET (Dublin Uveitis Evaluation Tool). Ann Rheum Dis. 2015;74(11):1990-5.
10. Rosenbaum JT. Evolving "Diagnostic" criteria for axial spondyloarthritis in the context of anterior uveitis. Ocul Immunol Inflamm. 2016;24(4):445-9.
11. Petty RE, Southwood TR, Manners P, et al. International League of Associations for Rheumatology classification of juvenile idiopathic arthritis: second revision, Edmonton, 2001. J Rheumatol. 2004;31(2):390-2.
12. Abu Samra K, Maghsoudlou A, Roohipoor R, et al. Current treatment modalities of JIA-associated uveitis and its complications: literature review. Ocul Immunol Inflamm. 2016;24(4):431-9.
13. Tugal-Tutkun I, Quartier P, Bodaghi B. Disease of the year: juvenile idiopathic arthritis-associated uveitis—classification and diagnostic approach. Ocul Immunol Inflamm. 2014;22(1):56-63.
14. Heiligenhaus A, Heinz C, Edelsten C, et al. Review for disease of the year: epidemiology of juvenile idiopathic arthritis and its associated uveitis: the probable risk factors. Ocul Immunol Inflamm. 2013;21(3):180-91.
15. Oray M, Tugal-Tutkun I. Treatment of juvenile idiopathic arthritis-associated uveitis. Turk J Ophthalmol. 2016;46(2):77-82.
16. Ramanan AV, Dick AD, Jones AP, et al. Adalimumab plus methotrexate for uveitis in juvenile idiopathic arthritis. N Engl J Med. 2017;376(17):1637-46.
17. Mandeville JT, Levinson RD, Holland GN. The tubulointerstitial nephritis and uveitis syndrome. Surv Ophthalmol. 2001;46(3):195-208.
18. Goda C, Kotake S, Ichiishi A, et al. Clinical features in tubulointerstitial nephritis and uveitis (TINU) syndrome. Am J Ophthalmol. 2005;140(4):637-41.
19. Mackensen F, Billing H. Tubulointerstitial nephritis and uveitis syndrome. Curr Opin Ophthalmol. 2009;20(6):525-31.
20. Jabs DA, Nussenblatt RB, Rosenbaum JT, Standardization of Uveitis Nomenclature Working G. Standardization of uveitis nomenclature for reporting clinical data. Results of the First International Workshop. Am J Ophthalmol. 2005;140(3):509-16.
21. Babu BM, Rathinam SR. Intermediate uveitis. Indian J Ophthalmol. 2010;58(1):21-7.
22. Ozdal PC, Berker N, Tugal-Tutkun I. Pars Planitis: epidemiology, clinical characteristics, management and visual prognosis. J Ophthalmic Vis Res. 2015;10(4):469-80.
23. Kempen JH, Gewaily DY, Newcomb CW, et al. Remission of intermediate uveitis: incidence and predictive factors. Am J Ophthalmol. 2016;164:110-7. e2.
24. de Boer J, Berendschot TT, van der Does P, et al. Long-term follow-up of intermediate uveitis in children. Am J Ophthalmol. 2006;141(4):616-21.
25. Gordon LK, Goldstein DA. Gender and uveitis in patients with multiple sclerosis. J Ophthalmol. 2014;2014:565262.
26. Quillen DA, Davis JB, Gottlieb JL, et al. The white dot syndromes. Am J Ophthalmol. 2004;137(3):538-50.
27. Raven ML, Ringeisen AL, Yonekawa Y, et al. Multi-modal imaging and anatomic classification of the white dot syndromes. Int J Retina Vitreous. 2017;3:12.
28. Crawford CM, Igboeli O. A review of the inflammatory chorioretinopathies: the white dot syndromes. ISRN Inflamm. 2013;2013:783190.
29. Minos E, Barry RJ, Southworth S, et al. Birdshot chorioretinopathy: current knowledge and new concepts in pathophysiology, diagnosis, monitoring and treatment. Orphanet J Rare Dis. 2016;11(1):61.
30. Vitale AT. Birdshot retinochoroidopathy. J Ophthalmic Vis Res. 2014;9(3):350-61.
31. Lim WK, Buggage RR, Nussenblatt RB. Serpiginous choroiditis. Surv Ophthalmol. 2005;50(3):231-44.
32. Cunningham ET Jr, Gupta A, Zierhut M. The creeping choroiditides - serpiginous and multifocal serpiginoid choroiditis. Ocul Immunol Inflamm. 2014;22(5):345-8.
33. Adan A, Sanmarti R, Bures A, Casaroli-Marano RP. Successful treatment with infliximab in a patient with Diffuse Subretinal Fibrosis syndrome. Am J Ophthalmol. 2007;143(3):533-4.
34. Cornish KS, Kuffova L, Forrester JV. Treatment of diffuse subretinal fibrosis uveitis with rituximab. Br J Ophthalmol. 2015;99(2):153-4.
35. Wang Q, Jiang L, Yan W, et al. Fundus autofluorescence imaging in the assessment of acute zonal occult outer retinopathy. Ophthalmologica. 2017;237(3):153-8.
36. Gass JD, Agarwal A, Scott IU. Acute zonal occult outer retinopathy: a long-term follow-up study. Am J Ophthalmol. 2002;134(3):329-39.
37. Jones N, Mochizuki M. Sarcoidosis: epidemiology and clinical features. Ocul Immunol Inflamm. 2010;18(2):72-9.
38. Pasadhika S, Rosenbaum JT. Ocular sarcoidosis. Clin Chest Med. 2015;36(4):669-83.
39. Papadia M, Herbort CP, Mochizuki M. Diagnosis of ocular sarcoidosis. Ocul Immunol Inflamm. 2010;18(6):432-41.
40. Liu D, Birnbaum AD. Update on sarcoidosis. Curr Opin Ophthalmol. 2015;26(6):512-6.
41. O'Keefe GA, Rao NA. Vogt-Koyanagi-Harada disease. Surv Ophthalmol. 2017;62(1):1-25.
42. Silpa-Archa S, Silpa-Archa N, Preble JM, et al. Vogt-Koyanagi-Harada syndrome: perspectives for immunogenetics, multimodal imaging, and therapeutic options. Autoimmun Rev. 2016;15(8):809-19.
43. Read RW, Holland GN, Rao NA, et al. Revised diagnostic criteria for Vogt-Koyanagi-Harada disease: report of an international committee on nomenclature. Am J Ophthalmol. 2001;131(5):647-52.
44. Herbort CP Jr, Abu El Asrar AM, Yamamoto JH, et al. Reappraisal of the management of Vogt-Koyanagi-Harada disease: sunset glow fundus is no more a fatality. Int ophthalmol; 2016.
45. Cunningham ET Jr, Kilmartin D, Agarwal M, et al. Sympathetic ophthalmia. Ocul Immunol Inflamm. 2017;25(2):149-51.

46. Chu XK, Chan CC. Sympathetic ophthalmia: to the twenty-first century and beyond. J Ophthalmic Inflamm Infect. 2013;3(1):49.
47. Chang GC, Young LH. Sympathetic ophthalmia. Semin Ophthalmol. 2011;26(4-5):316-20.
48. Damico FM, Kiss S, Young LH. Sympathetic ophthalmia. Semin Ophthalmol. 2005;20(3):191-7.
49. Tugal-Tutkun I. Behcet disease in the developing world. Int Ophthalmol Clin. 2010;50(2):87-98.
50. Criteria for diagnosis of Behcet's disease. International Study Group for Behcet's Disease. Lancet. 1990;335(8697):1078-80.
51. Tugal-Tutkun I, Onal S, Altan-Yaycioglu R, et al. Uveitis in Behcet disease: an analysis of 880 patients. Am J Ophthalmol. 2004;138(3):373-80.
52. Tugal-Tutkun I, Gupta V, Cunningham ET. Differential diagnosis of Behcet uveitis. Ocul Immunol Inflamm. 2013;21(5):337-50.
53. Oray M, Onal S, Bayraktar S, et al. Nonglaucomatous localized retinal nerve fiber layer defects in Behcet uveitis. Am J Ophthalmol. 2015;159(3):475-81. e1.
54. Tugal-Tutkun I. Imaging in the diagnosis and management of Behcet disease. Int Ophthalmol Clin. 2012;52(4):183-90.
55. Tugal-Tutkun I, Ozdal PC, Oray M, et al. Review for diagnostics of the year: multimodal imaging in Behçet uveitis. Ocul Immunol Inflamm. 2017;25(1):07-19.
56. Zierhut M, Abu El-Asrar AM, Bodaghi B, et al. Therapy of ocular Behçet disease. Ocul Immunol Inflamm. 2014;22(1):64-76.

Chapter 86 Uveitis Masquerades

Janet L Davis, Steven S Saraf

INTRODUCTION

Noninfectious uveitis, infectious uveitis, and masquerade syndromes were the three major subdivisions of the clinical classification of uveitis published by the International Uveitis Study Group in 2008.[1] In 2005, the Standardization of Uveitis Nomenclature (SUN) workshop reverted to an anatomic classification scheme of anterior, intermediate, posterior, and panuveitis with no mention of masquerades.[2] Later efforts by the same group to categorize uveitis into named, definable clinical patterns also did not consider masquerade syndromes.[3] The concept of masquerade syndromes nonetheless remains a useful one for clinicians who may be confronted with intraocular cellular infiltrations that mimic uveitis in lymphoma, leukemia or other intraocular malignancies. There may be a secondary component of a true anti-inflammatory or autoimmune uveitis that accompanies the malignancy and may further obscure the true diagnosis.[4] Other conditions such as ocular ischemia,[5] drug reactions,[6] and chronic retinal disease[7] can be considered masquerades even though they are mediated by typical inflammatory cells because they are initiated by distinct mechanisms and require diagnosis of the underlying cause. The focus of this chapter is therefore a review of conditions that have features of uveitis but for which uveitis is actually a misdiagnosis or a minor feature of the condition. Despite the heterogeneity of this group, there are certain clinical patterns that are useful to recognize and there are currently many imaging and laboratory techniques to assist in diagnosis.

NEOPLASTIC MASQUERADE SYNDROME

Lymphoproliferative Disorders

Neoplastic masquerade syndromes were identified in 21 of 853 (2.5%) patients attending a tertiary referral clinic at the National Eye Institute (NEI) in the United States.[8] The most common malignancy was primary vitreoretinal lymphoma (PVRL, 17 of the 21 lymphoid malignancies, 81%). Similarly, 16 of 19 (84%) neoplastic masquerade syndromes in a Dutch uveitis clinic population of 828 had lymphoid malignancy.[9] Unlike solid tumors, lymphomas and leukemias are more likely to present to the uveitis specialist. The intraocular cells, as in uveitis, are of lymphoid lineage and have no characteristics such as size or color to distinguish them from inflammatory cells at the slit lamp. Free-floating cells are more typical of lymphoma than leukemia, which is more likely to invade tissue such as iris, optic nerve or retina. The homogeneity of clonal lymphoma cells may create a distinctive pattern of evenly distributed vitreous cells that do not form small clumps as a mixed inflammatory reaction would do but may produce large sheets of proliferating cells. Because most lymphomas are B cells and secrete interleukin-10 (IL-10), an anti-inflammatory cytokine,[10] rather than proinflammatory cytokines, the hazy, quiet eye with good vision and without hyperemia, posterior synechiae, vitreous disorganization or cystoid macular edema is a common pattern of PVRL. Whereas leukemia is always metastatic to the eye, lymphoma may be isolated with no focus of lymphoma in the central nervous system or extraocular tissues at the time of the ocular diagnosis. Metastatic lymphoma to the eye usually localizes to the choroidal layers and requires a systemic diagnosis. There are case reports of chronic lymphocytic leukemias, B or T cell in origin, that involve the eye.[8-11]

Primary Vitreoretinal Lymphoma

Ocular involvement with lymphoma is rare, occurring in 15–25% of patients with primary central nervous system lymphoma.[12] Among neoplastic uveitis masquerades, primary vitreoretinal lymphoma is the most common.[8,9] Patients who present initially with ocular manifestations are considered to have primary vitreoretinal lymphoma, but up to 90% of these patients will eventually develop

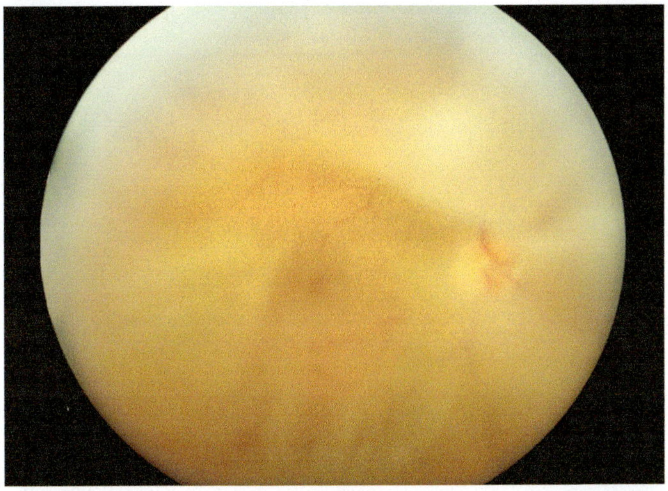

Fig. 86.1: Primary vitreoretinal lymphoma with vitreous infiltration. Fundus photograph, right eye, showing dense vitreous opacities in a patient confirmed to have diffuse large B cell lymphoma after vitreous biopsy. Vision was 20/30 and there was no CME. Clonal expansion within the vitreous cisterns may lead to the ray-like collections of cells. There is little vitreous stranding or clumping as the lymphoma cells do not produce inflammatory mediators. Focal retinal white lesions are barely visible in the posterior pole and indicate RPE level involvement.

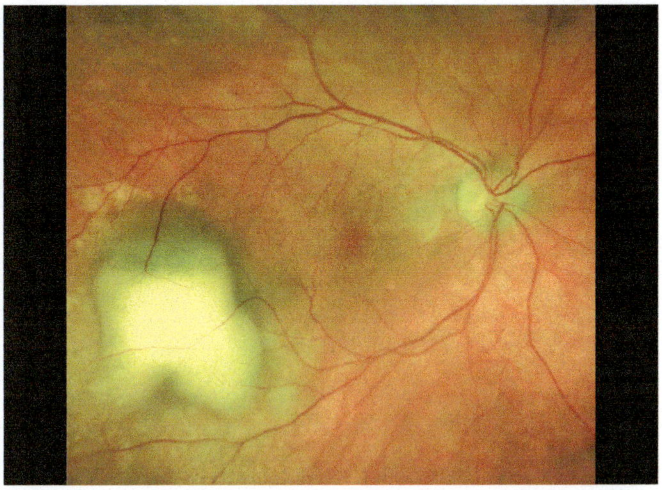

Fig. 86.2: Primary vitreoretinal lymphoma with subretinal pigment epithelial infiltration. Fundus photograph—right eye. The large solid RPED is the most prominent feature but there are additional white subretinal pigment epithelial infiltrates surrounding it and diffuse pigmentary changes. There was mild cellular infiltration in the vitreous with no haze.

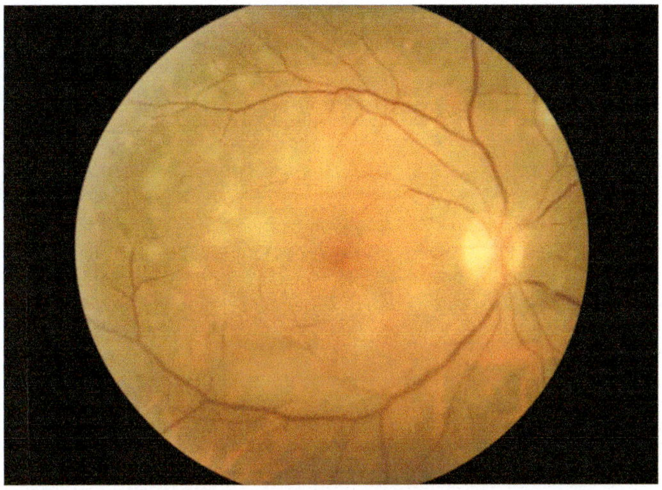

Fig. 86.3: Primary vitreoretinal lymphoma with retinal infiltrates. Fundus photograph—right eye. The patient presented with blurred vision and diffused involvement in both eyes 5 years following radiation and chemotherapy for primary central nervous system lymphoma with a large brain mass. The initial referral was for a "white dot syndrome". There is no pigmentary change indicating that the subretinal pigment epithelial space is free of tumor. Lesions line up along the retinal arterioles suggestive of hematogenous entry into the eye. CNS recurrence was not present but occurred later.

CNS lymphoma and PVRL is best considered as a subset of primary CNS lymphoma.[12] The best management for PVRL is early recognition and preemptive treatment to delay or prevent CNS disease although there is agreement as to the best protocol to accomplish this. Treatment of the eyes alone is ineffective to protect the CNS or even to reliably prevent ocular relapse.[13] Addition of systemic chemotherapy to local ocular therapy in patients without CNS involvement may also be ineffective to alter the course of disease but may prolong survival.[14-16] This pattern suggests that CNS and vitreoretinal lymphoma may arise asynchronously from a lymphoid source that seeds either the eye or the CNS because of a favorable microenvironment for proliferation. Treatment to eradicate all current evidence of active disease may be insufficient to ensure a durable remission.

Presentation

There are two distinctive growth patterns for PVRL. If the vitreous cavity is primarily involved with free-floating cells, the most common presenting symptom will be blurred vision and floaters. Clinically, the ophthalmologist notes haze out of proportion to the decrease in vision as well as a lack of other inflammatory signs (Fig. 86.1). The second growth pattern is in the subretinal pigment epithelial (RPE) space (Fig. 86.2). The patient may be asymptomatic, but usually the two growth patterns are combine, so they may notice floaters, or if the deposits are in the posterior pole, blurred vision. The ophthalmologist notes pigmentary changes, which may become more obvious with treatment or after vitrectomy. Less commonly, intraretinal proliferation may occur (Figs. 86.3 and 86.4). The lymphoma cells die off readily and large tumor masses are not usually seen,

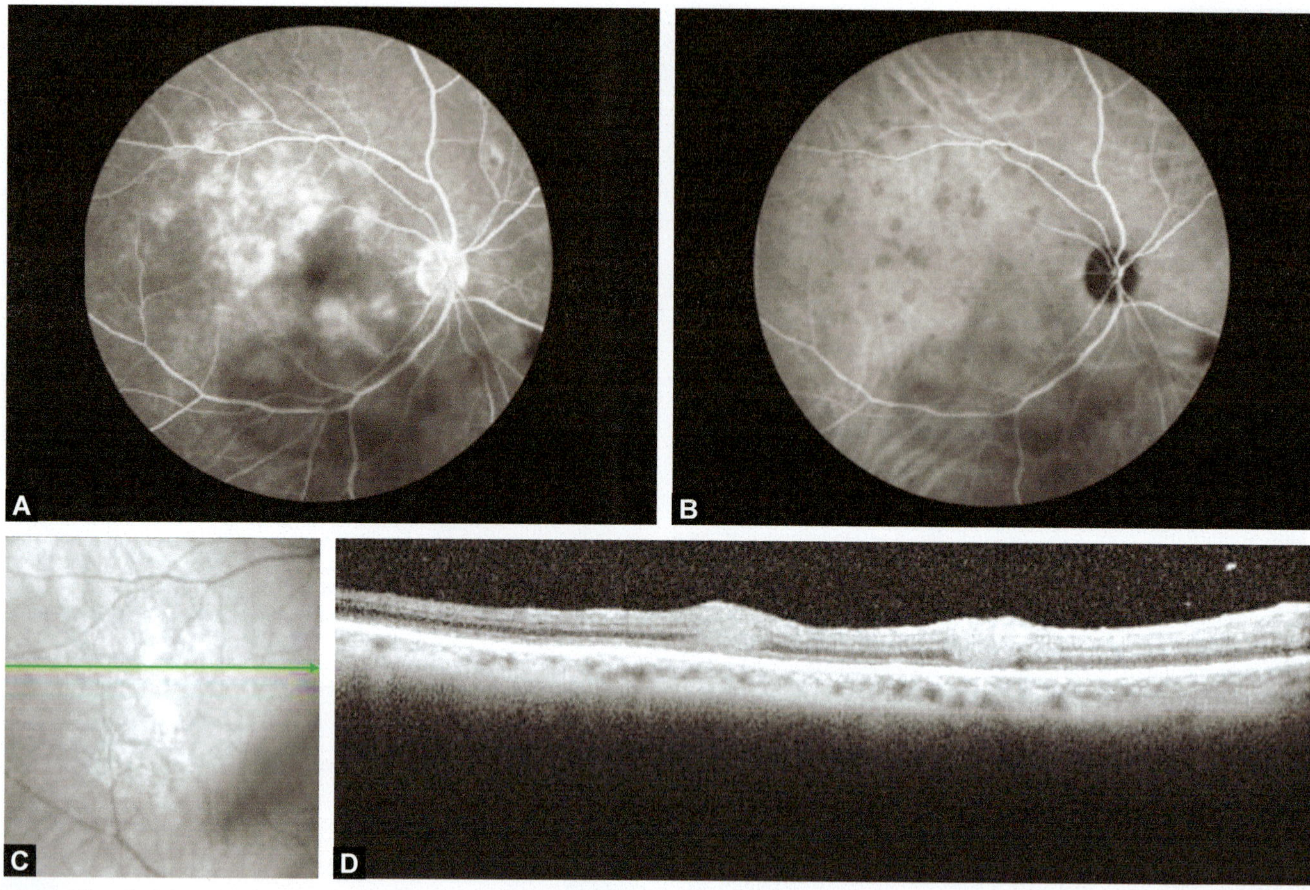

Figs. 86.4A to D: Primary vitreoretinal lymphoma with retinal infiltrates, same case as in Figure 86.1. (A) fluorescein angiography showing arteriolar leakage and retinal staining; (B) The indocyanine green angiogram (ICG) shows blockage from the denser retinal infiltrates. There is an amorphous dark artifact over the posterior pole related to vitreous opacities; (C) infrared image showing relatively normal RPE and choroid; (D) Optical coherence tomography (OCT) scan showing discrete retinal infiltrates without RPE involvement. There are a few vitreous cells seen.

however, this spontaneous regression creates difficulties in diagnosis when nonviable cells are biopsied or trials or corticosteroids seem to lead to improvement. Retinal or subretinal involvement can lead to permanent retinal damage and loss of function.

ANCILLARY DIAGNOSTIC IMAGING

Ancillary testing is increasingly used to enhance the clinical examination and to improve case selection for diagnostic vitrectomy.

Optical Coherence Tomography

Nodular hyper-reflective sub-RPE deposits are suspicious for PVRL, especially when present with abnormal fluorescence and indocyanine green (ICG) angiography.[17] Both untreated and treated eyes commonly show RPE and retinal changes on posterior polar optical coherence tomography (OCT) indicating that retinal-RPE involvement may be more diffuse than is obvious on clinical examination.[18] The sub-RPE lesions can be confused with drusen if the OCT is considered in isolation (Figs. 86.5A and B). Treatment can lead to rapid resolution of the sub-RPE deposits (Figs. 86.6A and B).

Fluorescein Angiography

Focal deposits of lymphoma cells can block the underlying fluorescence of normal structures on fluorescein angiography (FA). Window defects occur in areas where RPE atrophy has occurred after regression of sub-RPE deposits. The combination of blocking and window defects may produce the so-called leopard spot pattern on fluorescein angiography. Less blockage is detected on ICG angiography because the deposits are generally small and relatively thin.[17] Vascular leakage along retinal arterioles may occur. Cystoid macular edema is far less common than in intermediate uveitis, but can occur.

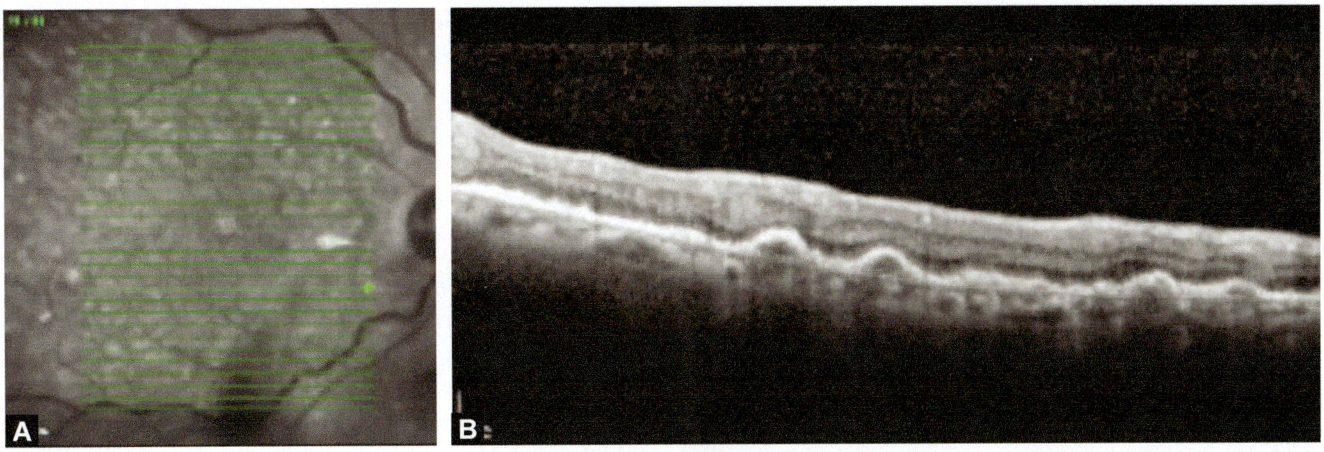

Figs. 86.5A and B: Primary vitreoretinal lymphoma. (A) Infrared image showing irregular RPE reflections; (B) Line scan with drusen-like elevations of the RPE. The lymphoid collections have variable reflectivity.

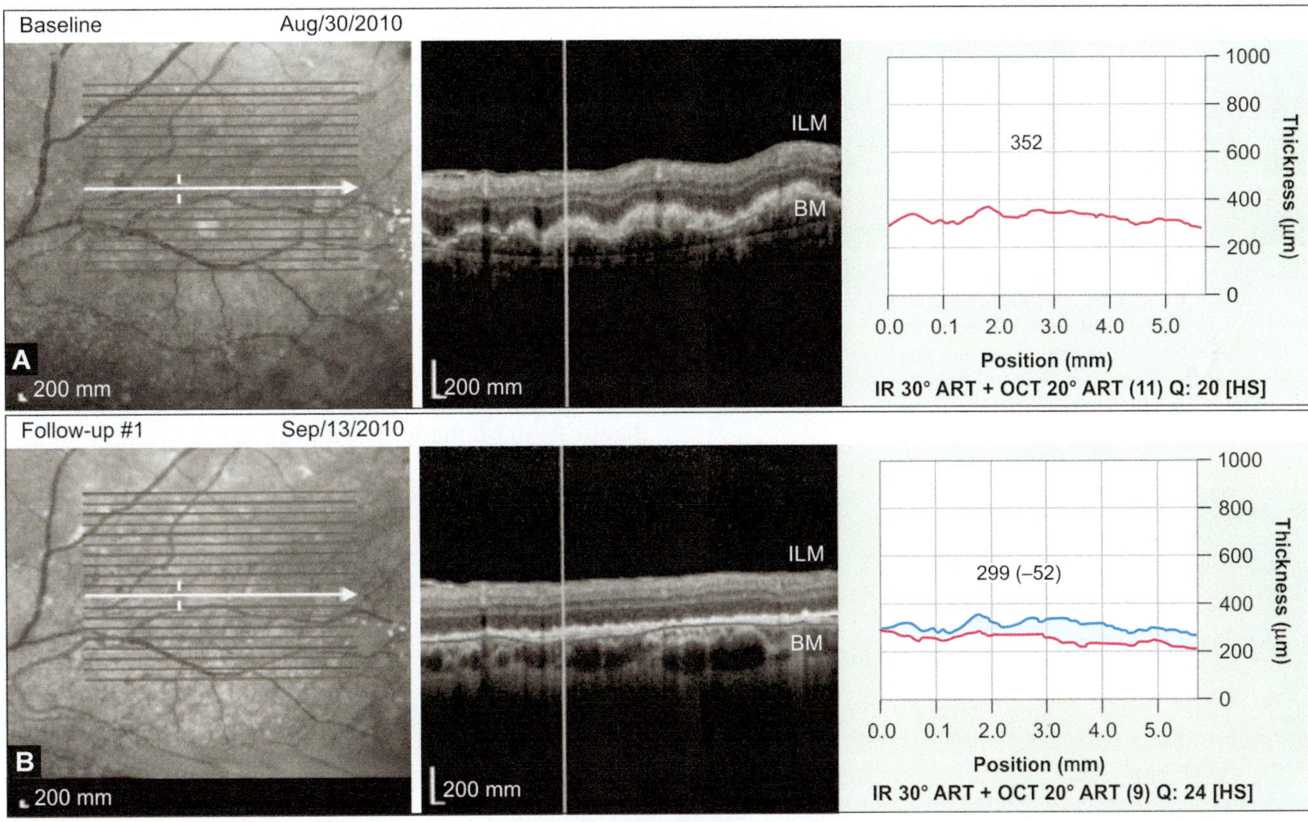

Figs. 86.6A and B: Primary vitreoretinal lymphoma. (A) Infrared, optical coherence tomography (OCT) line scan, and thickness profile performed prior to first injection of intravitreal methotrexate 400 µg/0.1 mL in a previously untreated patient. The vertical marker indicates the horizontal position through a visible lesion on the infrared image. Thickness is 352 µm in this area; (B) Corresponding images 2 weeks after treatment. Subretinal pigment epithelial deposits have flattened with a focal reduction in thickness to 299 µm. The gray zone on the bottom thickness profile indicates the reduction over the entire scan line.

Autofluorescence

Lymphoma cells possess intrinsic hyperautofluorescence in vitro compared to normal lymphocytes.[19] Blue autofluorescent photography also reveals focal deposits of lymphoma cells to be hyperautofluorescent.[20] When compared to OCT, the hyperautofluorescent patches correspond to the hyper-reflective subretinal nodules and when compared to FA, the patches may be either hyperfluorescent or hypofluorescent on FA (Fig. 86.7).[21] The hyperautofluorescent patches also correspond to fundus lesions that are lighter in color than background (Figs. 86.8A and B).

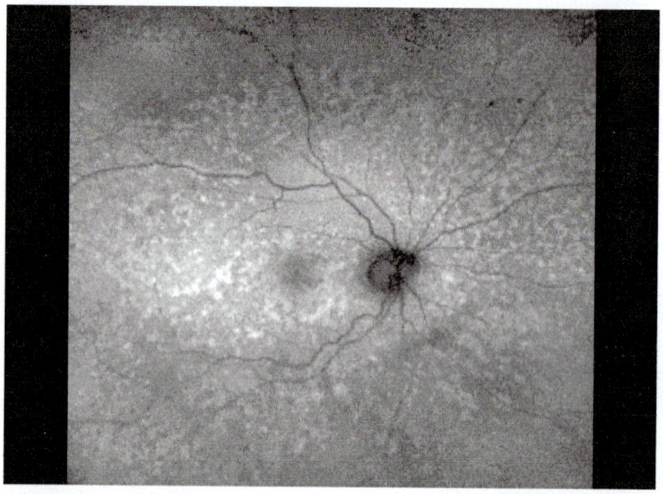

Fig. 86.7: Primary vitreoretinal lymphoma, same case as in Figure 86.5. Wide-angle autofluorescence image—right eye. Mottled hyperautofluorescence with few patches of hypoautofluorescence indicating little atrophy of the RPE and little infiltration of the retina with blockage of the underlying autofluorescence. When compared to optical coherence tomography (OCT) in Figure 86.5, the hyperautofluorescent patches correspond to the subretinal nodules.

Magnetic Resonance Imaging of Brain

Because of the frequent discordance between CNS and ocular findings, a normal magnetic resonance imaging (MRI) of the brain does not exclude intraocular lymphoma. It is therefore reasonable to pursue all diagnostic possibilities related to the eye, including diagnostic vitrectomy, before referring a patient for a hematologic work-up. If the ophthalmologist orders the MRI, the radiologist should be told that lymphoma is in the differential. Contrast imaging is necessary, and fluid attenuation inversion recovery (FLAIR) sequences and diffusion weighted imaging may increase the chance of detecting lymphoma. Lumbar puncture will occasionally yield lymphoma cells even if the MRI is normal. The consulting hematologist usually performs blood counts and chemistries, computerized tomography (CT) imaging with contrast of chest, abdomen and pelvis, and bone marrow biopsy.

INTRAOCULAR DIAGNOSTIC TESTING

As in the multimodal approach used with ancillary ocular imaging, use of multiple diagnostic tests to detect lymphoma cells in intraocular specimens is helpful.[22] There is no gold standard test that must be positive for a diagnosis to be made, but if cytology or histopathology is

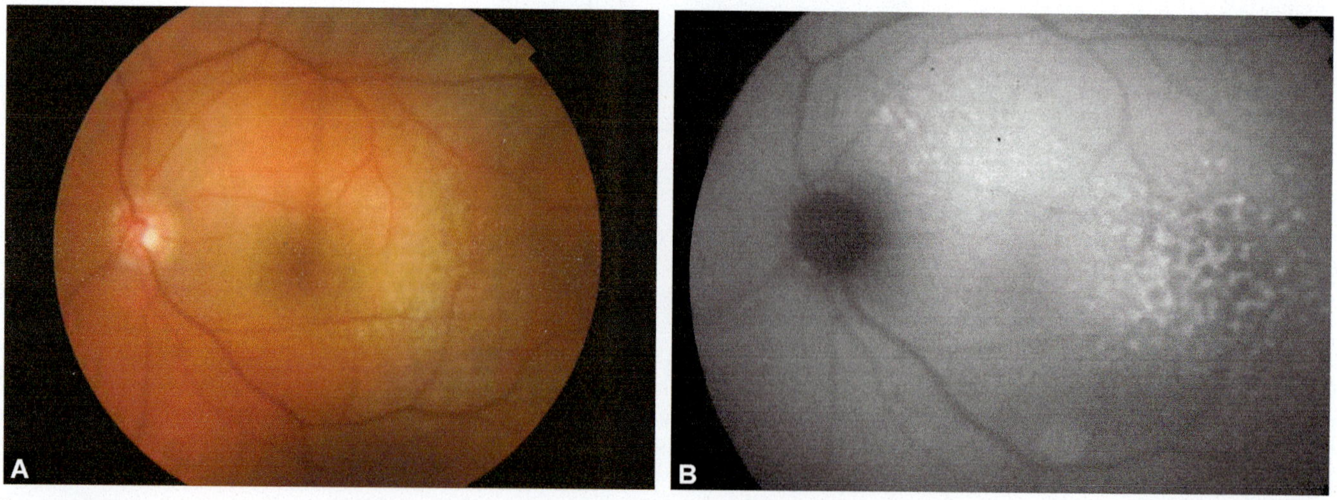

Figs. 86.8A and B: Primary vitreoretinal lymphoma. (A) Fundus photograph, left eye. The eye is status postvitrectomy 9 months previously. Biopsy findings were inconclusive and the patient refused treatment. There are new white subretinal lesions; (B) Hyperautofluorescence corresponds to the white retinal lesions. The spiculated and punctate pattern is associated with subretinal pigment epithelial growth.

negative, flow cytometry and genetic studies are essential to support a diagnosis of intraocular lymphoma. Multiple interventions for diagnosis may be needed.[23]

Specimen Collection

Vitreous sampling is the most common way to obtain tissue for analysis. Needle aspiration is usually superseded by pars plana vitrectomy, which allows more tests to be performed on a larger sample size.[24] Vitrectomy has the further advantage of allowing better vision and a clearer view of posterior structures. Manual aspiration of specimens into syringes reduces exposure to tubing and cassette bags that may jeopardize the sample. Gauge of vitrectomy instrument does not seem to influence results.[25] Other procedure-specific features that may reduce yield include poor cellular viability from prior corticosteroids or spontaneous regression and long operating room to pathologist time. Lymphoma cells have been observed to be fragile and undergo degradation within 60 minutes of collection.[26]

Biopsy of lymphoma infiltrates in the retina or sub-RPE space can be effective if the vitreous specimen is deemed insufficient or vitreous biopsy fails.[27] The easiest technique is manual aspiration of cells directly from lymphoma-filled RPE detachments followed by cytological examination (Figs. 86.2 and 86.9). Retinal dissection with scissors is useful to obtain tissue for histologic diagnosis (Figs. 86.3, 86.4 and 86.10).[28,29]

Cytology and Histopathology

Archival preservation of abnormal lymphoid cells with review of the specimen by an experienced cytopathologist or pathologist is the most accepted means of diagnosis, but can be difficult. Despite obtaining appropriate vitreous samples and proper handling, the false negative rate is estimated to be up to 30% in the literature, necessitating repeat biopsies when the clinical suspicion remains.[10] Observed morphologic features in diffuse large B cell lymphoma include large, pleomorphic cells with high nuclear/cytoplasmic ratios, and multiple nucleoli. T cell lymphomas are challenging to diagnose solely on morphologic grounds. Centrifugation of the specimen directly onto slides yields the best preparation for cytology. Centrifugation of the vitreous cassette and preparation of a cell block is an older technique that may provide larger cell numbers for studies. Interpretation of any cytologic or histologic specimen is greatly enhanced by immunohistochemical staining for cell identification, especially B cell markers such as CD19 and kappa and lambda.

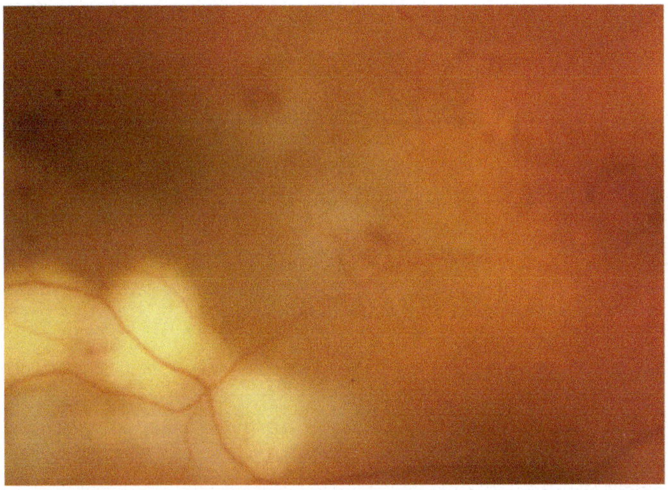

Fig. 86.9: Primary vitreoretinal lymphoma, case selected for subretinal aspiration. Fundus photograph right temporal macula. The domes of the RPED are incised with an MRI blade and the lymphoma cells are aspirated manually with a 20–23 gauge silicone tipped needle. The posterior hyaloid was previously removed during an inconclusive diagnostic vitrectomy. Air-fluid exchange and light laser photocoagulation prevent retinal detachment. See Figure 86.2 for another example of a case selected for aspiration biopsy.

Fig. 86.10: Primary vitreoretinal lymphoma, case selected for retinal biopsy. Fundus photograph of the left eye of same case as Figures 86.3 and 86.4. There are diffuse indistinct retinal infiltrates and evidence of periarteriolar vascular sheathing. Optical coherence tomography (OCT) scanning was performed to confirm the presence of intraretinal lesions in the biopsy site. The black and white inset is a section of the infrared image acquired with the OCT and shows the proposed site of biopsy.

Flow Cytometry

Flow cytometry can test for more cell surface markers than slide-based immunohistochemical techniques,[30] expanding the ability to distinguish T cell lymphomas from uveitis and from B cell lymphomas co-infiltrating with reactive T cells.[4] Uveitis is highly associated with an elevated CD4 + T cell to CD8+ T cell ratio.[4] Frequency distributions of cells bearing various cell surface markers can also identify monocyte/macrophage lineages that may be indicators of infection.

Gene Rearrangement

Amplification of the variable region of the *IgH gene* by polymerase chain reaction (PCR) can establish clonality of a predominantly B cell infiltrate by detecting a peak amplification product.[12,31,32] For T cell lymphomas amplification of the T cell receptor gene is used in the same way. PCR has also been useful to confirm HTLV-1 presence in adult T cell leukemias affecting the eye.[33,34] Mutation in myeloid differentiation primary response gene 88 (MYD88) is also detectable by PCR amplification and was highly associated with vitreoretinal B cell lymphoma in two large case series.[35,36]

Cytokine Analysis

Interleukin-10 is secreted by B cells, serving as an adaptive signal to suppress immune response and allow cellular proliferation. IL-6 is a proinflammatory cytokine found in most ocular fluids in uveitis. The IL-10 to IL-6 ratio in ocular fluid is biologically plausible as a test for the diagnosis of B cell intraocular lymphoma. Comparison of IL-10 and IL-6 levels in vitreous or aqueous specimens from 85 patients with endophthalmitis, lymphoma or uveitis showed IL-6 to be significantly higher in uveitis than in lymphoma and IL-10 to be significantly higher in lymphoma than uveitis; endophthalmitis had the highest IL-6 levels.[37] Vitreous IL-6 and IL-10 or aqueous IL-6 datasets had 100% predictive accuracy. Cytokine analysis of vitreous was positive in 18/22 cases of lymphoma in another series; gene rearrangement studies performed on the same cases had higher predictive values.[38] Cytokine assays are not generally accepted as diagnostic in isolation, but may be useful as screening tools and to monitor treatment.

TREATMENT OF INTRAOCULAR LYMPHOMA

In patients with concurrent CNS lymphoma, a high-dose methotrexate-based regimen is the most common treatment, often combined with other chemotherapeutic agents. Although early whole brain irradiation is usually deferred because of concerns for cognitive impairment,[39] radiation therapy is frequently used for local ocular control with a low rate of radiation retinopathy. Whole-brain irradiation or stem cell transplantation may be used for consolidation therapy or for salvage after CNS relapse.[40] For isolated ocular lymphoma, either ocular radiation or intravitreal chemotherapy with methotrexate or rituximab may be used. Predominant lymphoma involvement (retinal versus vitreous) does not seem to influence the development of CNS lymphoma.[41] Although deferral of systemic treatment for limited ocular disease may not influence overall outcomes,[13,14] early systemic chemotherapy may delay the onset of systemic disease.[15,41] Patients who have ocular-only disease at the time of diagnosis may have better survival.[16]

OTHER LYMPHOID MALIGNANCIES

In the US clinic-based series, 4 of 21 neoplastic masquerades were not primary vitreoretinal lymphoma but rather one case each of mucosal-associated lymphoid tissue lymphoma (MALT), chronic lymphocytic leukemia, HTLV-1 associated T cell leukemia, and non-Hodgkin's lymphoma.[8] In a Dutch series of similar size, there were seven non-PVRL lymphoid or leukemic malignant masquerades, three of which infiltrated iris.[9] History of lymphoid malignancy or leukemia is common, but may be absent.[9] Uveal infiltrates, retinal infiltrates that fail to clear with corticosteroids, abnormal white blood cell counts may be helpful but presentations are diverse enough that generalizations are difficult. Intraocular diagnostic procedures that include cell surface markers and genetic studies are helpful.

NON-LYMPHOPROLIFERATIVE MALIGNANCIES

Melanoma

Uveal melanoma is the most common primary intraocular tumor in adults, but accounts for few uveitis masquerades. Posterior masses may be mistaken for granulomas. Undetected tumors in peripheral retinal locations may produce intraocular inflammation before the tumor is recognized.[42] In the Dutch series previously cited,[9] one masquerade was attributed to melanoma metastatic to the iris. There are several other case reports of iridal and ciliary body melanomas presenting with anterior uveitis.[43,44] Metastasis of cutaneous melanoma to the vitreous is rare.[45]

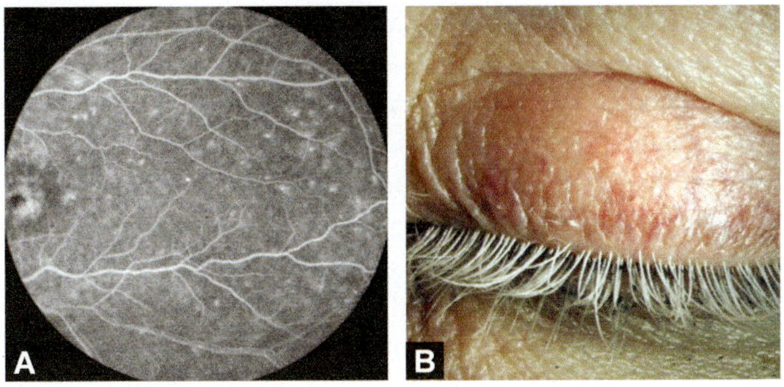

Figs. 86.11A and B: Vogt-Koyanagi-Harada (VKH) disease like uveitis in a patient with metastatic melanoma treated with tumor-infiltrating lymphocytes. (A) Multiple pinpoint leaks on FA and CME. There was intense anterior inflammation with posterior synechiae; (B) Poliosis. Brows, scalp hair and skin also were extensively depigmented. She improved with intravitreal corticosteroids and the eventual die-off of the engineered anti-tumor lymphocytes. Her metastatic melanoma was placed into remission.

Other than these exceptions, easily excluded by careful examination of the eye and ultrasonography, most uveitis associated with melanoma appears to be an autoimmune reaction directed against shared antigens on pigmented tissues. This can occur either spontaneously or associated with treatment (Figs. 86.11A and B). In a review of 450 eyes with choroidal and ciliary body melanoma, 22 (4.9%) had signs of ocular inflammation; seven cases demonstrated episcleritis, the remaining 14 demonstrated some form of uveitis, endophthalmitis, or panophthalmitis.[46] Treatment of cutaneous or metastatic melanoma with newer biologic agents such as checkpoint inhibitors, CTLA-4 blockades, programmed cell death receptor 1 inhibitors may be especially likely to produce uveitis, sometimes with a severe phenotype mimicking Vogt-Koyanagi-Harada (VKH).[47-51] Development of these secondary immune reactions has been associated with a favorable treatment prognosis.[52]

Retinoblastoma

Retinoblastoma is the most common intraocular malignancy of childhood. It is one of the most feared uveitis masquerades because death may occur with misdiagnosis.[53] Although some inflammation may occur from tumor necrosis in retinoblastoma, it is more common for the tumor cells to be mistaken for inflammatory cells. The tumor cells may form pseudohypopyon.[54] Posterior synechiae are either rare or nonexistent. If diagnostic vitrectomy is undertaken prior to recognition that retinoblastoma is active, there is concern for early dissemination. In a series of over 900 patients with retinoblastoma, Shields and colleagues reported 11 who had undergone prior pars plana vitrectomy; in five of these the indication was suspected uveitis.[55] Ten responded well to enucleation, radiation and chemotherapy. Diffuse infiltrating retinoblastoma presenting beyond the early childhood years is of special concern because it lacks a well-defined tumor mass and may mimic chorioretinitis or retinal detachment.[56]

Ancillary Testing

B-scan ultrasonography is an important step to check for posterior segment abnormalities in patients being evaluated for uveitis, especially in young children. A mass lesion with calcifications is a classic finding in retinoblastoma, but retinal thickening such as would be present in diffuse infiltrating retinoblastoma should raise clinical suspicion. If these signs are present, subspecialty consultation with an ocular oncologist may be helpful, especially if invasive diagnostic interventions such as vitrectomy or anterior chamber paracentesis are planned.

Metastatic Solid Tumors

As with uveal melanoma, choroidal metastases of solid tumors may be misdiagnosed as choroidal granulomas or exudative detachments. Secondary, true inflammation may arise in response to tumor necrosis or immune surveillance. Metastases to the vitreous are the most likely to be interpreted as uveitis, but are rare. No non-lymphoid malignant masquerades were reported in the NEI series[8] but the Dutch series reported a lung cancer metastasis producing vitritis[9] and there are two additional similar case reports (Fig. 86.12).[57,58] Diagnostic vitrectomy performed for retinal detachment without choroidal mass in a patient with known breast cancer resulted in seeding of two sclerotomy sites with tumor[59] indicating that intraocular diagnostic procedures should be undertaken with caution in metastatic tumors as well as in retinoblastoma.

NON-NEOPLASTIC MASQUERADE SYNDROMES

Retinitis Pigmentosa

Chronic inflammation is common in inherited retinal dystrophies, with 1+ or greater anterior vitreous cells occurring in 190 of 509 eyes (37.3%) in one series.[7] Vitreous cells are also common, as is cystoid macular edema. Some patients with RP may develop actual uveitis independent from the reactive inflammatory response to the retinal degeneration but this is uncommon. Uveitis was recorded in only 22 of 8,364 patients with retinitis pigmentosa (RP) at a tertiary eye hospital over a 30-year period.[60] Similar data to predict the number of patients who were initially diagnosed with uveitis but later determined to have an inherited retinal dystrophy are not available. Vascular narrowing, pigmentary changes and macular edema can be features of intermediate uveitis. Pigmentary changes and visual field loss can occur with posterior uveitis such as acute zonal occult outer retinopathy (AZOOR). Autoimmune retinopathy is a presumptive diagnosis in individuals who present with unexplained vision loss, but a substantial proportion of these patients likely have atypical inherited retinal dystrophies. Bilateral symmetric pigmentary changes on autofluorescence are suggestive of an inherited retinal dystrophy (Figs. 86.13A and B). Lack of response to corticosteroid treatment and immunosuppression may be helpful in suspecting a uveitis masquerade such as RP.

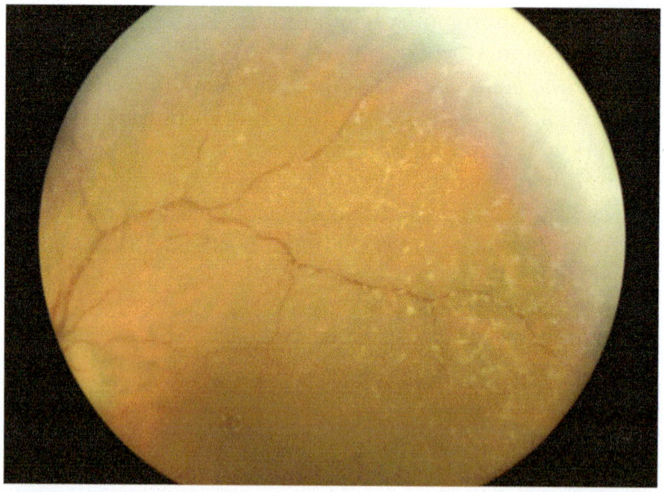

Fig. 86.12: Metastatic adenocarcinoma of lung. Fundus photograph—left eye. There were clumped vitreous opacities and diffuse scattered preretinal infiltrates. The perivascular sheathing could be related to tight vitreous adhesions along vessels or to "oxygen seeking" by the tumor cells. The patient was previously treated systemically with bevacizumab and it was hypothesized that this may have interfered with more typical metastatic growth such as a choroidal mass.

Ancillary Testing

Electroretinography (ERG) in uveitis patients is typically done for indications of birdshot chorioretinopathy or autoimmune retinopathy to assess the severity of disease. In typical RP and in some paraneoplastic retinopathies the ERG will be flat even with retained vision and field. Inflammatory disease usually produces less severe impairment of the ERG. Multifocal choroiditis, for example, often has amplitude reductions proportional to the surface area of diseased retina without alterations in timing latency such as would always be seen in a retinal dystrophy. Imaging studies may detect bilaterally symmetric autofluorescence abnormalities suggestive of dystrophy and unlikely to occur in uveitis. This class of uveitis masquerades is likely under diagnosed currently. With affordable genetic testing for disease-causing mutations, better diagnoses of atypical dystrophies will be possible in the future.

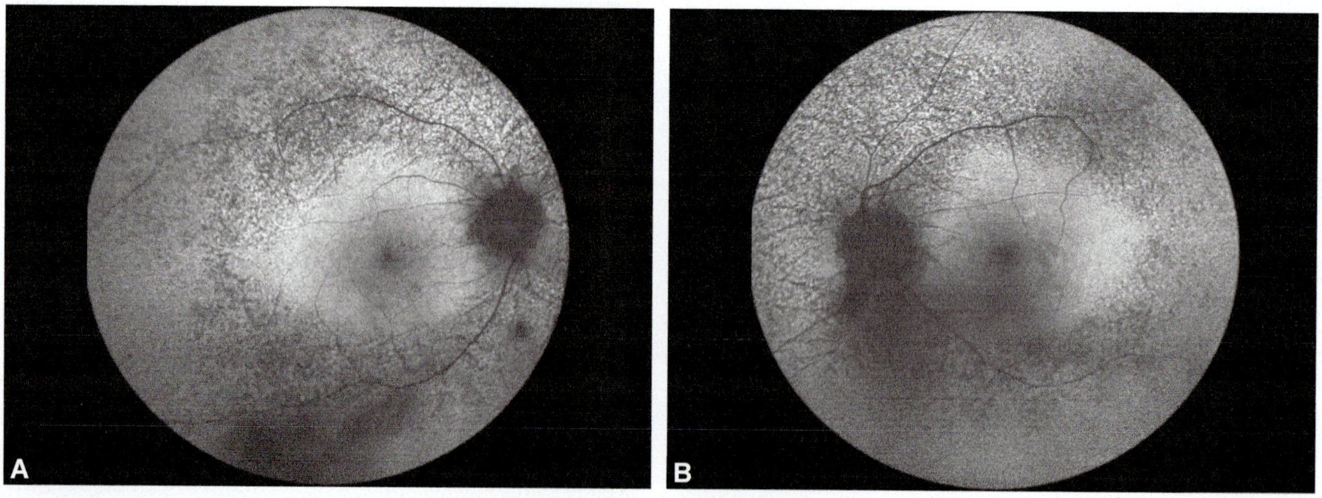

Figs. 86.13A and B: Probable late onset inherited retinal dystrophy masquerading as a uveitis or an autoimmune retinopathy. Autofluorescence, right and left posterior poles. There is a symmetric ring pattern of RPE loss and hypoautofluorescence that is more suggestive of a genetic than an acquired disorder. More accessible genetic testing would likely be helpful in confirming more cases of atypical retinal degenerations masquerading as inflammatory disorders.

Ocular Ischemic Syndrome

Ocular ischemic syndrome (OIS) is caused by ocular hypoperfusion due to occlusion of 90% or more of the carotid artery lumen.[5] The disease is associated with cardiovascular disease and is more common in men and the elderly. Vision loss is gradual in most patients over the course of weeks to months. In a minority of cases, the vision loss may be more acute. Patients may describe periocular pain or difficulty recovering from bright lights. In about 20% of cases, there are inflammatory cells in the anterior chamber, which are rarely higher than grade 2, and occasionally keratic precipitates or posterior synechiae. More common findings include neovascularization of the iris or angle. The intraocular pressure may be low due to hypoperfusion of the ciliary body, or high, due to extensive neovascularization of the angle and secondary neovascular glaucoma. Posterior segment signs include narrowed retinal vessels, retinal hemorrhages distributed in the mid-periphery (present in 80% of cases), microaneurysms, macular capillary telangiectasias, or macular edema.

Ancillary Testing

Fluorescein angiography should demonstrate a slow arm-to-retina perfusion time. Slow filling of all retinal arterial branches after the initial flush is also characteristic. There may be retinal vascular leakage. Doppler evaluation of the carotid artery is useful to demonstrate large vessel stenosis. Vascular stenosis may also be present in smaller vessels at the level of the ophthalmic artery or the retrobulbar vessels. Imaging of these vessels is rarely undertaken and interventions are available only for large vessel occlusions that meet certain criteria.

Rhegmatogenous Retinal Detachment

Rhegmatogenous retinal detachment may present with hyperemia, anterior uveitis including cell, flare, posterior synechiae, and fibrin. Choroidal detachments are common. The inflammation is a clinical dilemma because of the association of serous detachments with uveitis, however, all patients with retinal detachment and intraocular inflammation should be suspected of a rhegmatogenous retinal detachment even if the subretinal fluid is noted to shift. Shifting will occur the subretinal fluid is proteinaceous, which will be the case in any inflamed eye. Meticulous peripheral retinal examination and repeated examination for retinal hole are recommended. Fluorescein angiography will show leaking retinal vessels over any retinal detachment and this should not be considered a sign of inflammatory disease, however, choroidal leak points that may be feeding the retinal detachment are helpful to confirm a probable exudative detachment and support the use of a corticosteroid trial. B-scan ultrasonography can sometimes identify vitreoretinal adhesions or small flap tears.

Intraocular Hemorrhage

Careful examination of the eye will help distinguish hemorrhage from inflammatory cells. In the anterior segment of pseudophakic eyes, slit lamp examination may reveal areas of iris contact and pigment loss from malposition of the intraocular lens. This can produce a true uveitis, but in some cases the cells are just red blood cells. Gonioscopy may be helpful to visualize small hyphemas. In the vitreous cavity, red blood cells look darker than leukocytes and have different patterns of stranding. Patients without a known cause of vitreous bleeding such as trauma or diabetic retinopathy are the most likely to be misdiagnosed as uveitis, for example, other asymptomatic patients with sickle retinopathy. The hemorrhages of some patients decolorize rapidly and may be difficult to distinguish from inflammatory infiltrates.

Central Serous Chorioretinopathy

Central serous chorioretinopathy can be confused with inflammatory exudative retinal detachment despite the lack of cellular inflammation to support a diagnosis of VKH. Misdiagnosis is frequently accompanied by corticosteroid therapy, which makes the central serous worse. Withdrawal of corticosteroids is necessary for resolution.

Ancillary Testing

Ocular imaging studies are essential in making a correct diagnosis. There is some overlap between CSR and VKH: choroid will be thick in each disorder and there will likely be multiple pinpoint leaks. Discrete RPE detachments are not typical of VKH. The autofluorescence images will often show a gravitational distribution of damage to the RPE in CSR. Indocyanine green angiography shows an irregular pattern of mottled hyper- and hypofluorescence of the choroid in the late stages that is characteristic of CSR whereas ICG in active VKH is more likely to show multifocal hypofluorescent lesions of the choroid.

Intraocular Foreign Bodies

Copper foreign bodies can cause acute, intense inflammatory reactions. Siderosis from retention of an iron-containing foreign body may be accompanied by chronic anterior and intermediate inflammation.[61] Heterochromia iridis, mydriasis, pigmented deposits on the anterior lens capsule should prompt a search for an intraocular foreign body with scleral depression, gonioscopy, ultrasound, and computerized tomography imaging as needed. Inflammation can arise from retained foreign bodies without the distinctive signs of siderosis.[62] Imaging may be ineffective in detecting all foreign bodies, requiring repeated examinations in patients with a history of trauma or suspected trauma.

Drug-induced Uveitis

Uveitis produced by medications is worth considering as a masquerade syndrome because failure to recognize the underlying cause will lead to either excessive treatment, such as vitreous aspiration and culture for suspected endophthalmitis or inadequate treatment, which in many cases is as simple as drug withdrawal. Drugs that may cause uveitis have been recently reviewed.[6] Aromatase inhibitors for breast cancer prophylaxis and sulfonamides are relatively common medications that may cause ocular inflammation. Several other medications are notable, either because they are used for eye disease, or because they produce distinctive patterns of inflammation.

Topical Ocular Medications

Glaucoma medications are the most commonly associated with uveitic reactions, especially brimonidine and brimonidine containing fixed-combination products.[63,64] Duration of use before the uveitis is highly variable.[63] The prostaglandin analogs (PA, specifically latanoprost), were initially described to be proinflammatory but with greater clinical experience, iritis and macular edema following PA therapy seem to be rare. There is no need to avoid either brimonidine or PA in patients with uveitis. Those patients who are on therapy and are responding poorly to treatment should be considered for a simple trial of withdrawal to see if the inflammation can be reduced.

INTRAVITREAL OCULAR MEDICATIONS

Anti-Vascular Endothelial Growth Factor Agents

Anti-vascular endothelial growth factor agents—bevacizumab, ranibizumab, and aflibercept have each been reported to cause a transient intraocular inflammation after one or repeated injections. Prospective evaluation of incident iritis with a week of injection of aflibercept revealed a frequency of 19% versus 2% after ranibizumab.[65] The reactions were usually mild, transient and did not involve the vitreous or require intraocular culture. Series documenting the incidence of iritis after ranibizumab at more conventional intervals of 1 month after injection show a much lower rate of 0.026 per thousand injections.[66] Symptoms, if any, are controlled by topical corticosteroids; clinical judgment is necessary to determine if endophthalmitis is present.

Triamcinolone Acetonide

Sterile endophthalmitis following triamcinolone has been attributed to toxic reactions to preparations not intended for ocular use.[67] Alternatively, anterior migration of triamcinolone crystals can lead to pseudo-hyopyon. Serious infections with CMV retinitis have occurred in patients after triamcinolone injection without a prior history of CMV.[68]

SYSTEMIC MEDICATIONS

Rifabutin

Rifabutin was one of the first drugs in the modern era that was recognized to cause severe intraocular inflammation in HIV-infected patients receiving treatment for mycobacterial infection.[69] One of 205 patients experienced severe uveitis in a non-HIV population.[70] Toxicity is dose dependent and multiple drugs that interfere with metabolism through the P-450 pathway including clarithromycin, fluconazole, and protease inhibitors can interfere with metabolism and cause toxic reaction, which nonetheless responds well to drug withdrawal and topical corticosteroids.

Cidofovir

Direct toxicity to the eye with iritis and irreversible hypotony, were reported prior to the use of highly active

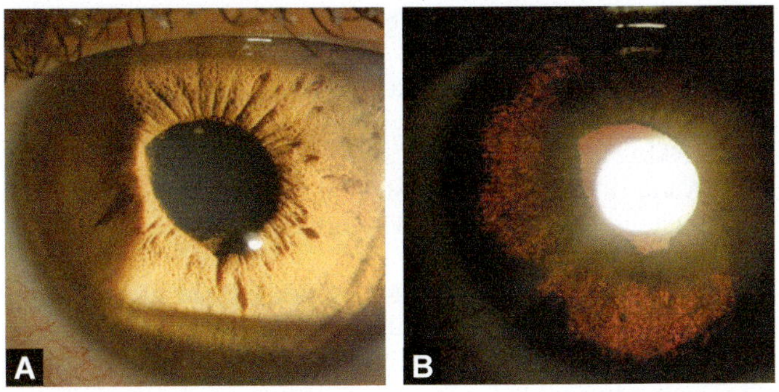

Figs. 86.14A and B: Possible drug-induced uveitis following moxifloxacin treatment for sinusitis. (A) Fundus photograph showing intact anterior iris stroma and irregular pupil after dilation. Areas of the pupil without synechiae. There are pigment clumps on the anterior lens surface and the cornea; (B) Large sectoral iris transillumination defect. Unlike herpetic iritis, the anterior iris pigment is preserved and the region between the collarette and pupillary ruff is not atrophic.

antiretroviral therapy (HAART) for HIV infection.[71,72] In the era of HAART, reactions are proportional to the CD4+ T lymphocyte count indicating that some may be due to an immune recovery uveitis,[73] although a toxic component cannot be excluded.

Bisphosphonates

A population-based retrospective cohort study in Canada documented an incidence rate of uveitis of 29/100,000 patient years and 63/100,000 patient years for scleritis among 10,827 persons using bisphosphonates for the first time during the study years and who visited an ophthalmologist.[74] Adjusted relative risk was 1.45 and 1.51 for uveitis and scleritis, respectively. Bisphosphonates include alendronate, risedronate, ibandronate, and zoledronic acid. Alternative agents with low or no risk of ocular inflammatory reactions include denosumab, teriparatide and abaloparatide.

Fluoroquinolones

Most clinicians feel that oral but not ocular fluoroquinolones are a possible cause of a stereotypical transient iritis with pigment dispersion, bilateral iris transillumination defects, and Adies-like pupils (Figs. 86.14A and B).[75,76] A controlled population-based study of 13,313 uveitis cases indicated an increased risk of uveitis diagnosis in first-time users of moxifloxacin (adjusted risk ratio, 2.98). Risk was also increased after ciprofloxacin but not levofloxacin.[77] Prolonged duration of moxifloxacin levels in the eye after oral administration may contribute to a direct toxicity reaction.[75,78]

CONCLUSION

Masquerade syndrome is not strictly a diagnosis, but an indication of misdiagnosis, ideally brief. Recognition that a patient presents clinical features atypical for noninfectious uveitis or responds inadequately to standard therapy should compel consideration first for infectious uveitis and second for a masquerade syndrome. Heuristics classic for masquerades such as primary vitreoretinal lymphoma and drug-reactions should be part of the working knowledge of all clinicians. Rare masquerades require strong suspicion, ancillary testing and careful therapeutic trials.

REFERENCES

1. Deschenes J, Murray PI, Rao NA, et al. International Uveitis Study G. International Uveitis Study Group (IUSG): clinical classification of uveitis. Ocul Immunol Inflamm. 2008;16(1):1-2.
2. Jabs DA, Nussenblatt RB, Rosenbaum JT. Standardization of Uveitis Nomenclature Working G. Standardization of uveitis nomenclature for reporting clinical data. Results of the First International Workshop. Am J Ophthalmol. 2005;140(3):509-16.
3. Jabs DA, Dick A, Doucette JT, et al. Inter-observer agreement among uveitis experts on uveitic diagnoses: the Standardization of Uveitis Nomenclature (SUN) experience. Am J Ophthalmol. 2017:S0002-9394(17)30459-2.
4. Davis JL, Ruiz P Jr, Shah M,et al. Evaluation of the reactive T-cell infiltrate in uveitis and intraocular lymphoma with flow cytometry of vitreous fluid (an American Ophthalmological Society thesis). Trans Am Ophthalmol Soc. 2012;110:117-29.
5. Terelak-Borys B, Skonieczna K, Grabska-Liberek I. Ocular ischemic syndrome—a systematic review. Med Sci Monit. 2012;18(8):RA138-44.
6. Cordero-Coma M, Salazar-Mendez R, Garzo-Garcia I, et al. Drug-induced uveitis. Expert Opin Drug Saf. 2015;14(1):111-26.
7. Yoshida N, Ikeda Y, Notomi S, et al. Clinical evidence of sustained chronic inflammatory reaction in retinitis pigmentosa. Ophthalmology. 2013;120(1):100-5.
8. Grange LK, Kouchouk A, Dalal MD, et al. Neoplastic masquerade syndromes in patients with uveitis. Am J Ophthalmol. 2014;157(3):526-31.
9. Rothova A, Ooijman F, Kerkhoff F, et al. Uveitis masquerade syndromes. Ophthalmology. 2001;108(2):386-99.
10. Chan CC, Whitcup SM, Solomon D, et al. Interleukin-10 in the vitreous of patients with primary intraocular lymphoma. Am J Ophthalmol. 1995;120(5):671-3.
11. Calfa CJ, Lossos IS, Ruiz P, et al. Ocular involvement as the initial manifestation of T-cell chronic lymphocytic leukemia. Am J Ophthalmol. 2007;144(2):326-9.
12. Chan CC, Rubenstein JL, Coupland SE, et al. Primary vitreoretinal lymphoma: a report from an International Primary Central Nervous System Lymphoma Collaborative Group symposium. Oncologist. 2011;16(11):1589-99.

13. Teckie S, Yahalom J. Primary intraocular lymphoma: treatment outcomes with ocular radiation therapy alone. Leuk Lymphoma. 2014;55(4):795-801.
14. Riemens A, Bromberg J, Touitou V, et al. Treatment strategies in primary vitreoretinal lymphoma: a 17-center European collaborative study. JAMA Ophthalmol. 2015;133(2):191-7.
15. Jahnke K, Korfel A, Komm J, et al. Intraocular lymphoma 2000-2005: results of a retrospective multicentre trial. Graefes Arch Clin Exp Ophthalmol. 2006;244(6):663-9.
16. Kim MM, Dabaja BS, Medeiros J, t al. Survival outcomes of primary intraocular lymphoma: a single-institution experience. Am J Clin Oncol. 2016;39(2):109-13.
17. Fardeau C, Lee CP, Merle-Beral H, et al. Retinal fluorescein, indocyanine green angiography, and optic coherence tomography in non-Hodgkin primary intraocular lymphoma. Am J Ophthalmol. 2009;147(5):886-941.
18. Saito T, Ohguro N, Iwahashi C, et al. Optical coherence tomography manifestations of primary vitreoretinal lymphoma. Graefes Arch Clin Exp Ophthalmol. 2016;254(12):2319-26.
19. Pantanelli SM, Li Z, Fariss R, et al. Differentiation of malignant B-lymphoma cells from normal and activated T-cell populations by their intrinsic autofluorescence. Cancer Res. 2009;69(11):4911-7.
20. Ishida T, Ohno-Matsui K, Kaneko Y, et al. Fundus autofluorescence patterns in eyes with primary intraocular lymphoma. Retina. 2010;30(1):23-32.
21. Casady M, Faia L, Nazemzadeh M, et al. Fundus autofluorescence patterns in primary intraocular lymphoma. Retina. 2014;34(2):366-72.
22. Chan CC, Sen HN. Current concepts in diagnosing and managing primary vitreoretinal (intraocular) lymphoma. Discov Med. 2013;15(81):93-100.
23. Dalal M, Casady M, Moriarty E, et al. Diagnostic procedures in vitreoretinal lymphoma. Ocul Immunol Inflamm. 2014;22(4):270-6.
24. Mudhar HS, Sheard R. Diagnostic cellular yield is superior with full pars plana vitrectomy compared with core vitreous biopsy. Eye. 2013;27(1):50-5.
25. Kanavi MR, Soheilian M, Hosseini SB, et al. 25-gauge transconjunctival diagnostic vitrectomy in suspected cases of intraocular lymphoma: a case series and review of the literature. Int J Ophthalmol. 2014;7(3):577-81.
26. Merle-Beral H, Davi F, Cassoux N, et al. Biological diagnosis of primary intraocular lymphoma. Br J Haematol. 2004;124(4):469-73.
27. Coupland SE, Bechrakis NE, Anastassiou G, et al. Evaluation of vitrectomy specimens and chorioretinal biopsies in the diagnosis of primary intraocular lymphoma in patients with Masquerade syndrome. Graefes Arch Clin Exp Ophthalmol. 2003;241(10):860-70.
28. Lim LL, Suhler EB, Rosenbaum JT, et al. The role of choroidal and retinal biopsies in the diagnosis and management of atypical presentations of uveitis. Trans Am Ophthalmol Soc. 2005;103:84-91.
29. Cassoux N, Giron A, Bodaghi B, et al. IL-10 measurement in aqueous humor for screening patients with suspicion of primary intraocular lymphoma. Invest Ophthalmol Vis Sci. 2007;48(7):3253-9.
30. Davis JL, Viciana AL, Ruiz P. Diagnosis of intraocular lymphoma by flow cytometry. Am J Ophthalmol. 1997;124(3):362-72.
31. Wang Y, Shen D, Wang VM, et al. Molecular biomarkers for the diagnosis of primary vitreoretinal lymphoma. Int J Mol Sci. 2011;12(9):5684-97.
32. Coupland SE, Hummel M, Muller HH, et al. Molecular analysis of immunoglobulin genes in primary intraocular lymphoma. Invest Ophthalmol Vis Sci. 2005;46(10):3507-14.
33. Levy-Clarke GA, Buggage RR, Shen D, et al. Human T-cell lymphotropic virus type-1 associated t-cell leukemia/lymphoma masquerading as necrotizing retinal vasculitis. Ophthalmology. 2002;109(9):1717-22.
34. Liu MM, Furusato E, Cao X, et al. Ocular manifestations and pathology of adult T-cell leukemia/lymphoma associated with human T-lymphotropic virus type 1. Rare Tumors. 2010;2(4):e63.
35. Bonzheim I, Giese S, Deuter C, et al. High frequency of MYD88 mutations in vitreoretinal B-cell lymphoma: a valuable tool to improve diagnostic yield of vitreous aspirates. Blood. 2015;126(1):76-9.
36. Raja H, Salomao DR, Viswanatha DS, Pulido JS. Prevalence of Myd88 L265p Mutation in Histologically Proven, Diffuse Large B-Cell Vitreoretinal Lymphoma. Retina. 2016;36(3):624-8.
37. Kuo DE, Wei MM, Armbrust KR, et al. Gradient Boosted Decision Tree Classification of Endophthalmitis Versus Uveitis and Lymphoma from Aqueous and Vitreous IL-6 and IL-10 Levels. J Ocul Pharmacol Ther. 2017;33(4):319-24.
38. Sugita S, Takase H, Sugamoto Y, et al. Diagnosis of intraocular lymphoma by polymerase chain reaction analysis and cytokine profiling of the vitreous fluid. Jpn J Ophthalmol. 2009;53(3):209-14.
39. Herrlinger U, Schafer N, Fimmers R, et al. Early whole brain radiotherapy in primary CNS lymphoma: negative impact on quality of life in the randomized G-PCNSL-SG1 trial. J Cancer Res Clin Oncol; 2017.
40. Ferreri AJ, Cwynarski K, Pulczynski E, et al. Whole-brain radiotherapy or autologous stem-cell transplantation as consolidation strategies after high-dose methotrexate-based chemoimmunotherapy in patients with primary CNS lymphoma: results of the second randomisation of the International Extranodal Lymphoma Study Group-32 phase 2 trial. Lancet Haematol. 2017;4(11):e510-23.
41. Hashida N, Nakai K, Saitoh N, et al. Association between ocular findings and preventive therapy with onset of central nervous system involvement in patients with primary vitreoretinal lymphoma. Graefes Arch Clin Exp Ophthalmol. 2014;252(4):687-93.
42. Feng L, Zhu J, Gao T, et al. Uveal melanoma in the peripheral choroid masquerading as chronic uveitis. Optom Vis Sci. 2014;91(9):e222-5.
43. al-Haddab S, Hidayat A, Tabbara KF. Ciliary body melanoma with optic nerve invasion. Br J Ophthalmol. 1990;74(2):123-4.

44. Nguyen QD, Foster CS. Ciliary body melanoma masquerading as chronic uveitis. Ocul Immunol Inflamm. 1998;6(4):253-6.
45. Soheilian M, Mirbabai F, Shahsavari M, et al. Metastatic cutaneous melanoma to the vitreous cavity masquerading as intermediate uveitis. Eur J Ophthalmol. 2002;12(4):324-7.
46. Fraser DJ Jr, Font RL. Ocular inflammation and hemorrhage as initial manifestations of uveal malignant melanoma. Incidence and prognosis. Arch Ophthalmol. 1979;97(7): 1311-4.
47. Arai T, Harada K, Usui Y, et al. Case of acute anterior uveitis and Vogt-Koyanagi-Harada syndrome-like eruptions induced by nivolumab in a melanoma patient. J Dermatol. 2017;44(8):975-6.
48. Baughman DM, Lee CS, Snydsman BE, et al. Bilateral uveitis and keratitis following nivolumab treatment for metastatic melanoma. Med Case Rep. 2017;3(2):8.
49. Hahn L, Pepple KL. Bilateral neuroretinitis and anterior uveitis following ipilimumab treatment for metastatic melanoma. J Ophthal Inflamm Infect. 2016;6(1):14.
50. Lim J, Lomax AJ, McNeil C, et al. Uveitis and papillitis in the setting of dabrafenib and trametinib therapy for metastatic melanoma: a case report. Ocul Immunol Inflamm. 2016:1-4.
51. Guedj M, Queant A, Funck-Brentano E, et al. Uveitis in patients with late-stage cutaneous melanoma treated with vemurafenib. JAMA Ophthalmol. 2014;132(12):1421-5.
52. Diem S, Keller F, Ruesch R, et al. Pembrolizumab-triggered Uveitis: An Additional Surrogate Marker for Responders in Melanoma Immunotherapy? J Immunother. 2016;39(9):379-82.
53. Shen T, Liu R, Lin J, et al. Pars Plana Vitrectomy and evisceration resulting in death due to misdiagnosis of retinoblastoma in children: a review of 3 cases. Medicine. 2015;94(32):e1338.
54. Fan RF, Ling YH. Pseudohypopyon—an unusual presenting sign in retinoblastoma. Singapore Med J. 1991;32(5):368-70.
55. Shields CL, Honavar S, Shields JA, et al. Vitrectomy in eyes with unsuspected retinoblastoma. Ophthalmology. 2000;107(12):2250-5.
56. Orellana ME, Brimo F, Auger M, et al. Cytopathological diagnosis of adult retinoblastoma in a vitrectomy specimen. Diagn Cytopathol. 2010;38(1):59-64.
57. Tan AH, Chee SP. Malignant uveitis masquerade syndrome. Am J Respir Crit Care Med. 2014;190(7):e24-5.
58. Mandelcorn ED, Palestine AG, Dubovy S, et al. Vascular co-option in lung cancer metastatic to the eye after treatment with bevacizumab. J Ophthal Inflamm Infect. 2010;1(1):35-8.
59. Kung YH, Wu TT, Lin CS. Tumor seeding after diagnostic vitrectomy for choroidal metastasis in breast cancer. J Chin Med Assoc. 2012;75(9):483-6.
60. Dutta Majumder P, Menia N, Roy R, et al. Uveitis in Patients with Retinitis Pigmentosa: 30 Years' Consecutive Data. Ocul Immunol Inflamm. 2017:1-6.
61. Politis M, Rosin B, Amer R. Ocular siderosis subsequent to a missed pars plana metallic foreign body that masqueraded as refractory intermediate uveitis. Ocul Immunol Inflamm. 2016:1-3.
62. Yeniad B, Beginoglu M, Ozgun C. Missed intraocular foreign body masquerading as intraocular inflammation: two cases. Int Ophthalmol. 2010;30(6):713-6.
63. Beltz J, Zamir E. Brimonidine induced anterior uveitis. Ocul Immunol Inflammat. 2016;24(2):128-33.
64. Carrasco MA, Schlaen BA, Zarate JO. Brimonidine-timolol fixed combination induced granulomatous inflammation of the eye. Int Ophthalmol. 2013;33(5):557-60.
65. Khanani AM, Cohen GL, Zawadzki R. A prospective masked clinical assessment of inflammation after intravitreal injection of ranibizumab or aflibercept. J Ocul Pharmacol Ther. 2016;32(4):216-8.
66. Hasler PW, Bloch SB, Villumsen J, et al. Safety study of 38,503 intravitreal ranibizumab injections performed mainly by physicians in training and nurses in a hospital setting. Acta Ophthalmologica. 2015;93(2):122-5.
67. Stepien KE, Eaton AM, Jaffe GJ, et al. Increased incidence of sterile endophthalmitis after intravitreal triamcinolone acetonide in spring 2006. Retina. 2009;29(2):207-13.
68. Tugal-Tutkun I, Araz B, Cagatay A. CMV retinitis after intravitreal triamcinolone acetonide injection in a patient with Behcet's uveitis. Int Ophthalmol. 2010;30(5):591-3.
69. Fraunfelder FW. Drug-induced ocular inflammatory diseases. Drugs Today (Barc). 2007;43(2):117-23.
70. Chien JY, Chien ST, Huang SY, et al. Safety of rifabutin replacing rifampicin in the treatment of tuberculosis: a single-centre retrospective cohort study. J Antimicrob Chemother. 2014;69(3):790-6.
71. Davis JL, Taskintuna I, Freeman WR, Weinberg DV, Feuer WJ, Leonard RE. Iritis and hypotony after treatment with intravenous cidofovir for cytomegalovirus retinitis. Archives of Ophthalmology. 1997;115(6):733-7.
72. Chavez-de la Paz E, Arevalo JF, Kirsch LS, et al. Anterior nongranulomatous uveitis after intravitreal HPMPC (cidofovir) for the treatment of cytomegalovirus retinitis. Analysis and prevention. Ophthalmology. 1997;104(3):539-44.
73. Berenguer J, Mallolas J. Intravenous cidofovir for compassionate use in AIDS patients with cytomegalovirus retinitis. Spanish Cidofovir Study Group. Clin Infect Dis. 2000;30(1):182-4.
74. Etminan M, Forooghian F, Maberley D. Inflammatory ocular adverse events with the use of oral bisphosphonates: a retrospective cohort study. CMAJ. 2012;184(8):E431-4.
75. Knape RM, Sayyad FE, Davis JL. Moxifloxacin and bilateral acute iris transillumination. J Ophthal Inflamm Infect. 2013;3(1):10.
76. Hinkle DM, Dacey MS, Mandelcorn E, et al. Bilateral uveitis associated with fluoroquinolone therapy. Cutan Ocul Toxicol. 2012;31(2):111-6.
77. Eadie B, Etminan M, Mikelberg FS. Risk for uveitis with oral moxifloxacin: a comparative safety study. JAMA Ophthalmol. 2015;133(1):81-4.
78. Hinkle DM, Kruh-Garcia NA, Kruh JN, et al. Moxifloxacin concentration and proteomic analysis of aqueous humor in human uveitis associated with oral moxifloxacin therapy. Open Ophthalmol J. 2017;11:107-16.

Chapter 87 Investigations in Uveitis

Aniruddha Agarwal, Kanika Aggarwal, K Srinivasarao, Vishali Gupta

INTRODUCTION

A number of infective or autoimmune etiologies can result in ocular inflammatory disease that may be associated with severe visual morbidity. Often, ocular findings may be the presenting feature of serious systemic conditions. A delay in the diagnosis of infectious uveitis and chorioretinitis may be associated with permanent visual impairment.[1] Similarly, lack of initiation of immunosuppressive therapy in autoimmune conditions may lead to sight-threatening ocular disease.

There are a number of reasons why ancillary investigations are necessary in uveitis. These have been listed in Box 87.1.

Ancillary investigations in uveitis are a backbone of uveitis practice, especially in atypical cases where diagnosis cannot be established without ancillary investigations. The most commonly used ancillary investigations in uveitis include laser flare photometer for anterior segment inflammation, ultrasound biomicroscopy (UBM) for ciliary body region, fundus photography and fundus fluorescein angiography (FA) for retinal diseases, indocyanine green angiography (ICGA) for choroidal pathologies, fundus autofluorescence (FAF) for retinal pigment epithelium (RPE) and optical coherence tomography (OCT) as well as ultrasonography for posterior segment. There are various considerations before such tests should be ordered.

With advancing biomedical engineering techniques, a number of state-of-the-art imaging devices have been introduced in the field of ophthalmology in the past few decades. With the help of multimodal imaging techniques, staging, treatment response, and prognosis of various uveitic entities can be accurately assessed. In the following sections, a comprehensive overview of ancillary investigative tools in uveitis has been described.

LABORATORY INVESTIGATIONS

Various laboratory investigations that are used in ocular inflammatory conditions include hematological, serological, cytological, microbiological, immunological, histopathological, radiological, and dermatological, among others. The laboratory investigations must be ordered on *tailored basis* to avoid unnecessary investigations that may be expensive, and more importantly, confuse the clinician (Box 87.2). Among the above listed investigations, hematological investigations are commonly performed to assess the systemic inflammatory cells (white cells) and basic hematological profile (such as hemoglobin and red blood cell count) that can be altered after initiation of therapy. Thus, these tests are largely independent of the type of uveitis. Additional tests include liver and renal function test, which play a role in patients who are already of therapy for monitoring their systemic profiles. Indications of hematological tests are provided in Box 87.3.

Box 87.1: Reasons to investigate a patient with uveitis.

- Establish a specific diagnosis (infection, autoimmunity, allergy or systemic association)
- Confirm the diagnosis
- Substantiate the institution of appropriate therapy
- To exclude other conditions such as tumors
- Identify complications
- Explain reasons for visual loss and why the vision has not improved
- Academic and Research purposes

Box 87.2: Various considerations before ordering investigations in uveitis.

- Age and gender of the patient
- Ethnic and geographic background
- Immigrant status
- Past or present medical history
- History of travel/exposure
- Anatomical location/type of uveitis
- Specific eye findings

Box 87.3: Indications for hematological investigations in uveitis.

- To rule out parasitic infections
- To rule out masquerade syndrome (leukemia/lymphoma)
- For specific investigations (e.g. serum ACE levels in sarcoidosis)
- For ruling out hematological diseases that may present as uveitis (factor V Leiden mutation, systemic lupus erythematosus)
- Prior to initiation of immunosuppressive or anti-infective therapy

Blood and Serum Analysis

Immunological investigations include serum analysis for toxoplasmosis, HIV, and other infectious diseases such as bartonella, cytomegalovirus, herpes virus, varicella zoster, and toxocariasis, among others. In addition, collagen vascular diseases such as systemic vasculitides (which are often associated with ocular manifestations such as retinal vasculitis or scleritis) can be diagnosed using immunological tests such as antinuclear antibody (ANA), anti-double stranded DNA (anti-dsDNA), and anti-neutrophil cytoplasmic antibody (ANCA), among others. Positive ANA is helpful in evaluating risk for uveitis in pauciarticular chronic arthritis and has an almost universal presence in systemic lupus erythematosus (SLE). Antibodies against dsDNA are found in 40–80% cases of SLE and only rarely in other connective tissue disorders. Hence, it is considered to be relatively specific for SLE. They may also be useful in monitoring disease activity in these patients. A combination of positive ANA test, dsDNA antibodies and hypocomplementemia is said to have a diagnostic specificity of 100% for SLE.

Most common conditions in ANCA as positive are Wegener's granulomatosis and microscopic polyarteritis nodosa. c-ANCA has a greater specificity than p-ANCA.

Systemic inflammatory markers include erythrocyte sedimentation rate (ESR) and C-reactive protein (CRP). ESR is affected by the hematological profile of the patients and may be falsely elevated or lower in certain patients depending upon various confounding factors. While the values of CRP generally parallel that of ESR, it is not influenced by factors such as anemia. CRP and ESR are nonspecific indicators of inflammatory activity in the body. CRP increases earlier and declines faster than ESR at the onset and resolution respectively of inflammation.

Serological investigations play an important role in uveitis. However, these must be carefully chosen since investigations testing for rheumatoid factor does not have any role in the diagnosis or management of uveitis, but it is the basis of dividing arthropathies into seropositive or seronegative. Serological tests that play an important role in diagnosing specific uveitic entities include ELISA tests for immunoglobulins against bartonella (Cat-scratch disease), toxoplasma, West Nile virus, and other such organisms.

Radiological Tests

Radiological methods for the diagnosis in uveitis usually target the chest because the lungs are the main site of involvement of conditions such as tuberculosis or sarcoidosis. CT and positron emission tomography (PET) scanning have demonstrated evidence of active tuberculosis remote to the eye with the most common site likely to be within the mediastinum when able to be defined. This compartment can now be targeted by techniques such as endobronchial ultrasound transbronchial needle aspiration (EBUS-TBNA).[2]

In immunosuppressed individuals, radiological findings are more often atypical. Moreover, it must be kept in mind that radiologic evidence of post-inflammatory lesions such as hilar lymphadenopathy and parenchymal scarring may not be specific of TB or sarcoidosis.[3] Furthermore, the pulmonary changes are not detected in many patients with extrapulmonary disease. Due to lower sensitivities, plain chest radiographies are no longer recommended in the initial workup of patients with uveitis. CT scans, which may help delineate concomitant hilar, parenchymal, or pleural disease, can be an effective diagnostic method, especially when plain chest radiographs are normal or inconclusive in highly suspected cases. However, the cost of CT scans and the increased exposure to radiation may preclude its use for routine investigation of all suspected cases.[4]

Microscopy and Culture

The diagnosis of uveitis can be confirmed in cases where the infective organisms can be identified under the microscope. In various uveitic entities, such as intraocular tuberculosis, syphilis and toxoplasmosis, actual detection of the organisms is very challenging due to the paucibacillary nature of the disease, or because the organisms may be very fastidious. In addition, difficulty in obtaining the adequate volume of the ocular sample limits the detection of microorganisms by conventional techniques like smear microscopy and culture. There are very few case series but several case reports where authors have demonstrated AFB either by microscopy or by culture from enucleated eyes, aqueous fluid, vitreous biopsy and sclera biopsy. In a series of 42 enucleated eyes, 1–2 bacilli were found close to areas of necrosis.[5] Another series described histopathological diagnosis in 5 eyes only.[6]

Molecular Biology

Several nucleic acid amplification tests (NAATs) have been used for diagnosis of uveitic entities such as viral uveitis, toxoplasmosis, intraocular tuberculosis and fungal endophthalmitis. Various techniques of NAAT include conventional and real-time polymerase chain reaction (PCR), Loop-mediated isothermal amplification (LAMP) and Gene Xpert TB/RIF. The limitation of these tools is that thus far, no controlled studies are available. For intraocular tuberculosis, available data shows that recently introduced multitarget PCR is more sensitive that Gene Xpert, though the latter can be useful for detection of drug resistance.[7-10] With further research, development of high throughput genomics approach may provide new tools to characterize the molecular events occurring in the several ocular inflammatory diseases including tuberculosis.

CLINICAL IMAGING INVESTIGATIONS

A number of novel imaging modalities are being used in the diagnosis and management of uveitis. In practice, one must make judicious use of these tools in order to fully understand the extent and severity of inflammatory damage resulting from the disease. Often, these imaging tools complement each other. Thus, use of multimodal imaging is essential in the practice of uveitis. A case example of such multimodal imaging is highlighted in Figures 87.1A to C.

Color Fundus Photography and Wide-Field Fundus Imaging

Fundus color photography helps in making a clinical diagnosis and serves as a very useful tool for monitoring the progression or regression of the inflammations of the retina and choroid. Since the diagnosis depends upon the clinical appearance and morphology of the choroiditis lesions, adequate assessment of the disease phenotype using high quality color fundus photography is essential. Serial fundus photography (from acute stage to the stage of healing) is very useful in assessment of morphological evolution of the lesions in conditions such as ocular tuberculosis.[11] In addition, color fundus photography can enable detection of vitreous haze among patients with posterior uveitis such as toxoplasmosis, viral retinitis and tuberculosis.

Few of conditions where fundus photography is useful include macular edema, epiretinal membranes, retinitis, choroiditis, parasitic infections such as toxocariasis, cysticercosis, onchocerciasis, etc., retinal vasculitis, masquerade syndromes and for assessing media clarity.

Ultra-wide field fundus imaging can provide new insights into the disease pathophysiology with a 200° panoramic view of the retina. For example, in a recent study, using ultra-wide field imaging, additional features such as peripheral choroiditis, active retinal vasculitis and neovascularization was observed among patients with intraocular tuberculosis compared to conventional imaging.[12] Using this technology, it is possible to simultaneously document posterior and peripheral retinochoroidal lesions in conditions such as viral retinitis,

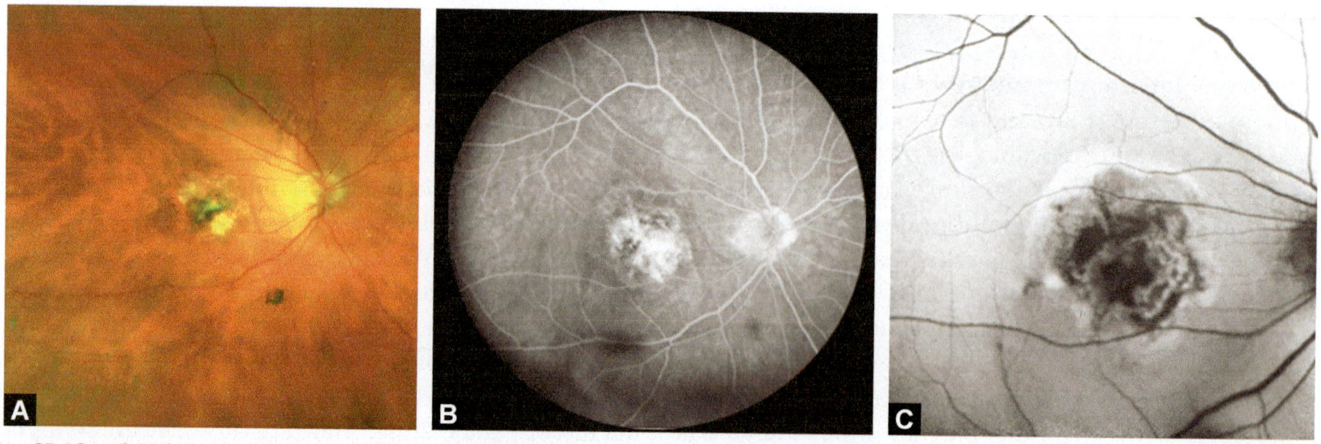

Figs. 87.1A to C: Multimodal imaging of a patient with punctate inner choroidopathy (PIC) complicated by development of choroidal neovascularization (CNV). (A) On color fundus photography, there is a choroidal lesion involving the center of the macula with pigmentation; (B) Fluorescein angiography (mid-phase) shows presence of hyperfluorescence in the macula suggestive of inflammatory CNV; (C) Fundus auto fluorescence imaging showed distinct areas of hyperautofluorescence due to the underlying CNV. The patient was treated with intraocular injection of antivascular endothelial growth factor antibody agent.

presumed ocular histoplasmosis, cytomegalovirus retinitis, toxoplasmosis and intraocular tuberculosis in one image and monitor the overall response to treatment on successive visits. Therefore, ultra-wide field imaging may be superior to conventional imaging in identifying changes (including worsening of disease) which may be otherwise missed.[12]

Fluorescein Angiography

Fluorescein angiography (FA) is the backbone of all investigations in uveitis. It is undoubtedly an indispensable investigation and an imaging modality of choice for most patients with ocular inflammation. It is quite useful in differentiating active from inactive uveitis, diagnosing coexistent pathologies such as cystoid macular edema (CME), choroidal neovascularization, monitor response to therapy and identifying areas of capillary nonperfusion as well as retinal neovascularization.

Choroiditis/Retinitis

Fluorescein angiography is useful in the evaluation of active retinochoroidal lesions to demonstrate active leakage from them. In white dot syndromes such as punctate inner choroidopathy. Birdshot chorioretinopathy (BSCR) tuberculosis, and sarcoidosis, active lesions are hypofluorescent in the early phase. Active lesions show late hyperfluorescence (*hypo to hyper*) (Figs. 87.2A and B). As the lesions progress and become confluent, the advancing edge shows early hypofluorescence with late hyperfluorescence. Areas of resolution show RPE transmission defects if there is underlying choriocapillaris atrophy. Choroidal granulomas are hypofluorescent in the early phase and become hyperfluorescent in the late frames. Retinitis lesions show early abnormal dye leakage.

Lesions of syphilis may show early central hypofluorescence or faint hyperfluorescence followed by progressive hyperfluorescence in the area of the lesion. Variable or punctate hypofluorescence producing a classic *leopard spot* pattern may be seen in later stages of the disease.

Retinal Vasculitis

Fluorescein angiography is very useful in determining presence of active retinal vasculitis, which may often be clinically undetectable (Figs. 87.3A and B). Thus, it is very useful in monitoring the response to therapy and titrating the dose of steroids/immunosuppressive agents. Retinal vasculitis occurs in several inflammatory conditions including Behçet's disease, tuberculosis, sarcoidosis, toxoplasmosis, syphilis, systemic lupus erythematosus, BSCR, acute retinal necrosis, idiopathic retinal vasculitis, aneurysms and neuroretinitis (IRVAN), and frosted branch angiitis.

Cystoid Macular Edema

Fluorescein angiography is very useful in determining presence of dye accumulation due to uveitic CME. CME is common in patients with pars planitis and intermediate uveitis, as well as an important sign of immune recovery uveitis. On FA, CME may appear as a classical petalloid pattern of dye accumulation due to the characteristic

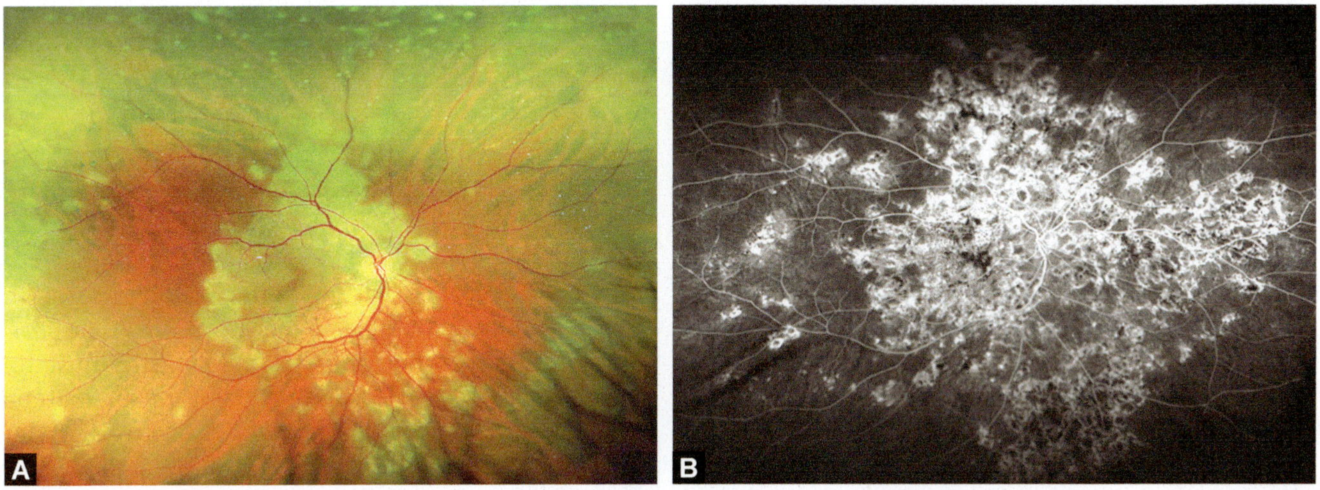

Figs. 87.2A and B: (A) A patient with acute posterior multifocal placoid pigment epitheliopathy (APMPPE) with outer retinal/choroiditis lesions on fundus photography; (B) Fluorescein angiography shows hyperfluorescence in the lesions in the late phase with diffuse spread indicating active choroiditis lesions.

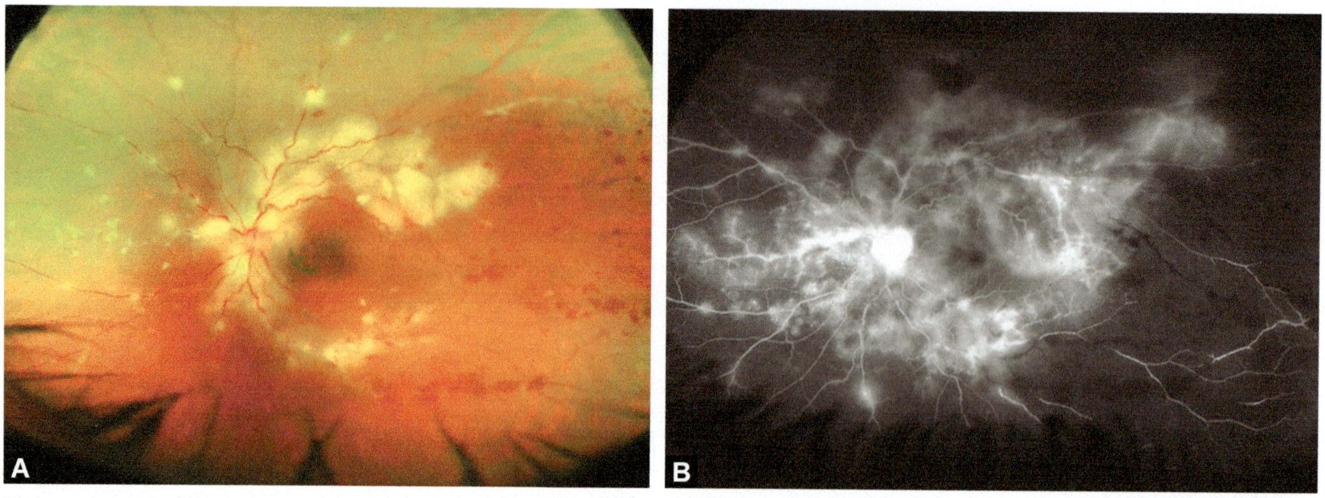

Figs. 87.3A and B: (A) Fundus photograph of a patient with active choroiditis and retinal vasculitis; (B) The fluorescein angiography performed during the active stage of the disease shows presence of diffuse retinal vascular leakage along with focal areas of periphlebitis.

anatomy of the parafoveal retina. Classification of CME on OCT is as follows:

Grade 0: No perifoveal hyperfluorescence

Grade 1: Incomplete perifoveal hyperfluorescence

Grade 2: Mild 360° hyperfluorescence

Grade 3: Moderate hyperfluorescent area being approximately 1-disc diameter across

Grade 4: Severe 360° hyperfluorescence with the hyperfluorescent area being approximately 1.5-disk diameter across.

Specific Patterns on Fluorescein Angiography

In addition, FA is useful in determining specific patterns of dye leakage that provide clues to the diagnosis. Examples include: starry sky pin point hyperfluorescence in Vogt-Koyanagi-Harada (VKH) disease or sympathetic ophthalmia, leopard skin pattern in lymphoma, fern-tree pattern of choriocapillaritis in Behcet's disease, and bacillary angiomatosis-like picture in cat-scratch disease, among others.

Ultra-wide Field Fluorescein Angiography

Ultra-wide field FA is very useful in the management of uveitis. In comparison with conventional FA, ultra-wide field imaging can reveal additional information such as peripheral capillary non-perfusion areas, retinal neovascularization, and retinal vascular leakage. Such findings may alter treatment decisions such as the need for additional immunosuppression or scatter laser photocoagulation.[12]

Indocyanine Green Angiography

Indocyanine green angiography (ICGA) is the imaging modality of choice for the analysis of choroidal inflammatory lesions including the choriocapillaris and the choroidal stroma. ICGA shows occult choroidal lesions that are subclinical and not seen clinically or on FA. The hypofluorescent lesions on ICGA can result from: (i) Choriocapillaris non-perfusion that shows patchy/geographic disposition in the early and intermediate phase and persists in the late frames; or (ii) Stromal inflammatory infiltration that show as more regular dots with an even distribution in the early phase. If these stromal lesions are full thickness (for example full thickness choroidal granulomas of sarcoidosis or tuberculosis), they shall remain hypofluorescent up to late frames, whereas partial thickness lesions become isofluorescent in late frames (such as choroidal granulomas of VKH disease) (Figs. 87.4A to D). Many a times, these lesions show fuzzy appearance of large choroidal vessels in the intermediate phase and may show diffuse choroidal fluorescence in the late phase.

Hyperfluorescence on ICGA may be (i) diffuse that results from increased leakage from large inflamed stromal choroidal vessels (ii) when seen at the level of disc indicates severe inflammation (iii) numerous late hyperfluorescent pinpoints are indicative of granulomatous disease.

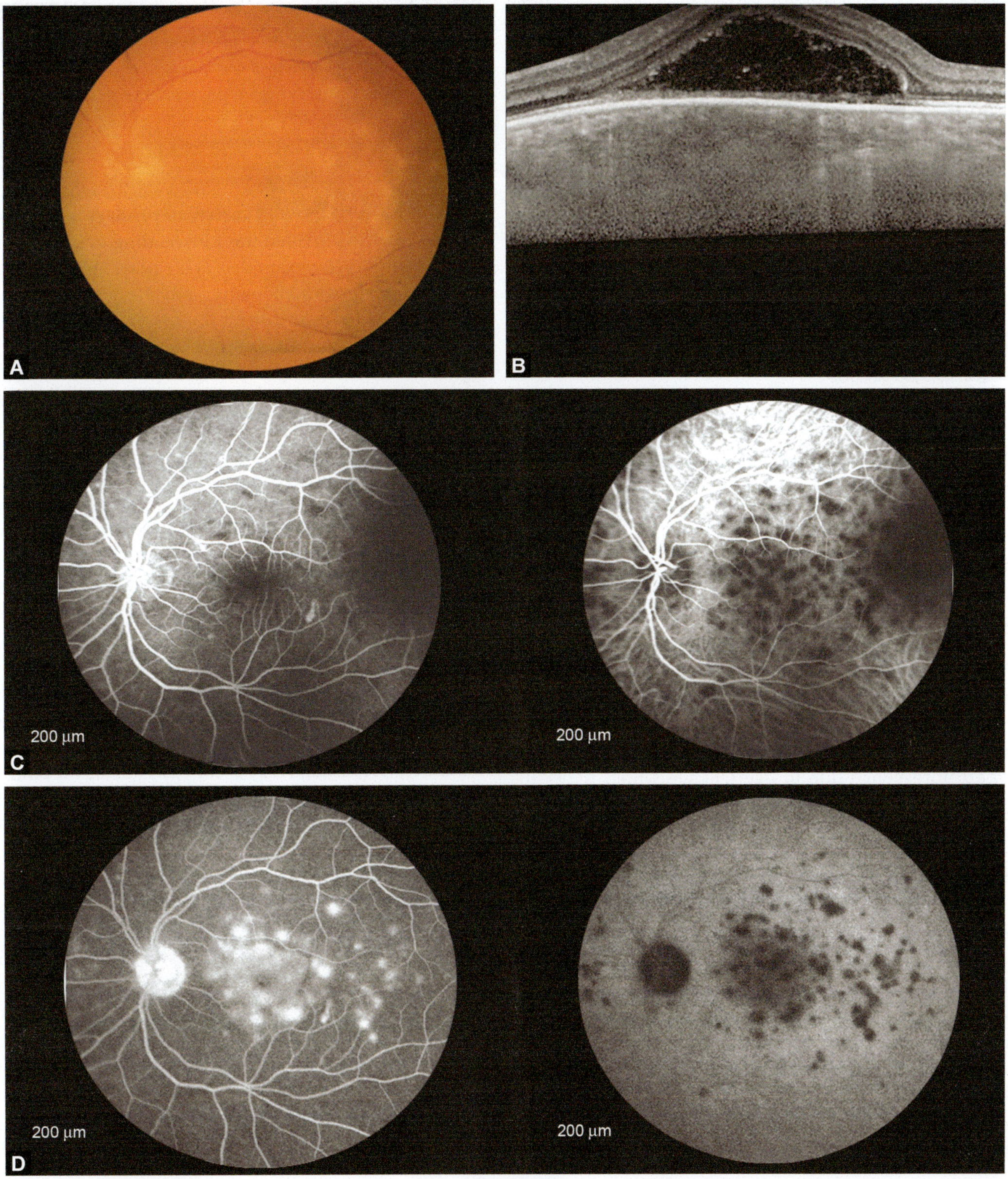

Figs. 87.4 A to D: Multimodal imaging analysis of a patient with acute Vogt-Koyanagi-Harada disease. (A) Fundus photography shows presence of vitritis and yellowish choroiditis lesions in the posterior pole and mid-periphery; (B) Optical coherence tomography shows presence of serous retinal detachment with septae suggestive of accumulation of exudative fluid; (C) Early phase fluorescein angiography (FA) and indocyanine green angiography (ICGA) shows hypofluorescent lesions (much more prominent on ICGA); (D) which become hyperfluorescent on FA in the late phase and remain hypofluorescent on ICGA in the late phase. These angiographic findings are suggestive of active choroidal granulomas consistent with Vogt-Koyanagi-Harada disease.

Table 87.1: Types of choroiditis based on indocyanine green angiography.

Choriocapillaritis	Stromal choroiditis
Multiple evanescent white dot syndrome	Vogt-Koyanagi-Harada disease
Acute idiopathic blind spot enlargement	Sympathetic ophthalmia
Acute posterior multifocal placoid pigment epitheliopathy	Birdshot chorioretinopathy
Multifocal choroiditis	Tuberculosis
Punctate inner choroidopathy	Syphilis
Serpiginous choroiditis	
Acute macular neuroretinopathy	
Acute zonal occult outer retinopathy	
Tuberculosis/sarcoidosis	

Based on ICGA, we can identify uveitic entities as choriocapillaritis or stromal choroiditis (Table 87. 1):

Indocyanine green angiography is very useful in detecting choriocapillaritis among patients with tubercular choroiditis. Active lesions remain hypofluorescence from early to late phase on ICGA. On the other hand, choroidal tubercles show early and intermediate hypofluorescence on ICGA. In the late phase, the lesions may become hyperfluorescent (Type 1) indicating active choroidal lesions or remain hypofluorescent (Type 2) indicating areas of atrophy. There may be presence of numerous hyperfluorescent spots, fuzzy appearance of choroidal vessels in the intermediate phase and late choroidal hyperfluorescence due to dye leakage which tends to regress after completion of treatment with antitubercular therapy and corticosteroids. The ICGA changes are usually reversible and may be used to monitor the response to therapy.[13-15]

Characteristic features of ICGA among patients with acute syphilitic posterior placoid chorioretinitis (ASPPC) have been described in various reports. Lesions of ASPPC show variable hypofluorescence in both early and late stages on ICGA. In some patients, there may be late hyperfluorescence on ICGA.[16,17] ICGA is a useful tool to demonstrate choroidal vascular involvement among patients with syphilitic posterior uveitis.

Fundus Autofluorescence

Fundus autofluorescence is a very useful noninvasive imaging modality in the management of ocular inflammatory conditions that involve the retinal pigment epithelium (RPE). A wide variety of primary/secondary choriocapillaritis involve the RPE leading to changes in the FAF patterns (for examples: acute posterior multifocal placoid pigment epitheliopathy, sarcoidosis, tuberculosis and serpiginous choroiditis). FAF allows detecting low intensity autofluorescence signals produced by fluorophores such as lipofuscin present in the RPE cells. The lipofuscin originates from the photoreceptor outer segments and its accumulation in the RPE cell lysosomes are an indicator of the quality of the RPE cell metabolism.

Table 87.2: Staging of lesions on autofluorescence.

Stage 1	Predominantly hyperautofluorescent
Stage 2	Hyperautofluorescent with hypoautofluorescent rim
Stage 3	Predominantly hypoautofluorescent with stippled hyperautofluorescent
Stage 4	Uniformly hypoautofluorescent

Fundus autofluorescence has wide applications in a number of diseases. Lesions of birdshot chorioretinopathy (BSCR) can be effectively studied using FAF. An interesting aspect of BSCR is that the lesions seen on FAF may not necessarily correspond to the chorioretinal lesions observed clinically[18] or on Goldmann visual field.[19] Often, greater extent of chorioretinal pathology may be noted on FAF compared to routine fundus imaging. Such a phenomenon in BSCR may be explained on the basis of greater involvement of outer retina, RPE-Bruch's complex in BSCR rather than choroidal stromal involvement. Therefore, RPE damage may occur early during the course of the disease resulting in greater damage visible on FAF. Thus, FAF is a relevant supplementary tool in the diagnosis and management of patients with BSCR.

Characteristic changes are observed on FAF as the lesions of serpiginous choroiditis, ampiginous choroiditis, placoid choroiditis and tuberculosis evolve from active to healed stage. Active evolving lesions correspond to the hyper-autofluorescence areas seen on FAF (Stage 1).[20] Lesions undergoing the healing process appear to have a hypoautofluorescent rim around the central hyperautofluorescence on FAF showing a rather stable lesion which is not increasing in size (Stage 2). Further resolution of the lesion demonstrates a hypoautofluorescent stippled pattern on FAF (Stage 3). It is possible to monitor the response of chorioretinal lesions to immunosuppressive therapy by periodic FAF imaging.[21] On complete healing, the lesions become uniformly hypoautofluorescent (Stage 4) (Table 87.2).[22]

Similarly, FAF imaging is an important investigation in patients with acute zonal occult outer retinopathy (AZOOR). In a study correlating FAF with OCT in patients with AZOOR, areas of hypoautofluorescence corresponded to decreased photoreceptor layer thickness, absent outer nuclear layer and abnormal photoreceptor inner segment-outer segment junction patterns (of absence or attenuation).[23,24]

Recently introduced wide-field FAF imaging has shown several peripheral abnormalities including multifocal hypofluorescent spots, hyperfluorescent spots and unique lattice-like pattern in patients with chronic VKH disease. In addition, wide-field FAF has recently been reported to correspond to visual field defect related to alterations of the RPE in uveitis cases.

Optical Coherence Tomography

Optical coherence tomography (OCT) is a novel tool in retinochoroidal imaging which can provide a near-histological cross-section of the retina in vivo without contact with the eye. OCT helps in establishing the diagnosis and monitoring response to therapy. It helps in the localization of the pathology by defining the extent, depth and thickness of the inflammatory lesion.

Cystoid Macular Edema

Similar to FA, OCT is very reliable in diagnosing various pathologies such as CME, retinitis, and subretinal fluid better than FA. There are three patterns of macular edema on OCT: (1) diffuse CME; (2) CME with well-defined cystoid spaces; (3) serous retinal detachment with subretinal fluid. A number of uveitic entities can be associated with CME, such as intermediate uveitis. Significant number of patients with Lyme disease may have CME that can be diagnosed and followed using OCT.[25,26]

Choroiditis Lesions

Optical coherence tomography plays a vital role in determining the nature of choroidal lesions. OCT features of active choroiditis include peripapillary retinal atrophy, disruption of the photoreceptor layer, thinning of the RPE, mild cystic changes as well as subretinal fibrosis in area of old choroidal neovascularization and marked attenuation of the interdigitation zone in the outer retina.[27,28] active edge of the lesions show a localized, fuzzy area of hyperreflectivity in the outer retinal layers involving the RPE, photoreceptor outer segment tips, ellipsoid and myoid zones, external limiting membrane, and the outer nuclear layer with no increased backscattering from the inner choroid. As the lesions begin to heal from the center, the hyper-reflective fuzzy areas begin to disappear from OCT scans and are replaced by irregular, hyperreflective knobbly elevations of the outer retinal layers. The RPE, ellipsoid and myoid zones, and the external limiting membrane cannot be distinguished at this stage. There is an increased reflectance from the choroidal layers due to attenuation of the RPE–photoreceptor complex. As the lesions continue to heal further, there is loss of RPE and outer retinal layers, and persistent increased reflectance from the choroid on OCT.[29]

Choroidal Granulomas

Findings on OCT among patients with subretinal granulomas correlate well with ICGA, obviating the need for an invasive procedure. In addition, OCT is useful in confirming the presence of exudative retinal detachment associated with choroidal granulomas. On EDI-OCT, active choroidal granulomas generate an increased transmission of the OCT signal towards the sclera. Using OCT, one can delineate the exact extent of the choroidal granulomas (full thickness versus partial thickness).

Retinitis

Optical coherence tomography is a useful imaging modality in determining the presence of retinitis lesions. Using OCT, characteristic of full-thickness necrotizing retinitis observed in herpetic infections can be well delineated. OCT also helps in the characterization of retinitis lesions in patients with Bartonellosis and helps in the detection of subretinal/choroidal neovascularization.[30] Retinitis lesions appear as hyperreflective disorganization of the inner retinal layers with shadowing on the posterior retinal layers and the choroid.

Choroidal Neovascularization

Posterior uveitis is often associated with development of type 2 choroidal neovascular membranes in conditions such as punctate inner choroidopathy, BSCR, tuberculosis, VKH disease and sarcoidosis, among others. OCT is very useful in determining the presence of choroidal neovascular membranes and associated intraretinal/subretinal fluid. OCT may have a higher sensitivity compared to FA in diagnosing these neovascular membranes and observing response to therapy.

Box 87.4: Newer optical coherence tomography technologies useful in uveitis.

- Enhanced-depth Imaging optical coherence tomography (OCT)
- Swept-source OCT
- Doppler OCT
- Combined-depth Imaging OCT
- En face OCT
- Anterior segment OCT
- Enhanced vitreous imaging OCT
- OCT angiography

Vitreoretinal Interface Disorders

Optical coherence tomography enables detection of various vitreoretinal interface disorders such as epiretinal membranes, tractional maculopathy, incomplete hyaloid detachment, and specific entities such as inner retinal projections in toxoplasma retinochoroiditis. Often, chronic posterior uveitis leads to development of epiretinal membranes that may result in distortion of vision.

The newer OCT technologies are listed in Box 87.4.

Ultrasound B-scan and Ultrasound Biomicroscopy

Ultrasonography (USG) is a very useful technique in the evaluation of ocular inflammatory conditions since there may be poor visualization of the retinochoroid due to various reasons such as presence of complicated cataract or vitreous haze. USG is useful in assessing the location, extent and density of vitritis. USG is also useful in the detection of other findings such as presence of posterior vitreous detachment, a common finding in eyes with vitreous inflammation. Using USG, exudative retinal detachment among patients with VKH disease, sympathetic ophthalmia and other cases of panuveitis can be diagnosed. Among patients with VKH and sympathetic ophthalmia, USG is very useful in detection of choroidal thickening in presence of media opacities precluding OCT scanning. USG is an important diagnostic modality in diffuse posterior scleritis where it shows high-reflective sclerochoroidal thickening. Scleral edema associated with fluid within Tenon's space results in a hypoechoic region just posterior to the sclera results in the classic *T* sign. Similarly, USG has a role in detection of suprachoroidal fluid in eyes of uveitis with chronic hypotony.

Ultrasound biomicroscopy is a noninvasive, quick to perform ancillary investigation that provides high resolution, cross-sectional biomicroscopic images of the anterior segment. It uses ultrasound of high frequency (35–100 MHz) than conventional ultrasound. Rotating the eye as far as possible can scan the conjunctiva, underlying sclera and peripheral retina as well. UBM is useful in patients with opaque media, patients with hypotony and toxocara uveitis. UBM plays a vital role in detection of ciliary body atrophy/cyclitic membranes. This assessment is important preoperatively in patients with complicated cataract and hypotony. UBM has been reported to show inflammatory cells in the anterior and posterior chamber, exudates as well as swelling of the ciliary body in patients with acute anterior uveitis and these signs resolved on treatment.

Laser Flare Photometer

The laser flare photometer (LFM) is an instrument that comprises of a constant power helium neon or diode laser light beam, which is directed into the anterior chamber at an angle of 45° to the anteroposterior axis. A photodetector unit then detects backscattered light from the incoming beam. LFM is an important quantitative method to measure intraocular inflammation and has been reported to be superior to slit lamp flare and slit lamp cells to assess and monitor anterior chamber inflammation. LFM is useful in diagnosing subclinical inflammation, especially among patients with anterior uveitis, monitoring response to an intervention as well as to detect the disease relapses. For instance, subtle relapses of anterior uveitis can be easily detected using LFM. An increase in more than 20% compared to the previous visit has a positive predictive value for disease relapse in uveitis.

Beside monitoring the disease response to therapy and helping titrating the dosage of anti-inflammatory therapy, early changes in LFM values following therapeutic intervention also help in establishing an early diagnosis. In addition, LFM can help in determining therapeutic efficacy of interventions by documenting early decrease in flare values prior to change in other clinical parameters.

Newer Diagnostic Tools

Newer imaging modalities such as OCTA are being increasingly used in the evaluation of posterior uveitides such as toxoplasmosis, tuberculosis, multifocal/placoid choroiditis, and punctate inner choroidopathy. OCTA enables early detection of complications such as choroidal neovascularization in these patients. In addition, in TB-related choroiditis, choriocapillaris hypoperfusion can be detected which correlates well with findings on ICGA. Thus, noninvasive tools such as OCTA may enable detailed evaluation of the retinochoroidal vasculature among patients with intraocular TB.[31] Thus, further advances in imaging may enhance our knowledge of pathogenesis of uveitis.

Other newer investigative tools that may be soon coming to our clinics include Doppler OCT, intraoperative OCT, and wide-field OCT, among several other technologies.

CONCLUSION

In the past decade, a number of advances have been made in the field of diagnosis in uveitis in order to help the clinician manage day-to-day as well as challenging cases. There has been an increasing trend towards the development of non-invasive and ultra-high speed imaging and laboratory tools that can provide novel information about various uveitic entities. With the introduction of newer laboratory tools such as NAATs, and imaging tools such as OCTA, diagnosis of ocular inflammation has improved significantly leading to better visual outcomes. In the presence of next-generation technologies and availability of advanced analysis software, it is important to order pertinent investigations rather than ordering a battery of irrelevant investigations to optimize management of uveitis patients. The choice of investigation should depend upon the site of inflammation and many a times, a number of ancillary tests may need to be performed in combination to get the useful information.

REFERENCES

1. Singh R, Gupta V, Gupta A. Pattern of uveitis in a referral eye clinic in north India. Indian J Ophthalmol. 2004;52(2):121-5.
2. Ye W, Zhang R, Xu X, et al. Diagnostic efficacy and safety of endobronchial ultrasound-guided transbronchial needle aspiration in intrathoracic tuberculosis: a meta-analysis. J Ultrasound Medicine. 2015;34(9):1645-50.
3. Marchiori E, Zanetti G, Barreto MM, et al. Atypical distribution of small nodules on high resolution CT studies: patterns and differentials. Respir Med. 2011;105(9):1263-67.
4. Ganesh SK, Roopleen, Biswas J, et al. Role of high-resolution computerized tomography (HRCT) of the chest in granulomatous uveitis: a tertiary uveitis clinic experience from India. Ocul Immunol Inflamm. 2011;19(1):51-7.
5. Wroblewski KJ, Hidayat AA, Neafie RC, et al. Ocular tuberculosis: a clinicopathologic and molecular study. Ophthalmology. 2011;118(4):772-7.
6. Biswas J, Madhavan HN, Gopal L, et al. Intraocular tuberculosis. Clinicopathologic study of five cases. Retina. 1995;15(6):461-8.
7. Sharma K, Gupta V, Bansal R, et al. Novel multi-targeted polymerase chain reaction for diagnosis of presumed tubercular uveitis. J Ophthalmic Inflamm Infect. 2013;3(1):25.
8. Balne PK, Modi RR, Choudhury N, et al. Factors influencing polymerase chain reaction outcomes in patients with clinically suspected ocular tuberculosis. J Ophthalmic Inflamm Infect. 2014;4(1):10.
9. Bansal R, Sharma K, Gupta A, et al. Detection of *Mycobacterium tuberculosis* genome in vitreous fluid of eyes with multifocal serpiginoid choroiditis. Ophthalmology. 2015;122(4):840-50.
10. Sharma K, Sharma A, Bansal R, et al. Drug-resistant tubercular uveitis. J Clin Microbiol. 2014;52(11):4113-4.
11. Bansal R, Gupta A, Gupta V, et al. Tubercular serpiginous-like choroiditis presenting as multifocal serpiginoid choroiditis. Ophthalmology. 2012;119(11):2334-42.
12. Aggarwal K, Mulkutkar S, Mahajan S, et al. Role of ultra-wide field imaging in the management of tubercular posterior uveitis. Ocul Immunol Inflamm. 2016;24(6):631-6.
13. Wolfensberger TJ, Piguet B, Herbort CP. Indocyanine green angiographic features in tuberculous chorioretinitis. Am J Ophthalmol. 1999;127(3):350-3.
14. De Luigi G, Mantovani A, Papadia M, et al. Tuberculosis-related choriocapillaritis (multifocal-serpiginous choroiditis): follow-up and precise monitoring of therapy by indocyanine green angiography. Int Ophthalmol. 2012;32(1):55-60.
15. Invernizzi A, Agarwal A, Cozzi M, et al. Enhanced depth imaging optical coherence tomography features in areas of choriocapillaris hypoperfusion. Retina. 2016;36(10): 2013-21.
16. Davis JL. Ocular syphilis. Curr Opin Ophthalmol. 2014;25(6):513-8.
17. Eandi CM, Neri P, Adelman RA, et al. Acute syphilitic posterior placoid chorioretinitis: report of a case series and comprehensive review of the literature. Retina. 2012;32(9):1915-41.
18. Giuliari G, Hinkle DM, Foster CS. The spectrum of fundus autofluorescence findings in birdshot chorioretinopathy. J Ophthalmol. 2009;2009:567693.
19. Jack LS, Agarwal A, Sepah Y, et al. Spatial agreement between goldmann visual field defects and fundus autofluorescence in patients with birdshot chorioretinopathy. J Ocular Inflamm Inf. 2016;6(1):18.
20. Samy A, Lightman S, Ismetova F, et al. Role of autofluorescence in inflammatory/infective diseases of the retina and choroid. J Ophthalmol. 2014;2014:418193.
21. Lee CS, Lee AY, Forooghian F, et al. Fundus autofluorescence features in the inflammatory maculopathies. Clin Ophthalmol. 2014;8:2001-12.
22. Gupta A, Bansal R, Gupta V, et al. Fundus autofluorescence in serpiginouslike choroiditis. Retina. 2012;32(4):814-25.
23. Fujiwara T, Imamura Y, Giovinazzo VJ, et al. Fundus autofluorescence and optical coherence tomographic

findings in acute zonal occult outer retinopathy. Retina. 2010;30(8):1206-16.
24. Gass JD. Are acute zonal occult outer retinopathy and the white spot syndromes (AZOOR complex) specific autoimmune diseases? Am J Ophthalmol. 2003;135(3):380-1.
25. Bergloff J, Gasser R, Feigl B. Ophthalmic manifestations in Lyme borreliosis. A review. J Neuroophthalmol. 1994;14(1):15-20.
26. Park M. Ocular manifestations of Lyme disease. J Am Optom Assoc. 1989;60(4):284-9.
27. Punjabi OS, Rich R, Davis JL, et al. Imaging serpiginous choroidopathy with spectral domain optical coherence tomography. Ophthalmic Surg Lasers Imaging. 2008;39(4 Suppl):S95-8.
28. Rifkin LM, Munk MR, Baddar D, et al. A new OCT finding in tuberculous serpiginous-like choroidopathy. Ocul Immunol Inflamm. 2015;23(1):53-8.
29. Bansal R, Kulkarni P, Gupta A, et al. High-resolution spectral domain optical coherence tomography and fundus autofluorescence correlation in tubercular serpiginous like choroiditis. J Ophthalmic Inflamm Infect. 2011;1(4):157-63.
30. Latanza L, Viscogliosi F, Solimeo A, et al. Choroidal neovascularisation as an unusual ophthalmic manifestation of cat-scratch disease in an 8-year-old girl. Int Ophthalmol. 2015;35(5):709-16.
31. Mandadi S, Agarwal A, Aggarwal K, et al. Novel findings on optical coherence tomography angiography in patients with tubercular serpiginous-like choroiditis. Retina. 2016;37(9):1647-59.

Chapter 88 Steroids, Immunosuppressives, and New Biologicals in Uveitis

John A Gonzales

CORTICOSTEROIDS

Commercially available, laboratory-produced corticosteroids used to treat systemic inflammatory diseases were introduced relatively recently in 1949 and originally for the treatment of rheumatoid arthritis.[1] Prior to this, corticosteroids were used on a limited basis and came from ox bile. Soon afterwards, topical corticosteroids for ophthalmic use were available and both systemic and topical corticosteroids (cortisone) were being used to treat uveitis.

Today, corticosteroids remain the usual first-line agents in managing noninfectious uveitis due to their rapid and effective action. Whether administered in topical, oral, parenteral, periocular, or intraocular forms, they can be effective and, particularly when used for short periods of time, safe. However, corticosteroids have important side effects. While many of the side effects of steroids resolve after discontinuation, chronic uveitis requires chronic management and the use of moderate to high doses of corticosteroids should be avoided. This is where corticosteroid-sparing immunomodulatory agents come into play. They provide a means to managing uveitis while having a better side effect profile than high-dose or frequent administration of corticosteroids.

Topical corticosteroids that are routinely used to treat anterior uveitis include prednisolone acetate 1% and dexamethasone 0.1%. Because prednisolone acetate 1% is a suspension, the patient must be instructed to shake the bottle well prior to instilling a drop in the eye otherwise the actual medication can sediment at the bottom of the bottle and only vehicle and very little medication get into the eye. Dexamethasone 0.1% is a solution and does not need to be shaken. For active anterior uveitis, these topical corticosteroids may be used every hour. Reductions in frequency (or tapering) can be made depending on how quickly the inflammation becomes controlled. Thus, frequent follow up with the uveitis patient is necessary to help guide the topical corticosteroid process. Intraocular pressure should be monitored when patients are taking topical corticosteroids as ocular hypertension is a side effect of topical corticosteroids, which left unmanaged, can evolve to glaucoma. A newer topical corticosteroid, difluprednate 0.05% (Durezol, Alcon Laboratories, Inc.) is a potent topical corticosteroid that may offer less frequent dosing compared to prednisolone acetate or dexamethasone, but close monitoring of intraocular pressure is necessary. Maintenance with topical corticosteroids alone may be considered in situations where the uveitis is anterior, is controlled with infrequent dosing, and provided that there are no complications including unmanaged ocular hypertension or glaucoma, or evolving posterior subcapsular cataract. In general, topical corticosteroid use less than or equal to 3 drops daily is associated with a lower risk of cataract development compared to using a topical corticosteroid more frequently.[2] It should be noted that long-term use of difluprednate is not recommended as it is more potent than prednisolone acetate and dexamethasone. Difluprednate has shown efficacy in improving or resolving uveitic cystoid macular edema.[3,4]

Periocular and intraocular corticosteroids can offer long-lasting management of noninfectious uveitis particularly for intermediate, posterior or panuveitis, which require more than topical corticosteroid drops alone. Periocular and intraocular corticosteroids can also be useful for uveitic macular edema.[5,6] The effects of periocular triamcinolone acetonide injection when administered to the sub-Tenon's space via the Nozik,[7] canula,[8,9] or orbital floor[8,9] methods can be seen for 4–6 weeks. Intraocular corticosteroids can also achieve control of active inflammation in noninfectious intermediate, posterior, and panuveitis.[10] For chronic uveitis, however, managing ocular inflammation with repeated peri- or intraocular injections is not ideal. In such cases, consideration should be made for longer lasting local therapy or systemic immunomodulatory therapy. With respect to longer lasting corticosteroids, the dexamethasone implant (Ozurdex, Allergan, Irvine, CA) and fluocinolone implant (Retisert, Bausch+Lomb, Inc,

Bridgewater, NJ) may be considered. Ozurdex can release steroid into the vitreous for up to 6 months. It should not be injected into eyes with compromised posterior lens capsules as the implant can migrate to the anterior segment.[11,12] Because many types of chronic anterior uveitis do not remit in 3–6 months, longer term therapy with the Retisert implant, which can release steroid into the vitreous for up to 30 months, can be achieved. With Retisert, most phakic patients will require cataract surgery due to steroid-induced cataract progression. Additionally, most patients will require topical ocular antihypertensive agents due to steroid-related ocular hypertension from the implant. Over one-third of patients will require glaucoma surgery in spite of using topical ocular antihypertensives. For bilateral uveitis, each eye would require a Retisert implant and discussion with the patient about the side effects and possible additional surgeries should be weighed against the systemic side effects of immunomodulatory or biologic therapy. However, in selected cases Retisert can be a good option in the chronic uveitis patient. While the Multicenter Uveitis Steroid Treatment Trial (MUST) demonstrated at 7-years of follow-up that patients with noninfectious intermediate, posterior, or panuveitis showed a greater proportion of patients on systemic immunosuppression achieving better visual acuity than those randomized to Retisert, both groups had visual acuity outcomes that were favorable.[13] The Retisert implant does achieve control of inflammation faster than systemic immunosuppression.[13] It should be noted that for chronic uveitis, placing a new implant after 30 months may be required and would be expected to control inflammation as long as an implant capable of eluting steroid is present.

Systemic corticosteroids (oral or intravenous) remain one of the most utilized initial therapies in the realm of uveitis. High-dose systemic steroids can be very effective in managing ocular inflammation, particularly because they have a rapid onset of action. However, systemic steroids have profound systemic side effects (Table 88.1) and are a poor

Table 88.1: Corticosteroids.

	Type	Frequency		Side effects
Topical	Prednisolone acetate 1%	Initial	1 drop every hour	Ocular hypertension; glaucoma; cataract; ocular surface irritation
		Maintenance	1 drop BID	
	Dexamethasone 0.1%	Initial	1 drop every hour	
		Maintenance	1 drop BID	
	Difluprednate 0.05%	Initial	1 drop QID	
		Maintenance	None	
Periocular	Triamcinolone acetonide 40 mg/mL	1 mL (40 mg) periocular injection		Ocular hypertension; glaucoma; cataract
Intraocular	Triamcinolone acetonide 4 mg/0.1 mL (preservative-free)	0.1 mL (4 mg) intraocular injection		Ocular hypertension; glaucoma; cataract; endophthalmitis; retinal detachment
	Dexamethasone implant 0.7 mg	One implant		
	Fluocinolone implant 0.59 mg	One implant		
Oral	Prednisone	Initial	1 mg/kg/day (typically no higher than 60 mg daily). Dose reduction/taper depending on course of uveitis	Weight gain; Cushingoid appearance; insomnia; mood lability; HTN; edema; acne; Cushing syndrome; diabetes
		Maintenance	7.5 mg daily or less	
	Prednisolone	Initial	1 mg/kg/day (typically no higher than 60 mg daily) Dose reduction/taper depending on course of uveitis	
		Maintenance	7.5 mg daily or less	
Intravenous	Methylprednisolone sodium succinate	1 g IV daily × 3 days then typically convert to high-dose oral corticosteroid		Weight gain; Cushingoid appearance; insomnia; mood lability; HTN; edema; acne; Cushing syndrome; diabetes

(BID: Twice a day; QID: Four times a day; HTN: Hypertension; IV: Intravenous)

long-term solution. Used appropriately, however, systemic steroids can allow for control of noninfectious uveitis especially when transitioning to an immunomodulatory or biologic agent that takes time (sometimes up to 3 or more months for some immunomodulatory medications) to become fully therapeutic. In some cases of very fulminant uveitis, for example VKH or sympathetic ophthalmia, intravenous methylprednisolone 1g IV daily for 3 days can be used prior to converting the patient to high-dose oral corticosteroids. Oral prednisone or prednisolone is typically dosed at 1 mg/kg/day, with maximum dosing typically being 60–80 mg daily. Prednisone should be decreased in a step-wise fashion with dose reductions occurring when control of inflammation is confirmed on clinical examination. Oral steroids are typically decreased by 10 or 5 mg increments every one to two weeks.[14] Suppression of the hypothalamic-pituitary-adrenal axis can occur if prednisone or prednisolone doses above 20 mg daily are used for greater than 3 weeks.[15,16] Calcium (1500 mg PO daily) and vitamin D (800 IU PO daily) should be taken as long as a patient is taking oral prednisone to prevent osteopenia that can occur with systemic corticosteroid use.

ANTIMETABOLITES

Interfering with metabolic pathways necessary for cell growth, the antimetabolites are typically first-line therapy when corticosteroid-sparing management of uveitis is required. In general, antimetabolites are well tolerated by patients and very familiar to most uveitis specialists. The dose, side effects and clinical monitoring of immunomodulatory medications are given in Table 88.2.

Azathioprine

Glutathione S-transferase converts azathioprine to 6-mercaptopurine (6-MP), which is a purine nucleoside analogue. 6-MP is then metabolized by hypoxanthine guanine phosphoribosyl transferase forming two active metabolites (thioinosinic and thioguanylic acid), which block purine metabolism and halt DNA synthesis. The enzyme thiopurine S-methyltransferase (TPMT) metabolizes 6-MP to the inactive metabolite, 6-methylmercaptopurine as well as metabolizing the active metabolites. Polymorphisms of the *TPMT* gene exist and in patients homozygous for mutations of *TPMT*, the enzyme is functionally inactive, which can lead to drug toxicity. In patients heterozygous for mutations of *TPMT*, the enzyme is partially functional and reduced doses of azathioprine should be used. Some specialists test for homo- or heterozygosity of *TPMT*, though others simply start a low dose and recheck monitoring tests (complete blood count with differential) prior to increasing to typical maintenance doses. Azathioprine seems to be particularly effective for intermediate uveitis.[17] Compared to methotrexate and mycophenolate mofetil, azathioprine was associated

Table 88.2: Immunomodulatory medications.

Medication		Dose		Side effects	Monitoring
Antimetabolites	Azathioprine	Initial	1 mg/kg/day PO	GI; hepatitis; BM suppression	CBC, CMP, AST, ALT every 4–6 weeks
		Maintenance/ maximum	2.5–4 mg/kg/day PO		
	Leflunomide	Initial	Loading dose: 100 mg PO daily × 3 days	GI; hepatitis; hepatotoxicity; BM suppression; pruritis	CBC, CMP, AST, ALT every 6 weeks
		Maintenance/ maximum	20 mg PO daily		
	Methotrexate	Initial	7.5–15 mg PO/SC weekly	GI; hepatitis; hair loss; stomatitis; pneumonitis	CBC, CMP, AST, ALT every 4–8 weeks
		Maintenance/ maximum	15–25 mg PO/SC weekly		
	Mycophenolate mofetil	Initial	500 mg PO BID	GI; fever; HA; tremor; HTN; infection	CBC, CMP, AST, ALT every 4–8 weeks.
		Maintenance/ maximum	1–1.5 g PO BID		

Contd...

Contd...

Medication		Dose		Side effects	Monitoring
Calcineurin inhibitors (T-cell inhibitors)	Cyclosporine	Initial	Modified: 2.5 mg/kg daily PO divided BID Non-modified: 2.5–5 mg/kg daily PO (divided BID)	HTN; nephrotoxicity; hirsutism; gingival hyperplasia; tremor; GI; paresthesias	CBC, CMP, AST, ALT every 4–8 weeks Check BP
		Maintenance/ maximum	Modified: 4 mg/kg daily PO Non-modified: 10 mg/kg daily PO		
	Tacrolimus	Initial	0.15–0.30 mg/kg daily PO	HTN; nephrotoxicity; tremor; GI; transaminitis	CBC, CMP, AST, ALT every 4–8 weeks Check BP
		Maintenance/ maximum	0.30 mg/kg daily PO		
Alkylating agents	Chlorambucil	Initial	0.1 mg/kg daily PO	BM suppression; sterility; infection; hemorrhagic cystitis; malignancy	CBC, CMP, AST, ALT weekly for first 6 weeks, then monthly
		Maintenance/ maximum	0.2 mg/kg daily PO		
	Cyclosporine	Initial	1.5–2 mg/kg daily PO	BM suppression; sterility; infection; hematuria hemorrhagic cystitis; malignancy	Check Cr and CBC prior to starting CBC and urinalysis weekly for first 6 weeks, then monthly
		Maintenance/ maximum	3 mg/kg daily PO		

[ALT, Alanine transaminase; AST: Aspartate transaminase; BM: Bone marrow; BP: Blood pressure; CBC: Complete blood count (with differential); CMP: Complete metabolic panel; CNS: Central nervous system; Cr: Creatinine; GI: Gastrointestinal side effects (abdominal pain, nausea, diarrhea, vomiting); HA: Headache; HTN: Hypertension; PO: Per OS (oral); SC: Subcutaneous; TB: Tuberculosis; URI: Upper respiratory infection; UTI: Urinary tract infection]

with a longer time (6.5 months) for achieving control of uveitis with doses of prednisone 10 mg PO daily or less.[18] Additionally, azathioprine has been combined with T-cell inhibitors and corticosteroids to achieve control of noninfectious uveitis, including serpiginous choroiditis[19] and sympathetic ophthalmia.[20-23]

Side Effects

Side effects of azathioprine include gastrointestinal upset, cytopenias due to bone marrow suppression (leukopenia and thrombocytopenia in particular).[24] Azathioprine is a pregnancy class D medication (human fetal risk). Breastfeeding is considered reasonable in lactating mothers taking azathioprine with very low levels of the medication being found in breast milk.[25]

Leflunomide

Leflunomide is converted to its active metabolite A77 1726 in the liver. Originally synthesized during the 1980s, leflunomide was approved by the United States Food and Drug Administration (FDA) for the treatment of rheumatoid arthritis in the 1990s. Leflunomide antagonizes lymphoproliferation by inhibiting dihydro-orotate dehydrogenase, leading to a reduction in the de novo synthesis of pyrimidines and, ultimately, halting DNA synthesis. Leflunomide has been shown to halt CD4+ T cell proliferation abrogate B-cell autoantibody synthesis, and decrease activation of NF-κ B.[26,27]

While leflunomide has been used in the treatment of uveitis,[28-30] it has been associated with more frequent rates of recurrences compared to methotrexate when used in the chronic anterior uveitis associated with juvenile idiopathic arthritis (JIA).[31] Others have shown that leflunomide has been effective at managing the chronic anterior uveitis associated with JIA. Molina and colleagues performed a retrospective review of 13 patients with JIA-associated uveitis using leflunomide for at least 7 months.[30] They found that 50% of patients achieved and maintained complete remission, 25% showed improvement, 25% exhibited persistent remission, and 38.5% showed no response to leflunomide. Thus, overall, 61% of the cohort exhibited a favorable response to leflunomide.

Leflunomide has been used effectively in combination with methotrexate, particularly in rheumatoid arthritis due to synergism.[32,33] While some antimetabolites are used with the biologic infliximab, to prevent human anti-chimeric antibody (neutralizing antibody) formation, using leflunomide with infliximab is associated with frequent adverse reactions.[34] The use of leflunomide with infliximab, then, is not recommended.

Side Effects

Side effects include nausea, diarrhea, rash, and reversible alopecia. Less frequent side effects include hypertension,[35] upper respiratory tract infections, and hepatotoxicity. Additionally, there has been an association with increasing total cholesterol and LDL cholesterol with increasing length of time patients take leflunomide.

Methotrexate

Methotrexate inhibits mammalian dihydrofolate reductase (DHFR). DHFR is important in de novo purine (adenine and guanine) synthesis.[33] Methotrexate also inhibits thymidylate synthase, which is involved in the de novo synthesis of pyrimidines. Other functions methotrexate exhibits include inhibition of the formation of polyamines,[36] which play a role in inflammation as seen in the synovial fluid and tissues in patients with rheumatoid arthritis.[37] Additionally, methotrexate promotes adenosine release,[38] which can have anti-inflammatory effects.[39,40]

In a large retrospective cohort study of 384 patients commenced on methotrexate for corticosteroid-sparing monotherapy of various types of ocular inflammation (including uveitis), 66% of patients were able to achieve inactivity of ocular inflammation that was sustained for at least 4 weeks within 1 year of therapy.[41] Approximately, 58% of patients were able to achieve corticosteroid-sparing control of inflammation (≤10 mg of oral prednisone daily).

Methotrexate is extensively used in the setting of JIA-associated uveitis and remains as a common first-line corticosteroid-sparing agent.[42-46]

If ocular inflammation is not responding to oral methotrexate, consideration should be made, if indicated, for subcutaneous administration. While many uveitis specialists routinely start all their patients on subcutaneous methotrexate, it is also very common to use methotrexate orally.

Side Effects

Methotrexate can be hepatotoxic, causing fibrosis and cirrhosis. Consequently, liver transaminases (including aspartate aminotransferase and alanine aminotransferase) should be routinely monitored. Methotrexate can rarely cause a direct toxic effect to lung parenchymal tissue, characterize by a non-productive cough and wheezing. Patients should be assessed for pulmonary symptoms while on methotrexate and, should complaints arise, be examined with auscultation of the lungs and consideration for pulmonary radiographic imaging, which can reveal a diffuse interstitial pattern.[47] An ulcerative stomatitis/mucositis can occur.[48]

Folic acid or folinic acid (Leucovorin) are typically administered to minimize the side effects of methotrexate without affecting methotrexate's efficacy.[49-51] Folic acid is typically dosed at 1 mg orally each day. While some hold folic acid on the day that methotrexate is administered, there is no data suggesting that taking folic acid on the day of methotrexate administration decreases methotrexate's efficacy. When side effects persist, the dose of folic acid may be increased to 3–5 mg daily. Folinic acid may be administered for especially recalcitrant side effects (10 mg orally taken 12 hours after methotrexate administration). Methotrexate is absolutely contraindicated in pregnancy (pregnancy class X) as it produces teratogenic effects and can induce fetal death. Methotrexate is detected in human breast milk and breastfeeding should cease if a mother is taking methotrexate.

Mycophenolate Mofetil

Mycophenolate mofetil is absorbed in the small intestine and metabolized to mycophenolic acid, which then undergoes glucuronidation via glucoronyl transferase to yield the phenolic glucoronide of mycophenolic acid (MPAG). MPAG is converted to mycophenolic acid during enterohepatic recirculation. As the morpholinoethyl ester of mycophenolic acid, mycophenolate mofetil exhibits more bioavailability than mycophenolic acid.[52] Carboxylesterases in the small intestine then convert mycophenolate mofetil to mycophenolic acid.[53] Mycophenolate mofetil is an inhibitor of inosine monophosphate dehydrogenase and block de novo purine synthesis preventing DNA synthesis.

The largest retrospective study involving the use of mycophenolate mofetil in uveitis comes from Siepmann and colleagues in Germany.[54] Nearly 87% experienced one or less recurrences of uveitis with good preservation of visual acuity particularly in those with anterior and intermediate uveitis. Others have shown effective corticosteroid-sparing control of uveitis with reduced recurrences as well.[55]

The median time to treatment success with mycophenolate mofetil 2 g daily was 3.5 months. In those patients requiring 3 g daily, the median time to treatment success was 4.7 months, though this was not statistically different from the lower-dosage.[56]

In one of the largest retrospective studies evaluating the use of mycophenolate mofetil in the setting of pediatric uveitis 88% were able to achieve ≤5 mg PO daily of prednisolone. While only 24% of patients during a mean follow-up of 3 years exhibited no relapses, all patients exhibited a reduction in relapses compared to the number experienced prior to starting mycophenolate mofetil.[57]

Mycophenolate mofetil has also been effective in controlling uveitis in patients failing methotrexate. Sobrin and colleagues performed a retrospective review of their patients with noninfectious ocular inflammation failing methotrexate (either due to efficacy or due to intolerance).[58] Approximately, half of their patients were able to achieve control of inflammation with mycophenolate. However, the odds of control of uveitis in patients with JIA-associated uveitis were lower than for those patients without this type of ocular inflammation.

Side Effects

The most common side effects of mycophenolate mofetil include gastric pain, diarrhea, and nausea.[54] Fatigue and pruritus are other common side effects. Gastrointestinal bleeding and perforations are rarely encountered. These cases have typically occurred in the organ transplantation literature. Additionally, infections involving opportunistic organisms as well as herpetic viral infections are more frequent than in azathioprine, but again, these instances have been reported typically in organ transplant patients. There is an increased risk of malignancy, particularly skin cancers, in transplant patients taking mycophenolate mofetil. Fetal loss and congenital malformations are noted with mycophenolate. Consequently, contraception must be practiced while taking mycophenolate mofetil. Additionally, patients taking oral contraceptives should be made aware that mycophenolate mofetil can decrease the serum levels of contraceptive hormones with a theoretically reduced efficacy of the contraceptive.

Considerations with the Antimetabolites

In a large retrospective study in which patients with noninfectious ocular inflammatory diseases were assessed, three of the most commonly used antimetabolites to control ocular inflammation (including uveitis) were assessed.[18] The median time to treatment success (on ≤10 mg prednisone PO daily) with methotrexate was 6.5 months compared to that of mycophenolate mofetil (4 months) and azathioprine (4.8 months). It was noted that methotrexate was frequently started at a low dose and increased over time, whereas mycophenolate mofetil and azathioprine were typically started at more therapeutic doses. After 6 months of therapy, the proportion of all ocular inflammation patients achieving treatment success with mycophenolate was 70% compared to 42% of those on methotrexate and 48% of those taking azathioprine. While these results are intriguing, there still remains the issue of determining the best antimetabolite to use as first-line therapy for corticosteroid sparing control of uveitis. To address this important issue, Acharya and colleagues compared methotrexate and mycophenolate mofetil (two of the most commonly used antimetabolites) for initial corticosteroid-sparing control of noninfectious intermediate, posterior, and panuveitis. While past retrospective studies have suggested that mycophenolate mofetil may be more effective in the management of uveitis, Acharya's RCT found that a higher proportion of those randomized to methotrexate achieved control of their uveitis compared to those randomized to mycophenolate mofetil.[59] Control of uveitis was defined as less than 1+ anterior chamber cell or vitreous haze or inactive retinal or choroidal lesions. However, while the maximum dose of methotrexate was used (25 mg PO weekly) the maximum dose for mycophenolate mofetil in the trial was 1 g PO BID rather than the typical maximum dose of 1.5 g PO BID. To address this issue, Acharya is currently conducting a National Eye Institute-sponsored randomized controlled trial, which is powered to detect a smaller difference (20%)

between the two randomization groups and utilizing the typical maximum doses of these medications. The data gathered from this pivotal study will provide uveitis specialists with much needed evidence to support the initial use of either methotrexate or mycophenolate mofetil as initial corticosteroid-sparing therapy.

Contraception should be practiced while on antimetabolites. Developing fetuses with their rapid cell turnover are especially vulnerable to the effects of antimetabolites that affect nucleic acid synthesis. In fact, high dose methotrexate is utilized as an abortive agent. It is recommended that in those wishing to become pregnant, they discontinue use and wait at least 3 months prior to conceiving.

Antimetabolites can be used in conjunction with other immunomodulatory agents, particularly from other classes such as the T-cell inhibitors (e.g. cyclosporine)[60,61] or with biologics. In the case of biologics, antimetabolites may help decrease the frequency of developing antibodies [e.g. human antichimeric antibodies, (HACAs)] against monoclonal antibodies (e.g. rituximab and infliximab).

In a retrospective cohort study evaluating nearly 8,000 patients with ocular inflammatory diseases (1,155 patients with uveitis), the antimetabolites were not associated with an increased risk in overall mortality and were not associated with an increased risk in cancer-related mortality.[62] Relating this information to patients when counseling them as they start antimetabolite therapy is important.

CALCINEURIN (OR T-CELL) INHIBITORS

Calcineurin is a phosphatase, an enzyme that is involved in the phosphorylation of the nuclear factor of activated T-cells (NFAT), allowing this transcription factor to translocate from the cytosol into the nucleus of T-cells. In the nucleus, NFAT can then transcribe mRNA to be utilized in the production of lymphokines including interleukin (IL) 2 and others.

Cyclosporine

Cyclosporine binds to cyclophilin, an intracellular cytoplasmic protein in T-cells. It is metabolized in the liver by the CYP3A4 enzymatic system. The microemulsion form of the original cyclosporine (Sandimmune, Novartis) is known as Neoral (also from Novartis) and has more consistent absorption rates and, thus, bioavailability.

Nussenblatt and colleagues were the first to use cyclosporine in the management of experimental autoimmune uveitis utilizing retinal S antigen in a murine model.[63]

Because of the encouraging results from murine models, Nussenblatt treated uveitis in eight humans.[64] Most patients exhibited a relatively rapid response in control of inflammation and improvement of visual acuity.

The systemic immunosuppressive therapy for eye diseases (SITE) cohort evaluated cyclosporine's efficacy in noninfectious ocular inflammation (including uveitis and scleritis). One definition of control of inflammation used by the SITE study was no inflammation (as defined by the SUN criteria) on ≤10 mg PO daily of prednisone. Using this definition, SITE found that inflammation was controlled in 22.1% of cohort participants (95% CI: 17.7–27.3) at 6 months and 36.1% of cohort participants (95% CI: 30.5–42.2) at 12 months.[65]

Side Effects

Common side effects with cyclosporine include fatigue, paresthesias, tremors, headaches, gum hyperplasia, and nausea.[65,66] Nephrotoxicity can be an issue, though in the SITE study, only 10.7% discontinued cyclosporine in the first year of starting the medication due to nephrotoxicity.[65] Additionally, the SITE study evaluating cyclosporine showed that patients older than 55 years of age were several-fold more likely to develop side effects limiting the use of cyclosporine compared to those aged 18–39 years.

Tacrolimus

The Fujisawa Pharmaceutical Company Ltd in Japan isolated a macrolide antibiotic from the fermentation broth of *Streptomyces tsukabensis*.[67] Tacrolimus was initially designated FK506 because it binds to the immunophilin-family-member, FK binding protein (FKBP), which functions as a protein folding chaperone. Tacrolimus suppressed human and murine cytotoxic T-cell generation and suppresses immune responses and suppress the expression of IL-2, IL-3, and interferon (IFN)-gamma.[68] Like cyclosporine, tacrolimus suppresses T-cell activity.

Mochizuki and colleagues studied tacrolimus and found it to be effective in the management posterior uveitis.[69] Eventually, Hogan et al. demonstrated the efficacy of tacrolimus in their uveitis patients.[70] Others have shown that tacrolimus is an effective and reliable immunosuppressive medication, particularly when uveitis patients had failed cyclosporine.[71,72]

Side Effects

Hypercholesterolemia, hypertension and nephrotoxicity are the most common side effects of tacrolimus.

ALKYLATING AGENTS

Colloquially known as the mustard gases (most of which were actually liquids) originally used during World War II, alkylating agents demonstrated their mutagenic effects in the fruit fly (*Drosophila melanogaster*).[73] Alkylation of DNA leads to its cross-linking, which results in inhibition of DNA synthesis.

Cyclophosphamide

Cyclophosphamide is activated by the liver enzyme cytochrome P450 yielding compounds with alkylating properties.[74]

In the retrospective SITE study of cyclophosphamide used to treat ocular inflammation (including uveitis), 76% of patients achieved control of inflammatory activity.[75] Most patients were also able to achieve a corticosteroid-sparing dose of prednisone (less than 10 mg daily of oral prednisone). Ocular inflammatory disease remission can be a benefit of cyclophosphamide treatment, though cyclophosphamide is typically reserved for especially sight-threatening inflammation given its significant side effect profile.

Side Effects

Side effects include gastrointestinal upset, myelosuppression with resultant cytopenias, gonadal failure, susceptibility for infections, hemorrhagic cystitis, and bladder cancer.[76]

Chlorambucil

Similar to cyclophosphamide, chlorambucil replaces a hydrogen ion for an alkyl group resulting in alkylated DNA that is unable to be replicated.

Similar to cyclophosphamide, chlorambucil has often been reserved for uveitis in which blindness is imminent, particularly in the setting of Behçet's disease and sympathetic ophthalmia. Because of its side effect profile, a preference has been to use it for a relatively short period of time,[77,78] but can be effective for recalcitrant uveitis.[79]

Side Effects

Gonadal dysfunction, secondary amenorrhea, and myelosuppression are important side effects.

BIOLOGICS

Immune responses are mediated by a variety of cell signaling proteins. Biologics are themselves proteins that are engineered to modulate the immune system in ways that tend to have more specific targets than antimetabolites, alkylating agents, and even calcineurin inhibitors. The biologics are made up of a variety of medications including monoclonal antibodies and fusion proteins. The dose, side effects and clinical monitoring of new biologic medications are given in Table 88.3.

Tumor Necrosis Factor Inhibitors

Tumor necrosis factor (TNF) is a cytokine produced by macrophages and lymphocytes. It is an important mediator of inflammation, septic shock, and cytotoxicity. However, TNF is also involved in autoimmune diseases.[80,81] Inhibiting TNF has been shown to be beneficial in the rheumatic diseases as well as uveitis.[82]

Adalimumab

Currently, adalimumab is the only nonsteroid pharmacologic agent that is approved by the US Food and Drug Administration for noninfectious intermediate, posterior, and panuveitis. With a half-life of 15–19 days, adalimumab is effective when administered every 14 days.

Adalimumab (Humira, AbbVie Inc.) is a fully humanized monoclonal antibody targeting TNF-alpha. Adalimumab has demonstrated efficacy for uveitis to other immunomodulatory medication in adults.[83] Uveitis associated with JIA has been shown to respond to adalimumab as well.[84,85] Additionally, in those with active JIA-associated uveitis and already on methotrexate, the addition of adalimumab lead to less frequent treatment failures compared to those that remained on their methotrexate alone.[86]

Side effects: Upper respiratory tract infection, rash, injection site reaction, transaminitis, and headache are more common reactions. Less common, but serious reactions include lymphoproliferative disorders (lymphoma and leukemia), reactivation of hepatitis B or latent tuberculosis, and opportunistic or nonopportunistic infections.

Table 88.3: Biologics.

Medication			Dose		Side effects	Monitoring
Biologics	Anti-TNF	Adalimumab	Initial	80 mg SC × 1	Injection site reaction; flu syndrome; abdominal pain; URI; HA; opportunistic infection; lymphoma; leukemia	Check TB, HBV prior to starting
			Maintenance/ maximum	40 mg SC every 14 days		CBC, CMP, AST, ALT every 4–8 weeks
		Infliximab	Initial	5 mg/kg IV q 2 weeks × 2, then monthly increasing to every 6–8 weeks	Infusion reaction; abdominal pain; URI; UTI; HA; opportunistic infection; malignancy	Check TB, HBV prior to starting CBC, CMP, AST, ALT every 4–8 weeks
			Maintenance/ maximum	7–15 mg/kg IV q 4–8 weeks		Anti-chimeric antibodies for lack of efficacy or serum sickness reaction
	IFN	Pegylated IFN alfa-2a	180 mg SC weekly		Fever; GI; depression; anxiety; irritability; pruritis	CBC, CMP, AST, ALT every 4–8 weeks
	Anti-CD20	Rituximab	1,000 mg IV q 14 days × 2 doses		Infusion reaction; fatigue; infection; GI; pulmonary toxicity; muscle spasms; leukopenia	CBC, CMP, AST, ALT every 4–8 weeks
	Anti-IL-6	Tocilizumab	Initial	4 mg/kg IV q 4 weeks	Infusion reaction; HA; URI; rash; demyelinating CNS disease; malignancy	CBC, CMP, AST, ALT every 4–8 weeks
			Maintenance/ maximum	8 mg/kg IV q 4 weeks		
	T-cell Costimu-latory blocker	Abatacept	Initial	750 mg IV ×1 on week 0, 2, 4	Infusion reaction; HA; URI; rash; demyelinating CNS disease; malignancy	CBC, CMP, AST, ALT every 4–8 weeks
			Maintenance/ maximum	750–1000 mg IV every 4 weeks		

[ALT, Alanine transaminase; AST: Aspartate transaminase; CBC: Complete blood count (with differential); CMP: Complete metabolic panel; CNS: Central nervous system; GI: Gastrointestinal side effects (abdominal pain, nausea, diarrhea, vomiting); HA: Headache; HBV: Hepatitis B virus; IV: Intravenous; SC: Subcutaneous; TB: Tuberculosis; URI: Upper respiratory infection; UTI: Urinary tract infection]

Infliximab

Infliximab (Remicade, Janssen Biotech, Inc.) is a chimeric monoclonal antibody that targets TNF-alpha. Fusion of the TNF-alpha binding site on the murine antibody A2 to the constant region of human IgG1 kappa immunoglobulin leads to the formation of this chimeric monoclonal antibody.

In a prospective study examining the use of infliximab in noninfectious uveitis refractory to systemic corticosteroids and at least one other immunomodulatory agent (or intolerance to such therapy) control of uveitis was achieved in most at 10 weeks.[87,88] Sarcoid uveitis failing conventional therapy with antimetabolites has been shown to achieve control of inflammation and improvement in macular edema with inflximab.[89] Infliximab has been useful in JIA-associated uveitis as well.[90,91]

An expert panel has suggested using anti-TNF agents (particularly adalimumab or infliximab) as first-line therapy for the uveitis associated with Behçet's disease and as second-line therapy for uveitis associated with juvenile inflammatory arthritis.[92] The French Uveitis Network has reported that adalimumab and infliximab exhibit similar efficacy in the management of uveitis.[93] However, randomized prospective trials comparing these two agents are needed.

Golimumab

There are small case reports that golimumab (Simponi, Janssen Biotech, Inc.) exhibits efficacy in uveitis. Golimumab has shown to be effective in patients with refractory recurrent anterior uveitis in the setting of ankylosing spondyloarthropathies with most patients achieving improvement or remission of uveitis.[94,95] While, in some cases patients had not previously tried infliximab, in other cases many patients had actually failed infliximab, but showed improvement in inflammation with golimumab.[96]

Etanercept

The fusion protein etanercept (Enbrel, Amgen, Inc. and Pfizer Inc.) targets both TNF-alpha and TNF-beta. Etanercept, however, exhibits minimal efficacy in ocular inflammation.[97] Historically, there was the thought that, unlike adalimumab and infliximab, etanercept did not bind membrane-bound (cell surface) TNF nor did it activate complement. In vitro studies have shown that while etanercept has superior binding of soluble TNF compared to adalimumab and infliximab, all three agents' exhibit similar affinity for membrane TNF.[98] Additionally, none of these agents were able to induce complement-dependent cytotoxicity in vitro.[98] Instead, the ability of one monoclonal antibody (either infliximab or adalimumab) to bind numerous membrane-bound TNF results in pro-apoptotic signaling that is not achieved when a single etanercept molecule binds to only one membrane TNF.[99]

Side Effects

The TNF-inhibitors have a 4–5% risk of serious infection (including reactivation of tuberculosis, fulminant hepatitis B, or fungal infections) as well as approximately a 1/1000 risk of lymphoma. There is at least a 15% risk of skin reaction, which is usually manageable with topical therapy. As these are antibodies, there is a risk of developing anti-drug antibodies (particularly with the chimeric antibodies) and increased clearance of the drug, which can lead to reduced effectiveness of the medication and possible side effects. In such cases, combining these medications with an antimetabolite can help decrease such reactions.

Interferon

Interferons are cytokines produced by host cells in the setting of viral infections. Their name comes from the fact that they exhibit the ability to interfere with viral replication (originally studied with influenza virus A).[100]

Pegylated IFN alpha is produced by recombinant DNA vector technology; it is produced gene expression in bacterial cells. There are two types of IFN, type I and type II. IFN alpha-2a and -2b belong to the type 1 family. Dendritic cells are major producers of interferon alpha in the setting of certain viral infections and tumor genesis inhibiting these destructive processes from progressing.[101,102] However, when IFN is aberrantly expressed autoimmune diseases, such as systemic lupus erythematosus to rheumatoid arthritis, may result.[103,104]

Studies

Interferon alpha was shown to be effective in animal models of experimental autoimmune uveitis, which lead to its consideration for use in uveitis in humans.[105-107]

In a Parisian study, IFN alpha-2a was used for uveitis patients experiencing a relapse on their prednisone/immunomodulatory combination. Behçet's disease-related uveitis made up just over half of the patients studied with

82.6% of cases exhibiting control after administration of interferon alpha-2a. Those with uveitis other than Behçet's in the study group exhibited control of their uveitis to the tune of 59%.[108] This same group has noted that interferon alpha-2a is especially effective for Behçet's disease uveitis[109]and in Turkey and Korea to interferon alpha-2a is useful in decreasing flare-ups of Behçet's disease uveitis when first-line immunomodulatory therapy has failed.[110,111] IFN alpha-2b has also been utilized for Behçet's disease, ocular sarcoidosis, and has demonstrated efficacy for refractory uveitic macular edema.[112-114]

Side Effects

Side effects of IFN therapy can commonly include flu-like symptoms, abdominal pain and diarrhea, headache, and rash. Less common, but more severe reactions include cardiomyopathy, myelosuppression, depression, psychosis, lupus-like reactions, and a severe skin reaction that resembles pemphigus.[115,116]

Anti-CD20

While T-cells are thought to play the largest role in mediating the inflammation involved in uveitis,[117-119] B-cells also play an important role in some ocular inflammatory diseases.

Rituximab (Rituxan, Genentech) is a chimeric monoclonal antibody originally developed to treat B-cell non-Hodgkin lymphomas.[120] Rituximab demonstrated it effectiveness in the setting of scleritis and orbital inflammation in granulomatosis with polyangiitis,[121] but rituximab has also been effective in a group of patients with refractory posterior uveitis.[122,123] Rituximab has also been effective in treating severe and refractory uveitis in JIA.[124,125]

Anti-interleukin-2

Daclizumab (Zinbryta, Biogen, Inc.) was originally introduced by Thomas Waldman, MD at the National Institutes of Health–National Cancer Institute. It is a humanized monoclonal antibody targeting the "Tac" portion of the IL-2 receptor. Collaborating with Laboratory of Immunology at the National Eye Institute, daclizumab was found to be effective in managing experimental autoimmune uveoretinitis in a primate model.[126] A collaboration between Dr Waldmann and Robert Nussenblatt, MD at the National Eye Institute lead to the demonstration of daclizumab's safety and efficacy in human uveitis patients.[127,128] Daclizumab has been effective in managing birdshot chorioretinopathy.[129]

Due to poor commercial performance, daclizumab was pulled off the market in 2009, but has recently re-emerged.

Anti-interleukin-6

Tocilizumab (Actemra, Genentech) is an IL 6 inhibitor. Inflammatory cells that mediate uveitis express IL-6 in high concentrations.[130,131]

Tocilizumab has been prospectively studied in the setting of JIA-associated uveitis refractory to other biologic therapy (including TNF inhibitors, T-cell costimulatory blockers, and anti-CD20 therapy).[132] Tocilizumab has also been effective in managing uveitic CME refractory to other therapies.[133]

T-cell Costimulatory Blockade

Abatacept (Orencia, Bristol-Myers Squibb Co.) is a fusion protein that inhibits the CD28 costimulatory molecule, which results in T-cell inactivation.[134,135] Abatacept has been shown to be effective when used as either first-line or second-line (after failing TNF-inhibitors) therapy in refractory JIA-associated uveitis.[136] However, further studies using abatacept in uveitis are required.

REFERENCES

1. Hench PS, Kendall EC, et al. The effect of a hormone of the adrenal cortex (17-hydroxy-11-dehydrocorticosterone; compound E) and of pituitary adrenocorticotropic hormone on rheumatoid arthritis. Proc Staff Meet Mayo Clin. 1949;24(8):181-97.
2. Thorne JE, Woreta FA, Dunn JP, et al. Risk of cataract development among children with juvenile idiopathic arthritis-related uveitis treated with topical corticosteroids. Ophthalmology. 2010;117(7):1436-41.
3. Slabaugh MA, Herlihy E, Ongchin S, et al. Efficacy and potential complications of difluprednate use for pediatric uveitis. Am J Ophthalmol. 2012;153(5):932-8.
4. Feiler DL, Srivastava SK, Pichi F, et al. Resolution of noninfectious uveitic cystoid macular edema with topical difluprednate. Retina. 2017;37(5):844-50.
5. Androudi S, Letko E, Meniconi M, et al. Safety and efficacy of intravitreal triamcinolone acetonide for uveitic macular edema. Ocul Immunol Inflamm. 2005;13(2-3):205-12.
6. Kok H, Lau C, Maycock N, et al. Outcome of intravitreal triamcinolone in uveitis. Ophthalmology. 2005;112(11):1916.e1-7.
7. Nozik RA. Periocular injection of steroids. Trans Am Acad Ophthalmol Otolaryngol. 1972;76(3):695-705.

8. Venkatesh P, Kumar CS, Abbas Z, et al. Comparison of the efficacy and safety of different methods of posterior subtenon injection. Ocul Immunol Inflamm. 2008;16(5): 217-23.
9. Ferrante P, Ramsey A, Bunce C, et al. Clinical trial to compare efficacy and side-effects of injection of posterior sub-Tenon triamcinolone versus orbital floor methylprednisolone in the management of posterior uveitis. Clin Exp Ophthalmol. 2004;32(6):563-8.
10. Benítez Del Castillo Sánchez JM, Garcia Sánchez J. Intravitreal injection of triamcinolone acetonide in non infectious uveitis. Arch Soc Esp Oftalmol. 2001;76(11):661-4.
11. Bernal L, Estevez B. Corneal toxicity after Ozurdex((®)) migration into anterior chamber. Arch Soc Esp Oftalmol. 2016;91(6):292-4.
12. Kang H, Lee MW, Byeon SH, et al. The clinical outcomes of surgical management of anterior chamber migration of a dexamethasone implant (Ozurdex(®)). Graefes Arch Clin Exp Ophthalmol. 2017.
13. Kempen JH, Altaweel MM, Holbrook JT, et al. Association between long-lasting intravitreous fluocinolone acetonide implant vs systemic anti-inflammatory therapy and visual acuity at 7 years among patients with intermediate, posterior, or panuveitis. JAMA. 2017;317(19):1993-2005.
14. Jabs DA, Rosenbaum JT, Foster CS, et al. Guidelines for the use of immunosuppressive drugs in patients with ocular inflammatory disorders: recommendations of an expert panel. Am J Ophthalmol. 2000;130(4):492-513.
15. LaRochelle GE Jr., LaRochelle AG, Ratner RE, et al. Recovery of the hypothalamic-pituitary-adrenal (HPA) axis in patients with rheumatic diseases receiving low-dose prednisone. Am J Med. 1993;95(3):258-64.
16. Krasner AS. Glucocorticoid-induced adrenal insufficiency. JAMA. 1999;282(7):671-6.
17. Pasadhika S, Kempen JH, Newcomb CW, et al. Azathioprine for ocular inflammatory diseases. Am J Ophthalmol. 2009;148(4):500-9.e502.
18. Galor A, Jabs DA, Leder HA, et al. Comparison of antimetabolite drugs as corticosteroid-sparing therapy for noninfectious ocular inflammation. Ophthalmology. 2008;115(10):1826-32.
19. Hooper PL, Kaplan HJ. Triple agent immunosuppression in serpiginous choroiditis. Ophthalmology. 1991;98(6):944-951; discussion 951-42.
20. Moore CE. Sympathetic ophthalmitis treated with azathioprine. Br J Ophthalmol. 1968;52(9):688-90.
21. Hakin KN, Pearson RV, Lightman SL. Sympathetic ophthalmia: visual results with modern immunosuppressive therapy. Eye (Lond). 1992;6(Pt 5):453-5.
22. Hellmund K, Fruhauf A, Seiler T, et al. Sympathetic ophthalmia 50 years after penetrating injury. A case report. Klin Monbl Augenheilkd. 1998;213(3):182-5.
23. Sisk RA, Davis JL, Dubovy SR, et al. Sympathetic ophthalmia following vitrectomy for endophthalmitis after intravitreal bevacizumab. Ocul Immunol Inflamm. 2008;16(5):236-8.
24. Liu H, Ding L, Zhang F, et al. The impact of glutathione S-transferase genotype and phenotype on the adverse drug reactions to azathioprine in patients with inflammatory bowel diseases. J Pharmacol Sci. 2015;129(2):95-100.
25. Nielsen OH, Maxwell C, Hendel J. IBD medications during pregnancy and lactation. Nat Rev Gastroenterol Hepatol. 2014;11(2):116-27.
26. Siemasko KF, Chong AS, Williams JW, et al. Regulation of B cell function by the immunosuppressive agent leflunomide. Transplantation. 1996;61(4):635-42.
27. Manna SK, Aggarwal BB. Immunosuppressive leflunomide metabolite (A77 1726) blocks TNF-dependent nuclear factor-kappa B activation and gene expression. J Immunol. 1999;162(4):2095-102.
28. Wang J, Xie QB, Zhao Y, et al. Flare up of rheumatoid arthritis associated with Vogt-Koyanagi-Harada syndrome treated with leflunomide. Int J Ophthalmol. 2014;7(5): 909-11.
29. Steigerwalt RD Jr, Bacci S, Valesini G. Severe uveitis successfully treated with leflunomide. Retin Cases Brief Rep. 2007;1(1):54-5.
30. Molina C, Modesto C, Martin-Begue N, et al. Leflunomide, a valid and safe drug for the treatment of chronic anterior uveitis associated with juvenile idiopathic arthritis. Clin Rheumatol. 2013;32(11):1673-5.
31. Bichler J, Benseler SM, Krumrey-Langkammerer M, et al. Leflunomide is associated with a higher flare rate compared to methotrexate in the treatment of chronic uveitis in juvenile idiopathic arthritis. Scand J Rheumatol. 2015;44(4):280-3.
32. Kremer JM, Genovese MC, Cannon GW, et al. Concomitant leflunomide therapy in patients with active rheumatoid arthritis despite stable doses of methotrexate. A randomized, double-blind, placebo-controlled trial. Ann Intern Med. 2002;137(9):726-33.
33. Fairbanks LD, Ruckemann K, Qiu Y, et al. Methotrexate inhibits the first committed step of purine biosynthesis in mitogen-stimulated human T-lymphocytes: a metabolic basis for efficacy in rheumatoid arthritis? Biochem J. 1999;342(Pt 1):143-52.
34. Kiely PD, Johnson DM. Infliximab and leflunomide combination therapy in rheumatoid arthritis: an open-label study. Rheumatology (Oxford). 2002;41(6):631-7.
35. Nurmohamed MT, van Halm VP, Dijkmans BA. Cardiovascular risk profile of antirheumatic agents in patients with osteoarthritis and rheumatoid arthritis. Drugs. 2002;62(11):1599-609.
36. Nesher G, Moore TL. The in vitro effects of methotrexate on peripheral blood mononuclear cells. Modulation by methyl donors and spermidine. Arthritis RheumArthritis and Rheumatism. 1990;33(7):954-9.
37. Yukioka K, Wakitani S, Yukioka M, et al. Polyamine levels in synovial tissues and synovial fluids of patients with rheumatoid arthritis. J Rheumatol. 1992;19(5):689-92.
38. Morabito L, Montesinos MC, Schreibman DM, et al. Methotrexate and sulfasalazine promote adenosine release by a mechanism that requires ecto-5'-nucleotidase-mediated conversion of adenine nucleotides. J Clin Invest. 1998;101(2):295-300.

39. Cronstein BN, Rosenstein ED, Kramer SB, et al. Adenosine; a physiologic modulator of superoxide anion generation by human neutrophils. Adenosine acts via an A2 receptor on human neutrophils. J Immunol. 1985;135(2):1366-71.
40. Cronstein BN, Daguma L, Nichols D, et al. The adenosine/neutrophil paradox resolved: human neutrophils possess both A1 and A2 receptors that promote chemotaxis and inhibit O_2 generation, respectively. J Clin Invest. 1990;85(4):1150-7.
41. Gangaputra S, Newcomb CW, Liesegang TL, et al. Methotrexate for ocular inflammatory diseases. Ophthalmology. 2009;116(11):2188-98.e2181.
42. Hemady RK, Baer JC, Foster CS. Immunosuppressive drugs in the management of progressive, corticosteroid-resistant uveitis associated with juvenile rheumatoid arthritis. Int Ophthalmol Clin. 1992;32(1):241-52.
43. Weiss AH, Wallace CA, Sherry DD. Methotrexate for resistant chronic uveitis in children with juvenile rheumatoid arthritis. J Pediatr. 1998;133(2):266-8.
44. Foeldvari I, Wierk A. Methotrexate is an effective treatment for chronic uveitis associated with juvenile idiopathic arthritis. J Rheumatol. 2005;32(2):362-5.
45. Malik AR, Pavesio C. The use of low dose methotrexate in children with chronic anterior and intermediate uveitis. Br J Ophthalmol. 2005;89(7):806-8.
46. Heiligenhaus A, Mingels A, Heinz C, et al. Methotrexate for uveitis associated with juvenile idiopathic arthritis: value and requirement for additional anti-inflammatory medication. Eur J Ophthalmol. 2007;17(5):743-8.
47. Jakubovic BD, Donovan A, Webster PM, et al. Methotrexate-induced pulmonary toxicity. Can Respir J . 2013;20(3):153-5.
48. Troeltzsch M, von Blohn G, Kriegelstein S, et al. Oral mucositis in patients receiving low-dose methotrexate therapy for rheumatoid arthritis: report of 2 cases and literature review. Oral Surg Oral Med Oral Pathol Oral Radiol. 2013;115(5): e28-33.
49. Morgan SL, Baggott JE, Vaughn WH, et al. Supplementation with folic acid during methotrexate therapy for rheumatoid arthritis. A double-blind, placebo-controlled trial. Ann Intern Med. 1994;121(11):833-41.
50. Morgan SL, Baggott JE, Vaughn WH, et al. The effect of folic acid supplementation on the toxicity of low-dose methotrexate in patients with rheumatoid arthritis. Arthritis Rheum. 1990;33(1):9-18.
51. Shea B, Swinden MV, Ghogomu ET, et al. Folic acid and folinic acid for reducing side effects in patients receiving methotrexate for rheumatoid arthritis. J Rheumatol. 2014;41(6):1049-60.
52. Lee WA, Gu L, Miksztal AR, et al. Bioavailability improvement of mycophenolic acid through amino ester derivatization. Pharm Res. 1990;7(2):161-6.
53. Staatz CE, Tett SE. Clinical pharmacokinetics and pharmacodynamics of mycophenolate in solid organ transplant recipients. Clin Pharmacokinet. 2007;46(1):13-58.
54. Siepmann K, Huber M, Stubiger N,. Mycophenolate mofetil is a highly effective and safe immunosuppressive agent for the treatment of uveitis : a retrospective analysis of 106 patients. Graefes Arch Clin Exp Ophthalmol. 2006;244(7):788-94.
55. Doycheva D, Zierhut M, Blumenstock G, et al. Long-term results of therapy with mycophenolate mofetil in chronic non-infectious uveitis. Graefes Arch Clin Exp Ophthalmol. 2011;249(8):1235-43.
56. Thorne JE, Jabs DA, Qazi FA, et al. Mycophenolate mofetil therapy for inflammatory eye disease. Ophthalmology. 2005;112(8):1472-7.
57. Doycheva D, Deuter C, Stuebiger N, et al. Mycophenolate mofetil in the treatment of uveitis in children. Br J Ophthalmo. 2007;91(2):180-4.
58. Sobrin L, Christen W, Foster CS. Mycophenolate mofetil after methotrexate failure or intolerance in the treatment of scleritis and uveitis. Ophthalmology. 2008;115(8):1416-21, 1421.e1411.
59. Rathinam SR, Babu M, Thundikandy R, et al. A randomized clinical trial comparing methotrexate and mycophenolate mofetil for noninfectious uveitis. Ophthalmology. 2014;121(10):1863-70.
60. Kaklamani VG, Kaklamanis PG. Treatment of Behcet's disease—an update. Semin Arthritis Rheum. 2001;30(5): 299-312.
61. Arcinue CA, Radwan A, Lebanan MO, et al. Comparison of two different combination immunosuppressive therapies in the treatment of Vogt-Koyonagi-Harada syndrome. Ocul Immunol Inflamm. 2013;21(1):47-52.
62. Kempen JH, Daniel E, Dunn JP, et al. Overall and cancer related mortality among patients with ocular inflammation treated with immunosuppressive drugs: retrospective cohort study. BMJ. 2009;339:b2480.
63. Nussenblatt RB, Rodrigues MM, Wacker WB, et al. Cyclosporine a. Inhibition of experimental autoimmune uveitis in Lewis rats. J Clin Invest. 1981;67(4):1228-31.
64. Nussenblatt RB, Palestine AG, Rook AH, et al. Treatment of intraocular inflammatory disease with cyclosporine A. Lancet. 1983;2(8344):235-8.
65. Kacmaz RO, Kempen JH, Newcomb C, et al. Cyclosporine for ocular inflammatory diseases. Ophthalmology. 2010;117(3):576-84.
66. Murphy CC, Greiner K, Plskova J, et al. Cyclosporine vs tacrolimus therapy for posterior and intermediate uveitis. Arch Ophthalmol. 2005;123(5):634-41.
67. Tanaka H, Kuroda A, Marusawa H, et al. Physicochemical properties of FK-506, a novel immunosuppressant isolated from Streptomyces tsukubaensis. Transplant Proc. 1987;19(5 Suppl 6):11-6.
68. Kino T, Hatanaka H, Hashimoto M, et al. FK-506, a novel immunosuppressant isolated from a Streptomyces. I. Fermentation, isolation, and physico-chemical and biological characteristics. J Antibiot (Tokyo). 1987;40(9):1249-55.
69. Mochizuki M, Masuda K, Sakane T, et al. A multicenter clinical open trial of FK 506 in refractory uveitis, including Behcet's disease. Japanese FK 506 Study Group on Refractory Uveitis. Transplant Proc. 1991;23(6):3343-6.

70. Hogan AC, McAvoy CE, Dick AD,. Long-term efficacy and tolerance of tacrolimus for the treatment of uveitis. Ophthalmology. 2007;114(5):1000-6.
71. Sloper CM, Powell RJ, Dua HS. Tacrolimus (FK506) in the treatment of posterior uveitis refractory to cyclosporine. Ophthalmology. 1999;106(4):723-8.
72. Kilmartin DJ, Forrester JV, Dick AD. Tacrolimus (FK506) in failed cyclosporine A therapy in endogenous posterior uveitis. Ocul Immunol Inflamm. 1998;6(2):101-9.
73. Auerbach C, Robson JM. Chemical production of mutations. Nature. 1946;157:302.
74. Arnold H, Bourseaux F, Brock N. Chemotherapeutic action of a cyclic nitrogen mustard phosphamide ester (B 518-ASTA) in experimental tumours of the rat. Nature. 1958;181(4613):931.
75. Pujari SS, Kempen JH, Newcomb CW, et al. Cyclophosphamide for ocular inflammatory diseases. Ophthalmology. 2010;117(2):356-65.
76. Houssiau FA. Cyclophosphamide in lupus nephritis. Lupus. 2005;14(1):53-8.
77. Tessler HH, Jennings T. High-dose short-term chlorambucil for intractable sympathetic ophthalmia and Behcet's disease. Br J Ophthalmo. 1990;74(6):353-7.
78. Goldstein DA, Fontanilla FA, Kaul S, et al. Long-term follow-up of patients treated with short-term high-dose chlorambucil for sight-threatening ocular inflammation. Ophthalmology. 2002;109(2):370-7.
79. Miserocchi E, Baltatzis S, Ekong A, et al. Efficacy and safety of chlorambucil in intractable noninfectious uveitis: the Massachusetts Eye and Ear Infirmary experience. Ophthalmology. 2002;109(1):137-42.
80. Fiers W. Tumor necrosis factor. Characterization at the molecular, cellular and in vivo level. FEBS Lett. 1991;285(2):199-212.
81. Heller RA, Kronke M. Tumor necrosis factor receptor-mediated signaling pathways. J Cell Biol. 1994;126(1):5-9.
82. Lerman MA, Burnham JM, Chang PY, et al. Response of pediatric uveitis to tumor necrosis factor-alpha inhibitors. J Rheumatol. 2013;40(8):1394-403.
83. Suhler EB, Lowder CY, Goldstein DA, et al. Adalimumab therapy for refractory uveitis: results of a multicentre, open-label, prospective trial. Br J Ophthalmo. 2013;97(4):481-6.
84. Biester S, Deuter C, Michels H, et al. Adalimumab in the therapy of uveitis in childhood. Br J Ophthalmo. 2007;91(3):319-24.
85. Diaz-Llopis M, Garcia-Delpech S, Salom D, et al. Adalimumab therapy for refractory uveitis: a pilot study. J Ocul Pharmacol Ther. 2008;24(3):351-61.
86. Ramanan AV, Dick AD, Jones AP, et al. Adalimumab plus methotrexate for uveitis in juvenile idiopathic arthritis. N Engl J Med. 2017;376(17):1637-46.
87. Suhler EB, Smith JR, Wertheim MS, et al. A prospective trial of infliximab therapy for refractory uveitis: preliminary safety and efficacy outcomes. Arch Ophthalmol. 2005;123(7): 903-12.
88. Suhler EB, Smith JR, Giles TR, et al. Infliximab therapy for refractory uveitis: 2-year results of a prospective trial. Arch Ophthalmol. 2009;127(6):819-22.
89. Riancho-Zarrabeitia L, Calvo-Rio V, Blanco R, et al. Anti-TNF-alpha therapy in refractory uveitis associated with sarcoidosis: Multicenter study of 17 patients. Semin Arthritis Rheum. 2015;45(3):361-8.
90. Ardoin SP, Kredich D, Rabinovich E, et al. Infliximab to treat chronic noninfectious uveitis in children: retrospective case series with long-term follow-up. Am J Ophthalmol. 2007;144(6):844-9.
91. Rajaraman RT, Kimura Y, Li S, et al. Retrospective case review of pediatric patients with uveitis treated with infliximab. Ophthalmology. 2006;113(2):308-14.
92. Levy-Clarke G, Jabs DA, Read RW, et al. Expert panel recommendations for the use of anti-tumor necrosis factor biologic agents in patients with ocular inflammatory disorders. Ophthalmology. 2014;121(3):785-96.e783.
93. Vallet H, Seve P, Biard L, et al. Infliximab versus adalimumab in the treatment of refractory inflammatory uveitis: a multicenter study from the French Uveitis Network. Arthritis Rheumatol. 2016;68(6):1522-30.
94. Yazgan S, Celik U, Isik M, et al. Efficacy of golimumab on recurrent uveitis in HLA-B27-positive ankylosing spondylitis. Int Ophthalmol. 2017;37(1):139-45.
95. Calvo-Rio V, Blanco R, Santos-Gomez M, et al. Golimumab in refractory uveitis related to spondyloarthritis. Multicenter study of 15 patients. Semin Arthritis Rheum. 2016;46(1): 95-101.
96. Miserocchi E, Modorati G, Pontikaki I, et al. Long-term treatment with golimumab for severe uveitis. Ocul Immunol Inflamm. 2014;22(2):90-5.
97. Galor A, Perez VL, Hammel JP, et al. Differential effectiveness of etanercept and infliximab in the treatment of ocular inflammation. Ophthalmology. 2006;113(12):2317-23.
98. Kaymakcalan Z, Sakorafas P, Bose S, et al. Comparisons of affinities, avidities, and complement activation of adalimumab, infliximab, and etanercept in binding to soluble and membrane tumor necrosis factor. Clin Immunol. 2009;131(2):308-16.
99. Van den Brande JM, Braat H, van den Brink GR, et al. Infliximab but not etanercept induces apoptosis in lamina propria T-lymphocytes from patients with Crohn's disease. Gastroenterology. 2003;124(7):1774-85.
100. Isaacs A, Lindenmann J. Virus interference. I. In: Isaacs A, Lindenmann J (Eds). The Interferon 1957. J Interferon Res. 1987;7(5):429-38.
101. Zou W, Machelon V, Coulomb-L'Hermin A, et al. Stromal-derived factor-1 in human tumors recruits and alters the function of plasmacytoid precursor dendritic cells. Nat Med 2001;7(12):1339-46.
102. Colonna M, Krug A, Cella M. Interferon-producing cells: on the front line in immune responses against pathogens. Curr Opin Immunol. 2002;14(3):373-9.
103. Vallin H, Perers A, Alm GV, et al. Anti-double-stranded DNA antibodies and immunostimulatory plasmid DNA in combination mimic the endogenous IFN-alpha inducer in systemic lupus erythematosus. J Immunol. 1999;163(11):6306-13.
104. Wampler Muskardin T, Vashisht P, Dorschner JM, et al. Increased pretreatment serum IFN-beta/alpha ratio predicts

non-response to tumour necrosis factor alpha inhibition in rheumatoid arthritis. Ann Rheum Dis. 2016;75(10):1757-62.
105. Okada AA, Keino H, Suzuki J, et al. Kinetics of intraocular cytokines in the suppression of experimental autoimmune uveoretinitis by type I IFN. Int Immunol. 1998;10(12): 1917-22.
106. Okada AA, Keino H, Fukai T, et al. Effect of type I interferon on experimental autoimmune uveoretinitis in rats. Ocul Immunol Inflamm.1998;6(4):215-26.
107. Stubiger N, Crane IJ, Kotter I, et al. Interferon alpha 2a in IRPB-derived peptide-induced EAU--part I. Adv Exp Med Biol. 2003;528:537-40.
108. Bodaghi B, Gendron G, Wechsler B, et al. Efficacy of interferon alpha in the treatment of refractory and sight threatening uveitis: a retrospective monocentric study of 45 patients. Br J Ophthalmol. 2007;91(3):335-9.
109. Gueudry J, Wechsler B, Terrada C, et al. Long-term efficacy and safety of low-dose interferon alpha 2a therapy in severe uveitis associated with Behcet disease. Am J Ophthalmol. 2008;146(6):837-44.e831.
110. Hasanreisoglu M, Cubuk MO, Ozdek S,. Interferon alpha-2a therapy in patients with refractory Behcet uveitis. Ocul Immunol Inflamm. 2017;25(1):71-5.
111. Park JY, Chung YR, Lee K,. Clinical experience of interferon alfa-2a treatment for refractory uveitis in Behcet's disease. Yonsei Med J. 2015;56(4):1158-62.
112. Butler NJ, Suhler EB, Rosenbaum JT. Interferon alpha 2b in the treatment of uveitic cystoid macular edema. Ocul Immunol Inflamm. 2012;20(2):86-90.
113. Doycheva D, Deuter C, Stuebiger N, et al. Interferon-alpha-associated presumed ocular sarcoidosis. Graefes Arch Clin Exp Ophthalmol. 2009;247(5):675-80.
114. Durand JM, Soubeyrand J. Interferon-alpha 2b for refractory ocular Behcet's disease. Lancet. 1994;344(8918):333.
115. Fleischmann M, Celerier P, Bernard P, et al. Long-term interferon-alpha therapy induces autoantibodies against epidermis. Dermatology. 1996;192(1):50-5.
116. Schilling PJ, Kurzrock R, Kantarjian H, et al. Development of systemic lupus erythematosus after interferon therapy for chronic myelogenous leukemia. Cancer. 1991;68(7):1536-7.
117. Becker MD, Adamus G, Davey MP, et al. The role of T cells in autoimmune uveitis. Ocul Immunol Inflamm. 2000;8(2): 93-100.
118. Caspi RR, Sun B, Agarwal RK, et al. T cell mechanisms in experimental autoimmune uveoretinitis: susceptibility is a function of the cytokine response profile. Eye (Lond). 1997;11(Pt 2):209-12.
119. Whitcup SM, Pleyer U, Lai JC, et al. Topical liposome-encapsulated FK506 for the treatment of endotoxin-induced uveitis. Ocul Immunol Inflamm. 1998;6(1):51-6.
120. Maloney DG, Grillo-Lopez AJ, White CA, et al. IDEC-C2B8 (Rituximab) anti-CD20 monoclonal antibody therapy in patients with relapsed low-grade non-Hodgkin's lymphoma. Blood. 1997;90(6):2188-95.
121. Keogh KA, Wylam ME, Stone JH, et al. Induction of remission by B lymphocyte depletion in eleven patients with refractory antineutrophil cytoplasmic antibody-associated vasculitis. Arthritis Rheum. 2005;52(1):262-8.
122. Lasave AF, You C, Ma L, et al. Long-term outcomes of rituximab therapy in patients with noninfectious posterior uveitis refractory to conventional immunosuppressive therapy. Retina. 2018;38(2):395-402.
123. Lopez-Gonzalez R, Loza E, Jover JA, et al. Treatment of refractory posterior uveitis with infliximab: a 7-year follow-up study. Scand J Rheumatol. 2009;38(1):58-62.
124. Miserocchi E, Modorati G, Berchicci L, et al. Long-term treatment with rituximab in severe juvenile idiopathic arthritis-associated uveitis. Br J Ophthalmo. 2016;100(6):782-6.
125. Heiligenhaus A, Miserocchi E, Heinz C, et al. Treatment of severe uveitis associated with juvenile idiopathic arthritis with anti-CD20 monoclonal antibody (rituximab). Rheumatology (Oxford). 2011;50(8):1390-4.
126. Guex-Crosier Y, Raber J, Chan CC, et al. Humanized antibodies against the alpha-chain of the IL-2 receptor and against the beta-chain shared by the IL-2 and IL-15 receptors in a monkey uveitis model of autoimmune diseases. J Immunol. 1997;158(1):452-8.
127. Nussenblatt RB, Thompson DJ, Li Z, et al. Humanized anti-interleukin-2 (IL-2) receptor alpha therapy: long-term results in uveitis patients and preliminary safety and activity data for establishing parameters for subcutaneous administration. J Autoimmun. 2003;21(3):283-93.
128. Nussenblatt RB, Peterson JS, Foster CS, et al. Initial evaluation of subcutaneous daclizumab treatments for noninfectious uveitis: a multicenter noncomparative interventional case series. Ophthalmology. 2005;112(5):764-70.
129. Sobrin L, Huang JJ, Christen W, et al. Daclizumab for treatment of birdshot chorioretinopathy. Arch Ophthalmol. 2008;126(2):186-91.
130. Murray PI, Hoekzema R, van Haren MA, et al. Aqueous humor interleukin-6 levels in uveitis. Invest Ophthalmol Vis Sci. 1990;31(5):917-20.
131. Kramer M, Monselise Y, Bahar I. Serum cytokine levels in active uveitis and remission. Curr Eye Res. 2007;32(7-8):669-75.
132. Calvo-Rio V, Santos-Gomez M, Calvo I, et al. Anti-interleukin-6 receptor tocilizumab for severe juvenile idiopathic arthritis-associated uveitis refractory to anti-tumor necrosis factor therapy: a multicenter study of twenty-five patients. Arthritis Rheumatol. 2017;69(3):668-75.
133. Adan A, Mesquida M, Llorenc V, et al. Tocilizumab treatment for refractory uveitis-related cystoid macular edema. Graefes Arch Clin Exp Ophthalmol. 2013;251(11):2627-32.
134. Yamada A, Salama AD, Sayegh MH. The role of novel T cell costimulatory pathways in autoimmunity and transplantation. J Am Soc Nephrol. 2002;13(2):559-75.
135. Sayegh MH, Turka LA. The role of T-cell costimulatory activation pathways in transplant rejection. N Engl J Med. 1998;338(25):1813-21.
136. Birolo C, Zannin ME, Arsenyeva S, et al. Comparable efficacy of abatacept used as first-line or second-line biological agent for severe juvenile idiopathic arthritis-related uveitis. J Rheumatol. 2016;43(11):2068-73.

Chapter 89 The Eye and Selected Rheumatic Diseases: A Rheumatology Perspective

Sung Jae Yang, Sherveen S Salek, James T Rosenbaum

INTRODUCTION

Rheumatology is the subspecialty within internal medicine that deals almost exclusively with immune-mediated diseases. Disorders evaluated in a rheumatology practice include: rheumatoid arthritis (RA), systemic lupus erythematosus (SLE), spondyloarthritis (including ankylosing spondylitis, reactive arthritis, psoriatic arthritis, and the arthritis associated with inflammatory bowel disease), juvenile idiopathic arthritis, Sjögren's syndrome, giant cell arteritis and polymyalgia rheumatica, polymyositis and dermatomyositis, Behçet's disease, vasculitis, and relapsing polychondritis. Each of these has a characteristic ocular manifestation and often some rare ocular manifestations. Conversely virtually any structure in or around the eye can be the target of an immune response. Examples include the uvea, the cornea, the conjunctiva, the lacrimal gland, the orbit, the optic nerve, the sclera and the episclera. Fibromyalgia reportedly is associated with ophthalmic disease in the form of reduction in corneal nerves.[1] Macular degeneration is clearly related to complement activation[2] and other aspects of inflammation.[3] Some forms of glaucoma[4] and cataract might be immunologically mediated.[5]

In this chapter, we summarize the ocular manifestations of selected immune-mediated diseases including RA, SLE, Sjögren's, spondyloarthritis, granulomatosis with polyangitis and relapsing polychondritis. The prototypical manifestations are summarized in Table 89.1. We also discuss the ocular toxicity of antimalarial therapy, since antimalarials are commonly prescribed by rheumatologists.

RHEUMATOID ARTHRITIS

Rheumatoid arthritis is a chronic autoimmune disease. It is an immune mediated inflammatory pathology. It manifests with painful and swollen joints. It characteristically presents with early morning stiffness and affects small joints (Figs. 89.1 to 89.3). It can also be associated with fever, malaise and rheumatoid nodules. Arthritis is potentially

Table 89.1: Important clinical manifestations of selected rheumatological disease.

	Diseases	Systemic manifestation	Ocular manifestation
1.	Rheumatoid arthritis	• Deforming small joint arthritis • Rheumatoid nodules	Scleritis, PUK, dry eye disease
2.	Ankylosing spondylitis	• Sacroiliitis • Inflammation of spine	Recurrent, unilateral, alternating anterior uveitis
3.	Psoriatic arthritis	• Skin—silvery white scaly lesion • Joint—recurrent erosive polyarthritis	U/L or B/L anterior uveitis
4.	Inflammatory bowel disease	• Recurrent/bloody diarrhea	U/L or B/L anterior uveitis
5.	Granulomatosis with polyangiitis	• Upper and lower respiratory tract inflammation • Necrotizing glomerulonephritis	Dry eye, scleritis, PUK, orbital disease
6.	SLE	• Skin lesion—malar rash, discoid rash • Nondeforming migratory polyarthritis, lupus nephritis, • Hematological abnormalities	• Dry eye syndrome, • SLE retinopathy • Choroidopathy
7.	Relapsing polychondritis	Ear and nasal chondritis	Scleritis

(U/L or B/L: Unilateral/Bilateral; PUK: Peripheral ulcerative keratitis; SLE: Systemic lupus erythematosus)
Note: The ocular manifestations listed here represent a selected list of the most common or most typical findings.

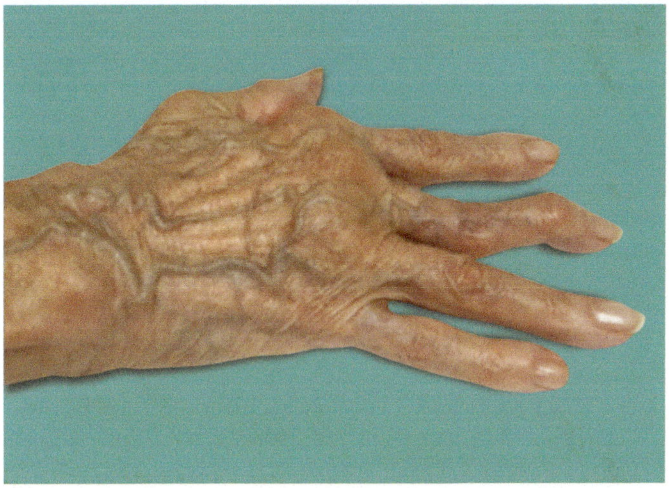

Fig. 89.1: Hand from a patient with rheumatoid arthritis. Multiple abnormalities are apparent including swelling of the metacarpal phalangeal joints, ulnar deviation of the fingers, atrophy of the intrinsic muscles of the hand, and a swan neck deformity of the third finger.

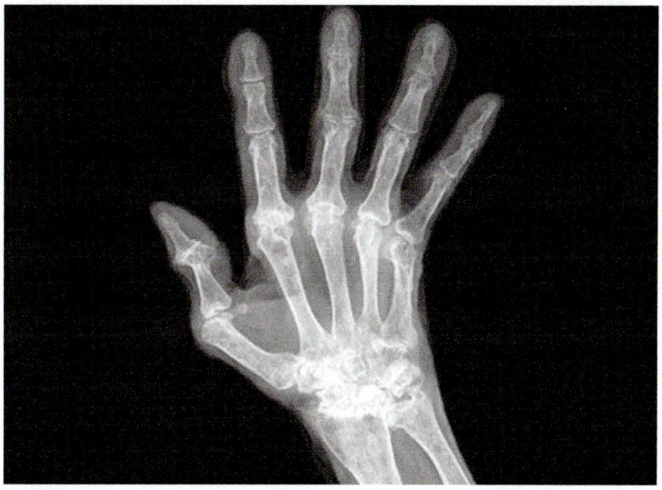

Fig. 89.2: X-ray of the hand shown in Fig. 89.1. Extensive carpal destruction and erosion of the metacarpal phalangeal joints are shown. The proximal interphalangeal joints also have erosions. The thumb has a "Z" deformity which is better appreciated on the X-ray than in the photograph of the hand itself.

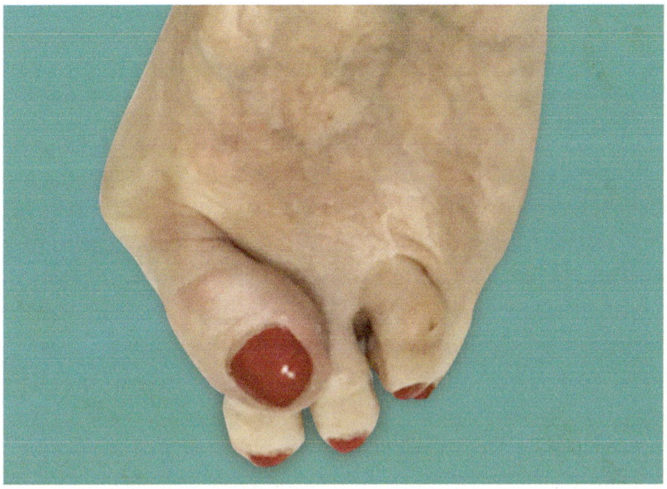

Fig. 89.3: Foot of a patient with rheumatoid arthritis. The great toe has a severe hallux valgus deformity and the fourth toe shows a cock-up deformity.

deforming, if not adequately treated. Ophthalmological manifestations can develop during the course of RA and more commonly affect the anterior part of the eye than the posterior part.[6] The associations include dry eye syndrome, episcleritis, scleritis and ulcerative keratitis.

Dry eye disease (DED) is the most common ocular manifestation of RA with an incidence up of to 90%.[7,8] The assessment of DED is based on symptoms (dryness, foreign body sensation) and signs (corneal staining, tear breakup time, and Schirmer test). Limited correlation between the symptoms and signs has been reported.[9] The correlation between the severity of dryness and the activity of RA is unclear.[10] But recent studies have reported there was a significant correlation between tear osmolarity and RA disease activity[7,8] Increased tear osmolarity indirectly reflects that the ocular surface inflammatory component is affecting the dry eye in RA patients.[11,12] Treatments of DED in RA include artificial tear substitutes and lubricating ointments. Preservative free preparations can be a more desirable choice for frequent use because the preservative can be toxic to the corneal epithelium. A mild topical corticosteroid, topical cyclosporine, or lifitegrast can help treat the underlying inflammation often associated with dry eye which is nonresponsive to topical lubrication alone.[13,14]

Episcleritis is a benign inflammation of the superficial layers overlying the sclera and presents as red eyes. The patient complains of discomfort rather than pain. The prevalence of episcleritis in RA patients has been reported to be 0.17–3.7%.[15] The redness of the eyes is blanched by the topical vasoconstrictor (phenylephrine). Nodular episcleritis is less frequent. Treatment of episcleritis is not usually necessary. Treatments of symptomatic patients include lubricants, topical nonsteroid anti-inflammatory drugs (NSAIDs) and topical corticosteroids.

Scleritis occurs in 1–6% of patients with RA (Fig. 89.4).[16,17] Conversely RA is observed in 10–19% of patients with scleritis and is generally considered the most frequently

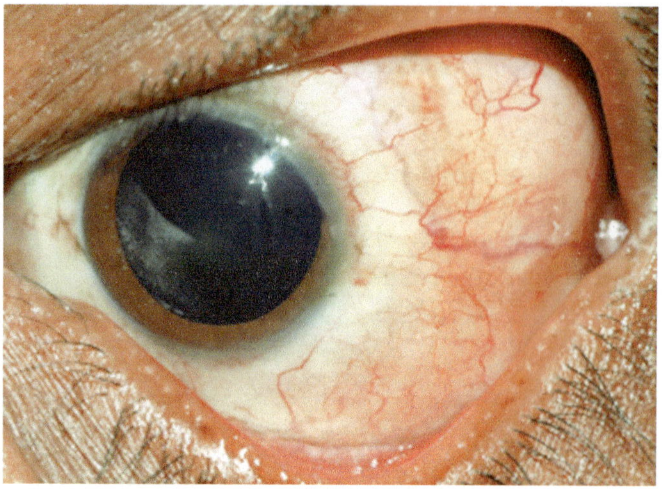

Fig. 89.4: Nodular scleritis in rheumatoid arthritis.
Source: SR Rathinam.

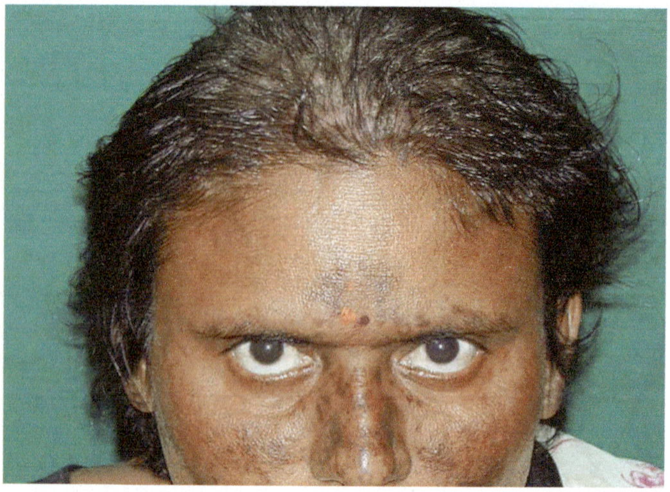

Fig. 89.5: Middle-aged woman with systemic lupus erythematosus.
Note: Alopecia and butterfly rashes.
Source: SR Rathinam.

associated systemic disease.[18,19] The pain of scleritis is typically severe, boring in nature, and can be retrobulbar (behind the eye) in location. Other symptoms include tearing, light sensitivity and visual loss. Redness of the eye persists after topical vasoconstrictor (phenylephrine) in contrast to what is observed for episcleritis. Treatment of scleritis includes systemic NSAIDs, oral corticosteroids and immunosuppressants (such as methotrexate or azathioprine) (Table 89.2). In general, scleritis in association with RA will respond to control of the underlying joint disease. Most rheumatologists will add a tumor necrosis factor (TNF) inhibitor other than etanercept if the patient is not already on biologic therapy (Table 89.3). For the occasional patient who fails to benefit adequately from a monoclonal antibody to TNF, options include a different class of biologic (such as rituximab, tocilizumab, or abatacept) or tofacitinib. Oral corticosteroids may be required until the biologic has had adequate time to control the joint disease and eye disease.

Corneal involvement often occurs along with anterior scleritis. Sclerosing keratitis occurs adjacent to the inflamed sclera and is characterized by corneal opacification and vascularization. Peripheral ulcerative keratitis (PUK) is an inflammatory condition of the peripheral cornea characterized by juxta-limbal corneal thinning and ulceration. The symptoms include ocular pain, redness, photophobia, tearing or even a loss of vision due to progressive astigmatism or corneal opacification. On clinical examination, crescent-shaped corneal ulceration is typically observed with epithelial breakdown, with a thinning of the underlying corneal stroma and congestion and elevation of adjacent conjunctiva. Corneal perforation is the most severe complication. PUK can be a complication of scleritis or independent of this condition. RA is observed in 34–42% of PUK cases.[15,20] The prevalence of PUK in patients with RA is now becoming uncommon, possibly because of improved treatment of RA.[21] PUK usually occurs in patients with a long standing RA and positive serology for both rheumatoid factor (RF) and anti-cyclic citrullinated peptide (CCP) antibody.[6] Studies have found upregulation of the inflammatory cytokines tumor necrosis factor-α and interleukin-6 from patients with rheumatoid associated PUK patients.[22] Systemic combination treatment with steroids, immunosuppressant and biologics can lead to rapid healing.[23]

SYSTEMIC LUPUS ERYTHEMATOSUS

Systemic lupus erythematosus is an autoimmune disease with multisystem involvement. The prevalence of SLE is 40 in 1,00,00 in North American population. Women are more affected than men with female to male ratio of 9:1. It is usually involves women in child bearing age. Systemic manifestations include cutaneous disease like malar/discoid rash (Fig. 89.5). Lupus arthritis usually presents as non-deforming migratory polyarthritis. Skin and articular manifestations are seen in nearly 85% of patients. Nearly 50% of patients have renal involvement either in the form of nephritis or nephrotic syndrome. Hematological abnormalities are frequently seen in these patients.

Table 89.2: Nonbiologic immunosuppressive medications often used for rheumatic diseases.

Medication	Dosage	Comments/Warnings
Antimetabolite		
Azathioprine	1.5–4.0 mg/kg/day	Relatively inexpensive. May cause flu-like symptoms in some. Do not use with allopurinol. Safest choice among antimetabolites during pregnancy. Some authorities check thiopurine methyl transferase polymorphisms before starting
Methotrexate	15–25 mg/week	May be subcutaneous or oral. Most popular antimetabolite for RA. Unique adverse effects include cirrhosis and pneumonitis
Mycophenolate mofetil	2000–3000 mg/day	Frequent bloating or loose stool. Avoid during pregnancy. Popular choice to treat lupus nephritis
Calcineurin antagonist		
Cyclosporine	2.5–5.0 mg/kg/day (divide dose with half dose every 12 hours)	Hypertension, renal disease, paresthesias, sore gums, hair growth. Has limited indications to treat rheumatic diseases; more popular for organ transplants and uveitis
Tacrolimus	0.1 mg/kg every 12 hours	Resembles cyclosporine in terms of benefits, risks, and indications
Alkylator		
Cyclophosphamide	1.0–2.5 mg/kg/day if given orally	Increased risk of malignancy and bladder cancer. Needs frequent monitoring for cytopenia. May cause hair loss, sterility, cystitis, fatigue. May be IV given so that risk of cytopenias is less but efficacy is also less. Mainly used for vasculitis and lupus nephritis and less toxic medications are often tried first

Table 89.3: Representative biologic therapies used to treat rheumatic diseases.

Drug or class of drug	Target	Representative indications
TNF inhibitor*	TNF	Rheumatoid arthritis, spondyloarthritis, psoriasis, juvenile idiopathic arthritis, Behçet's disease
Anakinra	IL-1	Rheumatoid arthritis, gout, Still's disease
Tocilizumab, Sarilumab	IL-6 receptor	Rheumatoid arthritis, giant cell arteritis, Still's disease
Abatacept	Co-stimulatory molecule	Rheumatoid arthritis
Rituximab	CD20 (B lymphocyte marker)	Rheumatoid arthritis, ANCA-associated vasculitis
Ustekinumab	IL-12/23	Psoriasis, psoriatic arthritis, inflammatory bowel disease
Secukinumab Ixekizumab	IL-17A	Psoriasis, ankylosing spondylitis

*The TNF inhibitors include etanercept (which is a soluble receptor) and several monoclonal antibodies including infliximab, adalimumab, certolizumab and golimumab. TNF inhibitors are roughly equivalent in treating RA or AS, but the antibodies tend to be superior in treating Behçet's disease, uveitis, or inflammatory bowel disease.

Ocular manifestations in SLE are common, and can lead to sight threatening conditions. SLE may affect almost any part of the eye and visual pathway. Eye disease can be the presenting manifestations of SLE. Dry eye syndrome (keratoconjunctivitis sicca) is the most common ocular feature of SLE and is termed secondary Sjögren's syndrome.[24] The prevalence of retinopathy varies among various populations, ranging from 3% in well controlled patients to 29% of patients with more active systemic disease.[25] The autoimmune process may affect the retina and choroid in two ways: directly, by immune complex-mediated vasculitis, and indirectly, by secondary hypertension from renal involvement. A strong correlation exists between the presence of retinopathy and central nervous system disease.[26] The major pathology of lupus retinopathy is attributed to vasculopathy, which may vary from mild lupus retinopathy showing cotton-wool spots, perivascular hard exudates, retinal hemorrhages and vascular tortuosity to severe vaso-occlusive retinopathy or retinal vasculitis (Fig. 89.6).[27]

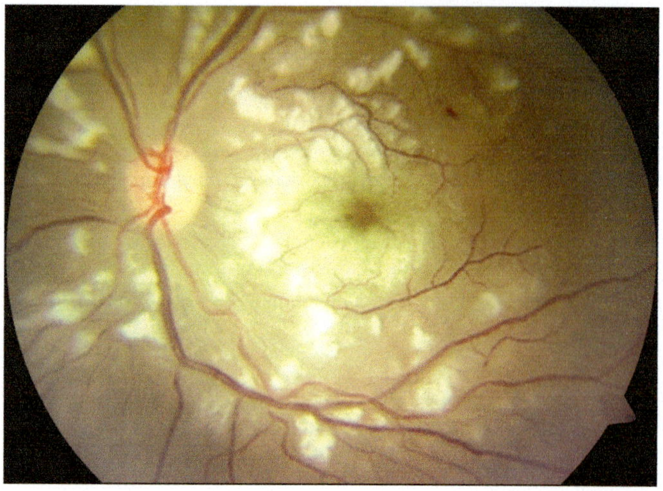

Fig. 89.6: Fundus photograph showing multiple cotton-wool spots in systemic lupus erythematosus vasculitis.
Source: SR Rathinam.

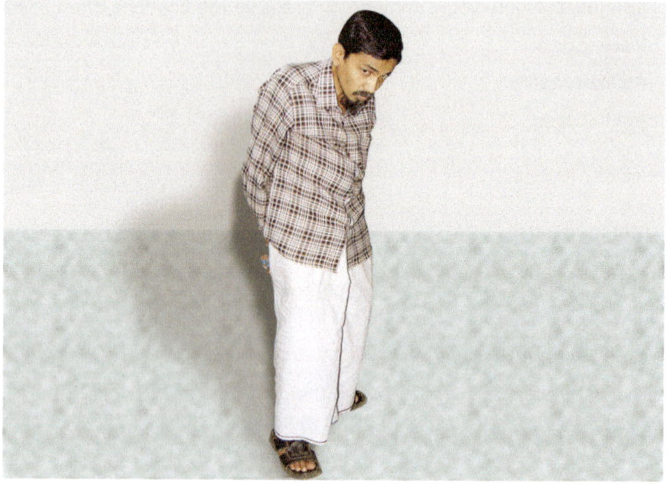

Fig. 89.7: Male patient with severe ankylosing spondylitis with multiple axial joint deformities.
Source: SR Rathinam.

Lupus choroidopathy also can occur either independently or with lupus retinopathy and may present with good visual acuity. The common manifestations include serous retinal detachment, detachment of the retinal pigment epithelium, or retinal pigment epitheliopathy due to choroidal ischemia.[28] Optic nerve disease occurs in around 1% of patients with SLE,[24,25] and includes optic neuritis and ischemic optic neuropathy (anterior or posterior).[27] The prognosis is worse in SLE associated optic neuritis, with more than half having a persistent central scotoma and progressing to optic atrophy. Optic neuropathy in SLE typically presents with bilateral, acute painless loss of vision associated with an altitudinal or arcuate field defect, with or without optic disk swelling.[27]

Treatment options for SLE associated eye disease depend on the specific manifestation. Dry eye, for example, can often be managed simply with preservative free artificial tears. A cotton wool spot is sometimes just observed without therapeutic intervention. Blood pressure, renal function, and anti-phospholipid antibodies should be checked. Optic neuritis, in contrast, is generally aggressively managed as with intravenous methylprednisolone and cyclophosphamide.[29]

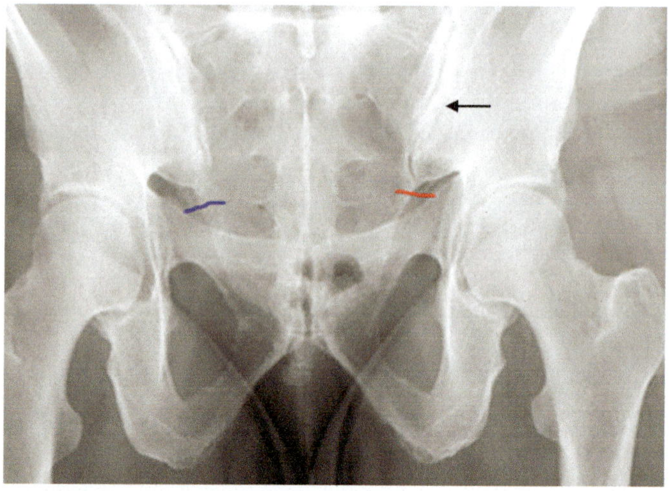

Fig. 89.8: X-ray of the sacroiliac joints and pelvis from a patient with ankylosing spondylitis. The margins of the sacroiliac joint on the right (superior to the blue line) are poorly seen due to the changes from chronic inflammation. The sacroiliac joint on the left is narrowed inferiorly (just above the red line). Both sacroiliac joints have abnormal adjacent sclerosis with the arrow indicating the sclerosis in the left ilium.

SPONDYLOARTHRITIS

Spondyloarthritis is a heterogeneous group of diseases that includes ankylosing spondylitis, reactive arthritis, psoriatic arthritis, and arthritis associated with inflammatory bowel disease. Ankylosing spondylitis is a chronic inflammatory arthritis that primarily affects the spine and sacroiliac joints (Figs. 89.7 and 89.8). Ocular involvement is seen in 25–50% of the patients. Anterior uveitis is the most common ocular manifestation. It is characteristically unilateral, alternating, recurrent, non-granulomatous, anterior uveitis with fibrinous exudation and even hypopyon. Other ocular manifestations, such as episcleritis and scleritis, may occur in spondyloarthritis patients, although less frequently. About 50% of all patients with acute anterior uveitis are

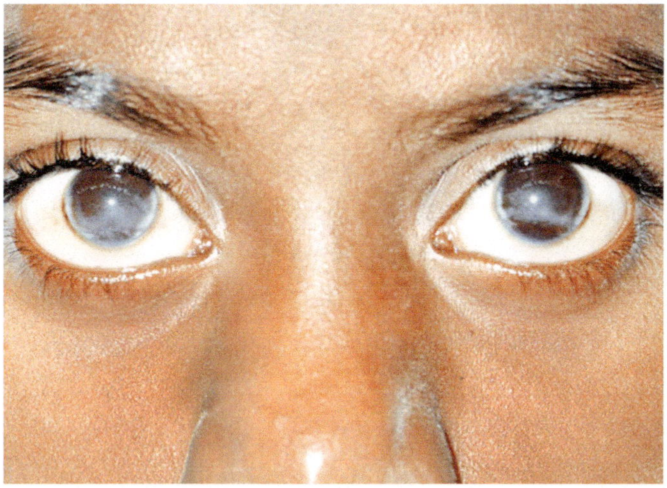

Fig. 89.9: Bilateral band keratopathy in a girl child with juvenile rheumatoid arthritis.
Source: SR Rathinam.

HLA-B27 positive.[30] Many patients with acute anterior uveitis are unaware that their chronic back pain may be related to the eye disease and results from previously undiagnosed spondyloarthritis.[31] It is usually associated with a good prognosis, but it requires early treatment to prevent sequelae. Other common spondyloarthropathies are psoriatic arthritis and inflammatory bowel disease.

Psoriatic arthritis is clinically characterized by skin and nail involvement with recurrent erosive polyarthritis. Distal interphalangeal joint is a commonly involved joint. Patients with ulcerative colitis and Crohn's disease systemically present with recurrent/bloody diarrhea and abdominal cramping. Ocular manifestations of inflammatory bowel disease (IBD) occur in less than 10% of cases. These manifestations include episcleritis, scleritis, uveitis, rarely optic neuritis and retinal vasculitis.[32] In IBD and psoriatic arthritis, uveitis tends to be more insidious in onset and/or chronic in duration, posterior to the lens and active bilaterally in comparison to the uveitis associated with ankylosing spondylitis.[33] Juvenile idiopathic arthritis in children can cause chronic bilateral uveitis with band-shaped keratopathy in both eyes (Fig. 89.9).

The management of uveitis in spondyloarthritis includes, corticosteroids (topically or by periocular injection and occasionally orally), and rarely immunomodulatory agents. Sulfasalazine has been effective in randomized controlled trials in reducing the frequency of recurrent attacks. Anti-TNF therapy with a monoclonal antibody will also reduce the frequency, duration and severity of recurrent attacks. Although adalimumab has been approved in many countries for the treatment of noninfectious, intermediate or posterior uveitis, it is rarely indicated simply to manage recurrent episodes of HLA B27-associated anterior uveitis.

GRANULOMATOSIS WITH POLYANGIITIS

Granulomatosis with polyangiitis (GPA, previously known as Wegener's granulomatosis) is a rare, multisystem inflammatory disorder characterized by both vasculitis and necrotizing granulomas.[34] Complete form of GPA includes the triad of necrotizing glomerulonephritis, necrotizing granulomas in respiratory tract and systemic vasculitis affecting small and medium-sized vessels. Limited form may involve isolated organ system without renal involvement and might have systemic vasculitis. 90% of patients present with upper respiratory tract involvement such as recurrent or chronic sinusitis, purulent nasal discharge, nasal mucosa ulceration, saddle nose (Fig. 89.10), epistaxis, cough, hemoptysis, dyspnea and chest pain due to pleural effusion. 11–20% can have renal involvement. Cutaneous manifestation includes purpuric rashes over trunk and extremities. In some cases subcutaneous nodules, papules, vesicles and ulcers can also be present. Neurologic features include most commonly mononeuritis multiplex, cranial nerve palsies commonly involving II, VI, VII cranial nerves, strokes and diabetes insipidus due to sinus inflammation extension to pituitary gland. Cardiac involvement can manifest as pericarditis and myocarditis. Other organs like breast, alimentary tract (mesenteric necrosis and gangrene) and urogenital involvement can also occur. The pediatric age group has similar features. However, nasal deformities and subglottic stenosis are more frequent in pediatric patients.

Ophthalmic manifestations have been reported in up to 58% of patients with GPA. Lacrimal disease resulting in keratoconjunctivitis is arguably the most common manifestation. Orbital disease is noted in around 15% of patients, and can manifest with proptosis and limitation of extraocular motility.[35] Orbital disease is usually contiguous from the ethmoid or maxillary sinuses, and can also arise de novo intraconally. Severe cases of necrotic inflammation involve erosion of bone. Scleritis (Fig. 89.11) and episcleritis are present in around 10% of patients, and can be distinguished from one another by the depth of vessel involvement on clinical examiation, as well as sectoral injection, which is more indicative of scleritis. Corneal involvement can also be present, including

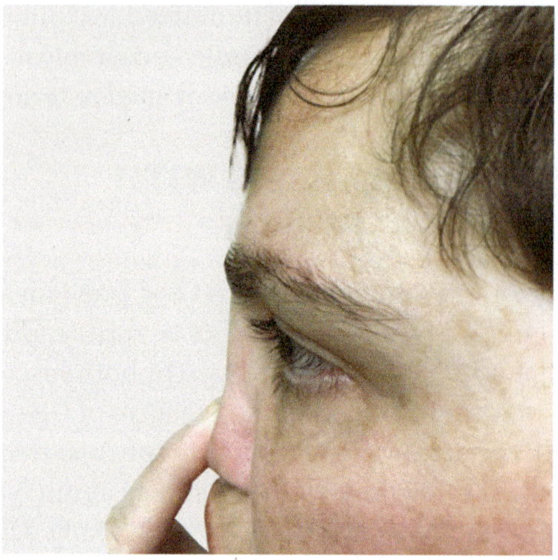

Fig. 89.10: Patient with granulomatosis with polyangiitis who has suffered nasal cartilage loss and collapse from the disease.

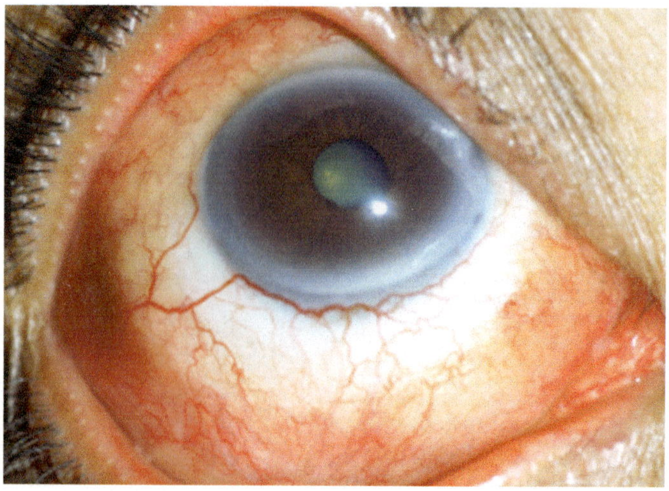

Fig. 89.11: Scleritis in granulomatosis with polyangiitis. *Source:* SR Rathinam.

peripheral ulcerative keratitis.[36,37] Posterior segment manifestations, such as retinal vasculitis, are exceedingly rare with GPA, with only a handful of cases reported in the literature.[38]

Over 90% of patients with active disease are seropositive for proteinase-3 anti-neutrophil cytoplasmic antibody (c-ANCA), although up to a third may be negative for the antibody until late in the disease course.[39,40] The recommended, initial laboratory workup for scleritis includes testing for ANCA.[41] However, patients with GPA whose disease spares the lung or kidney are often ANCA negative.

Granulomatosis with polyangiitis can be a life-threatening and sight-threatening disease, with a 2.75-fold increased risk of mortality in comparison with other forms of ocular inflammation.[41] Therefore, prompt treatment with corticosteroids and immunomodulatory therapy is necessary once the diagnosis has been made. While steroid-sparing therapy for GPA has traditionally consisted of cyclophosphamide, B-cell inhibition through use of rituximab has gained increased acceptance and shown comparable efficacy and reduced morbidity for treatment of both systemic and eye disease.[42] Methotrexate or other anti-metabolites are excellent options for patients whose disease does not involve either the lung or the kidney.[43]

RELAPSING POLYCHONDRITIS

Relapsing polychondritis (RP) is an autoimmune disease that affects tissues consisting of hyaline, elastic, and fibrous cartilage.[44] The pathophysiology of RP is thought to consist of an autoimmune reaction to components of cartilage, such as extracellular matrix, with subsequent spread of involvement to non-cartilaginous tissues.[45] The disease usually occurs between the ages of 30 and 60, with no gender predominance. It is exceedingly rare, with a reported incidence of as low as 0.71 per million per year.[46] In male patients above age 60, RP is associated with myelodysplastic syndrome.[47] Cardiac involvement is also more common in these older male patients, secondary to thoracic aortic aneurysm from progressive dilatation of the aortic root.

Relapsing polychondritis presents as a combination of chondritis along with inflammation of other tissues rich in proteoglycans, including the eyes, heart, blood vessels and inner ears (Fig. 89.12). Chondritis is initially present in only a third of cases. Therefore, familiarity with the other presenting manifestations is important.[48,49] Ear and nasal chondritis is present in 78% and 39% of patients, respectively, while half of patients have airway involvement that can threaten breathing.[44] Chondritis of the pinna of the ear sparing the earlobe is most common, and manifests as painful swelling and redness. The external auditory canal may be collapsed, leading to conductive hearing loss or otitis externa.[50] Eye involvement is present in up to 46% of patients. The disease course is chronic, with flares lasting up to several weeks and resolving spontaneously.

Familiarity with ophthalmic manifestations of RP is important as it can precede the development of chondritis. Scleritis is the most common ocular manifestation of RP, and can present as diffuse anterior, nodular, and necrotizing

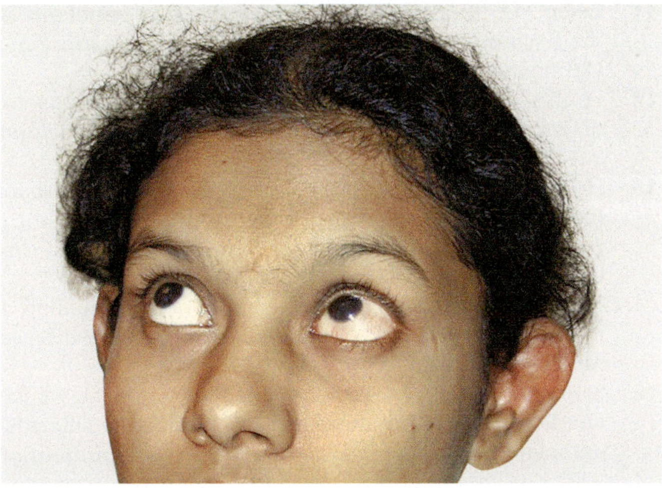

Fig. 89.12: Relapsing polychondritis severe auricular edema of the left ear along with scleritis of the left eye. The left ear shows inflammation of the pinna with edema and erythema. The earlobe is spared, which is typical of this disease.
Source: SR Rathinam.

forms. Most cases of scleritis associated with RP are diffuse (76.9%), bilateral (92.3%), and recurrent (84.6%).[51] Episcleritis, conjunctivitis, keratitis and anterior uveitis are less common with RP. Posterior segment manifestations such as retinal vasculitis and optic neuropathy are rare,[52] While inflammatory markers such as C-reactive protein may be elevated during flare-ups of RP, other serologic findings are nonspecific and not diagnostic of the disease. ANCA-associated vasculitides should remain in the differential for RP.

Treatment of RP consists of high dose systemic corticosteroids, and implementation of immunomodulatory therapy. The most commonly used steroid-sparing agents are methotrexate, mycophenolate mofetil, and azathioprine.[53] Biologics have gained increasing use for RP in the last decade, including TNF-alpha blockers such as adalimumab and infliximab, as well as additional agents such as tocilizumab, abatacept, and rituximab.[44] These are usually second-line agents after initial conventional steroid-sparing therapy fails to induce remission.

TOXICITY FROM CHLOROQUINE AND HYDROXYCHLOROQUINE

Chloroquine (CQ) is a commonly used antimalarial agent in the developing world, while hydroxychloroquine (HCQ, plaquenil) remains widely used for its effective treatment of rheumatoid arthritis and systemic lupus erythematosus, among other inflammatory conditions. Retinal toxicity associated with these medications has long been documented. Marmor and colleagues in conjunction with the American Academy of Ophthalmology released the first set of recommended screening guidelines for HCQ in 2002. Since the publication of these guidelines, additional data have emerged that have better delineated risk factors for retinal toxicity, and led to additional modifications of guidelines in 2011 and 2016.[54,55]

The exact mechanism of CQ and HCQ retinal toxicity remains unclear at the cellular level. Anatomically, damage is seen at the layer of the photoreceptors, also known as the ellipsoid layer or inner segment—outer segment junction. These findings are seen in later stages with the use of spectral domain optical coherence tomography (SD-OCT).[56] Later stages may also manifest with damage of the adjacent retinal pigment epithelium. Clinically, this may appear as a bullseye maculopathy on slit lamp biomicroscopy, although this finding may not be present until very late stages of toxicity, and is often absent in patients of Asian or Hispanic descent.[57]

In a recent study, HCQ retinal toxicity was present in approximately 7.5% of patients who were on therapy for more than five years.[58] Daily dose was most closely correlated with development of retinal toxicity. Patients who took 4.0–5.0 mg/kg of HCQ daily based on their real weight were at significantly less risk for toxicity than patients who took higher levels, with less than 1% toxicity at five years and 2% at ten years. Thus, 5 mg/kg of real body weight is the recommended dosing of HCQ (and 2.3 mg/kg for CQ). Given that dispensing of HCQ is usually limited to 200 mg tablets, splitting of the tablet or skipping the medication on certain days of the week is recommended in order to achieve ideal dosing.[54] Serum testing of HCQ levels does not correlate with toxicity, and is thus not recommended. Concomitant renal disease, tamoxifen use, and pre-existing retinal or macular pathology are correlated with development of toxicity. Less significant factors include age, liver disease, and genetic factors.

Screening recommendations for HCQ toxicity underwent significant revision in 2016.[55] All patients should undergo a careful baseline ophthalmologic examination within 1 year of starting therapy, with attention to underlying retinal or macular disease that would warrant closer follow-up. Baseline visual fields and SD-OCT can be helpful, but are not required. Annual screening should begin after 5 years of therapy, unless there are additional risk factors, such as renal or retinal/macular disease. SD-OCT and automated visual fields should be obtained as part of this annual screening. For most patients, Humphrey 10–2 visual fields are recommended for detection of parafoveal scotomas. However, Asian patients should receive 24–2 or 30–2 visual fields given their propensity for extra macular disease.[59] Multifocal electroretinography (MF-ERG) and autofluorescence (AF) photos are additional adjunctive tools besides the two core measures. Ultrawide field AF photos can be helpful in Asian eyes. Importantly, fundus photographs, older time domain OCT, fluorescein angiography, full-field ERG, and electro-oculograms are insufficient and ineffective screening tools.

Once HCQ or CQ toxicity is suspected, referral to a retinal specialist and additional testing such as MF-ERG is recommended. Depending on the level of suspicion, a discussion should be held with the patient, rheumatologist, primary care physician, and other providers regarding the need to stop therapy.

REFERENCES

1. Ramirez M, Martinez-Martinez LA, Hernandez-Quintela E, et al. Small fiber neuropathy in women with fibromyalgia. An in vivo assessment using corneal confocal bio-microscopy. Semin Arthritis Rheum. 2015;45(2):214-9.
2. Hughes AE, Bridgett S, Meng W, et al. Sequence and Expression of Complement Factor H Gene Cluster Variants and Their Roles in Age-Related Macular Degeneration Risk. Invest Ophthalmol Vis Sci. 2016;57(6):2763-9.
3. Rosenbaum JT. Eyeing macular degeneration: a few inflammatory remarks. N Engl J Med. 2012;367(8):768-70.
4. Vohra R, Tsai JC, Kolko M. The role of inflammation in the pathogenesis of glaucoma. Surv Ophthalmol. 2013;58(4):311-20.
5. Singh DP, Sueno T, Kikuchi T, et al. Antibodies to a microbial peptide sharing sequence homology with betaA3-crystallin damage lens epithelial cells in vitro and in vivo. Autoimmunity. 1999;29(4):311-22.
6. Artifoni M, Rothschild PR, Brezin A, et al. Ocular inflammatory diseases associated with rheumatoid arthritis. Nat Rev Rheumatol. 2014;10(2):108-16.
7. Schargus M, Wolf F, Tony HP, et al. Correlation between tear film osmolarity, dry eye disease, and rheumatoid arthritis. Cornea. 2014;33(12):1257-61.
8. Turkyilmaz K, Kucukali Turkyilmaz A, Kurt A, et al. Investigation of tear osmolarity in early rheumatoid arthritis: relation to disease activity. Can J Ophthalmol. 2013;48(4):235-9.
9. Schmidl D, Witkowska KJ, Kaya S, et al. The association between subjective and objective parameters for the assessment of dry-eye syndrome. Invest Ophthalmol Vis Sci. 2015;56(3):1467-72.
10. Fujita M, Igarashi T, Kurai T, et al. Correlation between dry eye and rheumatoid arthritis activity. Am J Ophthalmol. 2005;140(5):808-13.
11. Lemp MA, Bron AJ, Baudouin C, et al. Tear osmolarity in the diagnosis and management of dry eye disease. Am J Ophthalmol. 2011;151(5):792-8 e1.
12. Foulks GN, Pflugfelder SC. New testing options for diagnosing and grading dry eye disease. Am J Ophthalmol. 2014;157(6):1122-9.
13. Holland EJ, Luchs J, Karpecki PM, et al. Lifitegrast for the treatment of dry eye disease: results of a phase III, randomized, double-masked, placebo-controlled trial (OPUS-3). Ophthalmology. 2017;124(1):53-60.
14. Perry HD, Solomon R, Donnenfeld ED, et al. Evaluation of topical cyclosporine for the treatment of dry eye disease. Arch Ophthalmol. 2008;126(8):1046-50.
15. Sainz de la Maza M, Foster CS, Jabbur NS, et al. Ocular characteristics and disease associations in scleritis-associated peripheral keratopathy. Arch Ophthalmol. 2002;120(1):15-9.
16. Akpek EK, Thorne JE, Qazi FA, et.al. Evaluation of patients with scleritis for systemic disease. Ophthalmology. 2004;111(3):501-6.
17. Galor A, Thorne JE, Jabs DA. Rheumatic disease and scleritis. Ophthalmology. 2007;114(6):1232.
18. Sainz de la Maza M, Molina N, Gonzalez-Gonzalez LA, et al. Clinical characteristics of a large cohort of patients with scleritis and episcleritis. Ophthalmology. 2012;119(1):43-50.
19. Smith JR, Mackensen F, Rosenbaum JT. Therapy insight: scleritis and its relationship to systemic autoimmune disease. Nat Clin Pract Rheumatol. 2007;3(4):219-26.
20. Galor A, Thorne JE. Scleritis and peripheral ulcerative keratitis. Rheum Dis Clin North Am. 2007;33(4):835-54, vii.
21. Watanabe R, Ishii T, Yoshida M, et al. Ulcerative keratitis in patients with rheumatoid arthritis in the modern biologic era: a series of eight cases and literature review. Int J Rheum Dis. 2017;20(2):225-30.
22. Prada J, Noelle B, Baatz H, et al. Tumour necrosis factor alpha and interleukin 6 gene expression in keratocytes from patients with rheumatoid corneal ulcerations. Br J Ophthalmol. 2003;87(5):548-50.
23. Korsten P, Bahlmann D, Patschan SA. Rapid healing of peripheral ulcerative keratitis in rheumatoid arthritis with prednisone, methotrexate and adalimumab combination therapy. Rheumatology (Oxford). 2017;56(7):1094.
24. Read RW. Clinical mini-review: systemic lupus erythematosus and the eye. Ocul Immunol Inflamm. 2004;12(2):87-99.
25. Davies JB, Rao PK. Ocular manifestations of systemic lupus erythematosus. Curr Opin Ophthalmol. 2008;19(6):512-8.
26. Palejwala NV, Walia HS, Yeh S. Ocular manifestations of systemic lupus erythematosus: a review of the literature. Autoimmune Dis. 2012;2012:290898.
27. Sivaraj RR, Durrani OM, Denniston AK, et al. Ocular manifestations of systemic lupus erythematosus. Rheumatology (Oxford). 2007;46(12):1757-62.
28. Nguyen QD, Uy HS, Akpek EK, et al. Choroidopathy of systemic lupus erythematosus. Lupus. 2000;9(4):288-98.
29. Rosenbaum JT, Simpson J, Neuwelt EM. Successful treatment of optic neuritis in association with systemic

lupus erythematosus using intravenous cyclophosphamide. Br J Ophthalmol. 1997;81:130-2.
30. Rosenbaum JT. Evolving "diagnostic" criteria for axial spondyloarthritis in the context of anterior uveitis. Ocul Immunol Inflamm. 2016;24(4):445-9.
31. Haroon M, O'Rourke M, Ramasamy P, et al. A novel evidence-based detection of undiagnosed spondyloarthritis in patients presenting with acute anterior uveitis: the DUET (Dublin Uveitis Evaluation Tool). Ann Rheum Dis. 2015;74(11):1990-5.
32. Mintz R, Feller ER, Bahr RL, et al. Ocular manifestations of inflammatory bowel disease. Inflamm Bowel Dis. 2004;10(2):135-9.
33. Bacchiega AB, Balbi GG, Ochtrop ML, et al. Ocular involvement in patients with spondyloarthritis. Rheumatology (Oxford); 2017.
34. Watkins AS, Kempen JH, Choi D, et al. Ocular disease in patients with ANCA-positive vasculitis. J Ocul Biol Dis Infor. 2009;3(1):12-9.
35. Tarabishy AB, Schulte M, Papaliodis GN, et al. Wegener's granulomatosis: clinical manifestations, differential diagnosis, and management of ocular and systemic disease. Surv Ophthalmol. 2010;55(5):429-44.
36. Ebrahimiadib N, Modjtahedi BS, Roohipoor R, et al. successful treatment strategies in granulomatosis with polyangiitis-associated peripheral ulcerative keratitis. Cornea. 2016;35(11):1459-65.
37. Pakrou N, Selva D, Leibovitch I. Wegener's granulomatosis: ophthalmic manifestations and management. Semin Arthritis Rheum. 2006;35(5):284-92.
38. Sandhu RK, Adams T, Sibley C, et al. Granulomatosis with polyangiitis (GPA) presenting with frosted branch angiitis. Retinal Cases Brief Rep. 2016;10(3):249-51.
39. Sarraf P, Sneller MC. Pathogenesis of Wegener's granulomatosis: current concepts. Expert Rev Mol Med. 2005;7(8):1-19.
40. Cocho L, Gonzalez-Gonzalez LA, Molina-Prat N, et al. Scleritis in patients with granulomatosis with polyangiitis (Wegener). Br J Ophthalmol. 2016;100(8):1062-5.
41. Hoang LT, Lim LL, Vaillant B, et al. Antineutrophil Cytoplasmic Antibody-Associated Active Scleritis. Arch Ophthalmol. 2008;126(5):451-55.
42. Stone JH, Merkel PA, Spiera R, et al. Rituximab versus cyclophosphamide for ANCA-associated vasculitis. N Engl J Med. 2010;363(3):221-32.
43. Sneller MC, Hoffman GS, Talar-Williams C, et al. An analysis of forty-two Wegener's granulomatosis patients treated with methotrexate and prednisone. Arthritis Rheum. 1995;38(5):608-13.
44. Mathian A, Miyara M, Cohen-Aubart F, et al. Relapsing polychondritis: A 2016 update on clinical features, diagnostic tools, treatment and biological drug use. Best Pract Res Clin Rheumatol. 2016;30(2):316-33.
45. Arnaud L, Mathian A, Haroche J, et al. Pathogenesis of relapsing polychondritis: a 2013 update. Autoimmun Rev. 2014;13(2):90-5.
46. Hazra N, Dregan A, Charlton J, et al. Incidence and mortality of relapsing polychondritis in the UK: a population-based cohort study. Rheumatology (Oxford). 2015;54(12):2181-7.
47. Dion J, Costedoat-Chalumeau N, Sene D, et al. Relapsing polychondritis can be characterized by three different clinical phenotypes: analysis of a recent series of 142 patients. Arthritis Rheumatol. 2016;68(12):2992-3001.
48. Michet CJJ, McKenna CH, Luthra HS, et al. Relapsing polychondritis. Survival and predictive role of early disease manifestations. Ann Intern Med. 1986;104:74-8.
49. Trentham DE, Le CH. Relapsing polychondritis. Ann Intern Med. 1998;129(2):114-22.
50. Kent PD, Michet CJ, Jr., Luthra HS. Relapsing polychondritis. Curr Opin Rheumatol. 2004;16(1):56-61.
51. Sainz-de-la-Maza M, Molina N, Gonzalez-Gonzalez LA, et al. Scleritis associated with relapsing polychondritis. Br J Ophthalmol. 2016;100(9):1290-4.
52. Paroli MP, Priori R, Spinucci G, et al. Uveitis with retinal occlusive vasculitis and sensorineural hypoacusia as first symptoms of relapsing polychondritis. Clin Exp Rheumatol. 2012;30(1 Suppl 70):S101-3.
53. Lahmer T, Treiber M, von Werder A, et al. Relapsing polychondritis: an autoimmune disease with many faces. Autoimmun Rev. 2010;9(8):540-6.
54. Marmor MF, Kellner U, Lai TY, et al. American Academy of O. Revised recommendations on screening for chloroquine and hydroxychloroquine retinopathy. Ophthalmology. 2011;118(2):415-22.
55. Marmor MF, Kellner U, Lai TY, et al. American Academy of O. Recommendations on screening for chloroquine and hydroxychloroquine retinopathy (2016 Revision). Ophthalmology. 2016;123(6):1386-94.
56. Lee MG, Kim SJ, Ham DI, et al. Macular retinal ganglion cell-inner plexiform layer thickness in patients on hydroxychloroquine therapy. Invest Ophthalmol Vis Sci. 2014;56(1):396-402.
57. Melles RB, Marmor MF. Pericentral retinopathy and racial differences in hydroxychloroquine toxicity. Ophthalmology. 2015;122(1):110-6.
58. Melles RB, Marmor MF. The risk of toxic retinopathy in patients on long-term hydroxychloroquine therapy. JAMA Ophthalmol. 2014;132(12):1453-60.
59. Marmor MF, Melles RB. Disparity between visual fields and optical coherence tomography in hydroxychloroquine retinopathy. Ophthalmology. 2014;121(6):1257-62.

Part 11 Neuro-ophthalmology

Prem S Subramanian

OUTLINE

Chapter 90

The Neuro-ophthalmic Examination

Prem S Subramanian

INTRODUCTION

Neuro-ophthalmology, unlike other ophthalmic subspecialties such as glaucoma, retina, and cornea, is defined not by a single disease process or anatomic structure but rather by a broad categorization of the wide variety of ocular and systemic disorders that may be encountered by a clinician who is evaluating a patient with new visual symptoms. In this and subsequent chapters in this section, the diagnosis and management of various afferent and efferent visual disorders will be presented; although ancillary, laboratory, and radiographic tests often are used in the diagnosis and management of such patients, the initial neuro-ophthalmic examination must be performed thoroughly and systematically to direct an appropriate further workup. Indeed, the failure to obtain a complete patient history, as well as a cursory examination, will lead to inaccurate or missed diagnoses and delay the recognition and treatment of disease.

NEURO-OPHTHALMIC HISTORY

A complete medical and ophthalmic history must be obtained for every new patient, with particular attention to systemic disorders that are associated with optic nerve, orbital, and intracranial disease. These entities are discussed in greater detail in the chapter on systemic disease in neuro-ophthalmology, but a short list for inquiry of all patients would include prior neurologic disease (demyelinating, vascular, other), endocrine dysfunction (pituitary, thyroid), hematologic disorders (including lymphoma and leukemia), autoimmune diseases [systemic lupus erythematosus (SLE), sarcoidosis, vasculitides], and solid organ malignancies. The presence or absence of more common systemic disorders, such as hypertension, diabetes, atherosclerotic disease, and obesity, rarely will direct the ophthalmologist to a specific diagnosis, but the differential diagnosis and subsequent diagnostic workup will be shaped by this information. An informal axiom in neuro-ophthalmology (and perhaps medicine in general) states that if a patient has a history of malignancy, then new symptoms must be attributed to a recurrence or new manifestation of that malignancy until proven otherwise.

Family History

Family medical history requires more attention in neuro-ophthalmology than in other ophthalmic subspecialties. As described in the chapter on "Common Optic Neuropathies", there are a number of inherited disorders, often with mitochondrial inheritance patterns, which cause subacute and chronic vision loss. These conditions can mimic other disorders such as optic neuritis or may even be mistaken for functional problems in their early stages, so an accurate family history may assist in diagnosis. Patients with diplopia and/or ptosis should be questioned about other similar symptoms in other family members as well, as chronic progressive external ophthalmoplegia (CPEO), oculopharyngeal muscular dystrophy, and other inherited myopathies may present with symptoms identical to those of myasthenia gravis. The lack of a positive history should not, however, exclude a diagnosis of one of these conditions, as expressivity and penetrance of any of them can be variable. In addition, family history may be incomplete or even incorrect and must be considered in this context.

Social History

Social and behavioral history also contributes to the manifestation of neuro-ophthalmic diseases. Malnutrition may be unrecognized, particularly in patients who are following extremely restrictive diets for personal or medical reasons. Toxic chemical exposure can occur through occupations or hobbies, and these aspects of the patient's life must be explored as well. Finally, alcohol and drug consumption often go underreported by the patient, particularly if family members are present at the time of the examination, and careful private questioning may be necessary to ascertain the true extent of the use of these substances.

GENERAL MEDICAL EVALUATION

The ophthalmologist need not to perform a full medical examination on every patient, but routine assessment of height and weight (to allow calculation of body mass index) and blood pressure by medical assistants is quick and provides important ancillary information for diagnosis. If routine laboratory tests for blood glucose, serum chemistries, and lipids are available, they should be reviewed for abnormalities. Neuro-ophthalmologists who are trained in neurology rather than or in addition to ophthalmology may conduct a full neurological examination; however, the comprehensive ophthalmologist may not feel qualified to perform such an examination and should not feel compelled to do so.

Visual Acuity

Snellen visual acuity measurement at 6 m remains the typical manner in which central acuity is determined in neuro-ophthalmic patients. Some neuro-ophthalmologists will insist that the fellow eye is patched during testing to ensure only the tested eye is seeing the chart. In addition to the absolute acuity obtained, the speed and fluency of letter detection at each level of acuity should be considered. Patients with a visual field defect may need to scan the chart and/or use eccentric viewing. A patient with a homonymous hemianopia may read only one side of the chart. Subjects with nystagmus may have better binocular than monocular visual acuity.[1] Near visual acuity with appropriate age-related spectacle correction should be measured in all patients. Patients with cognitive disorders may report problems with reading, yet they may read single small letters or numbers without difficulty. In such cases, having the patient read a section of printed text (newspaper, magazine) and assessing their reading speed, fluency, and comprehension may assist in understanding the nature of the visual disorder.

Stereoacuity

Polarizing glasses are used with Titmus, Randot, or similar standardized tests to evaluate binocular fusion and the ability to fuse disparate targets into a simulated three-dimensional image (Fig. 90.1). Stereoacuity is measured in arc-seconds, and an estimation of binocular visual acuity can be made from this value. This value may be useful in patients with suspected unilateral functional vision loss (*see* Chapter 97), although there is some evidence that this estimate should be made with caution.[2]

Color Vision and Contrast Sensitivity

A number of studies demonstrate that patients with optic neuropathy (acute, chronic, or even resolved) will have deficits of pseudoisochromatic plate (PIP) color testing even in the setting of normal or near normal visual acuity.[3-6] Either Ishihara or Hardy-Rand-Rittler plates may be used, although the latter appear more sensitive in the diagnosis of optic nerve disease.[7] Reduced contrast sensitivity also occurs frequently in patients with optic neuropathy, and this phenomenon has been studied most extensively in patients with multiple sclerosis.[8-12] It is possible that reduced PIP identification is actually a function of reduced contrast sensitivity and not indicative of damage to color discrimination ability, as most patients

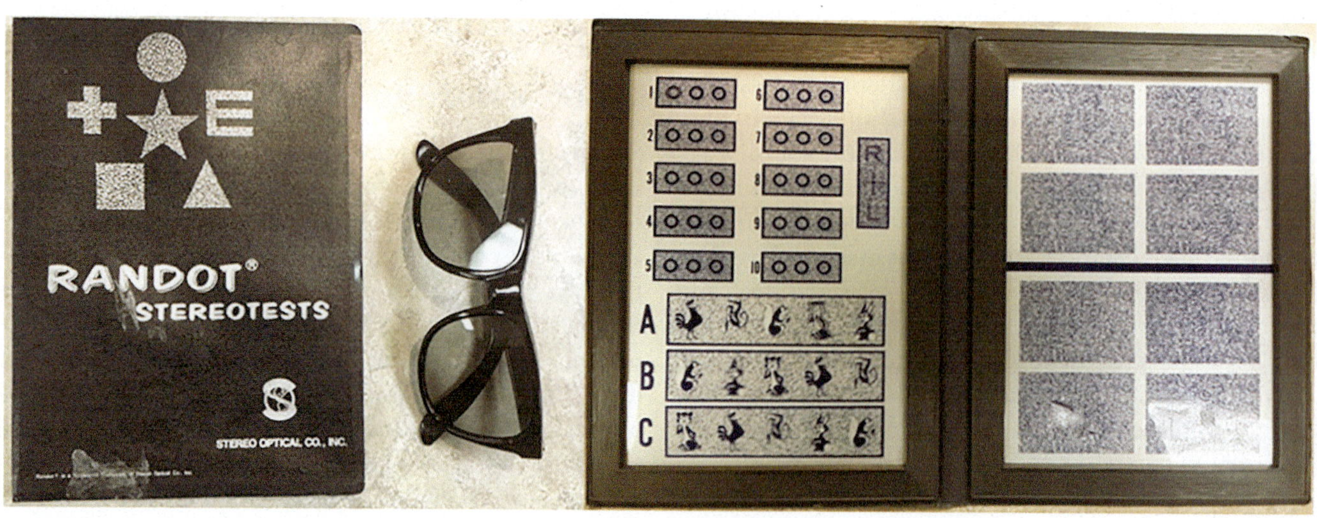

Fig. 90.1: Randot stereotest with polarizing glasses. The patient indicates which of the circles or animals appears to "pop up" out of the page on the left side, while the panels on the right side have embedded figures visible only when stereopsis is present (not visible in this 2-D photograph).

with optic neuropathy have normal color vision on color arrangement tests such as the D-15, despite having reduced PIP performance.[13] Nonetheless, the PIP plates remain an important diagnostic tool in the assessment of patients with suspected optic nerve disease.

VISUAL FIELD TESTING

Despite the utility and necessity of perimetric testing in the majority of patients with afferent visual pathway disease, office-based evaluation of peripheral vision still provides useful information for clinical diagnosis. Confrontation testing by finger counting is very insensitive but quick to conduct, and double simultaneous presentation of stimuli (Fig. 90.2) may reveal an extinction phenomenon in one hemifield (usually the left) that corresponds to a right parietal lobe lesion or stroke.[14] A small red object, such as a pinhead or the cap of a bottle of dilating drops (*see* Fig. 92.1), can be presented kinetically in various parts of the visual field and has been reported to detect up to 75% of clinically relevant field defects.[15] The Amsler grid (*see* Fig. 98.2) serves as a useful screening tool for visual field defects lying within the central 10°. It may be prudent to obtain automated perimetry on all patients presenting with afferent neuro-ophthalmologic complaints or suspected disorders, as several disorders such as suprasellar tumors may produce findings detectable only by these more sensitive techniques. [*See* Chapter 98, Topical Diagnosis of Visual Field Loss, for detailed information on automated perimetry and its interpretation].

Pupil Examination

It has been suggested that the relative afferent pupillary defect (RAPD) is among the most reliable and objective

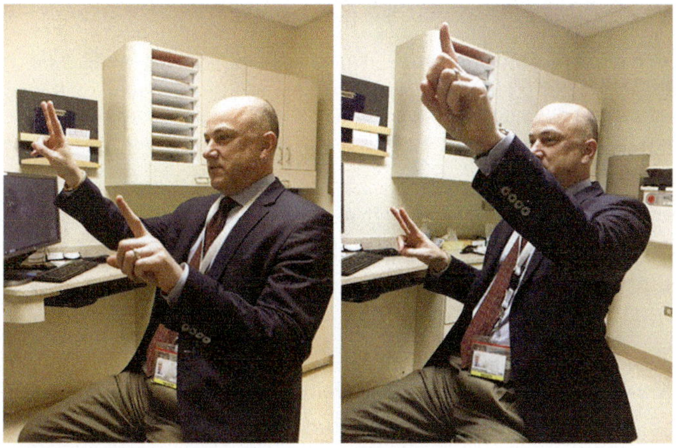

Fig. 90.2: Double simultaneous confrontation with fingers to determine if the stimulus is perceived equally on both sides of the vertical midline.

indicators of anterior visual pathway dysfunction. Anisocoria, a visible difference in pupil size, is a common reason for neuro-ophthalmic referral as well. The ophthalmologist must remember that afferent and efferent pupillary disorders are separate, and that involvement of one system does not affect the function of the other. To wit, optic neuropathy does not cause anisocoria, and unequal pupil size does not result in an RAPD. While some non-neuro-ophthalmic diseases, such as profound amblyopia or extensive retinal damage and/or scarring may produce an RAPD, such conditions can usually be diagnosed by history or examination and excluded from consideration. It is axiomatic that a patient with an acquired optic neuropathy will have an RAPD, unless the condition is extremely mild or there is prior or concurrent damage to the contralateral eye. Keys to the pupil examination include:

- Observe both pupils in both dim and bright lighting conditions.
- Illuminate both pupils simultaneously with a handheld light and observe constriction speed and symmetry, as well as redilation after light exposure.
- Illuminate each pupil individually for 1–3 seconds, observing the speed of constriction, maintenance of constriction, and speed of redilation.
- Illuminate one pupil for 1–2 seconds, then move the light to the fellow eye for the same amount of time ("swinging flashlight test") and observe if the second pupil constricts equally, does not constrict, or appears to dilate only (evidence for RAPD).

One of the keys in pupil examination is to ensure that each pupil is exposed to light for the same amount of time as the fellow eye; if one eye receives more light than the other, then an RAPD may be falsely induced by decreasing that eye's sensitivity to light exposure (light adaptation). Neutral density filters may be used to quantify the magnitude of the RAPD, while a 0.3 log unit filter may be used over each eye to help in the identification of a subtle RAPD (Fig. 90.3). The techniques of pupil examination and interpretation are presented in much greater detail in Chapter 100.

Fixation and Extraocular Movement

A standard ophthalmic examination includes the assessment of extraocular movement; in the neuro-ophthalmic examination, further testing of initiation and control of eye movements may be needed to aid in diagnosis of visual complaints. In addition to recording ductions (movements of each eye alone) and versions (binocular movements), the examiner should record fixation stability and any abnormalities of maintaining fixation such as nystagmus,

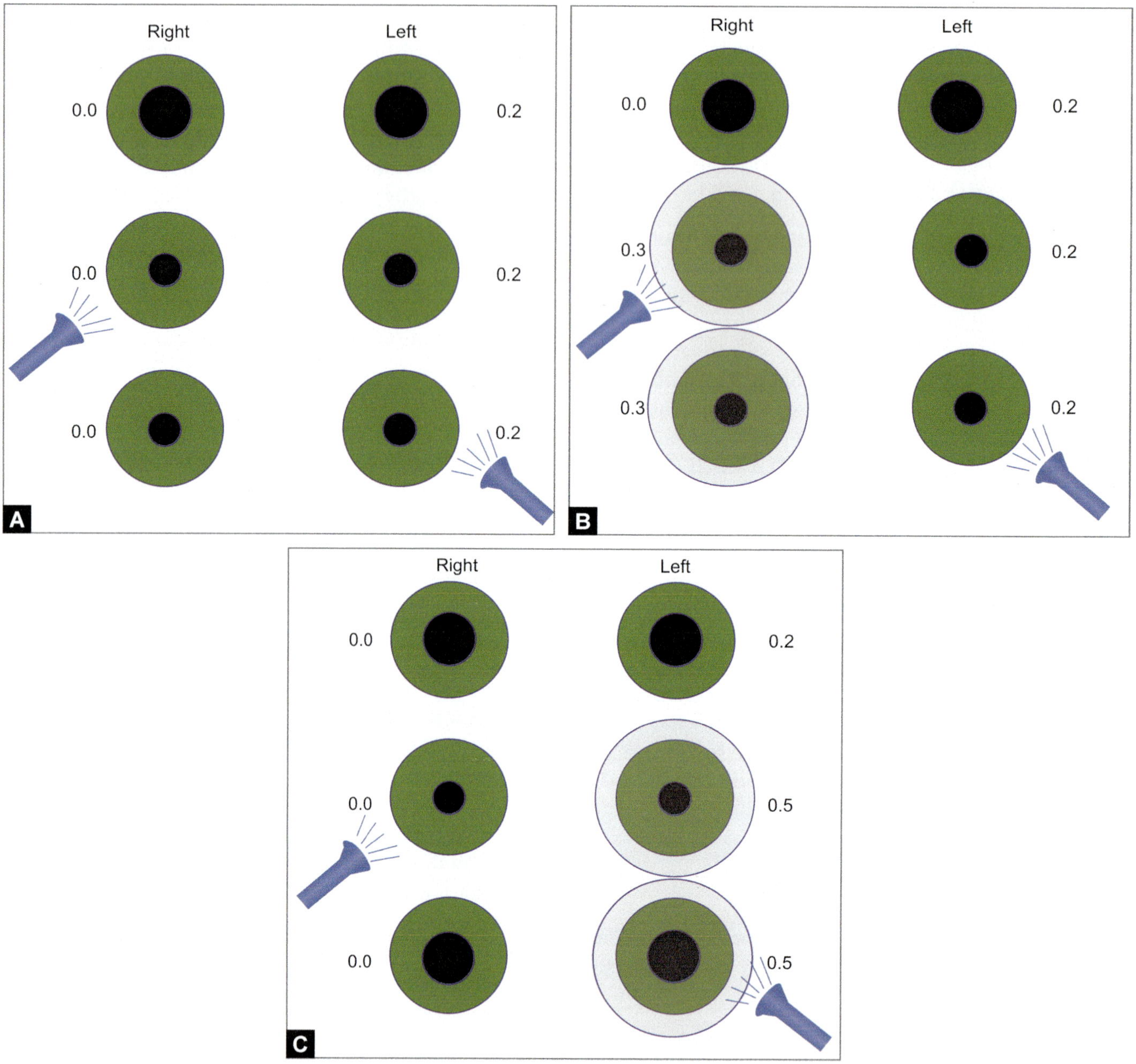

Fig. 90.3: Use of a 0.3 log filter to enhance a subtle RAPD. (A) The patient has a left optic neuropathy with a 0.2 log RAPD. With the swinging flashlight test, no RAPD is detected, and pupils appear to reach equally to light stimulus; (B) With a 0.3 log filter placed over the right (normal) eye, a difference of 0.1 log between the eyes is created. Thus, a brisk pupillary reaction still is seen when either eye is illuminated by the flashlight; (C) Placing the 0.3 log filter over the left eye gives a 0.5 log difference between the eyes, which now allows a left RAPD to be detected.

saccadic intrusions, and saccadic oscillations. Detailed methods of characterizing nystagmus and similar problems are provided in Chapter 96. It may be necessary to observe the patient for up to 2–3 minutes in order to identify correctly any instability of gaze. Furthermore, it may be instructive to have the patient hold an eccentric gaze and then return to primary position to unmask unusual conditions such as ocular neuromyotonia.[16] Both saccade and pursuit movements should be tested, and latency and accuracy of saccades as well as smoothness of pursuit should be noted. Delayed saccadic initiation may be seen with Parkinsonian disorders,[17,18] and saccadic inaccuracy may indicate vestibulocerebellar dysfunction.[19] Impaired smooth pursuit also may be a feature of Parkinson disease.[17]

Saccadic testing also should be correlated with visual field testing results; patients with a dense homonymous hemianopia will fail to see a peripheral target in the blind field and make no saccade or a delayed saccade after scanning into the blind field. Patients claiming visual field loss or constriction from functional disorders (*see* Chapter 97) may make accurate and rapid saccades to a target presented into the seemingly blind field, helping to confirm for the examiner that vision may be present in areas where blindness is claimed.

Ocular misalignment when present should be measured and recorded quantitatively. Cover testing or Maddox rod assessment in primary position, reading position, and in the 8 standard eccentric gaze positions should be performed. Some clinicians have advocated for the routine use of qualitative duction mapping with Hess screens[20,21] to assist in longitudinal assessments (Is the patient improving or not?) as well as for surgical planning. In general, the ophthalmologist should use the methods that he/she is most skilled in and endeavor to perform these tests with the greatest accuracy and consistency from visit to visit. Some variability in testing results is to be expected, both because the patient may perform differently on subsequent visits despite stable disease, and because of the inherent variability of standard testing protocols such as cover testing.[22]

Cranial Nerve Assessment and External Examination

The ophthalmologist typically will not perform a detailed neurologic examination but should evaluate the function of cranial nerves that traverse the skull base close to the ocular apparatus, including the ocular motor system. The trigeminal nerve supplies sensation to the ocular surface as well as the eyelids, face, and scalp (Fig. 90.4), and its function may be impaired by infiltrative or neoplastic processes

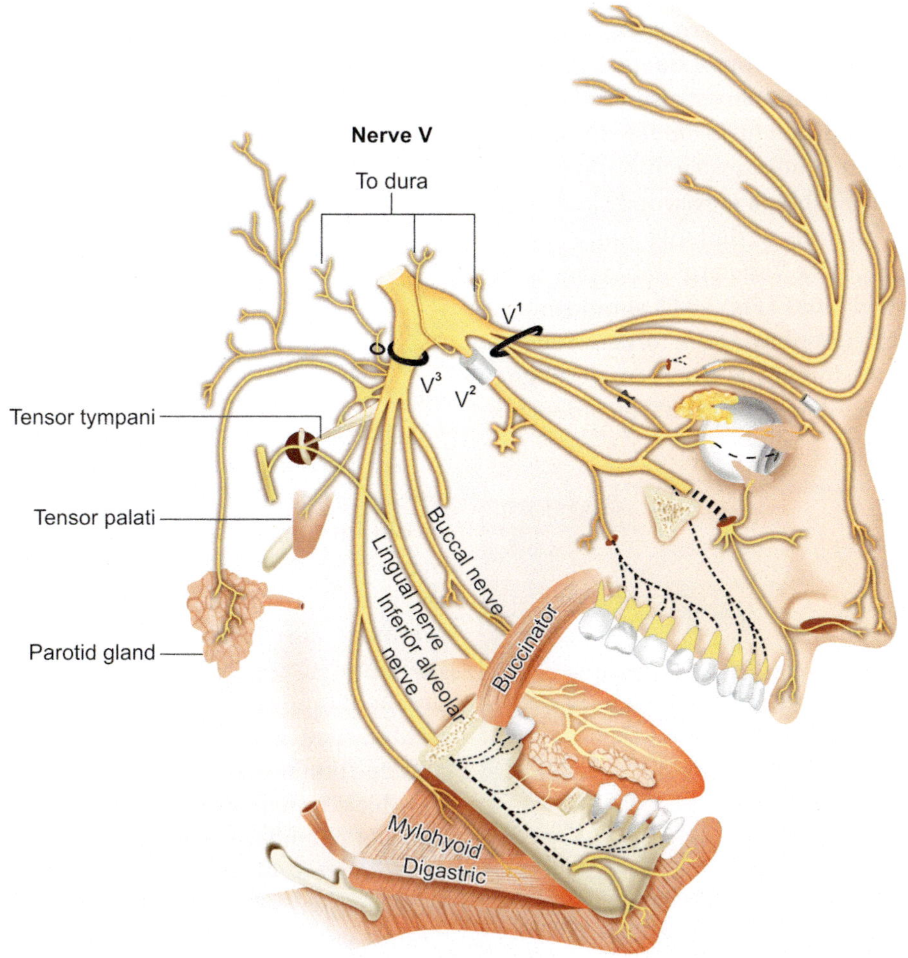

Fig. 90.4: Distribution of the sensory and motor branches of the trigeminal nerve.
Source: By Grant, John Charles Boileu. An Atlas of Anatomy/by regions 1962, Public Domain, https://commons.wikimedia.org/w/index.php?curid=30134811.

involving the orbit or cavernous sinus. The trigeminal nerve also has motor function, but it arises in an anatomically distinct pathway that is usually not affected by processes involving the eye and orbit; thus, the ophthalmologist is much more likely to identify impaired sensory function, if present, that is associated with afferent or efferent neuro-ophthalmic disease. A thin cotton fiber elongated from a cotton swab serves as a qualitative instrument for checking both corneal and facial sensation; an esthesiometer may be used if quantitative corneal sensation measurement is desired,[23] but is not typically employed in standard neuro-ophthalmic practice. Facial nerve function also may be affected in neuro-ophthalmic disorders with facial asymmetry or weakness noted. Orbicularis oculi strength may be reduced with neuromuscular disorders such as myasthenia gravis and CPEO,[24-26] and patients may complain of symptoms of ocular surface exposure. Excessive and/or repeated forceful blinking of both eyelids is characteristic of essential blepharospasm,[27] while purely unilateral symptoms are more likely to be from hemifacial spasm, a condition that may arise from inappropriate vascular contact with and irritation of the facial nerve at its root exit zone.[28] The ophthalmologist also should assess globe position and eyelid height in neuro-ophthalmic patients, as patients with conditions such as thyroid eye disease, orbit tumors, myasthenia gravis, and CPEO often present with initial symptoms of diplopia and/or ptosis, without any orbital symptoms. Vertical globe displacement (hypoglobus or hyperglobus) (Fig. 90.5) should not be mistaken for vertical heterophoria; the former does not result in diplopia, since the visual axes remain aligned between the eyes. Further details on orbital disorders may be found in Chapter 94, Systemic Disease and Neuro-Ophthalmology and Part Eleven, Orbit and Oculoplasty.

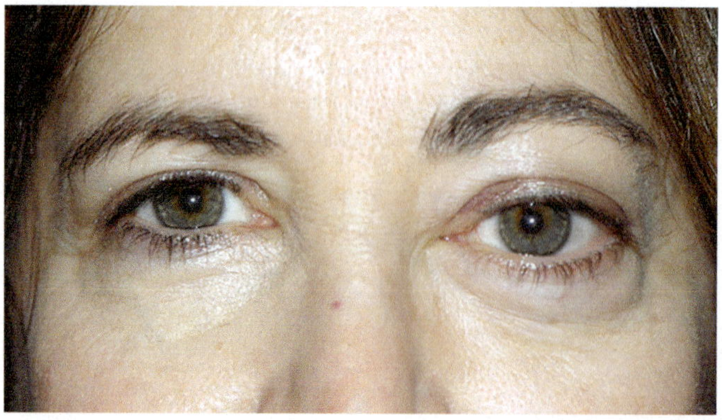

Fig. 90.5: External photograph of a patient with left eye hypoglobus from a spheno-orbital tumor invading the superior orbit. Note the pupillary light reflex is centered on both corneas, showing an absence of any vertical deviation of ocular alignment.

ANTERIOR SEGMENT AND POSTERIOR EVALUATION

In contrast with other areas of ophthalmology, the slit-lamp and fundus examinations often do not contain critical or distinctive findings to assist in the diagnosis and management of the patient's visual complaints. Classically, patients with retrobulbar optic neuritis will have a normal examination; in other patients with insidious or prior vision loss, the presence of optic disk pallor helps to confirm an optic neuropathy is present but does not provide additional diagnostic value. The recognition of the variation among "normal" optic disks and the differentiation of the swollen optic disk from one that is merely elevated often fall to the neuro-ophthalmologist (Table 90.1).

Anomalous Optic Disks

When a disk has an elevated appearance (Figs. 90.11A and B), the margins should be inspected carefully for any swelling within the peripapillary nerve fiber layer, obscuration of small blood vessels in the peripapillary zone, and presence of lipid or nerve fiber layer hemorrhages. The presence of spontaneous venous pulsations (SVP) may be used as evidence that the disk is not truly swollen,[29] although SVP may be absent for a variety of anatomic reasons, and their presence has been reported in patients with elevated intracranial pressure.[30] Ancillary testing such as optical coherence tomography may help in the differentiation of elevated and swollen optic disks.[31] The reader is directed to Chapter 91, The Swollen Optic Nerve, for further details.

All patients should be evaluated carefully for the presence of prior trauma and the presence of active or old intraocular inflammation. When a patient has a neurologic disorder such as MS, it is often presumed by the neurologist or other physicians that any new visual symptom must be related to the neurologic disease. During the examination, the ophthalmologist must look for other potential (and often more common) causes of vision loss or blur, such as ocular surface disease, incipient cataract, and epiretinal membrane. Patients with visual field loss may have unrecognized intraocular pressure elevation or anterior chamber angle abnormalities that could indicate glaucomatous optic neuropathy either in isolation or with another optic neuropathy that may confound the diagnosis. Critical assessment of the optic disk for pallor, cupping, and notching may help to distinguish these entities.

Table 90.1: Optic disk anomalies.

Ophthalmoscopic finding	Description	Visual impact/consequence
Myopic tilt/crescent (Figs. 90.6A and B)	• Usually in eyes with >6 D myopia • Baring of peripapillary choroidal vessels • Anomalous vascular branching pattern	None in isolation, but careful examination for any macular scarring or CNV needed
Optic disk hypoplasia (unilateral) (Figs. 90.7A and B)	• Small optic disk (less than 1,000 µm diameter) in otherwise normal sized eye • Scleral ring ("double ring sign") often present • Minimal or no optic cup • Disk may have normal color or pallor	• Acuity may be normal or reduced • Variable visual field defects • RAPD often present
Optic disk hypoplasia (bilateral)	• Bilateral findings similar to unilateral • Possible septo-optic dysplasia with agenesis of corpus callosum, absent septum pellucidum, chiasmal atrophy, hypothalamic and/or pituitary hypoplasia (Fig. 90.8).	Similar to unilateral hypoplasia
Optic disk coloboma (Fig. 90.9)	• Developmental abnormality that may be unilateral or bilateral • Can be in isolation or occur with retinochoroidal defects • Usually located inferomedially • May not be continuous with disk ("bridge coloboma")	• Typically reduced • Extent of visual impairment related in part to extend of the coloboma
Morning glory disk (Figs. 90.10A and B)	• Large optic nerve with excavated, deep cup • Vessels exit disk in a radial pattern • Usually unilateral	Moderate-to-severe visual impairment with RAPD and visual field defect present

(RAPD: Relative afferent pupillary defect; CNV: Choroidal neovascularization)

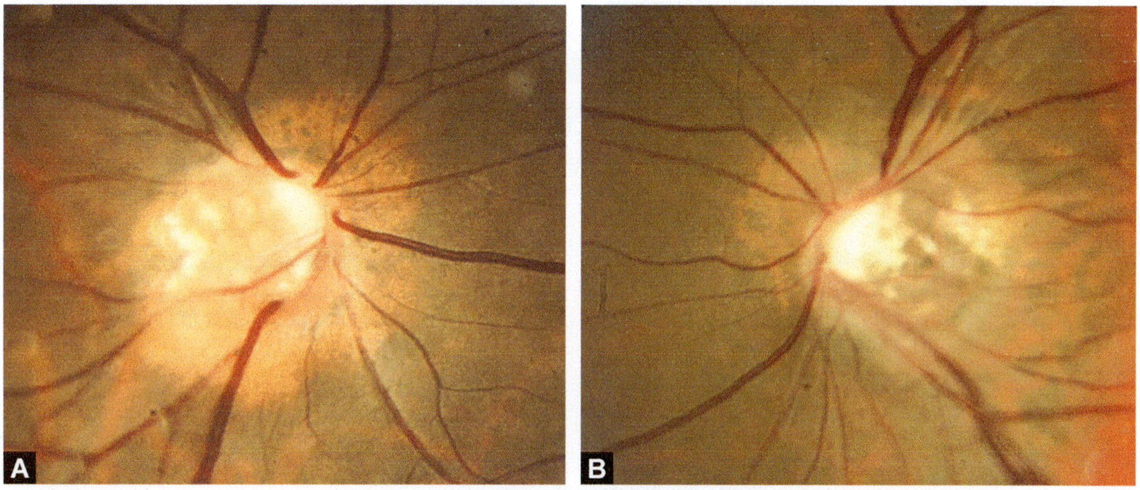

Figs. 90.6A and B: Severe myopic tilt of both optic disks in a patient with a refraction of –12 D in each eye and normal visual acuity. The temporal disk rim cannot be seen because of the tilted disk insertion.

CONCLUSION AND SUMMARY

The neuro-ophthalmologic assessment requires the ophthalmologist to obtain a detailed, often chronological, history of not only the patient's ophthalmic concerns but also their systemic medical disorders. Review of records from other ophthalmologists and physicians can help to establish the timeline of the symptoms and their change over time. Prior radiologic studies, if available, also should be obtained and interpreted either by the ophthalmologist or with the assistance of a local neuroradiologist skilled in modern neuroimaging techniques. Physical examination of the patient includes additional attention to ocular movement and visual function outside of foveal (central) visual acuity. Slit lamp and fundus examinations allow identification of other ophthalmic disease that may be contributing to the visual symptoms, in addition to providing a thorough assessment of the optic disk, its vasculature, and

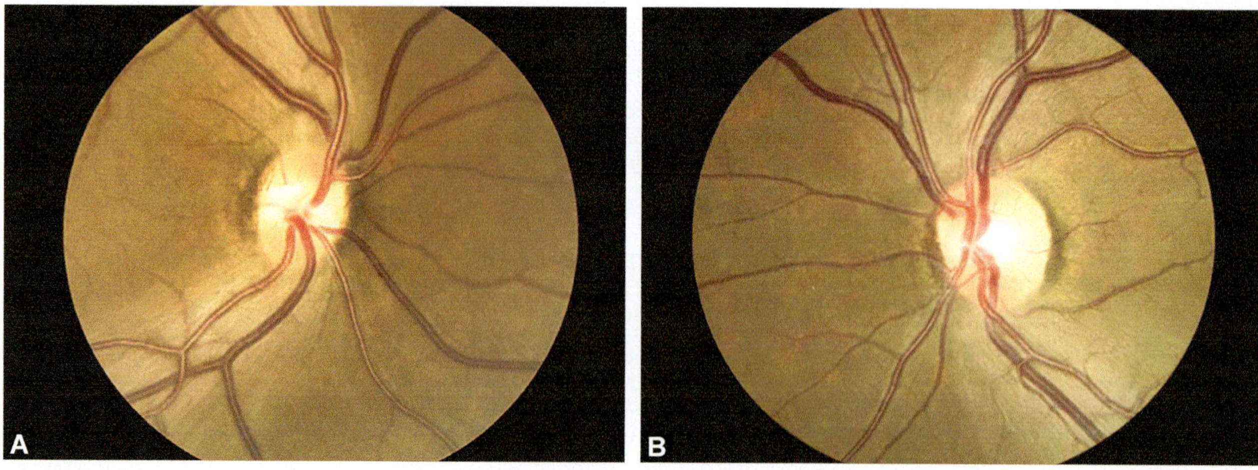

Figs. 90.7A and B: (A) Hypoplastic right optic nerve in a patient with unilateral loss of temporal visual field and mildly decreased (6/18) visual acuity right eye; (B) The left optic disk is normal.

Source: Reprinted with permission from Brooks DB, Subramanian PS. Monocular temporal hemianopia with septo-optic dysplasia. J Neuroophthalmol. 2006;26:195-6.

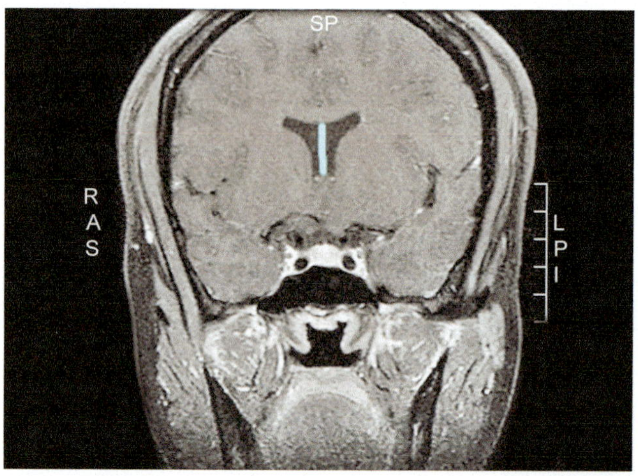

Fig. 90.8: T1-weighted coronal magnetic resonance imaging (MRI) brain from the patient in Fig. 90.7, showing an absent septum pellucidum (SP) (light blue line indicates where this structure normally would appear).

Source: Reprinted with permission from Brooks DB, Subramanian PS. Monocular temporal hemianopia with septo-optic dysplasia. J Neuroophthalmol. 2006;26:195-6.

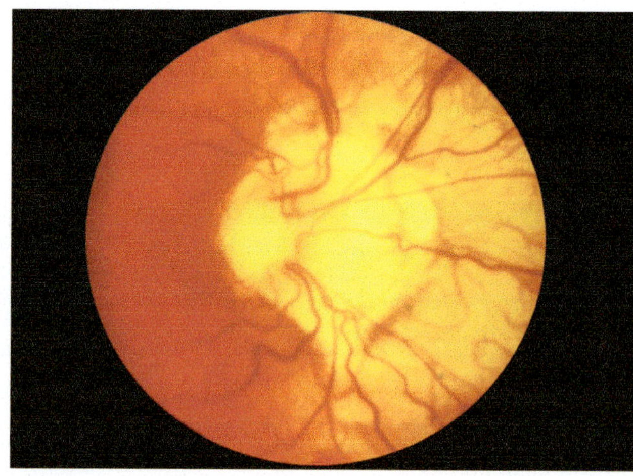

Fig. 90.9: Large retinochoroidal coloboma in the right eye of a patient with lifelong poor vision in that eye.

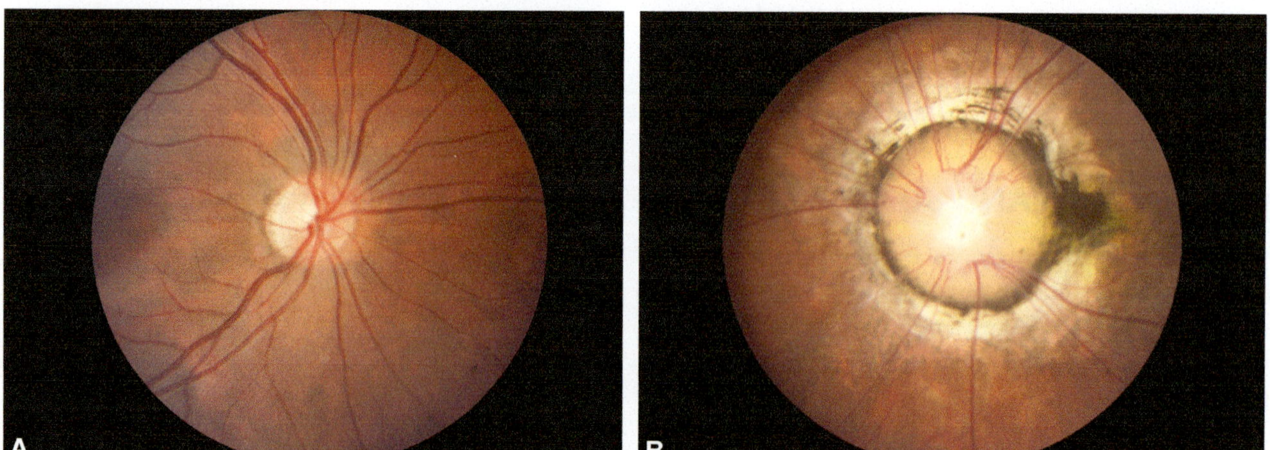

Figs. 90.10A and B: Normal right eye (A) and morning glory disk anomaly (B) in the left eye of a patient with lifelong decreased vision left eye. Note the much larger scleral opening for the optic disk in the left eye (photographs taken at the same magnification) and the anomalous vascular branching pattern.

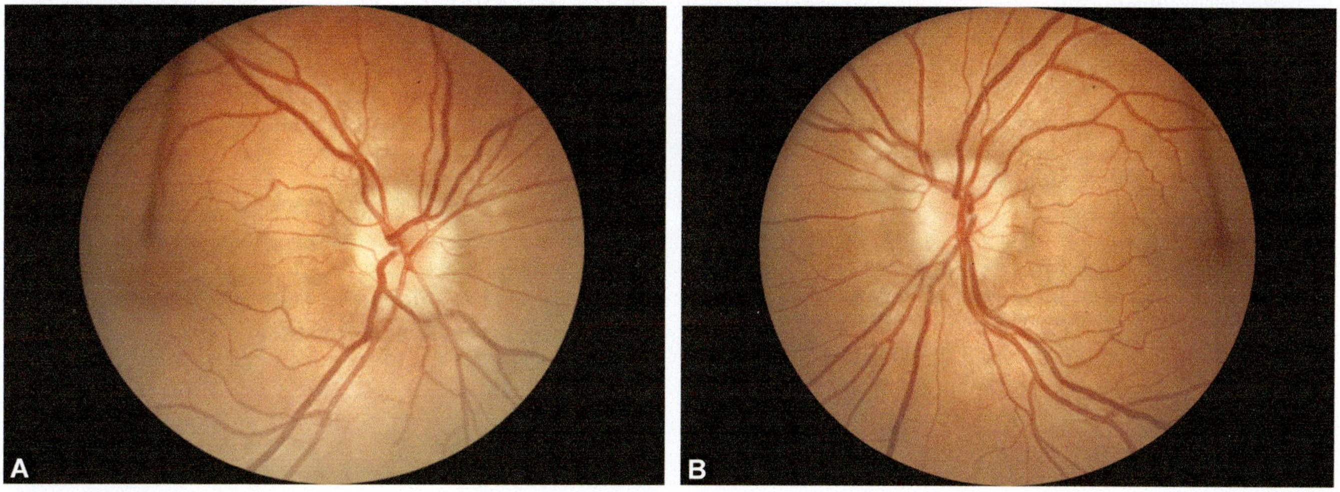

Figs. 90.11A and B: Optic disk photographs in an asymptomatic patient referred for evaluation because of optic disk elevation. Both optic disks are small and crowded, and (A) the right optic nerve has nasal elevation while the (B) left is elevated 360°. There is no obscuration of vessels at the optic disk margin and no true edema of the retinal nerve fiber layer in either eye.

the health of surrounding retinal tissue. At the conclusion of the neuro-ophthalmic examination, the ophthalmologist will be able to establish a complete and focused differential diagnosis that will permit an appropriate diagnostic and management plan to be formulated.

REFERENCES

1. Theodorou M, Clement R, Taylor D, et al. The development of infantile nystagmus. Br J Ophthalmol. BMJ Publishing Group Ltd; 2015;99(5):691-5.
2. Sitko KR, Peragallo JH, Bidot S, et al. Pitfalls in the use of stereoacuity in the diagnosis of nonorganic visual loss. Ophthalmology. 2016;123(1):198-202.
3. Almog Y, Nemet A. The correlation between visual acuity and color vision as an indicator of the cause of visual loss. Am J Ophthalmol. 2010;149(6):1000-4.
4. Martínez-Lapiscina EH, Ortiz-Pérez S, Fraga-Pumar E, et al. Colour vision impairment is associated with disease severity in multiple sclerosis. Mult Scler. SAGE Publications Sage UK: London, England. 2014;20(9):1207-16.
5. Felgueiras H, Parra J, Cruz S, et al. Dyschromatopsia in multiple sclerosis patients: a marker of subclinical involvement? J Neuroophthalmol. 2016;36(3):275-9.
6. Petzold A, Wattjes MP, Costello F,, et al. The investigation of acute optic neuritis: a review and proposed protocol. Nat Rev Neurol. 2014;10(8):447-58.
7. Aroichane M, Pieramici DJ, Miller NR, et al. A comparative study of Hardy-Rand-Rittler and Ishihara colour plates for the diagnosis of nonglaucomatous optic neuropathy. Can J Ophthalmol. 1996;31(7):350-5.
8. Balcer LJ, Frohman EM. Evaluating loss of visual function in multiple sclerosis as measured by low-contrast letter acuity. Neurology. 2010;74(Suppl 3):S16-23.
9. Rucker JC, Sheliga BM, Fitz Gibbon EJ, et al. Contrast sensitivity, first-order motion and Initial ocular following in demyelinating optic neuropathy. J Neurol. 2006;253(9): 1203-9.
10. Garcia-Martin E, Rodriguez-Mena D, Herrero R, et al. Neuro-ophthalmologic evaluation, quality of life, and functional disability in patients with MS. Neurology. 2013;81(1):76-83.
11. Fisher JB, Jacobs DA, Markowitz CE, et al. Relation of visual function to retinal nerve fiber layer thickness in multiple sclerosis. Ophthalmology. 2006;113(2):324-32.
12. Frohman EM, O'Suilleabhain P, Dewey RB, Jr, et al. A new measure of dysconjugacy in INO: the first-pass amplitude. J Neurol Sci. 2003;210(1-2):65-71.
13. Zhao J, Dave SB, Wang J, et al. Clinical color vision testing and correlation with visual function. Am J Ophthalmol. 2015;160(3):547-52.e1.
14. Karnath HO, Rorden C. The anatomy of spatial neglect. Neuropsychologia. 2012;50(6):1010-7.
15. Kerr NM, Chew SS, Eady EK, et al. Diagnostic accuracy of confrontation visual field tests. Neurology. 2010;74(15): 1184-90.
16. Cruz FM, Blitz AM, Subramanian PS. Partial third nerve palsy and ocular neuromyotonia from displacement of posterior communicating artery detected by high-resolution MRI. J Neuroophthalmol. 2013;33(3):263-5.
17. White OB, Saint-Cyr JA, Tomlinson RD, et al. Ocular motor deficits in Parkinson's disease. II. Control of the saccadic and smooth pursuit systems. Brain: a Journal of Neurology. 1983;106(Pt 3):571-87.
18. Pinkhardt EH, Jürgens R, Lulé D, et al. Eye movement impairments in Parkinson's disease: possible role of extradopaminergic mechanisms. BMC Neurol. 2012;12:5.
19. Beh SC, Frohman TC, Frohman EM. Cerebellar control of eye movements. J Neuroophthalmol. 2017;37(1):87-98.
20. Newman SA. Inferior oblique surgery for restrictive strabismus in patients with thyroid orbitopathy. Trans Am Ophthalmol Soc. 2009;107:72-90.

21. Grenga PL, Reale G, Cofone C, et al. Hess area ratio and diplopia: evaluation of 30 patients undergoing surgical repair for orbital blow-out fracture. Ophthal Plast Reconstr Surg. 2009;25(2):123-5.
22. Hatt SR, Leske DA, Liebermann L, et al. Variability of angle of deviation measurements in children with intermittent exotropia. J AAPOS. 2012;16(2):120-4.
23. Belmonte C, Acosta MC, Gallar J. Neural basis of sensation in intact and injured corneas. Exp Eye Res. 2004;78(3):513-25.
24. Kokotis P, Theodossiadis P, Bouros C, et al. Bilateral ocular myositis as a late complication of dermatomyositis. J Rheumatol. 2005;32(2):379-81.
25. Kusner LL, Puwanant A, Kaminski HJ. Ocular myasthenia: diagnosis, treatment, and pathogenesis. Neurologist. 2006;12(5):231-9.
26. Ziahosseini K, Nduka C, Malhotra R. Ophthalmic grading of facial paralysis: need for a closer look. Br J Ophthalmol. 2015;99(9):1171-5.
27. Defazio G, Hallett M, Jinnah HA, et al. Development and validation of a clinical guideline for diagnosing blepharospasm. Neurology. 2013;81(3):236-40.
28. Jariyakosol S, Hirunwiwatkul P, Lerdlum S, et al. Prevalence and associated factors of neurovascular contact in patients with hemifacial spasm. Asia Pac J Ophthalmol (Phila). 2015;4(4):212-5.
29. Donnelly SJ, Subramanian PS. Relationship of intraocular pulse pressure and spontaneous venous pulsations. Am J Ophthalmol. 2009;147(1):51-2.
30. Lascaratos G, Ahmed S, Madill SA. Pearls & Oysters: spontaneous venous pulsation and its role in differentiating papilledema from pseudopapilledema. Neurology. 2010;75(13):e53-4.
31. Fard MA, Fakhree S, Abdi P, et al. Quantification of peripapillary total retinal volume in pseudopapilledema and mild papilledema using spectral-domain optical coherence tomography. Am J Ophthalmol. 2014;158(1):136-43.

Chapter 91 The Swollen Optic Nerve

Michael Jordan, Collin M McClelland, Michael S Lee

INTRODUCTION

Optic nerve swelling represents a nonspecific finding that may indicate a response to a primary injury to the optic nerve, intraocular inflammation, diabetes, and increased intracranial pressure among other processes. Papilledema represents a subset of optic nerve edema secondary to elevated intracranial pressure (ICP). In some cases, increased ICP can cause optic disk edema along with an optic neuropathy, making the distinction of optic neuropathy from papilledema difficult. This chapter will focus on distinguishing papilledema and pseudopapilledema and the diagnostic algorithm when encountering this finding. Other causes of optic nerve swelling and optic neuropathies not associated with increased intracranial pressure are discussed elsewhere.

DISTINGUISHING TRUE PAPILLEDEMA FROM PSEUDOPAPILLEDEMA

In determining possible papilledema, the clinician utilizes a multifaceted approach including the history, clinical examination, and ancillary testing to differentiate papilledema from pseudopapilledema (Flowchart 91.1).

Flowchart 91.1: Papilledema evaluation.

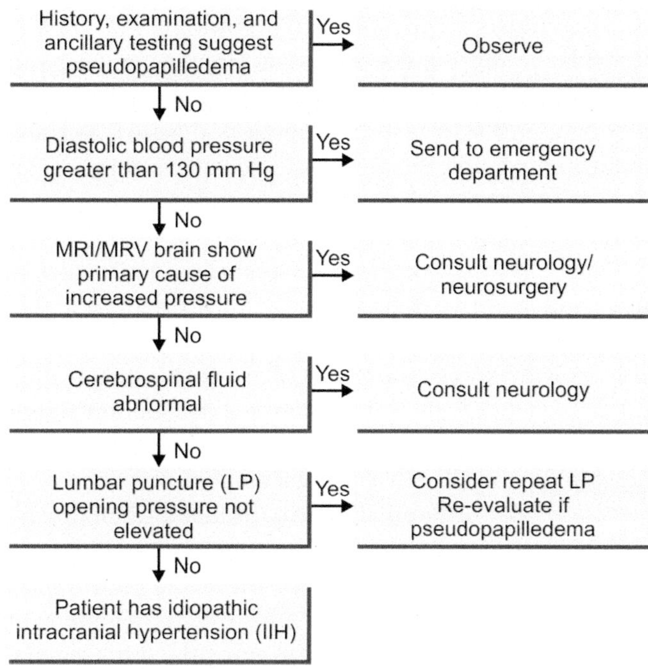

History

The most common cause of pseudopapilledema is optic disk drusen (ODD), but some patients merely have small, crowded optic disks which are often mistaken for papilledema. One of the most useful components of the history is the presence of a positive family history for ODD, which may be transmitted in an autosomal dominant fashion. Both pseudopapilledema and papilledema may present with transient visual obscurations (TVO), brief interruptions of vision lasting a few seconds that may occur when standing up from a seated position or with Valsalva maneuver. The absence of symptoms may be more suggestive of pseudopapilledema, but papilledema also may be asymptomatic. Other symptoms that may indicate the presence of increased intracranial pressure and true papilledema include headaches, diplopia, nausea, emesis, and pulse synchronous tinnitus.

While gathering the clinical history, specific questioning regarding medications known to be associated with papilledema should be undertaken. Specifically, the use of danazol, cyclosporine, growth hormone, levothyroxine, sulfonamides, tetracycline antibiotics, vitamin A or its derivatives, and corticosteroids should be assessed. Patients may fail to report these medications especially when they are being used topically and not orally.

The clinician should also perform a thorough review of the medical history including active and inactive medical conditions, surgical history, and other medications. Examples of associated conditions include cancer, sarcoidosis, syphilis, human immunodeficiency virus (HIV), tuberculosis and Lyme disease. Malignancy may metastasize to the brain and lead to a space occupying lesion or leptomeningeal infiltration causing optic disk edema and optic neuropathy. Infectious disorders can result in meningitis and subsequent papilledema and/or optic neuropathy.

A broad review of systems is crucial in narrowing the differential diagnosis.

Patients with exposure to individuals from endemic areas or those infected with tuberculosis should be asked about fever, night sweats, cough, and weight loss. These findings, while nonspecific, increase the pre-test probability of tuberculosis as the causative etiology. Patients, in particular young females of African-American or Hispanic ethnicity, should be questioned regarding the presence of cough, and skin rash (erythema nodosum), as these findings could indicate sarcoidosis. Recent weight gain may be consistent with idiopathic intracranial hypertension (IIH).

A patient with fever, malaise, nuchal rigidity, petechial rash, and positive Kernig's and/or Brudzinski's sign should be evaluated for meningitis. If a patient presents with clinical findings suggestive of meningitis then further history should be obtained regarding vaccination status, exposure to other people with meningitis or non-vaccinated individuals, and all active medical conditions.

A personal or familial history of bleeding diatheses or clotting disorders is important to ascertain. One may inquire about deep venous thrombosis, pulmonary embolism, or late miscarriage. A history of pregnancy or recent pregnancy, head trauma, sinusitis, otitis media, mastoiditis, use of oral contraceptives, or fertility inducing medications could predispose to dural venous sinus thrombosis as the cause of the increased ICP. Anemia has also been reported as a cause of papilledema.

Lyme meningitis may cause increased ICP. Clinicians should consider this diagnosis in patients from Lyme endemic areas such as the northeastern, mid-Atlantic, and Great Lakes regions of the United States,[1] as well as parts of Europe. The presence or history of erythema migrans, a bull's eye shaped rash, suggests Lyme disease as the responsible agent for new development of papilledema. Papilledema from Lyme is typically a late finding, and other historical features of early Lyme such as fatigue, myalgias, arthralgias, headache, fever and chills, and lymphadenopathy are typically absent. Other infections to consider include cysticercosis, toxoplasmosis, and *Cryptococcus*, which can all cause increased intracranial pressure.

Aside from erythema migrans, the development of new skin findings should be investigated. Erythema nodosum are painful, red nodules most commonly present on the legs, and they can be suggestive of sarcoidosis or Graves disease. Petechial rash in a patient with findings suggesting meningitis supports the diagnosis of bacterial meningitis. The presence of a painless genital ulcer, or history thereof, indicates that the patient may have syphilis or Behcet disease. The presence of a maculopapular rash is not entirely specific to syphilis but warrants further testing for the disease as the causative etiology of the optic disk swelling.

Examination

The examination begins the moment the clinician first lays eyes on the patient. Obesity in a young woman may increase suspicion for IIH, but this patient population may have pseudopapilledema as well. In contrast, a thin, male, very young, or very old patient may make the ophthalmologist consider pseudopapilledema more strongly. Evidence of an optic neuropathy (reduced acuity, dyschromatopsia, visual field defect, and afferent pupillary defect) may argue that the patient does not have papilledema at all, but a primary optic neuropathy. Fulminant IIH can present with potentially severe visual loss acutely and must be distinguished from a primary optic neuropathy. An abduction deficit can indicate a sixth cranial nerve palsy which suggests increased ICP in patients with possible papilledema. Other cranial neuropathies can also occur but are very uncommon. A bilateral facial nerve palsy may suggest Lyme disease or sarcoidosis.

Pseudopapilledema may manifest itself through a number of examination findings. These include: anomalous vascular branching such as arterial or venous trifurcation, cupless optic disks, elevated optic disks, surface refractile or partially visible ODD, and the absence of obscured optic disk margin and retinal nerve fibers (Figs. 91.1A to D).[2] Additionally, presence of spontaneous venous pulsations (SVPs) and absence of hyperemia are suggestive of pseudopapilledema. We have found that using the video mode on an optical coherence tomography (OCT) machine can help visualize SVPs. Clinicians should keep in mind that anatomic factors may cause normal individuals not to manifest SVPs, and that the absence of SVPs is not specific to papilledema.[3] The presence of a physiologic cup and/or retinal or choroidal folds is much more likely to indicate true papilledema rather than pseudopapilledema.[4]

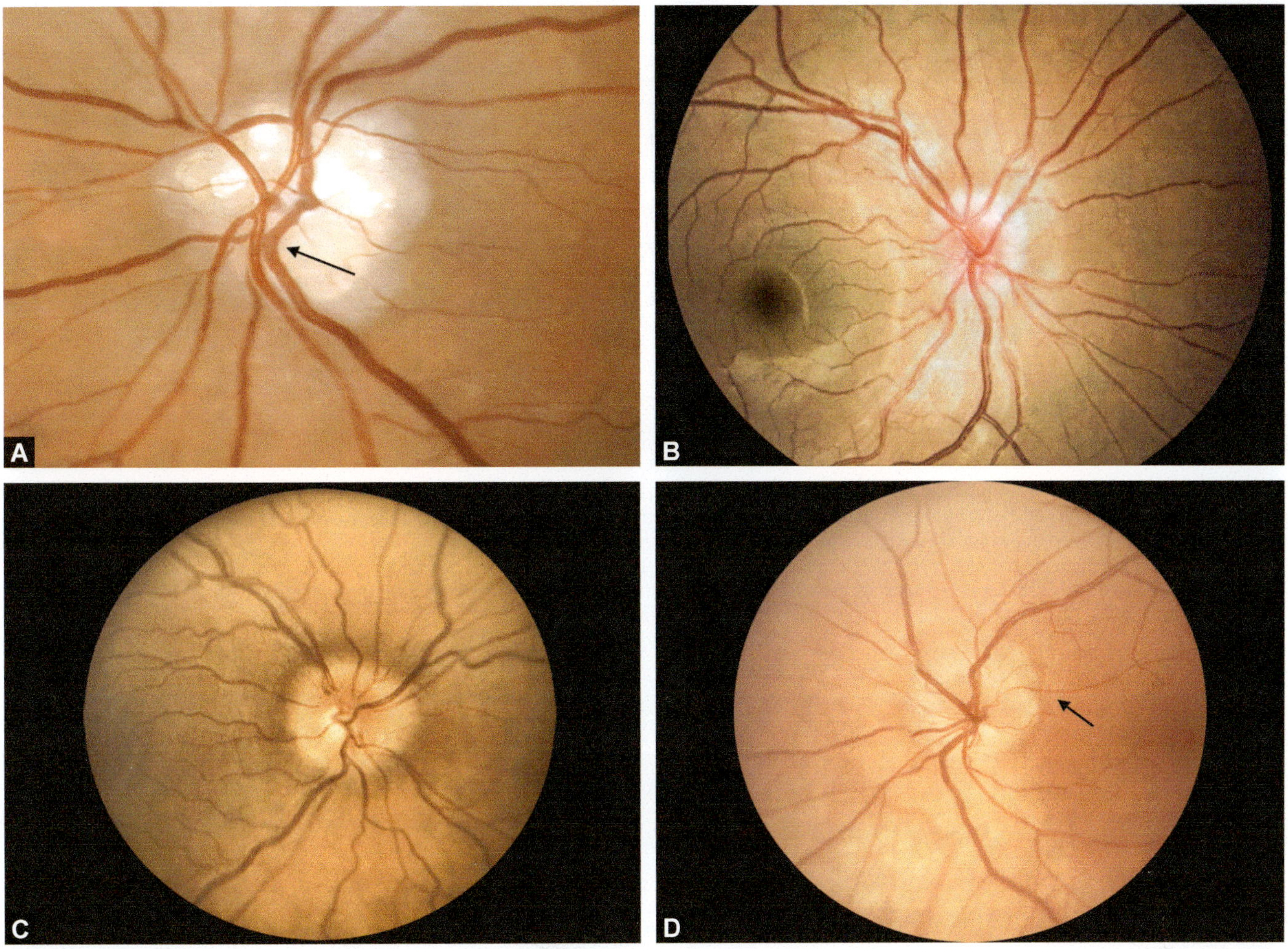

Figs. 91.1A to D: (A) Anomalous trifurcation of the veins (arrow) in a nerve with surface drusen. These are nonspecific but suggestive of pseudopapilledema; (B) Cupless optic disk consistent with pseudopapilledema; (C) Elevated optic disk. Note the presence of a cup strongly suggests true papilledema; (D) Cupless optic disk with peripapillary retinal folds (arrow), which support true papilledema.

Despite clues that may be present on history and clinical examination, it may not be possible even for the most seasoned clinicians to distinguish the two conditions, thus necessitating additional clinical testing.

ANCILLARY CLINICAL TESTING

B-scan may demonstrate acoustic shadowing at the junction of the optic nerve and globe consistent with ODD (Fig. 91.2A). The 30-degree test can differentiate intrinsic disk/sheath complex and pseudopapilledema from true optic disk edema. A B-scan with the eye in primary gaze may show an enlarged retrobulbar optic nerve/sheath from extracerebrospinal fluid (CSF), normal diameter, or intrinsic complex enlargement as in an optic nerve sheath tumor. When the patient looks laterally approximately 30°, eyes with papilledema will show compression of the CSF space with a resultant smaller nerve diameter. This is considered a positive 30-degree test.

Fundus autofluorescence (FAF) may be used to detect buried ODD not visible on clinical examination (Fig. 91.2B). FAF has been shown to have 88.5% sensitivity for detection of both buried and visible optic disk drusen.[5] FAF can be performed by either (1) placing the fluorescein filter on the camera and taking a picture of the optic disk without injecting fluorescein or (2) using the FAF feature on many digital cameras or OCT machines. Fluorescein angiography may also help evaluate for papilledema versus pseudopapilledema. Late leakage from the optic disk occurs in patients with papilledema as compared to patients with pseudopapilledema, in whom this leakage does not occur.

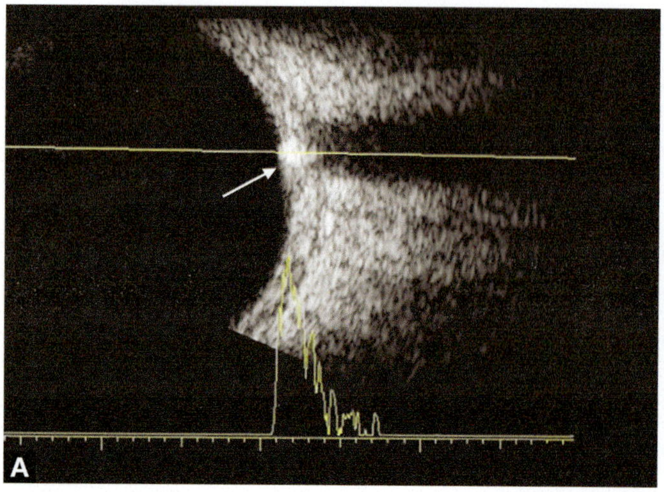

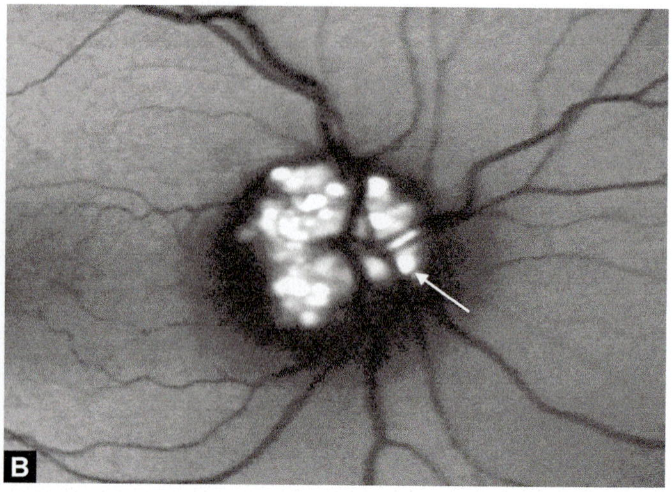

Figs. 91.2A and B: (A) B-scan ultrasound demonstrating acoustic shadowing at the junction of the optic nerve and retina showing optic disk drusen (ODD) (arrow). The corresponding A-scan shows a spike in reflectivity consistent with ODD; (B) Fundus autofluorescence image of the optic nerve demonstrating hyperautofluorescent buried optic disk drusen (ODD) (arrow).

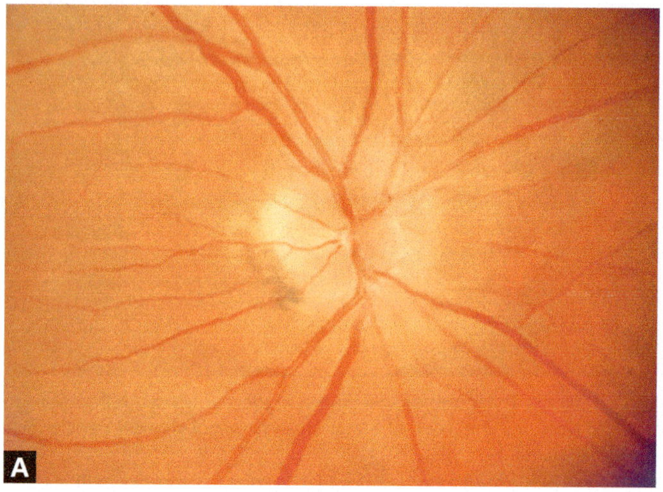

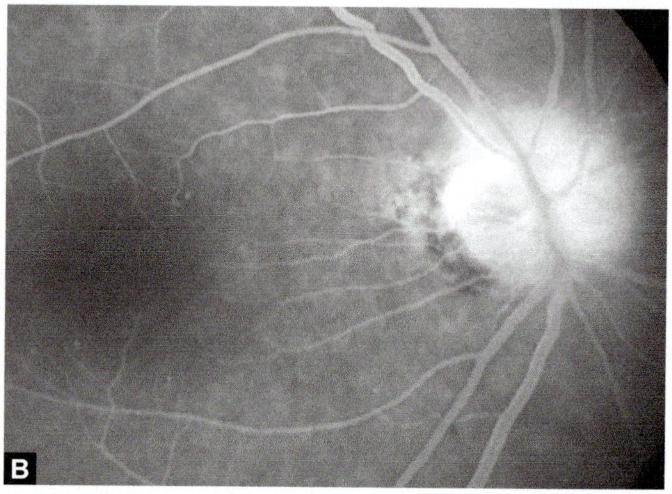

Figs. 91.3A and B: (A) Fundus photograph of an optic disk with blurred optic disk margins. It was uncertain if this represented pseudopapilledema or optic disk edema; (B) The nerve seen in the previous figure leaks late with fluorescein consistent with true optic disk edema.

Keep in mind that staining of the peripapillary region is common in normal individuals (Figs. 91.3A and B).

Enhanced depth imaging (EDI) OCT is another imaging modality that may be used to evaluate for the presence of ODD. As compared to spectral domain (SD) OCT, EDI-OCT provides deeper penetration of the retinal layers and optic disk. As such, EDI-OCT is an improvement over SD-OCT in imaging for ODD. ODD on EDI-OCT appear as hyporeflective tumefactions anterior to the lamina cribrosa with hyperreflective borders (Fig. 91.4).[5] Some authors have suggested that one can differentiate optic nerve drusen and papilledema when the nasal quadrant of the RNFL is thicker than 85 microns or the optic nerve shows a certain configuration of the subretinal hyporeflective space.

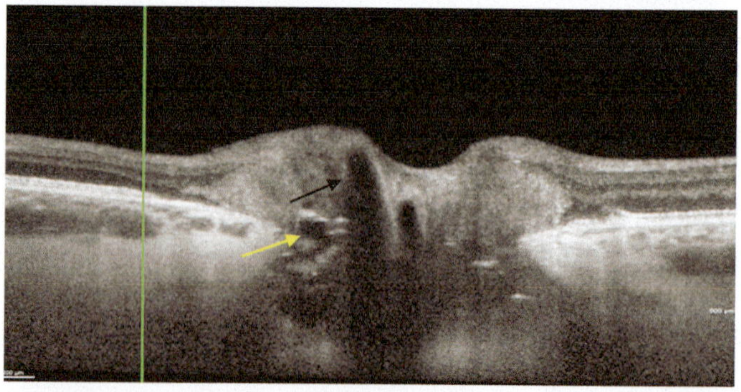

Fig. 91.4: Enhanced depth imaging (EDI) optical coherence tomography (OCT) demonstrating hyporeflective optic disk drusen (ODD) with a hyperreflective border present within the optic disk (yellow arrow). The black arrow points to a blood vessel. Note that the vessel does not have a hyperreflective border.

This has not been our experience, and we do not advocate this approach.

A line scan through the optic nerve head may show inward bowing of the retinal pigment epithelium (RPE) and basement membrane (BM) complex in patients with papilledema but not in patients with pseudopapilledema. This is thought to result from CSF pressure transmitted through the optic nerve that forces the complex to move anteriorly. As the ICP returns to normal, this inward bowing reverses, and the RPE-BM complex appears straighter. Orbital computed tomography (CT) may demonstrate optic nerve head calcifications in ODD, but in patients with true papilledema such a finding is absent (Fig. 91.5). However, CT may not show noncalcified ODD or small ODD. The sensitivity of orbital CT for detecting optic disk drusen may be as low as 43%.[6] However, these studies are older and were not performed with newer, higher-resolution technology. It is possible that the sensitivity of CT today would be higher than previously thought. Typically, a normal CT does not rule out ODD, and CT is not routinely used to diagnose ODD both because of the radiation exposure and extra time and expense needed to obtain this testing.

Visual fields do not distinguish papilledema from pseudopapilledema. Up to 71% of patients with visible ODD demonstrate visual field defects at the time of presentation. Amongst patients with buried ODD, 25–30% may have visual field defects initially.[7] Visual fields in patients with ODD typically remain stable throughout life; however, some may demonstrate mild-to-moderate visual field deficits that show subtle progression. One study found the rate of visual field progression to be 1.6% per year.[8] The most common visual field defects attributable to ODD include enlargement of the blind spot and nerve fiber bundle defects. The deficits in ODD often remain asymptomatic unless they occur in conjunction with other pathologic processes. Visual field defects are also common among patients with increased ICP regardless of etiology and often appear as nerve fiber bundle defects as well. The progression of visual fields may also occur in both conditions and limit the ability to distinguish between true papilledema and pseudopapilledema secondary to ODD.

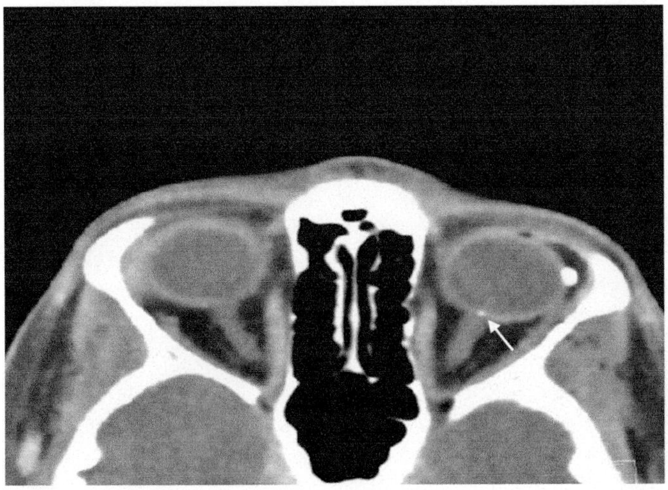

Fig. 91.5: Orbital coherence tomography (CT) demonstrating calcified optic disk drusen (ODD) at the junction of the optic nerve and globe (arrow) in the left eye.

Optical coherence tomography of the retinal nerve fiber layer (RNFL) is commonly performed in patients with an abnormal appearing optic disk. Both papilledema and pseudopapilledema may demonstrate thickening of the RNFL. A repeat mean RNFL measurement should not change by more than 6–7 microns with pseudopapilledema, but may demonstrate significant change, either thinning or thickening, in true optic disk edema after 4–6 weeks. With time, chronic papilledema may result in thinning of the nerve fiber layer as measurable by OCT. Nerve fiber layer thinning is not specific to papilledema. There may also be evidence of nerve fiber layer thinning amongst patients with ODD. A mixed pattern may also be seen with segmental thickening and thinning in the presence of ODD.

THE CLINICAL APPROACH AFTER THE DIAGNOSIS OF TRUE PAPILLEDEMA

Blood Pressure

In the office, the patient should have his/her blood pressure measured. Malignant hypertension can present with bilateral optic disk edema. Typically, the fundus shows other retinal and choroidal findings including lipid, cotton wool spots, hemorrhages, choroidal infarctions, and serous retinal detachments. The diastolic blood pressure generally measures over 130 mm Hg in cases of hypertension causing optic nerve swelling. This represents an urgency or an emergency and the clinician should send this patient to the emergency department.

Neuroimaging

The next critical step involves neuroimaging. Brain magnetic resonance imaging (MRI) and magnetic resonance venography (MRV) with and without contrast should be performed. Nonspecific findings of elevated ICP on MRI include a partially empty sella turcica, posterior globe flattening, transverse sinus stenosis, and distention of the perioptic CSF space. The presence of three or four of these findings strongly suggests increased ICP (Figs. 91.6A to D). One study concluded that transverse sinus stenosis was the most sensitive neuroimaging finding of IIH, although diagnosis typically requires a brain MRV.[9]

An intracranial neoplasm, if present as the cause of papilledema, may cause additional symptoms based on its anatomic location. A lesion in the frontal lobe compressing the optic nerve may result in Foster–Kennedy syndrome. A meningioma in the superior sulcus compressing the primary motor cortex may result in leg weakness. Metastasis of a systemic malignancy is commonly present at the gray-white matter junction and causes various cranial neuropathies or focal neurologic symptoms. Lesions compressing the foramen of Monro, the cerebral aqueduct, the foramen of Magendie or foramina of Luschka all may result in obstructive hydrocephalus (Figs. 91.7A and B). An ependymoma producing excessive CSF may cause nonobstructive hydrocephalus.

Brain MRV should be obtained at the same time as MRI to evaluate for dural venous sinus thrombosis (DVST), since this condition may present with signs and symptoms of increased ICP alone. MRV can be performed without contrast, but image quality improves with contrast. One study found that 9.4% of patients with presumed IIH had DVST.[10] In 90% of those cases, the DVST was not seen on MRI alone. The dural sinuses most commonly affected are the superior sagittal, transverse, and sigmoid sinuses, followed by the cavernous and straight sinuses.[11] MRV may demonstrate total or partial obstruction of laminar flow within one or more of the dural venous sinuses (Fig. 91.8).

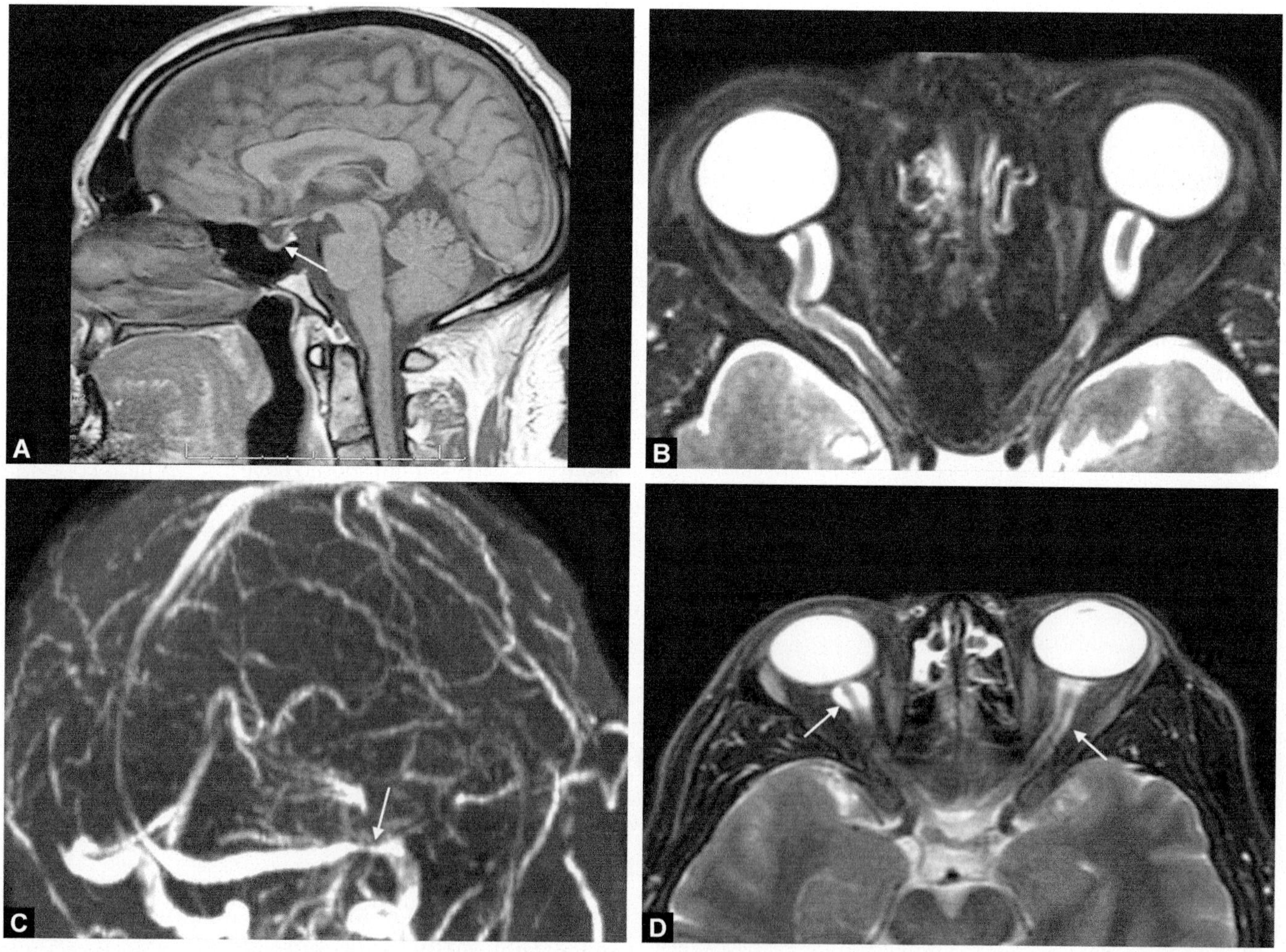

Figs. 91.6A to D: (A) Sagittal T1 MRI demonstrating a partially empty sella turcica (arrow); (B) Axial T2 MRI demonstrating posterior globe flattening; (C) Magnetic resonance venography (MRV) demonstrating transverse sinus stenosis (arrow); (D) Axial T2 MRI demonstrating distention of the peri-optic cerebrospinal fluid (CSF) spaces (arrows).

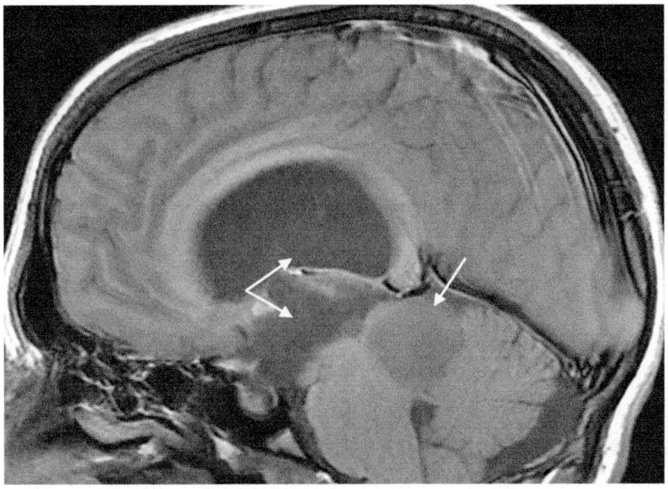

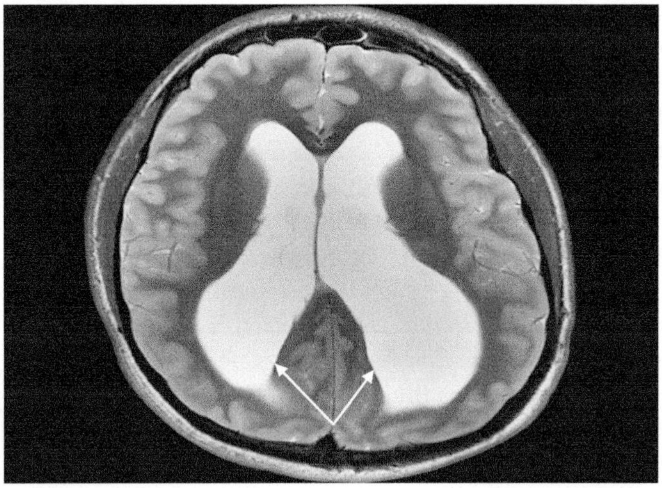

Figs. 91.7A and B: (A) Sagittal T1 MRI demonstrating a large tectal glioma (arrow) causing obstructive hydrocephalus as evidenced by enlargement of the lateral and third ventricles (arrows); (B) Axial T2 MRI demonstrating significant hydrocephalus and enlargement of the lateral ventricles (arrows) secondary to tectal glioma and aqueductal stenosis.

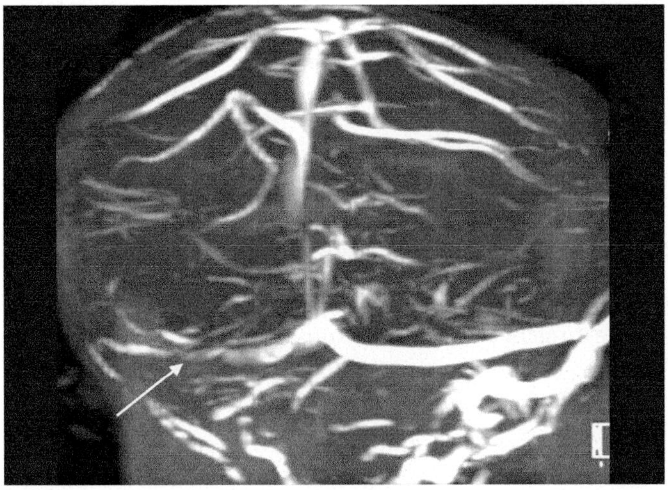

Fig. 91.8: MRV demonstrating partial obstruction of the right transverse sinus (arrow).

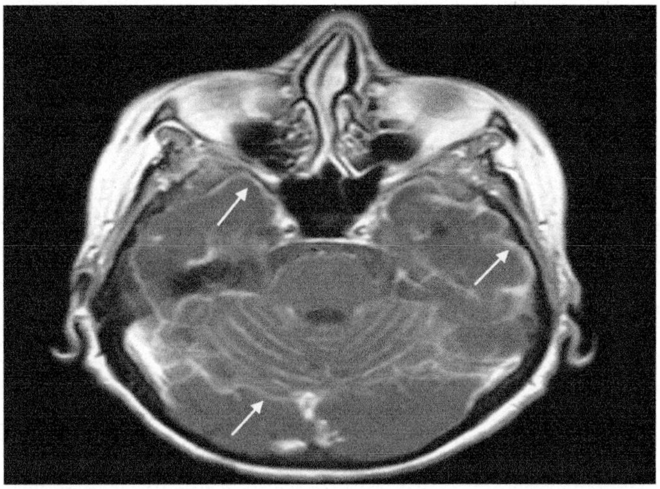

Fig. 91.9: Axial T2 MRI with gadolinium contrast demonstrating diffuse leptomeningeal enhancement consistent with leptomeningeal carcinomatosis (arrows).

The appearance of the venous sinus on MRV depends upon the timing of the thrombosis and the timing of the MRV, as the thrombosis undergoes changes in its composition with time.[12] We have also seen patients with meningioma compressing the posterior portion of the superior sagittal sinus leading to venous hypertension and intracranial hypertension. Such findings support the idea that cerebral venous sinus narrowing can result in elevated ICP.

In patients with a known history of malignancy, either active or in remission, one must consider leptomeningeal carcinomatosis as the cause of acute papilledema. Image findings suggestive of leptomeningeal carcinomatosis include enhancement of the leptomeninges, subependyma, cranial and spinal nerves, and communicating hydrocephalus (Fig. 91.9).[13] Solid tumors are more likely to result in abnormal neuroimaging (72–80%) as compared to hematologic malignancies (48–62%).[14] Abnormalities may only be seen after gadolinium is given, emphasizing the importance of contrast for all brain MRI studies in this circumstance.

Leptomeningeal enhancement also may be seen in patients with neurosarcoidosis. In a small subset of patients diagnosed with central nervous system (CNS) Lyme disease by clinical criteria, serology, and response to treatment, the presence of T2 prolongation, meningeal enhancement, and nerve root enhancement have been documented.[15]

Neuroimaging may be critical in confirming a diagnosis of meningitis when the clinical findings are not classic. Herpes simplex virus meningoencephalitis may produce focal enhancement of the temporal lobes on MRI, which may not be visible on CT. Tuberculous meningitis may manifest subclinically with nonspecific findings, but on MRI with gadolinium contrast may demonstrate diffuse basal enhancement.

It is unknown whether MR imaging affects a fetus. In our experience, gadolinium is not given to a pregnant patient at any stage. Some MRI units will not perform noncontrast scans for patients in their first trimester of pregnancy and others will do limited sequences. Because of radiation exposure, CT is not typically performed among pregnant individuals. We have ordered noncontrast brain MRI and MRV for patients in their second and third trimester without difficulty. One should inform the mother of the risks and benefits before ordering MR in a pregnant woman with papilledema.

Lumbar Puncture with Opening Pressure

Patients with normal neuroimaging should undergo lumbar puncture. Opening pressure (OP), CSF, protein, glucose, cytology and other laboratory tests should be ordered. Classically, the OP should be measured in the lateral decubitus position. Typically, a patient will curl into the fetal position to open the spinous processes. The pressure should be measured immediately after needle insertion with the patient in a fully extended position (legs and neck straight, with the head supported by a pillow) before any CSF is removed. The patient should be relaxed and not tensed, because this can artificially elevate the measured OP. Additionally, the pressure should be measured once the CSF has had an opportunity to equilibrate, which can take a few minutes. Some clinicians measure OP after the meniscus stops rising in the manometer.

Contrasting data have been published regarding positioning of the patient and OP. One study has shown no difference between OP in the lateral decubitus and prone position.[16] Zero pressure on the manometer should be at the level of the spinal canal. If the radiologist is placing the manometer on the needle, then the length of the needle needs to be added to the measurement on the manometer. Some radiologists use flexible tubing and zero should be brought down to the level of the spinal canal. In an adult patient, elevated OP is defined as exceeding 25 cm H_2O according to the modified Dandy criteria. In pediatric patients, an elevated OP is reportedly greater than 28 cm H_2O.[17] The difference between adult and pediatric opening pressure upper limits of normal likely relates to sedation. The decreased respiratory rate from sedation in children results in hypercapnia, and via autoregulation of cerebral blood flow, increased ICP results.

It is not only important to evaluate the opening pressure, but also the CSF analysis. As compared to bacterial meningitis, viral meningitis may have a normal or slightly elevated protein, normal glucose, and increased leukocytes with lymphocyte predominance. The OP may be elevated as well. In bacterial meningitis, the CSF protein may be significantly elevated, often above 200 mg/dL, while the CSF glucose is often markedly low, and the leukocyte differential typically shows a left shift with abundant neutrophils. Fungal meningitis may have mixed CSF findings that contain elements of both viral and bacterial meningitis. In this case, CSF protein and glucose are similar to that of bacterial meningitis; however, the cytology may show lymphocytic pleocytosis. In cases where suspicion for infection is low, as in obese young women without other concerning neurological features, we will often order a cell count, protein and glucose only and forego further analysis. Individuals with atypical features or symptoms should possibly undergo CSF cultures and Gram stain, cytology, and testing for various infectious causes. In endemic areas, cryptococcal antigen and acid-fast bacillus staining should be considered.

The presence of malignant cells within the CSF can be determined by cytology and flow cytometry. However, the sensitivity of high volume LPs is only 50%, and MRI enhancement of the leptomeninges is a more sensitive finding. In some cases, three serial LPs may need to be performed if suspicion is high. Cytology of the CSF will reveal the presence of cells allow their further characterization. Flow cytometry may be utilized to detect cell surface molecules that are known to be present in certain types of malignancy. Leptomeningeal carcinomatosis may be the first manifestation of a new primary malignancy that might be found upon subsequent systemic evaluation. Thus, a workup to identify the primary malignancy should be undertaken and then treated appropriately.

In patients where neurosyphilis is suspected, ordering venereal disease research laboratory (VDRL) testing of the CSF is warranted. Serum testing should also be obtained. Rapid plasmin reagent (RPR) and fluorescent treponemal antibody absorption (FTA-ABS) assays are warranted in addition. A positive RPR is indicative of active infection, while an isolated positive FTA-ABS may be present during active CNS infection or as a marker of previous infection. A negative RPR suggests either inactive treated syphilis or the absence of syphilis as the causative etiology.

Neurosarcoidosis (NS) may manifest with elevated OP, increased CSF protein, and decreased glucose. These findings have been found to correspond with NS with leptomeningeal enhancement as compared to diagnosed cases of NS without leptomeningeal enhancement.[18] A CSF CD4:CD8 greater than 5.0 may also be present in NS; however, this is nonspecific. Likewise, elevated CSF angiotensin-converting enzyme (ACE) is nonspecific and insensitive for NS. Patients diagnosed with NS have been found to have an elevated CSF ACE in 5–50% of patients. Additionally, falsely elevated CSF ACE levels may occur in patients with silicosis, diabetes, or cirrhosis.[19] Other moderately sensitive but nonspecific serum markers of sarcoid include chitotriosidase and serum IL-2 receptor.[20,21] Marangoni et al. have introduced the Marangoni-modified criteria to aid in the diagnosis of NS. Their criteria are as follows:

Certain NS:	Positive nervous system histology
Probable NS:	Signs of inflammation in the CNS, positive Histology for a systemic lesion, and/or positive test results for at least two of the following tests: Gallium scan, chest High resolution CT, bronchoalveolar lavage with a CD4:CD8 ratio >3.5 and a CD4: CD8 ratio >5 in the CSF
Possible NS:	Absence of histological confirmation and ruling out other inflammatory.[22]

In patients with history suggestive of Lyme disease, testing should include CSF Lyme IgM and IgG and serum Lyme serology. A CSF to serum antibody ratio greater than 1.0 indicates intrathecal antibody production. The misdiagnosis of neurosyphilis as neuroborreliosis may occur, as *Treponema pallidum* may cause falsely positive serum Lyme serology.[23]

DIAGNOSTIC CRITERIA FOR IDIOPATHIC INTRACRANIAL HYPERTENSION

The clinician should consider IIH among patients with papilledema without clinical examination findings suggestive of another disease process (including blood pressure), normal neuroimaging findings, and a LP with an elevated OP, but no other abnormalities. The updated diagnostic criteria as updated by Friedman and colleagues include the following:

- Papilledema (in almost all cases)
- A normal neurological examination aside from 6th cranial nerve palsy
- Normal CSF composition associated with an elevated opening pressure (>250 mm H_2O in adults and >280 mm H_2O in children)
- Neuroimaging (MRI typically, or CT if MRI is contraindicated) showing normal brain parenchyma and no evidence of mass or structural lesion, hydrocephalus, or meningeal enhancement
- In the absence of papilledema, a definitive diagnosis requires a 6th nerve palsy
- In the absence of papilledema and a 6th nerve palsy, a suggestive diagnosis requires 3 of 4 neuroimaging findings as described above
- A diagnosis is deemed "probable" if all other criteria are met but no lumbar puncture is performed to determine opening pressure.[24] (This should be determined cautiously, because the patient may have pseudopapilledema.)

MANAGEMENT OF IDIOPATHIC INTRACRANIAL HYPERTENSION

Patients with IIH are at risk of permanent and progressive visual loss. These patients deserve monitoring of their optic disk edema and automated visual fields. The optic nerve can be followed semi-quantitatively using the Frisen grading scale:

- *Grade 1:* Obscuration of the nasal border of the disk with temporal sparing without elevation of the disk
- *Grade 2:* Obscuration of all borders 360° around the disk with nasal elevation.
- *Grade 3:* Obscuration of all borders with obscuration of one or major segments of major blood vessels
- *Grade 4:* Elevation of the entire nerve head with obscuration of all borders and total obscuration of a segment of a major blood vessel
- *Grade 5:* Obliteration of the optic cup. Total obscuration of a segment of a major blood vessel may or may not be present (Figs. 91.10A to E).

Quantitative measurement of the optic nerves includes OCT RNFL and volume scans. These can be followed over time for change. In some cases, these parameters improve because the patient develops progressive optic atrophy and loss of retinal ganglion cells, and thus caution must be exercised in the interpretation of "improvement" on OCT. Macular segmentation on OCT can isolate the ganglion cell layer or the ganglion cell—inner plexiform complex and identify true loss before it is apparent on the OCT RNFL. It can also help determine if a new worsening of vision in

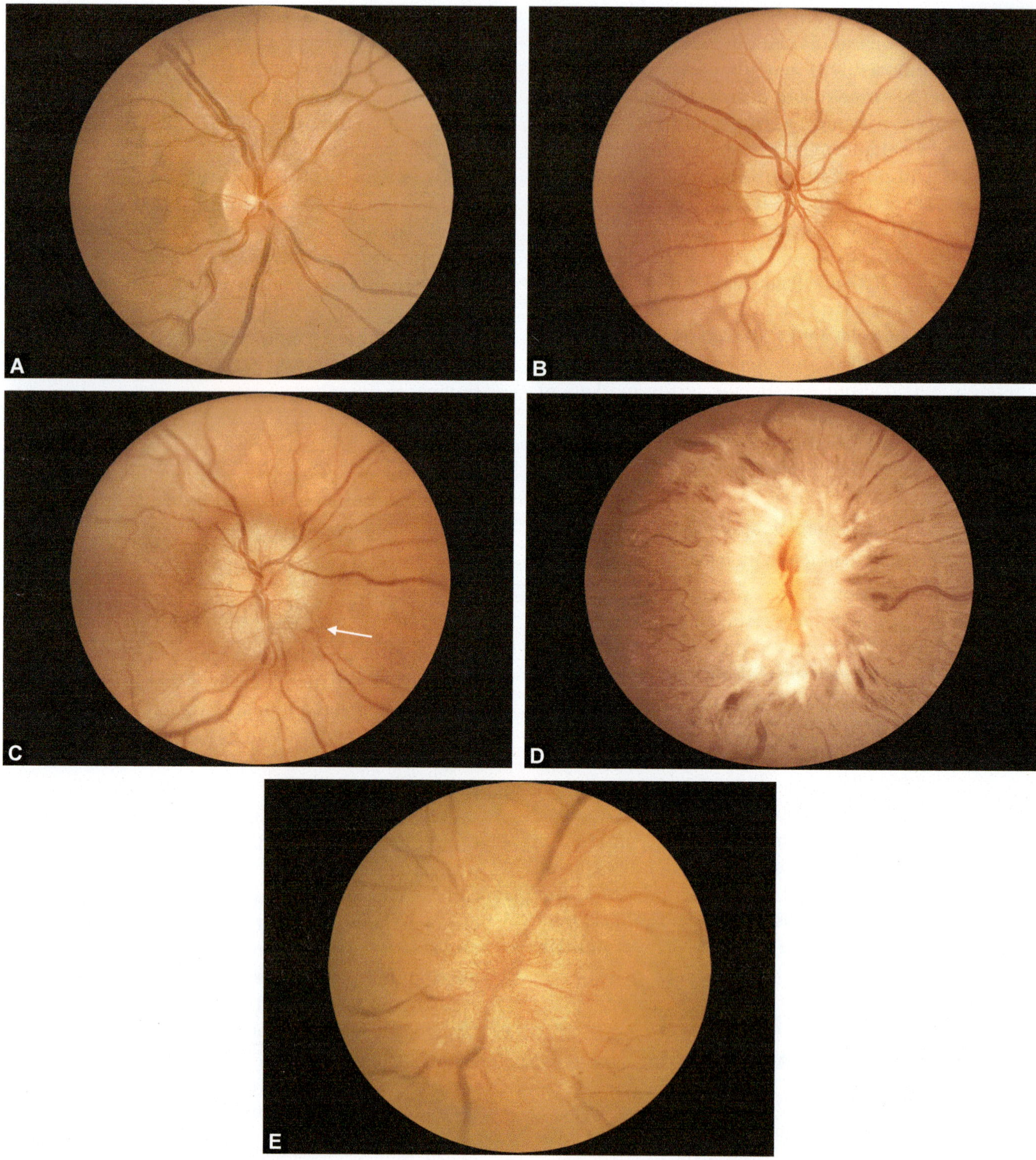

Figs. 91.10A to E: Fundus photographs demonstrating: (A) Grade 1 papilledema; (B) Grade 2 papilledema; (C) Grade 3 papilledema; (D) Grade 4 papilledema; (E) Grade 5 papilledema.

an eye is due to functional overlay as compared to true progression. Careful assessment of the pupils should also be performed in this scenario. A patient with very poor vision and briskly reactive pupils may have a nonphysiologic component of the vision loss, and this diagnosis can be particularly challenging to make.

Initial treatment of IIH involves correcting an underlying medical condition, such as anemia, or discontinuing a medication known to be associated with IIH. In the absence of such a condition, then weight loss is recommended along with oral diuretics. To monitor disease progress, serial visual fields and measurements of visual acuity should be followed.

Weight loss of 6–7% of total body weight may result in significant improvement in papilledema.[25] The initial therapeutic agent of choice for patients without hepatic or renal failure is acetazolamide. Acetazolamide inhibits carbonic anhydrase and thus reduces CSF production with resulting decrease in ICP. In patients with history of sulfonamide antibiotic allergy, patients may still be prescribed non-sulfonamide drugs including acetazolamide as evidenced by a study comparing the cross reactivity between sulfonamide antibiotics and sulfonamide nonantibiotics.[26] Initial dosing may vary, but up to 4,000 mg daily may be prescribed.[27] If the patient does not respond to treatment with acetazolamide or does not tolerate the side effects then an alternative agent may be used. Either topiramate or furosemide may be used as second line agents, either as monotherapy or in addition to acetazolamide. Nonetheless, evidence supporting their efficacy in directly lowering ICP is poor. In pregnant patients, topiramate is contraindicated. If pharmacologic treatment is needed during pregnancy, then acetazolamide or furosemide should be used. Active weight loss during pregnancy is not recommended, but obese patients may carry a pregnancy to term and deliver a healthy infant under appropriate obstetric management with minimal weight gain. Progressive loss of vision on one pharmacologic agent may necessitate the addition of a second agent or surgical intervention.

In patients with moderate, severe, or fulminant IIH and significantly worsening visual fields, surgical intervention to prevent irreversible vision loss is warranted (Flowchart 91.2). Patients with fulminant and sudden visual loss should receive rescue therapy of either intravenous Solu Medrol 250 mg four times daily or lumbar drain until further surgical therapy can take place. If vision loss is the primary concern for patients with medication resistant IIH or a fulminant course, then optic nerve sheath fenestration may be undertaken. If persistent and intolerable headaches are prominent, then a ventriculoperitoneal shunt should be considered after failing conservative and medical treatment, although long-term headache control may not occur with shunting, especially when headache symptoms have been present for more than 1 year.[28] Lastly, placement of a venous sinus stent represents another procedure available for relieving increased ICP. As discussed above, venous sinus stenosis may cause elevated ICP. Patients with stents can enjoy improvement in headache and resolution of papilledema, but may suffer from intracranial hemorrhage at the time of surgery or recurrent stenosis weeks to months later. Fewer long-term data exist for the safety and efficacy of venous sinus stenting in IIH.

SUMMARY

Distinguishing pseudopapilledema from papilledema can challenge even the most experienced clinicians. Clues to pseudopapilledema include lack of symptoms, spontaneous venous pulsation (SVP), cupless optic nerves, and evidence of ODD on ancillary testing. When

Flowchart 91.2: Idiopathic intracranial hypertension (IIH) management.

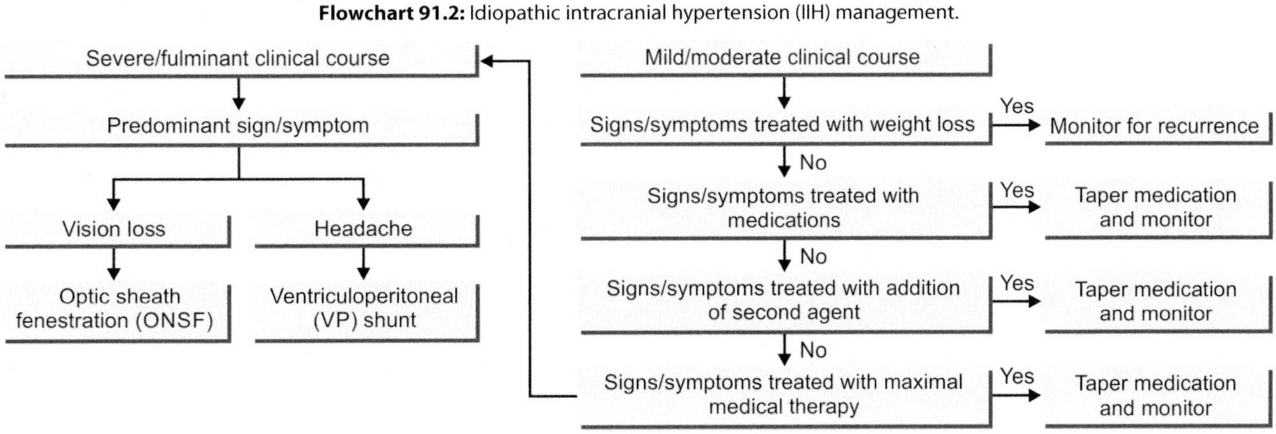

in doubt, neuroimaging findings may point to increased intracranial pressure. Alternatively, repeat OCT can show significant changes with RNFL testing. After the diagnosis of papilledema has been established, the clinician should assess blood pressure, brain MRI and MRV, and lumbar puncture with opening pressure. Patients with a diagnosis of IIH should be managed like glaucoma—little to no visual field loss then the pressure can be lowered medically versus significant visual field loss, then the pressure should be lowered surgically.

REFERENCES

1. Lyme disease maps. (2017). Lyme Disease. CDC Cdc. gov.2017 [online]. Available from: *https://www.cdc.gov/lyme/stat/maps.html.* [Accessed December 2017]
2. Brodsky M. The swollen optic disc in childhood. In: Brodsky M (Ed.). Pediatric Neuro Ophthalmology, 2nd edition. New York: Springer; 2010. pp. 97-154.
3. Lorentzen S. Incidence of spontaneous venous pulsation in the retina. Acta Ophthalmologica (Copenh). 1970;48: 765-76.
4. Sibony PA, Kupersmith MJ, Feldon SE, et al. Retinal and choroidal folds. Invest Ophthalmol Vis Sci. 2015;56(10); 5670-80.
5. Sato T, Mrejen S, Spaide R. Multimodal imaging of optic disc drusen. Am J Ophthalmol. 2013;156(2):275-82.e1.
6. Kurz-Levin M, Landau K. A comparison of imaging techniques for diagnosing drusen of the optic nerve head. Arch Ophthalmol. 1999;117(8):1045-9.
7. Tso M. Pathology and pathogenesis of drusen of the optic nerve head. Ophthalmology. 1981;88(10):1066-80.
8. Lee A, Zimmerman M. The rate of visual field loss in optic nerve head drusen. Am J Ophthalmol. 2005;139(6):1062-6.
9. Morris PP, Black DF, Port J, et al. Transverse sinus stenosis is the most sensitive MRI imaging correlate in idiopathic intracranial hypertension. AJNR. 2017;38(3):471-7.
10. Lin A, Foroozan R, Danesh-Meyer HV, et al. Occurrence of cerebral venous sinus thrombosis in patients with presumed idiopathic intracranial hypertension. Ophthalmology. 2006;113(12):2281-4.
11. Teasdale E. Cerberal venous thrombosis: making the most of imaging. J R Soc Med. 2000;93(5):234-7.
12. Ferro J, Canhão P, Stam J, et al. Prognosis of cerebral vein and dural sinus thrombosis: Results of the International Study on Cerebral Vein and Dural Sinus Thrombosis (ISCVT). Stroke. 2004;35(3):664-70.
13. Freilich RJ, Krol G, Deangelis LM. Neuroimaging and cerebrospinal fluid cytology in the diagnosis of leptomeningeal metastasis. Ann Neurol. 1995;38(1):51-7.
14. Clarke JL, Perez HR, Jacks L, et al. Leptomeningeal metastases in the MRI era. Neurology. 2010;74(18):1449-54.
15. Agarwal R, Sze. Neuro-lyme disease: MR imaging findings. Radiology. 2009;253(1):167-73.
16. Abel AS, Brace JR, McKinney AM, et al. Effect of patient positioning on cerebrospinal fluid opening pressure. J Neuroophthalmol. 2014;34(3):218-22.
17. Avery RA, Shah SS, Licht DJ, et al. Reference range for cerebrospinal fluid opening pressure in children. N Engl J Med. 2010;363(9):891-3.
18. Wengert O, Rothenfusser-Korber E, Vollrath B, et al. Neurosarcoidosis: correlation of cerebrospinal fluid findings with diffuse leptomeningeal gadolinium enhancement on MRI and clinical disease activity. J Neurol Sci. 2013;335(1-2):124-30.
19. Johns CJ, Michele TM. The clinical management of sarcoidosis. A 50-year experience at the Johns Hopkins Hospital. Medicine (Baltimore). 1999;78(2):65-111.
20. Bargagli E, Bennett D, Maggiorelli C, et al. Human chitotriosidase: a sensitive biomarker of sarcoidosis. J Clin Immunol. 2013;33(1):264-70.
21. Thi Hong Nguyen C, Kambe N, Kishimoto I. Serum soluble interleukin-2 receptor level is more sensitive than angiotensin-converting enzyme or lysozyme for diagnosis of sarcoidosis and may be a marker of multiple organ involvement. J Dermatol. 2017;44(7):789-97.
22. Marangoni S, Argentiero V, Tavolato B. Neurosarcoidosis. Clinical description of 7 cases with a proposal for a new diagnostic strategy. J Neurol. 2006;253(4):488-95.
23. Sibony P, Halperin J, Coyle PK, et al. Reactive lyme serology in optic neuritis. J Neuroophthalmol. 2005;5(2):71-82.
24. Friedman DI, Liu GT, Digre KB. Revised diagnostic criteria for the pseudotumor cerebri syndrome in adults and children. Neurology. 2013;81(13)1159-65.
25. Johnson LN, Korhel GB, Madsen RW, et al. The role of weight loss and acetazolamide in the treatment of idiopathic intracranial hypertension (pseudotumor cerebri). Ophthalmology. 1998;105(12):2313-7.
26. Strom BL, Schinnar R, Apter AJ, et al. Absence of cross-reactivity between sulfonamide antibiotics and sulfonamide nonantibiotics. N Engl J Med. 2003;349(17)1628-35.
27. The NORDIC Idiopathic Intracranial Hypertension Study Group Writing Committee. Effect of acetazolamide on visual function in patients with idiopathic intracranial hypertension and mild visual loss. The idiopathic intracranial hypertension treatment trial. JAMA. 2014;311(16):1641-51.
28. McGirt MJ, Woodworth G, Thomas G, et al. Cerebrospinal fluid shunt placement for pseudotumor cerebri-associated intractable headache: predictors of treatment response and an analysis of long-term outcomes. J Neurosurg. 2004;101(4):627-32.

Chapter 92 Common Optic Neuropathies

Kimberly K Gokoffski, Vivek R Patel

INTRODUCTION

The term optic neuropathy refers to all clinical entities which compromise the physiological structure and/or function of the optic nerve(s). Assessing for optic nerve dysfunction is a critical first step in subclassifying different causes of optic neuropathies. All patients should be assessed for decreased visual acuity, dyschromatopsia and visual field loss with formal testing. Detailed review of the character of visual field loss can be very useful in differentiating between various categories of optic neuropathies. If the process is unilateral, patients may be found to have decreased relative brightness sense, red color desaturation, and a relative afferent pupillary defect on the involved side (Figs. 92.1A and B). Optic neuropathies that generally do not lead to optic nerve dysfunction include: papilledema and pseudo-papilledema, papillophlebitis, optic nerve perineuritis, diabetic papillitis, hypertensive papillitis, and glaucoma (unless markedly asymmetric). In contrast, optic neuropathies that readily cause optic nerve dysfunction include ischemic optic neuropathies, traumatic optic neuropathy, optic neuritis, metabolic or nutritional deficiency or toxic optic neuropathies, hereditary optic neuropathies, and compressive lesions. Each of these etiologies will be reviewed here.

OPTIC NEUROPATHIES WITHOUT OPTIC NERVE DYSFUNCTION

Papilledema

True papilledema, or swelling of the retinal nerve fiber layer (RNFL), develops when there is obstruction of axoplasmic flow at the level of the lamina cribrosa, due to elevated intracranial pressure (ICP). Clinical manifestations of elevated ICP include positional headaches (worse when supine or with increased abdominal pressure, i.e. Valsalva maneuvers), nausea, vomiting, and pulsatile tinnitus. Patients may complain of bilateral transient visual obscurations lasting seconds as well as binocular horizontal diplopia. Magnetic resonance imaging (MRI) findings may include an empty sella or an enlarged remodeled sella from chronically elevated ICP, dilated perineural fluid cuff on T2 signaling, vertical tortuosity of optic nerve, flattening

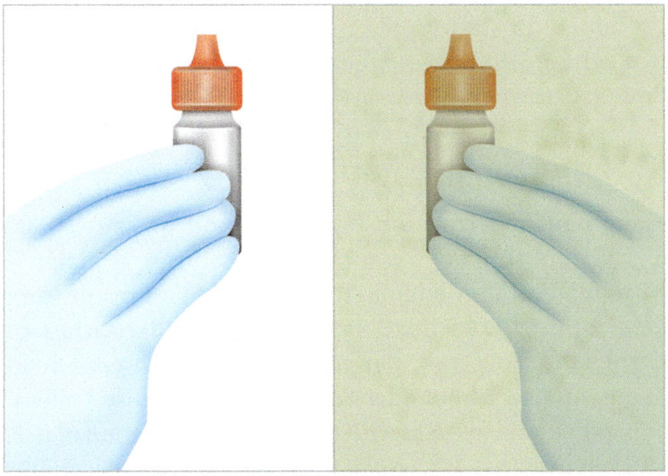

Fig. 92.1A: Relative subjective red desaturation experienced by patients with unilateral optic neuropathy. The sense of decreased brightness and "yellowing" on the visual scene is often described with the affected eye.

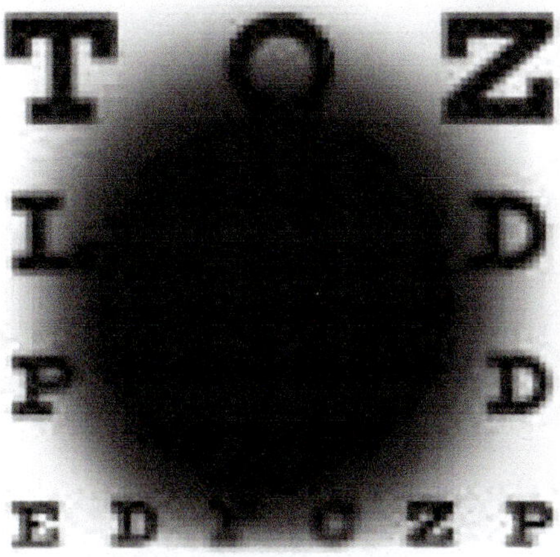

Fig. 92.1B: Central scotomas are classically seen–they may appear as a "fog" or "patch" of loss of vision with relative sparing of the periphery.

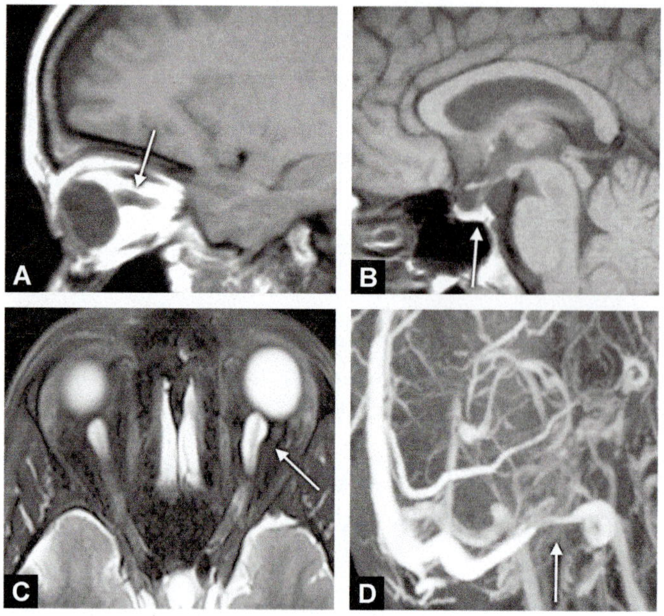

Figs. 92.2A to D: Imaging findings in pseudotumor cerebri syndrome. MRI orbits reveal vertical tortuosity of optic nerve (A); partially empty sella (B); dilated perioptic fluid cuff (best seen on T2 images) and flattening of posterior aspect of globe (C); and focal stenosis at distal portion of transverse sinus, at its intersection with the sigmoid sinus (D).

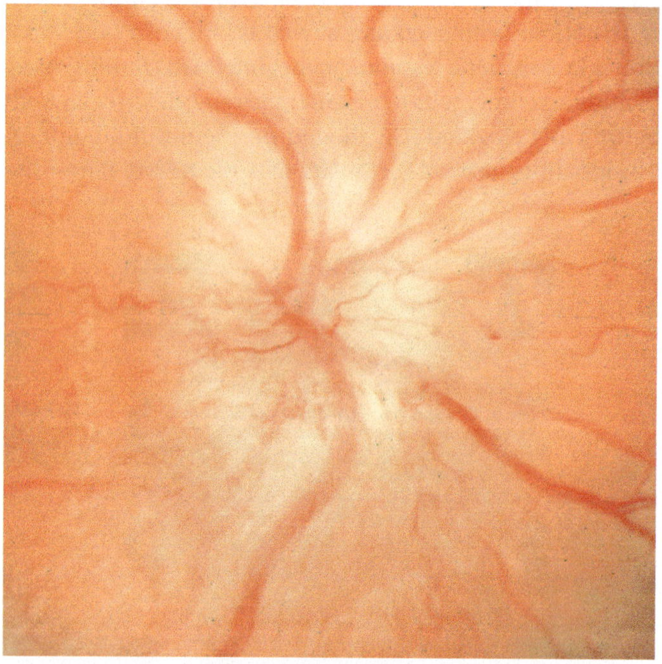

Fig. 92.3: Diabetic papillopathy. Right eye of a patient with diabetes mellitus (DM) type 1 revealing mild disk edema, hyperemia, and surface vessel telangiectasias. He had mild blurring of vision, and a minimally enlarged blind spot.

of the posterior globe, and distal transverse sinus stenosis on computed tomography (CT) or magnetic resonance (MR) venography (Figs. 92.2A to D).[1,2] *See* Chapter 91: The Swollen Disk, for additional details on this condition.

Diabetic Papillopathy

Young patients with type 1 diabetes mellitus (DM), although occasionally with type II DM, may present with swelling of the optic disk with minimal optic nerve dysfunction.[3,4] Diabetic papillopathy (Fig. 92.3) may occur with any degree of diabetic retinopathy (or lack thereof). Optic nerve swelling can be unilateral or bilateral, with dilated telangiectatic vessels on the disk surface, and may be considered on a spectrum of non-arteritic ischemic optic neuropathy (NAION, discussed further). However, unlike NAION, visual field findings are usually nonspecific, often presenting with an enlarged blind spot or mild diffuse decrease in sensitivity, but not a discrete altitudinal defect. Swelling usually resolves spontaneously within several weeks with no permanent visual dysfunction.

Papillophlebitis

Papillophlebitis is a diagnosis of exclusion applied to the clinical scenario where disk edema without optic nerve dysfunction is seen in an otherwise healthy young patient without significant vascular risk factors or MRI abnormalities.[5] Edema is thought to result from venous stasis, a subclinical variant of central retinal vein occlusion. Although we evaluate these patients for coagulopathies, this workup is usually unrevealing. In contrast to diabetic papillopathy, papillophlebitis tends to reveal more prominent posterior pole venous congestion, extending from the optic nerve, whereas congestion is typically limited to the nerve head in the former (Figs. 92.4A and B).

Hypertensive Papillopathy

Malignant hypertension (systolic blood pressure >180 or diastolic blood pressure >120) is often associated with bilateral disk edema. Disk swelling can result from local optic nerve head ischemia with disruption of axoplasmic flow, vascular congestion at the nerve head due to an overwhelmed vascular autoregulatory system, or papilledema in cases with concomitant elevation of ICP. Disk edema is usually associated with peripapillary splinter hemorrhages, cotton-wool spots, and retinal lipid exudates (Figs. 92.5A and B). Blood pressure should be checked on

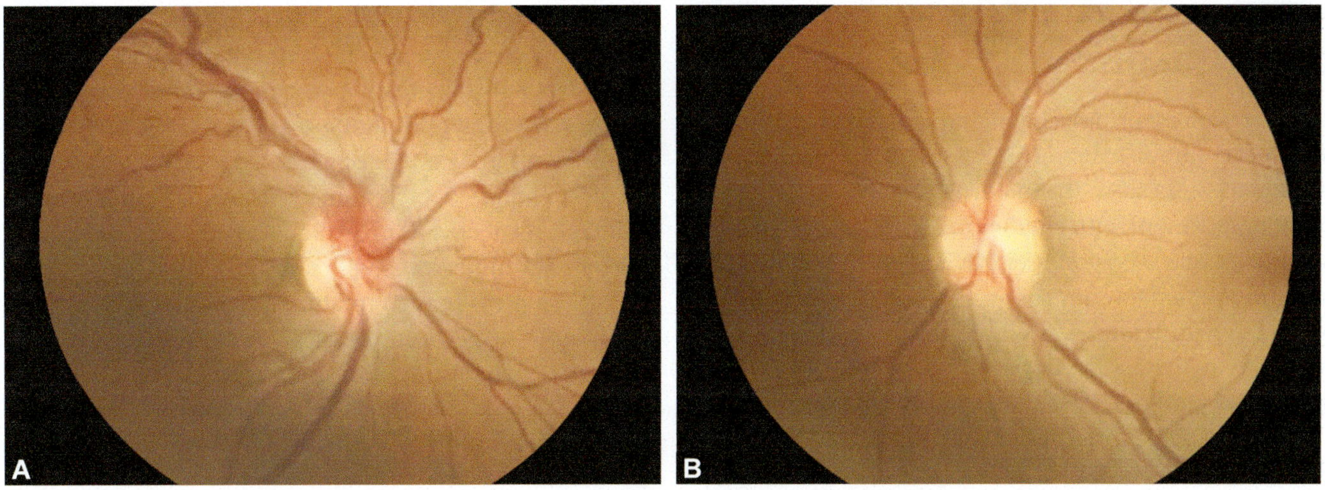

Figs. 92.4A and B: Papillophlebitis. (A) Right eye fundus photograph reveals relatively mild disk edema with venous congestion and tortuosity and minimal hemorrhages; (B) Left eye is normal.

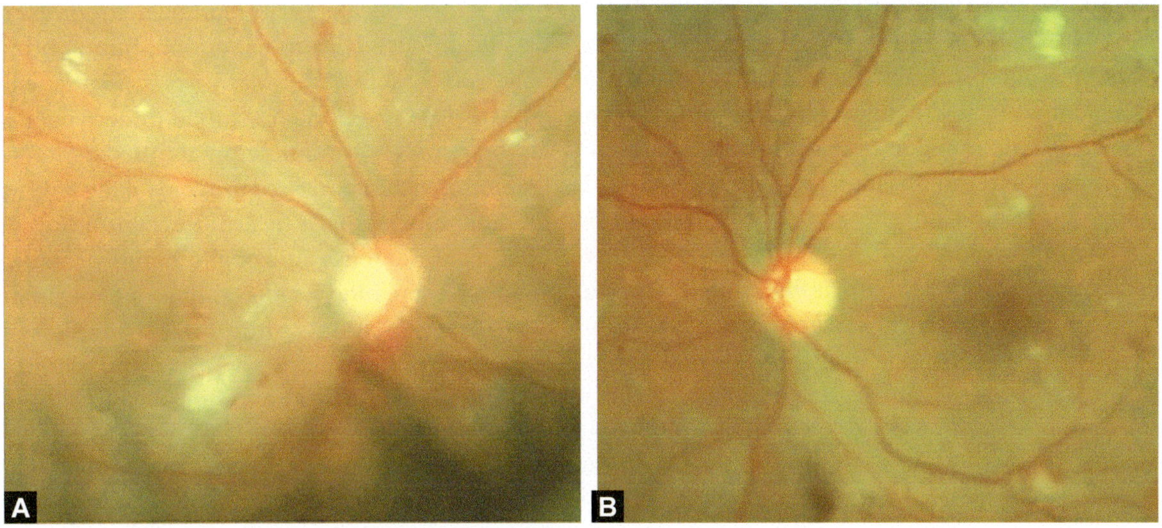

Figs. 92.5A and B: Hypertensive papillopathy/retinopathy. Bilateral disk edema with surrounding cotton wool spots, blot and retinal nerve fiber layer (RNFL) hemorrhages in patient presenting with blood pressure of 230/112 mm Hg.

all patients presenting with bilateral disk edema. Of note, these patients are at high risk for posterior reversible encephalopathy syndrome (PRES)[6] and thus should be comanaged with an internist. Mainstay of treatment involves careful blood pressure control.

OPTIC NEUROPATHIES WITH OPTIC NERVE DYSFUNCTION

Although, the differential diagnosis for optic neuropathies associated with optic nerve dysfunction is vast and can be overwhelming, the ophthalmologist will be able to significantly stratify his/her differential based on onset, nature, severity and evolution of vision loss and attention to the clinical signs described below.

Ischemic Optic Neuropathy

Ischemic optic neuropathies typically manifest with sudden loss of vision and are categorized by the involved portion of the optic nerve and etiology:

- *Optic nerve head:* Anterior ION (AION), either non-arteritic (NAION) or arteritic (AAION).
- *Retrobulbar optic nerve up to chiasm:* Posterior ION (PION) from hypotension, arteritis, or shock/severe blood loss.

Non-arteritic Anterior Ischemic Optic Neuropathy

Non-arteritic anterior ischemic optic neuropathy is by far the most common cause of unilateral AION, accounting for around 95% of cases. The majority of patients are age >50 years and present with sudden onset unilateral, painless, altitudinal loss of vision. Central acuity is variable with a nadir in the first few days of onset. Count fingers vision or worse is atypical for NAION, although may occur. Patients will have relative afferent pupillary defect (RAPD) in the involved eye unless the fellow eye was previously affected. Unlike in optic neuritis (discussed below), color vision loss is proportional to loss of visual acuity. Visual fields generally demonstrate dense altitudinal field loss, more commonly inferiorly. On exam, patients will have diffuse or segmental hyperemia of the disk (Fig. 92.6). There may be splinter hemorrhages in the RNFL and telangiectasias on the disk surface. Cotton wool spots or RNFL infarcts, however, are uncharacteristic and should suggest the possibility of an arteritic process. The prospective multicenter Ischemic Optic Neuropathy Decompression Trial (IONDT) found that by six months after onset, 42.7% of these patients will experience improvement in central visual acuity (≥3 lines), without improvement in visual field,[7] while 44.9% will experience no improvement and 12.4% will experience step-wise worsening in the first several weeks after onset.[8]

The etiology of NAION is still widely debated. A compartment-like syndrome incited by micro-infarcts may be causative, as the majority of NAION patients have small, crowded "disks at risk" (cup-to-disk ratio ≤0.2)[9] and a higher preponderance of vascular risk factors including hypertension, diabetes, hypercholesterolemia, sleep apnea, tobacco use, and phosphodiesterase inhibitor use.[10,11] Other theories propose a role of vitreo-papillary traction versus vitreo-papillary detachment as inducing focal ischemia or damage, respectively, to the RNFL at the optic nerve head,[12] as well as venous stasis with chronic ischemia.[13]

There is no proven treatment for NAION. The IONDT found that surgical decompression of the optic nerve lead to worse visual outcomes than observation alone.[8] Oral corticosteroids are postulated to decrease edema and have been proposed to improve visual outcomes in patients with moderate to severe central vision loss,[14] but these results have been widely criticized (REF editorials that followed). Intraocular pressure lowering eye drops, particularly brimonidine because of its reputed neuroprotective effects, have also received some attention, but no proven benefit has been established.[15] Many practitioners will prescribe daily aspirin given the presumed underlying vascular risk factors; studies to date show neither benefit nor harm. Patients may be counseled to avoid taking antihypertensive medications at night to avoid accentuating the normal nocturnal decrease in systolic blood pressure. Patients should be screened for sleep apnea and evaluated/treated accordingly. Patients should also be advised to avoid phosphodiesterase inhibitors[11] and amiodarone, the latter of which deposits at the optic nerve head and can lead to an NAION-like syndrome.[16] Finally, patients should be warned that they have a 14.7% risk of fellow eye NAION in the subsequent five years.[8]

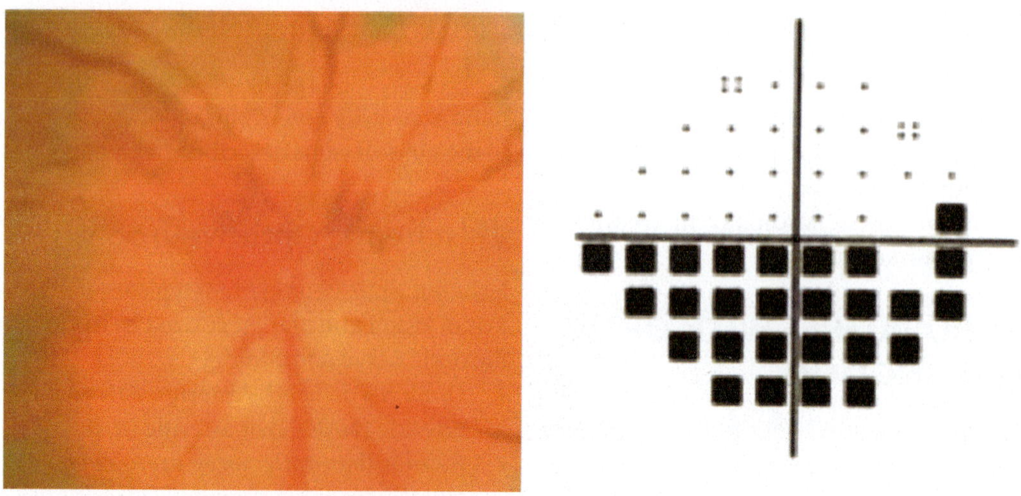

Fig. 92.6: Non-arteritic ischemic optic neuropathy (NAION). Right eye of patient presenting with acute painless vision loss. Fundus image reveals diffuse disk edema with superior segmental flame hemorrhages and corresponding dense inferior altitudinal visual field defect.

Arteritic Anterior Ischemic Optic Neuropathy

Arteritic anterior ischemic optic neuropathy is a less common but more devastating cause of unilateral AION than NAION, accounting for about 5% of cases. The most common form of AAION is associated with giant cell arteritis (GCA), a medium to large vessel vasculitis that typically affects older patients (average age 72) and is more common in females (3:1 F:M ratio) and Caucasians, rarely occurring in Blacks, Latinos, or Asians.[17,18] When vision loss occurs, it is severe, on the order of hand motions or worse, and results from infarction of the posterior ciliary arteries or even ophthalmic artery. Vision loss is often preceded by transient visual obscurations lasting seconds to minutes, a symptom that is uncharacteristic of NAION. On exam, the optic nerve is usually noted to have chalky-white, pallid edema with RNFL hemorrhages and infarcts (Figs. 92.7A to D). Fluorescein angiography may demonstrate patchy choroidal filling. There may also be associated or isolated cilioretinal, branch, or central retinal arterial occlusion.

Giant cell arteritis is not limited to the ophthalmic circulation and for this reason it is often accompanied by headaches, scalp tenderness, jaw claudication, and tongue ischemia arising from occlusion/hypoperfusion of the superficial temporal, facial, and lingual arteries respectively. GCA patients can present with cranial nerve palsies. GCA can affect the circulation of the heart and brain, and has a 7:1 predilection for the posterior cerebrovascular

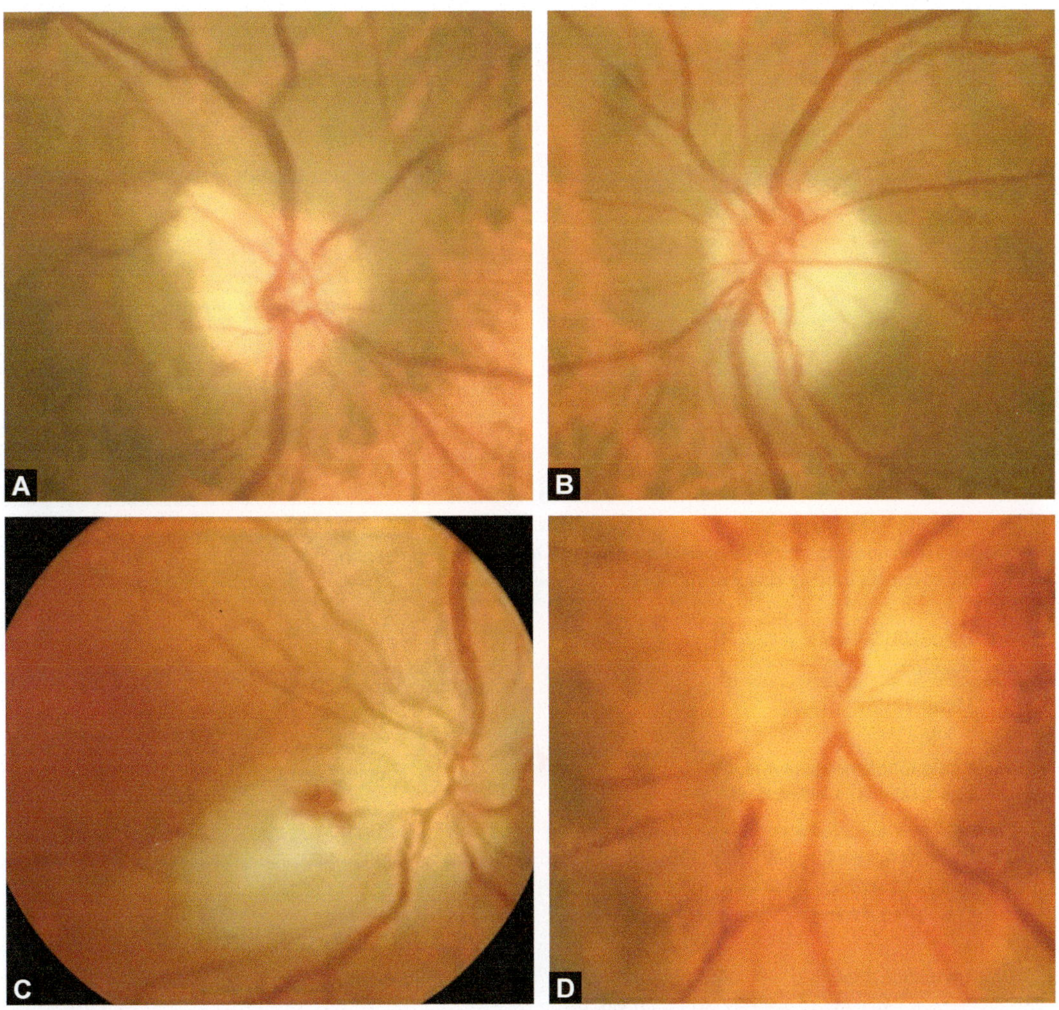

Figs. 92.7A to D: Arteritic anterior ischemic optic neuropathy (AAION) due to giant cell arteritis (GCA). Spectrum of potential presentations. (A and B) Represent right and left eye of a patient presenting with bilateral AAION, secondary to biopsy-proven GCA. Peripapillary pallid edema is seen bilaterally. Right eye of patient presenting with severe acute vision loss: AAION with associated cilioretinal artery occlusion (C). Classic appearance of pallid, chalky white disk edema and associated splinter hemorrhages in another patient with AAION (D).

circulation relative to the anterior circulation (internal carotid arteries) (Figs. 92.8A and B).[19]

Patients with GCA will generally have elevated acute phase reactants including erythrocyte sedimentation rate (ESR), C-reactive protein (CRP), and platelets with 97% specificity if ESR more than 47 [normal = age/2 for men, (age+10)/2 for women) and CRP >2.45 (normal <1).[20,21] However, the diagnostic gold standard is temporal artery biopsy (unilateral or bilateral), which, in addition to possible giant cell infiltration into the vessel wall, will show patchy destruction of the internal elastic lamina.[22,23] Suspicion for vision loss from GCA necessitates urgent initiation of steroids (preferably intravenous solumedrol, 1 g IV for 3 days, followed by oral prednisone 1 mg/kg/day), even before biopsy, as severe loss of vision in the fellow eye has been reported in 54–95% of untreated patients.[24] In biopsy proven patients, prednisone taper is subsequently guided by examination and laboratory results, with the typical treatment period being one year or longer.

As the acute edema resolves, the disk will remain pale and often develops an excavated appearance due to severe tissue destruction. This is in contrast to the chronic appearance of the nerve in NAION patients, where the disk will be pale but with minimal cupping (Table 92.1).

Other Ischemic Optic Neuropathies

Hypotensive ION ensues after severe systemic hypotension, anemia, or blood loss. Typical scenarios that can lead to this rare condition include severe, spontaneous GI or GU

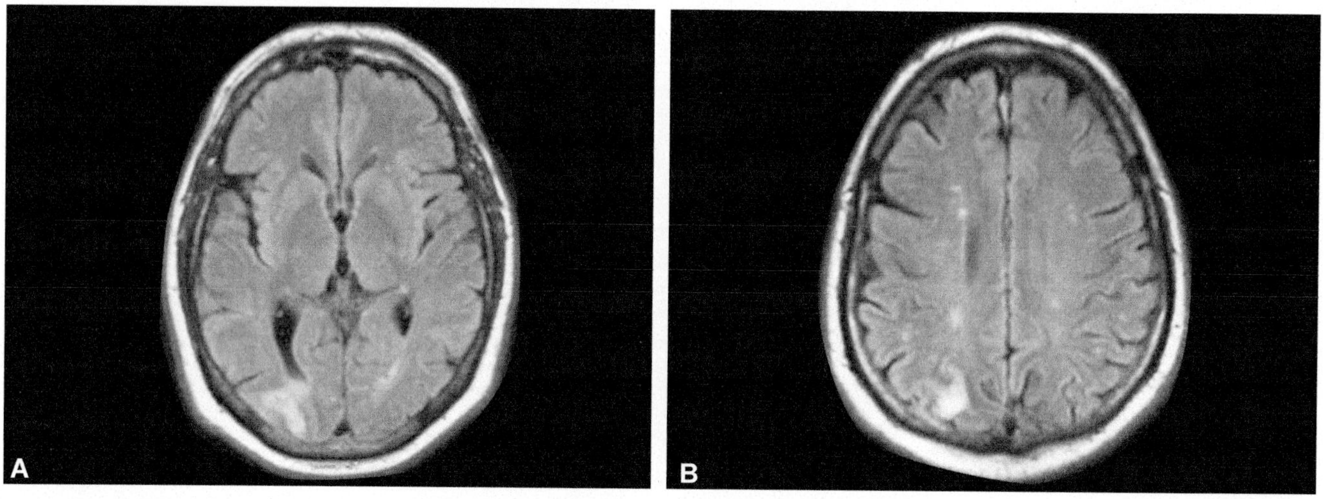

Figs. 92.8A and B: Cerebrovascular ischemia in giant cell arteritis (GCA). MRI T2-fluid-attenuated inversion recovery (FLAIR) images of a patient presenting with acute left homonymous hemianopsia and confusion. Patchy hyper-intensities representing focal vasculitic ischemia, are seen within posterior circulation, including the right occipital lobe in a patient with biopsy-proven GCA.

Table 92.1: Characteristics of NAION versus AAION.

	Arteritic	Non-arteritic
Age	Mean 72	Mean 60
Sex predominance	F > M (3:1)	F = M
ROS	Scalp tenderness, jaw claudication, transient visual obscurations, +/–diplopia	Painless, no transient visual obscurations
VA	<20/200	>20/200
DFE	Pallid disk swelling with cotton wool spots, splinter heme → chalky pallor with excavation	Diffuse or sectoral hyperemic disk → sectoral pallor without excavation
ESR	½ age (+5 if female)	Normal
CRP	↑	Normal
Platelets	Thrombocytosis	Normal
FA	Delayed disk filling, patchy choroidal filling	Early mild disk hyperfluorescence
Fellow eye	Normal	Crowded disk at risk

(ROS: Review of system; ESR: Erythrocyte sedimentation rate; VA: Visual acuity; CRP: C-reactive protein; DFE: Dilated fundus examination; FA: Fluorescein angiography)

hemorrhage, perioperative blood loss, or chronic anemia such as seen with renal dialysis.[25] Vision loss is usually sudden but can be delayed 2–3 weeks, presumably from vasoconstriction of ciliary arteries after activation of the renin-angiotensin system.

In terms of postsurgical hypotensive ION, spinal surgery in the prone position and surgery requiring cardiopulmonary bypass have been implicated most frequently, although this entity has been described following a wide variety of cases. It may manifest as anterior or posterior ION,[26] with PION differing only in the lack of acute disk swelling but otherwise following the same clinical course.

The American Society of Anesthesiology registry cites the following risk factors for post-surgical ischemic optic neuropathy:[27]

- Prolonged surgery (lasting ≥ 6 hours)
- Intraoperative hypotension
- Anemia
- Hypovolemia
- Hypoxia
- >1 L blood loss.

Recommendations include maintaining systolic blood pressure more than 100 mm Hg and hemoglobin more than 10 mg/dL, and using colloids in addition to crystalloids when replenishing blood loss. Most cases of perioperative ION result in severe bilateral vision loss, but unilateral cases have been reported as well.[28] Visual prognosis is typically poor.

Traumatic Optic Neuropathy

Traumatic optic neuropathies may occur from direct or indirect injury to the optic nerve. Direct trauma (i.e. impingement by a bony fragment or foreign body in the orbit or intracranially, surgical manipulation, etc.) causes sudden, severe vision loss, and prognosis is generally poor. More commonly, indirect optic nerve injury occurs when a blunt force injury to the ipsilateral forehead or temple is transmitted to the intra-orbital and intracanalicular portions of the optic nerve. This may cause focal axonal injury and/or swelling, shearing of small blood vessels feeding the optic nerve, or both. Vision loss may be immediate or delayed if swelling persists or worsens. Regardless, pallor ensues in the weeks following injury.

There is little consensus regarding the appropriate management of traumatic optic neuropathy. Treatment options range from observation to high dose steroids to surgical decompression of the optic canal. The International Optic Nerve Trauma Study showed no clear benefit with either steroids or surgery but a trend towards benefit if IV methylprednisolone was given within eight hours of injury.[29] However, the second National Acute Spinal Cord Injury Study (NASCIS II) demonstrated increased morbidity with megadose steroids started more than 8 hours after spinal cord injury,[30] and megadose steroid administration in head injury patients has been associated with increased mortality.[31] Furthermore, animal studies demonstrate decreased retinal ganglion cell survival with megadose corticosteroid administration after injury.[32] Surgical decompression of the optic nerve sheath or canal is not recommended unless a discrete intrasheath hematoma, foreign body, or compressive bony fragment is visualized and progressive visual loss in the first 24–48 hours after trauma can be documented.

Optic Neuritis

Optic neuritis (ON), or inflammation of the optic nerve, is categorized by anatomical location (anterior papillitis versus retrobulbar), as well as by etiology: demyelinating, inflammatory, or infectious.

Demyelinating ("Typical") Optic Neuritis

Demyelinating optic neuritis is a relatively common cause of unilateral optic neuropathy. Typically affecting females in their 20s and 30s, this condition is characterized by unilateral, subacute loss of vision associated with eye pain exacerbated by eye movements.[33] Bilateral simultaneous presentation is atypical in adults, but more common in pre-pubescent children. Vision loss is subacute and often progresses over several days, although severe vision loss (LP or NLP) is unusual. Patients usually note a "fog" or "cloud" over their vision and may also complain of photopsias. Dyschromatopsia and impaired contrast sensitivity may exceed the degree of visual acuity loss. This is in contrast to NAION where dyschromatopsia mirrors visual acuity and may be absent in cases with well-defined altitudinal field loss. Although any visual field defect can be seen in ON, the Optic Neuritis Treatment Trial (ONTT) found 42% of patients with demyelinating optic neuritis to have generalized depression, 20% nerve fiber layer defects (arcuate, altitudinal, nasal step), 8% cecocentral, and 5% hemianopic loss.[34,35] In retrobulbar ON, the optic nerve head will look normal, while about 30% of patients will have mild papillitis (anterior variant) (Fig. 92. 9), uncommonly with mild vitritis and sheathing of retinal veins. Evidence of peripapillary splinter hemorrhages and a macular star on exam is not typical of demyelinating ON and warrants a work up for other disorders. The involved nerve will demonstrate mild fusiform enlargement and enhancement on post-contrast T1-weighted orbital imaging.[36] These MRI findings are not specific for demyelinating ON (similar findings are expected in infectious, inflammatory and infiltrative causes) but are not seen in patients with ION.[37] Patients with isolated, demyelinating optic neuritis are at higher risk for developing multiple sclerosis (MS) than the general population. In fact, optic neuritis is the presenting sign in 20% of patients with MS. The ONTT showed that after their first episode of optic neuritis, if one or more subcortical/periventricular white matter lesions were seen on MRI T2-weighted fluid-attenuated inversion recovery (FLAIR) imaging, patients had a 72% 15-year risk of developing MS compared to 25% in patients with no white matter lesions, making brain MRI the most important prognostic test in the initial workup of patients with demyelinating optic neuritis (Figs. 92.10A and B).[38]

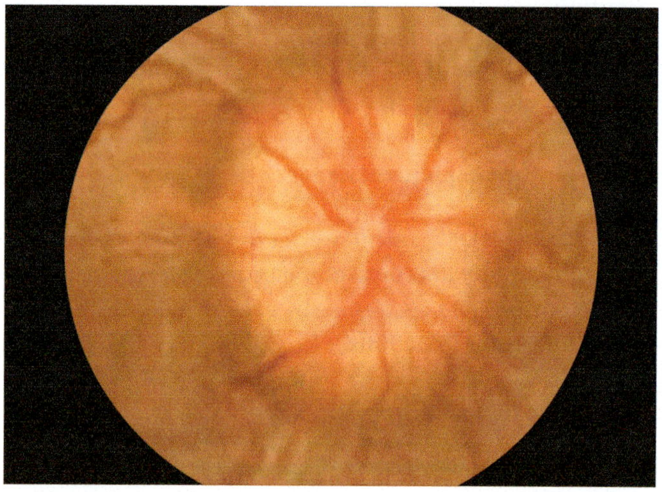

Fig. 92.9: Multiple sclerosis-associated (demyelinating) anterior optic neuritis. Right optic nerve of a patient presenting with acute optic neuritis, exhibiting diffuse hyperemic, nonhemorrhagic swelling.

In the ONTT, patients were randomized to treatment with IV methylprednisolone, oral prednisone 1 mg/kg/d, or placebo. Initial results showed that IV methylprednisolone (250 mg every 6 hours for 3 days) followed by an oral prednisone taper hastened visual recovery without impacting final visual acuity at 6 months. Although patients who received IV steroids had a lower rate of MS development at 2 years, this effect was not evident at 3 years and beyond. Importantly, the ONTT showed that treatment with prednisone 1 mg/kg/d alone was associated with an increased ON recurrence rate and is thus contraindicated. Patients with demyelinating ON, with or without treatment, typically recover visual acuity to nearly baseline over the course of weeks, but color vision and contrast sensitivity may remain impaired. The optic nerve may exhibit subsequent pallor, temporally or diffusely, with minimal excavation.

Pediatric Optic Neuritis

Optic neuritis in prepubescent children has many characteristics that distinguish it from its adult counterpart.[39]

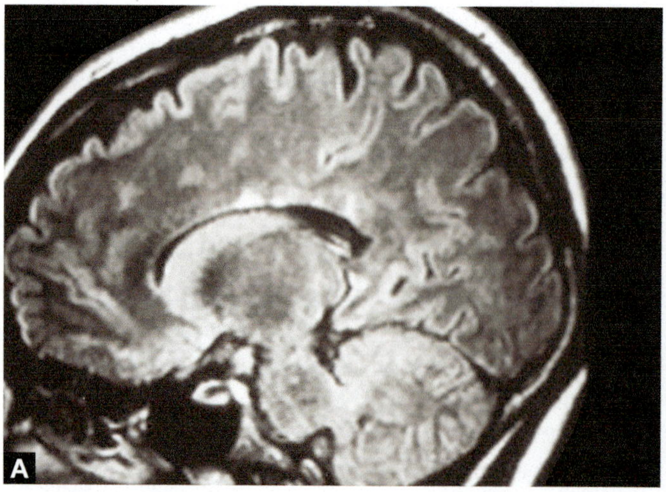

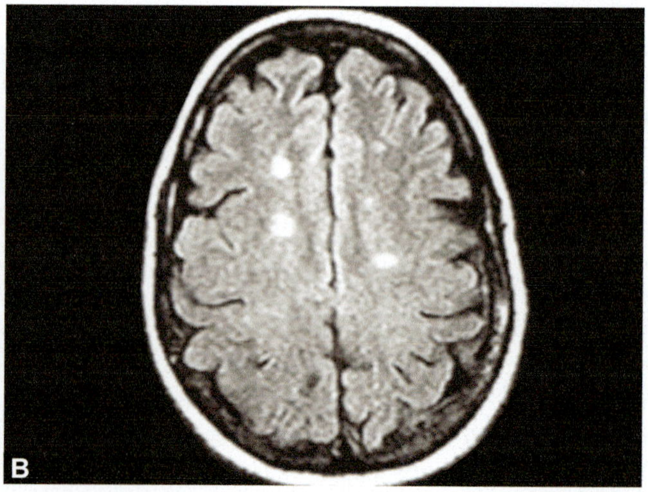

Figs. 92.10A and B: MRI T2-fluid-attenuated inversion recovery (FLAIR) images of a patient with multiple sclerosis (MS). (A) Sagittal image shows characteristic linear hyper-intensities extending from corpus callosum (Dawson's Fingers); (B) Axial image demonstrates the classical ovoid shape of MS demyelinating plaques.

Pediatric optic neuritis does not have a gender or ethnic predilection. Pediatric optic neuritis more commonly presents as anterior ON (papillitis) and is more likely to involve both optic nerves simultaneously. In children, the risk of developing MS after demyelinating optic neuritis is dichotomous: most have a self-limiting condition with a low risk of developing MS while a subset have markedly debilitating demyelinating disease. The best evidence suggests that MRI carries the same prognostic value for MS development as it does in adults.[40]

In children, acute demyelinating encephalomyelitis (ADEM) should be considered on the differential for optic neuritis with brain involvement. [41] ADEM is a transient, generally monophasic, parainfectious demyelinating disease with large, subcortical white matter lesions (Fig. 92.11). Unlike MS, these lesions are all of the same age and resolve months later, with remarkable recovery of function.

"Atypical" Optic Neuritis

Patients presenting with symptoms of ON (painful, subacute vision loss with or without optic disk swelling) but less common features such as:

- Male sex
- Age > 40
- Severe vision loss (counting fingers or worse)
- Bilateral simultaneous vision loss
- Moderate to severe optic disk swelling.

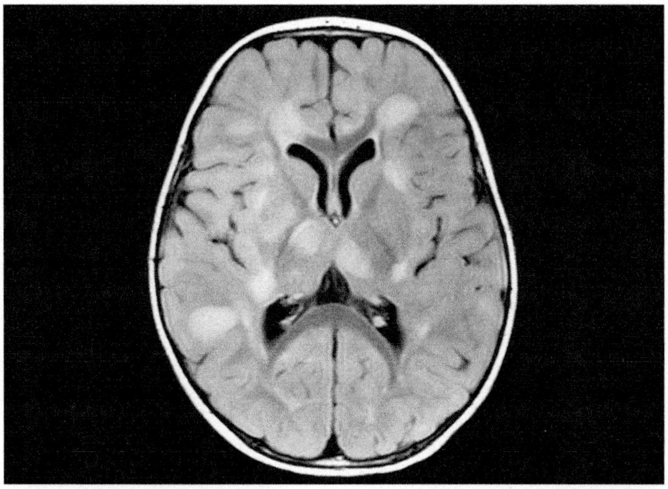

Fig. 92.11: MRI T2-fluid-attenuated inversion recovery (FLAIR) image of a young patient with ADEM. Bilateral asymmetric extensive "tumefactive" hyper-intensities involving the gray and white matter, without specific predilection for the corpus callosum, in contrast to MS. The lesions all tend to be in the same stage of evolution, as ADEM is typically a monophasic, post-viral illness.

And/or progressive spinal cord symptoms should be considered as having atypical ON and must be evaluated for alternative, non-demyelinating etiologies.

Neuromyelitis optica (NMO): It is an autoimmune disease that targets astrocytes, leading to destruction of both white and gray matter tissue in the CNS. Clinically, NMO is characterized by optic neuritis and transverse myelitis. Diagnosis includes two major criteria: optic neuritis and transverse myelitis; and two of three minor criteria: (1) Brain MRI without subcortical white matter changes characteristic of MS, (2) anti-aquaporin-4 antibody positivity, and (3) transverse myelitis that spans at least three vertebral segments.[42] Patients who do not satisfy these diagnostic criteria but whose clinical examination is more consistent with NMO are termed to have NMO-spectrum disorder (NMOSD).[43]

Neuromyelitis optica-spectrum disorder has no gender predilection and has a higher incidence in Asia and the Caribbean. Compared with MS-associated demyelinating ON patients, NMO patients are more likely to present with bilateral, simultaneous optic neuritis and/or more severe vision loss. Neuroimaging often reveals a longer segment of optic nerve enhancement than is typical for MS-associated optic neuritis (Figs. 92.12A to C). NMO patients can present with chiasmatic ON, which can also be seen in MS but is less typical. Although most NMO patients do not demonstrate periventricular white matter lesions typical of MS, observations of anti-NMO seropositive patients has revealed a large subset of patients with white matter lesions in the area postrema, brainstem, corpus callosum, and hypothalamus.[43] These lesions tend to be larger than MS lesions and demonstrate cavitary excavation. In fact, the optic nerve of patients with NMOSD also demonstrates cavitary excavation, along with marked pallor, as the episode of acute optic neuritis resolves—a characteristic that is not typical for MS associated ON (Figs. 92.13A and B). Involvement of the intracranial visual pathways is more common in NMO than it is MS, although can be seen in both conditions.

As noted earlier, MS-associated ON patients typically experience nearly full recovery of vision. Visual prognosis, however, is not as promising with NMO-associated ON, especially if treatment is delayed. Intravenous immunoglobulin and plasmapheresis may supplement steroids in the acute management of NMO-associated ON cases.

Despite differences in presentation, it can often be challenging to differentiate between MS and NMO-related ON at presentation. Serum anti-aquaporin-4 antibody

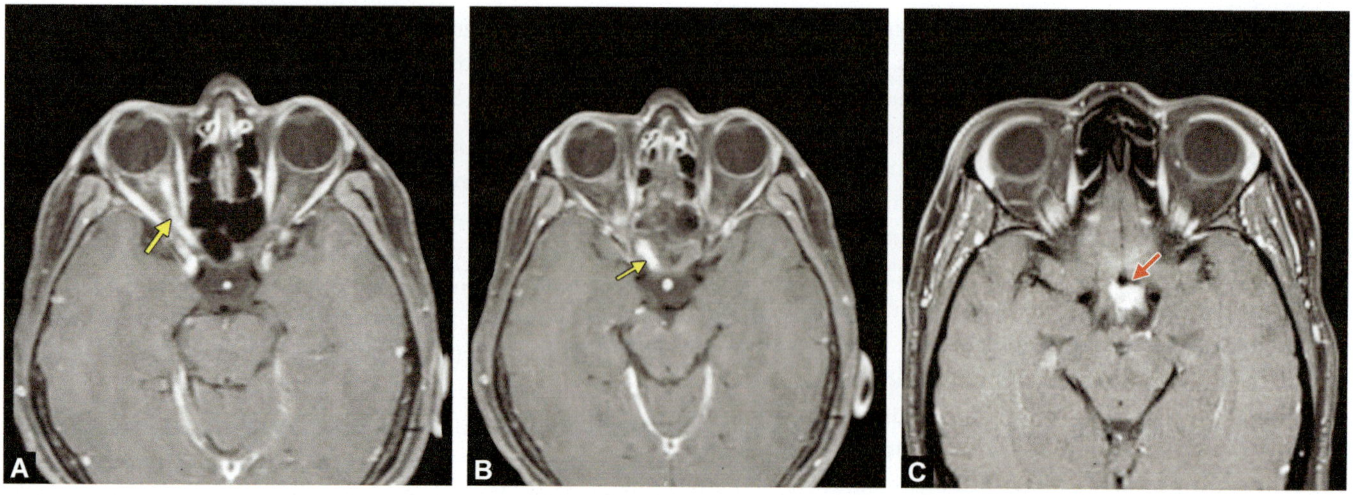

Figs. 92.12A to C: MRI orbits post-gadolinium infusion of a 21-year-old patient diagnosed with neuromyelitis optica (NMO), demonstrating a long segment of right optic nerve enhancement, extending from the anterior orbit to the pre-chiasmatic segment (A and B, yellow arrows); (C) A 36-year-old NMO patient demonstrating chiasmal involvement (red arrow).

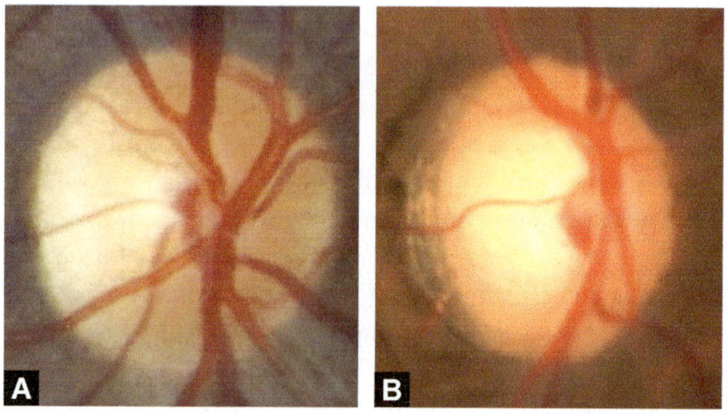

Figs. 92.13A and B: Optic atrophy following optic neuritis in MS versus NMO. (A) A patient with MS shows temporal pallor 6 weeks after acute optic neuritis, without significant cupping; (B) A patient with NMO-associated optic neuritis shows a greater degree of excavation of the optic nerve, 6 weeks after the acute episode. This can help differentiate between the two conditions.

Table 92.2: Multiple sclerosis versus neuromyelitis optica.

Multiple sclerosis	Neuromyelitis optica
White matter demyelination	White and gray matter
Unilateral optic neuritis (shorter segment) + typical periventricular brain lesions	Bilateral optic neuritis (longer segment) + transverse myelitis
Relapsing and remitting course	Single episode unless anti-NMO antibody (+)
Moderate vision loss → improve	Severe vision loss → little improvement*
CSF: oligoclonal bands, myelin basic protein	Serum: NMO*, MOG
VF: 42% generalized depression	VF: Cecocentral (papillomacular bundle), vertical respect if chiasmal or posterior
ON: temporal pallor, no excavation, gliosis	ON: pallor with significant excavation, no gliosis
White female (although broad range of ethnicities), 20s–30s	Asian/Caribbean (30s–40s)

*NMO-Ab positive patients generally have poorer recovery of vision than anti-MOG patients.

testing can be very helpful in the evaluation of patients presenting with their first episode of ON, especially when the above atypical features are noted. Although sensitivity of antibody testing is currently around 75%, it has added prognostic value: patients who demonstrate antibody positivity (mostly females) are more likely to have recurrent episodes of optic neuritis leading to additional optic nerve injury and to require long-term immunosuppression.[44,45] In contrast, a subset of NMOSD patients may test positive for anti-myelin oligodendrocyte associated glycoprotein (MOG) antibody. A retrospective study from Japan found no overlap between anti-NMO and anti-MOG positive patients.[46] Anti-MOG positive patients had milder disease and were more likely to be male and younger than the anti-NMO cohort. These patients have excellent visual prognosis and respond well to high dose steroids.

Differentiating between MS and NMO is important as immunomodulatory therapy for MS (interferon-β, natalizumab, and fingolimod) has been found to potentially aggravate NMOSD.[47] Immunosuppressants including azathioprine and mycophenylate mofetil, and rituximab are the current mainstay of NMO treatment (Table 92.2).[48]

Inflammatory optic neuropathies: Other inflammatory conditions that can cause ON include sarcoidosis, systemic lupus erythematosis, ANCA-associated vasculitides, and Sjogren disease. Patients may present with ON during the course of a systemic flare or as a presenting manifestation of disease. Visual acuity recovers rapidly with steroids but also rapidly declines as steroids are tapered. This relative steroid dependency is atypical of demyelinating ON and should suggest inflammatory etiologies as listed above.

Chronic relapsing inflammatory optic neuritis (CRION) refers to a form of inflammatory ON distinct from the conditions mentioned above.[49] Similar to inflammatory optic neuropathies, CRION is exquisitely sensitive to steroids with the exception that in these patients, vision tends to decline inexorably over time without long-term immunosuppression using a steroid-sparing agent. CRION also differs in that it occurs in isolation, without signs of underlying systemic inflammatory disease. Serologic work up is usually unremarkable; patients may demonstrate positive anti-nuclear or anticardiolipin antibodies, similar to autoimmune optic neuritis. Dermal biopsy of non-sun exposed skin may reveal inflammatory perivascular infiltration at the dermal/epidermal junction.

Bacteria, fungi, and viruses can directly infect the optic nerve or induce systemic inflammation that leads to optic neuritis or optic perineuritis (Figs. 92.14A and B). Bacterial disorders that have been more commonly implicated include syphilis, Lyme disease, Bartonella infection, leptospirosis and tuberculosis. Opportunistic infections including cryptococcus, cytomegalovirus, and herpes simplex virus, should be considered if the patient has underlying HIV. Lumbar puncture can be helpful in distinguishing infectious from demyelinating causes of optic neuritis, with the former potentially demonstrating growth of causal organisms, pleocytosis, or markedly elevated protein levels.

Neuroretinitis

If optic nerve swelling is associated with marked macular edema or a macular star, the condition is termed neuroretinitis. Neuroretinitis may affect people of all ages and is usually a self-limiting condition. Neuroretinitis has been associated with certain bacterial infections as listed above; however, no underlying etiology may be found in many cases (Figs. 92.15A and B). Most patients recover full visual acuity, although some are left with metamorphopsia from residual macular distortion. The ONTT reported that patients presenting with papillitis and associated retinal hemorrhages or exudates did not subsequently develop MS; such patients are more likely to have a form of neuroretinitis.[35]

Compressive Optic Neuropathy

Any lesion compressing the optic nerve, whether in the orbit or intracranially, can lead to optic nerve dysfunction and atrophy. Decreased central acuity may be a late sign of compressive optic neuropathy and is often preceded by visual field changes and dyschromatopsia. The differential diagnosis for compressive orbital lesions is large and includes tumors and mass lesions (e.g. cavernous hemangioma, lymphoma, optic nerve sheath meningioma, optic nerve gliomas, ICA aneurysm), choriostomas (e.g. dermoid cyst), as well as infectious/inflammatory conditions (e.g. thyroid eye disease, idiopathic orbital

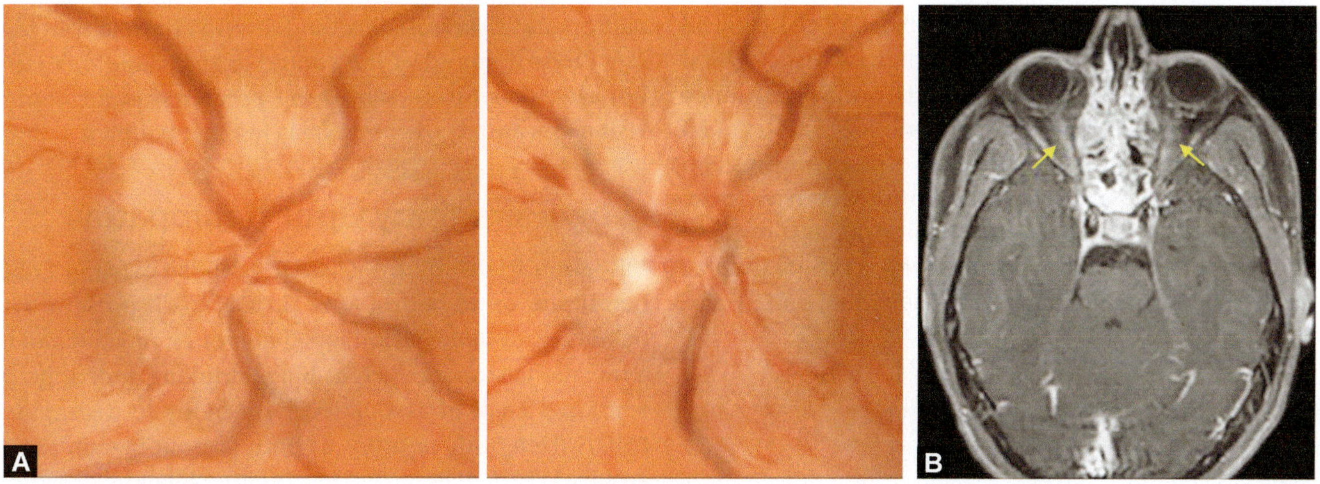

Figs. 92.14A and B: Optic perineuritis. (A) An 18-year-old boy presented with headaches, mild blurring of vision (20/25 OU, full visual fields), and markedly swollen optic nerves bilaterally; (B) MRI orbits post-gadolinium revealed severe pan-sinusitis, with extension of inflammation to the optic nerve sheaths (yellow arrows), without involvement of the optic nerves themselves, relatively sparing optic nerve function.

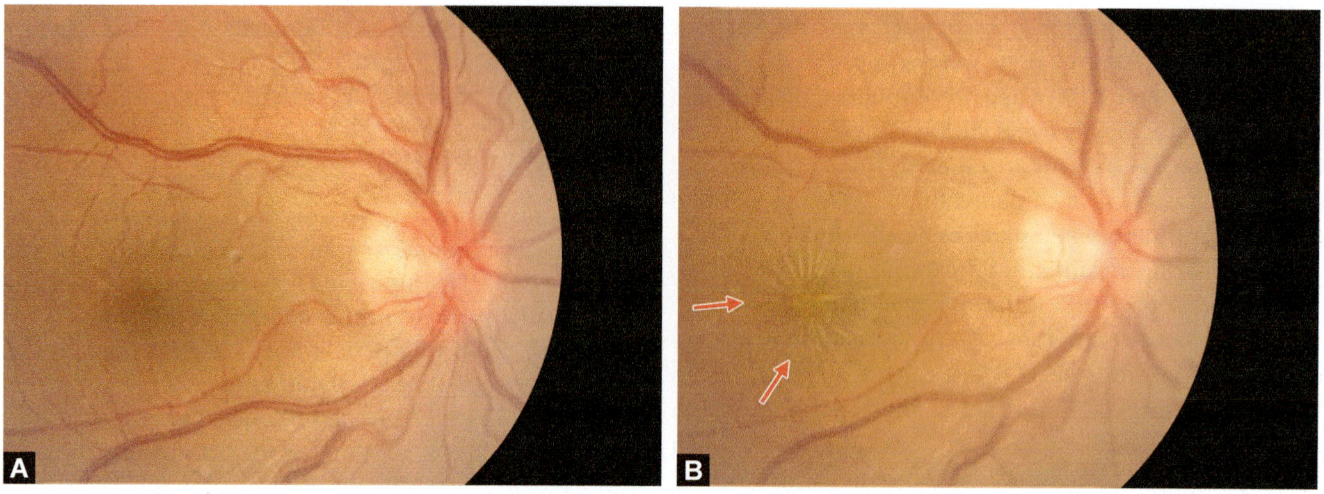

Figs. 92.15A and B: Neuroretinitis. A 26-year-old man presented with subacute blurring of vision in the right eye. (A) Shows mild disk edema and congestion with a normal appearing macula, 3 days after onset of symptoms; (B) 9 days after onset, the disk edema is similar; however, a macular star is clearly seen, as parafoveal exudates are left behind in Henle's layer (arrows). Laboratory testing revealed a high positive Bartonella henselae titer.

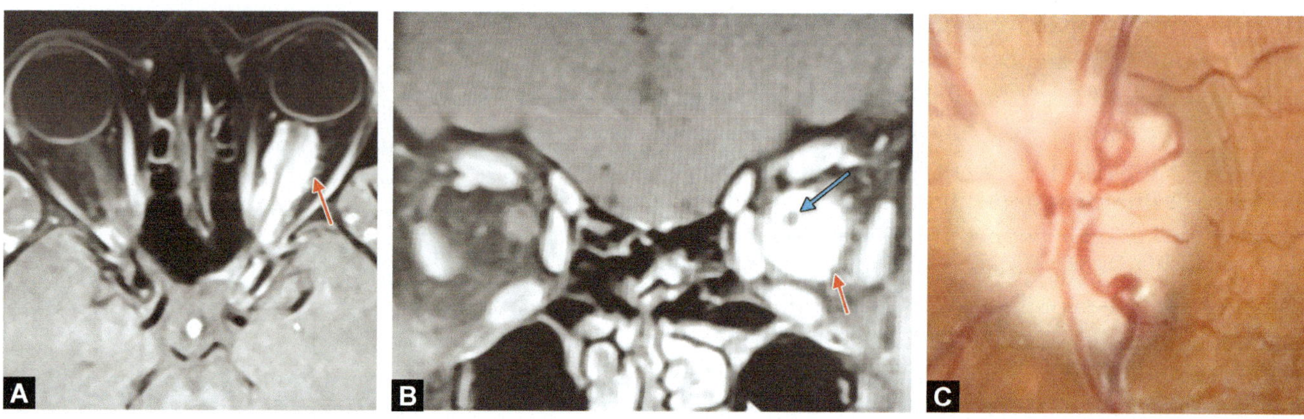

Figs. 92.16A to C: Compressive optic neuropathy due to an optic nerve sheath meningioma. A 56-year-old woman presented with slowly progressive vision loss and proptosis of the left eye over several years. MRI of orbits revealed a homogeneously enhancing tubular mass surrounding the left optic nerve (red arrows), compressing the optic nerve (blue arrow). The optic disk reveals signs of chronic venous congestion (optociliary shunt vessels).

inflammation, orbital cellulitis) (Figs. 92.16A to C). Clinical signs of a large orbital lesion include proptosis, orbital congestion, ophthalmoplegia, and increased resistance to retropulsion. Patients may experience gaze-evoked amaurosis, assumed to result from direct compression of the ophthalmic artery in different positions of gaze. On examination, disk swelling, venous congestion, and choroidal folds may be seen with anterior orbital lesions. Otherwise, the examination will demonstrate optic nerve pallor as atrophy ensues.

Hereditary/Metabolic Optic Neuropathies

Both somatic and mitochondrial genetic mutations may produce bilateral (simultaneous or sequential) optic neuropathy of variable onset and severity. The relatively high metabolic demand of the central axons (papillomacular bundle) likely underscores the predilection for central vision loss and dyschromatopsia in these patients.

Leber Hereditary Optic Neuropathy

Mitochondrial mutations, such as those causing Leber hereditary optic neuropathy (LHON), will present with painless, sub-acute vision loss that is often precipitated by a metabolic stressor such as binge drinking and/or heavy smoking. Lack of associated pain helps to distinguish LHON from optic neuritis, as both present in similar age groups. With LHON, vision loss is either bilateral or rapidly sequential, with the other eye becoming involved within months. LHON patients may not have an obvious RAPD at onset, likely the result of subtle preclinical involvement of the other eye, as well as relative sparing of melanopsin-containing retinal ganglion cells. Vision loss declines subacutely over the course of weeks, stabilizing to about 20/400 or worse three to six months after presentation. Light perception vision or worse is uncommon in patients with LHON. Visual fields demonstrate central or cecocentral scotomas. Fundus exam initially can be underwhelming, but often demonstrates mild optic nerve hyperemia with telangiectasia, and posterior pole arterial tortuosity (Figs. 92.17A and B). Fluorescein angiography reveals no evidence of disk leakage and serves to distinguish this entity from papillitis, where leakage would be expected. Weeks later, the optic nerve develops diffuse pallor with marked atrophy of the papillomacular bundle (Figs. 92.17A and B).

Leber hereditary optic neuropathy results from mitochondrial mutations that are maternally inherited but exhibit incomplete penetrance due to heteroplasmy. Men are more frequently symptomatic than women, with reports suggesting an 85% male predominance. Multiple mitochondrial mutations have been implicated in LHON, with G11778A being the most common.[50] Mutation T14484C has been associated with the best prognosis, as 37–65% of these patients spontaneously regain some vision one to two years after presentation.[51] LHON can be associated with other systemic findings including heart conduction defects (Wolff-Parkinson-White, Lown-Ganong-Levine, and QT prolongation), which are more common in patients with the G3460A mutation.[52] Promising clinical trials using gene therapy to correct the mitochondrial mutation are currently under way. At this time, patients are advised to avoid toxins including cigarette smoking and alcohol. Supplementation with antioxidants including idebenone, a coenzyme Q10 derivative, may be advised, but significant benefit is questionable, even in patients starting the medication shortly after presentation.[53]

Dominant Optic Neuropathy and Others Inherited Conditions

Other inherited optic neuropathies present with slowly progressive, bilateral, symmetric central loss in vision. The slow tempo of vision loss and family history are typically the only clinical characteristics that distinguish hereditary from other metabolic, toxic, and nutritional optic neuropathies, as clinical examination findings are otherwise similar. By the time the patient is symptomatic, temporal pallor and atrophy of the papillomacular bundle are usually apparent. Visual fields show central or cecocentral scotomas, and visual acuity loss is gradual and generally stabilizes to 20/200. Count fingers vision or worse would be uncharacteristic.

Autosomal dominant optic neuropathy (ADOA), or Kjer optic neuropathy, is the most common inherited optic neuropathy, with a prevalence as high as 1:10,000 in Danes and a high degree of penetrance. Vision loss is insidious and usually begins in childhood. Visual decline may progress relentlessly over decades to about 20/200 but may be better, with profound dyschromatopsia that occurs early in life. The nerves display symmetric temporal or diffuse pallor (Figs. 92.18A and B). Most patients have a mutation in the *OPA1* gene, a nuclear encoded mitochondrial gene.

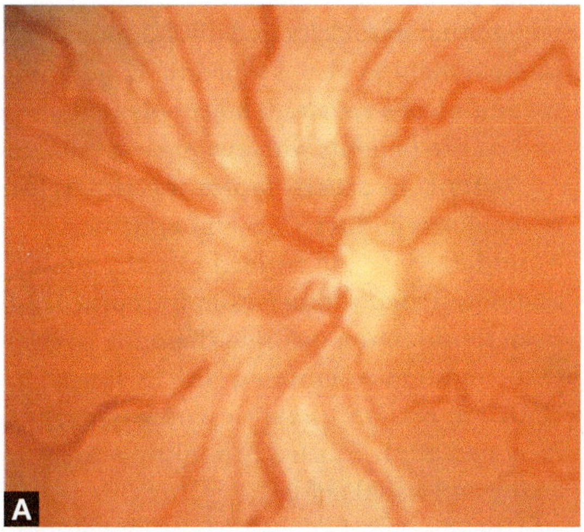

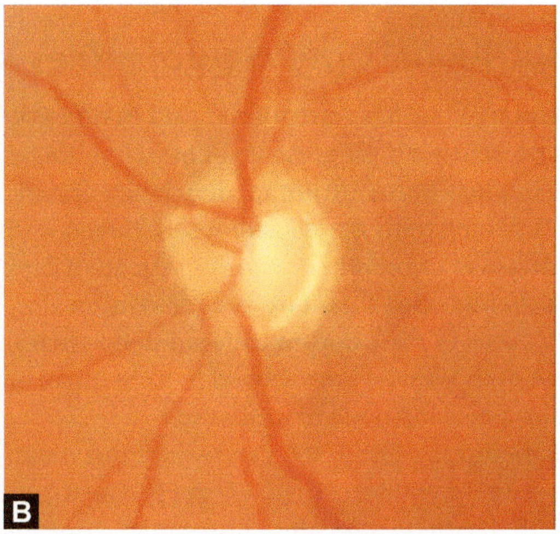

Figs. 92.17A and B: Leber's hereditary optic neuropathy (LHON). (A) A 26-year-old man presented with acute painless loss of vision in the left eye. Disk hyperemia, congestion, and posterior pole arterial tortuosity is appreciated; (B) An 18-year-old man presented with acute loss of vision in his left eye 8 months prior to the shown photograph. Note the temporal cupping and pallor as well lack of congestive features.

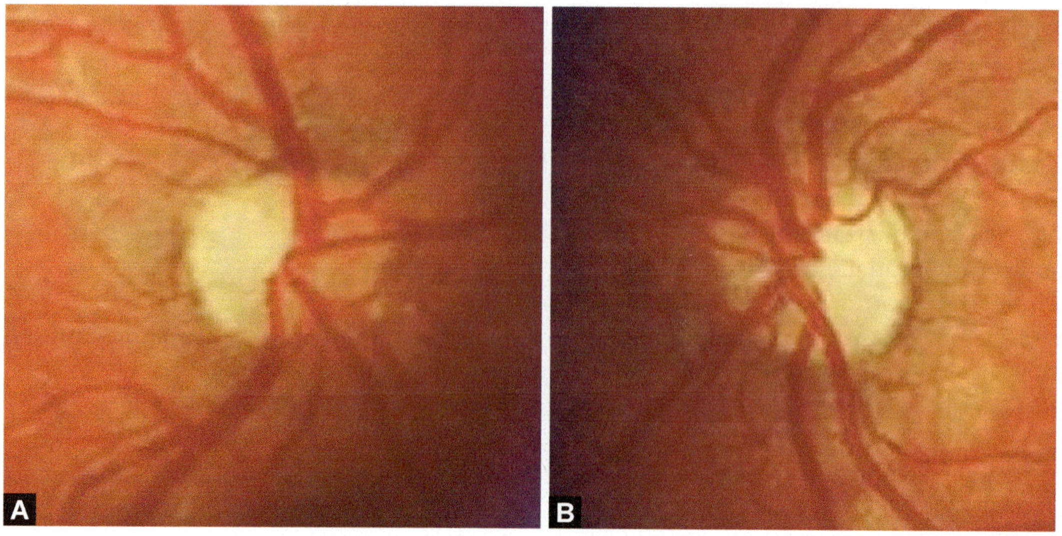

Figs. 92.18A and B: Autosomal dominant optic atrophy (ADOA). Fundus photographs of a 14-year-old girl with slowly progressive bilateral visual decline over years. Note the prominent temporal pallor bilaterally. She exhibited central scotomas and dyschromatopsia bilaterally from a young age.

Behr syndrome is an autosomal recessive optic neuropathy that begins in the first decade of life. Vision loss can be severe and often is associated with nystagmus. Imaging reveals diffuse white matter abnormalities. By the second decade of life, these patients develop chorea and spastic paraparesis.

Wolfram syndrome or DIDMOAD (diabetes insipidus, diabetes mellitus, optic atrophy, deafness) is an example of an inherited optic neuropathy with systemic associations. Patients usually present with diabetes mellitus in the first decade of life with variable onset of optic atrophy and neurosensory hearing loss. These patients demonstrate progressive degeneration of their brainstem with death at a median age of 30 years.

Toxic/Nutritional Optic Neuropathies

Similar to the above entities, nutritional and toxic optic neuropathies present with progressive bilateral, painless vision loss. Vision loss from nutritional deficiency or toxic optic neuropathy is generally more insidious than seen with LHON, occurring over the course of months instead of days to weeks. That being said, a genetic predisposition may underlie some cases of toxic and nutritional deficiencies, as only a subset of those who are exposed to a chemical or are malnourished develop optic neuropathy.

Toxic optic neuropathies (TON) can result from direct damage to the retinal ganglion cell (RGC), the RGC axon, or its myelin sheath. It can be difficult to prove that exposure to a chemical or medication is the cause of TON. Most data are anecdotal, citing animal studies and case reports of improvement in vision with cessation and decline with re-challenge. Untreated TONs can lead to vision loss on the order of 20/400. Methanol is a rare exception that can lead to no light perception vision bilaterally.

Ethambutol is one of the most widely implicated medications known to cause TON.[54] Ethambutol is a zinc chelator and is thought to damage RGC axons directly; central, cecocentral, and even bitemporal visual field defects may result. Toxicity was initially thought to occur with doses greater than 25 mg/kg/day with onset after a few months of use; however, the threshold may be as low as 18 mg/kg/day for some patients. Patients with underlying renal insufficiency may be at greater risk for toxicity given poor clearance of the medication and its metabolites. Early recognition of toxicity and discontinuation can lead to an improvement in visual function. In addition to cessation, we empirically recommend supplementation with copper and zinc in patients with evidence of ethambutol TON.

Tumor necrosis factor (TNF)-α inhibitors and toluene may induce CNS and optic nerve demyelination. Amiodarone is an antiarrhythmic medication that, in addition to depositing within the corneal epithelium, has been found to deposit into the optic nerve head, leading to a condition resembling NAION (Figs. 92.19A and B).[16] Unlike in NAION, involvement is typically bilateral, and drug cessation can lead to improvement in both visual acuity and visual fields.

The strongest evidence for nutritional optic neuropathies (NON) comes from observations during epidemics of mass famine, during which thousands of people developed vision

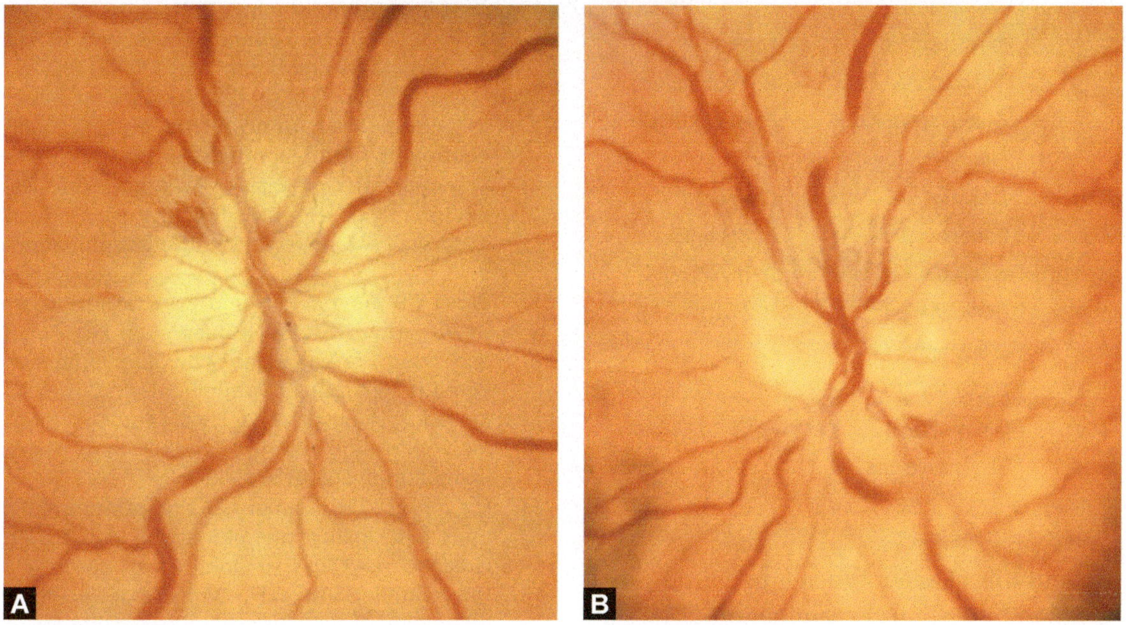

Figs. 92.19A and B: Amiodarone-associated optic neuropathy. A 62-year-old man on amiodarone for 6 months, presented with bilateral subacute optic neuropathy and concentric narrowing of the visual field in both eyes. Visual acuity was 20/80 right eye and 20/150 left eye. Note the bilateral disk edema, venous congestion and superficial hemorrhages.

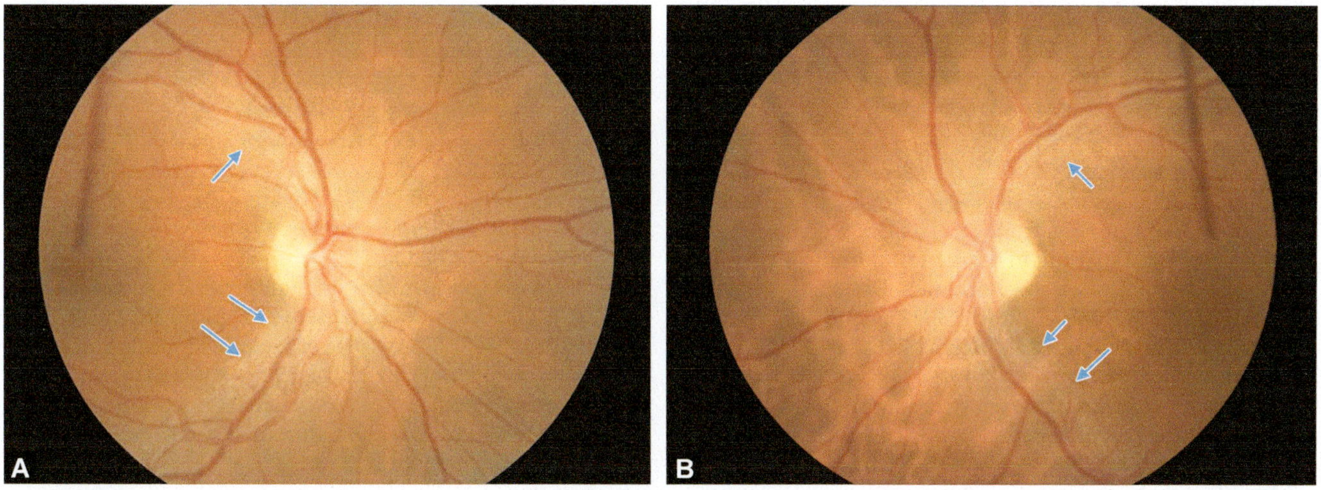

Figs. 92.20A and B: Vitamin B_{12} deficiency optic neuropathy. A 44-year-old man with progressive bilateral vision loss over several months. Visual acuities were 20/200 OD and 20/400 OS. He admitted to a poor diet, heavy consumption of alcohol and tobacco use. His B_{12} levels were very low. Temporal pallor OU, and a wedge of papillomacular bundle atrophy was observed, sharply demarcated (blue arrows) from the mildly congested superior and inferior arcuate nerve fiber bundles.

loss associated with dyschromatopsia and central scotomas that improved after vitamin supplementation. Today, patients at highest risk for NON include those with chronic alcoholism, eating disorders, malabsorption syndromes (including post-bariatric surgery), strict vegetarianism, and severe depression. With the exception of vitamin B_{12}, no deficiency in one nutrient has been proven to cause NON, although folate, pyridoxine, niacin, riboflavin, copper, and zinc are thought to play roles in a multifactorial manner (Fig. 92.20 and Table 92.3).

CONCLUSION

Optic nerve dysfunction may cause nearly any form and pattern of vision loss (acute vs. chronic, unilateral or bilateral) with variable accompanying symptoms as

Table 92.3: Toxic optic neuropathy.

Toxic	Medications	Nutrition
Lead	Amiodarone	B_{12} (cobalamin)
Arsenic	Chloramphenicol	Folate (RBC)
Cadmium	Linezolid	Zn
Methanol (NLP)	Cisplatin	Copper
Ethylene glycol	Ethambutol	B_1 (thiamine)
Tobacco	Isoniazid	B_6 (pyridoxine)
Cyanide	Penicillamine	B_3 (niacin)
Toluene*	Disulfram	
	Sildenafil	
	Streptomycin	
	TNFα inhibitors*	

*Induce demyelination.

noted throughout this chapter. When a patient presents with vision loss and the clinical examination directs the ophthalmologist to a diagnosis of optic neuropathy, it is usually not the eye examination itself that will allow the correct diagnosis to be reached. Rather, a synthesis of the medical and family history, ancillary testing results, and laboratory or radiographic investigations is required to determine the underlying cause and to initiate appropriate therapeutic interventions to preserve visual function.

REFERENCES

1. Bussiere M, Falero R, Nicolle D, et al. Unilateral transverse sinus stenting of patients with idiopathic intracranial hypertension. AJNR Am J Neuroradiol. 2010;31(4):645-50.
2. Agid R, Farb RI. Neuroimaging in the diagnosis of idiopathic intracranial hypertension. Minerva Med. 2006;97(4):365-70.
3. Regillo CD, Brown GC, Savino PJ, et al. Diabetic papillopathy. Patient characteristics and fundus findings. Arch Ophthalmol. 1995;113(7):889-95.
4. Appen RE, Chandra SR, Klein R, et al. Diabetic papillopathy. Am J Ophthalmol. 1980;90(2):203-9.
5. Ellenberger C Jr, Messner KH. Papillophlebitis: benign retinopathy resembling papilledema or papillitis. Ann Neurol. 1978;3(5):438-40.
6. Lamy C, Oppenheim C, Mas JL. Posterior reversible encephalopathy syndrome. Handb Clin Neurol. 2014;121: 1687-701.
7. Scherer RW, Feldon SE, Levin L, et al. Visual fields at follow-up in the Ischemic Optic Neuropathy Decompression Trial: evaluation of change in pattern defect and severity over time. Ophthalmology. 2008;115(10):1809-17.
8. Optic nerve decompression surgery for nonarteritic anterior ischemic optic neuropathy (NAION) is not effective and may be harmful. The Ischemic Optic Neuropathy Decompression Trial Research Group. JAMA. 1995;273(8):625-32.
9. Hayreh SS, Zimmerman MB. Nonarteritic anterior ischemic optic neuropathy: refractive error and its relationship to cup/disk ratio. Ophthalmology. 2008;115(12):2275-81.
10. Hayreh SS, Joos KM, Podhajsky PA, et al. Systemic diseases associated with nonarteritic anterior ischemic optic neuropathy. Am J Ophthalmol. 1994;118(6):766-80.
11. Pomeranz HD, Bhavsar AR. Nonarteritic ischemic optic neuropathy developing soon after use of sildenafil (viagra): a report of seven new cases. J Neuroophthalmol. 2005;25(1): 9-13.
12. Parsa CF, Hoyt WF. Nonarteritic anterior ischemic optic neuropathy (NAION): a misnomer. Rearranging pieces of a puzzle to reveal a nonischemic papillopathy caused by vitreous separation. Ophthalmology. 2015;122(3):439-42.
13. Levin LA, Danesh-Meyer HV. Hypothesis: a venous etiology for nonarteritic anterior ischemic optic neuropathy. Arch Ophthalmol. 2008;126:1582-5.
14. Hayreh SS, Zimmerman MB. Non-arteritic anterior ischemic optic neuropathy: role of systemic corticosteroid therapy. Graefes Arch Clin Exp Ophthalmol. 2008;246(7):1029-46.
15. Wilhelm B, Ludtke H, Wilhelm H, et al. Efficacy and tolerability of 0.2% brimonidine tartrate for the treatment of acute non-arteritic anterior ischemic optic neuropathy (NAION): a 3-month, double-masked, randomised, placebo-controlled trial. Graefes Arch Clin Exp Ophthalmol. 2006;244(5):551-8.
16. Macaluso DC, Shults WT, Fraunfelder FT. Features of amiodarone-induced optic neuropathy. Am J Ophthalmol. 1999;127(5):610-2.
17. Lam BL, Wirthlin RS, Gonzalez A, et al. Giant cell arteritis among Hispanic Americans. Am J Ophthalmol. 2007;143(1):161-3.
18. Pereira LS, Yoon MK, Hwang TN, et al. Giant cell arteritis in Asians: a comparative study. Br J Ophthalmol. 2011;95(2):214-6.
19. Gonzalez-Gay MA, Vazquez-Rodriguez TR, Gomez-Acebo I, et al. Strokes at time of disease diagnosis in a series of 287 patients with biopsy-proven giant cell arteritis. Medicine (Baltimore). 2009;88(4):227-35.
20. Hayreh SS, Podhajsky PA, Raman R, et al. Giant cell arteritis: validity and reliability of various diagnostic criteria. Am J Ophthalmol. 1997;123(3):285-96.
21. Gonzalez-Gay MA, Lopez-Diaz MJ, Barros S, et al. Giant cell arteritis: laboratory tests at the time of diagnosis in a series of 240 patients. Medicine (Baltimore). 2005;84(5):277-90.
22. Hunder GG, Bloch DA, Michel BA, et al. The American College of Rheumatology 1990 criteria for the classification of giant cell arteritis. Arthritis Rheum. 1990;33(8):1122-8.
23. Stacy RC, Rizzo JF, Cestari DM. Subtleties in the histopathology of giant cell arteritis. Semin Ophthalmol. 2011;26(4-5):342-8.
24. Liu GT, Glaser JS, Schatz NJ, et al. Visual morbidity in giant cell arteritis. Clinical characteristics and prognosis for vision. Ophthalmology. 1994;101(11):1779-85.
25. Jackson TL, Farmer CK, Kingswood C, et al. Hypotensive ischemic optic neuropathy and peritoneal dialysis. Am J Ophthalmol. 1999;128(1):109-11.

26. Barrier J, Pion P, Massari R, et al. Epidemiologic approach to Horton's disease in the department of Loire-Atlantique. 110 cases in 10 years (1970-1979). Rev Med Interne. 1982;3(1):13-20.
27. Lee LA, Roth S, Posner KL, et al. The American Society of Anesthesiologists Postoperative Visual Loss Registry: analysis of 93 spine surgery cases with postoperative visual loss. Anesthesiology. 2006;105(4):652-9; quiz 867-8.
28. Chang SH, Miller NR. The incidence of vision loss due to perioperative ischemic optic neuropathy associated with spine surgery: the Johns Hopkins Hospital Experience. Spine (Phila Pa 1976). 2005;30(11):1299-302.
29. Levin LA, Beck RW, Joseph MP, et al. The treatment of traumatic optic neuropathy: the International Optic Nerve Trauma Study. Ophthalmology. 1999;106(7):1268-77.
30. Bracken MB, Shepard MJ, Collins WF, et al. A randomized, controlled trial of methylprednisolone or naloxone in the treatment of acute spinal-cord injury. Results of the Second National Acute Spinal Cord Injury Study. N Engl J Med. 1990;322(20):1405-11.
31. Edwards P, Arango M, Balica L, et al. Final results of MRC CRASH, a randomised placebo-controlled trial of intravenous corticosteroid in adults with head injury-outcomes at 6 months. Lancet. 2005;365:1957-9.
32. Steinsapir KD, Goldberg RA. Traumatic optic neuropathy: an evolving understanding. Am J Ophthalmol. 2011;151: 928-33.e2.
33. Beck RW, Cleary PA, Anderson MM Jr, et al. A randomized, controlled trial of corticosteroids in the treatment of acute optic neuritis. The Optic Neuritis Study Group. N Engl J Med. 1992;326(9):581-8.
34. Keltner JL, Johnson CA, Spurr JO, et al. Baseline visual field profile of optic neuritis. The experience of the optic neuritis treatment trial. Optic Neuritis Study Group. Arch Ophthalmol. 1993;111(2):231-4.
35. Beck RW, Trobe JD. What we have learned from the Optic Neuritis Treatment Trial. Ophthalmology. 1995;102(10):1504-8.
36. Beck RW, Arrington J, Murtagh FR, et al. Brain magnetic resonance imaging in acute optic neuritis. Experience of the Optic Neuritis Study Group. Arch Neurol. 1993;50(8):841-6.
37. Rizzo JF, Andreoli CM, Rabinov JD. Use of magnetic resonance imaging to differentiate optic neuritis and nonarteritic anterior ischemic optic neuropathy. Ophthalmology. 2002;109:1679–84.
38. Optic Neuritis Study Group. Multiple sclerosis risk after optic neuritis: final optic neuritis treatment trial follow-up. Arch Neurol. 2008;65(6):727-32.
39. Chirapapaisan N, Borchert MS. Pediatric optic neuritis. J Med Assoc Thai. 2008;91(3):323-30.
40. Subramanian PS. Pediatric optic neuritis and multiple sclerosis: who is at risk for progression? J AAPOS. 2011;15: 419-20.
41. Tenembaum S, Chitnis T, Ness J, et al. Acute disseminated encephalomyelitis. Neurology. 2007;68(16 Suppl 2):S23-36.
42. Wingerchuk DM, Lennon VA, Pittock SJ, et al. Revised diagnostic criteria for neuromyelitis optica. Neurology. 2006;66(10):1485-9.
43. Wingerchuk DM, Banwell B, Bennett JL, et al. International consensus diagnostic criteria for neuromyelitis optica spectrum disorders. Neurology. 2015;85:177-89.
44. Jarius S, Frederikson J, Waters P, et al. Frequency and prognostic impact of antibodies to aquaporin-4 in patients with optic neuritis. J Neurol Sci. 2010;298(1-2):158-62.
45. Akman-Demir G, Tüzün E, Waters P, et al. Prognostic implications of aquaporin-4 antibody status in neuromyelitis optica patients. J Neurol. 2011;258(3):464-70.
46. Sato DK, Callegaro D, Lana-Peixoto MA, et al. Distinction between MOG antibody-positive and AQP4 antibody-positive NMO spectrum disorders. Neurology. 2014;82(6):474-81.
47. Min JH, Kim BJ, Lee KH. Development of extensive brain lesions following fingolimod (FTY720) treatment in a patient with neuromyelitis optica spectrum disorder. Mult Scler. 2012;18(1):113-5.
48. Trebst C, Jarius S, Berthele A, et al. Update on the diagnosis and treatment of neuromyelitis optica: recommendations of the Neuromyelitis Optica Study Group (NEMOS). J Neurol. 2014;261(1):1-16.
49. Kidd D, Burton B, Plant GT, et al. Chronic relapsing inflammatory optic neuropathy (CRION). Brain. 2003;126(Pt 2):276-84.
50. Newman NJ, Lott MT, Wallace DC. The clinical characteristics of pedigrees of Leber's hereditary optic neuropathy with the 11778 mutation. Am J Ophthalmol. 1991;111(6):750-62.
51. Johns DR, Heher KL, Miller NR. Leber's hereditary optic neuropathy. Clinical manifestations of the 14484 mutation. Arch Ophthalmol. 1993;111(4):495-8.
52. Johns DR, Smith KH, Miller NR. Leber's hereditary optic neuropathy. Clinical manifestations of the 3460 mutation. Arch Ophthalmol. 1992;110(11):1577-81.
53. Klopstock T, Yu-Wai-Man P, Dimitriadis K, et al. A randomized placebo-controlled trial of idebenone in Leber's hereditary optic neuropathy. Brain. 2011;134(Pt 9):2677-86.
54. Sharma P, Sharma R. Toxic optic neuropathy. Indian J of Ophthalmol. 2011;59(2):137-41.

Chapter 93 Neuroimaging in Neuro-ophthalmology

Zoë R Williams, Edward P Lin

INTRODUCTION

Although the location of a neuro-ophthalmic lesion is frequently apparent by examination, the etiology is often unknown. There are several diagnostic studies available in clinic including visual field testing, optical coherence tomography, fluorescein angiography and ultrasound, which can narrow the differential diagnosis of afferent visual pathway disorders. Orbital ultrasound can be useful for identifying optic disk drusen, assessing for papilledema with the 30° test[1,2] and distinguishing solid from fluid-filled orbital lesions. However, in many afferent and efferent visual disorders, neuroimaging is necessary to determine the etiology, exclude potentially life-threatening causes and provide prognostic information.

Orbital ultrasound is a noninvasive technique in which reflected sound waves can be used to determine the optic nerve width on a scan based on low optic nerve reflectivity and high reflectivity of the optic nerve sheath.[2] The 30° test requires a scan measurements in primary gaze followed by 30° of eccentric viewing to assess for a 10% decrease in optic nerve width reflecting cerebrospinal fluid space compression.[1,2] B scan can be used to assess for optic nerve head abnormalities such as hyper-reflective optic disk drusen or anterior optic nerve tumors.[1,2]

Beyond ultrasonography, computed tomography (CT) and magnetic resonance imaging (MRI) are cross-sectional imaging (CSI) modalities that provide a complete assessment of the orbits, skull base and intracranial contents. The objectives of CSI are to increase spatial resolution, maximize contrast between different types of tissues, amplify signal to noise, capture contrast agent enhancement, acquire images in a reasonable time, and adhere to as low as reasonably achievable (ALARA) principles minimizing radiation exposure. CT and MRI often complement each other and offer distinct advantages and disadvantages. CT, in general, offers greater spatial resolution, while MR provides superior contrast resolution.

COMPUTED TOMOGRAPHY

Overview

Computed tomography images are acquired by transmitting X-rays, a form of ionizing electromagnetic radiation, through the body and detecting the residual energy after exiting the body. The amount of residual energy in a volume of tissue is translated mathematically into an *attenuation coefficient*. Each CT image becomes a map of attenuation coefficients. Attenuations range from –1000 Hounsfield Units (HU) for air to more than 400 HU for bone (Table 93.1). Iodinated contrast may be given intravenously when needed.

The main disadvantage of CT is its use of ionizing radiation. The lenses are the dose-limiting structure of the head and neck and receive 50–100 mGy per CT. A lifetime accumulation of greater than 8 sieverts (Sv) may result in cataracts.[3] Current guidelines limit CT use in pediatric patients given their greater sensitivity to radiation effects. CT is also limited in evaluation of posterior fossa lesions due to beam hardening artifact.[4]

Clinical Application

Computed tomography is the preferred modality for evaluating bony structures and detecting calcifications.[5]

Table 93.1: Sample attenuation values (in Hounsfield Units—HU) in CT imaging.

Substance	Attenuation	
Air	–1000 HU	Dark ↑
Fat	–50–100 HU	
Water	0 HU	
Muscle	40 HU	↓ Bright
Blood	30–45 HU	
Contrast	130 HU	
Bone	400+ HU	

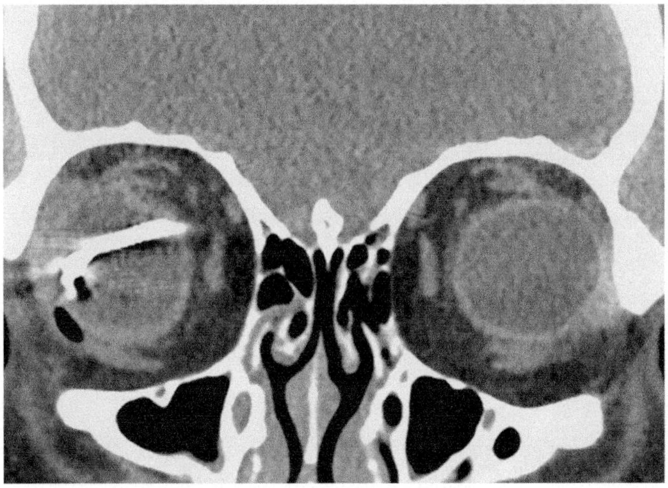

Fig. 93.1: Coronal CT image demonstrates an intraocular metallic foreign body with globe rupture, right eye.
Source: Mina Chung, MD.

In patients who are pacemaker dependent or have other implanted electronic devices, metallic aneurysm clips, or ferromagnetic foreign bodies (Fig. 93.1), CT is performed due to potential malfunction of the implanted device and propensity for heating and movement of ferromagnetic materials with MRI. CT is more accessible and inexpensive relative to MR, and can be acquired within seconds, reducing artifact caused by motion. As such, CT is most often employed in the acute setting, especially with trauma, stroke, intracranial hemorrhage and inflammation. Contrast administration is not required for evaluation of: orbital fractures (Figs. 93.2A to C), infarcts (Figs. 93.3A to C) (although CT perfusion and CT angiography (CTA) require contrast), intracranial hemorrhage (Fig. 93.4), extraocular muscle enlargement secondary to thyroid eye disease (Figs. 93.5A and B), optic neuropathy secondary to apical

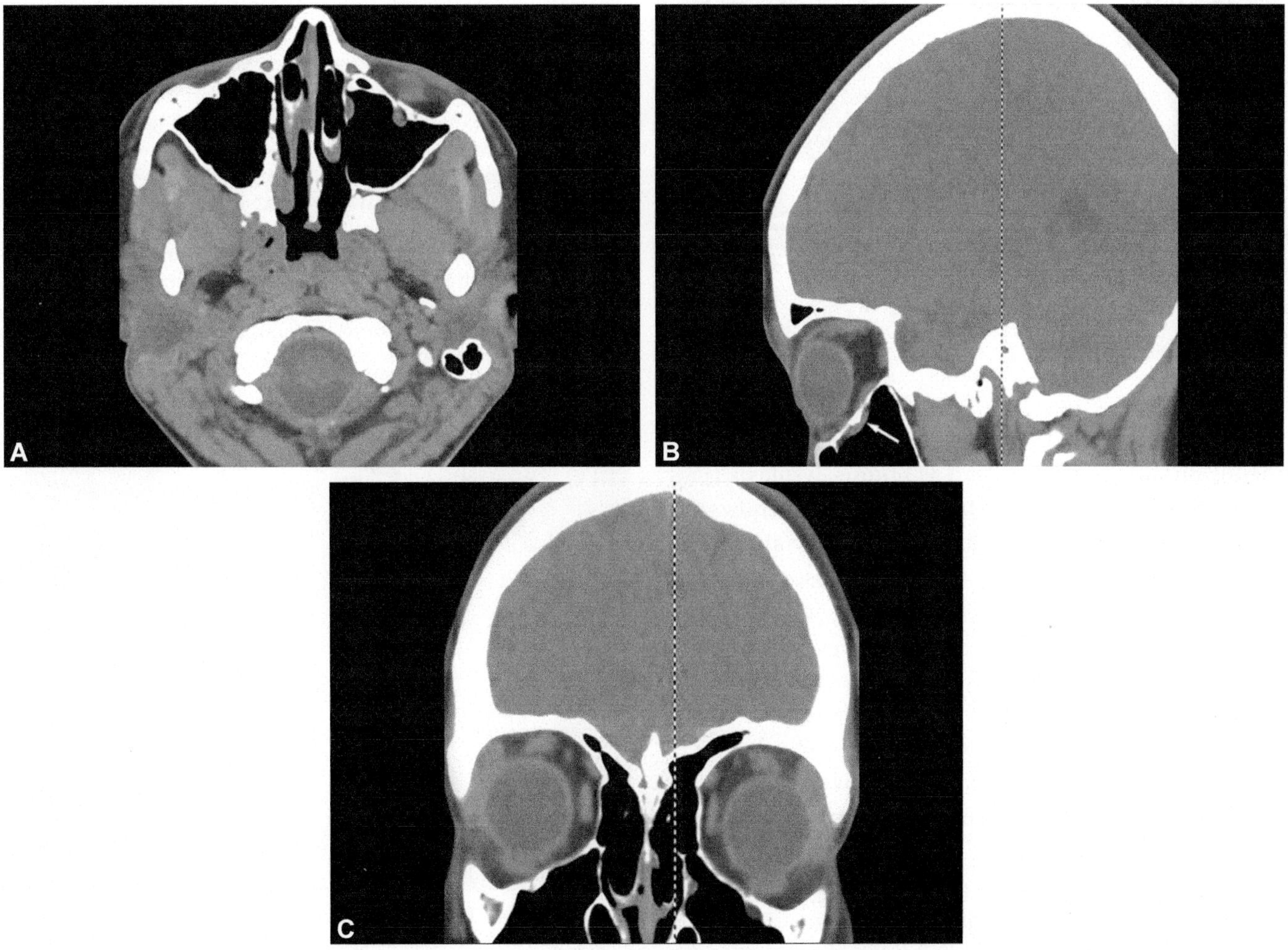

Figs. 93.2A to C: (A) Non-contrast orbital CT with axial; (B) Sagittal; and (C) Coronal views showing entrapment of the left inferior rectus muscle (arrow—B) in a patient with a white eyed blow-out fracture presenting with vertical diplopia.
Source: Mithra Gonzalez, MD.

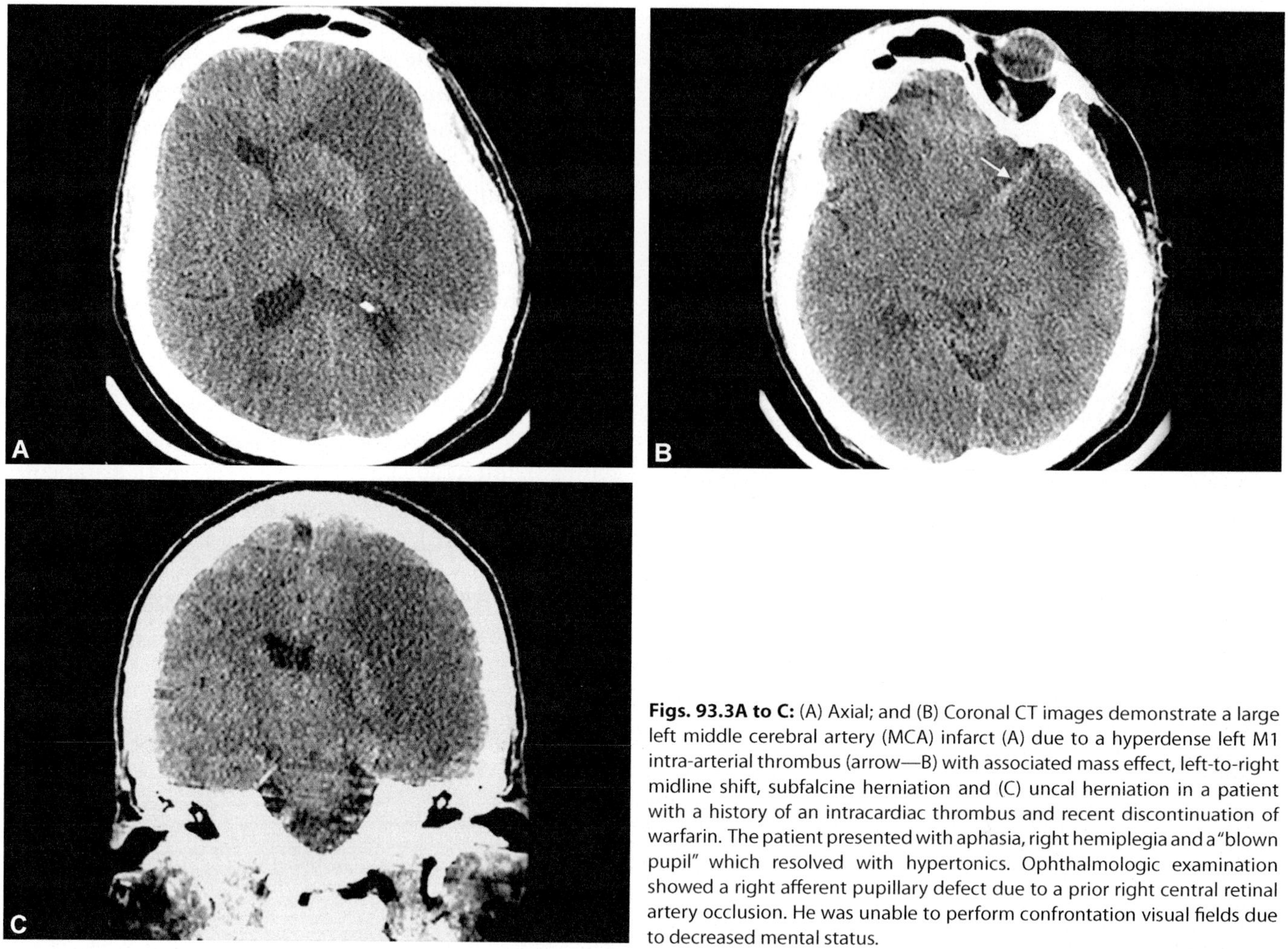

Figs. 93.3A to C: (A) Axial; and (B) Coronal CT images demonstrate a large left middle cerebral artery (MCA) infarct (A) due to a hyperdense left M1 intra-arterial thrombus (arrow—B) with associated mass effect, left-to-right midline shift, subfalcine herniation and (C) uncal herniation in a patient with a history of an intracardiac thrombus and recent discontinuation of warfarin. The patient presented with aphasia, right hemiplegia and a "blown pupil" which resolved with hypertonics. Ophthalmologic examination showed a right afferent pupillary defect due to a prior right central retinal artery occlusion. He was unable to perform confrontation visual fields due to decreased mental status.

compression from thyroid eye disease (Figs. 93.6A and B), osteodystrophic processes such as fibrous dysplasia (Figs. 93.7A and B) or sphenoid wing dysplasia, mineralization within tumors (Figs. 93.8A and B), or bony alterations (e.g. scalloping or destructive changes) associated with underlying neoplastic or infectious (especially fungal) disease processes. Thyroid eye disease (Figs. 93.5A and B) is distinguished from orbital myositis by sparing of the tendinous insertions; however, if there is a clinical suspicion for orbital pseudotumor based on associated eye pain or eyelid edema, use of contrast is indicated as orbital myositis will show diffuse enlargement and enhancement of the involved extraocular muscles.

Orbital inflammation or infection including subperiosteal abscess (Fig. 93.9) and orbital pseudotumor (Fig. 93.10) benefits from intravenous contrast administration, which improves contrast resolution and delineates vascular

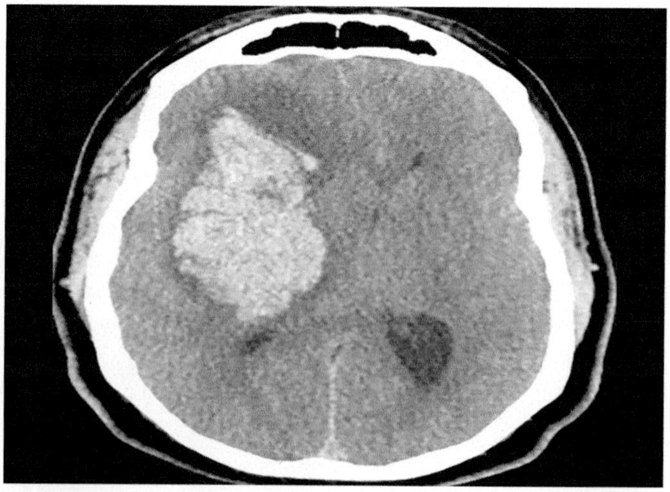

Fig. 93.4: Axial CT image reveals a large intraparenchymal hemorrhage arising from the left basal ganglia and extending into the left frontal and parietal lobes, with associated surrounding edema, midline shift and subfalcine herniation.

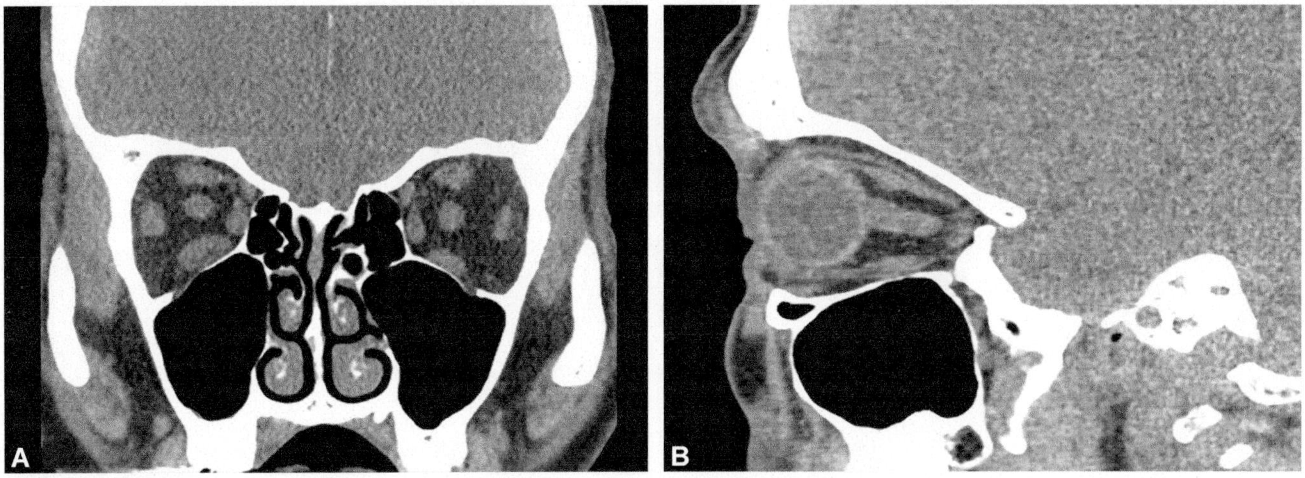

Figs. 93.5A and B: (A) Coronal; and (B) Sagittal CT images demonstrate enlargement of the right inferior rectus muscle with sparing of the tendinous insertion consistent with thyroid eye disease in a patient presenting with vertical diplopia.

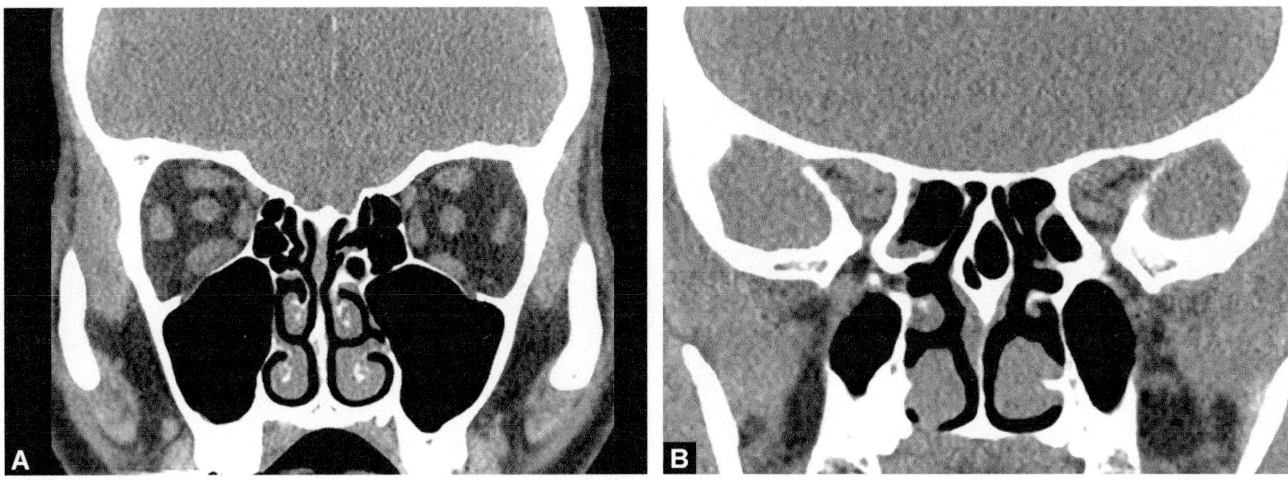

Figs. 93.6A and B: Two coronal CT images reveal bilateral extraocular muscle enlargement; greater on the right, with right apical compression causing a compressive right optic neuropathy. The patient had marked improvement in her vision after urgent orbital decompression.

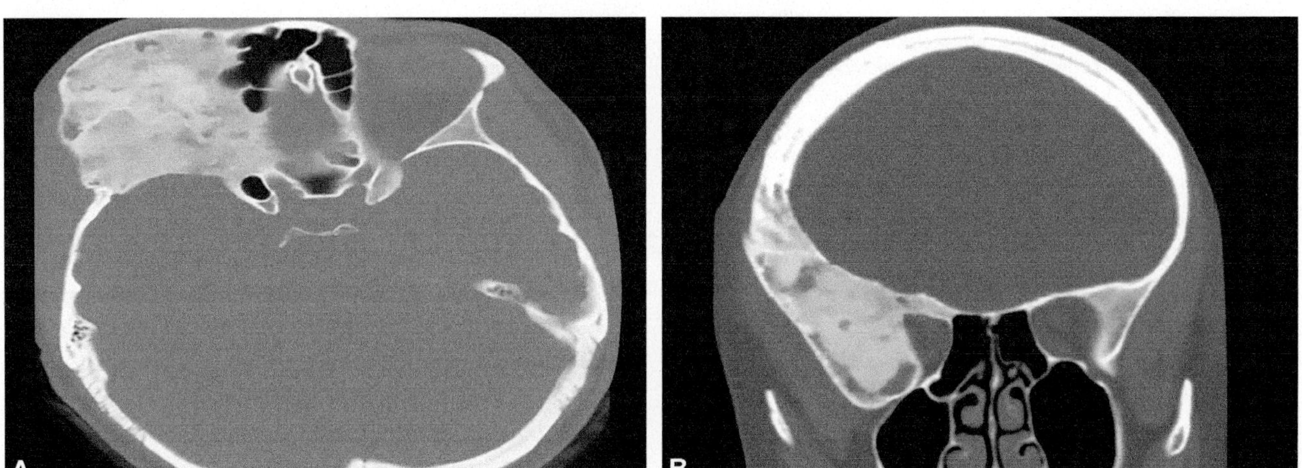

Figs. 93.7A and B: (A) Axial; and (B) Coronal CT images in a patient with fibrous dysplasia exhibit expansile ground-glass attenuation of the right frontal and sphenoid bones without narrowing of the optic canal. No clinical evidence of compressive optic neuropathy.

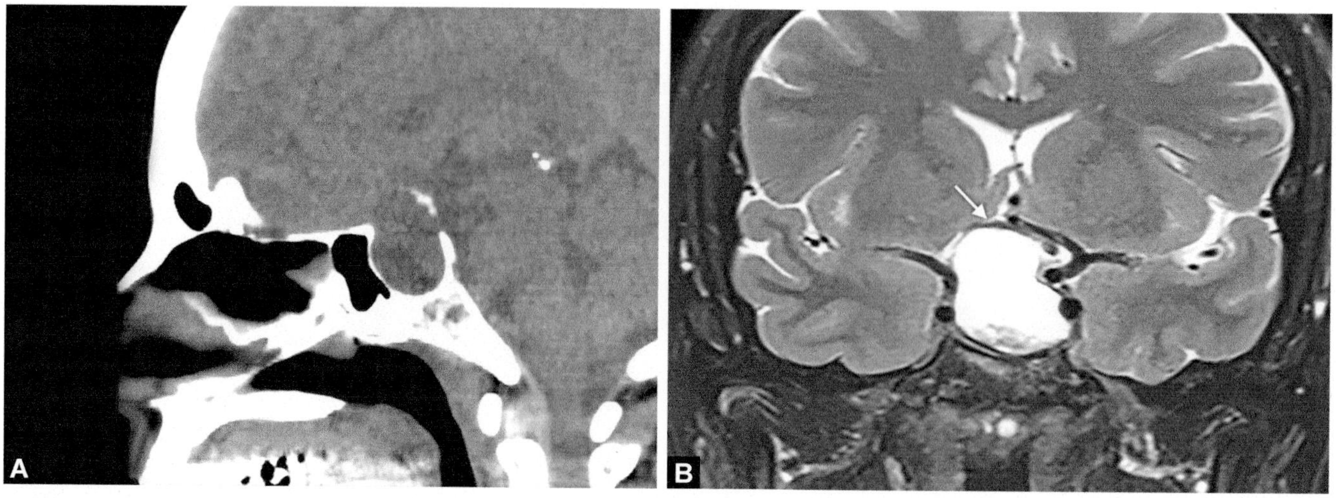

Figs. 93.8A and B: (A) Sagittal CT image and (B) coronal T2-weighted imaging (WI) reveals a sellar/suprasellar T2 hyperintense cystic adamantinomatous craniopharyngioma with peripheral calcifications, expansion of the sella turcica, and compression of the right optic nerve and optic chiasm (arrow-B) in a patient presenting with a right optic neuropathy and bitemporal visual field defects.

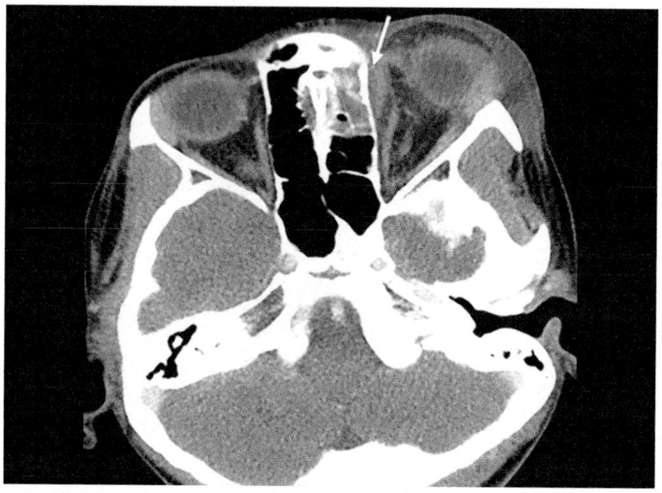

Fig. 93.9: Axial contrast-enhanced CT image demonstrates acute inflammatory changes of the left anterior ethmoid air cells with associated left subperiosteal abscess (arrow) and orbital cellulitis in an 11-year-old boy presenting with left eyelid edema, proptosis and restricted ocular motility.
Source: Mithra Gonzalez, MD.

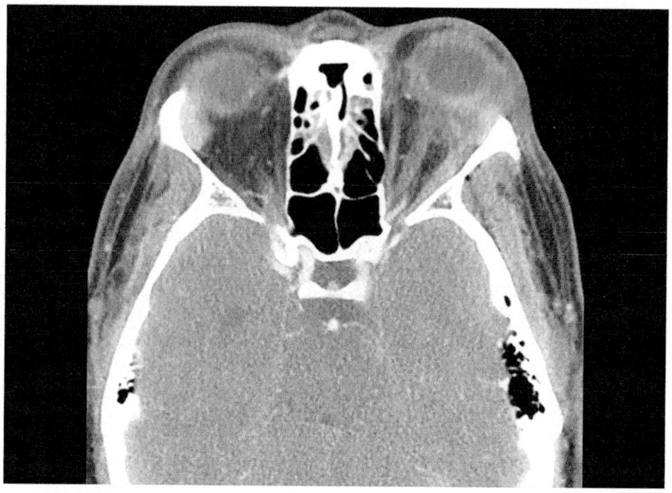

Fig. 93.10: Axial contrast-enhanced CT images reveals inflammatory changes centered around the left lateral rectus muscle and lacrimal gland in addition to the left orbital apex in a patient presenting with left eyelid edema and proptosis.
Source: Steven Feldon, MD.

structures. Contrast enhancement on neuroimaging denotes disruption of the blood brain barrier.[6] Contrast is also indicated for evaluation of orbital masses (Fig. 93.11), as enhancement properties can be useful in formulation of a differential diagnosis prior to biopsy, surgical resection, or radiation therapy. Optic nerve sheath meningiomas classically show the "tram track sign" with hyperdensity adjacent to the optic nerve (corresponding to the optic nerve sheath) and hypodensity of the nerve itself.[7,8] CT is useful in demonstrating bony erosion typical of adenoid cystic carcinoma of the lacrimal gland, rhabdomyosarcoma, metastases, and rarely high-grade lymphoma.[9] Bone window images on CT may show expansion of the optic canal in optic nerve glioma.[10,11] Perineural spread (Figs. 93.12A to C) typically manifests on CT as neural foraminal widening with or without loss of adjacent fat rather than enhancement along the affected nerve as demonstrated on contrast MRI.[12-14] CT and MRI are frequently used as parallel studies in evaluating perineural spread with tumor extension to the orbit and/or skull base.[14] For previously treated disease, positron emission tomography (PET) CT evaluating for increased metabolic activity serves as a useful adjunct in assessment of suspected recurrence or residual disease.[12]

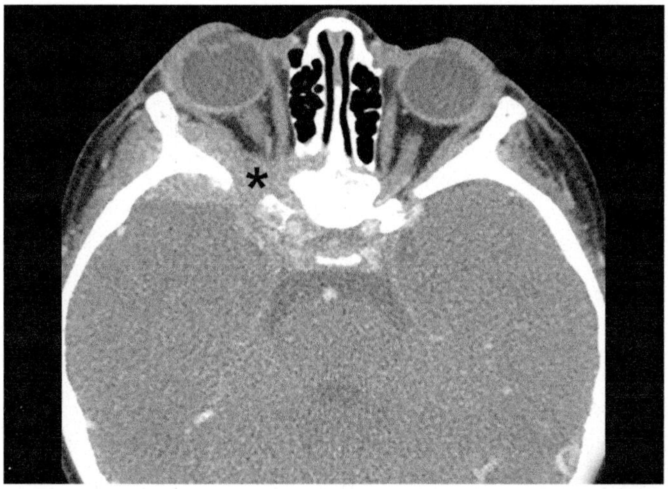

Fig. 93.11: Axial CT image in a 20-month-old male with metastatic neuroblastoma, presenting with proptosis and limited movement, reveals a transpatial soft tissue mass involving the sphenoid, with extension into the orbits bilaterally, greater on the right (asterisk).

MAGNETIC RESONANCE IMAGING

Overview

Magnetic resonance imaging creates images using nuclear magnetic resonance (NMR) principles which rely on protons (hydrogen nuclei) aligning in a magnetic field.[15] An antenna transmits nonionizing electromagnetic radiation to a patient lying within a high field strength magnet, whereupon the energy is absorbed causing excitation of the hydrogen nuclei, re-emitted by tissue as the nuclei relax, and received by the antenna.[15] A computer translates the raw data, which can be acquired slice by slice or by an entire volume (volumetric or three-dimensional (3-D) acquisition), into MR images. 3D acquisition creates isotropic voxels, which allow source images to be reformatted into different planes without compromising spatial resolution. Spin-echo (SE) MR sequences include

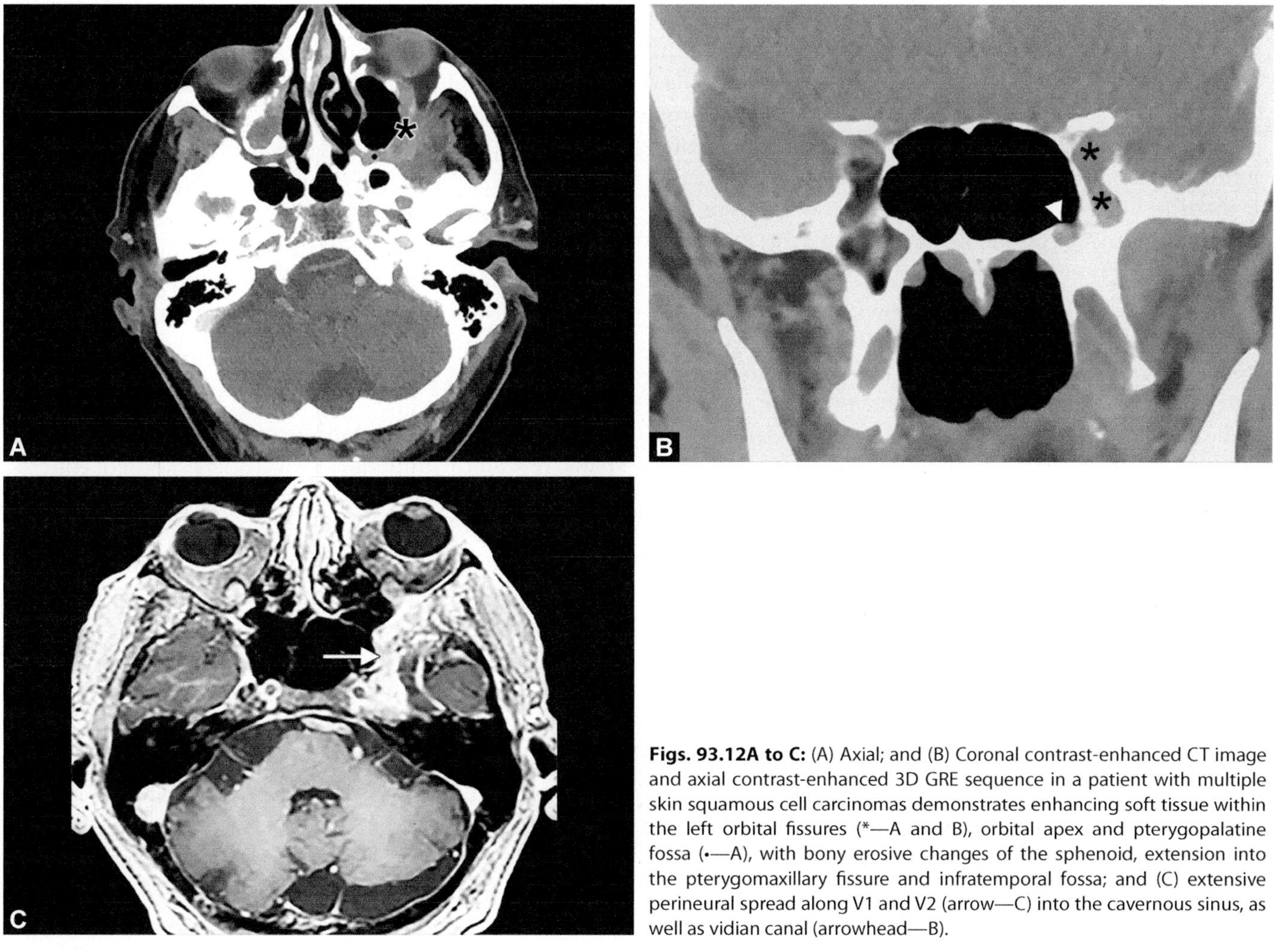

Figs. 93.12A to C: (A) Axial; and (B) Coronal contrast-enhanced CT image and axial contrast-enhanced 3D GRE sequence in a patient with multiple skin squamous cell carcinomas demonstrates enhancing soft tissue within the left orbital fissures (*—A and B), orbital apex and pterygopalatine fossa (•—A), with bony erosive changes of the sphenoid, extension into the pterygomaxillary fissure and infratemporal fossa; and (C) extensive perineural spread along V1 and V2 (arrow—C) into the cavernous sinus, as well as vidian canal (arrowhead—B).

Table 93.2: Sample MR protocols for orbital and intracranial imaging without and with contrast. Sequences in parentheses are an alternative to the Sag 3-D T1-fat suppression (FS).

Region	Orbits	Orbits	Brain
Indication	CN, diplopia, mass	Inflammation	Routine
Pre-contrast	Sag T1	Sag T1	Sag T1
	Cor T1	Ax T1	Ax T1
	Ax T2	Ax T2-FS	Ax T2
	Cor T2	Cor T2 FS	Ax T2 FLAIR
	Cor T2 FS	Sag 3D T2 FLAIR	Ax SWI
	Ax DWI	Ax DWI	Ax DTI
			Ax 3-D SS-GRE*
Post-contrast	Sag 3-D T1-FS	Sag 3-D T1-FS	Sag 3-D T1-FS
	(Ax and Cor T1-FS)	(Ax and Cor T1-FS)	Ax IR-SPGR

*3-D state gradient echo (SS-GRE) can be added to evaluate the cisternal segments of the cranial nerves.

T1, T2, T2 fluid-attenuated inversion recovery (FLAIR) and fat suppressed sequences (Table 93.2).

Other important MR sequences include gradient echo (GE) and diffusion weighted imaging (DWI) (Table 93.2). GE sequences obtain signal by manipulating local gradients as opposed to transmitting electromagnetic radiation. GE sequences are diverse and can capture T1 as well as T2 (more accurately T2*) signal, depending on how the sequence is created. GE sequences are useful in detecting mineralization and blood products, and can be constructed to provide high spatial resolution T1 and T2-weighted imaging (WI) using volumetric acquisition.

DWI reflects the diffusivity of hydrogen protons in tissue and can be measured by applying opposing gradients in at least 3 different directions. Highly mobile hydrogen molecules, such as in cerebrospinal fluid, will demonstrate high diffusivity, whereas stationary hydrogen molecules, such as in an acute infarct or abscess, will exhibit low diffusivity. DWI is useful in depicting acute or subacute infarcts, abscesses, epidermoid cysts, and hypercellular tumors, such as lymphoma, all of which show diffusion restriction. When assessing for infection or inflammation in suspected encephalitis, DWI and apparent diffusion coefficient (ADC) sequences are helpful in demonstrating restricted diffusion.[6] T2 hyperintensity of the optic nerve on DWI has been shown to be a specific although relatively insensitive marker for traumatic optic neuropathy,[16] which may show no abnormality on conventional MRI in the acute phase of vision loss.[17] Gadolinium, a paramagnetic contrast agent, may be administered intravenously when needed.

With its superior contrast resolution and tissue characterization, MRI is ideal for evaluation of most intraorbital and intracranial processes. MR orbit protocols can be tailored to specific indications, although for simplicity, most diseases can be assessed by two general protocols (Table 93.2). MR brain protocols are also designed to address specific indications, although a general protocol is found in Table 93.2. Certain sequences, such as 3-D steady state gradient echo (3-D SS-GRE) sequences, can be added to evaluate the cranial nerves.

MRI is more susceptible to artifact from motion, paramagnetic substances such as surgical hardware, and air/bone interfaces. Acquisition times are longer and sometimes require sedation in pediatric populations. Bony changes and calcifications may be more difficult to detect and interpret, although newer sequences such as susceptibility WI (SWI) are becoming increasingly sensitive.

Clinical Application

T1-WI provides great anatomical detail due to superior spatial resolution properties. T2-WI offers excellent contrast resolution and can be useful in detecting pathology, which often exhibits high T2 signal intensity. Sample T1 and T2 values are provided in Table 93.3. Contrast-enhanced (CE) T1-WI captures intravascular contrast enhancement and extravascular contrast leakage. Contrast enhancement is useful in evaluation of active inflammation, vascular diseases, tumors and perineural spread. These sequences can be modified to suppress fat or water signal with several techniques, such as chemical fat suppression and inversion recovery. While fat suppression reduces spatial resolution and increases susceptibility to artifact, it markedly improves contrast resolution, particularly for T2 and CE-T1 sequences. T2 FLAIR sequences suppress cerebrospinal fluid signal, creating greater contrast

Table 93.3: Examples of different signal intensities on T1 and T2-weighted imaging (WI).

	T1	T2
High	Fat, proteinaceous substances, subacute hemorrhage, mineralization, slow vascular flow, gadolinium contrast	Water, gliosis, late subacute hemorrhage, fat
Low	Water, calcifications, hemosiderin, high vascular flow	Proteinaceous substances, calcifications, hypercellular tumors, early subacute hemorrhage, hemosiderin, high vascular flow

resolution of abnormal white matter changes, especially adjacent to the ventricles. Performing T2 FLAIR sequences following contrast administration can also accentuate leptomeningeal and pachymeningeal enhancement.

Depending on the suspected location of optic nerve pathology, an appropriate imaging protocol would include MRI orbits without and with gadolinium (for intraocular, intraorbital or intracanalicular pathology) and/or MRI brain without and with gadolinium (for intracranial pathology). The angulation of the slices is different for MRI orbits (negative angulation) versus MRI brain (positive angulation); thus, an MRI brain does not include imaging of the entire course of the optic nerve within the orbit. Weber et al. describe the Massachusetts Eye and Ear Infirmary optic nerve imaging protocol as: 3 mm coronal short tau inverse recovery (STIR), axial T1, axial T1 fat suppressed with contrast, and coronal T1 non-fat suppressed images with contrast[10] to prevent artifact introduced by fat suppression from masking pathology.

Optic Nerve Tumors

Magnetic resonance imaging is the preferred imaging modality for optic nerve tumors as MRI can differentiate the optic nerve from the perioptic subarachnoid space and nerve sheath.[10] Optic nerve gliomas classically appear as a kinking or fusiform thickening of the optic nerve or, if there is extension through the optic canal, a dumbbell enlargement of the optic nerve which is hypo- or isointense on T1W and hyperintense on T2W MRI with variable degrees of enhancement.[8,10,11,18-20] In some studies, the degree of glioma enhancement has been correlated with propensity for tumor growth[8,10] although this is somewhat controversial.[18] Optic pathway gliomas may occur in the optic nerves, chiasm, optic tracts and rarely the optic radiations[19] with a higher incidence in the setting of neurofibromatosis type I (Figs. 93.13A and B). Calcification is atypical.[8,10,18] In contrast to histologically benign optic nerve gliomas that occur in the pediatric age group, malignant optic nerve gliomas usually present in adulthood.[11] Clinical suspicion is essential in guiding the need for biopsy as neuroimaging characteristics are nonspecific and include diffuse optic nerve enlargement and enhancement.[11] Optic nerve sheath meningiomas typically show hypointense signal on T1 and T2-WI,[10] nerve sheath enhancement with fine projections into the orbital fat, and no enhancement of the optic nerve itself.[7,8,10,21]

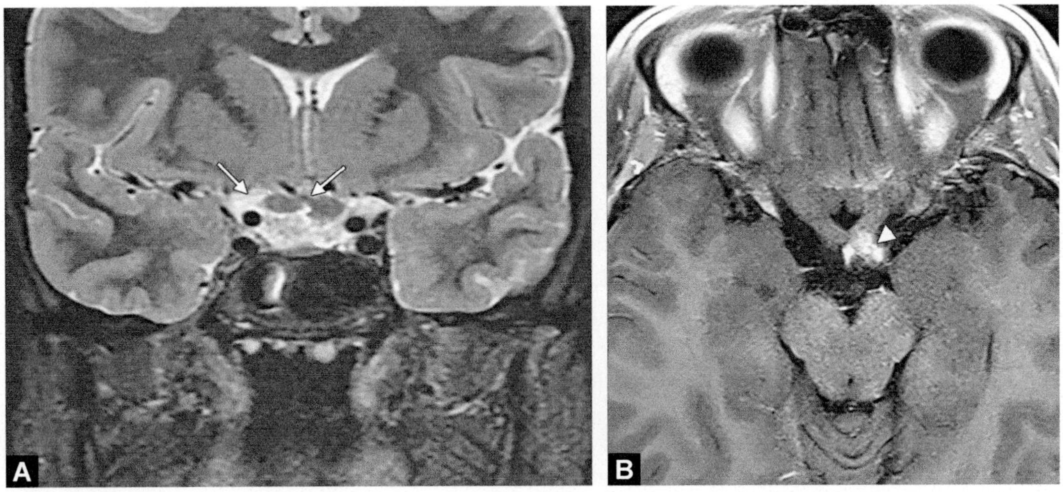

Figs. 93.13A and B: (A) Coronal short tau inverse recovery (STIR); and (B) Axial contrast-enhanced T1- weighted imaging (WI) exhibit bilateral asymmetric enlargement of the optic nerves, chiasm and tracts bilaterally, greater on the left (arrows—A), with associated enhancement of the left optic chiasm and tract (arrowhead—B) in a patient with NF1, bilateral optic neuropathy and a right homonymous hemianopsia.

They can be primary (Fig. 93.14), if arising from arachnoid cap cells within the optic nerve sheath, or secondary (Figs. 93.15A and B), if arising from intracranial dura along the planum sphenoidale.[7,8,11] Optic nerve sheath meningiomas can be associated with pneumosinus dilatans, an expanded adjacent posterior ethmoid and sphenoid sinus.[7]

Although choroidal metastases are not uncommon (Figs. 93.16A and B), metastasis to the optic nerve is quite rare and has been primarily reported with lung and breast cancer.[10,22,23] The appearance can be nonspecific with high T2 signal and diffuse enlargement and enhancement of the optic nerve.[22] More commonly optic nerve extension is

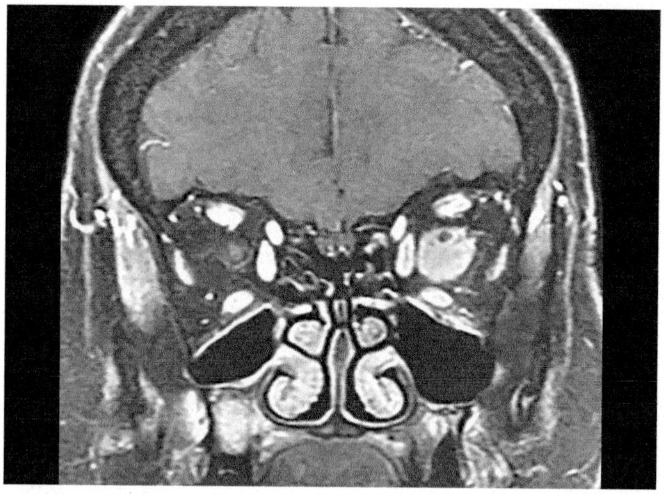

Fig. 93.14: Coronal contrast-enhanced T1-weighted imaging (WI) with fat suppression (FS) reveals an eccentric circumferential enhancing left anterior optic sheath meningioma in a patient presenting with left optic neuropathy, diffuse optic disk edema and macular striae.

seen from primary intraocular tumors such as peripapillary or juxtapapillary uveal melanoma or retinoblastoma (Figs. 93.17A to C).[10] Leukemia, lymphoma and multiple myeloma (Fig. 93.18) may involve the meninges and cause vision loss with radiographic evidence of optic nerve sheath and/or nerve enhancement.[10] Suspected meningeal carcinomatosis is optimally imaged using MRI with FLAIR and contrast enhancement to assess for meningeal enhancement (Figs. 93.19A and B).[10] In addition, lymphoma may involve the optic nerve alone or in association with systemic disease, primary CNS disease, or primary intraocular lymphoma, and demonstrates optic nerve enlargement or sheath enhancement.[23] Primary CNS lymphoma (PCNSL) usually presents as single or multifocal lesions of the thalamus, basal ganglia, periventricular regions, and gray-white matter junction which are either isointense or have an isointense peripheral ring with a hyperintense center on T2-WI and show diffuse or peripheral contrast enhancement (Figs. 93.20A to C).[24]

Chiasmal Lesions

Although clinical variables such as symptomatic vision loss, positive afferent pupillary defect, unilateral optic disk pallor, a complete visual field defect or a field defect denser inferiorly may help to diagnose conditions other than pituitary adenoma,[25] there are also clues on neuroimaging, particularly MRI, as to the underlying etiology of a chiasmal lesion. CT is useful for evaluating acute pituitary apoplexy or assessing for calcification

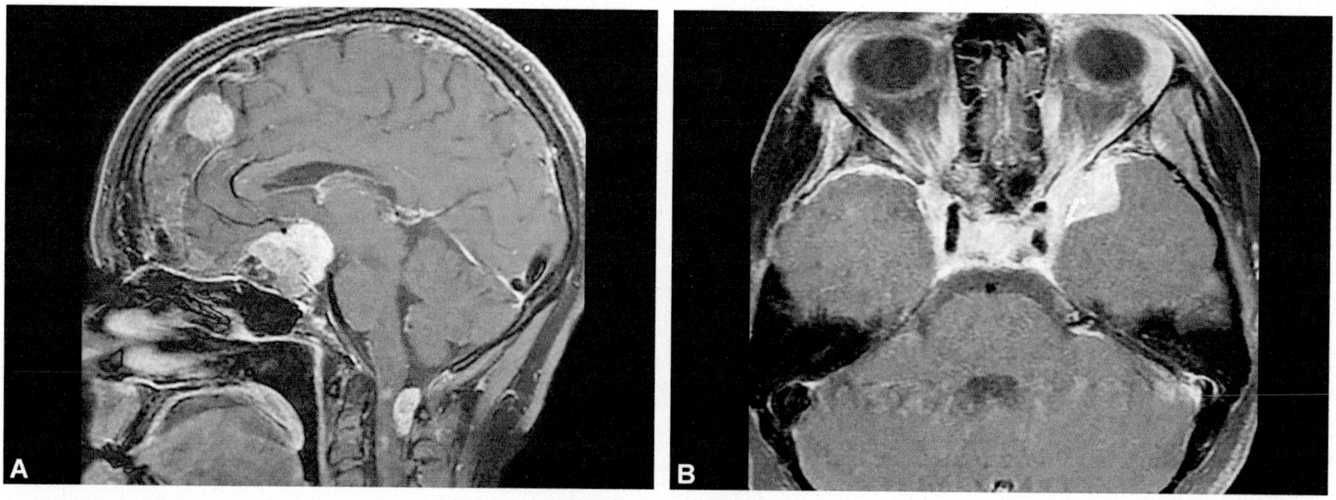

Figs. 93.15 A and B: (A) Sagittal; and (B) Axial T1-weighted imaging (WI) with fat suppression (FS) images demonstrate multiple enhancing meningiomas in a patient with neurofibromatosis type 2 (NF2). The sellar/suprasellar enhancing meningioma extends anteriorly along the planum sphenoidale as well as along the intraorbital optic sheaths bilaterally.

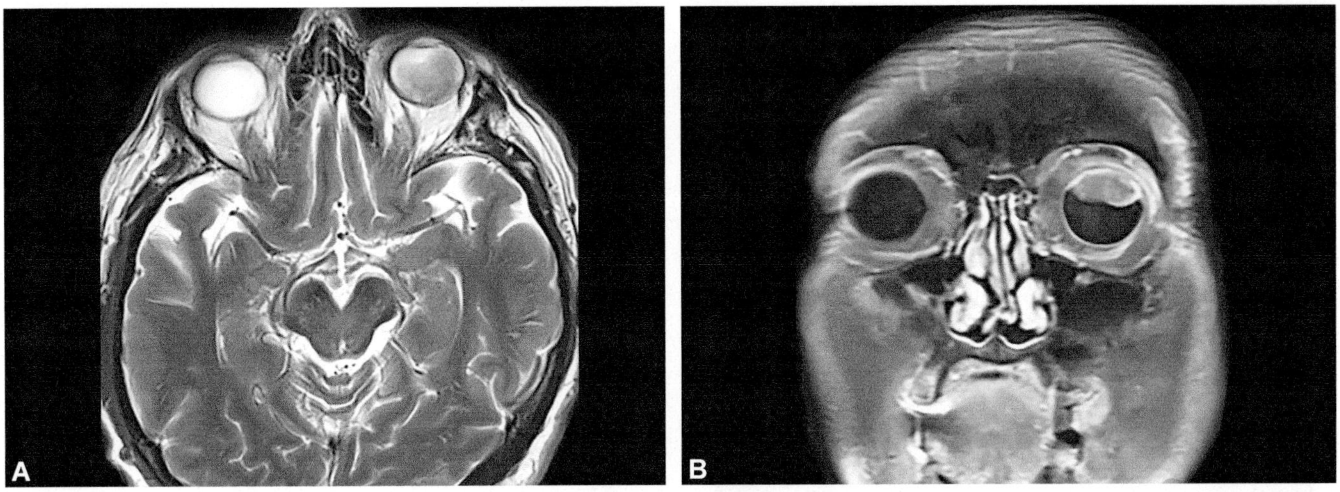

Figs. 93.16A and B: Axial T2-WI and post-contrast coronal T1-weighted imaging (WI) with fat suppression (FS) sequences reveal (A) a large left intraocular mass with T2 hypointense signal; and (B) Mild inhomogeneous enhancement in a patient with known metastatic adenosquamous carcinoma of lung.
Source: Edward Lin, MD.

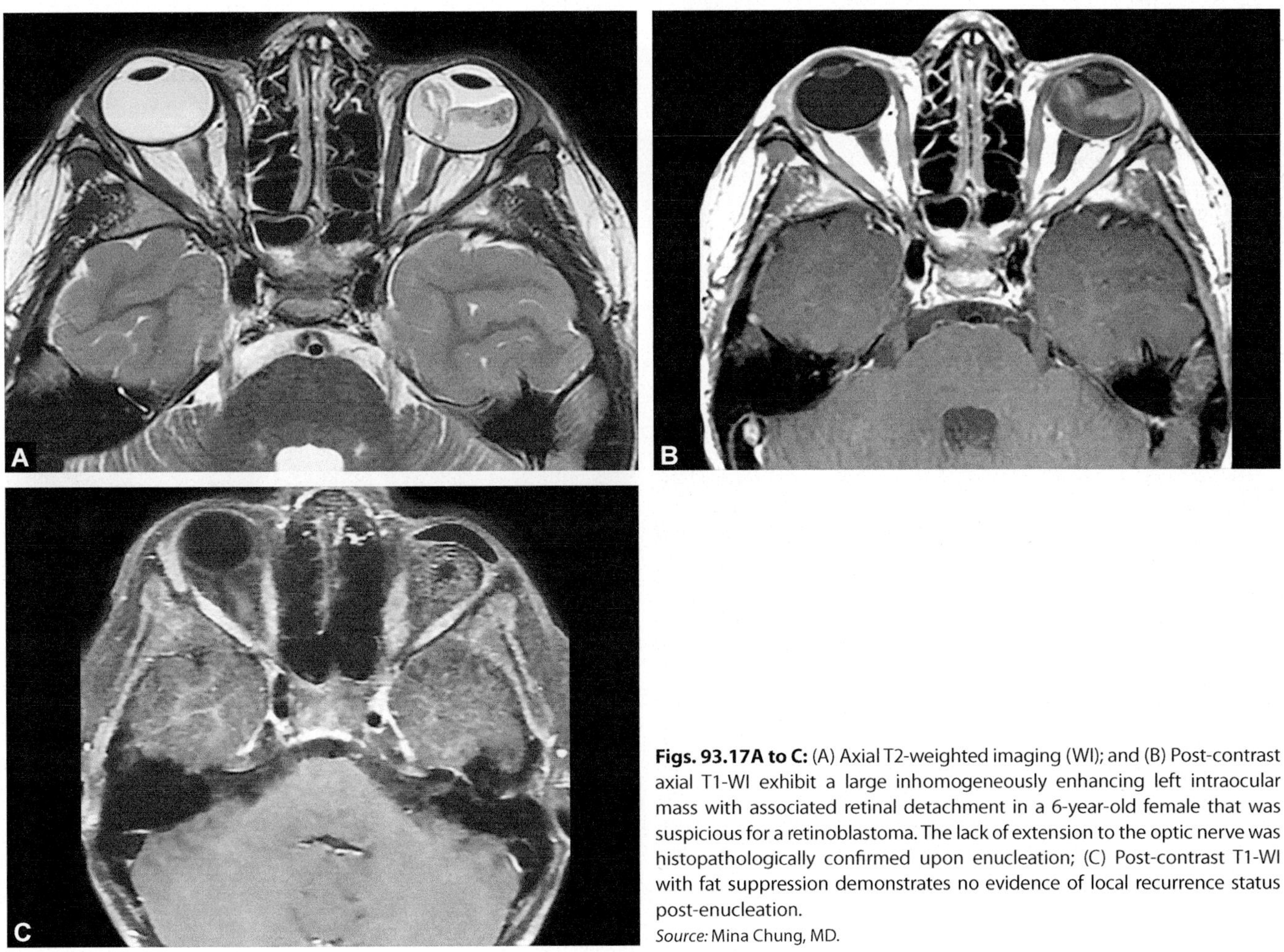

Figs. 93.17A to C: (A) Axial T2-weighted imaging (WI); and (B) Post-contrast axial T1-WI exhibit a large inhomogeneously enhancing left intraocular mass with associated retinal detachment in a 6-year-old female that was suspicious for a retinoblastoma. The lack of extension to the optic nerve was histopathologically confirmed upon enucleation; (C) Post-contrast T1-WI with fat suppression demonstrates no evidence of local recurrence status post-enucleation.
Source: Mina Chung, MD.

in suprasellar lesions such as craniopharyngioma or meningioma (*see* Fig. 93.8) but in general, MRI provides significantly more detail regarding intrinsic (neoplastic, demyelinating, infectious or inflammatory) versus extrinsic compressive (sella/suprasellar tumor, cyst or aneurysm) causes of chiasmal syndromes.[26] Lymphocytic hypophysitis usually demonstrates homogeneous enhancement and is associated with infundibular thickening in more than 90% patients (Figs. 93.21A and B).[27] In differentiating extrinsic tumors causing chiasmal compression, it is helpful to determine whether the pituitary gland can be identified separately from the tumor as in meningioma (Figs. 93.22A and B), assess the pattern of contrast enhancement (typically homogeneous in meningioma versus heterogeneous in pituitary adenoma) (Fig. 93.23) and assess for the presence of a dural tail (Figs. 93.22A and B). Craniopharyngiomas demonstrate calcification in 65% and cystic components in more than 90% of cases[28] and may show peripheral enhancement (Figs. 93.24A and B).[29] MRI enables assessment for optic nerve involvement or compression and tumor extension into the hypothalamus or cavernous sinus.

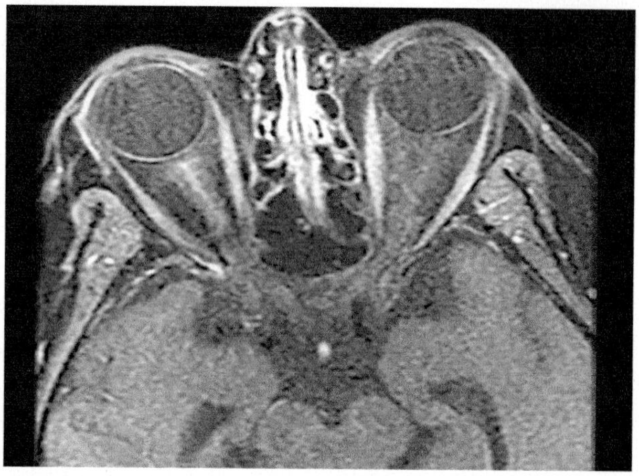

Fig. 93.18: Axial post-contrast T1-weighted imaging (WI) with fat suppression (FS) demonstrates thickening and mild enhancement of the right optic nerve sheath in a patient with a known history of meningeal involvement of multiple myeloma. The patient presented with rapid vision loss and diffuse left optic disk edema with peripapillary hemorrhage consistent with infiltrative optic neuropathy. She had significant visual improvement with orbital radiation but developed a subsequent right infiltrative optic neuropathy with similar imaging findings 7 months later.

Infectious/Inflammatory/ Demyelinating Optic Neuropathies

The imaging findings in optic neuropathies due to neoplastic, infectious, inflammatory and demyelinating processes have significant overlap.[23,30,31] Clinical history and examination therefore remain essential in directing diagnostic workup. Optic nerve and/or optic nerve sheath enhancement has been reported in syphilitic, tuberculous, viral (human immunodeficiency virus (HIV) and cytomegalovirus (CMV)) and fungal optic neuropathies[32-34] which may not be distinguishable by imaging alone from other causes of optic neuritis. Arteritic ischemic optic neuropathy due to giant cell arteritis (GCA) can also demonstrate optic nerve or nerve sheath enhancement and rarely chiasmal enhancement.[35] Neuroimaging is not warranted in suspected GCA, but anterior visual pathway enhancement should not deter clinicians from considering this condition.[35]

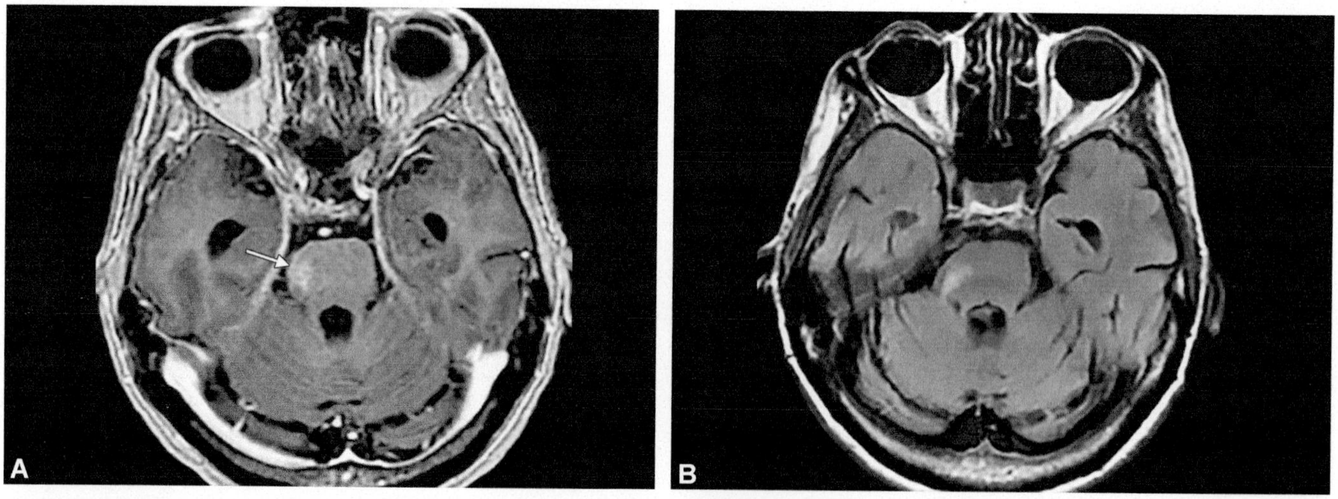

Figs. 93.19A and B: (A) Axial contrast-enhanced three-dimensional gradient recalled echo (3D GRE); and (B) Axial T2 fluid attenuation inversion recovery (FLAIR) images reveal an enhancing right pontine lesion with extension to the right lateral leptomeningeal surface (arrow—A) and corresponding vasogenic edema (B) in a patient with metastatic leptomeningeal carcinomatosis and multiple cranial neuropathies.

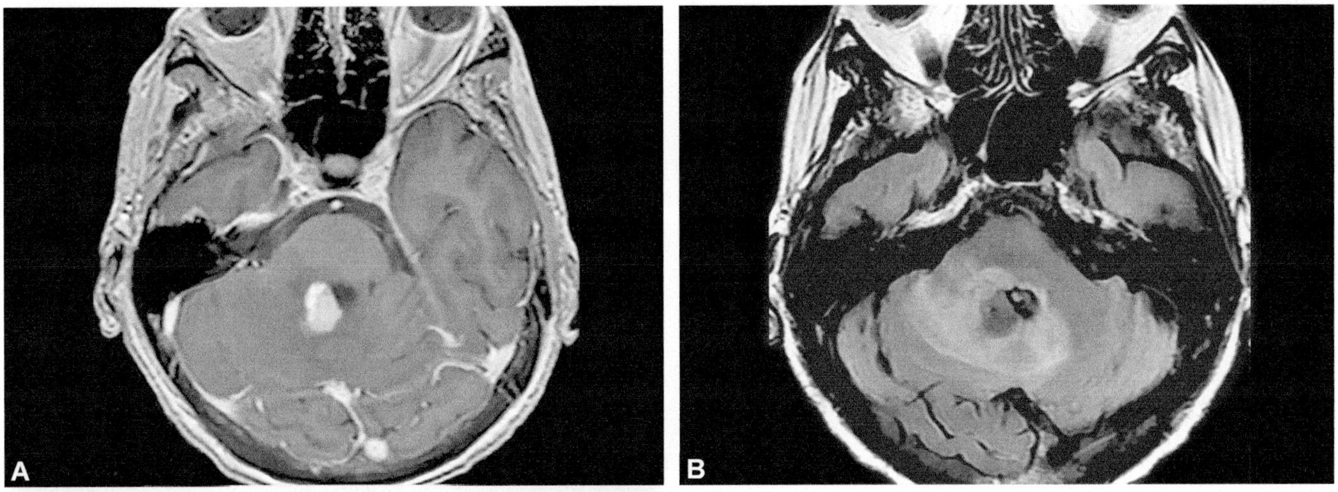

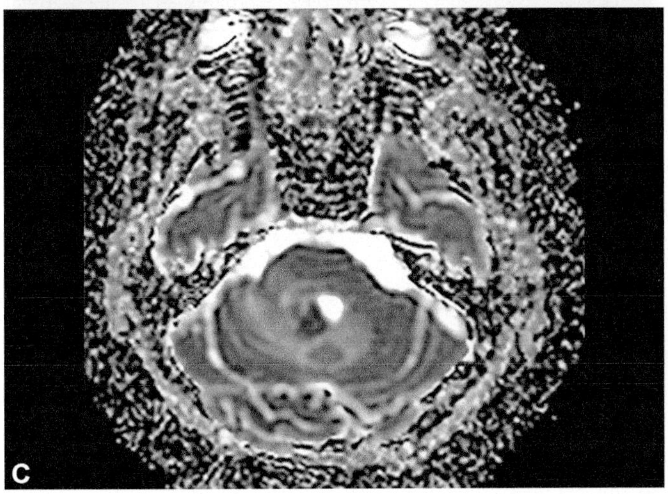

Figs. 93.20A to C: (A) Axial contrast-enhanced three-dimensional gradient recalled echo (3D GRE); (B) Axial T2 fluid attenuation inversion recovery (FLAIR); and (C) Axial apparent diffusion coefficients (ADC) map in a patient with central nervous system (CNS) lymphoma demonstrate an avidly inhomogeneously enhancing periventricular mass adjacent to the fourth ventricle, with surrounding vasogenic edema and corresponding decreased ADC values, reflecting the hypercellular nature of the tumor.
Source: David DiLoreto, MD.

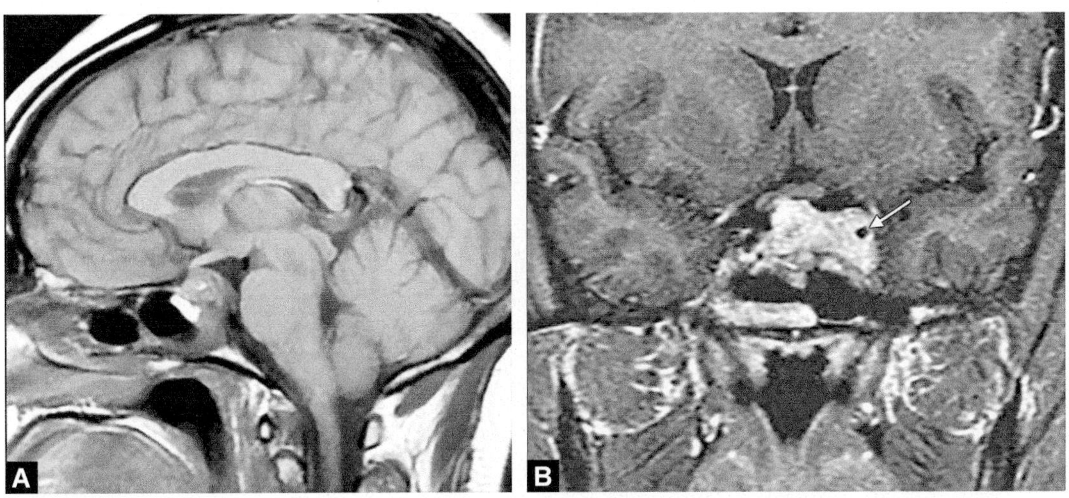

Figs. 93.21A and B: (A) Sagittal T1-weighted imaging (WI); and (B) Coronal post-contrast T1-WI with fat suppression (FS) images demonstrate a sellar/suprasellar inhomogeneously enhancing mass with left cavernous sinus extension, encasement of the left internal carotid artery (ICA) (arrow—B) and chiasmal compression in a patient presenting with diabetes insipidus secondary to lymphocytic hypophysitis.

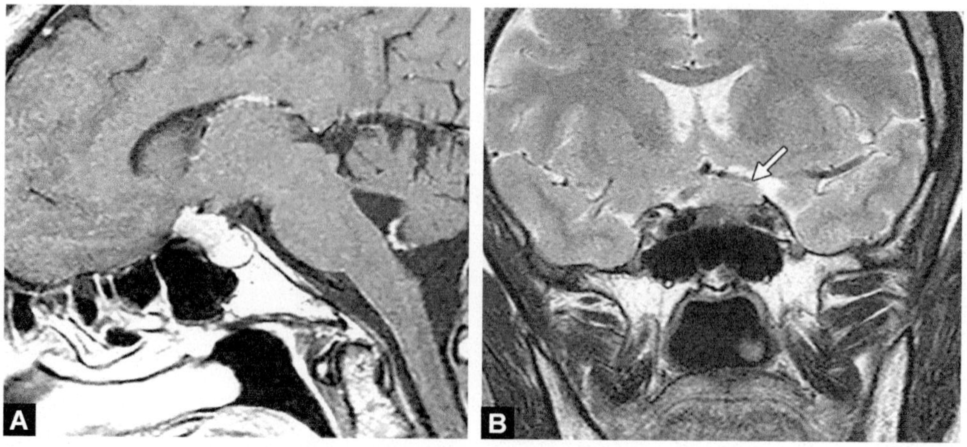

Figs. 93.22A and B: (A) A sagittal contrast-enhanced T1- weighted imaging (WI); and (B) Coronal T2-WI exhibit a sellar/suprasellar meningioma extending along the tuberculum sella with compression of the left optic nerve (arrow—B) in a patient presenting with left optic neuropathy, an inferior altitudinal visual field defect and left optic disk pallor. Pathology confirmed meningioma WHO grade I with atypical features.
Source: Babak Jahromi, MD

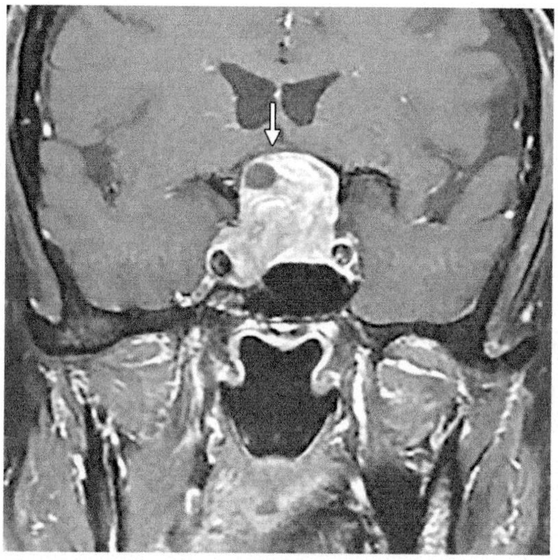

Fig. 93.23: Coronal contrast-enhanced T1-WI with FS images demonstrate a large sellar/suprasellar inhomogeneously enhancing mass with cystic component, extension into the right cavernous sinus, encasement of the right cavernous ICA and chiasmal compression (arrow) in a patient presenting with bitemporal hemianopsia and a left optic neuropathy due to pituitary adenoma.

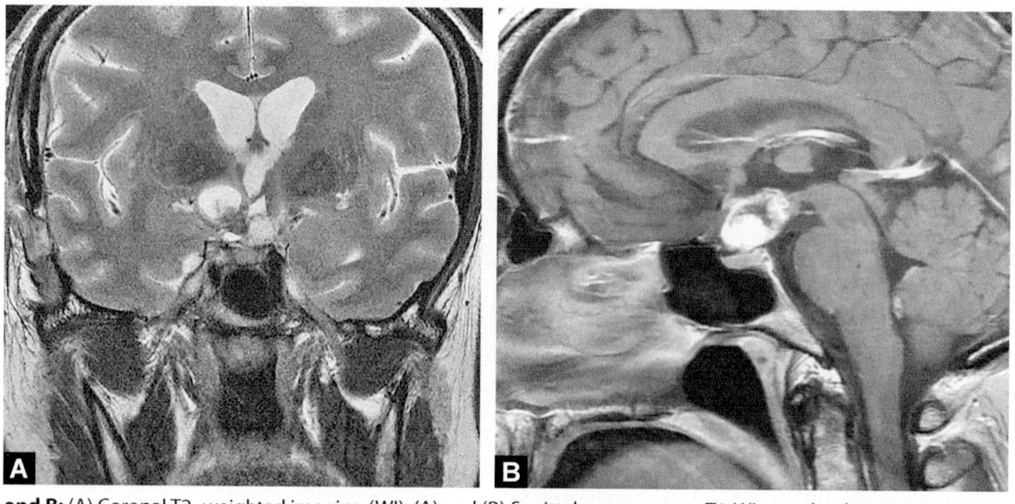

Figs. 93.24A and B: (A) Coronal T2- weighted imaging (WI); (A) and (B) Sagittal post-contrast T1-WI reveals a large complex sellar/suprasellar craniopharyngioma with solid and cystic components, nodular and peripheral enhancement and chiasmal compression.

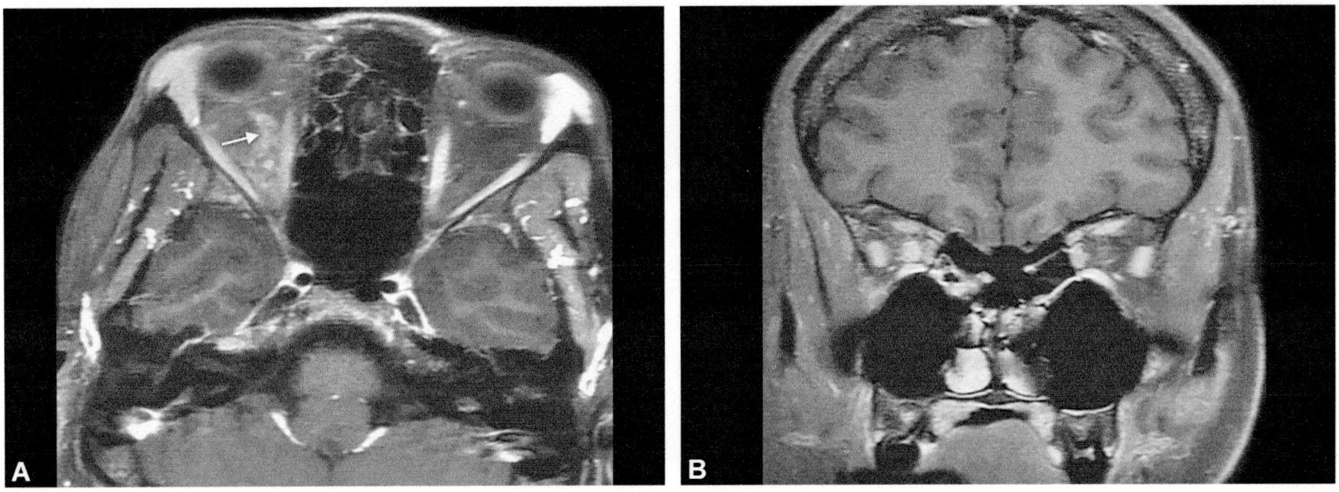

Figs. 93.25A and B: (A) Axial and (B) coronal contrast-enhanced T1-weighted imaging (WI) fat suppression (FS) images demonstrate diffuse enlargement and enhancement of the right optic nerve extending up to the chiasm (not shown) in a patient presenting with vision loss due to sarcoid optic neuropathy.

Often the extent of the optic nerve enhancement can be useful in differentiating typical optic neuritis from atypical cases due to sarcoidosis or neuromyelitis optica (NMO). Significant enlargement of the optic nerve may be seen with neoplastic and inflammatory conditions and is less commonly seen with demyelinating optic neuritis.[10,30] Dedicated orbital multiplanar imaging, including coronal views, is needed to assess for optic nerve enlargement due to volume averaging.[30] Enlargement and enhancement of the prechiasmal optic nerves and/or chiasm can also be seen with radiation induced optic neuropathy however, and is not specific to neoplastic or systemic inflammatory disease.[10]

In patients with optic disk swelling from any cause, lack of optic nerve enhancement is more compatible with posterior uveitis than optic neuritis.[36] Sarcoid optic neuropathy may present as diffuse enlargement of the optic nerve[10] or optic nerve sheath[37] in addition to extensive optic nerve enhancement (Figs. 93.25A and B).[8,37] Accompanying enhancement of the frontobasilar meninges supports a diagnosis of sarcoidosis.[8,37] Chiasmal and optic tract involvement has been reported and lacrimal gland enlargement and enhancement is frequent.[8,10,37] MRI brain with contrast and fat suppressed orbital views is recommended for suspected neurosarcoidosis.[37] Infectious/inflammatory disease presenting as neuroretinitis may show a range of neuroimaging abnormalities including:[38]

- Optic nerve head enhancement
- Retrobulbar optic nerve enhancement
- Diffuse optic nerve enhancement or optic nerve sheath enhancement.

MR findings of optic neuritis include increased T2 hyperintensity and contrast enhancement of the optic nerve without or with mild enlargement of the optic nerve (Figs. 93.26A and B)[8,10] and STIR hyperintensity.[31,39,40] Fast spin-echo (FSE) can be performed with fat saturation and improves resolution compared to STIR with more rapid acquisition time.[39,40] Three-dimensional T2 FLAIR sequences are used in evaluation of optic nerve signal abnormalities, as these are more sensitive than regular STIR and T2 FS sequences.[39-41] These sequences suppress fluid and fat as well.

There are several MR features which are useful in differentiating optic neuritis associated with multiple sclerosis (MS) from neuromyelitis optica (NMO) or neuromyelitis optica spectrum disorder (NMOSD) (*see* Chapter 92).[42] Bilateral optic neuritis or involvement of at least 3 combined segments (orbital, canalicular, cisternal) of both optic nerves, or involvement of the optic chiasm or tracts, and lack of white matter lesions characteristic of MS with dissemination in space supports a diagnosis of NMOSD with 69% sensitivity and 97% specificity.[43] Prior studies have also demonstrated a propensity for more posterior involvement of the visual pathway (i.e. distal optic nerve segment, chiasmal or tract involvement) and more "longitudinally extensive" visual pathway inflammation secondary to NMO (Figs. 93.27A and B) or NMOSD versus MS.[44-46]

White matter lesions due to MS are characteristically hyperintense on T2 or proton density imaging, more than 5 mm in diameter,[47,48] periventricular, juxtacortical or infratentorial,[48-52] and ovoid in appearance.[49,51,53] Similar white matter lesion distribution can be seen in LHON Plus disease, although the lesion characteristics differ in that Dawson fingers are not seen in LHON, and ovoid lesions

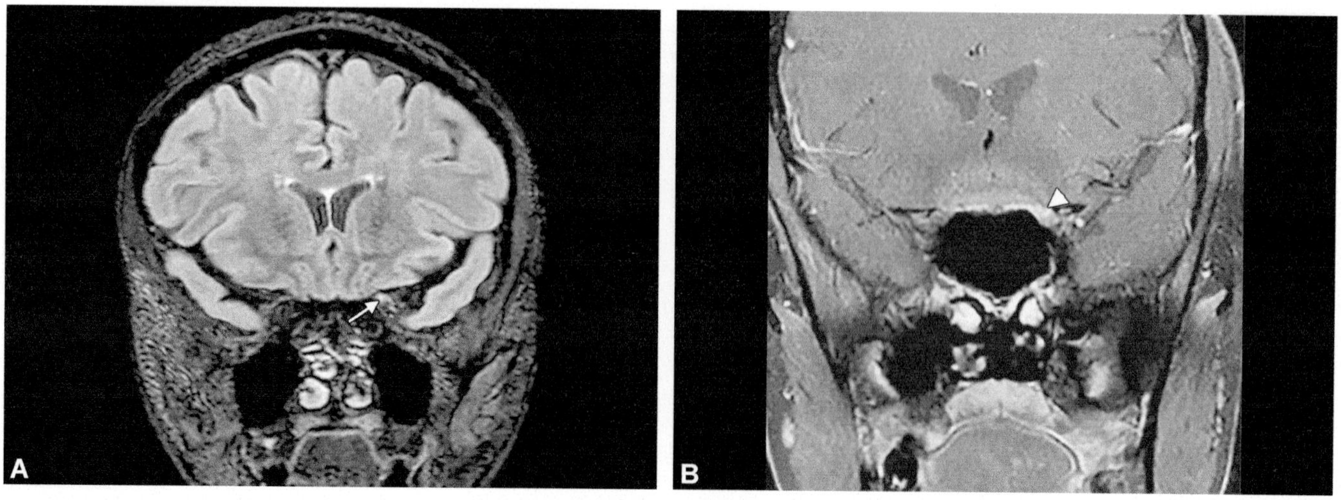

Figs. 93.26A and B: (A) Coronal three dimensional (3D) T2 fluid attenuation inversion recovery (FLAIR) and (B) coronal contrast-enhanced-T1 with fat suppression (FS) images reveal T2 FLAIR hyperintense signal (arrow—A) and enhancement of the left intraorbital optic nerve at the orbital apex extending to the intracanalicular segment (arrowhead—B) in a patient who met diagnostic criteria for multiple sclerosis two years later.

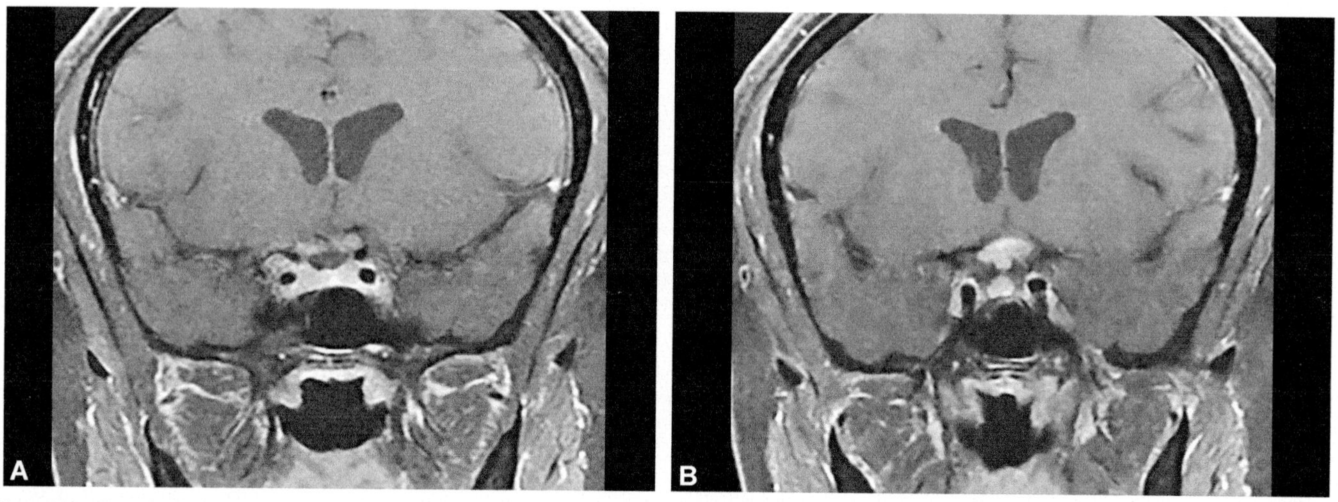

Figs. 93.27A and B: (A) Two coronal contrast-enhanced T1—weighted imaging (WI) with fat suppression (FS) demonstrates enhancement and (B) enlargement of the cisternal segments of the optic nerves bilaterally, extending to the optic chiasm in a patient presenting with bilateral subacute vision loss. Neuromyelitis optica (NMO) IgG was positive.

are less common.[54,55] Optic nerve enhancement and T2 hyperintensity has also been reported in association with acute vision loss from Leber's hereditary optic neuropathy (LHON) although the optic nerves often appear normal.[56] Periventricular and subcortical white matter T2 hyperintensities have also been demonstrated in patients with dominant optic atrophy (DOA) in addition to anterior visual pathway atrophy.[57]

By contrast, the white matter lesion distribution in NMO typically corresponds to regions with high levels of aquaporin 4 expression (regions adjacent to the third ventricle, cerebral aqueduct, and fourth ventricle, the thalamus and hypothalamus, and area postrema)[45,46,51,58-63] and whereas perpendicularly oriented lesions of the corpus callosum, "Dawson fingers", are characteristic of MS (Fig. 93.28),[45-47,64] periventricular lesions in NMO are typically oriented parallel to the ventricles.[45] Subcortical and extensive white matter lesions in the cerebral hemispheres can be seen in NMO[60,62] with "cloudlike enhancement" (Fig. 93.29)[58] described as faint heterogeneous enhancement with indistinct margins, in the vast majority of lesions showing enhancement.[45,58,60] Linear enhancement around the ventricles and leptomeningeal enhancement has also been described in NMO.[45] By contrast, ring or partial ring enhancement is more typical of MS.[45,61] Although cortical lesions are frequently identified in MS, to date studies have

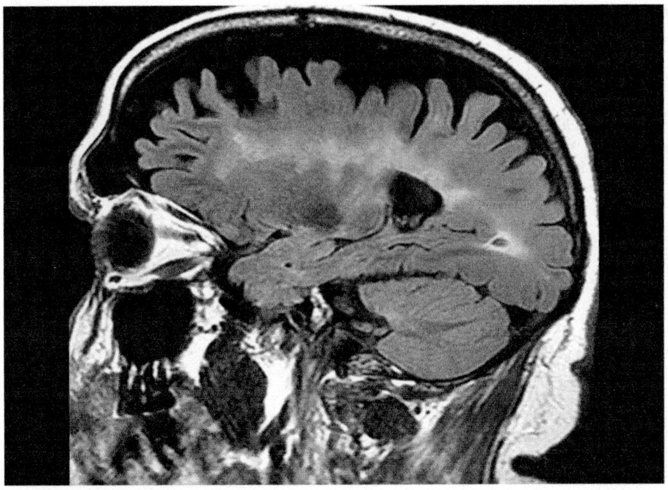

Fig. 93.28: Sagittal T2 fluid attenuation inversion recovery (FLAIR) exhibit numerous T2 FLAIR hyperintense periventricular white matter demyelinating lesions oriented perpendicular to the long axis of the lateral ventricles, depicting "Dawson fingers" in a patient with multiple sclerosis.

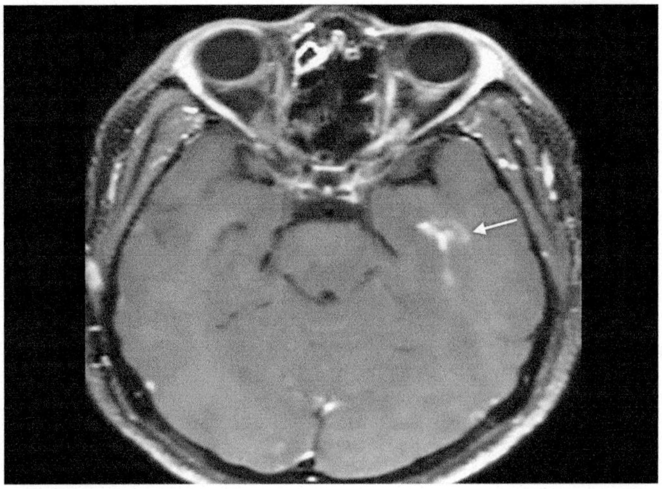

Fig. 93.29: Axial contrast-enhanced three-dimensional (3D) T1- weighted imaging WI with fat suppression (FS) reveals ill-defined peripherally enhancing ("cloud-like enhancement") demyelinating lesion (arrow) in the left temporal periventricular white matter in a patient with seropositive neuromyelitis optica (NMO).

not shown gray matter involvement in NMO.[46,52,53,60,65-67] In addition to longitudinally extensive transverse myelitis, central cord lesions[46,67,68] and "bright spotty lesions," described as T2 hyperintensities which are brighter than CSF on spine MRI, are characteristic of NMO.[68]

Consensus guidelines published by the MAGNIMS (Magnetic Resonance Imaging in MS) group in 2015 include repeat neuroimaging within 3–6 months of baseline MRI in patients presenting with a clinically or radiographically isolated syndrome but not meeting MS diagnostic criteria.[69] Use of low field strength "open" MRIs should be avoided, as higher strength magnets (3T) are superior for lesion detection.[70,71] The recommended brain MRI protocol includes sagittal T2 FLAIR (to assess for corpus callosum lesions), T2W, T1 with gadolinium and DWI images [to rule out alternate pathology and assess for progressive multifocal leukoencephalopathy (PML)].[69,70] As gadolinium enhancement due to active demyelinating lesions usually resolves within 2–6 weeks,[47,51,70] contrast can be useful to assess for evidence of dissemination in time.[52,69] Cervical spine MRI is recommended for all patients who have a nondiagnostic brain MRI, with possible extensive spinal imaging if suggestive symptomatology exists.[70] The orbital imaging protocol should include thin slices with coronal STIR or T2W fat suppression, and T1W with fat suppression and gadolinium.[70] Follow-up brain MRI should include proton density or T2 FLAIR and T2W FSE in addition to T1W with contrast.[69] A PML screening protocol necessitates T2 FLAIR (to assess for large subcortical hyperintense lesions) and DWI (to assess for hyperintensity) but does not require contrast as the majority of early lesions do not show contrast enhancement[70,72] (Figs. 93.30A and B).

Papilledema/Elevated Intracranial Pressure

In patients with suspected papilledema, neuroimaging is performed to exclude an intracranial mass lesion, noncommunicating hydrocephalus or venous sinus thrombosis (Figs. 93.31A and B) as the cause of elevated intracranial pressure. MRI brain without and with gadolinium is the ideal study to exclude an underlying structural etiology, but it is not always possible to obtain an MRI emergently. In cases where an MRI cannot be obtained with same day urgency, non-contrast head CT is sufficient to exclude a large mass lesion with potential to cause herniation (Figs. 93.32A and B). If CT is unrevealing, an MRI and MRV brain can be scheduled less urgently. Multiple radiographic signs of elevated intracranial pressure have been described including;[73-75]

- Empty or partially empty sella (Fig. 93.33A)
- Distended optic nerve sheaths
- Flattening of the posterior globes on MRI (Fig. 93.33B)
- Unilateral or bilateral transverse venous sinus stenosis on MRV (Figs. 93.34A and B)
- Enhancement and/or protrusion of the optic disk
- Optic canal and/or foramen ovale enlargement
- Optic nerve tortuosity
- Cerebellar tonsil herniation

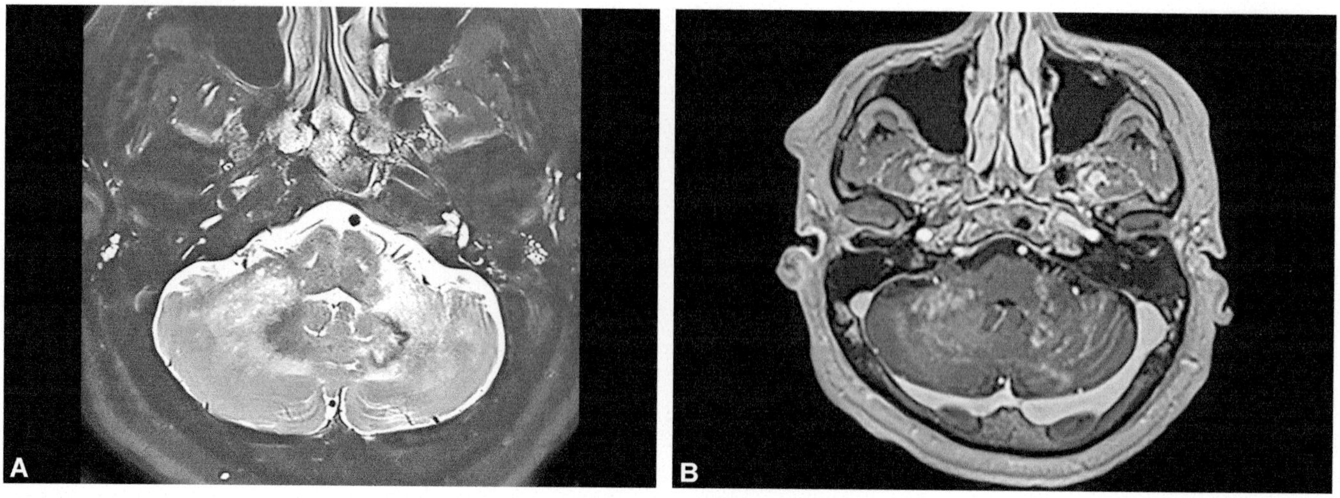

Figs. 93.30A and B: (A) Axial T2-weighted imaging (WI) with fat suppression (FS); and (B) Axial contrast-enhanced three-dimensional gradient recalled echo (3D GRE) demonstrate ill-defined confluent T2 hyperintense regions with associated ill-defined nodular enhancement in the cerebellar hemispheres bilaterally, extending into the cerebellar peduncles, medulla and pons, in a patient with multiple sclerosis and suspected progressive multifocal leukoencephalopathy and immune recovery inflammatory syndrome (IRIS).

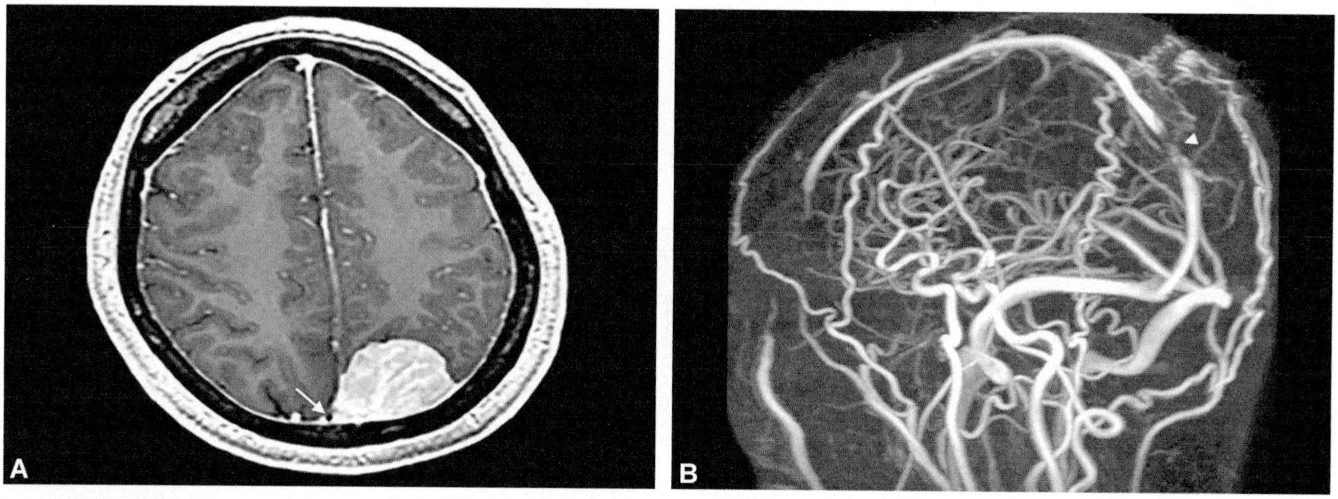

Figs. 93.31A and B: (A) Axial contrast-enhanced three-dimensional gradient recalled echo (3D GRE); and (B) 3D maximum intensity projection (MIP) rotational reconstruction from a contrast-enhanced magnetic resonance venography (MRV) reveals a large left parietal occipital convexity meningioma with invasion of the superior sagittal sinus and a small filling defect (arrow) within the sinus that represents a venous sinus thrombus. Decreased enhancement of the superior sagittal sinus is observed on the MRV 3D MIP (arrowhead). The patient presented with papilledema and a left cranial nerve (CN) VI paresis.

- Narrow (slit-like) ventricles
- Meningoceles
- Spontaneous CSF leaks.[74,75]

Although rare, bilateral transverse venous sinus stenosis can occur in the setting of normal intracranial pressure.[76]

Diplopia/Ocular Motility Disorders

Orbital Processes

The choice of appropriate neuroimaging for binocular diplopia and/or ocular motility disorders depends on the expected localization of the lesion (*see* Chapter 95). In patients with orbital signs such as proptosis, conjunctival injection, lid retraction, or lid lag, orbital imaging is indicated to assess for an orbital mass (Figs. 93.35A and B), extraocular muscle enlargement due to thyroid eye disease or orbital myositis (Figs. 93.36A to C), or in the case of pulsatile exophthalmos, sphenoid wing dysplasia with temporal lobe prolapse (Fig. 93.37). Although CT orbits are adequate to assess for extraocular muscle enlargement, if additional optic nerve pathology or cranial neuropathies are present, MRI is the preferred study (Figs. 93.36A to C). Quasi-coronal orbital MRI is advocated for assessment of sagging eye syndrome (SES) or heavy eye syndrome (HES).[77]

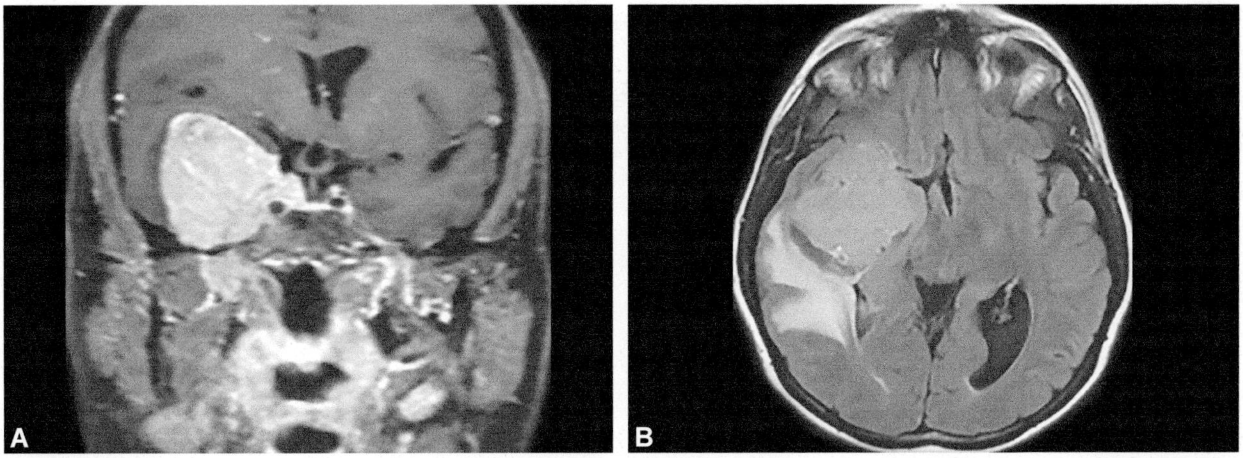

Figs. 93.32A and B: (A) Coronal contrast-enhanced 3D T1-weighted imaging (WI) with fat suppression (FS); and (B) Axial T2 fluid attenuation inversion recovery (FLAIR) demonstrates an avidly inhomogeneously enhancing right middle cranial fossa WHO II meningioma with extension into the right cavernous sinus and sella turcica, surrounding T2 FLAIR hyperintense vasogenic edema and midline shift from right to left in a patient presenting with mild papilledema.

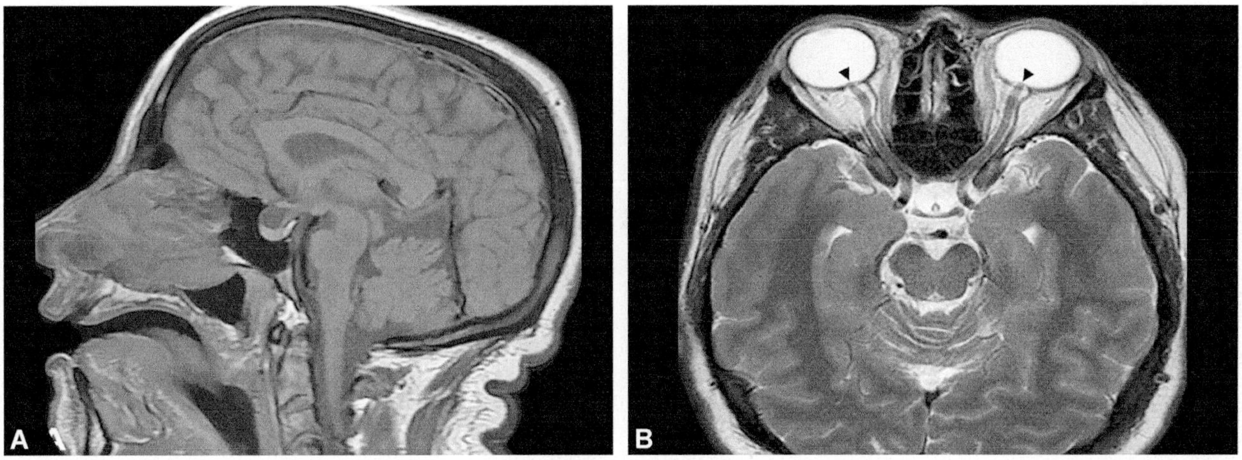

Figs. 93.33A and B: (A) Sagittal T1-weighted imaging (WI); and (B) Axial T2-WI reveals a partially empty sella and distended optic nerve sheaths with flattening of the posterior globes and intraocular disk protrusions (arrowheads) in a patient with idiopathic intracranial hypertension.

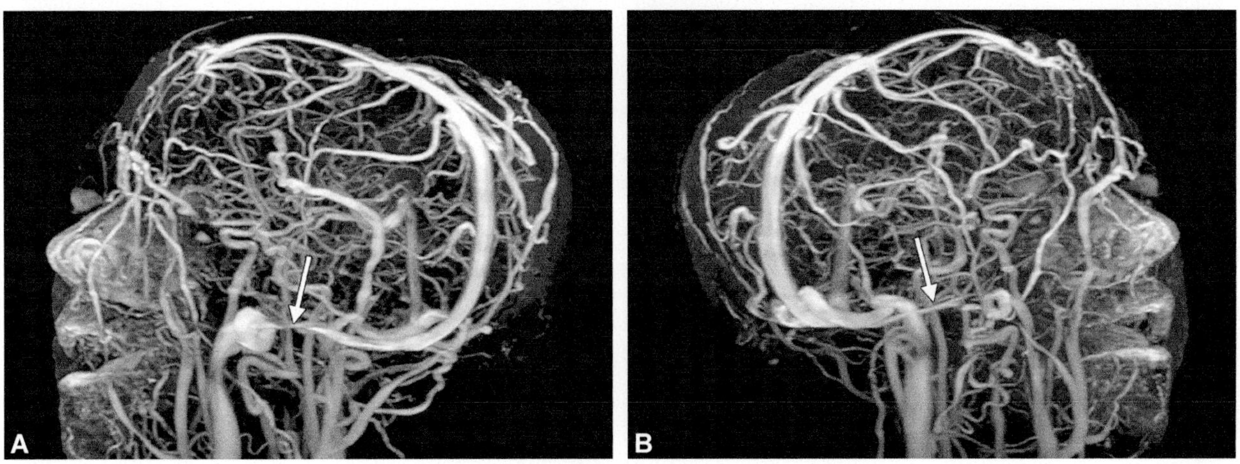

Figs. 93.34A and B: Magnetic resonance venography (MRV) brain with contrast with coronal views showing bilateral transverse venous sinus stenosis in a patient with idiopathic intracranial hypertension.

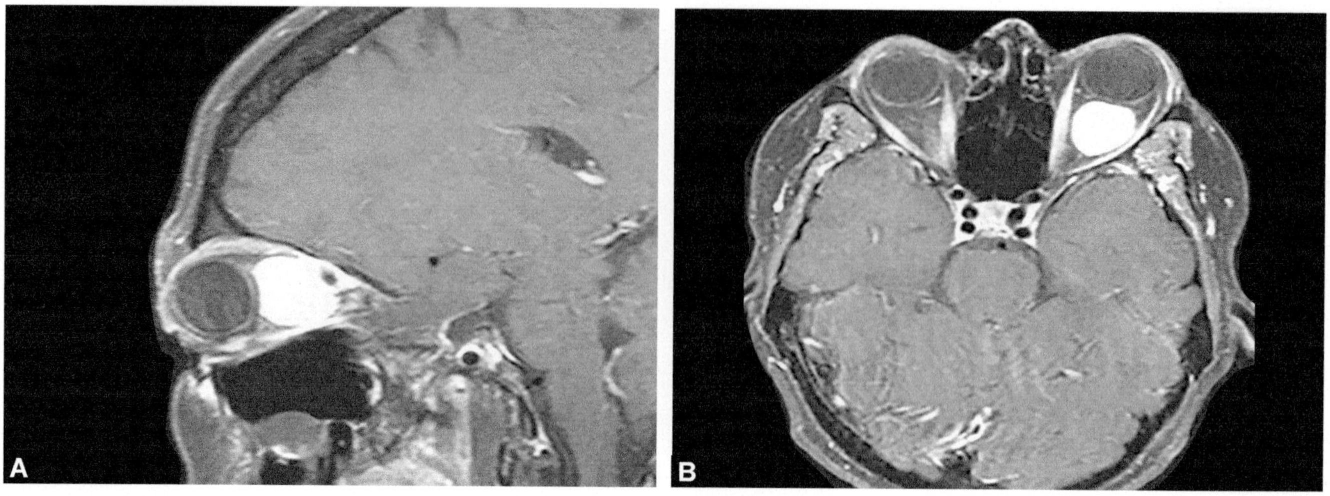

Figs. 93.35A and B: (A) Sagittal and (B) axial contrast-enhanced T1- weighted imaging WI with fat suppression (FS) images exhibit a large inhomogeneously enhancing retrobulbar intraconal malignant solitary fibrous tumor in a patient who presented with blurred vision, proptosis and diplopia.

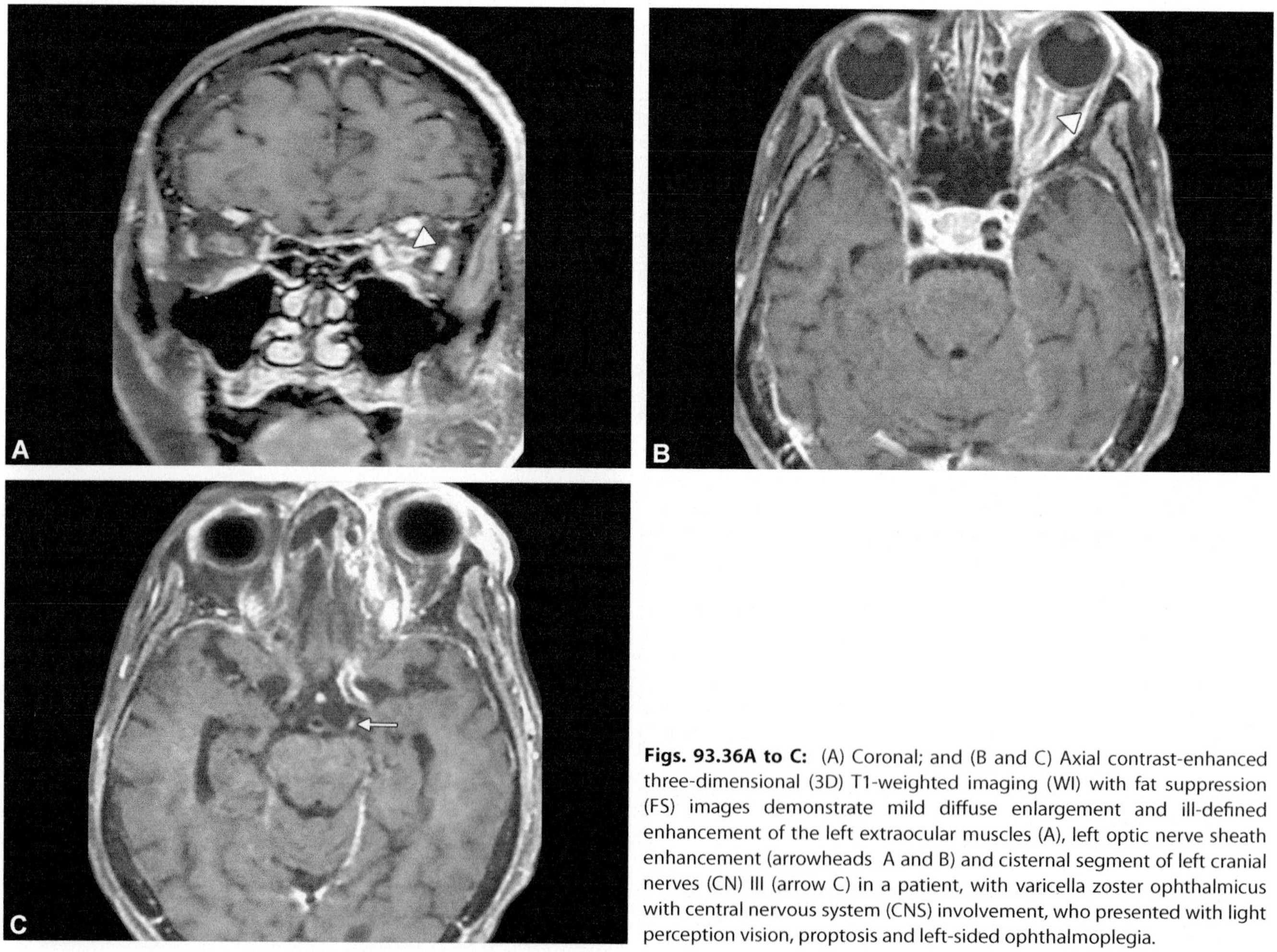

Figs. 93.36A to C: (A) Coronal; and (B and C) Axial contrast-enhanced three-dimensional (3D) T1-weighted imaging (WI) with fat suppression (FS) images demonstrate mild diffuse enlargement and ill-defined enhancement of the left extraocular muscles (A), left optic nerve sheath enhancement (arrowheads A and B) and cisternal segment of left cranial nerves (CN) III (arrow C) in a patient, with varicella zoster ophthalmicus with central nervous system (CNS) involvement, who presented with light perception vision, proptosis and left-sided ophthalmoplegia.

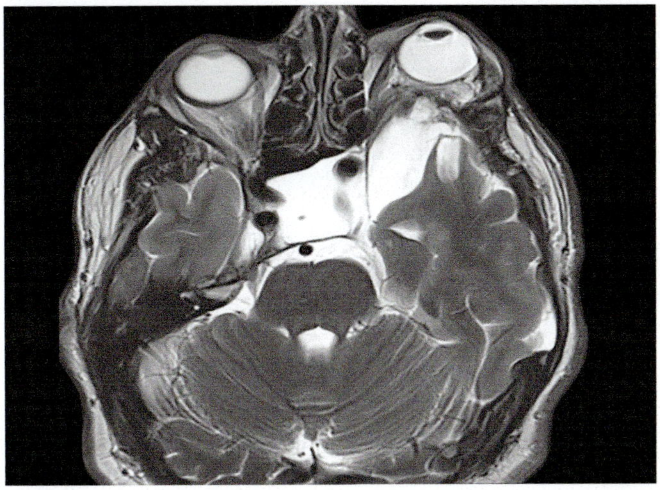

Fig. 93.37: Axial T2-weighted imaging (WI) demonstrates left sphenoid wing dysplasia with prolapse of an arachnoid cyst into the left orbit in a patient with neurofibromatosis (NF)1 who presented with pulsatile exophthalmos, and a large esotropia and left hypertropia.

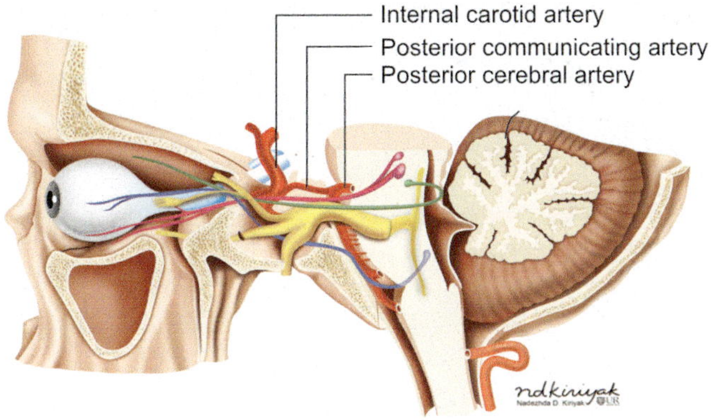

Fig. 93.38: Illustration of the course of cranial nerves III, IV and VI.

In SES, quasi-coronal images show stretch of the lateral rectus-superior rectus (LR-SR) connective tissue band, due to degenerative changes, inferiorly displacing the lateral rectus muscle.[77-79] Quasi-coronal cuts perpendicular to the orbital axis demonstrate an obtuse angle created by lines drawn from the centers of the superior and lateral rectus muscles to the center of the globe.[77] By contrast, HES shows superotemporal globe displacement and a more obtuse LR-SR displacement angle as there is additional medial displacement of the superior rectus muscle.[77,80]

Cranial Neuropathies

In order to determine the appropriate neuroimaging study, it is essential to be familiar with the course of each cranial nerve (CN) and potential additional localizing signs (Fig. 93.38). In the case of isolated CN III, CN IV or CN VI paresis, which either progresses or does not resolve within the expected time frame for a microvascular process, is inconsistent with a congenital etiology, or occurs in a patient with a history of malignancy or younger than age 50, MRI should include the entire course of the cranial nerve from brainstem to orbit. There are several sequences which optimize visualization of cranial nerves including:[81]

- 3-D T2-WI high resolution images performed with <1 mm slice thickness
- Constructive interference in steady state (CISS) or fast imaging employing steady state acquisition (FIESTA) which both decrease SNR by reducing imaging time
- 3D fast spin echo (FSE) or gradient echo
- Magnetization-prepared rapid acquisition with gradient echo (MPRAGE).

Three-dimensional T2W FLAIR sequences can also be useful to suppress CSF flow artifact, with contrast use to assess for neoplastic or inflammatory etiologies.[81]

Because of the propensity of the oculomotor nerve to be compressed by a PComm/ICA aneurysm, a pupil-involving CN III paresis or a progressive non-pupil involving partial CN III paresis is an indication for urgent vascular imaging (CTA or MRA brain)(Figs. 93.39A and B). Recurrent painful ophthalmoplegic neuropathy, formerly known as ophthalmoplegic migraine before re-designation under the International Classification of Headache Disorders, is a diagnosis of exclusion and requires neuroimaging. Indeed, 75% of patients with painful recurrent ophthalmoplegic neuropathy with CN III paresis showed contrast enhancement and/or thickening of the cisternal segment of the oculomotor nerve on MRI.[82] By contrast, additional neurologic symptoms such as weakness, numbness, ataxia, tremor or oscillopsia can be useful in localizing an oculomotor nerve paresis to the brainstem (fascicular portion)(Figs. 93.40A and B).

The trochlear nerve has a short intra-axial course but a long cisternal course due to its exit posteriorly from the brainstem. Signs that localize a CN IV palsy to the brainstem include an afferent pupillary defect (due to involvement of the brachium of the superior colliculus)[83]or a Horner syndrome.[84] The cisternal segment is a frequent site for trochlear schwannoma (Fig. 93.41).

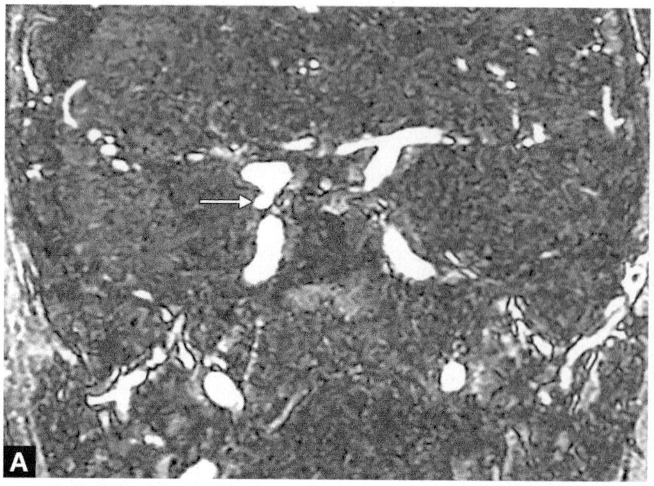

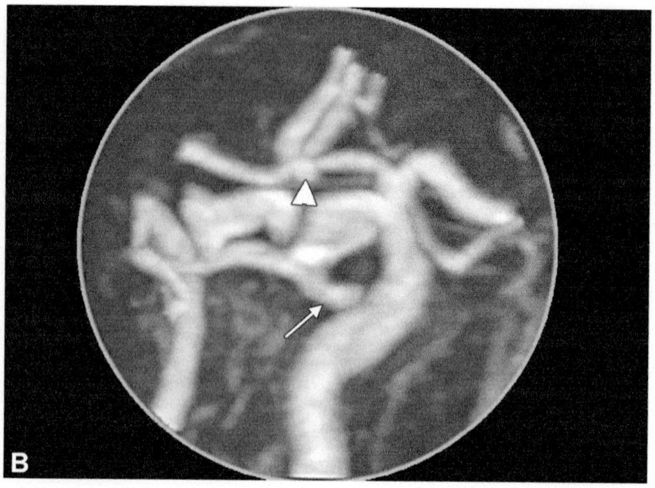

A B

Figs. 93.39A and B: (A) Coronal contrast-enhanced three-dimensional magnetic resonance angiography (3D MRA) with (B) corresponding 3D maximum intensity projection (MIP) rotational reconstruction demonstrates a saccular aneurysm arising inferiorly from the right posterior communicating artery (arrows—A and B) in a patient presenting with a right pupil-involving partial cranial nerve (CN) III paresis. A small anterior communicating artery aneurysm is also present (arrowhead—B).

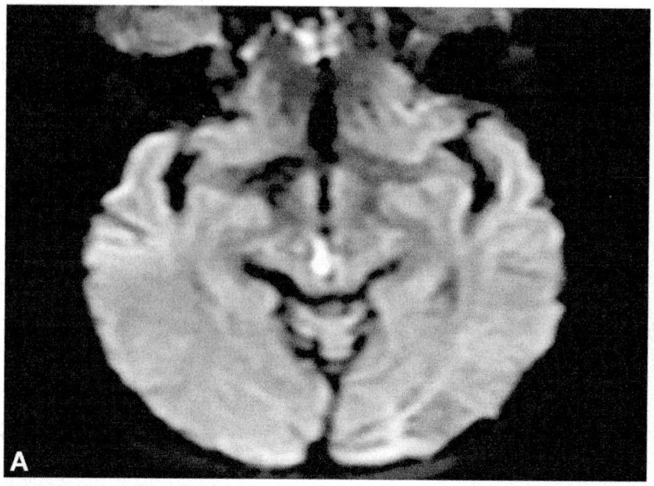

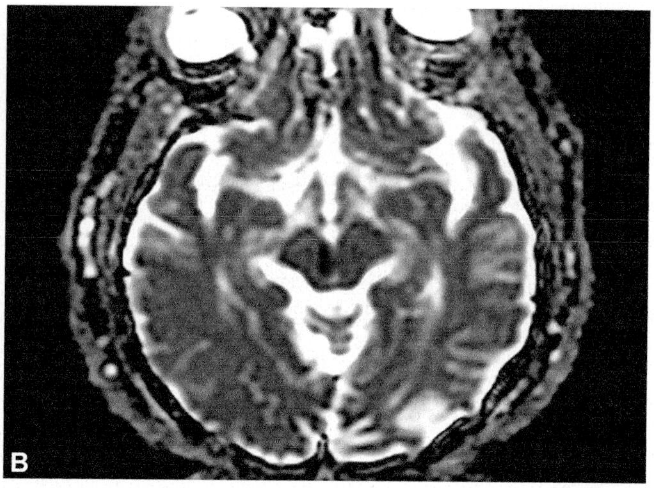

A B

Figs. 93.40A and B: (A) Axial diffusion tensor imaging; and (B) Axial apparent diffusion coefficients (ADC) map reveals an acute right midbrain infarct with corresponding decreased ADC values in a patient presenting with a right partial cranial nerve (CN) III paresis with limitation of contralateral supraduction and ataxia.

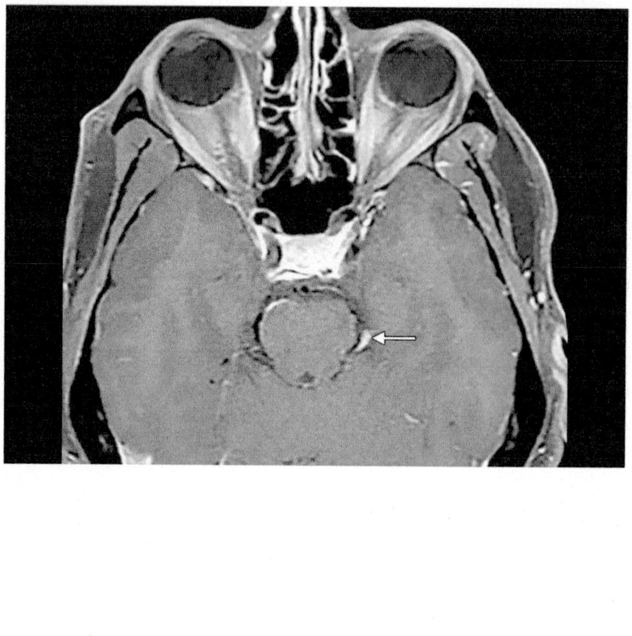

Fig. 93.41: Axial contrast-enhanced T1-weighted imaging (WI) with fat suppression (FS) demonstrates focal thickening and abnormal enhancement of the cisternal segment of the left trochlear nerve (arrow) consistent with a trochlear schwannoma.

The abducens nerve has an intra-axial, cisternal, and intradural course prior to reaching the cavernous sinus. In children, a frequent etiology of isolated CN VI paresis is brainstem tumor; therefore neuroimaging is almost always indicated.[85,86] Pontine gliomas are common but other lesions such as pontine cavernous malformation (Fig. 93.42) can be seen. Gradient recalled echo (GRE) T2* imaging, including SWI, is very sensitive in detection of blood products which appear hypointense and demonstrate "blooming effect", an artifact that increases the apparent radiographic size of the lesion (Figs. 93.42A to C).[87]

Multiple Cranial Neuropathies

The subarachnoid segments of the oculomotor and trochlear nerves and the intradural segment of the abducens nerve come in close proximity as they, along with the first and second divisions of the trigeminal nerve, enter the cavernous sinus (Fig. 93.43). In patients presenting with multiple cranial neuropathies, MRI brain with contrast is advised with attention to the cavernous sinus (Figs. 93.44 and Fig. 93.45) and skull base or cerebellopontine angle (Fig. 93.46) depending on which cranial nerves are involved. The 2004 revised diagnostic criteria for Tolosa Hunt syndrome (Fig. 93.44) require an inflammatory lesion in the cavernous sinus (most frequently), superior orbital fissure or orbit, detected by MRI or biopsy.[88,89] Optimal MRI sequences should include T1W, T2, FLAIR and T1W with contrast images with follow-up MRI after resolution of symptoms to ensure radiographic resolution.[88] The most common tumors seen in the cavernous sinus are pituitary adenoma, meningioma (Fig. 93.45), chordoma,

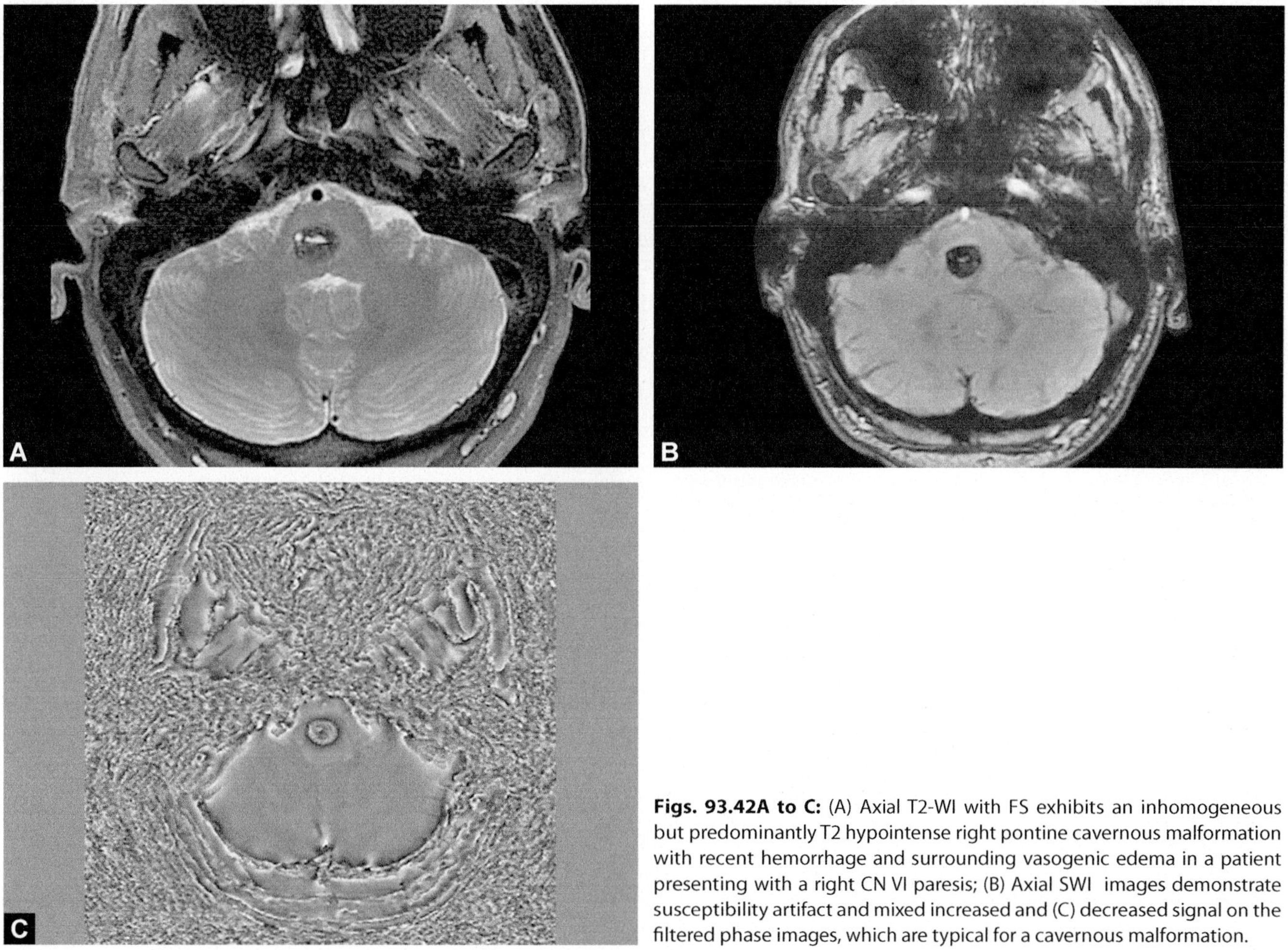

Figs. 93.42A to C: (A) Axial T2-WI with FS exhibits an inhomogeneous but predominantly T2 hypointense right pontine cavernous malformation with recent hemorrhage and surrounding vasogenic edema in a patient presenting with a right CN VI paresis; (B) Axial SWI images demonstrate susceptibility artifact and mixed increased and (C) decreased signal on the filtered phase images, which are typical for a cavernous malformation.

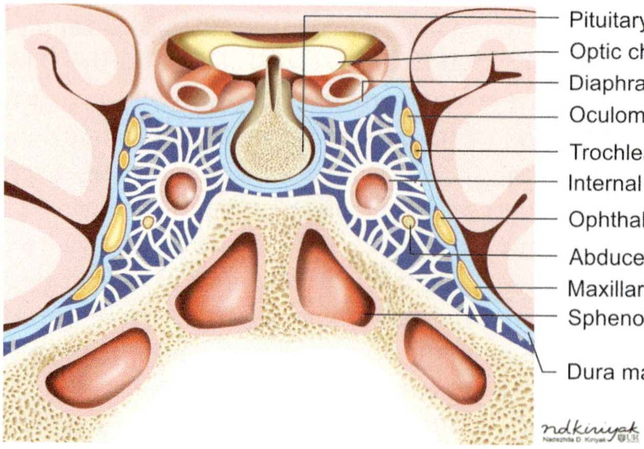

Fig. 93.43: Cavernous sinus/ parasellar anatomy.

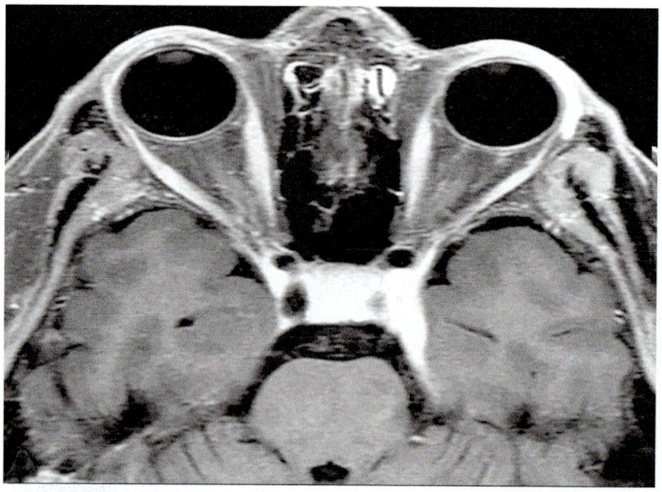

Fig. 93.44: Axial contrast-enhanced T1-weighted imaging (WI) with fat suppression (FS) demonstrates enhancing soft tissue within the left cavernous sinus extending along the left tentorium in a patient presenting with left periorbital pain and diplopia. Workup was consistent with Tolosa-Hunt syndrome with rapid resolution with corticosteroids.

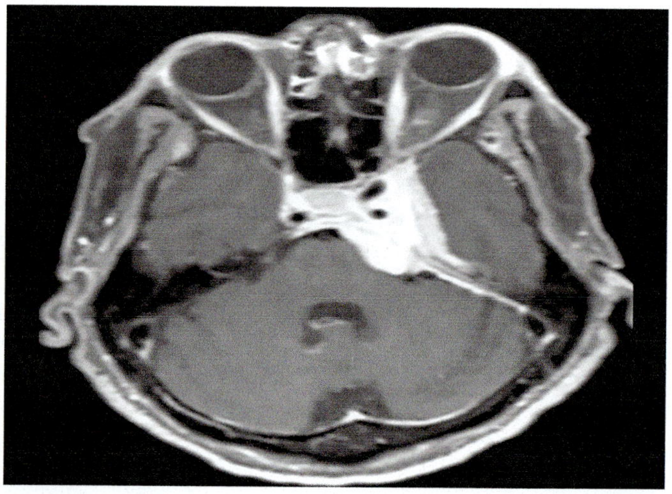

Fig. 93.45: Axial contrast-enhanced three-dimensional (3D) T1-weighted imaging (WI) reveals a large enhancing cavernous sinus meningioma extending into the superior orbital fissure in a patient who presented with left partial cranial nerve (CN) III, CN IV and CN VI paresis.
Source: Steven Feldon, MD.

nasopharyngeal carcinoma, lymphoma, and metastases, but vascular disorders (aneurysms and carotid cavernous fistulas) also cause a significant proportion of cavernous sinus syndromes.[89,90] The most common tumors of the cerebellopontine angle (CPA) (Fig. 93.46) are vestibular schwannomas and meningiomas,[91] which may present with facial weakness, hearing loss, and/or nystagmus (see below).

Internuclear Ophthalmoplegia

Patients presenting with internuclear ophthalmoplegia (INO) (Fig. 93.47) should have MRI brain either to assess for demyelinating disease involving the medial longitudinal fasciculus in young patients (Fig. 93.48) or stroke (including after DWI sequences)[92] in older patients. However, as a variety of brainstem lesions including tumors and hemorrhage[93] can cause INO, a contrast study is advised.

Nystagmus

Magnetic resonance imaging (MRI) is the superior imaging modality for evaluation of posterior fossa pathology causing nystagmus.[94,95] Although nystagmus is not always particularly localizing, structural lesions causing downbeat nystagmus tend to occur at the cervicomedullary junction

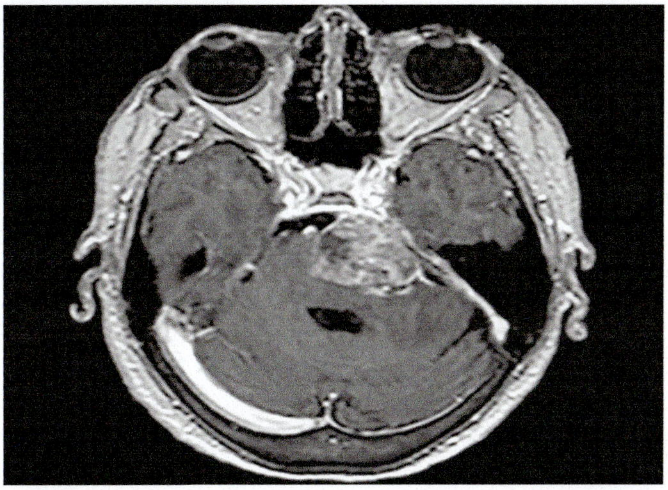

Fig. 93.46: Axial contrast-enhanced three-dimensional (3D) gradient recalled echo (GRE) exhibits a large inhomogeneously enhancing left petroclival anaplastic WHO III meningioma with brainstem compression in a patient presenting with left cranial nerve (CN) V, VI, VII, VIII paresis and poor vision due to a neurotrophic ulcer in her left eye.

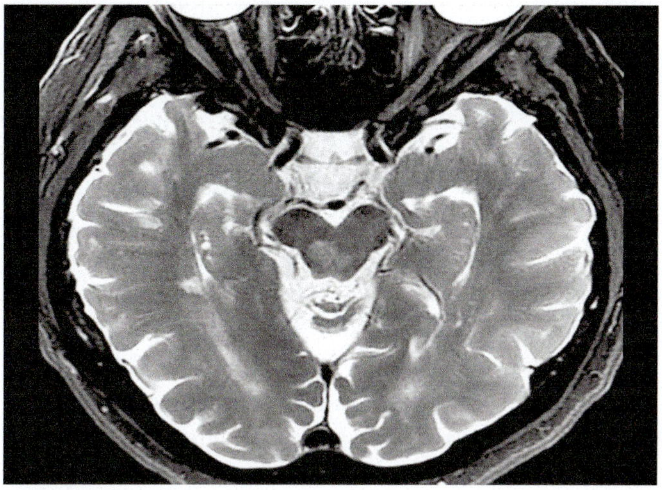

Fig. 93.48: Axial T2-weighted imaging (WI) with fat suppression (FS) reveals a T2 hyperintense demyelinating lesion in the right dorsal midbrain adjacent to the aqueduct of Sylvius in a patient with a long-standing internuclear ophthalmoplegia (INO) from multiple sclerosis.

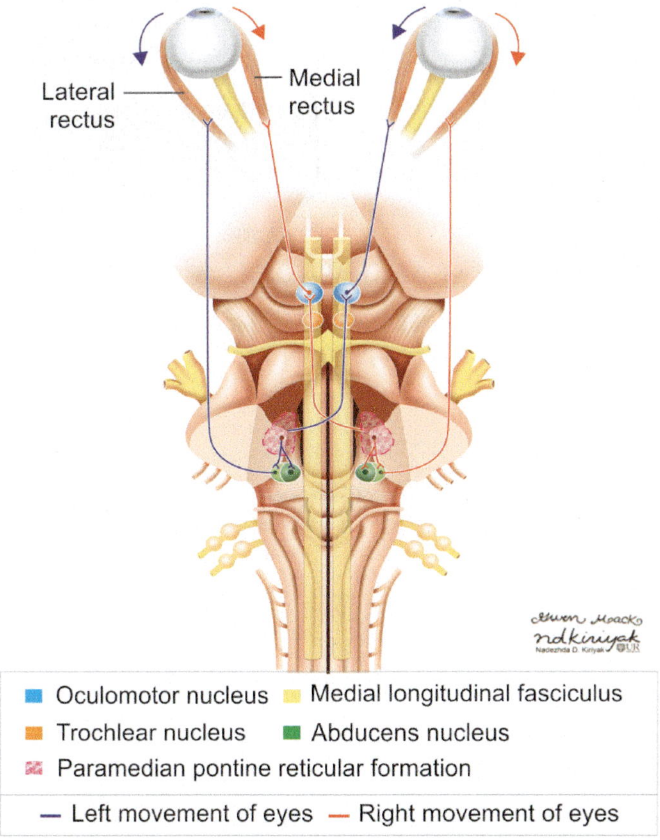

Fig. 93.47: Coordination of conjugate gaze via the medial longitudinal fasciculus.

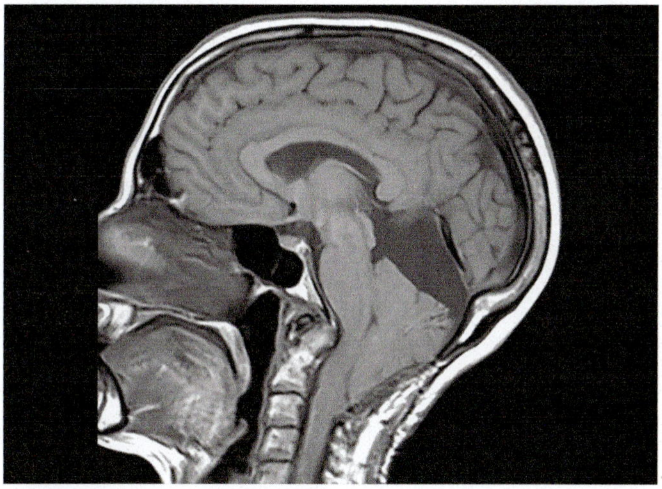

Fig. 93.49: Sagittal T1-weighted imaging (WI) reveals an enlarging posterior fossa cyst within the superior cerebellar cistern in a patient with a history of Chiari I malformation status post prior decompressive suboccipital craniectomy. The patient presented with downbeat nystagmus and a skew deviation.

with common causes including Arnold Chiari type I malformation (Fig. 93.49), demyelinating disease, stroke and neoplasm.

Computed Tomography/Magnetic Resonance Angiography

Contrast-enhanced CT angiography, similar to MR angiography, is used in evaluation of vascular diseases, such as stroke or transient ischemic attack, aneurysms, cavernous sinus thrombosis, carotid cavernous fistulas, vascular malformations and internal carotid artery dissection. The main advantage of CTA is rapid acquisition time but contrast is required. MRA can be performed as a time of flight (TOF) study without contrast.

The ability of 64-channel multidetector (MD) CTA and 3T 3-D TOF MRA to detect small aneurysms is roughly equivalent.[96] Digital subtraction angiography (DSA) remains the gold standard for diagnosis of cerebral aneurysms[96-99] although there have been significant advances in non-invasive techniques,[100] and DSA often is performed for therapeutic and not purely diagnostic purposes. *See* Chapter 99 for additional details and clinical cases.

Lee et al. described the high specificity of angiographic findings of enlarged superior ophthalmic vein, engorged cavernous sinus, comparable enhancement of ICA and cavernous sinus, and greater enhancement of the cavernous sinus than transverse sinus in diagnosis of carotid-cavernous fistulas (CCF) by CTA.[101] It has been shown that while orbital color Doppler imaging (CDI) has a more than 95% sensitivity for anteriorly draining CCFs, which demonstrate enlargement and arterialization of the superior ophthalmic vein, it is unable to diagnose posteriorly draining fistulas.[102] 3-DTOF MRA may show enlargement of the superior ophthalmic vein (Fig. 93.50B) whereas contrast MRA (Fig. 93.50A) demonstrates early enhancement of the cavernous sinus.[103] Indirect fistulas

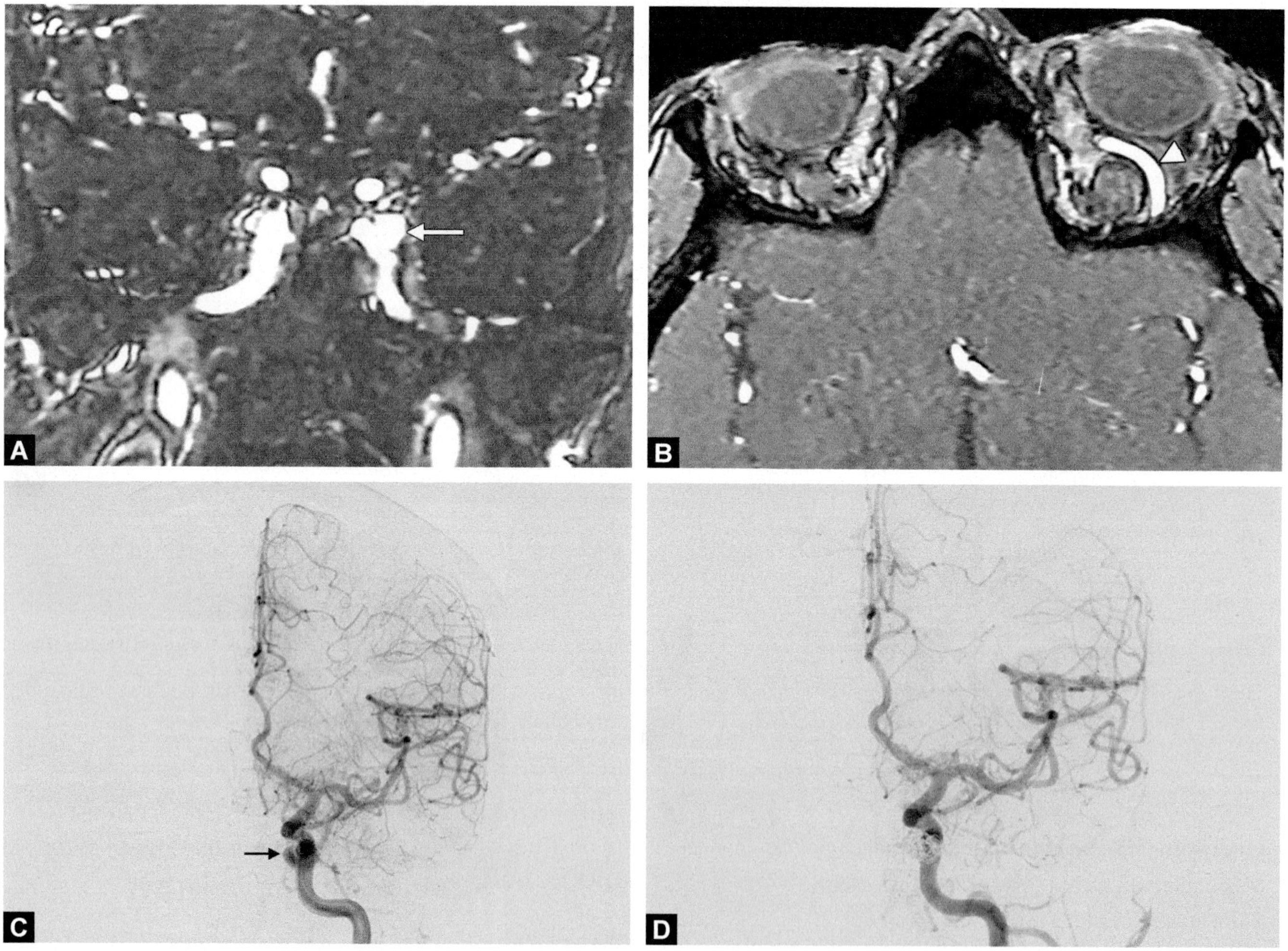

Figs. 93.50A to D: (A) A coronal contrast-enhanced three-dimensional (3D) magnetic resonance angiography (MRA) and (B) non-contrast time-of-flight MRA reveals a left direct carotid-cavernous fistula with early arterial filling of the left cavernous sinus (arrows—A and C) a dilated superior ophthalmic vein (arrowhead—B) in a patient presenting with a left partial cranial nerve (CN) III paresis and CN VI paresis, proptosis, conjunctival arteriolarization, elevated intraocular pressure and an audible bruit; (C) Pre- and (D) post-treatment digital subtraction angiographies demonstrate successful transvenous coil and Onyx embolization of the CCF.

are difficult to detect with conventional CSI, and DSA may be required for diagnosis. DSA also is used to characterize the arterial supply and venous drainage (Figs. 93.50C and D) for treatment planning.[103] Time-resolved contrast-enhanced MRA may improve detection of arteriovenous malformations.

Horner Syndrome

There are numerous protocols to accomplish imaging of the entire oculosympathetic pathway (Fig. 93.51) in patients with a non-localizing Horner syndrome (*see* Chapter 100), and no consensus exists. CT head and neck with contrast and CTA neck in the acute setting or in patients in whom MRI is contraindicated may be appropriate,[104] while MRI brain and neck with contrast extending down to T2 level to include the lung apices with or without an MRA neck to evaluate for carotid dissection should be considered with more chronic presentations and in cases of negative CT results (Figs. 93.52A and B).[104] Imaging of the entire oculosympathetic pathway for first or second order Horner syndrome versus MRI brain only for third order Horner syndrome also can be considered.[105] In pediatric patients with Horner syndrome, it is important to remember there is concern for neuroblastoma, and MRI of the chest and neck are indicated.[106,107]

Advanced Magnetic Resonance Imaging Techniques

Multiple advanced MRI techniques have been developed to address specific clinical indications and include diffusion tensor imaging (DTI), magnetization transfer (MT), MR perfusion, MR spectroscopy and functional MRI (fMRI). DTI applies diffusion weighted imaging principles in at least 6 different directions, allowing quantitative analysis of

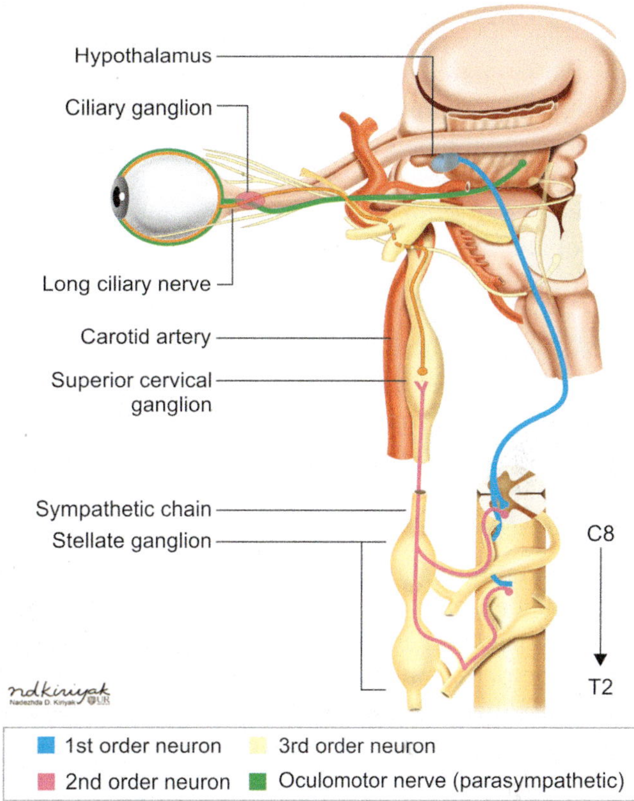

Fig. 93.51: Oculosympathetic pathway extending from the hypothalamus to the pupillary dilator muscle. A lesion along this pathway will cause an ipsilateral Horner syndrome.

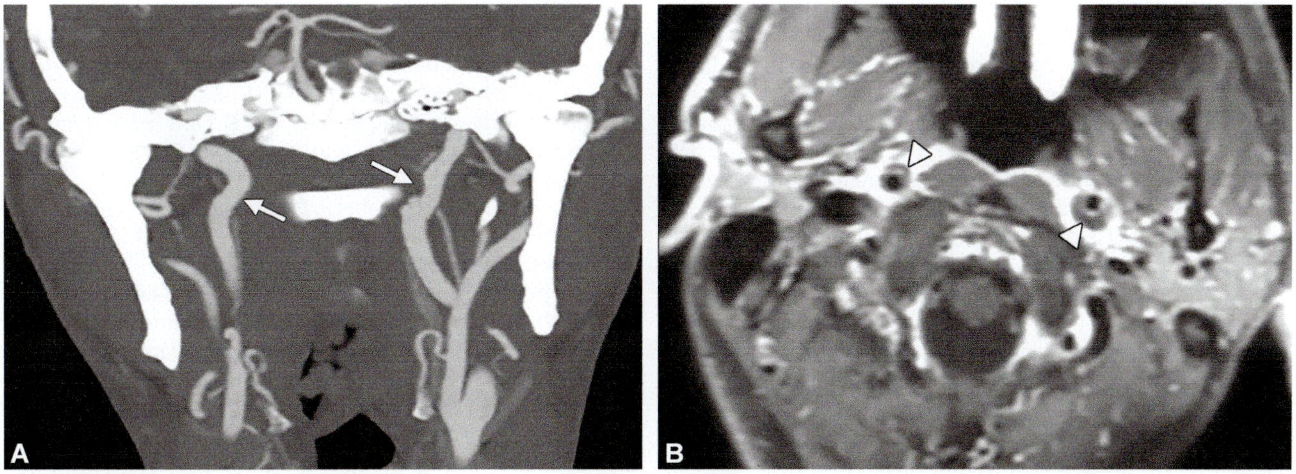

Figs. 93.52A and B: (A) Coronal maximum intensity projection (MIP) from a contrast-enhanced CTA and (B) axial contrast-enhanced three-dimensional (3D) T1-weighted imaging (WI) demonstrates a bilateral distal cervical ICA dissections (arrows—A) with wall irregularity, intraluminal narrowing and corresponding intramural hematomas (arrowheads—B) in a patient presenting with left-sided miosis and ptosis with pharmacologic confirmation of left Horner syndrome.

multidirectional diffusivity, magnitude of diffusion and of anisotropy, which is a reflection of local tissue organization. DTI can also be used to perform tractography, which is useful in brain tumor imaging and surgical planning. MT techniques measure interactions between protons in tissue and in free fluid. MT can reflect the degree of local tissue injury, such as in patients with multiple sclerosis.[47,67] MR perfusion is often applied in vascular and brain tumor imaging, and can provide semi-quantitative data such as relative cerebral blood volume and cerebral blood flow parameters. MR spectroscopy utilizes NMR principles to identify relative quantities of local brain parenchyma metabolites, and can be applied in a wide range of disease entities from white matter abnormalities to brain tumor imaging. fMRI is often used to map language and sensorimotor areas prior to tumor resection. fMRI derives information from differences in the magnetization properties of deoxyhemoglobin and oxyhemoglobin [blood oxygen level-dependent (BOLD) signal].[67]

CONCLUSION

The ophthalmologist must work closely with the neuroradiologist and provide sufficient history and exam findings to allow the most appropriate and sensitive CSI study to be performed, thus maximizing the yield and sparing the patient unnecessary time and expense. When in doubt about which test to order for a given clinical situation, consultation with Neuroradiology can be invaluable.

REFERENCES

1. Ossoinig KC, Cennamo G, Byrne SF. Echographic differential diagnosis of optic nerve lesions. Doc Ophthalmol Proc Ser. 1981:29:327-31.
2. Atta HR. Imaging of the optic nerve with standardised echography. Eye (Lond). 1988;2:358-66.
3. Suzuki S, Furui S, Ishitake T, et al. Lens exposure during brain scans using multidetector row CT scanners: methods for estimation of lens dose. AJNR Am J Neuroradiol. 2010;31:822-6.
4. Neuhaus V, Abdullayev N, Große Hokamp N, et al. Improvement of image quality in unenhanced dual-layer CT of the head using virtual monoenergetic images compared with polyenergetic single-energy CT. Invest Radiol. 2017; 52(8):470-6.
5. Brant-Zawadzki M, Badami JP, Mills CM, et al. Primary intracranial tumor imaging: a comparison of magnetic resonance and CT. Radiology. 1984;150:287-303.
6. Mullins ME. Emergent neuroimaging of intracranial infection/inflammation. Radiol Clin North Am. 2011;49(1):47-62.
7. Miller NR. New concepts in the diagnosis and management of optic nerve sheath meningioma. J Neuroophthalmol. 2006;26(3):200-8.
8. Jäger HR, Miszkiel KA. Pathology of the optic nerve. Neuroimaging Clin N Am. 2008;18(2):243-59.
9. Costello FE, Goyal M. Neuroimaging in neuro-ophthalmology. Neurol Clin. 2010;28(3):757-87.
10. Weber AL, Caruso P, Sabates NR. The optic nerve: radiologic, clinical, and pathologic evaluation. Neuroimaging Clin N Am. 2005;15(1):175-201.
11. Miller NR. Primary tumours of the optic nerve and its sheath. Eye (Lond). 2004;18(11):1026-37.
12. Yousem DM, Gad K, Tufano RP. Resectability issues with head and neck cancer. AJNR Am J Neuroradiol. 2006;27(10):2024-36.
13. Bhat V, Devere J, Ramakrishanan A, et al. Perineural spread in squamous cell carcinoma of the face: an overlooked facet of information on imaging. J Maxillofac Oral Surg. 2016;15(3):390-3.
14. Stambuk HE. Perineural tumor spread involving the central skull base region. Semin Ultrasound CT MR. 2013;34(5): 445-58.
15. Consensus conference. Magnetic resonance imaging. JAMA. 1988;259(14):2132-8.
16. Bodanapally UK, Shanmuganathan K, Shin RK, et al. Hyperintense optic nerve due to diffusion restriction: diffusion-weighted imaging in traumatic optic neuropathy. AJNR Am J Neuroradiol. 2015;36(8):1536-41.
17. Li J, Shi W, Li M, et al. Time-dependent diffusion tensor changes of optic nerve in patients with indirect traumatic optic neuropathy. Acta Radiol. 2014;55(7):855-63.
18. Pepin SM, Lessell S. Anterior visual pathway gliomas: The last 30 years. Semin Ophthalmol. 2006;21(3):117-24.
19. Liu GT. Optic gliomas of the anterior visual pathway. Curr Opin Ophthalmol. 2006;17(5):427-31.
20. Blanchard G, Lafforgue MP, Lion-François L, et al. Systematic MRI in NF1 children under six years of age for the diagnosis of optic pathway gliomas. Study and outcome of a French cohort. Eur J Paediatr Neurol. 2016;20(2):275-81.
21. Eddleman CS, Liu JK. Optic nerve sheath meningioma: current diagnosis and treatment. Neurosurg Focus. 2007;23(5):E4.
22. Cho HK, Park SH, Shin SY. Isolated optic nerve metastasis of breast cancer initially mimicking retrobulbar optic neuritis. Eur J Ophthalmol. 2011;21(4):513-5.
23. Kim JL, Mendoza PR, Rashid A, et al. Optic nerve lymphoma: report of two cases and review of the literature. Surv Ophthalmol. 2015;60(2):153-65.
24. Lee AG, Tang RA, Roberts D, et al. Primary central nervous system lymphoma involving the optic chiasm in AIDS. J Neuroophthalmol. 2001;21(2):95-8.
25. Mejico LJ, Miller NR, Dong LM. Clinical features associated with lesions other than pituitary adenoma in patients with an optic chiasmal syndrome. Am J Ophthalmol. 2004;137(5):908-13.
26. Foroozan R. Visual findings in chiasmal syndromes. Int Ophthalmol Clin. 2016;56(1):1-27.
27. Wang S, Wang L, Yao Y, et al. Primary lymphocytic hypophysitis: clinical characteristics and treatment of 50 cases in a single centre in China over 18 years. Clin Endocrinol (Oxf). 2017;87(2):177-84.

28. Mollá E, Martí-Bonmatí L, Revert A, et al. Craniopharyngiomas: identification of different semiological patterns with MRI. Eur Radiol. 2002;12(7):1829-36.
29. Mariotti S, Losa M, Mortini P, et al. The birth and rise of a craniopharyngioma: the radiological evolution of an incidental craniopharyngioma detected on serial MRI during medical treatment of a macroprolactinoma. Clin Case Rep. 2016;5(1):14-7.
30. Cornblath WT, Quint DJ. MRI of optic nerve enlargement in optic neuritis. Neurology. 1997;48(4):821-5.
31. Makhani N, Bigi S, Banwell B, et al. Diagnosing neuromyelitis optica. Neuroimaging Clin N Am. 2013;23(2):279-91.
32. Decanini-Mancera A, Lessell S, Lee MS, et al. Syphilis and the monk. Surv Ophthalmol. 2011;56(3):267-73.
33. Jaafar J, Hitam WH, Noor RA. Bilateral atypical optic neuritis associated with tuberculosis in an immunocompromised patient. Asian Pac J Trop Biomed. 2012;2(7):586-8.
34. Northey LC, Skalicky SE, Gurbaxani A, et al. Syphilitic uveitis and optic neuritis in Sydney, Australia. Br J Ophthalmol. 2015;99(9):1215-9.
35. D'Souza NM, Morgan ML, Almarzouqi SJ, et al. Magnetic resonance imaging findings in giant cell arteritis. Eye (Lond). 2016;30(5):758-62.
36. Koczman JJ, Rouleau J, Gaunt M, et al. Neuro-ophthalmic sarcoidosis: the University of Iowa experience. Semin Ophthalmol. 2008;23(3):157-68.
37. Frohman LP, Guirgis M, Turbin RE, et al. Sarcoidosis of the anterior visual pathway: 24 new cases. J Neuroophthalmol. 2003;23(3):190-7.
38. Vaphiades MS, Wigton EH, Ameri H, et al. Neuroretinitis with retrobulbar involvement. J Neuroophthalmol. 2011;31(1):12-5.
39. Rocca MA, Hickman SJ, Bö L, et al. Imaging the optic nerve in multiple sclerosis. Mult Scler. 2005;11(5):537-41.
40. Hickman SJ. Optic nerve imaging in multiple sclerosis. J Neuroimaging. 2007;17(Suppl 1):42S-5S.
41. Aiken AH, Mukherjee P, Green AJ, et al. MR imaging of optic neuropathy with extended echo-train acquisition fluid-attenuated inversion recovery. AJNR Am J Neuroradiol. 2011;32:301-5.
42. Wingerchuk DM, Lennon VA, Pittock SJ, et al. Revised diagnostic criteria for neuromyelitis optica. Neurology. 2006;66(10):1485-9.
43. Buch D, Savatovsky J, Gout O, et al. Combined brain and anterior visual pathways' MRIs assist in early identification of neuromyelitis optica spectrum disorder at onset of optic neuritis. Acta Neurol Belg. 2017;117(1):67-74.
44. Storoni M, Davagnanam I, Radon M, et al. Distinguishing optic neuritis in neuromyelitis optica spectrum disease from multiple sclerosis: a novel magnetic resonance imaging scoring system. J Neuroophthalmol. 2013;33(2):123-7.
45. Pekcevik Y, Orman G, Lee IH, et al. What do we know about brain contrast enhancement patterns in neuromyelitis optica? Clin Imaging. 2016;40(3):573-80.
46. Wingerchuk DM, Banwell B, Bennett JL, et al; International Panel for NMO Diagnosis. International consensus diagnostic criteria for neuromyelitis optica spectrum disorders. Neurology. 2015;85(2):177-89.
47. Arnold DL, Matthews PM. MRI in the diagnosis and management of multiple sclerosis. Neurology. 2002;58(8 Suppl 4):S23-31.
48. Kornek B, Schmitl B, Vass K, et al. Evaluation of the 2010 McDonald multiple sclerosis criteria in children with a clinically isolated syndrome. Mult Scler. 2012;18(12): 1768-74.
49. Barkhof F, Filippi M, Miller DH, et al. Comparison of MRI criteria at first presentation to predict conversion to clinically definite multiple sclerosis. Brain. 1997;120: 2059-69.
50. Ormerod I, Bronstein A, Rudge P, et al. Magnetic resonance imaging in clinically isolated lesions of the brain stem. J Neurol Neurosurg Psychiatry. 1986;49(7):737-43.
51. Fazekas F, Barkhof F, Filippi M, et al. The contribution of magnetic resonance imaging to the diagnosis of multiple sclerosis. Neurology. 1999;53(3):448-56.
52. Filippi M, Rocca MA, Ciccarelli O, et al. MRI criteria for the diagnosis of multiple sclerosis: MAGNIMS consensus guidelines. Lancet Neurol. 2016;15(3):292-303.
53. Trebst C, Jarius S, Berthele A, et al. Update on the diagnosis and treatment of neuromyelitis optica: recommendations of the Neuromyelitis Optica Study Group (NEMOS). J Neurol. 2014;261(1):1-16.
54. Tran M, Bhargava R, MacDonald IM. Leber hereditary optic neuropathy, progressive visual loss, and multiple-sclerosis-like symptoms. Am J Ophthalmol. 2001;132(4):591-3.
55. Matthews L, Enzinger C, Fazekas F, et al. MRI in Leber's hereditary optic neuropathy: the relationship to multiple sclerosis. J Neurol Neurosurg Psychiatry. 2015;86(5):537-42.
56. Lamirel C, Cassereau J, Cochereau I, et al. Papilloedema and MRI enhancement of the prechiasmal optic nerve at the acute stage of Leber hereditary optic neuropathy. J Neurol Neurosurg Psychiatry. 2010;81(5):578-80.
57. Rocca MA, Bianchi-Marzoli S, Messina R, et al. Distributed abnormalities of brain white matter architecture in patients with dominant optic atrophy and OPA1 mutations. J Neurol. 2015;262(5):1216-27.
58. Ito S, Mori M, Makino T, et al. "Cloud-like enhancement" is a magnetic resonance imaging abnormality specific to neuromyelitis optica. Ann Neurol. 2009;66(3):425-8.
59. Sahraian MA, Radue EW, Minagar A. Neuromyelitis optica: clinical manifestations and neuroimaging features. Neurol Clin. 2013;31(1):139-52.
60. Barnett Y, Sutton IJ, Ghadiri M, et al. Conventional and advanced imaging in neuromyelitis optica. Am J Neuroradiol. 2014;35(8):1458-66.
61. Cheng C, Jiang Y, Chen X, et al. Clinical, radiographic characteristics and immunomodulating changes in neuromyelitis optica with extensive brain lesions. BMC Neurol. 2013;13:72.
62. Matthews L, Marasco R, Jenkinson M, et al. Distinction of seropositive NMO spectrum disorder and MS brain lesion distribution. Neurology. 2013;80(14):1330-7.

63. Tillema JM, McKeon A. The spectrum of neuromyelitis optica (NMO) in childhood. J Child Neurol. 2012;27(11): 1437-47.
64. Hintzen RQ, Dale RC, Neuteboom RF, et al. Pediatric acquired CNS demyelinating syndromes: Features associated with multiple sclerosis. Neurology. 2016;87(9 Suppl 2):S67-73.
65. Calabrese M, Oh MS, Favaretto A, et al. No MRI evidence of cortical lesions in neuromyelitis optica. Neurology. 2012;79(16):1671-6.
66. Eshaghi A, Wottschel V, Cortese R, et al. Gray matter MRI differentiates neuromyelitis optica from multiple sclerosis using random forest. Neurology. 2016;87(23):2463-2470.
67. Kremer S, Renard F, Achard S, et al. Use of advanced magnetic resonance imaging techniques in neuromyelitis optica spectrum disorder. JAMA Neurol. 2015;72(7):815-22.
68. Yonezu T, Ito S, Mori M, et al. "Bright spotty lesions" on spinal magnetic resonance imaging differentiate neuromyelitis optica from multiple sclerosis. Mult Scler. 2014;20(3):331-7.
69. Rovira À, Wattjes MP, Tintoré M, et al. Evidence-based guidelines: MAGNIMS consensus guidelines on the use of MRI in multiple sclerosis-clinical implementation in the diagnostic process. Nat Rev Neurol. 2015;11(8):471-82.
70. Traboulsee A, Simon JH, Stone L, et al. Revised Recommendations of the Consortium of MS Centers Task Force for a Standardized MRI Protocol and Clinical Guidelines for the Diagnosis and Follow-Up of Multiple Sclerosis. AJNR Am J Neuroradiol. 2016;37(3):394-401.
71. Wattjes MP, Barkhof F. High field MRI in the diagnosis of multiple sclerosis: high field-high yield? Neuroradiology. 2009;51(5):279-92.
72. Yousry TA, Pelletier D, Cadavid D, et al. Magnetic resonance imaging pattern in natalizumab-associated progressive multifocal leukoencephalopathy. Ann Neurol. 2012;72(5):779-87.
73. Friedman DI, Liu GT, Digre KB. Revised diagnostic criteria for the pseudotumor cerebri syndrome in adults and children. Neurology. 2013;24;81(13):1159-65.
74. Bidot S, Saindane AM, Peragallo JH, et al. Brain imaging in idiopathic intracranial hypertension. J Neuroophthalmol. 2015;35(4):400-11.
75. Padhye LV, Van Stavern GP, Sharma A, et al. Association between visual parameters and neuroimaging features of idiopathic intracranial hypertension. J Neurol Sci. 2013;332(1-2):80-5.
76. Kelly LP, Saindane AM, Bruce BB, et al. Does bilateral transverse cerebral venous sinus stenosis exist in patients without increased intracranial pressure? Clin Neurol Neurosurg. 2013;115(8):1215-9.
77. Tan RJ, Demer JL. Heavy eye syndrome versus sagging eye syndrome in high myopia. J AAPOS. 2015;19(6):500-6.
78. Rutar T, Demer JL. "Heavy Eye" syndrome in the absence of high myopia: a connective tissue degeneration in elderly strabismic patients. J AAPOS. 2009;13(1):36-44.
79. Chaudhuri Z, Demer JL. Sagging eye syndrome: connective tissue involution as a cause of horizontal and vertical strabismus in older patients. JAMA Ophthalmol. 2013;131(5): 619-25.
80. Maiolo C, Fresina M, Campos EC. Role of magnetic resonance imaging in heavy eye syndrome. Eye (Lond). 2017; 31(8):1163-7
81. Hwang JY, Yoon HK, Lee JH, et al. Cranial nerve disorders in children: MR Imaging Findings. Radiographics. 2016;36(4):1178-94.
82. Gelfand AA, Gelfand JM, Prabakhar P, et al. Ophthalmoplegic "migraine" or recurrent ophthalmoplegic cranial neuropathy: new cases and a systematic review. J Child Neurol. 2012;27(6):759-66.
83. Miller NR. Pearls and oy-sters: central fourth nerve palsies. Neurology. 2013;81(6):603.
84. Guy J, Day AL, Mickle JP, et al. Contralateral trochlear nerve paresis and ipsilateral Horner's syndrome. Am J Ophthalmol. 1989;107(1):73-6.
85. Dotan G, Rosenfeld E, Stolovitch C, et al. The role of neuroimaging in the evaluation process of children with isolated sixth nerve palsy. Childs Nerv Syst. 2013;29(1): 89-92.
86. Teksam O, Keser AG, Konuskan B, et al. Abducens nerve paralysis in the pediatric emergency department: analysis of 14 patients. Pediatr Emerg Care. 2016;32(5):307-11.
87. Charidimou A, Jäger HR, Werring DJ. Cerebral microbleed detection and mapping: principles, methodological aspects and rationale in vascular dementia. Exp Gerontol. 2012;47(11):843-52.
88. La Mantia L, Curone M, Rapoport AM, et al. Tolosa-Hunt syndrome: critical literature review based on IHS 2004 criteria. Cephalalgia. 2006;26(7):772-81.
89. Fernández S, Godino O, Martínez-Yélamos S, et al. Cavernous sinus syndrome: a series of 126 patients. Medicine (Baltimore). 2007;86(5):278-81.
90. Keane JR. Multiple cranial nerve palsies: analysis of 979 cases. Arch Neurol. 2005;62(11):1714-7.
91. Thamburaj K, Radhakrishnan VV, Thomas B, et al. Intratumoral microhemorrhages on T2*-weighted gradient-echo imaging helps differentiate vestibular schwannoma from meningioma. AJNR Am J Neuroradiol. 2008;29(3):552-7.
92. Takeshige H, Ueno Y, Kamagata K, et al. Pathways linked to internuclear ophthalmoplegia on diffusion-tensor imaging in a case with midbrain infarction. J Stroke Cerebrovasc Dis. 2016;25(11):2575-9.
93. Virgo JD, Plant GT. Internuclear ophthalmoplegia. Pract Neurol. 2017;17(2):149-53.
94. Slamovits TL, Gardner TA. Neuroimaging in neuro-ophthalmology. Ophthalmology. 1989;96(4):555-68.
95. Rubenfeld M, Wirtschafter JD. The role of medical imaging in the practice of neuro-ophthalmology. Radiol Clin North Am. 1987;25(4):863-76.
96. Hiratsuka Y, Miki H, Kiriyama I, et al. Diagnosis of unruptured intracranial aneurysms: 3T MR angiography versus 64-channel multi-detector row CT angiography. Magn Reson Med Sci. 2008;7(4):169-78.

97. Mayberg MR, Batjer HH, Dacey R, et al. Guidelines for the management of aneurysmal subarachnoid hemorrhage. A statement for healthcare professionals from a special writing group of the Stroke Council, American Heart Association. Stroke. 1994;25(11):2315-28.
98. Galal A, ElSerry TH, Aziz MM. Is catheter diagnostic cerebral angiography still essential for patients with spontaneous perimesencephalic subarachnoid hemorrhage and negative computed tomography angiogram? Neurosurgery. 2016;63 (Suppl 1):188.
99. Walkoff L, Brinjikji W, Rouchaud A, et al. Comparing magnetic resonance angiography (MRA) and computed tomography angiography (CTA) with conventional angiography in the detection of distal territory cerebral mycotic and oncotic aneurysms. Interv Neuroradiol. 2016;22(5):524-8.
100. Zhang Q, Zhang Z, Yang J, et al. CBCT-based 3D MRA and angiographic image fusion and MRA image navigation for neuro interventions. Medicine (Baltimore). 2016;95(32):e4358.
101. Lee JY, Jung C, Ihn YK, et al. Multidetector CT angiography in the diagnosis and classification of carotid-cavernous fistula. Clin Radiol. 2016;71(1):e64-71.
102. Srinivasan A, Biro NG, Murchison AP, et al. Efficacy of orbital color Doppler imaging and neuroimaging in the diagnosis of carotid cavernous fistulas. Ophthal Plast Reconstr Surg. 2017;33(5):340-4.
103. Jindal G, Miller T, Raghavan P, et al. Imaging evaluation and treatment of vascular lesions at the skull base. Radiol Clin North Am. 2017;55(1):151-66.
104. Chen Y, Morgan ML, Barros Palau AE, et al. Evaluation and neuroimaging of the Horner syndrome. Can J Ophthalmol 2015;50(2):107-11.
105. Sadaka A, Schockman SL, Golnik KC. Evaluation of Horner syndrome in the MRI era. J Neuroophthalmol. 2013;37(3):268-72.
106. Trobe JD. The evaluation of horner syndrome. J Neuro-ophthalmol. 2010;30(1):1-2.
107. Barrea C, Vigouroux T, Karam J, et al. Horner syndrome in children: a clinical condition with serious underlying disease. Neuropediatrics. 2016;47(4):268-72.

Chapter 94 Systemic Diseases and Neuro-ophthalmology

Katy C Liu, M Tariq Bhatti

INTRODUCTION

The ability to see and move the eyes is linked inherently to central nervous system (CNS) function; therefore, many systemic diseases with neurological consequences can have important neuro-ophthalmic manifestations. The ophthalmologist can play a critical diagnostic role in a patient who presents with ocular symptoms or incidental findings heralding a previously undiagnosed systemic disease. In addition, systemic diseases may be significant risk factors for particular neuro-ophthalmic conditions that, if successfully modified or treated, can not only restore or prevent visual dysfunction but also lessen systemic morbidity and mortality. This chapter is not intended to be a comprehensive review, but rather is meant to provide an overview of the more common systemic diseases with neuro-ophthalmic manifestations that ophthalmologists may encounter in clinical practice.

VASCULAR DISEASES

Arterial Hypertension

Arterial hypertension is a significant and reversible cause of morbidity and mortality in the United States (US), affecting approximately 30% of adults.[1] Primary or essential hypertension is multifactorial in etiology associated with older age, obesity, positive family history, African-American race, high-salt diet, excessive alcohol intake, diabetes mellitus, and dyslipidemia. Secondary hypertension results from underlying medical conditions such as primary kidney disease, hyperaldosteronism, obstructive sleep apnea, and medications.

Neuro-ophthalmic Manifestations

Bilateral optic disk edema (with or without signs of encephalopathy) can occur in patients with severely elevated blood pressure (Figs. 94.1A and B). Signs of hypertensive retinopathy, such as vascular attenuation, cotton wool spots and flame hemorrhages, are often concurrently present. The etiopathogenesis of the optic disk edema can be either ischemia or elevated intracranial pressure (ICP) from cerebral edema.

Aside from causing a vasculopathy that can result in optic nerve edema (i.e. ischemic optic neuropathy), hypertension is a risk factor for nonarteritic anterior ischemic optic neuropathy (NAION). In addition, systemic hypertension is associated with microvascular ischemic ocular motor cranial neuropathies.

Diagnosis and Treatment

A diagnosis of hypertension requires two or more elevated blood pressure measurements greater than 140/90 in adults under 60 years of age, or greater than 150/90 in adults over 60 years of age. Beyond nonpharmacologic life style modifications, first-line therapies for uncomplicated hypertension include thiazide diuretics, long-acting calcium channels blockers, angiotensin-converting enzyme (ACE) inhibitors, and angiotensin II receptor blockers.[1]

Stroke

Stroke is the second leading cause of death worldwide and a very common reason for long-term disability in the United States. Broadly speaking, stroke is categorized as either ischemic or hemorrhagic. This section will discuss occlusion of the arterial and venous circulations affecting the visual pathway.

Arterial Stroke

Arterial infarctions can affect the anterior or posterior circulation of the brain. The classic visual symptom of anterior circulation infarction is amaurosis fugax (i.e. retinal transient ischemic attack) with the vision loss typically lasting minutes. Transient retinal ischemia or a retinal artery occlusion can be the result of an embolus originating from the carotid arteries, great vessels of the chest, or heart

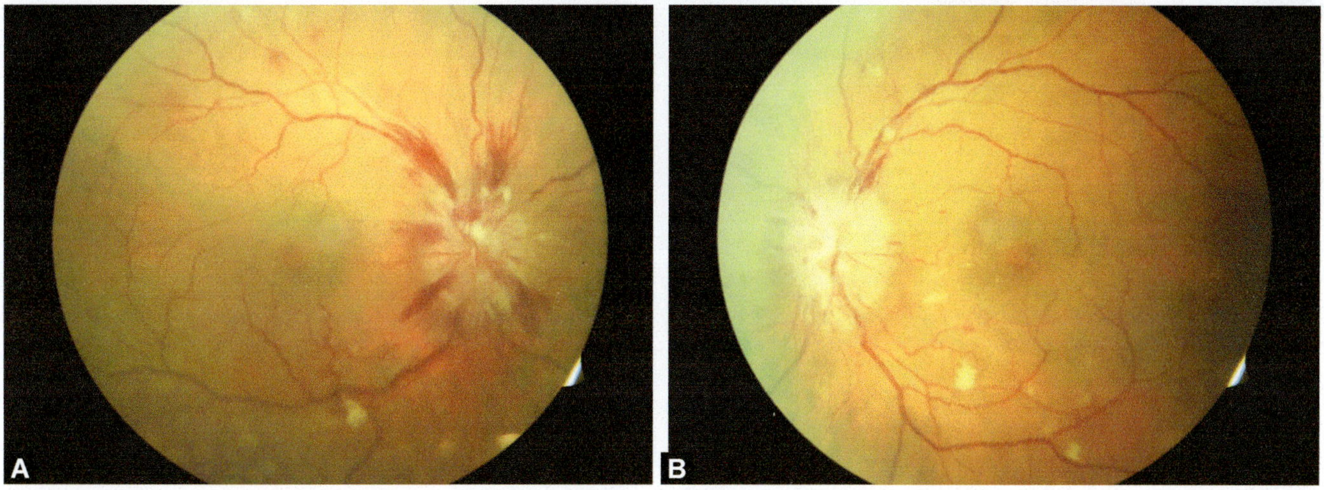

Figs. 94.1A and B: Bilateral optic disk edema in malignant hypertension. In addition to the bilateral optic disk edema, there are multiple cotton-wool spots, retinal hemorrhages and arteriolar attenuation. Blood pressure was measured to be 188/106.

and is associated with increased risk of cerebrovascular and cardiovascular disease.[2]

Infarctions of the posterior circulation comprise approximately 20% of ischemic strokes and are most often due to thromboembolism, followed by atherosclerosis. Interruption of the posterior circulation often results in binocular vision loss. Of note, migraine, epilepsy, and posterior reversible encephalopathy syndrome (PRES) can also result in bilateral visual loss.[3]

Diagnosis and Treatment

Initial stroke evaluation includes prompt neuroimaging to rule out hemorrhage, typically by noncontrast head computed tomography (CT) or brain magnetic resonance imaging (MRI). Diffusion-weighted imaging (DWI) has a very high sensitivity for detecting acute to early subacute infarctions but has suboptimal specificity.[4]

With confirmation of an ischemic stroke, intravenous (IV) thrombolysis with tissue plasminogen activator (tPA) can be administered within 4.5 hours of symptom onset.[5] In addition, appropriate diagnostic workup to ascertain any medically treatable etiologies (e.g. cardiac arrhythmias, carotid artery disease, and other embolic sources) should be performed immediately. With a posterior circulation stroke, the vertebrobasilar circulation is evaluated with either CT angiography (CTA), magnetic resonance angiography (MRA) or transcranial Doppler imaging. Secondary stroke prevention is focused on risk factor modification and treatment of hypertension, dyslipidemia, obesity, and cigarette smoking.[6]

Venous Sinus Thrombosis

Venous sinus thrombosis (VST) is a rare cerebrovascular disease that, unlike arterial stroke, generally affects younger patients. Thrombosis in the cerebral cortical veins can induce venous infarction and localized cerebral edema, while VST may cause ICP elevation by reducing cerebrospinal fluid (CSF) outflow. About 85% of patients with VST have prothrombotic risk factors such as genetic or acquired thrombophilias, infection, malignancy, trauma, or medications. The clinical presentation of VST can be variable, but most patients present with a severe headache.[7,8]

Neuro-ophthalmic Manifestations

Papilledema—defined as optic disk swelling due to increased ICP—is present in approximately 30–50% of patients with VST. Patients can be asymptomatic or complain of decreased vision, diplopia, and visual field deficits. All patients should be followed over time to monitor for visual loss in the presence of papilledema.

Diagnosis and Treatment

Either MRI with magnetic resonance venography (MRV) or CT with CT venography (CTV) are appropriate neuroimaging modalities for VST (Figs. 94.2A to C). Anticoagulation with unfractionated heparin or low molecular weight heparin in the acute phase of VST is followed by warfarin for long-term management. Progressive visual loss due to papilledema not responsive to medical therapy with anticoagulation

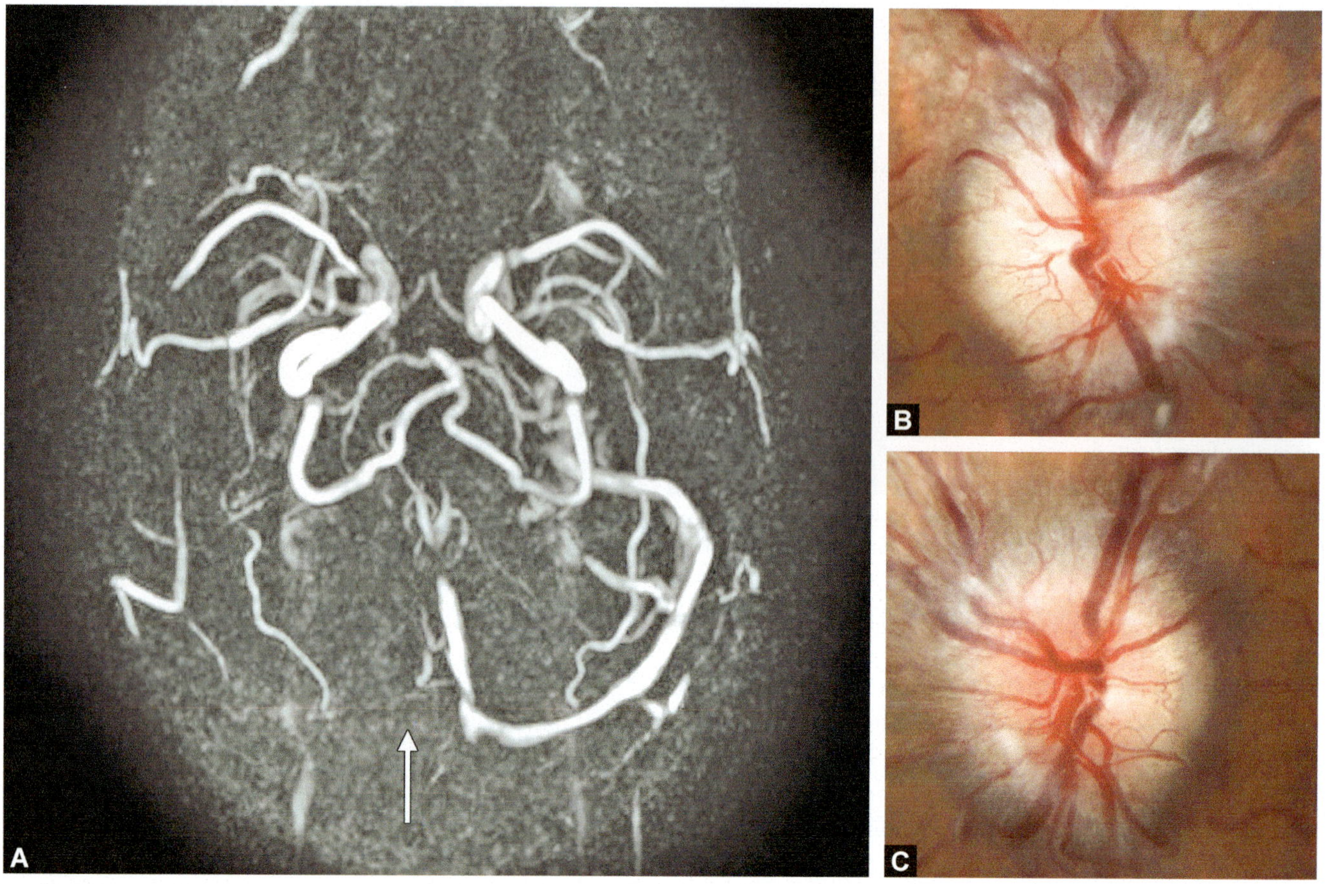

Figs. 94.2A to C: Venous sinus thrombosis with bilateral disk edema. (A) Magnetic resonance venography (MRV), axial view, demonstrating thrombosis of the right transverse sinus (arrow) resulting in (B and C) bilateral disk edema.

and acetazolamide may require an optic nerve sheath fenestration, endovascular thrombectomy or a CSF diversion procedure.

Cerebral Aneurysm

A cerebral aneurysm is a localized dilation of an arterial wall. Saccular aneurysms are localized outpouchings of the arterial wall, while fusiform aneurysms are circumferential arterial dilations. Intracranial aneurysms are found in about 5% of the US population. The majority of cerebral aneurysms are unruptured and asymptomatic. Approximately 90% of symptomatic aneurysms present at the time of rupture. The major risk factors for aneurysmal rupture are size (greater rate of rupture in aneurysms >10 mm in diameter), hypertension and smoking.[9]

Most aneurysms are located within the anterior cerebral artery circulation. About 25–40% of aneurysms arise at the internal carotid artery-posterior communicating artery bifurcation, with other common locations occurring at the anterior communicating artery (25–30%) and middle cerebral artery (13–30%). Ophthalmic artery aneurysms are rare (<5%).[10]

Neuro-ophthalmic Manifestations

A posterior communicating artery aneurysm can result in cranial nerve (CN) III palsy that generally is painful (Fig. 94.3). However, microvascular ischemic CN III palsies can also be painful; therefore, this symptom cannot be used to differentiate between an aneurysm or ischemia. Because the pupillomotor fibers are situated peripherally along the nerve, aneurysmal CN III palsies are often pupil involving but this "rule of the pupil" should not be considered absolute. Incomplete extraocular muscle involvement requires neuroimaging to rule out aneurysmal compression.

An anterior communicating artery aneurysm can result in vision loss from compression of the anterior visual pathways (e.g. optic nerve, chiasm or tract). Vision loss can

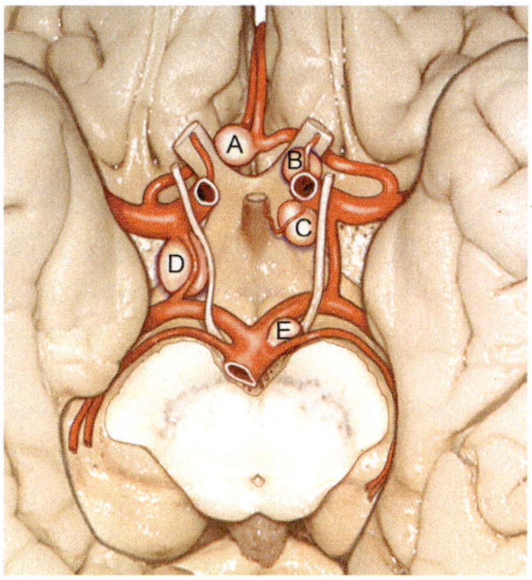

Fig. 94.3: Cerebral aneurysm sites within the circle of Willis causing neuro-ophthalmic manifestations. Aneurysms of (A) the anterior communicating artery and (B) ophthalmic artery can affect the optic chiasm and/or optic nerve. Aneurysms at the junction of (C) the superior hypophyseal artery, (D) posterior communicating artery, or at (E) the posterior cerebral artery can compress CN III.

Source: Reproduced with permission from Taravati P, Lee AG, Bhatti MT, et al. That's a wrap. Surv Ophthalmol. 2006;51(4):434-44.

also occur from subarachnoid hemorrhage, as aneurysms of the anterior communicating artery may rupture prior to direct compression on the visual pathway.

Ophthalmic artery aneurysm can present with acute onset or slowly progressive vision loss, headache, and orbital pain. The unilateral vision loss is associated with varying visual field defects; in some cases, there is an inferior defect due to compression of the superior optic nerve against the falciform ligament. If the anterior optic chiasm is compressed, there may be an ipsilateral optic neuropathy with a contralateral superotemporal field defect (i.e. junctional scotoma).

Aneurysmal subarachnoid hemorrhage can result in papilledema or CN VI palsy. Terson syndrome is defined as an intraocular hemorrhage in the presence of an intracranial hemorrhage (Figs. 94.4A and B).

Diagnosis and Treatment

If a cerebral aneurysm is suspected, urgent neuroimaging should be obtained. CTA or MRA is often adequate to detect a symptomatic aneurysm, but occasionally, conventional catheter angiography may be required to secure the diagnosis.

For small, asymptomatic cerebral aneurysms, expectant observation with blood pressure control is generally favored. For symptomatic aneurysms, treatment options include endovascular coil embolization, craniotomy with clipping, or very rarely wrapping with gauze (i.e. muslin).

INFLAMMATORY-IMMUNOLOGICAL DISEASES

Multiple Sclerosis

Multiple sclerosis (MS) is an immune-mediated, inflammatory, demyelinating disease of the CNS that most commonly affects young adults with women more frequently affected than men. The prevalence of MS varies geographically with Europe, southern Canada, the northern United States, New Zealand, and Southeast Australia having the highest prevalence rates.

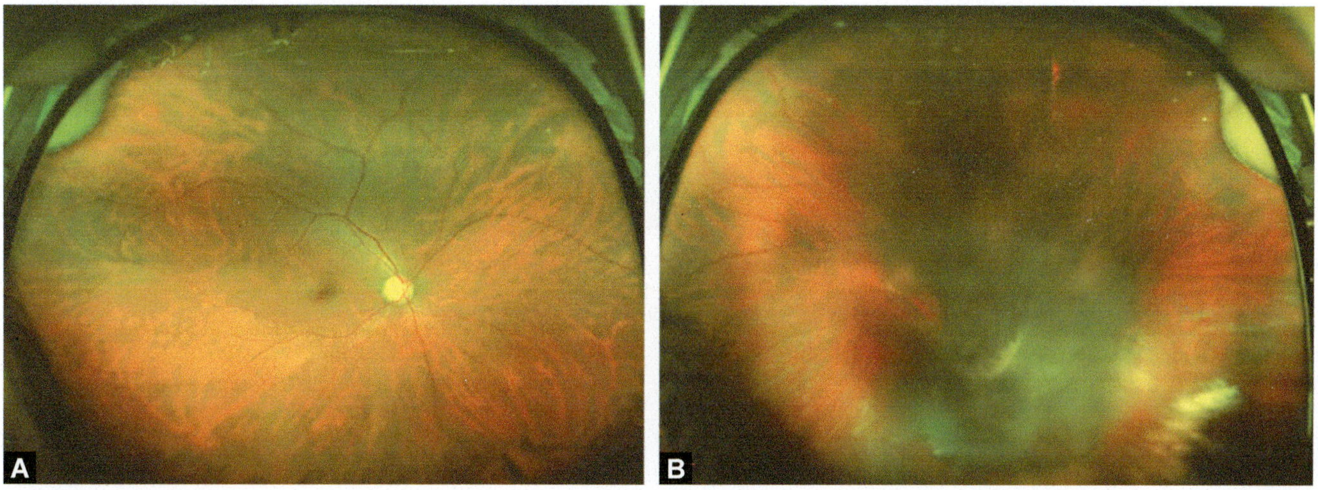

Figs. 94.4A and B: Terson syndrome. (A) Vitreous hemorrhage in the left eye in a patient with subarachnoid hemorrhage; (B) The right eye is normal.

It is believed that the oligodendrocyte is the primary target of the dysfunctional immune process. Focal demyelinating plaques are present in various areas of the CNS (e.g. cerebrum, cerebellum, brainstem or spinal cord), and are associated with inflammation, gliosis and axonal damage.

Neuro-ophthalmic Manifestations

Multiple sclerosis may present as a monosymptomatic or polysymptomatic disorder with neurological features of fatigue, paresthesias, vertigo, gait disturbance, motor weakness, or bowel and bladder dysfunction. Optic neuritis is the most common neuro-ophthalmic manifestation, characterized by acute, painful vision loss that typically resolves over weeks with or without treatment. After resolution of the visual loss, some patients may report transiently decreased vision with exercise or elevated body temperature, known as Uhthoff phenomenon. Approximately one-third of patients with optic neuritis have optic disk edema (i.e. papillitis). Infrequently, a demyelinating lesion can involve the optic chiasm, optic tracts, optic radiations or visual cortex, resulting in binocular visual field defects. A variety of supranuclear, nuclear, and fascicular ocular motility disturbances can be seen in the setting of MS. Internuclear ophthalmoplegia (INO) due to a lesion of the medial longitudinal fasciculus is the most common ocular motility syndrome, followed by CN VI palsy.

Diagnosis and Treatment

The diagnosis of MS is determined by the dissemination of CNS lesions in space and time based on clinical, CSF and MRI findings (Table 94.1).[11] MS lesions are typically seen in the periventricular region and corpus callosum. The lesions appear hyperintense on T2-weighted or fluid-attenuated inversion recovery (FLAIR) sequences, and hypointense (i.e. "black holes") or not visible on the precontrast T1-weighted sequences. Enhancement on the postcontrast T1-weighted images is indicative of acute inflammation.

Depending on the severity and location of the neurological deficit, acute MS exacerbations are generally treated with high-dose IV corticosteroids. The Optic Neuritis Treatment Trial (ONTT) showed that IV corticosteroids led to a faster visual recovery but did not affect the final visual outcome.

Based on the ONTT, the estimated 15-year risk of developing MS in a patient presenting with optic neuritis as their first demyelinating event (i.e. clinically isolated syndrome) is approximately 25% in the presence of a normal MRI, and approximately 70% with one or more brain lesions (Fig. 94.5).[12] Long-term treatments with disease-modifying immunomodulatory agents have been

Table 94.1: McDonald criteria for diagnosis of multiple sclerosis (MS).

Clinical presentation	Imaging	Additional information needed
≥2 MS attacks	Objective clinical evidence of ≥2 MRI lesions, or 1 MRI lesion with history of prior attack confirmed by objective findings	None
≥2 MS attacks	Objective clinical evidence of 1 MRI lesion	*Dissemination of lesions in space*: • ≥1 T2 lesion in at least 2 of 4 MS-typical regions (periventricular, juxtacortical, infratentorial, spinal cord) • Await clinical attack that implicates a different site
1 MS attack	Objective clinical evidence of ≥2 MRI lesions	*Dissemination of lesions in time*: • Simultaneous presence of asymptomatic contrast-enhancing and non-enhancing lesions at any time • New lesions on follow-up MRI
1 MS attack	Objective clinical evidence of 1 MRI lesion (clinically isolated syndrome)	• Dissemination of lesions in space • Dissemination of lesions in time
Insidious neurological progression suggestive of MS for 1+ years (primary progressive MS)		• Dissemination in space with ≥1 T2 lesion in at least 2 of 4 MS-typical regions • Dissemination in space with ≥2 T2 lesions in the spinal cord • CSF with oligoclonal bands or elevated IgG

(MRI: Magnetic resonance imaging; CSF: Cerebrospinal fluid)

Source: Adapted with permission from Polman CH, Reingold SC, Banwell B, et al. Diagnostic criteria for multiple sclerosis: 2010 revisions to the McDonald criteria. Ann Neurol. 2011;69(2):292-302.

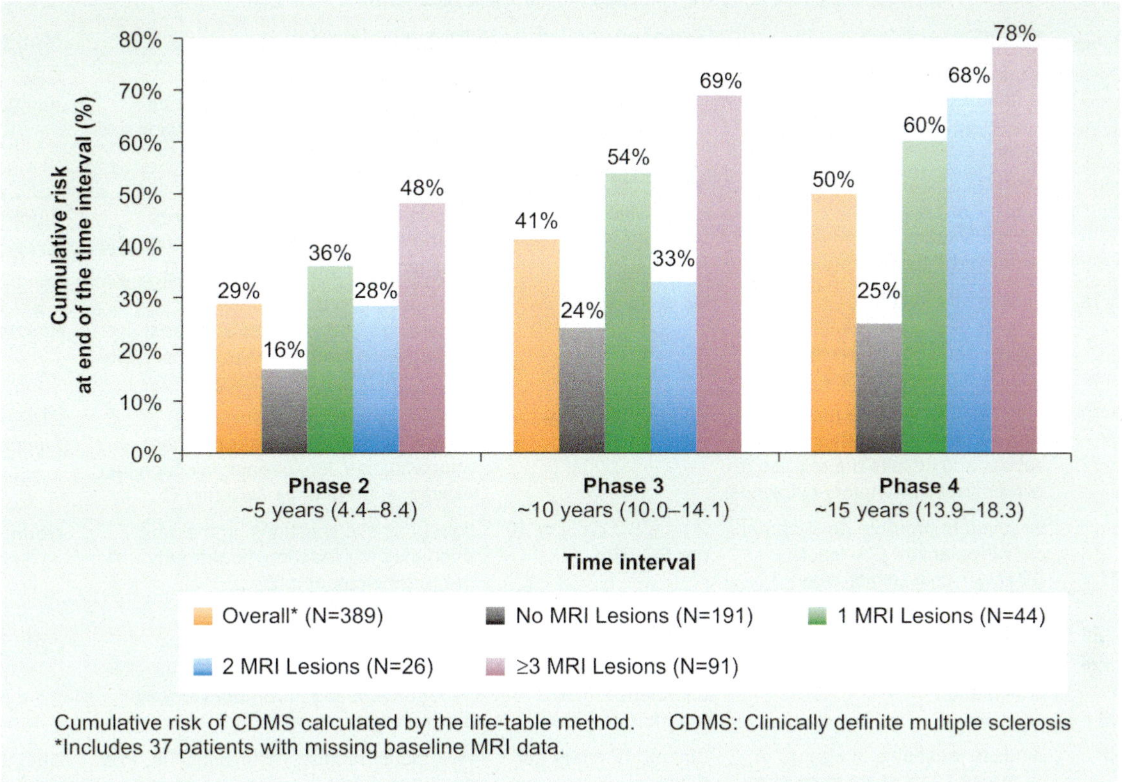

Fig. 94.5: Cumulative risk of developing multiple sclerosis (MS) after optic neuritis from the optic neuritis treatment trial. The cumulative 15-year risk of developing multiple sclerosis after an episode of optic neuritis is based on the initial brain neuroimaging findings. The risk of developing MS is approximately 25% in patients with a normal brain MRI and approximately 70% if there is 1 or more lesion.

Source: Reproduced with permission from Abou Zeid N, Bhatti MT. Acute inflammatory demyelinating optic neuritis: evidence-based visual and neurological considerations. Neurologist. 2008;14(4):207-23.

shown to delay the development of MS in patients with a clinically isolated syndrome and reduce the rate of relapses in patients with relapsing forms of MS (Table 94.2).

Neuromyelitis Optica

Neuromyelitis optica (NMO), or Devic disease, is an autoimmune inflammatory condition that preferentially affects the optic nerves and spinal cord. NMO has a strong female predilection, commonly presenting in young adults with a median age of onset of 31 years. NMO has been associated with other systemic autoimmune disorders such as systemic lupus erythematosus (SLE), Sjögren syndrome and rheumatoid arthritis.

Neuromyelitis optica is strongly associated with the NMO-immunoglobulin G (IgG) or anti-aquaporin-4 (AQP-4) antibody, which targets the astrocyte water channel protein AQP-4. NMO is within a spectrum of clinical presentations known as NMO spectrum of disorders (NMOSD) that includes AQP-IgG seronegative disease.

Neuro-ophthalmic Manifestations

Neuromyelitis optica can present with painful unilateral or bilateral optic neuritis (*see* Chapter 92, Common Optic Neuropathies, for details). Prior to, during, or after the optic neuritis, there may be spinal cord involvement (i.e. transverse myelitis). Brainstem involvement manifest by vomiting, hiccups, and nystagmus occurs in approximately one-third of patients and is thought to be due to the relative sensitivity of the area postrema to NMO-IgG.[13]

Diagnosis and Treatment

The current diagnostic criteria for NMOSD include the core clinical characteristics of optic neuritis and acute myelitis, AQP-IgG serologic testing, and MRI findings (Table 94.3). In the acute phase, NMO is treated with high-dose IV corticosteroids and/or plasma exchange. Chronic immunosuppression to reduce relapses can be accomplished with rituximab, mycophenolate mofetil or azathioprine.[14]

Table 94.2: Current US FDA-approved drugs for relapsing remitting multiple sclerosis (MS).

Drug	Mechanism of action	Dosage	Adverse effects	Monitoring
Interferon β-1a (Avonex®)	Modifies the cytokine production in favor of an anti-inflammatory subset and inhibits the release of certain proinflammatory cytokines	30 μg IM weekly	Flu-like symptoms, depression, thyroid dysfunction, liver enzymes abnormalities, leukopenia, injection site reactions; pregnancy-category C	CBC, LFT, thyroid function
Peginterferon β-1a (Plegridy®)	Modifies the cytokine production in favor of an anti-inflammatory subset and inhibits the release of certain proinflammatory cytokines	125 μg SQ every other week	Flu-like symptoms, depression, thyroid dysfunction, liver enzymes abnormalities, leukopenia, injection site reactions; pregnancy-category C	CBC, LFT, thyroid function
Interferon β-1a (Rebif®)	Modifies the cytokine production in favor of an anti-inflammatory subset and inhibits the release of certain proinflammatory cytokines	22 or 44 μg SQ tiw	Flu-like symptoms, depression, thyroid dysfunction, liver enzymes abnormalities, leukopenia, injection site reactions; pregnancy-category C	CBC, LFT, thyroid function
Interferon β-1b (Betaseron®/ Extavia®)	Modifies the cytokine production in favor of an anti-inflammatory subset and inhibits the release of certain proinflammatory cytokines	250 μg SQ every other day	Flu-like symptoms, depression, thyroid dysfunction, liver enzymes abnormalities, leukopenia, injection site reactions; pregnancy-category C	CBC, LFT, thyroid function
Glatiramer acetate (Copaxone®/ Glatopa®)	Believed to promote development of Th2-polarized GA-reactive CD4(+) T-cells, which may decrease additional inflammation	20 mg SQ daily or 40 mg SQ tiw	Injections site reactions, immediate post-injection reaction, lipoatrophy; pregnancy-category B	None
Mitoxantrone (Novantrone®)	Potent suppressor of T cell, B cell, and macrophage proliferation	12 mg/m^2 IV every 3 months with a lifetime cumulative dose ≤140 mg/mg/m^2	Hair loss, cardiotoxicity, leukemia, infertility, infection, leukopenia, anemia, nausea, vomiting, thrombocytopenia; pregnancy-category D	CBC, LFT, urinalysis, LVEF
Natalizumab (Tysabri®)	Binds to leukocyte integrins, impairing attachment to cerebral endothelial cells and reducing migration across the blood-brain barrier	300 mg IV every 28 days	Headache, fatigue, recurrent UTIs, PML, hypersensitivity reaction; pregnancy-category C	CBC, LFT, JC virus antibody index
Alemtuzumab (Lemtrada®)	Long-lasting depletion of circulating B and T lymphocytes followed by a slow repopulation from the unaffected hematopoietic precursor cells	12 mg IV daily for 5 days at month 0, then 12 mg IV daily for 3 days at month 12	Secondary autoimmunity, immune thrombocytopenic purpura, autoimmune thyroid disease, antiglomerular basement membrane disease, malignancy, infusion reactions, headaches, flushing; pregnancy-category C	CBC, serum creatinine, thyroid function, urinalysis
Fingolimod (Gilenya®)	Inhibits egress of lymphocytes from lymph nodes, reducing trafficking of pathogenic cells	0.5 mg PO daily	AV block, bradycardia, macular edema, zoster, liver enzyme abnormalities, PML; pregnancy-category C	Cardiac monitoring (initial dose only), CBC, LFT, macular edema screen
Teriflunomide (Aubagio®)	Inhibits DNA pyrimidine synthesis in dividing T and B cells	7 or 14 mg PO daily	Headache, diarrhea, fatigue, hair thinning, liver enzymes abnormalities; pregnancy-category X	CBC, LFT
Dimethyl fumarate (Tecfidera®)	Activation of Nrf-2 mediated antioxidative response pathways leading to innate anti-inflammatory effects	240 mg PO bid	Flushing, abdominal pain, diarrhea, lymphopenia, liver enzyme abnormalities, PML; pregnancy-category C	CBC, LFT
Ocrelizumab (Ocrevus™)	Selective depletion of CD20-expressing B cells	300 mg IV biweekly for 2 doses, then 600 mg IV every 6 months	Infection (upper respiratory tract, nasopharyngitis, UTI), infusion-related reaction, flu-like symptoms, headache, fatigue, depression, arthralgias, malignancy	Hepatitis B serologic testing

(AV: Atrioventricular; CBC: Complete blood count; GA: Glatiramer actetate; IM: Intramuscular; IV: Intravenous; LFT: Liver function test; LVEF: Left ventricular ejection fraction; PML: Progressive multifocal leukoencephlopathy; SQ: Subcutaneous; UTI: Urinary tract infection)

Source: Reproduced and modified with permission from Eckstein C, Bhatti MT. Currently approved and emerging oral therapies in multiple sclerosis: an update for the ophthalmologist. Surv Ophthalmol. 2016;61(3):3.

Table 94.3: Criteria for the diagnosis of NMOSD in adult patients.

Core clinical characteristics	Diagnostic criteria for NMOSD with AQP4-IgG	Diagnostic criteria for NMOSD without AQP4-IgG or unknown AQP4-IgG status	Additional MRI requirements for NMOSD without AQP4-IgG or unknown AQP4-IgG status
1. Optic neuritis 2. Acute myelitis 3. Area postrema syndrome (episode of hiccups or nausea and vomiting) 4. Acute brainstem syndrome 5. Symptomatic narcolepsy or acute diencephalic clinical syndrome with NMOSD-typical diencephalic MRI lesions 6. Symptomatic cerebral syndrome with NMOSD-typical brain lesions	1. At least 1 core clinical characteristic 2. Exclusion of alternative diagnoses	1. At least 2 core clinical characteristics during one or more clinical attacks and meeting all of the following requirements: a. At least 1 core clinical characteristic must be optic neuritis, acute myelitis, or area postrema syndrome b. Dissemination in space (2 or more core clinical characteristics) c. Fulfillment of additional MRI requirements (see right) 2. Exclusion of alternative diagnoses	1. *Acute optic neuritis*: A brain MRI showing normal findings (or only nonspecific white matter lesions), or an optic nerve MRI with lesion extending over more than one-half the optic nerve length or involving the optic chiasm 2. *Acute myelitis*: An associated intramedullary MRI lesion extending over either ≥3 contiguous segments or ≥3 contiguous segments of focal spinal cord atrophy in patients with a history compatible with acute myelitis 3. *Area postrema syndrome*: Associated dorsal medulla/area postrema lesions 4. *Acute brainstem syndrome*: Associated periependymal brainstem lesions

(AQP4: Aquaporin-4; IgG: Immunoglobulin G; MRI: Magnetic resonance imaging; NMOSD: Neuromyelitis optica spectrum disorder)
Source: Adapted with permission from Wingerchuk DM, Banwell B, Bennett JL, et al. International consensus diagnostic criteria for neuromyelitis optica spectrum disorders. Neurology. 2015;85(2):177-89.

Sarcoidosis

Sarcoidosis is a heterogeneous, multisystem inflammatory disease pathologically characterized by the formation of noncaseating granulomas. Sarcoidosis commonly affects younger women, with a high prevalence rate in Northern Europeans and African-Americans. The exact cause is unknown but is felt to be due to an immune response to unidentified antigen(s).

Neuro-ophthalmic Manifestations

Sarcoidosis most often affects the lungs but also commonly involves the skin and peripheral lymph nodes. Ocular manifestations of iritis, uveitis, retinal vasculitis, conjunctival nodules, and lacrimal gland enlargement occur in 10–30% of patients (Figs. 94.6A and B) and may be asymptomatic. Neurosarcoidosis occurs in approximately 5% of cases.

Cranial neuropathies are a common neurologic complication with CN VII most frequently involved. Heerfordt syndrome is the triad of CN VII palsy, uveitis and fever. An optic neuropathy can result from increased ICP, aseptic meningitis, optic neuritis, optic perineuritis, neuroretinitis, and less commonly, optic nerve granuloma. Other less frequent neuro-ophthalmic manifestations include Horner syndrome, Argyll-Robertson pupil, and tonic pupil.[15]

Diagnosis and Treatment

The diagnosis of sarcoidosis is predicated upon a detailed history, clinical examination and radiographic findings. Elevated serum ACE levels are nonspecific. Chest X-ray or chest CT can reveal bilateral hilar adenopathy and/or inflammatory lung disease. Generally, tissue biopsy is needed for histological confirmation (Figs. 94.6A and B).

Corticosteroids are first-line treatment. Methotrexate, cyclophosphamide, mycophenolate mofetil, and infliximab are the most common immunosuppressive agents used either in combination with or as alternatives to corticosteroid therapy.

Systemic Lupus Erythematosus

Systemic lupus erythematosus is a multisystem chronic inflammatory disease. In the United States, SLE is more prevalent in African-Americans, Asians, and Hispanics than in Caucasians. SLE has a female predominance with onset during the reproductive years.

Neuro-ophthalmic Manifestations

The ocular manifestations of SLE are broad but most commonly involve the posterior segment in the form of retinopathy or retinal vasculitis. Anterior segment manifestations include keratoconjunctivitis sicca, episcleritis and scleritis. SLE can rarely affect the orbit causing myositis or orbital inflammation.[16]

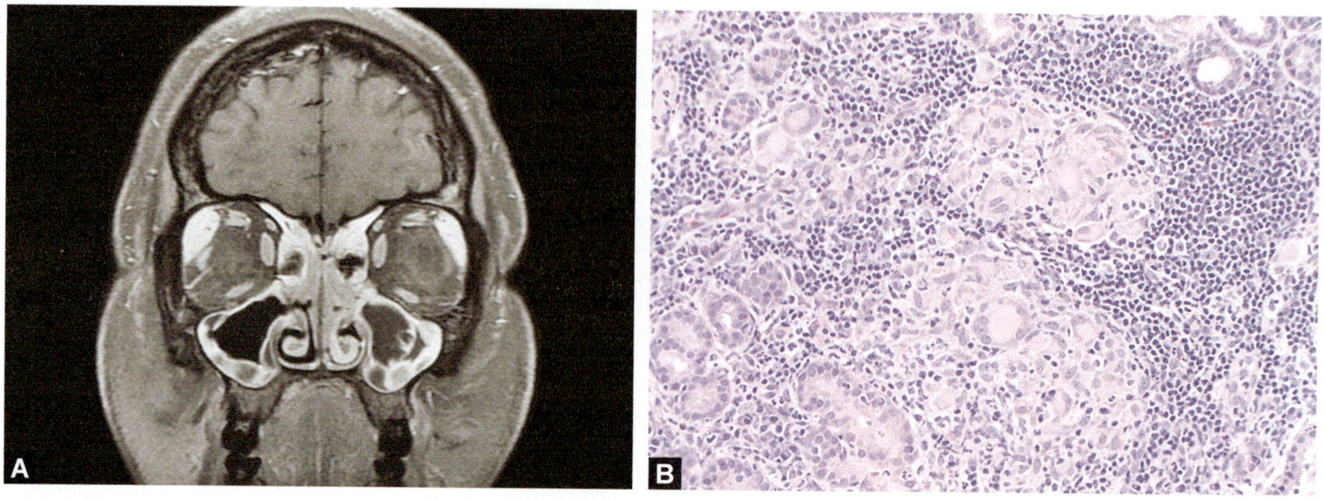

Figs. 94.6A and B: Sarcoid lacrimal gland enlargement. (A) Coronal T1-weighted fat-suppressed MRI shows enhancement of the both lacrimal glands; (B) Microphotograph (H&E stain) of the lacrimal gland biopsy demonstrates noncaseating granulomas and chronic inflammation within normal lacrimal gland alveoli.

Table 94.4: Criteria for the diagnosis of systemic lupus erythematosus (SLE).

Criterion	Definition
Malar rash	Flat or raised erythema in the malar distribution, tends to spare nasolabial folds
Discoid rash	Raised patches of erythema with adjacent keratotic scaling. Older lesions may show atrophic scarring
Photosensitivity	Skin rash due to reaction to sunlight
Oral ulcers	Painless oral or nasopharyngeal ulceration
Nonerosive arthritis	Arthritis that involves ≥2 peripheral joints, often with symptoms of tenderness and/or swelling
Pleuritis or pericarditis	Pleuritis: history of pleuritic pain, pleural friction rub, or pleural effusion Pericarditis: evidence on electrocardiogram, friction rub, or pericardial effusion
Renal disorder	Persistent proteinuria (>0.5 g/day) or cellular casts
Neurologic disorder	Seizures or psychosis (without medication effect or metabolic derangements)
Hematologic disorder	Hemolytic anemia, leukopenia or lymphopenia (≥2 occurrences), or thrombocytopenia (not medication-induced)
Immunologic disorder	Present of anti-DNA, anti-Smith, or antiphospholipid antibodies
Positive antinuclear antibody (ANA)	Abnormal ANA titer in the absence of drugs

Source: Adapted with permission from Hochberg MC. Updating the American College of Rheumatology revised criteria for the classification of systemic lupus erythematosus. Arthritis Rheum. 1997;40:1725; Tan EM, Cohen AS, Fries JF, et al. The 1982 revised criteria for the classification of systemic lupus erythematosus. Arthritis Rheum. 1982;25:1271-7.

Cranial neuropathies occur in 10–15% of cases, frequently affecting CN III, CN V and CN VII. An optic neuropathy is present in 1–2% of patients. Neurologic manifestations include headache, psychosis, cognitive dysfunction, meningitis, seizures and stroke.

Diagnosis and Treatment

The diagnostic criteria for SLE include a multitude of systemic clinical manifestations (e.g. malar rash, photosensitivity, discoid rash, oral ulcers, arthritis, serositis, proteinuria, seizures or psychosis), hematologic disorders, and abnormal serologic tests (Table 94.4).

Most patients are treated initially with hydroxychloroquine or chloroquine. Corticosteroids are used acutely in the setting of ocular or neurological involvement. Steroid-sparing immunomodulatory agents include methotrexate, mycophenolate mofetil, azathioprine and cyclophosphamide.

Giant Cell Arteritis

Giant cell arteritis (GCA) is the most common vasculitis in patients over the age of 50 years, affecting medium to large caliber vessels. GCA has a female predilection with the highest incidence in patients of Scandinavian descent and is associated with polymyalgia rheumatica (PMR). Histopathological analysis demonstrates inflammation within the vascular wall causing thickening of the intimal layer with subsequent arterial occlusion.

Neuro-ophthalmic Manifestations

The clinical presentation of GCA is variable and includes headache, jaw claudication, transient vision loss, scalp tenderness, fevers, weight loss and fatigue. Palpation of the temporal arteries can reveal tenderness, nodularity or beading, or absence of temporal pulses. Visual loss most frequently occurs from anterior ischemic optic neuropathy (Fig. 94.7). Other causes of visual loss include central retinal artery occlusion, ophthalmic artery occlusion, or posterior ischemic optic neuropathy. Fluorescein angiography may demonstrate delayed and patchy choroidal filling. In rare cases, GCA can cause ophthalmoplegia, ocular ischemia or orbital ischemia.

Diagnosis and Treatment

Because of its devastating effects on the eye and other organ systems, GCA is not only an ophthalmic emergency but also a medical emergency. Patients with suspected GCA should undergo a complete blood count (CBC), erythrocyte sedimentation rate (ESR) and C-reactive protein (CRP) (Flowchart 94.1). The gold standard for diagnosis is a temporal artery biopsy (TAB). The TAB should be at least 2 cm in length to avoid missing pathological "skip" lesions. Histologic examination can show transmural inflammation, internal elastic lamina disruption, multinucleated giant cells, and intima and media layer thickening (Figs. 94.8A and B). To ensure diagnostic accuracy of the TAB, the sample should be obtained within 2 weeks of starting corticosteroid therapy.

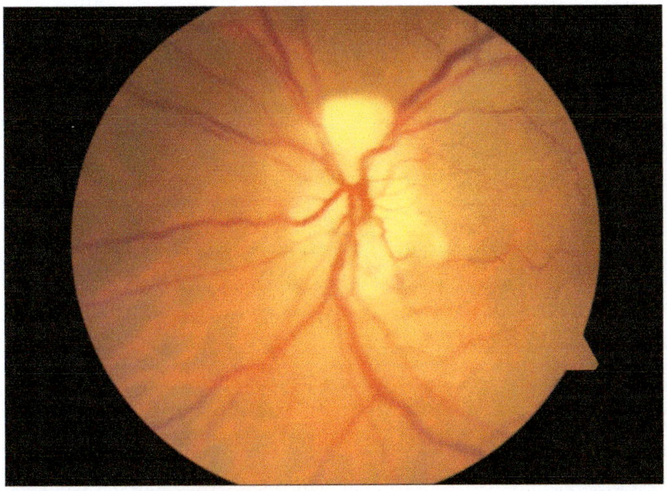

Fig. 94.7: Anterior ischemic optic neuropathy due to giant cell arteritis (GCA). There is a chalky white appearance of the optic disk edema with a cotton-wool spot superior to the disk.

Any patient with suspected GCA should be started immediately on corticosteroids. For those patients with visual loss, high-dose IV corticosteroids are recommended by most experts. Immunomodulatory treatment agents include methotrexate and the recently approved tocilizumab, a monoclonal antibody against interleukin 6.[17]

Myasthenia Gravis

Myasthenia gravis (MG) is an autoimmune neuromuscular junction disorder characterized by variable and fatigable muscle weakness. The age of onset of MG has a bimodal distribution with women less than 40 years and men greater than 50 years of age being affected. It is well established that the autoantibodies against the acetylcholine receptor are the pathogenic basis for the muscle weakness.

Neuro-ophthalmic Manifestations

In over half of patients, only ocular manifestations are present at disease onset (i.e. ocular MG). Approximately half of these patients will go on to develop systemic MG, frequently within the first 2 years of presentation. Ninety percent of patients with MG will have ocular symptoms at some time. Systemic manifestations include dysarthria, dysphagia, fatigable chewing, proximal limb weakness, and respiratory muscle weakness.

Ocular MG can present with unilateral or bilateral ptosis that worsens with prolonged upgaze. There may be overshoot of the upper eyelid from downgaze to upgaze (i.e. Cogan eyelid twitch). Eyelid curtaining can be elicited by elevation of one eyelid with observation of exaggerated ptosis of the contralateral eyelid. Diplopia is also common (*see* Chapter 95, Diplopia Diagnosis and Management).

Flowchart 94.1: Pretemporal artery biopsy risk factor assessment algorithm for giant cell arteritis (GCA).

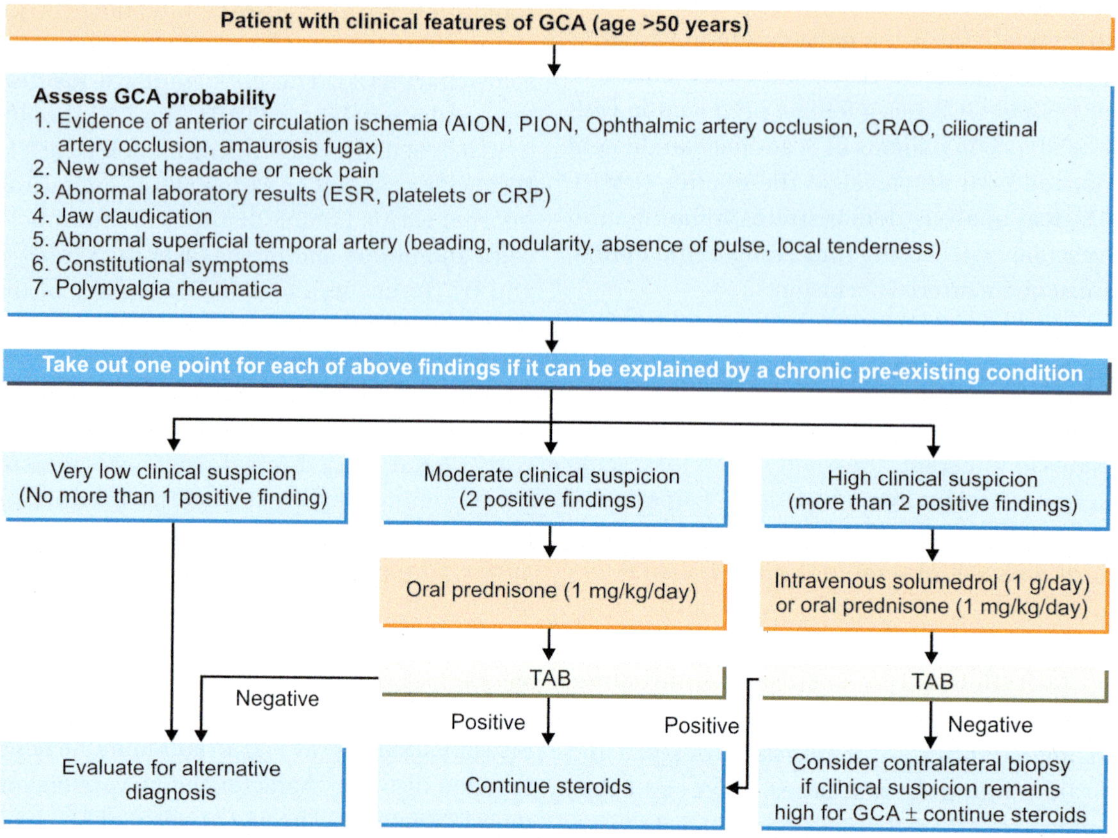

(AION: Anterior ischemic optic neuropathy; PION: Posterior ischemic optic neuropathy; CRAO: Central retinal artery occlusion; ESR: Erythrocyte sedimentation rate; CRP: C-reactive protein; TAB: Temporal artery biopsy)

Source: Reproduced with permission from El-Dairi MA, Chang L, Proia AD, et al. Diagnositc algorithm for patients with suspected giant cell arteritis. J Neuroophthalmol. 2015;35(3):246-53.

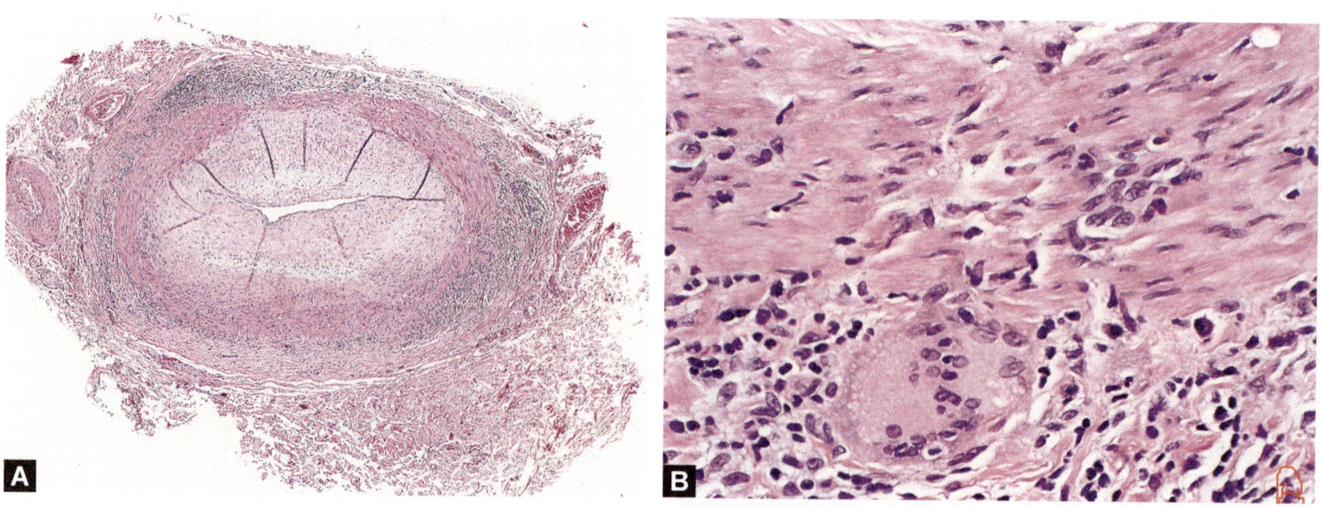

Figs. 94.8A and B: Histopathology of giant cell arteritis (H&E stain). (A) Low power microphotograph shows inflammation in all layers with thickening of the vessel wall and luminal stenosis; (B) High power view shows a multinucleated giant cell surrounded by inflammatory cells.

Diagnosis and Treatment

Diagnostic testing also is reviewed in Chapter 95. The goal of medical therapy includes both symptomatic relief and systemic remission and often starts with acetylcholinesterase inhibitors. For patients who remain symptomatic, corticosteroid therapy and/or immunosuppression with an agent such as mycophenolate mofetil is often required. Aminoglycosides, macrolides, fluoroquinolones, chloroquine, statins, and magnesium can worsen on "unmask" symptoms of MG. All patients with MG should undergo chest imaging to exclude the possibility of a thymoma.[18]

INFECTIOUS DISEASES

Syphilis

Syphilis is caused by the spirochete *Treponema pallidum* and is sexually acquired or congenitally transmitted through the birth canal. According to the World Health Organization, the global prevalence of syphilis in 2012 was estimated at 18 million in individuals aged 15–49 years. The highest prevalence rates are found in Africa, Southeast Asia, and the Western Pacific. In the United States, syphilis has been on the rise since the year 2000, in part, due to the increase in men who have sex with men.

Neuro-ophthalmic Manifestations

Syphilis can be classified into early (primary and secondary) or late (tertiary) stages. Following initial exposure and an incubation period of 3 weeks to 3 months, the hallmark of primary syphilis is a chancre, which is a painless papule at the inoculation site. The chancre resolves in 3–6 weeks without treatment. In secondary syphilis, patients develop a systemic illness with wide-ranging symptoms that include fever, malaise, skin rashes, aphthous ulcers, and lymphadenopathy. An optic neuropathy can develop in the secondary or tertiary stages of the disease. Early neurosyphilis can present as an aseptic meningitis with secondary cranial neuropathies, supranuclear palsies, or papilledema. Late neurosyphilis can affect the spinal cord (i.e. tabes dorsalis) and is classically associated with Argyll Robertson pupils (*see* Chapter 100). Five percent of patients may have a uveitis, vasculitis or chorioretinitis.

Diagnosis and Treatment

Diagnosis requires screening and reflex serologic testing of the blood. Nontreponemal tests include the Venereal Disease Research Laboratory (VDRL) test and rapid plasma reagin (RPR). Specific treponemal tests are the *T. pallidum* particle agglutination (TP-PA) test and fluorescent treponemal antibody absorption (FTA-ABS) test. A reactive CSF VDRL confirms neurosyphilis, but a nonreactive test is inconclusive. Patients testing positive for syphilis should also be tested for the human immunodeficiency virus (HIV) due to a high rate of coinfection. Treatment for syphilis is intramuscular or IV penicillin, with the dosage and route determined by the stage of infection (Table 94.5).[19]

Table 94.5: Syphilis treatment guidelines in adults.

Stage	Treatment regimen
Primary, secondary or early latent (<1 year)	2.4 million units of intramuscular (IM) benzathine penicillin G in a single dose
Late latent (>1 year), latent of unknown duration	7.2 million units of IM benzathine penicillin G total (administered in 3 doses of 2.4 million units weekly)
Tertiary syphilis (gummas and cardiovascular syphilis)	7.2 million units of IM benzathine penicillin G total (administered in 3 doses of 2.4 million units weekly)
Neurosyphilis	18–24 million units per day of aqueous crystalline penicillin G (administered as 3–4 million units every 4 hours or continuous infusion for 10–14 days)
Penicillin allergy	May undergo penicillin skin testing to confirm allergy Patients with positive skin test can undergo penicillin desensitization (limited data to support use of other medications such as doxycycline and tetracycline for primary or secondary stages)
Pregnant women	Penicillin treatment regimen appropriate for stage of disease

Source: Adapted with permission from Centers for Disease Control and Prevention. (2015). Syphilis. Sexually Transmitted Diseases Treatment Guidelines, 2015. [online] Available from: *https://www.cdc.gov/std/tg2015/syphilis.htm*. [Accessed December, 2017]

Cat Scratch Disease

Cat scratch disease (CSD) is an infection caused by *Bartonella henselae*, a gram-negative rod. Cats are the primary reservoir. CSD generally affects immunocompetent patients, more frequently children and young adults. Cats are infected by fleas carrying *B. henselae*. The bacterium is transmitted to humans by either inoculation indirectly from the cat flea or directly from a cat scratch or bite. Local infection leads to a regional lymphadenopathy, and sometimes there may be a papule or pustule at the primary site of skin inoculation.

Clinical Manifestations

Infected individuals often experience a flu-like illness. Ocular involvement occurs in 5–10% of cases. The most common ocular manifestation is Parinaud oculoglandular syndrome, a unilateral conjunctivitis with regional lymphadenopathy. Patients may have acute vision loss from neuroretinitis (Fig. 94.9). Other infectious causes of neuroretinitis include Lyme disease, syphilis and tuberculosis. Complications of neuroretinitis include serous retinal detachment, macular hole and arterial occlusion.

Diagnosis and Treatment

Cat scratch disease can be confirmed by serologic testing, polymerase chain reaction (PCR), blood culture, or histopathological examination of affected tissue. CSD is usually a self-limited infection. Doxycycline, azithromycin or trimethoprim-sulfamethoxazole can be given, depending on the severity of the illness. There is no evidence that treatment with antibiotics and/or corticosteroids improves the visual outcome in patients with CSD optic neuropathy.[20]

Zika Virus

Zika virus is a single-stranded ribonucleic acid (RNA) virus of the Flavivirus genus that includes dengue virus, West Nile virus, and yellow fever. Zika is most commonly transmitted by the mosquito *Aedes aegypti*, but it can also be acquired by sexual contact. Zika virus was first identified in the rhesus monkey in Uganda in 1947 and spread from a small area in Africa and Asia through the Western Pacific. In 2015, an outbreak occurred in Brazil and the America.[21]

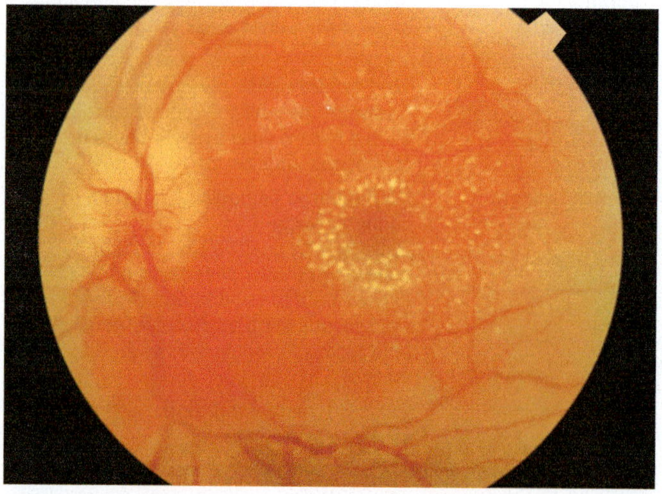

Fig. 94.9: Neuroretinitis in cat scratch disease. Optic disk edema associated with exudates in a macular star pattern of a patient with cat scratch disease.

Neuro-ophthalmic Manifestations

Zika infection can be asymptomatic or present with short-lived symptoms that include fever, maculopapular rash, and joint pain. Of great concern is infection in pregnant women during the first trimester. Infants born with congenital Zika infection have microcephaly amongst other neurologic sequelae.

Ophthalmic manifestations due to Zika infection are currently under intense investigation. In infants with microcephaly, posterior segment abnormalities can include pigmentary maculopathy, chorioretinal atrophy or scarring, vascular abnormalities, torpedo retinopathy consisting of lacunar hypopigmented macular or peripheral lesions, hemorrhagic retinopathy, and optic nerve abnormalities. At this time, controversy remains as to whether the ophthalmic findings are secondary to or independent of microcephaly. There has been one report of chorioretinal scarring in a confirmed case of an infant with Zika virus without microcephaly.[22,23]

Diagnosis and Treatment

Diagnosis of Zika infection is by PCR and serologic testing during the acute phase of the infection. Currently, there is no treatment, but a vaccine is under development. Prevention of Zika virus is critical, particularly in endemic areas, by mosquito control and safer sexual practices.

Prion Diseases

Human prion diseases comprise the sporadic, familial, iatrogenic and variant forms of Creutzfeldt-Jakob disease (CJD), Kuru, Gerstmann-Sträussler-Scheinker syndrome, and fatal familial insomnia. The misfolded prion protein causes a rapidly progressive neurodegenerative disease. Prion diseases are exceedingly rare with an incidence of 1–1.5 per million people. While sporadic CJD is the most common type, prion diseases became notorious for the 1994–1995 United Kingdom outbreak of "mad cow" disease, a bovine form transmissible to humans.

Neuro-ophthalmic Manifestations

Prion diseases can present with a psychiatric prodrome followed by neurologic symptoms such as cognitive decline, ataxia, cerebellar dysfunction, and myoclonus. Neuro-ophthalmic findings occur in approximately 30–40% of cases and include diplopia, homonymous visual field defects, visual disturbances, and cortical blindness.

Diagnosis and Treatment

Diagnosis can be aided by electroencephalogram (EEG) and cranial MRI. EEG demonstrates periodic sharp wave complexes, and DWI shows restricted diffusion in cortical and/or deep gray matter nuclei. CSF biomarkers such as 14-3-3, total tau (t-tau), and neuron-specific enolase (NSE) when positive are helpful in supporting the clinical diagnosis. Brain biopsy provides the definitive diagnosis. Prion diseases are rapidly progressive with a mean survival of 6 months for sporadic CJD. Unfortunately, no treatment is currently available.[24]

METABOLIC-TOXIC DISEASES

Thyroid Eye Disease

Thyroid eye disease (TED), also known as Graves' ophthalmopathy or thyroid-associated orbitopathy, is an autoimmune disorder that affects the extraocular muscles and orbital soft tissue. TED is most commonly associated with Graves' disease but can also occur in Hashimoto's autoimmune thyroiditis. About 20–50% of patients with Graves' disease will develop TED. Approximately 90% of patients with TED are hyperthyroid on diagnosis, with the remaining patients being either euthyroid or hypothyroid. Although thyroid hormone levels do not correlate with the severity of TED, thyroid-stimulating immunoglobulins (TSIs) have been shown to correlate with disease activity and severity.[25] Smoking is strongly associated with worsening of disease.

Neuro-ophthalmic Manifestations

Thyroid eye disease frequently presents with eyelid retraction with lateral flare and exposure of the superior and inferior sclera. TED patients can demonstrate lid lag, or delayed eyelid movement in downgaze. TED is the most common cause of unilateral and bilateral proptosis in adults. Axial proptosis can result in lagophthalmos and exposure keratopathy. Patients can also present with variable diplopia with restriction of eye movements. TED most commonly affects the inferior rectus and medial rectus muscles. Symptoms of orbital congestion include chemosis and periorbital edema. Orbital congestion can lead to glaucoma from increased episcleral venous pressure. Rarely, TED can result in visual loss due to a compressive optic neuropathy with or without optic disk edema (Figs. 94.10A to D).

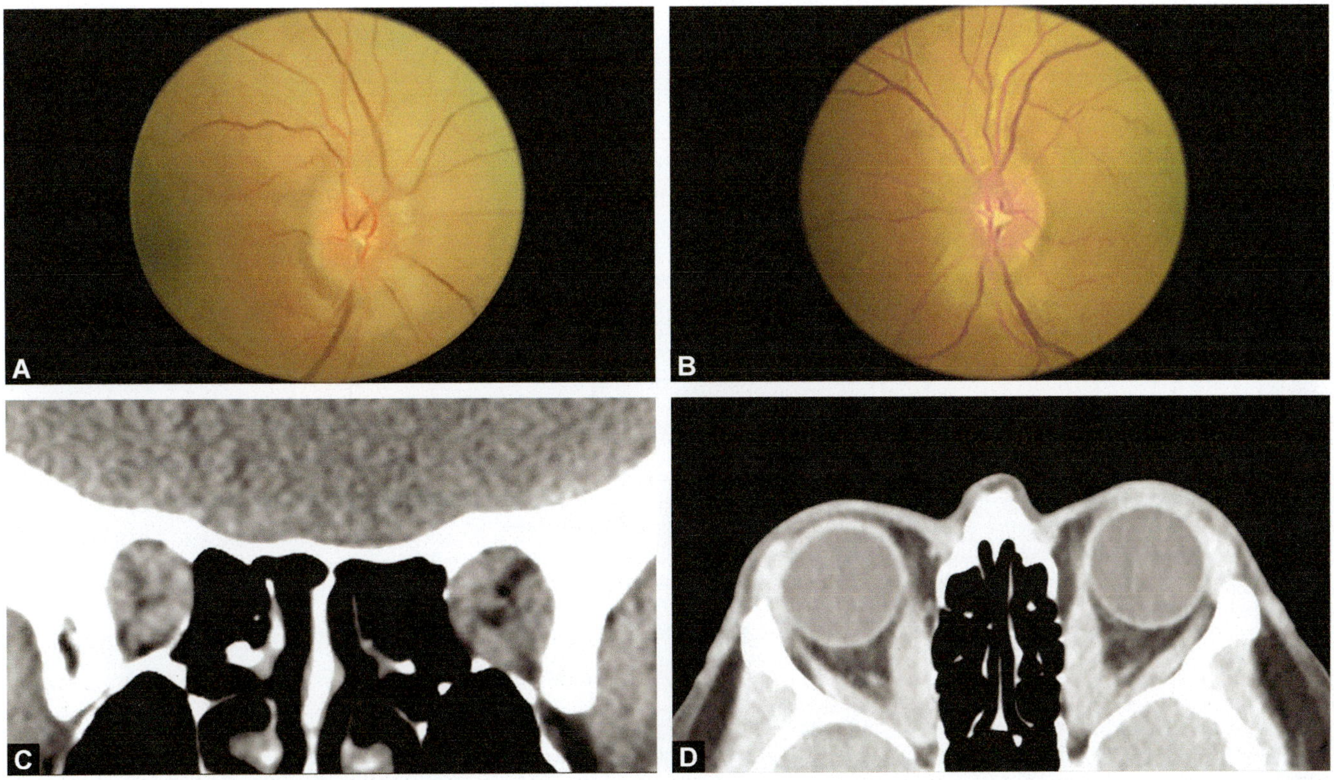

Figs. 94.10A to D: Compressive optic neuropathy in thyroid eye disease. (A) Bilateral optic disk edema due to compression of the optic nerve at (B) the orbital apex as seen on the coronal CT image; (C and D) Axial CT images show enlargement of the medial rectus muscles with sparing of the tendons.

Diagnosis and Treatment

The diagnosis of TED is based on the combination of clinical signs and neuroimaging findings of extraocular muscle enlargement with sparing of the tendons (Figs. 94.10A to D). TSI may be useful for diagnosis, especially in euthyroid patients or those without established Graves' disease.

Treatment of TED during the active phase requires a systemic approach and is based on the severity of the disease (Flowchart 94.2). Achieving a euthyroid endocrine status and smoking cessation can lessen the risk of worsening disease. TED can worsen during radioiodine therapy; therefore, concurrent oral steroids should be considered.

Nutritional Deficiencies

Nutritional deficiencies, toxins and medications can all result in an optic neuropathy (Table 94.6). Details of the clinical manifestations may be found in Chapter 92. Visual acuity does not often worsen beyond 20/400, with the exception of methanol toxicity. The prognosis for visual recovery is good if diagnosed promptly and a management plan instituted quickly.[26]

MITOCHONDRIAL DISEASES

Mitochondria are double membrane organelles involved in the metabolic function of nucleated cells. On a cellular

Flowchart 94.2: Thyroid eye disease (TED) treatment algorithm.

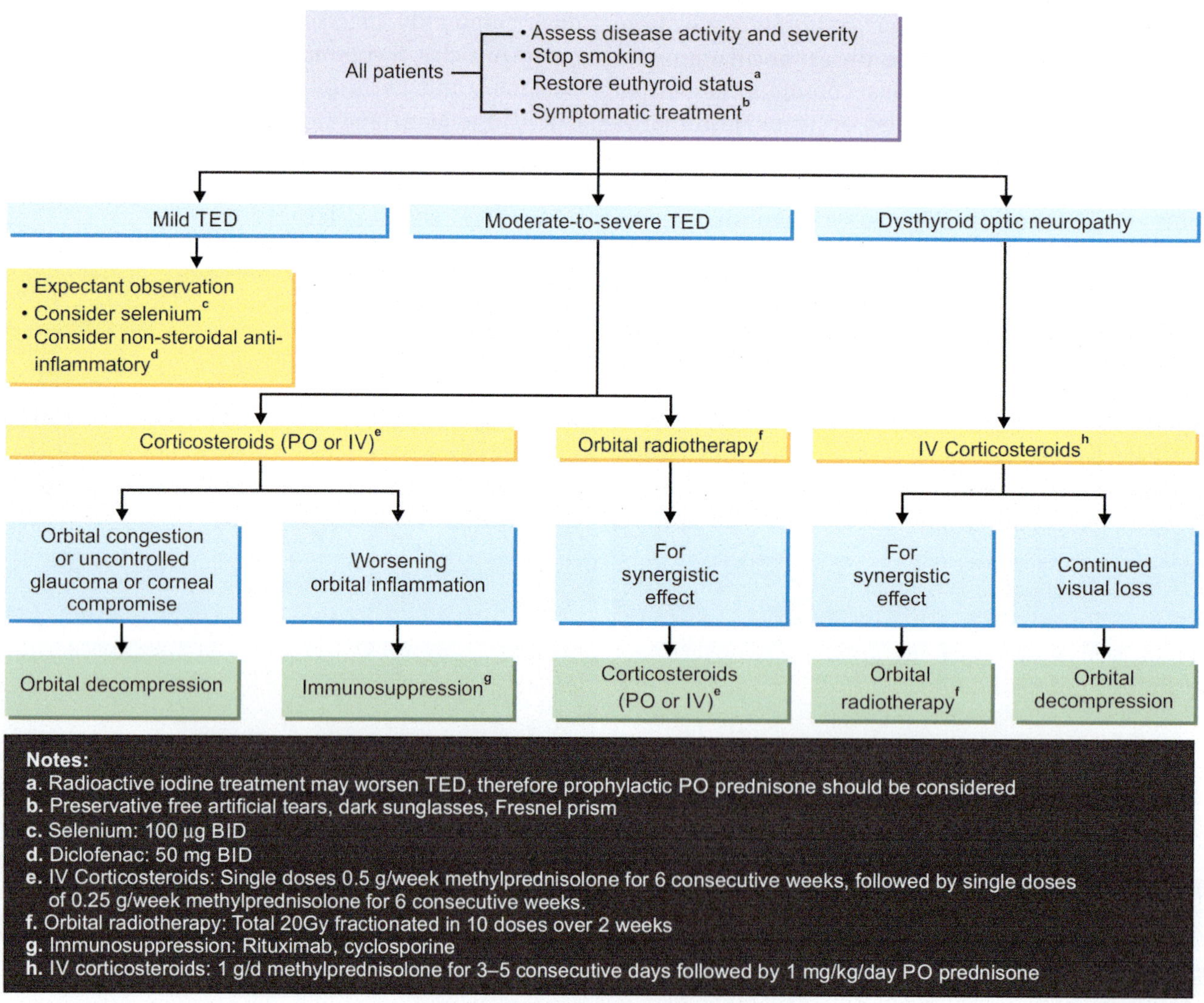

(PO: Oral; IV: Intravenous)

Source: Reprinted with permission from Bhatti MT, Dutton JJ. Thyroid eye disease: therapy in the active phase. J Neuroophthalmol. 2014;34(2):186-97.

Table 94.6: Selected list of toxic-nutritional optic neuropathy etiologies.

Nutritional deficiencies	• B_{12} • Folate • B_1
Toxins	• Methanol • Ethylene glycol • Lead, thallium • Arsenic • Carbon monoxide • Tobacco
Medications	*Antibiotics:* • Linezolid • Ciprofloxacin • Chloramphenicol • Streptomycin *Antimalarials:* • Chloroquine • Quinine *Antitubercular drugs:* • Ethambutol • Isoniazid *Antiarrhythmics:* • Digitalis • Amiodarone *Chemotherapeutics:* • Vincristine • Methotrexate • Tamoxifen • TNF-alpha inhibitors • Vigabatrin • Sildenafil

level, mitochondrial dysfunction can affect energy production, calcium homeostasis, reactive oxygen species production, and apoptosis. Mitochondrial diseases can often impair high-energy demand organs including cardiac and skeletal muscle, the nervous system, kidneys, liver, and the endocrine system. Thus, symptoms can include cardiac conduction defects, muscle weakness, stroke-like episodes, epilepsy, ataxia, developmental delay, and diabetes.[27]

Mitochondrial proteins are encoded by mitochondrial deoxyribonucleic acid (mtDNA) and nuclear DNA. Mitochondrial diseases can be sporadic or hereditary. Many mitochondrial diseases are due to mutations of the mtDNA, which are maternally transmitted. However, there are other mitochondrial diseases due to mutations of the nuclear DNA that are inherited in an autosomal dominant or autosomal recessive fashion.

Leber Hereditary Optic Neuropathy

Leber hereditary optic neuropathy (LHON) is characterized by rapid, painless vision loss in one eye with subsequent loss of vision in the fellow eye days to months following fellow eye involvement. Patients generally present with central or cecocentral visual field defects. Final visual acuity is poor (<20/200). *See* Chapter 92 for additional details on diagnosis and management.

Chronic Progressive External Ophthalmoplegia

Chronic progressive external ophthalmoplegia (CPEO) is a mitochondrial myopathy that causes slowly progressive bilateral ptosis and ophthalmoplegia. The onset of symptoms can occur at any age but most frequently occurs in childhood or young adulthood. Most patients with CPEO have a sporadic rearrangement of the mtDNA, but other cases occur due to either a mtDNA or nuclear DNA point mutation.

Ptosis is usually the initial manifestation of the disease, often associated with a chin-up posture and compensatory brow elevation. In addition, orbicularis oculi weakness can cause lagophthalmos and exposure keratopathy. Patients with ophthalmoplegia may not complain of diplopia, as the extraocular muscles are often symmetrically affected, and no ocular misalignment results in primary gaze. Diplopia at near is often due to convergence insufficiency. Kearns-Sayre disease, a "CPEO-plus" syndrome, is characterized by a pigmentary retinopathy, cardiac conduction abnormalities, and disease onset prior to 20 years of age.

Diagnosis and Treatment

The differential diagnosis for CPEO includes MG, idiopathic orbital inflammatory syndrome, myotonic dystrophy, congenital fibrosis of the extraocular muscles, and TED. Diagnosis by muscle biopsy (75% sensitivity) demonstrates ragged red fibers with Gomori trichrome stain. Additional mtDNA genetic testing may be needed either from blood or muscle tissue. Neuroimaging may show extraocular muscle atrophy. Systemic manifestations include cardiac conduction defects, respiratory insufficiency, and cerebellar ataxia. There is currently no treatment for CPEO. Symptomatic treatment with ptosis surgery and/or strabismus surgery can be helpful in some patients.[28,29]

NEOPLASTIC AND PARANEOPLASTIC DISEASES

Neoplastic Optic Neuropathies

Neoplastic optic neuropathies can be categorized as either compressive, infiltrative, or perineural. Compressive tumors generally present with slowly progressive visual loss. Examination may reveal dyschromatopsia, relative afferent pupillary defect (RAPD), and visual field defects. Proptosis and orbital congestion suggest an orbital process. The optic disk may appear swollen, pale or normal. Ocular motor CN palsies indicate either superior orbital fissure or cavernous sinus involvement.

Optic Nerve Sheath Meningioma

Intracranial meningiomas comprise approximately 20% of primary intracranial tumors. Meningiomas are derived from arachnoid cap cells found on the outer surface of the arachnoid layer, among other locations. Meningiomas often present in middle-aged adults and affect women more often than men. Of the meningiomas that occur in children, approximately 25% are associated with neurofibromatosis type 2 (NF2). In addition to NF2, prior brain radiation is a risk factor for the development of a meningioma.

Primary optic nerve sheath meningioma (ONSM) is the second most common optic nerve tumor. Visual loss on presentation varies, with approximately 45% of patients having a visual acuity of 20/40 or better and 25% of patients at count fingers or worse.[30] Classically, a primary ONSM results in optic disk pallor with optociliary shunt vessels (Fig. 94.11). Neuroimaging demonstrates a "tram-track sign" of enhancement along the optic nerve.

Intracranial meningiomas can extend into the optic canal. These secondary optic nerve sheath tumors are slow growing and typically originate from the sphenoid wing or tuberculum sellae. Patients may present with varying symptoms based on the location and degree of tumor involvement, including vision loss, globe displacement, orbital congestion, and/or impaired extraocular motility. Surgery often is needed to prevent spread of the intracranial component of the tumor.[31]

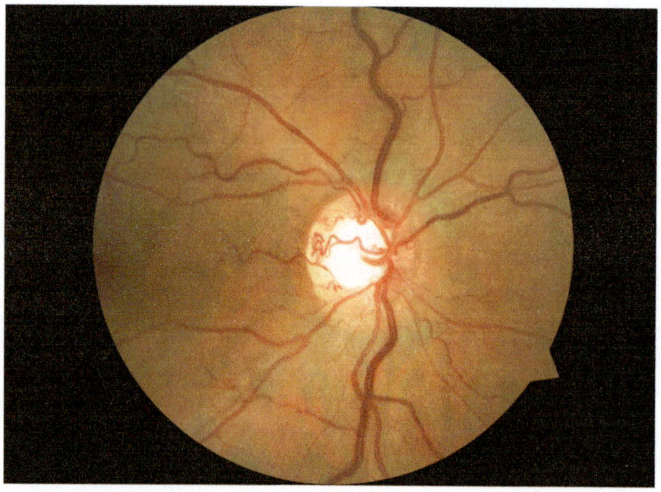

Fig. 94.11: Primary optic nerve sheath meningioma. There is mild temporal optic disk pallor and optociliary shunt vessels.

Optic Pathway Glioma

Optic pathway gliomas (OPGs) are the most common primary optic nerve tumor. Pilocytic astrocytoma occurs most commonly in children and may be associated with NF type 1. Pilocytic astrocytomas can involve the optic nerve and/or the optic chiasm. No treatment is needed for patients with relatively preserved visual function and no evidence of clinical or radiological progression. Chemotherapy (e.g. vincristine, vinblastine, carboplatin or temozolomide), rather than radiotherapy, is more appropriate for children with progressive visual loss. Malignant optic nerve glioblastoma of adults is a rare tumor that often presents in the seventh decade of life with rapidly progressive vision loss. Prognosis is poor with eventual death occurring in months despite medical or radiation therapy.

Optic Nerve Metastasis and Infiltration

Metastases to or infiltration of the optic nerve are rare conditions but can occur with solid tumors, leukemia, lymphoma, and carcinomatous meningitis. The most common cancers to metastasize to the optic nerve are breast in women and lung in men. Optic nerve metastasis may occur prior to diagnosis of the primary cancer. Leukemic optic nerve infiltration is seen with acute rather than chronic leukemia. Lymphomatous infiltration of the optic chiasm and optic nerve occurs more often in non-Hodgkin's lymphoma. In most cases, lymphoma spreads to the optic nerve from the CNS. In carcinomatous meningitis, meningeal spread of the malignant cells leads to cuffing of the subarachnoid space around the optic nerve, resulting in a compressive optic neuropathy, or less frequently, infiltration of the optic nerve. Diagnosis of a neoplastic optic neuropathy is based on neuroimaging (contrasted MRI with thin cuts through the orbits using fat-suppression techniques),[31] systemic evaluation with either CT or positron emission tomography (PET)-CT, CSF analysis and, in some cases, an optic nerve biopsy.

Neuroblastoma

Neuroblastomas are tumors derived from embryonic neuroblastic tissue, or cells of the sympathetic nervous system, and are therefore located in the adrenal medulla (most common site) or along the sympathetic chain (e.g. cervical, mediastinal, thoracic and pelvic ganglia). Frequent sites of metastasis are lymph nodes, bone and orbits.

Neuroblastoma almost exclusively occurs in infants and young children. Most cases are sporadic in origin with half the cases demonstrating chromosomal deletions, often as a partial deletion of chromosome 1p, which is associated with overexpression of the *N-myc* oncogene.

The clinical presentation of neuroblastoma varies and is based on the location of the tumor. Approximately 20% of patients with neuroblastoma can present with ophthalmic involvement, including opsoclonus or ocular flutter (*see* Chapter 96) and Horner syndrome (*see* Chapter 100). Neuroblastoma can metastasize to the orbit, leading to proptosis, periorbital ecchymosis, and/or ptosis. Neuroblastoma often metastasizes to the zygomatic bone, presenting as a mass in the temple and cheek region. An optic neuropathy can result from compression or increased ICP.

Measurements of urine and serum catecholamines, vanillylmandelic acid (VMA) and homovanillic acid (HVA) are an essential component of the evaluation of a patient suspected of harboring a neuroblastoma. Abdominal ultrasound, CT or MRI can identify the location of the tumor. Histopathological confirmation with either a biopsy of a specific lesion or bone marrow is needed for definitive diagnosis. After risk stratification, treatment includes surgery, chemotherapy or radiation therapy.

Paraneoplastic Diseases

Cancer-associated Retinopathy

Cancer-associated retinopathy (CAR) is the most common ocular paraneoplastic syndrome. The average age of presentation is 65 years. CAR can precede the diagnosis of the primary malignancy, most often small cell lung cancer. The pathogenesis involves molecular mimicry of retinal antigens, such as recoverin or enolase. Patients present with painless, progressive vision loss over weeks to months. CAR affects cone and rod photoreceptors with symptoms of photosensitivity, photopsias, dyschromatopsia, nyctalopia, and impaired dark adaptation. Visual field defects include ring scotomas and peripheral or central field loss. The retina may appear clinically normal, particularly early on in the disease course. Eventually, there is development of optic nerve pallor, vessel attenuation, retinal pigment epithelium (RPE) mottling and thinning, and in some cases, mild vitritis. Electroretinogram (ERG) will show reduced a- and b-waves. In general, the visual prognosis is poor, but corticosteroids, IV immunoglobulin and immunosuppressive therapy have been shown to be effective in some cases.

Melanoma-associated Retinopathy

Melanoma-associated retinopathy (MAR) typically presents in the sixth decade of life with painless vision loss, often with visual acuity of 20/60 or better. MAR has a male predilection and primarily affects rod bipolar cells. Patients present with symptoms of photopsias, nyctalopia, and peripheral field loss. The retinal examination can be normal on initial presentation with subsequent optic disk pallor, arteriolar attenuation, and RPE changes. ERG will classically show a normal a-wave but reduced b-wave. MAR is often associated with the presence of antibipolar cell antibodies. Similar to CAR, there is no proven treatment for MAR.

Paraneoplastic Optic Neuropathy

Paraneoplastic optic neuropathy (PON) is a rare disease that is most commonly associated with small cell lung cancer. Patients present with subacute, painless vision loss progressing over days to weeks. PON can have a variety of visual field defects. Patients with PON often have other neurologic signs including CNS and peripheral neuropathies, ataxia, and dementia. The optic nerve can appear normal, swollen or atrophic, and may be associated with vitritis. Fluorescein angiogram often demonstrates optic disk leakage. Antibodies against collapsin response-mediating protein-5 (CRMP-5) are frequently present. Therapy includes corticosteroids, immunosuppressive agents and treatment of the underlying malignancy.[32]

Radiation-induced Optic Neuropathy

Radiation-induced optic neuropathy (RION) is a devastating late complication of radiotherapy that invariably leads to irreversible visual loss due to vascular endothelium dysfunction. The visual loss may be unilateral or bilateral, depending on the location of the radiation exposure to the visual apparatus. RION occurs most frequently after irradiation of the paranasal sinuses, nasopharyngeal, and skull base malignancies, but can also develop after treatment of a pituitary adenoma, parasellar meningioma,

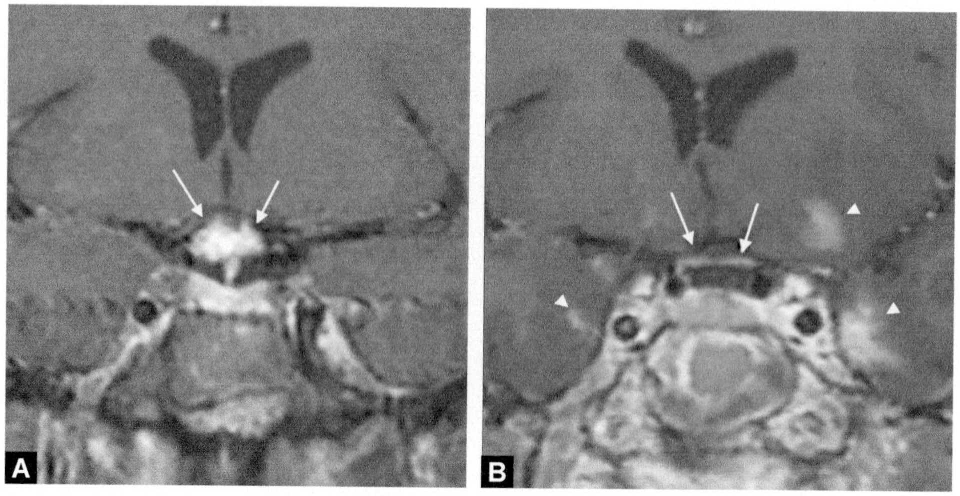

Figs. 94.12A and B: Radiation-induced chiasmal neuritis. (A) Gadolinium-enhanced T1-weighted image reveals marked enlargement and enhancement of the optic chiasm; (B) Six months later there is severe atrophy of the optic chiasm.
Source: Reproduced with permission from Bhatti MT, Schmalfuss I. Handbook of Neuro-Imaging for the Ophthalmologist, 1st edition. London: Jaypee Brothers Medical Publishers Pvt Ltd; 2014.

craniopharyngioma, and frontal and temporal lobe neoplasms. Cumulative doses of radiation that exceed 50 Gy or single doses of more than 10 Gy to the anterior visual pathways are most often associated with the development of RION. Several other factors predisposing to development of RION include older age, pre-existing tumor compression upon the anterior visual pathway, concurrent chemotherapy, and previous external beam radiation.

Radiation-induced optic neuropathy presents as painless visual loss commonly between 10 months and 20 months after treatment, but the onset may range from 3 months to 9 years. Episodes of transient visual loss may precede the onset of RION by several weeks. The progression of visual loss occurs over weeks to months. The visual field may show an altitudinal defect or a central scotoma. In some patients, the optic chiasm is also affected, leading to bilateral visual loss due to chiasmal neuritis (Figs. 94.12A and B). Spontaneous recovery is unusual. Treatment modalities that have been tried include corticosteroids, hyperbaric oxygen and pentoxifylline.[4]

NEURO-OPHTHALMIC CONDITIONS IN PREGNANCY

During pregnancy, increased progesterone levels lead to changes in the refractive power of the cornea resulting in a myopic shift. Women in pregnancy also experience reduced intraocular pressure, likely due to decreased episcleral venous pressure, increased aqueous outflow and/or reduced scleral rigidity. Pregnancy leads to physiologic changes in the volume of the brain with the pituitary gland enlarging nearly twofold.

Pituitary Gland

Pregnancy is associated with pituitary apoplexy and lymphocytic hypophysitis. Pituitary apoplexy is acute hemorrhage or infarction of the pituitary gland that is likely due to physiologic enlargement of the pituitary gland during pregnancy. Patients can present with sudden headache, nausea or vision loss. Pituitary apoplexy can also occur after an acute, large volume blood loss (Sheehan's syndrome) or from hemorrhage into an underlying pituitary tumor (Figs. 94.13A and B). Lymphocytic hypophysitis is a rare autoimmune disorder characterized by lymphocyte infiltration of the pituitary gland that can mimic the appearance of a mass, resulting in optic chiasm compression. Lymphocytic hypophysitis usually presents in the late stages of pregnancy or during the postpartum period.

Papilledema

Papilledema in pregnancy most often results from idiopathic intracranial hypertension or VST. Pregnancy may precipitate VST in patients with an underlying hypercoagulable state such as factor V Leiden mutation, or protein C or S deficiency. VST is treated by anticoagulation with heparin in pregnancy (warfarin is the US Food and Drug Administration (FDA) class X drug). MRI and MRV

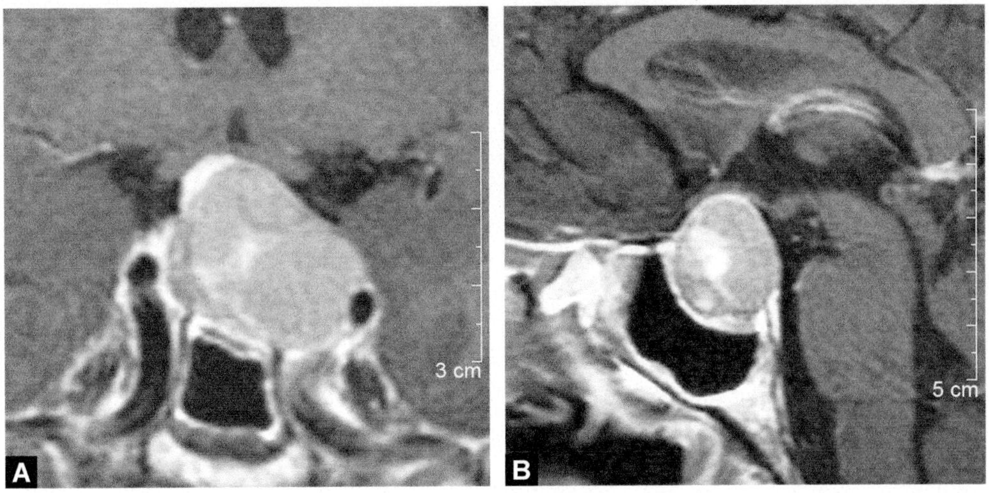

Figs. 94.13A and B: Pituitary apoplexy. (A) Coronal gadolinium-enhanced T1-weighted image demonstrates a large, heterogeneous sellar mass that markedly elevates and slightly flattens the optic chiasm; (B) Sagittal, noncontrasted T1-weighted image reveals that this lesion is spontaneously hyperintense due to hemorrhage into a pre-existing pituitary gland adenoma.

Source: Reproduced with permission from Bhatti MT, Schmalfuss I. Handbook of Neuro-Imaging for the Ophthalmologist, 1st edition. London: Jaypee Brothers Medical Publishers Pvt Ltd; 2014.

can be performed safely in pregnancy but gadolinium should not be administered.[33]

Posterior Reversible Encephalopathy Syndrome

Pregnancy-induced hypertension (PIH) can lead to PRES. Patients with severe PIH can experience visual disturbances such as scotomas, dyschromatopsia, or transient vision loss. Other symptoms include headache, nausea and vomiting, altered mental status, and seizures. MRI shows changes in the gray-white matter interface in the parieto-occipital lobes and basal ganglia. In general, prognosis for visual recovery is good with prompt diagnosis, blood pressure control, and supportive therapy.[34]

CONCLUSION

This chapter has provided an overview of the neuro-ophthalmic problems that may occur in patients with a variety of systemic disorders, and the ophthalmic symptoms may be the initial or only manifestation of the disease. Prompt recognition of symptoms and clinical signs will allow the ophthalmologist to refer the patient to the appropriate physician who can assist in the diagnosis and treatment of the underlying condition, thus preserving visual function and overall patient health.

REFERENCES

1. James PA, Oparil S, Carter BL, et al. 2014 evidence-based guideline for the management of high blood pressure in adults: report from the panel members appointed to the Eighth Joint National Committee (JNC 8). JAMA. 2014;311:507-20.
2. Zhou Y, Zhu W, Wang C. Relationship between retinal vascular occlusions and incident cerebrovascular diseases: a systematic review and meta-analysis. Medicine (Baltimore). 2016;95:e4075.
3. Lawlor M, Perry R, Hunt BJ, et al. Strokes and vision: the management of ischemic arterial disease affecting the retina and occipital lobe. Surv Ophthalmol. 2015;60: 296-309.
4. Bhatti MT, Schmalfuss I. Handbook of Neuro-Imaging for the Ophthalmologist, 1st edition. London: Jaypee Brothers Medical Publishers Pvt Ltd; 2014.
5. Catanese L, Tarsia J, Fisher M. Acute ischemic stroke therapy overview. Circ Res. 2017;120:541-58.
6. Kernan WN, Ovbiagele B, Black HR, et al. Guidelines for the prevention of stroke in patients with stroke and transient ischemic attack: a guideline for healthcare professionals from the American Heart Association/American Stroke Association. Stroke. 2014;45:2160-236.
7. Stam J. Thrombosis of the cerebral veins and sinuses. N Engl J Med. 2005;352:1791-8.
8. Saposnik G, Barinagarrementeria F, Brown RD, et al. Diagnosis and management of cerebral venous thrombosis: a statement for healthcare professionals from the American Heart Association/American Stroke Association. Stroke. 2011;42:1158-92.

9. International Study of Unruptured Intracranial Aneurysms Investigators. Unruptured intracranial aneurysms—risk of rupture and risks of surgical intervention. N Engl J Med. 1998;339:1725-33.
10. Day AL. Aneurysms of the ophthalmic segment. A clinical and anatomical analysis. J Neurosurg. 1990;72:677-91.
11. Polman CH, Reingold SC, Banwell B, et al. Diagnostic criteria for multiple sclerosis: 2010 revisions to the McDonald criteria. Ann Neurol. 2011;69:292-302.
12. Optic Neuritis Study Group. Multiple sclerosis risk after optic neuritis: final optic neuritis treatment trial follow-up. Arch Neurol. 2008;65:727-32.
13. Kremer L, Mealy M, Jacob A, et al. Brainstem manifestations in neuromyelitis optica: a multicenter study of 258 patients. Mult Scler. 2014;20:843-7.
14. Hazin R, Khan F, Bhatti MT. Neuromyelitis optica: current concepts and prospects for future management. Curr Opin Ophthalmol. 2009;20:434-9.
15. Hoitsma E, Faber CG, Drent M, et al. Neurosarcoidosis: a clinical dilemma. Lancet Neurol. 2004;3:397-407.
16. Preble JM, Silpa-Archa S, Foster CS. Ocular involvement in systemic lupus erythematosus. Curr Opin Ophthalmol. 2015;26:540-5.
17. Bhatti MT, Tabandeh H. Giant cell arteritis: diagnosis and management. Curr Opin Ophthalmol. 2001;12:393-9.
18. Gilbert ME, Savino PJ. Ocular myasthenia gravis. Int Ophthalmol Clin. 2007;47:93-103, ix.
19. Bhatti MT. Optic neuropathy from viruses and spirochetes. Int Ophthalmol Clin. 2007;47:37-66.
20. Chi SL, Stinnett S, Eggenberger E, et al. Clinical characteristics in 53 patients with cat scratch optic neuropathy. Ophthalmology. 2012;119:183-7.
21. World Health Organization. (2016). Zika virus. [online] Available from: *http://www.who.int/mediacentre/factsheets/zika/en/*. [Accessed December, 2017]
22. Miranda HA, Costa MC, Frazão MA, et al. Expanded spectrum of congenital ocular findings in microcephaly with presumed Zika infection. Ophthalmology. 2016;123:1788-94.
23. Ventura CV, Maia M, Dias N, et al. Zika: neurological and ocular findings in infant without microcephaly. Lancet. 2016;387:2502.
24. Geschwind MD. Prion diseases. Continuum (Minneap Minn). 2015;21:1612-38.
25. Ponto KA, Kanitz M, Olivo PD, et al. Clinical relevance of thyroid-stimulating immunoglobulins in graves' ophthalmopathy. Ophthalmology. 2011;118:2279-85.
26. Grzybowski A, Zülsdorff M, Wilhelm H, et al. Toxic optic neuropathies: an updated review. Acta Ophthalmol. 2015;93:402-10.
27. El-Hattab AW, Scaglia F. Mitochondrial cytopathies. Cell Calcium. 2016;60:199-206.
28. Fraser JA, Biousse V, Newman NJ. The neuro-ophthalmology of mitochondrial disease. Surv Ophthalmol. 2010;55:299-334.
29. McClelland C, Manousakis G, Lee MS. Progressive external ophthalmoplegia. Curr Neurol Neurosci Rep. 2016;16:53.
30. Dutton JJ. Optic nerve gliomas and meningiomas. Neurol Clin. 1991;9:163-77.
31. Volpe NJ. Compressive and infiltrative optic neuropathies. In: Miller NR, Newman NJ, Biousse V, Kerrison JB (Eds). Walsh and Hoyt's Clinical Neuro-Ophthalmology, 6th edition. Philadelphia: Lippincott Williams & Wilkins; 2005.
32. Rahimy E, Sarraf D. Paraneoplastic and non-paraneoplastic retinopathy and optic neuropathy: evaluation and management. Surv Ophthalmol. 2013;58:430-58.
33. Ray JG, Vermeulen MJ, Bharatha A, et al. Association between MRI exposure during pregnancy and fetal and childhood outcomes. JAMA. 2016;316:952-61.
34. Digre KB. Neuro-ophthalmology and pregnancy: what does a neuro-ophthalmologist need to know? J Neuroophthalmol. 2011;31:381-7.

Chapter 95 Diplopia

Marc A Bouffard, Dean Cestari

INTRODUCTION

Establishing a practical, simple, and comprehensive approach to diplopia is of paramount importance to the student of ophthalmology or neurology. The format of this chapter will follow that principle so that the student of neuro-ophthalmology at any level can learn how to approach diplopia in a rational manner, focusing on the cognitive approach to the patient with double vision. Though many texts provide excellent and exhaustive descriptions of pathology which may cause diplopia, few provide instruction as to the optimal approach to the patient complaining of double vision.

The first step in evaluating the patient with diplopia is to determine whether the complaint is monocular or not. Monocular diplopia, that which is perceived when viewing through one eye alone, is commonly due to refractive errors localizing to the cornea or lens. With few exceptions, binocular diplopia (diplopia which resolves upon occlusion of either eye but is present while viewing with both eyes simultaneously) is due to ocular misalignment. Patients with monocular diplopia may have binocular diplopia as well, but it is critically important to identify this early on as the focused examination may have a different emphasis depending on the binocularity or monocularity of the complaint.

The second step, provided the diplopia is binocular, is to identify the pattern of any eye movement abnormalities which may be present. This is done both by means of taking a detailed history (first by asking whether the diplopia is accentuated by viewing objects in a particular direction of gaze, head position, or at near versus far) and then with a careful examination. Testing pursuit is critical to localization. The alignment of the eyes should be examined in the 6 cardinal positions of gaze as well as primary gaze. However, it should be kept in mind that this will not capture defects of vergence (which are much more easily appreciated when employing cover-uncover testing with the patient fixating on a target) or other disorders such as skew deviations where there is no limitation of ductions.

The third step is to consider the structure whose dysfunction might be responsible for the observed pattern of abnormal eye movements. Some cases are straightforward, such as a patient presenting with a pattern of motility deficits compatible with dysfunction of the third cranial nerve. Frequently, the pattern of deficit does not so clearly reflect a single point of underlying neuroanatomical damage. For example, is an isolated adduction deficit representative of an internuclear ophthalmoplegia (INO) or a partial 3rd nerve palsy?

The fourth step is to consider the etiologies that might explain the anatomic dysfunction suspected, in so tailoring an appropriate workup. For example, if you have concluded that a patient's binocular diplopia is referable to a 6th nerve palsy, is the etiology of the 6th nerve palsy likely to be microvascular, compressive, etc.?

The above cognitive exercise should be followed on every diplopic patient. This allows for a comprehensive evaluation of the patient. All too often, students and house staff skip a step, leading to diagnostic confusion (for example, assuming that an abduction deficit is necessarily a 6th nerve palsy). By employing this cognitive framework, the reader will understand how the interview should be tailored, the importance and caveats of the physical examination (e.g. not all abduction deficits are 6th nerve palsies), and how a targeted workup can be pursued (e.g. "do I need to image the orbits as well as the brain?"). It should be kept in mind that there are several conditions, not discussed in depth here, in which eye movements are abnormal yet no diplopia results. This scenario is typically the result of conjugate disorders of gaze, such as gaze palsies, and symmetric myopathies (e.g. chronic progressive ophthalmoplegia).

MONOCULAR DIPLOPIA

The examiner should attempt to differentiate monocular from binocular symptoms as one of the first tasks in approaching the patient with diplopia. Because both monocular and binocular diplopia may coexist, the neuro-ophthalmic evaluation should not be cursory after discovery of monocular diplopia. However, approaching the patient without this information may lead to a great deal of confusion.

Monocular diplopia is the result of light reflected from a perceived target stimulating photoreceptors located in different areas of the retina. This most commonly occurs as the result of corneal irregularities (e.g. astigmatism, keratoconus, dystrophies) or of irregularities of the lens (e.g. dense cataracts, etc.). In most of these cases, the monocular diplopia should resolve when the patient is allowed to view a diplopic target through a pinhole, which eliminates the retinal perception of abnormally diffracted light.[1] Typically the second, diplopic image is more faint than the first.

BINOCULAR DIPLOPIA

Binocular diplopia is the realm of the neuro-ophthalmologist and almost always results from disconjugate eye movements, meaning those in which the eyes are no longer aligned. Maintaining an anatomic framework in mind is encouraged when approaching the patient with diplopia. Diplopia may occur as a result of processes affecting supranuclear inputs to cranial nerve nuclei (e.g. skew deviations, thalamic esotropia), the cranial nerve nuclei themselves, the cranial nerve nucleus outputs still within the brainstem (i.e. the fascicles), the cranial nerves in the subarachnoid space, nerves at the orbital apex, in the orbit, at the neuromuscular junction, or at the extraocular muscles themselves. Processes which physically distort the normal relationship of one globe to the other (e.g. structural abnormalities of the orbit) without any neurophysiologic efferent dysfunction should be kept in mind as well.

The history should be concerned with identifying the orientation of images (e.g. vertical, horizontal, or oblique), the extent of their separation, changes in orientation or extent of separation both over the course of a given day and in general since onset, whether the diplopia is intermittent or continuously present, whether it is elicited or maximized by gaze in a particular direction and conversely, whether it is minimized by gaze in a particular direction or by a particular head position. The patient should also be queried for other features of localizing value, such as brainstem symptoms (e.g. weakness, numbness, vertigo), meningeal symptoms (e.g. headache, neck pain, phono/photophobia), cavernous sinus symptoms (retro-orbital pain, evidence of multiple cranial neuropathies or sympathetic dysfunction), neuromuscular junction symptoms (variable ptosis, variable diplopia, head drop, proximal weakness, dysphonia, dysphagia, dysarthria, difficulty breathing), orbital symptoms (such as proptosis, pain, evidence of abnormal thyroid function), and importantly, evidence of vasculitides such as giant cell arteritis (GCA) (headache, temporal allodynia, jaw claudication, tongue pain, transient monocular vision loss, fevers, chills, diaphoresis, unintentional weight loss, proximal stiffness).

The discussion below proceeds according to various deficits of duction (or their absence). *It should be borne in mind that different patterns of deficits may be combined or isolated.*

Abduction Deficits

A commonly encountered cognitive error often demonstrated by students and house staff is the presentation of any patient with an abduction deficit as a patient "with a 6th nerve palsy." The key to a comprehensive cognitive framework for approaching diplopia is the consideration of all the pertinent localizations of pathology which might cause an abduction deficit. Though most abduction deficits are indeed due to 6th nerve palsies, a wide range of "pseudo-6th nerve palsies" exists and should be kept in mind (Box 95.1). In keeping with neurologic tradition, we will address the common causes of abduction deficits proceeding in a proximal-to-distal anatomic manner.

Box 95.1: Causes of abduction deficits.

- *Sixth nerve palsies*:
  - Nuclear 6th nerve palsies (typically without diplopia as MLF interneurons affected)
  - Fascicular 6th nerve palsies (often with accompanying long-tract signs)
  - Cisternal 6th nerve palsies (meningeal irritation or vascular lesions)
  - Damage at Dorello's canal (elevated intracranial pressure or clival lesions)
  - Cavernous sinus lesions (vascular, infectious, neoplastic, inflammatory)
  - Orbital apex lesions (often involvement of cranial nerves II, III, and IV)
  - Intraorbital lesions
- *Disorders of the neuromuscular junction*:
  - Myasthenia gravis
  - Botulism
- *Myopathies*:
  - Lateral rectus paresis (neoplasia, inflammation, ischemia)
  - Medial rectus sclerosis (thyroid eye disease, neoplasia, inflammation)
- *Nonpathologic causes*:
  - Duane's syndrome
  - Convergence spasm
  - Heavy eye syndrome
- *Uncommon supranuclear causes*:
  - Thalamic esotropia

The most proximal neuroanatomic area responsible for abduction of an eye is the frontal eye field (FEF), located in the contralateral frontal lobe of the abducting eye. The axons from FEF project to the pons, where they synapse on neurons in the contralateral paramedian pontine reticular formation (PPRF).[2] The PPRF contains excitatory burst neurons which project to the ipsilateral 6th nerve nucleus. Each 6th nerve nucleus is comprised of two populations of neurons, the first being interneurons whose axons ascend from the nucleus rostrally to form the medial longitudinal fasciculus (MLF) and eventually project to the subnucleus of the contralateral 3rd nerve whose neurons innervate the medial rectus (MR). The second population of neurons in the 6th nerve nucleus is of the motor neurons whose axons proceed ventrally through the medial pons to form the 6th nerve and eventually innervate the lateral rectus.[3] The net result of this is that pathology affecting the FEFs, PPRF, and 6th nerve nucleus generates conjugate eye movment abnormalities. A conjugate limitation of eye movements (i.e. the eyes do not move fully but they do remain aligned) is referred to as a gaze *palsy*, and it should be noted that diplopia does not result as there is no misalignment of the globes. Thus the most proximal point in the nervous system at which pathology can create diplopia from a deficit of abduction is at the point at which the axons of the 6th nerve motor nuclei exit the nucleus itself and are separate from those which form the MLF (Fig. 95.1). A few rare exceptions to this exist, the most common of which is Duane's syndrome. The most common type of Duane's syndrome (type 1) is typically encountered in the left eye of young women. Herein, there is a congenital absence of the neurons in the 6th nerve nucleus which would otherwise innervate the ipsilateral 6th nerve.[4]

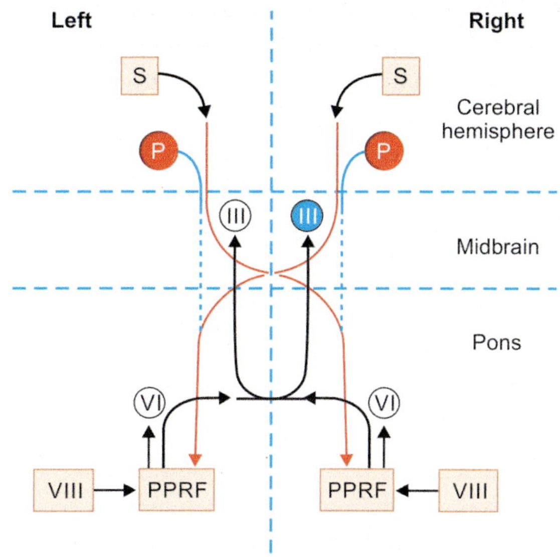

Fig. 95.1: Pathways for control of ocular movement.
(S: Saccade; P: Pursuit; PPRF: Paramedian pontine reticular formation)

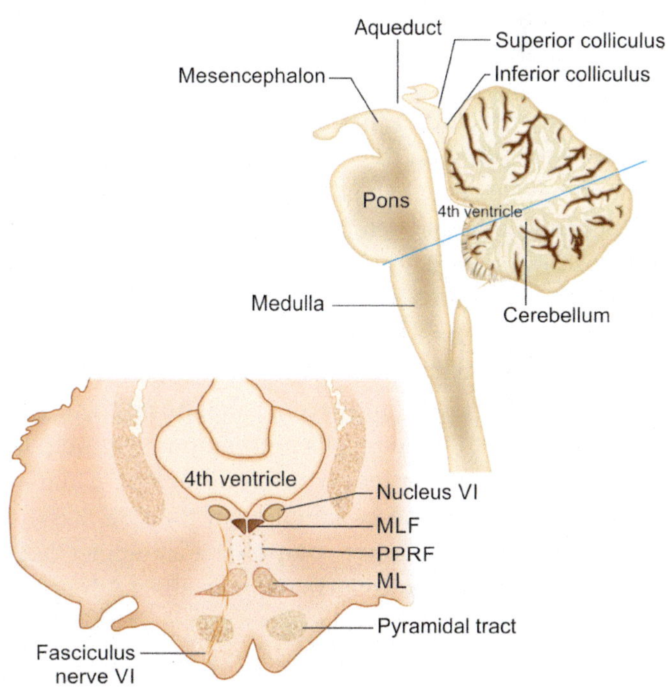

Fig. 95.2: Pontine section shows origin of sixth nerve and demonstrates medial longitudinal fasciculus (MLF) and paramedian pontine reticular formation (PPRF).
(ML: Medial lemniscus)

Fascicular 6th Nerve Palsies

Damage to the 6th nerve motor neuron's axons after they have exited the 6th nerve nucleus but while they remain in the brainstem results in a fascicular 6th nerve palsy. It is important to remember that the 6th nerve nucleus is located dorsally and medially in the pons; the fascicles which exit the nucleus remain medial as they proceed ventrally within the pons. Nearby structures include the medial lemniscus, which lies medially in the pons between the 6th nerve nucleus and the corticospinal tract, which travels at the ventral aspect of the pons (Fig. 95.2). The medial lemniscus is a tract formed by the second order neurons of the dorsal columns pathway, relaying proprioceptive and light touch information from the contralateral hemibody to the thalamus. As the 6th nerve fascicles proceed further ventrally, they pass through the corticospinal tract which relays motor information from the frontal lobe to the spinal cord. Damage to the corticospinal tract at the level of the pons results in an upper motor neuron pattern of weakness in the contralateral hemibody. Thus, assessment of proprioception, touch, and strength in the contralateral hemibody is of diagnostic utility when evaluating a patient with an abduction deficit. Though typically accompanied by other neurologic deficits, fascicular 6th nerve palsies may be isolated.[5,6]

Cisternal 6th Nerve Palsies

When the fascicles formed by the 6th nerve nucleus' axons exit the ventral pons, they form the 6th nerve proper. When the 6th nerve exits the pons, it lies in a cerebrospinal fluid (CSF) space referred to as the prepontine cistern. Here, it is susceptible to any meningeal pathology. Thus, a cisternal 6th nerve palsy may be caused by infectious meningitides (especially basilar meningitides, which include bacterial, viral, and fungal causes), autoimmune meningitides (e.g. sarcoidosis), and carcinomatous or lymphomatous meningitis.[7] Correspondingly, patients should be queried as to headache, neck pain, light and sound sensitivity, and pain with eye movements, all of which can be meningeal signs. However, the absence of these findings does not necessarily preclude a pathologic process in the CSF space. Depending on the exact pathologic process, the patient may be encephalopthic and in extremis (e.g. as a result of a fulminant bacterial meningitis) or completely asymptomatic aside from diplopia (half of patients with carcinomatous meningitis have no headache, for example).[8] The incorporation of other neurologic abnormalities (e.g. other cranial neuropathies), the presence or absence of alternate diagnoses, and the natural history of the patient's presentation will help to guide whether the patient with an otherwise isolated abduction deficit requires sampling of the CSF. Rarely, basilar aneurysms or other compressive etiologies (e.g. clival meningiomas or aneurysms) may effect 6th nerve palsies in the prepontine cistern.[7]

The 6th nerve then ascends rostrally along the clivus, passing through Dorello's canal to enter the cavernous sinus. Owing to the sharp angle which the 6th nerve takes to pass through Dorello's canal and the adherence of the connective tissue therein to the nerve, this is a common site of stretch injury in the setting of elevated or decreased intracranial pressure, which displace the brainstem caudally.[9] Patients with abduction deficits should be queried as to symptoms of elevated intracranial pressure as well as recent lumbar punctures or spinal procedures, and the fundus must be assessed for papilledema. Other clival lesions, such as chordomas, often affect the 6th nerve as it traverses Dorello's canal.[7]

Cavernous 6th Nerve Palsies

Within the cavernous sinus, the 6th nerve lies just lateral to the carotid artery. Herein, it may be affected by a wide variety of vascular, autoimmune, infectious, and neoplastic processes. The exhaustive differential diagnosis of cavernous sinus pathology is beyond the scope of this text, but a few points should be noted in particular:

- Other cranial nerve deficits may be present but are not required
- Abduction deficit + ipsilateral Horner's syndrome = cavernous sinus process until proven otherwise, as the sympathetic fibers travel with the carotid artery in its cavernous portion.[10,11]
- Painful 6th nerve palsies often localize to the cavernous sinus (i.e. Tolosa-Hunt syndrome) and may respond rapidly to steroids.[12,13]

Owing to the presence of the 2nd, 3rd, 4th, and 6th cranial nerves at the orbital apex, this is an uncommon localization for an isolated 6th nerve palsy. Within the orbit, the 6th nerve may be damaged as well.

Nonlocalizing 6th Nerve Palsies

Injury at a particular anatomic location may not be discernible from the examination, and the following points must be considered:

- Giant cell arteritis may cause 6th nerve and/or lateral rectus ischemia ("pseudo-6th nerve palsy") and should always be kept in mind in patients over the age of 50.[14]
- "Microvascular" or "ischemic" 6th nerve palsies are an extremely common etiology of isolated abduction deficits in patients over the age of 50 as well.[7]
- Approximately 90% of patients with a microvascular cranial neuropathy will recover within 90 days.[15]
- Cranial neuropathies failing to recover after 3 months must be investigated.
- Thorough face and scalp examination may be helpful, as cancers of the head and neck may have perineural spread tumor spread.[16,17]
- Some processes such as the Miller Fisher variant of Guillain-Barré do not localize per se,[18,19] in contrast other autoimmune process, such as sarcoidosis[20] (Box 95.2).

Box 95.2: Etiologies of 6th nerve palsies.

- *Ischemic*:
  - Small vessel disease
  - Giant cell arteritis
- *Trauma*:
  - Elevated intracranial pressure with traction at Dorello's canal
  - Moderate head trauma
- *Compressive*:
  - Compressive aneurysm
  - Intrinsic neoplasia
  - Extrinsic neoplasia
- *Infectious*:
  - Meningitis
  - Septic cavernous sinus thrombosis
  - Gradenigo's syndrome
- *Congenital*:
  - Duane's syndrome
  - Möbius syndrome
- *Autoimmune*:
  - Miller Fisher variant Guillain-Barré syndrome
  - Sarcoid
  - Tolosa-Hunt syndrome

Neuromuscular Junction Transmission Defects

Processes confined to the neuromuscular junction may similarly yield a "pseudo-6th nerve palsy". Myasthenia gravis (MG) is the most common example of this, and any patient with an abduction deficit should be questioned with regard to myasthenic symptoms such as variability in diplopia, variable ptosis, dysphonia, dysarthria, dysphagia, head drop, and proximal weakness, among others. Other, less common causes of abduction deficits exist, including botulism. Myasthenia will be discussed in more detail below.

Medial Rectus Restriction Resulting in Abduction Deficit

A fundamental distinction should be made between abduction deficits which are overcome with forced ductions (e.g. paresis of the nerve, neuromuscular junction, or muscle) and those which are not, thereby implying a restrictive abduction deficit:

- Thyroid eye disease commonly affects the inferior and medial recti before the superior and lateral recti and limits supraduction and abduction.[21,22]
- Other orbital inflammatory diseases may result in late MR scarring and restriction.
- Long-standing paretic processes may also have a restrictive component as the unopposed MR muscle shortens and scleroses.[23]

Nonpathologic Causes of Abduction Deficits

The following conditions should be considered in appropriate cases:

- Convergence spasm, in which spasm of the near reflex (accommodation, convergence, miosis), leads to the transient inability to abduct; it rarely has a pathologic cause such as thalamic esotropia.[24,25]
- Version testing alone with congenital esotropia may give a false impression of limited abduction of one or both eyes. Ductions are typically full (unless there is strong fixation preference of one eye and contralateral MR shortening/sclerosis occurs).[23]
- Duane's syndrome types 1 (abduction deficit with palpebral fissure widening on attempted abduction) and 3 (adduction and abduction deficits).[4,26,27]
- "Heavy eye syndrome" typical to high myopes,[28,29] usually with bilateral abduction deficits.

Adduction Deficits

Adduction, the movement of the eye nasally, is the result of activation of the MR muscle. The MR is innervated by the inferior division of the 3rd nerve. The presence of an adduction deficit should lead the examiner to closely scrutinize the other 3rd nerve-innervated muscles in order to determine whether there is a pattern suggestive of a 3rd nerve palsy. In straightforward cases, all of the muscles innervated by the 3rd nerve will be dysfunctional (Box 95.3). However, damage to the nerve frequently results in a *partial* 3rd nerve palsy, wherein only some of the innervated muscles are dysfunctional. All 3rd nerve palsies should be classified as to whether they are complete versus partial, pupil-sparing or not, painful or painless, and as to whether aberrant regeneration is seen (Box 95.4). Features of 3rd nerve paresis caused by lesions along its anatomic path are described below.

The MR subnucleus of the 3rd nerve, located in the ipsilateral dorsal midbrain, is innervated by the MLF interneurons, which originate from the contralateral 6th nerve nucleus and almost immediately decussate, ascending rostrally in the dorsomedial pons to reach the midbrain (Fig. 95.3). As described above, a lesion of the 6th nerve nucleus affects both the final input to the lateral rectus and the contralateral MR equally, resulting in a gaze palsy. Thus it is only at the MLF and more distally that a disconjugate adduction deficit can result rather than a gaze palsy (Box 95.5).

Box 95.3: Third nerve palsy patterns.

- *Complete 3rd nerve palsies*:
  - Supraduction deficit (superior rectus and inferior oblique)
  - Adduction deficit (medial rectus)
  - Infraduction deficit (inferior rectus)
  - Mydriasis (pupillary sphincter)
  - Ptosis (levator palpebrae)
- *Partial 3rd nerve palsies*:
  - Any combination of the above
- *Superior division 3rd nerve palsies*:
  - Supraduction deficit (superior rectus)
  - Ptosis (levator palpebrae)
- *Inferior division 3rd nerve palsies*:
  - Supraduction deficit in adduction (inferior oblique)
  - Adduction deficit (medial rectus)
  - Infraduction deficit (inferior rectus)
  - Mydriasis (pupillary sphincter)

Box 95.4: Common causes of 3rd nerve palsies with aberrant regeneration.

- Trauma
- Aneurysmal compression
- Neoplastic compression

Box 95.5: Common causes of adduction deficits.

- Internuclear ophthalmoplegia (with abducting nystagmus in the fellow eye)
- *3rd nerve palsies (partial or complete)*:
  - Central
  - Cisternal
  - Cavernous
- Myasthenia gravis
- *Myopathies*:
  - Medial rectus paresis
  - Lateral rectus sclerosis

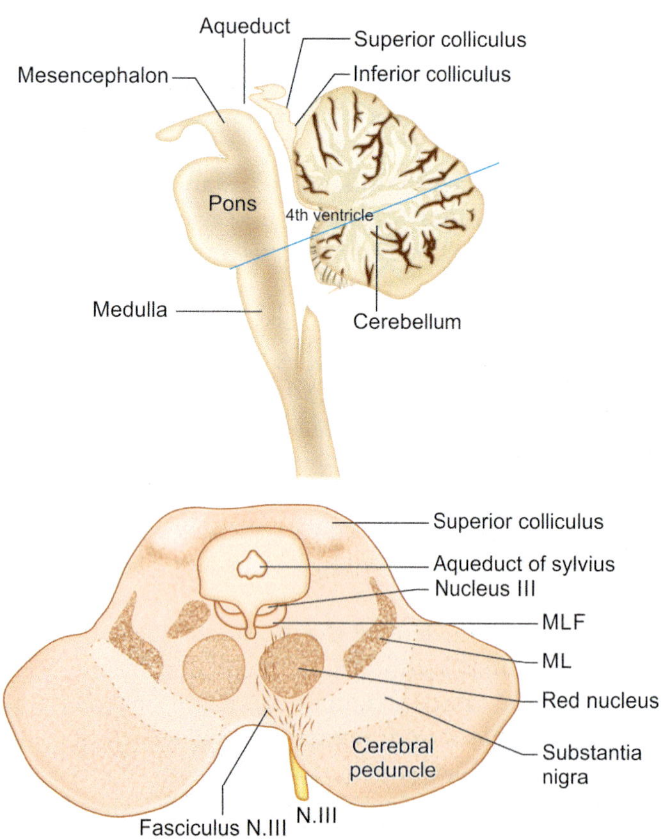

Fig. 95.3: Midbrain section shows origin of third nerve at level of superior colliculus.
(MLF: Medial longitudinal fasciculus; ML: Medial lemniscus)

Internuclear Ophthalmoplegia

Damage to the MLF results in the classic "INO" which is characterized by a supranuclear adduction deficit with slowed adducting saccades, almost always ipsilateral to the lesion (thus the laterality of the INO corresponds to the side of the adduction deficit), accompanied by a contralateral abducting nystagmus.[30] The abducting nystagmus in the nonparetic fellow eye is the result of Hering's Law, which stipulates the neuronal firing rates of PPRF neurons are uniform for both those that project to the 6th nerve nucleus motor neurons and the interneurons which form the MLF. Thus, when the contralateral eye fails to adduct as a result of MLF damage, the firing rate of the PPRF neurons increases, causing excess stimulation of the intact 6th nerve nucleus motor neurons and an over-activation of the intact 6th nerve which is visible to the examiner as abducting nystagmus. Depending on the anatomic extent of the lesion which causes the MLF, any combination of bilateral MLF lesions, skew deviations, medial lemniscus damage, and upbeat nystagmus may result.

Central 3rd Nerve Palsy

- Damage to the MR subnucleus itself or its axonal projections within the midbrain (its fascicles) may cause an ipsilateral adduction deficit but rarely in isolation.

- The 3rd nerve nucleus lies in the rostral midbrain and consists of a subnucleus for each muscle innervated.
- The inferior rectus (IR), MR, inferior oblique (IO), and pupillary sphincter (Edinger-Westphal) nuclei are located ipsilateral to the muscles they innervate.
- The superior rectus (SR) subnucleus innervates the contralateral SR muscle (fibers cross the midline and join the contralateral IR, MR, IO, and pupillomotor fibers to form the fascicle of the 3rd nerve.
- A midline levator papebrae nucleus projects fibers bilaterally to join each 3rd nerve (Fig. 95.4). Thus, ptosis resulting from a "nuclear" 3rd nerve palsy affects both eyes, while unilateral ptosis may occur with a "fascicular" 3rd nerve palsy.[31]

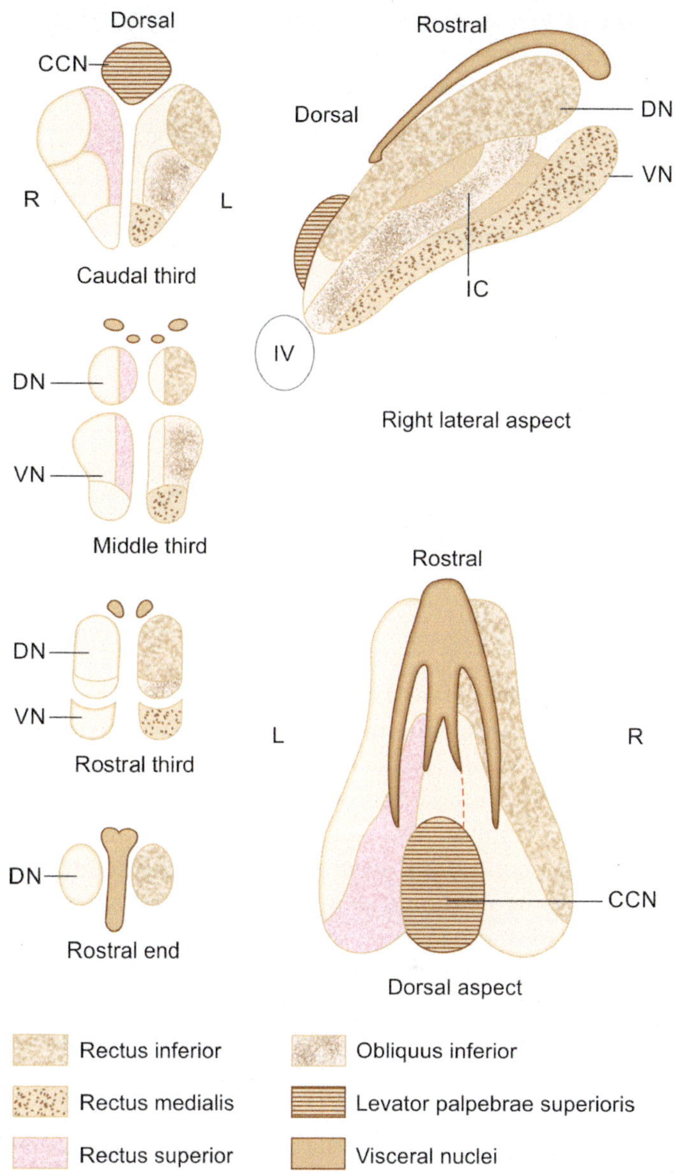

Fig. 95.4: Warwick's diagram of third nerve nuclear complex. (DN: Dorsal nucleus; VN: Ventral nucleus; CCN: Central caudal nucleus; IC: Intermediate complex)

Source: Reprinted with permission from Warwick.

Cisternal 3rd Nerve Palsy

The 3rd nerve exits the midbrain medially and briefly passes through the CSF space before entering the cavernous sinus.

- The 3rd nerve exits the midbrain just lateral to the basilar artery
  - Immediately inferior to the posterior cerebral artery
  - Immediately superior to the superior cerebellar artery.
- As the 3rd nerve passes anteriorly, is passes caudal to the posterior communicating artery, aneurysms of which are statistically the most likely to compress the 3rd nerve.[7]
- The same infectious, inflammatory, and neoplastic meningeal processes discussed with cisternal 6th nerve palsies apply here as well.

Most patients with compressive 3rd nerve lesions have pupillary mydriasis, as the pupillomotor fibers travel along the superficial, dorsal aspect of the 3rd nerve. But about 3% will not.[32] Thus, the lack of pupillary involvement in a new-onset 3rd nerve palsy does not immediately exonerate a compressive etiology.

Cavernous 3rd Nerve Palsy

After entering the cavernous sinus, the 3rd nerve travels at its superolateral aspect, just superior to the 4th nerve. As the 3rd nerve exits the cavernous sinus and enters the orbit via the orbital apex, it divides into a superior and inferior division. The superior division innervates the levator palpebrae and the SR. The inferior division subserves adduction as it innervates the MR, in addition to the IR, IO, and the pupillary constrictor. Dysfunction of the 3rd nerve proper or its inferior division are unlikely to result in an isolated adduction deficit, but the possibility of a partial 3rd nerve palsy should be considered.

Nonlocalizing 3rd Nerve Palsies

Giant cell arteritis should be kept in mind in patients over 50 with 3rd nerve palsies (the ischemia caused by GCA may

Box 95.6: Etiologies of 3rd nerve palsies.

- *Compressive*:
  - Aneurysm (most likely posterior communicating artery)
  - Uncal herniation
  - Intrinsic neoplasia (e.g. schwannomas, neurinomas)
  - Extrinsic neoplasia
- *Ischemic*:
  - Small vessel disease
  - Giant cell arteritis
  - Midbrain ischemia
- *Infectious*:
  - Meningitis
  - Septic cavernous sinus thrombosis
- *Trauma*:
  - Severe head injury
  - Skull base or orbital fracture
  - Midbrain hemorrhage
- *Autoimmune*:
  - Miller-Fisher variant Guillain-Barré syndrome
  - Tolosa-Hunt syndrome
  - Ophthalmoplegic migraine (in children)
  - Sarcoid
- Congenital

affect either the nerve or extraocular muscle). Just as with 6th nerve palsies, "microvascular" 3rd nerve palsies are very common, the risk factors being identical (diabetes, hypertension, etc.). Microvascular 3rd nerve palsies should not result in aberrant regeneration. Autoimmune neurologic conditions, such as Miller-Fisher syndrome and neurosarcoid should be kept in mind. Generally, more severe head trauma is required to cause a 3rd nerve palsy than to cause a 4th or 6th nerve palsy (Box 95.6).

Disorders of the Medial Rectus Muscle and Its Neuromuscular Junction

Myasthenia should always be maintained on the differential for painless, pupil-sparing ocular motor deficits. Long-standing or inflammatory (either autoimmune or neoplastic) myopathy may cause sclerosis of the lateral rectus, and restricted adduction. The lateral rectus is classically the last of the extraocular muscles to be affected by thyroid eye disease, and isolated adduction deficit from this condition is exceedingly rare.[21] Most myopathic processes causing MR weakness (e.g. chronic progressive external ophthalmoplegia) do not cause an isolated adduction deficit owing to the diffuse muscle involvement.

Supraduction Deficits

Supraduction, the movement of the eye upward, is achieved through the action of the SR (when the eye is abducted) and through the IO (when the eye is adducted), both of which are innervated by the 3rd nerve. The excitatory burst neurons for vertical gaze are located in the rostral interstitial nucleus of the MLF (riMLF). These project to the IO subnucleus, which lies ipsilateral to the muscle it innervates, and to the SR subnucleus of the 3rd nerve, which is unique among the 3rd nerve subnuclei as it is the only subnucleus that lies contralateral to the muscle it innervates (Box 95.7).

Box 95.7: Common causes of supraduction deficits.

- *Third nerve palsies (partial or complete)*:
  - Central
  - Cisternal
  - Cavernous
- Myasthenia gravis
- *Myopathies*:
  - Superior rectus (in abduction) or inferior oblique (in adduction) paresis
  - Inferior rectus or superior oblique sclerosis
- *Soft tissue disorders*:
  - Brown's syndrome (sclerosis of the superior oblique tendon sheath)

Third Nerve Palsies

As noted above, the axons originating from the SR nucleus decussate almost immediately and travel with the axons from the other 3rd nerve subnuclei to form the fascicular portion of the 3rd nerve before exiting the brainstem to contribute to the 3rd nerve proper. Lesions to the SR subnucleus causing a contralateral defect of supraduction are rare. The superior division of the 3rd nerve innervates only the SR and the levator palpebrae. Thus, the combination of ptosis and a defect of supraduction may localize a lesion to the anterior cavernous sinus or posterior orbit, but this pattern may be seen in any incomplete 3rd nerve palsy. Nonlocalizing causes of adduction deficits (above) also may cause supraduction abnormalities.

Disorders of the Orbit, Extraocular Muscles, and the Neuromuscular Junction

- A defect of supraduction in adduction may result from either restriction or paresis:
  - Inferior oblique paresis (rare)
  - Sclerosis of the tendon sheath of the superior oblique (Brown's syndrome[33]), which may be painful or painless.
- The most common restrictive process leading to incomplete supraduction is thyroid eye disease, with the IR typically the first muscle to be affected.

Box 95.8: Common causes of infraduction deficits.

- *Third nerve palsies (partial or complete)*:
  - Central
  - Cisternal
  - Cavernous
- Fourth nerve palsies
- Myasthenia gravis
- *Myopathies*:
  - Inferior rectus paresis (in abduction)
  - Superior oblique paresis (in adduction)
  - Superior rectus or inferior oblique paresis

Infraduction Deficits

Infraduction, the downward movement of the eye, is somewhat more complex than supraduction in that infraduction in abduction is accomplished by activating the IR muscle via the 3rd nerve whereas infraduction in adduction is achieved by activating the superior oblique muscle via the 4th nerve (Box 95.8). The axons of the excitatory burst neurons responsible for vertical gaze (which lie in the riMLF, as referenced above) project to both the IO subnucleus of the 3rd nerve and to the 4th nerve nucleus.

Third Nerve Palsy, Disorders of the Inferior Rectus, and Its Neuromuscular Junction

Isolated infraduction deficits from a 3rd nerve palsy are exceedingly rare, and function of the other muscles innervated by the 3rd nerve must be examined closely in patients with infraduction deficits. Neuromuscular junction disease can affect infraduction alone; SR tightness also may limit downward eye movement, as may IR contusion after acute orbital floor trauma.

Fourth Nerve Palsy

The 4th nerve nucleus lies in the dorsal midbrain contralateral to the superior oblique muscle its axons innervate. Its axons exit the contralateral midbrain dorsally. Its path both dorsal to the midbrain and in the ambient cistern make it particularly prone to trauma, wherein it may be compressed between the midbrain and the fibrous tentorium cerebelli.[34] Schwannomas also may affect the cisternal portion of the 4th nerve, as may the variety of inflammatory, infectious, and neoplastic processes referenced above. The 4th nerve enters the cavernous sinus and travels immediately inferior to the 3rd nerve and superior to the ophthalmic division of the 5th nerve. It enters the orbit through the superior orbital fissure and innervates the superior oblique. Nonlocalizing 4th nerve palsies, as seen with GCA, microvascular ischemia, and Miller-Fisher syndrome and pseudo-4th nerve palsies, such seen with MG or IO restrictive pathology, also may cause infraduction weakness. In addition, congenital 4th nerve palsies are seen with relative frequency, though they may not decompensate until well into adulthood.

Unlike deficits affecting the 3rd and 6th nerves, the impairment in ductions caused by 4th nerve lesions may be very subtle. As such, other diagnostic maneuvers have been developed to help diagnose 4th nerve palsies and differentiate them from other causes of vertical misalignments. These tests are predicated upon an understanding of the superior oblique's functions: depression in adduction, incyclotorsion, and weak abduction. The clinical result of superior oblique underaction is therefore an ipsilateral hypertropia worse in adduction and an excyclotorted globe. The Parks-Bielschowsky 3-step test is a means by which these features of superior oblique function may be assessed.[35,36]

- *Step 1:* Determine which eye is hyperdeviated.
- *Step 2:* Is the hyperdeviation greater in contraversive gaze (away from the side of the hypertropia) than ipsiversive gaze? (In 4th nerve palsy, it typically is).
- *Step 3:* Is the hyperdeviation greater in ipsilateral head tilt than in contralateral head tilt?
- A 4th step, comparison of the magnitude of the deviation in the upright versus supine positions, may help to distinguish 4th nerve palsy from skew deviation (see below).[37]

In cases of severe 3rd nerve injury, the eye may not adduct, and the examiner may be unable to determine whether the 4th nerve is able to perform its function of depressing the eye in adduction. This may be determined by closely observing the conjunctival vessels on the globe during attempted downgaze; if incyclotorsion is seen, then the function of the 4th nerve is preserved. Bilateral 4th nerve palsies may be difficult to identify; over 10° of excyclotorsion should raise the possibility of bilateral 4th nerve palsies. Finally, patients normally have a limited ability to fuse vertical deviations (often <4 prism diopters); the presence of a larger fusional amplitude is suggestive of a congenital etiology (Box 95.9). Despite the congenital nature of this issue, it may not become symptomatic until adulthood.[38]

Box 95.9: Common etiologies of the 4th nerve palsies.

- *Traumatic*:
  - Head injury, even relatively minor
- *Congenital*:
  - Decompensated congenital palsies
- *Compressive*:
  - Intrinsic neoplasia (e.g. schwannomas)
  - Extrinsic neoplasia (e.g. tentorial meningiomas)
- *Ischemic*:
  - Small vessel disease
  - Giant cell arteritis
- *Infectious*:
  - Meningitis
  - Septic cavernous sinus thrombosis
- *Autoimmune*:
  - Tolosa-Hunt syndrome
  - Miller Fisher variant Guillain-Barré syndrome
  - Sarcoid

Processes which May Cause Ocular Motor Deficits not Corresponding to a Single Cranial Nerve

Myasthenia Gravis

Myasthenia gravis is an autoimmune disorder wherein antibodies are generated which block neuromuscular transmission, the result of which is fatigable weakness. Ocular involvement is common in myasthenic patients, with 90% of patients having involvement of the eyelids and/or extraocular muscles at some point.[39] Approximately 50% of patients will have ocular symptoms in isolation, and 20–50% of pure ocular MG patients will progress to generalized MG over a median of 20–24 months.[39,40]

Myasthenia gravis may mimic any pupil-sparing, painless ocular motor neuropathy or may create an inscrutable pattern not mapping to any one ocular motor nerve (or pattern of nerves) with equal ease. The classic presentation of myasthenic diplopia is that of variable strabismus. A number of examination tests exist to assess for the presence of MG. Ocular myasthenia is very frequently accompanied by orbicularis oculi weakness; thus the strength of forced eye closure should be tested. Weakness of the orbicularis may lead to fatiguing of eye closure and resulting opening of the palpebral fissure, referred to as the "peek sign".[41] Upper eyelid ptosis, often fatigable, is a frequent manifestation; uninterrupted upgaze should be maintained for 60 seconds to look for appearance of ptosis and/or diplopia. Ptosis may be asymmetric. As discussed earlier, both levator palpebrae are innervated by a single, midline nucleus in the midbrain. Ptosis of one lid may trigger increased activity from the levator nucleus, resulting in overstimulation and retraction of the "nonblocked" lid.[42] The overstimulated lid may eventually fatigue, resulting in alternating ptosis. Patients with ptosis should also be maintained in downgaze for at least 5 seconds and directed to subsequently make a saccade back to primary position; this may result in flutter of the eyelids, presumably from transient overstimulation of the lids from acetylcholine (ACh) built up at the neuromuscular junction during rest (i.e. while in downgaze). This is referred to as Cogan's lid twitch.[43] Improvement with ice or rest should also be noted. Assessment of proximal weakness (including the neck flexors and extensors) and of the respiratory status of the patient is critical in those with identified myasthenia as these increase the urgency with which neurologic attention must be sought.

Several different autoantibodies may give rise to a similar myasthenic syndrome. The most common is the ACh receptor antibodies (AChR Abs). These are present in approximately 85% of cases of generalized myasthenia, but only in 50% of cases of ocular myasthenia.[44,45] Muscle-specific kinase (MuSK) and ligand-related peptide 4 (LRP4) antibodies may be present in some patients with negative AChR Abs, but many ocular myasthenic patients remain seronegative.[46,47]

Electromyography (EMG) can be an important neurophysiologic adjunct to the examination in cases where seronegative myasthenia is suspected or to confirm the diagnosis of myasthenia with borderline antibody titers. Ocular myasthenia often does not result in abnormal repetitive nerve stimulation in proximal muscles such as the deltoids.[44] Single fiber EMG of the orbicularis oculi, carries a higher yield, although the estimated sensitivity still varies from approximately 60–93% and requires technical expertise.[48-50] Incorporation of more technically difficult muscles, such as the SR, may raise the sensitivity, but these techniques are not widely performed.[49]

Giant Cell Arteritis

Giant cell arteritis has been referenced above and similarly can generate any eye movement limitation pattern. Its ocular manifestations are protean,[14] and it may cause cranial nerve and/or extraocular muscle ischemia. See Chapter 94, Systemic Disease and Neuro-Ophthalmology, for further details on the diagnosis and management of GCA.[51-53]

Wernicke's Encephalopathy

Wernicke's encephalopathy is a triad of encephalopathy, ophthalmoplegia, and ataxia due to a deficiency of thiamine (vitamin B_1). The ophthalmic manifestations of Wernicke's are variable, ranging from subtle nystagmus to gaze palsies or limitation of ductions which may mimic cranial nerve palsies. The full triad infrequently occurs.[54] A history of alcoholism, chronic diarrhea, gastric bypass, or poor nutritional status may raise suspicion for the diagnosis. Laboratory studies may demonstrate a mildly elevated lactate. Magnetic resonance imaging may show fluid attenuated inversion recovery (FLAIR) hyperintensities of the mammilary bodies (which may become hemorrhagic), medial thalami or periaqueductal gray as well as thinning of the corpus callosum.[55] Ophthalmoplegia is the first sign to resolve with adminstration of thiamine therapy.

Miller Fisher Variant of Guillain-Barré Syndrome

The Miller-Fisher variant of Guillain-Barré is an GQ1b autoantibody mediated disorder; patients may develop any combination of ophthalmoplegia, ataxia, and areflexia.[56] As with Wernicke's ophthalmoplegia, this may manifest as nystagmus, a gaze palsy, or as a cranial nerve palsy. Approximately 80–95% of patients have a positive GQ1b autoantibody from the serum.[57,58] Lumbar puncture classically reveals cytoalbuminologic dissociation, and neuroimaging should be normal. If this is suspected, prompt involvement of neurology is required.

Ocular Neuromyotonia

Ocular neuromyotonia is defined as the inability of an activated extraocular muscle to relax. This results in a clinical presentation diametrically opposite to that seen in ocular myasthenia; an activated muscle prevents the globe from moving in the direction of its antagonist. This may occur as a result of irradiation, tumor, vascular compression, or thyroid eye disease and is treatable with carbamazepine.[59] Though it is uncommon, its recognition is tremendously important given its treatability and the diagnostic uncertainty that is otherwise created.

Thyroid Eye Disease

Thyroid eye disease is an autoantibody mediated process with resulting fibroblast dysregulation and fibrous fatty infiltration of the extraocular muscles. This results in proptosis and lid retraction (Figs. 95.5A to C) as well as diplopia. Typically, the IR is affected first (causing a restrictive deficit of supraduction), followed by the MR, then the SR, and lastly the lateral rectus. See Chapter 94, Systemic Disease and Neuro-Ophthalmology, for further details on the diagnosis and management of thyroid eye disease.

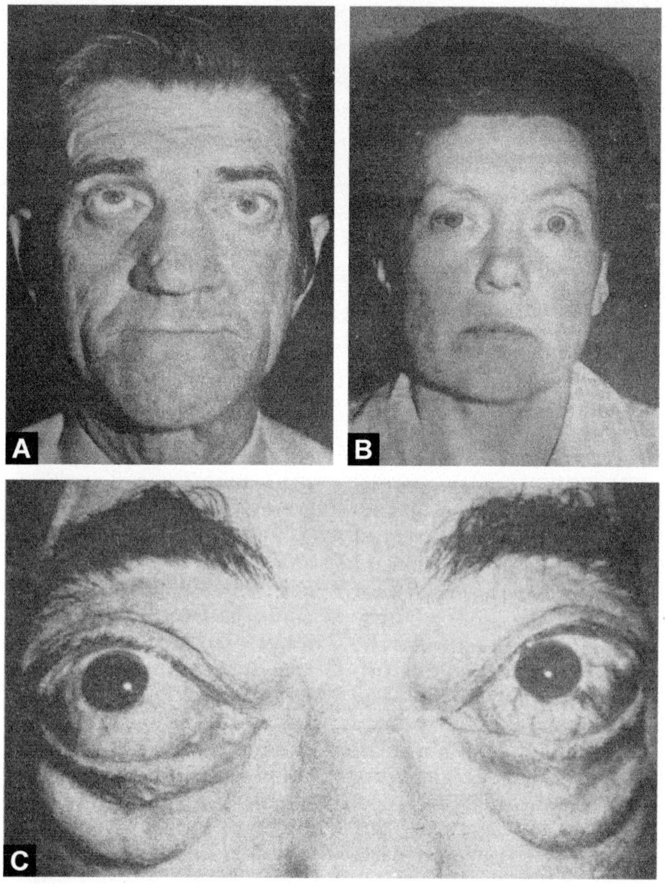

Figs. 95.5A to C: Thyroid ophthalmopathy. (A) Restricted upgaze in left eye; (B) Lid retraction in left eye; (C) Malignant exophthalmos.

Binocular Diplopia with Full Ductions

Convergence and Divergence Palsy

Disorders of vergence affect the ability of the eyes to maintain coordinated fixation on targets at various distances from the patient (i.e. the "z" plane) without affecting ductions (i.e. eye movement along the "x" and "y" planes). Convergence and divergence deficits are common causes of horizontal, binocular diplopia at near and far, respectively.

The normal point of convergence decreases with age but is approximately 10 cm for most adults. The most frequent symptom to result from convergence insufficiency is diplopia at near. The examination reveals full ductions with an exotropia larger at near than at far with the inability to converge normally. This may occur without any pathologic implications, although it may be associated with neurodegenerative disorders such as Parkinson's disease or other midbrain pathology. Patients may benefit from convergence training, though some require prism therapy or surgery.[60]

As the eyes normally diverge to view a target at distance, divergence palsy is manifest as a comitant esotropia which is larger (by 10 prism diopters or more) at distance than at near. Previously thought to arise from central nervous system dysfunction,[61] this condition may instead result from age-related orbital changes and has been dubbed the "sagging eye syndrome." The typical patient is a middle-aged or elderly Caucasian female; on examination, the ductions are full and there is evidence of soft tissue degenerative changes of the orbit, such as orbital fat atrophy and high lid creases.[62]

Skew Deviations

The ocular tilt reaction is a vestibular-mediated ocular reflex to aid the maintenance of the object of fixation on the fovea when the head moves in the roll plane. When leaning to one side, the head tilts contralaterally, the eye closer to the ground supraducts and intorts, and the eye closer to the sky infraducts and extorts. The afferent input to the ocular tilt reflex originates from each inner ear. When standing erect with the head straight, the input from each vestibular apparatus balances that of the other. Damage to one vestibular apparatus, vestibular nerve, or its central relays within the brainstem, will result in asymmetric input to the ocular motor centers. The net result is the brain's "perception" that the head has moved in the roll plane when it has not and the ocular tilt reflex emerges pathologically, causing a skew deviation. Because the disorder of ocular alignment is supranuclear, ductions are full.[63] Isolated hypertropias may be explained not only by skew deviations, but also by 4th nerve palsies and other mimics (e.g. myasthenia); these should be investigated using the Parks-Bielschowsky 3-step test with the added 4th step as suggested by Wong, in which a greater than 50% reduction in vertical deviation with supine positioning supports the diagnosis of skew deviation.[35-37]

Decompensation of Previously Latent or Suppressed Misalignments

An ocular misalignment only visible when binocular vision is interrupted is referred to as a phoria. This predisposition for the eyes to misalign may decompensate to the point where it is no longer kept in check by binocular viewing, becoming atropia and resulting in diplopia. Common triggers include illness, intoxication, fatigue, and advancing age. These patients do not have any pathology causing a limitation of ductions and thus the sensorimotor examination reveals a comitant deviation with full ductions.

Patients with congenital ocular misalignments often suppress one eye in order to prevent diplopia (amblyopia being the unfortunate corollary).[64] Diplopia may result if the eyes further misalign, eventually moving outside the zone of cortically mediated suppression. Diplopia in the setting of a congenital tropia with suppression may also occur if the previously suppressed eye is forced to take up fixation, often by asymmetric acuities (this is referred to as *fixation switch diplopia*).[65] These patients also have full ductions and a comitant deviation as the defective neural binding mechanisms responsible for the congenital ocular misalignment do not impair cranial nerve function.

Acute Acquired Comitant Esotropia in Adults

Acute acquired comitant esotropia developing in adulthood bears the same pattern as a decompensated phoria: full ductions, a comitant esotropia in all directions of gaze, and normal vergence. Despite its occurrence at a later age than typical to childhood esotropias, it too is usually a benign phenomenon. However, cases have been reported wherein a structural lesions was identified (Chiari I malformation) with resolution of the esotropia after surgical correction. Acute acquired comitant esotropia in the setting of neoplasia has been reported as well, though the majority of cases seem to be unassociated with pathology.[66]

Dragged Fovea

This uncommon condition arises when an epiretinal membrane physically dislocates the fovea from its normal location. As a result, the fovea in one eye no longer corresponds to the same visual field coordinates as its fellow eye.[67] Because wider retinal correspondence remains intact, intractable central diplopia arises from the foveal mismatch.

Binocular Diplopia by History but Not Present at the Time of Examination

This is a situation which must be approached with great caution. The first step is to consider the possibility that the patient may only have diplopia in one position of gaze, thus accurately but somewhat misleadingly reporting the diplopia as "intermittent." If truly intermittent, the differential diagnosis is broad and includes stroke with subsequent recovery, transient ischemic attack, deficits of cortical binding (e.g. intermittently decompensating phorias), transient compression of a cranial nerve (intracranial pressure related, aneurysmal, etc.), transient inflammation (e.g. Tolosa-Hunt), transient nerve ischemia (e.g. in GCA), MG, superior oblique myokymia, and transient muscle ischemia (e.g. GCA). Care should be taken to investigate the history all the more fully when the patient is examined interictally as the list of pathologic processes is replete with "high stakes" diagnoses.

CONCLUSION

Diplopia is an often challenging complaint for the trainee to evaluate. By first ascertaining the binocularity of the complaint, then identifying through history and examination the pattern of the misalignment, identifying the structures possibly involved, and then exploring potential etiologies, the examiner can maintain a logical and thorough approach to the complaint. Owing to the introductory nature of this text, this emphasis has been on establishing a clear cognitive framework for understanding and approaching diplopia. Many details regarding the pathologic processes responsible for diplopia and their management have largely been omitted due to space constraints, but the reader is directed to the references below for further information. This information only serves as an asset rather than a source of confusion during the diplopia evaluation when the above cognitive approach has already been clearly formed.

REFERENCES

1. Records RE. Monocular diplopia. Surv Ophthalmol. 1980;24(5):303-6.
2. Buttner-Ennever JA, Buttner U. Neuroanatomy of the oculomotor system. The reticular formation. Rev Oculomotor Res. 1988;2:119-76.
3. Baker R, Highstein SM. Physiologic identification of interneurons and motoneurons in the abducens nucleus. Brain Res. 1975;91:292-8.
4. Duane A. Congenital deficiency of abduction associated with impairment of adduction, retraction movements, contraction of the palpebral fissure and oblique movements of the eye. 1905. Arch Ophthalmol. 1996;114(10):1255-6; discussion 1257.
5. Donaldson D, Rosenberg NL. Infarction of abducens nerve fascicle as cause of isolated sixth nerve palsy related to hypertension. Neurology. 1988;38(10):1654.
6. Barr D, Kupersmith MJ, Turbin R, et al. Isolated sixth nerve palsy: an uncommon presenting sign of multiple sclerosis. J Neurol. 2000;247(9):701-4.
7. Richards DW, Jones FR, Younge BR. Causes and prognosis in 4,270 cases of paralysis of the oculomotor, trochlear, and abducens cranial nerves. Am J Ophthalmol. 1992;113: 489-96.
8. Balm M, Hammack J. Leptomeningeal carcinomatosis. Presenting features and prognostic factors. Arch Neurol. 1996;53:382-5.
9. Tubbs RS, Radcliff V, Shoja MM, et al. Dorello canal revisited: an observation that potentially explains the frequency of abducens nerve injury after head injury. World Neurosurg. 2012;77(1):119-21.
10. Keane JR. Cavernous sinus syndrome. Analysis of 151 cases. Arch Neurol. 1996;53:967-71.
11. Myles WM, Maxner CE. Localizing value of concurrent sixth nerve paresis and postganglionic Horner's syndrome. Can J Ophthalmol. 1994;29:39-42.
12. Smith JL, Taxdal D. Painful ophthalmoplegia: the Tolosa-Hunt syndrome. Am J Ophthalmol. 1966;61:1466-72.
13. Kline LB, Hoyt WF. The Tolosa-Hunt syndrome. J Neurol Neurosurg Psychiatry. 2001;71:577-82.
14. Hayreh SS, Podhajsky PA, Zimmerman B. Ocular manifestations of giant cell arteritis. Am J Ophthalmol. 1998;125(4):509-20.
15. Park UC, Kim SJ, Hwang JM, et al. Clinical features and natural history of acquired third, fourth, and sixth cranial nerve palsy. Eye (Lond). 2008;22(5):691-6.
16. Clouston PD, Sharpe DM, Corbett AJ, et al. Perineural spread of cutaneous head and neck cancer. Its orbital and central neurologic complications. Arch Neurol. 1990;47:73-7.
17. Catalano PF, Sen C, Biller HF. Cranial neuropathy secondary to perineural spread of cutaneous malignancies. Am J Otolol. 1995;16:772-7.
18. Yuki N, Odaka M, Hirata K. Acute ophthalmoparesis (without ataxia) associated with anti-GQ1b IgG antibody: clinical features. Ophthalmology. 2001;108:196-200.
19. Lee SH, Lim GH, Kim JS, et al. Acute ophthalmoparesis (without ataxia) associated with anti-GQ1b IgG antibody. Neurology. 2008;71:426-9.
20. Burns TM. Neurosarcoidosis. Arch Neurol. 2003;60:1166-8.
21. Khong JJ, McNab AA, Ebeling PR, et al. Pathogenesis of thyroid eye disease: review and update on molecular mechanisms. Br J Ophthalmol. 2016;100:142-50.
22. Bothun ED, Scheurer RA, Harrison AR, et al. Update on thyroid eye disease. Clin Ophthalmol. 2009;3:543-51.
23. Metz HS. Restrictive factors in strabismus. Surv Ophthalmol. 1983;28(2):71-83.
24. Dagi LR, Chrousos GA, Cogan DG. Spasm of the near reflex associated with organic disease. Am J Ophthalmol. 1987;103:582-5.

25. Goldstein JH, Schneekloth BB. Spasm of the near reflex: a spectrum of anomalies. Surv Ophthalmol. 1996;40:269-78.
26. Hoyt W, Nachtigaller H. Anomalies of ocular motor nerves: neuroanatomic correlates of paradoxical innervation in Duane's syndrome and related congenital ocular motor disorders. Am J Ophthalmol. 1965;60:443.
27. Parsa CF, Grant PE, Dillon WP, et al. Absence of the abducens nerve in Duane syndrome verified by magnetic resonance imaging. Am J Ophthalmol. 1998;125:399-401.
28. Ward DM. The heavy eye phenomenon. Trans Ophthalmol Soc UK. 1967;87:717-26.
29. Krzizok TH, Schroeder BU. Measurement of recti eye muscle paths by magnetic resonance imaging in highly myopic and normal subjects. Invest Ophthalmol Vis Sci. 1999;40:2554-60.
30. Leigh RJ, Zee DS. The Neurology of Eye Movements, 3rd edition. New York: Oxford University Press; 1999. pp. 502-9.
31. Growdon JH, Winkler GF, Wray SH. Midbrain ptosis: a case with clinicopathologic correlation. Arch Neurol. 1974;30(2):179-81.
32. Rucker CW. Paralysis of the third, fourth and sixth cranial nerves. Am J Ophthalmol. 1958;46(6):787-94.
33. Wilson ME, Eustis HS, Parks MM. Brown's syndrome. Surv Ophthalmol. 1989;34:153-72.
34. Keane JR. Fourth nerve palsy. Neurology. 1993;43(12): 2439-43.
35. Bielschowsky A. Lectures on motor anomalies. XI. Etiology, prognosis, and treatment of ocular paralysis. Am J Ophthalmol. 1939;22:723-34.
36. Parks MM. Isolated cyclovertical muscle palsy. AMA Arch Ophthalmol. 1958;60:1027-35.
37. Wong AM, Colpa L, Chandrakumar M. Ability of an upright-supine test to differentiate skew deviation from other vertical strabismus causes. Arch Ophthalmol. 2011;129(12):1570-5.
38. Mansour AM, Reinecke RD. Central trochlear palsy. Surv Ophthalmol. 1986;30:279-97.
39. Grob D, Arsura EL, Brunner G, et al. The course of myasthenia gravis and therapies affecting outcome. Ann NY Acad Sci. 1987;505:472-99.
40. Nagio L, Lemos J, Abusamra K, et al. Prognosis of ocular myasthenia gravis: retrospective multicenter analysis. Ophthalmology. 2015;122(7):1517-21.
41. Osher RH, Griggs RC. Orbicularis fatigue: the "peek" sign of myasthenia gravis. Arch Ophthalmol. 1979;97:677-9.
42. Schechter RJ. Ptosis with contralateral lid retraction due to excessive innervation of the levator palpebrae superioris. Ann Ophthalmol. 1978;10:1324-8.
43. Cogan DG. Myasthenia gravis: a review of the disease and a description of the lid twitch as a characteristic sign. Arch Ophthalmol. 1965;74:217-21.
44. Evoli A, Tonali P, Bartoccioni E, et al. Ocular myasthenia: diagnostic and therapeutic problems. Acta Neurol Scand. 1988;77(1):31.
45. Soliven BC, Lange DJ, Penn AS, et al. Seronegative myasthenia gravis. Neurology. 1988;38(4):514.
46. Caress JB, Hunt CH, Batish SD. Anti-MuSK myasthenia gravis presenting with purely ocular findings. Arch Neurol. 2005;62(6):1002-3.
47. Zisimopoulou P, Evangelakou P, Tzartos J, et al. A comprehensive analysis of the epidemiology and clinical characteristics of anti-LRP4 in myasthenia gravis. J Autoimm. 2014;52:139-45.
48. Mercelis R, Merckaert V. Diagnostic utility of stimulated single-fiber electromyography of the orbicularis oculi muscle in patients with suspected ocular myasthenia. Muscle Nerve. 2011;43(2):168.
49. Rivero A, Crovetto L, Lopez L, et al. Single fiber electromyography of extraocular muscles: a sensitive method for the diagnosis of ocular myasthenia gravis.Muscle Nerve. 1995;18(9):943.
50. Milone M, Monarco ML, Evoli A, et al. Ocular myasthenia: diagnostic value of single fiber EMG in the orbicularis oculi muscle. J Neurol Neurosurg Psychiatry. 1993;56:720-1.
51. Hayreh SS, Podhajsky PA, Zimmerman B. Occult giant cell arteritis: ocular manifestations. Am J Ophthalmol. 1998;125(4):521-6.
52. Danesh-Mayer H, Savino PJ, Gamble GD. Poor prognosis of visual outcome after visual loss from giant cell arteritis. Ophthalmology. 2005;112:1098-103.
53. Stone JH, Tuckwell K, Dimonaco S, et al. Trial of tocilizumab in giant-cell arteritis. New Engl J Med. 2017;277:317-28.
54. Charness ME, Simon RP, Greenberg DA. Ethanol and the nervous system. N Engl J Med. 1989;321:442-54.
55. Jung YC, Chanraud S, Sullivan EV. Neuroimaging of Wernicke's encephalopathy and Korsakoff's syndrome. Neuropsychol Rev. 2012;22(2):170-80.
56. Fisher M. An unusual variant of acute idiopathic polyneuritis (syndrome of ophthalmoplegia, ataxia, and areflexia). N Engl J Med. 1956;255:57-65.
57. Chiba A, Kusunoki S, Obata H, et al. Serum anti-GQ1b antibody is associated with ophthlamoplegia in Miller Fisher syndrome and Guillain-Barre syndrome. Neurology. 1993;43(10):1911.
58. Yuki N, Sato S, Tsuji S, et al. Frequent presence of anti-GQ1b antibody in Fisher's syndrome. Neurology. 1993;43(2): 414-7.
59. Frohman EM, Zee DS. Ocular neuromyotonia: clinical features, physiological mechanisms and response to therapy. Ann Neurol. 1995;37:620-6.
60. Lavich JB. Convergence insufficiency and its current treatment. Cur Opin Ophthalmol. 2010;21(5):356-60.
61. Lepore FE. Divergence paresis: a nonlocalizing cause of diplopia. J Neuroophthalmol. 1999;19(4):242-5.
62. Chaudhuri Z, Demer JL. Sagging eye syndrome: connective tissue involution as a cause of horizontal and vertical strabismus in older patients. JAMA Ophthalmol. 2013;131(5):619-25.
63. Brandt T, Dieterich M. Skew deviation with ocular torsion: a vestibular brainstem sign of topographic diagnostic value. Ann Neurol. 1993;33:528-34.
64. Pratt-Johnson JA, Tillson G. Suppression in strabismus—an update. Br J Ophthalmol. 1984;68:174-8.
65. Kushner BJ. Fixation switch diplopia. Arch Ophthalmol. 1995;113:896-9.
66. Legmann Simon A, Borchert M. Etiology and prognosis of acute, late-onset esotropia. Ophthalmology. 1997;104: 1348-52.
67. Barton JJ. "Retinal diplopia" associated with macular wrinkling. Neurology. 2004;63:925-7.

Chapter 96 Nystagmus and Disorders of Gaze

Roksolyana Tourkevich, Anthony Brune, Daniel Gold

WHAT IS NYSTAGMUS?

Nystagmus is an involuntary rhythmic movement of the eyes that leads to excessive movement of the visual environment. The slow phase is the pathologic phase of nystagmus and is responsible for the initial movement of the eyes and subsequent drift of the target of visual interest off the fovea. Nystagmus is seen by the examiner, while common symptoms experienced by the patient include blurry vision and oscillopsia. Oscillopsia is an illusory movement of the stationary environment and can be separated into two categories: (1) "sitting" oscillopsia—independent of head movements, usually the result of nystagmus or saccadic intrusions/oscillations and (2) "walking" oscillopsia—dependent on head movements, usually related to bilateral vestibular loss and experienced while walking or driving on a bumpy road (*see* Video 1; [online] Available from: *https://collections.lib.utah.edu/details?id=1213442)*. The localization and etiology can often be identified by observing the characteristics of the nystagmus itself in addition to associated neurologic and ophthalmic symptoms and signs (or lack thereof).

CHARACTERISTICS AND PATHOPHYSIOLOGY OF NYSTAGMUS

Nystagmus can be physiological, as in end-gaze nystagmus or induced by optokinetic tape or a drum, caloric testing or a rotating chair. Or, it can be pathological and indicate damage to the visual or vestibular pathways, or to the posterior fossa or other structures that contribute to normal eye movement function. There are three known mechanisms that hold the images steady on the retina:[1] (1) visual fixation—detects and corrects retinal image drift when eye movements are unwanted;[1] (2) vestibulo-ocular reflex (VOR)—holds the eyes steady during head movements to ensure retinal stability;[1,2] (3) gaze-holding system—sends a sustained signal to the extraocular muscles to maintain an eccentric eye position (usually following a saccadic burst) to counteract the elastic forces of the orbital tissue that would otherwise move the eyes back to the midline.[1,3,4] Impairment of any of these three mechanisms can result in drift of the visual target off the fovea—this *drift represents the slow or pathologic phase of nystagmus.*[1] When a *saccade initiates the movement, this is called a saccadic intrusion or oscillation,* with a square wave jerk (SWJ) being the most common example (see below).

The optokinetic reflex supplements the VOR during a sustained head movement and is activated by movement of the visual scene drifting across the retina. Eye movements in the direction of stimulus motion are periodically interrupted by rapid corrections in the opposite direction (the quick phases) to reset the eye position.[5] These alternating slow and fast phases make up optokinetic nystagmus (OKN). A typical example would be looking out the window of a moving train where the slow phase moves in the same direction as the passing scenery. When optokinetic tape is used at the bedside, this is not true full field visual stimulation; therefore, the pursuit and saccadic systems are mainly being evaluated as opposed to the optokinetic system. Both retinal and cerebral projections contribute to the optokinetic response.[6]

The two main types of nystagmus are: (1) pendular and (2) jerk (Fig. 96.1). Both are generated by the slow (pathologic) phase, but their corrective phase (the position reset mechanism) differs. In pendular nystagmus, the eyes move back and forth with about the same velocity and amplitude, similar to that of a pendulum. Patients with acquired pendular nystagmus almost always experience oscillopsia (unless severe vision loss is present), while those with congenital nystagmus almost never do, which is thought to be related to foveation periods and other factors.[7] Jerk nystagmus consists of alternating slow and fast phases and is named after the direction of the fast phase.

Jerk nystagmus can be further categorized by its slow phase velocity: (1) vestibular nystagmus—linear slow phase velocity (Fig. 96.1) due to VOR imbalance; (2) acquired

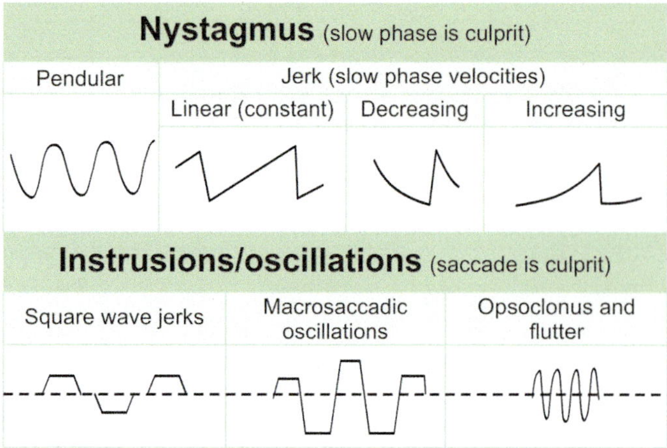

Fig. 96.1: Waveforms of nystagmus, intrusions and oscillations. The vertical axis reflects eye position and horizontal reflects time. Square wave jerks are small saccades that move the line of sight away from the target and then return it about 200 ms later.[1,8] Macrosaccadic oscillations are saccades that take the eye off target and oscillate the line of sight about the object of regard.[1,8] Ocular flutter is confined to the horizontal vector[8,9] whereas opsoclonus has horizontal, vertical and torsional vectors, and occurs in bursts lasting about a second.[8-10]

Source: Neuro-ophthalmology Virtual Education Library: NOVEL. [online] Available from: *https://collections.lib.utah.edu/details?id=1260009.* [Accessed December, 2017].

gaze-evoked nystagmus (GEN)—decreasing slow phase velocity (Fig. 96.1) due to an impaired neural integrator system (the gaze-holding machinery, see GEN section below); and (3) congenital nystagmus and occasionally cerebellar lesions that cause an unstable neural integrator system—increasing slow phase velocity (Fig. 96.1).

It is important to distinguish nystagmus from oscillations and intrusions, particularly given disparate localizations and etiologies. These include saccadic intrusions (SWJs) and saccadic oscillations (ocular flutter and opsoclonus). Saccadic intrusions consist of saccades with an intersaccadic interval (i.e. a brief pause between movements), while saccadic oscillations lack this interval (Fig. 96.1). These will be discussed later in this chapter.

TYPES OF NYSTAGMUS

Nystagmus Associated with Vestibular Imbalance

Peripheral vestibular nystagmus is the result of a unilateral lesion involving the labyrinth or vestibular (8th cranial) nerve.[11,12] A unilateral lesion of the VOR pathways causes a static vestibular imbalance. The most common types include horizontal-torsional nystagmus from vestibular neuritis and upbeat-torsional nystagmus (toward the affected ear) from posterior canal (PC) benign paroxysmal positional vertigo (BPPV). Spontaneous nystagmus that is pure torsional, upbeat or downbeat should alert the clinician to a central etiology. Peripheral vestibular nystagmus follows Alexander's law, where the nystagmus intensity is greatest when looking in the direction of the fast phase.[1] For example, a destructive lesion of the right labyrinth will result in right vestibular hypofunction with relative hyperactivity on the left side. The unopposed vestibular afferents from the left side create a rightward slow phase drift (the brain perceives a leftward head turn even though the head is still), with a resultant leftward fast phase. These alternating slow and fast movements produce left-beating nystagmus (LBN) (*see* Video 2; [online] Available from: *https://collections.lib.utah.edu/details?id=187732).* A torsional component is also seen with acute unilateral vestibular loss and results from vertical semicircular canals (SCs), since the anterior and PCs, when stimulated, normally cause conjugate vertical and torsional movements. While the spontaneous LBN (contralesional) is a consequence of static VOR imbalance, an abnormal head impulse test (HIT) to the right (ipsilesional) is a consequence of dynamic VOR impairment (*see* Video 3 for demonstration of normal HIT; [online] Available from: *https://collections.lib.utah.edu/details?id=187678).* When a patient presents with acute onset, continuous vertigo and spontaneous nystagmus, seeing an abnormal HIT (*see* Video 4; [online] Available from: *https://collections.lib.utah.edu/details?id=187723)* is a reassuring sign in that it strongly suggests a peripheral (ear) vestibulopathy rather than a stroke. The combination of prolonged vertigo with LBN and an abnormal HIT to the right in the absence of a skew deviation, for example, is highly suggestive of vestibular neuritis affecting the vestibular portion of the right 8th cranial nerve. Hearing loss (ipsilesional) occasionally accompanies this constellation of symptoms and signs, oftentimes related to inflammation or infection and referred to as labyrinthitis. However, the examiner should be cautious about making a benign (ear) diagnosis in patients with acute hearing loss, since labyrinthine ischemia is also a strong possibility.

Cold water in the right ear would similarly produce (albeit transient and reversible) right hypofunction and generate LBN for the same reasons. Peripheral vestibular nystagmus is suppressed by visual fixation[1] and therefore removal of fixation with occlusive ophthalmoscopy (occluding the fellow eye during ophthalmoscopy) or with Frenzel goggles (+20–30 D lenses that simultaneously inhibit fixation and magnify the eyes for the examiner) will accentuate nystagmus. When nystagmus and vertigo are brought on by loud noises (Tullio's phenomenon) and/or pressure changes (e.g. coughing, sneezing, straining, or glottic or pinched-nose Valsalva), superior canal dehiscence syndrome should be considered (*see* Video 5; [online] Available from: *https://collections.lib.utah.edu/details?id=1213443).* In this condition, patients may present to the ophthalmologist given concern for papilledema because of pulsatile tinnitus, or they may perceive internal noises such as hearing their own eye movements (autophony).

Central vestibular imbalance arises from lesions involving the brainstem, cerebellum (usually the vestibulocerebellum—the flocculus/paraflocculus and nodulus/uvula) and their connections, which have a role in modulation of the VOR.[1] While spontaneous nystagmus associated with central vestibular lesions can be purely horizontal, vertical or torsional, it can also be unidirectional, horizontal-torsional and follow Alexander's law. It is often not well suppressed with visual fixation, although it can be indistinguishable from "peripheral" nystagmus. Central nystagmus is commonly accompanied by other posterior fossa ocular motor (e.g. GEN, saccadic pursuit or dysmetric saccades, double vision) and neurologic symptoms and signs.

Downbeat Nystagmus

Downbeat nystagmus (DBN) is most commonly associated with cerebellar (flocculus/paraflocculus) pathology.[13] Multiple mechanisms may contribute to DBN including: (1) imbalance in the central vertical SC pathways;[14] (2) imbalance in the central utricular pathways;[15-18] (3) imbalance in the vertical smooth pursuit system;[18] and (4) impairment of the vertical gaze-holding network.[18] The most common explanation for the genesis of DBN involves asymmetry of the vertical SC pathways. The anterior canal (AC) sends signals via the superior vestibular nuclei to the elevator muscles (superior rectus and inferior oblique), while the PC sends signals via the medial vestibular nuclei [ascends the medial longitudinal fasciculus (MLF) only] to the depressor muscles (inferior rectus, superior oblique). Purkinje cells in the cerebellar flocculus/paraflocculus strongly inhibit the AC pathways.[1] Therefore, symmetric damage to the Purkinje cells [e.g. degeneration due to a spinocerebellar ataxia (SCA)] may result in disinhibition and resultant hyperactivity of the AC, leading to an upward drift (slow phase), with a corrective downward fast phase (*see* Video 6; [online] Available from: *https://collections.lib.utah.edu/details?id=187722).*[14]

Unlike the PC afferents which only travel through the MLF, the AC afferents have three pathways to the oculomotor nuclei: (1) MLF; (2) brachium conjunctivum, also known as the superior cerebellar peduncle; and (3) ventral tegmental tract. Therefore, in unilateral or bilateral MLF lesions which cause an internuclear ophthalmoplegia (INO), the PC pathways are more affected than the AC pathways. This causes vertical SC imbalance and relative VOR weakness in the planes of the PC and may produce "walking" oscillopsia or other head movement-induced vestibular and balance symptoms.

Downbeat nystagmus and GEN commonly coexist, causing nystagmus in down and lateral gaze that appears diagonal given horizontal and downward components, and this is referred to as "side pocket nystagmus". Patients with a DBN syndrome commonly present with oscillopsia and gait imbalance. Commonly associated ocular motor findings include a hypertropia in the abducting eye in lateral gaze (alternating skew deviation—e.g. right hypertropia in right gaze, left hypertropia in left gaze) and impaired smooth pursuit. DBN is poorly suppressed with fixation and may increase, decrease or convert to an upbeat with convergence.[1] Refer to Table 96.1 for common causes of DBN.

Upbeat Nystagmus

Upbeat nystagmus (UBN) is less common than DBN and usually results from brainstem disease (*see* Video 7; [online] Available from: *https://collections.lib.utah.edu/details?id=187754).*[13] Although most cases follow Alexander's law, a so-called "anti-Alexander's law" nystagmus may be seen with spontaneous UBN, where UBN increases in downgaze. This suggests an abnormal vertical gaze-holding mechanism.[1] Similar to DBN, mechanisms that have been proposed for UBN include imbalance in the central SC and utricle pathways, imbalance in the vertical smooth pathways and impaired vertical gaze holding. Refer to Table 96.1 for common causes of UBN.

Torsional Nystagmus

In *torsional jerk nystagmus*, the eyes move clockwise or counterclockwise, and pure torsional nystagmus results from asymmetry in the central vertical SC pathways (*see* Video 8; [online] Available from:

Table 96.1: Summary of etiologies, treatments and unique features of the various types of nystagmus.

	Treatment	Etiologies	Key points
Peripheral Vestibular Nystagmus			
Horizontal-torsional nystagmus	• Role of steroids is not well defined in acute vestibular neuritis[35,36] • Vestibular physical therapy	• Vestibular neuritis (no hearing loss) • Labyrinthitis (hearing loss present)[11,12]	• Constant velocity slow phases • Suppressed with visual fixation • Follows Alexander's law • No associated neurological or central ocular motor symptoms or signs
Positional nystagmus	Positional maneuvers[26,37]	BPPV[37] (posterior, horizontal, anterior canal variants)	• Mixed upbeat-torsional (triggered) nystagmus in PC BPPV, most common • Horizontal geotropic (beating toward the ground with right and left ear down) or apogeotropic (beating toward ceiling) in HC BPPV • Downbeat or downbeat-torsional nystagmus in AC BPPV—central etiologies should be excluded
Central Vestibular Nystagmus			
Downbeat	• 3,4-diaminopyridine (DAP)[38,39] • 4-aminopyridine (4-AP)[39-42] • Clonazepam[43,44] • Chlorzoxazone[45]	• Arnold-Chiari malformation[13,18] • Cerebellar disease[13,46] • Multiple sclerosis[47,48] • Medications (antiepileptics,[49] amiodarone,[50] opioids,[51] lithium[52]) • Thiamine and magnesium depletion[53] • Paraneoplastic disorders[54]	• May increase with convergence • Usually localizes to the flocculus/ paraflocculus • Commonly associated with GEN, impaired pursuit and other signs of cerebellar involvement
Upbeat	• 4-AP[44,55] • Memantine[44,56] • Baclofen[44]	• Medullary and midbrain lesions secondary to MS, stroke or tumors[13] • Tobacco[57]	• May increase with convergence, or transition to DBN • Usually related to brainstem disease • Usually increases on looking up
Torsional	Gabapentin[44,56]	• Lateral medullary syndrome (jerk)[58] • Multiple sclerosis (jerk or pendular)[1] • Oculopalatal tremor (pendular)[23]	• Commonly associated with ocular tilt reaction • Although mixed horizontal-torsional or vertical-torsional nystagmus may suggest a peripheral localization, pure torsional nystagmus suggests a central etiology
Seesaw	• Clonazepam[44] • Memantine[44,56]	• Jerk: unilateral midbrain, MLF,[48] Or lateral medullary lesions • Pendular: bitemporal hemianopia (e.g. pituitary adenoma, craniopharyngioma, head trauma), and chiasmal disorders	• Slow phase: one eye intorts and elevates, while the other extorts and depresses • Hemi-seesaw: conjugate torsional (toward the same ear) and vertical (upbeat in one eye, downbeat in the other eye)
Periodic alternating	• Baclofen[59,60] • Memantine[61]	• *Congenital:* Associated with albinism[62,63] • *Acquired:* MS,[48,64] anticonvulsants,[65] Arnold-Chiari,[66] spinocerebellar degeneration,[67,68] decreased vision (e.g. cataract[69,70])	• Usually horizontal • Reverses direction every 90–120 seconds • Head rotation or other vestibular stimuli may change or temporarily stop it • Not suppressed by fixation
Eccentric Gaze Nystagmus			
Gaze evoked	None	• Cerebellar lesions[1] • Antiepileptic medications and lithium intoxication[1] • Wernicke encephalopathy[53]	• May see centripetal and rebound • If downbeat nystagmus is present, may see "side pocket" nystagmus
Bruns	Usually there is minimal nystagmus in primary gaze so no medication is necessary	Cerebellopontine angle tumors (Schwannoma)[71,72]	• GEN in ipsilesional gaze • Vestibular nystagmus in contralesional gaze

Contd...

Contd...

	Treatment	Etiologies	Key points
Acquired Pendular Nystagmus			
Other acquired	• Gabapentin[56,73] • Memantine (may worsen MS symptoms)[56,73]	• Demyelinating diseases[48,74] (horizontal) • Whipple's disease[24,74] (convergent-divergent) • Hypoxic encephalopathy[74] • Serotonin syndrome[74] • Toluene sniffing[74] • Acquired blindness[74]	• Usually horizontal pendular in MS, although can be torsional or vertical • Sometimes vectors combine to form elliptical or other patterns
OPT	• Gabapentin[56,73] • Memantine[56,73]	Guillain-Mollaret triangle (dentato-rubro-olivary pathway) lesions[23]	• Associated with palatal or lower facial muscle tremor/contractions • Usually vertical, torsional, or vertical-torsional
Pediatric Nystagmus			
Congenital	If oscillopsia is experienced (usually later in life): • Gabapentin[59] • Memantine[59] • Acetazolamide[44] • Topical brinzolamide[44] • Base out prism to induce convergence[44]	• Cataracts[7] • Corneal opacities[7] • Retinopathy of prematurity[7] • Deficits of rod and cone systems[27] • Optic nerve hypoplasia[7] • Idiopathic	• Onset in the first 6 months of life • Over time, becomes mixed jerk and pendular • Stays horizontal in vertical gaze • Damps with convergence • Oscillopsia is rare • Head oscillation may be present • Reversal of OKN
Spasmus nutans	None	Unknown	• Starts in the first year of life, stops by 4 years of age • Intermittent • Usually horizontal and disconjugate • Can be suppressed with a head turn • Associated with head bobbing and tilting • Optic pathway glioma should be considered
Latent	None	Disrupted binocular vision[7]	• Horizontal jerk usually brought on when one eye is viewing, but may be "manifest" latent, which is spontaneous nystagmus • Associated with features of the congenital esotropia syndrome (inferior oblique overaction, DVD)

(BPPV: Benign paroxysmal positional vertigo; PC: Posterior semicircular canal; HC: Horizontal semicircular canal; AC: Anterior semicircular canal; GEN: Gaze-evoked nystagmus; DBN: Downbeat nystagmus; INO: Internuclear ophthalmoplegia; MLF: Medial longitudinal fasciculus; MS: Multiple sclerosis; OKN: Optokinetic nystagmus; DVD: Dissociated vertical divergence)

https://collections.lib.utah.edu/details?id=1209887).[19] Its direction is assigned based on whether the upper poles of the eyes beat toward the left or the right ear. Torsional jerk nystagmus is commonly seen with damage to the lateral medulla (Wallenberg syndrome), the MLF (usually with a vertical component), the rostral interstitial MLF (riMLF—torsional nystagmus beats toward the contralateral ear) and interstitial nucleus of Cajal (INC—torsional nystagmus beats toward the ipsilateral ear).[11,19] A complete or partial ocular tilt reaction can also be seen, consisting of (1) skew deviation, (2) head tilt and/or (3) ocular counter-roll.[1,11] *Torsional pendular nystagmus* is usually due to multiple sclerosis (MS) or oculopalatal tremor (OPT—commonly associated with a vertical pendular component, see below for details).

Seesaw Nystagmus

Seesaw nystagmus can either be jerk or pendular. In the slow phase, one eye intorts and elevates, while the other extorts and depresses.[13] Hemi- or "jerky" seesaw nystagmus is characterized by a conjugate torsional component (toward the same ear) and a disjunctive vertical component (upbeat in one eye, downbeat in the fellow eye). This is associated with vertical SC and/or utricle pathway imbalance (e.g. unilateral midbrain, MLF, or lateral medullary lesions). Pendular seesaw is often associated with bitemporal hemianopia (e.g. pituitary adenoma, craniopharyngioma, head trauma), visual loss and chiasmal disorders.[1,19] Visual inputs from the temporal visual fields contribute to the VOR in the roll plane (e.g. tilting the head to the right or left ear stimulates the utricle-ocular motor pathway), so it is thought that a bitemporal hemianopia may cause imbalance or dysregulation of the roll VOR pathways and subsequently pendular seesaw nystagmus.[1] However, pendular seesaw nystagmus is rare while bitemporal hemianopias are relatively common; therefore, the exact mechanisms that cause some patients with bitemporal loss to develop seesaw nystagmus while others do not has still not been completely worked out. In the congenital form of seesaw nystagmus, one eye elevates and extorts, while the other depresses and intorts.[1] This may be related to dissociated vertical deviation commonly encountered in the infantile strabismus syndrome.[20]

Acquired Pendular Nystagmus

Acquired pendular nystagmus can be horizontal, vertical, torsional, seesaw or a combination of these, and some asymmetry between the eyes is frequent (amplitudes differ and nystagmus may be monocular; *see* Video 9 [online] Available from: *https://collections.lib.utah.edu/details?id=1209724)*. Nystagmus can be temporarily suppressed by blinks or saccades (*see* Video 10; [online] Available from: *https://collections.lib.utah.edu/details?id=1209730)*. Oscillopsia is almost always experienced unless severe vision loss is present, and common etiologies include MS and OPT.[21] OPT is the result of a lesion involving the dentato-rubro-olivary pathway (Guillain-Mollaret triangle), and it is prudent to look for a palatal tremor in patients with pendular nystagmus.[22,23] A typical example would be a patient who develops nystagmus and palatal tremor several months after a pontine hemorrhage due to central tegmental tract injury (*see* Video 11; [online] Available from: *https://collections.lib.utah.edu/details?id=1209725)*.

In MS, possible mechanisms include asymmetric response times for visual processing since nystagmus is usually more prominent in the worse-seeing eye, or related to instability in the neural integrator related to posterior fossa involvement. Whipple's disease may cause a characteristic convergent-divergent pendular nystagmus, occasionally with the pathognomonic oculomasticatory myorhythmia (oscillatory movements of the jaw, face or limbs) and a supranuclear vertical gaze palsy.[24] Refer to Table 96.1 for other etiologies.

Periodic Alternating Nystagmus

Periodic alternating nystagmus (PAN) is a spontaneous horizontal nystagmus that reverses direction every 90–120 seconds,[1] with shorter or longer cycle lengths in some cases (as long as 6 min) (*see* Video 12; [online] Available from: *https://collections.lib.utah.edu/details?id=1209729)*.[25] It is thought to be related to dysfunction of the velocity storage mechanism, which normally augments the afferents coming from the vestibular apparatus. These signals would otherwise attenuate during sustained head movements given the mechanical properties of the SCs (e.g. flow of endolymph and deflection of the cupula). Refer to Table 96.1 for associated common diseases and treatment.

Positional Nystagmus

Peripheral (ear) disorders account for the majority of positional nystagmus. Upbeat-torsional nystagmus with the top pole beating toward the right ear during the right Dix-Hallpike maneuver (patient is seated on a table, head is turned 45° to the right, patient is quickly brought into a supine position with the head 30° extended) is due to right PC BPPV (*see* Video 13; [online] Available from: *https://collections.lib.utah.edu/details?id=187762)*.[26] Although DBN (with or without a torsional component) triggered by the Dix-Hallpike maneuver may suggest the AC variant of BPPV, central etiologies must be excluded. Horizontal canal BPPV causes either geotropic nystagmus (beats toward the ground with right and left ear down positions) or apogeotropic nystagmus (beats toward the ceiling with right and left ear down positions). The typical BPPV history is less than 60-second long episodes of vertigo triggered by head movements, such as turning over in bed. Features that are atypical for BPPV include: lack of a brief latency, lack of fatigability with repeated testing, atypical/unexpected vector depending the specific canal stimulated by diagnostic maneuvers, duration greater than 60 seconds, absence of response to properly performed therapeutic maneuvers and no attenuation with fixation. When atypical features are seen, a central etiology such as posterior fossa tumor, stroke or demyelinating lesion must be considered (*see* Video 14; [online] Available from: *https://collections.lib.utah.edu/details?id=187739)*; however, other posterior fossa symptoms and signs are usually present.[1]

Nystagmus in Eccentric Gaze

The most common form of nystagmus is GEN. Steady eccentric gaze is due to continuous contraction of the extraocular muscles, and the neural integrators send the commands that make this possible.[1] The neural integrator system is an eccentric gaze-holding network that is composed of the medial vestibular nucleus (MVN) and nucleus prepositus hypoglossi (NPH) in the medulla for horizontal gaze holding and the INC in the midbrain for vertical and torsional gaze holding. With disruption of the neural integrator, eccentric gaze cannot be maintained and the eyes drift back to the center. This is followed by corrective quick phases returning the eyes to the desired eccentric position. When GEN is present horizontally and vertically, this is typically due to cerebellar (or cerebellar connections) dysfunction. GEN is common with drug or alcohol intoxication and is commonly seen with antiepileptic medications and lithium.[1] When GEN is seen with acute prolonged vertigo, this indicates a central etiology. GEN is common with cerebellar flocculus and paraflocculus lesions.[1]

In addition to GEN, patients with impaired neural integrator function may also have: (1) rebound nystagmus—e.g. right-beating nystagmus (RBN) in right gaze, reverses direction to LBN when returning to primary position (*see* Video 15; [online] Available from: *https://collections.lib.utah.edu/details?id=187733)* and (2) centripetal nystagmus—e.g. RBN in right gaze may slow down and change direction to LBN while still in right gaze.[1] A few beats of rebound nystagmus can be seen in a healthy individual, but prominent rebound and centripetal nystagmus are pathologic.[1]

Cerebellopontine angle tumors (e.g. schwannoma of the 8th cranial nerve) can cause Bruns nystagmus. As an example, a left-sided tumor will cause (1) low frequency, large amplitude, left-beating GEN in left gaze due to neural integrator dysfunction on the left and (2) high frequency, small amplitude right-beating vestibular nystagmus in right gaze due to left cranial nerve VIII hypofunction (*see* Video 16; [online] Available from: *https://collections.lib.utah.edu/details?id=1248764).*

Mild direction-changing physiologic nystagmus is common and is referred to as end gaze or end point nystagmus. This nystagmus is not sustained and is symmetric in lateral gaze, often with a mild torsional component. Nystagmus typically resolves when the eyes are moved to 75% (or less) eccentric gaze position, or at least at the point where the adducting eye can see the eccentric target. If nystagmus direction changes in vertical gaze or if ocular motor abnormalities are appreciated, a central etiology should be excluded.

A patient with an INO will have an ipsilesional adduction lag or motility deficit with abducting nystagmus in the contralesional eye.[1] Vertical GEN may be seen with MLF injury as well, either relating to disruption of gaze-holding pathways between medulla and INC or from adjacent paramedian tract involvement (*see* Video 17; [online] Available from: *https://collections.lib.utah.edu/details?id=1278694).*"

Pediatric Nystagmus

Infantile nystagmus syndrome (congenital nystagmus) appears in the first 3–6 months of life.[7] Initially, movements are large amplitude, low frequency and horizontal. It is conjugate and damps with convergence and over time, jerk and pendular components become mixed—e.g. horizontal jerk in eccentric gaze and pendular in primary gaze (*see* Video 18; [online] Available from: *https://collections.lib.utah.edu/details?id=1209720).* A compensatory head turn may be adopted to keep the eyes in the null point, where nystagmus is minimal.[7] With an optokinetic stimulus, there can be reversal of the OKN. Infantile nystagmus can be idiopathic, but is commonly associated with albinism or with afferent pathology (retinopathy, maculopathy, optic neuropathy).[7] Red flags for typical infantile nystagmus include: onset after 6 months, asymmetric nystagmus (think about spasmus nutans) and an abnormal neurologic examination.[27]

Spasmus nutans starts in the first year of life. The associated pendular nystagmus is intermittent, asymmetric and (mainly) horizontal with low amplitude and high frequency. It tends to increase in intensity with convergence and in the abducting eye. It is accompanied by head tremor and head tilt. It dissipates by 1–4 years of age. Of note, the oscillations related to an optic pathway glioma can be indistinguishable from that produced by spasmus nutans.[1]

Fusional maldevelopment (latent) nystagmus is a horizontal jerk nystagmus which is conjugate and brought out by covering one eye. The fast phases beat toward the uncovered eye (*see* Video 19; [online] Available from: *https://collections.lib.utah.edu/details?id=187744).* Fusional maldevelopment nystagmus is postulated to arise from disrupted binocularity in the first 6 months of life (e.g. strabismus, cataract, optic nerve hypoplasia) and is commonly associated with congenital esotropia, inferior oblique overaction and dissociated vertical deviation.[7]

Pathologic Nystagmus Secondary to Visual Pathway Disorders

Nystagmus can also arise from lesions along the visual pathways, from retina to cortical visual areas and its projections to the pons and cerebellum.[1] Bilateral visual loss from retinal and optic nerve lesions may result in a continuous jerk nystagmus that is either horizontal, vertical, torsional or a combination of these.[1,7] Monocular pendular vertical nystagmus occurring in an eye with worse vision is called the Heimann-Bielschowsky phenomenon. Here, the nystagmus reflects a disruption of mechanisms that normally calibrate eye movements based on visual inputs.[1] It can occur with optic neuropathy, amblyopia and dense cataracts.[1] Commonly, the pendular nystagmus associated with MS is more prominent or only seen in the eye with worse vision, and this may relate to an asymmetric delay in visual inputs.

Voluntary Nystagmus

Nystagmus-like eye movements can be elicited voluntarily by some people (*see* Video 20; [online] Available from: *https://collections.lib.utah.edu/details?id=1209731*).[28-31] It occurs in bursts lasting 5–10 seconds (cannot be sustained for much longer) and appears as high frequency,[30,32] low amplitude, horizontal pendular oscillations.[30] This is not a true nystagmus, but rather an oscillation of saccades, produced during convergence.[28,30] Accompanying features include lid fluttering,[33] squinting, facial strain and miosis.[32] It has been reported to be a dominantly inherited trait with variable expression.[28,34]

INTRODUCTION TO GAZE

Eye movements can be divided into several classes: smooth pursuit, saccades, OKN, vergence and the VOR. Of these, disorders of pursuit and saccades will be emphasized in this section. Saccades are fast eye movements that quickly redirect gaze, which can be volitional or reflexive (*see* Video 21; [online] Available from: *https://collections.lib.utah.edu/details?id=187674*). Smooth pursuit allows one to follow a slow moving visual target (*see* Video 22; [online] Available from: *https://collections.lib.utah.edu/details?id=187673*).

NEUROANATOMY OF GAZE

To understand the different disorders of conjugate gaze, a general overview of the relevant neural pathways is necessary. These pathways differ for pursuit and saccades. In the case of voluntary horizontal saccades, a cortical brain area in the frontal lobe, the frontal eye field (FEF), sends the initial signal. In contrast, for reflexive saccades, the signal originates in parietal eye fields. These signals are processed by the basal ganglia and superior colliculus before traveling to the cerebellum and the contralateral pons. In the cerebellum, motor signals are modulated for increased accuracy. In the pons, the paramedian pontine reticular formation (PPRF) contains the burst neurons that control the activity of the abducens nucleus and allow for simultaneous excitation of the ipsilateral lateral rectus and contralateral medial rectus (MR) muscles (via interneurons that originating in the abducens nucleus) to make a conjugate saccade. The vertical (and torsional) correlate of the PPRF is the riMLF, which is the final common pathway for vertical and torsional saccade generation prior to the trochlear and oculomotor nuclei (Fig. 96.2). As discussed above, once the eyes are on target, the neural integrators ensure stimulation of appropriate ocular motor muscles for maintaining eccentric gaze.[1]

For smooth pursuit, the primary visual cortex is necessary for identification of targets in the contralateral

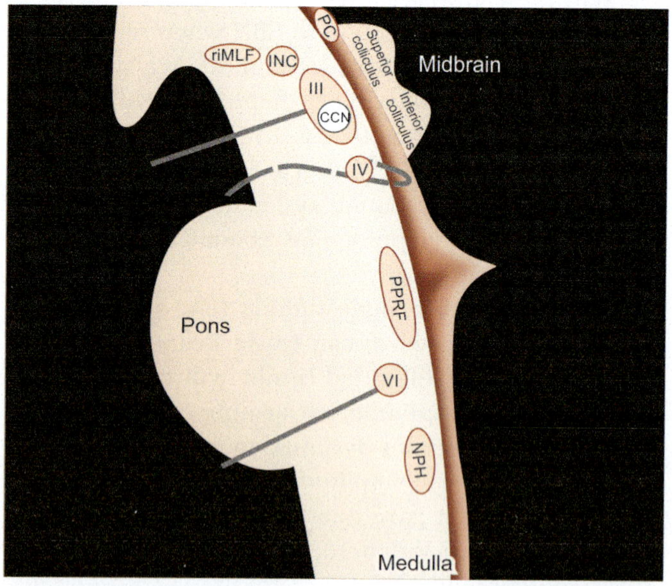

Fig. 96.2: The brainstem ocular motor machinery. Shown here is the brainstem anatomy relevant to the ocular motor system. Ocular motor nuclei for cranial nerves 3, 4, and 6 are shown here in addition to the neural integrators (NPH for horizontal and INC for vertical/torsional), and burst neuron cell groups (PPRF for horizontal and riMLF for vertical/torsional).
(PC: Posterior commissure; riMLF: Rostral interstitial medial longitudinal fasciculus; INC: Interstitial nucleus of Cajal; III: Oculomotor nucleus; CCN: Central caudal nucleus; IV: Trochlear nucleus; PPRF: Paramedian pontine reticular formation; VI: Abducens nucleus; NPH: Nucleus prepositus hypoglossi)
Source: Neuro-Ophthalmology Virtual Education Library: NOVEL. [online] Available from: *https://collections.lib.utah.edu/details?id=1256330* [Accessed December, 2017].

visual field. Projections to the posterior parieto-occipital region allow for detection of object motion including direction and velocity. Connections with the FEF allow the frontal lobe to play a role in the initiation of ipsilateral pursuit. Descending pathways reach the cerebellum via crossed pathways from pontine nuclei. The role of the cerebellum in smooth pursuit is complex, including integration of target and gaze motion, ensuring adequate ipsilateral pursuit gain. From the cerebellum, projections course via vestibular nuclei to the contralateral ocular motor neurons. When smooth pursuit is impaired or choppy in one direction (e.g. to the left), the combination of the aforementioned decussations to and from the cerebellum (i.e. doubly crossed fibers) allows the examiner to localize the pursuit deficit ipsilateral to the side of the lesion (e.g. left cerebral hemisphere). The pursuit system is also essential in suppressing the VOR, allowing for continued fixation with combined head and eye movements.[1,75]

An alternative pathway to the abducens nucleus comes directly from the vestibular apparatus of the inner ear, by way of the VOR. The SCs, which are angular acceleration detectors, send signals to the ocular motor nuclei via the vestibular (8th cranial) nerve allowing for finely tuned reflexive eye movements which maintain fixation and retinal stability during head movements.

GAZE DISORDERS

Gaze Deviation and Gaze Palsy

Gaze deviation can be seen with acute supratentorial or infratentorial strokes, or related to seizure activity. Due to an ischemic lesion involving the FEF, ipsilateral gaze deviation can be seen during stroke since the contralateral (unaffected) FEF drives the eyes away from the intact hemisphere. In the case of seizure, excitation of the affected FEF drives the eyes contralaterally. As with other similar presentations, localization is aided by the VOR. Lesions of the abducens nucleus lead to a loss of all ipsilesional horizontal eye movements and, in the acute setting, a contralateral gaze deviation (*see* Video 23; [online] Available from: *https://collections.lib.utah.edu/details?id=1209837* - second of the two patients in this video demonstrates gaze deviation). A conjugate unilateral deficit of horizontal gaze that cannot be overcome by the horizontal VOR localizes to the abducens nucleus (or PPRF and surrounding fibers that are destined for the 6th nucleus), as this sends fibers to the ipsilateral lateral rectus and contains the interneurons that send fibers (via the MLF) to the contralateral MR subnucleus and to the MR muscle itself. Caution should be taken here with hyperacute lesions, though, as the VOR may not be able to overcome cortical gaze deviation in this setting.[1] In contrast, a pontine lesion that involves only the fascicle of the 6th nerve will only affect ipsilateral abduction. Associated signs usually allow for pontine localization—e.g. in Foville's syndrome, there is ipsilateral lower motor neuron facial weakness and contralateral hemiparesis.[76] A gaze palsy associated with an INO in contralateral gaze is called a "one-and-a-half" syndrome (*see* Video 24; [online] Available from: *https://collections.lib.utah.edu/details?id=1209932*) and results from involvement of the 6th nerve nucleus and the adjacent MLF.

A prototypical vertical gaze disorder is the pretectal or Parinaud's syndrome. Parinaud's includes upgaze palsy, vergence abnormalities, convergence-retraction nystagmus, pseudoabducens palsy, SWJs, light-near dissociation, lid retraction (Collier's sign) and skew deviation (*see* Video 25; [online] Available from: *https://collections.lib.utah.edu/details?id=1251075*). Rarely are all features seen. Upgaze deficits may only been seen when attempting upward saccades. Attempted upward saccades, particularly those brought out by an optokinetic drum or tape directed downward (i.e. downward pursuit—slow phase, upward saccade—fast phase), are also used to elicit convergence-retraction nystagmus, during which the eyes converge and retract into the orbit. Causes of Parinaud's syndrome vary by age: obstructive hydrocephalus in infants, pineal region space occupying lesions in children and midbrain stroke in older adults.[77]

Limited vertical gaze is also seen in progressive supranuclear palsy (PSP), which gains its name from the ocular motor abnormalities. PSP is a parkinsonian syndrome with cardinal features of axial rigidity, early falls and gaze abnormality. The earliest ocular feature is slowed vertical saccades, with downward saccades affected before upward saccades. Again, evaluating OKN can be helpful in this situation, as loss of downward fast phases may be one of the first ocular motor signs. Limitation of downgaze is of greater significance as compared to loss of upgaze as normal aging itself results in at least some limitation of upgaze. It is not clear if these changes in normal aging are "supranuclear" or a result of age-related changes involving the orbital tissues.[78] Horizontal saccades in PSP are commonly hypometric and become slower as time passes,

Table 96.2: Ocular motor abnormalities associated with neurodegenerative movement disorders.[79-81]

Movement disorder	Ocular motor features
Parkinson's disease	• Hypometric saccades • Impaired inhibition of saccades
Progressive supranuclear palsy	• Impaired vertical before horizontal saccades • Saccadic pursuit • Frequent SWJ
Multiple system atrophy-cerebellar type	• Large SWJ • Saccadic pursuit • GEN and positional DBN
Huntington's disease	• Slow, hypometric saccades with increased latency • Impaired inhibition of saccades • Saccadic intrusions
Corticobasal degeneration	• Increased latency of saccades to apraxic side • Impaired smooth pursuit

and saccadic smooth pursuit is seen. Frequent SWJs are also a predominant feature (*see* Video 26; [online] Available from: *https://collections.lib.utah.edu/details?id=1213440).* Commonly, there is overlap between PSP and other neurodegenerative syndromes (including their ocular motor features), especially multiple system atrophy (MSA) and corticobasal degeneration (CBD)[1,79] (Table 96.2).

Disorders of Saccades

Saccades must be evaluated for several components: speed of initiation (latency), velocity, accuracy and conjugacy. As would be apparent from examination of the cortical contribution to saccade initiation discussed above, lesions of the FEF and PEF can lead to delays in initiation of contralateral volitional and reflexive visually guided saccades, respectively. Lesions of the PPRF can cause slowing or loss of horizontal saccades, and the riMLF can do the same for vertically directed saccades. Unilateral PPRF lesions will affect ipsilateral saccades.[82] Unilateral riMLF lesions cause impairment of primarily downward saccades, as the innervation of motoneurons responsible for elevation is from the bilateral riMLF (*see* Video 27; [online] Available from: *https://collections.lib.utah.edu/details?id=1209931*).[1] Metabolic disorders may selectively involve these structures, as in Niemann-Pick Type C (midbrain) and Gaucher disease (pons).[82]

There are disorders generally referred to as ocular motor apraxias, characterized by the inability to initiate saccades. Apraxia is defined as the loss of the ability to perform a learned skill, despite intact basic motor functions. In congenital cases, the term ocular motor apraxia may be a misnomer. A newer term, infantile-onset saccade initiation delay (ISID), appears more accurate, considering that reflexive visually guided saccades, which are not a "learned" movement, can also be impaired.[83] The underlying pathophysiology of these disorders may be more of a supranuclear deficit in saccade initiation.[84] ISID presents with a congenital impairment of horizontal saccades, which can be unilateral or asymmetric. Affected saccades are hypometric and of increased latency. Infants are identified when they are unable to follow moving objects or when neck motor control develops and compensatory head thrusts are seen. Large rapid head turns substitute the (normal) VOR for the (abnormal) saccadic system to reach an intended visual target. With later development, blinks are used to break fixation and assist in saccade initiation. Blinks are commonly used to initiate saccades in certain neurodegenerative conditions, especially in Huntington's disease. Motor and neurodevelopmental abnormalities are often associated with ISID, and imaging may identify abnormalities of cerebellar development. Joubert syndrome is a disease that presents with infantile hypotonia, motor and cognitive developmental delay and ataxia. It is associated with bidirectional head thrusts, hypometric saccades and prolonged saccade latencies, and different types of nystagmus may be seen. The classic neuroimaging finding is the "molar tooth sign" caused by elongation of the superior cerebellar peduncle. Ataxia-telangiectasia is associated with hypometric and delayed saccades, and prominent compensatory head movements are often seen.[85] Ocular motor apraxia may also be acquired due to bilateral frontal or frontoparietal lesions. Oculomotor apraxia is a feature of Bálint's syndrome. Other associated features include simultanagnosia (difficulty appreciating the big picture, as in the ability to identify the colors that make up the Ishihara plates, but inability to see the numbers made by the colors), optic ataxia (difficulty with accurate reaching for a target under visual guidance) and commonly bilateral inferior homonymous visual field defects given the parieto-occipital localization.[86]

Many disorders may have associated slow saccades, but the list can be narrowed substantially when considering conjugacy and directionality. Congenital myasthenia gravis can have subclinically slowed saccades with a normal initial velocity on quantitative testing.[82] Several muscle diseases also can have slowed saccades and are usually associated with ptosis among other neurologic features. In myotonic dystrophy type I, saccades tend to be slow and hypometric and occur with an increased latency. Impaired VOR suppression points toward a central contribution as well.[1] In oculopharyngeal muscular dystrophy, progressive ptosis, slowing of saccades and ophthalmoparesis accompany dysphagia as the primary presenting symptoms after the age of 40. Slow saccades can be seen even when the range of eye movements is normal and may contribute to the visual symptomatology.[87] Mitochondrial myopathies also present with progressive external ophthalmoplegia (PEO), characterized by orbicularis oculi weakness and bilateral ptosis accompanying the slowed saccades and limited range of eye movements. These diseases may be due either to mutations of mitochondrial DNA or of nuclear DNA responsible for producing proteins required for transcription/translation of mitochondrial DNA. Specific diseases can be identified by characteristic clinical features. Kearns-Sayre syndrome (KSS) is composed of a triad of PEO, cardiac conduction defects and pigmentary retinal degeneration. Disease onset is typically before age 20. Of note, long-term human immunodeficiency virus (HIV) treatment with nucleoside reverse transcriptase inhibitors can also precipitate a PEO.[88]

An uncommon complication of cardiac or aortic surgery is a saccadic abnormality. Slow or hypometric saccades, and even the complete loss of volitional saccades, have been reported. Typically, both horizontal and vertical saccades are affected. Pursuit and vergence are spared. The involvement of reflexive saccades differentiates this from an ocular motor apraxia; however, late adaptive responses may include head thrusts and blinks. Imaging has demonstrated cerebellar and pontine infarcts in one case, and the authors suggest these lesions may be pathologic.[89] Recent models also point toward involvement of pontine premotor neurons, particularly omnipause neurons, which normally inhibit saccades when fixation is desired.[90] Similar clinical features may be seen with Whipple's disease or anti-Ma2 paraneoplastic encephalitis.[82]

As dysmetric limb movements localize to the cerebellum (or its connections), so do dysmetric (abnormally calibrated) eye movements. These pathways are complex, but key features can be used to recognize the eye movement abnormalities indicating cerebellar lesions. Both hypermetric (overshoot) and hypometric (undershoot) saccades can be seen. The prototype for these disorders is Wallenberg syndrome, or lateral medullary syndrome, often caused by infarct in the distribution of the posterior inferior cerebellar artery. Wallenberg syndrome affects the resting tone between the PPRF (and subsequently the abducens nuclei) by affecting the projections that connect the medulla to the cerebellar vermis. The result is relative ipsilateral PPRF/abducens nucleus hyperactivity and contralateral PPRF/abducens nucleus hypoactivity, causing ipsilesional hypermetric saccades, contralesional hypometric saccades, and a tendency for the eyes to drift toward the side of the lesion [ipsipulsion (*see* Video 28; [online] Available from: *https://collections.lib.utah.edu/details?id=187724*)]. This imbalance also may be demonstrated by observing vertical saccades, which often have an elliptical trajectory that curves toward the side of the lesion. Associated neurologic features may include vertigo, sensory loss of the ipsilateral face and contralateral body, ipsilateral ataxia, dysarthria, dysphagia and an ipsilateral Horner's syndrome.[1,91] Dysmetric saccades, impaired smooth pursuit and other ocular motor abnormalities are commonly found in patients with SCA, although severe slowing of saccades should raise suspicion for SCA 2, while SCA 3 has a higher prevalence of ophthalmoparesis.[92]

Abnormalities of Smooth Pursuit

Lesions involving the temporo-occipital junction reduce smooth pursuit gain toward the side of the lesion regardless of the visual field in which the target falls (*see* Video 29; [online] Available from: *https://collections.lib.utah.edu/details?id=187721*). Clinically, this can be helpful in differentiation of pure occipital or parieto-occipital lesions causing a contralateral homonymous hemianopia. As optokinetic stimuli are presented to both visual fields, a unilateral lesion of the primary visual cortex will not affect the pursuit portion of the OKN response. However, involvement of the parietal lobe will cause an asymmetric OKN response with a weak or absent ipsilesional response.[93] Reduced gain is noted as saccadic pursuit, where saccades supplement the pursuit system to bring the target back onto the fovea. Lesions of the FEF or descending pathways may present similarly.[1] Cerebellar pathology commonly impairs smooth pursuit, and this can be unilateral or bilateral (usually horizontal and vertical). Gain is commonly reduced (i.e. "choppy" or saccadic pursuit) or initiation of pursuit can be delayed. The cerebellum also plays a role in integrating eye movements, head movements and relative motion of the visual target.[75,94]

SACCADIC INTRUSIONS AND INVOLUNTARY GAZE

Saccadic Intrusions

Of saccadic intrusions, SWJs are the most common. These are defined by horizontal saccadic interruptions of fixation of 0.5–5°, with an intersaccadic interval of 200–400 ms before returning to fixation. They are often seen as a part of normal aging and do not cause oscillopsia. However, SWJs that are more frequent than ~10/minute, larger than 5°, or that are disconjugate are usually pathologic. In addition to disorders discussed above, Huntington's chorea, cerebral lesions and Friedreich's ataxia have been associated with pathologic SWJ. Larger, asymmetric intrusions with shorter intersaccadic intervals, called square wave pulses or macrosquare wave jerks, are due to abnormal premotor inputs from the cerebellum or brainstem and can be seen in MS, PSP or MSA. Macrosaccadic oscillations are the result of dysmetric saccades that move back and forth laterally and straddle fixation. Intersaccadic intervals are around 200 ms, and these are seen with midline cerebellar lesions (*see* Video 30; [online] Available from: *https://collections.lib.utah.edu/details?id=1209728*).[8,95]

Ocular Flutter and Opsoclonus

While the intrusions and oscillations mentioned above all have an intersaccadic interval, ocular flutter and opsoclonus do not. Ocular flutter is defined by back-to-back horizontal saccades, whereas opsoclonus is defined by multidirectional (horizontal, torsional, vertical) saccades. Both disorders can be accompanied by myoclonus, ataxia and/or encephalopathy. The underlying pathophysiology may relate to omnipause cell damage in the brainstem (cannot suppress saccades), or perhaps disinhibition of the fastigial nucleus (the saccade-generating machinery is overactive). Whether a patient has flutter or opsoclonus does not significantly affect the differential diagnosis, workup or treatment. The most common causes of these disorders are paraneoplastic (older patients), viral encephalitis (younger patients) and toxic-metabolic derangements. The constellation of opsoclonus-myoclonus syndrome in children is associated with neuroblastoma.[8,95]

Oculogyric Crisis

Oculogyric crisis is a dystonic conjugate deviation of gaze, typically upward (*see* Video 31; [online] Available from: *https://collections.lib.utah.edu/details?id=1248766*). Accompanying features may include other dystonic craniocervical involvement or autonomic signs. Episodes can last seconds to hours. These are most often drug-induced by medications with antidopaminergic effects, such as neuroleptics or antiemetics, though antiepileptic medications have also been reported. Other associated diseases include hereditary movement disorders, disorders of dopamine metabolism and acquired or neurodegenerative movement disorders. Emergent treatment includes benztropine or diphenhydramine if removal of the provocative medications does not lead to resolution of symptoms.[96]

SUMMARY

A detailed evaluation of neurologic, neuro-ophthalmic, ocular motor and vestibular systems allows for accurate localization and generation of a differential diagnosis for nystagmus and gaze disorders. Nystagmus must be distinguished from saccadic intrusions and oscillations, which have different localizations and implications. Once nystagmus is identified, it should be determined whether it is congenital or acquired and then classified as jerk or pendular. Nystagmus is evaluated in all directions of gaze, and in certain cases where none is seen, it can be provoked (e.g. BPPV). Unidirectional mixed horizontal-torsional nystagmus increasing in intensity with visual fixation removed and with looking in the direction of the fast phase (Alexander's law) is usually peripheral vestibular in origin, but central vestibular disorders can behave similarly. Gaze-evoked or spontaneous vertical or torsional nystagmus is central in origin until proven otherwise. Conjugate ocular motor abnormalities can be better elucidated by identifying the particular classes of eye movements involved. If all classes are involved, possibilities include an ipsilateral brainstem or a large contralateral hemispheric lesion. The VOR can usually differentiate between the two localizations. Saccade deficits must be further divided into initiation, velocity or accuracy deficits, each of which has a specific differential diagnosis. Isolated deficits of smooth pursuit may be of cortical or cerebellar origin. As with nystagmus, the associated symptoms and signs are essential in reaching a specific diagnosis (Table 96.3).

Table 96.3: Gaze abnormalities by neuroanatomic localization.

Lesion localization	Ocular motor signs	Associated features	Common etiologies
Cerebral			
FEF	• Gaze deviation, can look like a palsy when acute • Impaired contralateral voluntary saccades	• Contralateral motor signs	• MCA stroke • Seizure
PEF	Impaired contralateral reflexive saccades	Inattention/neglect	MCA stroke
Visual cortex	Impaired pursuit to contralateral field	Homonymous visual field defects	PCA stroke
TPO junction	Impaired ipsilateral pursuit	Homonymous visual field defects	• PCA stroke • Mass lesions
Bilateral parietal	Delayed saccade initiation	Bálint's syndrome (simultanagnosia, optic ataxia, homonymous visual field defects)	Watershed infarcts
Basal ganglia	• Square wave jerks • Hypometric and/or delayed saccades	Parkinsonism and related movement disorders	Neurodegenerative disorders
Midbrain			
Pretectum	Parinaud's syndrome (upgaze palsy, convergence-retraction nystagmus)	Light-near dissociation	• Hydrocephalus • Neoplasm • Basilar stroke
riMLF	Impaired vertical (down worse than up) and torsional saccades	• Contralateral motor or sensory deficits if unilateral • Impaired consciousness if bilateral • Parkinsonism if neurodegenerative	• Vertebrobasilar or artery of Percheron stroke (bilateral involvement) • PSP (involved early)
Pons			
PPRF	Impaired ipsilateral saccades	• INO • Facial palsy	• Vertebrobasilar stroke • Demyelination
Omnipause neurons	• Ocular flutter • Opsoclonus	• Myoclonus • Encephalopathy	• Paraneoplastic • Viral encephalitis
Abducens nucleus	• Ipsilateral gaze palsy	• INO • Facial palsy • Foville's syndrome	• Vertebrobasilar stroke • Demyelination
Medulla			
Dorsolateral medulla	• Ipsilateral ocular lateropulsion • Dysmetric saccades	Wallenberg syndrome (Horner's, ataxia, crossed sensory findings)	• PICA infarcts • Demyelination
Cerebellum			
Flocculus/ Paraflocculus	• Saccadic pursuit • GEN, DBN	• Dizziness/vertigo • Gait imbalance	• PICA infarct • Cerebellar degeneration
Vermis	• Dysmetric saccades • Contralateral ocular lateropulsion • Saccadic pursuit	Truncal ataxia	• PICA or SCA infarct • Cerebellar degeneration

(FEF: Frontal eye field; MCA: Middle cerebral artery; PEF: Parietal eye field; PCA: Posterior cerebral artery; TPO: Temporoparietal occipital; riMLF: Rostral interstitial medial longitudinal fasciculus; PPRF: Paramedian pontine reticular formation; INO: Internuclear ophthalmoplegia; PICA: Posterior inferior cerebellar artery; GEN: Gaze-evoked nystagmus; DBN: Downbeat nystagmus; SCA: Superior cerebellar artery)

REFERENCES

1. Leigh RJ, Zee DS. The Neurology of Eye Movements, 5th edition. USA: Oxford University Press; 2015. p. 90.
2. Shaikh AG, Ghasia FF. Physiology and pathology of saccades and gaze holding. Neuro Rehabilitation. 2013;32: 493-505.
3. Cannon SC, Robinson DA. Loss of the neural integrator of the oculomotor system from brain stem lesions in monkey. J Neurophysiol. 1987;57:1383-409.
4. Crawford JD, Cadera W, Vilis T. Generation of torsional and vertical eye position signals by the interstitial nucleus of Cajal. Science. 1991;252:1551-3.
5. Cahill H, Nathans J. The optokinetic reflex as a tool for quantitative analyses of nervous system function in mice: application to genetic and drug-induced variation. PLoS One. 2008;3:e2055.
6. David NJ. Optokinetic nystagmus. A clinical review. J Clin Neuroophthalmol. 1989;9:258-66.
7. Papageorgiou E, McLean RJ, Gottlob I. Nystagmus in childhood. Pediatr Neonatol. 2014;55:341-51.
8. Lemos J, Eggenberger E. Saccadic intrusions: review and update. Curr Opin Neurol. 2013;26:59-66.
9. Cogan DG. Ocular dysmetria; flutter-like oscillations of the eyes, and opsoclonus. AMA Arch Ophthalmol. 1954;51:318-35.
10. Smith JL, Walsh FB. Opsoclonus—ataxic conjugate movements of the eyes. Arch Ophthalmol. 1960;64:244-50.
11. Brandt T, Dieterich M. The dizzy patient: don't forget disorders of the central vestibular system. Nat Rev Neurol. 2017;13(6):352-62.
12. Thompson TL, Amedee R. Vertigo: a review of common peripheral and central vestibular disorders. Ochsner J. 2009;9:20-6.
13. Strupp M, Kremmyda O, Adamczyk C, et al. Central ocular motor disorders, including gaze palsy and nystagmus. J Neurol. 2014;261 Suppl 2:S542-58.
14. Baloh RW, Spooner JW. Downbeat nystagmus: a type of central vestibular nystagmus. Neurology. 1981;31:304-10.
15. Barmack NH. A comparison of the horizontal and vertical vestibulo-ocular reflexes of the rabbit. J Physiol. 1981;314:547-64.
16. Gresty M, Barratt H, Rudge P, et al. Analysis of downbeat nystagmus: otolithic vs semicircular canal influences. Arch Neurol. 1986;43:52-5.
17. Marti S, Palla A, Straumann D. Gravity dependence of ocular drift in patients with cerebellar downbeat nystagmus. Ann Neurol. 2002;52:712-21.
18. Zee DS, Friendlich AR, Robinson DA. The mechanism of downbeat nystagmus. Arch Neurol. 1974;30:227-37.
19. Wong A. Eye Movement Disorders. USA: Oxford University Press; 2008.
20. Ten Tusscher MP. A neural model for cyclovertical eye movements and their disorders. Strabismus. 2011;19:162-5.
21. Tilikete C, Jasse L, Pelisson D, et al. Acquired pendular nystagmus in multiple sclerosis and oculopalatal tremor. Neurology. 2011;76:1650-7.
22. Nakada T, Kwee IL. Oculopalatal myoclonus. Brain. 1986;109 (Pt 3):431-41.
23. Tilikete C, Desestret V. Hypertrophic olivary degeneration and palatal or oculopalatal tremor. Front Neurol. 2017;8:302.
24. Simpson DA, Wishnow R, Gargulinski RB, et al. Oculofacial-skeletal myorhythmia in central nervous system Whipple's disease: additional case and review of the literature. Mov Disord. 1995;10:195-200.
25. Baloh RW, Honrubia V, Konrad HR. Periodic alternating nystagmus. Brain. 1976;99:11-26.
26. Gold DR, Morris L, Kheradmand A, et al. Repositioning maneuvers for benign paroxysmal positional vertigo. Curr Treat Options Neurol. 2014;16:307.
27. Ehrt O. Infantile and acquired nystagmus in childhood. Eur J Paediatr Neurol. 2012;16:567-72.
28. Zahn JR. Incidence and characteristics of voluntary nystagmus. J Neurol Neurosurg Psychiatry. 1978;41:617-23.
29. Lee J, Gresty M. A case of "voluntary nystagmus" and head tremor. J Neurol Neurosurg Psychiatry. 1993;56:1321-2.
30. Shults WT, Stark L, Hoyt WF, et al. Normal saccadic structure of voluntary nystagmus. Arch Ophthalmol. 1977;95: 1399-404.
31. Hotson JR. Convergence-initiated voluntary flutter: a normal intrinsic capability in man. Brain Res. 1984;294: 299-304.
32. Blair CJ. Voluntary nystagmus: electro-oculographic findings in four cases. Arch Ophthalmol. 1967;77:349.
33. Hain TC, Zee DS, Mordes M. Blink-induced saccadic oscillations. Ann Neurol. 1986;19:299-301.
34. Keyes MJ. Voluntary nystagmus in two generations. Arch Neurol. 1973;29:63-4.
35. Batuecas-Caletrío A, Yañez-Gonzalez R, Sanchez-Blanco C, et al. Glucocorticoids improve acute dizziness symptoms following acute unilateral vestibulopathy. J Neurol. 2015;262:2578-82.
36. Karlberg ML, Magnusson M. Treatment of acute vestibular neuronitis with glucocorticoids. Otol Neurotol. 2011;32: 1140-3.
37. Bhattacharyya N, Gubbels SP, Schwartz SR, et al. Clinical practice guideline: benign paroxysmal positional vertigo (update). Otolaryngol Head Neck Surg. 2017;156:S1-S47.
38. Strupp M, Schüler O, Krafczyk S, et al. Treatment of downbeat nystagmus with 3,4-diaminopyridine: a placebo-controlled study. Neurology. 2003;61:165-70.
39. Kalla R, Spiegel R, Claassen J, et al. Comparison of 10-mg doses of 4-aminopyridine and 3,4-diaminopyridine for the treatment of downbeat nystagmus. J Neuroophthalmol. 2011;31:320-5.
40. Claassen J, Spiegel R, Kalla R, et al. A randomised double-blind, cross-over trial of 4-aminopyridine for downbeat nystagmus—effects on slowphase eye velocity, postural stability, locomotion and symptoms. J Neurol Neurosurg Psychiatry. 2013;84:1392-9.
41. Strupp M, Teufel J, Zwergal A, et al. Aminopyridines for the treatment of neurologic disorders. Neurol Clin Pract. 2017;7:65-76.

42. Kalla R, Glasauer S, Buttner U, et al. 4-aminopyridine restores vertical and horizontal neural integrator function in downbeat nystagmus. Brain. 2007;130:2441-51.
43. Young YH, Huang TW. Role of clonazepam in the treatment of idiopathic downbeat nystagmus. Laryngoscope. 2001;111:1490-3.
44. Thurtell MJ, Leigh RJ. Treatment of nystagmus. Curr Treat Options Neurol. 2012;14:60-72.
45. Feil K, Claaßen J, Bardins S, et al. Effect of chlorzoxazone in patients with downbeat nystagmus: a pilot trial. Neurology. 2013;81:1152-8.
46. Strupp M, Hüfner K, Sandmann R, et al. Central oculomotor disturbances and nystagmus: a window into the brainstem and cerebellum. Dtsch Arztebl Int. 2011;108:197-204.
47. Nakamagoe K, Fujizuka N, Koganezawa T, et al. Downbeat nystagmus associated with damage to the medial longitudinal fasciculus of the pons: a vestibular balance control mechanism via the lower brainstem paramedian tract neurons. J Neurol Sci. 2013;328:98-101.
48. Nerrant E, Tilikete C. Ocular motor manifestations of multiple sclerosis. J Neuroophthalmol. 2017;37(3):332-40.
49. Wu D, Thijs RD. Anticonvulsant-induced downbeat nystagmus in epilepsy. Epilepsy Behav Case Rep. 2015;4: 74-5.
50. Arbusow V, Strupp M, Brandt T. Amiodarone-induced severe prolonged head-positional vertigo and vomiting. Neurology. 1998;51:917.
51. Korff C, Peter M, Burkhard PR. Downbeat nystagmus as a manifestation of intrathecal morphine toxicity. Eur J Anaesthesiol. 2007;24:201-2.
52. Halmagyi GM, Lessell I, Curthoys IS, et al. Lithium-induced downbeat nystagmus. Am J Ophthalmol. 1989;107:664-70.
53. Kattah JC. The spectrum of vestibular and ocular motor abnormalities in thiamine deficiency. Curr Neurol Neurosci Rep. 2017;5:1-9.
54. Bussière M, Al-Khotani A, Steckley JL, et al. Paraneoplastic downbeat nystagmus. Can J Ophthalmol. 2008;43:243-5.
55. Glasauer S, Kalla R, Büttner U, et al. 4-aminopyridine restores visual ocular motor function in upbeat nystagmus. J Neurol Neurosurg Psychiatry. 2005;76:451-3.
56. Thurtell MJ, Joshi AC, Leone AC, et al. Crossover trial of gabapentin and memantine as treatment for acquired nystagmus. Ann Neurol. 2010;67:676-80.
57. Sibony PA, Evinger C, Manning KA. Tobacco-induced primary-position upbeat nystagmus. Ann Neurol. 1987;21: 53-8.
58. Morrow MJ, Sharpe JA. Torsional nystagmus in the lateral medullary syndrome. Ann Neurol. 1988;24:390-8.
59. Strupp M, Kremmyda O, Brandt T. Pharmacotherapy of vestibular disorders and nystagmus. Semin Neurol. 2013;33:286-96.
60. Comer RM, Dawson EL, Lee JP. Baclofen for patients with congenital periodic alternating nystagmus. Strabismus. 2006;14:205-9.
61. Kumar A, Thomas S, McLean R, et al. Treatment of acquired periodic alternating nystagmus with memantine: a case report. Clin Neuropharmacol. 2009;32:109-10.
62. Abadi RV, Pascal E. Periodic alternating nystagmus in humans with albinism. Invest Ophthalmol Vis Sci. 1994;35:4080-6.
63. Guyer DR, Lessell S. Periodic alternating nystagmus associated with albinism. J Clin Neuroophthalmol. 1986;6:82-5.
64. Matsumoto S, Ohyagi Y, Inoue I, et al. Periodic alternating nystagmus in a patient with MS. Neurology. 2001;56:276-7.
65. Campbell WW. Periodic alternating nystagmus in phenytoin intoxication. Arch Neurol. 1980;37:178-80.
66. Korres S, Balatsouras DG, Zournas C, et al. Periodic alternating nystagmus associated with Arnold-Chiari malformation. J Laryngol Otol. 2001;115:1001-4.
67. Hashimoto T, Sasaki O, Yoshida K, et al. Periodic alternating nystagmus and rebound nystagmus in spinocerebellar ataxia type 6. Mov Disord. 2003;18:1201-4.
68. Colen CB, Ketko A, George E, et al. Periodic alternating nystagmus and periodic alternating skew deviation in spinocerebellar ataxia type 6. J Neuroophthalmol. 2008;28:287-8.
69. Jay WM, Williams BB, De Chicchis A. Periodic alternating nystagmus clearing after cataract surgery. J Clin Neuroophthalmol. 1985;5:149-52.
70. Chiu B, Hain TC. Periodic alternating nystagmus provoked by an attack of Meniere's disease. J Neuroophthalmol. 2002;22:107-9.
71. Lloyd SK, Baguley DM, Butler K, et al. Bruns' nystagmus in patients with vestibular schwannoma. Otol Neurotol. 2009;30:625-8.
72. Croxson GR, Moffat DA, Baguley D. Bruns bidirectional nystagmus in cerebellopontine angle tumours. Clin Otolaryngol Allied Sci. 1988;13:153-7.
73. Shaikh AG, Thurtell MJ, Optican LM, et al. Pharmacological tests of hypotheses for acquired pendular nystagmus. Ann N Y Acad Sci. 2011;1233:320-6.
74. Kang S, Shaikh AG. Acquired pendular nystagmus. J Neurol Sci. 2017;375:8-17.
75. Sharpe JA. Neurophysiology and neuroanatomy of smooth pursuit: lesion studies. Brain Cogn. 2008;68:241-54.
76. Silverman IE, Liu GT, Volpe NJ, et al. The crossed paralyses: the original brain-stem syndromes of Millard-Gubler, Foville, Weber, and Raymond-Cestan. Arch Neurol. 1995;52:635-8.
77. Shields M, Sinkar S, Chan W, et al. Parinaud syndrome: a 25-year (1991-2016) review of 40 consecutive adult cases. Acta Ophthalmol. 2017;95(8):e792-3.
78. Oguro H, Okada K, Suyama N, et al. Decline of vertical gaze and convergence with aging. Gerontology. 2004;50:177-81.
79. Gorges M, Pinkhardt EH, Kassubek J. Alterations of eye movement control in neurodegenerative movement disorders. J Ophthalmology. 2014;2014:658243.
80. Armstrong RA. Visual signs and symptoms of corticobasal degeneration. Clin Exp Optom. 2016;99:498-506.
81. Anderson T, Luxon L, Quinn N, et al. Oculomotor function in multiple system atrophy: clinical and laboratory features in 30 patients. Mov Disord. 2008;23:977-84.
82. Thurtell MJ, Tomsak RL, Leigh RJ. Disorders of saccades. Curr Neurol Neurosci Rep. 2007;7:407-16.

83. Shawkat FS, Kingsley D, Kendall B, et al. Neuroradiological and eye movement correlates in children with intermittent saccade failure. Neuropediatrics. 1995;26:298-305.
84. Harris CM, Hodgkins PR, Kriss A, et al. Familial congenital saccade initiation failure and isolated cerebellar vermis hypoplasia. Dev Med Child Neurol. 1998;40:775-9.
85. Salman MS. Infantile-onset saccade initiation delay (congenital ocular motor apraxia). Curr Neurol Neurosci Rep. 2015;15:24.
86. Rizzo M, Vecera SP. Psychoanatomical substrates of Balint's syndrome. J Neurol Neurosurg Psychiatry. 2002;72:162-78.
87. Renard D, Ferraro A, Lorenzini MC, et al. Orthoptic and video-oculographic analyses in oculopharyngeal muscular dystrophy. Muscle Nerve. 2015;52:554-8.
88. McClelland C, Manousakis G, Lee MS. Progressive external ophthalmoplegia. Curr Neurol Neurosci Rep. 2016;16:53.
89. Yee RD, Purvin VA. Acquired ocular motor apraxia after aortic surgery. Trans Am Ophthalmol Soc. 2007;105:152-8.
90. Solomon D, Ramat S, Tomsak RL, et al. Saccadic palsy after cardiac surgery: characteristics and pathogenesis. Ann Neurol. 2008;63:355-65.
91. Crevits L, vander Eecken H. Ocular lateropulsion in Wallenberg's syndrome: a prospective clinical study. Acta Neurol Scand. 1982;65:219-22.
92. Moscovich M, Okun MS, Favilla C, et al. Clinical evaluation of eye movements in spinocerebellar ataxias: a prospective multicenter study. J Neuroophthalmol. 2015;35:16-21.
93. Levenson DS, Smith JL. Optokinetic nystagmus and occipital lesions. Am J Ophthalmol. 1996;61:753-62.
94. Beh SC, Frohman TC, Frohman EM. Neuro-ophthalmic manifestations of cerebellar disease. Neurol Clin. 2014;32: 1009-80.
95. Thurtell MJ, Leigh RJ. Nystagmus and saccadic intrusions. Handb Clin Neurol. 2011;102:333-78.
96. Barow E, Schneider SA, Bhatia KP, et al. Oculogyric crises: etiology, pathophysiology and therapeutic approaches. Parkinsonism Relat Disord. 2017;36:3-9.

Chapter 97 Functional Vision Loss

Greg Van Stavern, Nathan Kung, James Liu

INTRODUCTION

Functional (nonorganic) vision loss (FVL) is a term used to refer to decreased visual function not caused by an organic lesion. Often, FVL is considered a diagnosis of exclusion. However, positive findings confirming normal or better than claimed vision are required to secure the diagnosis, so it may be thought of more as a diagnosis of CONclusion rather than EXclusion. Patients with FVL present a diagnostic challenge for the ophthalmologist and it is estimated that up to 5% of patients seen in a standard ophthalmology practice have FVL.[1] The presentation can be protean and may involve mild-to-severe visual dysfunction, including both afferent and efferent loss. Many ophthalmologists are reluctant to diagnose FVL, due in part to fear of missing a blinding disorder with an organic cause. This same fear often leads to unnecessary and costly testing, imaging, and consultations that may be avoided with a few clinical examination techniques and appropriate patient counseling. The primary focus of this chapter will be to review techniques that can help confirm a functional component to vision loss, highlighting techniques that prove normal or better than claimed visual function. We will also briefly discuss some management strategies for patients with FVL. We will focus primarily on afferent visual loss, but functional efferent presentations (convergence spasm, voluntary ptosis, voluntary nystagmus, and functional blepharospasm) can also occur and are discussed elsewhere.[2]

HISTORY AND TERMINOLOGY

The notion of FVL dates back to antiquity. Early examples of unexplained vision loss and often spontaneous return of vision can be seen in Biblical references, Greek and Roman mythology, and Shakespearean literature.[3] Given its long-standing history and presence in religious, mythological, and literary contexts, it is not surprising that FVL been described using different terms. Hysterical vision loss, factitious vision loss, ocular conversion reaction, psychogenic visual disturbances, and many other terms all share a common thread of attributing the process to a psychiatric cause.[4] The concept of conversion disorder originated with Sigmund Freud, who postulated that anxiety and psychological conflict manifested and converted into physical symptoms.[5]

More formalized characterization of the disease can be seen with the Diagnostic and Statistical Manual of Mental Disorders, Fifth Edition (DSM-5), which describes FVL as a functional vision disorder, falling into the category of somatoform conversion disorders.[6] This is distinct from factitious disorder, in which the visual symptoms are produced to maintain a sick role, and malingering, where secondary gain is involved (e.g. compensation from social welfare programs, insurance fraud, or a desire to avoid work-related duties).[7] In his description of FVL, Dr Stanley Thompson described a large spectrum of functional patients, which include the "suggestible innocent", "impressionable exaggerator", worried imposter", and the "deliberate malinger".[8]

We define FVL to include all of these different "types" of nonorganic vision loss. The goal of the clinician is not necessarily to provide a psychiatric diagnosis, but instead to clarify whether the nature of vision loss is nonorganic (FVL), organic, or some combination of both.

POTENTIAL PATHOPHYSIOLOGY

The exact pathophysiologic mechanisms underlying FVL are uncertain and theories vary, dependent in part upon whether one approaches FVL from a psychiatric, psychosocial or biologic perspective. Recent advances in technology have sought a physiologic explanation to certain aspects of FVL. Functional magnetic resonance imaging (fMRI) has produced some evidence that normal brain activity and function is altered under in patients with FVL. Several studies have shown reduced fMRI activation in the visual cortices of FVL patients compared to controls.[9,10]

However, these studies often lack controls and are limited by small sample sizes and variations in technique and image analysis between investigators. Some researchers argue that FVL reflects a complex interplay between neural, psychological, and social factors.[11]

Functional Vision Loss Coexisting with Organic Disease

Functional overlay on top of ocular pathology is also a common occurrence, further clouding the diagnosis. These confounding factors highlight the importance of proving normal or better than claimed vision to securely diagnose FVL. In a case review by Scott et al., 53% of patients had FVL superimposed upon organic pathology.[12] Patients with organic disease may demonstrate features of functional visual loss if they exaggerate their symptoms to "help" the examining physician. Although not always strictly factitious in etiology, patients with organic disease may also occasionally have decreased visual acuity, constricted visual fields, or other findings in the face of an otherwise stable or unremarkable examination. Because patient cooperation is crucial in psychophysical tests of visual function, the patient's fixation, cooperation, and reliability should always be monitored during testing. If the patient is fatigued, adequate rest and slower pacing may be needed in order to obtain the most accurate result. Simply repeating the test at a later time may also give a more reliable result. In the idiopathic intracranial hypertension treatment trial (IIHTT), approximately 21% of study patients were noted to have performance failures, defined as a worsening in visual field mean deviation by greater than 2–3 dB that subsequently resolved on repeat testing within 4 days, or as those tests which were judged to be due to performance failure after adjudication.[13]

Central diseases with involvement of the frontal lobes (Fig. 97.1) or hypothalamic-pituitary region may also result in concomitant visual abnormalities and psychiatric symptoms.[14] Patients with cortical visual dysfunction due to Alzheimer's disease, posterior cortical atrophy, or rarely, the visual variant of Creutzfeldt-Jakob disease, can also be mistaken for having FVL. These patients can also present with visuospatial and visuoperceptual impairments, including visual agnosias and visual hallucinations, sometimes in the setting of depression and anxiety.[15] Vague visual complaints are also common at presentation. Some of these patients may also perform paradoxically well on standard measures of visual function such as visual acuity or automated visual field testing, with deficits only noted on more detailed testing such as with double simultaneous stimulation, color plate testing, description of a complex scene, or clock drawing.[16] Therefore, a high index of suspicion is often required to make the diagnosis in these cases.

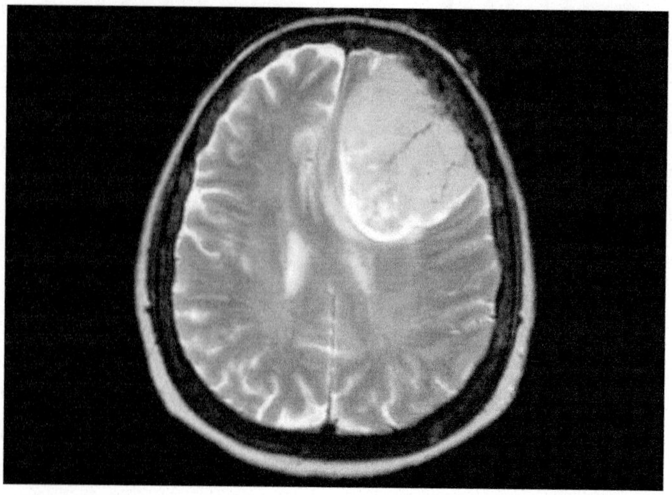

Fig. 97.1: Left frontal lobe tumor. Lesions involving the frontal lobes and pituitary-hypothalamic region of the brain may present with visual abnormalities and behavioral changes that may be misinterpreted as functional behavior.

CLINICAL EXAMINATION

History

The assessment of FVL begins with a thorough history, including a full review of records. Documentation that highlights inconsistencies between the history and physical examination may display an outside clinician's suspicion for FVL. This information can help tailor the examination toward establishing FVL early. Review testing and imaging that has already been obtained to ensure that an organic cause has not been missed.[17]

The best approach in obtaining history for FVL is to carry an attitude of sympathetic understanding.[18] A patient who feels secure that his or her symptoms are being taken seriously is less likely to exaggerate those symptoms in an effort to convince. Avoid blunt questions about depression, anxiety, or abuse early in the encounter. Avoid contradicting patient statements or using a confrontational tone. A patient is more likely to volunteer useful information if he/she does not feel threatened.

Descriptive features about the quality of vision loss should be documented. Establish the onset of symptoms and the time course to determine whether the visual dysfunction fits a known pathophysiologic process. Identify specific triggers that may have been present (e.g. physical or emotional trauma, illness, etc.) during times of vision loss. The patient may focus on what they can no longer do, but focusing on what they can still do may provide insight into their true visual potential.[11]

A history meticulously outlined by the patient may actually raise the suspicion for nonorganic etiology. One study found that a large number of written symptoms may be specific for somatization.[19] Other features early in the encounter may raise the suspicion for FVL as well. An observational study found that wearing of sunglasses into a neuro-ophthalmology clinic was highly correlated with nonorganic vision loss. The overall sensitivity of this "sunglasses sign" was 46% with 99% specificity.[20] Although "la bella indifference" (lack of interest or concern about the apparent visual loss) has been classically associated with FVL, recent studies and systematic reviews suggest that this is not a reliable "clinical sign" to discriminate between organic and nonorganic disease.[21]

Clinical Examination

The diagnosis of FVL depends on positive findings that prove normal or better than claimed visual acuity. These techniques rely upon aspects of the visual system with which the patient is often unfamiliar, including spatial resolution, stereopsis, and the parameters of a normal visual field. For patients who report no light perception in both eyes, any evidence of visual perception is enough to show some component of FVL. However, difficulty often arises when vision loss is only partial. It is important that examiner develops skill with at least some of these tests so that they can be deployed naturally, such that the patient does not recognize them as "special" tests.

Tests of Proprioception

Patients with FVL will often mistake tasks of proprioception and coordination with visual tasks, as those who are completely blind should still be able to reliably accomplish the tasks below. Although these tests do not provide any quantitative information regarding a patient's visual acuity, failure should greatly raise the clinician's suspicion for a functional component to vision loss. The exception to this would be an organic cause leading to deficiencies in both vision and proprioception, and the clinician must take care to not exclude this possibility.[22]

Burkhardt test: The patient is asked to bring his or her index fingers together. The ability to bring the fingertips of opposite hands together is a task based on proprioception, though patients with FVL will often perform the test poorly, mistaking it for a test of vision.[23]

Signature writing: Signature writing is a relatively automated process based largely on proprioception and coordination. Blind patients usually have no difficulty writing their signature when prompted with a starting point. Functional patients are more inclined to hesitate, move across the page, or write illegibly.[23]

Tests for Severe Bilateral Vision Loss

In scenarios where vision loss is reported as severe (count fingers vision to no light perception) tests based on visual reflexes may be sufficient to at least prove better than claimed vision and a functional component, although not necessarily normal vision.

Pupillary reaction: Poor pupil reactivity often indicates organic afferent visual pathway disease, but a normal pupillary response does not necessarily prove normal vision. The pupillary reflex will still be intact in patients with occipital lobe lesions.[24] However, in patients with severe, monocular visual loss, the absence of a relative afferent pupillary defect strongly suggests a functional etiology. One exception may be that of Leber's hereditary optic neuropathy (LHON), in which patients may have a subacute onset of unilateral central vision loss with an initially normal appearing optic disk and preserved ipsilateral pupillary reaction. In these instances, it has been suggested that there may be selective sparing of the melanopsin retinal ganglion cell fibers, which mediate the pupillary reaction.[25]

Mirror test: A large mirror is placed in front of a patient and rotated in different angles. The normal visual reflex is to exhibit nystagmoid movements as the eyes follow the moving reflections. The reflex should be present in cases where vision is better than hand motion. Sudden placement of the mirror close to the patient may also lead to reflexive accommodation, convergence, and miosis, again suggesting better than hand motion vision. Patients may try to suppress these reflexes by looking through the mirror.[23]

Optokinetic drum testing: A standard, but minimally quantitative, evaluation for visual acuity is with optokinetic drum testing. The presence of optokinetic nystagmus (OKN) suggests at least 20/400 vision (the minimum visual acuity necessary to resolve the alternating black and white stimuli).[26] Unfortunately, this technique is only useful when claimed visual acuity is severely diminished to the point of count fingers or worse vision, and does not prove normal vision. Furthermore, this reflex is relatively easy to suppress with voluntary defocus, and the lack of OKN response should not be used as evidence of organic vision loss.

Tests for Mild-to-Moderate Vision Loss: Correlates to Visual Acuity

For patients with partial vision loss (~20/40–20/200), more quantifiable measures must be used. Some of these tests are better suited for patients claiming monocular visual loss, but all can have some utility even with binocular FVL patients.

Bottom-up refraction: The simplest and in our experience the most useful method to document FVL and normal or near-normal visual acuity is with "bottom-up" or "toothpaste" refraction. The clinician begins with the 20/10 line and asks the patient to read the line. Slowly the patient is walked up the eye chart, with the clinician encouraging the patient to read each letter. This can be tedious (for patient and physician!), but if normal visual acuity is proven up front, this can ultimately be both cost and time saving. Showing multiple lines of 20/10 and then 20/15 letters may also help increase the likelihood of normal vision upon reaching the 20/20 line.

Counting acuity: The visual acuity chart can also be utilized by measuring "counting acuity". This relies upon the relationship between spatial resolution of single optotypes and overall visual acuity.[27] The patient is asked if they can at least see how many characters or "dots" there are on a single line. If a patient is able to accurately indicate the number of characters on the 20/20 line, this roughly corresponds to a Snellen acuity of 20/40. A counting level of 20/10 estimates to a visual acuity of 20/30 or better (Table 97.1).

Stereoscopic acuity: The Titmus stereotest is a commonly used contour stereotest that varies the amount of disparity between two polarized images seen through polarized lenses to produce stereoscopic images. At the most basic level, stereotesting can be used to rule out complete monocular vision loss, since binocular vision is required for stereopsis. In order to resolve the two polarized images into one stereoscopic image, however, a correlating minimum visual acuity in each eye is also necessary. One prior study correlated a 9/9 Titmus score (40 seconds of arc) with at worst 20/20 vision in each eye.[28] However a much larger recent study found that this likely overestimated the actual visual acuity due to interindividual variability.[29] The most recent data now suggest that a 9/9 Titmus score correlates with a Snellen acuity of at least 20/40 with 95% certainty, instead of 20/20 as previously described. Additional quantitative relationships based on the more conservative correlation established by Sitko et al. are provided (Table 97.2).

Threshold perimetry: isopters and foveal threshold: Visual field testing can also provide useful information regarding visual acuity. The Goldmann visual field can be used to correlate the size and brightness of a detectable stimulus to Snellen visual acuity. For example, a patient's ability to

Table 97.1: Correlation between counting and visual acuities. The ability to accurately count the number of characters shown on a Snellen visual acuity chart reliably estimates a corresponding visual acuity (with 95% confidence interval). Based on study of Levy et al., the visual acuity can be roughly estimated to be twice the counting acuity (counting acuity of 20/15 will correlate to a visual acuity of 20/30 or better in 50% of cases).

Counting acuity	Corresponding visual acuity
20/60	20/200
20/50	20/200
20/40	20/200
20/30	20/200
20/25	20/80
20/20	20/80
20/15	20/50
20/10	20/30

Source: Levy AH, McCulley TJ, Lam BL, et al. Estimating visual acuity by character counting using the Snellen visual acuity chart. Eye (Lond). 2005;19(6):622-4.

Table 97.2: Stereoscopic acuity as an indirect measure of visual acuity. Titmus score can provide a relatively accurate estimate for visual acuity (with 95% confidence interval) of the worse-seeing eye.

Titmus score	Snellen acuity correlate
1/9	20/5300
2/9	20/690
3/9	20/180
4/9	20/110
5/9	20/76
6/9	20/62
7/9	20/50
8/9	20/45
9/9	20/40

Source: Sitko KR, Peragallo JH, Bidot S, et al. Pitfalls in the use of stereoacuity in the diagnosis of nonorganic visual loss. Ophthalmology. 2016;123(1):198-202.

see the I1e stimulus correlates to a visual acuity of 20/30 or better, and the ability to see only the I2e stimulus correlates with 20/60 vision or better.[12]

In settings where Goldmann perimetry is not available, automated perimetry such as Humphrey visual field (HVF) testing can also provide quantitative measures using foveal threshold as a proxy for visual acuity. Foveal threshold is defined as the minimum amount of luminance on a uniform background that can be detected by a patient at central fixation. Although a foveal threshold takes only about 15 seconds to obtain, this feature is commonly turned off because of default settings and unfamiliarity with the utility of the measurement. A foveal threshold of 0–30 dB corresponds to a visual acuity worse than 20/50, whereas a foveal threshold better than 37 dB corresponds to a visual acuity of 20/20 or better.[30]

Four-Diopter prism testing: In this test, a 4-prism diopter loose prism is placed base-down over one eye to induce vertical diplopia. A letter from the 20/20–20/40 line is shown on the eye chart. If the patient reports that both images have similar clarity, this would prove the level of visual acuity.[31] The key component of this test is placing the prism over the *good* eye, so the patient is not aware that the poorer-seeing eye is being tested.

Red-green duochrome test: The patient is given red-green glasses and told that the following is a test of color vision. A red-green duochrome chart is then displayed and the patient is asked to read it. The eye behind the green lens will only perceive the green portion of the chart and the eye behind the red lens will only perceive the red portion of the chart. If the patient is able to read both sides of the chart, the Snellen acuity correlating with the displayed characters is confirmed for both eyes.[32]

Visual Field Loss

The previously described techniques assess only central visual acuity and may not useful or applicable when the primary issue is visual field loss. Heightened suspicion for FVL in these scenarios often can be gleaned by close observation of how the patient navigates the initial encounter and the clinic surroundings. The ability to grab a doorknob, find a hand to shake, or maneuver around a desk or chair may provide evidence for preserved peripheral vision. Visual field testing can be used both to confirm a functional component and to prove normal fields in each eye.

The classic pattern of functional visual field loss is "tubular" or "gun-barrel". This is nonphysiologic, as the normal field of vision is a cone, with highest sensitivity at the apex (fovea) and lowest sensitivity at the base (peripheral retina). So-called "tubular" visual fields can be demonstrated even with confrontation perimetry: the diameter of the visual field should expand with increased distance from the patient. Confrontation perimetry is performed at 1 m and then at 2–3 m. If the visual field remains severely constricted, this indicates a functional, nonphysiologic pattern.[23]

Static and kinetic perimetry: Visual field testing can be utilized to show incongruity between endorsed visual field loss and what the patient is able to perceive. Automated perimetry has limited utility for most patients with FVL, since functional patterns can mimic pathologic defects on HVF.[4,33] This can include hemifield defects, arcuate defects, and bitemporal hemianopias. In many of these cases, the reliability indices will be normal, and as such, they are not useful in differentiating functional from pathologic field loss. The one exception is central scotoma: Scott et al. showed that central scotoma only rarely occurs in FVL, and should raise suspicion for optic neuropathy or maculopathy (Figs. 97.2 and 97.3).[12]

Certain patterns highly suggestive of FVL are best seen with manual perimetry (usually Goldmann kinetic perimetry or a tangent screen) and a skilled technician operating the machine. Patterns such as spiraling, crossed, or inversion of isopters are classic functional patterns (Figs. 97.4 and 97.5), but manifest only as constricted visual fields on automated perimetry (Fig. 97.6).[4] Spiraling of isopters on Goldmann visual field describes the lack of constancy when the same isopter stimulus is retested in the same relative quadrant. Crossed isopters describe overlap between different stimuli of varying sizes and intensities, another indicator for nonorganic visual field loss. These findings are not consistent with organic visual field loss.

For suspected functional, bitemporal, or temporal hemianopic field loss, binocular visual fields can also prove a functional component, as most patients are unaware of the overlapping nasal fields between the two eyes. Persistence of a temporal hemianopic defect under binocular viewing conditions indicates nonphysiologic field loss (Figs. 97.7A to C).

Saccade testing and finger-to-nose perimetry: All of the above techniques indicate a functional, nonphysiologic pattern, but do not prove normal fields. Accurate saccades

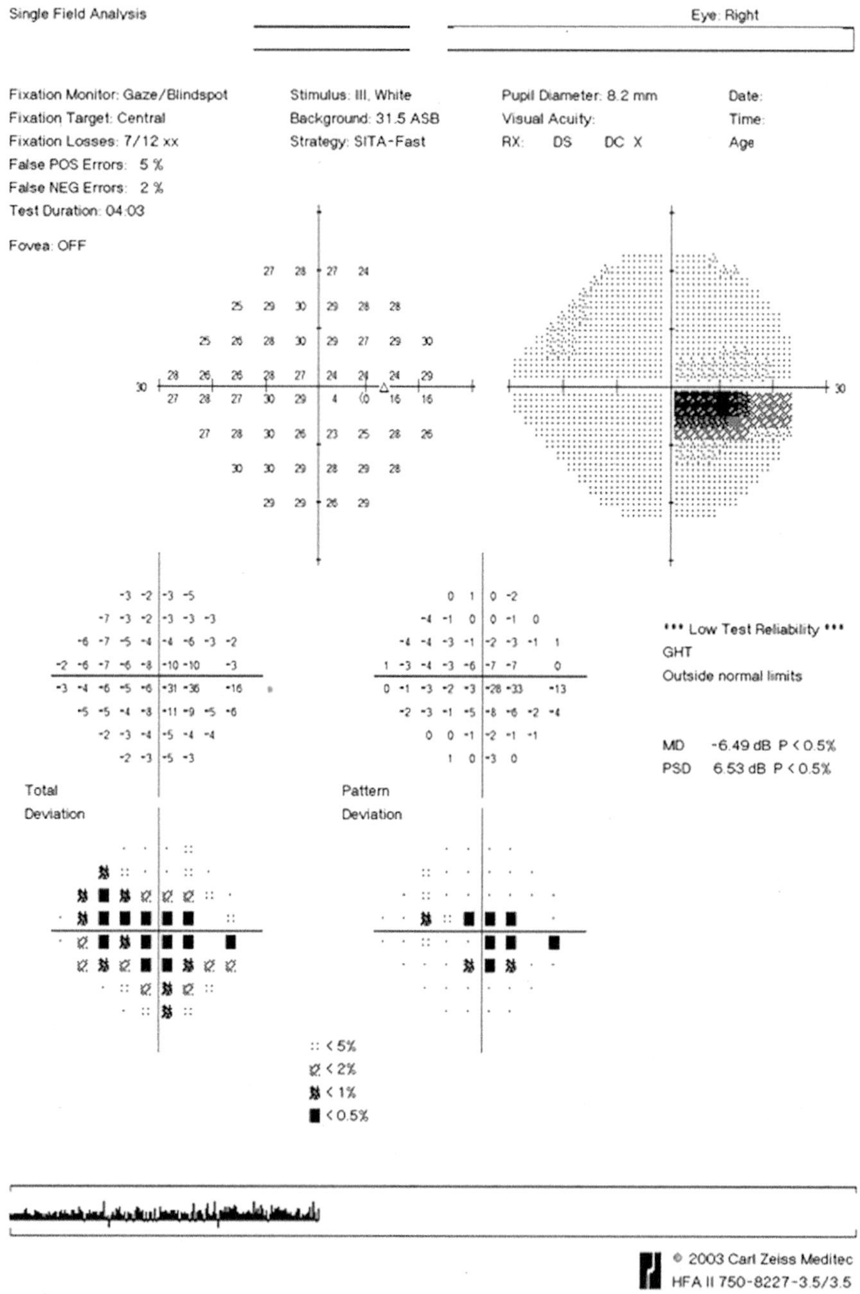

Fig. 97.2: Humphrey visual field (HVF) with central/cecocentral scotoma of the right eye. The visual field testing shows a central/cecocentral scotoma and multiple fixation losses with otherwise preserved peripheral vision.

to target in all four peripheral quadrants indicate grossly normal fields. This test should be performed monocularly for the most accurate results, with a reasonable premise being that the examiner is going to test how each eye moves independently.

Another option is to have the patient mimic hand movements (finger waggling, waving) in the periphery while staring ahead. The patient is told that you will be checking their coordination, and they may not realize that visual fields are being tested as well.

Finally, finger-to-nose perimetry can help verify normal fields. The patient is instructed to fixate on the clinician's nose, then to alternate touching the clinician's outstretched finger and the patient's nose, again after informing the patient you are testing coordination. Accurate finger-to-nose testing indicates grossly normal peripheral fields.

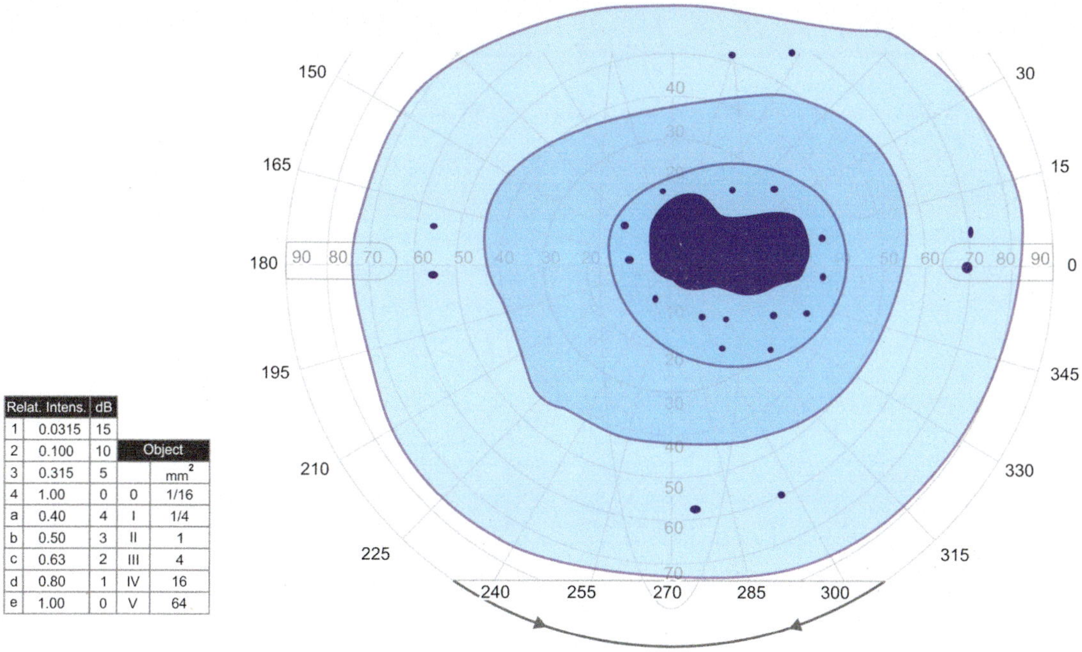

Fig. 97.3: Goldmann visual fields (GVF) with cecocentral scotoma of the left eye. The visual field testing is remarkable for a cecocentral scotoma with otherwise preserved peripheral vision.

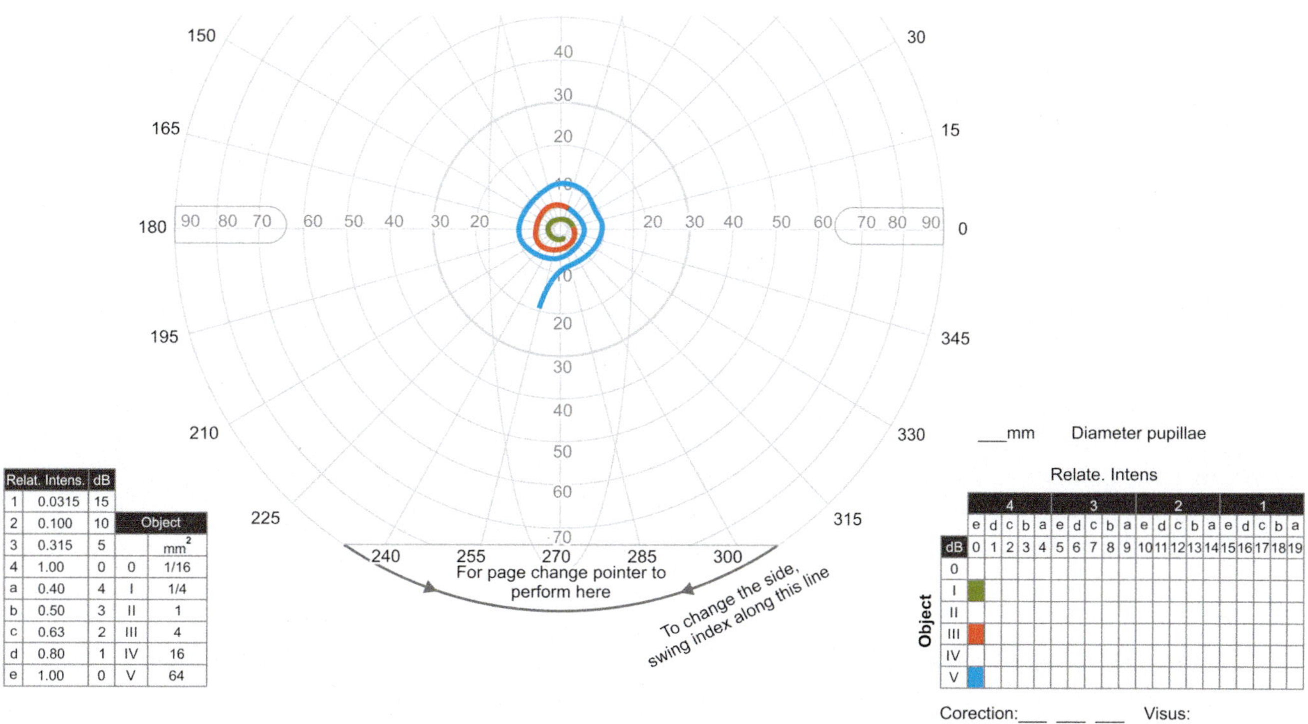

Fig. 97.4: Goldmann visual field with spiraling isopters of the right eye. Spiraling of isopters shows inconsistency with the same isopter tested in the same quadrant of vision. This pattern is not consistent with organic vision loss.

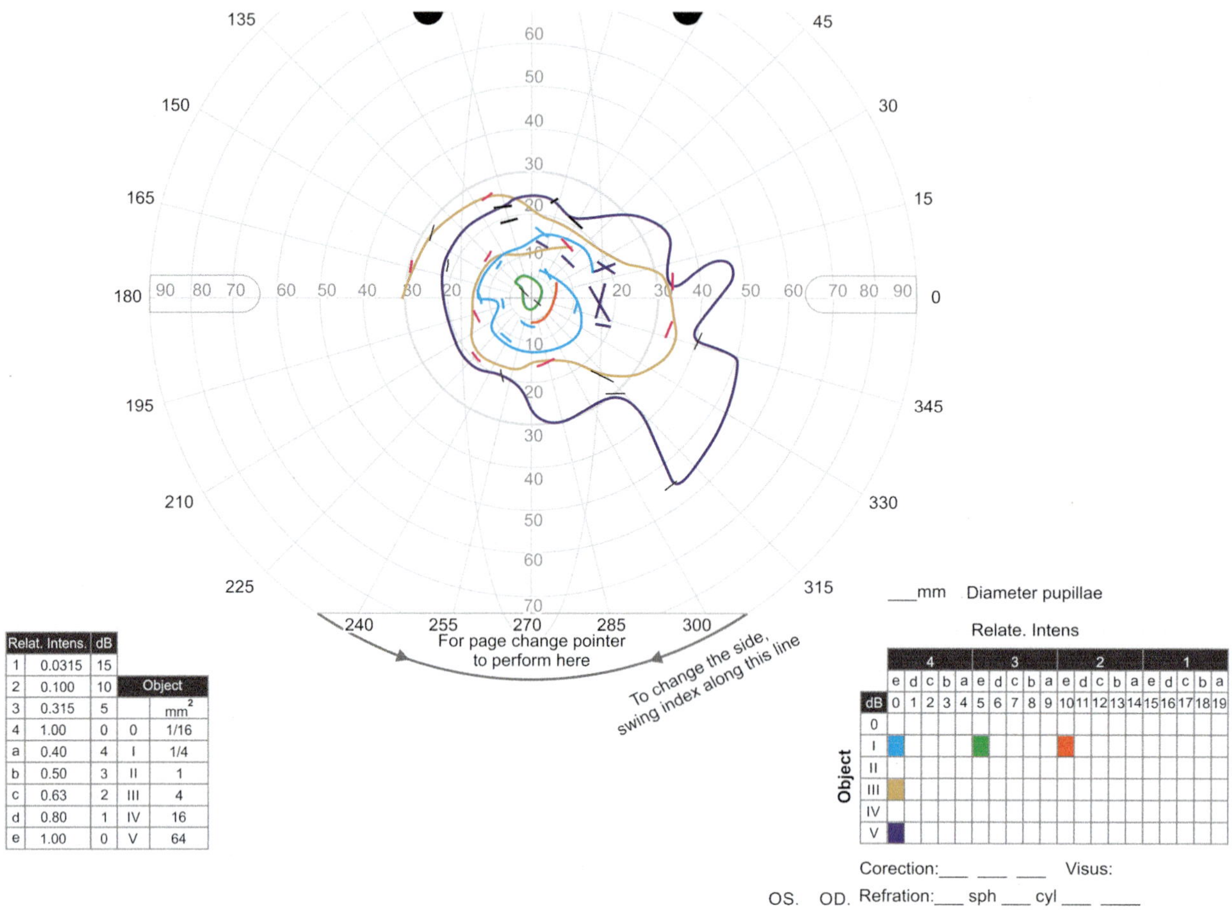

Fig. 97.5: Goldmann visual field with crossed and spiraling isopters of the right eye. The visual field testing shows multiple spiraling isopters (I4e and III4e) as well as crossing of multiple isopters. Physiologic visual field loss would demonstrate intraisopter constancy (no spiraling) and interisopter separation (no crossed isopters).

DIFFERENTIAL DIAGNOSIS

With careful observation, history taking, and the clinical examination techniques outlined above, the diagnosis of FVL can be confirmed in the majority of patients. However, in some patients, only better than claimed (not normal) visual function can be proven, and there is still the possibility of combined functional and organic visual loss.

Central lesions (e.g. neoplasm, stroke) that affect both the visual axis and behavioral centers may also produce a functional flavor to the examination, as previously discussed. Similarly, macular diseases can occasionally mimic optic neuropathy and present with a relatively normal fundus examination. Central serous chorioretinopathy may present with both visual and psychiatric symptoms, as vision loss is often preceded by some form of severe psychological stress.[34] Other retinal pathologies to consider include acute zonal occult outer retinopathy (AZOOR), cancer-associated retinopathy (CAR), and cone dystrophies. These can present with notable vision loss, but a normal fundus examination early on in the disease process.[35]

In these cases, a high index of suspicion combined with neuroimaging, optical coherence tomography (OCT), fundus autofluorescence (FAF), and retinal electrophysiology can often help to confirm the diagnosis, as described here.

Workup

Although some workup is indicated for many patients with FVL, the clinician must exercise caution and restrain when ordering ancillary tests. Doing so, limits the burden on the

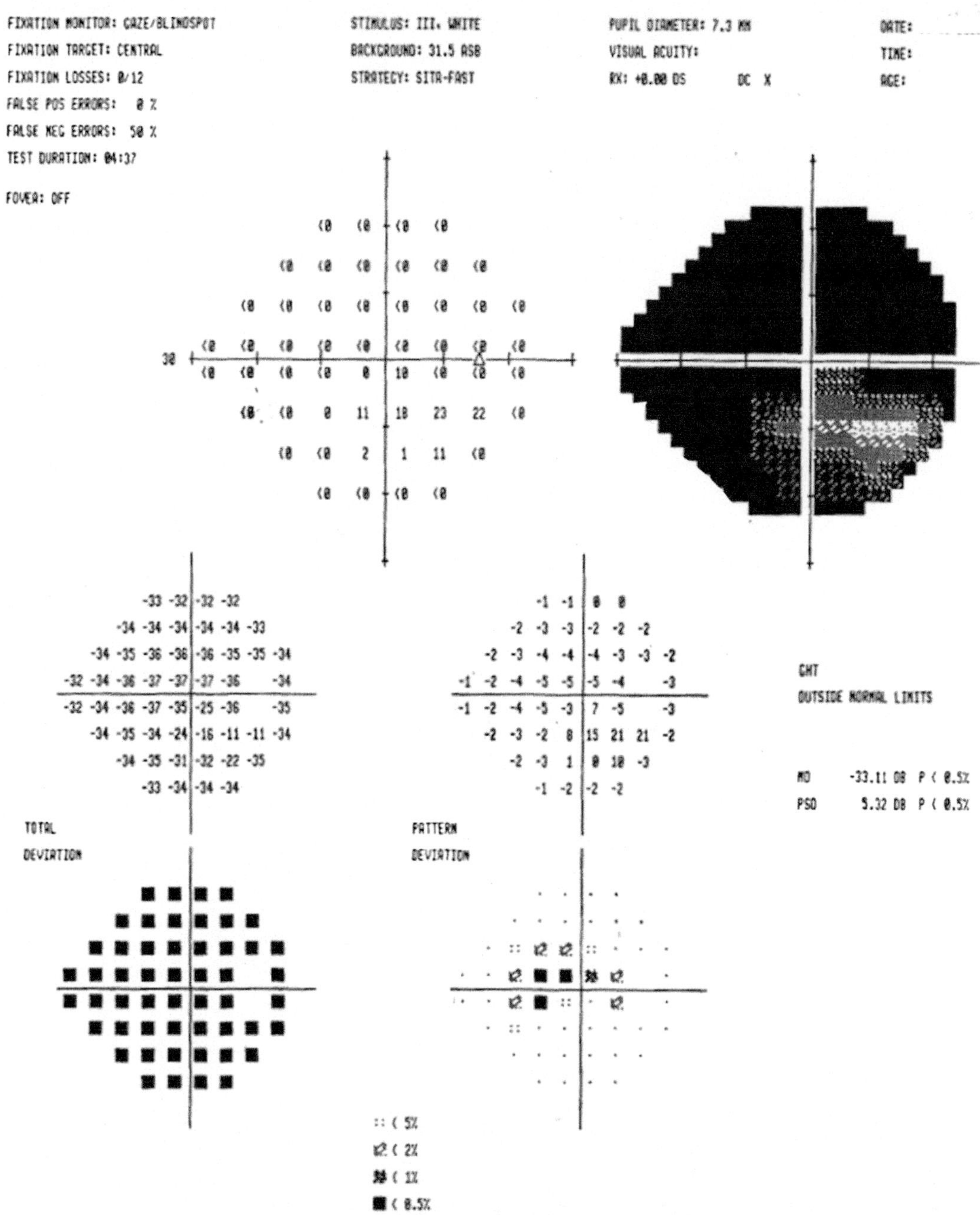

Fig. 97.6: Global depression on Humphrey visual field testing. Functional vision loss that presents with dense visual acuity or visual field deficits will tend to show global depression on automated perimetry. The utility of these testing results is minimal in such a setting and a Goldmann visual field may be more appropriate.

medical system as well as avoids reinforcing the "sick role", which may act as barrier to recovery. Over-testing may strengthen a patient's belief that their vision loss is due to a true organic cause, provoking anxiety and hindering recovery. An "exhaustive" workup is usually unnecessary and may result in false-positive results or insignificant incidental findings.

If normal visual acuity and visual fields are proven with a low suspicion for central disease, then no specific workup is indicated. If normal visual function cannot be proven, however, then selective testing may be warranted. Localizing the suspected source of vision loss (optic nerve, retina, visual cortex) will help guide the workup. An MRI of the brain and orbits with and without contrast is often the

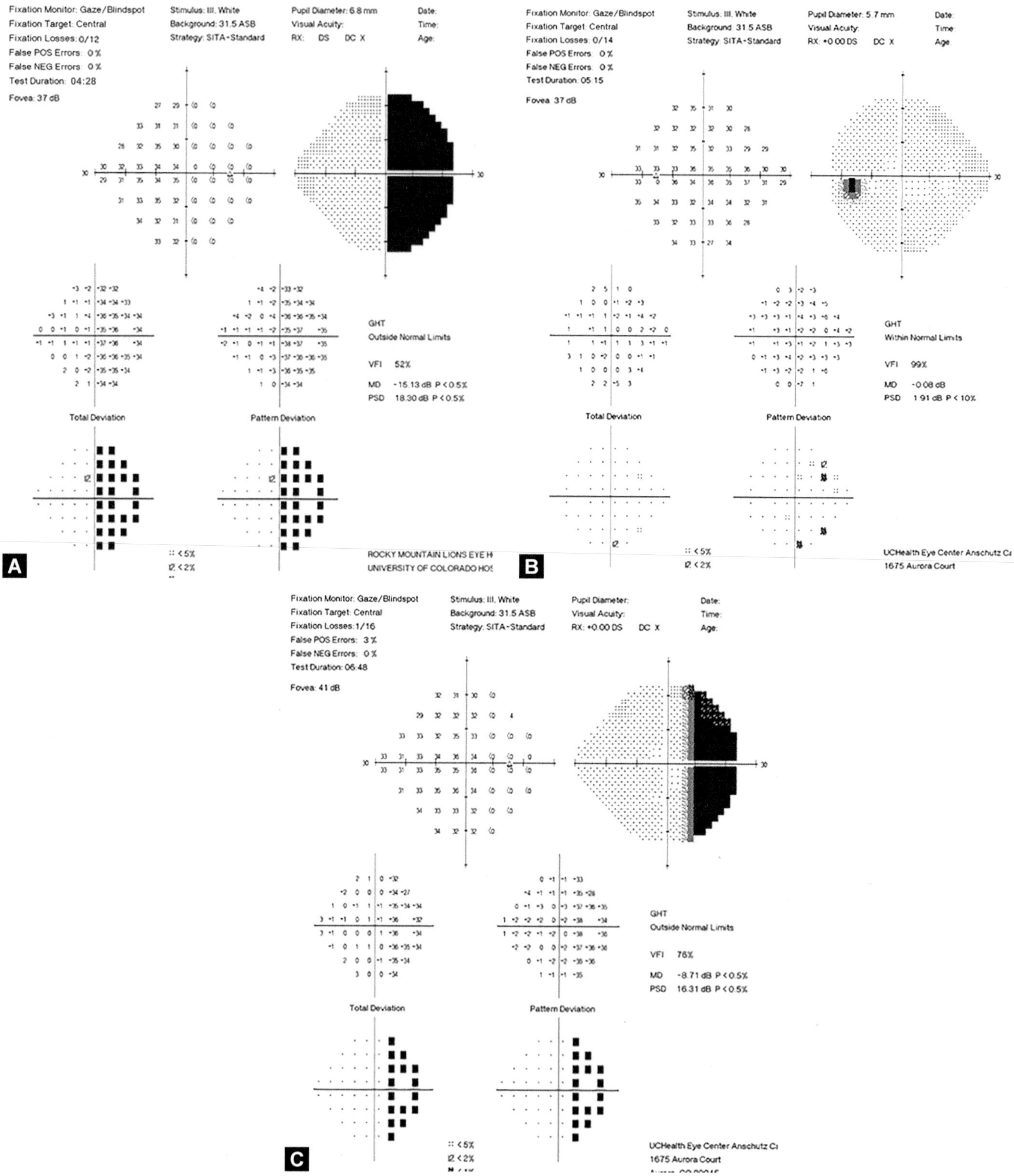

Figs. 97.7A to C: Monocular temporal hemianopia on HVF testing. (A) The patient had a complete temporal scotoma on HVF testing right eye and also claimed an identical defect on confrontation; (B) The left eye was normal on monocular testing; (C) When both eyes were tested together, a right-sided defect was seen as a nonphysiologic scotoma under binocular viewing conditions.

study of choice in these scenarios. If the study is abnormal, consider whether or not the findings explain the vision loss described.

Office-based testing such as OCT, FAF, and electroretinography (ERG) may be helpful to rule out optic nerve or retinal/macular pathology, particularly when stable and unchanged over time. For example, long-standing severe visual loss with normal retinal nerve fiber layer on OCT would argue against severe optic neuropathy. Normal FAF indicates a healthy retinal pigment epithelium and argues against widespread photoreceptor dysfunction. Some electrophysiologic tests (pattern visual evoked potential and multifocal ERG) are heavily dependent upon fixation and cooperation, so abnormal results must be viewed cautiously in patients with suspected FVL. These particular studies are most useful when completely normal.

MANAGEMENT/TREATMENT

The treatment of functional visual loss is generally supportive in nature. The exact methods for revealing the diagnosis and counseling the patient often vary among clinicians, but maintaining a strong physician-patient relationship is of the utmost importance. Patients should be given the opportunity to voice any recent stressors, whether related to relationships, finances, abuse, work, schooling, or recent trauma, as this may give insight into any psychosocial factors which may be provoking or perpetuating the patient's symptoms. Direct confrontation is typically not advised, as this may result in a loss of therapeutic relationship.

In our practice, we often begin by giving the patients their diagnosis, that of FVL. We reassure the patient that the visual system appears to be structurally intact or minimally damaged (if coexisting organic disease is present), but verbally validate that their symptoms are currently manifesting as more severe than expected. The portions of the examination that suggest better than perceived vision are reviewed and described as encouraging findings that suggest ongoing recovery or stability in their vision. Expressing experience and familiarity with the symptoms and prognosis of functional visual loss may also provide reassurance to the patient that their symptoms are not merely feigned or "made up". This is usually more productive than stating that there is "no explanation" for the symptoms they have. Expressing a reasonable expectation for gradual recovery may also help alleviate anxiety related to waiting for a rapid recovery, which is rare. We also suggest treatment of any comorbid conditions such as chronic migraine or ocular surface disease, if present, as patients with these conditions may also perceive their vision to be worse than actually measured.

Follow-up is important, as patients initially thought to have FVL may be later discovered to have an organic etiology on neuroimaging, or after additional symptoms evolve. For example, the optic atrophy found in LHON should develop in 4–8 weeks, with subsequent evolution of an afferent pupillary defect in the affected eye.[25]

Previous studies have explored the role of formal psychiatric intervention in patients with FVL. These studies have often shown inconsistent results, however, likely due to the variable underlying stressors and motivations provoking or perpetuating the patient's symptoms, as well as the heterogeneous nature of the provided therapies.[14] If undertaken, we suggest referring the patient to a trusted provider and formulating a specific diagnosis and treatment plan to be addressed based the patient's verbalized insight or psychiatric comorbidity, rather than referring simply for FVL.

CONCLUSION

In summary, we reiterate that the diagnosis of FVL should often be a diagnosis of CONclusion rather than one of EXclusion. By utilizing both direct and indirect quantitative and qualitative measures of vision, the examining physician should be able to arrive at an estimated level of true visual function, which should guide the next steps in imaging and ancillary testing. The management and treatment of functional visual loss is controversial, but often centers around patient reassurance and adequate follow-up to exclude comorbid conditions. We recommend becoming familiar with the various techniques described in this chapter so that they can be naturally deployed in the clinic setting as needed.

REFERENCES

1. Kathol RG, Cox TA, Corbett JJ, et al. Functional visual loss: I. A true psychiatric disorder? Psychol Med. 1983;13(2): 307-14.
2. Miller NR. Functional neuro-ophthalmology. Handb Clin Neurol. 2011;102:493-513.
3. Monbeck ME. The Meaning of Blindness: Attitudes Toward Blindness and Blind People. Bloomington: Indiana University Press, 1973.
4. Egan RA, LaFrance WC Jr. Functional vision disorder. Semin Neurol. 2015;35(5):557-63.

5. Bogousslavsky J, Dieguez S. Sigmund Freud and hysteria: the etiology of psychoanalysis? Front Neurol Neurosci. 2014;35:109-25.
6. American Psychiatric Association. Diagnostic and Statistical Manual of Mental Disorders, 5th edition. Arlington, VA: American Psychiatric Association Publishing; 2013.
7. Incesu AI, Sobaci G. Malingering or simulation in ophthalmology-visual acuity. Int J Ophthalmol. 2011;4(5):558-66.
8. Thompson HS. Functional visual loss. Am J Ophthalmol. 1985;100(1):209-13.
9. Schoenfeld MA, Hassa T, Hopf JM, et al. Neural correlates of hysterical blindness. Cereb Cortex. 2011;21(10):2394-8.
10. Werring DJ, Weston L, Bullmore ET, et al. Functional magnetic resonance imaging of the cerebral response to visual stimulation in medically unexplained visual loss. Psychol Med. 2004;34(4):583-9.
11. Stone J. The bare essentials: functional symptoms in neurology. Pract Neurol. 2009;9(3):179-89.
12. Scott JA, Egan RA. Prevalence of organic neuro-ophthalmologic disease in patients with functional visual loss. Am J Ophthalmol. 2003;135(5):670-5.
13. Cello KE, Keltner JL, Johnson CA, et al. Factors affecting visual field outcomes in the idiopathic intracranial hypertension treatment trial. J Neuroophthalmol. 2016;36(1):6-12.
14. Bruce BB, Newman NJ. Functional visual loss. Neurol Clin. 2010;28(3):789-802.
15. Crutch SJ, Lehmann M, Schott JM, et al. Posterior cortical atrophy. Lancet Neurol. 2012;11(2):170-8.
16. Beh SC, Muthusamy B, Calabresi P, et al. Hiding in plain sight: a closer look at posterior cortical atrophy. Pract Neurol. 2015;15(1):5-13.
17. McClelland C, Van Stavern GP, Shepherd JB, et al. Neuroimaging in patients referred to a neuro-ophthalmology service: the rates of appropriateness and concordance in interpretation. Ophthalmology. 2012;119(8):1701-4.
18. O'Hara M. Cracking the crock: how to deal with factitious eye disease. J Ophthalmic Nurs Technol. 1998;17(5):188-92.
19. Benbadis SR. Hypergraphia and the diagnosis of psychogenic attacks. Neurology. 2006;67(5):904.
20. Bengtzen R, Woodward M, Lynn MJ, et al. The "sunglasses sign" predicts nonorganic visual loss in neuro-ophthalmologic practice. Neurology. 2008;70(3):218-21.
21. Stone J, Smyth R, Carson A, et al. La belle indifférence in conversion symptoms and hysteria: systematic review. Br J Psychiatry. 2006;188:204-9.
22. Kung NH, Bartlett NL, Yaseen NR, et al. A young woman with blurred vision and distal paresthesias. JAMA Neurol. 2015;72(12):1519-23.
23. Enzenauer R, Morris W, O'Donnell T, Montrey J (Eds). Functional Ophthalmic Disorders: Ocular Malingering and Visual Hysteria. New York: Springer; 2014.
24. Gold AE, Marshall SM. Cortical blindness and cerebral infarction associated with severe hypoglycemia. Diabetes Care. 1996;19(9):1001-3.
25. Meyerson C, Van Stavern G, McClelland C. Leber hereditary optic neuropathy: current perspectives. Clin Ophthalmol. 2015;9:1165-76.
26. Millodot M, Miller D, Jernigan ME. Evaluation of an objective acuity device. Arch Ophthalmol. 1973;90(6): 449-52.
27. Levy AH, McCulley TJ, Lam BL, et al. Estimating visual acuity by character counting using the Snellen visual acuity chart. Eye (Lond). 2005;19(6):622-4.
28. Levy NS, Glick EB. Stereoscopic perception and Snellen visual acuity. Am J Ophthalmol. 1974;78:722-4.
29. Sitko KR, Peragallo JH, Bidot S, et al. Pitfalls in the use of stereoacuity in the diagnosis of nonorganic visual loss. Ophthalmology. 2016;123(1):198-202.
30. Flaxel CJ, Samples JR, Dustin L. Relationship between foveal threshold and visual acuity using the Humphrey visual field analyzer. Am J Ophthalmol. 2007;143(5):875-7.
31. Golnik KC, Lee AG, Eggenberger ER. The monocular vertical prism dissociation test. Am J Ophthalmol. 2004;137(1): 135-7.
32. Ing EB, Younge BR, Leavitt JA, et al. Functional visual loss and the duochrome test. Can J Ophthalmol. 1995;30:35-6.
33. Stewart JF. Automated perimetry and malingerers. Can the Humphrey be outwitted? Ophthalmology. 1995;102(1): 27-32.
34. Gelber GS, Schatz H. Loss of vision due to central serous chorioretinopathy following psychological stress. Am J Psychiatry. 1987;144:46-50.
35. Heckenlively JR, Ferreyra HA. Autoimmune retinopathy: a review and summary. Semin Immunopathol. 2008;30(2): 127-34.

Chapter 98 Topical Diagnosis of Visual Field Loss

Kimberly M Winges, Imran Jivraj

INTRODUCTION TO VISUAL FIELD TESTING

Visual field testing is an essential and highly localizing component of the neuro-ophthalmic examination. An understanding of the exquisite correlations between the neuroanatomy of the visual pathways and the corresponding patterns of visual field loss enables the clinician to identify the likely site of a lesion. While a patient may be aware of a decline in visual acuity, loss of peripheral visual field may not be as apparent to the patient, particularly when it is insidious. Patterns of visual field loss assist the clinician in localizing the site of pathology to the eye, optic nerve, or particular locations along the intracranial visual pathways. Thus, obtaining a formal visual field is often the clinician's "next step" in clarifying a patient's complaint of vision loss.

Formal visual field testing establishes the pattern of visual field loss, but it must be interpreted in the context of the clinical history and additional findings of the eye examination. A careful examination of the retina and optic nerve may clarify the etiology of the scotoma: an arcuate visual field defect with corresponding notching of the optic disk in a patient with elevated intraocular pressure would suggest a glaucomatous process. When no causative lesion is found on ophthalmic examination, the visual field is essential to localize the lesion more posteriorly in the visual pathways. For instance, the complaint of "difficulty reading" may present with normal visual acuities and a normal ophthalmic examination, but visual field testing may reveal a homonymous hemianopia, localizing the lesion posterior to the chiasm. Even when the clinician has identified an ophthalmic cause for visual field loss such as a visually significant cataract, correlation with the visual field results might suggest that another lesion is responsible for the patient's symptoms, such as a pituitary macroadenoma causing bitemporal hemianopia. Patients may also describe visual field loss that they interpret to be monocular in origin ("left eye") but in actuality represents bilateral visual field loss (left homonymous hemianopia). Thus, the clinician is encouraged, whenever possible, to test the visual field of each eye, even when the complaint appears to be monocular.

Visual fields are also commonly performed as part of clinical surveillance for retinal conditions, optic neuropathies, and lesions along the visual pathways. They are used to screen for treatment-related visual loss, as in the case of hydroxychloroquine or vigabatrin toxicity.[1,2] Visual field studies offer insight about a patient's suitability for certain work environments, driving, and eligibility for vision rehabilitation strategies or disability reimbursement. In addition, they allow the clinician to clarify the diagnosis of functional vision loss based on demonstration of nonphysiologic responses during testing.

Characteristics of the Human Visual Field

The human monocular visual field is best represented by the concept of a "hill of vision", which describes the variable sensitivity of the retina, highest at the fovea and declining toward the retinal periphery (Fig. 98.1). It is tested under predetermined background luminance, which is important because the sensitivity of the retina changes under different lighting conditions. The increased density of cone photoreceptors within the macula offers a heightened sensitivity to visual stimuli under photopic conditions. The fovea, the point of maximal retinal sensitivity under photopic conditions, is responsible for the resolution and clarity of central vision. In contrast, under scotopic conditions, the mid-peripheral retina has the highest sensitivity because of the increasing density of rod photoreceptors found 15–20° from the fovea.[3]

The monocular visual field extends approximately 90° temporally, 70° inferiorly, and 50–60° nasally and superiorly.[4] Approximately 15° temporally and slightly inferior to the point of fixation on the visual field lies the physiologic blind spot, which is an absolute scotoma of approximately 7.5° in diameter. This scotoma is produced

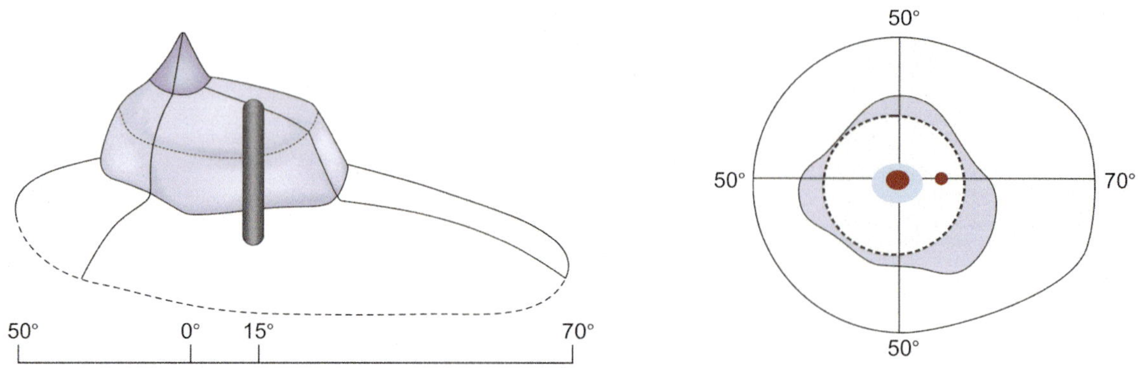

Fig. 98.1: Hill of vision. Traquair described the three-dimensional visual field as "an island of vision surrounded by a sea of blindness". The central area of the visual field is most sensitive; small dim objects are easily seen. The most peripheral portions of the visual field are least sensitive; objects must be large and bright to be visualized. Outside the borders of the visual field, no visual perception occurs. This figure illustrates Traquair's island of the right eye (OD) as viewed from the side (left image). The peak represents area of greatest sensitivity, as determined by perception of a dim and small stimulus. The base is the area of least sensitivity, as seen by perception of large and bright objects. Altitude from top to bottom is scale of increasing stimulation. The blind spot, an absolute scotoma, is depicted as a "well." Traquair's island as viewed from above appears as a topographic map (right image). Contours are mapped by concentric circles, each representing a single target. Blind spot (seen as a dark well) is 15° temporal of central fixation.

by the optic nerve head, where axons of the retinal nerve fiber layer (RNFL) exit the intraocular space, and where there are no photoreceptors.

Clinical Testing of the Visual Field: Testing to Confrontation

Visual field testing to confrontation should be performed routinely during the ophthalmic examination. It is particularly useful in patients who cannot position for a formal visual field, or who are too young, inattentive, or cognitively impaired to cooperate with automated testing. Visual field testing to confrontation is accomplished with the use of fingers, a red test object, or other moving targets; *see* Chapter 90, The Neuro-Ophthalmic Examination, for further details. An Amsler grid, when held 25–40 cm in front of the tested eye, is also an easily accessible office tool for identifying metamorphopsia or visual field loss within the central 8°, such as in small macular or posterior occipital lesions (Fig. 98.2).[5]

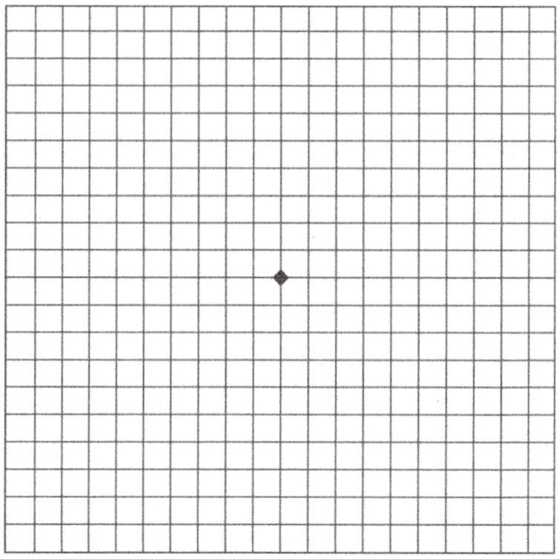

Fig. 98.2: Amsler grid. The Amsler grid displays a central point for fixation within a 10 cm square, enclosing a 20 × 20 grid of 5 mm squares. It is available in high contrast white on black (shown), black on white, red on black, and other variations. When viewed at approximately 1/3 of a meter, each small square subtends a visual angle of 1°. The patient is instructed to wear reading correction and cover one eye, while keeping the other fixated on the central point. The patient notes any scotoma, distortions, or metamorphopsia within the grid lines that indicate pathology within the central 20° of vision of each eye individually (Keeler Limited, Windsor, Berkshire).

Clinical Testing of the Visual Field: Perimetry

More sophisticated visual field testing is indicated among patients whose presenting complaint involves a loss of central or peripheral vision. There are three conceptual visual field testing strategies: threshold static and/or kinetic testing (quantitative) and suprathreshold static testing (screening). Static perimetry is performed by presenting stationary flashes of light stimuli of varying size and luminance at different points in the visual field, using age-appropriate near correction within the central 30°. The patient indicates a response using a handheld remote. By presenting stimuli of increasing brightness until a response is elicited, and then reducing the luminance in smaller increments until the response is lost, a threshold of sensitivity of each retinal location can be established. Various static automated perimetry algorithms have been designed to maximize the area of tested retina while minimizing the duration of the test to avoid fatigue and artifacts.[4] This chapter will provide an overview of the most commonly-used clinical perimetry modalities.

The Humphrey visual field (HVF) analyzer (Carl Zeiss Meditec Inc., Dublin, CA) is currently the most widely-used static automated perimetry device, with the Octopus automated perimeter (Haag-Streit USA) also performing similar tests. The threshold value is presented in units of decibels and indicates the stimulus intensity at which there is a 50% probability of perception, representing the lowest intensity a patient can detect. Since the fovea normally has the highest threshold intensity of any location across the retina, it will therefore detect the dimmest stimuli in a healthy eye (corresponding to higher decibel values).[4]

Humphrey visual field testing requires an alert and cooperative patient who has sufficient motor skills to be able to indicate a response during an automated test. HVF testing may be performed on the central 30° (30-2) or 24° (24-2) on either side of fixation (Fig. 98.3). The HVF 24-2 SITA Standard testing strategy was designed to identify and follow glaucomatous visual field loss and omits the inferior nasal and superior nasal rims of the full threshold 30-2 test that are especially prone to artifact, thereby increasing reliability and decreasing testing time.[6] These tests are sensitive in defining the pattern of visual field loss in the central field, which is affected by most disease processes, but they do not test the far periphery. A specialized test of the central 10° (10-2) on either side of fixation may be more useful when following central points among patients with advanced visual field loss encroaching upon fixation, particularly those in whom 30-2 or 24-2 tests already demonstrate severe peripheral loss. The HVF 10-2 strategy is also the visual field test of choice in identifying scotoma within the central 10°.

Kinetic visual field tests employ a moving target of a fixed luminance and size to trace the patient's entire visual field, starting from the nonseeing to seeing areas. The patient who maintains fixation centrally indicates that they have identified the target by clicking a remote

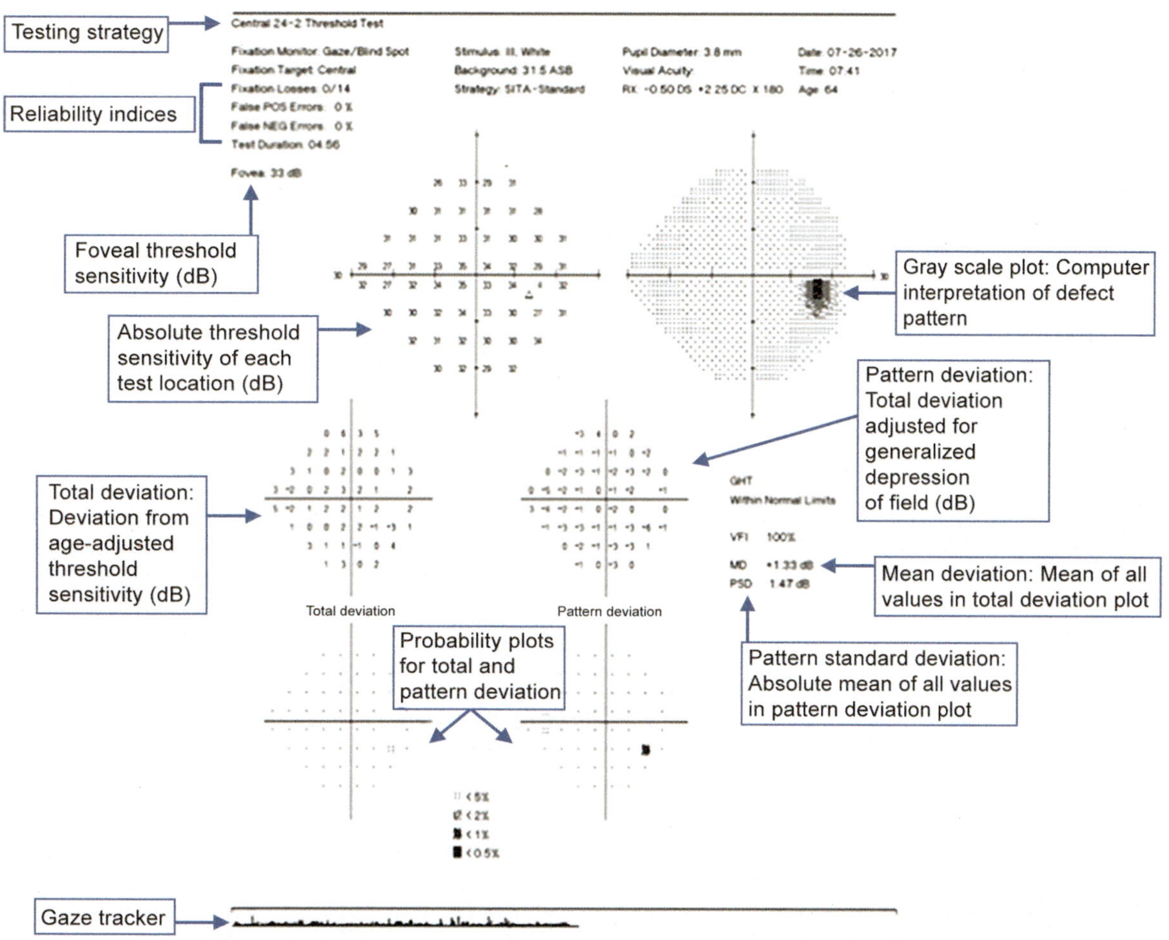

Fig. 98.3: Example of static automated perimetry. This Humphrey visual field (HVF) example shows a normal HVF 24-2 Sita Standard printout. Detailed are the various components for correct interpretation and assessment of field reliability.

or speaking. By projecting successively less intense targets, zones of similar retinal sensitivity (isopters) can be plotted to describe a patient's entire visual field.

Clinical visual field techniques incorporating a kinetic approach include the manual Goldmann perimeter, automated kinetic testing (e.g. Octopus Perimeter, Haag-Streit USA), and tangent screen.

Goldmann visual field (GVF) perimetry is a manual method of perimetry whereby a trained technician (perimetrist) uses both dynamic and static techniques (spot-checking) to produce a two-dimensional representation of a patient's entire "hill of vision", potentially identifying peripheral defects that would not be captured with a 24° or 30° HVF (Fig. 98.4). Targets of size and luminance that vary on a logarithmic scale are denoted by a combination of a Roman numeral indicating increasing stimulus size (I-V, corresponding to dots measuring 0.62–64 mm²) and an Arabic numeral and letter indicating increasing luminance (1-4, a-e) of the stimulus.[7] A very large and intense stimulus (e.g. V4e) can be used to map the remaining visual field of patient with advanced visual field depression who would be unable to detect a smaller (e.g. III4e) or dimmer (V3b) stimulus. GVF is invaluable in evaluating visual field loss among patients with reduced attention because the operator is constantly monitoring fixation and can provide encouragement or offer reinforcement throughout the test. Nonphysiologic patterns of visual field loss suggesting a functional disorder, such as "spiralling of isopters" may be more easily identified on GVFs (*see* Chapter 97, Functional Vision Loss). However, GVF perimetry is time-consuming and dependent on a skilled operator, and it does not provide quantitative output that can be statistically analyzed for longitudinal progression.

Reliability parameters: The interpretation of a visual field must take into consideration the reliability of the test. On HVF testing, four reliability indices should be reviewed (Fig. 98.3). "Fixation losses" are identified when the patient responds to a stimulus presented within the location of the physiologic blind spot; a rate of less than 20% is preferred.[7] "False-positive" responses occur when the patient indicates

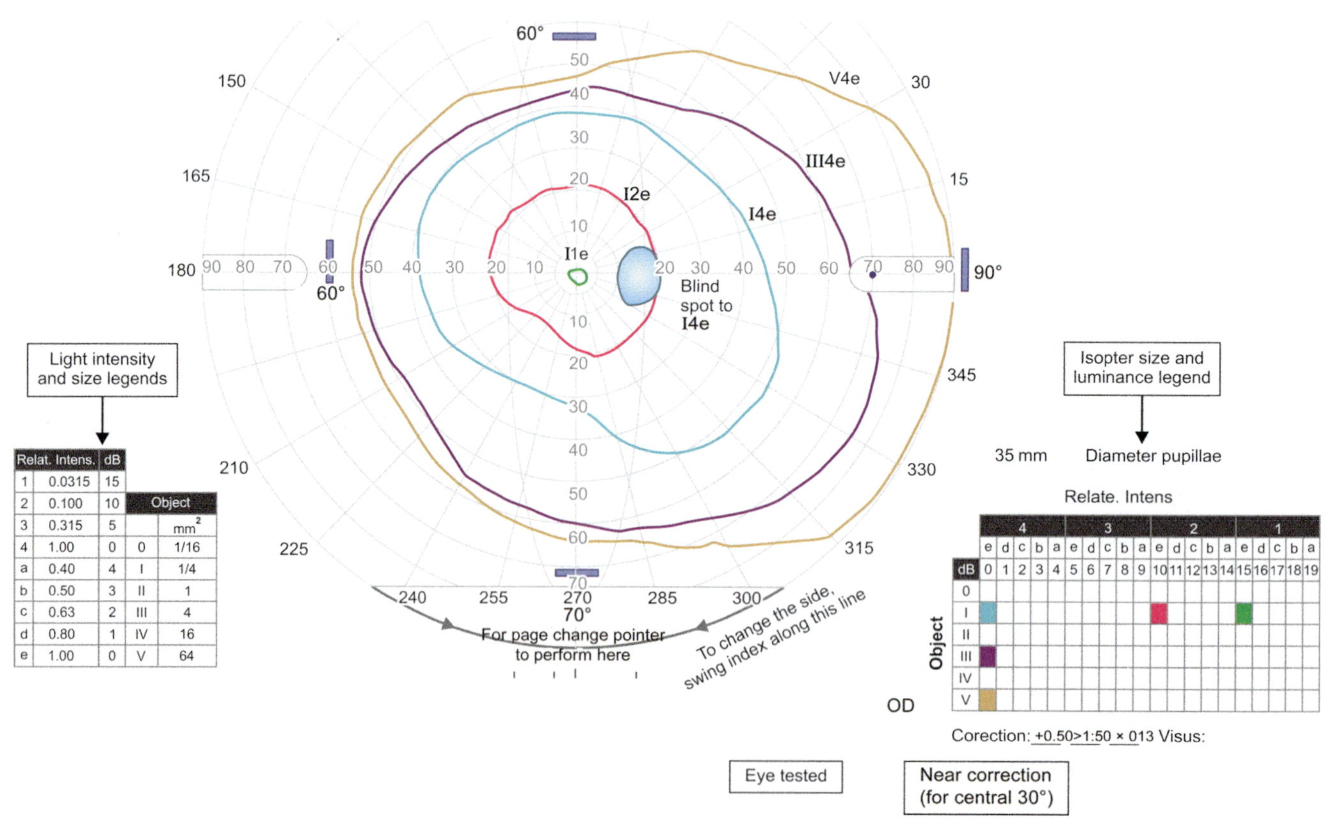

Fig. 98.4: Example of manual kinetic perimetry. This normal Goldmann visual field (GVF) details the various components for correct interpretation. Isopters of varying size and intensity trace the periphery of seeing field from non-seeing to seeing areas, with additional static testing as needed. Scotomas are colored in (example, blind spot). The full visual field subtends approximately 90° temporally, 70° inferiorly, and 60° nasally and superiorly to the largest and brightest target, the V4e isopter.

a response in the absence of a stimulus. "False-negative" responses occur when a patient fails to respond to a stimulus of greater intensity than the previously established threshold of sensitivity at the same retinal location.[6] For a test to be considered reliable, false-positive and false-negative errors should ideally occur at a rate of less than 33%, although false-negative errors are known to increase among patients with severe visual field loss, such as advanced glaucoma.[8] Finally, gaze tracking shows positive deflections during misalignment (such as fixation losses or head movement) and negative deflections during loss of the corneal light reflex (such as blinking, dry eye, or falling asleep).[6]

Artifacts in visual field testing: Artifacts may result in patterns of visual field loss that mimic true disease of the visual pathways. Upper eyelid ptosis or dermatochalasis may produce superior visual field loss. In such cases, repeating the visual field study after taping the eyelids or lifting the overhanging skin would provide clarification.[7,9] Improper refractive correction, significant miosis or mydriasis, and/or cataracts may produce global depression of a visual field. Rim artifact represents dense defects at the edge of the field from the trial lens rim, seen in decentered eyes, excessive vertex distance to the lens which decreases the effective lens aperture, or high hyperopic correction. High myopia may produce visual field defects that appear to be neurologic in origin by causing artificially decreased sensitivity or enlarged blind spots from significant associated peripapillary atrophy; thus, careful correction for refractive status and positioning at the time of testing is crucial (Fig. 98.5).[6]

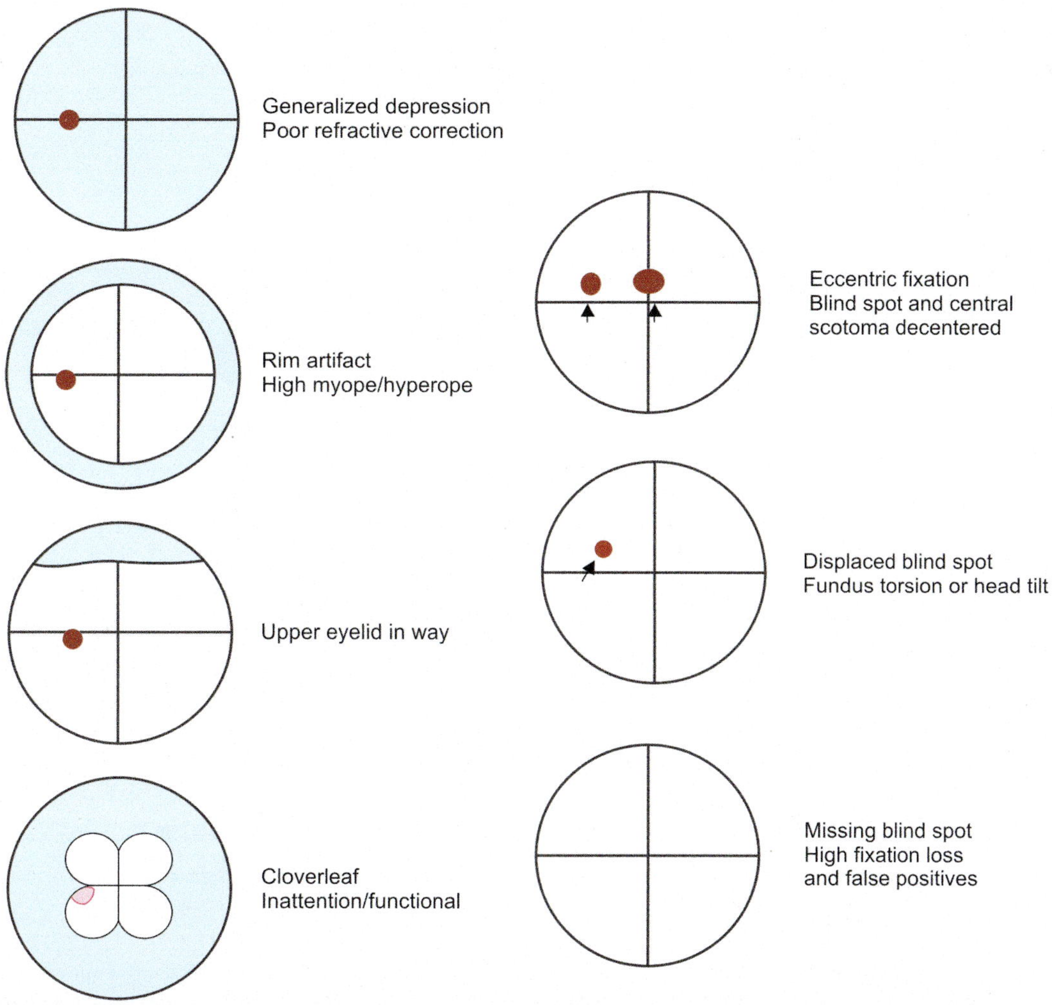

Fig. 98.5: Common artifacts on static automated perimetry. Several examples of non-physiologic visual field patterns that can be produced by patient inattention, poor refractive correction, obstruction of the visual axis by overlying eyelids, poor fixation, and displacement of the blind spot due to head or eye positioning.

PATTERNS OF VISUAL FIELD LOSS

In addition to the patient's history, including duration and tempo of vision loss, the pattern of visual field loss is key to diagnosis and assessment of progression, as the dilated fundus examination is not usually sufficient to localize a lesion behind the eye. Anatomical localization by visual field analysis allows the clinician to specifically target ophthalmic imaging and neuroimaging testing to the area of interest within the visual pathways (Fig. 98.6). This section will focus on specific visual field defects that relate to neuro-ophthalmic causes of vision loss. Field defects from glaucomatous optic neuropathies, functional vision loss, and retinal dystrophies are covered in other Chapters.

Optic Nerve

The ganglion cells axons of the retina lie within the RNFL and take a stereotypical course toward the optic disk to form the optic nerve (Fig. 98.7). Unilateral neuro-ophthalmic visual field defects arise within the eye, optic disk or optic nerve body anterior to the chiasm. There are often fundus findings corroborating the clinical suspicion of optic neuropathy, such as optic disk pallor or edema, although a normal appearing optic disk can be seen acutely in some conditions such as acute retrobulbar optic neuritis. The majority of these visual field defects can be detected within the central 24–30°.[8] The shape of the field defect often corresponds to the location of RNFL damage and mirrors

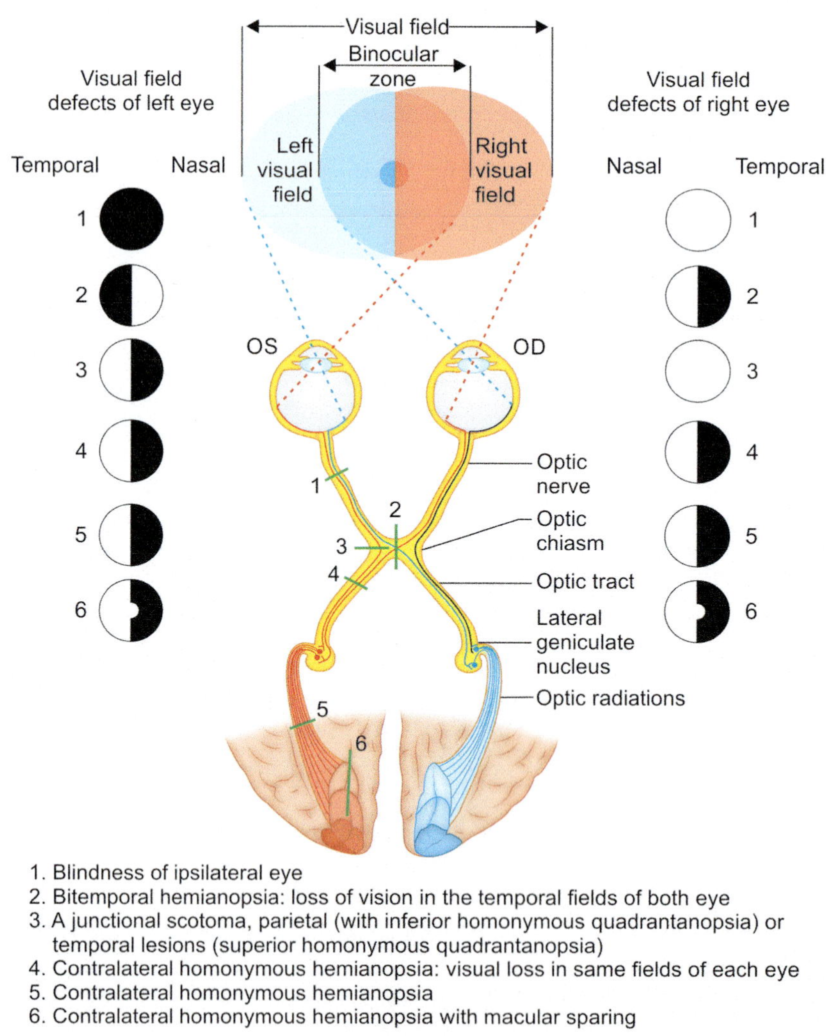

Fig. 98.6: Anatomy of the human visual field. Right and left visual fields have topographic consistency, with the nasal retina reflecting the temporal field and the temporal retina reflecting the nasal field of each eye. The central field is represented by a large area of occipital cortex starting at the posterior pole, while the far temporal field in each eye is represented by only the contralateral anterior occipital lobe.

Note: For clarity, this diagram presents the visual pathway as viewed from above, but conventional neuroimaging will show the brain and orbits as viewed from below.

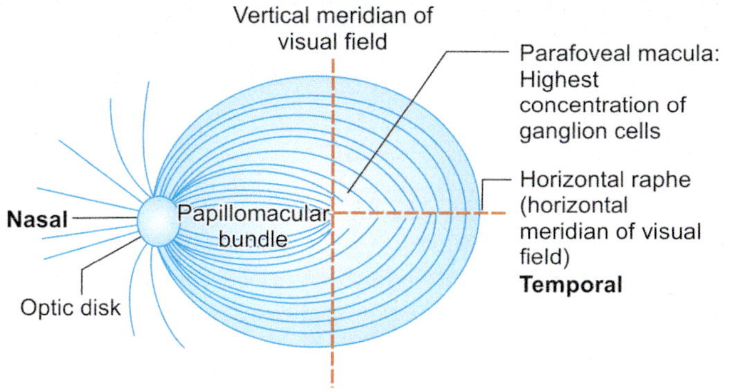

Fig. 98.7: Retinal nerve fiber layer distribution. General outline of ganglion cell axon course within the left eye. Retinal ganglion cell bodies originate within the inner retina and course in an arcuate pattern to insert radially at the optic nerve head in a stereotyped fashion. Focal damage to the optic nerve, disk, or ganglion cell is reflected in mirror image and inverted topographically on the visual field map.

the topographic pattern of macular ganglion cell layer loss seen on optical coherence tomography (OCT), such as in this example of nonarteritic anterior ischemic optic neuropathy (Figs. 98.8A and B).[10-13] In fact, visual fields may be more sensitive than OCT or fundus examination in diagnosis of an early occult optic neuropathy, when function is lost before structural damage is observed (Figs. 98.9A to C).[14,15]

Although characteristic RNFL defects such as arcuate/partial arcuate, nasal step, temporal wedge, and altitudinal defects are most often seen in glaucoma, optic nerve edema from inflammatory, vascular, infiltrative or infectious sources also may produce identical patterns of focal RNFL damage (Fig. 98.10).[8] RNFL defects from optic nerve disease often connect to the blind spot, respect the horizontal raphe, and have a gradual, sloping progression in severity to the center of the defect. In contrast, purely retinal lesions appear more "punched-out" on perimetric plots, with a steep divide between normal and abnormal test locations, and they may not respect the horizontal midline or extend to the blind spot (Fig. 98.11). Posterior segment examination thus may localize the pathology to optic nerve head or retina based on presence of sectoral optic nerve pallor, cavernous optic nerve cupping, optic rim notching, presence of hemorrhage or retinal changes. Often, focal absence of the RNFL can be visualized with red-free illumination at the slit lamp, or changes in optic disk or retinal layers demonstrated on OCT.

Altitudinal defects are commonly seen in nonarteritic anterior ischemic optic neuropathy as noted above (Fig. 98.8).[16] Unilateral central or diffuse depression are common patterns of visual field loss in compressive, inflammatory and demyelinating optic neuropathy (Figs. 98.12A to D), intrinsic or infiltrating optic nerve lesions (Figs. 98.13A to C), neuroretinitis, and optic perineuritis.[7,17-19] Acute ischemia to the ophthalmic artery causes severe visual field defects due to blockage of both choroidal and retinal circulations, and fluorescein angiogram showing choroidal filling defects may be helpful in the diagnostic evaluation to differentiate such a condition from disease in one circulatory system alone (Figs. 98.14A to C).[20,21] Cecocentral visual field loss occurs when the metabolically active papillomacular bundle is damaged, causing central visual field depression that connects to the blind spot. Optic neuropathy causing cecocentral visual field loss is associated with decreased visual acuity, dyschromatopsia and, with time, temporal optic disk pallor with temporal RNFL loss on OCT. Bilateral cecocentral visual field loss should prompt investigations for mitochondrial, nutritional, or toxic optic neuropathy (Figs. 98.15A and B).[22,23]

Anomalous optic nerve anatomy is also associated with visual field defects. Optic nerve head drusen often cause visual field loss mimicking that of glaucoma, including focal visual field pattern defects such as nasal step, arcuate scotoma, and peripheral loss with relative central sparing.[24,25] Corresponding focal RNFL defects may be present on OCT (Figs. 98.16A to C).[26] In contrast to glaucoma, however, field defects from optic nerve head drusen often do not progress; therefore, progression should prompt workup for alternative diagnoses such as coexisting glaucoma or compressive optic neuropathy. Highly myopic or staphylomatous eyes may have prominent temporal or inferonasal optic nerve tilt with peripapillary atrophy, causing enlarged blind spots and superotemporal field defects on visual field testing (Figs. 98.17A to D). Optic disk pits may cause neurosensory retinal detachments and macular scotomata. Occasionally, anomalous optic nerves and severe staphyloma or colobomas can produce a visual field pattern mimicking bitemporal hemianopia, but defects do not respect the vertical midline. Visual field defects are differentiated from concurrent neuro-ophthalmic disease by history and progression over time, and sometimes neuroimaging is necessary when an occult compressive optic neuropathy cannot be ruled out.

Increased intracranial pressure causes forward displacement and swelling of the optic nerve within the globe, causing axonal stasis and progressive damage to retinal ganglion cell axons.[18] Early papilledema causes enlargement of the blind spot bilaterally, representing photoreceptor displacement laterally from the swollen optic disk (Figs. 98.18A to D).[27,28] Papilledema is a dynamic process that typically resolves after the intracranial pressure has normalized but when protracted or severe, may be associated with progressive optic atrophy. When associated

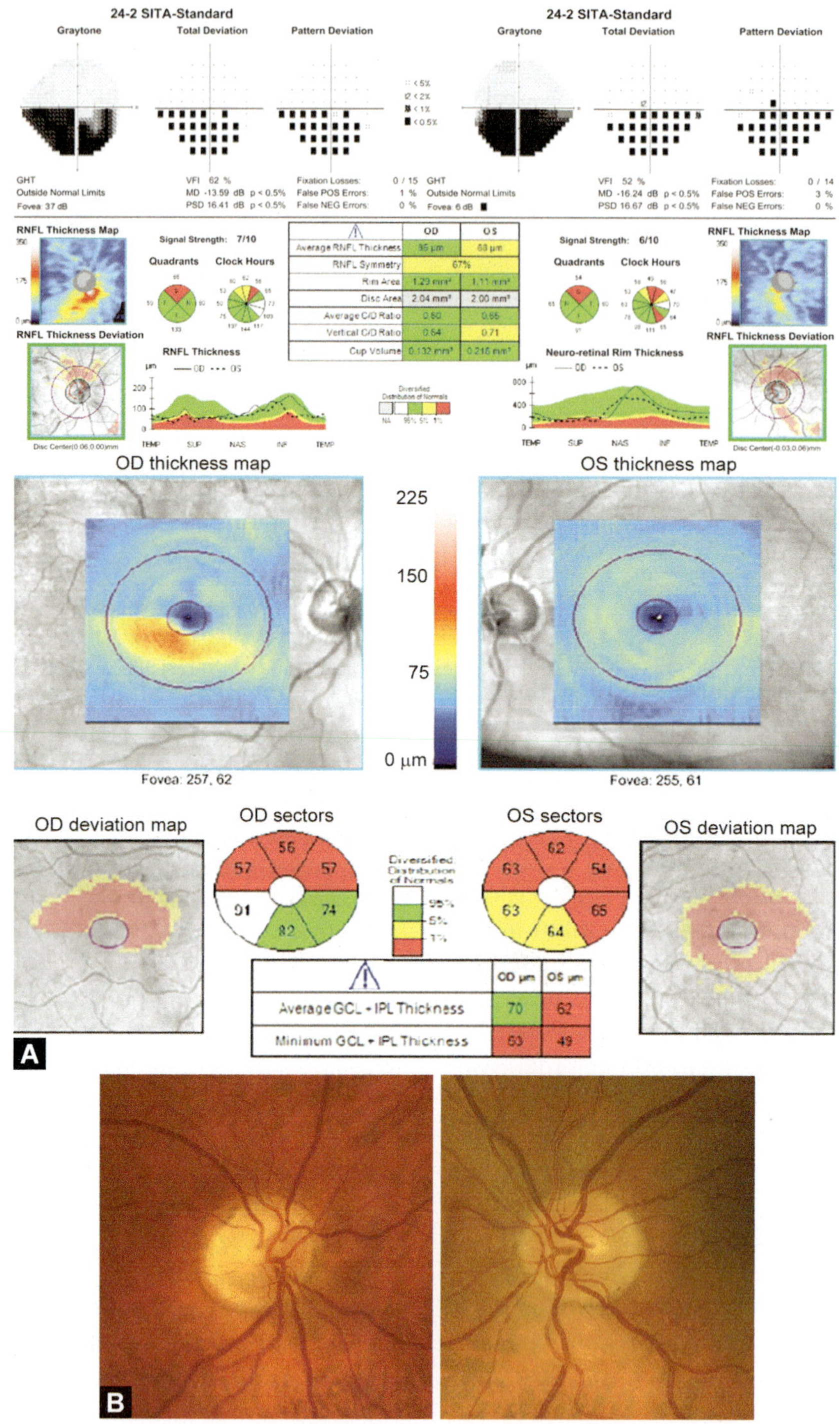

Figs. 98.8A and B: Nonarteritic anterior ischemic optic neuropathy (NAION) OU. A 75-year-old male with a past medical history of diabetes, hypertension and hyperlipidemia, as well as history of crowded optic disk and NAION OD, presented with acute inferior altitudinal vision loss OS with 20/200 BCVA (Vision OD was 20/20). He was found to have circumferential optic disk edema with subretinal fluid tracking into the macula OS. This visual field and OCT are captured 6 months after the event, showing excellent correlation between the visual field loss, RNFL, and macular ganglion cell layer loss in both eyes (A). Fundus examination showed superior sector pallor in the right eye and diffuse pallor in the left eye, worse superiorly than inferiorly (B).

with RNFL loss of function, diffuse central depression and nasal steps are the most common defects, but any pattern of RNFL loss can be observed.[28] Severe papilledema causes diffuse constriction and depression of the visual field with decreased reliability, as well as diminished visual acuity and color vision.

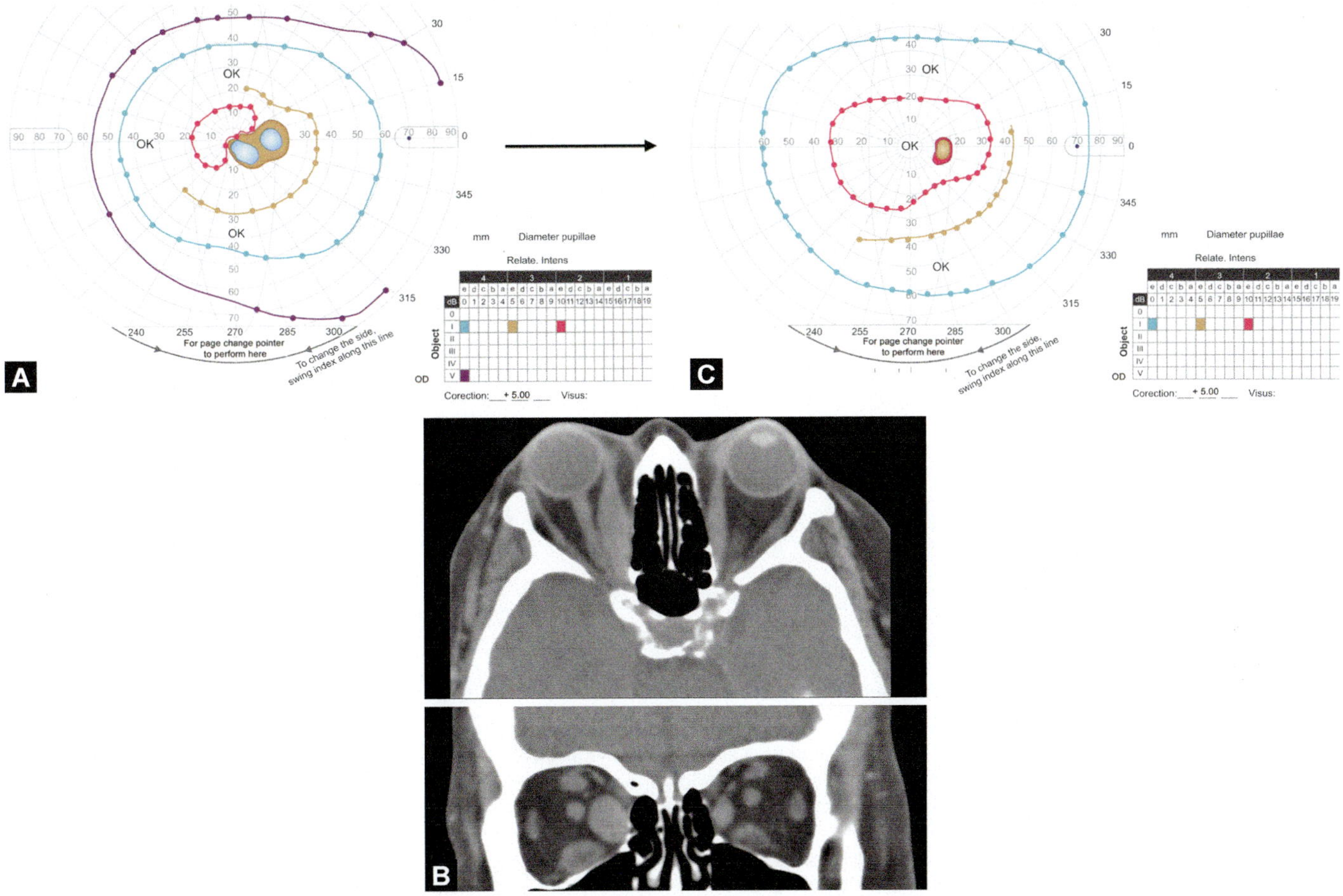

Figs. 98.9A to C: Central scotoma from thyroid eye disease. A 60-year-old female with 3 weeks of progressive central vision loss and chronic proptosis of the right eye presented with vision decreased to 20/60-2, and a central scotoma and enlarged blind spot was seen on GVF OD (A). CT orbits revealed fusiform thickening of the right medial and inferior rectus with compression at the optic nerve apex, consistent with compressive optic neuropathy from thyroid eye disease (B). She underwent radiation treatment and subsequently her vision improved to her baseline at 20/30+2, and GVF OD normalized (C).
Source: Randy Kardon, MD, PhD.

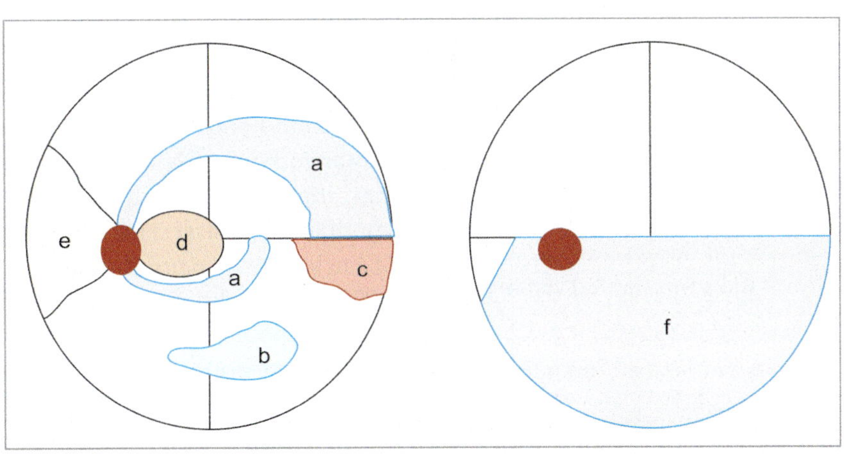

Fig. 98.10: General patterns seen in retinal nerve fiber layer (RNFL) defects. Shown on the 30° visual field, optic neuropathies produce focal damage to ganglion cell axons entering the optic nerve head in various quadrants and produce the following patterns: arcuate defect (a), partial arcuate defect (b), or nasal step (c), from partial superior or inferior RNFL loss; cecocentral or central defect from papillomacular bundle damage (d); temporal wedge defect from nasal RNFL loss (e); altitudinal defect from total superior or inferior RNFL loss (f). Colored regions refer to areas of decreased sensitivity to the visual stimulus.

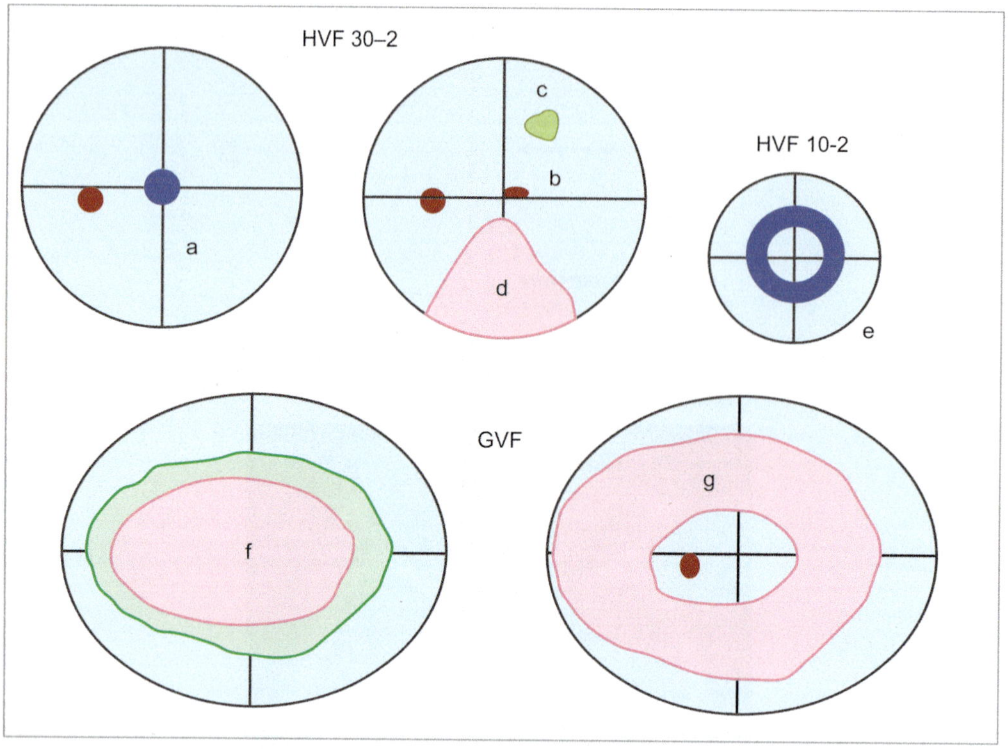

Fig. 98.11: General patterns seen in retinal defects. Retinal disease also produces visual field loss that is topographically correlated to the location of the lesion in the eye (upside-down and mirror image). Retinal lesions produce focal scotomas in the area of loss, with a sharp drop-off from normal to abnormal field. While not exclusive to retinal lesions, and most retinal lesions are visible on dilated fundus examination, some general patterns of field loss are as follows: Central scotoma seen in macular lesions (a); paracentral scotoma seen in small parafoveal lesions (b); small (c) or large (d) peripheral defect not extending to the blind spot or following RNFL course, which can be seen in some focal peripheral retinal lesions; ring scotoma on HVF 10-2 (e), seen in cone dystrophies or hydroxychloroquine toxicity; large central defect with relative peripheral sparing on GVF (f), seen in CRAO or other large macular scars; large ring scotoma/peripheral depression with central sparing on GVF (g), seen in rod bipolar cell dystrophies. Colored regions refer to areas of decreased sensitivity to the visual stimulus.

Junctional Scotoma

The cause of the junctional scotoma is contested, but the pattern of visual field loss is highly localizing to the junction of the optic nerve and chiasm.[29,30] A small anterior deflection of inferior nasal crossing fibers as they enter the chiasm has been described as "Wilbrand's knee".[31] Compression of the posterior optic nerve proximal to its insertion into the chiasm may cause an ipsilateral optic nerve pattern of visual field loss such as central depression, as well as superotemporal depression of the contralateral visual field (Figs. 98.19A to C).

Optic Chiasm

The optic chiasm contains ganglion cell axons from both eyes, and vision loss in this location is the most anterior location for bilateral vertical midline-respecting field defects. Approximately 55% of axons, those responsible for the temporal visual field, cross in this location, while axons subtending the nasal visual field run peripherally through the chiasm to the ipsilateral optic tract.[32,33] Thus, lesions of the optic chiasm characteristically involve the more central crossed fibers, producing a bitemporal hemianopia or quadrantanopia: temporal loss of both hemifields that respects the vertical midline. Pituitary adenoma is the most common causative lesion (Figs. 98.20A to C), although other pituitary tumors, hypothalamic masses, infundibular lesions, and intrinsic chiasm lesions also produce bitemporal hemianopia (Figs. 98.21A to C). Ophthalmoscopic examination of the patient with bitemporal hemianopia may show temporal or band-like pattern of optic disk atrophy. Macular OCT may mirror the visual field loss with binasal macular ganglion cell layer RNFL loss (Figs. 98.20A to C). Bitemporal hemianopias that are worse in the superior part of the visual field suggest a lesion compressing the optic chiasm from below, such as a pituitary adenoma; those that are worse inferiorly suggest a compressive lesion above the chiasm, such as a craniopharyngioma. Variations of visual field loss may be

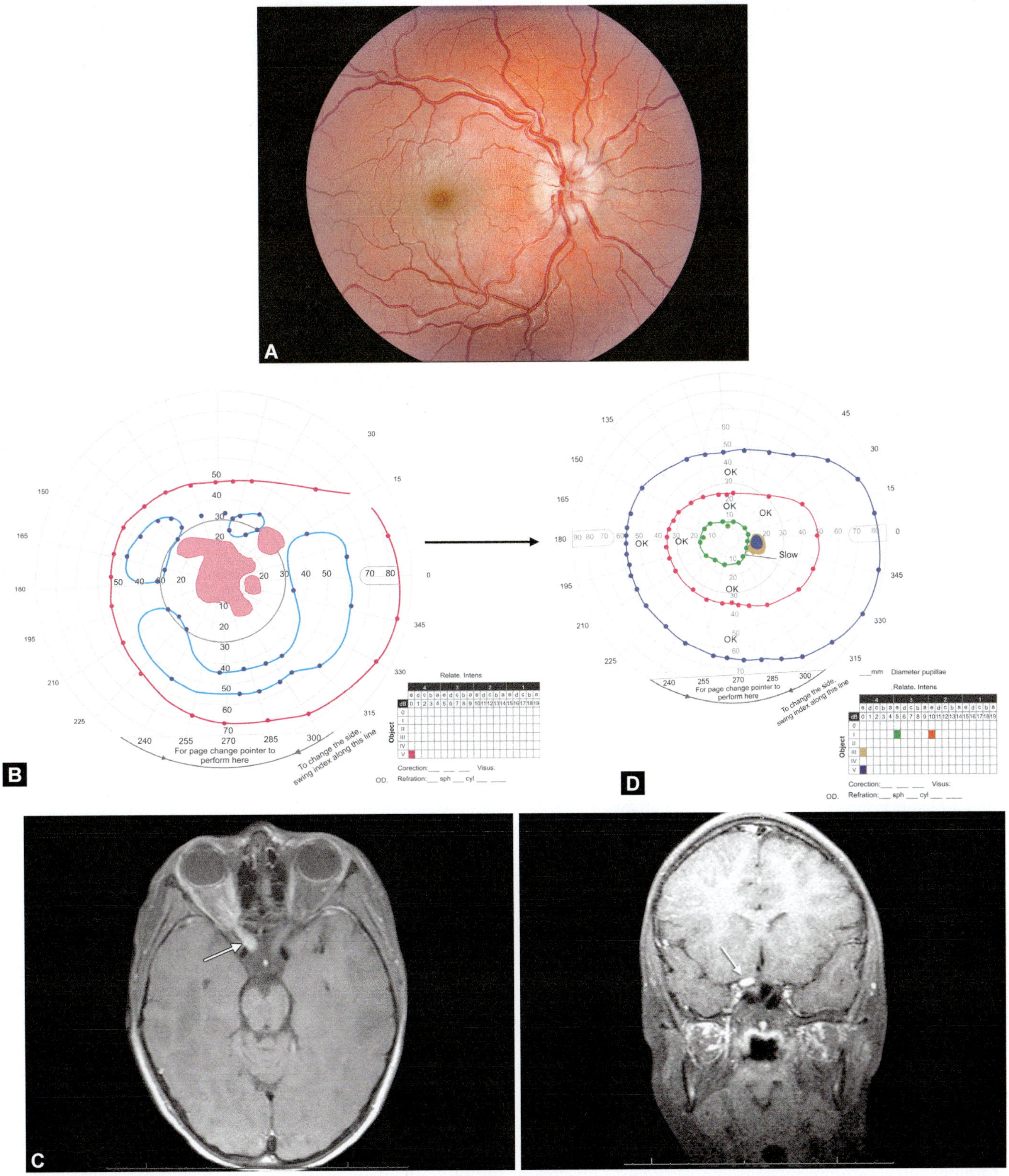

Figs. 98.12A to D: Central scotoma from optic neuritis. An 11-year-old female presented with acute painful right eye and central vision loss OD. Fundus examination revealed hyperemic optic disk edema of the right eye, with an otherwise normal fundus (A). Visual field testing revealed large and dense central scotoma in the right eye and normal visual field on the left (B). MRI revealed avid enhancement of the entire body of the right optic nerve (C) and she regained a normal visual field after IV steroid infusion (D).

Source: Matthew Thurtell, MBBS, MSc.

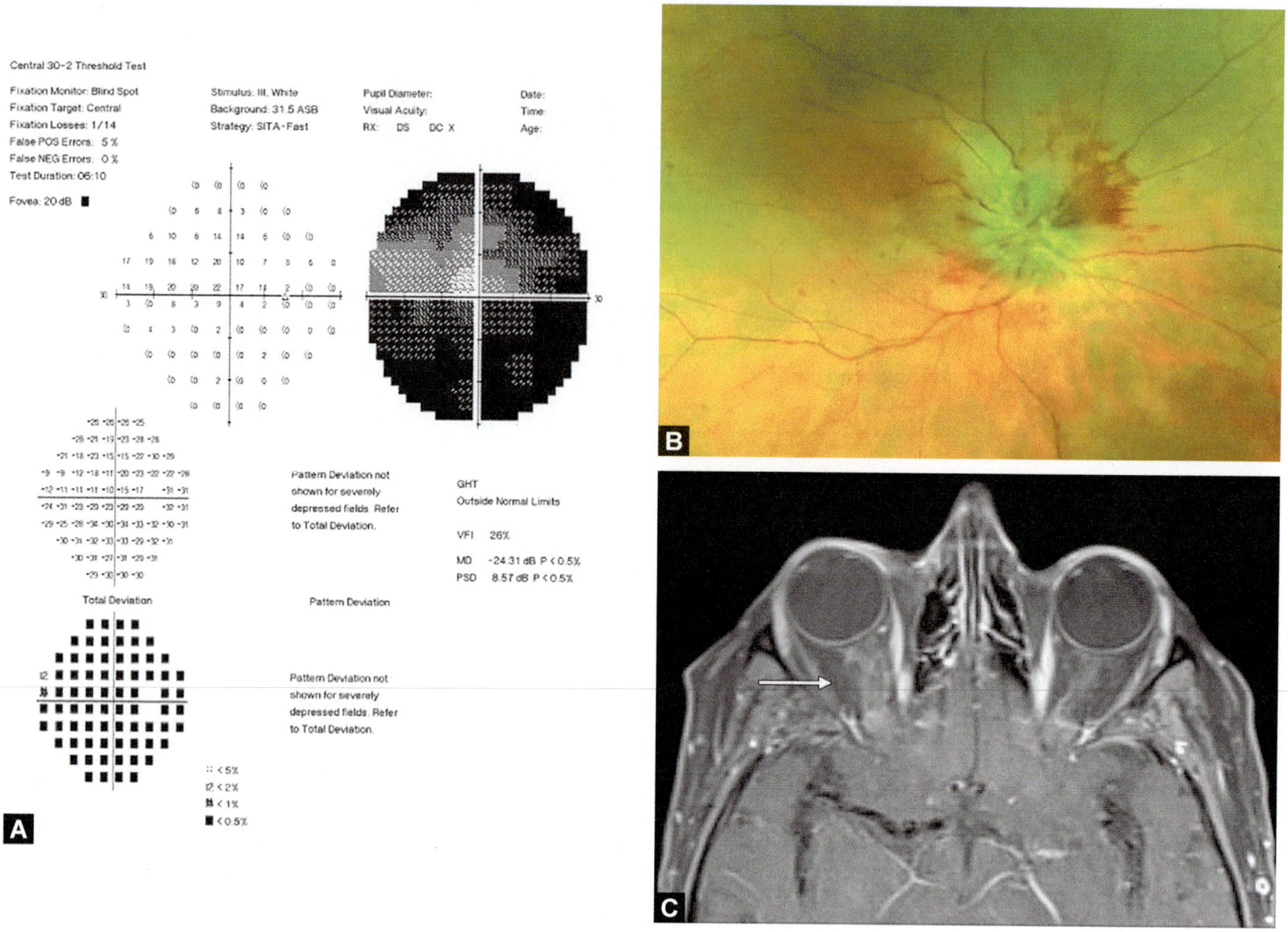

Figs. 98.13A to C: Infiltrative optic neuropathy. A 68-year-old woman with a past history of acute myeloid leukemia described painless vision loss in the right eye, malaise, and fatigue. She was found to have reduced visual acuity and dyschromatopsia on the right in addition to an afferent pupillary defect. Fundus examination revealed marked right optic nerve swelling and peripapillary hemorrhages (A). Her right visual field is diffusely depressed more inferiorly than superiorly (B). MRI of the brain and orbits demonstrated enhancement of the intraorbital portion of the right optic nerve and sheath (arrow), as well as multiple cranial nerves, consistent with leptomeningeal metastases (C). Her vision improved after receiving whole brain radiation and intrathecal chemotherapy.
Source: Robert Avery, DO, MSCE.

seen with different configurations of the chiasm relative to the pituitary gland. A prefixed chiasm is anteriorly situated relative to the pituitary gland, making the posterior chiasm and optic tracts are more susceptible to compression. A bitemporal hemianopia affecting the central visual field may result from compression of macular fibers, which cross most posteriorly in the chiasm, or homonymous visual field loss may result from optic tract compression. In contrast, a post-fixed chiasm is posteriorly situated relative to the sella. Compression of the post-fixed chiasm can produce typical bitemporal hemianopia but may also lead to optic nerve patterns of visual field loss or a junctional scotoma.

Optic Tract

Posterior to the optic chiasm, afferent visual fibers decussate to form the two optic tracts. Crossing visual fibers from the contralateral nasal retina that serve the temporal visual field, and the uncrossed fibers serving the ipsilateral temporal retina serving the nasal visual field, form each optic tract. For the first time in the visual pathway, the axons of both eyes serving the contralateral visual field are united. A lesion of the optic tract produces a contralateral homonymous hemianopia (Figs. 98.22A to C). Incomplete optic tract lesions produce characteristically incongruous (i.e. asymmetric between the two eyes) visual field defects.

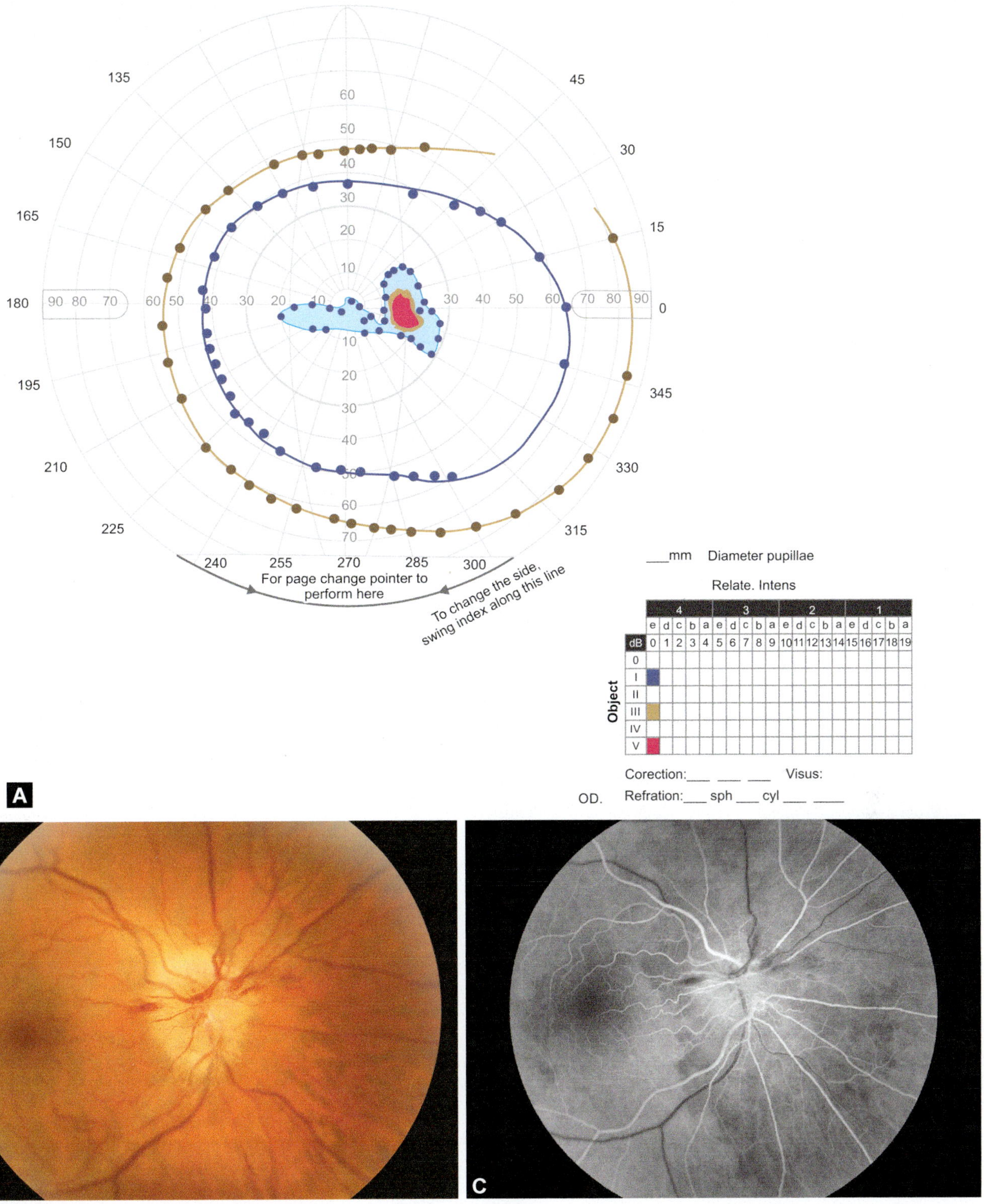

Figs. 98.14A to C: Central scotoma from arteritic anterior ischemic optic neuropathy. A 62-year-old female presented with 2 weeks of acute, painless, central vision loss of the right eye, associated with widespread joint pain, temporal headache and jaw claudication. She was placed on high-dose prednisone by the referring provider 1 week prior to presentation. Visual field by GVF showed a dense central/cecocentral scotoma of the right eye (A). Fundus examination showed pallid edema of the right eye (B) and subsequent fluorescein angiography revealed choroidal filling defect in the peripapillary watershed zone (C), raising suspicion of ophthalmic artery ischemia. Erythrocyte sedimentation rate and c-reactive protein labs were in normal range for age but temporal artery biopsy confirmed suspected active giant cell arteritis.

Source: Reid Longmuir, MD.

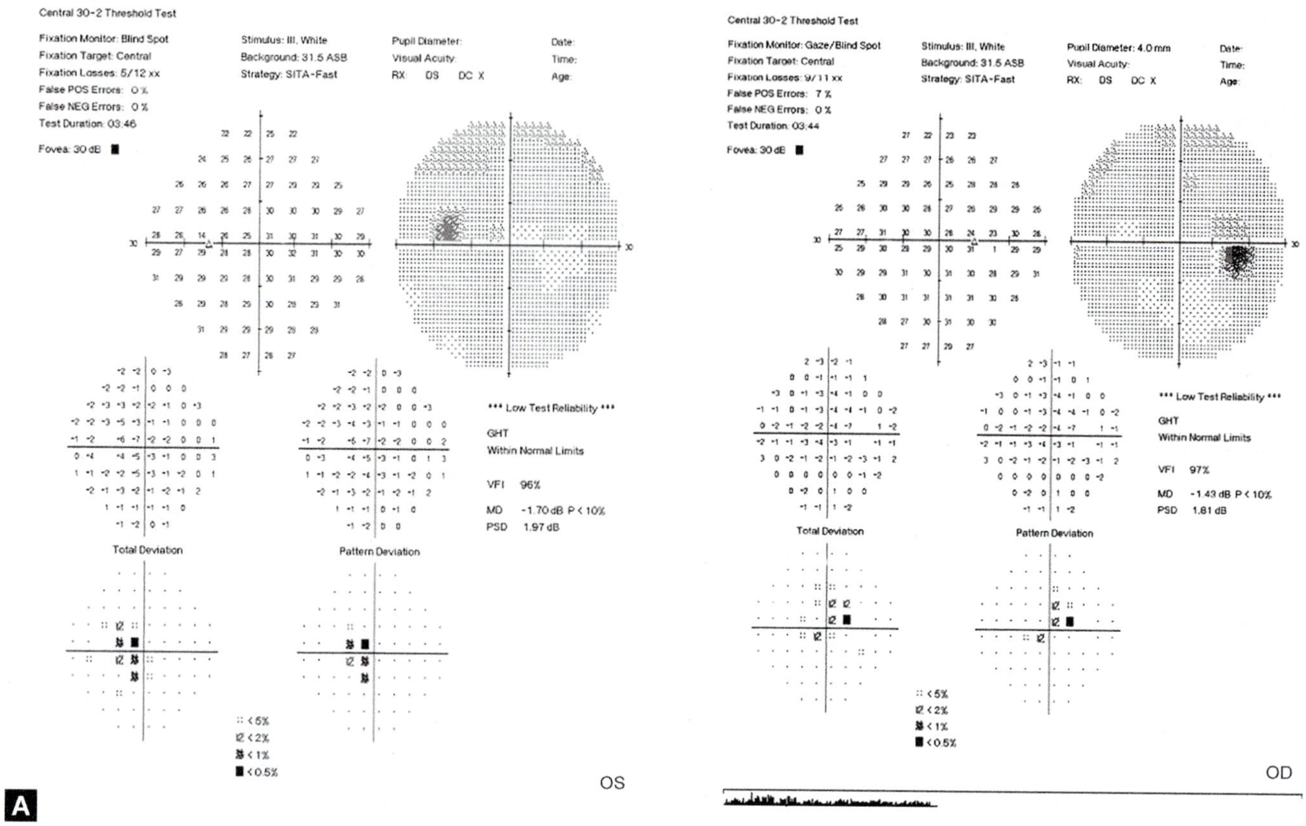

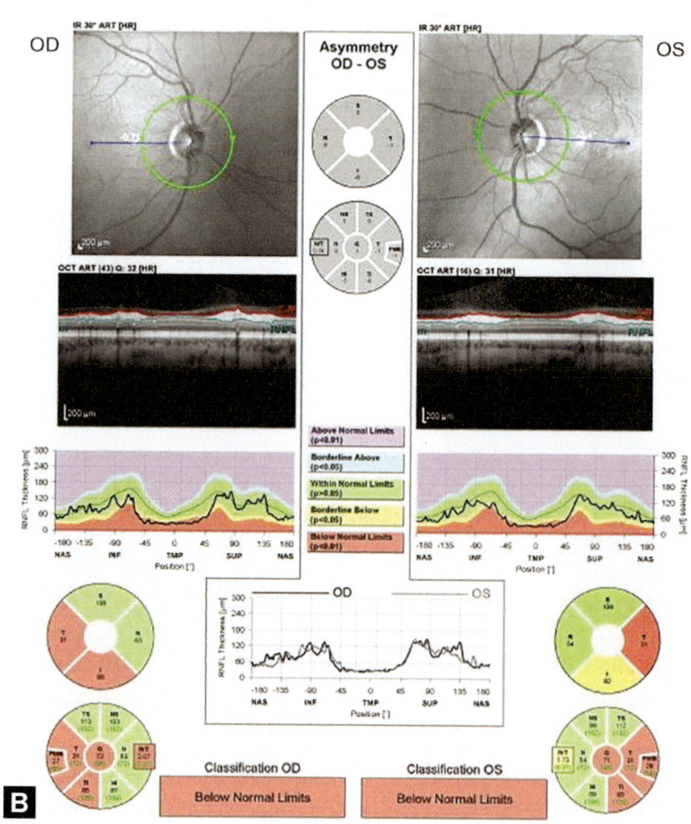

Figs. 98.15A and B: Bilateral cecocentral scotomas from toxic-nutritional optic neuropathy. The patient complained of subacute reduction in his central vision and had a long history of cigar smoking, alcohol consumption, and a limited diet and was found to have Vitamin B_{12} deficiency. Visual fields, while limited by significant fixation losses, demonstrate reduced sensitivity in the papillomacular bundle connecting the blind spot with fixation (A). The foveal threshold is reduced in both eyes which is consistent with his decreased central visual acuity. Because of the bitemporal appearance of the visual field loss, neuroimaging was performed and excluded chiasmal compression. OCT of the retinal nerve fiber layer confirmed temporal thinning of both optic nerves, consistent with the diagnosis of a toxic-nutritional optic neuropathy affecting the papillomacular bundles (B).

Source: Grant Liu, MD.

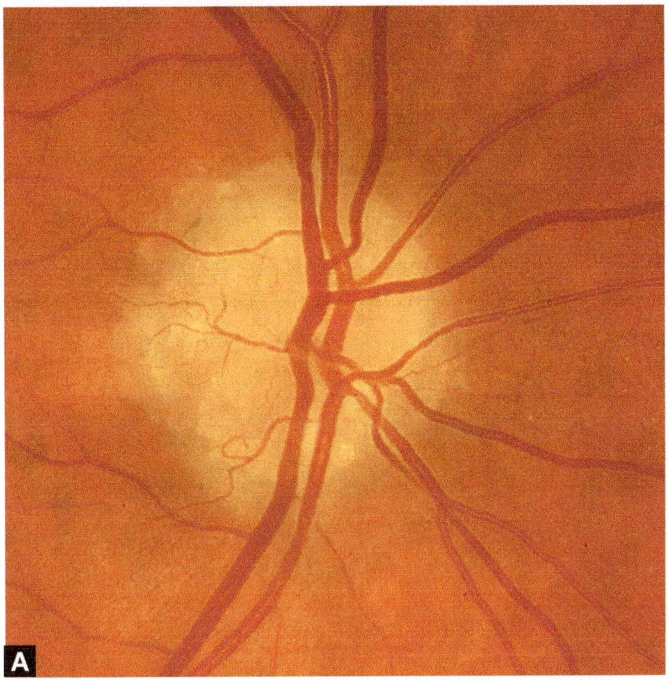

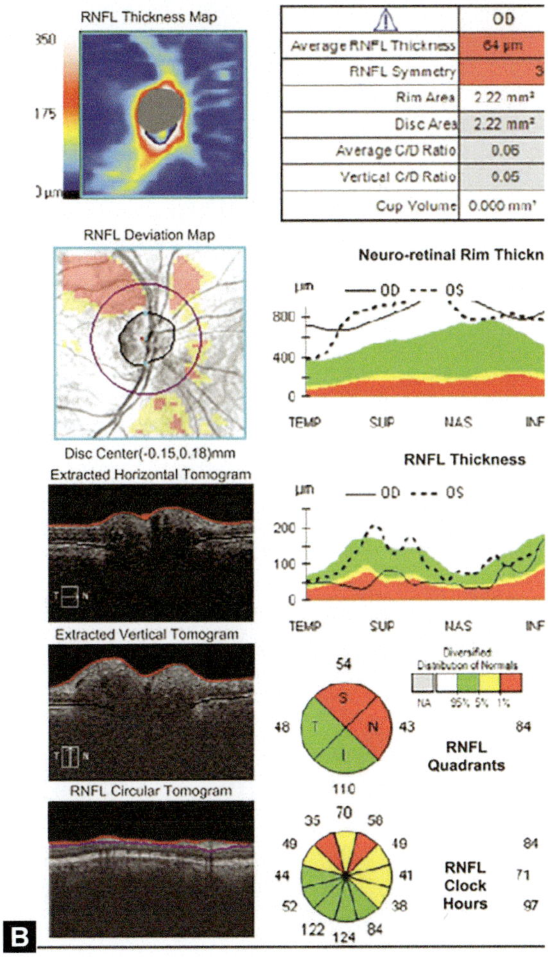

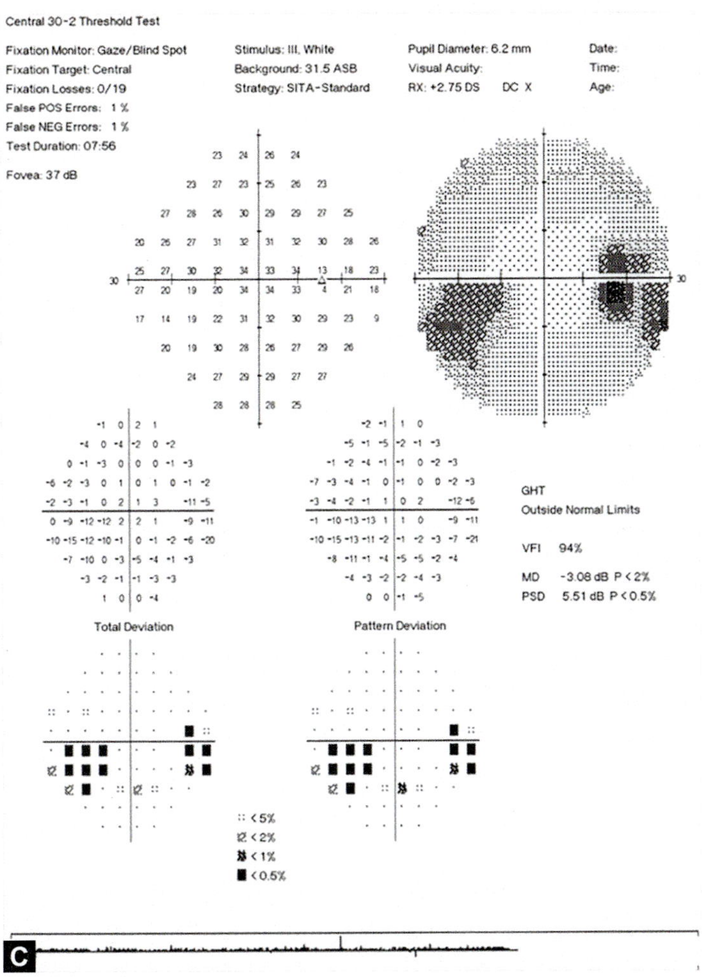

Figs. 98.16A to C: Optic nerve head drusen. A 52-year-old female who presented for routine dilated eye examination was found to have optic disk drusen OD (C). HVF 30-2 OD shows inferior nasal step and temporal wedge defects (B). OCT OD, showing superior and nasal retinal nerve fiber layer thinning correlates well to the pattern of vision loss (C). Visual fields remained stable in this patient over 15 years.

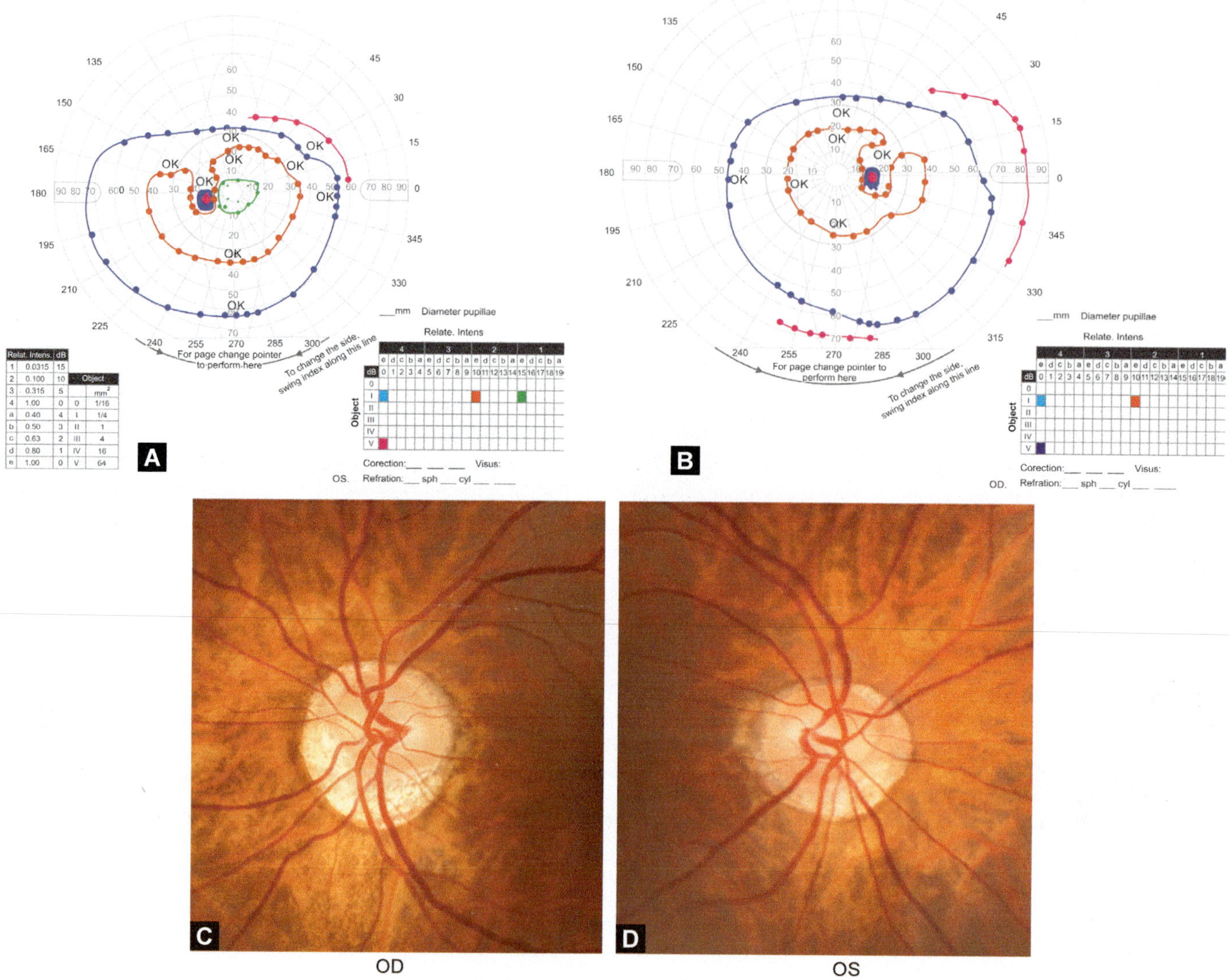

Figs. 98.17A to D: Pseudobitemporal hemianopsia from tilted optic disc OU. GVF OS (A) and GVF OD (B) show enlarged blind spot and superior temporal depression of the I2e isopter extending from the blind spot bilaterally, which did not respect the vertical midline. Fundus photograph OD (C) and OS (D) reveal situs inversus of both optic discs characterized by inferonasal disc tilt with anomalous vessel insertion angle and peripapillary atrophy.
Source: Reid Longmuir, MD.

Isolated unilateral retrochiasmal lesions should not affect patient's visual acuity, because the afferent visual pathway serving half of each retina remains preserved. Because of the pattern of retinal ganglion cell and axonal loss which results, optic tract lesions are associated with contralateral optic disk "bowtie atrophy" and ipsilateral temporal optic disk pallor. The optic tract contains afferent visual fibers that participate in the pupillary light reflex, with a slightly greater contribution from the contralateral eye. Thus, a mild contralateral relative afferent pupillary defect (RAPD) may be observed in optic tract lesions.[34,35]

An alternative explanation for the contralateral RAPD seen in some optic tract lesions is asymmetric contribution of axons to homonymous hemianopia, greater on the contralateral side that represents the larger temporal visual field.[36] Lesions which typically affect the optic tract include cranipharyngiomas or pituitary macroadenomas, particularly if the chiasm is prefixed. Aneurysms, trauma, iatrogenic injury from surgical manipulation to the adjacent temporal lobe, demyelination, ischemia, and a variety of intrinsic or extrinsic compressive lesions also may cause optic tract lesions.

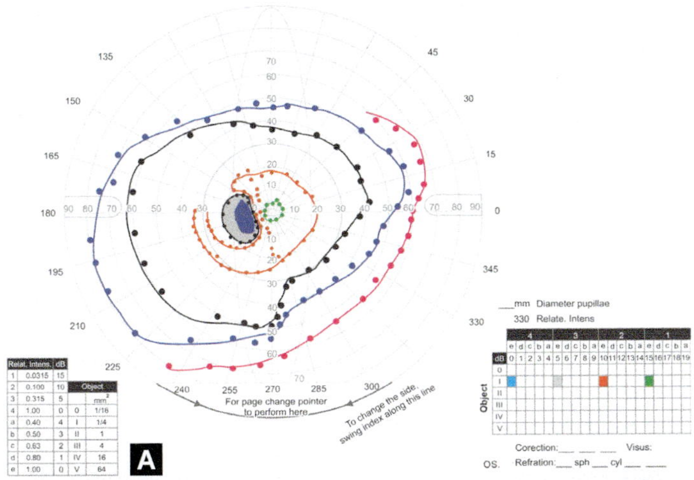

A

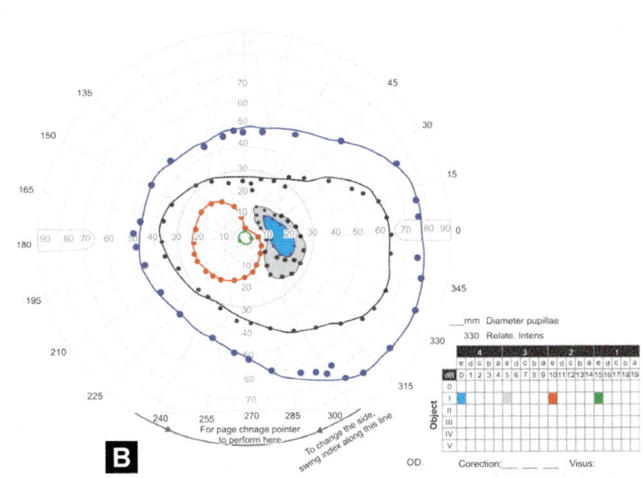

B

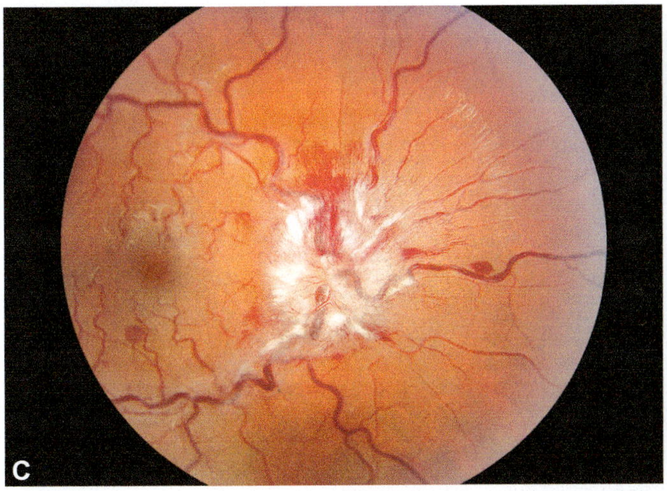

C

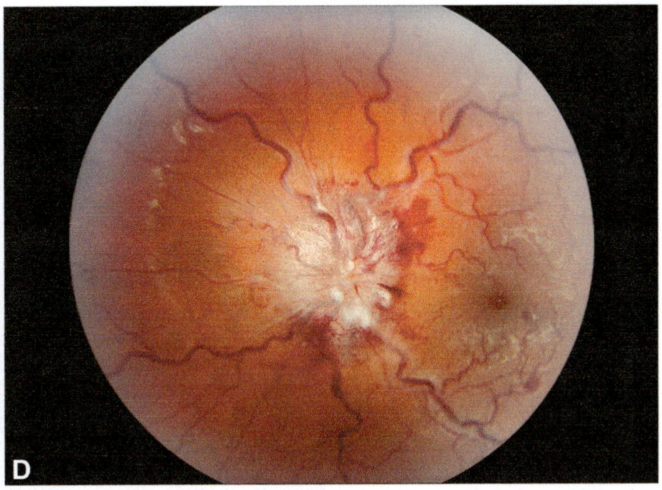

D

Figs. 98.18A to D: Enlarged blind spot from idiopathic intracranial hypertension. Goldmann visual field showing remarkable preservation of central vision to 20/20-2 OD, 20/30+2 OS, with enlarged blind spots OS (A) and OD (B) presenting in a 27-year-old morbidly obese male with worsening headache and Frisen grade IV papilledema (C and D). MRI and MRV were negative for alternative source, and lumbar puncture showed normal constituents but an opening pressure of 42 cm H_2O. The patient was diagnosed with idiopathic intracranial hypertension (IIH).
Source: Michael Wall, MD.

Lateral Geniculate Nucleus

Axons of the retinal ganglion cells reach the paired lateral geniculate nuclei (LGN) of the thalamus by way of the optic tracts. Here, they synapse with neurons that will form the optic radiations, which continue posteriorly and terminate at the calcarine fissure of the occipital lobe. The LGN is organized in layers dedicated to input from either the ipsilateral or contralateral eye. Lesions of the LGN are associated with contralateral homonymous hemianopias, but they may assume a peculiar sectoral shape when created by injury to one of the two vascular territories of the LGN. The anterior choroidal artery is a branch of the internal carotid artery (ICA), which supplies the medial and lateral horns of the LGN. Ischemia in the distribution of the anterior choroidal artery typically produces a superior and inferior contralateral homonymous visual field defect with a preserved central wedge (Fig. 98.23A). The middle hilum of the LGN is perfused by the posterior choroidal arteries, which are branches of the posterior cerebral artery (PCA); ischemia to the hilum may produce a homonymous contralateral central wedge defect affecting fixation but sparing the superior and inferior visual field (Fig. 98.23B). Lesions isolated to the LGN do not produce an afferent pupillary defect because the afferent input that causes light-induced pupillary constriction departs from the posterior optic tracts before they reach the LGN. Optic atrophy in a hemianopic pattern may be observed. Ischemic lesions of the LGN are rare because of its rich anastomotic blood supply, but may be seen after surgery; compressive, traumatic, and infiltrative lesions have been reported.

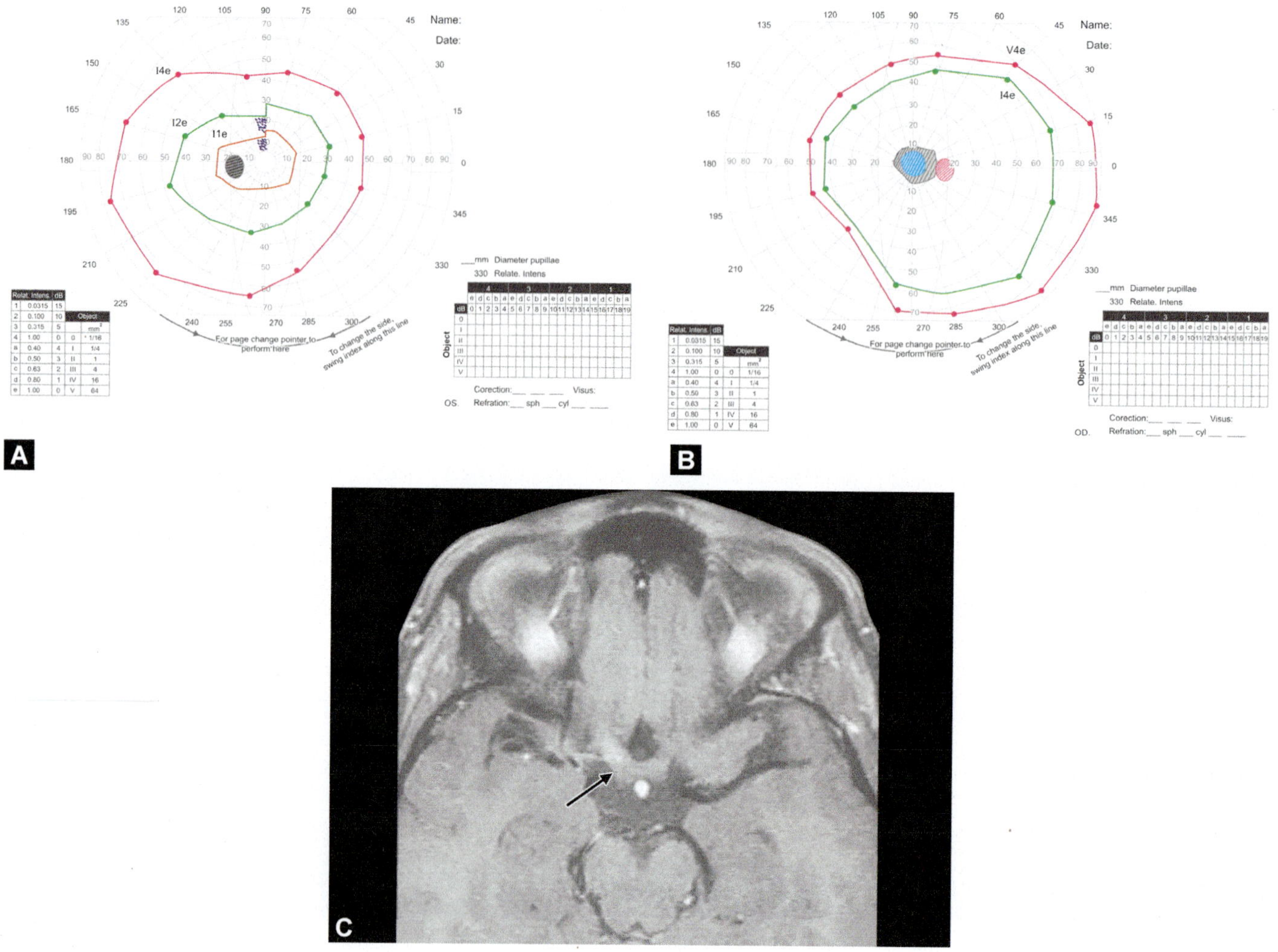

Figs. 98.19A to C: Junctional scotoma due to anterior chiasm inflammation. There is a central scotoma OD (B) and small superior temporal defect respecting the vertical midline OS (A), due to demyelination of the right anterior optic chiasm and extending into the right optic nerve, as shown on axial T1 post-contrast and coronal T2 FLAIR MRI views.
Source: Robert Egan, MD.

Optic Radiations

Axons leaving the LGN course through the optic radiations in two major bundles. Those carrying visual information from the superior visual field initially course inferiorly and anteriorly into the substance of the temporal lobe (Meyer's loop) before proceeding posteriorly to reach the occipital lobe. A lesion affecting Meyer's loop will often produce a contralateral superior quadrantanopia or a "pie in the sky" deficit (Figs. 98.24A and B). Temporal lobe lesions may be associated with other neurologic symptoms such as personality changes, seizures, memory impairment, hallucinations, and aphasia if the dominant side is lesioned.

Axons carrying visual information from the inferior visual field course superiorly and posteriorly into the parietal lobe. Thus, a lesion in this location usually produces a contralateral inferior homonymous quadrantanopia or hemianopia (Figs. 98.25A and B). Because descending parieto-occipitotemporal pursuit fibers are in close proximity, parietal lesions may be associated with ipsilesional slowed pursuit, and, therefore, impaired optokinetic responses when the drum is rotated toward the side of the lesion. A lesion affecting the angular gyrus of the dominant parietal lobe may cause Gerstmann syndrome (agraphia, acalculia, right-left confusion, and finger agnosia) or conduction aphasia, while a lesion of the

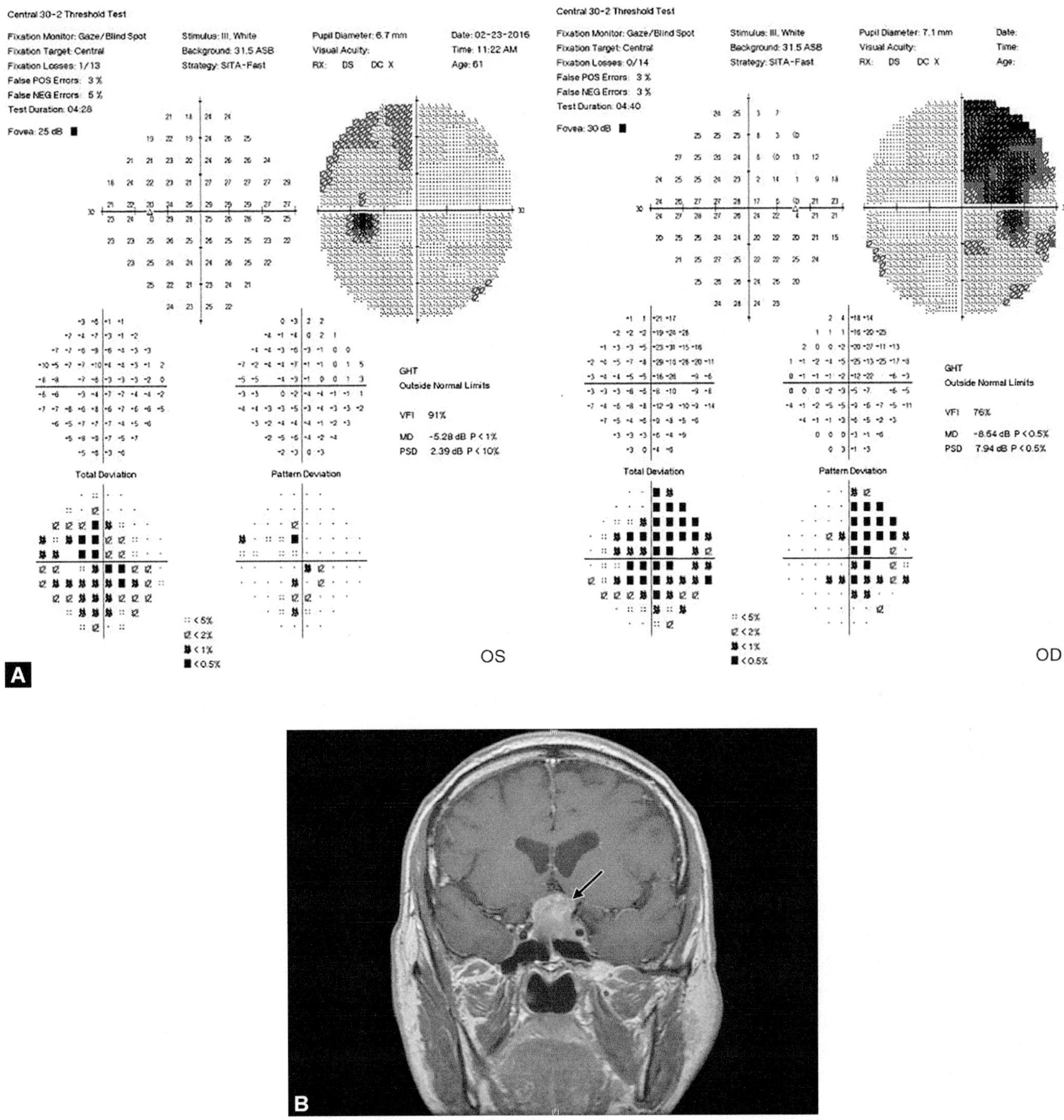

Figs. 98.20A and B

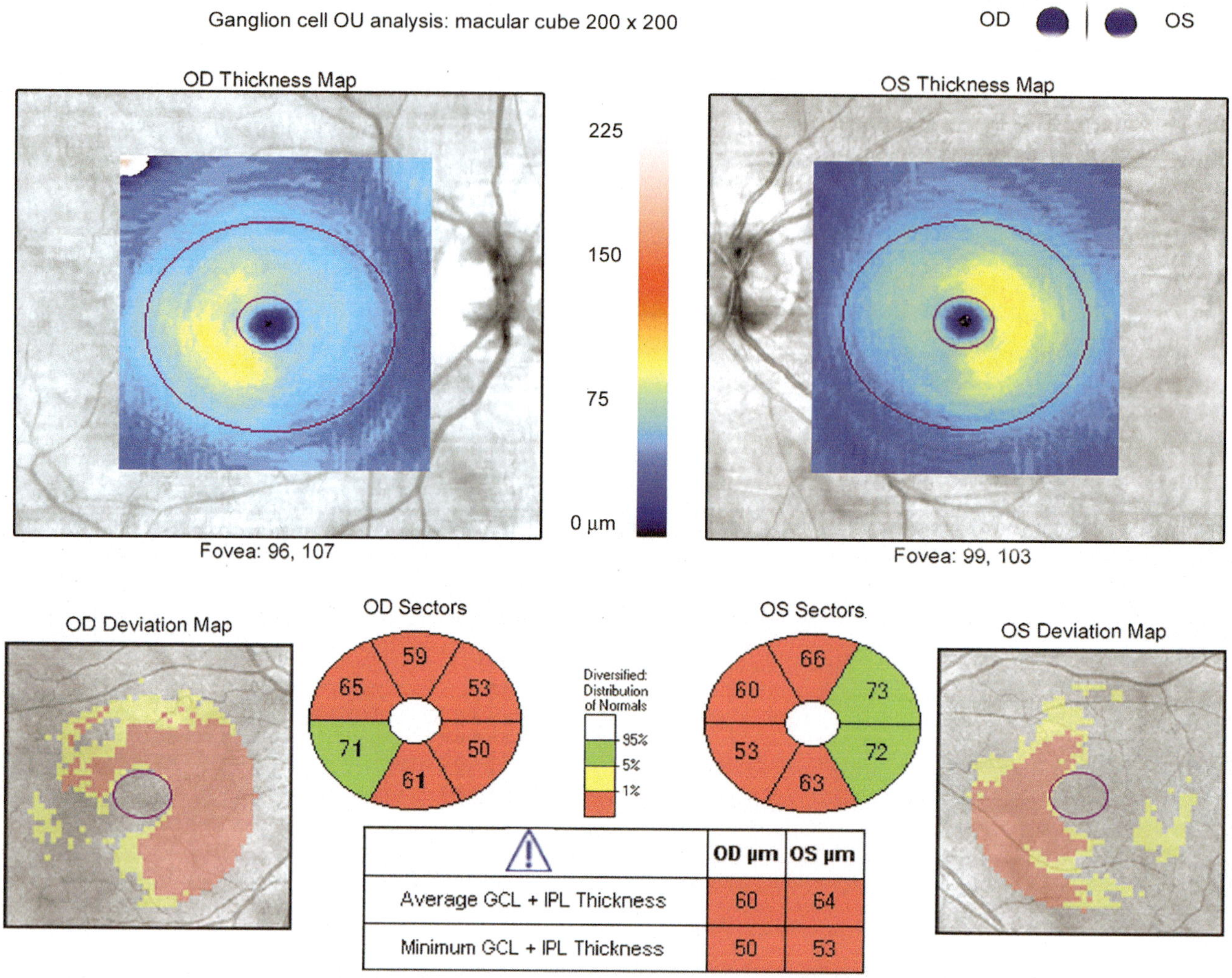

Fig. 98.20C

Figs. 98.20A to C: Incongruous superior bitemporal hemianopsia secondary to a 3 cm pituitary macroadenoma. Bitemporal visual field defects from inferior chiasmal compression start superiorly and may be subtle or incomplete. Nevertheless, they respect the vertical meridian, as shown in the HVF 30-2 gray scale plots (A). On the coronal T1 post-contrast enhanced MRI, the chiasm can be seen as a thin linear structure draped over the mass (B). OCT evidence of binasal macular ganglion cell layer thinning may mirror the bitemporal visual field defects (C).

Source: For Figures (A) and (B), Grant Liu, MD; for Figure (C), Randy Kardon, MD, PhD.

nondominant parietal lobe may cause contralateral neglect, in which an obvious visual field defect may not be present, but the patient will be unaware of visual or other stimuli in the affected hemifield. Unilateral lesions affecting the optic radiations will not impair visual acuity, and pupillary abnormalities would not be expected. Lesions affecting the optic radiations that occur prenatally or shortly after birth may be associated with trans-synaptic degeneration and a hemianopic pattern of optic atrophy, but the vast majority of lesions acquired later in life do not cause optic atrophy. Ischemia in the distribution of the middle cerebral artery (MCA), neoplasms, hemorrhages, trauma, infectious processes, surgical resection, and degenerative disease may affect the optic radiations in the parietal lobe.

Occipital Lobe

The occipital lobe is the final destination for the axons originating in the LGN. Here, they are organized along the banks of the calcarine sulcus, with those axons carrying visual information from the superior field terminating on the inferior bank, and vice versa. Occipital lobe lesions

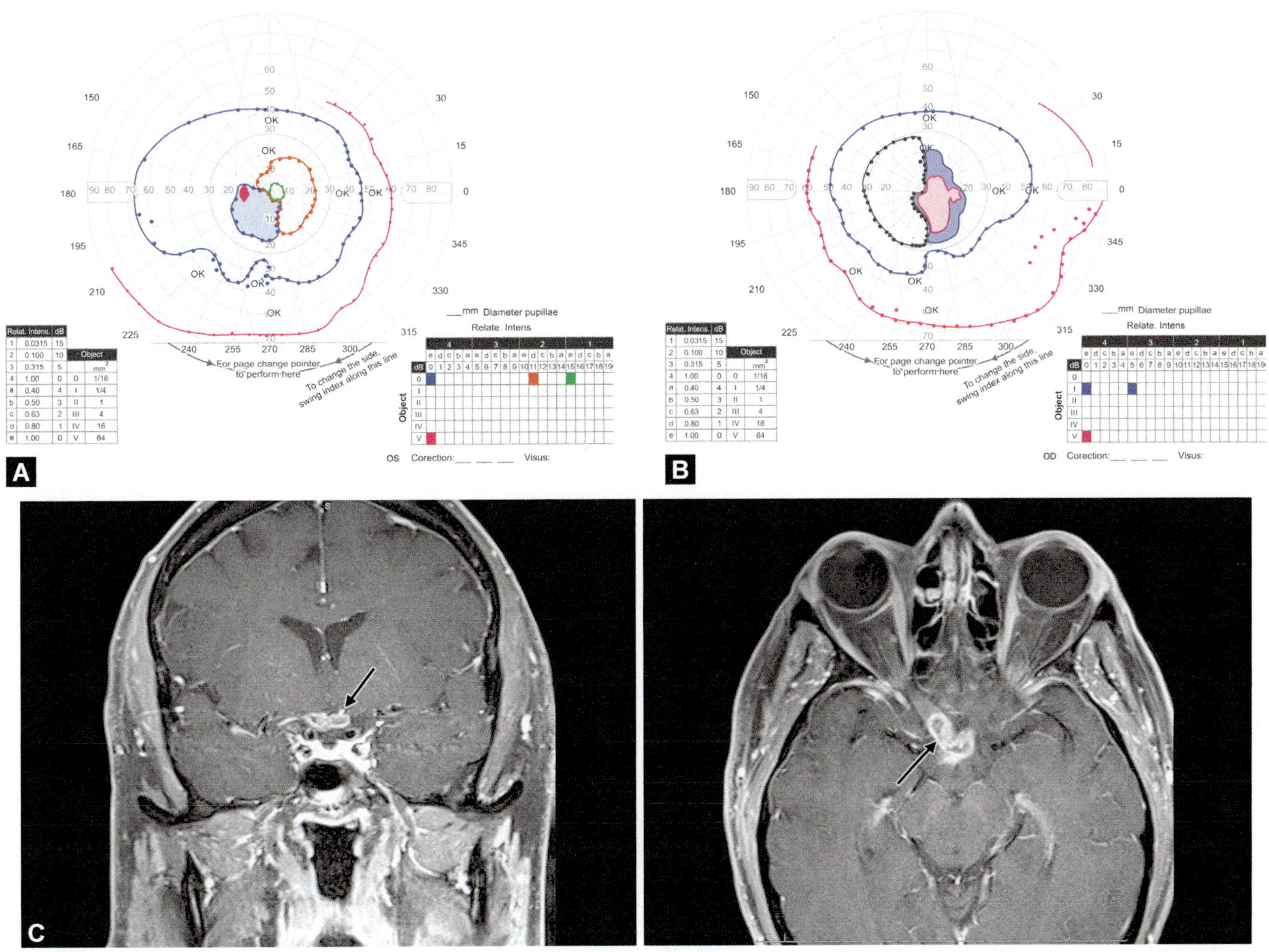

Figs. 98.21A to C: Bitemporal hemianopia. Bitemporal hemianopia secondary to chiasmal glioma. A 66-year-old male with 3 weeks of progressive vision loss, first in the right temporal field but progressing to both temporal fields, and eventually involving the central vision at 20/400 OD. Note the dense central scotoma to V4e isopter OD that respects the vertical midline (B). The left inferior temporal field is also involved, with preservation of visual acuity to 20/20 in the left eye (A). Presence of the bitemporal field defect prompted neuroimaging, showing a contrast-enhancing lesion in the posterior chiasm and extending into the right optic nerve (C), which was found to be a primary glioblastoma.
Source: Reid Longmuir, MD; Grant Liu, MD.

may therefore affect exclusively the superior or inferior homonymous visual field with great respect for the horizontal meridian. Visual information originating in the central macula terminates most posteriorly in the occipital lobe, and occupies an asymmetrically large proportion of the striate cortex.[37] More peripheral visual field information is organized more anteriorly in the occipital lobe. Because the monocular temporal visual field is approximately 30° larger than the nasal visual field, there exists a far anterior region of striate cortex that is dedicated to a monocular "temporal crescent" of contralateral peripheral visual field. Thus, a very anterior lesion in the occipital lobe may cause a unilateral far temporal crescentic defect; conversely, a posterior lesion in the occipital lobe may cause a homonymous hemianopia with contralateral sparing of the temporal crescent (Figs. 98.26A to C). These visual field defects are rare exceptions to the homonymous changes characteristically arising from retrochiasmal lesions, and they would not be captured by central HVF testing since the temporal crescent lies at least 50–60° temporal to fixation.

The occipital cortex receives the vast majority of its blood supply from the PCA, but a branch of the MCA provides additional perfusion to the occipital pole where

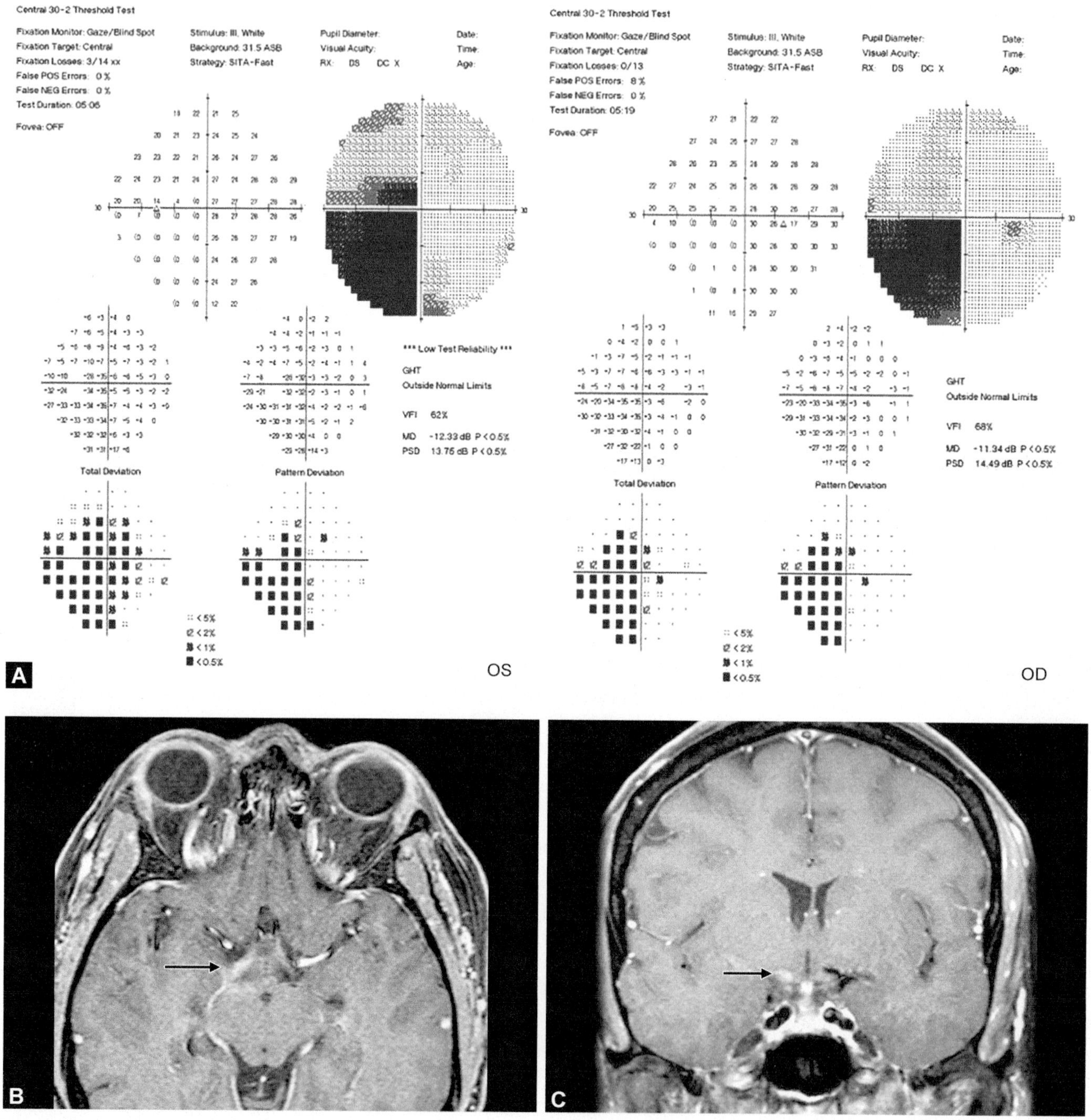

Figs. 98.22A to C: Optic tract demyelination. An incongruous left inferior homonymous hemianopsia from right optic tract demyelination in a patient with multiple sclerosis (A). Axial (B) and Coronal (C) T1 post-contrast MRI images demonstrate enlargement and enhancement of the right optic tract.
Source: Grant Liu, MD.

the central visual field is represented. Thus, homonymous visual field loss sparing the central visual field may be seen after ischemic occipital lobe injury from PCA occlusion (Fig. 98.27).[35] Bilateral PCA occlusion can therefore lead to bilateral homonymous visual field loss with a small preserved island of central vision. Conversely, a lesion selectively affecting the occipital pole, such as trauma, may produce a central homonymous visual field defect. Visual field loss from occipital lobe lesions is typically highly congruous because of the proximity of axons

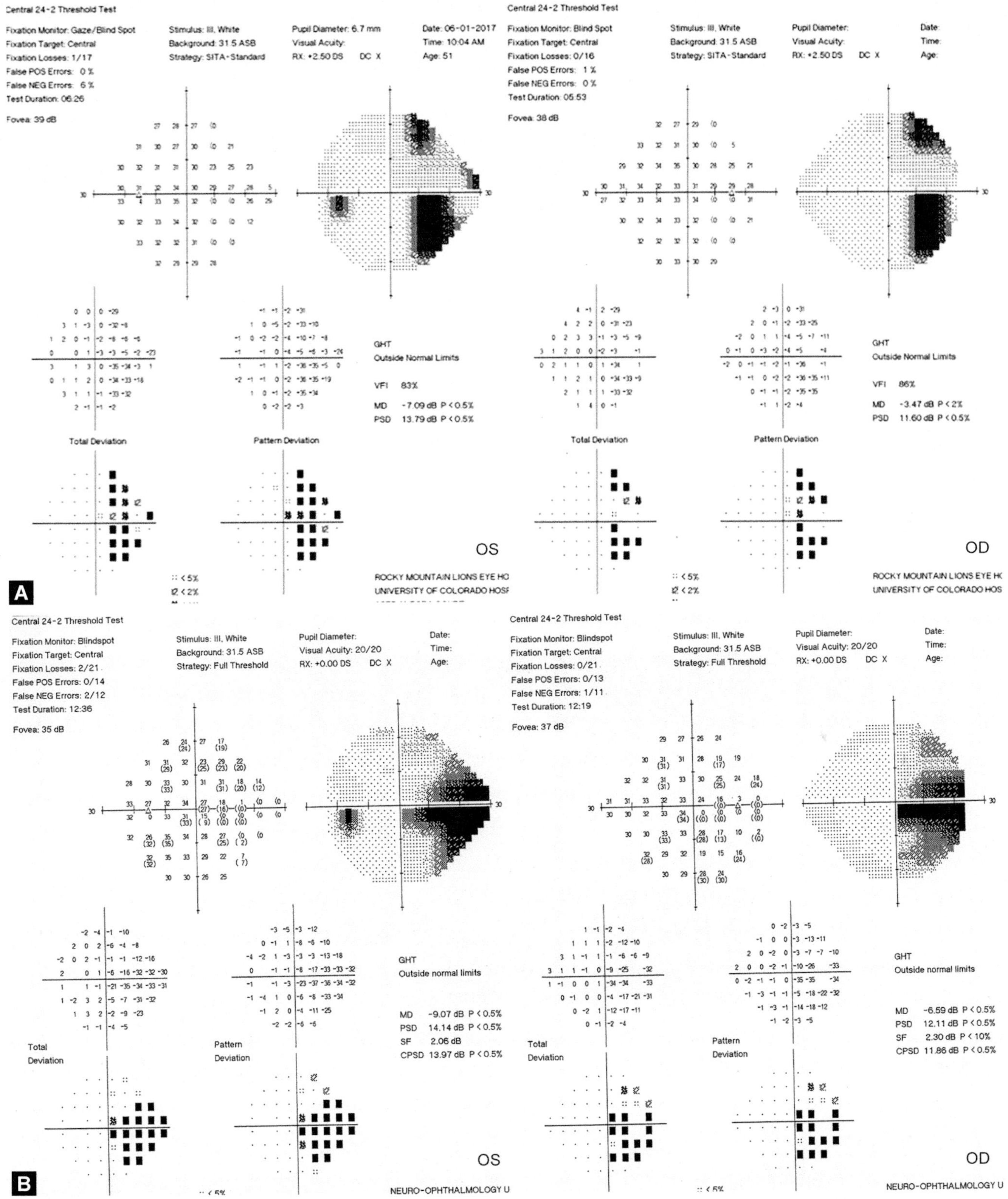

Figs. 98.23A and B: Visual field defects from ischemia to lateral geniculate nucleus (LGN). Right homonymous hemianopsia sparing the central sector, seen in stroke of the left anterior choroidal artery, a branch of the internal carotid artery (A). Right homonymous horizontal sectoranopia from stroke of the left posterior choroidal artery, a branch of the posterior cerebral artery (B). MRI not available.

Source: Prem Subramanian, MD, PhD.

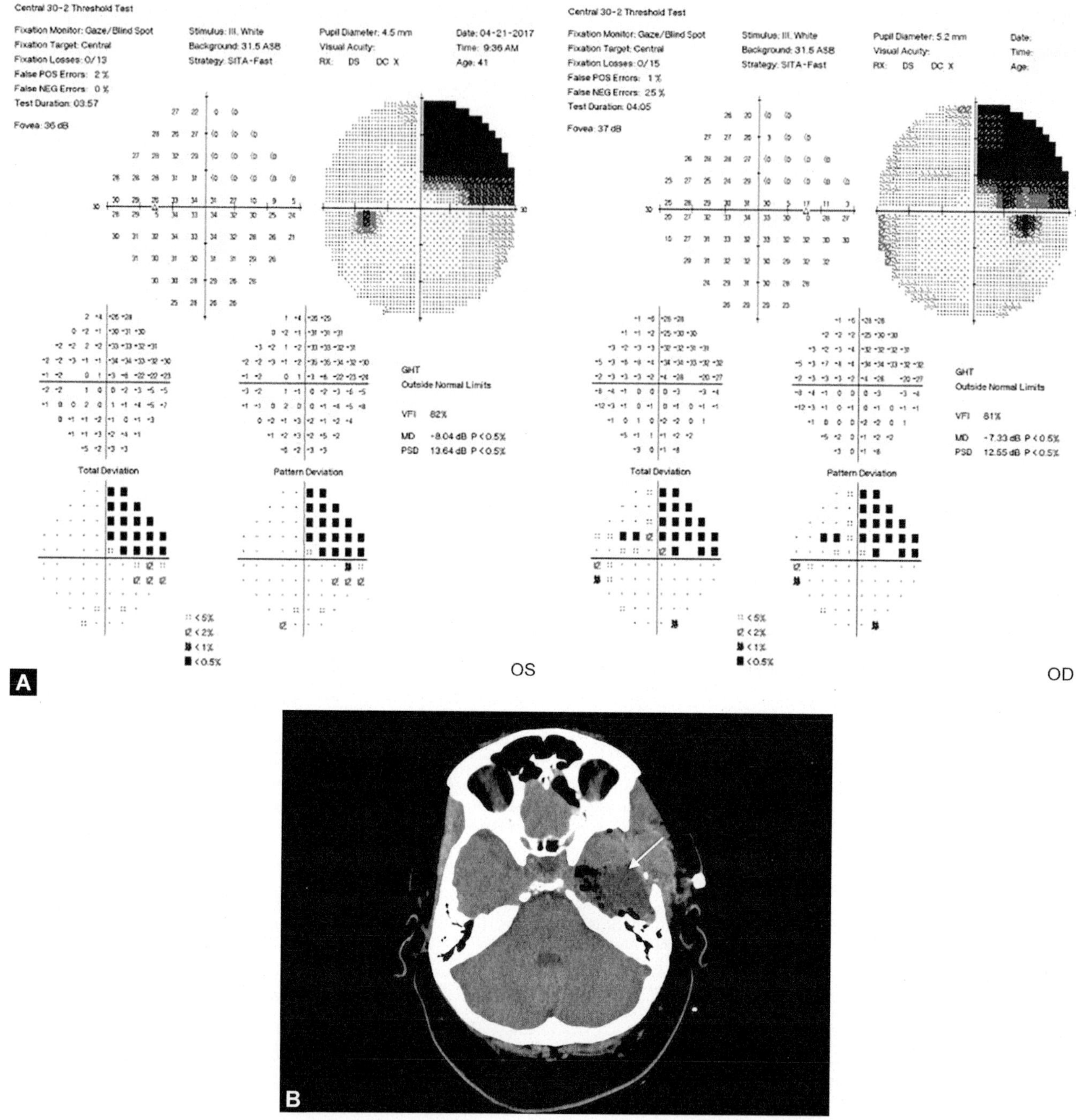

Figs. 98.24A and B: Right superior quadrantanopsia from left temporal lobectomy. HVF 30-2 demonstrates a congruous right superior homonymous quadrantanopsia ("pie in the sky", panel A) that developed after a left craniotomy and partial temporal lobectomy for epilepsy. Axial CT of the head demonstrates partial left temporal lobectomy (B).

Source: Grant Liu, MD.

carrying visual field information from similar areas of the visual field of each eye. Complex organization and processing of visual information occurs within the occipital lobe, and lesions in specific locations may affect higher-order aspects of vision such as color perception (hemiachromatopsia), face recognition (prosopagnosia), and many others. Ischemia in the distribution of the PCA is the most common cause among adults of visual field loss in this location, but neoplasms, hemorrhage, infectious processes, demyelination, trauma, malignant hypertension,

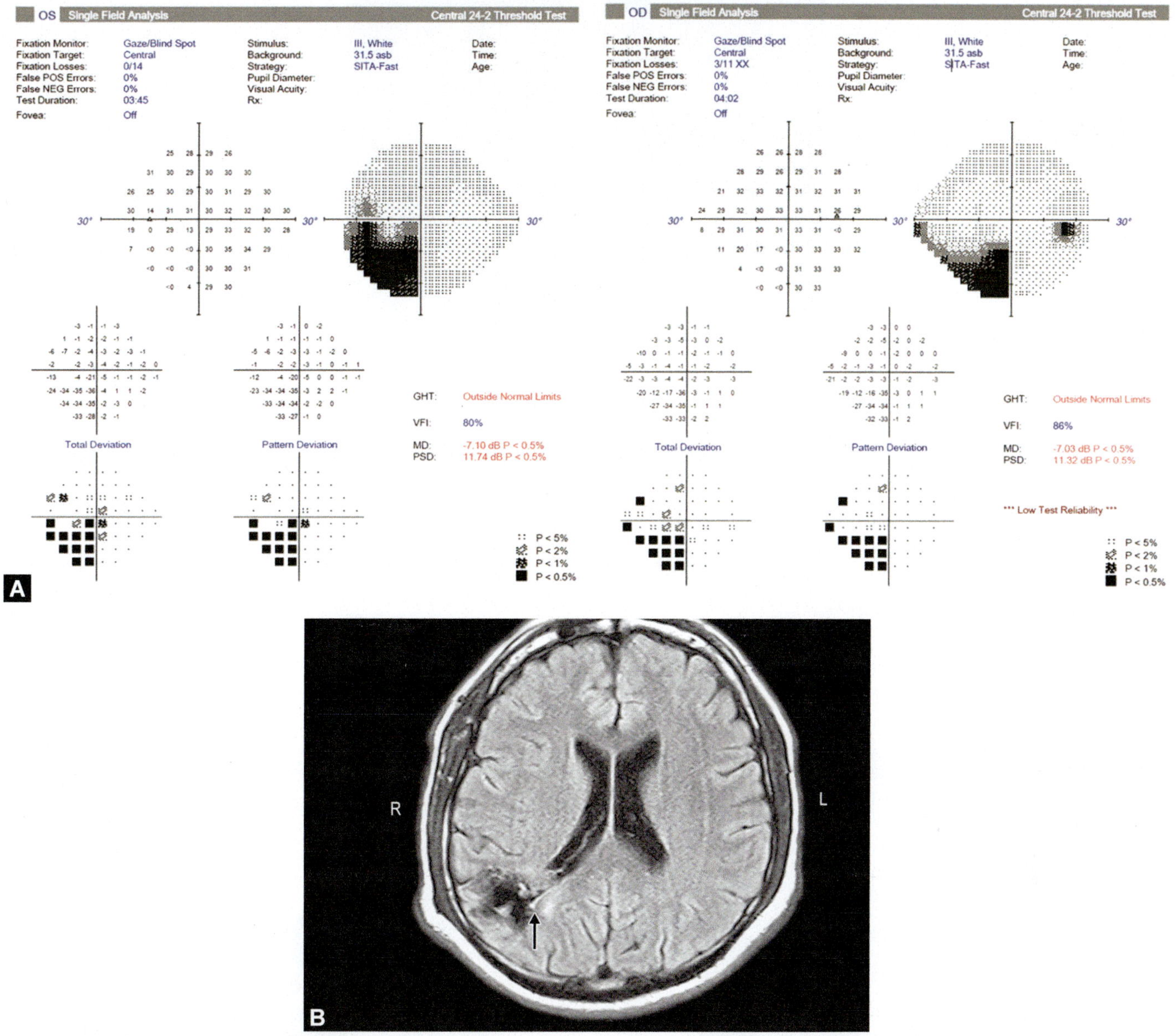

Figs. 98.25A and B: Left inferior quadrantanopsia from right parietal brain lesion. Left inferior quadrantanopsia resulting from intraparenchymal hemorrhage of the right parietal lobe (A). MRI and MRA showed cystic encephalomalacia and aging blood products at the site of the previous right temporoparietal hematoma, which resulted from an arteriovenous malformation of the middle cerebral artery at the same location (B).
Source: Fatema A Almannaei, MD.

medication toxicity, neurodegenerative disorders, seizures, perinatal hypoxia, and complex migraine also may cause similar patterns of visual field loss.

Select Retinal Visual Field Defects

Occasionally, patients will present with occult retinal disease mimicking a primary optic neuropathy. Central serous retinopathy causes impaired central acuity, metamorphopsia, and visual field loss resulting from neurosensory retinal detachments which may be visualized with careful fundus examination and OCT retinal imaging. Prior central retinal artery occlusions cause diffuse visual field loss, sometimes with peripheral sparing from peripheral predominance of choroidal blood flow, as well as optic atrophy, which may be confused with prior ischemic optic neuropathy;[38] demonstration of inner retinal

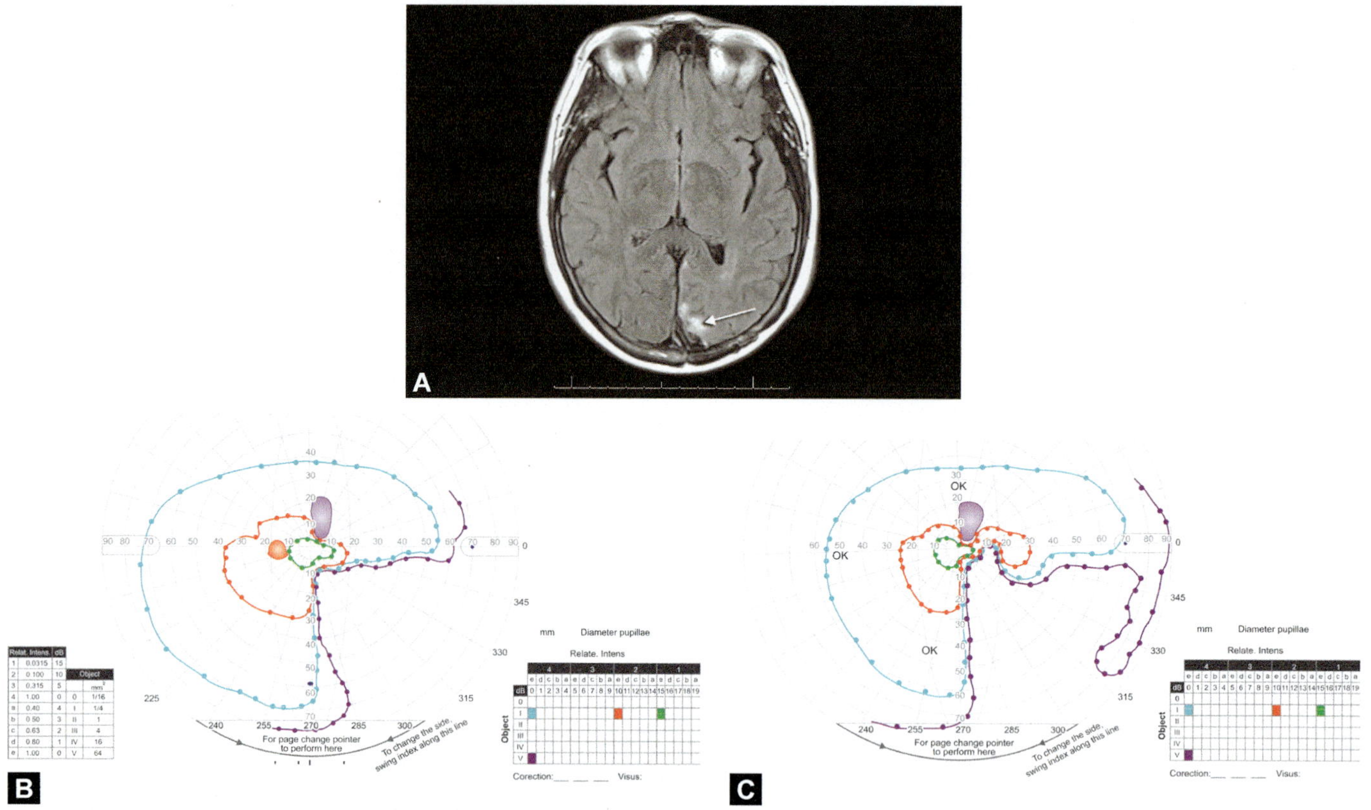

Figs. 98.26A to C: Right homonymous hemianopsia with unilateral sparing of the temporal crescent from posterior occipital lobe lesion. T1 post-contrast axial MRI showed left occipital lobe CVA (arrow, panel A). GVF shows a congruous, incomplete right homonymous hemianopsia sparing the central macula (OS panel B and OD panel C), as well as sparing of the unilateral far temporal crescent in the contralateral eye (OS panel C, purple temporal tracing), due to preserved anterior occipital cortex. BCVA is 20/20 OU.
Source: Randy Kardon, MD, PhD.

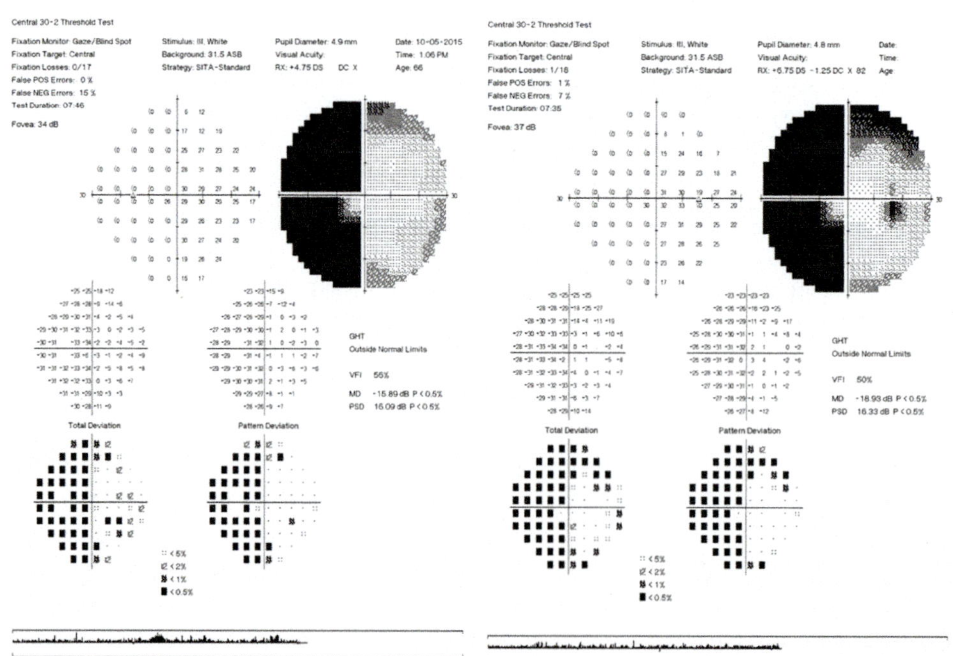

Fig. 98.27: Homonymous Hemianopsia with macular sparing from occipital lobe lesion. An 80-year-old male presented with acute vision loss of the left visual field of both eyes. Best-corrected visual acuity was 20/20 OU. HVF 30-2 revealed complete left homonymous hemianopsia with macular sparing. CT head revealed a right occipital lobe infarct within the posterior cerebral artery distribution with partial sparing of the occipital pole (not shown).

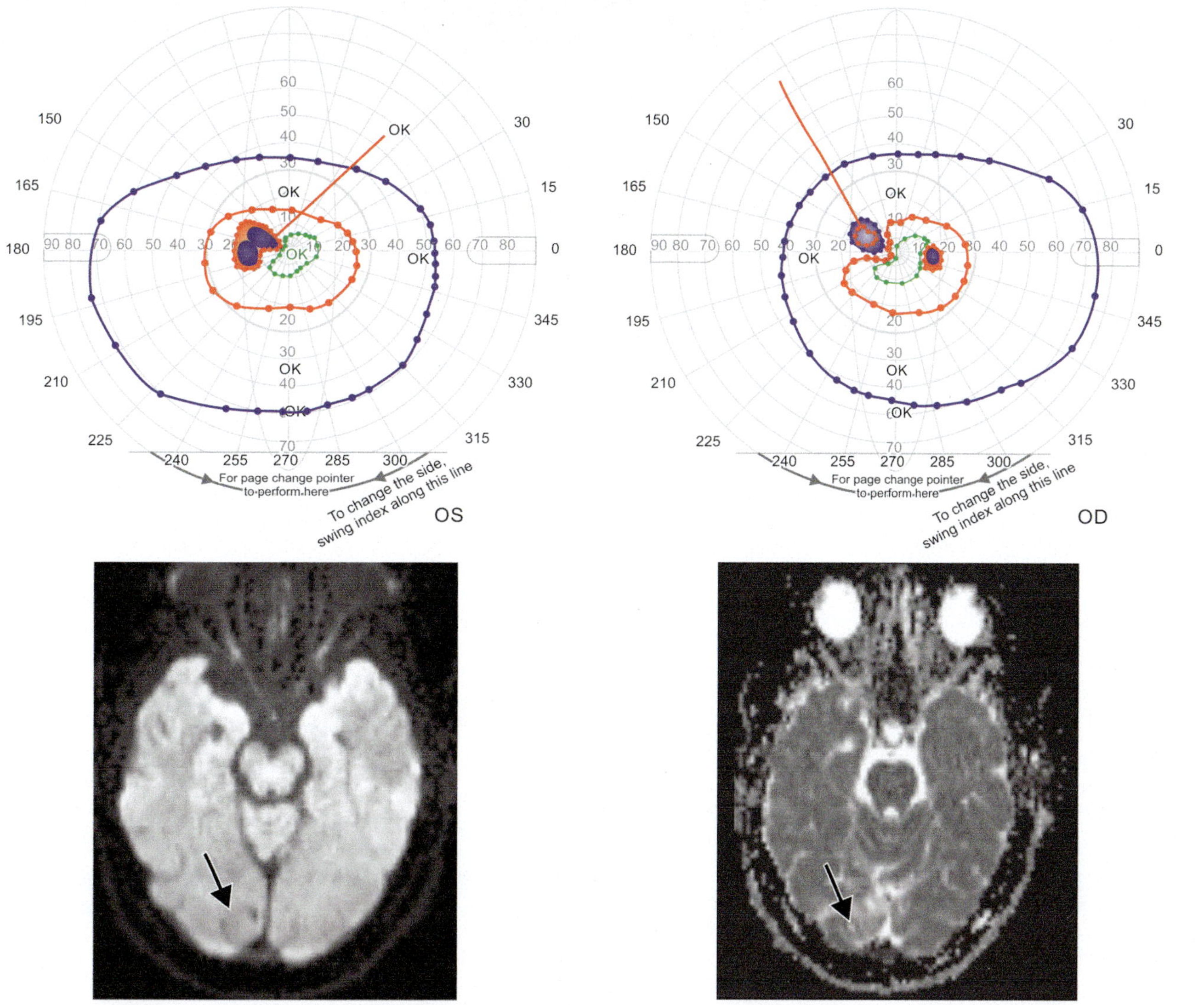

Fig. 98.28: A 70-year-old male presented to ophthalmology with an acute missing spot in his vision. Goldmann visual field revealed paracentral superior left homonymous scotoma and MRI confirmed acute right occipital lobe stroke (dark on ADC and bright on DWI on axial MRI). Note the high congruity of the scotoma between eyes, denoting its expected location in the occipital lobe.

atrophy on OCT may confirm prior retinal ischemia. Cone dystrophies such as Stargardt's disease cause progressive impairment of visual acuity and depressed central visual field from inherent photoreceptor dysfunction and may be identified with electroretinography (ERG) and genetic testing. Multiple evanescent white dot syndrome (MEWDS), acute idiopathic blind spot enlargement (AIBSE), acute macular neuroretinopathy (AMN) and acute zonal occult outer retinopathy (AZOOR) form part of a group of rare and incompletely understood retinal inflammatory conditions which are associated with enlarged blind spots and/or pericentral visual field loss and subtle fundus findings (Fig. 98.28).[7,39] With recent advances in ocular imaging, these focal visual field defects can be topographically correlated to OCT abnormalities and ERG findings consistent with photoreceptor outer segment dysfunction.[40] Degenerative retinal conditions such as retinitis pigmentosa, autoimmune, or paraneoplastic retinopathies may cause bilateral peripheral ring scotomas and retinal pigmentary changes which progress over time (Figs. 98.29A and B).[7,41] Retinal toxicity from hydroxychloroquine may cause early central visual field depression that is best identified with HVF 10-2.[2] Without cessation of the medication, a macular "bull's eye" pattern of damage may be visualized

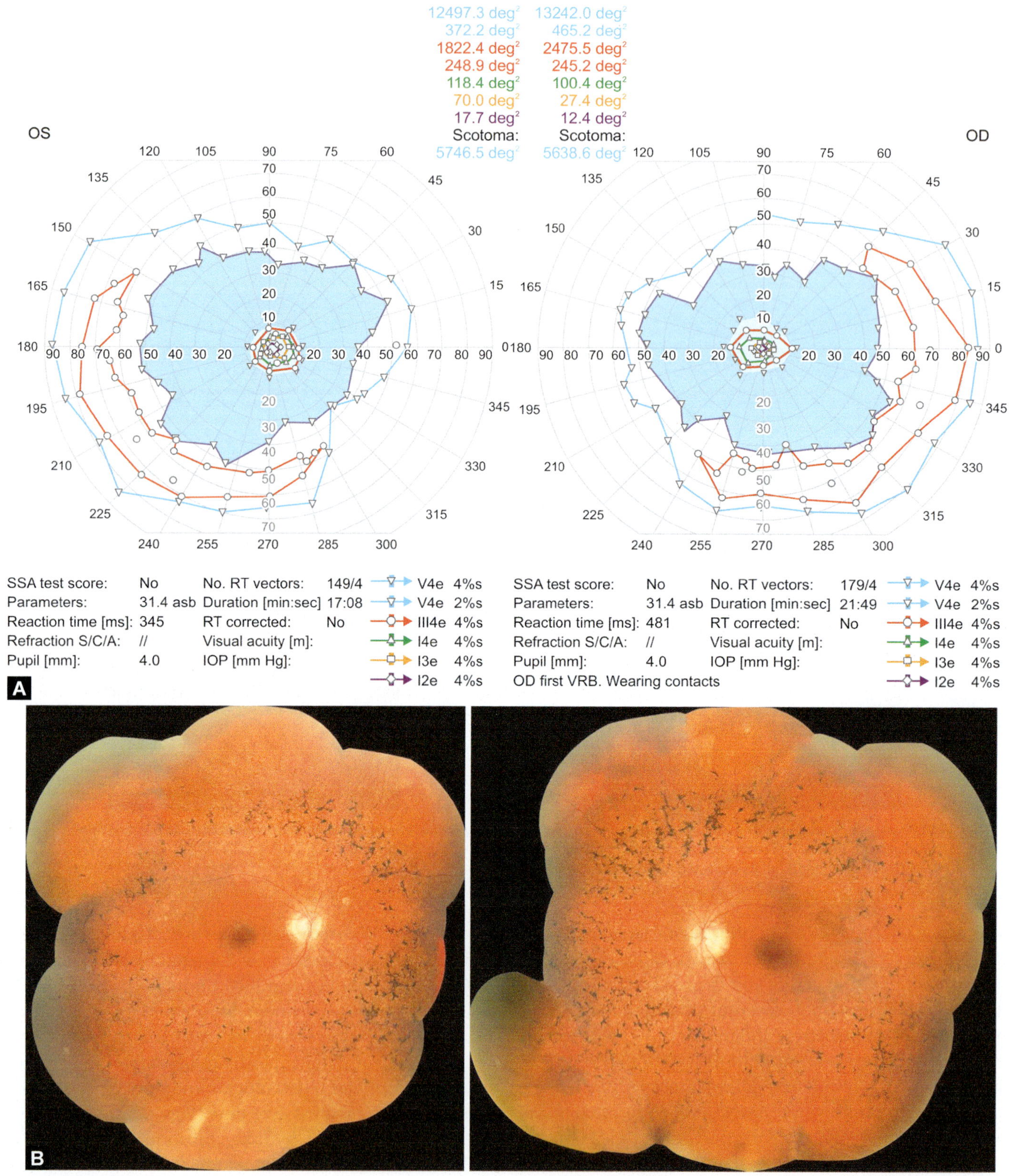

Figs. 98.29A and B: Severe concentric peripheral visual field defect on kinetic perimetry secondary to retinitis pigmentosa. Very far peripheral and central sparing remain on kinetic perimetry (A) in this patient with long-standing retinitis pigmentosa, which causes progressive loss of rod photoreceptors as seen on fundus examination (B) and loss of peripheral and low luminance vision. Octopus Kinetic Perimetry (Haag-Streit, USA).

Source: Mark Pennesi, MD, PhD.

on funduscopic examination with irreversible central ring scotomas and associated perifoveal photoreceptor loss on OCT.[42] These and a variety of other retinal lesions are covered more extensively in the retina sections of this text.

CONCLUSION

The human visual field is an essential part of any workup for vision loss if the abnormality is not readily visible on a thorough eye examination. It is extremely useful to follow natural history of disease, as well as to determine reponse to or toxicity from medical treatment. While visual acuity is a relatively sensitive detector of loss of vision from any cause, perimetry can be used to localize the pathology along the entire visual pathway, from the eye to the tip of the occipital lobes. It is important to remember that correct interpretation of visual fields takes an experienced clinician who can discern artifact from verifiable and repeatable defects. Visual fields should always be interpreted in clinical context and used in conjunction with the eye examination and other testing modalities to confirm or manage visual pathway lesions. As technology improves at an ever-increasing rate, there will no doubt be an increase in the ability of the clinician to match structural abnormalities to functional abnormalities, building confidence and credibility to diagnostic decision making.

REFERENCES

1. Murray JJ, Lee MS. Marmor RE, et al. American Academy of Ophthalmology Statement: Recommendations on screening for chloroquine and hydroxychloroquine retinopathy (2016 Revision). (Ophthalmology 2016;123:1386-94). Ophthalmology. 2017;124(3):e28-9.
2. Michaelides M, Stover NB, Francis PJ, et al. Retinal toxicity associated with hydroxychloroquine and chloroquine: risk factors, screening, and progression despite cessation of therapy. Arch Ophthalmol. 2011;129(1):30-9.
3. Hess RF. Early processing of spatial form. In: Levin L, Nilsson S, Ver Hoeve J, Wu S (Eds). Adler's Physiology of the Eye, 11th edition. Edinburgh: Elsevier; 2011. pp. 613-47.
4. Schiefer U, Patzold J, Dannheim F, et al. Conventional perimetry I: introduction—basic. Ophthalmologe. 2005; 102(6):627-46.
5. Amsler M. Earliest symptoms of diseases of the macula. Br J Ophthalmol. 1953;37(9):521-37.
6. Johnson C, Wall M. The visual field. In: Levin L, Nilsson S, Ver Hoeve J, Wu S (Eds). Adler's Physiology of the Eye, 11th edition. Edinburg: Elsevier; 2011. pp. 655-76.
7. Liu G, Volpe NJ, Galetta SL. Neuro-Ophthalmology, 2nd edition. Philadelphia, PA: Saunders; 2010.
8. Sadun AA, Agarwal MR. Topical diagnosis of acquired optic nerve disorders. In: Miller NR, Newman NJ, Biousse V, Kerrison JB (Eds). Walsh and Hoyt's Clinical Neuro-Ophthalmology, 6th edition. Philadelphia: Lipincott, Williams and Wilkins; 2005. pp. 197-236.
9. Heijl A, Asman P. Pitfalls of automated perimetry in glaucoma diagnosis. Curr Opin Ophthalmol. 1995;6(2):46-51.
10. Kardon RH. Role of the macular optical coherence tomography scan in neuro-ophthalmology. J Neuro-ophthalmol. 2011;31(4):353-61.
11. Brandao LM, Ledolter AA, Monhart M, et al. Ganglion cell layer segmentation and the two-flash multifocal electroretinogram improve structure function analysis in early glaucoma. Graefes Arch Clin Exp Ophthalmol. 2017; 255(10):1991-2000.
12. Moura AL, Raza AS, Lazow MA, et al. Retinal ganglion cell and inner plexiform layer thickness measurements in regions of severe visual field sensitivity loss in patients with glaucoma. Eye (Lond). 2012;26(9):1188-93.
13. Miraftabi A, Amini N, Morales E, et al. Macular SD-OCT outcome measures: comparison of local structure-function relationships and dynamic range. Invest Ophthalmol Vis Sci. 2016;57(11):4815-23.
14. Moon CH, Hwang SC, Ohn YH, et al. The time course of visual field recovery and changes of retinal ganglion cells after optic chiasmal decompression. Invest Ophthalmol Vis Sci. 2011;52(11):7966-73.
15. Choi CJ, Oropesa S, Callahan AB, et al. Patterns of visual field changes in thyroid eye disease. Orbit. 2017;36(4):201-7.
16. Gerling J, Meyer JH, Kommerell G. Visual field defects in optic neuritis and anterior ischemic optic neuropathy: distinctive features. Graefes Arch Clin Exp Ophthalmol. 1998;236(3):188-92.
17. Keltner JL, Johnson CA, Cello KE, et al. Visual field profile of optic neuritis: a final follow-up report from the optic neuritis treatment trial from baseline through 15 years. Arch Ophthalmol. 2010;128(3):330-7.
18. Foroozan R, Bhatti MT, Falardeau j, et al. Neuro-ophthalmology. In: Skutta GL, Cantor LB, Cioffi GA (Eds). 2013-2014 Basic and Clinical Science Course. San Francisco: American Academy of Ophthalmology; 2013.
19. Keltner JL, Johnson CA, Spurr JO, et al. Visual field profile of optic neuritis. One-year follow-up in the optic neuritis treatment trial. Arch Ophthalmol. 1994;112(7):946-53.
20. Hayreh SS, Zimmerman B, Kardon RH. Visual improvement with corticosteroid therapy in giant cell arteritis. Report of a large study and review of literature. Acta Ophthalmol Scand. 2002;80(4):355-67.
21. Hayreh SS. Posterior ischaemic optic neuropathy: clinical features, pathogenesis, and management. Eye (Lond). 2004; 18(11):1188-206.
22. Biousse V, Newman NJ. Neuro-ophthalmology of mitochondrial diseases. Curr Opin Neurol. 2003;16(1):35-43.
23. Woon C, Tang RA, Pardo G. Nutrition and optic nerve disease. Semin Ophthalmol. 1995;10(3):195-202.
24. Lam BL, Morais CG Jr, Pasol J. Drusen of the optic disc. Curr Neurol Neurosci Rep. 2008;8(5):404-8.

25. Auw-Haedrich C, Staubach F, Witschel H. Optic disk drusen. Surv Ophthalmol. 2002;47(6):515-32.
26. Pasol J. Neuro-ophthalmic disease and optical coherence tomography: glaucoma look-alikes. Curr Opin Ophthalmol. 2011;22(2):124-32.
27. Friedman DI. Papilledema and idiopathic intracranial hypertension. Continuum (Minneap Minn). 2014;20(4 Neuro-ophthalmology):857-76.
28. Keltner JL, Johnson CA, Cello KE, et al. Baseline visual field findings in the idiopathic intracranial hypertension treatment trial (IIHTT). Invest Ophthalmol Vis Sci. 2014; 55(5):3200-7.
29. Karanjia N, Jacobson DM. Compression of the prechiasmatic optic nerve produces a junctional scotoma. Am J Ophthalmol. 1999;128(2):256-8.
30. Horton JC. Wilbrand's knee of the primate optic chiasm is an artefact of monocular enucleation. Trans Am Ophthalmol Soc. 1997;95:579-609.
31. Wilbrand H, Saenger A. Die Neurologie des Auges: Ein Handbuch fur Nerven- und Augenarzte. Wiesbaden, Germany: Taschenbuch; 1904. pp. 98-120.
32. Kupfer C, Chumbley L, Downer JC. Quantitative histology of optic nerve, optic tract and lateral geniculate nucleus of man. J Anat. 1967;101(Pt 3):393-401.
33. Trobe JD. The Neurology of Vision. New York, NY: Oxford University Press; 2001.
34. Schmid R, Wilhelm B, Wilhelm H. Naso-temporal asymmetry and contraction anisocoria in the pupillomotor system. Graefes Arch Clin Exp Ophthalmol. 2000;238(2):123-8.
35. Levin L. Topical diagnosis of chiasmal and retrochiasmal disorders. In: Miller NR, Newman NJ, Biousse V, Kerrison JB (Eds). Walsh and Hoyt's Clinical Neuro-Ophthalmology, 6th edition. Philadelphia: Lippincott Williams and Wilkins; 2005. pp. 503-74.
36. Bell RA, Thompson HS. Relative afferent pupillary defect in optic tract hemianopias. Am J Ophthalmol. 1978;85(4):538-40.
37. Horton JC, Hoyt WF. The representation of the visual field in human striate cortex. A revision of the classic Holmes map. Arch Ophthalmol. 1991;109(6):816-24.
38. Hayreh SS. Ocular vascular occlusive disorders: natural history of visual outcome. Prog Retin Eye Res. 2014;41:1-25.
39. Heckenlively JR, Ferreyra HA. Autoimmune retinopathy: a review and summary. Semin Immunopathol. 2008;30(2):127-34.
40. Aleman TS, Sandhu HS, Serrano LW, et al. Acute zonal cone photoreceptor outer segment loss. JAMA Ophthalmol. 2017;135(5):487-90.
41. Rahimy E, Sarraf D. Paraneoplastic and non-paraneoplastic retinopathy and optic neuropathy: evaluation and management. Surv Ophthalmol. 2013;58(5):430-58.
42. Marmor MF, Kellner U, Lai TY, et al. Recommendations on screening for chloroquine and hydroxychloroquine retinopathy (2016 Revision). Ophthalmology. 2016;123(6): 1386-94.

Chapter 99 Vascular Diseases of the Central Nervous System and Orbit

Jocelyn Lam, Roberta Dalley, Courtney Francis

ANATOMY

Circle of Willis

The circle of Willis is an arterial system of anastomoses located on the ventral portion of the brain that supplies blood to the brain and surrounding structures. The circle of Willis receives blood from the internal carotid arteries and vertebral arteries, which are branches of the aortic arch. The internal carotid artery enters the skull bilaterally and divides into the anterior cerebral arteries and continues as the middle cerebral artery after it gives off the ophthalmic artery. The vertebral arteries join to form the basilar artery which then divides into the caudal branches of the circle of Willis, including the anterior inferior cerebellar arteries, superior cerebellar arteries, posterior cerebellar arteries and other vessels.

Venous Sinuses

Dural venous sinuses serve as the major drainage system of the brain. There are six major venous channels which drain into the internal jugular veins. Unpaired venous structures include the superior sagittal sinus, inferior sagittal sinus, straight sinus, occipital sinus, and intercavernous sinus. Paired structures include the transverse sinus, sigmoid sinus, superior petrosal and inferior petrosal sinuses, cavernous sinus, sphenoparietal sinus, and basilar venous plexus. They are located between the periosteum and dura mater and do not contain valves.

Cavernous Sinus

The cavernous sinus is a unique paired dural venous structure that resembles a cavity or sinus. It is located on either side of the sella turcica and bordered by the sphenoid and temporal bones of the skull. Important structures that course through the cavernous sinus include cranial nerves III, IV, V and VI, internal carotid arteries, and sympathetic nerves.

Orbit

The bony orbit serves to protect the globe. It is approximately 35 mm in height, 40–45 mm in width and has a volume of 30 mL. The roof of the orbit is composed of the frontal bone and lesser wing of the sphenoid. The lateral wall is comprised of the zygomatic bone and greater wing of the sphenoid. The medial wall contains the ethmoid, lacrimal, maxillary, and lesser wing of sphenoid bones. The orbital floor is composed of the maxillary, palatine and zygomatic bones.

ARTERIAL OCCLUSIVE DISEASE

Ophthalmic Signs and Symptoms

Cerebral vascular disease may present with vision loss, visual field deficits, diplopia, anisocoria, eye pain, neck pain and headache. Ophthalmic manifestations of stroke result from infarction of brain structures controlling visual, pupillary and ocular motor pathways. Occlusion typically results from thrombosis or embolus resulting from atherosclerotic disease. Other causes of arterial occlusion include vasculitis and vasospasm from migraines or drugs.

Amaurosis Fugax

Amaurosis fugax describes painless, transient monocular or binocular vision loss. Etiologies include: (1) thromboembolism leading to transient retinal ischemia, (2) retinal vascular insufficiency resulting from localized or generalized hypoperfusion, (3) vasospasm, and (4) idiopathic.[1] The term is derived from the Latin word fugax, which means fleeting, and the Greek word amaurosis, which means darkening, dark or obscured. Clinically, it suggests retinal ischemia, and workup for a cause should be initiated. Patients may not always present with total vision loss but may describe altitudinal or hemianopic transient field deficits. Episodes usually last between 1 minute and

15 minutes with complete recovery of vision. Amaurosis may be a sign of impending stroke due to thromboembolism and is considered clinically equivalent to a transient ischemic attack (TIA).[2] Therefore, all patients with symptoms of amaurosis should undergo urgent evaluation and risk stratification.

Ocular Ischemic Syndrome

Chronic arterial hypoperfusion to the eye can lead to ocular ischemic syndrome. Symptoms include vision loss and dull pain in or around the eye. Signs of ocular ischemic syndrome include corneal edema, mild anterior chamber cell and flare, asymmetric cataract, iris and retinal neovascularization, mid-peripheral retinal hemorrhages, cotton wool spots, and dilated retinal veins. Severe ipsilateral or bilateral carotid artery stenosis is the most common causes. The common carotid is most often affected, followed by internal carotid and external carotid. Vasculitis, including giant cell arteritis (GCA), may also cause ocular ischemic syndrome.

Vertebrobasilar Insufficiency

Hypoperfusion of the vertebral and basilar arteries can lead to vision loss due to reduced blood flow to the occipital lobes. Vision loss is typically sudden, simultaneous, and bilateral. Vision loss may be total or homonymous, hemianopic or altitudinal. Symptoms of vision loss may be transient and last less than minute if blood flow is restored, analogous to amaurosis fugax. Patients may also describe blurred vision, foggy vision or darkening of their vision. Other symptoms of decreased posterior circulation include vertigo and ataxia but may not always be present, and most patients do not experience any warning symptoms.

An isolated homonymous visual field defect of sudden onset is pathognomic for a vascular insult to the occipital lobe. Macular sparing occurs as the occipital lobe is also supplied by the middle cerebral artery. The anterior portion of the occipital lobe is responsible for the contralateral peripheral 30° of temporal field. An isolated unilateral anterior occipital lobe lesion will cause loss of the "temporal crescent" on the opposite side of the lesion.[3] Similarly, a unilateral lesion not affecting the anterior occipital lobe will cause a contralateral homonymous hemianopia with sparing of the contralateral temporal crescent. Goldmann perimetry is required for detection as Humphrey visual fields do not test the far periphery or temporal crescent.

Thrombosis and Embolism

Atherosclerosis is the most common cause of cerebral vascular disease and stroke. Thrombotic strokes are caused by occlusion of medium to small vessels. Embolic strokes often result from carotid artery plaques that dislodge and circulate in the intracranial vasculature. The other major source of emboli is the heart. Cardiac thrombi occurring from atrial fibrillation, atrial myxomas, impaired contractility from myocardial infarction, and vegetations from endocarditis or other valvular disease can introduce emboli into the carotid circulation. In young or pregnant patients, thrombosis due to hypercoagulability must be considered.

Vasculitis

Inflammatory disease of vessels supplying the brain, eye and orbit can cause vision loss. Other symptoms of central nervous system (CNS) vasculitis can include headache, seizure, stroke, encephalopathy, weakness, paralysis, and paresthesias.

Giant Cell Arteritis

Giant cell arteritis, also known as temporal arteritis, is a feared cause of blindness and presents with acute monocular vision loss or rarely binocular vision loss. *See* Chapter 94 for additional discussion of GCA. This inflammatory disease affects medium to large vessels and preferentially the branches of the temporal artery. The disease is exceedingly rare in individuals under age 50 and 80% of cases occur in patients over the age of 80.[4] Additionally, females and individuals of Scandinavian descent are at increased risk of developing GCA.[5] The condition is also strongly associated with polymyalgia rheumatic (PMR). Approximately 40–50% of patients with GCA have PMR and GCA is found in 15% of patients with PMR.[6] Vision loss occurs from occlusive vasculitis and may include:[7]

- Arteritic anterior ischemic optic neuropathy
- Central retinal artery occlusion (CRAO)
- Posterior ischemic optic neuropathy
- Cerebral ischemia.

The most feared complication is vision loss, as it is irreversible and can rapidly involve the fellow eye within days. It is estimated that this occurs in 25–50% of patients within 1 week without treatment.[8] Prompt initiation of high-dose steroids significantly reduces this risk. Thus, the diagnosis of GCA should be considered in all patients over the age of 50 presenting with ischemic optic neuropathy, CRAO or transient monocular vision loss with or without risk factors.

Granulomatosis with Polyangiitis

Granulomatosis with polyangiitis (GPA), formerly known as Wegener granulomatosis, is one of the antineutrophil cytoplasmic antibody (ANCA)-associated vasculitides. Systemic symptoms may include sinusitis, epistaxis, hematuria, hemoptysis, and arthritis. Ocular signs and symptoms can occur without systemic manifestations and may be the initial presentation in patients of all ages. Ophthalmic manifestations include dry eyes, conjunctivitis, ulcerative keratitis, episcleritis, scleritis, retinitis, eyelid swelling, proptosis, lacrimal gland enlargement, canalicular or nasolacrimal duct obstruction, and orbital inflammation that may mimic thyroid eye disease, immunoglobulin G4 (IgG4) orbitopathy or orbital pseudotumor.[9,10] Patients typically present with eye pain, foreign body sensation, epiphora, blurry vision and diplopia. Strabismus is often incomitant given the diffuse orbital involvement. Thus, it is important for the ophthalmologist to recognize signs and symptoms concerning for GPA. C-ANCA titers are positive in 90% of cases but may be negative in localized ocular disease. Orbital imaging may show diffuse inflammation and sinus involvement. Treatment of ocular disease involves anti-inflammatory agents, glucocorticoids, chemotherapeutics and ocular surface lubrication. Cyclophosphamide has been the mainstay of treatment for severe disease and azathioprine for maintaining remission.

Other Vasculitides

Other causes of CNS vasculitis important to ophthalmologists include systemic lupus erythematosus (SLE), Susac syndrome and acute multifocal placoid pigment epitheliopathy (AMPPE). Any ocular structure may be affected by SLE with keratoconjunctivitis sicca or dry eyes the most common manifestation.[11] This often results from lacrimal gland involvement from secondary Sjögren's syndrome. Ocular motility deficits are the most common neuro-ophthalmic manifestation of lupus occurring in up to 30% of patients[12] and may be caused by neuropathy or inflammation of extraocular muscles. Other less common manifestations include optic neuropathies and myasthenia gravis.[11] Patients with SLE and suspected optic neuritis with myelitis must be evaluated for neuromyelitis optica. Susac syndrome is a rare vasculitis that presents with the triad of multiple branch retinal artery occlusions, sensorineural hearing loss, and encephalopathy with findings of white matter lesions in the corpus callosum on magnetic resonance imaging (MRI). AMPPE is an acute self-limited, idiopathic inflammatory condition in young adults that presents with acute vision changes, scotomas or metamorphopsia and is bilateral is over 75%.[13] There are case reports of association between AMPPE with cerebral vasculitis and meningoencephalitis. Any patient diagnosed with AMPPE who develops neurologic symptoms including headache or stiff neck should be evaluated with neuroimaging.

Migraine

Many patients with migraines experience focal neurologic symptoms referred to as aura, which typically precede the headache. Visual aura is the most common form of migraine aura. Classically, the diagnosis of aura requires two of the following criteria to be met (1) gradual onset over 4 minutes, (2) aura lasts no more than 1 hour, (3) headache follows aura within 60 minutes onset or simultaneously with aura, and (4) is fully reversible.[14] Positive symptoms of aura include visual and auditory phenomenon, paresthesias, or motor disturbances. Visual aura is classically described as scintillating scotomas or arcs of light expanding across half of the visual field. Migraine auras without headache are known as acephalgic migraines. These are often referred to as ocular or retinal migraines, which are inaccurate, as the aura still originates from the brain as opposed to the eye.

Arterial vasospasm can cause transient ischemia and symptoms similar to stroke. Typically, symptoms last for over 20 minutes and may include transient binocular vision loss, homonymous visual field deficits, hemiplegia, cranial nerve palsies and ophthalmoplegia. Vasospasm of the ophthalmic or central retinal artery can cause transient monocular vision loss and is a diagnosis of exclusion.

Others

Some drugs and medications can cause arterial occlusion from thrombosis or vasospasm. Oral contraceptives and hormone therapies are known to cause hypercoagulability, which can lead to increased risk of CNS thrombosis. Cocaine causes vasoconstriction and can lead to stroke, myocardial infarction and vision loss.

INTRACRANIAL ANEURYSMS, DISSECTION AND HEMORRHAGE

Types

Saccular or berry aneurysms are outpouchings of arteries caused by a weakened portion of the vessel wall. These thinned outpouchings are at risk for spontaneous rupture causing subarachnoid hemorrhage. Septic aneurysms are caused by bacterial infection. Similarly, mycotic aneurysms are caused by fungal infection.

Locations and Incidence

The majority of intracranial aneurysms are located in the anterior cerebral circulation. The most common sites are at the junctions between arteries in the circle of Willis such as between the anterior communication artery with the anterior cerebral, between the posterior communicating and internal carotid, and at the bifurcation of the middle cerebral artery. There is a slight female predominance. Aneurysmal rupture is associated with subarachnoid hemorrhage and a high-mortality rate (Figs. 99.1A and B). When an aneurysm occurs in the cavernous portion of the carotid artery and ruptures, a carotid-cavernous fistula results instead of a subarachnoid hemorrhage. Common causes of aneurysms include hypertension, smoking and collagen vascular disease.

Ophthalmic Signs and Symptoms

Most aneurysms are asymptomatic until they exert mass effect or rupture. Symptoms and signs of intracerebral aneurysm depend on the location of the aneurysm and mass effect on adjacent structures. Symptoms may include headache, vision loss from compressive optic neuropathy or ischemia from interrupted flow to the ophthalmic artery, third nerve palsy, facial pain or paresthesias. Small aneurysms are often asymptomatic until enlargement prior to rupture. Noninvasive imaging is most reliable at detecting aneurysms 3 mm or larger. If clinical suspicion is high, the gold standard remains cerebral angiography.

Carotid Artery Dissection

Carotid artery dissection occurs from a tear in the inner wall of the carotid artery that leads to a separation between the vessel layers. The separation causes blood to accumulate between the vessel walls, forming a hematoma which can cause stenosis or pseudoaneurysm formation and leads to cerebral hypoperfusion. As a result, carotid dissection can lead to ischemic stroke, particularly in young adults. Trauma is the most common cause, typically from hyperextension of the neck. The most common symptom is head or neck pain, present in up to 80% of cases. Horner's syndrome occurs in 25% of cases due to interruption of sympathetic fibers traveling along the carotid artery.[15] Ptosis and miosis

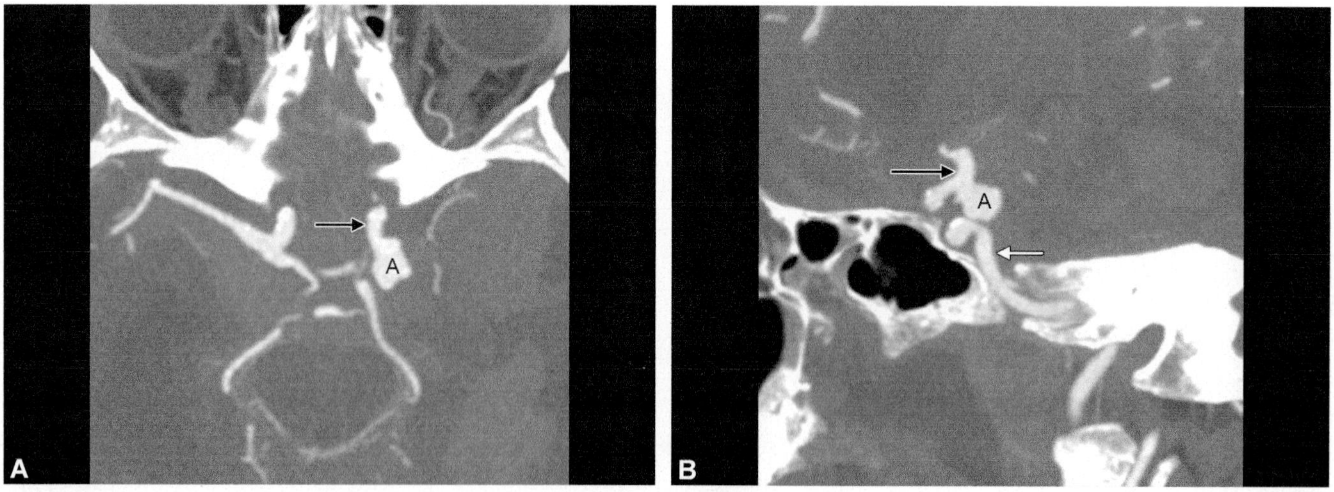

Figs. 99.1A and B: Posterior communicating aneurysm with acute subarachnoid hemorrhage. (A) Axial computed tomography angiography (CTA) image at the level of the supraclinoid internal carotid arteries (arrow) reveals a multilobulated aneurysm (A) projecting posteriorly. Associated large amount of acute subarachnoid blood is present in the adjacent cisterns; (B) Sagittal CTA reformation better shows the posterior communicating aneurysm (A) projecting posteriorly-inferiorly from the supraclinoid ICA (black arrow), and sitting just cranial to the cavernous left ICA (white arrow).

are present but anhidrosis is typically not seen as the fibers responsible for facial sweating travel along the external carotid artery. Other symptoms may include amaurosis fugax, pulsatile tinnitus, hemiparalysis, facial droop and aphasia. Orbital and eye pain are typically not seen in carotid artery dissection. Connective tissue disorders, most commonly fibromuscular dysplasia, have been associated with dissection. Computed tomography (CT) angiography is the gold standard for diagnosis of carotid artery dissection (Fig. 99.2) and should be considered immediately when the condition is suspected.

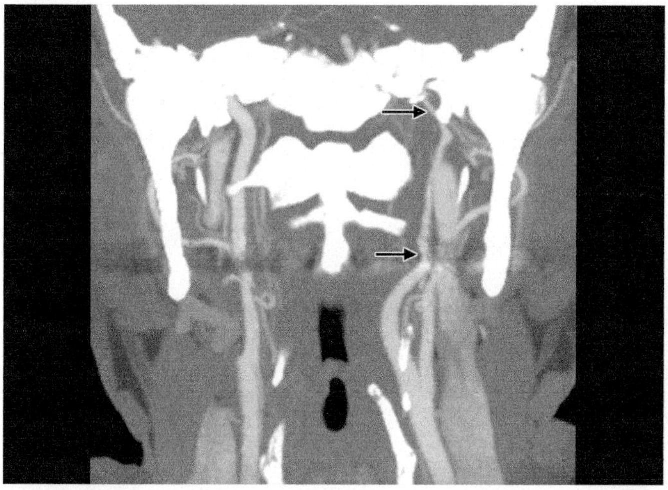

Fig. 99.2: Left ICA dissection. Coronal CTA shows a dissection (arrows) of the mid-to-distal ICA with irregularity and narrowing. Note the smooth uniform caliber of the right ICA.

Pituitary Apoplexy

This rare but life-threatening condition occurs after sudden hemorrhage into the pituitary gland, typically caused by rapid enlargement of a pituitary adenoma (Figs. 99.3A to D). Death occurs from sudden adrenocorticotropic hormone (ACTH) and cortisol deficiency leading to hypotension. Symptoms of apoplexy include acute onset of severe headache, decreased visual acuity or vision loss, visual field deficit, and diplopia due to cavernous sinus invasion. Surgical decompression is considered in patients with visual or neurologic impairments.

VENOUS OCCLUSIVE DISEASE

Dural Venous Thrombosis

Dural venous thrombosis is caused by acute clotting within a dural venous sinus (Figs. 99.4A to D). Classically, it causes an acute onset severe "thunderclap" headache. Intracranial pressure may be elevated from venous congestion and lack of drainage through the arachnoid meninges. In chronic thrombosis, papilledema may be seen but not necessarily in the acute phase. In younger patients, venous thrombosis should prompt systemic evaluation (*see* Chapter 94). Patients are treated with anticoagulation while monitoring for vision loss secondary to papilledema.

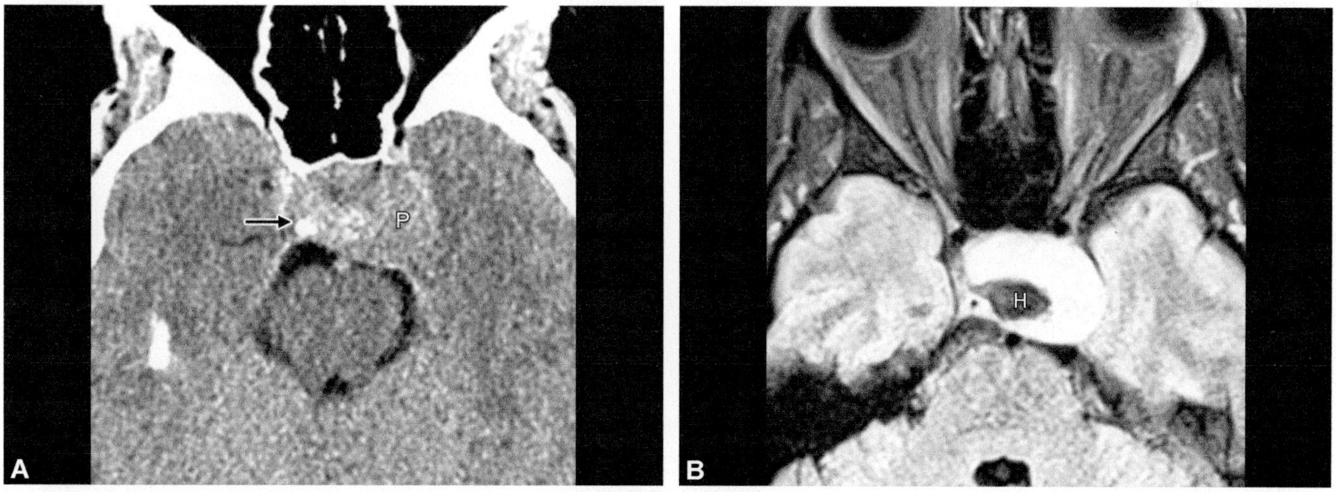

Figs. 99.3A and B: Pituitary apoplexy. (A) Axial noncontrast CT through an enlarged 3 × 2 cm pituitary adenoma (P) which invades the left cavernous sinus. Note the subtle higher density acute hemorrhage (arrow) in the right posterior aspect of the pituitary mass; (B) Axial noncontrast fat saturated FLAIR image better demonstrates the low signal deoxyhemoglobin (H) blood in the right posterior pituitary fossa, surrounded by the uniformly high T2 signal of the pituitary adenoma.

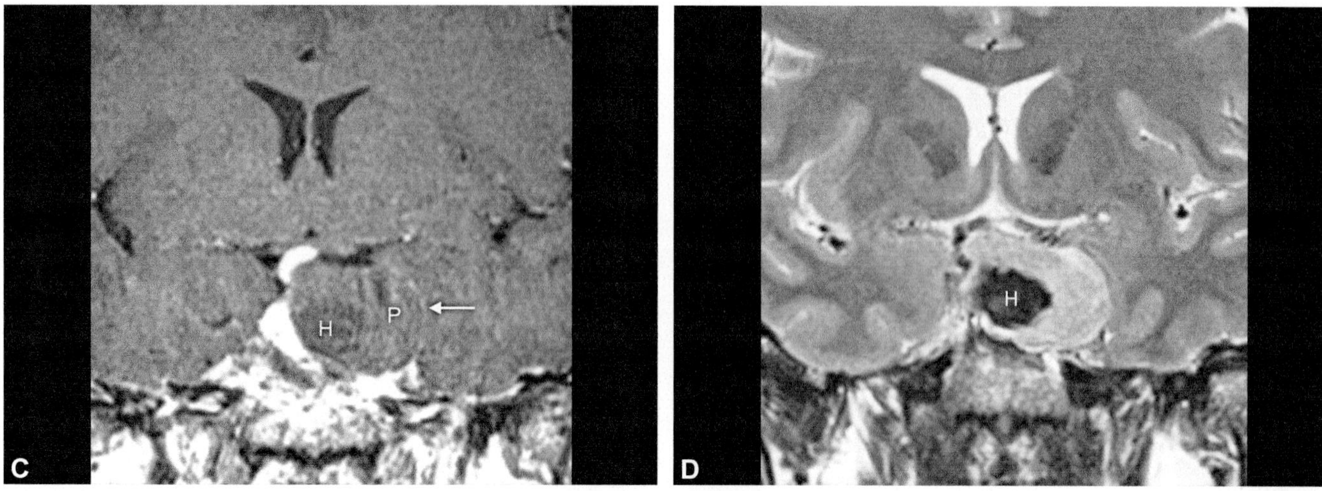

Figs. 99.3C and D: Pituitary apoplexy. (C) Coronal post-gadolinium enhanced T1 shows the relative subtle low signal deoxyhemoglobin (H) relative to the poorly enhancing surrounding pituitary mass (P). Note intensely enhancing normal pituitary tissue and the enhancing pituitary stalk pushed to the right by the adenoma; (D) Coronal T2 image better demonstrates the intrasellar and suprasellar pituitary adenoma with the internal bleed with low signal deoxyhemoglobin (H).

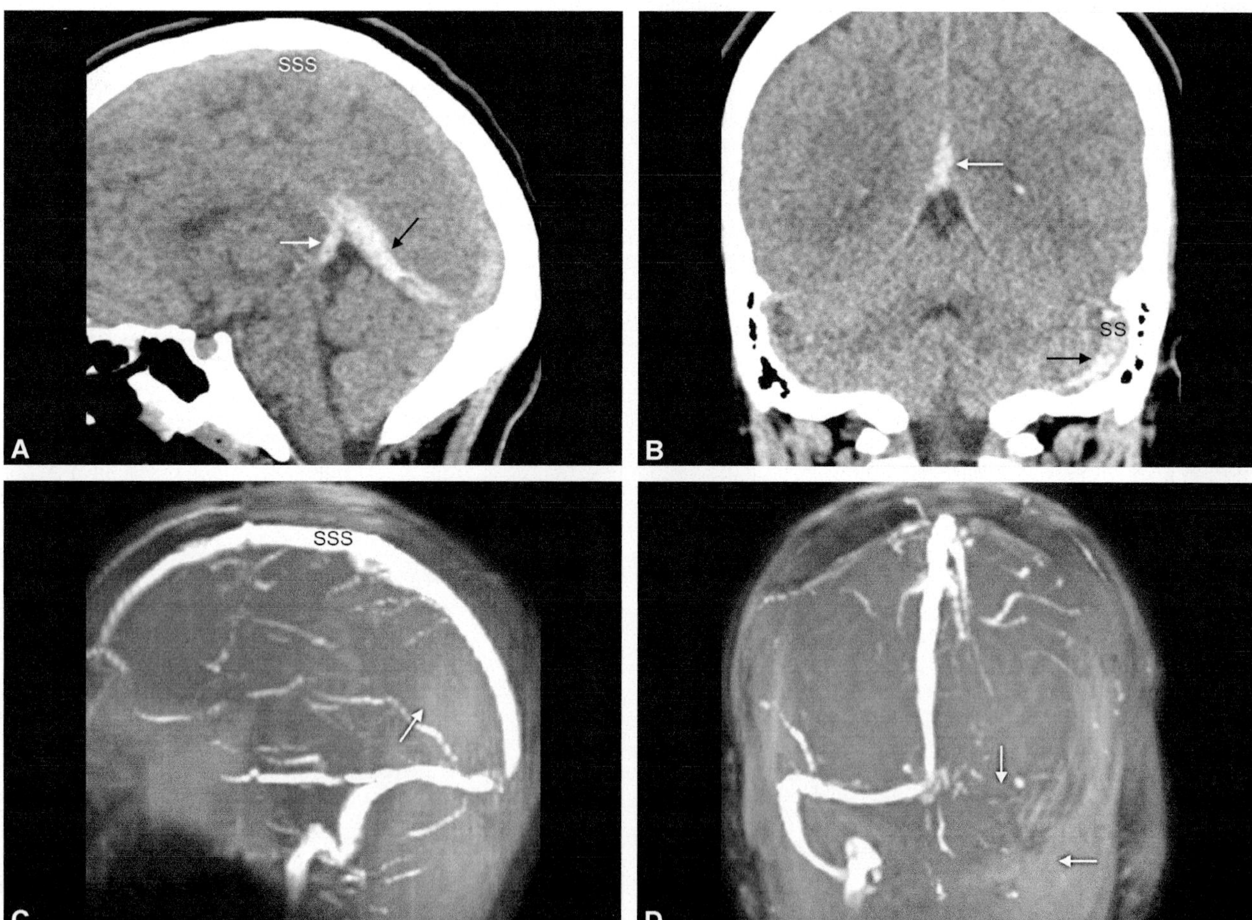

Figs. 99.4A to D: Pregnant woman with dural sinus thrombosis. (A) Sagittal noncontrast CT reveals hyperdense clot in the straight sinus (black arrow) and the vein of Galen (white arrow). The superior sagittal sinus (SSS) has normal density dural venous blood along the convexity; (B) Coronal noncontrast CT also shows the high-density clot in the straight sinus (white arrow), as well as in the lower portion of the sigmoid sinus (black arrow); (C) Lateral MR venogram has a normal superior sagittal sinus (SSS), right transverse sinus and right sigmoid sinus. However, the thrombosed straight sinus is absent (tip of white arrow); (D) MR angiogram AP view also demonstrates the complete absence of the left transverse (vertical arrow) and sigmoid (horizontal arrow) thrombosed dural sinuses.

Cavernous Sinus Thrombosis

Cavernous sinus thrombosis causes characteristic ophthalmic problems because of its effect on neurovascular structures that lie within its borders. Diplopia results from compression of cranial nerves III, IV or VI, and multiple cranial neuropathies with involvement of cranial nerve V should lead the ophthalmologist to search for a lesion in the cavernous sinus. Compression of the sympathetic nerves traveling along the internal carotid artery as it passes through the cavernous sinus may also cause a Horner's syndrome. Orbital signs include retrobulbar pain, proptosis and chemosis because of impaired venous outflow. Without treatment, thrombosis may spread to the contralateral cavernous sinus through communicating veins and cause signs in the fellow eye. Unilateral ophthalmoplegia progressing to bilateral involvement is highly suspicious for cavernous sinus thrombosis. Cavernous sinus thrombosis may result from hypercoagulability in younger patients. Orbital cellulitis may cause septic cavernous sinus thrombosis as venous drainage flows directly into the cavernous sinus. Mucormycosis is a life-threatening invasive fungal sinusitis that can rapidly invade the cavernous sinus and cause septic thrombosis. A patient who presents with headache and multiple cranial neuropathies should undergo imaging to include the cavernous sinus. MR venography is the most sensitive imaging method for demonstrating venous thrombosis, as head CT can be normal in many cases (Figs. 99.5A to C). CT venography also provides visualization of dural sinuses and may be an option for patients with contraindications for MRI scanning but provides lower resolution of venous structures.

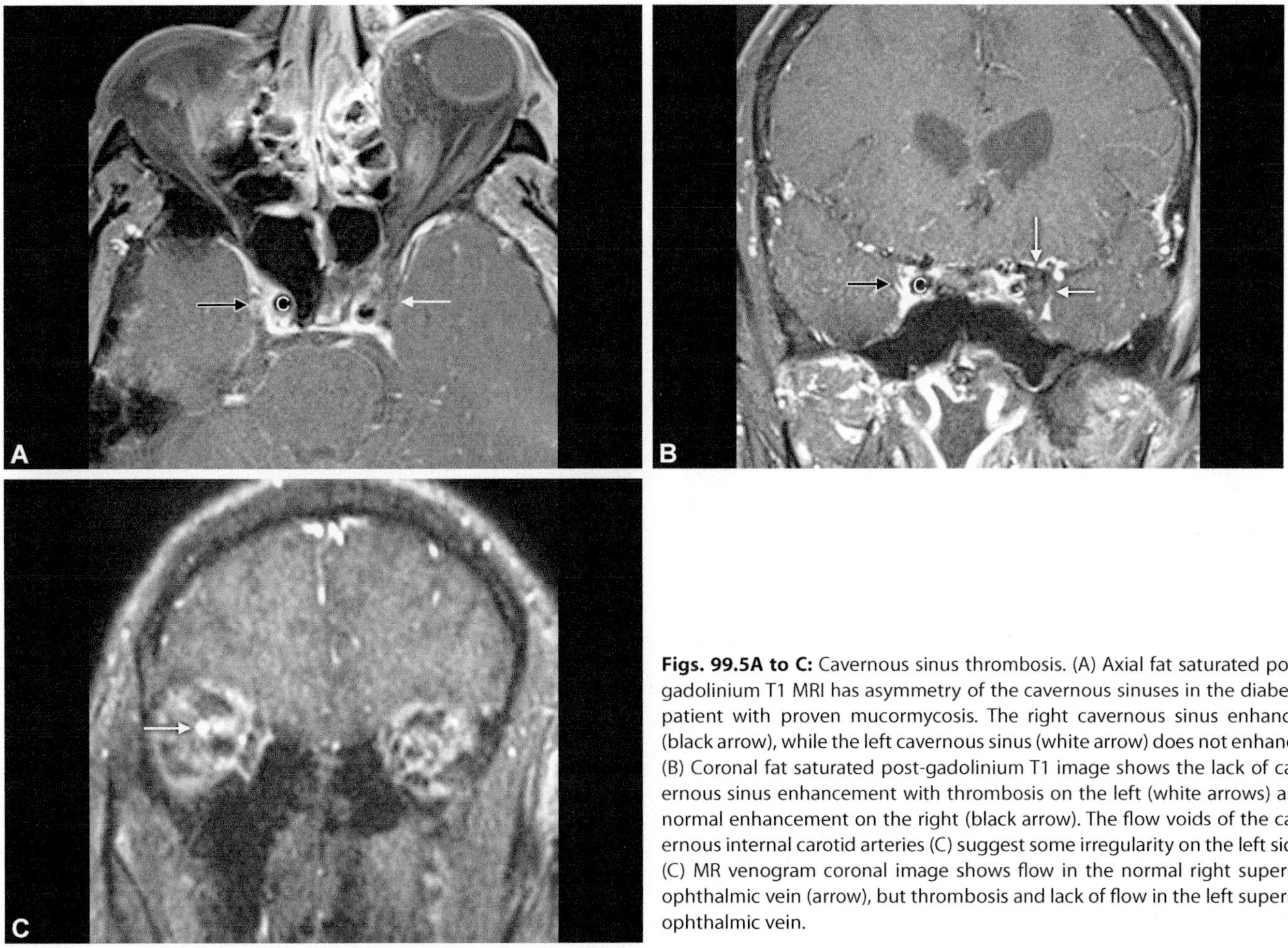

Figs. 99.5A to C: Cavernous sinus thrombosis. (A) Axial fat saturated post-gadolinium T1 MRI has asymmetry of the cavernous sinuses in the diabetic patient with proven mucormycosis. The right cavernous sinus enhances (black arrow), while the left cavernous sinus (white arrow) does not enhance; (B) Coronal fat saturated post-gadolinium T1 image shows the lack of cavernous sinus enhancement with thrombosis on the left (white arrows) and normal enhancement on the right (black arrow). The flow voids of the cavernous internal carotid arteries (C) suggest some irregularity on the left side; (C) MR venogram coronal image shows flow in the normal right superior ophthalmic vein (arrow), but thrombosis and lack of flow in the left superior ophthalmic vein.

Carotid-Cavernous Fistulas

Carotid-cavernous fistulas are acquired, abnormal communications between the carotid vasculature and the cavernous sinus. Low flow or indirect fistulas result from an abnormal connection between branches of the internal carotid artery into the cavernous sinus, while high flow or direct fistulas result from abnormal connection between the cavernous carotid itself and cavernous sinus.

High-flow carotid-cavernous fistulas typically result from trauma. These are referred to as Barrow type A fistulas.[16] A shearing force tears the arterial wall and permits rapid arterial flow into the cavernous sinus. Indirect fistulas are categorized in types B, C, and D based on the Barrow classification.[16] Type B fistulas arise from a defect in the dural branches of the cavernous (internal) carotid artery and type C from branches of the external carotid artery. Type D fistulas contain flow from branches of both internal and external carotid arteries. Low-flow fistulas often present in older patients with a history of hypertension and may occur spontaneously.

Symptoms of anterior draining fistulas may include retrobulbar pain and eye redness. Posterior draining fistulas may not exhibit anterior signs. Anterior and posterior draining fistulas may demonstrate cranial neuropathies and facial paresthesias. Ocular symptoms include:

- Vision changes
- Headache
- Orbital pain
- Diplopia.

Signs can include:

- Painful ophthalmoplegia
- Proptosis (potentially pulsatile if high flow)
- Orbital bruit
- Engorgement and arterialization of episcleral veins causing "corkscrew" vessels
- Subconjunctival hemorrhages
- Elevated intraocular pressure (IOP) with secondary glaucoma
- Vitreous hemorrhage
- Retinal hemorrhage
- Choroidal effusion (rare).[17]

Vision loss due to ischemic optic neuropathy has been reported caused by arterial steal syndrome from blood directed into the fistula and away from the optic nerve.[18] Cranial neuropathies may present with either anterior or posterior drainage. Abducens nerve palsy is the most commonly encountered cause of diplopia and occurs in 50–85% of cases followed by oculomotor nerve palsy in two-thirds and trochlear nerve palsy in about half of cases.[19] The differential diagnosis for painful ophthalmoplegia includes tumor, aneurysm, dissection, thrombosis, mucormycosis, sarcoid, syphilis, tuberculosis, Tolosa-Hunt syndrome, GPA and orbital cellulitis. Additionally, GCA and ophthalmoplegic migraine may also present with pain and abnormal motility. Imaging studies distinguish carotid-cavernous fistulas from other conditions. CT and MRI may show proptosis and dilation of superior ophthalmic vein in predominantly anterior draining fistulas (Figs. 99.6A to C). Cerebral angiography is the gold standard in patients with high clinical suspicion where noninvasive imaging is negative. Management involves serial examinations for optic neuropathy and elevated IOP which typically resolve with closure of the carotid-cavernous fistula. High-flow fistulas often require closure, while many indirect fistulas will close spontaneously without intervention. Ophthalmologic indications for closure include vision loss, severe proptosis and ophthalmoplegia.

Tolosa-Hunt Syndrome

Tolosa-Hunt syndrome is a rare disorder due to idiopathic granulomatous inflammation of the cavernous sinus, superior orbital fissure or orbital apex and presents clinically with episodic and painful ophthalmoplegia. The condition is rarely bilateral, which distinguishes it from cavernous thrombosis where progressive spread to bilateral ophthalmoplegia is pathognomonic. Symptoms also include severe periorbital headaches, diplopia, pain with eye movements, and facial paresthesias. Cranial nerve III is affected in 85% of cases followed by cranial nerve VI in 70%, cranial nerve VI in 30% and cranial nerve IV in 29%.[20] MRI is the preferred imaging modality and may show bilateral enhancement of the optic nerve sheaths and oculomotor nerve (Figs. 99.7A and B). Decreased vision from optic neuropathy can occur if the inflammation extends to the orbital apex. Other causes of cavernous sinus or orbital apex pathology must be excluded. Histology shows lymphocytic and plasma cell infiltration of the cavernous sinus walls along with giant cell granulomas. The condition rapidly responds to corticosteroids but tends to relapse and occur on an episodic basis. Without treatment, symptoms may resolve spontaneously. Tolosa-Hunt syndrome is a diagnosis of exclusion, therefore, it is important to rule out other causes of painful ophthalmoplegia.

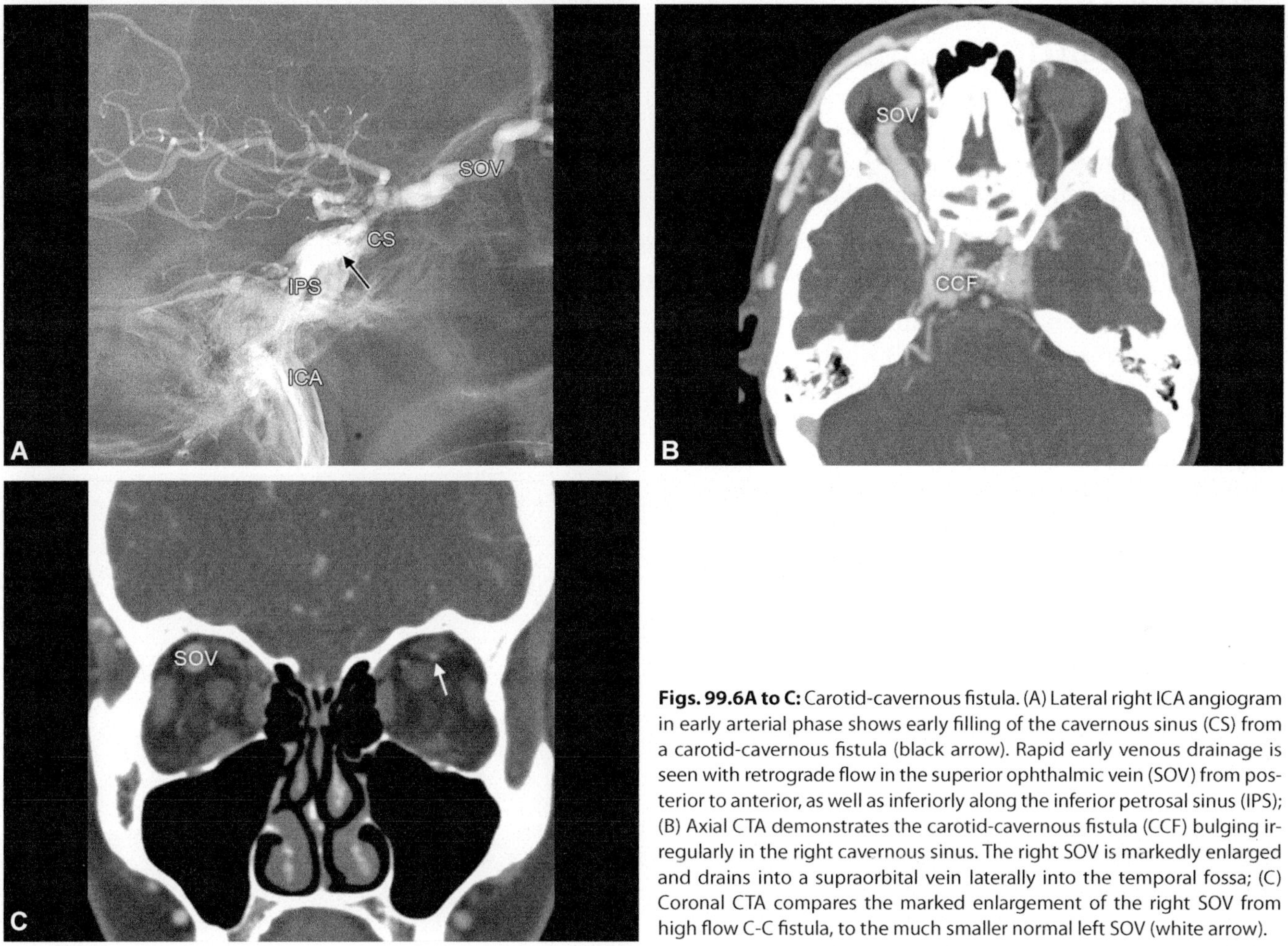

Figs. 99.6A to C: Carotid-cavernous fistula. (A) Lateral right ICA angiogram in early arterial phase shows early filling of the cavernous sinus (CS) from a carotid-cavernous fistula (black arrow). Rapid early venous drainage is seen with retrograde flow in the superior ophthalmic vein (SOV) from posterior to anterior, as well as inferiorly along the inferior petrosal sinus (IPS); (B) Axial CTA demonstrates the carotid-cavernous fistula (CCF) bulging irregularly in the right cavernous sinus. The right SOV is markedly enlarged and drains into a supraorbital vein laterally into the temporal fossa; (C) Coronal CTA compares the marked enlargement of the right SOV from high flow C-C fistula, to the much smaller normal left SOV (white arrow).

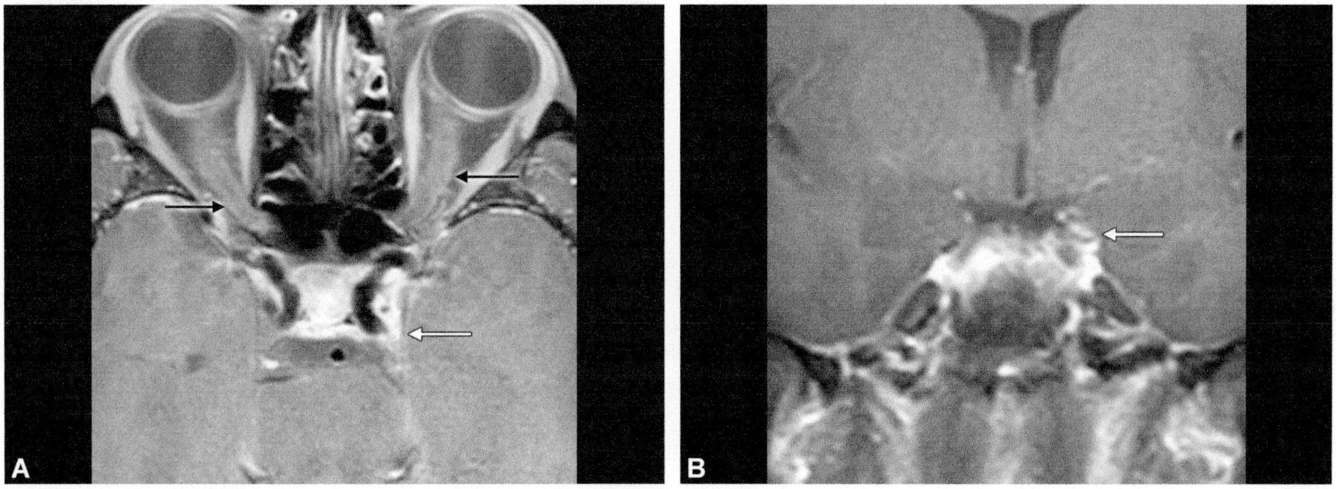

Figs. 99.7A and B: Tolosa-Hunt syndrome with optic neuritis and IIIrd cranial nerve palsy. (A) Axial fat saturated post-gadolinium T1 image highlights bilateral faint enhancement of the optic nerve sheaths (black arrows). Subtle asymmetric enhancement of the oculomotor nerve as it enters the superior-posterior aspect of the left cavernous sinus wall (white arrow); (B) Coronal fat saturated post-gadolinium T1 image shows abnormal asymmetric enhancement around the oculomotor nerve (arrow).

VASCULAR TUMORS AND MALFORMATIONS

Clinical Features

Vascular malformation is a general term used to describe anomalies of arterial, venous and lymphatic vessels or a combination of vessel types. They are typically congenital and share some features with vascular tumors. Cavernous malformations, previously called cavernous hemangiomas) are the most common vascular tumors in the orbit. Their new name recognizes that the vessels within the lesion do not proliferate, unlike true hemangiomas such as those occurring in early childhood. Lymphovenous malformations include lesions previously described as lymphangiomas and varices, while hemangiopericytomas have been reclassified as solitary fibrous tumors (SFTs) and remain rarer. Clinically, the most common presenting symptoms of orbital masses are proptosis, eyelid swelling, chemosis, and symptoms related to mass effect and displacement of globe such as diplopia and axial hyperopic shift. Additionally, patients may develop orbital apex syndrome and optic nerve compression, leading to monocular vision loss, visual field deficits, and gaze-evoked amaurosis. Additionally, some vascular tumors may rupture and cause acute painful proptosis.

Hemangiomas

Cavernous malformations are the most common benign orbital tumor in adults and continue to be called "hemangiomas" by many ophthalmologists (Figs. 99.8A to C). Patients are typically middle-aged females and present with painless, unilateral proptosis due to their slow and insidious growth. Some may present with acute painful proptosis if the lesion becomes hemorrhagic. Cavernous malformations in the orbital apex may lead to vision loss secondary to optic nerve compression. The lesions may be observed if asymptomatic or can be surgically excised.

Capillary hemangiomas are the most common benign orbital tumor in children and present early in life with often rapidly increasing unilateral, painless proptosis. There is usually a visible, superficial component in the eyelid or periocular area. Because they are proliferative (unlike cavernous malformations), change occurs on a much shorter timescale. Although spontaneous involution may occur, oral beta blockers such as propranolol are well-tolerated and frequently produce rapid regression of the lesion. Their use should be considered in patients with optic nerve compression or severe proptosis.

Solitary fibrous tumor, one histologic type of which has been called historically as hemangiopericytoma,

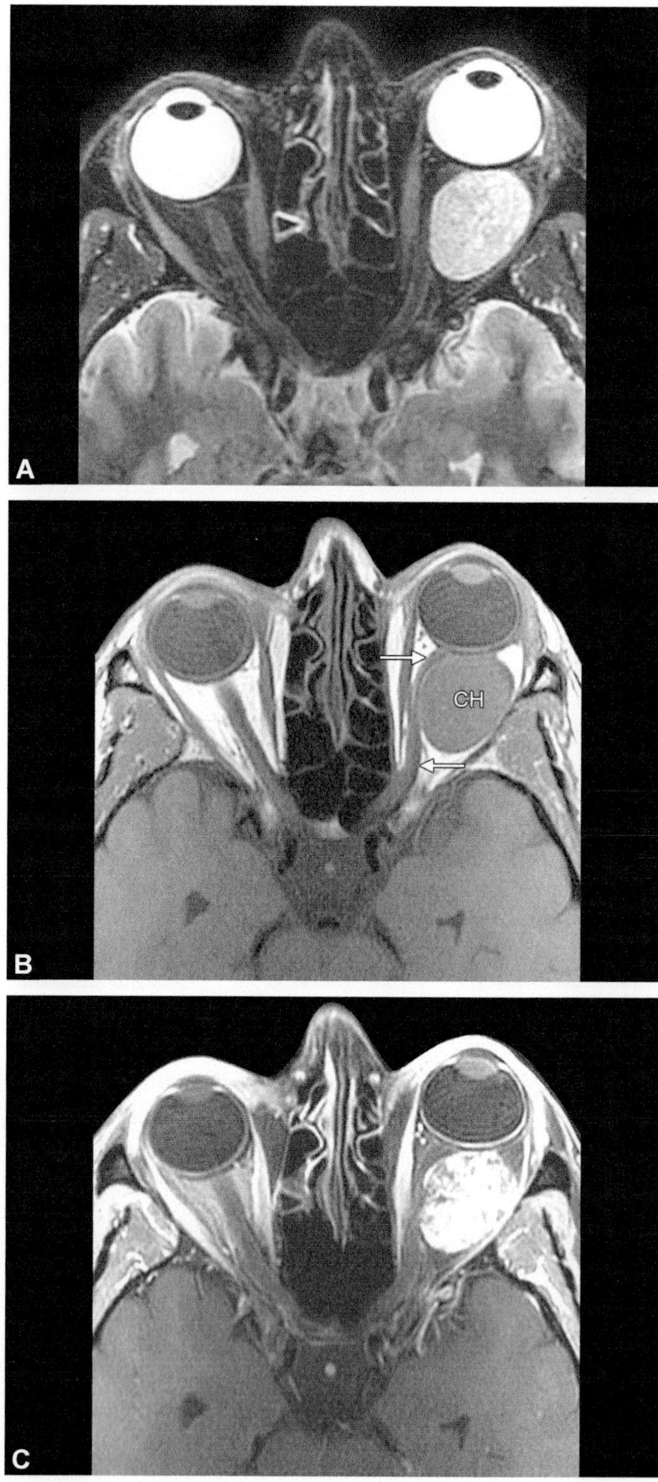

Figs. 99.8A to C: Intraconal cavernous malformation. (A) Axial STIR image has a well-defined moderately high signal mass posterior to the globe, deep to the lateral rectus and is causing axial proptosis; (B) Axial noncontrast T1 image shows the cavernous malformation (CS) is also displacing the left optic nerve (arrows) in the nasal direction; (C) Axial fat saturated post-gadolinium T1 image shows a typical mottled pattern of enhancement within the mass.

originates from mesenchymal cells and is considered a form of sarcoma when malignant. Benign SFT is the more common manifestation, but malignant transformation has been described after incomplete resection of these tumors.

Lymphovenous Malformations

Previous classification systems separated lymphatic and venous malformations into "lymphangiomas" and "orbital varices," but more recent studies have recommended that these lesions be considered on a continuum. Their clinical behavior is similar, since many lesions have mixed lymphatic and venous features. Predominantly lymphatic lesions may cause fluctuating orbital symptoms and signs (proptosis, pain, swelling) that worsen with upper respiratory infections or paranasal sinus congestion. CT imaging showing high signal fluid level is pathognomonic (Figs. 99.9A to C). Predominantly venous malformations may present with intermittent and dynamic proptosis exacerbated by Valsalva maneuver. Symptoms may also include diplopia due to globe displacement. Other signs include hyperintensity and enlargement of extraocular muscles on imaging due to increased venous engorgement (Figs. 99.10A to C). Treatment is indicated based on symptoms, and patients may consider endovascular or transcutaneous embolization and/or surgery.

Hereditary Diseases

Von Hippel-Lindau Disease

Von Hippel-Lindau (VHL) is an autosomal-dominant inherited disease characterized by the proliferation of various benign and malignant tumors throughout the body with mean age of presentation in young adulthood. A mutation occurs in the tumor suppressor VHL gene on chromosome 3. Common tumors include hemangioblastomas of the cerebellum and spine, retinal capillary angiomas, renal clear cell carcinoma, pheochromocytomas, middle endolymphatic sac tumors, neuroendocrine tumors, and others (Figs. 99.11A and B). The disease is categorized as type 1 or 2 based on the likelihood of developing pheochromocytoma, with type 2 disease at significantly higher risk. Retinal capillary angiomas are a common ophthalmic manifestation of VHL. They are found in up to 70% of patients. Vision loss is not common, but may occur from macular edema, epiretinal membrane, or distortion from tumor.[21,22] Tumors can be observed or treated depending on risk for vision loss with the exception of optic nerve hemangioblastomas which should not be treated. The mainstay of treatment of retinal

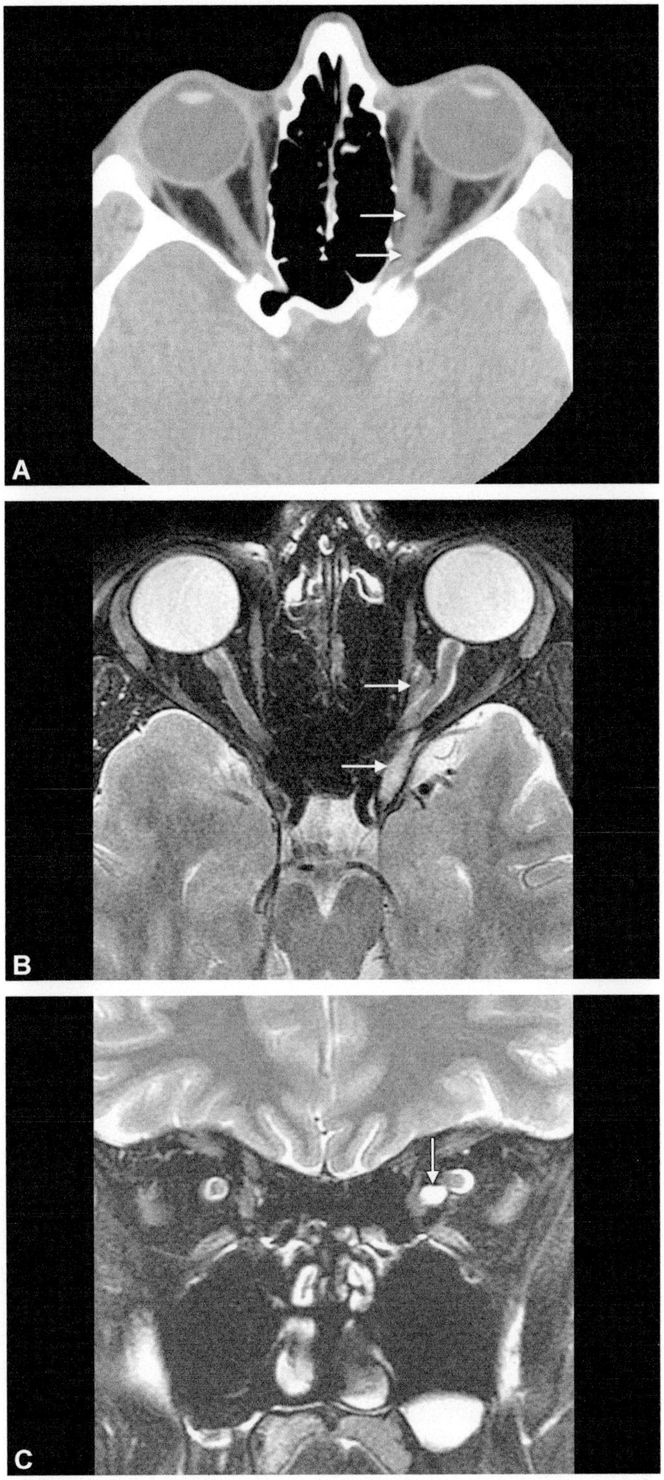

Figs. 99.9A to C: Orbital apex and cavernous sinus lymphatic malformation. (A) Axial noncontrast CT shows an elongated soft tissue mass (arrows) between the medial rectus muscle and the optic nerve extending to the orbital apex; (B) Axial STIR image better demonstrates that the apical soft tissue lesion contains high signal fluid and extends from the orbit into the left cavernous sinus (arrows); (C) Coronal STIR image reveals a tubular focus of high signal fluid (arrow) in between the medial rectus and left optic nerve.

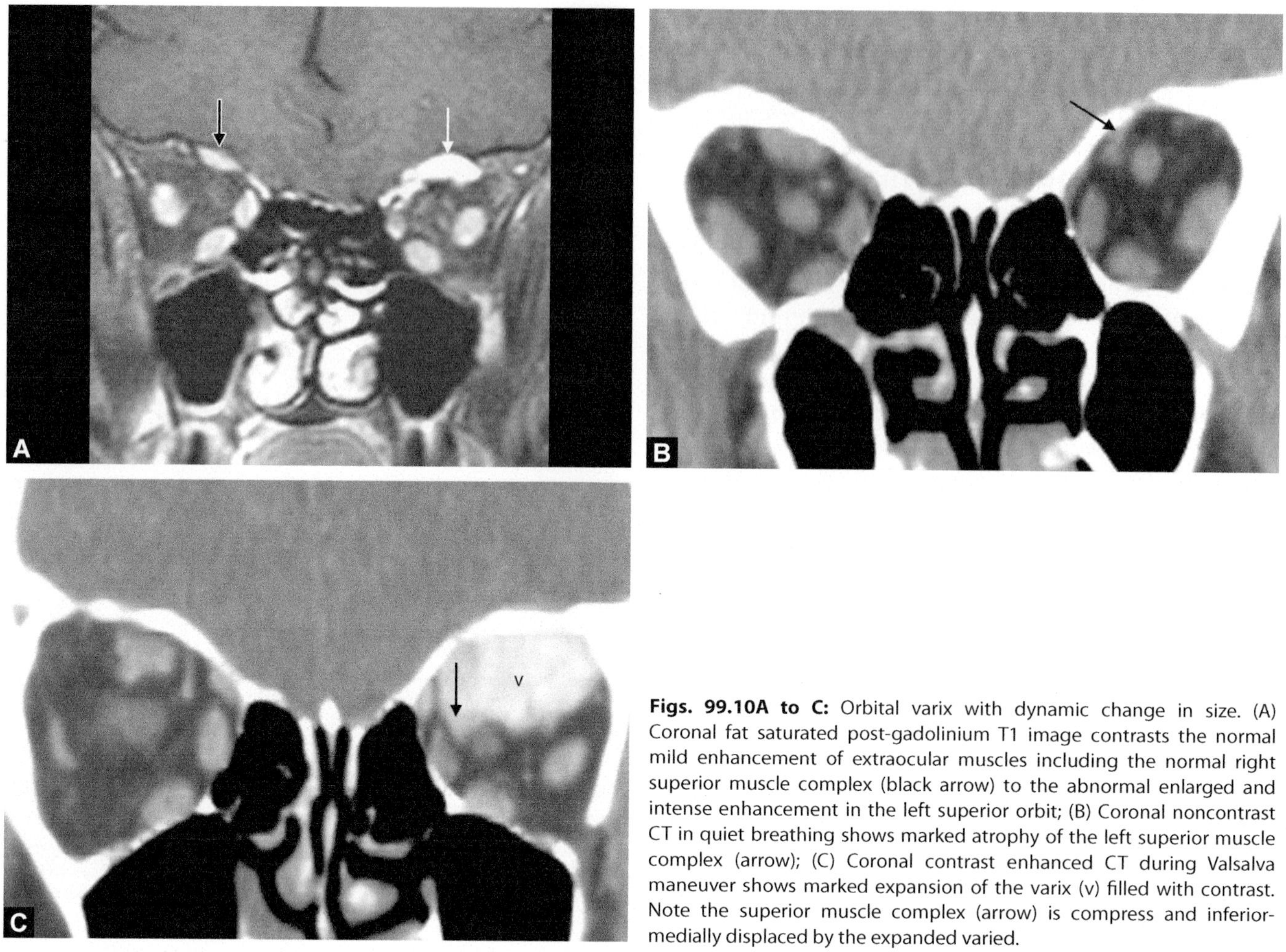

Figs. 99.10A to C: Orbital varix with dynamic change in size. (A) Coronal fat saturated post-gadolinium T1 image contrasts the normal mild enhancement of extraocular muscles including the normal right superior muscle complex (black arrow) to the abnormal enlarged and intense enhancement in the left superior orbit; (B) Coronal noncontrast CT in quiet breathing shows marked atrophy of the left superior muscle complex (arrow); (C) Coronal contrast enhanced CT during Valsalva maneuver shows marked expansion of the varix (v) filled with contrast. Note the superior muscle complex (arrow) is compress and inferior-medially displaced by the expanded varied.

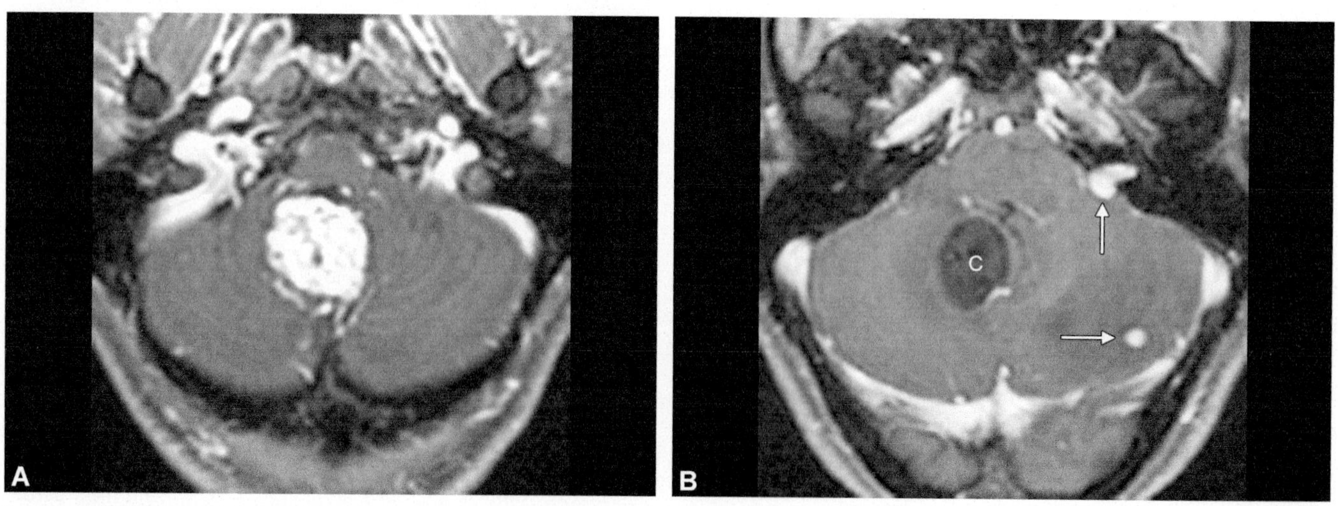

Figs. 99.11A and B: Hemangioblastomas in Von Hippel-Lindau disease. (A) Axial post-gadolinium T1 shows a 2 cm intensely enhancing cerebellar hemangioblastoma with internal flow voids along the posterior margin the 4th ventricle; (B) Slightly more superior slice showing cystic component (C) of the 4th ventricular hemangioblastoma. Two other smaller hemangioblastomas are present in the left internal auditory canal (vertical arrow) and in the left cerebellar hemisphere (horizontal arrow).

angiomas is laser photocoagulation and cryotherapy.[22] Genetic testing of children for VHL is important for early diagnosis and prompt evaluation of other systemic manifestations, treatment and ongoing surveillance.

Sturge-Weber Syndrome

Sturge-Weber syndrome (SWS), also known as encephalotrigeminal angiomatosis, is a congenital neurocutaneous disorder that presents with cerebral and unilateral facial vascular malformations known as port-wine stain or nevus flammeus. Occurrence is sporadic, and patients often present with seizures. The port-wine stain is usually found along the distribution of the V1 and V2 divisions of the trigeminal nerve unilaterally and may be associated with underlying leptomeningeal angiomas; thus, patients should undergo neuroimaging as part of their disease evaluation. Ocular manifestations include glaucoma or choroidal hemangiomas.[23] Glaucoma can be seen in 30–70% of patients, and risk is highest in the first decade.[24,25] Visual field deficits may occur in patients with leptomeningeal angiomas that compress the optic pathways or occipital lobes causing a homonymous hemianopia. Treatment for symptomatic patients includes anticonvulsants, glaucoma medications and laser treatment for the port-wine stain. All patients with port-wine lesion over the face should be evaluated for SWS for early diagnosis and to reduce complications from seizures and glaucoma.

Hereditary Hemorrhagic Telangiectasia

Hereditary hemorrhagic telangiectasia (HHT), also known as Osler-Weber-Rendu syndrome, is characterized by systemic arteriovenous malformations. Approximately 10% of patients with HHT manifest with cerebral arteriovenous malformations, fistulas and telangiectasias, particularly in the spinal cord.[26] The vascular malformations can become hemorrhagic and lead to stroke, vision loss and visual field deficits.

REFERENCES

1. Burde RM. Amaurosis fugax. An overview. J Clin Neuroophthalmol. 1989;9(3):185-9.
2. Current management of amaurosis fugax. The Amaurosis Fugax Study Group. Stroke. 1990;21(2):201-8.
3. Ali K. The temporal crescent syndrome. Pract Neurol. 2015;15(1):53-5.
4. Gonzalez-Gay MA, Vazquez-Rodriguez TR, Lopez-Diaz MJ, et al. Epidemiology of giant cell arteritis and polymyalgia rheumatica. Arthritis Rheum. 2009;61(10):1454-61.
5. Salvarani C, Crowson CS, O'Fallon WM, et al. Reappraisal of the epidemiology of giant cell arteritis in Olmsted County, Minnesota, over a fifty-year period. Arthritis Rheum. 2004;51(2):264-8.
6. Gonzalez-Gay MA, Barros S, Lopez-Diaz MJ, et al. Giant cell arteritis: disease patterns of clinical presentation in a series of 240 patients. Medicine (Baltimore). 2005;84(5):269-76.
7. Hayreh SS, Podhajsky PA, Zimmerman B. Ocular manifestations of giant cell arteritis. Am J Ophthalmol. 1998;125(4):509-20.
8. Jonasson F, Cullen JF, Elton RA. Temporal arteritis. A 14-year epidemiological, clinical and prognostic study. Scott Med J. 1979;24(2):111-7.
9. Harper SL, Letko E, Samson CM, et al. Wegener's granulomatosis: the relationship between ocular and systemic disease. J Rheumatol. 2001;28(5):1025-32.
10. Schmidt J, Pulido JS, Matteson EL. Ocular manifestations of systemic disease: antineutrophil cytoplasmic antibody-associated vasculitis. Curr Opin Ophthalmol. 2011;22(6):489-95.
11. Silpa-archa S, Lee JJ, Foster CS. Ocular manifestations in systemic lupus erythematosus. Br J Ophthalmol. 2016;100(1):135-41.
12. Keane JR. Eye movement abnormalities in systemic lupus erythematosus. Arch Neurol. 1995;52(12):1145-9.
13. Jones NP. Acute posterior multifocal placoid pigment epitheliopathy. Br J Ophthalmol. 1995;79:384-9.
14. Glaser JS. Neuro-Ophthalmology, 3rd edition. Philadelphia: Lippincott, Williams and Wilkins; 1999.
15. Lee VH, Brown RD Jr, Mandrekar JN, et al. Incidence and outcome of cervical artery dissection: a population-based study. Neurology. 2006;67(10):1809-12.
16. Barrow DL, Spector RH, Braun IF, et al. Classification and treatment of spontaneous carotid-cavernous sinus fistulas. J Neurosurg. 1985;62(2):248-56.
17. Stiebel-Kalish H, Setton A, Nimii Y, et al. Cavernous sinus dural arteriovenous malformations: patterns of venous drainage are related to clinical signs and symptoms. Ophthalmology. 2002;109(9):1685-91.
18. Hashimoto M, Ohtsuka K, Suzuki Y, et al. A case of posterior ischemic optic neuropathy in a posterior-draining dural cavernous sinus fistula. J Neuroophthalmol. 2005;25(3):176-9.
19. Kupersmith MJ, Berenstein A, Flamm E, et al. Neuroophthalmologic abnormalities and intravascular therapy of traumatic carotid cavernous fistulas. Ophthalmology. 1986;93(7):906-12.
20. Kline LB. The Tolosa-Hunt syndrome. Surv Ophthalmol. 1982;27(2):79-95.
21. Singh AD, Shields CL, Shields JA. Von Hippel-Lindau disease. Surv Ophthalmol. 2001;46(2):117-42.
22. Singh AD, Nouri M, Shields CL, et al. Treatment of retinal capillary hemangioma. Ophthalmology. 2002;109(10):1799-806.
23. Sullivan TJ, Clarke MP, Morin JD. The ocular manifestations of the Sturge-Weber syndrome. J Pediatr Ophthalmol Strabismus. 1992;29(6):349-56.
24. Javaid U, Ali MH, Jamal S, et al. Pathophysiology, diagnosis, and management of glaucoma associated with Sturge-Weber syndrome. Int Ophthalmol. 2017.
25. Sujansky E, Conradi S. Sturge-Weber syndrome: age of onset of seizures and glaucoma and the prognosis for affected children. J Child Neurol. 1995;10(1):49-58.
26. Haitjema T, Disch F, Overtoom TT, et al. Screening family members of patients with hereditary hemorrhagic telangiectasia. Am J Med. 1995;99(5):519-24.

Chapter 100 Disorders of the Pupil

Aki Kawasaki, Yanjun Chen

INTRODUCTION

Pupillary abnormalities can provide important clues to underlying neural or ocular pathology, and at times they may be the chief sign of a life-threatening condition such as cerebral aneurysm or carotid dissection. In addition, finding a relative afferent pupillary defect provides an objective evidence of optic nerve dysfunction. As such, a technical competence in the pupil examination combined with the ability to recognize the significance of an abnormal pupil response is a valuable clinical skill for ophthalmologists.

The pupillary light reflex is composed of an afferent limb and an efferent limb. Damage to either afferent or efferent limb of the light reflex can result in a subnormal pupillary constriction in response to a direct light stimulus, but only deficits in the efferent limb affect both the direct and consensual light response of the affected pupil and thus often result in anisocoria. This chapter addresses efferent (motor) pupillary defects and the evaluation of anisocoria.

Pupillary constriction is mediated by the oculoparasympathetic pathway that originates in the Edinger-Westphal subnucleus of the ocular motor nuclear complex in the midbrain (Fig. 100.1). This nucleus contains the preganglionic parasympathetic neurons whose fibers destined for the eye are carried with motor fibers in the oculomotor nerve. In the orbit, these parasympathetic fibers synapse in the ciliary ganglion. Postganglionic parasympathetic fibers are carried in the short ciliary nerves which pierce the sclera to reach the anterior segment, where they innervate the iris sphincter to mediate pupilloconstriction and the ciliary muscle to mediate accommodation.[1] Pupillary dilation is mediated by the oculosympathetic pathway, which is a three-neuron pathway (Fig. 100.2). In brief, the axons of the first-order neuron (central neuron) originate in the hypothalamus and descend in the brainstem and spinal cord to synapse in the lower cervical/upper thoracic spinal cord (C8-T2, also known as the ciliospinal center of Budge). The axons of the second-order neuron (preganglionic sympathetic neuron) pass across the apex of the lung and ascend the neck to synapse in the superior cervical ganglion. The third-order neuron (postganglionic neuron) supplies vasomotor and sudomotor function to the head and neck and innervates the pupil dilator muscle and tarsal muscles.[2,3] At the carotid bifurcation, the oculosympathetic fibers travel with the internal carotid artery as a plexus around its wall, whereas the sudomotor fibers course with the external carotid artery to the face. At the orbital apex, the oculosympathetic fibers follow the nasociliary nerve to the eye.

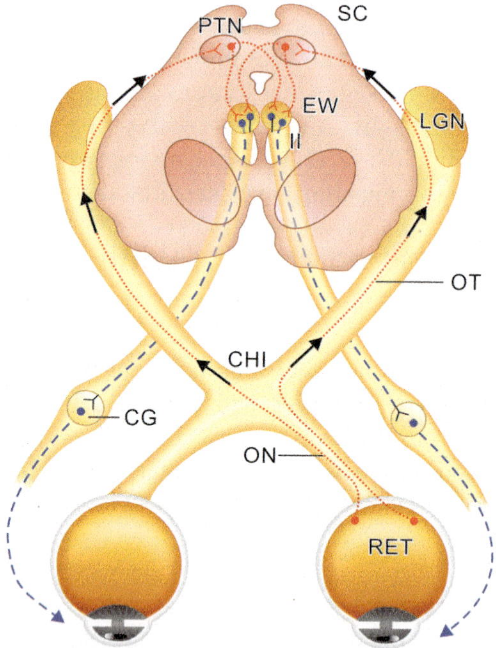

Fig. 100.1: Oculoparasympathetic pathway that mediates the pupil light reflex. The afferent pupillary fibers originate in the retinal ganglion cells (RET) and travel along the optic nerve (ON), partially decussate in the optic chiasm (CHI), and then depart from the optic tract (OT) and pass through the superior colliculus (SC) and reach the pretectal nucleus (PTN) in the dorsal midbrain. The pupil fibers then decussate and synapse with the Edinger-Westphal (EW) subnucleus of the third nerve nucleus complex located in the midbrain tegmentum. The pupillomotor fibers then travel with the third nerve to the orbits and innervate the iris sphincter muscle.
(LGN: Lateral geniculate nucleus; CG: Ciliary ganglion)
Source: Liu G, Volpe N, Galetta S. Pupillary disorders. In: Liu G, Volpe N, Galetta S (Eds). Neuro-Ophthalmology: Diagnosis and Management, 2nd edition. Philadelphia, PA: Saunders/Elsevier Inc.; 2010. p. 416.

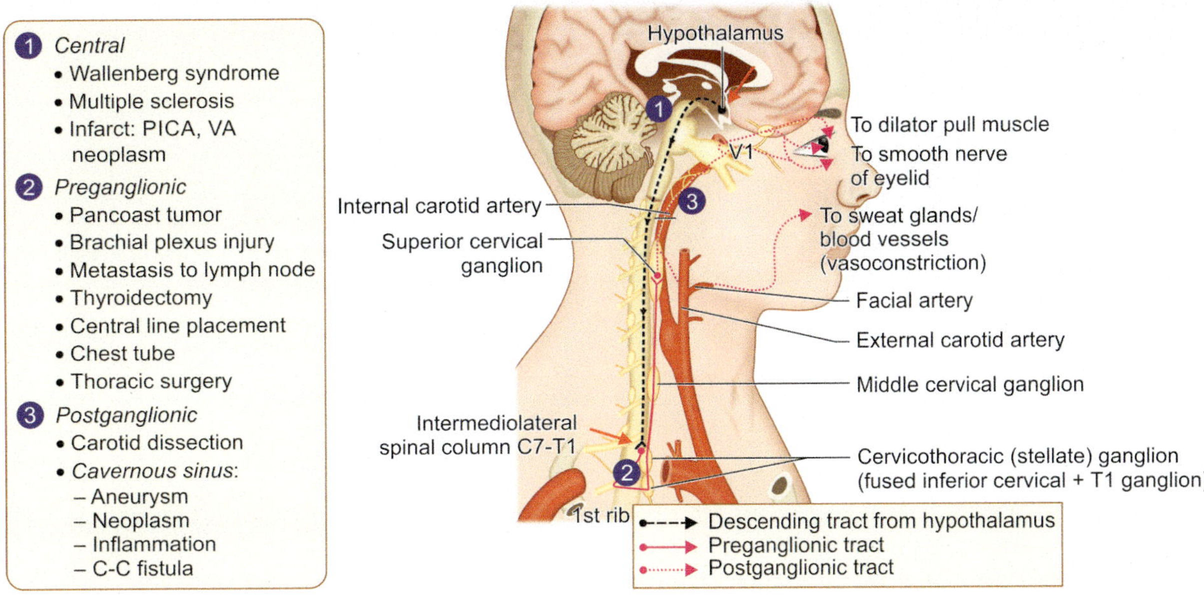

Fig. 100.2: Depiction of the three-neuron pathway of the oculosympathetic innervation and common causes of Horner's syndrome. (PICA: Posterior inferior cerebellar artery; VA: Vertebral artery; C-C fistula: Carotid-cavernous fistula) *Source:* http://www.physio-pedia.com/File:Horners_patho.jpg. [Accessed December, 2017]

EXAMINATION OF THE PUPILS

Examination of the pupil in an office setting includes inspection of pupil size and shape in conditions of darkness and light, pupil reactivity to light and near stimulation and slit-lamp examination of the iris (see also Chapter 90, The Neuro-ophthalmic Examination).

A normal pupil assumes a regular and round shape; any irregularity of pupil shape should be examined meticulously for evidence of acquired or congenital iris defects. The baseline pupil size varies with age. The pupil diameter in the darkness is greatest (7.0–7.5 mm) during the teenage years and then gradually decreases with increasing age, to an average of 4.5–5.0 mm in darkness at age 80 years.[4,5] In most patients, the right and left pupils are symmetric in size. An asymmetry of 0.4 mm or more between the two pupils is visible to the unaided eye and can be seen in about 20% of the normal population.

Baseline pupil size also is influenced by many systemic medications that can impact the autonomic nervous system. Agents that have a sympathomimetic or a parasympatholytic effect can increase baseline pupil size. Examples are inhalers for asthma treatment, central nervous system stimulants, cough and cold medications, decongestants (guaifenesin, pseudoephedrine), and illicit drugs (cocaine, marijuana, hallucinogens). On the other hand, those acting as parasympathomimetics or sympatholytics can decrease baseline pupil size; examples include nicotine lozenges, antipsychotics (clozapine), anxiolytics (benzodiazepine), and narcotics (morphine, oxycodone, or heroin). Furthermore, diseases affecting the autonomic nervous system can cause alteration of pupil size, often in both eyes and with manifestations of both sympathetic and parasympathetic dysfunction. Such conditions include diabetic neuropathy, multiple system atrophy, amyloidosis, Riley-Day syndrome, familial dysautonomia, and Sjögren syndrome.[6]

Normally the pupil is black due to minimally scattered light reflected back from the retina, as most of the light entering the eye is absorbed by the lens and pigmented layers outlining the eye, including retinal pigment epithelium and melanocytes embedded in the choroid and anterior uvea. Leukocoria, a white pupil, always signifies ocular pathology, such as retinoblastoma, persistent hyperplastic primary vitreous, retinopathy of prematurity (ROP), or cataract. A red pupil can be seen in eyes with albinism, or with trauma if there is a large amount of blood inside the eye.

The pupil light reflex should be examined under dim room light and with the subject fixating a distant target.[7] Light stimulation of one eye causes both pupils to constrict, the consensual pupil response owing to decussation of

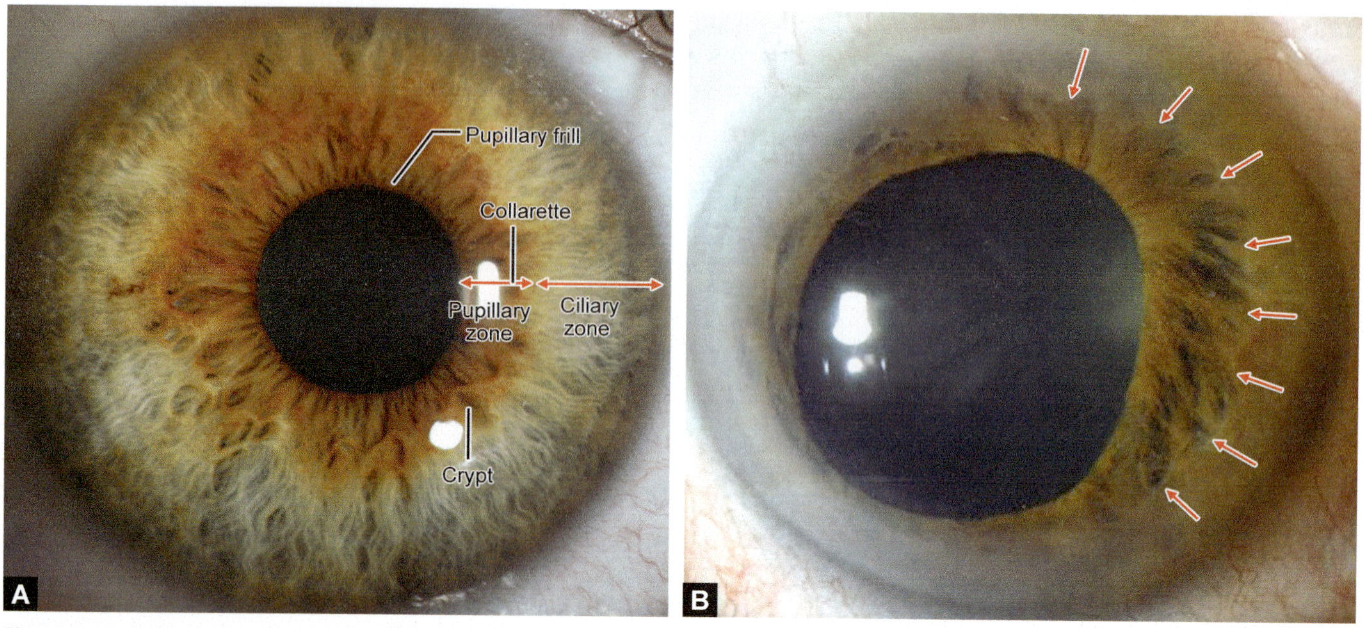

Figs. 100.3A and B: (A) Slit-lamp photograph of a normal pupil and (B) a pupil with distorted shape due to iris atrophy. A normal pupil is always round and centered on the iris. The pupil margin is wrapped around by the dark posterior pigment epithelium (pupillary frill). The iris surface is covered by a loose layer of iris stroma intermixed by a series openings (crypts) that allow free passage of aqueous humor. Collarette is the thickest region of the iris, separating the iris surface into the inner pupillary zone and outer ciliary zone. The pupil sphincter muscles are located in the pupillary zone encircling the pupil margin, whereas the pupil dilator muscles occupy the ciliary zone in a radial fashion; (B) The iris atrophy of the right eye in another patient was discovered as an incidental finding in a routine eye examination. Note that extensive iris atrophy affecting the temporal half and inferior nasal iris, resulting in the loss of normal surface landmarks such as collarettes and crypts, as well as a misshaped, dilated pupil along 4–12 o' clock hours. The iris is pulled towards the affected side due to unopposed dilator activity. Note some preservations of the collarette, crypts, and pupillary sphincter over 1–4 o'clock hours (red arrows).

pupillomotor signal at the chiasm and in the midbrain. Therefore, monocular blindness is never a cause of baseline anisocoria. Mental vigilance plays a role in pupillary constriction: the light reflex might appear sluggish in the both the sleepy subject and the overly excited one. Complete unresponsiveness of the pupils to light stimulation always signifies an underlying abnormality. Under constant and stable illumination, a normal pupil demonstrates small-amplitude alternation of spontaneous contractions and dilations, called *physiologic hippus* or *unrest*.[8] At times, this pupil oscillation could become prominent with a large amplitude of 1 mm, which can be readily visible on inspection.

The pupil response to a near target (accommodation) should be examined in dim-to-moderate room light, allowing the patient's pupils and the near object to be clearly visible without inducing significant pupillary constriction. The near response has a large volitional component and can appear reduced or even absent due to a lack of effort by the subject. A better response may be obtained in such cases by asking the subject to fixate on his/her own thumb placed close to forehead in between the eyes.

Slit-lamp examination of the anterior segment can help identify subtle pupillary abnormalities attributable to structural changes of the iris. First, inspect the integrity of the iris structure, pupillary frill, and the distribution of the iris epithelium (Figs. 100.3A and B). Then examine the iris sphincter muscle and the reactivity to a light stimulus at each clock hour to look for sectoral palsy or atrophy as seen in eyes with a tonic pupil or sphincter muscle tears. Iris transillumination can further define areas of iris damage.

ANISOCORIA

The evaluation of anisocoria should start with a careful history to determine the onset and duration of the inequality in pupil size. Reviewing old photos can sometimes estimate the duration of the pupil abnormality. Stroke-like symptoms accompanying the onset of the anisocoria, history of neck/head trauma, the presence of neck pain or headache, history of neoplasm or recent surgical intervention in the neck and chest area are important historical clues that can help to localize the lesion and to identify the etiology. In many cases of new onset anisocoria, only one pupil is faulty. In these cases, assessment of baseline pupil size in both bright light and darkness and comparison of pupillary constriction to light stimulation as well as its redilation to abrupt darkness between the two eyes are key components of the evaluation. Pharmacologic testing constitutes an adjunct step after the examination in select cases of anisocoria.

Ocular Causes of Anisocoria

Pupil asymmetry caused by ocular pathology is often signaled by an irregular pupil shape. A careful slit-lamp examination will reveal the majority of ocular causes of anisocoria. For example, pigment in the anterior iris and posterior cornea accompanied by spoke-like iris transillumination defects implicate pigment dispersion syndrome as the cause of a pupil that contracts and dilates poorly. Acute pigment dispersion, iris atrophy and bilateral mydriasis have been described as an adverse reaction to oral moxifloxacin, a synthetic broad-spectrum antibacterial agent.[9] Other causes are listed in Table 100.1.

Congenital anisocoria can be a result of an isolated developmental malformation in the eye or may be one component of a syndromic disorder. In aniridia, the underdeveloped eye has a hypoplastic iris and large pupil, cataracts, and impaired vision due to macular or optic nerve hypoplasia. Iris coloboma is a notch in the inferonasal iris due to incomplete closure of the embryonic fissure. It can occur in an otherwise healthy individual or as an ocular manifestation of a more extensive congenital malformation such as coloboma, heart disease, atresia or stenosis of the choanae, retardation, genital hypoplasia, and ear anomalies or deafness (CHARGE) syndrome. Patients with persistent pupillary membrane demonstrate strands of iris tissue crossing the pupil but otherwise have normal ocular function. Ectopia lentis et pupillae, misplaced pupils associated with dislocation of the lens, can have significant impact on visual function due to multiple ocular congenital malformations present in these patients. Ectopia lentis et pupillae is generally regarded as an autosomal recessive syndrome with uncertain pathogenesis.[10]

Table 100.1: Ocular conditions that may result in acquired anisocoria.

Condition	Clinical findings
Prior intraocular surgery	Tears in the pupillary margin or the sphincter muscle
Ocular trauma (acute or old)	Separation of the outer edge of the iris from its ciliary attachment (iridodialysis)
Intraocular inflammation	• *Acute*: Pupillary miosis due to ciliary spasm • *Late*: Mydriatic pupil with poor reactivity due to iris atrophy; deformation of pupillary shape and inability to dilate (synechiae)
Acute angle closure	Fixed, dilated pupil with eye pain, visual halos or redness
Iris ischemia and neovascularization	Loss of mechanical compliance (poor constriction and dilation)
Familial amyloidosis	Irregular, cup-shaped indentations (scalloping) in the pupillary margins

Pharmacologic Anisocoria

Either intentional or inadvertent ocular exposure to an agent that directly acts on one of the iris muscles can cause pharmacologic anisocoria.

Pharmacologic pupillary mydriasis is characterized by an extremely dilated, "blown" pupil that does not react to light or to near stimulation and is not associated with other ocular or neurologic deficits. A pharmacologically dilated pupil does not react to topical instillation of 1% pilocarpine, differentiating it from neurologic mydriasis seen in third nerve palsy or Adie's pupil, both of which invariably show strong pupillary constriction to 1% pilocarpine. Absence of constriction to 1% pilocarpine is also observed in eyes with mydriasis due to a traumatized iris. In such cases, a slit-lamp examination will distinguish the mechanical from pharmacologic cause of mydriasis. Common identifiable causes of pharmacologic mydriasis include scopolamine patch, certain asthma inhalers, allergy eye drops, and plants of the nightshade family which contain atropine-like substances. Pharmacologic mydriasis in one eye frequently prompts a visit to the emergency room, and if unrecognized, may lead to unnecessarily extensive imaging to look for life-threatening neurologic conditions. Therefore, patients presenting with an isolated, unilateral pupillary mydriasis should be carefully questioned about medications, drug exposure and gardening.

Anisocoria caused by pharmacologic miosis is rare compared to pharmacologic mydriasis and is usually associated with exposure to pilocarpine-like eye drops.

Physiologic Anisocoria

The most common cause of nontraumatic, non-pharmacologic pupil asymmetry is physiologic anisocoria (also called simple anisocoria, benign anisocoria, essential anisocoria). Using infrared pupillometry, a pupil asymmetry of 0.4 mm or greater can be observed in about 20% of healthy individuals.[5] Physiologic anisocoria is rarely greater than 0.6 mm; an anisocoria exceeding 1.0 mm should be carefully investigated for underlying pathology.

The pupil asymmetry is generally more noticeable in the dark, probably due to a generally smaller pupil size in light. Both pupils should constrict to light and dilate in the dark equally. The magnitude of physiologic anisocoria in an individual can vary from day to day.

Physiologic anisocoria is usually an incidental finding and is not associated with other systemic or neurologic symptoms. When pupil asymmetry is identified from previous photos, especially those which date back many years ago, the diagnosis could be made with fair certainty, and no further investigation is needed. However, it is not uncommon that patients with physiologic anisocoria will report coexisting but unrelated symptoms, such as a headache, neck pain, or droopy eyelids. In such cases, appropriate evaluation for pathologic causes of anisocoria is indicated, and the diagnosis of physiologic anisocoria becomes one of exclusion.

Neurologic Causes of Anisocoria

Large Pupil with Poor Light Reflex: Oculoparasympathetic Dysfunction

Insufficient parasympathetic signaling to the sphincter muscle leads to a larger pupil size and a slow and/or incomplete constriction to a light stimulus or a near effort. It follows naturally that the anisocoria is more apparent in light than in darkness. The location of the neurologic lesion is either the oculomotor nerve or the short ciliary nerve.

Oculomotor (third) nerve palsy: The clinical presentation of a complete third nerve palsy consists of pupillary mydriasis, ipsilateral ptosis, and loss of ipislateral adduction, supraduction, and infraduction. Partial oculomotor nerve paresis does not always involve the pupil, and the correct diagnosis may be overlooked. On the other hand, the presence of an obviously mydriatic pupil with poor light reflex without any accompanying motor deficit (lid or eye movements) is likely not a third nerve palsy.

Third nerve palsy can be caused by a variety of neurologic diseases affecting the third nerve nucleus in the midbrain or the third nerve fibers throughout its course through the midbrain, subarachnoid space, cavernous sinus, and orbit. The etiologies of third nerve palsy include stroke, intracranial space occupying lesions (tumor, vascular malformation, hematoma, and herniation), cerebral aneurysm, and leptomeningeal disease (from tuberculosis, sarcoidosis, and carcinomatous dissemination). Any patient with an oculomotor nerve palsy accompanied by acute neurologic symptoms or signs, such as imbalance, tremor, and weakness on one side of body, should have neuroimaging performed and be referred to a neurologist. An isolated oculomotor nerve palsy with pupillary involvement, especially associated with headache, is an emergency, and urgent imaging studies should be directed to the possibility of a posterior communicating artery aneurysm (Figs. 100.4A to C). On the other hand, a completely normal pupil (no anisocoria, normal light reflex) in the presence of complete ptosis and complete loss of adduction, supraduction and infraduction is most likely due to microvascular ischemia of the oculomotor nerve (Fig. 100.5). In developed nations, such patients will typically undergo neuroimaging studies despite the very low yield, while in countries with fewer resources, careful observation is more likely to occur. Patients with a microvascular or "vasculopathic" oculomotor nerve palsy usually experience significant spontaneous improvement of the ptosis and ocular motility deficits over a period of 3–4 months.

Adie's tonic pupil: An injury or lesion to the ciliary ganglion leads to a dilated and poorly reactive pupil. Commonly, the clinical diagnosis is Adie's tonic pupil. The exact cause of Adie's tonic pupil remains unclear, and a low-grade inflammation of the ciliary ganglion associated with viral infection has been proposed. Nonetheless, it is considered idiopathic in the vast majority of cases. Adie's tonic pupil tends to affect middle-aged women, with 80% of cases being unilateral. Acute symptoms include brow pain, accommodative difficulty and light sensitivity. Other times, Adie's tonic pupil is an incidental finding on a routine eye examination.

In the acute stage, an Adie's tonic pupil is dilated and reacts poorly to both light and near stimulation due to acute injury of the ciliary ganglion, causing parasympathetic denervation of both the iris sphincter muscle and the ciliary muscle. As the injury is often incomplete and sphincter palsy may be sectoral, contraction of the working segments of the sphincter can be observed at the slit lamp by observing each clock hour segment. As time goes by, the injured parasympathetic fibers regenerate. Because those fibers originally destined to the ciliary muscle are more abundant, there is often ample reinnervation of the ciliary muscle with recovery of accommodation. These fibers, however, also reinnervate the iris sphincter muscle (aberrant reinnervation) and this leads to the later finding of a slow, tonic and excessive constriction with near effort with equally slow redilation after near effort. However,

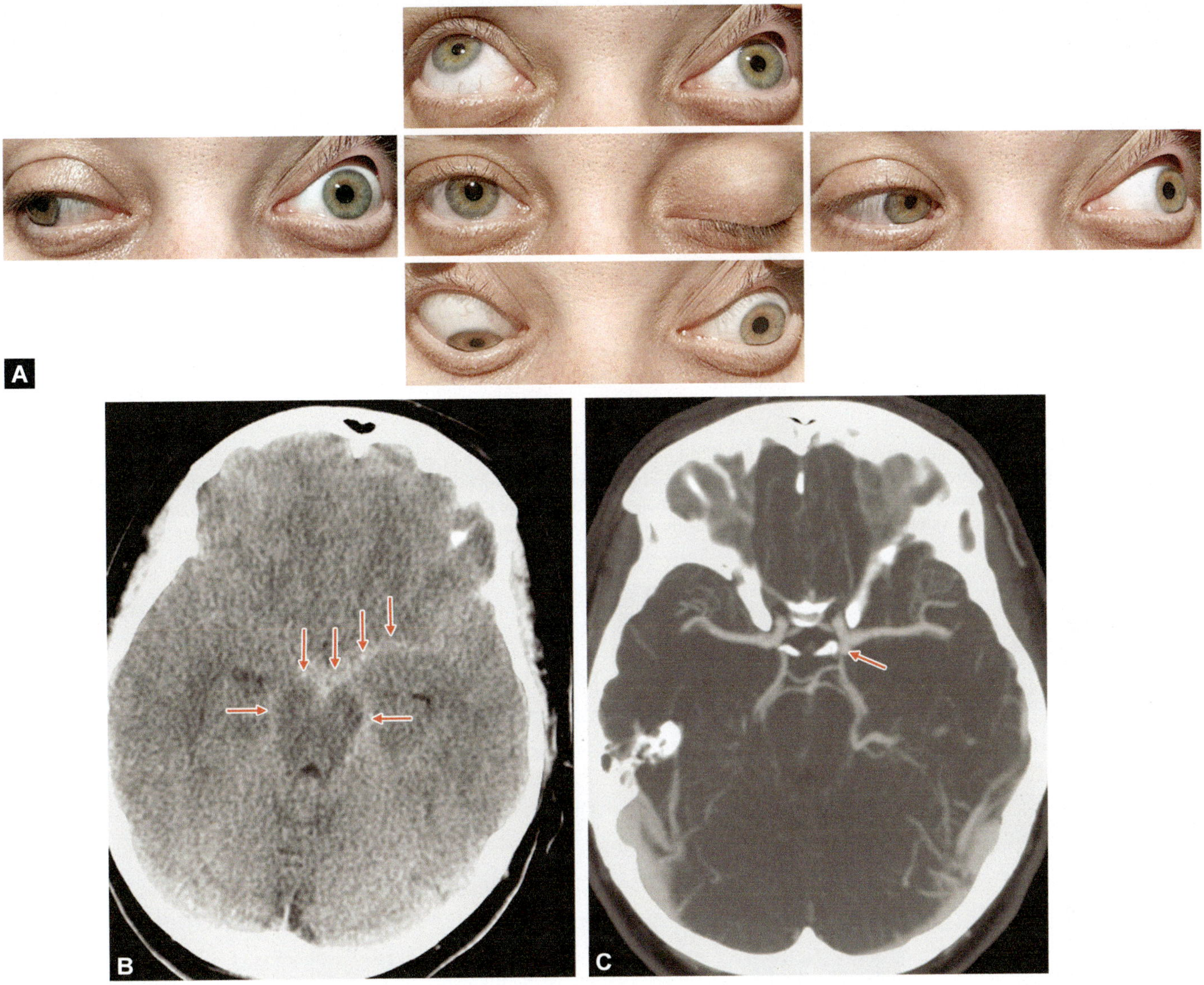

Figs. 100.4A to C: A 32-year-old woman had sudden onset of droopy eyelid in the left eye associated with severe headache and then loss of consciousness. (A) Examination showed a complete left ptosis and ophthalmoplegia involving adduction, supraduction and infraduction; the abduction was full. Note that the left pupil was larger with decreased constriction to light stimulation, consistent with a pupil-involving third nerve palsy in the left eye; (B) Head CT showed hyperdensity abnormalities within the Sylvian fissures (vertical arrows) and basilar cisterns (horizontal arrows), consistent with an acute subarachnoid hemorrhage; (C) CT angiogram of the head showed a left internal carotid artery aneurysm arising from the base of the posterior communicating artery (red arrow).

the affected pupil typically does not regain its light reflex, leading to a sign called light-near dissociation (Figs. 100.6A to C). Also at this later stage of tonic pupil, there may be segmental sphincter atrophy, where the involved iris appears pale and thin. When a large area of the iris is affected, the iris may be pulled toward the affected side due to unopposed pupil dilator muscle activity or toward the segment of preserved sphincter contraction, resulting in an irregularly shaped pupil (Fig. 100.3B).

Parasympathetic denervation hypersensitivity of the sphincter and ciliary muscles develops as early as 1–2 weeks following the acute onset of Adie's tonic pupil and forms the basis for the dilute pilocarpine test. A denervated sphincter demonstrates a significant pupillary constriction to dilute pilocarpine eye drops (0.1%), whereas the normal pupil does not react (Figs. 100.7A and B).[11]

Rarely, a unilateral tonic pupil can be seen in systemic illnesses, such as varicella-zoster, giant cell arteritis, syphilis, and sarcoidosis. Bilateral tonic pupils may be seen in patients with diabetes, alcoholism, syphilis, and dysautonomia associated with cancer or amyloidosis.

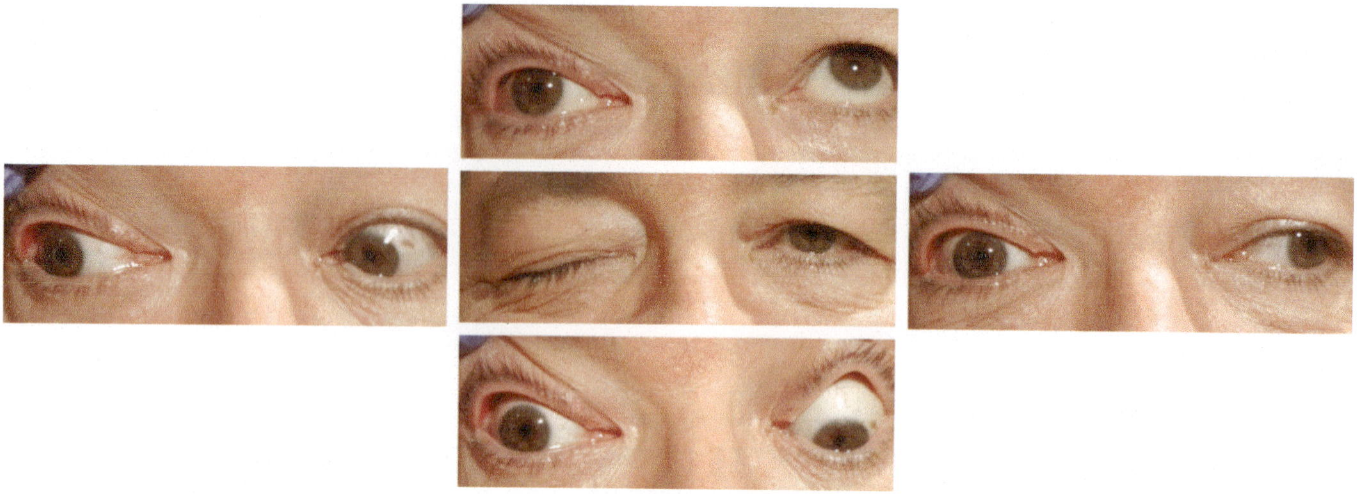

Fig. 100.5: A 69-year-old male presented with abrupt onset of double vision and droopy eyelid in the right eye. Examination showed a complete right ptosis and ophthalmoplegia involving adduction, supraduction and infraduction; the abduction was full. Note that his pupils are symmetric in size with normal pupil light reflex. The diagnosis was pupil-sparing third nerve palsy of ischemic (microvascular) origin in the right eye. The patient has hypertension and poorly controlled diabetes with the complication of renal insufficiency and recent partial toe amputation.

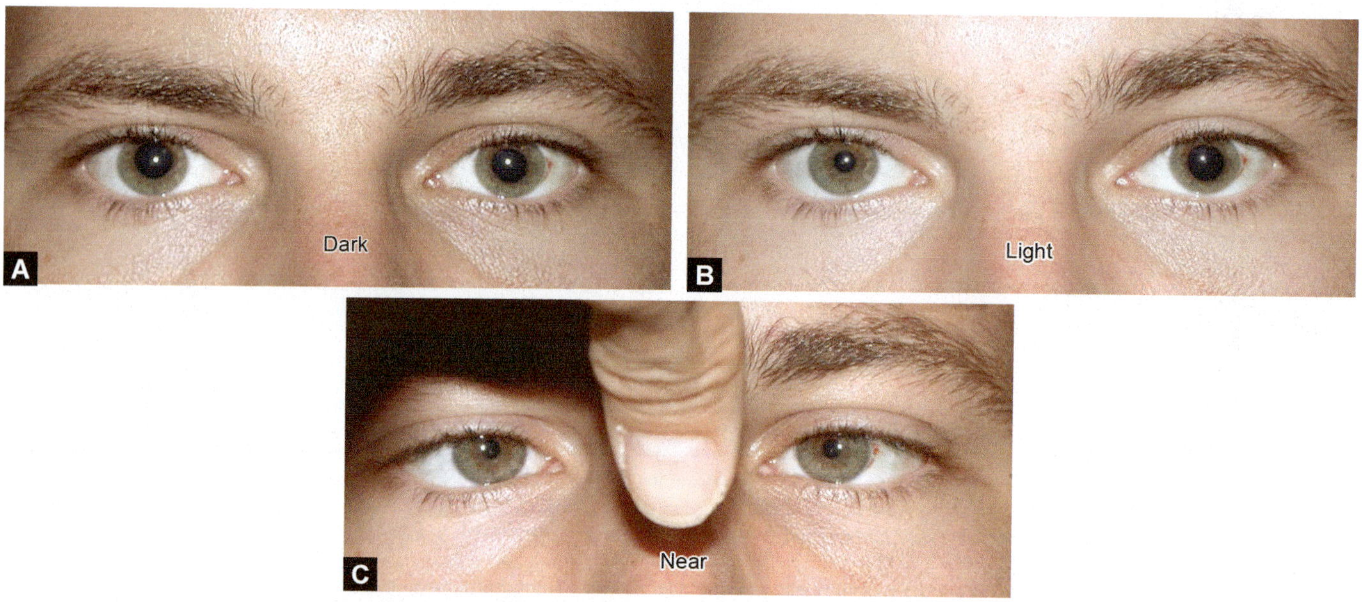

Figs. 100.6A to C: A 22-year-old student fell from his bicycle and noted a red eye. In the emergency room, a minor subconjunctival hemorrhage and a dilated unreactive left pupil was noted. (A) In darkness, the pupils were symmetrically dilated. But in bright light conditions, only the right pupil became constricted; (B) the left pupil was unreactive to light; (C) Upon a near effort, the left pupil showed a strong and tonic constriction. The presence of this light-near dissociation is a sign of aberrant regeneration and indicates that this tonic pupil should be at least several weeks old and thus unrelated to the bicycle accident. In retrospect, several months ago the patient had noted some difficulty with reading which has spontaneously improved. No further evaluation was needed for this idiopathic unilateral nonacute tonic pupil.

Small Pupil with Poor Dilation: Oculosympathetic Dysfunction

Horner's syndrome: Horner's syndrome is characterized by lid ptosis, pupillary miosis, and facial anhidrosis (Figs. 100.8A to E). Interruption of sympathetic innervation to the Müller (tarsal) muscles in the upper and lower eyelids produces upper and lower lid ptosis and a noticeable decrease of the palpebral fissure. The extent of facial anhidrosis depends on the site of the sympathetic defect. The more peripheral the lesion, the less extensive the anhidrosis such that postganglionic lesions are associated

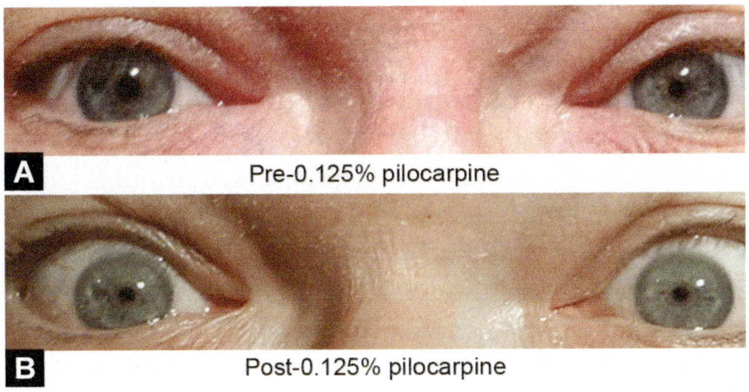

Figs. 100.7A and B: A 55-year-old man was referred to neuro-ophthalmology clinic after his eye doctor noticed that he had "unequal pupil and pupils were not reacting normally". Both pupils were small in size; the right pupil was slightly larger than the left. Both pupils constricted poorly to light stimulation, but demonstrated significant constriction when the patient attempted to focus on a near target. (A) Both pupils demonstrated significant degree of constriction following instillation of dilute pilocarpine (0.125%), consistent with a diagnosis of bilateral Adie's pupil (B). The small baseline size of the pupils indicates chronicity of the tonic pupils, the so-called "little old Adie's pupil".

with anhidrosis only on a patch on the forehead. Patients do not notice such minimal anhidrosis. Deficiency of sympathetic innervation to the iris dilator muscle leads to a small baseline pupil size and a slowness in pupillary redilation upon dark stimulation. When the room light is abruptly turned off, the pupil with an oculosympathetic defect shows slow redilation over 15–30 seconds compared to the normal pupil which promptly redilates back to baseline within 3–5 seconds. This is a clinical sign called dilation lag of the Horner's pupil.

Although dilation lag is diagnostic for Horner's syndrome, it is difficult to observe without pupillographic recording. Therefore, a diagnosis of Horner's syndrome usually relies on pharmacologic testing using either topical cocaine or apraclonidine. Cocaine acts at the terminal synapse as a norepinephrine reuptake inhibitor, causing accumulation of norepinephrine in the postsynaptic

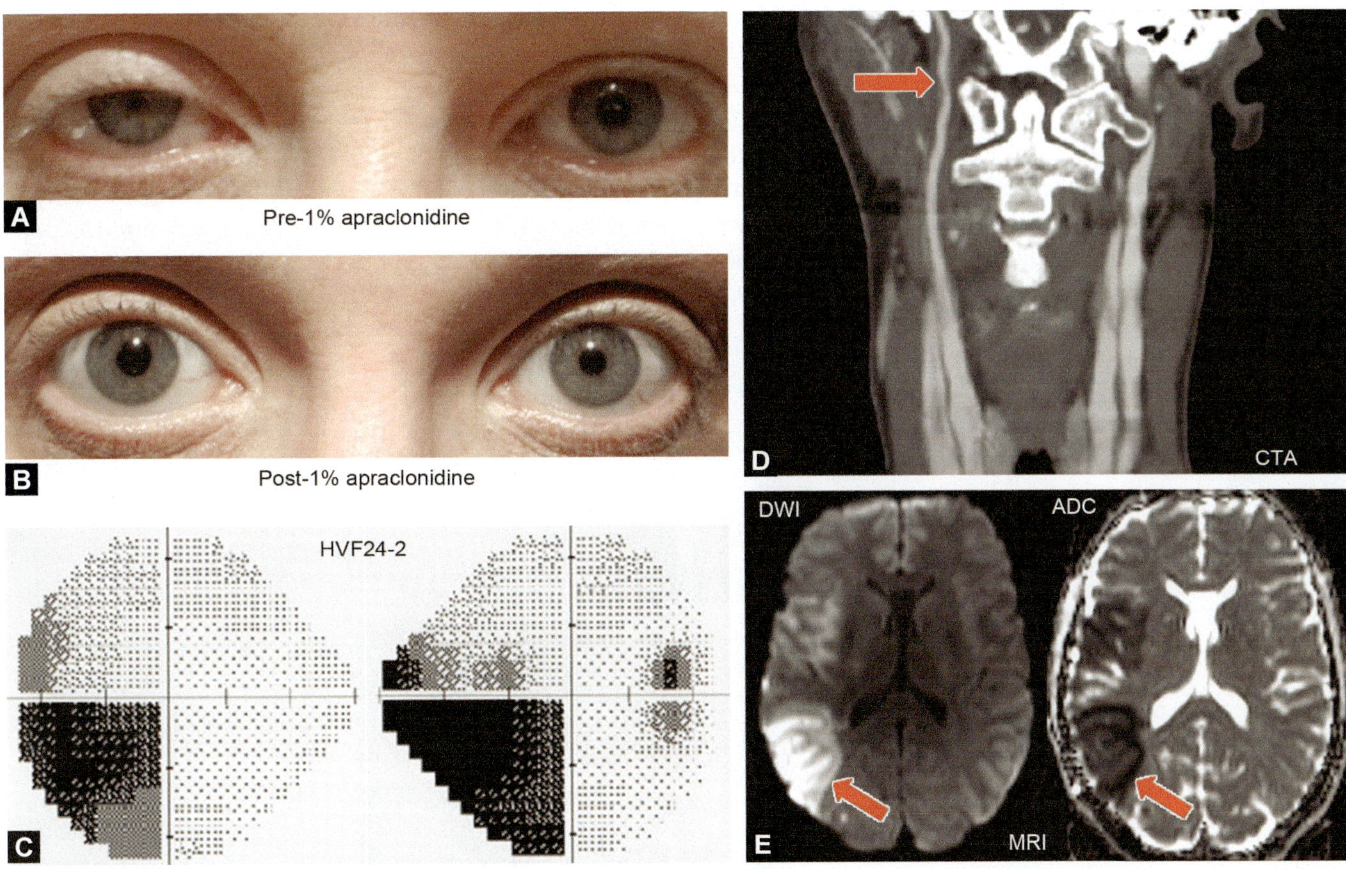

Figs. 100.8A to E: A 33-year-old female presented with acute onset of anisocoria, nausea/vomiting, slurred speech, left facial droop, weakness of the left arm and leg, and blurriness over the left side of her vision. The patient suffered from neck pain for about 2 months and had been going to chiropractor for the past month. Two weeks ago, she experienced a particularly painful "neck adjustment" after which her neck pain worsened. (A) Photograph shows her right-sided lid ptosis and pupillary miosis at baseline in room light, and then (B) reversal of anisocoria and ptosis after apraclonidine installation, consistent with a diagnosis of right Horner's syndrome. (C) The patient also had an incongruous left inferior quadrantanopia on automated perimetry testing (HVF24-2, Allergan-Humphrey, Inc., San Leandro, California). (D) A CT angiogram (CTA) of the head and neck showed a dissection involving the right distal internal carotid artery with abrupt narrowing at the level of C1 vertebrae extending into the petrous portion of the right carotid artery (red arrow); (E) A MRI of the brain showed diffusion restriction of the right middle cerebral artery distribution involving the right parietal and temporal lobe associated with corresponding ADC abnormalities, consistent with an acute infarction (red arrows).
(DWI: Diffusion-weighted image; ADC: Apparent diffusion coefficient)

junction. Instillation of 2 or 3 drops of 4% or 10% cocaine causes pupillary dilation in a normal eye. In a Horner's eye, there is minimal if any pupil dilation (Figs. 100.9A to C). Postcocaine anisocoria measuring 0.8 mm or greater is diagnostic for Horner's syndrome.[12] Apraclonidine is a α-2 adrenergic agonist with weak α-1 adrenergic agonist activity. The normal pupil constricts slightly to apraclonidine due to α-2 adrenergic receptor action inducing a downregulation of norepinephrine release. An eye with Horner's syndrome has adrenergic denervation hypersensitivity, and this causes the pupil to dilate and the lid to retract in response to the weak α-1 agonist action also present in apraclonidine. Reversal of anisocoria after apraclonidine instillation is regarded as a positive test for Horner's syndrome (*see* Figs. 100.8A to E).[13,14]

Hydroxyamphetamine eye drop testing is used to localize the site of the sympathetic defect. Hydroxyamphetamine enhances the release of norepinephrine from the postganglionic sympathetic nerve endings to synaptic junction. Whereas normal subjects and patients with a first (central) or second order, preganglionic Horner's syndrome show pupillary dilation in response to topical hydroxyamphetamine, patients with a third order, postganglionic Horner's syndrome demonstrate minimal to no pupil dilation due to damage of the terminal sympathetic nerve endings.[15,16] Inaccessibility to hydroxyamphetamine in the recent past has limited its use in the localization of Horner's syndrome.

The etiology of Horner's syndrome is influenced by the location of the oculosympathetic defect (Fig. 100.2). A common cause of first-order Horner's syndrome is lateral medullary syndrome (or Wallenberg syndrome) associated with occlusion of the posterior inferior cerebellar artery. Patients present with sudden onset dizziness, paresthesia of the ipsilateral face and contralateral body, ataxia, nausea/vomiting, and dysphagia. Ocular motor abnormalities are common and include skew deviation, nystagmus, lateropulsion, and abnormal smooth pursuit. Lateral medullary syndrome in young patients should prompt an investigation for vertebral dissection that is often associated with neck trauma. Second-order, or preganglionic, Horner's syndrome can present as an isolated finding without accompanying neurologic or systemic symptoms. An imaging study is warranted to look for soft tissue mass in the upper lungs (Pancoast tumor) or neck (thyroid goiter or tumor). Third-order neuron, or postganglionic, Horner's syndrome is commonly associated with lesions of or in close vicinity to the internal carotid artery or cavernous sinuses, such as carotid dissection, carotid-cavernous fistula, carotid aneurysm, meningioma, or inflammatory cavernous sinus syndrome. Patients with a postganglionic Horner's syndrome commonly report a new headache, periorbital

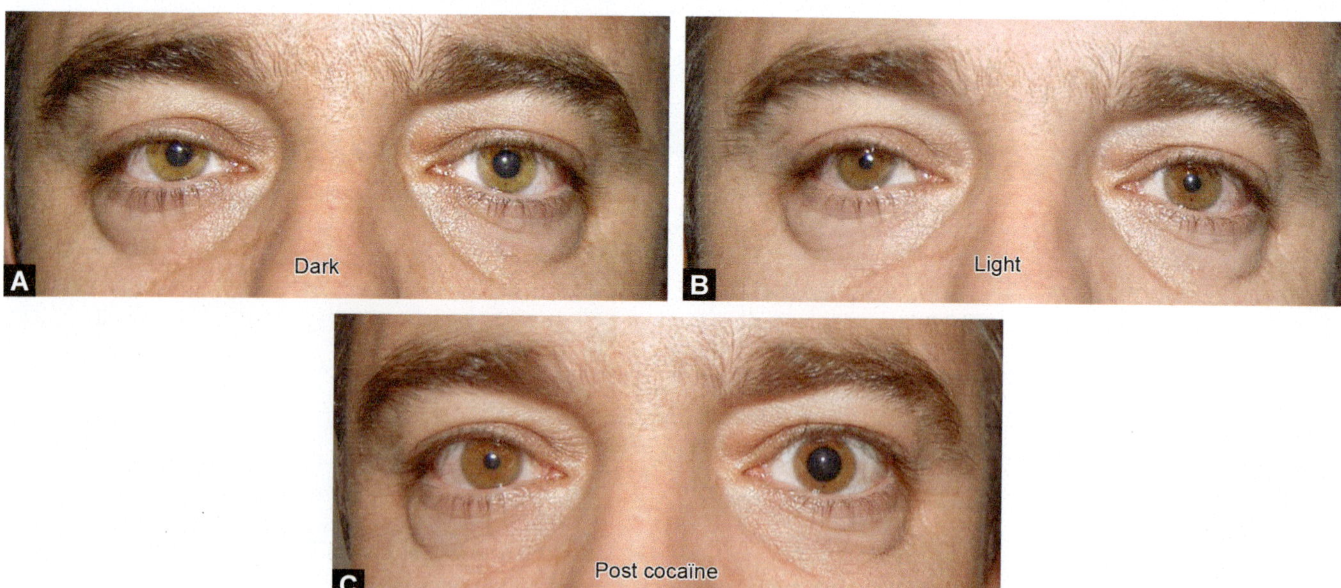

Figs. 100.9A to C: A 40-year-old construction worker had a mild ache around his right eye after returning from work. Upon self-examination in the mirror, he noted droopiness of the right upper lid and a smaller right pupil. The ache, redness and ptosis disappeared over the next few days. He was referred for further evaluation. (A and B) A subtle anisocoria was still present, particularly under dim light conditions; (C) Following instillation of topical cocaine to both eyes, the failure of the right pupil to dilate confirmed the presence of an oculosympathetic defect (Horner's syndrome). MRI and angiographic images of the carotid artery were negative. No specific cause of the Horner's syndrome was identified. He has remained stable over the next 1 year.

pain or neck pain. If the lesion is in the cavernous sinus and involves ocular motor cranial nerves as well, diplopia may accompany the Horner's syndrome.

Imaging is highly recommended in any patient with an acquired Horner's syndrome. If neurologic signs localizing to the brainstem are present, magnetic resonance imaging (MRI) of the head is sufficient. Otherwise, in an isolated Horner's syndrome, head, neck and chest imaging [computed tomography (CT) or MRI] is recommended. If Horner's syndrome is associated with eye pain or headache, especially in the setting of neck/head trauma or manipulation, then it is important to add a vascular study of the internal carotid artery (MR or CT angiogram of the head and neck) to rule out carotid dissection. Any acute and painful Horner's syndrome (2 weeks old or less) is considered a relative emergency in terms of neuroimaging. A delay in initiating therapy in acute carotid dissection can lead to carotid artery thrombosis and cerebral infarction.

Congenital Horner's syndrome is usually caused by birth trauma to the brachial plexus. Iris heterochromia with the lighter colored iris on the side of the lesion is a hallmark of congenital Horner's syndrome due to lack of sympathetic innervation to melanocytes of the iris during infancy. However, iris heterochromia is not pathognomonic of congenital Horner's syndrome and has been reported with acquired lesions of the sympathetic pathway. All infants and children with a nontraumatic Horner's syndrome should be evaluated for the possibility of a neuroblastoma arising in the sympathetic chain of the chest. Clinical analysis of the urine for determination of catecholamine excretion as well as imaging of the neck and chest are warranted.

LIGHT-NEAR DISSOCIATION

Pupillary light-near dissociation occurs when the pupil reacts poorly to bright light stimulation but its constriction to a near stimulus is better. There are several mechanisms for the development of light-near dissociation. The most common cause is injury to the afferent visual pathway which contains the pupillomotor signal, and bilateral optic neuropathy is the most common cause of bilateral light-near dissociation. Such patients are readily identified by their significant visual loss and optic atrophy. Their poor light reflex is related to the optic nerve damage, but the near response is a central reflex that can be induced by proprioceptive stimuli (asking the patient to look at his own thumb near the nose, even in the setting of complete blindness) and is thus preserved.

A second cause of light-near dissociation is selective injury of the light reflex fibers with sparing of the near fibers. Examples of this kind of light-near dissociation are Parinaud syndrome and Argyll Robertson pupils. A third mechanism leading to light-near dissociation is aberrant reinnervation of peripheral nerves, such as in case of aberrant regeneration of the third nerve.

Dorsal Midbrain Syndrome

The pupillomotor signal from the retina passes across the dorsal midbrain tectum. However, pupil constriction to near stimulus, as part of the near response of convergence, accommodation, and miosis, is mediated by near reflex whose fibers pass across the ventral aspect of the midbrain tegmentum. Dorsal midbrain syndrome, or Parinaud syndrome, is caused by intracranial lesions affecting the light reflex fibers passing in the midbrain tectum but sparing the near reflex neurons. Such patients have normal vision, midsize pupils and bilateral light-near dissociation. Closer examination will also reveal other signs of dorsal midbrain dysfunction such as lid retraction (Collier's sign), upgaze palsy, convergence-retraction nystagmus, and skew deviation. All patients with unexplained bilateral light-near dissociation should have neuroimaging of the upper brainstem. Common causes of dorsal midbrain syndrome are stroke in the elderly, pineoblastoma among children, and hydrocephalus.

Argyll Robertson Pupil

The Argyll Robertson pupil occurs in patients with tertiary syphilis involving the central nervous system. Unlike dorsal midbrain syndrome in which the pupils are midsized, patients with Argyll Robertson pupil have small pupils (< 2 mm) that are often irregular in shape. The pupils do not react to light, but the near response is brisk. Iris atrophy is frequently present, and portions of the iris transilluminate. Pupillary dilation is also poor, both in response to darkness and after instillation of mydriatics. This combination of pupillary findings is virtually pathognomonic of central nervous system syphilis but is rarely encountered. Mimickers of Argyll Robertson-like pupils are more common and seen in diabetes, chronic alcoholism, encephalitis, and following panretinal photocoagulation.

Aberrant Regeneration of Peripheral Nerves

Light-near dissociation is characteristic in chronic Adie's tonic pupil, owing to misdirected aberrant regeneration of the accommodative fibers of the short ciliary nerve to the pupil sphincters as described in Adie's tonic pupil. In the case of aberrant regeneration related to chronic compression of the third nerve, misdirected ocular motor fibers aberrantly innervate the iris sphincter. Thereafter, when the eye attempts to move in the direction of the regeneration fibers, there is a synchronized pupil coconstriction. For example, with aberrant regrowth of medial rectus fibers to the pupillary fibers, pupillary contraction will occur during adduction.

CONCLUSION

The efferent limb of the pupillary light and near responses follows defined anatomic pathways in the head, neck, and upper chest. Lesions along these paths may produce unilateral or bilateral pupillary deficits in pupillary reactivity, and anisocoria also may result. When coexisting findings of ptosis and/or ocular motility disturbances are present, then diagnosis of the underlying lesion(s) must take into account the multiple abnormalities observed. A thorough knowledge of the sympathetic, parasympathetic, and afferent pupillary light reflex pathways is essential in recognizing the presence and cause of pupillary dysfunction.

REFERENCES

1. Liu GT, Volpe NJ, Galetta SL. Pupillary disorders. In: Liu GT, Volpe NJ, Galetta SL (Eds). Neuro-Ophthalmology: diagnosis and management, 2nd edition. Philadelphia, PA: Saunders/ Elsevier Inc; 2010. pp. 415-6.
2. Giles CL, Henderson JW. Horner's syndrome: an analysis of 216 cases. Am J Ophthalmol. 1958;46:289-96.
3. Palumbo LT. A new concept of the sympathetic pathways to the eye; a new technique to avoid a Horner's syndrome. Surgery. 1957;42:740-8.
4. Birren JE, Casperson RC, Botwinick J. Age changes in pupil size. J Gerontol. 1950;5:216-21.
5. Loewenfeld IE. "Simple, central" anisocoria: a common condition, seldom recognized. Trans Sect Ophthalmol Am Acad Ophthalmol Otolaryngol. 1977;83:832-9.
6. Bremner FD, Smith SE. Pupil abnormalities in selected autonomic neuropathies. J Neuroophthalmol. 2006;26:209-19.
7. Kerrison JB. Examination of the pupils, accommodation, and lacrimation. In: Miller NR, Newman NJ, Biousse V, Kerrison JB (Eds). Walsh and Hoyt's Clinical Neuro-Ophthalmology: The Essentials, 2nd edition. Philadelphia, PA: Lippincott Williams and Wilkins; 2008. pp. 285-99.
8. Bouma H, Baghuis LC. Hippus of the pupil: periods of slow oscillations of unknown origin. Vision Res. 1971;11:1345-51.
9. Wefers Bettink-Remeijer M, Brouwers K, van Langenhove L, et al. Uveitis-like syndrome and iris transillumination after the use of oral moxifloxacin. Eye (Lond). 2009;23:2260-2.
10. Goldberg MF. Clinical manifestations of ectopia lentis et pupillae in 16 patients. Trans Am Ophthalmol Soc. 1988;86:158-77.
11. Younge BR, Buski ZJ. Tonic pupil: a simple screening test. Can J Ophthalmol. 1976;11:295-9.
12. Kardon RH, Denison CE, Brown CK, et al. Critical evaluation of the cocaine test in the diagnosis of Horner's syndrome. Arch Ophthalmol. 1990;108:384-7.
13. Brown SM. The utility of 0.5% apraclonidine in the diagnosis of Horner syndrome. Arch Ophthalmol. 2005;123:578; author reply p. 578.
14. Koc F, Kavuncu S, Kansu T, et al. The sensitivity and specificity of 0.5% apraclonidine in the diagnosis of oculosympathetic paresis. Br J Ophthalmol. 2005;89(11):1442-4.
15. Ing E. Hydroxyamphetamine drops for Horner's syndrome. Can J Ophthalmol. 2001;36:243.
16. Thompson HS, Mensher JH. Adrenergic mydriasis in Horner's syndrome. Hydroxyamphetamine test for diagnosis of postganglionic defects. Am J Ophthalmol. 1971;72:472-80.

Part 12 Orbit and Oculoplasty

Shannon S Joseph

OUTLINE

Chapter 101 Anatomy and Examination of the Eyelid, Orbit and Adnexa

Suzanne W van Landingham, Mark J Lucarelli

INTRODUCTION

A sound understanding of the anatomy of the eyelid, orbit, and adnexa is essential to the practice of ophthalmology. The ability to distinguish normal from abnormal findings may be crucial to diagnosing potentially disfiguring or life-threatening diseases, and helps to guide treatment and/or appropriate referral. An accurate anatomical framework is crucial to performing surgery on these structures, and to understanding their impact on the eye.

This chapter explains the detailed description of the anatomy of the orbit, lacrimal apparatus, eyebrows, and eyelids as well as techniques for examination. More detailed descriptions of disease processes that affect these structures and surgical procedures to correct them will follow in subsequent chapters.

ORBIT

Anatomy

Bony Structure

The orbit is surrounded by seven bones and can be described in shape as somewhere between a cone and a square pyramid (Fig. 101.1). The four walls: the roof, the lateral wall, the floor, and the medial wall, taper to a dull point at the orbital apex. The medial wall of the orbit is roughly parallel to the midline and forms a 45° angle with the lateral wall.

The anterior face of the bony orbit is called the orbital rim, and is generally thicker and stronger than the other areas of the orbital bones. This property serves to protect the eye from blunt trauma. The orbital rim forms a discontinuous spiral, starting at the anterior lacrimal crest of the maxilla and spiraling laterally and posteriorly until the posterior lacrimal crest of the lacrimal bone.[1] The lacrimal crests border the lacrimal sac fossa.

The orbital roof consists primarily of the frontal bone, with a small contribution from the lesser wing of the sphenoid bone (Table 101.1). It is bordered medially by the frontoethmoid suture and laterally by the superior orbital fissure. The roof is closely related to the frontal sinus anteriorly and the anterior cranial fossa posteriorly. For this reason, fractures of the orbital roof that involve the posterior table of the frontal sinus convey a risk of meningitis and are often managed collaboratively with otolaryngology and/or neurosurgery services.

The lateral orbital wall consists of the zygomatic bone anteriorly, the greater wing of the sphenoid posteriorly, and the zygomatic process of the frontal bone superiorly. It is separated from the orbital floor by the inferior orbital fissure. The temporalis muscle adheres tightly to its outer face. The lateral wall contains the tubercle of Whitnall, to which several important structures, including the lateral canthal tendon, attach.[2]

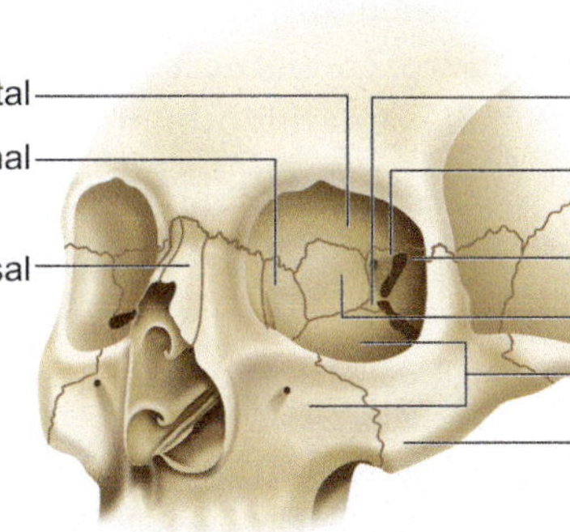

Fig. 101.1: The bony orbit, oblique view.
Source: Griepentrog GJ, Lucarelli MJ. Function of the Orbit and Eyelids. In: Kaufman PJ, Alm A (Eds). Adler's Physiology of the Eye: Clinical Application. St. Louis: © Mosby/Elsevier; 2002. pp. 333-9; used with permission.

Table 101.1: The seven bones of the four orbital walls. The bone listed first for each wall contributes the most area to that wall.

Wall	Bones
Roof	Frontal, sphenoid (lesser wing)
Lateral wall	Zygoma, frontal, sphenoid (greater wing)
Floor	Maxilla, palatine, zygoma
Medial wall	Ethmoid, maxilla, lacrimal, sphenoid (lesser wing)

The orbital floor consists primarily of the maxillary bone, with components of the palatine bone posteriorly and the zygoma anterolaterally. The floor forms the superior aspect of the maxillary sinus and is separated from the medial wall by the maxilloethmoidal suture. The infraorbital groove and canal run in the posteroanterior direction through the central portion of the floor, carrying the infraorbital branch of the maxillary nerve (V2), which supplies sensory innervation to the midface. The medial portion of the orbital floor is thin and is subject to fracture from blunt trauma (a "blow out" fracture).[3]

Finally, the medial wall of the orbit consists primarily of the ethmoid bone with contributions from the sphenoid, maxillary, and lacrimal bones. It separates the orbit from the ethmoid sinuses. The medial wall is the thinnest portion of the orbit, and is often involved in "blow out" fractures.

Orbital Apex

The orbital apex is the posterior-most portion of the orbit. It contains several openings—the optic canal, superior orbital fissure, and inferior orbital fissure—that transmit important nerves and blood vessels (Fig. 101.2).

The superior orbital fissure is located between the greater and lesser wings of the sphenoid bone and connects the orbit with the cavernous sinus. It is typically about 22 mm in length and traverses superotemporally to inferonasally.[4] From superolateral to inferomedial, it conveys the lacrimal and frontal nerves [branches of cranial nerve (CN) V-1], the trochlear nerve (CN IV), the superior orbital vein (SOV), the oculomotor nerve (CN III), and the abducens nerve (CN VI). The lacrimal, frontal, and trochlear nerves and SOV enter the orbit outside the annulus of Zinn, whereas the other structures listed above enter within the muscle cone. This is why torsional movement of the eye can be seen in a properly executed retrobulbar block—local anesthetic delivered within the cone will typically block the actions of CN III and CN VI but not CN IV.

The inferior orbital fissure is located inferotemporally in the orbit. It is about 20 mm long and bordered laterally by the greater wing of the sphenoid and medially by the maxillary and palatine bones. It separates the lateral orbital wall from the orbital floor and connects the orbit to the pterygopalatine fossa. It conveys the inferior ophthalmic veins to the pterygoid plexus, and the maxillary nerve (V2) into the orbit.

The optic canal is separated from the superior orbital fissure by the optic strut. It is bounded superolaterally by the lesser wing of the sphenoid and medially by the body of the sphenoid. It conveys the optic nerve, the ophthalmic artery, and sympathetic nerve fibers.

Because of this high density of critical structures, injuries to the orbital apex can have severe functional consequences.

Orbital Soft Tissue

Periorbital fascia: The periorbital fascia consists of a complex network of interconnecting structures.[5] The periorbita lines the orbital bones, meeting the facial periosteum at the arcus marginalis, a thicker fibrous band that encircles the orbital rim. It is tightly attached at the arcus marginalis, as well as

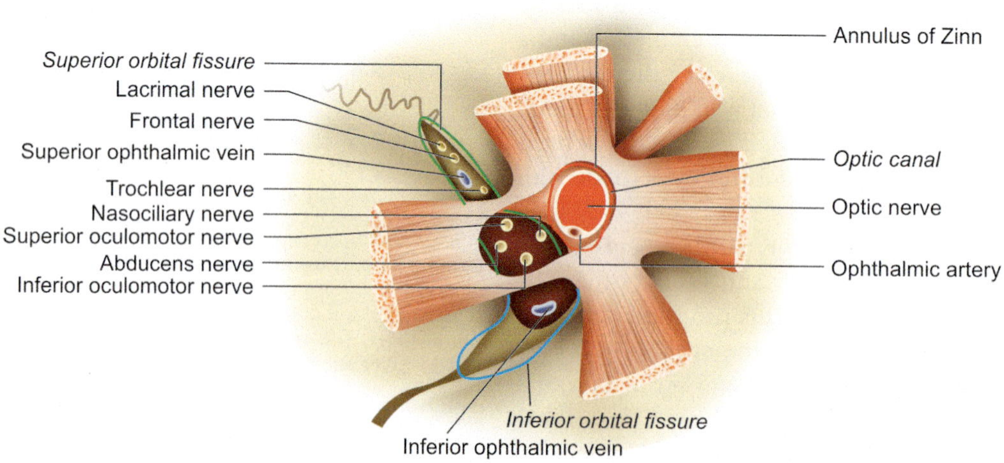

Fig. 101.2: Structures of the orbital apex. Foramina are outlined in color; their labels are italicized. Structures passing through each foramen are listed under the foramen's name. Note the extraocular muscles are included in the figure but are not labeled.
Source: Lemke BN, Lucarelli MJ. Anatomy of the Ocular Adnexa and Related Facial Structure. In: Nesi F, Levin M, Lisman R. Smith's Ophthalmic Plastic and Reconstructive Surgery. St. Louis: © Mosby/Elsevier; 1998. pp. 3-78; adapted with permission.

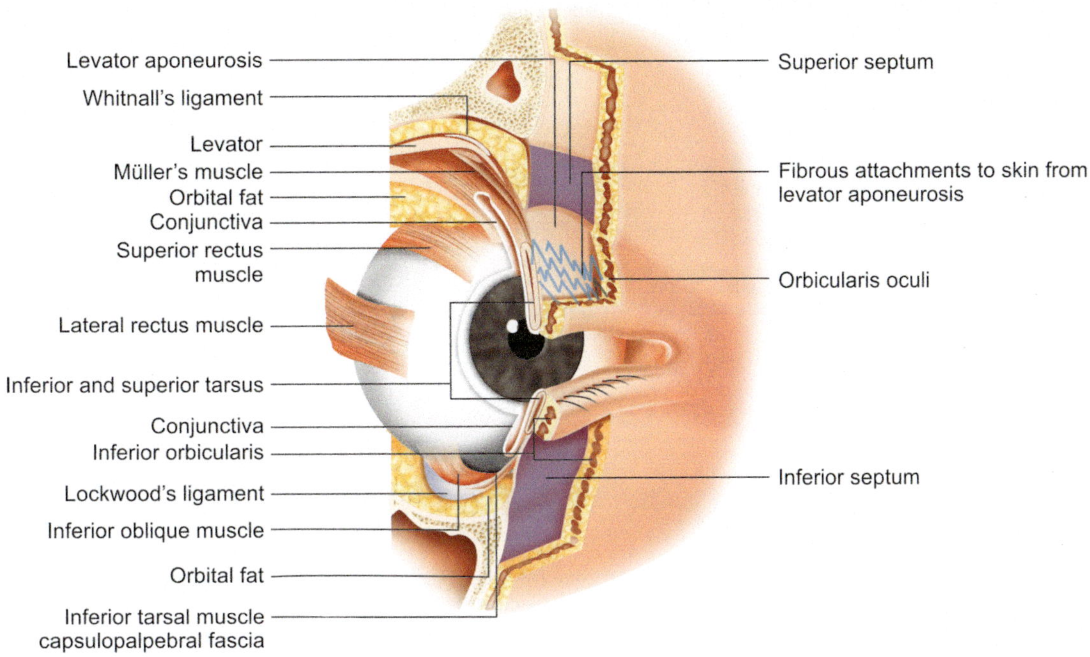

Fig. 101.3: Oblique section through the upper and lower eyelids, highlighting the eyelid musculature and orbital soft tissue.
Source: Lemke BN, Lucarelli MJ. Anatomy of the Ocular Adnexa and Related Facial Structure. In: Nesi F, Levin M, Lisman R. Smith's Ophthalmic Plastic and Reconstructive Surgery. St. Louis: © Mosby/Elsevier; 1998. pp. 3-78; adapted with permission.

the posterior lacrimal crest, suture lines, and foramina. It is more loosely attached elsewhere, which can allow for the accumulation of blood or pus. Tenon's capsule, also known as fascia bulbi, emanates from the dural sheath of the optic nerve, encompasses the globe deep to the conjunctiva, and fuses with the conjunctiva just posterior to the limbus. There are also check ligaments that connect the extraocular muscles to the bony orbit and sheaths that encircle the rectus muscles.

The orbital septum is an important landmark, dividing the orbit into "preseptal" and "retroseptal" spaces (Fig. 101.3). The septum extends from the inferior orbital rim, along the posterior lacrimal crest, upward to the canthal tendons and the inferior/anterior lower eyelid tarsus. The septum fuses with the lower eyelid retractors several millimeters below the inferior aspect of the tarsus.[6] Superiorly, the orbital septum extends from the superior orbital rim downward to the canthal tendons. It inserts onto the levator aponeurosis several millimeters above the superior tarsal border. In eyelids of Asian persons, the insertion point is lower.

Orbital fat: Orbital fat cushions and supports the globe and other orbital structures. Most orbital fat is retrobulbar, but some projects anteriorly as eyelid fat pads that can have an important impact on facial appearance (Fig. 101.4). There are two upper eyelid fat pads (nasal or medial and preaponeurotic fat pads) and three lower eyelid fat pads (medial, middle, and lateral). The preaponeurotic fat pad is an important landmark in upper eyelid surgery. In the lower eyelid, the medial and middle fat pads are separated by the inferior oblique.

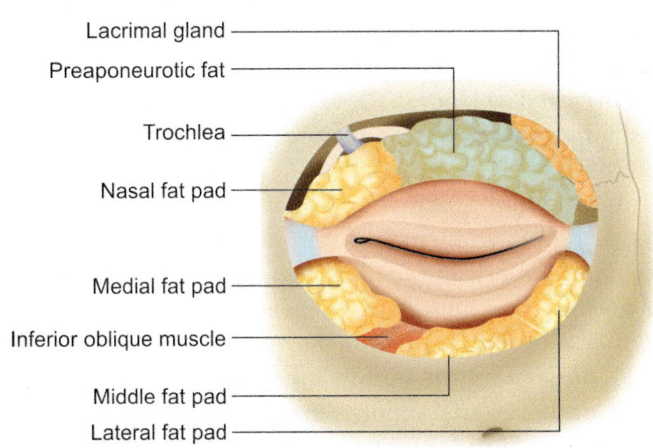

Fig. 101.4: Anterior orbital fat pads (septum removed).
Source: Griepentrog GJ, Lucarelli MJ. Surgical anatomy of the orbit, eyelids, and lacrimal system. In: Lucarelli MJ, Albert DM. Clinical Atlas of Procedures in Ophthalmic and Oculofacial Surgery, 2nd edition. Oxford: © Oxford University Press; 2011. pp. 647-57; adapted with permission.

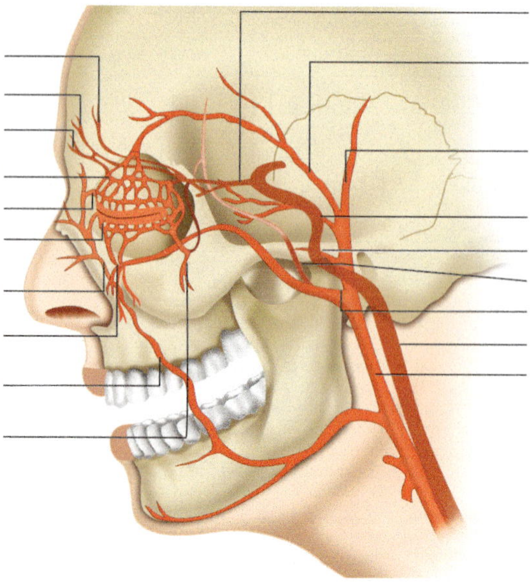

Fig. 101.5: Arterial supply of the orbit and periorbital region. The internal carotid and its branches are depicted in dark red; the external carotid and its branches are depicted in a lighter red.

Source: Nerad JA. Techniques in Ophthalmic Plastic Surgery: a Personal Tutorial. Philadelphia: © Saunders/Elsevier; 2009; used with permission.

Orbital blood supply: The orbit and periorbital tissues are supplied by branches of the carotid artery (Fig. 101.5). The external carotid supplies the face, including the eyelids and periorbital skin, and the internal carotid (via the ophthalmic artery) supplies the eye and orbit. There is extensive redundancy in the vascular supply of this region, and many anastomoses between the branches of the internal and external carotids.

In most individuals, the ophthalmic artery supplies the eye and orbit, with small contributions from the middle meningeal artery and the internal maxillary artery. In 3% of persons, the middle meningeal and the ophthalmic arteries contribute equally to the orbital blood supply and in 1% of persons, the middle meningeal contributes the entire orbital arterial supply.[7] The ophthalmic artery is the first branch of the internal carotid, and typically leaves the carotid just distal to the cavernous sinus. It enters the orbit via the optic canal, alongside the optic nerve. The subsequent branches vary quite a bit among individuals (Fig. 101.6). The central retinal artery is the first branch of the ophthalmic, and enters the optic nerve to supply the inner retina. Next, the ciliary arteries branch off to supply the globe: two long posterior ciliary arteries supply the ciliary muscle and iris, 15–20 short posterior ciliary arteries supply the choroid and optic nerve head, and the seven anterior ciliary arteries supply the rectus muscles.

The lacrimal artery supplies the lacrimal gland and then branches into the lateral palpebral arteries, the zygomaticofacial artery, and the zygomaticotemporal artery, which leave the orbit to supply the eyelids and periorbital tissues. The posterior and anterior ethmoid arteries leave the orbit to supply the soft tissues of the ethmoid sinuses and the nose, and both provide important landmarks in orbital surgery. Their foramina are located in the frontoethmoid suture, and damaging the bone superior to them (such as in an orbital decompression) risks intracranial damage and CSF leak. The supraorbital artery exits through the supraorbital foramen or notch to supply the eyebrow, forehead, and medial eyelid. The ophthalmic artery continues as the nasofrontal artery, which branches just posterior to the trochlea into the supratrochlear artery, which supplies the medial forehead and scalp, and the dorsal nasal artery, which supplies the nose and medial eyelids (via the medial palpebral arteries). In addition to the important branches described above, the ophthalmic artery and most of its named branches gives off smaller, unnamed branches that supply the deep orbit.

The relevant anatomy of the external carotid artery will be discussed later in this chapter.

Venous drainage of the orbit and periocular tissues does not follow arterial supply closely and is considerably less conserved. Venous drainage from the orbit occurs primarily via the superior ophthalmic vein (Figs. 101.7A and B), which travels through the superior orbital fissure into the cavernous sinus. This can be readily seen on orbital CT scans (coronal and axial cuts). Enlargement

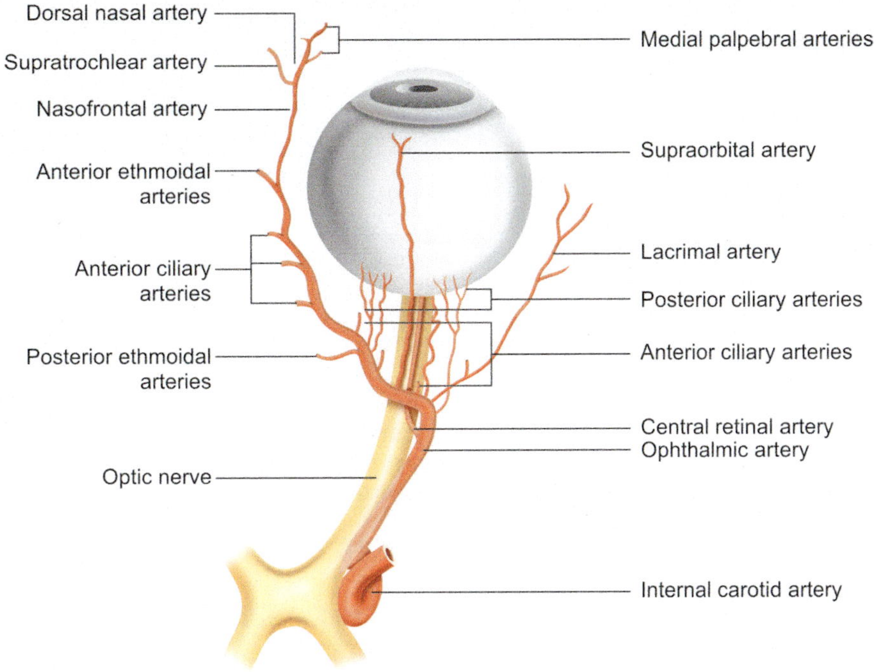

Fig. 101.6: Typical branching pattern of the ophthalmic artery.
Source: Lemke BN, Lucarelli MJ. Anatomy of the Ocular Adnexa and Related Facial Structure. In: Nesi F, Levin M, Lisman R. Smith's Ophthalmic Plastic and Reconstructive Surgery. St. Louis: © Mosby/Elsevier; 1998. pp. 3-78; adapted with permission.

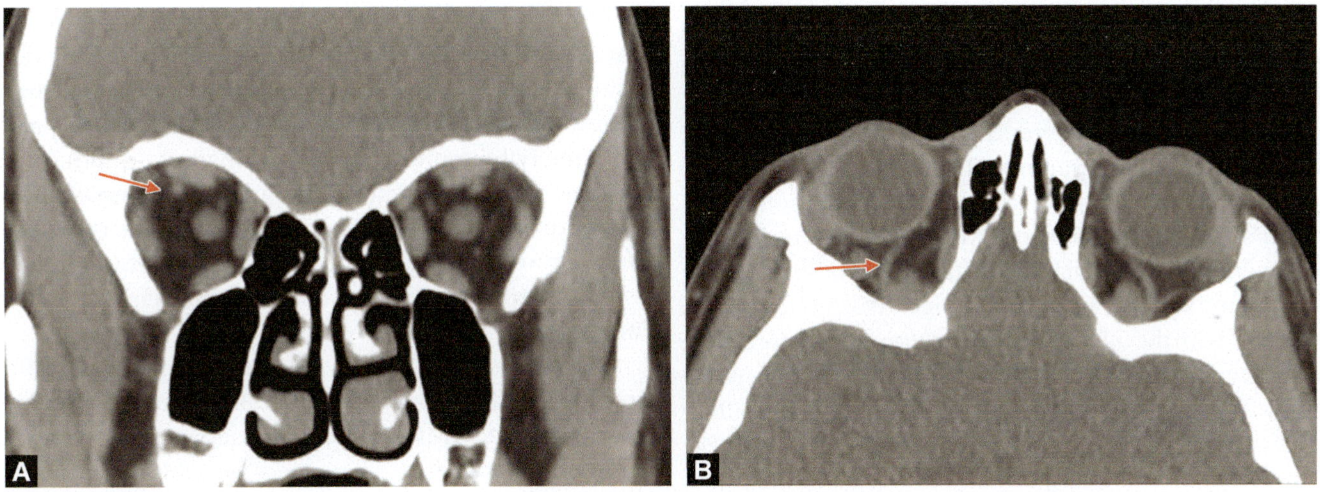

Figs. 101.7A and B: Superior ophthalmic vein. CT scan demonstrating a normal superior ophthalmic vein (red arrows)—(A) Coronal cut, and (B) Axial cut.
Source: Tabassum A Kennedy, MD.

may be indicative of carotid cavernous fistula or elevated intracranial pressure. Another major site of orbital venous drainage is the inferior ophthalmic vein, which exits the orbit via the inferior orbital fissure into the pterygoid venous plexus. Orbital and eyelid veins are valveless, which is thought to contribute to the spread of infections from the ethmoid to the orbit in cases of orbital cellulitis arising from sinusitis.

Orbital lymphatics: Orbital lymphatic drainage is sparse within the orbit.[8] It is likely that the posterior orbit drains toward the cavernous sinus and the anterior orbit drains similarly to the eyelids (described later).

Orbital innervation: The orbit's intricate innervation involves multiple cranial nerves and autonomic nerve fibers. The optic nerve arises from the retinal ganglion cell layer at the optic nerve head, which is approximately 1.5 mm in diameter. As it exits the globe into the orbit, it is coated in three layers of meninges and has a total diameter of 3.5 mm. The intraorbital portion of the optic nerve is approximately 25 mm long, and it travels approximately 18 mm from the globe to the orbital apex to exit the orbit via the optic canal. The "extra" length of intraorbital optic nerve allows the eye to move within the orbit and helps to prevent damage of the nerve with moderate degrees of proptosis. The intracanalicular portion of the optic nerve is tethered to periosteum, making it more susceptible to blunt or shearing type injury, which may lead to traumatic optic neuropathy. Finally, the intracranial portion of the optic nerve runs about 15 mm posterior to the orbit to the optic chiasm.[9]

Motor innervation of the orbit is supplied by CN III, IV, and VI, all of which enter the orbit via the superior orbital fissure (Fig. 101.2). Prior to entering the orbit, the oculomotor nerve (CN III) divides into superior and inferior branches. The superior branch innervates the superior rectus and levator palpebrae superioris muscles, allowing upgaze and eyelid elevation. The inferior branch innervates the medial rectus, inferior rectus, and inferior oblique, allowing globe adduction, downgaze, extorsion, and additional elevation (via the secondary action of the inferior oblique). The trochlear nerve (CN IV) innervates the superior oblique muscle, allowing for intorsion and depression of the globe. The abducens nerve causes globe abduction.

Sympathetic fibers enter the orbit via the optic canal and superior and inferior orbital fissures.[1] These allow for pupillary dilation, elevation of the eyelid via stimulation of Müller's muscle, and vasoconstriction. Parasympathetic nerves enter the orbit via several different paths including preganglionic fibers from the Edinger-Westphal nucleus that travel with the inferior division of the oculomotor nerve, synapse in the ciliary ganglion, and continue to the eye via the short ciliary nerves to innervate the pupil (pupillary constriction.) Other parasympathetics stimulate tear secretion by the lacrimal gland and choroidal vasodilation.

Sensory and motor innervation of the face and eyelids will be discussed later in this chapter.

Examination

Examination of the orbit starts with inspection. Asymmetry or gross deformity can indicate bony abnormalities or space-occupying lesions. Proptosis and enophthalmos can be assessed subjectively by worm's or ant's eye view, in which the examiner leans the patient back in their chair and positions himself below the patient in order to judge the axial position of the patient's globes (Figs. 101.8A and B). Hertel exophthalmometry can be used for objective measurement of the same: the exophthalmometer is rested on the orbital rims and the examiner uses the inset mirrors to measure the degree of proptosis.

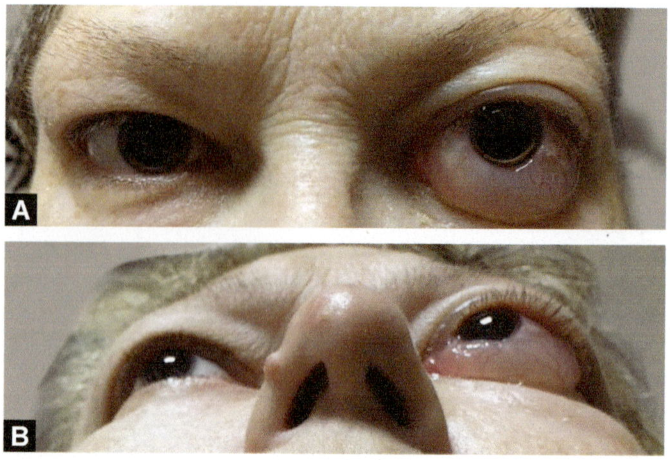

Figs. 101.8A and B: Gross evaluation of proptosis. This patient has left-sided proptosis due to an orbital mass. (A) Frontal view reveals left-sided chemosis; (B) Worm's or ant's eye view reveals several millimeters of left-sided proptosis.

Extraocular movements are an important component of the orbital exam. They may be impaired in inflammatory, traumatic, and neoplastic conditions. Visual acuity, color vision, visual field testing, and the pupillary exam can be helpful in assessing for compressive optic neuropathy, which may be found in space-occupying orbital lesions or thyroid orbitopathy. Pallor or edema of the optic nerve head can also be useful signs. Palpation of the orbital rim is important in patients with a history of orbital trauma, as bony step-offs, deformities, and point tenderness may indicate a fracture.

Computed tomography (CT) of the orbits with thin cuts is often the initial imaging modality for assessment of orbital disease. CT is excellent for assessing the bony orbit, for example, when there is concern for orbital fracture. It is also useful for evaluating the extraocular muscles (i.e. for diagnosis of thyroid eye disease), orbital inflammation (such as orbital cellulitis), and orbital abscesses or hematomas. CT is useful for diagnosing an orbital tumor, however, MRI may be needed to further characterize the lesion. CT has the advantage of being less expensive, quicker, and more readily available than MRI in most settings. Intravenous contrast should be used if there is concern for orbital abscess or mass, and is not necessary for evaluation of the orbital bones. Orbital ultrasound can also be used to evaluate the extraocular muscles, and has the advantage of being less expensive than CT scan and does not subject the patient to radiation exposure, however, the accuracy is very operator dependent.

LACRIMAL APPARATUS

Anatomy

Lacrimal Secretory System

The lacrimal secretory system consists of the lacrimal gland, the accessory lacrimal glands of Kraus and Wolfring, meibomian glands, and conjunctival goblet cells (Fig. 101.9). These glands together create the three layers of the tear film, listed here from outermost to innermost: aqueous, lipid, and mucinous.

The lacrimal gland is an exocrine gland. It is responsible for most of the aqueous tear secretion capacity. It is located in the superotemporal orbit and consists of the orbital and palpebral lobes, separated by the lateral horn of the levator muscle and connected by a band of parenchyma posteriorly. The orbital lobe is nestled within the lacrimal gland fossa of the frontal bone. Tears drain from the gland onto the ocular surface via many fine ductules. The ductules of the orbital lobe pass through the palpebral lobe to reach the ocular surface. Surgical trauma to the palpebral lobe, therefore, risks impairing the outflow from both lobes. This is why, despite the palpebral lobe being more easily accessible, the orbital lobe is preferred for biopsy.

Additional aqueous tear secretion comes from the small accessory glands of Kraus and Wolfring, located in the conjunctival fornices and at the upper border of the superior tarsus, respectively. Approximately 20 glands of Kraus are located in the superior fornix and about 10 in the inferior fornix. These accessory glands are thought to be important in basal tear secretion.

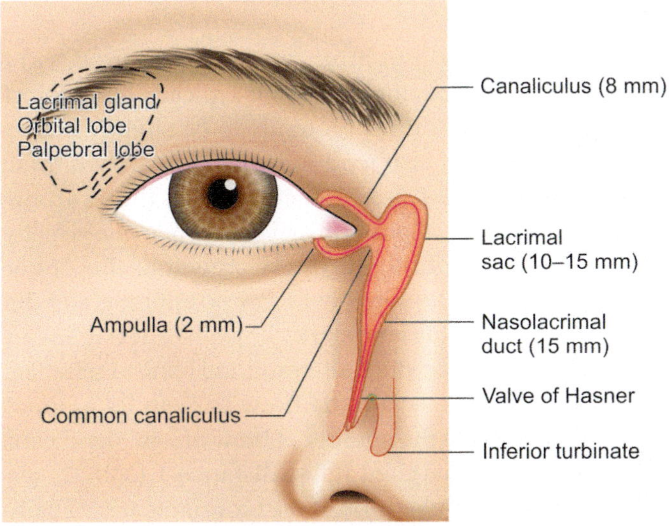

Fig. 101.9: Lacrimal apparatus.

The lipid layer of the tear film comes from the meibomian glands, which are modified sebaceous glands located within the tarsus. There are approximately 25 in the upper eyelid and 20 in the lower. Their orifices can be seen at the eyelid margin.

Finally, the goblet cells of the conjunctiva contribute the mucinous layer of the tear film.

Lacrimal Excretory System

Tears flow from the ocular surface to the nasal cavity via the lacrimal excretory system (Fig. 101.9). They pass first through the lacrimal puncta, which are located at the upper and lower eyelid margins about 5 mm from the medial canthus. The small area of elevated tissue around the punctum is called the lacrimal papilla. Subsequently, tears enter the 2 mm vertical portion of the canaliculus, flow through the ampulla (the dilated juncture of the vertical and horizontal portions of the canaliculi), and then through the 8 mm horizontal portion of the canaliculus. In more than 90% of eyes, the upper and lower canaliculi then join for 1–2 mm as the common canaliculus, which enters the lacrimal sac at the common internal punctum (in the remaining less than 10% of eyes, the canaliculi enter the sac separately). Of note, the canaliculi lie within pretarsal orbicularis oculi closely associated with the medial canthal tendon.

The lacrimal sac lies within the lacrimal sac fossa and is typically 10–15 mm in length. Tears flow out of the lacrimal sac into the nasolacrimal duct, a membranous, tubular structure that is usually about 15 mm in length. The membranous nasolacrimal duct lies within the bony nasolacrimal canal, which is formed by the maxilla and lacrimal bones. The duct enters the nasal cavity under the inferior turbinate. A small valve called the valve of Hasner limits the flow of tears into the nose.

Examination

Lacrimal Gland

The palpebral lobe of the lacrimal gland can be visualized in many patients by elevating the upper eyelid superotemporally and having the patient look inferonasally (Figs. 101.10A to C). The orbital lobe cannot be visualized on exam. A normal lacrimal gland will appear small and pink,

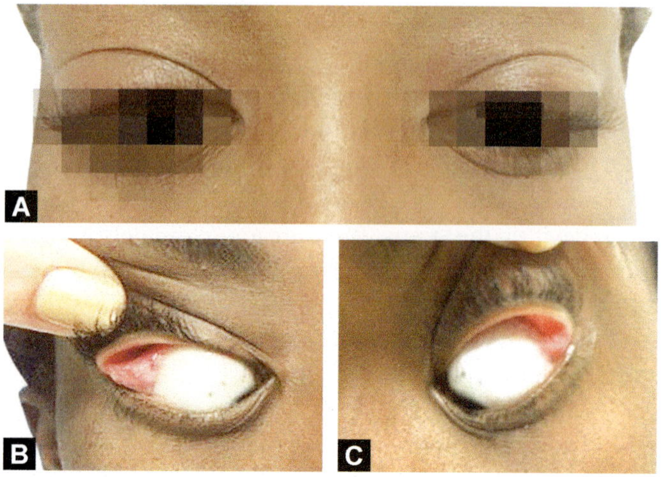

Figs. 101.10A to C: Lacrimal gland examination. This patient has a viral dacryoadenitis, right side worse than left. (A) Gross inspection reveals fullness in the superotemporal orbit, right greater than left; (B) The patient is looking down and to the left, revealing an erythematous and enlarged lacrimal gland (palpebral lobe); (C) The left lacrimal gland is visualized by having the patient look down and to the right.

and generally cannot be palpated through the eyelid skin. The gland may appear enlarged in cases of lacrimal gland tumor, or erythematous and purulent in dacryoadenitis. A patient with a large lacrimal gland tumor may have inferomedial displacement of the globe. CT is generally the best initial imaging modality for assessment of the lacrimal gland. It can show bony remodeling or erosion of the orbit and signs of inflammation. MRI with contrast may add additional soft tissue detail.

Lacrimal Drainage System

Examination of the lacrimal drainage system starts with inspection of the punctum, which should be patent and positioned toward the ocular surface. The healthy lacrimal drainage system is unremarkable on palpation, but an enlarged lacrimal sac (as in dacryocystitis or a dacryocystocele) can be palpated just medial to the medial commissure. Patency of the lacrimal drainage system can be assessed by probing and irrigation (Figs. 101.11A to D). First, the puncta are dilated. Then, the eyelid is stabilized with manual lateral traction, and 0 or 0-0 Bowman probe is introduced through the punctum into the canaliculus and advanced until it stops, approximately 10 mm. A "hard stop" indicates that the probe has reached the nasolacrimal sac and is pushing against the lacrimal sac fossa. A "soft stop" suggests an obstruction or stricture within the canaliculus. Next, the probe is removed. An irrigating syringe is prepared as follows: a 23 gauge irrigating cannula (blunt) is placed on a 3 cc syringe (or similar), which is then filled with tap water or eyewash solution. After stabilizing the eyelid with lateral traction, the cannula is introduced in the same manner as the probe. A small volume of fluid (about 1 cc) is injected until reflux from the other canaliculus is seen or the patient reports that they feel the fluid in their nasopharynx. The examiner then estimates the percentage of fluid that refluxed through the canaliculus onto the eye, if any, and the percentage that passed into the nose. A hard stop on probing followed by 100% canalicular reflux indicates complete nasolacrimal duct obstruction. The examiner should also look for purulence in the refluxed irrigation, as this may indicate infection. In rare instances, blood in the refluxed irrigation can indicate a lacrimal sac tumor. Jones testing is of historical interest but not routinely performed today, so it will not be described here.

EYEBROWS

Anatomy

The eyebrow is important to both facial appearance and facial expression. It consists of cilia, subcutaneous fibroadipose tissue, and underlying muscle and can be described as having a head, body, and tail.

Eyebrow movement is dictated by several facial muscles (Fig. 101.12). The frontalis muscle elevates the brows. The procerus depresses the glabellar region. The corrugator supercilii muscles lie deep to the frontalis and move the brows medially and inferiorly, resulting in a "furrowed brow." The depressor supercilii muscle, also deep to the frontalis, also depresses the brow. All of these muscles are innervated by the facial nerve.

Examination

Normal eyebrow position and appearance vary considerably. In men, the eyebrow is typically located just anterior to the orbital rim; it tends to be slightly higher in women. Women also tend to have more arched brow configuration. Brow ptosis occurs when the eyebrow droops below its usual position, which can become visually significant by weighting down or crowding the upper eyelid. Because of the variety in brow positioning and the relative lack of reliable landmarks, objective measurement of brow ptosis can be difficult in routine clinical practice. The examiner can elevate the brow back to its optimal position to estimate the amount of brow ptosis. Significant improvement of marginal reflex distance 1 (MRD1, see later) upon manual elevation of the brow indicates visually significant brow ptosis.

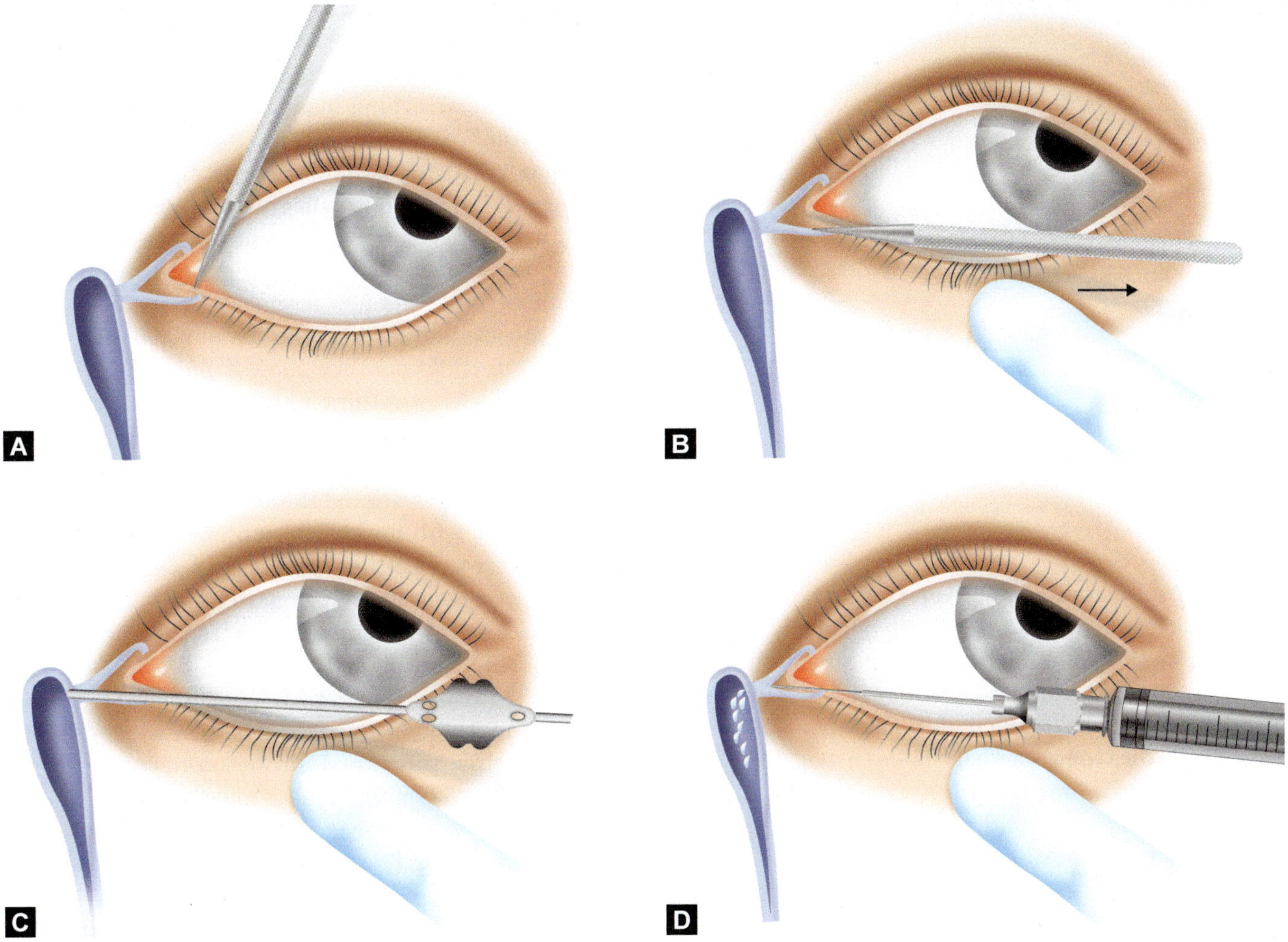

Figs. 101.11A to D: Lacrimal probing and irrigation. Used to assess patency of the lacrimal drainage system. (A) The punctal dilator is inserted into the punctum; (B) Manual lateral traction is applied, and the dilator is advanced to dilate the punctum and proximal canaliculus; (C) A 0-0 or 0 Bowman probe is inserted into the canaliculus and advanced until a stop is felt; (D) A 23-gauge irrigating cannula on a syringe is similarly advanced into the canaliculus. A small volume of fluid is injected.

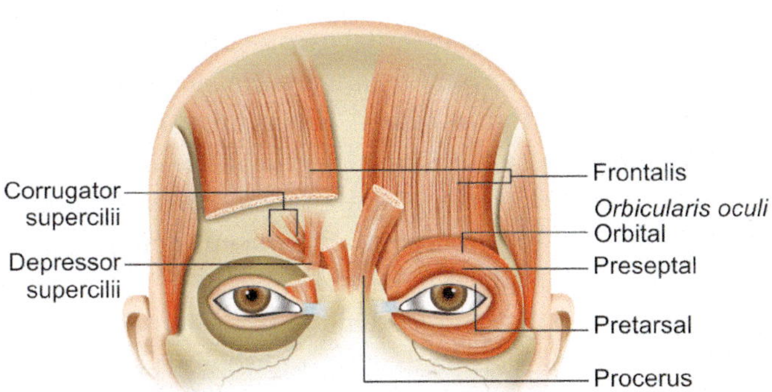

Fig. 101.12: Muscles of the eyebrow and forehead. The left side shows the superficial layer of muscles. The right shows these muscles cut away to reveal the deeper corrugator supercilii.

Source: Knize D. The forehead and temporal fossa: anatomy and technique. Philadelphia: © Lippincott Williams & Wilkins Inc.; 2001; adapted with permission.

EYELIDS

Anatomy

Eyelid Margin

The eyelid margin can divided into anterior and posterior lamellae, or layers. The anterior lamella consists of the eyelid skin, orbicularis, and adnexa (including hair follicles, glands of Zeis and Moll) (Fig. 101.13). The posterior lamella consists of tarsal plate and conjunctiva. The two layers of the eyelid are divided clinically at the center of the eyelid margin by the gray line, or muscle of Riolan, a fine extension of the orbicularis oculi muscle. Of note, the eyelid skin is the thinnest in the body and lacks a subcutaneous fat layer.

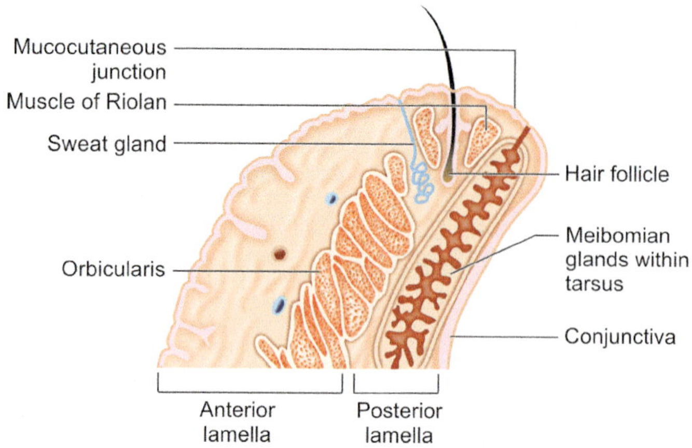

Fig. 101.13: Sagittal section of the eyelid margin.
Source: Lemke BN, Lucarelli MJ. Anatomy of the Ocular Adnexa and Related Facial Structure. In: Nesi F, Levin M, Lisman R. Smith's Ophthalmic Plastic and Reconstructive Surgery. St. Louis: © Mosby/Elsevier; 1998. pp. 3-78; adapted with permission.

The tarsal plates contain type I and III collagen and provide rigidity to the eyelids.[10] The upper tarsus measures approximately 10 mm tall centrally and the lower tarsus measures 3–4 mm centrally.[11] The upper and lower tarsal plates are connected to the periosteum of the orbital rim medially via the medial canthal tendon (*see* Fig. 101.3). This fibrous structure wraps around the canaliculi and lacrimal sac to attach anteriorly to the anterior lacrimal crest and posteriorly to the posterior lacrimal crest. The canthal tendon serves as the origin for the pretarsal orbicularis.[12] The lateral canthal tendon connects the tarsal plates to the periosteum of the lateral orbital wall at Whitnall's tubercle, just inside the orbital rim. It consists of an upper and a lower crus and serves as the insertion for the pretarsal orbicularis.

Eyelid Musculature

Eyelid movement is controlled by four main muscles/muscle groups: the orbicularis oculi, the levator palpebrae superioris, Müller's muscle, and the lower eyelid retractors. The orbicularis oculi is the main protractor of the eyelid, and allows for closure (Fig. 101.12). It can be divided into pretarsal, preseptal, and orbital components, moving away from the lid margin. It is innervated by the facial nerve.

The main retractor of the upper eyelid is the levator palpebrae superioris, which originates at the orbital apex on the lesser wing of the sphenoid bone, travels anteriorly just superior to the superior rectus muscle, and inserts onto the superior tarsal plate and into the upper eyelid skin (*see* Fig. 101.3). It is innervated by the oculomotor nerve. The levator palpebrae superioris can be divided into muscular and aponeurotic sections. The muscular section is approximately 36 mm long and transitions into the 14–20 mm fibrous aponeurosis at Whitnall's ligament, or the transverse orbital ligament.[13] Whitnall's may act as a fulcrum[13] or a sliding sling[14] for the action of the levator muscle. Disinsertion or attenuation of the levator aponeurosis is a common cause of involutional ptosis.

Müller's muscle, or the superior tarsal muscle, also retracts the upper eyelid. It is a smooth muscle with sympathetic innervation. It originates on the belly of the levator muscle and inserts onto the upper border of the tarsus.[15] It provides approximately 2 mm of upper eyelid elevation, which is why Horner's syndrome results in a mild ptosis.

The lower eyelid retractors originate at the inferior rectus muscle, pass around the inferior oblique muscle, and then fuse with the orbital septum before reaching the inferior aspect of the tarsus. They retract with the inferior rectus muscle in downgaze to prevent blockage of the pupil by the lower eyelid and receive their motor innervation from the oculomotor nerve. The retractors can be difficult to distinguish surgically, but can be divided into the capsulopalpebral fascia (outer layer, analogous to the levator palpebrae superioris) and the inferior tarsal muscle (inner layer, analogous to Muller's muscle).

Eyelid Vasculature and Lymphatics

The eyelids and periorbital tissues are supplied by the external carotid artery with many anastomoses with branches of the internal carotid artery (*see* Fig. 101.5). This robust blood supply allows for considerable flexibility in performing an eyelid or periorbital reconstruction: flaps and grafts tend to survive well.

The branches of the external carotid artery that supply the eyelids and periorbital region are the facial, maxillary, and superficial temporal artery. The facial artery, broadly, supplies the tissues anterior to the orbit via its terminal branch, the angular artery. The angular artery lies about 6–8 mm medial to the medial commissure, and can be encountered during dacryocystorhinostomy (DCR) surgery. The angular supplies the medial eyelids via anastomoses with the dorsal nasal branch of the ophthalmic artery. The maxillary artery supplies the jaws, palate, and interior of the nose, and also gives rise to the infraorbital artery. The infraorbital artery branches off within the pterygopalatine fossa, enters the orbit with the infraorbital nerve, and emerges from the infraorbital foramen to supply the cheek, lower eyelid and conjunctiva. The superficial temporal artery is the terminal branch of the external carotid. It can be palpated anterior to the tragus. This vessel is followed superiorly with a Doppler ultrasound to locate a site for temporal artery biopsy. Its branches supply the temple, lateral forehead, and, via the frontal artery, the upper eyelid.

The eyelids are supplied by rich anastomoses of the internal and external carotid arterial branches. The blood supply within the eyelid is organized into a double arcade system, supplied by the medial and lateral palpebral arteries. The medial palpebral artery is a branch of the dorsal nasal artery with contributions from the angular artery, and the lateral palpebral artery is a branch of the lacrimal artery (*see* Fig. 101.6). In the upper eyelid, the marginal arcade is found on the anterior tarsal surface 2–4 mm superior to the eyelid margin, and the peripheral arcade is found at the superior tarsal border between Müller's muscle and the levator aponeurosis. Both may be seen during external levator repair surgery, depending on the technique used. The lower eyelid has a similar but slightly less-developed arcade system.

As with the orbital veins, venous drainage of the eyelids is less well conserved. The small veins of the eyelid mostly drain into external jugular vein via the veins of the face. Much of this drainage occurs via the angular vein, which accompanies the angular artery and leads into the facial vein.

Eyelid lymphatic drainage occurs via the cervical system. The lateral two-thirds of the upper eyelid, lateral one-third of the lower eyelid, and the lateral conjunctiva drain into the preauricular nodes; the medial upper and lower eyelids and conjunctiva drain into the submandibular nodes.

Innervation

Motor innervation to the eyelids is supplied by cranial nerves III and VII as well as sympathetic nerve fibers. Eyelid elevation is mediated by the oculomotor nerve (CN III), which stimulates the levator palpebrae superioris; sympathetic fibers stimulate Müller's muscle. Most of the motor innervation of the face is supplied by the facial nerve (CN VII). The facial nerve divides into five main branches within the parotid gland, the two most superior (temporal and zygomatic) branches supply the periorbital region.

Sensory innervation to the face is supplied by the trigeminal nerve (CN V), whose ophthalmic (V1) and maxillary (V2) branches supply the periorbital region (Fig. 101.14). The ophthalmic nerve divides into three branches, the lacrimal, frontal, and nasociliary nerves, which enter the orbit via the superior orbital fissure (*see* Fig. 101.2). The lacrimal nerve supplies sensation to the lateral conjunctiva, lateral upper eyelid, and lacrimal gland. The frontal nerve branches into the supraorbital

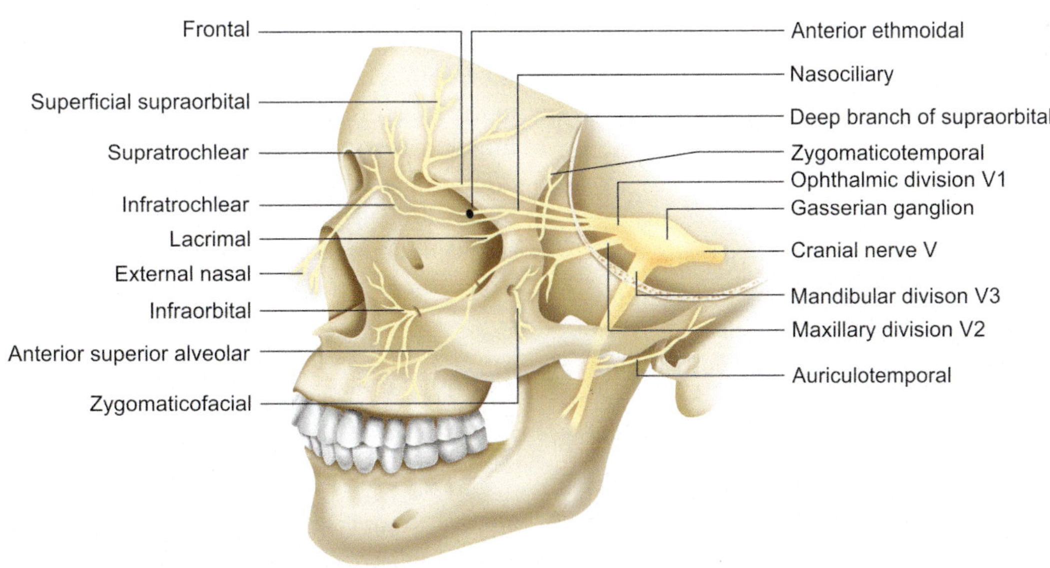

Fig. 101.14: Sensory innervation of the upper face.
Source: Lemke BN, Lucarelli MJ. Anatomy of the Ocular Adnexa and Related Facial Structure. In: Nesi F, Levin M, Lisman R. Smith's Ophthalmic Plastic and Reconstructive Surgery. St. Louis: © Mosby/Elsevier; 1998. pp. 3-78; adapted with permission.

and supratrochlear divisions. The supratrochlear supplies the glabella, medial upper eyelid, and lower forehead. The supraorbital passes through the supraorbital notch (or foramen) and supplies areas of the scalp and forehead. The nasociliary branch enters the orbit within the annulus of Zinn (unlike the other two branches of the ophthalmic nerve) and travels within the cone, giving off the long ciliary nerves to the globe, which supply the iris, cornea, and ciliary muscle. It then divides into the ethmoidal and infratrochlear braches, supplying the nasal mucosa and skin on the tip of the nose, and the side of the nose, respectively. Hutchinson's sign, herpes vesicles on the tip of the nose, indicates a higher likelihood of herpes zoster ophthalmicus owing to involvement of the nasociliary nerve.

The maxillary nerve (V2) enters the orbit via the inferior orbital fissure. Its terminal branch, the infraorbital nerve, enters the infraorbital groove about 30 mm posterior to the orbital rim. The infraorbital groove becomes the infraorbital canal, which ultimately exits the maxillary bone at the infraorbital foramen, about 6 mm inferior to the inferior orbital rim, to supply the anterior midface.

Examination

Examination of the eyelid relies on visual inspection as well as measurement of eyelid function.

Evaluation of Skin

A thorough examination of the eyelid may start with gross inspection of the eyelid and periorbital skin. Scars may shorten the anterior lamella, resulting in cicatricial ectropion (*see* Chapter 103; Other Eyelid Malpositions and Disorders). Excessive eyelid tissues and laxity may produce a mechanical ectropion or ptosis. A seventh CN palsy may produce paralytic ectropion, lagophthalmos, and brow ptosis.

Slit-lamp examination can aid in the diagnosis of eyelid margin diseases, such as rosacea or blepharitis, and in characterizing benign or malignant eyelid lesions. Malignancy is suggested by adjacent madarosis (loss of eyelashes), ulceration, and irregular borders, particularly if the patient reports intermittent bleeding or lack of healing. Further description of eyelid malignancies can be found in Chapter 104: Neoplasms of the Eyelid.

Lashes

Slit lamp examination can also reveal abnormalities in eyelash positioning. Many cases of trichiasis (misdirected lashes) are due to entropion, although some authors restrict trichiasis to misdirected eyelashes when the eyelid is in normal position. Trichiasis can occur following trauma or some severe forms of conjunctivitis. Distichiasis is a congenital (often autosomal dominant) or acquired eyelash disorder in which lashes are found to be growing ectopically from the meibomian gland orifices. Epiblepharon is a congenital condition in which an abnormal roll of the superior anterior lamella displaces normally positioned cilia posteriorly.

Eyelid Function

Several measurements are useful for evaluation of the eyelids. MRD1 (marginal reflex distance 1) is the distance between the corneal light reflex to the upper eyelid margin with the eyes in primary position (Fig. 101.15). It can be measured with a ruler as the patient fixates at a distant target with the examiner using a muscle light to create a corneal light reflex. Normal MRD1 is 3.5–5 mm: lower values may indicate blepharoptosis, higher values may indicate eyelid retraction. MRD2 is the distance between the corneal light reflex and the lower eyelid margin. Normal is 5 mm: higher values may indicate lower eyelid retraction. The palpebral fissure height is the distance between the two eyelid margins (normal is 8.5–10 mm).

In addition to MRD1, levator excursion is important to the diagnosis of blepharoptosis. Levator excursion is measured as the distance from the upper eyelid margin in downgaze to the upper eyelid margin in upgaze (normal is >12 mm). It is best to measure this with the eyebrow immobilized against the frontalis bone by the examiner's hand to avoid inflation of the measurement by frontalis recruitment. Poor levator function in a ptosis patient suggests myogenic or congenital etiology. Another useful finding in a ptosis evaluation is observation of the lid crease—a high lid crease is suggestive of levator dehiscence, whereas a poorly defined lid crease is

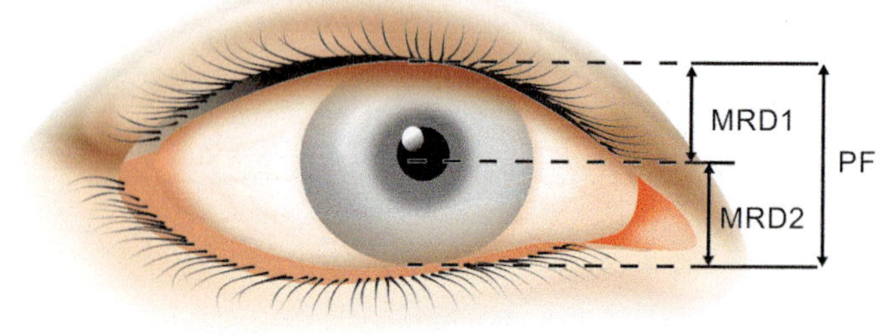

Fig. 101.15: Functional measurements of the eyelid. (MRD: Marginal reflex distance; PF: Palpebral fissure)

suggestive of congenital or myogenic etiology (*see* Chapter 102; The Droopy Eyelid for more detail).

To assess ocular surface protection, it is important to study eyelid closure and blink. Lagophthalmos, or a failure to close the eyelids completely, can result from problems with the eyelids (such as severe eyelid retraction) or orbit (such as severe proptosis). The patient may be asked to close the eyes gently, as though going to sleep. The amount of lagophthalmos is the measured distance between the eyelids. Subtle lagophthalmos can be seen by shining a muscle light at the patient's eyelashes from below—the reflection off the tear film will allow the examiner to identify lagophthalmos masked by eyelashes.

CONCLUSION

This chapter has described the anatomy of the eyelids and orbit, and introduced techniques for examination. The following chapters will build on these concepts and describe anatomy and examination techniques germane to specific diseases in more detail.

REFERENCES

1. Whitnall SE. The anatomy of the human orbit and accessory organs of vision, 2nd edition. New York: Oxford University Press; 1932.
2. Whitnall SE. On a tubercle on the malar bone, and on the lateral attachments of the tarsal plates. J Anat Physiol. 1911;45:426-32.
3. Jo A, Rizen V, Nikolić V, Banović B. The role of orbital wall morphological properties and their supporting structures in the etiology of "blow-out" fractures. Surg Radiol Anat SRA. 1989;11(3):241-8.
4. Natori Y, Rhoton AL. Microsurgical anatomy of the superior orbital fissure. Neurosurgery. 1995;36(4):762-75.
5. Koornneef L. Details of the orbital connective tissue system in the adult. In: Spatial aspect of orbital musclo-fibrous tissue in man. New York: Swets & Zweitlinger; 1977.
6. Hawes MJ, Dortzbach RK. The microscopic anatomy of the lower eyelid retractors. Arch Ophthalmol. 1982;100(8):1313-8.
7. Hayreh SS, Dass R. The ophthalmic artery: I. Origin and intra-cranial and intra-canalicular course. Br J Ophthalmol. 1962;46(2):65-98.
8. Gausas RE, Gonnering RS, Lemke BN, et al. Identification of human orbital lymphatics. Ophthal Plast Reconstr Surg. 1999;15(4):252-9.
9. Sarkies N. Traumatic optic neuropathy. Eye Lond Engl. 2004;18(11):1122-5.
10. Milz S, Neufang J, Higashiyama I, et al. An immunohistochemical study of the extracellular matrix of the tarsal plate in the upper eyelid in human beings. J Anat. 2005;206(1):37-45.
11. Wesley RE, McCord CD, Jones NA. Height of the tarsus of the lower eyelid. Am J Ophthalmol. 1980;90(1):102-5.
12. Anderson RL. Medial canthal tendon branches out. Arch Ophthalmol. 1977;95(11):2051-2.
13. Lemke BN, Stasior OG, Rosenberg PN. The surgical relations of the levator palpebrae superioris muscle. Ophthal Plast Reconstr Surg. 1988;4(1):25-30.
14. Goldberg RA, Wu JC, Jesmanowicz A, et al. Eyelid anatomy revisited. Dynamic high-resolution magnetic resonance images of Whitnall's ligament and upper eyelid structures with the use of a surface coil. Arch Ophthalmol. 1992;110(11):1598-600.
15. Kuwabara T, Cogan DG, Johnson CC. Structure of the muscles of the upper eyelid. Arch Ophthalmol. 1975;93(11):1189-97.

Chapter 102 The Droopy Eyelid

Natalie N Chung, Bobby S Korn, Don O Kikkawa

INTRODUCTION

The "droopy eyelid" is an increasingly ubiquitous problem, most commonly acquired with age, but also through prior trauma, inflammation, or infection.[1,2] Aging leads to loss of skin elasticity, and increased inflammatory and metalloproteinase activity, leading to accelerated degradation of structural and connective tissue.[2,3] The upper eyelid ages in three primary ways: (1) dermatochalasis, (2) blepharoptosis, and (3) fat atrophy. As the appearance of one's eyes significantly impacts social assessments of age and fatigue, addressing these issues can significantly enhance functional and psychosocial quality of life.[4] Oculofacial surgical rejuvenation has the unique ability to address these delicate areas effectively and safely (Table 102.1).

PREOPERATIVE EVALUATION AND DOCUMENTATION

Prior to undergoing any oculoplastic surgery, it is important to take a complete relevant history, including history of prior facial or ocular surgery, facial trauma, refractive surgery, dry eye symptoms, ocular disease, use of fillers, medications, use of anticoagulants, allergies, and coexistent systemic conditions, such as diabetes and high blood pressure. Due to possible corneal hypoesthesia, post-LASIK patients should wait at least three months after refractive surgery before considering any eyelid surgery. Third party payers require proper documentation of functional symptoms and office testing prior to surgery. Photo-documentation is essential and photos should be taken pre- and postoperatively in the frontal, three-fourths and profile planes.

Informed Consent

Detailed informed consent should be obtained and documented, including a thorough discussion of risks, benefits, and alternatives.

Surgical Preparation

Standard sterile technique should be used. Corneal protectors minimize exposure and inadvertent injury to

Table 102.1: Contributors to the "droopy eyelid", indications for surgery, and recommended surgical approaches.

Diagnosis/Problem	Description	Indications for surgery	Surgical approach
Dermatochalasis	Excess laxity or redundancy of upper eyelid skin.	• Functional visual field reduction • Cosmetically displeasing dermatochalasis and/or fullness • Lash ptosis, entropion, blepharitis or anophthalmic prosthetic instability • Use of redundant skin for grafting	*Upper blepharoplasty*: • Special consideration for different ethnicities
Fat Prolapse	Cosmetically displeasing lower eyelid fat prolapse	• Cosmetically displeasing lower eyelid fat prolapse without significant dermatochalasis • Obscuration of vision in reading position	*Lower blepharoplasty*: • Transconjunctival approach • Transcutaneous approach
Eyelid ptosis	Drooping of the upper eyelid with reduction in marginal reflex distance (MRD)	• Functional ptosis affecting vision • Cosmetically displeasing ptosis • Amblyopia in visually maturing children • Ptosis affecting anophthalmic prosthetic function	*Ptosis repair*: • External Levator Advancement • Internal Levator Advancement
Brow Ptosis	Drooping of the eyebrow below the superior orbital rim	• Brow ptosis affecting visual function • Cosmetic displeasing brow ptosis	*Brow ptosis repair*: • Direct, coronal, endoscopic, internal approaches

the eye. Most eyelid procedures can be performed under local anesthesia (2% lidocaine with 1:200,000 epinephrine) with IV sedation, when needed. Our preference is to inject prior to skin marking to reduce skin distortion.

Managing Expectations

Managing patient expectations is an integral component, especially in the discerning cosmetic patient. To optimize patient satisfaction, the surgeon should allow patients to point out focal areas of concern (using a handheld mirror). The surgeon must set realistic goals, making patients aware of limitations, and give ample discussion time to review benefits, risks, and the possible need for revision.

Surgical Approach

The choice of surgical approach is the most important factor in correcting these problems effectively. Consideration must be given to age, eyelid problem, ethnicity, as well as coexisting eye conditions or malformations that may affect outcomes. If a patient presents with upper and lower dermatochalasis, eyelid ptosis and brow ptosis, the general rule is to start with brow ptosis repair, followed by eyelid procedures. This will ensure optimal results and minimize complications.[1,5] A detailed description of every possible approach is, however, beyond the scope of this chapter.

BROW PTOSIS REPAIR

Depending on the degree of brow ptosis present, multiple approaches can be used to elevate the brow. Some approaches can decrease forehead rhytids, and this must be discussed with the patient in advance. Endoscopic and coronal approaches, for instance, elevate the entire forehead, and may have a more successful result, however, elevation of the hairline must also be considered. A pretrichial approach helps to reduce hairline elevation. Direct brow ptosis repair is generally more effective in elevating the brow, however it may leave visible incisions.[6] Internal browpexy through the upper eyelid is a reasonable alternative, however it may not be as long lasting as the direct approach. Assessment of the brows for brow ptosis is an aspect of addressing the "droopy eye," but the scope of this chapter will be limited to the eyelid.

UPPER BLEPHAROPLASTY

Upper blepharoplasty is one of the most common procedures performed globally. It is safe and effective with high patient satisfaction and should be a part of any rejuvenating surgical repertoire.[7,8] Additional preoperative evaluation should include visual field testing, if required by third-party payers; the degree of dermatochalasis and lateral hooding; any coexistent blepharoptosis or brow ptosis; symmetry and height of eyelid crease; the degree of eyelid fullness, including fat pads and any lacrimal gland prolapse; dry eye assessment, including quantitative or qualitative tear assessment and lagophthalmos; assessment of distinct ethnic characteristic, including epicanthal fold, pigmentation, and canthal position (Figs. 102.1A and B).

Procedure of Upper Blepharoplasty (Figs. 102.2A to H)

1. *Marking the crease:* Proper marking is critical. If preoperative crease height is asymmetrical, consider coexistent ptosis. To mark the incision line, the native crease is followed medially, and tapered superiorly prior to reaching the punctum. Similarly, the crease is followed laterally, and superior tapering is considered if lateral hooding is present. Symmetry should be confirmed by comparing both sides. If a crease is not present, the crease should measure 7–8 mm in men, and 8–10 mm in women.
2. *Marking redundant skin:* Toothless forceps are used to pinch redundant skin delineating maximum extent of skin removal. (At least 20 mm from brow to eyelid margin should remain to avoid anterior lamellar

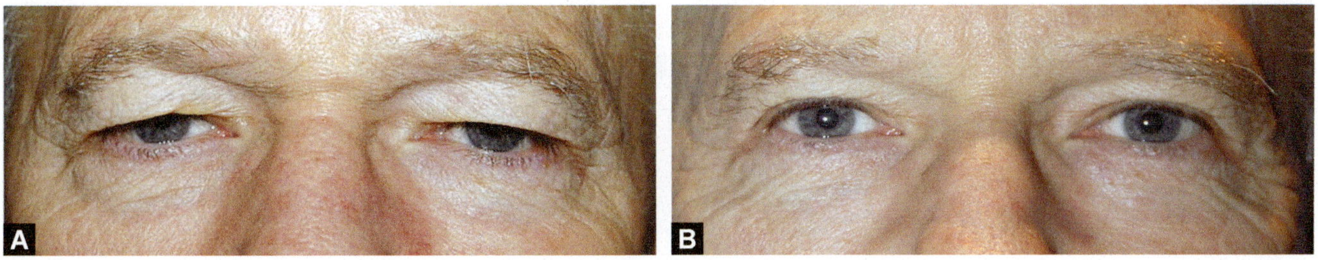

Figs. 102.1A and B: Before/after of upper blepharoplasty.

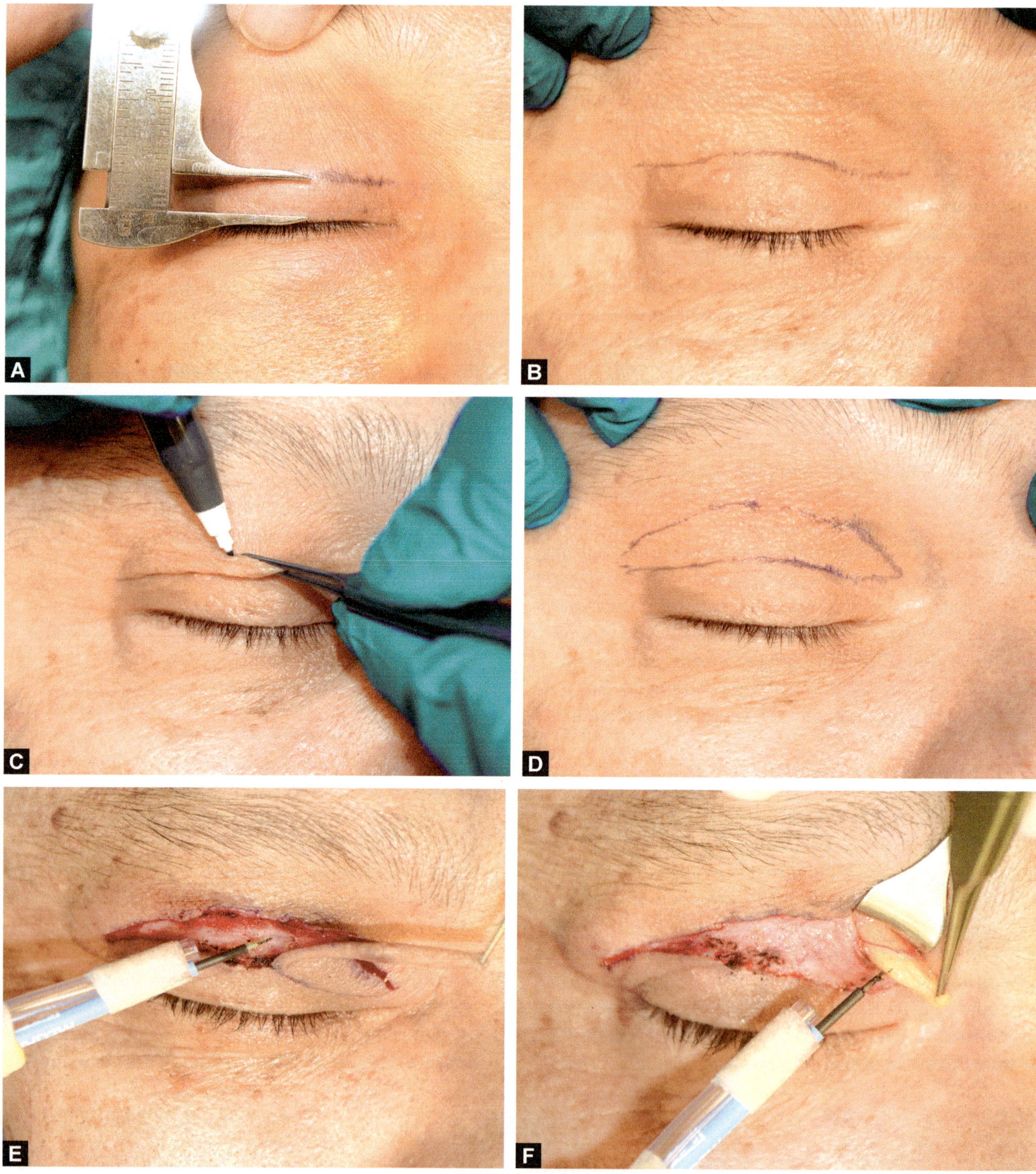

Figs. 102.2A to F

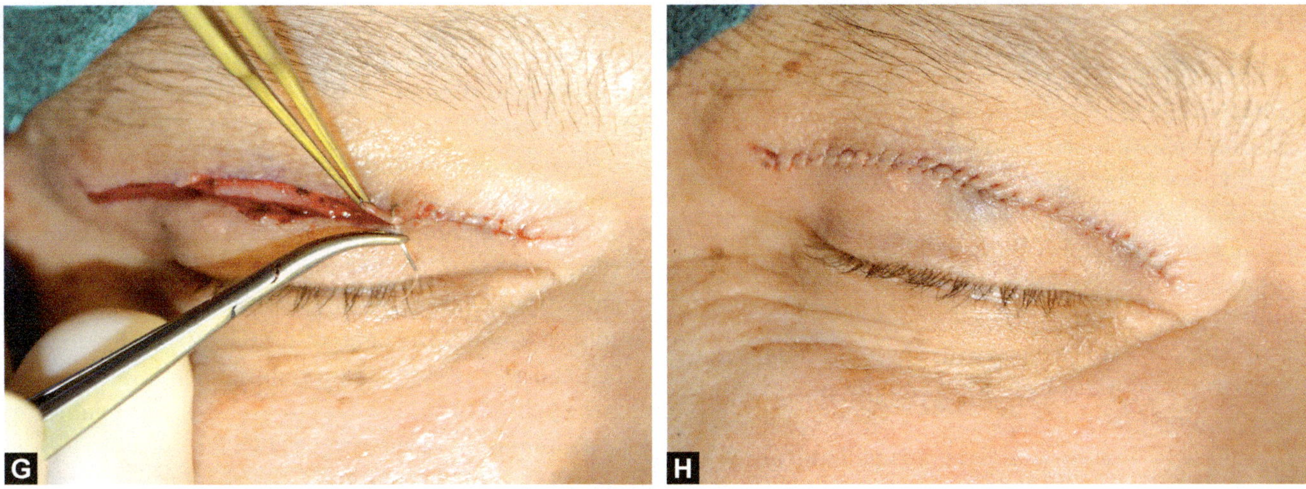

Figs. 102.2G and H

Figs. 102.2A to H: Intraoperative photo series of upper blepharoplasty—(A and B) Marking the crease; (C) Marking redundant skin; (D) Finished upper blepharoplasty marking; (E) Removal of skin; (F) Removal of excess fat pad; (G and H) Skin closure.

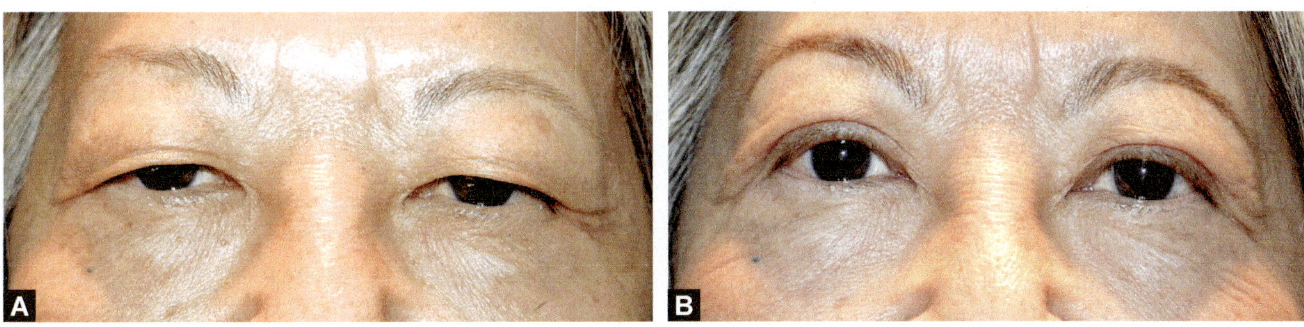

Figs. 102.3A and B: Before/after of Asian upper blepharoplasty.

shortage). Local anesthetic is injected subcutaneously, directed away from the globe.

3. *Removal of skin:* Skin incision can be made with surgical steel (#15 blade), laser, or radio frequency. Using countertraction, the lower mark is incised, followed by the upper marking. Our preference is to remove skin only with orbicularis preservation, using scissors or cutting cautery, to avoid lagophthalmos or thinning of the upper eyelid. Meticulous hemostasis should be achieved.
4. *Consider removal of excess fat pad:* To maintain fullness we typically preserve the preaponeurotic fat pad, which shows greatest loss over time through atrophy. The nasal fat pad, if redundant can be conservatively removed. Excessive deeper dissection should be avoided to preserve the trochlea, situated between the two upper eyelid fat pads, and if the lacrimal gland is prolapsed, it should be reposited and secured.
5. *Orbicularis and skin closure*: 7-0 polygalactin (Vicryl) is used to re-approximate the orbicularis (deep closure), and 6-0 polypropylene (Prolene) or nylon, or 6-0 fast absorbing gut suture is used to close the skin (Nonabsorbable suture should be removed within 5–7 days).

Ethnic Considerations

The Asian eyelid has distinct anatomical features. As such, distinctions in surgical approach should recognize and address these differences.[1,9] Patients with mixed ancestry may not fall into these categories, and choice of surgical approach should be made according to individual anatomic features and not solely the patient's stated ethnicity. In the Asian eyelid, the orbital septum fuses with the levator below the superior tarsal border, resulting in more inferior descent of the preaponeurotic fat pad, and possibly no apparent eyelid crease. Additional consideration inpatients of Asian heritage may include creation of the "double eyelid," or an entirely new crease. Consideration must also be given to the type of crease requested by the patient: nasal taper versus parallel configuration with or without lateral flare (Figs. 102.3A and B).

Extra Considerations for the Asian Patient

1. *Marking the inferior crease:* The most critical difference between Caucasian and Asian upper eyelid blepharoplasty is skin marking. In general, the Asian eyelid crease should be marked no higher than 6 mm above the superior eyelid margin. The crease mark should be tapered nasally to blend imperceptibly into the epicanthal fold. Laterally, the crease should flare superiorly.
2. *Marking for skin removal:* If a younger patient is receiving blepharoplasty for cosmetic purposes, we take minimal skin.
3. *Creation of orbicularis platform:* To facilitate formation of a new crease, a small 1–2 mm ellipsoid segment of pretarsal orbicularis muscle is excised parallel to the upper tarsal border.
4. *Crease formation:* Crease formation is achieved by securing the levator aponeurosis to the orbicularis platform just beneath the inferior skin incision. Three to four 7-0 Vicryl sutures with buried knots are placed, encouraging crease formation.
5. *Skin closure:* Identify areas of skin redundancy and remove dog ears. In general, nonabsorbable sutures are preferred due to increased inflammation in absorbable sutures, seen in Asian patients. Orbicularis is closed using 7-0 Vicryl, followed by skin closure with a running 6-0 polypropylene on a C-1 tapered needle (Tapered needles minimize bleeding during skin closure, which minimizes disruption of the formed crease). Remove nonabsorbable suture 1 week postoperatively.

LOWER EYELID BLEPHAROPLASTY

With age, the smooth transition from lower eyelid to midface is gradually lost with increased visibility of the inferior orbital rim and generation of the double convex deformity. These changes are caused by loss of orbital and cheek fat, and attenuation of the orbitomalar ligament with maxillary retrusion.[1,10] Lower eyelid blepharoplasty by the transconjunctival or transcutaneous approach can address these age-related changes (Table 102.2).[1,11,12]

Additional preoperative evaluation should include any history of fillers to the lower eyelid; the presence of eyelid malpositions (ectropion, entropion, lower eyelid retraction, lagophthalmos); presence of midfacial ptosis; degree of fat prolapse; amount of skin redundancy in lower eyelid; lower eyelid distraction test to assess lower eyelid tone; and examination of the conjunctiva for signs of cicatricial change (Figs. 102.4A and B).

Transconjunctival Lower Eyelid Blepharoplasty with Fat Redraping (Figs. 102.5A to D)

1. *Transconjunctival incision:* A transconjunctival incision is made 3–4 mm below the inferior tarsal border. Blunt preseptal dissection is performed in the avascular plane, directed toward the inferior orbital rim. (If fat redraping is planned, a preperiosteal dissection along the arcusmarginalis is also performed to expose the inferior orbital rim, leaving the periosteum intact.) In younger patients, a small 1–2 mm canthotomy and cantholysis can be performed for additional exposure.
2. *Development of fat pedicles for redraping:* Development of the lower fat pedicles involves identifying and dissecting free the medial and central fat pads (carefully avoiding the inferior oblique traversing between them). The orbital septum is opened over each fat pad, and the fat pedicle is developed with a cotton tip applicator.

Table 102.2: Comparison of the transconjunctival and transcutaneous approaches to lower eyelid blepharoplasty.

Approach	Pros	Cons	Best suited patient/adjunctive procedures
Transconjunctival Lower Blepharoplasty	• No skin incision • No incision of orbicularis (no potential for denervation)	• Smaller incision, poorer exposure (more technically demanding) • Increased risk of conjunctival chemosis and posterior lamellar shortening	• Patient in which the primary concern is lower eyelid fat prolapse with minimal skin redundancy • Patients with maxillary hypoplasia and prominent globes (this patient is at increased risk for lower eyelid retraction with the transcutaneous approach) *Adjunctive procedures:* Laser, chemical resurfacing, *fat redraping, lateral canthoplasty
Transcutaneous Lower Blepharoplasty	Improved exposure	• Skin incision can lead to scar • Orbicularis incision risks denervation	Patient with minimal fat prolapse and prominent eyelid rhytids *Adjunctive procedures*: *Fat redraping, canthoplasty, suborbicularis oculi fat (SOOF) lifting/orbitomalar suspension

*Fat redraping preserves the fullness of a youthful midface and addresses the double convex deformity of the lower eyelid by filling in the tear trough, and is preferred to subtractive lower eyelid blepharoplasty.

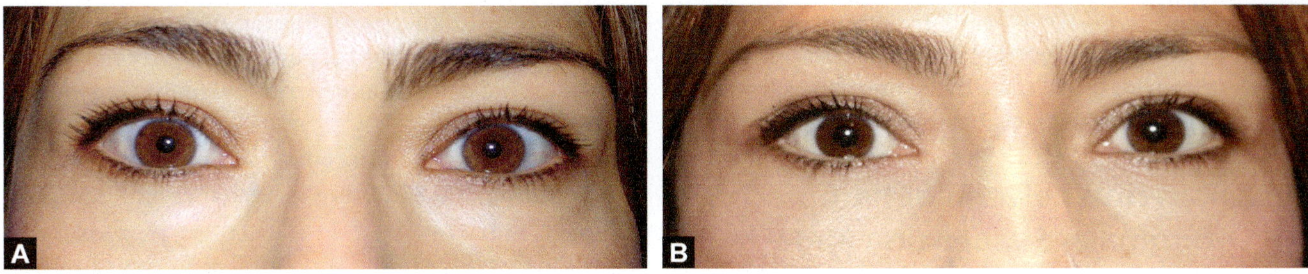

Figs. 102.4A and B: Before/after of lower blepharoplasty.

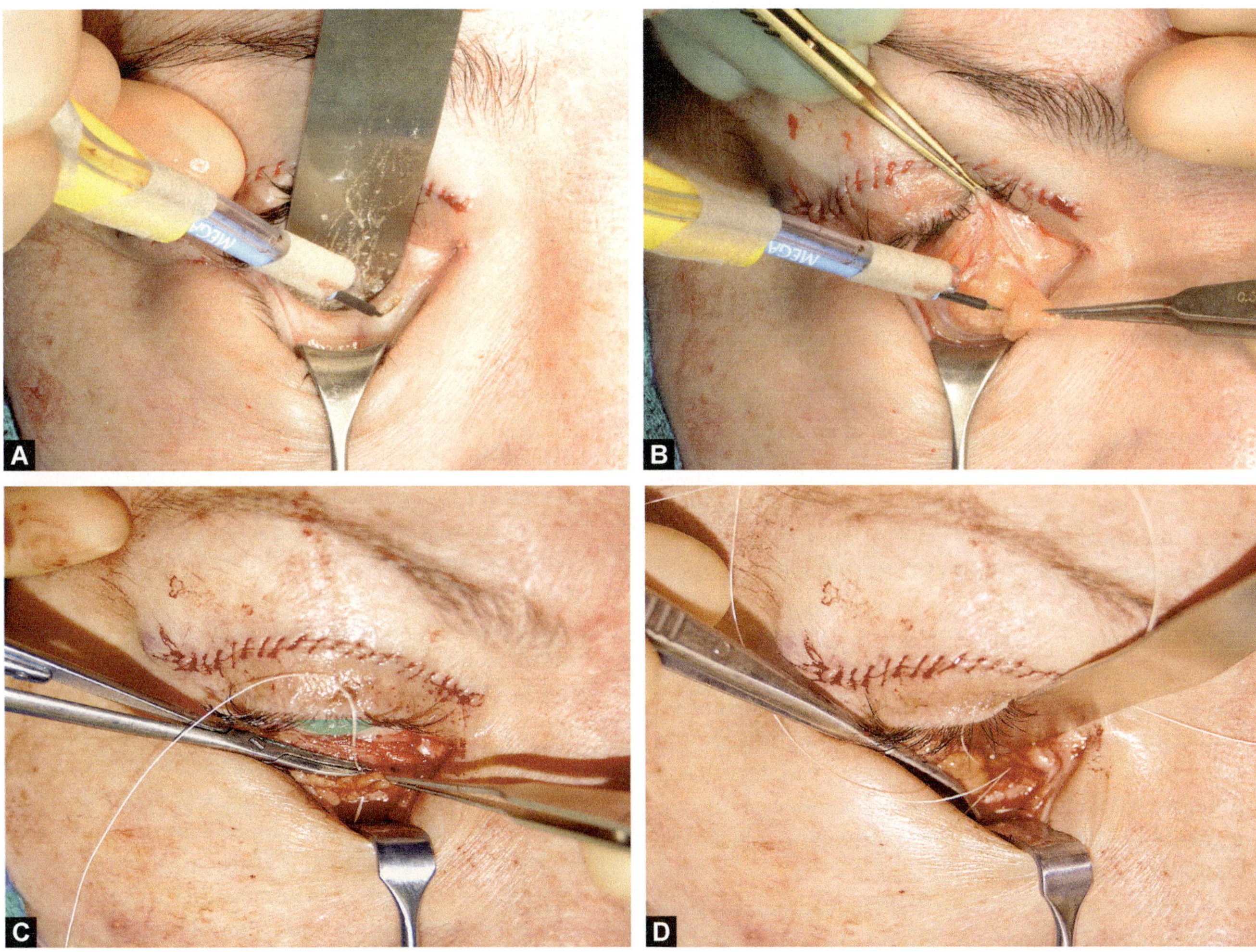

Figs. 102.5A to D: Intraoperative photograph series of the transconjunctival approach to lower blepharoplasty with fat redraping—(A) Transconjunctival incision; (B) Development and shaping of fat pedicles for redraping; (C and D) Fat redraping onto inferior orbital rim.

The nasal fat pedicle can conservatively be excised, and each fat pedicle can then be inferiorly redraped over the inferior orbital rim.

3. *Fat redraping:* Starting with the medial pedicle, moving laterally, the fat pedicles are redraped using a 5-0 Vicryl in a horizontal mattress fashion. The suture is passed through the center of each fat pedicle to avoid ripping through, and fat is re-draped along the inferior orbital rim. Avoid incarceration of the inferior oblique muscle, between the nasal and central fat pads. The lateral fat pad is usually excised judiciously without the need for re-draping. While our preference is for preperiosteal redraping, some surgeons prefer a subperiosteal plane for redraping with externalization of sutures.

4. *Lateral canthoplasty:* If laxity is present, the eyelid can be horizontally shortened and the canthus can be reinserted with 6-0 Vicryl. The skin at the canthus is then closed using 6-0 fast absorbing gut suture.

Transcutaneous Lower Blepharoplasty with Orbitomalar Suspension and Fat Redraping

1. *Incision planning:* An infraciliary mark is made within 0.5 mm of the ciliary line from the punctum to the lateral canthal angle. During anesthetic placement, the skin can be hydrodissected from the orbicularis. The skin incision is made as close to the lash line as possible.
2. *Preseptal dissection*: Sharp dissection is the performed at the level of the pretarsal and preseptal orbicularis extended medially and laterally to the inferior orbital rim. Blunt dissection with a peanut sponge can also be performed with inferior countertraction provided by a Senn retractor until the three lower eyelid fat pads are exposed.
3. *Orbitomalar ligament release:* The orbitomalar ligament, the one of the primary retaining ligament of the midface, is released. A malleable retractor is placed along the inferolateral rim and, using monopolarcautery, attachments of the orbitomalar ligament to the lateral orbital rim are lysed. Blunt dissection with a peanut sponge removes any residual attachments.
4. *Arcus marginalis release:* If fat redraping is to be performed, the arcus marginalis—the dense band of tissue along the orbital rim where the orbital septum originates—must be opened. The dissection should also remain outside the orbital rim to avoid the inferior oblique muscle. Blunt cotton-tip applicators can further expose the inferior orbital rim periosteum, where the orbital fat pedicles will be reposited.
5. *Development of fat pedicles:* The central and nasal fat pads are gently teased from behind the orbital septum. The central fat is more easily accessed while the medial fat pad (paler color) can be developed nasally with gentle pressure. If excessive fat is present, conservative debulking can be performed, however adequate fat pedicles should be preserved for re-draping. Hemostasis should be meticulously obtained.
6. *Re-draping of fat pedicles:* 5-0 Vicryl suture is used to secure the fat pedicles along the inferior orbital rim periosteum in a horizontal mattress fashion, starting with the nasal fat pedicle, and ending with the lateral pedicle. The inferior oblique muscle is meticulously avoided. The lateral fat pad is generally not excised, and is re-draped to address lateral fullness of the lower eyelid.
7. *Inspection of the lower eyelid fat pedicles:* Once fat redraping and sculpting has been completed, a final inspection is necessary to assess smoothness of contour when skin is overlaid. Ensure that inferior oblique is not inadvertently tethered, and identify any fullness or hollowness that may require further fat sculpting.
8. *SOOF Fixation:* SOOF elevation in conjunction with fat redraping helps to eliminate the double convex deformity. After release of the orbitomalar ligament (Step 4), the SOOF can be visualized. Toothed Adson forceps are used to elevate and secure the SOOF to evaluate the contour of the cheek. After the optimal fixation point of the SOOF is located, a 4-0 Vicryl suture secures the SOOF tissue within the midface. This should be adjusted if significant bunching or dimpling is seen.
9. *Orbitomalar suspension:* To achieve midfacial elevation, the SOOF suture is elevated superolaterally, and a small, curved hemostat is used to bluntly tunnel a pocket from the upper eyelid crease incision for SOOF suture retrieval. After retrieval through the tunnel, the suture is secured to the periosteum overlying the frontozygomatic suture line with a bite perpendicular to the lateral orbital rim to minimize "cheese-wiring" of the suture through the periosteum.
10. *Lower eyelid tightening:* If lower eyelid laxity is present, adjunct eyelid tightening should be performed and the canthus is reinserted.
11. *Skin removal and closure:* A small amount of excess skin may be present and can be conservatively excised. To address this, a triangular flap of excess skin with a small degree of redundant orbicularis can be marked and excised, and a small strip of skin (at most 2–3 mm) along the infraciliary edge, moving toward the punctum, can also be excised with it. Care should be taken medially to avoid punctal injury or punctalectropion. Skin closure with 6-0 fast absorbing gut suture is performed, lateral to nasal. Closure in this manner will minimize formation of dog ears.

EYELID PTOSIS REPAIR

Eyelid ptosis occurs when the eyelid migrates inferiorly, encroaching upon the visual axis, and obscuring vision. It is most commonly acquired through involutional changes or aponeurotic dehiscence. However, it is can

Table 102.3: Comparison of external and internal levator advancement for eyelid ptosis repair.

Approach	Pros	Cons	Best suited patient
External levator advancement (ELA)	• Effective for more severe ptosis • Early revision can be done in office • Can be used in event of unsatisfactory ILA	• Requires patient cooperation intraoperatively for symmetry • Cutaneous incision	• Patients with normal levator function and severe ptosis (MRD1 < 1.5 mm) • Patients with glaucoma filtration surgery, strabismus surgery, or cicatricial conjunctival disease with need to avoid conjunctiva incision
Internal levator advancement (ILA)/conjunctival Müller's muscle resection (CMMR)	• Conjunctival approach (no skin incision) • Tarsus is preserved • Favored in cosmetic patients for predictable outcomes and aesthetically pleasing contour • Does not require patient cooperation during surgery	• Less effective for more severe ptosis • Typically wait 3 months before revision	• Ptosis < 3 mm • Ptosis that develops after cataract surgery or contact lens related ptosis responds well to ILA • Patients with a positive response to phenylephrine test (The patient is given 2.5% phenylephrine on ptotic side. If the eyelid elevated sufficiently, patient likely a good candidate)

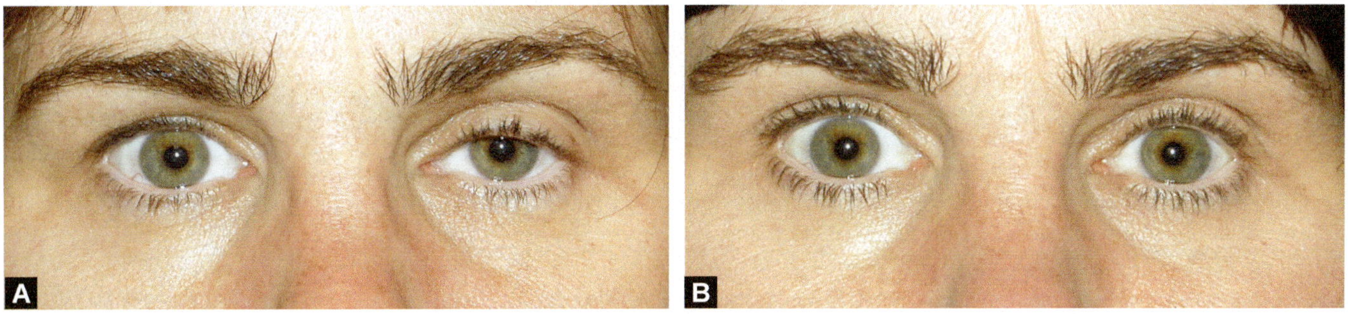

Figs. 102.6A and B: Before/after of ptosis repair.

also be caused by trauma, Horner's syndrome (neurogenic ptosis), myasthenia gravis or chronic progressive external ophthalmoplegia (myogenic ptosis), or mechanical ptosis secondary to a mass.[13]

The presence of ptosis can be determined through measurement of the marginal reflex distance (MRD1 and MRD2), the distance from the central corneal light reflex to the margin of the upper and lower eyelids, respectively. Note that the upper eyelid margin peaks nasally, while the lower eyelid margin's lowest point is lateral to the mid pupil in a normal eye. Sometimes, a patient may appear to have unilateral ptosis, when bilateral asymmetrical ptosis present. Assessing the presence of a Hering'slaw will help to clarify this, as outcomes are dependent on repairing both eyelids in bilateral ptosis.[1,14] We utilize two main surgical approaches for ptosis: external levator advancement (ELA) and conjunctival Müller's muscle resection (CMMR) (Table 102.3).[1,15]

Additional preoperative evaluation should emphasize: measurement of upper eyelid crease position (severe ptosis can result in a superiorly migrated crease) and presence of co-existent dermatochalasis; amount of levator function (normal levator function is at least 12 mm); MRD1 and MRD2; associated ocular surface issues, such as strabismus, glaucoma filtration surgery/drainage device, cicatricial conjunctival diseases, fornix shortening. Patients being considered for CMMR should have topical 2.5% phenylephrine testing, looking for elevation of the ptotic eyelid. To test for the presence of Hering's law the ptotic eyelid is manually elevated while examining the contralateral eyelid. If the contralateral eyelid falls, then asymmetric bilateral ptosis is present. Failure to treat a contralateral ptotic eyelid with a positive Hering's response can lead to unpredictable results, and all patients should be advised of the potential for revision (Figs. 102.6A and B).

Ptosis Repair by External Levator Advancement with or without Concurrent Blepharoplasty (Figs. 102.7A to K)

1. *Skin marking:* Levator surgery is performed under local anesthetic and minimal IV sedation to ensure maximal levator effort and patient cooperation in surgery. Infiltration of anesthetic is minimized (1.0–1.5 cc) to avoid diminishing levator function. If skin

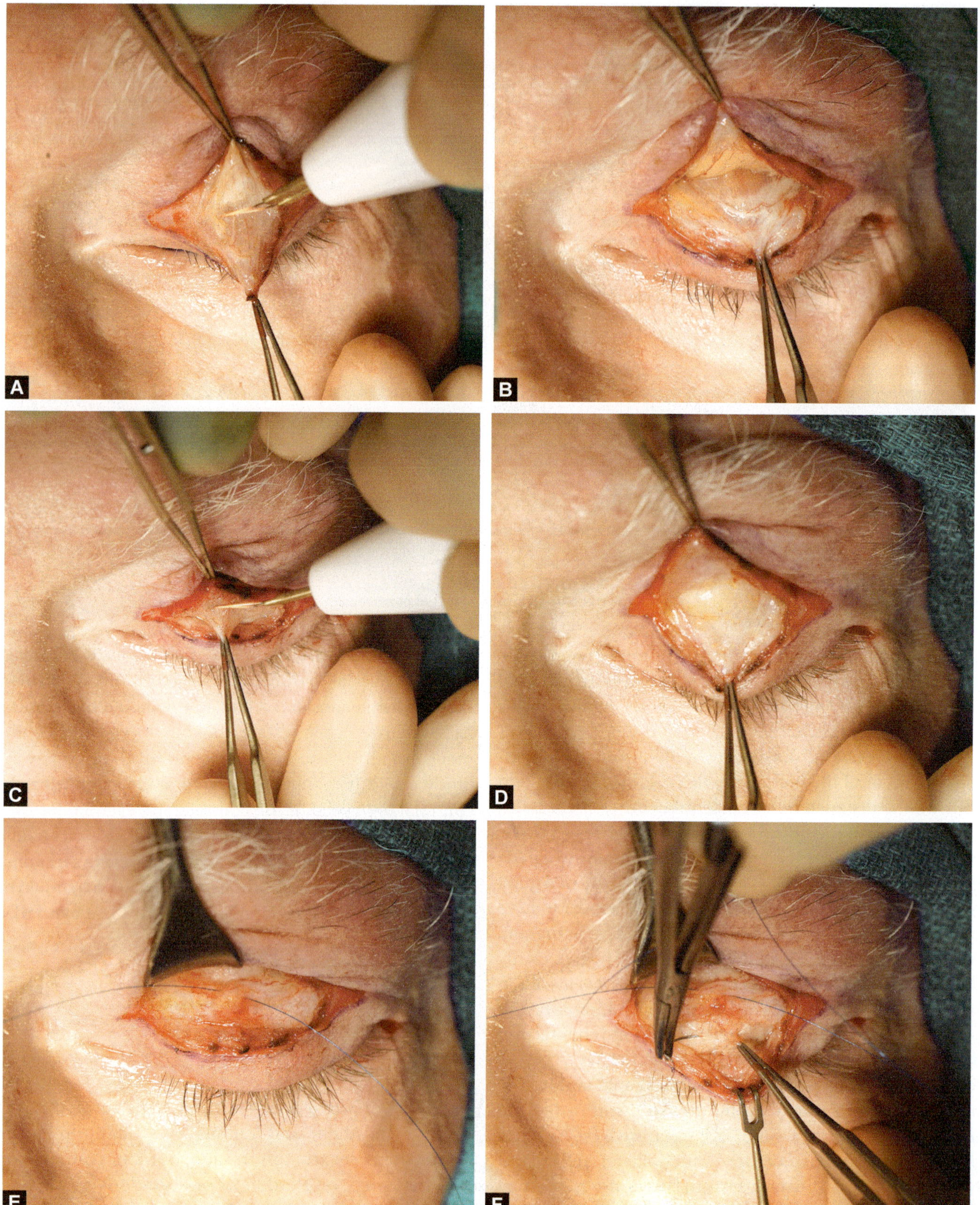

Figs. 102.7A to F

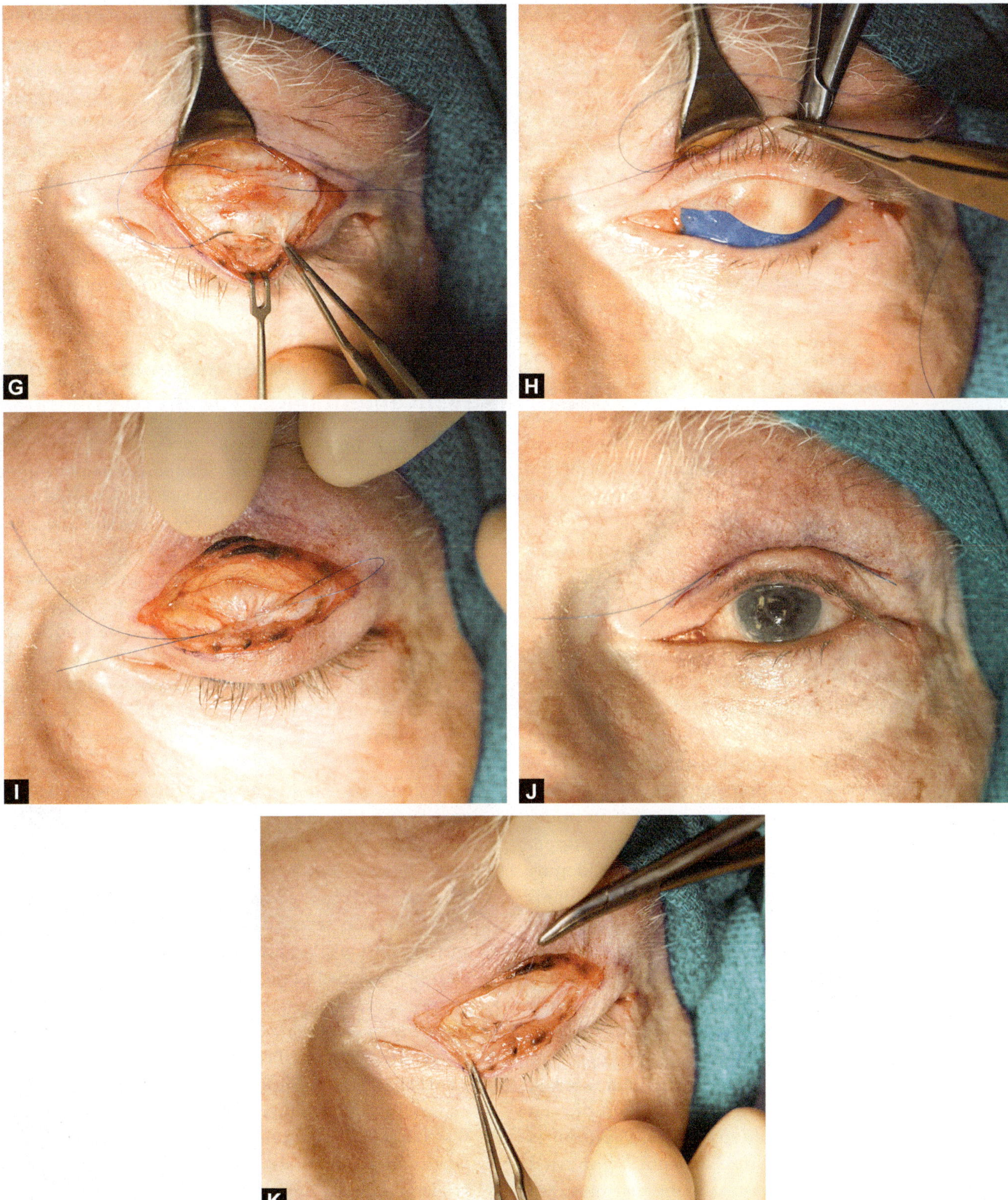

Figs. 102.7G to K

Figs. 102.7A to K: Intraoperative photograph series of ptosis repair by external levator advancement—(A) Dissection through the orbital septum; (B) Identification of the levator aponeurosis; (C and D) Creation of a pretarsal pocket; (E to G) Advancement of levator onto inferior tarsal border; (H) Checking for partial thickness bite; (I) Placement of temporary advancement suture; (J) Intraoperative eyelid assessment with patient cooperation; (K) Placement of permanent suture, and eyelid crease fixation.

removal is indicated, the upper eyelid crease is marked as described above for upper eyelid blepharoplasty. If blepharoplasty is not indicated, the marking is limited to the central third of the eyelid.

2. *Dissection through orbital septum:* After skin incision, the orbicularis is then incised, demonstrating the white, fibrous orbital septum underneath. The septum is opened centrally using cutting cautery or sharp dissection with meticulous hemostasis to avoid disrupting maximal levator effort.
3. *Identification of the levator aponeurosis:* The yellow preaponeurotic fat pad is typically the first structure visualized upon septum entry. Immediately posterior is the levator muscle and aponeurosis, which is white and avascular. If a true disinsertion is present, the aponeurosis is retracted superiorly, and the first structure to be visualized is the Müller's muscle and tightly adherent palpebral conjunctiva. The peripheral vascular arcade overlies the Müller's muscle, and should be preserved.
4. *Creation of pretarsal pocket:* A plane is then created between the tarsal plate and the overlying orbicularis for the upper third of the tarsus. Inadvertent trauma to the tarsus should be avoided, as it serves as the point of attachment for the levator aponeurosis. Careful dissection of the epitarsal tissues will facilitate suture passage. Excessive cautery on the tarsus can cause charring or discomfort to the patient, and is not preferred.
5. *Advancement of levator:* The levator aponeurosis is then advance with 6-0 polypropylene suture. A 4–5 mm of advancement is typically a good starting point. While providing gentle superior traction on the upper tarsal border, the eyelid contour is checked to identify a suitable location for suture placement. The suture is then passed horizontally in a lamellar fashion partial thickness through the upper third of the tarsal plate. The upper palpebral conjunctiva should be inspected to confirm a partial thickness. The suture is then brought back through the inferior portion of the levator and tied with a temporary knot.
6. *Intraoperative eyelid assessment:* The patient is asked to open the eyes, and the height and contour of each eye are compared for symmetry. If good contour is obtained with the central suture, the knot is converted to a permanent knot and no further sutures are placed. If the eyelid is too peaked, additional medial and lateral advancement sutures may also be placed until the desired contour is achieved. If the patient is too sedated, they can be sat upright to assist with adjustment. In general, the intraoperative level should be overcorrected by 1–1.5 mm to account for resumed orbicularis function.
7. *Eyelid crease fixation:* To restore the native eyelid crease, a 7-0 Vicryl suture can be used to attach the inferior cut edge of the pretarsal orbicularis is to the levator aponeurosis slightly higher than the fixation point of the levator advancement. Several fixation sutures can be placed evenly along the length of the inferior incision.
8. *Skin closure:* The skin incision is closed using either a running 6-0 polypropylene suture (and removed 1 week postoperatively) or a 6-0 fast-absorbing gut suture.

Ptosis Repair by Internal Levator Advancement (Figs. 102.8A to E)

1. *Exposure of the palpebral conjunctiva:* Local anesthetic should be administered subcutaneously over the upper eyelid near the superior tarsal border. A frontal nerve block can also be given which reduces the anesthetic volume. The upper eyelid is everted with a Desmarres retractor carefully exposing the palpebral conjunctiva.
2. *Marking of the conjunctiva:* Once the desired amount of Müller's muscle to be resection is determined, this amount is divided in half. A caliper is then used to mark this distance from the superior tarsal border centrally, laterally and medially. If an 8 mm correction is desired, then a 4 mm marking is made superior to the tarsal border.
3. *Traction suture placement:* A 6-0 silk suture is used to provide traction on the conjunctiva and Müller's muscle to elevate the tissue away from the superior tarsal border to assist with clamp placement.
4. *Placement of ptosis clamp:* A Müller's muscle resection clamp is then secured on the conjunctival/Müller's muscle flap, paying attention to not incorporate any part of the tarsal plate. The traction sutures are then removed.
5. *Suturing of conjunctiva and Müller's muscle:* Starting from the skin surface, a 6-0 polypropylene is internalized to the superior fornix medially above the clamp. The suture is then woven back and forth beneath the clamp in a horizontal fashion from medial to lateral. Once complete, the suture exits high in the fornix, and is secured on the upper eyelid skin.
6. *Excision of conjunctival Müller's muscle flap:* A #15 blade is then used to excise the excess tissue while exerting upward pressure on the ptosis clamp to minimize inadvertent cutting of the suture.

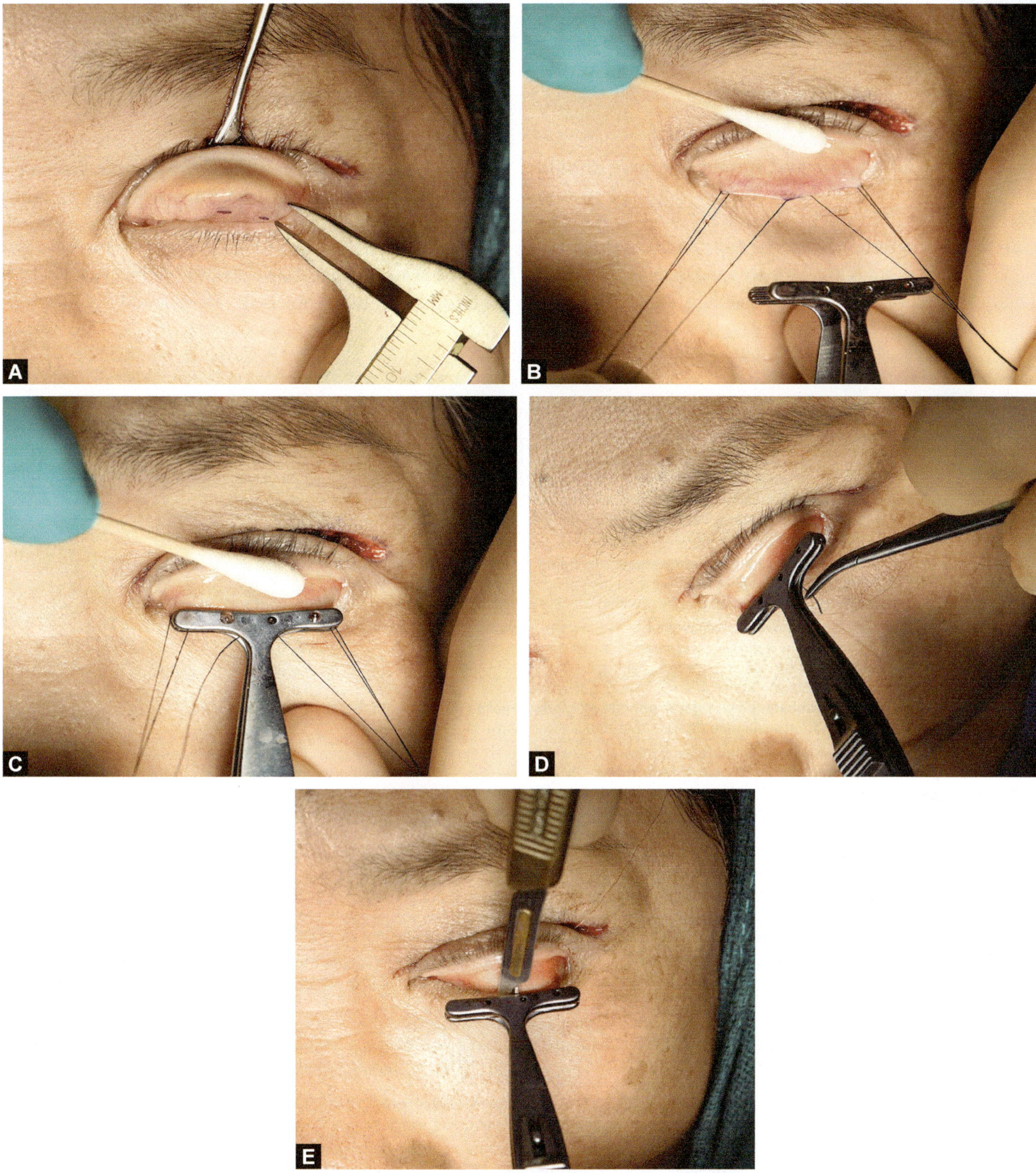

Figs. 102.8A to E: Intraoperative photo series of ptosis repair by internal levator advancement—(A) Exposure and marking of the conjunctiva; (B) Traction suture placement; (C) Placement of ptosis clamp; (D) Suturing of conjunctiva and Müller's muscle; (E) Excision of conjunctival Müller's muscle flap.

7. *Securing suture:* The suture is externalized to the upper eyelid and tied with minimal tension upon itself. The suture is removed at 1 week.

POSTOPERATIVE CARE

A combination antibiotic and steroid ointment should be applied twice daily over the incisions 2 weeks postoperatively. Ice packs should be used frequently at 20–30 minute intervals for the first 3 days to decrease swelling.[16] Patients may also be instructed to sleep with head of bed elevated to 30° to reduce swelling. Nonabsorbable sutures can be removed at 1 week postoperatively. Final postoperative results occur at 3–6 months.

COMPLICATIONS

As with any surgery, complications may occur despite careful planning.[13,17] Common complications, treatment and ways to minimize complications are listed in Tables 102.4 to 102.9. Although these procedures are routinely well tolerated, safe, and effective, untoward results may sometimes occur and these should be discussed during the informed consent process.

Table 102.4: General complications.

Complication	Suggestions to reduce risk/treatments
Asymmetry	• Careful preoperative assessment of co-existing ptosis, eyelid malpositions or globe prominence. • Careful measurement after skin marking; "measure twice, cut once" • Consider revision surgery at least 3 months postoperatively, or hyaluronic acid (HA) filler placement • Maximize patient cooperation in procedures that require it • Meticulous hemostasis intraoperatively
Corneal abrasion	• Use corneal shields, lubricating ointment, and/or lid plate during surgery • If CO_2 laser or radiofrequency ablation is being used, placement of a metallic corneal shield is warranted • Treat postoperatively by an eye-care specialist to prevent development of ulcer. • Most mechanical abrasions heal within quickly with proper monitoring and removal of any offending agent
Dry eyes/ lagophthalmos	• Minimize removal and dissection of orbicularis muscle • Minimize skin removal to retain at least 20 mm • Minimize chemical or laser resurfacing • Early temporary lagophthalmos can occur immediately postoperatively from swelling or anesthesia; reassure • Ocular lubricant; placement of punctal plug; tape eyelids shut at night, nightly topical ointment • Grafting from a suitable donor site to the anterior lamella
Postoperative hemorrhage	• Meticulous hemostasis intraoperatively, use of tapered needle for skin closure, ice packs postoperatively, and cessation of anticoagulants all help to reduce risk • Preseptal hematoma can be managed conservatively with ice, rest, elevation of the head of the bed • Retrobulbar hemorrhage may cause orbital compartment syndrome—educate patients on the warning signs and seek emergent attention • Treat retrobulbar hemorrhage by reopening the blepharoplasty incision; if inadequate, emergent lateral canthotomy and cantholysis are performed
Postoperative infection	• Uncommon; perform procedure under sterile preparation; be cognizant of immunosuppressed states; high suspicion for MRSA in nonresolving infection. • In a patient with proptosis, pain, decreased vision, and extraocular motility dysfunctions, consider orbital cellulitis
Postoperative diplopia	Differentiate monocular or binocular: Monocular—likely ocular surface changes from ointment, dry eye or refractive changes. Binocular—may be from trochlear injury or superior oblique (Brown's syndrome); inferior oblique injury can also cause diplopia
Postoperative blepharoptosis	• Assess preoperatively and consider treating concurrently • A risk in any surgery involving use of an eyelid speculum • Patient may have a pre-existing subclinical ptosis that increases risk of postoperative ptosis • Prevent surgical dissection induced levator injury by being aware of anatomy, located inferior and posterior to preaponeurotic fat pad, and avoiding excessive pretarsal dissection • Avoid excessive downward traction on the upper eyelid during surgery
Suture granuloma	• Use of removable nonabsorbable sutures (polypropylene or nylon) can significantly reduce risk. • Physician should have high index of suspicion for atypical mycobacterial infections that can present as delayed hyperemic nodules along incision lines and extension beyond the wound. • Recognize granulomas early if symptomatic and remove by excising in office and closure by secondary intent; give antibiotic/steroid ointment; culture if suspicious of atypical mycobacterial infection
Wound dehiscence	• Avoid eye rubbing heavy lifting; ice packs minimize hemorrhage and itching; protective eye shields; avoid use of contact lenses; use protective eye shields while sleeping • Smaller dehiscence may be observed • Requires repair if large or prolapsed deep tissues

Table 102.5: Additional complications of upper eyelid blepharoplasty.

Complication	Suggestions to reduce risk/treatments
Lacrimal gland injury	• Avoid lacrimal gland within redundant preaponeurotic fat; it is paler, located lateral to fat, and has greater sensory innervation (patient may feel pain if incised) • If prolapsed, the gland can be reposited along the periosteum
Canthal webbing	• Prevent by tapering the lateral and nasal incision markings superiorly, avoid extending the nasal marking medially to the punctum • Can be revised with Z-plasty
Superior sulcus deformity	• Preserve preaponeurotic fat pad and only addressing redundancy of nasal fat pad • Minimize damage to levator palpebrae muscle

Table 102.6: Additional complications of Asian upper eyelid blepharoplasty.

Complication	Suggestions to reduce risk/treatments
Unexpected formation of a high semilunar crease or hollow superior sulcus	• Keep superior marking flat and inferior marking low; avoid lateral and medial tapering; minimize removal of central fat • Consider revision or placement of HA filler
Multiple creases	• Careful marking, avoid excessive pretarsal dissection to preserve the central fat pad • HA filler to volumize areas of multiple creases
Loss of crease	• Careful creation of a pretarsal platform and meticulous crease fixation placement.
Medial – bifid crease	• Avoid superior tapering of the nasal marking and blend nasally to epicanthal fold.

Table 102.7: Additional complications of transconjunctival lower lid blepharoplasty with fat redraping.

Complication	Suggestions to reduce risk/treatments
Lower eyelid hollowing	Minimize fat removal; redrape fat instead of subtractive blepharoplasty; consider adjunctive HA filler
Conjunctival chemosis	• Minimize conjunctival trauma intraoperatively • Topical steroids postoperatively; reassurance • Needling of conjunctiva, placement of temporary tarsorrhaphy or thermal conjunctival tightening
Hardening/ nodule formation along inferior orbital rim	• Oral antibiotics (consider MRSA coverage) • Consider steroid injection along inferior orbital rim to address possible suture granuloma • Consider short PO steroid course

MRSA: Methicillin-resistant *Staphylococcus aureus*

Table 102.8: Additional complications of transcutaneous lower blepharoplasty with SOOF lift.

Complication	Suggestions to reduce risk/treatments
Lower eyelid retraction	Minimize fat removal, skin removal, cauterization to middle lamella; trauma/removal of pretarsal orbicularis; tighten lower lid
Lower eyelid ectropion	• Minimize skin removal • Upward massage of lower eyelid; consider steroid injection to pretarsal orbicularis
Punctal ectropion	• Minimize skin removal medially • Upwards massage of the eyelid; consider medial spindle procedure or full-thickness skin graft placement

SOOF: Suborbicularis oculi fat

Table 102.9: Additional complications of ptosis repair (ELA and ILA).

Complication	Suggestions to reduce risk/treatments
Contour deformity/ peaking	• Add additional advancement sutures medially and laterally, lengthen bite of the tarsal pass, tighten eyelid if laxity is present • Shift peak of excision nasally if excessive lateral tarsal distraction present
Overcorrection of eyelid	• Wait 3 months after surgery to re-evaluate; watch for contralateral ptosis and reflex upper eyelid retraction from Hering's law; if truly overcorrected, consider upper eyelid retractor recession
Increased dermatochalasis	• Counsel patients preoperatively of the potential for increased dermatochalasis if ptosis repair is performed in isolation; address with concurrent blepharoplasty if indicated
Under correction	• Common in first 1–2 weeks postoperatively from tissue edema—reassurance • If significantly under corrected occurs with ELA, consider early office adjustment if edema largely resolved; wait 3 months to reassess ILA; if ILA failed, consider performing ELA
Eyelid crease/ fold differences	• Placement crease fixation sutures, advance preaponeurotic fat to superior tarsus, or inject HA fillers
Conjunctival prolapse	• Avoid excessive levator dissection and resection superiorly. • Perform fornix repair if noted at the end of the case
Upper eyelid ectropion	• Replace advancement suture to a more superior position on the tarsal plate

(ELA: External levator advancement; ILA: Internal levator advancement)

SUMMARY

Multiple benefits are derived from improving the "droopy eyelid." In addition to functional benefits, patients often experience a feeling of youthful rejuvenation, and enhanced psychosocial morale. As the population ages, increasing need and demand for procedures to address the "droopy eyelid" necessitate familiarity with the breadth of rejuvenative options.

REFERENCES

1. Korn BS, Kikkawa DO. Video Atlas of Oculofacial Plastic and Reconstructive Surgery, 2nd edition. St. Louis: Elsevier Health Sciences; 2017.
2. Damasceno RW, Avgitidou G, Belfort R Jr, et al. Eyelid aging: pathophysiology and clinical management. Arq Bras Oftalmol. 2015;78:328-31.
3. Branham G, Holds JB. Brow/Upper lid anatomy, aging and aesthetic analysis. Facial Plast Surg Clin North Am. 2015;23:117-27.
4. Ko AC, Korn BS, Kikkawa DO. The aging face. Surv Ophthalmol. 2017;62:190-202.

5. Nakra T, Modjtahedi S, Vrcek I, et al. The effect of upper eyelid blepharoplasty on eyelid and brow position. Orbit. 2016;35:324-7.
6. Lee JW, Cho BC, Lee KY. Direct brow lift combined with suspension of the orbicularis oculi muscle. Arch Plast Surg. 2013;40:603-9.
7. Hahn S, Holds JB, Couch SM. Upper Lid Blepharoplasty. Facial Plast Surg Clin North Am. 2016;24:119-27.
8. An SH, Jin SW, Kwon YH, et al. Effects of upper lid blepharoplasty on visual quality in patients with lash ptosis and dermatochalasis. Int J Ophthalmol. 2016;9:1320-4.
9. Lee CK, Ahn ST, Kim N. Asian upper lid blepharoplasty surgery. Clin Plast Surg. 2013;40:167-78.
10. Baker S, LaFerriere K, Larrabee WFJ. Lower lid blepharoplasty: panel discussion, controversies, and techniques. Facial Plast Surg Clin North Am. 2014;22:97-118.
11. Davison SP, Irio M, Oh C. Transconjunctival lower lid blepharoplasty with and without fat repositioning. Clin Plast Surg. 2015;42:51-6.
12. Pepper JP, Baker SR. Transcutaneous lower blepharoplasty with fat transposition. Clin. Plast Surg. 2015;42:57-62.
13. Yang P, Ko AC, Kikkawa DO, et al. Upper eyelid blepharoplasty: evaluation, treatment, and complication minimization. Semin Plast Surg. 2017;31:51-7.
14. Nemet AY. The effect of Hering's law on different ptosis repair methods. Aesthetic Surg J. 2015;35:774-81.
15. Carruth BP, Meyer DR. Simplified Muller's muscle-conjunctival resection internal ptosis repair. Ophthal Plast Reconstr Surg. 2013;29:11-4.
16. Pool SMW, van Exsel DCE, Melenhorst WBW, et al. The effect of eyelid cooling on pain, edema, erythema, and hematoma after upper blepharoplasty: a randomized, controlled, observer-blinded evaluation study. Plast Reconstr Surg. 2015;135:277e-81e.
17. Godfrey KJ, Korn BS, Kikkawa DO. Blepharoptosis following ocular surgery: identifying risk factors. Curr Opin Ophthalmol. 2016;27:31-7.

Chapter 103 Eyelid Malposition

Monica Ertel, Gary J Lelli

INTRODUCTION

The eyelids are important for ocular health. They act as a barrier to protect the eyes from foreign bodies, play an integral role in proper maintenance of the tear film, are key for light regulation to the eye, and are important for facial expression. In order for the eyelids to serve their function, they must be properly positioned against the globe and the upper and lower eyelid should approximate with each blink. Disorders that result in malposition of the eyelids must be addressed to ensure ocular health. The eyelid consists of seven layers from superficial to deep: (1) skin and subcutaneous connective tissue, (2) muscles of protraction, (3) septum, (4) orbital fat, (5) muscles of retraction, (6) tarsus, and (7) conjunctiva (Figs. 103.1A and B). A thorough description of the eyelid anatomy can be found in Chapter 1. This chapter will focus on the relevant anatomy for proper eyelid positioning and diagnostic/treatment options for eyelid malposition (entropion, ectropion, eyelid retraction, floppy eyelid syndrome and eyelid imbrication).

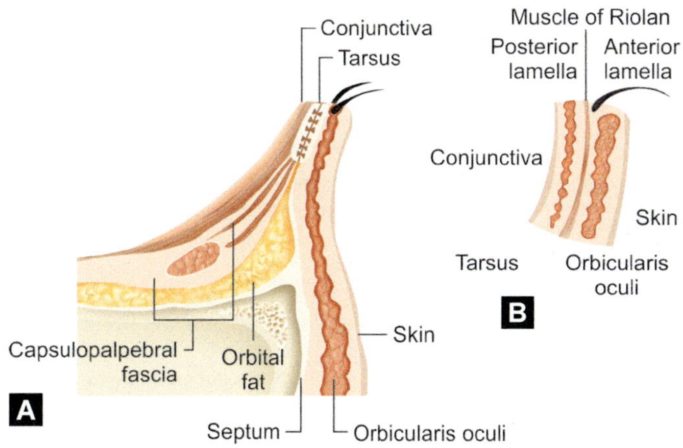

Figs. 103.1A and B: Eyelid anatomy. (A) The eyelid consists of seven layers, including: (1) the skin, (2) the orbicularis oculi, (3) the septum, (4) the orbital fat, (5) the retractors, (6) the tarsus, and (7) the conjunctiva; (B) The anatomy of the eyelid margin can be divided into the anterior lamella, which consists of the skin and orbicularis oculi muscle, and the posterior lamella, which consists of the tarsus and conjunctiva. The muscle of Riolan, which is a specialized portion of the pretarsal orbicularis oculi provides an anatomical division between the anterior and posterior lamella.

AGE-RELATED CHANGES IN NORMAL ANATOMY

There are several age-related changes that occur in the eyelid anatomy which predispose older patients to eyelid malposition syndromes. These changes are due to the effects of gravity, loss of muscle tone and the compounding effects of repetitive use. These changes affect all layers of the eyelid. In the skin, there is increased laxity from constant blinking. The orbital septum thins with aging, allowing the orbital fat to prolapse into the lower and upper eyelid that can result in eyelid malposition. There is stretching and lengthening of the tarsal strips, resulting in horizontal displacement of the tarsal strips with aging. Age-related changes to the muscles of the eyelids include attenuation, weakening and/or dehiscence of the retractor and protractor muscles which are responsible for maintaining the interpalpebral fissure and keeping the eyelids properly opposed to the globe.

EYELID MALPOSITION CATEGORIES

There are three primary types of eyelid malposition. The most commonly encountered eyelid malposition is blepharoptosis, which is an inferior displacement of the upper eyelid. Blepharoptosis is a broad topic with many underlying etiologies and several surgical approaches to its management. Chapter 2 focuses on this topic in depth.

Other eyelid malposition disorders include eyelid entropion and ectropion. Entropion refers to inward rotation of the eyelid and can be either congenital or acquired affecting either the upper or lower eyelid (Table 103.1). Ectropion refers to an outward rotation of the eyelid which can affect either the upper or lower eyelid and can be congenital or acquired in etiology (Table 103.2).

Eyelid retraction, floppy eyelid syndrome and eyelid imbrication syndrome are other eyelid malposition syndromes affecting the eyelid margin.

Table 103.1: Entropion.

		Cause	Treatment
Congenital	Congenital entropion	• Hypertrophy of the eyelid skin or orbicularis • Dysgenesis of the lower eyelid retractors • Structural defects in tarsal plate	Surgical correction
	Epiblepharon	Pretarsal orbicularis and skin override the eyelid margin	• Observation • Surgical correction, if corneal damage
Acquired	Involutional entropion	• Increased horizontal lid laxity from canthal tendon lengthening • Disinsertion, weakening of the lower eyelid retractors • Pretarsal orbicularis oculi overiding the retractors	Retractor reinsertion procedure +/– lateral tarsal strip
	Cicatricial entropion	Scarring resulting in shortening of the posterior lamella that produces an inward rotation of the eyelid margin	• *Mild:* Tarsotomy, tarsal fracture • *Moderate to severe:* Excision of scar tissue, mucous membrane grafts
	Marginal entropion	Anterior advancement of the mucocutaneous junction, rounding of the posterior aspect of the eyelid margin, scarring of the lid margin	Tarsotomy
	Spastic entropion	Intermittent, orbicularis overpowers retractors resulting in inward rotation of lid margin	• Treat ocular irritation • Quickert sutures

Table 103.2: Ectropion.

		Cause	Treatment
Congenital	Congenital ectropion	Congenital anomaly resulting in vertical insufficiency of the anterior lamella	• Observation • Skin graft to lengthen the anterior lamella +/– lateral tarsal strip
	Congenital eversion of the eyelids	Bilateral, symmetric; anterior lamella irritation resulting in lid eversion	• Lubrication and observation • Tarsorrhaphy
	Euryblepharon	Vertical shortening of the eyelid with horizontal eyelid lengthening and inferior displacement of the lateral tarsal tendon insertion	• Lateral canthal tendon reposition • +/– lateral tarsal strip • +/– skin graft
Acquired	Involutional ectropion	Horizontal eyelid laxity resulting in lengthening of the medial or lateral canthal tendon	• Lateral tarsal strip • Pentagonal wedge resection • Medial spindle procedure for medial entropion
	Cicatricial ectropion	Scarring of the anterior lamella resulting in shortening of the anterior lamella	• Release of tension on the anterior lamella • Lateral tarsal strip • Skin graft for anterior lamellar lengthening
	Paralytic ectropion	Loss of orbicularis oculi tone secondary to damage to the facial nerve	• Lubrication • Tarsorrhaphy • Lateral tarsal strip
	Mechanical ectropion	Outward eversion of the eyelid secondary to bulky tumors or mechanical effects of glasses	Removal of mechanical force causing lid eversion

EVALUATION OF THE PATIENT WITH EYELID MALPOSITION DISORDERS

When patients present to the clinic with concerns for eyelid malposition, it is important to start by assessing the health and integrity of the globe. All patients should have a complete examination of afferent and efferent visual function. A slit-lamp examination should be performed to evaluate the cornea. Focus should then be directed to the eyelid margin to assess for malposition.

If the eyelid margin is inverted, then gentle force should be applied with a fingertip to return it to its normal position. It should be noted if there is difficult returning the eyelid to the normal position or if the eyelid does not stay in this position after it is released. If there is laxity of the eyelid margin and the eyelid remains in its normal position for a short period of time after eversion, there are likely involutional changes to the lid. If the patient reports intermittent irritation and there is no evidence of eyelid inversion on examination, the patient should be asked to squeeze their eyelids to assess for spastic entropion.

If the eyelid margin is everted, the structure and laxity of the eyelids should also be assessed as well as tone of the muscles in the eyelid. The distraction tests should be performed by measuring the ability to pull the eyelid away from the globe. The test is positive if the eyelid can be pulled more than 6 mm from the globe. The snap back test should also be performed by applying inferior force on the lower eyelid and then releasing the lid. A lid without laxity will return to its normal position immediately after releasing the lid. A lid with laxity will require multiple blinks before the lid margin returns to its normal position. Another useful maneuver in assessing lower lid ectropion is to apply lateral force to the lateral aspect of the lid margin to assess for potential improvement with lateral canthal tendon tightening and elevation.

Eyelids should be assessed for excessive laxity which is a feature of floppy eyelid syndrome. Additionally, the margin reflex distance 1 (the distance from the pupillary light reflex to the upper eyelid margin) and the margin reflex distance 2 (the distance from the pupillary light reflex to the lower eyelid margin) should be measured to assess for upper and lower eyelid retraction. The proper position of the lower eyelid is at the inferior aspect of the limbus. Inferior displacement of the lower eyelid and the presence of inferior scleral show should be evaluated as these are signs of lower eyelid retraction.

ENTROPION

Entropion is an inward rotation, displacement or inversion of the eyelid (Table 103.1). Entropion changes occur most commonly in the lower eyelid. Entropion can result in misdirection of the eyelashes towards the globe, resulting in damage to the corneal surface. Eyelid misdirection can also disrupt the normal tear lake and can lead to epiphora and dry eye. Patients suffering from eyelid entropion often find it aesthetically unappealing. There are five categories of entropion: (1) congenital, (2) involutional, (3) cicatricial, (4) spastic, and (5) marginal.

Congenital Entropion

Congenital entropion can affect the upper or lower eyelid (Fig. 103.2A). Upper eyelid congenital entropion occurs most commonly in association with the mechanical effects of microphthalmos. Lower eyelid congenital entropion is more common than congenital entropion of the upper eyelid and is caused by anatomical changes that result in inward rotation of the eyelid margin. These anatomical changes include hypertrophy of the eyelid skin and of the orbicularis oculi, dysgenesis of the lower eyelid retractors or its aponeurosis, structural defects in the tarsal plate and shortening of the posterior lamella. Congenital lower eyelid entropion does not spontaneously improve and requires surgical intervention. Surgical correction is performed by removing the skin and orbicularis oculi muscle from the subciliary aspect of the eyelid with advancement of the lower eyelid retractors.

A rare form of congenital upper eyelid entropion is tarsal kink in which there is an inward folding of the upper eyelid tarsal plate. Tarsal kink is managed through surgical repair which involves flattening of the tarsus and rotation of the lid margin with possible skin grafting for lengthening of the anterior lamella.

Epiblepharon: Another congenital eyelid malposition that is easily mistaken as congenital entropion is epiblepharon. An epiblepharon occurs when the eyelashes are vertically oriented but the eyelid margin maintains its normal position at the globe (Fig. 103.2B). The pretarsal orbicularis and skin override the eyelid margin which creates a horizontal fold of skin that pushes the eyelashes posteriorly against the globe. The vertically orientation of the eyelashes can result in corneal touch which is usually seen only in downgaze.

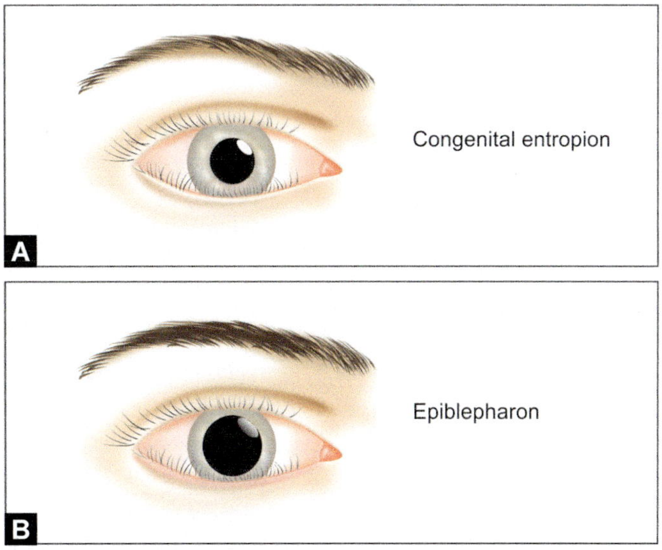

Figs. 103.2A and B: (A) Congenital forms of entropion. In congenital entropion, there are abnormalities in normal eyelid anatomy that result in inward rotation of the eyelid margin; (B) Conversely, in epiblepharon, the eyelid margin maintains its normal position against the globe but there is malposition of the lashes secondary to the force from the overriding skin and orbicularis oculi.

Treatment of epiblepharon is often observation; however, if the misdirected lashes result in corneal damage, surgical intervention may be necessary. This procedure involves removal of the excess muscle and skin that override the eyelid margin.

Acquired Entropion

There are four causes of acquired entropion: involutional, cicatricial, spastic and marginal (Figs. 103.3A and B).[1] Entropion formation of the lower eyelid is the result of changes to normal anatomy: age-related horizontal lid laxity and disinsertion or weakness of the eyelid retractors and cicatricial changes resulting in shortening of the posterior lamella. Entropion of the upper eyelid is the result of cicatricial changes of the posterior lamella.

Involutional Entropion

Involutional entropion is the most common eyelid malposition and only affects the lower eyelids (Fig. 103.3A). This is an age-related condition and can result in pseudotrichiasis or misdirection of the lashes from inversion of the lid margin. The lashes and the inverted keratinized skin of the eyelid can rub on the cornea and cause irritation or damage to the corneal surface. Involutional entropion occurs because of anatomical changes from aging that disrupt the stability of the lower eyelid, including: (1) increased horizontal lid laxity from canthal tendon or tarsal plate lengthening, (2) disinsertion, dehiscence, or weakening of the lower eyelid retractors muscles, (3) pretarsal orbicularis oculi overriding the retractors, and (4) prolapse of orbital fat into the lower lid causing laxity of the orbital septum. These changes weaken the normal tension on the tarsus provided by the lower lid retractors and allow the pretarsal orbicularis to push the eyelid margin inward. Surgical correction of this condition focuses on techniques to: (1) tighten and elevate the lower eyelid via a lateral tarsal strip procedure, (2) reattach the eyelid retractors to the inferior tarsal border of the tarsal plate, and/or (3) correct the overriding pretarsal orbicular muscle (Wheeler procedure). Additionally, rotational sutures to evert the eyelid margin may be combined with these techniques to achieve optimal results.[13,16]

The surgical treatment of choice for involutional entropion typically involves addressing the horizontal laxity of the lower eyelid via a tarsal strip procedure. This is typically coupled with one of the following: (1) reinsertion of the lower eyelid retractors through a subciliary or transconjunctival approach, (2) Quickert rotational sutures, (3) transfer of the pretarsal orbicularis muscle inferiorly (Wheeler procedure). Please note that the lateral tarsal strip procedure is described in more detail in the involutional ectropion section of this chapter.

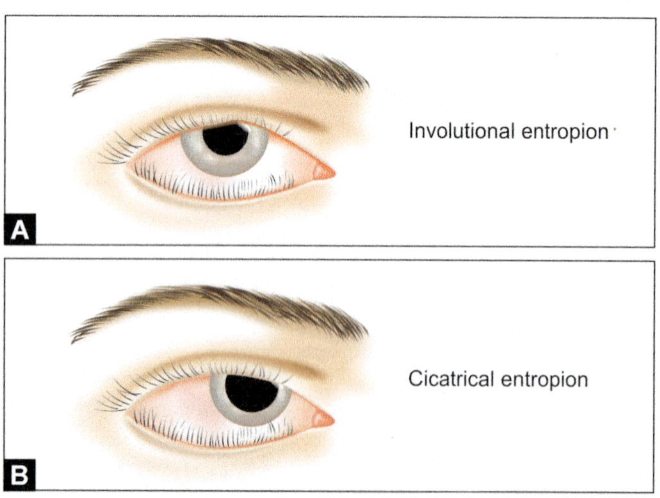

Figs. 103.3A and B: (A) Acquired entropion. There are four types of acquired entropion. The most commonly encountered form is involutional entropion, which results from age-related changes to the normal anatomy; (B) Cicatricial entropion results from shortening of the posterior lamella resulting in inward rotation of the eyelid margin. Margin entropion results from mild cicatrical changes at the lid margin from chronic lid irritation (not depicted here). Spastic entropion results from squeezing of the eyelid and is intermittent (not depicted here).

Cicatricial Entropion

Cicatricial entropion occurs because of shortening of the posterior lamella as a result of chronic irritation and scar formation (Fig. 103.3B). The shortened posterior lamella produces a posterior force that pulls the eyelid margin towards the globe and results in an inward rotation of the eyelid margin. Common causes include: Stevens-Johnson syndrome, thermal or chemical burns of the eyelids, trauma, previous surgery, infections, ocular cicatricial pemphigoid, Sjögren's and trachoma. Upper eyelid entropion almost always involves a cicatricial etiology. The first step in treatment of cicatricial entropion is to identify the underlying cause of scarring or inflammation and to treat these causes, if possible.

Surgical management of cicatricial entropion involves lengthening of the posterior lamella and depends on the severity of the disease. Mild cicatricial changes can be addressed with a tarsotomy or tarsal fracture operation. This procedure involves making a full-thickness incision through the superior aspect of the tarsus and using rotational sutures to maintain the wound in an open position. This allows for a small degree of posterior lamellar lengthening. Moderate-to-severe cicatricial entropion require greater lengthening of the posterior lamella than can be achieved with a tarsotomy. In these cases, the scar tissue is excised from the posterior lamella and mucous membrane grafts are placed to allow for lengthening of the posterior lamella. Mucosal graft tissue can be obtained from the mouth, either the buccal mucosa or the labial mucosa.

Marginal Entropion

Marginal entropion is a form of cicatricial entropion that results from chronic irritation and inflammation of the eyelid margin. Eyelid margin changes include anterior advancement of the mucocutaneous junction, rounding of the posterior aspect of the lid margin and scarring of the lid margin. These changes result in mild shortening of the posterior lamella which results in inward lid marginal rotation and potential corneal-lash touch. Treatment of marginal entropion can be achieved through a tarsotomy, as mentioned earlier. This operation allows for a minimal degree of posterior lamella lengthening which frees the eyelid from inward forces causing lid margin inversion.

Spastic Entropion

Spastic entropion is usually intermittent in nature and results from squeezing of the eyelids in response to ocular irritation or pain. The contraction of the orbicularis muscles overrides the retractors and results in inward rotation of the lid margin. If the source of ocular irritation is temporary, spastic entropion should resolve with the irritation. Otherwise, the first step in treatment of spastic entropion should focus on any modifiable causes of ocular irritation. If pain control cannot be achieved, Quickert sutures can be used to treat spastic entropion.[15] Full thickness sutures are placed from the inferior fornix through the eyelid exiting under the lash line. These sutures are left to dissolve and provide structural support to the retractors through the fibrotic changes that occur from the trauma of suture placement. Botulinum toxin injection to the pretarsal and preseptal orbicularis muscle is another option for relief of spastic entropion.[5]

ECTROPION

Ectropion is defined as an outward turning of the eyelid margin which results in loss of apposition of the eyelid to the globe (Table 103.2). This can result in chronic irritation of the conjunctiva leading to hypertrophy and keratinization. It can also result in loss of appropriate punctum positioning and can cause epiphora. Finally, loss of eyelid apposition disrupts the normal tear lake resulting in ocular surface disease and exposure keratopathy. Moreover, patients find the presence of ectropion cosmetically undesirable. Ectropion can be congenital or acquired in nature and the acquired forms are further classified based on etiology as involutional, cicatricial, paralytic, and mechanical.

Congenital Ectropion

Congenital ectropion is associated with other congenital syndromes, including blepharophimosis-ptosis-epicanthus inversus syndrome, Down syndrome or ichthyosis (Fig. 103.4A). Affected children present with epiphora and ocular surface disease. There is abnormal eyelid anatomy with vertical insufficiency of the anterior lamella. Mild cases do not require intervention. More severe cases can be treated with lengthening of the anterior lamella with full-thickness skin grafting and horizontal tightening of the lateral canthal tendon.

Congenital eversion of the eyelid: Complete eversion of the upper eyelids can be seen in newborn children. It may be secondary to conjunctivitis or anterior lamellar

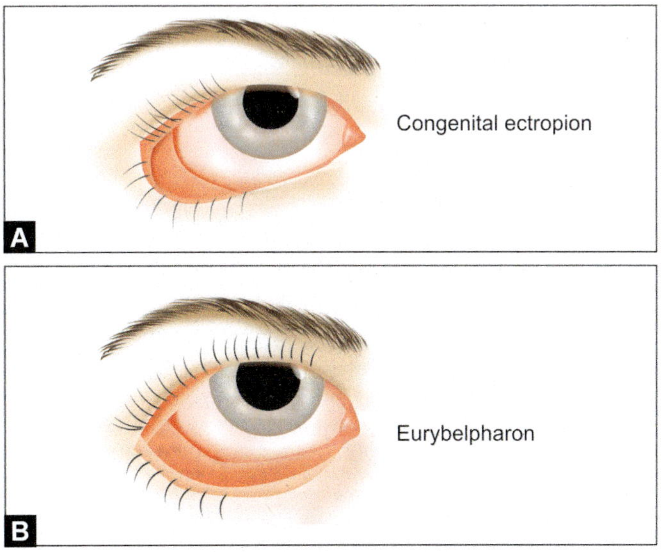

Figs. 103.4A and B: (A) Congenital ectropion. In true congenital ectropion, there is a vertical insufficiency of the anterior lamella which results in eversion of the eyelid margin; (B) Euryblepharon is a congenital eyelid malposition that results from vertical shortening of the eyelid, horizontal eyelid lengthening, and inferior displacement of the lateral canthal tendon insertion.

inflammation. Eversion of the eyelids can be associated with Down syndrome or ichthyosis. When it occurs, it is typically bilateral and symmetric. Treatment involves lubrication of the eye and the exposed conjunctiva as the condition is typically self-limiting. In more severe cases, tarsorrhaphy may be necessary.

Euryblepharon: Euryblepharon is a congenital eyelid malposition that results from vertical shortening of the eyelid in the presence of horizontal eyelid lengthening (Fig. 103.4B). There is also inferior displacement of the lateral canthal tendon insertion. Children appear to have a down-slanting inferior eyelid margin and an enlarged interpalpebral distance. It is associated with blepharophimosis-ptosis-epicanthus inversus syndrome and children typically present with ocular surface disease and exposure keratopathy due to abnormal blinking and lagophthalmos.

Treatment of euryblepharon is surgical in nature and can involve a combination of multiple approaches. Lateral canthal tendon reposition may be employed to correct inferior displacement. A lateral tarsal strip procedure may be necessary if there is horizontal lengthening of the lid. Finally, any anterior lamellar shortening may be addressed with skin grafts to achieve lengthening.

Acquired Ectropion

Acquired ectropion results from factors that disrupt the stability of the eyelid and produce an outward force on the lid margin that results in its eversion (Figs. 103.5A to D). These changes can be from the impact of age-related horizontal lid laxity causing involutional ectropion. Cicatricial ectropion results from shortening of the anterior lamella which produces an outward pull on the eyelid margin and results in lid margin eversion. Paralytic ectropion is the result of loss of innervation to the orbicularis oculi which disrupts lid stability and allows the lid margin to evert.

Involutional Ectropion

Involutional ectropion is the most commonly encountered form of ectropion. It results from horizontal eyelid laxity, which is the result of lengthening of medial or lateral canthal tendons (Fig. 103.5A). Lateral canthal tendon laxity is more common but medial canthal tendon laxity can occur and is demonstrated by excessive lateral movement of the lower punctum with lateral eyelid traction.

The preferred procedure for surgical treatment of involutional ectropion is the lateral tarsal strip, which involves horizontal shortening of the lower lid. The procedure involves releasing the lateral canthal tendon from its insertion in the lateral orbital rim via a lateral canthotomy and cantholysis. A tarsal strip is then formed by dissecting away the anterior lamella and shaving away the conjunctival epithelium from the posterior aspect of the tarsus, if necessary, the tarsal strip is shortened by approximating the edge of the tarsal strip to the lateral orbital rim and conservatively removing any excess tarsus.[2]

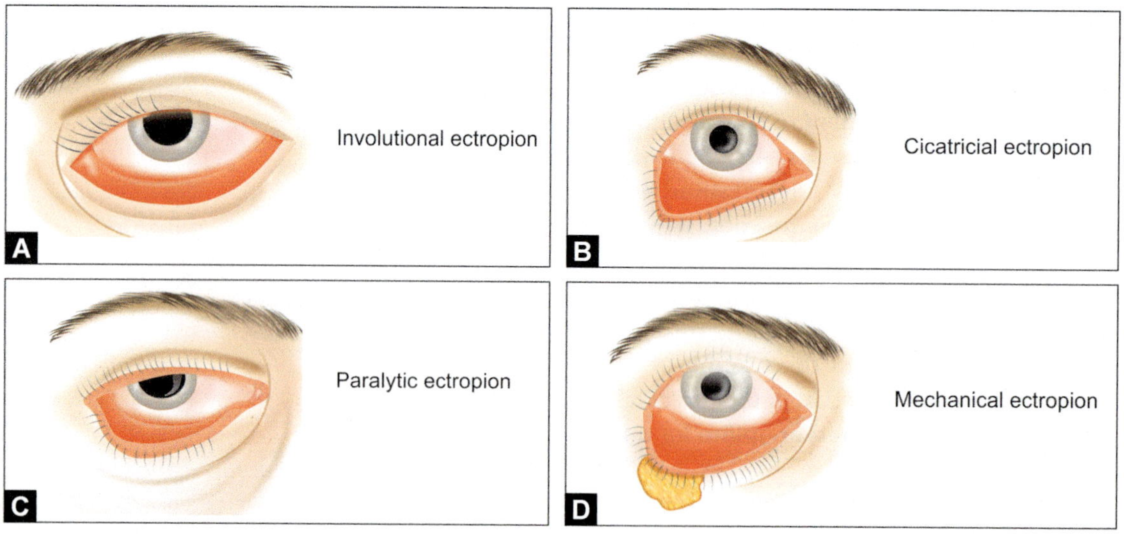

Figs. 103.5A to D: Acquired ectropion. There are four forms of acquired ectropion. (A) Involutional ectropion results from age-related horizontal eyelid laxity causing eversion of the eyelid margin; (B) Cicatricial ectropion results from shortening of the anterior lamella secondary to scarring; (C) Paralytic ectropion is eyelid eversion caused by paralysis of the orbicularis oculi from facial nerve damage; (D) Mechanical ectropion is due to the effects or bulky tumors or other external objects exerting force on the lid resulting in its eversion.

The tarsal strip is reattached to the periosteum of the lateral orbital rim. Any excess anterior lamella is removed. The canthus is reformed and the skin incision is closed. Variations of this procedure have been described as well, with similarly excellent results, such as the Bick Strip procedure.[3]

Alternative surgical interventions include a pentagonal wedge resection, which involves full-thickness excision of the eyelid margin to shorten the lid margin. This procedure is not preferred because it results in rounding of the lateral canthal angle and is not as effective at correcting the laxity of the lower eyelid.[10]

Lower lid ectropion resulting from the laxity of the medial canthal tendon is less common. In these patients, a medial spindle procedure is helpful for reapproximating the punctum to the globe. The procedure involves excision of a diamond shaped piece of palpebral conjunctiva followed by closure of the resulting defect with mattress sutures to invert the punctum. The medial spindle procedure can also be used in conjunction with the lateral tarsal strip to correct ectropion from lateral or medial canthal tendon laxity. For more severe cases of medial ectropion, medial canthoplasty can be performed, as described by Lee et al.[9]

Cicatricial Ectropion

Cicatricial ectropion arises from shortening of the anterior lamella as a result of scarring (Fig. 103.5B). Common etiologies of scar formation include chemical or thermal burns involving the periorbital skin or postsurgical scar formation. Other common cicatrizing diseases include Stevens-Johnson's syndrome, rosacea, atopic dermatitis, and herpes zoster. It is important to identify any underlying cause of chronic inflammation and scarring so that these can be addressed as a first approach to treatment.

Surgical intervention may also be necessary depending on disease severity. The first step in surgical management is to release tension on the anterior lamella by lysis of the scar tissue. Next, a lateral tarsal strip may be performed to correct any horizontal lid laxity and to return the eyelid margin to its proper position. A skin graft is used to lengthen the anterior lamella. Donor skin may be harvested from the upper eyelid, if there is dermatochalasis, or from the postauricular, preauricular, supraclavicular area, or the brachial aspect of the upper arm.

Paralytic Ectropion

Paralytic ectropion is an outward eversion of the lower eyelid that results from loss of orbicularis oculi tone due to damage of the facial nerve (CN VII). This leads to laxity and eversion of the lower eyelid (Fig. 103.5C). It is important to determine the cause of facial nerve paralysis, as these may be life-threatening conditions such as stroke, intracranial masses or paraneoplastic disease. Other etiologies include infectious and idiopathic causes. All patients should have a thorough neurological evaluation to rule out systemic disease.

Risk of corneal exposure is high in these patients because of dysfunction of the eyelids. These patients are at increased risk of neurotrophic keratitis if the underlying cause of the cranial neuropathy also affects the trigeminal nerve. Physical examination should focus on assessment of orbicularis oculi strength, presence of lagophthalmos, and evaluation of corneal sensation and corneal reflex.

Treatment varies based on severity of ocular surface involvement. All patients should receive prophylactic treatment for ocular surface disease with some combination of lubricating drop and ointment, moisture chambers and/or tape tarsorrhaphy. This may be sufficient in cases of temporary facial nerve paralysis such as Bell's palsy. More permanent tarsorrhaphy options can also be considered including: botulinum toxin tarsorrhaphy, temporary suture tarsorrhaphy or permanent tarsorrhaphy. Lower lid ectropion from facial nerve paralysis can be treated with a lateral tarsal strip with the possible addition of a medial spindle procedure, as previously described for involutional ectropion repair. Additional midface elevation may be required.[6]

Mechanical Ectropion

Mechanical ectropion is an outward turning of the lower lid secondary to the effect of bulky tumors of the lower eyelid and may also be secondary to herniated orbital fat or poorly fitted spectacles (Fig. 103.5D). In these cases, treatment should be directed at removal of the secondary forces causing eversion of the eyelid.

OTHER EYELID MALPOSITIONS

Eyelid Retraction

Eyelid retraction can affect the upper or lower eyelids. In the upper eyelids, eyelid retraction is present when the upper eyelid sits at or above the superior limbus. In the lower eyelids, retraction is diagnosed with the presence of inferior scleral show (Fig. 103.6A). The most common cause of eyelid retraction in adults is thyroid eye disease. Thyroid function should be evaluated in patients presenting with

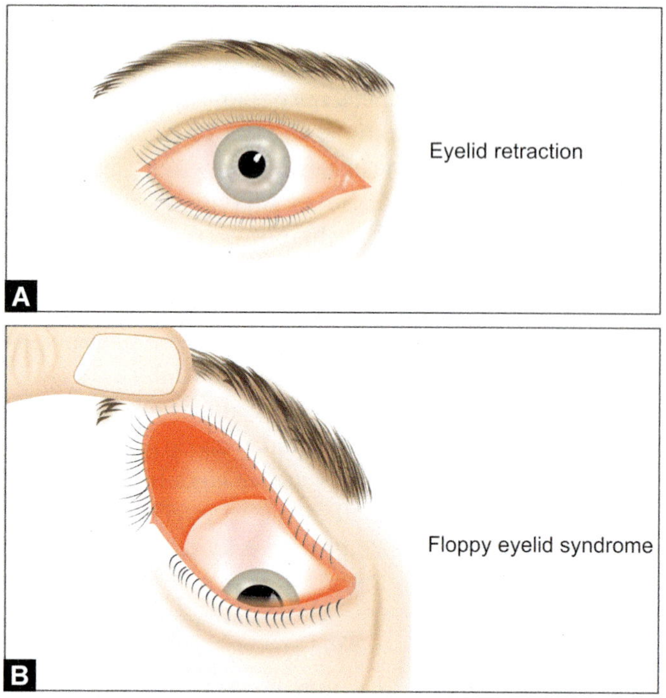

Figs. 103.6A and B: Other eyelid malposition. (A) Eyelid retraction can affect the upper eyelids, evidenced when the upper eyelid sits above the superior limbus. Eyelid retraction is present in the lower eyelid when there is inferior scleral show. The most common cause of eyelid retraction is thyroid eye disease; (B) Floppy eyelid syndrome results from excessive laxity of the eyelids from mechanical eversion of the eyelid on the pillow during sleep. There is a strong correlation with sleep apnea.

unilateral or bilateral eyelid retraction. Other causes of eyelid retraction can be divided into neurogenic, mechanical, and congenital causes. Neurogenic causes include facial nerve palsy, Marcus Gunn jaw-winking syndrome, or Parinaud syndrome. Mechanical causes of lid retraction include cicatricial changes and surgical overcorrection of ptosis. Congenital lid retraction can occur with Duane syndrome and is associated with Down's syndrome.

Surgical treatments of upper eyelid retraction is best accomplished with a Koornneef full-thickness blepharotomy, or a variation of the initially described procedure.[6-8] Surgical treatment of lower eyelid retraction includes a lateral tarsal strip to raise the eyelid or an inferior retractor recession with placement of a posterior lamellar spacer.

Floppy Eyelid Syndrome

Floppy eyelid syndrome results from excessive laxity of the eyelids (Fig. 103.6B). It is a common cause of ocular irritation than can be either unilateral or bilateral. Patients are often obese, middle-aged or older men. There is a strong correlation with obstructive sleep apnea. The underlying etiology of floppy eyelid syndrome is eversion of the eyelids on the pillow during sleep. On examination, there is extreme laxity of the eyelids and the presence of excess eyelid skin. The eyelids of these patients can be everted with minimal effort. Other diagnostic clues include the presence of papillary conjunctivitis and evidence of exposure keratopathy. If patients do not have a pre-existing diagnosis of obstructive sleep apnea, they should be asked about snoring and daytime sleepiness and referred for evaluation if these symptoms exist.

Treatment of floppy eyelid syndrome should first be directed at obtaining treatment for obstructive sleep apnea if present. Mild cases of floppy eyelid syndrome can usually be treated with ocular surface lubrication and the use of a nocturnal eye shield. More severe cases require surgical intervention with a pentagonal wedge resection. This involves excision of a pentagonal wedge of tarsus and eyelid tissue at the lateral third of the lid margin. The amount of excised tissue is case-dependent but usually is 10 mm or more in length.

Eyelid Imbrication Syndrome

Eyelid imbrication syndrome results in improper closure of the eyelids due to overlap of the lower eyelid by the upper eyelid. This results in irritation of the upper eyelid palpebral conjunctiva from rubbing on the eyelashes of the lower eyelid. Eyelid imbrication can be unilateral or bilateral and is often associated with floppy eyelid syndrome. Surgical treatment includes pentagon wedge resection of the upper eyelid, as previously mentioned for treatment of floppy eyelids. Lateral canthal tendon tightening via a lateral tarsal strip may also be necessary for complete treatment.

Blepharospasm

Benign essential blepharospasm is the involuntary contraction of the orbicularis oculi and upper facial muscles. Blepharospasm often presents in female patients in the 6th decade of life. The disease is progressive and often starts with involuntary blinking, but evolves to include more prolonged and forceful contraction of the facial muscles. Spasms are precipitated by ocular surface disease, stress and exposure to bright light. By definition, this condition is bilateral and does not occur while the patient is asleep. It is thought to be due to an abnormality in the basal ganglia.

The treatment of blepharospasm first involves removing any precipitating factors such as treating ocular surface disease, if present, or using sunglasses. If these simple approaches are unsuccessful, botulinum toxin injections can be used to paralyze the spastic muscles. Injections typically need to be repeated every three months. Surgical treatment with a myectomy is uncommon today, and represents a last resort in patients intolerant or unresponsive to injections.[12]

Hemifacial Spasms

Hemifacial spasm is another facial muscle disorder that should be differentiated from benign essential blepharospasm. Hemifacial spasm involves involuntary contraction of the facial muscles on one side of the face. Movements can vary from short quick spasms to longer sustained contracture of the muscles and commonly start in the periorbital area and progress to involve the rest of the face. Unlike blepharospasm, they are almost always unilateral and persist during sleep. Ipsilateral facial nerve weakness is commonly present. Most cases of hemifacial spasms are secondary to vascular compression of the facial nerve where it leaves the brainstem. Less commonly (in less than 1% of cases) cerebellopontine angle masses are the cause. Hemifacial spasm can also be seen with aberrant regeneration after a facial nerve palsy.

The evaluation of patients with hemifacial spasm should include asking about any other neurological deficits or a history of Bell's palsy and a clinical examination. All patients should undergo MRI of the brain to evaluate for masses, cerebellopontine angle lesions or the presence of a dilated basilar artery adjacent to facial nerve as it exits the brainstem.

Vascular decompression of the nerve in healthy patients can be considered as the surgery is low-risk and has a high rate of success (up to 75%). In patients without vascular compression or who are poor surgical candidates, botulinum toxin is the treatment of choice and often has extended treatment duration, up to 4–6 months, due to concurrent facial nerve weakness.[5]

SUGGESTED READING

1. American Academy of Ophthalmology. Orbit, Eyelids and Lacrimal System. In: 2016-2017 Basic and Clinical Science Course. San Francisco, CA: American Academy of Ophthalmology; 2016.
2. Anderson RL, Gordy DD. The tarsal strip procedure. Arch Ophthalmol. 1979;97(11):2192-6.
3. Barret RV, Meyer DR. The modified Bick quick strip procedure for surgical treatment of eyelid malposition. Opthal Plast Reconst Surg. 2012;28(4):294-9.
4. Bowling B. Kanski's Clinical Ophthalmology: A Systematic Approach, 8th edition. Philadelphia: Elsevier; 2016.
5. Dutton J, Fowler A. Botulinum toxin in ophthalmology. Surv Ophthalmol. 2007;52(1):13-31.
6. Elner VM, Hassan AS, Frueh BR. Graded full-thickness anterior blepharotomy for upper eyelid retraction. Arch Ophthalmol. 2004;122(1):55-60.
7. Elner VM, Mauffray RO, Fante RG, et al. Comprehensive midfacial elevation for ocular complications of facial nerve palsy. Arch Facial Plast Surg. 2003;5(5):427-33.
8. Kazim M, Gold KG. A review of surgical techniques to correct upper eyelid retraction associated with thyroid eye disease. Curr Opin Ophthalmol. 2001;22(5):391-3.
9. Lee BJ, Elner SG, Douglas RD, et al. Island pedicle and horizontal advancement cheek flaps for medial canthal reconstruction. Ophthal Plast Reconstr Surg. 2001;27(5): 376-9.
10. Nerad J. Techniques in Ophthalmic Plastic Surgery: A Personal Tutorial. Philadelphia: Saunders/Elsevier; 2009.
11. Nimitwongsakul A, Zoumalan CI, Kazim M. Modified full-thickness blepharotomy for treatment of thyroid eye disease. Ophthal Plast Reconstr Surg. 2013;29(1):44-7.
12. Pariseau B, Worley M, Anderson R. Myectomy for blepharospasm. Curr Opin Ophthalmol. 2013;24(5):488-93.
13. Perira M, Rodrigues M, Rodrigues S. Eyelid entropion. Semin Ophthalmol. 2010;25(3):52-8.
14. Piskiniene R. Eyelid malposition: lower lid entropion and ectropion. Medicina. 2006;(42):11.
15. Quickert M, Rathbun E. Suture repair of entropion. Arch Ophthal. 1971;85(3):304-5.
16. Van den Bosch W, Rosman M, Stijnen T. Involutional lower eyelid entropion: results of a combined approach. Ophthalmic Surg Lasers. 1998;29 (7):581-6.

Chapter 104 Eyelid Neoplasms: Evaluation and Management

Oded Sagiv, Thomas J Kandl, Sudip D Thakar,
Stephanie Ding, Bita Esmaeli

INTRODUCTION

Eyelid and periocular skin lesions are frequently encountered by ophthalmologists. The more common benign lesions, are usually managed by observation, or by simple excision, if there is doubt about their nature or for functional or aesthetic reasons. Malignant neoplasms in the eyelid present additional management considerations that are discussed in this chapter.

TYPES OF MALIGNANT EYELID NEOPLASMS

Basal Cell Carcinoma

Basal cell carcinoma is the most common malignant neoplasm accounting for over 90% of all eyelid cancers.[1-3] Known risk factors for BCC include ultraviolet light exposure, fair skin type, increased age, immunosuppression and pre-existing scars and ulcers. People with xeroderma pigmentosum or basal cell nevus syndrome (BCNS, also Gorlin-Goltz syndrome) are predisposed to developing multiple BCCs from an early age.[4,5] BCCs arise from the basal cell layer, stratum basale, of the epidermis and can present in a number of ways, most commonly as a pearly nodule with overlying telangiectasia and ulceration (Figs. 104.1 and 104.2). Histologic characteristics include cells with large hyperchromatic nuclei, scant cytoplasm which forms cords and nests in the dermis with peripheral palisading of nuclei. A cleft-like artifact between the nests and surrounding stroma is frequently present. Several pathologic variants of BCC exist with nodular and morpheaform being the most prevalent. Nodular BCC is the most common variant and shows the distinctive round nests with palisading nuclei. Morpheaform BCC is the second most common variant and characteristically has irregular borders and a more aggressive behavior. Metastasis is uncommon, however, local invasive growth is possible, if left untreated. Perineural invasion is also possible with large and locally advanced BCC.

Squamous Cell Carcinoma

Accounting for 5–10% of all eyelid neoplasms, squamous cell carcinoma (SCC) is the second most common eyelid

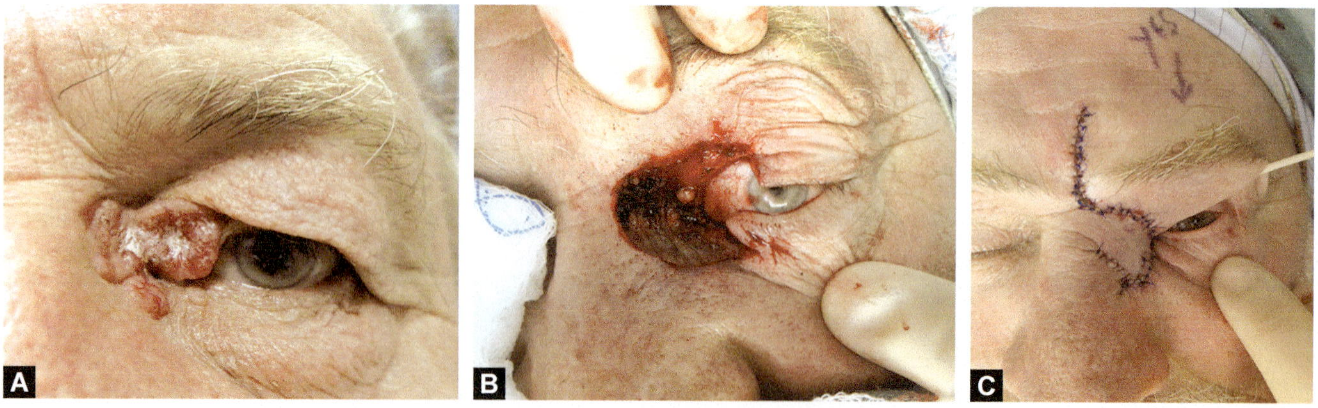

Figs. 104.1A to C: Clinical and intraoperative photographs of a patient with nodular basal cell carcinoma. (A) The lesion has pearly borders with some ulceration and overlying telangiectasia and involves the left medial canthus with extension onto the upper and lower eyelids and with involvement of the upper canaliculus and partial involvement of the lower canaliculus; (B) Intraoperative defect after complete surgical excision (defect size—3.5 cm x 4.0 cm); (C) The defect was repaired using a glabellar rotational flap with local advancement flaps for repair of the left upper and lower eyelids and repair of the partial defect in the left lower canaliculus.

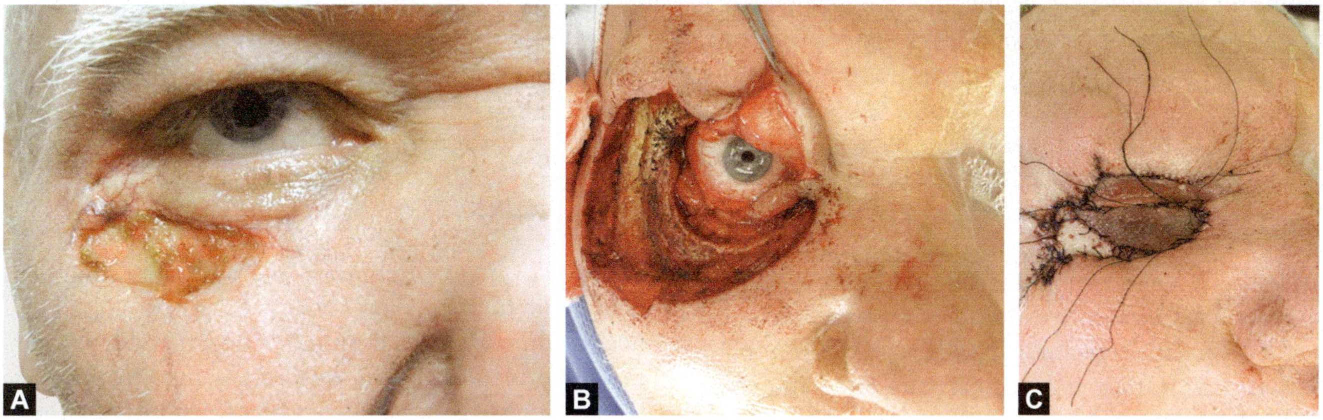

Figs. 104.2A to C: Clinical and intraoperative photographs of a patient with recurrent infiltrative basal cell carcinoma. (A) The lesion involved the right lower eyelid and lateral canthal area and was adherent to the orbital floor and zygoma; (B) The patient underwent a wide excision of the upper and lower eyelid and the periorbital soft tissue (defect size—6.5 cm x 4.0 cm); (C) The defect was repaired using a combination of flaps including a tarsoconjunctival flap and a harvested skin graft from the right upper eyelid and a facial flap.

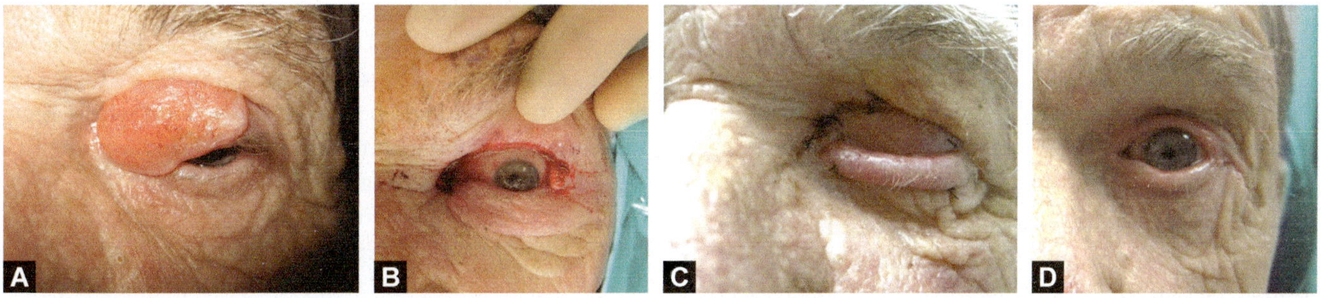

Figs. 104.3A to D: Clinical, intraoperative, and postoperative photographs of a patient with squamous cell carcinoma. (A) Large squamous cell carcinoma spanning most of the left upper eyelid with medial canthal involvement; (B) Intraoperative defect after resection of the lesion (defect size—3.5 cm x 2.5 cm); (C) The left upper eyelid defect was repaired using a Cutler-beard conjunctival and skin muscle flap from the left lower eyelid; (D) The flap was divided 3 months later. This photograph shows the reconstructed upper eyelid and the lower eyelid donor site after the second stage surgery.

malignancy.[6,7] As in BCC, ultraviolet light exposure and fair complexion are the two most common risk factors, with chronic ulcers, infection, immunosuppression and radiation also playing a role. Patients with genetic skin disorders also show higher rates of SCC.[8-10] SCCs arise from keratinocytes either from a premalignant lesion, such as actinic keratosis or squamous cell carcinoma in situ, or de novo. Clinically, SCC can present in a variety of ways. Most typically a lesion will appear as an ulcer, plaque, or nodule with scaling, and erythema most commonly in the lower eyelid but it can also occur in the upper eyelid (Figs. 104.3A to D). On pathology, the characteristic appearance is fingerlike extensions invading the dermis. These are made up of large cells with eosinophilic cytoplasm, hyperchromatic nuclei, high mitotic activity with formation of keratin pearls.[11] SCCs which arise de novo have a higher metastatic potential. The parotid and submandibular lymph nodes are the most common site of metastasis with hematogenous spread to distant sites possible.[12] Nodal metastasis rates can be as high as 24% in advanced, large neoplasms. Perineural invasion portends the worst prognosis with 47.2% of lesions having local recurrence and 47.3% becoming metastatic. Additional poor prognostic indicators include tumor size (>2 cm), depth of invasion (>4 mm), poor differentiation, occurrence in scar tissue, and recurrent disease.[13]

Melanoma

Melanoma represents the 5th most common cancer, however, primary melanomas of the eyelid only represent less than 1% of eyelid malignancies.[3,14] While relatively uncommon in the periorbital region, melanoma is a life-threatening condition requiring close attention. Melanoma patients typically present between the years of 55–74 with a median age at diagnosis of 64. It is more common in men and is more typically seen in people of fair complexion with significant exposure to UV light, either natural or artificial (tanning beds).[14] Also geographical location has been linked to a higher incidence with individuals closer to the equator having a higher incidence of melanoma of the eyelid.[15] Like BCC and SCC, people with xeroderma pigmentosum have a higher risk of developing multiple melanomas.[16]

Melanoma typically presents as a change in size and color of a pre-existing pigmented lesion (Fig. 104.4).[17,18] It results from malignant proliferation of melanocytes and has been classified into multiple categories. Melanoma in situ indicates there are neoplastic cells present but no dermal penetration. Superficial spreading melanoma accounts for two-third of all cutaneous melanomas. In this type, the radial growth phase predominates. Nodular melanoma arises de novo and only has a vertical growth phase. Lentigo maligna melanoma arises from a lentigo maligna (a melanoma in situ) that has been present in skin with sun damage. Amelanotic melanoma is typically a nodular melanoma that has lost its pigment. Desmoplastic melanoma is frequently located on the head and neck and is comprised of melanoma cells in a dense desmoplastic stroma.[19,20] Histologically, the malignant cells are described as spindle, shaped, epithelioid or nevus like with neoplasms frequently showing a mixture of these cells. Important factors in establishing prognosis include Clark level, Breslow thickness, ulceration, vascular invasion and number of mitoses. Clark level describes the depth of invasion using anatomic relationships (I–IV) and Breslow thickness describes depth in terms of millimeters.[19] Prognosis varies considerably according to the existence of regional lymph nodes or distant metastasis. Sentinel lymph node status is considered one of the most important prognostic indicators for cutaneous melanomas.[21,22] Early detection is key as localized 5-year survival rate is 98.5% with regional spread survival rate decreasing to 62.9% and distant metastasis decreasing the 5-year survival rate to 19.9%.[14]

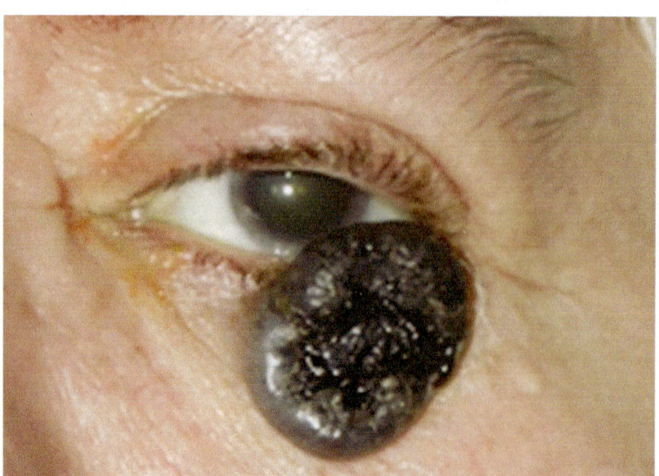

Fig. 104.4: External photograph of a patient with a large, exophytic melanoma of the left lower eyelid, with central ulceration.

Sebaceous Gland Carcinoma

Sebaceous gland carcinoma (SGC) is a rare, potentially fatal eyelid tumor arising from the sebaceous glands of the ocular adnexa. Due to the abundance of sebaceous glands in the periocular region, this area is the most common location for SGC typically arising from the Meibomian glands, glands of Zeis or caruncle. These lesions typically present as a nodule or diffuse eyelid thickening, most commonly in the upper eyelid. Diagnosis is often delayed due to neoplasms masquerading as benign lesions. In one study, over 2/3 of SGCs were initially diagnosed as another, less serious, lesion.[23] In a different study, median time from symptom onset to diagnosis was 24 months.[24] Mean age of presentation is between 64 and 72 years old with a higher incidence in Asian populations, accounting for 30% of all eyelid malignant neoplasms in studies from Asia versus only 1–3% in US and Europe.[7,23,25,26] Risk factors include prior radiation treatment as well as a history of Muir-Torre syndrome although the latter is most often associated with non-ocular sebaceous carcinoma.[27-30]

In addition to being difficult to diagnose clinically, SGC is also difficult to diagnose on pathology due to poor differentiation and expression of characteristic features. Histologically, the cells feature foamy cytoplasm and are classified by level of differentiation and growth pattern. Diagnosis is often aided by the use of special stains such as Oil Red O or adipophilin.[23,31] SGC has the propensity for intraepithelial spread, also described as pagetoid spread (Figs. 104.5A to C).[25] This type of spread has been found in approximately 50% of patients who have SGC which is associated with an increased risk of local recurrence.[23,32]

Sebaceous gland carcinoma has a significant risk of metastasis with an estimated risk of 10–15% for both nodal and distant organ metastases, with lung and liver the most common distant site. Unlike melanoma, depth of invasion has not been correlated with rate of metastasis, rather tumor size is correlative. According to the 7th edition of the American Joint Committee on Cancer (AJCC) Staging Manual tumors greater than or equal to T2b (i.e. tumor >10 mm but not >20 mm in greatest dimension, or involves full thickness of eyelid) had an increased risk of nodal metastasis with tumors greater than or equal to T3b (i.e. tumor

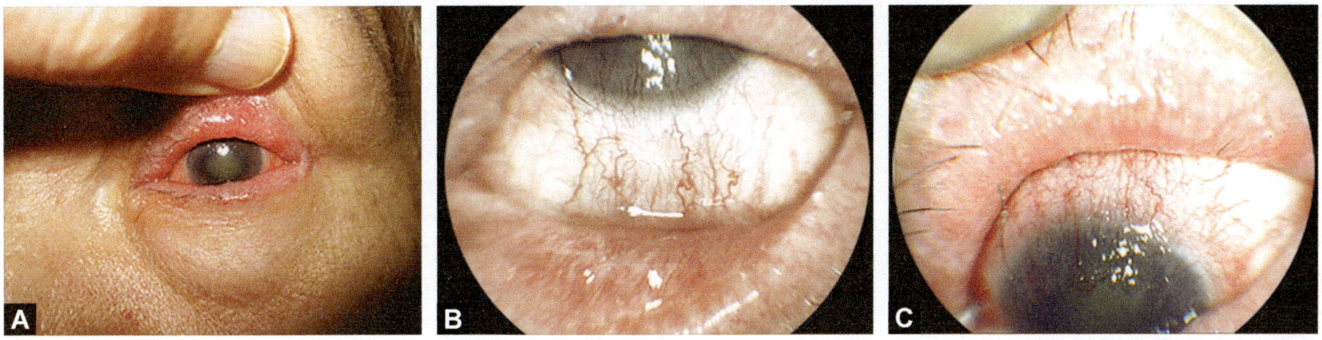

Figs. 104.5A to C: Clinical and anterior segment photographs of a patient with sebaceous carcinoma. (A and B) There is diffuse involvement of the left upper and lower eyelids and the ocular surface; (B and C) Circumferential corneal neovascularization and haze suggests corneal and bulbar conjunctival involvement.

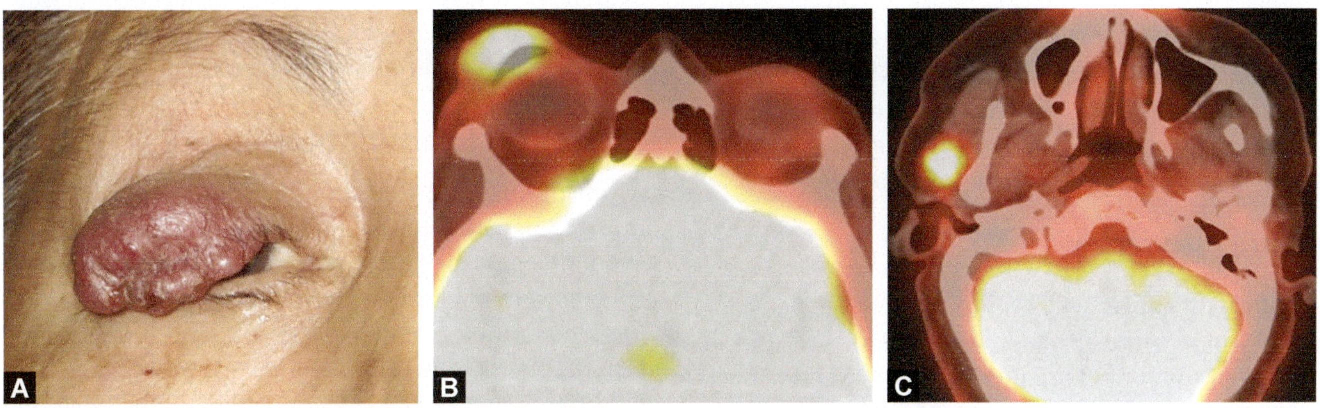

Figs. 104.6A to C: (A) External photograph of a patient with Merkel cell carcinoma of the right upper eyelid; (B and C) A PET/CT scan demonstrates high metabolic activity of the eyelid mass and also uptake in a metastatic parotid node.

complete resection requires enucleation, exenteration or bone resection) associated with an increased risk of distant metastasis.[33]

Sweat Gland Tumors

Malignant sweat gland carcinomas in the eyelid are rare neoplasms with multiple overlapping classification systems. These tumors are often heterogeneous, have variable histologic features and include eccrine carcinoma, apocrine carcinoma, mucinous carcinoma and microcystic carcinoma. They present as growth in a nodular, cystic, papillary or diffuse lesion. According to a report of 22 patients with sweat gland carcinoma, the median age was 69 years with 59% of these patients being female. Perineural invasion was present in a quarter of the cases with local recurrence present in 23% of the cases. Of the 22 cases, only one case had nodal metastasis. An AJCC classification (7th edition) of greater than T2b was associated with a more aggressive behavior. Microcystic adnexal carcinoma showed more aggressive behavior in contrast to mucinous carcinoma.[34]

Merkel Cell Carcinoma

Merkel cell carcinoma is a rare cutaneous neuroendocrine carcinoma arising from mechanoreceptors in the basal layer of the epidermis and is most typically seen in the head and neck region. These lesions typically present as a firm purple or violaceous nodule (Figs. 104.6A to C). Risk factors include ultraviolet light exposure and immunosuppressive therapy after organ transplantation.[35,36] These neoplasms have a high rate of metastasis with nodal metastasis between 15 and 66% at the time of diagnosis.[37,38] Five-year survival rate is 67.5% with tumor thickness, large tumor size, infiltrative growth pattern, lymphovascular invasion and tumor infiltrating lymphocytes all portending a worse prognosis.[39]

Vascular Tumors

Cutaneous angiosarcoma is a malignant neoplasm and a form of soft tissue mesenchymal sarcoma with a poor prognosis which develops from lymphatic or vascular endothelial cells.[40,41] The most common presentation is a reddish maculopapular lesion which often appears benign.[42,43] Risk factors include radiation therapy and chronic lymphedema.[44,45] The 5-year survival rate is 13–50% and recurrences are common.[41,46]

Lymphoma

Lymphoma of the eyelid can be both B- and T- cell, but primary lymphoma of the eyelid is rare, with cases of eyelid involving lymphoma most frequently occurring in cases of systemic involvement.[47]

Metastatic Lesions

Isolated metastasis to the eyelid is a rare event. Neoplasms that have been reported to metastasize to the eyelid include melanoma, breast cancer, renal cell carcinoma, prostate cancer, lung cancer, leiomyosarcoma, salivary gland carcinoma and hepatocellular carcinoma.[48-50]

EVALUATION

Although diagnosis will eventually rely on pathologic analysis of a surgical biopsy specimen, a careful and detailed evaluation of a patient with an eyelid cancer is essential. This includes a detailed medical history, clinical examination and ancillary tests as needed.

History

Prior history of skin cancer and sun exposure should be noted.[51] Multiple previous BCCs, especially at a young age, should raise the possibility of BCNS or xeroderma pigmentosum.[4, 5] Skin type can be assessed by physical examination but also by asking the patient whether he or she normally reacts to sun exposure with a burn with no subsequent tan, a risk factor for melanoma.[52] The number of previous painful sunburns is probably more significant than the lifetime exposure to the sun.[53] History of trauma or chronic ulcers are risk factors for developing BCC or SCC and should be sought. Other risk factors including human papilloma virus infection, previous radiation treatment, exposure to various chemical agents or pesticides, immunosuppression (such as HIV-positive patients) and albinism should be noted.[9,10,54] History of other visceral cancers (specifically colorectal, urogenital, small intestine, and breast cancers) should raise concern for Muir-Torre syndrome that is associated also with sebaceous gland tumors.[29] Race may also play a role, with higher prevalence of SGC among Asian population, and higher prevalence of melanoma among Whites, compared to Blacks and Hispanics.[26,55]

Recent history regarding the lesion should be taken and specifically note rapid growth, associated pain (suggestive of perineural invasion) and ulceration. History of chronic blepharitis, especially a unilateral disease, or a chronic inflammatory lesion treated as a chalazion, should raise concern for SGC. If in doubt, previous pictures, readily accessible today through smartphones and social media, can aid to assess progression of a lesion.

Detailed general medical history should be obtained, including factors that can impact surgery or post-surgical healing, such as other comorbidities, history of poor wound healing, smoking, coagulation disorders, the use of blood-thinners, cardiac pacemaker and more.

Clinical Examination

A full ophthalmic examination should be carried out in every patient with an eyelid tumor. Special attention should be paid for skin type, tumor size and location with specific reference to key structures such as lateral and medial canthus, puncta, canaliculi, and eyelid margin. Clinical photographs are essential. Any mass effect caused by the tumor affecting eyelid position, globe position or movement should be noted. On palpation, the physician should try to determine if the tumor is superficial and can be easily mobilized, or if it may involve deeper tissues such as the orbit or lacrimal sac. Extension to adjacent structures such as brow, cheek or temporal region should be noted. Both eyelids should be everted to determine the extent of the lesion and rule-out conjunctival or forniceal involvement. Palpation of the lymph nodes in the preauricular, submandibular and cervical regions is critical for detection of nodal metastases. Sensation of V1 and V2 branches of cranial nerve V should be checked, as well as facial nerve function, to evaluate for perineural invasion.

Ancillary Tests

Once the diagnosis of an eyelid malignant lesion has been confirmed via a biopsy, radiologic studies may be appropriate when there is clinical suspicion for tumor infiltration in the orbit, lacrimal sac and duct, paranasal sinuses, cheek, forehead or temporal region. If there is clinical suspicion of perineural spread magnetic resonance imaging (MRI) of the orbits and adjacent structures should be obtained with specific comments regarding cranial neuropathies to the radiologist. Computed tomography

(CT) of the orbits can be useful to assess gross tumor extension and bony destruction, but MRI is superior in identifying soft tissue involvement, perineural invasion and recurrences in post-surgical patients with large soft tissue flaps. Extending imaging to the neck area is prudent in case of tumors with propensity for lymphatic spread.

For all eyelid cancers with a propensity for lymphatic spread, baseline ultrasound of the lymph nodes should be obtained, and any suspicious lymph nodes or mass biopsied. This is true for most eyelid cancers other than BCC, including: melanoma, SCC, SGC Merkel cell carcinoma, lymphoma. If an enlarged lymph node is palpated on clinical examination, it should be evaluated by ultrasonography and biopsied either using fine needle aspiration (FNA) or directly through an open biopsy. Sentinel lymph node biopsy (SLNB) for the same eyelid cancers is discussed later in this chapter.

Metastatic work-up should be performed for eyelid cancers with aggressive biology. Brain MRI and CT of chest abdomen and pelvis should be done at baseline in patients with eyelid or conjunctival melanoma to rule out metastasis.[56] Gastrointestinal and gynecologic evaluation are recommended for all patients with a new diagnosis of eyelid SGC due to the rare association with Muir-Torre syndrome. Generally, the presence of an eyelid cancer should prompt the search for skin cancers elsewhere and a full-body skin check by a dermatologist is recommended.

MANAGEMENT

Surgical excision with margins that are free of tumor is the most common treatment for eyelid cancers. However, other treatment modalities may play a role, depending on the type, location and extent of the cancer. An incisional or excisional biopsy may be appropriate prior to definitive surgery.

Excision/Biopsy

Control of margins is critical due to propensity of eyelid tumors for subclinical spread, which can be difficult to identify clinically.[57] Previously published large series found that incomplete excision of BCC (i.e. margins positive for tumor) was associated with as much as 27% of patients experiencing local recurrence.[58] Simple wide local excision of a grossly-visible tumor have been shown to result in 25% of incomplete excision, even with 3 mm of clinical margins planned for BCC and 5 mm for SCC.[57] Control of margins is accomplished by either intraoperative analysis on frozen section or permanent section evaluation, or by Mohs micrographic surgery (MMS) which also uses frozen section.

Mohs micrographic surgery is a surgical technique for excision and analysis of skin cancers, which is performed by especially trained dermatologists. The tumor is excised and the especimen and margins are examined by frozen sections with slicing of the specimen in an en-face direction. The examination is done by a specifically trained Mohs dermatologic surgeon. The excision area is marked carefully so that additional tissue can be resected from locations correlating with areas of tumor-positive margins. This technique was developed to enable removal of tumors while minimizing the removal of surrounding healthy tissue, and is therefore favored in body areas the lack redundant skin or near functional organs such as the periocular region. MMS has been shown to be highly effective in the excision of BCC and SCC of the eyelids.[59-61] However, the use of MMS for removal of melanoma, MCC, and SGC is controversial.[24,62-65] MMS is not the procedure of choice for removal of melanocytic lesions in the eyelid, since frozen sections are unreliable to identify atypical melanocytes. An alternative method in these cases could be a "slow-Mohs", in which rush-permanent sections are used, analyzed by a pathologist.[66]

The authors treat eyelid carcinomas with excision and intraoperative frozen section control of margins using the same principles as Mohs surgery, i.e. evaluation of en-face adjacent tissue in all directions, with the analysis of the sections performed by an experienced dermatopathologist. Typical margins taken for BCC and SCC are 2 mm of tumor-free tissue based on microscopic immediate evaluation on frozen section. If margins are found to harbor tumor cells, additional tissue is excised, guided by the location of the involved margins, until clear margins are achieved all the way around the tumor.

In cases of melanoma, we only use permanent section for margin assessment. WHO guidelines recommend clinical margins of 1 cm for lesions under 2 mm thickness, and 2 cm for lesions 2 mm or thicker.[67] A retrospective study of eyelid melanomas found that rates of recurrences and metastasis were significantly different between patients with margins of excision under 5 mm or over 5 mm.[68] The authors typically use margins of 4–5 mm for excision of periocular melanomas.

Frozen sections are not reliable for confirming clear margins in melanomas. Thus, we typically repair the eyelid defect after melanoma excision in a delayed fashion after rush permanent (paraffin) evaluation of margins allowing for additional tissue removal the following day in case of positive margins. In a study from our center, we demonstrated that using this approach there is a need for a second consecutive excision to achieve negative margins in approximately 1/3 of patients with eyelid melanoma.[21]

Sebaceous gland carcinoma presents a special situation due to its propensity for intraepithelial (pagetoid) spread in noncontiguous tissues ("skip lesions"). Several studies have reported local control rates to be 82–90% for both traditional WLE and MMS for sebaceous carcinoma of eyelid.[23,33,69] Conjunctival map biopsies can be considered; however, the yield of map biopsies is higher when done in a targeted fashion in the areas around the lesion and in areas with clinical signs of inflammation or involvement. The map biopsies are usually small and are not appropriate for frozen section evaluation. They can help with consideration of postoperative adjuvant topical chemotherapy or other secondary surgical procedures, if positive.[70]

Eyelid tumors may invade the orbit or globe, and an orbital exenteration may be needed to achieve local control. In a large series of 429 orbital exenterations, 40% were performed for eyelid tumors.[71] Another series found BCC to be responsible for 90% of orbital exenterations.[72] These numbers may significantly decrease in the era of targeted therapy for BCC (see below). Neoadjuvant therapy with sonic hedgehog inhibitors will likely decrease the number of orbital exenteration performed in patients with locally advanced BCC. Furthermore, some locally advanced invasive eyelid tumors can be managed with eye-preserving surgery and judicious use of postoperative radiation therapy with or without systemic chemotherapy.[73]

Surgical Specimen Handling

Handling of the surgical specimen and direct communication with the pathologist is a critical and practical matter that is often overlooked. The pathologist should be made aware of the proper orientation of the specimen and the surgical margins of interest. A drawing of the eye and periocular structures with clear labels is helpful (Fig. 104.7).

Specimens suspected for lymphoproliferative tumors should be sent fresh. For lesions suspected to be sebaceous carcinoma, recent availability of adipophilin immunohistochemical stain which can be done on paraffin embedded tissue has eliminated the need for fresh tissue harvest.[74] As stated previously, margins for melanoma have to be requested on "rush" paraffin section to allow for timely reconstruction of the periocular defect.

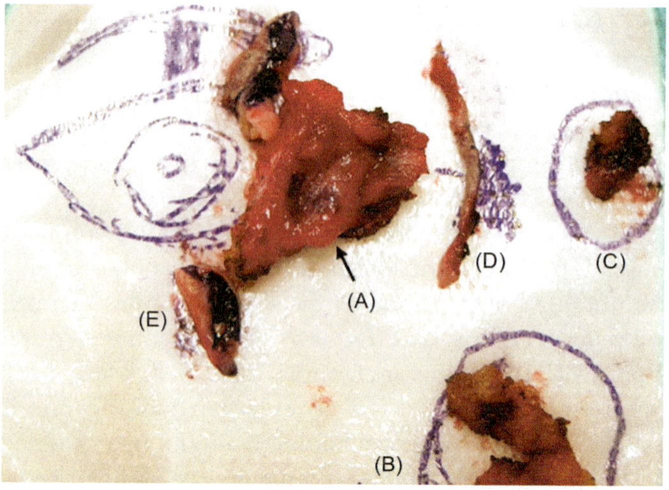

Fig. 104.7: Photograph of the surgical specimen from a patient with squamous cell carcinoma of the right medial canthus (A), medial upper (B) and lower (C) eyelids, canaliculi (D) and lacrimal sac (E). The surgical specimen is positioned on the drawing with proper orientation. The margins are positioned in each side with the true margin inked and clearly labelled.

Reconstruction

After complete microscopic removal of the eyelid cancer, reconstruction is carried out aiming to achieve good functional and cosmetic outcome. Functionally, the goal is to achieve sufficient coverage of the eye without impairing vision. Details of the various reconstructive techniques will be discussed elsewhere in this book. Generally, for small defects in the eyelid, primary closure is appropriate. For larger lower eyelid defects our preferred method is a modified Hughes flap with skin graft usually taken from the upper eyelid. The flap will usually be divided in 4–6 weeks. For larger upper eyelid defects, a Cutler-Beard technique is used.

Sentinel Lymph Node Biopsy

Some eyelid malignancies can spread to the regional lymph nodes prior to systemic metastasis.[75] Sentinel lymph node biopsy (SLNB) is a procedure that aims at localization and biopsy of the first draining node (i.e. sentinel node) in a patient that has no clinical or radiologic evidence of regional lymph node metastasis. It can identify early microscopic metastasis that would otherwise go undetected on conventional imaging studies or palpation. It is a surgical procedure that is typically performed on the same day as the eyelid tumor resection. The authors use preoperative lymphoscintigraphy by injecting a Technetium-labeled sulfur colloid into the dermal or subconjunctival space around the tumor on the day before surgery. A SPECT/CT

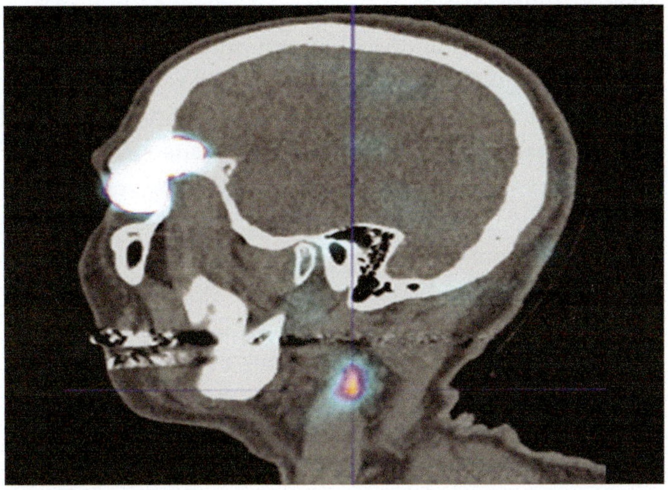

Fig. 104.8: Preoperative lymphoscintigraphy (SPECT/CT scan) of a patient with upper eyelid and brow melanoma after injection of a 0.52 nCi unfiltered technetium-99m sulfur colloid. The sentinel lymph node was localized as a level IIB lymph node.

scan provides a higher resolution anatomic localization for the draining lymph nodes compared with traditional lymphoscintigraphy and enables preoperative planning for SLNB (Fig. 104.8). During surgery, a handheld gamma probe is used to localize the nodes to be excised.

Sentinel lymph node biopsy should be considered for the following eyelid tumors: melanomas of intermediate thickness (greater than 1.5 mm Breslow thickness) or evidence of ulceration, any case of eyelid Merkel cell carcinoma, sebaceous carcinoma that is more than or equal to T2b (AJCC 7th edition staging manual), i.e. larger than 10 mm or involves the full thickness of the eyelid.

NON-SURGICAL TREATMENTS FOR LOCALLY ADVANCED TUMORS

Topical Treatments

Topical treatments have been reported with various degrees of success and could be considered in patients who are poor surgical candidates or who refuse surgery. However, with the availability of newer and safer systemic therapy (targeted therapy and immune therapy), topical modalities are used less frequently. Topical imiquimod 5% had been reported to successfully treat eyelid BCC, SCC and melanoma in situ.[76-78] Topical 5-FU and interferon were used to treat actinic keratosis. Mitomycin C is used topically to treat sebaceous carcinoma invading the conjunctiva.[79] Topical tazarotene, a retinoid, was used to treat BCC with 31% of tumors healing with no recurrence in 3 years.[80] Photodynamic therapy and cryotherapy have also been used to treat eyelid BCC and SCC.[81]

Radiation Therapy

Radiation therapy (RT) can be used as a primary treatment modality for eyelid tumors, but is most frequently used as an adjuvant therapy after surgical resection. This is mainly due to higher success rate for surgical resection, and significant ocular toxicity from radiation. RT can be sometimes combined with chemotherapy to enhance the effect of treatment. Primary RT was suggested for locally-advanced periocular BCC, with local control of 94% for primary and 67% for recurrent tumors, and for periocular SCC with local control rates of 89–93%.[82,83] It can also be considered as an adjuvant therapy in BCC or SCC with microscopic perineural invasion or positive surgical margins. A positive SLNB in a patient with SCC with no other metastasis is often treated with lymphadenectomy and adjuvant RT to the nodal basin.[84] Sebaceous carcinoma has low radiosensitivity, but RT has been used anecdotally when surgery was not possible, and as an adjuvant therapy for patients with regional lymphnode metastases after undergoing neck dissection. RT has been reported in extensive or recurrent eyelid melanoma and eyelid sweat gland tumors as adjuvant treatment after surgery or for treatment of regional nodal metastasis when patient may not be a good surgical candidate.[85-87] Adjuvant RT was shown to achieve better locoregional control and improved overall survival compared to surgical excision alone, in patients with Merkel cell tumor.[88, 89] The relatively high radiosensitivity of Merkel cell carcinoma, and its propensity for nodal metastasis, have led to the practice of empiric prophylactic adjuvant RT to the regional lymph node basins, whether nodal metastases was diagnosed or not; however, the National Comprehensive Cancer Network (NCCN) guidelines recommend sentinel lymph node biopsy as part of staging of Merkel cell carcinoma and radiation therapy to nodal basins only in the case of a positive SLN.[90] Lymphoma localized to the eyelid can be controlled with RT. Isolated metastases to the eyelid are not common, and can also be treated with surgery versus local RT, in addition to any other systemic treatment given for the primary cancer.

Chemotherapy

Various chemotherapeutic drugs have been used or treatment of metastatic tumors such as SCC, SGC and more.

Treating cutaneous angiosarcoma of the head-and-neck region with neoadjuvant chemotherapy was reported to have a complete response rate of 93%, and made definitive surgery unnecessary in 60% of patients.[46]

Targeted Biologic Therapy

Targeted therapy is an emerging modality of cancer therapy, which target specific molecules that are needed for carcinogenesis and tumor growth, in contrast with traditional chemotherapy that inhibits all rapidly-dividing cells. In the recent years, some of these drugs have been used to treat locally advanced eyelid tumors as well, specifically BCC, SCC and melanoma.

The Sonic Hedgehog (SHH) pathway was found to be mutated and abnormally active in multiple cancers, including sporadic BCC, BCC in patients with BCNS, and SCC. SHH inhibitors are a group of drugs that target the protein smoothened (smo), which is part of this pathway, thus blocking activation of transcription factors. Vismodegib (Erivedge™, Genentech, given orally at 150 mg daily) was the first drug approved by the FDA in 2012 for the treatment of metastatic and locally advanced BCC that has recurred after surgery or for patients who are not candidates for surgery or radiation therapy[91] Sonidegib (Odomzo®, Novartis, given orally at 200 mg daily) is another HHI approved by the FDA in 2015 for locally advanced BCC that has recurred after surgery or radiation, or not amenable for surgery or radiation.[92] In small series published on patients with eyelid BCC, response rate to vismodegib was 86% for locally advanced BCC, 100% for BCNS, and 33% for metastatic BCC.[93-95] Drug resistance has been reported in as much as 21% of patients with tumor progression occurring after a mean of 56 weeks of good initial response.[96] Side effects occur in 98–00% of patients, but are mostly mild, and include: muscle spasms (that can be alleviated by treatment with calcium-channel blockers), weight loss, changes in taste, decreased appetite and fatigue. The neoadjuvant use of SHH inhibitors prior to surgery is most intriguing and currently under study (Figs. 104.9A to C).

Cetuximab (Erbitux, Lilly) is an epidermal growth-factor receptor (EGFR) antagonist that is FDA-approved to treat locally or regionally advanced H&N SCC in combination with radiation or with platinum-based therapy with 5-FU. It has been used to treat SCC locally advanced periocular SCC invading the orbit.[97]

BRAF gene mutation V600E was found in up to 90% of cutaneous melanomas.[98] Vemurafenib and dabrafenib are selective BRAF inhibitors that target the BRAF V600E mutant kinase. Vemurafenib (Zelboraf, Genentech) is FDA-approved since 2011 for treatment of unresectable or metastatic melanomas that are positive for the V600E mutation.[99] Dabrafenib (Taflinar, Novartis) is FDA approved since 2013 for treatment of patients with unresectable or metastatic melanoma that is positive for V600E mutation, and also in combination with trametinib (Mekinist, Novartis, a MEK inhibitor) for V600K or V600E mutations.[100,101] We did not find reports of these drugs used for treatment of eyelid melanomas specifically but we have experienced positive responses in patients with melanoma metastatic to the orbit.

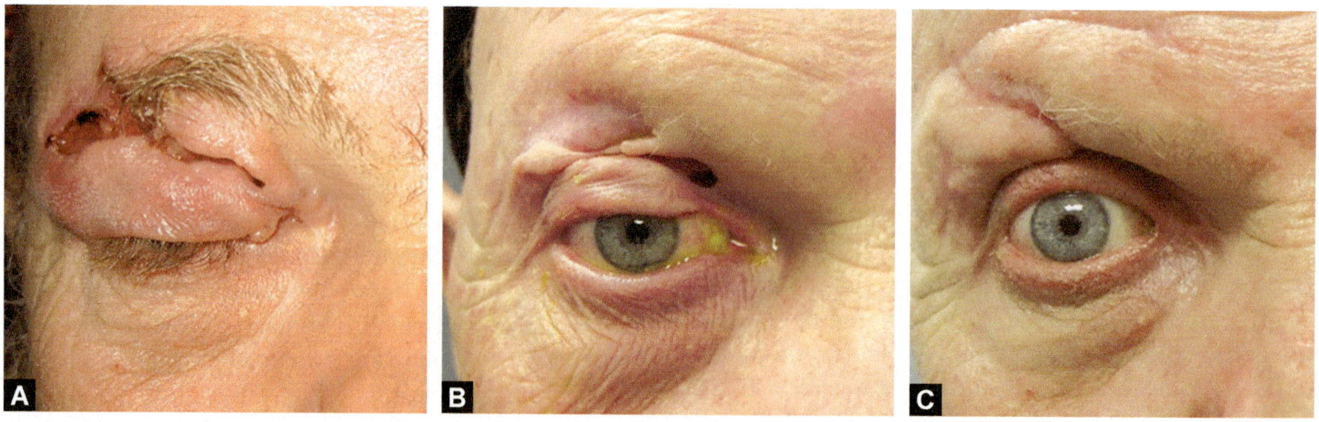

Figs. 104.9A to C: Clinical and postoperative photographs of a patient treated with neoadjuvant vismodegib for a recurrent, locally advanced basal cell carcinoma. (A) External photograph shows a large and deeply ulcerated basal cell carcinoma involving the right upper eyelid, brow, and anterior orbit with extension onto the lateral canthal soft tissue with areas of necrosis; (B) Clinically obvious positive response of tumor after an 18 months of treatment with daily oral vismodegib; (C) Postoperative outcome 5 months after surgical excision of small amount of residual BCC.

Immune Checkpoint Inhibitors

Cytotoxic T-lymphocyte antigen 4 (CTLA-4) and programmed cell death protein 1 (PD-1) are found on the surface of activated T-lymphocytes, and when activated, they inhibit the proliferation of T-lymphocytes. This new class of drugs block inhibitory checkpoints used by cancer cells to "hide" s from the immune system and currently include five FDA-approved drugs, four of which can be considered for patients with metastatic eyelid melanoma and for locally advanced squamous carcinomas of the periocular region.

Ipilimumab (Yervoy, Bristol-Myers Squibb), a CTLA-4 inhibitor, was FDA-approved in 2011 for the treatment of unresectable or metastatic melanoma, and as adjuvant treatment for patients with melanoma with lymph node metastasis of more than 1 mm, after total lymphadenectomy.[102] Nivolumab (Opdivo, Bristol-Myers Squibb) and pembrolizumab (Keytruda, Merck) are anti-PD-1 agents. Pembrolizumab, was approved in 2014, and is currently indicated for the treatment of metastatic melanoma, and recurrent or metastatic head and neck squamous cell carcinoma (HNSCC).[103] Nivolumab was approved in 2014 for patients with unresectable or metastatic melanoma and is indicated for recurrent or metastatic HNSCC.[104] Avelumab (BAVENCIO, EMD Serono), an anti-PD ligand-1 agent, was approved in 2017 for the treatment of metastatic Merkel cell carcinoma.[105] We have reported positive responses to Nivolumab and pembrolizumab in patients with metastatic eyelid or conjunctival melanoma and with cutaneous melanoma metastatic to the orbit.[106] We also have observed preliminary positive results for locally advanced recurrent SCC of the periocular region in response to immune check point inhibitors.

RECOMMENDATIONS FOR SURVEILLANCE

Patients with eyelid cancer require long-term surveillance after treatment, which is tailored according to the specific histologic type and stage of eyelid tumor at presentation. All patients should be instructed about and to report any signs of recurrence. For patients with BCC excised with negative margins, the authors usually do follow-up visits once a year for 5 years. Patients with other histologic types, such as melanoma, invasive SCC, or SGC require more frequent and longer follow-up. With recent advances in therapy, and the use of neoadjuvant or adjuvant medical and surgical treatments, patients may need shorter interval follow-ups and imaging studies to assess treatment response and to check for recurrence. The exact frequency of surveillance and the types of ancillary tests to order for each type of eyelid cancer is outside the scope of this chapter; we refer the reader to a recent Focal Points publication on this topic.[56]

REFERENCES

1. English DR, Kricker A, Heenan PJ, et al. Incidence of non-melanocytic skin cancer in Geraldton, Western Australia. Int J Cancer. 1997;73(5):629-33.
2. Bielsa I, Soria X, Esteve M, Ferrandiz C. Population-based incidence of basal cell carcinoma in a Spanish Mediterranean area. Br J Dermatol. 2009;161(6):1341-6.
3. Cook BE Jr., Bartley GB. Epidemiologic characteristics and clinical course of patients with malignant eyelid tumors in an incidence cohort in Olmsted County, Minnesota. Ophthalmology. 1999;106(4):746-50.
4. Malhotra AK, Gupta S, Khaitan BK, et al. Multiple basal cell carcinomas in xeroderma pigmentosum treated with imiquimod 5% cream. Pediatr Dermatol. 2008;25(4):488-91.
5. Honavar SG, Shields JA, Shields CL, et al. Basal cell carcinoma of the eyelid associated with Gorlin-Goltz syndrome. Ophthalmology. 2001;108(6):1115-23.
6. Limawararut V, Leibovitch I, Sullivan T, et al. Periocular squamous cell carcinoma. Clin Exp Ophthalmol. 2007;35(2):174-85.
7. Deprez M, Uffer S. Clinicopathological features of eyelid skin tumors. A retrospective study of 5504 cases and review of literature. Am J Dermatopathol. 2009;31(3):256-62.
8. Gallagher RP, Hill GB, Bajdik CD, et al. Sunlight exposure, pigmentation factors, and risk of nonmelanocytic skin cancer. II. Squamous cell carcinoma. Arch Dermatol. 1995;131(2):164-9.
9. Asuquo ME, Ngim O, Ebughe G, Bassey EE. Skin cancers amongst four Nigerian albinos. Int J Dermatol. 2009;48(6):636-8.
10. Herman S, Rogers HD, Ratner D. Immunosuppression and squamous cell carcinoma: a focus on solid organ transplant recipients. Skinmed. 2007;6(5):234-8.
11. Lohmann CM, Solomon AR. Clinicopathologic variants of cutaneous squamous cell carcinoma. Adv Anat Pathol. 2001;8(1):27-36.
12. Faustina M, Diba R, Ahmadi MA, et al. Patterns of regional and distant metastasis in patients with eyelid and periocular squamous cell carcinoma. Ophthalmology. 2004;111(10):1930-2.
13. Rowe DE, Carroll RJ, Day CL, Jr. Prognostic factors for local recurrence, metastasis, and survival rates in squamous cell carcinoma of the skin, ear, and lip. Implications for treatment modality selection. J Am Acad Dermatol. 1992;26(6):976-90.

14. Sheets SSF. (2015) Melanoma of the Skin. National Cancer Insitute Surveillance, Epidemiology and End Results Program. [online] Available from http://seer cancer gov/ statfacts/html/melan html. [Accessed December 2017]
15. Yu GP, Hu DN, McCormick SA. Latitude and incidence of ocular melanoma. Photochem Photobiol. 2006;82(6): 1621-6.
16. Wang Y, Digiovanna JJ, Stern JB, et al. Evidence of ultraviolet type mutations in xeroderma pigmentosum melanomas. Proc Natl Acad Sci USA. 2009;106(15):6279-84.
17. Chan FM, O'Donnell BA, Whitehead K, et al. Treatment and outcomes of malignant melanoma of the eyelid: a review of 29 cases in Australia. Ophthalmology. 2007;114(1):187-92.
18. Wick MM, Sober AJ, Fitzpatrick TB, et al. Clinical characteristics of early cutaneous melanoma. Cancer. 1980;45(10):2684-6.
19. Sanchez R, Ivan D, Esmaeli B. Eyelid and periorbital cutaneous malignant melanoma. Int Ophthalmol Clin. 2009 Fall;49(4):25-43.
20. Thakar S, Kandl TJ, Sagiv O, et al. Desmoplastic Melanoma of the Periorbital Region. Ophthal Plast Reconstr Surg. 2017.
21. Yin VT, Warneke CL, Merritt HA, et al. Number of excisions required to obtain clear surgical margins and prognostic value of AJCC T category for patients with eyelid melanoma. Br J Ophthalmol. 2014;98(12):1681-5.
22. Morton DL, Thompson JF, Cochran AJ, et al. Sentinel-node biopsy or nodal observation in melanoma. N Engl J Med. 2006;355(13):1307-17.
23. Shields JA, Demirci H, Marr BP, et al. Sebaceous carcinoma of the eyelids: personal experience with 60 cases. Ophthalmology. 2004;111(12):2151-7.
24. Song A, Carter KD, Syed NA, et al. Sebaceous cell carcinoma of the ocular adnexa: clinical presentations, histopathology, and outcomes. Ophthal Plast Reconstr Surg. 2008;24(3): 194-200.
25. Rao NA, Hidayat AA, McLean IW, et al. Sebaceous carcinomas of the ocular adnexa: A clinicopathologic study of 104 cases, with five-year follow-up data. Hum Pathol. 1982;13(2):113-22.
26. Takamura H, Yamashita H. Clinicopathological analysis of malignant eyelid tumor cases at Yamagata university hospital: statistical comparison of tumor incidence in Japan and in other countries. Jpn J Ophthalmol. 2005;49(5): 349-54.
27. Howrey RP, Lipham WJ, Schultz WH, et al. Sebaceous gland carcinoma: a subtle second malignancy following radiation therapy in patients with bilateral retinoblastoma. Cancer. 1998;83(4):767-71.
28. Rumelt S, Hogan NR, Rubin PA, Jakobiec FA. Four-eyelid sebaceous cell carcinoma following irradiation. Arch Ophthalmol. 1998;116(12):1670-2.
29. Rishi K, Font RL. Sebaceous gland tumors of the eyelids and conjunctiva in the Muir-Torre syndrome: a clinicopathologic study of five cases and literature review. Ophthal Plast Reconstr Surg. 2004;20(1):31-6.
30. Tetzlaff MT, Singh RR, Seviour EG, et al. Next-generation sequencing identifies high frequency of mutations in potentially clinically actionable genes in sebaceous carcinoma. The Journal of Pathology. 2016;240(1):84-95.
31. Ostler DA, Prieto VG, Reed JA, et al. Adipophilin expression in sebaceous tumors and other cutaneous lesions with clear cell histology: an immunohistochemical study of 117 cases. Modern pathology: an Official Journal of the United States and Canadian Academy of Pathology, Inc. 2010;23(4): 567-73.
32. Tan KC, Lee ST, Cheah ST. Surgical treatment of sebaceous carcinoma of eyelids with clinicopathological correlation. British Journal of Plastic Surgery. 1991;44(2):117-21.
33. Savar A, Oellers P, Myers J, et al. Positive sentinel node in sebaceous carcinoma of the eyelid. Ophthal Plast Reconstr Surg. 2011;27(1):e4-6.
34. Baker MS, Yin VT, Ivan D, et al. Epidemiology and Prognosis of Primary Periocular Sweat Gland Carcinomas. Ophthal Plast Reconstr Surg. 2017;33(2):101-5.
35. Miller RW, Rabkin CS. Merkel cell carcinoma and melanoma: etiological similarities and differences. Cancer epidemiology, biomarkers and prevention: a publication of the American Association for Cancer Research, cosponsored by the American Society of Preventive Oncology. 1999;8(2):153-8.
36. Buell JF, Trofe J, Hanaway MJ, et al. Immunosuppression and Merkel cell cancer. Transplant Proc. 2002;34(5):1780-1.
37. Eng TY, Boersma MG, Fuller CD, et al. A comprehensive review of the treatment of Merkel cell carcinoma. Am J Clin Oncol. 2007;30(6):624-36.
38. Missotten GS, de Wolff-Rouendaal D, de Keizer RJ. Merkel cell carcinoma of the eyelid review of the literature and report of patients with Merkel cell carcinoma showing spontaneous regression. Ophthalmology. 2008;115(1): 195-201.
39. Andea AA, Coit DG, Amin B, et al. Merkel cell carcinoma: histologic features and prognosis. Cancer. 2008;113(9): 2549-58.
40. Morrison WH, Byers RM, Garden AS, et al. Cutaneous angiosarcoma of the head and neck. A therapeutic dilemma. Cancer. 1995;76(2):319-27.
41. Tran LM, Mark R, Meier R, et al. Sarcomas of the head and neck. Prognostic factors and treatment strategies. Cancer. 1992;70(1):169-77.
42. Lapidus CS, Sutula FC, Stadecker MJ, et al. Angiosarcoma of the eyelid: yellow plaques causing ptosis. J Am Acad Dermatol. 1996;34(2 Pt 1):308-10.
43. Ettl T, Kleinheinz J, Mehrotra R, et al. Infraorbital cutaneous angiosarcoma: a diagnostic and therapeutic dilemma. Head Face Med. 2008;4:18.
44. Billings SD, McKenney JK, Folpe AL, et al. Cutaneous angiosarcoma following breast-conserving surgery and radiation: an analysis of 27 cases. Am J Surg Pathol. 2004;28(6):781-8.
45. Cabo H, Cohen ES, Casas GJ, et al. Cutaneous angiosarcoma arising on the radiation site of a congenital facial hemangioma. Int J Dermatol. 1998;37(8):638-9.
46. DeMartelaere SL1, Roberts D, Burgess MA,, et al. Neoadjuvant chemotherapy-specific and overall treatment outcomes in

patients with cutaneous angiosarcoma of the face with periorbital involvement. Head Neck. 2008;30(5):639-46.
47. Margo CE, Mulla ZD. Malignant tumors of the eyelid: a population-based study of non-basal cell and non-squamous cell malignant neoplasms. Arch Ophthalmol (Chicago, Ill : 1960). 1998;116(2):195-8.
48. Esmaeli B, Cleary KL, Ho L, et al. Leiomyosarcoma of the esophagus metastatic to the eyelid: a clinicopathologic report. Ophthal Plast Reconstr Surg. 2002;18(2):159-61.
49. Bianciotto C, Demirci H, Shields CL, et al. Metastatic tumors to the eyelid: report of 20 cases and review of the literature. Arch Ophthalmol (Chicago, Ill: 1960). 2009;127(8):999-1005.
50. Yeung SN, Blicker JA, Buffam FV, et al. Metastatic eyelid disease associated with hepatocellular carcinoma. Can J Ophthalmol. 2007;42(5):752-4.
51. Zanetti R, Rosso S, Martinez C, et al. The multicentre south European study 'Helios.' I: Skin characteristics and sunburns in basal cell and squamous cell carcinomas of the skin. Br J Cancer. 1996;73(11):1440-6.
52. Marrett LD, King WD, Walter SD, et al. Use of host factors to identify people at high risk for cutaneous malignant melanoma. CMAJ. 1992;147(4):445-53.
53. Kennedy C, Bajdik CD, Willemze R, et al. The influence of painful sunburns and lifetime sun exposure on the risk of actinic keratoses, seborrheic warts, melanocytic nevi, atypical nevi, and skin cancer. J Invest Dermatol. 2003;120(6):1087-93.
54. Fortes C, Mastroeni S, Melchi F, et al. The association between residential pesticide use and cutaneous melanoma. Eur J Cancer. 2007;43(6):1066-75.
55. Tsai T, Vu C, Henson DE. Cutaneous, ocular and visceral melanoma in African Americans and Caucasians. Melanoma Res. 2005;15(3):213-7.
56. Vivian T, Yin BE. Staging for Patients With Ocular, Orbital, and Ocular Adnexal Malignancies. American Academy of Ophthalmology; 2016.
57. Nemet AY, Deckel Y, Martin PA, et al. Management of periocular basal and squamous cell carcinoma: a series of 485 cases. Am J Ophthalmol. 2006;142(2):293-7.
58. Auw-Haedrich C, Frick S, Boehringer D, et al. Histologic safety margin in basal cell carcinoma of the eyelid: correlation with recurrence rate. Ophthalmology. 2009;116(4):802-6.
59. Malhotra R, Huilgol SC, Huynh NT, et al. The Australian Mohs database, part II: periocular basal cell carcinoma outcome at 5-year follow-up. Ophthalmology. 2004;111(4):631-6.
60. Bernardini FP. Management of malignant and benign eyelid lesions. Curr Opin Ophthalmol. 2006;17(5):480-4.
61. Pennington BE, Leffell DJ. Mohs micrographic surgery: established uses and emerging trends. Oncology (Williston Park). 2005;19(9):1165-71; discussion 1171-2, 1175.
62. Boulos PR, Rubin PA. Cutaneous melanomas of the eyelid. Semin Ophthalmol. 2006;21(3):195-206.
63. Pathai S, Barlow R, Williams G, et al. Mohs' micrographic surgery for Merkel cell carcinomas of the eyelid. Orbit. 2005;24(4):273-5.
64. Boyer JD, Zitelli JA, Brodland DG, et al. Local control of primary Merkel cell carcinoma: review of 45 cases treated with Mohs micrographic surgery with and without adjuvant radiation. J Am Acad Dermatol. 2002;47(6):885-92.
65. O'Connor WJ, Roenigk RK, Brodland DG. Merkel cell carcinoma. Comparison of Mohs micrographic surgery and wide excision in eighty-six patients. Dermatol Surg. 1997;23(10):929-33.
66. Whalen J, Leone D. Mohs micrographic surgery for the treatment of malignant melanoma. Clin Dermatol. 2009;27(6):597-602.
67. Cook J. Surgical margins for resection of primary cutaneous melanoma. Clin Dermatol. 2004;22(3):228-33.
68. Esmaeli B, Youssef A, Naderi A, et al. Margins of excision for cutaneous melanoma of the eyelid skin: the Collaborative Eyelid Skin Melanoma Group Report. Ophthal Plast Reconstr Surg. 2003;19(2):96-101.
69. Chao AN, Shields CL, Krema H, et al. Outcome of patients with periocular sebaceous gland carcinoma with and without conjunctival intraepithelial invasion. Ophthalmology. 2001;108(10):1877-83.
70. Shields JA, Demirci H, Marr BP, et al. Conjunctival epithelial involvement by eyelid sebaceous carcinoma. The 2003 J. Howard Stokes lecture. Ophthal Plast Reconstr Surg. 2005;21(2):92-6.
71. Gunalp I, Gunduz K, Duruk K. Orbital exenteration: a review of 429 cases. Int Ophthalmol. 1995-1996;19(3):177-84.
72. Tyers AG. Orbital exenteration for invasive skin tumours. Eye (Lond). 2006;20(10):1165-70.
73. Hsu A, Frank SJ, Ballo MT, et al. Postoperative adjuvant external-beam radiation therapy for cancers of the eyelid and conjunctiva. Ophthal Plast Reconstr Surg. 2008;24(6):444-9.
74. Prieto-Granada C, Rodriguez-Waitkus P. Sebaceous Carcinoma of the Eyelid. Cancer control: Journal of the Moffitt Cancer Center. 2016;23(2):126-32.
75. Esmaeli B. Sentinel node biopsy as a tool for accurate staging of eyelid and conjunctival malignancies. Current Opinion in Ophthalmology. 2002;13(5):317-23.
76. Brannan PA, Anderson HK, Kersten RC, Kulwin DR. Bowen disease of the eyelid successfully treated with imiquimod. Ophthal Plast Reconstr Surg. 2005;21(4):321-2.
77. Prokosch V, Thanos S, Spaniol K, et al. Long-term outcome after treatment with 5% topical imiquimod cream in patients with basal cell carcinoma of the eyelids. Graefe's archive for clinical and experimental ophthalmology = Albrecht von Graefes Archiv fur klinische und experimentelle Ophthalmologie. 2011;249(1):121-5.
78. Murchison AP, Washington CV, Soloman AR, Bernardino CR. Ocular effects of imiquimod with treatment of eyelid melanoma in situ. Dermatol Surg. 2007;33(9):1136-8.
79. Shields CL, Naseripour M, Shields JA, et al. Topical mitomycin-C for pagetoid invasion of the conjunctiva by eyelid sebaceous gland carcinoma. Ophthalmology. 2002;109(11):2129-33.
80. Peris K, Ferrari A, Fargnoli MC, et al. Dermoscopic monitoring of tazarotene treatment of superficial basal cell carcinoma. Dermatol Surg. 2005;31(2):217-20.

81. Puccioni M, Santoro N, Giansanti F, et al. Photodynamic therapy using methyl aminolevulinate acid in eyelid basal cell carcinoma: a 5-year follow-up study. Ophthal Plast Reconstr Surg. 2009;25(2):115-8.
82. Swanson EL, Amdur RJ, Mendenhall WM, et al. Radiotherapy for basal cell carcinoma of the medial canthus region. Laryngoscope. 2009;119(12):2366-8.
83. Petsuksiri J, Frank SJ, Garden AS, et al. Outcomes after radiotherapy for squamous cell carcinoma of the eyelid. Cancer. 2008;112(1):111-8.
84. Hinerman RW, Indelicato DJ, Amdur RJ, et al. Cutaneous squamous cell carcinoma metastatic to parotid-area lymph nodes. Laryngoscope. 2008;118(11):1989-96.
85. Durairaj VD, Hink EM, Kahook MY, et al. Mucinous eccrine adenocarcinoma of the periocular region. Ophthal Plast Reconstr Surg. 2006;22(1):30-5.
86. Auw-Haedrich C, Boehm N, Weissenberger C. Signet ring carcinoma of the eccrine sweat gland in the eyelid, treated by radiotherapy alone. Br J Ophthalmol. 2001;85(1):112-3.
87. Stannard CE, Sealy GR, Hering ER, et al. Malignant melanoma of the eyelid and palpebral conjunctiva treated with iodine-125 brachytherapy. Ophthalmology. 2000;107(5):951-8.
88. Gillenwater AM, Hessel AC, Morrison WH, et al. Merkel cell carcinoma of the head and neck: effect of surgical excision and radiation on recurrence and survival. Arch Otolaryngol Head Neck Surg. 2001;127(2):149-54.
89. Clark JR, Veness MJ, Gilbert R, et al. Merkel cell carcinoma of the head and neck: is adjuvant radiotherapy necessary? Head Neck. 2007;29(3):249-57.
90. NCCN Clinical Practice Guidelines in Oncology, Merkel Cell Carcinoma. Version 1.2017. 10/3/2016. NCCN website. Online: *https://www.nccn.org/professionals/physician_gls/pdf/mcc.pdf2017.*
91. US-FDA. FDA labeling information - ERIVEDGE. FDA website. Online: *https://www.accessdata.fda.gov/drugsatfda_docs/label/2012/203388lbl.pdf2012.*
92. US-FDA. FDA labeling information - ODOMZO. FDA website. Online: *https://www.accessdata.fda.gov/drugsatfda_docs/label/2015/205266s000lbl.pdf2015.*
93. Ozgur OK, Yin V, Chou E, et al. Hedgehog Pathway Inhibition for Locally Advanced Periocular Basal Cell Carcinoma and Basal Cell Nevus Syndrome. Am J Ophthalmol. 2015;160(2):220-7.e2.
94. Yin VT, Esmaeli B. Targeting the Hedgehog Pathway for Locally Advanced and Metastatic Basal Cell Carcinoma. Curr Pharm Des. 2017;23(4):655-9.
95. Demirci H, Worden F, Nelson CC, et al. Efficacy of Vismodegib (Erivedge) for Basal Cell Carcinoma Involving the Orbit and Periocular Area. Ophthal Plast Reconstr Surg. 2015;31(6):463-6.
96. Chang AL, Oro AE. Initial assessment of tumor regrowth after vismodegib in advanced basal cell carcinoma. Archives of Dermatology. 2012;148(11):1324-5.
97. El-Sawy T, Sabichi AL, Myers JN, et al. Epidermal growth factor receptor inhibitors for treatment of orbital squamous cell carcinoma. Arch Ophthalmol (Chicago, Ill : 1960). 2012;130(12):1608-11.
98. Chapman PB, Hauschild A, Robert C, et al. Improved survival with vemurafenib in melanoma with BRAF V600E mutation. N Engl J Med. 2011;364(26):2507-16.
99. US-FDA. FDA labeling information—ZELBORAF. FDA website. Online: *https://www.accessdata.fda.gov/drugsatfda_docs/label/2017/202429s012lbl.pdf2011.*
100. US-FDA. FDA labeling information—TAFLINAR. FDA website. Online: *https://www.accessdata.fda.gov/drugsatfda_docs/label/2014/202806s002lbl.pdf2013.*
101. US-FDA. FDA labeling information—MEKINIST. FDA website. Online: *https://www.accessdata.fda.gov/drugsatfda_docs/label/2014/204114s001lbl.pdf2013.*
102. US-FDA. FDA labeling information—YERVOY. FDA website. Online: *https://www.accessdata.fda.gov/drugsatfda_docs/label/2015/125377s074lbl.pdf. 2015.*
103. US-FDA. FDA labeling information—KEYTRUDA. FDA website. Online: *https://www.accessdata.fda.gov/drugsatfda_docs/label/2017/125514s015lbl.pdf. 2017.*
104. US-FDA. FDA labeling information—OPDIVO. FDA website. Online: *https://www.accessdata.fda.gov/drugsatfda_docs/label/2017/125554s024lbl.pdf. 2017.*
105. US-FDA. FDA labeling information—BAVENCIO. FDA website. Online: *https://www.accessdata.fda.gov/drugsatfda_docs/label/2017/761049s000lbl.pdf. 2017.*
106. Ford J, Thuro BA, Thakar S, et al. Immune Checkpoint Inhibitors for Treatment of Metastatic Melanoma of the Orbit and Ocular Adnexa. Ophthal Plast Reconstr Surg. 2017;33(4):e82-5.

Chapter 105 Orbital Tumors and Vascular Abnormalities

Honeylen Maryl T Teo, Hakan Demirci

INTRODUCTION

Orbital tumors can be classified based on their location within the orbit, clinical behavior, and site and tissue of origin. In this chapter, we will discuss orbital tumors based on their tissue of origin. These include vascular tumors and malformations or abnormalities, soft tissue tumors, neural tumors, lymphoproliferative disorders, and metastatic tumors. While most orbital tumors are benign, the constant possibility of visual decline and life-threatening sequelae with a delay in management always makes having an early, correct diagnosis imperative.

VASCULAR TUMORS AND MALFORMATIONS

Capillary Hemangioma

Capillary hemangioma, also known as infantile hemangioma, is the most common vascular orbital tumor in infants and children. It may be present at birth or develop a few weeks after birth, with a proliferative phase of rapid growth from 6 months to 1 year of age.[1,2] Studies reveal a higher incidence among newborns from mothers who underwent chorionic villous sampling.[3]

The pathogenesis by which capillary hemangioma occurs remains unknown. Immunohistochemical studies show glucose transporter 1 (GLUT1), which is normally expressed in the placenta, to also be present in capillary hemangioma. Placental microtrauma from the procedure is hypothesized to cause trophoblast embolization which leads to capillary hemangioma.[4] However, the absence of fetal-maternal chimerism in the lesion, and the fetal rather than maternal origin of the vascular endothelial cells[5,6] challenge the theory.

Most periorbital capillary hemangioma involves the skin and eyelid, but it may extend to adjacent ocular structures and into the orbit. Isolated orbital capillary hemangioma is less common, but may also occur.[1] Capillary hemangioma that involves the orbit and periocular tissue usually has no systemic involvement. However, a large facial capillary hemangioma may be associated with Kasabach-Merritt syndrome, a condition that involves superficial systemic and visceral hemangiomas with thrombocytopenia.[1,7]

Symptoms and Signs

Isolated deep orbital capillary hemangioma may be intraconal or extraconal.[8] An enlarging retrobulbar lesion may lead to hyperopia, painless axial proptosis, diplopia with restricted extraocular motility, and optic neuropathy with mass effect.[7] A capillary hemangioma in the anterior orbit may present as a reddish to bluish painless palpable mass that is usually located in the superior or superonasal quadrant, and may cause astigmatism and globe displacement with further tumor growth.[1,7]

Imaging

Orbital computed tomography (CT) reveals a homogeneous markedly enhancing irregular to well-defined mass.[8] Early imaging is important to distinguish capillary hemangioma from rhabdomyosarcoma. In orbital CT, orbital capillary hemangioma opacifies rapidly and more profusely than rhabdomyosarcoma due to a more direct expanded arterial supply.[7] Chronic lesions may lead to orbital expansion with bone remodeling, while rhabdomyosarcoma may have bone erosion.[1,8] Capillary hemangioma is heterogeneous on T1- and T2-weighted magnetic resonance imaging (MRI). It is hyperintense on T1, but hypointense to extraocular muscle on T2-weighted MRI due to high blood flow.[8]

Management

Because majority of capillary hemangioma spontaneously regress by age 5–7, an asymptomatic orbital capillary hemangioma is observed with periodic monitoring.[9] Management includes correction of refractive error and amblyopia therapy.[1]

Treatment options for a nonregressing anterior orbital and deep orbital capillary hemangioma include systemic beta-blocker (1–3 mg/kg/day) with 96% success rate,[10] intralesional steroid injection, and oral steroid (2 mg/kg/day) for cases unresponsive to intralesional injection. Surgery is reserved for cases with significant threat to vision and severe complications from initial pharmacologic treatment.[11]

Histopathology

Pericytes support the endothelial cells of capillary hemangioma. This is in contrast to the smooth muscle cells that support the endothelial cells of cavernous hemangioma.[12]

Cavernous Hemangioma

Cavernous hemangioma is the most common benign orbital neoplasm among adults.[13] It is a unilateral lesion that usually affects females in their fourth decade of life.[14] Although the tumor grows gradually, its enlargement is accelerated with pregnancy.[15] Cases of multiple cavernous hemangioma in the same orbit[16] and bilateral orbits have also been reported.[17] These have been associated with Maffucci syndrome[18] and blue rubber bleb nevus syndrome.[19]

Symptoms and Signs

Cavernous hemangioma is usually intraconal, but extraconal tumors may occur.[20] Depending on its location and extent, symptoms may include hyperopia from mass effect, diplopia, gaze-evoked amaurosis fugax from an ischemic optic nerve,[21] and scotoma and visual loss from optic atrophy.[22] The lesion is painless, but reported headache and periorbital pain may be associated with the enlargement of the tumor within the confined bony orbital cavity.[7]

The most common sign is slowly progressive, painless, nonpulsatile axial proptosis from mass effect.[14] Other ophthalmologic findings include retinal striae, choroidal folds, optic disc edema or pallor, relative afferent pupillary defect (RAPD), globe displacement, and strabismus.[22]

Imaging

Orbital CT reveals a well-circumscribed, homogeneous, round to ovoid hyperdense mass compared to extraocular muscle.[23] They show variable mild to moderate contrast enhancement.[8] Hyperdense phleboliths and bone remodeling can be seen in large, chronic lesions.[14,20] Cavernous hemangioma is isointense to extraocular muscle on T1-weighted MRI, but it is hyperintense to extraocular muscle on T2-weighted MRI (*see* Figs. 105.1 to 105.4).[14]

Management

Although spontaneous involution is rare, asymptomatic incidental findings may be observed and regularly followed up.[24] The main indications for surgery include functional visual decline, pain, and disfigurement.[25] The definitive treatment involves complete surgical excision. However,

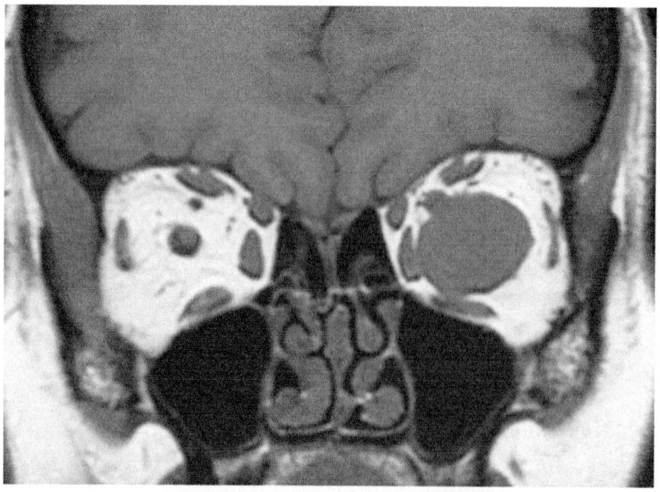

Fig. 105.1: Cavernous hemangioma seen via coronal T1-weighted magnetic resonance imaging (MRI) without contrast. There is a well-circumscribed, homogeneous left intraconal mass that is isointense to extraocular muscles, but hypointense to fat.

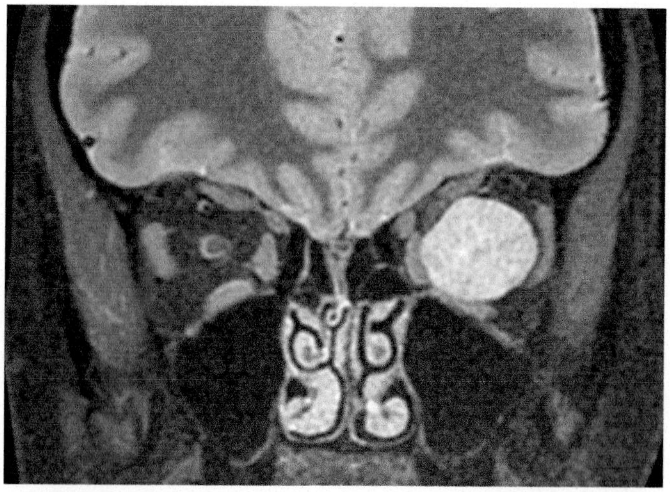

Fig. 105.2: Cavernous hemangioma seen via coronal T2-weighted MRI without contrast. The mass is hyperintense to extraocular muscles.

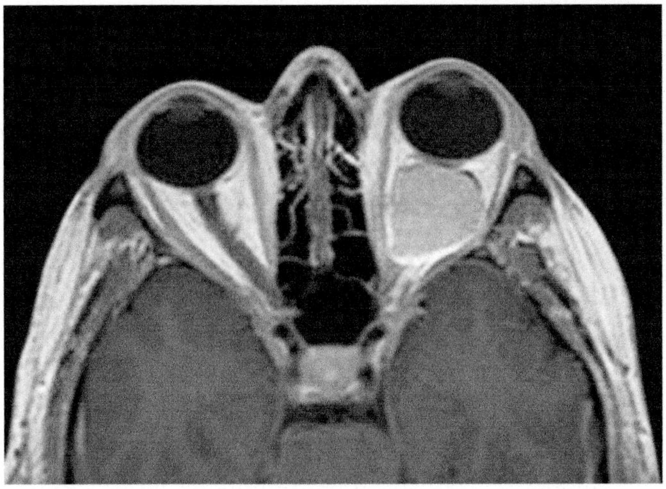

Fig. 105.3: Cavernous hemangioma seen via axial T1-weighted MRI with contrast. The mass mildly enhances with contrast in the left orbit of the same patient.

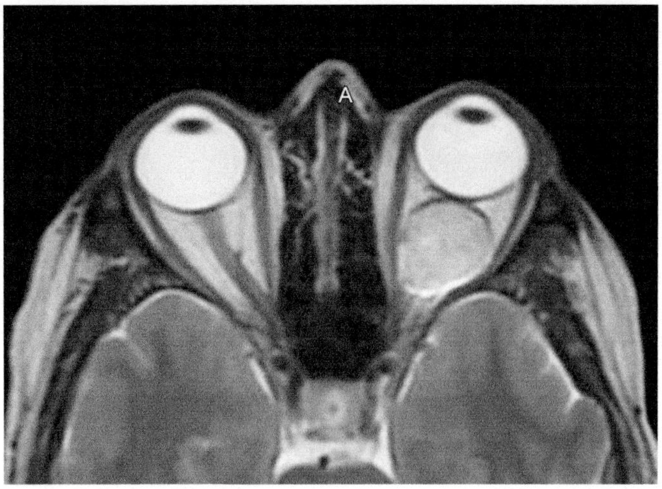

Fig. 105.4: Cavernous hemangioma seen via axial T2-weighted MRI with contrast. The mass mildly enhances with contrast in the left orbit of the same patient.

an incomplete excision does not always necessarily require immediate secondary surgery due to the indolent nature of the tumor.

Histopathology

The lesions are encapsulated and are composed of large cavernous spaces containing red blood cells (RBCs), and the walls of the spaces contain smooth muscle.[12]

Lymphatic Malformation

Lymphatic malformation, previously known as lymphangioma, is a congenital malformation that arises from pluripotent vascular anlage,[26] and often clinically presents in the first decade of life. It may occur solitarily or as part of an extensive lesion that diffusely involves adjacent structures in the orbit, eyelid, conjunctiva, oropharynx, sinuses, or brain.[27] Rarely, lymphatic malformation may be associated with noncontiguous intracranial vascular anomalies such as developmental venous anomalies and arteriovenous malformation (AVM).[28,29]

Symptoms and Signs

The usual feature is a painless, slowly progressive proptosis.[28] There may be a history of upper respiratory tract infection or trauma.[27] A large extraconal or anterior orbital lesion may lead to globe displacement.[28] Eyelid involvement may present with blepharoptosis and amblyopia,[30] while conjunctival involvement may present with clear or hemorrhagic lymph channels.[31] Deep orbital lesions may be asymptomatic.[28]

The dreaded complications are associated with bleeding in the lymphatic channels that form "chocolate cysts",[32] which may compress adjacent orbital structures. This may lead to acute proptosis, exposure keratopathy, increased intraocular pressure, ophthalmoplegia, eyelid ecchymosis, subconjunctival hemorrhage, and optic neuropathy with visual deterioration.[30-32]

Unlike orbital varices, lymphatic malformation is isolated from orbital arterial and venous systems. Thus, it is not affected by Valsalva maneuver and postural changes such as inversion.[33]

Imaging

A fluid-fluid layering on MRI is pathognomonic of lymphatic malformation.[33] MRI reveals a heterogeneous, diffuse, infiltrating, multicystic lesion with varying signal intensity depending on the age of the blood within the cysts. In both T1-weighted and T2-weighted MRI, deoxyhemoglobin in the acute hemorrhage is hypointense; paramagnetic methemoglobin from RBC lysis is hyperintense; while hemosiderin and ferritin from methemoglobin degradation are hypointense compared to extraocular muscle (*see* Figs. 105.5 to 105.7).[8,34]

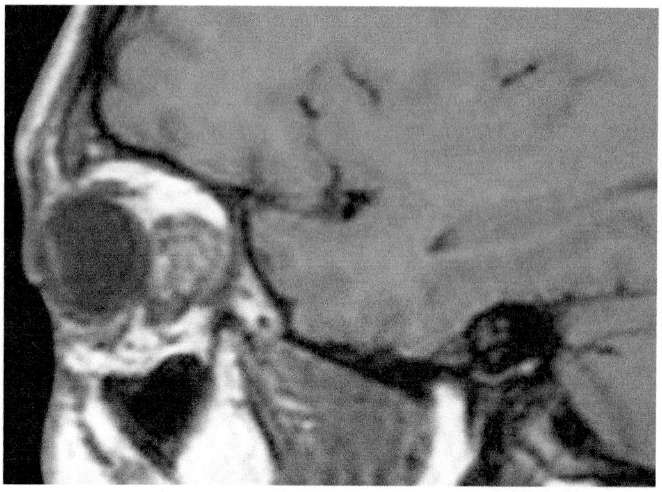

Fig. 105.5: Lymphangioma seen via sagittal T1-weighted MRI without contrast. There is a heterogeneous multicystic intraconal mass of varying signal intensity that denotes the presence of different blood degradation products.

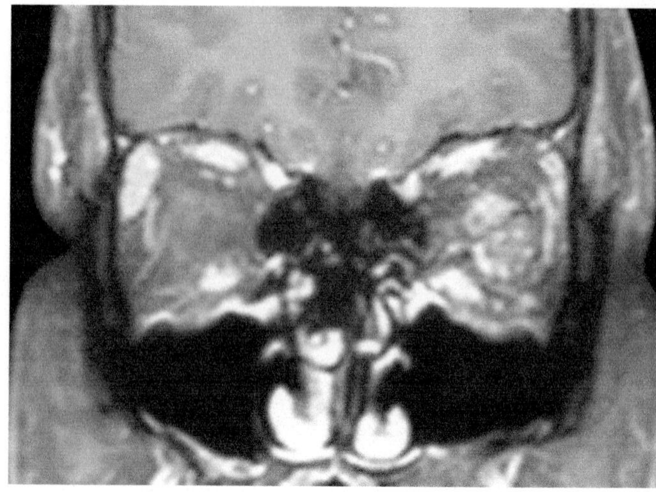

Fig. 105.6: Lymphangioma seen via coronal T1-weighted MRI with contrast and fat suppression. The septations of the multicystic lesion is seen in the left orbit of the same patient.

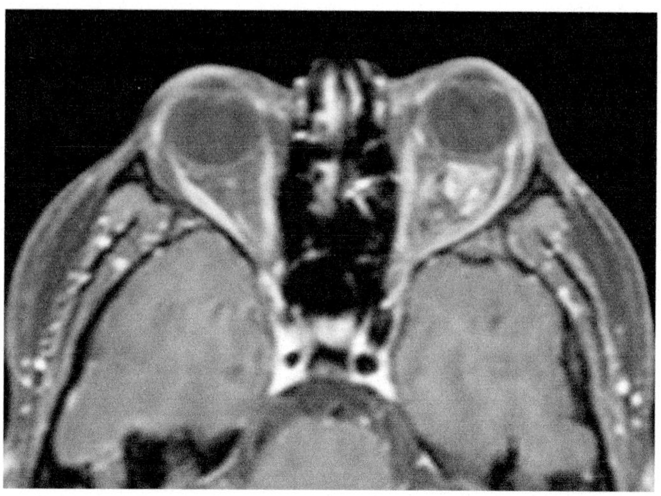

Fig. 105.7: Lymphangioma seen via axial T1-weighted MRI with contrast and fat suppression. The pathognomonic fluid-fluid layering is evident in the intraconal lymphangioma in the left orbit of the same patient.

Orbital CT scan reveals an ill-defined heterogeneous infiltrative lesion that crosses anatomic septa and fascial layers. Bone remodeling may be noted for large, slow growing lesions. Intracystic phleboliths may be present for chronic lesions.[23]

Management

The management ranges from observation to medical treatment of acute episodes, embolization, sclerotherapy, and surgery. Deep, asymptomatic lesions may be observed. Acute episodes associated with viral infections may be managed with prophylactic oral antibiotics and steroids to prevent bacterial coinfection and to decrease inflammation, respectively. Orbital hemorrhage may be allowed to resorb spontaneously or temporarily decompressed through surgical aspiration.[30,31] The indications for surgery include visual deterioration from compressive orbital signs, risk of amblyopia from blepharoptosis, and facial disfigurement or unacceptable cosmesis.[30-32] Embolization or sclerotherapy has been performed to induce intralesional fibrosis prior to surgery. However, visual loss from increased orbital pressure and chemical toxicity has been reported. If complete excision could not be performed, large lesions may be surgically debulked, albeit with a higher risk of hemorrhage and recurrence.[31]

Venous Malformation

Venous malformation of the orbit, also known as orbital varix, is a congenital vascular dysgenesis that presents from the second to third decade of life.[35] Venous malformation is characterized by congenitally weak veins with abnormal venous tangles, which distinguishes this lesion from venous ectasia.[36] It may be associated with intracranial venous malformation or hemifacial malformation that involves the scalp, temple, eyelid, cheek, and mouth.[7,37]

Symptoms and Signs

Slow blood flow from thrombosis and recanalization through the valveless lesion to the cavernous sinus and systemic veins lead to its clinical presentation. Proptosis or exophthalmos with increased intravenous pressure during Valsalva maneuver, or with dependent head position during head inversion or prone position, is a classic feature of venous malformation.[36,38,39] Large, chronic lesions may cause gradual orbit enlargement and fat atrophy, with notable enophthalmos at rest when the lesion is not engorged.[38] Other features include compressive optic neuropathy, exposure keratopathy, ophthalmoplegia, blepharoptosis, amblyopia, astigmatism, vermiform conjunctival mass,[40] and chemosis. Venous malformation has a relentless, unpredictable enlargement.[7] Complications include orbital compartment syndrome and pain from thrombosis and hemorrhage.[35]

Imaging

In some cases with narrow or fewer outflow vessels, venous distention is only seen via imaging.[38] Orbital MRI and CT scan with contrast performed during Valsalva maneuver or in prone position reveal engorged veins.[33,39] MRI is preferred over CT to show the heterogeneity, distensibility, and extent of the lesion. Both T1-weighted and T2-weighted MRI reveal a hypointense to isointense lesion compared to extraocular muscle. Signal intensity depends on the presence of blood degradation products such as deoxyhemoglobin, paramagnetic methemoglobin, hemosiderin, and ferritin.[8]

Computed tomography scan may reveal phleboliths from the low flow.[35] Contrast shows enhancement in patent venous areas, but without enhancement in thrombotic areas.

Management

Surgery is indicated for orbital pain, compressive optic neuropathy, and disfigurement.[38] Complete surgical excision, especially for lesions located deep in the orbit, is difficult due to involvement of normal adjacent structures, direct communication with venous reservoir, and rupture of intralesional thin-walled veins intraoperatively.[36] A Trendelenburg position, increased intrathoracic pressure through medication, and jugular compression may be performed during surgery for an easier identification and dissection of the malformation that is usually collapsed in the supine position.[41]

Due to the risk of severe bleeding, embolization and sclerotherapy may be performed prior to, during, or as an alternative to surgery.[38] The use of sclerosants may be monitored with intraoperative venography to prevent complications such as cavernous sinus thrombosis.

Arteriovenous Malformation

Arteriovenous malformation (AVM) is a congenital vascular dysgenesis that directly connects high flow arteries to low resistance veins. It is usually present at birth and childhood,[42] but may remain asymptomatic until the second to fourth decade of life. AVM may present as a gradually enlarging to a rapidly enlarging lesion. Aggravating factors include puberty, pregnancy, and trauma.[43,44]

Pure orbital AVM is rare.[45] Similar to venous malformation, orbital and periocular AVM may occur in isolation or may have hemifacial involvement that includes the maxilla, ears, nose, and forehead. Ipsilateral orbital AVM may be associated with retinal or cerebral AVM in Wyburn-Mason syndrome.[45,46]

Symptoms and Signs

Anterior orbital AVM may present as a bluish pulsatile subcutaneous mass. Although rarer, AVM is more destructive compared to other vascular malformation. Dystrophic skin changes secondary to tissue hypoxia include ulceration, bleeding, and necrosis.[47]

Small, deep orbital AVM may be asymptomatic.[42] Larger orbital AVM may present with pulsatile exophthalmos with bruit or thrill.[33] Orbital congestion may be evident as lid swelling, blepharoptosis, chemosis, and dilated corkscrewing of episcleral vessels with increased episcleral venous pressure and intraocular pressure.[45] Optic neuropathy with visual loss may result from diversion of blood flow from the ophthalmic artery.[44]

Imaging

Arteriography is preferred as both a diagnostic and therapeutic tool to identify the rapid filling of feeder arteries and opacification of the enlarged veins.[42,45]

Computed tomography scan and T1-weighted MRI reveal AVM as a serpiginous hypodense and hypointense lesion due to high flowing blood. T2-weighted MRI signal intensity varies depending on the state of blood degradation products.[8] Contrast reveals marked enhancement on imaging.[33]

Management

Management includes observation, embolization, and surgery. Small lesions may be observed and regularly followed up.[42,45] The low resistance shunt from the feeding arteries to the draining veins may cause rapid enlargement of the lesion.

The main treatment for orbital AVM is surgical resection with preoperative angiography and embolization to decrease perioperative bleeding.[45,48] Indications include pain, visual loss, disfigurement,[45] and life-threatening congestive heart failure.[47] In most cases, complete surgical excision of a large AVM and visual loss from either embolism or from destruction of normal orbital structures make the surgery difficult. It may also be challenging to differentiate the AVM from the collateral vessels, which may increase the risk for recurrence from incomplete surgical excision.[43]

SOFT TISSUE TUMORS

Solitary Fibrous Tumor

Solitary fibrous tumor is an indolent benign spindle cell neoplasm that usually affects the pleura, but may affect extrapleural sites such as the orbit. It commonly affects adults, with a few reported cases among children.[49,50] The diagnosis is confirmed through histopathologic and immunohistochemistry examination. It is differentiated from other orbital space-occupying lesions via a strong and diffuse positive staining for CD34[51] and STAT6.[52] It also stains positively for bcl2[53] and CD99,[54] while it stains mostly negatively for keratin, S-100 protein, and smooth muscle-specific actin.[55]

Since the characterization of its immunohistochemistry properties in 1994, some orbital tumors have been reclassified as solitary fibrous tumor. Tumors once considered distinct entities such as hemangiopericytoma, giant cell angiofibroma, and fibrous histiocytoma are now categorized as variants of solitary fibrous tumor.[56-58]

Symptoms and Signs

Solitary fibrous tumor may involve any part of the orbit including the extraconal and intraconal space, lacrimal gland fossa,[59] lacrimal sac,[60,61] and eyelids.[62] It commonly presents as a unilateral, gradual, painless proptosis.[63] Other signs include globe displacement, palpable mass, restricted extraocular motility, blepharoptosis, and lid swelling.[63]

Imaging

Orbital CT scan reveals an oval, well-defined, moderately to markedly enhancing mass that is isodense to extraocular muscles. Orbital bone remodeling may be seen in chronic lesions (*see* Figs. 105.8 and 105.9).

T1-weighted MRI shows a homogeneous isointense lesion compared to gray matter. T2-weighted MRI shows a heterogeneously hypointense to isointense mass with marked enhancement from its high vascularity.[64]

Management

Complete excision is the definitive treatment. Incomplete excision is the most important factor associated with local recurrence and malignant transformation. The management becomes difficult as a recurrent tumor infiltrates adjacent tissues, bone, and extends to the intracranial region.[65]

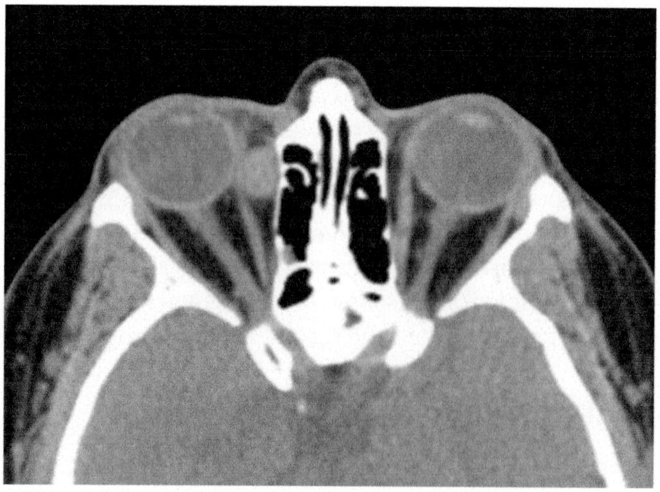

Fig. 105.8: Solitary fibrous tumor seen via axial computed tomography (CT) scan without contrast. There is an oval, well-defined extraconal mass that is isodense to extraocular muscles in the right orbit.

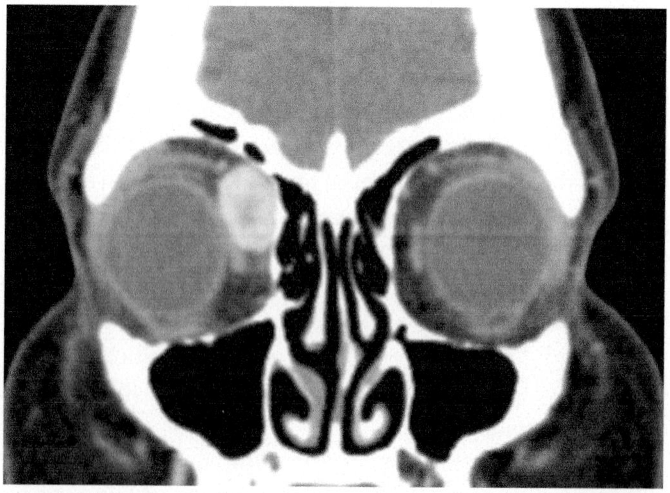

Fig. 105.9: Solitary fibrous tumor seen via coronal CT scan with contrast. The mass moderately enhances in the right medial orbit of the same patient.

Regular long-term follow-up is important due to the poor correlation between the histologic morphology and malignant potential of this tumor.[63]

Rhabdomyosarcoma

Rhabdomyosarcoma is the most common primary orbital malignancy in childhood.[66] It commonly occurs among boys between 7 years and 9 years of age. Primary rhabdomyosarcoma is usually unilateral, but tumors from the paranasal sinuses may be bilateral.[8,67] It is mostly sporadic, but it can be seen in syndromes such as neurofibromatosis[68] and Wilms tumor.[69] In some cases, an association with prior trauma usually contributes to a delay in the diagnosis and treatment.[67,70]

Symptoms and Signs

The clinical feature depends on the site of origin and location of the tumor. Eyelid involvement may reveal ptosis, lid edema, and bluish or reddish skin discoloration that resembles ecchymosis and acute infection.[7]

An abrupt onset and progression of proptosis and globe displacement are the hallmark of rhabdomyosarcoma.[66,71] These occur over days to weeks. However, rhabdomyosarcomas that arise in the orbit and those in older children may initially present insidiously over weeks to months, and may mimic other orbital tumors. Choroidal folds, visual loss from optic neuropathy and atrophy, and ophthalmoplegia may be noted.[66,71] The initially painless proptosis in orbital rhabdomyosarcoma may become painful with orbital bone erosion[72] that may metastasize to the central nervous system, lung, and bone.[67]

Imaging

Computed tomography and MRI reveal an initially well-circumscribed, enhancing, homogeneous mass that becomes irregular and heterogeneous with tumor enlargement. Rhabdomyosarcoma is isodense to extraocular muscle on CT. T1-weighted MRI reveals isointensity, while T2-weighted MRI reveals hyperintensity to extraocular muscles.[72]

Most tumors may conform to adjacent bony walls and orbital structures. Large tumors may lead to bony erosion with subsequent intracranial extension.[72]

Evaluation of lymph nodes, chest CT scan, bone scan, and bilateral bone marrow aspiration biopsy must be performed at the time of biopsy to rule out metastasis.[7]

Management

Early histopathologic diagnosis via biopsy is imperative for proper treatment to prevent metastasis.[70] Pleomorphic, embryonal, and alveolar have the best to worst prognosis, respectively. Embryonal is the most common histologic type, and is commonly located in the superonasal orbit. Alveolar type is commonly located in the inferior orbit.[73] Botryoid secondarily affects the orbit from the conjunctiva or epibulbar tissue.[7]

Orbital rhabdomyosarcoma has a 91% survival rate if the tumor has not invaded beyond the bony orbit.[74,75] Chemotherapy and radiotherapy are the main treatment. Surgical excision alone may be performed for biopsy or tumor debulking. However, it often leaves microscopic residual tissue with subsequent tumor recurrence, so adjunctive chemotherapy with or without radiotherapy is required.[76] In the case of recurrence, exenteration is usually performed.

NEURAL TUMORS

Optic Nerve Glioma

Optic nerve glioma is the most common primary benign neural tumor in children within their first decade of life. It is either isolated or a part of neurofibromatosis type 1. Tumors associated with neurofibromatosis type 1 are more commonly bilateral.[77]

Symptoms and Signs

A gradual, painless, unilateral axial proptosis is the main feature.[77] Optic nerve edema followed by optic nerve pallor may lead to visual deterioration. RAPD, ophthalmoplegia, and nystagmus may be present.[77,78] Optic nerve glioma may extend posteriorly to the chiasm, optic tract, and the rest of the optic pathway. In this case, it is called optic pathway glioma. The other features depend on the extent of the tumor within the optic pathway. A chiasmal lesion may have bitemporal hemianopsia, while a more posterior lesion may lead to homonymous hemianopsia, increased intracranial pressure, and endocrine signs.[77,78]

Imaging

Orbital and cranial MRI is preferred over CT to identify the extent in the optic pathway.[78] Furthermore, MRI does not expose young children to irradiation so serial imaging can be performed.[77] The hallmark of optic nerve glioma is fusiform or lobulated enlargement of the optic nerve with frequent kinking and cystic areas. This allows for a presumptive diagnosis on neuroimaging.

The lesion is isointense and hyperintense on T1-weighted and T2-weighted MRI, respectively. Cystic degeneration and cerebrospinal fluid (CSF) are hypointense on T1-weighted MRI, but hyperintense on T2-weighted MRI.[8]

Management

Biopsy is unnecessary for proper management. It may lead to further visual loss from nerve destruction or to misdiagnosis when tissue specimen is taken too peripheral in the lesion.

Due to its slow-growing behavior and some reported cases of spontaneous regression,[77,79,80] optic nerve glioma is often initially observed to preserve vision. However, periodic MRI is important for early detection of posterior extension.[77,80]

Complete surgical resection is performed for a rapidly growing tumor prior to chiasmal involvement. Indications include visual loss, proptosis with severe discomfort, and unacceptable cosmesis.[77,78,80] Surgery does not improve survival in those with optic pathway gliomas, but shunt insertion may be performed to control hydrocephalus.[77,78]

Radiotherapy is reserved for gliomas that could not be completely resected, for those with continued posterior invasion despite surgery, and for older children. Radiotherapy is reserved for optic pathway gliomas in older children to avoid radiation-induced complications such as pituitary insufficiency, secondary tumor development, and bone hypoplasia.[77,78]

Chemotherapy is currently the main treatment for younger children with large optic pathway glioma. Unlike radiotherapy, chemotherapy allows further neuroendocrine development in children. However, adverse effects still occur so risks versus benefits should be weighed.[78,80]

Optic Nerve Sheath Meningioma

Optic nerve sheath meningioma arises from meningothelial cells of the arachnoid villi of the optic nerve sheath. It is common among females in their third to sixth decade of life. Most are unilateral, but bilateral cases usually associated with neurofibromatosis type 2 occur.[81] Bilaterality can be from two distinct tumors, from spread of a planum sphenoidale meningioma to both optic canals, or from a unilateral tumor spreading across the planum to the contralateral optic canal.[82] The tumor gradually enlarges over years, but pregnancy has been associated with rapid growth.[83]

Symptoms and Signs

The triad of optic nerve sheath meningioma includes visual loss, optic atrophy, and optociliary shunt. The triad is not invariably present as the optociliary shunt only occurs in 25–30% of cases.[82,83] The optic disc may initially be normal. Further nerve compression may lead to optic disc edema, the initial and most common optic nerve change. Optic atrophy with visual loss and visual field defect gradually worsens over years. Axial proptosis follows visual deterioration. Other clinical features include RAPD, ophthalmoplegia, lower eyelid edema, and chemosis. There may also be a nonspecific boring headache and periorbital pain.[83]

Imaging

Magnetic resonance imaging is preferred over CT scan to identify its intracanalicular and intracranial extent,[82] to monitor for recurrence, and to evaluate the lesion prior to radiotherapy. T1-weighted MRI shows an isointense tumor compared to the extraocular muscle and optic nerve, while T2-weighted MRI shows a heterogeneous tumor that is slightly hypointense (calcified areas) to slightly hyperintense (CSF or cysts) to the cerebral gray matter.[84] With contrast, diffuse tubular enhancement of the tumor around the optic nerve is the most common pattern.[82] CT scan may reveal the characteristic finding of tram-track sign in 25% of cases.[82,85] This represents calcification within the tumor that usually implies chronicity.[82]

Other radiologic patterns include a fusiform, globular, or focal knobby (en plaque variant) exophytic tumor that breaks through the dura.[82] These enhance with contrast on both CT and MRI.

Management

Treatment depends on the clinical signs and extent of the tumor. Biopsy is reserved for atypical cases. Due to its indolent nature, observation via regular clinical examination with serial imaging is the first line of management for those with good vision.[82,83] Radiotherapy is given for continual visual deterioration, posterior tumor extent that is beyond resection, or postresection with posterior intracanalicular invasion. Surgical tumor resection is technically difficult and often leads to visual loss from compromised pial blood supply to the optic nerve. It is reserved for those with severe visual loss, prechiasmal or parachiasmal lesion with risks of intracranial tumor extent, and proptosis with unacceptable cosmesis.[82,84]

Sphenoid Wing Meningioma

This is the most common tumor of the sphenoid wing.[86] Sphenoid wing meningioma is a slow-growing tumor that arises from the dura of the sphenoid bone and extends into the orbit via the sphenoid bone itself, or via the superior orbital fissure or optic canal.[87] It commonly occurs among women in their fifth decade of life.[88]

Symptoms and Signs

The clinical presentation depends on the location and extent of the tumor. Tumors from the lateral part that involve the greater wing of the sphenoid may lead to temporal fossa enlargement and nonaxial proptosis, which is the most common feature.[87] Tumors from the medial part that involve the lesser wing of the sphenoid may affect the optic nerve through the superior orbital fissure and optic canal. These may present with optic disc edema, optic atrophy, visual loss, visual field defect, ophthalmoplegia, and venous congestion with subsequent lower lid edema and chemosis.[86,89]

Imaging

Magnetic resonance imaging is preferred over CT scan to locate the tumor and to delineate any posterior intracanalicular and intracranial dural extension.[90] T1-weighted and T2-weighted MRI show an isointense to slightly hypointense enhancing tumor compared to extraocular muscle.[8,88] In T1-weighted MRI, the intra-osseous tumor is more homogeneous and hyperintense; in T2-weighted MRI, the intraosseous tumor remains hypointense. Contrast enhancement defines the tumor extent along the dura.[90]

Orbital CT scan delineates hyperostosis in sphenoid wing meningioma.[90] It shows a well-defined isodense to slightly hyperdense enhancing lesion compared to extraocular muscle. There may be bone hyperostosis with hyperdensity from hyperplasia of soft tissues.[8] Periodic neuroimaging is important to monitor for intracranial extension, tumor enlargement, and recurrence (*see* Figs. 105.10 and 105.11).[87]

Management

Observation is the primary management for tumors without visual deterioration and neuro-ophthalmologic deficits. Surgical tumor resection is performed to relieve its compressive effects. However, complete removal may be difficult in the presence of dural tail and posterior tumor extension beyond the orbit. In such cases, near-

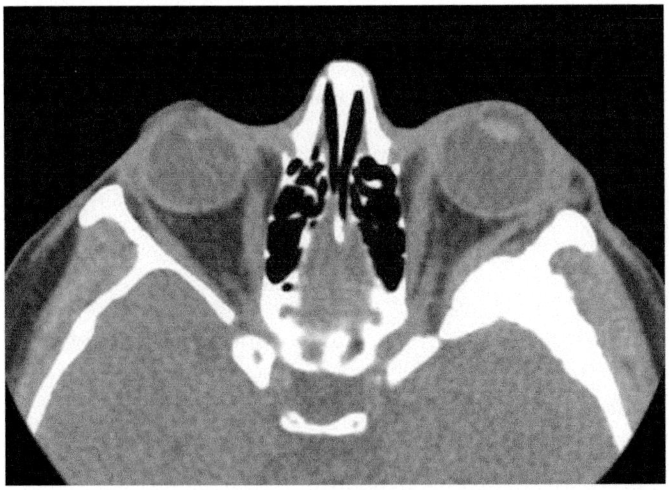

Fig. 105.10: Sphenoid wing meningioma seen via axial CT scan without contrast. There is a hyperdense hyperostosis of the left sphenoid bone.

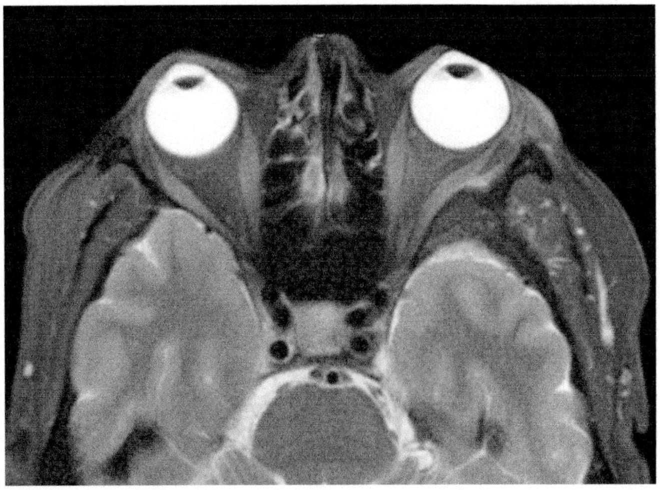

Fig. 105.11: Sphenoid wing meningioma seen via axial T2-weighted MRI without contrast. There is a slightly hypointense sphenoid wing meningioma in the left orbit of the same patient.

total tumor resection with removal of the hyperostotic bone, with or without orbital wall reconstruction,[91] must be performed. Aggressive tumor resection in the cavernous sinus, superior orbital fissure, and intracanalicular region is not recommended due to risks of serious morbidities.[86] Adjuvant radiotherapy may be given to decrease the risk of tumor invasion and recurrence, and increase the 10-year survival to 81% over 8 years.[92]

Neurofibroma

Neurofibroma is the most common peripheral nerve tumor of the orbit. This tumor arises from Schwann cells, axons, perineural cells, and fibroblasts.[93] The three types of neurofibroma include: (1) solitary, isolated, or localized; (2) plexiform; and (3) diffuse.[94] The clinical features of plexiform and diffuse neurofibromas are similar, but diffuse neurofibroma rarely occurs in the orbit.[95] In this chapter, we will focus on localized neurofibroma.

Localized Neurofibroma

Localized neurofibroma, also known as solitary or isolated neurofibroma, is a rare, benign, slow-growing tumor that affects middle-aged adults in their third to fifth decade of life. It commonly affects the supraorbital and supratrochlear branches of the ophthalmic division of the trigeminal nerve in the superior orbit.[96] Neurofibroma may also affect the lacrimal gland and may be difficult to distinguish from a primary lacrimal gland tumor.[97]

Localized neurofibroma is often unilateral. In rare cases, multiple solitary neurofibromas located in a unilateral orbit have been reported. These have been more appropriately referred to as localized, instead of solitary or isolated, neurofibroma.[94,98] Compared to plexiform neurofibroma, localized neurofibroma is less commonly associated with neurofibromatosis type 1.[94,95]

Symptoms and Signs

The clinical features of localized neurofibroma may be similar to the mass effect of other well-defined orbital tumors such as schwannoma. There may be gradually progressive proptosis, downward globe displacement, and paresthesia or pain along the distribution of the affected sensory nerves.[96]

Imaging

Orbital CT scan reveals an ovoid, well-defined, homogeneously isodense to slightly hyperdense tumor compared to extraocular muscle.[95] The radiologic features may appear similar to orbital schwannoma and cavernous hemangioma. Compared to cavernous hemangioma, however, localized neurofibroma is usually elongated anteroposteriorly along the involved nerve. T1-weighted MRI shows a homogeneous to heterogeneous lesion that is isointense, while T2-weighted MRI shows a hyperintense lesion compared to extraocular muscle.[96,99] Cystic degeneration is hypodense on CT, hypointense on T1-weighted MRI, hyperintense on T2-weighted MRI, and does not enhance on contrast. Contrast shows moderate to marked tumor enhancement on MRI, and is important to identify the intracranial extension.[100]

Management

Complete excision of the tumor is the definitive treatment. Although localized neurofibroma has no capsule, it acquires a pseudocapsule through compressive effects on adjacent tissues.[99] The pseudocapsule and low vascularity allows surgical excision to be bloodless and easily performed.[95] Recurrence is rare even with incomplete excision. However, localized neurofibroma poses a small risk of malignant transformation.[101]

Schwannoma

Schwannoma, previously known as neurilemmoma, is a benign, encapsulated tumor that arises from the proliferation of Schwann cells of neural crest cell origin.[102,103] It is composed of solid areas of palisading nuclei (Antoni A) with a loose myxomatous background (Antoni B).[96]

Schwannoma often occurs from the second to the fifth decade of life,[103] but it has been reported in older age groups. This tumor may be extraconal or intraconal. It more commonly affects sensory nerves than motor nerves.[99] Orbital schwannoma frequently arises from the supratrochlear and supraorbital nerves of the ophthalmic branch of trigeminal nerve located in the superior orbit.[99,103,104] In some cases, orbital schwannoma can arise from nerves within the extraocular muscle[105] and epibulbar conjunctiva.[106,107] A few cases are associated with neurofibromatosis.

Symptoms and Signs

Clinical signs depend on the location and extent of the tumor. The most common signs include gradual painless proptosis and globe displacement. There may be paresthesia or pain in the distribution of the involved nerve.[103,104] Intraconal tumor may lead to optic disc edema with subsequent optic atrophy and visual loss.[99,103,108] Ophthalmoplegia may result from mechanical restriction secondary to mass effect,[102] or from involvement of cranial nerves that innervate the extraocular muscles.[8]

Imaging

Orbital CT scan shows a smooth, well-defined, ovoid to elongated or fusiform lesion that may, on rare occasions, reveal hypodense cysts that mimic mucocele. Large tumors may show some calcification[102] and bone remodeling.[8]

The cellular part (Antoni A) is isointense and slightly hyperintense compared to extraocular muscle on T1-weighted and T2-weighted MRI, respectively. The myxomatous part (Antoni B) is hyperintense on both T1-weighted and T2-weighted MRI. Contrast shows enhancement of both the cellular and myxomatous parts.[8,96,99]

Management

Complete surgical excision with an intact capsule is the treatment for schwannoma.[102] This is surgically feasible due to the relatively tough capsule of the tumor. Any incomplete removal may lead to tumor recurrence and rare malignant transformation.[109]

LYMPHOPROLIFERATIVE TUMORS

Lymphoid Hyperplasia and Lymphoma

Lymphoproliferative lesions are the most common tumors that affect the orbit in the elderly population above the age of 60.[110,111] They represent a continuum of benign lymphoid hyperplasia, atypical hyperplasia, to malignant lymphoma[112] that is either isolated in the adnexa and orbit, or more extensive in involvement.[113] Approximately 5% of those with systemic lymphoma will develop ocular adnexal or orbital metastases.[111]

Lymphoma

Majority of lymphoproliferative lesions in the orbit are non-Hodgkin B cell lymphomas,[111,114] which are associated with chronic autoimmune disease[115] and immunodeficiency including acquired immunodeficiency syndrome (AIDS).[112] Lymphomas can arise from B cells or T cells. T cell lymphomas are rare and lethal. Hodgkin B cell lymphoma rarely occurs in the orbit.[115]

The most common type of orbital lymphoma is the extranodal marginal zone B cell lymphoma (mucosa-associated lymphoid tissue type). Follicular lymphoma is the second most common lymphoma, and is the most common secondary orbital lymphoma. The most common type that arises from adjacent structures of the orbit is the diffuse large B cell lymphoma.[115,116] Other less common types include chronic lymphocytic lymphoma and mantle cell lymphoma.[117]

Most lymphomas occur from the fourth to sixth decade of life. The tumor is most commonly located in the superior and anterior orbit.[112,116] About 33% of orbital lymphomas have systemic spread at 10 years.[113] Clinical findings associated with systemic spread include the initial anatomic involvement of the eyelid and lacrimal gland,[118,119] bilaterality,[113] and monoclonality. However, the risk of systemic spread increases with chronicity of the tumor regardless of its initial anatomic site, bilaterality, or clonality.

Symptoms and Signs

The clinical presentation depends on the histologic type and tumor location. A gradually progressive painless proptosis is the most common feature,[112] especially for indolent histologic types. Globe displacement may occur for bulkier tumors. Superior orbital lesions may feel firm and less defined, while inferior orbital lesions may feel nodular or rubbery. Superior or anterior orbital lesions may have lid swelling and ptosis.[116] Restricted extraocular motility and visual deterioration suggest involvement of the optic nerve and orbital apex,[112] or represent late signs of advanced cases. Pain and inflammation are often associated with more aggressive histologies.[117]

Imaging

Putty-like or pancake-like molding to adjacent orbital structures is the typical presentation of benign to malignant lymphoproliferative lesions. Orbital CT reveals a diffuse to well-circumscribed, moderately enhancing homogeneous mass that is hyperdense to brain.[120] Bone erosion and tissue infiltration may occur in highly malignant lymphomas and lesions that invade the orbit from paranasal sinuses such as diffuse large B cell lymphoma.[113] T1-weighted and T2-weighted MRI reveal an isointense lesion with moderate enhancement on contrast (*see* Figs. 105.12 to 105.14).[120]

Management

Biopsy is required to establish the diagnosis. Due to the overlap in clinical behavior and risk of metastasis, systemic

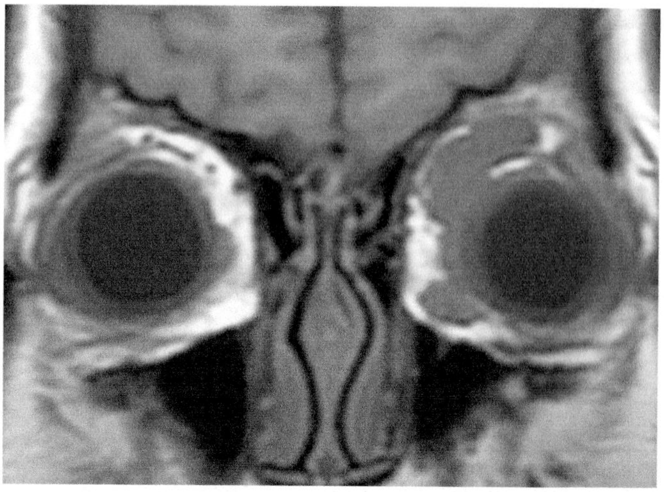

Fig. 105.12: Lymphoma seen via coronal T1-weighted MRI without contrast. There is an isointense mass that molds onto the superonasal part of the globe in the left orbit.

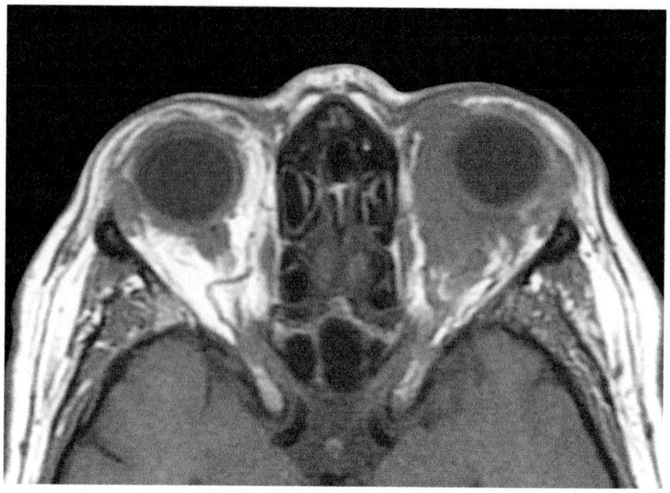

Fig. 105.13: Lymphoma seen via axial T1-weighted MRI without contrast. There is molding of the isointense mass that extends from the intraconal to the retrobulbar and anterior globe in the left orbit of the same patient.

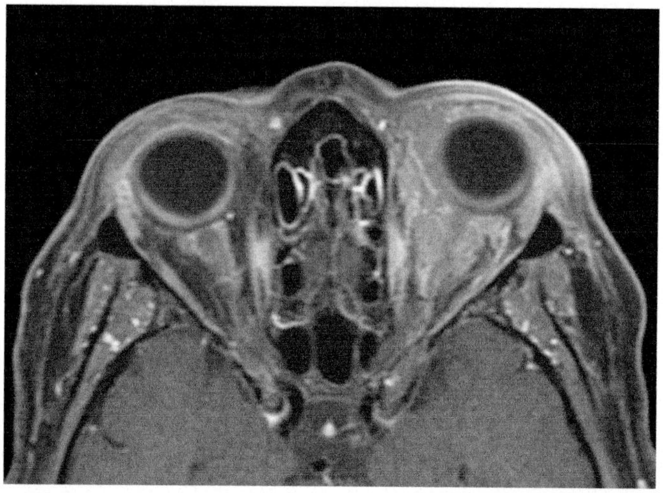

Fig. 105.14: Lymphoma seen via axial T1-weighted MRI with contrast and fat suppression. The mass moderately enhances with contrast in the left orbit of the same patient.

workup for lymphoproliferative lesions must be performed. This includes clinical palpation of lymph nodes; complete blood count; liver function test; bone marrow biopsy; and CT scan of the neck, chest, abdomen, and pelvis.[116] Periodic systemic re-evaluation is required since systemic lymphoma may occur years after an isolated orbital lymphoma presents.[119]

Depending on the size, location, and systemic involvement, management includes chemotherapy, radiotherapy, immunotherapy, and surgical excision. In the absence of systemic spread, lymphoma in the anterior orbit or lacrimal gland can be surgically excised. A poorly-defined localized lymphoma or those located in the posterior orbit can be treated with radiotherapy with almost complete local control rate. Systemic chemotherapy may be used as the primary treatment for cases with systemic involvement.[113] Recently, immunotherapy or monoclonal antibodies, such as rituximab, administered systemically and/or intralesionally have shown good results.[121] However, their specific role in the treatment must be further elucidated.

METASTATIC ORBITAL TUMORS

Neuroblastoma

Neuroblastoma is the most common tumor that metastasizes to the orbit during childhood.[122] There is only one reported case of primary orbital tumor, which was found in an adult.[123] It is a rapidly progressing tumor that commonly affects children at the age of 2 years. Most cases originate from the abdomen, with the primary tumor located in the adrenal medulla. Other primary sites include the mediastinal and cervical sympathetic ganglia.[124] These tumors spread hematogeneously to the orbit.

Symptoms and Signs

Metastasis occurs late in the course of neuroblastoma. In most cases, the presence of the primary tumor is known prior to orbital involvement.[125] Ophthalmic features are secondary to the mass effect, bone involvement, or periorbital soft tissue infiltration of the tumor.[126]

The most common signs include painless proptosis and periorbital ecchymosis.[127-129] Periorbital ecchymosis, also known as "raccoon eye", results from blood deposition within the eyelids and may be mistaken for injury.[130] Other features include ptosis, globe displacement, ophthalmoplegia, optic disc edema, dilated retinal vessels, and subconjunctival hemorrhage.[127,128] Unilateral Horner syndrome occurs with a primary mediastinal tumor. Opsoclonus occurs with a cervical sympathetic ganglion tumor, but may not always be present in orbital neuroblastoma.[131]

Approximately 20% of neuroblastoma cases present with ophthalmic features, so a correct diagnosis is imperative for early management.[130,132]

Imaging

Orbital CT scan reveals an ill-defined hyperdense lesion compared to extraocular muscle, with hypodense necrotic areas and lytic bone erosion. T1-weighted and T2-weighted MRI reveal an ill-defined homogeneous or heterogeneous lesion with variable signal intensity that depends on the state of blood degradation products. Contrast enhancement also varies.[131]

Management

Orbital neuroblastoma is considered a high risk, stage IV disease based on the International Neuroblastoma Staging System.[126] Thus, treatment begins with intensive chemotherapy to decrease the tumor burden, to render it resectable, and to improve bone marrow involvement to harvest either bone marrow or peripheral blood stem cells. This is followed by surgical excision or debulking, myeloablative chemotherapy with stem cell transplant, immunotherapy, and differentiation therapy with isotretinoin. Radiotherapy is reserved for visual loss from compressive optic neuropathy. Unfortunately, although complete remission can initially be achieved, death from subsequent relapse usually occurs.

Metastatic Tumors in Adults

Metastatic orbital tumor is rare. It is usually unilateral and affects adults who are at least in their fourth decade,[133] or children within their first decade of life. The most common orbital metastatic tumor among adults and women is breast cancer.[133-135] This is followed interchangeably by lung cancer and prostate cancer.[133] The most common orbital metastatic tumor among children is neuroblastoma, which has been previously discussed.

Symptoms and Signs

Metastatic tumor in the orbit can present with a mass effect, diffuse or localized tissue infiltration, cranial nerve II–VI dysfunction, and inflammation. Some are asymptomatic, while others may have combined features. The clinical presentation depends on the type of primary tumor and its distinct tissue preference for metastasis. Breast cancer is predisposed to affect extraocular muscles and fat, while prostate carcinoma tends to affect orbital bone.[134]

Proptosis and motility disorder are the most common features.[134] Other signs include a palpable mass, early onset of pain, blepharoptosis, enophthalmos, and diplopia.[133-135] Pulsation may occur from orbital bone destruction with subsequent transmission of brain pulsation.[134]

Imaging

The patterns seen in CT and MRI may vary depending on the primary tumor.[133] These may range from an ill-defined infiltrating lesion to a well-circumscribed enhancing mass. Orbital CT scan may reveal bone erosion or hyperostosis, while MRI may show the extent of orbital tissue involvement (*see* Figs. 105.15 to 105.19).[134] Neuroimaging is important to identify concomitant brain metastasis.[135]

Management

An orbital metastatic tumor is the initial manifestation in at least one-third of systemic cancer cases[135] so a high clinical suspicion and good history taking are imperative

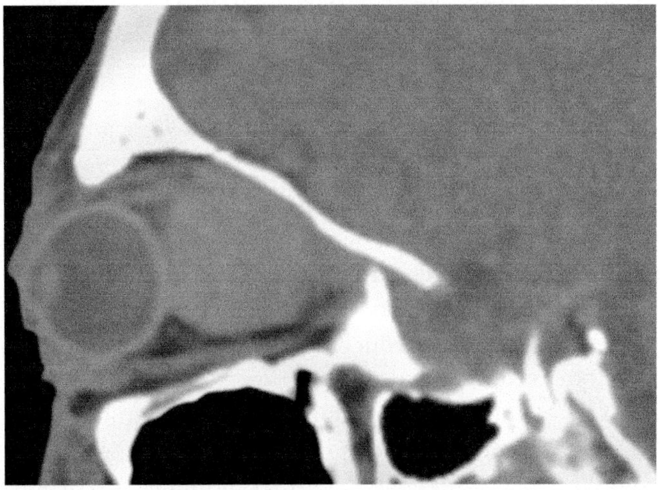

Fig. 105.15: Metastatic orbital tumor from a primary stage IV lung adenocarcinoma seen via sagittal CT scan without contrast. There is a moderately well-defined intraconal mass that is isodense to extraocular muscles.

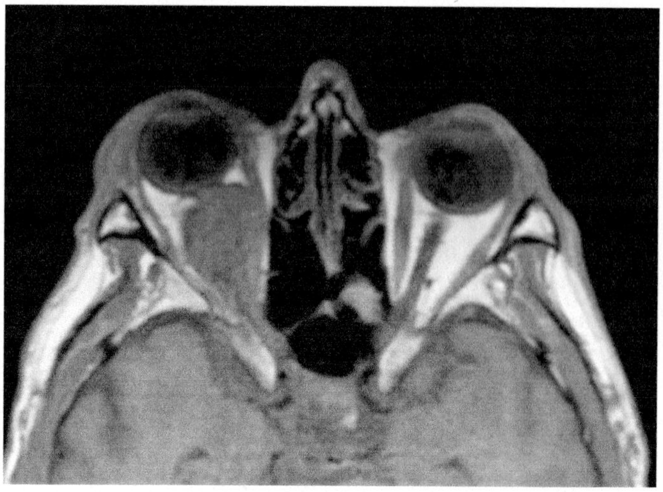

Fig. 105.16: Metastatic orbital tumor from a primary stage IV lung adenocarcinoma seen via axial T1-weighted MRI without contrast. The intraconal mass is isointense to extraocular muscles in the right orbit of the same patient.

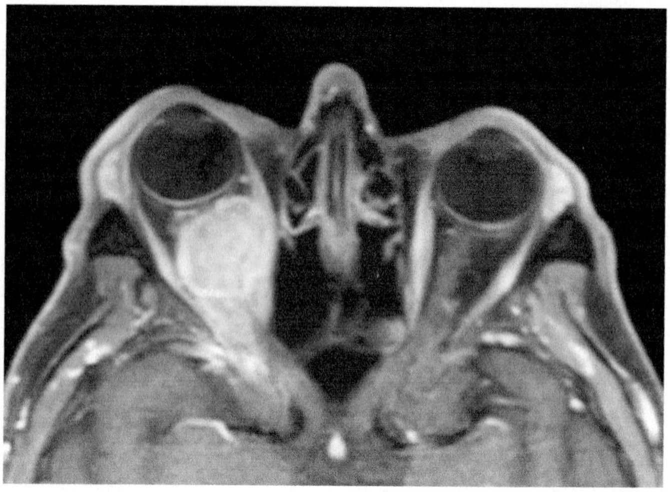

Fig. 105.17: Metastatic orbital tumor from a primary stage IV lung adenocarcinoma seen via axial T1-weighted MRI with contrast and fat suppression. The mass mildly to moderately enhances with contrast in the same patient.

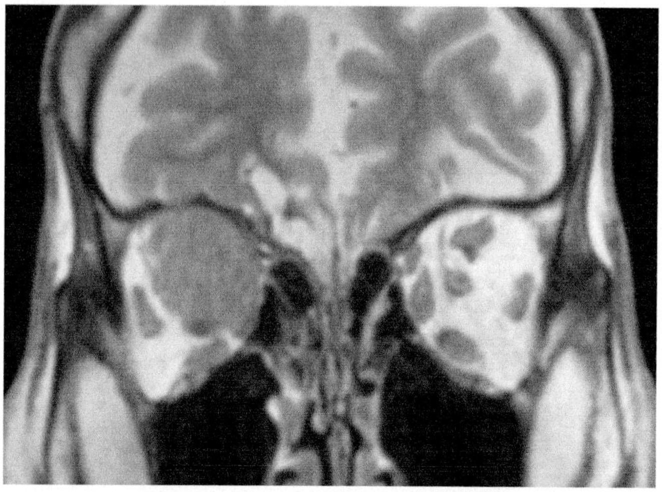

Fig. 105.18: Metastatic orbital tumor from a primary stage IV lung adenocarcinoma seen via coronal T2-weighted MRI without contrast. The mass is isointense to extraocular muscles, but hypointense to fat in the right orbit of the same patient.

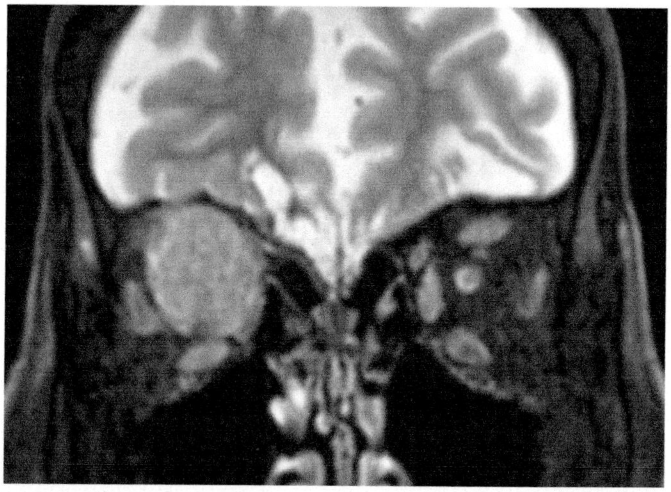

Fig. 105.19: Metastatic orbital tumor from a primary stage IV lung adenocarcinoma seen via coronal T2-weighted MRI with contrast and fat suppression. The mass mildly to moderately enhances with contrast in the same patient.

to avoid further diagnostic delay. Although an elevated carcinoembryogenic antigen may suggest metastasis, definitive diagnosis is done through a fine needle aspiration biopsy or open biopsy which may also provide samples for hormone receptor assays.[134]

An asymptomatic or mildly symptomatic tumor may be observed. Although majority carry a poor prognosis, some live years after the diagnosis of metastatic orbital tumor. Radiotherapy, hormonal therapy, chemotherapy, or surgery may be employed for palliation. Orbitotomy with excision biopsy is both diagnostic and palliative to preserve vision and relieve pain. Because majority have coexistent metastasis to other sites, a general evaluation through the help of an oncologist is prudent.[134]

REFERENCES

1. Haik BG, Karcioglu ZA, Gordon RA, et al. Capillary hemangioma (infantile periocular hemangioma). Surv Ophthalmol. 1994;38(5):399-426.
2. Mulliken JB, Glowacki J. Hemangiomas and vascular malformations in infants and children: a classification based on endothelial characteristics. Plast Reconstr Surg. 1982;69(3):412-22.

3. Burton BK, Schulz CJ, Angle B, et al. An increased incidence of haemangiomas in infants born following chorionic villus sampling (CVS). Prenat Diagn. 1995;15(3):209-14.
4. Campbell S, Park JH, Rowe J, et al. Chorionic villus sampling as a source of trophoblasts. Placenta. 2007;28(11-12):1118-22.
5. Barnes CM, Huang S, Kaipainen A, et al. Evidence of molecular profiling for a placental origin of infantile hemangioma. Proc Natl Acad Sci USA. 2005;102(52):19097-102.
6. Regnier S, Dupin N, Le Danff C, et al. Endothelial cells in infantile haemangiomas originate from the child and not from the mother (a fluorescence in situ hybridization-based study). Br J Dermatol. 2007;157(1):158-60.
7. Garrity JA, Henderson JW, Cameron JD. Henderson's Orbital Tumors, 4th edition. Philadelphia: Lippincott Williams and Wilkins; 2007.
8. Dutton JJ. Radiology of the Orbit and Visual Pathways. London: Elsevier Health Sciences; 2010.
9. Margileth AM, Museles M. Cutaneous hemangiomas in children. Diagnosis and conservative management. JAMA. 1965;194(5):523-6.
10. Spiteri Cornish K, Reddy AR. The use of propranolol in the management of periocular capillary haemangioma—a systematic review. Eye (Lond). 2011;25(10):1277-83.
11. Durairaj VD. Treatment of deep orbital hemangiomas of infancy: an overview. Arch Facial Plast Surg. 2006;8(3):217-20.
12. Iwamoto T, Jakobiec FA. Ultrastructural comparison of capillary and cavernous hemangioma of the orbit. Arch Ophthalmol. 1979;97(6):1144-53.
13. Gunalp I, Gunduz K. Biopsy-proven orbital lesions in Turkey. A survey of 1,092 cases over 30 years. Orbit. 1994;13(2):67-79.
14. Ansari SA, Mafee MF. Orbital cavernous hemangioma: role of imaging. Neuroimaging Clin N Am. 2005;15(1):137-58.
15. Zauberman H, Feinsod M. Orbital hemangioma growth during pregnancy. Acta Ophthalmol. 1970;48(5):929-33.
16. McNab AA, Wright JE. Cavernous hemangiomas of the orbit. Aust NZ J Ophthalmol. 1989;17(4):337-45.
17. Sullivan TJ, Aylward GW, Wright JE, et al. Bilateral multiple cavernous haemangiomas of the orbit. Br J Ophthalmol. 1992;75(10):627-9.
18. Johnson TE, Nasr AM, Nalbandian RM, et al. Enchondromatosis and hemangioma (Maffucci's Syndrome) with orbital involvement. Am J Ophthalmol. 1990;110(2):153-9.
19. Chang EL, Rubin PA. Bilateral multifocal hemangiomas of the orbit in the blue rubber bleb nevus syndrome. Ophthalmology. 2002;109(3):537-41.
20. Davis KR, Hesselink JR, Dallow RL, et al. CT and ultrasound in the diagnosis of cavernous hemangioma and lymphangioma of the orbit. J Comput Tomogr. 1980;4(2):98-104.
21. Rootman DB, Heran MK, Rootman J, et al. Cavernous venous malformations of the orbit (so-called cavernous haemangioma): a comprehensive evaluation of their clinical, imaging and histologic nature. Br J Ophthalmol. 2014;98(7):880-8.
22. Harris GJ, Jakobiec FA. Cavernous hemangioma of the orbit. J Neurosurg. 1979;51(2):219-28.
23. Bilaniuk LT. Orbital vascular lesions: role of imaging. Radiol Clin North Am. 1999;37(1):169-83.
24. Scheuerle AF, Steiner HH, Kolling G, et al. Treatment and long-term outcome of patients with orbital cavernomas. Am J Ophthalmol. 2004;138(2):237-44.
25. Boari N, Gagliardi F, Castellazzi P, et al. Surgical treatment of orbital cavernomas: clinical and functional outcome in a series of 20 patients. Acta Neurochir (Wien). 2011;153(3): 491-8.
26. Graeb DA, Rootman J, Robertson WD, et al. Orbital lymphangiomas: clinical, radiologic, and pathologic characteristics. Radiology. 1990;175(2):417-21.
27. Jones IS. Lymphangiomas of the ocular adnexa: an analysis of 62 cases. Trans Am Ophthalmol Soc. 1959;57:602-65.
28. Katz SE, Rootman J, Vangveeravong S, et al. Combined venous lymphatic malformations of the orbit (so-called lymphangiomas): association with noncontiguous intracranial vascular anomalies. Ophthalmology. 1998;105(1):176-84.
29. Bisdorff A, Mulliken JB, Carrico J, et al. Intracranial vascular anomalies in patients with periorbital lymphatic and lymphaticovenous malformations. Am J Neuroradiol. 2007;28(2):335-41.
30. Greene AK, Burrows PE, Smith L, et al. Periorbital lymphatic malformation: clinical course and management in 42 patients. Plast Reconstr Surg. 2005;115(1):22-30.
31. Wiegand S, Eivazi B, Bloch LM, et al. Lymphatic malformations of the orbit. Clin Exp Otorhinolaryngol. 2013;6(1):30-5.
32. Tunc M, Sadri E, Char DH. Orbital lymphangioma: an analysis of 26 patients. Br J Ophthalmol. 1999;83(1):76-80.
33. Harris GJ. Orbital vascular malformations: a consensus statement on terminology and its clinical implications. Am J Ophthalmol. 1999;127(4):453-5.
34. Kazim M, Kennerdell JS, Rothfus W, et al. Orbital lymphangioma: correlation of magnetic resonance images and intraoperative findings. Ophthalmology. 1992;99(10):1588-94.
35. Rubin PA, Remulla HD. Orbital venous anomalies demonstrated by spiral computed tomography. Ophthalmology. 1997;104(9):1463-70.
36. Lacey B, Rootman J, Marotta TR. Distensible venous malformations of the orbit: clinical and hemodynamic features and a new technique of management. Ophthalmology. 1999;106(6):1197-209.
37. Osaki TH, Fay A, Waner M. Vascular malformations. In: Fay A, Dolman PJ (Eds). Diseases and Disorders of the Orbit and Ocular Adnexa. Edinburgh: Elsevier Health Sciences; 2017. pp. 447-72.
38. Rootman J, Heran MK, Graeb DA. Vascular malformations of the orbit: classification and the role of imaging in diagnosis and treatment strategies. Ophthal Plast Reconstr Surg. 2014;30(2):91-104.
39. Shields JA, Dolinskas C, Augsburger JJ, et al. Demonstration of orbital varix with computed tomography and valsalva maneuver. Am J Ophthalmol. 1984;97(1):108-10.

40. Shields JA, Eagle RC Jr, Shields CL. Orbital varix presenting as a subconjunctival mass. Ophthal Plast Reconstr Surg. 1995;11(1):37-8.
41. Gunduz K, Karcioglu ZA. Vascular tumors. In: Karcioglu ZA (Ed.) Orbital Tumors: Diagnosis and Treatment. New York: Springer Science + Business Media, Inc.; 2005. pp. 141-62.
42. Rootman J. Vascular malformations of the orbit: hemodynamic concepts. Orbit. 2003;22(2):103-20.
43. Trout HH, McAllister HA, Giordano JM. Vascular anomalies. J Vasc Surg. 1986;3(5):833-6.
44. Hayes BH, Shore JW, Westfall CT, et al. Management of orbital and periorbital arteriovenous malformations. Ophthalmic Surg. 1995;26(2):145-52.
45. Warrier S, Prabhakaran VC, Valenzuela A, et al. Orbital arteriovenous malformations. Arch Ophthalmol. 2008;126(12):1669-75.
46. Ponce FA, Han PP, Spetzler RF, et al. Associated arteriovenous malformation of the orbit and brain: a case of Wyburn-Mason syndrome without retinal involvement. Case report. J Neurosurg. 2001;95(2):346-9.
47. Mulligan PR, Prajapati HJ, Martin LG, et al. Vascular anomalies: classification, imaging characteristics and implications for interventional radiology treatment approaches. Br J Radiol. 2013;87(1035):1-18.
48. Christie DB, Kwon YH, Choi I, et al. Sequential embolization and excision of an orbital arteriovenous malformation. Arch Ophthalmol. 1994;112(10):1377-9.
49. Alexandrakis G, Johnson TE. Recurrent orbital solitary fibrous tumor in a 14-year-old girl. Am J Ophthalmol. 2000;130(3):373-6.
50. Lucci LM, Anderson RL, Harrie RP, et al. Solitary fibrous tumor of the orbit in a child. Ophthal Plast Reconstr Surg. 2001;17(5):369-73.
51. Westra WH, Gerald WL, Rosai J. Solitary fibrous tumor consistent CD34 immunoreactivity and occurrence in the orbit. Am J Surg Pathol. 1994;18(10):992-8.
52. Geramizadeh B, Marzban M, Churg A. Role of immunohistochemistry in the diagnosis of solitary fibrous tumor, a review. Iran J Pathol. 2016;11(3):195-203.
53. Suster S, Fisher C, Moran C. Expression of bcl-2 oncoprotein in benign and malignant spindle cell tumors of soft tissue, skin, serosal surfaces, and gastrointestinal tract. Am J Surg Pathol. 1998;22(7):863-72.
54. Renshaw AA. O13 (CD99) in spindle cell tumors: reactivity with hemangiopericytoma, solitary fibrous tumor, synovial sarcoma, and meningioma but rarely with sarcomatoid mesothelioma. Appl Immunohistochem. 1995;3(4):250-6.
55. Fukunaga M, Ushigome S, Nomura K, et al. Solitary fibrous tumor of the nasal cavity and orbit. Pathol Int. 1995;45(12):952-7.
56. Gengler C, Guillou L. Solitary fibrous tumour and haemangiopericytoma: evolution of a concept. Histopathology. 2006;48(1):63-74.
57. Leoncini G, Maio V, Puccioni M, et al. Orbital solitary fibrous tumor: a case report and review of literature. Pathol Oncol Res. 2008;14(2):213-7.
58. Furusato E, Valenzuela IA, Fanburg-Smith JC, et al. Orbital solitary fibrous tumor: encompassing terminology for hemangiopericytoma, giant cell angiofibroma, and fibrous histiocytoma of the orbit: reappraisal of 41 cases. Hum Pathol. 2011;42(1):120-8.
59. Scott IU, Tanenbaum M, Rubin D, et al. Solitary fibrous tumor of the lacrimal gland fossa. Ophthalmology. 1996;103(10):1613-8.
60. McElvanney AM, O'Donovan DG, Banerjee SS. Solitary fibrous tumour: an atypical presentation within the orbit. Eye (Lond). 1996;10(3):396-9.
61. Woo KI, Suh YL, Kim YD. Solitary fibrous tumor of the lacrimal sac. Ophthal Plast Reconstr Surg. 1999;15(6):450-3.
62. Bernardini FP, de Conciliis C, Schneider S, et al. Solitary fibrous tumor of the orbit: is it rare? Report of a case series and review of the literature. Ophthalmology. 2003;110(7):1442-8.
63. Krishnakumar S, Subramanian N, Mohan R, et al. Solitary fibrous tumor of the orbit: a clinicopathologic study of six cases with review of the literature. Surv Ophthalmol. 2003;48(5):544-54.
64. Yang BT, Wang YZ, Dong JY, et al. MRI study of solitary fibrous tumor in the orbit. Am J Roentgenol. 2012;199(4):W506-11.
65. Hayashi S, Kurihara H, Hirato J, et al. Solitary fibrous tumor of the orbit with extraorbital extension: case report. Neurosurgery. 2001;49(5):1241-5.
66. Warner MA, Weber AL, Jakobiec FA. Benign and malignant tumors of the orbital cavity including the lacrimal gland. Neuroimaging Clin N Am. 1996;6(1):123-42.
67. Shields JA, Shields CL. Rhabdomyosarcoma: review for the ophthalmologist. Surv Ophthalmol. 2003;48(1):39-57.
68. McKeen EA, Bodurtha J, Meadows AT, et al. Rhabdomyosarcoma complicating multiple neurofibromatosis. J Pediatr. 1978;93(6):992-3.
69. Muwakkit S, Antillon F, Jenkins JJ 3rd, et al. Simultaneous occurrence of Wilms tumor and rhabdomyosarcoma in two patients. Med Pediatr Oncol. 2002;39(2):143-5.
70. Frezzotti R, Hadjistilianou T, Tosi P, et al. Rhabdomyosarcoma of the orbit: clinical and histopathological analysis of a personal series of 19 cases. Orbit. 1990;9(4):307-12.
71. Shields CL, Shields JA, Honavar SG, et al. Clinical spectrum of primary ophthalmic rhabdomyosarcoma. Ophthalmology. 2001;108(12):2284-92.
72. Sohaib SA, Moseley I, Wright JE. Orbital rhabdomyosarcoma—the radiological characteristics. Clin Radiol. 1998;53(5):357-62.
73. Porterfield JF, Zimmerman LE. Rhabdomyosarcoma of the orbit; a clinicopathologic study of 55 cases. Virchows Arch Pathol Anat Physiol Klin Med. 1962;335:329-44.
74. Grosfeld JL, Weber TR, Weetman RM, et al. Rhabdomyosarcoma in childhood: analysis of survival in 98 cases. J Pediatr Surg. 1983;18(2):141-6.
75. Crist WM, Anderson JR, Meza JL, et al. Intergroup Rhabdomyosarcoma Study-IV: results for patients with nonmetastatic disease. J Clin Oncol. 2001;19(12):3091-102.

76. Kodet R, Newton WA Jr, Hamoudi AB, et al. Orbital rhabdomyosarcomas and related tumors in childhood: relationship of morphology to prognosis—an Intergroup Rhabdomyosarcoma Study. Med Pediatr Oncol. 1997;29(1): 51-60.
77. Dutton JJ. Gliomas of the anterior visual pathway. Surv Ophthalmol. 1994;38(5):427-52.
78. Lee AG. Neuroophthalmological management of optic pathway gliomas. Neurosurg Focus. 2007;23(5):E1-6.
79. Parsa CF, Hoyt CS, Lesser RL, et al. Spontaneous regression of optic gliomas. Thirteen cases documented by serial neuroimaging. Arch Ophthalmol. 2001;119(4):516-29.
80. Astrup J. Natural history and clinical management of optic pathway glioma. Br J Neurosurg. 2003;17(4):327-35.
81. Bosch MM, Wichmann WW, Boltshauser E, et al. Optic nerve sheath meningiomas in patients with neurofibromatosis type 2. Arch Ophthalmol. 2006;124(3):379-85.
82. Saeed P, Rootman J, Nugent RA, et al. Optic nerve sheath meningiomas. Ophthalmology. 2003;110(10):2019-30.
83. Dutton JJ. Optic nerve sheath meningiomas. Surv Ophthalmol. 1992;37(3):167-83.
84. Turbin RE, Pokorny K. Diagnosis and treatment of orbital optic nerve sheath meningioma. Cancer Control. 2004;11(5): 334-41.
85. Jakobiec FA, Depot MJ, Kennerdell JS, et al. Combined clinical and computed tomographic diagnosis of orbital glioma and meningioma. Ophthalmology. 1984;91(2):137-55.
86. Sughrue ME, Rutkowski MJ, Chen CJ, et al. Modern surgical outcomes following surgery for sphenoid wing meningiomas. J Neurosurg. 2013;119(1):86-93.
87. Saeed P, van Furth WR, Tanck M, et al. Natural history of spheno-orbital meningiomas. Acta Neurochir (Wien). 2011;153(2):395-402.
88. Roser F, Nakamura M, Jacobs C, et al. Sphenoid wing meningiomas with osseous involvement. Surg Neurol. 2005;64(1):37-43.
89. Verma SK, Sinha S, Sawarkar DP, et al. Medical sphenoid wing meningiomas: experience with microsurgical resection over 5 years and a review of literature. Neurol India. 2016;64(3):465-75.
90. Bikmaz K, Mrak R, Al-Mefty O. Management of bone-invasive, hyperostotic sphenoid wing meningiomas. J Neurosurg. 2007;107(5):905-12.
91. Saeed P, van Furth WR, Tanck M, et al. Surgical treatment of sphenoorbital meningiomas. Br J Ophthalmol. 2011;95(7):996-1000.
92. Taylor BW Jr, Marcus RB Jr, Friedman WA, et al. The meningioma controversy: postoperative radiation therapy. Int J Radiat Oncol Biol Phys. 1988;15(2):299-304.
93. Kottler UB, Conway RM, Schlotzer-Schrehardt U, et al. Isolated neurofibroma of the orbit with extensive myxoid changes: a clinicopathologic study including MRI and electron microscopic findings. Orbit. 2004;23(1):59-64.
94. Shields JA, Shields CL, Lieb WE, et al. Multiple orbital neurofibromas unassociated with von Recklinghausen's disease. Arch Ophthalmol. 1990;108(1);80-3.
95. Lee LR, Gigantelli JW, Kincaid MC. Localized neurofibroma of the orbit: a radiographic and histopathologic study. Ophthal Plast Reconstr Surg. 2000;16(3):241-6.
96. Carroll GS, Haik BG, Fleming JC, et al. Peripheral nerve tumors of the orbit. Radiol Clin N Am. 1999;37(1):195-202.
97. McDonald P, Jakobiec FA, Hornblass A, et al. Benign peripheral nerve sheath tumors (neurofibromas) of the lacrimal gland. Ophthalmology. 1983;90(12):1403-13.
98. Meyer DR, Wobig JL. Bilateral localized orbital neurofibromas. Ophthalmology. 1992;99(8):1313-7.
99. Kapur R, Mafee MF, Lamba R, et al. Orbital schwannoma and neurofibroma: role of imaging. Neuroimaging Clin N Am. 2005;15(1):159-74.
100. Dervin JE, Beaconsfield M, Wright JE, et al. CT findings in orbital tumours of nerve sheath origin. Clin Radiol. 1989;40(5):475-9.
101. Lyons CJ, McNab AA, Garner A, et al. Orbital malignant peripheral nerve sheath tumours. Br J Ophthalmol. 1989;73(9):731-8.
102. Rootman J, Golberg C, Robertson W. Primary orbital schwannomas. Br J Ophthalmol. 1982;66(3):194-204.
103. Rose GE, Wright JE. Isolated peripheral nerve sheath tumours of the orbit. Eye (Lond). 1991;5 (Pt 6):668-73.
104. Konrad EA, Thiel HJ. Schwannoma of the orbit. Ophthalmologica. 1984;188(2):118-27.
105. Capps DH, Brodsky MC, Rice CD, et al. Orbital intramuscular schwannoma. Am J Ophthalmol. 1990;110(5):535-9.
106. Le Marc'hadour F, Romanet JP, Fdili A, et al. Schwannoma of the bulbar conjunctiva. Arch Ophthalmol. 1996;114(10): 1258-60.
107. Vincent NJ, Cleasby GW. Schwannoma of the bulbar conjunctiva. Arch Ophthalmol. 1968;80(5):641-2.
108. Mafee MF, Putterman A, Valvassori GE, et al. Orbital space-occupying lesions: role of computed tomography and magnetic resonance imaging: an analysis of 145 cases. Radiol Clin N Am. 1987;25(3):529-59.
109. Schatz H. Benign orbital neurilemoma: sarcomatous transformation in von Recklinghausen's disease. Arch Ophthalmol. 1971;86(3):268-73.
110. Demirci H, Shields CL, Shields J, et al. Orbital tumors in the older adult population. Ophthalmology. 2002;109(2):243-8.
111. Bairey O, Kremer I, Rakowsky E, et al. Orbital and adnexal involvement in systemic non-Hodgkin's lymphoma. Cancer. 1994;73(9):2395-9.
112. Cockerham GC, Jakobiec JA. Lymphoproliferative disorders of the ocular adnexa. Int Ophthalmol Clin. 1997;37(4):39-59.
113. Demirci H, Shields CL, Karaza EC, et al. Orbital lymphoproliferative tumors: analysis of clinical features and systemic involvement in 160 cases. Ophthalmology. 2008;115(9):1626-31.
114. Shields JA, Shields CL, Scartozzi R. Survey of 1,262 patients with orbital tumors and simulating lesions. Ophthalmology. 2004;111(5):997-1008.
115. Ferry JA, Fung CY, Zukerberg L, et al. Lymphoma of the ocular adnexa: a study of 353 cases. Am J Surg Pathol. 2007;31(2):170-84.

116. White WL, Ferry JA, Harris NL, et al. Ocular adnexal lymphoma: a clinicopathologic study with identification of lymphomas of mucosa-associated lymphoid tissue type. Ophthalmology. 1995;102(12):1994-2006.
117. Sullivan TJ, Whitehead K, Williamson R, et al. Lymphoproliferative disease of the ocular adnexa: a clinical and pathologic study with statistical analysis of 69 patients. Ophthal Plast Reconstr Surg. 2005;21(3):177-88.
118. Jenkins C, Rose GE, Bunce C, et al. Clinical features associated with survival of patients with lymphoma of the ocular adnexa. Eye (Lond). 2003;17(7):809-20.
119. Knowles DM, Jakobiec FA, McNally L, et al. Lymphoid hyperplasia and malignant lymphoma occurring in the ocular adnexa (orbit, conjunctiva, and eyelids): a prospective multiparametric analysis of 108 cases during 1977-1987. Hum Pathol. 1990;21(9):959-73.
120. Sullivan TJ, Valenzuela AA. Imaging features of ocular adnexal lymphoproliferative disease. Eye (Lond). 2006;20(10):1189-95.
121. Esmaeli B, Murray JL, Naderi A, et al. Immunotherapy for low-grade non-Hodgkin secondary lymphoma of the orbit. Arch Ophthalmol. 2002;120(9):1225-7.
122. Chung EM, Murphey MD, Specht CS, et al. From the Archives of the AFIP. Pediatric orbit tumors and tumorlike lesions: osseous lesions of the orbit. Radiographics. 2008; 28(4):1193-214.
123. Jakobiec FA, Klepach GL, Crissman JD, et al. Primary differentiated neuroblastoma of the orbit. Ophthalmology. 1987;94(3):255-66.
124. Matthay KK. Neuroblastoma: a clinical challenge and biologic puzzle. CA Cancer J Clin. 1995;45(3):179-92.
125. Khanna G, Sato Y, Smith RJ, et al. Causes of facial swelling in pediatric patients: correlation of clinical and radiologic findings. Radiographics. 2006;26(1):157-71.
126. Ahmed S, Goel S, Khandwala M, et al. Neuroblastoma with orbital metastasis: ophthalmic presentation and role of ophthalmologists. Eye (Lond). 2006;20(4):466-70.
127. Albert DM, Rubenstein RA, Scheie HG. Tumor metastasis to the eye. II. Clinical study in infants and children. Am J Ophthalmol. 1967;63(4):727-32.
128. Musarella MA, Chan HS, DeBoer G, et al. Ocular involvement in neuroblastoma: prognostic implications. Ophthalmology. 1984;91(8):939-40.
129. Alfano JE. Ophthalmological aspects of neuroblastomatosis: a study of 53 verified cases. Trans Am Acad Ophthalmol Otolaryngol. 1968;72(6):830-48.
130. D'Ambrosio N, Lyo J, Young R, et al. Common and unusual craniofacial manifestations of metastatic neuroblastoma. Neuroradiology. 2010;52(6):549-53.
131. Rao AA, Naheedy JH, Chen JY, et al. A clinical update and radiologic review of pediatric orbital and ocular tumors. J Oncol. 2013;2013:975908.
132. Gunalp I, Gunduz K. Metastatic orbital tumors. Jpn J Ophthalmol. 1995;39(1):65-70.
133. Shields JA, Shields CL, Brotman HK, et al. Cancer metastatic to the orbit: the 2000 Robert M. Curts Lecture. Ophthal Plast Reconstr Surg. 2001;17(5):346-54.
134. Goldberg RA, Rootman J, Cline RA. Tumors metastatic to the orbit: a changing picture. Surv Ophthalmol. 1990;35(1):1-24.
135. Char DH, Miller T, Kroll S. Orbital metastases: diagnosis and course. Br J Ophthalmol. 1997;81(5):386-90.

Chapter 106 Lacrimal Gland Tumors: Evaluation and Management

Catherine J Choi, David T Tse

INTRODUCTION

Lacrimal gland (LG) is located in the superolateral orbit within the bony concavity of the lacrimal fossa. It is a non-encapsulated eccrine gland composed of orbital and palpebral lobes. LG is responsible for secreting the aqueous layer of the tear film containing an array of soluble proteins essential for maintaining a healthy ocular surface. LG secretions reach the ocular surface via the interlobular ductules that empty into the superior fornix.

A wide spectrum of neoplastic and inflammatory processes can affect the LG. Lesions of the LG overall are rare, estimated to represent approximately 10% of all space-occupying orbital lesions,[1] and an estimated annual incidence of 1.3/million.[2] The oft-cited survey by Reese in 1956 of 112 consecutive expanding lesions of the LG reported that 50% are epithelial and 50% are nonepithelial in origin. Of the epithelial tumors, approximately 50% were benign and 50% were malignant, 50% of which was adenoid cystic carcinoma (ACC). Of the nonepithelial tumors, 50% were lymphoid in nature, and the remaining 50% consisted of various infectious and inflammatory etiologies.[3]

The clinical history, physical examination, and radiographic findings will often provide clues for determining the type of LG lesion. An acute presentation with significant pain, edema, erythema, and tenderness of the LG region in a younger patient typically suggests an infectious or inflammatory etiology. A more slow-growing, insidious, and painless onset in an older patient with appearance of the LG lesion molding around the orbit and ocular structures on imaging is highly suggestive of a lymphoproliferative lesion. A subacute onset with pain, adjacent bony destruction, and infiltration of surrounding structures, orbital apex, or intracranial extension is consistent with a malignant epithelial tumor, while a painless chronic expansion of the lacrimal fossa with bony remodeling is characteristic of benign epithelial tumors.[4]

The infectious and inflammatory disorders of the orbit are discussed in Chapters 107 and 108. The clinical evaluation, management, and current understanding of the pathophysiology of the most common LG tumors will be presented in this chapter.

LYMPHOID TUMORS OF THE LACRIMAL GLAND

Lymphoid tumors of the LG are examples of extranodal lymphoproliferative disease originating from the population of lymphocytes within the interstitium of the LG. They can range from benign or reactive lymphoid hyperplasia to various types of malignant lymphomas. The latter constitutes 58% of all malignant LG tumors, with a median age of 63 and a female predominance.[5,6] Patients present with slow, insidious onset of painless proptosis, ptosis, restricted motility, and inferonasal globe displacement over a mean duration of 6 months.[4,6,7] A firm, nontender mass can be palpated in the region of the lacrimal fossa. Anterior extension beyond the orbit is suggestive of palpebral lobe involvement, which is more typical of a lymphoid rather than an epithelial tumor, and serves as a useful distinguishing feature.[4] The tumor involvement may be limited to the LG or occur with diffuse orbital, conjunctival, or eyelid involvement. While eyelid involvement is the least common (14%), it is associated with the highest rate of systemic lymphoma.[8]

Orbital computed tomography (CT) and magnetic resonance imaging (MRI) show a homogeneous mass that molds to the contour of the lacrimal fossa and adjacent orbital structures without evidence of bony erosion or destruction. The lesion is typically isodense with extraocular muscles, enhances brightly with contrast, and a posterior perpendicular take-off from the lateral wall of the orbit has been described (Figs. 106.1A and B).[4,9]

Neither the clinical presentation nor the imaging studies are specific enough to distinguish between benign lymphoid hyperplasia and malignant lymphoid tumors. Incisional biopsy with histopathology, flow cytometry, and immunohistochemistry are required for diagnosis.[4] A trans-

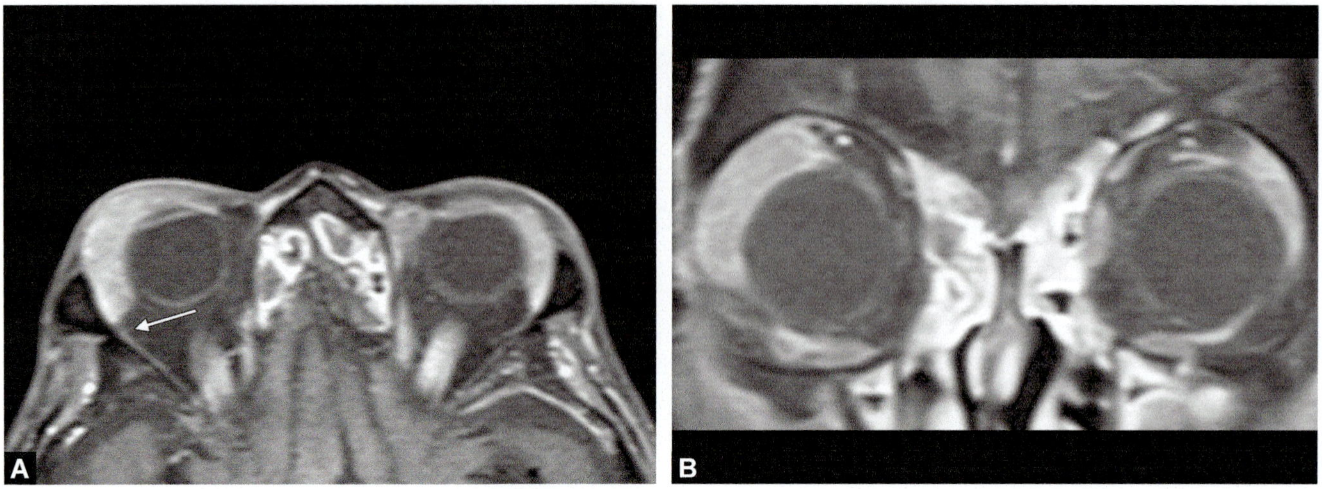

Figs. 106.1A and B: Extranodal marginal zone lymphoma. T1-weighted, contrast-enhanced fat suppression MRI images in (A) axial and (B) coronal views demonstrate a homogeneous mass that molds to the contour of the lacrimal fossa and adjacent orbital structures without evidence of bony destruction. A sharp angulation of perpendicular take-off from the lateral orbital wall is noted, resulting from proliferation of lymphoid cells along the septations of the orbital fat (arrow).

septal anterior orbitotomy via a lid crease incision provides direct access to the LG for biopsy.

Benign or reactive lymphoid hyperplasia appears similar to normal lymph node structure with small mature B- and T- lymphocytes and mitotic figures that are limited to germinal centers. The lymphocytes are polyclonal, with a mix of kappa and lambda chains. There is a 15–25% chance of association with systemic disease at 5 years.[4,7] Atypical lymphoid hyperplasia describes intermediate differentiation between benign and malignant states and is associated with 40% chance of systemic disease at 5 years.[4,10]

A large retrospective chart review by Bonavolonta et al. reported that non-Hodgkin lymphoma constitutes up to 7% of all LG lesions. (1) Approximately 37–40% of these cases are extranodal marginal zone lymphoma (EMZL) (Fig. 106.2), followed by follicular lymphoma (19–28%) and diffuse large B-cell lymphoma (DLBCL) (15%).[6,7,10] The malignant lymphoid tumors of the LG are characterized by monoclonal B-cell proliferation with atypical, immature lymphocytes showing nuclear pleomorphism and lack of organized follicle or germinal center formation.[7] Malignant lymphoma of the LG has 60% chance of being associated with systemic disease.[4,10]

Patients diagnosed with malignant lymphoid tumor of the LG should undergo a complete systemic workup with a medical oncologist. The workup typically consists of a complete physical examination, staging scans (CT of chest/abdomen/pelvis), bone marrow biopsy, serum and urine electrophoresis, complete blood count, liver function tests, and metabolic panel. Central nervous system involvement is ruled out with imaging and lumbar puncture in the presence of neurologic symptoms.[4]

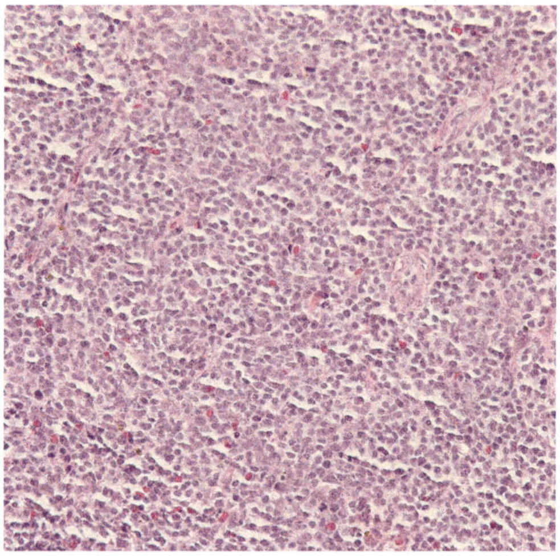

Fig. 106.2: Extranodal marginal zone lymphoma. Hematoxylin and eosin (H&E) stain demonstrating predominantly small lymphoid cells with mature nuclear chromatin in a diffuse distribution (400X).

Treatment of lymphoid lesions of the LG varies with the extent of systemic involvement. Benign lymphoid hyperplasia can be treated with high dose steroids alone or with low dose external beam radiation therapy (EBRT) in the 15–20 Gy range.[4,7] For malignant lymphoid tumors limited to the LG only without evidence of systemic disease, EBRT alone in the 25–30 Gy range in

10–15 fractions provides sufficient control. Lens-sparing protocol can be used to minimize the most common late toxicity of cataract formation, but acute radiation toxicities such as conjunctivitis and dermatitis can still be seen in approximately 50% of patients.[11] In the presence of concurrent systemic lymphoma, chemotherapy is recommended. Current guidelines recommend R-CHOP, which combines the anti-CD20 monoclonal antibody rituximab with cyclophosphamide, hydroxydaunorubicin, vincristine, and prednisone. After induction chemotherapy, rituximab maintenance for 2 years is recommended in cases of high tumor burden.[7,12] Bilateral LG involvement does not confer a higher risk of systemic disease and is also treated with EBRT alone.[4]

Prognosis for primary LG lymphoma limited to the LG is generally favorable for EMZL and follicular lymphoma, and more guarded for DLBCL. The 10-year disease-specific survival of all LG lymphoma from the Surveillance, Epidemiology, and End Results (SEER) database has been reported to be as high as 79%.[5] Other studies indicate that the degree of concurrent systemic involvement likely determines the overall survival. In follicular lymphoma of all ocular adnexa, although the 10-year overall survival was 60%, the rate among those with primary ocular adnexal disease treated with EBRT alone was 94% compared to 40% in those requiring EBRT and chemotherapy.[13] For ocular adnexal DLBCL, on the other hand, 5-year overall survival was only 36%.[14] Following remission, close follow-up is warranted as relapse has been reported in 58% of ocular adnexal follicular lymphoma and 44% of ocular adnexal DLBCL.[6,13,14]

Benign Pleomorphic Adenoma

Benign pleomorphic adenoma, or benign mixed tumor (BMT) of LG is the most common LG lesion overall, constituting approximately 50% of epithelial lesions.[2,4,15,16] The mean age of diagnosis ranges from 38 to 44 with a slight male predilection.[2,16,17] Patients typically present with a very slow-growing, painless welling of the superotemporal orbit and eyelid with varying degrees of proptosis, and a nontender, firm, round mass arising from the orbital lobe of the LG. Due to the nonspecific and limited nature of initial symptoms, patients often report progression over 12 or more months prior to presentation.[18] Large BMT can cause globe dystopia or even globe indentation, and in rare cases, secondary dacryoadenitis or tumor necrosis can also cause atypical pain.[4] BMT can also arise from the palpebral, accessory, or ectopic LG tissue.[4,19] Orbital CT and MRI can provide valuable diagnostic information and will demonstrate a well-circumscribed, solid, round mass with bony expansion (rather than destruction or infiltration) of the lacrimal fossa and curved contact with the bony surface (Figs. 106.3A to C).[9]

Histologically, BMT is a pseudoencapsulated tumor consisting of bland epithelial and mesenchymal tissue. Duct-like lumen are lined by double-layered cuboidal to columnar epithelium surrounded by an outer myoepithelial layer that extends into stroma. The stromal component can undergo metaplasia into hyaline, osteoid, or cartilaginous material, with characteristic "mixed" appearance (Fig.106.4).[20,21] Pseudocapsules range from few microns to few hundred microns in thickness and can demonstrate bosselations.[4,15] Mitotic figures are rare and Ki-67 proliferative index is low, consistent with the typically benign course.[15,20] Cytogenetic studies of BMT have demonstrated a t(5;8)(p13;q12) translocation leading to overexpression of transcription factor PLAG1 (pleomorphic adenoma gene 1).[22] PLAG1 immunohistochemistry has been proposed as a useful diagnostic marker for differentiating BMT from ACC.[20]

The standard management of BMT of the LG is complete surgical excision with intact pseudocapsule via a lateral orbitotomy. Removal of normal tissue in the surrounding area is also recommended in cases of incomplete or dehiscent pseudocapsules, and some advocate for removal of periosteum in all cases.[23] BMT of the palpebral lobe can be removed anteriorly from a transcutaneous or transconjunctival approach.[4,19] Classical teaching is that an incisional biopsy is contraindicated because violation of the pseudocapsule is likely to lead to spilling of malignant cells into the surrounding tissue with subsequent recurrence. This no-biopsy approach has been challenged, however, given the lack of clear evidence and from extrapolation of extensive data from salivary gland ACC.[24] While many cases of BMT can be diagnosed correctly based on clinical history, examination, and imaging studies, the less typical cases can be misdiagnosed, and undergoing resection via lateral orbitotomy may be harmful to the patient. For those with ACC misdiagnosed as BMT, such cases would preclude the patient from benefiting from certain treatment options (e.g. neoadjuvant intra-arterial cytoreductive chemotherapy) and potentially lead to dire consequences for the patient's overall prognosis. For those with other benign lesions, lateral orbitotomy may be a surgery that

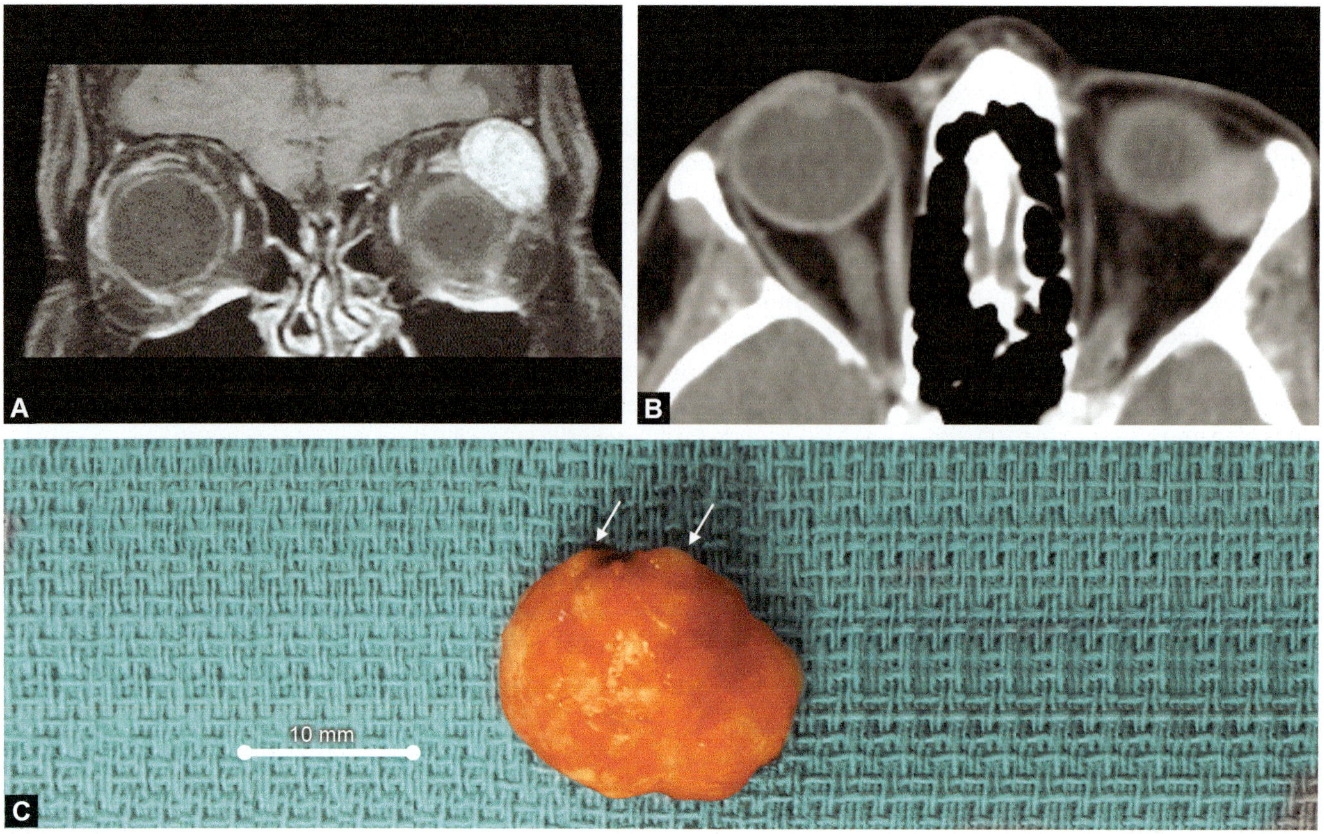

Figs. 106.3A to C: Benign pleomorphic adenoma. (A) T1-weighted, contrast-enhanced fat suppression MRI image in coronal view; (B) Axial view of CT with contrast showing a well-circumscribed, round mass with bony expansion of the lacrimal fossa and curved contact with the bony surface; (C) Completely excised specimen with intact pseudocapsule. Arrows demonstrate surface bosselations, which are irregular projections beyond the surface contour.

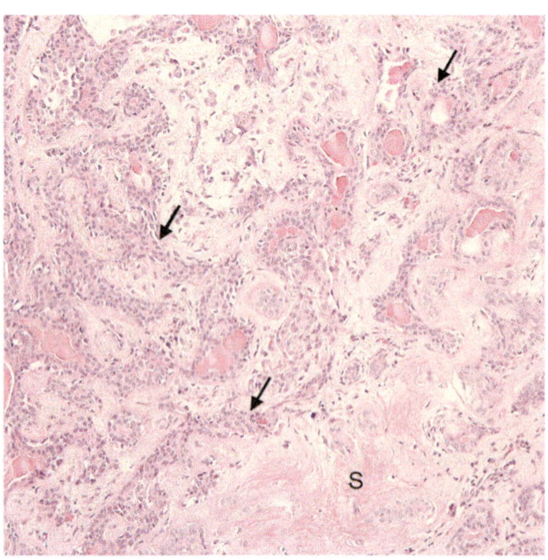

Fig. 106.4: Benign pleomorphic adenoma. Hematoxylin and eosin (H&E) stain demonstrating a mixture of cytologically benign myoepithelial elements that are present in glands and cords (arrows) interspersed with foci of variably basophilic stroma and mesenchymal elements (labeled S) (200X).

is unnecessarily extensive. Incisional biopsy is therefore no longer considered an absolute contraindication and routinely recommended by some surgeons for all LG masses.[4] Tse et al. also reported a technique of using butyl-2-cyanoacrylate glue at the incision site to avoid tumor spillage in the event of occult malignancy, which can be used as an adjunct during incisional biopsies.[25]

It is thought that recurrence is more likely related to incomplete removal of BMT at the time of excision rather than from tumor cell seeding. Font and Gamel reported a 3% 5-year recurrence rate for a completely excised BMT compared to 32% in incompletely excised BMT.[26] Given the slow-growing nature of BMT, recurrences typically take a long time to manifest (up to 60 years postresection).[27] However, recurrent cases of BMT can be more infiltrative with less clear demarcation of pseudocapsule or malignant transformation into carcinoma ex-pleomorphic adenoma (CEPA).[15,18,23,28]

Adenoid Cystic Carcinoma

Adenoid cystic carcinoma (ACC) of the LG is the most common epithelial malignancy of the LG constituting 32% of all epithelial tumors of the LG and 60% of all malignant epithelial tumors of the LG.[15,28,29] The mean age of presentation is 40, with slight female predilection.[30] Compared to salivary gland or breast ACC, ACC of the LG occurs less frequently, but is more often fatal.

Patients typically present with ptosis, proptosis, diplopia, and inferonasal displacement of the globe as can be expected from the location of the LG. Periocular pain is also a very characteristic symptom, occurring more frequently and earlier than in other LG tumors. This pain is thought to be secondary to the tendency for perineural spread and bony invasion. Involvement of sensory nerves (e.g. lacrimal nerve) can also result in frontotemporal hypesthesia. Diagnosis of ACC is typically made within 6 months of onset of symptoms. Both CT and MRI provide useful information for clinical diagnosis, management, and post-treatment surveillance. Given the propensity for infiltrative growth with bony destruction, CT is useful for demonstrating the integrity of the bony margins of the lacrimal fossa and assessing the risk or the extent of tumor extension into the intracranial space or temporalis fossa. MRI provides essential soft tissue anatomic details of the orbital structures and can demonstrate the presence of posterior extension through the orbital apex and superior orbital fissure, which can have significant implications for treatment plan and prognosis (Figs. 106.5A to D).[4,29,30]

The histopathologic characteristics of ACC result from mutated ductal epithelial and myoepithelial components

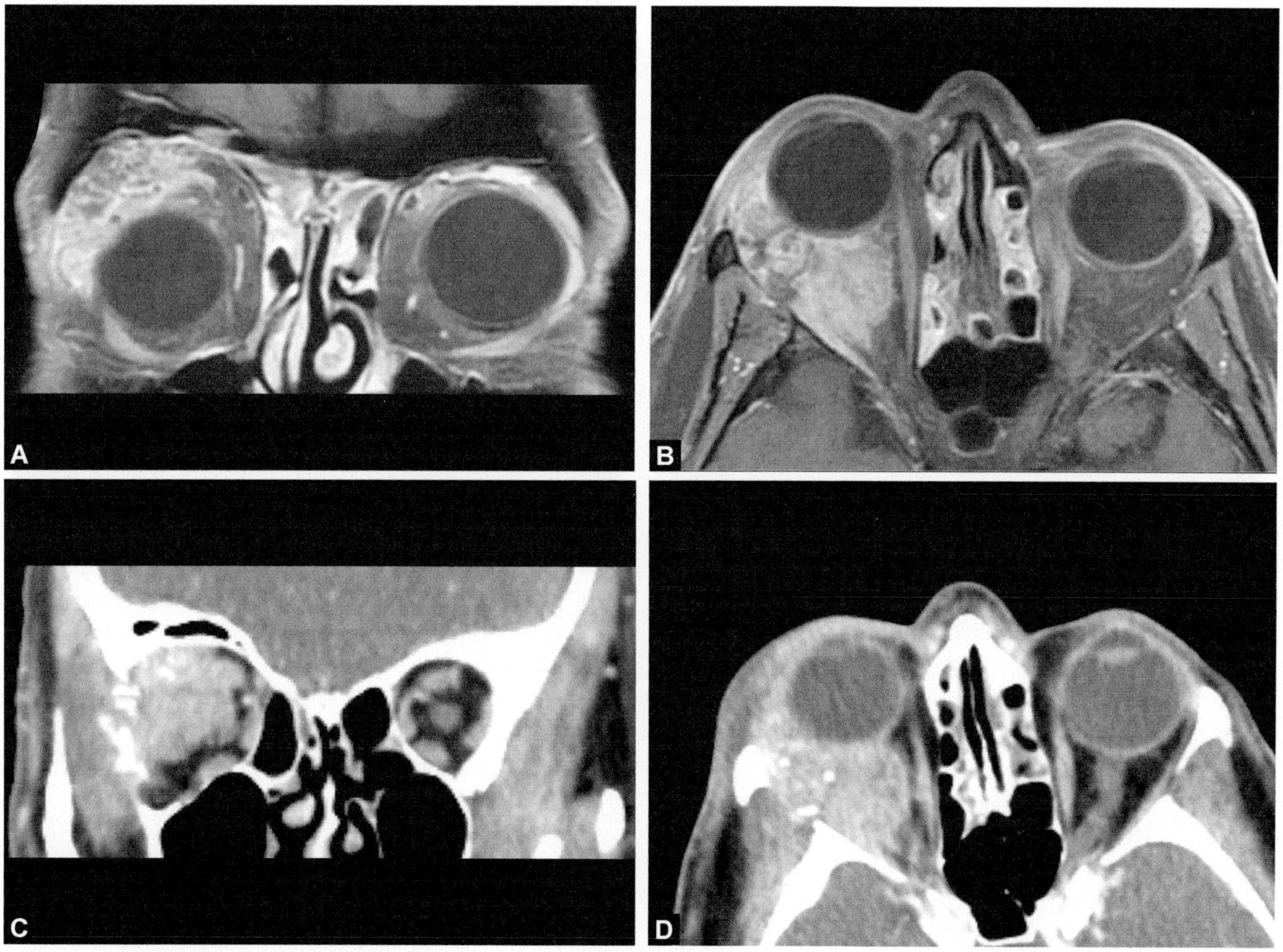

Figs. 106.5A to D: Adenoid cystic carcinoma. T1-weighted, contrast-enhanced fat suppression MRI images in (A) coronal and (B) axial views and CT with contrast in (C) coronal; (D) axial views demonstrating a large, heterogeneously enhancing infiltrative mass with extraconal and intraconal extension and adjacent bony destruction.

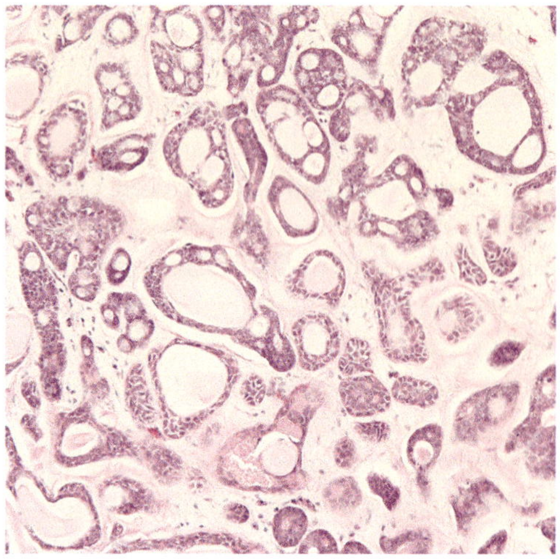

Fig. 106.6: Adenoid cystic carcinoma. Hematoxylin and eosin (H & E) stain demonstrating basophilic cells in a cribriform (Swiss cheese) architecture (200X).

that mimic normal glandular structures. The three predominant histopathologic subtypes are cribriform (55%), solid/basaloid (18%), and tubular/ductal (5%).[15] Cribriform or "Swiss cheese" pattern is generally associated with lower mitotic activity and more favorable survival rate (Fig. 106.6), while those with any component of solid/basaloid subtype are associated with higher mitotic activity and worse prognosis.[15,29] On histologic sections, perineural invasion was present in up to 85% of cases, and Ahmad et al. reported presence of perineural invasion in the initial surgical specimen of 93% of patients who experienced subsequent local recurrence.[29-31] Interestingly, perineural invasion itself did not correlate with higher mitotic activity or histologic subtype.[15] Due to the infiltrative nature of ACC, microscopic metastases are thought to exist at the time of diagnosis in many cases. Rates of distant metastasis have been reported to range from 50% to 80% and the most common sites of distant metastasis are lung (45%), bone (20%), liver (20%), and lymph nodes (10%).[23,26,30] The principal cause of death, however, is frequently intracranial extension from local recurrence rather than from distant metastasis.[4]

ACC is a slow-growing but aggressive disease, with unfavorable prognosis for many patients. The most commonly cited actuarial survival rates are from Font and Gamel who reported a survival rate of 50% at 5 years and 20% at 10 years regardless of type of treatment regimen.[26] A retrospective case series of 20 patients over 50 years showed local recurrence in 7 patients (35%), distant metastasis in 16 patients (80%), disease-related deaths in 13 patients (65%) and overall median disease-free survival of 18 months.[30] A review of 53 patients from 8 institutions using the American Joint Committee on Cancer (AJCC) classification demonstrated that tumor stage at the time of initial diagnosis correlates with outcome, with 17 of 38 patients (45%) with more than T3 tumors and 1 of 15 patients (7%) with less than T3 tumors dying of disease during the study period.[31] Age of disease onset also has a prognostic value, as patients younger than 19 years tend to have a low-grade, nonbasaloid type ACC with higher survival rates compared to older patients.[29,32] However, for those that do survive, long-term follow-up is essential, as demonstrated by reports of recurrences occurring 7–9 years post-treatment.[32]

No standardized consensus treatment based on staging exists for LG ACC and patients may be offered different surgical, chemotherapeutic, or radiation therapy depending on the institution. First, an incisional biopsy via trans-septal approach is recommended to establish a definitive diagnosis. Once confirmed, local surgical control has traditionally been in the form of orbital exenteration with or without adjacent bone removal. Despite such radical surgery, the infiltrative nature of ACC often makes it challenging to achieve clear surgical margins. In such cases, adjuvant external beam radiotherapy can be delivered up to a total dose of 60–65 Gy.[29,30] Brachytherapy, proton beam therapy, and neutron therapy have also been reported with variable results. Adjuvant intravenous chemotherapy is not considered part of standard treatment and is thought to have limited and short-lived effect even in metastatic disease. In cases of radiotherapy, however, cisplatin can be delivered as a radio sensitizer, and can be combined with additional cytotoxic therapy (e.g. doxorubicin) for added effect.[33] In cases of early detection with relatively confined tumor extent, globe-sparing resection has also been proposed in lieu of radical resection.[31,34] A number of studies have demonstrated lack of clear survival benefit from radical surgery, especially when globe-sparing surgery is paired with adjuvant radiotherapy.[31,35] Preferred surgical approach is via lateral orbitotomy, and superior or transfrontal orbitotomy is not recommended given the risk of intracranial seeding of malignant cells.[4]

Another approach to treatment of ACC is via neoadjuvant intra-arterial cytoreductive chemotherapy (IACC) proposed by Tse et al.[36-38] This protocol consists of three cycles of intra-arterial cisplatin 100 mg/m^2 on day 1 and intravenous (IV) doxorubicin 25 mg/m^2 on days 1–3 every 3 weeks. Repeat imaging is obtained at the conclusion of third cycle, which typically shows visible shrinkage of tumor volume, downstaging advanced cases into surgically resectable cases. 3–4 weeks are allowed for hematologic recovery, and orbital exenteration is then performed. Surgery is followed by adjuvant radiotherapy with concomitant weekly IV cisplatin 20 mg/m^2 for radio sensitization. Three cycles of adjuvant IV cisplatin 100 mg/m^2 on day 1 and IV doxorubicin 20 mg/m^2 on days 1–3 every 3 weeks are given. Tse et al. reported 100% 10-year disease-free survival rate with the neoadjuvant IACC protocol compared to 14.3% in conventional treatment group.[38] The longest surviving patient treated with this protocol was 24 years post-treatment in 2013 at the time of publication of the long-term outcomes.[38]

Potential advantages of neoadjuvant IACC include the ability to deliver a high concentration of chemotherapeutic agent to the area of interest while minimizing systemic toxicity. Treatment prior to surgery can also achieve tumor shrinkage, and potentially minimizes dissemination or seeding of malignant cells during surgical manipulation. LG's arterial supply is via the lacrimal artery, which is a branch off of the ophthalmic artery. IACC is delivered via the external carotid circulation through the anastomotic branches to avoid any untoward side effects to the intracranial circulation.[36,37] The most common complications of the IACC protocol include myelosuppression, nausea, vomiting, fever, sepsis, hair loss, and potential for cardiac damage, renal dysfunction, ototoxicity, and thrombotic or vascular compromise due to the intra-arterial approach. One case of ophthalmic artery occlusion, anterior segment ischemia, and partial skin nonperfusion and hyperpigmentation after administration of intra-arterial chemotherapy via the ophthalmic artery has been reported.[38] It is therefore recommended that the neoadjuvant IACC be offered and administered in a tertiary care center with appropriate support services and experienced medical and radiation oncologists.[4]

Most recent efforts in genetic and molecular profiling of ACC have demonstrated an overexpression of oncogene MYB, frequently as a result of a translocation t(6;9) (q22-23; p23-24) leading to a fusion transcript MYB-NFIB.[39] The translocation has been shown to juxtapose super-enhancers to the MYB locus leading to a positive feedback loop that drives MYB overexpression.[40] One of the downstream targets of MYB has been identified as the notch signaling pathway via whole-genome sequencing of LG ACC.[40,41] These molecular components of the oncogenic pathway of ACC have potential implications for targeted therapy for the disease in the future—notch inhibitors and bromodomain (MYB enhancer-associated protein) inhibitors, for instance, have been studied in vitro and in mouse xenograft models with some promising results.[40,42] MYB has also been proposed as an immunohistochemical marker for ACC for its ability to discriminate ACC from BMT with high specificity.[20,43]

OTHER TUMORS OF THE LACRIMAL GLAND

Primary Adenocarcinoma

Primary adenocarcinoma of the LG is an aggressive tumor comprising 5–10% of malignant epithelial tumors of the LG and 3% of all malignant tumors of the LG.[5,15,26,28,35] Histopathologically, ductal or glandular cells in sheets and cords with varying degrees of differentiation can be seen with high pleomorphism and mitotic activity.[15,28] Mean age at presentation has been reported between 56 and 63, with a male predilection.[5,15,26,28] Clinical symptoms and presentation are similar to those of ACC with palpable mass, proptosis, and pain. Early lymphatic metastasis can be seen, with distant metastasis to liver, lung, bone, and spinal cord.[4] Treatment consists of exenteration and adjuvant radiation, with or without radical neck dissection. Prognosis is poor, however, with 50–80% mortality.[15,26,32]

Pleomorphic Adenocarcinoma (Malignant Mixed Tumor, Carcinoma Ex Pleomorphic Adenoma)

Malignant mixed tumor, or pleomorphic adenocarcinoma can arise de novo, or as a result of malignant transformation of incompletely excised BMT (carcinoma ex pleomorphic adenoma, or CEPA). Reported incidence ranges from 4% to 19% of malignant epithelial tumors of the LG with male predominance and mean age of presentation of 52 years.[4,28] Histopathologically, areas of BMT can be seen adjacent to variable proportions of malignant transformation. Treatment consists of complete surgical resection. Prognosis is guarded, however, with 50% mortality by 12 years.[26] Patients with pleomorphic adenocarcinomas arising from BMT show longer survival (mean 19.2 years) compared to patients with de novo type (mean 7.7 years).[44]

Mucoepidermoid Carcinoma

Mucoepidermoid carcinoma makes up 2% of all LG tumors and approximately 4% of malignant epithelial tumors of the LG.[1,28] Histopathologically, the tumor is composed of mucous, epidermoid-squamous, intermediate, columnar, clear, and oncocytic cells in cords and islands. Mucin stains with mucicarmine and Alcian blue. The clinical presentation is generally less aggressive than that of ACC or primary adenocarcinoma with a mean age at presentation of 49–61 years with a female predilection.[5,28,45] Treatment consists of excision with or without adjuvant radiation for grade 1 and 2 tumor, and exenteration with radiation in grade 3. While a 10-year disease-specific survival of 79% has been reported, it should be noted that prognosis varies with tumor grade, with greater than 50% mortality in grade 3 with lung and mediastinal metastasis.[5,15]

CONCLUSION

Lacrimal gland tumors are relatively rare entities compared to the gland's involvement with inflammatory disorders. The three most common types of LG tumors are lymphoma, benign pleomorphic adenoma, and adenoid cystic carcinoma. While rare, it is essential to recognize and manage these conditions appropriately, as delayed or missed diagnosis can have dire consequences for the patient. Lymphoma of the LG may uncover systemic lymphoma requiring chemotherapy and radiation. Benign pleomorphic adenoma versus adenoid cystic carcinoma is an important bifurcation point in the evaluation of LG tumors with two vastly different treatment algorithms and prognosis. As with any orbital process, every patient should be approached with a thorough history and physical examination to formulate a differential diagnosis. Imaging studies, and ultimately tissue biopsy confirms the diagnosis of the type of LG tumor.

REFERENCES

1. Bonavolontà G, Strianese D, Grassi P, et al. An analysis of 2,480 space-occupying lesions of the orbit from 1976 to 2011.Ophthal Plast Reconstr Surg. 2013;29(2):79-86.
2. von Holstein SL. Tumours of the lacrimal gland. Epidemiological, clinical and genetic characteristics.Acta Ophthalmol (Copenh). 2013;916:1-28.
3. Reese AB. The treatment of expanding lesions of the orbit with particular regard to those arising in the lacrimal gland; the seventh Arthur J. Bedell lecture. Am J Ophthalmol. 1956;41(1):3-11.
4. Tse DT, Neff AG, Onofrey CB. Recent developments in the evaluation and treatment of lacrimal gland tumors. Ophthalmol Clin. 2000;13(4):663-81.
5. Andreoli MT, Aakalu V, Setabutr P. Epidemiological trends in malignant lacrimal gland tumors. Otolaryngol Head Neck Surg. 2015;152(2):279-83.
6. Rasmussen P, Ralfkiaer E, Prause JU, et al. Malignant lymphoma of the lacrimal gland: a nation-based study. Arch Ophthalmol. 2011;129(10):1275-80.
7. Andreasen S, Esmaeli B, Holstein SL von, et al. An Update on Tumors of the Lacrimal Gland. Asia-Pac J OphthalmolPhila Pa. 2017;6(2):159-72.
8. Verdijk RM. Lymphoproliferative tumors of the ocular adnexa. Asia-Pac J Ophthalmol Phila. 2017;6(2):132-42.
9. Jakobiec FA, Yeo JH, Trokel SL, et al. Combined clinical and computed tomographic diagnosis of primary lacrimal fossa lesions. Am J Ophthalmol. 1982;94(6):785-807.
10. Jakobiec FA, Knowles DM. An overview of ocular adnexal lymphoid tumors. Trans Am Ophthalmol Soc. 1989;87:420-42; discussion 442-4.
11. Woolf DK, Kuhan H, Shoffren O, et al. Outcomes of primary lymphoma of the ocular adnexa (orbital lymphoma) treated with radiotherapy. Clin Oncol R CollRadiol GB. 2015;27(3):153-9.
12. Salles G, Seymour JF, Offner F, et al. Rituximab maintenance for 2 years in patients with high tumour burden follicular lymphoma responding to rituximab plus chemotherapy (PRIMA): a phase 3, randomised controlled trial. Lancet Lond Engl. 2011;377(9759):42-51.
13. Rasmussen PK, Ralfkiaer E, Prause JU, et al. Follicular lymphoma of the ocular adnexal region: a nation-based study. Acta Ophthalmol (Copenh). 2015;93(2):184-91.
14. Munch-Petersen HD, Rasmussen PK, Coupland SE, et al. Ocular adnexal diffuse large B-cell lymphoma: a multicenter international study. JAMA Ophthalmol. 2015;133(2):165-73.
15. Weis E, Rootman J, Joly TJ, et al. Epithelial lacrimal gland tumors: pathologic classification and current understanding. Arch Ophthalmol. 2009;127(8):1016-28.
16. Chawla B, Kashyap S, Sen S, et al. Clinicopathologic review of epithelial tumors of the lacrimal gland. Ophthal Plast Reconstr Surg. 2013;29(6):440-5.
17. von Holstein SL, Fehr A, Persson M, et al. Lacrimal gland pleomorphic adenoma and carcinoma ex pleomorphic adenoma: genomic profiles, gene fusions, and clinical characteristics. Ophthalmology. 2014;121(5):1125-33.
18. Rose GE, Wright JE. Pleomorphic adenoma of the lacrimal gland. Br J Ophthalmol. 1992;76(7):395-400.
19. Auran J, Jakobiec FA, Krebs W. Benign mixed tumor of the palpebral lobe of the lacrimal gland. Clinical diagnosis and appropriate surgical management. Ophthalmology. 1988;95(1):90-9.
20. Mendoza PR, Jakobiec FA, Krane JF. Immunohistochemical features of lacrimal gland epithelial tumors. Am J Ophthalmol. 2013;156(6):1147-58.e1.
21. Rashid A, Jakobiec FA. Avoiding the major complication of ophthalmic pathology: misdiagnosis. A review of three

common diagnostic challenges. Semin Ophthalmol. 2014;29(5-6):468-74.
22. Voz ML, Aström AK, Kas K, et al. The recurrent translocation t(5;8)(p13;q12) in pleomorphic adenomas results in upregulation of PLAG1 gene expression under control of the LIFR promoter. Oncogene. 1998;16(11):1409-16.
23. Wright JE, Stewart WB, Krohel GB. Clinical presentation and management of lacrimal gland tumours. Br J Ophthalmol. 1979;63(9):600-6.
24. Lai T, Prabhakaran VC, Malhotra R, et al. Pleomorphic adenoma of the lacrimal gland: is there a role for biopsy? Eye Lond Engl. 2009;23(1):2-6.
25. Tse DT, Folberg R. Technique for incisional biopsy of a lacrimal gland mass when the diagnosis of benign mixed tumor cannot be excluded clinically. Ophthalmic Surg. 1988;19(5):321-4.
26. Font RL, Gamel JW. Epithelial tumors of the lacrimal gland: an analysis of 265 cases. In: Jakobiec FA (Ed). Ocular and adnexal tumors. Birmingham, Alabama: Aesculapius Publishing Co.; 1978. pp. 787-805.
27. Shields JA, Shields CL. Malignant transformation of presumed pleomorphic adenoma of lacrimal gland after 60 years. Arch Ophthalmol. 1987;105(10):1403-5.
28. Shields JA, Shields CL, Epstein JA, et al. Review: primary epithelial malignancies of the lacrimal gland: the 2003 Ramon L. Font lecture. Ophthal Plast Reconstr Surg. 2004;20(1):10-21.
29. Woo KI, Yeom A, Esmaeli B. Management of lacrimal gland carcinoma: lessons from the literature in the past 40 years. Ophthal Plast Reconstr Surg. 2016;32(1):1-10.
30. Esmaeli B, Ahmadi MA, Youssef A, et al. Outcomes in patients with adenoid cystic carcinoma of the lacrimal gland. Ophthal Plast Reconstr Surg. 2004;20(1):22-6.
31. Ahmad SM, Esmaeli B, Williams M, et al. American Joint Committee on Cancer classification predicts outcome of patients with lacrimal gland adenoid cystic carcinoma. Ophthalmology. 2009;116(6):1210-5.
32. Wright JE, Rose GE, Garner A. Primary malignant neoplasms of the lacrimal gland. Br J Ophthalmol. 1992;76(7):401-7.
33. Le Tourneau C, Razak AR, Levy C, et al. Role of chemotherapy and molecularly targeted agents in the treatment of adenoid cystic carcinoma of the lacrimal gland. Br J Ophthalmol. 2011;95(11):1483-9.
34. Esmaeli B, Yin VT, Hanna EY, et al. Eye-sparing multidisciplinary approach for the management of lacrimal gland carcinoma. Head Neck. 2016;38(8):1258-62.
35. Polito E, Leccisotti A. Epithelial malignancies of the lacrimal gland: survival rates after extensive and conservative therapy. Ann Ophthalmol. 1993;25(11):422-6.
36. Meldrum ML, Tse DT, Benedetto P. Neoadjuvant intracarotid chemotherapy for treatment of advanced adenocystic carcinoma of the lacrimal gland. Arch Ophthalmol. 1998;116(3):315-21.
37. Tse DT, Benedetto P, Dubovy S, et al. Clinical analysis of the effect of intra-arterial cytoreductive chemotherapy in the treatment of lacrimal gland adenoid cystic carcinoma. Am J Ophthalmol. 2006;141(1):44-53.
38. Tse DT, Kossler AL, Feuer WJ, et al. Long-term outcomes of neoadjuvant intra-arterial cytoreductive chemotherapy for lacrimal gland adenoid cystic carcinoma. Ophthalmology. 2013;120(7):1313-23.
39. von Holstein SL, Fehr A, Persson M, et al. Adenoid cystic carcinoma of the lacrimal gland: MYB gene activation, genomic imbalances, and clinical characteristics. Ophthalmology. 2013;120(10):2130-8.
40. Drier Y, Cotton MJ, Williamson KE, et al. An oncogenic MYB feedback loop drives alternate cell fates in adenoid cystic carcinoma. Nat Genet. 2016;48(3):265-72.
41. Sant DW, Tao W, Field MG, et al. Whole Exome Sequencing of Lacrimal Gland Adenoid Cystic Carcinoma. Invest Ophthalmol Vis Sci. 2017;58(6):BIO240-6.
42. Ferrarotto R, Heymach JV, Glisson BS. MYB-fusions and other potential actionable targets in adenoid cystic carcinoma. Curr Opin Oncol. 2016;28(3):195-200.
43. Moon A, Cohen C, Siddiqui MT. MYB expression: Potential role in separating adenoid cystic carcinoma (ACC) from pleomorphic adenoma (PA). Diagn Cytopathol. 2016;44(10):799-804.
44. Henderson JW, Farrow GM. Primary malignant mixed tumors of the lacrimal gland. Report of 10 cases. Ophthalmology. 1980;87(6):466-75.
45. Eviatar JA, Hornblass A. Mucoepidermoid carcinoma of the lacrimal gland: 25 cases and a review and update of the literature. Ophthal Plast Reconstr Surg. 1993;9(3):170-81.

Chapter 107 Orbital and Periorbital Infections: Evaluation and Management

Md Shahid Alam, Bipasha Mukherjee

INTRODUCTION

The orbit is a closed space surrounded by bony walls and the overlying periorbita. There are several anatomical factors which are responsible for orbital infections:

- Close proximity to the paranasal sinuses
- Thin bone of lamina papyracea forming the medial wall of the orbits
- The valveless veins of the midface.

Orbital infections most commonly result from spread from the surrounding structures.

Various pathogenic organisms (bacteria, fungi, viruses) or parasites (rhinosporidia, cysticerci) are found to infect the orbits.

The diverse clinical features and management protocols are outlined below for each of them.

BACTERIAL INFECTIONS

Bacteria are the most common causative organisms for orbital infections amongst all age groups. Bacterial infections in the orbit can be secondary to trauma,[1] endogenous spread,[2,3] sinusitis,[4] dental infections,[5] postsurgery[6] and intraocular infection.[7]

Classification and Management

Chandlers classified orbital cellulitis into five distinct stages.[8] These are based upon the evolution of disease process, but patients may not necessarily follow the disease sequence and can present at any stage.

Stage 1: Preseptal Cellulitis (Fig. 107.1)

Preseptal cellulitis refers to inflammation which is limited anterior to the orbital septum. Patients usually present with erythema, edema, and tenderness of the eyelid and periorbital tissues. There can be associated redness and watering from the eyes. Patient can have mild to moderate temperature elevation. The condition should be differentiated from orbital cellulitis which needs treatment on an emergent basis (Table 107.1).

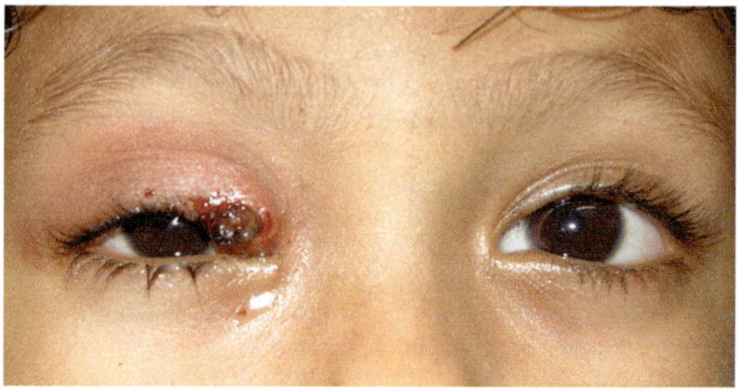

Fig. 107.1: External photograph showing erythema and edema of right upper lid along with crusting and excoriation suggestive of external hordeolum with preseptal cellulitis.

Table 107.1: Differentiating clinical features between preseptal and orbital cellulitis.

Clinical features	Preseptal cellulitis	Orbital cellulitis
Vision	Normal	Decreased
Pain	Absent/Mild	Present
Proptosis	Absent	Present
Pupillary involvement	Absent	Variable
Chemosis	Absent/Mild	Present
Ophthalmoplegia	Absent	Present
Systemic features	Absent	Present

Management: Preseptal cellulitis, either in adults or pediatric population, can be treated on an outpatient basis with broad-spectrum oral antibiotics and anti-inflammatory medication. A penicillin-clavulanic acid combination is the preferred choice. Hot fomentation helps in symptomatic relief. Topical antibiotic ointment for local application can be prescribed for any visible foci of infection. The patients should be under close follow-up especially if children. Imaging and blood investigations are generally not required.

Stage 2: Orbital Cellulitis (Figs. 107.2A to C)

Orbital cellulitis is when the inflammation extends beyond the orbital septum. These patients generally present with proptosis, blurring of vision, pupillary involvement, and decreased extraocular motility. These patients can have associated fever. Orbital cellulitis is an emergency and all such patients need to be admitted and treated immediately. If not managed promptly and properly, patients of orbital cellulitis can develop sight, or life-threatening complications (Box 107.1).

Ethmoidal sinusitis is the most common cause of orbital cellulitis at all ages and results from septic thrombophlebitis of the valveless veins between the orbit and the sinuses.[8] The sphenoid sinus may also get involved by contiguous spread from the ethmoid sinus. Patients with sphenoethmoidalis can present with marked visual loss with or without ophthalmoplegia even before proptosis and other orbital signs develop.[9]

Box 107.1: Complications of orbital cellulitis.

Orbital cellulitis complications:[10,11]
- Permanent blindness
- Cavernous sinus thrombosis
- Optic neuropathy
- Exposure or neurotrophic keratitis
- Carotid occlusion
- Exudative retinal detachment
- Central retinal artery occlusion
- Septic embolus
- Meningitis
- Brain abscess

A retrospective review of pediatric orbital cellulitis found that *Staphylococcus* species was the most common organism isolated followed by *Streptococcus*. This study found that 73% of *Staphylococcus aureus* isolates were methicillin-resistant *S. aureus* (MRSA).[10] Nonhemolytic *Streptococcus*, group A β-hemolytic *Streptococcus*, *S. aureus* and *Haemophilus influenzae*, were the most common isolated organisms in a cohort of 41 pediatric cases of postseptal cellulitis studied by Nageswaran et al.[11] The number of *H. influenzae* cases has decreased significantly after introduction of *H. influenzae* type b vaccine.[12] In adults, most cases of orbital cellulitis are caused by *Staphylococcus* and *Streptococcus* species,[13] but unlike children, adults are more likely to harbor polymicrobial infections. This is understandable, given the difference in sinus anatomy between the adult and pediatric population. In adults, the sinus ostia are smaller and the sinuses are well developed leading to a poorer drainage and better chances of colonization by polymicrobial and anaerobic organisms.[14]

Investigations:
- *Hematological:* Routine hemogram (total and differential blood count, hemoglobin), blood sugar and blood culture.
- *Imaging:* Computed tomography (CT) is the imaging of choice.[15] CT scans help in identifying extent of sinusitis and delineate subperiosteal abscess (SPA). Use of contrast helps to differentiate an abscess from an inflammatory phlegmon. It also rules out conditions

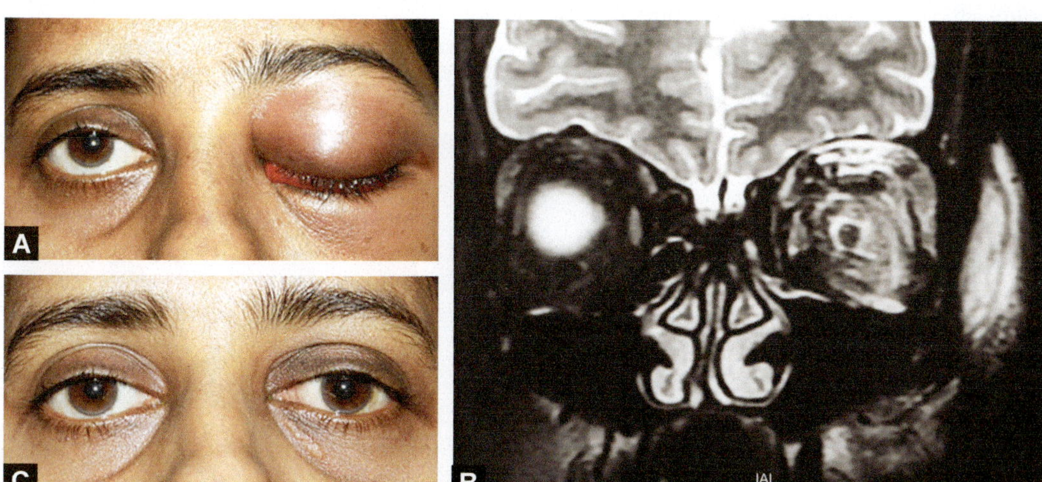

Figs. 107.2A to C: (A) External photograph showing left eye upper lid edema, proptosis, and mechanical ptosis in a patient of orbital cellulitis; (B) MRI coronal section, T2-weighted sequence of the same patient showing ill-defined mixed intensity soft tissue lesion of the left orbit with fat stranding suggestive of orbital inflammation; (C) Complete resolution of left eye orbital cellulitis with systemic antibiotics.

which can masquerade as orbital cellulitis in children (retinoblastoma and rhabdomyosarcoma).
- *Microbiological investigation:* Any purulent discharge from the orbits, lids or sinuses should be sent for microbiological evaluation.

Management: Orbital cellulitis either in an adult or a child warrants urgent admission and broad-spectrum intravenous antibiotics. Parenteral cefuroxime 1.5 g or amoxicillin-clavulanic acid combination 1.2 g with metronidazole 500 mg thrice daily can be started on an empirical basis until culture results are available. In areas of high incidence of MRSA, patients can be given vancomycin, cefotaxime and either metronidazole or clindamycin.[16] A nasal decongestant like oxymetazoline helps in drainage of the sinus.[17] Consultation with an Otolaryngologist is desirable in patients with documented sinusitis on CT scan. Unresponsive patients ultimately will need sinus drainage. Vision, ocular motility, and pupillary reaction of the patient should be closely monitored. Any patient of orbital cellulitis with suspected orbital compartment syndrome should undergo emergency canthotomy and cantholysis to prevent compressive neuropathy.

Neutropenic patients are especially susceptible to get infected with *Pseudomonas aeruginosa. Pseudomonas* is a rare cause of orbital infection and can present with eyelid necrosis, extensive soft tissue necrosis and can be life threatening. Early reversal of neutropenia is vital in management of these patients.[18]

The use of steroids in orbital cellulitis remains controversial. Fungal infections and immunocompromised patients may further deteriorate. However, studies show that addition of steroids, after ruling out fungal infection, hasten solution of inflammation with a low risk of exacerbating infection.[19]

Stage 3: Subperiosteal Abscess (Figs. 107.3A and B)

Subperiosteal abscess refers to collection of pus in the space between the orbital bones and periosteum. Clinically orbital SPA may resemble orbital cellulitis and it may be difficult to differentiate between the two unless imaging is done.

Imaging: CT scan typically shows a dome-shaped lesion along one of the orbital walls. The corresponding sinus would often be opacified.

Management: Garcia and Harris have laid down the criteria for the management of SPA. Expectant observation on broad-spectrum intravenous antibiotics is recommended if there are no indications for abscess drainage[20] (Box 107.2).

Stage 4: Orbital Abscess (Figs. 107.4A to C)

Approximately 29–52% of all orbital cellulitis progress to orbital abscess wherein coalescence of the inflammatory response occurs leading to suppuration in the orbital fat

Box 107.2: Criteria for draining subperiosteal abscess (SPA).

Subperiosteal abscess drainage criteria:[21]
- Age more than 9 years
- Presence of frontal sinusitis
- Nonmedial location of SPA
- Large SPA
- Suspicion of anaerobic subperiosteal infection (e.g. presence of gas within the abscess as visualized on CT scan)
- Recurrence of SPA after previous drainage
- Evidence of chronic sinusitis
- Acute optic nerve or retinal compromise
- Infections of dental origin

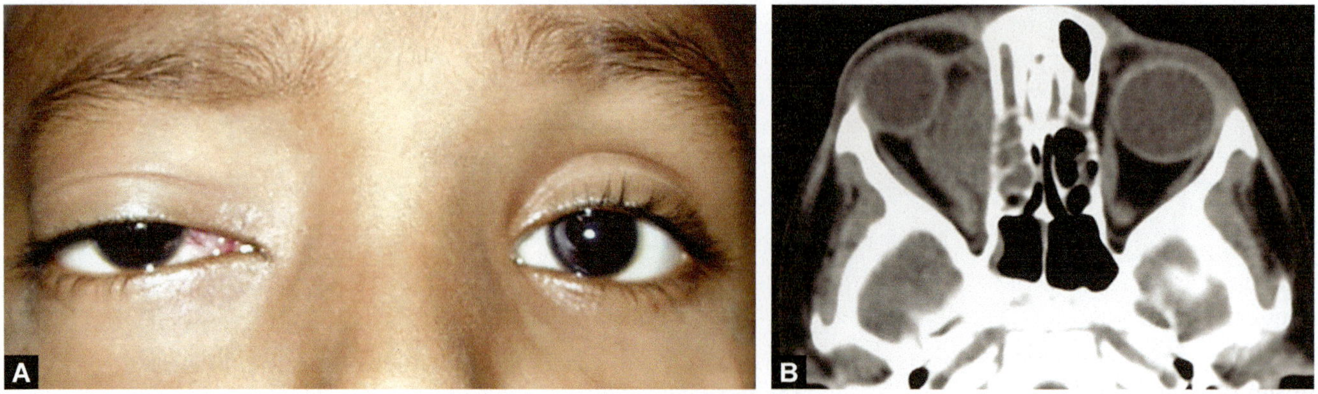

Figs. 107.3A and B: (A) External photograph showing fullness of right upper eyelid with proptosis; (B) CT scan of the same patient showing a dome-shaped hyperdense lesion in the medial orbit along with right ethmoid sinusitis suggestive of subperiosteal abscess.

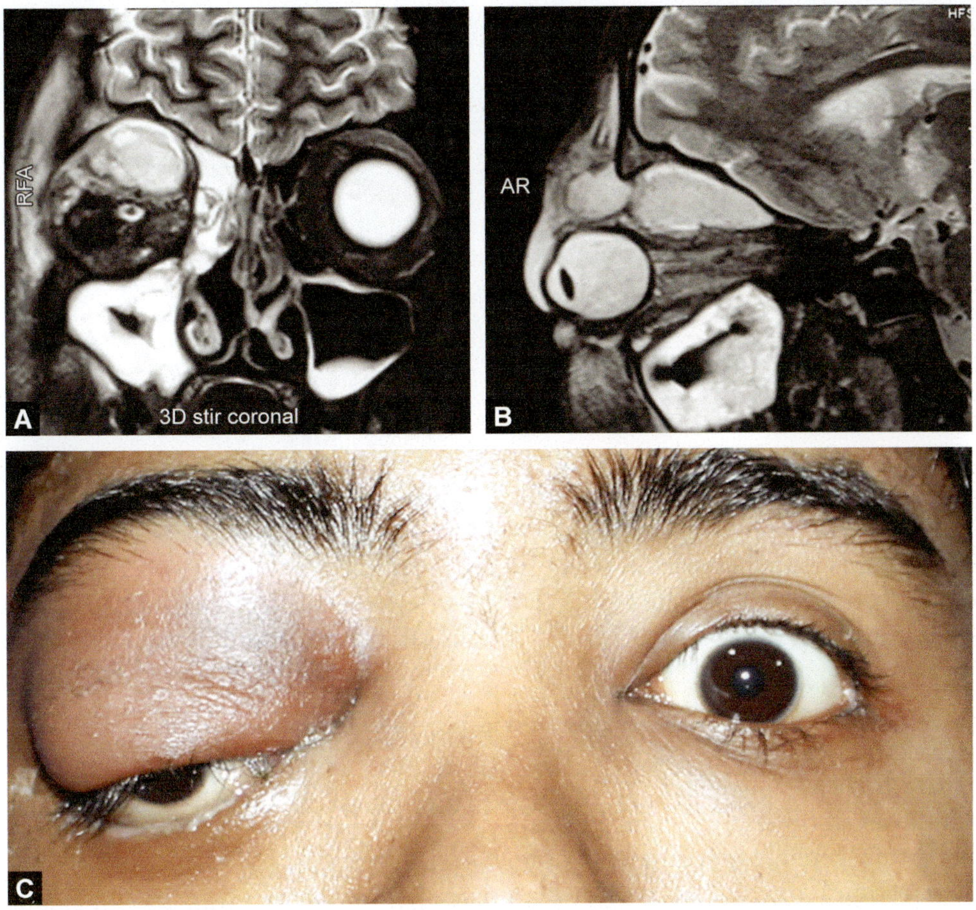

Figs. 107.4A to C: (A and B) MRI coronal and axial section, T2 sequence showing well-defined multiple cystic hyperintense lesion in the superior extraconal space with a peripheral rim, suggestive of multiple intraorbital abscesses; (C) External clinical photograph of the same patient showing proptosis, and inferior dystopia of right eye, suggesting a mass in the superior extraconal space.

inside or outside the muscle cone. Orbital abscesses can lead to both sight and life-threatening complications and blindness in known to ensue in 10–20% of these cases.[22]

Imaging: Orbital abscesses are more readily diagnosed on magnetic resonance imaging (MRI) and are better delineated compared to CT scan. They appear as well defined single or multiple orbital lesions with thick walls and central necrotic areas which are hypointense on T1 and hyperintense on T2-weighted sequences.

Management: All orbital abscesses irrespective of age and orbital location need an emergency drainage via orbitotomy. The patient can rapidly loose his vision if the abscess is not drained on an emergency basis. *Streptococcus milleri* is generally associated with multiple abscesses and a more fulminant course. In patients presenting with multiple intraorbital abscesses, *S. milleri* should be suspected and patient should be put on aggressive antibiotic coverage.[21,23]

Stage 5: Cavernous Sinus Thrombosis (Figs. 107.5A and B)

Cavernous sinus thrombosis (CST) is defined as thrombophlebitis of the cavernous sinus. CST is a rapidly progressing potentially life-threatening condition. It is usually heralded by progressive headache which precedes fever and cranial nerve palsies. Patients exhibit features of orbital infection including proptosis, chemosis, limited extraocular motility, pupillary involvement and visual compromise.[24] The process can become bilateral in the setting of CST, with infection spreading to other cavernous sinus via the intercavernous sinus and then to the fellow orbit. Lateral gaze palsy is usually the first sign to develop since 6th cranial nerve lies within the sinus.

Imaging: MRI and MR venography are better in identifying CST as compared to CT scan. MRI displays heterogeneous

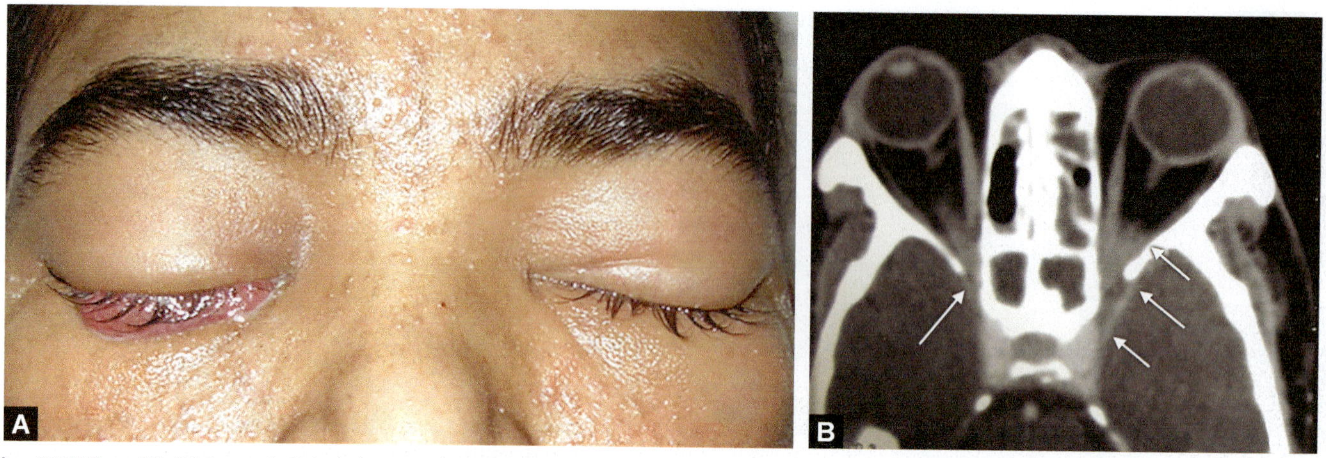

Figs. 107.5A and B: (A) External clinical photograph showing bilateral proptosis and complete ptosis; (B) CT scan axial cut of the same patient showing soft tissue lesion in the bilateral superior orbital fissure and cavernous sinus (arrows) suggestive of cavernous sinus thrombosis.

signal in the cavernous sinus with hyperintensity along the thrombosed portion.[25] There may be associated dilation of the superior ophthalmic vein.

Management:

- Broad-spectrum intravenous antibiotics with good central nervous system (CNS) penetration for 3–4 weeks are the mainstay of treatment for CST. The most commonly employed antibiotic regimen consists of a third-generation cephalosporin (cefotaxime, ceftriaxone, ceftazidime) and vancomycin in high doses (e.g. ceftazidime adult dose of 6 g/day in divided doses every 8 hours, vancomycin adult dose of 2–3 g/day in divided dose every 6–12 hours).[26] Administration of intravenous metronidazole is recommended if intracranial abscess is present.[26]
- *Anticoagulants:* Use of anticoagulants as a therapy in CST is controversial with studies citing both beneficial and adverse effects. Decreased thrombus formation and increased clot lysis prevent bacterial sequestration and less chances of relapses after cessation of antibiotic therapy.[27]
- *Steroids:* Corticosteroids may be beneficial for patients of CST by reducing intraorbital congestion and edema. They are absolutely indicated in cases of Addisonian crisis caused by pituitary ischemia. Corticosteroids also reduce cranial nerve inflammation in patients with cranial dysfunction.[28]

NECROTIZING FASCIITIS

Necrotizing fasciitis is a fulminant subcutaneous infection caused most commonly by group A β-hemolytic streptococci.[29] However, other organisms such as *Staphylococcus*, *Pseudomonas*, other anaerobes and many fungal and viral infections have also been reported to cause necrotizing fasciitis.[30] Necrotizing fasciitis is an emergency and should be differentiated from simple cellulitis or periorbital abscess.

Risk Factors[30]

Trauma is the most common risk factor. Even a minor incidental trauma is sufficient enough to incite the tissue destructive process.

- Diabetes mellitus
- Malignancy
- Sinusitis
- Immunocompromised state.

Pathophysiology[30]

Periorbital necrotizing fasciitis results from liquefactive necrosis caused by enzymes released both by the offending bacteria and inflammatory cells. Thrombosis of vessels invaded by bacteria cause tissue ischemia which further worsens the condition. As the condition progresses, ischemic necrosis of the skin, along with gangrene of the subcutaneous fat and dermis develops.

Clinical Features (Figs. 107.6A and B)

Diagnosis of necrotizing fasciitis is purely clinical. There is intense periorbital edema along with violaceous, tense skin. The patient is generally febrile. It is difficult to differentiate necrotizing fasciitis from simple cellulitis

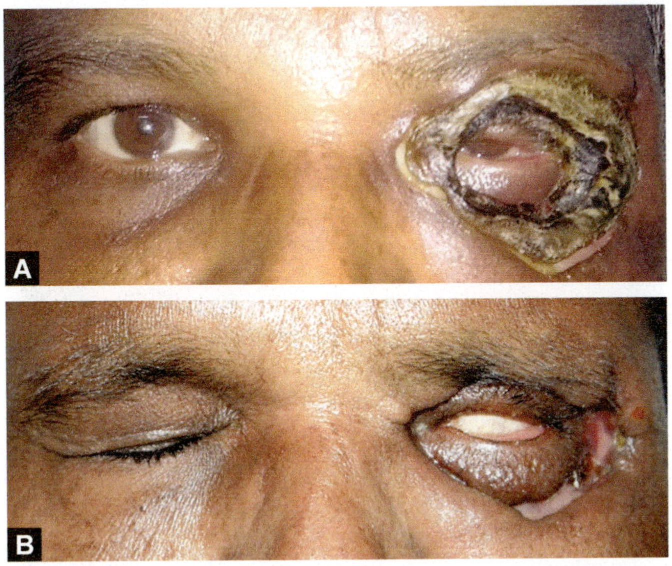

Figs. 107.6A and B: (A) Periorbital necrotizing fasciitis of the left eye with gangrenous necrotic periocular skin with purulent discharge; (B) External photograph showing lagophthalmos and lower lid cicatricial ectropion after surgical debridement.

in the initial stages. Severe pain disproportionate to the clinical findings and crepitus are clinical hallmarks of necrotizing fasciitis.

Investigations

- *Laboratory risk indicator in necrotizing fasciitis (LRINEC) score:* Laboratory investigations include total white blood cell count, C-reactive protein, hemoglobin level, serum sodium, serum creatinine, and the blood glucose level. Score of more than or equal to 6 is indicative of necrotizing fasciitis.[31]
- *Imaging:* CT scan with contrast is the imaging modality of choice. The hallmark feature is presence of air in soft tissue with fluid collection. CT is also helpful in demonstrating the extent of osseous involvement.[32]
- *Microbiology:* All debrided tissue should be sent for microbiological evaluation to identify the organism and its sensitivity to antibiotics.

Management

- *Surgical debridement:* Emergency surgical debridement is indicated in all cases of necrotizing fasciitis. Early surgical intervention is life-saving and a delay beyond 12 hours can prove fatal.[33]
- *Systemic antibiotics:* Intravenous broad-spectrum antibiotic coverage which includes a β-lactam (penicillin or cephalosporin), a protein synthesis inhibitor (clindamycin) and antianaerobe (metronidazole) should be prescribed.[30]
- *Hyperbaric oxygen:* Hypoxia present in the wound tissue resulting from vascular compromise can prove detrimental in wound healing.[29] Hyperbaric oxygen can increase the oxygen tension locally by up to 400 mm Hg which can hasten wound healing. However, its role still remains controversial.

FUNGAL INFECTIONS

Fungal infections are the second most common cause of orbital and periorbital infections. They are potentially vision and life threatening if timely intervention is not taken. The most common isolates in the orbit are Zygomycota and Ascomycota. Both classes have different clinical presentations, risk factors and virulence potential.[34]

Zygomycosis

The orbital fungal infection by this class of fungi is referred to as rhino-orbital-cerebral-zygomycosis (ROCZ), rhino-orbital-cerebral-mucormycosis (ROCM), zygomycosis, phycomycosis, mucormycosis and hyphomycosis.[34,35] The most common species is *Rhizopus oryzae*. It is the cause of roughly 90% of all ROCZ infections. It is a nonseptate filamentous fungus and is generally found in soil, decaying fruit and vegetables, animal feces and old bread.[35]

Routes of Spread to Orbit

- Infections from adjacent paranasal sinuses (most common)
- Hematogenous spread
- Spread from primary respiratory infection.

Risk Factors

- *Immunocompromised status:* Acquired immunodeficiency syndrome (AIDS), diabetes, organ transplant patients
- Neutropenia
- *Iron overload:* Hemodialysis and hemochromatosis
- Desferrioxamine therapy
- Intravenous drug abuse
- Systemic steroids.

Clinical Features

- Early sign and symptoms of ROCM include fever, sinusitis, nasal discharge, epistaxis, orbital and periorbital pain, nasal mucosal, ulceration, crusting and necrosis.[34]

- A black eschar of skin, nasal mucosa or palate is characteristic of mucormycosis.
- Decreased vision, proptosis, periorbital edema and complete external ophthalmoplegia are the most common ophthalmic features.
- Other ophthalmic sign and symptoms include ptosis, chemosis, congestion, internal ophthalmoplegia, and corneal anesthesia.
- Sudden blindness can occur due to central retinal artery occlusion, thrombosis of post ciliary arteries, infarction of the intraorbital part of optic nerve, or direct fungal invasion of the intracranial part of the optic nerve or optic chiasm.
- From the orbit the infection can spread to brain through cribriform plate, orbital apex and ophthalmic vessels.
- Features associated with a poorer prognosis include periorbital necrosis, CST and hemiplegia.

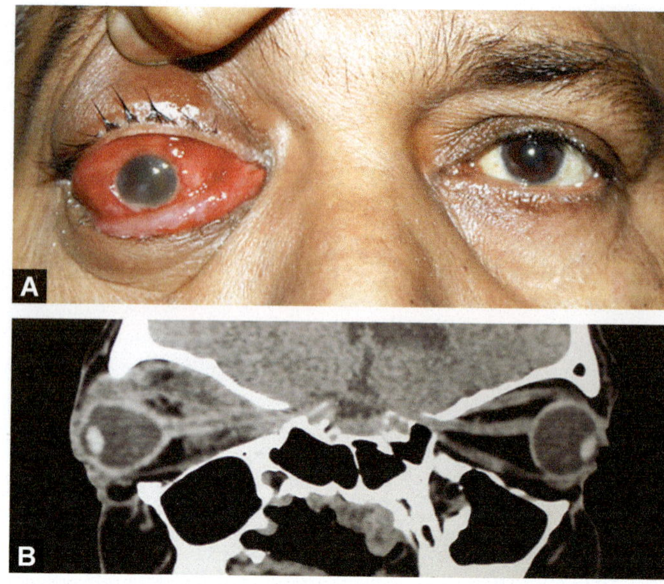

Figs. 107.7A and B: (A) External clinical photograph showing eye proptosis and chemosis; (B) CT scan parasagittal section showing proptosed right globe with fat stranding and ill-defined mass in the posterior and superior orbit.

Orbital Aspergillosis

Orbital aspergillosis is an uncommon orbital fungal infection which can affect both immunocompetent and immunocompromised individuals. Similar to mucormycosis, the infection commonly spreads from the paranasal sinuses.

Common species: *Aspergillus fumigatus, Aspergillus flavus, Aspergillus niger.*

Risk Factors[34,36]

- Immunocompromised state (AIDS, organ transplant)
- Diabetes
- Neutropenia
- Hematologic malignancy
- Trauma
- Marijuana intake
- Environmental exposure (nearby demolition of restoration of buildings, yardwork, compost heaps)
- Residence in endemic areas like Sudan
- Advanced age.

Clinical Features (Figs. 107.7A and B)

Clinical features of orbital aspergillosis are similar to mucormycosis but are somewhat less severe and less rapid as compared to the later. Clinical signs are quite variable and might mimic idiopathic orbital inflammation or orbital malignancy.[37] Patients present with proptosis, limited extraocular motility and visual loss with minimal orbital inflammation. Visual loss is often absent and the presentation is very subtle in patients with AIDS.[38]

Investigations in Fungal Infections

- *Blood investigations*: Blood investigations include a routine hemogram (total and differential blood count, hemoglobin), and blood sugar. Blood culture should be ordered. Newer serological investigations for diagnosis of orbital aspergillosis include estimation of serum galactomannan and β-D glucan.[39]
- *Histopathological and microbiological investigation*: Nasal and oral mucosa should be thoroughly examined and specimens should be sent for microbiological evaluation. Open orbital biopsy provides adequate specimen for examination. Histopathological examination with Gomori Methenamine Silver (GMS) stain would reveal the fungal hyphae.

The potassium hydroxide (KOH) mount shows nonseptate branched fungal hyphae arranged at right angles in mucormycosis and septate hyphae arranged at 45° in aspergillosis. Sabouraud's agar without cycloheximide is used for culture. Newer alternate techniques to diagnose the causative agent present in the tissue samples include immunohistochemistry, in situ hybridization, and polymerase chain reaction (PCR).

- *Imaging*: CT scan is the preferred initial imaging of choice because of its ability to image bone and also to differentiate tissues (air, mycetoma, and hemorrhage), which otherwise give almost a similar low intensities on T1- and T2-weighted MRI images. CT scans show heterogeneous soft tissue masses with calcification and bony erosion. This heterogeneous image may be due to the presence of iron, calcium, or manganese in the fungal concretions. In ROCZ, the scan may demonstrate sinusitis, mucosal thickening, bone necrosis with involvement of pterygoid and infratemporal fossa and thrombosis of superior ophthalmic vein. Intracerebral fungi appear as hypodense masses with peripheral enhancement (ring abscess).[40]

Management of ROCZ

Rhino-orbital-cerebral-zygomycosis is a dangerous infection with more than 50% mortality rate.[41] Proper treatment of mucormycosis requires early diagnosis, reversal of the predisposing and systemic factors, wide local excision of the necrotic tissues, establishment of adequate sinus drainage, and systemic antifungals.

- *Amphotericin B*: The dosage of amphotericin B is slowly increase from 0.7 mg/kg to 1 mg/kg intravenous to a cumulative dose of 2–4 g over a period of weeks to months, after giving an initial test dose of 1 mg. Nephrotoxicity is the major dose limiting side effect hence patients' renal function test should be continuously monitored. Amphotericin B can also be used topically for irrigating and packing the involved sinuses in a dose of 1 mg/mL.[42]
- *Liposomal amphotericin B*: Lipid formulations of amphotericin B (amphotericin B lipid complex and liposomal amphotericin B) are newer preparations of amphotericin B. They appear to enhance its delivery to fungi, infected organs and phagocytes, thus accounting for its increased efficacy. Conversely the renal delivery is decreased with fewer side effects.[43] They are now the first drug of choice for treatment of ROCM.
- *Surgery and local debridement*: Wide local excision of the necrotic orbital tissues and sinuses should be carried out to decrease the fungal burden. Repeated surgical debridement is necessary in many cases.[44] Many authors agree that in the presence of active fungal infections exenteration may be life-saving.[45] In general, exenteration should be carried in the presence of an actively inflamed orbit with a blind eye.[46]
- *Hyperbaric oxygen*: Hyperbaric oxygen acts by increasing oxygenation and thereby decreasing acidosis and increasing the phagocytic activity. Its role is not clearly defined and expensive and cumbersome.
- *Newer modalities*:
  - *Posaconazole:* An oral agent which can be used in combination with amphotericin B.[47]
  - *Caspofungin:* It is an echinocandin which has shown increased survival when given in combination with amphotericin B.[48]
  - *Immune augmentation therapies:* Granulocyte-colony stimulating factor (G-CSF), granulocyte-monocyte-colony stimulating factor (GM-CSF), interferon-γ.[47]

Management of Orbital Aspergillosis

- At present, there is no universal guideline for management for orbital aspergillosis. Conventional therapy suggests the use of amphotericin B followed by azoles. Recently it has been found that primary therapy with voriconazole is more effective with fewer side effects as compared to amphotericin B.[49] The recommended regimen consists of intravenous voriconazole in a dose of 6 mg/kg twice daily on day 1, followed by 4 mg/kg for 1 week and then switching over to oral voriconazole 200 mg twice daily for 12 weeks.
- The primary goal of management in immunosuppressed individuals is reversal of the immunosuppressed state. The management protocol is otherwise similar. Exenteration might be required in advanced and unresponsive cases.

ORBITAL VIRAL INFECTIONS (FIGS. 107.8A AND B)

Viral infections due to adenovirus, herpes simplex, or herpes zoster can cause preseptal cellulitis. Adenovirus infection is usually secondary to viral conjunctivitis.

Vesicular or crusted lesions of the eyelids along with keratouveitis may be present in herpetic infections. Herpes zoster ophthalmicus may also present as orbital cellulitis.[50] It results from ischemia and the resultant inflammatory mass.[51] Enophthalmos, miosis, and contracture of palpebral fissure can all be possible due to a disturbance of sympathetic nervous system.[52]

Management

Oral acyclovir in a dose of 800 mg five times a day is the treatment of choice. Oral steroids can be used in case of extensive inflammation but their role is controversial.

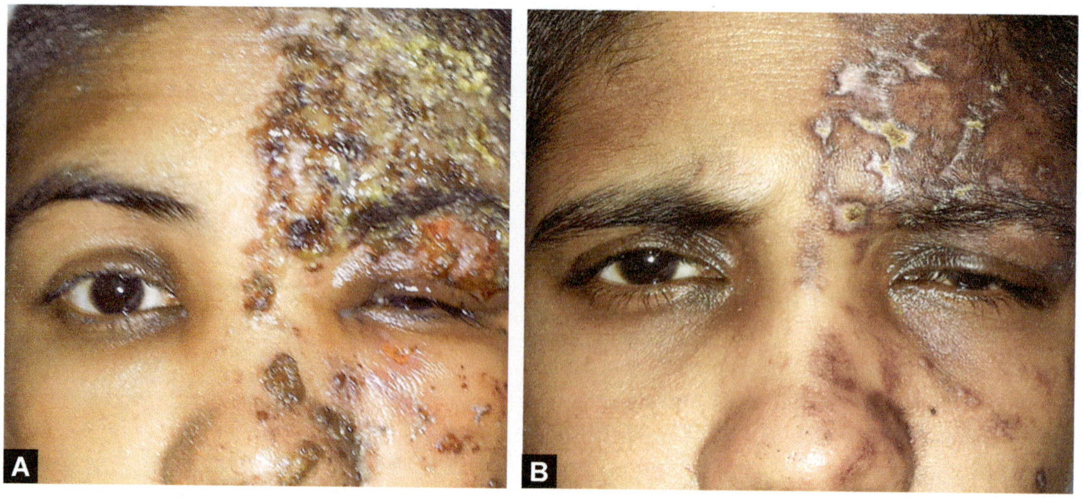

Figs. 107.8A and B: (A) Left periorbital herpes zoster ophthalmicus in patient with uncontrolled diabetes; (B) Resolution of lesion with scarring after treatment with oral acyclovir in another patient.

Later in the course of disease, lagophthalmos may develop secondary to cicatricial changes in the eyelid and palsy of orbicularis oculi. The lagophthalmos can be managed with copious lubricants, tarsorrhaphy and gold weight implant.[53]

Human immunodeficiency virus (HIV) and AIDS: Ophthalmic manifestations of HIV infection may involve the orbit and the adnexa. A number of opportunistic infections and tumors of the periocular tissues are associated with HIV.[54] The most common complications include orbital lymphoma and orbital cellulitis due to *Aspergillus* infection. HIV-associated aspergillosis typically occurs in patients with $CD4^+$ cell counts below 100/μL.

Kaposi sarcoma (KS): In approximately 20% of individuals with HIV-associated KS, the tumor involves the eyelids, conjunctiva, and, in rare cases, the orbit. It may appear as persistent subconjunctival hemorrhage or a raised, purplish-red mass.

INFECTIVE DACRYOADENITIS (FIGS. 107.9A TO C)

Possible infectious causes of dacryoadenitis comprise a wide range of pathogens. They include viruses, bacteria, fungi, and parasites. Among these viruses are thought to be the most common infectious agents and include mumps, Epstein-Barr virus (EBV), infectious mononucleosis, herpes zoster, cytomegalovirus, echovirus, and Coxsackie A virus. The common bacterial agents are *S. aureus* and *Streptococcus, Neisseria gonorrhoeae, Treponema pallidum, Chlamydia trachomatis, Mycobacterium tuberculosis*, and *Borrelia burgdorferi*.

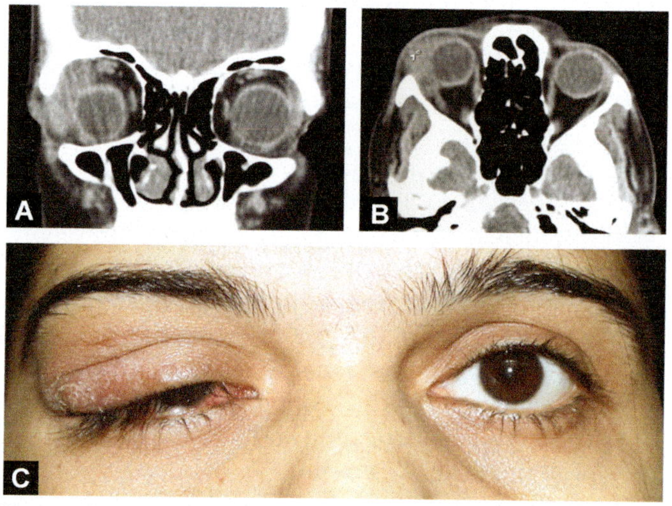

Figs. 107.9A to C: (A and B) CT scan coronal and axial cuts showing enlargement and inflammation of right lacrimal gland suggestive of dacryoadenitis; (C) External clinical photograph of the same patient showing right upper lid S-shaped ptosis with edema, erythema, and crusting of upper lid with fullness along superotemporal orbit.

Rarely, it can be associated with *Acanthamoeba*.[55] Mumps and brucellosis are recognized causes of bilateral dacryoadenitis.[56,57]

The clinical features include an inflamed S-shaped swelling of the upper eyelid. The palpebral lobe of the lacrimal gland is commonly enlarged and there may be a downward and inward dystopia of the globe. It is important to look for associated submandibular and preauricular lymphadenopathy. Pharyngitis and tonsillitis may be present. A routine hematological evaluation with serology for suspected viral infections should be ordered.

Bacterial dacryoadenitis is very well managed with oral antibiotics and anti-inflammatory drugs.

Viral dacryoadenitis is best managed with cool compresses, antipyretics and analgesics until resolution. EBV infection has been reported to respond well to oral steroids.[58]

DACRYOCYSTITIS (FIG. 107.10)

Dacryocystitis is inflammation of the lacrimal sac which can be acute or chronic. The mucous membrane lined tract of the lacrimal sac is contiguous with the conjunctival and nasal mucosa, both normally colonized with bacteria. Hence it is at risk of being infected. Accumulation of tear in a stenosed nasolacrimal duct can result in dacryocystitis. Chronic dacryocystitis commonly presents with complaints of watering, discharge or a mucocele formation.

Acute dacryocystitis presents with painful swelling in the region of the lacrimal sac with or without periorbital edema. The swelling characteristically does not extend above the medial canthal tendon and is an important feature which distinguishes it from lacrimal sac masses which may extend above it. The most common pathogens responsible are *S. aureus* and *Streptococcus pneumoniae*.[59] Acute dacryocystitis can be complicated by formation of lacrimal abscess, lacrimal fistula, lacrimal bone osteomyelitis, and orbital cellulitis.

Management

Acute dacryocystitis is managed with warm compresses, oral and topical antibiotics and anti-inflammatory drugs. The patient ultimately requires an external dacryocystorhinostomy (DCR) once the acute infection resolves. Kamal et al. have reported good results after primary powered endoscopic DCR in cases of acute dacryocystitis and lacrimal abscess, leading to rapid resolution of the condition.[60]

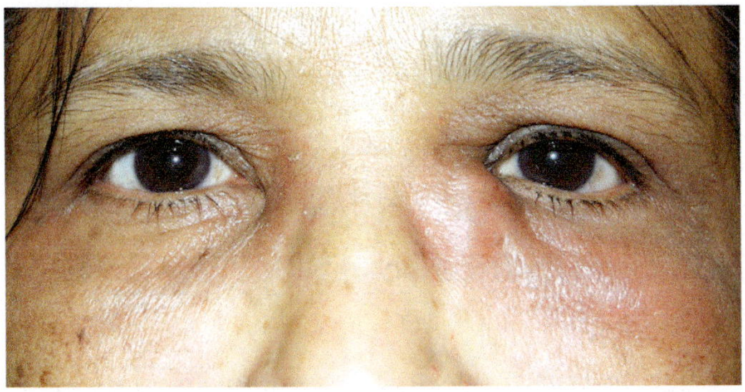

Fig. 107.10: External clinical photograph showing swelling and erythema along left lacrimal sac suggestive of acute dacryocystitis. Note that the swelling is not extending above medial canthal tendon.

ORBITAL TUBERCULOSIS (FIGS. 107.11A AND B)

Orbital tuberculosis is a rare form of extrapulmonary tuberculosis which afflicts the orbit and its surrounding structures either by hematogenous spread or from paranasal sinuses. Clinically it presents as one of the following five characteristic presentations:[61]

1. *Classical periostitis:* It presents as chronic ulceration or a discharging sinus from the periorbital region with or without cold abscess formation and soft tissue swelling.
2. *Orbital soft tissue tuberculoma with cold abscess with no bony destruction:* This group of patients present with pain, proptosis, palpable orbital mass and diplopia. There can be visual loss because of total destruction of globe or direct involvement of the optic nerve by the disease process.
3. *Orbital tuberculosis with bony involvement not classified as classical periostitis:* There is evidence of bony destruction radiologically with erosion, osteomyelitis, and rarely, bony sclerosis.
4. Orbital tuberculosis secondary to spread from paranasal sinuses.
5. Tubercular dacryoadenitis.

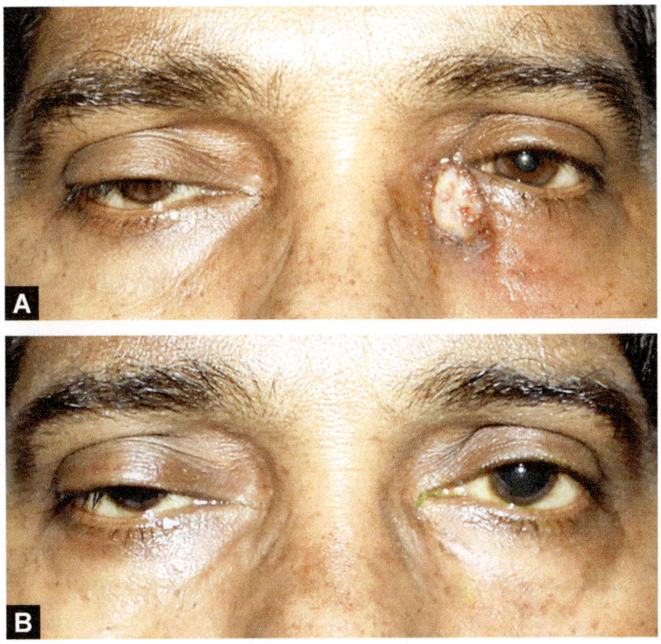

Figs. 107.11A and B: (A) External clinical photograph showing an ulcerated lesion along left medial canthal area. Incisional biopsy showed caseating necrosis and multinucleated giant cells suggestive of tuberculosis; (B) Complete resolution of the lesion with antitubercular treatment.

Investigations and Diagnosis

- Diagnosis is based on high index of suspicion. CT scan is the preferred modality of imaging
- To rule out systemic involvement
  - Chest X-ray/CT scan chest
- Orbital biopsy
- Demonstration of acid-fast bacilli along with culture
- Automated commercial broth culture system utilizing colorimetric and radiometric method
- Polymerase chain reaction.

Management

In general, the regimen for orbital tuberculosis is same as that of pulmonary tuberculosis. A 6- to 9-month course of antitubercular treatment (ATT) is recommended preferably under the care of an infectious disease specialist. Surgery is needed for excising the fistulous tract, debriding the affected bone[62] and clearing of the paranasal sinuses.

PARASITIC INFESTATIONS (TABLES 107.2 AND 107.3)

In recent times, the study of parasitology has been considerably refined and enhanced by the use of sophisticated tools, and by the interdisciplinary approach of the human and veterinary medical sciences. Increase in awareness may have led to increased rates of reporting of these infections. Parasitic infestations of the human eyes are mainly caused by the helminths. These helminths can be nematodes, cestodes, or trematodes, which may be transmitted by vectors (dirofilariasis, onchocerciasis, thelaziasis), food consumption (sparganosis, trichinellosis) and those acquired indirectly from the environment (ascariasis, echinococcosis).[56,63,64]

- *Nematodes*: Orbital infestations by nematodes can be due to *Trichinella spiralis, Wuchereria bancrofti, Thelazia callipaeda*, and *Thelazia californiensis*.[65] Treatment for *Trichinella* infestation includes oral mebendazole and corticosteroids. Treatment of choice for *Wuchereria* involvement is diethylcarbamazine and surgery in selected cases. Mechanical surgical removal of the lesion is the treatment of choice for *Thelazia* infestation.
- *Cestodes*: The two most common cestodal orbital infestations are cysticercosis and echinococosis. Both these entities are discussed in detail later.
- *Trematodes*: The most common trematodes to infest the orbit are *Schistosoma haematobium* and *Schistosoma japonicum*. Both of these can cause orbital tumor like lesions and orbital granulomas. Whereas *S. haematobium* is mainly found in Africa and Middle East, *S. japonicum* is mainly seen in China, Japan, and Philippines. The Center for Disease Control (CDC) advises avoiding drinking or coming into contact with contaminated water in areas where schistosomiasis is common. The treatment of choice is oral praziquantel.[63]

Table 107.2: Parasites affecting the human eye.

Order	Family and species
Nematodes	• Strongylida (*Angiostrongylus cantonensis*) • Trichiroids (*Trichinella* spp.) • Ascarids (*Toxocara canis, Toxocara cati, Baylisascaris procyonis*) • Spirurida (*Gnathostoma, Thelazia*) • Filaroids (*Wuchereria bancrofti, Loa loa, Brugia malayi, Dirofilaria, Onchocerca*)
Cestodes	• *Taenia crassiceps, Taenia multiceps* • *Spirometra* • *Echinococcus*
Trematodes (Flukes)	• Fasciola

Source: Otranto D, Eberhard ML. Zoonotic helminths affecting the human eye. Parasit Vectors. 2011;4:41.

Table 107.3: Common parasitic infestations of the orbit and periorbital tissues.

Affected site	Signs	Causative parasite
Eyelids	Eyelid edema	*Taenia solium* (cysticercus), *Toxocara, Trichinella, Dirofilaria*
Lacrimal ducts and glands	Lacrimation	*Thelazia* (oriental eye worm)
Orbit	Exophthalmos	*Echinococcus*, Coenurus, *Taenia solium* (cysticercus), *Trichinella, Dirofilaria, Gnathostoma*
Ocular muscles	Diplopia	*Trichinella, Taenia*
Conjunctiva	Subconjunctival cysts/mass	*Taenia, Dirofilaria, Rhinosporidiosis*
	Chemosis and conjunctivitis	*Thelazia, Trichinella, Onchocerca*
	Hemorrhages	*Trichinella*

Source: Ash LR, Orihel TC. Ash and Orihel's Atlas of Human Parasitology, 5th edition. Chicago, IL: American Society for Clinical Pathology Press; 2007.

Orbital Cysticercosis (Figs. 107.12A to C)

Cysticercosis is a parasitic infestation by cysticercus cellulosae, the larval form of pork tapeworm, *Taenia solium*. Infection occurs by drinking contaminated water, eating raw uncooked vegetables infested with eggs of the

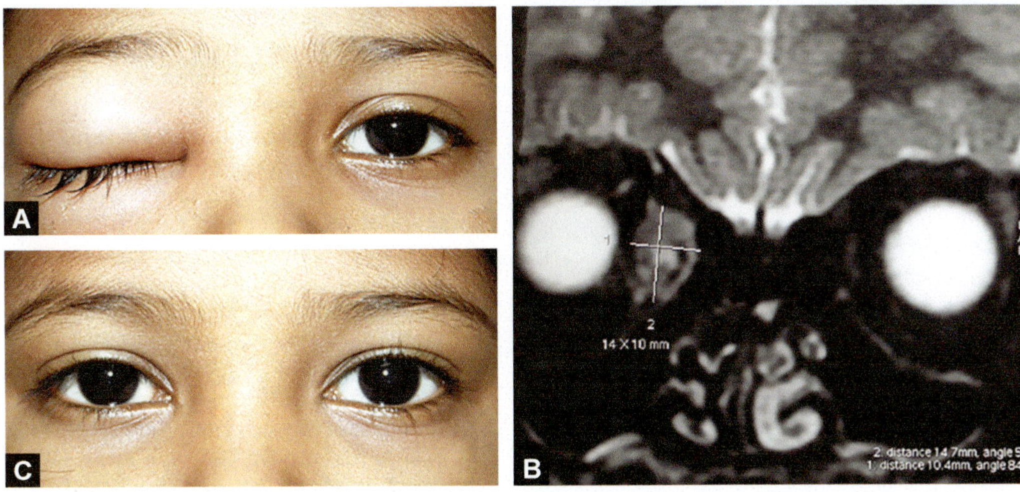

Figs. 107.12A to C: (A) Clinical picture showing right orbital cellulitis secondary to cysticercosis of right medial rectus muscles as evidenced by (B) presence of scolex on MRI; (C) Complete resolution of signs and symptoms after medical management of cysticercosis.

worm and by autoinfection. Cysticerci larva travel via hematogenous route and lodge themselves at sites with high glycogen content.[66] The extraocular muscle form is the most common form of orbital cysticercosis.[67] Inferior rectus and medial rectus are the most common muscles to be involved.[67] The varied presentations of orbital cysticercosis include pain, diplopia, proptosis, restriction of ocular motility, subconjunctival cyst, lid nodule, acquired ptosis, and optic neuritis.[68] If the parasite is left untreated it eventually dies after 2–4 years, releasing toxins which induce intense inflammatory reaction and can lead to alarming sequelae. Ultrasonography (USG) and CT scan are useful in demonstrating cyst with scolex. Higher resolution scans with 1 mm cuts and spiral CT scans with image reconstruction can be used for better visualization of the scolex. Serial ultrasounds can be used for documentation of response to therapy.[67] The standard medical management for orbital cysticercosis includes oral albendazole 15 mg/kg body weight for 4 weeks along with oral steroids in a dose of 1 mg/kg body weight tapered over 4–6 weeks.[69] Oral praziquantel in a dose of 40 mg/kg body weight for 4 weeks can also be used. CT scan brain should be done to rule out neurocysticercosis before starting cysticidal drugs. Surgical excision is indicated in case of failure of medical treatment.[69]

Orbital Echinococcosis

Orbital echinococcosis or hydatid disease is caused by *Echinococcus granulosus*. It resides in dogs' intestines and after being shed in the dog's feces, the eggs of the tapeworm then get ingested by the intermediate hosts, cow and sheep. The hydatid cyst then hematogenously spread to a wide variety of tissues in these animals. Ingestion of these tissues leads to hydatid disease different organs in man (liver, lungs, heart). Though orbital hydatid disease accounts for 0.3–0.8% of all cases, in endemic areas it accounts for up to a quarter of all orbital cystic lesions.[70-72] It presents as painless proptosis with motility restriction and an orbital mass. CT shows a well-defined cyst of aqueous density with contrast-enhancing rim.[73]

The most appropriate treatment for orbital hydatid cyst is surgical removal. Dissemination of the disease after cyst rupture is the most feared complication.[74] The typical surgical technique used is known as puncture-aspiration-injection-reaspiration technique. Herein the cyst content is aspirated gently after puncture with a fine needle, and then a scolicidal agent in the form of hypertonic saline solution is injected into the cyst; left there for a few minutes and then reaspirated.[74] The collapsed cyst wall is then removed with the help of forceps. The other scolicidal solutions include absolute alcohol, silver nitrate, and mebendazole.[74] Some authors recommend a preoperative course of oral albendazole 14–28 days before surgery.[75] The patient should be put on oral albendazole or praziquantel in the postoperative period to prevent relapse.[76]

Rhinosporidiosis

Rhinosporidium seeberi has been reclassified as an aquatic protistan parasite, the natural host being fish and amphibians. Rhinosporidiosis is endemic in South India, Sri Lanka, parts of East Africa and South America. It typically presents as a polypoidal mass in the conjunctiva,

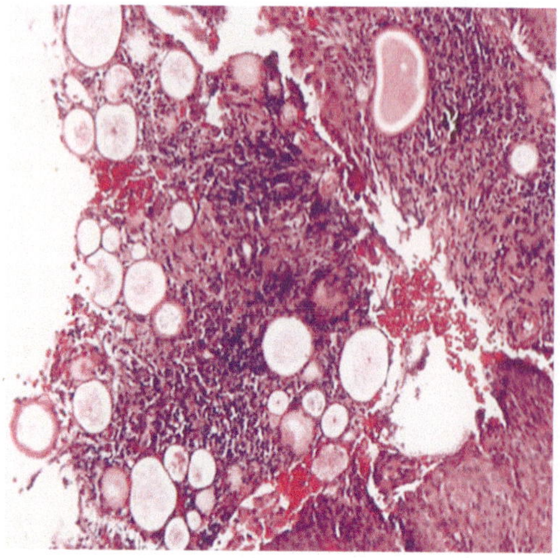

Fig. 107.13: Microphotograph showing multiple sporangia and sporocysts of rhinosporidiosis (hematoxylin and eosin stain; 100x).

but can involve the lacrimal sac, and rarely, eyelids and sclera. The mode of infection and transmission is thought to be waterborne, with the patients usually giving history of swimming in lakes or ponds.[77] Microscopically, rhinosporidial lesions have a distinctive morphology (Fig. 107.13).

The treatment of choice remains surgical, with complete removal of the lesions and electrocautery of the base. The lacrimal sac involvement is suggested by presence of a doughy swelling and the preferred mode of management is dacryocystectomy. However, Nuruddin et al. have reported successful outcomes after modified DCR surgery in these cases.[78] Postoperative dapsone (4, 4-diaminodiphenyl sulfone) therapy (100 mg once/twice daily for 3–6 months) may prevent recurrence. Antiseptics such as cetrimide-chlorhexidine, povidone-iodine and silver nitrate solutions have antirhinosporidial activity and can be used for topical application.[77]

CONCLUSION

Orbit is at risk of getting infected by a variety of pathogens because of its close proximity to paranasal sinuses, and spread of midfacial infection by valveless veins. Orbital infections are potentially vision and life threatening. Timely diagnosis and management may help in improving the prognosis.

REFERENCES

1. Goldfarb MS, Hoffman DS, Rosenbrg S. Orbital cellulitis and orbital fractures. Ann Ophthalmol. 1987;19:97-9.
2. Fiandaca MS, Specter RH, Hartman TM, et al. Unilateral septic cavernous sinus thrombosis: a case report with digital orbital venographic documentation. J Clin Neuro-ophthalmol. 1986;6:35-8.
3. Hornblass A, To K, Coden DJ, et al. Endogenous orbital cellulitis an endogenous endophthalmitis in subacute bacterial endocarditis. Am J Ophthalmol. 1989;108:196-7.
4. Jackson KJ, Baker SR. Clinical implications of orbital cellulitis. Laryngoscope. 1986;96:568-73.
5. Bullock JD, Fleishman JA. The spread of odontogenic infections to the orbit: diagnosis and management. J Oral Maxillofac Surg. 1985;43:749-55.
6. Rumelt S, Rubin PA. Potential sources for orbital cellulitis. Int Ophthalmol Clin. 1996;36:207-21.
7. Ullman S, Pflugfelder SC, Hughes R, et al. *Bacillus cereus* panophthalmitis manifesting as an orbital cellulitis. Am J Ophthalmol. 1987;103:105-6.
8. Chandler JR, Langenbrunner DJ, Stevens ER. The pathogenesis of orbital complications in acute sinusitis. Laryngoscope. 1970;80:1414.
9. Slavin ML, Glaser JS. Acute severe irreversible visual loss with sphenoehtmoiditis-"posterior" orbital cellulitis. Arch Ophthalmol. 1987;105:345-8.
10. McKinley SH, Yen MT, Miller AM, et al. Microbiology of pediatric orbital cellulitis. Am J Ophthalmol. 2007;144: 497-501.
11. Nageswaran S, Woods C, Benjamin D, et al. Orbital cellulitis in children. Pediatr Infect Dis J. 2006;25:695-9.
12. Weiss A, Friendly D, Eglin K, et al. Bacterial periorbital and orbital cellulitis in childhood. Ophthalmology. 1983;90: 195-203.
13. Ferguson MP, McNab AA. Current treatment and outcome in orbital cellulitis. Aust NZJ Ophthalmol. 1999;27:375-9.
14. Harris GJ. Subperiosteal abscess of the orbit. Age as a factor in the bacteriology and response to treatment. Ophthalmology. 1994;101:585-95.
15. Davis PC, Hopkins KL. Imaging of the pediatric orbit and visual pathways: Computed tomography and magnetic resonance imaging. Neuroimaging Clin North Am. 1999;9:93-114.
16. Yen MT. Current techniques for the management of orbital cellulitis. Tech Ophthalmol. 2006;4:45-9.
17. Benninger MS, Anon J, Mabry RL. The medical management of rhinosinusitis. Otolaryngol Head Neck Surg. 1997;117: S41-49.
18. Watkins LM, Pasternack MS, Banks M, et al. Bilateral cavernous sinus thromboses and intraorbital abscesses secondary to *Streptococcus milleri*. Ophthalmology. 2003;110:569-74.
19. Pushker N, Tejwani LK, Bajaj MS, et al. Role of oral corticosteroids in orbital cellulitis. Am J Ophthalmol. 2013;156:178-83.
20. Garcia GH, Harris GJ. Criteria for nonsurgical management of subperiosteal abscess of the orbit: analysis of outcomes 1988–1998. Ophthalmology. 2000;107:1454-8.
21. Udaondo P, Garcia-Delpech S, Díaz-Llopis M, et al. Bilateral intraorbital abscesses and cavernous sinus thromboses

secondary to *Streptococcus milleri* with a favorable outcome. Ophthal Plast Reconstr Surg. 2008;24:408-10.

22. Chaudhry IA, Shamsi FA, Elzaridi, et al. Outcome of treated orbital cellulitis in a tertiary eye care center in the Middle East. Ophthalmology. 2007;114(2):345-54.
23. Lattman J, Massry GG, Hornblass A. Pseudomonal eyelid necrosis: clinical characteristics and review of the literature. Ophthal Plast Reconstr Surg. 1998;14:290-4.
24. Nair AG, Naik MN. Life threatening infection. In: Mukherjee B, Yuen H (Eds). Emergencies of the Orbit and Adnexa. New Delhi: Springer. 2017;35:303-4.
25. Feldman DP, Picerno NA, Porubsky ES. Cavernous sinus thrombosis complicating odontogenic parapharyngeal space neck abscess: a case report and discussion. Otolaryngol Head Neck Surg. 2000;123:744-5.
26. Mandell GL, Bennett JE, Dolin R. Principles and Practice of Infectious Disease, 6th edition. Philadelphia: Elsevier/Churchill Livingstone; 2005.
27. Shaw RE. Cavernous sinus thrombophlebitis: a review. Br J Surg. 1952;40:40-8.
28. Yarrington CT. Cavernous sinus thrombosis revisited. Proc R Soc Med. 1977;70:456-9.
29. Singam NV, Rusia D, Prakash R. An eye popping case of orbital necrotizing fasciitis treated with antibiotics, surgery, and hyperbaric oxygen therapy. Am J Case Rep. 2017;18: 329-33.
30. Amrith S, Hosdurga Pai V, Ling WW. Periorbital necrotizing fasciitis–a review. Acta Ophthalmol. 2013;91(7):596-603.
31. Wong CH. The LRINEC (Laboratory Risk Indicator for Necrotizing Fasciitis) score: a tool for distinguishing necrotizing fasciitis from other soft tissue infections. Crit Care Med. 2004;32:1535-41.
32. Zacharias N, Velmahos GC, Salama A, et al. Diagnosis of necrotizing soft tissue infections by computed tomography. Arch Surg. 2010;145:452-5.
33. Misiakos EP, Bagias G, Patapis P, et al. Current concepts in the management of necrotizing fasciitis. Front Surg. 2014;29;1:36.
34. Mukherjee B, Raichura ND, Alam MS. Fungal infections of the orbit. Indian J Ophthalmol. 2016;64:337-45.
35. Kirszrot J, Rubin PA. Invasive fungal infection of the orbit. Int Ophthalmol Clin. 2007;47:117-32.
36. Lehrer RI, Howard DH, Sypherd PS, et al. Mucormycosis. Ann Intern Med. 1980;93:93-10837.
37. Mody KH, Ali MJ, Vemuganti GK, et al. Orbital aspergillosis in immunocompetent patients. Br J Ophthalmol. 2014;98:1379-84.
38. Johnson TE, Casiano RR, Kronish JW, et al. Sinoorbital aspergillosis in acquired immunodeficiency syndrome. Arch Ophthalmol. 1999;117:57-64.
39. Arvanitis M, Mylonakis E. Diagnosis of invasive aspergillosis: recent developments and ongoing challenges. Eur J Clin Invest. 2015;45:646-52.
40. Gamba JL, Woodruff WW, Djang WT, et al. Craniofacial mucormycosis: assessment with CT. Radiology. 1986;160: 207-12.
41. Reed C, Bryant R, Ibrahim AS, et al. Combination polyene-caspofungin treatment of rhino-orbital-cerebral mucormycosis. Clin Infect Dis. 2008;47:364-71.
42. Kohn R, Hepler R. Management of limited rhino-orbital mucormycosis without exenteration. Ophthalmology. 1985;92:1440-4.
43. Hay R. Liposomal amphotericin B, AmBisome. J Infect. 1994;28(S):35.
44. Lehrer RI, Howard DH, Sypherd PS, et al. Mucormycosis. Ann Intern Med. 1980;93:93-108.
45. Gregory JL, Golden A, Haymaher W. Mucormycosis of the central nervous system: a report of three cases. Bull Johns Hopkins Hosp. 1943;73:405-19.
46. Yohai RA, Bullock JD, Aziz AA, et al. Survival factors in rhino-orbital-cerebral-mucormycosis. Surv Ophthalmol. 1994;39:3-22.
47. Gamaletsou MN, Sipsas NV, Roilides E, et al. Rhino-orbital-cerebral mucormycosis. Curr Infect Dis Rep. 2012;14:423-34.
48. Reed C, Bryant R, Ibrahim AS, et al. Combination polyene-caspofungin treatment of rhino-orbital-cerebral mucormycosis. Clin Infect Dis. 2008;47:364-71.
49. Herbrecht R, Denning DW, Patterson TF, et al. Voriconazole versus amphotericin B for primary therapy of invasive aspergillosis. N Engl J Med. 2002;347:408-15.
50. Karbassi M, Raizman MB, Schuman JS. Herpes zoster ophthalmicus. Surv Ophthalmol. 1992;36:395-410.
51. Carmody RF. Herpes zoster ophthalmia complicated by ophthalmoplegia and exophthalmos. Arch Ophthalmol. 1937;18:707-11.
52. Edgerton AE. Herpes zoster ophthalmicus. Report of cases and review of literature. Arch Ophthalmol. 1945;34:40-62 and 114-153.
53. Kaufman SC. Anterior segment complications of herpes zoster ophthalmicus. Ophthalmology. 2008;115:S24-S32.
54. Ai E, Wong KL. Ophthalmic manifestations of AIDS. Ophthalmol Clin North Am 1988;1:53.
55. Tomita M, Shimmura S, Tsubota K, et al. Dacryoadenitis associated with *Acanthamoeba keratitis*. Arch Ophthalmol. 2006;124:1239-42.
56. Krishna N, Lyda W. Acute suppurative dacryoadenitis as a sequel to mumps. Arch Ophthalmol. 1958;59:350-1.
57. Bekir NA, Gungor K. Bilateral dacryoadenitis associated with brucellosis. Acta Ophthalmol Scand. 1999;77:357-8.
58. Aburn NS, Sullivan TJ. Infectious mononucleosis presenting with dacryoadenitis. Ophthalmology. 1996;103:776-8.
59. Mills DM, Bodman MG, Meyer DR, et al. The microbiologic spectrum of dacryocystitis: a national study of acute versus chronic infection. Ophthal Plast Reconstr Surg. 2007;23: 302-6.
60. Kamal S, Ali MJ, Pujari A, et al. Primary powered endoscopic dacryocystorhinostomy in the setting of acute dacryocystitis and lacrimal abscess. Ophthal Plast Reconstr Surg. 2015;31(4):293-5.
61. Madge SN, Shome D, Kim U, et al. Orbital tuberculosis: a review of the literature. Orbit. 2008;27:267-77.
62. Agrawal PK, Nath J, Jain BS. Orbital involvement in tuberculosis. Ind J Ophthalmol. 1977;25:12-6.

63. Nimir AR, Saliem A, Ibrahim IA. Ophthalmic parasitosis: a review article. Interdisci Perspec Infect Dis. 2012;2012:1-12.
64. Otranto D, Eberhard ML. Zoonotic helminths affecting the human eye. Parasit Vectors. 2011;4:41.
65. Gould SE. The eye and orbit in trichinosis. Bull NY Acad Med. 1954;30:726-9.
66. Miller NR. Diseases caused by helminths. In: Miller NR (Ed). Walsh and Hoyt's Clinical Neuroophthalmology. Philadelphia: William and Wilkins; 1995. pp. 3318-43.
67. Sekhar GC, Honavar SG. Myocysticercosis: experience with imaging and therapy. Ophthalmology. 1999;106:2336-40.
68. Pushker N, Bajaj MS, Chandra M, et al. Ocular and orbital cysticercosis. Acta Ophthalmol Scand. 2001;79:408-13.
69. Rath S, Honavar SG, Naik M, et al. Orbital cysticercosis: clinical manifestations, diagnosis, management and outcome. Ophthalmology. 2010;117:600-5.
70. Morales AG, Croxatto JO, Crovetto L, et al. Hydatid cysts of the orbit: a review of 35 cases. Ophthalmology. 1988;95:1027-32.
71. Abbassioun K, Amirjamshidi A. Diagnosis and management of hydatid cyst of the central nervous system. Part 2. Hydatid cysts of the skull, orbit, and spine. Neurosurg Quart. 2001;11:10-6.
72. Talib H. Orbital hydatid disease in Iraq. Br J Surg. 1972;59:391-4.
73. Kars Z, Kansu T, Ozcan OE, et al. Orbital echinococcosis: report of two cases studied by computerized tomography. J Clin Neuro-ophthalmol. 1982;2:197-9.
74. Kahveci R, Sanli AM, Gurer B, et al. Orbital hydatid cyst. J Neurosurg Pediatrics. 2012;9:42-4.
75. Al-Muala HD, Sami SM, Shukri MA, et al. Orbital hydatid cyst. Ann Maxillofac Surg. 2012;2:197-9.
76. Jimenez-Mejios ME, Alarcon-Cruz JC, Marquez-Rivas FJ, et al. Orbital hydatid cyst: treatment and prevention of recurrences with albendazole plus praziquntel. J Infect. 2000:41:105-7.
77. Mukherjee B, Mohan A, Sumathi V, et al. Infestation of the lacrimal sac by *Rhinosporidium seeberi:* a clinicopathological case report. Indian J Ophthalmol. 2013;61:588-90.
78. Nuruddin M, Mudhar HS, Osmani M, et al. Lacrimal sac rhinosporidiosis: clinical profile and surgical management by modified dacryocystorhinostomy. Orbit. 2014; 33:29-32.

Chapter 108 Orbital Inflammatory Disorders: Evaluation and Management

Natalie Wolkow, Suzanne K Freitag

INTRODUCTION

Orbital inflammation encompasses a broad range of diseases that present with varied signs and symptoms. Many of these are nonspecific and overlap with those of orbital infection and neoplasm (*see* Chapters 104 and 107). Thus, one challenge facing the orbital surgeon is to make the distinction between infection, neoplasm and inflammation. Computed tomography (CT) or magnetic resonance imaging (MRI) of the orbits may be helpful, as orbital inflammation may produce characteristic patterns that are easily identified. More often, however, a definitive diagnosis hinges upon tissue biopsy.

Here we review orbital inflammatory disorders. The most common orbital inflammatory disorder, thyroid eye disease, is covered in a separate chapter, while mimickers of orbital inflammation, neoplasm and infection, are discussed in Chapters 104 and 107.

INFLAMMATORY DISEASES

Sarcoidosis

Sarcoidosis is a systemic inflammatory disease of unknown etiology that is characterized by noncaseating granulomas on histopathologic examination. It can affect almost any organ, but most commonly affects the lungs, skin and eyes. It is more frequent in women, African Americans and Northern Europeans, and often presents between ages 20 and 40.[1-3]

In ocular structures, sarcoid most commonly causes anterior uveitis or conjunctival nodules. Orbital involvement is less common. Any ocular adnexal structure, including the lacrimal gland, lacrimal sac and extraocular muscles may be affected,[4,5] but the lacrimal gland is the most frequently involved.[2,5,6] Lacrimal gland sarcoidosis may present with eyelid swelling, a palpable nontender nodule, eyelid ptosis or eyelid erythema (Figs. 108.1A and B).[2,5] Patients with orbital involvement often do not have a history of systemic sarcoid, and biopsy is frequently needed to identify the underlying disease process. In addition, systemic testing for sarcoid, such as blood work for angiotensin converting enzyme (ACE) and lysozyme, and CT of the chest for hilar lymphadenopathy, is often needed.[1,3] Histopathologic examination of tissues affected by sarcoidosis reveals noncaseating granulomas composed of epithelioid histiocytes.[6]

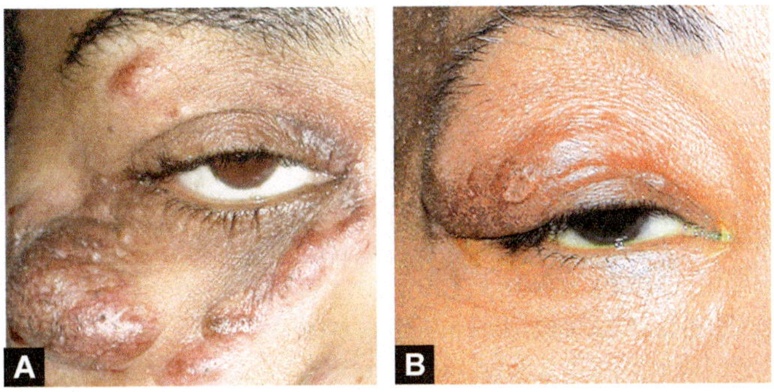

Figs. 108.1A and B: Sarcoidosis. (A) Clinical photograph of facial skin nodules from sarcoidosis; (B) Clinical photograph of an S-shaped erythematous and edematous upper eyelid secondary to sarcoidosis involving the lacrimal gland.

Some patients with orbital sarcoidosis do not require therapy and are observed; however, those with more severe orbital or systemic involvement may need to be treated with systemic corticosteroids or immunosuppressive agents.[5] Tuberculosis and fungal infection must be ruled out prior to initiating immunosuppression. Intralesional corticosteroids may be considered if indicated. In most patients, orbital sarcoid lesions resolve and do not recur after systemic steroid therapy.[5]

Histiocytic Disorders

The histiocytic disorders are a large group of diverse but overlapping diseases which are undergoing reclassification as more genetic information becomes available.[7-10] These diseases are unified by their common cell of origin, the histiocyte, a mononuclear cell. Mononuclear cells originate in the bone marrow, then migrate to tissues to become histiocytes, also known as tissue phagocytes, macrophages, antigen-presenting Langerhans cells and follicular dendritic cells.

Earlier classifications divided the histiocytic disorders based upon histopathologic differences, separating them into Langerhans cell histiocytoses and non-Langerhans cell histiocytoses (which include the xanthogranulomatous diseases).[9,10] Recent genetic studies, however, have found that these separations may not be as distinct as they were previously thought. For example, Langerhans cell histiocytosis and Erdheim-Chester disease are now both known to harbor the same mutations in the RAF-MEK-ERK pathway and may respond to similar drugs.[7,8] Moreover, recent studies have revealed that some histocytic proliferations, such as Langerhans cell histiocytosis and Erdheim–Chester disease, are monoclonal, and may in fact be inflammatory neoplasms.[7,8] For the purposes of this chapter, the histiocytic disorders are still organized according to their histopathologic appearance, with the caveat that these divisions are artificial and subject to change as more knowledge is gained from research.

Langerhans Cell Histiocytosis

Langerhans cell histiocytosis is a proliferation of unknown etiology of Langerhans-type cells. Although classically thought of as an inflammatory disease, recent evidence of monoclonality and conserved mutations in B-RAF in the RAF-MEK-ERK pathway suggest that Langerhans cell histiocytosis may instead be an inflammatory neoplasm.[7,8,11] Langerhans cells are mononuclear antigen-presenting immune cells of hematopoietic origin that reside in the epidermis and lymph nodes. They can be recognized immunohistochemically by the expression of CD1a, S100 and CD207, and recognized on electron microscopy by the presence of Birbeck granules.[7,8,11]

Langerhans cell histiocytosis was previously called histiocytosis X before the Langerhans cell was identified as the histiocyte of interest. The current name unites under one umbrella several conditions which were previously considered separate diseases: eosinophilic granuloma, Hand–Schüller–Christian and Abt-Letterer–Siwe diseases.[12] Eosinophilic granuloma refers to histocytic disease that is confined to one or several bony foci without systemic manifestations (Figs. 108.2A to C).[12] Hand–Schüller–Christian refers to orbital disease along with multifocal lytic lesions of the skull and diabetes insipidus secondary to pituitary gland infiltration.[12] Abt-Letterer–Siwe refers to disease with prominent diffuse systemic involvement, including a generalized skin rash, anemia and hepatosplenomegaly.[12]

Children between ages 1 and 4 and young adults are most commonly affected by Langerhans cell histiocytosis.[12] In the ocular adnexa, the eosinophilic granuloma-type of involvement, a single bone lesion with an associated soft tissue mass, is most common. The lesion is typically in the superior or superolateral orbit and may cause a reactive dacryoadenitis. Presenting symptoms vary depending upon the location of the mass. An anterior mass presents with eyelid swelling, ptosis and erythema, while a posterior mass presents more typically with proptosis. If muscles are infiltrated, diplopia can be seen. CT and MRI imaging studies typically demonstrate punched-out bony lesions (Figs. 108.2A to C).[12]

Biopsy of the orbital mass will demonstrate a proliferation of CD1a- and S100-positive histiocytes

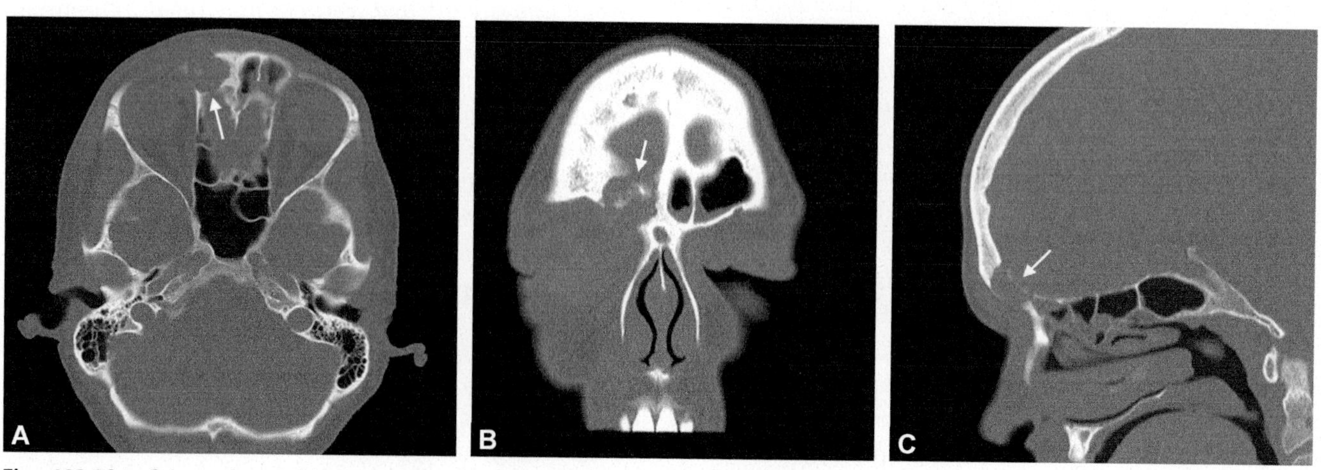

Figs. 108.2A to C: Langerhans cell histiocytosis, eosinophilic granuloma. CT scan of the head without contrast demonstrating bony erosion (arrows) secondary to localized Langerhans cell histiocytosis (also known as eosinophilic granuloma). (A) Axial; (B) Coronal; (C) Sagittal.

(therefore of Langerhans lineage), which may be accompanied by giant cells, eosinophils, plasma cells, histiocytes, abundant vascularity and hemorrhage.[12]

Treatment depends upon the extent of the disease. Isolated orbital lesions may be observed, excised, treated with a combination of excision and steroid injection, or with radiation. Multisystemic and recurrent disease may require chemotherapy or bone marrow transplant. Newer drugs targeting the RAF-MEK-ERK pathway may be beneficial. Although some recent guidelines recommend treating orbital disease with 6 months of systemic chemotherapy post-tumor excision, this is an area of great debate as many children do well with local therapy alone and systemic chemotherapy has significant long-term side effects.[11]

Adult Xanthogranulomatous Diseases

The adult xanthogranulomatous diseases are characterized histopathologically by a proliferation of non-Langerhans xanthomatous histiocytes and Touton giant cells. These histiocytes, unlike Langerhans cells, are S100- and CD1a-negative, and are CD68- and CD163-positive. Four diseases are typically grouped under the adult xanthogranulomatous disease category because of their histopathologic similarities; adult onset xanthogranuloma, adult onset asthma with periocular xanthogranuloma, necrobiotic xanthogranuloma and Erdheim–Chester disease. Although similar histopathologically, these diseases affect various organs to very different degrees, and have extremely different prognoses.[9,10] The former three diseases tend to be restricted to the anterior orbit and have less systemic involvement, while Erdheim–Chester disease tends to affect the posterior orbit and is associated with severe systemic involvement and a high mortality rate.[9,10] Most of these diseases affect adult men and women equally, with an average age of 50 years at onset.[9,10]

Adult onset xanthogranuloma: Adult onset xanthogranuloma is the least common and the most benign of the xanthogranulomatous diseases. It presents with yellowish swelling of the anterior orbital structures caused by infiltration with xanthomatous non-Langerhans histiocytes. It does not have systemic associations, is often self-limiting, and is not associated with increased mortality. Excision or corticosteroids are the typical treatments (Figs. 108.3A and B).[9,10]

Adult onset asthma with periocular xanthogranuloma: Adult onset asthma with periocular xanthogranuloma was described as a unique entity by Jakobiec in 1993.[13] It is characterized by the development of asthma in adulthood, typically a few months or years prior to the appearance of yellow nonulcerated infiltrative masses in the eyelids and anterior orbits.[13] Histopathologic examination is notable for prominent lymphoid follicles, as compared to the other xanthogranulomatous diseases. It can be associated with prominent systemic lymphadenopathy and occasionally with lymphoproliferative disorders. Treatment varies and may consist of surgical excision, systemic corticosteroids, systemic immunosuppressive agents or low dose radiation.[13-15]

Necrobiotic xanthogranuloma: Necrobiotic xanthogranuloma also presents with yellowish or violaceous subcutaneous papules in the eyelids which coalesce into plaques

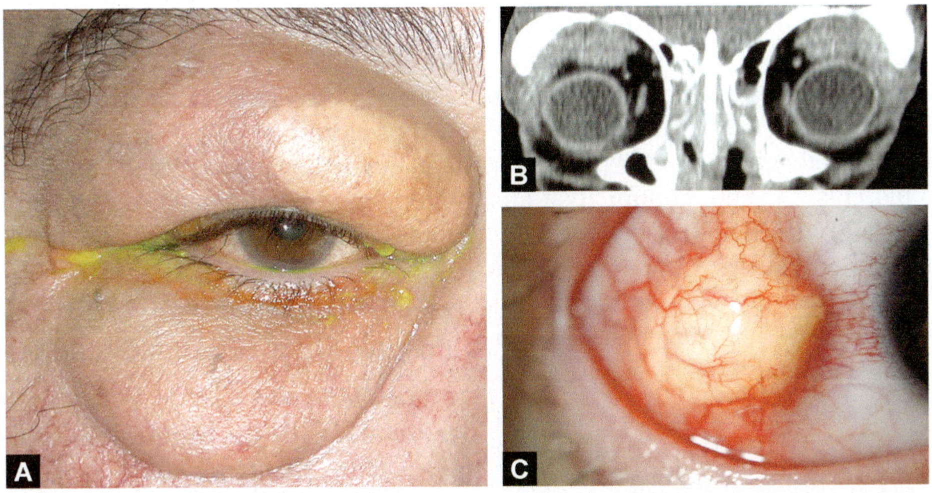

Figs. 108.3A to C: Xanthogranulomatous disease. (A) External photograph demonstrating eyelid infiltration with a characteristic cutaneous yellow patch in the medial upper eyelid in a patient with adult onset xanthogranuloma; (B) CT scan with contrast from a different patient with adult onset xanthogranuloma demonstrating mass lesions involving bilateral lacrimal glands and superior orbits; (C) External photograph of subconjunctival xanthomatous accumulations in a patient with Erdheim–Chester disease.

that ulcerate and become fibrotic.[9,16] Histopathologic examination is notable for necrobiosis, with histiocytes surrounding areas of necrosis in a palisading pattern.[9] This disorder is associated with the development of monoclonal gammopathy and multiple myeloma, so patients need to be closely monitored.[9] Treatment consists of systemic corticosteroids or immunosuppressive agents, but surgical debulking is not recommended.[9]

Erdheim–Chester disease: Erdheim–Chester disease is a systemic xanthogranulomatous disease that may present with proptosis from posterior orbital xanthogranulomatous involvement (Fig. 108.3C). It is characterized by pathognomonic osteosclerosis lesions, pericardial disease, ensheathing of the aorta, vascular infiltrates, lung and retroperitoneal infiltration.[9,10,17] The disease is associated with a high mortality rate. Posterior orbital disease can cause compressive optic neuropathy, leading to vision loss.[9,10] Histopathologic examination is notable for more fibrosis than the other xanthogranulomatous diseases.[9]

Therapies have historically consisted of corticosteroids, alkylating agents, and bone marrow transplant, with a poor response and high mortality. The recent discovery of the B-RAF mutation and activation of the RAF-MEK-ERK pathway in many patients has lead to the use of interferon alpha and B-RAF inhibitors, with improved patient survival.[7,8,17]

Juvenile Xanthogranuloma

Juvenile xanthogranuloma, like the adult xanthogranulomas, is characterized histopathologically by a proliferation of xanthomatous non-Langerhans histiocytes with Touton giant cells. It is generally limited to the skin where it presents as red/yellow nodules. It may, however, affect the eyelids, globe and orbit. Iris involvement is the most common ocular manifestation, and is responsible for the spontaneous hyphemas that are often the presenting symptom in these patients.[18] Eyelid, conjunctival and orbital lesions are typically excised and do not recur. The clinician should remember that there is an association between juvenile xanthogranuloma, neurofibromatosis type 1, and juvenile myleomonocytic leukemia. Children should be appropriately screened.[18]

Rosai–Dorfman Syndrome

Rosai–Dorfman syndrome is a rare systemic histiocytosis, most often affecting children and teenagers, frequently of African descent. It presents with large lymphadenopathy of the neck, often involves the paranasal sinuses, and may occasionally infiltrate the orbit. The pathognomonic histopathologic finding of biopsied lesions is emperipoleisis (engulfment of entire lymphocytes within the histiocyte, without their degradation). The histiocytes are CD68-positive and CD1a-negative, but unlike the histiocytes in adult xanthogranulomatous diseases, they are often S100-positive. Currently there is no good treatment option available. Observation is often elected, and corticosteroids, surgery or radiotherapy are used for orbital disease that is causing functional problems. Chemotherapy is poorly effective.[8]

Vasculitides

Granulomatosis with Polyangiitis (formerly known as Wegener's Granulomatosis)

Granulomatosis with polyangiitis (GPA) is a systemic granulomatous necrotizing vasculitis that affects many organs, most commonly the respiratory tract and kidneys. Ocular involvement occurs in 50–60% of patients, while orbital involvement in particular is present in 10–20%. Of all the vasculitides affecting the orbit, GPA is the most common. It can affect any part of the orbit, including the soft tissues, muscles, fat and optic nerve, and may present primarily in the orbit or as an extension from the sinuses (Figs. 108.4A to C).[19,20]

Histopathologic examination demonstrates small and medium vessel vasculitis, tissue necrosis and granulomatous inflammation. The orbital inflammation can lead to orbital fibrosis and enophthalmos, which can result in compressive optic neuropathy and vision loss.[19-21] Laboratory testing is often positive (90%) for c-ANCA, which is very specific for GPA. ESR and CRP can also be elevated. Patients traditionally have been treated with corticosteroids, cyclophosphamide, methotrexate or azathioprine, but now more commonly rituximab is used.[19-21]

Eosinophilic Granulomatosis with Polyangiitis (Churg-Strauss)

Churg-Strauss is a systemic allergic disease, characterized by asthma, allergic rhinitis, blood eosinophilia, and a necrotizing granulomatous vasculitis of the small and medium blood vessels. The disease affects mostly the lungs, sinuses and peripheral nervous system, with ocular and orbital involvement being extremely rare.[22]

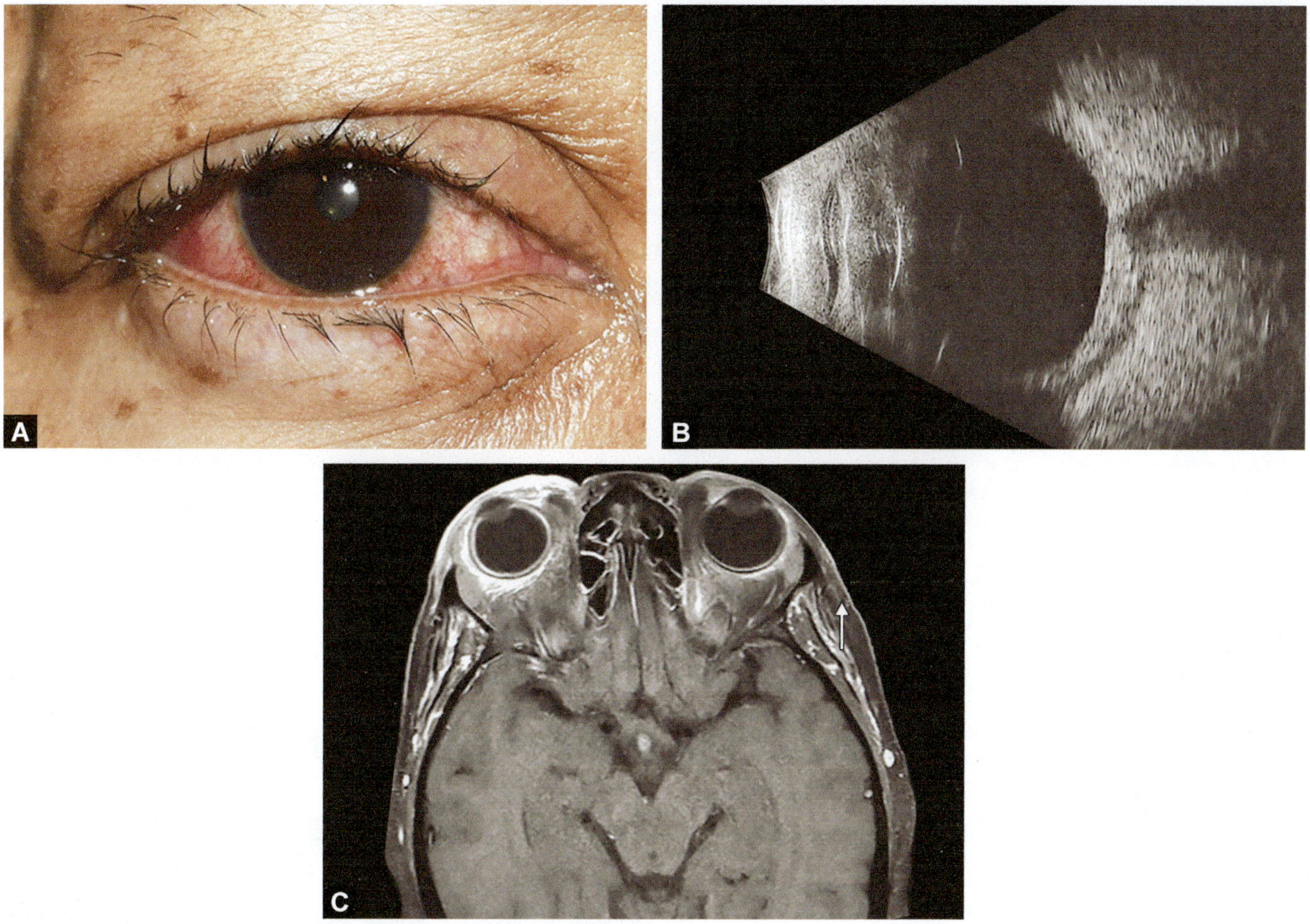

Figs. 108.4A to C: Granulomatosis with polyangiitis. (A) External photograph demonstrating scleral injection in a patient with scleritis secondary to GPA; (B) B-scan ultrasonography in the same patient reveals a T-sign, indicative of posterior scleritis; (C) Axial T1-weighted MRI of the orbits reveals contrast enhancement of the right sclera (arrow) as well as the preseptal soft tissues.

Orbital inflammation may involve any part of the orbit, and typically one of two patterns of involvement is seen, either an ischemic-type pattern or an inflammatory pseudotumor type. Histopathologic examination of the affected tissue reveals a necrotizing vasculitis of small and medium-sized vessels. The involved blood vessels are typically full of eosinophils, and there is extravascular infiltration of eosinophils into the tissues. Blood eosinophilia is also usually present, and a p-ANCA test is positive in 70% of affected individuals; serum IgE levels may also be elevated.[19,21 22]

Sjögren's Syndrome

Sjögren's syndrome is a systemic autoimmune condition of unknown cause, characterized by infiltration and destruction of major and minor salivary glands. The infiltrating cells are mostly CD4-positive T-lymphocytes.[23,24] Destruction of salivary and lacrimal glands leads to dry mouth and dry eyes. Diagnosis is typically made through elevated anti-Ro/SSA antibodies and anti-La/SSB antibodies, as well as signs of salivary gland inflammation and destruction on biopsy. The minor salivary glands of the lips are biopsied more frequently than the lacrimal gland because they are easier to access and the biopsy is less invasive. Treatment of the ocular component of Sjögren's syndrome consists of ocular surface lubrication, corticosteroids, cyclosporine and serum tears.[23,24]

Melkersson–Rosenthal Syndrome

Melkersson-Rosenthal syndrome is a very rare condition characterized by painless eyelid edema which is often unilateral (Figs. 108.5A and B). Histopathologic

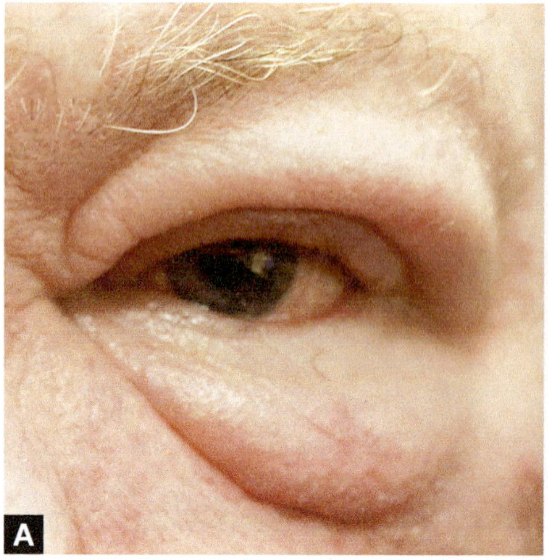

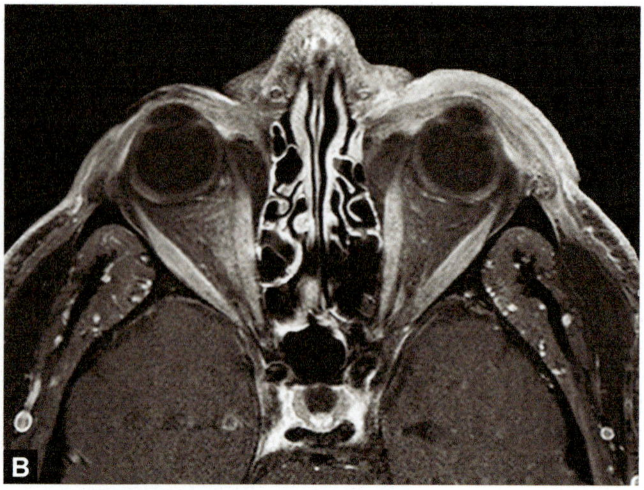

Figs. 108.5A and B: Melkersson-Rosenthal syndrome. (A) External photograph demonstrating unilateral upper and lower eyelid edema; (B) Axial T1-weighted fat-saturated postcontrast MRI image in the same patient revealed significant inflammation and edema of the preseptal soft tissues on the left.
Source (Figure 108.5A): Michael K Yoon, MD.

examination reveals that the eyelid edema is due to dermal inflammation with T-lymphocytes as well as noncaseating granulomatous inflammation. The epithelioid histiocytes in this disease often surround blood vessels and lymphatics, and granulomas may be present within lymphatics, plugging them and causing decreased lymphatic drainage which is responsible for the clinically apparent edema.[25]

IgG4-related Orbital Inflammation

IgG4-related orbital inflammation is a new category of orbital inflammation, with an unknown etiology. First described in the pancreas, it is known to affect almost every organ in the body, and is frequently encountered in the orbit.[26,27] Any structure within the orbit may be affected, including the lacrimal gland, extraocular muscles, periorbital soft tissues, cranial nerves and sclera (Fig. 108.6). Orbital disease often presents with painless proptosis, and may be difficult to distinguish from Sjögren syndrome, sarcoid, GPA and lymphoma. Both males and females are affected and the average age at presentation is in the sixth decade. The lacrimal gland is the most common orbital structure affected. There is a propensity for infraorbital nerve involvement. Diagnosis depends on tissue examination. The typical histopathologic appearance consists of a lymphoplasmocytic infiltrate with storiform fibrosis and an obliterative vasculitis. The infiltrating lymphocytes are often predominantly T lymphocytes and more than 40% of the plasma cells are IgG4 positive.[26,27] In the orbit, the lymphoplasmocytic infiltrate and partial storiform fibrosis are the major findings, with obliterative vasculitis rarely seen. Treatment currently is either with corticosteroids or rituximab.[26-28]

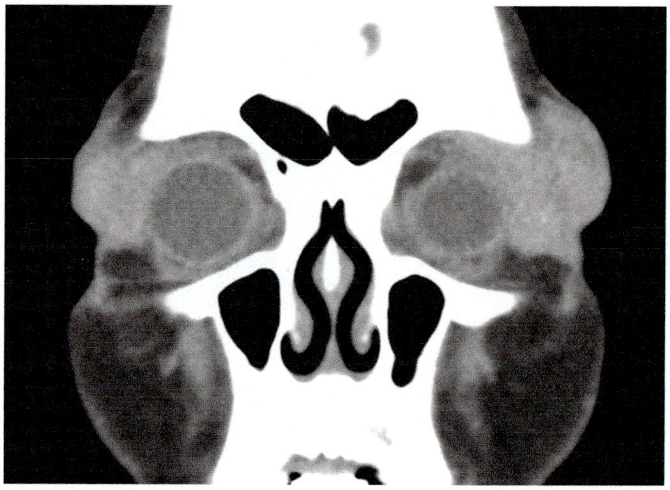

Fig. 108.6: IgG4-related orbital inflammation. Coronal CT scan demonstrating massive bilateral lacrimal gland enlargement and inflammation.

Drugs and Chemical-induced Orbital Inflammation

A small number of drugs and chemicals have been associated with the development of orbital inflammation, and the clinician should always remember to include this possibility in the differential diagnosis. Local injection of hyaluronidase,[29-32] alcohol and chlorpromazine[33,34] have been found to incite orbital inflammation. Systemic therapy with bisphosphonates, in particular after intravenous administration,[35,36] has been associated with orbital inflammation (Figs. 108.7A and B). Systemic therapy with monoclonal antibodies ipulimumab[37] and adalimumab,[38] as well as intravesicular BCG vaccine have also been associated with orbital inflammation.

Orbital Inflammation Secondary to Foreign Materials

Orbital foreign bodies may cause inflammation that ranges from an almost immediate response to a delayed response decades after implantation of the offending agent. Thus, a careful history of prior orbital surgery, procedures and trauma is important to elicit when evaluating a patient with orbital inflammation.

Reports of orbital inflammation in response to surgically-implanted devices are not uncommon in the literature. Delayed orbital inflammation a decade after the implantation of a hydrogel scleral buckle is a well-known sequela, especially of the MIRAgel variety, which was in use in the 1980s and 1990s (Figs. 108.8A to C).[39,40] Similar inflammation has also been described in response to silicone scleral buckle components.[41] Lipogranulomatous orbital inflammation has been reported in response to leaking silicone oil after retinal surgery.[42] Orbital inflammation has also been described in response to porous polyethylene, silicone and supramid implants used for orbital fracture repair,[43-45] as well as to hydroxyapatite orbital implants[46] and glaucoma implants (Fig. 108.9).[47]

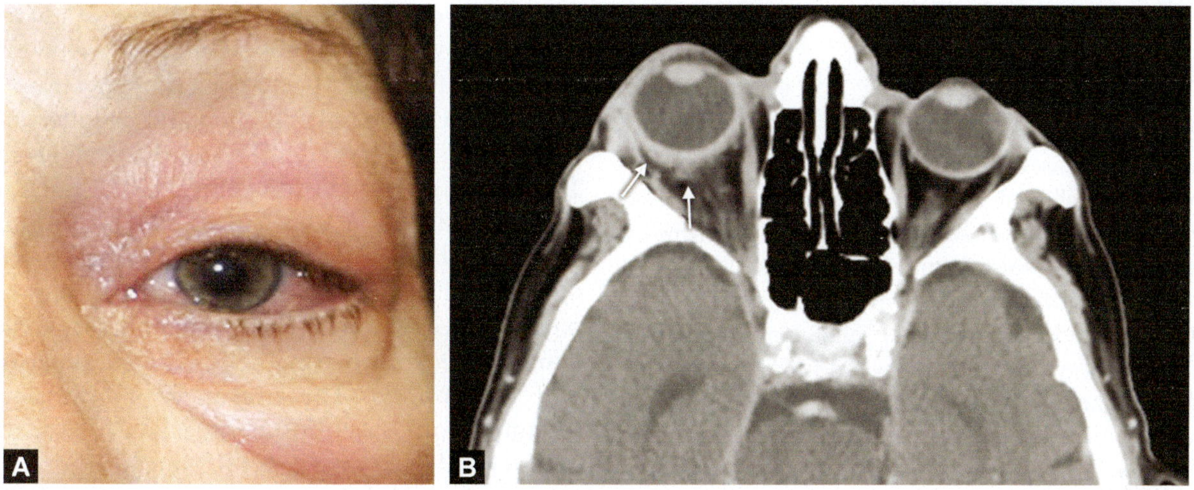

Figs. 108.7A and B: Bisphosphonate-related orbital inflammation. (A) External photograph demonstrating eyelid edema and erythema as well as scleral injection and mild chemosis in a patient with orbital inflammation after a bisphosphonate infusion; (B) Axial CT scan with contrast in another patient with orbital inflammation after a bisphosphonate infusion, demonstrating proptosis and fat stranding near the posterior aspect of the right globe.
Source: Nahyoung Grace Lee, MD.

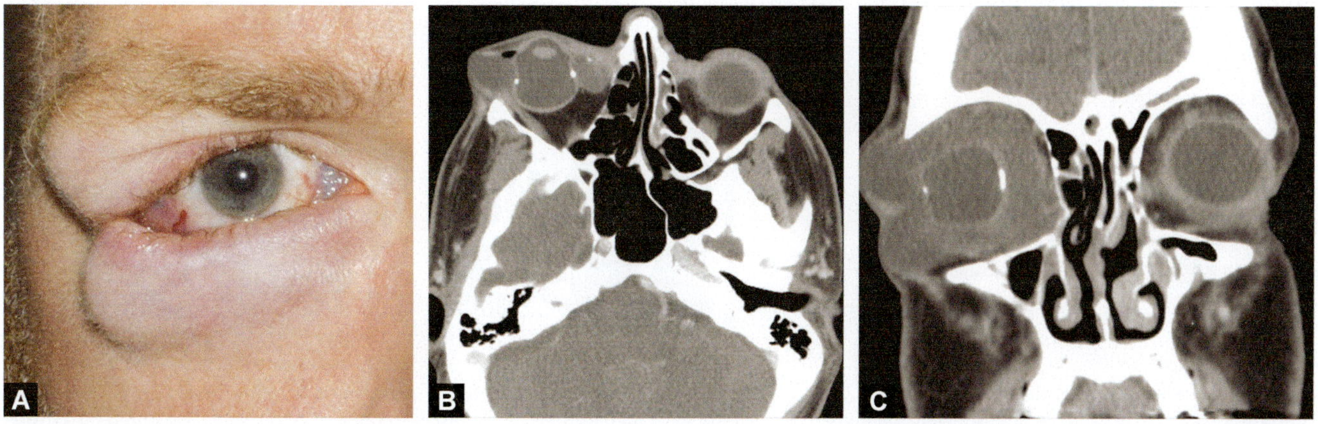

Figs. 108.8A to C: Hydrolyzed MIRAgel scleral buckle. External photograph demonstrating stretching of upper and lower eyelid skin secondary to a grossly enlarged underlying hydrolyzed MIRAgel scleral buckle. A small portion of the buckle is exposed and visible inside the medial commissure of the eyelids. (A) Axial; (B) Coronal; (C) CT scan with showing the hydrolyzed MIRAgel scleral buckle encircling the globe and filling the anterior orbit.
Source: Michael K Yoon, MD.

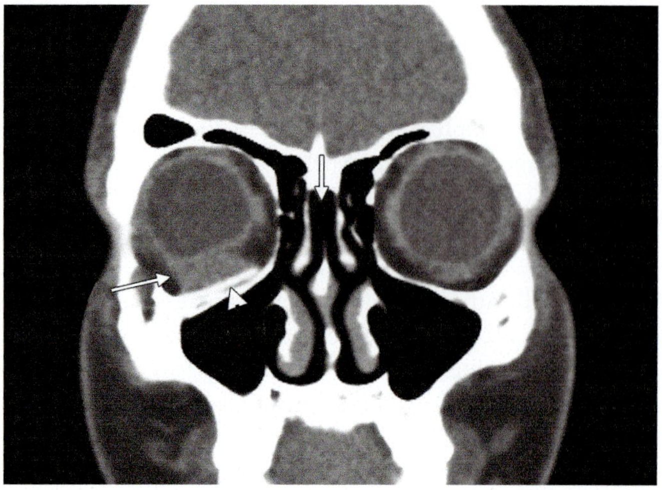

Fig. 108.9: Supramid orbital implant-related inflammation. Coronal CT scan demonstrating a supramid orbital implant along the right orbital floor (arrowhead) with an inflammatory capsule (arrow) seen above the implant and displacing the globe superiorly.

Inflammatory reactions may also occur in association with materials that are used intraoperatively, such as suture[48] and bone wax,[49] as well as talc from gloves, cotton fibers and Gelfilm.[47] Petroleum-based ophthalmic ointments that are used postoperatively may also incite inflammatory reactions in the form of ointment granulomas.[50]

Almost all types of injectable facial filler materials have been associated with orbital or eyelid inflammation.[51-53] LipoDissolve, an injectable material that is meant to nonsurgically induce fat melting, may also cause inflammation.[54]

Exogenous materials, such as textile fibers,[55] diesel fuel,[56] wood,[57,58] and material from grease guns[59] are all known to incite inflammation.

Ruptured dermoid cysts also cause orbital inflammation. Although the material they produce is native to the body, it is foreign to the orbit and may incite a robust inflammatory response.[60,61]

Nongranulomatous Idiopathic Orbital Inflammation

This common inflammatory condition is also called orbital pseudotumor or idiopathic orbital inflammation. The etiology is unknown, and it is diagnosed when other diseases have been ruled out.[62]

The disease is often unilateral and occurs in patients of all ages. Patients typically have no history of a systemic condition that could cause orbital inflammation, and may present with an acute or subacute onset of orbital pain. Almost any orbital structure may be affected, and depending on the location and degree of involvement patients may also have proptosis, ptosis, eyelid erythema or edema (Figs. 108.10A to C).[62] Nomenclature reflects the location of the inflammation and includes: myositis, perineuritis, dacryoadenitis, and posterior scleritis. Tolosa-Hunt describes idiopathic orbital inflammation of the orbital apex. Bony changes on CT or MRI imaging are atypical and should lead the clinician to consider other diagnoses. Histopathologic examination of tissue biopsies reveals a nonspecific inflammatory infiltrate of lymphocytes and plasma cells, as well as eosinophils and neutrophils. The presence of granulomatous inflammation, vasculitis or necrosis points to other etiologies. Fibrosis may be present in the sclerosing pseudotumor variant, and immunohistochemial staining to determine an IgG4 to IgG ratio may aide in distinguishing this disease from IgG4-related orbital inflammation.[62] Patients are typically treated with systemic corticosteroids.

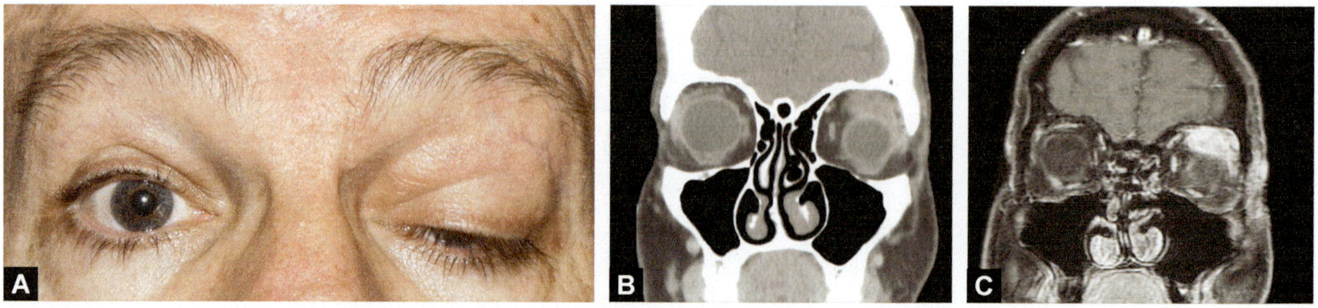

Figs. 108.10A to C: Idiopathic orbital inflammation. (A) External photograph demonstrating nearly complete left upper eyelid ptosis with edema; (B) Coronal CT scan in the same patient showing inflammation of the superior rectus and levator muscle complex; (C) Coronal T1-weighted fat-saturated postcontrast MRI in the same patient demonstrating inflammation in the left superior orbit.
Source: Michael K Yoon, MD.

CONCLUSION

Orbital inflammatory conditions are still in many ways mysterious to us, and we are only beginning to understand their biology. As our understanding of the molecular bases and functioning of these diseases expands, we can expect that there will be more re-classifications, as well as the welcome addition of new therapies.

REFERENCES

1. Bokhari SR, Mansur A. Sarcoidosis. Treasure Island (FL): StatPearls Publishing LLC; 2017.
2. Mavrikakis I, Rootman J. Diverse clinical presentations of orbital sarcoid. Am J Ophthalmol. 2007;144:769-75.
3. Iannuzzi MC, Rybicki BA, Teirstein AS. Sarcoidosis. N Engl J Med. 2007;357:2153-65.
4. Pasadhika S, Rosenbaum JT. Ocular sarcoidosis. Clin Chest Med. 2015;36:669-83.
5. Demirci H, Christianson MD. Orbital and adnexal involvement in sarcoidosis: analysis of clinical features and systemic disease in 30 cases. Am J Ophthalmol. 2011;151:1074-80.e1.
6. Collison JM, Miller NR, Green WR. Involvement of orbital tissues by sarcoid. Am J Ophthalmol. 1986;102:302-7.
7. Emile JF, Abla O, Fraitag S, et al. Revised classification of histiocytoses and neoplasms of the macrophage-dendritic cell lineages. Blood. 2016;127:2672-81.
8. Haroche J, Cohen-Aubart F, Rollins BJ, et al. Histiocytoses: emerging neoplasia behind inflammation. Lancet Oncol. 2017;18:e113-e125.
9. Kerstetter J, Wang J. Adult orbital xanthogranulomatous disease: a review with emphasis on etiology, systemic associations, diagnostic tools, and treatment. Dermatol Clin. 2015;33:457-63.
10. Sivak-Callcott JA, Rootman J, Rasmussen SL, et al. Adult xanthogranulomatous disease of the orbit and ocular adnexa: new immunohistochemical findings and clinical review. Br J Ophthalmol. 2006;90:602-8.
11. Esmaili N, Harris GJ. Langerhans cell histiocytosis of the orbit: spectrum of disease and risk of central nervous system sequelae in unifocal cases. Ophthal Plast Reconstr Surg. 2016;32:28-34.
12. Herwig MC, Wojno T, Zhang Q, et al. Langerhans cell histiocytosis of the orbit: five clinicopathologic cases and review of the literature. Surv Ophthalmol. 2013;58:330-40.
13. Jakobiec FA, Mills MD, Hidayat AA, et al. Periocular xanthogranulomas associated with severe adult-onset asthma. Trans Am Ophthalmol Soc. 1993;91:99-125; discussion 125-9.
14. Mukherjee B, Shrirao N. Adult-onset asthma and periocular xanthogranuloma with orbital involvement: a rare entity. Ann Allergy Asthma Immunol. 2016;116:466-7.
15. Hammond MD, Niemi EW, Ward TP, et al. Adult orbital xanthogranuloma with associated adult-onset asthma. Ophthal Plast Reconstr Surg. 2004;20:329-32.
16. Luck J, Layton A, Noble BA. Necrobiotic xanthogranuloma with orbital involvement. J R Soc Med. 1992;85:357-8.
17. Haroun F, Millado K, Tabbara I. Erdheim-Chester disease: comprehensive review of molecular profiling and therapeutic advances. Anticancer Res. 2017;37:2777-83.
18. Samara WA, Khoo CT, Say EA, et al. Juvenile xanthogranuloma involving the eye and ocular adnexa: tumor control, visual outcomes, and globe salvage in 30 patients. Ophthalmology. 2015;122:2130-8.
19. Rothschild PR, Pagnoux C, Seror R, et al. Ophthalmologic manifestations of systemic necrotizing vasculitides at diagnosis: a retrospective study of 1,286 patients and review of the literature. Semin Arthritis Rheum. 2013;42:507-14.
20. Santiago YM, Fay A. Wegener's granulomatosis of the orbit: a review of clinical features and updates in diagnosis and treatment. Semin Ophthalmol. 2011;26:349-55.
21. Perumal B, Black EH, Levin F, et al. Non-infectious orbital vasculitides. Eye (Lond). 2012;26:630-9.
22. Takanashi T, Uchida S, Arita M, et al. Orbital inflammatory pseudotumor and ischemic vasculitis in Churg-Strauss syndrome: report of two cases and review of the literature. Ophthalmology. 2001;108:1129-33.
23. Both T, Dalm VA, van Hagen PM, et al. Reviewing primary Sjogren's syndrome: beyond the dryness—from pathophysiology to diagnosis and treatment. Int J Med Sci. 2017;14:191-200.
24. Tabbara KF, Vera-Cristo CL. Sjogren syndrome. Curr Opin Ophthalmol. 2000;11:449-54.
25. Chen X, Jakobiec FA, Yadav P, et al. Melkersson-Rosenthal syndrome with isolated unilateral eyelid edema: an immunopathologic study. Ophthal Plast Reconstr Surg. 2015;31:e70-7.
26. Deshpande V. IgG4-related disease of the head and neck. Head Neck Pathol. 2015;9:24-31.
27. Wallace ZS, Deshpande V, Stone JH. Ophthalmic manifestations of IgG4-related disease: single-center experience and literature review. Semin Arthritis Rheum. 2014;43:806-17.
28. Mulay K, Wick MR. Ophthalmic immunoglobulin G4-related disease IgG4-RD Current concepts. Semin Diagn Pathol. 2016;33:148-55.
29. Zamora-Alejo K, Moore S, Leatherbarrow B, et al. Hyaluronidase toxicity: a possible cause of postoperative periorbital inflammation. Clin Exp Ophthalmol. 2013;41:122-6.
30. Park S, Lim LT. Orbital inflammation secondary to a delayed hypersensitivity reaction to sub-Tenon's hyaluronidase. Semin Ophthalmol. 2014;29:57-8.
31. Mukherji S, Esakowitz L. Orbital inflammation after sub-Tenon's anesthesia. J Cataract Refract Surg. 2005;31:2221-3.
32. Borchard K, Puy R, Nixon R. Hyaluronidase allergy: a rare cause of periorbital inflammation. Australas J Dermatol. 2010;51:49-51.
33. Cotliar JM, Shields CL, Meyer DR. Chronic orbital inflammation and fibrosis after retrobulbar alcohol and chlorpromazine injections in a patient with choroidal melanoma. Ophthal Plast Reconstr Surg. 2008;24:410-1.

34. Eftekhari K, Shindler KS, Lee V, et al. Histologic evidence of orbital inflammation from retrobulbar alcohol and chlorpromazine injection: a clinicopathologic study in human & rat orbits. Ophthal Plast Reconstr Surg. 2016;32:302-4.
35. Lefebvre DR, Mandeville JT, Yonekawa Y, et al. A case series and review of bisphosphonate-associated orbital inflammation. Ocul Immunol Inflamm. 2016;24:134-9.
36. Pirbhai A, Rajak SN, Goold LA, et al. Bisphosphonate-induced orbital inflammation: a case series and review. Orbit. 2015;34:331-5.
37. Papavasileiou E, Prasad S, Freitag SK, et al. Ipilimumab-induced ocular and orbital inflammation—a case series and review of the literature. Ocul Immunol Inflamm. 2016;24:140-6.
38. Wladis EJ, Tarasen AJ, Roth ZJ, et al. Orbital sarcoid-like granulomatosis after inhibition of tumor necrosis factor-alpha. Ophthal Plast Reconstr Surg. 2016;32:e30-2.
39. Bernardino CR, Mihora LD, Fay AM, et al. Orbital complications of hydrogel scleral buckles. Ophthal Plast Reconstr Surg. 2006;22:206-8.
40. Shields CL, Demirci H, Marr BP, et al. Expanding MIRAgel scleral buckle simulating an orbital tumor in four cases. Ophthal Plast Reconstr Surg. 2005;21:32-8.
41. Rubinstein TJ, Clemett J, Birnbach CD, et al. Clinical-radiological correlation of retained silicone sponge presenting as orbital inflammation. Case Rep Ophthalmol Med. 2016;2016:5291587.
42. Donker DL, Paridaens D, Mooy CM, et al. Blepharoptosis and upper eyelid swelling due to lipogranulomatous inflammation caused by silicone oil. Am J Ophthalmol. 2005;140:934-6.
43. Aryasit O, Ng DS, Goh AS, et al. Delayed onset porous polyethylene implant-related inflammation after orbital blowout fracture repair: four case reports. BMC Ophthalmol. 2016;16:94.
44. Custer PL, Lind A, Trinkaus KM. Complications of supramid orbital implants. Ophthal Plast Reconstr Surg. 2003;19:62-7.
45. Warrier S, Prabhakaran VC, Davis G, Selva D. Delayed complications of silicone implants used in orbital fracture repairs. Orbit. 2008;27:147-51.
46. Rosner M, Edward DP, Tso MO. Foreign-body giant-cell reaction to the hydroxyapatite orbital implant. Arch Ophthalmol. 1992;110:173-4.
47. Karcioglu ZA, Nasr AM. Diagnosis and management of orbital inflammation and infections secondary to foreign bodies: a clinical review. Orbit. 1998;17:247-69.
48. Callahan AB, Scofield SM, Gallin PF, et al. Retained strabismus suture material masquerading as nonspecific orbital inflammation. J AAPOS. 2016;20:280-2.
49. Katz SE, Rootman J. Adverse effects of bone wax in surgery of the orbit. Ophthal Plast Reconstr Surg. 1996;12:121-6.
50. Merkur AB, Jardeleza MS, Iliff NT, et al. Periocular petrolatum. Ophthal Plast Reconstr Surg. 2005;21:23-31.
51. Nathoo NA, Rasmussen S, Dolman PJ, et al. Periocular mass lesions secondary to dermatologic fillers: report of 3 cases. Can J Ophthalmol. 2014;49:468-72.
52. Jakobiec FA, Rai R, Rashid A, et al. Bilateral eyelid pseudoptosis from lipogranulomas of the preaponeurotic fat pads. Ophthal Plast Reconstr Surg. 2015;31:e125-31.
53. Ross AH, Malhotra R. Long-term orbitofacial complications of polyalkylimide 4% (Bio-Alcamid). Ophthal Plast Reconstr Surg. 2009;25:394-7.
54. Nabavi CB, Minckler DS, Tao JP. Histologic features of mesotherapy-induced orbital fat inflammation. Ophthal Plast Reconstr Surg. 2009;25:69-70.
55. Chappelow AV, McMahon JT, Jones CL, et al. Granulomatous orbital inflammation associated with intraorbital titanium-impregnated acetate fiber. Orbit. 2010;29:171-3.
56. Rabinowitz MP, Goldstein SM. Diesel fuel injury to the orbit. Ophthal Plast Reconstr Surg. 2013;29:e31-3.
57. Mayo GL, Long LS, Fitzsimmons T, et al. Delayed orbital foreign body reaction to dicotyledon (hardwood) libriform fibers. Arch Ophthalmol. 2002;120:1770-1.
58. Liu D. Common denominators in retained orbital wooden foreign body. Ophthal Plast Reconstr Surg. 2010;26:454-8.
59. Gekeler F, Cruz AA, de Paula SA, et al. Intraconal grease-gun injury: a therapeutic dilemma. Ophthal Plast Reconstr Surg. 2005;21:393-5.
60. Colombo F, Holbach LM, Naumann GO. Chronic inflammation in dermoid cysts: a clinicopathologic study of 115 patients. Orbit. 2000;19:97-107.
61. Abou-Rayyah Y, Rose GE, Konrad H, et al. Clinical, radiological and pathological examination of periocular dermoid cysts: evidence of inflammation from an early age. Eye (Lond). 2002;16:507-12.
62. Mombaerts I, Bilyk JR, Rose GE, et al. Consensus on diagnostic criteria of idiopathic orbital inflammation using a modified delphi approach. JAMA Ophthalmol. 2017;135:769-76.

Chapter 109 Thyroid Eye Disease: Evaluation and Management

Pimkwan Jaru-ampornpan, Raymond S Douglas, Shannon S Joseph

INTRODUCTION

Thyroid eye disease (TED) is one of the most common orbital inflammatory disorders. It is an autoimmune condition that can often be associated with Graves' disease. TED can have devastating consequences including facial disfigurement and vision loss. In this chapter, we review the epidemiology, pathophysiology, diagnosis, and management of this important condition.

EPIDEMIOLOGY

TED is an autoimmune condition that can be sight threatening. It is strongly associated with autoimmune thyroid disorders. Nearly, 90% of TED cases are associated with hyperthyroidism in the setting of Graves' disease (GD), 5% with euthyroidism, 3% with Hashimoto's thyroiditis, and 1% with primary hypothyroidism.[1-4] TED is the most common orbital disease in Europe and North America, affecting women more than men, with the age-adjusted incidence rate of 14–16 per 100,000 in women and one-fifth of that in men.[1,5] TED affects all ages but the peak incidences occur in a bimodal distribution, with age groups in the 4th and 6th decades being the most affected.[1] The estimated prevalence of TED is 0.25% among the US population.[4] The prevalence of TED among those with GD is higher at 20–50%.[4,6] Subclinical TED with extraocular muscle (EOM) enlargement on imaging is present in up to two-thirds of GD individuals.[7] Declining trend in cigarette smoking may have contributed to a decrease in the prevalence and severity of TED in recent decades.[4,6]

PATHOPHYSIOLOGY

Anatomically, individuals affected by TED are found to have enlarged EOMs and expansion of orbital fat.[8] Histopathological changes in TED orbits consist of inflamed orbital tissues, as evidenced by mononuclear cell infiltration, interstitial edema, and an overabundance of cytokines.[9,10] Additionally, hyaluronan, a hydrophilic glycosaminoglycan is found to accumulate in EOMs and orbital fat in TED.[11,12] The accumulation of hyaluronan is believed to contribute to the enlargement of the orbital soft tissue in TED. Nonetheless, the cellular and molecular underpinnings for these findings are only recently becoming better understood.

The underlying pathogenesis of TED involves a complex interplay of immune system responses and site-specific cellular responses that lead to inflammatory cascades affecting the orbital soft tissues[13-15] (Fig. 109.1). Recent studies have shown that orbital fibroblasts (OFs) are key players in TED pathogenesis.[14,16-18] The orbital fibroblasts (OFs) display distinct phenotypes of receptors and ligands as well as unique regulatory mechanism of hyaluronan synthesis compared to fibroblasts in other anatomical regions.[16] OFs become abnormally activated in TED, which leads to upregulation of hyaluronan and collagen synthesis, causing edema and fibrosis.[19-26] Production of inflammatory cytokines from activated OFs can also perpetuate the cascade of inflammatory responses by attracting T-cells to the orbit.[27-35] T-cells then interact with OFs, activating both cell types.[31] Once T-cells are activated, they may become autoreactive T-cells or trigger B-cell differentiation and monocyte-macrophage activation. Additionally, a subpopulation of OFs can differentiate into myofibroblasts and adipocytes,[36-40] leading to fibrosis and orbital fat expansion, respectively. Fibrocytes, which are bone marrow-derived monocyte progenitor cells, share similar phenotypic and functional characteristics with OFs, and may be an important link between the systemic immune response and site-specific disease.[15,41] In TED, fibrocytes leave the bloodstream and migrate to the orbit and behave such as OFs, contributing to TED pathogenesis.[42]

Abnormal activation of OFs in TED involves autoantigens, including thyrotropin receptor (TSHR) and insulin-like growth factor-1 receptor (IGF-1R). As a membrane-spanning tyrosine kinase receptor, IGF-1R is known for its role in development and metabolism.[43] In GD, IGF-1R can synergistically enhance the action of

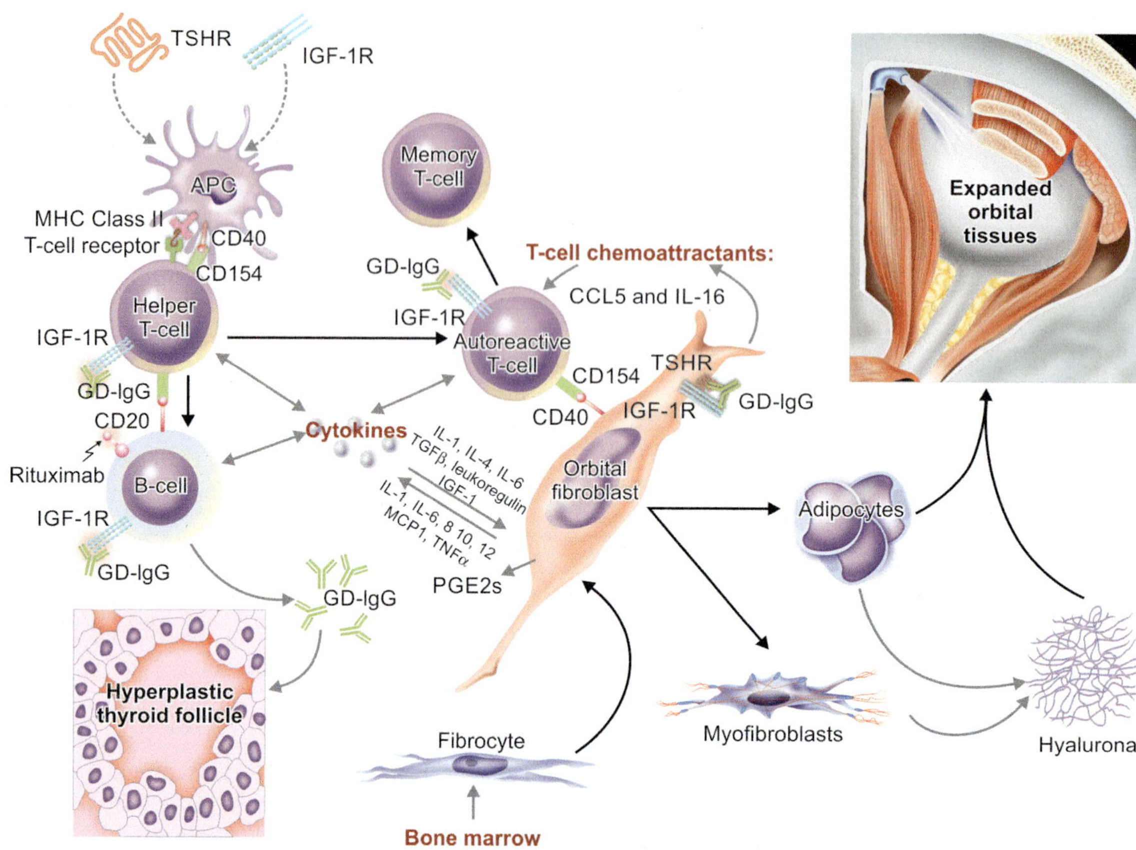

Fig. 109.1: Pathophysiology of thyroid eye disease. Autoantigens, TSHR and IGF-1R, are internalized by antigen-presenting cells (APC), and presented to helper T-cells, leading to cellular activation. Activated helper T-cells may either induce B-cells' autoantibodies (GD-IgGs) production or transform to autoreactive T-cells. Attracted by chemoattractants, autoreactive T-cells then travel to orbital tissues, and interact with orbital fibroblasts (OFs), resulting in mutual activation of both cell types. Activated T- and B-cells and OFs then secrete various inflammatory cytokines, which perpetuates the vicious inflammatory cycle. IGF-1R, which is overexpressed on these cell types, can interact with GD-IgGs and lead to cellular activation. IGF-1R can synergistically interact with TSHR on OF surface to create a physical and functional complex that may interact with GD-IgGs. Some of the OFs may be derived from infiltrating fibrocytes, which are progenitor cells that travel from the bone marrow. Activated OFs can differentiate into either adipocytes or myofibroblasts and can increase hyaluronan synthesis. Overall, the inflammatory cascades and OF differentiation result in the orbital soft tissue expansion and congestion in TED.

(TSHR: Thyrotropin-stimulating hormone receptor; IGF-1R: Insulin-like growth factor-1 receptor; TED: Thyroid eye disease; MCP1: Monocyte chemoattractant protein-1; TNF-α: Tumor necrosis factor-alpha; TGF-β: Transforming growth factor-beta; GD-IgG: Graves' disease immunoglobulin)

Source: Shan SJ, Douglas RS. The pathophysiology of thyroid eye disease. J Neuroophthalmol. 2014;34(2):177-85. with permission.

thyrotropin, and may be responsible, in part, for TED pathogenesis.[44,45] TSHR and IGF-1R are highly expressed on cell surface of OFs and fibrocytes in patients with TED.[19,46] Studies also revealed upregulation of IGF-1R on cell surface of B-and T-cells from GD patients.[47,48] In addition to autoantigen upregulation, antibodies to these receptors are also identified in patients with TED. TSHR-activating antibodies, known as thyroid-stimulating immunoglobulin (TSI), are detectable in up to 98% of individuals with GD and usually correlates with TED activity and severity.[49-54] Similarly, immunoglobulin that activates IGF-R signaling pathway has been detected in patients with TED.[33] In vitro and in vivo studies have supported the synergistic roles of TSHR and IGF-1R signaling pathways in the activation of OFs as part of TED pathogenesis.[19,33,36,37,51,55-59]

Recent understanding of the role of the IGF-1R signaling pathway in TED pathogenesis allowed researchers to develop a novel-targeted therapy against TED. Teprotumumab, an inhibitory immunoglobulin against IGF-1R, has been shown to result in significant clinical improvement in patients with active, moderate-to-severe disease by dramatically reversing proptosis. Since teprotumumab has been the first drug to reverse the end organ damage it has been recognized by Food and Drug Administration (FDA) as a 'breakthrough therapy' for TED, and is currently undergoing phase III clinical trials.[60]

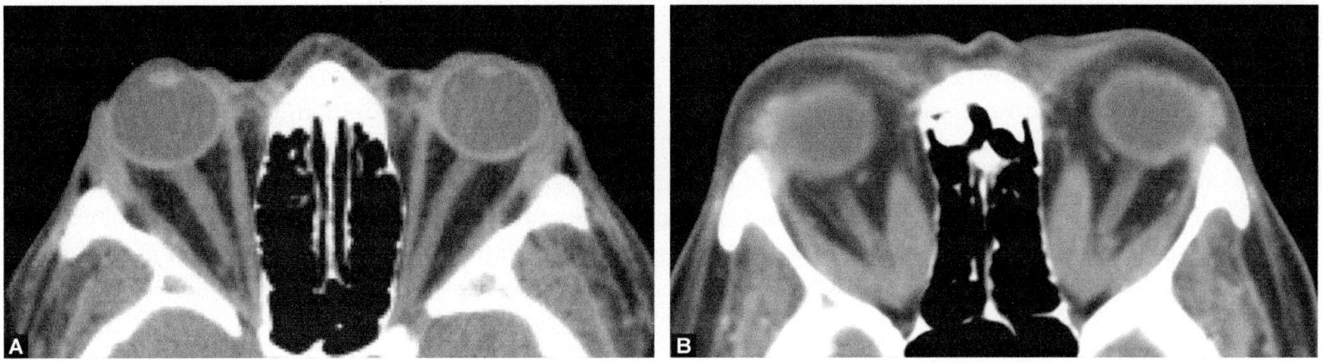

Figs. 109.2A and B: Axial view of computed tomography scans of (A) type I TED with fat predominant disease and (B) type II TED with EOMs enlargement.
(TED: Thyroid eye disease)

CLINICAL PRESENTATION AND DIAGNOSIS

The inflammatory cascades in TED lead to orbital tissue enlargement. Because the expansion of the soft tissues is limited by the bony structure of the orbit, it results in elevated intraorbital pressure and orbital congestion. Common clinical manifestations of TED include eyelid retraction with lateral flare, exophthalmos, lagophthalmos, lid lag upon downgaze, conjunctival injection, chemosis, periorbital edema, and strabismus. Eyelid retraction is one of the most common findings in TED.[61] Lagophthalmos and eyelid retraction can cause exposure keratopathy, which may result in ocular surface breakdown and even corneal perforation in severe cases. Compressive optic neuropathy (CON) occurs when the increased intraorbital pressure and physical crowding affects the optic nerve, which can cause decreased visual acuity, dyschromatopsia, relative afferent pupillary defect in unilateral cases, and optic disc edema or atrophy.[62,63] Visual field loss can be found in approximately two-thirds of patients with CON but is not required to diagnose CON.[62-67]

If TED is suspected in patients with suggestive clinical findings, laboratory testing including thyroid function tests [T3, free T4, and thyroid-stimulating hormone (TSH) should be obtained. TSI titer is also useful as this antibody is present in up to 98% of individuals affected by TED.[50,68] However, false negatives may occur, particularly in long-standing TED, and normal test results do not necessarily exclude the diagnosis of TED.

Orbital imaging is helpful in aiding the diagnosis of TED. In particular, computed tomography (CT) of the orbit allows visualization of the orbital bony structures as well as orbital apex region. Based on orbital imaging findings,

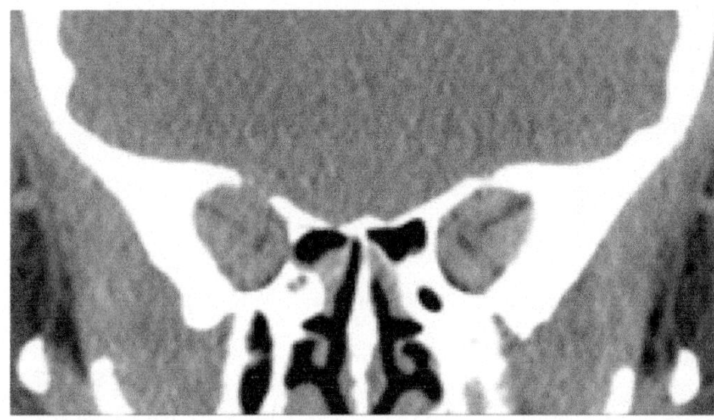

Fig. 109.3: Coronal view of computed tomography scan is showing obliteration of the fat plane around the optic nerve near the orbital apex in congested TED orbits.
(TED: Thyroid eye disease)

TED patients may be classified as type I or type II, with predominantly fat or EOM enlargement, respectively (Figs. 109.2A and B).[69] Apical crowding is secondary to enlarged EOMs and may suggest possible CON. In severe cases, obliteration of the fat plane around optic nerve near the orbital apex is observed (Fig. 109.3). Long-standing TED may lead to a medial bowing of the lamina papyracea in normally parallel medial orbital walls as a form of self-decompression.[70] Additionally, presurgical planning prior to orbital decompression relies upon both orbital CT and clinical findings. Magnetic resonance imaging (MRI) provides better soft tissue details but is usually insufficient in rendering details of the bony anatomy.[71] Ultrasound can be used to help identify and measure the enlarged EOMs in TED patients. However, it does not address the bony structure and its quality can be technician-dependent.[71] Therefore, orbital CT is the preferred imaging modality for TED.

Several scoring systems have been utilized to describe the extent and severity of TED. Based on the European Group on Graves' Orbitopathy (EUGOGO) classification, TED can be categorized into three groups—mild, moderate-to-severe, and sight-threatening disease—depending on the subjective symptoms and objective findings[72] (Table 109.1). Most of TED patients exhibit symptoms and signs in the mild category (Figs. 109.4A and B). Nevertheless, 15–25% of patients with mild TED can progress to more severe disease.[6,68,73] Up to 30% of TED patients may present with moderate-to-severe disease (Figs. 109.5A and B).[1,74] Sight-threatening disease is present in 4–8.6% of TED cases (Figs. 109.6A to C).[1,62,75] NO SPECS is another classification system used to document the severity of TED, which generates a global severity score (Table 109.2).[76] One disadvantage of the global severity score is that it may obscure the details of how a patient is specifically affected, and does not include sufficient information to document disease progression between visits.[5] TED can also be classified by phases based on disease activity: active

Table 109.1: Classification of disease severity of patients with TED by European Group on Graves' Orbitopathy (EUGOGO).

Mild	• Signs and symptoms only minor impact on daily life, insufficient to justify risks of immunosuppressive or surgical treatment • Patients usually have one or more of the following: minor lid retraction (<2 mm), mild soft tissue involvement, exophthalmos <3 mm above normal for race and gender, transient or no diplopia, and corneal exposure responsive to lubricants
Moderate-to-severe	• Lack of sight-threatening disease but the disease has sufficient impact on daily life to justify risks of immunosuppressive (if active) or surgical treatment (if inactive) • Patients usually have one or more of the following: lid retraction ≥2 mm, moderate or severe soft tissue involvement, exophthalmos ≥3 mm above normal for race and gender, inconstant or constant diplopia
Sight-threatening	Patients with CON and/or corneal breakdown warranting immediate intervention

(TED: Thyroid eye disease; CON: Compressive optic neuropathy)

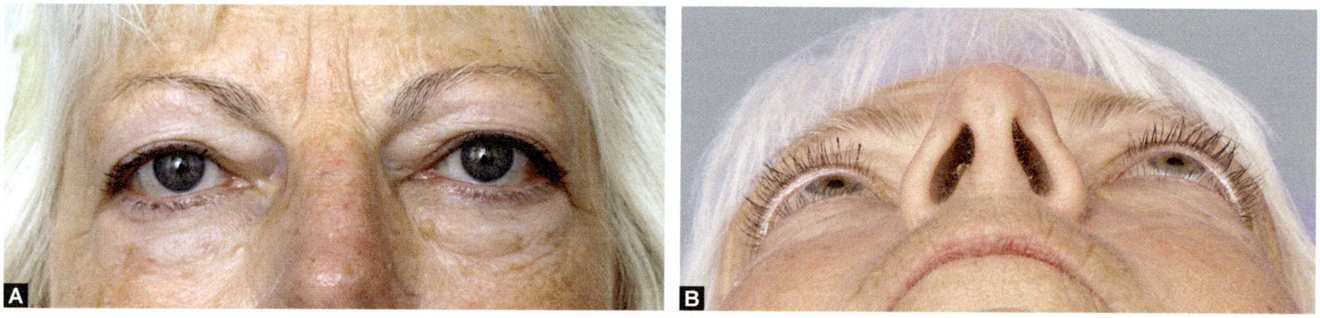

Figs. 109.4A and B: External photograph of a patient with mild TED demonstrating—(A) minimal lower eyelid retraction; and (B) slight exophthalmos without significant inflammatory findings.
(TED: Thyroid eye disease)

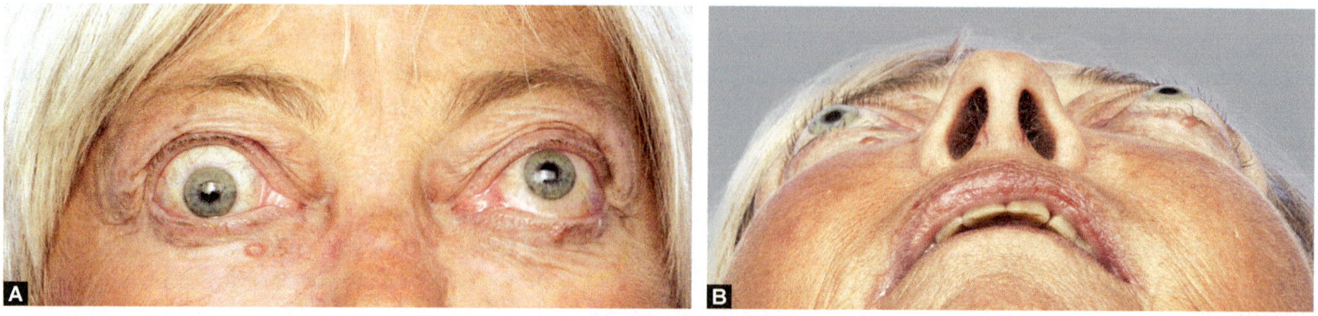

Figs. 109.5A and B: External photograph of a patient with moderate-to-severe TED is demonstrating (A) significant upper and lower eyelid retraction and strabismus, and (B) severe bilateral exophthalmos.
(TED: Thyroid eye disease)

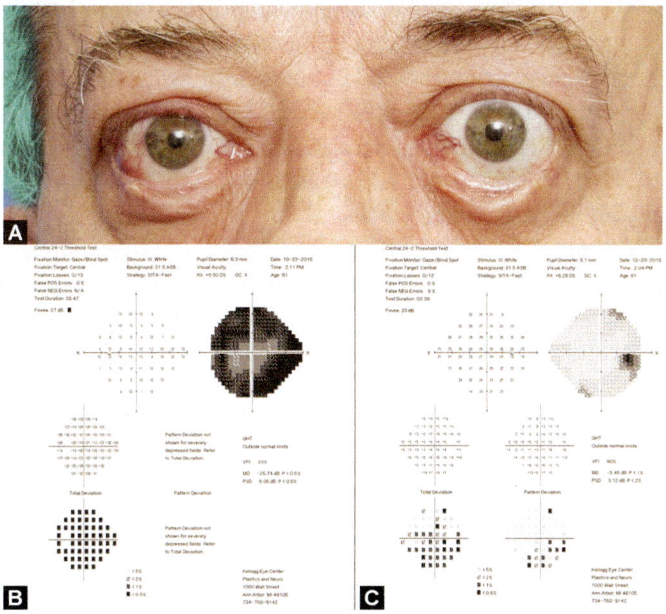

Figs. 109.6A to C: (A) External photograph of a patient with sight-threatening TED with eyelid retraction and conjunctival injection, and Humphrey visual fields of the left eye; and (B and C) right eye of the same patient showing constricted visual fields consistent with severe compressive optic neuropathy (CON) on the left and mild CON on the right. (TED: Thyroid eye disease)

versus inactive phases. Based on the Rundle's curve, TED begins in an active phase as evidenced by soft tissue inflammation that lasts 6 months–2 years before reaching a peak of maximum severity. The disease then improves and reaches a plateau of an inactive phase where fibrosis occurs.[77] The clinical activity score (CAS) was introduced in 1989 to classify the activity of the disease and to help identify active TED patients who are likely to respond to therapy (Table 109.3). It is now widely used. A CAS score of more than equal to 4 out of 10 points was shown to be associated with a positive predictive value of 80% in responding to immunosuppressive treatment.[78] Lastly, the vision, inflammation, strabismus, and appearance (VISA) classification was developed based on both subjective and objective parameters, and assesses for both disease severity and activity.

Table 109.2: NO SPECS classification.

Class	Grade
0	*N*o physical signs or symptoms
I	*O*nly signs (eyelid retraction)
II	*S*oft tissue involvement 0, absent; a, minimal; b, moderate; c, marked
III	*P*roptosis 0, absent; a, minimal; b, moderate; c, marked
IV	*E*xtraocular muscle signs 0, absent; a, limitation in extremes of gaze; b, evident restriction; c, fixation of globe(s)
V	*C*orneal involvement 0, absent; a, stippling; b, ulceration; c, clouding, necrosis, perforation
VI	*S*ight loss 0, VA better than 20/25; (a) VA 20/30–20/60; (b) VA 20/70–20/150; c, 20/200 or worse

Table 109.3: Clinical activity score (CAS). One point is given for each item using a binary scale. The sum of points is the clinical activity score.

Pain	• Painful feeling behind globe within the last 4 weeks • Pain on attempted gaze within the last 4 weeks
Redness	• Redness of eyelid(s) • Redness of conjunctiva
Swelling	• Chemosis • Swelling of eyelid(s) • Swelling of caruncles • Increase of proptosis ≥2 mm within the last 1–3 months
Impaired function	• Decrease in visual acuity of ≥1 line(s) on the Snellen chart within the last 1–3 months • Decrease in eye movement of ≥5 degrees within the last 1–3 months

MANAGEMENT

Risk Factor Modification

Smoking, diabetes mellitus (DM), and dysthyroidism are the three main modifiable risk factors known to be associated with new development or worsening of TED. Smoking is the most significant modifiable risk factor for TED.[79-81] Active smokers with GD carry about 3–4 times higher risk of developing TED as well as higher degree of disease severity and treatment unresponsiveness compared to nonsmokers.[6,80-83] Smoking cessation should thus be counseled at every visit for patients with GD or TED who are active smokers. DM is another important modifiable risk factor especially for the development of CON. Its association with vasculopathy may cause the optic nerve to be sensitized to the increased intraorbital pressure in TED, leading to CON.[84] Studies have shown that patients with CON are more likely to have DM, and TED individuals with DM are more likely to develop more severe CON.[64,75,84] Therefore, it is important to counsel patients with DM and TED on the importance of glycemic control.

Poorly controlled thyroid function is another modifiable risk factor for more severe TED.[85] Euthyroidism should be achieved and maintained as soon as possible in all TED patients to prevent worsening of TED and/or lessen the disease severity.[6] Three treatment modalities exist for dysthyroidism: anti-thyroid medication, radioablation with iodine-131 (RAI), and surgical thyroidectomy. The mainstay of medical therapy in the management of hyperthyroidism is antithyroid drugs, including propylthiouracil, methimazole, and carbimazole.[86] These drugs suppress the production of thyroid hormone by inhibiting the coupling of iodothyronines.[87] In most studies, antithyroid drugs have not been associated with worsening of TED.[88] Some experts believe that there are theoretical benefits of antithyroid drugs because they were shown to result in a more rapid reduction of TSHR antibody level compared to surgery or RAI.[89,90] However, these drugs are not without side effects, and long-term use should be monitored closely. RAI has become a popular modality among endocrinologists as a first-line treatment for uncomplicated GD or in cases of antithyroid drug failure. It is, however, contraindicated in pregnancy and breastfeeding. It uses the radioactive isotope ^{131}I to destroy the thyroid follicular cells and suppress thyroid hormone production. Studies have shown that RAI treatment can lead to the development or progression of TED in 15–35% of patients, possibly associated with post-treatment hypothyroid state and increased antithyroid antibody levels from the release of autoantigens.[89-91] Low-dose prophylactic oral corticosteroids (0.2 mg/kg/day) can be used in conjunction with RAI to prevent the progression of TED: starting 1 day after RAI treatment and tapered off over 6 weeks.[80,88,92] Surgical thyroidectomy is a definitive and effective means to treat hyperthyroidism in GD. Removal of the thyroid gland can be total or partial. Thyroidectomy has a theoretical advantage of reducing antithyroid antibody levels and removing the autoantigens in thyroid glands.[90] Thyroid hormone supplementation is generally required after surgical thyroidectomy due to postoperative hypothyroidism.

Mild Disease

Although most TED patients exhibit mild clinical symptoms and findings, these symptoms can significantly affect the patient's quality of life.[93] Conservative measures are the mainstay treatment in this group. For exposure keratopathy and dry eyes, ocular surface lubrication with artificial tears, ointment, and moisture chamber at night should be implemented. Punctal plugs or cauterization should be considered. Surgical tarsorrhaphy may be necessary in sight-threatening corneal exposure. Cold compresses, low-sodium diet, and head elevation during sleep may help improve periorbital edema.[2,72,80] For symptomatic diplopia, Fresnel prisms or unilateral ocular patching may be helpful.

Selenium supplementation has been shown to alleviate mild TED symptoms and improving the quality of life in some TED patients.[94] Selenium is a trace element found in soil that works as an antioxidant and has immunomodulating effects.[68,80] Taking sodium selenite 100 mg twice daily by mouth has been shown to improve the disease severity, clinical activity, and quality of life in mild TED patients. Selenium has also been shown to lower the rate of progression to more severe TED in a randomized clinical trial.[95] However, this study was conducted in European countries where selenium was marginally deficient. Therefore, it is unclear if selenium supplementation for mild TED in selenium-sufficient areas, such as North America, will be as beneficial. Higher dose of selenium supplement (exceeding 400 µg daily) has also been associated with increased risk of type II diabetes, and it is important to discuss this information with patients prior to starting therapy.[96]

Moderate-to-severe or Sight-threatening Disease

Management of moderate-to-severe or sight-threatening TED varies depending on disease activity. In active disease, the first-line therapy is systemic glucocorticoids with or without adjunctive low-dose orbital radiation to mitigate the risk of vision loss. The main goal of treatment is to abort or shorten the duration of active inflammatory phase. In those with CON or who are refractory to steroids, urgent orbital decompression is recommended. On the contrary, systemic glucocorticoids, and orbital radiation are usually not effective in inactive TED. Instead, surgical rehabilitation should be considered in this population.

Active Disease

- *Systemic glucocorticoids:* Systemic glucocorticoids are the first-line treatment for active moderate-to-severe and sight-threatening disease.[72,97] Glucocorticoids have anti-inflammatory and immunosuppressive properties, as well as the ability to reduce hyaluronan synthesis by OFs.[98] The mode of steroids administration is important. Pulse therapy of intravenous (IV) glucocorticoids has been proven to be better tolerated and superior in efficacy to the oral form in treating moderate-to-severe and sight-threatening TED, with a response rate of 80% and 60%, respectively.[99] Optimal dosing for IV glucocorticoid regimen has not been well established. A recent study used 500 mg of IV methylprednisone weekly for 6 weeks followed by 250 mg weekly doses for 6 weeks.[100] For patients with sight-threatening TED, IV pulse steroids are typically given in 1 g daily doses for 3 consecutive days and repeated in the second week if needed.[101] Potential side effects of high-dose IV steroids include acute hepatic failure, cerebrovascular, and cardiovascular events.[94,102-106] Therefore, the total cumulative doses of methylprednisone should not exceed 8 g in each 12 week-course and the side effects should be carefully monitored during the treatment period. Oral steroids taper can then be initiated, if there is a clinical response to the IV steroids course. However, orbital decompression should be performed in refractory cases, or if steroids are contraindicated.[94,107,108]

- *Orbital radiotherapy:* Radiation therapy (RT) has also been used to treat active TED. The effect of RT may be secondary to alteration of the nitric oxide pathway,[97,109] impairment of lymphocytic function,[109] and reduction of hyaluronan synthesis by OFs.[110] The most common dosing regimen is a cumulative dose of 20 Gy per eye divided into 10 fractions over 10 days. The radiation is aimed at the retrobulbar tissue of each orbit.[111] Comparing to steroids, the effect of which is rapid, RT takes weeks to months to achieve maximal clinical effect. Therefore, it is usually not the first-line therapy in active TED but rather an adjunctive treatment to IV glucocorticoids therapy. RT is a viable option when steroid therapy is contraindicated, when the steroid side effects are poorly tolerated, or in poor surgical candidates. Matthiesen et al. reported that, among patients with active TED, 96% of those who received orbital RT had stabilization of disease, and 46% reported complete resolution of symptoms.[112] Shams et al. compared the efficacy of corticosteroids with or without orbital radiotherapy and showed that the TED patients who received orbital RT in addition to corticosteroids had significantly lower rates of CON and greater improvement in ocular motility.[113] Overall, RT is a relatively safe regimen with well-tolerated transient side effects including periorbital edema, alopecia at entry ports, and conjunctival injection. Other rare side effects to be monitored consist of radiation retinopathy, optic neuropathy, cataract, and scleral necrosis.[114-118] Uncontrolled systemic hypertension and DM are contraindications to RT due to elevated risk of developing or worsening retinopathy.[116]" Lastly, there is a theoretical lifetime risk of developing secondary malignancies in the radiated field from low-dose RT.[116,117,119] Thus, orbital RT should be avoided in patients under age 35 years due to the long latency of these tumors.
- *Novel therapeutic agents:* Immunomodulatory therapies employ disease-modifying agents that target the underlying molecular pathogenesis of the disease. Rituximab and teprotumumab have been tested in randomized clinical trials for their efficacy in TED treatment.[60,120]

Rituximab is a monoclonal chimeric antibody to CD20 on mature B-cells and effectively depletes the CD20+ B-cell population for 6–9 months.[121] It has been approved for the treatment of non-Hodgkin lymphomas, rheumatoid arthritis, and chronic lymphocytic leukemia. Several prospective and retrospective studies have examined the efficacy of rituximab in treating moderate-to-severe and sight-threatening TED, and the findings are equivocal.[122-130] Silkiss *et al.* treated 12 patients with active TED with 1000 mg of rituximab on days 1 and 18, and showed that the CAS significantly improved from baseline at each follow-up visit.[129] On the contrary, a randomized clinical trial by Stan et al. showed that rituximab offered no additional benefit over placebo to subjects with active and moderate-to-severe TED.[120] However, both treatment groups in the latter study had received prior corticosteroid treatment, and thus the improvement experienced in the control group may have been influenced by persistent benefit from prior corticosteroid treatment.[120] Side effects of rituximab include infusion-related reactions, which has been reported in one-third of the patients.[131] No other significant adverse events have been reported in TED patients treated with rituximab.[124] Current recommendation for the use of rituximab in TED is in patients with severe, active disease, and for whom steroids are refractory or contraindicated.

Teprotumumab is an IGF-1R inhibitory antibody that has also been shown to have a promising role as disease-modifying therapy for TED.[19] A multicenter, randomized-controlled trial was conducted by Smith et al. to determine the efficacy of teprotumumab in treating active TED.[60] Inclusion criteria were recent onset of active moderate-to-severe TED and a CAS of 4 or more. The regimen used in the clinical trial consisted of eight IV infusions, one every 3 weeks, starting with an initial dose of 10 mg/kg of body weight, followed by 20 mg/kg for the remaining seven infusions. The trial showed that teprotumumab was more effective than placebo in reducing proptosis and

CAS; with 69% of patients who received teprotumumab, as compared with 20% of patients who received placebo, having a clinical response at week 24 after the initiation of treatment.[60] Teprotumumab was also shown in this trial to improve the quality of life in TED patients.[60] The only drug-related adverse event was hyperglycemia in patients with diabetes, which was corrected with diabetic medication adjustment. In August 2016, teprotumumab received a "breakthrough therapy" designation from the FDA and is currently undergoing a phase III clinical trial.

- *Urgent surgical management:* Surgical management in TED is usually performed when the disease is stable and inactive. However, when sight-threatening TED is present, and the response to IV glucocorticoids treatment or other treatments are incomplete or the medical treatment itself is contraindicated, urgent surgical intervention is usually necessary to prevent further vision loss.[132]
- *Orbital decompression surgery:* The goal of orbital decompression surgery is to remove orbital fat or parts of the orbital walls to allow the enlarged orbital soft tissue to expand into new effective orbital space, thus relieving intraorbital pressure and congestion.[132,133] In CON, if the patient does not response to IV glucocorticoids, urgent orbital wall decompression is indicated. Bony decompression near the posteromedial orbital apex allows rapid improvement in vision.[134-138] The most common approach for medial orbital wall decompression is the transcaruncular approach, which avoids cutaneous scarring that can be caused by transcutaneous and coronal techniques.[139] It is important to remove the posterior two-thirds of the inframedial orbital strut as well as part of the palatine bone to allow maximal medial wall decompression in CON cases. Sparing the anterior inframedial orbital strut reduces the risk of postoperative diplopia.[140] The deep lateral wall, or part of the greater wing of the sphenoid bone, can be further removed to relieve the compression of the posterior orbit.

In severe exposure, keratopathy cases due to significant exophthalmos, several approaches to surgical orbital decompression are available. The degree of desired proptosis reduction dictates the amount of orbital fat as well as the number of orbital walls to be removed. Orbital fat removal should be considered in all cases undergoing orbital decompression. Transconjunctival approach via an inferior fornix incision is the most common technique used to remove orbital fat, if no additional bony walls need to be decompressed. Removal of orbital fat alone allows for mild exophthalmos reduction as well as relief in intraorbital pressure.[111,141] Bony decompression should be considered next if a higher degree of proptosis reduction is desired, especially in severe exposure keratopathy cases. In the absence of CON, lateral orbital wall decompression is preferred over medial and floor decompressions as the first choice because of a lower risk of postoperative diplopia.[142-144] Traditional technique for lateral orbital wall decompression involved removal of the zygoma from the frontozygomatic suture to slightly above the zygomatic arch. However, a modified technique has been developed to allow axial reduction of the globe position by removing the "deep" lateral wall, which includes the bone marrow of the greater wing of the sphenoid extending to the inferior and superior orbital fissures and anteriorly to the orbital rim.[134,139,145] This technique reduces the risk of postoperative diplopia.[134,142] In more severe cases of lagophthalmos, a "balanced" orbital decompression (removing both medial and lateral walls) or a three-wall decompression (removing medial, lateral walls, and orbital floor) may be considered.[145-147]

Potential complications after orbital decompression include diplopia, sinusitis, cerebrospinal fluid (CSF) leak, and hypoesthesia of the cheek and lower eyelid. The development of new diplopia or exacerbation of existing diplopia can be observed in 10–30% of patients after orbital decompression.[148] This is mostly due to the displacement of rectus muscles away from the orbital axis.[149-151] The risk of postoperative diplopia is higher in medial wall and orbital floor decompression (up to 66%), compared to deep lateral wall decompression (up to 7%).[142-143] Postoperative hypoesthesia due to injury to the infraorbital neurovascular bundle may be presented after orbital floor decompression. Stereotactic guidance during orbital decompression can be employed to improve localization and visualization of the extent of bone removal, and minimize the risk of intraoperative complication.[110,152]

- *Temporizing eyelid procedures:* In cases of severe exposure, keratopathy due to proptosis and eyelid retraction, emergent eyelid retractor recession with or without temporary suture tarsorrhaphy may be required, in addition to orbital decompression, to prevent further deterioration of the ocular surface. Aggressive lubrication with moisture chamber should be implemented immediately. In nonsurgical candidates, botulinum toxin injection to the levator palpebrae superioris muscle may be considered as a temporizing measure to lower the upper eyelid in severe upper eyelid retraction.[153,154] However, there is a delay in the effect of botulinum toxin for up to 48 hours. Further, inadvertent injection into the superior rectus muscle can reduce the Bell's phenomenon and worsen ocular surface exposure.[68] Subconjunctival or periocular triamcinolone (TA) injection has also been shown to improve upper eyelid retraction within 6 months of symptom onset in TED, before the onset of the fibrotic phase.[155-158] It should be cautioned that periocular TA injection can result in elevated intraocular pressure (IOP), and treated patients should be closely monitored. Shorter needles, smaller injection volumes, and a more distant injection site from the globe could prevent severe IOP elevation. In addition, although the TA injection is administered locally, systemic side effects of corticosteroids have been observed in some patients.[159]

Inactive Disease

Surgical rehabilitation in inactive TED may be indicated to restore patients' predisease appearance and function. TED should be stable for at least 6 months prior to any rehabilitative procedures. The sequence of TED surgical rehabilitation is as followed: first orbital decompression, second strabismus surgery, and third eyelid surgery. Orbital decompression is the first step to reduce exophthalmos and exposure keratopathy. Strabismus is usually performed at least 3 months after orbital decompression, and ocular alignment measurements should be stable for at least 6 months prior to strabismus surgery. Eyelid retraction repair is performed as the last step, at least 2 months after strabismus surgery, because strabismus surgery can affect eyelid positioning.

- *Orbital decompression surgery:* The guidelines for orbital decompression surgery in inactive TED are similar to those in active disease as discussed in the previous section.
- *Extraocular muscle surgery:* The EOMs in TED are usually enlarged and fibrotic, especially in type II disease, resulting in incomitant restrictive strabismus, and binocular diplopia. The most commonly affected muscle is the inferior rectus. The main goal for strabismus surgery in TED patients is to restore binocular single vision in primary gaze at distant and near.[132] Surgical repair usually involves recessing the fibrotic muscles. It is important to note that inferior rectus recession may subsequently cause lower eyelid retraction. In addition, recession surgery may worsen exophthalmos. Therefore, orbital decompression should be performed in anticipation for worsened exophthalmos after the recession surgery in TED patients who require both orbital decompression and EOM recession surgery. Patients should be counseled that numerous strabismus surgeries may be necessary to achieve the desired results.
- *Eyelid procedures:* When there is more than 1 mm of either upper or lower eyelid retraction, lateral flare, or asymmetry between the eyelid positions, surgical intervention may be indicated. Upper eyelid retraction in TED is likely related to fibrosis and sympathetic stimulation of the levator palpebrae superioris and Mueller's muscle.[160] Two common approaches for surgical repair of upper eyelid retraction are anterior approach (eyelid crease incision) and posterior approach (conjunctival incision) to recess the upper eyelid retractor muscles. To correct the lateral flare, the lateral horn of the levator aponeurosis can be disinserted from the tarsus.

Lower eyelid retraction in TED is also thought to be related to the fibrosis of the lower eyelid retractors, or may occur postoperatively after inferior rectus recession surgery. Surgical repair of lower eyelid retraction usually involves recessing the lower eyelid retractor via a transconjunctival incision. In more severe cases, various types of spacer grafts can be used to provide support and lengthen the lower eyelids vertically. The graft placement is between the inferior edge of the tarsus and the surgically recessed lower eyelid retractors. The size of the spacer graft is determined by the degree of eyelid retraction. Materials used as spacer grafts can range from synthetic materials to autologous tissues such as hard palate or ear cartilage.[161-169] The effect of lower eyelid retraction repair can be improved with a lateral tarsal strip or lateral canthopexy and/or tarsorrhaphy.[163,170]

Blepharoplasty with fat excision may be indicated in TED patients with the appearance of bulging eyelids secondary to the enlargement and fibrosis of preaponeurotic fat pads and subdermal brow fat. However, conservative amount of skin excision in blepharoplasty is advised in TED due to the risk of worsening eyelid retraction, lagophthalmos, and exposure keratopathy.[171] If there is no excess skin then enlarged fibrotic fatty tissue may be removed via a transconjunctival approach.

Nonsurgical modalities are also available as alternatives for the treatment of eyelid malposition in TED. This includes the use of hyaluronic acid (HA) and botulinum toxin.[172] HA products are the most frequently used in the periocular region among other types of fillers, due to their reversibility and safety profiles. The effect of HA lasts about 6–12 months in the periocular region and is reversible with the administration of hyaluronidase. HA can serve as a temporary weight to reduce upper eyelid retraction and lagophthalmos. As for the lower eyelid, HA can be used to lengthen the lower eyelid retractors and provide structural support over the inferior orbital rim to improve lower eyelid position and reduce retraction.[173] The use of botulinum toxin was as discussed in the previous section for addressing upper eyelid retraction.

REFERENCES

1. Bartley GB. The epidemiologic characteristics and clinical course of ophthalmopathy associated with autoimmune thyroid disease in Olmsted County, Minnesota. Trans Am Ophthalmol Soc. 1994;92:477-588.
2. Dolman PJ. Evaluating Graves' orbitopathy. Best Pract Res Clin Endocrinol Metab. 2012;26(3):229-48.
3. Marcocci C, Bartalena L, Bogazzi F, et al. Studies on the occurrence of ophthalmopathy in Graves' disease. Acta Endocrinol (Copenh). 1989;120(4):473-8.
4. Lazarus JH. Epidemiology of Graves' orbitopathy (GO) and relationship with thyroid disease. Best Pract Res Clin Endocrinol Metab. 2012;26(3):273-9.
5. Dolman PJ. Natural History of Thyroid Eye Disease. In: Douglas RS, McCoy AN, Gupta S (Eds). Thyroid Eye Disease. New York: Springer; 2015. pp. 13-22.
6. Tanda ML, Piantanida E, Liparulo L, et al. Prevalence and natural history of Graves' orbitopathy in a large series of patients with newly diagnosed Graves' hyperthyroidism seen at a single center. J Clin Endocrinol Metab. 2013;98(4):1443-9.
7. Enzmann DR, Donaldson SS, Kriss JP. Appearance of Graves' disease on orbital computed tomography. J Comput Assist Tomogr. 1979.;3(6):815-9.
8. Forbes G, Gorman CA, Brennan MD, et al. Ophthalmopathy of Graves' disease: computerized volume measurements of the orbital fat and muscle. Am J Neuroradiol. 1986;7(4):651-6.
9. Wang Y, Smith TJ. Current concepts in the molecular pathogenesis of thyroid-associated ophthalmopathy. Invest Ophthalmol Vis Sci. 2014;55(3):1735-48.
10. Hufnagel TJ, Hickey WF, Cobbs WH, et al. Immunohistochemical and ultrastructural studies on the exenterated orbital tissues of a patient with Graves' disease. Ophthalmology. 1984;91(11):1411-9.
11. Smith TJ, Bahn RS, Gorman CA. Connective tissue, glycosaminoglycans, and diseases of the thyroid. Endocr Rev. 1989;10(3):366-91.
12. Prabhakar BS, Bahn RS, Smith TJ. Current perspective on the pathogenesis of Graves' disease and ophthalmopathy. Endocr Rev. 2003;24(6):802-35.
13. Bahn RS. Graves' ophthalmopathy. N Engl J Med. 2010;362(8):726-38.
14. Smith TJ. Emerging Role of Fibrocytes in the Pathogenesis of Thyroid Eye Disease. In: Douglas RS, McCoy AN, Gupta S (Eds). Thyroid Eye Disease. New York: Springer; 2015. pp. 23-32.
15. Joseph SS, Douglas RS. Thyroid Eye Disease: A Comprehensive Review. In: Demirci H (Ed). Orbital Inflammatory Diseases and Their Differential Diagnosis Berlin, Heidelberg: Springer; 2015. pp. 73–89.
16. Smith TJ, Koumas L, Gagnon A, et al. Orbital fibroblast heterogeneity may determine the clinical presentation of thyroid-associated ophthalmopathy. J Clin Endocrinol Metab. 2002;87(1):385-92.
17. Smith TJ, Tsai CC, Shih M-J, et al. Unique attributes of orbital fibroblasts and global alterations in IGF-1 receptor signaling could explain thyroid-associated ophthalmopathy. Thyroid Off J Am Thyroid Assoc. 2008;18(9):983-8.
18. Smith RS, Smith TJ, Blieden TM, et al. Fibroblasts as sentinel cells. Synthesis of chemokines and regulation of inflammation. Am J Pathol. 1997;151(2):317-22.
19. Smith TJ, Hoa N. Immunoglobulins from patients with Graves' disease induce hyaluronan synthesis in their orbital fibroblasts through the self-antigen, insulin-like growth factor-I receptor. J Clin Endocrinol Metab. 2004;89(10):5076-80.
20. Korducki JM, Loftus SJ, Bahn RS. Stimulation of glycosaminoglycan production in cultured human retroocular fibroblasts. Invest Ophthalmol Vis Sci. 1992;33(6):2037-42.
21. Smith TJ, Wang HS, Evans CH. Leukoregulin is a potent inducer of hyaluronan synthesis in cultured human orbital fibroblasts. Am J Physiol. 1995;268(2 Pt 1):C382-8.
22. Cao HJ, Wang HS, Zhang Y, et al. Activation of human orbital fibroblasts through CD40 engagement results in a dramatic induction of hyaluronan synthesis and prostaglandin endoperoxide H synthase-2 expression. Insights into potential pathogenic mechanisms of thyroid-associated ophthalmopathy. J Biol Chem. 1998;273(45):29615-25.
23. Kaback LA, Smith TJ. Expression of hyaluronan synthase messenger ribonucleic acids and their induction by interleukin-1beta in human orbital fibroblasts: potential insight into the molecular pathogenesis of thyroid-associated ophthalmopathy. J Clin Endocrinol Metab. 1999;84(11):4079-84.
24. Han R, Smith TJ. T helper type 1 and type 2 cytokines exert divergent influence on the induction of prostaglandin E2 and hyaluronan synthesis by interleukin-1beta in orbital fibroblasts: implications for the pathogenesis of thyroid-associated ophthalmopathy. Endocrinology. 2006;147(1):13-9.
25. Krieger CC, Gershengorn MC. A modified ELISA accurately measures secretion of high molecular weight hyaluronan (HA) by Graves' disease orbital cells. Endocrinology. 2014;155(2):627-34.
26. Tan GH, Dutton CM, Bahn RS. Interleukin-1 (IL-1) receptor antagonist and soluble IL-1 receptor inhibit IL-1-induced glycosaminoglycan production in cultured human orbital

fibroblasts from patients with Graves' ophthalmopathy. J Clin Endocrinol Metab. 1996;81(2):449-52.

27. Han R, Tsui S, Smith TJ. Up-regulation of prostaglandin E2 synthesis by interleukin-1beta in human orbital fibroblasts involves coordinate induction of prostaglandin-endoperoxide H synthase-2 and glutathione-dependent prostaglandin E2 synthase expression. J Biol Chem. 2002;277(19):16355-64.
28. Wang HS, Cao HJ, Winn VD, et al. Leukoregulin induction of prostaglandin-endoperoxide H synthase-2 in human orbital fibroblasts. An in vitro model for connective tissue inflammation. J Biol Chem. 1996;271(37):22718-28.
29. Cao HJ, Smith TJ. Leukoregulin upregulation of prostaglandin endoperoxide H synthase-2 expression in human orbital fibroblasts. Am J Physiol. 1999;277(6 Pt 1):C1075-85.
30. Young DA, Evans CH, Smith TJ. Leukoregulin induction of protein expression in human orbital fibroblasts: evidence for anatomical site-restricted cytokine-target cell interactions. Proc Natl Acad Sci USA. 1998;95(15):8904-9.
31. Hwang CJ, Afifiyan N, Sand D, et al. Orbital fibroblasts from patients with thyroid-associated ophthalmopathy overexpress CD40: CD154 hyperinduces IL-6, IL-8, and MCP-1. Invest Ophthalmol Vis Sci. 2009;50(5):2262-8.
32. Sciaky D, Brazer W, Center DM, et al. Cultured human fibroblasts express constitutive IL-16 mRNA: cytokine induction of active IL-16 protein synthesis through a caspase-3-dependent mechanism. J Immunol. 2000;164(7):3806-14.
33. Pritchard J, Han R, Horst N, et al. Immunoglobulin activation of T cell chemoattractant expression in fibroblasts from patients with Graves' disease is mediated through the insulin-like growth factor I receptor pathway. J Immunol. 2003;170(12):6348-54.
34. Cao HJ, Han R, Smith TJ. Robust induction of PGHS-2 by IL-1 in orbital fibroblasts results from low levels of IL-1 receptor antagonist expression. Am J Physiol Cell Physiol. 2003;284(6):C1429-37.
35. Heufelder AE, Bahn RS. Modulation of Graves' orbital fibroblast proliferation by cytokines and glucocorticoid receptor agonists. Invest Ophthalmol Vis Sci. 1994;35(1): 120-7.
36. Valyasevi RW, Erickson DZ, Harteneck DA, et al. Differentiation of human orbital preadipocyte fibroblasts induces expression of functional thyrotropin receptor. J Clin Endocrinol Metab. 1999;84(7):2557-62.
37. Valyasevi RW, Harteneck DA, Dutton CM, et al. Stimulation of adipogenesis, peroxisome proliferator-activated receptor-gamma (PPAR gamma), and thyrotropin receptor by PPAR gamma agonist in human orbital preadipocyte fibroblasts. J Clin Endocrinol Metab. 2002;87(5):2352-8.
38. Sorisky A, Pardasani D, Gagnon A, et al. Evidence of adipocyte differentiation in human orbital fibroblasts in primary culture. J Clin Endocrinol Metab. 1996;81(9):3428-31.
39. Feldon SE, O'loughlin CW, Ray DM, et al. Activated human T lymphocytes express cyclooxygenase-2 and produce proadipogenic prostaglandins that drive human orbital fibroblast differentiation to adipocytes. Am J Pathol. 2006;169(4):1183-93.
40. Koumas L, Smith TJ, Feldon S, et al. Thy-1 expression in human fibroblast subsets defines myofibroblastic or lipofibroblastic phenotypes. Am J Pathol. 2003;163(4):1291-300.
41. Douglas RS, Afifiyan NF, Hwang CJ, et al. Increased Generation of Fibrocytes in Thyroid-Associated Ophthalmopathy. J Clin Endocrinol Metab. 2010;95(1):430-8.
42. Hong KM, Belperio JA, Keane MP, et al. Differentiation of human circulating fibrocytes as mediated by transforming growth factor-beta and peroxisome proliferator-activated receptor gamma. J Biol Chem. 2007;282(31):22910-20.
43. Gallagher EJ, LeRoith D. Minireview: IGF, Insulin, and Cancer. Endocrinology. 2011;152(7):2546-51.
44. Tramontano D, Cushing GW, Moses AC, et al. Insulin-like growth factor-I stimulates the growth of rat thyroid cells in culture and synergizes the stimulation of DNA synthesis induced by TSH and Graves'-IgG. Endocrinology. 1986;119(2):940-2.
45. Song D, Wang R, Zhong Y, et al. Locally produced insulin-like growth factor-1 by orbital fibroblasts as implicative pathogenic factor rather than systemically circulated IGF-1 for patients with thyroid-associated ophthalmopathy. Graefes Arch Clin Exp Ophthalmol. 2012;250(3):433-40.
46. Wakelkamp IM, Bakker O, Baldeschi L, et al. TSH-R expression and cytokine profile in orbital tissue of active vs. inactive Graves' ophthalmopathy patients. Clin Endocrinol (Oxf). 2003;58(3):280-7.
47. Douglas RS, Gianoukakis AG, Kamat S, et al Aberrant expression of the insulin-like growth factor-1 receptor by T cells from patients with Graves' disease may carry functional consequences for disease pathogenesis. J Immunol. 2007;178(5):3281-7.
48. Douglas RS, Naik V, Hwang CJ, et al. B cells from patients with Graves' disease aberrantly express the IGF-1 receptor: implications for disease pathogenesis. J Immunol. 2008;181(8):5768-74.
49. Weetman AP. Graves' disease. N Engl J Med. 2000;343(17):1236-48.
50. Ponto KA, Kanitz M, Olivo PD, et al. Clinical relevance of thyroid-stimulating immunoglobulins in Graves' ophthalmopathy. Ophthalmology. 2011;118(11):2279–85.
51. Gerding MN, van der Meer JW, Broenink M, et al. Association of thyrotrophin receptor antibodies with the clinical features of Graves' ophthalmopathy. Clin Endocrinol (Oxf). 2000;52(3):267-71.
52. Eckstein AK, Plicht M, Lax H, et al. Clinical results of anti-inflammatory therapy in Graves' ophthalmopathy and association with thyroidal autoantibodies. Clin Endocrinol (Oxf). 2004;61(5):612-8.
53. Eckstein AK, Plicht M, Lax H, et al. Thyrotropin receptor autoantibodies are independent risk factors for Graves' ophthalmopathy and help to predict severity and outcome of the disease. J Clin Endocrinol Metab. 2006;91(9):3464-70.
54. Lytton SD, Ponto KA, Kanitz M, et al. A novel thyroid stimulating immunoglobulin bioassay is a functional

indicator of activity and severity of Graves' orbitopathy. J Clin Endocrinol Metab. 2010;95(5):2123-31.
55. Moshkelgosha S, So P-W, Deasy N, et al. Cutting edge: retrobulbar inflammation, adipogenesis, and acute orbital congestion in a preclinical female mouse model of Graves' orbitopathy induced by thyrotropin receptor plasmid-in vivo electroporation. Endocrinology. 2013;154(9):3008-15.
56. Jyonouchi SC, Valyasevi RW, Harteneck DA, et al. Interleukin-6 stimulates thyrotropin receptor expression in human orbital preadipocyte fibroblasts from patients with Graves' ophthalmopathy. Thyroid. 2001;11(10):929-34.
57. Starkey KJ, Janezic A, Jones G, et al. Adipose thyrotrophin receptor expression is elevated in Graves' and thyroid eye diseases ex vivo and indicates adipogenesis in progress in vivo. J Mol Endocrinol. 2003;30(3):369-80.
58. Kumar S, Nadeem S, Stan MN, et al. A stimulatory TSH receptor antibody enhances adipogenesis via phosphoinositide 3-kinase activation in orbital preadipocytes from patients with Graves' ophthalmopathy. J Mol Endocrinol. 2011;46(3):155-63.
59. Tsui S, Naik V, Hoa N, et al. Evidence for an association between thyroid-stimulating hormone and insulin-like growth factor 1 receptors: a tale of two antigens implicated in Graves' disease. J Immunol. 2008;181(6):4397-405.
60. Smith TJ, Kahaly GJ, Ezra DG, et al. Teprotumumab for Thyroid-Associated Ophthalmopathy. N Engl J Med. 2017; 376(18):1748-61.
61. Goldberg RA, Rootman DB. Noninvasive, Minimally Invasive, and Surgical Pearls for Cosmetic Rejuvenation of the Thyroid Eye Disease Patient. In: Douglas RS, McCoy AN, Gupta S (Eds). Thyroid Eye Disease. New York: Springer; 2015. pp. 127-42.
62. McKeag D, Lane C, Lazarus JH, et al. Clinical features of dysthyroid optic neuropathy: a European Group on Graves' Orbitopathy (EUGOGO) survey. Br J Ophthalmol. 2007;91(4):455-8.
63. Trobe JD, Glaser JS, Laflamme P. Dysthyroid optic neuropathy. Clinical profile and rationale for management. Arch Ophthalmol. 1978;96(7):1199-209.
64. Day RM, Carroll FD. Optic nerve involvement associated with thyroid dysfunction. Trans Am Ophthalmol Soc. 1961;59:220-38.
65. Henderson JW. Optic neuropathy of exophthalmic goiter (Graves' disease). AMA Arch Ophthalmol. 1958;59(4):471-80.
66. Hedges TR, Scheie HG. Visual field defects in exophthalmos associated with thyroid disease. AMA Arch Ophthalmol. 1955;54(6):885-92.
67. Igersheimer J. Visual changes in progressive exophthalmos. AMA Arch Ophthalmol. 1955;53(1):94-104.
68. Verity DH, Rose GE. Acute thyroid eye disease (TED): principles of medical and surgical management. Eye Lond Engl. 2013;27(3):308-19.
69. Kuriyan AE, Woeller CF, O'Loughlin CW, et al. Orbital fibroblasts from thyroid eye disease patients differ in proliferative and adipogenic responses depending on disease subtype. Invest Ophthalmol Vis Sci. 2013;54(12):7370-7.
70. Jun B, Subramanian PS. Strabismus in Thyroid Eye Disease. In: Douglas RS, McCoy AN, Gupta S (Eds). Thyroid Eye Disease. New York: Springer; 2015. pp. 99-114.
71. Müller-Forell W, Kahaly GJ. Neuroimaging of Graves' orbitopathy. Best Pract Res Clin Endocrinol Metab. 2012;26(3):259-71.
72. Bartalena L, Baldeschi L, Dickinson A, et al. Consensus statement of the European Group on Graves' orbitopathy (EUGOGO) on management of GO. Eur J Endocrinol. 2008;158(3):273-85.
73. Bartley GB, Fatourechi V, Kadrmas EF, et al. Long-term follow-up of Graves' ophthalmopathy in an incidence cohort. Ophthalmology. 1996;103(6):958-62.
74. Perros P, Kendall-Taylor P. Natural History of Thyroid Eye Disease. Thyroid. 1998;8(5):423-5.
75. Neigel JM, Rootman J, Belkin RI, et al. Dysthyroid Optic Neuropathy. Ophthalmology. 1988;95(11):1515-21.
76. Werner SC. Modification of the classification of the eye changes of Graves' disease: recommendations of the Ad Hoc Committee of the American Thyroid Association. J Clin Endocrinol Metab. 1977;44(1):203-4.
77. Menconi F, Profilo MA, Leo M, et al. Spontaneous improvement of untreated mild Graves' ophthalmopathy: Rundle's curve revisited. Thyroid Off J Am Thyroid Assoc. 2014;24(1):60-6.
78. Mourits MP, Prummel MF, Wiersinga WM, et al. Clinical activity score as a guide in the management of patients with Graves' ophthalmopathy. Clin Endocrinol (Oxf). 1997;47(1):9-14.
79. Wiersinga WM. Management of Graves' ophthalmopathy. Nat Clin Pract Endocrinol Metab. 2007;3(5):396-404.
80. Bartalena L. Prevention of Graves' ophthalmopathy. Best Pract Res Clin Endocrinol Metab. 2012;26(3):371-9.
81. Prummel MF, Wiersinga WM. Smoking and risk of Graves' disease. JAMA. 1993;269(4):479-82.
82. Bartalena L, Marcocci C, Tanda ML, et al. Cigarette smoking and treatment outcomes in Graves ophthalmopathy. Ann Intern Med. 1998;129(8):632-5.
83. Eckstein A, Quadbeck B, Mueller G, et al. Impact of smoking on the response to treatment of thyroid associated ophthalmopathy. Br J Ophthalmol. 2003;87(6):773-6.
84. Kalmann R, Mourits MP. Diabetes mellitus: a risk factor in patients with Graves' orbitopathy. Br J Ophthalmol. 1999;83(4):463-5.
85. Prummel MF, Wiersinga WM, Mourits MP, et al. Effect of abnormal thyroid function on the severity of Graves' ophthalmopathy. Arch Intern Med. 1990;150(5):1098-101.
86. Rajaii F, Gupta S, Douglas RS. Management of Hyperthyroidism in the Setting of Thyroid Eye Disease. In: Douglas RS, McCoy AN, Gupta S (Eds).Thyroid Eye Disease. New York: Springer; 2015. pp. 33–7.
87. Hegedüs L, Bonnema SJ, Smith TJ, et al. Treating the thyroid in the presence of Graves' ophthalmopathy. Best Pract Res Clin Endocrinol Metab. 2012;26(3):313-24.
88. Bartalena L. The dilemma of how to manage Graves' hyperthyroidism in patients with associated orbitopathy. J Clin Endocrinol Metab. 2011;96(3):592-9.

89. Tallstedt L, Lundell G, Tørring O, et al. Occurrence of ophthalmopathy after treatment for Graves' hyperthyroidism. The Thyroid Study Group. N Engl J Med. 1992;326(26):1733-8.
90. Laurberg P, Wallin G, Tallstedt L, et al. TSH-receptor autoimmunity in Graves' disease after therapy with anti-thyroid drugs, surgery, or radioiodine: a 5-year prospective randomized study. Eur J Endocrinol. 2008;158(1):69-75.
91. Träisk F, Tallstedt L, Abraham-Nordling M, et al. Thyroid-associated ophthalmopathy after treatment for Graves' hyperthyroidism with antithyroid drugs or iodine-131. J Clin Endocrinol Metab. 2009;94(10):3700-7.
92. Lai A, Sassi L, Compri E, et al. Lower dose prednisone prevents radioiodine-associated exacerbation of initially mild or absent Graves' orbitopathy: a retrospective cohort study. J Clin Endocrinol Metab. 2010;95(3):1333-7.
93. Wiersinga WM. Quality of life in Graves' ophthalmopathy. Best Pract Res Clin Endocrinol Metab. 2012;26(3):359-70.
94. Marcocci C, Marinò M. Treatment of mild, moderate-to-severe and very severe Graves' orbitopathy. Best Pract Res Clin Endocrinol Metab. 2012;26(3):325-37.
95. Marcocci C, Kahaly GJ, Krassas GE, et al. Selenium and the course of mild Graves' orbitopathy. N Engl J Med. 2011;364(20):1920-31.
96. Laclaustra M, Navas-Acien A, Stranges S, et al. Serum Selenium Concentrations and Diabetes in US. Adults: National Health and Nutrition Examination Survey (NHANES) 2003–2004. Environ Health Perspect. 2009;117(9):1409-13.
97. Bartalena L, Pinchera A, Marcocci C. Management of Graves' ophthalmopathy: reality and perspectives. Endocr Rev. 2000;21(2):168-99.
98. Smith TJ. Dexamethasone regulation of glycosaminoglycan synthesis in cultured human skin fibroblasts. Similar effects of glucocorticoid and thyroid hormones. J Clin Invest. 1984;74(6):2157-63.
99. Zang S, Ponto KA, Kahaly GJ. Clinical review: Intravenous glucocorticoids for Graves' orbitopathy: efficacy and morbidity. J Clin Endocrinol Metab. 2011 ;96(2):320-32.
100. Bartalena L, Krassas GE, Wiersinga W, et al. Efficacy and safety of three different cumulative doses of intravenous methylprednisolone for moderate to severe and active Graves' orbitopathy. J Clin Endocrinol Metab. 2012;97(12):4454-63.
101. Macchia PE, Bagattini M, Lupoli G, et al. High-dose intravenous corticosteroid therapy for Graves' ophthalmopathy. J Endocrinol Invest. 2001;24(3):152-8.
102. Weissel M, Hauff W. Fatal liver failure after high-dose glucocorticoid pulse therapy in a patient with severe thyroid eye disease. Thyroid. 2000;10(6):521.
103. Marinó M, Morabito E, Brunetto MR, et al. Acute and severe liver damage associated with intravenous glucocorticoid pulse therapy in patients with Graves' ophthalmopathy. Thyroid Off J Am Thyroid Assoc. 2004;14(5):403-6.
104. Lendorf ME, Rasmussen AK, Fledelius HC, et al. Cardiovascular and cerebrovascular events in temporal relationship to intravenous glucocorticoid pulse therapy in patients with severe endocrine ophthalmopathy. Thyroid. 2009;19(12):1431-2.
105. Gursoy A, Cesur M, Erdogan MF, et al. New-onset acute heart failure after intravenous glucocorticoid pulse therapy in a patient with Graves' ophthalmopathy. Endocrine. 2006;29(3):513-6.
106. Salvi M, Vannucchi G, Sbrozzi F, et al. Onset of autoimmune hepatitis during intravenous steroid therapy for thyroid-associated ophthalmopathy in a patient with Hashimoto's thyroiditis: case report. Thyroid Off J Am Thyroid Assoc. 2004;14(8):631-4.
107. Bartalena L, Marcocci C, Chiovato L, et al. Orbital cobalt irradiation combined with systemic corticosteroids for Graves' ophthalmopathy: comparison with systemic corticosteroids alone. J Clin Endocrinol Metab. 1983;56(6):1139-44.
108. Marcocci C, Bartalena L, Bogazzi F, et al. Orbital radiotherapy combined with high dose systemic glucocorticoids for Graves' ophthalmopathy is more effective than radiotherapy alone: results of a prospective randomized study. J Endocrinol Invest. 1991;14(10):853-60.
109. Dolman PJ, Rath S. Orbital radiotherapy for thyroid eye disease. Curr Opin Ophthalmol. 2012;23(5):427-32.
110. Tanda ML, Bartalena L. Efficacy and safety of orbital radiotherapy for graves' orbitopathy. J Clin Endocrinol Metab. 2012;97(11):3857-65.
111. Trokel S, Kazim M, Moore S. Orbital Fat Removal. Decompression for Graves' orbitopathy. Ophthalmology. 1993;100(5):674-82.
112. Matthiesen C, Thompson JS, Thompson D, et al. The efficacy of radiation therapy in the treatment of Graves' orbitopathy. Int J Radiat Oncol Biol Phys. 2012;82(1):117-23.
113. Shams PN, Ma R, Pickles T, et al. Reduced risk of compressive optic neuropathy using orbital radiotherapy in patients with active thyroid eye disease. Am J Ophthalmol. 2014;157(6):1299-305.
114. Prummel MF, Mourits MP, Blank L, et al. Randomized double-blind trial of prednisone versus radiotherapy in Graves' ophthalmopathy. Lancet Lond Engl. 1993;342(8877):949-54.
115. Chundury RV, Weber AC, Perry JD. Orbital Radiation Therapy in Thyroid Eye Disease. Ophthal Plast Reconstr Surg. 2016;32(2):83-9.
116. Marcocci C, Bartalena L, Rocchi R, et al. Long-Term Safety of Orbital Radiotherapy for Graves' Ophthalmopathy. J Clin Endocrinol Metab. 2003;88(8):3561-6.
117. Wakelkamp IM, Tan H, Saeed P, et al. Orbital irradiation for Graves' ophthalmopathy: Is it safe? A long-term follow-up study. Ophthalmology. 2004;111(8):1557-62.
118. Kahaly GJ, Rösler H-P, Pitz S, et al. Low-Versus High-Dose Radiotherapy for Graves' Ophthalmopathy: A Randomized, Single Blind Trial. J Clin Endocrinol Metab. 2000;85(1):102-8.
119. Snijders-Keilholz A, De Keizer RJW, Goslings BM, et al. Probable risk of tumour induction after retro-orbital irradiation for Graves' ophthalmopathy. Radiother Oncol. 1996;38(1):69-71.

120. Stan MN, Garrity JA, Carranza Leon BG, et al. Randomized controlled trial of rituximab in patients with Graves' orbitopathy. J Clin Endocrinol Metab. 2015;100(2):432-41.
121. Leandro MJ, Cambridge G, Ehrenstein MR, et al. Reconstitution of peripheral blood B cells after depletion with rituximab in patients with rheumatoid arthritis. Arthritis Rheum. 2006;54(2):613-20.
122. Salvi M, Vannucchi G, Campi I, et al. Treatment of Graves' disease and associated ophthalmopathy with the anti-CD20 monoclonal antibody rituximab: an open study. Eur J Endocrinol. 2007;156(1):33-40.
123. Salvi M, Vannucchi G, Campi I, et al. Rituximab treatment in a patient with severe thyroid-associated ophthalmopathy: effects on orbital lymphocytic infiltrates. Clin Immunol Orlando Fla. 2009;131(2):360-5.
124. Salvi M, Vannucchi G, Currò N, et al. Small dose of rituximab for Graves' orbitopathy: new insights into the mechanism of action. Arch Ophthalmol. 2012;130(1):122-4.
125. Salvi M, Vannucchi G, Campi I, et al. Efficacy of rituximab treatment for thyroid-associated ophthalmopathy as a result of intraorbital B-cell depletion in one patient unresponsive to steroid immunosuppression. Eur J Endocrinol. 2006;154(4):511-7.
126. Fassi DE, Nielsen CH, Hasselbalch HC, et al. Treatment-resistant severe, active Graves' ophthalmopathy successfully treated with B lymphocyte depletion. Thyroid. 2006;16(7):709-10.
127. Khanna D, Chong KKL, Afifiyan NF, et al. Rituximab treatment of patients with severe, corticosteroid-resistant thyroid-associated ophthalmopathy. Ophthalmology. 2010;117(1):133-9.
128. Krassas GE, Stafilidou A, Boboridis KG. Failure of rituximab treatment in a case of severe thyroid ophthalmopathy unresponsive to steroids. Clin Endocrinol (Oxf). 2010;72(6):853-5.
129. Silkiss RZ, Reier A, Coleman M, et al. Rituximab for thyroid eye disease. Ophthal Plast Reconstr Surg. 2010;26(5):310-4.
130. Madaschi S, Rossini A, Formenti I, et al. Treatment of thyroid-associated orbitopathy with rituximab: a novel therapy for an old disease: case report and literature review. Endocr Pract. 2010;16(4):677-85.
131. Salvi M, Vannucchi G, Beck-Peccoz P. Potential Utility of Rituximab for Graves' Orbitopathy. J Clin Endocrinol Metab. 2013;98(11):4291-9.
132. Eckstein A, Schittkowski M, Esser J. Surgical treatment of Graves' ophthalmopathy. Best Pract Res Clin Endocrinol Metab. 2012;26(3):339-58.
133. Otto AJ, Koornneef L, Mourits MP, et al. Retrobulbar pressures measured during surgical decompression of the orbit. Br J Ophthalmol. 1996;80(12):1042-5.
134. Goldberg RA. The Evolving Paradigm of Orbital Decompression Surgery. Arch Ophthalmol. 1998;116(1):95-6.
135. Liao SL, Chang TC, Lin LL-K. Transcaruncular orbital decompression: an alternate procedure for Graves' ophthalmopathy with compressive optic neuropathy. Am J Ophthalmol. 2006;141(5):810-8.
136. McCann JD, Goldberg RA, Anderson RL. Medial Wall Decompression For Optic Neuropathy But Lateral Wall Decompression With Fat Removal For Non Vision-Threatening Indications. Am J Ophthalmol. 2006;141(5):916-7.
137. Metson R, Pletcher SD. Endoscopic Orbital and Optic Nerve Decompression. Otolaryngol Clin North Am. 2006;39(3):551-61.
138. Siracuse-Lee DE, Kazim M. Orbital decompression: current concepts. Curr Opin Ophthalmol. 2002;13(5):310-6.
139. Rootman DB. Orbital decompression for thyroid eye disease. Surv Ophthalmol. 2018;63(1):86-104.
140. Gupta S, McCoy AN, Douglas RS. Customized Minimally Invasive Orbital Decompression for Thyroid Eye Disease. In: Douglas RS, McCoy AN, Gupta S (Eds). Thyroid Eye Disease. New York: Springer; 2015. pp. 115-26.
141. Olivari N. Transpalpebral decompression of endocrine ophthalmopathy (Graves' disease) by removal of intraorbital fat: experience with 147 operations over 5 years. Plast Reconstr Surg. 1991;87(4):627-41;
142. Goldberg RA, Perry JD, Hortaleza V, et al. Strabismus after balanced medial plus lateral wall versus lateral wall only orbital decompression for dysthyroid orbitopathy. Ophthal Plast Reconstr Surg. 2000;16(4):271-7.
143. Garrity JA, Fatourechi V, Bergstralh EJ, et al. Results of transantral orbital decompression in 428 patients with severe Graves' ophthalmopathy. Am J Ophthalmol. 1993;116(5):533-47.
144. Ben Simon GJ, Wang L, McCann JD, et al. Primary-gaze diplopia in patients with thyroid-related orbitopathy undergoing deep lateral orbital decompression with intraconal fat debulking: a retrospective analysis of treatment outcome. Thyroid. 2004;14(5):379-83.
145. Goldberg RA, Weinberg DA, Shorr N, et al. Maximal, three-wall, orbital decompression through a coronal approach. Ophthalmic Surg Lasers. 1997;28(10):832-43.
146. Graham SM, Brown CL, Carter KD, et al. Medial and lateral orbital wall surgery for balanced decompression in thyroid eye disease. Laryngoscope. 2003;113(7):1206-9.
147. Cansiz H, Yilmaz S, Karaman E, et al. Three-wall orbital decompression superiority to 2-wall orbital decompression in thyroid-associated ophthalmopathy. J Oral Maxillofac Surg. 2006;64(5):763-9.
148. Boulos PR, Hardy I. Thyroid-associated orbitopathy: a clinicopathologic and therapeutic review. Curr Opin Ophthalmol. 2004;15(5):389-400.
149. Trokel SL, Cooper WC. Symposium: extraocular muscle problems associated with Graves' disease. Orbital decompression: effect on motility and globe position. Ophthalmology. 1979;86(12):2064-70.
150. Abràmoff MD, Kalmann R, de Graaf MEL, et al. Rectus extraocular muscle paths and decompression surgery for Graves orbitopathy: mechanism of motility disturbances. Invest Ophthalmol Vis Sci. 2002;43(2):300-7.
151. Inoue Y, Tsuboi T, Kouzaki A, et al. Ophthalmic surgery in dysthyroid ophthalmopathy. Thyroid. 2002;12(3):257-63.

152. Millar MJ, Maloof AJ. The application of stereotactic navigation surgery to orbital decompression for thyroid-associated orbitopathy. Eye (Lond). 2009;23(7):1565-71.
153. Kikkawa DO, Cruz RC, Christian WK, et al. Botulinum A toxin injection for restrictive myopathy of thyroid-related orbitopathy: effects on intraocular pressure. Am J Ophthalmol. 2003;135(4):427-31.
154. Uddin JM, Davies PD. Treatment of upper eyelid retraction associated with thyroid eye disease with subconjunctival botulinum toxin injection. Ophthalmology. 2002;109(6):1183-7.
155. Chee E, Chee SP. Subconjunctival injection of triamcinolone in the treatment of lid retraction of patients with thyroid eye disease: a case series. Eye (Lond). 2008;22(2):311-5.
156. Xu D, Liu Y, Xu H, et al. Repeated triamcinolone acetonide injection in the treatment of upper-lid retraction in patients with thyroid-associated ophthalmopathy. Can J Ophthalmol. 2012;47(1):34-41.
157. Lee SJ, Rim THT, Jang SY, et al. Treatment of upper eyelid retraction related to thyroid-associated ophthalmopathy using subconjunctival triamcinolone injections. Graefes Arch Clin Exp Ophthalmol. 2013;251(1):261-70.
158. Lee JM, Lee H, Park M, et al. Subconjunctival injection of triamcinolone for the treatment of upper lid retraction associated with thyroid eye disease. J Craniofac Surg. 2012;23(6):1755-8.
159. Goldberg RA. Orbital steroid injections. Br J Ophthalmol. 2004;88(11):1359-60.
160. Shih MJ, Liao SL, Kuo KT, et al. Molecular pathology of Muller's muscle in Graves' ophthalmopathy. J Clin Endocrinol Metab. 2006;91(3):1159-67.
161. Cohen MS, Shorr N. Eyelid reconstruction with hard palate mucosa grafts. Ophthal Plast Reconstr Surg. 1992;8(3):183-95.
162. Doxanas MT, Dryden RM. The use of sclera in the treatment of dysthyroid eyelid retraction. Ophthalmology. 1981;88(9):887-94.
163. Feldman KA, Putterman AM, Farber MD. Surgical treatment of thyroid-related lower eyelid retraction: a modified approach. Ophthal Plast Reconstr Surg. 1992;8(4):278-86.
164. McCord CD. Current trends in orbital decompression. Ophthalmology. 1985;92(1):21-33.
165. Mourits MP, Koornneef L. Lid lengthening by sclera interposition for eyelid retraction in Graves' ophthalmopathy. Br J Ophthalmol. 1991;75(6):344-7.
166. Oestreicher JH, Pang NK, Liao W. Treatment of lower eyelid retraction by retractor release and posterior lamellar grafting: an analysis of 659 eyelids in 400 patients. Ophthal Plast Reconstr Surg. 2008;24(3):207-12.
167. Olver JM, Rose GE, Khaw PT, et al. Correction of lower eyelid retraction in thyroid eye disease: a randomised controlled trial of retractor tenotomy with adjuvant anti metabolite versus scleral graft. Br J Ophthalmol. 1998;82(2): 174-80.
168. Tan J, Olver J, Wright M, et al. The use of porous polyethylene (Medpor) lower eyelid spacers in lid heightening and stabilisation. Br J Ophthalmol. 2004;88(9):1197-200.
169. Waller RR. Lower eyelid retraction: management. Ophthalmic Surg. 1978;9(3):41-7.
170. Yoo DB, Griffin GR, Azizzadeh B, et al. The minimally invasive, orbicularis-sparing, lower eyelid recession for mild-to-moderate lower eyelid retraction with reduced orbicularis strength. JAMA Facial Plast Surg. 2014;16(2):140-6.
171. Baldeschi L. Correction of lid retraction and exophthalmos. Dev Ophthalmol. 2008;41:103-26.
172. Grisolia ABD, Couso RC, Matayoshi S, et al. Non-surgical treatment for eyelid retraction in thyroid eye disease (TED). Br J Ophthalmol. 2017:II
173. Goldberg RA, Lee S, Jayasundera T, et al. Treatment of lower eyelid retraction by expansion of the lower eyelid with hyaluronic Acid gel. Ophthal Plast Reconstr Surg. 2007;23(5):343-8.

Chapter 110 Orbitofacial Trauma

Marie Somogyi, Ivan Vrcek, Vikram Durairaj

INTRODUCTION AND BACKGROUND

Orbitofacial traumas, including blunt and penetrating trauma to the eyelids and orbit, are common presentations to emergency departments and outpatient ophthalmology clinics.[1] Following a thorough assessment of the patient's vital signs and overall medical stability, a comprehensive examination, including a complete ophthalmic examination, is required. Orbital fractures, orbital hemorrhage, and intraorbital foreign bodies (IOrbFB) are all common sequelae of facial trauma. It is estimated that 10% of all facial fractures are isolated orbital wall fractures, the majority of which are the orbital floor. Furthermore, approximately 30–40% of all facial fractures involve the orbit.[2-4] Treatment of these injuries requires careful identification of the anatomical structures involved, and recognizing the need and timing for appropriate intervention. In this chapter, we will discuss these injuries in detail with an emphasis on the diagnosis, treatment, and postoperative care of these often challenging patients.

PREOPERATIVE EVALUATION AND DIAGNOSTIC APPROACH

Systemic Stabilization

The evaluation and treatment of any orbitofacial trauma begins after a complete and thorough examination to assure that life-threatening injuries have been adequately assessed and managed before the orbital region is addressed.

History

Once the patient has been cleared of life-threatening injuries, it is important to obtain a thorough history from the patient. This should include the time and mechanism of the injury. Most commonly, the patient will report a traumatic event; however, in both children and the elderly, consideration must be given to nonaccidental trauma potentially related to abuse. A history consistent with injuries from high-speed projectile particles typically requires the appropriate imaging studies to determine the presence of intraocular or IOrbFB. A complete medical and surgical history also should be gathered to effectively plan perioperative care.

Examination

Once the patient is medically stable, a complete ophthalmic examination is necessary in all facial trauma patients. It has been shown that 11–15% of orbital fractures are associated with ophthalmic injuries, including the development of an orbital compartment syndrome due to acute hemorrhage or soft tissue swelling.[5] We recommend a methodical approach to the orbital and ophthalmic examination. In the case of trauma, it is necessary to first evaluate the integrity of the globe; as all life and vision-threatening injuries should take precedent. Visual acuity should be recorded, which is often best done with a near card at the bedside in trauma patients. The pupillary examination should include the size, shape, and reactivity of the pupils, as well as the presence of a relative afferent pupillary defect, which may suggest a traumatic optic neuropathy.

A slit-lamp examination should be performed to thoroughly evaluate the anterior segment, including the conjunctiva, sclera, and cornea. Fluorescein staining is a useful tool, both for the detection of abrasions as well as evaluating for Seidel positivity, which may be indicative of a globe rupture. The depth of the anterior chamber and the presence of cell, flare, or red blood cells should be noted. Once the globe is cleared of injury, the intraocular pressure should also be carefully measured. If no contraindication exists, such as an abnormal pupillary examination or elevated intraocular pressure, a dilated funduscopic examination should be performed.

After the integrity of the globe is confirmed, attention is turned to the periorbital and ocular adnexal examination. Beginning with the skin envelope, attention is directed to the presence, location, and depth of any lacerations to the skin and subcutaneous tissues. Particular emphasis is placed on a thorough examination of the eyelid margin as well as the medial and lateral canthal regions, as lacerations in these areas can be difficult to immediately identify. Injuries to the skin and soft tissue must be carefully documented and their dimensions recorded. Eyelid and canalicular lacerations are covered in more detail in other chapters.

Many patients with orbital fractures will demonstrate ecchymosis and edema of the periorbital tissue. If the patient recounts a history of a high-velocity projectile injury, the clinician should maintain a high level of suspicion for orbital foreign bodies. Furthermore, subcutaneous emphysema may be present as a result of a new connection with the aerated sinuses.

Following a careful examination of the skin and adnexa, the bony anatomy is next assessed clinically. A detailed knowledge of the bony orbital anatomy is critical to understanding the natural history of orbital trauma, and is presented in depth later in this chapter. The integrity of the bony orbit can be carefully assessed by palpating the superior, lateral, and inferior orbital rims. The nasal sidewall should also be assessed for step-offs and deformities. A low threshold for obtaining radiographic studies should be maintained as bony orbital trauma may not be immediately obvious; as is the case of orbital "blow-out" fractures where the inferior orbital rim remains intact, but the more posterior orbital floor has fractured downward into the maxillary sinus. Orbital floor fractures can occur in isolation or in association with other orbital or facial fractures, which may include the zygomatic bone as part of a zygomaticomaxillary complex (ZMC) fracture, nasal, and ethmoidal fractures as seen in naso-orbital-ethmoidal (NOE) fractures, mandibular fracture, or Le Fort fractures, all of which involve the pterygoid plates.

The globe position should also be carefully evaluated. In the setting of orbitofacial trauma and significant soft tissue swelling and/or lateral orbital rim fracture, the use of a Hertel exophthalmometer may be unreliable. Alternatively, the patient can be viewed from either a worm's eye view, where the clinician evaluates the globe position from the angle of the patient's chin, or the bird's eye view, where the clinician views from the patient's forehead looking down. Hyper- and hypoglobus, as well as other globe dystopias, should be noted at the initial consultation.

Lastly, the cranial nerves must be carefully examined with particular attention to the frontal and zygomatic branches of the facial nerve. It is important to assess sensation in the territories of the first (V1) and second divisions (V2) of cranial nerve V as these are often compromised in orbital fractures. Cranial nerves III, IV, and VI may be evaluated through extraocular motility.

Imaging in Orbitofacial Trauma

In patients with orbitofacial trauma, there is a low threshold to obtain imaging as bony trauma, as well as orbital and intraocular foreign bodies can often go undetected.[6] Computed tomography (CT) is the preferred imaging modality in the setting of trauma over magnetic resonance imaging (MRI) for many reasons. CT provides faster acquisition times, superior imaging of the bony structures, improved cost-effectiveness, and readily aides in the identification of orbital and intraocular foreign bodies. MRI maintains superiority in its imaging of the soft tissues and orbital apex; however, these are often less relevant in an acute trauma situation. Furthermore, MRI is contraindicated in the case of a retained metallic foreign body.

More specifically, a facial CT scan should be ordered with thin cuts, which provides approximately 1.5 mm slices. It is also necessary to obtain multiple views, including axial, coronal, and sagittal views. Orbital floor fractures are best evaluated on coronal and sagittal views, whereas a ZMC fracture benefits especially from the coronal and axial views. In the case of an orbital floor fracture, coronal views provide the best assessment of the medial wall and lateral floor involvement of the fracture (Fig. 110.1), whereas the sagittal views demonstrate the anterior and posterior aspects of the floor fracture. Furthermore, the sagittal views also provide a view of the posterior ledge of the fracture

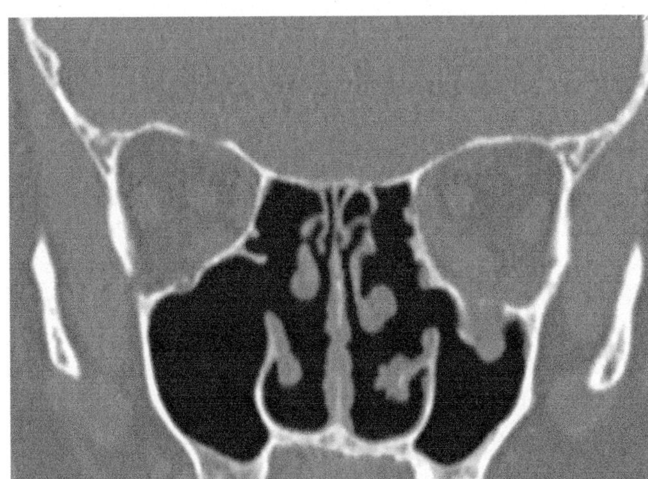

Fig. 110.1: CT orbit (bone window, coronal view). Left orbital floor fracture involving the infraorbital canal with herniation of soft tissue into the maxillary sinus.

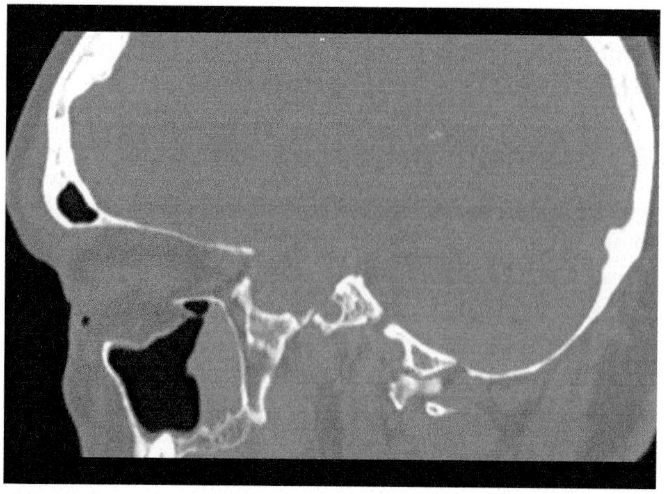

Fig. 110.2: CT orbit (bone window, sagittal view). Left orbital floor fracture with herniation of orbital contents into the maxillary sinus. Posterior ledge evident.

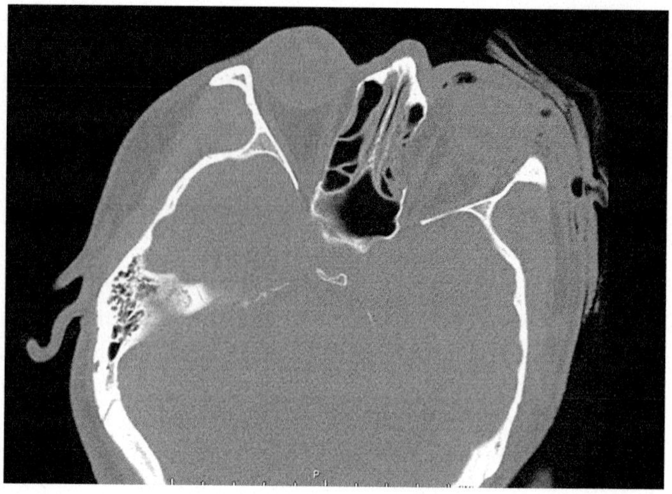

Fig. 110.3: CT orbit (bone window, axial view). Left medial wall fracture with soft tissue herniation into the ethmoid sinus without muscle entrapment.

that may be used for stabilization of the orbital implant (Fig. 110.2). In contrast, medial wall fractures are more readily apparent and visualized in the axial views (Fig. 110.3).

ORBITAL FLOOR FRACTURES

Orbital floor fractures are common sequelae of orbitofacial trauma, and may be managed by a variety of surgical subspecialists, including oculofacial plastic surgeons, oral and maxillofacial surgeons (OMFS), otolaryngologist, and plastic surgeons. The management of orbital floor fractures may depend on the surgeon's training background, clinical experience, and finally, on published literature.

As stated previously, a thorough knowledge of the anatomy of the orbital floor is paramount to understanding the mechanisms, evaluation, and surgical management of orbital floor fractures. The medial orbital floor averages 0.37 mm thick and is thinnest over the infraorbital canal, whereas the lateral orbital floor typically 1.25 mm in thickness.[7] Blunt injury to the periorbital region increases intraorbital pressure and may result in a fracture at the thinnest portion of the floor. The blunt force may also be directly transmitted to the weakest point of orbital bone, which is typically along the infraorbital canal. Isolated inferior orbital wall fractures occur typically over the very thin area of the infraorbital canal.[7] The bone medial and/or lateral to the canal may also fracture and become displaced downward into the maxillary sinus, resulting in the classic "blow-out" fracture. Orbital soft tissue may herniate downward into the sinus and musculofibrous tissue such as the inferior rectus and associated pulley structures, may become tethered to bone fragments (entrapped), resulting in diplopia, and the potential for the oculocardiac reflex.

The hydraulic and the buckling theories are the two commonly accepted theories regarding the mechanism of orbital blow-out fractures.[7] The hydraulic theory proposes that the elevation in intraorbital pressure transmits force to the orbital walls creating a fracture at the weakest point.[8] In contrast, the buckling theory hypothesizes that direct trauma to the thick infraorbital rim transmits the force posteriorly and creates a compression fracture at the floor's weakest point.[9] The energy required to fracture the orbital floor in the hydraulic theory is 71 mJ, whereas the predicted theoretical energy for the buckling theory is 68 mJ.[7] Recent cadaveric studies suggest that both theories are valid and each mechanism may be occurring to different degrees depending on the mechanism and location of the injury.

Once an orbital floor fracture has been diagnosed following a thorough clinical evaluation and review of CT imaging, the management is primarily guided by the surgeon's individual clinical training and experience.[10] In 2003, Burnstine[11] provided clinical recommendations that have helped to establish a standard of care when determining the timing for surgical repair (Table 110.1).

In most circumstances, orbital fractures can be medically managed for the first 5–7 days to allow for improvement in edema. Most patients benefit from a short course of oral steroids and nasal decongestants, if there are no contraindications. All patients should be provided with instructions to apply ice packs to the affected orbit for the first 2–3 days, sleep with the head of the bed elevated, and

Table 110.1: Clinical recommendations to establish a standard of care for surgical repair.

Intervention	Clinical presentation
Immediate	• Diplopia with CT and clinical evidence of entrapped muscle are associated with oculocardiac reflex (i.e. bradycardia, heart block, nausea, vomiting, and syncope) • "White eyed blow-out" fracture. Young patient with significant limitation in upgaze, "white eye", and CT imaging with orbital floor fracture with entrapment of orbital tissue • Early enophthalmos or hypoglobus is causing distinct facial asymmetry
Within 2 weeks	• Persistent diplopia with limitation in extraocular motility and no improvement overtime • Large floor fracture (>50%) • Early enophthalmos (>2 mm) • Significant hypoglobus • Progressive infraorbital hypesthesia
Observation	• No diplopia in primary or downgaze • Good ocular motility • No significant enophthalmos or hypoglobus

Source: Burnstine MA. Clinical recommendations for repair of orbital facial fractures. Curr Opin Ophthalmol. 2003;14(5):236-40.

avoid nose blowing, as this can lead to orbital emphysema with potential for serious sequelae.[12]

The optimal timing for surgical intervention in nonemergent orbital fractures is approximately 7–14 days following the injury to allow for improvement in edema. The generally accepted indications for nonimmediate surgical repair include patients with unresolved diplopia in primary and downgaze, early enophthalmos (>2 mm), large fracture size (>50% of the orbital floor on CT scan), and significant hypoglobus.[11] Infraorbital nerve hypesthesia alone is not typically an independent indication for surgical intervention; however, progression of hypesthesia or failure to resolve may prompt intervention.[13] Patients that present with intact ocular motility, a small fracture size, and absence of diplopia can often be observed without surgical intervention.

Special Considerations—Pediatric Orbital Floor Fractures

Pediatric orbital floor fractures represent a distinct subclass of orbital trauma. "Trapdoor" fractures are more common in younger patients and may present in a distinct clinical and radiographic fashion. Specifically, children may present with an orbital floor fracture with minimal signs of external trauma. However, they may demonstrate significant restriction of extraocular motility in upgaze, and occasionally in downgaze, associated with diplopia. Furthermore, movement of the eye may illicit nausea, vomiting, and bradycardia consistent with the oculocardiac reflex. As a result, these fractures in children have been termed "white-eyed blow-out" fractures. Immediate repair of orbital fractures is indicated primarily in children with "white-eyed blow-out" fractures to avoid extraocular muscle ischemia from entrapment and prevent permanent motility deficits.[14]

Surgical Approaches

There are a variety of surgical approaches to the orbital floor described in the literature, including subciliary transcutaneous, subtarsal transcutaneous, transantral, and transconjunctival technique. Our preferred approach to the orbital floor is the transconjunctival approach due to its ability to provide excellent exposure and access to the orbit, low rate of complications, ease of dissection, and superior aesthetic outcome in comparison to a transcutaneous incision.[15]

After local anesthetic infiltration of the lower eyelid palpebral conjunctiva, an incision is made across the length of the conjunctiva approximately 3 mm inferior to the inferior border of the tarsus. The dissection is then carried out in a bloodless, preseptal plane to the inferior orbital rim. The monopolar cautery is then used to score the periosteum and a subperiosteal dissection can be initiated using an elevator. The subperiosteal dissection proceeds along the orbital floor towards the fracture using a hand-over-hand dissection technique to retract orbital soft tissues with a malleable retractor. The dissection should continue along areas of stable bone to expose the defect 360 degree around the fracture site. It is imperative to identify the posterior ledge of the fracture site since this may serve as the location for posterior fixation of the orbital implant. In some cases, a posterior ledge is either involved in the fracture, is unstable, or is too small to support an implant. In these cases, the orbital implant can be fixated to the anterior orbital rim with screws.

Orbital Implant Choices

There are several implant materials available for reconstructing the orbital floor. Broadly, these fall into two categories being autologous and alloplastic materials. As the options for alloplastic implants have improved, autologous materials, such as iliac, mandibular, maxillary, and calvarial bone grafts, have fallen out of favor. Similarly, there are many options available for alloplastic materials including silicone, polytetrafluorethylene, nylon, porous polyethylene, titanium, hyaluronic acid gel sheets, and hydroxyapatite. The individual advantages and disadvantages to each are outside the scope of this chapter; however, in general, alloplastic materials are readily available, cost-effective, and easily conform to the contour of the orbital floor. Our preference in most cases is to use a porous polyethylene implant (with or without titanium) that is either 0.85 mm or 1.0 mm thick. We have found these to be well tolerated and an excellent substitute for reforming the orbital floor and prefer this over autologous materials due to the ease of use, low complication rate, avoidance of donor site morbidity, and overall surgical predictability.

Postoperative Management

Orbital fracture repair is typically outpatient surgery that can be performed safely in either a hospital setting or surgery center. Although the use and timing of systemic steroids and antibiotics varies, a recent survey of American Society of Ophthalmic Plastic and Reconstructive Surgery (ASOPRS) members helped to clarify common practices—95% reported using intraoperative steroids and, similarly, 75% elected to use intraoperative antibiotics, and 69% used postoperative antibiotics.[16] Similarly, nearly all surgeons checked visual acuity and any signs of orbital compartment syndrome in the recovery room. Most surgeons avoid patching the eye after surgery to allow for prompt recognition of increased proptosis or decreased vision suggestive of an orbital compartment syndrome.[16]

The patient is typically discharged from surgery with antibiotic ointment for the eye, anti-inflammatory medication (i.e. Solu-Medrol dose pack), pain medication, and antinausea medication. It is recommended that the patient ice the eye for 20 minutes out of every hour for the first 2–3 days, avoid nose blowing, and limit activity that may raise the blood pressure or heart rate to avoid a risk of bleeding. Furthermore, the patient should always be provided a contact number to reach a doctor if he/she experiences an increase in pain, bleeding, swelling, or decrease in vision. The patient should be instructed to call immediately with any of these signs or symptoms. The patient would typically be scheduled to follow-up in the office 3–7 days following surgery.

MEDIAL WALL FRACTURES

Medial orbital wall fractures can occur in isolation, or more commonly, they may occur in the presence of other fracture patterns, including an extension of an orbital floor fracture, NOE fracture, or Le Fort fractures.[17] Blow-out fractures of the medial wall were first recognized clinically in the 1960s,[18] but have become increasingly identified with advances in imaging techniques.

A thorough understanding of the anatomy of the medial wall aides in comprehending the mechanism of fracture, as well as the surgical repair. The medial wall is composed of the frontal process of the maxilla, lacrimal bone, ethmoidal bone, and the lesser wing of the sphenoid through with the optic nerve traverses the optic canal. The majority of the medial wall is comprised of the lamina papyracea, which is only 0.2–0.4 mm in thickness.[19] Similar to the orbital floor, there are two theories to explain the mechanism of medial wall fractures. Medial wall fractures are primarily explained by the hydraulic pressure theory,[20,21] in which increased orbital pressure transmits to the weak and thin medial orbital wall, and is less commonly explained by the buckling theory.[22]

As mentioned previously, CT imaging is preferred with special attention to the coronal and axial views in which the structure of the medial wall can be most directly examined (Fig. 110.3). The surgeon must main a high level of suspicion of a medial wall fracture in the presence of orbitofacial trauma since the immediate symptoms associated with a medial wall fracture are not as serious as those of an orbital floor fracture. Entrapment of the medial rectus is less common than the inferior rectus, and also varies in its clinical manifestation with muscle paresis rather than restrictive limitation. Motility dysfunction associated with the medial rectus entrapment also has delayed onset from the trauma, which has been hypothesized to be secondary to muscle ischemia.[23]

Indications for surgical repair of a medial wall fracture as not as well defined as orbital floor fractures; however, the clinical guidelines outlined by Burnstine et al.[11] (Table 110.1) can be extrapolated to medial wall fractures as well. Specifically, immediate surgical repair should be considered in a patient with nonresolving oculocardiac reflex or marked extraocular restriction secondary to an entrapped muscle. Beyond that, surgical repair should ideally be undertaken within the first 2 weeks for patients with symptomatic diplopia, motility restriction, or a large fracture with enophthalmos.

Surgical Approaches

There are multiple surgical approaches available to access the medial orbital wall, including the transcaruncular, transcutaneous, or transnasal endoscopic approach. Our preferred approach is transcaruncular as it affords direct, reliable access to the medial wall without a cutaneous scar.[24] Furthermore, this approach can be combined with a transconjunctival approach for wide access to the orbit for repair of combined medial and orbital floor fractures.

The transcaruncular approach is initiated with a vertical incision through the lateral portion of the caruncle using Stevens tenotomy scissors. The incision should extend superiorly and inferiorly for a total of 8–10 mm, with care taken to preserve the canalicular system. The dissection is then taken down to the posterior lacrimal crest, with the plane of dissection passing between the medial orbital septum and the Horner muscle.[25] The periosteum along the posterior lacrimal crest can be incised using the monopolar cautery and a subperiosteal dissection initiated using an elevator. The subperiosteal dissection should proceed on stable bone 360 degree around the fracture site and can be accomplished with thin ribbon retractors. An implant can then be placed over the fracture site, taking care not to incarcerate any orbital tissues. The caruncle should be closed with a buried, absorbable suture of choice.

Orbital Implant Choices

Similar to the orbital floor, there are various implant options available to use for the medial wall including both autologous and alloplastic materials. Our preferred implant for most medial wall fractures is porous polyethylene, but unlike an orbital floor fracture, the thickness of the implant is typically only 0.4 mm, as there is less gravitational strain on a medial wall implant than a floor implant. Thinner material can be used that more closely simulates the thickness of the fractured medial orbital wall (i.e. lamina papyracea).

Postoperative Management

See "Orbital Floor Fractures" section of this chapter.

ORBITAL ROOF FRACTURES

Orbital roof fractures are relatively uncommon orbital fractures accounting for only 1–9% of all facial fractures, but up to 30% of orbital fractures in the pediatric population.[26,27] They are typically the result of high-energy blunt trauma, such as a motor vehicle accident, falls, or assault; however, in young children they can result from relatively low-energy blunt trauma.[28] Unlike adults, the frontal sinus does not pneumatize until approximately the age of 7, leaving nothing to absorb the energy as it extends along the roof.[26,27] Along with absent pneumatization of the frontal sinus, newborns, and infants also have an increased cranium to face ratio and a relatively prominent brow that make the pediatric population more susceptible to orbital roof fractures in comparison to the rare occurrence in the adult population.[27,29,30]

Isolated orbital roof fractures in an adult are uncommon and may be associated with potentially serious concomitant craniofacial injuries, including the frontal sinus, NOE, and Le Fort fractures, as well as intracranial injury, most commonly presenting with cerebrospinal fluid (CSF) rhinorrhea.[28,31] These often involve the management with many specialists, including neurosurgery, otolaryngologists, oral maxillofacial surgeons, and ophthalmologists.[32] Life-threatening injuries should always be addressed first, followed by any vision-threatening injuries and stabilization of facial fractures.

Computed tomography imaging should be utilized in the diagnosis of orbital roof fractures, particularly the coronal and sagittal views provide the best visualization for fracture involvement (Figs. 110.4 and 110.5). Orbital roof fractures can be generally classified into three different fracture patterns, including nondisplaced fractures, isolated "blow-in" fractures, and isolated "blow-up" (or blow-out) fractures. An isolated "blow-in" fracture is characterized by the inferior displacement of the orbital roof without involvement of the superior orbital rim, which may result from a sudden increase in intracranial

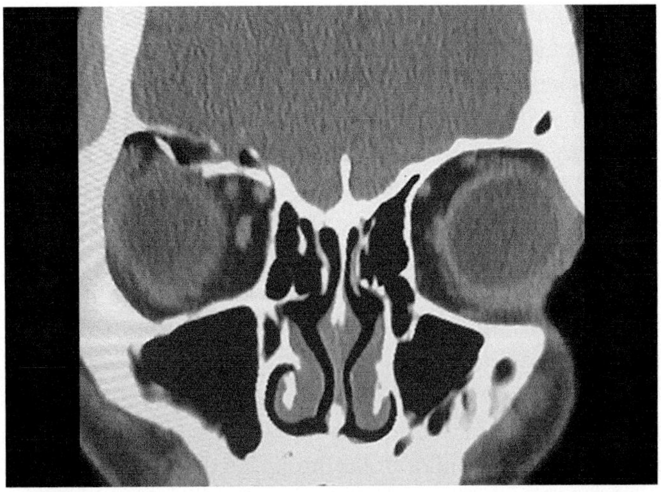

Fig. 110.4: CT orbit (soft tissue window, coronal view). Right displaced, blow-in orbital roof fracture.

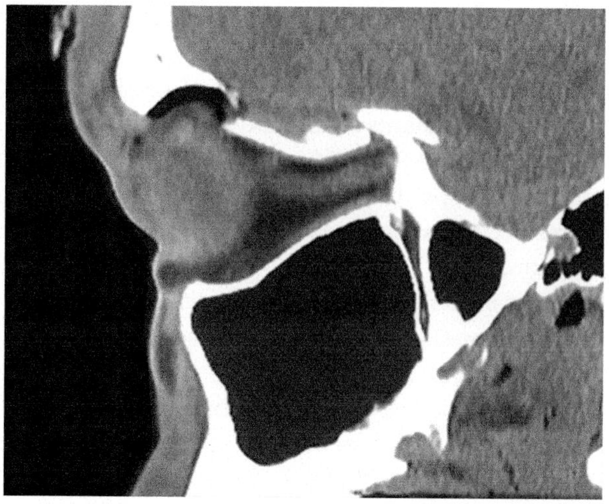

Fig. 110.5: CT orbit (soft tissue window, sagittal view). Same patient with a right displaced, blow-in orbital roof fracture. Note the intraparenchymal hemorrhage just above the fracture.

pressure.[33,34] Alternatively, a "blow-up" or "blow-out" fracture is characterized by the displacement of the orbital roof superiorly into the anterior cranial fossa without involvement of the superior orbital rim. These fractures are typically the result of a direct orbital blunt force with subsequent increase in intraorbital pressure.[34]

There are many clinical features specific to orbital roof fractures that must be carefully examined, including decreased vision, color vision, or pupillary defects suggestive of a traumatic optic neuropathy, decreased extraocular motility from entrapped muscles or palsies of cranial nerves III, IV, or VI, a developing upper eyelid hematoma, which may indicate intracranial bleeding, lacerations to the eyebrow or upper eyelid resulting from a penetrating injury, CSF rhinorrhea, superior orbital rim bony step-offs, and/or altered mental status. It has been shown that intraocular injuries have been associated with orbital roof fractures in 14–29% of cases, which emphasizes the importance of a thorough and comprehensive ophthalmology evaluation.[35]

Unlike other orbital fractures, orbital roof fractures can often be managed conservatively without surgical intervention. Early surgical intervention had previously been thought necessary to prevent meningitis and brain abscess formation, however, more recent studies have suggested that medical management or delayed repair does not increase morbidity.[32] The decision to intervene surgically is often made with neurosurgical consultation, given potential concomitant intracranial issues. However, urgent surgical repair of orbital roof fractures is indicated in the case of direct optic nerve compression, expanding orbital hemorrhage, perforating eye injury, and/or early evidence of meningitis (Table 110.2).[32] Delayed repair can be reserved for enophthalmos, persistent CSF fistula, or when bony impingement causes diplopia or ptosis (Table 110.2).[32] Despite the timing, the goals of surgical intervention include reduction of a roof fracture with placement of a titanium plate or implant, repair of a dural tear if present, obliteration or cranialization of the frontal sinus as needed, and optic canal decompression if necessary.[32]

Table 110.2: Clinical presentation of orbital roof fractures.

Intervention	Clinical presentation
Immediate	• Displaced fracture with direct optic nerve compromise • Expanding orbital hemorrhage • Perforating eye injury • Early evidence of meningitis or brain abscess
Delayed	• Foreign body present • Bony impingement causing vertical diplopia, torsional diplopia, ptosis, or lagophthalmos • Large dural defect resulting in persistent CSF leak • Frontal sinus fracture • Enophthalmos

(CSF: Cerebrospinal fluid)

Source: Fulcher TP, Sullivan TJ. Orbital roof fractures: management of ophthalmic complications. Ophthal Plast Reconstr Surg. 2003;19(5):359-63.

Surgical Approaches

When surgical intervention is indicated, there are multiple approaches available to access the orbital roof including extracranial, intracranial, and endonasal endoscopic approaches. Among the extracranial approaches, there are multiple incision options including an upper lid crease incision, brow incision, Lynch, bicoronal, or through an existing laceration from the trauma.[36] Intracranial approaches are performed via craniotomy in conjunction with neurosurgery. Endonasal endoscopic approaches are reserved for decompression of the optic canal and are not useful for fracture reduction itself.[37]

Postoperative Management

Postoperative management for the orbital roof fracture is similar to other fracture repairs as detailed above; however, in the case of orbital fractures with concomitant intracranial injury, the systemic management is often governed per neurosurgery recommendations.

NASO-ORBITAL-ETHMOIDAL FRACTURES

Naso-orbital-ethmoidal fractures are seen commonly following high-impact trauma, such as a motor vehicle accident or assault. An NOE fracture refers to a delicate three-dimensional structure that centers on the frontal process of the maxilla and may involve the ethmoid bone, lacrimal bone, nasal bone, or frontal bone. NOE fractures can occur in isolation or as part of other named fracture patterns, including high Le Fort II and Le Fort III fractures (see later—*Le Fort Fractures*). Notably, this area contains the medial canthal tendon, whose integrity is essential for the function of the eyelids. As such, NOE fractures are most commonly classified according to the comminution of the fracture and involvement of the medial canthal tendon as described by Markowitz.[38] Classically, NOE fractures can be divided into three subtypes (Fig. 110.6):

1. *Type 1 NOE*: Minimal comminution with the medial canthal tendon attached to a large bone segment
2. *Type 2 NOE*: More severe comminution of the bone fragments with the medial canthal tendon remaining attached to a bone fragment
3. *Type 3 NOE*: Severe comminution with disinsertion or disruption of the medial canthal tendon.

In addition to the clinical signs seen in other fracture patterns previously described, there are clinical findings evident on the examination, which are suggestive of NOE fractures. Specifically, telecanthus (i.e. greater than 40 mm intercanthal distance), flattened nose with widened nasal dorsum, nasal bone instability when pinching the dorsum, upturned nasal tip, epistaxis or rhinorrhea on intranasal

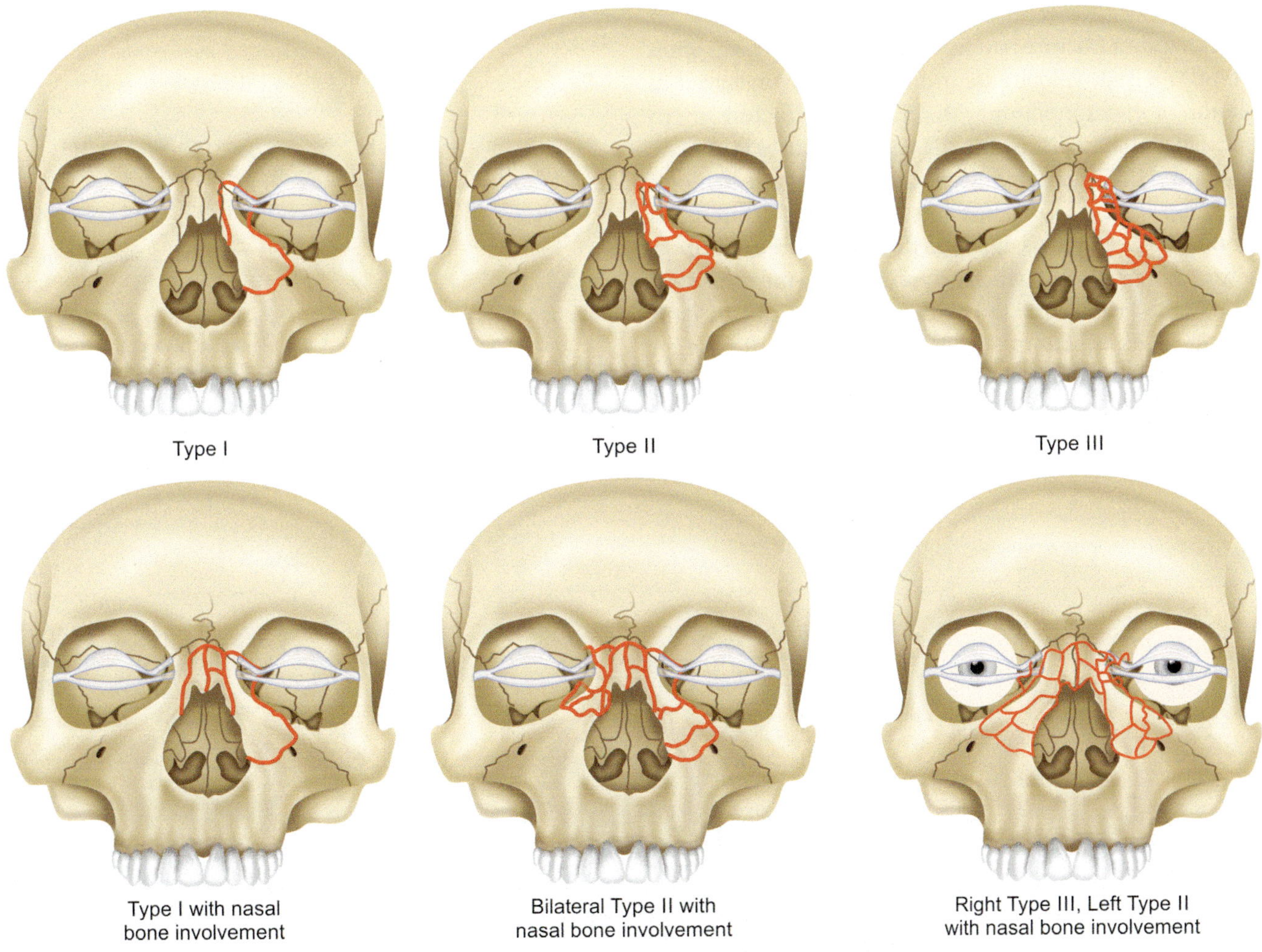

Fig. 110.6: Classification of naso-orbito-ethmoidal (NOE) fractures.
Source: AO Foundation. (2016). AO Surgery Reference. [online] Available from: *https://www2.aofoundation.org*. [Accessed December, 2017]

examination, mobility on palpation of the medial canthal tendon, and signs of nasolacrimal duct obstruction are suggestive of NOE fractures.[39]

The NOE fractures typically require surgical reduction with internal fixation with microplates. Although a detailed discussion of surgical repair is outside the scope of this chapter, it is important to note that general principles for surgical repair. A type I NOE fracture requires plating of the unstable segment, whereas type II and III injuries more frequently require transnasal wiring for stabilization of the medial canthal tendon.[40] The bony nasolacrimal duct may be traumatized in the setting of an NOE fracture, and it is typically recommended to properly reduce the bony fragments in the initial repair and consider a dacryocystorhinostomy as a second stage procedure at least 3 months after the primary repair, if indicated.[41]

Le Fort Fractures

Similar to other fracture patterns, Le Fort fractures are often seen after a high-velocity trauma and can be observed in isolation or in conjunction with other facial fractures.[42] An extensive, detailed discussion of Le Fort fractures is outside the scope of this chapter; however, the injury pattern is one that is important to recognize in the setting of orbitofacial trauma. The Le Fort classification describes three common fracture patterns, all of which extend through the pterygoid plates, and are associated with maxillary trauma and craniofacial dysfunction (Fig. 110.7). Le Fort fractures often occur in the presence of other well-established fracture patterns; Le Fort II and III fractures both involve an NOE fracture, and a Le Fort II includes the frontozygomatic suture as seen in many ZMC fractures.

The classic Le Fort fracture patterns are the following (Fig. 110.8):

- *Le Fort I (Guerin fracture)*: Low transverse fracture through the maxillary alveolus, separating the teeth from the upper face. *No orbital involvement*
- *Le Fort II (pyramidal fracture)*: Fracture through the nasal bridge, lacrimal, and maxillary bones extending through the medial orbital floor and inferior orbital rim near the infraorbital canal

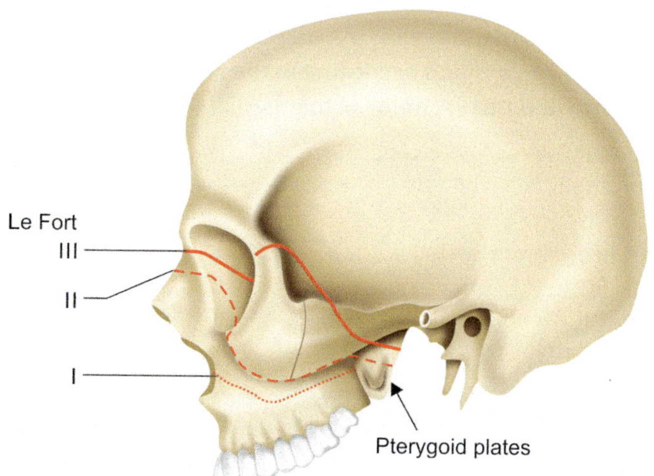

Fig. 110.7: Lateral view of Le Fort fractures. Note that all the fractures extend posteriorly through the pterygoid plates (arrow).[50]
Source: Converse JM. Reconstructive Plastic Surgery: Principles and Procedures in Correction, Reconstruction, and Transplantation, 2nd edition. Philadelphia: Saunders; 1977. pp. 2.

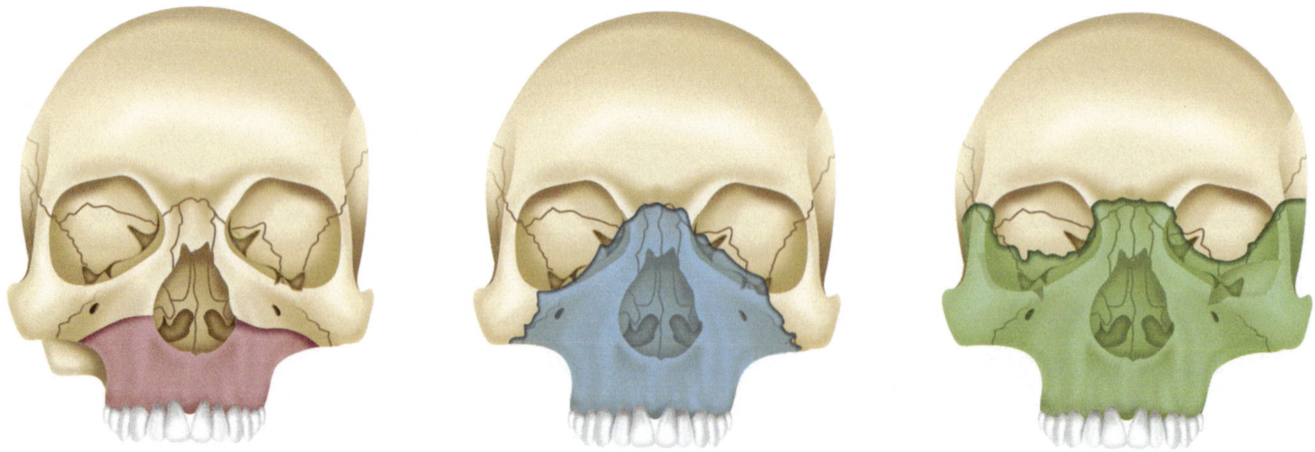

Fig. 110.8: Classification of midfacial fractures as described by Le Fort.[50]
Source: Converse JM. Reconstructive Plastic Surgery: Principles and Procedures in Correction, Reconstruction, and Transplantation, 2nd edition. Philadelphia: Saunders; 1977. pp. 2.

- *Le Fort III (craniofacial dysjunction):* Fracture through the nasal bridge, entire orbit, and laterally through the frontozygomatic suture. This completely detaches the lower facial skeleton.

It is important to note that any combination of Le Fort fractures is possible and the fracture should be named independently on each side based on the highest fracture line.[43]

Examination features that should be specifically assessed in patients with Le Fort fractures include dental occlusion abnormalities, Battle's sign (bruising over the mastoid), nasal examination for bleeding for CSF rhinorrhea, and midface segment mobility and retrusion assessment.

Orbital Hemorrhage

Orbital hemorrhage is one of the few oculoplastic surgery emergencies as bleeding within the orbit can quickly cause vision loss as a result of an orbital compartment syndrome. An orbital hemorrhage most commonly occurs following trauma or recent orbital, lacrimal, or sinus surgery. Special attention is warranted in patients on blood thinning agents, especially in the setting of trauma.

If an orbital compartment syndrome is identified, the surgical team must act promptly to decompress the hemorrhage. Intraocular pressure readings, visual acuity testing, a pupillary assessment, and extraocular motility can guide the decision-making process. If there is evidence of a vision threatening orbital compartment syndrome, the initial intervention of choice is lateral canthotomy with inferior cantholysis. A superior cantholysis can be added if needed for further decompression. Care must be taken to ensure that the cantholysis is complete as a simply canthotomy is often insufficient.

If a canthotomy and cantholysis performed at the bedside is inadequate in decompressing the orbital compartment syndrome, emergent decompression of the orbit can be performed surgically with orbital floor or medial wall decompression. Typically, the presence of an orbital floor fracture or medial wall fracture naturally allows an egress for the hemorrhage, and may reduce the risk of orbital compartment syndrome.

Intraorbital Foreign Bodies

Similar to other orbitofacial trauma, IOrbFB are typically the result of a high-velocity injury, including projectiles, occupational trauma (i.e. nail guns), or blast injuries, but can also occur from organic materials, such as tree branches.[44,45] The surgeon must maintain a high index of suspicion for an IOrbFB in the setting of trauma, especially since the patient may be incapacitated on initial examination and the external injury may seem inconsequential on initial examination. A retained IOrbFB may create significant orbital complications, with inorganic foreign bodies causing visual loss from the direct trauma, whereas organic material may result in a severe orbital infection.[46]

A thorough ophthalmic examination must be performed, with particular attention to potential entry wounds, globe integrity, presenting visual acuity, pupillary reflexes, and extraocular motility. CT imaging should be performed in this setting given the excellent visualization of many foreign bodies, including metal and glass. Furthermore, MRI is contraindicated in the presence of suspected metallic foreign bodies. Wooden foreign bodies may be misdiagnosed as intraorbital air; therefore, an MRI can be performed after a CT scan if there is possibility of a wooden foreign body.[47]

The decision to proceed with surgical removal is dependent upon the location and material of the IOrbFB. Foreign bodies that are located in the anterior orbit and those patients presenting with good initial visual acuity are associated with a better outcome. Metallic and nonmetallic inert IOrbFB located posteriorly in the orbit are often well tolerated without urgent need for surgical removal.[48,49] The exception to this is iron and copper; iron IOrbFB can result in siderosis and slow retinal deterioration and foreign bodies comprised of more than 85% copper can create chalcosis. Both of these can be monitored with serial electroretinograms (ERGs).[49]

Definitive surgical intervention is indicated for foreign bodies composed of organic or vegetative matter, toxic foreign bodies (i.e. copper and iron), location near the optic nerve causing decreased vision, causing intracranial penetration, and/or readily accessible metallic foreign bodies that would prevent future MRI studies. Fulcher et al.[44] developed an algorithm for surgical management of IOrbFB (Flowchart 110.1).

SUMMARY

Orbitofacial trauma, including orbital fractures, orbital hemorrhage, and IOrbFB, are all common sequelae of facial trauma that commonly presents to emergency departments. In this review, we have identified many of the common fracture patterns and other associated injuries as well as the pertinent and relevant anatomy that is necessary to properly diagnose and treat these injuries.

Flowchart 110.1: Algorithm for removal of intraorbital foreign bodies.

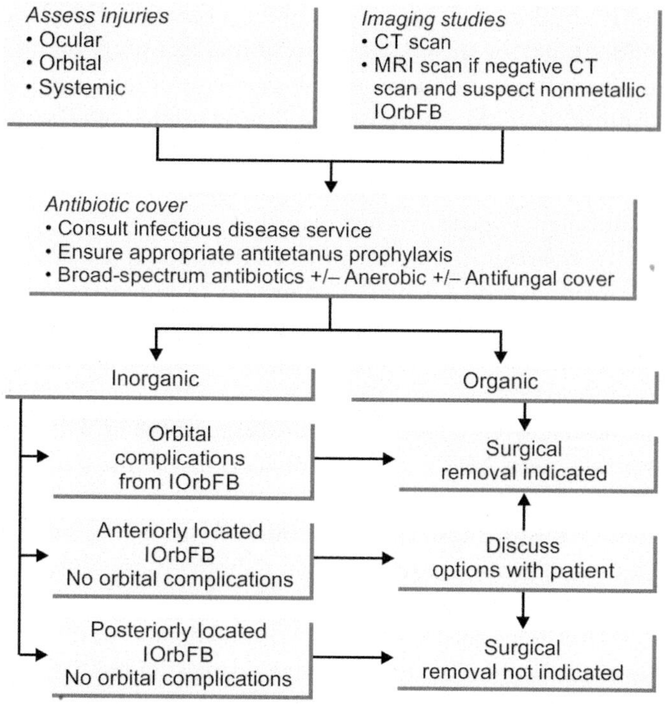

(CT: Computed tomography; MRI: Magnetic resonance imaging; IOrbFB: Intraorbital foreign bodies)

Source: Fulcher TP, McNab AA, Sullivan TJ. Clinical features and management of intraorbital foreign bodies. Ophthalmology. 2002;109(3):494-500.

REFERENCES

1. Hatton MP, Thakker MM, Ray S. Orbital and adnexal trauma associated with open-globe injuries. Ophthal Plast Reconstr Surg. 2002;18(6):458-61.
2. Erdmann D, Follmar KE, Debruijn M, et al. A retrospective analysis of facial fracture etiologies. Ann Plast Surg. 2008;60(4):398-403.
3. Scherer M, Sullivan WG, Smith DJ Jr, et al. An analysis of 1,423 facial fractures in 788 patients at an urban trauma center. J Trauma. 1989;29(3):388-90.
4. Kelley P, Crawford M, Higuera S, et al. Two hundred ninety-four consecutive facial fractures in an urban trauma center: lessons learned. Plast Reconstr Surg. 2005;116(3):42e-49e.
5. Mellema PA, Dewan MA, Lee MS, et al. Incidence of ocular injury in visually asymptomatic orbital fractures. Ophthal Plast Reconstr Surg. 2009;25(4):306-8
6. Wei LA, Chen HH, Hink EM, et al. Pediatric facial fractures from dog bites. Ophthal Plast Reconstr Surg. 2013;29(3):179-82.
7. Warwar RE, Bullock JD, Ballal DR, et al. Mechanisms of orbital floor fractures: a clinical, experimental, and theoretical study. Ophthal Plast Reconstr Surg. 2000;16(3):188-200.
8. Smith, B, Regan WF Jr. Blow-out fracture of the orbit (mechanism and correction of internal orbital fracture). Am J Ophthalmol. 1957;44(6):733-79.
9. Fujino T, Sato TB. Mechanisms, tolerance limit curve and theoretical analysis in blow-out fractures of two and three-dimensional orbital wall models. Proceedings of the Third International Symposium on Orbital Disorders, Amsterdam. 1977. pp. 240-7.
10. Desner, SC. Discussion by Steve C. Dresner. Ophthalmology. 2002;109(7):1210-1.
11. Burnstine MA. Clinical recommendations for repair of orbital facial fractures. Curr Opin Ophthalmol. 2003; 14(5):236-40.
12. Harmer SG, Ethunandan M, Zaki GA, et al. Sudden transient complete loss of vision caused by nose blowing after a fracture of the orbital floor. Br J Oral Maxillofac Surg. 2007;45(2):154-5
13. Boush BA, Lemke BN. Progressive infraorbital nerve hypesthesia as a primary indication for blow-out fracture repair. Ophthal Plast Reconstr Surg. 1994;10(4):271-5.
14. Jordan DR, Allen LH, White J, et al. Intervention within days for some orbital floor fractures: the white-eyed blowout. Ophthal Plast Reconstr Surg. 1998;14(6):379-90.
15. Davies BW, Hink EM, Durairaj VD. Transconjunctival inferior orbitotomy: indications, surgical technique, and complications. Craniomaxillofac Trauma Reconstr. 2014;7(3):169-74.
16. Vrcek I, Bratton E, Amato M, et al. Orbit Fracture Management: Toward a Consensus. Chicago, IL: ASOPRS 47th Annual Fall Scientific Symposium; 2016.
17. Blaydon SM, Shore JW, Neuhaus RW. Medial Orbital Wall Fractures. In: Holck D, Ng J (Eds). Evaluation and Treatment of Orbital Fractures a Multidisciplinary Approach. Philadelphia, Pennsylvania: Elsevier Saunders; 2006. pp. 103-17.
18. Fischbein FI, Lesko WS, Blowout fracture of the medial orbital wall. Arch Ophthalmol. 1969;81(2):162-3.
19. Rodriguez ED, Dorafshar AH, Manson PN. Facial Fractures. In: Neligan P, Rodriguez ED, Losee JE (Eds). Plastic surgery. Philadelphia; Elsevier Saunders; 2013. pp. 53-7.
20. Fujino T, Makino K. Entrapment mechanism and ocular injury in orbital blowout fracture. Plast Reconstr Surg. 1980;65(5):571-6.
21. Fujino T. Experimental "blowout" fracture of the orbit. Plast Reconstr Surg. 1974;54(1):81-2.
22. Rhee JS, Kilde J, Yoganadan N, et al. Orbital blowout fractures: experimental evidence for the pure hydraulic theory. Arch Facial Plast Surg. 2002;4(2):98-101.
23. Brannan PA, Kersten RC, Kulwin DR. Isolated medial orbital wall fractures with medial rectus muscle incarceration. Ophthal Plast Reconstr Surg. 2006;22(3):178-83.
24. Choi M, Flores RL. Medial orbital wall fractures and the transcaruncular approach. J Craniofac Surg. 2012;23(3): 696-701
25. Goldberg RA, Mancini R, Demer JL. The transcaruncular approach: surgical anatomy and technique. Arch Facial Plast Surg. 2007;9(6):443-7.
26. Greenwald MJ, Boston D, Pensler JM, et al. Orbital roof fractures in childhood. Ophthalmology. 1989;96(4):491-6.

27. Hink EM, Wei LA, Durairaj VD. Clinical features and treatment of pediatric orbit fractures. Ophthal Plast Reconstr Surg. 2014;30(2):124-31.
28. Cossman JP, Morrison CS, Taylor HO, et al. Traumatic orbital roof fractures: Interdisciplinary evaluation and management. Plast Reconstr Surg. 2014;133(3):335e-43e.
29. Alcalá-Galiano A, Arribas-García IJ, Martín-Pérez MA, et al. Pediatric facial fractures: children are not just small adults. Radiographics. 2008;28(2):441-61.
30. Chandler DB, Rubin PA. Developments in the understanding and management of pediatric orbital fractures. Int Ophthalmol Clin. 2001;41(4):87-104.
31. Antonelli V, Cremonini AM, Campobassi A, et al. Traumatic encephalocele related to orbital roof fractures: report of six cases and literature review. Surg Neurol. 2002;57(2):117-25.
32. Fulcher TP, Sullivan TJ. Orbital roof fractures: management of ophthalmic complications. Ophthal Plast Reconstr Surg. 2003;19(5):359-63.
33. Jones AL, Jones KE. Orbital Roof "blow-in" fracture: a case report and review. J Radiol Case Rep. 2009;3(12):25-30
34. Haug RH, Van Sickels JE, Jenkins WS. Demographics and treatment options for orbital roof fractures. Oral Surg Oral Med Oral Pathol Oral Radiol Endod. 2002;93(3):238-46.
35. Miller GR, Tenzel RR. Ocular complications of mid-facial fractures. Plast Reconstr Surg. 1967;39(1):37-42.
36. Markiewicz MR, Bell RB. Traditional and contemporary surgical approaches to the orbit. Oral Maxillofac Surg Clin North Am. 2012;24(4):573-607.
37. Kuppersmith RB, Alford EL, Patrinely JR, et al. Combined transconjunctival/intranasal endoscopic approach to the optic canal in traumatic optic neuropathy. Laryngoscope. 1997;107(3):311-5.
38. Markowitz BL, Manson PN, Sargent L, et al. Management of the medial canthal tendon in nasoethmoid orbital fractures: the importance of the central fragment in classification and treatment. Plast Reconstr Surg. 1991;87(5):843-53.
39. Sargent LA. Nasoethmoid orbital fractures: diagnosis and treatment. Plast Reconstr Surg. 2007;120(7 Suppl 2):16S-31S.
40. Shibuya TY, Chen VY, Oh YS. Nasoorbito-ethmoid fracture management. Oper Tech Otolaryngol. 2008;19:140e-144.
41. Gruss JS, Hurwitz JJ, Nik NA, et al. The pattern and incidence of nasolacrimal injury in naso-orbital-ethmoid fractures: the role of delayed assessment and dacryocystorhinostomy. Br J Plast Surg. 1985;38(1):116-21.
42. Richards AM. Le Fort Fractures. In: Key Notes on Plastic Surgery. Oxford: Blackwell Science (Wiley); 2002. pp. 132-3.
43. Fraioli RE, Branstetter BF 4th, Deleyiannis FW. Facial fractures: beyond Le Fort. Otolaryngol Clin North Am. 2008;41(1):51-76.
44. Fulcher TP, McNab AA, Sullivan TJ. Clinical features and management of intraorbital foreign bodies. Ophthalmology. 2002;109(3):494-500.
45. Finkelstein M, Legmann A, Rubin PA. Projectile metallic foreign bodies in the orbit. A retrospective study of epidemiologic factors, management, and outcomes. Ophthalmology. 1997;104(1):96-103.
46. Elkington AR, Khaw PT. Injuries around the orbit: more than meets the eye. Br Med J (Clin Res Ed). 1987;295:1652.
47. Green BF, Kraft SP, Carter KD, et al. Intraorbital wood. Detection by magnetic resonance imaging. Ophthalmology. 1990;97(5):608-11.
48. Ho VH, Wilson MW, Fleming JC, et al. Retained intraorbital metallic foreign bodies. Ophthal Plast Reconstr Surg. 2004;20(3):232-6.
49. Callahan AB, Yoon MK. Intraorbital foreign bodies: retrospective chart review and review of literature. Int Ophthalmol Clin. 2013;53(4):157-65.
50. Converse JM. Reconstructive plastic surgery: principles and procedures in correction, reconstruction, and transplantation, 2nd edition. Philadelphia: Saunders; 1977. pp. 2.

Chapter 111 The Anophthalmic Socket

Nina M Farivari, Louise A Mawn

INTRODUCTION

Acquired anophthalmia describes the condition in which the eye is no longer present, whether through surgery or due to trauma. Evisceration, enucleation, and exenteration are the main surgical techniques by which orbital contents are removed. Evisceration involves removal of the entire intraocular contents and leaving intact sclera. Enucleation refers to removal of the entire globe, and exenteration requires removal of the globe and some or all orbital contents. Indications for enucleation are most commonly tumor, trauma, and glaucoma, whereas nonmalignant etiologies including infection may be more likely managed by evisceration.[1-6] Exenterations are performed in the rare setting of potentially life-threatening or otherwise progressive orbital pathologies unresponsive to conservative management.[7] In the anophthalmic socket, volume is replaced by an orbital implant (either autologous tissue or synthetic) and aesthetic appearance is maintained by a prosthesis. This chapter will describe considerations for long-term management of the anophthalmic socket as well as care of the prosthesis.

PATIENT EVALUATION

History

The examiner first should identify what type of eye removal surgery the patient has undergone, and for what reason. Etiologies can include tumor, traumatic or chemical injury, glaucoma, chronic uveitis, infection, retinal detachment, congenital anomalies, and other diseases;[1-6] this determination may affect the health of the remaining socket and guide future management. Information regarding the prosthesis age and care regimen, including frequency of removal and cleaning, and last ocularist evaluation are valuable components of the history.

In addition to the objective components of the history, the clinician should understand that the removal of an eye can have a profound physical and psychological impact on a person. Many patients experience depression, stress, anxiety, and lower health-related quality of life. It is valuable to consider a multi-disciplinary approach to management in these circumstances, possibly involving both psychological care and also cognitive behavioral management.[8]

Examination

The ideal anophthalmic socket provides a symmetric appearance relative to the remaining, seeing eye. A number of features can lend to this appearance (Table 111.1). The aim of postoperative management is to maintain a noninfected and noninflamed socket that is painless and fits a prosthesis with the appearance and motility of a normal eye.

Table 111.1: Features of the ideal anophthalmic socket.

Component	Features
Implant	• Centrally placed • Well covered • Inert material • Transmits motility to overlying prosthesis

Socket	• Healthy conjunctival lining
	• Minimal discharge
	• *Deep fornices*:
	  – Retain prosthesis
	  – Allow for horizontal and vertical movement of prosthesis

Eyelids, eyelashes	• *Normal eyelid position and tone*:
	  – Absence of ptosis or retraction
	  – Absence of ectropion or entropion
	  – Absence of lagophthalmos
	• Normal lash position
	• Supratarsal eyelid fold symmetric with other eye

Ocular prosthesis	• Comfortable
	• *Similar appearance to contralateral globe*:
	  – Painted appearance
	  – Lack of enophthalmos or proptosis
	  – Horizontal and vertical globe position
	  – Motility
	• Smooth and clean surface

The initial assessment should begin with external examination of the prosthesis, eyelids, and periorbital region. Comparison of the anophthalmic socket to the nonoperative side should include evaluation of relative globe position (with specific attention to enophthalmos, proptosis, or hyper or hypoglobus). The eyelids should next be evaluated, and presence of ptosis or lid retraction, lower lid position including laxity, ectropion or entropion, or lagophthalmos should be noted.

Slit-lamp examination of the prosthesis should ideally reveal a glossy surface with an adequate tear film. The prosthesis surface should be smooth and without chips, scratches, or deposition of debris.

Next, the prosthesis should be removed to examine the conjunctival lining of the socket under the slit lamp. The fornices should be deep and the orbital implant well covered by overlying conjunctiva and Tenon capsule (in instances of enucleation) or scleral shell (following evisceration). Conjunctival edema, injection, giant papillary conjunctivitis (GPC), and purulence or ropey mucous discharge should notably be absent.[9,10]

Attention should be then turned to the fellow eye for completion of a thorough examination.

Care of the Prosthesis

There is a wide range of recommendations among both ocularists and oculoplastic surgeons regarding the care of the ocular prosthesis. This vast array of often-conflicting information can lead to confusion and frustration for the patient.

The American Society of Ocularists recommends a patient-specific approach to prosthetic hygiene, but advises once- or twice-yearly polishing of the prosthesis depending on the frequency of removal.[11] The United Kingdom National Artificial Eye Service similarly advises a personalized approach, but recommends removal of the prosthesis at minimum every 30 days for cleaning.[12]

Conversely, The National Association of Ocularists has a number of blanket recommendations including minimizing removal of the prosthesis to only when necessary, and avoidance of alcohol and suggests use of soap for cleaning.[13] These recommendations are in line with those of the British Oculoplastic Surgery Society, which promotes infrequent removal, annual polishing, and replacement of the prosthesis within 5–7 years of placement.[14]

Although there is no consensus statement on ocular prosthesis care, most sources agree that close collaboration between the clinician and/or surgeon and ocularist is necessary.[15]

Care of the Remaining Eye

In the monocular patient, utmost precaution should be taken in the care of the remaining eye. Annual eye examinations are recommended. Shatterproof and polycarbonate lenses should be worn at all times regardless of the need for corrective lenses. High-risk activities for the safety of the remaining eye, including projectile sports, lawn mowing, metalworking, and other related activities should be avoided.

SOCKET COMPLICATIONS

Mucoid Discharge

Second only to concerns regarding the health of their remaining eye, patients cite increased mucous discharge as their most distressing complaint (Fig. 111.1). A number of known conditions can lead to increased mucoid discharge from the anophthalmic socket, including GPC, pyogenic granuloma, infection, environmental allergens, and orbital implant exposure. However, even in the absence of these findings patients continue to experience this bothersome symptom. Pine et al. have proposed a three-phase model to describe the homeostatic response of the socket to a prosthesis. Phase 1 describes the initial period following introduction of the prosthesis to the socket, during which homeostasis is being established. Irritation from socket manipulation and introduction of foreign materials are

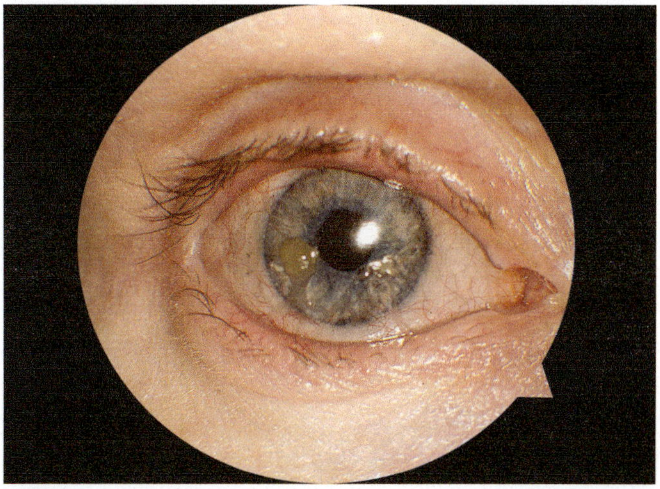

Fig. 111.1: Mucoid discharge. Increased mucoid discharge from the anophthalmic socket can be seen covering the anterior surface of the prosthesis.

balanced by the development of a tear film and deposit build-up on the prosthesis surface. Phase 2, equilibrium, describes a stable homeostasis in which mucous substrate forms and surface deposits facilitate lubrication. Phase 3, or breakdown, is a loss of homeostasis. It is postulated to result from excessive build-up of deposits, which can lead to physical irritation as well as an immune-mediated inflammatory response. Cleaning of the prosthesis is recommended at this phase.[9]

Inflammation and Infection

Chronic irritation and inflammation should prompt the examiner to look for an inciting pathology. GPC can develop in patients with prolonged prosthetic use in a similar fashion to contact lens wearers. The development of giant papillae is mediated by a type I hypersensitivity reaction of the conjunctiva to antigenic protein deposits on the surface of the prosthesis. Additional trauma may be inflicted upon the conjunctiva as it rubs against the prosthesis edge. In addition to conjunctival hyperemia, discomfort, and increased discharge, examination reveals large pretarsal conjunctival papillae upon eversion of the upper lid. Management includes polishing of the prosthesis, topical steroid or nonsteroidal anti-inflammatory drops, or mast-cell stabilizers.[8,16]

A pyogenic granuloma may also be found in cases of chronic socket discharge (Figs. 111.2A to D). Pyogenic granulomas are a vasoproliferative response to tissue irritation or inflammation, and can bleed intermittently.

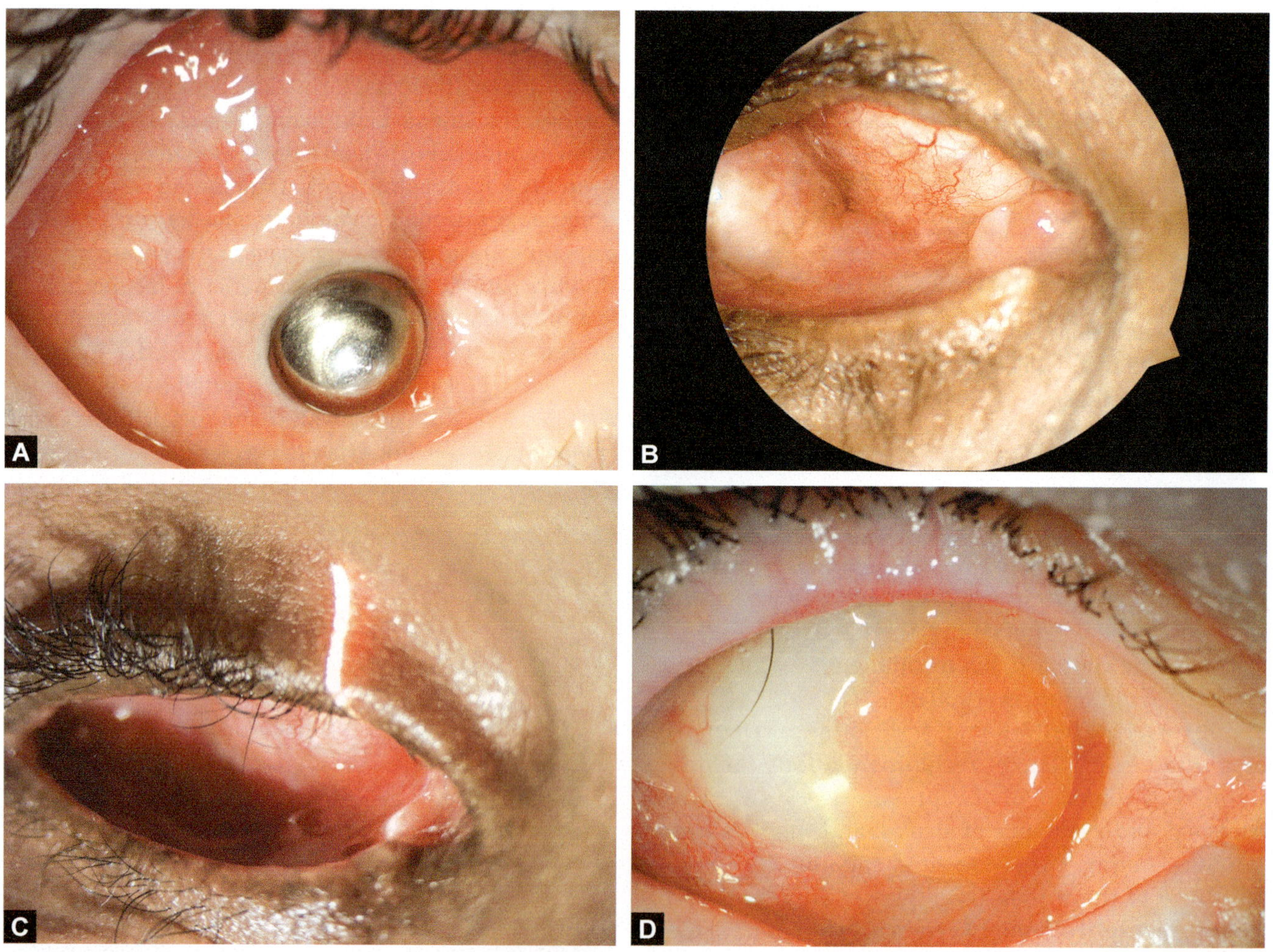

Figs. 111.2A to D: Pyogenic granuloma. (A) Recurrent pyogenic granuloma adjacent to implant peg site. This patient had a chronic low-grade infection of the orbital implant, unresponsive to antibiotics and ultimately required implant exchange; (B) Inferonasal pyogenic granuloma related to poor prosthesis fit; (C) The same socket as (B), showing dramatic improvement following four months of topical steroids; (D) A large pyogenic granuloma adjacent to an area of implant exposure.

They can develop in response to a suture, implant infection or exposure, or another irritating agent. Removal of inciting agent and use of topical anti-inflammatory medications may be helpful in these circumstances.[8]

Deposits on the retropalpebral surface of the ocular prosthesis, which are in constant contact with the palpebral conjunctiva, are suggested to reduce inflammation and promote the health of the socket. These deposits have been associated with improved socket lubrication, less mucoid discharge, and reduction of friction between the prosthesis and the conjunctiva.[17,18]

Infection in the anophthalmic socket can also be a cause of persistent erythema, irritation, and increased discharge. Infectious conjunctivitis can develop in the anophthalmic socket in a similar fashion to in a normal socket with the globe intact. These cases are often accompanied by eyelid edema, chemosis, or hyperemia. Cultures of the discharge may guide management. Infection of the orbital implant should also be considered in instances of discharge resistant to therapy, tenderness upon palpation of the implant, or persistent pyogenic granulomas. The risk of implant infection increases with recent implant placement, exposure, chemotherapy, or radiation therapy, and may ultimately require explantation.[19,20]

Tear Film

There are a number of factors that lead to more severe dryness of the anophthalmic socket compared to normal eyes. One generally accepted principle is that the absent corneal reflex leads to decreased tear production. The sensation of dryness can be further aggravated by decreased blink, as well as lagophthalmos or abnormal eyelid position.[8] It has been shown that prosthetic wearers have 50% decreased reflex tearing by Schirmer testing in the anophthalmic socket compared to the fellow eye, accompanied by symptoms of stringy mucous, dragging eyelids, or bloody tears. Additionally, among all sockets with prostheses, those with the aforementioned symptoms had less reflex tearing than asymptomatic sockets.[21] A more recent study using Fourier domain optical coherence tomography (FD OCT) found prosthetic eyes to have decreased tear meniscus height, depth, area, and volume with respect to normal eyes.[22] A loss of meibomian glands has been also demonstrated in the lids of anophthalmic sockets, possibly related to eyelid margin irritation due to a poor-fitting prosthesis.

These symptoms can be managed with aqueous or oil-based artificial tears, punctal plug insertion, or even applying a small amount of mineral oil to the prosthetic surface.[8]

Bacterial Environment

Anophthalmic sockets as well as ocular prostheses have a unique pattern of bacterial colonization distinct from normal eyes. It has been extensively demonstrated that anophthalmic sockets have higher rates of bacterial pathogens compared to the normal conjunctival flora, including a predominance of gram negative and anaerobic bacteria. Frequent prosthesis manipulation and removal have been associated with a greater degree of bacterial colonization as well.[23,24] The formation of biofilms around spherical orbital implants, in a similar fashion to nasolacrimal implants, contact lenses, and intraocular implants, allows for antibiotic-resistant growth of bacteria.[25] A relationship between increased socket colonization and infection risk has not yet been demonstrated.

Anatomical Changes

Orbital volume loss after enucleation or evisceration surgery can result in a redistribution of intraorbital contents and poor fit of a prosthesis (Figs. 111.3A and B). Shortening of orbital tissues leads to socket contracture and conjunctival fornices with insufficient space to retain a prosthesis (Fig. 111.4). A number of processes can lead to socket contracture including—scarring associated with original injury, including chemical burns; iatrogenic including damage and scarring to the conjunctiva and orbital tissues during enucleation or evisceration surgery or multiple socket surgeries leading to worsening scarring and decreased vascular supply; radiation therapy; chronic socket inflammation; poor compliance with prosthesis use; and poorly fitting prosthesis.[26-28]

In addition to forniceal shallowing, lower-lid laxity can develop or worsen in these patients due to the weight of the prosthesis. "Postenucleation socket syndrome" describes a characteristic constellation of enophthalmos, a deep superior sulcus, lower lid laxity, and upper lid ptosis as a result of these anatomical changes (Figs. 111.5A to C). A larger prosthesis may be able to quell this problem, but eventually surgical interventions aimed at volume replacement, forniceal deepening, and lower lid laxity may be indicated.[26,27]

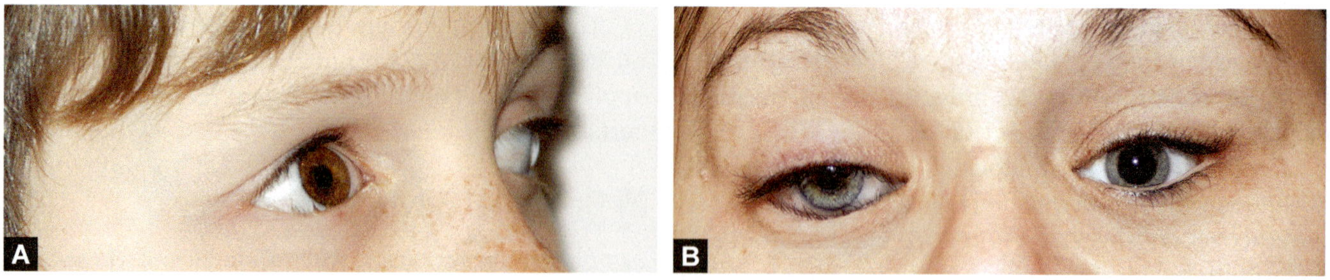

Figs. 111.3A and B: Orbital Volume Loss. (A) A pediatric patient following right eye enucleation with dermis fat grafting to the orbit with prosthesis in place. This patient has malpositioning of the prosthesis and right lower lid entropion related to volume loss. A spherical implant was later placed along with entropion repair; (B) An anophthalmic adult patient with right upper lid ptosis and right lower lid entropion, secondary to orbital volume loss.

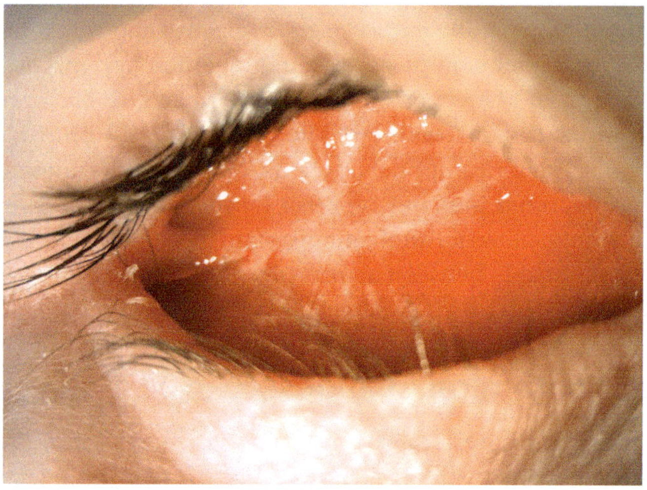

Fig. 111.4: Socket contracture. This patient underwent enucleation years following chemical injury to the right eye. The socket has developed scarring and contracture with difficulty fitting a prosthesis.

Implant Migration and Exposure

Implant migration can occur secondary to contracture or changes in distribution of orbital volume. This can lead to poor motility and malpositioning of the prosthesis, resulting in enophthalmos, and deep superior sulcus deformity. Refitting with a new prosthesis is a more conservative measure to improve comfort and motility, alternatively an implant exchange may be required.[9, 29-31]

Orbital implant exposure can result in implant infection or extrusion, and may require surgical wound revision or even implant replacement (Fig. 111.6). Reported rates of exposure range from 1.5% to 58%, and can occur at any point after surgery. Delayed exposure can be related to conjunctival abrasion against the prosthesis with continuous erosion; as a result, long-term or even lifelong follow-up of the anophthalmic socket may be necessary.[31,32]

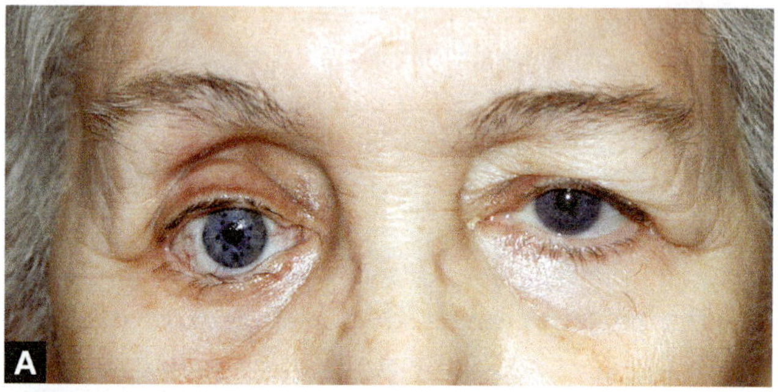

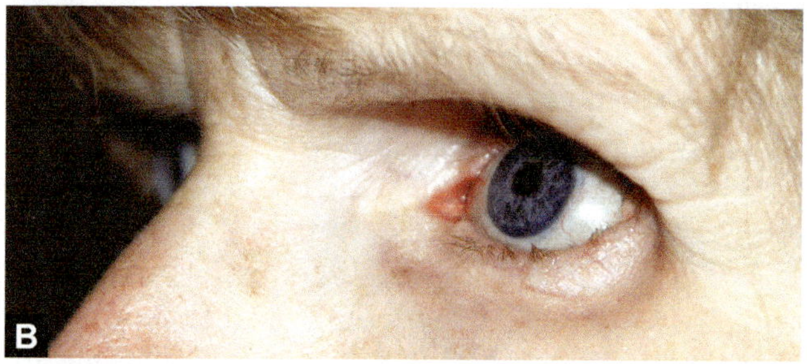

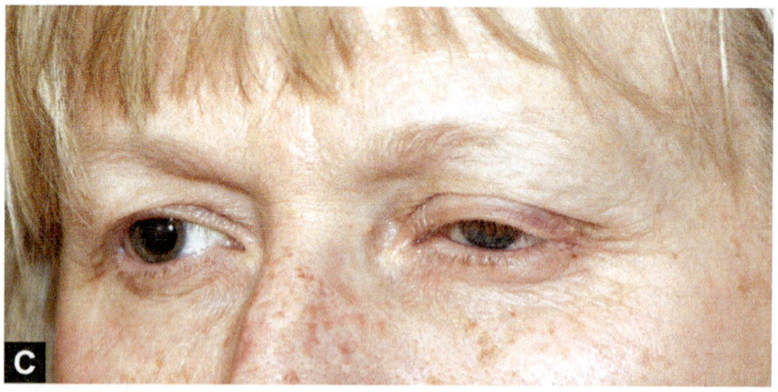

Figs. 111.5A to C: Postenucleation socket syndrome. (A) Right anophthalmia with deep superior sulcus deformity and right lower eyelid laxity, in part related to weight of prosthesis; (B) Left anophthalmos with very deep left superior sulcus and apparent enophthalmos of the prosthesis compared to the right eye; (C) Left anophthalmos with upper lid ptosis, lower lid laxity, and enophthalmos.

Socket Pain

Pain in the anophthalmic socket can be attributed to a wide array of etiologies (Table 111.2). In the healthy-appearing

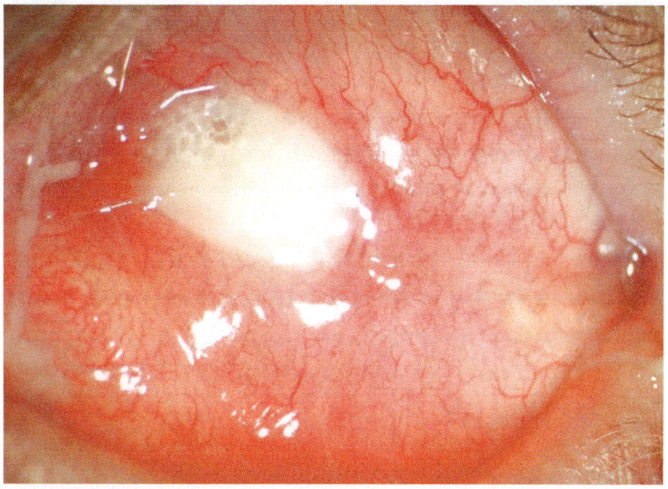

Fig. 111.6: Orbital implant exposure. Porous orbital implant exposure with surrounding conjunctival injection and increased mucous discharge. The area of exposure was closed with a temporalis fascia graft and conjunctivoplasty.

Table 111.2: Causes for socket pain.

Problem		Management
Prosthesis related	• Poor fit • Coarse anterior surface – Debris – Chips, cracks, and scratches	• Ocularist evaluation or socket revision • Removal with polishing • Change of prosthesis
Dry socket	• Decreased tear production • Decreased blink • Meibomian gland dysfunction	• Artificial tears • Punctal plugs • Eyelid hygiene
Inflammation or infection	• Giant papillary conjunctivitis • Pyogenic granuloma • Infectious conjunctivitis	• Topical steroids • Mast cell stabilizer • Prosthesis hygiene • Surgical excision +/– steroids
Surgery related	• Epithelial inclusion cyst • Implant exposure or infection • Implant migration • Socket contraction	• Observation • Excision • Antibiotics • Covering of exposed implant • Prosthesis modification • Implant removal • Prosthesis modification • Implant exchange • Surgical socket revision
Other	• Phantom eye pain • Tumor	• Conventional analgesia • Multidisciplinary approach • History • Examination • Imaging

socket, phantom eye pain should be considered. Phantom eye pain is defined as a painful sensation that the patient refers to his or her removed eye. It results from damage or interruption of sensory nerves during surgery, with up to 28% reported incidence with high correlation to the presence of preoperative pain. Phantom eye pain can be difficult to treat; reported approaches include rest, heat, firm pressure, distraction, and conventional analgesics and opioids. No treatment has been shown to completely eliminate the pain, however,[8] persistent or intractable socket pain may require imaging for complete evaluation.

EVISCERATION, ENUCLEATION, AND EXENTERATION: AN OVERVIEW

Evisceration

Evisceration involves removal of the intraocular contents with replacement of intraocular volume. The sclera remains intact. Historically, there has been a concern for the development of sympathetic ophthalmia (SO) following disruption of the globe and theoretical exposure of uveal antigens. Numerous recent studies; however, have found the risk of SO to be remarkably low, especially in the advent of developments in uveitis treatment.[1,33-35] While a controversial issue, orbital surgeons generally consider SO to be less of a concern in present times.

Indications include a blind and painful eye with either infectious or other nonmalignant disease. Many surgeons prefer evisceration to enucleation in instances of severe endophthalmitis. Contraindications to evisceration exist in cases of intraocular malignancy or if histopathology of the globe in its entirety is required. Severe phthisis bulbi is a relative contraindication.[1,35-37]

In recent years, evisceration has been gaining favor over enucleation both internationally and in the United States, most notably in cases of nonmalignancy. Because evisceration is less disruptive to the extraocular muscles and other orbital soft tissue, the surgery typically is shorter and less complex and can confer better ocular motility. Additional advantages include less patient exposure to anesthesia, superior cosmesis, possible decreased implant exposure rate, and improved socket health.[1,2,33,36,37]

Enucleation

Enucleation surgery involves removal of the entire globe, with preservation of other orbital contents.

A primary indication for enucleation is an intraocular malignancy that is not amenable to alternative management, and threatens the health or life of the patient. A corollary indication is the inability to evaluate for the presence of intraocular tumor (e.g. inability to evaluate the posterior pole) in an otherwise blind and painful eye with unknown etiology. Enucleation may also be indicated over evisceration in cases of severe phthisis, or if complete histopathologic evaluation of the globe is required.

Exenteration

Orbital exenteration involves removal of all orbital tissues, including the globe, optic nerve, extraocular muscles, periorbita, and some or all of the eyelids. While total exenteration requires removal of all orbital contents, a subtotal exenteration can spare the eyelids and conjunctiva. Extended exenteration requires the additional removal of bone and adjacent soft tissue. Orbital exenteration is a significantly psychologically and anatomically disfiguring surgery, and generally is reserved for the treatment of life-threatening or progressively destructive disease processes that are unresponsive to more conservative management. Indications can include eyelid or ocular neoplasms with orbital extension; some primary orbital tumors including lacrimal gland malignancies; sinonasal masses invading the orbit; conjunctival tumors; and aggressive fungal infections such as mucormycosis or aspergillosis of the orbit and sinuses.[7,35,38] Other indications can include exenteration for palliative debulking of a large tumor burden for pain control, as well as management of severe trauma, meningioma, or congenital deformities.

Aesthetic rehabilitation options are limited and primarily involve custom-made silicone prostheses, which can be spectacle-retained or adhesive. Newer advances utilize osseointegration and magnetic coupling, a process that can provide improved cosmesis and eliminate the need for adhesive. Alternatively, patients may elect to wear opaque spectacle lenses or an occlusive eye patch.[38-41]

NONSURGICAL MANAGEMENT OF THE BLIND AND PAINFUL EYE

For patients with a nonmalignant etiology of their blind and painful eye who are unable to undergo surgery or who are otherwise unwilling to have their eye removed, management options include topical therapy, bandage contact lens, and retrobulbar injection of ethanol or chlorpromazine. Historically, retrobulbar ethanol has provided adequate pain relief; however, its duration of effect is temporary averaging only about 6 months. Retrobulbar chlorpromazine, an antipsychotic medication, has been shown to provide superior pain control with longer duration of action and fewer reported side effects. Following use of both of these agents, however, orbital fibrosis has been reported, which can pose challenges for future removal of the eye and ultimate socket health postenucleation surgery.[42]

SUMMARY

Surgically acquired anophthalmia is achieved via either enucleation, evisceration, or exenteration. The orbital implant replaces volume while the prosthesis maintains aesthetic similarity to the remaining eye. Ophthalmologic examination should include evaluation first of the ocular prosthesis condition and position in the socket, followed by removal of prosthesis with evaluation of the socket itself. Though there are varying recommendations on care of the prosthesis, the socket homeostasis model and recent literature provide insight into an ideal regimen. Removal of the prosthesis at maximum every 30 days and at least once every 6 months can minimize socket discharge and inflammation, allowing maintenance of socket homeostasis. A close relationship between the patient, the ocularist, and the surgeon is invaluable to prosthesis care and socket health. Furthermore, monitoring of the socket long-term by either a general ophthalmologist or oculoplastic surgeon may be indicated as numerous complications can arise at any point. Lastly, care of the remaining eye is of utmost importance; monocular precautions should be reviewed and regular examinations are vital.

The clinician should note the presence or absence of the above features during evaluation of the anophthalmic socket.

Common etiologies of pain in the anophthalmic socket, to be considered and evaluated by the examiner.

REFERENCES

1. Yousuf SJ, Jones LS, Kidwell ED Jr. Enucleation and evisceration: 20 years of experience. Orbit. 2012;31(4):211-5.
2. Koh V, Chiam N, Sundar G. Survey of Common Practices Among Oculofacial Surgeons In The Asia-Pacific Region: Evisceration, Enucleation and Management of Anophthalmic Sockets. Orbit. 2014;33(6):477.

3. Zhang Y, Zhang MN, Wang X, et al. Removal of the eye in a tertiary care center of China: a retrospective study on 573 cases in 20 years. Int J Ophthalmol. 2015;8(5):1024-30.
4. Erie JC, Nevitt MP, Hodge D, et al. Incidence of enucleation in a defined population. Am J Ophthalmol. 1992;113(2):138-44.
5. Koylu MT, Gokce G, Uysal Y, et al. Indications for eye removal surgeries: A 15-year experience at a tertiary military hospital. Saudi Med J. 2015;36(10):1205-9.
6. Setlur VJ, Parikh JG, Rao NA. Changing causes of enucleation over the past 60 years. Graefes Arch Clin Exp Ophthalmol. 2010;248(4):593-7.
7. Soysal HG. Orbital exenteration: a 10-year experience of a general oncology hospital. Orbit. 2010. 1;29(3):135-9.
8. Bohman E, Rassmusen ML, Kopp ED. Pain and discomfort in the anophthalmic socket. Curr Opin Ophthalmol. 2014;25(5):455-60.
9. Pine KR, Sloan BH, Jacobs RJ. A proposed model of the response of the anophthalmic socket to prosthetic eye wear and its application to the management of mucoid discharge. Med Hypotheses. 2013;81(2):300-5.
10. Nerad JA. Enucleation, Evisceration, and Exenteration: The Care of the Eye Socket. In Nerad JA (Ed.). Techniques in Ophthalmic Plastic Surgery, 1st edition. China: El Sevier; 2010. pp. 463-86.
11. American Society of Ocularists. (2017). When Should You See an Ocularist. [online] Avialable from: *http://www.ocularist.org/resources_see_ocularist.asp*. [Accessed January 2018].
12. The National Artifical Eye Service. (2017). Artificial Eye Care. [online] Available from: *http://www.naes.nhs.uk/eye-care/artificial-eye-care/*. [Accessed January 2018].
13. National Association of Ocularists. (2017). FAQs. [online] Available from: *http://nationalassociationofocularists.org/faqs.htm*. [Accessed January 2018].
14. British Oculoplastic Surgery Society. (2017). Removal of an Eye, Artificial Eyes, and Socket Care. [online]. Available from: *http://www.bopss.co.uk/public-information/common-conditions/removal-of-an-eye-artificial-eyes-and-socket-care/*. [Accessed January 2018].
15. Bonaque-González S, Amigó A, Rodríguez-Luna C. Recommendations for post-adaption care of an ocular prosthesis: A review. Cont Lens Anterior Eye. 2015;38(6):397-401.
16. Bozkurt B, Akyurek N, Irkec M, et al. Immunohistochemical findings in prosthesis-associated giant papillary conjunctivitis. Clin Exp Ophthalmol. 2007;35(6):535-40.
17. Pine KR, Sloan B, Jacobs RJ. Deposit buildup on prosthetic eyes and implications for conjunctival inflammation and mucoid discharge. Clin Ophthalmol. 2012;6:1755-62.
18. Pine KR, Sloan B, Stewart J, et al. The response of the anophthalmic socket to prosthetic eye wear. Clin Exp Optom. 2013;96(4):388-93.
19. Wladis EJ, Aakalu VK, Sobel RK, et al. Orbital Implants in Enucleation Surgery: A Report by the American Academy of Ophthalmology. Ophthalmology. 2017; pii: S0161-6420(17)32438-7.
20. Karslioglu S, Serin D, Simsek I, et al. Implant infection in porous orbital implants. Ophthal Plast Reconstr Surg. 2006;22(6):461-6.
21. Allen L, Kolder HE, Bulgarelli EM, et al. Artificial eyes and tear measurements. Ophthalmology. 1980;87(2):155-7.
22. Kim SE, Yoon JS, Lee SY. Tear measurement in prosthetic eye users with fourier-domain optical coherence tomography. Am J Ophthalmol. 2010;149(4):602-7.
23. Toribio A, Marrodán T, Fernández-Natal I, et al. Study of conjunctival flora in anophthalmic patients: influence on the comfort of the socket. Graefes Arch Clin Exp Ophthalmol. 2017;255(8):1669-79.
24. Vasquez RJ, Linberg JV. The anophthalmic socket and the prosthetic eye: a clinical and bacteriologic study. Ophthal Plast Reconstr Surg. 1989;5(4):277-80.
25. Samimi DB, Bielory BP, Miller D, et al. Microbiologic trends and biofilm growth on explanted periorbital biomaterials: a 30-year review. Ophthal Plast Reconstr Surg. 2013;29(5):376-81.
26. Kim HE, Jang SY, Yoon JS. Combined Orbital Floor Wedge Implant and Fornix Reconstruction for Postenucleation Sunken Socket Syndrome. Plastic Reconstr Surg. 2014;133(6):1469-75.
27. Ibrahiem MF, Abdelaziz ST. Shallow inferior conjunctival fornix in contracted socket and anophthalmic socket syndrome: a novel technique to deepen the fornix using fascia lata strips. J ophthalmol. 2016;2016.
28. Tawfik HA, Raslan AO, Talib N. Surgical management of acquired socket contracture. Curr Opin Ophthalmol. 2009;20(5);406-11.
29. Baino F, Potestio I. Orbital implants: state-of-the-art review with emphasis on biomaterials and recent advances. Mater Sci Eng C Mater Biol Appl. 2016;69:1410-28.
30. Jordan DR. Localization of Extraocular muscles during secondary orbital implantation surgery. The tunnel technique: experience with 100 patients. Ophthalmology. 2004;111(5);1048-54.
31. Trichopoulos N, Augsburger JJ. Enucleation with unwrapped porous and nonporous orbital implants: a 15-year experience. Ophthal Plast Reconstr Surg. 2005;21(5):331-6.
32. Lin CW, Liao SL. Long-term complications of different porous orbital implants: a 21-year review. Br J Ophthalmol. 2017;101(5):681-5.
33. Chu XK, Chan CC. Sympathetic ophthalmia: to the twenty-first century and beyond. J ophthalmic Inflamm Infect. 2013;3(1):49.
34. Levine MR, Pou CR Lesh RH. The 1998 Wendell Hughes lecture. Evisceration: is sympathetic ophthalmia a concern in the new millenium? Ophthal Plast Reconstr Surg. 1999;15(1):4-8.
35. Jordan DR, Mawn L. Enucleation, Evisceration, and Exenteration. In: JP Dunn, PD Langer (Eds). Basic Techniques of Ophthalmic Surgery, American Academy of Ophthalmology Manual. San Francisco: American Academy of Ophthalmology; 2015. pp. 305-28.

36. Phan LT, Hwang TN, McCulley TJ. Evisceration in the modern age. Middle East Afr J Ophthalmol. 2012;19(1):24-33.
37. Shah RD, Singa RM, Aakalu VK, et al. Evisceration and enucleation: a national survey of practice patterns in the United States. Ophthalmic Surg Lasers Imaging. 2012;43(5):425-30.
38. Taylor A, Roberts F, Kemp EG. Orbital exenteration: a retrospective study over an 11-year period analyzing all cases from a single unit. Orbit. 2006;25(3):185-93.
39. Rahman I, Cook AE, Leatherbarrow B. Orbital exenteration: a 13-year Manchester experience. Br J Ophthalmol. 2005;89(10):1335-40.
40. Pruthi G, Jain V, Rajendiran S, et al. Prosthetic rehabilitation after orbital exenteration: a case series. Indian J Ophthalmol. 2014;62(5):629-32.
41. Larson JSM, Nerad JA. The use of osseointegration and rare earth magnetic couling for oculofacial prosthesis retention in the exenterated orbit. Curr Opin Ophthalmol. 2009;20(5):412-6.
42. Eftekhari K, Shindler KS, Lee V, et al. Histologic evidence of orbital inflammation from retrobulbar alcohol and chlorpromazine injection: a Clinicopathologic Study in human and rat orbits. Ophthal Plast Reconstr Surg. 2016;32(4):302-4.

Chapter 112 Diseases of the Lacrimal Drainage System

Mohammad Javed Ali

INTRODUCTION

The lacrimal drainage system is one of the most marvelous examples of biophysical and biochemical integration with the physiological process to facilitate tears drainage from the ocular surface to the nasal cavity. In addition to their actions as tear conduits, they play vital roles in the resorption of the tears from the nasolacrimal ducts (NLDs), defenses, and immunomodulation. Diseases of the lacrimal drainage are not uncommon and epiphora is one of the common presentations to an ophthalmologist. The science dealing with this is called dacryology and it has come a long way to be established now as a focused subspecialty of ophthalmology. Lacrimal disorders have a wide spectrum and outside the purview of this chapter, hence we will address the common conditions, their symptomatology, investigations, and managements.

CONGENITAL NASOLACRIMAL DUCT OBSTRUCTION

Congenital nasolacrimal duct obstruction (CNLDO) is amongst the most common causes of epiphora in pediatric age group and the incidence of symptoms range from 1.2% to 30%.[1-10] It is believed to occur secondary to noncanalization of the NLD at its distal end in the nasal cavity. In the embryonic life, lacrimal excretory system starts developing at Carnegie stage 16, with a formation of lacrimal groove between the nasal and maxillary processes which subsequently thicken to form the lacrimal lamina. Subsequent development into a chord-like structure continues and, three significant changes occur at 10th week of fetal life: epithelia of the canaliculi and conjunctiva forms continuous lamina, development of cavitation at the caudal end of lacrimal cord and inferior meatal lamina, and appearance of lumen in lacrimal system. The last portion to canalize is the distal end of the NLD and aberrations in this process results in a CNLDO.[1,2]

Kushner first described the types of CNLDO into simple and complex based on the intraoperative findings.[2] A simple obstruction is characterized by the lack of resistance, while passing the probe through the NLD until a point of an easily perforable membranous obstruction. Numerous aberrations of development like nondevelopment of NLD with a bony obstruction, buried probet, variable misdirections of NLD in the nasal cavity, and anlages or those associated with syndromes or systemic abnormalities.[5-10] Box 112.1 lists the various entities constituting the complex CNLDOs and Box 112.2 lists the common syndromic and systemic associations with CNLDO.

The characteristic triad includes epiphora, discharge, and matting of eyelashes (Fig. 112.1). The onset of watery eye is within the 1st month of age and can be unilateral or bilateral. Objective assessment may reveal an increased tear meniscus height, delayed fluorescein dye disappearance test (FDDT) (Fig. 112.2), and regurgitation on pressure

Box 112.1: Entities constituting the complex CNLDO.

- Non-canalization of bony nasolacrimal duct (Bony obstruction)
- Various embryonic misdirection of the NLD
- Buried probe
- Dacryocele with or without intranasal cyst
- Pediatric acute dacryocystitis
- Anlage tracts
- Multiple level sausage stenosis
- Atonic sac
- Craniofacial syndromes
- Associated intranasal abnormalities

(CNLDO: Congenital nasolacrimal duct obstruction, NLD: Nasolacrimal duct)

Box 112.2: Common syndromic and systemic associations of CNLDO

- Down's syndrome
- Ectodermal ectrodactyly clefting syndrome
- Treacher Collins syndrome
- Hay-Wells syndrome
- Lacrimo-auriculo-dento-digital syndrome
- Rubinstein Taybi syndrome
- ADULT syndrome
- Facial clefting
- Craniofacial dysplasia
- Auricular abnormalities and preauricular sinus

(CNLDO: Congenital nasolacrimal duct obstruction, EEC: Ectrodermal ectrodactyly clefting, LADD: Lacrimo-auriculo-dento-digital, ADULT: Acro-dermato-ungual-lacrimal-tooth)

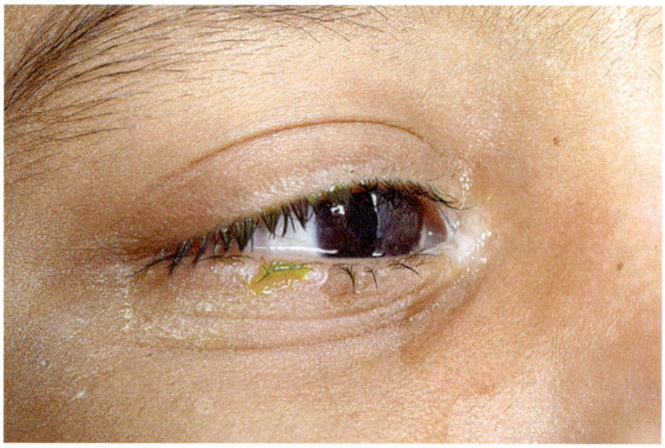

Fig. 112.1: Signs of congenital nasolacrimal duct obstruction.

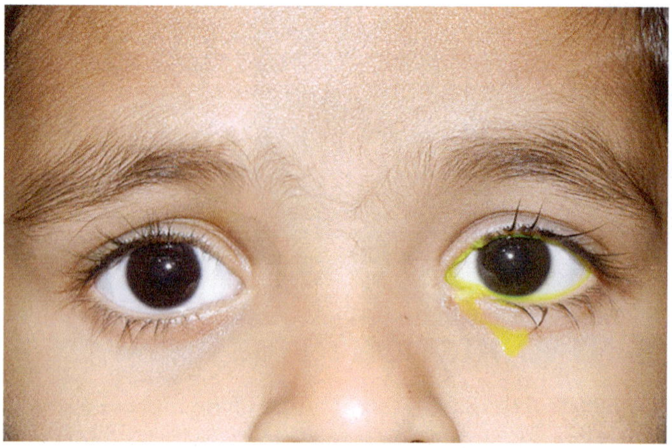

Fig. 112.2: A left-sided CNLDO with gross delay upon FDDT test.
(CNLDO: Congenital nasolacrimal duct obstruction;
FDDT: Fluorescein dye disappearance test)

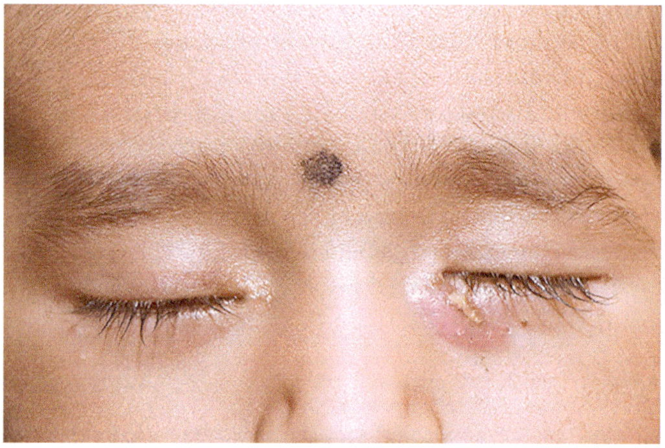

Fig. 112.3: A left-sided pediatric acute dacryocystitis.

over lacrimal sac (ROPLAS). The spectrum of CNLDO can occasionally include acute dacryocystitis at presentation (Fig. 112.3), dacryocystocele, preseptal, and orbital cellulitis.

Dacryocystocele or dacryocele is a swelling of the lacrimal sac, which presents in the neonatal life, below the medial canthal tendon (Fig. 112.4). These can be associated with intranasal cysts (cystic dilatation of the NLD) and can occasionally be life-threatening since neonates are obligate nasal breathers.[8]

The management options for a case of a simple CNLDO is conservative, which includes lacrimal sac compression (up to the age of 1 year) aimed to enhance the hydrostatic pressure within the lacrimal sac, which can overcome the usual thin perforable membranous obstruction at the distal end of NLD. It is important to perform this technique in a right way by placing contralateral index finger at the medial canthus of the baby and compressing it inwards medial to the anterior lacrimal crest (Fig. 112.5). The strokes are

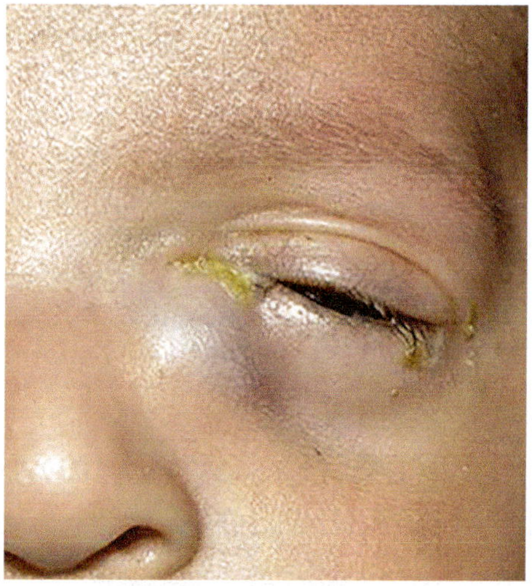

Fig. 112.4: A left-sided dacryocystocele in a neonate.

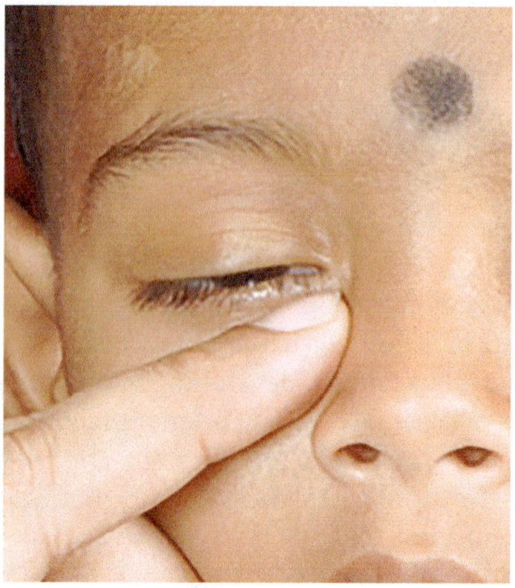

Fig. 112.5: Technique of Criggler's lacrimal sac compression.

directed inwards and should not be downwards towards the lateral nasal wall, since pressure over bones cannot generate the desired hydrostatic pressure within the lacrimal sac. Suggested frequency is 10 times/session and 4 sessions/day. Most of the cases of simple CNLDO would resolve spontaneously.

The standard of care for nonresolving cases includes irrigation and probing. The probing may be alone or combined with a silicone intubation. The usual age at which probing is contemplated is 12 months. Earlier indications for a probing include dacryoceles, acute dacryocystitis, progressively dilating lacrimal sac, earlier attempts of probing, various complex CNLDOs, and associated ocular comorbidities such as congenital glaucoma.[2]

The principle of probing is to pass a rigid probe into the lacrimal drainage system and directed towards the distal end of NLD with an aim of overcoming the membranous obstruction (Figs. 112.6A to G). Probe of appropriate size (size "0" or "1" at 1 year of age) is passed gently, along vertical canaliculus and then along the horizontal canaliculus with the lid out stretched. The probe is then directed into the lacrimal sac till it touches the medial wall and a hard stop is noticed. The probe is then turned 90° so as to be flat on the forehead and is subsequently advanced towards the NLD in a gentle fashion till the membranous obstruction at its distal end can be overcome with use of minimal force. This entire procedure should preferably be performed under endoscopic visualization to confirm the recanalization. Fluorescein-stained fluid can be used for subsequent irrigation to assess the patency.

Although silicone intubation can also be used as a primary treatment modality, more common indications include cases with complex CNLDO and previous failed probings.[2-5] Other modes of management that are employed for specific cases include balloon dacryoplasty for certain syndromic CNLDOs and cruciate marsupialization for dacryoceles with intranasal cysts.[8,9] The general outcomes in simple CNLDOs are excellent and beyond 95%, however, this drops to as low as 40–50% in complex CNLDOs necessitating further measures such as dacryocystorhinostomy (DCR).[5]

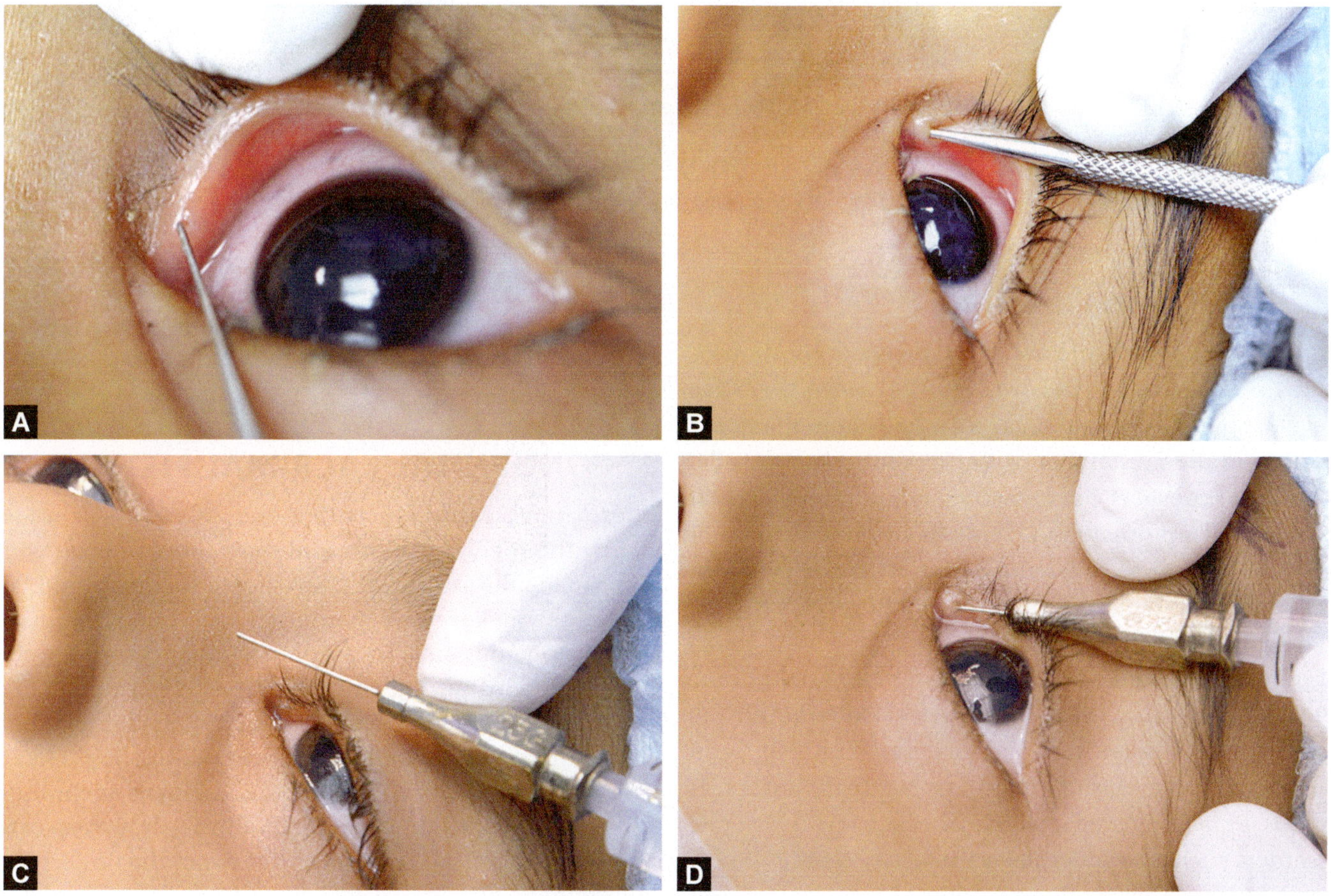

Figs. 112.6A to D

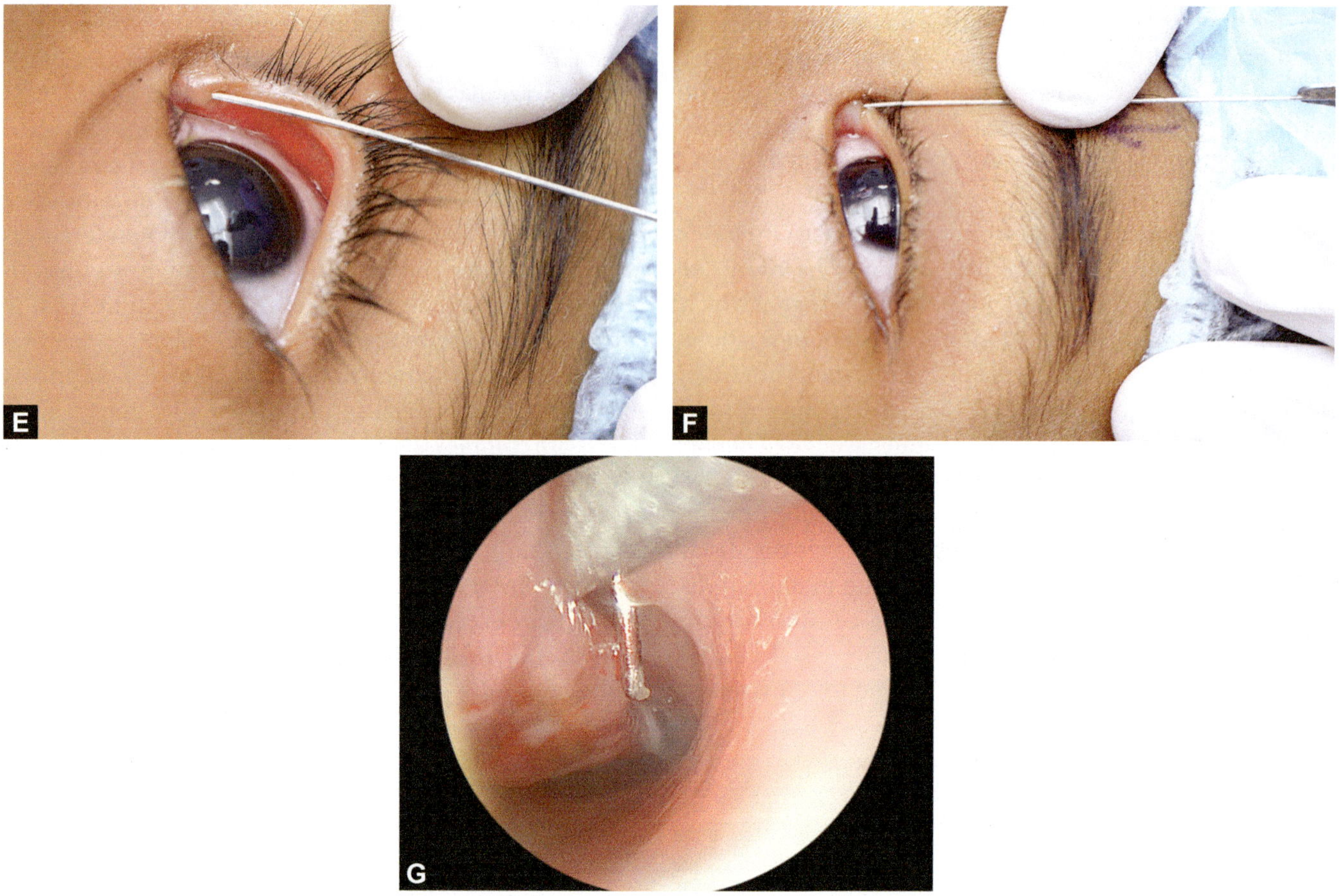

Figs. 112.6E to G

Figs. 112.6A to G: Steps of irrigation and probing for a case of congenital nasolacrimal duct obstruction.

PUNCTAL AGENESIS

Punctal agenesis refers to nondevelopment of one or more puncta. This is widely believed to occur when there is a developmental failure of canalicular buds from the upper portion of the lacrimal cord during embryogenesis.[11,12] Punctal agenesis is hence associated with canalicular agenesis. Symptomatology depends on whether one or both the puncta are agenetic. Epiphora is the common complaint. Slit-lamp examination would reveal absence of the papilla of the punctum or any dimple in the area of punctum, absence of any transilluminant membrane (this differentiates it from another closely mimicking condition, incomplete punctal canalization or IPC),[13] and the presence of eyelashes in the pars lacrimalis portion of eyelids. Punctal agenesis may be associated with systemic disorders such as ectodermal ectrodactyly clefting (EEC), Hay-Wells, and Levy-Hollister syndromes.[10] Most cases with single punctal agenesis are not very symptomatic and are observed. For those with more symptoms, a conjunctivo-DCR with Lester-Jones or Gladstone-Putterman's tubes is the standard for care.

CONGENITAL LACRIMAL FISTULA

These are accessory ducts that open on to the skin just below the medial canthus and may communicate with the canaliculus or the lacrimal sac on the other end.[11,14] The widely believed etiopathology is out budding of an extracanaliculus such as arm from the upper end of the lacrimal chord during embryogenesis.[15] Symptoms can be visible opening in the skin near the medial canthus and epiphora or discharge from the opening (Fig. 112.7). The treatment option of choice is a closed technique of fistulectomy as described by Sullivan, however, care should be exercised to prevent trauma to the underlying communicating lacrimal apparatus.[11,14,15]

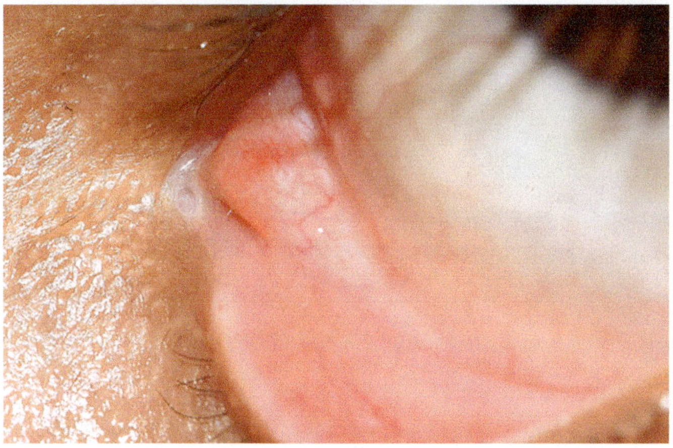

Fig. 112.7: A left side congenital lacrimal sac fistula at the medial canthus.

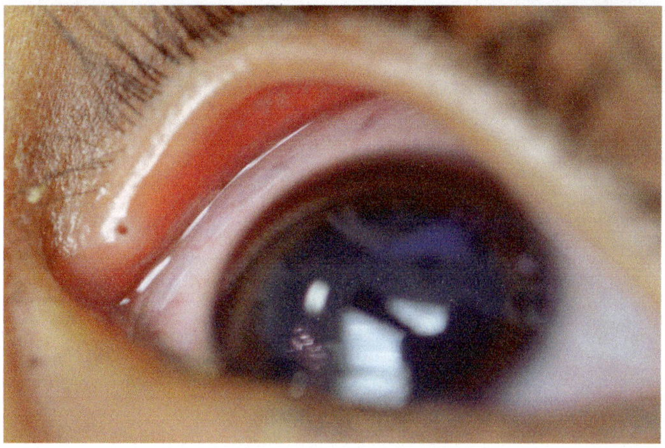

Fig. 112.8: A normal punctum.

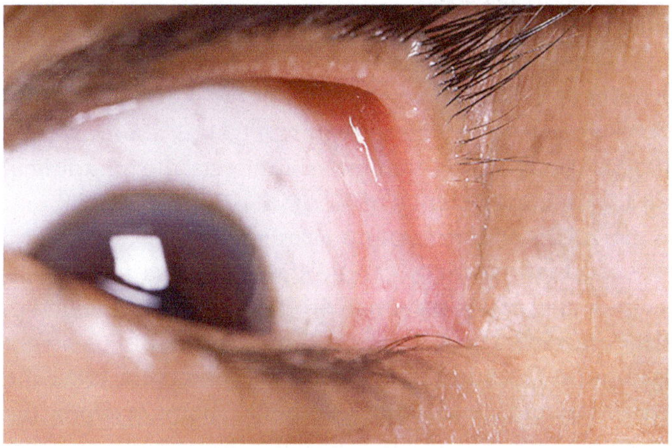

Fig. 112.9: Right upper punctal stenosis.

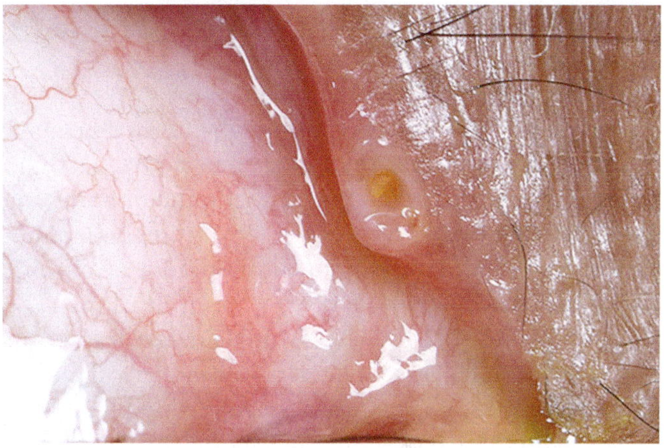

Fig. 112.10: Post-Monoka intubation photograph of the patient in Figure 112.9. Note the well-dilated upper punctum.

Box 112.3: Grades of punctal narrowing.

Grade 0 – Punctal agenesis
Grade 1 – Incomplete punctal canalization (IPC-EM and IPC-IM)
Grade 2 – Stenosis—recognizable but less than normal
Grade 3 – Normal, round punctum (admits 26G canula)
Grade 4 – Slit punctum <2 mm in size

PUNCTAL STENOSIS

Punctal stenosis accounts for 8% of presentations with epiphora and hence is not uncommon.[11] The widespread belief with regards to its etiopathogenesis is chronic inflammation, circumferential fibrosis and subsequent stenosis.[16] Box 112.3 depicts various grades of punctal narrowing. Figure 112.8 demonstrates a normal punctal opening. Most common symptom is epiphora, which can be troublesome. 1–3 snip punctoplasty are commonly used for managing punctal stenosis, however, recent mounting evidence suggests noncutting procedures such as punctal dilatation and use of Monoka stents, to have better functional outcomes (Figs. 112.9 and 112.10).[11,17]

CANALICULITIS

The term canaliculitis usually refers to an acute infection of the canaliculus. It has been reported to account for 2% of lacrimal disorders with a female gender and lower lid preponderance.[18] Common etiological factors include *Staphylococcus* species, *Streptococcus* species, *Actinomyces,* and *Nocardia* species. Common presentations include epiphora, discharge, pain, and swelling over the canalicular areas of the eyelids (Fig. 112.11). Treatment is initially conservative and includes antibiotics and canalicular expression of the retained discharge or concretions. Nonresponsive cases or those with advanced presentations may require surgical modalities in the form of snip punctoplasties or canaliculotomy with canalicular curettage.[18]

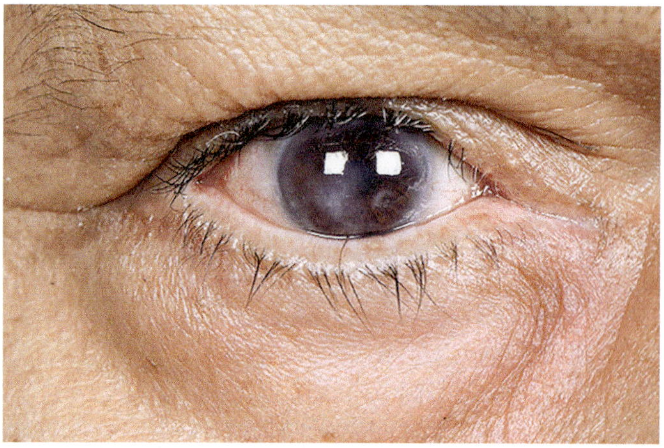

Fig. 112.11: A right-sided upper and lower canaliculitis. Note the medial eyelid swelling and epiphora.

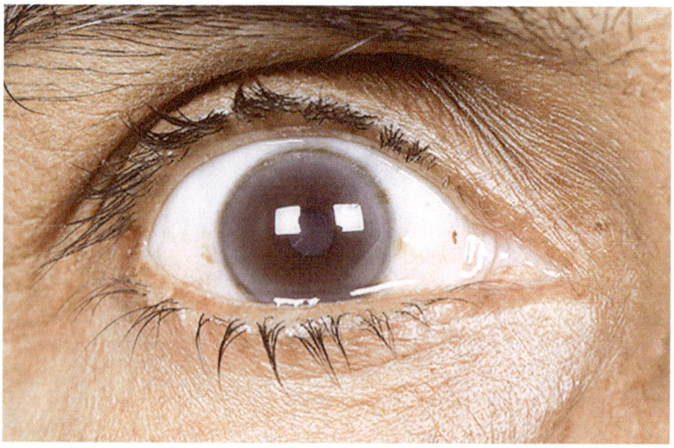

Fig. 112.12: Signs in a case of right-sided primary acquired nasolacrimal duct obstruction.

PRIMARY ACQUIRED NASOLACRIMAL DUCT OBSTRUCTION

Linberg and McCormick coined the term "primary acquired nasolacrimal duct obstruction (PANDO)" in 1986.[19] They described a clinical syndrome of epiphora, usual onset beyond 40 years of age, female preponderance, and if untreated, subsequent development of chronic or acute dacryocystitis and their complications. The etiopathogenesis of PANDO is unclear but numerous factors proposed include infections, hormonal influences, derangement of lacrimal drainage associated lymphoid tissues, anatomical configurations of bony NLD, sinusitis or ascending infections from the nasal cavity, and cavernous body malfunctions.[20] However, the common pathway noted is inflammation, fibrosis, and obstruction of the NLD.

Symptoms of NLD obstruction manifest as epiphora discharge, and excoriation at the medial canthus, with occasional tear fluid induced blurred vision (Fig. 112.12). Continuous dilatation of the lacrimal sac may lead to development of a mucocele, which presents classically as a swelling below the medial palpebral ligament (MPL).

Evaluation should always include a detailed past history, facial examination, periocular and eyelid examination, and ocular surface assessment to determine the cause of epiphora and additional causes other than lacrimal drainage, if any, contributing to it. Lacrimal sac area should be palpated (avoid it or very carefully in acute dacryocystitis) to assess the dilated lacrimal sac or rarely lacrimal sac masses. ROPLAS can indirectly confirming a diagnosis of PANDO or chronic dacryocystitis or lacrimal mucocele. It is important to document the type of the regurgitated material (mucoid, purulent, watery, mucopurulent, or blood stained). Slit-lamp examination of the punctum, canaliculus, and ocular surface is very helpful.

Fluorescein dye disappearance test is a noninvasive diagnostic modality that grossly reflects the anatomical and functional patency of lacrimal drainage system and is useful in pediatric populations (*see* Fig. 112.2). The existing tear meniscus can be stained with a fluorescein strip or alternatively a single drop of the dye is instilled in the conjunctival cul-de-sac and the tear meniscus height is noted at 1, 3, and 5 minutes using a cobalt blue filter. The patient should blink normally without rubbing or wiping the tears. Normal individuals drain away the entire fluorescein from the ocular surface within 5 minutes and any retention beyond this time indicates a possible anatomical or functional obstruction in the outflow pathway. However, it is important to understand that this test is not confirmatory in nature and does not help in differentiating the levels of obstructions.

Lacrimal irrigation and diagnostic probing is the most common clinical investigation performed for the confirmation of NLD obstruction. Following conjunctival anesthesia with suitable topical agents, the patient can lie down or reclined on a chair. It is preferable to use the upper punctum and canaliculus, since that facilitates intrasac irrigation owing to anatomical make up. 24G or 25G straight cannulas are preferable (*see* Fig. 112.6C). Following dilatation with a punctum dilator (*see* Figs. 112.6A and 6B), the cannula is inserted gently into the punctum, vertical and horizontal canaliculus and the on a stretched lid, till a gentle hard stop is felt (*see* Fig. 112.6D). The cannula is retracted by 1–2 mm and gently irrigated, slowly. The fluid passes into the nasal cavity in cases of patent lacrimal systems and regurgitates from the opposite punctum in cases of distal obstructions. The advantage of using straight cannulas is the possibility of simultaneous probing during irrigation.

Nasal endoscopic evaluation (*see* Fig. 112.6G) is an essential part of any PANDO management. Endoscopic examination provides useful clues with regards to associated intranasal pathologies such as deviated septum, concha bullosa, or nasal mucosal diseases, all of which may have bearing on the outcomes of surgery. Imaging modalities such as dacryocystography (DCG), computed tomography (CT)-DCG and magnetic resonance (MR)-DCG are used uncommonly in cases of trauma, suspected mass lesions within the lacrimal system or in the vicinity, and for planning navigation-guided surgeries. Dacryoscintigraphy reflects the functional drainage aspects of the lacrimal drainage but is rarely used in view of its cumbersome nature and with the advent of simpler investigations such as FDDT or dacryoendoscopy.

The most common modality of managing a PANDO is by DCR. Various approaches such as the external, endoscopic endonasal, nonendoscopic endonasal, and transcanalicular laser have been used, however, the external and the standard endoscopic DCRs are more favored. The principle of any DCR is to create an anastomosis between the lacrimal sac and the nasal cavity. A brief discussion of each technique will help the readers in understanding the surgical management better.

External Dacryocystorhinostomy

The two major goals of external DCRs are to make a wide osteotomy and to create a mucosal-lined anastomosis between the nasal cavity and the lacrimal sac.[21] Anesthesia can be local infiltrative or a general anesthesia. The local infiltration includes an infratrochlear, infraorbital, and infiltration over the anterior lacrimal crest (Figs. 112.13A and B). A nasal packing with neuropathies soaked in 2% xylocaine with decongestant of choice (adrenaline, cocaine or xylometazoline or oxymetazoline) is applied. A curvilinear incision is taken just anterior to the surface marking of the anterior lacrimal crest (Fig. 112.13C),

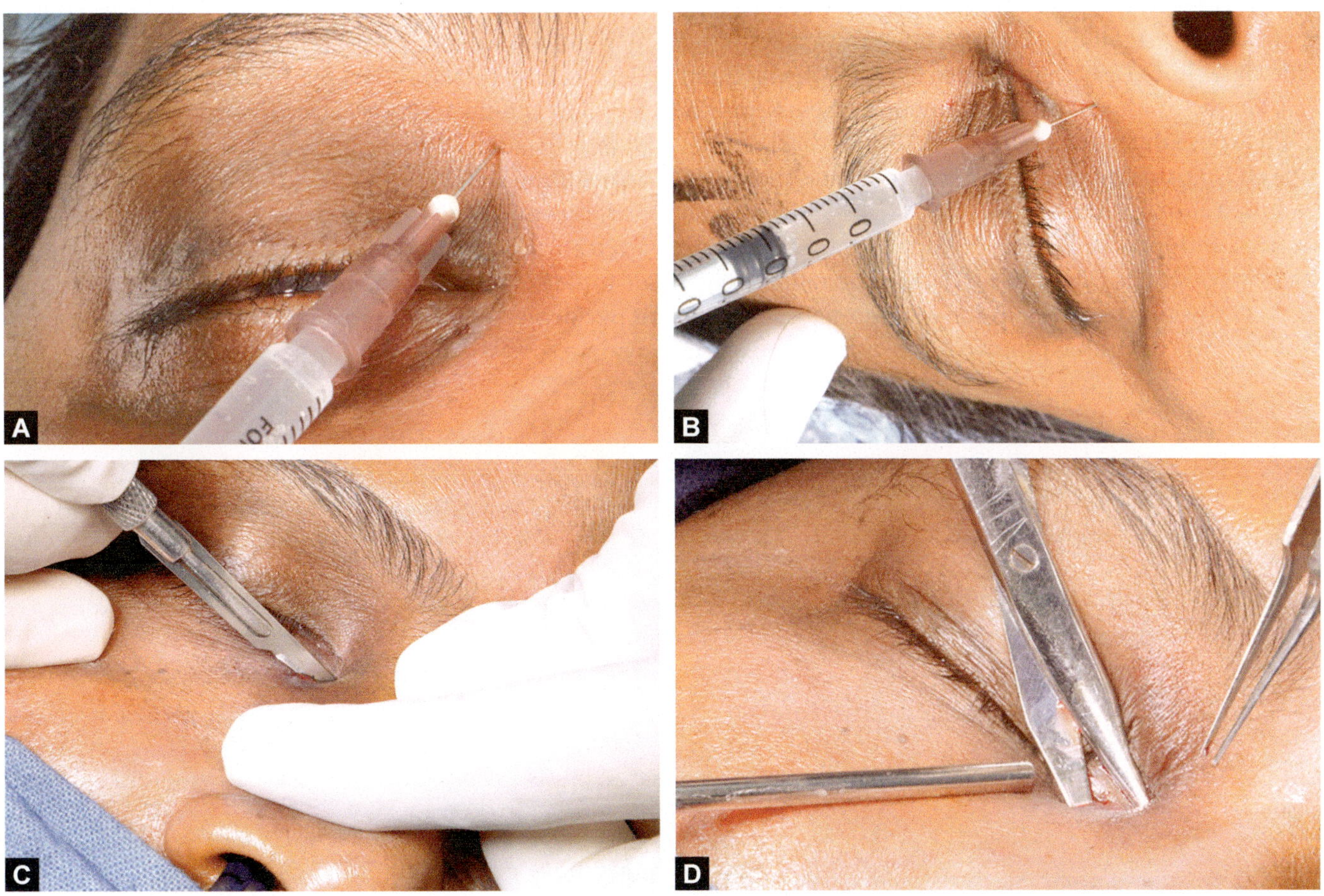

Figs. 112.13A to D

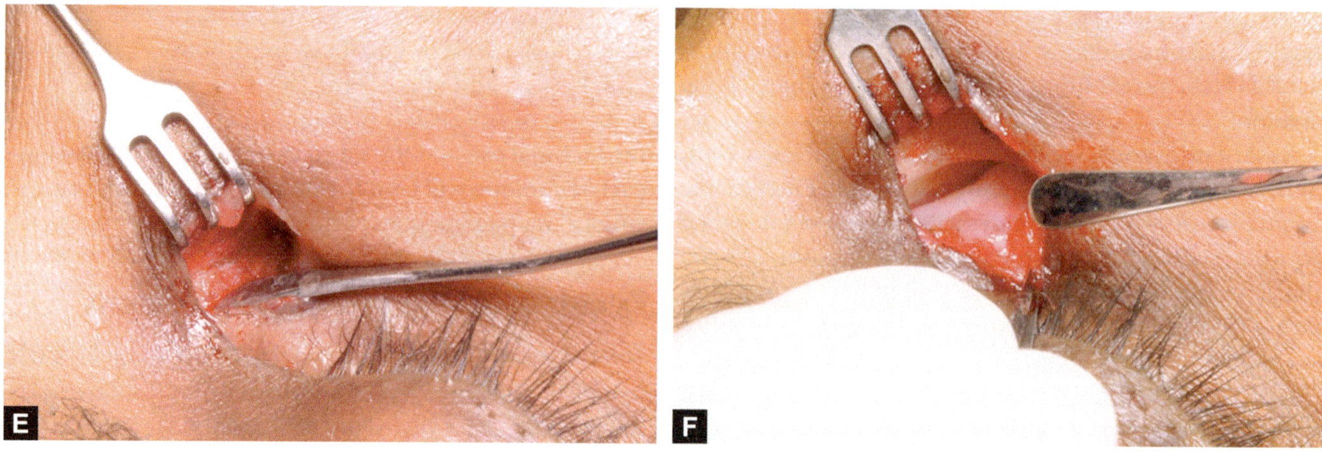

Figs. 112.13E and F

Figs. 112.13A to F: Operative steps of an external dacryocystorhinostomy-I (DCR-I).

orbicularis is dissected (Fig. 112.13D), and a periosteal incision is taken to expose the frontal process of maxilla (Fig. 112.13E). The lacrimal sac along with its fascia is then reflected laterally (Fig. 112.13F). A small opening is made in the thin lacrimal component of the bony fossa (Fig. 112.14A) and serial Kerrison bone punches are used to create a large osteotomy (Fig. 112.14B). The extent of the osteotomy should match the whole length of the lacrimal sac from the fundus to the NLD junction. The osteotomy would expose the taut nasal mucosa. The medial lacrimal sac wall is pushed medially a probe and is incised along the longitudinal sac axis (Fig. 112.14C), followed by a superior and inferior cut to create "H" shaped anterior and posterior flaps (Fig. 112.14D). One can either excise the posterior flap or use both the anterior and posterior flaps for mucosal anastomosis. The nasal mucosa is similarly fashioned in a rectangular shape (Fig. 112.14E). The use of adjuvants such as mitomycin C and intubation (Fig. 112.14F) is controversial but if planned, need to be used at this step.[22,23] The lacrimal sac and nasal mucosal flaps are sutured together with vicryl 6-0 to create a taut anastomosis (Fig. 112.14G). The orbicularis and the skin are approximated by sutures (of surgeon's choice) (Fig. 112.14H). Nasal packing is performed in a gentler way and is only anterior packing to soak any blood. The patient is advised oral antibiotics (controversial)[24] and anti-inflammatory drugs. Next day, the Merocel® pack is removed from the nasal cavity and the patient is advised with regards to wound dressing and the use of topical antibiotic-steroid combination. Intubation, if performed is best removed at 4 weeks as per current evidence.[25,26]

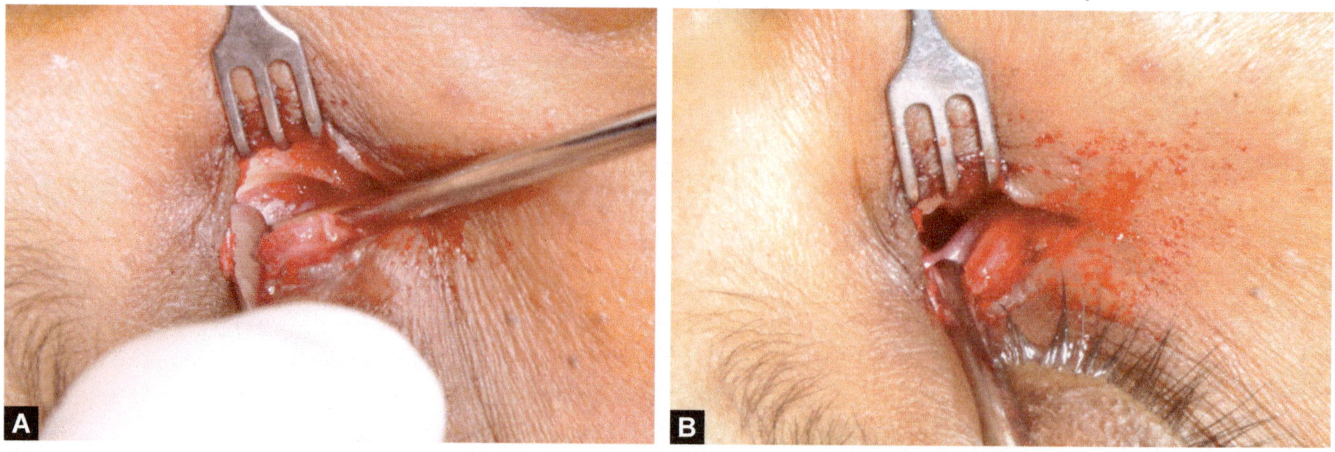

Figs. 112.14A and B

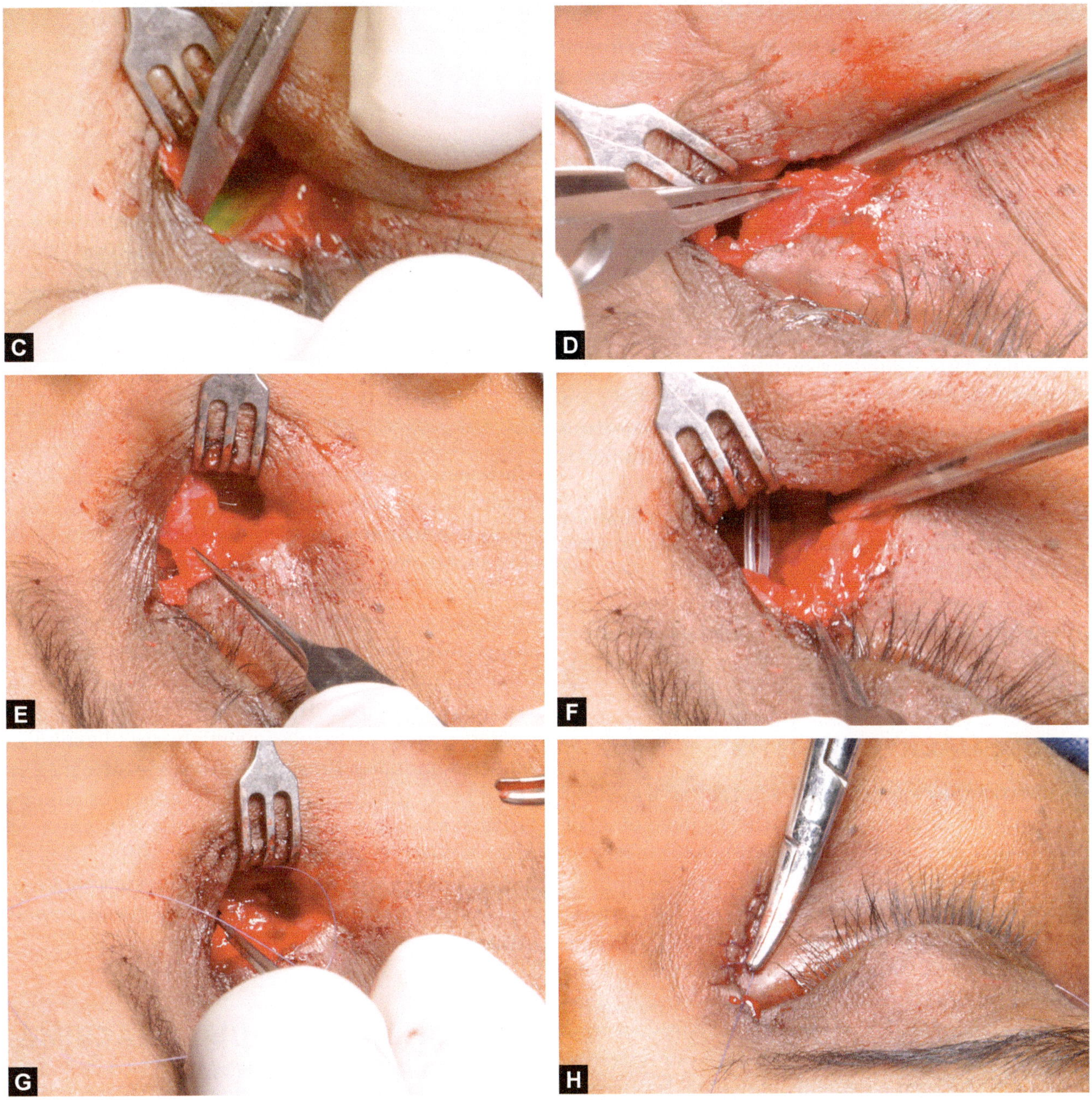

Figs. 112.14C to H

Figs. 112.14A to H: Operative steps of an external dacryocystorhinostomy-II (DCR-II).

Endoscopic Dacryocystorhinostomy

The principle of an endoscopic DCR remains the same as an external DCR but the technique is inside out![27,28] A local infiltration anterior to the axilla of the middle turbinate is performed followed by nasal packing as in external DCR. A horizontal incision of 10–12 mm is taken at about 8–10 mm above and in front of the axilla of the middle turbinate. From the anterior end of horizontal incision, a vertical one is taken down to the junction of upper two-thirds and lower one-third of the middle turbinate and taken backwards towards the middle turbinate to reflect a rectangular flap. These incisions may vary based on specific anatomical variants. Once the flap is reflected, the frontal process of maxilla is exposed. A periosteum elevator is used to make a small opening into the lacrimal bone just like in external DCR. The endoscopic Kerrison bone punches are used to create the osteotomy to facilitate complete exposure of the lacrimal sac from the fundus to the NLD junction. The exposure of agger nasi is a good landmark for the fundus of lacrimal sac. The medial lacrimal sac wall is then pushed with a probe and the medial wall is incised along its longitudinal axis with relaxing cuts at the superior and inferior ends to create "H" shaped anterior and posterior flaps. Adjuvants such as mitomycin C and intubation, if needed are used at this stage. The flaps are then reflected like an open book on to the lateral wall of the nasal cavity and the nasal mucosal flap created is trimmed, in such a way that the nasal mucosal and lacrimal sac flaps approximate each other for a whole 360º. This facilitates a 360º approximation of mucosae and facilitates a primary intention healing thereby resulting in large patent ostia.[27,28] The postoperative management remains the same as that of an external DCR. Both the approaches have excellent result and the choice is based on surgeon's comfort and patient's wish.

ACUTE DACRYOCYSTITIS

Acute dacryocystitis was defined by Ali et al.[29] as "a medical urgency which is clinically characterized by rapid onset of pain, erythema, and swelling, classically below the medial canthal tendon with or without preexisting epiphora mainly resulting from the acute infection of the lacrimal sac and perisac tissues". The common sequences of events that occur include NLD obstruction, followed by stagnation of tear fluids, bacterial overgrowth, and an acute infection. In one of the largest series on acute dacryocystitis over two decades, its prevalence was noted to be 2.4% of all lacrimal disorders, encountered commonly in the 3rd–5th decade of life with a female and unilateral preponderance. The common etiological factors isolated include *Staphylococcus aureus, Streptococcus* species, *Haemophilus influenzae, Pseudomonas aeruginosa* and *Escherichia coli*.[30] Patients usually complain of swelling and pain in the lacrimal sac area with or without past history of epiphora. A tender distended lacrimal sac with induration below the medial canthal tendon is usual (Fig. 112.15). There may be a regurgitation of purulent material either from the punctum or from a spontaneous fistula. Occasionally, patients may have constitutional symptoms like fever and malaise.

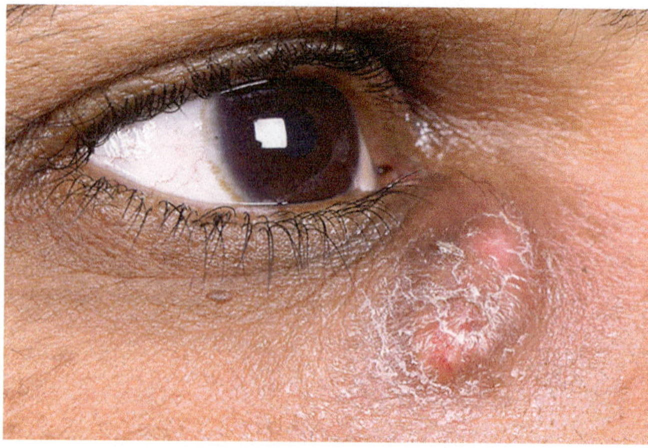

Fig. 112.15: A right-sided acute dacryocystitis with evolving lacrimal abscess.

Untreated case may present with complications, which commonly includes orbital cellulitis, orbital abscess, and rarely may manifest as cavernous sinus thrombosis, vision loss, meningitis, and necrotizing fasciitis.[29,31]

The treatment initially is *conservative and include* warm compresses, oral antibiotics and anti-inflammatory drugs. Advance presentation may need admission and intravenous medications.[29,31] Antibiotics are guided initially by empirical treatment based on geographical microbial isolates and subsequently by specific culture and sensitivity profiling. The surgical modalities of management could be incision and drainage in cases presenting with lacrimal or orbital abscess or DCR following conservative management. Evidence is mounting with regards to the benefits of performing an endoscopic DCR in an acute stage and has been reported to decrease the morbidity and quicken the patient recovery with good outcomes even at long-term.[32,33]

SECONDARY ACQUIRED LACRIMAL DUCT OBSTRUCTION

The term "secondary acquired lacrimal duct obstruction (SALDO)" was described by Bartley[34] to include five classes of secondary causes of lacrimal duct obstructions. In this spectrum, specific causes can be identified and if treatment strategies are used in a targeted manner, these can help in either recanalization or improved symptomatology. The five categories of SALDO include inflammatory, infectious, mechanical (Fig. 112.16), traumatic, and neoplastic with each category having multiple disorders.[34,35] Box 112.4 describes the common etiological factors under each category of SALDO.

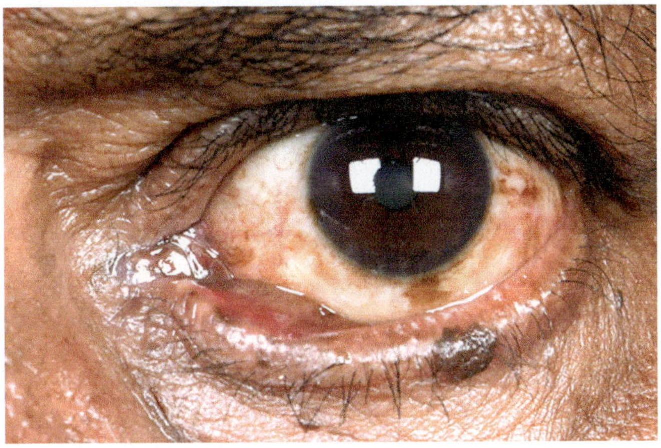

Fig. 112.16: Example of a mechanical secondary acquired lacrimal duct obstruction.

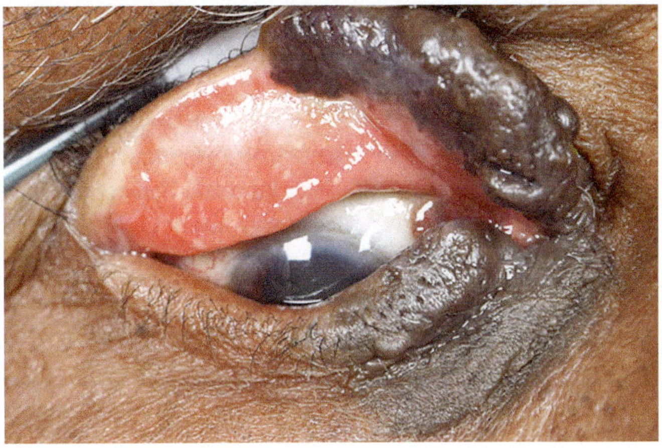

Fig. 112.17: Gross punctal and peripunctal involvement by a nevus.

Box 112.4: Common etiological factors in SALDO.

- **Infectious SALDO**
  - Punctal abscess
  - Canaliculitis
  - Acute viral dacryocystitis
- **Inflammatory SALDO**
  - Allergies
  - Stevens-Johnson syndrome
  - Cicatrical pemphigoid
  - Burns
  - Chemotherapy drugs such as 5FU and paclitaxel
  - Antiviral and antiglaucoma medications
- **Mechanical SALDO**
  - Conjunctivochalasis
  - Caruncular masses
  - Dacryoliths
  - Migrated punctal plugs
  - Compressive sinus mucoceles
- **Traumatic SALDO**
  - Soft tissue trauma
  - Bony trauma
  - Iatrogenic trauma like during probing, intubation, sinus surgeries
- **Neoplastic SALDO**
  - Primary malignancies like papillomas, squamous carcinoma and melanoma
  - Secondary malignancies from adjacent infiltration of basal cell, squamous and sebaceous carcinomas
  - Metastatic

(SALDO: Secondary acquired lacrimal duct obstruction)

TUMORS OF THE LACRIMAL DRAINAGE SYSTEM

The involvement of the lacrimal drainage system by tumors is rare but notorious for delayed presentations, local spread, and metastasis because of the intricate anatomy. The proximal lacrimal system is usually affected by benign tumors like nevi involving the punctum or canalicular papillomas (Fig. 112.17). Lacrimal sac is the most common site for primary malignancies. Box 112.5 lists the commonly encountered malignancies. Clinical symptoms that should raise suspicion include bloody epiphora, partial or complete obstruction of lacrimal drainage, and a medial canthal swelling, which may not necessarily be below the medial canthus.[36] A contrast-enhanced CT or MRI with or without additional DCG are very useful investigations that aid in diagnosis. A careful incision biopsy with histopathology and immunohistochemistry are confirmatory.[37] Management depends on the type of malignancy, local spread, and disease staging. Surgical options include a complete dacryocystectomy or extended dacryocystectomy with various combinations (depending on the tumor and its spread) such as medial maxillectomy, lateral wall rhinotomy, and orbital exenteration.[37,38] In addition, the role of radiotherapy and chemotherapy is important and decided based on the type of tumor.

Box 112.5: Commonly encountered lacrimal drainage malignancies.

- Inflammatory, transitional and squamous papillomas
- Transitional cell carcinoma
- Squamous cell carcinoma
- Non-Hodgkin's lymphomas
- Adenoma and adenocarcinomas
- Malignant melanona
- Secondary invasion by tumors from orbit, sinuses and periocular skin
- Metastasis from head and neck tumors

QUALITY OF LIFE AND LACRIMAL DRAINAGE DISORDERS

Lacrimal disorders are known to have negative emotional, social, and economic impacts and hence only treatment of these disorders in not enough. Numerous scales have been used to assess the impact of lacrimal disorders on the quality of life and include general ones like the "Glasgow Benefit Inventory questionnaire" and specific ones like the "Holmes questionnaire", "NLDO symptom score", and the "LAC-Q scales".[39] Although, each have their advantages and disadvantages, the take home message is that the social and emotional aspects of lacrimal diseases can be measured objectively and the improvement in them can be monitored after the desired interventions.[40]

REFERENCES

1. Macewen CJ, Young JD. Epiphora during the first year of life. Eye (Lond). 1991;5(Pt 5):596-600.
2. Kamal S, Ali MJ, Gauba V, et al. Congenital nasolacrimal duct obstruction. In: Ali MJ (Ed). Principles and Practice of Lacrimal Surgery. New Delhi: Springer; 2015. pp. 117-32.
3. Paediatric Eye Disease Investigator Group. Resolution of congenital nasolacrimal duct obstruction with nonsurgical management. Arch Ophthalmol. 2012;130(6):730-4.
4. PEDIG. Primary treatment of nasolacrimal duct obstruction with probing in children less than four years. Ophthalmology. 2008;115(3):577-84.
5. Ali MJ, Kamal S, Gupta A, et al. Simple versus complex congenital nasolacrimal duct obstruction: etiology, management and outcomes. Int Forum Allergy Rhinol. 2015;5(2):174-7.
6. Gupta A, Kamal S, Ali MJ, et al. Buried probe in complex congenital nasolacrimal duct obstruction: clinical profiles and outcomes. Ophthal Plast Reconstr Surg. 2015;31(4): 318-20.
7. Kamal S, Ali MJ, Gupta A, et al. Lacrimal and nasal masquerades of congenital nasolacrimal duct obstruction: etiology, management and outcomes. Int Ophthalmol. 2015;35(6):807-10.
8. Ali MJ, Psaltis AJ, Brunworth J, et al. Congenital dacryocele with large intranasal cysts. Efficacy of cruciate marsupialization, adjunctive procedures and outcomes. Ophthal Plast Reconstr Surg. 2014;30(4):346-51.
9. Ali MJ, Naik MN, Honavar SG. Balloon dacryoplasty: ushering the new and routine era in minimally invasive lacrimal surgeries. Int Ophthalmol. 2013;33(2):203-10.
10. Ali MJ, Paulsen F. Syndromic and non-syndromic systemic associations of congenital lacrimal drainage anomalies: a major review. Ophthal Plast Reconstr Surg. 2017;33(6): 399-407.
11. Ali MJ. Disorders of the upper lacrimal system. In: Ali MJ (Ed). Principles and Practice of Lacrimal Surgery. New Delhi: Springer; 2015. pp. 103-16.
12. Lyons CJ, Rosser PM, Welham RAN. The management of punctal agenesis. Ophthalmology. 1993;100(12):1851-5.
13. Ali MJ, Mohapatra S, Mulay K, et al. Incomplete punctal canalization: The external and internal punctal membranes. Outcomes of membranotomy and adjunctive procedures. Br J Ophthalmol. 2013;97(1):92-5.
14. Ali MJ, Mishra DK, Naik MN. Histopathology and immunophenotyping of congenital lacrimal (anlage) fistulae. Ophthal Plast Reconstr Surg. 2016;32(1):17-9.
15. Chaung JQ, Sundar G, Ali MJ. Congenital lacrimal fistula: a major review. Orbit. 2016;35(4):212-20.
16. Ali MJ, Mishra DK, Baig F, et al. Punctal stenosis: histopathology, immunology and electron microscopic features: a step towards unraveling the mysterious etio-pathogenesis. Ophthal Plast Reconstr Surg. 2015;31(12): 98-102.
17. Ali MJ, Ayyar A, Naik MN. Outcomes of rectangular 3-snip punctoplasty in acquired punctal stenosis: is there a need to be minimally invasive? Eye (Lond). 2015;29(4):515-8.
18. Kaliki S, Ali MJ, Honavar SG, et al. Primary canaliculitis: clinical features, microbiological profile, and management outcome. Ophthal Plast Reconstr Surg. 2012;28(5):355-60.
19. Linberg JV, McCormick SA. Primary acquired nasolacrimal duct obstruction: a clinicopathologic report and biopsy technique. Ophthalmology. 1986;93(8):1055-63.
20. Paulsen F. The human nasolacrimal ducts. Adv Anat Embryol Cell Biol. 2003;170:1-106.
21. Ali MJ, Naik MN, Honavar SG. External dacryocystorhino-stomy: tips and tricks. Oman J Ophthalmol. 2012;5(3):191-5.
22. Feng YF, Yu JG, Shi JL, et al. A meta-analysis of primary external dacryocystorhinostomy with and without mitomycin C. Ophthalmic Epidemiol. 2012;19(6):364-70.
23. Sarode D, Bari DA, Cain AC, et al. The benefit of silicone stents in primary endonasal dacryocystorhinostomy: a systematic review and meta-analysis. Clin Otolaryngol. 2017;42(2):307-14.
24. Ali MJ, Ayyar A, Motukupally SR, et al. Bacteremia during dacryocystorhinostomy: results of intraoperative blood cultures. J Ophthalmic Inflamm Infect. 2014;4:27-30.
25. Ali MJ, Psaltis AJ, Ali MH, et al. Endoscopic assessment of the dacryocystorhinostomy ostium after powered endoscopic surgery: behaviour beyond 4 weeks. Clin Exp Ophthalmol. 2015;43(2):152-5.
26. Murphy J, Ali MJ, Psaltis AJ. Biofilm quantification on nasolacrimal silastic stents after dacryocystorhinostomy. Ophthal Plast Reconstr Surg. 2015;31(5):396-400.
27. Ali MJ, Psaltis AJ, Bassiouni A, et al. Long-term outcomes in primary powered endoscopic dacryocystorhinostomy. Br J Ophthalmol. 2014;98(12):1678-80.
28. Ali MJ, Psaltis AJ, Murphy J, et al. Outcomes in primary powered endoscopic dacryocystorhinostomy: comparison between experienced versus less experienced surgeons. Am J Rhinol Allergy. 2014;28(6):514-6.
29. Ali MJ, Joshi SD, Naik MN, et al. Clinical profile and management outcome of acute dacryocystitis: two decades of experience in a tertiary eye care center. Semin Ophthalmol. 2015;30(2):118-23.
30. Ali MJ, Motukupally SR, Joshi SD, et al. The microbiological profile of lacrimal abscess: two decades of experience from a tertiary eye care center. J Ophthalmol Inflamm Infect. 2013;3:57-61.

31. Ali MJ. Pediatric acute dacryocystitis. Ophthal Plast Reconstr Surg. 2016;31(5):341-7.
32. Kamal S, Ali MJ, Pujari A, et al. Primary powered endoscopic dacryocystorhinostomy in the setting of acute dacryocystitis and lacrimal abscess. Ophthal Plast Reconstr Surg. 2015;31(4):293-5.
33. Chisty N, Singh M, Ali MJ, et al. Long-term outcomes of powered endoscopic dacryocystorhinostomy in acute dacryocystitis. Laryngoscope. 2016;126(3):551-3.
34. Bartley GB. Acquired lacrimal drainage obstruction: an etiologic classification system, case reports, and a review of the literature. Part 1. Ophthal Plast Reconstr Surg. 1992;8(4):237-42.
35. Bartley GB. Acquired lacrimal drainage obstruction: an etiologic classification system, case reports and a review of literature. Part 2. Ophthal Plast Reconstr Surg 1992;8(4): 243-9.
36. Sundar G. Tumors of the lacrimal drainage system. In: Ali MJ (ed). Principles and Practice of Lacrimal Surgery. New Delhi: Springer; 2015. pp. 319-26.
37. Pujari A, Ali MJ, Mulay K, et al. The black lacrimal sac: a clinicopathological correlation of a malignant melanoma with anterior lacrimal crest infiltration. Int Ophthalmol. 2014;34(1):111-5.
38. Ali MJ. Dacryocystectomy: goals, indications, techniques and complications. Ophthal Plast Reconstr Surg. 2014;30(6):512-6.
39. Ali MJ. Quality of life in lacrimal disorders and patient satisfaction following management. In: Ali MJ (Ed). Principles and Practice of Lacrimal Surgery. New Delhi: Springer; 2015. pp. 359-62.
40. Ali MJ, Iram S, Ali MH, et al. Assessing the outcomes of powered endoscopic dacryocystorhinostomy in adults using the lacrimal symptom (Lac-Q) questionnaire. Ophthal Plast Reconstr Surg. 2017;33(1):65-8.

Chapter 113 Congenital Disorders of the Eyelid, Orbit, and Adnexa

Jessica R Chang

INTRODUCTION

The purpose of this chapter is to provide ophthalmologists with an overview that will guide the diagnosis, treatment, and counseling of patients with congenital disorders of the eyelids, orbit, and adnexa. Careful observation and an appropriate index of suspicion, based on a solid foundation of knowledge are needed for diagnosis of many syndromes. Body size and proportion, gait and posture, head size and shape, anomalies of scalp hair, ear position, and skeletal deformities may often be more revealing than the findings of a detailed ophthalmic examination. Familiarity with the constellation of physical findings associated with a syndrome facilitates detection of subtle pathology.

Anomalies may result from direct damage to the ocular or adnexal tissues during embryologic development, whether mechanical (such as amniotic bands) or chemical (teratogens), or from chromosomal anomalies or specific gene mutations. Many ophthalmic signs and symptoms occur as early or late complications of the disturbed anatomy in the surrounding structures. The problems manifested by this latter group of signs are not static but change with the growth of the skull and facial bones. Not only will treatment depend on the pathology detected at the initial examination but it will also include preventive therapy for anticipated pathologic conditions that may occur in future months or years.

The first part of this chapter will describe the various findings in congenital eyelid, orbital, and lacrimal conditions, as well as specific congenital tumors. Several of these findings are repeatedly observed in patients with specific systemic and craniofacial syndromes. A comprehensive description of all such syndromes is beyond the scope of this chapter but the relatively common conditions with significant ophthalmic findings are reviewed, and some of the less common syndromes are summarized in Table 113.1.

EYELID

Ablepharon is a rare congenital absence of eyelids, and may be associated with cryptophthalmos, in which the eye is abnormal but present under the skin, or with ablepharon-macrostomia syndrome, where the eye is exposed.[1] Fraser syndrome may include cryptophthalmos, as well as syndactyly and genitourinary anomalies (Table 113.1). Microblepharon (small eyelids with vertical shortening) may be associated with anophthalmos (Fig. 113.1), in which no eye is present. Ankyloblepharon (Fig. 113.2A) refers to the persistent fusion of the upper and lower eyelids, which normally separate by 7 months gestation.[1] Broad or fine strands are treated with surgical separation of the eyelids; the underlying eye may or may not be normal.

Epiblepharon is a very common finding in otherwise normal healthy children, often of east Asian descent and most often affecting the lower eyelid (Figs. 113.3A and B). A horizontal fold of skin causes the eyelashes to be turned inwards and to contact the cornea. In infancy, this is usually well tolerated, and the condition usually resolves spontaneously as the child's face grows but surgical repair may be needed if there is ocular surface irritation or injury.[2] In contrast, congenital entropion with true inversion of the eyelid margin is much less common and always requires surgical intervention.

Distichiasis is a separate condition in which another row of eyelashes emerges from the posterior lamella, at the level of the meibomian gland orifices. When congenital, this finding may be sporadic or autosomal dominant, in conditions such as lymphedema-distichiasis syndrome.[3] If causing ocular surface irritation or injury, the involved lashes may be removed (through electrolysis, cryotherapy, etc.) but if extensive, the entire eyelid margin must be rotated with tarsotomy.

In euryblepharon, the width of the lower eyelid is greater than average, with a characteristic downward curve of the

Table 113.1: Ophthalmic findings in congenital syndromes.

Syndrome	Etiology	Ophthalmic features	Non-ophthalmic features
Cri-du-chat syndrome	Sporadic; deletion on short arm of chromosome 5	Downslanting palpebral fissures, epicanthal folds, strabismus, hypertelorism, and iris colobomas	Weak, high-pitched cry, moon facies, hypoplastic mandible, low-set ears, and intellectual disability
Rubinstein-Taybi syndrome	Autosomal dominant	Downslanting palpebral fissures, epicanthal folds, strabismus, ptosis, and nasolacrimal duct obstruction	Intellectual disability, broad thumbs, great toes, short stature, microcephaly, and beaked nose with broad nasal bridge
Marden-Walker syndrome	Autosomal recessive	Blepharophimosis, strabismus, and deep-set eyes	Muscular hypotonia, joint contractions, micrognathia, cleft palate, and kyphoscoliosis
Whistling face syndrome (Freeman-Sheldon syndrome and craniocarpotarsal dysplasia)	Autosomal dominant and rarely recessive (more severe)	Epicanthal folds, strabismus, blepharophimosis, ptosis, and down-slanting fissures	Microstomia sometimes requiring tracheostomy, flat face, equinus-varus-supine clubfoot, flexion contractions of figures, and paramedian grooves from lip to chin
Waardenburg syndrome	Autosomal dominant	Dystopia canthorum (telecanthus) usually with normal interpupillary distance, blepharophimosis, laterally displaced inferior punctal, confluent brows, iris heterochromia from hypoplasia, microphthalmia, ptosis, and retina pigmentary changes	Hypopigmentation of hair and skin (white forelock), sensorineural deafness, cleft palate/lip, nasal hypoplasia, and skeletal anomalies
De Lange syndrome	Sporadic	Confluent eyebrows, long curly eyelashes, optic atrophy, telecanthus, and high myopia	Low birthweight, dysphagia, gastroesophageal reflux disease, severe intellectual disability, brachycephaly, hirsutism, and low-set ears and short forehead
Smith-Lemli-Opitz syndrome	Autosomal recessive defect in 7-dehydrocholesterol reductase (7-DHC)[44]	Epicanthal folds, ptosis, strabismus, cataract, hypertelorism, optic atrophy, downslanting palpebral fissures, iris deformities, retinal pigment defects, and nystagmus	Microcephaly, intellectual disability, cleft palate, broad nasal tip with antiverted nostrils, cardiac defects, micrognathia, anomalies of male genitalia, and polydactyly and syndactyly
Blepharonasofacial syndrome (Pashayan syndrome)	Autosomal dominant	Primary telecanthus, lateral displacement and stenosis of puncta, nasolacrimal duct obstruction, downslanting palpebral fissures, blepharophimosis, and strabismus	Intellectual disability, midface hypoplasia, prominent nose, hypotonia, mask-like facies, and torsion dystonia
Craniometaphyseal dysplasia	Autosomal dominant or recessive	Optic atrophy, hypertelorism, and exophthalmos	Skull hyperostosis with obliteration of sinuses, narrowing of foramina, broad flat nose, and abnormal bones
Osteopetrosis (Albers-Schönberg syndrome)	Autosomal recessive or dominant (less severe)	Exophthalmos, optic atrophy, and cranial nerve palsies	Dense thickened brittle bones with encroachment on marrow causing anemia, hepatosplenomegaly, and raised intracranial pressure
Rieger syndrome (oligodontia and primary mesodermal dysgenesis of the iris)	Autosomal dominant	Posterior embryotoxon, iris, angle and corneal defects, telecanthus, strabismus, and glaucoma	Brachycephaly, prognathism, hypodontia, oligodontia, microdontia, and umbilicus abnormalities
Lowe syndrome (oculocerebral renal syndrome)	X-linked recessive	Cataract, glaucoma, nystagmus, and malformations of the anterior chamber or angle	Renal tubular dysfunction, hypotonia, growth retardation, skeletal anomalies, and intellectual disability
Edwards syndrome	Trisomy 18	Ptosis, epicanthal folds, corneal and lens opacities, glaucoma, and optic atrophy	Intellectual disability, polyhydramnios, intrauterine growth restriction, hyper-tonicity, flexion contraction of fingers, rocker-bottom foot, cardiac anomalies, low-set ears, and small mouth

Contd...

Contd...

Syndrome	Etiology	Ophthalmic features	Non-ophthalmic features
Turner syndrome	XO	Ptosis, epicanthal folds, hypertelorism, glaucoma, corneal and lens opacities, blue sclera, few have red-green color blindness, and strabismus	Genital anomalies, pterygium colli, cubitus valgus, hearing deficiencies, and peripheral lymphedema
Weill Marchesani syndrome	Autosomal dominant or recessive	Microspherophakia, refractive error, and pupillary block glaucoma	Brachydactyly, small stature, broad skull, and dental anomalies
Cockayne syndrome	Autosomal recessive	Exophthalmos, retinal pigmentary degeneration, optic atrophy, and cataract	Cachexia, microcephaly, dwarfism, sensorineural deafness, premature aging, intracranial calcification, and intellectual impairment
Chondrodystrophia punctata	Autosomal dominant or X-linked dominant (Conradi-Hünermann-Happle syndrome)	Upward slanting palpebral fissures, cataract, hypertelorism, and optic atrophy	Malar hypoplasia, flat facies, punctate calcification in vertebral bones and epiphyses, and saddle nose
Laurence-Moon-Biedl syndrome	Autosomal recessive	Retinitis pigmentosa, ptosis, nystagmus, epicanthus, strabismus, iris coloboma, and optic atrophy	Obesity, polydactyly, syndactyly, genital hypoplasia, and mental impairment
Fraser syndrome	Autosomal recessive	Cryptophthalmos	Syndactyly, respiratory, genital, and urinary tract anomalies
Wildervanck syndrome	Autosomal dominant with incomplete penetrance, 10:1 female:male	Duane retraction syndrome	Deafness, vertebral anomalies (Klippel-Feil anomaly), and variably ear deformities, facial asymmetry, short stature, intellectual disability, and cleft palate

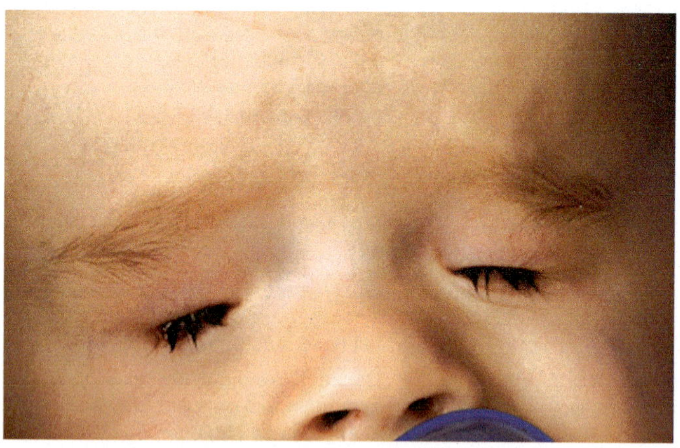

Fig. 113.1: Bilateral anophthalmos and microblepharon.
Source: Dr. Shannon Joseph, University of Michigan, Ann Arbor, USA.

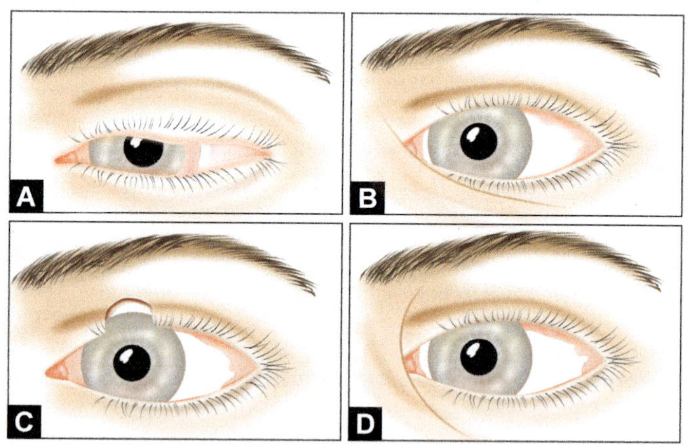

Figs. 113.2A to D: *Diagrams of eyelid anomalies*: (A) Ankyloblepharon; (B) Epicanthus inversus; (C) Eyelid coloboma; (D) Epicanthus superciliaris.

eyelid margin in the lateral half of the lower lid (Fig. 113.3C). The lateral canthus, however, is not displaced downwards. Most patients are otherwise normal and asymptomatic, but it may also be a feature in syndromes, such as Kabuki syndrome. Congenital ectropion is a separate disorder in which the lower eyelid is everted due to vertical tension from a shortage of skin, as in ichthyosis, and requires surgical treatment.[1] Another rare condition is congenital tarsal kink, usually presenting as a fold in the upper eyelid. Like ectropion, this may cause exposure keratopathy and often requires surgical intervention.

Other characteristic eyelid skin folds commonly seen in young children cover part of the medial canthus and are collectively called epicanthal folds. These include epicanthus tarsalis (a fold extending over the superior eyelid, Figures 113.3A and B), epicanthus palpebralis (a fold extending equally over the superior and inferior eyelids, Figure 113.3D) and epicanthus superciliaris

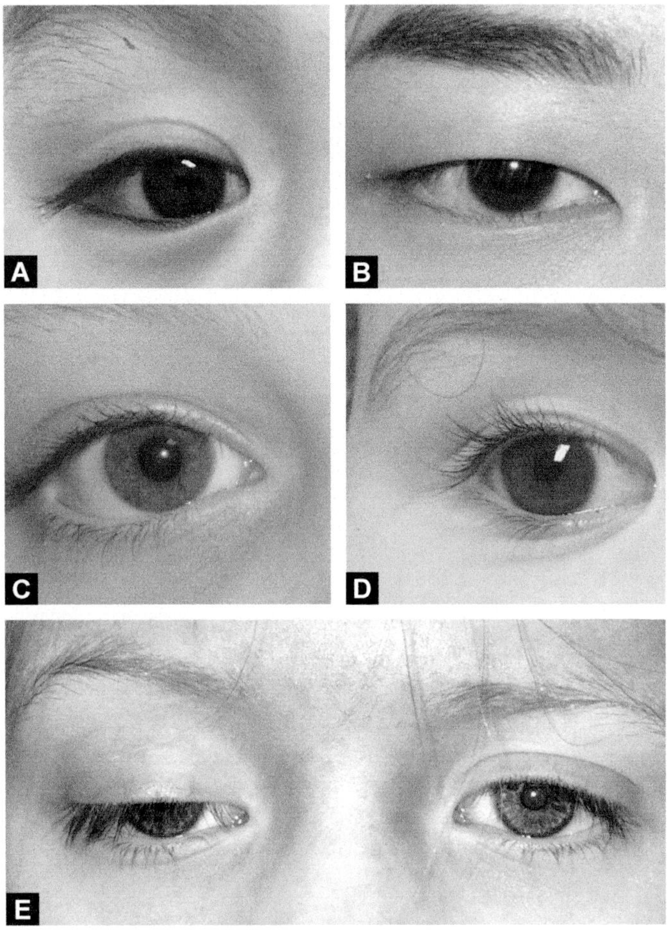

Figs. 113.3A to E: *Photographs of eyelid anomalies*: (A and B) Varying degrees of epicanthus tarsalis and epiblepharon; (C) Euryblepharon; (D) Epicanthus palpebralis; (E) Congenital ptosis right upper eyelid with characteristic lack of eyelid crease and compensatory frontalis overaction.
Source: Dr Timothy J McCulley, Wilmer Eye Institute, Baltimore, USA.

(a fold extending from the lower eyelid to the eyebrow, Figure 113.2D). These do not usually require intervention, although they may be associated with pseudo-esotropia. Epicanthus inversus (a fold extending predominantly across the lower eyelid, Figure 113.2B) is a characteristic finding in blepharophimosis syndrome, and can be addressed with Z-plasty or similar procedures.

Eyelid coloboma refers to a congenital absence of a portion of the eyelid; the etiology is thought to be similar to other facial clefts, or from amniotic bands (Fig. 113.2C).[1] The upper eyelid is more often involved in Goldenhar syndrome, and the lower eyelid may be involved in Treacher Collins syndrome. Severity varies from a small notch or focal absence of lashes to complete absence of an eyelid. Surgical repair is often needed, and there may be associated astigmatism, exposure, or other ocular abnormalities.

Congenital blepharoptosis is relatively common (as high as 0.18% in some studies) and may be sporadic, familial, or associated with syndromes such as Noonan or Smith-Lemli-Opitz syndrome (Fig. 113.3E).[1,4] Most commonly there is congenital fibrosis or underdevelopment of the levator palpebralis, which may affect one or both eyes, but a thorough history and examination is needed to evaluate for other causes of ptosis in an infant: Congenital Horner's syndrome is usually associated with anisocoria, iris heterochromia, and birth trauma, but an acquired Horner's syndrome is also possible in a child, due to trauma, infection, vascular malformation, or neoplasm (such as neuroblastoma). Marcus-Gunn jaw-winking, or congenital trigemino-oculomotor synkinesis, is another etiology that can be elicited with proper history and clinical examination. Monocular elevation deficiency (previously known as double elevator palsy) describes hypotropia related to inferior rectus restriction and associated true or pseudoptosis. Congenital fibrosis syndrome includes ptosis and variable ophthalmoplegia related to defective innervation of the muscles; it is also called congenital fibrosis of the extraocular muscles, and has autosomal dominant and recessive forms. Congenital third nerve palsy will also demonstrate abnormal motility. Mechanical ptosis may result from congenital lesions such plexiform neurofibroma or capillary hemangioma.[2]

Intervention for congenital ptosis depends on the etiology and the severity. Even relatively mild ptosis may cause astigmatism therefore cycloplegic refraction and monitoring for amblyopia is required. Depending on levator function, age, and etiology, frontalis sling, levator advancement, or mullerectomy can be performed.[2]

The angle of the palpebral fissures, or the height of the lateral versus medial canthus, is another feature commonly affected in craniofacial syndromes. In Caucasians the palpebral fissure usually assumes a nearly horizontal position, while in East Asians the outer canthus may be higher than the inner canthus, producing an upward slant of the palpebral aperture. Patients with Down syndrome and Conradi syndrome often have such an upward slant.

A downward slanting lateral canthus may occur secondary to a local anomaly of the lateral canthal ligament or may be associated with skeletal malformations of the face. The most striking example occurs in mandibulofacial dysostosis (Treacher-Collins syndrome, Fig. 113.4), but it is also found in other syndrome complexes (e.g. cri du chat and Rubinstein-Taybi syndromes). In these patients, the fissure position is related to the hypoplastic or absent malar bones and poorly developed zygomatic arches.

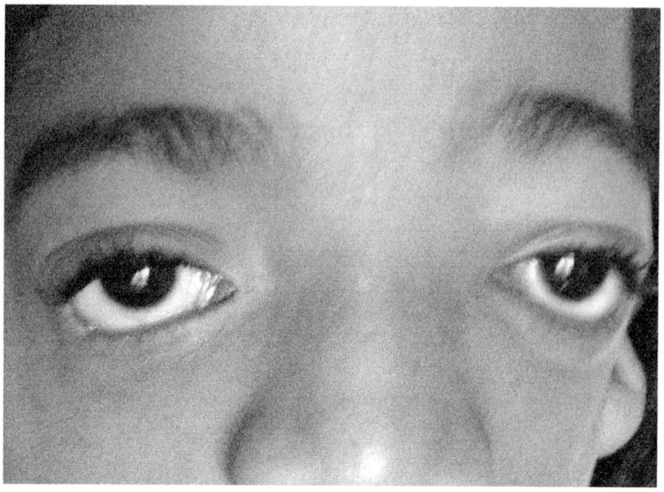

Fig. 113.4: Mandibulofacial dysostosis (Treacher-Collins syndrome).

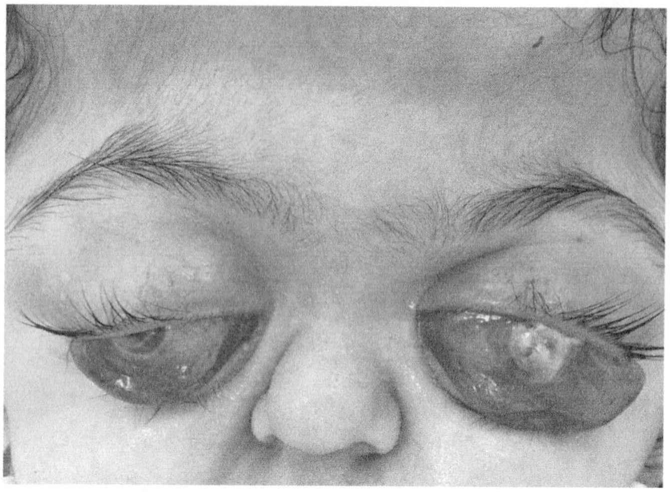

Fig. 113.5: Exophthalmos and severe exposure keratopathy in the setting of craniosynostosis.

ORBIT

Anophthalmos and the more common microphthalmos are often associated with impaired orbital development. Microphthalmos refers to a malformed eye (unlike nanophthalmos where the eye is formed but small); microphthalmic eyes are usually smaller than normal eyes but can be associated with a cyst (also known as colobomatous cyst) that can grow to be as large as or even larger than a normal eye. Sometimes this can be helpful to promote orbital development, as otherwise the bony orbit will also tend to be smaller than average, but the abnormal eye and cyst often need to be surgically removed.

In craniosynostosis syndromes, the bony orbit may be relatively small in volume despite normal globe size, leading to exophthalmos, also described as proptosis or exorbitism—forward protrusion of the globe relative to the orbit. With severe proptosis, the eyelids cannot cover the globe leading to exposure keratopathy (Fig. 113.5) and sometimes even globe luxation (where the globe equator is anterior to the eyelids). In addition to influencing the volume of the bony orbit, craniofacial disorders can also impact their relative orientation; for example, rotation of the bony orbit contributes to V-pattern strabismus in Apert syndrome by altering the usual alignment of extraocular muscles. Another metric is the distance between the orbits (usually measured as distance between the medial walls of the orbit)—many syndromes show increased distance, or hypertelorism. Abnormally decreased distance between the orbits, hypotelorism is found in conditions such as holoprosencephaly spectrum disorders. Hypertelorism is usually associated with telecanthus, with greater than average distance between the medial canthi and also between the lateral canthi, and it may also be detected by measuring the interpupillary distance.[5,6] Lateral displacement of the medial canthi is also known as dystopia canthorum, a specific finding in Waardenburg syndrome.[7]

LACRIMAL SYSTEM

By far the most common congenital abnormality is congenital nasolacrimal duct obstruction (NLDO), occurring in 5% of full-term newborns. Most often the obstruction is an imperforate valve of Hasner, and approximately 70% resolve spontaneously by 12 months. Affected infants have tearing and mucus discharge; initial treatment is lacrimal sac massage, and some patients require probing or other surgical intervention. Severe forms of NLDO may be associated with congenital dacryocele (also called dacryocystocele), a distended lacrimal sac presenting as a swelling below the medial canthal tendon. The stagnant mucus and tears in the sac can become infected leading to dacryocystitis, which is treated with systemic antibiotics and sometimes probing to decompress the sac contents. The differential for a dacryocele includes meningocele/encephalocele (which are more likely to bulge above the medial canthal tendon or cause proptosis), hemangiomas, and dermoid cysts.

The proximal portion of the lacrimal system can also have congenital anomalies, such as punctal atresia—a failure of the punctum to form. In mild forms there may be just a membranous covering that can be opened with simple puncture and dilation, with or without stenting. It is also possible to have extra or supernumerary puncta, which is usually asymptomatic. Congenital lacrimal fistula occurs when the tear drainage system connects to the surface of the skin via an epithelialized tract usually extending from the common canaliculus or the sac. This tract will have discharge, if there is NLDO; and if there is discharge even with a patent normal drainage route, the fistula tract requires surgical excision.

Several syndromes have associated lacrimal drainage system anomalies, including Down syndrome, ectrodactyly-ectodermal dysplasia-clefting (EEC), mandibulofacial dysostosis, Rubinstein-Taybi, and several other syndromes (*see* Table 113.1).[8]

CONGENITAL TUMORS

Hamartomas are abnormal proliferations of tissue in the organs where that tissue type is usually found. Neurocutaneous syndromes or phakomatoses include several disorders that involve hamartomas of the skin and the central nervous system. Neurofibromatosis (NF) type 1 and 2 are both autosomal dominant disorders with high penetrance, but there is also a high rate of sporadic cases. Up to 4% of NF1 patients may have plexiform neurofibroma, which involves the orbit and upper eyelid, causing characteristic S-shape deformity and enlargement of the surrounding soft tissue (Figs. 113.6A to C), and associated glaucoma in half of cases. Treatment is difficult and often requires several surgeries to address ptosis and debulk the tumor.[9] Another orbital finding

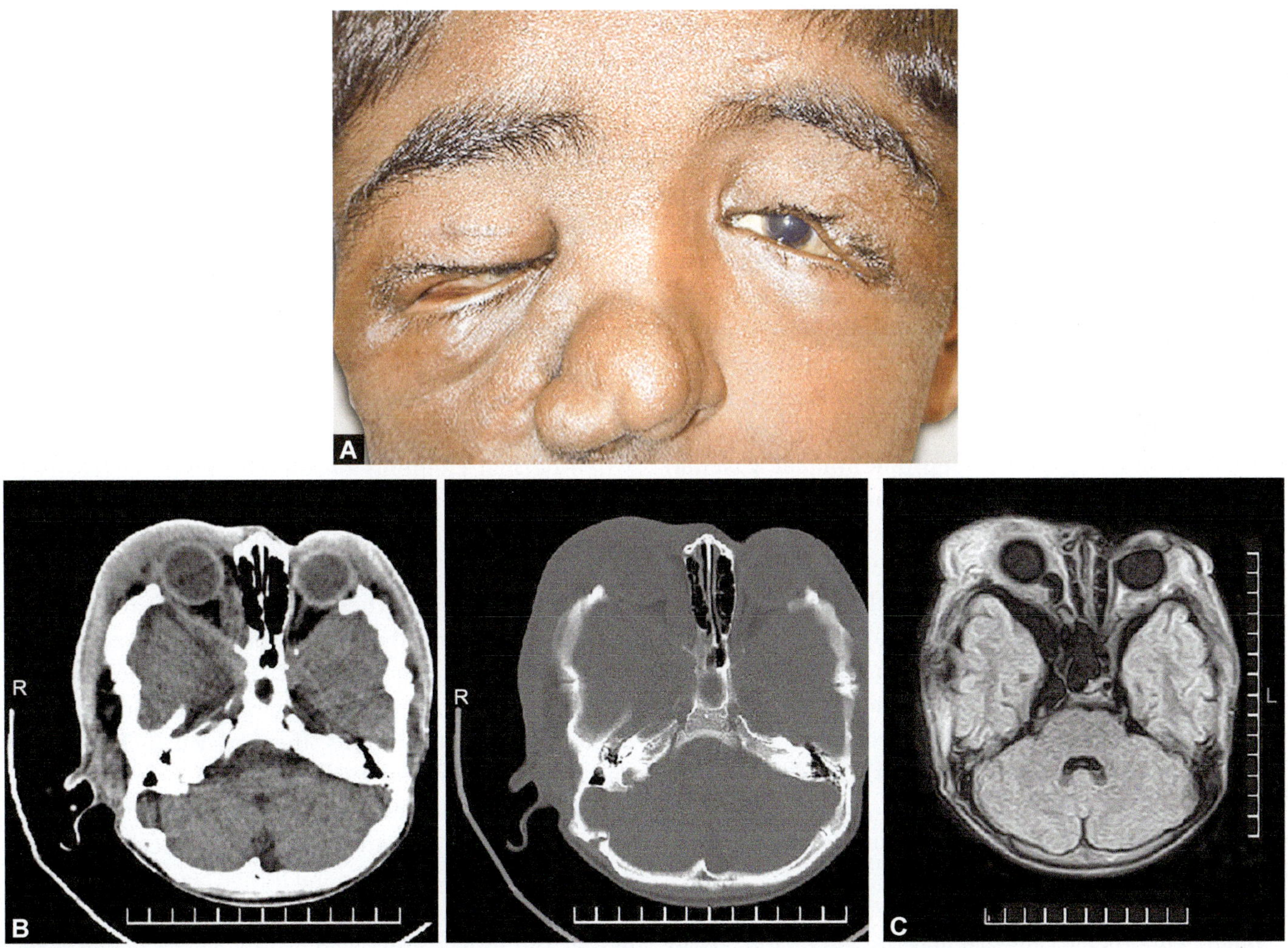

Figs. 113.6A to C: (A) Bilateral plexiform neurofibroma in a patient with neurofibromatosis type 1. CT images (B) demonstrate characteristic bony changes such as sphenoid dysplasia; MRI image (C) highlights the soft tissue tumor.

(CT: Computed tomography; MRI: Magnetic resonance imaging)

Source: Dr Mahesh Kumar, Aravind Eye Hospital, Madurai, Tamil Nadu, India.

associated with NF1 is sphenoid wing dysplasia, causing pulsatile proptosis. Optic nerve glioma is another tumor that can be associated with NF1, causing proptosis, optic neuropathy, and if there is extension to the chiasm, hydrocephalus, hypopituitarism, and other morbidity. Treatment is challenging, and includes chemotherapy, radiation, and surgical resection.[9] NF2 is less common and is characterized by acoustic neuromas, meningiomas, schwannomas, gliomas, and posterior subcapsular cataracts in addition to neurofibromas.

Congenital melanocytic (nevocellular) nevi are usually large patches of hyperpigmented, thickened skin that may cause amblyopia when present on the eyelids. Larger lesions (>20 cm projected size in adulthood) carry risk of malignant transformation, although lesions of any size may show atypia on biopsy, and often have extracutaneous extension, along nerves, vessels, and other subcutaneous structures.[10] Oculodermal melanocytosis (nevus of Ota) is a melanocytic hamartoma that presents with slate-gray coloration of the sclera, increased intraocular pigment, and hyperpigmentation of the eyelids and surrounding skin without thickening. It carries an increased risk of glaucoma and melanoma, and is most common in Asian populations.[11]

Port-wine stain (nevus flammeus, a cutaneous vascular malformation) is a common finding, occurring in approximately 1 in 300 births, usually located on the head. When present in the ophthalmic distribution of the trigeminal nerve, there is up to 26% chance of having encephalofacial angiomatosis (Sturge–Weber syndrome), which includes ipsilateral leptomeningeal vascular malformation that cause seizures and other neurologic deficits. Encephalofacial angiomatosis is not inherited, unlike other phakomatoses. A somatic mutation in *GNAQ* causes isolated port-wine stain and also encephalofacial angiomatosis, depending on the developmental timing and location.[12] The soft tissue and bone underlying the port-wine stain is often hypertrophied. Ipsilateral glaucoma and diffuse choroidal hemangioma are common, especially when the lesion involves the upper eyelid. Port-wine stains are also a feature of Proteus syndrome, along with macrodactyly, cranial exostoses, and other bone, soft tissue, and skin hamartomatous tumors.[13]

Capillary hemangiomas are common hamartomas of capillary endothelial cells that may present on the face or elsewhere in up to 3% of full-term infants and more often in low birthweight infants.[14] Periocular hemangiomas may induce deprivational or anisometropic amblyopia; treatment involves topical or systemic beta blockers, or local or systemic steroids; spontaneous regression begins after 1 year of age. Kassabach-Merritt syndrome describes sequestration of platelets in extensive hemangioma-like lesions (kaposiform hemangioendothelioma or tufted angioma) leading to thrombocytopenic coagulopathy.[15] When hemangioma covers more than one dermatome, think of PHACES (*p*osterior fossa malformations, *h*emangiomas, *a*rterial anomalies, *c*oarctation of aorta, cardiac defects, *e*ye abnormalities, and *s*ternal clefting/supraumbilical raphe syndrome).[16] If an infant has more than three apparent hemangiomas, consider multifocal infantile hemangioma (diffuse neonatal hemangiomatosis) or multifocal lymphangioendotheliomatosis with thrombocytopenia, which can be fatal due to visceral lesions and heart failure.[17] Hemangiopericytoma is another orbital hamartoma of pericytes that can manifest with gradual proptosis; while usually benign, malignant transformation is possible.

Lymphangioma is a lymphatic vascular malformation that may cause intermittent proptosis by enlarging during systemic infections or because of intralesional hemorrhage. Other congenital vascular malformations include venous malformations (varix), some of which are associated with intracranial arteriovenous malformations.[18]

Choristomas are collections of normal tissue outside of their normal location. The most common choristoma of the orbit is the dermoid cyst (Fig. 113.7A), which occurs when dermal elements become entrapped, usually in suture lines resulting in lesions in the superotemporal or superonasal orbit, sometimes trapped within the actual bony sutures.[19]

Teratomas occur when all three germinal layers are present in a tumor; these rarely present in the orbit but may cause significant proptosis. Limbal dermoid tumors are also hamartomas but distinct from dermoid cysts, and often present on the limbus. They are usually keratinized and may have dermal elements like hair and fat; they may cause irritation and astigmatism and can be shaved down. Lipodermoids are lesions on the ocular surface, usually located in the temporal fornix, covered by normal conjunctiva (Fig. 113.7B). They consist of fat and connective tissue, and unlike prolapsed orbital fat the lesion is not mobile. Both epibulbar limbal dermoids and lipodermoids are associated with Goldenhar syndrome.

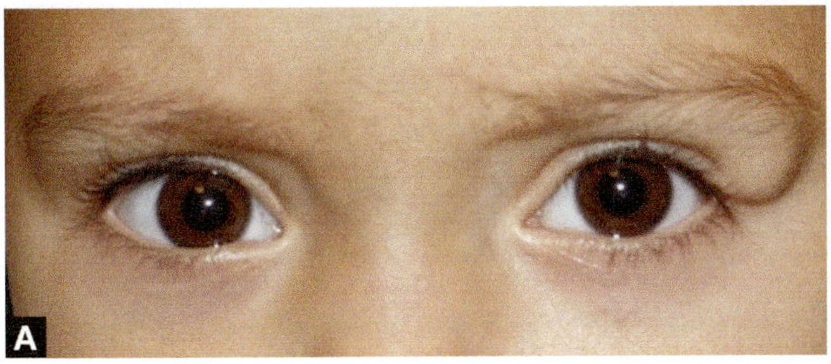

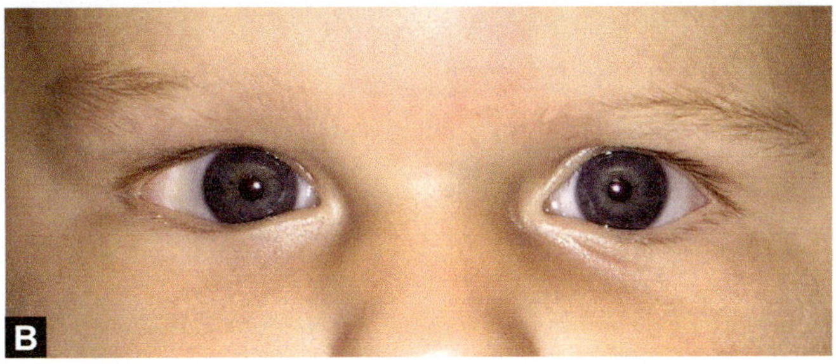

Figs. 113.7A and B: (A) Orbital dermoid in the left zygomaticofrontal suture; (B) Right lipodermoid on the temporal bulbar conjunctiva and asymmetry of lateral canthi and palpebral fissure width.
Source: Dr Timothy J McCulley, Wilmer Eye Institute, Baltimore, USA.

REVIEW OF SPECIFIC SYNDROMES

Down syndrome is a common condition (1 in ~1500 live births) with a characteristic appearance marked by upward-slanting palpebral fissures, epicanthal folds, broad nasal bridge, and low-set ears;[20] other ophthalmic findings include nasolacrimal obstruction, blepharitis, cataract, keratoconus, and strabismus. Systemically, affected patients have hypotonia, brachycephaly, short stature, "simian" crease on palms, developmental delay, and some may have cardiac abnormalities and increased risk of Alzheimer's disease.[21]

Blepharophimosis describes a condition with shortening of both horizontal and vertical dimensions of the eyelids. Blepharophimosis syndrome is autosomal dominant and includes blepharophimosis, ptosis, and epicanthus inversus (*See* diagrams of epicanthal folds, Fig. 113.2B). Telecanthus, or abnormally wide distance between the medial canthi, is another finding common in blepharophimosis syndrome. Type I also includes premature ovarian insufficiency and type II requires only the ophthalmic findings. Fetal alcohol syndrome is the most common cause of blepharophimosis, and may also be associated with strabismus, and optic nerve or retinal abnormalities.[1,22] Affected patient characteristically have a broad or absent philtrum, flat midface, and low nasal bridge.[23]

Ectodermal dysplasia encompasses over 100 inherited nonprogressive syndromes affecting tissues derived from ectoderm. Patients often have dry thickened skin with loss of sweat glands and hair follicles. In EEC syndrome, absence of the meibomian orifices has been observed in a number of cases.[24] Ophthalmic findings often include severe blepharitis with secondary thickening of the eyelids, loss of cilia, and recurrent corneal pathology. Many patients tolerate severe symptoms without complaint and are reluctant to accept the necessity of lifelong attention to eyelid hygiene and medication. Systemic findings beyond skin changes include abnormal nails, teeth, and disorders of the respiratory and genitourinary tracts.

CRANIOSYNOSTOSIS SYNDROMES

Synostosis refers to abnormal closure of the bony sutures, which leads to deformities of the skull. Involvement of the coronal or lambdoidal suture prevents growth in the anteroposterior axis, leading to a wide skull (brachycephaly). A high skull (oxycephaly and acrocephaly) results from coronal suture closure, which is usually associated with involvement of the other sutures. If the sagittal suture alone fuses prematurely, the skull assumes a long, narrow appearance (scaphocephaly, Figs. 113.8A to G). Asymmetric involvement of the sutures results in a condition termed plagiocephaly.

Crouzon syndrome may be autosomal dominant or sporadic. Although cranial abnormality may be present at birth, the signs may not become fully apparent until the first few years of life. A variety of sutures may be affected. With extensive sutural synostosis, increased intracranial pressure may result in neurologic deficits, mental retardation, and optic nerve damage. Exophthalmos is frequent and often severe, leading to corneal complications and, in a few patients, to spontaneous luxation of the eye (*see* Fig. 113.5). Strabismus is usually present: a V-pattern exotropia with overacting inferior oblique muscles. Hypertelorism is another characteristic finding, along with maxillary hypoplasia, parrot-beak nose, and highly arched palate.[25,26]

In 1906, Apert described the association of misshapen skull and syndactyly of the hands and feet, utilizing the term acrocephalosyndactyly.[27] Most cases of Apert syndrome occur sporadically but rarely it may be autosomal dominant. The characteristic findings include irregular,

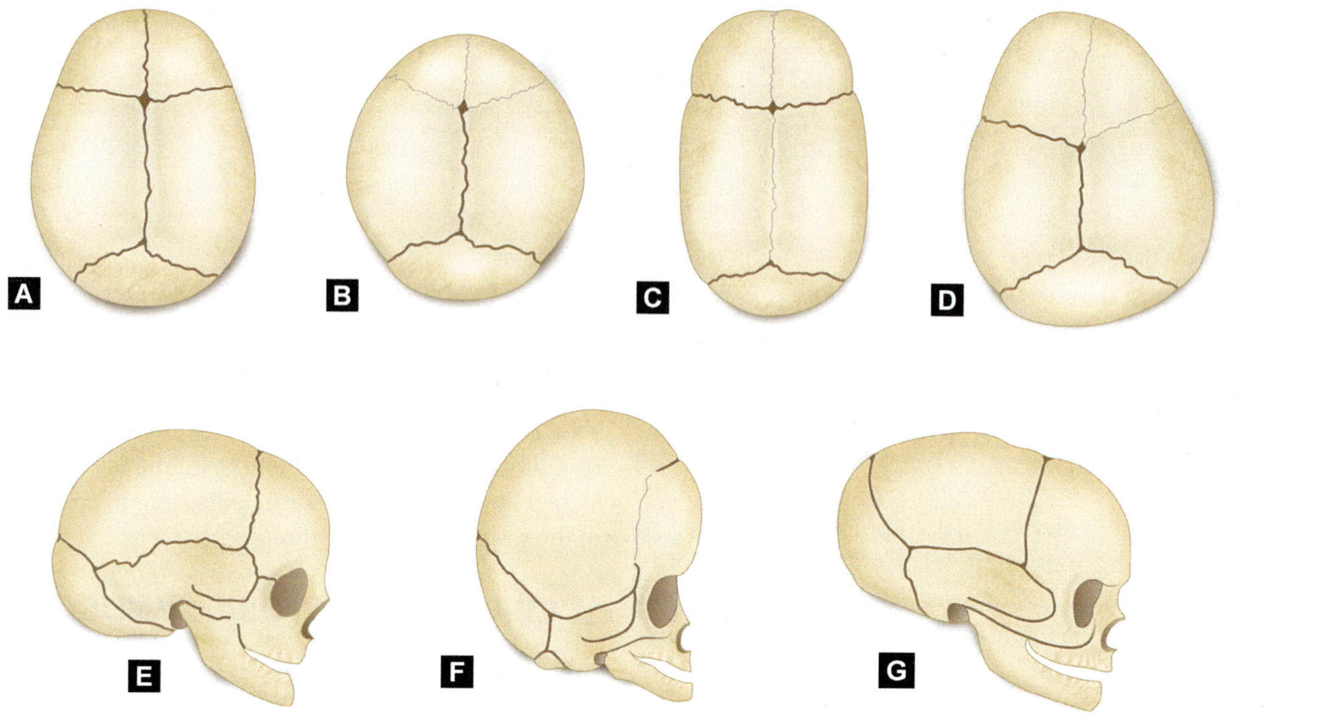

Figs. 113.8 A to G: *Craniosynostosis*: (A) Superior view of cranial sutures with normal morphology: metopic and coronal sutures join at the anterior fontanelle, sagittal and lambdoid sutures join at the posterior fontanelle; (B) Fusion of coronal sutures results in widening of the skull as growth proceeds parallel to the remaining sutures; (C) Fusion of sagittal sutures results in elongation of the skull; (D) Asymmetric fusion of sutures causing plagiocephaly; (E) Side view of normal skull morphology, showing the sphenoid fontanelle between the coronal and parietotemporal sutures, and posterolateral fontanelle between lambdoidal and parietotemporal sutures; (F) Brachycephaly with coronal suture fusion; (G) Side view of scaphocephaly from sagittal suture fusion.

premature closure of the cranial sutures resulting in a broad (brachycephalic) head with the high point near the junction of the coronal and sagittal sutures (bregma). There is a prominent forehead, often with transverse grooves over the eyebrow in the young child, as well as ptosis, proptosis, and downward slanting lateral canthi. Inadequate lid protection of the eye predisposes to corneal complications. Other features include a hypoplastic maxilla, highly arched palate, hypertelorism, and low-set ears. Hearing is often affected. Like Crouzon syndrome, most patients show a V-pattern exotropia on upgaze but on down there may be esotropia. Raised intracranial pressure (ICP) is less common than in Crouzon but also may occur, with or without papilledema and optic atrophy. Other ophthalmic findings include keratoconus, ectopic lens, congenital glaucoma, high astigmatism, pigmentary disturbances of the retina, tortuous retinal vessels, staphyloma, nystagmus, and eccentric pupils.[28,29]

Acrocephalosyndactyly also includes Carpenter (Figs. 113.9A and B), Pfeiffer, and Saethre-Chotzen syndromes, which manifest craniosynostosis and deformities of the extremities. Patients with Saethre-Chotzen syndrome do not manifest the marked maxillary hypoplasia that is so prominent in Apert syndrome.[30,31]

FIRST AND SECOND BRANCHIAL ARCH SYNDROMES

A number of syndromes involve structures derived from the first and second branchial arches: predominantly unilateral anomalies such as hemifacial microsomia (hemifacial hypoplasia) or oculoauriculovertebral spectrum (Goldenhar syndrome); and invariably bilateral syndromes such as mandibulofacial dysostosis (Treacher-Collins syndrome) or oculomandibulodyscephaly (Hallermann-Streiff syndrome).

Patients with hemifacial microsomia may demonstrate microtia (small ears), failure of formation of the mandibular ramus and condyle, and macrostomia. Branchial pits and ear tags are common. The palpebral fissure on the affected side is smaller and lower. Severity varies widely—from mild asymmetry to microphthalmia or anophthalmia in

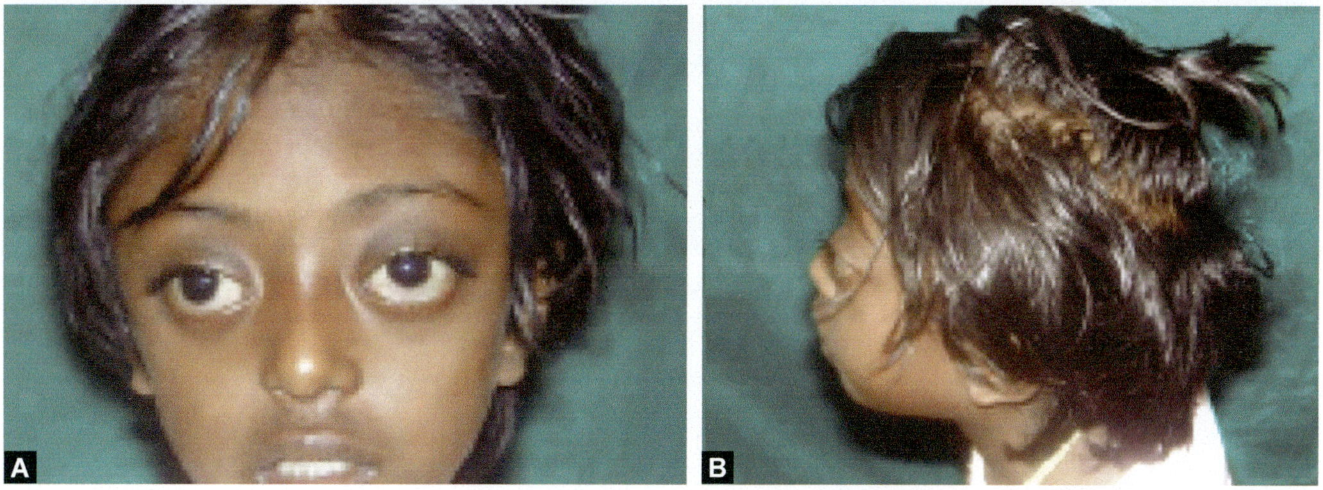

Figs. 113.9A and B: Carpenter syndrome with bilateral exophthalmos.
Source: Dr Mahesh Kumar, Aravind Eye Hospital, Madurai, Tamil Nadu, India.

the more severe cases. Often the anomalies involve not only the first and second branchial arch derivatives but also the visceral and skeletal structures. Most cases occur sporadically, although examples of familial inheritance have been reported. Interestingly the right side of the face is more often involved.[32,33]

Goldenhar syndrome, the severe manifestation of oculoauriculovertebral spectrum disorder, describes patients with hemifacial microsomia, epibulbar dermoids and/or lipodermoids, and vertebral anomalies.[34] Epibulbar dermoids are present in 75% of affected patients, and may be bilateral in up to 25% of patients. They are usually at the inferotemporal limbus. Lipodermoids are less frequent, and are located subconjunctivally some distance from the limbus in the temporal quadrants. Upper lid colobomas occur in nearly 25% and are rarely bilateral. Less frequently reported anomalies include microphthalmia, cataract, iris anomalies, decrease in corneal sensation, and anophthalmia. Patients with Goldenhar syndrome may also have cardiac and kidney defects, as well as fused vertebrae.[35]

Mandibulofacial dysostosis is also known as Treacher-Collins syndrome or Franceschetti (Franceschetti-Zwahlen-Klein) syndrome.[36,37] The disorder shows a very wide range of expressivity and involves structures primarily derived from the first branchial arch (*see* Fig. 113.4). The complete form is characterized by (1) coloboma of the lower lid; (2) hypoplasia of the malar bone and mandible; (3) downward slanting palpebral fissures; (4) large mouth (macrostomia), highly arched palate, and anomalies of dentition; (5) malformations of the external and middle ear; and (6) atypical hairline with projections toward the cheek. They share features of Pierre Robin sequence, such as micrognathia, glossoptosis, cleft palate, and dental abnormalities. The condition is almost always bilateral, and genetic transmission is autosomal dominant. Aside from eyelid colobomas, which may cause astigmatism or exposure requiring repair, patients have good vision and require little ophthalmic intervention. Infants may have breathing and feeding difficulties, and lacrimal drainage abnormalities may exist as well.[38]

The Hallermann-Streiff syndrome (also known as oculomandibulodyscephaly or Francois syndrome) is a rare sporadic syndrome that involves frequent and severe eye defects and poor vision.[39-41] Patients frequently have microphthalmia, congenital cataracts, microcornea, downward slanting fissures, iris and chorioretinal atrophy, optic disc coloboma, and vitreous opacities. Nonophthalmologic findings include dwarfism (nanism), mandibular hypoplasia, dyscephaly (malformation of head and face), beaked nose, hypotrichosis or alopecia (decreased hair), dental anomalies, and atrophy of the skin. Normal intelligence and life expectancy can be expected in the majority of patients.

SYNDROMES WITH LATERAL RECTUS DYSFUNCTION

Duane syndrome is a relatively common type of strabismus, usually sporadic and affecting the left more often than the right. The classic picture was described by Duane in 1905, consisting of limitation of abduction and a narrowing of the fissure with retraction and up-shoot or down-shoot of the

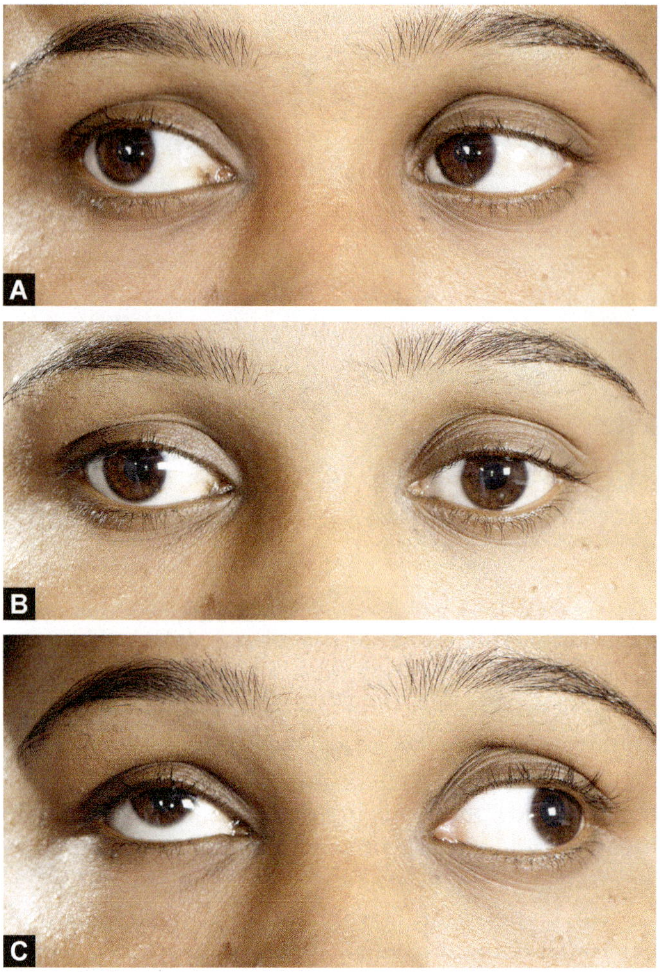

Figs. 113.10A to C: *Duane syndrome*: (A) Right eye demonstrates limitation of attempted abduction and widening of palpebral fissure in right eye on right gaze; (B) Right exotropia in primary gaze; (C) Up-shoot on attempted adduction with retraction and narrowing of the right palpebral fissure, while the left eye movements are intact.

Source: Dr P Vijayalakshmi, Aravind Eye Hospital, Madurai, Tamil Nadu, India.

eye on adduction (Figs. 113.10A to C). Electromyographic data suggest that there is a paradoxic innervation with co-contraction of the medial and lateral rectus muscles on adduction. Duane syndrome has been associated with an increasingly wide variety of anomalies and syndromes, including: Smith-Lemli-Opitz syndrome and Wildervanck syndrome (cervical-ocular-acoustic dysmorphia), Klippel-Feil anomaly of the neck, Goldenhar syndrome, deafness, nevus of Ota, Brown tendon sheath syndrome, microcornea, and iris flocculi.[42]

Mobius syndrome (congenital facial diplegia) classically involves congenital paralysis of the sixth and seventh cranial nerves due to aplasia or hypoplasia of the nuclei, although the exact etiology remains unknown. The mask-like facial appearance is characteristic, although the facial nerve paresis is incomplete, affecting the muscles of the lower face less severely. The ocular muscle findings characteristically include limitation not only in abduction but also in adduction, though to a lesser extent. Medial rectus function may be better in convergence than in ductions. Vertical muscle movements are usually normal, as is Bell's phenomenon. A large number of patients with Mobius syndrome also show malformations of the limbs and oral structures.[43]

REFERENCES

1. Dollfus H, Verloes A. Dysmorphology and the orbital region: a practical clinical approach. Sur Ophthalmol. 2004;49(6):547-61.
2. Lin LK, Martin J. State of the art in congenital eyelid deformity management. Facial Plast Surg. 2016;32(2):142-9.
3. Sadiq MA, Ur-Rehman M. Genetics of strabismus and lid diseases. J Pediatr Genet. 2014;3(4):281-90.
4. SooHoo JR, Davies BW, Allard FD, et al. Congenital ptosis. Surv Ophthalmol. 2014;59(5):483-92.
5. Pryor HB. Objective measurement of interpupillary distance. Pediatrics. 1969;44(6):973-7.
6. Gerber FR, Taylor FH, DeLevie M, et al. Normal standards for exophthalmometry in children 10 to 14 years of age: relation to age, height, weight, and sexual maturation. J Pediatr. 1972;81(12):327-9.
7. Waardenburg PJ. A new syndrome combining developmental anomalies of the eyelids, eyebrows and nose root with pigmentary defects of the iris and head hair and with congenital deafness. Am J Hum Genet. 1951;3(3):195-253.
8. Ali MJ, Paulsen F. Syndromic and nonsyndromic systemic associations of congenital lacrimal drainage anomalies: a major review. Ophthal Plast Reconstr Surg. 2017;33(6):399-407.
9. Gandhi NG. Treatment of neuro-ophthalmic and orbitofacial manifestations of neurofibromatosis type 1. Curr Opin Ophthalmol. 2013;24(5):506-11.
10. Simons EA, Huang JT, Schmidt B. Congenital melanocytic nevi in young children: Histopathologic features and clinical outcomes. J Am Acad Dermatol. 2017;76(5):941-7.
11. Radhadevi CV, Charles KS, Lathika VK. Orbital malignant melanoma associated with nevus of Ota. Indian J Ophthalmol. 2013;61(6):306-9.
12. Shirley MD, Tang H, Gallione CJ, et al. Sturge-Weber syndrome and port-wine stains caused by somatic mutation in GNAQ. N Eng J Med. 2013;368(21):1971-9.
13. Tattelbaum AG, Dufresne CR. Proteus syndrome: a newly recognized hamartomatous syndrome with significant craniofacial dysmorphology. J Craniofac Surg. 1995;6(2):151-60.
14. Painter SL, Hildebrand GD. Review of topical beta blockers as treatment for infantile hemangiomas. Surv Ophthalmol. 2016;61(1):51-8.
15. Mahajan P, Margolin J, Iacobas I. Kasabach-Merritt Phenomenon: Classic Presentation and Management

Options. Clin Med Insights Blood disord. 2017;10:1179545X 17699849.
16. Heyer GL. PHACE(S) syndrome. Handb Clin Neurol. 2015;132:169-83.
17. Glick ZR, Frieden IJ, Garzon MC, et al. Diffuse neonatal hemangiomatosis: an evidence-based review of case reports in the literature. J Am Acad Dermatol. 2012;67(5):898-903.
18. Shields JA, Shields CL. Orbital cysts of childhood--classification, clinical features, and management. Surv Ophthalmol. 2004;49(3):281-99.
19. Shields JA, Kaden IH, Eagle RC Jr, et al. Orbital dermoid cysts: clinicopathologic correlations, classification, and management. The 1997 Josephine E. Schueler Lecture. Ophthal Plast Reconstr Surg. 1997;13(4):265-76.
20. de Graaf G, Buckley F, Dever J, et al. Estimation of live birth and population prevalence of Down syndrome in nine U.S. states. Am J Med Genet A. 2017;173(10):2710-19.
21. Zigman WB. Atypical aging in Down syndrome. Dev Disabil Res Rev. 2013;18(1):51-67.
22. Clarren SK, Smith DW. The fetal alcohol syndrome. N Eng J Med. 1978;298:1063-7.
23. Del Campo M, Jones KL. A review of the physical features of the fetal alcohol spectrum disorders. Eur J Med Genet. 2017;60(1):55-64.
24. Di Iorio E, Kaye SB, Ponzin D, et al. Limbal stem cell deficiency and ocular phenotype in ectrodactyly-ectodermal dysplasia-clefting syndrome caused by p63 mutations. Ophthalmology. 2012;119(1):74-83.
25. Parks MM, Costenbader FD. Craniofacial dysostosis (Crouzon's disease). Am J Ophthalmol. 1950;33(1):77-82.
26. Gray TL, Casey T, Selva D, et al. Ophthalmic sequelae of Crouzon syndrome. Ophthalmology. 2005;112(6):1129-34.
27. Apert E. De l'acrocephalosyndactylie. Bull Soc Med Hop Paris. 1906;23:1310.
28. Buckley RW, Yakovlev PI. Dysostosis of skull, face and extremities. Am J Dis Child. 1948;75(5):688-94.
29. Khong JJ, Anderson P, Gray TL, et al. Ophthalmic findings in Apert syndrome prior to craniofacial surgery. Am J Ophthalmol. 2006;142(2):328-30.
30. Buchanan EP, Xue AS, Hollier LH Jr. Craniofacial syndromes. Plast Reconstr Surg. 2014;134(1):128e-53e.
31. Sharma N, Greenwell T, Hammerton M, et al. The ophthalmic sequelae of Pfeiffer syndrome and the long-term visual outcomes after craniofacial surgery. Journal of AAPOS. 2016;20(4):315-9.
32. Birgfeld CB, Heike C. Craniofacial microsomia. Semin Plast Surg. 2012;26(2):91-104.
33. Brandstetter KA, Patel KG. Craniofacial microsomia. Facial Plast Surg Clin North Am. 2016;24(4):495-515.
34. Goldenhar M. Association malformations de l'oeil et de l'oreille: En particulier le syndrome dermoid epibulbaire appendices auricularies-fistula, airis congenita et ses relations avec la dysostose mandibulo-faciale. J Human Genetics. 1952;243.
35. Tuin J, Tahiri Y, Paliga JT, et al. Distinguishing Goldenhar syndrome from craniofacial microsomia. J Craniofac Surg. 2015;26(6):1887-92.
36. Zwahlen AFP. Un syndrome nouveau, la dysostose mandibulo-faciale. Bull Schweiz Acad Med Wissensch. 1944;1.
37. Collins E. Cases with symmetrical congenital notches in the outer part of each lid and defective development of the malar bones. Trans Ophthalmol Soc UK. 1900;20:190.
38. Hertle RW, Ziylan S, Katowitz JA. Ophthalmic features and visual prognosis in the Treacher-Collins syndrome. BrJ Ophthalmol. 1993;77(10):642-5.
39. Hallermann W. Vogelgesult und cataracta congenita. Klin Monatsbl Augenheilkd. 1948;113:315.
40. Streiff. Dysmorphie mandibulo-faciale (tete d'oiseau) et alterations oculaires. Ophthalmologica. 1950;12079-83.
41. Francois J. A new syndrome; dyscephalia with bird face and dental anomalies, nanism, hypotrichosis, cutaneous atrophy, microphthalmia, and congenital cataract. AMA Arch Ophthalmol. 1958;60(5):842-62.
42. Pfaffenbach DD, Cross HE, Kearns TP. Congenital anomalies in Duane's retraction syndrome. Arch ophthalmol. 1972;88:635-9.
43. MacKinnon S, Oystreck DT, Andrews C, et al. Diagnostic distinctions and genetic analysis of patients diagnosed with moebius syndrome. Ophthalmology. 2014;121(7):1461-8.
44. Nowaczyk MJ. Smith-Lemli-Opitz Syndrome. In: Pagon RA, Adam MP, Ardinger HH (Eds). Gene Reviews. Seattle, WA: University of Washington; 2013.

Part 13 Miscellaneous

N Venkatesh Prajna

OUTLINE

Chapter 114 Sterilization and Aseptic Practices in an Ophthalmic Operation Theater

Lalitha Prajna

INTRODUCTION

Cataract surgery is the most commonly performed surgery worldwide and has become a safe surgical procedure with the advent of modern surgical techniques and instrumentation. However, postoperative endophthalmitis following cataract surgery is the most dreaded complication. The reported rates of postoperative endophthalmitis are about 0.01–0.05%.[1] The important aspects of prevention of postoperative endophthalmitis are multifactorial and involve meticulous care in the preoperative patient preparation, and intraoperative aseptic protocols. Proper and adequate instrument cleaning and sterilization are other very important aspects in the prevention of both postoperative endophthalmitis and postoperative inflammation such as toxic anterior segment syndrome (TASS).

This chapter describes the various protocols for aseptic process for any intraocular surgical procedure as well as sterilization and cleaning of instruments that are mandatory. As cataract surgery is the most commonly performed surgery most of the procedures described are pertaining to cataract surgery. This chapter also has a section describing TASS, its etiology and prevention.

DEFINITIONS

Sterilization

Sterilization is the process of destroying all microorganisms, including bacterial endospores. Instruments and other consumables that have direct contact with the eye and other sterile body sites must be sterilized. Steam under high pressure is known to be the most effective sterilization method. All sterilization processes must be regularly monitored by chemical and biological methods.

Disinfection

Disinfection is the process that inactivates most pathogenic microorganisms with help of chemical agents. The required disinfection may be low, intermediate, or high-level depending on the degree of disinfection required. Disinfectants are mostly used for floor cleaning and hand hygiene. The efficacy of the disinfectant depends on the optimum concentration, adequate time of contact with the surface to be disinfected and adherence to the instructions and precautions advised by the manufacturer. Disinfection is not a substitute for sterilization and should be considered as an adjuvant step in infection prevention.

Asepsis and Aseptic Practices in an Ophthalmic Operation Theater

Asepsis is the process of removing pathogenic microorganism either from the skin or from the environment. An antiseptic is a chemical agent for use on skin or tissue to achieve asepsis. The important aseptic practices before any ophthalmic surgery are the use of povidone-iodine for skin scrub as well as for conjunctival application.

ASEPTIC PRACTICES FOR THE PREVENTION OF POSTOPERATIVE ENDOPHTHALMITIS

The first and foremost principle is to ensure that the entire team in the operation theater understands the importance of adherence to protocols with regard to the process of sterilization and disinfection. It should not just be the responsibility of the operating surgeon or the assisting theater nurse. Aseptic protocol for surgical team members include proper surgical scrub according to the World Health Organization (WHO) recommendations for hand scrubbing[2] and proper theater attire include sterile gown, gloves, cap and mask. Periodic review of the protocol and audits of the processes should be done at regular intervals with utmost discipline.

Preoperative Ocular Examination and Antibiotics

- Preoperative clinical examination of the ocular surface is performed prior to surgery to check for any infections. If there is an obvious infection such as conjunctivitis or lid infections, the same must be treated before scheduling the patient for surgery.
- Preoperative topical broad-spectrum antibiotics such as ofloxacin or moxifloxacin can be initiated a day prior to surgery.
- *Povidone-iodine skin scrub:* The preoperative prophylaxis that has been proven beyond doubt to be the most effective in the prevention of postoperative endophthalmitis is the use *10% povidone-iodine skin preparation and 5% povidone-iodine eye drops into the eye before surgery.* Povidone-iodine is a broad-spectrum microbicide that has a very quick onset of action and acts by destroying microbial protein and DNA. Within the operating theater, the periocular region (lids, brow, and cheeks) should be treated with 10% povidone-iodine before the drape is applied and then a further dose of 5% povidone-iodine applied to the ocular surface after retracting the lids with a speculum. The povidone-iodine should have a contact time of at least 3 minutes before irrigating the conjunctival sac with saline.

It is now well established that 5% povidone-iodine reduces both the variety and number of bacteria present on the conjunctival and corneal surface by nearly a 100-fold. A meta-analysis of an evidence-based update of bacterial endophthalmitis prophylaxis for cataract surgery highlights the benefits of povidone-iodine antisepsis.[3]

Intraoperative Prophylaxis

- *Intracameral antibiotics:* Use of intracameral (IC) antibiotics such as cefuroxime and moxifloxacin have helped reduce the incidence of endophthalmitis. The European Society of Cataract and Refractive Surgeon (ESCRS) Endophthalmitis Study Group has shown that the use of IC cefuroxime brings down the endophthalmitis rates from 0.59% to 0.039%.[4] IC moxifloxacin has also shown to significantly reduce the rates of postoperative infection.[5] Studies were conducted at Aravind Eye Hosptial, India by Haripriya et al. to compare the rate of postoperative endophthalmitis before and after initiation of IC moxifloxacin for endophthalmitis prophylaxis in patients undergoing cataract surgery. It was found that routine IC moxifloxacin prophylaxis achieved a highly significant, four-fold reduction in postoperative endophthalmitis in patients undergoing cataract surgery. This study provides strong evidence that moxifloxacin is an effective IC prophylactic antibiotic against the development of postoperative endophthalmitis.

In recent times, ready to use prefilled syringes or vials containing 1 mL of preservative free 0.5% moxifloxacin meant for ophthalmic use (Auromox®, manufactured by Aurolab, India) is available.

STERILIZATION OF SURGICAL INSTRUMENTS

Cleaning and Drying of Surgical Instruments

Physical removal of all visible dust, dried blood, and viscoelastic from the surgical instruments is the first and most important step before disinfection and sterilization of the surgical instruments. It is important to presoak the entire instrument set in water immediately after use to prevent proteins and viscoelastic from drying on surgical instruments. After any surgical procedure contaminated instruments such as phaco handpieces, microscope handles, cannulas, etc. should be collected into a covered container and transported to the decontamination area. Soiled disposable items should be collected into a trash bag and disposed as per hospital policy. Disposable sharp items (such as blades, suture needles, etc.) must be disposed in an approved sharps container.

Instruments can be cleaned manually and in an ultrasonic cleaner.

Manual Cleaning

All surgical instruments must be rinsed in distilled water immediately after the surgery. They should be kept soaked in the water till the cleaning starts. Instruments are washed while still submerged in the water.

Precautions to be undertaken during cleaning of surgical instruments:

- A toothbrush or any soft brush is used for cleaning the instruments.
- If any cleaning agents are used, then the directions on the label must be carefully followed.

- Only distilled water should be used for soaking and cleaning the instruments and not balanced salt solution, which can damage delicate surgical instruments.
- Instruments must be inspected for cleanliness and for any defects before sterilization.
- Proper attire like gloves and mask must be adhered to even during the cleaning process.
  - If any detergents are used for cleaning the instruments, the cleaning agent must be washed off completely as any residual agents may lead to TASS.

Ultrasonic Cleaning

Ultrasonic cleaning instruments work by subjecting instruments to high-frequency, high-energy sound waves, which produce tiny bubbles that implode, resulting in a scouring action that cleans.

- Ultrasonic cleaning and instrument washers supplement manual cleaning of delicate tubes or other hollow instruments, such as special syringes or needles. (Fig. 114.1)
- They are especially effective in removing dust particles from areas which are hard to reach.
- When using an ultrasonic cleaning process, instruments made of similar metals only should be combined in the ultrasonic cleaner to avoid ion transfer, which may result in instrument etching and pitting.
- The handpieces of the phacoemulsification machine should not be placed in the ultrasonic cleaner.
- Before placing instrument in the ultrasonic cleaner the instruments must be cleaned manually.
- Ultrasonic unit must be emptied, cleaned and dried at the end of the day.

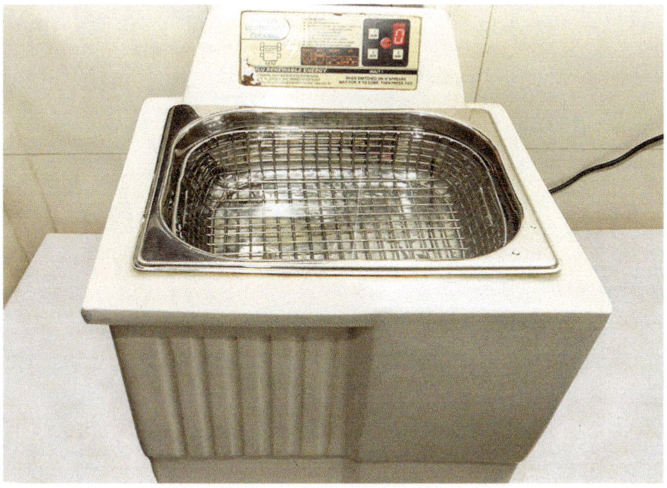

Fig. 114.1: Ultrasonic cleaner.

Drying

After the cleaning, the instruments must be absolutely dry in order to reduce the risk of contamination and minimize rusting and staining. Residual moisture will also interfere with the sterilization process and can damage instruments. Instruments can be dried with either a particle-free cloth or an air-drying machine.

Instruments must be inspected visually or under a microspore to check for:

- Cleanliness
- Proper functioning and alignment
- Any rusting, cracks or breaks
- Dullness of cutting edge.

The recommendations for the cleaning and sterilization of intraocular surgical instruments from the American Society of Cataract and Refractive Surgery and the American Society of Ophthalmic Registered Nurses are very useful and can serve as a guide in developing hospital protocols.[6,7]

Packing of the Instruments for Sterilization

The packing of the instruments that are used for ophthalmic surgeries can be performed using either wrapped or unwrapped techniques. If a central sterilization unit is used, then the instruments must be wrapped. However, if the sterilization area is adjacent to the operating room and especially so if it is a dedicated ophthalmic facility, then "unwrapped instruments" can be used. A recent study compared these two techniques (wrapped and unwrapped) and found both the procedures were equally efficacious in preventing postoperative infections.[8] If instruments have to be wrapped, items may be double wrapped, for porous loads only, and marked with autoclave indicator tape, date of autoclaving and the name of the person who has packed the instruments. The advantage of packing the instruments is that they can have a longer shelf life of about 8 weeks. If dampness of drapes and gowns is noted when they are removed from the autoclaves they must not be used as this indicates a faulty cycle where sterility has not been achieved.

Sterilization Procedures

All items and instruments that are used for ocular surgeries need to be sterile. This is achieved by either steam sterilization in an autoclave or gas sterilization depending on the item or instrument sterilized. In recent times, plasma sterilizers are also used in many ophthalmic surgical centers as sterilizers for rapid sterilization.

cleaning and sterilization of intraocular surgical instruments is very well described in the publication by Chang DF et al.[9]

Steam Sterilization in Autoclave

Majority of the instruments and linen are sterilized in a steam sterilizer (Fig. 114.2). Autoclaving under high pressure with steam is the best method of achieving absolute sterilization. Table 114.1 describes the different types of sterilization techniques, the materials that are sterilized in each and the conditions that need to be maintained.

The temperature setting and sterilizing time is dependent on the type of autoclave and articles being treated. It is important to follow the specific manufacturer's instructions very carefully. All the instruments are sterilized in a full cycle autoclave. The term "flash sterilizer" is no longer recommended and is replaced by "Immediate Use Steam Sterilization" (IUSS). The IUSS is recommended for use on an emergency basis. This is different from "short-cycle" sterilization that includes a complete dry time and the instruments are wrapped so that they can be used at a later date. This cycle can be used in centers that perform eye surgery. These latest recommendation and guidelines for the

Ethylene Oxide Sterilization

Ethylene oxide (ETO) sterilization uses a toxic gas to alkalinize microorganisms and kill them. It is used for moisture-sensitive instruments that cannot be steam sterilized. ETO gas is the most common and effective method of terminal sterilization for medical instruments that cannot be autoclaved. This method is the preferred alternative for equipment that must be stored sterile and ready for use, although the time necessary to process through an entire sterilization cycle can be up to 14 hours. The instruments which are sterilized using this technique will have a lengthy aeration time after each cycle to allow removal of harmful residuals before opening the chamber door. The aeration time varies by manufacturer, but can be between 12 hours and 24 hours. Compatibility of materials with ETO sterilization should be established before using this method. Instruments such as cryoprobe, vitrectomy cutter, and cautery wire can be sterilized using this method of sterilization (Fig. 114.3).

Table 114.1: Type of autoclaves and associated minimum exposure time and temperature.

S. No.	Type of autoclave	Pressure	Temperature (°C)	Time	Items that can be sterilized
1.	Steam autoclave (long cycle)	20 psi	121°C	30–45 minutes	Gowns, dressings, drapes, vessels, and wiper, Bed and bandage, and metal instruments
2.	High speed autoclave (short cycle)	30 psi	134°C	7–10 minutes	Subtenon, scope cup, and metal instruments
3.	ETO sterilization	—	30–60°C	7–8 hours	Heat labile tubings, cryo and laser probes, scope cup, infusion set, forceps, and Buckle band

(ETO: Ethylene oxide)

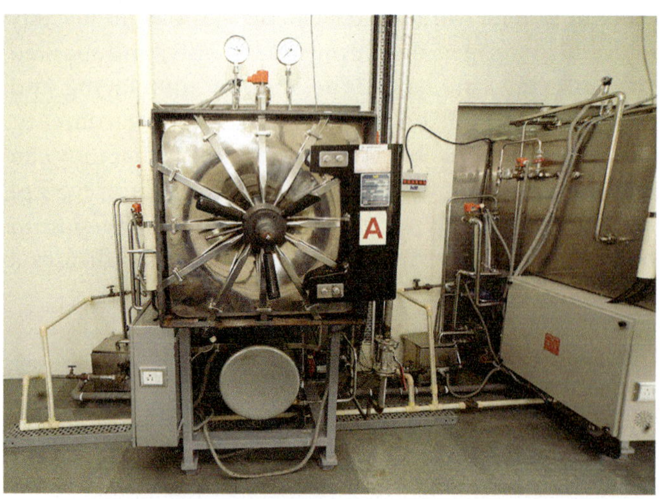

Fig. 114.2: Steam sterilization—double door autoclave.

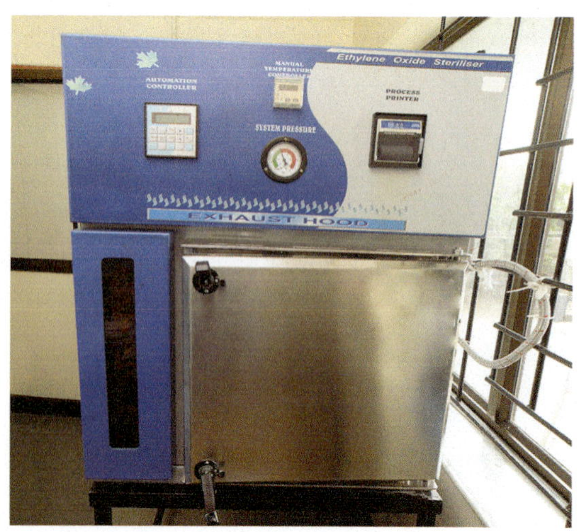

Fig. 114.3: Ethylene oxide gas sterilizer.

Mechanical monitors of ETO sterilizers should record the parameters for sterilization, including temperature, exposure time, relative humidity, and sterilant concentration. ETO is a known carcinogen and can have harmful effects on patients and personnel. If instruments are not completely dry before ETO sterilization, a potent hemolytic (destructive to red blood cells) agent can form, which also can have ill effects on the patient.

The US Occupational Safety and Health Administration (OSHA) has very strict guidelines for ETO exposure, and policies and instructions, such as training on alarms and ventilation, are essential for ETO use. Regular exposure testing of areas and personnel is necessary. The instruments are packed in special polythene bags with an indicator tape inside the bag. Due to their toxic nature, an aeration period of minimum 72 hours for the sterilized items is a mandatory requirement before they are used.[10]

Plasma Sterilization

Definition

Plasma is defined as an ionized (or energized) gas with an equal number of positively and negatively charged particles. It is often regarded as the "fourth state of matter" (the other three being solids, liquids, and gases) because, while plasma is neither a gas nor a liquid, its properties are similar to those of both gases and liquids. Plasma can be categorized as either high-temperature- or low-temperature-based. Low-temperature plasmas, used in surface modification, cleaning, decontamination, and sterilization applications, are ionized gases generated under deep vacuum (low-pressure) conditions. The temperature of this sterilization method is maintained in the 40–50°C range, which makes it particularly well suited for use with heat-sensitive and moisture-sensitive medical devices. The instruments are wrapped prior to sterilization, and can either be stored or used immediately.

The sterilization of surgical items by plasma sterilizer acts by destruction by ultraviolet (UV) irradiation of the genetic material of the microorganism or erosion of the microorganism, atom by atom, through *intrinsic photo-desorption*.[11,12]

Application of Plasma Sterilization

Common applications for hydrogen peroxide plasma sterilizers include sterilizing non-hollow loads, such as electrocautery instruments, dopplers, laser probes, defibrillator paddles, thermometers, ophthalmic lenses, and harmonic cables. Hollow loads, such as laryngoscopes and their blades, fiber optic light cables, surgical power drills and endoscopes can also be sterilized by this technique.

Advantages of Plasma Sterilization

Low-temperature hydrogen peroxide gas plasma sterilization has the following advantages:

- A short (1–4 hours) sterilization cycle,
- Low temperature and humidity,
- No aeration requirement,
- No toxic residues or environmental impact and
- Broad compatibility with materials.

Biological indicators such as *Bacillus atrophaeus* and *Bacillus stearothermophilus* spores can be used for quality control.

Disadvantages of using Plasma Sterilization for Sterilizer Surgical Instruments

The major disadvantages include weak penetrating power and inability to sterilize liquids, powders, and strong absorbers. It requires specific synthetic packaging of the load. Sterilization chamber is relatively smaller than that of an ETO gas sterilizer.

Monitoring Steam Sterilization

All sterilizers must be monitored for their effectiveness with regards to the various parameters like time, pressure, and steam penetration. Validation does not assure that the items are completely sterile, but it furnishes a documented proof of the ongoing effectiveness of the sterilization process under the operating conditions prevailing inside the autoclave. Various classes and types of indicators are available that monitor and validate these parameters.[13] Chemical indicators, biological indicators, and mechanical monitors are available and their periodicity of use must be determined (Figs. 114.4A to E). The different types of indicators and frequency of use are described in Table 114.2.

ENVIRONMENT IN THE OPERATING ROOM

Guidelines for Air Conditioning System for Operation Theaters

Proper ventilation and air conditioning are required for the comfort of the staff inside the operation theater as

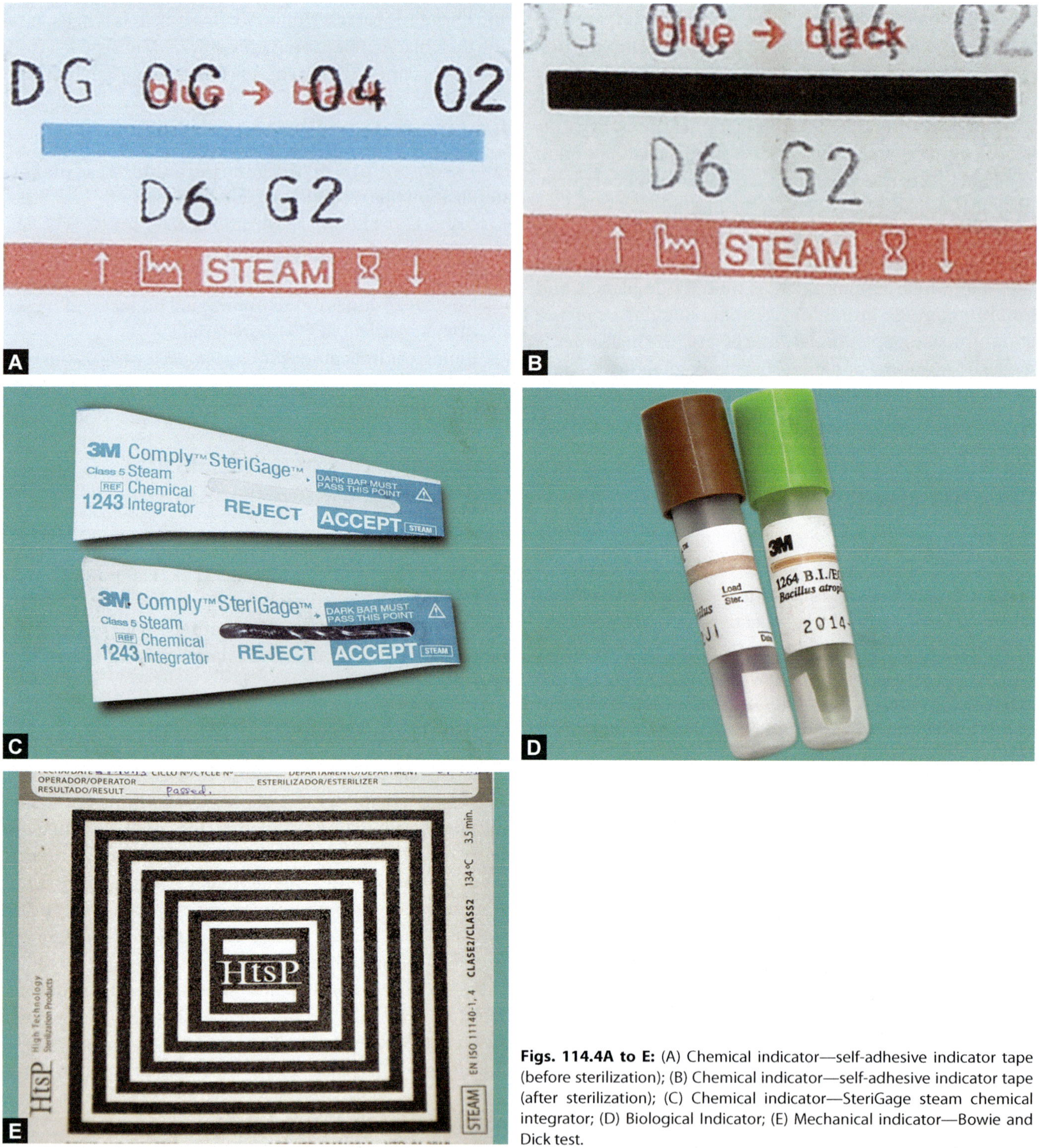

Figs. 114.4A to E: (A) Chemical indicator—self-adhesive indicator tape (before sterilization); (B) Chemical indicator—self-adhesive indicator tape (after sterilization); (C) Chemical indicator—SteriGage steam chemical integrator; (D) Biological Indicator; (E) Mechanical indicator—Bowie and Dick test.

well as the patients. Adequate and proper ventilation and air-flow systems inside the operation theater also helps in reducing contamination arising from airborne organisms. However, airborne organisms are a very negligible source of postoperative infection. There are specific guidelines for proper ventilation and airflow. Ambient temperature and humidity inside the operation theater must be considered taking into account the size of the operating room and also

Table 114.2: Methods of sterilization monitoring, type of indicators usage, and frequency.

S. No.	Type of indicators	Methods of monitoring	Testing methodology	Frequency (as per ANSI/AAMI ST66 standard)
1.	Mechanical indicator	Equipment control	• Bowie-Dick test packs • Bowie-Dick test sheets • Monitors the performance of sterilizer prior to and during the sterilization cycle • To detect air pockets in sterilizer during sterilization process	• Each day, before the first processed load in an empty chamber or • During initial installation or after relocation or malfunction or major repair
2.	Chemical indicator	Exposure control	*Indicator tape:* To identify processed from unprocessed medical devices at a glance	Should be used with every package
		Pack control	*Chemical indicators and chemical integrators:* To confirm that sufficient exposure conditions have been met or not	• Should be used within each package in the area least accessible to steam penetration • This might or might not be center of the pack • ETO–chemical indicators must be on or in each package
3.	Biological indicator	Load control	Biological indicator	• Should be used at least weekly • But preferably daily, each load that contains an implantable • Sterilizer tested when installed and after any major repair • Test 3 consecutive cycles with a biological indicator in a test tray

(ETO: Ethylene oxide, ANSI: American National Standards Institute; AAMI: Association for the Advancement of Medical Instrumentation)

Table 114.3: Parameters for operating room ventilation.

S. No	Parameter	Desired range
1.	Temperature	20–23°C
2.	Relative humidity	30–60%
3.	Air movement	From clean to less clean areas and laminar flow
4.	Air changes	Minimum 15 total air changes per hour

the expected occupancy and equipment load.[14] Table 114.3 describes the parameters that have to be monitored and documented such as the air change per hour, air velocity, positive pressure, temperature, humidity and air filtration.

Guidelines for Water Quality and Monitoring

Water is used in many of the process involved in the cleaning and sterilization of instruments. Most often distilled water is used for cleaning instruments and for the running of the autoclave. The quality of the water must be verified on a periodic interval. This should include both the microbial sterility check as well as the chemical content of the water. The water filtration systems should also be checked and validated at least yearly.[15]

MICROBIOLOGY SURVEILLANCE

Surveillance of Aseptic and Sterilization Practices

Routine surveillance of activities pertaining to the aseptic and sterilization process must be undertaken. Hospital and healthcare facilities must develop protocols and frequency depending on the surgical load, frequency of operating, etc. Some recommendations are described in Table 114.4. Frequent monitoring of microbiological samples from various sources is very important to know about the microbial contamination sources.[16]

The document from the American Academy of Ophthalmology describes various current protocols for the prevention of infection in eye care services and operating areas, and also describes regulation required by the various federal agencies as well as current literature of surgical site prevention of infection. Recommendations and standards by organization and instructions on equipment cleaning and disinfection by manufacturers are also described. This document has useful links to the resources with this information.[17]

Table 114.4: Microbiological surveillance and sampling frequency of ophthalmology operating theater (OT) environment.

Test details	Sampling frequency	Suggested normal values
Air samples from OT environment by passive air sampling method (Settle Plate 30 minutes)	Once in a month (during busy hours)	Not more than 30 colonies. Free from pathogenic organisms
RO water sample from OT environment	Once in a month	• RO water—not more than 100 cfu/mL • Free from pathogenic organisms
Filtered water or boiled water for instrument cleaning purpose (if any)	Once in a month	Not more than 1 cfu/mL (Should be "no growth")

(cfu: Colony forming unit)

TOXIC ANTERIOR SEGMENT SYNDROME

Introduction

Toxic anterior segment syndrome is an acute postoperative intraocular inflammation caused by the introduction of a noninfectious toxic agent into the anterior chamber of the eye at the time of surgery. The syndrome was first named by Monson et al. in 1992.[18] TASS, although an uncommon complication of eye surgery, can have devastating effects. This is most commonly associated with inadequate or improper cleaning and sterilization of instruments. This inflammatory response can lead to severe visual impairment. Cleaning agent residues, endotoxins, bioburden (residual biological tissue living on a surface), denatured ophthalmic viscoelastic agents, preservatives, and residues from sterilization processing all can induce TASS and the subsequent intraocular inflammation can damage ocular tissue severely.[19-23]

The TASS can present as either sporadic cases or in outbreaks. The incidence of TASS is estimated to range from 2% to less than 0.1%.[24] It is difficult to get an accurate estimate of the number of cases of TASS that occur because of the inadequate reporting as well as the difficulty in establishing an accurate diagnosis. In an effort to better understand the incidence of TASS and prevent outbreaks, surveillance programs are undertaken to monitor medical devices used in cataract surgery and to aid in identification of a TASS outbreak.

Clinical Signs and Symptoms

The clinical hallmark of the syndrome is immediate or early onset of the inflammation, usually within 12–48 hours of surgery. The early onset (within 24 hours compared with 4–7 days for bacterial endophthalmitis), the favorable response to steroids and the lack of posterior segment inflammation are helpful to differentiate TASS from bacterial endophthalmitis. Delayed onset of TASS has also been reported.[25]

Patients diagnosed with TASS often have symptoms of blurred vision and redness of the operated eye; if pain is present, it is usually very mild. The most common clinical findings in TASS are diffuse "limbus-to-limbus" corneal edema and anterior segment inflammation. In severe case of TASS, fibrin formation may also be noted in the anterior chamber and or on the surface of the iris and intraocular lens (IOL). Iris and trabecular meshwork might be damaged resulting in refractory glaucoma.[26]

Etiology

The etiology of TASS is relatively broad and may include any substance that has access into the eye at the time of surgery. Irrigating solutions such as balanced saline solution (BSS), any ophthalmic solutions used during surgery, especially those which contain preservatives or stabilizing agents may cause toxicity to corneal endothelium and precipitate TASS. Medications such as antibiotics and anesthetics which are injected into the eye may also be associated with TASS. Additionally, residues of ophthalmic viscosurgical devices may cause significant postoperative inflammation. Lastly, any enzymes or detergents that are used in the cleaning of instruments used in anterior-segment surgery may leave behind a residue which could cause TASS. Table 114.5 describes all the different etiological agents that have been reported to cause TASS.

Preventive Measures

Since TASS has the possibility of causing significant ocular morbidity, major effort should be focused on the prevention of TASS. It is crucial that the entire surgical team including nurses, operating room technicians, physicians, and pharmacists are aware of what is appropriate for use

Table 114.5: Etiology of toxic anterior segment syndrome.

S. No.	Chemical agents	Etiologic agents
1.	Preservatives	Benzalkonium chloride (BAC) 0.01% and hydroxypropyl methylcellulose (HPMC) 2%
2.	Intraocular anesthetics	High concentrations of lidocaine
3.	Chemical impurities in sterilizers	Chemical impurities such as sulfates, copper, zinc, nickel, and silica
4.	Detergent solutions in ultrasonic bath	The 10-folds increase of a detergent solution
5.	Endotoxin in microkeratome blades	Contamination observed in microkeratome blades
6.	Endotoxin contamination in BSS solutions	BSS exceeding the endotoxin limit (0.5 EU/mL)
7.	Sterilized by plasma gas (low-temperature *peracetic acid)*	Plazlyte degraded brass to copper and zinc on cannulated surgical instruments
8.	Intraocular lens	A polishing compound on the memory lens
9.	Ophthalmic ointment	Antibiotic/steroid ointment and pilocarpine gel
10.	Viscoelastic	A residue of the viscoelastic substance remains inside the cannula
11.	Ophthalmic dyes—trypan blue	0.1 mL of 0.1% trypan blue ophthalmic injection
12.	Surgical glove powder	Surgical gloves are commonly coated with dusting powders that have severe toxic effects on the eye

(BSS: Balanced saline solution

in ophthalmic surgery and that they be educated about protocols that are in place. In the event of an outbreak of TASS in a facility, documentation may aid in identification of the cause for the outbreak. Policies and procedures for processing ophthalmic instruments should be written and reviewed annually. These policies must be readily available and accessible on all shifts. Personnel should receive education and training in the care and handling of ophthalmic instruments prior to processing these instruments.

When an outbreak of TASS occurs, a thorough investigation of possible causes should be undertaken. Investigation should include checking solutions, medications, detergents used, operating room protocols, and adherence to manufacturer's instructions for processing instruments. Guidelines are available (www.ascrs.org) that can help surgeons and their staff in the critical process of cleaning and sterilization of instruments with the goal of preventing further TASS outbreaks.[27]

CONCLUSION

Postoperative endophthalmitis after cataract surgery is largely preventable. Healthcare workers must ensure compliance with infection prevention and aseptic practices. Knowing and understanding the scientific principles and various sterilization methods and their proper applications, as well as the monitoring and record-keeping requirements can help to ensure effective sterilization, patient safety, and cost-effectiveness.

REFERENCES

1. Tyson SL, Bailey R, Roman JS, et al. Clinical outcomes after injection of a compounded pharmaceutical for prophylaxis after cataract surgery: a large-scale review. Curr Opin Ophthalmol. 2017;28(1):73-80.
2. World Health Organization. WHO guidelines on hand hygiene in health care: first global patient safety challenge: clean care is safer care. Geneva, Switzerland: World Health Organization (Patient Safety); 2009.
3. Ciulla TA, Starr MB, Masket S. Bacterial endophthalmitis prophylaxis for cataract surgery: an evidence-based update. Ophthalmology. 2002;109(1):13-24.
4. Endophthalmitis Study Group, European Society of Cataract & Refractive Surgeons. Prophylaxis of postoperative endophthalmitis following cataract surgery: results of the ESCRS multicenter study and identification of risk factors. J Cataract Refract Surg. 2007;33(6):978-88.
5. Haripriya A, Chang DF, Namburar S, et al. Efficacy of Intracameral Moxifloxacin Endophthalmitis Prophylaxis at Aravind Eye Hospital. Ophthalmology. 2016;123(2): 302-8.
6. Hellinger WC, Bacalis LP, Edelhauser HF, et al. Recommended practices for cleaning and sterilizing intraocular surgical instruments. J Cataract Refract Surg. 2007;33(6):1095-100.
7. American Ophthalmic Registered Nurses. Recommended practices for cleaning and caring for surgical instrumentation and powered equipment. In: Association of operating room nurses: standards, recommended practices and guidelines. Denver, CO: AORN; 2006. pp. 555-63.
8. Carpel EF, Mancera AD, Rowan LL, et al. Full-cycle steam sterilization in ophthalmic surgery-the effect of wrapping instruments. Am J Ophthalmol. 2012;153(3):405-11.
9. Chang DF, Hurley N, Mamalis N, et al. Evaluation of ophthalmic surgical instrument sterility using short-cycle

sterilization for sequential same-day use. Ophthalmology. 2018. pii: S0161-6420(18)30341-5.
10. Shintani H, Sakudo A, Burke P, et al. Gas plasma sterilization of microorganisms and mechanisms of action. Exp Ther Med. 2010;1(5):731-8.
11. Shintani H. Ethylene Oxide Gas Sterilization of Medical Devices. Biocontrol Sci. 2017;22(1):1-16.
12. Moisan M, Barbeau J, Crevier M, et al. Plasma sterilization: methods and mechanisms. Pure Appl Chem. 2002;74(3): 349-58.
13. Schneider PM, Reich RR, Kirckof SS, et al. Performance of various steam sterilization indicators under optimum and sub-optimum exposure conditions. Am J Infect Control. 2005;33(5 Suppl 2):S55-67.
14. American Society of Heating Refrigerating and Air Conditioning Engineers. (2013). Standard Ventilation for Acceptable Indoor Air Quality. [online] Available from: *http://rahmannejad.ir/uploads/posts/ASHRAE-ANSI-ASHRAE%20Standard%2062.1-2013%20Ventilation%20for%20Acceptable%20Indoor%20Air%20Quality.pdf* [Accessed December 2017].
15. Spagnolo AM, Ottria G, Amicizia D, et al. Operating theatre quality and prevention of surgical site infections. J Prev Med Hyg. 2013;54(3):131-7.
16. Kelkar U, Kelkar S, Bal AM, et al. Microbiological evaluation of various parameters in ophthalmic operating rooms. The need to establish guidelines. Indian J Ophthalmol. 2003;51(2):171-6.
17. American Academy of Ophthalmology. (2012). Infection Prevention in Eye Care Services and Operating Areas and Operating Rooms-2012. [online] Available from: https://*www.aao.org/clinical-statement/infection-prevention-in-eye-care-services-operatin.* [Accessed December 2017]
18. Monson MC, Mamalis N, Olson RJ. Toxic anterior segment inflammation following cataract surgery. J Cataract Refract Surg. 1992;18(2):184-9.
19. Breebaart AC, Nuyts RM, Pels E, et al. Toxic endothelial cell destruction of the cornea after routine extracapsular cataract surgery. Arch Ophthalmol. 1990;108(8):1121-5.
20. Holland SP, Mathias RG, Morck DW, et al. Diffuse lamellar keratitis related to endotoxins released from sterilizer reservoir biofilms. Ophthalmology. 2000;107(7):1227-33; discussion 34.
21. Hellinger WC, Hasan SA, Bacalis LP, et al. Outbreak of toxic anterior segment syndrome following cataract surgery associated with impurities in autoclave steam moisture. Infect Control Hosp Epidemiol. 2006;27(3):294-8.
22. Liu H, Routley I, Teichmann KD. Toxic endothelial cell destruction from intraocular benzalkonium chloride. J Cataract Refract Surg. 2001;27(11):1746-50.
23. Kim JH. Intraocular inflammation of denatured viscoelastic substance in cases of cataract extraction and lens implantation. J Cataract Refract Surg. 1987;13(5):537-42.
24. Duffy RE, Brown SE, Caldwell KL, et al. An epidemic of corneal destruction caused by plasma gas sterilization. The Toxic Cell Destruction Syndrome Investigative Team. Arch Ophthalmol. 2000;118(9):1167-76.
25. Lee SN. Mild toxic anterior segment syndrome mimicking delayed onset toxic anterior segment syndrome after cataract surgery. Indian J Ophthalmol 2014;62(8):890-2.
26. Parikh CH, Edelhauser HF. Ocular surgical pharmacology: corneal endothelial safety and toxicity. Curr Opin Ophthalmol. 2003;14(4):178-85.
27. American Society of Cataract and Refractive Surgery. ACSRS. [online] Available from: *http://www.ascrs.org/* [Accessed December 2017].

Chapter 115 Management of Ophthalmic Trauma

Fasika A Woreta, James T Banta, Ferenc Kuhn, Nicholas R Mahoney

EPIDEMIOLOGY OF OCULAR TRAUMA

Epidemiology and Demographics

Ocular trauma is an important public health problem, as it is a significant cause of preventable vision loss. The World Health Organization estimates that approximately 55 million eye injuries restricting activities for 1 or more days occur each year.[1] Furthermore, an estimated 19 million people are unilaterally blind and 1.6 million are bilaterally blind from eye injuries. Eye injuries are the most frequent cause of eye-related emergency department visits[2] and approximately 200,000 open globes injuries occur each year.[1]

Ocular trauma has a bimodal age distribution, with the first peak in young adults under the age of 30 years. A second peak occurs in the elderly after the age of 70 and is more associated with falls and globe rupture.[3] Severe eye injuries are more common among males, with a male: female prevalence ratio of 4:1.[3] Other risk factors for ocular trauma include lower socioeconomic status,[4] cigarette smoking,[5] alcohol consumption,[6] nonwhite race,[7] and a previous history of eye injury.[8]

Location and Source of Injury

The majority of ocular injuries occur in either the workplace or home environment. In developed countries, the number of eye injuries occurring in the workplace has decreased for a variety of reasons including required use of proper eye protective devices and fewer workers in industrial settings. However, in developing countries, the workplace remains the most frequent setting of ocular trauma. In rural areas, trauma from vegetable matter is the most common cause of injury, reflecting the fact that agriculture is the primary occupation in this setting.[9,10] In industrialized areas, workplace injuries are largely due to grinding, cutting metal, or drilling.[11] When occupational injuries do occur, the majority of workers are not wearing eye protection devices at the time of injury, highlighting the importance of continuing to improve safety standards and education in the workplace.

The rate of injuries occurring in the home has increased dramatically and in both the United States Eye Injury Registry (USEIR) and the Hungarian Eye Injury Registry (HEIR), the home was the most frequent place of injury (USEIR 41% and HEIR 35%).[12] Children are at particular risk in this setting, with most injuries occurring at home with a sharp object during unsupervised play.[13]

Sports and recreational activities are an increasing cause of ocular trauma worldwide. In the United States, the most common injuries are from playing basketball, baseball, or softball,[14] while soccer ball injuries are more common in other parts of the world.[15] Small, fast projectiles fired from a paintball, air, or BB gun are associated with more devastating eye injuries. Other high risk sports include hockey, squash or racquetball, cricket, fencing, and lacrosse.[16] Proper eye protection has resulted in a dramatic reduction in sports-related eye injuries and should always be utilized as specified by professional organizations.

In urban environments, assault is a major cause of eye injury and can be responsible for up to 40% of ocular and adnexal trauma.[17] In industrialized countries, motor vehicle accidents are an important source of eye trauma, but this risk can be decreased two-fold with seatbelt use.[18] In USEIR, fireworks accounted for 4% of eye injuries, with bystanders at greatest risk.[19] Legislation that prohibits consumer fireworks results in a significant decrease in firework-related eye injuries.

Conclusion

Ocular trauma has a devastating impact on both the individual and society. Beyond the direct cost associated

Conflicts of interest and source of funding: The authors have no conflicts of interest or financial disclosures.

with medical care, indirect costs such as lost days of work and long-term disability are tremendous. The prevention of eye trauma should be a major public health goal for all eye care providers.

DEFINITIONS AND CLASSIFICATION IN OCULAR TRAUMA

Using standardized language when describing ocular traumatology is imperative to avoid miscommunication between healthcare professionals. The Birmingham Eye Trauma Terminology (BETT) is an unambiguous and comprehensive classification scheme to describe any type of mechanical globe trauma.[20] Figure 115.1 outlines this classification system and Table 115.1 defines the terminology. For example, the terms *open globe* and *ruptured globe* are often incorrectly used interchangeably. It is important to remember that the term *open globe* refers to a full-thickness wound of the cornea or sclera and can be due to either a *laceration* caused by a sharp object or a *rupture* caused by a blunt object. Lacerations can be further classified into one of three categories:

1. *Penetrating injury:* The entry and exit wound are the same; if more than one wound is present, each must have been caused by a separate object.
2. *Perforating injury:* There are separate entry and exit wounds caused by the same object.
3. *Intraocular foreign body (IOFB):* An entry wound is present and the object remains within the eye.

An IOFB is a type of penetrating injury, but is classified separately due to differences in management and prognosis.

Table 115.1: Terms and definitions in Birmingham eye trauma terminology (BETT)

Eyewall	Sclera and cornea
Open globe injury	Full-thickness wound of eyewall
Laceration	Full-thickness wound of eyewall caused by a sharp object
Penetrating injury	Entrance wound
Perforating injury	Entrance and exit wound caused by the same object
Intraocular foreign body	Retained foreign object
Rupture	Full-thickness wound of the eye cause by a blunt object
Closed globe injury	No full-thickness wound of eyewall
Contusion	Injury results from direct energy delivered by the object (e.g. choroidal rupture) or changes to the shape of the globe (e.g. angle recession)
Lamellar laceration	Partial-thickness wound of eyewall

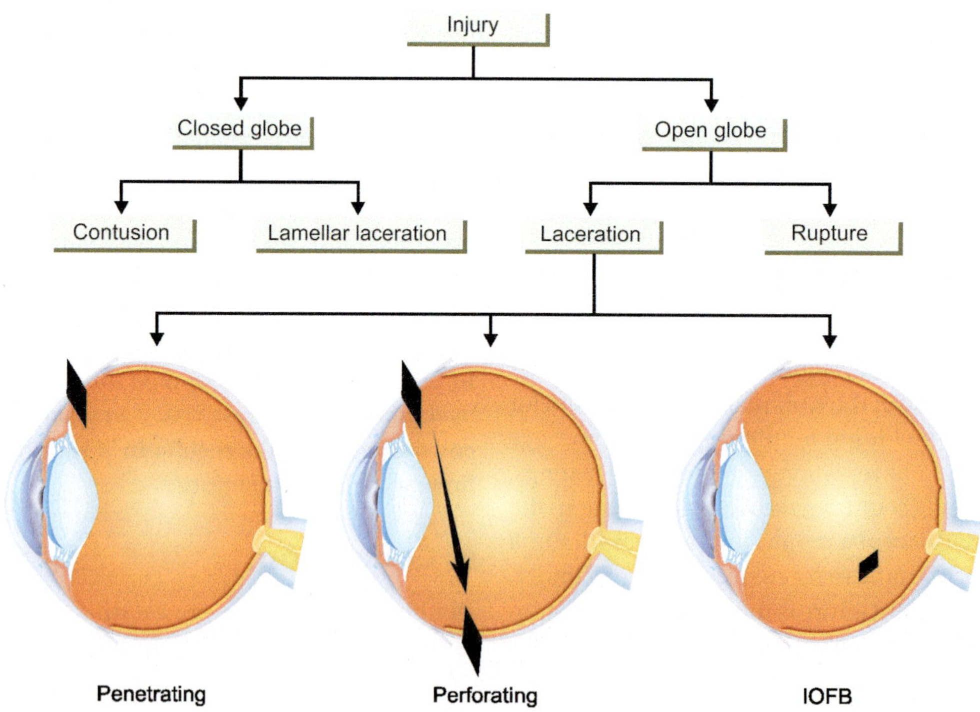

Fig. 115.1: Birmingham Eye Trauma Terminology (BETT): Classification of mechanical eye injuries.

Table 115.2: Open and closed globe injury classification.

Grade
Visual acuity:
- >20/40
- 20/50–20/100
- 19/100–5/200
- 4/200 to light perception.

Pupil
Positive: Relative afferent pupillary defect present in affected eye
Negative: Relative afferent pupillary defect absent in affected eye.

For open globes	For closed globes
Type	
A. Rupture	A. Contusion
B. Penetrating	B. Lamellar laceration
C. Intraocular	C. Superficial foreign body
D. Perforating	D. Mixed
E. Mixed	
Zone	
I: Cornea, including limbus	I: External (bulbar conjunctiva, cornea, or sclera)
II: Limbus to 5 mm posterior into sclera	II: Anterior segment to the posterior capsule of lens
III: Posterior to the anterior 5 mm of sclera	III: Posterior segment

Source: Adapted from Pieramici DJ, Sternberg P Jr, Aaberg TM Sr, et al. A system for classifying mechanical injuries of the eye (globe). Ocular Trauma Classification Group. Am J Ophthalmology. 1997;123(6):820-31.

A closed globe injury lacks a full-thickness wound of the eyewall. It is further classified as a *lamellar laceration* if a partial-thickness defect of the cornea or sclera is present or a *contusion* if the injury is caused by direct energy delivered by an object with deformation of the globe.

A separate classification system, also based on BETT, can be used for open and closed globe injuries, based on four variables[21] (Table 115.2):

1. Grade (based on initial visual acuity)
2. Pupil [based on absence or present of a relative afferent pupillary defect (RAPD)]
3. Type (based on mechanism of injury)
4. Zone (based on the location of wound in open globe injuries and the most posterior tissue damaged in closed globe injuries).

All four variables were found to be significant in the prediction of final visual outcome following an open globe injury with initial visual acuity and presence of a RAPD being most the most significant predictors of final visual acuity.[22]

For open globe injuries, Zone I injuries involve the cornea or limbus, Zone II injures involve the anterior 5 mm of the sclera, and Zone III injuries involve sclera more than 5 mm posterior to the limbus (Fig. 115.2). If more than one zone is involved, the zone is defined by the most posterior full-thickness aspect of the globe opening. For closed globe juries, the zone of the injury is defined by the location of

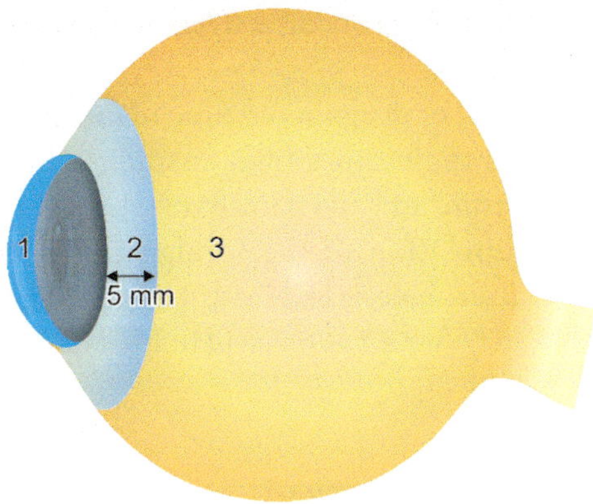

Fig. 115.2: Classification of open globe injuries by zone of involvement. Injury involving: (1) cornea (including limbus), (2) limbus to 5 mm posterior in sclera, and (3) posterior to the anterior 5 mm of sclera.

the tissue injured. When more than one zone is involved, the injury is classified by the zone of the most posterior involvement.

HISTORY AND EXAMINATION

Systemic Evaluation

The first step in evaluating a patient with ocular trauma is to make sure there are no other life-threatening injuries and that the patient is medically stable. In the case of chemical injuries, the history should be delayed until copious irrigation is performed. A brief general medical history should then ensue, documenting current and past medical conditions, previous major surgeries, and current medications. Drug allergies, tetanus immunization status, and the last time the patient ate or drank should also be documented.

Ocular History

The primary goal of the evaluation is to identify the most important injuries so any intervention can be optimally planned with respect to timing and type of surgery. A directed ocular history should address prior ocular surgeries and any pre-existing ocular conditions. Details of the injury should be well documented in the medical record and include:

- Date and time of incident
- Mechanism of injury (fall, hammering, motor vehicle accident, chemical splash, etc.)
- Object causing injury (glass, metal, nail, paintball, etc.)
- Location of incident (work, home, sports-related, etc.)
- Nature of injury (accidental, intentional, or self-inflicted)

- Use of safety glasses or corrective eyeglasses at the time of injury
- Use of alcohol or drugs at the time of the injury.

One should maintain a high suspicion for an IOFB based on the nature and mechanism of injury. If suspected, the exact composition of the foreign body should be documented. If an object is involved, the speed and distance traveled should be noted as this will help in understanding the severity of the injury.

Ocular Examination

The examination of a patient with an ocular injury can be challenging, as the patient is often in significant pain and anxious. Thus, it is important to approach the patient with a calm and reassuring manner. If an open globe is suspected, it is important to minimize manipulation of the eye as forceful eyelid opening could lead to an expulsive hemorrhage. Any drops administered should be from an unopened sterile bottle. If there is extensive periorbital swelling and the patient is unable to open the eye, Desmarres retractors should be used to gently open the eyelids to allow for proper examination without putting pressure on the globe. Once the diagnosis of an open globe is confirmed, the eye should be covered with a protective shield.

Documenting an accurate visual acuity is important for counseling the patient regarding prognosis. The visual acuity in the fellow eye should also be documented. If the patient is found to have no light perception, this should be confirmed with the brightest light source available. It is critical to document an RAPD if present, as this also has prognostic implications. If the pupil is affected in the injured eye but the other eye reacts normally, the presence of an RAPD by reverse testing should be performed. Extraocular motility testing is important in cases when an orbital fracture is suspected. In the setting of an open globe injury, intraocular pressure (IOP) measurement should be deferred.

A careful slit-lamp examination is critical in the patient with ocular trauma and should be performed in a stepwise fashion. The posterior segment may be difficult to examine in the setting of significant anterior chamber trauma, and ancillary testing such as ultrasonography may be warranted. Scleral depression should not be performed in the presence of an open globe injury. It is important to perform a dilated examination of the uninjured eye as well.

Special attention should be paid to a child with a potential open globe injury, as the examination can be particularly challenging. If the child is uncooperative and there is a high suspicion of an open globe, an examination under anesthesia should be performed with subsequent repair of the open globe as necessary.

Radiologic Imaging

Computed tomography (CT) is the preferred imaging modality for ocular and orbital trauma. CT scans are indicated in cases of suspected open globe injuries, intraorbital or intraocular foreign bodies, or orbital fractures. Findings suggestive of an open globe include eyewall deformity and intraocular emphysema. Magnetic resonance imaging (MRI) is contraindicated in patients with suspected magnetic foreign bodies. CT is also advantageous in that it is faster and less expensive than an MRI. CT can visualize soft tissues, bony structures, and foreign bodies without intravenous contrast (Fig. 115.3). Plain radiography can be performed if CT is not available, although soft tissue structures and radiolucent foreign bodies are not visualized as well. B-scan ultrasonography can also be used to localize IOFBs and assess the posterior segment when there is no view. Since contact with the eyelid is required, B-scan should be performed with great caution in the setting of open globe injures. In addition, an experienced technician is needed to pick up subtle findings such as a retinal tear or scleral rupture.

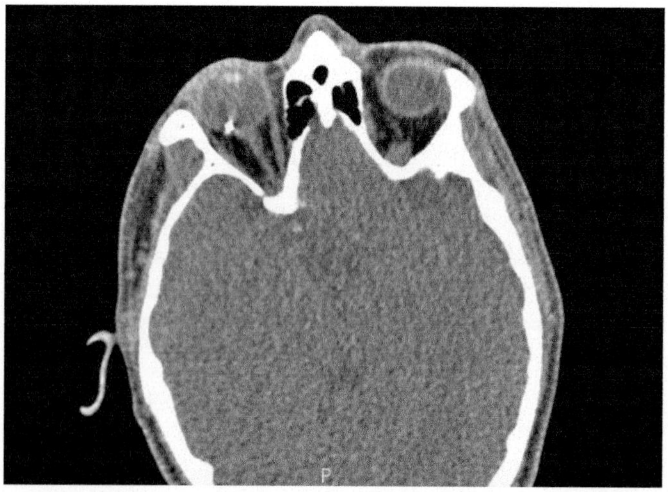

Fig. 115.3: A metallic foreign body is readily visible on this axial computed tomography scan.

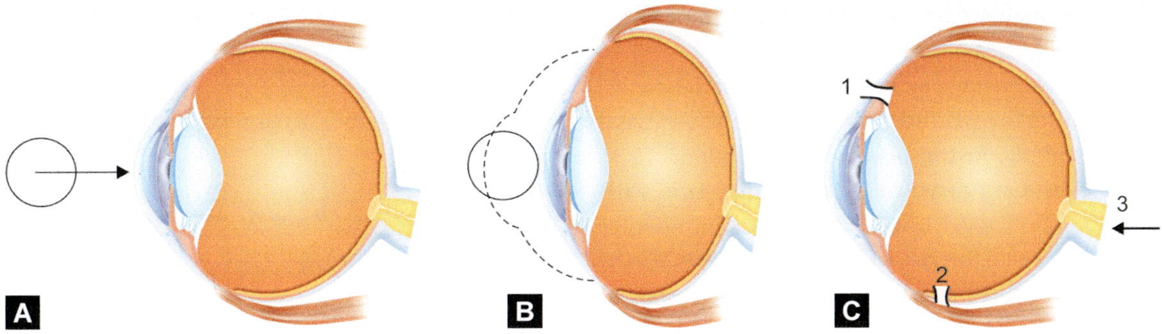

Figs. 115.4A to C: When a blunt object approaches the eye at high speed, anteroposterior decompression of the globe occurs, which can lead to rupture at points of weakness such as the (1) limbus; (2) under the insertion of the rectus muscles, where the sclera is thinnest at about 0. 3 mm; and (3) optic nerve.

OPEN GLOBE INJURIES

An open globe injury can be classified into laceration or rupture. A laceration is a full-thickness violation of the eyewall caused by a sharp object. A rupture occurs when a blunt object hits the eye with enough force to cause a rapid rise in IOP and equatorial expansion of the globe. Ruptures most commonly occur at the weakest points of the sclera, which are just under the insertion of the rectus muscles, the limbus, or at the optic nerve head. Sites of prior surgery, such as an extracapsular cataract surgery or penetrating keratoplasty wound, are particularly vulnerable to ruptures (Figs. 115.4A to C).

Signs of an open globe injury include:

- 360° of hemorrhagic chemosis
- Conjunctival laceration
- Peaked pupil
- Low IOP compared to the fellow eye
- Shallow anterior chamber
- Violation of the lens capsule.

Although low IOP is suggestive of an open globe injury, it is important to note that a normal or high IOP does not rule out the possibility of an open globe injury, as this can occur if the wound is plugged by uveal tissue.

A Seidel test can be used to determine whether a laceration of the cornea or sclera is full-thickness or partial-thickness. A fluorescein strip is wet with a few drops of sterile saline or topical anesthetic and used to paint the fluorescein over the wound. If the wound is leaking, the fluorescein will be diluted with aqueous and turn bright green under the cobalt blue filter (Fig. 115.5). Once the diagnosis of an open globe is confirmed, a Fox shield should be placed over the eye and the patient should be instructed to remain nil per os (NPO). Tetanus prophylaxis should be given if not up to date. Systemic antibiotics such as vancomycin and a third generation cephalosporin or a fluoroquinolone should be administered.[23] Intracameral or intravitreal antibiotics can be given at the time of open globe repair and are indicated in injuries with a high risk for contamination (such as those occurring in a rural setting) or if an IOFB is present.

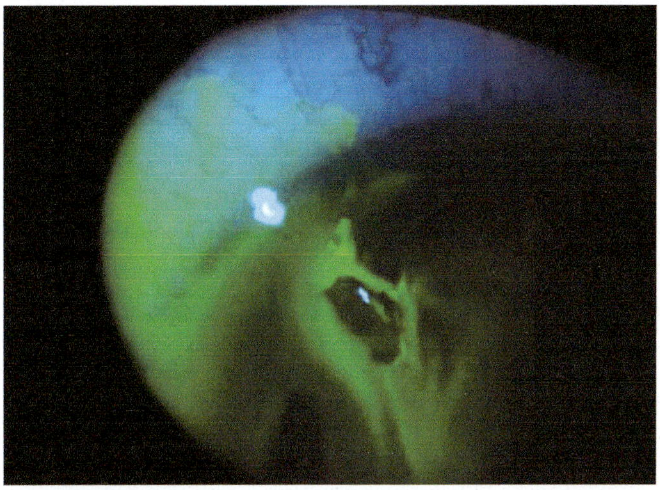

Fig. 115.5: A sterile fluorescein strip wet with a few drops of saline is used to paint the area suspicious for a full-thickness injury. The area is then examined with a cobalt blue filter. Aqueous exiting through the wound appears as bright green, indicating a positive Seidel test.

Surgical Management

Primary repair of open globe injuries should be performed as soon as possible, but may depend on factors such as anesthesia clearance of the patient and operating room availability. If possible, the repair should occur immediately but no later than 24 hours after the initial injury, as each day of delay may be associated with a worse visual prognosis.[24]

Extensive open globe injuries and pediatric patients require general anesthesia for repair.

Periocular anesthesia may be used in selected cases, such as small anterior wounds without extensive uveal prolapse or if general anesthesia is contraindicated.[25]

The goals of the surgery are to close the globe with minimal manipulation, reposit or excise exposed intraocular contents, and minimize the risk of endophthalmitis.[26]

The following sutures should be used in the repair of tissue:

- *Cornea:* 10-0 nylon
- *Limbus:* 9-0 nylon
- *Sclera:* 8-0 or 9-0 nylon or 7-0 or 8-0 polyglactin
- *Conjunctiva:* 7-0 or 8-0 polyglactin.

When suturing a laceration, the first step is to clean the edges of the wound. Avoid cutting any cornea or sclera as this will make closure difficult without extremely tight sutures. The next step is to make a paracentesis at a distant location and reposit prolapsed iris with a blunt spatula. A minimal amount of viscoelastic can be used if needed to maintain anterior chamber depth. When suturing, a 3-1-1 or "slip" knot can be used, as demonstrated in Figures 115.6 and 115.7.

Principles for corneal suturing are outlined in Figures 115.8 and 115.9. All sutures should be buried into the cornea. In children, corneal sutures can be removed within 6–8 weeks and in adults within 2–6 months.[27]

For corneoscleral lacerations, the limbus is first approximated, followed by closure of the cornea and then the sclera. For scleral lacerations, it is important to carefully dissect overlying conjunctiva and Tenon's capsule. Scleral sutures should be approximately 80% deep, avoiding full thickness bites. For more posterior lacerations, the sutures can be placed from anterior to posterior until the posterior edge of the wound is identified. Care should be taken to avoid pressure on the globe.

With injuries that extend posterior to the equator, it may be difficult to achieve complete closure as manipulation may lead to expulsion of ocular contents. In these cases, the wound may be left to heal by secondary intention. If a scleral laceration extends underneath a rectus muscle, the rectus muscle should be secured with a double-armed 5-0 polyglactin suture and disinserted as performed in standard strabismus surgery. The laceration can then be repaired and the muscle then reattached. Scleral knots should be buried or rotated posteriorly.

Ruptures are often more challenging to repair than lacerations, as they can be associated with irregular wounds

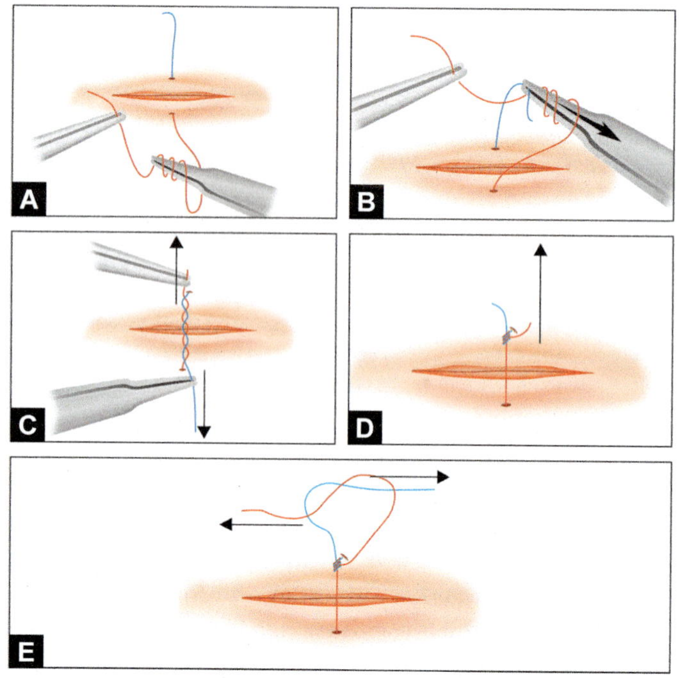

Figs. 115.6A to E: A surgeon's knot (3-1-1) is the primary knot of anterior segment surgeons and should be used in any corneal wounds under tension. (A to C) The first knot is a square knot consisting of three throws. The sutures are pulled in opposite directions, parallel to the initial throw; (D) The knot can be locked by pulling the short end towards the long end, while holding the long end still; (E) The second square knot is thrown in the opposite direction and tightened at right angles to the suture plane. The final securing square knot is thrown in the original direction and tightened parallel to the suture plane (not shown).

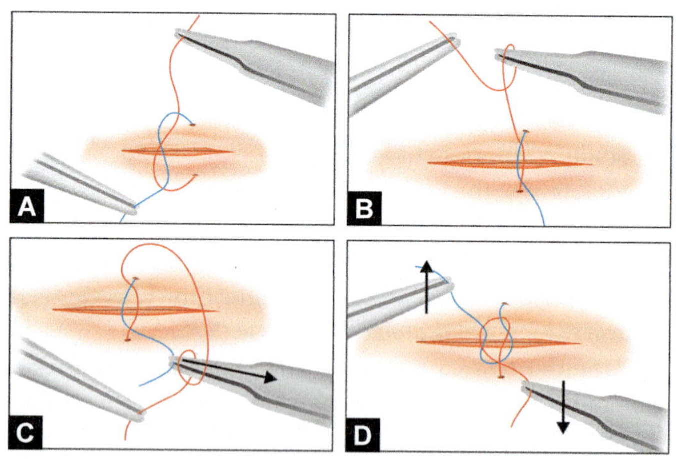

Figs. 115.7A to D: A slip knot (1-1-1) is an adjustable knot that can be used to minimize tension when suturing. If the suture if too tight, it can be loosened to the desired tension. (A) The first throw is a standard square knot; (B and C) For the second throw, a granny knot is performed by placing the forceps external to the proximal suture and bringing the forceps around the back of the knot, towards the free end of the suture; (D) Once the free end is grabbed, the suture is tied in the same direction as the first throw, with the free pulled towards the surgeon. The knot is now a sliding knot, and can be adjusted to the desired tension. Once the desired tension is achieved, one or two square knots are placed to lock the suture into place.

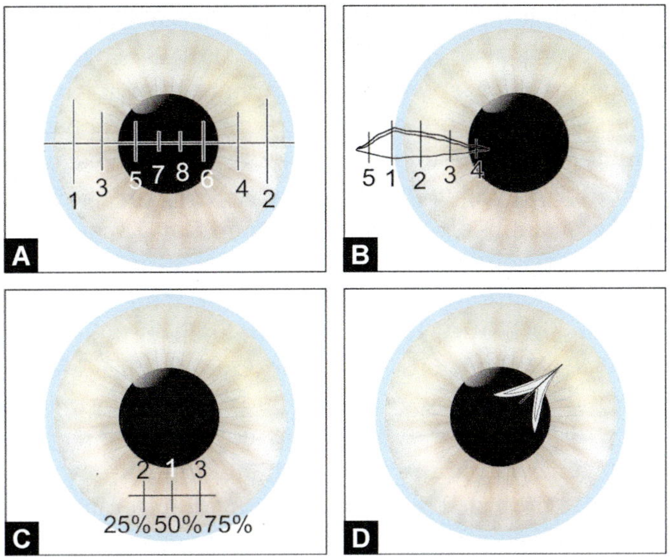

Figs. 115.8A to D: Order of suture placement for corneal wounds. (A) If the wound is long and transects the cornea, sutures should start from the periphery with long bites and get progressively shorter as the center is approached in order to minimize postoperative astigmatism. Avoid placing sutures in the visual axis when possible; (B) If the wound crosses the limbus, the limbus should be approximated first as this is the most critical step in restoring the proper anatomy. The corneal wound should then be closed, followed by the sclera. In a wound with multiple angles, the angle should be aligned first and then each part should be considered a separate wound; (C) Simple wounds can be closed with the 50% divide rule, bisecting the wound with each pass; (D) For wounds involving an angle, the suture should be placed away from, as opposed to towards, the angle.

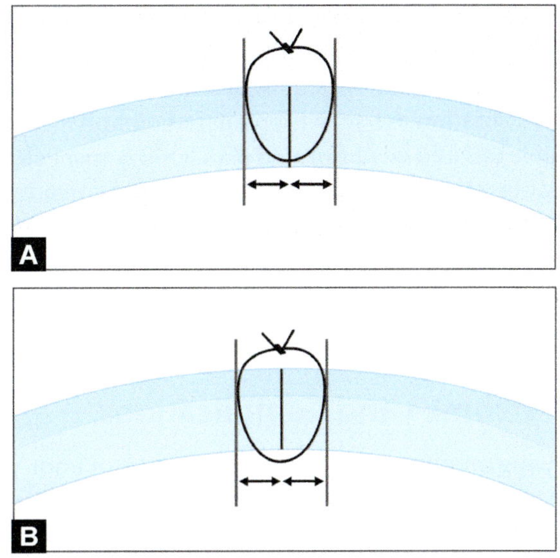

Figs. 115.9A and B: Appropriate depth of corneal sutures. (A) Traditionally, corneal sutures are recommended to be 90% deep, with the bite length equidistant on both sides. Entry and exit with the needle should be perpendicular to the surface. Practically, it may difficult to achieve an exact depth of 90%; (B) Sutures of 100% depth have several advantages. Misalignment caused by uneven suture depth is prevented. In addition, immediate closure of the wound is achieved, preventing the entry of aqueous into the stroma and thus allowing the cornea to clear more quickly. However, when you remove full-thickness sutures, this must be done under sterile conditions using 5% betadine as rotating the suture through the anterior chamber is a potential source of contamination.

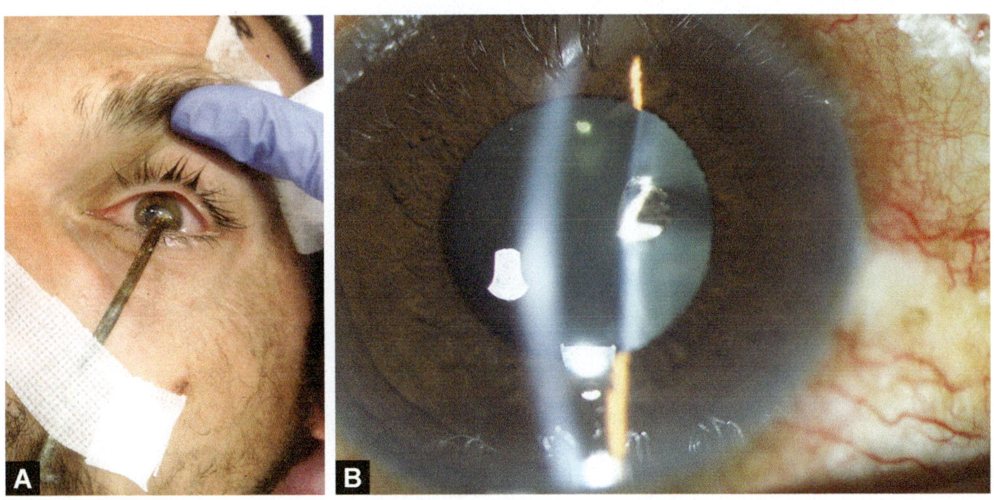

Figs. 115.10A and B: (A) A 25-year-old patient presents with a nail in the eye after hammering at work without eye protection; (B) Intralenticular foreign body. A corneal entry wound can often be visualized. Other more subtle signs include focal cataract and iris transillumination defects, particularly when associated with a penetrating wound.

and expulsion of intraocular contents. The rupture site may be hidden by extensive chemosis and hemorrhage; thus it is critical to proceed with exploration in the operating room if there is suspicion for an open globe injury. At times, a 360 degree peritomy is necessary to localize the rupture site.

Finally, IOFBs are a type of penetrating injury which deserve special attention. This injury most commonly occurs in young men who are hammering without eye protection (Figs. 115.10A and B).[28] The majority of IOFBs involve the posterior segment, but they can also be found lodged in the anterior chamber or in the lens. Signs of an IOFB include iris transillumination defects or focal cataract, particularly when associated with a corneal or scleral laceration. CT scan (or plain radiograph if CT is not available) should be performed if an IOFB is suspected but cannot be visualized on exam. An IOFB is considered a surgical emergency and should be removed immediately to decrease the risk of endophthalmitis. An IOFB involving the posterior segment should be managed by a vitreoretinal surgeon, as there is a high risk of retinal detachment.

Outcomes and Complications

Following an open globe injury, predictors of poor visual outcome include poor preoperative visual acuity, the presence of an RAPD, retinal detachment, posterior location, and contusive mechanism of injury.[22,29] Based on over 2,500 cases from USEIR, Kuhn, and colleagues developed an ocular trauma score (OTS) based on six variables found to be of prognostic significance[30] (Tables 115.3 and 115.4). Each variable is assigned a point value and the sum of the numbers relates to an OTS category allowing the physician to estimate the probability of visual recovery.

Post-traumatic endophthalmitis after an open globe injury occurs in less than 5% of cases, and most commonly occurs within the 1st week following trauma. The risk is higher when an IOFB is present, so intracameral or intravitreal antibiotics should always be given in the presence of an IOFB. The most common organisms causing post-traumatic endophthalmitis are *Staphylococcus* and *Bacillus* species.

Sympathetic ophthalmia is another rare but feared complication following an open globe injury, with an incidence of about 0.4%.[31] In this condition, the injured eye incites a granulomatous inflammatory response in the fellow eye. In the past, primary enucleation of a severely injured eye with no visual potential was often recommended. However, with improvement in immunosuppressive therapies the visual prognosis of sympathetic ophthalmia is generally good and thus enucleation as a prophylactic measure is not recommended.

Retinal detachment has been reported in up to 30% of patients following open globe surgery and can be an early or late complication. The presence of vitreous hemorrhage, higher zone of injury, and poor visual acuity at initial presentation were found to be associated with an increased risk of retinal detachment.[32]

Table 115.3: Calculating the ocular trauma score (OTS): The variables and the raw points.

Variable	Raw points
Initial vision	
NLP	60
LP/HM	70
1/200–19/200	80
20/200–20/50	90
≥20/40	100
Rupture	– 23
Endophthalmitis	– 17
Perforating injury	– 14
Retinal detachment	– 11
Afferent pupillary defect	– 10

(NLP: No light perception; LP: Light perception; HM: Hand motion)

Table 115.4: Calculating the OTS. Conversion of raw points into an OTS category and calculating the likelihood of the final visual acuity in five categories.

Sum of raw points	OTS	No light perception	Light perception/hand motion	1/200–19/200	20/200–20/50	≥20/40
0–44	1	74	15	7	3	1
45–65	2	27	26	18	15	15
66–80	3	2	11	15	31	41
81–91	4	1	2	3	22	73
92–100	5	0	1	1	5	94

OTS: Ocular trauma score.

CLOSED GLOBE INJURIES

A closed globe injury can be classified into a lamellar laceration, in which there is a partial-thickness wound of the cornea or sclera, or a contusion, in which direct energy causes deformation of the globe. Both will be covered in the following sections, along with superficial injuries of the conjunctiva and cornea.

Anterior Segment

Ocular Surface

The conjunctiva, cornea, and sclera should be systematically examined in the setting of ocular trauma. Significant subconjunctival hemorrhage or chemosis may obscure an open globe injury, so meticulous ocular examination is mandatory. If a conjunctival laceration is present, the underlying sclera should be carefully examined for a defect and remaining debris should be irrigated or removed. Small conjunctival lacerations (<1 cm) can be left to heal without sutures. Large lacerations can be closed with 7-0 or 8-0 polyglactin sutures.

The cornea should be examined for abrasions, foreign bodies, or lamellar lacerations. Vertical linear corneal abrasions indicate the presence of a subtarsal foreign body, and the upper eyelid should be everted and the conjunctival fornices swept in search of the foreign body.

Corneal abrasions are typically treated with prophylactic topical antibiotics. An abrasion associated with organic matter or possible contamination should never be patched. Superficial metallic corneal foreign bodies are very common and can be removed easily at the slit-lamp with a 27-or 30-gauge needle. If a rust ring is present, this can be removed with a corneal burr. Partial-thickness or lamellar lacerations of the cornea should be examined with a Seidel test and light pressure to rule out a small full-thickness wound. The wound should be cleaned of any foreign material. Broad spectrum topical antibiotics should be prescribed, as the risk of infection is high. Surface injuries associated with organic material should be followed closely for the development of fungal keratitis.

Anterior Chamber

Traumatic hyphema, circulating red blood cells in the anterior chamber, and traumatic iritis, circulating white blood cells in the anterior chamber, are commonly seen after trauma. Symptoms may include photophobia and the treatment is cycloplegia and a short course of topical steroids.

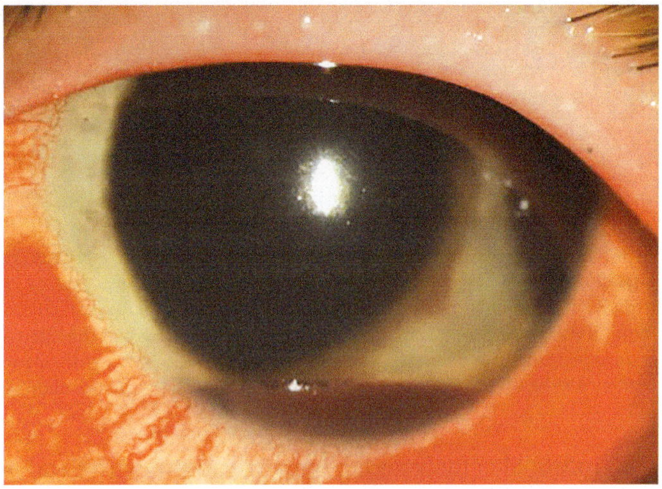

Fig. 115.11: A 16-year-old presents with hyphema after being hit in the eye with a baseball.

Table 115.5: Grading of hyphema.

Grade	Size of hyphema
0	Microhyphema (circulating red cells)
I	≤1/3 of anterior chamber
II	1/3–1/2 of anterior chamber
III	>1/2 but less than total anterior chamber
IV	Total filling anterior chamber or "eight ball" hyphema

Traumatic hyphema occurs when there is gross layering of the red blood cells in the anterior chamber (Fig. 115.11). Following a contusive injury to the eye, anteroposterior compression of the globe and equatorial expansion leads to shearing of the major arterial circle of the iris or its branches. The clinical grading system for hyphema is shown in Table 115.5. Elevated IOP is common in patients with hyphema and if prolonged, can lead to corneal blood staining. All patients who are of African or Mediterranean descent or have a positive family history of a sickling hemoglobinopathy should be screened with sickle cell prep, as patients with sickle cell trait or disease are at higher risk for uncontrolled IOP and optic nerve damage. Rebleeding can occur 3–5 days after the initial injury so patients should be seen frequently in the first week after injury. Systemic aminocaproic acid, an antifibrinolytic agent, has been used to prevent rebleeds but its use has been limited by systemic side effects. Patients should be told to maintain bed rest

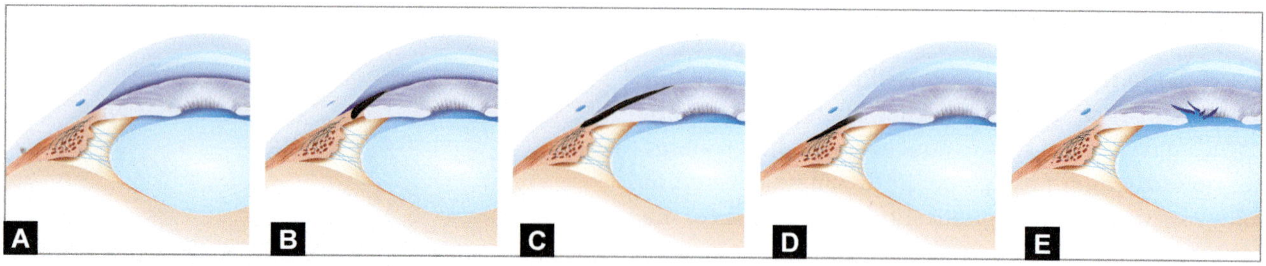

Figs. 115.12A to E: Anterior segment abnormalities following trauma. (A) Normal anterior chamber anatomy; (B) Iridodialysis—disinsertion of the iris from its attachment to the ciliary body at the iris root; (C) Angle recession—tear between the longitudinal and circular muscle of the ciliary body. The longitudinal muscle remains attached to the sclera spur, while the circular muscle and the iris root are separated; (D) Cyclodialysis cleft—ciliary body is disinserted from the sclera, allowing a direct route of aqueous entry into the suprachoroidal space and leading to hypotony; (E) Iris sphincter tears-tears in the iris sphincter at the pupillary margin may lead to traumatic mydriasis and disabling glare.

with minimal activity and to remain upright (with head of bead of at least 45 degrees) even while sleeping. Medical therapy includes topical steroids, cycloplegia, and IOP-lowering agents as needed. Carbonic anhydrase inhibitors (both oral and topical) should be avoided in patients with sickle cell trait or disease, as they lower oxygen tension and can lead to more sickling of red blood cells in the anterior chamber. The majority of cases can be managed medically. Indications for surgical intervention include:[33]

- Microscopic corneal blood staining, regardless of IOP values
- Total hyphema with IOP rather than or equal to 50 mm Hg for more than 5 days (to prevent optic nerve damage)
- Hyphema that is initially total and does not resolve below 50% at 6 days of with IOP > 25 mm Hg (to prevent corneal blood staining)
- Hyphema that does not resolve after 9 days (to prevent peripheral anterior synechiae).

In the presence of sickle cell trait or disease, even mild elevations of IOP can lead to optic atrophy because vascular perfusion is already compromised in these patients. Surgical intervention is thus indicated for:

- Average IOP > 24 mm Hg for more than 24 hours ("24 for 24 rule")
- Repeat IOP spiking > 30 mm Hg.

Surgical intervention is anterior chamber washout with clot removal. In certain cases, trabeculectomy can be a useful adjunct to the washout.

A summary of trauma to the iris, ciliary body, and angle is summarized in Figures 115.12A to E.

Iris sphincter tears and iridodialysis are commonly seen after contusive trauma. Iris sphincter tears may lead to traumatic mydriasis and the patient may suffer from glare. Iridodialysis, a disinsertion of the iris from its attachment to the ciliary body at the iris root, can cause glare and monocular diplopia (Fig. 115.13). Surgical intervention (pupilloplasty for traumatic mydriasis and suturing the peripheral iris to sclera for iridodialysis) is indicated for refractory symptoms or during future cataract surgery.

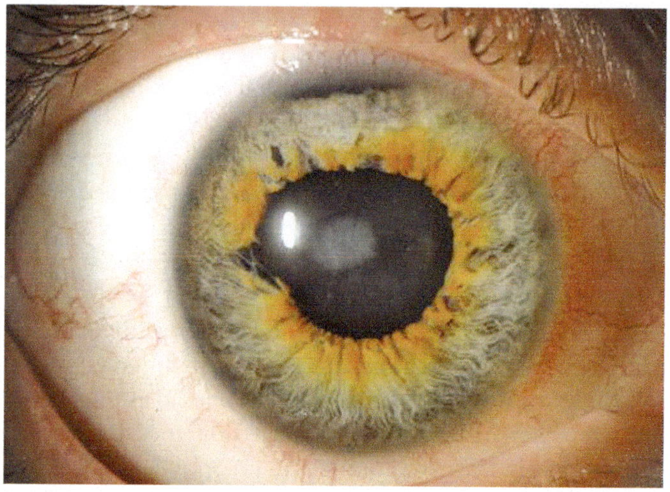

Fig. 115.13: A superior iridodialysis, iris sphincter tear, and traumatic cataract are seen in a 28-year-old patient after contusive trauma.

Angle recession is a tear between the longitudinal and circular muscle of the ciliary body that can occur after contusive trauma. The longitudinal muscle remains attached to the scleral spur, while the circular muscle and the iris root are separated. About 5–20% of eyes with angle recession will develop glaucoma and the greater degree of angle recession, the higher the risk. Up to 50% of patients with angle recession will develop glaucoma in the other eye, suggesting these patients may have predisposition to glaucoma. Thus, all patients with contusive trauma causing a microhyphema, hyphema, iris sphincter tears, or iridodialysis should be checked yearly with gonioscopy to assess for angle recession and future glaucoma development.

Traumatic cyclodialysis is rare and occurs when the ciliary body is disinserted from the sclera, allowing a direct route of aqueous entry into the suprachoroidal space and subsequent hypotony. The dialysis is visualized as a gap between the sclera and ciliary body on gonioscopy. Ultrasound biomicroscopy can be used to confirm and localize the cleft. Initial treatment should include atropine to rotate the ciliary body closer to the scleral spur to promote closure. If medical managements fail after 4–6 weeks, Argon laser can be applied to the ciliary body and scleral sides of the cleft. Direct cyclopexy, in which the ciliary body is sutured to the cleft under a scleral flap, can be attempted if the laser fails. Successful closure of a cyclodialysis cleft typically leads to an acute rise in IOP, so close monitoring is important.

Trauma to the lens is also common after both open and closed globe injuries. After a contusive injury, the most common type of cataract that develops is a sunflower cataract, which consists of radiating spokes in the anterior or posterior cortex. This may develop immediately or years following the injury. It is important to examine carefully for anterior or posterior capsular violation at the time of the initial trauma. If a violation is present, cortical material will often escape into the anterior chamber and will necessitate removal. Primary intraocular lens implantation can be considered if the inflammation is well controlled. Intraocular retinal scissors are useful in the creation of a capsulorrhexis when fibrosis of the anterior capsule is encountered. If there is posterior violation, a vitreoretinal surgeon is preferred for the removal of the lens. Lens subluxation or dislocation can occur immediately or years after the initial injury, and thus one should carefully look for evidence of phacodonesis or zonular weakness if there is any history of trauma.

Posterior Segment Injuries

The vitreous is tightly adherent to the retina at the vitreous base, the retinal vessels, and the optic nerve head. Following contusive trauma, all patients should have a scleral depressed exam to visual the ora serrata for 360 degrees when the eye is stable.

Vitreous base avulsion, visualized as vitreous draped over the peripheral retina with a "bucket handle" appearance, is pathognomonic for contusive trauma. Although alone it does not require treatment, it should alert the clinician to the possibility of a dialysis or peripheral retinal tear. Traction at the vitreous base can lead to retinal dialysis giant retinal tears, and horseshoe tears. Retinal dialysis is the most frequent traumatic retinal break (Fig. 115.14). The most common location is the inferotemporal quadrant, followed by the superotemporal quadrant. The vitreous base remains attached to the ora serrata, thus making a detachment less likely and the progression to a retinal detachment may take years. Prophylactic laser retinopexy should be performed when diagnosed. Giant retinal tears extend for at least 3 clocks hours circumferentially and are more common in myopic patients after contusive injury. Both giant retinal tears and horseshoe tears after trauma are almost always associated with a posterior vitreous detachment and can rapidly progress to a retinal detachment. Necrotic retinal breaks, which occur posterior to the ora serrata at the sight of direct ocular contusion, may also rapidly progress to retinal detachment.

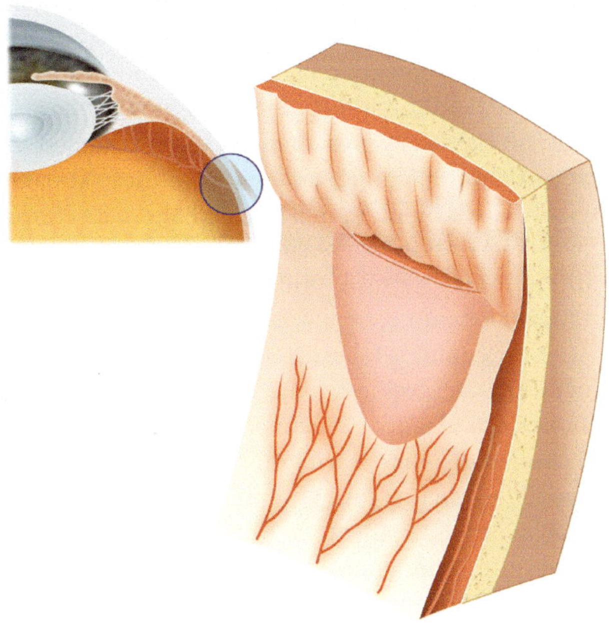

Fig. 115.14: Retinal dialysis is a disinsertion of the retina from the nonpigmented pars plana epithelium at the ora serrata.

Commotio retinae, a retinal whitening also known as Berlin's edema, is the most common retinal manifestation after contusive trauma. When isolated to the peripheral retina, the visual prognosis is excellent. Foveal involvement may lead to long-term retinal pigment epithelium (RPE) changes and visual loss.

A traumatic macular hole, a full-thickness defect in the neurosensory retina at the fovea, can occur instantly or years following contusive trauma. The natural history is variable and spontaneous closure has been reported.

Surgical intervention offers improved closure rates, but it is unclear whether final visual acuity is improved by surgery.

Choroidal rupture, a break in the choroid, Bruch's membrane, and the RPE, can occur following contusive injury and classically presents as a crescent-shaped streak concentric to the optic nerve. Initially, these streaks are often obscured by subretinal hemorrhage. Late choroidal neovascularization can occur in up to 1/3rd of patients with choroidal rupture, underlying the importance of long-term follow-up.

Chorioretinitis sclopetaria is rare and occurs following injury with a high-velocity projectile. The shock wave forces of the projectile lead to simultaneous retraction of the retina and choroid together, leaving an area of bare sclera. There is usually extensive retinal and choroidal hemorrhage initially. Fibrous proliferation during the healing process anchors the retinochoroidal margin to the underlying sclera and thus retinal detachment is rare.

Finally, traumatic suprachoroidal hemorrhage (SCH) is rare injury that can happen following sudden decompression of the globe following contusive trauma. The patient will present classically with severe pain and increased IOP. On examination, dark, dome-shaped elevations of the retina and choroid will be visible. B-scan ultrasound can confirm the diagnosis. The outcome is poor regardless of any surgical intervention.

CHEMICAL INJURIES

Chemical injuries are true ocular emergencies and immediate irrigation is critical, as the extent of tissue damage is related to the duration of contact between the chemical agent and the eye. A history and examination should be deferred until proper irrigation is performed, as each second after the injury is vital. It is important to document the chemical causing the injury. Alkaline agents generally cause more severe ocular damage than acids, as they readily penetrate the eye and cause saponification of cell membranes. Acids denature proteins, typically preventing deeper penetration into the eye. Steps of management are as follows:

- Irrigate copiously with normal saline or lactate Ringer's solution or balanced salt solution
- Evert the lid upper lid, sweep the fornices looking for particulate matter, and irrigate the fornices
- Wait 5 minutes and check the pH
- Continue irrigation until the pH is 7.0 (may take over 1 hour, can compare pH to the other side).

Table 115.6: Roper-Hall classification for ocular surface burns.

Grade	Cornea	Limbal ischemia	Prognosis
I	Corneal epithelial damage and no haze	None	Excellent
II	Corneal haze and iris details visible	<1/3	Good
III	Total corneal epithelial loss and stromal haze obscuring iris details	1/3–1/2	Guarded
IV	Cornea opaque, iris, and pupil obscured	>1/2	Poor

After irrigation is complete, visual acuity, IOP, and a detailed anterior segment examination with attention to limbal ischemia and stromal haze should be performed. The Roper–Hall modification of the Hughes classification for ocular surface burns (Table 115.6) can be used as an assessment and prognostic indicator. Grade I injuries can be treated with topical antibiotic ointment. Topical steroids can also be used but should be limited to the first 7–10 days after the injury to avoid delayed wound healing. More severe injuries should also be treated with high-dose vitamin C (total of 2 g orally a day) and doxycycline (100 mg orally twice a day) in adults. If available, 10% sodium ascorbate or 10% citrate drops every 2 hours can be used.

The IOP may be elevated and should be managed with glaucoma drops. In Grade III or IV injuries (Fig. 115.15), amniotic membrane transplantation should be used and may need to be replaced every few days until re-epithelialization occurs.

OCULOPLASTIC TRAUMA

Eyelid Lacerations

Eyelid lacerations are a common finding in periocular trauma. Violation of periocular soft tissue can be categorized as a true laceration, a tissue puncture, or an avulsion. Injuries can be superficial involving only skin or deep involving functional and supportive elements of the eyelid. Special care is taken to repair injuries that otherwise would result in loss of the normal protective function of the eyelid.

Relevant Anatomy

The eyelids are divided into two layers: the *anterior lamella,* which consists of the skin and orbicularis oculi muscle, and the *posterior lamella,* which consists of the tarsal plate and

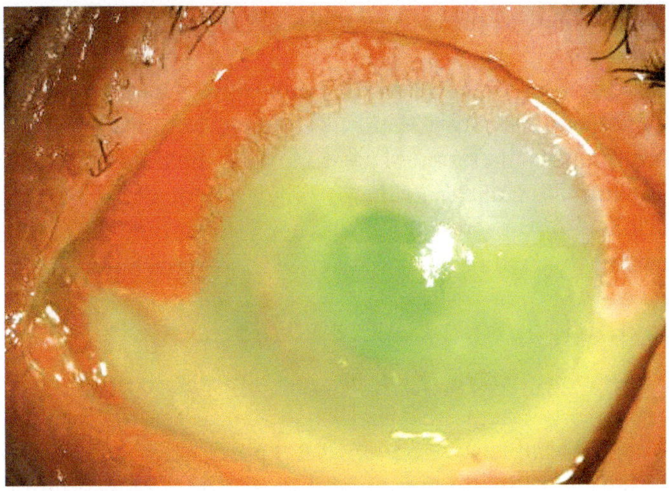

Fig. 115.15: A 70-year-old-female was splashed with alkali fluid (sodium hydroxide) while cleaning. Slit-lamp examination of the affected eye demonstrates six clocks-hours of limbal ischemia seen as blanching of the limbal vessels. A large corneal and conjunctival epithelial defect is present.

palpebral conjunctiva. The tarsal plate provides structural support to the eyelid, vertically measuring 10–12 mm and serves as the insertion point for the levator aponeurosis and Müller's muscle. The inferior tarsus is 4 mm in height and is the insertion point for the lower eyelid retractors. The orbital septum is a membranous sheet that extends from the orbital rim periosteum and blends with the tendon of the levator palpebrae in the upper eyelid and with the tarsal plate in the lower eyelid. Behind the septum are the two extraconal fat pads of the upper eyelid and the three extraconal fat pads of the lower eyelid.

The eyelid margins meet laterally at the lateral canthal angle and the orbicularis oculi condenses into the inferior and superior lateral canthal tendons which insert on the zygomatic bone. Medially, the orbicularis oculi condenses into an anterior and posterior leaflet (medial canthal tendon) which insert on the anterior and posterior lacrimal crests, respectively. The lacrimal sac sits between these two crests and the canaliculi are channels found within the two canthal tendon leaflets, making this portion of the eyelid margin weaker. The medial canthal tendon is thus important for lacrimal pump function and lid-globe apposition. The upper and lower eyelid puncta are found on the medial eyelid margin and are connected to the lacrimal sac by the canaliculi.

Evaluation

A complete history should be obtained, focusing on the *timing, mechanism*, and *location* of injury. The wound should be inspected to determine the injury *type, location, depth*, and *length*. The wound types include:

- *Abrasion:* Superficial scraping of skin
- *Laceration:* Cutting of tissue, typically caused by a sharp object, such as a knife
- *Puncture:* Passage of a sharp object through tissue planes, such as an animal bite
- *Avulsion:* It occurs when the eyelid is pulled forcefully, often disrupting the canalicular-containing medial canthal tendon since this area is natural weak.

A complete ocular examination should be performed to assess any damage to the globe. If an open globe injury is present, the lid laceration repair should be delayed until the globe is closed to avoid any pressure on the eye. All patients should have an up-to-date tetanus immunization.

Tips for examining lid lacerations include:

- Anesthetize and clean the wound properly to allow for complete examination
- Inspect for foreign bodies
- Look for fat prolapse which indicates violation of the orbital septum and raises concern for a levator aponeurosis laceration, increased risk of infection, and occult globe injury
- If an upper eyelid laceration is present, ptosis and levator function should be assessed
- Inspect the eyelid margin and evert the lid to look for posterior tarsal lacerations
- Canalicular lacerations are identified by direct observation of a laceration medial to the punctum, or by gentle probing of the canalicular system with a 00 Bowman probe. A visible probe within the soft tissue laceration confirms the presence of a canalicular injury
- If there is injury to the canalicular system, suspect a medial canthal tendon injury as the lacrimal sac lies between the anterior and posterior limbs of the medial canthal tendon. Look for rounding of the canthal angle or acquired telecanthus
- Assess for deeper involvement of lacerations even if it appears superficial, particularly in the case of puncture wounds from animal bites.

General Principles of Lid Lacerations Repair

If significant periorbital swelling is present, the repair can be delayed by 1–2 days as the eyelid is a highly vascularized tissue. Ice packs should be applied to decrease swelling. General anesthesia may be indicated for children. For adults, the repair can often be performed with local injection of lidocaine 2% with epinephrine. Sedation may be needed for adults who are anxious or with complicated lacerations. After numbing the area, the wound should be cleaned and irrigated. Povidone-iodine should be used to sterilize the area. Tissue loss is rare so thin eyelid skin that may be rolled up can often be flattened and reapproximated. Frankly necrotic skin should be debrided. Antibiotics are prescribed topically and systemically as indicated by the mechanism of injury. For example, animal bites are at high risk of infection and therefore oral antibiotics should always be prescribed.

Simple Laceration Repair

For deep wounds above the brow, layered closure can be performed with deep absorbable sutures such as 5-0 polyglactin. Deep suturing below the orbital rim should be avoided to prevent septal scarring and resultant lid retraction.

The overlying eyelid skin can be closed with 7-0 nylon, which can be removed after 7–10 days. Nylon is preferred over polyglactin for the skin, as it causes the least amount of inflammation and scarring. 7-0 polyglactic acid may be used if follow-up for suture removal is not possible or in the case of young child who would not tolerate suture removal.

Eyelid Margin Laceration Repair

Lacerations involving the eyelid margin are closed in a layered manner. The steps are described in Figures 115.16A to D.

Dissolvable suture such as 6-0 polyglactin can be very irritating to the lid margin and should only be used for a patient who will not likely return for suture removal or a young child who will not tolerate suture removal.

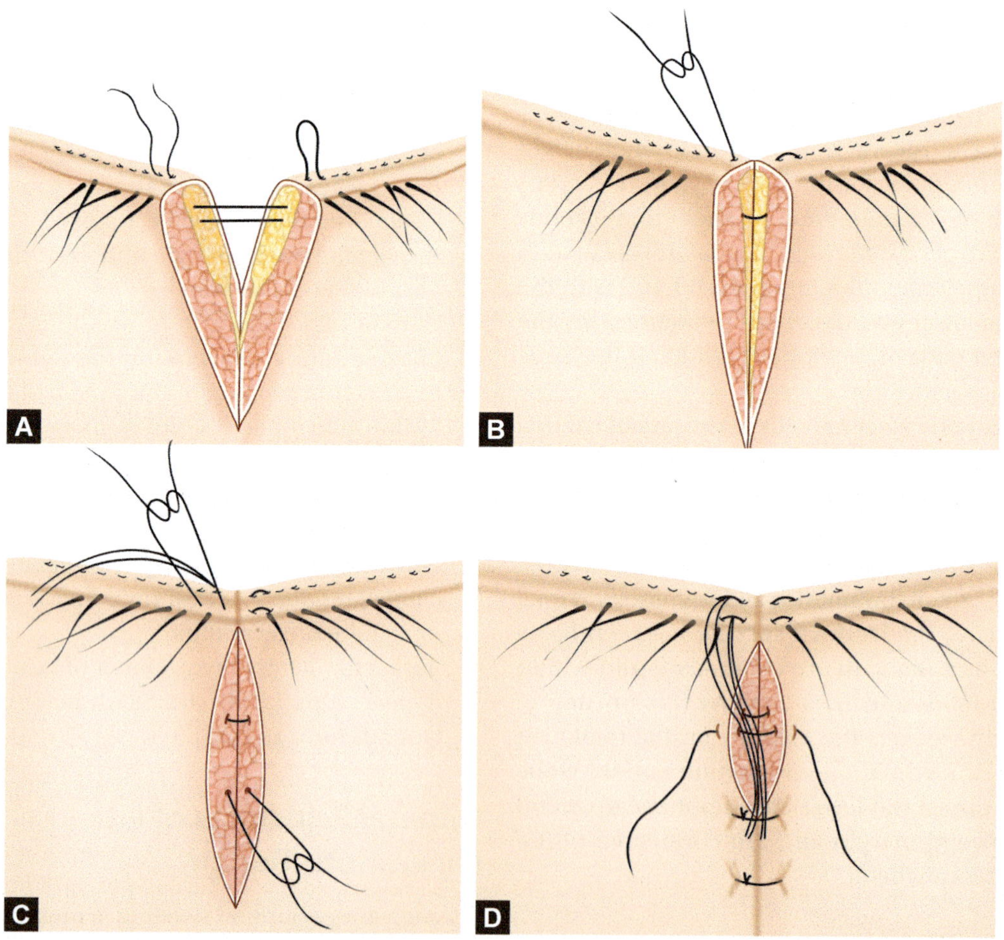

Figs. 115.16A to D: Margin lid laceration repair. (A) Align the lid margin using a vertical mattress suture placed through the meibomian gland orifices with a 6-0 silk suture; (B and C) Approximate the tarsus by passing two or three interrupted partial-thickness sutures through the tarsal plate horizontally (6-0 polyglactin). Tie the silk vertical mattress suture and cut the suture long. Add additional vertical mattress sutures anterior to the gray line if needed for additional alignment of the lid margin; (D) Close the overlying skin with 7-0 nylon, incorporating the ends of the 6-0 silk to keep it away from the cornea.

Canalicular and Medial Canthal Tendon Repair

As the canaliculus and medial canthus are intimately related, avulsions nearly always necessitate repair of both structures. The canaliculus should be repaired with a stent to align the cut edges properly and promote healing. The first step is to identify the cut edges of the canaliculus.

The nasal or distal edge of the canaliculus may be difficult to identify and the surgeon should clean the wound and look for a small white cuff of epithelial tissue. If this is not visualized, diluted fluorescein, air, or viscoelastic may be injected via a cannula through the intact punctum. A pigtail probe with lubricating ointment also can be rotated through the intact punctum, though care is needed to avoid creating a false passage.

A variety of lacrimal stents are available for repair of canalicular lacerations, which are left in place as long as 3–6 months to allow healing of canalicular edges. For simple monocanalicular lacerations, the Mini Monoka (FCI Ophthalmics) monocanalicular stent is a popular choice. Bicanalicular lacerations may be repaired with two Mini Monoka stents or a bicanalicular stent. Bicanalicular tubes are passed through the upper and lower canaliculi, through the nasolacrimal duct, and then retrieved in the nose. They should be secured together to prevent prolapse. The Crawford and the Ritleng are two of the most popular examples of bicanalicular stents. Bicanalicular stents generally require sedation, but are less likely to be dislodged than monocanalicular stents. Once stented, the canaliculus should be closed with absorbable suture such as 5-0 polyglactin on one or both sides of the tubes. Figures 115.17A to E illustrates placement of a Crawford stent.

The medial canthal tendon should be repaired using a large braided suture such as a 4-0 polyglactin. If available, a heavy, small 1/2 circle or 5/8 circle needle facilitates grasping the periosteum at the superior anterior lacrimal crest where the residual canthal tendon can be secured. The lower eyelid should be over corrected to be "too high" and "too deep" if possible to account for natural descent and to prevent medial ectropion. Bicanalicular tubes, particularly when used as cerclage, can facilitate proper canthal tendon restoration.

Orbital Trauma

Orbital fractures are among the most common facial fractures and should be suspected in all cases of contusive periocular trauma. The most common causes of orbital trauma are motor vehicle accidents, assaults, falls, and sports injuries involving impact with a ball.

Relevant Anatomy

The orbit is pyramidal in shape and the bony walls protect the globe. The roof and lateral wall are the thickest and least prone to fractures. The orbital floor is composed of the maxillary, zygomatic, and palatine bones and is 0.5–1 mm thick. The infraorbital nerve, which provides sensation to the lower eyelid, side of the nose, and upper lip, travels along the orbital floor. The medial wall is composed of the maxillary, lacrimal, ethmoid, and lesser wing of the sphenoid bones. The ethmoid bone, also known as the lamina papyracea, is the thinnest bone in the orbit (0.2–0.4 mm). The maxillary sinus is located beneath the orbital floor and the ethmoid sinus medial to the medial wall. The cribriform plate is part of the ethmoid bone and houses the olfactory fibers as they travel from the nose to the brain.

Orbital Blowout Fractures

Internal orbital fractures involve the orbital floor and/or medial wall and spare the orbital rim. The most common fracture locations are in the orbital floor medial to the infraorbital groove and lamina papyracea. Contusive ocular trauma can lead to a "blowout" of these thin bones. Signs of a fracture include subcutaneous emphysema, hypoesthesia of the cheek, side of nose, and teeth, or a "step-off" in the inferior orbital room. The inferior rectus runs along the orbital floor and the muscle or its surrounding fibers can be entrapped within the fracture bones leading to upgaze restriction and diplopia. If the muscle is entrapped in a nondisplaced fracture, the muscle is at risk for necrosis in as little as 8 hours and emergent surgery is indicated. When an orbital fracture is suspected, CT scan of the orbits with 1–2 mm slices and axial and coronal cuts should be performed to confirm the diagnosis.

In addition to diplopia, enophthalmos can occur with orbital fractures from expansion of the orbital cavity and dislocation of intraconal orbital fat. This may be hard to identify early because of swelling, thus Hertel measurements should be performed at follow-up visits. The indications for surgical intervention include diplopia that persists for 7–10 days after trauma, significant enophthalmos (>1 mm), or large fractures of the floor or medial wall. Repair is typically done after the swelling resolves and before scarring develops, ideally within about 2 weeks after injury.

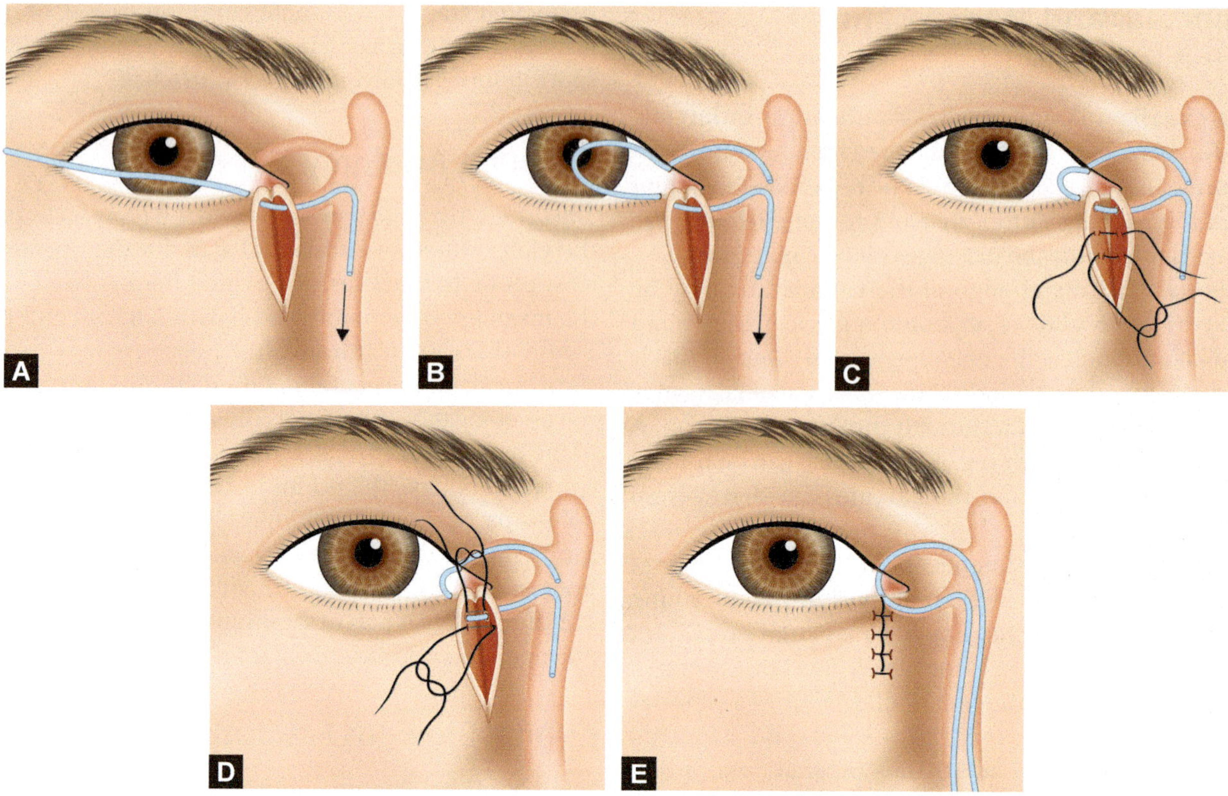

Figs. 115.17A to E: Canalicular laceration repair with Crawford stents. (A) Pass the stent though cut end of the canaliculus until a hard stop is encountered. Redirect the stent vertically and through the nasolacrimal duct. Retrieve the stent under the inferior turbinate; (B) Place the other end of the Crawford stent through the uninjured punctum, through the canaliculus and down the nasolacrimal duct, and retrieve the stent underneath the inferior turbinate; (C) Reinforce the medial canthal tendon with 4-0 polyglactin; (D) Reapproximate the canalicular mucosa and surrounding tissues with 6-0 polyglactin; (E) Use additional sutures in the orbicularis muscle as needed to reinforce the wound. Suture the skin with 7-0 nylon and anchor the stents in the nose.

Patients should be instructed to avoid nose blowing to prevent orbital emphysema. Oral antibiotics should be given to patients with medial wall fractures and ethmoid sinus disease.

Corticosteroids have no proven benefit but may be helpful in swelling reduction for patients without medical contraindications undergoing surgery. Surgical repair involves release of any entrapped tissues and placement of an orbital implant to span the fracture defect.

As above, the entrapment of extraocular muscle in a nondisplaced fracture is a surgical emergency and deserves special attention. These are known at the "trapdoor" or "white-eyed" blowout fracture. This fracture pattern most often occurs in children owing to the increased elasticity of their bones. In children the bones fracture and bend, but the bone springs back into anatomic position and entraps the extraocular muscle (Figs. 115.18A and B). This may tamponade bleeding and patients may present with a very quiet examination. Patients present with severe restriction on upgaze. The oculocardiac reflex may be elicited with nausea, vomiting, and bradycardia in upgaze. This is a surgical emergency as the inferior rectus can rapidly become ischemic and necrotic leading to permanent dysfunction.

Rim Involving Orbital Fractures

Several common midfacial fracture patterns involve the orbital rim:

- *Zygomaticomaxillary complex fractures* (also known as tripod fractures) involve the zygomatic bone. Clinically, patients present with a widened face, depressed cheekbone, and depression of the lateral canthal angle.
- *Naso-orbital-ethmoid fractures* involve the nose, medial wall, and inferomedial orbital rim. They are often centered on the lacrimal sac and may be comminuted. The medial canthal tendon and nasolacrimal duct may be disrupted. Clinically, patients present with medial canthal rounding and telecanthus.

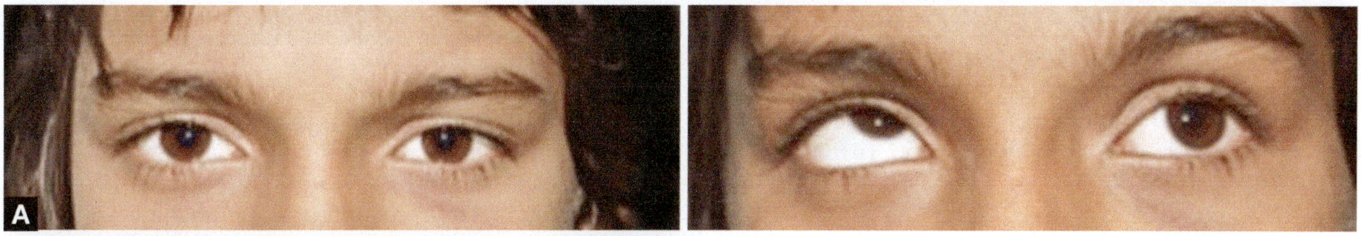

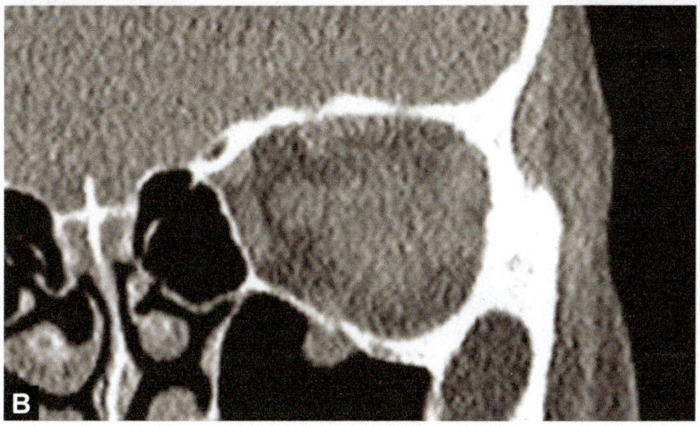

Figs. 115.18A and B: (A) A 10-year-old girl presenting after blunt trauma to the left eye. She has severe restriction on attempted upgaze with her left eye; (B) Coronal CT scan reveals a trapdoor fracture, where the bone has snapped back into place, incarcerating the inferior rectus muscle.
Source: Dr Usha, Aravind Eye Hospital, Madurai, Tamil Nadu, India.

- *Orbital roof fractures* are often associated with severe head trauma and can present with cerebrospinal fluid leaks.
- *Le Fort* fractures are various fractures that involve the pterygoid plates posteriorly and extend anteriorly to disassociate the maxillary teeth from the calvarium. *Le Fort I* fractures extend just above the teeth, *Le Fort II* fractures extend across the nasal dorsum in a manner similar to a naso-orbital-ethmoid fracture, and *Le Fort III* fractures extend across the medial and lateral orbital walls just below the roof. Patients present with poor teeth apposition in addition to other signs of complex facial trauma.

Intraorbital Foreign Bodies

The majority of intraorbital foreign bodies are a result of gunshot wounds or industrial accidents. The composition of the foreign body should be obtained as some are inert like glass and steel, where others like copper and organic material are poorly tolerated. Indications for removal include if the object is organic matter or copper, causing an inflammatory reaction, or is impinging on critical structures like extraocular muscles or nerves. MRI should not be performed in the presence of a metallic foreign body.

Vision Loss in Orbital Trauma: Retrobulbar Hemorrhage and Traumatic Optic Neuropathy

Retrobulbar hemorrhage can create a compartment syndrome in the orbit where increasing orbital tension prevents blood flow to the eye or optic nerve. Patients typically present with obvious periorbital ecchymosis, severe pain, and elevated intraocular pressure. They may have a history of anticoagulation. Vision loss and an afferent pupillary defect in the setting of swelling and increased IOP warrant emergent intervention. Initial management includes a lateral canthotomy as well as an inferior and/or superior cantholysis. Intravenous mannitol or topical IOP-lowering agents may be necessary. In cases with persistent bleeds that continue to cause pressure elevations, orbital decompression may be needed.

Traumatic optic neuropathy can occur with or without optic canal fractures. Vision loss can be profound and is accompanied by an afferent pupillary defect. Corticosteroids and surgical decompression of the optic canal have not been proven to improve visual outcomes when compared to observation alone and are associated with additional risks.[34] Novel neuroprotective therapies such as erythropoietin are being investigated and may prove worthwhile.

REFERENCES

1. Negrel AD, Thylefors B. The global impact of eye injuries. Ophthalmic Epidemiol. 1998;5(3):143-69.
2. Edwards RS. Ophthalmic emergencies in a district general hospital casualty department. Br J Ophthalmol. 1987;71(12):938-42.
3. Wong TY, Tielsch JM. A population-based study on the incidence of severe ocular trauma in Singapore. Am J Ophthalmol. 1999;128(3):345-51.
4. Moreira CA Jr, Debert-Ribeiro M, Belfort R Jr. Epidemiological study of eye injuries in Brazilian children. Arch Ophthalmol. 1988;106(6):781-4.
5. Chua D, Wong W, Lamoureux EL, et al. The prevalence and risk factors of ocular trauma: the Singapore Indian eye study. Ophthalmic Epidemiol. 2011;18(6):281-7.
6. Loon SC, Tay WT, Saw SM, et al. Prevalence and risk factors of ocular trauma in an urban south-east Asian population: the Singapore Malay Eye Study. Clin Exp Ophthalmol. 2009;37(4):362-7.
7. Tielsch JM, Parver L, Shankar B. Time trends in the incidence of hospitalized ocular trauma. Arch Ophthalmol. 1989;107(4):519-23.
8. Wong TY, Klein BE, Klein R. The prevalence and 5-year incidence of ocular trauma. The Beaver Dam Eye Study. Ophthalmology. 2000;107(12):2196-202.
9. Krishnaiah S, Nirmalan PK, Shamanna BR, et al. Ocular trauma in a rural population of southern India: the Andhra Pradesh Eye Disease Study. Ophthalmology. 2006;113(7):1159-64.
10. Nirmalan PK, Katz J, Tielsch JM, et al. Ocular trauma in a rural south Indian population: the Aravind Comprehensive Eye Survey. Ophthalmology. 2004;111(9):1778-81.
11. Voon LW, See J, Wong TY. The epidemiology of ocular trauma in Singapore: perspective from the emergency service of a large tertiary hospital. Eye (Lond). 2001;15 (Pt 1):75-81.
12. Kuhn F, Mester V, Berta A, et al. Epidemiology of severe eye injuries. United States Eye Injury Registry (USEIR) and Hungarian Eye Injury Registry (HEIR). Ophthalmologe. 1998;95(5):332-43.
13. Grieshaber MC, Stegmann R. Penetrating eye injuries in South African children: aetiology and visual outcome. Eye (Lond). 2006;20(7):789-95.
14. Haring RS, Sheffield ID, Canner JK, et al. Epidemiology of sports-related eye injuries in the United States. JAMA Ophthalmol. 2016;134(12):1382-90.
15. Capao Filipe JA, Rocha-Sousa A, Falcao-Reis F, et al. Modern sports eye injuries. Br J Ophthalmol. 2003;87(11):1336-9.
16. Vinger PF. A practical guide for sports eye protection. Phys Sportsmed. 2000;28(6):49-69.
17. Liggett PE, Pince KJ, Barlow W, et al. Ocular trauma in an urban population. Review of 1132 cases. Ophthalmology. 1990;97(5):581-4.
18. McGwin G Jr., Owsley C. Risk factors for motor vehicle collision-related eye injuries. Arch Ophthalmol. 2005;123(1):89-95.
19. Kuhn FC, Morris RC, Witherspoon DC, et al. Serious fireworks-related eye injuries. Ophthalmic Epidemiol. 2000;7(2):139-48.
20. Kuhn F, Morris R, Witherspoon CD. Birmingham Eye Trauma Terminology (BETT): terminology and classification of mechanical eye injuries. Ophthalmol Clin North Am. 2002;15(2):139-43.
21. Pieramici DJ, Sternberg P Jr, Aaberg TM, et al. A system for classifying mechanical injuries of the eye (globe). The Ocular Trauma Classification Group. Am J Ophthalmol. 1997;123(6):820-31.
22. Pieramici DJ, Au Eong KG, Sternberg P Jr, et al. The prognostic significance of a system for classifying mechanical injuries of the eye (globe) in open-globe injuries. J Trauma. 2003;54(4):750-4.
23. Ahmed Y, Schimel AM, Pathengay A, et al. Endophthalmitis following open-globe injuries. Eye (Lond). 2012;26(2):212-7.
24. Cruvinel Isaac DL, Ghanem VC, Nascimento MA, et al. Prognostic factors in open globe injuries. Ophthalmologica. 2003;217(6):431-5.
25. Scott IU, McCabe CM, Flynn HW, et al. Local anesthesia with intravenous sedation for surgical repair of selected open globe injuries. Am J Ophthalmol. 2002;134(5):707-11.
26. Banta JT. Ocular trauma. Edinburgh: Saunders Elsevier; 2007.
27. Kuhn F, SpringerLink (Online service). Ocular Traumatology. Berlin, Heidelberg: Springer-Verlag; 2008. Available from: http://dx.doi.org/10.1007/978-3-540-33825-3.
28. Behrens-Baumann W, Praetorius G. Intraocular foreign bodies. 297 consecutive cases. Ophthalmologica. 1989;198(2):84-8.
29. Esmaeli B, Elner SG, Schork MA, et al. Visual outcome and ocular survival after penetrating trauma. A clinicopathologic study. Ophthalmology. 1995;102(3):393-400.
30. Kuhn F, Maisiak R, Mann L, et al. The Ocular Trauma Score (OTS). Ophthalmol Clin North Am. 2002;15(2):163-5.
31. Zhang Y, Zhang MN, Jiang CH. Development of sympathetic ophthalmia following globe injury. Chin Med J (Engl). 2009;122(24):2961-6.
32. Stryjewski TP, Andreoli CM, Eliott D. Retinal detachment after open globe injury. Ophthalmology. 2014;121(1):327-33.
33. Read J. Traumatic hyphema: surgical vs medical management. Ann Ophthalmol. 1975;7(5):659-62, 64-6, 68-70.
34. Chaon BC, Lee MS. Is there treatment for traumatic optic neuropathy? Curr Opin Ophthalmol. 2015;26(6):445-9.

Chapter 116 Community Perspectives to Ophthalmology

Thulasiraj Ravilla, Allen Foster

INTRODUCTION: POPULATION HEALTH AND EYE HEALTH

The core components of clinical medicine are taking a history, undertaking a clinical examination, and followed by appropriate investigations, which leads to a diagnosis and then treatment. Applying these principles to a population (village, city, state, or country) is population health.

- How many people have what diseases (surveys or registers)?
- What are the priorities for intervention (preventive or therapeutic) based upon evidence and cost (intervention trials and studies)?
- How can these interventions be implemented through the health system (health system management)?
- What are the results and what can we learn (evaluation)?

So, Community Ophthalmology (eye health), starts with defining visual loss, estimates its magnitude, asks why people have visual loss and different eye diseases, and then most importantly asks how the eye health of the population can be improved. It identifies trends in disease occurrence, health-seeking behavior, and service delivery so as to improve intervention strategies.

For example, a study in north-west Nigeria in 2005 showed that only 55 in every 100-people aged 50 years and over had a visual acuity of 6/18 or better with cataract being the major cause of visual loss. A population eye care service was planned and implemented. 10 years later, 75 in every 100-people had visual acuity 6/18 or better—the eye health of the population had improved.[1]

GLOBAL MAGNITUDE OF BLINDNESS AND VISUAL IMPAIRMENT

Vision Categories

The World Health Organization (WHO) classifies visual acuity into four categories shown in Table 116.1. Categories 2 and 3 are grouped under the term *"low vision"* and also referred as moderate-to-severe visual impairment (MSVI). The broad term of "visual impairment" includes categories 2, 3, and 4.

Table 116.1: Categories of visual loss.[2]

Sl. No.	Category	From	To
1.	Normal vision	6/6	6/18
2.	Moderate visual impairment	<6/18	6/60
3.	Severe visual impairment	<6/60	3/60
4	Blindness	<3/60	No light perception

Prevalence

Based on this classification, the number of people with visual impairment (prevalence) can be estimated from population based surveys (Fig. 116.1).[3]

The most recent estimates of blindness and visual impairment come from the Global Burden of Disease. Globally, there were an estimated 36 million blind people in 2015 and 216.6 million people had MSVI.[4]

Incidence

The incidence of visual impairment is more difficult to estimate as it requires time consuming expensive cohort studies.[5,6]

Causes

The causes of blindness and moderate or severe visual impairment are classified by disease entity and shown in Table 116.2.[7] Cataract is the major cause globally of blindness and uncorrected refractive error of moderate or severe visual impairment. Cataract and uncorrected refractive error together are estimated to be responsible for 75% of all visual impairment [<6/18—no light perception (NLP)].

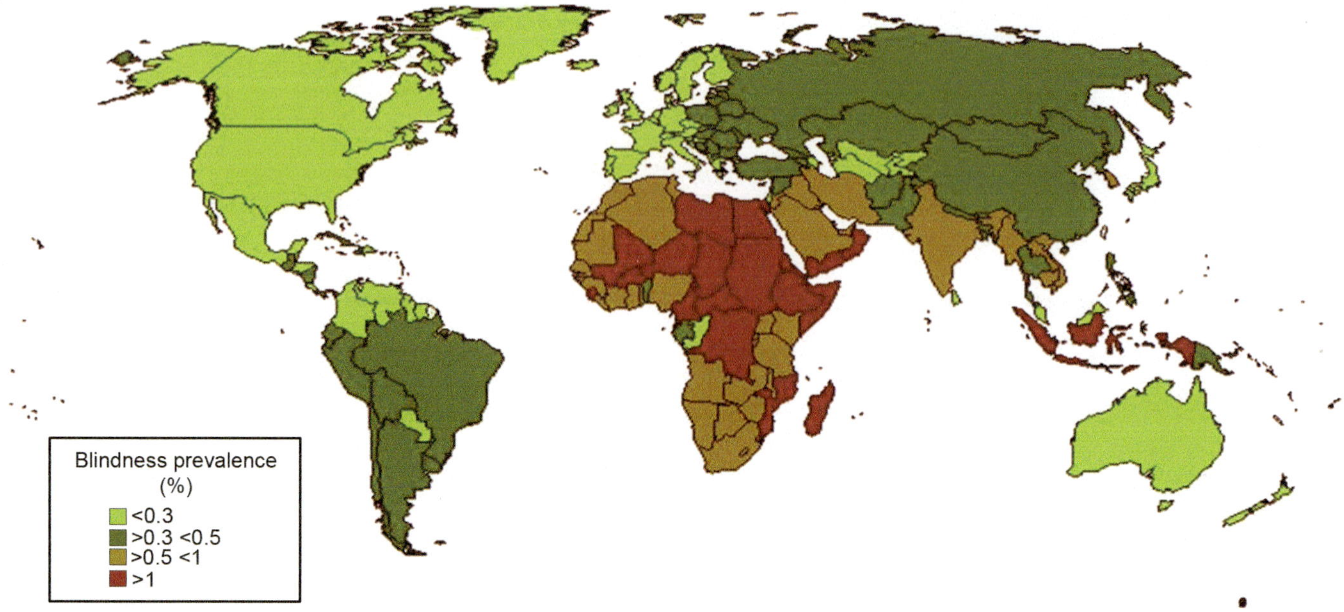

World Health Organization

The boundaries and names shown and the designations used on this map do not imply the expression of any opinion whatsoever on the part of the World Health Organization concerning the legal status of any country, territory, city or area or of its authorities, or concerning the delimitation of its frontiers or boundaries. Dotted lines on maps represent approximate border lines for which there may not yet be full agreement.

Fig. 116.1: Prevalence of blindness.

Table 116.2: Global causes of visual impairment (2015).

	Blind <3/60—NLP		Moderate or Severe Visual Impairment <6/18–3/60		All Visual Impairment <6/18—NLP	
Cause	**No (Millions)**	**%**	**No (Millions)**	**%**	**No (Millions)**	**%**
Cataract	12.6	35	52.6	24	65.2	26
Uncorrected ref. error	7.4	21	116.3	54	123.7	49
The glaucomas	3.0	8	4.0	2	7.0	3
Macula degeneration	2.0	5	8.4	4	10.4	4
Corneal opacity	1.3	4	2.9	1	4.2	2
Trachoma	0.4	1	1.6	1	2.0	1
Diabetic retinopathy	0.4	1	2.6	1	3.0	1
All other causes	8.9	25	28.2	13	37.1	14
Total	36.0	100	216.6	100	252.6	100

(NLP: No light perception)

Risk Factors

The causes of visual impairment vary by age group, gender, ethnicity, socioeconomic status, and therefore geographic region. Table 116.3 highlights some of the major differences.

The causes of visual impairment also change over time as the demography and socioeconomic status change in a community. Before the year 2000, communicable diseases (trachoma, onchocerciasis, and measles) and nutritional conditions (vitamin A deficiency) were important causes of blindness in areas of the world with low economy and inadequate health services. With increasing longevity, noncommunicable diseases (NCD) (cataract, glaucoma, and age-related macular degeneration) have become

Table 116.3: Patterns of visual impairment.

Cause	Comment
Adult cataract	• Increases with age • Cataract blindness related to low socio-economic status
Refractive error	• Myopia increases from around puberty • Associated with near work • High prevalence in China and SE Asia
Corneal scar	• Various infective and nutritional causes • More common with low socioeconomic status • Maybe seen in children
Trachoma	• Associated with inadequate WASH facilities • More common in females
Glaucomas	*Different types:* • Open-angle more common in Africa • Closed-angle more common in South East Asia
Diabetic retinopathy	Increasing problem associated with lifestyle and overweight
Retinopathy of prematurity	Increasing problem in upper and middle economy settings
Macula degeneration	• Two types • Increases with age

(WASH: Water, sanitation and hygiene)

increasingly important, and with increasing socioeconomic status diabetic eye disease in adults and retinopathy of prematurity (ROP) in children are emerging as new problems.

Assessment Tools

As in clinical medicine, there are various investigations, so in population health there are tools, which can be used to make a "community diagnosis". In eye health, the most comprehensive investigation is a total population-based survey of eye disease and visual impairment. This is a resource intensive exercise although the information gathered can be very important in long-term planning of eye services. Approximately, 80% of all blindness occurs in people age 50 years and over and therefore a focused population-based survey of people in this age group will provide important information at a much lower cost than a total population-based survey as the sample and survey are much smaller.

The Rapid Assessment of Avoidable Blindness (RAAB) is a standard methodology to examine a random sample of the population aged 50 years and over for the prevalence and causes of blindness and visual impairment. A sample size in the order of 3,000 people is required and the study can usually be completed in several weeks at a reasonable

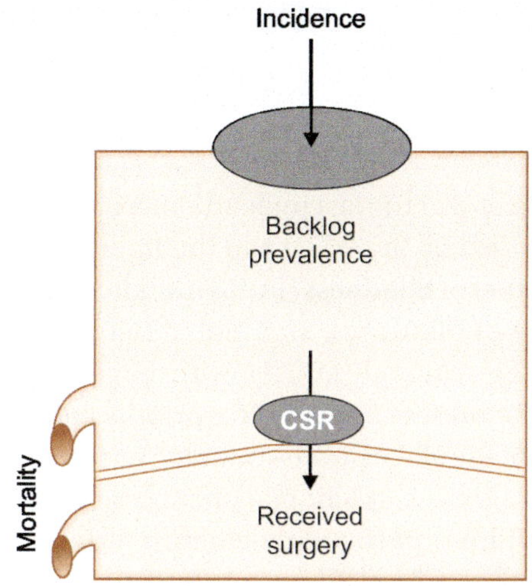

Fig. 116.2: Schematic illustration of cataract services.
(CSR: Cataract surgical rate)

cost. Over 100 RAABs have been conducted in the world.[8] RAAB does not give information on the prevalence and causes of blindness and visual impairment in people aged under 50 years of age; and does not give any information on eye diseases in people with a visual acuity of 6/18 or better, e.g. earlier stages of glaucoma.

Other disease targeted population-based surveys can also be performed, for example refractive error in school children, and trachoma infection in suspected endemic communities. The Global Trachoma Mapping Project is an example of the assessment of one blinding disease using a standardized methodology.[9]

With a RAAB survey, important information on the need and delivery of cataract service provision can be obtained:

- Number of people with visual impairment or blindness from the prevalence of cataract
- Number of people with operated cataract
- The visual acuity after cataract surgery—outcome
- The reasons why people with cataract have not had surgery—barriers
- The cataract surgical coverage (CSC)—proportion operated of all those who needed surgery (at different visual acuity levels).

An estimate of the number of cataract operations done in a year for a given population can be obtained from operation records, which allows for the cataract surgical rate (CSR) to be estimated (CSR = cataract ops/million pop/year).[10]

The prevalence of cataract, CSC and CSR allow a picture to be built up of the cataract services in the population, which can be monitored and evaluated as services are provided (Fig. 116.2). Across countries, CSR has wide variation ranging from under 1,000 in many sub-Saharan countries to over 6,000 in high income countries.

SPECIFIC BLINDING DISEASES

Toward the end of the last millennium a coordinated effort was developed by the WHO and the International Agency for Prevention of Blindness (IAPB) to address the increasing magnitude of blindness. This global initiative was called *"Vision 2020—The Right to Sight"* with the goal of eliminating avoidable blindness. Initially, five priority conditions were identified at the global level—cataract, refractive errors and low vision services, trachoma, onchocerciasis, and visual loss in children, particularly vitamin A deficiency; later diabetic retinopathy (DR) and glaucoma were also added.

Trachoma

Trachoma is an infection of the conjunctiva caused by *Chlamydia trachomatis* serotypes A, B, and C. The bacteria are transmitted in ocular and facial discharges from child to child by flies, fingers, and cloths. Repeated infection in young children produces a local immune response in the upper eyelid conjunctiva with follicle formation and inflammation. Years of repeated infection and inflammation lead to cicatricial conjunctival scarring, which in the upper eyelid causes the eyelashes to turn in (trichiasis and entropion). The lashes damage the cornea leading to ulceration and scarring with visual loss. The simplified grading of trachoma is given in Table 116.4 and Figures 116.3A to D.

- Trachomatous inflammation—follicular (TF)
- Trachomatous inflammation—intense (TI)
- Trachomatous conjunctival scarring (TS)
- Trachomatous trichiasis (TT) and corneal opacity (CO)

Trachoma occurs in situations with inadequate water supply and poor sanitation, which predispose to children having unclean faces with ocular discharge, and often a preponderance of flies. The control of trachoma is known by the acronym surgery for trichiasis, antibiotics, facial cleanliness, and environmental improvement (SAFE) (Table 116.5).

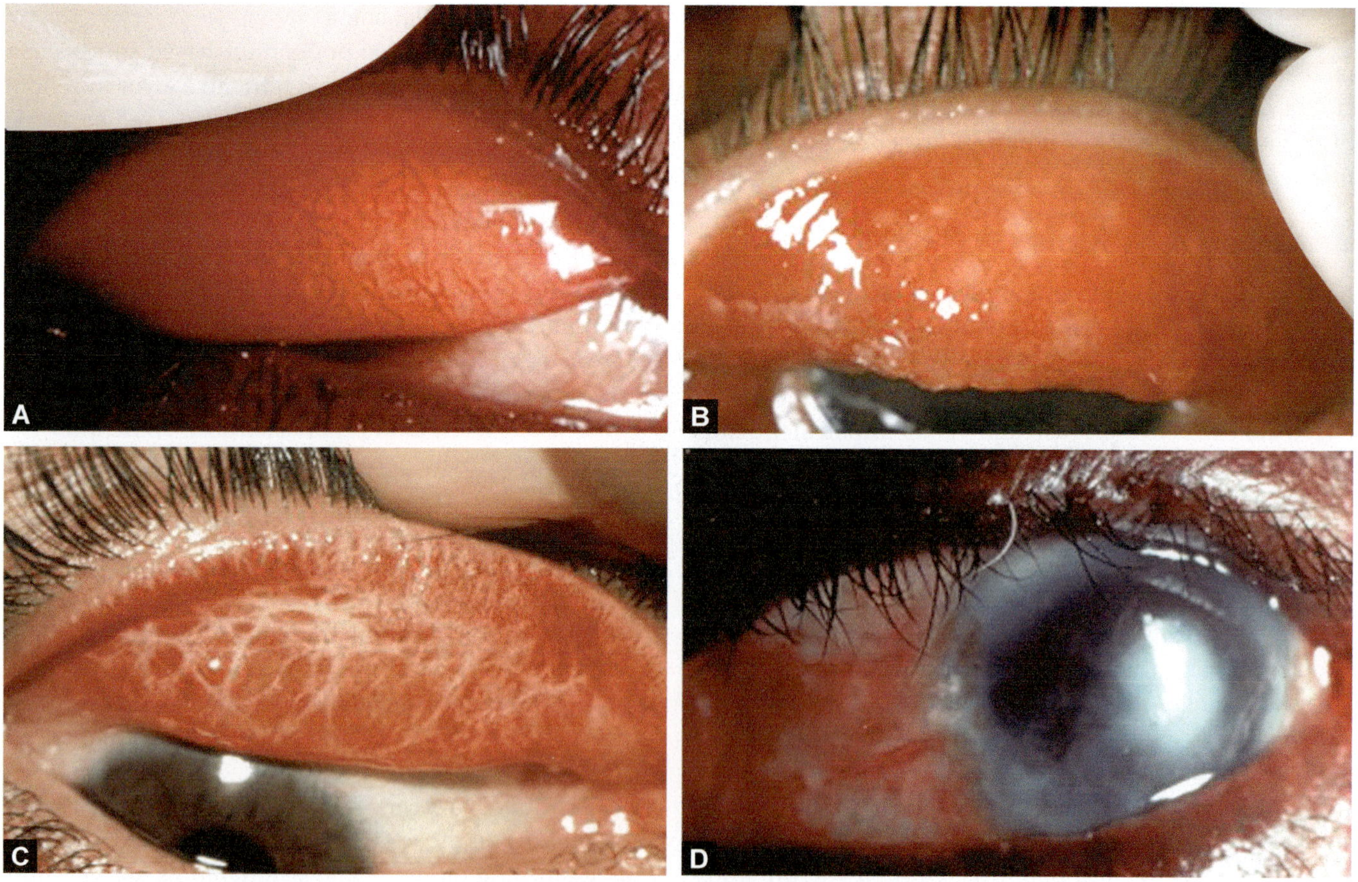

Figs. 116.3A to D: The simplified grading of trachoma.

Table 116.4: Simplified Trachoma Grading Scheme.

Grade	Name	Definition
TF	Trachomatous inflammation—follicular	Five or more follicles at least 0.5 mm in diameter, in the central part of the upper tarsal conjunctiva
TI	Trachomatous inflammation—intense	Pronounced inflammatory thickening of the upper tarsal conjunctiva obscuring more than half the normal deep tarsal vessels
TS	Trachomatous conjunctival scarring	Easily visible scars in the tarsal conjunctiva.
TT	Trachomatous trichiasis	At least one eyelash rubs on the eyeball, or evidence of recent removal of inturned eyelashes.
CO	Corneal opacity	Easily visible corneal opacity over the pupil, so dense that at least part of the pupil margin is blurred when viewed through the opacity

Table 116.5: Control of trachoma through SAFE.

SAFE	Objective	Intervention
S	Surgery for trichiasis	Tarsal rotation procedure
A	Antibiotics to reduce transmission of *Chlamydia*	Mass distribution of azithromycin to communities with TF 10% or greater in children aged 1–9 years: an annual dose for 3 years then reassess
F	Facial cleanliness	Encourage mothers and carers to keep children's faces clean
E	Environmental improvement	Promote better sanitation and water supply

(TF: Trachomatous inflammation—follicular)

Approximately, 50 countries are endemic for trachoma with an estimated 80 million children having active disease. A major initiative, the Global Elimination of Trachoma by 2020 (GET2020) is underway in many countries to eliminate blindness from trachoma and control transmission of trachoma infection (Fig. 116.4).

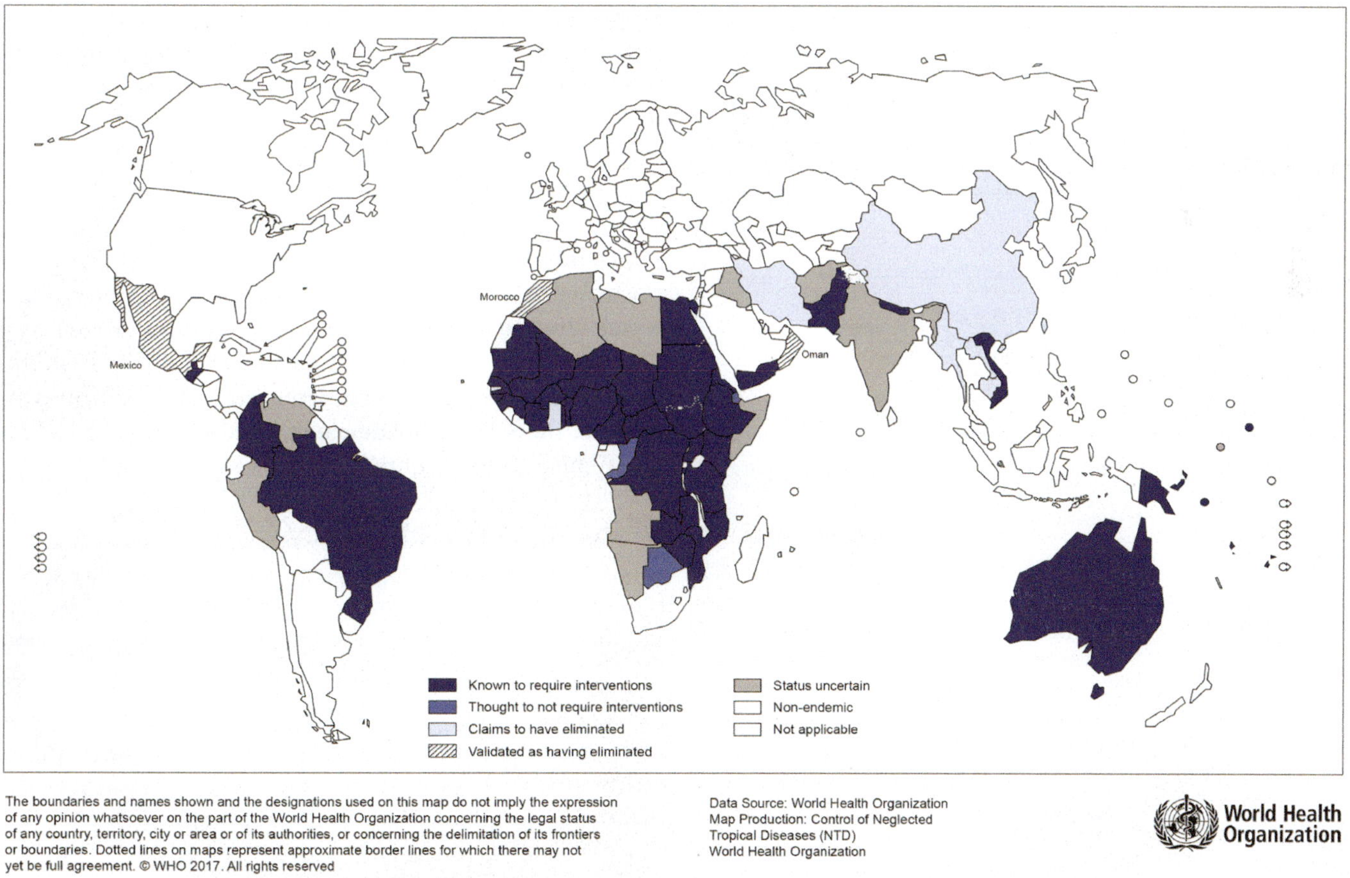

Fig. 116.4: Status of elimination of trachoma as a public health problem, 2017.

The WHO leads an international alliance, which supports Ministries of Health in carrying out essential activities such as epidemiological assessment, baseline mapping, project implementation, coordination, monitoring, surveillance, project evaluation, and resource mobilization. It is open to all parties—governments, international organizations, and nongovernmental organizations, which are willing and ready to contribute to international efforts' (http://www.who.int/trachoma/partnership/en/).

Onchocerciasis

Onchocerciasis is a skin and eye disease caused by infection with a parasitic worm—*Onchocerca volvulus* (Flowchart 116.1). This is also commonly referred to as the river blindness. The adult worms in humans are macroscopic and live for more than 10 years, producing millions of microscopic microfilariae, which are motile and attracted to the pigment in skin and eyes. If the infected human is bitten by a blackfly (*Simulium* species) the microfilaria can be ingested into the fly and develop through several larval stages before being injected into another human by the fly, where it develops into an adult worm so completing the cycle.

If the microfilaria migrates to the eye, they can be seen on high-power slit-lamp microscopy in the anterior chamber and cornea. If the microfilaria dies in the eye, then they produce an inflammatory response, seen in the anterior part of the eye as punctate keratitis and/or low-grade iritis. After many years of onchocerca infection the ocular signs of long-standing disease are sclerosing keratitis, chronic iritis with secondary glaucoma, and chorioretinal atrophy with optic atrophy (Fig. 116.5).

Flowchart 116.1: Life cycle of *Onchocerca volvulus.*

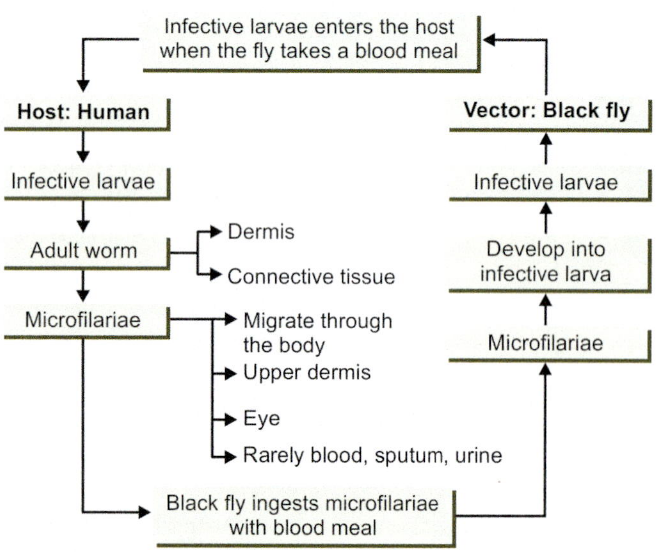

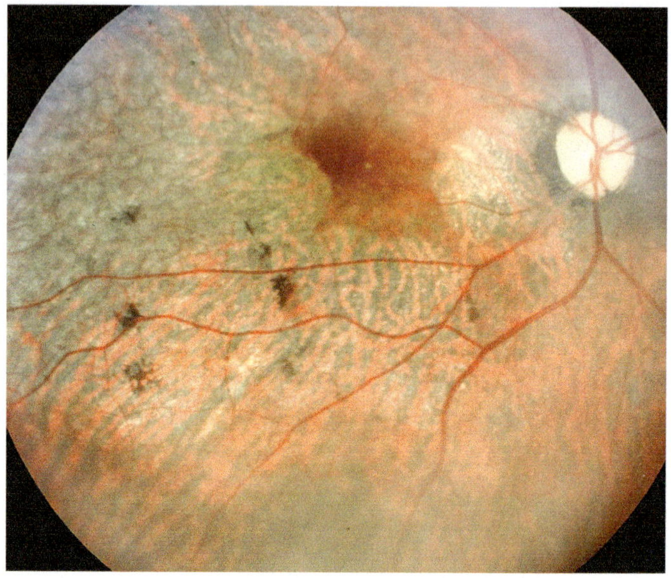

Fig. 116.5: Chorioretinal atrophy and optic atrophy due to chronic onchocerciasis.

Approximately, 36 countries in Africa, Latin America, and Yemen were endemic. Ivermectin (Mectizan) is provided free of charge by Merck Inc. for national onchocerciasis programs and is usually given once a year to all eligible subjects (some programmes treat every 6 months). Mectizan reduces the microfilarial load in the body, resulting in a decrease in morbidity from skin and eye disease. There is also evidence that over many years, it can also reduce and even eliminate transmission of the parasite.

Vitamin A Deficiency

Vitamin A (retinol) is essential for various processes in the body including embryo development, immunity, epithelial function, and vision. Vitamin A is fat-soluble and the body requirements come from food. Food rich in vitamin A (or its precursors) includes breast milk, papaya, mangoes, green leafy vegetables, carrots, fish, and liver. After absorption retinol is stored in the liver and released to the tissues via the blood bound to retinal-binding protein.

Vitamin A is required for the formation of rhodopsin in rod photoreceptors. Rhodopsin is made of retinal and the protein opsin. Rod cells are especially important for night vision. Vitamin A is also essential for normal functioning of goblet cells, which produce mucus in the conjunctiva and other mucous membranes. Lack of vitamin A deficiency produces loss of goblet cells and a poor tear film, resulting in dry eye with conjunctival and corneal xerosis. A typical sign in children aged 3–10 years of chronic vitamin A deficiency is a Bitot spot. The classification of ocular xerophthalmia (vitamin A deficiency) is given in Table 116.6 and some signs are shown in Figures 116.6A and B.

The major risk factors for vitamin A deficiency are:

- Inadequate maternal education
- Malnutrition
- Malabsorption
- Measles.

The treatment for a child with xerophthalmia is given in Table 116.7, and the prevention of vitamin A deficiency through vitamin A supplementation is shown in Table 116.8. Vitamin A is best given orally as a liquid or capsule containing either oil-based retinyl palmitate or retinyl acetate.

Table 116.6: Classification of xerophthalmia.

Sign	Definition	Comment
XN	Night blindness	Common symptom in older children and adults
X1a	Conjunctival xerosis	Loss of goblet cells, mucin, and poor tear film with dry wrinkled conjunctiva
X1b	Bitot spots	• Children aged 3+ • White raised foamy lesion on exposed temporal conjunctiva
X2	Corneal xerosis	Poor tear film with loss of clear corneal reflex
X3a	Corneal ulceration <1/3 of cornea	• Often bilateral • Children 6 months–5 years
X3b	Corneal ulceration >1/3 of cornea	• Often bilateral • Children 6 months–5 years • May result in adherent leucoma. Staphyloma or phthisis bulbi
XS	Corneal scar from X3	Usually dense, white, and well demarcated.

Table 116.7: Treatment of vitamin A deficiency.

Target age group	Oral dose	Frequency
6–11 months	1,00,000 IU	Immediately, again after 24 hours and again after 10 days
12 months and above	2,00,000 IU	Immediately, again after 24 hours and again after 10 days

Table 116.8: Prevention of vitamin A deficiency through supplementation (only in areas where vitamin A deficiency is a severe public health problem).

Target age group	Oral dose	Frequency
6–11 months	100,000 IU	Once
12–59 months	200,000 IU	Every 4–6 months
Pregnant women	Up to 10,000 IU or Up to 25,000 IU	Daily dose or Weekly dose
	For a minimum of 12 weeks during pregnancy up to delivery	

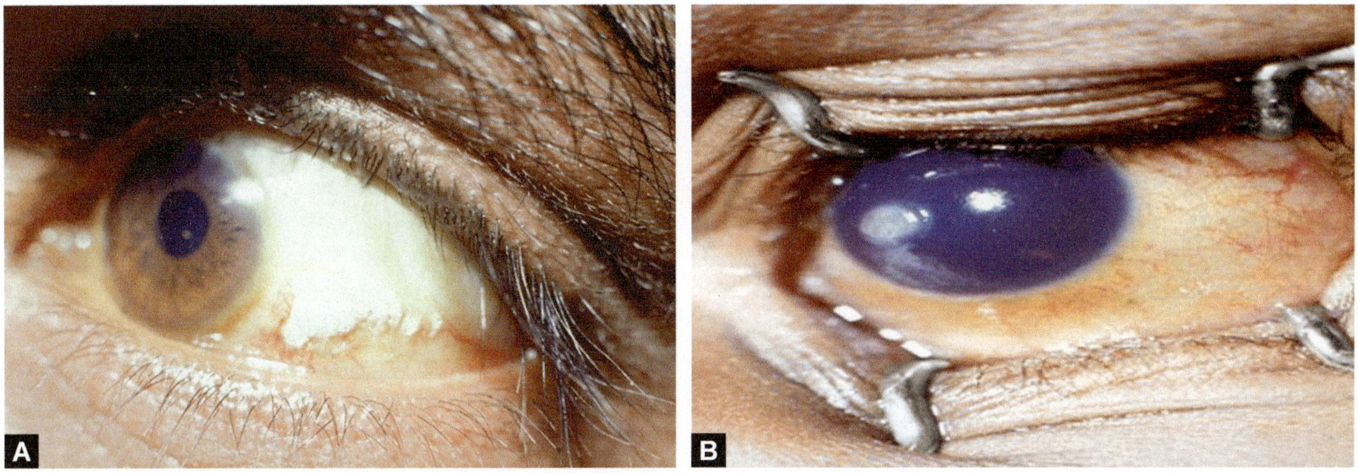

Figs. 116.6A and B: (A) Bitot spot due to vitamin A deficiency (X1B); (B) Corneal ulcer due to vitamin A deficiency (X3A).

Cataract

Cataract continues to be the leading cause of blindness and visual impairment. In developing countries, cataract accounts for over 50% of all blindness; while in developed countries, cataract continues to be the leading cause of "treatable" blindness.

In some sense, this is the challenge to the whole ophthalmic community because treatment for cataract has existed for centuries. The visual results and quality of surgery have evolved over the years with rapid technological advances in the past 3 decades. Cataract now is listed amongst the highest performed surgical procedures and one of the safest surgeries with good visual outcome when performed well. In one of its publications, the World Bank determined cataract surgery to be one of the most cost-effective surgical interventions[11] and in the mid 1990s in India made a healthcare investment for a cataract blindness control program. This together with the availability of low-cost intraocular lenses (IOLs) led to the quadrupling of the surgical output to about 5 million cataract surgeries a year and a significant improvement in quality. In spite of having proven technology and successful intervention models, cataract continues to account for over 50% of blindness in developing countries including in India. This is the reason for this being a paradox and a challenge to the whole ophthalmic community.

Addressing this paradox requires a deep understanding of the various challenges. It is not sufficient to just have a cost-effective intervention since it already exists, so other factors such as the distribution and effective use of resources need to be considered. The available evidence suggests that the challenges to delivering a cataract service are multifaceted.

Resources

In most developing countries, there is an acute shortage of resources. Since there are many dimensions to resources, the number of ophthalmologists[12] and cataract surgeons per million population will be used as a key indicator, since other resources such as buildings, equipment, and support staff are usually developed around the ophthalmologist, especially in the context of cataract surgery. The recommended density of ophthalmologist is 20 per million population.[13] For the sub-Saharan region; however, the initial benchmark is set at four ophthalmologist per million people in recognition of the current human resource (HR) status, which stands at 2 per million. In many African countries, insufficient general doctors are trained each year, so that few take up ophthalmology as their area of specialization.[14] To address this situation several years ago a separate cadre of "cataract surgeon" was developed whereby experienced ophthalmic assistants were specifically trained in cataract surgery. While this measure continued to be practiced particularly in east and central Africa gradually the training of this cadre has decreased.

In most developing countries, the ophthalmologists are essentially concentrated in large urban towns. In small countries, almost all of the ophthalmologists are in the capital city. This maldistribution, significantly accentuates the challenges faced by cataract patients in accessing surgery.

Addressing the challenges resulting from lack of resources and its maldistribution has been the most daunting one for eye care planners and international agencies working in eye care. Recognizing the long gestation period of about 10 years or more (post-high school) to produce an ophthalmologist, a short-term approach has been to employ ophthalmologists from other countries. International funding agencies brought in expatriate ophthalmologists to staff the local hospitals. Till recently, this was possible because of relatively low wages in their own countries and safe work environments. However, this has changed rapidly in the recent years with security becoming an issue in some countries and the long training period and costs entailed in becoming a skilled ophthalmic surgeon.

Quality

Though cataract surgery has good outcomes when done well, the visual results remain a concern in some situations. In one of the meetings of the technical advisory group, WHO recommended the following post-operative visual acuity (anytime between discharge and 12 weeks) as the desirable bench mark (Table 116.9).[15]

While this was arrived by consensus as something feasible, what is achieved by way of quality often falls short. The following table gives the postoperative visual activity of 3,708 cataract surgeries done at 40 surgical centers spread across 10 countries in Asia, Africa, and Latin America. Of these surgeries, 63% received manual small incision cataract surgery, 21% phacoemulsification, and 16% extracapsular cataract extraction, all with IOL implant (Table 116.10).[16]

For want of hard evidence, this could be attributed to various factors such as basic training during ophthalmology

Table 116.9: Categories of postoperative visual acuity.

Postoperative visual acuity categorization		Available correction	Best correction
Good	≥6/18 (≥20/60)	80% +	90% +
Borderline	< 6/18–6/60 (< 20/60–20/200)	15% –	5% –
Poor	< 6/60 (< 20/200)	5% –	5% –

Table 116.10: Postoperative visual activity of cataract surgeries.

Acuity	Pre-operative (%)	Post-operative 1–3 days (%)	Post-operative 40 days: Presenting acuity (%)	Post-operative 40 days: Best correction (%)
6/6–6/18	3	46	64	85
<6/18–6/60	11	32	26	10
<6/60	85	22	10	5
Missing data	37	21	278	369

residency, availability of appropriate equipment and their regular maintenance, supplies (IOLs of desired powers), and support staff. In most hospitals, the quality monitoring is not part of the standard protocol. Though important, very few providers insist on longer term follow-up to get a feedback on final outcomes, residual refractive errors, etc. Ensuring good outcomes and continually improving the patient experience is critical to sustaining the demand and growing it.

Metrics and Monitoring

The only matrix that continues to be used to define the magnitude of cataract continues to be prevalence data. As with any prevalence data, this is determined only through population-based studies. In the recent years, such studies are more commonly done using the RAAB protocol. These surveys essentially cover the population above the age of 50 and hence, the estimates of cataract causing visual impairment could be slightly understated, to the extent of not including this condition in those under 50 years of age. Such prevalence data, when done periodically could inform the eye care planners about the impact of the intervention programs that are in place. However, such prevalence estimates are grossly inadequate for planning of cataract services, beyond understanding geographically, where this problem is higher or lower. Since cataract blindness is a treatable condition with potential for restoration of normal vision (in most instances), the prevalence of cataract blindness should be viewed essentially as an indicator of "system failure" in delivering the surgical intervention to the person requiring it at the appropriate time. Today, we lack a robust methodology or a process to determine the number of cataract surgeries that would need to be performed to preempt people from transitioning from mild to MSVI and finally blindness due to cataract.

The performance of a cataract program and target setting is commonly done using a metric called CSR. This is fairly simple to compute, robust, and accurate (to the extent that the data is complete and reliable). Thus this has become the most widely used performance indicator often to compare performance across countries or regions. CSR, however, cannot be related to prevalence of blindness since not all surgeries are done on blind eyes or blind persons. Increasingly, people are opting for early intervention and also surgery on both eyes.

The third metric that is used is the CSC. This is often computed from the same population-based prevalence surveys that estimate the prevalence of blindness. Here, all operated persons are added to those who are blind to form the denominator. This then is used to calculate the surgical coverage. This inherently assumes that all those operated were blind at the time of surgery, which increasingly is not the case. Hence, this estimate tends to somewhat overestimate the CSC.

When it comes to monitoring, some gross national level figures around performance (CSR) and resources (number of ophthalmologists) are periodically made available or estimated. There is a paucity of information at field level to help with planning and for enhancing performance and quality. Robust monitoring and review is critical for continuous improvement of programs as well as care to individual patients.

Productivity

Since surgical intervention is the only option to deal with cataract, the logical inference would be that more cataract surgeries should be performed to address significant backlog and the growing need for this service. It is in this context that productivity becomes important. Though there is not a standardized definition of productivity, a useful proxy has been the number of cataract surgeries per year by an ophthalmologist or cataract surgeon.

This metric becomes important in the context of the scarce resources as described earlier. When we look at productivity across countries one sees a huge variation. While it is high in Nepal, it is low in parts of sub-Saharan Africa and Latin America. Strategies that can leverage the underutilized capacity can go a long way in reducing the cataract blindness. The reasons for low productivity, again is varied ranging from the density of population, cost of service, issues with equipment, and supplies as well as leadership and work ethics.

Role of Cataract in Financial Viability

Cataract formation is gradual, the decision of when to intervene is at an individual level. It is an elective procedure. Cataract also occurs across all economic strata, affecting the rich and the poor. The intervention is very-well proven resulting in improved vision immediately following the surgery. This allows people to continue in their economic vocation or return to it.[17] Because of this, those who have the resources are very willing to pay for the service. Thus, cataract surgeries along with correction of refractive errors, offer a significant opportunity for generating revenues to cover the cost of the intervention as well as significant surplus either to cross subsidize those who cannot pay or to meet some of the developmental costs. The scale of the activity and the efficiency with which it is done are drivers of the revenue and the surplus, respectively. This concept of achieving financial viability has been widely promoted and there are several charitable eye care institutions, which serve the poor for free or at very subsidized fees, that have become financially viable through a robust-cataract service. Providing cataract surgery at the right time when, the person is still gainfully employed will ensure that he or she will continue to earn and the possibility that they can pay for the services. Delaying the surgery often leads to losing their job and dependency in getting the treatment.

Diabetic Retinopathy

Diabetic retinopathy is a condition of the eye, which can afflict people with diabetes mellitus. With the increasing prevalence of diabetes and improved life expectancy the number of people who develop DR will increase. It is estimated that DR could affect as many as 191 million people globally by 2030.[18]

Pathogenesis and Prevention

The main pathogenic mechanism is abnormality of the retinal capillaries due to high blood glucose leading to increased permeability of the capillaries and later ischemia of the retina with new vessel formation. The risk of developing DR can be minimized through proper glycemic control and by reducing blood lipids and controlling any hypertension.

Classification

Diabetic retinopathy (DR) is broadly classified as nonproliferative DR (NPDR) and proliferative DR (PDR).

International Classification of Diabetic Retinopathy and Diabetic Macular Edema

International Classification of Diabetic Retinopathy and Diabetic Macular Edema has been given in Tables 116.11 and 116.12.

Screening for Diabetic Retinopathy

Integral to prevention of visual loss is the early detection of DR. Some countries have robust diabetes management program and mandated eye examinations. However, in the majority of countries national DR screening programs do not exist.

In India only 50% of the diabetics are diagnosed and only a very small proportion of them actually end up having a detailed retinal examination. The awareness that diabetic patients have a high risk of developing DR and that they must have regular eye examinations is not known even to many health professionals.

The DR is diagnosed by visualizing the retina using an ophthalmoscope or by taking a photo with a fundus camera, which are becoming cheaper and portable. Image recognition technology is being developed to automatically analyze the images for the presence of DR and its severity. In the future, one can anticipate significant technological advances that will enhance access and affordability leading to more universal screening of diabetics and case finding of DR.

A challenge for programs is the periodic follow-up eye examination. Organizations such as the International Council of Ophthalmology (ICO) have brought out guidelines[19] for the re-examination schedule based on the severity of the condition for different eyecare-resource setting, as well as the management of DR.

International Council of Ophthalmology Guidelines for Diabetic Eye Care

Follow-up schedule and management based on DR severity for high-resource settings (Tables 116.13 and 116.14).

Table 116.11: International Classification of Diabetic Retinopathy.

Diabetic retinopathy	Findings observable on dilated ophthalmoscopy
No apparent DR	No abnormalities
Mild nonproliferative DR	Microaneurysms only
Moderate nonproliferative DR	Microaneurysms and other signs (e.g. dot and blot hemorrhages, hard exudates, and cotton-wool spots), but less than severe nonproliferative DR
Severe non-proliferative DR	Moderate nonproliferative DR with any of the following: • Intraretinal hemorrhages (≥20 in each quadrant); • Definite venous beading (in 2 quadrants); • Intraretinal microvascular abnormalities (in 1 quadrant); and • No signs of proliferative retinopathy
Proliferative DR	Severe nonproliferative DR and 1 or more of the following: • Neovascularization • Vitreous or preretinal hemorrhage

(DR: Diabetic retinopathy)

Table 116.12: International Classification of Diabetic Macular Edema.

Diabetic macular edema	Findings observable on dilated ophthalmoscopy
No DME	No retinal thickening or hard exudates in the macula
Noncentral-involved DME	Retinal thickening in the macula that does not involve the central subfield zone that is 1 mm in diameter
Central-involved DME	Retinal thickening in the macula that does involve the central subfield zone that is 1 mm in diameter

(DME: Diabetic macular edema)

Follow-up schedule and management based on DR severity for low- or intermediate-resource settings (Tables 116.15 and 116.16).

Treatment of Diabetic Retinopathy

Sight-threatening DR, whether, proliferative DR or macular edema requires treatment to stop progression and visual loss. Different modes of treatment are available including pan-retinal laser and/or antivascular endothelial growth factor (anti-VEGF) intravitreous injection. Occasionally, surgery for vitreous hemorrhage and/or retinal detachment may also be indicated. Since, this also involves adequate metabolic control, an integrated coordinated approach between the ophthalmologist and a physician is important.

Table 116.13: Follow-up schedule for management of diabetic retinopathy severity.

Diabetic retinopathy severity	Follow-up schedule for management by ophthalmologists
No apparent DR	Re-examination in 1–2 years; this may not require reexamination by an ophthalmologist
Mild nonproliferative DR	6–12 months; this may not require reexamination by an ophthalmologist
Moderate nonproliferative DR	3–6 month
Severe nonproliferative DR	<3 months; consider early panretinal photocoagulation
Proliferative DR	<1 month; consider panretinal photocoagulation.
Stable (treated) PDR	6–12 months

(DR: Diabetic retinopathy; PDR: Proliferative diabetic retinopathy)

Table 116.14: Follow-up schedule for management of diabetic macular edema severity.

Diabetic macular edema severity	Follow-up schedule for management by ophthalmologists
Noncentral-involved DME	3–6 month; consider focal laser photocoagulation
Central-involved DME	1–3 month; consider focal laser photocoagulation or anti-VEGF therapy
Stable DME	3–6 month

(DME: Diabetic macular edema; VEGR: Vascular endothelial growth factor)

Table 116.15: Follow-up schedule and management based on diabetic retinopathy severity for low- or intermediate-resource settings.

Diabetic retinopathy severity	Follow-up schedule for management by ophthalmologists
No apparent DR	Re-examination in 1–2 years; this may not require re-examination by an ophthalmologist
Mild nonproliferative DR	1–2 years; This may not require re-examination by an ophthalmologist
Moderate nonproliferative DR	6–12 months
Severe nonproliferative DR	<3 month
Proliferative DR	<1 month; consider panretinal photocoagulation
Stable (Treated) PDR	6–12 month

(DR: Diabetic retinopathy; PDR: Proliferative diabetic retinopathy)

Table 116.16: Follow-up schedule and management based on diabetic macular edema severity for low- or intermediate-resource settings.

Diabetic macular edema severity	Follow-up schedule for management by ophthalmologists
Noncentral-involved DME	3–6 month
Central-involved DME	1–3 month; consider focal laser photocoagulation or anti-VEGF therapy
Stable DME	3–6 month

(DME: Diabetic macular edema; VEGF: Vascular endothelial growth factor)

Refractive Error

Refractive error is a common disorder where the eye cannot focus on an object to get a clear image. The result of refractive error is blurred vision leading in severe cases to visual impairment. Refractive errors include:

- Myopia (short-sightedness)
- Hyperopia (long-sightedness)
- Astigmatism (the eye does not create a sharp single focus and causes distorted vision)
- Presbyopia (difficulty in reading or near vision, it is linked to aging).

Prevalence

Refractive error can usually be effectively managed using spectacles, contact lenses, or refractive surgery. However, WHO estimates that 124 million people worldwide live with visual impairment due to uncorrected refractive errors (even while excluding those with uncorrected presbyopia).[7,20]

The prevalence of refractive error differs in different age groups; as does the type of refractive error. The prevalence of refractive error also varies greatly by geographic region. Europe has a 30% prevalence of myopia among its adult population.[21] In Taiwan, over 70% of the adults are myopic.[22]

Several studies point out that with rapid urbanization, decreased outdoor exposure and increased near vision activity, the likelihood of developing myopia or short-sightedness increases. Thus it is estimated that about a third of the world's population will be myopic by 2020.[23]

As presbyopia is related to aging, almost everyone is prone to develop this condition. An estimated 1.1 billion people aged 35 years and above have functional presbyopia (those requiring a correction of at least +1.00 D).[4]

Despite the widespread prevalence of the condition and the seemingly simple solution for it, uncorrected refractive error remains the leading cause of visual impairment (53%) and the second leading cause of blindness (21%).[7] This is reported to have resulted in a total loss of productivity of an estimated $121 billion.[24]

Management

Refractive errors cannot be prevented, but they can be diagnosed by a simple examination and corrected using spectacles, contact lenses, or refractive surgery. Of these spectacles are the most affordable and easiest to make available.[25] If corrected in time, this can prevent loss of visual function and the resulting productivity.

Considerations

Unlike other eye disorders, the correction of refractive error is not entirely dependent on the presence of an ophthalmologist to manage the condition. Optometrists or vision technicians can screen for, evaluate, prescribe, and dispense the corrective lenses for refractive error. Well-trained allied ophthalmic personnel (refractionists, opticians, spectacle technicians, contact lens dispensers, etc.) can also contribute significantly in various roles throughout this process.[26,27] Also, it is not essential to have sophisticated equipment or infrastructure for this; implying that refractive services can be incorporated even at primary levels of care.

Given the widespread prevalence of refractive error, it is essential that refractive services are made widely available. At the least, they should be integrated at all levels of care, and the refractive services should be comprehensive—including not only screening and evaluation of refractive error but also spectacle dispensing. Many developing countries adopt outreach camps as a common strategy to create access for eye care services—especially for cataract screening. With well-trained allied ophthalmic personnel, it is possible to successfully integrate comprehensive refractive services along with such camps.[28]

For successful integration of refractive services, it is important to have in place a minimum of a well-trained team and basic equipment. In addition, it is necessary to ensure procurement and access to a steady supply of spectacle lenses and frames. The latter is taken for granted, yet in many countries trade regulations and market forces restrict the import of such essential goods, which then become only available at very-high prices.

Pediatric Ophthalmology

Pediatric eye care encompasses prevention and treatment of eye diseases in children. Examining and assessing vision in small children requires considerable expertise and hence mandates special training.

It is often mentioned that though the percentage of childhood blindness appears small; the impact is much more in terms of blind years. According to review of available data in 2009,[29] the prevalence of blindness in children varies according to socioeconomic development and under 5 mortality rates. In low-income countries with high under 5 mortality rates, the prevalence may be as high as 1.5 per 1,000 children.

Common Treatable Eye Conditions in Children

Common treatable eye conditions in this age group are refractive errors, allergic and infective conjunctivitis, amblyopia, strabismus, and eye injuries. Important but less common conditions include retinoblastoma, congenital cataract, and ROP. Refractive error and amblyopia are often missed in children as they are unaware of their symptoms. It is critical to identify amblyopia early to reverse the vision loss. Large scale school screening programs will help in identifying significant refractive error in children. Focus also needs to be given to ensure spectacle compliance amongst school children.

The management of cataract in children differs from that in adults. There are challenges in anesthesia, IOL calculation in a growing eye; and the high incidence of thick posterior capsular opacification (PCO). The children also require long-term follow-up to maintain the correct refraction, screening for glaucoma and amblyopia prevention.

Prevention and Rehabilitation

The major causes of childhood blindness vary between developed and developing countries. In situations, with very poor primary health Care (PHC) the leading cause of visual impairment used to be corneal opacification caused by measles, xerophthalmia, and use of traditional eye medicine.[30] With improved neonatal care, vitamin A supplementation and measles immunization, there seems to be a shift in the spectrum of eye diseases. ROP and cerebral visual impairment (CVI) are now amongst the most prevalent causes in middle and high economy situations.[31] Vision loss due to ROP can be prevented, if identified and treated early. This can be done by creating awareness, training of staff in neonatal units on protocols and efficient networking amongst obstetricians, neonatologists, and pediatricians.

Cataract in childhood occurs in all situations although cataract occurring as part of the congenital rubella syndrome seems to be on the decline with widespread immunization. Heredity retinal dystrophies are important where consanguinity is common.[32]

Children with congenital globe anomalies, retinal dystrophies and CVI need to be identified early as visual impairment in the first few years of life can adversely impact a child's overall development. They need early stimulation and appropriate low vision services with training on sensory skills for better long-term independence.

The Glaucomas

Glaucoma is a significant irreversible cause of blindness worldwide. It is a much underdiagnosed condition. There are several distinct types of glaucoma. At the global level primary chronic open-angle glaucoma is the most common followed by primary closed angle (either chronic or acute). The distribution of these two forms varies considerably geographically and by ethnicity; open-angle is more common in Africa and western countries, while closed-angle glaucoma is more prevalent in East Asia.[33]

Prevalence

The prevalence of glaucoma increases with age, particularly after the age of 40 year and varies by ethnicity. Worldwide the current estimate is that 70 million people have glaucoma and this number is projected to rise to over 110 million by the year 2040 with Asia accounting for 60% of all glaucoma.[34] However, this may be an underestimate as many people with glaucoma are undiagnosed.

Screening

High intraocular pressure (IOP) is a major risk factor for chronic open-angle glaucoma and is often used as a test for screening; however, a raised IOP (for example 24 mm Hg or above) suffers from both low sensitivity and specificity. A definitive diagnosis of glaucoma is based on full clinical assessment including visual acuity, refraction, pupil reaction to light, assessment of anterior chamber depth and angle structures, IOP measurement, assessment of the optic nerve, and visual field. This full examination on which to make a definitive diagnosis makes it impractical to carryout population screening to diagnose glaucoma. The practical alternative is to assess the visual acuity, optic disk, and measure the IOP of everyone over 40 who presents for an eye examination, either for refraction for reading spectacles or an eye clinic appointment. Raised IOP above 24 mm Hg and/or a vertical cup or disk ratio of more than 0.5 indicates that the patient needs referral for a full clinical assessment of glaucoma.

Treatment

High intraocular pressure which is strongly associated with glaucoma is modifiable through intervention with medications, laser or surgery and most glaucoma management is aimed at reducing the IOP to a level which no longer damages the optic nerve. However, there are several major challenges to effective treatment. First glaucoma is a chronic condition and requires life-long treatment and monitoring of the response to treatment. Second in resource poor settings, facilities for comprehensive glaucoma examinations are limited. Third in low income countries, the availability and cost of glaucoma medications combined with the fact that these medications do not improve the vision, results in very poor compliance to medication. The overall result in many settings is inadequate control of IOP by medication with further visual loss leading to blindness. For this reason, one time treatment, either surgery or laser if available, may be an alternative cost-effective treatment.

Glaucoma is a major challenge and innovative solutions are required to address both diagnosis and treatment, if a successful public health strategy is to be promoted and implemented.

FUNCTIONAL LOW VISION

Definition

There are two different definitions of low vision. A visual acuity in the better eye of less than 6/18 but equal or better than 3/60 can be called low vision (or moderate or severe visual impairment). The second definition (discussed here) is usually called functional low vision (FLV) is "a person who has impairment of visual functioning even after treatment and/or standard refractive correction, and has a visual acuity of less than 6/18 to perception of light (PL) in the better eye, or a visual field of less than 10° from the point of fixation, but who uses, or is potentially able to use vision for the planning and/or execution of a task".[35] Using this FLV definition, low vision services are used to enable the person to improve function and participation in everyday activities, e.g. reading.

Magnitude

There have been few population-based surveys to assess the magnitude of FLV; however, a thumb rule is that it is of the same order as the prevalence of blindness.[36]

Common Causes

The causes of FLV vary according to country and age. In children the causes will be similar to the causes for blindness with corneal scar being important in low resource settings, ROP in middle and high-resource settings and postcataract surgery, microphthalmos, and retinal diseases in all countries.

In adults age-related macular degeneration, other retinal diseases, glaucoma, and DR are the major causes.

Low Vision Services

The aim of low vision services is to optimally use any residual vision for maximal functioning. Low vision services include both optical devices, e.g. magnifiers (near and distant) and nonoptical devices, e.g. better lighting, reading rulers, etc.[37]

All people with low vision should first have a full refraction and correction. This refraction may be difficult to undertake, for example in children after cataract surgery.

The clinical diagnosis will give guidance as to what are likely to be the visual problems, e.g. distortion and reading difficulties with macular diseases, field defects and mobility problems with glaucoma, and peripheral retinal dystrophies. It is important to ask the patient about their visual problems and needs and undertake a full assessment of visual function including distance and near vision, visual fields, and sometimes contrast sensitivity. Find out what the person can do and the difficulties they have.

For people with central visual field loss magnification (including electronic devices) or training in eccentric viewing may help. For those with peripheral visual field loss, adaptation of the environment may be important to assist mobility.

Each person has their own visual problems and capabilities; also each person has their own visual needs, so it is important that an individual plan of low vision services, both optical and nonoptical) is developed for each person and follow-up ensured to continue to provide services, particularly if their condition is progressive.

Technology

Until 1970's, technology for diagnostics and treatment in eye care was very minimal. In most settings, it was essentially limited to torchlight, ophthalmoscope, and a trial set or phoropter for refraction. Having a slit lamp or a surgical microscope was a rare luxury, especially in low- and middle-income countries (LMIC). This scenario has completely changed now with new technologies being introduced literally on a daily basis. This at one hand has increased the complexity but at the same time has brought in the benefit of better early diagnosis and treatment for many conditions. Technology has also significantly enhanced the quality and outcomes.

The technology is keeping pace with the rapidly increasing need for eye care due to literacy, functional needs, and longevity. The proliferation of information technology (IT), Internet, and smart phones has also resulted in a lot of innovations in eye care. The technology development around existing equipment continues to happen, often resulting in incremental capabilities leading to refinements in diagnosis or treatment. However, the new breed of innovations that are powered by IT, increasing Internet connectivity, and mobile technologies, could bring about paradigm shifts and be disruptive of current practices. They also have the potential to address several fundamental issues such as access, coverage, and affordability. It is not the medical professionals or the traditional medical industry that is ushering in this technology revolution. A lot of the technology development is being driven by engineers and IT professionals who see the potential of their expertise in medicine. It is this outside perspective that is powering the disruptive potential. The people involved range from individuals with little or no resources to giant companies such as Google and Microsoft. Certain broad trends are emerging with these rapid advancements in technology and we need to be aware of them and their potential in eye care.

Portability

With the advent of smartphones and miniaturization, many of the equipment, which were large and bulky, are now becoming very small. For instance, now fundus images can be taken using a smartphone with an appropriate lens adapter; visual fields can be assessed using a smartphone or a tablet. The quality of diagnostics using such portable devices is steadily improving and will soon match or exceed what is considered as a gold standard today by equipment, which are often large and not easily transportable. The trend toward portability and miniaturization is accompanied by significant drop in prices often at very disruptive levels. This combination of portability and reducing investments has the twin opportunity of creating better access and being able to do it in a cost-effective manner. Today, it is possible for an eye health worker to carry in the shirt pocket a fundus imaging or visual field testing technology and perform these tests at household level. Hence, this has the opportunity to reach out to more people and bring them into appropriate level of eye care services, in a very cost-effective manner.

Information Anywhere

With widespread digital connectivity, information exchange is becoming instantaneous. Information exchange is happening increasingly through smartphones thereby eliminating the high investments in computer hardware, which otherwise would have been necessary. This real-time information exchange and competence, available anywhere, will significantly help in the care giving process and in field research. The field worker will no more be lonely or isolated, but will have the benefit of being connected at demand.

Intelligent and Connected Equipment

In the past and even today, most equipment essentially collect data or images but do not have the capacity to interpret. Interpretation remains in the domain of appropriately trained technician, ophthalmologist, or subspecialist. Today, this is being replaced by sophisticated algorithms driven by technologies such as image recognition, artificial intelligence, and deep learning. So, we are likely to see many of the newer equipment coming with such intelligence inbuilt within the equipment or by automatically connecting to the information cloud and getting such feedback. The fundus cameras will soon be able to give fairly definitive diagnosis and recommended intervention, just as it takes the images. There will be autorefractors, which can give the perfect prescription for most patients, with minimal training for the person using the equipment.

Such paradigm shifting technologies are already happening and will redefine the practice of eye care. This redefining will include eye care becoming more accessible, reduce the cost of care, and reduce the learning curve for carrying out many of the very advanced diagnostics and treatments.

PROGRAMMATIC INITIATIVES

At the global level, the concerted efforts of WHO, International Agency for the Prevention of Blindness (IAPB), ICO, International Nongovernmental Organizations (INGOs), and national eye care organizations led to the global initiative, "Vision 2020—The Right to Sight". The global launch in 1999 at WHO, Geneva was followed by regional and national launches across the world. This initiative defined the priority disease conditions as well as the three essential strategies to address them—disease control, HRs development, and infrastructure. This broad action framework has helped various stakeholders to target their efforts.

Intersectoral Collaboration

In many countries, the school education system includes eye health as a component. This has resulted in many countries having either programmatic or voluntary school eye health programs. Just as the schools, the workforce in the organized sector again offers relatively easy access to screen and provide needed eye care.

Integration

The 2011 WHO declaration on NCD, states "*Promote the inclusion of NCD prevention and control within sexual and reproductive health and maternal and child health programs, especially at the PHC level, as well as other programs, as appropriate, and also integrate interventions in these areas into NCD prevention programs*". This declaration which has been adopted by the member countries is resulting in the scope of PHC being expanded to include NCDs. In a parallel development, in order to bring down the infant mortality rate, several countries are establishing neonatal intensive care units (NICU) at district levels to ensure the survival of preterm and low-birth weight babies. These developments are opening up opportunities for integrating DR at PHC level as well as the management of ROP at the NICUs.

National Plans

Many countries now have a national plan for eye care. This is reviewed periodically and some of the countries have also made budgetary allocations for priority interventions. Many LMICs have introduced a healthcare safety net through insurance schemes, with the government paying all or most of the annual premiums. This is both to reduce the financial barrier to healthcare and avoid families from slipping into poverty due to high costs associated with catastrophic health incidents. Several countries have launched targeted programs to reduce blindness due to cataract, which continues to be the leading cause of blindness in LMICs. Vitamin-A supplementation and elimination of Trachoma and Onchocerciasis are some of the other targeted approaches.

International Nongovernmental Organizations

International Nongovernmental Organizations have been involved in eye care worldwide since the 1950s. They continue to make significant contribution aligning with the national agenda. The focus of such support includes direct service delivery, developing HRs, and building local capacity.

Primary Eye Care and Universal Eye Health Coverage

Eye care infrastructure and services seem to have developed largely around cataract services. This probably is a reflection of cataract accounting for over 50% of the blindness and the fact that we have an effective intervention. This concentration at the secondary level of care slowly gave rise to the development of tertiary care services. However, at the primary level eye care (PEC) has been confined to "first-aid" and referral. Over the last decade PEC has evolved significantly to provide comprehensive eye examinations and address the common refractive errors. With deployment of technologies such as electronic medical records in the cloud and telemedicine and real-time face-to-face consultations with an ophthalmologist has become possible. This has enlarged the scope of PEC to detect or monitor conditions like DR and glaucoma. The comprehensiveness of care, easy access, and its affordability is encouraging all those with any eye condition to seek care. For the first time, we seem to have a viable approach toward universal eye health coverage.

RELEVANCE IN CLINICAL PRACTICE

While, it is seldom taught in residency programs or in medical schools, a public health perspective is fundamental to effective and equitable clinical practice. It is integral to clinical care and should not be kept in isolation. We first need to understand, what "effective and equitable clinical practice" is? Routine clinical practice is when diagnosis and prescription of treatment happens essentially to those who present themselves. The actual provision of surgery or recommended treatment is to the subset of those who comply with the advice. This "reactive" approach to providing care, essentially excludes those who would benefit by intervention but who are not seeking it due to whatever reasons and those who are unable to comply with the recommended intervention—surgery or treatment.

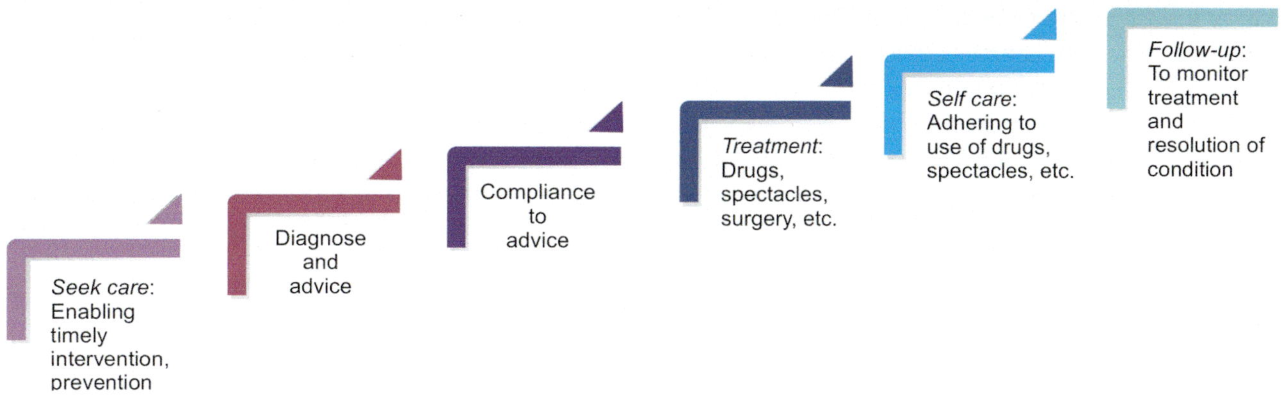

Fig. 116.7: Continuum of care.

Thus, current clinical practice is often not "effective and equitable clinical practice". Effective and equitable care should attempt to reach everyone with a good quality clinical care, being able to diagnose and treat, and know that the intervention worked. The following diagram depicts the continuum of care as it ought to be (Fig. 116.7).

An effective care giving program needs a deep understanding of those who will benefit from eye care interventions and what it will take to convert this latent need into demand. It would also design the program in a manner so as to eliminate barriers such as access, information, empowerment, and financial capacity.

Generating Demand

In most settings, eye hospitals tend to under-perform with respect to their capacity. While there could be a number of reasons for this, a significant reason is low demand. Such low demand, especially in developing countries, is not reflective of low need but rather of issues relating to awareness, access, and affordability. To find the right solutions, these challenges will need to be owned by the clinician or the eye hospital. Otherwise they often get quoted as reasons to explain under-performance—*"our population is too scattered; we don't have good roads and transport facilities; people do not appreciate eye care and give it a priority, etc."* The programs, which have taken these challenges head-on, have found innovative ways to effectively address them—outreach mechanisms, case finders, key informants, free care, etc.

Care-giving Process

This public health orientation and understanding would equally influence the design of the care giving protocol to individual patients to make it very patient centric and thus effective. The following are some examples that stem out of understanding the needs of the community that they serve.

Prescribing Medicines

Since affordability as well as availability of specialized ophthalmic medications would be a significant issue, both of these will need to be kept in mind while prescribing. Otherwise, it is unlikely that the patient will be able comply and follow through. For chronic conditions such as glaucoma, it is helpful to have at hand an estimate of annual cost of medications for various prescriptions. This information can guide the physician to make a judgment about the patient's financial ability to comply and this will help in moderating the prescription accordingly. Fortunately, for most conditions multiple options exist including lower priced generics. The challenge relating to availability should also be addressed since local drug stores are unlikely to be carrying specialized ophthalmic drugs. In India, in the recent years, a novel scheme has evolved for glaucoma medication. Since these glaucoma patients are often advised to come once in 6 months for regular monitoring, they are encouraged to buy the medications required for the 6 month period at one go. To facilitate this, some pharma companies have instituted a scheme of one bottle free for every two bottles of medications purchased, enough to last till the next visit. Such innovative approaches are required to address cost and supply chain challenges.

Prescribing Glasses

In most developing country settings, prescription glasses are available essentially in large towns. Thus, when a patient receives a glass prescription in a rural area at an eye camp or a PEC center, the patient will have to go to the nearest town, which sometimes could be quite far, to buy the glasses. More often than not, this may involve two or three trips, with each trip costing significantly on account of lost wages and travel. Thus the cost associated with buying the glasses could sometimes be more than the cost of the glasses themselves. When one has this understanding ways for delivering the glasses immediately, whether it is in the hospital setting or in outreach, can be found. This is a win-win for both—reducing the procurement cost to zero for the patients and the hospital having the satisfaction that the entire care loop is complete and potentially make a small surplus in the sale of glasses.

Completing Care in Single Visit

Countless studies have shown that access and cost to be the most significant barriers to healthcare. Logically, this would apply not only to initial access but to subsequent visits as well. An eye care provider who fully internalizes this, will be more inclined to design services so as to complete the full care cycle—investigations, diagnosis, and prescription or treatment—on the same day or in a single visit. For instance, a patient needing cataract surgery could be diagnosed, all preoperative investigations done and admitted for surgery on the same day, subject to the willingness of the patient. With surgery performed the following day, the entire care cycle including surgery could thus be completed on a single visit. The cost and efforts saved for the patient would be enormous and this also reduces work to the hospital as well.

Enhancing Compliance

The patient's condition never gets resolved by sophisticated investigations or excellence in diagnosis, but only when the patients follow through with the intervention advised. Most patients do not fully understand and appreciate the nuances or consequences of noncompliance or they may need a lot more information to become adequately empowered to make the decision. Recognizing this dynamic will encourage the inclusion of patient counseling as a standard part of the care giving process.

Quality

For more reasons than one, it is important to get the quality right every time and for every patient. While we may or may not succeed 100% of the time, the aspiration and the protocols have to reflect this. Two important reasons are—good outcomes makes the process cost effective both for the patients and the providers; good outcomes, combine with good experience with the care process is what sustains and reinforces demand.

Thus, having a public health perspective to eye care will influence the right design from demand generation to care giving, resulting in effective delivery of eye care services.

REFERENCES

1. Muhammad N, Mansur RM, Dantani AM, et al. Prevalence and causes of blindness and visual impairment in Sokoto state, Nigeria: baseline data for vision 2020: the right to sight eye care programme. Middle East Afr J Ophthalmol. 2011;18(2):123-8.
2. *http://www.who.int/blindness/Change%20the%20Definition%20of%20Blindness.pdf.*
3. IAPB Vision Atlas. (2017). Global Vision Database Maps. [online] Available from: *http://atlas.iapb.org/gvd-maps/#AllAges* [Accessed January 2018].
4. Bourne RRA, Flaxman SR, Braithwaite T, et al. Magnitude, temporal trends, and projections of the global prevalence of blindness and distance and near vision impairment: a systematic review and meta-analysis. Lancet Glob Health. 2017;5(9):e888-97.
5. Khanna RC, Murthy GV, Marmamula S, et al. Longitudinal Andhra Pradesh Eye Disease Study: rationale, study design and research methodology. Clin Exp Ophthalmol. 2016;44(2):95-105.
6. Bastawrous A, Mathenge W, Wing K, et al. Six-Year Incidence of Blindness and Visual Impairment in Kenya: The Nakuru Eye Disease Cohort Study. Invest Ophthalmol Vis Sci. 2016;57(14):5974-83.
7. Flaxman SR1, Bourne RRA2, Resnikoff S, et al; Vision Loss Expert Group of the Global Burden of Disease Study. Global causes of blindness and distance vision impairment 1990-2020: a systematic review and meta-analysis. Lancet Glob Health. 2017;5(12):e1221-34.
8. RAAB repository. (2016). Rapid Assessment of Avoidable Blindness database. [online] Available from: *http://raabdata.info* [Accessed January 2018].
9. Solomon AW, Kurylo E. The global trachoma mapping project. Community Eye Health. 2014;27(85):18.
10. IAPB Vision Atlas. (2017). GAP Implementation Progress-Cataract Surgery. [online] Available from: *http://atlas.iapb.org/global-action-plan/gap-implementation/gap-implementation-cataract-surgery* [Accessed January 2018].
11. Prajna NV, Thulasiraj RD, Srinivasan S. Cataract Surgery. In: Debas HT (Ed). Disease Control Priorities-Essential Surgery Volume. 1, 3rd edition. Washington: World Bank Group; 2015. pp. 197-219.
12. Resnikoff S, Felch W, Gauthier TM, et al. The number of ophthalmologists in practice and training worldwide: a growing gap despite more than 200,000 practitioners. Br J Ophthalmol. 2012;96(6):783-7.

13. World Health Organization (2000). Global Initiative for the elimination of avoidable blindness. Available from: *www.who.int/iris/handle/10665/63748* [Accessed January 2018].
14. Courtright P, Mathenge W, Kello AB, et al. Setting targets for human resources for eye health in sub-Saharan Africa: what evidence should be used? Hum Resour Health. 2016;14:11.
15. World Health Organization (1998). Informal Consultation on Analysis of Blindness Prevention Outcomes, Geneva, 16-18 February 1998. [online] Available from: *http://www.who.int/iris/handle/10665/67843* [Accessed January 2018].
16. Congdon N, Yan X, Lansingh V, et al. Assessment of cataract surgical outcomes in settings where follow-up is poor: PRECOG, a multicentre observational study. Lancet Glob Health. 2013;1(1):e37-45.
17. Polack S, Eusebio C, Mathenge W, et al. The impact of cataract surgery on activities and time-use: results from a longitudinal study in Kenya, Bangladesh and the Philippines. PLoS One. 2010;5(6):e10913.
18. Zheng Y, He M, Congdon N. The worldwide epidemic of diabetic retinopathy. Indian J Ophthalmol. 2012;60(5):428-31.
19. International Council of Ophthalmology (2017). ICO guidelines for Diabetic retinopathy. [online] Available from: *www.icoph.org/downloads/ICO Guidelines for Diabetic Eye Care* [Accessed January 2018].
20. Resnikoff S, Pascolini D, Mariotti SP, et al. Global magnitude of visual impairment caused by uncorrected refractive errors in 2004. Bull World Health Organ. 2008;86(1):63-70.
21. Williams KM, Verhoeven VJ, Cumberland P, et al. Prevalence of refractive error in Europe: the European eye epidemiology (E3) Consortium. Eur J Epidemiol. 2015;30(4):305-15.
22. Guo YH, Lin HY, Lin LLK, et al. Self-reported myopia in Taiwan: 2005 Taiwan National Health Interview Survey. Eye (Lond). 2012;26(5):684.
23. Holden BA, Fricke TR, Wilson DA, et al. Global Prevalence of Myopia and High Myopia and Temporal Trends from 2000 through 2050. Ophthalmology. 2016;123(5):1036-42.
24. Smith TST, Frick KD, Holden BA, et al. Potential lost productivity resulting from the global burden of uncorrected refractive error. Bull World Health Organ. 2009;87(6):431-7.
25. Berdeaux G, Alió JL, Martinez JM, et al. Socioeconomic aspects of laser in situ keratomileusis, eyeglasses, and contact lenses in mild to moderate myopia. J Cataract Refract Surg. 2002;28(11):1914-23.
26. De Souza N, Cui Y, Looi S, et al. The role of optometrists in India: An integral part of an eye health team. Indian J Ophthalmol. 2012;60(5):401-5.
27. Naidoo K, Govender P. A team approach to providing refractive error services. Community Eye Health. 2014;27(86):29-30.
28. Ramasamy D, Joseph S, Valaguru V, et al. Cluster randomized trial to compare spectacle delivery systems at outreach eye camps in South India. Ophthalmic Epidemiology. 2013;20(5):308-14.
29. Gilbert CE, Anderton L, Dandona L, et al. Prevalence of visual impairment in children: a review of available data. Ophthalmic Epidemiol. 1999;6(1):73-82.
30. Steinkuller PG, Du L, Gilbert C, et al. Childhood blindness. J AAPOS. 1999;3(1):26-32.
31. Hatton DD, Ivy SE, Boyer C. Severe visual impairments in infants and toddlers in the United States. J Vis Impairment Blindness. 2013;107(5):325.
32. Kong L, Fry M, Al-Samarraie M, Gilbert C, Steinkuller PG. An update on progress and the changing epidemiology of causes of childhood blindness worldwide. J AAPOS. 2012;16(6):501-7.
33. International Council of Ophthalmology. (2016) Glaucoma Guidelines. [online] Available from: *http://www.icoph.org/ICOGlaucomaGuidelines.pdf* [Accessed January 2018].
34. Tham YC, Li X, Wong TY,. Global prevalence of glaucoma and projections of glaucoma burden through 2040: a systematic review and meta-analysis. Ophthalmology. 2014;121(11):2081-90.
35. World Health Organization (1993). Management of low vision in children: report of a WHO consultation; (Bangkok, 23-24 July 1992). [online] Available from: *http://www.who.int/iris/handle/10665/61105* [Accessed January 2018].
36. World Health Organization. (2001). Asia Pacific Regional Low Vision Workshop. (Hong Kong, 28-30 May 2001.). [online] Available from: *whqlibdoc.who.int/hq/2002/WHO_PBL_02.87.pdf* [Accessed January 2018].
37. Lee SM, Cho JC. Low vision devices for children. Community Eye Health. 2007;20(62):28-9.

Index

Page numbers followed by, *b* refer to box, *f* refer to figure, *fc* refer to flowchart, and *t* refer to table

A

B

C

D

E

F

G

H

I

J

K

L

M

N

O

Q

R

S

T

U

V

W

X

Y

Z